Brain Injury Medicine
Principles and Practice

Second Edition

EDITORS

NATHAN D. ZASLER, MD
DOUGLAS I. KATZ, MD
ROSS D. ZAFONTE, DO

ASSOCIATE EDITORS

DAVID B. ARCINIEGAS, MD
M. ROSS BULLOCK, MD, PhD
JEFFREY S. KREUTZER, PhD

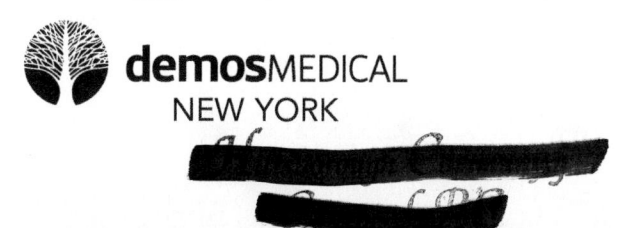

demosMEDICAL
NEW YORK

Visit our website at www.demosmedpub.com

ISBN: 9781936287277
e-book ISBN: 9781617050572

Cover image: Pathway tractography based on diffusion tensor imaging in traumatic brain injury, courtesy of Erin D. Bigler and Tracy J. Abildskov, Brain Imaging and Behavior Laboratory, Brigham Young University

Acquisitions Editor: Beth Barry
Compositor: Absolute Service, Inc.

Medicine is an ever-changing science. Research and clinical experience are continually expanding our knowledge, in particular our understanding of proper treatment and drug therapy. The authors, editors, and publisher have made every effort to ensure that all information in this book is in accordance with the state of knowledge at the time of production of the book. Nevertheless, the authors, editors, and publisher are not responsible for errors or omissions or for any consequences from application of the information in this book and make no warranty, express or implied, with respect to the contents of the publication. Every reader should examine carefully the package inserts accompanying each drug and should carefully check whether the dosage schedules mentioned therein or the contraindications stated by the manufacturer differ from the statements made in this book. Such examination is particularly important with drugs that are either rarely used or have been newly released on the market.

Library of Congress Cataloging-in-Publication Data

Brain injury medicine : principles and practice / editors, Nathan D. Zasler,
Douglas I. Katz, Ross D. Zafonte ; associate editors, David B. Arciniegas,
M. Ross Bullock, Jeffrey S. Kreutzer. — 2nd ed.
   p. ; cm.
Includes bibliographical references and index.
ISBN 978-1-936287-27-7 — ISBN 978-1-61705-057-2 (e-book)
I. Zasler, Nathan D., 1958- II. Katz, Douglas I. III. Zafonte, Ross D.
[DNLM: 1. Brain Injuries. 2. Continuity of Patient Care. WL 354]

617.4'810443—dc23
                    2012029354

Special discounts on bulk quantities of Demos Medical Publishing books are available to corporations, professional associations, pharmaceutical companies, health care organizations, and other qualifying groups. For details, please contact:

Special Sales Department
Demos Medical Publishing, LLC
11 West 42nd Street, 15th Floor
New York, NY 10036
Phone: 800-532-8663 or 212-683-0072
Fax: 212-941-7842
E-mail: specialsales@demosmedpub.com

Printed in the United States of America by Courier.

15 16 17 18 19 / 6 5 4 3 2

I must first acknowledge my wife Lisa for her love, understanding, and support in the work that I do and the time it takes me away from her and my family. I would also like to thank my parents for instilling in me my sense of intellectual curiosity and exploration. My children—Aaron, Anya, Maia, and Maytal—may not fully grasp what drives my commitment to educating and helping others, but I hope that someday when perusing this volume, they too will understand what drove their father and have a similar desire to reach out and better the lives of their fellow man each in their own unique way. I would like to thank my role models and mentors and especially all the patients and families I have worked with over the years who have all taught me one way or another . . . this book is dedicated to all of you. A special thanks to my coeditors, Drs. Katz and Zafonte, as well as our three associate editors without whose help this text would not have met the high standards we strove for when we considered proceeding with the second edition.

Nathan D. Zasler

I also thank my coeditors and our associate editors for their effort and dedication to this project. Kudos to Dr. Nathan Zasler for his leadership in once again setting high standards and keeping us on track to complete this second edition. I would also like to acknowledge all those who have influenced, instructed, supported, inspired, and collaborated with me throughout my career, including my mentors, teachers, neurorehabilitation fellows, residents, students, colleagues, and my professional partners and fellow staff at Braintree Rehabilitation Hospital and Boston University. I would also like to acknowledge my patients and their families who have inspired me and taught me so much over the years. Most importantly, I thank my wonderful family, my wife Kim, my children Rachel and Daniel, who are now developing their own professional lives, and my deceased parents Carol and Warner, who have been never-ending sources of love and support over the years.

Douglas I. Katz

Foremost I would like to thank my co-editors and associate especially Drs. Zasler and Katz whose vision and friendship helped make this edition happen. I would also like to acknowledge my wife Cheryl and son Alexander who in a selfless manner support me in my academic efforts. For my parents Albert and Grace who are now deceased but touch me each day with their lifelong lesson of trying "to make a difference." I am forever grateful for those with brain injury and their families who have done so much to help enhance the awareness of this disease. I also wish to acknowledge my colleagues; residents and fellows at Spaulding Rehabilitation Hospital, Massachusetts General Hospital and Harvard Medical School, their questions, collaboration, and enthusiasm make each day a positive experience.

Ross D. Zafonte

Acknowledgments

It has been 5 years since the publication of the first edition of *Brain Injury Medicine: Principles and Practice*. We are very pleased to have completed the expanded second edition and share it with our readers—current and future. As coeditors, we are very grateful for the contributions of our associate editors—Dr. Jeffery Kreutzer, Dr. David Arciniegas, and Dr. Ross Bullock—who have added an additional quality dimension to the text inherent in their respective backgrounds in neuropsychology, neuropsychiatry, and neurosurgery, respectively.

We, once again, have aimed for a multidisciplinary comprehensive volume with not only transdisciplinary neurorehabilitation involvement but also—just as importantly, if not more importantly—cross-disciplinary medical involvement and, as possible, transdisciplinary authorship of individual chapters. Several new features to the text have been added to increase practical use of the information herein and, of course, the second edition is also available as an e-book with additional added content relative to the hard cover volume.

We would be remiss if we did not thank the individuals at Demos Medical Publishing for their patience with this daunting project. Special thanks to Beth Barry for her guidance and advocacy with this project. Most importantly, this text would not have come to fruition were it not for the help of our managing editor, Mary Alice Hanford, who through immaculate organizational skills, patience, and perseverance, made sure all authors had what they needed, when they needed it.

Obviously, a project like this would not have been possible without the contributions of many busy professionals from around the world. We are very pleased to have had the participation of so many excellent contributors. We believe that their clinical acumen will clearly shine through the pages as you read this volume.

We would like to dedicate this text to all individuals with brain injuries, their families, and the professionals who are committed to assisting them in optimizing their potential for a better quality of life as an integrated member of society seeking all those things that make us human including love and social relationships, work identities and roles, as well as leisure opportunities.

Contents

Preface

Brain Injury Medicine: Principles and Practice is designed as a comprehensive text for all clinicians dealing with the assessment, management, and rehabilitation of patients with traumatic brain injury (TBI) from coma to community. This text is also a resource for nonclinicians who interface with persons with TBI, family members, and attorneys. As with the first edition, we hope that the second edition continues to serve as the "go-to reference" for practitioners on TBI to use in their day-to-day practice, as well as when confounded by less common clinical occurrences. We believe this text will also serve as an excellent core resource for students, trainees, and physicians pursing brain injury medicine certification, and for that matter, any professionals who need to learn more about TBI relative to assessment and management.

We have tried to further broaden the scope of the second edition with the inclusion of several new topics such as health policy, international systems of care and research, concepts and issues in conducting research, biomechanics, electrophysiological techniques, acute care neurosurgical and neurological issues, military TBI, and pediatric issues, to name but a few. Our goal is to present the relevant information using a disease state management approach, but at the same time convey the importance of biopsychosocial issues in both assessment and management of persons with TBI. . . . We believe that we have accomplished that goal.

Ultimately, the 86 chapters in this comprehensive text will provide readers with a full complement of neurological, neuropsychiatric, neurosurgical, and interdisciplinary neurorehabilitation perspectives dealing with management of persons (both pediatric and adult) with mild to severe TBI. We have sought to bring together in this volume knowledge, experience, and evidence-based medicine in a manner that will promote further cross- and trans-disciplinary practice and research in the field at large. Most of all, we hope that this book will result in individuals with TBI and their families receiving more timely and accurate assessments and consequentially more appropriate management to optimize their functional and neurological outcomes, as well as their quality of life.

Nathan D. Zasler, MD
Douglas I. Katz, MD
Ross D. Zafonte, DO

Foreword

Brain Injury Medicine: Principles and Practice, Second Edition represents the translation of neuroscience and biomechanics to clinical practice, especially rehabilitation. The second edition brings together leading multidisciplinary and interdisciplinary internationally known clinicians and researchers in areas dealing with all aspects of traumatic brain injury (TBI) including, but not limited to, prevention, biomechanics, pathophysiology, functional mobility and adjustment to daily activities (ADLs), neuroimaging, neuropharmacology and neurotechnology, complementary and alternative medicine, psychosocial functioning/community reentry/productivity, and medicolegal and ethical issues. This volume has been significantly expanded in scope and features in comparison to the first edition and is recommended for all professionals—health care and otherwise—involved with persons with TBI.

Drs. Zasler, Zafonte, and Katz have assembled a cadre of leading clinician-investigators in their respective subspecialties of brain injury medicine. Although most chapters are multiauthored and many interdisciplinary, the review subsequently mentions only the lead author of various chapters. The approach of the editors emphasizes the mechanisms involved in various interventions. For example, the section on Functional Mobility and ADLs is introduced by Dr. Randy Nudo's chapter on the Neuroscientific Basis for Occupational and Physical Therapy, which provides a foundation of neuroplasticity based on translational research using animal models that has guided development of novel therapies to enhance motor function. This section also includes chapters on Impairments and Motor Skill Acquisition (Katherine Sullivan), Therapy for ADL (Joan Toglia), and Rehabilitation Equipment (Rory Cooper).Similarly, the mechanisms of neuropharmacology in relation to brain injury (Jay Meythaler) introduce the section on Neuropharmacology and Neurotechnology, which includes chapters on the Pharmacotherapy of Cognitive Impairment and Neuropsychiatric Disturbances (David Arciniegas) and Neurotechnology (Paolo Bonato). The section on Complementary and Alternative Medicine (Jacinta McElligott) addresses emerging therapies that have become increasingly part of the rehabilitation toolbox. The review of postacute rehabilitation (James Malec) provides an overview for the chapters on domains that are especially salient in this later phase of rehabilitation, including driving (Megan Pierce), substance abuse (John Corrigan), family assessment and intervention (Jeffrey Kreutzer), returning to work (Michael West), and therapeutic recreation (Ann French). The final section on Medicolegal and Ethical Issues begins with an overview of medical ethics issues in TBI (John Banja), which introduces key chapters including A Clinicolegal Primer for Professionals Working with Persons with TBI (Arthur Ameis), Assessment of Response Bias and Forensic Evaluations of Impairment (Michael Martelli), and Life Care Planning: Clinical and Forensic Issues (Roger Weed).

This second edition of *Brain Injury Medicine: Principles and Practice* provides up-to-date, scholarly integration of major areas of brain injury care and neurorehabilitation, from coma to community, encompassing biomedical, neurobehavioral, psychosocial, medicolegal, and ethical aspects. The content is timely and highly relevant to researchers and clinicians engaged in the care and rehabilitation of persons with acquired brain injury, particularly TBI. In this second edition of *Brain Injury Medicine: Principles and Practice*, Drs. Zasler, Zafonte, and Katz extend their scholarly, translational approach to this burgeoning field.

Harvey Levin, PhD
Professor and Director of Research
Department of Physical Medicine & Rehabilitation
Baylor College of Medicine
Director, Center of Excellence on Traumatic Brain Injury
Michael E. DeBakey Veterans Affairs Medical Center
Houston, Texas

Contributors

Arthur Ameis, BSC(HONS), MD, FRCPC, FAAPM&R [Subcert Pain Medicine], CMLE
Lecturer, Certification Program in Insurance Medicine and Medicolegal Expertise
Faculty of Medicine
University of Montreal
Montreal, Quebec, Canada
Chapter 84: Clinicolegal Issues

Peter S. Amenta, MD
Resident
Department of Neurological Surgery
Thomas Jefferson University Hospital
Philadelphia, PA
Chapter 24: The Surgical Management of Traumatic Brain Injury

David B. Arciniegas, MD
Beth K. and Stuart C. Yudofsky Chair in Brain Injury Medicine
Menninger Department of Psychiatry & Behavioral Sciences
Baylor College of Medicine
Medical Director for Brain Injury Research
Brain Injury Research Center
TIRR Memorial Hermann Hospital
Houston, TX
Chapter 73: Pharmacotherapy of Cognitive Impairment
Chapter 74: Pharmacotheraphy of Neuropsychiatric Disturbances

Patricia M. Arenth, PhD
Assistant Professor
Department of Physical Medicine and Rehabilitation
University of Pittsburgh School of Medicine
Pittsburgh, PA
Chapter 16: Functional Neuroimaging

Lynn Babcock, MD, MS
Associate Professor
Department of Pediatrics, Division of Emergency Medicine
Cincinnati Children's Hospital Medical Center
Cincinnati, OH
Chapter 34: Pediatric Traumatic Brain Injury: Special Considerations

Ian J. Baguley, MBBS, PhD
Associate Professor
Brain Injury Rehabilitation Service
Westmead Hospital
Sydney, New South Wales, Australia
Sydney Medical School
The University of Sydney
Camperdown, New South Wales, Australia
Chapter 52: Autonomic Dysfunction

Keith Baldwin, MD, MSPT, MPH
Assistant Professor
Department of Orthopaedic Surgery
Children's Hospital of Philadelphia
Philadelphia, PA
Hospital of the University of Pennsylvania
Pennsylvania
Chapter 51: Neuro-Orthopedics

John D. Banja, PhD
Professor
Department of Rehabilitation Medicine
Medical Ethicist
Center for Ethics
Emory University
Atlanta, GA
Chapter 83: Ethics in Brain Injury Medicine

Anna M. Barrett, MD
Director
Stroke Rehabilitation Research
Kessler Foundation
West Orange, NJ
Professor
Department of Physical Medicine and Rehabilitation
The University of Medicine and Dentistry—New Jersey Medical School
Newark, NJ
Chapter 59: Cognitive Impairments

Shahid Bashir, PhD
Instructor
Berenson-Allen Center for Noninvasive Brain Stimulation
Beth Israel Deaconess Medical Center
Harvard Medical School
Boston, MA
Department of Physiology
Faculty of Medicine, KSU-Autism Research and Treatment Center
King Saud University
Riyadh, Saudi Arabia
Chapter 17: Electrophysiologic Techniques

Simon Beaulieu-Bonneau, PhD
Research Associate
École de psychologie
Université Laval
Research Professional
Centre interdisciplinaire de recherche en réadaptation et intégration sociale
Québec, Canada
Chapter 43: Sleep-Awake Disturbances

Kathleen R. Bell, MD
Professor and Chief of Service
Department of Rehabilitation Medicine
University of Washington
Seattle, WA
Chapter 49: Complications Associated With Immobility

Mark C. Bender, PhD
Rehabilitation Neurophysiologist
Hunter Holmes McGuire VA Medical Center
Affiliate Associate Professor
Psychology Department
Virginia Commonwealth University
Richmond, VA
Chapter 85: Assessing and Addressing Response Bias

Debra E. Berens, BS, MS, PhD
Rehabilitation Consultant and Life Care Planner
Atlanta, GA
Chapter 86: Life Care Planning After Traumatic Brain Injury: Clinical and Forensic Issues

Jean E. Bérubé, JD
President
Bérubé & Associates
New Market, MD
Chapter 3: Health Policy: United States and International Perspectives

Erin D. Bigler, PhD
Professor of Psychology
Department of Psychological Science and Neuroscience Center
Brigham Young University
Provo, UT
Adjunct Professor of Psychiatry
Department of Psychiatry
University of Utah
Salt Lake City, UT
Chapter 19: Neuroimaging Correlates of Functional Outcome

Paolo Bonato, PhD
Assistant Professor
Department of Physical Medicine and Rehabilitation
Harvard Medical School
Boston, MA
Affiliated Faculty Member
Harvard-MIT Division of Health Science and Technology
Massachusetts Institute of Technology
Cambridge, MA
Chapter 75: Neurotechnology in Traumatic Brain Injury Rehabilitation

Allen W. Brown, MD
Director
Brain Rehabilitation Services
Department of Physical Medicine and Rehabilitation
Associate Professor
College of Medicine
Mayo Clinic
Rochester, MN
Chapter 21: Life Expectancy and Wellness

M. Ross Bullock, MD, PhD
Professor
Department of Neurosurgery
University of Miami Miller School of Medicine
Miami, FL
Chapter 4: International Systems of Care and Research Agendas
Chapter 11: Pathobiology of Primary Traumatic Brain Injury
Chapter 25: Development of Acute Care Guidelines and Effect on Outcome

Shane S. Bush, PhD, ABPP, ABN
Neuropsychologist
Long Island Neuropsychology, P.C.
Lake Ronkonkoma, NY
Clinical Assistant Professor
Department of Psychiatry & Behavioral Sciences
Stony Brook University School of Medicine
Stony Brook, NY
Chapter 84: Clinicolegal Issues

Dominic A. Carone, PhD, ABPP-CN
Coordinator
Neuropsychology Assessment Program
Department of Physical Medicine and Rehabilitation
SUNY Upstate Medical University
Syracuse, NY
Chapter 5: Education, Training, and Certification for Health Care Providers

Freeman Chakara, PsyD, ABPP-CN
Chief of Neuropsychology and Behavioral Medicine
Department of Psychology
Providence Behavioral Health
Neuropsychologist
Department of Psychiatry
Lancaster Regional Medical Center
Lancaster, PA
Chapter 59: Cognitive Impairments

Jeffrey P. Cheng, BS
Student
Department of Physical Medicine & Rehabilitation
University of Pittsburgh
Pittsburgh, PA
Experimental Therapeutic Approaches for Traumatic Brain Injury

Keith D. Cicerone, PhD
Director of Neuropsychology
Department of Physical Medicine and Rehabilitation
JFK – Johnson Rehabilitation Institute
Edison, NJ
Clinical Professor
Department of Physical Medicine and Rehabilitation
Robert Wood Johnson Medical School
New Brunswick, NJ
Chapter 61: Cognitive Rehabilitation

Robert S.B. Clark, MD
Chief
Division of Pediatric Critical Care Medicine
Children's Hospital of Pittsburgh of UPMC
Professor
Department of Critical Care Medicine and Pediatrics
University of Pittsburgh School of Medicine
Pittsburgh, PA
Chapter 12: Pathobiology of Secondary Brain Injury

Richard A. Clendaniel, PT, PhD
Assistant Professor
Department of Community and Family Medicine
Duke University School of Medicine
Durham, NC
Chapter 47: Balance and Dizziness

Carl A. Coelho, PhD
Professor
Speech, Language, and Hearing Sciences
University of Connecticut
Storrs, CT
Chapter 67: Cognitive-Communication Deficits Following Traumatic Brain Injury

Daniel H. Coelho, MD
Assistant Professor
Department of Otolaryngology—Head and Neck Surgery
Virginia Commonwealth University
Richmond, VA
Chapter 46: Daniel H. Coelho

Jennifer L. Collinger, PhD
Assistant Professor
Department of Physical Medicine & Rehabilitation
University of Pittsburgh
Pittsburgh, PA
*Chapter 71: Assistive Technology for People With Traumatic Brain
    Injuries*

Michael W. Collins, PhD
Associate Professor
Departments of Orthopaedic and Neurological Surgery
Program Director
Sports Medicine Concussion Program
University of Pittsburgh Medical Center
Pittsburgh, PA
Chapter 31: Sport-Related Concussion

Rosemarie Cooper, MPT, ATP
Assistant Professor
Department of Rehabilitation Science and Technology
University of Pittsburgh
Director of Clinical Services
UPMC Center for Assistive Technology
Pittsburgh, PA
*Chapter 71: Assistive Technology for People With Traumatic Brain
    Injuries*

Rory A. Cooper, PhD
FISA & Paralyzed Veterans of America (PVA) Chair and
    Distinguished Professor
Department of Rehabilitation Science and Technology
University of Pittsburgh
Founding Director and VA Senior Research Career Scientist
VA Rehabilitation Research and Development Center of
    Excellence, VA
Pittsburgh Healthcare System
Pittsburgh, PA
*Chapter 71: Assistive Technology for People With Traumatic Brain
    Injuries*

Victor G. Coronado, MD, MPH
Medical Officer
Division of Injury Response
National Center for Injury Prevention and Control, Centers for
    Disease Control and Prevention
Atlanta, GA
*Chapter 8: Traumatic Brain Injury Epidemiology and Public Health
    Issues*

John D. Corrigan, PhD
Professor
Department of Physical Medicine & Rehabilitation
The Ohio State University Wexner Medical Center
Columbus, OH
*Chapter 79: Substance Misuse Among Persons With Traumatic Brain
    Injury*

Richard M. Costanzo, PhD
Professor
Department of Physiology and Biophysics
Department of Otolaryngology – Head and Neck Surgery
Virginia Commonwealth University
Richmond, VA
Chapter 48: Smell and Taste

Linda Creasey, BS
Clinical Nutrition Supervisor
Department of Clinical Nutrition
VCU Health System
Richmond, VA
Chapter 54: Gastrointestinal and Nutritional Issues

Satoko Y. Crockatt, PhD
Research Associate
Rehabilitation Research and Training Center
Virginia Commonwealth University
Richmond, VA
Chapter 81: Return to Work Following Traumatic Brain Injury

Numa Dancause, PT, PhD
Assistant Professor
Groupe de Recherche sur le Système Nerveux Central (GRSNC),
    Département de Physiologie
Université de Montréal
Montréal, Quebec, Canada
*Chapter 68: Neuroscientific Basis for Occupational and Physical
    Therapy Interventions*

Richard Delmonico, PhD
Chief, Neuropsychology
Department of Physical Medicine and Rehabilitation
Vallejo, CA
Associate Clinical Professor
Department of Physical Medicine and Rehabilitation
University of California, Davis School of Medicine
Sacramento, CA
Chapter 55: Sexuality and Intimacy Following Traumatic Brain Injury

Roberta DePompei, PhD
Interim Dean
Distinguished Professor
College of Health Professions
The University of Akron
Akron, OH
Chapter 38: Family Assessment and Intervention

Michael J. DeVivo, DrPH
Professor
Department of Physical Medicine and Rehabilitation
University of Alabama at Birmingham
Birmingham, AL
Chapter 21: Life Expectancy and Wellness

Marcel P.J.M. Dijkers, PhD
Professor
Department of Rehabilitation Medicine
Mount Sinai School of Medicine
New York, NY
*Chapter 20: Functional Assessment in Traumatic Brain Injury
    Rehabilitation*

Dan Ding, PhD
Assistant Professor
Department of Rehabilitation Science and Technology
University of Pittsburgh
Pittsburgh, PA
*Chapter 71: Assistive Technology for People With Traumatic Brain
    Injuries*

Craig DiTommaso, MD
Resident Physician
Department of Physical Medicine and Rehabilitation
Baylor College of Medicine
Houston, TX
*Chapter 18: Prognosis After Severe Traumatic Brain Injury: A
    Practical, Evidence-Based Approach*

C. Edward Dixon, PhD
Professor and Vice Chair
Department of Neurological Surgery
University of Pittsburgh
Research Scientist
Geriatric Research Education and Clinical Center
Veterans Affairs Pittsburgh Health Care System
Pittsburgh, PA
Chapter 14: Experimental Therapeutic Approaches for Traumatic Brain Injury

Matthew B. Dodson, OTD, OTR/L
Occupational Therapist
Supervisor
TBI Section of the Occupational Therapy Department
Walter Reed National Military Medical Center
Bethesda, MD
Chapter 71: Assistive Technology for People With Traumatic Brain Injury

Ana Durand-Sanchez, MD
Advanced Brain Injury Rehabilitation Fellow
Department of Physical Medicine and Rehabilitation
Baylor College of Medicine/University of Texas Health Science Center-Houston PM&R Alliance
Houston, TX
Physician and Assistant Professor
Department of Physical Medicine and Rehabilitation
Indiana University
Indianapolis, IN
Chapter 26: Acute Rehabilitation

Elie P. Elovic, MD
Program Director
Healthsouth Rehabilitation Hospital
Sandy, UT
Chapter 9: Primary Prevention
Chapter 42: Fatigue: Assessment and Treatment

Syed Faaiz Enam
Student
Beth Israel Deaconess Medical Center
Harvard Medical School
Boston, MA
Medical Student
Medical College
Aga Khan University Hospital
Karachi, Pakistan
Chapter 17: Electrophysiologic Techniques

Paul J. Eslinger, PhD
Professor and Director of Clinical Neuropsychology and Cognitive Neuroscience Programs
Department of Neurology
Neural & Behavioral Sciences
Pediatrics, Radiology, and Public Health Sciences
Penn State Hershey Medical Center and Rehabilitation Hospital
Hershey, PA
Chapter 59: Cognitive Impairments

Alberto Esquenazi, MD
Professor
Department of Physical Medicine and Rehabilitation
Temple University School of Medicine
Philadelphia, PA
Chief Medical Officer, MossRehab
Director, Gait and Motion Analysis Laboratory
Department of Physical Medicine and Rehabilitation
MossRehab Einstein at Elkins Park
Elkins Park, PA
Chapter 50: Managing Upper Motoneuron Muscle Overactivity

Deborah Ettel, PhD
Associate Fellow
Center on Brain Injury Research and Training
Teaching Research Institute, Western Oregon University
Eugene, OR
Educational Issues and School Reentry for Students With Traumatic Brain Injury

Mark Faul, PhD, MA
Senior Health Scientist
National Center for Injury Prevention and Control
Centers for Disease Control and Prevention
Atlanta, GA
Chapter 8: Traumatic Brain Injury Epidemiology and Public Health Issues

Anne M. Fenech, DipCOT, Dip Geront, MSc, MBA
International Fellow in Recreation and Leisure/ Lecturer
Faculty of Health Sciences
University of Southampton
Southampton
Hampshire, UK
Chapter 82: Lifelong and Therapeutic Recreation and Leisure

Joseph J. Fins, MD, MACP
Chief, Division of Medical Ethics
The E. William Davis, Jr., MD Professor of Medical Ethics
Professor of Medicine, Public Health, and Medicine in Psychiatry
Division of Medical Ethics
Weill Cornell Medical College
Director of Medical Ethics & Attending Physician (Medicine)
Department of Medical Ethics
New York Presbyterian Hospital-Weill Cornell Medical Center
New York, NY
Chapter 83: Ethics in Brain Injury Medicine

Kelly L. Shaw Fisher, Certified Therapeutic Recreation Specialist
Recreational Therapist
Rehabilitation Department
Tree of Life Services
Richmond, VA
Chapter 82: Lifelong and Therapeutic Recreation and Leisure

Steven R. Flanagan, MD
Howard A. Rusk Professor of Rehabilitation Medicine
Chairman
Department of Rehabilitation Medicine
Department of Physical Medicine and Rehabilitation
Rusk Institute of Rehabilitation Medicine
NYU-Langone Medical Center
New York, NY
Chapter 28: Traumatic Brain Injury in the Elderly

Samson Sujit Kumar Gaddam, MBBS
Senior Research Assistant
Department of Neurosurgery
Baylor College of Medicine
Houston, TX

Michael B. Gaetz, BA, MSc, PhD
Professor
Department of Kinesiology and Physical Education
University of the Fraser Valley
Chilliwack, British Columbia, Canada
Chapter 29: Mild Traumatic Brain Injury
Chapter 31: Sport-Related Concussion

Caron Gan, RN, MScN, AAMFT
Clinical Fellow & Approved Supervisor
Registered Marriage and Family Therapist
Family Support Service
Brain Injury Rehabilitation Team
Holland Bloorview Kids Rehabilitation Hospital
Toronto, Ontario, Canada
Chapter 28: Family Assessment and Intervention

Kent Garber, BA
Spaulding Rehabilitation Hospital
Boston, MA
*Chapter 32: Assessment and Rehabilitive Management of Individuals
    With Disorders of Consciousness*

Alisa D. Gean, MD
Professor of Radiology, Neurology, and Neurosurgery
University of California, San Francisco
San Francisco, CA
Chapter 15: Structural Neuroimaging

Joseph T. Giacino, PhD
Associate Professor
Physical Medicine and Rehabilitation
Harvard Medical School
Director of Rehabilitation Neuropsychology
Spaulding Rehabilitation Hospital
Boston, MA
*Chapter 32: Assessment and Rehabilitive Management of Individuals
    With Disorders of Consciousness*

Christopher C. Giza, MD
Associate Professor
Division of Pediatric Neurology
Department of Pediatrics
Mattel Children's Hospital - UCLA
UCLA Brain Injury Research Center
Department of Neurosurgery
David Geffen School of Medicine at UCLA
Los Angeles, CA
Chapter 35: Pediatric Neurocritical Care: Special Considerations

Ann Glang, PhD
Senior Fellow
Center on Brain Injury Research and Training
Research Scientist, ORCAS
Eugene, OR
*Chapter 37: Educational Issues and School Reentry for Students With
    Traumatic Brain Injury*

Emilie E. Godwin, PhD
Faculty Instructor
Department of Physical Medicine & Rehabilitation
Virginia Commonwealth University
Richmond, VA
Chapter 60: Neuropsychological Assessment and Treatment Planning
*Chapter 80: Practical Approaches to Family Assessment and
    Intervention*

Kathleen Golisz, OTD, OTR
Professor
Graduate Occupational Therapy Program
Mercy College
Dobbs Ferry, NY
*Chapter 70: Therapy for Activities of Daily Living: Theoretical and
    Practical Perspectives*

Mary Goonan, RN, BSN, CRRN
Clinical Nurse III
Department of Rehabilitation Nursing
Virginia Commonwealth University Health System
Richmond, VA
Chapter 27: Neurorehabilitation Nursing

Brian D. Greenwald, MD
Assistant Professor
Department of Rehabilitation Medicine
Mount Sinai School of Medicine
New York, NY
*Chapter 20: Functional Assessment in Traumatic Brain Injury
    Rehabilitataion*

Col. Jamie Grimes, MD
National Director
Defense & Veterans Brain Injury Center
Rockville, MD
Assistant Professor
Department of Neurology
Uniformed Services University of Health Sciences
Bethesda, MD
Chapter 33: Military Traumatic Brain Injury: Special Considerations

Kristin Guilliams, MD
Fellow
Department of Neurology
Division of Pediatric and Developmental Neurology
Department of Pediatrics
Division of Critical Care
Washington University
St. Louis, MO
Chapter 35: Pediatric Neurocritical Care: Special Considerations

Flora M. Hammond, MD
Chair
Department of Physical Medicine & Rehabilitation
Indiana University School of Medicine
Indianapolis, IN
Chapter 41: Cranial Nerve Disorders

Jaynee A. Handelsman, PhD
Director of Pediatric Audiology
Department of Otolaryngology–Head and Neck Surgery
University of Michigan Health System
Ann Arbor, MI
Chapter 47: Balance and Dizziness

Cynthia L. Harrison-Felix, PhD
Assistant Director of Research
Craig Hospital
Research Department
Englewood, CO
Assistant Clinical Professor
Department of Physical Medicine and Rehabilitation
University of Colorado Denver
Denver, CO
Chapter 21: Life Expectancy and Wellness

Lenore A. Hawley, MSSW, LCSW, CBIST
Clinical Professional in Research
Craig Hospital
Research Department
Englewood, CO
Chapter 21: Life Expectancy and Wellness

Michael Henrie, MO
Assistant Professor
Department of Physical Medicine and Rehabilitation
University of Utah
Salt Lake City, UT
Chapter 42: Fatigue: Assessment and Treatment

Holly E. Hinson, MD
Assistant Professor
Department of Neurology
Oregon Health and Science Center
Portland, OR
Chapter 22: Prehospital Assessment and Care

Shivayogi Hiremath, MS
Graduate Student/Researcher
Department of Rehabilitation Science and Technology
University of Pittsburgh
Pittsburgh, PA
*Chapter 71: Assistive Technology for People With Traumatic Brain
   Injuries*

Michael Hoffer, CAPT MC USN, MD
Director Spatial Orientation Center
Department of Otolaryngology
Navy Medical Center San Diego
San Diego, CA
Chapter 46: Audiologic Impairment

Lawrence J. Horn, MD, MRM
Professor and Interim Chair
Department of Physical Medicine & Rehabilitation/Rehabilitation
   Institute of Michigan
Wayne State University School of Medicine
Detroit, MI
Chapter 56: Post-Traumatic Headache
*Chapter 57: Post-Traumatic Pain Disorders: Medical Assessment and
   Management*

Harish Hosalkar, MD
Attending Orthopedic Surgeon
Co-Director International Hip Center
Director Hip Research Program
Hip and Trauma Specialist
AO-North America Faculty for Orthopedic Traumatology
Rady Children's Hospital, UCSD
San Diego, CA
Chapter 51: Neuro-Orthopedics

**Ming-Yun Hsieh, B Soc Sc (Hons)i, M Soc Sci, PGDip (Clinical
   Psychology), D. Psych (Clin Neuropsych)**
Clinical Psychologist and Clinical Neuropsychologist
Neuropsychological Assessment & Intervention Services,
   (NPAIS)
ARBIAS
Brunswick, Victoria, Australia
*Chapter 64: Psychological Interventions for Emotional and Behavioral
   Problems Following Traumatic Brain Injury*

Nancy H. Hsu, PsyD
Assistant Professor
Department of Physical Medicine & Rehabilitation
Virginia Commonwealth University
Richmond, VA
Chapter 60: Neuropsychological Assessment and Treatment Planning

Cindy B. Ivanhoe, MD
Chief Medical Officer
Mentis Neurorehabilitation
Associate Professor
Baylor College of Medicine–University of Texas
Physical Medicine and Rehabilitation Alliance
Houston, TX
Chapter 26: Acute Rehabilitation

Grant L. Iverson, PhD
Professor
Department of Psychiatry
University of British Columbia
Vancouver
British Columbia, Canada
Chapter 29: Mild Traumatic Brain Injury
*Chapter 30: Conceptualizing Outcome from Mild Traumatic Brain
   Injury*
Chapter 31: Sport-Related Concussion

Col. Michael S. Jaffee, MD
Associate Professor
Department of Neurology
Uniformed Services University of the Health Sciences
Bethesda, MD
University of Texas
San Antonio, TX
Chapter 33: Military Traumatic Brain Injury: Special Considerations

Jack I. Jallo, MD, PhD
Professor
Thomas Jefferson University Hospital—Department of
   Neurological Surgery
Philadelphia, PA
Chapter 24: The Surgical Management of Traumatic Brain Injury

Joseph Jankovic, MD
Director
Parkinson's Disease Center and Movement Disorders Clinic
Professor of Neurology
Department of Neurology
Baylor College of Medicine
Houston, TX
Chapter 40: Movement Disorders After Traumatic Brain Injury

Larry W. Jenkins, PhD
Professor
Department of Neurosurgery
University of Pittsburgh School of Medicine
Pittsburgh, PA
Chapter 12: Pathobiology of Secondary Brain Injury

Andrew Jinks, MA, CCC-SLP, ATP
Speech-Language Pathologist
UPMC Center for Assistive Technology
Adjunct Instructor
Department of Rehabilitation Science and Technology
University of Pittsburgh
Pittsburgh, PA
*Chapter 71: Assistive Technology for People With Traumatic Brain
   Injuries*

Melinda Kahn, RN, BSN, CRRN
Clinical Coordinator
Department of Rehabilitation Nursing
Virginia Commonwealth University Health System
Richmond, VA
Chapter 27: Neurorehabilitation Nursing

David E. Kahn, DO
Neuro Critical Care Fellow
Department of Neurology
University of Miami Miller School of Medicine/Jackson
 Memorial Hospital
Miami, FL
*Chapter 25: Development of Acute Care Guidelines and Effect on
 Outcome*

Robert L. Karol, PhD, ABPP, CBIST
President
Karol Neuropsychological Services & Consulting
Vice President of Brain Injury Services
Mission Healthcare
Minneapolis, MN
Chapter 63: Principles of Behavioral Analysis and Treatment

Douglas I. Katz, MD
Associate Professor
Department of Neurology
Boston University School of Medicine
Boston, MA
Medical Director
Acquired Brain Injury Program
Braintree Rehabilitation Hospital
Braintree, MA
Chapter 1: Clinical Continuum of Care and Natural History
*Chapter 32: Assessment and Rehabilitive Management of Individuals
 With Disorders of Consciousness*

Mary Ann Keenan, MD
Professor
Department of Orthopaedic Surgery
University of Pennsylvania School of Medicine
Philadelphia, PA
Chapter 51: Neuro-Orthopedics

**Donald F. Kirby, MD, FACP, FACN, FACG, AGAF, CNSP,
CPNS**
Director, Center for Human Nutrition
Digestive Disease Institute/ Gastroenterology
Cleveland Clinic
Cleveland, OH
Chapter 54: Gastrointestinal and Nutritional Issues

Anthony E. Kline, PhD
Associate Professor
Department of Physical Medicine & Rehabilitation
Associate Director of Rehabilitation Research
Safar Center for Resuscitation Research
University of Pittsburgh
Pittsburgh, PA
*Chapter 14: Experimental Therapeutic Approaches for Traumatic Brain
 Injury*

Lee M. Kneer, MD, BA Biology
Rehabilitation Associates of Indiana
Indianapolis, IN
Chief Resident
Department of Physical Medicine and Rehabilitation
University of Utah
Salt Lake City, UT
Chapter 9: Primary Prevention

Christina Knuepffer, MSc
Centre for Neurogenic Communication Disorders Research,
 School of Health and Rehabilitation Sciences
The University of Queensland
Brisbane, Queensland, Australia
*Chpater 65: Assessment and Treatment of Speech and Language
 Disorders in Traumatic Brain Injury*

Patrick M. Kochanek, MD, MCCM
Professor and Vice Chairman, Director, Safar Center for
 Resuscitation Research
Critical Care Medicine
Professor of Anesthesiology, Pediatrics, and Clinical and
 Translational Science
University of Pittsburgh School of Medicine
Pittsburgh, PA
Chapter 12: Pathobiology of Secondary Brain Injury

Mary Jean Kotch, BSN, MSN, CRRN
Clinical Nurse Specialist
Department of Nursing
Kaiser Foundation Rehabilitation Center
Vallejo, CA
Chapter 55: Sexuality and Intimacy Following Traumatic Brain Injury

Sunil Kothari, MD
Assistant Professor
Department of Physical Medicine and Rehabilitation
Baylor College of Medicine
Houston, TX
*Chapter 18: Prognosis After Severe Traumatic Brain Injury: A
 Practical, Evidence-Based Approach*
Chapter 76: Complementary and Alternative Medicine

Joachim K. Krauss, MD
Chairman and Director
Professor of Neurology
Department of Neurology
Medical University Hannover, MHH
Hannover, Germany
Chapter 40: Movement Disorders After Traumatic Brain Injury

Jeffrey S. Kreutzer, PhD, ABPP, FACRM
Rosa Schwarz Cifu Professor
Department of Physical Medicine and Rehabilitation,
 Neurosurgery, and Psychiatry
Virginia Commonwealth University
Richmond, VA
Chapter 60: Neuropsychological Assessment and Treatment Planning
*Chapter 80: Practical Approaches to Family Assessment and
 Intervention*

Hatice Kumru, MD, PhD
Institut Guttmann
Institut Universitari de Neurorehabilitació adscrit a la UAB -
 Univ Autonoma de Barcelona
Barcelona, Spain
Chapter 17: Electrophysiologic Techniques

Brad G. Kurowski, MD, MS
Instructor
Clinical PM&R and Clinical Pediatrics
Cincinnati Children's Hospital Medical Center, University of
 Cincinnati College of Medicine
Cincinnati, OH
Chapter 34: Pediatric Traumatic Brain Injury: Special Considerations

Rael T. Lange, PhD
Research Director & Senior Scientist
Defense and Veterans Brain Injury Center, Walter Reed National
 Military Medical Center
North Bethesda, MD
Clinical Assistant Professor
Department of Psychiatry
University of British Columbia
Vancouver, British Columbia, Canada
Chapter 29: Mild Traumatic Brain Injury
*Chapter 30: Conceptualizing Outcome from Mild Traumatic Brain
 Injury*

Marilyn Lash, MSW
President
Lash & Associates Publishing/Training, Inc.
Youngsville, NC
Chapter 38: Family Assessment and Intervention

Jaime M. Levine, DO
Medical Director, Brain Injury Rehabilitation
Clinical Instructor
Department of Physical Medicine and Rehabilitation
Rusk Institute of Rehabilitation Medicine, NYU-Langone Medical
    Center
New York, NY
Chapter 28: Traumatic Brain Injury in the Elderly

Fiona Lewis, PhD, B Sp Path, BA
Centre for Neurogenic Communication Disorders Research,
    School of Health and Rehabilitation Sciences
The University of Queensland
Brisbane, Queensland, Australia
*Chapter 65: Assessment and treatment of Speech and Language
    Disorders in Traumatic Brain Injury*

Allen Lewis, PhD
Associate Professor
Department of Rehabilitation Science and Technology
University of Pittsburgh
Pittsburgh, PA
*Chapter 71: Assistive Technology for People With Traumatic Brain
    Injuries*

Geoffrey S. F. Ling, MD, PhD
Professor and Interim Chair
Department of Neurology
Uniformed Services University of the Health Sciences
Bethesda, MD
Chapter 22: Prehospital Assessment and Care

Jeri A. Logemann, PhD, CCC-SLP, BRS-S
Ralph and Jean Sundin Professor
Department of Communication Sciences and Disorders
Northwestern University
Evanston, IL
Director, Speech and Voice Services
Communication Sciences and Disorders
Northwestern Memorial Hospital
Chicago, IL
Chapter 66: Evaluation and Treatment of Swallowing Problems

David F. Long, MD
Medical Director, Brain Injury Program
Bryn Mawr Rehab Hospital
Malvern, PA
*Chapter 44: Diagnosis and Management of Late Intracranial
    Complication*

Edmund LoPresti, PhD
President, AT Sciences, LLC
Pittsburgh, PA
*Chapter 71: Assistive Technology for People With Traumatic Brain
    Injuries*

Mark R. Lovell, BS, PhD
Chairman and Chief Executive Officer
ImPACT Applications, Inc.
Pittsburgh, PA
Chapter 31: Sport-Related Concussion

Christine M. MacDonell, BS Occupational Therapy
Managing Director
Medical Rehabilitation and International Aging Services/Medical
    Rehabilitation
Commission on Accreditation Rehabilitation Facilities (CARF)
Washington, DC
*Chapter 6: Commission on Accreditation of Rehabilitation Facilities
    Accreditation for Brain Injury Programs*

Andranik Madikians, MD
Associate Professor of Pediatrics
Pediatrics Division of Critical Care
Mattel Children's Hospital at UCLA
Los Angeles, CA
Chapter 35: Pediatric Neurocritical Care: Special Considerations

W. Michael Magrun, BS
Vice President and CE Administrator
Clinician's View
Las Cruces, NM
Chapter 45: Evaluating and Treating Visual Dysfunction

James F. Malec, PhD
Professor and Research Director
Department of Physical Medicine and Rehabilitation
Indiana University School of Medicine
Research Director
Rehabilitation Hospital of Indiana
Indianapolis, IN
Chapter 77: Posthospital Rehabilitation

Michael F. Martelli, PhD
Rehabilitation Neuropsychologist
NeuroLife Rehab
Senior Services
Chapman Senior Care
Richmond, VA
*Chapter 57: Post-Traumatic Pain Disorders: Medical Assessment and
    Management*
*Chapter 58: Psychological Assessment and Management of Post-
    Traumatic Pain*
Chapter 84: Clinicolegal Issues
Chapter 85: Assessing and Addressing Response Bias

Brent E. Masel, MD
President
Transitional Learning Center at Galveston
Clinical Professor
Department of Neurology
University of Texas Medical Branch
Galveston, TX
*Chapter 53: Neuroendocrine Dysfunction After Traumatic Brain
    Injury*

Todd Masel, MD
Assistant Professor of Neurology
Department of Neurology
University of Texas Medical Branch
Galveston, TX
Chapter 41: Cranial Nerve Disorders

Nathaniel H. Mayer, MD
Emeritus Professor of Physical Medicine and Rehabilitation
Department of Physical Medicine & Rehabilitation
Temple University School of Medicine
Philadelphia, PA
Emeritus Director, Drucker Brain Injury Center
Director, Motor Control Analysis Laboratory
PM&R
MossRehab Einstein at Elkins Park
Elkins Park, PA
Chapter 50: Managing Upper Motoneuron Muscle Overactivity

William L. Maxwell, BSc (Hons), PhD, DSc
Senior Lecturer in Human Anatomy
Department of Anatomy, School of Biological Sciences, College of
    Medicine, Veterinary and Biology
University of Glasgow
Glasgow, Scotland, United Kingdom
Chapter 19: *Neuroimaging Correlates of Functional Outcome*

Thomas W. McAllister, MD
Millennium Professor of Psychiatry & Neurology, Vice Chair for
    Neuroscience Research, Director Section of Neuropsychiatry
Department of Psychiatry
Geisel School of Medicine at Dartmouth
Lebanon, NH
Chapter 62: *Emotional and Behavioral Sequelae of Traumatic Brain
    Injury*

Laura McClure, PhD
Visiting Assistant Professor
Department of Kinesiology
University of Illinois at Urbana-Champaign
Physical Therapist
Carle Foundation Hospital
Urbana, IL
Chapter 71: *Assistive Technology for People With Traumatic Brain
    Injuries*

Michael McCue, PhD
Associate Professor and Vice-Chair
Department of Rehabilitation Science and Technology
University of Pittsburgh
Pittsburgh, PA
Chapter 71: *Assistive Technology for People With Traumatic Brain
    Injuries*

Karen McCulloch, PT, PhD, NCS
Professor
Division of Physical Therapy, Department of Allied Health
    Sciences, School of Medicine
University of North Carolina at Chapel Hill
Chapel Hill, NC
Chapter 69: *Movement Rehabilitation*

**Jacinta McElligott, MB Bch BAO, Board Certification PM&R,
    Subspecialty Spinal Cord Injury**
Consultant in Rehabilitation Medicine
Department of Rehabilitation Medicine
National Rehabilitation Hospital
Dublin, Ireland
Clinical Associate Professor
Department of Physical and Rehabilitation Medicine
East Carolina University, Brody School of Medicine
Greenville, NC
Chapter 76: *Complementary and Alternative Medicine*

Lisa C. McGuire, PhD
Lead Health Scientist & Research Team Leader
Division of Injury Response, National Center for Injury
    Prevention and Control
Centers for Disease Control and Prevention
Atlanta, GA
Chapter 8: *Traumatic Brain Injury Epidemiology and Public Health
    Issues*

William P. Meehan III, MD
Sport-Related Concussion
Departments of Pediatrics and Orthopedics
Children's Hospital Boston
Boston, MA
Chapter 31: *Sport-Related Concussion*

Kimberly S. Meyer, MSN, ACNP-BC
Nurse Practitioner
Division of Clinical Initiatives
Defense & Veterans Brain Injury Center
Rockville, MD
Neurosurgery Nurse Practitioner
Trauma Institute
University of Louisville Hospital
Louisville, KY
Chapter 33: *Military Traumatic Brain Injury: Special Considerations*

Jay Meythaler, MD, JD
Professor and Chair
Department of Physical Medicine and Rehabilitation – Oakwood
Wayne State University
Dearborn, MI
Chapter 72: *Neuropharmacology: A Rehabilitation Perspective*

Linda Michaud, MD
Director, Pediatric Physical Medicine and Rehabilitation
Aaron W. Perlman Professor of Pediatric PM&R
Professor of Clinical PM&R and Clinical Pediatrics
Cincinnati Children's Hospital Medical Center
University of Cincinnati College of Medicine
Cincinnati, OH
Chapter 34: *Pediatric Traumatic Brain Injury: Special Considerations*

Charles M. Morin, PhD
Professor
École de psychologie
Université Laval
Québec, Canada
Chapter 43: *Sleep-Wake Disturbances*

Raquel Munitz, MS
Psychologist
Department of Vision Development
Colegio Senda
Mexico City, Mexico
Padula Vision Institute
Guilford, CT
Chapter 45: *Evaluating and Treating Visual Dysfunction*

Bruce E. Murdoch, BSc(Hons), PhD, DSc
Professor
Centre for Neurogenic Communication Disorders Research,
    School of Health and Rehabilitation Sciences
The University of Queensland
Brisbane, Queensland, Australia
Chapter 65: *Assessment and Treatment of Speech and Language
    Disorders in Traumatic Brain Injury*

W. Jerry Mysiw, MD
Associate Professor
The Ohio State University Wexner Medical Center
Columbus, OH
Chapter 79: *Substance Misuse Among Persons With Traumatic Brain
    Injury*

Keith Nicholson, PhD
Psychologist
Comprehensive Pain Program
Toronto Western Hospital
Toronto, Ontario, Canada
Chapter 57: *Post-Traumatic Pain Disorders: Medical Assessment and
    Management*
Chapter 58: *Psychological Assessment and Management of Post-
    Traumatic Pain*
Chapter 85: *Assessing and Addressing Response Bias*

Melissa T. Nott, BAppSc, PhD
Occupational Therapy Lecturer
School of Community Health
Charles Sturt University
Albury, New South Wales, Australia
Research Consultant
Brain Injury Rehabilitation Service
Westmead Hospital
Sydney, New South Wales, Australia
Chapter 52: Autonomic Dysfunction

Randolph J. Nudo, PhD
Marion Merrell Dow Distinguished Professor in Aging
Director, Landon Center on Aging
Department of Molecular and Integrative Physiology
University of Kansas Medical Center
Kansas City, KS
*Chapter 68: Neuroscientific Basis for Occupational and Physical
Therapy Interventions*

Morris Odell, MBBS, FRACGP, DMJ FFFLM
Clinical Forensic Medicine
Victorian Institute of Forensic Medicine, Department of Forensic
Medicine
Monash University
Melbourne, Victoria, Australia
Chapter 78: Driving After Traumatic Brain Injury

Marie-Christine Ouellet, PhD
Assistant Professor
École de psychologie
Université Laval
Researcher
Centre interdisciplinaire de recherche en réadaptation et
intégration sociale
Québec, Canada
Chapter 43: Sleep-Wake Disturbances

William V. Padula, OD, FNAP, FAAO, FNORA
Adjunct Associate Professor
Salus University of Health Sciences
College of Optometry
Padula Institute of Vision Rehabilitation
Guilford, CT
Chapter 45: Evaluating and Treating Visual Dysfunction

Nirav K. Pandya, MD
Attending Pediatric Orthopedic Surgeon
Department of Orthopedics
Children's Hospital of Oakland/University of California San
Francisco
Oakland, CA
Chapter 51: Neuro-Orthopedics

Keely R. Parisian, MD
Gastroenterology and Hepatology Fellow
Digestive Disease Institute
The Cleveland Clinic
Cleveland, OH
Chapter 54: Gastrointestinal and Nutritional Issues

Alvaro Pascual-Leone, MD, PhD
Professor
Department of Neurology
Harvard Medical School and Beth Israel Deaconess
Medical Center
Boston, MA
Institut Universitari de Neurorehabilitació Guttmann
Universidad Autónoma de Barcelona
Barcelona, Spain
Chapter 17: Electrophysiologic Techniques

Neil Patel, DO
Resident
Department of Physical Medicine & Rehabilitation/Rehabilitation
Institute of Michigan
Wayne State University School of Medicine
Detroit, MI
Chapter 56: Post-Traumatic Headache

Peter Patrick, PhD
Neuropsychologist
Department of Pediatrics
University of Virginia
Charlottesville, VA
*Chapter 36: Pediatric Neuropsychological Issues and Cognitive
Rehabilitation*

William S. Pearson, PhD, MHA
Epidemiologist
Division of Injury Response
Centers for Disease Control and Prevention
Atlanta, GA
*Chapter 8: Traumatic Brain Injury Epidemiology and Public Health
Issues*

Jose Pineda, MD, MSc
Assistant Professor
Department of Pediatrics and Neurology
Washington University School of Medicine
St. Louis, MI
Chapter 35: Pediatric Neurocritical Care: Special Considerations

Jennie Ponsford, BA (Hons), MA (Clin Neuropsych), PhD
Professor of Neuropsychology
School of Psychology and Psychiatry
Monash University
Clayton, Victoria, Australia
*Chapter 64: Psychological Interventions for Emotional and Behavioral
Problems Following Traumatic Brain Injury*

Megan Preece, BSc BA(Hons), MS
School of Psychology
The University of Queensland
School of Applied Psychology
Griffith University
Brisbane, Queensland, Australia
Chapter 78: Driving After Traumatic Brain Injury

Amanda M. Reinsfelder, MS, ATP
Assistive Technology Specialist
TBI Section of the Occupational Therapy Department
Bethesda, MD
*Chapter 71: Assistive Technology for People With Traumatic Brain
Injuries*

Evan R. Reiter, MD, FACS
Associate Professor, Vice Chair, Residency Program Director
Department of Otolaryngology – Head and Neck Surgery
Virginia Commonwealth University Health System
Richmond, VA
Chapter 48: Smell and Taste

Tara Rhine, MD
Clinical Fellow
Department of Pediatrics, Division of Emergency Medicine
Cincinnati Children's Hospital Medical Center
Cincinnati, OH
Chapter 34: Pediatric Traumatic Brain Injury: Special Considerations

Joseph H. Ricker, PhD
Associate Professor
Department of Physical Medicine and Rehabilitation
University of Pittsburgh School of Medicine
Pittsburgh, PA
Chapter 16: Functional Neuroimaging

Claudia S. Robertson, MD
Professor
Department of Neurosurgery
Baylor College of Medicine
Houston, TX
Chapter 23: Critical Care

Bradford Ross, PhD
Neuropsychologist
Department of Neurorehabilitation and Neuropsychology
Children's Specialized Hospital
Mountainside, NJ
*Chapter 36: Pediatric Neuropsychological Issues and Cognitive
    Rehabilitation*

Jose J. Sanchez, MD
Head Trauma/Neuro Critical Care Fellow
University of Miami Miller School of Medicine/Jackson
    Memorial Hospital
Miami, FL
*Chapter 25: Development of Acute Care Guidelines and Effect on
    Outcome*

M. Elizabeth Sandel, MD
Chief, Physical Medicine and Rehabilitation, Napa/Solano
    Service Area and Director, Research and Training
Department of Physical Medicine and Rehabilitation
Kaiser Foundation Rehabilitation Center
Vallejo, CA
Clinical Professor (Adjunct)
Department of Physical Medicine and Rehabilitation
University of California, Davis School of Medicine
Sacramento, CA
Chapter 55: Sexuality and Intimacy Following Traumatic Brain Injury

Joanne Scandale, PhD, CRC. CCM, LMHC
Rehabilitation Counselor
Department of Physical Medicine & Rehabilitation
Upstate University Hospital
Syracuse, NY
Chapter 5: Education, Training, and Certification

Kathryn Wilder Schaaf, PhD
Postdoctoral Fellow
Department of Physical Medicine & Rehabilitation
Virginia Commonwealth University
Richmond, VA
Chapter 60: Neuropsychological Assessment and Treatment Planning
*Chapter 80: Practical Approaches to Family Assessment and
    Intervention*

Richard M. Schein, PhD
Research Scientist
Department of Rehabilitation Science and Technology
University of Pittsburgh
Pittsburgh, PA
*Chapter 71: Assistive Technology for People With Traumatic Brain
    Injuries*

Nicholas Schiff, MD
Professor of Neurology and Neuroscience
Professor of Public Health
Well Cornell Medical College
Attending Neurologist
New York-Presbyterian Hospital
New York, NY
*Chapter 32: Assessment and Rehabilitive Management of Individuals
    With Disorders of Consciousness*

Christian N. Shenouda, MD
Physician
Center for Neuroscience and Regenerative Medicine (CNRM)
National Institutes of Health (NIH)
Bethesda, MD
Chapter 49: Complications Associated With Immobility

Neil T. Shepard, PhD
Professor of Audiology
Mayo Clinic
Mayo Medical School
Rochester, MN
Chapter 47: Balance and Dizziness

Capt. Benjamin Siebert, MD
Chief Resident
Department of Physical Medicine & Rehabilitation/Rehabilitation
    Institute of Michigan
Wayne State University School of Medicine
Detroit, MI
Chapter 56: Post-Traumatic Headache

Jonathan M. Silver, MD
Clinical Professor of Psychiatry
Department of Psychiatry
New York University School of Medicine
New York, NY
Chapter 73: Pharmacotherapy of Cognitive Impairment
Chapter 74: Pharmacotherapy of Neuropsychiatric Disturbances

Noah Silverberg, PhD
Psychologist
Department of Acquired Brain Injury
GF Strong Rehab Centre
Clinical Assistant Professor
Department of Medicine, Division of Physical Medicine &
    Rehabilitation
University of British Columbia
Vancouver, British Columbia, Canada
*Chapter 30: Conceptualizing Outcome from Mild Traumatic Brain
    Injury*

Eric Singman, MD, PhD
Division Chief, General Eye Services Clinic
Wilmer Eye Institute
Johns Hopkins University School of Medicine
Baltimore, MD
Chapter 45: Evaluating and Treating Visual Dysfunction

Stephen W. Smith, PhD
ARRT Postdoctoral Fellow
Department of Physical Medicine and Rehabilitation
Virginia Commonwealth University
Richmond, VA
Chapter 60: Neuropsychological Assessment and Treatment Planning

Eric T. Spier, MD
Medical Director
Department of Rehabilitation
Highlands Regional Rehabilitation Hospital
Department of Neuro Rehabilitation
Mentis El Paso, LLP
El Paso, TX
Chapter 26: Acute Rehabilitation

Michelle L. Sporner, MS, CRC
Instructor, Rehabilitation Counseling
Department of Rehabilitation Science and Technology
University of Pittsburgh
Pittsburgh, PA
*Chapter 71: Assistive Technology for People With Traumatic Brain
   Injuries*

Donald G. Stein, PhD
Asa G. Candler Professor and Distinguished Professor
Department of Emergency Medicine
Emory University
Atlanta, GA
*Chapter 13: Concepts of Central Nervous System Plasticity and Their
   Implications for Recovery After Brain Damage*

Harriet Straus, BSN, MAOM
Nurse Manager Rehabilitation Units, VCUHS
Department of Rehabilitation Nursing
Virginia Commonwealth University Health System
Richmond, VA
Chapter 27: Neurorehabilitation Nursing

David E. Sugerman, MD, MPH
Medical Officer
LCDR U.S. Public Health Service
Division of Injury Response
Centers for Disease Control and Prevention
Atlanta, GA
*Chapter 8: Traumatic Brain Injury Epidemiology and Public Health
   Issues*

Katherine J. Sullivan, PhD, PT
Associate Professor of Clinical Physical Therapy
Division of Biokinesiology & Physical Therapy at the Ostrow
   School of Dentistry
University of Southern California
Los Angeles, CA
Chapter 69: Movement Rehabilitation

Pamela S. Targett, Med
Director of Special Projects
Rehabilitation Research and Training Center
Virginia Commonwealth University
Richmond, VA
Chapter 81: Return to Work Following Traumatic Brain Injury

Laura A. Taylor, PhD
Licensed Clinical Psychologist
Village Family Psychiatry
Richmond, VA
Chapter 60: Neuropsychological Assessment and Treatment Planning

**Sir Graham Teasdale, MB, BS, MD, FRCS, FRCP,
   F Med Sci, FRSE**
Emeritus Professor of Neurosurgery
Department of Mental Health and Well Being
University of Glasgow
Glasgow, Scotland
Chapter 2: History of Acute Care and Rehabilitation and Head Injury

Olli Tenovuo, MD, PhD
Adjunct Professor of Neurology and Neurotraumatology
Finnish Brain Injury Research and Development
University of Turku and Turku University Hospital
Turku, Finland
Chapter 4: International Systems of Care and Research Agendas

Bonnie Todis, PhD
Senior Fellow
Center on Brain Injury Research and Training
Teaching Research Institute, Western Oregon University
Eugene, OR
*Chapter 37: Educational Issues and School Reentry for Students With
   Traumatic Brain Injury*

Joan Toglia, PhD, OTR/L
Professor and Program Director
Graduate Occupational Therapy Program
Mercy College
Dobbs Ferry, NY
Professional Associate
Department of Rehabilitation Medicine
New York Presbyterian–Weill Cornell Medical
New York, NY
*Chapter 70: Therapy for Activities of Daily Living: Theoretical and
   Practical Perspectives*

Alan R. Towne, MD, MPH
Professor of Neurology, Epidemiology and Community
   Health/Director, Epilepsy Center of Excellence
Department of Neurology
Virginia Commonwealth University/McGuire Veterans
   Affairs Hospital
Richmond, VA
Chapter 39: Post-Traumatic Seizures and Epilepsy

Margaret A. Turk, MD
Professor
Department of Physical Medicine & Rehabilitation and Pediatrics
Vice Chairman
Department of Physical Medicine & Rehabilitation
SUNY Upstate Medical University
Syracuse, NY
*Chapter 5: Education, Training, and Certification for Health Care
   Providers*

Lynne Turner-Stokes, ARCM, MA, MBBS, DM, FRCP
Herbert Dunhill Professor of Rehabilitation
Department of Palliative Care Policy and Rehabilitation
King's College London
London, UK
Consultant Physician in Rehabilitation Medicine, Clinical
   Director
Regional Rehabilitation Unit
Northwick Park Hospital
London, Middlesex, UK
Chapter 3: Health Policy: United States and International Perspectives

Janet Siantz Tyler, PhD
Brain Injury Education Consultant/Trainer
Private Practice
Kansas City, KS
*Chapter 37: Educational Issues and School Reentry for Students With
   Traumatic Brain Injury*

Carolyn A. Unsworth, PhD, AccOT, OTR
Professor
Department of Occupational Therapy
La Trobe University
Melbourne, Victoria, Australia
Adjunct Visiting Professor
Department of Rehabilitation
Jönköping University
Jönköping, Sweden
Chapter 78: Driving After Traumatic Brain Injury

Marine Vernet, PhD
Research Fellow
Berenson-Allen Center for Noninvasive Brain Stimulation
Beth Israel Deaconess Medical Center, Harvard Medical School
Boston, MA
Chapter 17: Functional Neuroimaging

David C. Viano, MD, PhD
Principal
ProBiomechanis LLC
Bloomfield, MI
Adjunct Professor
Biomedical Engineering, Wayne State University
Detroit, MI
Chapter 10: Biomechanics of Brain Injury

Vincent Vicci, OD
Clinical Directo
Neuro-optometric Rehabilitation Clinic
Kessler Institute
West Orang, NJ
Chapter 45: Evaluating and Treating Visual Dysfunction

Amy K. Wagner, MD
Associate Professor and Vice-Chair Research
Department of Physical Medicine and Rehabilitation
University of Pittsburgh School of Medicine
Pittsburgh, PA
Chapter 7: Conducting Research in Traumatic Brain Injury: Current Concepts and Issues
Chapter 16: Functional Neuroimaging

Hongwu Wang, PhD
Post-Doctoral Researcher
Department of Rehabilitation Science and Technology
University of Pittsburgh
Pittsburgh, PA
Chapter 71: Assistive Technology for People With Traumatic Brain Injuries

Roger O. Weed, BS, MS, PhD
Professor Retired
Counseling & Psychological Services
Georgia State University
Atlanta, GA
Chapter 86: Life Care Planning After Traumatic Brain Injury: Clinical and Forensic Issues

Paul H. Wehman, PhD
Director
Rehabilitation Research and Training Center
Virginia Commonwealth University
Richmond, VA
Chapter 81: Return to Work Following Traumatic Brain Injury

Michael D. West, PhD
Research Associate
Rehabilitation Research and Training Center
Virginia Commonwealth University
Richmond, VA
Chapter 81: Return to Work Following Traumatic Brain Injury

Stuart A. Yablon, MD
Associate Professor
Division of Physical Medicine & Rehabilitation
University of Alberta
Medical Lead
Brain Injury Program
Glenrose Rehabilitation Hospital
Chapter 39: Post-Traumatic Seizures and Epilepsy

Arthur F. Yeager, MS, OTR/L
Occupational Therapist
Department of Orthopedics & Rehabilitation
Walter Reed National Military Medical Center
Bethesda, MD
Chapter 71: Assistive Technology for People With Traumatic Brain Injuries

Joshua C. Yelverton, MD
Resident
Department of Otolaryngology–Head and Neck Surgery
Virginia Commonwealth University Health System
Richmond, VA
Chapter 48: Smell and Taste

Shoji Yokobori, MD, PhD
Visiting Researcher
Department of Neurosurgery
University of Miami Miller School of Medicine
Miami, FL
Chapter 11: Pathobiology of Primary Traumatic Brain Injury

Esther L. Yuh, MD, PhD
Assistant Professor in Residence
Department of Radiology and Biomedical Imaging
University of California at San Francisco
San Francisco, CA
Chapter 15: Structural Neuroimaging

Ross D. Zafonte, DO
Earle P. and Ida S. Charlton Professor and Chair
Department of Physical Medicine and Rehabilitation
Harvard Medical School
Vice President of Medical Affairs, Research and Education
Spaulding Rehabilitation Network
Chief, Physical Medicine and Rehabilitation
Massachusetts General Hospital
Boston, MA
Chapter 1: Clinical Continuum of Care and Natural History
Chapter 4: International Systems of Care and Research Agendas
Chapter 72: Neuropharmacology: A Rehabilitation Perspective

Giuseppe Zappalà, MD
Behavioral Neurologist
Behavioral Neurology Unit–Alzheimer's Center Cognitive Rehabilitation Unit
Garibaldi Hospital–Nesima
Catania, Italy
Chapter 59: Cognitive Impairments

Nathan D. Zasler, MD, FAAPM&R, FAADEP, DAAPM, CBIST
CEO and Medical Director
Concussion Care Centre of Virginia, Ltd.
CEO & Medical Director
Tree of Life Services, Inc.
Medical Director, iWalk Program
Sheltering Arms Hospitals
Professor, Affiliate
VCU Department of Physical Medicine and Rehabilitation
Richmond, VA
Associate Professor, Adjunct
Department of Physical Medicine and Rehabilitation
University of Virginia
Charlottesville, VA
Chairperson, International Brain Injury Association
Chapter 1: Clinical Continuum of Care and Natural History
Chapter 29: Mild Traumatic Brain Injury
*Chapter 30: Conceptualizing Outcome from Mild Traumatic Brain
    Injury*
Chapter 56: Post-Traumatic Headache
*Chapter 57: Post-Traumatic Pain Disorders: Medical Assessment and
    Management*
*Chapter 58: Psychological Assessment and Managemen of Post-
    Traumatic Pain*
Chapter 84: Clinicolegal Issues
Chapter 85: Assessing and Addressing Response Bias

George A. Zitnay, BS, MS, PhD
Professor
Department of Health and Rehabilitation
University of Pittsburgh
Pittsburgh, PA
Department of Physical Therapy
St. Francis University
Lorretto, PA
Chapter 2: History of Acute Care and Rehabilitation of Head Injury

Felise S. Zollman, MD
Director, Memory & Cognitive Disorders Program
Department of Neurology
NorthShore University Health System
Glenview, IL
Chapter 76: Complementary and Alternative Medicine

I

PERSPECTIVES ON CLINICAL CARE, PUBLIC HEALTH, AND RESEARCH

1

Clinical Continuum of Care and Natural History

Douglas I. Katz, Nathan D. Zasler, and Ross D. Zafonte

INTRODUCTION

Systems of care for patients with traumatic brain injury (TBI) should account for the particular characteristics of this disorder. First, TBI is a large problem. TBI is among the most common of serious, disabling neurological disorders. It is a major problem in all societies. In the United States, it is estimated that 1.7 million TBIs occur every year, and there are an estimated 3.2 million people living with disability from TBI (1,2) (see Coronado et al., Chapter 8, for a full discussion of epidemiology of TBI). Systems of care must allocate resources for the large number of people who are affected by the disorder.

Second, TBI is more commonly a younger and older person's disorder (3). Individuals younger than 30 years old, mostly males, make up the largest proportion of those affected by TBI. TBI frequently impacts people in the later stages of adolescent development or early adulthood. Therefore, TBI typically disrupts important periods of the life cycle that involve completing formal education, maturing social development, emerging vocational productivity, achieving adult independence, beginning spousal relationships, and child rearing. Older persons present particular problems related to aging, including comorbidities, slower and less complete recovery and vulnerability to complications of injury and treatment (4) (see Levine and Flanagan, Chapter 28). Systems of care must address needs that include special educational requirements, independent living, vocational training and supports, and supports for family members.

Third, TBI commonly affects people with preexisting problems such as substance abuse, learning disability, behavioral disorders, psychiatric disorders, and other risk factors that may make people more prone to injuries. In addition, persons with brain injury are more prone to psychiatric comorbidities and psychosocial difficulties following injury. Systems of care must consider these preinjury and postinjury issues with respect to injury prevention, their interactions with the clinical effects of injury, and potential detrimental influence on recovery from TBI.

Fourth, the most important and consistent effects of TBI involve cognitive, emotional, and behavioral functioning. Motor and sensory perceptual problems also occur in varying amounts, more likely in those with more severe injuries. Cognitive and behavioral problems present more challenges

to the health care system because they are often more difficult to recognize, characterize, and treat than traditional medical and physical problems. Persons with TBI may not have any physical markers or obvious signs of injury, although there may be profound effects on the individual's ability to function, resulting from cognitive and behavioral problems. Criteria for medical rehabilitation reimbursement, length of stay, and utilization decisions are often centered more on physical and motor issues that affect function and less on cognitive and behavioral treatment issues. Some insurance payers even exclude coverage for cognitive rehabilitation, although there is expanding evidence to support the efficacy of a variety of cognitive rehabilitation strategies and models (5,6) (see Cicerone, Chapter 61 on cognitive rehabilitation). Systems of care must support proper assessment and treatment of cognitive and behavioral problems after TBI, even though they may not fit the characteristics of medical rehabilitative systems that were originally developed for medical and physical disabilities (see Chapters 59–64).

Fifth, TBI, especially more severe injuries, can have a relatively extended natural history and lifelong effects. Recovery from TBI may be more protracted and extend over a relatively longer portion of the life span than most other acquired injuries or neurological disorders that evolve more quickly or affect persons at later stages of life. The natural history of TBI has a longer horizon than most other acquired injuries or neurological disorders of similar severity and systems of care for TBI need to recognize the potentially prolonged recovery timetable. Further, recovery after TBI has a somewhat predictable and characteristic course, with a variety of recognizable cognitive, behavioral, and sensorimotor syndromes at different stages of recovery. An appreciation of the natural history of TBI is essential in assessing the individual with TBI, applying treatment and services effectively and appropriately at different stages of recovery, and/or avoiding treatment that may be unnecessary or ineffective (see discussion on natural history subsequently).

Finally, TBI is a disorder with a wide variety of pathophysiological effects, a broad range of severities, and a multitude of problems that can occur as the result of injury. Persons with apparently similar injuries may have significant variation in their presentation, course of recovery, secondary problems, response to interventions, and ability to reintegrate into community. Systems of care should have a breadth of treatments and services to intervene for the variety of problems that can occur after TBI and the flexibility to move persons with TBI through the system as their needs change and evolve at different times postinjury.

THE DEVELOPMENT OF SYSTEMS OF CARE

The provision of a comprehensive continuum of care for persons with TBI is an enormous challenge given the characteristics of TBI outlined earlier and the wide range of services that should be provided to large numbers of people over relatively longer periods than most other disorders. This challenge is shared by consumers (persons with TBI and their families), providers (clinicians and facilities attempting to provide effective and efficient care), payers (health insurers—public and private—balancing coverage needs with financial pressures), and society, making choices about resource allocation and costs. Resources for patients with TBI include acute and postacute medical care; rehabilitative services in the hospital, at home, in the community, and in residential settings; psychosocial services; educational and vocational services; and a variety of other support services.

The development of systems of care for persons with TBI evolved in the 1970s and 1980s. In part, the systems that developed for care of patients with TBI were influenced by systems of care that were developed for those with spinal cord injury (SCI). Prior to development of specific programs for persons with TBI, patients were frequently treated in psychiatric facilities, nursing homes, or more general rehabilitation facilities. The Rehabilitation Services Administration and National Institute on Disability and Health Research (NIDHR) (which was to become NIDRR) that had funded SCI model systems in the early 1970s also funded 2 model system projects for TBI in 1978 at Stanford and New York Universities (7). The recommendations from these projects helped promote the development of interdisciplinary, dedicated TBI programs with services across the continuum of recovery. As programs began to develop, the lack of organized planning led to an initiative by the NIDRR under the Department of Education in 1987 to fund 5 TBI model systems demonstration projects (8). This has expanded to 16 TBI Model Systems Projects throughout the country in part aimed at gathering information to improve comprehensive systems of care for patients with TBI. The components of these model systems of care includes emergency medical services, acute neurosurgical care, comprehensive rehabilitation services, long-term interdisciplinary follow-up and rehabilitation services, as well as what were termed *optional services*, including behavior modification programs, home rehabilitation services, case management, and community living options (8). A key portion of this program has been longitudinal and project-specific–based research.

Beginning in the mid-1980s, the Commission on Accreditation of Rehabilitation Facilities (CARF), now known as CARF International, developed standards for TBI rehabilitative care by establishing specialized accreditation for TBI programs. CARF International provides accreditation for brain injury programs among five categories: comprehensive integrated inpatient rehabilitative program, outpatient medical rehabilitation program, home and community services, residential rehabilitation program, and vocational services.

An important development in TBI care was the TBI Act of 1996 passed by the Congress (P.L. 104-66) to "provide for the conduct of expanded studies and the establishment of innovative programs with respect to traumatic brain injury." Four provisions of the act included surveillance and prevention under the CDC; basic and applied research to improve diagnosis, therapeutics, and the continuum of clinical care conducted by the National Institutes of Health (NIH); a planning and implementation grant program to the states under the Health Resources and Services Administration (HRSA); and a consensus conference conducted by the National Center for Medical Rehabilitation and Research (NCMRR) at the NIH (9). The NIH consensus conference panel addressed the continuum of care for TBI in their conclusions. The recommendations included that "persons with TBI should have access to rehabilitation services through the entire course of recovery, which may last for many years after the injury" and that "community-based, nonmedical services should be components of the extended care and rehabilitation available to persons with TBI"(10).

Another important development in the care of persons with TBI in the United States has arisen from the needs of active duty military and veterans of the wars in Afghanistan and Iraq with TBI and post-traumatic stress disorder (PTSD). Systems of care have been developed and expanded among military centers and Veterans Affairs hospitals to screen, diagnose, and treat the large number or military personnel returning from the wars with TBI and PTSD. In 1992, the Congress created the Defense and Veterans Brain Injury Center (DVBIC) (originally the Defense and Veterans Head Injury Program) to integrate specialized TBI care, research, and education across military and veteran medical care systems and the role of DVBIC in TBI surveillance, care, and research has grown enormously in recent years. The Departments of Defense and Veterans Affairs have also played a major role in expanding support of research for TBI and clinical care practices and guidelines (e.g., Guidelines for Management of Concussion/mild TBI [11]) that will benefit both military and civilian care. (See Meyer et al., Chapter 33, for a discussion of TBI in the military.)

REALITIES OF THE MARKETPLACE

Although demonstration projects such as the TBI Model Systems have presented apparently effective systems of care for persons with TBI, the realities of the marketplace in the United States have presented challenges to providing such care and services to all those in need. Corrigan outlined 20 important challenges to meeting the needs of persons with TBI, within the categories of access, availability, appropriateness, and acceptability (9). Regarding access, the problems involve identifying and using services, even if they are available. There may be difficulties accessing information about available resources. Sometimes, it is difficult to determine what resources are covered by health insurance, and sometimes coverage is denied even after services are delivered. Families and care providers usually lack road maps to guide access to appropriate resources and points of entry into publicly funded system may be unclear. Service systems may have artificial barriers created by narrow eligibility criteria. Services are often fragmented and not well coordinated.

Corrigan pointed out several availability issues for which the main limiting factor is funding. In the United States, even if available, health insurance may not cover needed services, or may direct individuals to centers that are less familiar with the care of persons with TBI. Further, lack of payer support may limit the availability of some services to begin with. Many persons with TBI have no health care funding at all at the time of injury and present state budget constraints are further threatening the Medicaid program. When available, health insurance typically covers acute care more fully than rehabilitative care. Coverage usually becomes incrementally more difficult across the continuum of care, from inpatient to outpatient to residential and community services. Health insurance coverage also tends to be more restrictive for cognitive and behavioral services as opposed to more traditional physical, rehabilitative, and medical treatment. For many cases in the United States, coverage for services has to shift from private to public sources such as Medicaid and Medicare over the course of recovery because of limits in coverage for longer term care in many policies. Public funding has further restraints on long-term coverage. Several states have developed a system of Medicaid waivers to provide long-term home and community-based services that would otherwise be covered only for institutional settings, such as nursing homes. The fragmentation and limitations in financing of care and services can create a nightmare of coordination for persons with brain injury, their families, and service providers. Clinicians who coordinate care for persons with brain injury must become aware of the complexities of reimbursement and the array of alternative sources of funding for TBI care and support in their community.

Other issues affecting the availability of services include geographic limitations, lack of transportation, paucity of appropriate, affordable housing, limitations in resources for children with special needs, and a lack of resources for behavioral and other long-term problems after TBI (9). Patients with TBI in rural communities have special challenges in finding services within a reasonable distance. Even when available in a nearby area, transport to and from these services can be a major problem and home services may not be sufficiently expert or available at all for this population. The ability to provide the full array of services, to all age groups, within a reasonable proximity to a person with TBI, with full funding support is an enormous challenge that may never be fully satisfied.

The appropriateness of available resources is also a common problem. Sometimes, the reason for inappropriate services is dictated by payer constraints. For instance, since the main payer for long-term care services is Medicaid, if waivers to support home and community services are not available, patients with TBI who cannot return home may be placed in nursing homes, even though community-based services may be more appropriate. Even if services are available, programs and professional providers may lack the knowledge and expertise to serve this population. Generalists in a particular discipline or specialty may not have the skills for proper assessment or treatment of the patient with TBI. Accreditation programs such as CARF and the American Academy of Certified Brain Injury Specialists (AACBIS) have attempted to set standards and credentialing to assure appropriateness of programming and expertise in treating persons with TBI (see also Chapter 6 on training and certification). Nevertheless, such expertise may simply not be available in some geographic areas or at certain levels of care. Sometimes, erroneous services are applied because of

this lack of expertise, but at times services may be improperly or needlessly applied even by those with expertise. Inaccurate diagnosis, inappropriate application of treatment at a particular stage of recovery, use of unproven or ineffective treatments, or application of effective treatment to those for whom it would not be of benefit are examples. Use of accurate diagnosis and prognosis is necessary to avoid some of these problems of inappropriate treatment (see section on Natural History). Sometimes, even appropriate services are not fully relevant to a person's and family's needs at a particular time or in a particular environment. The acceptability of these services to the goals of the individual with the TBI and their caretakers and how services promote a person's self-actualization is another challenge to the TBI service marketplace (9).

ESSENTIAL COMPONENTS OF THE CLINICAL CONTINUUM

The continuum of care for patients with TBI occurs in a variety of settings. Figure 1-1 illustrates the different types of care and how patients may move through these components. The flow through these services may not be linear, and patients may enter or leave the system of care at different points or reverse directions, based on injury severity, individual needs, and the dictates of the marketplace.

Prevention

The earliest aspect of the care continuum involves public health issues prior to injury occurrence. Injury prevention is an essential part of trauma care systems. The TBI Act of 1996 charged the CDC with the responsibility for prevention, in addition to surveillance, to assess factors that increase risk of TBI and those that are protective. At the international level, the World Health Organization has played a major role in surveillance and prevention. Injury prevention programs generally include 3 components: programs designed to alter behavior and improve decision making to increase self-protection; product improvement to minimize chance of injury or protect the individual in an accident; and legislation and public policies that require individuals to follow safety guidelines. Prevention of TBI includes several efforts such as reducing alcohol-related injuries, preventing falls, preventing violence, promoting safe practices in sports, promoting helmet and seatbelt use, enhancing safe driving practices, and improving vehicle safety (see Kneer and Elovic, Chapter 9, for a discussion of primary prevention).

Emergency Medical Services

Since the 1980s, emergency trauma systems have developed throughout the United States and have led to improved survival and recovery (12–14). Mortality for those who reach the hospital has been reduced from nearly 50% to less than 18% (1). Regional trauma systems have developed to promote quick evacuation using ground or air transport to Level I and Level II trauma centers from the field or from Level III and IV trauma centers when necessary for more serious injuries. The Level I and II trauma centers have full-time

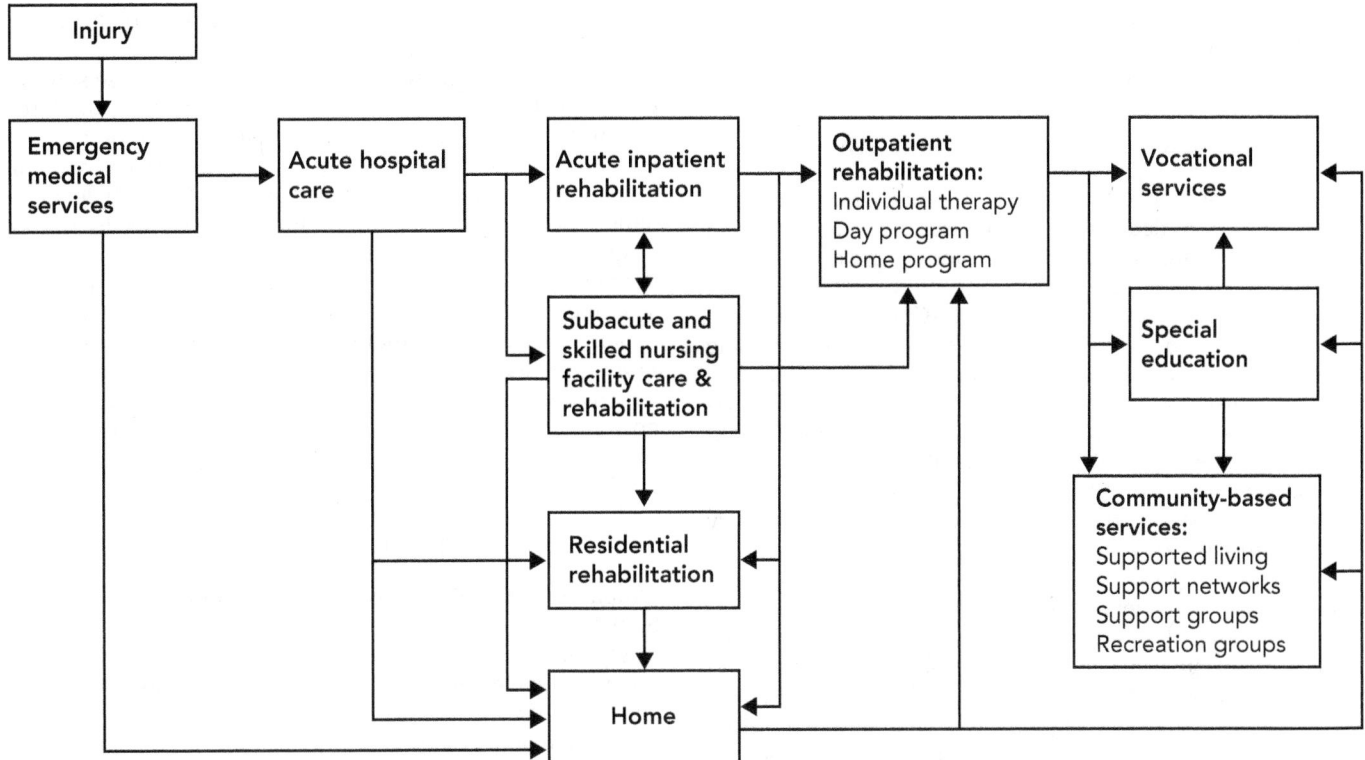

FIGURE 1-1 Usual flow of patients through the clinical continuum of care. Choices of services and direction of flow will be based on severity, stage of recovery, patient's needs, availability of resources, availability of home and community supports, and constraints of the marketplace.

intensive care, imaging, neurosurgical, and other trauma subspecialists. The Brain Trauma Foundation (BTF) Guidelines for Prehospital Management of Traumatic Brain Injury have played a role in improving emergency prehospital care (13,15). Recognition of mild TBI and patient education and follow-up have improved, but proper diagnosis, patient education, and referral for proper follow-up is still lacking for many patients (16) (see Chapters 29–31 for further discussion of diagnosis and treatment of mild TBI.)

Acute Hospital Care

Patients with TBI who are admitted for acute hospital care range from those who need a period of observation to recognize secondary neurological deterioration and neurosurgical complications that may ensue after a delay to those with comorbidities that require hospital care and to those with more severe brain injury that may require intensive care management. Acute neurosurgical and intensive care for patients with TBI have improved over the last 2 decades with better survival and outcomes (17). Evidence-based guidelines for acute TBI care, including the use of intracranial pressure monitoring, have contributed to better outcomes (18–21) (see also Chapters 22–24 on acute care).

   Rehabilitation assessment and early interventions should take place a short time after admission in the acute hospital setting. Subsequent decisions for rehabilitative care are made as the patient progresses toward medical and surgical stability, when the severity of injury and clinical rehabilitation needs become more apparent. The pathway toward acute

inpatient rehabilitation vs outpatient or subacute care is largely based on injury severity and pace of recovery. Generally, patients with severe injuries (e.g., unconsciousness of a day or more or post-traumatic amnesia [PTA] and confusional states of at least days to weeks or patients with large focal lesions [see section on Natural History subsequently]) move to acute inpatient rehabilitation facilities (IRFs). Constraints related to marketplace issues may affect this decision. For instance, some health care plans in the United States will not support admission to IRFs if a patient has few traditional physical rehabilitation needs (e.g., needs little or no help ambulating) even if the patient has profound cognitive and behavioral disturbances related to the injury. Patients with less severe injuries generally return home and may need outpatient rehabilitation services. A proportion of patients with moderate injury may benefit from at least a brief inpatient rehabilitation stay, depending on their circumstances. Patients who are slower to recover and who typically have more prolonged disorders of consciousness may require extended care in the acute hospital. Some patients with more severe injuries and prolonged disorders of consciousness are transferred to subacute or skilled nursing facility (SNF) care instead of inpatient rehabilitation. In many systems, such persons may be lost to the follow-up with clinicians who have expertise in caring for patients with very severe TBI and disorders of consciousness. Strong consideration should be given to transferring such patients to facilities with special expertise in the assessment and care of patients who are unconscious or minimally conscious (usually in acute inpatient rehabilitation or specialized subacute facilities) because these patients are vulnerable to secondary complications and may have significant potential for further recovery, albeit at a slower pace (22).

Acute Inpatient Rehabilitation

Acute inpatient rehabilitation may occur on general rehabilitation units or in dedicated brain injury units that are within acute care facilities or part of freestanding postacute hospitals (usually either an inpatient rehabilitation facility [IRF] or a long-term acute care hospital [LTACH]). Admission criteria to IRFs involve (a) an intensity of medical and nursing care needs that requires full-time physician and rehabilitation specialist monitoring and specialized rehabilitative nursing expertise and (b) functional deficits that would benefit from higher level of rehabilitation treatment intensity (usually designated at a minimum duration of 3 hours a day). Patients are best served in programs dedicated to brain injury care or those with a significant proportion of staff with expertise in managing brain injury. Rehabilitation teams usually include case managers; physical, occupational, and speech therapy staff; rehabilitation nurses; nursing assistants; psychologists; neuropsychologists; rehabilitation physicians (usually physiatrist, rehabilitation neurologist, or neuropsychiatrist); primary care physicians; and a variety of other consultant medical specialists. Other disciplines such as social workers, rehabilitation technicians, therapy assistants, behavior specialists, recreation therapists, other subspecialty therapists, chaplains, and attorneys may also contribute to care. Expertise in managing behavioral problems and assuring patient, family, and staff safety is important in managing patients at this level of care because patients in agitated confusional states are usually managed at this level of care (see the following texts). Family education to familiarize them with the problems and needs of persons with brain injury is essential at this level of care, especially for those that will transition home from acute inpatient rehabilitation. The decision regarding the next level of care depends on the patient's medical stability, level of dependency, safety, and whether the person's needs can be adequately met at home or requires further care in a facility. Patients with severe TBI typically still require some supervision and perhaps physical assistance for self-care and mobility when they are ready to be discharged from acute inpatient rehabilitation (see Chapter 26).

Subacute and Skilled Nursing Facility Rehabilitation

Patients with TBI are usually admitted to this level of care from acute hospital care or acute inpatient rehabilitation. Therapies are provided at a lower level of intensity than in acute inpatient rehabilitation, and the level of medical monitoring is less frequent than acute inpatient rehabilitation. There are many programs at this level that specialize in neurorehabilitation, and it is certainly preferable if this level of care occurs in programs with special expertise in brain injury management. Specialized neurobehavioral treatment units in SNFs are available in some areas for patients with more persistent behavioral regulation problems. As noted earlier, some SNFs may offer specialized care for patients with TBI with prolonged impairments of conscious-

ness. The availability of specialized subacute and SNF facilities may be limited in some areas because of market constraints. Care for the needs of TBI patients in these settings may be costly, exceeding the usual reimbursement standards for this level of care. Alternative funding sources or variance in reimbursement standards may be necessary to maintain more specialized subacute or SNF care. Often, SNF level rehabilitation care takes place in more general facilities and, frequently, younger patients with TBI are in the minority among an older group of patients with other disorders such as dementia. Lengths of stay at this level of care varies but usually lasts 1 or more months; a minority of patients transition to unskilled residential levels of care at the same facilities. A large proportion of patients transition home and may go on to outpatient rehabilitation or other outpatient services.

Outpatient Rehabilitation

Outpatient rehabilitation can take on several different forms. Sometimes, it consists of individual therapies involving physical, occupational, and speech therapists. There may be other available services, including psychology, neuropsychology, and therapeutic recreation. The team may be led by a case manager, and they may provide other coordinated activities such as group treatments. Usually, rehabilitation at this level is less coordinated than inpatient treatment, and therapists provide care more autonomously. This type of care may occur in the setting of the home through visiting nurses or other agencies, on the premises of an acute hospital, a rehabilitation hospital, or in a distinct outpatient rehabilitation facility.

A more coordinated form of outpatient rehabilitation may take place in a day program, with a full array of therapies, group treatments and group activities, case management, and regular team meetings to set goals and review progress. More holistic programs may include a psychotherapeutic milieu associated with the therapy programming. These programs are often in naturalistic community settings and take advantage of this location to set up activities to foster community reentry treatment goals.

The length and intensity of treatment is determined by the patient's needs but is largely constrained by health insurance payer contracts and public funding policies limiting duration of care and range of covered services. Following outpatient rehabilitation, additional community-based services may be provided.

Residential Rehabilitation

Group residence programs may provide services at various stages after injury. These programs may offer individual therapies and group therapies, as well as resources to foster independent living skills. Residential programs may be aimed at patients just discharged from acute hospital settings, acute inpatient rehabilitation, or for those later in the process of recovery who require more structured supervised setting, more specialized programming, and cannot be in their own home setting. There are usually only part-time nursing services and programs may or may not provide physician services. Those states with more generous auto insurance benefits tend to have more extensive residential programs. Staffing includes a mix of professional therapists, other professional disciplines, and lay staff. Patients may progress in levels of independence in these settings and go back home or to other long-term living arrangements, such as supported living (see Other Community-based Services section subsequently) after this level of care.

Vocational Services

For most persons with TBI, return to work is the most important long-term rehabilitation goal and measure of treatment success. Return to some sort of productive activity is an essential part of societal reintegration and life satisfaction after brain injury and an important part of the continuum of care. In the United States, the states receive federal money to operate vocational rehabilitation programs to provide vocational rehabilitation services to individuals with disabilities. Services support reeducation, training, and worksite-related support services. Even those with severe injuries, who may not qualify for regular marketplace jobs, are eligible for services under this mandate. Supported employment has become one of the important vocational rehabilitation strategies for getting persons with disabilities back to employment in regular worksites. These services are most successful when coordinated with outpatient rehabilitative care and assessments. Many of these programs have been underfunded, and it has been a problem to provide intensive ongoing supports that are necessary to keep some persons with TBI employed. Many states have adopted innovative programs to extend funding using resources such as Medicaid waivers to improve services and employment retention (23) (see Chapter 81).

Special Education

Education services are a necessary component of the continuum of care for children and adolescents with TBI. TBI became a part of the federal Individuals with Disability Education Act in 1990. This federal law mandates that the education needs of school-age children with TBI, among other disabilities, will be provided by the public schools by mainstreaming in the classroom, in special classrooms, or in specialized schools. Programming must include any necessary rehabilitation services. Services should be planned and monitored using an individualized educational program (IEP). Students often transition from inpatient or outpatient rehabilitation to school-based services, sometimes beginning with home tutoring. Ylvisaker and colleagues have made several recommendations for assessment, intervention, student support, educator training, family support, and system flexibility to better serve the particular educational and rehabilitative needs of students after TBI (24) (see Glang, Chapter 37, for a discussion of education issues.)

Other Community-Based Services

Persons with TBI may require other ongoing care and supports after formal rehabilitative care has ended. These home-based and community-based services are more fragmented and less readily available. Patients who are unable to live independently and are not relying on home supervision by family or friends require supported living environments. Previously, this usually meant placement in nursing homes, generably a less desirable alternative for younger persons with TBI. A growing number of states with Medicaid waiver programs have been able to provide supported living services in the community using such models as supervised group homes, foster homes, and personal care attendants. Several other models have been developed.

Community support networks and support groups for persons with TBI and their families are important resources. One such support network, the Clubhouse Model, adapted for persons with TBI in the 1980s from the psychiatric community, provides a setting for members and volunteers to participate in social, recreational, and work-related activities. Such models provide a cost-effective method to promote practical, functional living skills. Support groups for persons with TBI and their families are often sponsored by state chapters of the Brain Injury Association of America (BIAA).

Other necessary community services include provisions for transportation for those who are unable to drive or ride public transportation. Respite care to provide time-off for full-time caretakers of persons with severe disability or other particularly taxing impairments (i.e., neurobehavioral disorders) after TBI is another important need. Legal services, financial and estate planning, recreational and diversional activities, mental health services, and treatment of substance abuse must also be considered part of community-based system of care for people with TBI.

Case Management

Fragmentation and lack of coordination of care is one of the major problems in finding and applying proper services for the individual with TBI. Case managers within institutions and in the community play an essential role in coordinating services. Case managers collaborate with others, including patients, families, providers, and payers to assess, plan, implement, coordinate, and monitor services to meet an individual's needs and promote favorable outcomes in a cost-effective manner. In addition to coordinating care within the TBI system, case managers must coordinate treatment in other areas such as chronic pain, mental health, and other medical specialty areas. Case managers and life care planners may develop proposals outlining the anticipated, life-long care needs of persons with TBI (see Weed and Berens, Chapter 86 on life care planning).

SERVICE DELIVERY IN RELATION TO NATURAL HISTORY OF TRAUMATIC BRAIN INJURY

Accurate diagnosis and an appreciation of the natural history of TBI are useful in formulating treatment plans and assuring appropriateness of services along the continuum of care. This effort involves assessing a person's brain injury in the context of pathophysiologic damage, associated clinical neurobehavioral syndromes, stage of recovery, and anticipated course of recovery based on knowledge of brain–behavior relationships and natural history (25). The formulation must also consider interaction with noninjury factors such as age and psychosocial issues, associated injuries, premorbid problems, comorbidities, and later complications. This understanding helps in determining where the patient is along the path of recovery and in projecting expectations for subsequent recovery to inform treatment planning with respect to treatment setting, treatment strategies, treatment goals, and length of stay. It may also help avoid unnecessary treatment for problems that may be expected to resolve as part of the natural course of recovery (e.g., PTA or confusional agitation) or problems with worse prognosis that may be more difficult to treat (e.g., amnesia after extensive, bilateral hippocampal injury, or behavior dysregulation after massive bilateral, orbital, prefrontal, and temporal polar damage). Such an understanding of natural history also helps determine when clinical syndromes do not fit the expected path of recovery, suggesting possible secondary neurological complications (e.g., hydrocephalus, chronic subdural hematomas), the influence of noninjury factors (medical, iatrogenic, psychogenic, or secondary gain), or misdiagnosis of injury type and severity. The clinical natural history of TBI can be defined in the context of focal or diffuse neuropathologic events (see Yokobori and Bullock Chapter 11; Kochanek et al., Chapter 12; Kothari, Chapter 18; and Bigler, Chapter 19 for extended discussions of TBI neuropathology and outcome). The critical pathophysiologic factors are the type, distribution, severity, and location of these combined neuropathological events after brain injury. Although focal and diffuse pathological processes are often intermingled and have common secondary injury consequences, it is useful to consider them separately for the purposes of clinical diagnosis. Precise clinical pathophysiologic diagnosis is challenging, especially with respect to diffuse and secondary injuries, for which there are as yet no standardized, direct clinical, diagnostic probes. Protein biomarkers and neuroimaging techniques such as diffusion tensor imaging and MR spectroscopy hold promise as clinical diagnostic biomarkers of diffuse and secondary injury (see Bigler, Chapter 19 and Ricker, Chapter 16).

Diffuse Injury

Diffuse axonal injury represents the main diffuse pathological process, but it is associated with a host of secondary pathophysiological phenomena (see Chapter 12). The natural history of diffuse injury is characterized by a recognizable pattern of stages of recovery that occur across the wide spectrum of severity. Injury severity determines the duration of recovery stages and levels of impairment at each stage of recovery. These stages can be combined into 3 principal phases of recovery from the acute to chronic stages: (a) loss of consciousness (LOC), (b) post-traumatic confusion and PTA, and (c) postconfusional restoration of cognitive function. These form the basis for the main indices of clinical severity for TBI, and these indices can help project rough approximations for time course of recovery and probabilities for outcome (26–30) (see Kothari, Chapter 18). These 3 phases of recovery appear to be proportionally related in patients with diffuse injury; each subsequent phase is typically several fold longer than the previous one (26). Their proportionality in patients with diffuse injury, although variable, can contribute to predicting time course of recovery. For instance, there was a

predictable relationship between the duration of unconsciousness (i.e., LOC) and duration of confusion/PTA in a series of patients with diffuse injury defined by a linear regression model that predicted nearly 60% of the variance—PTA (weeks) = 0.4 × LOC (days) + 3.6 (26). This model was confirmed in a separate cohort of 228 patients (31). Longer PTA was observed in older patients, especially those older than age 40, or if a focal frontal lesion was present. Predicting PTA may aid rehabilitative treatment planning with respect to length of stay decisions, treatment choices for confusional agitation, and other treatment issues at this stage of recovery. The severity of post-traumatic confusion and presence of certain components of confusion, such as psychotic-like features, have predictive value for rehabilitation outcomes and employability (32–34).

Patients with the least severe diffuse injuries (mild concussion) evolve through LOC (if complete LOC occurs at all) in seconds to minutes and through PTA usually in minutes to hours, followed by a postconfusional phase typically lasting days to weeks. In mild TBI, the transition through the earliest stages may be brief, unwitnessed, and difficult to document. Patients with severe TBI may require days to weeks to evolve through LOC, weeks to months to resolve confusion and PTA, and months to years to evolve through the postconfusional residual recovery phase. The course of recovery after severe TBI is among the longest observed after neurological damage. Dynamic changes in neuropsychological functioning have been observed as long as 5 years postinjury (35–38). Some patients with very severe injuries may stall in recovery at some stage in this process (e.g., permanent vegetative state [39,40] or minimally conscious state [41,42]) (see Giacino et al., Chapter 32 for a discussion of disorders of consciousness).

This pattern of recovery has been delineated in stages according to various schemas. The most widely used is the Rancho Los Amigos levels of cognitive functioning (43)(see Table 1-1). Another schema, first proposed by Alexander (44) and further modified (referred to as the Braintree scale) (25,45), tracks similar stages using more familiar neurological nomenclature and transition criteria (see Table 1-2). As patients progress through these stages, the principal defining cognitive limitations evolve from deficits in arousal and consciousness to basic attention and anterograde amnesia to higher level attention, memory, executive functioning, processing speed, insight, and social awareness (46).

The first stage of recovery is *coma*, a state of unconsciousness without spontaneous eye opening. This corresponds to Rancho Level I. Patients with diffuse axonal injury

---

TABLE 1–1 Rancho Los Amigos Levels of Cognitive Functioning After Traumatic Brain Injury

I. No response
II. Generalized responses
III. Localized responses
IV. Confused—agitated
V. Confused—inappropriate
VI. Confused—appropriate
VII. Automatic—appropriate
VIII. Purposeful and appropriate

Source: Ref 43.

TABLE 1-2 Braintree Neurologic Stages of Recovery from Diffuse TBI and Corresponding Rancho Los Amigos Scale Levels (typical settings of care)

1. *Coma*: unresponsive, eyes closed, no sign of wakefulness (Rancho Level I) (emergency medical services; acute inpatient hospital)
2. *Vegetative state (VS)/wakeful unconsciousness*: no cognitive awareness; transition marked by beginning spontaneous eye opening and sleep–wake cycles (Rancho Level II) (acute hospital)
3. *Minimally conscious state (MCS)*: inconsistent, simple purposeful behavior, inconsistent response to commands begin; transition can be documented using Coma Recovery Scale-Revised (CRS-R) subscale criteria for MCS (47); often mute (Rancho Level III) (acute hospital; acute inpatient rehabilitation; subacute rehabilitation)
4. *Confusional state*: interactive communication and appropriate object use begin; transition can be documented using CRS-R subscale criteria for emergence from MCS (47); amnesic (PTA), severe basic attentional deficits, hypokinetic or agitated, labile behavior; later more appropriate goal-directed behavior with continuing anterograde amnesia (Rancho Level IV, V, and partly VI) (acute inpatient rehabilitation; acute hospital)
5. *Post-confusional/emerging independence*: marked by resolution of PTA; transition can be marked using scales such as the Galveston Orientation and Amnesia Test (GOAT) (48); cognitive impairments in higher level attention, memory retrieval, and executive functioning; deficits in self-awareness, social awareness, behavioral, and emotional regulation; achieving functional independence in daily self care; improving social interaction; developing independence at home (Rancho Level VI and partly VII) (acute inpatient rehabilitation, subacute inpatient rehabilitation, outpatient rehabilitation, residential treatment, outpatient day hospital and community reentry)
6. *Social competence/community reentry*: marked by resumption of basic household independence and ability to be left home unsupervised for the better part of a day; developing independence in community, household management skills, and later returning to academic or vocational pursuits; recovering higher level cognitive abilities (divided attention, cognitive speed, executive functioning), self-awareness, and social skills; developing effective adaptation and compensation for residual problems (Rancho Level VII and VIII) (outpatient community reentry programs, community-based services—vocational, special education, supported living services, mental health services)

are unconscious at the outset, without lucid interval. The depth of coma in the period shortly after injury, as measured by the Glasgow Coma Scale (GCS), is one of the common markers of injury severity and prognosis.

Almost all persons with severe TBI who survive resume spontaneous eye opening and sleep–wake cycles while still unconscious, a condition termed VS or Rancho Level II. Except for the small percentage of very severely injured patients who remain *permanently* vegetative, evidence of awareness and purposeful behavior resume, often heralded by visual fixation and tracking. The ability to follow commands is the usual convincing marker of restored consciousness. Almost all patients with some LOS will be evaluated and treated by emergency medical services. Those with brief

alterations of consciousness (e.g., seconds or minutes) may be discharged home. Patients with more prolonged LOC or more complicated injuries (e.g., focal lesions, other injuries) will likely be admitted for acute inpatient care, often beginning in surgical intensive care units, usually supervised by neurosurgical or surgical trauma specialists.

For patients recovering slowly, cognitive responsiveness may begin erratically and inconsistently, without any reliable interactive communication. This stage may be termed MCS and corresponds to Rancho Level III (41). Many patients at this stage will continue in acute medical care settings and some who are slower to recover will transition to rehabilitation facilities, including acute IRFs or LTACH facilities, subacute rehabilitation, long-term care hospitals, or SNFs (see also Chapter 32 on disorders of consciousness).

When purposeful cognition is unequivocally established, basic attention and new learning remain severely impaired; this clinical condition may be labeled a post-traumatic *confusional state* and corresponds to Rancho Levels IV, V, and part of VI. At this stage, patients are often highly distractible, with poorly regulated behavior. They may rapidly escalate to agitated behavior (Rancho Level IV). Less often, patients may remain in a state of underactivated, hypokinetic, withdrawn behavior. Dense anterograde amnesia also defines this stage; patients are disoriented, have little or no moment-to-moment episodic recall, and display little or no ability to learn new information after even a brief delay (*PTA*). As this stage evolves, patients are better able to focus attention and regulate behavior (Rancho Level V). The end of this stage is characterized by a significant improvement in focused and sustained attention, reliable orientation, and resumption of continuous, day-to-day memory, albeit still somewhat defective and inefficient. (Rancho Level VI). Patients at this period of recovery are appropriate for care in dedicated TBI units in acute inpatient rehabilitation. Toward the end of this period of recovery, transition to home and outpatient rehabilitation programs should be contemplated. Patients who are transitioning slowly or who still require significant amounts of supervision and assistance that may not be feasible at home, may require continued treatment in a supervised care facility, perhaps at an SNF or a residential treatment facility. Some may transition to an outpatient day program.

The *post-confusional stages* of recovery are characterized by a gradual improvement in cognitive and behavioral functioning in those with more severe injuries. This phase of recovery may be further broken into stages of *emerging independence*, as patients' cognitive abilities, self awareness, and insight allow independence in self-care and safe unsupervised activity at home (Rancho Level VII) and a stage of *social competence* and *community reentry*, with the ability to manage independently at home for an extended time during the day and restorating the capacity for independent functioning in the community or at the higher level demands of school or the workplace (Rancho Level VIII). Services at these stages of care include outpatient therapies, day programs, community reentry programs, residential treatment, and a variety of community-based services.

Focal Injury

Focal cortical contusions, deep cerebral hemorrhages, and extra-axial (subdural and epidural) hemorrhages make up most focal lesions after TBI. The time course of natural history of focal injury resembles that of vascular lesions of other causes, particularly hemorrhagic stroke, but the clinical consequences of focal injury after TBI are characteristic, owing to the predilection of lesions in the anterior and inferior portions of the frontal and temporal lobes. The acute phase involves edema and other early secondary pathophysiological phenomena, which are maximal over the first few days postinjury. The resulting effects may include confusion and, perhaps, decreased arousal, especially if mass effect compromises diencephalic and mesencephalic structures. Otherwise, primary focal pathology is not directly associated with LOC.

As edema and other secondary effects wane over the first 1–3 weeks, more specific localizing effects of focal damage may become more apparent. Recovery during this subacute phase is maximal over the first 3 months, but improvement may continue at a slower rate over many months. The size and depth of focal lesions, their laterality, and the potential for reorganization within the neural network affected by the damage, in large part determines the time course and outcome.

Damage to limbic neocortical and heteromodal areas of the frontal and temporal lobes determine the usual effects of focal TBI on cognitive and behavioral functioning. The residual syndromes of prefrontal lesions include alterations in affect and behavior (e.g., disinhibition or apathy) impairment in attention, working memory and memory retrieval, and dysfunctional higher level cognition (e.g., executive functions, insight, social awareness). Lesions in anterior and inferior temporal areas may also contribute to affective and behavioral disturbances. Larger lesions extending to medial temporal areas may produce specific impairments in memory encoding and retrieval (amnesia). Other localizing temporal syndromes involve extension of lesions into auditory association areas (e.g., aphasia, with left hemisphere lesions) and visual association areas (e.g., visual agnosias, especially with bilateral lesions).

The clinical syndromes associated with focal lesions are often embedded in the evolving effects of diffuse injury—if both types of injury are combined. Particularly, with more severe diffuse injuries, overall outcome is driven largely by the effects of diffuse rather than focal injury (49). In patients with mild-to-moderate diffuse injury, large focal lesions may have more influence on recovery (50–52). Characterization of the localizing syndromes associated with focal lesions may be difficult until unmasked after resolution of posttraumatic confusion. Further, the clinical syndromes associated with focal damage may go beyond that expected with a focal lesion on structural neuroimaging because of more widespread functional network disruption and distal secondary damage (see Bigler, Chapter 19 for a more complete discussion). Another difficulty in isolating the effects of focal lesions is that neurobehavioral syndromes may be identical to those related to diffuse injury (e.g., dysexecutive syndrome, behavioral dysregulation) because these same areas, especially their axonal projections, are affected by diffuse pathology (53). Although problems are similar, recovery and prognosis may be different. For instance, features of the frontal lobe syndrome may be more persistent in patients with frontal focal cortical contusion (54,55). Levin et al. (56) observed that although other aspects of recovery were similar, unilateral frontal lesions adversely affect psychosocial outcome in children with TBI compared to those without

focal frontal lesions. These aspects of diagnosis and prognosis related to focal lesions should also help inform rehabilitation planning. For example, behavioral regulation problems related to bilateral frontal and temporal focal lesions might be more persistent and thus demand more active early intervention and treatment planning over a longer horizon than similar problems that might occur after diffuse injury that might be expected to resolve more successfully as the stages of recovery evolve.

A more complete picture of the relationship between clinical effects, natural history, and pathophysiology—diffuse, focal, and secondary—requires an overall assessment of preinjury personal factors (e.g., age, education, premorbid problems, psychosocial issues), injury mechanism, early clinical markers (e.g., GCS, duration of unconsciousness, and PTA), neuroimaging, secondary complications, and clinical assessment including neuropsychological profile. Investigations have demonstrated the benefits of combining multiple structural imaging, functional imaging, and clinical assessment modalities to enhance understanding of brain–behavior relationships in TBI (57). As newer neuroimaging and other technologies come on line for clinical use, pathophysiologic–clinical correlations and predictions of natural history and outcome will improve.

CONCLUSION

TBI is a major health care problem in the United States and internationally. Systems of care for persons with TBI have evolved since the 1970s but have not done so in a geographically symmetrical fashion. Components of ideal systems of care include prevention, emergency medical services, acute hospital care, acute inpatient rehabilitation, subacute/SNF, outpatient rehabilitation, residential rehabilitation, avocational and vocational services, special education, community-based services, long-term care, and case management. The development and ability to sustain such systems relies on an interaction between multiple variables, agencies, and interfaces that often have conflicting agendas and interests. Advocacy in multiple forms, including scientific, political, ethical, and societal remain important drivers of such systems of care.

An understanding of brain injury, its clinical consequences, associated problems and complications, and natural history of recovery aids in applying proper services for patients along the continuum of care and helps assure more effective and efficient use of resources.

Further research on the cost efficacy of such systems of care, including how they impact long-term neurological, functional, and quality of life outcomes clearly remains indicated. Additionally, continued research is needed to optimize our understanding of the natural history of recovery from TBI and interventions that may positively impact prognosis, recovery expediency and quality and ultimately biopsychosocial outcomes.

KEY CLINICAL POINTS

1. The provision of systems of care for persons with TBI needs to account for the high incidence and prevalence of TBI; potential long-term course of recovery; possible

lifelong effects, often beginning at an earlier stage of life that affect not only patients but also families and others in patient's circle; common occurrence of preexisting problems such as substance abuse and learning disability; typical effects on cognition and behavior; and the wide variety in range of severity, types of brain damage, clinical effects, and associated problems.

2. Systems of care for TBI must involve coordination of numerous services involving many disciplines across the range of severities and over the course of recovery.

3. Several marketplace factors constrain the full development and availability of components of these systems in many countries for persons in need after TBI, most notably cost, payer support, and availability of resources. These constraints become progressively restrictive for services and supports beyond the acute treatment period.

4. Patients may have various combinations of diffuse, focal, and secondary brain injury. The natural history of TBI, particularly diffuse injury, is characterized by a recognizable pattern across a range of severities involving loss or alteration of consciousness, post-traumatic confusion and PTA, and postconfusional restoration of cognitive function.

5. Focal lesions may add to the clinical consequences and affect outcome based on their disruption of neural networks, typically prefrontal and temporal lobe cognitive, emotional, and behavioral networks. The individual clinical effects of focal lesions may be difficult to distinguish from the effects of diffuse and secondary injuries and vary considerably depending how focal lesions and other combinations of pathology disrupt these neural networks.

As newer imaging and other diagnostic technologies become clinical tools for assessment, relationships and predictions regarding brain damage, clinical consequences, natural history, and prognosis will improve for patients with TBI. Ongoing efforts at high-quality research to determine what interventions are most effective, for who, at particular stages of recovery, will be essential to refine best clinical practices along the continuum of care.

KEY REFERENCES

1. Badjatia N, Carney N, Crocco TJ, et al. Guidelines for prehospital management of traumatic brain injury 2nd edition. *Prehosp Emerg Care*. 2008;12(suppl 1):S1–S52.
2. Brain Trauma Foundation, American Association of Neurological Surgeons; Congress of Neurological Surgeons. Guidelines for the management of severe traumatic brain injury. *J Neurotrauma*. 2007;24(suppl 1):S1–S106.
3. Cope DN, Mayer NH, Cervelli L. Development of systems of care for persons with traumatic brain injury. *J Head Trauma Rehabil*. 2005;20(2):128–142.
4. Corrigan JD. Conducting statewide needs assessments for persons with traumatic brain injury. *J Head Trauma Rehabil*. 2001;16(1):1–19.
5. Povlishock JT, Katz DI. Update of neuropathology and neurological recovery after traumatic brain injury. *J Head Trauma Rehabil*. 2005;20(1):76–94.
6. Ragnarsson KT, Thomas JP, Zasler ND. Model systems of care for individuals with traumatic brain injury. *J Head Trauma Rehabil*. 1993;8:1–11.
7. Rehabilitation of persons with traumatic brain injury. *NIH Consens Statement*. 1998;16(1):1–41.
8. Zaloshnja E, Miller T, Langlois JA, Selassie AW. Prevalence of long-term disability from traumatic brain injury in the civilian population of the United States, 2005. *J Head Trauma Rehabil*. 2008;23(6):394–400.

References

1. Faul M XL, Wald MM, Coronado VG. *Traumatic Brain Injury in the United States: Emergency Department Visits, Hospitalizations and Deaths 2002–2006*. Atlanta, GA: Centers for Disease Control and Prevention, National Center for Injury Prevention and Control; 2010.
2. Zaloshnja E, Miller T, Langlois JA, Selassie AW. Prevalence of long-term disability from traumatic brain injury in the civilian population of the United States, 2005. *J Head Trauma Rehabil*. 2008;23:394–400.
3. Langlois JA, Marr A, Mitchko J, Johnson RL. Tracking the silent epidemic and educating the public: CDC's traumatic brain injury-associated activities under the TBI Act of 1996 and the Children's Health Act of 2000. *J Head Trauma Rehabil*. 2005;20(3):196–204.
4. Coronado VG, Thomas KE, Sattin RW, Johnson RL. The CDC traumatic brain injury surveillance system: characteristics of persons aged 65 years and older hospitalized with a TBI. *J Head Trauma Rehabil*. 2005;20(3):215–228.
5. Cicerone KD, Dahlberg C, Kalmar K, et al. Evidence-based cognitive rehabilitation: recommendations for clinical practice. *Arch Phys Med Rehabil*. 2000;81(12):1596–1615.
6. Cicerone KD, Dahlberg C, Malec JF, et al. Evidence-based cognitive rehabilitation: updated review of the literature from 1998 through 2002. *Arch Phys Med Rehabil*. 2005;86(8):1681–1692.
7. Cope DN, Mayer NH, Cervelli L. Development of systems of care for persons with traumatic brain injury. *J Head Trauma Rehabil*. 2005;20(2):128–142.
8. Ragnarsson KT, Thomas JP, Zasler ND. Model systems of care for individuals with traumatic brain injury. *J Head Trauma Rehabil*. 1993;8:1–11.
9. Corrigan JD. Conducting statewide needs assessments for persons with traumatic brain injury. *J Head Trauma Rehabil*. 2001;16(1):1–19.
10. Rehabilitation of persons with traumatic brain injury. *NIH Consens Statement*. 1998;16(1):1–41.
11. Management of Concussion/mTBI Working Group. VA/DoD clinical practice guideline for management of concussion/mild traumatic brain injury. *J Rehabil Res Dev*. 2009;46(6):CP1–CP68.
12. Rudehill A, Bellander BM, Weitzberg E, Bredbacka S, Backheden M, Gordon E. Outcome of traumatic brain injuries in 1,508 patients: impact of prehospital care. *J Neurotrauma*. 2002;19(7):855–868.
13. Watts DD, Hanfling D, Waller MA, Gilmore C, Fakhry SM, Trask AL. An evaluation of the use of guidelines in prehospital management of brain injury. *Prehosp Emerg Care*. 2004;8(3):254–261.
14. Zink BJ. Traumatic brain injury outcome: concepts for emergency care. *Ann Emerg Med*. 2001;37(3):318–332.
15. Badjatia N, Carney N, Crocco TJ, et al. Guidelines for prehospital management of traumatic brain injury 2nd edition. *Prehosp Emerg Care*. 2008;12(suppl 1):S1–S52.
16. von Wild K, Terwey S. Diagnostic confusion in mild traumatic brain injury (MTBI). Lessons from clinical practice and EFNS—inquiry. European Federation of Neurological Societies. *Brain Inj*. 2001;15(3):273–277.
17. Sumann G, Kampfl A, Wenzel V, Schobersberger W. Early intensive care unit intervention for trauma care: what alters the outcome? *Curr Opin Crit Care*. 2002;8(6):587–592.
18. The Brain Trauma Foundation. The American Association of Neurological Surgeons. The Joint Section on Neurotrauma and Critical Care. Recommendations for intracranial pressure monitoring technology. *J Neurotrauma*. 2000;17(6–7):479–506.

19. Bulger EM, Nathens AB, Rivara FP, Moore M, MacKenzie EJ, Jurkovich GJ. Management of severe head injury: institutional variations in care and effect on outcome. *Crit Care Med.* 2002;30(8):1870–1876.

20. Guidelines for the management of severe head injury. Brain Trauma Foundation, American Association of Neurological Surgeons, Joint Section on Neurotrauma and Critical Care. *J Neurotrauma.* 1996;13(11):641–734.

21. Brain Trauma Foundation, American Association of Neurological Surgeons, Congress of Neurological Surgeons. Guidelines for the management of severe traumatic brain injury. *J Neurotrauma.* 2007;24(suppl 1):S1–S106.

22. Katz DI, Polyak M, Coughlan D, Nichols M, Roche A. Natural history of recovery from brain injury after prolonged disorders of consciousness: outcome of patients admitted to inpatient rehabilitation with 1–4 year follow-up. *Prog Brain Res.* 2009;177:73–88.

23. Goodall P, Ghiloni CT. The changing face of publicly funded employment services. *J Head Trauma Rehabil.* 2001;16(1):94–106.

24. Ylvisaker M, Todis B, Glang A, et al. Educating students with TBI: themes and recommendations. *J Head Trauma Rehabil.* 2001;16(1):76–93.

25. Povlishock JT, Katz DI. Update of neuropathology and neurological recovery after traumatic brain injury. *J Head Trauma Rehabil.* 2005;20(1):76–94.

26. Katz DI, Alexander MP. Traumatic brain injury. Predicting course of recovery and outcome for patients admitted to rehabilitation. *Arch Neurol.* 1994;51(7):661–670.

27. Haslam C, Batchelor J, Fearnside MR, Haslam SA, Hawkins S, Kenway E. Post-coma disturbance and post-traumatic amnesia as non-linear predictors of cognitive outcome following severe closed head injury: findings from the Westmead Head Injury Project. *Brain Inj.* 1994;8(6):519–528.

28. Tate RL, Perdices M, Pfaff A, Jurjevic L. Predicting duration of post-traumatic amnesia (PTA) from early PTA measurements. *J Head Trauma Rehabil.* 2001;16(6):525–542.

29. Zafonte RD, Mann NR, Millis SR, Black KL, Wood DL, Hammond F. Posttraumatic amnesia: its relation to functional outcome. *Arch Phys Med Rehabil.* 1997;78(10):1103–1106.

30. Whyte J, Cifu D, Dikmen S, Temkin N. Prediction of functional outcomes after traumatic brain injury: a comparison of 2 measures of duration of unconsciousness. *Arch Phys Med Rehabil.* 2001;82(10):1355–1359.

31. Katz DI, Otto RM, Agosti RM, MacKinnon DJ, Alexander MP. Factors affecting duration of posttraumatic amnesia after traumatic brain injury. *J Int Neuropsychol Soc.* 1999;5:139.

32. Sherer M, Yablon SA, Nakase-Richardson R, Nick TG. Effect of severity of post-traumatic confusion and its constituent symptoms on outcome after traumatic brain injury. *Arch Phys Med Rehabil.* 2008;89(1):42–47.

33. Sherer M, Yablon SA, Nakase-Richardson R. Patterns of recovery of posttraumatic confusional state in neurorehabilitation admissions after traumatic brain injury. *Arch Phys Med Rehabil.* 2009;90(10):1749–1754.

34. Nakase-Richardson R, Yablon SA, Sherer M. Prospective comparison of acute confusion severity with duration of post-traumatic amnesia in predicting employment outcome after traumatic brain injury. *J Neurol Neurosurg Psychiatry.* 2007;78(8):872–876.

35. Hammond FM, Hart T, Bushnik T, Corrigan JD, Sasser H. Change and predictors of change in communication, cognition, and social function between 1 and 5 years after traumatic brain injury. *J Head Trauma Rehabil.* 2004;19(4):314–328.

36. Millis SR, Rosenthal M, Novack TA, et al. Long-term neuropsychological outcome after traumatic brain injury. *J Head Trauma Rehabil.* 2001;16(4):343–355.

37. Olver JH, Ponsford JL, Curran CA. Outcome following traumatic brain injury: a comparison between 2 and 5 years after injury. *Brain Inj.* 1996;10(11):841–848.

38. Corrigan JD, Smith-Knapp K, Granger CV. Outcomes in the first 5 years after traumatic brain injury. *Arch Phys Med Rehabil.* 1998;79(3):298–305.

39. Medical aspects of the persistent vegetative state (1). The Multi-Society Task Force on PVS. *N Engl J Med.* 1994;330(21):1499–1508.

40. Estraneo A, Moretta P, Loreto V, Lanzillo B, Santoro L, Trojano L. Late recovery after traumatic, anoxic, or hemorrhagic long-lasting vegetative state. *Neurology.* 2010;75(3):239–245.

41. Giacino JT, Ashwal S, Childs N, et al. The minimally conscious state: definition and diagnostic criteria. *Neurology.* 2002;58(3):349–353.

42. Luauté J, Maucort-Boulch D, Tell L, et al. Long-term outcomes of chronic minimally conscious and vegetative states. *Neurology.* 2010;75(3):246–252.

43. Hagen C, Malkmus D, Durham P. *Levels of Cognitive Functioning.* Downey, CA: Ranchos Los Amigos Hospital; 1972.

44. Alexander MP. Traumatic brain injury. In: DF B, Blumer D, eds. *Psychiatric Aspects of Neurologic Disease.* New York, NY: McGraw-Hill; 1982:251–278.

45. Katz DI. Neuropathology and neurobehavioral recovery from closed head injury. *J Head Trauma Rehabil.* 1992;7:1–15.

46. Stuss DT, Buckle BA. Traumatic brain injury: neruopsychological deficits and evaluation at different stages of recovery and in different pathological subtypes. *J Head Trauma Rehabil.* 1992;7:40–49.

47. Giacino JT, Kalmar K, Whyte J. The JFK Coma Recovery Scale-Revised: measurement characteristics and diagnostic utility. *Arch Phys Med Rehabil.* 2004;85(12):2020–2029.

48. Levin HS, O'Donnell VM, Grossman RG. The Galveston orientation and amnesia test. A practical scale to assess cognition after head injury. *J Nerv Ment Dis.* 1979;167(11):675–684.

49. Ross BL, Temkin NR, Newell D, Dikmen SS. Neuropsychological outcome in relation to head injury severity. Contributions of coma length and focal abnormalities. *Am J Phys Med Rehabil.* 1994;73(5):341–347.

50. van der Naalt J, Hew JM, van Zomeren AH, Sluiter WJ, Minderhoud JM. Computed tomography and magnetic resonance imaging in mild to moderate head injury: early and late imaging related to outcome. *Ann Neurol.* 1999;46(1):70–78.

51. Levin HS, Williams DH, Eisenberg HM, High WM Jr, Guinto FC Jr. Serial MRI and neurobehavioural findings after mild to moderate closed head injury. *J Neurol Neurosurg Psychiatry.* 1992;55(4):255–262.

52. Wilson JT, Hadley DM, Wiedmann KD, Teasdale GM. Neuro-psychological consequences of two patterns of brain damage shown by MRI in survivors of severe head injury. *J Neurol Neurosurg Psychiatry.* 1995;59(3):328–331.

53. Wallesch CW, Curio N, Galazky I, Jost S, Synowitz H. The neuropsychology of blunt head injury in the early postacute stage: effects of focal lesions and diffuse axonal injury. *J Neurotrauma.* 2001;18(1):11–20.

54. Bigler ED. Quantitative magnetic resonance imaging in traumatic brain injury. *J Head Trauma Rehabil.* 2001;16(2):117–134.

55. Wallesch CW, Curio N, Kutz S, Jost S, Bartels C, Synowitz H. Outcome after mild-to-moderate blunt head injury: effects of focal lesions and diffuse axonal injury. *Brain Inj.* 2001;15(5):401–412.

56. Levin HS, Zhang L, Dennis M, et al. Psychosocial outcome of TBI in children with unilateral frontal lesions. *J Int Neuropsychol Soc.* 2004;10(3):305–316.

57. Wilde EA, Newsome MR, Bigler ED, et al. Brain imaging correlates of verbal working memory in children following traumatic brain injury. *Int J Psychophysiol.* 2011;82(1):86–96.

2

History of Acute Care and Rehabilitation of Head Injury

Graham Teasdale and George Zitnay

INTRODUCTION

For much of recorded history, the main interest in head injuries lay in open wounds of the head and battlefield experiences repeatedly highlighted the lethal complications of penetrating injury of the brain. Civilian closed head injuries became the focus when their occurrence increased dramatically as a consequence of the growth of road traffic and urbanization throughout the world in the second half of the 20th century. The many advances in acute care of head injuries over this period are built on principles derived from military experiences expressed through modern scientific, technological, and organizational progress.

The work of Sir Hugh Cairns and colleagues in Oxford was especially influential during World War II (WWII) (1) and in later developments. Like Harvey Cushing in the First World War, with whom he had worked, Cairns recognized the need for early specialized care of head injuries. His response was the creation of Mobile Neurosurgical Units, staffed by surgeons with neurosurgical experience and supported by skilled trained staff and with specialized neurosurgical equipment. These operated close to the front lines and set the pattern for the acute care of injuries in subsequent conflicts from Korea to Afghanistan. Alongside this, the expectation of casualties in the United Kingdom arising from bombing stimulated the development of a system of emergency medical services, anticipating later trauma systems. Cairns also saw the importance of specialized care after the acute phase and at St. Hugh's Hospital in Oxford, a commandeered lady's college, created a base for the mobile units and for continuing multidisciplinary care and rehabilitation of military head injuries. Alongside this clinical work, experimental research initiated at that time in Oxford also had long lasting influence on understanding the fundamental mechanisms of traumatic brain injury (TBI).

Substantial improvements in the care of head injuries have been achieved in the last 5 decades. Nevertheless, this was not a continuous process and 3 main, overlapping phases in approaches to acute care can be identified. Thus, in the 2 decades after the end of WWII, the care of head injuries attracted little attention and management was directed by what can be regarded as traditional approaches. Then, beginning in the late 1960s and accelerating in 1970s and 1980s, there was a growing recognition of the importance of head injuries accompanied by many advances in understanding. Improved approaches to care were instituted, applying Cushing and Cairns' principles of early, proactive specialized care. The benefits were evident in the finding of a recent overview that progress in reducing mortality of head injury was most pronounced in the 1970s and 1980s (2). The period since then has seen these gains consolidated through organizational and educational efforts, while the search for further improvements continues.

ACUTE CARE IN THE POST-WAR ERA: 1945–1960S

The enormous challenges of reconstruction that most countries faced in the post-war years meant that the management of head injuries did not receive prominent attention. Neurosurgery was just becoming established as a distinct speciality. The creation of the National Health Service instituted regional systems of care in Britain but neurosurgeons were in short supply: their numbers were greater in North America yet the distribution was uneven. Shortages were even greater in most of the rest of the world. Moreover, the treatment of "nontraumatic" pathology such as tumors and vascular lesions claimed most attention among the neurosurgeons of the day and much of head injury care was provided by general or orthopedic surgeons. In Britain, Sir Norman Dott in 1945 referred to "the care of head injuries" as "a Cinderella of medical science" (e1).

Contemporary accounts (e1,e2,e3) show that management of head injuries was based on concepts of diagnosis and treatment guided largely from clinical features. Apart from skull x-rays, there was little use of investigations. Surgical intervention in closed injuries was typically undertaken only when prompted by prolonged and deep worsening of clinical responsiveness, even awaiting features of impending brain herniation. Operations usually began with "exploratory" burr holes, guided by scalp wound, skull fracture, or neurological signs but often led to a sequence of 8 sites—frontal, temporal, parietal, and posterior fossa on both sides of the head. Such "woodpecker" surgery was often negative and failed to detect many significant clots. If the exploration was positive, the burr hole was enlarged by craniectomy, but this often was too small to achieve complete evacuation of the clot.

What was clearly recognized was the need to address the extracranial disorders, especially affecting respiration, that could complicate severe brain injury. Early establishment of airway patency through positioning and suctioning, followed by tracheostomy, and the administration of oxygen were seen to be important but were conducted without recourse to physiological guidance.

The main targets of "nonoperative" management of severe brain injury were the raised cerebrospinal fluid (CSF) pressure and cerebral edema, which were deduced to be important from the frequent appearance of a swollen brain at operation or autopsy. The treatments that were used drew on concepts put forward decades previously by workers such as Heinrich Quincke (e4) and Harvey Cushing (e5) to reduce intracranial pressure (ICP) by repeated lumbar puncture or subtemporal decompression and by Lewis Weed (e6) to shrink the brain by administration of hypertonic solutions like urea, mannitol, sucrose, saline, and magnesium sulphate. The approach was essentially empirical and the lack of clear evidence of benefit was acknowledged.

Publications on head injuries consisted of retrospective accounts of the experiences of a single center. The mortality of patients admitted in "coma" was typically reported to be almost 70% (3) and in all sizeable series of patients with an extradural hematoma, the mortality exceeded 20%. Wylie McKissock's analysis (4) that in a half of these cases death could be attributed to mistakes in management was an early signpost to the benefit that could come from improved care.

RECOGNIZING AND RESPONDING TO THE IMPORTANCE OF HEAD INJURIES: 1960s–1980s

During the 1960s, several factors began to focus public, political, and professional attention on head injuries and to promote interest in improving their care. A major influence was the escalating occurrence of motor vehicle accidents (MVA) and their toll in the developed world. In the mid 1960s, it was estimated that annually in the United States, there were 3 million MVAs leading to 30,000 deaths. Head injury was the leading cause of death—accounting for some 60% of fatalities. Moreover, the preponderance of young adult males among the victims made head injury the leading cause of loss of years of life and of lifelong disability in some survivors.

Social, clinical, and academic developments were creating more favorable circumstances to address the concerns. Recovering economies supported expanded numbers of doctors with consequent increasing specialization and research. In Europe, the pattern of regionalized deployment of neurosurgery, with responsibility to the care of a defined population, was well advanced. In the United States, where there were several times more neurosurgeons, they were affiliated to many more hospitals and educated in formal training programs. These were often in an academic research environment where pioneers, such as Thomas Langfitt at the University of Pennsylvania, led fundamental programs of work on the effects of mass lesions and raised ICP (5). Furthermore, technical developments were opening new possibilities in clinical monitoring, including the introduction by

Neils Lundberg of continuous recording of ICP in patients with head injury in Lund (6).

The new status of head injuries was clearly evident by the mid 1960s. In 1964, the National Institute of Neurological Diseases and Blindness in the United States designated craniocerebral trauma a program area of major interest, and in response, in February the next year, the first of the influential Chicago Head Injury Conferences (e7) was organized by Dr Joe Evans. Also in 1965, head injury was the major topic at the Third International Congress of Neurological Surgery in Copenhagen (e8). The World Federation of Neurosurgical Societies then wrote to the governments of all its members to emphasize the national importance of head injury and set up an ad hoc group that became its Neurotraumatology Committee in 1971. This went on to promote knowledge of injuries in many countries and was followed by the birth of national and continental neurotrauma societies.

Opening the Possibility of Improvement and Promoting Change

A key catalyst came in the early 1970s from the work in the group that formed around Bryan Jennett in Glasgow. Jennett's interest in head injuries had arisen while a young trainee with Cairns in Oxford. After appointment to the Chair of Neurosurgery in Glasgow in 1967, he initiated a far reaching program that engaged colleagues from many disciplines and from many parts of the world.

Insights From Clinical–Pathological Interactions

For many years, neuropathological studies had yielded very limited insights into head injury because ownership lay with forensic pathologists who prioritized prompt examination of the unfixed brain. In a key initiative, special arrangements were established in Glasgow to allow academic neuropathologists to assemble a unique bank of fixed brains—eventually 1,500 cases—on which they were able to perform innovative, detailed, quantitative studies. A highly influential early output from the collaboration was the identification in 1971 by David Graham and Hume Adams (7) of a high rate (91%) of ischemic brain damage—indicating that it had developed as a secondary event and hence was potentially avoidable or remediable. Many patients clearly had not sustained fatal brain damage at the time of the injury—as judged by them not having been deeply unconscious and not having neuropathological findings of severe primary brain damage. This sequence was highlighted in the term "Talked and Died" (8) and further work identified that there were several potentially "avoidable factors" in these cases, which made up almost a third of deaths at that time. The most striking was the delayed recognition of a traumatic intracranial hematoma; others were hypoxia, hypotension, and multiple injuries.

The Clinical Response

It was obvious that neurosurgeons could make most impact on reducing mortality and morbidity by ensuring early detection and evacuation of significant intracranial clots. Delayed recognition of neurological worsening as a result of a clot was identified as a frequent problem (e9) so that first step was to improve clinical assessment.

In early 1970s, there was a lack of a widely accepted standard approach to the assessment of alterations of responsiveness, as expressed in so called conscious level, even though this was recognized to be the most important index of the initial effects of head injury and of subsequent changes. Proposals had been set out by many clinics and organizations; most depended on presumed clinicopathological mechanistic correlations and on terms about which Earl Walker in 1965 (e10) had commented there was "no unanimity of opinion on the precise meaning." The Glasgow Coma Scale (GCS) was described by Graham Teasdale and Bryan Jennett in 1974 (9) to meet this need. Its simple objective approach, based on describing and recording 3 separate features, eye, verbal, and motor responsiveness, was developed through close involvement of nurses and junior doctors in an effort to achieve consistent observation. The scale was found to promote reliable monitoring, communication, and decision making. Gradual worldwide acceptance followed, promoted by its incorporation in statements of good practice such as the Advanced Trauma Life Support (ATLS) and later guidelines.

Intracranial Hematoma, Imaging, and Guidelines

The invention of the computed tomography (CT) scan in the early 1970s and its application to head injuries (10) (Figure 2-1) was the greatest single factor in genesis of the modern management of head injuries. Scanning made it possible to replace fallible clinical concepts in the diagnosis of intracranial lesions by effective, noninvasive, and easily repeated imaging. "Pre- and post-CT eras" are recognized. However, experience in the first few years of the scanner, when availability was very limited, showed that outcomes were not improving as hoped because scanning was still not being done soon enough. Improvement depended on making organizational changes in the proactive spirit of Cushing and Cairns to ensure that patients at risk of a clot could have early scanning and prompt and skilled surgical intervention.

The challenge of realizing the benefits of CT posed different issues depending on the ease of access to scanning. For many years, there were many fewer scanners in Europe and other parts of the world than in the United States; moreover, most were in regional units so that investigation required agreement about triage for transfer. Because a compressive hematoma is such an infrequent complication—for example 1:6,000 of attendees at hospital—it became essential to identify factors associated with the risk that a patient would develop this complication. Studies of several thousand patients in Scotland quantified the influence on the risk of a skull fracture and level of consciousness (e11). The information guided a change in transfer policies (e12) that led to more patients being scanned sooner with improved outcomes (11). On this basis, the first guidelines for head injury management were agreed nationally by neurosurgeons in Britain—for x-raying the skull, for observation, for CT scanning, and neurosurgical consultation (12). Admissions for observation fell and detection of hematoma increased. Mortality from an extradural hematoma became rare—a dramatic reduction from the era reported by McKissock (4).

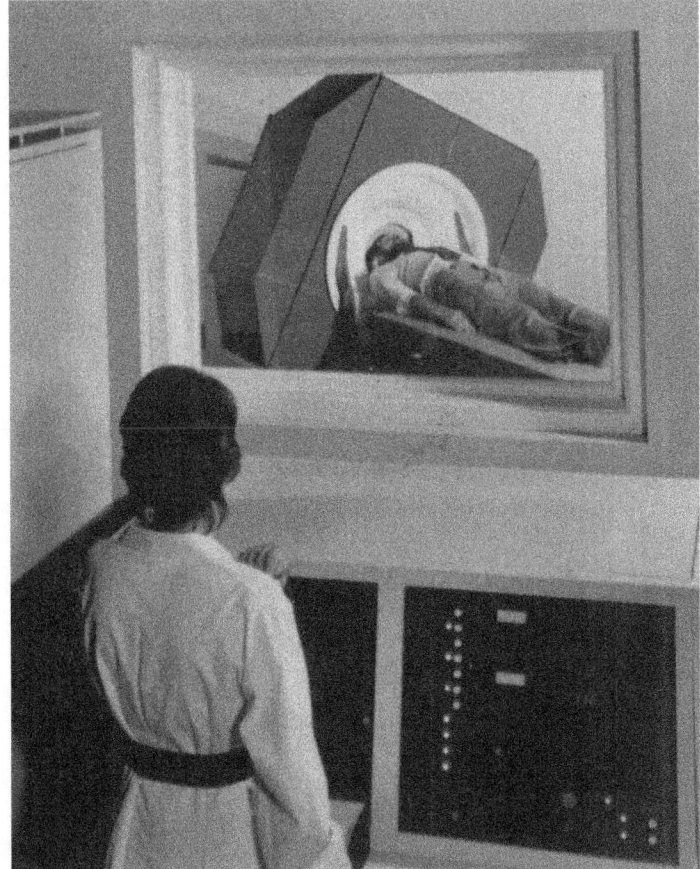

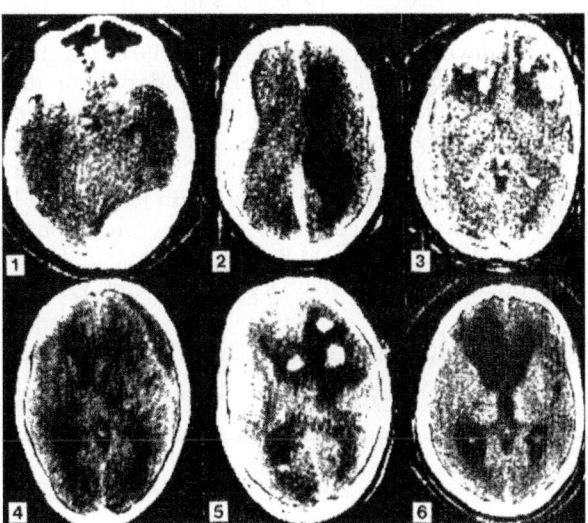

FIGURE 2-1 (A) Patient in first commercially available CT scan produced by EMI in 1976 and **(B)** images of extradural hematoma, acute subdural hematoma, bifrontal contusions, chronic subdural hematoma, ICHs and edema, post-traumatic hydrocephalus. Reprinted from Ambrose, Gooding, Uttley, (10) with permission. (Figure 2-1A kindly provided by Drs. Sue Edyvean and Jonathan Turner ImPACT group, Medical Physics Department, St George's Hospital, London).

After the 1980s, availability of CT expanded throughout the developed world and rapid access is now considered an essential feature of any hospital caring for acute head injuries. Nevertheless, the need for guidelines for CT scanning continues—although they are now more directed at limiting overuse in minor injuries. Current recommendations come from a range of bodies (e13,e14) and increasingly are based on decision rules tested in prospective cohorts. They differ in detail—depending in part on local circumstances—and what is important is that there is agreement about the criteria within a local trauma system.

As the technology advanced, CT increasingly showed abnormalities previously unsuspected in life. Many were intracranial hemorrhagic lesions for which the need for evacuation was unclear. Criteria for deciding which could be safely managed conservatively were developed using clinical and radiological features and the findings of measurements of the ICP. Other findings included cerebral contusions, indicators of diffuse primary brain injury, of subarachnoid hemorrhage and intracranial volume pressure status; these become the basis for the development of a new system for classifying injury by Lawrence Marshall of San Diego (e15).

Despite the introduction of magnetic resonance imaging (MRI), CT has remained the primary diagnostic test in the acute evaluation of head injury. MRI is superior to CT in the detection of the small traumatic parenchymal abnormalities that occur in diffuse injury, but CT is superior to MRI in delineating the types of acute hemorrhagic lesions important in early management.

Secondary Insults in Life

The third development in the 1970s and 1980s was the linking of the pathological findings of secondary brain damage in fatal cases to the detection in life of a high frequency of what were tellingly referred to as "early" (e16) or "secondary" insults to the injured brain (13). The terms were coined by Douglas Miller, who had trained with Jennett and Langfitt and later became a Professor in Edinburgh, while he was working in the team Donald Becker brought together at Virginia Commonwealth University in Richmond, VA. The em-

phasis this group placed on monitoring and treating raised ICP and other insults (e17,e18) was reinforced by the careful prospective work of the North American Traumatic Coma Data Bank study (14). This collected data from 1,030 patients in 4 clinical head injury centers between 1984 and 1987 on the occurrence and impact on outcome of factors such as clinical and investigative indices of injury severity, complications, and management. The findings documented the extremely frequent occurrence of intracranial and extracranial abnormalities (Table 2-1) and their adverse effects.

The Potential for Benefit From Intensive Treatment of Severe Injuries

During the 1960s, the view developed that recovery from coma from severe injury might be promoted by what was then termed intensive care, the forerunner of modern neurocritical care. This was at a time that intensive care units were mushrooming from almost 0 in 1960 to 55,000 in1980 in the United States. This development built on the intensive monitoring of cardiac patients and followed the use of mechanical ventilation for respiratory insufficiency that had been pioneered in Copenhagen in the polio epidemics of the 1950s. By the late 1960s, the fall in polio following the introduction of vaccination freed these facilities for other uses, including head injuries with respiratory problems associated with severe brain damage.

Work in Newcastle (e19) had linked an increasing focus on care of the airway, tracheostomy, and the adequacy of ventilation to improved survival but concerns developed that a risk of intensive treatment was of an increased survival with disability (e20). Addressing this was hampered by the perception that the course followed by patients with head injury was capricious—some who initially looked to be hopeless survived, whereas others, apparently less serious, failed to make a satisfactory recovery. This prompted efforts to develop prognostic criteria for the likely outcome and so to help decision making in the acute stage.

In 1967, Jennett instituted prospective collection of information of early severity and later outcome. The work began in Glasgow but then expanded to the Netherlands

---

TABLE 2-1 Secondary Problems in Severely Head Injured Patients in the North American Traumatic Coma Data Bank

EXTRACRANIAL DISTURBANCES BEFORE OR ON ARRIVAL AT NEUROCENTER		DURING TREATMENT	
Hypotension (SBP < 90 mm Hg)	35%	Electrolyte imbalance	59%
Hypoxia (PaO$_2$ < 60 mm Hg)	46%	Pulmonary infection	41%
		Coagulopathy	19%
		Septicemia	10%
LESIONS ON CT BRAIN SCAN		**ABNORMALITIES DURING MONITORING**	
Abnormal CT	93%	Raised ICP (> 20mm Hg)	81%
Mass lesion	42%	Hypotension (SBP < 80 mm Hg)	84%
Diffuse injury	55%		
with brain swelling	21%		
+ shift > 5mm	4%		

SBP, systolic blood pressure; PaO$_2$, partial pressure of arterial oxygen; CT, computed tomography; ICP, intracranial pressure.
Reprinted from Marshall (14), Marmarou (15), Chesnut (16), and Piek (17) with permission.

through collaboration with Reinder Braakman in Rotterdam and Jan Minderhoud in Groningen and to the United States through collaboration with Thomas Kurze in Los Angeles and Laurence Pitts in San Francisco. This International Data Bank (18) focused on patients who had been in coma—defined as no eye opening, not uttering understandable words, and not obeying commands—for at least 6 hours so that the patients were both severe and resistant to early resuscitation. In most subsequent reports, patients were included on the basis of their state at admission, some of whom recovered in the next 6 hours with a corresponding better outcome.

To codify the data charting a patient's course, the components of the GCS were allocated digits that were then summed, creating the Glasgow Coma Score which proved a useful summary of severity (e21). The Glasgow Outcome Scale (GOS) (19) was also described as a way to summarize outcome in large numbers, rather than changes in an individual—a contrast to the Coma Scale. The 2 papers became the most highly cited Neurosurgical publications over the next 30 years (e22).

Results from the data bank and many similar studies identified the age of the victim, clinical indices of severity—GCS and pupil reaction—and results of CT scans and measurements of ICP as the most powerful prognostic factors (e23). Unfortunately, reliable predictions about individuals could be made only at extremes—that is, very high likelihood of death or of good recovery—and early identification of survival with severe disability was very difficult. Clinical predictive tools are now available online (e23,e24) but the main use of the work became in resolving controversies about care by supporting more valid comparisons between groups of patients—either treated according to different views about "conventional" care or in formal research designs.

Intensive Management of Severe Head Injuries

The scale of the adverse effects of secondary insults emphasized the importance of the quality of surgery and intensive care in avoiding or rapidly correcting adverse factors. Such care became progressively more feasible and available through technical developments that enabled continuous monitoring of indices of cardiovascular and respiratory function and their response to treatment and also by the emergence of a cadre of trained intensivists—drawn usually from the ranks of anesthesia. There is no debate about the benefit this yielded through detecting and minimizing the adverse effects of extracranial disorders or of expansive intracranial lesions. What emerged as less clear was the benefit from measures aimed primarily at control of raised ICP, irrespective of its cause.

Initially, the picture seemed straightforward. An early finding from continuous monitoring was that an elevated ICP was common in severe injuries and that there was a link between the degree and duration of the increase and mortality (15,e18). Monitoring and management of raised ICP received strong advocacy from Becker, Miller, Marmarou, and many others. However, the relationships were neither simple nor predictable; raised ICP could be a consequence as well as a cause of damage and other pathophysiological factors could be critical. These included the difference

between arterial pressure and ICP—the cerebral perfusion pressure, along with the autoregulatory capacity of the cerebral circulation and its responsiveness to CO_2 and other physiological influences. Efforts to unravel the complexities of these interrelationships through clinical and laboratory studies have continued for many years and are chronicled in the proceedings of successive International Symposia on ICP, commencing in Hannover in 1972, to the 14th in Tubingen in 2012 (e25).

There was little debate that if a raised ICP is caused by an identifiable complication such as a newly evolving mass lesion or disordered systemic conditions, monitoring could provide early warning and prompt correction. What has been controversial has been the value of responding to a raised ICP through deliberately inducing a departure from normal physiological conditions with the aim of improving intracranial volume pressure relationships. Benefits were reported, usually in single center studies with historical controls, from packages that included hyperventilation; hypertension; the use of barbiturates, steroids, osmotic agents, and CSF drainage; hypothermia; and external decompressive craniectomy. Each component had an apparent rationale in experimentally derived concepts but randomized comparative studies largely failed to find benefit.

Thus, in prospective randomized studies in Richmond, neither barbiturates (e26) nor prophylactic hyperventilation (e27) were beneficial. Work in Houston showed that a focus on raising blood pressure to produce a high cerebral perfusion pressure (CPP) as against lowering ICP did not improve outcome and indeed led to a higher incidence of acute respiratory distress syndrome (e28). After encouraging results in small studies, a large trial of induced hypothermia led from Houston did not improve outcome (e29). These and subsequent studies made clear that the potential for benefit could be counterbalanced by unintended adverse consequences and that improved control of ICP might not be reflected in an improved outcome.

Among the reasons put forward for the disappointing findings was that the variability between patients and in the same patient over time meant that developments were needed to make it possible for interventions to be tailored to the individual. Another view was that effort should be put into standardizing care through the use of guidelines. These approaches were taken forward in next decades which also saw advances in the organization of care for injured people and an explosion of research into basic mechanisms of neural injury.

IMPLEMENTATION AND CONTINUING INVESTIGATION: 1980s–2010

Organization of Trauma Care and Guidelines for Severe Head Injuries

In the late 1970s, after the Vietnam War, a cohort of well-trained and experienced trauma surgeons returned to the United States to find a disorganized and highly variable civilian trauma care infrastructure. The wide range in size, facilities, staffing, presence of relevant subspecialties, catchment area, and experience found in hospitals potentially providing care for victims of injuries seemed likely to be associated with variations in outcome. Studies led by Donald

Trunkrey in Orange County California (e30) showed that this variation could be reduced by an organized, stratified approach. The American College of Surgeons and the US Department of Health and Human Services then implemented and formalized a pre-hospital care infrastructure and tiered referral system. This was successfully refined over the ensuing 40 years in order that the most severe trauma victims are triaged to "level one" facilities that are equipped to provide for them. The approach has been progressively taken up in many countries in the developed world.

The need for guidance to achieve consistency in the care of severe head injuries was highlighted by a survey of practices in 261 randomly selected intensive care units in the United States (20). Tremendous variability in management was disclosed in the use of ICP monitoring, CSF drainage, barbiturates, hyperventilation, osmotic diuretics, and corticosteroids. Almost a third of centers reported aiming for $PaCO_2$ values of < 25 mm Hg despite the evidence referred to previously (e27) against the use of such marked hyperventilation.

The Brain Trauma Foundation and the Neurotrauma Foundation, in collaboration with the American Association of Neurologic Surgeons and the Congress of Neurologic Surgeons, formed groups to review the available literature and develop guidance for the management of severely head injured patients (21). There was recognition that the quality of evidence available would vary and that this should be linked to the strength of a recommendation: Class I data from randomized studies supporting a grade A treatment standard, Class II from prospective cohorts supporting a grade B recommendation, and Class III from expert opinion supporting a grade C option. To the surprise of most neurosurgeons involved, high quality evidence was in very short supply; few grade A recommendations could be made and these were not to do something.

Through continuing work, an immense amount of evidence has been brought together and critically assessed. The early guidelines have been revised, translated into more than a dozen languages, and recommendations produced for most aspects of management of adult and pediatric head injuries (Table 2-2). Nevertheless, the shortage of high quality supporting data continues, and in a review covering 83 treatment topics, Class I evidence was found only for 4 of the 277 recommendations (e31).

Even without evidence for the value of specific components, guidelines can improve care by focusing attention on "the basics," standardizing what is "good practice" and making achievement of this more reliable. Surveys have shown that increasing numbers of head injury centers report the adoption of the guidelines. Most evaluations indicate that their introduction is associated with a reduction in mortality, but these are usually based on historical comparisons of cohorts in a single center (e32). As for many aspects of neurotrauma care, rigorous evidence from prospective randomized comparisons has not been produced, but this standard of evaluation of complex "packages" may be very difficult to achieve. A fuller account of management guidelines can be found in Chapter 25 by Bullock.

Advances in Monitoring

Advances in technology have enabled experimental and clinical investigations that have given a clearer perception of

TABLE 2-2 Management Topics Covered in Current Guidelines

MINOR AND MODERATE INJURIES IN ADULTS AND IN CHILDREN

Prehospital initial assessment, referral to hospital, transfer to hospital

Assessment in the emergency department, head CT and timing, cervical spine imaging

Admission to hospital, observation, referral to neurosurgery

Discharge advice, outpatient follow-up, long-term problems

SEVERE HEAD INJURIES IN ADULTS AND IN CHILDREN

Prehospital care: assessment, oxygenation, blood pressure, GCS, pupils. Treatment: airway ventilation, oxygenation, fluid resuscitation, brain specific therapies

Hospital care: blood pressure and oxygenation, hyperosmolar therapy, prophylactic hypothermia prophylaxis of seizures, infection, DVT

Monitoring ICP: indications, methodology, thresholds, CPP, and brain oxygen

Anesthetics, analgesic, sedatives, nutrition hyperventilation, steroids

SURGICAL MANAGEMENT

Indications timing methods for EDH, SDH, ICH, posterior fossa, depressed cranial fractures

COMBAT

Triage and transport, algorithm for field management

CT, computed tomography; GCS, Glasgow Coma Scale; DVT, deep vein thrombosis; ICP, intracranial pressure; CPP, cerebral perfusion pressure; EDH, epidural hemorrhage; SDH, subdural hemorrhage; ICH, intracerebral hemorrhage. Reprinted from SIGN (e13), NICE (e14), and BTF (21) with permission.

intracranial events in individual patients and how best to apply the findings to management. ICP has remained a focus and monitoring by intraparenchymal devices has removed the need for ventricular puncture—a step requiring neurosurgical skills. However, the major change has been the replacement of "eyeballing" a tracing or a single digit display by more accurate and informative computerized acquisition and analysis of its findings. An early finding (22) was that secondary insults were more common than previously appreciated—even in patients considered to be stable in intensive care. Analyses of changes in ICP in response to various manipulations, such as the effect of small changes in intracranial volume or blood pressure on components of the ICP wave form and their transmission, have cast light on ICP volume dynamics and cerebrovascular reactivity and regulation.

In view of the importance of secondary ischemic damage, the search for direct indicators of cerebral blood flow (CBF) and oxygenation has been natural but challenging. Complexities come from the balance between the utility of indices reflecting total, overall or net conditions in the brain, which can miss critical local inadequacies, and of local data, which can be very variable and unrepresentative at any one site. The transient nature of many insults adds the need for frequent or continuous acquisition. Invasiveness also needs to be minimized.

Techniques used include measurement of oxygenation in jugular venous samples, transcranial doppler, and near infrared spectroscopy, implanted devices for sensing tissue Po_2, and microdialysis probes to obtain extracellular fluid in which levels of chemicals including neurotransmitters such as glutamate, glucose, lactate, pyruvate, and other metabolites have been measured. Some of the most definitive insights have come from the comprehensive pictures provided by research combining positron emission tomography (PET) scanning of local and global oxygenation and intracerebral metabolic monitoring. These have displayed the heterogeneity of local conditions and their response to therapeutic maneuvers (e30,e31).

The findings from these techniques have been of great research interest, yielding many insights into the complexities of damage and, in some academic centers, have been incorporated into practical care with apparent benefit over previous methods (23). However, distillation into messages that have been taken up into routine, individually tailored management in less specialized circumstances has not so far been evident. Instead, the more generally used approach is to use interventions against raised ICP in a sequential, "tiered" way (16). Initially, a patient is sedated and mildly hyperventilated; hyperthermia is avoided and cardiovascular stability established. If ICP remains or becomes raised, successive steps are drainage of CSF and administration of mannitol. If ICP remains high, one measure is administration of barbiturates, but their action in lowering ICP by reducing metabolic requirements and hence CBF needs to be set against side effects such as hypotension. Another option is the creation of an external decompression by removal of a large bone flap. This procedure was in vogue in the 1960s and 1970s and, after falling out of use, has seen resurgence in use in the last decade, despite lack of rigorous evidence. The search for evidence through prospective randomized studies has been difficult because of problems in recruitment. A recent disturbing finding has been that patients randomized to undergo bifrontal craniectomy have a worse outcome, especially a high rate of survival with severe disability (e35), echoing the concerns of the 1960s (e20). Efforts to clarify the benefits of decompressive operations continue through ongoing trials (e36,e37).

Cellular and Molecular Mechanisms as Targets of Treatment—Neuroprotection

Extensive experimental research during the later years of the 20th century resulted in much being learnt about the fundamental cellular and molecular mechanisms of brain damage. The primary focus was often the ischemic damage of stroke. Nevertheless, the implications for head injuries were clear. First, there was the abundant evidence of the importance of secondary ischemic damage in severe and fatal injuries. Second, experimentally, the consequences of primary and secondary injury were additive, the extent of brain damage being greater when traumatic injury and hypotension were combined than after either insult alone (e38). This made it likely that there were interactions and overlaps between the processes of traumatic and ischemic damage. A full account of the work in ischemia is beyond the remit

of this chapter and the application of the findings to brain and spinal cord injury has been set out in a sequence of Neurotrauma symposia (e39) that have brought basic and clinical researchers together in North America and internationally. The outputs have been regularly reported in the *Journal of Neurotrauma*; since this was founded in 1983, its development into a high "impact" publication has promoted the quality and repute of central nervous system injury research. (See also Chapters 11 and 12 in this text.)

The damaging processes and mediators identified in experimental and clinical research included excessive intracellular calcium, excess action of a range of neurotransmitters, oxidative damage from "free radicals," mitochondrial dysfunction, and inflammation. A range of interventions, with varying specific targeting, has been developed in the pharmaceutical industry and shown to reduce the extent of damage in various experimental models. Attention expanded to the processes of recovery from damage and the potential for benefit from biological agents such as trophic factors and genetic influences.

The need to promote safe, valid evaluations of these new treatments in patients with head injury led to the formation of academically led clinical collaborative groups such as the American Brain Injury Consortium (e40) and the European Brain Injury Consortium (e4). Working in partnership with industry, these consortia brought the influence of experienced clinical investigators to the design, conduct, and analysis of studies, in particular in trials aimed to test efficacy. In spite of these efforts, and so far more than 30 "Phase III" randomized trials, none have provided clear evidence of benefit in head injury (24) or indeed in stroke. The reasons for these failures continue to be debated, in particular the "jump" between the controlled circumstances of the experimental laboratory and clinical treatment of patients and limitations in the design and analysis of clinical trials.

New Approaches to Clinical Trials

Trials of neuroprotection have been criticized as based on exaggerated expectations of the likely size of the effect of the treatment and the study of too few patients (e42). One response was the advocacy of the need for simple, "mega trials" of many thousands of subjects. The only such study so far, the MRC CRASH trial (e43), concerned a steroid, methylprednisone. In any event, the trial was discontinued because of evidence that treatment actually increased mortality. A more promising path has been to seek methods of design and analysis that enhance the sensitivity of a trial. This appears to have been achieved through work of IMPACT (25). This European/North American collaboration, led by Andrew Maas from Rotterdam and Antwerp, Gordon Murray from Edinburgh, and Tony Marmarou from Richmond, and funded by the National Institute of Health (NIH) is descended from the International Data Bank and incorporates data from 43,678 patients in previous studies. The group predicted that analysis using the ordered nature of components of GOS and incorporating prognostic weighting could double the sensitivity of the trial (e44). This appears to have been be confirmed by the finding that application of the method to the data from MRC CRASH Trial showed the adverse effects of methylprednisone in only a half of the number recruited (e45). The approach is now being used in most studies in acute brain injury.

Understanding the Primary Effects of a Head Injury

The apparent lack of benefit from treatments aimed at the mechanisms of secondary damage redirected attention to the importance of understanding the mechanisms of primary injury and their potential for treatment. Work in Oxford in WWII by Denny Brown and Ritchie Russell (e6) had showed that the immediate loss of consciousness that is characteristic of a head injury, despite little to see in the brain, was produced experimentally by dynamic head movement, not static compression. Ayub Ommaya, a neurosurgeon who had been a Rhodes fellow in Oxford in 1956, then implemented biomechanically based experimental investigations of concussion and coma at the National Institute of Neurological Disorders and Stroke (NINDS) in Baltimore (e47). These were subsequently continued in Philadelphia at the University of Pennsylvania when Ommaya's collaborator, Thomas Gennarelli moved to join Langfitt's team.

The picture that emerged was of brain injury produced by rotational forces, especially coronal, and occurring without the necessity of head contact or any rise in ICP, leading to shear strain damage of the kind originally identified by AHS Holbourne in Oxford (e48) using gelatin models. The concept elaborated was of damage developing in a centripetal sequence—starting in the outer layers of the cerebral hemisphere and descending with increasing severity of input through white matter to deep structures, with the brain stem involved only at the ultimate stage. This pattern was also expressed in increasing neurological and behavioral impairments (26).

Observations by Adams and colleagues in Glasgow (27) in the bank of brains from fatal human head injuries reinforced the experimental findings in Philadelphia. They identified a pattern of damage characterized by macroscopic lesions in the corpus callosum and dorsolateral brain stem accompanied by widespread microscopic damage in the white matter in patients who had been rendered unconscious from the instant of injury. The pattern was subsequently termed diffuse axonal injury and graded I–III according to the location of the macroscopic lesion (e49). In accord with the Omaya/Gennarelli concept, the brain stem was never the only site of damage and deep coma could occur without brain stem involvement. Collaboration between the Glasgow neuropathologists and the University of Pennsylvania researchers showed that the human findings were fully replicated in the primate experimental model.

Diffuse axonal injury can be found at autopsy in people who had been unconscious for matters of only a few minutes in the acute stage (e50). Conversely, recent findings in the Glasgow brain bank point to diffuse axonal injury as also having a key role in late outcome. In contrast to early deaths, in which secondary ischemic damage seems to dominate, the main finding in groups of patients who had initially survived but died later after remaining in either a vegetative or severely disabled state was of severe diffuse axonal injury (e51).

Although, for biomechanical reasons, the full picture of diffuse axonal injury cannot be replicated in small brains,

studies in rodents have been important in dissecting the cellular and molecular mechanisms of damage and their time course. From extensive histological work, John Povlishock's group in Richmond discovered that axonal disconnection, which had been assumed to be a reflection of instantaneous shearing, usually develop secondarily as a delayed event (28). The interval to disconnection may last several hours, potentially opening a window for treatment (e52).

TRENDS IN OUTCOME

Mortality

The report of Stein and colleagues (2) presents average mortality rates in 176 series containing at least 60 patients from 1930 to 2006. This showed 3 distinct phases (Figure 2-2).

Mortality fell sharply in the 1970s and 1980s, by an average of 5% per decade, but there was not a significant change in the preceding or following periods. This pattern broadly corresponds with the foregoing account of evolution in approaches to management but many factors may lie behind findings over such a long term and there is a need for caution in comparisons. The causes of injury have been altering, victims are older, documentation of severity has evolved, and varying criteria used for inclusion in reports. Nevertheless, studies in which case selection and severity have been matched have also reported declines in mortality between 1984 and 1996 (e53) but that case fatality did not improve between 1994 and 2003 (e54).

Disability in Survivors

The outcomes in survivors are particularly relevant to practitioners and providers of rehabilitation services. The frequency of disability after severe injury does not appear to have decreased over time and, instead, data from cohort studies (Table 2-3) indicate that the proportion judged still to have severe disability 6 months after a severe head injury

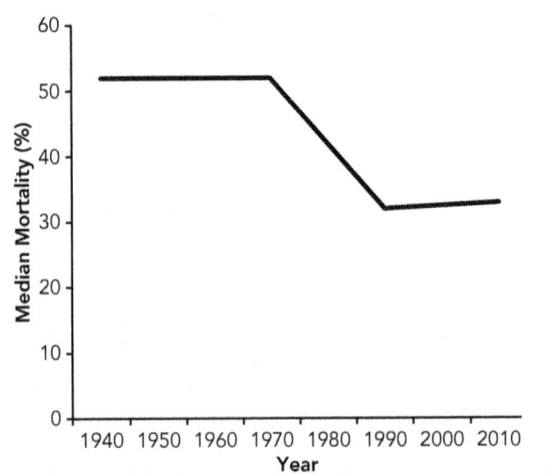

FIGURE 2-2 Composite diagrams of average mortality rates in 176 series containing at least 60 victims reported between 1930 and 2006. Reprinted from Stein, Georgoff, Meghan, Mizra, Sonnad (2) with permission.

TABLE 2-3 Severe Disability in Survivors of Severe Head Injury

SERIES	DATE	TOTAL	MORTALITY	SEVERE DISABILITY IN SURVIVORS
International Data Bank (19)	1977	2959	49%	29%
North American Traumatic Coma Data Bank (15)	1983	746	36%	27%
Four UK Neurosurgical Centers (30)	1993	976	40%	28%
European Brain Injury Survey (31)	1999	481	40%	29%

has remained remarkably similar over time at around 25%. Thus, although mortality has fallen and achievement of independent recovery has correspondingly increased, in between lies a consistent, enduring group of victims who require the benefits of the advances in rehabilitation that are the subject of the next part of this history.

HISTORY OF TRAUMATIC BRAIN INJURY NEUROREHABILITATION

World War II

WWII marked the real beginning of modern rehabilitation. One of the most significant contributors to rehabilitation of brain injury during the 1940s was Professor Oliver L. Zangwill, a professor of Experimental Psychology at the University of Cambridge in the United Kingdom. He made valuable contributions to the understanding of localization in the cerebral cortex, to the changes in memory following brain injury, and to the long-standing idea that language and handedness are necessarily co-located. He also made valuable contributions to the study of retrograde amnesia. He provided a solid basis for the inclusion of psychology within biological science (31). In the United States, Professor Noel Kephart, a physical therapist, began treating children and adults with TBI based on his experience in treating WWII veterans utilizing a wide range of therapies, including physical therapy, occupational therapy, speech therapy, and aqua therapy (32).

Ritchie Russell, a physician in Edinburgh, later a Professor in Oxford, joined the Army during the war and developed a keen interest in head injuries among soldiers injured in the war. He studied thousands of wounded warriors that produced a better understanding of head trauma caused by war and, in later years, contributed greatly to our understanding of speech and memory problems resulting from head injury (33).

WWII made a huge difference not only in the way in which Americans perceived persons with disability but also in the formalization of Physical Medicine and Rehabilitation as a medical specialty. Dr Howard Kessler was a strong advocate of rehabilitation of veterans. It was he who implemented the concept of a comprehensive medical-social-psychological-vocational approach to disability. It was during this time that Howard Rush, MD, a colonel in the Air Force, demonstrated the effectiveness of physical medicine with injured pilots. After WWII, when rehabilitation began to falter, it was Howard Kessler and Howard Rush (34) who persisted, resulting in the American Medical Association creating a specialty board in Physical Medicine in 1947.

Post–World War II Through the 1970s

Looking back on the history of rehabilitation, we see the emergence of neurorehabilitation of persons with TBI in the earliest stages of recovery. The early treatment of persons with TBI was also influenced by the discovery of new drugs. These psychopharmacological discoveries included lithium in 1949, chlorpromazine in 1952, and the discovery of the antidepressant properties of iproniazid and imipramine in 1957, and the introduction of chlordiazepoxide in 1960.

During the 1960s and 1970s, there was shift from rehabilitation and disability program expansion to disability rights. Independent living, the concept of normalization, community-based rehabilitation, class action suits, and personal advocacy grew into a movement (35).

The Vietnam War made its mark on the history of disability rehabilitation as better medicine and the use of medevac helicopters resulted in more soldiers surviving more severe injuries. Unfortunately, many of the Vietnam survivors with TBI went unrecognized and untreated. Andres Salazar, MD conducted a longitudinal study of a large cohort of veterans with TBI sustained in the Vietnam War. He found large numbers of homeless men, a high frequency of drug problems, as well as high rates of suicide and unemployment (36).

Brain Injury Rehabilitation Pioneers
The development of the GCS and the GOS (9,19) created a standardized method for assessing the severity of injury and predicting long-term outcomes and helped to push brain injury rehabilitation to the forefront. Henry Stonnington, Sheldon Berrol, Leonard Diller, Anne-Lise Christensen, and Yehuda Ben Yishay were pioneers in innovative rehabilitation and treatment. These men and women began the movement of "community-based rehabilitation for persons with TBI." This new concept led to the development of holistic treatment programs and new venues for providing rehabilitation. Yehuda Ben Yishay began a specialized vocational program which was both academic, psychological, and work oriented (37). Professor Anne-Lise Christensen in Denmark started a program at the University of Copenhagen, which combined academic training, music, and psychological therapy with a firm foundation based in neuropsychological principles (38). George Prigatano began his seminal work on understanding the role of emotions and caring in the rehabilitation process (39). This marked the beginning of patients being referred to specialized brain injury rehabilitation centers rather than being sent to nursing homes (40). According to Mitchell Rosenthal, this paradigm shift in care of persons with TBI occurred between 1975 and 1977. During this time,

an influential association was established for professionals by Henry Stonnington, MD and Sheldon Berrol, MD—the International Association for the Study of Traumatic Brain Injury (IASTBI). This marked the beginning of international research cooperation and sharing of treatment and training ideas and methods.

TBI Rehabilitation in the 1980s

National Head Injury Foundation, Brain Injury Association, International Brain Injury Association, and Other Brain Injury Organizations

In April 1980, Marilyn Spivak and her husband Martin hosted the first meeting of what was to become the National Head Injury Foundation (NHIF) at their home in Massachusetts (41). The purpose of the meeting was to discuss forming an organization to serve people who had survived TBI. During that year, a Board of Directors was selected and NHIF was incorporated as a not-for-profit organization. The founding goals have relevance even to this day. The goals of the NHIF were as follows:

1. To stimulate public and professional awareness of the problem of head injury—the silent epidemic. To make the public aware of the nature and causes of head injury and the necessary steps that needs to be taken to prevent them.
2. To provide a central clearinghouse for information and resources for individuals with head injury and their families. To provide these individuals and their families with necessary information and support during and after crises.
3. To develop a support group network for individuals with head injury and their families.
4. To establish and promote specialized head injury rehabilitation programs. To help educate health care professionals about the unique needs of individuals with head injury.
5. To advocate for increased research funding and more appropriate care for individuals with brain injury.
6. In 1983, the goal of prevention was added.

It was during this time that the consumer movement in TBI really took hold. The establishment of "chapters of NHIF" across the country helped fuel this movement. NHIF moved from Massachusetts to Washington, DC to begin a new era of expansion. Soon, the name was changed to the Brain Injury Association (BIA). Although BIA was expanding into research and public policy, George A. Zitnay, PhD and Martin B. Foil Jr founded a new international organization in 1992 (32). The International Brain Injury Association (IBIA) rapidly grew with the support of the World Health Organization (WHO). IBIA became a leader in multidisciplinary and interdisciplinary training and treatment with the establishment of the World Congress on Brain Injury, which has since been held in 7 countries around the world, truly an international movement.

Similar family and consumer organizations sprung up in other countries led by HEADWAY in England. In Europe, the formation of the European Brain Injury Society led the way for cooperative research, sharing of date, and expansion of community-based treatment programs.

During the 1980s, with increasing interest by professionals in brain injury rehabilitation, the American Congress of Rehabilitation Medicine created the Head Injury Interdisciplinary Special Interest Group (HI-ISIG). In the late 1980s, 2 journals—*Brain Injury* and the *Journal of Head Trauma Rehabilitation*—began publishing, greatly expanding the scientific literature in TBI (40).

Commission on Accreditation of Rehabilitation Facilities, National Institute on Disability and Rehabilitation Research Model Systems, and Growth of Brain Injury Rehabilitation Programs

In 1985, standards of care for brain injury rehabilitation were adopted by the Commission on Accreditation of Rehabilitation Facilities (CARF) (42). These standards resulted from the work of the HI-ISIG. A milestone in brain injury rehabilitation was reached in 1987 when the US Department of Education's National Institute on Disability and Rehabilitation Research (NIDRR) funded 5 TBI model systems of care (43).

The 1980s were a tumultuous time for brain injury rehabilitation. In the early 1980s, there was a huge increase in the development of for-profit rehabilitation programs aimed at attracting those families of persons with brain injury that had insurance, court settlements, or the ability to pay. Glossy brochures, recruiting techniques that included bringing whole families by private jet to visit programs, and facilities that looked terrific but lacked professionally trained staff. Some call this the "golden age" but others, particularly persons with brain injury, called it a time of shame. The 1980s can be classified as a period of ups and downs, growth, investigation of fraud, decline, and then reemergence as the 1980s closed into a period of downsizing, buyouts, closures, and finally settling into a period of insurance companies questioning the value of rehabilitation and limiting the amount and time for rehabilitation services. As the 1980s ended, change was taking place in the delivery systems of rehabilitation. Emphasis was placed on home treatment, community-based rehabilitation, day services, independent living, and advocacy.

1990s to the Present

In 1990, the Americans with Disabilities Act (ADA) was passed and signed into law by President George H. Bush. The Act proclaims participation in the mainstream of daily life as an American right and calls for accommodation in housing and public spaces. The ADA was intended to foster independence and integration, providing persons with disability antidiscrimination protection. Similar laws were passed around the world. Change was again propelling the TBI system of care to demonstrate effectiveness and efficacy.

Research and Evidence-Based Guidelines

An article on the State of Rehabilitation by Denise Tate (44) was published in the *Archives of Physical Medicine and Rehabilitation* (Vol. 87, No. 2 Feb. 2006). The author used quantitative methods to determine if rehabilitation research adequately stood up to the rigors of scientific methods to be called "science." She stated that the field of rehabilitation had been portrayed as slow to promote its scientific achievements and to include them under the rubric of evidence-based rehabilitation. Her findings suggested that, as a field, rehabilitation had made a contribution to science. She pointed out the difficulties associated with the use of the scientific method in rehabilitation research and suggested that the field needed to devise new ways in which to bolster science and develop greater research capacity in rehabilitation. The question whether successful rehabilitation is science or art was not answered.

The demand for scientific support for treatment has led to the development of evidence-based guidelines in all areas of health care. Guidelines are specific formulations of the traditional standard of care concept. Although physicians have followed clinical protocols for years, those protocols were not based on a rigorous review of the scientific evidence of their appropriateness. The process of guideline development distinguishes the current movement from historical methods of promoting science-driven practice. In response to increasing concerns of physicians, third-party payers, and patients about the quality and costs of medical care in the United States, the American Association of Neurological Surgeons (AANS) and the societies supporting rehabilitation have strongly supported the development of guidelines and/or practice parameters.

More needs to be done to study the effect of guidelines in TBI care and rehabilitation. Currently, in addition to those already described for acute management, practice guidelines exist for prognosis in TBI, mild TBI, and, most recently, the Defense and Veterans Brain Injury Center work in the development of guidelines for the management of neurobehavioral consequences following TBI (45).

Finally, the late 1990s and into early 2000 have come to be seen as a period of cost reduction, accountability, managed care, and the closing or merging of many programs in TBI rehabilitation. Length of stay, payment, and reimbursement constraints have become real problems in the rehabilitation of persons with TBI. The move toward empowering persons with disabilities has led to greater expectations for quality of life and consequently greater efforts at finding innovative rehabilitation techniques and programs. This, combined with a better understanding of how the brain can heal, has helped shape the evolution of TBI rehabilitation.

As stated earlier, outcomes, evidence-based practice guidelines for management of acute care, penetrating brain injury, and neurobehavioral sequelae of TBI have been developed by the Neurotrauma Foundation (NTF) and the National Brain Injury Research, Treatment, and Training Foundation (NBIRTT) and various professional societies throughout Europe. Recognizing there were no specific guidelines or tools for measuring quality of life issues in persons with TBI, an international group of rehabilitation specialists under the leadership of Edmund Neugebauer and Jean Luc-Truelle, MD of France, et al, as created a new assessment tool to measure quality of life for persons with TBI. The Quality of Life after Brain Injury (QOLIBRI) is available for widespread distribution.

What is the future of TBI neurorehabilitation? Traditionally, rehabilitation has been a reactive rather than proactive profession. Rehabilitation education and similar activities have been based on past experience, often with little thought given to future needs. There is agreement in rehabilitation that several issues will profoundly affect the future. Those issues include changes in the nature of work in the United States and around the world, growing diversity in the workforce, changes in the nature of disability, advances in rehabilitation and medical technology, and alterations in the nature of strategies of service delivery and payment for same.

Ongoing research into existing and new methodologies offers new hope for improving outcomes in TBI neurorehabilitation. Many of the most recent lessons learned have come from the war experiences in Iraq and Afghanistan. Blast injury research, electronic psychological evaluation, battlefield triage, and better imaging and more powerful imaging tools are leading to a better understanding of the cascade of events following TBI, as well as to better outcomes.

To respond to the injured with brain trauma coming from the wars, Defense Centers of Excellence for Psychological Health and Traumatic Brain Injury (DCoE) was established by the United States Congress in November 1977 to bring together disparate programs providing health care, training, research, and education for wounded warriors. The purpose was to develop a coordinating center under the Assistant Secretary of Defense for Health Affairs that would consolidate purpose and direction for psychological health, TBI and smaller centers for the study of traumatic stress, telehealth, clinical health, and the center for deployment psychology.

The Congress was looking for a way forward to provide leadership to address the growing numbers of wounded warriors coming from the wars in Iraq and Afghanistan with TBI, post-traumatic stress disorder, and other stress related health issues. In addition, suicide was on the increase. To bring about this effort, the Congress mandated that all of the branches of the military—Army, Navy, Air Force, and Marines—support the new DCoE with personnel. In addition, the Department of Veterans Affairs (VA) was asked to provide support through a liaison officer assigned to DCoE.

Under the leadership of the first Director of the DCoE, Brigadier General Loree Sutton, MD, the mission was defined as follows: to assess, validate, oversee, and facilitate prevention, resilience, identification, treatment, outreach, rehabilitation, and reintegration programs for psychological health (PH) to ensure the Department of Defense meets the needs of the nation's military communities, warriors, and families. DCoE works across the entire "continuum of care" including a collaborative effort that includes the VA, civilian agencies, community leaders, advocacy groups, clinical efforts, and academic institutions.

It was during the initial period of organization that the Fisher family and the Intrepid Fallen Heroes Fund approached the Department of Defense and DCoE to create a new center, the National Intrepid Center of Excellence (NICoE).

NICoE was dedicated in June 2010. It is designed to be the leader in advancing world-class psychological health and TBI research, treatment, and education for servicemembers, veterans, and their families. NICoE is located on the grounds of the National Naval Medical Center campus in Bethesda, MD. The NICoE provides the best in assessment, diagnosis, treatment planning, and long-term follow-up for PH and TBI. It will be a proving ground for the initiatives, guidelines, and trainings developed by DCoE and provide a base for clinical research into the PH and TBI issues that impact on servicemembers and their families.

In addition, NICoE, through a Fisher House (home) on the campus, provides families to come and live and learn while their family member is being diagnosed or treated. Dr James Kelly, a noted expert in concussion and TBI, serves as the first Director of NICoE (46).

Constant changes in rehabilitation can be predicted with certainty. History suggests that rehabilitation practitioners, especially those working in brain injury, will continue to face budget cutbacks resulting in staffing shortages, growing caseloads, and changes in the structure and function of the rehabilitation system. To respond, the field must become proactive. This will involve networking with other rehabilitation professionals, facilities, agencies, and consumers. There is and will continue to be a need to deliver efficient and effective rehabilitation services that can be measured and evaluated.

Finally, we must continue to provide for continued learning and education of professionals, consumers, and policymakers (47).

CONCLUSION

Because there are few demonstrable effective treatments for TBI, we must look to the future. It holds great promise because of emerging advanced microtechnology, new drugs that could prove extremely beneficial, the development of neuroprosthesis, the promise of the study of proteins, implantation of devices to stimulate damaged parts of the brain, new advanced imaging, and the hope of clinical research in the use of genetic therapy.

The ongoing wars and growing numbers of wounded warriors is forcing governments to rethink funding priorities for clinical, applied, and experimental research in brain injury, which may lead to more effective treatments and outcomes. These changes are being driven by increased awareness of the consequences of TBI as portrayed daily on television, social media, and in other new forms of instant communication. Showing wounded warriors with TBI on the battlefield or in the struggle to overthrow a dictator or on the sports field has not only increased public awareness but also a growing understanding of the public health concerns regarding the impact of TBI on society. The public is now demanding the government and political leaders to provide resources for research, treatment, and for community and family support.

KEY CLINICAL POINTS

1. The many advances in acute care of head injuries since WWII are built on principles derived from military experiences and expressed through modern scientific, technological, and organizational progress.
2. The dramatic increase in civilian closed head injuries throughout the world in the second half of the 20th century, as a consequence of the growth of road traffic and urbanization, stimulated growing recognition of the importance of head injuries.
3. In the early 1970s the group that formed around Bryan Jennett in Glasgow drew attention to the importance of

secondary ischemic brain damage and established assessment of the severity of damage by the Glasgow Coma Scale and the use of CT scanning as the basis of management in the acute stage and in comparing early severity with outcome.
4. Data acquired by such studies as the North American Traumatic Coma Data Bank study further spurred the advancement of prevention and treatment of intra and extra-cranial "secondary" insults through organised approaches, based on rigorous guidelines, from pre-hospital to modern neuro-critical intensive care systems.
5. Although successful in limiting brain damage in experimental models, "neuroprotective" pharmacological treatment has so far been not shown to improve outcome in patients.
6. The advances in management since 1960s have reduced mortality significantly but the perisisting incidence of late disability reflects the occurence of severe primary damage in the most seriously affected survivors.
7. Rehabilitation efforts for brain injury also grew out of treatment of war injuries during World War II with the efforts of Dr. Howard Kessler, a strong advocate of rehabilitaion of veterans and Dr. Howard Rush, an Air Force colonel who demonstrated the effectiveness of physical medicine with injured pilots.
8. In the 1970s and 1980s, pioneers in brain injury rehabilitation such as Henry Stonnington, Sheldon Berrol, Leonard Diller, Anne-Lise Christensen, and Yehuda Ben Yishay developed specialized programs beginning the movement of "community-based rehabilitation for persons with TBI."
9. The 1980s saw the growth of organizations for TBI advocacy, research, and professional association including NHIF, BIA, IBIA, ACRM-BIISIG), CARF, NIDRR Model Systems, as well as huge growth of rehabilitation treatment programs.
10. The late 1990s and 2000s have come to be seen as a period of cost reduction, accountability, managed care, and the closing or merging of many programs in TBI rehabilitation, as well as a period of growth of research and push to develop evidence-based practice guidelines for treatment and rehabilitation. The large number of injuries associated with the wars in Iraq and Afghanistan after 2001 has been a catalyst to expand efforts in research, prevention, assessment and treatment in rehabilitation of persons with TBI in military and civilian settings.

KEY REFERENCES

1. Bullock R, Chesnut RM, Clifton G, et al. Guidelines for the management of severe head injury. Brain Trauma Foundation. *Eur J Emerg Med.* 1996;3(2):109–127.
2. Graham DI, Adams JH. Ischaemic brain damage in fatal head injuries. *Lancet.* 1971;1(7693):265–266.
3. Jennett B, Bond M. Assessment of outcome after severe brain damage. *Lancet.* 1975;1(7905):480–484.
4. Jennett B, Teasdale G, Galbraith S, et al. Severe head injuries in three countries. *J Neurol Neurosurg Psychiatry.* 1977;40(3):291–298.

5. Langfitt TW, Tannanbaum HM, Kassell NF. The etiology of acute brain swelling following experimental head injury. *J Neurosurg.* 1966;24(1):47–56.

6. Marshall LF, Gautille T, Klauber M, et al. The outcome of severe closed head injury. *J Neurosurg.* 1991;75:S28–S36.

7. Ommaya AK, Gennarelli TA. Cerebral concussion and traumatic unconsciousness. Correlation of experimental and clinical observations of blunt head injuries. *Brain.* 1974;97(4):633–654.

8. Povlishock JT. Traumatically induced axonal injury: pathogenesis and pathobiological implications. *Brain Pathol.* 1992;2(1):1–12.

9. Prigatano GP, Klonoff PS. Psychotherapy and neuropsychological assessment after brain injury. *J Head Trauma Rehabil.* 1988;3:45–56.

10. Teasdale G, Jennett B. Assessment of coma and impaired consciousness. A practical scale. *Lancet.* 1974;2(7872): 81–84.

References

1. Cairns H. Neurosurgery in the British Army, 1939–1945. *Br J Surg.* 1947;55(suppl 1):9–26.

2. Stein SC, Georgoff P, Meghan S, Mizra K, Sonnad SS. 150 years of treating severe traumatic brain injury: a systematic review of progress in mortality. *J Neurotrauma.* 2010;27(7):1343–1353.

3. Rowbotham GF, Maciver IN, Dickson J, Bousfield ME. Analysis of 1,400 cases of acute injury to the head. *Br Med J.* 1954;1(4864): 726–730.

4. McKissock W, Taylor JC, Bloom WH, Till K. Extradural haematoma: observations on 125 cases. *Lancet.* 1960;2:167–172.

5. Langfitt TW, Tannanbaum HM, Kassell NF. The etiology of acute brain swelling following experimental head injury. *J Neurosurg.* 1966;24(1):47–56.

6. Lundberg N, Troupp H, Lorin H. Continuous recording of the ventricular-fluid pressure in patients with severe acute traumatic brain injury. A preliminary report. *J Neurosurg.* 1965;22(6):581–590.

7. Graham DI, Adams JH. Ischaemic brain damage in fatal head injuries. *Lancet.* 1971;1(7693):265–266.

8. Reilly PL, Graham DI, Adams JH, Jennett B. Patients with head injury who talk and die. *Lancet.* 1975;2(7931):375–377.

9. Teasdale G, Jennett B. Assessment of coma and impaired consciousness. A practical scale. *Lancet.* 1974;2(7872):81–84.

10. Ambrose J, Gooding MR, Uttley D. E.M.I. scan in the management of head injuries. *Lancet.* 1976;1(7964):847–848.

11. Teasdale G, Galbraith S, Murray L, Ward P, Gentleman D, McKean M. Management of traumatic intracranial haematoma. *Br Med J (Clin Res Ed).* 1982;285(6356):1695–1697.

12. Guidelines for initial management after head injury in adults. Suggestions from a group of neurosurgeons. *Br Med J (Clin Res Ed).* 1984;288(6422):983–985.

13. Miller JD, Becker DP. Secondary insults to the injured brain. *J R Coll Surg Edinb.* 1982;27(5):292–298.

14. Marshall LF, Gautille T, Klauber M, et al. The outcome of severe closed head injury. *J Neurosurg.* 1991;75:S28–S36.

15. Marmarou A, Anderson RL, Ward JD, Choi SC, Young HF. Impact of ICP instability and hypotension on outcome in patients with severe head trauma. *J Neurosurg.* 1991;75:S59–S66.

16. Chesnut RM, Marshall LF, Klauber MR, et al. The role of secondary brain injury in determining outcome from severe head injury. *J Trauma.* 1993;34(2):216–222.

17. Piek J, Chesnut RM, Marshall LF, et al. Extracranial complications of severe head injury. *J Neurosurg.* 1992;77(6):901–907.

18. Jennett B, Teasdale G, Galbraith S, et al. Severe head injuries in three countries. *J Neurol Neurosurg Psychiatry.* 1977;40(3):291–298.

19. Jennett B, Bond M. Assessment of outcome after severe brain damage. *Lancet.* 1975;1(7905):480–484.

20. Ghajar J, Hariri RJ, Narayan RK, Iacono LA, Firlik K, Patterson RH. Survey of critical care management of comatose, head-injured patients in the United States. *Crit Care Med.* 1995;23(3):560–567.

21. Bullock R, Chesnut RM, Clifton G, et al. Guidelines for the management of severe head injury. Brain Trauma Foundation. *Eur J Emerg Med.* 1996;3(2):109–127.

22. Jones PA, Andrews PJ, Midgley S, et al. Measuring the burden of secondary insults in head-injured patients during intensive care. *J Neurosurg Anesthesiol.* 1994;6(1):4–14.

23. Patel HC, Menon DK, Tebbs S, Hawker R, Hutchinson PJ, Kirkpatrick PJ. Specialist neurocritical care and outcome from head injury. *Intensive Care Med.* 2002;28(5):547–553.

24. Tolias CM, Bullock MR. Critical appraisal of neuroprotection trials in head injury: what have we learned? *NeuroRx.* 2004;1(1):71–79.

25. Maas AI, Marmarou A, Murray GD, Teasdale SG, Steyerberg EW. Prognosis and clinical trial design in traumatic brain injury: the IMPACT study. *J Neurotrauma.* 2007;24(2):232–238.

26. Ommaya AK, Gennarelli TA. Cerebral concussion and traumatic unconsciousness. Correlation of experimental and clinical observations of blunt head injuries. *Brain.* 1974;97(4):633–654.

27. Adams H, Mitchell DE, Graham DI, Doyle D. Diffuse brain injury of immediate impact type. Its relationship to 'primary brain-stem damage' in head injury. *Brain.* 1977;100(3):489–502.

28. Povlishock JT. Traumatically induced axonal injury: pathogenesis and pathobiological implications. *Brain Pathol.* 1992;2(1):1–12.

29. Murray LS, Teasdale GM, Murray GD, Miller DJ, Pickard JD, Shaw MD. Head injuries in four British neurosurgical centres. *Br J Neurosurg.* 1999;13(6):564–569.

30. Murray GD, Teasdale GM, Braakman R, et al. The European Brain Injury Consortium survey of head injuries. *Acta Neurochir* (Wien). 1999;141(3):223–236.

31. Zangwill OL. Psychological aspects of rehabilitation in cases of brain injury. *Br J Psychol Gen Sect.* 1947;37(2):60–69.

32. Zitnay G. Head Injury. In: Dell Orto AE, Marinelli RP, eds. *Encyclopedia of Disability and Rehabilitation.* New York, NY: McMillan; 1995: 361–366.

33. Russell R. *Neurotimes.* London, UK: 2009.

34. Kessler HH. Principles and practices of rehabilitation. *Am J Med Sci.* 1950;219.

35. Owens MJ. Consumer perspectives on the preparation of rehabilitation professions. *J Vocat Rehabil.* 1992;2:4–11.

36. Salazar AM, Zitnay GA, Warden DL, Schwab KA. Defense and Veterans Brain Injury Program. *J Head Trauma Rehabil.* 2000;15: 1081–1091.

37. Yishay YG. In: Bigler ED, ed. *Traumatic Brain Injury: Mechanisms of Damage, Assessment, Intervention, and Outcome.* Austin, TX: Pro-Ed; 1990.

38. Christensen AL. *Luria's Neuropsychological Investigation: Text.* New York, NY: Spectrum Publications; 1975.

39. Prigatano GP, Klonoff PS. Psychotherapy and neuropsychological assessment after brain injury. *J Head Trauma Rehabil.* 1988;3:45–56.

40. Rosenthal M. 1995 Sheldon Berrol, MD senior lectureship: the ethics and efficacy of traumatic brain injury rehabilitation—myths, measurements, and meaning. *J Head Trauma Rehabil.* 1996;11:88–95.

41. Spivak M. A perspective of National Head Injury Foundation (NHIF) from 1980–1990. *TBI Challenge.* 2000;4(1).

42. Switzer MD. Report of the U.S. Social and Rehabilitation Services Commission. Washington, DC: US Government Printing Office; 1966.

43. US Department of Education. *Creation of the National Institute on Disability and Rehabilitation Research (NIDRD).* Washington, DC: US Government Printing Office; 1980.

44. Frontera WR, Fuhrer MJ, Jette AM, et al. Rehabilitation Medicine Summit: Building Research Capacity: executive summary. *Am J Occup Ther.* 2006;60(2):165–176.

45. Department of Defense and Department of Veterans Affairs, Traumatic Brain Injury Task Force, 2008.

46. Defense Centers of Excellence of Psychological Health and Traumatic Brain Injury, US Government Document, December 2011.

47. Ward MJ, Halloran W. Transition issues for the 1990s. *OSERS News in Print.* 1993;6(1):4–5.

3

Health Policy: United States and International Perspectives

Jean E. Bérubé and Lynne Turner-Stokes

INTRODUCTION

The World Health Organization (WHO) states that "good health is essential to human welfare and to sustained economic and social development" (1). The dimensions of health can encompass "a state of complete physical, mental, and social well-being and not merely the absence of disease or infirmity" (2).

Most governments now recognize the importance of public health programs in reducing the incidence of disease, disability, and the effects of aging and other physical and mental health conditions. "Public health" is the science and art of preventing disease, prolonging life, and promoting health through the organized efforts and informed choices of society, organizations (public and private), communities, and individuals.

WHAT IS HEALTH POLICY?

The WHO defines "health policy" as follows:

> Decisions, plans, and actions that are undertaken to achieve specific health care goals within a society. An explicit health policy can achieve several things: it defines a vision for the future which in turn helps establish targets and points of reference for the short and medium term; it outlines priorities and the expected roles of different groups; and it builds consensus and informs people (3).

Mosby's Medical Dictionary defines health policy as (a) a statement of a decision regarding a goal in health care and a plan for achieving that goal, for example, to prevent an epidemic, a program for inoculating a population is developed and implemented; and (b) a field of study and practice in which the priorities and values underlying health resource allocation are determined (4).

The term health policy often means different things to different people. To the economist, health policy is about the allocation of resources; to the law maker, it concerns the improvement of public health; and to the physician, it may be about health services. Health policy is often considered in terms of content, but it is also the process of determining what actions are to be taken (5).

In this chapter we will address the role of government in establishing health policy with respect to brain injury and discuss the various drivers of health policy: culture, science, politics, and economics. Health policy is developed as a product of the tensions between political, cultural, and economic drivers. Those factors vary in different parts of the world, and as a result, different countries around the world have very different approaches to health policy.

The US Institute of Medicine (IOM) says that "public policy can be one of the most effective approaches to protecting and improving the health of the population." "Healthy" public policy is particularly important in a time of scarce resources because it can diminish or preclude the need for other, more costly and potentially less effective interventions" (6).

In the case of brain injury, there are unique factors that differentiate it from other public health care policy. In particular, there has been a long-standing lack of awareness of brain injury as a major public health problem. It has often been referred to as a "silent epidemic" in large part because of unapparent problems, mostly invisible cognitive/behavioral problems, especially with more mild injuries. In addition, it is a relatively new phenomenon—past 20–30 years —that survival after severe traumatic brain injury (TBI) is more likely than not. As a result of advanced medical interventions and improved outcomes, many of the factors that have historically applied to the development of general public health policy do not apply to brain injury. Using the example from Mosby's, a government may develop and implement a program to inoculate a population to prevent an epidemic, but that usually involves contagion—affecting large swaths of the population. Except in recent cases of blast injury in warfare, brain injury usually does not occur en masse but rather in individual instances. There is a further bias against intervention on a large scale for injuries that may occur as a result of multitude of causes. Public policy advocates in recent years have been successful in addressing those causes in preventive ways: urging the use of seatbelts and advocating for lower speed limits to reduce highway and traffic crashes, lobbying for greater motorcycle and bike helmet use, and so forth. However, resistance from individual rights advocates, the lack of public understanding of brain injury diagnosis, treatment and rehabilitation along with the absence of a consistent coherent health care financing policy have contributed to the challenges of improving health policy in the United States.

The following is an explanation of some of the drivers of health policy as they pertain to brain injury in the United States. We will conclude with a comparison of international approaches to financing brain injury rehabilitation.

DRIVER OF HEALTH POLICY: CULTURE

In many countries, human rights philosophy is integrated into health care policy. The Universal Declaration of Human Rights (UDHR) asserts that medical care is a right of all people. UDHR Article 25 states that:

> Everyone has the right to a standard of living adequate for the health and well-being of himself and of his family, including food, clothing, housing and medical care, and necessary social services, and the right to security in the event of unemployment, illness, disability, widowhood, old age, or other lack of livelihood in circumstances beyond his control (7).

According to the WHO, "people have different expectations of their health and therefore different perceptions of their health care needs" and "the rich often report greater need than the poor, even though the poor are in generally worse health using objective criteria" (8). This is evident in the United States where per capita spending on health care is the highest among Organisation for Economic Cooperation and Development (OECD) countries* and consumes 16% of the national gross domestic product (GDP). Despite this high level of spending, the United States does not achieve better outcomes on various health care measures (9).

The United States is the only industrialized nation that does not recognize health care as a right (10). According to a Congressional Research Service report, "almost 51 million people or 16.7% of the US population had no health insurance for at least some of 2009. In fact, the aggregate uninsurance rate over the past decade was never less than 13.4%" (11). Despite the inequality of access to health insurance, there is a common expectation that the most advanced technological medical interventions should be used for emergency medical care and diagnosis, acute care and rehabilitation after brain injury, and that all means necessary will be used for the injured to return to life similar to the one before the brain injury. This dichotomy persists as sentiments of the United States having the best medical care in the world are embraced.

The Centers for Disease Control and Prevention (CDC) estimates that 1.7 million Americans sustain a TBI each year: of those, 52,000 die, 275,000 are hospitalized, and 1.365 million, nearly 80%, are treated and released from an emergency department. This does not include the number of people with TBI who are not seen in an emergency department or who receive no care. The number of undiagnosed TBIs is also unknown (12). More than 3 million Americans live with a lifelong disability as a result of brain injury, but there are no reliable data on the prevalence of survivors of brain injury living in the minimally conscious or vegetative state. Despite the enormous impact TBI has on society, it does not command the same level of public interest and federal funding as many other health issues.

For a long time, TBI was considered a silent epidemic because those with the most severe injuries were out of sight and those with mild and moderate TBIs recovered or were stifled by stigma and would not self-identify as having a brain injury. The brain injury advocacy movement began in earnest in the United States in 1980 with the creation of the National Head Injury Foundation which was later renamed the Brain Injury Association of America (BIAA). The advocates that participated in BIAA activities were family members, clinicians, rehabilitation specialists, educators, and people with brain injury who shared the common goals of improving public awareness, research and treatment, and services to support individuals and their families after injury. Despite the involvement of well-known public figures, including former Assistant to the President and White House Press Secretary James S. Brady who survived a gunshot to the head in an assassination attempt on the life of President Ronald Reagan in 1981, the brain injury advocacy community struggled for the limelight of mainstream media. Advocates sought greater public awareness and understanding of brain injury but stigma and fear prevailed (13). In 2000, a poll commissioned by the BIAA found that 1 in 3 Americans were unfamiliar with the term *brain injury* (14).

Nevertheless, brain injury advocates were successful in getting a federal law enacted specifically addressing brain injury. The Traumatic Brain Injury (TBI) Act was first enacted in 1996 (P.L. 104–166) and reauthorized in 2000 (P.L. 106–310) and again in 2008 (P.L. 110–206). The TBI Act authorized the CDC to study the incidence and prevalence of brain injury in the United States, engage in public awareness and educational activities, and support prevention initiatives. The law established a state grant program to assist states in developing and improving access to health services and it authorized the National Institutes of Health (NIH) to support grants for basic and applied research. The data and information that resulted made a significant difference in brain injury policy on both the state and federal level.

At the same time that the brain injury advocacy movement was picking up steam, researchers and public health advocates were developing data on the impact of injury on society and urging greater leadership by government. Medical advances were resulting in increased survival rates and the costs of rehabilitation were climbing. In 1985, the National Academy of Sciences published a report entitled *Injury in America: A Continuing Public Health Problem*, which called for injuries to be addressed as any other major public health issue that contributes to a significant number of deaths and disabilities. The report highlighted the need for a federal coordinating agency to address injury prevention, research, treatment and rehabilitation, and improved systems to ameliorate or reduce the extent of disability following a brain injury (15). The report led to the Department of Health and Human Services (DHHS) adding the term *prevention* to the CDC, and in 1990 created the National Center for Injury Prevention and Control (NCIPC) (16). The DHHS has since included prevention in its Healthy People 2000, 2010, and 2020 strategic plans. Prior to the creation of the NCIPC, the

---

* OECD countries include Australia, Austria, Belgium, Canada, France, Germany, Italy, Japan, Netherlands, Norway, Spain, Sweden, Switzerland, the United Kingdom, and the United States.

Department of Transportation's National Highway Traffic Safety Administration (NHTSA) was the lead federal agency responsible for reducing the number of injuries and deaths on US highways and supporting national Emergency Medical Services System development.

The US culture of taking pride in innovation, medical advances, and reducing mortality contributed to the progress advocates made in shaping brain injury policy. But there were many challenges. The lack of understanding and acceptance of disability in mainstream society continued to distract advocacy efforts. For example, James Brady is best known as a gun control advocate, not a survivor of brain injury. In addition, although advocates lobby for emergency medical services and trauma care systems and push for full recovery, they also urge acceptance, understanding, and accommodations of disability and limitations. Although some advocates tried to lobby for a "cure" for brain injury to increase research efforts and gain public attention and increase willingness of survivors to speak out, (17) others, such as BIAA, has argued that brain injury is a "neurological disease" requiring "lifelong disease management and individualized services and supports" (18). Because of the enormous breadth of brain injury—from concussion to coma from various causes (shaking, falling, anoxia, motor vehicle crashes, violence, war)—the brain injury advocacy community has faced formidable challenges and has suffered from a lack of a clear, succinct public message.

Great Expectations

On January 8, 2011, United States Congresswoman Gabrielle Giffords was shot at point blank range on the left side of her head in an assassination attempt. After being provided with state-of-the-art acute and post care rehabilitation, on August 1, 2011 she returned to the House floor to vote in favor of raising the US debt ceiling. Her recovery may possibly serve as one of the single most significant events to improve brain injury policy in recent years. The last was the case of ABC News Anchor Bob Woodruff in 2006. Woodruff had just been named to replace Peter Jennings when he sustained a severe TBI while embedded with US troops in Iraq (19). Woodruff is credited with shining a bright public light on the need for the US Congress and the Department of Defense (DOD) and Department of Veterans' Affairs (DVA) to acknowledge the severity of the instances of brain injury in Iraq and Afghanistan and the needs for ongoing treatment and rehabilitation for military personnel and veterans. Soon after Woodruff's report, the Congress appropriated hundreds of millions of dollars for research and treatment in TBI at the DOD and DVA.

After 15 years, the US Congress continues to fund the TBI Act at less than $20 million per year, and the state grant program remains limited because of the ideological tension between state and federal responsibilities and tight economic conditions. Brain injury advocates are hopeful that Congresswoman Giffords can deliver significant improvements to public awareness and increased funding.

Individual Rights vs Public Health Policy and Prevention

The United States claims to have "the best medical care in the world" (20). At the same time, there is what is known as the American Creed by which individual rights and freedoms are considered a foundation of the nation itself (21). Much of the resistance to health system overhaul has been caused by the desire to protect individual rights (to choose doctors, to sue for noneconomic damages in medical malpractice and automobile crash cases). The United States is defined by its desire for individual rights and freedoms. As a culture, individual rights are chosen over collective goals (22).

This conflict of public health vs individual rights and freedoms has been illustrated best by the debate regarding the enactment of the Patient Protection and Affordable Care Act of 2010 (PPACA) (23) that includes a mandate that individuals purchase health care coverage. In response to legal challenges, various federal courts have ruled both in favor and against the premise that the provision violates the US Constitution by requiring individuals to purchase health insurance or pay a penalty.

It has been well established in various arenas that government can compel citizen compliance for the good of society (e.g., pay taxes, obey laws, some states require the purchase of auto insurance) but the connection is missing between individual health status and insurance and the impact on society as a whole.

Much of the debate about enacting the PPACA was centered on the philosophy that health care should be a "right" for all Americans, although others believe that whether or not it is a right, it is not the responsibility of the government to provide or protect it.

Although there is a clear acceptance on the part of the government to take responsibility for the health of military personnel and veterans, this is not the case in the civilian sector. During the mid-1990s, a popular mantra of "personal responsibility" permeated the national dialogue resulting in reducing welfare and social services and extended to issues of injury. The sentiment that accidents will happen and that they are inevitable and health insurance should be purchased by individuals and families to use when the need arises, prevented large scale interventions. As a result, efforts to reduce injuries such as reducing highway speed limits and mandating the use of motorcycle and bike helmets were repealed. The fact that prevention requires behavioral changes and interventions provides a challenge not realized in health conditions that can be inoculated or ameliorated with pharmaceutics.

Motorcycle Helmet Laws

Although TBI is the most common diagnosis for hospitalized motor vehicle injury (24), there continues to be a strong lobby against laws mandating motorcycle helmet use. On July 3, 2011, while engaging in a protest against helmet laws, a motorcyclist crashed, sustained a severe TBI, and died (25). In response, representatives of the group "American Bikers Aimed Toward Education" (ABATE) claimed that they were advocating for the choice not to wear a helmet (26). Although ABATE claims that "mandatory helmet laws do nothing to prevent accidents," the Governors Highway Safety Association (GHSA) claims that "helmets meeting federal standards reduce the chances of fatality in an accident by more than 40%." NHTSA estimates that if all motorcyclists wore helmets in 2008, 823 lives would have been saved (27).

This debate is being played out in the states. From 1992 to 1995, as an incentive for states to enact all rider helmet laws, the federal Intermodal Surface Transportation Efficiency Act permitted states to transfer highway construction funds to highway safety accounts. The National Highway System Designation Act repealed this provision in 1995. States have enacted mandatory helmet laws and faced legal challenges. More than 25 states have upheld motorcycle helmet laws to be constitutional. Courts often cite the Massachusetts case, *Simon v Sargent*, (28), which was affirmed by the US Supreme Court. There, the court stated:

> From the moment of the injury, society picks the person up off the highway; delivers him to a municipal hospital and municipal doctors; provides him with unemployment compensation if, after recovery, he cannot replace his lost job, and, if the injury causes permanent disability, may assume the responsibility for his and his family's continued subsistence. We do not understand a state of mind that permits [the motorcyclist] to think that only he himself is concerned.

A few courts, however, have ruled in favor of personal freedom, such as the Supreme Court of Illinois in *People v Fries* (42 Ill 2d 446 250 NE 2d 149). Illinois continues to be what advocates call "helmet law free" (29). The helmet free lobby is also supported by rights advocates in the US Congress who have introduced legislation forbidding NHTSA to encourage states to mandate helmet use.[†]

Sports Concussion Laws

Where there has been progress is in state laws governing children's sports. In 2006, 16-year-old Zackery Lystedt sustained a life-threatening brain injury after he returned to play football following a concussion. His father then successfully advocated for legislation in his home state of Washington to prevent other student athletes from similar consequences. Signed into law in 2009 by Governor Chris Gregoire, Washington became the first state to pass legislation regulating sports-related concussions occurring in public school sports. The law prohibits athletes younger than 18 years, who are suspected of sustaining a concussion, from returning to play without a licensed health care provider's written approval. Since then, 22 states and the District of Columbia have passed similar laws. In addition, the Congressional Brain Injury Task Force introduced legislation in the 111th Congress (HR 1347) directing CDC to assist states in the development of concussion guidelines to be used in schools.

Increased media attention has also been paid to the incidence of chronic traumatic encephalopathy among professional boxers and football players (30). Whether or not this publicity will translate into policy change remains to be seen, but hearings and briefings have been held on Capitol Hill to illuminate the issues, and in July 2011, 75 former professional football players sued the National Football League (NFL) claiming that the dangers of concussion were known since the 1920s and the NFL concealed the information and failed to protect its players (31).

[†] H.Res. 1498 introduced July 1, 2010 in the 111th Congress by US Congressman James Sensenbrenner (R-WI), cosponsored by Representatives Lamborn, Rehberg, Petri, and Ryan, to retain the ban on the NHTSA's ability to lobby State legislators using Federal funds.

DRIVER OF HEALTH POLICY: SCIENCE

As medical innovation progresses and there is greater understanding of the state-of-the-art diagnosis, treatment, and rehabilitation, policy makers are better informed and have the opportunity to develop better public policy. In the spring of 2011, to commemorate the 50th anniversary of President John F. Kennedy's challenge to put a man on the moon, his nephew, former United States Congressman from Rhode Island Patrick Kennedy, held a conference about the brain and presented a 10-year plan to achieve greater understanding of brain conditions and new treatments. Brain issues including TBI and post-traumatic stress disorder (PTSD) experienced by veterans in the wars in Iraq and Afghanistan were at the top of the agenda. Cochairman of the One Mind for Research Scientific Forum, Kennedy speaking before an audience of high-level government officials and well-known scientists, said "science is the only means to taking care of the people we love" (32).

According to the Congressional Budget Office, the private sector does not conduct enough research relative to the needs of society, and therefore, strong Federal Government support is needed. Private firms need financial incentives to support research because they must recoup investment costs (33). In 2007, 84% of federal funding for biomedical research was conducted by the NIH, a component of the DHHS (34). Although considerable brain injury research has been conducted by the NIH through the National Institute on Neurological Disorders and Stroke (NINDS) and the National Center for Medical Rehabilitation Research (NCMRR), critics have argued that there has been too great a focus on "cures" rather than the complexities of rehabilitation research which includes consideration of the individual, disability, and the environment (35). Since 1997, the IOM has advocated for an increase in visibility of rehabilitation research within federal research agencies (36).

As far as return on investment, DOD has the most to gain with investing in brain injury research because it is responsible for funding prevention, mitigation, diagnosis, and treatment, followed by the DVA which is responsible for funding rehabilitation and community reentry initiatives. TBI has become known as the "signature injury" of the wars in Iraq and Afghanistan. In a 2008 RAND report, it was noted that TBI is still poorly understood, leaving a large gap in knowledge related to how extensive the problem is or how to address it (37).

Unlike many countries with centralized health care systems, the US research community relies on investigator initiated research. This means that with the exception of responding to specific federal agency program announcements or requests for proposals, the focus of research is based upon investigator interest, not necessarily the needs of society. The exceptions are the DOD and DVA, which engage in their own research and as such, are better able to adhere to clearly defined goals and principles. Even though the experience of war has led the way in realizing new medical interventions, particularly with respect to acute care, the translation from military medical care to the civilian sector has been slow. With estimates as high as 320,000 military personnel having sustained brain injury as a result of blasts in the wars in Afghanistan and Iraq (37), the DOD and DVA have invested hundreds of millions of dollars in research into the mechanisms of blast injury, new and improved diagnostics, and innovative rehabilitation efforts.

Although military research has proliferated, brain injury research advocates have continued to seek greater civilian efforts to advance rehabilitation science and have urged the NIH to elevate its NCMRR to the level of an institute and to include brain injury rehabilitation in efforts to increase translational research (38). Prior to the creation of the NCMRR in 1990 at the direction of Congress, there was no rehabilitation agency at NIH, and research was spread over 5 NIH institutes. Another roadblock to increasing federal focus and funding on brain injury research and rehabilitation is that a good deal of brain injury rehabilitation research has been conducted not within DHHS but instead by the Department of Education in the National Institute of Disability Rehabilitation Research, which funds TBI Model Systems of Care. This provides a challenge to advocacy because there is greater support in Congress for medical research than for a federal role in education. Many members of Congress who have strongly supported research have called for the elimination of the Department of Education.

The US Congress has urged an exchange of information and collaboration between and among federal agencies and the private sector, and there are many examples of cooperation resulting from efforts of brain injury advocates such as the creation of Interagency Task Forces. Another collaborative effort is the Warfighter Head Injury Study, a clinical trial sponsored by NIH and DOD to examine the long-term outcome of brain injuries, the effects of treatment on outcome, and the effects of brain injury on people's behavior and abilities (39).

Evidence-Based Guidelines

In rallying support for enactment of the PPACA, President Obama touted the use of evidence-based guidelines (40). As brain injury medicine evolves, advocates continue to urge greater use of evidence-based guidelines for severe TBI, penetrating injury, post-acute care, pediatric brain injury, and concussion guidelines to be used in school sports settings (41).

Acute Care Guidelines

The CDC has urged greater use of guidelines for in-hospital treatment of adults with severe TBI as adopted by the American Association of Neurological Surgeons (AANS) and in a study published in the *Journal of Trauma* found that widespread adoption of the guidelines could result in a 50% decrease in deaths, a savings of some $288 million in medical and rehabilitation costs, and overall could save $3.8 billion in the estimated lifelong savings in annual societal costs for patients sustaining severe brain trauma (42). At this time, two-thirds of all trauma centers in the United States do not comply with the AANS guidelines. An actuarial estimate of Medicaid cost savings in the State of New York found that the implementation of a computerized system to assist with guideline compliance at 6 New York hospitals resulted in increased compliance with the AANS guidelines, from an average of 58% to 71%, peaking at 80%. The estimate further found that if all 44 New York State health care facilities were to implement the system over the next 10 years, the state

could potentially save nearly $500 million (43). New York and Michigan funded demonstration projects with such a system but could no longer sustain the investment after 2 years.

Post-Acute Care Guidelines and Cognitive Rehabilitation

According to BIAA, "medical treatment guidelines for post-acute rehabilitation of moderate and severe TBI do not exist" (44). BIAA has lobbied the US Congress to direct the DOD to fund the development of such guidelines, and veterans' service organizations such as American Veterans (AMVETS) seek to have the DVA's separate treatment guidelines for the management of mild TBI consistent with DOD care coordination for improved transition from DOD to DVA (45).

BIAA has also urged Congress to direct the DOD to cover cognitive rehabilitation through its Tricare insurance program. There is a dearth of understanding of which cognitive rehabilitation interventions are most effective. This gap in knowledge has been used by Tricare and private insurance companies to avoid having to pay for costly rehabilitation. As a result, the services available to ABC Anchor Bob Woodruff and Congresswoman Giffords are not generally available to the average citizen (46).

DRIVER OF HEALTH POLICY: POLITICS

Politics often provides the theater where conflicts between culture and values, economics, and science play out. Although one would hope that good policy is made as the result of reasoned, logical decisions being made by educated, well-informed lawmakers, it is not always the case. How individual lawmakers perceive their role to "uphold the Constitution of the United States" varies widely. A significant faction of lawmakers believes they must reduce the size and scope of government interference. Others view government as a means to protect and serve the most vulnerable of populations. The variety of ideological differences along with the structure of the federal and state systems requires a great deal of political will and focus to change existing or create new policies.‡

The case of Terri Schiavo is an example of the struggle between religion and the values of the right to life movement, the inadequacy of understanding of disorders of consciousness, and the unfortunate attempts by lawmakers to intervene. The Schiavo case involved a 39-year-old woman in a persistent vegetative state as the result of anoxic brain injury whose husband urged her feeding tube be removed (based on evidence of her desire to cease life support) against the wishes of her parents. The parents' position was supported by right to life advocates who succeeded in getting the legislature of the state of Florida to pass a law authorizing the Governor of Florida to intervene. The order of Governor Jeb Bush for Schiavo's feeding tube to be replaced was pub-

---

‡ The US federal system is made of 3 branches: the legislature (Congress), the executive branch (President and the Administration), and the courts (Supreme Court and federal district and appellate courts). Each of the 50 states has similar systems. The federal and state systems are designed to provide a balance of power so that no one branch becomes too powerful.

licly endorsed by US President George W. Bush. The Supreme Court of the State of Florida ruled that the Governor's action was unconstitutional and a violation of the separation of powers (47). Ms. Schiavo's parents continued legal challenges and with the help of the larger right to life movement maintained public pressure and lobbied for the US Congress to draft a federal law that would mandate review of the Schiavo case by a federal court to investigate whether Ms. Schiavo's civil rights were protected.

What was most alarming to professional brain injury specialists was the diagnostic assessments offered by Senate Majority Leader Bill Frist, a cardiologist, that were "infused by ideology and departed from accepted clinical norms" (48). As a result, "important diagnostic distinctions amongst disorders of consciousness were confused and conflated" (48). The media frenzy, supported by politicians taking advantage of the situation to appease their base, led to an untrained public offering medical opinions that were contrary to clinical assessments. Nevertheless, the Congress passed the Act and President Bush signed it into law. The US District Court reviewed the case and denied the request of Ms. Schiavo's parents to have the tube re-inserted. On appeal, the US Circuit Court as well as the US Supreme Court upheld the District Court decision. Ms. Schiavo died on March 31, 2005 (48).

This case highlights the enormous power of special interest lobbying efforts and the need for greater understanding of brain injuries as well as respect for science. Fortunately, the courts were successful in restraining actions based on ideology but the conflicts between religion and science remain.

Although the US system was designed to protect against the unruly whim of the majority or the very loud minority, the courts are not always the protectors of human rights or good science. One of the most infamous of cases in 1927, *Buck v Bell* (49), the US Supreme Court upheld a Virginia statute instituting the eugenic "sterilization of the unfit" for the "protection and health of the state." In his opinion, Chief Justice Oliver Wendell Holmes stated that "3 generations of imbeciles are enough." This case led to a proliferation of state sterilization laws that stayed on the books for many years (50). The Virginia statute was not officially overturned until 1974.

Some would argue that politicians and lawmakers have legal and moral responsibilities to protect and preserve public health. But as both the Schiavo and Buck cases illustrate, there are differences of opinion regarding what that means. The late Senator Edward M. Kennedy stated at the 2008 Democratic Convention that it is the role of the government to "guarantee that every American . . . will have decent quality health care as a fundamental right and not a privilege" (51). Former presidential candidate Congressman Dennis Kucinich (D-OH), among others, argues that "health care is a civil right," relying on the Preamble and Article 1, Section 8 of the Constitution of the United States, which defines a purpose of government "to promote the general welfare" (52).

Other lawmakers put more emphasis on the Doctrine of Enumerated Powers that limits the role of the Federal Government to only those enumerated in the US Constitution (53). Politicians in this camp view government interference in the provision of health care and insurance as a threat to individual freedom and the free market (54). Specifically, they argue that a competitive health care market place is needed to protect the physician–patient relationship and individual choice in choosing health care services (55). The argument against government-supported health care has been made at times using strong rhetoric, such as the frequently cited quote of former President Ronald Reagan who said that (if Medicare is not stopped), "You and I are going to spend our sunset years telling our children and our children's children what it once was like in America when men were free" (56).

Although ideological differences may always exist between a right to health care and insurance, ideally there should be respect and deference for what state of the art medicine has to offer. In a democracy, the will of the people does not always provide for society's long-term well-being and instead seeks short-term solutions. Politicians will often choose the most expedient means to an end. Therefore, it is critical that good science and reliable data assist and inform the policy process. Greater awareness and public understanding must continually grow regarding what brain injury is (from concussion to coma); how it can be treated; what can be expected as possible outcomes; what might be the costs to the individual, the family, the community, and the society; and how systems can be developed and improved to best serve the individual and the public.

Health policy does not change in the United States unless there is media attention and sustained concern, the political will, and sufficient economic resources. Otherwise, individual cases continue to be considered as individual cases. It is incumbent on brain injury specialists, researchers, clinicians, and providers to improve education and awareness of best practices and the latest scientifically based understanding of brain injuries of all types. However, data does not drive policy. The incidence of brain injury is greater than that of breast cancer, multiple sclerosis, spinal cord injury, and HIV combined (57). Clearly, if numbers were to rule, there would be similar levels of public interest and funding, but there is not. Policy is the end result of timing (culture), evidence (science), funding (economics), and political will (public outrage).

DRIVER OF HEALTH POLICY: ECONOMICS

Universal health care is a term referring to organized health systems built around the principle of universal coverage for all members of society, combining mechanisms for health financing and service provision. Government spending on health care is sometimes used as a global indicator of a particular government's commitment to the health of its people. Many types of health policy focus on the financing of health care services to spread the economic risks of ill health.

All the best science and public understanding of brain injury and recovery cannot improve health policy regarding brain injury without adequate financial resources. In recent years, many countries around the world have experienced what is called the "Great Recession," and as governments look to balance their budgets, the cost of health care is often at the top of the agenda for reform.

The United States puts a significant financial emphasis on health care because 23% of all federal spending is for Medicare and Medicaid, which insure more than 100 million people (58). The Federal Government and states also jointly fund the Children's Health Insurance Program that began in 1997 and covers some 7 million children whose family incomes are low but not low enough to qualify for Medicaid (59). This does not include the hundreds of millions spent on health care for military personnel, their families, and veterans. What is referred to as the "US health system" is really a mix of private insurance with government filling in the gaps for the very poor (Medicaid) and the elderly (Medicare) and varying standards for prevention and standards of care by state augmented by federal health programs. Public health agencies are financed primarily by federal, state, and local governments. Government budgets draw from different sources, including different types of taxes and fees (tobacco lawsuit settlement funds), depending on jurisdiction, and allocate resources to public health based on priorities set by the executive and legislative branches. Additional funding sources support public health activities in the community such as community-based organizations, not-for-profit clinical care providers, and other stakeholders that provide health and medical care activities (6).

The Federal Government shares the costs of Medicaid—a program for very low-income individuals and children—with the states. Medicaid coverage varies widely by state. The State of Arizona, for example, in the summer of 2011, began denying health insurance coverage through Medicaid for childless adults. Some 100,000 residents were to be affected in the first year (60). In addition, the state is taxing smokers, those with diabetes, and the obese. In 2010, Arizona changed its policy to deny Medicaid coverage for transplants of the heart, liver, pancreas, and bone marrow, affecting some 100 patients already on the transplant list (61).

There simply has not been the political will to pool resources and provide for a societal system for equal access to health care for all. As a result, not all brain injuries are treated equally. Acute care, post-acute care, and rehabilitation will vary depending on the economics of the individual, the region and community in which the injury occurred, or where the injured lives. The lack of a uniform policy for brain injury prevention, care, and rehabilitation leaves a large disparity of treatment (62) as well as outcomes, particularly for minority populations (63).

COST-EFFECTIVENESS OF BRAIN INJURY REHABILITATION

Effective rehabilitation may produce cost benefits to society by restoring long-term independence (so reducing the costs of ongoing care), and, where possible, supporting people into work and financial independence. There is now a strong body of research evidence for the effectiveness of rehabilitation following acquired brain injury (64). The trial-based evidence is strongest for early, intensive multidisciplinary rehabilitation in the post-acute stage but there is also good evidence from cohort studies to support vocational and community-based programs. However, for this process to be "cost-efficient," the initial investment in rehabilitation must be offset by the ongoing savings on care within a reasonably short time frame.

Several studies, both from the United Kingdom and the United States, have specifically examined cost-effectiveness following brain injury rehabilitation (65) and demonstrated

that the costs of providing post-acute rehabilitation are offset by long-term savings within 1–3 years (66,67), with estimated lifetime savings of between 1.5 and 6 million US dollars. Importantly, the benefits are not confined to higher level patients who make a good recovery and return to work. In the United Kingdom and other socially supported systems of health care (where state-funded social services provide life-long care and support), reduction in long-term care costs is a critical outcome. Cost-benefit analysis across a range of dependency demonstrates that inpatient rehabilitation can be highly cost-efficient for the most dependent group of patients (68) even though they require longer lengths of stay to maximize the gains (69).

Attitudes of health policy makers to investment in rehabilitation for brain injury will depend on the extent of their responsibilities for long-term support. It is a weakness of many health care systems around the world that health and social welfare are separately funded. Even though investment in excellent rehabilitation for brain injury may reap substantial savings in respect of ongoing social care, this investment is likely to be given low priority if the savings only accrue to another sector.

WHO PAYS FOR HEALTH CARE?

Universal health care systems vary according to the extent of government involvement in providing care and/or health insurance. In some countries, such as the United Kingdom and the Nordic countries, access to health care is based on residence rights through central taxation; and the government (through its Department of Health) is closely involved in the commissioning and delivery of health care services. Others have a more pluralistic delivery system with health funds derived from a variety of sources including insurance premiums, salary-related mandatory contributions by employees and/or employers to regulated sickness funds, and by government taxes. These insurance-based systems tend to reimburse private or public medical providers, often at heavily regulated rates, through mutual or publicly owned medical insurers.

A few countries (e.g., the Netherlands and Switzerland) operate via privately owned, but heavily regulated private insurers that are not allowed to make a profit from the mandatory element of insurance but can profit by selling supplemental insurance.

Debate continues regarding which of these offers the best quality of health care services and how to ensure allocated funds are used effectively, efficiently, and equitably. There are arguments in favor of both public and private health financing policies summarized in Table 3-1.

HEALTH CARE FUNDING MODELS

A range of different funding models have been applied to the purchase of health care services.

Health care funding models take several different forms.

- In a *block contract* model, a hospital or provider is allocated a set sum to provide health care services over a set period (usually 1 year) regardless of activity. In a centrally funded health care system with a tightly fixed

TABLE 3-1 Arguments for Publicly and Privately Funded Health Care

ARGUMENTS FOR PUBLICLY FUNDED HEALTH CARE	ARGUMENTS FOR PRIVATELY FUNDED HEALTH CARE
Government funding underpins and sustains an appropriate range of programs.	Privately funded health care offers freedom to invest in new technologies that enhance health care and efficiencies.
Commissioning/contracting arrangements can include quality parameters to ensure that service delivery meets certain standards.	Competition between providers drives up quality and efficiencies.
Individuals on lower income have access to services that they could not otherwise afford.	Limiting the allocation of public funds for personal health care does not curtail the ability of uninsured citizens to pay for their own health care. Scarce public funds can then be reserved for certain services such as emergency and intensive care.
Because people consider health services to be free, they are more likely to seek preventive health care reducing disease burden and overall health care costs in the longer term.	The perception that publicly funded health care is *free* can lead to overuse of medical services and hence raise overall costs compared to private health financing.
Single-payer systems reduce wastefulness in time and resources by cutting out the middle man (e.g., insurance company) to concentrate resources on the treatment itself.	Large bureaucratic systems, particularly if multiple government agencies are involved, may compound inefficiencies.

budget, this system has the advantage of simplicity. It is relatively risk-free because the provider can plan expenditure based on a predictable income and the commissioner can set the expected activity levels as a condition of the contract. However, the contracted level of activity may not meet the health care demands of the population served, and patient choice is limited to the contracted provider(s).

- The *fixed and variable* model involves a fixed grant for hospital overhead costs and a payment for each patient treated, covering only variable costs.
- The *integrated (activity-based)* model provides an integrated payment to hospitals for each patient treated, covering both the fixed and variable costs.

Activity-based contracts offer the advantage that payment is provided for each patient treated, encouraging providers to increase their activity and drop their prices to capture contracts. However, the challenge is to ensure that different providers are offering services that are "like for like," and that the "case mix" and "commissioning currencies" reflect the true costs of treating patients. For example, in a health system where privately funded elective services exist alongside state-run hospitals with a duty of care for a population of patients, it is possible that entrepreneurial private providers may be tempted to cream-skim the simple cases leaving more complex (expensive to treat) cases to the statutory providers.

The term *case mix* is used variously to describe the type of mix of patients treated (70) in terms of prognosis or resources, depending on the parameter of interest. In the context of health care funding models, case-mix systems classify people into groups that are homogeneous in their use of resources, but a good case-mix system also gives meaningful clinical descriptions of these individuals (71).

Case-mix information has several uses—it can provide the basis for reimbursement and also for comparing facilities or programs, practice patterns, and patient outcomes. Case-mix information is collected as a standard minimum data set and, depending on the content of the data set, it may also be used to benchmark quality and efficiency and for internal management purposes. As well as informing resource allocation, it therefore serves as an information tool that allows policy makers to understand the nature and complexity of health care delivery (70).

DEVELOPMENT OF CASE MIX AND COMMISSIONING CURRENCIES IN HEALTH CARE

Case-mix classification was first pioneered in the United States some 40 years ago (72) and Medicare introduced a "prospective payment system" for short-stay acute care hospitals in 1983. The system was based on Diagnosis Related Groups (DRGs), which were designed to measure and classify health care activity, based primarily on the diagnosis and the procedures carried out (73). DRGs classify acute inpatient episodes into several manageable categories based on clinical condition and resource consumption. A single acute episode of inpatient care is allocated to one DRG using coded clinical information derived from the patient's medical record. Other countries that have since followed on similar lines to introduce DRG-equivalent systems include Australia, Canada, Nordic Countries, and several European countries including Italy, Germany, Hungary, and Denmark (74).

The options for commissioning currencies range from a single fixed tariff payment for each episode, regardless of length of stay ("episode rates" or "prospective payments"), to payment at a daily rate ("bed-day" or "per diem" rates). Both systems present potential opportunities for gaming.

- Fixed episode payments tend to place the greater share of risk on the provider and may encourage them to "cream-skim" the easy cases and to discharge too early.
- Per diem payments may contain insufficient incentives to move the patient on and so result in unnecessarily long admissions (75).

The principal argument for episode payments is that most active treatment costs are incurred during the early part of the episode—longer-staying patients mainly incurring only "hotel costs" because of largely avoidable delays—so restriction of payment to within a few days either side of the average length of stay provides an incentive toward efficient case throughput. However, although this may be true for acute medical and surgical treatments, it does not necessarily hold good for other areas of health care. Different payment models are required for longer-term (or subacute) service areas such as rehabilitation or palliative care.

Case Mix in Rehabilitation—International Models

Rehabilitation poses some particular challenges for the development of case mix design.

- Diagnosis alone is a relatively poor indicator of costs for inpatient rehabilitation (76,77) where nursing and therapy staff input (as opposed to medical treatments) are the major cost indicators (78,79,80).
- Cost-efficiency does not always equate with shorter stay. Evidence from the United States and other countries has shown that the introduction of fixed episode payment schemes in rehabilitation may lead to poorer functional outcomes (81) and increased rates of discharge to institutional care (82) because of pressure for early discharge when reimbursement ceases.
- As noted earlier, some patients need longer time to achieve maximal independence but there is also evidence that the resulting savings in the cost of ongoing care can offset the initial investment in rehabilitation by several fold (68,69).

As a result, some health care systems have recognized that rigid episode-based reimbursement may be unsuitable for rehabilitation and alternative case mix and payment models are required, which are fair to both purchasers and providers and still reward efficiency. For example:

- Italy has explored a system that links reimbursement to effective stay (83,84) based on the time to reach peak improvement for different groups of conditions.
- Australia has developed a "weighted blended payment model" for rehabilitation, which applies a mixture of episode and per diem rates (described in more detail subsequently).

The United States System

When the US case-mix system was first introduced for health care in the 1980s, medical rehabilitation was excluded from the US-DRGs because it was recognized that rehabilitation inpatients could not be classified reliably by diagnosis alone (85). The level of functional dependency was considered to be a better cost-indicator, and in the 1990s, a classification system based on function (as defined by the Functional Independence Measure [FIM]) (86) was developed instead (87). This system of "FIM–function-related groups" (FRGs) was subsequently rederived to predict total rehabilitation costs and renamed "case-mix groups" (CMGs). These form the current basis for reimbursement by Medicare for inpatient rehabilitation in the United States. Medicare requires completion of a standardized data set consisting of diagnostic and demographic information (the Inpatient Rehabilitation Facility Patient Assessment Instrument [IRF-PAI]) to be completed for each patient within 72 hours of admission to

qualify for reimbursement. The FIM is embedded in this tool. Twenty-one rehabilitation impairment categories are broken down into CMGs classified by the FIM motor score and, in some instances, also the FIM cognitive score and age of the patient where these are required to provide further definition of costs.

The Australian System

Development of case mix in Australia followed a broadly similar pattern to the United States. Case mix funding for health care was first introduced in the state of Victoria in 1993–1994, and since then most states have moved toward either case-mix–based funding or using case mix to inform the commissioning and budget-setting process (88). When Australian National Diagnosis-Related Groups (AN-DRGs) were introduced, it was similarly recognized that the costs of subacute care (including rehabilitation medicine, palliative care, psychogeriatric, and elderly care evaluation) were not well described by this system (77). As in the United States, function-related groups were identified as a better way to determine the differential cost of rehabilitation episodes (89).

Two separate function-related case-mix systems have been developed to classify patient episodes for different levels of reimbursement for rehabilitation. The first, published in 1996, is the Casemix Rehabilitation and Funding Tree (CRAFT) system, which is based on 12 functional categories determined by the modified Barthel Index (90). The second, published 3 years later, is the Australian National Sub-Acute and Non-Acute Patient (AN-SNAP) Classification, which is based on the FIM (91).

Although the AN-SNAP classification was originally developed as an episode classification, a more sophisticated "blended payment model" for funding was subsequently developed, which is illustrated in Figure 3-1. Episode and per diem cost weights are derived from analysis of resource use within each of the AN-SNAP classes (92). The model is designed to provide incentive to move patients on (because bringing in a new patient will attract a new episode weight), but still provides payment above simple hotel costs for longer episodes.

The InterRAI Network

The InterRAI network (71) is an international collaborative group of researchers in more than 30 countries developing case-mix systems in areas of health care for persons who are elderly, frail, or disabled. The network is not linked to any particular health care system or payment model but has developed a family of instruments with the aim of providing a common language that will produce integrated health care information across a range of settings and across international borders.

The best known of the InterRAI case-mix systems is the Resource Utilization Groups Version III (RUG-III) which is used in institutional long-term care settings and skilled nursing facilities in the United States and Canada. In all, there are currently 12 related assessment systems in the interRAI network, spanning areas that include post-acute, mental health, palliative, and long-term care facilities.

Episode range for rehabilitation

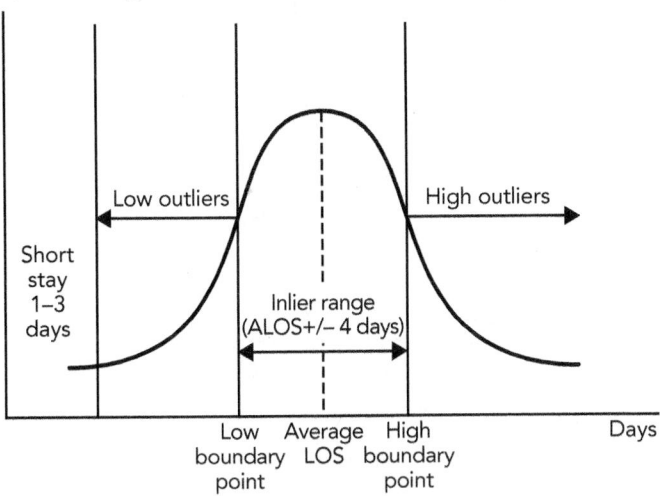

FIGURE 3-1 A blended payment model. (LOS, lengths of stay; ALOS, average length of stay)

- Patients staying for very short admissions are reimbursed at a standard short-stay rate.
- Those below the low trim point are reimbursed at the "low outlier" per diem rate.
- Those with lengths of stay (LOS) within the episode range attract the weighted episode rate plus an "inlier per diem" payment for each day.
- Those staying beyond the episode period attract the episode rate plus inlier per diem payment for the whole episode period plus the days beyond the high trim point at the outlier per diem rate.

Case Mix Development in the United Kingdom

The United Kingdom has a very different health culture from that in Australia or the United States. The National Health Service (NHS) provides the most comprehensive publicly funded health care system in the world, with most health care being provided free at the point of delivery. In addition, a closely integrated social services system provides life-long care and support, which is free to all individuals who are unable to pay for it themselves. In the light of this ongoing responsibility, maximizing functional independence is highly valued.

The NHS is now moving toward a standard "fixed tariff" payment system along similar lines to the US-style prospective payment system. Introduction of the Department of Health's Payment by Results program (93) in England represents the biggest change in financial flows in the history of the NHS and introduces some particular challenges as payment systems change from a block contract to an activity-based payment model.

The UK scheme introduces a national episode-based tariff for health care treatments based on a case-mix classification of Healthcare Resource Groups (HRGs). Like DRGs, HRGs are groups of conditions and interventions that are intended to have similar resource implications. As in other episode-based funding models, the system is intended to reward additional activity and give an incentive to reduce length of stay, so driving up cost-efficiency. However, many specialties have recognized the need for increased "granu-

larity" of the classification to account for the additional costs of treating people with more complex needs.

Accepting the evidence that shorter lengths of stay do not always equate with efficiency (68,69), the Department of Health of England has also started to explore alternative payment models for management of long-term conditions, for example, in the areas of mental health, palliative care, and rehabilitation.

The Challenges for Case Mix in Rehabilitation

The implementation of standard tariffs for rehabilitation in the United Kingdom poses several specific challenges, including limited data on rehabilitation derived from the standard coding systems and high variance in treatment costs, because of the marked diversity of needs for rehabilitation among patients within each diagnostic grouping.

A further challenge is presented by variation in caseload across different levels of service specialization. Since the 1980s (94), rehabilitation services have developed in the United Kingdom on a 3-tiered model of local, district, and regional services. To gain the advantage of critical mass, complex cases have been clustered into regional (tertiary) centers with specialized staff and facilities (95). This clustering is feasible in the United Kingdom because of the relatively small geographic distances involved. However, it distorts the reference costs because caseload complexity varies across the different levels of service. These 3 levels are now formally defined (96) as follows:

- Level 1 services—are discrete tertiary specialized rehabilitation services serving a regional catchment of greater than 1 million population.
- Level 2 services—are discrete specialist rehabilitation services led/supported by a consultant specialist in rehabilitation medicine but operating within a more local, district-level catchment population (typically 350,000 –500,000).
- Level 3 services—are local nonspecialist rehabilitation services, often provided in the context of acute or intermediate care as opposed to a discrete rehabilitation unit.

In general, level 1 services have been shown to carry a greater proportion of complex cases (97). However, because of the scarcity of such services, level 2 services in many areas have evolved to serve a supradistrict population (e.g., 600,000–1,000,000) and also carry a relatively high proportion of complex cases. This has led to calls for more accurate "patient level costing" (98) and a case-mix classification based on complexity of needs for rehabilitation as opposed to simply categorizing by service type.

Preliminary exploration of the various existing international models revealed that none were immediately suitable for implementation in the United Kingdom. Case-mix classifications based on measures of physical dependency (e.g., the FIM or the RUG-III system) may work reasonably well in the context of short-stay level 3 services where acute stroke and orthopedic rehabilitation form the bulk of the case load; patients have reasonably predictable requirements for intervention. However, they work less well in specialist level 1 and 2 programs, where the predominant focus in the United Kingdom is on neurological rehabilitation. For patients with

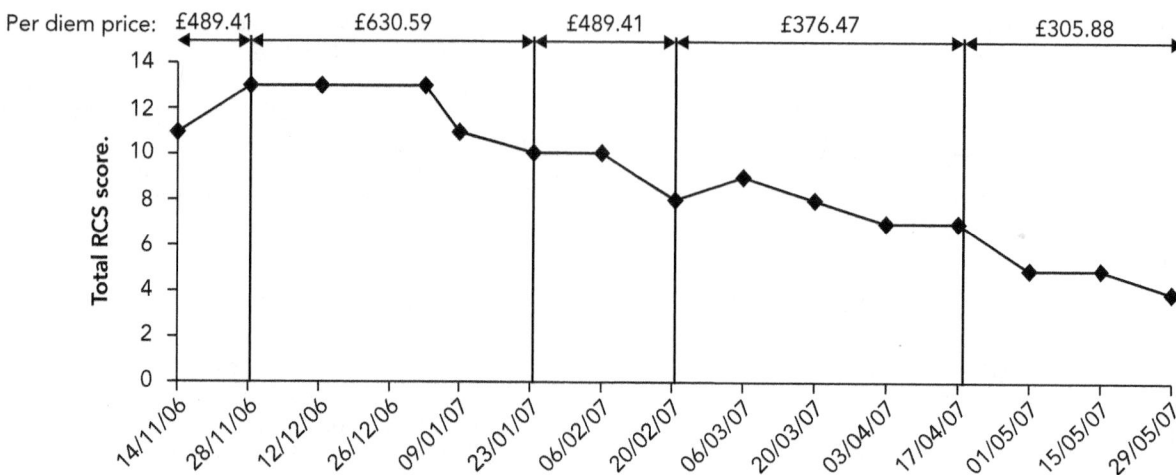

FIGURE 3–2 Illustration of a multilevel weighted per diem payment model (RCS, rehabilitation complexity score). Reproduced from Turner-Stokes (99) with permission.

brain injury and other complex neurological disabilities, physical dependency is a much less good predictor of rehabilitation needs.

Therefore, although existing classifications provided a useful model to build on, they were not in themselves fit for purpose as a case-mix and costing model for the United Kingdom. Instead, a different case-mix classification is proposed based on complexity of needs for rehabilitation (96,97,98).

The weighted per diem payment model has been developed in the context of neurological rehabilitation, but application is expected in other areas of rehabilitation once it has been validated in this context. The weighted per diem payment model applies a simple 5-tier multilevel tariff through serial complexity ratings so that the level of reimbursement changes with the requirement for intervention as the episode progresses (see Figure 3-2) (99). The model is based on serial complexity ratings measured using the Rehabilitation Complexity Scale (100), a simple 5-item scale encompassing needs for care, nursing therapy, and medical treatment.

The critical feature of this case-mix and payment model is that it is fair to both payer and provider. The provider receives reimbursement to meet the additional costs of providing for patients with complex needs. However, the payer does not continue to pay high rates for a patient who had very complex needs on admission but who progresses to lower levels of need in the course of their recovery. Complexity may go up or down, but is expected to fall for most patients over time as they regain independence, and the corresponding reduction in payment provides an incentive toward early discharge.

Figure 3-2 illustrates the application of the multilevel per diem payment model in a single case.

- The payment is weighted in proportion to the differential costs of treating patients in 5 bands of complexity based on the total RCS score.
- The daily payment rate is adjusted according to the level of complexity and so allows for change over time.
- Payment for the overall episode is calculated at discharge depending on the number of days the patient spent at any given complexity level.

- In this illustrative case, the total episode of 194 days was made up of 42 "very heavy," 48 "heavy," 70 "medium," and 34 "light" days at a total cost of £86,730.

To claim the higher-rate payments for patients with complex needs, specialist services must also be able to demonstrate that they provide the additional *inputs* to meet those needs. Similarly, payers who meet those extra costs are entitled to ask for evidence that their investment has led to meaningful *outcomes* in terms of improved independence, reduced ongoing care costs, or at least the attainment of individual goals for rehabilitation. Therefore, a national data set (the UK Rehabilitation Outcomes Collaborative [UKROC] data set) has been established to record *needs, inputs,* and *outcomes*. Service designation is contingent on data set reporting for all specialist inpatient neurorehabilitation episodes (101). Further information about the UK case-mix and funding model is published elsewhere (99,102,103).

In summary, the development of case mix in rehabilitation poses similar challenges for health care systems all around the world. Well-established case-mix systems in the United States and Australia have afforded valuable lessons for other countries to learn from but have not provided all the answers. A range of case-mix and payment models is required to cater for different health care cultures. Case-mix tools must be simple and timely for clinicians to apply in routine practice but must also capture *all* the key cost-determinants to allow fair payment for treatment of patients with complex needs. The UK approach may have wider application in other socially supported systems of health care.

CONCLUSION

There are many drivers of health policy—culture, science, politics, and economics—and as a result, policy changes with time along with scientific and medical advances. To create better health policy, it is critical that good science and reliable data assist and inform the policy process. Therefore, it is incumbent on persons with brain injury, family members, care givers, brain injury specialists, researchers, clinicians, and providers to improve education and awareness of brain injury, to advance best practices, and inform policy-makers of the latest scientifically based understanding of brain injuries of all types. Greater awareness and public understanding must continually grow regarding what brain injury is (from concussion to coma); how it can be treated; what can be expected as possible outcomes; what might be the costs to the individual, the family, the community, and the society; and how systems can be developed and improved to best serve the individual and the public.

In the United States, the debate about whether health care is a right and the extent of government responsibility to provide access to care or insurance will likely continue and affect health care policy and funding decisions. Even though the United Kingdom provides the most comprehensive publicly funded health care system in the world and highly values maximizing functional independence, there are still challenges with policy decisions regarding providing the most cost-effective rehabilitation. These challenges are echoed in other countries all around the globe. Effective rehabilitation may produce cost-benefits to society by restoring long-term independence (so reducing the costs of ongoing care), and where possible supporting people into work and financial independence. Attitudes of health policy makers to investment in rehabilitation for brain injury will depend on the extent of their responsibilities for long-term support. Even though investment in excellent rehabilitation for brain injury may reap substantial savings with respect to ongoing social care, this investment is likely to be given low priority if the savings only accrue to another sector. International collaborative work is underway to develop common approaches to systematic cohort data analysis in order to quantify the benefits of rehabilitation in different groups of patients and identify models of effective and cost-efficient service provision to suit individual needs.

KEY CLINICAL POINTS

1. Health policy is developed as a product of the tensions between political, cultural, and economic drivers. Those factors vary in different parts of the world, and as a result, different countries around the world have very different approaches to health policy.
2. Attitudes of health policy makers to investment in rehabilitation for brain injury will depend on the extent of their responsibilities for long-term support.
3. Effective rehabilitation may produce cost-benefits to society by restoring long-term independence (so reducing the costs of ongoing care), and where possible supporting people into work and financial independence.
4. Even though investment in excellent rehabilitation for brain injury may reap substantial savings in respect of ongoing social care, this investment is likely to be given low priority if the savings only accrue to another sector.
5. It is incumbent on persons with brain injury, family members, care givers, brain injury specialists, researchers, clinicians, and providers to improve education and awareness of brain injury to advance best practices and inform policymakers of the latest scientifically based understanding of brain injuries of all types.
6. It is critical that good science and reliable data assist and inform the policy process. Greater awareness and public

understanding must continually grow regarding what brain injury is (from concussion to coma); how it can be treated; what can be expected as possible outcomes; what might be the costs to the individual, the family, the community, and the society; and how systems can be developed and improved to best serve the individual and the public.

KEY REFERENCES

1. Institute of Medicine. *For the Public's Health: Revitalizing Law and Policy to Meet New Challenges.* Washington, DC: The National Academies Press; 2011.
2. National Prevention Council. *National Prevention Strategy.* Washington, DC: US Department of Health and Human Services, Office of the Surgeon General; 2011.
3. Turner-Stokes L. Evidence for the effectiveness of multidisciplinary rehabilitation following acquired brain injury: a synthesis of two systematic approaches. *J Rehabil Med.* 2008;40(9):691–701.
4. Turner-Stokes L, Sutch S, Dredge R, Eagar K. International casemix and funding models: lessons for rehabilitation. *Clin Rehabil.* 2012;26(3):195–208.
5. Turner-Stokes L, Sutch S, Dredge R. Healthcare tariffs for specialist inpatient neurorehabilitation services: rationale and development of a UK casemix and costing methodology. *Clin Rehabil.* 2012;26(3):264–279.

ACKNOWLEDGMENTS

Many thanks to Susan L. Vaughn, MEd of SLVaughn & Associates, Jefferson City, MO.

References

1. World Health Organization. The World Health Report - Health Systems Financing: The Path to Universal Coverage. Geneva, Switzerland: World Health Organization; 2010.
2. World Health Organization. Preamble to the Constitution of the World Health Organization. International Health Conference; June 19–22, 1946; New York, NY.
3. World Health Organization. Health policy. 2011. WHO Web site. http://www.who.int/topics/health_policy/en/. Accessed July 4, 2011.
4. *Mosby's Medical Dictionary.* 8th ed. St. Louis, MO: Elsevier; 2009.
5. Walt G. *Health Policy: An Introduction to Process and Power: People, Governments and International Agencies—Who Drives Policy and How It is Made.* London, United Kingdom: Zed Books; 1994.
6. Institute of Medicine. *For the Public's Health: Revitalizing Law and Policy to Meet New Challenges.* Washington, DC: The National Academies Press; 2011.
7. United Nations. The Universal Declaration of Human Rights. Adapted on December 10, 1948 by the General Assembly of the United Nations. 1948.
8. Xu K, Saksena P, Evans D. *Health Financing and Access to Effective Interventions. World Health Report, Background Paper # 8.* Geneva, Switzerland: World Health Organization; 2010.
9. Kaiser Family Foundation. Health care spending in the United States and other OECD countries. 2011. Kaiser Family Foundation Web site. http://www.kff.org. Accessed August 5, 2011.
10. Bodenheimer T, Grumbach K. *Understanding Health Policy: A Clinical Approach.* 5th ed. New York, NY: McGraw-Hill; 2008.
11. Rapaport C. *Characteristics of Individuals With and Without Health Insurance, 2009.* Congressional Research Service Report; March 2, 2011. CRS Report R41665.

12. US Centers for Disease Control and Prevention. How many people have TBI? CDC Web site. http://www.cdc.gov/TraumaticBrain Injury/statistics.html. Updated March 23, 2012. Accessed August 10, 2011.

13. Bérubé JE. Brain injury advocacy. *J Head Trauma Rehabil*. 1998;13(5): 99–102.

14. Brain Injury Association of America. 30th Anniversary of THE Challenge! 2010. BIAA Web site. http://www.biausa.org. Accessed July 5, 2010.

15. Institute of Medicine, Committee on Trauma Research, National Research Council. *Injury in America: A Continuing Public Health Problem*. Washington, DC: National Academies Press; 1985.

16. US Centers for Disease Control and Prevention. About CDC's Injury Center. CDC Web site. http://www.cdc.gov/injury/about/ index.html. Updated January 27, 2009. Accessed August 1, 2011.

17. Bérubé JE. A campaign for a "cure". *J Head Trauma Rehabil*. 2003; 18(2):204–206.

18. Masel B. Conceptualizing Brain Injury as a Chronic Disease. BIAA position paper. Published February 2009. http://www.biausa.org. Accessed August 2, 2011.

19. Leaders and Board of the Bob Woodruff Foundation. REMIND Web site. http://www.remind.org. Accessed July 5, 2011.

20. National Prevention Council. *National Prevention Strategy*. Washington, DC: US Department of Health and Human Services, Office of the Surgeon General; 2011.

21. Samuelson RJ. Radicals, reactionaries and an unhappy Fourth. *The Washington Post*. http://www.washingtonpost.com/opinions/ radicals-reactionaries-and-an-unhappy-fourth/2011/07/02/ AGx3dvwH_story.html. Accessed July 3, 2011.

22. MacGillis A. The rise of zombie liberalism: half-dead, half-alive. *The Washington Post*. http://www.washingtonpost.com/opinions /the-rise-of-zombie-liberalism-half-dead-half-alive/2011/06/29/ AG0934tH_story.html. Accessed July 3, 2011.

23. Patient Protection and Affordable Care Act, Pub L No. 111–148, 124 Stat 119 (2010), Health Care and Education Reconciliation Act, Pub L No. 111–152, 124 Stat 1029 (2010).

24. Miller T, Langston E, Lawrence B, et al. *Rehabilitation Costs and Long-Term Consequences of Motor Vehicle Injury*. DOT HS 810 581. Washington, DC: National Highway Traffic Safety Administration; 2006; contract no. DTNH22-98-D-35079.

25. NY Motorcyclist Dies After Hitting Head on Pavement During Protest Against Helmet Laws. *The Washington Post*. July 3, 2011. http://www.washingtonpost.com/national/upstate-ny-motorcyclist -dies-after-hitting-head-on-pavement-during-protest-against-helmet -laws/2011/07/03/AGNicNwH_story.html. Accessed July 5, 2011.

26. American Bikers Aimed Toward Education. Position statement on mandated helmet use. ABATE of NY Web site. http://abateny .org/leg/ny/helmets.pdf. Accessed July 5, 2011.

27. Governors Highway Safety Association. Motorcycle safety. GHSA Web site. http://statehighwaysafety.org/html/issues/motorcy-clesafety.html. Accessed August 1, 2011.

28. *Simon v. Sargent*, 346 F Supp 277 (DC Mass), *aff'd*, 93 SCt 463, 409 US 1020, 34 LEd2d 312 (1972).

29. Illinois motorcycle helmet law. Bikers Rights Web site. http:// www.bikersrights.com/states/illinois/illinois.html. Accessed August 1, 2011.

30. Center for the Study of Traumatic Encephalopathy. Boston University Web site. http://www.bu.edu/cste/news/media. Accessed August 3, 2011.

31. CNN. Former NFL players: league concealed concussion risks. CNN Web site. http://www.cnn.com/2011/HEALTH/07/20/ nfl.lawsuit.concussions/index.html. Accessed August 3, 2011.

32. Brophy M. Brain research new "moon shot" Patrick Kennedy says. *USA TODAY*. http://www.usatoday.com/news/health/medical /story/2011/05/Brain-research-new-moon-shot-Patrick-Kennedy -says/47399244/1. Accessed August 3, 2011.

33. Congressional Budget Office. *Research and Development in the Pharmaceutical Industry*. Washington, DC: Congressional Budget Office; 2006.

34. Johnson JA, Smith PW. *The National Institutes of Health (NIH): Organization, Funding, and Congressional Issues*. Washington, DC: Congressional Research Service; 2011.

35. Thomas PW, Silverstein R. Memorandum. Washington, DC: Disability and Rehabilitation Research Coalition; 2011. The future of disability and medical rehabilitation research at NIH. http:// www.aapmr.org/advocacy/health-policy/DRRC/Documents/ nih-meeting-statement-020711.pdf. Accessed August 9, 2011.

36. Institute of Medicine. *Enabling America: Assessing the Role of Rehabilitation Science and Engineering, Institute of Medicine*. In: Brandt E Jr, Pope A, eds. Washington, DC: The National Academies Press; 1997.

37. Tanielian T, Jaycox LH, eds. *Invisible Wounds of War: Psychological and Cognitive Injuries, Their Consequences, and Services to Assist Recovery*. Washington, DC: RAND; 2008.

38. Institute of Medicine. *The Future of Disability in America*. In: Field M, Jette AM, eds. Washington, DC: The National Academies Press; 2007.

39. National Institutes of Neurological Disorders and Stroke, Department of Defense, National Institutes of Health Clinical Center, Center for Neuroscience and Regenerative Medicine. *Warfighter Head Injury Study*. http://clinicaltrials.gov/ct2/show/NCT00754169. Accessed August 7, 2011.

40. Stephanie Condon. *Obama: More Health Care Should Be Based on Science*. http://www.cbsnews.com/8301-503544_162-5111374-503544.html?tag=mncol;lst;2. Accessed August 10, 2011.

41. BIAA Legislative Priorities. http://www.biausa.org/biaa-legisla tive-priorities.htm. Accessed August 10, 2011. BTF Guidelines. https://www.braintrauma.org/coma-guidelines/. Accessed August 10, 2011. Gradual Return to Play Protocol. http://www .sportsconcussions.org/return-to-play.html. Accessed August 10, 2011.

42. Faul M, Wald M, Rutland-Brown W, Sullivent E, Sattin R. Using a cost-benefit analysis to estimate outcomes of a clinical treatment guideline: testing the Brain Trauma Foundation guidelines for the treatment of severe traumatic brain injury. *J Trauma*. 2007;63(6): 1271–1278.

43. Puroshotham M, Vadiveloo, J. *Actuarial Estimate of Medicaid Healthcare Cost Savings in the State of New York With CarePath Program Implementation*. Watson Wyatt Worldwide. May 13, 2009.

44. House Armed Services Committee adopts TBI amendment. Brain Injury Association of America Web site. http://www.biausa.org. May 12, 2011. Accessed August 8, 2011.

45. Roof C. AMVETS legislative priorities for the 112th Congress. American Veterans Web site. http://www.amvets.org/pdfs/AM-VETS-LegislativePriorities.pdf. Accessed August 8, 2011.

46. Tate C. Giffords' recovery renews focus on coverage gap for veterans. McClatchy News. http://www.mcclatchydc.com/2011/08/ 10/120215/giffords-recovery-renews-focus.html. Accessed August 11, 2011.

47. Supreme Court of Florida. No. SC04-925 Jeb Bush, Governor of Florida, et. al. *Appellants v Schiavo*, Guardian of Theresa Schiavo, Appellee. September 23, 2004.

48. Fins J. *A Palliative Ethic of Care: Clinical Wisdom at Life's End*. Sudbury, MA: Jones & Bartlett Learning; 2006.

49. Holmes, J. Opinion of the Court, Supreme Court of the United States. *Buck v Bell*, 274US200(1927).

50. *Skinner v. Oklahoma*, 316 US 535 (1942), the US Supreme Court ruled compulsory sterilization as a punishment violated the Equal Protection Clause of the Fourteenth Amendment of the US Constitution.

51. Kennedy, EM. *The Cause of My Life: Inside the Fight for Universal Health Care*. http://www.thedailybeast.com/newsweek/2009/ 07/17/the-cause-of-my-life.html. Accessed July 18, 2011.

52. Change.org. *Sign the Petition Establishing Health Care as a Civil Right*. http://www.change.org/petitions/sign-the-petition-establishing-health-care-as-a-civil-right. Accessed August 1, 2011.

53. Pilon R. *Cato's Letter #13: The Purpose and Limits of Government*. Washington, DC: Cato Institute; 1999.

54. Leonhardt D. Opposition to health law is steeped in tradition. *New York Times*. December 14, 2010:A1.

55. Turner G, Capretta JC, Miller TP, Moffitt RE. *Why ObamaCare is Wrong For America: How the New Health Care Law Drives Up Costs, Puts Government In Charge of Your Decisions, and Threatens Your Constitutional Rights*. New York, NY: HarperCollins; 2011.

56. Volsky I. Flashback: Republicans opposed medicare in 1960s by warning of rationing, "socialized medicine." ThinkProgress Web site. http://thinkprogress.org/health/2009/07/29/170887/medicare-44/. Published July 29, 2009. Accessed August 9, 2011.

57. Centers for Disease Control and Prevention. Traumatic brain injury. CDC Web site. http://www.cdc.gov/traumaticbraininjury/index.html. Updated February 28, 2012. Accessed August 2, 2011.

58. Pear R. Administration offers health care cuts as part of budget negotiations. *The New York Times.* July 4, 2011:A1.

59. Robert Wood Johnson Foundation. Health policy brief: key issues of health reform. *Health Affairs.* August 20, 2009.

60. Gramlich J. Arizona Medicaid Cuts Go Into Effect. *Stateline.* July 5, 2011. http://stateline.org/live/details/story?contentId=585687 (accessed August 11, 2011).

61. Sack K. Arizona's Medicaid cuts seen as a sign of the Times. *The New York Times.* December 4, 2010:A1.

62. Sternberg S. For brain injuries a treatment gap. *USA Today.* March 3, 2011:A1.

63. Arango-Lasparilla JC, Rosenthal M, Deluca J, Komaroff E, Sherer M, Cifu D, Hanks R. Traumatic brain injury and functional outcomes: does minority status matter? *Brain Inj.* 2007;21(7);701–708.

64. Turner-Stokes L. Evidence for the effectiveness of multidisciplinary rehabilitation following acquired brain injury: a synthesis of two systematic approaches. *J Rehabil Med.* 2008;40:691–701.

65. Turner-Stokes L. The evidence for the cost-effectiveness of rehabilitation following acquired brain injury. *Clinl Med.* 2004;4:10–12.

66. Aronow H. Rehabilitation effectiveness with severe brain injury: translating research into policy. *J Head Traum Rehabil.* 1987;2:24–36.

67. Nyein K, Turner-Stokes L, Robinson I. The Northwick park care needs assessment (NPCNA): a measure of community care needs: sensitivity to change during rehabilitation. *Clin Rehabil.* 1999;13:482–491.

68. Turner-Stokes L, Paul S, Williams H. Efficiency of specialist rehabilitation in reducing dependency and costs of continuing care for adults with complex acquired brain injuries. *J Neurol Neurosurg Psychiatr.* 2006;77:634–639.

69. Turner-Stokes L. Cost-efficiency of longer-stay rehabilitation programmes: can they provide value for money? *Brain Inj.* 2007;21:1015–1021.

70. Wikipedia. Case mix. 2010. http://en.wikipedia.org/wiki/Case_mix. Updated August 28, 2010. Accessed November 27, 2010.

71. InterRAI. InterRAI network. 2006. http://www.interrai.org/section/view/. Accessed November 27, 2010.

72. Fetter R, ed. *DRGs, Their Design and Development.* Ann Arbour, MI: Health Administration Press; 1991.

73. Vladeck BC, Kramer PS. Case mix measures: DRGs and alternatives. *Ann Rev Public Health.* 1988;9:333–359.

74. Schreyögg J, Stargardt T, Velasco-Garrido M, Busse R. Defining the "Health Benefit Basket" in nine European countries. Evidence from the European Union Health BASKET Project. *Eur J Health Econ.* 2005;(suppl):2–10.

75. Stineman MG, Kallen MA, Thompson C, Gage B. Challenges in paying for effective stays. *Med Care.* 2005;43:841–843.

76. Sutherland JM, Walker J. Challenges of rehabilitation case mix measurement in Ontario hospitals. *Health Policy.* 2008;85:336–348.

77. Lee LA, Eagar KM, Smith MC. Subacute and non-acute case mix in Australia. *Med J Aust.* 1998;169:19.

78. Heinemann AW, Hamilton B, Linacre JM, et al. Functional status and therapeutic intensity during inpatient rehabilitation. *Am J Phys Med Rehabil.* 1995;74:315–326.

79. Heinemann AW, Kirk P, Hastie BA, et al. Relationships between disability measures and nursing effort during medical rehabilitation for patients with traumatic brain and spinal cord injury. *Arch Phys Med Rehabil.* 1997;78:143–149.

80. Disler PB, Roy CW, Smith BP. Predicting hours of care needed. *Arch Phys Med Rehabil.* 1993;74:139–143.

81. Hoffman JM, Doctor JN, Chan L, Whyte J, Jha A, Dikmen S. Potential impact of the new Medicare prospective payment system on reimbursement for traumatic brain injury inpatient rehabilitation. *Arch Phys Med Rehabil.* 2003;84(8):1165–1172.

82. Evans RL, Halar EM, Hendricks RD, Lawrence KV, Kirk C, Bishop DS. Effects of prospective payment financing on rehabilitation outcome. *Int J Rehabil Res.* 1990;13(1):27–35.

83. Saitto C, Marino C, Fusco D, Arcà M, Perucci CA; for Prospective Payment in Rehabilitation Collaborative Group. Toward a new payment system for inpatient rehabilitation. Part II: reimbursing providers. *Med Care.* 2005;43(9):856–864.

84. Saitto C, Marino C, Fusco D, Arcà M, Perucci CA; for Prospective Payment in Rehabilitation Collaborative Group. Toward a new payment system for inpatient rehabilitation. Part I: predicting resource consumption. *Med Care.* 2005;43(9):844–855.

85. Batavia AI, DeJong G. Prospective payment for medical rehabilitation: the DHHS report to congress. *Arch Phys Med Rehabil.* 1988;69:377.

86. Heinemann AW, Linacre JM, Wright BD, Hamilton BB, Granger C. Relationships between impairment and physical disability as measured by the Functional Independence Measure. *Arch Phys Med Rehabil.* 1993;74(6):566–573.

87. Stineman MG, Tassoni CJ, Escarce JJ, et al. Development of function-related groups version 2.0: a classification system for medical rehabilitation. *Health Serv Res.* 1997;32(4):529–548.

88. Duckett SJ. Case mix funding for acute hospital inpatient services in Australia. *Med J Aust.* 1998;169:17S–21S.

89. Eagar K, Cromwell D, Kennedy C, Lee L. Classifying sub-acute and non-acute patients: results of the New South Wales Casemix Area Network study. *Aust Health Rev.* 1997;20(2):26–42.

90. Webster F. Development of a case mix classification system for inpatient rehabilitation services: stage 1 of the Victorian rehabilitation project. *Aust Health Rev.* 1996;19:81–92.

91. Eagar K. The Australian national sub-acute and non-acute patient case mix classification. *Aust Health Rev.* 1999;22:180–196.

92. Green J, Gordon R. The development of version 2 of the AN-SNAP casemix classification system. *Aust Health Rev.* 2007;31(suppl 1):S68–S78.

93. Department of Health. Reforming NHS Financial Flows Introducing Payment by Results. London, United Kingdom: Department of Health; 2002.

94. Royal College of Physicians in London. Physical disability in 1986 and beyond. London: Royal College of Physicians. 1986. London, United Kingdom: Royal College of Physicians in London; 1986.

95. Nyein K, Thu A, Turner-Stokes L. Complex specialized rehabilitation following severe brain injury: a UK perspective. *J Head Traum Rehabil.* 2007;22:239–247.

96. Department of Health. *National Definition Set for Specialised Services No 7: Complex Specialised Rehabilitation for Brain Injury and Complex Disability (Adult).* 3rd ed. London, United Kingdom: Department of Health; 2009.

97. Turner-Stokes L, Disler R, Williams H. The Rehabilitation Complexity Scale: a simple, practical tool to identify 'complex specialised' services in neurological rehabilitation. *Clin Med.* 2007;7:593–599.

98. Department of Health. *Options for the Future of Payment by Results: 2008/09 to 2010/11.* London, United Kingdom: Department of Health; 2007.

99. Turner-Stokes L, Sutch S, Dredge R. Healthcare tariffs for specialist inpatient neurorehabilitation services: rationale and development of a UK case mix and costing methodology. *Clin Rehabil.* 2012;26(3):264–279.

100. Turner-Stokes L, Williams H, Siegert RJ. The Rehabilitation Complexity Scale version 2: a clinimetric evaluation inpatients with severe complex neurodisability. *J Neurol Neurosurg Psychiatr.* 2010;81:146–153.

101. Department of Health. *National Definition Set for Specialised Services No 7: Complex Specialised Rehabilitation for Brain Injury and Complex Disability (Adult).* London, United Kingdom: Department of Health; 2002.

102. Turner-Stokes L, Bill A, Dredge R. A cost analysis of specialist inpatient neurorehabilitation services in the UK. *Clin Rehabil.* 2012;26(3):256–263.

103. Turner-Stokes L, Sutch S, Dredge R. International case mix and costing models: lessons for rehabilitation in the UK. *Clin Rehabil.* 2012;26(3):195–208.

International Systems of Care and Research Agendas

Olli Tenovuo, M. Ross Bullock, and Ross D. Zafonte

INTRODUCTION

Traumatic brain injury (TBI) is a global health problem, and no one is immune to the risk of severe injury. There are significant differences in the frequency and causes of TBI among various cultures because of the types of activities in which people engage. Because of the availability or lack thereof of health care resources around the world, the epidemiology, causes and care of TBI are as varied as the injury itself. In addition to complicating the care of the individual with a TBI, this international variability poses a great challenge in creating solutions for brain injury medicine in general.

OVERVIEW OF GLOBAL EPIDEMIOLOGY

Information on the epidemiology of TBI on a global scale is unreliable. Researching the epidemiology of TBI is notoriously difficult as there are several sources of potential error (see Table 4-1). There are only a few reliable studies of epidemiology done at the national level within the global community, which makes comparing these studies difficult. Most studies are based on hospital admissions, records, or national registries, but there are marked differences even within a nation in how patients are admitted and treated. Moreover, studies have suggested that significant numbers of these injuries remain undiagnosed (1–3), unrecorded (4,5), falsely coded (6,7), or underestimated (8), and these issues may vary considerably even between neighboring hospitals.

In principle, the more severe the TBI is, the more reliable the epidemiological data are. This is evidenced by the fact that almost all individuals with severe TBI are admitted to the hospital. Epidemiological data for milder injuries is unreliable because not all patients sustaining these injuries are admitted to in-patient wards. Several studies have shown, however, that up to 90% of all TBI are mild (9). The definition of "mild TBI" is unclear (8), so this percentage is questionable. Furthermore, in many studies, mortality figures do not include subjects who die from their injuries before reaching the hospital. In many cultures, victims are not admitted to the hospital and their true mechanism of death has not been determined by forensic medicine; however, most TBI-related deaths caused by motor vehicle accidents (MVAs) occur at the scene or during the pre-hospital period (10,11).

Available studies of TBI epidemiology have almost exclusively focused on incidence. Figures obtained from various sources vary considerably, ranging from less than 100 to more than 3,000 per 100,000 inhabitants (12,13). Most studies have been done in developed countries; there is little published data from many population-rich countries (14). Because there are discrepancies in how the study population is defined in these, it is difficult to ascertain the exact range of injuries per 100,000 people. Studies that include subjects who have been admitted to hospitals yield figures within 100 to 300 per 100,000 (15,16); whereas, studies that include patients who visit emergency departments or general practitioners, or who do not seek medical attention at all yield figures from 500 per 100,000 (17,18).

The prevalence of TBI, defined as chronic symptoms from an earlier TBI, is not widely studied. An oft-quoted estimate from the United States is that 2% of the population has suffered a TBI (19). If this statistic is extrapolated to a global scale, approximately 140 million people experience chronic symptoms caused by TBI; however, there are major discrepancies with this figure (20). Some studies suggest that as many as 10% of adults have sustained a TBI (21,22). Exact percentages are difficult to ascertain because of unreliable data, and a dearth of studies from developing countries and in some of the most populated countries, such as India and China. The incidence of TBI in these countries may be higher than in the United States, but the number of those who survive more severe injuries may be lower. The results of these studies are presented in Table 4-2.

Consequently, the true prevalence of TBI on a global scale is unknown. In addition, these studies do not necessarily separate the symptoms of TBI from those caused by other illnesses or injuries, and there is a possibility that the diagnosis of TBI is overestimated or underestimated. Reliable studies of the severity and long-term consequences of TBI are strongly needed. Recently published reports on the follow-up of long-term studies suggest that chronic symptoms may occur more frequently than initially reported and may appear long after the injury was sustained; although, there are also contradictory results (31).

Determining the occurrence and prevalence of TBI and an approximate number of TBI-related fatalities worldwide is difficult; however, a moderate estimate of 150 per 100,000 of TBI-related hospitalizations, based on several studies and, 600 per 100,000 of mild TBI based on reports from the World Health Organization (WHO) Task Force (9), would result in 10.5 million hospitalizations and 43 million mild TBI each year. These numbers are uncertain because studies yield

TABLE 4-1 Potential Sources of Error in Epidemiological Studies of Traumatic Brain Injury

Registry studies	Undiagnosed TBI (multitraumas, inebriated subjects, etc.) Diagnosis made but not recorded (especially as a second diagnosis) Severity misclassified (if selection based on severity) Invalid coding Technical registry problems
Population studies	Recruitment bias (not seeking medical care) Admission bias (not following local guidelines) False diagnoses
Prevalence studies	Lost from follow-up Diagnostic uncertainty

figures between 15.1 and 162.5 million people (15,27), with an average estimate of 68.5 million people who require hospitalization because of TBI. An oft-quoted estimate of mortality, derived mainly from European studies, is 15 per 100,000 (15), which means there are more than 1 million TBI-related deaths annually. However, the mortality rate may be much higher in many population-rich countries that have less developed health care resources, more chaotic traffic, and more frequent natural disasters. The unknown number of prehospital deaths in these countries contributes to this rate.

COSTS

The costs of TBI are as unreliable as the epidemiological data. Costs are influenced by epidemiological patterns, the use and availability of health care resources and the various ways to calculate financial loss caused by death or disability in different societies. For example, from a purely financial perspective, the death of a young American causes more economic hardship than the death of a young Nigerian because of the estimated loss of the individual's earnings. Emigration could considerably change the predicted income of the individual. Consequently, lost human potential has to

be calculated based on the average income in developed countries. Cost estimates that are based on hospital fees may be problematic because these fees vary widely within systems of care.

Fewer studies concerning TBI-related costs are available than epidemiological studies. In addition, most of these studies have been done in developed countries (30,32–34). The Center for Disease Control and Prevention (CDC) reported that estimated direct and indirect costs of TBI in the United States were $60 billion in the year 2000 (35). Extrapolating this figure to a global scale would result in $1,340 billion per year. Sweden estimates that the average cost of a TBI-related death is €375,000 (34). Again, on a global scale this would be between €375 billion and €1,125 billion ($540–$1,620 billion) from TBI-related deaths. This estimate does not include costs of caring for those who survive.

Although the actual costs of TBI are unknown, it is probable that TBI annual costs are higher than 1 trillion dollars—more than $142 per person worldwide. This figure is close to the average yearly income per capita in many poorly developed countries. The actual costs may be considerably higher, which will be discussed later in this chapter.

TRENDS

Several studies have reported considerable change in the epidemiology of TBI. A common finding in studies that have been done in developed countries is the increase in the number of TBI in the elderly. A Finnish study reported an increase exceeding 200% in age-related incidences of severe TBI between 1970 and 2004, with the total number increasing more than 1,000% (36). Similar trends have been reported in other studies (37).

MVAs are a major cause of TBI and contribute to the rise in the incidence of TBI. Although many developed countries have reported a decrease in MVAs because of legislation and improved safety regulations (19,38–39), globally the view is less positive. In many developing countries with large populations, the number of cars is increasing rapidly, road and highway infrastructure is poor, legislation is lacking, and vehicles are old or of poor quality and have no modern safety features. Accordingly, WHO statistics show that MVAs are a major cause of fatalities in low- and middle-income countries, and the number of MVAs is predicted to steeply in-

TABLE 4-2 Prevalence Figures (/100,000) of Symptomatic Traumatic Brain Injury Sequels in Various Studies

STUDY	POPULATION	PREVALENCE	NOTES	REFERENCE
Yang et al. 1987	Urban areas, China	783.3	Door survey	23
Zhu et al. 1989	Rural areas, China	442.2	Door survey	24
Engberg 1995	Denmark	317.0	Work-precluding	25
Langlois et al. 2004	United States	1,893.0		26
Whiteneck et al. 2004	Colorado	2,000.0		27
Shukri et al. 2006	Yemen	219.0		28
Tagliaferri et al. 2006	Europe	2,356.0		15
Winqvist et al. 2007	Northern Finland	269.0	< 35 yrs	29
Mar et al. 2011	Northern Spain	657.0		30

crease by 2030, making this the number five cause of death worldwide (40). This predicted increase will affect the number of TBI, which is the most common cause of death or chronic disability in MVAs (41).

Other trends in the epidemiology of TBI are less clear. Contributing factors may include population growth, climate change, and increasing economical inequality, which is likely to result in a higher number of refugees and violent conflicts or wars. Extreme weather conditions because of global warming may contribute to the incidence of TBI. Developed countries are not excluded from these trends and risks; current lifestyles in these nations seem to contribute to the number of TBI. Although the number of TBI sustained in MVAs has diminished, other causes have increased. In addition to the increasing number of falls in the elderly, such factors as drug abuse, extreme sports, and violence contribute to the alarming rise in the incidence of TBI. A recent study conducted in the United States reported an increase of almost 20% between the years 2002 and 2006—about 4 times greater than the rate of increase in population (42). Despite modern safety devices and advanced technology, it appears that the need for improved clinical and effective preventive care of TBI is greater than ever (see Chapter 7).

INDIRECT CONSEQUENCES OF TRAUMATIC BRAIN INJURY

Too often, TBI has been regarded as an accidental, momentary incident, which will either cause some persistent handicap or, in many cases, only transient harm. The true nature of TBI is much more complicated, and it meets all of the criteria of a chronic condition (43). Within the category of chronic diseases, TBI has many unique features that have been underreported and seldom discussed in the medical literature. Moreover, these issues have not been taken into account in any studies that have tried to clarify the cost of TBI.

TBI affects not only the patient, but also his or her family and friends. TBI is often an "invisible" injury. The patient may seem well and recovered; however, TBI regularly affects higher brain function that impacts cognitive ability and personality. The loss of self-awareness, self-esteem, previous emotional balance, and higher cognitive and social abilities puts the patient, his or her family, friends, and colleagues under considerable stress (44,45). Not surprisingly, patients with TBI are at risk for divorce (46) and suicide (47,48). One study reports that families of patients with TBI are willing to pay more for restoring the injured person to his or her former self than for paying for medical treatment for a relative with a terminal illness (49). Clinical care providers often see and feel the considerable stress of the family, but it is not widely known how this stress impacts the caregivers' ability to work outside the home and their health and psychosocial well-being or the development of children in the family.

Cross-sectional studies suggest a connection between TBI and Alzheimer disease (AD) (50,51); although, the causality remains questionable. Whether TBI is actually able to trigger an AD process is still unknown, but it is apparent that TBI, by decreasing the cognitive reserve, contributes to an earlier manifestation of degeneration (52,53) (see Figure

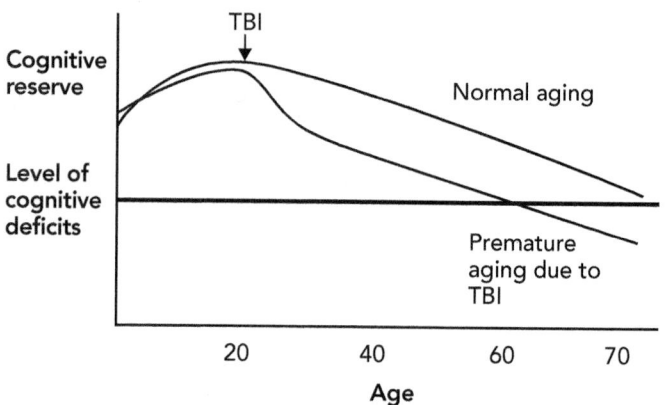

FIGURE 4-1 During normal aging, the level of cognitive deficits that impair everyday functioning is reached at about 80 years of age. A TBI sustained at the age of 20 lowers the cognitive reserve, causing the age-related cognitive deficits to appear earlier.

4-1). The role of TBI in premature aging is important to clarify because of the significant impact it would have on public health and the economy. It has been suggested that moderate or severe TBI hastens the aging phenomena by several years (53). For example, the loss of brain tissue in severe TBI is about 50 cc (54), which is equal to 3.5 billion neurons, and in normal aging, the loss is about 31 million neurons annually (55).

TBI contributes to increased risk of many late sequelae, such as aging phenomena, psychiatric illness, epilepsy, and premature death (43). A person with TBI is also at risk for new injuries; the likelihood of another TBI increases threefold to tenfold (2,56). This is only partially explained by the fact that certain persons, such as those who abuse drugs or engaging in risky behavior, are generally at increased risk for TBI. It seems logical that some of the consequences of TBI, such as impaired balance and coordination, slower reactions, lower tolerance to centrally acting agents, and deficient executive functions contribute to an increased risk of new injuries.

The literature that addresses the social consequences for persons shows that an unmarried person with TBI who lives alone and is unable to work is at considerable risk for alienation (57,58). This risk also exists for persons with TBI and subsequent sequelae who are divorced. Although the financial impact caused by social exclusion is difficult to assess, many studies suggest it is significant (59). When determining the financial impact of TBI on society, costs of litigation that result from accidents involving TBI and social security benefits for those who are unable to return to work should be taken into consideration. Because disability benefits vary significantly from country to country, it is very difficult to provide an international comparison of the cost of TBI.

Finally, the concept that pediatric TBI is benign has radically changed. Several studies suggest that TBI sustained in childhood and adolescence impairs psychosocial development, increases the risk of learning difficulties and cognitive deficits, predisposes to epilepsy and attention deficit hyperactivity disorder (ADHD), increases the risk of antisocial behavior and drug abuse, and puts children with TBI at risk for psychiatric illness (60–65). Currently, there are no reliable studies that examine long-term consequences of TBI in pediatric patients. It is apparent that the developing central nervous system is more vulnerable to the deleterious effects of TBI than previously thought (66), and the implications from pediatric TBI may be very significant in society.

In summary, future discussions of the financial consequences of TBI should examine the indirect costs affecting the individual, the individual's family, and society. The frequency of, the costs incurred by, and ways to prevent or minimize TBI require much more research.

GEOGRAPHICAL AND CULTURAL ASPECTS OF TRAUMATIC BRAIN INJURY

Globally, there is remarkable inequality in the availability of natural resources, social support, and health care. In part this inequality stems from geographical and cultural factors. Historical and political factors also play a role. On a global scale, these different circumstances affect the causative epidemiology of TBI, and the outcome and effects on society.

Variable Risk Factors and Causes of Traumatic Brain Injury

As discussed briefly earlier, the epidemiology of TBI greatly varies among countries, continents, and cultures. In this section, the causative epidemiology of TBI from a global viewpoint will be discussed.

Causative epidemiology can be divided into *risk factors* and *causes of injury*. Table 4-3 lists common risk factors for TBI. Some of these show little geographical or cultural variation (such as gender); whereas, some are unevenly distributed worldwide. For example, elderly people or people who participate in winter sports are at greater risk for TBI. On a global scale, some risk factors, such as snowboarding are of little importance, although they may be locally significant. This section will focus on those risk factors that are generally

---

TABLE 4-3 Common Risk Factors of Traumatic Brain Injury

Young or advanced age (< 25 or > 70 years)

Male gender

Abuse of alcohol or other psychoactive substances

Risk-taking personality

Certain sports (e.g., professional boxing, alpine skiing, snowboarding, roller skating, ice hockey, American football, many motor sports)

Speeding or other negligence in traffic

Cycling without a helmet

Car driving without a seatbelt

Low social class

Psychiatric disorders

Proneness to violence

Low intelligence

Previous brain injuries

---

important and that cause significant geographical or cultural variability in the epidemiology of TBI.

The use of alcohol and/or illicit drugs is a major contributor to TBI morbidity. There are few cultures that do not use any psychoactive substances for entertainment. There are several studies that report the use of alcohol as a significant risk factor for TBI, and in many studies about 50% of victims have been under the influence of alcohol when sustaining a TBI (67,68). Blood alcohol level is the major determinant, and the risk of TBI increases 1.64-fold when levels are 100–149 mg/dl and increases 9.23-fold when levels exceed 199 mg/dl (69). Consequently, the number of alcohol-related TBI is not clearly associated with the amount of alcohol used per capita but prevailing drinking habits within countries. In countries such as Ireland, Finland, and Russia, where inebriation is common, the number of fall-related TBI seems to be high (70–72). In areas such as the Arabian Peninsula where alcohol use is negligible, the total incidence of TBI is similar to other countries where inebriation is not prevalent (28). In some instances, the role of alcohol as a risk factor is difficult to assess because blood alcohol levels are not measured or recorded. Regardless of whether or not records kept, it is evident that alcohol use contributes to TBI sustained in traffic accidents, falls, and violence.

The use of other psychoactive substances as a risk factor for TBI has not been widely studied, and current data is fragmented. It is difficult to obtain accurate data because of the criminalization of these substances as well as the unreliability of self-reporting by users and the fact that some users combine alcohol with illicit drugs. It can be asserted, however, that the more an intoxicant affects brain function, the higher the risk of TBI.

As discussed earlier, the number of elderly people with TBI is on the rise in many countries. Epidemiological studies have shown that the age-related risk curve of TBI is U-shaped, with young adults and the elderly being at higher risk than the rest of the adult population (73). The number of elderly people has markedly increased in countries with good standards of living and easy access to quality medical care; the percentage of those who are 65 years and older is commonly around 15% (74). In many low- and middle-income countries, however, life expectancy is shorter, so TBI in the elderly population is not as prevalent. Advanced age and the incidence of TBI involve several factors, including impaired senses and balance, slower reaction time, and the impact of polypharmacy on the elderly. In addition, elderly people are more physically active than they have been in the past. The use of alcohol is also on the rise among the elderly (75).

Risk taking behavior has long been a factor in TBI (76,77). This is likely the most important single factor that explains the occurrence of TBI in young men. Little is known about the cultural differences regarding young men, risk taking behavior, and subsequent TBI; however, it is likely that biological and hormonal factors contribute to this type of behavior in young men.

Major cultural differences, not related to age, contribute to the number of TBI sustained in MVAs. Safety constraints for automobile drivers and helmets for bicyclists are universally available, and their use has been shown to considerably reduce the risk of TBI. It has been reported that the use of safety constraints decreases the risk of TBI sustained in a

MVA by almost 50% (78,79), and the use of bicycle helmets reduces the risk of TBI up to 88% (80). Although data on whether or not these safety devices are used in many countries is not available, it is likely that chaotic traffic patterns, speeding, and mechanically unsound motor vehicles contribute to death and permanent disability each year.

Several sports, particularly winter and motor sports that involve high speed, increase the risk for TBI (81). Therefore, protective equipment has been mandatory in ice hockey for several years but in general regulations vary considerably by country. In many popular sports such as skateboarding and roller-skating/blading, the use of protection is not "fashionable." Moreover, in professional boxing, the goal is to knock out one's opponent, which increases the risk of TBI.

Studies show that lack of education is a risk factor in TBI (82). This is intimately connected to many of the factors discussed earlier because besides legislative measures, education or lack thereof impacts these risks. Because risk profiles and levels of education in preventing TBI vary from country to country, increasing global efforts to improve disseminating information may reduce the risks of injury and advance clinical care.

Typically, there are only a few major causes of TBI commonly seen across countries. Table 4-4 reflects these causes and the frequency with which they occur around the world. It is important to note that current data is difficult to obtain and that percentages shown may be very different than actual numbers.

In general, MVAs and falls are the most prevalent causes of TBI worldwide; however, the prevalence varies from country to country. For example, some countries may see a higher frequency of MVAs than falls when assessing the cause of TBI (14). In countries where winter temperatures sink below freezing, falls because of slipping on ice are significant. The percentage of falls is greater in northern countries, especially in cultures where heavy drinking is common (70,72). In countries with warmer climates, MVAs and vio-lence tend to cause TBI (14,74). Natural disasters, especially earthquakes, may result in a considerable number of TBI, with up to 50% of casualties sustaining significant head injury (95). Thus, disastrous earthquakes may cause hundreds of thousands TBI, posing an insurmountable challenge to any health care system.

Differing Outcome and Effects of Traumatic Brain Injury

The outcome of TBI is an extremely complex issue and depends on such factors as the individual, the extent of the injury, the type and length of treatment, and the social support. From an international perspective, some aspects of outcome deserve a closer look.

As previously discussed, it is difficult to ascertain actual mortality rates because data presented in numerous studies significantly vary. The causes of TBI play a significant role, because the mortality from MVAs is much higher than from falls. Interestingly, a Scandinavian study reports that even between neighboring countries with similar cultures and access to health care, the difference in the rate of mortality may be significant (96). The reasons for this kind of disparity are not apparent, but may be related to the severity of TBI. Similarly, in countries where MVAs and penetrating injuries caused by violence are predominant, mortality rates are above average. Access to quality health care plays a role in mortality rates, as evidenced in comparative studies and by the decrease in in-hospital mortality in developed countries in recent decades. Consequently, TBI mortality rates vary considerably among countries and cultures, and when combined with poor level of care, the results can be devastating (14,97).

Patients with mild, nonfatal TBI encounter societal challenges that patients with similar injuries did not face a few decades ago. Technological advances, competitive job mar-

---

TABLE 4-4 Common Causes of Traumatic Brain Injury in Different Countries and Continents

CONTINENT/COUNTRY	TRAFFIC	FALLS	VIOLENCE	YEAR	REFERENCE
Europe					
England	25.0%	47.0%	16.0%	1990–2001	83
Germany	26.3%	52.5%	14.2%	2000	84
North America					
United Sates	19.0%	32.0%	10.0%	2003	85
Canada	77.6%	13.0%	4.4%	1986–2007	86
South America					
Argentina	37.6%	26.8%	11.0%	2001	87
Brazil	41.0%	24.0%	25.0%	2001	88
Asia					
Taiwan	55.0%	28.0%	13.0%	2001	89
Pakistan	52.8%	28.0%	14.0%	1995–1999	90
The Middle East					
Israel	35.7%	51.0%	9.0%	1984–1988	91
Qatar	45.7%	34.3%	?	2007	92
Africa					
South-Africa	36.5%	3.4%	43.6%	1987	93
Australia & New Zealand	61.4%	24.9%	8.0%	2001	94

kets, and hectic lifestyles are factors that impact society as a whole, but persons with slight cognitive impairments may have more difficulty keeping up with constant changes at work and elsewhere. Studies show that only a few decades ago, vocational prospects of persons with TBI were much better than they are today (98). Although not widely studied, there is data that suggests that persons with mild TBI have better vocational success in cultures with less demanding lifestyles (99,100).

There has been little discussion about the burden of persons with TBI on society. As mentioned earlier in this chapter, TBI frequently affects children, young adults, and others who are in their prime. Diminished intellectual capacity and productivity because of TBI is undoubtedly high but the true burden on society remains unknown. It is likely, however, that a person who sustains a TBI as a child may not perform well in school or have great success during years of employment, and may be at increased risk of cognitive decline in later years. Caring for a person with TBI may also be a considerable burden on relatives and friends. The societal effects of TBI remain an unexplored issue, but in countries where traffic accidents are abundant, level of health care is low, and general educational level is poor, TBI combined with other factors that may harm brain development and functions may cause a remarkable burden for the society.

SYSTEMS OF CARE FROM A GLOBAL PERSPECTIVE

Global Inequality of Resources

Medical care of patients with TBI is twofold. In mild TBI, there are not many therapeutic options available, irrespective of the standard of health care. On the other hand, the treatment of severe TBI is quite sophisticated and requires physicians with high levels of expertise, cutting edge technology, and considerable financial resources. Consequently, outcomes from mild TBI may be similar regardless of the availability of medical care, but a severe TBI may be fatal or disastrous without effective health care.

Treating a patient with TBI requires access to appropriate diagnostic tools. Assessing clinical neurological signs is not as helpful (101) as using modern brain imaging and other current diagnostic measures to determine the extent of and best course of treatment for a patient with TBI. There are still several areas in the world with limited or no access to computed tomography (CT) scans and magnetic resonance imaging (MRI), and it is unlikely that this situation will improve anytime in the near future.

The current standard of care for TBI taxes health care systems. Patients who have sustained potentially severe TBI should be admitted to a neurosurgical unit with ICU facilities and have diagnostic brain imaging as soon as possible.

The number of TBI fatalities resulting because of lack of accessibility to health care is unclear; however, a rough estimate can be obtained by comparing current mortality figures with those from the era before the advent of modern brain imaging. Studies show that mortality from a severe TBI decreased by about 18% between 1970 and 1990, with no additional decrease thereafter (102). Reliable mortality rate comparisons are difficult to ascertain even among devel-

oped countries; however, it can be assumed that in countries with excellent access to health care the mortality rate is lowest, in poorly developed countries the rate is similar to that of the 1970s, and in middle-income countries the rate is somewhere in between. Based on this assumption, it is probable that 120,000 people who sustain TBI die because of inadequate access to health care.

Future Visions

It is unrealistic to expect that there will be equality of care for persons with TBI on a global scale given the lack of financial, political, and natural resources in most low- and middle-income countries. One solution to this conundrum would be to develop innovative and reliable diagnostic tools for use in developing countries, which are not dependent on high technology. For example, a way to assess blood biomarkers at the scene of an accident might be very useful. In general, common terminology and comparative statistics based on standardized data such as Common Data Elements (http://www.tbi-impact.org/cde/) would further the stand of care internationally.

INTERNATIONAL ORGANIZATIONS AND SOCIETIES WITHIN THE FIELD OF TRAUMATIC BRAIN INJURY

The underrepresented nature of TBI in medicine is reflected also in the fairly limited number of organizations that are devoted to brain trauma. This may be due in part to the nature of TBI, where chronic sequelae diminish the ability of the victims to found or organize these organizations. Indeed, most existing international organizations are founded by and geared toward professionals who specialize in TBI. Following is a brief description of these organizations (in alphabetical order). It is important to note that there are several other international organizations that pertain to the fields of neurosurgery, neurology, and neuropsychology that also address TBI. Moreover, there are numerous organizations that function solely or mainly at a national level.

Academy for Multidisciplinary Neurotraumatology (AMN) was founded in 2003 to advance research, teaching, and the practical application of neurotraumatology. The academy organizes of world congresses and workshops and engenders cooperation among scientific academies, societies, associations, research institutions, and companies concerned neurotraumatology. AMN members come from a variety of fields, including neurosurgery, neurorehabilitation, basic research, education, health care administration, and public policy. The 2012 World Congress was held in Taipie, Taiwan.

Brain Injured and Families—European Confederation (BIF-EC) (www.bif-ec.eu) was founded in 1999 and raises awareness about TBI. BIF-EC consists of national patient organizations from 18 European countries and it held its first biennial multidisciplinary conference (TBI-Challenge.eu) in Vienna in 2011. This organization is also affiliated with the European Disability Forum.

Brain Trauma Foundation (BTF) (www.braintrauma.org) was founded in 1986 to support TBI research. BTF develops best practice guidelines, conducts clinical research, and educates both medical professionals and patients. It is based in the United States, but it has established international guidelines in Eastern Europe. BTF is funded by donations and federal and industry grants and awards.

Euroacademia Multidisciplinaria Neurotraumatologica (EMN) (http://www.emn-neurotrauma.de/start.htm) is the European version of the AMN, with similar goals and offerings. This organization offered its 16th annual congress in Newcastle, United Kingdom in May 2011. The 17th annual conference will be held in Romania in 2012. EMN has approximately 130 members from different disciplines.

European Brain Injury Consortium (EBIC) (www.ebic.nl) is a charitable organization founded in 1994. Its members consist of European neurotrauma centers and investigators who focus on the management of TBI and other acute brain injuries. The EBIC advises its members about the practical and theoretical issues pertaining to brain injury studies. It has conducted or collaborated in clinical trials and created guidelines to standardize treatment across the participating centers. EBIC membership is open to all neurotrauma centers.

European Brain Injury Society (EBIS) (http://www.ebis society.org/) was founded in 1989 and members include persons with TBI and other cerebral lesions such as stroke, anoxia, encephalitis, and brain neoplasms. Currently, EBIS has about 165 individual and institutional members from most European countries, with the majority being from France and neighboring countries. EBIS organizes seminars and symposia, provides training and education, conducts research especially within the field of TBI epidemiology, and promotes patient and family organizations. Membership requires support from 2 existing members.

International Brain Injury Association (IBIA) (www.internationalbrain.org) was founded in 1993. It was established to encourage international exchange of information, to support research, to provide training especially in developing countries, and to advocate for brain injury. Since 1995, IBIA has held its "World Congresses on Brain Injury" in Denmark, Spain, Canada, Italy, Sweden, Australia, Portugal, and in the United States every second year. The most recent world congress was held in Edinburgh, Scotland in March 2012. IBIA has organized professional training programs in several developing countries and worked with other organizations to develop evidence-based guidelines for the care, treatment, and management of TBI. IBIA has also collaborated with the WHO to create prevention programs, implement guidelines, and promote education of TBI.

International Association for the Study of Traumatic Brain Injury merged with IBIA in 1998. As a result of this collaboration, the peer-reviewed journal *Brain Injury* became the official journal of IBIA. A more informal quarterly "International NeuroTrauma Letter" is e-mailed to more than 75,000 brain injury professionals around the world.

International Neurotrauma Research Organization (INRO) (http://www.igeh.org) is a collaborative organization based in Vienna and consists mainly of researchers in Central Europe. Its mission is to improve the recovery of victims of neurotrauma through implementing evidence-based care, reengineering trauma systems, and collaborating in clinical research.

International Neurotrauma Society (INS) organizes international conferences that occur every few years. The next conference will be in Budapest in March 2014. This society does not yet have a website.

International Pediatric Brain Injury Society (IPBIS) (http://www.ipbis.org) was founded in 2009 and is a collaborative group of health care professionals from a variety of specialties whose main interest is pediatric brain injury. Their mission is to educate others about the prevention, treatment, rehabilitation, and long-term management of pediatric acquired brain injuries. They host an online community called Headspace.

Latin American Brain Injury Consortium (LABIC) (www.labic.org) is the South American counterpart for the European and American Brain Injury Consortiums. It was founded in 2003 and actively participates in international trials and promotes the implementation of TBI guidelines in Latin America.

Women in NeuroTrauma Research (WiNTR) (www.wintr.org) is an organization that promotes international gender equality in neurotrauma research. It was founded in the late 1990s and is a subdivision of the National Neurotrauma Society (www.neurotraumasociety.org), which is a national society in the United States, but it has an increasing number of international members. These societies organize an annual symposium that attracts an international audience.

INTERNATIONAL EFFORTS WITHIN TRAUMATIC BRAIN INJURY RESEARCH AND CLINICAL CARE

Recently, there have been international efforts to promote research, solve problems, or develop treatments within TBI medicine. The following is a noncomprehensive description of the major international efforts within the field. The line between organizations/societies and other collaborations in the field of TBI research is often arbitrary and needs to become more transparent.

Past Efforts

Clinical Trials

The following is not a comprehensive list of all internationally conducted clinical trials in TBI, and some minor, phase II, or interrupted studies have been excluded. The studies are in chronological order.

HIT I and II were multicenter studies investigating the efficacy of *nimodipine* in patients with severe head injury between the years 1987 and 1991 in 13 European countries (103,104). They enrolled a total of 1,203 subjects within 24 hours of injury. The HIT I reported an absolute difference of 4% and HIT II of 1% in patients treated with nimodipine. In a subgroup of patients with traumatic subarachnoid hemorrhage (tSAH), the difference was 8%.

TINT and TIUS were international and North American trials that were conducted simultaneously from 1991 to1994 and that examined the effect of the lipid peroxidation inhibitor *tirilazad*. These studies enrolled a total of 2,286 patients with severe or moderate closed TBI within 4 hours of injury from 86 centers in 17 countries (105). Both studies found a slight 2%–3% difference in outcome in favor of the placebo. TIUS was not completed because of preliminary concerns of excess mortality with the use of tirilazad, which was not corroborated on full analysis.

SLIN (1994–1996) studied the effect of the competitive N-methl-D-aparatate (NMDA) receptor antagonist *Selfotel* in 2 parallel studies in several countries and 5 continents (106). The international arm included 409 patients with severe TBI enrolled in 50 centers and the treatment was initiated within 8 hours of injury. The studies were stopped prematurely because of concerns of excess mortality and severe brain-related adverse events that were seen in 2 stroke trials that were using the same agent. The data analysis from the TBI subjects did not show an excess of adverse events in the treatment group, but there were no major benefits either. The trial was never completed.

The Saphir study (SAP) evaluated the efficacy of the competitive NMDA antagonist *DCPP-ene* from 1995 to 1997 in 57 European centers. The study recruited 924 patients with severe TBI and treatment was initiated within 12 hours of injury. Study results have never been published, so there is no information available about the effects of the drug.

Cerestat (*aptiganel*), a noncompetitive NMDA blocker, was used in an international study from 1996 to 1997 in subjects with acute severe TBI. The goal of the study was to enroll 700 patients at approximately 40 North American sites and 30 European sites. The study, which had 532 patients, was terminated prematurely because an interim analysis showed insufficient evidence of a positive clinical effect.

The CRASH study (1999–2004) aimed to resolve the role of steroids in treating acute TBI, and it is the only mega-trial conducted within TBI medicine (107,108). The study recruited 10,008 patients in 239 centers from 49 countries and included subjects with mild TBI. Intravenous *methylprednisolone* was started within 8 hours of injury. The risk of death and severe disability were high in the treatment arm, and as a result of this study, steroids are contraindicated in the treatment of acute TBI.

The Pharmos Dexanabiol trial recruited 861 patients with severe TBI from 86 centers in 15 countries from 2001 to 2004 (109). Patients received *dexanabinol* or placebo within 6 hours of injury. The outcome at 6 months did not differ between the groups, and a subgroup analysis failed to show differential treatment effects. It was concluded that dexanabinol is safe but ineffective in the treatment of TBI.

Amantadine was tested for the treatment of severe TBI in an international multicenter trial from 2003 to 2010. This trial included 8 centers from the United States and 3 from Europe. The 184 subjects were enrolled and were in a vegetative or a minimally conscious state at 4–16 weeks postinjury. Study subjects received a 4-week treatment of amantadine or placebo. The results have not yet been published.

Recombinant activated factor VII was studied in subjects with TBI in an international trial from 2005 to 2006. There were 11 centers in as many countries that participated in this study, and 96 subjects were enrolled. The purpose was to study the safety and preliminary efficacy of this compound within the first 15 days of injury. The study was completed but the results have not been published.

Genotropin, a synthetic growth hormone analog, was tested to treat growth hormone deficiency in adults after TBI. This international study in 6 European countries started in autumn 2007 but was terminated in December 2008 because of an inability to recruit the appropriate patient population.

Armodafinil was tested to treat excessive sleepiness caused by mild or moderate TBI in a randomized placebo-controlled international study, which started in 2009. There were 65 study sites, which were mostly located in the United States. Study sponsors terminated the trial at the end of 2010. Results or the causes for termination have not been published.

SLV334 is a combined neutral endopeptidase inhibitor and endothelin converting enzyme inhibitor. In spring 2009, a multicenter study in 5 countries began to study the safety and pharmacokinetics of SLV334 in patients with moderate or severe TBI. The study was terminated after 1 year because of strategic considerations of the sponsor. No results have been published.

Other Studies and Efforts

The EBIC surveyed 1,005 subjects with moderate or severe TBI from 67 centers throughout Europe (74). These subjects answered questions pertaining to demographics, clinical features, investigations, management, and early complications at admission, at discharge, and at 6 months after injury. Of the centers, 55 have provided the 6-month outcome data.

Trauma Audit and Research Network (TARN) has a large dataset of acute trauma subjects that includes more than 20,000 patients with TBI (110). It began as an initiative of emergency specialists in the United Kingdom. In 2002, 14 European countries joined TARN to form EuroTARN. EuroTARN seeks to promote high standards of care for trauma victims in Europe, to establish a common international comparable dataset, and to use the database to develop clinical guidelines and performance indicators. In addition, the network examines the epidemiology of trauma in an effort to contribute to targeted injury prevention. Recently, EuroTARN activities have waned, but the UK TARN Network is active.

Current Projects

The following lists ongoing significant international studies and efforts within the field of TBI. These have been listed in alphabetical order and either a clinical trials identifier or a link to the study webpage has been provided.

Clinical Trials

EPO-TBI (ClinicalTrials.gov NCT00987454) is a randomized controlled trial (RCT) that began in May 2012 and is being conducted in Australia, New Zealand, and Saudi Arabia. This RCT plans to recruit 606 subjects and to determine if *erythropoietin* given within 24 hours of injury improves long-term neurological function in patients with moderate or severe TBI.

Hypothermia in Children after Trauma (ClinicalTrials.gov NCT00222742) is an international effort that began in 2007 and is being conducted in 30 centers in 6 countries. This study plans to enroll 340 subjects before October 2013 and to determine whether moderate hypothermia, started within 6 hours after a severe TBI, improves survival and functional outcome.

NeuroSTAT (cyclosporine-A) is considered potentially beneficial in the treatment of TBI because it has neuroprotective properties. EBIC has signed an agreement to start a multicenter European clinical trial to study the safety and efficacy of NeuroSTAT. This study will begin in 2012.

RESCUEicp (www.rescueicp.com) is a large international multicenter trial, consisting of 48 centers in 19 countries, aims to clarify the role of decompressive craniectomy in treating refractory intracranial hypertension. This RCT, which began in 2006, is recruiting 400 subjects who will receive either decompressive craniectomy or conservative medical treatment.

STOP-TBI (ClinicalTrials.gov NCT00908063) is a multicenter international study, which began in 2009, involving centers from India, Israel, and Switzerland. The goal of this study is to examine the safety and tolerability of *perfluorocarbon-enhanced oxygen* (Oxycyte) in patients with TBI. Ninety subjects with severe TBI caused by closed head injury are participating in this study. Recruitment has ended but the trial is ongoing.

The *STITCH Trauma Trial* (http://research.ncl.ac.uk/trauma.STITCH) is a randomized study, which began in 2009, that seeks to clarify whether surgical removal of intraparenchymal traumatic hemorrhage is more beneficial than conservative treatment. Patients have to be enrolled in the study within 48 hours of injury. Currently, the study involves 37 centers from 17 countries; many of the centers are in Asia. The goal is to enroll 840 patients before March 2013.

SyNAPSe (ClinicalTrials.gov NCT01143064) is a large international randomized controlled phase III study investigating the efficacy and safety of *progesterone* in patients with severe TBI. This 2-year study began in June 2010 in more than 100 centers in 15 countries and 5 continents. The aim is to enroll 1,180 patients with closed TBI within 8 hours of injury. Progesterone is supposed to treat brain edema in acute TBI.

Other Studies and Efforts

Biomarkers of Mild and Moderate TBI (ClinicalTrials.gov NCT 01295346) is a remarkable international effort that started in January 2011. The goal of the trial is to see if putative blood biomarkers of brain injury are clinically useful as diagnostic and monitoring tools of TBI. The study planned to enroll 900 subjects in 10 centers in 3 countries during a 1 year period.

BRAIN-IT (www.brain-it.eu) or The Brain Monitoring with Information Technology group is a multidisciplinary international collaboration that aims to improve the intensive care of patients with TBI. It develops and tests tools to collect and analyze more standardized and accurate patient information from the monitoring devices in an intensive care unit (ICU). It has created a core dataset from 22 ICUs in 11 European countries.

COSBID-TBI (ClinicalTrials.gov NCT00803036) is an international study, which began in January 2009, being conducted in the United States and United Kingdom. Its primary objective is to determine whether the occurrence or severity of *spreading depression* is related to poor neurologic recovery from TBI. The study is also evaluating whether monitoring spreading depression should be used to inform treatment options in subjects with TBI. The study accepts subjects who require craniotomy because spreading depression can only be reliably monitored with corticography. The study aims to enroll 180 subjects until September 2013.

The *EU-NIH workshops* are a transatlantic effort of the European commission and National Institutes of Health aiming to promote clinical TBI research. Both organizations are aware of the significance of the impact of TBI on public health and of the problems in conducting productive clinical research in this extremely heterogeneous patient population. The first workshop was held at the National Neurotrauma Symposium in Las Vegas in June 2010. This collaboration aims to unite the efforts of these 2 major funding organizations to create significant progress in clinical TBI research. Currently, this research is being done as a collaborative effort that calls itself International Initiative in Traumatic Brain Injury Research (InTBIR).

The *IMPACT* project (www.tbi-impact.org) is an international effort funded by the National Institutes of Health, which focuses on conducting more powerful trials in the field of TBI. IMPACT has established and analyzed an enormous database that consists of several randomized controlled TBI studies that have been done during the last 2 decades and includes 40,000 patients. IMPACT has developed and validated prognostic models, participated in developing the Common Data Elements recommendation, and provided recommendations for improving sensitivity and efficiency of TBI trials. This ongoing project is one of the major achievements in current TBI medicine, and it will surely result in more productive clinical research efforts.

QOLIBRI (www.qolibrinet.com) is an instrument developed specifically to assess the quality of life after TBI, and it was developed and is maintained by an international collaboration founded in 1999 (the QOLIBRI Task Force). It is freely available in several languages.

TBIcare (www.tbicare.eu) is a European international EU-funded effort, which began in February 2011. They are creating software that is able to provide an individual with an evidence-based assessment of the injury and recommendations for appropriate treatments. The project analyzes large TBI datasets (including the IMPACT database, see earlier texts) using data mining, system simulation modeling, and modern statistical methodology and collects prospective validation material.

Future Needs and Visions

The Unmet Needs Within International Traumatic Brain Injury Research

- Although the etiology of TBI is well known, the pathophysiological mechanisms are just being discovered and treatment of this injury is in its infancy. From an international perspective, the major needs in TBI education and research are more effective prevention of and public awareness about TBI.
- Development of reliable and accessible diagnostic tools
- Development of effective and targeted treatments for the pathophysiological mechanisms of TBI
- Equalizing diagnostic and treatment resources on a global basis

Development of Diagnostic Methodologies

Emergency care clinicians around the world face difficulties diagnosing TBI. Differential diagnosis of an acute TBI is much more complicated than generally thought. Although there are plenty of injuries that are straightforward, a large number of milder yet significant injuries are still overlooked because they are difficult to diagnose (1). Currently, there is no reliable method for ruling out acute TBI. The diagnosis is based on unspecific clinical signs such as lowered consciousness, amnesia, or other neurological signs. These symptoms may also be caused by several other factors, including the use of alcohol or drugs, other injuries, or preexisting conditions. Brain imaging is often used as a diagnostic tool; although its primary role is to reveal lesions requiring surgical measures. In addition, the radiological diagnosis of acute TBI is quite complicated (111).

In addition to the lack of tools needed to rule out acute TBI, there are not ways to determine pathophysiological mechanisms. With brain imaging, major lesions such as hemorrhages, contusions, and edema can be seen, but there are no methods to classify injuries in pathophysiological categories. This complicates how physicians can choose to treat the patient with TBI, which could guide our treatment efforts in the right direction for a particular individual. Current classification techniques are crude and outdated, and there is ongoing debate about how to define terms such as "mild" when diagnosing TBI.

Modern MRI is a promising tool used to reliably diagnose and classify TBI; however, few places even in well-developed countries have MRI available for acute on-call imaging, and MRI of an acutely injured subject requires experts trained in this technology. It is uncertain as to what extent MRI is able to reveal pathophysiological processes such as neuroinflammation or apoptosis, which in turn complicate determining appropriate therapeutic interventions. Consequently, the development a tool to measure blood biomarkers of brain pathophysiology that is widely available for use internationally may make accurately ruling out, detecting, and classifying TBI possible.

Previous studies of brain biomarkers in blood have largely relied on a simplistic view that a single substance could reflect the ongoing extremely complicated phenomena. Consequently, the markers studied have been both unspecific and insensitive. The blood-brain barrier (BBB) is a major obstacle in developing blood biomarkers of brain injury. As such, measuring the degree of BBB injury or the substances that are brain-specific or sufficiently small molecules that are able to penetrate an intact BBB may help with the development of this method. If a tool is developed that can reliably measure blood biomarkers, they may be used in the following ways:

- To verify or exclude the presence of brain tissue injury
- To assess the true severity and nature of the injury
- To inform necessary treatments
- To determine the effectiveness of prescribed treatments
- To more effectively and reliably monitor the state of the patient
- To reliably predict outcomes

It is likely that no single substance can provide all necessary information, and that laboratory diagnostics of TBI will be comprised of different sets of biomarkers to reflect the current state and processes of the brain.

Developing laboratory diagnostics for TBI is a major challenge and the development of these tools should be strongly supported and funded. The development process is complicated and demanding and requires (a) detection of substances that alone or in combination reflect brain phenomena, (b) assessment of specificity and sensitivity, (c) validation for clinical use in authentic TBI populations, and (d) development of reliable assays for clinical use. Reliable blood biomarkers for diagnosing and monitoring TBI pathophysiology would be revolutionary and major laboratory and clinical efforts are clearly warranted.

Development of Targeted Treatments

No other major public health problem is as devoid of targeted treatments as TBI. Thus far, not a single drug is indicated for treating the acute or chronic consequences of TBI. The results of RCTs have not been widely discussed (112–115). A successful drug trial requires knowledge of the pathophysiological process as a specific target of the agent and a way to enroll subjects in a trial within an appropriate timeframe. Despite the history of TBI trials, it is likely that breakthroughs in specific treatments of TBI will emerge in the foreseeable future.

The main prerequisite for the development of effective targeted treatments is improved diagnostics—determining ongoing pathophysiological processes in patients with TBI is critical. This requires the development of blood biomarkers, possibly combined with modern imaging. To what extent targeted treatments can improve the outcome of TBI in general remains to be seen. Changing one portion of the pathophysiologic cascade may or may not be beneficial based on the time course and other metabolic processes that are impacted. Indeed, a wide array of biomarkers to describe the complicated brain phenomena and a variety of concomitant treatments to tackle the ongoing detrimental processes effectively in TBI are needed.

In summary, the need for individual diagnostics and tailored treatments is essential to provide patients with TBI optimal care. When tools of this nature are developed, it would be beneficial to have an international online repository containing data from successful clinical trials for physicians to use to determine the best course of treatment for their patients. Although expert knowledge is necessary and useful, technology-based solutions would be useful in sorting out the approximate 100 variables that can affect the course and outcome of TBI.

Leveling the Global Inequality

TBI is a global health problem, increasingly so in low- and middle-income countries. A clear discrepancy exists between research and development efforts that are done almost exclusively in first world countries, and access to current treatment options in the rest of the world. Global responsibility is imperative, and there have been instances of productive collaboration between scientists in developed countries and clinicians in developing countries that have resulted in increased knowledge or improved outcomes (116,117).

The main obstacle in TBI medicine from a global perspective is the increasing polarity between research progress and everyday needs and resources in most parts of the world. Although there are technological advances in diagnosing and treating TBI, this progress benefits only a small portion of patients with TBI worldwide because of lack of accessibility to the most up to date treatment options. In theory, diagnosing and treating all patients with TBI equally around the world would require the following:

Developing diagnostics based on simple laboratory analytics and not sophisticated brain imaging.

Developing online networks and databases to provide remote centers in low-income countries access to critical clinical information to guide treatments.

Creating affordable targeted treatments for use in any country.

CONCLUSION

Although TBI is a major global health issue causing considerable death, permanent invalidity, and great expense, knowledge of many important TBI-related issues is still fragmented. More reliable data of the epidemiology, including causative epidemiology of TBI is strongly needed, particularly in low- and middle-income countries. Without reliable epidemiological data, it is difficult to prevent TBI. Prevention of TBI requires more effort from health care professionals, government officials, and the media.

International collaboration in the field of TBI is the key to a better future. Creating large international, multicenter studies that address highly complex issues surrounding TBI may prove useful in preventing and treating these injuries and in developing accessible, affordable targeted treatments across the globe.

KEY CLINICAL POINTS

1. A wide variation in care occurs between developed and undeveloped nations, outcomes vary a great deal because of this.
2. Numerous agencies and clinical trials groups exist to examine the issue of TBI, however a universal data set is lacking.
3. The Future will require multinational cooperation on diagnostic and therapeutic interventions for those with TBI.

KEY REFERENCES

1. Cassidy JD, Carroll LJ, Peloso PM, et al; for WHO Collaborating Centre Task Force on Mild Traumatic Brain injury. Incidence, risk factors and prevention of mild traumatic brain injury: results of The WHO Collaborating Centre Task Force on Mild Traumatic Brain Injury. *J Rehabil Med.* 2004;43(suppl):28–60.
2. Faul M, Xu L, Wald MM, Coronado VG. *Traumatic Brain Injury in the United States: Emergency Department Visits, Hospitalizations and Deaths 2002–2006.* Atlanta, GA: Centers for Disease Control and Prevention, National Center for Injury Prevention and Control; 2010.
3. Murray GD, Teasdale GM, Braakman R, et al. The European Brain Injury Consortium survey of head injuries. *Acta Neurochir (Wien).* 1999;141(3):223–236.

References

1. Powell JM, Ferraro JV, Dikmen SS, Temkin NR, Bell KR. Accuracy of mild traumatic brain injury diagnosis. *Arch Phys Med Rehabil.* 2008;89(8):1550–1555.
2. Thornhill S, Teasdale GM, Murray GD, McEwen, Roy CW, Penny KI. Disability in young people and adults one year after head injury: prospective cohort study. *BMJ.* 2000;320(7250):1631–1635.
3. Sommers MS. Missed injuries: a case of trauma hide and seek. *AACN Clin Issues.* 1995;6(2):187–195.
4. Moss NE, Wade DT. Admission after head injury: how many occur and how many are recorded? *Injury.* 1996;27(3):159–161.
5. Whedon JM, Fulton G, Herr CH, von Recklinghausen FM. Trauma patients without a trauma diagnosis: the data gap at a level one trauma center. *J Trauma.* 2009;67(4):822–888.
6. Bazarian JJ, Veazie P, Mookerjee S, Lerner EB. Accuracy of mild traumatic brain injury case ascertainment using ICD-9 codes. *Acad Emerg Med.* 2006;13:31–38.
7. Deb S. ICD-10 codes detect only a proportion of all head injury admissions. *Brain Inj.* 1999;13:369–373.
8. Carroll LJ, Cassidy JD, Holm L, Kraus J, Coronado VG; for WHO Collaborating Centre Task Force on Mild Traumatic Brain injury. Methodological issues and research recommendations for mild traumatic brain injury: The WHO Collaborating Centre Task Force on Mild Traumatic Brain Injury. *J Rehabil Med.* 2004;43(suppl): 113–125.
9. Cassidy JD, Carroll LJ, Peloso PM, et al; for WHO Collaborating Centre Task Force on Mild Traumatic Brain injury. Incidence, risk factors and prevention of mild traumatic brain injury: results of The WHO Collaborating Centre Task Force on Mild Traumatic Brain Injury. *J Rehabil Med.* 2004;43(suppl):28–60.
10. Conroy C, Kraus JF. Survival after brain injury. Cause of death, length of survival, and prognostic variables in a cohort of brain-injured people. *Neuroepidemiology.* 1988;7(1):13–22.
11. Evans JA, van Wessem KJ, McDougall D, Lee KA, Lyons T, Balogh ZJ. Epidemiology of traumatic deaths: comprehensive population-based assessment. *World J Surg.* 2010;34(1):158–163.
12. Caveness WF. Incidence of craniocerebral trauma in the United States in 1976 with trend from 1970 to 1975. *Adv Neurol.* 1979;23: 1–3.
13. Reilly P. The impact of neurotrauma on society: an international perspective. *Prog Brain Res.* 2007;161:3–9.
14. Hyder AA, Wunderlich CA, Puvanachandra P, Gururaj G, Kobusingye OC. The impact of traumatic brain injuries: A global perspective. *NeuroRehabilitation.* 2007;22(5):341–353.
15. Tagliaferri F, Compagnone C, Korsic M, Servadei F, Kraus J. A systematic review of brain injury epidemiology in Europe. *Acta Neurochir (Wien).* 2006;148:255–268.
16. Corrigan JD, Selassie AW, Orman JA. The epidemiology of traumatic brain injury. *J Head Trauma Rehabil.* 2010;25:72–80.
17. Andersson EH, Björklund R, Emanuelson I, Stålhammar D. Epidemiology of traumatic brain injury: a population based study in western Sweden. *Acta Neurol Scand.* 2003;107:256–259.
18. Sosin DM, Sniezek JE, Thurman DJ. Incidence of mild and moderate brain injury in the United States, 1991. *Brain Inj.* 1996;10:47–54.
19. Thurman DJ, Alverson C, Dunn KA, Guerrero J, Sniezek JE. Traumatic brain injury in the United States: a public health perspective. *J Head Trauma Rehabil.* 1999;14:602–615.
20. Corrigan JD, Harrison-Felix C, Bogner J, Dijkers M, Terrill MS, Whiteneck G. Systematic bias in traumatic brain injury outcome studies because of loss to follow-up. *Arch Phys Med Rehabil.* 2003; 84(2):153–160.
21. Carlsson GS, Svardsudd K, Welin L. Long-term effects of head injuries sustained during life in three male populations. *J Neurosurg.* 1987;67:197–205.
22. Annegers JF, Grabow JD, Kurland LT, Laws ER Jr. The incidence, causes, and secular trends of head trauma in Olmstead County, Minnesota, 1935–1974. *Neurology.* 1980;30:912–919.
23. Yang YC, Li SZ, Chung XM, Wang WZ, Wu SP. The epidemiology of craniocerebral injury in 6 cities of China. *Chin J Neurosurg.* 1987; 3:23.
24. Zhu GL, Song JR, Zhang DX, Wang WZ, Xu ZL. The epidemiology of head injury in rural and minority areas of China. *Chin J Neurosurg.* 1989;5(suppl):44.
25. Engberg A. Severe traumatic brain injury: epidemiology, external causes, prevention, and rehabilitation of mental and physical sequelae. *Acta Neurol Scand.* 1995;164(Suppl):1–151.

26. Langlois J, Rutland-Brown W, Thomas K. *Traumatic Brain Injury in the United States: Emergency Department Visits, Hospitalizations, and Deaths.* Atlanta, GA: Centers for Disease Control and Prevention, National Center for Injury Prevention and Control; 2004.

27. Whiteneck G, Brooks CA, Mellick D, Harrison-Felix C, Terrill MS, Noble K. Population-based estimates of outcomes after hospitalization for traumatic brain injury in Colorado. *Arch PhysMed Rehabil.* 2004;85(4)(suppl 2):S73–S81.

28. Shukri AA, Bersnev VP, Riabukha NP. The epidemiology of brain injury and the organization of health care to victims in Aden (Yemen) [in Russian]. *Zh Vopr Neirokhir Im N N Burdenko.* 2006;(2):40–42.

29. Winqvist S, Lehtilahti M, Jokelainen J, Luukinen H, Hillbom M. Traumatic brain injuries in children and young adults: a birth cohort study from Northern Finland. *Neuroepidemiology.* 2007;29:136–142.

30. Mar J, Arrospide A, Begiristain JM, Larrañaga I, Elosegui E, Oliva-Moreno J. The impact of acquired brain damage in terms of epidemiology, economics and loss in quality of life. *BMC Neurology.* 2011;11:46.

31. Brown A, Leibson C, Malec J, Perkins P, Diehl N, Larson D. Long-term survival after traumatic brain injury: a population-based analysis. *NeuroRehabilitation.* 2004;19:37–43.

32. McGarry L, Thompson D, Millham FH, et al. Outcomes and costs of acute treatment of traumatic brain injury. *J Trauma.* 2002;53:1152–1159.

33. Kayani NA, Homan S, Yun S, Zhu BP. Health and economic burden of traumatic brain injury: Missouri, 2001–2005. *Public Health Rep.* 2009;124:551–560.

34. Berg J, Tagliaferri F, Servadei F. Cost of trauma in Europe. *Eur J Neurol.* 2005;12(suppl 1):85–90.

35. Finkelstein EA, Corso PS, Miller TR. *The Incidence and Economic Burden of Injuries in the United States.* New York, NY: Oxford University Press; 2006.

36. Kannus P, Niemi S, Parkkari J, Palvanen M, Sievänen H. Alarming rise in fall-induced severe head injuries among elderly people. *Injury.* 2007;38:81–83.

37. Steudel WI, Cortbus F, Schwerdtfeger K. Epidemiology and prevention of fatal head injuries in Germany—trends and the impact of reunification. *Acta Neurochir (Wien).* 2005;147:231–242.

38. http://ec.europa.eu/transport/road_safety/pdf/observatory/trends_figures.pdf. Accessed June 22, 2012.

39. World Health Organization. *Global Status Report on Road Safety: Time for Action.* Geneva, Switzerland: World Health Organization; 2009. http://www.who.int/violence_injury_prevention/road_safety_status/2009. Accessed June 22, 2012.

40. Murray CJ, Lopez AD. *The Global Burden of Disease: A Comprehensive Assessment of Mortality and Disability from Diseases, Injuries and Risk Factors in 1990 And Projected To 2020.* Vol 1. Cambridge, MA: Harvard School of Public Health; 1996.

41. Salgado MS, Colombage SM. Analysis of fatalities in road accidents. *Forensic Sci Int.* 1988;36:91–96.

42. Faul M, Xu L, Wald MM, Coronado VG. *Traumatic Brain Injury in the United States: Emergency Department Visits, Hospitalizations and Deaths 2002–2006.* Atlanta, GA: Centers for Disease Control and Prevention, National Center for Injury Prevention and Control; 2010.

43. Masel BE, DeWitt DS. Traumatic brain injury: a disease process, not an event. *J Neurotrauma.* 2010;27:1529–1540.

44. Hall KM, Karzmark P, Stevens M, Englander J, O'Hare P, Wright J. Family stressors in traumatic brain injury: a two-year follow-up. *Arch Phys Med Rehabil.* 1994;75:876–884.

45. Ergh TC, Rapport LJ, Coleman RD, Hanks RA. Predictors of caregiver and family functioning following traumatic brain injury: social support moderates caregiver distress. *J Head Trauma Rehabil.* 2002;17:155–174.

46. Wood RL, Yurdakul LK. Change in relationship status following traumatic brain injury. *Brain Inj.* 1997;11:491–501.

47. Teasdale TW, Engberg AW. Suicide after traumatic brain injury: a population study. *J Neurol Neurosurg Psychiatry.* 2001;71:436–440.

48. Simpson G, Tate R. Suicidality after traumatic brain injury: demographic, injury and clinical correlates. *Psychol Med.* 2002;32:687–697.

49. Hashimoto K, Nakamura T, Wada I, et al. How great is willingness to pay for recovery from sequelae after severe traumatic brain injury in Japan? *J Rehabil Med.* 2006;38:141–143.

50. Mortimer JA, French LR, Hutton JT, Schuman LM. Head injury as a risk factor for Alzheimer's disease. *Neurology.* 1985;35:264–267.

51. Guo Z, Cupples LA, Kurz A, et al. Head injury and the risk of AD in the MIRAGE study. *Neurology.* 2000;54:1316–1323.

52. Gedye A, Beattie BL, Tuokko H, Horton A, Korsarek E. Severe head injury hastens age of onset of Alzheimer's disease. *J Am Geriatr Soc.* 1989;37:970–973.

53. Nemetz PN, Leibson C, Naessens JM, et al. Traumatic brain injury and time to onset of Alzheimer's disease: a population-based study. *Am J Epidemiol.* 1999;149:32–40.

54. Bigler ED. The lesion(s) in traumatic brain injury: implications for clinical neuropsychology. *Arch Clin Neuropsychol.* 2001;16:95–131.

55. Pakkenberg B, Gundersen HJ. Neocortical neuron number in humans: effect of sex and age. *J Comp Neurol.* 1997;384:312–320.

56. Guskiewicz KM, McCrea M, Marshall SW, et al. Cumulative effects associated with recurrent concussion in collegiate football players: the NCAA Concussion Study. *JAMA.* 2003;290:2549–2555.

57. Hawthorne G, Gruen RL, Kaye AH. Traumatic brain injury and long-term quality of life: findings from an Australian study. *J Neurotrauma.* 2009;26:1623–1633.

58. Whitnall L, McMillan TM, Murray GD, Teasdale GM. Disability in young people and adults after head injury: 5–7 year follow-up of a prospective cohort study. *J Neurol Neurosurg Psychiatry.* 2006;77:640–645.

59. Scott S, Knapp M, Henderson J, Maughan B. Financial cost of social exclusion: follow up study of antisocial children into adulthood. *BMJ.* 2001;323:191.

60. Anderson V, Brown S, Newitt H, Hoile H. Educational, vocational, psychosocial, and quality-of-life outcomes for adult survivors of childhood traumatic brain injury. *J Head Trauma Rehabil.* 2009;24:303–312.

61. Donders J, Warschausky S. Neurobehavioral outcomes after early versus late childhood traumatic brain injury. *J Head Trauma Rehabil.* 2007;22:296–302.

62. Max JE, Schachar RJ, Levin HS, et al. Predictors of secondary attention-deficit/hyperactivity disorder in children and adolescents 6 to 24 months after traumatic brain injury. *J Am Acad Child Adolesc Psychiatry.* 2005;44:1041–1049.

63. Emanuelson I, Uvebrant P. Occurrence of epilepsy during the first 10 years after traumatic brain injury acquired in childhood up to the age of 18 years in the south western Swedish population-based series. *Brain Inj.* 2009;23:612–616.

64. Schwartz L, Taylor HG, Drotar D, Yeates KO, Wade SL, Stancin T. Long-term behavior problems following pediatric traumatic brain injury: prevalence, predictors, and correlates. *J Pediatr Psychol.* 2003;28:251–263.

65. McKinlay A, Grace R, Horwood J, Fergusson D, MacFarlane M. Adolescent psychiatric symptoms following preschool childhood mild traumatic brain injury: evidence from a birth cohort. *J Head Trauma Rehabil.* 2009;24:221–227.

66. Anderson V, Spencer-Smith M, Leventer R, et al. Childhood brain insult: can age at insult help us predict outcome? *Brain.* 2009;132(pt 1):45–56.

67. Bombardier CH, Rimmele CT, Zintel H. The magnitude and correlates of alcohol and drug use before traumatic brain injury. *Arch Phys Med Rehabil.* 2002;83:1765–1773.

68. Parry-Jones BL, Vaughan FL, Miles Cox W. Traumatic brain injury and substance misuse: a systematic review of prevalence and outcomes research (1994–2004). *Neuropsychol Rehabil.* 2006;16:537–560.

69. Savola O, Niemelä O, Hillbom M. Alcohol intake and the pattern of trauma in young adults and working aged people admitted after trauma. *Alcohol Alcohol.* 2005;40:269–273.

70. Murray GD, Teasdale GM, Braakman R, et al. The European Brain Injury Consortium survey of head injuries. *Acta Neurochir (Wien).* 1999;141(3):223–236.

71. McNicholl B, Cooke RS. The epidemiology of major trauma in Northern Ireland. *Ulster Med J.* 1995;64:142–146.

72. Baker TD, Baker SP, Haack SA. Trauma in the Russian Federation: then and now. *J Trauma.* 2011;70:991–995.

73. Bruns J Jr, Hauser WA. The epidemiology of traumatic brain injury: a review. *Epilepsia*. 2003;44(suppl 10):2–10.

74. United Nations. *World Population Ageing 2009*. New York, NY: United Nations Publication; 2010. http://www.un.org/esa/population/publications/WPA2009/WPA2009-report.pdf. Accessed June 22, 2012.

75. Hallgren MÅ, Högberg P, Andréasson S. Alcohol consumption and harm among elderly Europeans: falling between the cracks. *Eur J Public Health*. 2010;20(6):616–617.

76. Alexander CS, Ensminger ME, Somerfield MR, Kim YJ, Johnson KE. Behavioral risk factors for injury among rural adolescents. *Am J Epidemiol*. 1992;15:673–685.

77. Soderstrom CA, Ballesteros MF, Dischinger PC, Kerns TJ, Flint RD, Smith GS. Alcohol/drug abuse, driving convictions, and risk-taking dispositions among trauma center patients. *Accid Anal Prev*. 2001;33:771–782.

78. Tolonen J, Kiviluoto O, Santavirta S, Slätis P. The effects of vehicle mass, speed and safety belt wearing on the causes of death in road traffic accidents. *Ann Chir Gynaecol*. 1984;73:14–20.

79. Allen S, Zhu S, Sauter C, Layde P, Hargarten S. A comprehensive statewide analysis of seatbelt non-use with injury and hospital admissions: new data, old problem. *Acad Emerg Med*. 2006;13:427–434.

80. Thompson DC, Rivara FP, Thompson R. Helmets for preventing head and facial injuries in bicyclists. *Cochrane Database Syst Rev*. 2000;(2):CD001855.

81. McBeth PB, Ball CG, Mulloy RH, Kirkpatrick AW. Alpine ski and snowboarding traumatic injuries: incidence, injury patterns, and risk factors for 10 years. *Am J Surg*. 2009;197:560–563.

82. Haas JF, Cope DN, Hall K. Premorbid prevalence of poor academic performance in severe head injury. *J Neurol Neurosurg Psychiatry*. 1987;50:52–56.

83. Wittenberg MD, Sloan JP, Barlow IF. Head injuries in Leeds: changes in epidemiology and survival over 12 years. *Emerg Med J*. 2004;21:429–432.

84. Rickels E, Von Wild K, Wenzlaff P. Head injury in Germany: a population-based prospective study on epidemiology, causes, treatment and outcome of all degrees of head-injury severity in two distinct areas. *Brain Inj*. 2010; 24:1491–1504.

85. Rutland-Brown W, Langlois JA, Thomas KE, Lily Y. Incidence of traumatic brain injury in the United States, 2003. *J Head Trauma Rehabil*. 2006;21(6):544–548.

86. Cadotte DW, Vachhrajani S, Pirouzmand F. The epidemiological trends of head injury in the largest Canadian adult trauma center from 1986 to 2007. *J Neurosurg*. 2011;114:1502–1509.

87. Marchio PS, Previgliano IJ, Goldini CE, Murillo-Cabezas F. Head injury in Buenos Aires city: a prospective, population based, epidemiologic study. *Neurocirugia*. 2006;17:14–22.

88. Melo JR, Silva RA, Moreira ED Jr. Characteristics of patients with head injury at Salvador City (Bahia – Brazil) [in Portuguese]. *Arq Neuropsiquiatr*. 2004;62(3A):711–715.

89. Chiu WT, Huang SJ, Tsai SH, et al. The impact of time, legislation, and geography on the epidemiology of traumatic brain injury. *J Clin Neurosci*. 2007;14(10):930–935.

90. Raja IA, Vohra AH, Ahmed M. Neurotrauma in Pakistan. *World J Surg*. 2001;25:1230–1237.

91. Levi L, Linn S, Revach M, Feinsod M. Head trauma in Northern Israel: incidence and types. *Neuroepidemiology*. 1990;9:278–284.

92. Bener A, Omar AOK, Ahmad AE, Al-Mulla FH, Rahman YS. The pattern of traumatic brain injuries: a country undergoing rapid development. *Brain Inj*. 2010;24(2):74–80.

93. Nell V, Brown DS. Epidemiology of traumatic brain injury in Johannesburg – II. Morbidity, mortality and etiology. *Soc Sci Med*. 1991;33(3):289–296.

94. Myburgh JA, Cooper DJ, Finfer SR, et al. Epidemiology and 12-month outcomes from traumatic brain injury in Australia and New Zealand. *J Trauma*. 2008;64:854–862.

95. Papadopoulos IN, Kanakaris N, Triantafillidis A, Stefanakos J, Kainourgios A, Leukidis C. Autopsy findings from 111 deaths in the 1999 Athens earthquake as a basis for auditing the emergency response. *Br J Surg*. 2004;91:1633–1640.

96. Sundstrøm T, Sollid S, Wentzel-Larsen T, Wester K. Head injury mortality in the Nordic countries. *J Neurotrauma*. 2007;24(1):147–153.

97. Adeleye AO, Olowookere KG, Olayemi OO. Clinicoepidemiological profiles and outcomes during first hospital admission of head injury patients in Ikeja, Nigeria. A prospective cohort study. *Neuroepidemiology*. 2009;32(2):136–141.

98. Groswasser Z, Mutin M, Cherkasky T, Hart J. Temporal change in rehabilitation outcome of patients following severe traumatic brain injury [in Hebrew]. *Harefuah*. 2008;147(11):847–850.

99. De Silva MJ, Roberts I, Perel P, et al; CRASH Trial Collaborators. Patient outcome after traumatic brain injury in high-, middle- and low-income countries: analysis of data on 8927 patients in 46 countries. *Int J Epidemiol*. 2009;38(2):452–458.

100. Ferrari R, Constantoyannis C, Papadakis N. Cross-cultural study of symptom expectation following minor head injury in Canada and Greece. *Clin Neurol Neurosurg*. 2001;103:254–259.

101. Vilke GM, Chan TC, Guss DA. Use of a complete neurological examination to screen for significant intracranial abnormalities in minor head injury. *Am J Emerg Med*. 2000;18:159–163.

102. Stein SC, Georgoff P, Meghan S, Mizra K, Sonnad SS. 150 years of treating severe traumatic brain injury: a systematic review of progress in mortality. *J Neurotrauma*. 2010;27:1343–1353.

103. Bailey I, Bell A, Gray J, et al. A trial of the effect of nimodipine on outcome after head injury. *Acta Neurochir (Wien)*. 1991;110:97–105.

104. The European Study Group on Nimodipine in Severe Brain Injury. A multicenter trial of the efficacy of nimodipine on outcome after severe head injury. *J Neurosurg*. 1994;80(5):797–804.

105. Marshall LF, Maas AI, Marshall SB, et al. A multicenter trial on the efficacy of using tirilazad mesylate in cases of head injury. *J Neurosurg*. 1998;89:519–25.

106. Morris GF, Bullock R, Marshall SB, Marmarou A, Maas A, Marshall LF. Failure of the competitive N-methyl-D-aspartate antagonist Selfotel (CGS 19755) in the treatment of severe head injury: results of two phase III clinical trials. The Selfotel Investigators. *J Neurosurg*. 1999;91(5):737–743.

107. Roberts I, Yates D, Sandercock P, et al; CRASH trial collaborators. Effect of intravenous corticosteroids on death within 14 days in 10008 adults with clinically significant head injury (MRC CRASH trial): randomised placebo-controlled trial. *Lancet*. 2004;364(9442):1321–1328.

108. Edwards P, Arango M, Balica L, et al; CRASH trial collaborators. Final results of MRC CRASH, a randomised placebo-controlled trial of intravenous corticosteroid in adults with head injury-outcomes at 6 months. *Lancet*. 2005;365(9475):1957–1959.

109. Maas AI, Murray G, Henney H III, et al; Pharmos TBI investigators. Efficacy and safety of dexanabinol in severe traumatic brain injury: results of a phase III randomized, placebo-controlled, clinical trial. *Lancet Neurol*. 2006;5(1):38–45.

110. Patel HC, Bouamra O, Woodford M, King AT, Yates DW, Lecky FE. Trends in head injury outcome from 1989 to 2003 and the effect of neurosurgical care: an observational study. *Lancet*. 2005;366:1538–1544.

111. Laalo J, Kurki T, Tenovuo O, Sonninen P. Reliability of diagnosis of traumatic brain injury by computed tomography in acute phase. *J Neurotrauma*. 2009;26:2169–2178.

112. Stein DG, Glasier MM, Hoffman SW. Conceptual and practical issues in the pharmacological treatment of brain injury. *J Neural Transplant Plast*. 1993;4:227–237.

113. Narayan RK, Michel ME, Ansell B, et al. Clinical trials in head injury. *J Neurotrauma*. 2002;19:503–57.

114. Farin A, Marshall LF. Lessons from epidemiologic studies in clinical trials of traumatic brain injury. *Acta Neurochir Suppl*. 2004;89:101–107.

115. Maas AI, Roozenbeek B, Manley GT. Clinical trials in traumatic brain injury: past experience and current developments. *Neurotherapeutics*. 2010;7:115–126.

116. Vukic M, Negovetic L, Kovac D, Ghajar J, Glavic Z, Gopcevic A. The effect of implementation of guidelines for the management of severe head injury on patient treatment and outcome. *Acta Neurochir (Wien)*. 1999;141:1203–1208.

117. Petroni G, Quaglino M, Lujan S, et al. Early prognosis of severe traumatic brain injury in an urban argentinian trauma center. *J Trauma*. 2010;68:564–570.

Education, Training, and Certification for Health Care Providers

Margaret A. Turk, Dominic A. Carone, and Joanne Scandale

INTRODUCTION

An increasing number of individuals survive traumatic brain injury (TBI) as a result of advances in medical technology, emergency medical procedures, and neurosurgical techniques (1–3). About 1.7 million people sustain a TBI annually (4), and US emergency departments treated an estimated 135,000 sports and recreation related TBIs, including concussions, among children 5–18 years (5). Between 70% and 90% of all TBIs occurring annually are concussions (6,7). An estimated 5.3 million Americans currently live with disabilities resulting from brain injury, which is about 80,000–90,000 new cases per year. This means that more than 2% of the American population is living with disabilities caused by TBI (6). TBI is one of the most common childhood injuries (8). The prevalence and total impact of war-related brain injuries has not yet been realized, with the Department of Veterans Affairs (VA) and Department of Defense (DoD) pouring resources into the diagnosis and treatment of brain injury and its sequelae.

As noted throughout this textbook, TBI can significantly affect many physical, cognitive, behavioral, and psychological processes, significantly disrupting the lives of individuals who experience such injuries. This is particularly evident at the moderate to severe end of the TBI spectrum where more services are required. Survivors and their families require an increasing amount of support along this continuum of disability. Early needs are usually provided within the emergency department and/or acute care hospitalization followed by acute rehabilitation. Medical and health care professionals are the primary providers of service interacting daily with patients and their families. Restorative goal-based rehabilitation services are delivered by interdisciplinary or multidisciplinary teams. Specialized programs and providers are sought to deliver quality care. With more recognition of concussion and post-traumatic stress disorder symptoms, outpatient programs are expected to provide expert diagnosis and treatment of mild brain injury sequelae. Subacute and longer term postacute care needs may continue to be very high for those with more moderate to severe brain injury, and at some point, the care can be provided at the community level. Many different agencies and multiple health professionals often provide community and outpatient services, making coordination and continuity of services difficult. Postacute care may focus on specific impairments that limit independence for return to work/school or on more general impairment, such as cognitive impairments or behavior dysregulation requiring behavioral plans, daily structure, and routinized tasks implemented by trained aides. Support aides require communication skills and at least a knowledge base about implementation of behavior modifications and strategies. With increasing numbers of survivors, there is a greater need for trained and experienced providers for the acute through postacute continuum.

The VA and DoD have recognized the importance of early recognition, expert clinicians, coordination of care, and multidisciplinary support services for soldiers returning with combat-related brain injuries, especially mild TBI. They have developed screening and treatment programs for these service members, the VA Polytrauma System of Care (9), and recognized the importance of education, training, and certification for health care providers through their guidelines for care (10–12).

Families are usually unprepared for the long term needs of their family member post-TBI, despite the education and support received during the acute care and rehabilitation processes. The diminishing psychosocial support noted after discharge to home can result in increased family stress and difficulties providing all medical, behavioral, and cognitive assists. Return to work and other previously held social roles might not be possible for those who have survived brain injury, which further contributes to pressures within the family (13). Soldiers returning from conflicts overseas may have additional sequelae that require recognition and ongoing support from family (12). There is a need for trained community aide services to improve the success of individuals with post brain injury sequellae to live in the community.

Clinical practice, programs, and research in TBI medicine have grown significantly for the past 40 years. However, a study in South Carolina noted that persons with TBI and their families have described the service system as "unorganized, uneducated, unresponsive, and uncaring" (14). A parent of a child with brain injury writes,

> Another area of concern is the insufficient numbers of caregivers with training in ways brain injury differs from other neurologically impairing conditions. Until caregivers better understand the cognitive and behavioral changes and learn

more effective methods of dealing with deficits resulting from injury to the brain, we'll still be where we are today (15).

On a national and more general level, the Institute of Medicine (IOM) report, "To Err Is Human: Building a Safer Health System," notes the importance of communication among multiple providers and the need for standards for training and certification, especially regarding safety and prevention of medical errors (16). This call for improved education for care providers is also echoed in the 2007 IOM report "The Future of Disability in America" (17) and the World Health Organization/World Bank sponsored "World Report on Disability" (18). Although there has been advancement in formal training and certification for medical health care providers within the field of brain injury medicine in recent years, there continues to be only small numbers of clinicians providing specialty services (relative to larger medical, rehabilitation, and therapy services such as musculoskeletal care) and lack of recognition in certain disciplines. Additionally, primary care and triage medical services may not be well versed in recognition of brain injury symptoms, related medical conditions, treatment, or referral standards of care.

There are many disciplines involved in the ongoing care, medical management, and rehabilitation of persons who have sustained brain injury. Although there are expert clinicians in the field, formal certification for professionals or paraprofessionals is inconsistent. Consumers and their families have made a strong case for the requirement of well trained and certified health care providers in the field of brain injury medicine. The rationale for the establishment of brain injury medicine (BIM) subspecialization for various health care professionals and paraprofessionals are

- provision of a high level of care for patients with acquired brain injury and their families in hospitals, postacute settings, and for the continuum of care to facilitate the process of recovery and improve medical and functional outcomes;
- increasing the number of expert health care providers, teachers, researchers, and advocates dedicated to the care of individuals with post–brain injury;
- development of core competency standards for health personnel training involved in the evaluation, treatment, and management of patients with brain injuries;
- assurance of administrative skills sensitive to the needs of patients and consumers who have sustained brain injuries for program development, quality assurance, facilities planning, and standards setting;
- promotion and strengthening of research for the advancement of the clinical science of BIM, including prevention, treatment, restoration of function, outcomes research, and advocacy; and
- improvement in education opportunities and resources in BIM for college undergraduate and graduate, health professional, and medical/surgical students.

This chapter will review the state of the field regarding training and certification of health care professionals and paraprofessionals providing frontline care and support in the community.

HEALTH CARE PROVIDERS

Brain injury rehabilitation has been provided for at least the past 4 decades in the United States initially as a part of a larger rehabilitation program, and, increasingly since about the 1980s, as dedicated programs. Service provision has moved beyond hospitals and clinics and into residences and communities. Advancements of medical science and vast improvements in medical and surgical care have foreshadowed the growth of specialized practice. Patients often require the services of an interdisciplinary treatment team consisting of physicians, occupational and physical therapists, nurses, speech and language pathologists, rehabilitation counselors, psychologists, and social workers among other professional and paraprofessional staff. Interdisciplinary rehabilitation team members are typically guided by a set of standards of ethical practice for their particular professions (19).

To practice within a specific discipline, practitioners are required to attain licensure. This is conferred by a government agency, is not voluntary, and requirements are not common across states. Certification, on the other hand, is usually voluntary and follows national standards; professional certification or accrediting bodies define standards and requirements. Certification implies a standard of skill and knowledge mastery beyond minimum requirements and within a specified scope but does not infer any legal standing. The public has become more aware of the differences between the two, with increasing expectations for expert care. Physicians and health care professionals have risen to the challenge to provide high quality care, with expertise recognized through experience and practice; only recently has subspecialization been acknowledged by certification in some disciplines.

Health care professionals require standard education, training, and licensure. Requirements for education and training regarding TBI within disciplines now exist, although implementation is inconsistent depending on the profession, educational institution, and training site. Health professionals often gain experience by sharing information through team interactions, mentorship, courses, or years of practice and experience. Training, certification, and/or licensure for most professionals do not require specialization in the care of individuals with post–brain injury. However, the need for subspecialty training and certification in BIM has been recognized increasingly, nationally and internationally (20–23).

Physician Training and Certification

Physicians must obtain licensure for practice, and requirements are defined by each state. Certification, although not required, has become the standard, and is based on training and examination, with national requirements. Physicians must maintain both licensure and specialty certification in response to the national call for protection of the public. State medical boards maintain oversight of licensure, and each state determines time requirements and needed documentation to determine relicensure. Two national medical organizations provide some infrastructure and oversight for certification: (*a*) The Accreditation Council for Graduate Medical Education (ACGME) is responsible for the accreditation of post–medical degree in medical training programs through development of standards and guidelines of training and a peer review process of training sites; (*b*) The American Board for Medical Specialties[1] (ABMS) is an organization of 24 medical specialty member boards with shared goals and standards for initial certification, admission of new specialties and subspecialties, and maintenance of certification. Since 2000, all physicians with certification must provide evidence of ongoing professionalism, lifelong learning and self-assessment, cognitive expertise, and practice performance assessment to achieve the status of maintenance of certification (MOC) (24); each member board has determined specific time lines and components within their specialty for their diplomates to assure continuous professional development. ABMS assists member boards in the development and implementation of educational, examination, and professional standards for all certification processes. Both ABMS and ACGME have organized a subspecialty development process, involving proposal development, review, vetting, and training program and certification requirements development.

Multiple medical specialties are involved in health care for persons who have sustained brain injury, including emergency medicine, neurosurgery, otolaryngology, physical medicine and rehabilitation, neurology, psychiatry, internal medicine (including subspecialties), and pediatrics, to name a few. Physicians provide the most care during the acute phase of care and lead the team of rehabilitation professionals during early and later care. There are a variety of medical conditions and management issues that require the expertise of a clinician well versed in typical conditions encountered in brain injury both early and late (e.g., increased intraventricular pressures, seizures, agitations, neuroendocrine axis abnormalities, spasticity, brachial plexus injuries, heterotopic ossifications, neurogenic bladder). Additionally, the clinician must be aware of the typical evolution of recovery and points of rehabilitation intervention. A supplementary knowledge base of less traditional medicine concepts (e.g., team process, aging and development, function, biomechanics, orthotics/prosthetics, neurophysiology, assistive devices and equipment, systems of care, health care financing) is also required to provide optimum care.

Although many training programs in a variety of specialties and their subspecialties provide experiences with patients with brain injury and survivors, only physical medicine and rehabilitation (PMR) and psychiatry specifically name brain injury as an area of required study within the ACGME training requirements for initial general certification (25). Further, PMR has developed formal BIM training within the general training programs. PMR residency programs developed this formal training during the 1980s and 1990s. As early as 1991, two-thirds of PMR residency programs either offered a formal rotation or required residents to participate in a clinical rotation in BIM including experiences across the continuum of care (23,26). Currently, all

PMR residents must have formal training and competency in BIM. Because PMR trainings and examinations require substantive coverage of BIM, certification in PMR conveys a basic competence in BIM.

Until recently, there was no formal subspecialty certification for physicians providing care for patients with and survivors of brain injury. However, non-ACGME approved brain injury fellowships within the PMR field and non-ACGME approved neurorehabilitation fellowships within the field of neurology have existed for some time. The American Board of Physical Medicine and Rehabilitation (ABPMR) proposed BIM subspecialization to ABMS in conjunction with the American Board of Psychiatry and Neurology (ABPN). The vetting process required review of the proposal and agreement by all 24 member boards and was approved in September, 2011. ACGME will develop fellowship training requirements, with PMR in conjunction with neurology, again requiring a vetting process. ABPMR is the lead board for certifying purposes, and the examination will be developed jointly with ABPN. For the first 5 years the exam is offered, candidates applying for the exam must meet initial requirements of active specialty board certification and licensure and practice experience or non-ACGME approved training. After this first 5 years, the requirement of board certification and licensure will continue, with the addition of successful completion of an ACGME-accredited fellowship, to be accepted to sit for the examination. The first BIM subspecialty certification examination will be held in the fall of 2014. MOC requirements will be developed for this subspecialty.

Although the medical community has responded to the "call to action" by the brain injury disability community with this new certification, physicians are not required to obtain subspecialization to provide health care services to individuals with brain injury. There will continue to be physicians with expertise in BIM supporting the needs of people who have sustained brain injuries without this additional subspecialty certification, just as there are many today. As noted, some general specialty board certifications and/or training programs require knowledge and experience in BIM. However, the new subspecialty certification provides the opportunity to increase the level of medical care and improve resources and responses to the needs of individuals post–brain injury and their families.

Psychology Training and Certification

Psychology is the study of behavior and mental processes (e.g., social and cognitive processes). Most psychologists are involved in therapeutic roles (e.g., clinical, counseling, education), often focusing on mental health, substance abuse, adjustment to disability or rehabilitation, anger management, and sports, to name a few. In general, psychologists are an integral part of rehabilitation and brain injury rehabilitation programs.

Within the field of psychology, the specialization area that is well suited to evaluate and provide treatment guidance for persons with TBI is clinical neuropsychology. Neuropsychologists use many specialized tests, procedures, and methods to assess various aspects of cognition (e.g., memory, attention, language), emotions, behaviors, personality, efforts, motivations, and symptoms validity. The tests compare the individual's performance against a set of normative

---

[1] ABMS Member Boards certify both allopathic (MD) and osteopathic (DO) physicians, with application for certification dependent on successfully completing ACGME-accredited residency training programs. Osteopathic medical students can participate in the application process for ACGME accredited training programs or osteopathic training programs; the latter programs are not accredited through ACGME.

data (i.e., healthy volunteers) that controls for the effects of demographic variables (e.g., age, education) on test performance, with the neuropsychologist determining the degree to which the test performance deviates from expected norms and whether the level and pattern of performance is consistent with the clinical history, behavioral observations, and known or suspected neuropathology. This specialized psychologist can uncover the influence of additional contexts encountered in persons who have sustained brain injuries, such as emotional states from changing life circumstances (e.g., depression, anxiety), medical comorbities (e.g., substance abuse, heart disease), and social contextual factors (e.g., litigation, financial distress) that can complicate the clinical presentation and impact neuropsychological test performance. Thus, the neuropsychologist can account for these contexts and explain their potential influence to the injured person, family members, and other health care providers. Specific additional education, training, and mentoring/experience are required for competent neuropsychologic practice. Formal neuropsychology internships and fellowships have been more readily available since the 1990s.

Clinical and counseling psychologists must receive a doctorate degree, participate in an accredited internship experience, and achieve licensure by passing state specific examination(s) to practice. Some states require continuing education for license renewal. Most states (exclusions are Louisiana and Texas) have generic psychology licensing laws, which allow psychologists to practice in self-identified specialized areas in which they declare expertise based on appropriate education and training. Psychologists can identify themselves as "neuropsychologists" in these states depending on personal standards of declaration, which can lead to a great deal of confusion among the public and other health care professionals.

Board certification in psychology was designed to be similar to that of the medical profession with established standards of competency, evaluation of educational background and training, and development of formal written and/or oral evaluations to be deemed competent to provide specialized services. There are currently 3 national certifying boards in neuropsychology. The American Board of Clinical Neuropsychology (ABCN; initially established 1981) was admitted to the American Board of Professional Psychology (ABPP; the largest unifying certification entity within psy-

chology) in 1984 as the first new specialty area since 1968 (27). ABCN has the largest number of diplomates in neuropsychology and is the only 1 of the 3 board certification organizations in neuropsychology that is part of ABPP (see Figure 5-1). The American Board of Professional Neuropsychology (ABN) has the second largest diplomate membership and was established in 1982 by individuals who already held ABPP diplomate status but with differing philosophical views. Thus, ABN and ABCN serve as competing national neuropsychological certification organizations. Attempts to merge the two organizations have proven unsuccessful.

Although both ABCN and ABPN certify neuropsychologists who work with children and/or adults, there is a third board certifying organization specific to pediatric neuropsychology known as the American Board of Pediatric Neuropsychology (ABPdN). ABPdN began in 1996, and diplomate membership has tripled in size for the past 10 years. ABPdN is the smallest of the 3 national neuropsychological certification boards owing to the more specialized nature of the certification (i.e., pediatrics only) and the age of the organization.

All 3 boards in clinical neuropsychology share common aspects of peer review of training and education, a written examination, and an oral examination. In clinical neuropsychology, the candidates most likely to be successful in pursuit of board certification are those whose training and education is consistent with the Houston Conference guidelines established through a collaboration among multiple national neuropsychological organizations (28). There continue to be many neuropsychologists who are not board certified or who are pursuing board certification who can also provide an excellent service by virtue of practice and experience. However, board certification credentials allow ease of recognition by the public and other health care providers. There is currently no maintenance of certification or recertification requirement, although this concept is being explored.

Clinical and counseling psychologists, not neuropsychologically trained or certified, often interface with persons who have sustained TBI in inpatient (e.g., rehabilitation units) and outpatient settings usually for psychotherapy. Some psychologists refer to themselves as rehabilitation psychologists. Rehabilitation psychology is a specialty area of psychology that assists the individual (and family) with *any* injury, illness, or disability that may be chronic, traumatic,

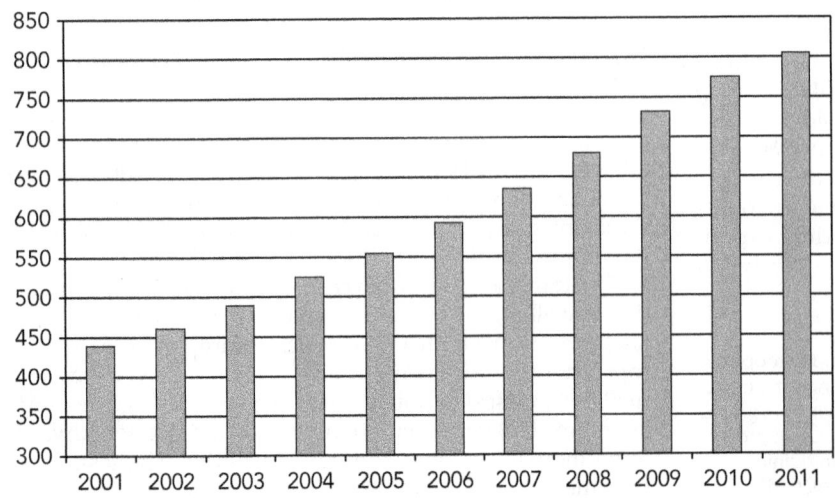

FIGURE 5-1 Total number of ABCN diplomates awarded per year in the past decade. Note that 2011 information is current as of May 2011 and does not include data from the November 2011 examination. The information provided is courtesy of the ABCN office, specifically Dr. John Lucas, ABPP-CN.

and/or congenital in achieving optimal physical, psychological, and interpersonal functioning (29). Rehabilitation psychology involves assessment and intervention that is tailored to the person's level of impairment and is set within an interdisciplinary framework. Rehabilitation psychologists are expected to be knowledgeable about how disability and medical issues affect their diverse patient clientele, although there are no specific requirements for education or training. Board certification in rehabilitation psychology identifies those individuals who have demonstrated a specialized level of competence in that area. The American Board of Rehabilitation Psychology (ABRP) became affiliated with ABPP in 1997 with relatively slow growth over the years since (30). Some psychologists are board certified in both clinical neuropsychology and rehabilitation psychology, although most pursue certification in only 1 of these 2 areas. The 2 professions sometimes work within the same department in rehabilitation settings.

Rehabilitation Nurse, Social Worker, Counselor, and Therapist Education and Certification

Within the care provision schema for patients and consumers who have sustained brain injuries, nurses, therapists, social workers, and counselors play an important role. Subspecialty education and recognition in these areas is not as well developed as for physicians and psychologists. Licensure is required, although requirements vary by state. Certification within the discipline may or may not be required. Certification or licensure renewal is determined by each certifying organization or state and usually includes some declaration or documentation of at least continuing education, but may also include participation in professional development, discipline specific experience, or community service.

Rehabilitation nurses provide more than the traditional acute medical and surgical care; they are versed in typical medical conditions seen in disability and treatment strategies (e.g., environmental changes to help manage agitation) and provide needed education for patients/consumers and families. They are certified through the Certified Registered Rehabilitation Nurse (CRRN) program administered by the Rehabilitation Nursing Certification Board, accredited by the American Board of Nursing Specialties. An unrestricted nurse license is required along with experience in rehabilitation nursing or advanced degree education. There is no specialty designation for brain injury; however, care issues for people who have sustained brain injuries are included in the suggested resources and examination content outline (31).

Social workers engage with patients/consumers and families and can provide a variety of services within brain injury programs, such as coordination of services, referral to community agencies and services, guidance regarding insurance and benefits, and family and individual counseling. Within rehabilitation centers and programs, they are typically required to have master's level training, which is overseen by the Council on Social Work Education (CSWE). The CSWE defines the components for social work programs, but the individually accredited MSW programs specify specialty areas. There is no specific brain injury specialty training or certification (32).

Rehabilitation counselors (also known as vocational counselors) assist persons with both physical and mental disabilities, and cover the areas of vocational, psychological, social, and medical aspects of disability, through a partnership with the individuals served. Within the field of BIM, rehabilitation counselors can evaluate and coordinate the services needed, provide counseling to assist people in coping with limitations caused by brain injury, and provide advocacy for needs. There is no focused BIM curriculum, and training is primarily at the graduate level, with employment entry-level positions in rehabilitation programs at a master's or doctorate level. The Council on Rehabilitation Education (CORE) accredits qualifying institutions; however, not all programs are CORE accredited. Rehabilitation counselors are certified by the Commission on Rehabilitation Counselor Certification, a member of the National Commission for Certifying Agencies. To become certified, rehabilitation counselors must meet eligibility requirements including advanced education and work experience and achieve a passing score on an examination (33).

Typical rehabilitation therapists seen in brain injury programs include occupational, physical, speech and language, and recreation therapists. Each has specific educational requirements for professional education completion, which includes some components related to BIM. All therapy professions require licensure, and each state determines licensure requirements for practice. There are requirements for renewal of license and/or general certification and are determined by each state or certifying board. There are no specialty certificates or credentials specifically for BIM.

- Occupational therapists (OTs) typically work with patients/consumers to participate in living and working environments, using a variety of techniques including exercise, cognitive strategies, vision, or adaptive equipment. The academic programs are accredited by the Accreditation Council for Occupational Therapy Education, and a master's level or higher are required to join the workforce. The profession requires that a therapist hold a registration certificate and use the title of Occupational Therapist Registered (OTR) through the National Board for Certification in Occupational Therapy achieved through examination. The American Occupational Therapy Association (AOTA), which is the OT professional organization, offers board certification (4 discrete areas) and specialty certification (4 discrete areas) all through provision of evidence of experience and competency. Many of these topics are areas of expertise needed in providing care and services for individuals with post–brain injury, although there is no specific brain injury designation (34,35).
- Physical therapists assess movement dysfunction and use treatment interventions, such as exercise, functional training, manual therapy techniques, assistive and adaptive devices and equipments, and physical agents to progress mobility. Currently, only graduate degree physical therapist programs are accredited through the Commission on Accreditation of Physical Therapy Education associated with the professional organization, which is the American Physical Therapy Association (APTA). Practice requires passing a national or specific state examination. There is no focused education and training regarding BIM; however, the advanced degrees can allow focused areas of education and training. In addition, there is specialization offered through the

American Board of Physical Therapy Specialists, another APTA organized entity, requiring eligibility and examination. Of the 8 specialty areas offered, the neurology specialist certificate is the most aligned with BIM (36,37).

- Speech and language pathology education consists of undergraduate college education in communication sciences and disorders followed by additional graduate study to achieve a master's degree. Speech and language pathologists assess, treat, and help to prevent disorders related to speech, language, cognitive communication, voice, swallowing, and fluency. The Council on Academic Accreditation in Audiology and Speech-Language Pathology, associated with the national professional society, accredits programs of study, and graduates of these programs must successfully complete the required clinical experiences and pass a national examination. The professional association, which is the American Speech and Hearing Association (ASHA), in collaboration with the Educational Testing Service, develops the certification of clinical competence (CCC-SLP) examination. Although there are 3 areas of specialization offered that can be helpful in treating people who have sustained brain injuries, there are no BIM specialty educations or training programs (38,39).

- Recreational therapists, also referred to as therapeutic recreation specialists, provide treatment services and recreation activities for individuals with disabilities or illnesses, and use a variety of techniques to improve and maintain the physical, mental, and emotional well-being of their clients. There are no specialty educations and training programs focused on brain injury services for recreation therapists; however, the typical patient goals of greater independence and integration into the community resonate with people who have sustained brain injuries. The National Council for Therapeutic Recreation Certification established standards for certification, including education, experience, and continuing professional development. The Certified Therapeutic Recreation Specialist (CTRS) credential is offered to qualified individuals who must also document experience and complete an examination (40,41).

- Additional specific interventions may have defined programs of education that cross disciplines and are organized by individual entities. Each has standards for education courses and some type of examination or documentation of experience, conferring credentialing. None names brain injury as the condition of focus, but the techniques may prove beneficial for patients and consumers post–brain injury. These include such techniques as vestibular rehabilitation, neuro-developmental treatment (NDT), functional capacity evaluation (FCE), and Pilates education and certification/credentialing.

COMMUNITY CARERS AND PARAPROFESSIONALS

Following discharge from the acute or subacute setting into the community, many persons with moderate or severe brain injury require ongoing postacute care often for a lifetime. Outpatient rehabilitation interventions may be focused on specific functions (e.g., improving balance) or conditions (e.g., tone management), depending on the level of impairment and functional disability, and are time limited. Support needs may typically be very high for behavior programs. Oftentimes, persons with brain injury of significant severity continue to require the services of a multidisciplinary treatment team or focused services of cognitive rehabilitation strategies (42). Unfortunately, these services may be unavailable, spread among several different provider agencies, or fall to family members and personal service providers (14), making coordination and continuity of service a significant challenge, especially in rural areas (43). Preexisting community service models (i.e., those for persons with developmental disabilities or mental illness) usually do not meet the needs of individuals who have sustained brain injuries. These factors contribute to the serious need for specialized training to meet the various needs of persons with brain injuries, caregivers, and their families.

Although professional education, certification, and licensure requirements continue in the outpatient and postacute phase, there is limited literature discussing the need for formalized training of direct care workers providing TBI services in the postacute phase. A national US survey of 565 acute, subacute, and postacute programs (45% response rate) noted that 75% of respondents indicated the need for specialized training for licensed staff, and 84% for nonlicensed staff (22). The specific educational needs areas that have been identified are those concepts integral to the provision of rehabilitation services to persons with moderate to severe brain injury and include treatments and management of cognitive deficits, strategies to deal with family and social issues, behavior modification techniques, and approaches to adjustment to brain injury (20,22). The individuals who provide care to persons with TBI residing in the community are usually family members and direct care staff. Families often receive general education and training within acute and subacute rehabilitation programs in preparation for discharge to home (44). The education and information, however, may not be generalizable to home, and contextual strategies usually are of more benefit (43,45). Home- or community-based programs (46,47) and web-based videoconferencing (43) have proven effective.

Direct care or paid staff are often at the forefront of care, receive the least training, and yet are recognized as the most helpful by families and consumers (48). One of the major challenges faced by provider agencies has been the difficulty to attract and retain qualified staff. It has been suggested that agencies should increase efforts to train and orient new staff to the types of challenges encountered working with persons with brain injury (49) and that closer contact between professionals and paid caregivers may improve care provision (50).

A discussion of long term or lifelong care issues would not be complete without mentioning care costs and funding. The lifelong sequelae of TBI often exhaust private insurance funding streams early in the rehabilitation process. Return to work or school is often not an option for the moderately to severely brain injured individual, and therefore, public programs such as Medicaid and Medicare often become the primary sources of service payment. Several states have established waiver programs for persons with TBI. These programs offer opportunities for designing integrated service plans for individuals with brain injury who might otherwise require some type of institutionalized care. Care usually includes support for specialists in case coordination and behavior management and not otherwise funded through typical private insurance. A demonstration project through the New York State Department of Health developed support and contextualized training/coaching for family members, friends, and community support staff and suggested that this community support could be provided in a cost-effective manner (51). The waiver services are based in a philosophy of individual choice while accounting for the accompanying realities of needs, health and welfare issues, and budgets. However, within the present economic and health care reform climate, it is unclear how these programs will function in years to come.

American Academy of Certified Brain Injury Specialists

In response to the need for education and training of frontline care providers, the Brain Injury Association of America (BIAA) established the American Academy of Certified Brain Injury Specialists (ACBIS) in 1996 as a standing committee of the association to address training needs. More specifically, ACBIS was established to improve the quality of care given to individuals with brain injury through the education and training of those who provide community- and home-based brain injury services.

The ACBIS program is divided into 2 levels: Certified Brain Injury Specialist (CBIS) and Certified Brain Injury Specialist Trainer (CBIST). There is a specified curriculum for each, with certification deemed through eligibility requirements documenting hours of experience and passing a written examination. Additionally, the program has been expanded to include a certification category called Provisional Certified Brain Injury Specialist (PCBIS). This certification process is open to graduate students who are enrolled in an accredited university program, with the intent to provide in-depth training for those preprofessionals who intend having a career working with individuals with acquired or traumatic brain injury. Full certification (CBIS) requires clinical or academic employment experience working with individuals who have a brain injury within a 3-year period from the date of original PCBIS certification (52).

Despite the name "Certified Brain Injury Specialist," ACBIS is clear that the credential does not imply or warrant that the certified individual is an expert in brain injury rehabilitation, is qualified to offer professional services without the appropriate licensure, or able to provide unsupervised treatment. The ACBIS certification program is especially designed to address specific training issues in brain injury services and may *complement* other credentials.

In regard to the testing offered by ACBIS, critics of the examination focus on it being knowledge based when many of the skills integral for effective work with this population rely on technique. A model has been developed that is both knowledge and practice based, and uses a mobile team approach, educating caregivers and persons with brain injury on how to implement and sustain home-based behavior management programs (53). This model operates in the natural environment (e.g., home, community), which has brought to light the importance of flexible interventions that address both client and caregiver needs. Therefore, ideally, at least a portion of training must be contextualized to increase the likelihood of positive influence given the cognitive and behavioral sequelae of TBI. Training programs specifically fashioned to provide knowledge and skills training regarding brain injury are needed to facilitate both the caregiver's and the person with brain injury's adjustment to providing/receiving services. To further the dissemination of knowledge in the field, all new applicants receive a 1-year subscription to the *Journal of Head Trauma Rehabilitation* as part of their initial application fee. More than the past five years, the number of certificants has grown substantially by 10 fold.

In addition to affording individuals the opportunity for certification as providers of brain injury services, ACBIS now provides certification services to agencies through the ACBIS Alliance program. The ACBIS Alliance provides public recognition to a brain injury services provider or designated facility that has achieved the benchmark of having 20% of its staff (who are eligible for national certification) certified as CBIS or CBIST. ACBIS established the Alliance Member Award to recognize and honor providers of brain injury services that support and encourage national certification of their staff and thereby demonstrate a commitment to provide higher quality services to persons with brain injury. Alliance members achieving this minimum benchmark in any given application year receive recognition with successive years at silver (first year), gold (second year), and platinum (third and successive years) levels. This expansion of ACBIS certification opportunities in the field of brain injury rehabilitation furthers the mission to improve the quality of care given to individuals with brain injury through the education and training of those who work in brain injury services (52).

CONCLUSION

With advancements in research and science, there have been improvements in acute and emergency medical care, with a significant increase in the numbers of persons who survive brain injury. Residual impairments from the brain injury include a variety of conditions; however, cognitive, behavioral, and emotional impairments are often the most difficult to manage. Health professionals with expertise in BIM are required to provide ongoing services and support. Consumers and professionals recognize the importance of subspecialty training and certification.

Professionals and paraprofessionals providing services should receive appropriate training, and ultimately certification, to further assure high quality care and avoidance of medical errors (see Table 5-1). Physicians and psychologists have new and long-standing established board certification programs for specialization and subspecialization areas that directly relate to TBI and other neurological conditions. Physicians are now further required to participate in ongoing professional education and development programs to maintain certification. Physical, occupational, and speech therapy have some additional certifications that align with BIM, but do not focus there. The establishment of the ACBIS is a dynamic step toward addressing the needs and concerns of the brain injury community.

Subspecialty training and certification in BIM and rehabilitation should be considered across all disciplines serving the needs of persons with brain injury. Programs offering such training narrow the information gap between health

TABLE 5-1 Summary of Specialized Training and Certification for Providing High Quality Brain Injury Medicine Services*

DISCIPLINE	REHABILITATION TRAINING	BIM SUBSPECIALTY TRAINING	CERTIFICATION WITHIN SUBSPECIALIZATION
Physician	Specialty residency training: PMR—specifies rehabilitation and brain injury experience Psychiatry—specifies brain injury experience	ACGME directed, Residency Review Committees must approve guidelines for training (in process)	Approval ABMS 2011 Planned first examination 2014 Maintenance of certification is required
Psychology	Postdoctoral residency training programs available in rehabilitation psychology	Neuropsychology training fellowships available; joint rehabilitation and neuropsychology are also available	Neuropsychology: ABCN, ABN, ABPdN No required recertification
Nurse	Experience only, not required during general training	—	—
Social worker	None required	—	—
Rehabilitation counselor	Required in formal training	—	—
Occupational therapist	Part of formal training	—	—
Physical therapist	Part of formal training	—	—
Speech and language pathologist	Part of formal training	—	—
Recreational therapist	Part of formal training	—	—
Community care providers	NA	Specialized BIM training for community workers; also meant to complement other training or certification	CBIS or CBIST

*BIM, brain injury medicine; PMR, physical medicine and rehabilitation; ACGME, Accreditation Council for Graduate Medical Education; ABMS, American Board for Medical Specialties; ABCN, American Board of Clinical Neuropsychology; ABN, American board of Professional Neuropsychology; ABPdN, American Board of Pediatric Neuropsychology; NA, Not Applicable; CBIS, Certified Brain Injury Specialist; CBIST, Certified Brain Injury Specialist Trainer.

care professionals in the tertiary care hospitals and those in the long-term care facilities or communities, contributing to the integration of brain injury services across the continuum of care. Partnerships among professional organizations, credentialing bodies, service agencies, and accrediting bodies must be forged to further integration of knowledge and skills set into community-based brain injury services.

KEY CLINICAL POINTS

1. The care and management of the specific and unique sequelae of brain injury require expert knowledge, skills, and attitudes, usually not a part of routine medical or health care education.
2. Licensing and certification are not the same. Licensing is usually mandated by regulating bodies and is not voluntary; requirements to achieve a license are usually minimal standards and may not be similar across regulating bodies. Certification is usually voluntary and is defined by a professional organization; requirements to achieve certification are considered to be beyond minimal standards and are consistent within professional organizations. Only licensing provides legal standing.
3. Board certification is generally accepted as the most objective method to identify a practitioner who is capable of providing specialized services within the health care community.

4. Physician and psychology services are currently the only disciplines that confer subspecialty certification for providers who specialize in brain injury medicine health care.
5. Because there are significant care needs for those with more moderate to severe brain injuries, especially regarding the need for cognitive and behavioral support, there is specialized training and certification for both community care providers and the health care community in general to support community living.

KEY REFERENCES

1. American Board of Rehabilitation Psychology. *Periodic Comprehensive Review, 2010.* American Board of Rehabilitation Psychology.
2. Field MJ, Jette AM, eds. *The Future of Disability in America.* Washington, DC: The National Academies Press; 2007.
3. Officer AM, Posarac A, eds. *World Report on Disability.* Geneva, Switzerland: WHO Press; 2011.
4. Sandel ME, Finch M. The case for comprehensive residency training in traumatic brain injury. A commentary. *Am J Phys Med Rehabil.* 1993;72(5):325–326.

References

1. Colantonio A, Dawson DR, McLellan BA. Head injury in young adults: long-term outcome. *Arch Phys Med Rehabil.* 1998;79(5):550–558.

2. Dixon TM, Layton BS. Traumatic brain injury. In: Eisenberg MG, Glueckauf RL, Zaretsky HH, eds. *Medical Aspects of Disability: A Handbook for the Rehabilitation Professional*. 2nd ed. New York, NY: Springer Publishing; 1999:98–120.

3. Thurman DJ, Alverson C, Dunn KA, Guerrero J, Sniezek JE. Traumatic brain injury in the United States: a public health perspective. *J Head Trauma Rehabil*. 1999;14(6):602–615.

4. Injury Prevention & Control. Centers for Disease Control and Prevention Web site. http://www.cdc.gov/traumaticbraininjury/. Accessed June 10, 2011.

5. Centers for Disease Control and Prevention. Nonfatal traumatic brain injuries from sports and recreation activities—United States, 2001–2005. *MMWR Morb Mortal Wkly Rep*. 2007;56(29):733–737.

6. Centers for Disease Control and Prevention. National Center for Injury Prevention and Control. *Report to Congress on Mild Traumatic Brain Injury in the United States: Steps to Prevent a Serious Public Health Problem*. Atlanta, GA: Centers for Disease Control and Prevention; 2003.

7. Cassidy JD, Carroll LJ, Peloso PM, et al. Incidence, risk factors and prevention of mild traumatic brain injury: results of the WHO Collaborating Centre Task Force on Mild Traumatic Brain Injury. *J Rehabil Med*. 2004;(suppl 43):28–60.

8. Gruskin KD, Schutzman SA. Head trauma in children younger than 2 years: are there predictors for complications? *Arch Pediatr Adolesc Med*. 1999;153(1):15–20.

9. US Department of Veterans Affairs. *VA Polytrauma System of Care*. Washington, DC: U.S. Department of Veterans Affairs. http://www.polytrauma.va.gov/system-of-care/. Accessed September 30, 2011.

10. Department of Veterans Affairs. *Polytrauma-Traumatic Brain Injury (TBI) System of Care*. Washington, DC: Veterans Health Administration; 2009. http://www.va.gov/vhapublications/ViewPublication.asp?pub_ID=2032. Accessed September 30, 2011.

11. Department of Veterans Affairs. *Management of Concussion/Mild Traumatic Brain Injury*. http://www.healthquality.va.gov/mtbi/concussion_mtbi_full_1_0.pdf. Accessed September 30, 2011.

12. http://www.pdhealth.mil/TBI.asp#eat. Accessed September 30, 2011.

13. Osberg JS, Brooke MM, Baryza MJ, Rowe K, Lash M, Kahn P. Impact of childhood brain injury on work and family finances. *Brain Inj*. 1997;11(1):11–24.

14. Leith KH, Phillips L, Sample PL. Exploring the service needs and experiences of persons with TBI and their families: the South Carolina experience. *Brain Inj*. 2004;18(12):1191–1208.

15. Rocchio A. Where do we go from here? *Family News and Views*. 1997; 4(6).

16. Kohn LT, Corrigan JM, Donaldson MS, eds. *To Err is Human: Building a Safer Health System*. Washington DC: National Academy Press; 2000.

17. Field MJ, Jette AM, eds. *The Future of Disability in America*. Washington DC: The National Academies Press; 2007.

18. Officer AM, Posarac A, eds. *World Report on Disability*. Geneva, Switzerland: WHO Press; 2011.

19. Niemeier JP, Burnett DM, Whitaker DA. Cultural competence in the multidisciplinary rehabilitation setting: are we falling short of meeting needs? *Arch Phys Med Rehabil*. 2003;84(8):1240–1245.

20. Jackson H, Manchester D. Towards the development of brain injury specialists. *NeuroRehabilitation*. 2001;16(1):27–40.

21. Swan IJ, Walker A. Who cares for the patient with head injury now? *Emerg Med J*. 2001;18(5):352–357.

22. Becker H, Harrell W, Keller L. A survey of professional and paraprofessional training needs for traumatic brain injury rehabilitation. *J Head Trauma Rehabil*. 1993;8:88–101.

23. Bell K, Massagli TL. Subacute brain injury rehabilitation: an opportunity for medical education and training. *Brain Inj*. 1996;10(12): 875–881.

24. ABMS Maintenance of Certification. American Board of Medical Specialties Web site. http://www.abms.org/Maintenance_of_Certification/MOC.aspx. Accessed September 26, 2011.

25. Physical Medicine & Rehabilitation Program Requirements. ACGME Website. http://www.acgme.org/acWebsite/RRC_340/340_prIndex.asp. Accessed July 15, 2011.

26. Sandel ME, Finch M. The case for comprehensive residency training in traumatic brain injury. A commentary. *Am J Phys Med Rehabil*. 1993;72(5):325–326.

27. Goldstein G. Board certification in clinical neuropsychology: some history, facts, and opinions. *J Forensic Neuropsychology*. 2001;2:57–65.

28. Hannay HJ, Bieliauskas LA, Crosson BA, Hammeke TA, Hamsher K. deS, Koffler SP. Proceedings: the Houston Conference on specialty education and training in clinical neuropsychology. *Arch Clin Neuropsychol*. 1998;13(2):157–249.

29. Scherer MJ, Blair KL, Banks ME, Brucker B, Corrigan J, Wegener JH. Rehabilitation psychology. In: Craighead WE, Nemeroff CB, eds. *The Concise Corsini Encyclopedia of Psychology and Behavioral Science*. 3rd ed. Hoboken, NJ: John Wiley & Sons, Inc. 2004:801–802.

30. American Board of Rehabilitation Psychology. *Periodic Comprehensive Review, 2010*. American Board of Rehabilitation Psychology.

31. http://www.rehabnurse.org/certification/content/index.html. Accessed July 7, 2011.

32. U.S. Bureau of Labor Statistics, U.S. Department of Labor. *Occupational Outlook Handbook, 2010–11 Edition*. Washington, DC: U.S. Bureau of Labor Statistics. http://www.bls.gov/oco/ocos060.htm. Accessed July 18, 2011.

33. Commission on Rehabilitation Counselor Certification Web site. http://www.crccertification.com/. Accessed July 19, 2011.

34. The American Occupational Therapy Association Web site. http://www.aota.org/. Accessed July 7, 2011.

35. http://www.bls.gov/oco/ocos078.htm. Accessed July 18, 2011.

36. American Physical Therapy Association Web site. http://www.apta.org/. Accessed July 7, 2011.

37. http://www.bls.gov/oco/ocos080.htm. Accessed July 18, 2011.

38. American Speech-Language-Hearing Association Web site. http://www.asha.org/. Accessed July 8, 2011.

39. http://www.bls.gov/oco/ocos099.htm. Accessed July 18, 2011.

40. National Council for Therapeutic Recreation Certification Web site. http://www.nctrc.org/aboutnctrc.htm. Accessed July 10, 2011.

41. http://www.bls.gov/oco/ocos082.htm. Accessed July 18, 2011.

42. Cicerone KD, Dahlberg C, Malec JF, et al. Evidence-based cognitive rehabilitation: updated review of the literature from 1998 through 2002. *Arch Phys Med Rehabil*. 2005;86(8):1681–1692.

43. Sanders AM, Clark AN, Atchison TB, Rueda M. A web-based videoconferencing approach to training caregivers in rural areas to compensate for problems related to traumatic brain injury. *J Head Trauma Rehabil*. 2009;24(4):248–261.

44. Pressley M. More about the development of self-regulation: complex, long-term, and thoroughly social. *Educ Psychol*. 1995;30(4): 207–212.

45. Braga LW, Da Paz AC, Ylvisaker M. Direct clinician-delivered versus indirect family-supported rehabilitation of children with traumatic brain injury: a randomized controlled study. *Brain Inj*. 2005; 19(10):819–831.

46. Carnevale GJ, Anselmi V, Busichio K, Millis SR. Changes in ratings of caregiver burden following a community-based behavior management program for persons with traumatic brain injury. *J Head Trauma Rehabil*. 2002;17(2):83–95.

47. Carnevale GJ, Anselmi V, Johnston MV, Busichio K, Walsh V. A natural setting behavior management program for persons with acquired brain injury: a randomized controlled trial. *Arch Phys Med Rehabil*. 2008;87(10):1289–1297.

48. Fisher J. Cognitive and behavioral consequences of closed head injury. *Sem Neuro*. 1985;5(3):197–204.

49. McCluskey A. Paid attendant carers hold important and unexpected roles which contribute to the lives of people with brain injury. *Brain Inj*. 2000;14(11):943–957.

50. Sohlberg MM, Glang A, Todis B. Improvement during baseline: three case studies encouraging collaborative research when evaluating caregiver training. *Brain Inj*. 1998;12(4):333–346.

51. Feeney TJ, Ylvisaker M, Rosen BH, Greene P. Community supports for individuals with challenging behavior after brain injury: an analysis of the New York state behavioral resource project. *J Head Trauma Rehabil*. 2001;16(1):61–75.

52. http://www.crccertification.com/. Accessed July 11, 2011.

53. Carnevale GJ. Natural-setting behavior management for individuals with traumatic brain injury: results of a three-year caregiver training program. *J Head Trauma Rehabil*. 1996;11:27–38.

Commission on Accreditation of Rehabilitation Facilities Accreditation for Brain Injury Programs

Christine M. MacDonell

INTRODUCTION

The Commission on Accreditation of Rehabilitation Facilities (CARF) accreditation process is a voluntary, peer review, external evaluation process that health and human service providers choose as a means to review the functioning and practices of their organizations, programs, and services. CARF has engaged with brain injury service providers and individuals with brain injuries since the early 1980s to ensure quality and accountability throughout the continuum of services provided for individuals with acquired brain injuries (ABIs). Providers around the world have chosen to pursue accreditation because "it is well recognized that application of the principles of accreditation on an ongoing basis facilitates continuous quality improvement" (1).

Accreditation can create a social capital, provide a learning environment for change in practice, encourage both formal and informal relationships and communication, and, through shared values, enhance care for individuals with acute brain injury (ABI) (2). CARF accreditation standards and the survey process provide programs with a template to organize a quality rehabilitation program. Using CARF standards can also produce results in a number of areas that determine overall organizational quality. In a Veterans Health Administration (VHA) study, preparing for a CARF survey appeared to have had significant positive impacts on the programs surveyed: communication with members of the rehabilitation team, overall program quality, medical record documentation practices, communication with Veterans Administration Medical Center (VAMC) management regarding mission and/or actual performance of the rehabilitation program, and quality of information provided the patient and family regarding the care plan (3).

Although researchers have not established a direct link between accreditation and service quality or client outcomes, there is evidence that the activities associated with accreditation promote positive change in health care organizations, such as improvements in the physical facilities and safety, the dissemination and quality of health care guidelines, and the opportunity to reflect on practice (2). These changes have the potential to improve client outcomes. In reporting the results of his phenomenological study of the experience of accreditation from the perspective of the frontline worker, Bates (4) concluded that the self-study process, which is a key component of the accreditation process, "involves many concurrent developmental changes to the existing operations in the agency." He also identified "stakeholder feedback" as a component of the accreditation process that promotes developmental change in the organization.

THE COMMISSION ON ACCREDITATION OF REHABILITATION FACILITIES' ACCREDITATION SCOPE

CARF International is a private, nonprofit organization that accredits health and human services across the lifespan and continuum of care. CARF was formed in 1966 by 2 national organizations—the Association of Rehabilitation Centers (ARC) and the National Association of Sheltered Workshops and Homebound Programs (NASWHP)—that had been developing standards for their respective memberships for about a decade. In September 1966, the 2 organizations agreed to pool their interests in setting standards and formed the Commission on Accreditation of Rehabilitation Facilities, now known as CARF International or simply CARF.

CARF accreditation opportunities are available in the fields of aging services, behavioral health, child and youth services, employment and community services, medical rehabilitation, opioid treatment programs, and vision rehabilitation services. CARF also accredits one-stop career centers; business networks, services management networks; continuing care retirement communities; aging services networks; and durable medical equipment, prosthetics, orthotics, and supplies (DMEPOS) suppliers. Accreditation is based on application of practical and relevant standards of quality through a peer review process to determine how well an organization is implementing practices designed to result in quality services to consumers. The standards are developed with the input of the persons served, professionals, purchasers of services, and other stakeholders with relevant expertise and experience and refined through external field review.

CARF currently accredits more than 47,000 programs at more than 20,000 locations internationally. In 2010, more than 8.7 million persons of all ages were served annually by more than 6,100 CARF-accredited providers in the United States, Canada, Europe, the Middle East, Southeast Asia,

Africa, Mexico, and South America. CARF conducts more than 2,400 surveys annually. The CARF International family includes CARF, CARF Canada, CARF Continuing Care Accreditation Commission (CARF–CCAC), and CARF Europe with offices in Tucson, Arizona; Washington, DC; Edmonton, Alberta, Canada; and Toronto, Ontario, Canada. CARF Europe's office will be located in London, England.

Hundreds of governmental agencies, insurers, and workers' compensation and private entities have accepted, mandated, or endorsed accreditation by CARF. An example is the Irish "National Policy and Strategy for the Provision of Neuro-rehabilitation Services in Ireland 2011–2015." This work was jointly commissioned by the Secretary General of the Department of Health and the Chief Executive Officer of the Health Services Executive. It states, "Accreditation of services is a positive driver endorsing provision of high quality services according to internationally accepted norms. The Commission on Accreditation of Rehabilitation Facilities (CARF) is a relevant instrument in this regard" (5).

CARF is financed by fees from accreditation surveys, workshops and conferences, sales of publications, and grants from public entities. In 2012, approximate costs associated with the application and survey fees range between $6,875 and $8,875 (US dollars [USD]). The fee is determined by the size and number of locations for which the organization is seeking accreditation, as well as the country in which the organization is located. These fees include all costs associated with the surveyors' travel, lodging, and meals. The fee also covers the survey itself, the survey report, and the certificate of accreditation if accreditation is achieved. There are no annual fees. The CARF standards manuals are available in printed and electronic versions. The manuals are necessary for the survey and prices start at $225 (USD). Additional fees that might be incurred while preparing for and maintaining accreditation include CARF face-to-face trainings and webinars in the price range of $200–$900 (USD), depending on the length and type of training. Indirect costs depend on an organization's consistent use of the standards and appreciation that a CARF survey is not an event but an ongoing process. Organizations that prepare well in advance of their surveys, maintain currency with the standards, and use the standards as business and clinical tools report less indirect preparation costs. The organizations that report high indirect accreditation costs are usually organizations that work with consultants before attempting to prepare for the survey themselves, have decreasing census, have high turnover of staff, or are merging with organizations that are not CARF accredited.

THE STRUCTURE OF THE COMMISSION ON ACCREDITATION OF REHABILITATION FACILITIES

Since its inception in 1966, CARF has benefited from national organizations joining together in support of the goals of accreditation. These organizations, representing a broad range of expertise, sponsor CARF by providing input on standards and other related matters through membership in CARF's International Advisory Council (IAC). A list of current IAC members is available on the CARF website: http://www.carf.org/members.

The world of brain injury has been engaged with CARF since the early 1980s. Beginning in 1984, the American Congress of Rehabilitation Medicine Brain Injury Interdisciplinary Special Interest Group (ACRM BI-ISIG) and the National Head Injury Foundation (NHIF) were instrumental and the leading associations to assist CARF in developing the first set of brain injury standards.

CARF published its initial brain injury standards in 1985. As associations change and new ones emerge, other associations have been diligent in assisting CARF in its mission to enhance the lives of persons served in CARF-accredited brain injury programs. These associations include the Brain Injury Association of America (BIAA), North American Brain Injury Society (NABIS), International Brain Injury Association (IBIA), and the European Brain Injury Society (EBIS).

Insurers, governmental agencies, providers, and consumers of services have also been engaged in developing and revising the CARF standards in the brain injury arena since the standards' initial development.

CARF is governed by an international board of directors composed of individuals elected based on their expertise, experience, and perspective on matters of importance to CARF. The board develops the strategic direction of CARF in conjunction with CARF leadership and approves corporate policies, including policies regarding standards development, the accreditation process, and fiscal matters.

Mission

The mission of CARF is to promote the quality, value, and optimal outcomes of services through a consultative accreditation process that centers on enhancing the lives of the persons served.

Vision

Through responsiveness to a dynamic and diverse environment, CARF serves as a catalyst for improving the quality of life of the persons served by CARF-accredited organizations and the programs and services they provide.

Values

The CARF board of directors has identified that the persons served shall be the moral owners of CARF. Persons served are the primary consumers of services, which may be referred to as clients, participants, or residents. When these persons are unable to exercise self-representation at any point in the decision-making process, persons served is interpreted to also refer to those persons willing and able to make decisions on behalf of the primary consumer. The persons served as the moral owners of CARF means that CARF cannot fail to protect those owners through the CARF accreditation process. CARF believes in the following core values:

- All people have the right to be treated with dignity and respect.
- All people should have access to needed services that achieve optimal outcomes.
- All people should be empowered to exercise informed choice.

CARF's accreditation, research, and educational activities are conducted in accordance with these core values and with the utmost integrity.

In addition, CARF is committed to

- the continuous improvement of both organizational management and service delivery;
- diversity and cultural competence in all CARF activities and associations;
- enhancing the involvement of persons served in all of CARF's activities;
- having persons served be active participants in the development and application of standards for accreditation; and
- enhancing the meaning, value, and relevance of accreditation to the persons served.

Purposes

In support of our mission, vision, and values, CARF's purposes are the following:

- To develop and maintain current, field-driven standards that improve the value and responsiveness of the programs and services delivered to people in need of rehabilitation and other life enhancement services.
- To seek input and to be responsive to persons served and other stakeholders.
- To provide information and education to persons served and other stakeholders on the value of accreditation.
- To recognize organizations that achieve accreditation through a consultative peer review process and demonstrate their commitment to the continuous improvement of their programs and services with a focus on the needs and outcomes of the persons served.
- To conduct accreditation research emphasizing outcomes measurement and management and to provide information on common program strengths and areas for improvement.
- To provide consultation, education, training, and publications that support organizations in achieving and maintaining accreditation of their programs and services.

STANDARDS DEVELOPMENT

The CARF standards are central to the accreditation process, and CARF recognizes and accepts its responsibility to assess and review the continuing applicability and relevance of its standards. CARF convenes its IAC; International Standards Advisory Committees (ISACs); and regional, national, and international focus groups to systematically review and revise CARF's standards and to develop standards in new areas as warranted by the needs of the field. Composed of individuals with acknowledged expertise and a broad base of experiences, including persons served, these committees and groups make recommendations to CARF concerning the adequacy and appropriateness of the standards. Individuals involved with standards development use their knowledge and expertise to inform CARF of leading clinical research, clinical practices, and leading business strategies to generate new and revised standards.

The work of these groups is a starting point in standards development and revision. Recommendations from the standards development and revision process are consolidated and made available to persons served, accredited organizations, surveyors, regulatory agencies, national professional groups, advocacy groups, third-party purchasers, and other stakeholders for review and comment.

Field review is a critical component of the CARF standards development process. Respondents do not need to be in a CARF-accredited organization to participate in field review of proposed standards. Organizations or individuals interested in participating in field reviews should contact CARF. Field reviews are generally open 2–4 weeks and are posted on the CARF website at http://www.carf.org.

The field review process is electronic. The format includes general demographic information and the proposed standards. Each proposed standard is rated on a 4-point scale (strongly agree, agree, disagree, strongly disagree). If the standard is rated disagree or strongly disagree, CARF expects to receive comments about how to improve the standard or the reasons the standard is not appropriate. If disagree or strongly disagree is designated with no feedback or suggestions, it is extremely difficult for CARF to address that dissatisfaction. The more information provided on field review, the better the standards become. Field input can range from suggested wording changes to clarify the standards to evidence supporting the addition or deletion of a standard.

Field input is reviewed by CARF, and changes are made if necessary from input received. At the completion of this standards development process, a new or revised set of standards is published and copyrighted by CARF.

THE COMMISSION ON ACCREDITATION OF REHABILITATION FACILITIES BRAIN INJURY STANDARDS

The CARF medical rehabilitation standards from 1966 focused on inpatient and outpatient programs without any specialization being noted. In the early 1980s, as brain injury groups such as the NHIF and the ACRM BI-ISIG became more active and began to address the quality issues with the plethora of developing brain injury programs, CARF began to take interest in this specialized component of medical rehabilitation. In 1984, the chief executive officer (CEO) of CARF contacted both NHIF and ACRM BI-ISIG leadership and coordinated the first brain injury standards advisory group to formulate the initial set of CARF brain injury standards. These standards were published in the 1985 *Standards Manual for Organizations Serving People With Disabilities*.

The 1985 brain injury standards applied only to brain injury inpatient programs. In 1988, the first set of postacute brain injury standards was developed. In 1991, postacute programs were redefined, and in 1992, changes included a set of brain injury standards that applied to both inpatient and community integrative programs—a new definition of community integrated programs, standards for designated pediatric brain injury programs, brain injury comprehensive inpatient standards, standards for residential services, and standards for vocational services.

Standards developed from 1988 to 1992 addressed a field that was rapidly expanding and morphing into a variety of different services and sites. When brain injury standards were reviewed in 1995, substantive changes were occurring in the field of medical rehabilitation, payment structures, and continuums in the inpatient (acute, subacute) and postacute arenas. The field of brain injury was undergoing growth pains and became the topic of many investigative news stories in the early 1990s. The for-profit industry in medical rehabilitation was rapidly expanding. CARF was experiencing major growth in many areas and at the same time settling in with a new CEO. In January 1995, CARF published the first stand-alone *CARF Medical Rehabilitation Standards Manual*. As the dust settled with multiple changes in the field and in CARF, it was determined that it was again time to revisit and revise the brain injury standards in 1996. During this review, CARF took into account the expansion of both acute and postacute brain injury programs.

In 1996, the wording *acquired brain injury* was used for the first time in the CARF standards. In the CARF Glossary, ABI is defined as:

> Acquired brain injury (ABI) is an insult to the brain that affects its structure or function, resulting in impairments of cognition, communication, physical function, or psychosocial behavior. ABI includes both traumatic and nontraumatic brain injury. Traumatic brain injuries may include open head injuries (e.g., gunshot wound, other penetrating injuries) or closed head injuries (e.g., blunt trauma, acceleration/deceleration injury, and blast injury). Nontraumatic brain injuries may include those caused by strokes, nontraumatic hemorrhage (e.g., ruptured arteriovenous malformation, aneurysm), tumors, infectious diseases (e.g., encephalitis, meningitis), hypoxic injuries (e.g., asphyxiation, near drowning, anesthetic incidents, hypovolemia), metabolic disorders (e.g., insulin shock, liver or kidney disease), and toxin exposure (e.g., inhalation, ingestion). ABI does not include brain injuries that are congenital, degenerative, or induced by birth trauma. (6) (p. 317)

In defining brain injury programs, the concept "outcomes-driven" was introduced. Outcome is defined by CARF as a result or end point of care or status achieved by a defined point following delivery of services (7). Results were beginning to be demanded by consumers as well as payers. Results of services became important factors for both consumers and payers in determining where they would receive services and how much service providers would be paid. CARF since 1973 has required organizations to be engaged with program evaluation and performance improvement. It was becoming imperative that programs be able to communicate their results and share that information with the persons they serve, their families and support systems, personnel, and key stakeholders.

The other concept introduced in the 1996 standards was the International Classification of Function (ICF) from the World Health Organization (WHO). This leading rehabilitation framework establishes the preferences of the person served as key to the development of rehabilitation services that address the total needs of the person. Standards reflect that services need to address the ICF.

In 1996, when an organization was seeking accreditation as a Brain Injury Community Integrative Program, all portions of the program (day treatment, residential, vocational, etc.) that an organization provided were to be included in the application and the site survey. This was an important change brought forth by consumer input. This was the first time that CARF required that if the organization provided the program and met the CARF program definition, the organization must seek accreditation for those programs. Consumers were very clear that if an organization provided the service, it should not be allowed to opt out of seeking accreditation for 1 or more components of the continuum that the organization offered.

The 1996 standards advisory committee also developed 2 levels of standards for children and adolescents. The first level identified programs that occasionally saw children or adolescents. The second level identified designated pediatric brain injury programs.

In 1997, CARF developed a new rating system to rate standards conformance during a survey. The rating system is a 4-point scale of conformance. The standards use the following scale: 0 = nonconformance, 1 = partial conformance, 2 = conformance, and 3 = exemplary. Standards are unidimensional (one component reviewed at a time) to facilitate accurate rating of conformance. This allows organizations to better understand what specific components of a standard they still need to improve on. Consistency of the use of the phrase *person served* also became mandatory throughout the CARF manuals in 1997.

The 1996 brain injury standards remained in use until June 2000. The year 2000 set of brain injury standards introduced the importance of case management and the development of a full continuum of brain injury programs and services.

The next major change occurred in 2008 when the *CARF Medical Rehabilitation Standards Manual* was reorganized. The brain injury program definition stayed the same, but 5 locations and/or components of brain injury services were defined. These 5 are comprehensive integrated inpatient rehabilitation, which can be offered in a freestanding rehabilitation hospital, a unit within a larger entity, a skilled nursing facility, and/or a long-term acute hospital; outpatient medical rehabilitation (single service or interdisciplinary); home and community services; residential rehabilitation; and vocational services.

Brain injury program standards can be applied to any of these components, and if they are offered by the organization and the organization meets the program description of these components, they must seek accreditation in them. An organization may also apply the specialty brain injury standards to the case management standards.

The field of brain injury has matured and changed over the 26 years that CARF has developed, revised, and maintained brain injury standards. The brain injury standards reflect the systematic reviews of cognitive rehabilitation, development of more research and professional consensus of clinical practice, and the sophistication of consumer and payer demands. The first set of brain injury standards from 1985 had 23 standards to meet and only inpatient programs could seek accreditation. In contrast, the 2012 standards reflect a full continuum of brain injury programs/services. An adult brain injury program would now meet more than 124 standards.

The most recent revision of CARF's brain injury standards occurred in February 2012 when an ISAC met. The ISAC's work will be submitted to the IAC, which includes BIAA and ACRM BI-ISIG, as well as professional groups such as American Speech Language and Hearing Association (ASHA), American Physical Therapy Association (APTA), American Psychological Association (APA), American Occupational Therapy Association (AOTA), Association of Rehabilitation Nurses (ARN), American Academy of Physical Medicine and Rehabilitation (AAPMR), and American Academy of Neurology (AAN) among its members. These groups will receive the ISAC work and submit it to their constituents for review before there is general field review. In this phase of the standards revision process, substantive changes can occur prior to general field review.

THE COMMISSION ON ACCREDITATION OF REHABILITATION FACILITIES ACCREDITATION AND USING THE STANDARDS

Achieving CARF accreditation involves demonstrating conformance to standards of quality in the provision of programs and services as evidenced through observable practices, verifiable results over time, and comprehensive supporting documentation. To determine conformance to the CARF standards, CARF peer surveyors

- observe the environment and interactions among staff members, management, and the persons served;
- conduct interviews with persons served, personnel, and other stakeholders;
- study the organization's policies and procedures;
- observe practices and service provision;
- review documentation; and
- provide consultation.

The role of the CARF peer surveyor is not that of an inspector or auditor, but rather a consultant. The goal is not only to gather and assess information to determine conformance to the standards but also to assist the organization in improving its programs and services and its business operations. The entire CARF accreditation process is focused on continuous improvement of the organization, programs, and service delivery.

Brain injury organizations that seek accreditation must demonstrate conformance to a variety of standards. The first section of standards is the ASPIRE to Excellence standards, which apply to all organizations seeking CARF accreditation. Since CARF's inception in 1966, the standards have focused not just only on clinical/service practices but also on running the organization using robust business and performance improvement models. CARF's ASPIRE to Excellence model crosswalks with International Organization for Standardization (ISO) 9001, Six Sigma, LEAN, and Baldrige criteria. The advantage for brain injury service providers is that the language of the CARF standards reflects the daily practices of brain injury service providers as well as the concepts of most modern quality frameworks. Many CARF-accredited organizations use multiple systems (CARF, ISO, Baldrige, etc.). Providers using more than 1 quality system express that the CARF standards make the intentions of the quality framework become practical in the provision of services, make sense to personnel on all levels of the organization, and require them to look at their results and not just their processes.

The ASPIRE to Excellence business model includes the structure of leadership and governance; development and use of an integrated strategic planning process; and dynamic listening to the individuals, the organization served, personnel, and stakeholders to analyze and use ideas and thoughts in organizational functions. The listening process engages all parties in a sense of shared future that promotes long-term organizational excellence.

The organization demonstrates compliance with legal requirements; financial planning and management; human resource requirements that promote the competency of staff and their performance reviews; an active risk management plan; a healthy and safe environment for persons served, personnel, and stakeholders; and a strong technology plan. The rights of the persons served and the promotion and practice of these rights is a critical component of the ASPIRE standards. CARF standards promote the removal of all barriers for persons served, personnel, and stakeholders in the key domains of architecture, environment, attitude, communication, financial, transportation, community integration, and any other area where anyone from the key groups (persons served, personnel, or stakeholders) identifies a barrier. This is a dynamic process that is also linked with reducing potential risks and improving performance.

The last 2 sections of the ASPIRE standards cover establishing and measuring key performance indicators in business and clinical practices. It also sets the stage to review data collected with the filters of reliability, validity, completeness, and accuracy. CARF standards require an organization to establish targets for their performance and measure against them. If targets are not met, performance improvement plans are developed and implemented. Performance measurement is repeated to see if improvement is gained. There is no finish line with quality, only the raising of the bar for the delivery of optimal quality. CARF standards require organizations to be transparent with their results and share this information with persons served, personnel, and stakeholders in meaningful ways.

Brain injury programs that are CARF accredited should be able to share their results using a variety of mechanisms. This can be done via web, handouts, charts, focus groups, newsletters, one-on-one discussions, town hall meetings, residential councils, staff meetings, and so on.

The second section of CARF standards, applied to all medical rehabilitation programs, is "The rehabilitation and service process for the persons served." This section devotes itself to standards that formulate the day-to-day process of providing case-managed care for persons in medical rehabilitation programs. It addresses scope of services, admission, transition and discharge criteria, the role of the interdisciplinary team, communication and collaboration of the team, education and training for persons served and families/support systems, equipment, supplies, physical plant, behavior programs, medical records, conferencing, and a variety of other topics related to the rehabilitation process.

The third section of CARF standards includes the specific location standards (e.g., residential rehabilitation) and the specific diagnostic category standards (e.g., brain injury).

BENEFITS OF THE COMMISSION ON ACCREDITATION OF REHABILITATION FACILITIES ACCREDITATION—WHY SEEK ACCREDITATION?

CARF accreditation affords many benefits to an organization, consumers, payers, and regulators of services, including the following:

- Identification as an organization meeting internationally developed standards in the provision of quality services.
- Assurance to persons seeking services that a provider meets internationally accepted standards.
- Assurance to funding sources, referral agencies, payers, regulators, other providers, and the community of the quality of programs and services provided.
- Standards based on and integrating a quality framework for business and service delivery.
- Guidance for providing high-quality services focused on the persons served that emphasize an integrated and individualized approach to services and outcomes.
- An independent, external review to identify strengths and areas for improvement based on objective program expectations and guidelines.
- Consultation and education focused on integration of business functions with service delivery.
- Guidance for responsible management that promotes active, dynamic planning focused on
  - positive outcomes for persons served and other stakeholders,
  - the impact of strategies on persons served and key stakeholders, and
  - organizational development of existing or new services to meet the needs and expectations of the community served.
- Enhanced safety and risk management.
- Increased funding and reimbursement opportunities created by stronger relationships and partnership with purchasers and regulatory bodies.
- Practices that demonstrate
  - accountability,
  - positive outcomes,
  - a person-centered and interdisciplinary approach to service delivery,
  - teamwork within the organization,
  - ongoing professional growth of personnel,
  - networking with other providers and resources,
  - comprehensive financial management, and
  - an overall focus on service to the persons served.
- Techniques for designing and implementing organizational and financial systems that are efficient, cost-effective, and based on outcomes and satisfaction of the persons served and other stakeholders.
- Evidence of practice and performance that can be used in
  - marketing programs and services to consumers, referral sources, and third-party funders;
  - seeking grants;
  - public education; and
  - advocacy activities.
- Involvement of the persons served as active participants in planning, selecting, evaluating, and improving the services provided.
- Improved communication with personnel, persons served, and other stakeholders.
- Support from CARF through consultation, publications, conferences, training opportunities, and newsletters.
- Participation in insurance programs that offer discounted premiums to eligible providers.

- Access to free courses for persons served and personnel through EditU, a consortium of public and private partners that include IBM, SkillSoft, the Association of Rehabilitation Programs in Computer Technology (ARPCT), the National Science Foundation, the Educational Leadership, Research and Technology Department at Western Michigan University, and CARF.

INFLUENCE OF ACCREDITATION ON ORGANIZATIONAL IMPROVEMENT

In September 2011, the British Columbia Ministry of Children and Family Development, Modeling, Evaluation, and Analysis Branch published the *Review of the Ministry of Children and Family Development's Accreditation Program*. The ministry requires accreditation. When evaluating the influence of accreditation at the operational level, respondents used a 4-point scale (not at all, slightly, moderately, a great deal) to describe the extent to which they thought accreditation had influenced areas related to the operations of the agency. These included areas addressing communication of the vision, mission and values of the agency, organizational planning, resource allocation, staff engagement in service decisions, efforts to improve service quality, client rights, health and safety, and risk mitigation. Only 4% or fewer of the respondents indicated that they did not know the extent to which accreditation had influenced the agency in all of the areas related to operations. Of those who felt they knew, 60% or more indicated that, in all of the areas listed, accreditation had influenced the agency moderately or a great deal. The study found that 56% thought accreditation had a great deal of influence on the agency in terms of collecting and analyzing client outcome and client satisfaction data for the purpose of improving the quality of programs and services. Another 53% indicated that accreditation had a great deal of influence in terms of the agency having a structured process that collects and analyzes data for the purpose of improving quality as a system. These were the 2 areas of operations in which the highest number of participants thought accreditation had a great deal of influence (8).

The CARF Performance Report measures a variety of indicators of its performance ranging from "Why did you choose to seek or maintain CARF accreditation?" to "Involvement with CARF helped improved organization's performance." Results in 2010 from provider surveys are included in Tables 6-1 and 6-2 (9).

Other results from the 2011 CARF Performance Report include 97.3% state that the on-site survey was a beneficial process, 91% state that the on-site consultation was helpful, and 97.3% state that the recommendations in the survey report gave adequate guidance to address areas needing improvement.

Although CARF has many successes, some organizations choose to drop their accreditation. The attrition rate in 2010 was 5.6% across all of CARF's business units. In medical rehabilitation, the top 3 reasons for dropping accreditation were merged with another accredited organization, change in organization's funding/resources, and program closed (10). These reasons are difficult to address because closures

TABLE 6–1 Statistical Report on Accreditation Surveys and Organizational Characteristics Standards Manual Year 2010 (July 2010–June 2011)

WHY DID YOU CHOOSE TO SEEK OR MAINTAIN CARF ACCREDITATION?	N	PERCENT OF TOTAL RESPONSES
Accreditation process	341	56.3%
Belief in accreditation	374	61.7%
CARF's reputation	282	46.5%
CARF fits us best	304	50.2%
History with CARF	295	48.7%
Cost	72	11.9%
Hallmark of quality	232	38.3%
Help sell our business	141	23.3%
Mandated	233	38.4%
Required for funding	264	43.6%
Other	41	6.8%

Abbreviations: CARF, Commission on Accreditation of Rehabilitation Facilities; N, total number of participants.

and mergers are out of CARF's control. CARF addresses changes in funding and resources by working with payers and governmental agencies on the importance of quality rehabilitation programs that are CARF accredited.

CARF also sees many organizations that drop their accreditation return. The range for return is from 6 months to 32 years after the organization's last survey. Reasons stated include administration now supports CARF accreditation; when no longer CARF accredited, quality of services not maintained; not competitive with local market; and no external review has lessened demand for change in practice (11).

THE COMMISSION ON ACCREDITATION OF REHABILITATION FACILITIES-ACCREDITED BRAIN INJURY ORGANIZATIONS

More than 900 brain injury organizations seek CARF accreditation, including for-profit and nonprofit corporations; sole proprietorships; small businesses; individual service providers; partnerships; coalitions; units of larger entities; private

TABLE 6–2 Statistical Report on Accreditation Surveys and Organizational Characteristics Standards Manual Year 2010 (July 2010–June 2011)

INVOLVEMENT WITH CARF HAS HELP IMPROVED PERFORMANCE	N	PERCENT OF TOTAL RESPONSES
Customer/consumer relations	249	41.1%
Documentation/policies and procedures	489	80.7%
Health and safety	424	70.0%
Information management	276	45.5%
Performance improvement activities	394	65.0%
Provided direction for improvement	359	59.2%
Rehab process/program	99	16.3%
Other	53	8.7%

Abbreviation: N, total number of participants.

and governmental entities; local, city, and county service organizations; educational institutions; health centers; and networks of service providers.

Each type of organization may have special considerations and questions in preparing for accreditation. Achieving accreditation is easier when an organization prepares systematically for the CARF survey. An introduction to and an overview of the accreditation process is provided subsequently.

Step 1: Consult with a designated CARF resource specialist.

An organization contacts CARF and a resource specialist is designated to provide guidance and technical assistance.

- For an organization preparing for its first survey, it is important to make this contact early in the process. The resource specialist is available to answer questions in preparation for a survey and throughout the tenure of the accreditation.
- For an organization preparing for a resurvey, the designated resource specialist may already be known. It is suggested that contact still be made early in the reaccreditation process to update relevant organizational or program information.
- The resource specialist provides the organization access to Customer Connect—CARF's secure website for transmitting documents and maintaining ongoing communication with accredited organizations and organizations seeking accreditation.
- The organization orders the standards manual in which its programs and services best fit. Visit http://www.carf.org/catalog.
- The organization maintains ongoing contact with CARF for assistance.

Step 2: Conduct a self-evaluation.

The organization conducts a self-study and evaluation of its conformance to the standards using the standards manual and its companion publication, the survey preparation workbook. The self-evaluation is part of the organization's internal preparation process and is not submitted to CARF.

Step 3: Submit the intent to survey.

The organization submits the intent to survey via Customer Connect.

- The intent to survey requests detailed information about leadership, programs, and services that the organization is seeking to accredit and the service delivery location(s).
- The organization submits the intent to survey, required supporting documents, and a nonrefundable intent fee at least 3 full calendar months before the 2-month time frame in which it is requesting a survey. Organizations undergoing resurvey submit their intent to survey on the date that corresponds with their accreditation expiration month.
- The submission of the completed intent to survey indicates the organization's desire for the survey and its agreement to all terms and conditions contained therein.
- If any information in the intent to survey changes after submission, CARF should be notified immediately.

Step 4: CARF invoices for the survey fees.

After reviewing all information, CARF invoices the organization for the survey fee.

- The fee is based on the number of surveyors and days needed to complete the survey.
- Scheduling of the survey begins immediately on invoicing. Any changes in problem dates must be communicated in writing to CARF by this time.

Step 5: CARF selects the survey team.
CARF selects a survey team with the appropriate expertise.

- Surveyors are selected by matching their program or administrative expertise and relevant field experience with the organization's unique requirements.
- CARF notifies the organization of the names of team members and the dates of the survey at least 30 days before the survey.

Step 6: The survey team conducts the survey.
The survey team determines the organization's conformance to all applicable standards on site through observation of services, interviews with persons served and other stakeholders, and review of documentation.

- Surveyors also provide consultation to organization personnel.
- The organization is informed of the survey team's findings related to the standards at an exit conference before the team leaves the site. The survey team submits its findings to CARF, but the team does not determine the accreditation decision.

Step 7: CARF renders the accreditation decision.
CARF reviews the survey findings and renders one of the following accreditation decisions:

- 3-year accreditation
- 1-year accreditation
- provisional accreditation
- nonaccreditation

Approximately 6–8 weeks after the survey, the organization is notified of the accreditation decision and receives a written report. The organization is also awarded a certificate of accreditation that lists the programs and services included in the accreditation award.
Step 8: Submit a quality improvement plan (QIF).
Within 90 days after notification of an accreditation award, the organization fulfills an accreditation condition by submitting to CARF a QIP outlining the actions that have been or will be taken in response to the areas identified in the report.
Step 9: Submit the annual conformance to quality reports (ACQRs).
An organization that achieves a 3-year accreditation award submits a signed ACQR to CARF on the accreditation anniversary date in each of the 2 years following the award. This is a condition of accreditation.

- CARF sends the organization the form for this report approximately 10 weeks before it is due.
- The ACQR reaffirms the organization's ongoing conformance to the CARF standards.

Step 10: CARF maintains contact with the organization.

CARF maintains contact with the organization during the tenure of accreditation. Organizations are also encouraged to contact CARF as needed to help maintain conformance to the CARF standards.

- CARF offers publications to help organizations provide quality programs and services.
- CARF's public website, http://www.carf.org, and its secure customer website, Customer Connect, provide news, information, and resources.
- CARF seminars and conferences are excellent ways to receive updates and other information about the accreditation process and the standards.

INTERNATONAL MARKETS

CARF has a long history of working with organizations in different countries to prepare for surveys and accreditation. CARF accreditation in Canada dates back to 1969 and now includes a wide spectrum of programs and services, including brain injury programs. In 2002, the CARF Canada office was opened in Edmonton, Alberta and soon after an office in Ontario, first in Ottawa, and later moved to Toronto.

CARF has developed accreditation opportunities that meet the unique needs of Canadian providers. Some provincial government organizations in Canada use CARF accreditation as a tool to assess the quality of providers. Workers' Compensation Boards in some provinces mandate CARF accreditation for specialty programs in brain injury that are community based. Canadian third-party payers also are exploring and using accreditation to assist in assessing the effectiveness and efficiency of providers. The fields of human services and technology have made the world a smaller place and CARF continues to expand its accreditation borders. Since 1996, CARF has accredited a growing number of organizations and programs outside of North America. The first brain injury program to become accredited outside of North America was the Comprehensive Inpatient Program, which was accredited in 1996 in Lund, Sweden at the University of Lund. In 2010, CARF-accredited organizations and programs included providers in Europe, the Middle East, Africa, Southeast Asia, and South America.

There is an increased interest from the international community to review and participate in CARF activities. CARF regularly conducts training sessions in Europe and elsewhere to meet the growing demand for accreditation information. Individuals from the international community participate in CARF standards development and contribute to a global emphasis on quality service provision.

Brain injury service providers are currently accredited in England, Ireland, Northern Ireland, Denmark, Sweden, Norway, New Zealand, and Saudi Arabia. Brain injury providers are preparing for a CARF survey in Spain, Italy, France, and Australia.

CARF's work in international markets has demonstrated that the differences in services are minor and the processes of person-centered services, good business practices, outcomes management systems, and performance improvement are global in scope. CARF is committed to continuing its work with international communities that embrace quality and demonstrate value for all persons served. For international brain injury service providers, the use of standards can be a tool to assist with the development of continuums of care for brain injury services, establish links with providers outside of their countries to increase learning opportunities, and establish partnerships and collaborations for research and clinical practice.

International providers have many reasons for seeking CARF accreditation. Most are related to the intrinsic value of the accreditation process to the development of their programs and organizational structures. These providers continually state that peer review, consultation, and the ability to participate in the revision of the standards are critical components.

There are few external requirements to seek CARF accreditation internationally. The Swedish Physical Rehabilitation and Medicine physicians have recommended that rehabilitation providers should be CARF accredited. Ireland, in its newest neuro-rehab strategy, recommends that neuro-rehab service providers seek CARF accreditation. In the United Kingdom, the Care Quality Commission (CQC) has put out a request for a quality system for community-based providers, including ones that serve the brain injury population.

Some countries with no-fault insurance have contacted CARF to explore potential acceptances or mandates. A uniqueness of the international market is that there may be only 1or 2 rehabilitation hospitals or limited community-based providers in a country, so there are few providers to seek accreditation. In countries outside of the United States, there is an eagerness to be part of an international network of similar providers, have outside review and consultation, and develop a continuum of services. The ability to tap into multiple resources is the driver for seeking accreditation outside of the United States.

CARF is committed to ensuring that all surveyors who travel internationally are well prepared and educated about the markets they will be surveying. Surveyors from other countries who conduct surveys in the United States also are provided with information to assist them in the survey process. There are more than 1,500 peer review CARF surveyors. These surveyors represent 9 countries.

SURVEYORS

Individuals who are selected, trained, and assigned to conduct site surveys for CARF are designated as surveyors. They are selected based on their professional experience, expertise, and program leadership. CARF surveyors are committed to the principle that accreditation is essential in ensuring that organizations offer programs and services of demonstrated value to the persons served. Surveyors are employees of CARF only during the survey process. They pursue other professional endeavors during the remainder of their time. As a condition of their continuing roles as CARF surveyors, they are required to maintain the highest standards of ethical conduct and to participate in continuing education sessions. Either while a surveyor is on site or after the survey, any questions the organization may have about the conduct of a surveyor or the survey process should be directed to CARF.

The role of a CARF surveyor is consultative while applying the standards. He or she encourages the organization in its efforts, asks questions to help generate new ideas, provides information, and makes suggestions for improvement.

A CARF surveyor is not an inspector or auditor and does not tell the organization what to do. There are many ways to achieve conformance to the standards, and the CARF surveyor will support an organization's originality in discovering ways to apply the standards that fit the particular organization.

Currently, there are more than 1,500 CARF surveyors throughout all 50 states, Canada, Europe, South America, and the Middle East. They have expertise in all program and service areas in which CARF accredits. CARF surveyors are expected to conduct at least 3 surveys each year. All surveyors receive ongoing feedback from fellow surveyors, CARF, and the organizations surveyed. To stay current with the standards and CARF's procedures, surveyors are also required to participate in continuing education provided by CARF.

Persons interested in becoming CARF surveyors should check the CARF website for more information and to request an application. Each applicant is required to submit several items, including a résumé and professional references. After all required materials have been received, the candidate is considered for acceptance into the pool of applicants. If an applicant is accepted into the pool, CARF keeps the individual's file active for up to 2 years. Many factors, including the needs of CARF for surveyors with certain expertise, the expertise of the applicant, and the location of the applicant, are considered when inviting applicants from the pool to attend surveyor training.

CONCLUSION

CARF International is the accreditor of choice for providers around the world working with individuals with ABIs. More than 900 CARF-accredited brain injury service providers are motivated to enhance the lives of individuals with ABI who are receiving services in many treatment settings. They provide and improve their business and clinical practices though a peer review, on-site survey process. CARF recognizes the dedication and quest for excellence of all CARF-accredited programs. CARF encourages all brain injury providers to interact with CARF and the standards development process to improve, revise, and update brain injury practices to reflect the needs of consumers, providers, payers, and government agencies. CARF looks forward to future collaborations with experts in the field of brain injury around the world to continue to enhance the lives of persons with ABIs.

KEY CLINICAL POINTS

1. CARF focuses on development of quality systems for health and human service providers.
2. CARF standards are developed by the field of brain injury to ensure relevance of the accreditation survey process.
3. CARF standards are guides for good business practices and good clinical practice.
4. CARF accreditation brings benefits to providers as supported by feedback from accredited providers.
5. CARF has an international presence that continues to expand and is being recognized by government officials and payer groups outside of North America.

KEY REFERENCES

1. Commission on Accreditation of Rehabilitation Facilities. *Accreditation Sourcebook*. Commission on Accreditation of Rehabilitation Facilities; 2012.
2. Commission on Accrediation of Rehabilitation Facilities. *CARF Medical Rehabilitation Standards Manual*. Commission on Accreditation of Rehabilitation Facilities; 2012.
3. http://www.carf.org
4. http://www.uspeq.org

References

1. Nicklin WL, McLellan T, Robblee JA. Aim for excellence: integrating accreditation standards into the continuous quality improvement framework. *Healthc Q*. 2004;7(4):44–48.
2. Pomey MP, Contandriopoulus AP, Francois P, Bertrand D. Accreditation: a tool for organizational change in hospitals? *Int J Health Care Qual Assur Inc Leadersh Health Serv*. 2004;17(3):113–124.
3. Jacobson JM. The effect of external accreditation on perceived rehabilitation program, quality, physical medicine and rehabilitation. *VACO Newsletter*. June, 2003:8–9.
4. Bates R. *Reframing the "A" Word: Front Line Worker Perceptions of Organizational Change and Personal Transitions Through the Process of Child and Family Services Accreditation* [master's thesis]. 2005. Available at: http://hdl.handle.net/1828/858. Accessed July 2011.
5. Secretary General of the Department of Health, Chief Executive Officer of the Health Service Executive. *National Policy and Strategy for the Provision of Neuro-rehabilitation Services in Ireland 2011–2015*. Dublin, Ireland: Minister for Health; 2011:91.
6. Commission on Accreditation of Rehabilitation Facilities. Glossary. In: *CARF Medical Rehabilitation Standards Manual*. Commission on Accreditation of Rehabilitation Facilities; 2012:317.
7. Commission on Accreditation of Rehabilitation Facilities. Glossary. In: *CARF Medical Rehabilitation Standards Manual*. Commission on Accreditation of Rehabilitation Facilities; 2012:325.
8. Ministry of Children and Family Development: Modeling, Evaluation and Analysis Branch. *A Review of the Ministry of Children and Family Development's Accreditation Program: Final Report*. British Columbia, Canada: Ministry of Children and Family Development; 2011:37.
9. Commission on Accreditation of Rehabilitation Facilities. *2010 CARF Performance Report*. Commission on Accreditation of Rehabilitation Facilities; 2011:87–90.
10. Commission on Accreditation of Rehabilitation Facilities. *CARF Survey Attrition Report Q4 2011*. Commission on Accreditation of Rehabilitation Facilities; 2012:1–2.
11. Commission on Accreditation of Rehabilitation Facilities. *CARF Survey Attrition Report Q4 2011*. Commission on Accreditation of Rehabilitation Facilities; 2012:5–6.

Conducting Research in Traumatic Brain Injury: Current Concepts and Issues

Amy K. Wagner

INTRODUCTION

The National Center for Injury Prevention and Control (NCIPC) suggests that injuries have a substantial impact on the lives of individual Americans, their families, and society. The consequences of injuries can be extensive and wide ranging. They are physical, emotional, and financial; in the case of disabling injuries, the consequences are enduring (1). Traumatic brain injury (TBI) is no exception to these consequences. Approximately 1.4 million TBIs occur each year in the United States (2). It has been well established that TBI causes chronic debilitation and functional loss over a lifetime. Unlike other disease processes with later onset, survivors of TBI often have many decades of productive life loss, costing themselves, their families, and society much with loss of the capability for competitive employment and other meaningful community roles. An estimated 5.3 million Americans, or 2% of the population, currently live with disabilities resulting from brain injury. The costs of TBI in the United States, including direct medical costs and lost productivity, were estimated to total $60 billion in 2000 (3). Injury is the leading cause of years of potential life lost before age 65 years, and TBI is responsible for a greater proportion of this mortality rate than most other types of injury (1). For survivors, TBI often results in cognitive, behavioral, emotional, and physical functioning deficits. Impairments within these domains can be a persistent and debilitating problem. Mild TBI is often undiagnosed, making the public health burden even larger than reported estimates indicate.

The magnitude of TBI-related public health burden mandates that TBI researchers delineate the contributing mechanisms of injury and recovery, evaluate and implement effective treatments, and accurately prognosticate outcome with effective assessment tools. In the population with TBI, patients can have markedly different outcomes, despite similarities in the extent of the initial insult and in type of clinical management. Additionally, the population sustaining TBI is diverse, and a broad and complex range of internal and external factors can influence injury and recovery. These factors make accurate prognostication, sensitive outcome assessment, and effective conduct of clinical trials and comparative effectiveness studies challenging issues in TBI research. To date, there is a paucity of proven interventions that significantly reduce morbidity and mortality or improve recovery

and quality of life. Mechanisms of injury, neuroplasticity, and recovery are not fully understood, and outcome prognostication is unrefined. In this chapter, we discuss unique issues with conducting research in the population with TBI and appropriate outcome assessment in this population. We also highlight the importance of translational research and preclinical trials, evaluate challenges with conducting clinical trial and comparative effectiveness research (CER) in this population, and outline issues with statistical approach and research design. Finally, we will discuss contemporary trends and new directions for the field of TBI research.

UNIQUE ASPECTS ASSOCIATED WITH TBI RESEARCH

TBI is a complex disease involving both primary (focal and diffuse injuries) and secondary injury, with secondary injury involving complex biochemical cascades that lead to excitotoxicity (4–6), brain swelling (7), loss of cerebral blood flow autoregulation (8), oxidative injury (9,10), inflammation (11,12), and cellular necrosis and apoptosis (13,14). Overlaid on this complex myriad of pathophysiological cascades are the influences of genetic makeup, and other premorbid and demographic characteristics that can influence the extent of injury or recovery. Further, there is variability in the type and intensity of both acute and rehabilitation care that patients may receive. These factors are often influenced by treatment location, social supports, and payor source (15–17). The multidisciplinary approach to therapies also creates issues in understanding what components of the rehabilitation process are crucial in improving a particular individual's recovery course. All of the differences in injury variables, personal characteristics, and treatments outlined earlier can create variability in recovery from TBI. This variability creates unique challenges for researchers in TBI to tease out the important mechanisms associated with injury and recovery, identify appropriate and effective therapeutic targets, and accurately prognosticate outcome.

RESEARCHING THE POPULATION WITH TRAUMATIC BRAIN INJURY

Researching the population with TBI poses other unique methodological challenges to researchers regarding recruitment, diagnostic criteria, subject grouping and population characteristics, and follow-up. Biases with recruitment may introduce other systematic bias into the study population. One study evaluated this issue in mild TBI by comparing demographic, premorbid, and injury-related characteristics of their population. Those who had more severe injuries, who were hospitalized, and who had a significant additional major injury were more likely to consent to participate in the study (18). In studies requiring the evaluation of patients who are unable to consent themselves for enrollment in a research study and/or the immediate implementation of a treatment intervention, obtaining consent can be a challenging issue that impacts recruitment and study design. A multicenter trial investigated the efficacy of early hypothermia treatment implemented within the first 6 hours from injury for patients with severe TBI. At the beginning of the study, informed consent was required for each study patient. During the course of the study, federal regulations change to allow waived informed consent. Post-hoc analysis of this study population showed that with waived inform consent, time to randomization and treatment implementation decreased, patient accrual increased, and minority representation in the study population increased (19). Since then, other studies have incorporated a waiver of consent process as a part of their study design (20).

There are several criteria and scoring systems for classifying degree or severity of mild TBI. Concussion severity nomenclature has been developed for the purposes of injury characterization and injury management (21–23), but the definitions and criteria for mild injury vary across scales. Also, the types of symptoms, proportion of patients who have persistent symptoms, and the duration of symptoms required to define symptoms as persistent vary (24). From a research perspective, the variation in clinical definitions and terminology present challenges regarding grouping subjects for treatment/analyses and for generalizing and relating findings to clinical care. In the populations with moderate-to-severe injury, the Glasgow Coma Scale is a key measure for grouping subjects for treatment intervention studies (20) as well as prognosis (25,26). However, recent reviews support the inclusion of other or additional approaches for TBI grouping or classification strategies such as those that incorporate molecular markers as well as other constructs like subject symptomatology, pathoanatomic criteria, and prognostic markers (27). In TBI rehabilitation, markers of activity, participation, and functional status may be particularly relevant to use as grouping variables within the research design.

Systematic biases may be introduced into a clinical data set through loss to follow-up, an inherent problem when conducting research in the population with TBI. One study evaluating loss to follow-up using a variety of data sets, including a single-center, multicenter, and statewide surveillance data set, found a loss to follow-up rate of approximately 37% and 58% 1 year and 2 years after injury respectively. Additionally, there was a selective bias to lose those who were socioeconomically disadvantaged, with violent etiologies of injury, and with a history of substance abuse (28). Systematic bias with loss to follow-up can significantly decrease the generalizability of study findings and potentially confound apparent treatment efficacy with clinical trials. Response bias, regarding effort, comorbidity influ-

ences, secondary gain, and proxy variability response can also impact the veracity of the data collected from those who do follow-up.

A myriad of variables, including patient comorbidities and complications (15,29), gender (30–32) cognitive reserve (33), injury severity (30,33,34), injury-type (35–38) minority status (39), social supports (40), and acute discharge location (15) may all influence outcomes. Also, payor status may influence rehabilitation services received (41). Additionally, patient recovery can occur over a prolonged period (42–44), and outcome assessment may vary with the type of individual (patient, caregiver, clinician) interviewed (45). More recently, blast-induced TBI has received increased attention as a common phenomenon impacting military populations, and the mechanisms of this injury and its associated deficits, as well as risk for repetitive injury and concomitant post-traumatic stress disorder (PTSD), create unique issues with researching this population with TBI (46–50). Each of these issues must be considered carefully when designing studies. The appropriate use of covariate analysis, including time variables for longitudinal studies and stratification, is often necessary to avoid confounders obscuring research results. Time postinjury is also an important consideration when designing clinical trials to minimize the effects of natural recovery on the apparent treatment effect.

OUTCOME ASSESSMENT TOOLS IN TBI RESEARCH

The World Health Organization (WHO) has provided widely accepted definitions of impairment, disability, and handicap that have resulted in a conceptual framework by which worldwide research has been conducted, investigating the impact of injury and illness on individual function (51). This system has been replaced by the International Classification of Functioning, Disability and Health (ICF) (52), providing an updated framework for rehabilitation research, including information regarding body function, ability to perform activities, and social participation (53). Several TBI assessments measure outcome within more than one of these domains. Commonly used TBI outcome assessments vary in scope and mode of measurement. An ICF core set of outcomes for TBI is being developed, particularly within European rehabilitation and research communities for use in tracking patient outcomes (54). Some widely used outcome assessments are general and designed to provide a global index of outcome, (e.g., Glasgow Outcome Scale-Extended [GOS-E] [55], Disability Rating Scale [DRS] [56]). Others are meant to measure functional abilities for daily activities (Functional Independence Measure [FIM] [57]) or community integration (Community Integration Questionnaire [CIQ] [58]). Assessments may also focus on quality of life (42,59,60), caregiver needs (61,62), whereas others focus specifically on neuropsychological performance (43) or psychiatric dysfunction (63,64). The *Patient Health Questionnaire* (PHQ-9) is a brief depression measure that is derived from the *Diagnostic and Statistical Manual of Mental Disorders* (*DSM-IV*) criteria for major depressive disorder and has been specifically validated for TBI (65–67). Validation of this measure for the TBI population include specialized criteria to ensure that subjects classified as depressed have symptoms across several DSM categories (66). Finally, measurement tools may target specific populations, such as those with mild TBI (68). Increasingly, computerized assessment tools evaluating neuropsychological functioning are gaining increasing attention for both clinical care and research, particularly for those at risk for repetitive injury. However, caution should be used in understanding their limitations regarding test–retest reliability and the validity of generalized use across populations that include a broad range of injury severity (69–71).

Outcomes assessment is an important aspect of TBI rehabilitation research. However, studies often published in rehabilitation journals do not report the validity and reliability of the outcome measures used (72). Variable definitions and operationalization, as well as associated social values and target population, can be difficult to address when developing new or using existing TBI outcomes assessments (73). Multimodal assessments are often necessary to effectively reflect the complex range of factors affecting TBI outcome. Yet, no single measurement tool can encompass all relevant areas of TBI outcome. Additionally, there are limitations with the collection and analysis of many existing measurements. There are ceiling effects associated with some measures as individuals with TBI improve over time (74,75), and some outcome measures have a limited ability to measure group differences in function over long evaluation intervals (76). Attention to cultural-, minority-, age-, and gender-related differences in response range for outcome assessments should also be considered when selecting assessments and interpreting results (77–81). Some measures, including FIM (82) and CIQ (58,83) have been validated for administration over the telephone, but many other measures have not been validated for multiple modes of administration, despite their widespread use in this manner. In part to address some of these difficulties, the National Institutes of Health (NIH) has been working in concert with multiple institutes at the NIH, several offices that comprise the NIH Blueprint for Neuroscience Research, as well as other federal funding agencies like the National Institute on Disability and Rehabilitation Research (NIDRR) and the NIH Toolbox initiative. This initiative seeks generate and compile a comprehensive set of assessment tools that can be used by both clinicians and researchers to measure outcomes in longitudinal cohort studies as well as with clinical trial and comparative effectiveness studies across the life span (84). Other groups have proposed a battery of common data elements for TBI research studies in order to better pool data for meta-analyses and to compare treatment effects across multiple studies (85,86). As TBI research includes evaluation and study of injury related complications (e.g., seizures), the incorporation of available common data elements for these related conditions may also be useful to compare and contrast these conditions to those found in the uninjured population (87).

Choosing an appropriate primary outcome measure is of critical importance when designing clinical trials, selecting a proposed treatment effect size, and for developing effective models for prognostication. Appropriate and well-validated outcome measures are often most effective when they target a population with a varied demographic profile and broad range of injury severity, are able to accurately place subjects in appropriate outcome categories at given time intervals, and are sensitive to change over time. For clinical trials, the

GOS-E has gained popularity as a primary outcome assessment tool and is thought to be more sensitive than the standard GOS (55). However, the *Functional Status Examination* (FSE) is a well-validated newer instrument that has been used in long-term studies for the population with moderate and severe TBI (42,88). Its measurement properties are linked with other constructs such as family burden, depression, and satisfaction with functioning that make it an effective multimodal assessment (42) that could also be considered when designing clinical studies.

More recently, outcomes focused on neuropsychological domains of cognitive functioning are being developed (89) and may complement the use of other functional or global outcomes batteries. In addition to the assessment of individual neuropsychological tests and scales, cognitive composite scores are being more frequently used as an overall index of cognitive functioning or function within a specific range of neuropsychological domains (90). Recently, cognitive composite methods have been incorporated into large multicentered research designs (91). Effort, malingering, exaggeration, somatization, concurrent affective disorders, pain, and stress can influence neuropsychological testing performance (92). Although these issues are commonly considered regarding testing interpretation and clinical patient management, these issues potentially may also present themselves as confounds when administering these tests for research.

The cognitive impairments of persons with TBI often make the use of proxies for outcome assessment and evaluation attractive. However, self-awareness of deficits for people with TBI (93) and participant-proxy differences in disability perceptions and quality of life (94) may preclude participant-proxy responses from being interchangeable. Some measures have been specifically evaluated for their reliability and accuracy when administered to both individuals with TBI and their proxies (82,95), whereas others have not been evaluated for participant-proxy agreement. Previously, the intraclass correlations between participants with TBI and participant-selected proxies on the Craig Handicap Assessment and Reporting Technique (CHART), the CIQ, and the FIM were evaluated. Results showed a high intraclass correlation for participants and proxies, with the highest values occurring on items assessing concrete or observable information (96). Other studies in a variety of patient populations also indicate that patient-proxy agreement is generally better for questions regarding physical dimensions of functional status, and agreement is less consistent for questions regarding subjective or affective aspects of outcome assessment (94). Investigators should take time to carefully consider their primary outcome measure and choose their criteria for considering persons with TBI to be a capable respondent. The agreement between patient and proxy responses should be evaluated prior to an outcome assessment's inclusion in a study in order to avoid overestimation or underestimation of treatment effects or invalid conclusions. Further, consistent criteria for the selection of a knowledgeable caregiver or significant other should be considered in the research design.

CLINICAL TRIALS IN TRAUMATIC BRAIN INJURY

Randomized clinical trials are the gold standard by which researchers in any field of medicine test the efficacy and safety of treatment interventions. Clinical trials, particularly randomized clinical trials, provide a strong foundation for evidence-based clinical practice and justification of payors to reimburse for treatments and therapies (97). However, in the area of TBI, there have been few clinical trials that have definitively identified any effective treatments for reducing morbidity or improving recovery. Numerous TBI clinical trials of acute pharmacological interventions, intended to improve functional and neuropsychological outcomes, have been conducted over previous decades, with often disappointing results (98–105). The justification for virtually all of these trials were positive findings in animal studies, using rodent models, testing the trial drug or intervention that could not capture variables that may influence treatment outcome such as gender, age, and genetic variability (106,107). Other issues like concomitant extracranial injury can impact human TBI pathophysiology, yet experimental models to capture these components of injury are just emerging (108). Also, unique mechanisms of injury—for example, shaken baby syndrome—may be associated with worse outcomes and may respond differently to therapeutic intervention (109–111).

For TBI rehabilitation research, double-blind randomized control trials are particularly difficult to carry out. Sample sizes tend to be small and the number of confounding variables is often quite high. There can be a lack of consensus on appropriate outcome measures to use, how to objectively quantify rehabilitation-based interventions, and how to operationalize and implement intervention algorithms that are based on functional progress. Recently, participation and barriers to participation in therapy has also become a variable of interest regarding clinical trial design for those with both cognitive and physical deficits (112,113). In addition to functional abilities, rehabilitation research also focuses on participation in the community and quality of life (53). For instance, social interventions such as caregiver education may improve community integration and quality of life for the population with TBI. Rehabilitation outcome often can be context specific and affected by a patient's physical environment, social environment, and personal attitudes and expectations (114). These contextual factors may influence rehabilitation outcome and decrease the generalizability of clinical study results. Despite these challenges, some high-quality rehabilitation-based randomized clinical trials have occurred in the areas of seizure prophylaxis (115,116), community-based rehabilitation for long-term survivors of TBI (117), methylphenidate treatment (118), and cognitive rehabilitation (119). Contemporary modalities, like computer-based cognitive training strategies are being explored (120,121). However, replication studies, studies with large population numbers, and the generalizability of findings to a large population are difficult to find in any area of TBI rehabilitation research.

A recent analysis regarding clinical trials in rehabilitation (122) suggests that characterizing (and appropriately grouping) participants in rehabilitation research studies is of critical importance to eliminate confounding factors, to ensure comparability across treatment conditions, and to adjust for differences in prognosis among participants. Additionally, the treatment or intervention must be adequately and objectively characterized in terms of mechanism of action, dose, route, intensity, and subject participation. In-vestigators should identify the appropriate target of their outcome assessment (e.g., disease, impairment, activity, participation, quality of life) and ensure the measurability of their outcome target with the treatment intervention. Often, broadly defined outcomes such as quality of life have several factors that affect it. As such, a single intervention may impact specific impairments after TBI, but those changes may not be large enough to translate into a meaningful change in quality of life (122). Additional challenges in rehabilitation research occur with blinding of physical treatments and with limitations of crossover designs when significant contamination of the study population from cross-training might dilute the effectiveness of the treatment intervention (123).

Multicenter clinical trials in TBI are considered necessary because the ability of a single center to recruit enough subjects to provide adequate statistical power is often limited. However, several statistical and design issues have been identified by investigators directing multicenter clinical trials that begin during emergency and intensive care. Intercenter variance in patient care and adherence to the research protocol has been a fatal flaw in some multicenter clinical trials. For example, it has been reported that intercenter variation, not explicable by injury severity or type, was responsible for approximately 40% of the variation in a multicenter clinical trial evaluating the effectiveness of tirilazad mesylate (101,124). Intercenter variation was noted in a multicenter clinical trial evaluating the efficacy of hypothermia with a variety of intensive care treatments, including narcotic use for sedation, and several physiological variables (125). Interestingly, experimental TBI studies suggest that choice of anesthesia or sedation, including fentanyl and isoflurane, can have marked effects on outcome and in the context of hypothermia treatment (126,127). Centers who enroll small numbers of patients may contribute the most variability to standard care treatment regimens because they may be less likely to follow consensus recommendations for standard treatment (124). Misclassification of outcomes can also influence study results. One study reports that as the numbers of outcome categories increase, the greater the likelihood of outcome misclassification and erroneous results (128). Although dichotomous outcomes are not reasonable for all clinical trials, care must be taken to create effective algorithms for accurate data collection, and the use of pilot data may be helpful in determining an effective outcome measure with a minimum necessary requirement of categories. Subset analysis of data, even in negative multicenter trials, is recommended to identify potential subpopulations who might benefit from a particular treatment (129).

Over the last 5 years and with support from the NIH, the International Mission for Prognosis and Clinical Trial (IMPACT) database of TBI was formed and contains the complete dataset from several clinical trials and organized epidemiologic studies conducted over the last several years (130). When analyzing this data set, investigators have demonstrated significant intercenter variability with respect to TBI outcome. In addition to differences in patient management, population characteristics were different across centers (131). Among patient characteristics affecting outcome were variables related to both anatomic and physiologic injury parameters (132). Recommendations to mitigate variability within multisite clinical trials include the incorporation and measurement of baseline, validated prognostic variables, broad inclusion of patients with varied mechanisms and types of injury, and covariate adjusted assessment of treatment effects (133).

Previously, the NINDS May 2000 Clinical Trials in Head Injury Study Group also identified and discussed many of the issues associated with failure to produce positive results with several recent trials (124). The study group concluded that in order for clinical trials to be effective, it is essential to (a) establish that a drug or proposed intervention is having the desired effect on a specific mechanism of injury in vivo, (b) to obtain adequate preclinical data, (c) target subpopulations of patients most likely to benefit from the treatment, (d) standardize clinical care, (e) choose appropriate outcome measures or endpoints, and (f) have reasonable expectations for treatment effect (124). Priority should be placed on conducting preliminary experimental and clinical studies aimed at understanding mechanisms of injury and recovery. Evaluating the most effective window of treatment, dose response curves, drug pharmacokinetics and drug delivery to the brain, and multiple models of experimental TBI are needed for adequate preclinical trial data (124). Using injury-related prognostic variables in the selection criteria for studies may allow investigators to effectively target subpopulations for particular interventions. Strict adherence to clinical care guidelines, centralization of some study variables (e.g., CT scan interpretation), collection of concurrent medications, and collection of only essential study variables may improve the clinical management of clinical trials. Smaller effect sizes (5%–7.5%), the careful design, and use of sensitive outcomes as well as the judicious use of relevant proxy variables may allow investigators to appreciate subtle treatment effects for specific interventions (124). Also, functional status at the time of entry into rehabilitation trials may be more prognostic of outcome and a relevant way to group patients than injury variables (124). Other intrinsic variables such as age, gender, and genetic makeup are emerging as important variables to consider in trial design (134,135).

ALTERNATIVES TO CLINICAL TRIALS AND RESEARCH DESIGN

Although randomized clinical trials are considered the gold standard for clinical research, they are not always feasible or practical for each research question. Ethical issues and the inability to obtain the resources necessary to conduct a full-scale randomized clinical trial may preclude this study design (136). However, randomized clinical trials may have their own limitations in that they may not provide a representative measure of the effectiveness of the treatment in common clinical practice settings (137). CER studies have become increasingly popular as a method for establishing treatment effects in the clinical setting, delineating how treatments and interventions work best across outcome domains and for whom. Currently, there is little literature available regarding CER in TBI (138). Interestingly, CER studies are priorities for TBI research across funding organizations to assess treatment approaches for effective rehabilitation (139) and with TBI-related conditions and complications that exist for persons with TBI, including post-traumatic depression (140).

Observational studies are another alternative to clinical trials research by which to study necessary research questions, particularly when treatment variables of interest are not assigned based on prognostic factors influencing outcome (136). Some reports suggest that effect sizes generated from well-done observational studies can be comparable to those obtained from randomized clinical trials (141). However, observational studies are vulnerable to confounding variables affecting the outcome variable of interest and require the use of covariate analysis. Common issues associated with exploratory analyses or observational studies such as appropriate correction for multiple comparisons, avoiding type II experimental error, and appropriate sample size also need to be considered in the study design (142,143) in order to provide accurate conclusions and a solid foundation for the design of a future clinical trial. Single subject research designs can be valuable, particularly in clinical practice, to determine effectiveness of treatments and lay the groundwork for larger studies (144).

TRANSLATIONAL RESEARCH IN TRAUMATIC BRAIN INJURY

Translational research is an important area of focus for TBI in that it identifies mechanisms of injury and recovery and lays the groundwork for the conduct of clinical trials incorporating these mechanisms as targets for treatment. Advances in genomics and proteomics can provide a novel approach to identifying and exploring therapeutic targets (145,146). Using functional imaging technology (147–149) or quantitative electroencephalography (EEG) (150) are contemporary avenues by which to explore injury and recovery mechanisms directly in the clinical population with TBI. Experimental models of TBI provide a reproducible model to characterize injury mechanisms to assess potential therapies and interventions in the context of behavioral outcome.

Clinical Biomarkers and TBI Research: A Rehabilomics Framework

Biomarkers are increasingly used in medicine to monitor biological and pathological processes that ultimately aid in patient management and care. Biomarkers can also serve as effective proxy variables that reflect treatment response. Biomarker profiles are molecular fingerprints that have the potential to assist rehabilitation researchers in determining how long-term outcome can be linked to plasticity, treatment response, and natural recovery. Increasing focus has been placed on rehabilomics research as an approach to TBI research, where rehabilitation relevant outcomes, in conjunction with the incorporation of biomarkers into the study design, are used to better understand the biology, function, prognosis, complications, treatments, adaptation, and recovery for persons with disabilities (151,152). For example, multiple genetic studies have been published recently implicating apolipoprotein E4 (APOE4), neprilysin, and the prosurvival factor BCL2 in long-term TBI pathology and recovery (153,154). Adenosine systems have been linked to the development of post-traumatic seizures (155). Other markers linked to structural damage, cell death, and hormone status has been studied in relation to TBI outcome prognostication (109,153,154,156–160). As the pool of relevant rehabilomics studies increase, the use of these biomarkers as grouping variables for clinical trials may be attainable (27).

Experimental Models of Traumatic Brain Injury

Most translational research requires the effective use of experimental models that reproduce the physiological and behavioral sequelae associated with injury. Several models, including fluid percussion (161) and controlled cortical impact (CCI) (162), are commonly used in rodents. Characteristics of the CCI model include not only a representative contusion but also reproducible brain edema and marked changes in cerebral blood flow in surrounding cortex (163). Rodent models are cost effective, can provide a relevant and reproducible injury, and are effective in studying a variety of behavioral paradigms (164–167). Rodents, however, are not gyrocephalic animals, and the use of larger animal models, including primate models, may be necessary to fully characterize pathology associated with diffuse axonal injury. Experimental models of TBI have largely been used to study acute pathology and neuroprotection; however, they can be a useful approach for examining long-term outcome, mechanisms of recovery, and relevant rehabilitation interventions. For example, the CCI model recently was used to study the differential effects of gender and environmental enrichment, an experimental correlate to therapy, on behavioral recovery (167), and mechanisms for neurostimulant effects on recovery (168,169). Research is increasingly being conducted to develop relevant blast injury models of TBI to examine and characterize mechanisms of primary and secondary injury for blast TBI and to assess behavioral effects (170,171). As TBI rehabilitation research moves forward, collaborative efforts with other basic science disciplines, such as neuroscience and psychology, to tackle complex issues such as cortical reorganization, neural plasticity, and the effects of rehabilitation strategies like forced use will be required (172). Future work will also require that researchers find ways to actively link studies involving acute mechanisms of injury and treatment inventions with central nervous system repair and recovery.

PRIORITY AREAS FOR TBI REHABILITATION RESEARCH

In 1999, an NIH consensus group identified and published some research priorities in the area of TBI (173). Highlighted among these priorities include a need for epidemiological studies targeting different demographic groups and to study mild TBI. The therapeutic window for treatment interventions and the neurobiology of clinical TBI were highlighted as need areas. Prognostic equations and the relationship between impairments and global outcome were highlighted as key areas requiring further evaluation. Finally, the long-term consequences of TBI and the developmental impact of TBI on children were identified as focus areas of study (173). Over a decade later, these priorities remain relevant despite recent research on these topics. The incidence of TBI due to combat-related injuries has increased sharply over the last decade and affects health and outcome among military casualties (174–177). Initiatives to address TBI and discern how it differs/overlaps with post-traumatic stress disorder(PTSD) in the warfighter have been lead by several Department of Defense (DOD) research programs (178).

Several priority areas for TBI, injury prevention, and rehabilitation research have been set by primary federal organizations that fund TBI research. The NIDRR has research priorities in the areas of employment outcomes, individual health and function, technology for access and function, and independent living and community integration that have been a part of their previous long-range plan (LRP) (179) and remain focus areas for the 2010–2014 LRP (180). The development of sensitive and effective outcome measures is a priority. Research in rehabilitation science, disability studies, and disability policy are also current NIDRR research priorities. Investigators, particularly in the field of TBI rehabilitation research, have had a long history of using NIDRR funding to evaluate important questions in the area of TBI outcome. The TBI model system centers have been an important part of this endeavor (181,182). NIDRR-based collaborative networks for TBI research also foster increased interactions between varied groups of investigators and allow for the recruitment of large samples to answer important TBI rehabilitation research questions.

The Centers for Disease Control's (CDC) injury centers (183) have provided priorities in the area of TBI for 2009–2018. Highlighted among their many priorities relevant to TBI are to (*a*) improve TBI identification, assessment, and management; (*b*) determine the best estimates of the number of TBI cases treated in outpatient settings among those who do not seek immediate medical evaluation; (*c*) examine long-term outcomes and disability among the military population with TBI; (*d*) provide a contemporary needs assessment for services after TBI and identify barriers that restrict access to support services and programs for this population; and (*e*) determine which interventions are effective in reducing disability from TBI and in eliminating postinjury symptoms and long-term effects.

The national health objectives highlighted by the NIH as research priorities in Healthy People 2010 report (184) has been replaced with Healthy People 2020 (185). The goals of the Healthy People initiative are designed to identify significant threats to national health and to establish goals aimed at reducing these threats. One priority of Healthy People 2010 has been to eliminate health disparities among different segments of the population, including those with disabilities. In particular, Healthy People 2010 aims to "promote the health of people with disabilities, prevent secondary conditions, and eliminate disparities between people with and without disabilities in the US population" (184). The Healthy People 2020 priorities build upon milestones attained with the Healthy People 2010 initiative and continue to focus on quality of life and health as well as both individual and aggregate social determinants of health (186). These particular aims suggest that NIH views disability-related research, including research on assessing and preventing secondary conditions associated with TBI and quality of life and health, as important priority areas of research. However, compared to other conditions, TBI research is relatively underfunded when compared to the large number of people affected by TBI each year (Figure 7-1). Continued work to increase funding and research capacity in the field TBI is necessary to achieve the medical breakthroughs in TBI care required to optimize recovery.

In 2002, the NIH began developing its roadmap for medical research in the 21st century and identifying new pathways to discovery, research teams of the future, and reengineering the clinical research enterprise (187). Since

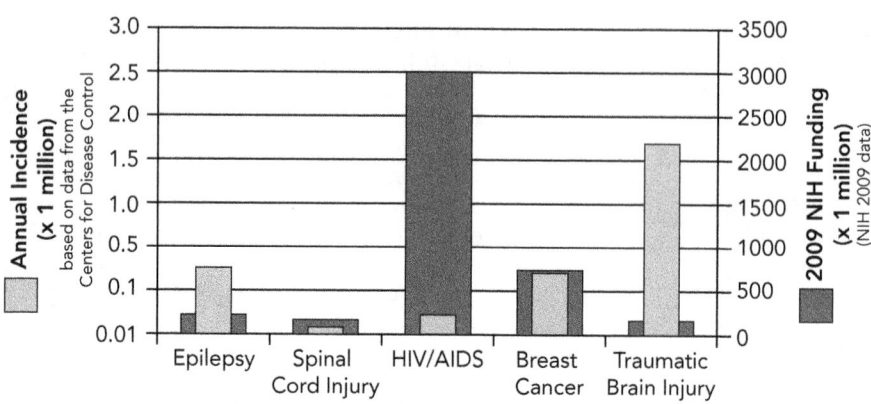

FIGURE 7-1 Funding versus incidence for traumatic brain injury (TBI) and other disorders. NIH fundings dollars spent per person affected are significantly less for TBI than for other diseases listed.

then, large-scale Institutional Clinical and Translational Science Awards have done much to help increase accessibility to cutting edge techniques and to appropriate expertise, wherein the technology is "brought to the masses" of clinician scientists who can leverage these resources for conducting innovative and contemporary research with hight-ranslational impact to patients and clinical care. Also, entities like the nonprofit foundation for NIH have helped facilitate groundbreaking findings in biomarker research as a part of its mission and regularly partner with small business entities to help translate these biomarkers research discoveries into clinically useful assays and technology (http://www.fnih.org/). As mentioned earlier, institutions like the AHRQ have TBI relevant priorities that are designed with the overarching goal of creating an environment for more effective health care (188).

KEY CLINICAL POINTS

1. TBI outcomes research needs to address recovery across multiple functional domains. The NIH toolbox and the Common Data Elements initiatives are helpful resources to allow study findings to be more easily generalized across multiple study populations.
2. Systemic biases that lead to loss to follow-up or biases in measurement response may limit generalizability of the findings to other populations.
3. Clinical trials to date in the area of neuroprotection have not been successful in identifying clear evidence for beneficial agents, in part because of the heterogeneity of the disease, limitations with outcomes analyzed, variations in standard of care provided, and limited consideration of how subjects should be grouped to best assess treatment effects.
4. Rehabilitation intervention studies show promise for some TBI-specific treatments, yet for the most part, TBI rehabilitation-focused interventions are small and underpowered. Comparative effectiveness studies are needed within the TBI rehabilitation field to better understand what works best for whom in order to translate findings to clinical practice.
5. Biomarkers may provide unique information that helps accurately stratify patients for clinical trials, shed new light on pathophysiology, and aid in prognostication. Rehabilitation specific or rehabilomics studies can use

biomarkers to uniquely study the neurobiology of recovery, efficacy of exercise and other rehabilitation relevant treatments, and aid in the management of post-TBI complications.
6. Translational research, including the use of preclinical models, is important when assessing the viability of new therapies to study in clinical populations.
7. The Healthy People 2020 priorities and focus on quality of life and health suggests that NIH views disability-related research as important priority areas of research. DOD funding focuses on military TBI and related disorders, whereas NIDRR and CDC continue to support TBI research within established priority areas.

KEY REFERENCES

1. Agency for Healthcare Research and Quality. *Comparative Effectiveness of Multidisciplinary Postacute Rehabilitation for Moderate to Severe Traumatic Brain Injury.* Rockville, MD: Agency for Healthcare Research and Quality; 2011. http://www.effectivehealthcare.ahrq.gov/index.cfm/search-for-guides-reviews-and-reports/?pageaction=displayproduct&productid=726. Accessed April 19, 2012.
2. Dahl TH. International classification of functioning, disability and health: an introduction and discussion of its potential impact on rehabilitation services and research. *J Rehabil Med.* 2002;34(5):201–204.
3. Faul M, Xu L, Wald MM, Coronado VG. *Traumatic Brain Injury in the United States: Emergency Department Visits, Hospitalizations, and Deaths 2002–2006.* Atlanta, GA: Centers for Disease Control and Prevention; 2006. http://www.cdc.gov/traumaticbraininjury/tbi_ed.html. Accessed April 19, 2012.
4. NIH Toolbox: Assessment of Neurological and Behavioral Function Website. http://www.nihtoolbox.org/. Accessed April 19, 2012.
5. Rosenfeld JV, Ford NL. Bomb blast, mild traumatic brain injury and psychiatric morbidity: a review. *Injury.* 2010; 41(5):437–443.
6. Traumatic Brain Injury. NINDS Common Data Elements Website. http://www.commondataelements.ninds.nih.gov/TBI.aspx. Accessed April 19, 2012.
7. Wagner AK. TBI translational rehabilitation research in the 21st Century: exploring a Rehabilomics research model. *Eur J Phys Rehabil Med.* 2010;46(4):549–556.

8. Wright DW, Kellermann AL, Hertzberg VS, et al. ProTECT: a randomized clinical trial of progesterone for acute traumatic brain injury. *Ann Emerg Med.* 2007;49(4): 391–402.

References

1. Jurkovich GJ, Rivara FP, Johansen JM, Maier RV. Centers for Disease Control and Prevention injury research agenda: identification of acute care research topics of interest to the Centers for Disease Control and Prevention—National Center for Injury Prevention and Control. *J Trauma.* 2004;56(5):1166–1170.
2. Faul M, Xu L, Wald MM, Coronado VG. *Traumatic Brain Injury in the United States: Emergency Department Visits, Hospitalizations, and Deaths 2002–2006.* Atlanta, GA: Centers for Disease Control and Prevention; 2006. http://www.cdc.gov/traumaticbraininjury/tbi_ed.html. Accessed April 19, 2012.
3. Finkelstein E, Corso P, Miller T. *The Incidence and Economic Burden of Injuries in the United States.* New York, NY: Oxford University Press; 2006.
4. Danbolt NC. Glutamate uptake. *Prog Neurobiol.* 2001;65(1):1–105.
5. Globus MY, Alonso O, Dietrich WD, Busto R, Ginsberg MD. Glutamate release and free radical production following brain injury: effects of posttraumatic hypothermia. *J Neurochem.* 1995;65(4): 1704–1711.
6. Zipfel GJ, Babcock DJ, Lee JM, Choi DW. Neuronal apoptosis after CNS injury: the roles of glutamate and calcium. *J Neurotrauma.* 2000;17(10):857–869.
7. Roof RL, Duvdevani R, Heyburn JW, Stein DG. Progesterone rapidly decreases brain edema: treatment delayed up to 24 hours is still effective. *Exp Neurol.* 1996;138(2):246–251.
8. Roof RL, Hall ED. Estrogen-related gender difference in survival rate and cortical blood flow after impact-acceleration head injury in rats. *J Neurotrauma.* 2000;17(12):1155–1169.
9. Kontos HA, Povlishock JT. Oxygen radicals in brain injury. *Cent Nerv Syst Trauma.* 1986;3(4):257–263.
10. Bayir H, Kagan VE, Tyurina YY, et al. Assessment of antioxidant reserves and oxidative stress in cerebrospinal fluid after severe traumatic brain injury in infants and children. *Pediatr Res.* 2002; 51(5):571–578.
11. Kushi H, Saito T, Makino K, Hayashi N. IL-8 is a key mediator of neuroinflammation in severe traumatic brain injuries. *Acta Neurochir Suppl.* 2003;86:347–350.
12. Frati A, Salvati M, Mainiero F, et al. Inflammation markers and risk factors for recurrence in 35 patients with a posttraumatic chronic subdural hematoma: a prospective study. *J Neurosurg.* 2004;100(1): 24–32.
13. Yakovlev AG, Faden AI. Caspase-dependent apoptotic pathways in CNS injury. *Mol Neurobiol.* 2001;24(1–3):131–144.
14. Raghupathi R, Conti AC, Graham DI, et al. Mild traumatic brain injury induces apoptotic cell death in the cortex that is preceded by decreases in cellular Bcl-2 immunoreactivity. *Neuroscience.* 2002; 110(4):605–616.
15. Wagner AK, Hammond FM, Grigsby JH, Norton HJ. The value of trauma scores: predicting discharge after traumatic brain injury. *Am J Phys Med Rehabil.* 2000;79(3):235–242.
16. Mullins RJ, Veum-Stone J, Helfand M, et al. Outcome of hospitalized injured patients after institution of a trauma system in an urban area. *JAMA.* 1994;271(24):1919–1924.
17. Mullins RJ, Hedges JR, Rowland DJ, et al. Survival of seriously injured patients first treated in rural hospitals. *J Trauma.* 2002;52(6): 1019–1029.
18. McCullagh S, Feinstein A. Outcome after mild traumatic brain injury: an examination of recruitment bias. *J Neurol Neurosurg Psychiatry.* 2003;74(1):39–43.
19. Clifton GL, Knudson P, McDonald M. Waiver of consent in studies of acute brain injury. *J Neurotrauma.* 2002;19(10):1121–1126.
20. Wright DW, Kellermann AL, Hertzberg VS, et al. ProTECT: a randomized clinical trial of progesterone for acute traumatic brain injury. *Ann Emerg Med.* 2007;49(4):391–402.e1–e2.

21. Collins MW, Iverson GL, Gaetz M, Lovell MR. Sport-related concussion. In: Zasler ND, Katz DI, Zafonte RD, eds. *Brain Injury Medicine: Principles and Practice.* New York, NY: Demos; 2007:407–421.
22. Kelly JP, Nichols JS, Filley CM, Lillehei KO, Rubinstein D, Kleinschmidt-DeMasters BK. Concussion in sports. Guidelines for the prevention of catastrophic outcome. *JAMA.* 1991;266(20): 2867–2869.
23. Cantu RC. Posttraumatic retrograde and anterograde amnesia: pathophysiology and implications in grading and safe return to play. *J Athl Train.* 2001;36(3):244–248.
24. World Health Organization. *International Statistical Classification of Diseases and Related Health Problems.* 10th ed. Geneva, Switzerland: Author; 1992.
25. Wagner AK, Amin KB, Niyonkuru C, et al. CSF Bcl-2 and cytochrome C temporal profiles in outcome prediction for adults with severe TBI. *J Cereb Blood Flow Metab.* 2011;31(9):1886–1896.
26. Wagner AK, McCullough EH, Niyonkuru C, et al. Acute serum hormone levels: characterization and prognosis after severe traumatic brain injury. *J Neurotrauma.* 2011;28(6):871–888.
27. Saatman KE, Duhaime AC, Bullock R, Maas AI, Valadka A, Manley GT. Classification of traumatic brain injury for targeted therapies. *J Neurotrauma.* 2008;25(7):719–738.
28. Corrigan JD, Harrison-Felix C, Bogner J, Dijkers M, Terrill MS, Whiteneck G. Systematic bias in traumatic brain injury outcome studies because of loss to follow-up. *Arch Phys Med Rehabil.* 2003; 84(2):153–160.
29. Lew HL, Lee E, Date ES, Zeiner H. Influence of medical comorbidities and complications on FIM change and length of stay during inpatient rehabilitation. *Am J Phys Med Rehabil.* 2002;81(11): 830–837.
30. Wagner AK, Hammond FM, Sasser HC, Wiercisiewski D, Norton HJ. Use of injury severity variables in determining disability and community integration after traumatic brain injury. *J Trauma.* 2000; 49(3):411–419.
31. Farace E, Alves WM. Do women fare worse: a metaanalysis of gender differences in traumatic brain injury outcome. *J Neurosurg.* 2000;93(4):539–545.
32. Wagner AK, Sasser H. Gender associations with disability and community integration after TBI. *Arch Phys Med Rehabil.* 2000;81(9): 1267–1268.
33. Kesler SR, Adams HF, Blasey CM, Bigler ED. Premorbid intellectual functioning, education, and brain size in traumatic brain injury: an investigation of the cognitive reserve hypothesis. *Appl Neuropsychol.* 2003;10(3):153–162.
34. Zafonte RD, Mann NR, Millis SR, Black KL, Wood DL, Hammond F. Posttraumatic amnesia: its relation to functional outcome. *Arch Phys Med Rehabil.* 1997;78(10):1103–1106.
35. Zafonte RD, Wood DL, Harrison-Felix CL, Valena NV, Black K. Penetrating head injury: a prospective study of outcomes. *Neurol Res.* 2001;23(2–3):219–226.
36. Wagner AK, Sasser HC, Hammond FM, Wiercisiewski D, Alexander J. Intentional traumatic brain injury: epidemiology, risk factors, and associations with injury severity and mortality. *J Trauma.* 2000; 49(3):404–410.
37. Hanks RA, Wood DL, Millis S, et al. Violent traumatic brain injury: occurrence, patient characteristics, and risk factors from the Traumatic Brain Injury Model Systems project. *Arch Phys Med Rehabil.* 2003;84(2):249–254.
38. Bushnik T, Hanks RA, Kreutzer J, Rosenthal M. Etiology of traumatic brain injury: characterization of differential outcomes up to 1 year postinjury. *Arch Phys Med Rehabil.* 2003;84(2):255–262.
39. Sherer M, Nick TG, Sander AM, et al. Race and productivity outcome after traumatic brain injury: influence of confounding factors. *J Head Trauma Rehabil.* 2003;18(5):408–424.
40. Hibbard MR, Cantor J, Charatz H, et al. Peer support in the community: initial findings of a mentoring program for individuals with traumatic brain injury and their families. *J Head Trauma Rehabil.* 2002;17(2):112–131.
41. Paddock SM, Escarce JJ, Hayden O, Buntin MB. Did the Medicare inpatient rehabilitation facility prospective payment system result in changes in relative patient severity and relative resource use? *Med Care.* 2007;45(2):123–130.

42. Dikmen SS, Machamer JE, Powell JM, Temkin NR. Outcome 3 to 5 years after moderate to severe traumatic brain injury. *Arch Phys Med Rehabil.* 2003;84(10):1449–1457.

43. Millis SR, Rosenthal M, Novack TA, et al. Long-term neuropsychological outcome after traumatic brain injury. *J Head Trauma Rehabil.* 2001;16(4):343–355.

44. Novack TA, Alderson AL, Bush BA, Meythaler JM, Canupp K. Cognitive and functional recovery at 6 and 12 months post-TBI. *Brain Inj.* 2000;14(11):987–996.

45. Powell JM, Machamer JE, Temkin NR, Dikmen SS. Self-report of extent of recovery and barriers to recovery after traumatic brain injury: a longitudinal study. *Arch Phys Med Rehabil.* 2001;82(8):1025–1030.

46. Tanielian T, Jaycox LH, eds. *Invisible Wounds of War: Psychological and Cognitive Injuries, Their Consequences, and Services to Assist Recovery.* Santa Monica, CA: RAND Corporation; 2008.

47. Chafi MS, Karami G, Ziejewski M. Biomechanical assessment of brain dynamic responses due to blast pressure waves. *Ann Biomed Eng.* 2010;38(2):490–504.

48. Luethcke CA, Bryan CJ, Morrow CE, Isler WC. Comparison of concussive symptoms, cognitive performance, and psychological symptoms between acute blast-versus nonblast-induced mild traumatic brain injury. *J Int Neuropsychol Soc.* 2011;17(1):36–45.

49. Ropper A. Brain injuries from blasts. *N Engl J Med.* 2011;364(22):2156–2157.

50. Rosenfeld JV, Ford NL. Bomb blast, mild traumatic brain injury and psychiatric morbidity: a review. *Injury.* 2010;41(5):437–443.

51. Schuntermann MF. The International Classification of Impairments, Disabilities and Handicaps (ICIDH)—results and problems. *Int J Rehabil Res.* 1996;19(1):1–11.

52. Bornman J. The World Health Organisation's terminology and classification: application to severe disability. *Disabil Rehabil.* 2004;26(3):182–188.

53. Dahl TH. International classification of functioning, disability and health: an introduction and discussion of its potential impact on rehabilitation services and research. *J Rehabil Med.* 2002;34(5):201–204.

54. Koskinen S, Hokkinen EM, Wilson L, Sarajuuri J, Von Steinbüchel N, Truelle JL. Comparison of subjective and objective assessments of outcome after traumatic brain injury using the International Classification of Functioning, Disability and Health (ICF). *Disabil Rehabil.* 2011;33(25–26):2464–2478.

55. Wilson JT, Pettigrew LE, Teasdale GM. Structured interviews for the Glasgow Outcome Scale and the extended Glasgow Outcome Scale: guidelines for their use. *J Neurotrauma.* 1998;15(8):573–585.

56. Hall K, Cope DN, Rappaport M. Glasgow Outcome Scale and Disability Rating Scale: comparative usefulness in following recovery in traumatic head injury. *Arch Phys Med Rehabil.* 1985;66(1):35–37.

57. Cook L, Smith DS, Truman G. Using Functional Independence Measure profiles as an index of outcome in the rehabilitation of brain-injured patients. *Arch Phys Med Rehabil.* 1994;75(4):390–393.

58. Willer B, Ottenbacher KJ, Coad ML. The community integration questionnaire. A comparative examination. *Am J Phys Med Rehabil.* 1994;73(2):103–111.

59. Dikmen S, Machamer J, Miller B, Doctor J, Temkin N. Functional status examination: a new instrument for assessing outcome in traumatic brain injury. *J Neurotrauma.* 2001;18(2):127–140.

60. Corrigan JD, Bogner JA, Mysiw WJ, Clinchot D, Fugate L. Life satisfaction after traumatic brain injury. *J Head Trauma Rehabil.* 2001;16(6):543–555.

61. Struchen MA, Atchison TB, Roebuck TM, Caroselli JS, Sander AM. A multidimensional measure of caregiving appraisal: validation of the Caregiver Appraisal Scale in traumatic brain injury. *J Head Trauma Rehabil.* 2002;17(2):132–154.

62. Sander AM, High WM Jr, Hannay HJ, Sherer M. Predictors of psychological health in caregivers of patients with closed head injury. *Brain Inj.* 1997;11(4):235–249.

63. Glenn MB, O'Neil-Pirozzi T, Goldstein R, Burke D, Jacob L. Depression amongst outpatients with traumatic brain injury. *Brain Inj.* 2001;15(9):811–818.

64. Levin HS, Goldstein FC, MacKenzie EJ. Depression as a secondary condition following mild and moderate traumatic brain injury. *Semin Clin Neuropsychiatry.* 1997;2(3):207–215.

65. Cook KF, Bombardier CH, Bamer AM, Choi SW, Kroenke K, Fann JR. Do somatic and cognitive symptoms of traumatic brain injury confound depression screening? *Arch Phys Med Rehabil.* 2011;92(5):818–823.

66. Fann JR, Bombardier CH, Dikmen S, et al. Validity of the Patient Health Questionnaire-9 in assessing depression following traumatic brain injury. *J Head Trauma Rehabil.* 2005;20(6):501–511.

67. Bombardier CH, Fann JR, Temkin NR, Esselman PC, Barber J, Dikmen SS. Rates of major depressive disorder and clinical outcomes following traumatic brain injury. *JAMA.* 2010;303(19):1938–1945.

68. Collins MW, Iverson GL, Lovell MR, McKeag DB, Norwig J, Maroon J. On-field predictors of neuropsychological and symptom deficit following sports-related concussion. *Clin J Sport Med.* 2003;13(4):222–229.

69. Donovan NJ, Heaton SC, Kimberg CI, et al. Conceptualizing functional cognition in traumatic brain injury rehabilitation. *Brain Inj.* 2011;25(4):348–364.

70. Broglio SP, Ferrara MS, Macciocchi SN, Baumgartner TA, Elliott R. Test–retest reliability of computerized concussion assessment programs. *J Athl Train.* 2007;42(4):509–514.

71. Webbe FM, Barth JT. Short-term and long-term outcome of athletic closed head injuries. *Clin Sports Med.* 2003;22(3):577–592.

72. Dijkers MP, Kropp GC, Esper RM, Yavuzer G, Cullen N, Bakdalieh Y. Reporting on reliability and validity of outcome measures in medical rehabilitation research. *Disabil Rehabil.* 2002;24(16):819–827.

73. Dijkers M. Measuring quality of life: methodological issues. *Am J Phys Med Rehabil.* 1999;78(3):286–300.

74. Hall K, Mann N, High W, Wright J, Kreutzer JS, Wood D. Functional measures after traumatic brain injury: ceiling effects of FIM, FIM + FAM, DRS, and CIQ. *J Head Trauma Rehabil.* 1996;11(5):27–39.

75. Hall K, Mann N, High W, Wright J, Kreutzer JS, Wood D. Functional measures after traumatic brain injury: ceiling effects of FIM, FIM + FAM, DRS, and CIQ. *J Head Trauma Rehabil.* 1996;11(5), 27–39.

76. Hammond FM, Grattan KD, Sasser H, Corrigan JD, Bushnik T, Zafonte RD. Long-term recovery course after traumatic brain injury: a comparison of the functional independence measure and disability rating scale. *J Head Trauma Rehabil.* 2001;16(4):318–329.

77. Fenton G, McClelland R, Montgomery A, MacFlynn G, Rutherford W. The postconcussional syndrome: social antecedents and psychological sequelae. *Br J Psychiatry.* 1993;162:493–497.

78. O'Bryant SE, Hilsabeck RC, McCaffrey RJ, Drew Gouvier W. The Recognition Memory Test Examination of ethnic differences and norm validity. *Arch Clin Neuropsychol.* 2003;18(2):135–143.

79. Rosenthal M, Dijkers M, Harrison-Felix C, et al. Impact of minority status on functional outcome and community integration following traumatic brain injury. *J Head Trauma Rehabil.* 1996;11(5):40–57.

80. Rosselli M, Ardila A. The impact of culture and education on nonverbal neuropsychological measurements: a critical review. *Brain Cogn.* 2003;52(3):326–333.

81. Schopp L, Shigaki C, Johnstone B, Kirkpatrick H. Gender differences in cognitive and emotional adjustment to traumatic brain injury. *J Clin Psychol.* 2001;8(3):181–188.

82. Segal ME, Gillard M, Schall R. Telephone and in-person proxy agreement between stroke patients and caregivers for the functional independence measure. *Am J Phys Med Rehabil.* 1996;75(3):208–212.

83. Willer B, Ottenbacher KJ, Coad ML. The community integration questionnaire. A comparative examination. *Am J Phys Med Rehabil.* 1994;73(2):103–111.

84. NIH Toolbox: Assessment of Neurological and Behavioral Function Web site. http://www.nihtoolbox.org/. Accessed April 19, 2012.

85. Maas AI, Harrison-Felix CL, Menon D, et al. Standardizing data collection in traumatic brain injury. *J Neurotrauma.* 2011;28(2):177–187.

86. Traumatic Brain Injury. NINDS Common Data Elements Web site. http://www.commondataelements.ninds.nih.gov/TBI.aspx. Accessed April 19, 2012.

87. Loring DW, Lowenstein DH, Barbaro NM, et al. Common data elements in epilepsy research: development and implementation of the NINDS epilepsy CDE project. *Epilepsia.* 2011;52(6):1186–1191.

88. Temkin NR, Machamer JE, Dikmen SS. Correlates of functional status 3–5 years after traumatic brain injury with CT abnormalities. *J Neurotrauma.* 2003;20(3):229–241.

89. Hart T, Whyte J, Ellis C, Chervoneva I. Construct validity of an attention rating scale for traumatic brain injury. *Neuropsychology.* 2009;23(6):729–735.

90. Bell KR, Temkin NR, Esselman PC, et al. The effect of a scheduled telephone intervention on outcome after moderate to severe traumatic brain injury: a randomized trial. *Arch Phys Med Rehabil.* 2005; 86(5):851–856.

91. Zafonte R, Friedewald WT, Lee SM, et al. The citicoline brain injury treatment (COBRIT) trial: design and methods. *J Neurotrauma.* 2009; 26(12):2207–2216.

92. Lynch WJ. Determination of effort level, exaggeration, and malingering in neurocognitive assessment. *J Head Trauma Rehabil.* 2004; 19(3):277–283.

93. Flashman LA, McAllister TW. Lack of awareness and its impact in traumatic brain injury. *NeuroRehabilitation.* 2002;17(4):285–296.

94. Weinfurt KP, Trucco SM, Willke RJ, Schulman KA. Measuring agreement between patient and proxy responses to multidimensional health-related quality-of-life measures in clinical trials. An application of psychometric profile analysis. *J Clin Epidemiol.* 2002; 55(6):608–618.

95. Tepper S, Beatty P, DeJong G. Outcomes in traumatic brain injury: self-report versus report of significant others. *Brain Inj.* 1996;10(8): 575–581.

96. Cusick CP, Gerhart KA, Mellick DC. Participant-proxy reliability in traumatic brain injury outcome research. *J Head Trauma Rehabil.* 2000;15(1):739–749.

97. Fuhrer MJ. Overview of clinical trials in medical rehabilitation: impetuses, challenges, and needed future directions. *Am J Phys Med Rehabil.* 2003;82(suppl 10):S8–S15.

98. Bullock MR, Lyeth BG, Muizelaar JP. Current status of neuroprotection trials for traumatic brain injury: lessons from animal models and clinical studies. *Neurosurgery.* 1999;45(2):207–220.

99. Clifton GL, Miller ER, Choi SC, et al. Lack of effect of induction of hypothermia after acute brain injury. *N Engl J Med.* 2001;344(8): 556–563.

100. Ikonomidou C, Turski L. Why did NMDA receptor antagonists fail clinical trials for stroke and traumatic brain injury? *Lancet Neurol.* 2002;1(6):383–386.

101. Marshall LF, Maas AI, Marshall SB, et al. A multicenter trial on the efficacy of using tirilazad mesylate in cases of head injury. *J Neurosurg.* 1998;89(4):519–525.

102. McIntyre LA, Fergusson DA, Hébert PC, Moher D, Hutchison JS. Prolonged therapeutic hypothermia after traumatic brain injury in adults: a systematic review. *JAMA.* 2003;289(22):2992–2999.

103. Muizelaar JP, Marmarou A, Ward JD, et al. Adverse effects of prolonged hyperventilation in patients with severe head injury: a randomized clinical trial. *J Neurosurg.* 1991;75(5):731–739.

104. Muizelaar JP, Marmarou A, Young HF, et al. Improving the outcome of severe head injury with the oxygen radical scavenger polyethylene glycol-conjugated superoxide dismutase: a phase II trial. *J Neurosurg.* 1993;78(3):375–382.

105. Wolf AL, Levi L, Marmarou A, et al. Effect of THAM upon outcome in severe head injury: a randomized prospective clinical trial. *J Neurosurg.* 1993;78(1):54–59.

106. Clifton GL, Jiang JY, Lyeth BG, Jenkins LW, Hamm RJ, Hayes RL. Marked protection by moderate hypothermia after experimental traumatic brain injury. *J Cereb Blood Flow Metab.* 1991;11(1):114–121.

107. Marion DW, White MJ. Treatment of experimental brain injury with moderate hypothermia and 21-aminosteroids. *J Neurotrauma.* 1996;13(3):139–147.

108. Kochanek PM, Bauman RA, Long JB, Dixon CR, Jenkins LW. A critical problem begging for new insight and new therapies. *J Neurotrauma.* 2009;26(6):813–814.

109. Berger RP, Ta'asan S, Rand A, Lokshin A, Kochanek P. Multiplex assessment of serum biomarker concentrations in well-appearing children with inflicted traumatic brain injury. *Pediatr Res.* 2009; 65(1):97–102.

110. Beers SR, Berger RP, Adelson PD. Neurocognitive outcome and serum biomarkers in inflicted versus non-inflicted traumatic brain injury in young children. *J Neurotrauma.* 2007;24(1):97–105.

111. Shore PM, Berger RP, Varma S, et al. Cerebrospinal fluid biomarkers versus glasgow coma scale and glasgow outcome scale in pediatric traumatic brain injury: the role of young age and inflicted injury. *J Neurotrauma.* 2007;24(1):75–86.

112. Lenze EJ, Munin MC, Quear T, et al. The Pittsburgh Rehabilitation Participation Scale: reliability and validity of a clinician-rated measure of participation in acute rehabilitation. *Arch Phys Med Rehabil.* 2004;85(3):380–384.

113. Skidmore ER, Whyte EM, Holm MB, et al. Cognitive and affective predictors of rehabilitation participation after stroke. *Arch Phys Med Rehabil.* 2010;91(2):203–207.

114. Wade DT. Outcome measures for clinical rehabilitation trials: impairment, function, quality of life, or value? *Am J Phys Med Rehabil.* 2003;82(suppl 10):S26–S31.

115. Temkin NR, Dikmen SS, Anderson GD, et al. Valproate therapy for prevention of posttraumatic seizures: a randomized trial. *J Neurosurg.* 1999;91(4):593–600.

116. Temkin NR, Dikmen SS, Wilensky AJ, Keihm J, Chabal S, Winn HR. A randomized, double-blind study of phenytoin for the prevention of post-traumatic seizures. *N Engl J Med.* 1990;323(8): 497–502.

117. Powell J, Heslin J, Greenwood R. Community based rehabilitation after severe traumatic brain injury: a randomised controlled trial. *J Neurol Neurosurg Psychiatry.* 2002;72(2):193–202.

118. Whyte J, Hart T, Schuster K, Fleming M, Polansky M, Coslett HB. Effects of methylphenidate on attentional function after traumatic brain injury. A randomized, placebo-controlled trial. *Am J Phys Med Rehabil.* 1997;76(6):440–450.

119. Carney N, Chesnut RM, Maynard H, Mann NC, Patterson P, Helfand M. Effect of cognitive rehabilitation on outcomes for persons with traumatic brain injury: a systematic review. *J Head Trauma Rehabil.* 1999;14(3):277–307.

120. Wade SL, Walz NC, Carey J, et al. A randomized trial of teen online problem solving for improving executive function deficits following pediatric traumatic brain injury. *J Head Trauma Rehabil.* 2010; 25(6):409–415.

121. Lundqvist A, Grundström K, Samuelsson K, Rönnberg J. Computerized training of working memory in a group of patients suffering from acquired brain injury. *Brain Inj.* 2010;24(10):1173–1183.

122. Whyte J. Clinical trials in rehabilitation: what are the obstacles? *Am J Phys Med Rehabil.* 2003;82(suppl 10):S16–S21.

123. Terrin M. Fundamentals of clinical trials for medical rehabilitation. *Am J Phys Med Rehabil.* 2003;82(suppl 10):S22–S25.

124. Narayan RK, Michel ME, Ansell B, et al. Clinical trials in head injury. *J Neurotrauma.* 2002;19(5):503–557.

125. Clifton GL, Choi SC, Miller ER, et al. Intercenter variance in clinical trials of head trauma—experience of the National Acute Brain Injury Study: Hypothermia. *J Neurosurg.* 2001;95(5):751–755.

126. Statler KD, Alexander HL, Vagni VA, et al. Moderate hypothermia may be detrimental after traumatic brain injury in fentanyl-anesthetized rats. *Crit Care Med.* 2003;31(4):1134–1139.

127. Statler KD, Kochanek PM, Dixon CE, et al. Isoflurane improves long-term neurologic outcome versus fentanyl after traumatic brain injury in rats. *J Neurotrauma.* 2000;17(12):1179–1189.

128. Choi SC, Clifton GL, Marmarou A, Miller ER. Misclassification and treatment effect on primary outcome measures in clinical trials of severe neurotrauma. *J Neurotrauma.* 2002;19(1):17–22.

129. Choi SC, Bullock R. Design and statistical issues in multicenter trials of severe head injury. *Neurol Res.* 2001;23(2–3):190–192.

130. Marmarou A, Lu J, Butcher I, et al. IMPACT database of traumatic brain injury: design and description. *J Neurotrauma.* 2007;24(2): 239–250.

131. Lingsma HF, Roozenbeek B, Li B, et al. Large between-center differences in outcome after moderate and severe traumatic brain injury in the international mission on prognosis and clinical trial design in

traumatic brain injury (IMPACT) study. *Neurosurgery*. 2011;68(3): 601–608.

132. Murray GD, Butcher I, McHugh GS, et al. Multivariable prognostic analysis in traumatic brain injury: results from the IMPACT study. *J Neurotrauma*. 2007;24(2):329–337.

133. Maas AI, Steyerberg EW, Marmarou A, et al. IMPACT recommendations for improving the design and analysis of clinical trials in moderate to severe traumatic brain injury. *Neurotherapeutics*. 2010; 7(1):127–134.

134. Wagner AK, Bayir H, Ren D, Puccio A, Zafonte RD, Kochanek PM. Relationships between cerebrospinal fluid markers of excitotoxicity, ischemia, and oxidative damage after severe TBI: the impact of gender, age, and hypothermia. *J Neurotrauma*. 2004;21(2):125–136.

135. Friedman G, Froom P, Sazbon L, et al. Apolipoprotein E-epsilon4 genotype predicts a poor outcome in survivors of traumatic brain injury. *Neurology*. 1999;52(2):244–248.

136. Whyte J. Traumatic brain injury rehabilitation: are there alternatives to randomized clinical trials? *Arch Phys Med Rehabil*. 2002; 83(9):1320–1322.

137. D'Agostino RB, Kwan H. Measuring effectiveness. What to expect without a randomized control group. *Med Care*. 1995;33(suppl 4): AS95–AS105.

138. Maas A, Menon D, Lingsma H, Pineda J, Sandel M, Manley GT. Re-orientation of clinical research in traumatic brain injury: report of a international workshop on comparative effectiveness research. *J Neurotrauma*. 2012;29(1):32–46.

139. Agency for Healthcare Research and Quality. *Comparative Effectiveness of Postacute Rehabilitation for Moderate to Severe Traumatic Brain Injury*. Rockville, MD: Agency for Healthcare Research and Quality; 2011. http://www.effectivehealthcare.ahrq.gov/index.cfm/search-for-guides-reviews-and-reports/?pageaction=displayproduct&productide=726. Accessed April 19, 2012.

140. Guillamondegui OD, Montgomery SA, Phibbs FT, et al. *Traumatic Brain Injury and Depression: Executive Summary No. 25*. Rockville, MD: Agency for Healthcare Research and Quality (US); 2011. http://www.effectivehealthcare.ahrq.gov/index.cfm/search-for-guides-reviews-and-reports/?productide=657&pageaction=displayproduct. Accessed April 19, 2012.

141. Benson K, Hartz AJ. A comparison of observational studies and randomized, controlled trials. *N Engl J Med*. 2000;342(25):1878–1886.

142. Ottenbacher KJ. Statistical conclusion validity. Multiple inferences in rehabilitation research. *Am J Phys Med Rehabil*. 1991;70(6): 317–322.

143. Ottenbacher KJ, Barrett KA. Statistical conclusion validity of rehabilitation research. A quantitative analysis. *Am J Phys Med Rehabil*. 1990;69(2):102–107.

144. Zhan S, Ottenbacher KJ. Single subject research designs for disability research. *Disabil Rehabil*. 2001;23(1):1–8.

145. Jenkins LW, Peters GW, Dixon CE, et al. Conventional and functional proteomics using large format two-dimensional gel electrophoresis 24 hours after controlled cortical impact in postnatal day 17 rats. *J Neurotrauma*. 2002;19(6):715–740.

146. Marciano P, Eberwine JH, Raghupathi R, McIntosh TK. The assessment of genomic alterations using DNA arrays following traumatic brain injury: a review. *Restor Neurol Neurosci*. 2001;18(2–3):105113.

147. Ricker JH, Hillary FG, DeLuca J. Functionally activated brain imaging (O-15 PET and fMRI) in the study of learning and memory after traumatic brain injury. *J Head Trauma Rehabil*. 2001;16(2):191–205.

148. Bigler ED. Quantitative magnetic resonance imaging in traumatic brain injury. *J Head Trauma Rehabil*. 2001;16(2):117–134.

149. Bergsneider M, Hovda DA, McArthur DL, et al. Metabolic recovery following human traumatic brain injury based on FDG-PET: time course and relationship to neurological disability. *J Head Trauma Rehabil*. 2001;16(2):135–148.

150. Wallace BE, Wagner AK, Wagner EP, McDeavitt JT. A history and review of quantitative electroencephalography in traumatic brain injury. *J Head Trauma Rehabil*. 2001;16(2):165–190.

151. Wagner AK. Rehabilomics: a conceptual framework to drive biologis research. *PMR* 2011;3(6 suppl 1):S28–S30.

152. Wagner AK. TBI translational rehabilitation research in the 21st century: exploring a Rehabilomics research model. *Eur J Phys Rehabil Med*. 2010;46(4):549–556.

153. Hoh NZ, Wagner AK, Alexander SA, et al. BCL2 genotypes: functional and neurobehavioral outcomes after severe traumatic brain injury. *J Neurotrauma*. 2010;27(8):1413–1427.

154. Wagner AK, Amin KB, Niyonkuru C, et al. CSF Bcl-2 and cytochrome C temporal profiles in outcome prediction for adults with severe TBI. *J Cereb Blood Flow Metab*. 2011;31(9):1886–1896.

155. Wagner AK, Miller MA, Scanlon J, Ren D, Kochanek PM, Conley YP. Adenosine A1 receptor gene variants associated with posttraumatic seizures after severe TBI. *Epilepsy Res*. 2010;90(3): 259–272.

156. Berger RP, Kochanek PM, Pierce MC. Biochemical markers of brain injury: could they be used as diagnostic adjuncts in cases of inflicted traumatic brain injury? *Child Abuse Negl*. 2004;28(7):739–754.

157. Berger RP, Adelson PD, Pierce MC, Dulani T, Cassidy LD, Kochanek PM. Serum neuron-specific enolase, S100B, and myelin basic protein concentrations after inflicted and noninflicted traumatic brain injury in children. *J Neurosurg*. 2005;103(suppl 1):61–68.

158. Berger RP. The use of serum biomarkers to predict outcome after traumatic brain injury in adults and children. *J Head Trauma Rehabil*. 2006;21(4):315–333.

159. Berger RP, Beers SR, Richichi R, Wiesman D, Adelson PD. Serum biomarker concentrations and outcome after pediatric traumatic brain injury. *J Neurotrauma*. 2007;24(12):1793–1801.

160. Buttram SD, Wisniewski SR, Jackson EK, et al. Multiplex assessment of cytokine and chemokine levels in cerebrospinal fluid following severe pediatric traumatic brain injury: effects of moderate hypothermia. *J Neurotrauma*. 2007;24(11):1707–1717.

161. Dixon CE, Lighthall JW, Anderson TE. Physiologic, histopathologic, and cineradiographic characterization of a new fluid-percussion model of experimental brain injury in the rat. *J Neurotrauma*. 1988;5(2):91–104.

162. Dixon CE, Clifton GL, Lighthall JW, Yaghmai AA, Hayes RL. A controlled cortical impact model of traumatic brain injury in the rat. *J Neurosci Methods*. 1991;39(3):253–262.

163. Kochanek PM, Marion DW, Zhang W, et al. Severe controlled cortical impact in rats: assessment of cerebral edema, blood flow, and contusion volume. *J Neurotrauma*. 1995;12(6):1015–1025.

164. Hamm RJ, Dixon CE, Gbadebo DM, et al. Cognitive deficits following traumatic brain injury produced by controlled cortical impact. *J Neurotrauma*. 1992;9(1):11–20.

165. Whalen MJ, Clark RS, Dixon CE, et al. Reduction of cognitive and motor deficits after traumatic brain injury in mice deficient in poly(-ADP-ribose) polymerase. *J Cereb Blood Flow Metab*. 1999;19(8): 835–842.

166. Kline AE, Massucci JL, Marion DW, Dixon CE. Attenuation of working memory and spatial acquisition deficits after a delayed and chronic bromocriptine treatment regimen in rats subjected to traumatic brain injury by controlled cortical impact. *J Neurotrauma* 2002;19(4):415–425.

167. Wagner AK, Willard LA, Kline AE, et al. Evaluation of estrous cycle stage and gender on behavioral outcome after experimental traumatic brain injury. *Brain Res*. 2004;998(1):113–121.

168. Wagner AK, Sokoloski JE, Chen X, et al. Controlled cortical impact injury influences methylphenidate-induced changes in striatal dopamine neurotransmission. *J Neurochem*. 2009;110(3):801–810.

169. Wagner AK, Drewencki LL, Chen X, et al. Chronic methylphenidate treatment enhances striatal dopamine neurotransmission after experimental traumatic brain injury. *J Neurochem*. 2009;108(4): 986–997.

170. Bauman RA, Ling G, Tong L, et al. An introductory characterization of a combat-casualty-care relevant swine model of closed head injury resulting from exposure to explosive blast. *J Neurotrauma*. 2009;26(6):841–860.

171. Long JB, Bentley TL, Wessner KA, Cerone C, Sweeney S, Bauman RA. Blast overpressure in rats: recreating a battlefield injury in the laboratory. *J Neurotrauma*. 2009;26(6):827–840.

172. Taub E, Uswatte G, Elbert T. New treatments in neurorehabilitation founded on basic research. *Nat Rev Neurosci*. 2002;3(3):228–236.

173. Consensus conference. Rehabilitation of persons with traumatic brain injury. NIH Consensus Development Panel on Rehabilitation of Persons With Traumatic Brain Injury. *JAMA*. 1999;282(10): 974–983.

174. Heltemes KJ, Holbrook TL, Macgregor AJ, Galarneau MR. Blast-related mild traumatic brain injury is associated with a decline in self-rated health amongst US military personnel. *Injury.* 2011.

175. Heltemes KJ, Dougherty AL, Macgregor AJ, Galarneau MR. Inpatient hospitalizations of U.S. military personnel medically evacuated from Iraq and Afghanistan with combat-related traumatic brain injury. *Mil Med.* 2011;176(2):132–135.

176. MacGregor AJ, Shaffer RA, Dougherty AL, et al. Prevalence and psychological correlates of traumatic brain injury in operation iraqi freedom. *J Head Trauma Rehabil.* 2010;25(1):1–8.

177. Warden D. Military TBI during the Iraq and Afghanistan wars. *J Head Trauma Rehabil.* 2006;21(5):398–402.

178. U.S. Department of Defense. The Budget for Fiscal Year 2012. http://www.whitehouse.gov/sites/default/files/omb/budget/fy2012/assets/budget.pdf. Accessed April 19, 2012.

179. National Institute on Disability and Rehabilitation Research. National Institute on Disability and Rehabilitation Research (NIDRR) Long Range Plan for Fiscal Years 1999–2003. http://www2.ed.gov/rschstat/research/pubs/nidrr-lrp-99-03.pdf. Accessed April 19, 2012.

180. Sherwood AM. Development of the NIDRR Long-range Plan: 2010–2014. Washington, DC: U.S. Department of Education; 2011. http://www2.ed.gov/rschstat/research/pubs/nidrr-lrp-10-14-draft-overview.ppt. Accessed April 19, 2012.

181. Craig Hospital Research Department. *Traumatic Brain Injury Model Systems National Data and Statistical Center (TBINDSC).* Englewood, CO: Craig Hospital Research Department; 2011. http://www.tbindsc.org/. Accessed April 19, 2012.

182. Bushnik T. Introduction: the Traumatic Brain Injury Model Systems of Care. *Arch Phys Med Rehabil.* 2003;84(2):151–152.

183. Centers for Disease Control and Prevention. CDC Injury Research Agenda, 2009–2018. Centers for Disease Control and Prevention Web site. http://www.cdc.gov/injury/ResearchAgenda/. Accessed April 19, 2012.

184. Healthy People 2010. *What are Its Goals?* Washington, DC: U.S. Department of Health and Human Services. http://www.healthypeople.gov/2010/?visit=1. Accessed April 19, 2012.

185. Healthy People 2020: Improving the Health of American. Washington, DC: U. S. Department of Health and Human Services. http://www.healthypeople.gov/2020/default.aspx. Accessed April 19, 2012.

186. Koh HK. A 2020 vision for healthy people. *N Engl J Med.* 2010; 362(18):1653–1656.

187. Division of Program Coordination, Planning, and Strategic Initiatives (DPCPSI). *The NIH Common Fund.* Bethesda, MD: National Institutes of Health; 2011. http://commonfund.nih.gov/. Accessed April 19, 2012.

188. Agency for Healthcare Research and Quality. *Effective Health Care Program: Helping You Make Better Treatment Choices.* Rockville, MD: Agency for Healthcare Research and Quality; 2011. http://www.effectivehealthcare.ahrq.gov/index.cfm/. Accessed April 19, 2012.

Traumatic Brain Injury Epidemiology and Public Health Issues

Victor G. Coronado, Lisa C. McGuire, Mark Faul, David E. Sugerman, and William S. Pearson

INTRODUCTION

Traumatic brain injury (TBI), an often preventable injury, is a leading cause of morbidity and mortality in the United States and the world. In this chapter, we describe the epidemiology of TBI in terms of frequency, demographics, mechanism of injury, risk factors, severity, outcomes, and economic impact. Most of the US data presented in this chapter were estimated by researchers from the Centers for Disease Control and Prevention (CDC) and National Center for Injury Prevention and Control (NCIPC) using standard TBI definitions developed by CDC in the mid 1990s. Epidemiological data are essential for developing effective prevention programs directed to those at highest risk and to plan for providing appropriate health care and rehabilitation services to survivors.

TRAUMATIC BRAIN INJURY EPIDEMIOLOGY

Traumatic Brain Injury Definition

Estimating the burden of TBI requires standard definitions (1). Yet, over the past 3 decades, disparate case definitions have been used to study TBI, making epidemiologic and clinical research difficult (1,2), especially when studying less severe TBI (1). Since 1995, the CDC has defined TBI as an injury to the head arising from blunt or penetrating trauma or from acceleration/deceleration forces resulting in one or more of the following: decreased level of consciousness, amnesia, objective neurologic or neuropsychological abnormality(s), skull fracture(s), diagnosed intracranial lesion(s), or head injury listed as a cause of death in the death certificate (3). The CDC has established surveillance case definitions for obtaining data from different sources, including data using codes of the International Classification of Diseases (ICD) (1,3–4). A limitation of the CDC definition is that it does not include injuries from blasts or explosions, which can also produce TBI through multiple mechanisms, including overpressure or shock waves (5). The International and Interagency Initiative toward Common Data Elements of Research on TBI and Psychological Health group—a Federal initiative that includes CDC—produced a definition that includes injuries because of this and other energy sources (6).

Classification of Traumatic Brain Injury

Classifying TBI is essential to improving clinical management and to facilitating epidemiological and scientific research. Many classifications exist for TBI; the most common methods used by researchers include: (*a*) Abbreviated Injury Scale (AIS), which classifies injuries by body region according to relative severity (7); (*b*) Revised Trauma Score (RTS), which uses systolic blood pressure, respiratory rate, and scores of the Glasgow Coma Scale (GCS) (8); and (*c*) the GCS, a clinical tool designed to assess coma and impaired consciousness after TBI (9,10). The GCS, one of the most commonly used methods, has scores ranging from 3 to 15 based on verbal, motor, and eye-opening reactions to stimuli. Patients with TBI with GCS scores of 3–8 are categorized as severe TBI; 9–12 as moderate TBI; and 13–15 as mild TBI. Despite that this classification system has been widely adopted because of its high interobserver reliability, reasonably good prognostic capabilities (11), and value for inpatient assessment (10,12), serious concerns have arisen about its low accuracy and reliability (12–14) and utility for TBI classification (15). Moreover, medical management has changed since the development of the GCS, and most patients who appear to have serious injuries now receive intubation, sedation, and pharmacologic paralysis prior to clinical evaluation, which interferes with accurate assessment and GCS scoring. Similarly, it is difficult to apply the GCS to people who are intoxicated or incapacitated from drug use or to infants, young children, and patients who have preexisting neurologic impairment. The GCS is also a poor discriminator for the spectrum of less severe TBI because most people with a mild TBI do not exhibit signs that impact the scoring of the GCS. Despite these and other limitations, the GCS is used widely worldwide as a standard for classifying TBI severity.

Traumatic Brain Injury Severity: Current Classification Schemes

The CDC defines a case of mild TBI as a brain injury with one or more of the following conditions: any period of observed or self-reported transient confusion, disorientation,

TABLE 8-1 Department of Defense/Department of Veterans Affairs Severity Stratification for Non-Penetrating Traumatic Brain Injury

CHARACTERISTIC	MILD	MODERATE	SEVERE
Brain imaging	Normal	Normal or abnormal	Normal or abnormal
Length of time of loss of consciousness	0–30 min	> 30 min and < 24 hours	> 24 hours
Alternation of consciousness/mental state	Lasting up to 24 hours	> 24 hours. Severity based on other criteria	
Post-traumatic amnesia	0–1 day	> 1 and < 7 days	> 7 days
Glasgow Coma Scale[a]	13–15	9–12	3–8

[a] For purposes of injury stratification, the GCS is measured at or after 24 hours.
Reprinted from Centers for Disease Control and Prevention, National Institutes of Health, Department of Defense, Department of Veterans Affairs Leadership Panel (16) with permission.

or impaired consciousness; amnesia around the time of injury; loss of consciousness (LOC) lasting < 30 minutes; post-traumatic amnesia (PTA) lasting up to 24 hours; GCS scores of 13–15; and an AIS score of 2 for the head region (1). According to CDC, persons with intracranial lesions demonstrated by neuroimaging or with focal neurological deficits (e.g., hemiplegia) may still be considered mild if the criteria described earlier are met. Mild TBI clinical screening indicators are, however, limited in consistently predicting TBI severity and clinical outcomes. For example, persons with GCS scores of 13–15 and intracranial injury (e.g., focal cerebral contusion) and/or depressed skull fractures may have comparable outcomes to patients with more severe TBI (16).

Other classification methods exist, including a model to classify TBI severity recently developed by the Departments of Defense (DOD) and Veterans Affairs (VA) (17) (Table 8-1). The sensitivity and specificity of this model for mild, moderate, and severe TBI has yet to be determined.

Surveillance Methods

In the United States, TBI surveillance is associated with some challenges. TBI information is obtained from multiple sources, including hospitals, emergency departments (EDs), doctors' offices, outpatient facilities, and vital statistics. TBI surveillance does not include persons who had a TBI while serving abroad in the US military or those who did not seek medical care (18–22), which, in 1991, accounted for almost 25% of people who self-reported TBI (23).

Because there is no single unified system for TBI surveillance, TBI researchers use a variety of methods for TBI-related epidemiologic research in terms of key measures (1,3,4,18,22).

Assessing Traumatic Brain Injury Incidence
With respect to the incidence of non-fatal TBI, many TBI surveillance systems in the United States, including CDC's, rely on surveillance data based on ICD-9-CM (International Classification of Diseases, Ninth Revision, Clinical Modification) coded administrative/billing records related to services rendered to patients during their hospitalizations, ED visits, outpatient care, and visits to doctors' offices; most of these data are collected via surveys by the National Center for Health Statistics (NCHS) (http://www.cdc.gov/nchs/surveys.htm) and the Agency for Health Care Research and Quality's (AHRQ) Health Care Cost and Utilization Project

(HCUP) (http://www.ahrq.gov/data/). To assess TBI-related mortality in the United States, CDC uses data from NCHS' Multiple Cause-of-Death Mortality Data Public Use Data files (22); which are coded using ICD-9 (ICD-Ninth Revision) codes for years prior to 1999, and ICD-10 (ICD-Tenth Revision) codes from 1999 to present (4,24). The death certificates submitted by all 50 states and the District of Columbia contain diagnoses and external cause of injury codes; these are identified from parts I and II and from the underlying cause-of-death field on the death certificate. These files exclude deaths that occurred abroad among US residents and members of the active duty US military.

Assessing Traumatic Brain Injury–Related Hospitalizations
To estimate the number of TBI hospitalizations in the United States, CDC uses ICD-9-CM coded administrative/billing data from NCHS' National Hospital Discharge Survey (NHDS) (18) and from the AHRQ's HCUP Nationwide Inpatient Sample (HCUP-NIS). HCUP also includes the Kids' Inpatient Database (HCUP-KID) that can be used to study the epidemiology of TBI in children. An additional source is the CDC TBI Surveillance System (CDC-TBI-SS) that started in the mid 1990s (19). This system has two aspects. The first is the "core" aspect, which during 2005–2011 was conducted by 30 states. This aspect relies on ICD-9-CM coded hospital-based administrative/billing and ICD-10 coded vital statistics data. The second aspect is called "extended." Through this aspect, 4 states collect selected clinical data (e.g., GCS scores) abstracted from a representative sample of medical records identified through the core aspect (4). Two of these 30 states conduct core TBI surveillance in EDs. More severe TBI can be studied using the National Trauma Data Bank (NTDB) and NTDB's National Sample Program (NSP), which provides baseline estimates of TBI-related incidence and care in trauma centers (http://facs.org/trauma/ntdb/nsp.html).

Assessing Traumatic Brain Injury–Related Visits to Emergency Departments and Ambulatory Care
To study TBI in EDs, CDC relies on data from NCHS' National Hospital Ambulatory Medical Care Survey (NHAMCS) (18) and the National Electronic Injury Surveillance System-All Injury Program (NEISS-AIP) (25). The NEISS-AIP is a Consumer Product Safety Commission (CPSC) and CDC sponsored national survey of all US hospitals with EDs. Other

sources include the CDC-TBI-SS extended aspect and the HCUP's Nationwide Emergency Department Sample (NEDS) and HCUP's State Emergency Department Databases (SEDD); the latter may yield selected TBI-related state level statistics.

In ambulatory care settings, TBI researchers (21) have used data from NCHS' NHAMCS-Outpatient Department module and from the National Ambulatory Medical Care Survey (NAMCS).

Other Sources of Traumatic Brain Injury Incidence Data

To study the epidemiology of TBI by intent, researchers rely on data from multiple sources. For violence-related TBI, researchers use data from the National Violent Death Reporting System (NVDRS), an 18-state CDC-funded system that collects information from death certificates, police reports, and coroner or medical examiner reports about violent deaths (e.g., child maltreatment). To study work-related TBI, researchers use data from state employee and workers' compensation insurance programs. To study motor vehicle crash-related TBI, 2 systems can be used: the Fatality Analysis Reporting System (FARS) and FARS' General Estimates System (GES); FARS/GES allows estimating fatal and nonfatal motor vehicle crash-related TBIs in the United States (http://www.nhtsa.gov/NCSA). Sports-related TBI data can be obtained from the NEISS-AIP (25) and from the National Collegiate Athletic Association (NCAA) Injury Surveillance System, which contains data from a representative sample of NCAA colleges only, although it excludes some contact sports (http://www.ncaa.org/wps/wcm/connect/public/ncaa/resources). Information on TBI among US military personnel and veterans can be obtained from the Department of Defense website (http://www.health.mil/Research/TBI_Numbers.aspx) and the Armed Forces Health Surveillance Report (http://afhsc.army.mil/dmss).

Registries

TBI registries capture population-based information over time on patient demographics, medical history, diagnoses, treatment, outcomes, and status at discharge for every injured patient locally or nationally (26). The aim of TBI registries varies. Population-based registries may help to determine the incidence of TBI or identify risks, whereas hospital-based registries may help to identify the best therapies. Funded by the US Department of Education, the TBI Model Systems (TBIMS) is a registry that aims to advance medical rehabilitation of individuals with TBI. Two CDC-funded 4-year longitudinal follow-up registries were conducted by state public health agencies: one in Colorado, in the late 1990s (27); and the other in South Carolina, in the early 2000s (28). Other states have implemented registries, for example in response to a state law. For example, since July 1, 2007, the Rhode Island Department of Health (RI-DoH) maintains a TBI Registry. RI hospitals are mandated to report to the RI-DoH within 14 days of diagnosis—all cases of TBI diagnosed through inpatient and EDs. Reported data include principal diagnosis, cause of injury, place of incident, type of discharge, dates of admission/discharge, and patient demographics including name, address, social security number, date of birth, gender, ethnicity, and race (http://www

.health.state.ri.us/injury/traumaticbrain). These registries provided answers to unique questions about the acute and long-term health and prevalence of patients with TBI and the impact of the injury on society.

Methodological Issues and Limitations of Traumatic Brain Injury Surveillance in the United States

The United States lacks a uniform national surveillance system to study TBI-related morbidity and mortality at the national and state levels; thus, researchers must mainly rely on data sources with ICD coded databases and death certificates. The data quality and completeness of ICD coded databases used by CDC and others (e.g., NHDS, NHAMCS, HCUP-NIS, etc.) depends on hospital coding practices, coders' knowledge and expertise, the effects of attaining maximum reimbursement by providers, or provider's failure to properly document findings. Moreover, because these surveillance systems obtain data from ICD-9-CM coded administrative/billing databases, they may provide limited information. These systems may omit clinical and prevention-related information, such as outcome indicators like GCS (29) or external causes of injury codes (E-codes) (18–19). By design, some of these surveillance systems do not collect all ICD coded diagnostic codes reported by providers. For example, the NHAMCS collects up to 3 ICD-9-CM diagnostic codes, leading to underreporting of mild TBI cases, which, unless a unique diagnosis, tend to be reported last. With the exception of vital statistics, most surveys do not allow the estimation of patient level data. They yield hospital discharge- or visit-related TBI statistics because they cannot distinguish first admissions or visits from readmissions or follow up visits (18). Additionally, the validity of certain ICD-9-CM codes, for example 959.01 (head injury, unspecified), needs to be determined. This code, added to ICD-9-CM in 1997, was not intended to be assigned to TBI cases; however, in the United States it has been assigned incorrectly to a substantial proportion of cases previously coded as 854 (intracranial injury of other and unspecified nature). Data from the CDC-TBI-SS suggest that the sensitivity for this code in EDs ranges from 60% to 70% and in hospital wards from 70% to 80% (CDC unpublished data).

Questions have been raised about the accuracy of TBI reporting using death certificates. A study of TBI-related death using surveillance data from death certificates in Oklahoma, reported a sensitivity of 78%. Most missed cases (62%) listed "multiple trauma" as the cause of death. Death certificate surveillance in this state was more likely to miss TBI-related deaths in traffic crashes, falls, and among persons aged 65 years and older (30). Furthermore, until 2011, only 30 states were funded to participate in the ICD coded-based CDC surveillance system; of these, only 4 conducted medical record review and abstraction.

THE BURDEN OF TRAUMATIC BRAIN INJURY IN THE UNITED STATES

The Overall Incidence of Traumatic Brain Injury in the United States

During 2002–2006, approximately 1.7 million TBI-related hospitalizations, ED visits, and deaths occur every year; of

TABLE 8-2 Estimated Average Annual Numbers, Rates, and Percentages of Traumatic Brain Injury–Related Emergency Department Visits, Hospitalizations, and Deaths, by Age Group—United States, 2002–2006

Age (years)	HOSPITALIZATIONS[b]			EMERGENCY DEPARTMENT VISITS[a]			DEATHS[c]			TOTAL	
	Number	Rate[d]	Row %	Number	Rate[d]	Row %	Number	Rate[d]	Row %	Number	Rate[d]
0–4	15,239	76.1	5.7	251,546	1,256.2	93.9	998	5.0	0.4	267,783	1,337.3
5–9	8,799	44.7	7.7	105,015	532.9	91.9	450	2.3	0.4	114,264	579.9
10–14	11,098	52.9	8.6	117,387	559.8	90.8	726	3.5	0.6	129,211	616.2
15–19	24,896	119.9	13.4	157,198	757.0	84.5	3,995	19.2	2.1	186,089	896.2
20–24	20,683	99.7	12.8	136,079	655.8	84.1	5,048	24.3	3.1	161,810	779.8
25–34	28,953	72.6	13.7	174,811	438.3	83.0	6,826	17.1	3.2	210,591	528.0
35–44	32,310	73.3	19.9	123,436	279.9	75.8	6,995	15.9	4.3	162,741	369.1
45–54	29,068	69.9	21.4	99,715	239.7	73.4	7,125	17.1	5.2	135,908	326.7
55–64	22,600	77.7	26.5	57,612	198.2	67.6	5,028	17.3	5.9	85,240	293.2
65–74	20,990	113.3	29.3	46,365	250.2	64.7	4,252	22.9	5.9	71,607	386.4
≥ 75	60,510	339.3	36.4	95,633	536.2	57.5	10,095	56.6	6.1	166,237	932.0
Total	275,146	93.8	16.3	1,364,797	465.4	80.7	51,538	17.6	3.0	1,691,481	576.8
Adj.[e]		93.0			468.0			17.4			579.0

[a] Persons who were hospitalized, died, or transferred to another facility were excluded.
[b] Based on part I of the cause of death section of the death certificate. In-hospital deaths and patients who transferred from another hospital were excluded.
[c] 128 mortality records (from 2002–2006) were omitted because of missing age information.
[d] Average annual rate per 100,000 population.
[e] Age-adjusted to the 2000 U.S. standard population.
Reprinted from Faul M, Xu L, Wald MM, Coronado VG. *Traumatic Brain Injury in the United States: Emergency Department Visits, Hospitalizations, and Deaths, 2002–2006*. Atlanta, GA: Centers for Disease Control and Prevention, National Center for Injury Prevention and Control; 2010.

these, 1.4 million were treated and released from EDs, 275,000 were hospitalized and discharged alive, and 52,000 died (based on part I of the cause of death section of the death certificate) (18) (Table 8-2). These statistics, however, do not include persons treated in physicians' offices and outpatient facilities, those who did not seek medical care, and US military personnel serving abroad.

Traumatic Brain Injury–Related Mortality
Nearly one-third of all injury related deaths involve a TBI (31). Using parts I and II of the cause of death section of the death certificate, CDC data for 1997–2007 indicates that approximately 53,000 US residents die every year with a TBI-related injury (22). The rate of TBI deaths among males was 3 times that of females, and among males, rates were highest among non-Hispanic American Indian/Alaska Natives and lowest among Hispanics. For the general US population—firearm, motor-vehicle traffic (MVT) accidents, and falls were the leading causes of TBI-related death. In trauma centers, where more severe TBI might be treated, TBI-related mortality was reported to be as high as 50% of all trauma-related deaths (32).

Traumatic Brain Injury–Related Morbidity
Traumatic Brain Injury–Related Hospitalizations
TBI-related hospitalizations represent 16% of the 1.7 million people reported with a TBI in the United States; males accounted for 62% of these TBI hospitalizations (18). The highest rates of TBI hospitalizations occurred among older adults aged 75 years and older (339.3/100,000 population) and children aged 15–19 years (119.9/100,000 population) (Table 8-

2) (Figure 8-1). Falls and MVT accidents were the leading causes of TBI hospitalizations in the United States (Figure 8-2). In 2005, rates of TBI-related hospitalizations varied by state. Data from the CDC-TBI-SS indicate that these rates ranged from 43.1/100,000 population in Rhode Island to 127.9/100,000 population in Pennsylvania (33); the reported overall rate for the 30 states participating in this system was 84.3/100,000 population.

Traumatic Brain Injury–Related Emergency Department Visits
During the mid-2000s, approximately 5% of the 28.7 million injury-related visits to EDs in the United States were cases of TBI-treated and released from those settings (Table 8-2) (18). This statistic represents approximately 80% of the 1.7 million people diagnosed annually with a TBI in the United States. These data suggest that most TBIs in the United States are mild with males accounting for 58% of these TBI-related visits. The highest rates of TBI-related ED visits occurred among older adults aged 75 years and older (536.2/100,000 population) and children aged 0–4 years (1256.2/100,000 population). Falls and being struck by or against objects were the leading causes of TBI among those treated and released from EDs in the United States.

Traumatic Brain Injury–Related Visits to Physician Offices and Outpatient Facilities
According to the 1991 NCHS' National Health Interview Study (NHIS), an estimated 1.5 million noninstitutionalized US civilians sustained nonfatal brain injuries that did not result in hospitalization; of these, 25% (*n* = 381,000) never sought medical care and 14% (*n* = 221,000) were treated in clinics and offices (23). Data from NCHS' NAMCS and NHAMCS for 1995–1997 indicated that 439,000 TBI-related

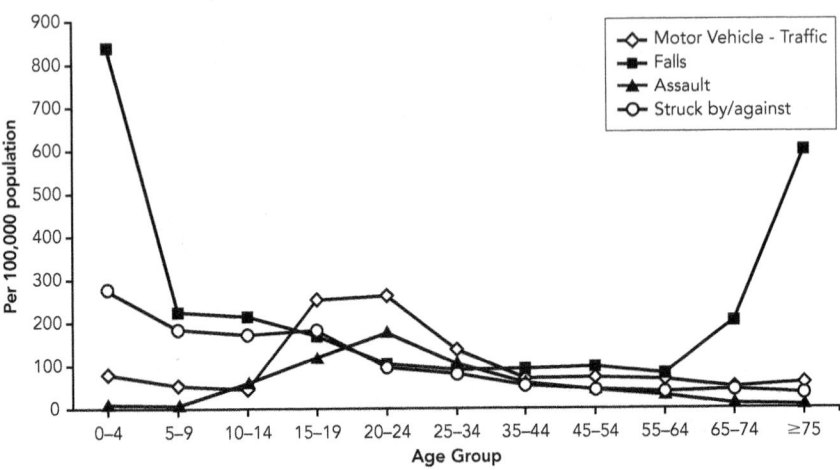

FIGURE 8–1 Estimated average annual rates of traumatic brain injury–combined emergency department visits, hospitalizations, and deaths by age group and external cause—United States, 2002–2006.
Reprinted from Faul M, Xu L, Wald MM, Coronado VG. *Traumatic Brain Injury in the United States: Emergency Department Visits, Hospitalizations, and Deaths, 2002–2006.* Atlanta, GA: Centers for Disease Control and Prevention, National Center for Injury Prevention and Control; 2010.

visits were made to physicians' offices and another 89,000 visits to various outpatient facilities (21). Because an undetermined number of patients were seen more than once by their health care providers for the same or a recurrent TBI, these statistics are not comparable. NHIS weighted data reflect all noninstitutionalized civilians in the United States (i.e., person/patient level data); in contrast, both NAMCS and NHAMCS reflect the number of encounters/visits to those facilities.

Trends in Morbidity and Mortality

Trends in TBI morbidity vary by site of medical care. TBI-related visits to EDs and hospitalizations in the United States have steadily increased over time. During periods of 1995–2001 and 2002–2006, the rate of TBI-related ED visits increased from 401.2 to 468.0 per 100,000 population, respectively (34,18). In those periods, the increases were especially higher in children aged 0–4 years (from 1,035.0 to 1,256.2 per 100,000 population, respectively) and in older adults aged 75 years and older (from 336.4 to 536.2 per 100,000 population, respectively), largely reflecting the increases of fall-related TBI-related visits to EDs (from 229.9 to 440.2 per 100,000 population, respectively). During the same periods, TBI-related hospitalization increased from 85.2 to 93.8 per 100,000 population; these increases were higher in older adults aged

65–74 years and 75 years and older, largely reflecting the increases of fall-caused (from 108.1 to 126.0/100,000, respectively) and motor vehicle collision (MVC)-caused (from 19.2 to 22.6/100,000, respectively) TBI-related hospitalizations in those age groups (Figure 8-3). During the same periods, the rate of TBI-related hospitalization because of MVC among 15–19 year olds—the group with the highest MVC TBI rates—decreased from 55.4 to 46.2 per 100,000 population, respectively (34,18).

From 1997 to 2007, the rates of TBI-related death in the United States have declined 7.6% (from 19.3 to 17.8 per 100,000 population, respectively). These decreases were greatest in persons aged 0–44 years and among those aged 75 years and older (22); in the latter age group, these rates increased with increasing age. These trends follow the declines reported by CDC for periods 1979–1992 and 1989–1998 (from 22% to 11.4%, respectively) (35,36,22). Except for falls, during 1997–2007, the rates for all causes of TBI-related deaths decreased (22). Although firearms are the leading cause of TBI-related death in the United States since the 1980s (35–36), the rates declined from 7.2 (in 1997) to 6.2 (in 2007) per 100,000 population (22). In contrast, from 1997 to 2007, fall-related TBI deaths (especially among older adults) increased from 2.4 to 3.8 per 100,000 population, respectively, offsetting some of the declines observed in MVT-related

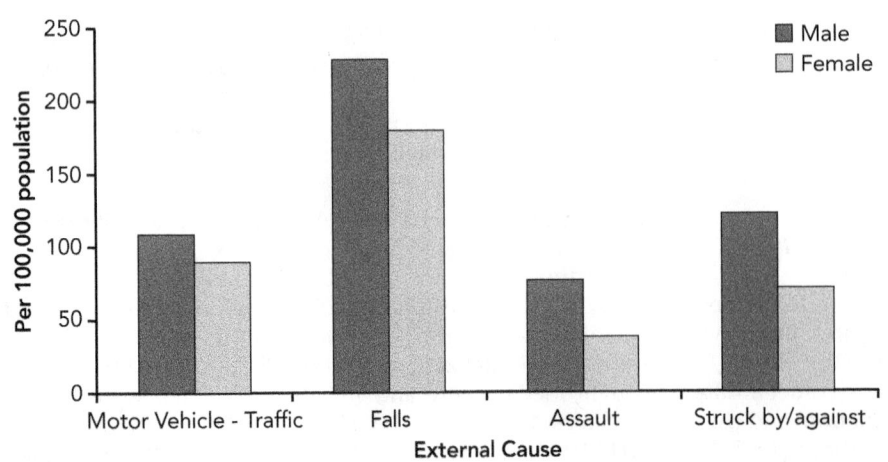

FIGURE 8–2 Estimated average annual age-adjusted rates of traumatic brain injury-combined emergency department visits, hospitalizations, and deaths, by external cause and sex—United States, 2002–2006. Reprinted from Faul M, Xu L, Wald MM, Coronado V. *Traumatic Brain Injury in the United States: Emergency Department Visits, Hospitalizations, and Deaths, 2002–2006.* Atlanta, GA: Centers for Disease Control and Prevention, National Center for Injury Prevention and Control; 2010.

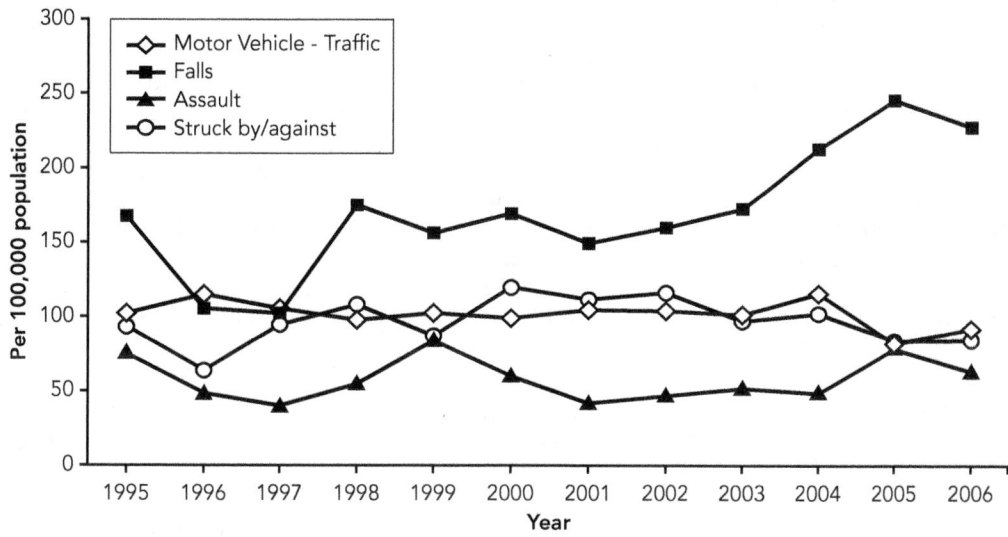

FIGURE 8–3 Estimated annual age-adjusted rates of traumatic brain injury-combined emergency department visits, hospitalizations, and death, by year and external cause of injury—United States, 1995–2006.
Reprinted from Faul M, Xu L, Wald MM, Coronado V. *Traumatic Brain Injury in the United States: Emergency Department Visits, Hospitalizations, and Deaths, 2002–2006.* Atlanta, GA: Centers for Disease Control and Prevention, National Center for Injury Prevention and Control; 2010.

(from 6.4 to 5.8 per 100,000 population, respectively) and firearm-related TBI (from 7.2 to 6.2 per 100,000 population, respectively) TBI (22). Additionally, there was a significant decrease in the rates of TBI-related death among persons who were dead on arrival to hospitals and those who died in EDs or in outpatient facilities (22).

Traumatic Brain Injury in the United States Military and in Zones of Conflict

TBI has been called the signature injury of the Iraq and Afghanistan wars and is a critically important health issue affecting survivors of these and other previous wars. Since October 2001, approximately 2 million US service members have served at least 1 tour of duty in Iraq or Afghanistan (37). Of the 497,300 veterans who sought care from VA Medical Centers from 2004 to 2009, 34,700 veterans were identified as having been evaluated or treated for a condition possibly related to a TBI (38). Compared to previous wars, the use of improved protective equipment (e.g., Kevlar body armor) and timely access to trauma care in these theaters may have contributed to a decrease in injury-related mortality among US soldiers (39). Among surviving soldiers wounded in combat in Iraq and Afghanistan, TBI accounts for a larger proportion of casualties than in other recent US wars. Approximately 25% of all soldiers who were evacuated alive from those theaters had head and neck injuries, including severe TBIs (39–40). In contrast, in Vietnam, this figure ranged from 12% to 14%; and an additional 2% to 4% had a TBI and a lethal wound to the chest or abdomen. Because mortality from TBI among US combatants in Vietnam was at least 75%, soldiers with nonfatal TBIs made up only a small fraction of the casualties treated in hospitals (39).

Overall, from 2000 to the 4th quarter of 2010, 202,281 TBIs were identified in the US military; of these, approximately 77% were mild, 17% were moderate, and 1% were severe, 2% penetrating, and 3% not classifiable (41). The numbers of US soldiers with TBI, however, have steadily increased during this decade from 10,963 in 2000 to 29,252 in 2009 (41). These increases in non-fatal TBI may be related to blasts from improvised explosive devices (IEDs) (42), increased awareness of TBI, better surveillance, and improved

combat lifesaving techniques. According to a study of 8,687 soldiers with TBIs in 2008, 54% were caused by blasts, 27% because of multiple causes, 6% from falls, 6% vehicular, 2% from bullets, and 5% from other causes (Defense and Veterans Brain Injury Center. Data from January through October 31, 2008).

TBI is also a public health problem among civilians living near war or conflict zones. Unprotected civilians are victims of war-related violence; for example, the United Nations Assistance Mission in Afghanistan (UNAMA) reported that, in 2009, almost 6,000 civilians were killed or injured because of hostilities (43). This UNAMA report, however, does not present data on the burden of TBI. Without information on the incidence of TBI among civilians caught in war zones, it will be difficult to address current and future rehabilitation needs of survivors.

Traumatic Brain Injury in Sports and Recreation

Sports and recreation (SR) injuries constitute an additional public health problem in the United States. In the United States, approximately 44 million boys and girls participate in organized sports (44); and 7.6 million United States high school students participate in sports-related activities each year. Of these, approximately 1 million play 11-man football and 500,000 each play basketball and baseball (45). It has been estimated that 1.6 to 3.8 million SR-related TBIs occur in the United States every year (46,47). These SR TBI numbers, however, are at least equal or almost double the TBI numbers for the US population—highlighting the magnitude of the public health problem and the need for better surveillance to develop sound prevention interventions.

Using NEISS data, CDC estimated that during 2001–2005, on average, approximately 207,830 persons were treated in EDs for SR-related TBIs annually; of these, children aged 10–19 years had the highest rates of SR-related TBI visits to EDs. Almost 90% of these patients were treated and released, suggesting that most of these cases were mild (25). Football ($N = 22,689$), basketball ($N = 14,680$), and baseball ($N = 10,103$) were the organized sports with the greatest proportion of TBI visits to EDs. Bicycling, however, ranked highest in the number of TBIs seen in EDs for all ages at

40,424 cases. However, when comparing the number of TBIs to the total number of injuries for each SR activity, horseback riding was the activity with the greatest number of TBIs per injury episode (12/100; $N = 6,650$). These data suggest that younger children and high school aged athletes may be most at risk because of their high levels of sports participation and because of their levels of brain development and other anatomical and developmental differences.

Mild TBIs are the most common athletic head injury (48) and can occur in any SR activity (25); these account for up to 9% of all high school athletic injuries and 6% of injuries in college (49). Among high school soccer players, boys had higher concussion rates than girls (50). At the high school and collegiate levels, girls sustained higher concussion rates than boys while playing basketball, soccer, and baseball/softball (49).

It is important to note that the true burden of SR-related TBI potentially is underestimated because of lack of risk data documentation and the fact that many people do not seek care after the injury (1–51).

Brain Injury in Childhood

TBI is one of the leading causes of morbidity and mortality in children and young adults (18–22). From 2002 to 2006, approximately 697,347 TBIs occurred among children aged 0–19 years. Of these, 631,146 were TBI-related ED visits, 60,032 hospitalizations, and 6,169 deaths (Table 8-2) (18). For children aged 15–19 years and 0–4 years, the rates of TBI-associated hospitalizations (119.9 and 76.1 per 100,000 population, respectively) and deaths (19.2 and 5.0 per 100,000 population, respectively) were highest compared to children in other age groups.

External Causes and Intentionality

During 2002–2006, the leading external causes of TBI in the United States were falls (35.2%), MVT accidents (17.3%), being struck by or against objects (16.5%), and assaults (10.2%) (Figure 8-2); most of these injuries were unintentional (CDC unpublished data). Unfortunately, for approximately 12% of these cases, information on the mechanisms of injury was missing (18).

Knowledge about the external causes and intentionality are crucial for understanding the epidemiology and prevention of TBI (22); researchers obtain this information mainly from administrative/billing based databases using the external cause of injury ICD-9-CM codes, also known as E-codes. These codes allow researchers to identify populations at risk (e.g., TBI caused by falls in older adults) and injury locale (e.g., abusive TBI in inner city children) that can be used to develop prevention strategies (e.g., helmet give-away programs to school-aged children), to evaluate the effectiveness of interventions (52), and to determine the intent (e.g., suicide among youths). Thus, it is of extreme importance that health care providers document diagnoses, external causes, and information on the circumstances of injury—and that ICD coding is complete.

Falls

During 2002–2006, falls were the leading cause of TBI in the United States (Figure 8-2) (18). On average, falls accounted for almost 35% of the 1.7 million reported TBIs in the United States; of these, 523,043 were treated and released from EDs, 62,334 were hospitalized, and 9,718 died. Falls caused 50.2% of the TBIs among children aged 0–4 years and 60.7% of the TBIs among older adults aged 65 years or older. The rates of fall-related TBI increased after 65 years of age (Figure 8-1).

During 1997–2007, falls were the second leading cause of TBI-related death in the United States (22). Overall, males had 1.5 times higher rates of fall-related TBI death than females (3.7 vs 2.5 per 100,000 population, respectively). These fall-related TBI rates in all age groups were higher among males than females and increased significantly with age for both sexes.

Motor Vehicle Traffic

During 2002–2006, MVT accidents were the second leading cause of TBI in the United States (18). Overall, rates of MVT-related TBIs were higher among teens and younger adults aged 15–24 years; these rates slightly increased with age after 65 years of age (Figure 8-1). The rates of TBI among motor vehicle (MV)-occupants were at least 4 times higher than those of motorcyclists, pedestrians, and pedal cyclists who were seen in EDs or were hospitalized or died (18). These statistics may partially reflect the large number of persons at risk. According to the US Bureau of Transportation Statistics, in 2008, for example, there were approximately 137 million passenger cars compared to 7.7 million motorcycles (available at: http://www.bts.gov/publications/national_transportation_statistics/html/table_01_11.html).

During 1997–2007, males had 2.4 times higher rates of MVT-related TBI deaths than females (8.2 vs 3.5 per 100,000 population, respectively) (22). These rates were higher among males in every age group; especially among males aged 15–19, 20–24, and 85 years and older (15.3, 17.9, and 13.0 per 100,000 population, respectively). From 1997 to 2007, the annual overall rates of MVT–related TBI deaths decreased significantly for MV-occupants (from 3.7 to 2.0 per 100,000 population, respectively), pedestrians (from 0.8 to 0.5 per 100,000 population, respectively), and pedal cyclists (from 0.2 to 0.1 per 100,000 population, respectively); in contrast, motorcycle-related TBI death rates increased 133.1%, from 0.3 to 0.6 per 100,000 population (22).

Assaults, Suicides, and Homicides

During 2002–2006, assaults accounted for almost 10% (169,625) of the 1.7 million annually reported TBIs in the United States (18); of these, 148,471 were treated and released from EDs, 15,341 were hospitalized, and 5,813 died. Overall, persons aged 15–34 years, especially 20–24 year olds, had the highest rates of assault-related TBIs.

During 1997–2007, firearm-related events (34.8%) were the leading cause of TBI-related death in the United States; of these, 74.2% were suicides and 22.2% were homicides (22). In this period, firearm-related TBI suicides decreased 11.5%, from 5.1 to 4.7 per 100,000 population whereas firearm-related homicides decreased 21.8%, from 1.7 to 1.4 per 100,000 population. Overall, males had more than 6 times higher rates of firearm-related TBI deaths than females (11.2 vs 1.8 per 100,000 population). Among males, these rates were highest among persons aged 20–24 years and 75 years and older; especially among black males aged 20–34 year old (22). CDC unpublished data indicated that among older adult males, excess risk for self-inflicted TBI was associated with the age range 72–84 years, not living in the Northeast of the United States, and comorbid conditions of depression and cancer. Among older adult females, excess risk was associated with age range 65–78 years and comorbid condition of depression only. These data indicate that self-inflicted TBI is rare but when it occurs, older men aged 72–84 years are more likely to be the victims and that the injury is usually life threatening.

Risk Factors

Risk factors associated with TBI are multiple, complex, and interdependent. In this section, we will discuss the risk factors of age, sex, race/ethnicity, and recurrent TBI.

Age

The CDC data indicated that children aged 0–4 years, youths aged 15–24 years, and older adults aged 65 years and older had the highest rates of TBI in the United States (18–22). For older adults, the TBI rates increased with increasing age. These high age-related TBI rates mostly reflect exposure to falls and MV incidents in children, youths, and older adults. The high rates of TBI in these age groups may be caused by body and brain anatomical differences in children; and among older adults, the effects of aging, the high prevalence of comorbidities, and the frequent use of medications, including those that may affect brain function (19,32).

Sex

Overall and in almost every age group, TBI morbidity and mortality were higher for males than for females. These differences may reflect the higher rates of general injury among males (available at http://www.cdc.gov/injury/wisqars/index.html) and perhaps differences between males and females in risk-taking behavior and the traditional societal roles and activities (53). Other factors may also contribute to these differences because these statistics vary by age group and by external mechanism. For example, in soccer, boys have higher levels of concussion than girls (50), and girls sustain higher rates of concussion than boys while playing basketball, soccer, and baseball/softball at high school and collegiate levels (49).

Race/Ethnicity

Information on race/ethnicity helps to identify populations at risk that can be used to design and evaluate interventions. The incidence of TBI varies by race or ethnic group (18,22). During 2002–2006, blacks and whites had the highest rates of TBI-related ED visits, followed by American Indian, Alaska Native, Asian, or Pacific Islanders (618.6, 448.3, and 334.7 per 100,000 population, respectively) (18). These rates vary by age group, mechanism, and intent. For example, although firearm-related TBI suicides were high among whites compared to blacks (5.6 vs 2.4 per 100,000 population), firearm-related TBI homicides were lower among whites compared to blacks (0.7 vs 4.9 per 100,000 population) (22). These differences were substantially higher among black men aged 20–24 years and 25–34 years who had the highest annual

average rates of firearm-related TBI death than other racial/ethnic and age groups (22). These racial differences may be related to socioeconomic and educational status (54).

Clinical outcomes may also vary by race/ethnicity. Compared with whites, in-hospital mortality is higher for blacks (odds ratio [OR] = 1.19, P = .026) and Asians (OR = 1.41, P = .005). Among those who survived moderate or severe TBIs, blacks and Hispanics were less likely to be discharged to a rehabilitation center when compared to whites (OR = 0.68, P < .001, and OR = 0.67, P = .002, respectively) (55).

Recurrent Traumatic Brain Injury

Research suggests that the risk of recurrent TBI progressively increases after a first or a second brain injury (56–58). The risk for having a second TBI after a first brain injury increases approximately 3 times compared to the general noninjured population, and the risk for a third TBI after a second brain injury increases between 7.8 and 9.3 times (56). Among many potential factors, recurrent TBI may be related to alcohol abuse (59–60) or to internal and/or external factors that make the individuals more vulnerable (59) to recurrent TBI.

Athletes who experience repetitive brain injuries, including subconcussive blows to the head, may be at risk of developing a more severe and chronic form of this condition known as chronic traumatic encephalopathy (CTE), which is mostly reported in boxers (61). More recently, in case-series studies of brains of deceased National Football League (NFL) athletes with history of concussion CTE has been reported (62). Patients with CTE may present a constellation of symptoms, including those of dementia (61).

Another form of recurrent TBI is the *repeat impact syndrome* or *second-impact syndrome*. This is a rarely reported condition in which the brain is thought to swell catastrophically after a person suffers a repeat concussion before symptoms from an earlier one have resolved that can lead to permanent brain damage or even death (63,64). The recurrent TBI may occur minutes, days, or weeks after an initial concussion of any severity (64). Young athletes may be especially vulnerable (65) as are people with a history of multiple brain injuries (66). Although controversy exists about the validity of this diagnosis, it is recognized by physicians. To reduce the likelihood of this condition and the risk of more severe outcomes, CDC and other organizations have recommended training for coaches and trainers, removal from play, the use of guidelines to return-to-play, and proper medical evaluation and care (available at: http://www.cdc.gov/concussion/HeadsUp).

Comorbidities and Prescription Drugs

Several medical comorbidities and prescription drugs are known TBI risk factors, especially among older adults (19). Comorbidities that increase the risk of TBI mainly because of falls and MVT accidents among older adults include diabetes mellitus, cardiac arrhythmias, dementias, depression, and Parkinson disease (19). Prescription drugs may also play a role; for example, drugs that affect brain functioning or that cause postural hypotension may increase the risk for falls. Anticoagulants also may increase the risk of intracranial bleeding after head trauma with long-term disability and fatal consequences occurring more frequently (19,67–69).

Socioeconomic Factors

Along with age and gender, socioeconomic status is also considered a major risk factor for TBI morbidity (2,70) and mortality (71) in the United States. Higher rates of TBI are often seen in geographical areas with lower mean incomes and in metropolitan areas (72), predominantly because of intentional mechanisms (73). Single, young, male, minorities who are unemployed and have only completed a high school education are at a higher risk for TBI (54). Significant factors associated with the risk for developing major depression following a TBI includes socioeconomic factors, minority status, unemployment and low income (74), and premorbid characteristics including less than 12 years of education and a history of alcohol abuse (75).

Alcohol Use

Despite a study that revealed a neuroprotective effect of alcohol for moderate to severe TBI (76), alcohol use is a major risk factor for overall injury morbidity (77–78) and mortality, including TBI morbidity, hospital length of stay, and mortality (79–80). One-quarter to one-half of all patients with acute TBI were intoxicated at the time of injury (81). CDC data for 1997 indicated that approximately 21% of MV occupants, 19% of motorcycle riders, and 10% of persons who fell and who had a TBI, had consumed alcohol or had blood alcohol concentration levels $\geq$ 0.01 g/dL (82). In a CDC study of older adults with TBI, approximately 6% tested positive for alcohol use, 42% tested negative, and for 52%, this information was missing (19). In this study, approximately 6% of those who fell and 8% of those who had an MVT accident tested positive for alcohol use at the time of TBI injury (19). In the years following a TBI, patients may experience increasing levels of substance abuse (75).

Use of Protective Equipment

The use of protective equipment (PE) such as helmets, mouth guards, and face shields does provide protection against some head, neck, and facial injuries. However, the evidence is not substantial to demonstrate that the use of this equipment reduces the incidence of concussion (83–84). TBI data from the late 1990s indicate that 41%–53% of MV-occupants, motorcyclists, and pedal cyclists injured in collisions were not using PE at the time of the injury (82) suggesting that these persons were at higher risk for more severe TBIs.

Recreational activities such as cycling and motorcycling also pose a risk for head and brain injury. Proper helmet use provides a significant amount of protection from head injuries during these activities. Deaths resulting from TBI are common among motorcyclists because of the high velocity of impact and the quick change in the principle direction of force encountered during a crash. Helmet use can reduce both morbidity and mortality among motorcycle riders (85). Bicycle helmet laws have produced significant decreases in head injury among children; unfortunately, adoption of helmet use among adults is lacking (86). These findings suggest that the use of PE can be useful in preventing head and brain injuries depending on the activity.

The Prevalence of Traumatic Brain Injury–Related Disability

The prevalence of TBI-related disability refers to the number of TBI survivors who are living with the physical, cognitive/ behavioral, and psychosocial consequences of TBI. Researchers have estimated that between 3.2 million (87,88) and 5.3 million (89) people live with the consequences of TBI in the United States. These estimates, however, may underestimate the true prevalence of TBI because they do not account for those treated in nonhospital settings or those who did not receive medical care or those serving in the US military abroad.

The Socioeconomic and Medical Consequences of Traumatic Brain Injury

The acute and long-term consequences of TBI result in a reduced quality of life and in prolonged medical and socioeconomic costs to patients and society (90,91). An estimated 43% of Americans have disabilities related to TBI 1 year after injury (2). Depending on severity, it is likely that TBI survivors experience cognitive and emotional impairments (92) negatively affecting everyday life even 10 years after injury (93). A study of financial and vocational outcomes among adult TBI survivors found that nearly 50% of previously employed individuals were unemployed 2 years postinjury and at the time of the interview, many were receiving public assistance and financial assistance from their families (94). A study of families with a child who survived a TBI found that there was a significant impact on family members who reported issues with perceived unmet health needs for their TBI children, stress, and interruptions of their daily routines, including having altered work schedules (95). Current research is focusing on the less easily measured psychosocial consequences of TBI that frequently affect all levels of society.

Other medical consequences of TBI may include increased risk of dementia after a single TBI as suggested by a study of 550 World War II veterans who were hospitalized for nonpenetrating TBI (96). In this study, researchers found that the risk of dementia after a single TBI increased with the initial TBI severity (96). TBI may also contribute to reduce life expectancy as evidenced by TBI survivors who had approximately 2.5 times the risk of death compared with the general population (72). A study of causes of death 1 year post moderate or severe TBI (97) found that when compared to the general population of similar age, gender, and race—TBI survivors were more likely to die of seizures (37 more times), septicemia (12 more times), and pneumonia (4 more times). Additionally, brain injury may increase the risk of suicidality among TBI survivors (98).

Consequences of Traumatic Brain Injury by Severity

After mild TBI, 50%–80% of the patients reported mild TBI-related signs and symptoms for days or weeks following injury. Approximately 50% of persons with a mild TBI present signs and symptoms for up to 3 months, and 10%–15% present signs and symptoms for more than a year after the injury (1, 99). If these signs and symptoms persist from 1 (99) to 3 (100) months after the injury, the condition is known as postconcussion syndrome (PCS); if symptoms persist > 3 months, it is called persistent PCS (99).

TBI sequelae can affect aspects of daily living such as employment, social integration, and family functioning (101); however, it is controversial which outcomes are a better predictor of the survivor's level of functioning in these areas. Himanen et al. found that the age at injury, independent of TBI severity, was a significant predictor of job performance 2 years postinjury or of mortality later in life; in contrast, TBI severity was a significant predictor of only job performance (79). Sendroy-Terril et al. found that cognitive, physical, and social functioning were all significantly impacted by injury severity and the age at injury was also a significant predictor of the same outcomes (102). Additionally, a study of 620 patients with multiple injuries, including TBI, found that injury severity was not a significant predictor of either physical or psychological measures and the age at injury was a significant predictor of both measures (103). Each of these studies suggests that age at injury may be a significant predictor of outcomes after a TBI, which may have implications for age as a factor in the recovery process. Interestingly, research has shown that recovery time may be longer for children and adolescents (104,105).

Other factors that may affect outcomes in TBI are advancements in acute care and rehabilitation that may yield better outcomes (106), even after severe injuries are sustained. Cases of severe TBI may require more intensive care upfront such as emergent surgery and medical management during resuscitation compared to less severe cases, but better outcomes for all levels of severity have been achieved over the past several decades (107).

Prevalence-Related Methodological Issues

Although there are estimates of the prevalence of TBI (87–89), there is no ongoing follow-up study or surveillance system that exists at the state or national level in the United States that may allow for periodically estimating the prevalence of TBI or TBI-related disability. Some studies have attempted to assess prognosis and sequelae of TBI; however, these studies (108,109) were conducted in small, selected clinical samples using different methodologies, so their findings are not comparable and cannot be generalized to the US population.

Economic Cost of Traumatic Brain Injury

Data on the economic cost of TBI are important to properly allocate resources for injury surveillance, prevention, acute care, and rehabilitation. Knowledge of the economic impact of TBI in the United States, however, is limited. According to Finkelstein et al., in year 2000 dollars, the lifetime costs of TBI in the United States was $60.4 billion; of these, $9.1 billion were direct medical costs and $51.2 billion were indirect costs (90). We adjusted these estimates for inflation, yielding $76.5 billion in 2010; of these, $11.5 billion were direct medical costs and $64.8 billion were indirect costs. Other researchers have estimated that the lifetime costs of TBI in year 2009 dollars, including expenditures related to lost quality of life, among civilians in the United States that were medically treated in the year 2000 totaled more than $221 billion; of these, $14.6 billion were for medical costs, $69.2 billion were for work loss costs, and $137 billion were for the value of lost quality of life (110). Among children who suffer TBI, hospitalization costs have been estimated at $2.5 billion annually (111). All the estimates mentioned earlier, however, only account for persons who received medical treatment and do not fully account for the costs of ex-

tended rehabilitation, services, and supportive services (e.g., formal and informal caregiving), or the value of lost quality of life, or productivity losses for informal caregivers including parents.

GAPS IN TRAUMATIC BRAIN INJURY EPIDEMIOLOGY IN THE UNITED STATES

The United States lacks a system that can determine the incidence, prevalence, and the long-term consequences of TBI at the patient level. The incidence and prevalence statistics of those who seek care in doctors' offices, outpatient facilities, or those who do not seek medical care needs to be elucidated. To understand the long-term consequences of TBI and the impact of newer medical and rehabilitation management, prospective rigorous patient level incidence and prevalence studies are needed; these should include people formerly in the military who do not seek medical care in the military or in the VA systems. As medical management and technology (e.g., neuroimaging) advance, studies of the natural history of this condition that may allow researchers to better understand TBI-related impairment and disability are also needed. Among children, these studies should account for developmental milestones. To improve clinical and epidemiological research and to design cost-effective and evidence-based prevention interventions, sound data collection systems need to be designed and implemented.

Researchers and practitioners also use different definitions, especially for mild TBI. In an attempt to address this deficiency, US Federal agencies, including CDC, have launched the *Common Data Elements for TBI Initiative* to harmonize clinical and epidemiological data standards, including clinical and surveillance definitions (available at: http://www.commondataelements.ninds.nih.gov/TBI.aspx). Under this umbrella, CDC and other Federal agencies are developing a standard definition for concussion for use in clinical and research settings.

THE INCIDENCE AND PREVALENCE OF TRAUMATIC BRAIN INJURY IN THE WORLD

According to a 2006 systematic review of the epidemiology of TBI in Europe, there were many scientific reports on this topic but the data in the reports were not comparable (112). Despite these methodological limitations, the authors of this study provided a picture of the incidence, prevalence, and mortality of TBI in Europe and selected countries of the world. The authors estimated that the incidence of TBI was highest in Asia (344 per 100,000) followed by Europe (235 per 100,000), Australia (226 per 100,000), India (160 per 100,000) and the United States (103 per 100,000). The prevalence of TBI was estimated for the United States, Asia, and India (1,893; 709; and 97 per 100,000 population, respectively). The mortality related to TBI was estimated for Europe, United States, Asia, and India (15.4, 18.1, 38.0, and 20.0 per 100,000) (112).

Other authors have also attempted to estimate the burden of TBI worldwide. One such study used data from the 1996 Global Health Statistics (113) to produce an approximation of the burden of TBI in the world; these approximations were succinctly disseminated in 2009 (91). To produce global

TBI-related incidence and prevalence estimates, Coronado et al. (91) combined the following TBI-related diagnoses reported in the 1996 Global Health Statistics: fractured skulls (including fracture of facial bones) and intracranial injuries with short- and long-term consequences. These conditions were severe enough to require medical attention or lead immediately to death. Because regional TBI data were available, estimates of the TBI-related incidence and prevalence were produced for the following 8 geographic regions: established market economies (EME); formerly socialist economies of Europe (FSE); India; China; Latin America and the Caribbean (LAC); other Asian countries and islands (OAI); the Middle Eastern Crescent (MEC); and Sub-Saharan Africa (SSA) (Tables 8-3 and 8-4). Estimates of the global and regional TBI incidence and prevalence by external cause and by intentionality, not disseminated previously, are presented in this section (Tables 8-3 and 8-4).

Global and Regional Estimates of Traumatic Brain Injury–Related Incidence by External Causes and Intentionality

Approximately 10 million TBIs that were severe enough to require medical attention or leading immediately to death (184.6 per 100,000) occurred worldwide in 1990 (Table 8-3); the rate ranged from 110.1 to 361.6 per 100,000 population in China and in the Sub-Saharan Africa (SSA), respectively

(Table 8-3). Overall and in every region of the world, road traffic accidents (RTA) were the leading cause of TBI and violence was the second leading cause. The global rate of RTA-related TBI was 111.7 per 100,000 population (range = 66.6–172.2 per 100,000 population; Table 8-3). The global rate of violence-related TBI was 45.8 per 100,000 population (range = 8.3–153.3 per 100,000). Falls were the third leading global cause of TBI (rate = 16.1 per 100,000 population). India, however, had at least twice the rates of fall-related TBI than any other region in the world (48.5 per 100,000 population; Table 8-3). Overall, the rates for unintentional causes of TBI were higher than those of intentional causes of TBI (135.0 vs 49.6 per 100,000, respectively; Table 8-3). Except in SSA, with intentional and unintentional causes of TBI were nearly the equivalent, all the other regions of the world had this intentional/unintentional global pattern. These global and regional approximations, potentially underestimate the incidence of TBI because they do not include injured people who did not receive medical care.

Global Estimates of Traumatic Brain Injury–Related Mortality

Although the 1996 Global Health Statistics did not present separate TBI-related mortality estimates, the magnitude of TBI mortality may be inferred assuming that the worldwide injury mortality patterns are comparable to those of the

TABLE 8-3 Estimated Numbers of Incident Cases[a] and Incidence Rates per 100,000 Population for Traumatic Brain Injury in the World, by Region, Intent, and External Cause, 1990.

INTENT	ESTIMATES	SSA[b]	LAC[c]	INDIA	FSE[d]	OAI[e]	EME[f]	MEC[g]	CHINA	WORLD TOTAL[h]
Unintentional										
Road traffic accidents	Number[i]	843	765	1,067	451	764	822	418	755	5,885
	Rate[j]	165.2	172.2	125.6	130.3	111.9	103.0	83.1	66.6	111.7
Falls	Number[i]	46	36	412	28	123	42	51	111	849
	Rate[j]	9.0	8.1	48.5	8.1	18.0	5.3	10.1	9.8	16.1
Other unintentional	Number[i]	68	32	83	18	53	20	28	78	379
	Rate[j]	13.3	7.2	9.8	5.2	7.8	2.5	5.6	6.9	7.2
Total unintentional	Number[i]	957	833	1,562	497	878	884	497	944	7,113
	Rate[j]	187.5	187.5	183.9	143.5	137.7	110.8	98.8	83.3	135.0
Intentional										
Violence	Number[i]	782	314	251	199	251	268	42	304	2,413
	Rate[j]	153.3	70.7	29.5	57.5	36.8	33.6	8.3	26.8	45.8
War	Number[i]	106	7	0	12	6	0	67	0	198
	Rate[j]	20.8	1.6	0.0	3.5	0.9	0.0	13.3	0.0	3.8
Total intentional	Number[i]	888	321	251	211	257	268	109	304	2611
	Rate[j]	174.0	72.2	29.5	60.9	37.7	33.6	21.7	26.8	49.6
World Total[i]	Number[i]	1,845	1,154	1,813	708	1,197	1,152	606	1,248	9,724
	Rate[j]	361.6	259.7	213.4	204.5	175.4	144.4	120.5	110.1	184.6

[a] Based on any traumatic brain injury severe enough to result in death or hospitalized medical care.
[b] Sub-Saharan Africa.
[c] Latin America and the Caribbean.
[d] Former socialist economies.
[e] Other Asian countries and islands.
[f] Established market economies.
[g] Middle Eastern Crescent.
[h] Totals may not add precisely due to rounding.
[i] Numbers in thousands.
[j] Rate per 100,000 population.
Reprinted from Murray CJL, Lopez AD (111) with permission.

TABLE 8-4 Estimated Number of Prevalent Cases[a] and Prevalence Rates per 100,000 Population for Traumatic Brain Injury in the World, by Region, Intent and External Cause, 1990.

INTENT	ESTIMATES	SSA[b]	LAC[c]	INDIA	FSE[d]	OAI[e]	EME[f]	MEC[g]	CHINA	WORLD TOTAL[h]
Unintentional										
Road traffic accidents	Number[i]	1,139	1,224	1,736	872	1,238	1,726	609	1,368	9,914
	Rate[j]	223.2	275.5	204.4	251.9	181.4	216.3	121.1	120.7	188.2
Falls	Number[i]	1,067	1,095	13,063	1,026	4,014	1,551	1,398	4,161	27,375
	Rate[j]	209.1	246.5	1,537.7	296.3	588.1	194.4	277.9	367.0	519.7
Other unintentional	Number[i]	1,572	873	2,363	590	1,498	601	710	2,666	10,873
	Rate[j]	308.1	196.5	278.2	170.4	219.5	75.3	141.1	235.2	206.4
Total unintentional	Number[i]	3,778	3,192	17,162	2,488	6,750	3,878	2,717	8,195	48,162
	Rate[j]	740.4	718.4	2020.2	718.6	989.0	486.1	540.1	722.9	914.3
Intentional										
Violence	Number[i]	1,080	469	405	355	380	542	56	612	3,898
	Rate[j]	211.7	105.6	47.7	102.5	55.7	67.9	11.1	54.0	74.0
War	Number[i]	2,415	180	3	441	151	1	1,629	8	4,829
	Rate[j]	473.3	40.5	0.4	127.4	22.1	0.1	323.8	0.7	91.7
Total intentional	Number[i]	3,495	649	408	796	531	543	1,685	620	8,727
	Rate[j]	684.9	146.1	48.0	229.9	77.8	68.1	334.9	54.7	165.7
World Total[h] ††	Number[i]	7,273	3,841	17,570	3,284	7,281	4,421	4,402	8,815	56,889
	Rate[j]	1,425.3	864.5	2,068.2	948.5	1,066.8	554.2	875.0	777.5	1,080.0

[a] Based on any traumatic brain injury severe enough to result in death or in hospitalized medical care.
[b] Sub-Saharan Africa.
[c] Latin America and the Caribbean.
[d] Former socialist economies.
[e] Other Asian countries and islands.
[f] Established market economies.
[g] Middle Eastern Crescent.
[h] Totals may not add precisely due to rounding.
[i] Numbers in thousands.
[j] Rate per 100,000 population.
Reprinted from Murray CJL, Lopez AD (111) with permission.

United States. According to CDC, approximately one-third of all injury-related deaths in the United States are TBI-related (114). Applying this proportion to a worldwide estimate of 5 million deaths from all injuries in 1990 (113), we estimated that about one-third of these—or 1.7 million—were TBI-related deaths. This approximation of TBI-related mortality must be interpreted with caution because reporting practices, cultural differences, external causes of injury, and the availability and quality of medical care vary substantially and throughout the world.

Global and Regional Estimates of Traumatic Brain Injury–Related Prevalence by External Causes and Intentionality

The prevalence of TBI worldwide is approximately 1,080.0 per 100,000 population (57 million people worldwide; Table 8-4). TBI-related prevalence ranged from 554.2 to 2068.2 per 100,000 population in EME region and India, respectively (Table 8-4). TBI prevalence was highest for fall-related injuries (519.7 per 100,000 population), accounting for about 50% of the TBI prevalence globally. The prevalence of fall-related TBI ranged from 194.4 to 1,537.7 per 100,000 population in the EME region and India, respectively. RTAs were the second leading cause of TBI prevalence (188.2 per 100,000 population). Overall, the prevalence of unintentional causes of

TBI was significantly higher than that for intentional causes of TBI (Table 8-4).

Gaps in the Traumatic Brain Injury Epidemiology Worldwide

Although TBI-related research from developed countries is abundant, comparisons between these countries is marred with methodological differences (112). In contrast, consistent and periodic TBI-related epidemiological data are lacking from developing countries (112,91). Although it is difficult to compare the data compiled by Tagliaferri et al. (112) and the authors of these studies, their approximations indicate that the incidence and prevalence of TBI is a public health problem that varies by region or by country; and that the estimated incidence and prevalence of TBI in developing regions (e.g., SSA, LAC, India) or countries tend to be higher than in the EME and MEC regions and China. These findings highlight the need for better and more complete surveillance for a condition that clearly constitutes a global public health problem. Better TBI surveillance systems may allow public health practitioners and clinicians globally to timely disseminate findings, to augment its importance on the public health agenda, and to increase awareness of this potentially preventable condition through the implementation of proven and cost-effective preventive measures that focus on its leading causes: motor vehicles, unintentional injury, falls, and violence. For maximum effectiveness, public health practitioners should work in an integrated and coordinated manner taking into account the social and cultural characteristics of the population to improve the acceptability and adoption of interventions. Findings from successful surveillance and injury prevention programs around the world need to be widely disseminated so that others can benefit from this knowledge and choose from an array of proven programs that best suit regionally specific needs.

PREVENTION

Translating Data Into Action

The evidence presented in this chapter indicates that TBI is a public health problem in the United States and the world. To lessen the burden of injury, we must recognize that these injuries are often preventable and are usually not the result of random events. Practitioners and scientists need to vigilantly determine the magnitude of TBI, the particular groups at most risk, the effectiveness of protective interventions, and additional risk factors. To prevent injury, it is also necessary to explore options by designing, implementing, and evaluating interventions; and once these interventions are identified, they should actively promote their adoption (91). For example, the large decline of MVC-related TBI deaths observed among 15–24 year olds (22) may partially reflect the implementation of graduated licensing of new drivers and education programs by the states (more information is available at: http://www.cdc.gov/Motorvehiclesafety/Teen_Drivers/index.html).

The Haddon Matrix is often used in injury prevention to devise targeted intervention, describing the influence of personal, vector/agent, physical environmental, and social environmental factors before, during, and after an injury event. For example, the agent or vector could be a speeding driver under the influence of alcohol or drugs, the host is an injured pedestrian, and the environment may be a poorly lit and maintained road (Table 8-5) (115–117). In the preevent phase, examination of the physical and medical condition of a driver (e.g., use of alcohol), knowledge of the activity and skill (e.g., licensed driver), and usage of protective equipment (e.g., seat belt) can help determine the most effective prevention strategies. In the event phase, examination of the preexisting physical and medical condition of the individual (e.g., use of anticoagulants) or the circumstances of the event (e.g., use of seat belt) help to determine the extent and severity of the injury. In the postevent phase, examination of the emergency response, quality of care, and any environmental factors that may slow the treatment and rehabilitation may be used to prevent potential long-term or permanent consequences of the injury. Worldwide, practitioners and researchers should use surveillance data and the elements of this matrix to translate science into effective health practice.

Through the implementation of prevention interventions, thousands of injuries and deaths could be prevented because of falls and MVC accidents—the leading causes of TBI in the United States. These interventions, ideally, should be evidence-based and cost-effective, and should be aimed to prevent or reduce the occurrence of TBI and its severity and to decrease the long-term medical and socioeconomic consequences of this condition. CDC also promotes capacity building at the state level by increasing understanding about the injury problem, sharing effective strategies, and assisting states in implementing prevention programs. In sports and recreation activities, CDC recommends the education of coaches and staff on concussion monitoring, adherence to the rules to return to play and proper medical care. More information on TBI prevention is available elsewhere in this textbook and at: http://www.cdc.gov/injury/.

CONCLUSION

Despite the significant improvements in the field in the recent years, 4 areas require additional exploration for advancement of TBI efforts. First, although the current knowledge of the TBI epidemiology and periodic dissemination of TBI data at the national level have improved compared to

TABLE 8-5 Examples of the Haddon Matrix Applied to the Prevention of Traumatic Brain Injury

	AGENT (VEHICLE)	HOST (CONDUCTOR)	PHYSICAL ENVIRONMENT	SOCIAL ENVIRONMENT
Preevent phase	Velocity Maintenance of tires and brakes	Licensed driver Medical examination: - Vision - Alcohol use	Adequate roadway: - Lighting - Traffic signs/markings - Shoulders	Speed limits Laws: - Graduated licensing - Impaired driving
Event phase	Vehicle size Safety rating	Seat belts Child restraints Air bags	Presence of: - Median barriers - Guard rails - Embankments	Laws enforcing use of: - Seat belt and child restraint - Helmet use
Postevent phase	Redesign/improve - Braking systems - Gas tank for fire prevention	Survivors' - Age - Previous health status	Availability of adequate: - Emergency medical services (EMS) - Rehabilitation services - Distance to trauma center	Public support for - trauma care - rehabilitation - EMS training

Produced using concepts from Haddon W Jr (113,114), Runyan CW (115) with permission.

past decades, the United States still lacks a surveillance system able to produce reliable patient-level estimates of the incidence and prevalence of TBI at the state and national levels. To address the public health problem of TBI in the United States, such surveillance system needs to be designed, implemented, and properly funded to ensure its sustainability. Second, definitions, especially those for the mild forms of this condition and for concussion are not standard yet, producing confusion among researchers and clinicians. These definitions need to be standardized and—because knowledge is acquired—periodically updated. Third, adequate funding and better design of epidemiological research, including follow-up studies to characterize the natural course of this condition, as well as the medical and rehabilitation needs of civilian and military TBI survivors in the United States, are needed to overcome these limitations. Standardized measures for TBI outcomes are also needed to identify those most amenable to prevention via adoption of low cost integrated interventions. Fourth, technological advances, including those related to TBI diagnosis (e.g., neuroimaging, neuropathology, serum biomarkers) and the widespread adoption of standard electronic medical records in the United States are likely to advance and facilitate epidemiological and clinical research.

TBI is an often preventable public health problem in the United States. Most importantly, if we are to prevent TBI—a potentially disabling condition—we need to understand the causes, magnitude, and impact of TBI at the individual and societal levels. Continued collaboration between public and clinical health providers and stakeholders, including promotion of individual and societal responsibilities, are needed to reduce the burden of this condition in the United States.

KEY CLINICAL POINTS

1. TBI is an important public health problem in the United States that affects people regardless of age, sex, or race/ethnicity.

  - Approximately 1.7 million TBI-related hospitalizations, ED visits, and deaths occur every year in the United States.
  - Between 3.6 and 5.3 million Americans live with the consequences of TBI.
  - From 2000 to the fourth quarter of 2010, 202,281 TBIs were identified in the US military.
    - The numbers of US soldiers with TBI have steadily increased during this decade from 10,963 in 2000 to 29,252 in 20
    - From October 1, 2001 when the war started in Afghanistan to March 31, 2009, 25,737 war veterans were identified in the VA system as having been evaluated or treated for a condition possibly related to a TBI.
  - In the United States, the major overall causes of TBI are falls (affecting mainly young children and older adults) and MVT accidents (affecting mainly teens and young adults).
  - The estimated cost of TBI in 2010 dollars is approximately $76.5 billion; of these:
    - $11.5 billion were caused by direct medical costs.
    - $64.8 billion were caused by indirect costs.

  - These dollar figures do not account for the current and life time cost incurred by TBI survivors of the Iraq and Afghanistan wars.
2. Globally, the incidence and prevalence of TBI varies by country and region.
  - Both, the incidence and prevalence of TBI is higher in developing regions or countries (e.g., SSA, LAC, India) than in the EME and MEC regions and China. Worldwide, countries, including the United States, lack surveillance systems able to produce timely and reliable patient-level estimates of the incidence and prevalence of TBI.
  - Countries should consider strengthening or developing and implementing such systems to prevent this potentially disabling condition.

Prevention efforts should be directed to the entire population. Special attention, however, should be placed on groups at risk for TBI.

DISCLAIMER

The findings and conclusions in this chapter are those of the authors alone and do not necessarily represent the official views or policies of the Centers for Disease Control and Prevention (CDC) or any agency of the US government. Inclusion of individuals, programs, or organizations in this chapter does not constitute endorsement by the US government.

KEY REFERENCES

1. Coronado VG, Xu L, Basavaraju SV, et al. Surveillance for traumatic brain injury-related deaths—United States, 1997–2007. *MMWR Surveill Summ.* 2011;60(5):1–32.
2. Faul M, Xu L, Wald MM, Coronado VG. *Traumatic Brain Injury in the United States: Emergency Department Visits, Hospitalizations, and Deaths, 2002–2006.* Atlanta, GA: Centers for Disease Control and Prevention, National Center for Injury Prevention and Control; 2010.
3. Injury prevention & control: traumatic brain injury. Centers for Disease Control and Prevention Web site. http://www.cdc.gov/traumaticbraininjury/. Accessed December 12, 2011.
4. Marr A, Coronado VG. *Annual Data Submission Standards. Central Nervous System Injury Surveillance.* Atlanta, GA: US Department of Health and Human Services, Public Health Service, CDC; 2001.

References

1. National Center for Injury Prevention and Control. *Report to Congress on Mild Traumatic Brain Injury in the United States: Steps to Prevent a Serious Public Health Problem.* Atlanta, GA: Centers for Disease Control and Prevention; 2003.
2. Corrigan JD, Selassie AW, Orman JA. The epidemiology of traumatic brain injury. *J Head Trauma Rehabil.* 2010;25(2):72–80.
3. Thurman DJ, Sniezek JE, Johnson D, Greenspan A, Smith SM. Guidelines for surveillance of central nervous system injury. Atlanta, GA: US Department of Health and Human Services, Public Health Service, Centers for Disease Control and Prevention; 1995.

4. Marr A, Coronado VG. *Annual Data Submission Standards. Central Nervous System Injury Surveillance.* Atlanta, GA: US Department of Health and Human Services, Public Health Service, CDC; 2001.

5. DeWitt DS, Prough DS. Blast-induced brain injury and posttraumatic hypotension and hypoxemia. *J Neurotrauma.* 2009;26(6):877–887.

6. Menon DK, Schwab K, Wright DW, Maas AI; Demographics and Clinical Assessment Working Group of the International and Interagency Initiative toward Common Data Elements of Research on Traumatic Brain Injury and Psychological Health. Position Statement: Definition of traumatic brain injury. *Arch Phys Med Rehabil.* 2010;91(11):1637–1640.

7. Association for the Advancement of Automotive Medicine. *Abbreviated Injury Scale. What is the Abbreviated Injury Scale?* Available at: http://www.aaam1.org/ais/. Accessed March 03, 2011.

8. Champion HR, Sacco WJ, Copes WS, Gann DS, Gennarelli TA, Flanagan ME. A revision of the trauma score. *J Trauma.* 1989;29(5):623–629.

9. Teasdale G, Jennett B. Assessment of coma and impaired consciousness. A practical scale. *Lancet.* 1974;304(7872):81–84.

10. Bastos PG, Sun X, Wagner DP, Wu AW, Knaus WA. Glasgow coma scale score in the evaluation of outcome in the intensive care unit: findings from the Acute Physiology and Chronic Health Evaluation III Study. *Crit Care Med.* 1993;21(10):1459–1465.

11. Narayan RK, Michel ME, Ansell B. Clinical trials in head injury. J Neurotrauma. 2002;19:503–557.

12. Mullie A, Buylaert W, Michem N, et al. Predictive value of Glasgow Coma score for awakening after out-of-hospital cardiac arrest. Cerebral Resuscitation Study Group of the Belgian Society for intensive care. *Lancet.* 1998;1(8578):137–140.

13. Segatore M, Way C. The Glasgow Coma Score: Time for change. Heart Lung. 1992;21(6):548–57.

14. Crossman J, Bankes M, Bhan A, Crockard HA. The Glasgow Coma Score: Reliable evidence? *Injury.* 1998;29(6):435–437.

15. Saatman KE, Duhaime AC, Bullock R, et al. Classification of Traumatic Brain Injury for Targeted Therapies. J Neurotrauma. 2008;25:719–38.

16. Williams DH, Levin HS, Eisenberg HM. Mild head injury classification. *Neurosurgery.* 1990;27(3):422–428.

17. Department of Veterans Affairs/Department of Defense Management of Concussion/mTBI Working Group. VA/DoD Clinical Practice Guideline: Management of Concussion/Mild Traumatic Brain Injury (mTBI). April, 2009. Page 17. Available from: http://www.healthquality.va.gov/mtbi/concussion_mtbi_full_1_0.pdf. Accessed May 21, 2012.

18. Faul M, Xu L, Wald MM, Coronado VG. *Traumatic Brain Injury in the United States: Emergency Department Visits, Hospitalizations, and Deaths, 2002–2006.* Atlanta, GA: Centers for Disease Control and Prevention, National Center for Injury Prevention and Control; 2010.

19. Coronado VG, Thomas KE, Sattin RW, Johnson RL. The CDC traumatic brain injury surveillance system: characteristics of persons aged 65 years and older hospitalized with a TBI. *J Head Trauma Rehabil.* 2005;20(3):215–228.

20. Coronado VG, McGuire LC, Basavaraju SV, Corrigan JD, Xu L. TBI hospitalizations among older adults: clinical and epidemiological characteristics. Paper presented at: 3rd Inter Federal Conference on Traumatic Brain Injury (oral presentation); June 2011; Washington, DC.

21. Schootman M, Fuortes LJ. Ambulatory care for traumatic brain injuries in the US, 1995–1997. *Brain Inj.* 2000;14(4):373–381.

22. Coronado VG, Xu L, Basavaraju SV, et al. Surveillance for traumatic brain injury-related deaths—United States, 1997–2007. *MMWR Surveill Summ.* 2011;60(5):1–32.

23. Sosin DM, Sniezek JE, Thurman DJ. Incidence of mild and moderate brain injury in the United States, 1991. *Brain Injury.* 1996;10(1):47–54.

24. Centers for Disease Control and Prevention. *National Center for Health Statistics Multiple Cause of Death Public Use Data, 1996–2006.* Hyattsville, MD: US Department of Health and Human Services, Centers for Disease Control and Prevention; 2009.

25. Centers for Disease Control and Prevention. Nonfatal traumatic brain injuries from sports and recreation activities—United States, 2001–2005. *MMWR Morb Mortal Wkly Rep.* 2007;56(29):733–737.

26. Reid SR, Roesler JS, Gaichas AM, Tsai AK. The epidemiology of pediatric traumatic brain injury in Minnesota. *Arch Pediatr Adolesc Med.* 2001;155(7):784–789.

27. Whiteneck G, Brooks CA, Mellick D, Harrison-Felix C, Terrill MS, Noble K. Population-based estimates of outcomes after hospitalization for traumatic brain injury in Colorado. *Arch Phys Med Rehabil.* 2004;85(4)(suppl 2):S73–S81.

28. Pickelsimer EE, Selassie AW, Gu JK, Langlois JA. A population-based outcomes study of persons hospitalized with traumatic brain injury: operations of the South Carolina Traumatic Brain Injury Follow-up Registry. *J Head Trauma Rehabil.* 2006;21(6):491–504.

29. Thurman DJ, Coronado V, Selassie A. The epidemiology of TBI: implications for public health. In: Zasler ND, Katz DI, Zafonte RD, eds. *Brain Injury Medicine: Principles and Practice.* New York, NY: Demos Medical Publishing; 2007:45–56.

30. Rodriguez SR, Mallonee S, Archer P, Gofton J. Evaluation of death certificate-based surveillance for traumatic brain injury—Oklahoma 2002. *Public Health Rep.* 2006;121(3):282–289.

31. Centers for Disease Control and Prevention. Quickstats: injury and traumatic brain injury (TBI)-related death rates, by age group—United States, 2006. *MMWR Morb Mortal Wkly Rep.* 2010;59(10):303.

32. Dutton RP, Stansbury G, Leone S, Kramer E, Hess JR, Scalea TM. Trauma mortality in mature trauma systems: are we doing better? An analysis of trauma mortality patterns, 1997–2008. *J Trauma.* 2010;69(3):620–626.

33. Johnson RL, Thomas RG, Thomas KE, Sarmiento K. *State Injury Indicators Report: Fourth Edition—2005 Data.* Atlanta, GA: Centers for Disease Control and Prevention, National Center for Injury Prevention and Control; 2009.

34. Langlois JA, Rutland-Brown W, Thomas KE. *Traumatic Brain Injury in the United States: Emergency Department Visits, Hospitalizations, and Deaths.* Atlanta, GA: Centers for Disease Control and Prevention, National Center for Injury Prevention and Control; 2006.

35. Sosin DM, Sacks JJ, Smith SM. Head injury-associated deaths in the United States from 1979 to 1986. *JAMA.* 1989;262(16):2251–2255.

36. Adekoya N, Thurman DJ, White DD, Webb KW. Surveillance for traumatic brain injury deaths—United States, 1989–1998. *MMWR Surveill Summ.* 2002;51(10):1–14.

37. Armed Forces Health Surveillance Center. Cause of medical evacuations from Operations Iraqi Freedom (OIF), New Dawn (OND) and Enduring Freedom (OEF), active and reserve components, U.S. Armed Forces, October 2001-September 2010. *MSMR.* 2011;18(2):2–7.

38. The Congress of the United States. Congressional Budget Office. *A CBO Study: The Veterans Health Administration's Treatment of PTSD and Traumatic Brain Injury among Recent Combat Veterans. February 2012.* Available from: http://www.cbo.gov/sites/default/files/cbo files/attachments/02-09-PTSD.pdf. Accessed: May 12, 2012.

39. Okie S. *Traumatic brain injury in the war zone.* N Engl J Med. 2005; 352(20):2043–2047.

40. Xydakis MS, Fravell MD, Nasser KE, Casler JD. Analysis of battlefield head and neck injuries in Iraq and Afghanistan. *Otolaryngol Head Neck Surg.* 2005;133(4):497–504.

41. Defense and Veterans Brain Injury Center. DoD worldwide numbers for traumatic brain injury. DVBIC Web site. http://www.dvbic.org/TBI-Numbers.aspx. Accessed February 17, 2011.

42. Mayorga MA. The pathology of primary blast overpressure injury. *Toxicology.* 1997;121(1):17–28.

43. United Nations. Security Council. Report of the Secretary General on the protection of civilians in armed conflict. United Nations Nov 11, 2010; S/2010/579. Available at: http://unispal.un.org /UNISPAL.NSF/0/3005D1DCED28C57A852577E000587882. Accessed May 21, 2011.

44. National Federation of State High School Associations. 2009–2010 High School Athletic Participation Survey results: based on competition at the high school level in the 2009–2010 school year. National Federation of State High School Associations Web site. http://www.nfhs.org/content.aspx?id = 3282&linkidentifier = id&itemid = 3282. Accessed March 2, 2011.

45. National Council of Youth Sports. *Report on Trends and Participation in Organized Youth Sports*. Stuart, FL: National Council of Youth Sports; 2008. Available at: http://www.ncys.org/pdfs/2008/2008-ncys-market-research-report.pdf. Accessed January 3, 2011.

46. Halstead ME, Walter KD; for Council on Sports Medicine and Fitness. American Academy of Pediatrics. Clinical report—sport-related concussion in children and adolescents. *Pediatrics*. 2010; 126(3):597–615.

47. Langlois JA, Rutland-Brown W, Wald MM. The epidemiology and impact of traumatic brain injury: a brief overview. *J Head Trauma Rehabil*. 2006;21(5):375–378.

48. Guskiewicz KM, Weaver NL, Padua DA, Garrett WE Jr. Epidemiology of concussion in collegiate and high school football players. *Am J Sports Med*. 2000;28(5):643–650.

49. Gessel LM, Fields SK, Collins CL, Dick RW, Comstock RD. Concussions among United States high school and collegiate athletes. *J Athl Train*. 2007;42(4):495–503.

50. Schulz MR, Marshall SW, Mueller FO, et al. Incidence and risk factors for concussion in high school athletes, North Carolina, 1996–1999. *Am J Epidemiol*. 2004;160(10):937–944.

51. Bazarian JJ, McClung J, Shah MN, Cheng YT, Flesher W, Kraus J. Mild traumatic brain injury in the United States, 1998–2000. *Brain Inj*. 2005;19(2):85–91.

52. Abellera JP, Annest JL, Conn JM, Kohn MA. *How States are Collecting and Using External Cause of Injury Data: 2004 Update to the 1997 Report*. Atlanta, GA: Council of State and Territorial Epidemiologists; 2005.

53. Baker SP, O'Neill B, Ginsburg MJ, et al., eds. *The Injury Fact Book*. 2nd ed. New York, NY: Oxford University Press; 1982.

54. Burnett DM, Kolakowsky-Hayner SA, Slater D, Stringer A, Bushnik T, Zafonte R, Cifu DX. Ethnographic analysis of traumatic brain injury patients in the national model systems database. *Arch Phys Med Rehabil*. 2003;84(2):263–267.

55. Bowman SM, Martin DP, Sharar SR, Zimmerman FJ. Racial disparities in outcomes of persons with moderate to severe traumatic brain injury. *Med Care*. 2007;45(7):686–690.

56. Annegers JF, Grabow JD, Kurland LT, Laws ER Jr. The incidence, causes, and secular trends of head trauma in Olmstead County, Minnesota, 1935–1974. *Neurology*. 1980;30(9):912–919.

57. Guskiewicz K, McCrea M, Marshall SW, et al. Cumulative effects associated with recurrent concussion in collegiate football players: the NCAA Concussion Study. *JAMA*. 2003;290(19):2549–2555.

58. Guskiewicz KM, Marshall SW, Bailes J, et al. Recurrent concussion and risk of depression in retired professional football players. *Med Sci Sports Exerc*. 2007;39(6):903–909.

59. Salcido R, Costich JF. Recurrent traumatic brain injury. *Brain Injury*. 1992;6(3):293–298.

60. Kreutzer JS, Doherty KR, Harris JA. Zasler ND. Alcohol use among persons with traumatic brain injury. *J Head Trauma Rehabil*. 1990; 5(3):9–20.

61. Erlanger DM, Kutner KC, Barth JT, Barnes R. Neuropsychology of sports-related head injury: dementia pugilistica to post concussion syndrome. *Clin Neuropsychol*. 1999;13(2):193–209.

62. McKee AC, Cantu RC, Nowinski CJ, et al. Chronic traumatic encephalopathy in athletes: progressive tauopathy after repetitive head injury. *J Neuropathol Exp Neurol*. 2009;68(7):709–735.

63. Centers for Disease Control and Prevention. Sports-related recurrent brain injuries—United States. *MMWR Morb Mortal Wkly Rep*. 1997;46(10):224–227.

64. Cifu DX, Steinmetz BD, Drake DF. Repetitive head injury syndrome. eMedicine.com. http://emedicine.medscape.com/article/92189-overview. Updated November 16, 2010. Accessed February 3, 2011.

65. Kirkwood MW, Yeates KO, Wilson PE. Pediatric sport-related concussion: a review of the clinical management of an oft-neglected population. *Pediatrics*. 2006;117(4):1359–1371.

66. MacReady N. Study leading some experts to question the existence of "second-impact syndrome." *Clinical Psychiatry News*. 2004; 32(10):55.

67. Cumming RG. Epidemiology of medication-related falls and fractures in the elderly. *Drugs Aging*. 1998;12(1):43–53.

68. Wong DK, Lurie F, Wong LL. The effects of clopidogrel on elderly traumatic brain injured patients. *J Trauma*. 2008;65(6):1303–1308.

69. Williams TM, Sadjadi J, Harken AH, Victorino GP. The necessity to assess anticoagulation status in elderly injured patients. *J Trauma*. 2008;65(4):772–777.

70. Ahmed N, Andersson R. Unintentional injury mortality and socioeconomic development among 15–44 year-olds: in a health transition perspective. *Public Health*. 2000;114(5):416–422.

71. Cubbin C, LeClere FB, Smith GS. Socioeconomic status and injury mortality: individual and neighbourhood determinants. *J Epidemiol Community Health*. 2000;54(7):517–524.

72. Ventura T, Harrison-Felix C, Carlson N, et al. Mortality after discharge from acute care hospitalization with traumatic brain injury: a population-based study. *Arch Phys Med Rehabil*. 2010;91(1):20–29.

73. Wagner AK, Sasser HC, Hammond FM, Wiercisiewski D, Alexander J. Intentional traumatic brain injury: epidemiology, risk factors, and associations with injury severity and mortality. *J Trauma*. 2000; 49(3):404–410.

74. Seel RT, Kreutzer JS, Rosenthal M, Hammond FM, Corrigan JD, Black K. Depression after traumatic brain injury: a national institute on disability and rehabilitation research model systems multicenter investigation. *Arch Phys Med Rehabil*. 2003;84(2):177–184.

75. Ashman TA, Spielman LA, Hibbard MR, Silver JM, Chandna T, Gordon WA. Psychiatric challenges in the first 6 years after traumatic brain injury: cross-sequential analyses of Axis I disorders. *Arch Phys Med Rehabil*. 2004;85(4)(suppl 2):S36–S42.

76. Berry C, Salim A, Alban R, Mirocha J, Margulies DR, Ley EJ. Serum ethanol levels in patients with moderate to severe traumatic brain injury influence outcomes: a surprising finding. *Am Surg*. 2010; 76(10):1067–1070.

77. Maier RV. Controlling alcohol problems among hospitalized trauma patients. *J Trauma*. 2005;59(suppl 2):S1–S2.

78. Macdonald S, Cherpitel CJ, Borges G, DeSouza A, Giesbrecht N, Stockwell T. The criteria for causation of alcohol in violent injuries based on emergency room data from six countries. *Addict Behav*. 2005;30(1):103–113.

79. Himanen L, Portin R, Hämäläinen P, Hurme S, Hiekkanen H, Tenovuo O. Risk factors for reduced survival after traumatic brain injury: a 30-year follow-up study. *Brain Inj*. 2011;25(5):443–452.

80. Heffernan DS, Vera RM, Monaghan SF, et al. Impact of socioethnic factors on outcomes following traumatic brain injury. *J Trauma*. 2011;70(3):527–534.

81. Shandro JR, Rivara FP, Wang J, Jurkovich GJ, Nathens AB, Mac Kenzie EJ. Alcohol and risk of mortality in patients with traumatic brain injury. *J Trauma*. 2009;66(6):1584–1590.

82. Langlois JA, Kegler SR, Butler JA, et al. Traumatic brain injury-related hospital discharges. Results from a 14-state surveillance system, 1997. *MMWR Surveill Summ*. 2003;27;52(4):1–20.

83. Daneshvar DH, Baugh CM, Nowinski CJ, McKee AC, Stern RA, Cantu RC. Helmets and mouth guards: the role of personal equipment in preventing sport-related concussions. *Clin Sports Med*. 2011;30(1):145–163.

84. Navarro RR. Protective equipment and the prevention of concussion—what is the evidence? *Curr Sports Med Rep*. 2011;10(1):27–31.

85. Liu BC, Ivers R, Norton R, Boufous S, Blows S, Lo SK. Helmets for preventing injury in motorcycle riders. *Cochrane Database of Syst Rev*. 2008;(1).

86. Macpherson A, Spinks A. Bicycle helmet legislation for the uptake of helmet use and prevention of head injuries. *Cochrane Database of Syst Rev*. 2008;(3).

87. Zaloshnja E, Miller T, Langlois JA, Selassie AW. Prevalence of long term disability from traumatic brain injury in the civilian population of the United States, 2005. *J Head Trauma Rehabil*. 2008;23(6): 394–400.

88. Selassie AW, Zaloshnja E, Langlois JA, Miller T, Jones P, Steiner C. Incidence of long-term disability following traumatic brain injury hospitalization, United States, 2003. *J Head Trauma Rehab*. 2008; 23(2):123–131.

89. Thurman DJ, Alverson CA, Dunn KA, Guerrero J, Sniezek JE. Traumatic brain injury in the United States: a public health perspective. *J Head Trauma Rehabil*. 1999;14(6):602–615.

90. Finkelstein EA, Corso PS, Miller TR. *The Incidence and Economic Burden of Injuries in the United States.* New York, NY: Oxford University Press; 2006.

91. Coronado VG, Thurman DJ, Greenspan AI, Weissman BM. Epidemiology. In: Jallo J, Loftus CM, eds. *Neurotrauma and Critical Care of the Brain.* New York, NY: Thieme; 2009:3–19.

92. Draper K, Ponsford J. Cognitive functioning ten years following traumatic brain injury and rehabilitation. *Neuropsychology.* 2008; 22(5):618–625.

93. Konrad C, Geburek AJ, Rist F, et al. Long-term cognitive and emotional consequences of mild traumatic brain injury. *Psychol Med.* 2011;41(6):1197–211.

94. Shigaki CL, Johnstone B, Schopp LH. Financial and vocational outcomes 2 years after traumatic brain injury. *Disabil Rehabil.* 2009; 31(6):484–489.

95. Aitken ME, McCarthy ML, Slomine BS, et al. Family burden after traumatic brain injury in children. *Pediatrics.* 2009;123(1):199–206.

96. Plassman BL, Havlik RJ, Steffens DC, et al. Documented head injury in early adulthood and risk of Alzheimer's disease and other dementias. *Neurology.* 2000;55(8):1158–1166.

97. Harrison-Felix C, Whiteneck G, Devivo MJ, Hammond FM, Jha A. Causes of death following 1 year postinjury among individuals with traumatic brain injury. *J Head Trauma Rehabil.* 2006;21(1):22–23.

98. Simpson G, Tate R. Suicidality in people surviving a traumatic brain injury: Prevalence, risk factors and implications for clinical management. *Brain Injury.* 2007;21(13–14):1335–51.

99. Miele VJ, Bailes JE. Mild Brain Injury. In: Jallo J, Loftus CM, eds. *Neurotrauma and Critical Care of the Brain.* New York, NY: Thieme; 2009.

100. Kashluba S, Casey JE, Paniak C. Evaluating the utility of ICD-10 diagnostic criteria for postconcussion syndrome following mild traumatic brain injury. *J Int Neuropsychol Soc.* 2006;12(1):111–118.

101. Shames J, Treger J, Ring H, Giaquinto S. Return to work following traumatic brain injury: trends and challenges. *Disabil Rehabil.* 2007; 29(17):1387–1395.

102. Sendroy-Terrill M, Whiteneck GG, Brooks CA. Aging with traumatic brain injury: cross-sectional follow-up of people receiving inpatient rehabilitation over more than 3 decades. *Arch Phys Med Rehabil.* 2010;91(3):489–497.

103. Steel J, Youssef M, Pfeifer R, et al. Health-related quality of life in patients with multiple injuries and traumatic brain injury 10 + years postinjury. *J Trauma.* 2010;69(3):523–531.

104. Field M, Collins MW, Lovell MR, Maroon J. Does age play a role in recovery from sports-related concussion? A comparison of high school and collegiate athletes. *J Pediatr.* 2003;142(5):546–553.

105. Pellman EJ, Lovell MR, Viano DC, Casson IR. Concussion in professional football: recovery of NFL and high school athletes assessed by computerized neuropsychological testing—Part 12. *Neurosurgery.* 2006;58(2):263–274.

106. Summers CR, Ivins B, Schwab KA. Traumatic brain injury in the United States: an epidemiologic overview. *Mt Sinai J Med.* 2009; 76(2):105–110.

107. Losiniecki L, Shutter L. Management of traumatic brain injury. *Curr Treat Options Neurol.* 2010;12(2):142–54.

108. Dikmen SS, Levin HS. Methodological issues in the study of mild head injury. *J Head Trauma Rehabil.* 1993;8(3):30–37.

109. Bohnen N, Twijnstra A, Jolles J. Post-traumatic and emotional symptoms in different subgroups of patients with mild head injury. *Brain Inj.* 1992;6(6):481–487.

110. Langlois Orman JA, Kraus JF, Zaloshnja E, Miller T. Epidemiology. In: Silver JM, McAllister TW, Yudofsky SC, eds. *Textbook of Traumatic Brain Injury.* 2nd ed. Washington, DC: American Psychiatric Association; 2011:3–22.

111. Shi J, Xiang H, Wheeler K, et al. Costs, mortality likelihood and outcomes of hospitalized US children with traumatic brain injuries. *Brain Inj.* 2009;23(7):602–611.

112. Tagliaferri F, Compagnone C, Korsic M, Servadei F, Kraus J. A systematic review of brain injury epidemiology in Europe. *Acta Neurochi* (Wien). 2006;148:255–268.

113. Murray CJL, Lopez AD. *Global Health Statistics: A Compendium of Incidence, Prevalence, and Mortality Estimates for Over 200 Conditions.* Boston, MA: Harvard School of Public Health on behalf of the World Health Organization and the World Bank; 1996.

114. Centers for Disease Control and Prevention. *Traumatic Brain Injury in the United States: A Report to Congress.* US Department of Health and Human Services. Atlanta, GA: Centers for Disease Control and Prevention; 1999.

115. Haddon W Jr. A logical framework for categorizing highway safety phenomena and activity. *J Trauma.* 1972;12(3):193–207.

116. Haddon W Jr. Advances in the epidemiology of injuries as a basis for public policy. *Public Health Rep.* 1980;95(5):411–441.

117. Runyan CW. Introduction: back to the future—revisiting Haddon's conceptualization of injury epidemiology and prevention. *Epidemiol Rev.* 2003;25(1):60–64.

9

Primary Prevention

Lee M. Kneer and Elie P. Elovic

INTRODUCTION

The intent of this chapter is to review common prevention strategies and their overall effectiveness in this patient population, with an emphasis on the need for further preventative measures. The importance of these efforts will be obvious to readers after the following discussion that addresses the data on the incidence, severity, and consequences of traumatic brain injury (TBI).

Accidental injury is the fifth leading cause of death overall in the United States and the leading cause of mortality among Americans younger than 44 years old (1). Nearly one-third of all injury-related deaths from 2002 to 2006 were TBI-associated, with the highest incidence in the pediatric and elderly populations (2). Numerous estimates exist regarding the number of Americans who present to the emergency departments secondary to TBI annually, with two of the more recent being 1.1 (3) and 1.7 million (2). This does not include those who seek other treatment or no care at all (2). Of those seen, an estimated 52,000 die and 275,000 are hospitalized (2). Furthermore, significant prolonged disability can result from TBI. The 43.3% of those who sustain a brain injury will have some disability as a result, and an estimated 3.2 million Americans are currently living with TBI-related disability (3). The annual cost of medical treatment and lost productivity because of TBI in the United States was estimated to be $60 billion in 2000 (4).

The incidence of emergency room encounters for TBI has risen in recent years (2,3). This may not only result from population growth or indicate an increase in TBI incidence and severity, but may also suggest an improved awareness in recognizing the symptoms of TBI and of the importance of seeking medical attention. Regardless, the morbidity and mortality associated with TBI places a substantial and, in large part preventable, burden on the health care system (5–7). For a more complete discussion of TBI Epidemiology, see Chapter 8 of this book.

TRAUMATIC BRAIN INJURY VS OTHER DISABLING CONDITIONS

TBI has often been referred to as the *silent* or *invisible epidemic*, both caused by the vagueness of its sequelae and the relatively nominal amount of financial resources dedicated to its prevention, diagnosis, and treatment. This is unfortunate because mortality related to TBI nearly equals that of diseases with aggressive prevention campaigns such as colon cancer and diabetes and surpasses mortality associated with HIV/AIDS, influenza/pneumonia, Parkinson disease, as well as cancer of the breast, skin, and prostate (2,7–10). The mortality rate for HIV/AIDS has steadily declined since its apex in 1995 (11), thought to be in large part because of increased public awareness and dedication to preventative measures, research, and treatment. The same trend is possible regarding TBI if efforts are similarly directed toward awareness and prevention, the groundwork for which was laid in the 1970s and 1980s (12–14).

ECONOMICS OF TRAUMATIC BRAIN INJURY: COSTS, BURDEN, AND ITS PREVENTION

The economic costs associated with TBI are monumental, especially when one considers not only direct medical care but also indirect costs such as loss of productivity of the TBI-injured patient and their support system, which often consists of family and friends whose time spent caring for their loved one often precludes them from pursuing employment (4,5,7). Despite increased prevention efforts, the economic burden on the US economy resulting from TBI is increasing. This is not necessarily an indictment on current prevention strategies because studies abound illustrating the success rate of various interventions. Rather, this affirms the importance of continued research directed at brain injury epidemiology and the development of effective prevention strategies.

WHAT IS PREVENTION?

Prevention can be subdivided into primary, secondary, and tertiary components. Although the scope of this chapter will be confined to primary prevention, an understanding of all aspects of prevention will further delineate the role of primary prevention in reducing the incidence and severity of acquired brain injury.

Primary prevention efforts are designed to prevent the initial injury. Examples of primary prevention include screening tests, fall-proofing homes, traffic laws and their enforcement, salting of ice-covered roads, and education on topics such as the dangers of driving while impaired. Primary preventative measures have been shown to work with other conditions. For example, the effect of lowering blood pressure in hypertensive individuals, independent of other factors, has shown to reduce the incidence of cerebrovascular accidents (15).

Once an event has occurred, secondary prevention strategies aim to reduce event recurrence and prevent complications stemming from the initial event. To illustrate, once a patient has suffered an embolic cerebrovascular event, the use of aspirin to prevent a recurrent stroke in the future, albeit with associated risk, is clear (16). In addition, the prevention of sequelae resulting from the initial event is demonstrated in the projection reduction exposure with variable axis immersion lens (PREVAIL) study, which compared the efficacy of enoxaparin and low-molecular-weight heparin in preventing the incidence of venous thromboembolism in a population of patient who had suffered an ischemic stroke (17).

INJURY CONTROL THEORY

Originally, the general belief was that TBI resulted from accidents, with the implication that all persons had equal probability of sustaining injury (18,19). After a review of TBI epidemiology literature, it appears that this may not be the case. Careful consideration must be made of a person's age, sex, and other individual risk factors that increase the likelihood of sustaining an injury (20). For example, falls among the elderly may be secondary to sedatives, antidepressants, lower extremity disability, or balance impairments (21). In addition, environmental factors associated with an increased incidence of brain injury have been identified, and there is now also a focus on injury-preventive environments, such as the increase in roof-crush standards for automobiles set to take place in 2012 (22,23). There has been substantial work devoted to the identification of environmental hazards and individual qualities associated with increased risk of brain injury and developing effective preventive countermeasures (18,24). As a result, there has been a substantial increase in the science of injury control theory over the last 50 years.

THE HADDON MATRIX

The *Haddon Matrix* is a model that facilitates the identification of injury risk factors. It was developed by William Haddon Jr. in the 1970s, and although it was initially devised to classify the factors leading to motor vehicle collisions, it has far-reaching applications including infectious disease and other injury epidemiology and prevention as well (25–29).

A basic understanding of the Haddon Matrix will facilitate brain injury primary prevention efforts.

Haddon identified temporal phases surrounding injuries. The preinjury phase examines risk factors that led to the initial injurious event. This would be the area of interest to one seeking primary prevention. The second phase is the injury phase, where factors are identified that may increase or decrease the severity of the initial event, such as seat belts in a motor vehicle collision. Finally, the postinjury phase seeks to describe factors that may predispose or prevent the occurrence of the same event in the future. The preinjury, injury, and postinjury phases correlate with primary, secondary, and tertiary events, respectively.

Haddon described the categories of risk leading to injury as they relate to the host, vector, and the social and physical environment (28) as illustrated in Tables 9-1a and 9-1b.

Using these sets of variables, a table can be created where each cell represents an area and a temporal component. All the different variables that contribute to an injury can be placed into one of the table's cells, and from this table, injury prevention targets are organized.

To best illustrate this concept, consider the factors related to a motor vehicle accident (MVA) in the preinjury phase. Age and alcohol use would be placed in the host precrash or preinjury cell, and the vector would include the condition of the vehicle. The physical environment cell would describe the roadway design and the public acceptance that not wearing seatbelts is "normal" would reflect the social environment. Precrash socioeconomic environmental factors include the social stigma of driving while impaired, as well as public perception on the importance of purchasing vehicles with modern safety features. Event factors may reflect the use of a child safety seat. Host variables such as proper positioning, vector factors including a seat not meeting accepted standards, even social environmental factors such as the nonuse of these seats with celebrities being photographed holding their children on their lap in the front seat can be examined. Postevent, the injured person's ability to tolerate rehabilitation, an exploding gas tank, the importance a society places on standards for medical care, and the availability of paramedics complete the matrix.

By studying the epidemiology of injury, efforts can be made at identifying and remedying various injury patterns. Potentially, the most efficacious way to prevent an injury is to target the vector or injuring agent and thereby alter the mechanism of energy transmission. Designing safer cars, better engineered roads, and improving conditions of the vehicle would greatly impact injury prevention.

TABLE 9-1a Haddon Matrix As It Applies to Falls in the Elderly

	HOST	VECTOR	SOCIAL ENVIRONMENT	PHYSICAL ENVIRONMENT
Pre-event	Visual impairment	Crowd	Acceptance of falls as "normal"	Ice
Event	Hypocoagulability	Presence of headgear	Soft flooring requirements	Surface fallen onto
Postevent	Ability to tolerate rehabilitation	Personal alarm	Financial support for rehabilitation	EMS availability

TABLE 9-1b Haddon Matrix As It Applies to Motor Vehicle Accidents

	HOST	VECTOR	SOCIAL ENVIRONMENT	PHYSICAL ENVIRONMENT
Pre-event	Alcohol consumption	Brakes worn out	Now wearing a seatbelt is "normal"	Poor state of road repair/lighting
Event	Child safety seat in front seat	Child safety seat not up to specifications	Lack of enforcement of safety regulations	Fallen tree on road
Postevent	Ability to tolerate rehabilitation	Exploding gas tank	Extremely limited automobile insurance to fund care	EMS availability

APPROACH TO HEALTH MAINTENANCE

The maintenance of health as it refers to TBI requires a comprehensive approach. It must include passive and active strategies implemented via education and, at times, legislation. Passive strategies require no effort on the part of the host and as a result offer protection to a larger percentage of the population than active strategies (30,31). Some examples of passive strategies include automotive air bags, road barriers, fingerprint-based gunlocks, and improved child safety seat design. Active strategies require the host's participation, such as donning a seat belt, avoiding driving when under the influence of alcohol or other drugs, and helmet usage. Active prevention strategies depend on the public's awareness of such measures and their overall compliance. It may take a tremendous amount of societal effort and financial support to encourage the host to adopt these active measures of prevention. Although cost and continued educational efforts are disadvantages of active strategies, they have been shown to be efficacious when used in combination with passive measures in preventing TBI (32–35).

The responsibility of educating the public, advocating for increased awareness, and promoting legislative action has largely fallen on professional health organizations. These organizations use their position and expertise to promote research that identifies targets for injury prevention, which guides public education efforts and lends credence to testimonials given to legislative groups. The Brain Injury Association of America (formerly National Head Injury Foundation) or BIAA is an example of such an organization. Founded in 1980, its mission is "to be the voice of brain injury" and boasts individual associations in 39 of the United States (36). The BIAA works closely with the Congressional Brain Injury Task Force to promote legislation to ensure funding for TBI prevention and treatment efforts, and with state associations such as the National Association of State Head Injury Administrators to further TBI awareness and prevention efforts.

In general, changing human behavior can be a very challenging endeavor and there is still some controversy on the appropriate approach. Haddon stated that targeting the vector with passive interventions and the environment may be the most effective in decreasing death and injury (28). This does not negate the potential benefit of using a combined approach of active and passive measures of intervention, such as using seatbelts in combination with air bags. Each prevention method has shown efficacy in reducing crash-related injuries; however, concomitant use of each has been shown to be more effective than either in isolation.

If one factors in legislation to increase compliance with active prevention efforts, further benefits can be attained.

States that strengthened existing seatbelt laws and adopted primary enforcement seatbelt legislation had an estimated 79% compliance with belt use in 1998—a 17% increase over just 6 years following the introduction of primary enforcement legislation (37,38).

DEVELOPMENT OF A COMPREHENSIVE INJURY PREVENTION PROGRAM

The components critical to development of a comprehensive injury prevention program are active and passive strategies, education, and legislation. Engineering solutions are an important component of the passive interventions and include items such as energy-absorbing car bodies, road barriers, and air bags. Active strategies, such as education, are also critical, both at the individual and community level (37). Some of the most effective interventions include hands-on demonstrations and reinforcement at subsequent visits (39). However, the listener is more inclined to change their behavior if there is some incentive to do so.

It has been shown that if only education is used, then the general public may not change their overall behavior (40). Community-based intervention programs combining education with legislative action has been shown to be effective in increasing bicycle helmet usage (41). A study carried out in 3 separate Maryland counties explored bike helmet usage by children under 3 separate conditions. In one county, helmet use increased by 43% when education and legislation were combined. Another county, which used education alone, showed only an 11% increase, which was not statistically significant (42). The third county, which did nothing, actually demonstrated a decreased rate of helmet use from 19% to 4%.

Enforcement of legislation is critical to maximize its potential benefit, with seatbelts being an example. By 1984, passenger cars were required to have seatbelts, but only 15% of people used them while driving. By 1987, education combined with seatbelt legislation increased this rate to 42%. This was further increased to 62% when secondary enforcement laws were enacted, which allow citation of a driver for seatbelt noncompliance although they were pulled over for another offense. This rate stayed the same through 1998 in the states that used secondary enforcement laws. When some states increased legislation and enforcement efforts with the enactment of primary enforcement legislation allowing ticketing when the only infraction was seatbelt nonuse, compliance increased to 79% (43).

In summary, a comprehensive approach to injury control, including active and passive measures, education at both the community and individual level, and appropriate legislation is the most efficacious way to facilitate injury prevention. It is necessary to take a multifaceted approach, targeting as many components of the Haddon Matrix as possible to promote injury prevention.

MOTOR VEHICLE ACCIDENT PREVENTION

To begin the exploration of TBI prevention efforts, it is most fitting to approach this issue by examining the leading cause of TBI-related death in the United States—MVA (2). It is well established that younger, inexperienced drivers are more commonly involved in MVA (44). An increasingly popular strategy to decrease accident rates in this population involves limiting adolescents' ability to operate a vehicle in a graduated fashion, and these programs have proven efficacy (45,46). All states have adopted graduated drivers' license programs with varying restrictions of driving during certain hours and the ability to transport passengers (47). Multiple studies have illustrated the concomitant decrease in MVA in teenage drivers after implementation of a graduated drivers' licensing program (48,49). This rate of decrease was greater than that observed in older drivers with unrestricted licenses and advocates for allowing novice drivers the opportunity to hone their skills in safer environments prior to prevent motor vehicle collisions and, therefore, TBI. These efforts may be further tailored in the future, as factors have been identified that are associated with an increased incidence of motor vehicle collisions in the teenage population (50).

Efforts at improving pedestrian safety have also proven efficacious in MVA prevention. In addition to improved vehicle design, targets for prevention include driver and pedestrian behaviors such as increasing required stops, speed humps, and promoting crossing only in crosswalks after ensuring a clear path (51–54). Publicly funded prevention efforts are promoted through programs established by The National Highway Traffic Safety Administration (NHTSA) (55) and Centers for Disease Control and Prevention (CDC), and recent passage of the Pedestrian Safety Enhancement Act of 2010 suggests that primary prevention of traffic accidents will remain a priority.

One area of intense research, legislation, and public funding surrounds the use of cell phones while operating a motor vehicle. Cellular phones are nearly ubiquitous, and using a phone to make calls or text while driving is rampant among US drivers (56). Distracted driving has been implicated in up to 16% of motor vehicle collisions resulting in fatalities and 39 states have implemented laws requiring cellular phone users to use a hands-free device while driving, although using any communication device while operating a motor vehicle is a distraction to drivers (57–62). In 2 year-long pilot projects carried out by the NHTSA and funded with both state and federal monies, motorists were cited for using a cell phone illegally while driving (63). This resulted in a significant reduction in the number of people using cell phones while driving, and may indicate a possible target for a motor vehicle collision and thus TBI active prevention strategy.

The incidence of both death and injury because of MVAs declined in the decade ending in 2009 (59). This likely results from programs such as graduated driving privileges and improved pedestrian safety targets, in addition to the issues of seatbelts, air bags, and alcohol consumption, which will be addressed in later discussion.

Air Bags and Seatbelts

Air bags are designed to rapidly and automatically deploy during a frontal vehicle collision, creating an absorptive impact barrier between the vehicle's occupants and the automobile's front interior paneling. This barrier allows for safer transfer of the energy resulting from impact. Complete deployment and subsequent deflation of air bags occurs within 1 second, ostensibly allowing the driver to maintain control of the vehicle and also prevent the trapping of passengers (64).

Advocacy for air bags resulted in their installation as standard equipment in all passenger cars and light trucks in 1997 (65). This requirement mandated only front-impact protection, which when used in conjunction with a lap-shoulder belt has an estimated reduction in head injuries of 83% compared to unrestrained drivers (66). In 2007, however, legislation mandating air bags to deploy in side-impact collisions passed and went into effect in 2009, allowing 4 years for compliance. Side-impact protection testing estimates that torso and head air bag devices reduce fatality risk in near-side occupants by 24% (67).

The use of both air bag systems and lap-shoulder restraints illustrates a strategy of injury prevention using passive strategies synergistically. The NHTSA's Crashworthiness Data System estimated that the effects of air bags alone do not demonstrate a statistically significant result, as moderate and severe injuries to all organ systems decreased by merely 18% and 7%, respectively, with their use independent of lap-shoulder restraints. Similar injuries were reduced by 49% with the use of a lap-shoulder belt system. Interestingly, the combination of both systems reduced risk by 60%. From this information, one might conclude that air bags provide only moderate benefit to the use of lap-shoulder belt system restraints. However, although injury severity to different body systems must be taken into consideration, TBI has been shown to be the major source of mortality in the multiple trauma occupant (68). With this in mind, a restraint system that protects against head and brain injury is of great importance. The use of manual lap-shoulder belt and air bags in combination resulted in an 83% and 75% reduction in moderate and severe head injuries, respectively. This data is significant when compared to the risk reduction of 59% and 38% with the use of a lap-shoulder belt alone. Although much of the risk reduction results from the use of the lap-shoulder belt alone, it is important to remember that lap-shoulder belts must be "used," which differs from the automatic deployment of an air bag restraint system.

The preventative benefits of seatbelts and air bags are clearly demonstrable. However, there have been several injuries associated with their use. Case reports abound associating air bag use with spinal cord injury, brachial plexopathy, liver laceration, small bowel perforation, traumatic hernia, aortic dissection, ocular and facial trauma, neck sprain, kidney trauma, sternal fracture, pneumothorax, and placental/fetal injury (69–87). Air bags have also been implicated in several injuries, including skull fracture and facial injury (88–90), ocular trauma (91–95), burn injuries (96–98), reflex sympathetic dystrophy (99,100), extremity fracture (101,102), cervical spine injuries (103,104), auricular trauma, and hearing loss (105,106).

There is substantial evidence that children are most susceptible to injury because of air bag deployment (91,103,107–113). Severe and fatal injuries have occurred in situations where children have been both properly and improperly positioned (91,103,107,109,114,115). In the 1990s, advocacy for air bag safety led to legislation mandating child seating in the rear seat only and in approved child car seats for children younger than a certain age. This led to a decline in the front seating of children in vehicles involved in fatal collisions, although studies have estimated that an additional 500 deaths could be prevented with full compliance of child safety seating laws (110,116). This is an excellent example, however, of education and legislation leading to active and passive preventative strategies to decrease brain injury risk.

MOTORCYCLE INJURY PREVENTION

TBI resulting from motorcycle accidents is a serious problem in the United States. Although injuries related to passenger car collisions have steadily declined over the past 2 decades, injury incidence in motorcycle collisions has increased by 14%, and motorcycle-related fatalities increased by a staggering 144%, a rate that exceeds the increase in motorcycle registrations during that time (117,118). Motorcyclists are also more likely to sustain a TBI in a collision compared to passenger car or truck occupants (118). As one might expect, motorcyclists with TBI have a disproportionately poorer outcome than those without TBI. They account for only 17% of those seeking treatment for motorcycle collision-related injuries, but represent 54% of admitted riders who did not survive, are more likely to discharge to a long-term care facility, and incur 13 times the costs of hospitalizations of helmeted motorcyclists (117).

The demographics of motorcycle injury victims have changed over the past 2 decades. In 1988, nearly two-thirds of motorcycle fatalities involved riders younger than 30 years old (117). By 2007, however, as baby boomers aged, this decreased to approximately one-third, whereas the number of fatalities affecting riders aged 40 and older increased to include nearly half of all fatalities. This has important implications because motorcycle accident prevention efforts will be most effective when targeting the appropriate demographics.

Possibly, the most critical mitigating factor relating to TBI and fatalities caused by motorcycle accidents is the use of helmets. A 1994 study of the efficacy of helmet use reported a 37.5% decrease in motorcycle fatalities and a statistically significant decrease in TBIs among both fatally and nonfatally injured riders, and several studies have confirmed the decrease in TBI incidence and severity among helmeted motorcyclists (119–122). In addition, and despite a popular myth to the contrary that led to the repeal of helmet laws in some states, helmeted motorcycle riders have a lower risk of cervical spine injury(123,124). The overwhelming result of legislation mandating helmet use is a reduced rate of overall fatalities, TBI-related fatalities, overall TBI incidence, injury severity, length of hospitalization, and overall cost to society (124–127).

Motorcycle Helmet Design

Improved helmet design also plays a role in brain injury prevention. Once made of cloth or leather, today's helmets are composed of synthetic materials that work to absorb forces on impact and distribute them over a wide area. In states with mandatory helmet use laws, head protection must meet standards set forth by the US Department of Transportation. Features of approved helmets include a dense foam internal liner and rigid external materials, including Kevlar, ABS plastic, carbon fiber, and fiberglass (128). Studies have shown the effectiveness of helmets meeting these standards and the ineffectiveness of unapproved helmets (128,129).

Despite this strong evidence from countries around the world, there are still several states across the United States that have not enacted mandatory helmet laws. In 2011, there remain 3 states with no helmet legislation, 20 states with helmets required solely for teenage riders, and only 21 states with mandatory helmet use for all motorcycle riders (130). As stated earlier, several states have enacted motorcycle helmet laws as early as the 1970s only to repeal them on the basis of case reports of helmet-induced injury that we now know occurs rarely and is outweighed by the substantial fatality, injury risk, and societal cost reduction (131,132).

In 1967, the Federal Government required states to pass a motorcycle helmet law in order to continue to receive federal safety funds. As a result, by 1975, 47 states had passed legislation requiring the use of helmets. However, as opposition mounted against the use of helmets, Congress overturned the helmet requirement. Following this action, more than half of all states with mandatory helmet laws revised their laws (127), with a resultant decrease use of helmets in those states. Within 9 months of the repeal, the states of Texas and Arkansas saw a decline in helmet usage from 97% to 66% and 52%, respectively. There was a concomitant increase in overall motorcycle injuries, head injuries, and an increased proportion of those injured having suffered head injuries according to data obtained from the Arkansas Trauma Registry (127). This trend was also seen in Miami Dade County with an increased incidence of TBI and fatalities in the post-repeal era that saw helmet usage drop from 83% to 56% (133). Bledsoe et al. reported on the Arkansas experience of helmet law repeal (134). A 6-year retrospective review of the trauma registry compared the results of the 3 years prior to repeal as compared to the 3 years afterward. There was no statistical change in total and fatal collisions; however, there was a significant increase in nonhelmeted deaths at the scene of the accident. The nonhelmeted had significantly higher Abbreviated Injury scores involving the head and neck, more expensive, longer ICU stays, and substantially higher non-reimbursed hospital charges.

As mentioned earlier, the financial costs to society following the repeals of mandatory helmet laws have been substantial. A study in Texas concluded the median cost of motorcycle-related injury increased 300% to $22,531 per event, with TBI costs increasing 75% to more than $32,000, and subsequent studies report similar results (135,136). In addition to the loss of life, function, and emotional trauma sustained by the patient and their loved ones, these costs (up to $250 million annually) represent a significant financial burden (136).

Another issue that also arises is the relationship between alcohol consumption and the operation of motorcycles. The consequences of motorcycle collisions are typically more severe, yet among both fatal and nonfatal crash victims, motorcyclists are more likely to have alcohol in their system (137, 138). Although difficult to test in real-world scenarios, in controlled conditions, experienced riders have been shown to exhibit delayed responses even at the per se 0.05% alcohol level, well lower than the accepted limit in any state (139). Since handling a motorcycle requires more balance and coordination, lowering the blood alcohol content (BAC) that classifies a motorcyclist as being under the influence may be a target for prevention.

Roadway Design

Accident prevention can also be achieved by identifying hazardous road locations with specific collision patterns. Various approaches can be used to correct these accident-prone areas through road engineering and technology. Attempts to engineer safer driving surfaces date back to the 1930s when skidding resistance was added to wet roads (140). However, more than 40 years passed before a major push to develop safer roads was initiated. *The Road Safety Code of Good Practice* was a publication from the Local Authority Associations that included engineering in addition to education and enforcement, the three E's (education, enforcement, and engineering), for better road safety (141). One study attempted to identify crash problems on various urban arterial streets in Washington, DC (142). Police reports of more than 2,000 crashes yielded crash data, and the locations that had a large number of crashes were analyzed to identify precrash movements and travel directions of the involved vehicles. At some intersections, drivers had difficulty turning left from a private driveway, whereas some intersections had extremely high traffic speeds with crashes likely to occur at the end of a ramp. In addition, many intersections lacked left turn signals. These targets for prevention were identified by researchers and implemented by authorities. Changes included the addition of left turn signals, prohibition of left turns from a driveway, improvement of storm drainage, increased pavement skid resistance, as well as the initiation of pavement milling. It was also noted that stopped buses obstructed drivers' visual fields. Relocating bus stops, as well as removing large fixed objects, was a simple intervention that was effective in reducing accidents.

Sabey suggested that the use of 4 investigative techniques could be the foundation for intervention and treatment of the problem (140). These 4 areas included *single sites* where accidents cluster or "blackspots," *mass action* or locations that have common accident factors, *route action* or lengths of road with above-average accident rates, and *area action* including areas requiring a more global approach aimed at dealing with scattered accidents. He also provided examples of proposed treatments for each of the 4 variables. For instance, route action could be addressed with road marking to deter overtaking, increasing skidding resistance, or installing roundabouts at key junctions to provide access to adjacent neighborhoods. In one trial of a 3-km road with a large number of accidents per year, a roundabout was added as well as a new light to control crossings in addition to right turn bans. This resulted in a 12% reduction in accidents that resulted in injury.

Improved roadway design does not have to be expensive. For instance, the US Department of Transportation's Federal Highway Administration recently experimented with adding a *safety edge* to pavement-shoulder drop-offs in 3 states undergoing roadway resurfacing (143). They proposed that drivers who leave the roadway encounter abruptly increased resistance when tires remount the pavement when there is a steep drop-off. To remedy this, the edges of resurfaced roads were sloped at an angle of 30°, leading to a more gradual transition from off-road to on-road. This inexpensive strategy was associated with a 5.7% estimated crash rate reduction.

One technique engineers and urban planners use to reduce the incidence and severity of motor vehicle collisions is traffic calming. Traffic calming aims to slow vehicle speed by physically altering roadways. Speed bumps, chicanes, median islands, and curb extensions are all techniques used to encourage slower speeds. The number of roundabouts in the United States has increased by 1000% from 1997 to 2007. Several studies highlight the effectiveness in reducing both collisions and fatalities after converting conventional stop sign–controlled intersections into roundabouts (144–146). In contrast to modifying roadway edges, however, roundabouts are costly and usually require the intersection to be closed to traffic for several months for construction (146). In addition, motorists must have the knowledge of how to navigate through a roundabout regarding lane changes and right-of-way. Regardless, they have proven efficacy, and recent research has explored ways of making these intersections even safer, namely by increasing the deviation angle or the angle at which a driver must turn to enter the roundabout (147).

A 2003 Cochrane Review touted the benefits of areawide traffic calming measures in reducing traffic-related injuries and fatalities (53). There remains, however, a consistent call for further funding for research to identify roadway characteristics that put motorists at increased risk for collision and injury. These targets can then be addressed via legislation, increased public awareness, and urban planning in this critical area of injury prevention in the United States.

FALLS

As the incidence of TBI from motor vehicle collisions has tapered, falls have become the leading cause of TBI in the United States (2). More than 35% of brain injuries result from falls in a bimodal distribution that is well-established (18). Children aged 0–4 years and those aged 75 and older account for 40% of all falls despite representing a much smaller percentage of the populace (2). Younger children have a much larger head-to-body ratio, and thus, the head strikes the ground more frequently during play even though they may fall only a few feet (148,149). More than 2 decades ago, falls from extreme heights accounted for 12% of all unintentional traumatic deaths in New York City children. Overall, in the United States, it has been estimated that falls comprise almost 9% of pediatric trauma deaths and account for up to 41% of pediatric hospital admissions (116,150).

Turning our attention to the elderly, fatalities as a result of TBI are most common for those older than 65 years and are implicated in 61% of TBIs in this population (2). Jagger et al. found that there was a stable pattern of occurrence of fall-related TBI up to about 59 years old. However, in the seventh decade, a dramatic increase in TBI resulting from falls occurred, and incidence rates continued to rise in those aged 70 years and older (13). The financial burden from falls in the elderly is enormous. In 2000, direct medical costs totaled $200 million for fatal and $19 billion for nonfatal falls—numbers that obviously don't affect the productivity lost by both the patient and their caregivers (151).

Efforts at fall prevention via legislation and education have been effective. In 1972, the New York City Department of Health developed a health education program termed "Children Can't Fly." This initiated installment of window guards in all New York City apartments that had children younger than 11 years old residing in them. This resulted in a 96% decrease in falls from windows after implementation (116). The use of safety devices for windows in suburban areas has also shown to be helpful, and from 1990 to 2008, a study revealed a statistically significant decrease in falls from windows (150,152). There have been positive results in fall prevention both abroad such as in Sweden (153), as well as in American urban neighborhoods (152,154,155).

The issue of playground-related falls can be addressed by the use of protective surfaces, including adding a safe 12-inch border of a soft material such as wood chips, sand, or rubber around play areas (155). A study adopting a holistic approach found that the risk of playground injury decreased without affecting enjoyment when playground features emphasized lower body strength, coordination, and lower free fall heights predominated (156). Parental supervision and education is critical, and efforts directed at educating children, their parents, and the community at large have been shown to be effective at reducing playground-related injury (157,158).

Fall prevention in the elderly requires several strategies that often require physician input. Health care providers must be vigilant to identify various factors that may contribute to falls in the elderly. Miller et al. (159) identified four common issues that have been implicated in increasing the risk of falls in the elderly. They are postural hypotension, gait and balance instability, polypharmacy, and the use of sedating medications. Other host-related risk factors that have been associated with falls include musculoskeletal or neurological abnormalities, visual disturbances, dementia, alcohol consumption, frailty, and a history of prior falls (160,161).

Balance deficits in the elderly appear to be related to the deterioration of various input systems necessary for postural control. It has been demonstrated that in subjects older than 70 years of age, there is a 40% reduction in sensory cells of the vestibular system (162). These older adults are more likely to fall if other systems required for postural control, such as vision and proprioception, are impaired (163). Impaired balance in the elderly can also be attributed to multiple deficits in the neuromuscular system. It has been consistently shown that disuse atrophy, motor weakness, abnormal tone, and posturing contribute to impaired balance in the elderly (164, 165). There may be generalized slowing of central-processing areas in the elderly that involve integration and coordination of multiple inputs and outputs in the brain including the motor cortex, basal ganglia, and cerebellum (164). Lesions within these pathways, such as that sustained by an ischemic stroke or intracerebral hemorrhage, may compound the problem.

Assessing patients for imbalance is an important component to brain injury prevention. Various means of measuring body sway have been looked at for reliability and repeatability in assessing our elderly population. One method, such as the posturographic quiet standing test, has been referred to in the literature. Helbostad et al. (166) evaluated subjects after asking them to stand as still as possible for 30 seconds. Task conditions were performed in random order among the subjects and included eyes open or closed, wide or narrow stance, and firm or compliant surface. Some patients were also asked to perform a cognitive task. It appears across all domains that one can consistently and appropriately assess the frail elderly with repeated testing. Clinicians need to develop simple assessment measures, such as those described, that can be taken into the office setting to identify elderly patients at risk for balance instability and falls who may benefit from preventative measures (166).

Prevention must then be aimed at the various contributing factors. Balance training in physical therapy can be directed at lower extremity strengthening as well as proprioceptive and visual system training with repetitive feedback and continual cueing. Various approaches have been employed to enhance balance in therapy. The use of force-plate biofeedback system to improve standing ability has been reported to have positive effects (167). One study looked at the addition of jumping to rehabilitation programs in elderly residence of a long-term care facility (168). The experimental group experienced decreased fall frequency and improved balance over controls, although such an intervention would clearly require careful patient selection. There is no standard physical therapy program or protocol for balance training, and more research in this area is warranted.

In addition to targeting the physical aspects, one must address polypharmacy, a common and, in many cases, avoidable cause of balance impairment in the aged population. The estimated prevalence of inappropriate medication use in the elderly is 20% in the United States and various countries in Europe (169). The result may lead to balance instability, sedation, and confusion in our elderly population. Physician awareness of those at increased risk, such as elders treated with psychotropic medications and those with depression is important because it allows for targeting modifiable variables as well as avoidance of inappropriate prescription writing. Physicians must constantly readdress prescription and nonprescription medications to avoid both inappropriate use and polypharmacy and may benefit from an electronic medical record to reduce reliance on patients for this information (169,170).

The environment plays an important part in falls of the elderly. Speechley and Tinetti (161) found in a sample community of older persons that 15% of those experiencing falls did not have a chronic intrinsic risk factor and would not be considered frail. Environmental risk factors were identified that led to a higher risk of falls. These factors include poor lighting, failing to avoid temporary hazards, distraction, poor friction between shoes and flooring, attempting to navigate unsafe obstacles, habitual environmental use despite a change in ability, and inappropriate use of environmental objects (171). Fall prevention strategies, especially those involving home modifications and closer monitoring of psychotropic medications, have been shown to be effective at reducing fall frequency and health care costs (172). Programs such as the CDC's "Help Seniors Live Better, Longer: Prevent Brain Injury" initiative to prevent fall-related TBI demonstrate how legislation leads to federal funding toward effective active prevention measures (173).

Physicians can play an important role in fall prevention, especially after a first fall. More aggressive efforts at assessing the cause of falls are needed by physicians. Risk factors for osteoporosis should be identified, as low bone mineral density (BMD) has been shown to increase the risk of fracture resulting from falls (174). BMD screening must be considered in high-risk patients such as chronic steroid users, those with a sedentary lifestyle, and patients on antiepileptic medications.

Primary TBI prevention, as it relates to falls involves identifying a complex range of potential risk factors. As Haddon described, these factors can relate to the host (poor vision), vector (inappropriate shoe), physical environment (tall playground equipment), and social environment (assuming that falling is a part of "being a kid"), and successful fall prevention programs will incorporate many of these factors.

SPORTS AND RECREATIONAL INJURY

Recreational and sporting activities cause 1.6 to 3.8 million TBIs in the United States annually, with most injuries classified as concussions (12,14,18,175,176). See Chapter 31 for a more comprehensive discussion of sports-related concussion. Unlike musculoskeletal training, the brain cannot be conditioned to withstand the energy assault, which is the cause of concussion (177). Therefore, preventative efforts must instead be directed at improving equipment safety, awareness and behavior modification of the athlete, development of rules to mitigate risks, and rigorous enforcement of rules and regulations to promote safety and prevent injury. This includes proper equipment design such as helmets for contact sports, rules that discourage dangerous activities, and training and educational efforts for coaches and participants.

Cycling

TBI resulting from bicycle accidents is a significant concern given their frequency. In 2009, 51,000 bicyclists were injured in traffic in the United States, and 630 people died from injuries sustained in bicycle accidents (59). Boufous et al. showed that adolescents had the highest rates of cycling accidents and crashes resulting in hospitalization, whereas younger children were more likely to suffer a TBI as a result of bicycle accidents (178). Financially, the cost of nonfatal bicycle injuries in those younger than 19 years of age alone approaches $4.7 billion annually (179).

The aforementioned injury statistics from 2009 represent a decrease in the number of fatalities from bicycle accidents, whereas the incidence of non-TBI injuries increased by nearly 19% (59). This may be caused by increased helmet usage because helmets have been estimated to prevent up to 85% of bicycle accident-related fatalities (180). In addition to preventing fatalities, wearing a bicycle helmet has been correlated with a decrease in the risk of brain injury by 88%, severe brain injury by at least 75%, and facial injury, particularly in the upper and midfacial regions, by 65% (181).

Thompson et al. performed 2 separate extensive reviews of the literature to evaluate risk reduction for cyclists and helmet use during riding (181,182). The authors found that helmets were beneficial in the reduction of head, brain, and severe brain injury in all-age group by nearly 70%. This is a conservative value when compared to the numbers suggested by Koplan et al. in their CDC-sponsored work, which reported a risk difference of 85% for head injury and 88% for TBI (183).

Helmet usage is only one component of the Haddon Matrix regarding cycling injuries. As stated previously, a comprehensive approach is the most effective intervention for injury control, and this must be incorporated for bicycle injuries. Passive measures such as wearing helmets and conspicuous clothing, road engineering, bicycle lanes, and speed bumps must be employed (184). Active strategies such as modifying cyclists' behavior and counseling children on safety skills while riding have proven efficacy and must be aggressively pursued (185). Finally, legislation mandating helmet use for certain bicyclists appears to effectively increase helmet compliance and decrease the incidence of TBI (186).

Fighting Sports

Boxing has long been associated with TBI. Atha et al. (187) compared the force of a heavyweight's punch to a 13-pound mallet swung at 20 miles an hour. Unfortunately, record keeping regarding brain injury has not been as precise as in football, but between 1945 and 1979, 335 deaths from boxing-related head injury were documented (188). One must be cautious not to associate the boxing environment of yesteryear with today, although. Clausen et al. examined the exposures of today's generation of boxers and found that a professional boxer's career lasts 5 years on average, down from 19 years in the era between 1900 and 1955 (189).

Preventing brain injuries in boxing is a difficult proposition since the objective is to inflict injury upon your opponent. Several strategies have been proposed, including altering the weight of gloves, disallowing blows to the head, and requiring the use of helmets, but this may have an effect on the popularity and thus the profitability of the sport, and boxing is as much pageantry as pugilism (190,191). Instead of primary TBI prevention, efforts have been directed at preventing repeat brain injuries through improved recognition of the signs of impairment after concussion and enforcement of regulations prohibiting a boxer from fighting until symptoms have resolved (192). On a molecular level, serum markers, including S-100B neuron-specific enolase and cortisol have been identified to be elevated in those sustaining blows to the head, and the presence of the APOE epsilon 4 allele has been associated with increased risk of chronic brain injury in high-exposure boxers (193,194).

Over the past 2 decades, mixed martial arts (MMA) has gained significant popularity such that it now rivals boxing in revenue generation (195). From a safety perspective, proponents tout a decreased concussion rate compared to boxing. Indeed, Ngai et al. (196) found the concussion rate to be 16.5 per 1,000 exposures or 3.3% of all matches, significantly lower than that of boxing, where up to 11.3% of matches had to be stopped because of knockout (concussion) or other serious injury (134,196–198). MMA fighters use thinner, lighter gloves that offer less protection from hand injury than the heavily padded gloves worn by boxers and would ostensibly discourage repetitive punching an opponent's hard skull. Also, in MMA bouts, grappling to force the opponent to forfeit is a common outcome, leading to alternative means by which a fight can end. Forfeiture, either by the fighter or his or her trainer, occurs much less frequently in boxing.

Boxing remains a popular spectator sport, and MMA viewership and participation continues to skyrocket. Although the emphasis on financial gain is strong in both enterprises, there are rules in place to protect the combatants. Injury prevention efforts will need to be creative to ensure continued enjoyment by spectators while offering participants protection against TBI. In addition, continued education efforts must emphasize the short- and long-term risks of TBI, altering what some may deem acceptable entertainment.

American Football

Professional football is the most popular spectator sport in the United States. Five of the top 6 most-watched programs of all time are Super Bowl telecasts, and the National Football League (NFL) set attendance records for the sixth consecutive year in 2007(199,200). Unfortunately, TBIs are commonplace in American football, from youth leagues to the professional ranks (201–205). The National Football Head and Neck Injury Registry reported 59 intracranial football injuries that resulted in death between the years of 1971 and 1975. In 1974, Blyth and Mueller (206) reported that although TBI accounted for only 5% of overall football injuries, it accounted for 70% of football-related fatalities, with 75% of those occurring during tackling. Even when nonfatal, recurrent concussions have been associated with chronic traumatic encephalopathy, highlighting the need for primary prevention (207–209).

In 1996, the NFL began a 6-year study to assess the circumstances, causes, and effects of concussions with the aim of improving and updating helmets (210). Newer, safer helmet designs did emerge as a result of this study, and this technology has trickled down to the amateur level (211). In addition to helmet design changes, other proposed interventions to limit the incidence of brain injuries include the use of mandibular orthotics, limiting the number of players on the field, eliminating the 3-point stance, concussion-prevention education for coaches and parents, and limiting or even eliminating intentional head contact (212–214). The NFL has made concussion prevention a priority and has enacted rules to limit head-to-head contact and hits above the head of receivers in vulnerable positions, although research supporting the efficacy of these rule changes is lacking.

Given the popularity of the sport and interest to play among high school athletes, football will likely continue to have many fans and participants. The focus must therefore be on injury prevention in addition to good clinical judgment in removing players from play at the greatest risk. The highest percentage of head and cervical spine fatalities associated with football occurred between 1965 and 1974. There was a significant decrease in head fatalities from 1985 through 1994 (215). This is attributed to increased awareness in the multidisciplinary team involved in the football family, including coaches, administrators, athletic trainers, physicians, national organizations, all of whom have been provided education and public awareness.

Prevention efforts used for football have been effective. The issue of legislation and enforcement as well as passive and active strategies should again be revisited. With immediate punishment and consequences from illegal plays called by the officials, illegal dangerous plays can be discouraged, and their incidence greatly reduced. There was a key rule change in 1976 that played a role in reducing head and spine fatalities. The rule prohibited initial contact with the helmet, also known as "head butting," or face mask, also known as "face tackling," when tackling or blocking. Tackling was responsible for 40.6% of all head fatalities from 1985 to 1994, and it is therefore imperative to adhere to this rule because a violation of it may result in a serious injury (206).

Soccer

Although football is the most popular spectator sport in the United States, in the rest of the world, soccer is king. Unfortunately, just as in football, concussion in soccer is prevalent, and this risk is magnified by the number of participants, 265 million worldwide according to a recent Fédération Internationale de Football Association (FIFA) report (204,216). According to a 2011 study, concussions represent 3.9% of injuries in male high school soccer players and 7.4% of soccer-related injuries in females (204). Because of the large number of participants worldwide, the number of potential injuries can be significant, even if the rate of injury may be lower than that of other higher contact sports (217).

As in football, recurrent concussion in soccer players has been associated with changes in cerebral architecture and long-term neuropsychological sequelae. Tysvaer and Storli looked at 69 active soccer players and 37 former players of a Norwegian national team and found that one-third of the players had central cerebral atrophy, and 81% had some form of neuropsychological impairment (218,219). Dvorak et al. established a risk analysis for prediction of injuries and promoted the development of a prevention program focusing on the trainers, medical professionals, and players. Recommendations included structured training, better medical supervision, player reaction time, rule design, and enforcement that could result in an overall decrease in injury (217).

The use of controlled head contact with the ball is an integral part of soccer. Some would argue that it plays a major role in TBI, but this remains a controversial issue (220–222). Long ago, soccer balls were manufactured with leather panels. It has been shown that older leather balls absorb water and increase the weight of the ball by 20% or more, making them more dangerous (223). Soccer balls are now made of waterproof synthetic leather covered with urethane that repels water, which has decreased the injury potential (172). Headgear designed to decrease the incidence of concussion has promise but suffers from limited use (224,225). A review of the literature suggests that heading the ball plays a very small part of in soccer–related TBI (220,221). Instead, accidental unplanned contact against goalposts, head-to-head contact, elbow contact, and a ball kicked directly at the head are more likely to be the source of problems (220,221). Tysvaer and Storli (219) also noted that younger players with less experience heading the ball had greater electroencephalogram (EEG), radiographic, and neuropsychologic changes than their older, more experienced counterparts, possibly because of incomplete brain development and weak cervical stabilizing musculature (218,226).

Prevention efforts therefore should be directed to better training techniques, proper coaching, adhering to return to play guidelines, medical supervision postinjury, rule changes, and enforcement. These strategies would minimize unintentional head contact. The use of protective headgear by goalies and development of better head protection has also been proposed as a target for injury prevention (221,227).

Hockey

Like American football and soccer, hockey is a high-speed sport where collisions are inevitable and, in men's hockey, an integral component of gameplay. Accordingly, TBI among hockey players is common. A recent 7-year review of collegiate men's and women's hockey-related injuries reported concussions to be the most commonly sustained injury (228). Interestingly, in women's collegiate hockey, where checking is prohibited, concussions were only attributable to player contact 41% of the time vs 72% of the concussions sustained by males (228). In contrast to football, where the incidence of concussions increases with age, concussions occur with alarming frequency in all ages in hockey (229,230).

Most concussions occur during checking, both legal and illegal (230,231). In one study, it was found that 57% of children with ice hockey-related injuries resulted from checking and that more than half of these injuries were subjectively considered significant (232). It was apparent that children were not educated on safety and injury prevention because 45% stated they could not sustain a TBI while wearing a helmet.

Attempts have been made at decreasing injury risk associated with the game of hockey. The American Academy of Pediatrics recommends that checking be prohibited in children younger than 16 based on the significant size discrepancies among children of the same age (233). In addition, many leagues have instituted a ''fair-play'' scoring system, whereby teams are awarded points not only for victories but also for limiting penalties (234). This has shown to lead to a decrease in hockey-related collisions, the primary means by which concussions occur (235).

There was some thought, previously, that the use of face masks by hockey players could actually increase head and neck injuries because it may lead to perceptions of invincibility and more aggressive play. A review of the literature does not support this belief because no significant increase in concussion or neck injuries with the use of face masks was detected. There was a decrease in the incidence of overall head injuries and, specifically, facial injuries with the use of facial protection (236). It has been demonstrated that more hockey injuries occur early in the season, late in the periods, and in the final period of games, suggesting that conditioning may assist in injury prevention (230).

Concussion education of younger hockey players and coaches is imperative and has shown promise (237). A prospective interventional trial by which youth hockey players were assigned to watch a DVD highlighting the importance of concussion prevention led to a significant decrease in body checking-related penalties in the experimental group (238). This finding is important, especially when considering attitudes toward violent behavior in hockey. Alarmingly, in one study, nearly one-third of children polled would check illegally to win and 6% would intentionally injure another player to win (232). Legislation and mandatory education are not sufficient, however. Parents should encourage nonviolence so these behaviors can be learned by their children and taken into adolescence and adulthood.

On the professional level, the National Hockey League recently implemented Rule 48, prohibiting ''blind side'' hits to the head (239). This resulted in a 75% decrease in concussions resulting from these types of hits in midway through its first year of enforcement (240). It would behoove teams to encourage compliance with the new rule because statistics show that in the Stanley Cup Finals, the team with the least penalties secondary to violent behavior wins most championships (241).

Mouthguards

The use of mouthguards to prevent concussion in sports is widely debated. Mouth protection is mandatory in many sports, but although their ability to prevent oral trauma is well-established, the ability to prevent even mild TBI has not been established by large randomized controlled trials (RCTs), and in fact, RCTs have shown a lack of such efficacy (242–244). A systematic review of the literature evaluating the effectiveness of different types of protective equipment found no evidence to support the claim that mouthguards play a role in concussion prevention (245). Indeed, recent studies have shown no ability of current mouthguard materials to attenuate football concussion risk (246). Despite claims to the contrary, the role of mouthguards in TBI prevention has been deemed ''neuromythology'' (247).

In summary, sport-related injuries account for a significant number of head injuries. These can be severe, fatal, result in long-term debility, and lead to the termination of a player's career and long-term neuropsychological effects. It is important to stress a multifaceted approach to prevention of injury, including education, rule enforcement, improvement in safety equipment, and better conditioned athletes with encouragement of nonviolent behaviors.

VIOLENCE AND SUICIDE

Violence in the United States is a major cause of morbidity and mortality. The most recent data available from the National Violent Death Reporting System indicates the yearly incidence of violent death was nearly 20 per 100,000 population in the 16 reporting states (248). Youth violence is of particular concern. The 2007 CDC data shows that 16 patients, 10–24 years old, died daily from violent causes, 84% of those as a result of firearms (249). Acts of violence account for 10% of all TBI (2).

Upon review of the literature, self-inflicted injuries range from 11% to 50%, with an unclear percentage being accidental (250,251). Survivors of self-inflicted gunshot wounds have poorer outcomes than patients with TBI from other causes, highlighting an increased need for preventive measures (252). Findings predictive of positive outcomes include an initial Glasgow Outcome Score of at least 8, computerized tomography findings of injury limited to a single lobe of the brain, and normal pupil reaction (253,254).

Gun Control and Safety

By numbers, there is a firearm for every adult in the United States (255). In a 2007 national survey, 38% of US households contained a firearm, with 40% of gun owners owning at least one handgun (255). Interestingly, married men reported significantly higher household firearm ownership rates than married women. Firearm violence led to nearly 60,000 deaths in the United States in 2006–2007 (256). Attempts at gun control frequently run into political opposition, although the presence of a gun in the home has been shown to increase the risk of homicide in the home, suicide, and accidental death of a child (257–259).

Given their prevalence and lethal capabilities, gun safety is of paramount significance. Education programs have shown promise, although large-scale studies correlating this education with decreased rates of injury are lacking. In one smaller study, parents gave their child education regarding how to react to finding a gun, and the child's response in such a situation was monitored (260). Multimodal programs, including modeling, rehearsal, and feedback have been shown to have improved efficacy in teaching safety skills compared to other educational strategies, although both can be significantly enhanced with in situ training (261). Clearly, parents play a key role in their children's knowledge of safe handling of firearms and attitudes toward gun safety. More controversial is the idea of gun safety education in schools (262).

Different technological approaches have been tried to improve handgun safety. Safety locks (trigger locks being the most common), cable locks, manual thumb safeties, loaded chamber indicators, magazine disconnectors, drop safeties, and decockers are all attempts to prevent unintentional injuries (263). However, these devices do not protect from intentional injuries such as suicide or homicide. A grip safety feature is a passive preventative method designed to protect children from using the gun. Young children do not have the strength, coordination, or hand size to press the safety lever and pull the trigger at the same time. Personalized handguns discourage unauthorized use by requiring a magnetic "key" to render the firearm operational. Low-tech safety measures such as disassembling firearms when not in use as well as storing the empty gun in a separate, locked location from the locked-away ammunition also have been associated with a decreased risk of handgun-related injuries (264).

The role of the government in gun control remains controversial. Federal funding for education programs to encourage gun safety is universally supported, but regulating the sale of firearms, mandating safety precautions, and banning certain types of firearms draws the ire of those with liberal interpretations of the second amendment. There is evidence that access to firearms leads to increased rates of gun violence, both as stated earlier and as the following examples will illustrate.

A 2004 review of youth suicide rates found that child access prevention (CAP) laws, which mandate safe storage of firearms, were associated with 8.3% fewer suicides among children aged 14–17 years old, although no association existed between minimum age requirements for firearm purchase and suicide (265). A 2003 study that categorized states' gun laws as restrictive, modest, or unrestrictive found that states with loose firearm regulation had higher suicide incidence rate ratios (IRR) than states with modest or stringent restrictions (266). Regarding homicide, areas of higher firearm ownership rates have been associated with a disproportionate amount of homicide deaths (267), and instituting a ban on carrying handguns has been associated with a decrease in the homicide rate (268). To be clear, studies finding causation do not claim causal relationships, and large-scale studies are lacking. Efforts to curb the incidence of TBI will be augmented by such research and will require passive and active interventions, funding for these programs and increased education, and legislative measures to promote safety while protecting constitutional rights.

DEPRESSION, SUICIDE, AND TRAUMATIC BRAIN INJURY

Self-inflicted TBI has been associated with gender, minority status, age, substance abuse, and low socioeconomic status, with the most predictive of these variables being minority status and substance abuse (269). Additionally, a major concern is the risk of suicide among those with TBI. A systematic review of the literature found that 18% of persons affected by brain injury had attempted suicide and were successful 3–4 times more often than the general population (270,271). In contrast, CDC statistics from 2007 delineate a suicide rate of 11.5 per 100,000 in the general populations (8). This affects even those with mild TBI, as having suffered a concussion was associated with an increased rate of suicide (271). Risk factors, including an increased incidence of suicidal ideation (21%–22%) and depression (33%) have also been reported in the TBI population (270,272).

There is considerable variability in TBI prevention strategies worldwide. Goals, including regular follow-up to assess for signs of depression, education of general knowledge about suicide, and development of skills in suicide risk assessment and management are ubiquitous, but prevention programs have a wide range of variability in training requirements and interventions used to achieve these goals. The biopsychosocial model is a comprehensive approach, but assessing efficacy has been difficult given the current body of research, which consists of largely underpowered studies (273). Physicians are trained to recognize symptoms of depression in patients, but often, these encounters involve therapists and disability workers with less training in evaluating for signs and symptoms of depression. Programs to train these providers in recognition and counseling of TBI-affected patients with depression range from 1 to 16 hours in length and show variable efficacy and retention (274–277). Instructional materials used include anything from written materials, self-instructional videos to other methods such as didactic sessions, and simulation exercises.

Whether depression results from brain injury or was antecedent to the traumatic event, physicians should consider pharmacologic intervention. Unfortunately, randomized, high-powered studies are lacking regarding choice of antidepressant, dosage, and timing. A 2009 review by Fann et al. highlighted data examining the effect of serotonin-specific reuptake inhibitors (SSRIs), serotonin-norepinephrine reuptake inhibitors (SNRIs), tricyclic antidepressants (TCAs), monoamine oxidase inhibitors (MAOIs), atypical antipsychotics, stimulants, cholinesterase inhibitors, and anticonvulsants (278). Although no firm guidelines were established, the favorable side effect profile led authors to recommend SSRIs as first-line therapy of depression in the TBI population. Sertraline, with its dopaminergic features, was specifically recommended. Chapter 74 of this book discussed these topics in greater detail.

DRUGS AND ALCOHOL

Recreational pharmaceutical agents greatly complicate the problem of TBI from both an incidence and severity perspective (279,280). In its seminal "White Paper" released in 1988, the National Head Injury Foundation Substance Abuse Task Force stated, "Neither age, nor occupation, nor any other factors place an individual at a greater risk of a TBI than does alcohol" (281). Many factors contribute to alcohol's exacerbation of TBI risk. First, retrospective analysis of patients with TBI reveals increased preinjury rates of heavy drinking (282). Alcohol consumption at the time of injury has been associated with decreased initial Functional Independence Measure (FIM) scores at the time of admission to acute rehabilitation and a two-and-a-half–fold higher risk for trauma readmission after discharge (283,284).

Prevention of alcohol consumption by teenagers as a target for TBI primary prevention was highlighted by a study by Hingson et al. (285). A survey of college students demonstrated a relationship between alcohol intoxication for the first time before the age of 19 and driving while intoxicated, riding with a driver who was under the influence and, after drinking, sustaining injuries that required medical attention. In addition, drinking as a teenager tripled the likelihood that an individual would be involved in a physical fight in the past year and was associated with a higher risk of heavy drinking later in life (286,287).

These factors lead to increase risk of TBI. Fortunately, community programs such as Mothers Against Drunk Driving (MADD) have been instrumental in raising awareness of the problem of teenage drunk driving and were pivotal in the push to raise the drinking age to 21 years (18). This has not eliminated the problem as the latest NHTSA statistics reported BACs greater than 0.01% in 31% of underage drivers killed in crashes; 26% of young drivers had BACs greater than 0.08% (59). Control of access clearly is not sufficient to address the problem of alcohol-related MVAs and resultant risk of TBI. Other interventions with promise and public support include increased police patrols and enforcement, limiting marketing to teenagers, in-vehicle alcohol detection systems, and even allowing young drivers to experience drunk driving in a controlled environment to show the effects of impairment (288–291).

Although a clear relationship has been established between alcohol and brain injury in the literature, questions still arise about the most effective means of preventing alcohol-related TBI. Ideally, prevention efforts will use both passive and active measures. Passive efforts such as BAC testing, mental status, or coordination testing prior to starting a car have been discussed but have not become reality except where mandatory after a driving while intoxicated conviction (292). A combination of passive and active interventions involve modification of the alcohol server's behavior based on the concept that many people who drink and drive are consuming alcohol at bars, clubs, and restaurants

(293–295). Efforts that focus on educating servers to carefully screen underage drinkers, refuse service to intoxicated persons, call taxi services for consumers that seem unfit to drive, and offer food to those drinking are all potential strategies to prevent driving under the influence (DUI). Many states have such educational programs, although they are not standardized across the country and address different issues such as legislation regarding intoxication, DUI, recognizing the signs of intoxication, and liability issues. However, many states do not have these programs despite clear evidence that such programs lead to decreased levels of patron intoxication, decreased rates of alcohol-related traffic accidents, and reduced frequency with which minors were able to obtain alcohol (296–300). The fear of litigation may assist the management structure of these establishments to be supportive of their employees' efforts to mitigate this national problem and run a safer establishment (295).

Significant progress has been achieved because of alcohol-related prevention programs (301). In 1995, mandatory alcohol testing programs went into effect for operators of large (>26,000 lbs) commercial motor vehicles and has been associated with a 23% reduction in alcohol-related fatalities in these motor carrier operators (302). Similar random testing is not done on automobile drivers in the United States because of lack of probable cause. In Europe, however, random testing has been shown to be effective, as the frequency of alcohol-related accidents has leveled off after decreasing steadily from 1982 to 1995 (303,304). This has also led some to promote reducing legal BAC limits to 0.05% or lower, as studies have shown significant impairment even at a legal level of BAC (305,306).

Despite proven efficacy and cost-effectiveness, random breath testing programs face resistance as a possible violation of Fourth Amendment rights (34). The US Supreme Court weighed in and ruled that selective breath testing (i.e., police checkpoints), but not random breath testing, is a minor intrusion on personal freedoms that is outweighed by public benefit of reducing DUI (307). This example highlights the important interplay between public advocacy groups promoting legislature balanced with civil rights jurisprudence to promote primary TBI prevention. Chapter 79 of this book discussed substance abuse more completely.

ELDER ABUSE

In 2002, a research council for the World Health Organization defined elder abuse and mistreatment as "a single or repeated act, or lack of appropriate action, occurring within any relationship where there is an expectation of trust which causes harm or distress to an older person" (308). Furthermore, it can be of various forms: physical, psychological, emotional, sexual, financial, or simply reflect intentional or unintentional neglect (308). This same group lamented the fact that there were no efforts "to develop, implement, and evaluate interventions based on scientifically grounded hypotheses about the causes of elder mistreatment, and no systematic research has been conducted to measure and evaluate the effects of existing interventions."

In a recent review article (309), the authors performed an in-depth evaluation of the elder abuse literature. They were able to identify 590 publications that discussed this issue. Of these, 492 were quantitative, 78 were qualitative, and 20 were case studies. None of these papers consisted of a meta-analysis, 14 of them reported evidence from well-designed clinical trials, 484 were observational in nature, and 93 were either expert opinion or case studies. There has been an increasing awareness and attention dedicated to the issue because there were only 55 articles from 1975 to 1999, followed by an increase to 332 between 2000 and 2008. The work of Clark et al. (310) was one of the first articles discussing the topic and included a description of the poor living conditions, finances, and nutritional experienced in a geriatric inpatient unit. They concluded that elder neglect is a significant issue and that a patient's permission is required to administer care. In 1979, Lau and Kosberg (311) examined issues at "chronic illness center." They identified 39 cases of abuse during that time. In 7% of these cases, the abuse was physical, and in 90% of cases, the abuse came from a relative. What may be most troubling is that 26% of those abused were resigned to the abuse and 33% denied it occurred.

In the 14 controlled trials, issues addressed included evaluating the efficacy of intervention on the victims of abuse (312), the effect of education on clinicians and staff in their handling of the person who could be a victim of elder abuse (313–319), the effect of education on nonclinicians (319,320), the ability to recognize that elder abuse is occurring (313,316–320), society's general perception of the believability of the victim and the abuser (321), the importance of the crime (322), and, finally, the efficacy of interventions to lessen the occurrence of abuse (315–317,323,324). The literature itself is very limited and interventions have also been ineffective in improving recognition (318,320) or demonstrating significant treatment effect (312,317).

Prevalence of Elder Abuse

Information regarding the prevalence of elder abuse can be obtained from several different sources. For the sake of this discussion, data obtained from epidemiological studies and reports from government agencies will be reviewed. When looking at the data from epidemiological studies, there are clear differences noted likely secondary to cultural and socioeconomic issues. The numbers reported vary substantially from 2.6% in the United Kingdom (325) to 14% in Chennai, India (326). Looking at data collected from US Adult Protective Services from 1999, 242,430 reported investigations into domestic abuse were reported from 47 states. This worked out to a rate of 5.5 per 1,000, and 2.7 per 1,000 were substantiated (327). This number is thought to understate the severity of domestic abuse considering the lack of close oversight and victim factors, including resignation or even a lack of the ability to perceive or report the abuse.

Elder Abuse in Nursing Homes

The issue of elder abuse in care facilities, although often difficult to assess, is an important issue. Pillemer and Moore (328) reported in 1989 a survey of nursing home nurses and assistants, of whom 36% reported witnessing an act of physical abuse and 81% noted witnessing psychological abuse. A staggering 10% admitted that they themselves had committed the abusive act. Although dated, the issue persists, as

recent literature shows that elder abuse is a significant current issue as well. Zhang's group (329) elicited data from family members of residents of a nursing home population in Michigan. They reported neglect in 21% and a 24% rate of physical abuse (330). In particular, abuse from aides seems related to the stress level experienced by the staff member (331). Dr Flanagan's Chapter 28 of this book addresses the special issues associated with the older adult and TBI.

PEDIATRIC HEAD TRAUMA

Pediatric head injuries are the leading cause of trauma-related morbidity and mortality in the United States, with nearly half a million children aged 0–14 years presenting to emergency departments annually (2,332). The annual costs for those admitted to the hospital exceed more than $1 billion annually, and significant caregiver burden and loss of productivity adds to this cost and highlights the need for primary preventative measures (333,334). The incidence of pediatric head trauma has been declining over the past 2 decades, however, thought to be caused by primary prevention efforts such as compulsory helmet usage, car safety improvements, and roadway design as stated previously (335). Other targets for pediatric primary brain injury prevention include child abuse, playground design, and recreational issues.

CHILD ABUSE

Nearly 1,800 children died in the United States in 2009 from child abuse or neglect, and there are estimates that more than half of such fatalities go unreported (336,337). Most infant and young child deaths related to abuse or neglect involve abusive head trauma, identifying a significant need for primary preventative measures (338). In addition to preventing fatalities, prevention of nonfatal child abuse is a worthwhile goal as abuse in childhood has been associated with early pregnancy, drug abuse, school failure, mental illness, suicidal, and aggressive behavior and violence later in life (339).

Fatal and nonfatal child abuse often results in subdural hemorrhage, retinal hemorrhage, and encephalopathy, a triad commonly referred to as "Shaken Baby" syndrome (SBS). There are a myriad of educational and interventional programs addressing SBS and child abuse in general, including home visitation, parent training programs addressing commonly frustrating childcare issues, enhanced pediatric medical care, and reporting of suspected child abuse (340). These interventions have had varying success as child abuse rates continue to climb (337,341,342). This only highlights the need for further primary preventative efforts, including physician education regarding identification, management, and possible outcomes of child abuse and intervention, as well as the role of Child Protective Services. There currently is only one state that mandates such education for all physicians, and this may be an active preventive strategy worth targeting (343). Chapters 34–38 of this book address the special issues regarding TBI in the pediatric population.

CONCLUSION

TBI is associated with significant morbidity, mortality, and financial cost to society. Successful prevention strategies have been identified and can make a substantial difference in overall public health. These efforts must be directed at many different components that include passive and active strategies, legislation, education, and motivation of the public to control this area of injury. Significant progress in TBI prevention has been made, although there is still a large amount of work needed to target all the different aspects or "cells" in the Haddon Matrix. Health care providers must continue to educate the lay public and assist politicians in recognizing the benefits of injury control. There has been a growing awareness of the value of prevention efforts required to minimize the prevalence and sequelae that may result from TBI. This can be seen in the areas of sports and recreation as well as everyday decision making by people living their daily lives. Increased public awareness will hopefully lead to continued technological advancements, legislation, enforcement, compliance, and a decreased rate of TBI incidence worldwide.

KEY CLINICAL POINTS

1. Nearly one-third of all injury-related deaths from 2002 to 2006 were associated with a TBI, with the highest incidence in the pediatric and elderly populations.
2. The maintenance of health as it refers to TBI requires a comprehensive approach. It must include passive and active strategies implemented via education and, at times, legislation.
3. Distracted driving has been implicated in up to 16% of motor vehicle collisions resulting in fatalities.
4. Mandated front-impact air bag protection, which when used in conjunction with a lap-shoulder belt has an estimated reduction in head injuries of 83% compared to unrestrained drivers.
5. The most critical mitigating factor relating to TBI and fatalities caused by motorcycle accidents is the use of helmets.
6. Neither age, nor occupation, nor any other factors place an individual at a greater risk of a TBI than does alcohol.
7. Experienced motorcycle riders have been shown to exhibit delayed responses even at the per se 0.05% alcohol level.
8. More than 35% of TBIs result from falls, in a bimodal distribution that is well-established. Children aged 0–4 years and those aged 75 and older account for 40% of all falls despite representing a much smaller percentage of the populace.
9. One must address polypharmacy, an avoidable cause of balance impairment in the aged population.
10. Prevention efforts used for football have been effective in reducing the incidence and severity of football-related injuries.

KEY REFERENCES

1. Brady JE, Baker SP, Dimaggio C, McCarthy ML, Rebok GW, Li G. Effectiveness of mandatory alcohol testing programs in reducing alcohol involvement in fatal motor carrier crashes. *Am J Epidemiol.* 2009;170(6):775–782.
2. Faul M, Xu L, Wald MM, Coronado VG. *Traumatic Brain Injury in the United States: Emergency Department Visits, Hospitalizations and Deaths 2002–2006.* Atlanta, GA: Centers for Disease Control and Prevention, National Center for Injury Prevention and Control; 2010.
3. Liu BC, Ivers R, Norton R, Boufous S, Blows S, Lo SK. Helmets for preventing injury in motorcycle riders. *Cochrane Database Syst Rev.* 2008;(1):CD004333.
4. Macpherson A, Spinks A. Bicycle helmet legislation for the uptake of helmet use and prevention of head injuries. *Cochrane Database Syst Rev.* 2008;(3):CD005401.
5. National Highway Traffic Safety Administration. Fifth/sixth report to Congress: effectiveness of occupant protection systems and their use. Washington, DC: US Department of Transportation; 2001. Report No. DOT HS 809-442.

References

1. Kochanek KD, Smith BL, Anderson RN. Deaths: preliminary data for 1999. *Natl Vital Stat Rep.* 2001;49(3):1–48.
2. Faul M, Xu L, Wald MM, Coronado VG. *Traumatic Brain Injury in the United States: Emergency Department Visits, Hospitalizations and Deaths 2002–2006.* Atlanta, GA: Centers for Disease Control and Prevention, National Center for Injury Prevention and Control; 2010.
3. Corrigan JD, Selassie AW, Orman JA. The epidemiology of traumatic brain injury. *J Head Trauma Rehabil.* 2010;25(2):72–80.
4. Finkelstein E, Corso P, Miller T. *The Incidence and Economic Burden of Injuries in the United States.* New York, NY: Oxford Unviersity Press; 2006.
5. Mar J, Arrospide A, Begiristain JM, Larrañaga I, Elosegui E, Oliva-Moreno J. The impact of acquired brain damage in terms of epidemiology, economics and loss in quality of life. *BMC Neurol.* 2011; 11:46.
6. van Heugten CM, Geurtsen GJ, Derksen RE, Martina JD, Geurts AC, Evers SM. Intervention and societal costs of residential community reintegration for patients with acquired brain injury: a cost-analysis of the Brain Integration Programme. *J Rehabil Med.* 2011; 43(7):647–652.
7. Zaloshnja E, Miller T, Langlois JA, Selassie AW. Prevalence of long-term disability from traumatic brain injury in the civilian population of the United States, 2005. *J Head Trauma Rehabil.* 2008;23(6): 394–400.
8. Xu J, Kochanek KD, Murphy SL, Tejada-Vera B. Deaths: final data for 2007. *Natl Vital Stat Rep.* 2010;58(24):1–135.
9. Posada IJ, Benito-León J, Louis ED, et al. Mortality from Parkinson's disease: a population-based prospective study (NEDICES). *Mov Disord.* 2011;26(14):2522–2529.
10. DeSantis C, Siegel R, Bandi P, Jemal A. Breast cancer statistics, 2011. *CA Cancer J Clin.* 2011;61(6):409–418.
11. Palella FJ Jr, Delaney KM, Moorman AC, et al. Declining morbidity and mortality among patients with advanced human immunodeficiency virus infection. HIV outpatient study investigators. *N Engl J Med.* 1998;338(13):853–860.
12. Annegers JF, Grabow JD, Kurland LT, Laws ER Jr. The incidence, causes, and secular trends of head trauma in Olmsted County, Minnesota, 1935–1974. *Neurology.* 1980;30(9):912–919.
13. Jagger J, Levine JI, Jane JA, Rimel RW. Epidemiologic features of head injury in a predominantly rural population. *J Trauma.* 1984; 24(1):40–44.
14. Kraus JF, Black MA, Hessol N, et al. The incidence of acute brain injury and serious impairment in a defined population. *Am J Epidemiol.* 1984;119(2):186–201.
15. Hypertension detection and follow-up program. Baseline characteristics of the enumerated, screened, and hypertensive participants. The Hypertension Detection and Follow-up Program Cooperative Group. *Hypertension.* 1983;5(6, pt 2):IV1–IV205.
16. Sandercock PA, Counsell C, Kamal AK. Anticoagulants for acute ischaemic stroke. *Cochrane Database Syst Rev.* 2008;(4):CD000024.

17. Sherman DG, Albers GW, Bladin C, et al. The efficacy and safety of enoxaparin versus unfractionated heparin for the prevention of venous thromboembolism after acute ischaemic stroke (PREVAIL Study): an open-label randomised comparison. *Lancet*. 2007; 369(9570):1347–1355.

18. Elovic E, Antoinette T. Epidemiology and primary prevention of traumatic brain injury. In: Horn LJ, Zasler ND, eds. *Medical Rehabilitation of Traumatic Brain Injury*. Philadelphia, PA: Hanley & Belfus; 1996:1–28.

19. Guyer B, Gallagher SS. An approach to the epidemiology of childhood injuries. *Pediatr Clin North Am*. 1985;32(1):5–15.

20. US Preventative Services Task Force. *Guide to Clinical Preventative Services: Report on the US Preventative Services Task Force*. Baltimore, MD: Williams and Wilkins; 1989.

21. Thurman DJ, Alverson C, Dunn KA, Guerrero J, Sniezek JE. Traumatic brain injury in the United States: a public health perspective. *J Head Trauma Rehabil*. 1999;14(6):602–615.

22. US Preventative Services Task Force (USPSTF). U.S. Department of Health and Human Services: Agency for Healthcare Research and Quality. Washington, D.C.; 2011.

23. Stokols D. Establishing and maintaining healthy environments. Toward a social ecology of health promotion. *Am Psychol*. 1992;47(1): 6–22.

24. Teutsch SM. A framework for assessing the effectiveness of disease and injury prevention. *MMWR Recomm Rep*. 1992;41:1–12.

25. Short D. Using science to prevent injuries: dissecting an event using the Haddon Matrix. *JEMS*. 1999;24(9):68–70, 72–74.

26. Patel MS, Phillips CB, Pearce C, Kljakovic M, Dugdale P, Glasgow N. General practice and pandemic influenza: a framework for planning and comparison of plans in five countries. *PLoS One*. 2008; 3(5):e2269.

27. Haddon W Jr. On the escape of tigers: an ecologic note. *Am J Public Health Nations Health*. 1970;60(12):2229–2234.

28. Haddon W Jr. A logical framework for categorizing highway safety phenomena and activity. *J Trauma*. 1972;12(3):193–207.

29. Gruen RL. Crocodile attacks in Australia: challenges for injury prevention and trauma care. *World J Surg*. 2009;33(8):1554–1561.

30. Gielen AC, Girasek DC. Integrating perspectives on the prevention of unintentional injuries. In: Schneiderman N, Speers MA, Silva JM, Tomes H, Gentry JH, eds. *Integrating Behavioral and Social Sciences with Public Health*. Washington DC: American Psychological Association; 2001:203–230.

31. Karlson TA. Injury control and public policy. *Crit Rev Environ Contr*. 1992;195–241.

32. Liu BC, Ivers R, Norton R, Boufous S, Blows S, Lo SK. Helmets for preventing injury in motorcycle riders. *Cochrane Database Syst Rev*. 2008;(1):CD004333.

33. Macpherson AK, To TM, Macarthur C, Chipman ML, Wright JG, Parkin PC. Impact of mandatory helmet legislation on bicycle-related head injuries in children: a population-based study. *Pediatrics*. 2002;110(5):e60.

34. Miller TR, Galbraith MS, Lawrence BA. Costs and benefits of a community sobriety checkpoint program. *J Stud Alcohol*. 1998;59(4): 462–468.

35. Voas RB, Holder HD, Gruenewald PJ. The effect of drinking and driving interventions on alcohol-involved traffic crashes within a comprehensive community trial. *Addiction*. 1997;92(suppl 2): S221–S236.

36. Brain Injury Association of America. *Brain Injury Association of America*. Vienna, VA: Brain Injury Association of America. www.biausa.org/About-Us/about-brain-injury-association.htm. Accessed May 6, 2011.

37. Nguyen VQC, Cruz TH, McDeavitt JT. Traumatic brain injury and the science of injury control. *State of the Art Reviews: PM&R*. 2001; 213–227.

38. US Preventative Services Task Force. *Guide to Clinical Preventative Services: Report on the US Preventative Services Task Force*. Baltimore, MD: Williams and Williams; 1989.

39. DiGuiseppi C, Roberts IG. Individual-level injury prevention strategies in the clinical setting. *Future Child*. 2000;10(1):53–82.

40. Robertson LS, Kelley AB, O'Neill B, Wixom CW, Eiswirth RS, Haddon W Jr. A controlled study of the effect of television messages on safety belt use. *Am J Public Health*. 1974;64(11):1071–1080.

41. Klassen TP, MacKay JM, Moher D, Walker A, Jones AL. Community-based injury prevention interventions. *Future Child*. 2000;10(1): 83–110.

42. Coté TR, Sacks JJ, Lambert-Huber DA, et al. Bicycle helmet use among Maryland children: effect of legislation and education. *Pediatrics*. 1992;89(6, pt 2):1216–1220.

43. US Department of Transportation. *National Highway Traffic Safety Administration. Standard enforcement saves lives; the case for strong seatbelt laws*. Washington, DC: Author; 1999.

44. US Census Bureau. U.S. Census Bureau, Statistical Abstract of the United States: 2012. Licensed drivers and number in accidents by Age: 2009. http://www.census.gov/compendia/statab/2012/tables/12s1114.pdf. Accessed August 30, 2011.

45. Preusser DF, Williams AF, Zador PL, Blomberg RD. The effect of curfew laws on motor vehicle crashes. *Law & Policy*. 1984;6: 115–128.

46. Ferguson SA, Leaf WA, Williams AF, Preusser DF. Differences in young driver crash involvement in states with varying licensure practices. *Accid Anal Prev*. 1996;28(2):171–180.

47. Insurance Institute for Highway Safety. Young driver licensing systems in the U.S. http://www.iihs.org/laws/graduatedlicenseintro.aspx. Accessed June 10, 2011.

48. McCartt AT, Teoh ER. Strengthening driver licensing systems for teenaged drivers. *JAMA*. 2011;306(10):1142–1143.

49. Chen LH, Baker SP, Li G. Graduated driver licensing programs and fatal crashes of 16-year-old drivers: a national evaluation. *Pediatrics*. 2006;118(1):56–62.

50. Martín FS, Estévez MA. Prevention of traffic accidents: the assessment of perceptual-motor alterations before obtaining a driving license. A longitudinal study of the first years of driving. *Brain Inj*. 2005;19(3):189–196.

51. Matsui Y, Hitosugi M, Mizuno K. Severity of vehicle bumper location in vehicle-to-pedestrian impact accidents. *Forensic Sci Int*. 2011; 212(1–3):205–209.

52. Duperrex O, Roberts I, Bunn F. Safety education of pedestrians for injury prevention. *Cochrane Database Syst Rev*. 2002;(2):CD001531.

53. Bunn F, Collier T, Frost C, Ker K, Roberts I, Wentz R. Area-wide traffic calming for preventing traffic related injuries. *Cochrane Database Syst Rev*. 2003;(1)CD003110.

54. Aeron-Thomas AS, Hess S. Red-light cameras for the prevention of road traffic crashes. *Cochrane Database Syst Rev*. 2005;(2):CD003862.

55. National Highway Traffic Safety Administration. Fatality Analysis Reporting System. http://www.nhtsa.gov/FARS. Accessed August 30, 2011.

56. Pickrell TM, Ye TJ. *Driver Electronic Device Use in 2009. Traffic Safety Facts Research Note*. Washington, DC: National Highway Traffic Safety Administration, US Department of Transportation; 2010.

57. Klauer SG, Dingus TA, Neal VL, Sudweeks J, Ramsey D. *The Impact of Driver Inattention on Near-Crash/Crash Risk: An Analysis Using the 100-Car Naturalistic Driving Study Data*. Washington, DC: National Highway Traffic Safety Administration,US Department of Transportation; 2006. Report No. DOT HS 810-594.

58. National Highway Traffic Safety Administration. *Overview of the National Highway Traffic Safety Administration's Driver Distraction Program*. Washington, DC: US Department of Transportation; 2010. Report No. DOT HS 811-299.

59. National Highway Traffic Safety Administration. *Traffic Safety Facts 2009*. Washington, DC: US Department of Transportation; 2010. Report No. DOT HS 811-402.

60. Ishigami Y, Klein RM. Is a hands-free phone safer than a handheld phone? *J Safety Res*. 2009;40(2):157–164.

61. Ibrahim JK, Anderson ED, Burris SC, Wagenaar AC. State laws restricting driver use of mobile communications devices distracted-driving provisions, 1992–2010. *Am J Prev Med*. 2011;40(6): 659–665.

62. Dula CS, Martin BA, Fox RT, Leonard RL. Differing types of cellular phone conversations and dangerous driving. *Accid Anal Prev*. 2011; 43(1):187–193.

63. National Highway Traffic Safety Administration. *New Research Shows Enforcement Cuts Distracted Driving*; 2011. Press Release Report No. DOT 82-11.

64. National Highway Traffic Safety Administration. *Fifth/Sixth Report to Congress: Effectiveness of Occupant Protection Systems and Their Use*. Washington, DC: US Department of Transportation; 2001. Report No. DOT HS 809-442.

65. National Highway Traffic Safety Administration. Federal motor vehicle safety standards. US Department of Transportation 1998. http://www.nhtsa.gov/cars/rules/import/fmvss/index.html#SN208. Accessed August 30, 2011.

66. National Highway Traffic Safety Administration. *Third Report to Congress: Effectiveness of Occupant Protection Systems and Their Use*. Washington, DC: US Department of Transportation; 1996. Report No. DOT HS 808-470.

67. National Highway Traffic Safety Administration. *An Evaluation of Side Impact Protection*. Washington, DC: US Department of Transportation; 2007. Report No. DOT HS 810-748.

68. Gennarelli TA, Champion HR, Sacco WJ, Copes WS, Alves WM. Mortality of patients with head injury and extracranial injury treated in trauma centers. *J Trauma*. 1989;29(9):1193–1201.

69. Agran PF, Dunkle DE, Winn DG. Injuries to a sample of seatbelted children evaluated and treated in a hospital emergency room. *J Trauma*. 1987;27(1):58–64.

70. Appleby JP, Nagy AG. Abdominal injuries associated with the use of seatbelts. *Am J Surg*. 1989;157(5):457–458.

71. Arajärvi E, Santavirta S, Tolonen J. Abdominal injuries sustained in severe traffic accidents by seatbelt wearers. *J Trauma*. 1987;27(4):393–397.

72. Blacksin MF. Patterns of fracture after air bag deployment. *J Trauma*. 1993;35(6):840–843.

73. Bourbeau R, Desjardins D, Maag U, Laberge-Nadeau C. Neck injuries among belted and unbelted occupants of the front seat of cars. *J Trauma*. 1993;35(5):794–799.

74. Chandler CF, Lane JS, Waxman KS. Seatbelt sign following blunt trauma is associated with increased incidence of abdominal injury. *Am Surg*. 1997;63(10):885–888.

75. Hall CE, Norton SA, Dixon AR. Complete small bowel transection following lap-belt injury. *Injury*. 2001;32(8):640–641.

76. Holbrook JL, Bennett JB. Brachial plexus injury associated with chest restraint seatbelt: case report. *J Trauma*. 1990;30(11):1413–1414.

77. Immega G. Whiplash injuries increase with seatbelt use. *Can Fam Physician*. 1995;41(41):203–204.

78. Johnson DL, Falci S. The diagnosis and treatment of pediatric lumbar spine injuries caused by rear seat lap belts. *Neurosurgery*. 1990;26(3):434–441.

79. Kaplan BH, Cowley RA. Seatbelt effectiveness and cost of noncompliance among drivers admitted to a trauma center. *Am J Emerg Med*. 1991;9(1):4–10.

80. Lubbers EJ. Injury of the duodenum caused by a fixed three-point seatbelt. *J Trauma*. 1977;17(12):960.

81. May AK, Chan B, Daniel TM, Young JS. Anterior lung herniation: another aspect of the seatbelt syndrome. *J Trauma*. 1995;38(4):587–589.

82. Restifo KM, Kelen GD. Case report: sternal fracture from a seatbelt. *J Emerg Med*. 1994;12(3):321–323.

83. Santavirta S, Arajärvi E. Ruptures of the heart in seatbelt wearers. *J Trauma*. 1992;32(3):275–279.

84. Shoemaker BL, Ose M. Pediatric lap belt injuries: care and prevention. *Orthop Nurs*. 1997;16(5):15–22.

85. Verdant A. Abdominal injuries sustained in severe traffic accidents by seatbelt wearers. *J Trauma*. 1988;28(6):880–881.

86. Warrian RK, Shoenut JP, Iannicello CM, Sharma GP, Trenholm BG. Seatbelt injury to the abdominal aorta. *J Trauma*. 1988;28(10):1505–1507.

87. Yarbrough BE, Hendey GW. Hangman's fracture resulting from improper seat belt use. *South Med J*. 1990;83(7):843–845.

88. Bandstra RA, Carbone LS. Unusual basal skull fracture in a vehicle equipped with an air bag. *Am J Forensic Med Pathol*. 2001;22(3):253–255.

89. Murphy RX Jr, Birmingham KL, Okunski WJ, Wasser T. The influence of airbag and restraining devices on the patterns of facial trauma in motor vehicle collisions. *Plast Reconstr Surg*. 2000;105(2):516–520.

90. Rozner L. Air bag-bruised face. *Plast Reconstr Surg*. 1996;97(7):1517–1519.

91. Lueder GT. Air bag-associated ocular trauma in children. *Ophthalmology*. 2000;107(8):1472–1475.

92. Stein JD, Jaeger EA, Jeffers JB. Air bags and ocular injuries. *Trans Am Ophthalmol Soc*. 1999;97:59–82.

93. Ruiz-Moreno JM. Air bag-associated retinal tear. *Eur J Ophthalmol*. 1998;8(1):52–53.

94. Zabriskie NA, Hwang IP, Ramsey JF, Crandall AS. Anterior lens capsule rupture caused by air bag trauma. *Am J Ophthalmol*. 1997;123(6):832–833.

95. Ghafouri A, Burgess SK, Hrdlicka ZK, Zagelbaum BM. Air bag-related ocular trauma. *Am J Emerg Med*. 1997;15(4):389–392.

96. Ulrich D, Noah EM, Fuchs P, Pallua N. Burn injuries caused by air bag deployment. *Burns*. 2001;27(2):196–199.

97. White JE, McClafferty K, Orton RB, Tokarewicz AC, Nowak ES. Ocular alkali burn associated with automobile air-bag activation. *CMAJ*. 1995;153(7):933–934.

98. Conover K. Chemical burn from automotive air bag. *Ann Emerg Med*. 1992;21(6):770.

99. Guarino AH. More on reflex sympathetic dystrophy syndrome following air-bag inflation. *N Engl J Med*. 1998;338(5):335.

100. Shah N, Weinstein A. Reflex sympathetic dystrophy syndrome following air-bag inflation. *N Engl J Med*. 1997;337(8):574.

101. Kirchhoff R, Rasmussen SW. Forearm fracture due to the release of an automobile air bag. *Acta Orthop Scand*. 1995;66(5):483.

102. Ong CF, Kumar VP. Colles fracture from air bag deployment. *Injury*. 1998;29(8):629–631.

103. Giguère JF, St-Vil D, Turmel A, et al. Airbags and children: a spectrum of C-spine injuries. *J Pediatr Surg*. 1998;33(6):811–816.

104. Traynelis VC, Gold M. Cervical spine injury in an air-bag-equipped vehicle. *J Spinal Disord*. 1993;6(1):60–61.

105. Morris MS, Borja LP. Air bag deployment and hearing loss. *Am Fam Physician*. 1998;57(11):2627–2628.

106. Kramer MB, Shattuck TG, Charnock DR. Traumatic hearing loss following air-bag inflation. *N Engl J Med*. 1997;337(8):574–575.

107. Centers for Disease Control and Prevention. Air-bag-associated fatal injuries to infants and children riding in front passenger seats—United States. *MMWR Morb Mortal Wkly Rep*. 1995;44(45):845–847.

108. From the Centers for Disease Control and Prevention. Update: fatal air bag-related injuries to children—United States, 1993–1996. *JAMA*. 1997;277(1):11–12.

109. McCaffrey M, German A, Lalonde F, Letts M. Air bags and children: a potentially lethal combination. *J Pediatr Orthop*. 1999;19(1):60–64.

110. Wittenberg E, Goldie SJ, Graham JD. Predictors of hazardous child seating behavior in fatal motor vehicle crashes: 1990 to 1998. *Pediatrics*. 2001;108(2):438–442.

111. Angel CA, Ehlers RA. Images in clinical medicine. Atloido-occipital dislocation in a small child after air-bag deployment. *N Engl J Med*. 2001;345(17):1256.

112. Marshall KW, Koch BL, Egelhoff JC. Air bag-related deaths and serious injuries in children: injury patterns and imaging findings. *AJNR Am J Neuroradiol*. 1998;19(9):1599–1607.

113. Totten VY, Fani-Salek MH, Chandramohan K. Hyphema associated with air bag deployment in a pediatric trauma patient. *Am J Emerg Med*. 1998;16(1):102–103.

114. Morrison AL, Chute D, Radentz S, Golle M, Troncoso JC, Smialek JE. Air bag-associated injury to a child in the front passenger seat. *Am J Forensic Med Pathol*. 1998;19(3):218–222.

115. Willis BK, Smith JL, Falkner LD, Vernon DD, Walker ML. Fatal air bag mediated craniocervical trauma in a child. *Pediatr Neurosurg*. 1996;24(6):323–327.

116. Stylianos S, Eichelberger MR. Pediatric trauma. Prevention strategies. *Pediatr Clin North Am*. 1993;40(6):1359–1368.

117. National Highway Traffic Safety Administration. Motorcycle helmet use and head and facial injuries: crash outcomes in CODES-

linked data. National Highway Traffic Safety Administration; 2009. Report No. DOT HS 811-208.

118. Research and Innovative Technology Administration: Bureau of Transportation Statistics. *National Transportation Statistics 2010, Table 2-2: Injured Persons by Transportation Mode*. Washington, DC: US Department of Transportation. http://www.bts.gov/publications/national_transportation_statistics/2010/html/table_02_02.html. Accessed July 14, 2011.

119. Bachulis BL, Sangster W, Gorrell GW, Long WB. Patterns of injury in helmeted and nonhelmeted motorcyclists. *Am J Surg*. 1988; 155(5):708–711.

120. Christian WJ, Carroll M, Meyer K, Vitaz TW, Franklin GA. Motorcycle helmets and head injuries in Kentucky, 1995–2000. *J Ky Med Assoc*. 2003;101(1):21–26.

121. Kraus JF, Peek C, McArthur DL, Williams A. The effect of the 1992 California motorcycle helmet use law on motorcycle crash fatalities and injuries. *JAMA*. 1994;272(19):1506–1511.

122. Sauter C, Zhu S, Allen S, Hargarten S, Layde PM. Increased risk of death or disability in unhelmeted Wisconsin motorcyclists. *WMJ*. 2005;104(2):39–44.

123. Crompton JG, Bone C, Oyetunji T, et al. Motorcycle helmets associated with lower risk of cervical spine injury: debunking the myth. *J Am Coll Surg*. 2011;212(3):295–300.

124. Vaca F. National Highway Traffic Safety Administration (NHTSA) notes. Evaluation of the repeal of the all-rider motorcycle helmet law in Florida. *Ann Emerg Med*. 2006;47(2):203–206.

125. Muelleman RL, Mlinek EJ, Collicott PE. Motorcycle crash injuries and costs: effect of a reenacted comprehensive helmet use law. *Ann Emerg Med*. 1992;21(3):266–272.

126. Rowland J, Rivara F, Salzberg P, Soderberg R, Maier R, Koepsell T. Motorcycle helmet use and injury outcome and hospitalization costs from crashes in Washington State. *Am J Public Health*. 1996; 86(1):41–45.

127. Vaca F, Berns SD, Harris JS, Jolly BT, Runge JW, Todd KH. National Highway Traffic Safety Administration. Evaluation of the repeal of motorcycle helmet laws. *Ann Emerg Med*. 2001;37(2):229–230.

128. DeMarco AL, Chimich DD, Gardiner JC, Nightingale RW, Siegmund GP. The impact response of motorcycle helmets at different impact severities. *Accid Anal Prev*. 2010;42(6):1778–1784.

129. Peek-Asa C, McArthur DL, Kraus JF. The prevalence of non-standard helmet use and head injuries among motorcycle riders. *Accid Anal Prev*. 1999;31(3):229–233.

130. Insurance Institute for Highway Safety. Motorcycle and bicycle helmet use laws. http://www.iihs.org/laws/helmetusecurrent.aspx. Accessed June 30, 2011.

131. Doi A, Deguchi J, Yamada M, et al. Traumatic internal carotid artery dissection due to compression by a helmet strap [in Japanese]. *No Shinkei Geka*. 2004;32(12):1279–1282.

132. Kuo LC, Lin HL, Chen CW, Lee WC. Traumatic hyoid bone fracture in patient wearing a helmet: a case report. *Am J Emerg Med*. 2008; 26(2):251.e1–e2.

133. Hotz GA, Cohn SM, Popkin C, et al. The impact of a repealed motorcycle helmet law in Miami-Dade County. *J Trauma*. 2002; 52(3):469–474.

134. Bledsoe GH, Schexnayder SM, Carey MJ, et al. The negative impact of the repeal of the Arkansas motorcycle helmet law. *J Trauma*. 2002;53(6):1078–1086.

135. Brandt MM, Ahrns KS, Corpron CA, Franklin GA, Wahl WL. Hospital cost is reduced by motorcycle helmet use. *J Trauma*. 2002; 53(3):469–471.

136. Eastridge BJ, Shafi S, Minei JP, Culica D, McConnel C, Gentilello L. Economic impact of motorcycle helmets: from impact to discharge. *J Trauma*. 2006;60(5):978–983.

137. McLellan BA, Vingilis E, Larkin E, Stoduto G, Macartney-Filgate M, Sharkey PW. Psychosocial characteristics and follow-up of drinking and non-drinking drivers in motor vehicle crashes. *J Trauma*. 1993;35(2):245–250.

138. National Highway Traffic Safety Administration. *Traffic Safety Facts 2005: Motorcycles*. Washington, DC: US Department of Transportation; 2007. Report No. DOT HS 810-631.

139. Creaser JI, Ward NJ, Rakauskas ME, Shankwitz C, Boer ER. Effects of alcohol impairment on motorcycle riding skills. *Accid Anal Prev*. 2009;41(5):906–913.

140. Sabey B. Engineering safety on the road. *Inj Prev*. 1995;1(3):182–186.

141. Local Authority Associations. *Road Safety Code of Good Practice*. London, UK: Association of County Councils; 1989.

142. Retting RA, Weinstein HB, Williams AF, Preusser DF. A simple method for identifying and correcting crash problems on urban arterial streets. *Accid Anal Prev*. 2001;33(6):723–734.

143. Federal Highway Administration. *Safety Evaluation of the Safety Edge Treatment*. Washington, DC: US Department of Transportation; 2011. Publication No. FHWA-HRT-11-025.

144. Rodegerdts L, Cibor A, Pochowski A. *Status of Roundabouts in North America*. Kansas City, MO: Transportation Research Board; 2008.

145. Lenters MS. *Safety auditing roundabouts. National Roundabout Conference: 2005 Proceedings*. Washington, DC: Transportation Research Board; 2005.

146. US Department of Transportation: Federal Highway Administration. Roundabouts can improve safety at stop sign-controlled intersections. http://safety.fhwa.dot.gov/intersection/resources/casestudies/fhwasa09018/md_rdabt_article.cfm. Accessed June 5, 2011.

147. Montella A. Identifying crash contributory factors at urban roundabouts and using association rules to explore their relationships to different crash types. *Accid Anal Prev*. 2011;43(4):1451–1463.

148. Kotch JB, Chalmers DJ, Langley JD, Marshall SW. Child day care and home injuries involving playground equipment. *J Paediatr Child Health*. 1993;29(3):222–227.

149. Lillis KA, Jaffe DM. Playground injuries in children. *Pediatr Emerg Care*. 1997;13(2):149–153.

150. Benoit R, Watts DD, Dwyer K, Kaufmann C, Fakhry S. Windows 99: a source of suburban pediatric trauma. *J Trauma*. 2000;49(3):477–481.

151. Stevens JA, Corso PS, Finkelstein EA, Miller TR. The costs of fatal and non-fatal falls among older adults. *Inj Prev*. 2006;12(5):290–295.

152. Harris VA, Rochette LM, Smith GA. Pediatric injuries attributable to falls from windows in the United States in 1990–2008. *Pediatrics*. 2011.

153. Bjerre B, Schelp L. The community safety approach in Falun, Sweden—is it possible to characterise the most effective prevention endeavours and how long-lasting are the results? *Accid Anal Prev*. 2000;32(3):461–470.

154. Davidson LL, Durkin MS, Kuhn L, O'Connor P, Barlow B, Heagarty MC. The impact of the Safe Kids/Healthy Neighborhoods Injury Prevention Program in Harlem, 1988 through 1991. *Am J Public Health*. 1994;84(4):580–586.

155. Durkin MS, Olsen S, Barlow B, Virella A, Connolly ES Jr. The epidemiology of urban pediatric neurological trauma: evaluation of, and implications for, injury prevention programs. *Neurosurgery*. 1998; 42(3):300–310.

156. Wakes S, Beukes A. Height, fun and safety in the design of children's playground equipment. *Int J Inj Contr Saf Promot*. 2011.

157. Gresham LS, Zirkle DL, Tolchin S, Jones C, Maroufi A, Miranda J. Partnering for injury prevention: evaluation of a curriculum-based intervention program among elementary school children. *J Pediatr Nurs*. 2001;16(2):79–87.

158. Jeffs D, Booth D, Calvert D. Local injury information, community participation and injury reduction. *Aust J Public Health*. 1993;17(4):365–372.

159. Miller KE, Zylstra RG, Standridge JB. The geriatric patient: a systematic approach to maintaining health. *Am Fam Physician*. 2000; 61(4):1089–1104.

160. Bell AJ, Talbot-Stern JK, Hennessy A. Characteristics and outcomes of older patients presenting to the emergency department after a fall: a retrospective analysis. *Med J Aust*. 2000;173(4):179–182.

161. Speechley M, Tinetti M. Falls and injuries in frail and vigorous community elderly persons. *J Am Geriatr Soc*. 1991;39(1):46–52.

162. Rosenhall U, Rubin W. Degenerative changes in the human vestibular sensory epithelia. *Acta Otolaryngol*. 1975;79(1–2):67–80.

163. Manchester D, Woollacott M, Zederbauer-Hylton N, Marin O. Visual, vestibular and somatosensory contributions to balance control in the older adult. *J Gerontol*. 1989;44(4):M118–M127.

164. Hasselkus BR. Aging and the human nervous system. *Am J Occup Ther*. 1974;28(1):16–21.

165. Sinclair AJ, Nayak US. Age-related changes in postural sway. *Compr Ther.* 1990;16(9):44–48.

166. Helbostad JL, Askim T, Moe-Nilssen R. Short-term repeatability of body sway during quiet standing in people with hemiparesis and in frail older adults. *Arch Phys Med Rehabil.* 2004;85(6):993–999.

167. Shumway-Cook A, Anson D, Haller S. Postural sway biofeedback: its effect on reestablishing stance stability in hemiplegic patients. *Arch Phys Med Rehabil.* 1988;69(6):395–400.

168. Cakar E, Dincer U, Kiralp MZ, et al. Jumping combined exercise programs reduce fall risk and improve balance and life quality of elderly people who live in a long-term care facility. *Eur J Phys Rehabil Med.* 2010;46(1):59–67.

169. Fialová D, Topinková E, Gambassi G, et al. Potentially inappropriate medication use among elderly home care patients in Europe. *JAMA.* 2005;293(11):1348–1358.

170. Weber V, White A, McIlvried R. An electronic medical record (EMR)-based intervention to reduce polypharmacy and falls in an ambulatory rural elderly population. *J Gen Intern Med.* 2008;23(4): 399–404.

171. Connell BR, Wolf SL. Environmental and behavioral circumstances associated with falls at home among healthy elderly individuals. Atlanta FICSIT Group. *Arch Phys Med Rehabil.* 1997;78(2):179–186.

172. Frick KD, Kung JY, Parrish JM, Narrett MJ. Evaluating the cost-effectiveness of fall prevention programs that reduce fall-related hip fractures in older adults. *J Am Geriatr Soc.* 2010;58(1):136–141.

173. Sarmiento K, Langlois JA, Mitchko J. "Help seniors live better, longer: prevent brain injury": an overview of CDC's education initiative to prevent fall-related TBI among older adults. *J Head Trauma Rehabil.* 2008;23(3):164–167.

174. Smeltzer SC, Zimmerman V, Capriotti T. Osteoporosis risk and low bone mineral density in women with physical disabilities. *Arch Phys Med Rehabil.* 2005;86(3):582–586.

175. Whitman S, Coonley-Hoganson R, Desai BT. Comparative head trauma experiences in two socioeconomically different Chicago-area communities: a population study. *Am J Epidemiol.* 1984;119: 570–580.

176. Langlois JA, Rutland-Brown W, Wald MM. The epidemiology and impact of traumatic brain injury: a brief overview. *J Head Trauma Rehabil.* 2006;21(5):375–378.

177. Johnston KM, McCrory P, Mohtadi NG, Meeuwisse W. Evidence-based review of sport-related concussion: clinical science. *Clin J Sport Med.* 2001;11(3):150–159.

178. Boufous S, Rome LD, Senserrick T, Ivers R. Cycling crashes in children, adolescents, and adults—a comparative analysis. *Traffic Inj Prev.* 2011;12(3):244–250.

179. Sheppard MA, Taylor D. Medical, work loss, and quality of life costs for fatal and hospital-admitted bicycle injuries to children 0–19 in 2004 dollars. Calverton, MD: Pacific Institute for Research and Evaluation; 2011.

180. Noakes TD. Fatal cycling injuries. *Sports Med.* 1995;20(5):348–362.

181. Thompson DC, Rivara FP, Thompson R. Helmets for preventing head and facial injuries in bicyclists. http://www2.cochrane.org/reviews/en/ab001855.html. Updated November 8, 2006. Accessed November 2, 2011.

182. Thompson DC, Rivara FP, Thompson R. Helmets for preventing head and facial injuries in bicyclists. *Cochrane Database Syst Rev.* 2000;(2):CD001855.

183. Koplan JP, Thacker SB. Working to prevent and control injury in the United States. *Fact Book for the Year 2000.* Centers for Disease Control and Prevention National Center for Inquiry Prevention and Control; 2000. http://www.cdc.gov/Injury/publications/FactBook/InjuryBook2006.pdf 2000. Accessed November 2, 2011.

184. Thornley SJ, Woodward A, Langley JD, Ameratunga SN, Rodgers A. Conspicuity and bicycle crashes: preliminary findings of the Taupo Bicycle Study. *Inj Prev.* 2008;14(1):11–18.

185. Blake G, Velikonja D, Pepper V, Jilderda I, Georgiou G. Evaluating an in-school injury prevention programme's effect on children's helmet wearing habits. *Brain Inj.* 2008;22(6):501–507.

186. Macpherson A, Spinks A. Bicycle helmet legislation for the uptake of helmet use and prevention of head injuries. *Cochrane Database Syst Rev.* 2008;(3):CD005401.

187. Atha J, Yeadon MR, Sandover J, Parsons KC. The damaging punch. *Br Med J.* 1985;291(6511):1756–1757.

188. Wilberger JE Jr, Maroon JC. Head injuries in athletes. *Clin Sports Med.* 1989;8(1):1–9.

189. Clausen H, McCrory P, Anderson V. The risk of chronic traumatic brain injury in professional boxing: change in exposure variables over the past century. *Br J Sports Med.* 2005;39(9):661–664.

190. Schmidt-Olsen S, Jensen SK, Mortensen V. Amateur boxing in Denmark. The effect of some preventive measures. *Am J Sports Med.* 1990;18(1):98–100.

191. Silfverskiöld B. Protection against blows must be put in the boxers' gloves! [in Swedish]. *Lakartidningen.* 1990;87(13):1036.

192. Heilbronner RL, Bush SS, Ravdin LD, et al. Neuropsychological consequences of boxing and recommendations to improve safety: a National Academy of Neuropsychology education paper. *Arch Clin Neuropsychol.* 2009;24(1):11–19.

193. Graham MR, Myers T, Evans P, et al. Direct hits to the head during amateur boxing is associated with a rise in serum biomarkers for brain injury. *Int J Immunopathol Pharmacol.* 2011;24(1):119–125.

194. Jordan BD, Relkin NR, Ravdin LD, Jacobs AR, Bennett A, Gandy S. Apolipoprotein E epsilon4 associated with chronic traumatic brain injury in boxing. *JAMA.* 1997;278(2):136–140.

195. HR&A. UFC event impacts: economic study for New York State: upstate (Buffalo) and downstate (NYC). http://www.mmafacts.com/images/FE/chain226siteType8/site195/client/HR&A-ImpactStudy-11-10-08.pdf. Accessed July 13, 2011.

196. Ngai KM, Levy F, Hsu EB. Injury trends in sanctioned mixed martial arts competition: a 5-year review from 2002 to 2007. *Br J Sports Med.* 2008;42(8):686–689.

197. Bledsoe GH, Li G, Levy F. Injury risk in professional boxing. *South Med J.* 2005;98(10):994–998.

198. Jako P. Boxing. In: Kordi R, Maffulli N, Wroble RR, eds. *Combat Sports Medicine.* London, UK: Springer; 2011:193–213.

199. Nielsen Wire. Super Bowl XLV most viewed telecast in U.S. broadcast history. http://blog.nielsen.com/nielsenwire/media_entertainment/super-bowl-xlv-most-viewed-telecast-in-broadcast-history/. Accessed May 26, 2011.

200. National Football League. NFL sets attendance record in 2007. NFL Web site. http://www.nfl.com/news/story?confirm = true&id = 09000d5d8077f84d&template = without-video. Accessed May 26, 2011.

201. Pellman EJ, Powell JW, Viano DC, et al. Concussion in professional football: epidemiological features of game injuries and review of the literature—part 3. *Neurosurgery.* 2004;54(1):81–94.

202. Nation AD, Nelson NG, Yard EE, Comstock RD, McKenzie LB. Football-related injuries among 6- to 17-year-olds treated in US emergency departments, 1990–2007. *Clin Pediatr.* 2011;50(3): 200–207.

203. Meehan WP III, d'Hemecourt P, Comstock RD. High school concussions in the 2008–2009 academic year: mechanism, symptoms, and management. *Am J Sports Med.* 2010;38(12):2405–2409.

204. Lincoln AE, Caswell SV, Almquist JL, Dunn RE, Norris JB, Hinton RY. Trends in concussion incidence in high school sports: a prospective 11-year study. *Am J Sports Med.* 2011;39(5):958–963.

205. Gessel LM, Fields SK, Collins CL, Dick RW, Comstock RD. Concussions among United States high school and collegiate athletes. *J Athl Train.* 2007;42(4):495–503.

206. Blyth CS, Mueller F. Football injury survey, part 1: when and where players get hurt. *Phys Sports Med.* 1974;45–52.

207. Omalu BI, DeKosky ST, Minster RL, Kamboh MI, Hamilton RL, Wecht CH. Chronic traumatic encephalopathy in a National Football League player. *Neurosurgery.* 2005;57(1):128–134.

208. Omalu BI, DeKosky ST, Hamilton RL, et al. Chronic traumatic encephalopathy in a national football league player: part II. *Neurosurgery.* 2006;59(5):1086–1092.

209. Omalu BI, Hamilton RL, Kamboh MI, DeKosky ST, Bailes J. Chronic traumatic encephalopathy (CTE) in a National Football League Player: case report and emerging medicolegal practice questions. *J Forensic Nurs.* 2010;6(1):40–46.

210. Pellman EJ, Viano DC. Concussion in professional football: summary of the research conducted by the National Football League's

Committee on Mild Traumatic Brain Injury. *Neurosurg Focus.* 2006; 21(4):E12.

211. Collins M, Lovell MR, Iverson GL, Ide T, Maroon J. Examining concussion rates and return to play in high school football players wearing newer helmet technology: a three-year prospective cohort study. *Neurosurgery.* 2006;58(2):275–286.

212. Singh GD, Maher GJ, Padilla RR. Customized mandibular orthotics in the prevention of concussion/mild traumatic brain injury in football players: a preliminary study. *Dent Traumatol.* 2009;25(5): 515–521.

213. Gregory S. The problem with football: how to make it safer. Time magazine online. http://www.time.com/time/magazine/article/ 0,9171,1957459-3,00.html. Accessed May 27, 2011.

214. Crisco JJ, Greenwald RM. Let's get the head further out of the game: a proposal for reducing brain injuries in helmeted contact sports. *Curr Sports Med Rep.* 2011;10:7–9.

215. Mueller FO. Fatalities from head and cervical spine injuries occurring in tackle football: 50 years' experience. *Clin Sports Med.* 1998; 17:169–182.

216. Kunz M. 265 Million playing footbal. *FIFA Magazine: BIG COUNT.* http://www.fifa.com/mm/document/fifafacts/bcoffsurv/emaga_9384_10704.pdf. Accessed October 24, 2010.

217. Dvorak J, Junge A. Football injuries and physical symptoms. A review of the literature. *Am J Sports Med.* 2000;28:S3–S9.

218. Tysvaer AT. Head and neck injuries in soccer. Impact of minor trauma. *Sports Med.* 1992;14(3):200–213.

219. Tysvaer A, Storli O. Association football injuries to the brain. A preliminary report. *Br J Sports Med.* 1981;15(3):163–166.

220. Fuller CW, Junge A, Dvorak J. A six year prospective study of the incidence and causes of head and neck injuries in international football. *Br J Sports Med.* 2005;39(suppl 1):i3–i9.

221. Kirkendall DT, Jordan SE, Garrett WE. Heading and head injuries in soccer. *Sports Med.* 2001;31(5):369–386.

222. Kontos AP, Dolese A, Elbin RJ, Covassin T, Warren BL. Relationship of soccer heading to computerized neurocognitive performance and symptoms among female and male youth soccer players. *Brain Inj.* 2011;25(12):1234–1241.

223. Smodlaka VN. Medical aspects of heading the ball in soccer. *Phys Sports Med.* 1984;12:127–131.

224. Delaney JS, Al-Kashmiri A, Drummond R, Correa JA. The effect of protective headgear on head injuries and concussions in adolescent football (soccer) players. *Br J Sports Med.* 2008;42(2):110–115.

225. Navarro RR. Protective equipment and the prevention of concussion—what is the evidence? *Curr Sports Med Rep.* 2011;10(1):27–31.

226. Lenroot RK, Giedd JN. Brain development in children and adolescents: insights from anatomical magnetic resonance imaging. *Neurosci Biobehav Rev.* 2006;30(6):718–729.

227. Dailey SW, Barsan WG. Head injuries in soccer: a case for protective headgear? *Phys Sports Med.* 1992;20:79–82.

228. Agel J, Harvey EJ. A 7-year review of men's and women's ice hockey injuries in the NCAA. *Can J Surg.* 2010;53(5):319–323.

229. Benson BW, Meeuwisse WH, Rizos J, Kang J, Burke CJ. A prospective study of concussions among National Hockey League players during regular season games: the NHL-NHLPA Concussion Program. *CMAJ.* 2011;183(8):905–911.

230. Emery CA, Meeuwisse WH. Injury rates, risk factors, and mechanisms of injury in minor hockey. *Am J Sports Med.* 2006;34(12): 1960–1969.

231. Dryden DM, Francescutti LH, Rowe BH, Spence JC, Voaklander DC. Epidemiology of women's recreational ice hockey injuries. *Med Sci Sports Exerc.* 2000;32(8):1378–1383.

232. Reid SR, Losek JD. Factors associated with significant injuries in youth ice hockey players. *Pediatr Emerg Care.* 1999;15(5):310–313.

233. Safety in youth ice hockey: the effects of body checking. American Academy of Pediatrics. Committee on Sports Medicine and Fitness. *Pediatrics.* 2000;105(3, pt 1):657–658.

234. Marcotte G, Simard D. Fair-play: an approach to hockey for the 1990s. In: Castaldi CR, Bishop PJ, Hoerner ER, eds. *Safety in Ice Hockey.* 2nd ed. Philadelphia, PA: American Society for Testing and Materials; 1993:103–108.

235. Warsh JM, Constantin SA, Howard A, Macpherson A. A systematic review of the association between body checking and injury in youth ice hockey. *Clin J Sport Med.* 2009;19(2):134–144.

236. Asplund C, Bettcher S, Borchers J. Facial protection and head injuries in ice hockey: a systematic review. *Br J Sports Med.* 2009;43(13): 993–999.

237. Echlin PS, Johnson AM, Riverin S, et al. A prospective study of concussion education in 2 junior ice hockey teams: implications for sports concussion education. *Neurosurg Focus.* 2010;29(5):E6.

238. Cook DJ, Cusimano MD, Tator CH, Chipman ML. Evaluation of the ThinkFirst Canada, Smart Hockey, brain and spinal cord injury prevention video. *Inj Prev.* 2003;9(4):361–366.

239. NHL.com. Rules. National Hockey League Web site. http://www.nhl.com/ice/page.htm?id=64063. Accessed July 1, 2011.

240. Roarke SP. NHL.com. NHL Insider. Bettman discusses concussions, player safety. http://www.nhl.com/ice/news.htm?id=556046#&navid=nhl-search. Accessed July 2, 2011.

241. McCaw ST, Walker JD. Winning the Stanley Cup Final Series is related to incurring fewer penalties for violent behavior. *Tex Med.* 1999;95(4):66–69.

242. Newsome PR, Tran DC, Cooke MS. The role of the mouthguard in the prevention of sports-related dental injuries: a review. *Int J Paediatr Dent.* 2001;11(6):396–404.

243. Daneshvar DH, Baugh CM, Nowinski CJ, McKee AC, Stern RA, Cantu RC. Helmets and mouth guards: the role of personal equipment in preventing sport-related concussions. *Clin Sports Med.* 2011;30(1):145–63, x.

244. Barbic D, Pater J, Brison RJ. Comparison of mouth guard designs and concussion prevention in contact sports: a multicenter randomized controlled trial. *Clin J Sport Med.* 2005;15(5):294–298.

245. Benson BW, Hamilton GM, Meeuwisse WH, McCrory P, Dvorak J. Is protective equipment useful in preventing concussion? A systematic review of the literature. *Br J Sports Med.* 2009;43(suppl 1): i56–i67.

246. Viano DC, Withnall C, Wonnacott M. Effect of mouthguards on head responses and mandible forces in football helmet impacts. *Ann Biomed Eng.* 2012;40(1):47–69.

247. McCrory P. Do mouthguards prevent concussion? *Br J Sports Med.* 2001;35(2):81–82.

248. National Violent Death Reporting System. Injury prevention and control: data and statistics (WISQARS). Centers for Disease Control and Prevention Web site. http://www.cdc.gov/injury/wisqars/nvdrs.html. Accessed January 28, 2011.

249. Centers for Disease Control and Prevention, National Center for Injury Prevention and Control. Youth violence: facts at a glance 2010. http://www.cdc.gov/ViolencePrevention/pdf/YV-Data Sheet-a.pdf. Accessed January 28, 2011.

250. Krieger MD, Levy ML, Apuzzo ML. Gunshot wounds to the head in an urban setting. *Neurosurg Clin N Am.* 1995;6(4):605–610.

251. Nagib MG, Rockswold GL, Sherman RS, Lagaard MW. Civilian gunshot wounds to the brain: prognosis and management. *Neurosurgery.* 1986;18(5):533–537.

252. Pruitt BA Jr. Part 2: prognosis in penetrating brain injury. *J Trauma.* 2001;51:S44–S86.

253. Tsuei YS, Sun MH, Lee HD, et al. Civilian gunshot wounds to the brain. *J Chin Med Assoc.* 2005;68(3):126–130.

254. Hofbauer M, Kdolsky R, Figl M, et al. Predictive factors influencing the outcome after gunshot injuries to the head-a retrospective cohort study. *J Trauma.* 2010;69(4):770–775.

255. Hepburn L, Miller M, Azrael D, Hemenway D. The US gun stock: results from the 2004 national firearms survey. *Inj Prev.* 2007;13(1): 15–19.

256. Centers for Disease Control and Prevention. Violence-related firearm deaths among residents of metropolitan areas and cities—United States, 2006–2007. *MMWR Morb Mortal Wkly Rep.* 2011; 60(18):573–578.

257. Dahlberg LL, Ikeda RM, Kresnow MJ. Guns in the home and risk of a violent death in the home: findings from a national study. *Am J Epidemiol.* 2004;160(10):929–936.

258. Grossman DC, Reay DT, Baker SA. Self-inflicted and unintentional firearm injuries among children and adolescents: the source of the firearm. *Arch Pediatr Adolesc Med.* 1999;153(8):875–878.

259. Kellermann AL, Rivara FP, Somes G, et al. Suicide in the home in relation to gun ownership. *N Engl J Med*. 1992;327(7):467–472.

260. Gross A, Miltenberger R, Knudson P, Bosch A, Breitwieser CB. Preliminary evaluation of a parent training program to prevent gun play. *J Appl Behav Anal*. 2007;40(4):691–695.

261. Gatheridge BJ, Miltenberger RG, Huneke DF, et al. Comparison of two programs to teach firearm injury prevention skills to 6- and 7-year-old children. *Pediatrics*. 2004;114(3):e294–e299.

262. Obeng C. Should gun safety be taught in schools? Perspectives of teachers. *J Sch Health*. 2010;80(8):394–398.

263. Milne JS, Hargarten SW. Handgun safety features: a review for physicians. *J Trauma*. 1999;47(1):145–150.

264. Grossman DC, Mueller BA, Riedy C, et al. Gun storage practices and risk of youth suicide and unintentional firearm injuries. *JAMA*. 2005;293(6):707–714.

265. Webster DW, Vernick JS, Zeoli AM, Manganello JA. Association between youth-focused firearm laws and youth suicides. *JAMA*. 2004;292(5):594–601.

266. Conner KR, Zhong Y. State firearm laws and rates of suicide in men and women. *Am J Prev Med*. 2003;25(4):320–324.

267. Miller M, Azrael D, Hemenway D. Rates of household firearm ownership and homicide across US regions and states, 1988–1997. *Am J Public Health*. 2002;92(12):1988–1993.

268. Villaveces A, Cummings P, Espitia VE, Koepsell TD, McKnight B, Kellermann AL. Effect of a ban on carrying firearms on homicide rates in 2 Colombian cities. *JAMA*. 2000;283:1205–1209.

269. Wagner AK, Sasser HC, Hammond FM, Wiercisiewski D, Alexander J. Intentional traumatic brain injury: epidemiology, risk factors, and associations with injury severity and mortality. *J Trauma*. 2000; 49(3):404–410.

270. Simpson G, Tate R. Suicidality in people surviving a traumatic brain injury: prevalence, risk factors and implications for clinical management. *Brain Inj*. 2007;21(13–14):1335–1351.

271. Teasdale TW, Engberg AW. Suicide after traumatic brain injury: a population study. *J Neurol Neurosurg Psychiatry*. 2001;71(4): 436–440.

272. Jorge RE, Robinson RG, Moser D, Tateno A, Crespo-Facorro B, Arndt S. Major depression following traumatic brain injury. *Arch Gen Psychiatry*. 2004;61(1):42–50.

273. Gaynes BN, West SL, Ford CA, Frame P, Klein J, Lohr KN. Screening for suicide risk in adults: a summary of the evidence for the U.S. Preventive Services Task Force. *Ann Intern Med*. 2004;140(10): 822–835.

274. Pentland B, Hutton L, Macmillan A, Mayer V. Training in brain injury rehabilitation. *Disabil Rehabil*. 2003;25(10):544–548.

275. Simpson G, Winstanley J, Bertapelle T. Suicide prevention training after traumatic brain injury: evaluation of a staff training workshop. *J Head Trauma Rehabil*. 2003;18(5):445–456.

276. Simpson G, Franke B, Gillett L. Suicide prevention training outside the mental health service system: evaluation of a state-wide program in Australia for rehabilitation and disability staff in the field of traumatic brain injury. *Crisis*. 2007;28(1):35–43.

277. Wilson FC, Nelson S, Downes C, McQuigg H, Lockhart C, Robinson H. Effectiveness of neurodisability simulation training for NHS staff working in brain injury rehabilitation. *Disabil Rehabil*. 2009; 31(17):1418–1423.

278. Fann JR, Hart T, Schomer KG. Treatment for depression after traumatic brain injury: a systematic review. *J Neurotrauma*. 2009;26(12): 2383–2402.

279. Bombardier CH, Rimmele CT, Zintel H. The magnitude and correlates of alcohol and drug use before traumatic brain injury. *Arch Phys Med Rehabil*. 2002;83(12):1765–1773.

280. Gerhart KA, Mellick DC, Weintraub AH. Violence-related traumatic brain injury: a population-based study. *J Trauma*. 2003;55(6): 1045–1053.

281. NHIF Professional Council Substance Abuse Task Force. *NHIF Professional Council Substance Abuse Task Force White Paper*. Washington, DC: National Head Injury Foundation; 1988.

282. Kolakowsky-Hayner SA, Gourley EV III, Kreutzer JS, Marwitz JH, Cifu DX, Mckinley WO. Pre-injury substance abuse among persons with brain injury and persons with spinal cord injury. *Brain Inj*. 1999;13(8):571–581.

283. Rivara FP, Koepsell TD, Jurkovich GJ, Gurney JG, Soderberg R. The effects of alcohol abuse on readmission for trauma. *JAMA*. 1993;270(16):1962–1964.

284. Schutte C, Hanks R. Impact of the presence of alcohol at the time of injury on acute and one-year cognitive and functional recovery after traumatic brain injury. *Int J Neurosci*. 2010;120(8):551–556.

285. Hingson R, Heeren T, Zakocs R, Winter M, Wechsler H. Age of first intoxication, heavy drinking, driving after drinking and risk of unintentional injury among U.S. college students. *J Stud Alcohol*. 2003;64(1):23–31.

286. Henry KL, McDonald JN, Oetting ER, Walker PS, Walker RD, Beauvais F. Age of onset of first alcohol intoxication and subsequent alcohol use among urban American Indian adolescents. *Psychol Addict Behav*. 2011;25(1):48–56.

287. Hingson R, Heeren T, Zakocs R. Age of drinking onset and involvement in physical fights after drinking. *Pediatrics*. 2001;108(4): 872–877.

288. Brookhuis KA, de Waard D, Steyvers FJ, Bijsterveld H. Let them experience a ride under the influence of alcohol; a successful intervention program? *Accid Anal Prev*. 2011;43(3):906–910.

289. Goss CW, Van Bramer LD, Gliner JA, Porter TR, Roberts IG, Diguiseppi C. Increased police patrols for preventing alcohol-impaired driving. *Cochrane Database Syst Rev*. 2008;CD005242.

290. McCartt AT, Wells JK, Teoh ER. Attitudes toward in-vehicle advanced alcohol detection technology. *Traffic Inj Prev*. 2010;11(2): 156–164.

291. Paschall MJ, Grube JW, Kypri K. Alcohol control policies and alcohol consumption by youth: a multi-national study. *Addiction*. 2009; 104(11):1849–1855.

292. Elder RW, Voas R, Beirness D, et al. Effectiveness of ignition interlocks for preventing alcohol-impaired driving and alcohol-related crashes: a Community Guide systematic review. *Am J Prev Med*. 2011;40(3):362–376.

293. Lang E, Stockwell T. Drinking locations of drink-drivers: a comparative analysis of accident and nonaccident cases. *Accid Anal Prev*. 1991;23(6):573–584.

294. O'Donnell MA. Research on drinking locations of alcohol-impaired drivers: implications for prevention policies. *J Public Health Policy*. 1985;6(4):510–525.

295. Shults RA, Elder RW, Sleet DA, et al. Reviews of evidence regarding interventions to reduce alcohol-impaired driving. *Am J Prev Med*. 2001;21:66–88.

296. Gliksman L, McKenzie D, Single E, Douglas R, Brunet S, Moffatt K. The role of alcohol providers in prevention: an evaluation of a server intervention programme. *Addiction*. 1993;88(9):1195–1203.

297. Holder HD, Saltz RF, Grube JW, et al. Summing up: lessons from a comprehensive community prevention trial. *Addiction*. 1997; 92(suppl 2):S293–S301.

298. Lang E, Stockwell T, Rydon P, Beel A. Can training bar staff in responsible serving practices reduce alcohol-related harm? *Drug Alcohol Rev*. 1998;17(1):39–50.

299. Russ NW, Geller ES. Training bar personnel to prevent drunken driving: a field evaluation. *Am J Public Health*. 1987;77(8):952–954.

300. Saltz RF. The role of bars and restaurants in preventing alcohol-impaired driving: an evaluation of server intervention. *Eval Health Professions*. 1987;10:5–27.

301. U.S. Preventive Services Task Force. Counseling about proper use of motor vehicle occupant restraints and avoidance of alcohol use while driving: U.S. Preventive Services Task Force recommendation statement. *Ann Intern Med*. 2007;147(3):187–193.

302. Brady JE, Baker SP, Dimaggio C, McCarthy ML, Rebok GW, Li G. Effectiveness of mandatory alcohol testing programs in reducing alcohol involvement in fatal motor carrier crashes. *Am J Epidemiol*. 2009;170(6):775–782.

303. Fell JC, Tippetts AS, Voas RB. Fatal traffic crashes involving drinking drivers: what have we learned? *Ann Adv Automot Med*. 2009; 53:63–76.

304. Solomon R, Chamberlain E, Abdoullaeva M, Tinholt B. Random breath testing: a Canadian perspective. *Traffic Inj Prev*. 2011;12(2): 111–119.

305. Compton RP, Blomberg RD, Moskowitz H, Burns M, Peck RC, Fiorentino D. Crash risk of alcohol impaired driving. In: Mayhew

DR, Dussault C., eds. *Proceedings of Alcohol, Drugs & Traffic Safety—T2002: 16thInternational Conference on Alcohol, Drugs & Traffic Safety, Agust 4–9, 2002.* Montreal, Canada: International Council on Alcohol, Drugs, and Traffic Safety (ICADTS); 2002:39–44.

306. Fell JC, Voas RB. The effectiveness of reducing illegal blood alcohol concentration (BAC) limits for driving: evidence for lowering the limit to .05 BAC. *J Safety Res.* 2006;37(3):233–243.

307. Supreme Court Ruling. Michigan Department of State Police v Sitz, 496 US 444, 110 LEd 2d 412, 1990 US LEXIS 3144, 110 SCt 2481, 58 USLW 4781 (1990).

308. World Health Organization. The Toronto Declaration on the Global Prevention of Elder Abuse. Geneva, Switzerland: World Health Organization; 2002. http://www.who.int/ageing/projects/elder_abuse/alc_toronto_declaration_en.pdf. Accessed December 31, 2011.

309. Daly JM, Merchant ML, Jogerst GJ. Elder abuse research: a systematic review. *J Elder Abuse Negl.* 2011;23(4):348–365.

310. Clark AN, Mankikar GD, Gray I. Diogenes syndrome. A clinical study of gross neglect in old age. *Lancet.* 1975;1(7903):366–368.

311. Lau EE, Kosberg JI. Abuse of the elderly by informal care providers. *Aging.* 1979;279:10–15.

312. Brownell P, Heiser D. Psycho-educational support groups for older women victims of family mistreatment: a pilot study. *J Gerontol Soc Work.* 2006;46(3–4):145–160.

313. Désy PM, Prohaska TR. The Geriatric Emergency Nursing Education (GENE) course: an evaluation. *J Emerg Nurs.* 2008;34(5):396–402.

314. Goodridge D, Johnston P, Thompson M. Impact of a nursing assistant training program on job performance, attitudes, and relationships with residents. *Educational Gerontology.* 1997;23:37–51.

315. Pillemer K, Hudson B. A model abuse prevention program for nursing assistants. *Gerontologist.* 1993;33(1):128–131.

316. Richardson B, Kitchen G, Livingston G. What staff know about elder abuse in dementia and the effect of training. *Dementia.* 2004;3(3):377–384.

317. Richardson B, Kitchen G, Livingston G. The effect of education on knowledge and management of elder abuse: a randomized controlled trial. *Age Ageing.* 2002;31(5):335–341.

318. Uva JL, Guttman T. Elder abuse education in an emergency medicine residency program. *Acad Emerg Med.* 1996;3(8):817–819.

319. Vinton L. Educating case managers about elder abuse and neglect. *J Case Manag.* 1993;2:101–105.

320. Nusbaum NJ, Mistretta M, Wegner J. An educational intervention for police and firefighters for elders at risk: limits of education alone as a strategy for behavior change. *Educational Gerontology.* 2007;33:801–809.

321. Golding JM, Yozwiak JA, Kinstle TL, Marsil DF. The effect of gender in the perception of elder physical abuse in court. *Law Hum Behav.* 2005;29(5):605–614.

322. Leedahl SN, Ferraro FR. Why is elder abuse overlooked? Media and ageism. *Psychology and Education.* 2007;44:1–9.

323. Hsieh HF, Wang JJ, Yen M, Liu TT. Educational support group in changing caregivers' psychological elder abuse behavior toward caring for institutionalized elders. *Adv Health Sci Educ Theory Pract.* 2009;14(3):377–386.

324. Reay AM, Browne KD. The effectiveness of psychological interventions with individuals who physically abuse or neglect their elderly dependents. *J Interpers Violence.* 2002;17:416–431.

325. Manthorpe J, Biggs S, McCreadie C, et al. The U.K. national study of abuse and neglect among older people. *Nurs Older People.* 2007;19(8):24–26.

326. Chokkanathan S, Lee AE. Elder mistreatment in urban India: a community based study. *J Elder Abuse Negl.* 2005;17(2):45–61.

327. Jogerst GJ, Daly JM, Brinig MF, Dawson JD, Schmuch GA, Ingram JG. Domestic elder abuse and the law. *Am J Public Health.* 2003;93(12):2131–2136.

328. Pillemer K, Moore DW. Abuse of patients in nursing homes: findings from a survey of staff. *Gerontologist.* 1989;29(3):314–320.

329. Zhang Z, Schiamberg LB, Oehmke J, et al. Neglect of older adults in Michigan nursing homes. *J Elder Abuse Negl.* 2011;23(1):58–74.

330. Schiamberg LB, Oehmke J, Zhang Z, et al. Physical abuse of older adults in nursing homes: a random sample survey of adults with an elderly family member in a nursing home. *J Elder Abuse Negl.* 2012;24(1):65–83.

331. Cohen M, Shinan-Altman S. A cross-cultural study of nursing aides' attitudes to elder abuse in nursing homes. *Int Psychogeriatr.* 2011;23(8):1213–1221.

332. Inaba AS, Seward PN. An approach to paediatric trauma. Unique anatomic and pathophysiologic aspects of the pediatric patient. *Emerg Med Clin North Am.* 1991;9(3):523–548.

333. Stancin T, Wade SL, Walz NC, Yeates KO, Taylor HG. Traumatic brain injuries in early childhood: initial impact on the family. *J Dev Behav Pediatr.* 2008;29(4):253–261.

334. Schneier AJ, Shields BJ, Hostetler SG, Xiang H, Smith GA. Incidence of pediatric traumatic brain injury and associated hospital resource utilization in the United States. *Pediatrics.* 2006;118(2):483–492.

335. Kumar R, Mahapatra AK. The changing "epidemiology" of pediatric head injury and its impact on the daily clinical practice. *Childs Nerv Syst.* 2009;25(7):813–823.

336. Crume TL, DiGuiseppi C, Byers T, Sirotnak AP, Garrett CJ. Underascertainment of child maltreatment fatalities by death certificates, 1990–1998. *Pediatrics.* 2002;110(2, pt 1):e18.

337. Child Welfare Information Gateway. *Child Abuse and Neglect Fatalities 2009: Statistics and Interventions.* Washington, DC: U.S. Department of Health and Human Services, Children's Bureau; 2011.

338. Klevens J, Leeb RT. Child maltreatment fatalities in children under 5: findings from the National Violence Death Reporting System. *Child Abuse Negl.* 2010;34(4):262–266.

339. Hahn RA, Bilukha OO, Crosby A; for Task Force on Community Preventative Services. First reports evaluating the effectiveness of strategies for preventing violence: firearms laws. *MMWR.* 2003;52(RR-14):11–20. http://www.cdc.gov/mmwr/preview/mmwr html/rr5214a2.htm. Updated October 3, 2003. Accessed November 3, 2011.

340. Scribano PV. Prevention strategies in child maltreatment. *Curr Opin Pediatr.* 2010;22(5):616–620.

341. Gomby DS. The promise and limitations of home visiting: implementing effective programs. *Child Abuse Negl.* 2007;31(8):793–799.

342. Olds DL. The nurse–family partnership: an evidence-based preventive intervention. *Infant Ment Health J.* 2006;27:5–25.

343. Flaherty EG, Sege R. Barriers to physician identification and reporting of child abuse. *Pediatr Ann.* 2005;34(5):349–356.

II

BIOMECHANICS, PATHOPHYSIOLOGY, AND NEURAL RECOVERY

Biomechanics of Brain Injury

David C. Viano

INTRODUCTION

Severe impact to the head deforms the skull and loads the brain with a potential for skull fracture and brain injury. The underlying risk depends on the concentration of the loading area, the velocity of impact, and the kinematics of the head. The most relevant biomechanical parameter of a head response is the "effective" acceleration (a_{eff}) and duration (T) of a head impact. Gadd (1) found that when combined as $a_{eff}^{2.5}T$, the product was related to the risk of brain injury and skull fracture. Hard surface impacts cause short duration loads with high accelerations, which pose the greatest risk for skull fracture. Longer duration loads with softer, deforming surfaces decrease the risk for skull fracture but do not eliminate the risk for brain contusion or diffuse axonal injury if $a_{eff}^{2.5}T$ is sufficient. What represents a sufficient violence to cause brain injury has been the subject of considerable research and reasonable means are available to assess head injury risks in laboratory tests. This understanding is based on evaluations of human volunteers, crash tests dummies, mathematical simulations, and crash victims (2–9).

This chapter summarizes the current understandings of the biomechanics of brain injury. The key biomechanical responses are actually more complex than merely the a_{eff} and duration of a head impact. They involve the triaxial or 3-dimensional, translational (A_x, A_y, and A_z), and rotational (α_x, α_y, and α_z) acceleration of the head, which provides a complete description of the head dynamics in an impact. Head acceleration is usually reported as the resultant translational acceleration from the triaxial acceleration of the head in 3 orthogonal directions (fore–aft, x or [AP]; up–down, z or [SI]; and left–right, y or [LR]) measured at the center of gravity (CG) of the head. Acceleration is measured in units of m/s^2, but is commonly reported in g, where the measured acceleration is normalized by the acceleration of gravity ($1\,g = 9.8\,m/s^2$). When integrated, the accelerations determine the change in translational triaxial velocity, when combined gives the resultant change in velocity (ΔV); and angular triaxial velocity, when combined gives the resultant rotational velocity (ω). With double integration, the displacement and rotation of the head is determined. These responses also have triaxial components where the resultant value is usually reported. What do we know about the biomechanics of head responses and brain injuries?

HEAD ACCELERATIONS DURING ACTIVITIES OF DAILY LIVING

Allen et al. (10) evaluated head accelerations in 13 different daily activities of 8 volunteers wearing a tightly fit helmet with 3 biaxial accelerometers attached to determine the triaxial responses of the head in the x, y, and z directions. Figure 10-1 summarizes the peak resultant accelerations in 7 of the activities, including sitting in a chair, coughing, sneezing, and a slap on the back. These activities involved peak accelerations of 2.5–4.1 g. Hopping off a step involved 8.1 g. The highest head accelerations occurred by plopping in a chair with responses up to 10.5 g. Ng et al. (11) evaluated 7 daily activities with a biteplate in 18 volunteer's mouth to measure head accelerations. They reported the average, standard deviation, and peak head accelerations. Walking at 1.3 m/s (2.9 mph) involved 0.71 ± 0.13 g head accelerations, and running at 2.7 m/s (6.0 mph) involved 1.70 ± 0.35 g. The highest responses occurred with a vertical leap at 4.8 ± 2.2 g and a jump off a step at 3.3 ± 0.9 g with peak accelerations of 9.5 and 5.0 g, paralleling the earlier data from Allen et al. (10) with peaks of 10.5 g.

Funk et al. (12) extended the information of head accelerations during daily activities by adding drops from heights of 5–10 cm, tipping a chair 5–15 cm, and jumps of 30–90 cm. These activities involved average head accelerations of 3.9–6.4 g with peaks of 5.7–10 g measured by an instrumented biteplate used by 20 volunteers. They tested a plop on a chair and found 3.7 ± 2.1 g with peaks up to 12 g. The 3 different series of volunteer tests demonstrate head accelerations of 2–6 g in low-level daily activities up to 6–12 g with more dynamic activities. None of the activities involved muscle pain or brain injury, and all activities were well tolerated by the volunteers.

In vivo movement of the brain has been studied. Bayly et al. (13) measured brain displacements in volunteers exposed to head deceleration in a magnetic resonance imaging machine. The deceleration was obtained by dropping the back of the volunteer's head 2 cm (0.81 in) onto a padded surface. The head accelerations peaked at 2–3 g over 40 milliseconds and were compared to the head acceleration levels when jumping vertically a few inches and landing flat-footed. Strains of 2%–5% were observed in the brain tissue. There was compression in frontal regions and stretching in posterior regions of the brain. The motion appeared to be constrained by structures at the frontal base of the skull. The

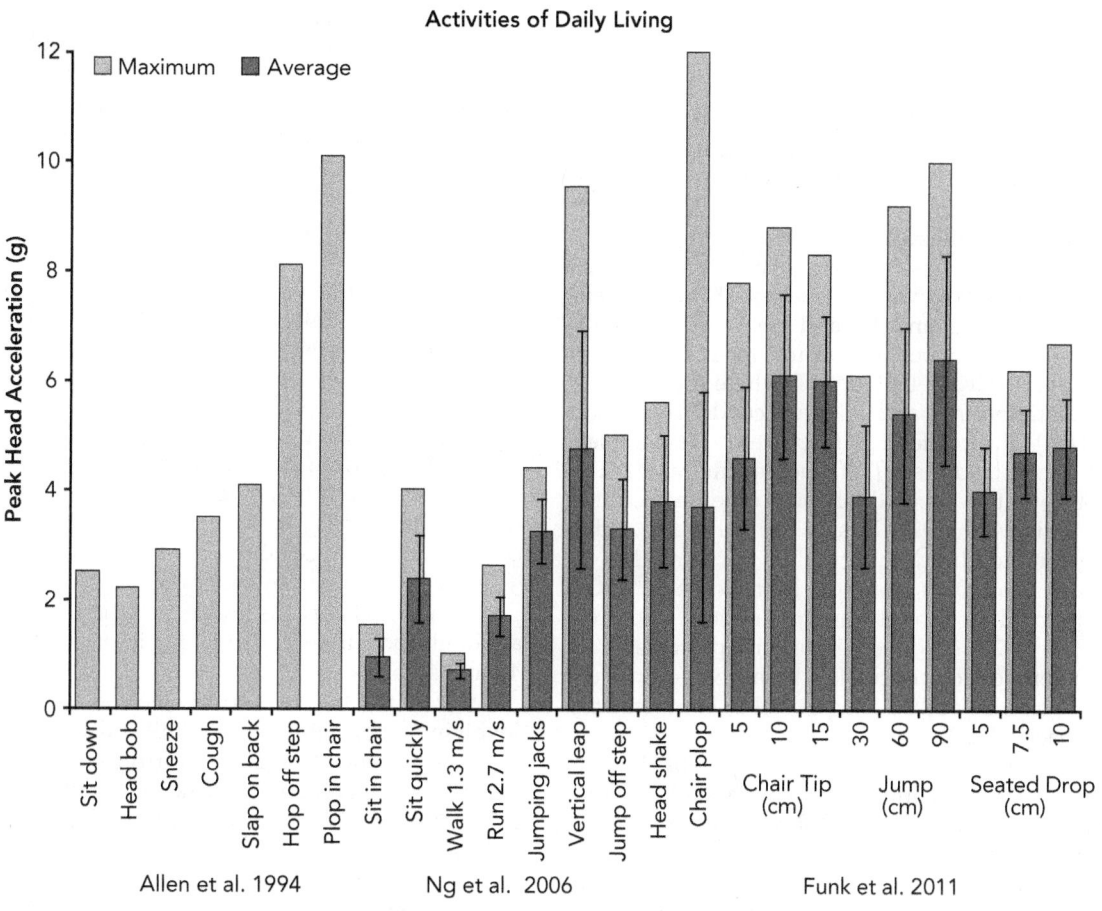

FIGURE 10-1 Head accelerations in activities of daily living.

brain had to pull away from the constraint before it could compress against the occipital bone.

MEASURES OF HEAD INJURY RISK

For head impacts beyond the activities of daily living, there can be risks for brain injury. The assessment of head injury risks has been extensively studied, and there are several comprehensive reviews (4,7,14–24). Lissner et al. (25) developed the Wayne State University (WSU) concussion tolerance curve relating the tolerable effective head acceleration to the impact duration. Gadd (1) showed that $a_{eff}^{2.5}T$ fit the experimental data. In the original work, a_{eff} was the average head acceleration. As laboratory data increased and computational power to collect and analyze data developed, the peak head acceleration (A) and duration (T) became more widely used in the study of head injury. This chapter reports data on peak head acceleration (A). The original Wayne State tolerance curve is redrawn using peak accelerations based on a half-sine fit to the original a_{eff} for a given duration.

The early experimental work emphasized skull fracture, since concussion occurred in 80% of the clinical cases with skull fracture. The tolerance curve was determined from cadaver head drops onto a flat steel plate causing high accelerations of 1–10 milliseconds impact duration (25). The tolerance curve was extended to longer durations by animal experiments with dynamic pressure applied to the brain

causing concussion and similar tests with cadavers (26). Tolerance for acceleration of about 40 milliseconds duration was estimated from human volunteer tests. Stapp (27) originally suggested a 42-g tolerance for long duration exposures. Patrick (28) recommended 80 g.

Gadd (1) was the first to present a time-weighted tolerance for head acceleration based on the WSU concussion tolerance curve and other human tolerance data summarized by Eiband (29). He recommended the severity index (SI), which fit the decreasing tolerance to head acceleration as the duration of the impact increased. SI is determined by integrating the acceleration raised to the 2.5 power:

$$SI = {}^{T}\!\int a(t)^{2.5}\, dt \tag{1}$$

where a(t) is the resultant translational acceleration at the head CG in g, and T is the duration of the acceleration in seconds. SI depended on the time history of the resultant translational acceleration. An SI = 1,000 represented the tolerance level for serious brain injury and skull fracture. The SI function nicely fit the available experimental data on head injury biomechanics.

The National Highway Traffic Safety Administration (NHTSA) adopted a variation of SI for its evaluation of head protection in car crashes. The Head Injury Criterion (HIC) was proposed by Versace (30) and has been in effect since 1975:

$$HIC = \{(t_2 - t_1)[\int_{t_1}^{t_2} a(t)dt / (t_2 - t_1)^{2.5}]\}_{max} \qquad (2)$$

where t_1 and t_2 give the maximum value to the HIC function and a(t) is the resultant translational acceleration of the head CG. HIC essentially searches for the maximum SI over all durations of an impact. In practice, a maximum time limit of T $t_2 - t_1$ 15 or 36 milliseconds is used.

Figure 10-2 summarizes the tolerable head accelerations and impact durations from various sources. The curves represent HIC = 1,000, 700, and 250 and are based on a half-sine acceleration waveshape. The formula for HIC based on a half-sine impact is HIC = $0.4146A^{2.5}T$, where A is the peak resultant acceleration in g and T is in seconds from Chou and Nyquist (31). The 3 different HIC curves represent tolerances for the midsized male (50th percentile male). The HIC_{36} = 1,000 was the accepted tolerance criterion from the issuance by NHTSA in 1975. It is still widely used today to limit long-duration head impacts. This curve reaches an asymptote of 82 g at 40-ms duration. More recently, HIC_{15} = 700 was adopted for shorter duration impacts. The third curve with HIC = 250 is added because it represents a recommended tolerance for concussion based on reconstructions of the National Football League (NFL) game injuries in helmet impacts (32,33).

Mertz and Prasad (34) summarized available biomechanical data on 25 head impact tests with skull fracture and 22 with brain injury. Figure 10-2 shows the average and standard deviation bars for the peak head acceleration and duration with skull fracture and brain injury. These data show the relevance of the short-duration portion of the tolerance curve and involve impacts against nearly rigid surfaces. Skull fracture occurred with HIC of 1,485 ± 743, average accelerations of 176 ± 57 g, and 4.4 ± 2.5 milliseconds dura-

tion. Based on a half-sine fit to the reported HIC and duration, the peak head accelerations were 244 ± 74 g. There were 29 tests without skull fracture with HIC of 846 ± 524, average accelerations of 143 ± 42 g, and duration of 3.5 ± 2.1 milliseconds. The peak head acceleration was 211 ± 62 g based on the half-sine waveshape. Brain injuries occurred with HIC ± 1,218 ± 669, average acceleration of 158 ± 60 g, and 5.3 ± 3.6 milliseconds duration. The peak half-sine acceleration was 225 ± 86 g. There were 21 tests without serious brain injury. The HIC was 970 ± 557, average acceleration 140 ± 43 g and duration 4.5 ± 2.4 milliseconds with a calculated peak acceleration of 200 ± 62 g.

Figure 10-2 also shows the WSU concussion tolerance curve adjusted for half-sine waveforms. The original data was approximated by an effective or average head acceleration and duration. In this variation of the curve, the responses involve a half-sine with a peak head acceleration (A) and duration (T) as shown. For short durations, the WSU concussion tolerance curve and HIC = 1,000 closely fit the skull fracture and brain injury data. For longer duration impacts, the WSU curve is lower than the HIC = 700 or 1,000 although the curves converge for impact durations beyond 40 milliseconds.

When the head is struck, there is complex dynamics involving deformation of the skull and surrounding soft tissues, displacement of the skull from the translational and rotational accelerations of the head impact, and deformation of the brain. The translational accelerations can involve curvilinear motion of the head as the x, y, and z acceleration can cause the head to move in a circular or arcing motion. The rotational acceleration is the angular change of the head about its centroidal axes. A combination of translational and rotational acceleration occurs in any head impact. The historic and current tolerance criteria involve the translational

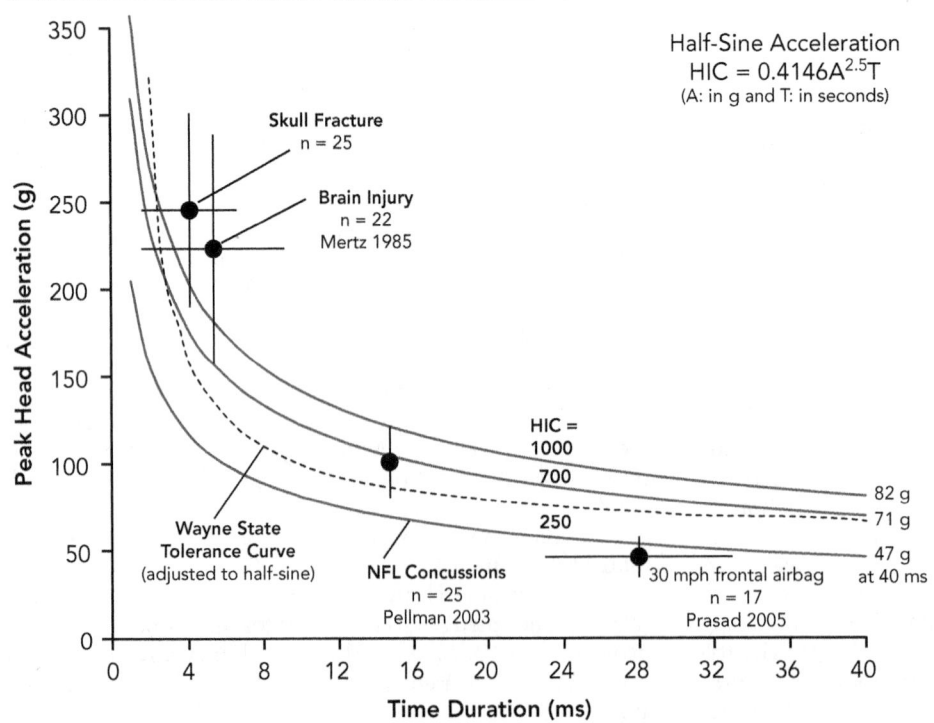

FIGURE 10-2 Tolerable head acceleration vs impact duration, including HIC, the Wayne State tolerance curve, and various biomechanical data on head responses.

acceleration of the head. However, some researchers believe rotational acceleration is an important factor related to brain injury (21,35–39). Various tolerance limits have been proposed, but there is no consensus on an acceptable limit for rotational acceleration.

FRONTAL CRASH TESTING OF VEHICLES

Vehicles equipped with frontal air bags are routinely crash tested to measure responses in instrumented dummies. The data from these tests on head accelerations provides a glimpse of levels occurring in field accidents. Prasad et al. (40) reported on a series of tests conducted by the NHTSA. The tests involved 2003–2004 model year vehicles equipped with advanced driver air bags. Nine different vehicles were tested with dummies in the front outboard seating positions. Figure 10-2 shows the results on the tolerance data and curves. The peak head acceleration was 49 ± 16 g, with a 91 g maximum. The HIC was 208 ± 137 with a maximum of 523. The duration was 28 ± 5 milliseconds based on a half-sine approximation of the measured HIC and peak head acceleration. The crash tests involve head responses that are well lower than the tolerance of $HIC_{36} = 1,000$.

Mertz et al. (41) evaluated driver and right-front passenger HIC in frontal barrier crash tests conducted by Transport Canada and NHTSA to determine brain injury risks. For belted occupants without head contact on the interior in 30-mph barrier crashes, the risk of life-threatening brain injury was <2%. For the more severe NCAP tests at 35 mph, 27% of the drivers and 21% of the passengers had brain injury risks greater than 16% with belt use only. For belts and air bags, the brain injury risk was <7%.

HEAD ACCELERATIONS IN CRASH TESTING WITH HUMAN VOLUNTEERS

Figure 10-3 summarizes peak head accelerations measured in human volunteers subjected to frontal sled tests. Ewing

et al. (42) ran a series of frontal sled tests with military volunteers restrained by seat belts to study head and neck kinematics. The highest severity frontal tests resulted in up to 47.8 g peak head acceleration with an average of 20.7 ± 14.7 g measured on a biteplate in the volunteer's mouth. In 8 of the 18 tests, the peak head acceleration was more than 20 g. Ewing et al. (43) conducted other sled series with volunteers but the exposures were less severe as they studied the effects of chin up (CU) or chin down (CD) and the neck forward (NF) or neck upright (NU) on head–neck kinematics. The highest responses were with the NU and CU. In 13 tests, the average head acceleration was 10.3 ± 2.4 g with a peak of 14.3 g.

The most severe volunteer exposures were run at Southwest Research Institute in San Antonio, Texas during the development of the driver's frontal air bag. Smith et al. (44) reported on head accelerations in 40 volunteer tests from 13 to 30 mph. The sled tests involved an inflating driver air bag. The volunteers were lap-shoulder belted and braced against the steering wheel. For the 27 tests greater than 20 mph, the average peak head acceleration was 42.8 ± 10.0 g with a 71.0 g maximum acceleration. Fifteen of these tests involved peak head accelerations greater than 40 g and none were lower than 20 g. HIC was 243 ± 76 with a maximum of 460. None of the volunteers experienced central nervous system (CNS) effects.

Wagner (45) staged actual crashes with volunteer drivers where head accelerations of 9.1 ± 0.5 g were measured in three 30 mph car-to-car collisions. He also conducted 8 tests with belted volunteers in 15–16 mph frontal sleds, where peak head acceleration were 7.9 ± 1.6 g with a peak of 11 g. Begeman et al. (46) ran university student volunteers in frontal sled tests where head accelerations of about 10 g occurred with lap-shoulder belt restraints.

Figure 10-4 summarizes head accelerations from 7 series of rear sled testing with volunteers. Some of the tests involved male and female volunteers in similar exposures. The early rear impact testing of Severy et al. (47) involved head accelerations of 3–7 g with peaks up to 16.6 g. Seigmund et al. (48,49) ran rear crash tests with 1.1 m/s (2.5 mph) and 2.2 m/s (5 mph) change in velocity of the vehicle. The head responses were reported as components in the x or fore–aft (AP) and the z or up–down (SI) directions. The female responses were slightly higher than those in the males, but the differences were not statistically significant. Linder et al. (50) conducted additional low-speed rear tests and found similar results as Seigmund et al. (48,49). The testing was limited by concerns for neck injuries in the volunteers, so the head responses are conservative and did not involve head injury. The highest responses were found by Szabo et al. (51) with peak head accelerations of 16.6 g.

HEAD ACCELERATIONS IN SPORTS

Figure 10-5 summarizes measurements of head accelerations during different sport activities. Because of the higher levels of head acceleration and dynamics of the activities, more elaborate techniques are required to measure head accelerations at the CG of the head. In some case, the translational and rotational accelerations were measured, giving a more complete picture of the head response. Funk et al. (12)

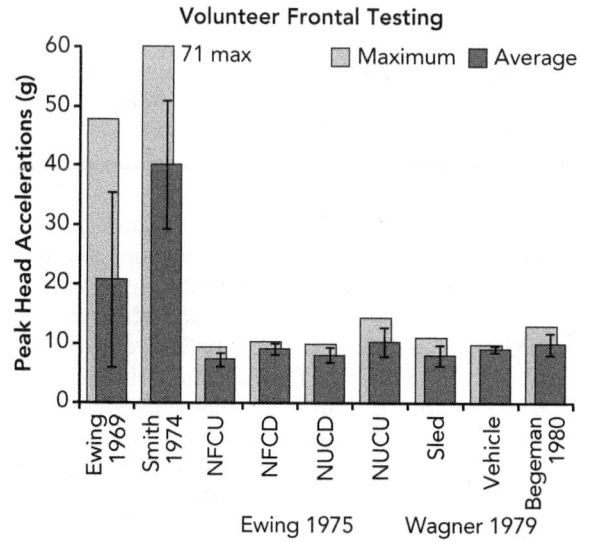

FIGURE 10-3 Head accelerations in human volunteers exposed to frontal crash tests (NF, neck forward; CU, chin up; NU, neck upright; CD, chin down).

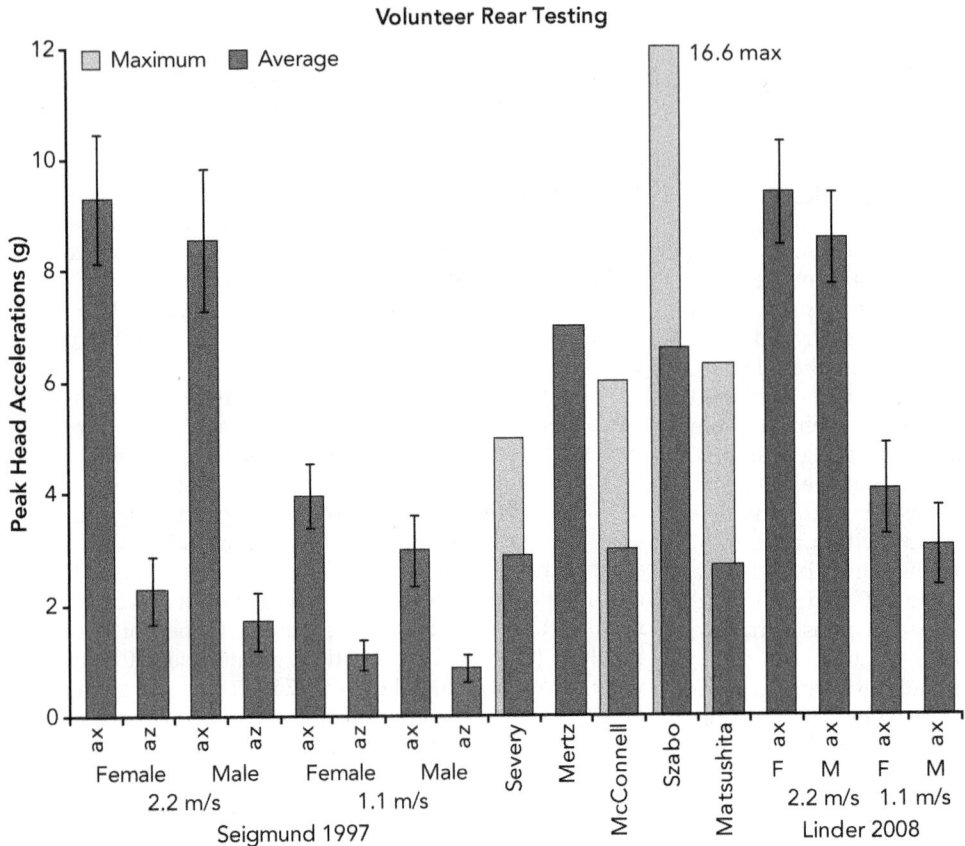

FIGURE 10-4 Head accelerations in human volunteers exposed to rear crash tests.

measured head accelerations with a soccer ball impacts at 5–11.5 m/s (11.2–25.7 mph). The average head accelerations were 10–14 g with peaks greater than 25 g. The average rotational acceleration was 2,000 r/s^2 with peaks approaching 3,000 r/s^2.

Naunheim et al. (52) measure head accelerations in football, hockey, and soccer games using an instrumented helmet and found head accelerations of 29.2 ± 1.0 g in football, 35.0 ± 1.7 g in hockey, and 54.7 ± 4.1 g in soccer. The responses in actual soccer games were higher than in the staged impacts measured by Funk et al. (12) on hockey and football, however, the heading involved impacts to the instrumented helmet, which may influence the accuracy of the reported accelerations. Duma et al. (53) used an instrumented football helmet from Simbex called the head impact telemetry (HIT) system, which uses an accelerometer array pressed against the player's head to calculate head acceleration at the CG. The calculations showed 32 ± 25 g from 3,311 recorded helmet impacts. The rotational acceleration was 2,020 ± 2,042 r/s^2 in one plane.

Pellman et al. (32,33) reported on head accelerations from 31 reconstructed NFL game impacts involving 25 concussions. Head accelerations were measured in the Hybrid III dummy wearing a football helmet experiencing the same impact velocity and head kinematics as found in NFL players. Head impacts causing concussion averaged 98 ± 28 g with a peak of 138 g. The struck players who were not concussed had accelerations of 60 ± 24 g with a peak of 85 g and the player striking the injured player had head accelerations of 56 ± 22 g with a peak of 102 g. None of the striking players was injured in the helmet-to-helmet collision. The

peak rotational accelerations with concussion were 6,432 ± 1,813 r/s^2 with a 9,678 r/s^2 peak. The delta V for with concussion was 15.8 ± 4.2 mph (7.2 ± 1.8 m/s) with a 22.6 mph (10.1 m/s) peak. The rotational velocity was 34.8 ± 15.2 r/s with a 80.9 r/s peak. Biomechanics of the striking and struck player's head has been determined, including features of the head dynamics associated with concussion (54–57). This includes the motion sequence of the head, including rotation about the z and x axes and translation involving deformation of the neck.

Viano et al. (55) measured 4 different punches from 11 Olympic-level boxers weighing 51–130 kg (112–285 lb). The boxers delivered 78 blows to the hybrid III dummy head, including hooks, uppercuts, and straight punches to the forehead and jaw. The hook produced the highest head accelerations of 71.2 ± 32.2 g and 9,306 ± 4,485 r/s^2, but the associated HIC was low at 79 ± 70. The head accelerations were consistent with those causing concussion in NFL impacts, but the HIC was considerably lower with boxing punches because of the shorter duration of the impact.

The boxers delivered punches with a velocity of 24.6 ± 7.6 mph (11.0 ± 3.4 m/s). The punch involved proportionately more rotational than translational acceleration of the head than in football concussion. The punch had a 65-mm effective distance from the head CG compared to 34 mm in football. A smaller radius in football prevents the helmets from sliding off each other in a tackle. Olympic boxers deliver punches with high impact velocity but lower HIC and translational acceleration than in football impacts because of a lower effective mass of the hand at 3.67 ± 0.62 lb (1.67 ±

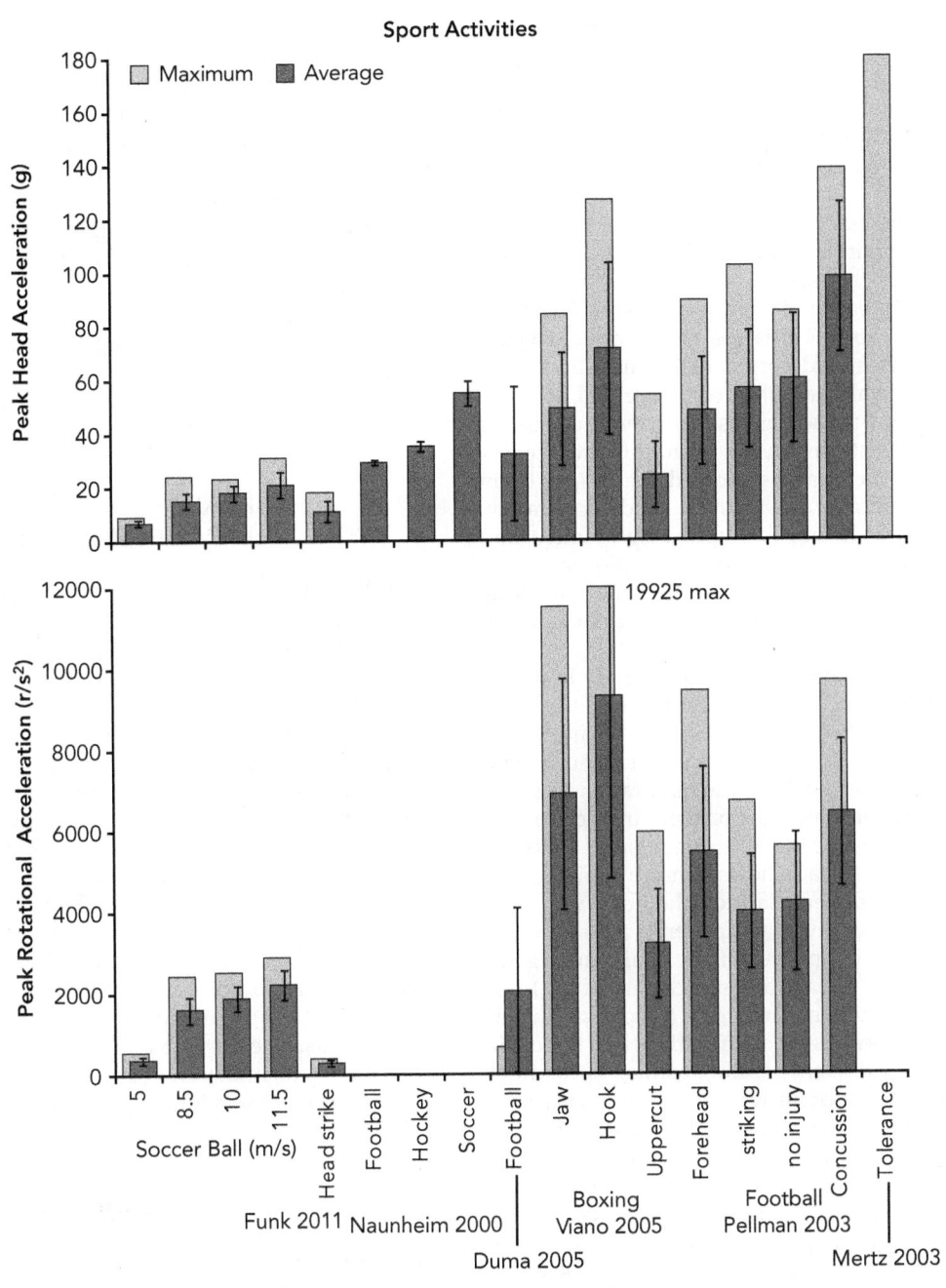

FIGURE 10-5 Head accelerations in sports.

0.28 kg) compared to 30.8 lb (14.0 kg) with the striking player in a football impact to the helmet (54–57).

There are probably 2 means by which boxers deliver concussive blows. The first involves enough translational acceleration. The hook involves a blow to the temple, which is just above the head CG. The forehead punch delivers force frontally above the head CG and the jaw impact applies force below the head CG. These impacts translate the head, and the forces can reach levels consistent with NFL concussions. The second involves rotational acceleration, which occurs with the impacts taking advantage of the offset from the head CG. During the punch, the axis of impact moves away from the head CG and introduces proportionally more rotational acceleration during the punch. The hook, for example,

is thrown with the elbow bent resulting in the axis of impact moving away from the CG during impact and causing rotational acceleration. Analysis of high-speed movies of the punches shows that the lighter weight of the hand causes it to stop on contact with the head.

Viano et al. (54,55) used the WSU finite element model of the brain developed by Zhang et al. (58) to analyze head impacts in football and boxing. The model has fine anatomic detail of the cranium and brain involving more than 300,000 elements. Fifteen different material properties were used representing various brains and surrounding tissues. The model included viscoelastic gray and white brain matter, membranes, ventricles, cranium and facial bones, soft tissues, and slip interface conditions between the brain and dura. The cranium of the finite element model was loaded by the translational and rotational accelerations measured in the Hybrid III dummies from 28 laboratory reconstructions of NFL impacts involving 22 concussions (32,33). Brain responses were determined using a nonlinear, finite element code to simulate the large deformation response of white and gray matter.

With concussion, strain concentration "hot spots" migrated through the brain with time (54). In 9 of 22 concussions, the early strain "hot spots" occurred in the temporal lobe adjacent to the impact and migrated to the far temporal lobe after head acceleration. The largest strains occurred later in the fornix, midbrain, and corpus callosum. The strains correlated with removal from play, cognitive and memory problems, and loss of consciousness; however, dizziness correlated with early strains in the orbital–frontal cortex and temporal lobe. The analysis showed the largest brain deformations occurred after the primary head acceleration. Concussions occurred during the rapid displacement and rotation of the head after peak head acceleration and momentum transfer in helmet impacts. Rotation about the long axis of the neck (eyes right or left) was a consistent factor in injury.

The finite element model was used to study brain responses from a hook punch (55). The brain responses were similar to the patterns of strain hot spots and timing found with football concussions. The strain migrated from the temporal lobes early in the response to the midbrain, where the largest strain occurred late after the primary impact force of the punch. Because most of the NFL concussions involved lateral acceleration of the head, the hook had a similar direction of head loading. Boxers claimed the hook was their knockout blow, but it was hard to deliver in a bout.

The biomechanical responses of the brain during the sport impacts showed a pattern of displacement of the brain and local tissue deformation. The strain (ε) and strain-rate ($\dot{\varepsilon}$) were measures of local tissue deformations and were critical to injury of brain tissue. For slow-loading rates, much more deformation of the brain was required to crush the tissue and cause injury. For high-loading rates, very little deformation of brain tissue was needed to cause either contusions of diffuse axonal injury. Viano and Lovsund (59) found the product of strain and strain-rate ($\varepsilon\dot{\varepsilon}$) was an important biomechanical measure of brain and spinal cord injury, much like the viscous response (VC) was related to soft-tissue injuries of the chest and abdomen (60). The use of finite element modeling offered a means of considering the local effects of a head impact on the complex geometry of the human brain.

Mertz et al. (61) summarized human tolerances for children to adults of different sizes for use in setting limits for the family of Hybrid III dummies. The peak head acceleration was 180 g at the threshold for serious head injury in the mid-sized male (50th percentile male). The threshold represented a 16% risk for serious brain injury or skull fracture. The sport-related head acceleration data indicated a concussion threshold of about 70 g in professional football players.

IMPACTS CAUSING BRAIN INJURY

Table 10-1 summarizes impacts causing brain injury in children to adults based on the tolerable HIC and a half-sine acceleration pulse. Six different size children and 3 adult

sizes are included using the calculations of Chou and Nyquist (31). For example, the mid-sized male (50% M) weighs 172 lb, stands 68.9 in tall, and has a head weight of 10 lb. Using the HIC_{15} tolerance of 700, the allowable peak head acceleration, force, change in head velocity, and impact distance moved by the head CG are listed for impact durations of 3, 5, and up to 20 milliseconds. The peak accelerations fall on the HIC = 700 curve in Figure 10-2. The table includes other information about the head impacts. With a 10 millisecond impact, the peak force is 1,234 lb with a 17.2 mph velocity change of the head and the impact involves 1.52 in of head CG displacement during the loading. The tolerable forces and accelerations decrease with younger children, where the lighter head mass and lower tolerances are factors in the lower tolerable responses.

FEDERAL TESTING FOR HEAD IMPACT PROTECTION

In addition to the NHTSA crash testing of vehicles with the Hybrid III dummy, the safety standard Federal Motor Vehicle Safety Standard (FMVSS) 201 is used to address head impact protection on the upper interior of the vehicle (62). The original standard included impacts on the instrument panel, seatback, glove box, sunvisor, and armrest; but in 1993, NHTSA reported that head impacts with the upper interior of vehicles were the leading cause of fatal head injury for nonejected occupants in motor vehicle crashes.

FMVSS 201 was upgraded in 1995 to include head impacts on upper interior surfaces above the beltline (63). The impact locations were chosen as the most likely head impact areas causing serious injury. The revised test requirements involve a 15 mph head impact using an instrumented head form, which is a modification of the Hybrid III dummy head. The original requirement consisted of an 80 g limit for 3 milliseconds. The current requirement limits the HIC(d) to 1,000 for any 36 millisecond period, where HIC(d) is a variation of HIC that takes into account the lack of neck structures (HIC[d] = 0.754HIC + 166.4).

HEAD INJURY RISKS

The most comprehensive evaluation of head injury risks was conducted by Mertz and Prasad (34,41,64) with further analysis performed on the data by Mertz et al. (61). Head injury risk curves were developed for HIC and peak head acceleration involving skull fracture and/or brain injury. The risks follow a sigmoidal function with increasing HIC or peak head acceleration. For low responses, the risk asymptotically approaches zero. For very high responses, the risk asymptotically approaches 100%. In the transition region, there is a steady increase in risk with increasing response. The risk for head injury can be described by a 2-parameter Logist function relating the response, x, to the risk of injury, p(x), shown by the following equation:

$$p(x)[1 + \exp(\alpha - \beta x]^{-1} \tag{3}$$

where α and β are parameters fitting the biomechanical data to injury risks. For the risk of AIS 4 + F head injury, the biomechanical data on HIC versus injury from the certainty

TABLE 10-1 Tolerable Head Impacts for Different Children Through Adults

Age/Size/Gender	Child Age and Adult Size								
	6 mo	12 mo	18 mo	3 yo	6 yo	10 yo	5%F	50%M	95%M
Body Weight (lb)	17.2	21.3	24.6	31.9	45.9	71.3	102.8	172.0	225.5
Head mass (lb)	4.6	5.5	6.0	6.7	7.7	8.1	8.1	10.0	10.9
Standing Height (in)	26.4	29.4	32.0	37.5	46.0	54.1	59.6	68.9	73.4
Tolerances (Mertz 2003)									
Acceleration (g)	156	154	160	175	189	189	193	180	175
HIC_{15}	377	389	440	568	723	741	779	700	670
Acceleration (g)	Tolerances for Head Injury and Skull Fracture Based on Impact Duration								
3 ms duration	156	158	166	184	202	204	208	200	196
5 ms	127	129	135	150	165	166	170	163	160
10 ms	96	97	102	113	125	126	129	123	121
15 ms	82	83	87	96	106	107	109	105	103
20 ms	73	74	78	86	95	96	98	93	92
Force (lb)									
3 ms duration	724	865	993	1,233	1,550	1,646	1,689	1,998	2,140
5 ms	590	705	809	1,005	1,263	1,342	1,377	1,629	1,744
10 ms	447	535	613	762	957	1,017	1,043	1,234	1,322
15 ms	380	455	522	648	814	865	887	1,050	1,124
20 ms	339	405	465	577	725	771	791	935	1,002
Velocity change (mph)									
3 ms duration	6.5	6.6	7.0	7.7	8.5	8.6	8.7	8.4	8.2
5 ms	8.9	9.0	9.4	10.5	11.5	11.6	11.9	11.4	11.2
10 ms	13.5	13.6	14.3	15.9	17.5	17.6	18.0	17.2	16.9
15 ms	17.2	17.4	18.3	20.2	22.3	22.5	23.0	22.0	21.6
20 ms	20.4	20.7	21.7	24.0	26.5	26.7	27.3	26.1	25.7
Displacement (in)									
3 ms duration	0.17	0.17	0.18	0.20	0.22	0.23	0.23	0.22	0.22
5 ms	0.39	0.40	0.42	0.46	0.51	0.51	0.52	0.50	0.49
10 ms	1.18	1.20	1.26	1.40	1.54	1.55	1.58	1.52	1.49
15 ms	2.27	2.29	2.41	2.67	2.94	2.97	3.03	2.90	2.85
20 ms	3.59	3.63	3.82	4.23	4.66	4.70	4.80	4.60	4.52

groups of Mertz et al. (41) involve $\alpha = 5.45701$ and $\beta = 0.00380$. This gives a 16% risk for severe brain injury with HIC = 1,000 and 56% risk with HIC = 1,500. The risk for skull fracture vs peak head acceleration involves $\alpha = 7.35989$ and $\beta = 0.026850$. This gives a 7% risk for skull fracture with A = 180 g and 67% risk with A = 300.

Khalil and Viano (65) summarized 16 studies on the variation in skull fracture force vs the effective area of head contact. Most of the biomechanical data involves head drops on rigid surfaces, so most information in the 0.2–1.2 in² area of contact. Figure 10-6 summarizes the finding that the tolerable impact load to the frontal bone increases with contact area. The fracture force depends on contact area with F = 608(Area + 1.70), R = 0.74. The linear fit is plotted with the ± 95% confidence interval (CI) for skull fracture, where the force is in lb and area in in². The clustering of data at the lower contact areas is consistent with the findings of Hodgson and Thomas (5) that in order to produce skull fracture or concussion, the duration of the effective part of the impact must be less than 15 milliseconds in duration. The shortest duration impacts involve relatively stiff contact surfaces and relatively small contact areas as the skin and skull deform.

Yoganandan et al. (66) conducted 6 static and 6 dynamic head impacts with a 48-mm (1.89 in) radius anvil. Skull frac-

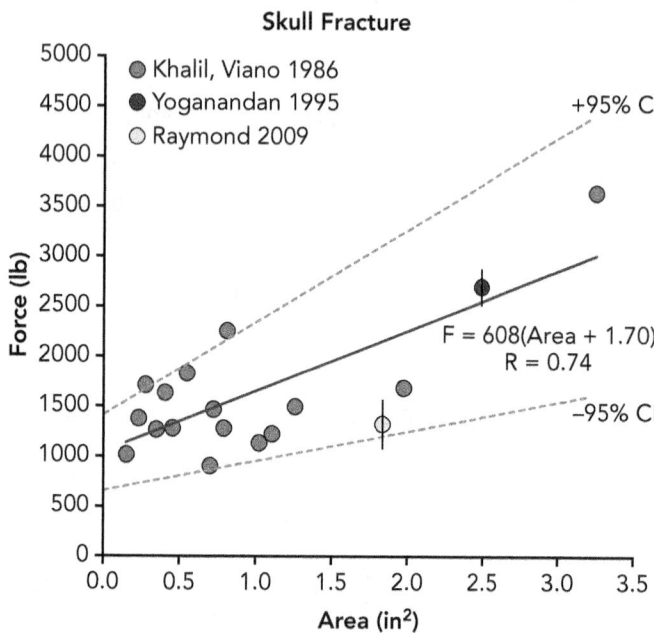

FIGURE 10-6 Skull fracture force vs the effective contact area with head impacts.

Yoganandan and Pintar (67) reviewed test data on temporoparietal skull fractures and compared them to frontal bone fractures. They found the fracture data overlapped with a tendency for lower tolerance to loads on the side of the skull. Gurdjian (3,4) showed that the stiffness of the side of the skull was less than at the front, indicating more skull deformation occurred on side loading of the head at failure. Raymond et al. (68,69) conducted ballistic impacts at 40–83 mph (18–37 m/s) to the side of the head and found skull fractures occurred at 1,266 ± 471 lb peak force in 7 tests with 0.31 in ± 0.13 in displacement and 562 ± 260 g peak head acceleration. The fracture loads are shown in Figure 10-6. No fracture occurred in 7 other tests with 862 ± 274 lb peak force, 0.37 in ± 0.07 in displacement and 334 ± 144 g.

HEAD INJURY RISKS IN MOTOR VEHICLE CAR CRASHES

Figure 10-7 shows the risk for serious (AIS 3+) head injury in motor vehicle crashes based on a study by Parenteau and Viano (70). It summarizes 15 years of accident data from the 1993 to the 2008 National Automotive Sampling System Crashworthiness Data System (NASS-CDS) (www.nhtsa .gov) for front outboard-seated occupants by the type of crash and seat belt use. The largest fraction of head injuries occur in side impacts (40%) and rollovers (32%) with only 3% occurring in rear impacts. The greatest risk for head injury is with unbelted occupants. The risk is highest in rollovers (20.0%) followed by side impacts (14.2%). It is lowest in frontal crashes (3.4%). Seat belt use significantly reduces the risk for serious head injury. The effectiveness is greatest in rear impacts and gives a 95% reduction in head injury risk. Seat belt use is effective in all crashes. The lowest risk for head injury is with belted occupants in rear impacts (0.28%). This indicated only 1 occupant out of 360 involved in rear impacts experiences serious head injury when lap-shoulder belted.

ture occurred at 2,683 ± 199 lb, with a displacement of 0.228 ± 0.039 in in dynamic impacts at 16.8 ± 0.8 mph (7.5 ± 0.4 m/s). Based on the hemispherical shape of the anvil and the peak displacement, the average contact area was 2.5 in² at fracture. The impact data fits nicely on the analysis of earlier cadaver testing shown in Figure 10-6. In contrast, the static tests involved skull fractures with lower loads and more displacement of the anvil. The fracture load was 1,438 ± 255 lb with a displacement of 0.472 in ± 0.063 in and 4.9 in² area of contact at fracture. The fracture load was 46.4% lower with static loading. This demonstrates the dynamic strength of skull structures is significantly greater during head impact than the static strength. A slow, crushing force involved more skull deformation at fracture.

Much is known about the biomechanics of brain injury, but more information is needed on the role of translational and rotational accelerations in the rapid movement of the

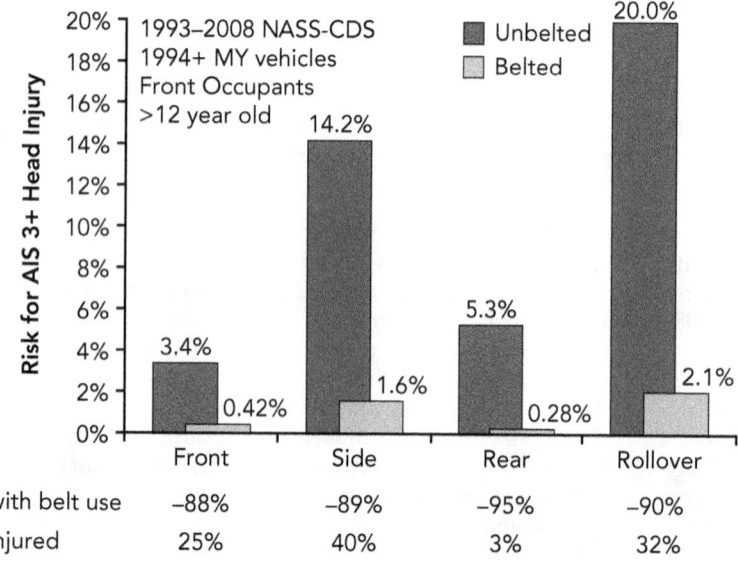

FIGURE 10-7 Risk for serious head injury (AIS 3+) in motor vehicle car crashes.

head and production of concussion and more severe brain injury. The available information summarized in this chapter provides a basis for future research to build on in an effort to reduce head impact injuries.

WEARABLE TECHNOLOGIES TO MEASURE HEAD ACCELERATIONS

There are several technologies that can be worn to measure head impact acceleration. One is the HIT, which was developed by Simbex (Lebanon, NH) using an instrumented helmet worn in football practices and games (71). HIT uses accelerometers mounted in the helmet and held against the head using spring pads. The spring pads were designed to maintain contact with the head and couple the accelerometers to the head. This is intended to decouple head acceleration from helmet acceleration. Once an impact occurs, data is time-stamped and transmitted to the sideline using a wireless link to a computer for each impact above a selected threshold.

Although the HIT technology offers an opportunity to measure on-field impacts to the head, there remains a need to make sure the technology is accurate. Linear impact tests were conducted with the Hybrid III wearing an HIT-instrumented football helmet following the established methods (32,33,72,73). Table 10-2 shows 68 tests at velocities of 5.0–11.2 m/s. Figure 10-8 shows the impacts at 3 locations on the shell (B, C, and D) and 3 on the face mask (A, A′, and A″). The head acceleration from the Hybrid III was considered the "gold standard" to compare with the HIT measurement.

Table 10-2 summarizes the average difference between the 2 measurements and the average absolute difference. Very large differences were found for the face mask impacts. The B impact condition is on the front corner of the helmet shell attachment to the face mask. Peak head acceleration was 10% higher on average with HIT than the Hybrid III

but the average absolute difference was 16% for B impacts. The differences were larger for HIC_{15}.

Based on the analysis of NFL game impacts (32,33), impacts on the face mask represented 29.3% with another 30.5% on the face mask attachment to the helmet shell. In total 59.8% of impacts were to the front half of the helmet. The evaluation of HIT shows some impacts involve very large errors from what is measured by the Hybrid III. This supports the conclusion that for any given game impact, the reported head acceleration from HIT cannot be considered accurate.

Broglio et al. (74) reported on a high school football impact causing C6 fracture and showed head accelerations from the Simbex HIT system, which has accelerometers installed in the football helmet. There are several reasons the acceleration shown is inconsistent with what is known about head impacts causing compression fractures of the neck. The most authoritative study of neck compression injuries in football with head-first impacts into a tackling block was conducted by Mertz et al. (75). They reconstructed 3 injuries to high school football players with the Hybrid III dummy wearing a football helmet and being struck by a padded tackling block. The helmet impacts were at 3.0, 4.1, and 5.2 m/s and resulted in peak head accelerations of 3.9 ± 1.9 g, 18.2 ± 5.8 g, and 42.9 ± 5.6 g and neck compression forces of 2.3 ± 0.8 kN, 4.3 ± 0.4 kN, and 6.6 ± 0.2 kN, respectively. The acceleration traces involved a single peak that rose then fell with 5–7 milliseconds duration. The overall duration of the collision and neck loading was 30–40 milliseconds. The most authoritative study on the head impact velocity to cause flexion-compression injury of the neck was by McElhaney et al. (76). They reported neck fractures occur with head impacts of 3.1–3.8 m/s.

Rowson et al. (77) impacted the crown of a football helmet causing compressive loads in the Hybrid III neck. The low speed impacts caused peak head accelerations of 28.5 ± 3.3 g and lower neck forces of 3.37 ± 0.21 kN. The higher

---

TABLE 10-2 Comparison of HIT and Hybrid III Head Responses in Linear Impact Tests

	SIMBEX HIT COMPARISON WITH THE HYBRID III										ANALYSIS OF NFL GAME IMPACTS		
	NUMBER OF LINEAR IMPACT TESTS						PEAK ACCELERATION		HIC_{15}					
SITE	IMPACT VELOCITY (M/S)				TOTAL	%	% DIFF	% ABS DIFF	% DIFF	% ABS DIFF	%	# CASES	SITE
	5.0	7.4	9.3	11.2									
A″	4	3	3	—	10	14.7%	−182%	182%	−482%	482%	5.2%	9	A″
A′	3	4	2	—	9	13.2%	−186%	186%	−315%	315%	6.3%	11	A′
A	3	3	3	3	12	17.6%	−6%	13%	−9%	93%	17.8%	31	A
											8.6%	15	F
B	3	3	3	3	12	17.6%	−10%	16%	19%	19%	21.8%	38	B, UT
C	3	3	3	3	12	17.6%	−8%	9%	−14%	31%	19.5%	34	C
D	4	3	3	3	13	19.1%	−2%	18%	4%	37%	20.7%	36	D,R
total	20	19	17	12	68	100.0%					100.0 %	174	subtotal
												8	indeterminant
												182	total
	Facemask (A,A′,A″)			31	45.6%						29.3%	51	Facemask (A,A′,A″)
	Facemask-Shell (B)			12	17.6%						30.5%	53	Facemask-Shell (F,B,UT)
	Shell (C,D)			25	36.8%						40.2%	70	Shell (C,D,R)
	subtotal			68	100.0%						100.0 %	174	subtotal

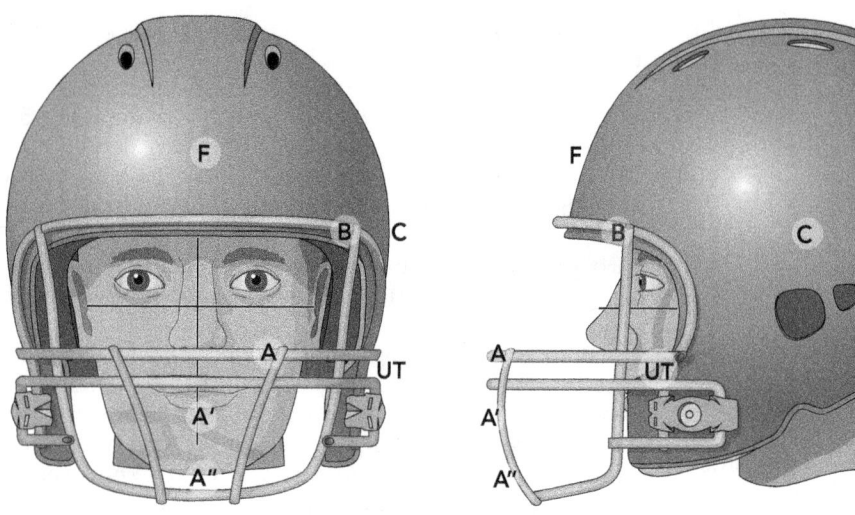

FIGURE 10-8 Impact locations on the facemask and shell (73).

speed tests resulted in 37.8 ± 4.3 g and 4.41 ± 0.27 kN. Viano et al. (56) reconstructed helmet-to-helmet impacts in the NFL. For 27 collisions, the peak head acceleration was 56.1 ± 22.1 g and 3,983 ± 1,402 r/s² in the striking player, resulting in a change in head velocity of 4.1 ± 1.2 m/s and 4.22 ± 1.89 kN upper neck compression (32).

These various studies establish a range of 20–50 g peak head acceleration with crown or frontal crown impacts to the helmet causing sufficient neck load for cervical fractures with the tackler's head into the body of another player. The typical change of velocity of the head is 3–5 m/s with injury. The acceleration trace from the HIT measurement (74) is a 3-peaked waveshape with a peak acceleration of 114 g and duration of about 20 milliseconds. The acceleration trace looks like a resultant acceleration. It was digitized and integrated to determine the change in velocity in the game impact. This resulted in a velocity change of 11.4 m/s (25.5 mph). The video clip from the game collision shows a relatively low-velocity tackle that resulted in the neck fracture. The collision was probably less than 3.6 m/s (8 mph), clearly not 11.4 m/s (25.5 mph). One would not expect an oscillation in the head acceleration for the type and duration of the game impact shown. The literature shows head accelerations with injury are less than half of what is reported by HIT in this injury (73,75,77). The change in velocity cannot be as large as what the helmet instrumentation reports.

Since Broglio et al. (78) describe 16 other instrumented impacts in football games that are typical, but somewhat less severe than this one, it is understandable that they have not found a correlation between HIT head responses and concussion symptoms. However, it is not that a correlation between head accelerations and concussion does not exist; the fundamental principles of biomechanics tell us that it must exist. It seems clear, the HIT data on the injury are not accurate and that HIT is an imprecise measurement technique that does not accurately record accelerations of the head in football.

CONCLUSION

Much is known about the causes and prevention of traumatic brain injury (TBI) after more than 50 years of biomechanics research on head impacts. The HIC standard used by NHTSA has proven successful in reducing serious brain injury to occupants in car crashes. Furthermore, the use of cycling and sport-related helmets has dramatically reduced serious brain injuries in children and young adults. Over the past 10 years, attention has been directed at mild traumatic brain injury (mTBI) and repetitive mild traumatic brain injury (rmTBI), where the underlying mechanisms of injury, long-term effects, and prevention require more research. In the meantime, the reduction of head accelerations and HIC provide a means of reducing forces on the head and risks for brain injury as the complex interaction of translational and rotational acceleration of the head becomes further understood to cause brain injuries of all severities.

KEY CLINICAL POINTS

1. Biomechanical criteria for serious brain injury (TBI) are well known and are related to head acceleration and HIC based on years of volunteer and laboratory testing. These are clinically identifiable bleedings and other observable effects on the brain.
2. The tolerance to TBI is related to the age, size, and physical condition of an individual. Scaling techniques provide a range of tolerable head accelerations and HIC for children through adults for impacts to the front, side, and back of the head.
3. The prevention of TBI is well understood. The use of energy-absorbing padding lowers forces on the head and the risks for brain injury by reducing head acceleration and HIC.
4. Concussion (mTBI) can occur without the loss of consciousness in sports, motor vehicle crashes, and military–police situations. They are subclinical injuries that cannot be visualized by current imaging techniques. Concussion risks can be controlled by reducing head accelerations and HIC.
5. More research is needed on the causes, diagnosis, and prevention of mTBI and rmTBI because of concerns for immediate and long-term effects on the brain.

KEY REFERENCES

1. Mertz HJ, Irwin AL, Prasad P. Biomechanical and scaling bases for frontal and side impact injury assessment reference values. *Stapp Car Crash J.* 2003;47:155–188.
2. Mertz HJ, Prasad P, Nusholtz G. *Head Injury Risk Assessment for Forehead Impacts.* Warrendale, PA: Society of Automotive Engineers; 1996. SAE technical paper 960099.
3. Pellman EJ, Viano DC, Tucker AM, Casson IR, Waeckerle JF. Concussion in professional football: reconstruction of game impacts and injuries. *Neurosurgery.* 2003;53(4): 799–814.
4. Viano DC, Casson IR, Pellman EJ. Concussion in professional football: biomechanics of the struck player—part 14. *Neurosurgery.* 2007;61(2):313–328.

References

1. Gadd CW. Use of a weighted impulse criterion for estimating injury hazard. In: proceedings of the 10th Stapp Car Crash Conference, Society of Automotive Engineers, Paper No. 660793, Warrendale, PA, 1966, pp. 164–174.
2. Gurdjian ES, Webster JE, Lissner HR. Observations on the mechanism of brain concussion, contusion and laceration. *Surg Gynecol Obstet.* 1955;101(6):688–690.
3. Gurdjian ES. *Impact Head Injury: Mechanistic, Clinical, and Preventative Correlations.* Springfield, IL: Thomas; 1975.
4. Gurdjian ES. Re-evaluation of the biomechanics of blunt impact injury of the head. *Surg Gynecol Obstet.* 1975;140(6):845–850.
5. Hodgson VR, Thomas LM. *Effect of Long-Duration Impact on Head. SAE 720956, 16th Stapp Car Crash Conference.* Warrendale, PA: SAE International; 1972.
6. Viano DC, King AI, Melvin JW, Weber K. Injury biomechanics research: an essential element in the prevention of trauma. *J Biomech.* 1989;22(5):403–417.
7. King AI, Viano DC. Mechanics of Head and Neck. In: Bronzino JD, eds. *The Biomedical Engineering Handbook.* Boca Raton, FL: CRC Press, Inc. and IEEE Press; 1995.
8. Goldsmith W, Monson KL. The state of head injury biomechanics: past, present, and future part 2: physical experimentation. *Crit Rev Biomed Eng.* 2005;33(2):105–207.
9. Goldsmith W. The state of head injury biomechanics: past, present, and future: part 1. *Crit Rev Biomed Eng.* 2001;29(5–6):441–600.
10. Allen ME, Weir-Jones I, Motiuk DR, et al. Acceleration perturbations of daily living. A comparison to "whiplash." *Spine.* 1994; 19(11):1285–1290.
11. Ng TP, Bussone WR, Duma SM, Kress TA. Thoracic and lumbar spine accelerations in everyday activities. *Biomed Sci Instrum.* 2006; 42:410–415.
12. Funk JR, Cormier JM, Bain CE, Guzman H, Bonugli E, Manoogian SJ. Head and neck loading in everyday and vigorous activities. *Ann Biomed Eng.* 2011;39(2):766–776.
13. Bayly PV, Cohen TS, Leister EP, Ajo D, Leuthardt EC, Genin GM. Deformation of the human brain induced by mild acceleration. *J Neurotrauma.* 2005;22(8):845–856.
14. Patrick LM, Lissner HR, Gurdjian ES. *Survival by Design-Head Protection. 7th Stapp Car Crash Conference.* Warrendale, PA: Society of Automotive Engineers; 1965.
15. Snyder RG. *State of the Art: Human Impact Tolerance.* Warrendale, PA: SAE International; 1970, updated in 1972. SAE technical paper 700398.
16. Goldsmith W, Ommaya AK. Head and neck injury criteria and tolerance levels. In: Aldman B, Chapon A, eds. *The Biomechanics of Impact Trauma, International Center for Transportation Studies.* New York, NY: Elsevier Science Publisher; 1984:149–190.

17. Society of Automotive Engineers. *Human Tolerance to Impact Conditions as Related to Motor Vehicle Design.* Warrendale, PA: Society of Automotive Engineers; 1986. SAE technical paper J885.
18. Newman JA. Biomechanics of human trauma: head protection. In: Nahum AM, Melvin JW, eds. *Accidental Injury Biomechanics and Prevention.* New York, NY: Spinger-Verlag; 1993:292–310.
19. Newman JA. *Head Injury Criteria in Automotive Crash Testing. SAE 801317, 24th Stapp Car Crash Conference.* Warrendale, PA: SAE International; 1980.
20. Newman JA. *On the Use of the Head Injury Criterion (HIC) in Protective Headgear Evaluation. SAE 751162, 19th Stapp Car Crash Conference.* Warrendale, PA: SAE International; 1975.
21. Ommaya AK, Gennarelli TA. Cerebral concussion and traumatic unconsciousness. Correlation of experimental and clinical observations of blunt head injuries. *Brain.* 1974;97(4):633–654.
22. Ommaya AK, Goldsmith W, Thibault L. Biomechanics and neuropathology of adult and paediatric head injury. *Br J Neurosurg.* 2002; 16(3):220–242.
23. Ommaya AK. Biomechanics of Head Injury: Experimental Aspects. In: Nahum AM, Melvin J, eds. *The Biomechanics of Trauma.* East Norwalk, CT: Appleton-Century-Croft, Prentice-Hall; 1985:245–270.
24. Ommaya AK. Head injury mechanisms and the concept of preventive management: a review and critical synthesis. *J Neurotrauma.* 1995;12(4):527–546.
25. Lissner HR, Lebow M, Evans FG. Experimental studies on the relation between acceleration and intracranial pressure changes in man. *Surg Gynecol Obstet.* 1960;111:329–338.
26. Gurdjian ES, Lissner HR, Evans FG, Patrick LM, Hardy WG. Intracranial pressure and acceleration accompanying head impacts in human cadavers. *Surg Gynecol Obstet.* 1961;113:185–190.
27. Stapp JP. Human tolerance to severe, abrupt deceleration. In: Gauer OH, Zuidema GD, eds. *Gravitational Stress in Aerospace Medicine.* Boston, MA: Little, Brown; 1961:165–188.
28. Patrick LM, Kroell CK, Mertz HJ. *Forces on the Human Body in Simulated Crashes. SAE 650961, Ninth Stapp Car Crash Conference.* Warrendale, PA: SAE International; 1965.
29. Eiband AM. Human tolerance to rapidly applied accelerations: A summary of the literature. In: NASA Memorandum 5-19-59E, National Aeronautics and Space Administration; June, 1959; Washington, DC.
30. Versace J. *A Review of the Severity Index. SAE 710881, 15th Stapp Car Crash Conference.* Warrendale, PA: SAE International; 1971.
31. Chou CC, Nyquist GW. *Analytical Studies of the Head Injury Criterion (HIC).* Warrendale, PA: Society of Automotive Engineers; 1974. SAE technical paper 740082.
32. Pellman EJ, Viano DC, Tucker AM, Casson IR, Waeckerle JF. Concussion in professional football: reconstruction of game impacts and injuries. *Neurosurgery.* 2003;53:799–814.
33. Pellman EJ, Viano DC, Tucker AM, Casson IR. Concussion in professional football: location and direction of helmet impacts—part 2. *Neurosurgery.* 2003;53(6):1328–1341.
34. Mertz HJ, Prasad P. The Position of the United States Delegation to the ISO Working Group 6 on the Use of HIC in the Automotive Environment. In: SAE Government Industry Meeting and Exposition, SAE International, 1985; Warrendale, PA. SAE 851246.
35. Holbourn AHS. Mechanics of head injuries. *Lancet.* 1943;245: 438–441.
36. Ommaya AK. Trauma to the nervous system. *Ann R Coll Surg Engl.* 1966;39(6):317–347.
37. Gennarelli TA, Adams JH, Graham DI. Acceleration induced head injury in the monkey. I. The model, its mechanical and physiological correlates. *Acta Neuropathol Suppl.* 1981;7:23–25.
38. Gennarelli TA, Ommaya AK, Thibault LE. *Comparison of Translational and Rotational Head Motions in Experimental Cerebral Concussions. 15th Stapp Car Crash Conference.* Warrendale, PA: Society of Automotive Engineers;1971.
39. Gennarelli TA, Thibault LE, Adams JH, Graham DI, Thompson CJ, Marcincin RP. Diffuse axonal injury and traumatic coma in the primate. *Ann Neurol.* 1982;12(6):564–574.
40. Prasad AK, Louden AE, Pack R. Evaluation of frontal airbag perfor-

mance. No. 05-0395, ESV Conference, NHTSA, USDOT, 2005. http://www.nhtsa.org/ESV

41. Mertz HJ, Irwin AL, Prasad P. Biomechanical and scaling bases for frontal and side impact injury assessment reference values. *Stapp Car Crash J*. 2003;47:155–188. SAE technical paper 2003-22-0009.

42. Ewing CL, Thomas DJ, Patrick LM, Beeler GW, Smith MJ. *Living Human Dynamic Response to -Gx Impact Acceleration ~ Accelerations Measured on Head and Neck*. 13th Stapp Car Crash Conference. Warrendale, PA: SAE International; 1969. SAE technical paper 690817.

43. Ewing CL, Thomas DJ, Lustick L. *The Effect of the Initial Position of the Head and Neck on the Dynamic Response of the Human Head and Neck to -Gx Impact Acceleration*. Warrendale, PA: Society of Automotive Engineers; 1975. SAE technical paper 751157.

44. Smith GR, Gulash EC, Baker RG. *Human Volunteer and Anthropometric Dummy Tests of General Motors Driver Air Cushion System*. Warrendale, PA: Society of Automotive Engineers; 1974. SAE technical paper 740578.

45. Wagner R. *A 30 mph Front / Rear Crash with Human Test Persons*. 23rd Stapp Car Crash Conference. Warrendale, PA: SAE International; 1979. SAE technical paper 791030.

46. Begeman PC, King AI, Levine RS, Viano DC. *Biodynamic Response of the Musculoskeletal System to Impact Acceleration*. 24th Stapp Car Crash Conference, Warrendale, PA: SAE International; 1980. SAE technical paper 801312.

47. Severy DM, Mathewson JH, Bechtol CO. Controlled automobile rearend collisions, an investigation of related engineering and medical phenomena. *Can Serv Med J*. 1955;11(10):727–759.

48. Siegmund GP, King DJ, Lawrence JM, Wheeler JB, Brault JR, Smith TA. *Head / Neck Kinematic Response of Human Subjects in Low-Speed Rear-End Collisions*. Warrendale, PA: Society of Automotive Engineers; 1997. SAE technical paper 973341.

49. Siegmund GP, Heinrichs BE, Lawrence JM, Philippens MM. *Kinetic and Kinematic Responses of the RID2a, Hybrid III and Human Volunteers in Low-Speed Rear-End Collisions*. Warrendale, PA. Society of Automotive Engineers; 2001. SAE technical paper 2001-22-0011.

50. Linder A, Carlsson A, Svensson MY, Siegmund GP. Dynamic responses of female and male volunteers in rear impacts. *Traffic Inj Prev*. 2008;9(6):592–599.

51. Szabo TJ, Welcher JB, Anderson RD, et al. *Human Occupant Kinematic Response to Low Speed Rear-End Impacts*. Warrendale, PA: Society of Automotive Engineers; 1994. SAE technical paper 940532.

52. Naunheim RS, Standeven J, Richter C, Lewis LM. Comparison of impact data in hockey, football, and soccer. *J Trauma*. 2000;48(5): 938–941.

53. Duma SM, Manoogian SJ, Bussone WR, et al. Analysis of real-time head accelerations in collegiate football players. *Clin J Sport Med*. 2005;15(1):3–8.

54. Viano DC, Casson IR, Pellman EJ, Zhang L, King AI, Yang KH. Concussion in professional football: brain responses by finite element analysis—part 9. *Neurosurgery*. 2005;57(5):891–916.

55. Viano DC, Casson IR, Pellman EJ, et al. Concussion in professional football: comparison with boxing head impacts—part 10. *Neurosurgery*. 2005;57(6):1154–1172.

56. Viano DC, Pellman EJ. Concussion in professional football: biomechanics of the striking player—part 8. *Neurosurgery*. 2005;56(2): 266–280.

57. Viano DC, Casson IR, Pellman EJ. Concussion in professional football: biomechanics of the struck player—part 14. *Neurosurgery*. 2007;61(2):313–328.

58. Zhang L, Yang KH, Dwarampudi R, et al. *Recent Advances in Brain Injury Research: A New Human Head Model Development and Valida-

tion*. Ann Arbor, MI: The Stapp Association; 2001. SAE technical paper 2001-22-0017.

59. Viano DC, Lovsund P. Biomechanics of the brain and spinal cord: analysis of neurophysiological experiments. *Crash Prev Inj Control*. 1999;1(1):35–43.

60. Viano DC, Lau IV. A viscous tolerance criterion for soft tissue injury assessment. *J Biomech*. 1988;21(5):387–399.

61. Mertz HJ, Prasad P, Nusholtz G. *Head Injury Risk Assessment for Forehead Impacts*. Warrendale, PA: Society of Automotive Engineers; 1996. SAE technical paper 960099.

62. Kahane CJ, Tarbet MJ. *HIC test results before and after the 1999–2003 Head Impact Upgrade of FMVSS 201* (Report No. DOT HS 810 739). Washington, DC: National Highway Traffic Safety Administration; 2006.

63. National Highway Traffic Safety Administration. *Final Economic Assessment, FMVSS No. 201, Upper Interior Head Protection*. Washington, DC: Office of Regulatory Analysis, Plans and Policy; 1995.

64. Mertz HJ, Irwin AL. *Brain Injury Risk Assessment of Frontal Crash Test Results*. Warrendale, PA: SAE International; 1994. SAE technical paper 941056.

65. Khalil TB, Viano DC. Finite element analysis of head impact. In: Sances A, Thomas D, eds. *Mechanisms of Head and Spine Trauma*. Goshen, NY: Aloray Publishers. 1986:717–736.

66. Yoganandan N, Pintar FA, Sances A Jr, et al. Biomechanics of skull fracture. *J Neurotrauma*. 1995;12(4):659–668.

67. Yoganandan N, Pintar FA. Biomechanics of temporo-parietal skull fracture. *Clin Biomech*. 2004;19(3):225–239.

68. Raymond D, Crawford G, Van Ee C, Bir C. Development of biomechanical response corridors of the head to blunt ballistic temporo-parietal impact. *J Biomech Eng*. 2009;131(9):094506.

69. Raymond D, Van Ee C, Crawford G, Bir C. Tolerance of the skull to blunt ballistic temporo-parietal impact. *J Biomech*. 2009;42(15): 2479–2485.

70. Parenteau CS, Viano DC. Basilar Skull Fractures by Crash Type and Injury Source. Warrendale, PA: Society of Automotive Engineers; 2011. SAE technical paper 2011-01-1126.

71. Head Impact Telemetry. Simbex Solutions Web site. http://www.simbex.com/HIT_system.htm. Accessed April 16, 2012.

72. Pellman EJ, Viano DC, Withnall C, Shewchenko N, Bir CA, Halstead PD. Concussion in professional football: helmet testing to assess impact performance—part 11. *Neurosurgery*. 2006;58(1): 78–96.

73. Viano DC, Withnall C, Halstead D. Impact performance of modern football helmets. *Ann Biomed Eng*. 2012;40(1):160–174. doi:10.1007/s10439-011-0384-4.

74. Broglio SP, Swartz EE, Crisco JJ, Cantu RC. In vivo biomechanical measurements of a football player's C6 spine fracture. *N Engl J Med*. 2011;365(3):279–281.

75. Mertz HJ, Hodgson VR, Thomas LM, Nyquist GW. An assessment of compressive neck loads under injury producing conditions. *Phys Sportsmed*. 1978;6:95–106.

76. McElhaney JH, Snyder RG, States JD, Gabrielsen MA. *Biomechanical Analysis of Swimming Pool Injuries*. Warrendale, PA: Society of Automotive Engineers; 1979. SAE technical paper 790137, 47-53.

77. Rowson S, McNeely DE, Brolinson PG, Duma SM. Biomechanical Analysis of Football Neck Collars. *Clin J Sport Med*. 2008;18(4): 316–321.

78. Broglio SP, Eckner JT, Surma T, Kutcher JS. Post-concussion cognitive declines and symptomatology are not related to concussion biomechanics in high school football players. *J Neurotrauma*. 2011; 28(10):2061–2068.

Pathobiology of Primary Traumatic Brain Injury

Shoji Yokobori and M. Ross Bullock

INTRODUCTION

Primary brain injury is a principal determinate of prognosis after traumatic brain injury (TBI), although secondary brain damage, which evolves after the primary events following impact, has an additional important influence on outcome. Historically, classification of TBI has been divided into focal and diffuse injury and so-called primary and secondary brain injury.

Primary brain injury (i.e., diffuse axonal injury, vascular tears, focal cortical contusions, intracranial hemorrhage, etc.) results from the forces of impact, and these pathobiological events evolve in the early period after impact. Secondary brain injury occurs when complex pathways are triggered shortly after the impact and continue to evolve and magnify the extent of damage. Examples include ischemia, edema, necrosis, apoptosis, inflammation, seizures, and meningitis. Most TBI treatments are aimed at these complex secondary pathways leading to secondary brain injury. This chapter will review and summarize TBI pathophysiology and pathobiology relating to the primary damage mechanisms for both focal and diffuse primary brain injury. Secondary injury and its treatment will be covered in more detail in Chapter 12.

CLASSIFICATION OF TRAUMATIC BRAIN INJURY: PRIMARY AND SECONDARY, FOCAL AND DIFFUSE

There have been many studies on the classification of TBI (1–4). As mentioned earlier, primary brain injury is caused by the immediate effects of the unavoidable direct mechanical forces occurring at the time of traumatic impact. Both primary and secondary brain injury can be further classified by focal or diffuse mechanisms (Table 11-1). The clinical distinction of focal and diffuse injuries is historically derived from the computed tomography (CT) findings of radiographic mass lesions to diagnose focal injury or the finding of edema, petechial white matter, callosal or upper brainstem hemorrhages, and subarachnoid or intraventricular hemorrhage to support the diagnosis of diffuse injury. This distinction has now evolved to consider the pathological mechanisms imparted by the trauma in regions local to and remote from the focal lesions apparent on neuroimaging. Although these classifications are widely accepted, most TBIs consist of a heterogenous admixture of focal and diffuse damage. Further, some argue that this emphasis on focal vs diffuse injury does not reflect patients' severity of injury satisfactorily (5) and that it does not take adequate account of secondary damage mechanisms. As has been recognized by the Marshall score for CT findings, particularly in severe and moderate TBI, focal and diffuse pathologies both contribute to morbidity (6). The definition and classification of TBI is also important for targeted TBI treatments (7).

Although focal and diffuse pathological process are often intermingled, making it difficult to divide into focal, diffuse, primary, and secondary categories, it is useful to consider them separately for the purpose of understanding pathophysiology and pathobiology (Table 11-1)

PRIMARY DIFFUSE BRAIN INJURY

Diffuse Axonal Injury

The best example of primary diffuse injury is diffuse axonal injury (DAI). DAI was first described by Strich (8) as a clinical pathological syndrome in patients who were unconscious from the time of trauma, with microscopic traumatic axonal damage involving the whole of the brain and without intraparenchymal lesions (9). In a very recent clinical study of 122 patients with diffusion tensor imaging (DTI) data in US military personnel, blast-related TBI was also shown to cause DAI (10).

In DAI, traumatic lesions most commonly affect white matter in areas including brainstem, corpus callosum, basal ganglia, thalamus, and the cerebral hemispheres (Figure 11-1).

DAI is now recognized to typically involve a more progressive response involving a transient traumatically induced disruption of the axonal membrane over 24–48 hours in humans, primarily caused by uncontrolled calcium influx (11) at ion channels near the nodes of Ranvier of axons (Figure 11-2) (12).

The cytoskeletal components of axons include 3 main protein: microtubules, neurofilaments, and microfilaments. After suffering TBI, calcium-related activation of the calpain system results in proteolysis of the cytoskeletal structure and may play an integral role in delayed neuronal degeneration of calpain-mediated spectrin proteolysis (CMSP) (13). In axonal distortion injury, within minutes, there is malalignment and distortion of the cytoskeletal components (14), which leads to loss of microtubules and increased spacing of neurofilaments, especially at the node of Ranvier. In addition

TABLE 11-1 A Neuropathological Classification of Traumatic Brain Injury

	DIFFUSE BRAIN INJURY	FOCAL BRAIN INJURY
Primary brain injury[a]	• Diffuse axonal injury • Petechial white matter hemorrhage with diffuse vascular injury	• Focal cortical contusion • Intracerebral hemorrhage • Extracerebral hemorrhage
Secondary brain injury[b]	• Delayed neuronal injury • Diffuse brain swelling • Diffuse ischemic injury • Diffuse hypoxic injury • Diffuse metabolic dysfunction	• Delayed neuronal injury • Focal brain swelling • Focal ischemic injury • Focal hypoxic injury • Regional metabolic dysfunction

[a]In traumatic brain injury (TBI) cases, several types of injury coexist at the same time—ex nerve and vessel injury or diffuse and focal injury.
[b]These will be covered in more details in Chapter 12 by Kochanek, et al.
Adapted from Povlishock and Katz (5) with permission.

to trauma, the proteolysis of MAP2 (a type of membrane-associated protein contained in microtubules) is also limited by the inhibition of calpain after ischemia (15,16).

These mechanisms induce a subsequent failure of axoplasmic transportation, pooling of intra-axonal contents, and disconnection of the axon from its distal part. This disconnection occurs over 24–72 hours after the traumatic impact and is termed delayed or secondary axotomy. The primary impact thus causes axotomy by secondary biochemical processes, and this phenomenon makes the so-called "retraction ball"—the characteristic signature of DAI on microscopy (see also Figure 11-2). These delayed pathophysiologic processes suggest that DAI might be also characterized as a secondary brain injury.

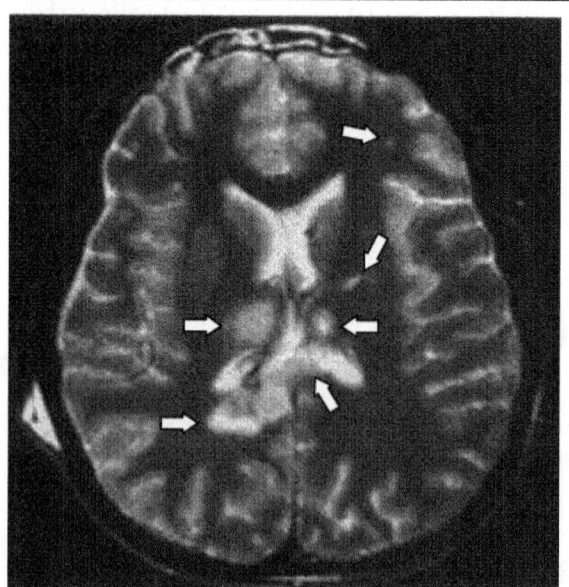

FIGURE 11-1 Typical image of diffuse axonal injury (DAI) in T2-weighted MRI. In DAI patients, traumatic lesions exist in the white matter, brainstem, corpus callosum, basal ganglia, thalamus, and the cerebral hemispheres. This image indicates the small shear lesions (*white arrows*) in the frontal lobe and basal ganglia, including the globus pallidus, bilateral thalamus, corpus callosum, and posterior commissure.

At the molecular level, trauma-inducing calcium influx initiates calpain activation (17–20) and mitochondrial injury/swelling (21) with cytochrome c release and caspase activation (22). This worsens axonal injury and may also cause neuronal death by apoptosis (23). In recent studies of DAI pathophysiology, the mechanical perturbation of integrins, which are transmembrane proteins that couple the cytoskeleton to the intracellular space, was clarified as one of the pathobiological mechanisms in a mild DAI in vitro model (24). This mechanical integrin-related change thus directly influences neural function. Arrest of axonal flow continues to progress to the proximal and distal Wallerian degeneration. Distally, the axon degenerates, fragments disappears within weeks to months, thereby resulting in deafferentation of the affected neuronal fields. The functional influences of this mechanism may include seizures with excitatory electric potentials because of lack of inhibitory effects, spasticity, cognitive and intellectual decline, unmodulated behavior patterns and, in the worst cases, a persistent vegetative state (25,26). When this process is widespread and Wallerian degeneration destroys a great number of neurons, the whole brain becomes atrophic with ventriculomegaly.

Repair/Recovery From Diffuse Axonal Injury and Its Treatment

The injured brain also possesses a robust program for repair and recovery. These mechanisms can be reduced to 3 basic mechanisms: plasticity of intact networks, repair of damaged circuitry, and replacement of lost neurons.

Plasticity occurs when following an injury, goal-directed activity induces neural reorganization, including processes such as unmasking of dormant circuits, synaptic sprouting, and the development of new polysynaptic connections to restore functioning. Plasticity does not always reconstitute neural connections to achieve adequate functional recovery. Neural reorganization may also restrict function as occurs when maladaptive plasticity produces problems, such as a traumatic epileptic focus or neuropathic (27). (See Chapter 68 for more discussion on neuroplasticity.)

DAI can be associated with delayed neuronal damage in a wide area. Neuronal reduction may occur as a result of both rapid necrosis and slow apoptosis (28,29). Although

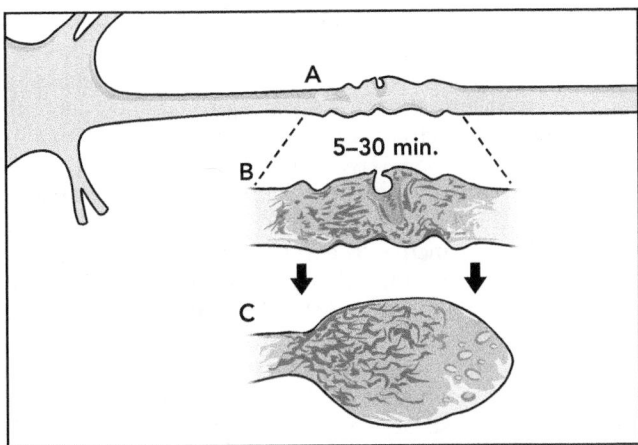 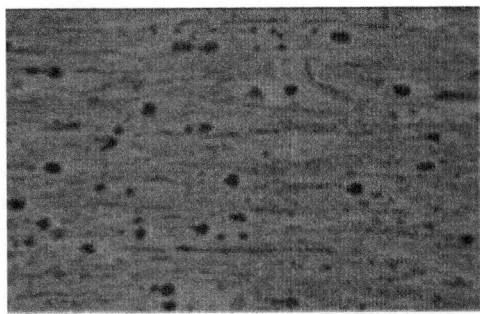

FIGURE 11-2 Microscopic characteristics in diffuse axonal injury (DAI)
A, Schematic illustration that shows the fate of the axon subjected to focal cytoskeletal perturbation. At the site of injury (*A*), traumatically induced neurofilamentous misalignment detectable after a brief period of survival and depicted in this enlargement (*B*) results in focal impairment of axonal transport. The subsequent accumulation of organelles results in formation of a reactive axonal swelling, its continued expansion, and its eventual disconnection (*C*) from the distal segment of the axon, often by 6 hours. **B**, Microscopic image of retraction balls (silver stain × 800). This is the most representative, microscopic feature of DAI. Figure 11-2A reproduced from Povlishock and Christman (12) with permission.

irreversible neuronal damage after primary axotomy was once thought to be inevitable, more recent studies of DAI have demonstrated that neuronal cell death is not inevitable and that, in fact, some neurons and axons exhibit reorganization and repair (30).

Petechial White Matter Hemorrhage With Diffuse Vascular Injury

Mechanical change with shearing force, compression, and tension will cause injuries of blood vessel walls and hemorrhage into the perivascular tissue provided there is sufficient moving blood in the circulatory system. Injury to the intra-axial capillary vessels causes numerous petechial hemorrhages and microhemorrhages (31) (see Figure 11-3). The volume of the hemorrhage in the neural tissue depends greatly on systemic factors such as blood pressure, body temperature (e.g., hyperthermia or hypothermia), hypoxia, coagulation factor changes, age, alcohol intoxication, effects of medications, or substance abuse.(e.g., cocaine).

PRIMARY FOCAL BRAIN INJURY

Focal brain injuries usually relate to tissue strains at sites of contact of the brain against the cranial coverings, particularly the more confining ridges of the anterior and middle cranial fossa against the anterior and inferior surfaces of the frontal and temporal lobes. Focal brain injury may also occur at points of impact with or without fracture, although depressed, compound fractures add to the chance of brain contusion and laceration. This type of injury very frequently occurs in combination with diffuse brain injury described previously when the rapidly decelerating brain is displaced within the skull. In some instances, focal brain injuries result from a stationary cranium being struck by moving objects with relatively small mass such as sticks, baseball bats, or

golf clubs. In such cases, the impact of focal brain injury do not usually cause prolonged coma but might cause focal damage with consequent neurological deficits related to the area of brain disruption. Impaired consciousness and other clinical effects related to damage apart from primary focal lesions may occur because of the delayed consequences of

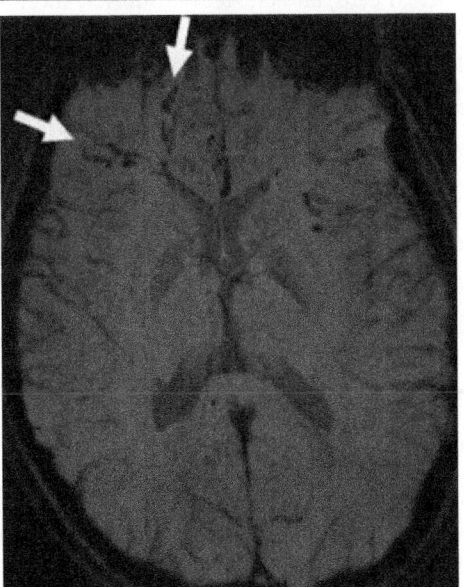

FIGURE 11-3 SWI (susceptibility-weighted image) of a 17-year-old girl 10 days after injury caused by a traffic accident. SWI, which uses a fully flow compensated, long echo, gradient echo scan to acquire images, is one of the most sensitive methods to detect microbleeding because it can identify susceptibility differences between tissues. On SWI, small hemorrhagic lesions are visualized as low signals in the white matter. SWI shows convergent-type hemorrhage in the right frontal lobe (*arrows*). Reproduced from Iwamura et al. (31) with permission.

cerebral contusion or intracranial hematoma, such as swelling, brain herniation, and a variety of secondary injury processes.

Focal Cortical Contusion

Focal cortical contusion is usually caused by shearing forces, which injure the blood vessels (arteries, veins, and large capillaries) and other structures of the parenchyma (neural cells and glial cells). Contusions are usually surface lesions of the cerebrum, but some also include larger hemorrhages in the deeper areas of the cerebrum.

In a usual type of contusion, the glial–pial membrane is intact. Injury of this membrane with tearing of underlying tissue constitutes a brain laceration or "burst lobe." Surface contusion of the cerebrum may vary from microhemorrhages visible only under the microscope to confluent hemorrhagic necrotic lesions extending through the cortex into the subcortical white matter. Contusions on the surface of the cerebrum injure the gyri and are usually associated with subarachnoid hemorrhages either focally or diffusely over the hemisphere.

Contusions often progress within hours to days with evolving events related to the interplay of hemorrhage, vasogenic edema, and ischemic necrosis. In the first 24 hours, contused brain tissue biopsies show an inflammatory response, which is predominantly intravascular and consists of vascular margination of polymorphonuclear leukocytes. Extravascular polymorphonuclear leukocytes can be demonstrated in injured brain tissue only a few minutes after TBI. Within 3–5 days, the inflammation is in the parenchyma and consists of reactive microglia monocyte/macrophages, polymorphonuclear cells, and cluster of differentiation (CD8) and CD4 T cells (32) relating with further neuronal swelling. Inflammatory cells also produce free radicals and cytokines, such as tumor necrosis factor α (TNF-α) and interleukin-1β

(IL-1β)—mediator of blood–brain barrier injury that leads to brain swelling and induce DNA fragmentation in oligodendrocytes (33) and neurons.

Several reports have also provided evidence that, in addition to necrosis, apoptosis also occurs with human cerebral contusions (23,34). Apoptosis, necrosis, and autophagy are different mechanisms leading to secondary tissue destruction (Figure 11-4 , see also Chapter 12). In living neurons after TBI, increased expression of the antiapoptotic protein B-cell lymphoma 2 (Bcl-2), which works in the intrinsic pathway of apoptotic mechanism, has been observed (Figure 11-5). Bcl-2 proteins might take part in the control of cell death and living with regulating the release of mitochondrial cytochrome c, which is involved in the activation of caspases, such as caspase-3, which cleaves substrates associated with DNA damage and repair, including DNA fragmentation factor (DFF45/40), poly adenosine diphosphate (ADP)-ribose polymerase (PARP), and the cytoskeletal proteins actin and laminin (Figure 11-5). (For more details, see Chapter 12.)

As with ischemic injury, a cerebral contusion may have a characteristic necrotic core and a perilesional penumbral zone. In addition, any insult below the threshold to induce necrosis may progress to apoptosis (35). Moreover, terminal deoxynucleotidyl transferase deoxyuridine triphosphate (dUTP) nick end labeling (TUNEL) staining documented a direct relationship between the number of apoptotic cells and the duration of ischemia (36). Therapy might be directed toward antiapoptotic strategies for mild-to-moderate ischemic damage and antinecrotic strategies for more severe and prolonged ischemic insults. Apoptosis exhibits a window of opportunity to reverse the harmful effects of the perilesional area.

Focal contusions are associated with increased metabolic activity in the surrounding tissues. In the rat fluid percussion model study, increase in glucose metabolism occurs immediately and is maximally localized to regions of the brain that are maximally deformed by the impact of injury

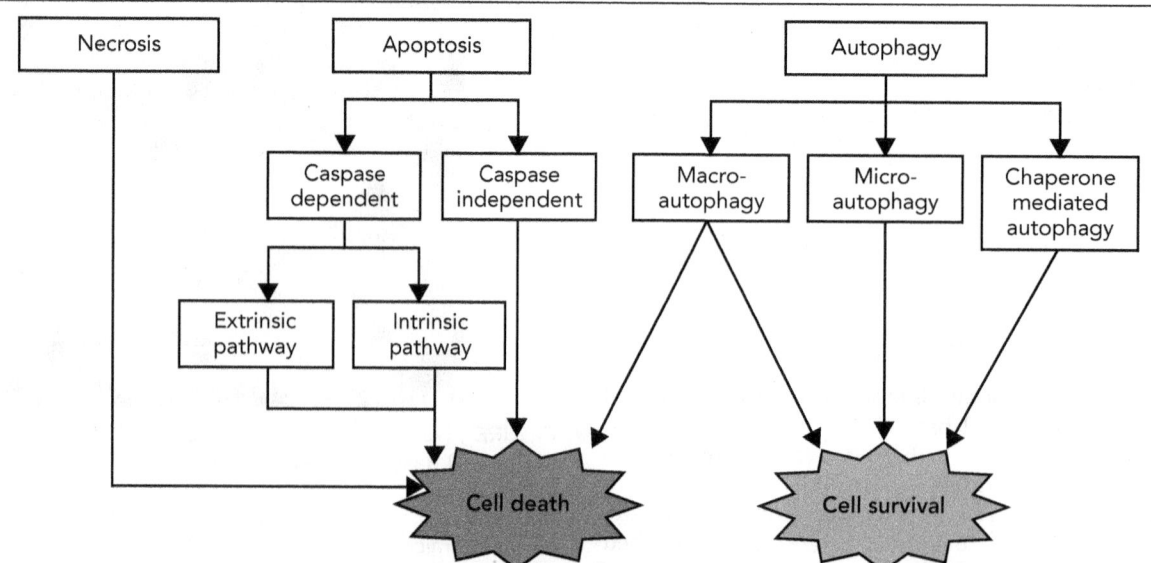

FIGURE 11-4 Overview over the 3 different modes of cell death (necrosis, apoptosis, and autophagy) that can be morphologically distinguished within the cell. Although debated, this classification is now generally accepted. Adapted from *Prog Histochem Cytochem*. 2009;44(1):1–27.

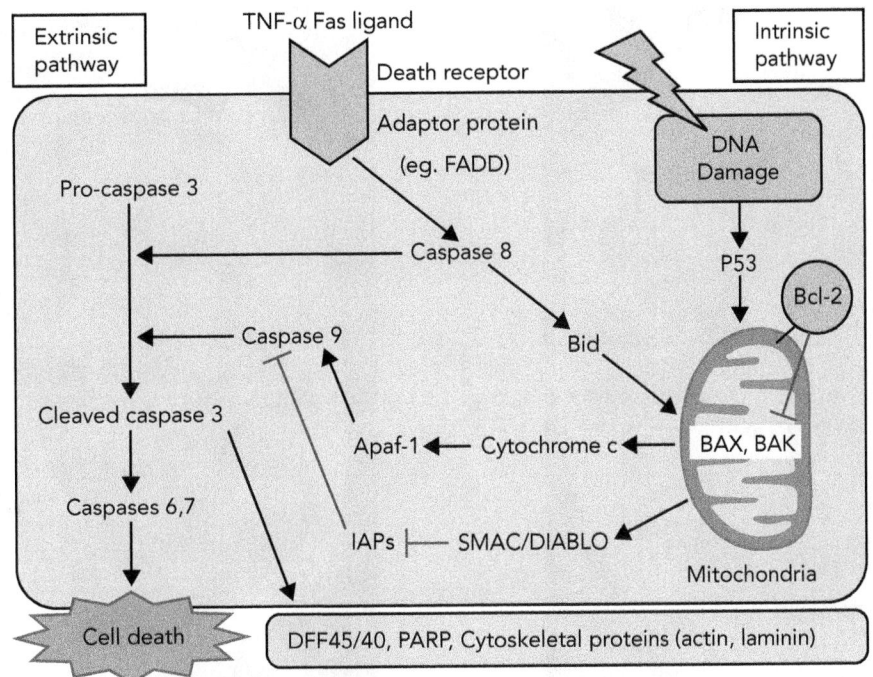

FIGURE 11-5 Extrinsic and intrinsic caspase-dependent apoptotic pathways. Apoptosis can be initiated by external or internal signals that lead to a final common pathway. The extrinsic pathway can be activated when death ligands such as Fas or tumor necrosis factor-α (TNF-α) bind to their corresponding death receptor. On binding of ligand, an adaptor protein such as Fas-associated death domain (FADD) is recruited. This leads to the activation of caspase 8. The intrinsic pathway is initiated by pathologic intracellular processes such as DNA damage or increased levels of proapoptotic proteins, such as Bcl-2 –associated X protein (BAX) or Bcl-2 antagonist killer (BAK) (B-cell lymphoma 2 [Bcl-2] family of proteins). These processes trigger the release of cytochrome c from the mitochondria, which binds and activates actin filament-associated protein 1 (Apaf-1); in turn, Apaf-1 can bind and activate caspase 9. Active caspase 8 or caspase 9 can cleave caspase 3, which triggers apoptosis. For apoptosis to proceed, inhibitor of apoptosis proteins (IAP) must be inactivated. *BID*, Bcl2 interacting protein; *DIABLO*, direct IAP binding protein with low pl; *DFF*, DNA fragmentation factor; *PARP*, poly ADP-ribose polymerase; *P53*, protein 53; *SMAC*, secondary mitochondria-derived activator of caspases.

(37). One study suggested that anaerobic glycolysis occurred as a result of both increased ionic pumping and excessive glutamate release (38). These series of reactions exhaust glucose in extracellular space. In the setting of focal injury (e.g., subdural hematoma, cerebral infarction, or cerebral contusion), glucose exhaustion increases for a longer period in the penumbra around the ischemic core (39,40). In rat experiments, glucose exhaustion persists for 2–4 hours; in human clinical study, it persists for 5–7 days (39,41). In basic and clinical research, the exhaustion of glucose metabolism gradually decreases from several days to weeks after impact (42).

Clinical positron emission tomography (PET) studies also demonstrate that this increase in glucose usage is largest in the penumbra of injured brain and in the hemisphere underlying hematomas when this area of brain is viable (41). These PET studies have clarified that glucose and oxygen metabolisms were decreased for 1–4 weeks after injury (41).

Deep Intracerebral Hemorrhage

Traumatic hematoma defined as intracerebral hemorrhage refers to a lesion 2 cm or larger and not in contact with the brain surface parenchyma. Deep intracerebral hemorrhages are present in 15% of autopsy cases of severe head injury (Figure 11-6). The pathology of intracerebral hemorrhage is caused by the rupture of the intraparenchymal vessels at the moment of impact. Multiple small vessel injuries may result in the combination of many small hemorrhages into a larger deep hemorrhage. Hemorrhage sometimes expands with time, and the speed and range of increase are related to elements such as the size and type of injured vessel, blood pressure, and the bleeding tendency.

The location of traumatic intracerebral hemorrhages and their features are also discussed in several examinations. Boto et al. (43,44) reviewed 37 records of basal ganglia hematoma (BGH) in patients with severe head injury , and they found that BGH is contralateral to the side of impact in 28 cases (76%). Hematoma enlargement over the first few post-traumatic days was found in 65% of the patients in whom control CT scans had been obtained (22 of 34 patients). Their final outcomes were poor: 22 patients (59%) died, 2 (5%) became vegetative, 7 (19%) experienced severe disabilities, and only 6 patients (16%) made a favorable recovery. This data showed that deep traumatic intracerebral hemorrhage including BGH must be one of the feature of poor prognosis in patients with TBIs.

Delayed traumatic intracerebral hemorrhage (DTICH) is one of the problems leading to neurological worsening after TBI, and increases in the size of intracranial hemorrhage has been reported in up to 51% of patients on a repeat

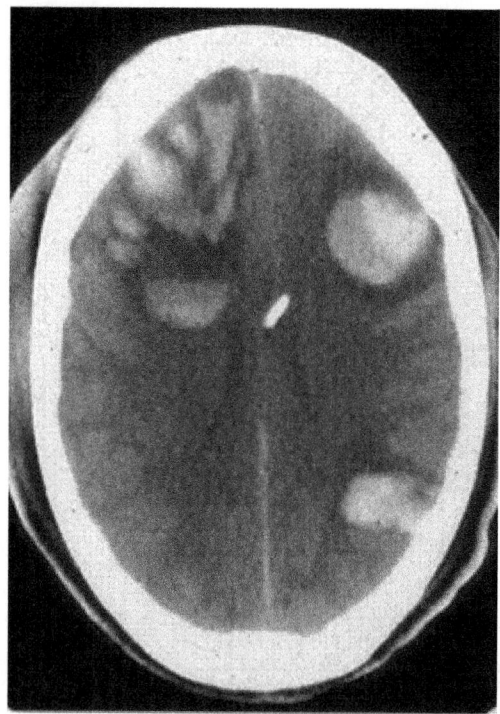

FIGURE 11-6 Multiple cerebral contusion. In patients with cerebral contusion, sometimes contusional hematoma with perifocal edema exists in subcortical, gray–white matter border zone. In some cases, increase in the size of the hematoma and edema cause elevation of intracranial hypertension. This patient with cerebral contusion received a ventricular drainage for the aim of intracranial pressure (ICP) reduction.

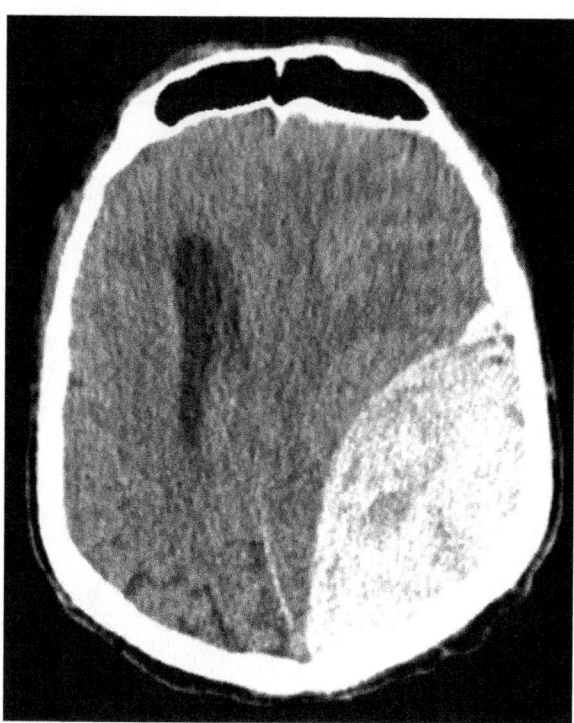

FIGURE 11-7 Epidural hematoma. Epidural hematomas usually present as convex shape because their expansion stops at skull sutures where the dura is attached to the skull tightly. This is sometimes called "lentiform hemorrhage."

CT scan in the first 24 hours (45). DTICH can occur in patients with severe TBI as well as in patients who initially appeared to have relatively less severe injuries. In some cases, new hemorrhage may be discovered days to weeks after suffering head injury. Sometimes angiography is indicated to exclude the possibility of a hemorrhage caused by the rupture of an arteriovenous malformation (AVM) or aneurysm. Several biomarkers of endothelial damage that may lead to DTICH have been proposed, such as a thrombomodulin, which is also located on the surface of the endothelium in the arteries (45).

Extracerebral Hemorrhage

Epidural Hematoma

Epidural hematoma, which is defined as a hematoma in the epidural space (Figure 11-7), occurs in almost 2% of TBI and in up to 15% of severe TBI. The usual pathogenesis of epidural hematoma is the tearing of middle meningeal arteries often associated with skull fracture in adults. The size and severity of epidural hematoma depends on the size of the injured vessels and the degree of adhesion between the dura and the skull. The dura mater of infants is strongly adherent to the developing skull, and the meningeal vessels are not embedded in the skull as in the more mature cranium. Therefore, epidural hematomas are not common in the baby and toddler ages. In the adolescents or younger adults, deformation of the elastic skulls may strip the dura mater from the

bone, without fracturing the bone, and may produce a hemorrhage. In older populations, the meningeal vessels become embedded in the bone and are, therefore, at a greater risk for being damaged with bone trauma than in younger populations.

As with other expanding focal lesions, some patients with epidural hematoma will have a "lucid interval," which is a delay in the onset of unconsciousness.

Subdural Hematoma

Subdural hematomas are usually caused by rupture of the veins that bridge the subdural space where they connect the brain surface of the cerebrum to the superior sagittal sinus (bridging vein).

Because blood can spread freely throughout the subdural space, subdural hematomas tend to cover more of the cerebral hemisphere and are more extensive than extradural hematomas (see Figure 11-8). About 50% of subdural hematomas are arterial in origin, with the hemorrhage stemming from a cortical artery, injured as a part of contusion, or by tearing of adhesions to the overlying dural arachnoid.

The reported mortality of subdural hematoma is from 30% to 90%. Early intervention is critical for larger subdural hematomas that may lead to greater morbidity or death. The timing of operation within 4 hours of injury is sometimes referred to as the "golden time" that provides lower mortality (46). Worse outcome has been correlated with pathological findings of ischemic brain damage in the hemisphere underlying the hematoma. One of the important causes of ischemia is increased intracranial pressure (ICP), which pro-

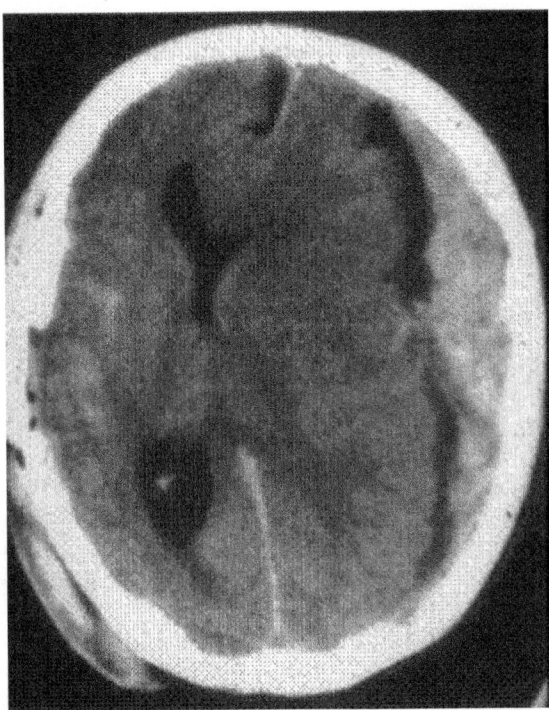

FIGURE 11-8 Acute subdural hematoma (SDH). In SDH, hemorrhage is spreading below the inner layer of the dura (subdural space). A large crescent-shaped clot is the most likely pattern on CT scan.

duces cerebral hypoperfusion. Increased ICP reduces the volume of cerebral blood circulation. Removal of the subdural hematoma may cause the immediate recovery from the global cerebral hypoperfusion preventing further ischemic injury; however, sudden reperfusion may also lead to secondary injury after abrupt reduction of a mass lesion (39,47,48). Thus, removal of the subdural hematoma may be associated with ischemic/reperfusion (I/R) injury (49) (see section on I/R injury subsequently).

Focal Vascular Injury

The cerebral vasculature is more resistant to shear damage than axons. In most significant head injuries, however, focal concentrations of impact developing at the tips of the frontal and temporal poles disrupt these pial surface vessels and induce a focal contusion. In other words, focal injury might be superimposed on diffuse injury (50).

Penetrating injuries also may be caused by missiles or projectiles, which have low mass but strike the cranium with high or very high velocity, or by stab wounds, in which sharp objects moving at low velocity are driven into the cranial cavity. Stab wounds usually damage vascular structures. Delayed conventional or CT angiography are suggested for diagnosis after stab wounds (51). These vascular injuries also may cause traumatic aneurysm formation in larger part of cerebral vessels. These pseudoaneurysms sometimes rupture and may dramatically worsen the prognosis (52,53). Such lesions have recently been demonstrated in 18% of military victims of penetrating TBI (54).

PATHOBIOLOGICAL ASPECT OF SECONDARY BRAIN INJURY

Secondary brain injury arises immediately and continues to evolve after the primary events described in the previous sections. Secondary damage is most often associated with delayed neuronal injury, inflammatory response, brain swelling, microvascular injury, ischemia, hypoxia, metabolic failure, and elevated ICP. However, primary biochemical events, such as ionic flux and microporation, set these processes in motion immediately after suffering injury. (Secondary brain injury will be discussed more fully in Chapter 12.)

Ischemic/Hypoxic Neuronal Damage

The incidence of ischemic brain damage seen at postmortem in patients with severe injuries who die is extremely high, with estimates ranging between 60% and 90% of patients (55). During life, most of these patients do not manifest the long periods of low cerebral perfusion pressure (e.g. <30 mm Hg for 30 minutes or more) that are known to be necessary for the generation of ischemic damage.

Similarly, in animal models of impact-type head injuries, such as fluid percussion, weight drop, and contusional impact, widespread ischemic damage is not seen other than around the periphery of focal contusions. Thus, there is a fundamental paradox, and the high incidence of ischemic brain damage is not easily explained.

Until recently, numerous studies using various cerebral blood flow (CBF) measurement techniques had failed to demonstrate levels of blood flow sufficiently low to cause ischemic neuronal damage. However, tomographic regional blood flow measurements early after severe injury have now clearly demonstrated flow levels <18 mL/100 g/min—sufficient to generate neuronal ischemic necrosis in about 34% of severely injured patients (56–58). These were predominantly patients with fixed dilated pupils, acute subdural hematoma, or early acute brain swelling. Other studies using these same techniques have revealed profound regional flow reductions around intraparenchymal lesions, such as contusions and intracerebral hematomas, where blood flow is about 18 mL/100 g/min (57–59). This is in accordance with the uniform neuropathological observation in humans that pyknotic neuronal degeneration and astrocytic swelling is seen in the tissues surrounding focal contusions (25) and that this develops within a few hours of injury.

In the healthy normally autoregulating brain, cortical flow reduction decreased to levels around 20 mL/100 g/min may be tolerated without functional consequences, although the electroencephalography (EEG) may begin to slow, and the subject may develop anxiety and drowsiness. Abruptly, at around 20 mL/100 g/min, consciousness is lost and the brain loses the capacity to make neurotransmitter substances, therefore coma ensues.

When flow falls below 18 mL/100 g/min, ionic homeostasis becomes jeopardized because the energy-dependent Na^+-/K^+-ATPase (adenosine triphosphatase) pump system, which maintains ionic gradient across the cell wall, cannot function. At this level, neurons move to anaerobic metabolism, and lactate begins to be generated in large amounts. When flow falls further to levels around 10 mL/100 g/min, membrane integrity is lost, massive calcium influx begins, and the biochemical cascade of neuronal destruction becomes irreversible. The ultrastructural hallmarks of this process are mitochondrial swelling and perineuronal astrocytic process vacuolation, followed by swelling of the Golgi apparatus and intracellular cytoplasmic vesicles. Eventually, nuclear definition is lost (55). Many of these postischemic events are synergistic with the loss of ionic homeostasis seen after trauma and can be demonstrated within minutes to hours after injury (Figure 11-9).

Several studies have shown that CBF may be markedly reduced within the first few minutes to hours after severe brain injury in both human and animal models (56,60). In zones of focal cerebral contusion and beneath intracranial hematomas, flow may fall to levels close to or below the thresholds for ischemic brain damage (39,58,61). When there is a concomitant increase in glucose metabolism, cerebral tissue is placed at an increased risk of damage to intracellular structures dependent on continuous oxygen delivery, such as mitrochondria and various enzyme systems. These include, in particular, the enzyme systems that break down free radicals, thus leading to delayed damage in the hours that follow, especially during the reperfusion phase (62–64).

Therefore, the most severely damaged tissue that sustains the greatest magnitude of shearing injury will be unable to restore ionic homeostasis despite of maximally increasing glycolytic activity. If tissue blood flow is reduced during this time of maximal metabolic need, tissue glucose and oxygen levels will fall to subthreshold levels. Tissue swelling will be exacerbated and ischemic necrosis will occur. The vulnerability of brain regions to ischemia varies; hence, the process is not uniform. CBF may be further reduced at the tissue level by such processes as astrocytic swelling and generally by low blood pressure, high ICP (itself generated by cytotoxic swelling) or intracranial hematomas causing distortion. Probably the effects of all these insults may be cumulative and occur to a varying extent in most patients with severe head injury.

This can explain the relative success of therapies such as metabolic suppression using barbiturates or hypothermia or raising cerebral perfusion and CBF by the use of pressors. Diuretics and rheological agents, such as mannitol, may help to improve tissue perfusion during these crucial early periods (65). Ion channel blockade using agents directed at both voltage-dependent and agonist-operated channels may be important avenues for future therapy as may be the use of hemoglobin substitutes, which augment the oxygen carrying capacity of the microcirculation to damaged tissue (66).

Ischemic/Reperfusion Injury

As mentioned previously, recovery from ischemia may induce I/R injury. The processes leading to cellular damage

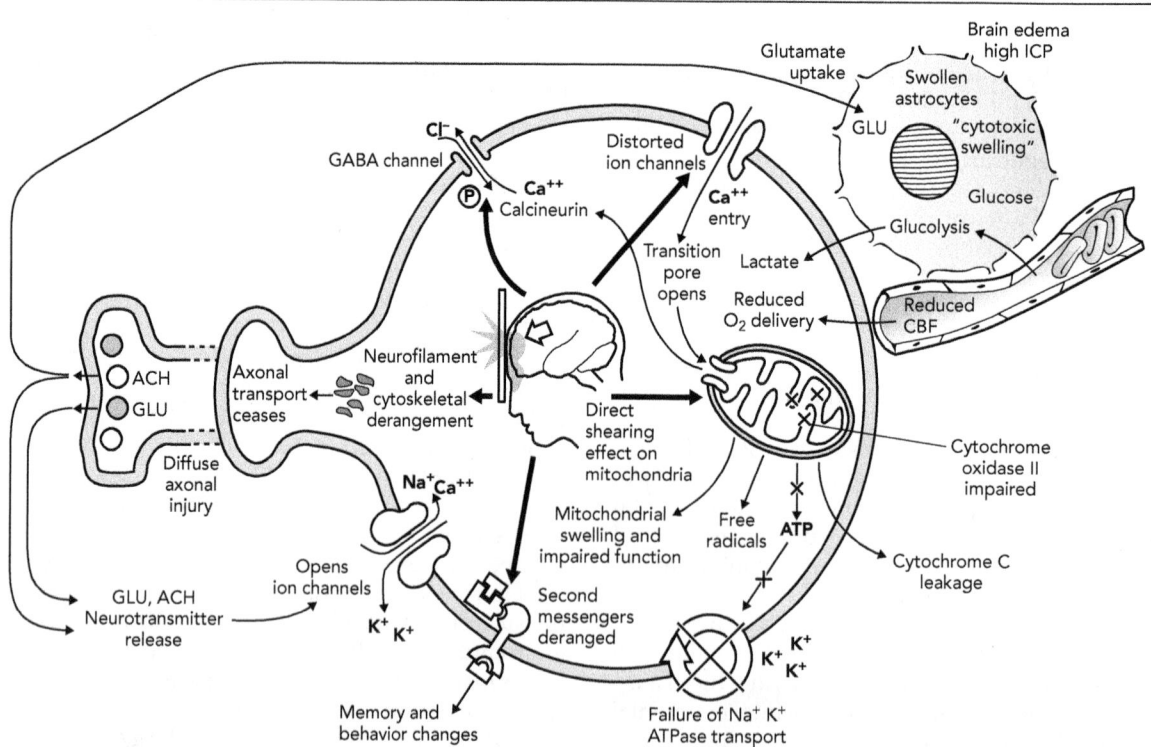

FIGURE 11-9 Neuromembrane events in post-traumatic phase. Neurotransmitter release causes the opening of ion channels and influx of Na^+ and Ca^{++}. The resultant combination of intracellular volume and Ca^{2+} overload induces cell swelling, plasma membrane swelling, necrosis, and apoptosis and leads to the activation of destructive enzymes. ACH, acetylcholine; ATP, adenosine triphosphate; ATPase, adenosine triphophatase; CBF, cerebral blood flow; GABA, gamma-aminobutyric acid; GLU, glutamate; ICP, intracranial pressure; TBI, traumatic brain injury. Reprinted from Bullock R, Nathoo N. Injury and cell function. In: Reilly PL, Bullock R, eds. *Head Injury Pathophysiology and Management.* 2nd ed. London, United Kingdom: Hodder Arnold Publication; 2005.

after I/R injury are complex and multifactorial. At this point, the pathology of I/R injury has been separated into 2 distinct mechanisms. First is the cell death following cellular dysfunction, that is, excitotoxicity, acidotoxicity, and ionic imbalance. This first process is seen primarily very early in the ischemic phase. The second type of early I/R injury comes from free radical production, and this becomes particularly bad during the reperfusion phase (67). Together, these mechanisms create a complicated picture of injury.

In the early ischemic phase, brain ischemia initiates a cascade of destructive and often irreversible processes that destroy brain cells and tissue. One example of this is the intracellular conversion to anaerobic metabolism (68). Depletion of adenosine triphosphate (ATP) in the absence of oxidative metabolism leads to failure of the Na^+-/K^+- ATPase pump. This causes depolarization of the cell membrane leading to activation of voltage-gated calcium channels and an influx of intracellular calcium (69). Moreover, with the anaerobic metabolism induced, intracellular and extracellular acidosis contributes to the calcium influx. This rapid increase in intracellular calcium causes release of large amounts of the excitatory neurotransmitter glutamate, which further stimulates calcium influx in postsynaptic cells (70). Among other things, calcium triggers activation of phospholipase, nitric oxide synthase, proteases, endonucleases, and oxidase enzymes (71). These activated molecules can easily damage other cell proteins and lipid membranes causing necrosis (72). These processes have been shown to be present within minutes to hours after the injury and probably peak at between 4 and 6 hours (69,73). Recent studies have also demonstrated the production of superoxide radicals by N-methyl-D-aspartate (NMDA) receptor-mediated nicotinamide adenine dinucleotide phosphate (NADPH) oxidase activation (74). Such events amplify reactive oxygen species (ROS) production, mitochondrial dysfunction, and proapoptotic protein activation. Intracellular calcium accumulation itself also triggers initiation of mitochondrial dysfunction and fragmentation leading to activation of proapoptotic proteins such as the caspases (75).

Reperfusion to this ischemic tissue results in a short period of excessive free radical production (76). Experimental measurements of the reperfusion phase demonstrate that oxygen- and carbon-centered free radicals peak within 5 minutes of reperfusion (77) and that hydroxyl generation peaks within 15 minutes (78). This oxidative stress can damage proteins, lipids, and DNA, possibly leading to necrosis and apoptosis (79,80). Oxidants also modulate neuroinflammation (73) leading to increased levels of neuronal apoptosis in adjacent cells (81–83). (See also Chapter 12 for additional discussions of ischemic damage.)

CONCLUSION

TBI pathobiology can be classified as primary and secondary, focal and diffuse injury. Almost all the responsible mechanisms are now targeted for the prevention of further secondary brain damage. In this chapter, we summarized the mechanisms of neural tissue damage relating to primary TBI. The mechanisms are heterogeneous, complex, synergistic, and still inadequately understood.

In the near future, bioscience technologies will improve our understanding of the pathobiology of TBI. Future translational research will also give us more innovations in the treatment of TBI, with better prevention of primary injury and therapy to limit the extent of primary and secondary damage. With such efforts, prognosis for severe TBI will almost certainly improve.

KEY CLINICAL POINTS

1. Primary brain injury is caused by the immediate effects of the unavoidable direct mechanical forces occurring at the time of traumatic impact.
2. Secondary brain injury occurs when complex pathways are triggered shortly after the impact and continue to evolve and magnify the extent of damage.
3. Both primary and secondary brain injury can be further classified by focal or diffuse mechanisms.
4. Each type of primary brain injury has their own features relating injury mechanisms, severity, and their prognosis.
5. In DAI, traumatic lesions most commonly affect white matter in areas including brainstem, corpus callosum, basal ganglia, thalamus, and the cerebral hemispheres.
6. Mechanical change with shearing force, compression, and tension will cause injuries of blood vessel walls and hemorrhage.
7. Brain contusions often progress within hours to days with evolving events related to the interplay of hemorrhage, vasogenic edema, and ischemic necrosis.
8. DTICH can occur in patients with severe TBI as well as in patients who initially appeared to have relatively less severe injuries.
9. Some patients with epidural hematoma have a "lucid interval," which is a delay in the onset of unconsciousness.
10. Removal of the subdural hematoma may be associated with I/R injury, which results in a short period of excessive free radical production.

KEY REFERENCES

1. Pellerin L, Magistretti PJ. Glutamate uptake into astrocytes stimulates aerobic glycolysis: a mechanism coupling neuronal activity to glucose utilization. *Proc Natl Acad Sci U S A.* 1994;91(22):10625–10629.
2. Polderman KH. Mechanisms of action, physiological effects, and complications of hypothermia. *Crit Care Med.* 2009;37(7)(suppl):S186–S202.
3. Povlishock JT, Katz DI. Update of neuropathology and neurological recovery after traumatic brain injury. *J Head Trauma Rehabil.* 2005;20(1):76–94.
4. Raghupathi R, Graham DI, McIntosh TK. Apoptosis after traumatic brain injury. *J Neurotrauma.* 2000;17:927–938.
5. Saatman KE, Duhaime AC, Bullock R, Maas AI, Valadka A, Manley GT. Classification of traumatic brain injury for targeted therapies. *J Neurotrauma.* 2008;25(7):719–738.

References

1. Lindenberg R, Freytag E. The mechanism of cerebral contusions. A pathologic-anatomic study. *Arch Pathol.* 1960;69:440–469.
2. Maloney AF, Whatmore WJ. Clinical and pathological observations in fatal head injuries. A 5-year survey of 173 cases. *Br J Surg.* 1969;56(1):23–31.
3. Freytag E. Autopsy findings in head injuries from firearms. Statistical evaluation of 254 cases. *Arch Pathol.* 1963;76:215–225.

4. Adams JH, Graham DI, Scott G, Parker LS, Doyle D. Brain damage in fatal non-missile head injury. *J Clin Pathol*. 1980;33(12): 1132–1145.

5. Povlishock JT, Katz DI. Update of neuropathology and neurological recovery after traumatic brain injury. *J Head Trauma Rehabil*. 2005;20(1):76–94.

6. Marshall LF, Marshall SB, Klauber MR, et al. The diagnosis of head injury requires a classification based on computed axial tomography. *J Neurotrauma*. 1992;9(suppl 1):S287–S292.

7. Saatman KE, Duhaime AC, Bullock R, Maas AI, Valadka A, Manley GT. Classification of traumatic brain injury for targeted therapies. *J Neurotrauma*. 2008;25(7):719–738.

8. Strich SJ. Diffuse degeneration of the cerebral white matter in severe dementia following head injury. *J Neurol Neurosurg Psychiatry*. 1956;19(3):163–185.

9. Gennarelli TA. Mechanisms of brain injury. *J Emerg Med*. 1993; 11(suppl 1):5–11.

10. Mac Donald CL, Johnson AM, Cooper D, et al. Detection of blast-related traumatic brain injury in U.S. military personnel. *N Engl J Med*. 2011;364(22):2091–2100.

11. Pettus EH, Christman CW, Giebel ML, Povlishock JT. Traumatically induced altered membrane permeability: its relationship to traumatically induced reactive axonal change. *J Neurotrauma*. 1994; 11(5):507–522.

12. Povlishock JT, Christman CW. The pathobiology of traumatically induced axonal injury in animals and humans: a review of current thoughts. *J Neurotrauma*. 1995;12(4):555–564.

13. Kampfl A, Posmantur RM, Zhao X, Schmutzhard E, Clifton GL, Hayes RL. Mechanisms of calpain proteolysis following traumatic brain injury: implications for pathology and therapy: implications for pathology and therapy: a review and update. *J Neurotrauma*. 1997;14(3):121–134.

14. Maxwell WL, Povlishock JT, Graham DL. A mechanistic analysis of nondisruptive axonal injury: a review. *J Neurotrauma*. 1997;14(7): 419–440.

15. Inuzuka T, Tamura A, Sato S, Kirino T, Toyoshima I, Miyatake T. Suppressive effect of E-64c on ischemic degradation of cerebral proteins following occlusion of the middle cerebral artery in rats. *Brain Res*. 1990;526(1):177–179.

16. Inuzuka T, Tamura A, Sato S, et al. Changes in the concentrations of cerebral proteins following occlusion of the middle cerebral artery in rats. *Stroke*. 1990;21(6):917–922.

17. Buki A, Siman R, Trojanowski JQ, Povlishock JT. The role of calpain-mediated spectrin proteolysis in traumatically induced axonal injury. *J Neuropathol Exp Neurol*. 1999;58(4):365–375.

18. Shields DC, Schaecher KE, Hogan EL, Banik NL. Calpain activity and expression increased in activated glial and inflammatory cells in penumbra of spinal cord injury lesion. *J Neurosci Res*. 2000;61(2): 146–150.

19. Saatman KE, Creed J, Raghupathi R. Calpain as a therapeutic target in traumatic brain injury. *Neurotherapeutics*. 2010;7(1):31–42.

20. Kilinc D, Gallo G, Barbee KA. Mechanical membrane injury induces axonal beading through localized activation of calpain. *Exp Neurol*. 2009;219(2):553–561.

21. Okonkwo DO, Povlishock JT. An intrathecal bolus of cyclosporin A before injury preserves mitochondrial integrity and attenuates axonal disruption in traumatic brain injury. *J Cereb Blood Flow Metab*. 1999;19(4):443–451.

22. Buki A, Okonkwo DO, Wang KK, Povlishock JT. Cytochrome c release and caspase activation in traumatic axonal injury. *J Neurosci*. 2000;20(8):2825–2834.

23. Raghupathi R. Cell death mechanisms following traumatic brain injury. *Brain Pathol*. 2004;14(2):215–222.

24. Hemphill MA, Dabiri BE, Gabriele S, et al. A possible role for integrin signaling in diffuse axonal injury. *PLoS One*. 2011;6(7):e22899.

25. Adams JH, Doyle D, Ford I, Gennarelli TA, Graham DI, McLellan DR. Diffuse axonal injury in head injury: definition, diagnosis and grading. *Histopathology*. 1989;15(1):49–59.

26. Ding K, Marquez de la Plata C, Wang JY, et al. Cerebral atrophy after traumatic white matter injury: correlation with acute neuroimaging and outcome. *J Neurotrauma*. 2008;25(12):1433–1440.

27. Kwakkel G, Kollen B, Lindeman E. Understanding the pattern of functional recovery after stroke: facts and theories. *Restor Neurol Neurosci*. 2004;22(3–5):281–299.

28. Smith FM, Raghupathi R, MacKinnon MA, et al. TUNEL-positive staining of surface contusions after fatal head injury in man. *Acta Neuropathol*. 2000;100(5):537–545.

29. Clark RS, Kochanek PM, Watkins SC, et al. Caspase-3 mediated neuronal death after traumatic brain injury in rats. *J Neurochem*. 2000;74(2):740–753.

30. Singleton RH, Zhu J, Stone JR, Povlishock JT. Traumatically induced axotomy adjacent to the soma does not result in acute neuronal death. *J Neurosci*. 2002;22(3):791–802.

31. Iwamura A, Taoka T, Fukusumi A, et al. Diffuse vascular injury: convergent-type hemorrhage in the supratentorial white matter on susceptibility-weighted image in cases of severe traumatic brain damage. *Neuroradiology*. 2012;54(4):335–343.

32. Clausen F, Lorant T, Lewén A, Hillered L. T lymphocyte trafficking: a novel target for neuroprotection in traumatic brain injury. *J Neurotrauma*. 2007;24(8):1295–1307.

33. Lu J, Goh SJ, Tng PY, Deng YY, Ling EA, Moochhala S. Systemic inflammatory response following acute traumatic brain injury. *Front Biosci*. 2009;14:3795–3813.

34. Raghupathi R, Graham DI, McIntosh TK. Apoptosis after traumatic brain injury. *J Neurotrauma*. 2000;17(10):927–938.

35. Bonfoco E, Krainc D, Ankarcrona M, Nicotera P, Lipton SA. Apoptosis and necrosis: two distinct events induced, respectively, by mild and intense insults with N-methyl-D-aspartate or nitric oxide/superoxide in cortical cell cultures. *Proc Natl Acad Sci U S A*. 1995;92(16):7162–7166.

36. Li Y, Chopp M, Jiang N, Zhang ZG, Zaloga C. Induction of DNA fragmentation after 10 to 120 minutes of focal cerebral ischemia in rats. *Stroke*. 1995;26(7):1252–1257; discussion 7–8.

37. Kawamata T, Katayama Y, Hovda DA, Yoshino A, Becker DP. Lactate accumulation following concussive brain injury: the role of ionic fluxes induced by excitatory amino acids. *Brain Res*. 1995; 674(2):196–204.

38. Pellerin L, Magistretti PJ. Glutamate uptake into astrocytes stimulates aerobic glycolysis: a mechanism coupling neuronal activity to glucose utilization. *Proc Natl Acad Sci U S A*. 1994;91(22): 10625–10629.

39. Kuroda Y, Bullock R. Local cerebral blood flow mapping before and after removal of acute subdural hematoma in the rat. *Neurosurgery*. 1992;30(5):687–691.

40. Sutton RL, Hovda DA, Adelson PD, Benzel EC, Becker DP. Metabolic changes following cortical contusion: relationships to edema and morphological changes. *Acta Neurochir Suppl (Wien)*. 1994;60: 446–448.

41. Bergsneider M, Hovda DA, Shalmon E, et al. Cerebral hyperglycolysis following severe traumatic brain injury in humans: a positron emission tomography study. *J Neurosurg*. 1997;86(2):241–251.

42. Yoshino A, Hovda DA, Kawamata T, Katayama Y, Becker DP. Dynamic changes in local cerebral glucose utilization following cerebral conclusion in rats: evidence of a hyper- and subsequent hypometabolic state. *Brain Res*. 1991;561(1):106–119.

43. Katz DI, Alexander MP, Seliger GM, Bellas DN. Traumatic basal ganglia hemorrhage: clinicopathologic features and outcome. *Neurology*. 1989;39(7):897–904.

44. Boto GR, Lobato RD, Rivas JJ, Gomez PA, de la Lama A, Lagares A. Basal ganglia hematomas in severely head injured patients: clinicoradiological analysis of 37 cases. *J Neurosurg*. 2001;94(2):224–232.

45. Yokota H, Naoe Y, Nakabayashi M, et al. Cerebral endothelial injury in severe head injury: the significance of measurements of serum thrombomodulin and the von Willebrand factor. *J Neurotrauma*. 2002;19(9):1007–1015.

46. Seelig JM, Becker DP, Miller JD, Greenberg RP, Ward JD, Choi SC. Traumatic acute subdural hematoma: major mortality reduction in comatose patients treated within four hours. *N Engl J Med*. 1981; 304(25):1511–1518.

47. Miller JD, Bullock R, Graham DI, Chen MH, Teasdale GM. Ischemic brain damage in a model of acute subdural hematoma. *Neurosurgery*. 1990;27(3):433–439.

48. Burger R, Bendszus M, Vince GH, Solymosi L, Roosen K. Neurophysiological monitoring, magnetic resonance imaging, and

histological assays confirm the beneficial effects of moderate hypothermia after epidural focal mass lesion development in rodents. *Neurosurgery.* 2004;54(3):701–711; discussion 711–712.

49. Kuroda Y, Fujisawa H, Strebel S, Graham DI, Bullock R. Effect of neuroprotective N-methyl-D-aspartate antagonists on increased intracranial pressure: studies in the rat acute subdural hematoma model. *Neurosurgery.* 1994;35(1):106–112.

50. Kuijpers AH, Claessens MH, Sauren AA. The influence of different boundary conditions on the response of the head to impact: a two-dimensional finite element study. *J Neurotrauma.* 1995;12(4):715–724.

51. du Trevou MD, van Dellen JR. Penetrating stab wounds to the brain: the timing of angiography in patients presenting with the weapon already removed. *Neurosurgery.* 1992;31(5):905–911; discussion 911–912.

52. Risdall JE, Menon DK. Traumatic brain injury. *Philos Trans R Soc Lond B Biol Sci.* 2011;366(1562):241–250.

53. Litvack ZN, Hunt MA, Weinstein JS, West GA. Self-inflicted nail-gun injury with 12 cranial penetrations and associated cerebral trauma. Case report and review of the literature. *J Neurosurg.* 2006;104(5):828–834.

54. Bell RS, Ecker RD, Severson MA III, Wanebo JE, Crandall B, Armonda RA. The evolution of the treatment of traumatic cerebrovascular injury during wartime. *Neurosurg Focus.* 2010;28(5):E5.

55. Graham DI. The pathology of brain ischaemia and possibilities for therapeutic intervention. *Br J Anaesth.* 1985;57(1):3–17.

56. Bouma GJ, Muizelaar JP, Stringer WA, Choi SC, Fatouros P, Young HF. Ultra-early evaluation of regional cerebral blood flow in severely head-injured patients using xenon-enhanced computerized tomography. *J Neurosurg.* 1992;77(3):360–368.

57. Schroder ML, Muizelaar JP, Bullock MR, Salvant JB, Povlishock JT. Focal ischemia due to traumatic contusions documented by stable xenon-CT and ultrastructural studies. *J Neurosurg.* 1995;82(6):966–971.

58. Schroder ML, Muizelaar JP, Kuta AJ. Documented reversal of global ischemia immediately after removal of an acute subdural hematoma. Report of two cases. *J Neurosurg.* 1994;80(2):324–327.

59. Zauner A, Bullock R, Kuta AJ, Woodward J, Young HF. Glutamate release and cerebral blood flow after severe human head injury. *Acta Neurochir Suppl.* 1996;67:40–44.

60. Obrist WD, Langfitt TW, Jaggi JL, Cruz J, Gennarelli TA. Cerebral blood flow and metabolism in comatose patients with acute head injury. Relationship to intracranial hypertension. *J Neurosurg.* 1984;61(2):241–253.

61. Jones TH, Morawetz RB, Crowell RM, et al. Thresholds of focal cerebral ischemia in awake monkeys. *J Neurosurg.* 1981;54(6):773–782.

62. Kontos HA. George E. Brown memorial lecture. Oxygen radicals in cerebral vascular injury. *Circ Res.* 1985;57(4):508–516.

63. Siesjö BK. Pathophysiology and treatment of focal cerebral ischemia. Part II: mechanisms of damage and treatment. *J Neurosurg.* 1992;77(3):337–354.

64. Siesjö BK. Pathophysiology and treatment of focal cerebral ischemia. Part I: pathophysiology. *J Neurosurg.* 1992;77(2):169–184.

65. Muizelaar JP, Wei EP, Kontos HA, Becker DP. Mannitol causes compensatory cerebral vasoconstriction and vasodilation in response to blood viscosity changes. *J Neurosurg.* 1983;59(5):822–828.

66. Di X, Harpold T, Watson JC, Bullock MR. Excitotoxic damage in neurotrauma: fact or fiction. *Restor Neurol Neurosci.* 1996;9(4):231–41.

67. Lampe JW, Becker LB. State of the art in therapeutic hypothermia. *Annu Rev Med.* 2011;62:79–93.

68. Polderman KH. Mechanisms of action, physiological effects, and complications of hypothermia. *Crit Care Med.* 2009;37(7)(suppl):S186–S202.

69. Badruddin A, Taqi MA, Abraham MG, Dani D, Zaidat OO. Neurocritical care of a reperfused brain. *Curr Neurol Neurosci Rep.* 2011;11(1):104–110.

70. Simon RP. Acidotoxicity trumps excitotoxicity in ischemic brain. *Arch Neurol.* 2006;63(10):1368–1371.

71. Wahlgren NG, Ahmed N. Neuroprotection in cerebral ischaemia: facts and fancies—the need for new approaches. *Cerebrovasc Dis.* 2004;17(suppl 1):153–166.

72. Leker RR, Shohami E. Cerebral ischemia and trauma-different etiologies yet similar mechanisms: neuroprotective opportunities. *Brain Res Brain Res Rev.* 2002;39(1):55–73.

73. Wong CH, Crack PJ. Modulation of neuro-inflammation and vascular response by oxidative stress following cerebral ischemia-reperfusion injury. *Curr Med Chem.* 2008;15(1):1–14.

74. Brennan AM, Suh SW, Won SJ, et al. NADPH oxidase is the primary source of superoxide induced by NMDA receptor activation. *Nat Neurosci.* 2009;12(7):857–863.

75. Eldadah BA, Faden AI. Caspase pathways, neuronal apoptosis, and CNS injury. *J Neurotrauma.* 2000;17(10):811–829.

76. Tuttolomondo A, Di Sciacca R, Di Raimondo D, et al. Neuron protection as a therapeutic target in acute ischemic stroke. *Curr Top Med Chem.* 2009;9(14):1317–1334.

77. Bolli R, Jeroudi MO, Patel BS, et al. Marked reduction of free radical generation and contractile dysfunction by antioxidant therapy begun at the time of reperfusion. Evidence that myocardial "stunning" is a manifestation of reperfusion injury. *Circ Res.* 1989;65(3):607–622.

78. Khalid MA, Ashraf M. Direct detection of endogenous hydroxyl radical production in cultured adult cardiomyocytes during anoxia and reoxygenation. Is the hydroxyl radical really the most damaging radical species? *Circ Res.* 1993;72(4):725–736.

79. Halliwell B. Free radicals, antioxidants, and human disease: curiosity, cause, or consequence? *Lancet.* 1994;344(8924):721–724.

80. Sugawara T, Chan PH. Reactive oxygen radicals and pathogenesis of neuronal death after cerebral ischemia. *Antioxid Redox Signal.* 2003;5(5):597–607.

81. Huang Y, Rabb H, Womer KL. Ischemia-reperfusion and immediate T cell responses. *Cell Immunol.* 2007;248(1):4–11.

82. Jung JE, Kim GS, Chen H, et al. Reperfusion and neurovascular dysfunction in stroke: from basic mechanisms to potential strategies for neuroprotection. *Mol Neurobiol.* 2010;41(2–3):172–179.

83. Lv M, Liu Y, Zhang J, et al. Roles of inflammation response in microglia cell through toll-like receptors 2/interleukin-23/interleukin-17 pathway in cerebral ischemia/reperfusion injury. *Neuroscience.* 2011;176:162–172.

Pathobiology of Secondary Brain Injury

Patrick M. Kochanek, Robert S.B. Clark, and Larry W. Jenkins

INTRODUCTION

In the United States, more than 50,000 people die and more than 200,000 are hospitalized each year from traumatic brain injury (TBI) (1). Severe TBI is an important contributor to both this mortality and the associated morbidity. Treatment remains supportive neurointensive care focused on the control of intracranial hypertension. The development of breakthroughs in the treatment of TBI have been hampered by a lack of understanding of the key mechanisms operating in the injured brain.

TBI involves a *primary injury*, which includes direct disruption of brain parenchyma and *secondary injury*, characterized by a cascade of biochemical, cellular, and molecular events involved in the evolution of secondary damage. This chapter focuses mostly on the pathobiology of secondary injury. (See Chapter 11 by Yokobori and Bullock for a more detailed discussion of primary brain injury.)

PRIMARY INJURY

Primary injury has traditionally been characterized as the damage that results directly from the shear forces at impact. Consequently, this topic has been of greater interest to investigators in the fields of injury prevention and biomechanics than those focused on the treatment of the evolution of secondary damage. (See Chapter 10 for a detailed discussion of the biomechanics of primary injury.) Nevertheless, some insight into the components of primary injury is valuable. Key components of primary injury include cortical disruption, axonal injury, vascular injury, hemorrhage, and unusual, albeit important, miscellaneous forms of primary injury.

Primary injury has been modeled in vitro using approaches such as mechanical stretch of cultured neurons (2). Clinically, several aspects of primary injury can be appreciated when viewing the initial postinjury cranial computed tomographic (CT) scan or cranial magnetic resonance imaging (MRI) of patients. Direct cortical disruption seen in the initial minutes to hours after the insult represents primary injury that is not likely to be amenable to resuscitative therapy. In addition to direct cortical disruption, axonal injury and vascular disruption can result from primary injury. Indeed, likely related to the anatomical association between axons and blood vessels, primary injury often results in coupled injury to these structures—and the commonly observed clinical picture of petechial hemorrhages in white matter signaling diffuse axonal injury (DAI) (3). Interestingly, classically, axonal disruption with retraction was believed to result only from direct shearing. However, work from the laboratory of Povlishock (4) over the past 3 decades has identified a parallel secondary injury cascade in axons. Thus, as with gray matter injury, both primary and secondary axonal damage can occur after severe TBI. The concept of secondary axonal damage will be discussed in greater detail later in this chapter. Finally, there are several miscellaneous forms of primary injury—and several of these can have critical consequences in the setting of acute injury. For example, pituitary stalk transation from shear forces has been reported (5) and leads to acute pituitary failure. Primary injury to the brain stem can also occur and often is associated with poor outcome (6). Similarly, primary injury from violent shaking in the setting of inflicted childhood neurotrauma (Shaken baby syndrome) can include direct shearing of nerve roots in the upper cervical spine (7).

Another important aspect of primary injury is impact depolarization. At the time of severe injury, impact depolarization occurs, with massive increases in extracellular potassium ion and the indiscriminate release of the excitatory neurotransmitter glutamate (8). This immediate event initiates excitotoxicity—a key secondary mechanism that is discussed in detail latter in this chapter.

Although by definition, primary injury is not likely to be responsive to resuscitative approaches; it is interesting that our thinking on the lack of therapeutic approaches to primary injury may require reconsideration in the emerging era of tissue engineering and stem cell therapeutics (9). It is possible that tissue replacement therapy in the future may allow successful therapeutic avenues even to lesions produced by primary injury and previously felt to lack therapeutic options. This could be particularly important as an adjunctive therapy in rehabilitation.

EVOLUTION OF SECONDARY INJURY

Secondary injury includes both the endogenous evolution of damage within the brain and the effects of secondary extracerebral insults (i.e., hypotension, hypoxemia) from the injury scene through the intensive care unit (ICU).

Studies in models of TBI have begun to unravel the mechanisms producing secondary damage. Four categories of mechanisms can be defined (Figure 12-1), those associated

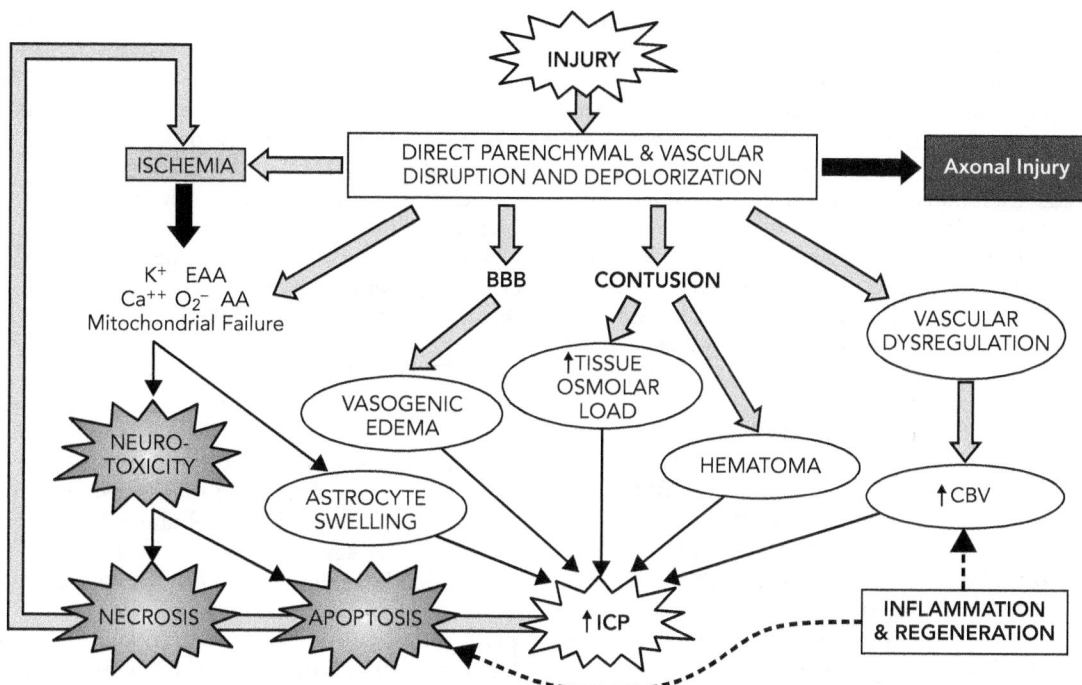

FIGURE 12–1 Categories of mechanisms proposed to be involved in the evolution of secondary damage after severe TBI in infants and children. Three major categories for these secondary mechanisms include (a) ischemia, excitotoxicity, energy failure, and cell death cascades; (b) cerebral swelling; and (c) axonal injury. A fourth category, inflammation and regeneration, contributes to each of these cascades.

with (a) ischemia, excitotoxicity, energy failure, and resultant cell death cascades; (b) secondary cerebral swelling; (c) axonal injury; and (d) inflammation and regeneration. Within each category, a constellation of mediators of secondary damage, endogenous neuroprotection repair, and regeneration are involved. The quantitative contribution of each mediator to outcome and the interplay between these mediators remains poorly defined.

A variety of methods have been used to study the evolution of secondary damage in human head injury including (a) the analysis of brain biochemistry and molecular biology via ventricular cerebrospinal fluid (CSF) drained in the treatment of intracranial hypertension, (b) assessment of brain interstitial fluid by cerebral microdialysis, (c) imaging techniques linked to assessment of cerebral blood flow (CBF) and cerebral metabolism, and (d) the assessment of molecular markers in brain tissue obtained from patients treated with surgical decompression for refractory intracranial hypertension. We discuss these studies and cite the clinical evidence supporting proposed mechanisms of secondary damage. It is impossible to address all of the mediators that may be involved; however, key mechanisms will be considered.

INJURY SEVERITY

Figure 12-1 outlines all of the major mechanisms of secondary injury that are known to participate in severe TBI—which is the focus of this chapter. As severity of TBI decreases, neuronal death, tissue destruction and intracranial hypertension, and brain edema become less important to the overall pathobiology. Thus, in mild TBI and concussion,

major ionic alterations, metabolic depression, CBF alterations, and axonal perturbations predominate. For a review of secondary injury mechanisms in mild TBI, the reader is referred to the review of Giza and Hovda (10).

POST-TRAUMATIC ISCHEMIA

Clinical studies in adults indicated that early after severe TBI, CBF is reduced and suggest that early post-traumatic ischemia might represent a therapeutic target (11,12). Clinical studies applying the stable xenon CT method of CBF assessment in the initial hours after severe TBI have been the most important in this regard. Early hypoperfusion or ischemia after severe TBI appears to represent a finding that is seen in most cases and is associated with poor outcome. The devastating consequences of secondary extra-cerebral insults early after injury (i.e., hypotension, hypoxemia) and early post-trauma are also consistent with this possibility—because a hypoperfused brain is at high risk and may be incapable of mounting an appropriate vasodilatory response during these added insults (13). This is not to suggest that secondary insults are limited to the field or emergency department. Secondary ischemic insults can also occur in the ICU. This was best described in the classic report of Gopinath et al. (14) who used a jugular venous catheter to identify episodes of jugular venous desaturation (SjvO2 < 50% for more than 10 minutes) in the ICU in 116 patients with severe TBI. In that study, 46 of the 116 patients had at least 1 episode of desaturation—suggesting ischemia. The causes of these episodes were either systemic such as hypotension or cerebral such as refractory intracranial hypertension. Episodes of desaturation were strongly associated with a poor neurological outcome. Just a single desaturation increased the incidence of poor outcome from 55% to 74%.

Numerous mechanisms may underlie the early post-traumatic hypoperfusion. Armstead reported reductions in the vasodilatory response to nitric oxide (NO), cGMP, cAMP, and prostanoids after experimental TBI in pigs, along with the release of superoxide anion (15,16). Also, greater injury-induced release of the potent vasoconstrictor peptide endothelin-1 in the newborn vs the juvenile pig was posed to mediate the hypoperfusion (17). Others have suggested a loss of either endothelial NO production, or vascular responsivity to NO as mediating hypoperfusion. Treatment with L-arginine (the substrate for NO production) improved CBF after TBI in rats (18). Similarly, treatment with L-arginine improved CBF and reduced contusion volume after TBI in rats (19). L-arginine is being tested in a clinical TBI trail in adults (personal communication, C. Robertson MD). Loss of vasodilators and elaboration of vasoconstrictors, or other mechanisms, could be involved in producing early post-traumatic hypoperfusion (Figure 12-2).

Increases in metabolic demands, related to uptake of glutamate, as reflected by increases in brain tissue and CSF lactate, early after TBI have been reported in both models (20) and humans (21–23). Thus, reduced metabolic demands with a coupled CBF reduction in severely injured brain regions, early after injury, is an unlikely explanation for the hypoperfusion.

At more delayed times after injury (several hours to days), oxidative metabolism has been noted to be reduced to levels of ~50% of baseline for most of the ICU course (21). The complex issue of alterations in metabolic demands after severe TBI is discussed in greater detail in the section on brain swelling later in this chapter.

EXCITOTOXICITY

Excitoxicity describes the process by which glutamate and other excitatory amino acids (EAAs) cause neuronal damage. Lucas and Newhouse (24) first described the toxicity of glutamate. Olney (25) subsequently reported that intraperitoneal administration of glutamate produces brain injury. Although glutamate is the most abundant neurotransmitter in the brain, exposure to toxic levels produces neuronal death (26).

Glutamate exposure produces neuronal injury in 2 phases. Minutes after exposure, sodium-dependent neuronal swelling occurs (27). This is followed by delayed, calcium-dependent degeneration. These effects are mediated through both ionophore-linked receptors, labeled according to specific agonists (N-methyl-D-aspartate [NMDA], kainate and α-amino-3-hydroxy-5-methyl-4-isoxazolepropionic acid [AMPA]), and receptors linked to second messenger systems called metabotropic receptors. Activation of these receptors leads to calcium influx through receptor-gated or voltage-gated channels, or through the release of intracellular calcium stores. Increased intracellular calcium concentration is the trigger for several processes that can lead to cellular injury or death (Figure 12-3). One mechanism involves activation of constitutive NO synthase, leading to NO production, peroxynitrite formation, and resultant DNA damage. Poly (ADP-ribose) polymerase (PARP) is an enzyme operative in DNA repair, and in the face of DNA damage, PARP activation leads to ATP depletion, metabolic failure, and cell death (28). This may be important because PARP knockout mice exhibit improved outcome vs controls (29). Recent evidence suggests that activation of PARP within mitochondria may contribute importantly to their failure (30).

Faden et al. (31) first reported an increase in interstitial EAAs to neurotoxic levels after experimental TBI. Anti-excitotoxic therapies improve outcome after experimental TBI. Pretreatment with NMDA antagonists (phencyclidine, MK-801) attenuate behavioral deficits after TBI in rats (32,33). Other therapies that modify the glutamate-NMDA receptor interaction and improve outcome following experimental TBI are magnesium (34), glycine site antagonists (35), hypothermia (36), and pentobarbital (37).

Palmer et al. (38) first demonstrated increased concentrations of EAAs in ventricular CSF from adult patients with TBI. Glutamate concentrations were about 5-fold greater than in control patients (up to 7 μM)—levels sufficient to cause neuronal death in cell culture (39). However, CSF glutamate concentrations do not correlate to outcome after TBI in adults (40). Bullock et al. (41) characterized patterns of glutamate release by measuring EAAs by microdialysis after adult TBI. Patients with a normal head CT and no secondary ischemic events had interstitial concentrations of glutamate that were increased early in their course, then returned to normal, similar to the pattern seen in most experimental models. A second group of patients had an intermediate increase in glutamate concentration (5–20 μM) that declined over time, but remained higher than normal. Most of these patients had ischemic events or intracranial hypertension. A third group of patients had markedly increased concentrations of glutamate (more than 20 μM). All patients with a progressively rising level of glutamate died.

Despite these findings, clinical trials with anti-excitotoxic therapies have been unsuccessful. This may be caused by the fact that most therapies have been applied to all patients with TBI rather than those with excitotoxicity (42). Also, treatment may have been initiated too late. Inhibition

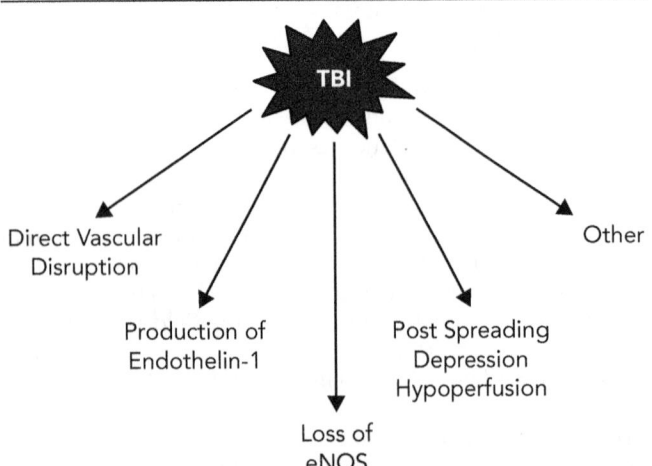

FIGURE 12–2 Schematic outlining putative mediators involved in the production of early post-traumatic hypoperfusion and/or ischemia after severe TBI. NOS, NO synthase. (See text for details.)

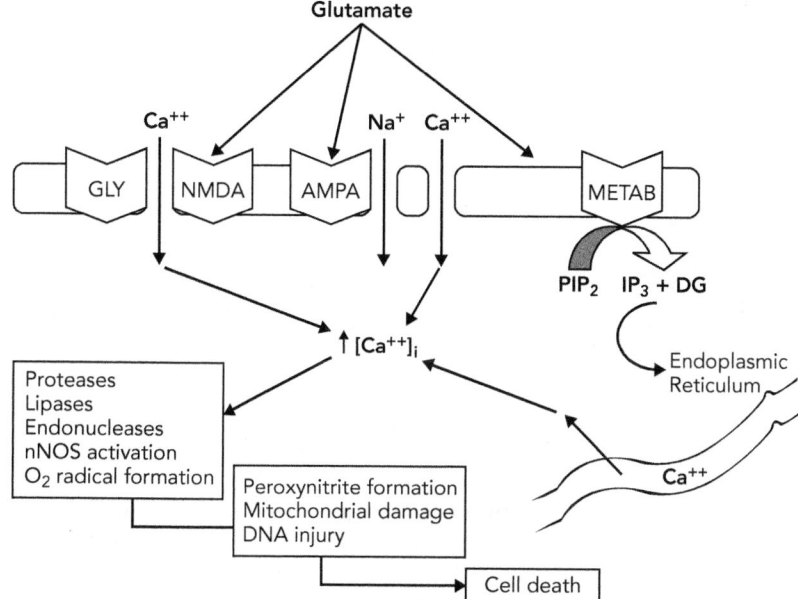

FIGURE 12–3 Mechanisms involved in excitotoxicity. Glutamate causes an increase in intracellular calcium concentration through stimulation of (*a*) the NMDA receptor with opening of the receptor-linked calcium ionophore, (*b*) the AMPA receptor with opening of the voltage-gated calcium channels, and (*c*) the metabotropic receptor, with the release of intracellular calcium stores via the second messenger's inositol triphosphate and diacylglycerol. Increased intracellular calcium concentration leads to activation of proteases, lipases, and endonucleases, along with neuronal NOS stimulation and production of oxygen radicals. This results in peroxynitrite formation, mitochondrial damage, and DNA injury with subsequent cellular injury and death. GLY, glycine coagonist site; NMDA, α-amino-3-hydroxy-5-methylisoazole-4-pro-prionic acid receptor; METAB, glutamate metabotropic receptor; PIP_2, phosphoinositide; IP_3, inositol triphosphate; DG, diacylglycerol.

of plasticity by anti-excitotoxic therapies may limit their efficacy—especially at the interface between the acute and subacute periods after injury (43). Related to this possibility, contemporary approaches to targeting excitotoxicity have focused on a novel target, namely, the extrasynaptic NMDA receptors. Recent evidence suggests that synaptic NMDA receptors are innocuous and linked to plasticity, while extrasynaptic NMDA receptors are coupled to loss of mitochondrial membrane potential and neuronal death (44). Whether antagonists of these receptors could attenuate neuronal death after experimental or clinical TBI remains to be determined.

Endogenous Neuroprotectants

Ischemia, excitotoxicity, or their combination is a key facet of secondary injury. These mechanisms are linked to calcium overload, oxidative stress, and mitochondrial failure. Studies have begun to define, in infants and children with severe TBI, the endogenous retaliatory response to these ischemic and excitotoxic insults. Space limitations have directed us to focus on 2 examples of this cascade—namely, adenosine and heat shock protein 70 (HSP 70). Endogenous neuroprotective responses related to the apoptosis, cell signaling, and inflammatory cascades are discussed later.

Adenosine is an endogenous neuroprotectant produced in response to both ischemia and excitotoxicity. Adenosine antagonizes several events thought to mediate neuronal death (45). Breakdown of adenosine triphosphate (ATP) leads to formation of adenosine, a purine nucleoside that decreases neuronal metabolism and increasing CBF, among other mechanisms. Adenosine binding to A1 receptors decreases metabolism by increasing K^+ and Cl^- and decreasing Ca^{++} conductances in the neuronal membrane. A1 receptors are located on neurons in brain regions that are susceptible to injury (i.e., hippocampus) and are spatially associated with NMDA receptors (46). Thus, released adenosine minimizes excitotoxicity. Binding of adenosine to A2 receptors (on cere-

brovascular smooth muscle) causes vasodilation, although binding to A2a receptors on neurons may be detrimental. Brain interstitial levels of adenosine are increased early after TBI in rats (47–49). In experimental TBI, brain interstitial adenosine increases immediately after injury to levels 50- to 100-fold greater than baseline (49). In clinical studies, marked increases in brain interstitial levels of adenosine in adults with TBI, were seen during episodes of jugular venous desaturation (secondary insults), supporting a role of adenosine as a "retaliatory" defense metabolite (50).

Another putative endogenous neuroprotectant that plays a role after severe TBI is HSP 70. This protein is induced as part of the classic preconditioning response in brain and has recently been shown to be increased in both CSF and brain tissue after severe TBI in humans (51–53). HSP 70 is believed to play an important role in optimizing protein folding as a molecular chaperone. It also inhibits pro-inflammatory signaling (54). Thus, the brain mounts an important endogenous defense response to TBI. Therapies designed to augment these pathways have not been examined adequately.

APOPTOSIS CASCADES

It is now increasingly clear from experimental models and human data that cells dying after TBI can be categorized on a morphological continuum ranging from necrosis to apoptosis (55,56). *Apoptosis* is a morphological description of cell death defined by cell shrinkage and nuclear condensation, internucleosomal DNA fragmentation, and the formation of apoptotic bodies (57). In contrast, cells dying of necrosis display cellular and nuclear swelling with dissolution of membranes. Apoptosis requires a cascade of intracellular events for completion of cell death; thus, "programmed-cell death" is the currently accepted term for the process of cell death that leads to apoptosis (58). In diseases with complex and multiple mechanisms, such as TBI, it is typically difficult to distinguish clinical apoptotic vs necrotic cell

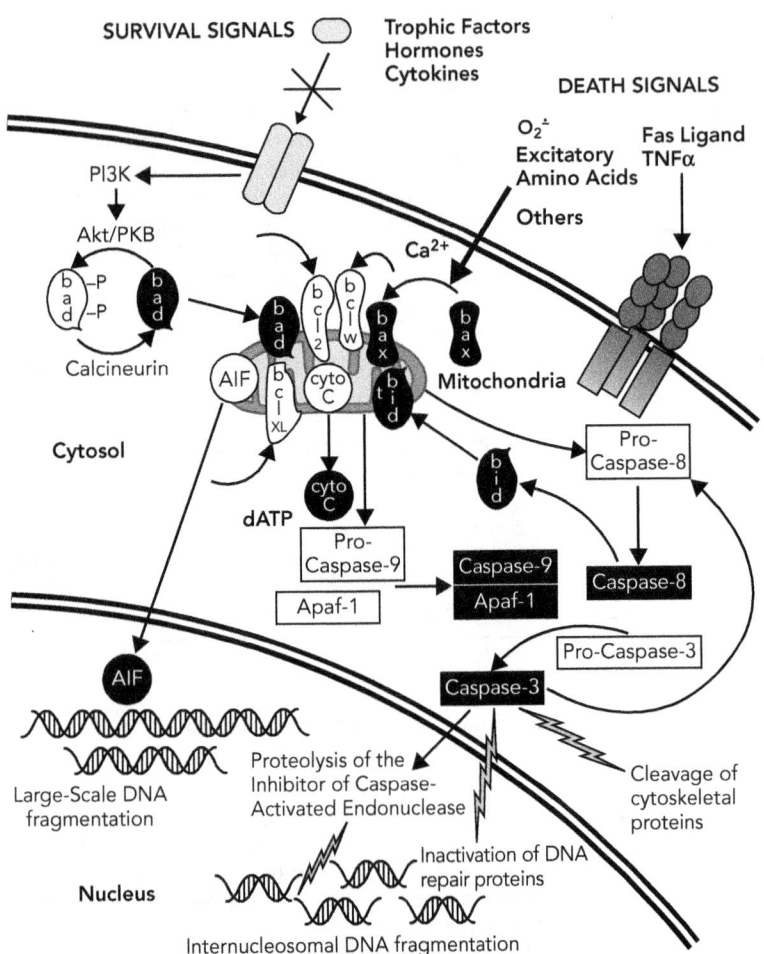

FIGURE 12–4 Simplified schematic depicting intracellular and extracellular pathways for programmed cell death. Mitochondrial dysfunction caused by injurious stimuli such as oxidative stress or calcium fluxes can trigger release of cytochrome c or apoptosis inducing factor (AIF). Cytochrome c in the cytosol along with other enzymes and cofactors initiates activation of a cascade of caspases, culminating in apoptosis, with nucleosomal DNA cleavage. AIF triggers caspase-independent large-scale DNA fragmentation (see text for details). Programmed cell death can also be initiated by cell death receptors on the cell surface. Fas-ligand (Fas-L), either presented by an effector cell or in soluble form, binding to Fas-receptor (Fas-Rc), or TNFα binding to TNF-receptor (TNF-Rc), can also initiate a cascade of caspases via intracellular death domains.

death as classically defined (59). Some cells may display DNA fragmentation and activation of proteases involved in programmed-cell death, despite having nuclear and cellular swelling. Dying cells with mixed phenotypes may represent particularly difficult therapeutic targets after TBI.

In mature tissues, programmed-cell death requires initiation via either intracellular or extracellular signals (see Figure 12-4). These signals have now been well characterized in vitro and are becoming better characterized in vivo. Intracellular signaling appears to be initiated in mitochondria, triggered by disturbances in cellular homeostasis such as ATP depletion, oxidative stress, or calcium fluxes (60). Mitochondrial dysfunction leads to egress of cytochrome c from the inner mitochondrial membrane into the cytosol. Cytochrome c release can be blocked by anti-apoptotic members of the bcl-2 family (e.g., bcl-2, bcl-xL, bcl-w, and Mcl-1), and promoted by pro-apoptotic members of the bcl-2 family (e.g., bax, bcl-xS, Bad, and bid) (61). Cytochrome c in the presence of dATP and a specific apoptotic-protease activating factor (Apaf-1) in cytosol activates the initiator cysteine protease caspase-9 (62). Caspase-9 then activates the effector cysteine protease caspase-3, a key apoptosis effector that cleaves cytoskeletal proteins, DNA repair proteins, and activators of endonucleases (63).

An additional intracellular cascade of programmed cell death linked to mitochondrial injury is the apoptosis-inducing factor (AIF) pathway (64–68). This caspase-independent

pathway is activated by mitochondrial permeability transition and results in the release of AIF from the mitochondrial membrane. AIF release leads to large-scale DNA fragmentation (50–700 kilo-base-pair in size). Recently, Zhang et al. (69) reported that the AIF pathway is activated in experimental TBI. To date, specific pharmacologic inhibitors of this pathway are lacking, however, this alternative form of delayed neuronal death may represent an important therapeutic target.

Extracellular signaling of apoptosis occurs through the TNF superfamily of cell surface death receptors which include TNFR1 and Fas/Apo1/CD95 (70). Receptor-ligand binding of TNFR1-TNFα or Fas-FasL promotes formation of a trimeric complex of TNF- or Fas-associated death domains, respectively. These death domains contain caspase recruitment domains. The proximity of multiple caspases, in this case caspase-8, allows for activation of the effector cysteine protease followed by activation of caspase-3, where the mitochondrial- and cell death receptor-pathways converge. The cell death receptor pathway can also be regulated by soluble receptors and ligands that prevent and promote apoptosis, respectively, and by receptors lacking death domains. Finally, there is cross-talk between mitochondrial- and cell death receptor-pathways (71).

Bcl-2 is an important endogenous inhibitor of programmed-cell death in vitro (72). It is induced after experimental TBI (73) and reduces cortical tissue loss (74). Bcl-2 is increased in injured brain after severe TBI in humans (56). CSF levels of bcl-2 were increased, approximately 4-fold in TBI compared with control patients. Moreover, CSF bcl-2 was associated with patient survival (75).

Clearly there is now substantial evidence, even in the clinical setting, for an important role for delayed neuronal death by apoptosis or mixed "apo-necrotic" phenotypes after severe TBI. This may represent a valuable opportunity for the development of new therapeutic approaches in the future.

CELL SIGNALING ABNORMALITIES IN NEURONAL DEATH

Neuronal death occurs after both experimental and clinical TBI. In addition to regions of brain directly contused, the hippocampus appears particularly vulnerable to TBI (76–80). As previously discussed, cell death execution pathways are activated by a sufficient severity of TBI involving mitochondrial injury, cytochrome C release with caspase activation, AIF release, and receptor-coupled pro-death pathways. Neurotransmitters, neurotrophins, cytokines, other growth factors, and oxidative stress activate multiple upstream signaling pathways linked to either pro-survival or pro-death activities (81). These receptors couple to signal transduction pathways involving interactions and cross-talk between multiple serine or threonine and tyrosine protein kinase cascades.

Many kinases involved in cell death process are serine or threonine protein kinases. Important participants in the cell death cascades include the mitogen activated protein kinases (MAPK). MAPKs cascades are complex and are mediated by successive protein kinases that sequentially activate each other by phosphorylation. They are importantly linked to 2 key components of the cell death cascade—jun kinase (JNK) and P38 MAPK (Figure 12-5). JNK and p38 MAPK pathways activate caspase-3 (81–83). Activation of JNK leads to induction of pro-death genes including FasL (81,83,84). JNK increases p53 and Bax levels which increase cell death. JNK and p38 function in different stress signaling pathways and both target similar nuclear transcription factors that can be activated by pro-death stimuli such as oxidative stress (85). Studies in various TBI models have documented significant changes in both JNK, and p38 MAPKs that may be related to cell death and functional impairment after injury (86–88). MAPKs are also linked to survival signals through the ERK pathway, highlighting the complex cross-talk between these cascades (Figure 12-5).

Several protein kinase cascades play a major survival role. Phosphoinositide 3-kinase (PI3K), protein kinase B (PKB), and protein kinase A (PKA) pathways are prototype examples (Figure 12-6). PKB is also called akt; the complex nomenclature of these kinases has evolved across many disease processes. PKB is activated upstream by PI3K in response to survival signals, and have numerous pro-survival, growth, differentiation, and synaptic plasticity actions (89, 90). PKB affects survival by several mechanisms including the phosphorylation and inactivation of several pro-death mediators such as Bad. *Bad*, a member of the bcl-2 family, is phosphorylated by PKB at ser136 resulting in Bad dissociation from bcl-xL and binding to 14-3-3 proteins inhibiting cell death (Figure 12-6) (91). CAMP-mediated activation of

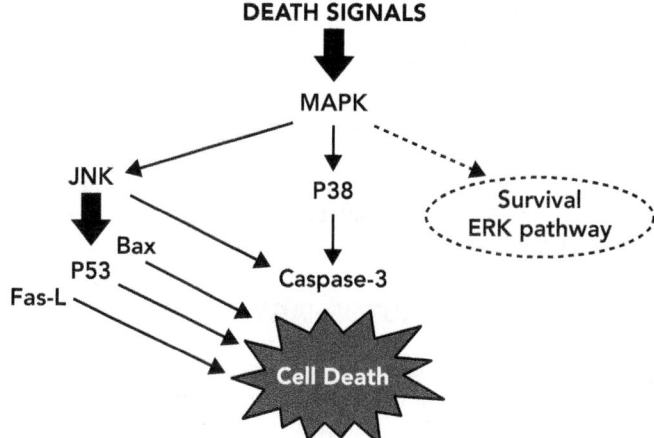

FIGURE 12–5 Cartoon showing the role of mitogen-activated protein kinases (MAPK) in transducing the signals involved in neuronal death. For example, oxidative stress triggers MAPK activation with resultant activation of jun kinase (JNK), which facilitates neuronal death mediated by several mechanisms including death receptors (Fas-Fas-L), P53, and Bax. MAPK also involves cross talk with some survival pathways such as ERK.

PKA can also lead to formation of the transcription factor "cAMP response element binding protein" (CREB), which is similarly associated with cell survival. These pro-survival kinase pathways are outlined in Figure 12-6 (84). Survival signals are exemplified by growth factors, cytokines, hormones, cell–cell interactions, as well as extracellular matrix adhesion molecules. Of course, inactivation of 2 pro-death members of the MAPK family—p38 and JNK/SAPK—have also been proposed as promoting survival by extracellular stimuli (92). Finally, activation of some PKC isoforms by

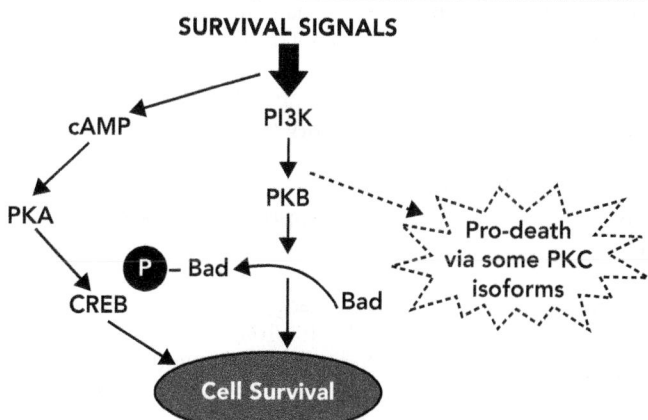

FIGURE 12–6 Cartoon showing the role of important survival signal-mediated kinase activation in promoting neuronal survival. Phosphoinositide 3-kinase (PI3K), protein kinase B (PKB), and protein kinase A (PKA) pathways are involved. PKB affects survival by several mechanisms including the phosphorylation and inactivation of the pro-death mediator Bad. Phosphorylation of Bad results in its dissociation from bcl-xL inhibiting cell death. CAMP-mediated activation of PKA can also lead to formation of the transcription factor "cAMP response element binding protein" (CREB), which also promotes cell survival.

PI3K can transduce pro-death signals, once again highlighting the complexity of these kinase cascades (Figure 12-6).

In summary, the complex but important kinase pathways are critically involved in the control of neuronal death and plasticity. Further insight into these cascades will likely lead to the development of powerful new tools to manipulate both neuronal death and rewiring after injury. Proteomics approaches may be essential to unraveling the cybernetic nature of these kinase pathways (93).

AUTOPHAGY

In addition to necrosis and apoptosis, a third "cell death" pathway, *autophagy*, is involved in the evolution of secondary injury after TBI. Autophagy was classically described in the setting of starvation or nutrient deprivation and in that setting represents a survival pathway that is involved in mobilizing energy substrates essential for cell survival. Although a detailed discussion of autophagy is beyond the scope of this chapter, it involves a highly regulated process that involves a series of autophagy-associated proteins (Atgs) that orchestrate the formation of an autophagosomal vesicle around material and/or organelles (i.e., mitochondria) that are destined to be digested to amino acids by lysosomes (reviewed in 95). This process is gender dependent, with male neurons tending to break down mitochondria during starvation whereas female neurons target membrane lipids. In the setting of experimental TBI, recent studies suggest that autophagy may be detrimental because inhibiting it has been associated with enhanced outcomes (95). The role of autophagy in TBI is likely complex given that impairment in this process is linked to accumulation of damaged proteins that may be linked as neurodegenerative diseases (94).

AXONAL INJURY

Traumatic axonal injury (TAI), also known as DIA, encompasses the spectrum of mild-to-severe TBI, both clinically (96–99) and in models (100–102). The extent and distribution of TAI depend on injury severity and category (focal vs diffuse) (103). (See also Chapter 11, by Yokobori and Bullock on Pathobiology of Primary Injury for additional discussion of axonal injury.)

The classical view that TAI occurs because of immediate physical shearing is represented primarily in severe injury where frank axonal tears occur (96,97,104,105). However, recent experimental studies suggest that TAI predominantly occurs as a secondary phenomenon by a delayed process termed "secondary axotomy" (101,106,107). Two hypothetical sequences have attempted to explain secondary axotomy, one attributing axolemmal permeability and calcium influx as the initiating event (Figure 12-7) and the other a direct cytoskeletal abnormality impairing axoplasmic flow (101, 107,108). It has been posited that both forms of reactive axonal swelling take place but in different proportions depending on the severity of injury. Superimposed on these theories is the finding that hypoxic/ischemic insults can also produce axonal swelling that resembles retraction balls. As a result, differing as well as unifying theories for axonal injuries in brain injury have been proposed (101,107–110). Common mechanistic features include focal ion flux, calcium dysregulation, and mitochondrial and cytoskeletal dysfunction.

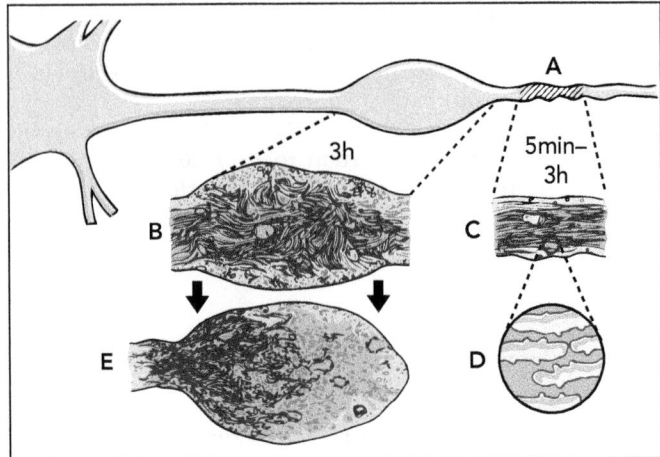

FIGURE 12–7 Reactive axonal swellings have been proposed to result from focal axolemmal disruption, ionic shifts, and neurofilamentous compaction at site (*A*) results in a reactive swelling at site (*B*) in an upstream region of the axon. At the site of ionic influx, neurofilamentous compaction and mitochondrial swelling is seen (*C*). Neurofilament compaction is associated with neurofilament sidearm loss (*D*). Obstructed axonal transport results in upstream axonal enlargement, neurofilament misalignment, organelle accumulation, and formation of the typical reactive axonal swelling (*E*).

TAI contributes to the morbidity after TBI (101,103–105). Until recently, the contributions of TAI to morbidity have remained speculative because TAI has remained refractory to treatment even in the laboratory. However, recent studies in experimental TBI models have shown that hypothermia, cyclosporin A, FK 506, docosahexanoic acid, and, possibly, other therapies can reduce TAI (111–114). In contradistinction, hypothermia reduces growth factor signaling after experimental TBI (115,116) that could blunt regeneration. These therapeutic advances should help determine more definitively the contributions of TAI to secondary damage. Recent application of diffusion tensor MRI to the study of TAI (117,118) and axonal connectivity (119,120) may improve our understanding of TAI and regeneration.

A recent area of great interest in the field is blast TBI that occurs in combat casualty care of soldiers wounded in terrorist attacks from improvised explosive devices, and also in civilians with similar exposures. Blast injury appears to highlight axonal injury, particularly in deep white matter structures such as cerebellum and brainstem, and has been the subject of considerable investigation in clinical models (Figure 12-8). Therapies targeting axonal injury could thus also be of special importance to this form of TBI.

CEREBRAL SWELLING

In addition to cascades of neuronal death and axonal damage, *brain swelling* is a hallmark finding in severe TBI and results in the development of intracranial hypertension, which can have devastating consequences. Cerebral swelling and accompanying intracranial hypertension contributes to secondary damage in 2 ways. Intracranial hypertension can compromise cerebral perfusion leading to secondary is-

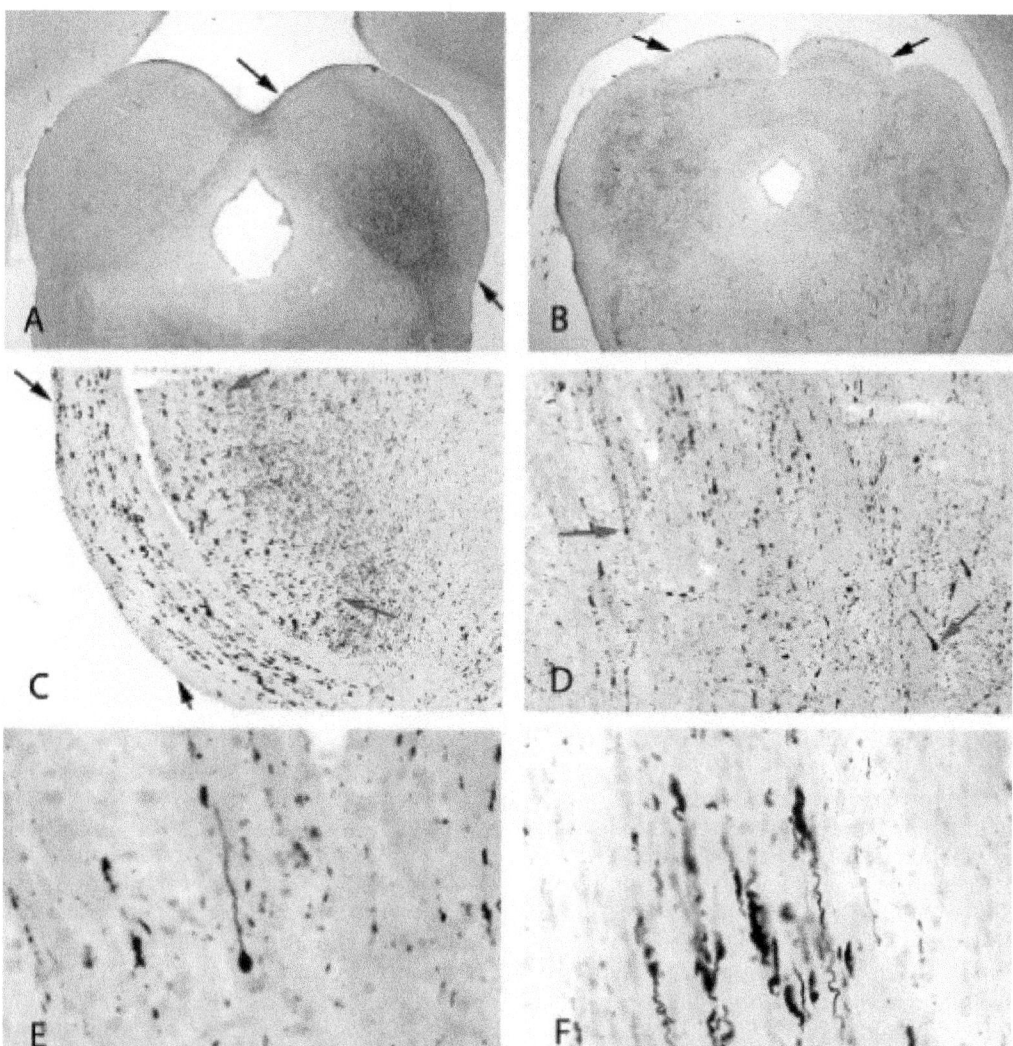

FIGURE 12–8 *See color insert.* Amino cupric silver-stained sections depicting axonal injury in brainstem and other regions of rats exposed to experimental blast TBI. Affected regions included the inferior colliculus (*between the arrows* in Panel **A**), numerous tracts within the midbrain (Panel **B**, in which the *arrows* point to the superior colliculus), sensory root of the trigeminal nerve (*red arrows* in Panel **C**) and trapezoid (*black arrows* in Panel **C**). Panels **D**, **E**, and **F** all show silver-stained axons that have irregular contours and/or swellings (spheroids) that are consistent with a diagnosis of diffuse axonal injury. Panel **E** is a higher magnification of Panel **D**; Panel **F**, at the same magnification, is of the optic tract. (Magnification bars for Panels **E** and **F** = 50 μm). Reprinted from Garman et al. (153) with permission.

chemia. In addition, it can produce the devastating consequences of deformation through herniation syndromes. Intracranial hypertension results from increases in intracranial volume from a variety of sources, which are outlined in Figure 12-1. In some cases, such as with epidural, subdural, or parenchymal hematoma formation, an extra-axial or parenchymal blood collection is the key culprit and is generally addressed by surgical evacuation (121). However, there are several important mechanisms that are more uniformly involved in the development of intracranial hypertension. These are related to either brain swelling from vasogenic edema, astrocyte swelling, and an increase in tissue osmolar load, or vascular dysregulation with swelling secondary to an increase in cerebral blood volume (CBV).

Recent data suggest that brain swelling after severe TBI results from edema rather than increased CBV. Marmarou

et al. (122) measured both CBV and brain water in adults with TBI. Using a dye indicator technique (coupled to CT) to measure CBV and MRI to quantify brain water, increases in brain water were commonly observed but were generally associated with reduced (not increased) CBV (Figure 12-9).

Thus, edema rather than increased CBV appears to be the predominant contributor to cerebral swelling after TBI. Both cytotoxic and vasogenic edema may play important roles in cerebral swelling. However, our traditional concept of cytotoxic and vasogenic edema is evolving. There appear to be four putative mechanisms for edema formation in the injured brain. First, vasogenic edema may form in the extracellular space as a result of blood-brain barrier (BBB) disruption. Second, cellular swelling can be produced in 2 ways. Astrocyte swelling can occur as part of the homeostatic uptake of substances such as glutamate. Glutamate uptake

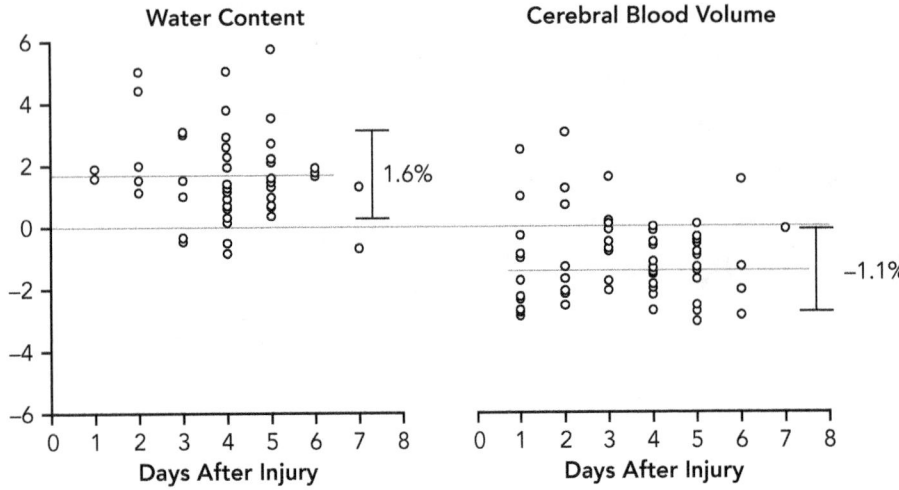

FIGURE 12–9 The percentage change in brain water content as assessed by MRI and cerebral blood volume (CBV) as measured by CT and indicatory dilution technique in 109 studies of adults with TBI. Brain water is increased and CBV is reduced in adults with severe TBI. Reprinted from Marmarou, Barzo, Fatouros, Yamamoto, Bullock, Young (122) with permission.

is coupled to glucose utilization via a sodium/potassium ATPase, with sodium and water accumulation in astrocytes. Swelling of both neurons and other cells in the neutrophil can also result from ischemia- or trauma-induced ionic pump failure. Finally, osmolar swelling may also contribute to edema formation in the extracellular space, particularly in contusions. Osmolar swelling, however, is actually dependent on an intact BBB or an alternative solute barrier.

Cellular swelling may be of greatest importance. Using a model of diffuse TBI in rats, Barzo et al. (123) applied diffusion-weighted MRI to localize the increase in brain water. A decrease in the apparent diffuse coefficient after injury suggested predominantly cellular swelling, rather than vasogenic edema, in the development of intracranial hypertension. Cellular swelling may be of even greater importance in the setting of TBI with a secondary hypoxemic-ischemic insult (124).

Katayama et al. (125) also suggested that the role of BBB in the development of post-traumatic edema may have been overstated—even in the setting of cerebral contusion. One intriguing possibility is that as macromolecules are degraded within injured brain regions, the osmolar load in the con-

tused tissue increases. As the BBB reconstitutes (or as other osmolar barriers are formed), a considerable osmolar driving force for the local accumulation of water develops, resulting in the marked swelling so often seen in and around cerebral contusions (Figure 12-10).

In some cases, increases in CBV can be seen after TBI and contribute to intracranial hypertension. When an increase in CBV is seen, it may result from local increases in cerebral glycolysis—"hyperglycolysis"—as described by Bergsneider et al. (23). In regions with increases in glutamate levels, such as in contusions, increases in glycolysis, are observed because astrocyte uptake of glutamate is coupled to glycolysis rather than oxidative metabolism. Recall that oxidative metabolism is generally depressed by ~50% in comatose victims of severe TBI in the ICU (21). Hyperglycolysis results in a marked local increase in cerebral glucose utilization with a coupled increase in CBF and CBV and resultant local brain swelling. Recent studies suggest that an important component of this hyperglycolysis represents shunting of glucose into the pentose phosphate pathway which may occur in response to oxidative stress to restore antioxidant defenses (126). Further study of the fates of glucose in the injured

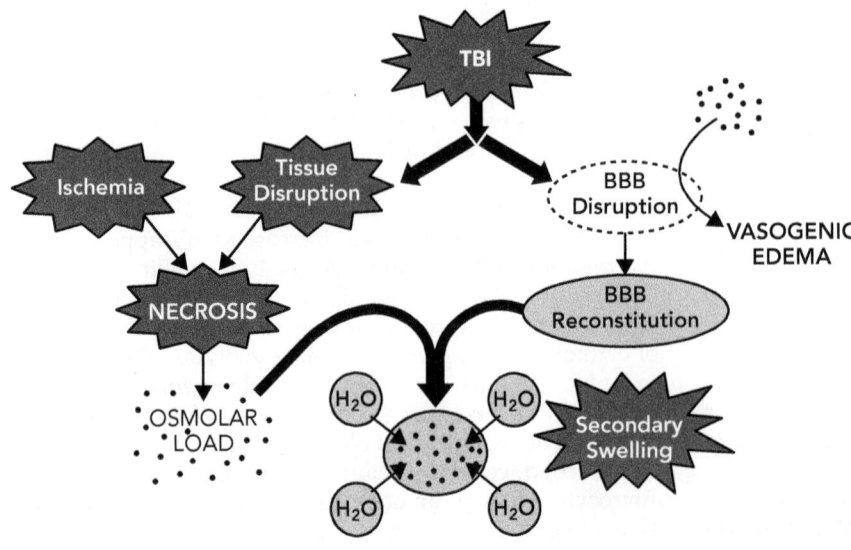

FIGURE 12–10 Schematic based on hypothesis of Katayama et al. (125) suggesting that as the osmolar load increases (breakdown of macromolecules in the region of contusion necrosis), a considerable driving force develops for the accumulation of water, resulting in the secondary swelling so often seen in and around cerebral contusions.

brain could be important given the possibility that alternative fuels such as lactate or ketones might represent preferred energy substrates in the traumatically injured brain.

As MRI and MR-spectroscopic methods continue to develop and become applied to critically ill patients (127) our "black box" knowledge of the mechanisms involved in cerebral swelling should greatly advance. It must be remembered that although neuronal and axonal injury are key downstream events in the evolution of damage after severe TBI, brain swelling and resultant intracranial hypertension is still the principal target for titration of therapy in the ICU.

INFLAMMATION AND REGENERATION

There appear to be both acute detrimental and sub-acute/ chronic beneficial aspects of inflammation. There is robust acute inflammation after TBI. This has been shown in models of TBI (128–130), and in adult patients (131–134). NF-κB (135), TNFα (136,137), IL-1β (138,139), eicosanoids (140), neutrophils (129,141), and macrophages (142,143) contribute to both secondary damage and repair.

Markers of inflammation after TBI have been assessed in humans using 2 general strategies: (*a*) examination of inflammation in contused brain tissue resected from patients with refractory intracranial hypertension and (*b*) study of mediator levels in CSF. Consistent with a role for IL-1β in the evolution of tissue damage in human TBI, Clark et al. (56) performed western analysis of brain samples resected from adults with refractory intracranial hypertension secondary to severe contusion. Interleukin-1β-converting enzyme (ICE) was activated, as evidenced by specific cleavage in patients with TBI. ICE activation is critical to the production of IL-1β. ICE activation was not detected in patients that died of non-CNS etiologies (Figure 12-11). This supports the production of IL-1β, a pivotal pro-inflammatory mediator, in the traumatically injured brain in humans.

Studies of CSF further support a role for inflammation in TBI. Marion et al. (132) demonstrated increases in IL-1β in CSF after severe TBI in adults. These increases were attenuated by the use of moderate therapeutic hypothermia. Similarly, there are increases of several cytokines in CSF after severe TBI including IL-6, and IL-8 (134,144). Contusion and local tissue necrosis appear to be important to trigger neutrophil influx with resultant secondary tissue damage (129).

Neutrophil influx is accompanied by increases in inducible nitric oxide synthase (iNOS) levels in brain (130) and is followed by macrophage infiltration, which peaks between 24 and 72 hours after injury (145). Macrophage infiltration and the differentiation of endogenous microglia into resident macrophages may signal the link between inflammation and regeneration, with elaboration of several trophic factors (i.e., nerve growth factor [NGF], nitrosothiols, vascular endothelial growth factor) (139,144,146,147).

Kossmann et al. (144) reported a link between IL-6 production and the production of neurotrophins such as NGF. Cultured astrocytes treated with either IL-6, IL-8 or CSF from brain-injured adults, produced NGF. Cytokine production after TBI may be important to neuronal plasticity and repair, as discussed subsequently.

Studies in models of TBI (137,148) suggest beneficial aspects of inflammation on long-term outcome. Mice deficient in TNFα exhibit improved functional outcome (vs wild-type) early after TBI. However, the long-term consequences of TNFα deficiency on outcome are detrimental (137). Similarly, despite a detrimental role for iNOS in the initial 72 hours post-trauma (149), iNOS deficient mice demonstrated impaired long-term outcome vs controls (148). iNOS is important in wound healing and iNOS-derived nitrosylation of proteins may play a role (147,150). Regeneration and plasticity play important roles in mediating beneficial long-term effects on recovery, and these responses are linked to inflammation.

The contribution of the inflammatory response to TBI remains to be determined. Although there are a few promising reports in models of the use of anti-inflammatory therapies in TBI and ischemia (targeting IL-1β, ICE, and TNFα), it is unclear whether anti-inflammatory therapies will improve outcome after clinical TBI. If inhibition of the inflammatory response is considered, exacerbation of infection risk must also be anticipated (151). Also, the link between inflammation and regeneration must be recognized.

CONCLUSION

Mechanisms involved in the evolution of secondary brain injury after TBI have been reviewed. Particular attention has been paid to studies at the bedside. Our understanding of the biochemical, cellular, and molecular responses has pro-

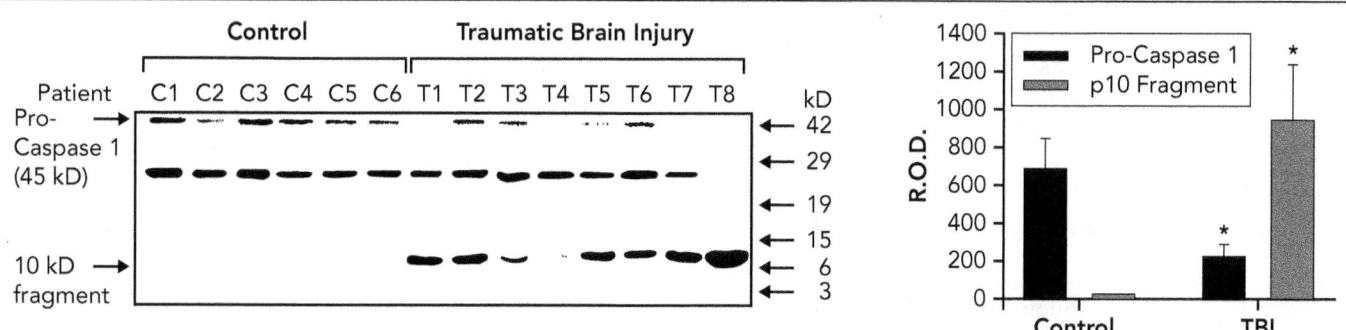

FIGURE 12–11 Evidence for activation of IL-1β converting enzyme (ICE) activation in cerebral contusions resected from adult patients with severe TBI and refractory intracranial hypertension. Western analysis demonstrating cleavage of the intact 45 kD pro-caspase-1 to the 10 kD fragment in each of 8 victims of severe TBI but in none of 6 control brain samples from patients that died of non-CNS causes. Reprinted from Clark et al. (63) with permission.

gressed—particularly with the application of molecular biology methods to human materials. Additional details on these mechanisms have also been reviewed in a companion article to this chapter which addresses the unique setting of pediatric TBI (152). Future investigation should integrate these findings with bedside physiology and an improved assessment of outcome. Finally, novel imaging and diagnostic methods, particularly MRI and MRS must be coupled with biochemical and molecular methods to clarify the mechanisms involved in secondary damage and the local effects of novel therapies.

KEY CLINICAL POINTS

1. Studies of the most relevant secondary injury mechanisms that have been carried out at the bench in experimental models of TBI have been generally confirmed by transitional studies in patients through the use of biological samples such as cerebrospinal fluid and brain tissue samples.
2. Contemporary techniques in neuromonitoring such as microdialysis have provided bedside evidence of key secondary injury mechanisms in TBI and some of these biomarkers may represent therapeutic targets.
3. Based on the findings presented in this chapter, novel therapeutic approaches targets neuronal death, axonal injury, brain edema, neuroinflammation, and cellular dysfunction and/or disruptions in cell signaling are needed to develop new therapies for TBI neuroprotection.

KEY REFERENCES

1. Chesnut RM, Marshall LF, Klauber MR, et al. The role of secondary brain injury in determining outcome from severe head injury. *J Trauma*. 1993;34(2):216–222.
2. Clark RS, Kochanek PM, Chen M, et al. Increases in Bcl-2 and cleavage of caspase-1 and caspase-3 in human brain after head injury. *FASEB J*. 1999;13(8):813–821.
3. Hovda DA, Lee SM, Smith ML, et al. The neurochemical and metabolic cascade following brain injury: moving from animal models to man. *J Neurotrauma*. 1995;12(5): 903–906.
4. Kochanek PM, Clark RSB, Ruppel RA, et al. Biochemical, cellular, and molecular mechanisms in the evolution of secondary damage after severe traumatic brain injury in infants and children: lessons learned from the bedside. *Pediatr Crit Care Med*. 2000;1(1):4–19.
5. Povlishock JT. Traumatically induced axonal injury: pathogenesis and pathobiological implications. *Brain Pathol*. 1992;2(1):1–12.

ACKNOWLEDGMENTS

The authors dedicate this chapter to the late Dr. Peter Safar for his vision and inspiration. We thank the National Institutes of Health/NINDS NS38087 (PMK), NS38620 (RSBC), NS 40049 (LJ), and NS30318 (PMK, RSBC); and Dr. Kochanek is also supported by the US Army W81XWH-09-2-0187 (PMK). We thank Marci Provins, Cara Boyer, Trudy Clark, and Fran Mistrick for the preparation of the manuscript.

References

1. Waxweiler RJ, Thurman D, Sniezek J, Sosin D, O'Neil J. Monitoring the impact of traumatic brain injury: a review and update. *J Neurotrauma*. 1995;12(4):509–516.
2. Engel DC, Slemmer JE, Vlug AS, Maas AI, Weber JT. Combined effects of mechanical and ischemic injury to cortical cells: secondary ischemia increases damage and decreases effects of neuroprotective agents. *Neuropharmacology*. 2005;49(7):985–995.
3. Pittella JE, Gusmão SN. Diffuse vascular injury in fatal road traffic accident victims: its relationship to diffuse axonal injury. *J Forensic Sci*. 2003;48(3):626–630.
4. Povlishock JT. Pathophysiology of neural injury: therapeutic opportunities and challenges. *Clin Neurosurg*. 2000;46:113–126.
5. Mark AS, Phister SH, Jackson DE Jr, Kolsky MP. Traumatic lesions of the suprasellar region: MR imaging. *Radiology*. 1992;182(1): 49–52.
6. Hashimoto T, Nakamura N, Richard KE, Frowein RA. Primary brain stem lesions caused by closed head injuries. *Neurosurg Rev*. 1993;16(4):291–298.
7. Ghatan S, Ellenbogen RG. Pediatric spine and spinal cord injury after inflicted trauma. *Neurosurg Clin N Am*. 2002;13(2):227–233.
8. Katayama Y, Becker DP, Tamura T, Hovda DA. Massive increases in extracellular potassium and the indiscriminate release of glutamate following concussive brain injury. *J Neurosurg*. 1990;73(6): 889–900.
9. Atala A. Tissue engineering for the replacement of organ function in the genitourinary system. *Am J Transplant*. 2004;4(suppl 6):58–73.
10. Giza CC, Hovda DA. The neurometabolic cascade of concussion. *J Athl Train*. 2001;36(3):228–235.
11. Marion DW, Darby J, Yonas H. Acute regional cerebral blood flow changes caused by severe head injuries. *J Neurosurg*. 1991;74(3): 407–414.
12. Bouma GJ, Muizelaar JP, Stringer WA, Choi SC, Fatouros P, Young HF. Ultra-early evaluation of regional cerebral blood flow in severely head-injured patients using xenon-enhanced computerized tomography. *J Neurosurg*. 1992;77(3):360–368.
13. Chesnut RM, Marshall LF, Klauber MR, et al. The role of secondary brain injury in determining outcome from severe head injury. *J Trauma*. 1993;34(2):216–222.
14. Gopinath SP, Robertson CS, Contant CF, et al. Jugular venous desaturation and outcome after head injury. *J Neurol Neurosurg Psychiatry*. 1994;57(6):717–723.
15. Armstead WM. Superoxide generation links protein kinase C activation to impaired ATP-sensitive K+ channel function after brain injury. *Stroke*. 1999;30(1):153–159.
16. Armstead WM. Brain injury impairs prostaglandin cerebrovasodilation. *J Neurotrauma*. 1998;15(9):721–729.
17. Armstead WM. Role of endothelin-1 in age-dependent cerebrovascular hypotensive responses after brain injury. *Am J Physiol*. 1999; 277(5, pt 2):H1884–H1894.
18. DeWitt DS, Smith TG, Deyo DJ, Miller KR, Uchida T, Prough DS. L-arginine and superoxide dismutase prevent or reverse cerebral hypoperfusion after fluid-percussion traumatic brain injury. *J Neurotrauma*. 1997;14(4):223–233.
19. Cherian L, Chacko G, Goodman JC, Robertson CS. Cerebral hemodynamic effects of phenylephrine and L-arginine after cortical impact injury. *Crit Care Med*. 1999;27(11):2512–2517.
20. Hovda DA, Lee SM, Smith ML, et al. The neurochemical and metabolic cascade following brain injury: moving from animal models to man. *J Neurotrauma*. 1995;12(5):903–906.
21. Obrist WD, Langfitt TW, Jaggi JL, Cruz J, Gennarelli TA. Cerebral blood flow and metabolism in comatose patients with acute head injury. Relationship to intracranial hypertension. *J Neurosurg*. 1984; 61(2):241–253.
22. DeSalles AA, Kontos HA, Becker DP, et al. Prognostic significance of ventricular CSF lactic acidosis in severe head injury. *J Neurosurg*. 1986;65(5):615–624.
23. Bergsneider M, Hovda DA, Shalmon E, et al. Cerebral hyperglycolysis following severe traumatic brain injury in humans: a positron emission tomography study. *J Neurosurg*. 1997;86(2):241–251.

24. Lucas DR, Newhouse JP. The toxic effect of sodium L-glutamate on the inner layers of the retina. *AMA Arch Ophthalmol.* 1957;58(2): 193–201.

25. Olney JW. Brain lesions, obesity, and other disturbances in mice treated with monosodium glutamate. *Science.* 1969;164(3880): 719–721.

26. Choi DW, Maulucci-Gedde M, Kriegstein AR. Glutamate neurotoxicity in cortical cell culture. *J Neurosci.* 1987;7(2):357–368.

27. Choi DW. Ionic dependence of glutamate neurotoxicity. *J Neurosci.* 1987;7(2):369–379.

28. Zhang J, Dawson VL, Dawson TM, Snyder SH. Nitric oxide activation of poly(ADP-ribose) synthetase in neurotoxicity. *Science.* 1994; 263(5147):687–689.

29. Whalen MJ, Clark RSB, Dixon CE, et al. Reduction of cognitive and motor deficits after traumatic brain injury in mice deficient in poly (ADP-ribose) polymerase. *J Cereb Blood Flow Metab.* 1999;19(8): 835–842.

30. Du L, Zhang X, Han YY, et al. Intra-mitochondrial poly (ADP-ribosylation) contributes to NAD+ depletion and cell death induced by oxidative stress. *J Biol Chem.* 2003;278(20):18426–18433.

31. Faden AI, Demediuk P, Panter SS, Vink R. The role of excitatory amino acids and NMDA receptors in traumatic brain injury. *Science.* 1989;244(4906):798–800.

32. Hayes RL, Jenkins LW, Lyeth BG, et al. Pretreatment with phencyclidine, an N-methyl-D-aspartate receptor antagonist, attenuates long-term behavioral deficits in the rat produced by traumatic brain injury. *J Neurotrauma.* 1988;5(4):287–302.

33. McIntosh TK, Vink R, Soares H, Hayes R, Simon R. Effects of the N-methyl-D-aspartate receptor blocker MK-801 on neurologic function after experimental brain injury. *J Neurotrauma.* 1989;6(4): 247–259.

34. Smith DH, Okiyama K, Gennarelli TA, McIntosh TK. Magnesium and ketamine attenuate cognitive dysfunction following experimental brain injury. *Neurosci Lett.* 1993;157(2):211–214.

35. Huettner J. Indole-2-carboxylic acid: a competitive antagonist of potentiation by glycine at the NMDA receptor. *Science.* 1989; 243(4898):1611–1613.

36. Suehiro E, Fujisawa H, Ito H, Ishikawa T, Maekawa T. Brain temperature modifies glutamate neurotoxicity in vivo. *J Neurotrauma.* 1999;16(4):285–297.

37. Goodman JC, Valadka AB, Gopinath SP, Cormio M, Robertson CS. Lactate and excitatory amino acids measured by microdialysis are decreased by pentobarbital coma in head-injured patients. *J Neurotrauma.* 1996;13(10):549–556.

38. Palmer AM, Marion DW, Botscheller ML, Bowen DM, DeKosky ST. Increased transmitter amino acid concentration in human ventricular CSF after brain trauma. *NeuroReport.* 1994;6(1):153–156.

39. Meldrum BS, Garthwaite J. Excitatory amino acid neurotoxicity and neurodegenerative disease. *Trends Pharmacol Sci.* 1990;11(9): 379–387.

40. Brown JI, Baker AJ, Konasiewicz SJ, Moulton RJ. Clinical significance of CSF glutamate concentrations following severe traumatic brain injury in humans. *J Neurotrauma.* 1998;15(4):253–263.

41. Bullock R, Zauner A, Woodward JJ, et al. Factors affecting excitatory amino acid release following severe human head injury. *J Neurosurg.* 1998;89(4):507–518.

42. Doppenberg EM, Choi SC, Bullock R. Clinical trials in traumatic brain injury. What can we learn from previous studies? *Ann N Y Acad Sci.* 1997;825:305–322.

43. Hendricson AW, Thomas MP, Lippmann MJ, Morrisett RA. Suppression of L-type voltage-gated calcium channel-dependent synaptic plasticity by ethanol: analysis of miniature synaptic currents and dendritic calcium transients. *J Pharmacol Exp Ther.* 2003; 307(2):550–558.

44. Léveillé F, El Gaamouch F, Gouix E, et al. Neuronal viability is controlled by a functional relation between synaptic and extrasynaptic NMDA receptors. *FASEB J.* 2008;22(12):4258–4271.

45. Rudolphi KA, Schubert P, Parkinson FE, Fredholm BB. Neuroprotective role of adenosine in cerebral ischaemia. *Trends Pharmacol Sci.* 1992;13(12):439–445.

46. Deckert J, Jorgensen MB. Evidence for pre- and postsynpatic localization of adenosine A1 receptors in the CA1 region of rat hippocampus: a quantitative autoradiographic study. *Brain Res.* 1988; 446(1):161–164.

47. Nilsson P, Hillered L, Pontén U, Ungerstedt U. Changes in cortical extracellular levels of energy-related metabolites and amino acids following concussive brain injury in rats. *J Cereb Blood Flow Metab.* 1990;10(5):631–637.

48. Headrick JP, Bendall MR, Faden AI, Vink R. Dissociation of adenosine levels from bioenergetic state in experimental brain trauma: potential role in secondary injury. *J Cereb Blood Flow Metab.* 1994; 14(5):853–861.

49. Bell MJ, Kochanek PM, Carcillo JA, et al. Interstitial adenosine, inosine, and hypoxanthine, are increased after experimental traumatic brain injury in the rat. *J Neurotrauma.* 1998;15(3):163–170.

50. Bell M, Robertson C, Kochanek P, et al. Interstitial purine metabolites after traumatic brain injury in humans: evidence for energy failure during jugular venous desaturation. *J Neurotrauma.* 1997; 14:791.

51. Dutcher SA, Underwood BD, Michael DB, Diaz FG, Walker PD. Heat-shock protein 72 expression in excitotoxic versus penetrating injuries of the rodent cerebral cortex. *J Neurotrauma.* 1998;15(6): 421–432.

52. Seidberg NA, Clark RS, Zhang X, et al. Alterations in inducible 72-kDa heat shock protein and the chaperone cofactor BAG-1 in human brain after head injury. *J Neurochem.* 2003;84(3):514–521.

53. Lai Y, Kochanek PM, Adelson PD, Janesko K, Ruppel RA, Clark RSB. Induction of the stress response after inflicted and non-inflicted traumatic brain injury in infants and children. *J Neurotrauma.* 2004;21(3):229–237.

54. Simon MM, Reikerstorfer A, Schwarz A, et al. Heat shock protein 70 overexpression affects the response to ultraviolet light in murine fibroblasts. Evidence for increased cell viability and suppression of cytokine release. *J Clin Invest.* 1995;95(3):926–933.

55. Rink A, Fung KM, Trojanowski JQ, Lee VM, Neugebauer E, McIntosh TK. Evidence of apoptotic cell death after experimental traumatic brain injury in the rat. *Am J Pathol.* 1995;147(6):1575–1583.

56. Clark RS, Kochanek PM, Chen M, et al. Increases in Bcl-2 and cleavage of caspase-1 and caspase-3 in human brain after head injury. *FASEB J.* 1999;13(8):813–821.

57. Kerr JF, Wyllie AH, Currie AR. Apoptosis: a basic biological phenomenon with wide-ranging implications in tissue kinetics. *Br J Cancer.* 1972;26(4):239–257.

58. Steller H. Mechanisms and genes of cellular suicide. *Science.* 1995; 267(5203):1445–1449.

59. Portera-Cailliau C, Price DL, Martin LJ. Excitotoxic neuronal death in the immature brain is an apoptosis-necrosis morphological continuum. *J Comp Neurol.* 1997;378(1):70–87.

60. Zamzami N, Susin SA, Marchetti P, et al. Mitochondrial control of nuclear apoptosis. *J Exp Med.* 1996;183(4):1533–1544.

61. Adams JM, Cory S. The Bcl-2 protein family: arbiters of cell survival. *Science.* 1998;281(5381):1322–1326.

62. Li P, Nijhawan D, Budihardjo I, et al. Cytochrome c and dATP-dependent formation of Apaf-1/caspase-9 complex initiates an apoptotic protease cascade. *Cell.* 1997;91(4):479–489.

63. Clark RSB, Kochanek PM, Watkins SC, et al. Caspase-3 mediated neuronal death after traumatic brain injury in rats. *J Neurochem.* 2000;74(2):740–753.

64. Susin SA, Zamzami N, Castedo M, et al. Bcl-2 inhibits the mitochondrial release of an apoptogenic protease. *J Exp Med.* 1996; 184(4):1331–1341.

65. Susin SA, Lorenzo HK, Zamzami N, et al. Molecular characterization of mitochondrial apoptosis-inducing factor. *Nature.* 1999; 397(6718):441–446.

66. Susin SA, Daugas E, Ravagnan L, et al. Two distinct pathways leading to nuclear apoptosis. *J Exp Med.* 2000;192(4):571–580.

67. Hill IE, Murray C, Richard J, Rasquinha I, MacManus JP. Despite the internucleosomal cleavage of DNA, reactive oxygen species do not produce other markers of apoptosis in cultured neurons. *Exp Neurol.* 2000;162(1):73–88.

68. Dumont C, Dürrbach A, Bidere N, et al. Caspase-independent commitment phase to apoptosis in activated blood T lymphocytes: reversibility at low apoptotic insult. *Blood*. 2000;96(3):1030–1038.

69. Zhang X, Chen J, Graham SH, et al. Intranuclear localization of apoptosis-inducing factor (AIF) and large scale DNA fragmentation after traumatic brain injury in rats and in neuronal cultures exposed to peroxynitrite. *J Neurochem*. 2002;82(1):181–191.

70. Ashkenazi A, Dixit VM. Death receptors: signaling and modulation. *Science*. 1998;281(5381):1305–1308.

71. Li H, Zhu H, Xu CJ, Yuan J. Cleavage of BID by caspase 8 mediates the mitochondrial damage in the Fas pathway of apoptosis. *Cell*. 1998;94(4):491–501.

72. Hockenbery D, Nunez G, Milliman C, Schreiber RD, Korsmeyer SJ. Bcl-2 is an inner mitochondrial membrane protein that blocks programmed cell death. *Nature*. 1990;348(6299):334–336.

73. Clark RSB, Chen J, Watkins SC, et al. Apoptosis-suppressor gene bcl-2 expression after traumatic brain injury in rats. *J Neurosci*. 1997;17(23):9172–9182.

74. Raghupathi R, Fernandez SC, Murai H, et al. BCL-2 overexpression attenuates cortical cell loss after traumatic brain injury in transgenic mice. *J Cereb Blood Flow Metab*. 1998;18(11):1259–1269.

75. Clark RSB, Kochanek PM, Adelson PD, et al. Increases in bcl-2 protein in cerebrospinal fluid and evidence for programmed cell death in infants and children after severe traumatic brain injury. *J Pediatr*. 2000;137(2):197–204.

76. Kotapka MJ, Graham DI, Adams JH, Gennarelli TA. Hippocampal pathology in fatal human head injury without high intracranial pressure. *J Neurotrauma*. 1994;11:317–324.

77. Jenkins LW, Lyeth BG, Lewelt W, et al. Combined pretrauma scopolamine and phencyclidine attenuate posttraumatic increased sensitivity to delayed secondary ischemia. *J Neurotrauma*. 1988;5(4):275–287.

78. Forbes ML, Clark RS, Dixon CE, et al. Augmented neuronal death in CA3 hippocampus following hyperventilation early after controlled cortical impact. *J Neurosurg*. 1998;88(3):549–556.

79. Colicos MA, Dixon CE, Dash PK. Delayed, selective neuronal death following experimental cortical impact injury in rats: possible role in memory deficits. *Brain Res*. 1996;739(1):111–119.

80. Graham DI, McIntosh TK, Maxwell WL, Nicoll JA. Recent advances in neurotrauma. *J Neuropathol Exp Neurol*. 2000;59(8):641–651.

81. Cross TG, Scheel-Toellner D, Henriquez NV, Deacon E, Salmon M, Lord JM. Serine/threonine protein kinases and apoptosis. *Exp Cell Res*. 2000;256(1):34–41.

82. Orban PC, Chapman PF, Brambilla R. Is the Ras-MAPK signalling pathway necessary for long-term memory formation? *Trends Neurosci*. 1999;22(1):38–44.

83. Naor Z, Benard O, Seger R. Activation of MAPK cascades by G-protein-coupled receptors: the case of gonadotropin-releasing hormone receptor. *Trends Endocrinol Metab*. 2000;11(3):91–99.

84. Kaplan DR, Miller FD. Neurotrophin signal transduction in the nervous system. *Curr Opin Neurobiol*. 2000;10(3):381–391.

85. Ono K, Han J. The p38 signal transduction pathway: activation and function. *Cell Signal*. 2000;12(1):1–13.

86. Dash PK, Mach SA, Moore AN. The role of extracellular signal-regulated kinase in cognitive and motor deficits following experimental traumatic brain injury. *Neuroscience*. 2002;114(3):755–767.

87. Otani N, Nawashiro H, Fukui S, Nomura N, Shima K. Temporal and spatial profile of phosphorylated mitogen-activated protein kinase pathways after lateral fluid percussion injury in the cortex of the rat brain. *J Neurotrauma*. 2002;19(12):1587–1596.

88. Mori T, Wang X, Jung JC, et al. Mitogen-activated protein kinase inhibition in traumatic brain injury: in vitro and in vivo effects. *J Cereb Blood Flow Metab*. 2002;22(4):444–452.

89. Nuñez G, del Peso L. Linking extracellular survival signals and the apoptotic machinery. *Curr Opin Neurobiol*. 1998;8(5):613–618.

90. Konishi H, Matsuzaki H, Takaishi H, et al. Opposing effects of protein kinase C delta and protein kinase B alpha on H(2)O(2)-induced apoptosis in CHO cells. *Biochem Biophys Res Commun*. 1999;264(3):840–846.

91. Coffer PJ, Jin J, Woodgett JR. Protein kinase B (c-Akt): a multifunctional mediator of phosphatidylinositol 3-kinase activation. *Biochem J*. 1998;335(pt 1):1–13.

92. Xia Z, Dickens M, Raingeaud J, Davis RJ, Greenberg ME. Opposing effects of ERK and JNK-p38 MAP kinases on apoptosis. *Science*. 1995;270(5240):1326–1331.

93. Jenkins LW, Peters GW, Dixon CE, et al. Conventional and functional proteomics using large format two-dimensional gel electrophoresis 24 hours after controlled cortical impact in postnatal day 17 rats. *J Neurotrauma*. 2002;19(6):715–740.

94. Au AK, Bayir H, Kochanek PM, Clark R. Evaluation of autophagy using mouse models of brain injury. *Biochimica et Biophysica Acta*. 2010;1802:918–923.

95. Lai Y, Hickey RW, Chen Y, et al. Autophagy is increased after traumatic brain injury in mice and is partially inhibited by the antioxidant gamma-glutamycysteinyl ethyl ester. *J Cereb Blood Flow Metab*. 2008;28(3):540–550.

96. Adams JH, Graham DI, Murray LS, Scott G. Diffuse axonal injury due to nonmissile head injury in humans: an analysis of 45 cases. *Ann Neurol*. 1982;12(6):557–563.

97. Adams JH, Doyle D, Ford I, Gennarelli TA, Graham DI, McLellan DR. Diffuse axonal injury in head injury: definition, diagnosis and grading. *Histopathology*. 1989;15(1):49–59.

98. Christman CW, Grady MS, Walker SA, Holloway KL, Povlishock JT. Ultrastructural studies of diffuse axonal injury in humans. *J Neurotrauma*. 1994;11(2):173–186.

99. Gennarelli TA, Thibault LE, Adams JH, Graham DI, Thompson CJ, Marcincin RP. Diffuse axonal injury and traumatic coma in the primate. *Ann Neurol*. 1982;12(6):564–574.

100. Povlishock JT. Traumatically induced axonal injury: pathogenesis and pathobiological implications. *Brain Pathol*. 1992;2(1):1–12.

101. Fitzpatrick MO, Maxwell WL, Graham DI. The role of the axolemma in the initiation of traumatically induced axonal injury. *J Neurol Neurosurg Psychiatry*. 1998;64(3):285–287.

102. Smith DH, Chen XH, Xu BN, McIntosh TK, Gennarelli TA, Meaney DF. Characterization of diffuse axonal pathology and selective hippocampal damage following inertial brain trauma in the pig. *J Neuropathol Exp Neurol*. 1997;56(7):822–834.

103. Gennarelli TA. Mechanisms of brain injury. *J Emerg Med*. 1993;11(suppl 1):5–11.

104. Graham DI, Lawrence AE, Adams JH, Doyle D, McLellan DR. Brain damage in fatal non-missile head injury without high intracranial pressure. *J Clin Pathol*. 1988;41(1):34–37.

105. Graham DI, Ford I, Adams JH, et al. Fatal head injury in children. *J Clin Pathol*. 1989;42(1):18–22.

106. Povlishock JT, Buki A, Koiziumi H, Stone J, Okonkwo DO. Initiating mechanisms involved in the pathobiology of traumatically induced axonal injury and interventions targeted at blunting their progression. *Acta Neurochir Suppl*. 1999;73:15–20.

107. Povlishock JT, Jenkins LW. Are the pathobiological changes evoked by traumatic brain injury immediate and irreversible? *Brain Pathol*. 1995;5(4):415–426.

108. Maxwell WL, Povlishock JT, Graham DL. A mechanistic analysis of nondisruptive axonal injury: a review. *J Neurotrauma*. 1997;14(7):419–440.

109. Stys PK. Anoxic and ischemic injury of myelinated axons in CNS white matter: from mechanistic concepts to therapeutics. *J Cereb Blood Flow Metab*. 1998;18(1):2–25.

110. Kampfl A, Posmantur RM, Zhao X, Schmutzhard E, Clifton GL, Hayes RL. Mechanisms of calpain proteolysis following traumatic brain injury: implications for pathology and therapy: implications for pathology and therapy: a review and update. *J Neurotrauma*. 1997;14(3):121–134.

111. Büki A, Koizumi H, Povlishock JT. Moderate posttraumatic hypothermia decreases early calpain-mediated proteolysis and concomitant cytoskeletal compromise in traumatic axonal injury. *Exp Neurol*. 1999;159(1):319–328.

112. Reeves TM, Phillips LL, Lee NN, Povlishock JT. Preferential neuroprotective effect of tacrolimus (FK506) on unmyelinated axons following traumatic brain injury. *Brain Res*. 2007;1154:225–236.

113. Mills JD, Bailes JE, Sedney CL, Hutchins H, Sears B. Omega-3 fatty acid supplementation and reduction of traumatic axonal injury in a rodent head injury model. *J Neurosurg*. 2011;114(1):77–84.

114. Büki A, Okonkwo DO, Povlishock JT. Postinjury cyclosporin A administration limits axonal damage and disconnection in traumatic brain injury. *J Neurotrauma*. 1999;16(6):511–521.

115. Goss JR, Styren SD, Miller PD, et al. Hypothermia attenuates the normal increase in interleukin 1 beta RNA and nerve growth factor following traumatic brain injury in the rat. *J Neurotrauma.* 1995; 12(2):159–167.

116. DeKosky ST, Goss JR, Miller PD, Styren SD, Kochanek PM, Marion D. Upregulation of nerve growth factor following cortical trauma. *Exp Neurol.* 1994;130(2):173–177.

117. Cecil KM, Hills EC, Sandel ME, et al. Proton magnetic resonance spectroscopy for detection of axonal injury in the splenium of the corpus callosum of brain-injured patients. *J Neurosurg.* 1998;88(5): 795–801.

118. McGowan JC, McCormack TM, Grossman RI, et al. Diffuse axonal pathology detected with magnetization transfer imaging following brain injury in the pig. *Magn Reson Med.* 1999;41(4):727–733.

119. Xue R, van Zijl PC, Crain BJ, Crain BJ, Solaiyappan M, Mori S. In vivo three-dimensional reconstruction of rat brain axonal projections by diffusion tensor imaging. *Magn Reson Med.* 1999;42(6): 1123–1127.

120. Pajevic S, Pierpaoli C. Color schemes to represent the orientation of anisotropic tissues from diffusion tensor data: application to white matter fiber tract mapping in the human brain. *Magn Reson Med.* 1999;42:526–540.

121. Seelig JM, Becker DP, Miller JD, Greenberg RP, Ward JD, Choi SC. Traumatic acute subdural hematoma: major mortality reduction in comatose patients treated within four hours. *N Engl J Med.* 1981; 304(25):1511–1518.

122. Marmarou A, Barzo P, Fatouros P, Yamamoto T, Bullock R, Young H. Traumatic brain swelling in head injured patients: brain edema or vascular engorgement? *Acta Neurochir Suppl.* 1997;70:68–70.

123. Barzó P, Marmarou A, Fatouros P, Hayasaki K, Corwin F. Contribution of vasogenic and cellular edema to traumatic brain swelling measured by diffusion-weighted imaging. *J Neurosurg.* 1997;87(6): 900–907.

124. Barzó P, Marmarou A, Fatouros P, Ito J, Corwin F. MRI diffusion-weighted spectroscopy of reversible and irreversible ischemic injury following closed head injury. *Acta Neurochir Suppl.* 1997;70: 115–118.

125. Katayama Y, Mori T, Maeda T, Kawamata T. Pathogenesis of the mass effect of cerebral contusions: rapid increase in osmolality within the contusion necrosis. *Acta Neurochir Suppl.* 1998;71: 289–292.

126. Dusick JR, Glenn TC, Lee WN, et al. Increased pentose phosphate pathway flux after clinical traumatic brain injury: a [1,2–13C2]glucose labeling study in humans. *J Cereb Blood Flow Metab.* 2007;27(9): 1593–1602.

127. Ashwal S, Holshouser BA, Shu SK, et al. Predictive value of proton magnetic resonance spectroscopy in pediatric closed head injury. *Pediatr Neurol.* 2000;23(2):114–125.

128. Rosomoff HL, Clasen RA, Hartstock R, Bebin J. Brain reaction to experimental injury after hypothermia. *Arch Neurol.* 1965;13(4): 337–345.

129. Schoettle RJ, Kochanek PM, Magargee MJ, Uhl MW, Nimoto EM. Early polymorphonuclear leukocyte accumulation correlates with the development of posttraumatic cerebral edema in rats. *J Neurotrauma.* 1990;7(4):207–217.

130. Clark RSB, Schiding JK, Kaczorowski SL, Marion DW, Kochanek PM. Neutrophil accumulation after traumatic brain injury in rats: comparison of weight drop and controlled cortical impact models. *J Neurotrauma.* 1994;11(5):499–506.

131. McClain C, Cohen D, Phillips R, Ott L, Young B. Increased plasma and ventricular fluid interleukin-6 levels in patients with head injury. *J Lab Clin Med.* 1991;118(3):225–231.

132. Marion DW, Penrod LE, Kelsey SF, et al. Treatment of traumatic brain injury with moderate hypothermia. *N Engl J Med.* 1997;336(8): 540–546.

133. Kossmann T, Hans VH, Imhof HG, et al. Intrathecal and serum interleukin-6 and the acute-phase response in patients with severe traumatic brain injuries. *Shock.* 1995;4(5):311–317.

134. Kossmann T, Stahel PF, Lenzlinger PM, et al. Interleukin-8 released into the cerebrospinal fluid after brain injury is associated with blood-brain barrier dysfunction and nerve growth factor production. *J Cereb Blood Flow Metab.* 1997;17(3):280–289.

135. Bethea JR, Castro M, Keane RW, Lee TT, Dietrich WD, Yezierski RP. Traumatic spinal cord injury induces nuclear factor-kappaB activation. *J Neurosci.* 1998;18(9):3251–3260.

136. Shohami E, Bass R, Wallach D, Yamin A, Gallily R. Inhibition of tumor necrosis factor alpha (TNFalpha) activity in rat brain is associated with cerebroprotection after closed head injury. *J Cereb Blood Flow Metab.* 1996;16(3):378–384.

137. Scherbel U, Raghupathi R, Nakamura M, et al. Differential acute and chronic responses of tumor necrosis factor-deficient mice to experimental brain injury. *Proc Natl Acad Sci U S A.* 1999;96(15): 8721–8726.

138. Toulmond S, Rothwell NJ. Interleukin-1 receptor antagonist inhibits neuronal damage caused by fluid percussion injury in the rat. *Brain Res* 1995;671(2):261–266.

139. DeKosky ST, Styren SD, O'Malley ME, et al. Interleukin-1 receptor antagonist suppresses neurotrophin response in injured rat brain. *Ann Neurol.* 1996;39(1):123–127.

140. Shapira Y, Artru AA, Yadid G, et al. Methylprednisolone does not decrease eicosanoid concentrations or edema in brain tissue or improve neurologic outcome after head trauma in rats. *Anesth Analg.* 1992;75:238–244.

141. Uhl MW, Biagas KV, Grundl PD, et al. Effects of neutropenia on edema, histology, and cerebral blood flow after traumatic brain injury in rats. *J Neurotrauma.* 1994;11(3):303–315.

142. Blight AR. Effects of silica on the outcome from experimental spinal cord injury: implication of macrophages in secondary tissue damage. *Neuroscience.* 1994;60(1):263–273.

143. Popovich PG, Guan Z, Wei P, Huitinga I, Van Rooijen N, Stokes BT. Depletion of hematogenous macrophages promotes partial hindlimb recovery and neuroanatomical repair after experimental spinal cord injury. *Exp Neurol.* 1999;158(2):351–365.

144. Kossmann T, Hans V, Imhof HG, Trentz O, Morganti-Kossann MC. Interleukin-6 released in human cerebrospinal fluid following traumatic brain injury may trigger nerve growth factor production in astrocytes. *Brain Res.* 1996;713(1–2):143–152.

145. Sinz EH, Kochanek PM, Heyes MP, et al. Quinolinic acid is increased in CSF and associated with mortality after traumatic brain injury in humans. *J Cereb Blood Flow Metab.* 1998;18(6):610–615.

146. Shore PM, Jackson EK, Wisniewski SR, Clark RS, Adelson PK, Kochanek PM. Vascular endothelial growth factor is increased in cerebrospinal fluid after traumatic brain injury in infants and children. *Neurosurgery.* 2004;54(3):605–611.

147. Bayır H, Kochanek PM, Siu SX, et al. Increased S-nitrosothiols and S-nitrosoalbumin in cerebrospinal fluid after severe traumatic brain injury in infants and children: indirect association with intracranial pressure. *J Cereb Blood Flow Metab.* 2003;23(1):51–61.

148. Sinz EH, Kochanek PM, Dixon CE, et al. Inducible nitric oxide synthase is an endogenous neuroprotectant after traumatic brain injury in rats and mice. *J Clin Invest.* 1999;104(5):647–656.

149. Wada K, Chatzipanteli K, Kraydieh S, Busto R, Dietrich WD. Inducible nitric oxide synthase expression after traumatic brain injury and neuroprotection with aminoguanidine treatment in rats. *Neurosurgery.* 1998;43(6):1427–1436.

150. Yamasaki K, Edington HD, McClosky C, et al. Reversal of impaired wound repair in iNOS-deficient mice by topical adenoviral-mediated iNOS gene transfer. *J Clin Invest.* 1998;101(5):967–971.

151. Heard SO, Fink MP, Gamelli RL, et al. Effect of prophylactic administration of recombinant human granulocyte colony-stimulating factor (filgrastim) on the frequency of nosocomial infections in patients with acute traumatic brain injury or cerebral hemorrhage. The Filgrastim Study Group. *Crit Care Med.* 1998;26(4):748–754.

152. Kochanek PM, Clark RSB, Ruppel RA, et al. Biochemical, cellular, and molecular mechanisms in the evolution of secondary damage after severe traumatic brain injury in infants and children: lessons learned from the bedside. *Pediatr Crit Care Med.* 2000;1(1):4–19.

153. Garman RH, Jenkins LW, Switzer RC III, et al. Blast exposure in rats with body shielding is characterized primarily by diffuse axonal injury. *J Neurotrauma.* 2011;28(6):947–959.

Concepts of Central Nervous System Plasticity and Their Implications for Recovery After Brain Damage

Donald G. Stein

If the facts don't fit the theory, change the facts.—Albert Einstein

INTRODUCTION

It is now accepted that after brain injury, "plasticity" and recovery may be possible, but their underlying mechanisms remain a matter of debate. The term plasticity is seldom explicitly defined in reports on brain injury or neurorehabilitation. When any functional restitution or recovery after brain injury is observed, the assumption is that the inherent plasticity of the brain is responsible. But what does this explain about what is actually taking place in response to brain damage?

Until the late 1960s, few people in neurorehabilitation supported the idea that the adult central nervous system (CNS) was capable of substantial reorganization in response to brain damage. Recovery by definition entailed resumption of the same function by the same irreplaceable anatomical structures, and so was impossible. Therefore, any "recovery" was attributed to strategic behavioral tricks—compensatory strategies—that subjects with brain injuries were able to master to overcome their deficits (1). But the argument was circular: you had behavioral recovery because of compensatory strategies, which were inferred because you had behavioral recovery—hardly a meaningful explanation of mechanism!

The term "compensation" implicitly assumes that an organism with brain injury accomplishes some goal (e.g., turning on a light switch or opening a door) without necessarily considering the means by which the goal is achieved. A seeing-eye dog is an example of this type of compensation for someone who has lost visual function. Crossing the street is still accomplished (the goal) but *the means* of doing so are very different from what a sighted person might do (see 2 and 3 for interesting discussions of this issue). On the one hand, although different cues, motor movements and behavioral strategies are used in this type of compensation, there is no need to posit any neuronal regeneration or restructuring. The alternative view, first formulated by some of the earliest pioneers in neuroscience and now being developed

in the light of new concepts and technologies, holds that changes in brain organization and function can be mediated by structural alterations in brain maps, and rehabilitation and training can initiate morphological and biochemical changes in the brain that can be sustained over long periods.

One of the dogmas that blocked research on the mechanisms of recovery after brain damage was promoted by the Nobel laureate neuroanatomist Santiago Ramón y Cajal (4), who forcefully argued that once development was over, any regeneration in the adult brain would be very limited, if it occurred at all. During the first half of the 20th century, some neuroanatomists who observed structural changes in the injured adult brain such as axonal or dendritic sprouting, or even neurogenesis—now considered characteristic of neuronal repair—often reported such changes as artifacts of histological techniques rather than as evidence of CNS structural plasticity.

The paradigm shift that led to acceptance of the idea of CNS plasticity in response to injury began with the work of Raisman (5). Using then state-of-the-art electron microscopic techniques, Raisman mapped the 2 primary afferent pathways into the subcortical structure he called the "septal nuclear complex" in adult rats. Once the pathways were identified, Raisman made separate, selective knife-cuts to disrupt 1 of the 2 paths and observe changes in the intact pathway in response to the injury. After a suitable time, he observed that (*a*) degenerating fibers caused by the cut left synapses in the septal nucleus vacated, and (*b*) fibers from the surviving pathway reoccupied the vacated synapses. Particularly interesting was that the new afferents were "heterotypic": they did not provide the same neurotransmitter to the septal cells as had the original fibers. Raisman concluded that

the finding that the distribution of one fiber pathway to the septum is altered by the destruction of another system of septal afferents suggests that synapses in the central nervous system of adult mammals may be far more labile than had been previously suspected. It is interesting to speculate why, in view of this anatomical plasticity, so little functional recovery accompanies lesions of the brain. (5, p. 45)

Raisman and his colleagues did not follow up his remarkable observations with behavioral studies, but his work did lead others to change the view of the adult CNS from a static, phrenological collection of structures with fixed functions to a much more dynamic system capable of reorganization in response to injury (see, e.g., 6 and 7).

Although studies on promoting recovery of function appeared as early as the first decades of the 20th century (see, e.g., 8), until the early 1970s they were largely dismissed by the field as describing anomalous events not worthy of serious study. At the behavioral level, adherents of the more static view of the adult CNS could claim that when functional recovery was observed, it was because the tests being used were not sensitive enough to detect the underlying deficits. The idea that recovery of function can be promoted by pharmacological agents, the transplantation of fetal or stem cell tissues, environmental stimulation, hormonal factors, and other means, is still a relatively new concept in the history of the science.

The remainder of this chapter reviews several concepts of recovery that were proposed in the fields of neuropsychology and neurorehabilitation before there was much empirical and clinical data to support them. Given the large body of evidence we now have for dramatic reorganization and repair after injury, are these early concepts of functional recovery consistent with the principle of functional localization in the brain? Are plasticity concepts and localization theory mutually consistent? Is recovery of function supported by the evidence, both modern high-tech data and the older intuitive clinical approach (9)?

WHAT IS NEUROPLASTICITY?

What do we mean by "neuroplasticity"? Is it a well-defined phenomenon that can be applied as an explanatory construct? Over the last several decades, there has been an explosion of interest in neuroplasticity, and it is often taken for granted that what the term implies is well understood. PubMed, the National Institutes of Health's search engine, is a powerful tool for finding articles in biomedical sciences. Search for neuroplasticity and 30,850 articles appear. Neuroplasticity is applied to the symptoms of Parkinson disease, Alzheimer disease, interactions between steroid hormones and neurotrophins, alterations in apolipoprotein E synthesis, chronic pain, mood disorders, recovery from stroke, long-term potentiation in the hippocampus, changes in memory in development and aging, neurogenesis during development and aging, allodynia, interactions between glia and neurons, presynaptic neurotransmitter vesicle release, changes in synaptic terminal arborization, changes in voltage-sensitive ion channels, epigenetic regulation of gene expression, insulinlike signaling pathways in worms, changes in memory caused by alterations in the levels of brain aquaporin-4 expression, alterations during critical periods of development, alterations in glutamate receptors, alterations in sensory-cortical maps, alterations in dynamical network organization, stem cell effects, axonal sprouting, amphetamine addiction, epileptic seizure activity, and augmentation of immune-induced neural inflammatory response, all in the first 40 references. How can such a ubiquitous term be of use in understanding what happens in the damaged nervous system in response to injury? One argument is that plasticity has manifold ways of expressing itself in both the intact and the damaged nervous system. But if every type of change in neural, or any other tissue for that matter, is seen as plasticity, what then is *not* an example of the phenomenon? Is using neuroplasticity as an explanatory concept any different from saying that if you do something to the nervous system of an organism, you will produce a change?

In a recent review, Dietz (10) defines neuronal plasticity as "the neuronal changes occurring after spinal cord injury with and without functional training." The way neuroplasticity is used here can be confusing because neuronal changes in response to injury can lead to adaptive *or* maladaptive functional outcomes such as spasticity. What do we learn about the specific mechanism(s) causing a specific outcome? Unless specific mechanisms of action are described (e.g., genomic, molecular, physiological, or anatomical), the term neuroplasticity could be seen as only a descriptive placeholder signifying that some change—beneficial or detrimental—may be occurring.

Here is an example from the field of neurogenesis that illustrates how neuroplasticity can perhaps be overused as an explanatory construct. Parent and Lowenstein (11) reviewed the literature on the effects of stem cell proliferation in the adult nervous system of rodents. These authors reported that there is, indeed, a fivefold to tenfold increase in the number of dentate granule cells in the hippocampus following chemotoxic injury to the brain, and this proliferation is taken as an example of injury-induced neuroplasticity even though the results are detrimental to the organism. However, their review of the literature also showed that the neurogenesis was associated with increases in kindling and seizure activity in the hippocampus and with a later increase in apoptotic cell death. This is not to imply that, under all conditions, injury-induced neurogenesis would be detrimental. But this is a typical example of using neuroplasticity to explain a negative outcome. But if such a phenomenon (i.e., neurogenesis as a cause for post-traumatic epilepsy) is an example of "plasticity," how useful is that concept for explaining recovery of function? Perhaps one ought to distinguish between negative or maladaptive and positive or adaptive plasticity and to think more critically about how we use the term to describe events in the CNS associated with functional recovery and rehabilitation.

In this chapter, neuroplasticity will be used only for verifiable examples of functional and adaptive recovery after brain injury. Behaviorally, after a CNS injury, cognitive, sensory, or motor impairments gradually diminish or are eliminated over time rather than getting worse. Limiting the term in this way implies that acute or chronic deficits can disappear spontaneously, or can be reduced by pharmacological, physiological, surgical, or behavioral treatments (11–15). Here, neuroplasticity is descriptive and phenomenological—a catch-all term to denote improvements in behavioral outcomes without necessarily specifying the underlying molecular or physiological mechanisms responsible for the improved behaviors. The goal of rehabilitation, in this context, is to teach the patient new strategies to replace functions lost by the injury, and plasticity is defined by the extent to which such substitution of function(s) is possible. The brain tissue remaining after an injury just does what it does to varying degrees of effectiveness, so it is not required that the brain add neurons or rebuild damaged circuits. Thus, it is suggested that although the patient who has suffered brain injury may eventually accomplish the same goals as an intact individual, the means by which the task is accomplished may be very different.

LOCALIZATION OF FUNCTION AND NEUROPLASTICITY

In the clinic, it may be difficult to accept a more limited definition of plasticity because it is often necessary for patients with a brain injury to succeed in a variety of activities of daily living by substituting new behavioral strategies. This strategy substitution is a form of "compensation" or adaptation to a deficit. As noted, some critics of the idea that recovery of function is possible argue that all recovery is only a type of compensation (see 1 and 12 for good discussions of this issue). This view is an offshoot of the idea that specific areas of the brain are genetically programmed to control or mediate behaviors, so the destruction or perturbation of a center in which a function is localized leads to the permanent loss (or serious impairment) of that function.

The battle between adherents of precise localization of functions and those who think that functions are distributed throughout the brain has been going on for well over a hundred years, and despite breakthroughs in brain imaging techniques, no resolution is in sight. The definitions and extent of localization, as well as what brain structures are supposed to do, seem to shift with advances in technology, but in the final analysis they amount to an advanced form of 19th century phrenology. For example, cortical maps grow or shrink according to how imaging methods are applied, and this determines how the loci of control are defined. As imaging studies proliferate, structures are added or subtracted at will to the number required to mediate a particular function, with the expansion said to be taking place in the serial or parallel circuits so popular in earlier computer-based metaphors of the brain. The more recovery observed, especially in the case of bilateral structural damage, the more structures have to be postulated to account for the observed plasticity. The arguments for this scenario tend to be circular; that is, the greater the extent of the parallel circuitry proposed to mediate function, the greater the functional plasticity/recovery and likewise, the more the recovery, the greater the parallel circuitry there is to subsume it. It would be hard to come up with experiments to support or disprove this hypothesis. It is a good example of reification—explanation by naming. This issue is discussed further below.

Providing technical support for the parallel or multiple circuitry approach to brain function is the rapid progress in molecular biological assays, which has led to a plethora of functional activities being assigned to the expression or inhibition of specific genes, a form of localization doctrine gone wild—a molecular biology of phrenology, so to speak, which is of growing concern to some investigators in this field. In an excellent brief review of the issue, Kosik (13) cautions that

genes, neurons and brain regions are annotated with func-

tional descriptors that fail to capture the interactive nature of these units. The temptation is strong to jump beyond what a biological unit actually does, to a more encompassing functional label. For example, a mutant gene does not cause a disease, it merely encodes a mutant protein that leads to a cascade of events and, eventually, to a disease. The methodology to ascertain function can also be limiting. Just as the carpenter, whose only tool is a hammer, treats all objects like nails, so neurophysiologists and brain "imagers" probe the brain with their own hammers and have cobbled a picture of brain function that is not explicitly integrated. (p. 235)

The notion that single genes or a set of a few genes can be "responsible for complex behavioral disorders following a brain injury" is beginning to be questioned more rigorously. As Villoslada and colleagues (14) write, "Under the reductionist paradigm, a positive correlation between a single biological parameter and the occurrence of a disease is often considered a major success, even though the complete pathogenic mechanism may remain largely unknown" (p. 125). I take this to mean that individual genes or sets of genes can play multiple roles in driving multiple processes producing functional deficits or their repair. Furthermore, as these different systems are called into play as a result of environmental inputs, disease, or internal homeostatic demands, "certain properties emerge from [the aggregate] that cannot be derived from the individual analysis of each of the components"—that is, each separate gene (p. 128). Extrapolating from the emergent properties of gene combinations to how different brain areas interact to produce deficits or repair is not a great leap. After all, when a brain area is damaged and ceases to function, it is the activity of the remaining brain tissue producing the symptoms and syndromes—not the tissue that has been removed.

The Serial Lesion Effect

One of the most interesting forms of spontaneous recovery in both animals and humans is seen in the serial lesion effect (see 8 for a review). John Hughlings Jackson, a pioneer of neurology in the late 19th and early 20th century, named this the "momentum of the lesion" effect. In this type of injury, brain lesions develop slowly or are experimentally inflicted in stages so that, for example, the left frontal cortex may be extirpated and then a second operation takes the homologous right frontal cortex 30 days later. Under these conditions, both animals and humans show remarkable and robust postinjury sparing of function compared to counterparts with the same damage inflicted in 1 stage (8). In humans, slow-growing injuries often do not lead to either the severity or sometimes even the appearance of the functional impairments seen when the same extent of injury occurs after a stroke or acute traumatic damage (15). Although there are numerous replications of the serial lesion effect in fully mature subjects, the research has not received much attention in contemporary neuroscience, probably because instances of plasticity as demonstrated by considerable sparing of function *in the absence of special training or treatment* are problematic for current theories of highly organized modular function (see, e.g., 8, 16–19). In the face of bilateral removal of a structure with no loss of function, it is difficult to sustain the notion that individual aggregates of cells or structures are critical for the expression of that function. Fortunately, the literature is beginning to take another look at what such plasticity implies for concepts about the organization of function in the adult CNS.

Several years ago, Seitz and Freund (20) reviewed human studies showing that some slowly progressive lesions remain asymptomatic for years because space-occupying tumors cause a substantial reorganization of function as measured by regional cerebral blood flow (rCBF) studies. These investigators studied a group of patients with brain tumors that had invaded the entire hand/arm motor cortex. They had developed seizures but were normal on neurologic examination. The rCBF showed that during finger movements, the areas of activation were substantially displaced to more lateral positions, even to cortical areas outside the motor strip. The authors concluded that "the astonishing discrepancy between the functional consequences of acute versus chronic lesions of the nervous system raises the possibility that reorganization (of function) is not restricted to within-system recovery in the motor cortex" (p. 329). This type of slowly developing reorganization can be considered evidence for equipotentiality or vicarious function (see below) in the broad sense. The authors also point out that over time, the patients learn to use and refine other behavioral strategies often seen in normal subjects. It is thought that such patients can be given substantial skill training to recruit other cortical areas into the functional reorganization produced by the demands on the damaged CNS.

Substitution of Function Concepts

The assumption of substitution rather than restitution of function after brain damage fits well with the idea that intact parts of the brain can take over the functions of tissue lost or destroyed after injury or disease. In this paradigm, remaining healthy tissue is said to modulate its physiological activities to compensate for the damage to a specific area. But there is evidence to support a different model for response to injury. As Finger noted in a recent review (21), "The theories of behavioral compensation, 'shock,' and redundancy share a common feature: none requires rewiring the nervous system in a new way or rearranging the functions normally associated with specific parts of the brain" (p. 833). Thus, in laboratory rats and monkeys, if injury occurs during certain critical periods in early development, recovery of cognitive and motor functions can sometimes be greater than that seen in adults with similar kinds of CNS damage. Is this merely a form of compensatory strategy or is structural reorganization of the brain a major factor in plasticity?

Development, Brain Injury, and Plasticity
In the 1960s, the developmental psychologist Eric Lenneberg (22) proposed that, at birth, the two cerebral hemispheres are equipotential for cognitive and language functions, and only gradually become specialized as the child matures. This idea seemed to be supported by the now classic studies of Margaret Kennard in monkeys. She showed that animals with large cortical lesions inflicted early in life showed none of the extensive deficits seen when the same type of damage was inflicted at a later age (23). Subsequently, Patricia Goldman was able to show that early brain lesions in monkeys

led to substantially more sparing of cognitive functions than when the damage was inflicted in later life. Goldman and Galkin (24) reported that lesions of the frontal cortex in a fetal rhesus monkey operated on and returned to the womb until term not only showed complete sparing of cognitive function, but also demonstrated a radical reorganization of the entire cortical mantle evidenced by numerous ectopic gyri and sulci not seen in the intact animal.

A more recent approach challenging the ideas of limited plasticity and discrete localization has been proposed by Goldberg (25, pp. 56–59), who suggests that training and experience can subtly modify brain areas so that there is a gradient of overlap between them, especially in the cerebral cortex. Taking this one step further, Goldberg suggests that the changes produced by experience (including injury or illness) could lead to a constant state of flux incorporating brain areas into a temporary system for the performance of a task and then changing configuration to incorporate other disparate brain areas when task demands or physiological needs (e.g., hormonal or metabolic state) change. Depending on conditions at the time of injury, it is also possible that injury or stroke to a brain in one state of organization could "lock in" that particular organizational pattern, leading to a localization of symptoms that might dissipate over time, or remain permanent if the gradient of plasticity is more limited, as might be the case if thalamic or brain stem structures were implicated.

It has become increasingly clear that neither strict localization nor complete equipotentiality explain how the brain is organized in normal and pathological conditions. In an excellent brief review of this literature, Vargha-Khadem et al. (26) reported that better testing of children has revealed residual deficits after early hemispheric removals. They note that some of these residual deficits could have been caused by medications, seizures, and nutritional and other environmental factors. When such variables are controlled, the authors observe that, as equipotentiality theory would predict, the deficits are extremely mild considering the extent of tissue loss. According to Vargha-Khadem et al., either hemisphere appears to be able to subserve linguistic and cognitive functions during the early stages of development; however, the cost of such compensation may be a generally reduced level of such functions as visuospatial behaviors caused by "crowding" of the supposedly lateralized functions into the one remaining hemisphere (27).

In humans with early brain injury, the issues are more complex and controversial than for adult brain injury, especially with respect to intellectual skills, language, and cognition. For example, many studies in both animals and children provide strong substantiation that early brain damage is associated with long-term deficits and intellectual impairments (28,29). Other studies support what has been called the Kennard principle (30), that early brain lesions lead to much more sparing than the same injury in a more mature organism (31,32). How is it possible to reconcile these divergent findings? Factors have now been identified that can predispose to better or worse outcomes after injury during early development. In particular, there appears to be a very specific, critical period for plasticity such that an early-occurring injury to the brain may be much worse than a comparable injury sustained just a few weeks or months later (33). Bryan Kolb and his colleagues have repeatedly demonstrated this phenomenon in laboratory rats. They also review evidence in human infants that a cortical injury in the first months of life can be devastating, but if the same cortical area is damaged at around 1–2 years of age, there is much better recovery. Kolb and Cioe (34) found that as little as 1 week of difference in age could have a dramatic impact on morphogenesis and sparing of function after medial frontal cortical lesions in rats. Thus, if the lesions were created on postnatal day 2, animals tested as adults on spatial learning and reaching tasks were very impaired. If the same surgery was done on postnatal day 9, there was extensive recovery and apparently substantial generation of new neurons to replace neurons removed by the surgery.

More recently, Nemati and Kolb (35) created unilateral motor cortex lesions in rats at either 35 or 55 days of age, then tested the rats on a variety of motor tasks as adults and compared them to age-matched, sham-operated counterparts. The animals brain-injured at 35 days of age had substantial motor impairments, whereas those given brain damage at 55 days of age had almost complete functional recovery. In addition, this latter group showed bilateral hypertrophy of dendritic fields in the sensorimotor cortex—an effect not seen in the younger-operated rats. In development, then, the precise timing of the injury may be critical in determining whether recovery, and/or the rebuilding of neuronal circuits, will be observed. Injuries sustained slightly or moderately later than immediately after birth, when one might assume the most plasticity, could lead to much better outcomes. This calls for a more modulated interpretation of the Kennard principle that the earlier the injury, the better the outcome.

Equipotentiality and Vicariation

When sparing of function is observed, it is often attributed to the equipotentiality or vicarious function of cerebral (usually cortical) areas. Equipotentiality refers to the capacity of anatomically distinct areas of the brain to mediate a rather wide variety of functions. In a sense, the concept of equipotentiality was the forerunner of the more contemporary notion of serial and parallel circuits, whereby several different structures "cooperate" to mediate various kinds of motor and cognitive performance. Equipotentiality is thought more likely to be expressed when the brain is developing and not yet specialized for particular activities such as speech or patterned movement, but there is both historical and contemporary evidence to suggest that (*a*) equipotentiality may not be seen in every part of the brain to the same extent and (*b*) both equipotentiality and vicarious function can be expressed in the adult organism as well.

The concept of neural vicariation implies that even the mature CNS has redundant or backup subsystems that participate in this takeover of function (27). Although equipotentiality implies that different brain structures can mediate a variety of functions without any loss of an ongoing functional activity, vicariation implies that another structure can take over the function of a damaged area but the original function as well as the new one may be less than fully normal. Again, the idea of serial and parallel structure–function relationships is the contemporary version. In the older version, however, the mechanisms by which area *a* could take over the function of damaged area *b* and still perform func-

tion *a* were not described, creating once more a kind of circular reasoning. The more important problem is: If there is substitution or vicarious function, how can it be identified at the physiological and/or behavioral levels of analysis? In one study, Xerri, Merzenich, Peterson, and Jenkins (36) trained adult squirrels and owl monkeys to retrieve small objects, used microelectrode techniques to map responsivity to afferent activity when the animals performed the tactile discrimination tasks, and then selectively damaged specific parts of the sensorimotor cortex by electrocoagulation of surface blood vessels. The brain tissue was then checked to make sure that it was completely unresponsive to any peripheral stimulation. Immediately after the lesions, the monkeys were retrained on the tasks and cortical mapping was repeated. Performance initially deteriorated, then started to get better with retraining, and appeared to be proportional to the difficulty of the task. In some cases, animals with large lesions actually recovered better than those with less damage. The resulting changes in postinjury behaviors were complex and highly individualistic, suggesting that the individual monkey's experience and environment play a role in shaping the behavior and cortical map organization. Most striking was the fact that the postlesion reorganization of the cortex was very variable across monkeys; completely new cortical fields representing the fingers emerged and were enlarged in cortical areas that are not normally responsive to cutaneous stimulation. The changes appeared to be caused both by the lesion and by the training procedures. According to the authors, the representation of the hands in the S1 region of the somatosensory cortex is topographically organized into discrete cytoarchitectonic and functional regions, so that when these regions are damaged, area-specific deficits can be observed. For example, damage to area 1 leads to deficits in the discrimination of textures, whereas damage to area 2 impairs recognition of size and shape. Damage to area 3 causes significant deficits in texture, size, and shape discriminations. These observations suggest that areas not normally involved in mediating certain behaviors can take over those functions under the right circumstances—an example of vicarious function as we have used it here. This means that when behavioral substitution occurs, specific physiological mechanisms subserve the changes. More important, it means that the brain is not just functioning as it did before but without a part. Rather, extensive permissive reorganization of neuronal activity (and structure) underlies vicarious function.

The extent of vicarious function and equipotentiality is subject to several conditions that can vary over the spectrum of development. Kolb, Teskey, and Gibb (16) recently pointed out that this type of plasticity varies across brain structures, environmental experiences (e.g., drug and medical history, nutritional factors, exposure to early or maternal stress), and critical periods of development (e.g., exposure to drugs or brain damage at one stage of development can have completely different effects from the same exposure earlier or later in life). In another example of how functional brain organization can be affected by development (17), Qi and colleagues sectioned the dorsal columns of the spinal cord between C3 and C5 in 3- to 12-day-old rhesus monkeys and then studied the organizational map of the motor cortex by microelectrode stimulation when the animals reached 5 years of age. Interestingly, large spinal cord lesions did not alter the "basic organization of the motor cortex," but there were abnormalities in hand and forelimb representations indicative of lesion-induced changes in cortical activity. Five years after injury, deprivation of sensory inputs into the motor cortex led not to a nonfunctional state but rather to a representation of new muscle movements not seen in normal animals of the same age.

Examples of this kind of reorganization (vicariation or equipotentiality) can be even more dramatic. Muckli, Naumer, and Singer (18) studied the organization of retinotopic maps in the lateral geniculate nucleus (LGN) and visual areas (V1–V3) in a female patient born with the complete loss of the right cerebral hemisphere and almost complete loss of the right eye. At 10 years of age, the child was tested using structural magnetic resonance imaging (MRI), functional MRI (fMRI) (to measure retinotopic maps), perimetry, and functional visual field mapping of the LGN. The investigators found a dramatic reorganization of optic pathways and rerouting of optic fibers into the intact hemisphere. "There was a surprising capacity of visual projections and processing centers to adapt to the early loss of an entire cerebral hemisphere that normally processes information of the whole contralateral visual hemifield" (p. 13,036). The authors concluded that "the fact that the rerouted projections support absolutely normal perceptual functions as well as visuomotor coordination strongly indicates the action of highly efficient adaptation mechanisms beyond early visual cortices that are capable of extracting useful information from maps that—because of rerouted axons and molecular cuing—exhibit markedly abnormal topologies" (p. 13,039). Taken together, all these findings also highlight the importance of applying the right rehabilitation strategies at the right time to enhance adaptive cortical reorganization (19,37).

Yet such reorganization may demand a high price: the emerging patterns can prevent true restitution of function by encumbering the brain with an experience-induced reorganization that may be difficult or impossible to undo. Until the recent development of sophisticated imaging and electrophysiological techniques, it was not possible to determine whether such equipotential, vicarious, or pluripotent systems exist. Recent studies using fMRI, positron emission tomography (PET) and other new technologies show that functional compensation may be caused by extensive reorganization of activity in the damaged brain. For instance, after an infarct in the striatum of human patients, several subcortical areas both ipsilateral and contralateral to the injury site become activated as behavioral recovery progresses. The activation, measured by increases in CBF and glucose metabolism, is not observed when normal, healthy volunteers are asked to perform the same motor tasks. If "tricks" are being used to compensate for lost functions, they could be mediated by shifts in the activity of cerebral structures that are not initially involved in the behaviors (or at least not in the same way) under normal circumstances. This type of reorganization can take weeks, months, or years to occur (38).

In an earlier report typical of studies on compensation, Castro-Alamancos, Garcia Segura, and Borrell (39) showed that after bilateral injury of the sensory-motor cortex in rats, there is a substantial deficit in bar-pressing response to prevent aversive stimulation. If the injury is followed by direct-brain stimulation of the ventral tegmental nucleus, substan-

tial recovery of the bar-press behavior is observed. Under these conditions, if the hind limb sensory cortex in the recovered animals is ablated, the deficit returns. It is important to note that the ablation of this area in the first place does not cause the same deficit, and this is taken as evidence of compensatory shifts in cortical function; the hind limb area "assumes the role of another area after induced recovery from brain damage."

In another example of shifts in function thought to be compensatory, Buckner et al. (40) used PET and fMRI scanning techniques to examine the preservation of speech using a variety of linguistic and cognitive tests in a 72-year-old patient 1 month after a stroke in the left inferior frontal cortex. Although the patient was impaired in speech generation tasks, he was able to access words when given partial words as cues, a task that usually depends (according to the authors) on an intact left inferior frontal cortex. The scanning during performance showed that the right inferior prefrontal area was activated during the tasks. "This area is not typically activated by normal subjects performing word-stem completion and appears to be used (by the patient) to compensate for his damaged cortex" (p. 1,253).

WHAT DOES FUNCTIONAL IMAGING ACTUALLY MEASURE?

Despite the many scientific and clinical benefits derived from imaging technologies and the resulting growth of studies on structure/function relationships using those techniques, there is still some controversy about what is actually being measured with respect to functional changes in the brain. A growing number of recent, still controversial studies report that MRI and PET techniques are recording the metabolic activity of glial cells perhaps even more than neurons. Figley and Stroman argue strongly that much imaging data following "brain activation" is actually measuring oxidate and glycolytic astrocyte metabolism, not neuronal activity. Because glial cells vastly outnumber neurons in the brain, it is highly likely that their activation would overwhelm signals coming from neurons. Glial cells are known to modulate neurotransmitter activity as well as cerebral blood flow, especially astrocytes in close proximity to blood vessels and capillaries in the brain (see 41 and 42 for reviews). Figley and colleagues (41) conclude their excellent review: "[M]ost functional neuroimaging techniques . . . are, in fact, more closely tied to the underlying function and metabolic activity of astrocytes than of neurons" (p. 586). Is it conceivable that glial activity could mask that of neurons and lead to a false reading of what is happening in the neurons? This might be a tough pill to swallow because it could have important implications for using imaging for neuronal localization of complex cognitive and behavioral functions.

Another growing concern arises because most MRI technology currently assumes that increased glucose metabolism, oxygen use, and blood flow in a specific part of the brain while the organism is performing some task is a direct reflection of the neural activity that "mediates" that task. The measurements are usually taken by subtracting background activity from the area of interest and adding false color to represent the range of localized activity higher than baseline levels. Such studies can be interpreted to indicate that those areas with activity at baseline (or even lower) are not active during task performance and therefore not implicated in the functional localization. Marcus Raichle, a leading investigator in brain imaging, has recently questioned whether this approach is valid (43,44). He argues that ongoing intrinsic activity of the brain involves high-energy consumption and that changes in brain activation triggered by external stimuli (or performing tasks) represents less than 5% of additional energy consumption. Thus, "it is clear that the brain's enormous energy consumption is *little affected by task performance,* an observation made 50 years ago" (italics mine; 43, p. 12 729). I take this to mean that current imaging of structure/function relationships (i.e., hard localization) is likely to be misleading for understanding brain organization. Subtle but widespread changes in energy and blood flow in both neurons and glia may be contributing to changes in the patterning of activities throughout the brain but largely ignored by subtraction techniques. As Raichle notes, the brain is constantly busy but in ways that are not always indicative of higher levels of activity.

In the 1990s, Raichle showed that during the performance of a task (reading aloud), some brain regions underwent a *decreased* level of activity (relative to a baseline resting state) associated with the task. If measurement of functional activities assumes that only *increases* in metabolism are representative of function, it will fail to take into account that decreases in activity are also parts of cognitive processing. Most researchers today still look for "hot spots" and effectively ignore low-level metabolic activity that could also contribute to the overall patterns of brain activity associated with cognitive processing. Current imaging approaches may be giving only part of the story of how ensembles of brain structures work together to mediate complex behaviors. "The idea that the brain might exhibit such internal activity across multiple regions while at rest had escaped the neuroimaging establishment" (44, p. 47). If Raichle's findings and conclusion are correct, what is the best way to image locality of function? Might functions be more widely distributed than previously thought? Could complex cognitive functions be the result of subtle system-wide changes in "dark" activity that include and require inhibiting some regions to create the overall pattern of brain activity associated with the task?

DIASCHISIS AND FUNCTIONAL INHIBITION

Sophisticated imaging and electrophysiological techniques have been employed with increasing frequency to support the idea of diaschisis, proposed by von Monakow at the beginning of the last century (45). In this early concept, brain injury triggers long-lasting inhibition of neural activity that is not limited to the site of injury but can spread to distal regions by means that were not clearly understood. Now we know that injury-induced biochemical and genomic alterations in protein synthesis can generate actions that are many synapses removed from the initial site of damage. The changes occur not only in the affected hemisphere, but also in the intact contralateral homologues (see 46). Von Monakow postulated that recovery of function occurred as diaschisis dissipated over time, whereas permanent deficits were the result of permanent diaschisis.

Current research shows that injury to the brain can produce chronic suppression of activity in regions that may be spatially quite distal to the lesion itself (47–50). Agonist drugs that increase neurotransmitter activity or block inhibitory neurotransmitters have been used to promote functional recovery after stroke in both animal (51) and human (52) subjects. However, clinical trials with these agents have had apparently limited success (53). Can behavioral therapy (e.g., the forced-use paradigm) or treatment with stimulants (e.g., amphetamine) reduce or eliminate diaschisis caused by injury? Do other brain areas "take over the function" of the area of stroke? Current evidence can be interpreted to suggest that this may be the case. A stroke (experimental or naturally induced) often leads to functional reorganization in brain tissue immediately adjacent to the injured area, but there are also significant changes in the contralateral homologous regions. In one study, 12 patients with acute strokes had unilateral arm weakness and some ability to move the arm after 1 month. Six of the patients showed good recovery and 6 did not. The 6 with good recovery showed much more activation of the cerebellar hemisphere opposite the damaged corticospinal tract than did the poorly recovered patients (54). The authors suggest that the recovery could have been caused by diaschisis, or as it might now be termed, unmasking of existing but latent pathways for the functions in the contralateral cerebellum.

In a recent review, Price and colleagues (55) introduce the concept of dynamic diaschisis. They suggest that the environmental context as well as the locus of damage can play a role in determining functional outcome. Price et al. propose that

> the basic idea behind dynamic diaschisis is that an otherwise viable cortical region expresses aberrant neuronal responses when those responses depend on interactions with a damaged region. This effect might arise because normal responses in any given region depend upon driving and modulatory inputs from, and reciprocal interactions with, many other regions. The regions involved will depend on the cognitive and sensorimotor operation engaged in at any particular time. (p. 419)

In other words, areas of the brain that are distant from the area of injury, including the contralateral hemisphere, can show abnormal responses when the functional demand on the damaged tissue increases. The authors conclude that dynamic diaschisis can be measured only with whole-brain functional imaging because one has to take into consideration the functional integration of many different brain regions. More important, "pathophysiological expression depends on the functional brain state *at the time the measurements are made*" (55, p. 426, my italics). This can be taken to mean that brain structures may move in and out of a state of diaschisis, depending on the functional demands made on them at a given time in the patient's experience. It is interesting to note that, well before there was sophisticated imaging, this same point was made by the neuropsychologist Alexander Luria in 1966 (46).

REORGANIZATION, UNMASKING, SPARING, AND LATENT SYNAPSES

Because of refinements in microelectrode recording techniques, it has now been amply demonstrated in primates that certain brain areas such as the sensory motor cortex are capable of very rapid electrophysiological reorganization in response to injury. Within a very short time after lesions of the afferent pathways or even after cortical damage, tissue adjacent to the affected areas reorganizes or expands its receptive fields to capture and mediate at least some of the original physiological activities that were destroyed by the injury. There is no doubt that such rapid reorganization occurs in several sensory and motor areas, but as noted earlier, it must be emphasized that not all the reorganization is necessarily adaptive or beneficial to the organism. Plow et al. (56) point out that spontaneous reorganizational processes following a stroke or traumatic brain injury (TBI) are complex and dependent on multiple mechanisms including (a) reorganization of neural activity immediately surrounding the damaged tissue, (b) recruitment of more distal neural tissue on the same side as the brain damage, (c) recruitment of brain cells on the side of the brain opposite the lesion, and (d) organizational shifts of neural activity and interhemispheric connections leading to novel forms of interactions between the hemispheres. Plow and colleagues argue that "rehabilitation modulates 1 or more of these mechanisms, enhancing some and suppressing others, to improve function" (p. 1,926). From their perspective, different types of rehabilitation therapy produce highly specific changes in brain region activities, so the type of therapy has to be matched to the specific deficit. So, for example, hand and forelimb training as well as language therapy for aphasia in humans leads to specific reorganization of the area surrounding the lesion. Virtual reality training stimulates the activation of sensorimotor cortex on the same side as the injury, whereas bilateral training and constraint induced therapies "help return interhemispheric balance." The authors emphasize that, despite best efforts, most rehabilitation training leaves patients with residual deficits that can be relatively permanent without additional chronic noninvasive or invasive (implanted electrodes) brain stimulation.

Although proponents of electrical stimulation therapy might like to believe that the stimulation is localized to the injury, such optimism is probably not warranted. It is more likely that chronic electrical brain stimulation produces both biochemical and morphological changes at a distance, and functional activity resulting from such stimulation would likely be modified by timing, sex differences in brain, and hormonal and chemical changes throughout the CNS. The story gets even more complex. Gong, He, and Evans (57) note that male and female brains display marked differences in CNS organization and "network topology" across the entire brain. If this is the case, cortical reorganization therapies must take into account gender, hormonal status, local as well as widespread cortical and subcortical changes in connectivity and function (see 58–60 for more discussion of sex differences), and age of the patient in interpreting any results based on a neural connectivity paradigm.

Among the first to demonstrate dramatic but maladaptive injury-induced plasticity in the adult nervous system were Patrick D. Wall and his colleagues (61). Wall's group first mapped the body surface of the ventral posterior lateral (VPL) nucleus of the thalamus by tactile stimulation on the surface of the arms and legs of laboratory animals. In a normal animal, the arm takes up two-thirds of the medial VPL and the leg occupies the lateral third. When inputs to the leg area were removed by unilateral excision of the gracile nucleus, the arm area expanded to "occupy two-thirds of the area previously responding to stimulation of the leg." This change was noted within 3 days of the lesion. Although this is an example of reorganization and cellular plasticity in response to injury, it is hardly an adaptive response to have an area that previously subserved inputs from the leg area now responding primarily to stimulation of the arm. Using other forms of temporary deafferentation such as blockage of nerve conduction by ice, Wall's group was able to produce instantaneous remapping of cells in the lateral nucleus gracilis (LNG). Thus, the cells in the leg, normally activated by stimulation of the paws, now responded only to stimulation of the abdomen. In this case, the unmasking of latent pathways was almost instantaneous, but again, hardly adaptive with respect to behavioral utility. Wall's data could be taken to suggest that not all forms of "plasticity" are necessarily beneficial—a point I raised earlier in this review.

Such changes in reorganization may be very long-lasting and dependent on postinjury experience. Some years after the Wall experiments, Pons et al. showed that up to 11 years after a dorsal rhizotomy in adult rhesus monkeys, the brain region responding to stimulation of the hand (area 3b) responded instead to tactile stimulation of the face (62). In human patients, similar reorganization can be seen in phantom limb phenomena in response to amputation. This too has been taken as an example of maladaptive neural plasticity in the adult nervous system (63,64). These investigators found that tactile stimulation of the face often led to referred sensations somewhere out on the phantom limb. Thus, "there was a topographically organized map of the hand on the lower face region and the referred sensations were modality specific," for example, heat, cold, vibration, rubbing, and so forth were felt as these same sensations at specific points on the phantom limb. The authors noted that this modality-specific referral from the face to the limb could occur only within a few hours after amputation, implying that the reorganized "localization" of sensations must have been caused by unmasking of previously silent pathways rather than structural or morphological changes.

Some patients report that, after a time, their phantom limb feels as if it is paralyzed or frozen into an excruciatingly painful clench with the fingers digging deeply into the palm. The patient cannot will the fingers to open and relieve the pain. Ramachandran (63) and his group developed an ingeniously simple technique to provide relief, and in doing so, again demonstrated the rapid reorganization of function that can occur under some conditions. Investigators asked patients to put their unaffected hand into a box with a mirror in the sagittal plane of the hand. This gave a mirror image of the normal hand, so it looked to the patients as if they had 2 hands opposing one another in the mirror-box. Now the investigators asked the patients to slowly open and close the normal hand while looking at the image in the mirror so it would seem as if the phantom hand was now opening and closing. Several patients reported that seeing what appeared to be the phantom hand paradoxically unclench (because it was in fact the normal hand they were seeing) relieved the cramping pain. Thus, amputation-induced reorganization may be undone by training and experience, with a novel engram replacing the maladaptive one, and the effects can be very long-lasting if not permanent.

Phantom limb effects are dramatic examples of reorganizational plasticity that can be very disruptive in the adult brain, but similar mechanisms can be seen in the visual and auditory systems when injuries are inflicted during early development. Rauschecker (65,66) has shown that if the visual (occipital) cortex is deprived of its inputs from the optic nerves, it can then be stimulated by auditory input. The visual cells are taken over by the auditory and somatosensory nerve fibers, and thus both the auditory and somatosensory cortex could be said to expand into the territory previously controlled and occupied by visual inputs. Likewise, if the auditory cortex is destroyed or the auditory nerve is cut, the auditory cortex will be captured by visual inputs that have expanded into the deafferented zone. It would be interesting to study whether these neuronal alterations have beneficial or detrimental effects.

Rapid reorganization tends to be more robust during early development, which may be one reason young subjects with brain damage recover better than older counterparts with the same injury. Rauschecker asks what the postrecovery perception of animals brain-damaged during early development is like. Do they "see" sounds and touches as in purported synesthesias, or does the visual cortex "change" its functions to become auditory and/or somatosensory? What are the implications for concepts of localization of function in the CNS during development and later in life?

Investigators have shown that reorganization and expansion of functional cortical maps can be induced by intensive training experience in normal animals. Specific kinds of sensory training may be beneficial as rehabilitation therapy in subjects with brain damage because they directly enhance the extent of rapid reorganization and functional plasticity. Nudo and his colleagues reported that injury-induced reorganization and recovery of function can occur in the adult organism (67). Such recovery often requires experience-induced modifications in synaptic and cellular systems throughout remaining healthy brain tissue that may not necessarily be contiguous to, or immediately involved in, the affected area and its functions. Functions are widely distributed and in a constant state of dynamic interaction and change, not fixed and static as they are often represented in neuroscience texts.

It is clearly time to accept the idea that dynamic reorganization of functions is an ongoing process, not only in the damaged brain but also in the course of normal activity and learning. Indeed, these changes may well serve as the basis for recovery mechanisms when there is an attack on the brain. For example, in accomplished musicians and athletes, somatosensory fields are markedly expanded compared to nontrained individuals. According to Nudo et al., highly repetitive practice on a tactile task in humans leads to marked expansion of the receptive field in the motor cortex, which can persist for several months after the training is terminated. Maps also expand during the initial phases of training when the procedures are unfamiliar, and then shrink once explicit knowledge of the task has become habitual.

There are also apparently marked individual differences in the location and size of cortical receptive fields in normal individuals, which vary in their degree of modifiability according to the subject's experiential history (68,69). The notion that neuronal pathways can be rewired by drugs or stimulation needs to be approached carefully because the wiring for each individual may be influenced by early experience and training (69). In designing rehabilitation therapy, it should be noted that some routinely used therapies could result in the formation of inappropriate connections and the prevention of functional recovery, even a form of learned helplessness (70). For instance, if the current paradigm of structure–function relationships is valid, it is hard to imagine how the capture of auditory input by visual fibers would automatically lead to an adaptive outcome.

In conjunction with electrophysiological experiments in primates, computer-assisted rapid fMRI studies in humans have shown that multiple systems throughout the brain are activated during selected cognitive tasks, such as naming objects or performing simple mathematical calculations. Many neuroscientists now accept the view that widely distributed neural modules are involved in even simple cognitive or sensory processing. However, there is much less agreement about the number of modules (brain areas) required to mediate even a simple behavior like reaching for a piece of food. Over the last 10 years or so, the number of CNS structures in the network said to be in control of vision has increased from about 12 to well more than 50. A corollary of this assumption is that very localized damage would cause very widespread changes both serially and in parallel throughout the brain. Therefore, recovery of behavioral functions may depend on equally widespread changes in synaptic connectivity and their metabolic consequences.

WHAT HAVE WE LEARNED ABOUT THE CONCEPTUAL ISSUES SURROUNDING NEURAL PLASTICITY?

"Those who forget history are condemned to repeat it" means as much in neuroscience as it does in political and social philosophy. Theories and hypotheses now in vogue rarely acknowledge early 20th-century literature that pleaded for a more dynamic and modular view of function to replace the idea that the adult nervous system is fixed and immutable in its structure–function relationships. In the 1960s, 1970s, and 1980s, many neurobiologists, focusing on molecular and reductionistic techniques, derided the ideas of Karl Lashley, who wrote in 1937 that "the function of cells may be deduced from their position and connections, but their position is not therefore a necessary consequence of their function." He went on to say that "the mere existence of specialized regions in the brain is not conclusive evidence that the specialization is necessary or important for the integrative functions" (71). In one series of studies (72), Lashley examined visual discrimination learning after lesions of the visual (occipital) cortex in rats. Following the injury, the rats lost their ability to perform the task, but they were able to relearn the visual discrimination in the same number of trials as it took for the original learning, despite bilateral damage to the visual cortex. For Lashley, if visual specialization was hardwired, how were the animals able to relearn the task and in the same amount of time as it took for the original learning? Given the subsequent observations of reorganizational changes in response to brain injury discussed here, Lashley's position now has a contemporary ring. Writing a few years later, Kurt Goldstein (73), a German neurologist, stressed that

[T]he destruction of one part of the brain never leaves unchanged the activity of the rest of the organism, especially the rest of the brain. On the contrary, there usually occurs a widespread change of the distribution of excitation. Whether a certain symptom will appear on account of a local injury, especially whether it will become a permanent symptom, certainly depends on many other factors: the nature of the disease process, the condition of the rest of the brain, the difficulty of the performance requirements and the reaction of the entire organism to the defect. The localization of a performance (after an injury) no longer means an excitation in a certain place, but a dynamic process which occurs in the entire nervous system, even in the whole organism. (pp. 258–259)

Thirty years after Goldstein, Alexander Luria argued that "the facts suggest that a disturbance of a particular form of activity may arise in far more extensive lesions than was hitherto supposed. Consequently, the performance of a given function necessitates the integrity of far more extensive and far more structurally varied zones of the cortex than was assumed by classical neurology" (46). Thus, almost 4 decades ago, Luria was arguing for a more dynamic view of nervous system function to explain how recovery from brain injury might occur. Luria felt it would eventually be recognized that "complex forms of psychological functions are never localized in isolated areas of the brain, but are always dependent on entire working constellations of cerebral zones, appearing in the course of postnatal development and changing dynamically as a particular functional system reaches a higher level of development" (p. 70). He predicted that the loss of any 1 link must inevitably lead to a disturbance of the normal working of the functional system as a whole. Luria's, Goldstein's, and Lashley's views were essentially ignored by cerebral cartographers, who continued to add to the complexity of their diagrams without offering much account of how the parts worked together in the intact and the damaged brain. It was as if drawing the lines between anatomical components was a sufficient explanatory tool.

Contemporary research on localization of complex functions to specific areas of the cerebral cortex marshals some of neuroscience's most elegant techniques in support of its paradigm. This often entails careful testing of complex behaviors or components of behaviors using high-resolution brain imaging or microelectrodes to record from individual cells in anatomically defined loci. Some of the most elegant work in this domain was done by Goldman-Rakic and her colleagues, who defined and elaborated the role of the prefrontal cortex in spatial performance, memory, and cognition. Goldman-Rakic tested the hypothesis that highly discrete areas of the frontal cortex are critical in the mediation of spatial and object cognition (74–77). Monkeys showed significant increases in electrophysical activity in individual neurons in circumscribed areas of the prefrontal cortex. During object recognition, 1 set of neurons is activated, whereas in a spatial cognition task, other cells in a different anatomical region become more active. Both electrophysiological and metabolic recording techniques were used to demonstrate changes in activity. In Goldman-Rakic's view, "a signal advance attributable to research in nonhuman primates over the past decades has been the fine-grained functional mapping of the cerebral cortex and the realization that cytoarchitectonically defined areas are not homogenous with respect to circuitry or to

physiology.... It is to be confidently expected that functional specializations will surely follow the lines of these anatomical divisions when the appropriate tests are applied." She concludes, "In view of the parcellation of these fundamental information processing domains, it is far too early to reject cortical specialization so well grounded in cytoarchitectonic, hodological, and neurochemical parcellation ..." (74, p. 454). To be sure, the rigorous and refined techniques employed and the elegance of the results make for compelling support for localization, but such findings and interpretations do not address the plasticity and reorganization seen after injury and are difficult to explain in the context of behavioral sparing or recovery of function in the adult organism. Studies not supporting parcellation theory are still sometimes dismissed as lacking technical sophistication or as using inadequate behavioral tests.

Moreover, where plasticity of function is acknowledged, it is often limited to the idea that immediately adjacent *cortical* tissue, where the most dynamic changes in maps are registered, can be reorganized to mediate behaviors. Wall and Wang refer to these notions as "corticocentric theories" (77). In a more radical approach, these authors argue that changes in response to injury are far more ubiquitous in both subcortical and cortical substrates and include molecular, morphological, neurochemical, and anatomical changes that reorganize basically the entire functioning of the organism. The authors take a position similar to that of neurologists of the mid-20th century who believed that deficits as well as recovery were the result of such total organization, rather than the result of loss of a particular part in the brain.

In response to injury, initial multilevel changes emerge surprisingly rapidly. Functional changes can appear concurrently within minutes in spinal, brainstem, thalamic, and cortical substrates. With the passage of time during the subsequent days, weeks, months, and longer, acute changes in normal substrates apparently continue, spread, and are further supplemented by subcortical and cortical abilities to regenerate and sprout new connections. (pp. 204–205)

The views of Wall et al. are consistent with the work of Jones (78) and Nudo (67). Jones presents evidence that even very small changes in subcortical organization caused by a peripheral or CNS injury can lead to highly amplified changes in the organizational maps of the cerebral cortex. Others such as Chen et al. (79) argue that the brain is constantly being modified by experience and that fixed wiring diagrams do not represent the kinds of rapid and long-lasting injury-induced plasticity seen in developmental and adult brain damage. The authors also note that not all types of "plastic" reorganization are beneficial and that one must distinguish between those changes that lead to recovery and those plastic changes that result in permanent impairments. Finally, discussing motor cortex damage, Nudo et al. (67) conclude a review of the literature by stating that "both human and animal studies have demonstrated both acute and chronic changes in functional topography and anatomy of intact cortical tissue adjacent to the injury, and of more remote cortical areas, including those of the contralateral (uninjured) hemisphere" (p. 1,013). Although not always given the credit they deserve, the early investigators into plasticity of function—Lashley, Goldstein, and Luria—had only their clinical and observational skills to evaluate patient behavior and draw conclusions that today are based on a wide variety of sophisticated molecular and physiological techniques. Nonetheless, their conclusions resonate well with those of contemporary neuroscientists.

Considering the implications of his own work on phantom limb plasticity for theories of brain organization, Ramachandran (64) concluded that new findings on reorganization after amputation "allow us to test some of the most widely accepted assumptions of sensory psychology and neurophysiology, such as Müller's law of specific nerve energies, 'pattern coding' versus 'place coding' (i.e., the notion that perception depends exclusively on which particular neuron fires rather than the overall pattern of activity)." Furthermore, the work showing that training-induced sensations associated with phantom limbs "suggests that the modular, hierarchical 'bucket brigade' model of the brain popularized by computer engineers needs to be replaced by a more dynamic view of the brain in which there is a tremendous amount of back-and-forth interaction between different levels in the hierarchy and across different modules" (p. 319). Ramachandran's "mirror therapy" for phantom limb pain tested the view of a hardwired, highly localized nervous system that, once damaged, cannot change in response to environmental inputs (80). Ramachandran and colleagues have recently begun to use the mirror therapy in stroke rehabilitation and other CNS disorders (81,82). They have found varying degrees of success in restoring hand control and, to a more limited extent, recovery of lower limb hemiparesis. Ramachandran's ideas sound similar to von Monakow's discussion of diaschisis about a century ago when he notes that

> instead of thinking of brain modules as hardwired and autonomous, we should think of them as being in a state of dynamic equilibrium with each other and with the environment (including the body), with connections being constantly formed and re-formed in response to changing environmental needs. Neurological dysfunction, at least in some instances, may be caused not so much by irreversible destruction of a module but by a functional shift in equilibrium. (45, p. 1708)

ACKNOWLEDGMENT

I would like to thank Leslie McCann for her incalculable help in working through the many drafts of this chapter.

KEY CLINICAL POINTS

1. Recent findings and the revised concepts of how adaptive and maladaptive plasticity occur in the adult human brain after injury clearly demonstrate that the adult CNS is capable of much more dynamic change in function and structure than has been believed during the last few decades.
2. Despite the attempts to support a modern phrenology found in many imaging studies, molecular, genomic, and functional assessments of brain activity are revealing a much more dynamic perspective on the consequences of brain injury based on the critical feedback mechanisms between different brain areas, and between brain and other organ systems in both normal and pathological functions.

3. Brain injuries like stroke and trauma and neurodegenerative diseases like Alzheimer or Parkinson are beginning to be seen as caused by large-scale neural network dysfunctions that may start out localized to a given region but then spread to more distal regions through signaling errors, biochemical dysregulation, protein conformational changes, and perturbations in neuron/glia interactions (see Refs. 83 and 84 for discussion).
4. It is not easy to change scientific paradigms, especially when the tools available are designed at great cost and effort specifically to support the prevailing view of how nature works, but it may be time for a more holistic and dynamic perspective. Many of the early thinkers discussed here may have been on to something, even though they did not have the advantage of our newer techniques.
5. Parcellation doctrine, whatever its current guise, leaves many unanswered questions and unsolved issues, which can hinder progress in developing treatments for brain injuries and other CNS disorders. In science, as it should be, change can come slowly but it will eventually come as researchers begin to recognize the complex and systemic and holistic nature of brain disorders.

KEY REFERENCES

1. Plow EB, Carey JR, Nudo RJ, Pascual-Leone A. Invasive cortical stimulation to promote recovery of function after stroke: a critical appraisal. *Stroke.* 2009;40(5):1926–1931.
2. Raichle ME. A paradigm shift in functional brain imaging. *J Neurosci.* 2009;29(41):12729–12734.
3. Ramachandran VS, Altschuler EL. The use of visual feedback, in particular mirror visual feedback, in restoring brain function. *Brain.* 2009;132(7):1693–1710.
4. Seitz RJ, Freund HJ. Plasticity of the human motor cortex. *Adv Neurol.* 1997;73:321–333.
5. Wolf SL, Blanton S, Baer H, Breshears J, Butler AJ. Repetitive task practice: a critical review of constraint-induced movement therapy in stroke. *Neurologist.* 2002;8(6): 325–338.

References

1. Goldberger ME. Recovery of movement after CNS lesions in monkeys. In: Stein DG, Rosen JJ, Butters N, eds. *Plasticity and Recovery of Function in the Central Nervous System.* New York, NY: Academic Press; 1974:265–338.
2. Greenblatt SH. Hughlings Jackson's theory of localization and compensation. In: Finger S, LeVere TE, Almli CR, Stein DG, eds. *Brain Injury and Recovery: Theoretical and Controversial Issues.* New York, NY: Plenum; 1988:181–190.
3. Almli CR, Finger S. Toward a definition of recovery of function. In: Finger S, LeVere TE, Almli CR, Stein DG, eds. *Brain Injury and Recovery: Theoretical and Controversial Issues.* New York, NY: Plenum; 1988: 1–14.
4. Cajal SR. *Degeneration and Regeneration of the Nervous System.* London, United Kingdom: Oxford University Press; 1928.
5. Raisman G. Neuronal plasticity in the septal nuclei of the adult rat. *Brain Res.* 1969;14(1):25–48.
6. Cotman CW, ed. *Neuronal Plasticity.* New York, NY: Raven Press; 1978.
7. Steward O. Reorganization of neuronal connections following CNS trauma: principles and experimental paradigms. *J Neurotrauma.* 1989;6(2):99–152.
8. Finger S, Stein DG. *Brain Damage and Recovery: Research and Clinical Perspectives.* New York, NY: Academic Press; 1982.

9. Finger S. *Origins of Neuroscience*. New York, NY: Oxford University Press; 1994.

10. Dietz V. Neuronal plasticity after a human spinal cord injury: positive and negative effects [published online ahead of print April 20, 2011]. *Exp Neurol*. doi:10.1016/j.expneurol.2011.04.007.

11. Parent JM, Lowenstein DH. Seizure-induced neurogenesis: are more new neurons good for an adult brain? *Prog Brain Res*. 2002;135: 121–131.

12. LeVere N, Gray-Silvia S, LeVere TE. Neural system imbalances and the consequence of large brain injuries. In: Finger S, LeVere TE, Almli R, Stein DG, eds. *Brain Injury and Recovery: Theoretical and Controversial Issues*. New York, NY: Plenum; 1988:15–27.

13. Kosik KS. Beyond phrenology, at last. *Nat Rev Neurosci*. 2003;4(3): 234–239.

14. Villoslada P, Steinman L, Baranzini SE. Systems biology and its application to the understanding of neurological diseases. *Ann Neurol*. 2009;65(2):124–139.

15. Stein DG, Finger S, Hart T. Brain damage and recovery: problems and perspectives. *Behav Neural Biol*. 1983;37(2):185–222.

16. Kolb B, Teskey GC, Gibb R. Factors influencing cerebral plasticity in the normal and injured brain. *Front Hum Neurosci*. 2010;4:204.

17. Qi HX, Jain N, Collins CE, Lyon DC, Kaas JH. Functional organization of motor cortex of adult macaque monkeys is altered by sensory loss in infancy. *Proc Natl Acad Sci USA*. 2010;107(7):3192–3197.

18. Muckli L, Naumer MJ, Singer W. Bilateral visual field maps in a patient with only one hemisphere. *Proc Natl Acad Sci USA*. 2009; 106(31):13034–13039.

19. Beaulieu CL. Rehabilitation and outcome following pediatric traumatic brain injury. *Surg Clin North Am*. 2002;82(2):393–408.

20. Seitz RJ, Freund HJ. Plasticity of the human motor cortex. *Adv Neurol*. 1997;73:321–333.

21. Finger S. Recovery of function: redundancy and vicariation theories. In: Aminoff MJ, Boller F, Swaab DF, eds. *Handbook of Clinical Neurology*. Amsterdam, United Kingdom: Elsevier; 2009:833–841.

22. Lennberg EH. *Biological Foundations of Language*. New York, NY: Wiley; 1967.

23. Kennard MA. Cortical reorganization of motor function. Studies on series of monkeys of various ages from infancy to maturity. *Arch of Neurol Psychiatry*. 1942;48(2):227–240.

24. Goldman PS, Galkin TW. Prenatal removal of frontal association cortex in the fetal rhesus monkey: anatomical and functional consequences in postnatal life. *Brain Res*. 1978;152(3):451–485.

25. Goldberg E. *The New Executive Brain: Frontal Lobes in a Complex World*. New York, NY: Oxford University Press; 2009.

26. Vargha-Khadem F, Isaacs E, Muter V. A review of cognitive outcome after unilateral lesions sustained during childhood. *J Child Neurol*. 1994;9(suppl 2):67–73.

27. Slavin MD, Laurence S, Stein DG. Another look at vicariation. In: Finger S, LeVere TE, Almli CR, Stein DG, eds. *Brain Injury and Recovery: Theoretical and Controversial Issues*. New York, NY: Plenum; 1988: 165–178.

28. Jordan FM, Murdoch BE. Linguistic status following closed head injury in children: a follow-up study. *Brain Inj*. 1990;4(2):147–154.

29. Anderson VA, Catroppa C, Rosenfeld J, Haritou F, Morse SA. Recovery of memory function following traumatic brain injury in preschool children. *Brain Inj*. 2000;14(8):679–692.

30. Finger S, LeVere TE, Almli CR, Stein DG, eds. *Brain Injury and Recovery: Theoretical and Controversial Issues*. New York, NY: Plenum; 1988.

31. Prins ML, Hovda DA. Mapping cerebral glucose metabolism during spatial learning: interactions of development and traumatic brain injury. *J Neurotrauma*. 2001;18(1):31–46.

32. Trudeau N, Poulin-Dubois D, Joanette Y. Language development following brain injury in early childhood: a longitudinal case study. *Int J Lang Commun Disord*. 2000;35(2):227–249.

33. Kolb B, Gibb R, Gorny G. Cortical plasticity and the development of behavior after early frontal cortical injury. *Dev Neuropsychol*. 2000; 18(3):423–444.

34. Kolb B, Cioe J. Recovery from early cortical damage in rats, VIII. Earlier may be worse: behavioural dysfunction and abnormal cerebral morphogenesis following perinatal frontal cortical lesions in the rat. *Neuropharmacology*. 2000;39(5):756–764.

35. Nemati F, Kolb B. Motor cortex injury has different behavioral and anatomical effects in early and late adolescence. *Behav Neurosci*. 2010; 124(5):612–622.

36. Xerri C, Merzenich MM, Peterson BE, Jenkins W. Plasticity of primary somatosensory cortex paralleling sensorimotor skill recovery from stroke in adult monkeys. *J Neurophysiol*. 1998;79(4):2119–2148.

37. Kolb B, Gibb R, Gonzales CL. Cortical injury and neuroplasticity during development. In: Shaw C, McEachern JC, eds. *Toward a Theory of Neuroplasticity*. Philadelphia, PA: Taylor & Francis; 2001: 223–243.

38. York GK, Steinberg DA. Hughlings Jackson's theory of recovery. *Neurology*. 1995;45(4):834–838.

39. Castro-Alamancos MA, García-Segura LM, Borrell J. Transfer of function to a specific area of the cortex after induced recovery from brain damage. *Eur J Neurosci*. 1992;4(9):853–863.

40. Buckner RL, Corbetta M, Schatz J, Raichle ME, Petersen SE. Preserved speech abilities and compensation following prefrontal damage. *Proc Natl Acad Sci USA*. 1996;93(3):1249–1253.

41. Figley CR, Stroman PW. The role(s) of astrocytes and astrocyte activity in neurometabolism, neurovascular coupling, and the production of functional neuroimaging signals. *Eur J Neurosci*. 2011;33(4): 577–588.

42. Koehler RC, Roman RJ, Harder DR. Astrocytes and the regulation of cerebral blood flow. *Trends Neurosci*. 2009;32(3):160–169.

43. Raichle ME. A paradigm shift in functional brain imaging. *J Neurosci*. 2009;29(41):12729–12734.

44. Raichle ME. The brain's dark energy. *Sci Am*. 2010;302(3):44–49.

45. von Monakow C. *Die lokalisation im grosshirn und der abbau der funktion durch kortikale herde*. Wiesbaden, Germany: JF Bergmann; 1914.

46. Luria AR. *Higher Cortical Functions in Man*. New York, NY: Basic Books; 1966.

47. Hausen HS, Lachmann EA, Nagler W. Cerebral diaschisis following cerebellar hemorrhage. *Arch Phys Med Rehabil*. 1997;78(5):546–549.

48. Imahori Y, Fujii R, Kondo M, Ohmori Y, Nakajima K. Neural features of recovery from CNS injury revealed by PET in human brain. *Neuroreport*. 1999;10(1):117–121.

49. Laatsch L, Jobe T, Sychra J, Lin Q, Blend M. Impact of cognitive rehabilitation therapy on neuropsychological impairments as measured by brain perfusion SPECT: a longitudinal study. *Brain Inj*. 1997;11(12):851–863.

50. Rosen HJ, Petersen SE, Linenweber MR, et al. Neural correlates of recovery from aphasia after damage to left inferior frontal cortex. *Neurology*. 2000;55(12):1883–1894.

51. Feeney DM, Sutton RL. Pharmacotherapy for recovery of function after brain injury. *Crit Rev Neurobiol*. 1987;3(2):135–197.

52. Goldstein G, Beers SR. *Rehabilitation*. New York, NY: Plenum; 1998.

53. Gladstone DJ, Black SE. Enhancing recovery after stroke with noradrenergic pharmacotherapy: a new frontier? *Can J Neurol Sci*. 2000; 27(2):97–105.

54. Small SL, Hlustik P, Noll DC, Genovese C, Solodkin A. Cerebellar hemispheric activation ipsilateral to the paretic hand correlates with functional recovery after stroke. *Brain*. 2002;125(pt 7):1544–1557.

55. Price CJ, Warburton EA, Moore CJ, Frackowiak RS, Friston KJ. Dynamic diaschisis: anatomically remote and context-sensitive human brain lesions. *J Cogn Neurosci*. 2001;13(4):419–429.

56. Plow EB, Carey JR, Nudo RJ, Pascual-Leone A. Invasive cortical stimulation to promote recovery of function after stroke: a critical appraisal. *Stroke*. 2009;40(5):1926–1931.

57. Gong G, He Y, Evans AC. Brain connectivity: gender makes a difference [published online ahead of print April 28, 2011]. *Neuroscientist*. 2011;17(5):575–591. doi:10.1177/1073858410.

58. Lopez-Larson MP, Anderson JS, Ferguson MA, Yurgelun-Todd D. Local brain connectivity and associations with gender and age. *Dev Cogn Neurosci*. 2011;1(2):187–197.

59. Tomasi D, Volkow ND. Gender differences in brain functional connectivity density [published online ahead of print March 21, 2011]. *Human Brain Mapp*. 2011;. doi:10.1002/hbm.21252.

60. Menzler K, Belke M, Wehrmann E, et al. Men and women are different: diffusion tensor imaging reveals sexual dimorphism in the microstructure of the thalamus, corpus callosum and cingulum. *Neuroimage*. 2011;54(4):2557–2562.

61. Merrill EG, Wall PD. Plasticity of connection in the adult nervous system. In: Cotman CW, ed. *Neuronal Plasticity*. New York, NY: Raven Press; 1978:97–111.

62. Pons TP, Garraghty PE, Ommaya AK, Kaas JH, Taub E, Mishkin M. Massive cortical reorganization after sensory deafferentation in adult macaques. *Science*. 1991;252(5014):1857–1860.

63. Ramachandran VS, Blakeslee S. *Phantoms in the Brain: Probing the Mysteries of the Human Mind*. New York, NY: William Morrow; 1998.

64. Ramachandran VS, Rogers-Ramachandran D. Phantom limbs and neural plasticity. *Arch Neurol*. 2000;57(3):317–320.

65. Rauschecker JP. Compensatory plasticity and sensory substitution in the cerebral cortex. *Trends Neurosci*. 1995;18(1):36–43.

66. Rauschecker JP. Mechanisms of compensatory plasticity in the cerebral cortex. *Adv Neurol*. 1997;73:137–146.

67. Nudo RJ, Plautz EJ, Frost SB. Role of adaptive plasticity in recovery of function after damage to motor cortex. *Muscle Nerve*. 2001;24(8):1000–1019.

68. Jenkins WM, Merzenich MM. Reorganization of neocortical representations after brain injury: a neurophysiological model of the bases of recovery from stroke. *Prog Brain Res*. 1987;71:249–266.

69. Merzenich M, Wright B, Jenkins W, et al. Cortical plasticity underlying perceptual, motor, and cognitive skill development: implications for neurorehabilitation. *Cold Spring Harb Symp Quant Biol*. 1996;61:1–8.

70. Wolf SL, Blanton S, Baer H, Breshears J, Butler AJ. Repetitive task practice: a critical review of constraint-induced movement therapy in stroke. *Neurologist*. 2002;8(6):325–338.

71. Lashley K. Functional determinants of cerebral localization. *Arch Neurol Psychiatry*. 1937;38(2):371–387.

72. Lashley KS. Factors limiting recovery after central nervous lesions. *J Nerv Mental Disease*. 1938;88:733–755.

73. Goldstein K. *The Organism: A Holistic Approach to Biology Derived from Pathological Data in Man*. New York, NY: American Book Company; 1939.

74. Goldman-Rakic P. Localization of function all over again. *Neuroimage*. 2000;11(5, pt 1):451–457.

75. Levy R, Goldman-Rakic PS. Segregation of working memory functions within the dorsolateral prefrontal cortex. *Exp Brain Res*. 2000;133(1):23–32.

76. Adcock RA, Constable RT, Gore JC, Goldman-Rakic PS. Functional neuroanatomy of executive processes involved in dual-task performance. *Proc Natl Acad Sci USA*. 2000;97(7):3567–3572.

77. Wall JT, Xu J, Wang X. Human brain plasticity: an emerging view of the multiple substrates and mechanisms that cause cortical changes and related sensory dysfunctions after injuries of sensory inputs from the body. *Brain Res Brain Res Rev*. 2002;39(2–3):181–215.

78. Jones EG. Cortical and subcortical contributions to activity-dependent plasticity in primate somatosensory cortex. *Annu Rev Neurosci*. 2000;23:1–37.

79. Chen R, Cohen LG, Hallett M. Nervous system reorganization following injury. *Neuroscience*. 2002;111(4):761–773.

80. Ramachandran VS, Altschuler EL. The use of visual feedback, in particular mirror visual feedback, in restoring brain function. *Brain*. 2009;132(7):1693–1710.

81. Altschuler EL, Wisdom SB, Stone L, et al. Rehabilitation of hemiparesis after stroke with a mirror. *Lancet*. 1999;353(9169):2035–2036.

82. Sathian K, Greenspan AI, Wolf SL. Doing it with mirrors: a case study of a novel approach to neurorehabilitation. *Neurorehabil Neural Repair*. 2000;14(1):73–76.

83. Seeley WW, Crawford RK, Zhou J, Miller BL, Greicius MD. Neurodegenerative diseases target large-scale human brain networks. *Neuron*. 2009;62(1):42–52.

84. Goh KI, Cusick ME, Valle D, Childs B, Vidal M, Barabási AL. The human disease network. *Proc Natl Acad Sci USA*. 2007;104(21):8685–8690.

Experimental Therapeutic Approaches for Traumatic Brain Injury

Anthony E. Kline, Jeffrey P. Cheng, and C. Edward Dixon

INTRODUCTION

The aim of this chapter is to provide a summary of experimental therapeutics that have demonstrated enhancement in behavioral outcome, reduction of functional deficits, and/or attenuation of histopathology after traumatic brain injury (TBI). The various categories of discussion are not necessarily mutually exclusive but have consistently been targets for therapeutic manipulation after TBI. Pharmacological agents that are routinely provided to patients with TBI, but that exert deleterious behavioral effects in animal models are also briefly discussed. This review focuses on exogenous treatments rather than genetically induced manipulations (i.e., transgenic modification). Lastly, because it is possible that the beneficial effects of some treatments may be model-dependent (e.g., rat vs mouse and cortical impact vs fluid percussion injury), this review is not intended to distinguish between them (1).

Excitotoxicity

Excitotoxicity plays an important role in secondary neuronal injury after TBI. Glutamate, aspartate, and glycine are 3 of the most abundant excitatory neurotransmitters and the most commonly implicated in excitotoxic injury. Glutamate, the most prominent of these amino acids, activates receptors that are classified according to specific agonists. Receptors that modulate ionic channels are divided into those stimulated by N-methyl-D-aspartate (NMDA receptors) or those stimulated by [alpha]-amino-3-hydroxy-5-methylisoazole-4-proprionic acid (AMPA) or kainic acid (together referred to as non-NMDA receptors). Glutamate also acts at metabotropic receptors that produce effects via second messenger systems (2). Excitotoxicity resulting from the TBI-induced release of excitatory amino acids and the damaging effects of increased intracellular calcium associated with glutamate receptor activation has been one of the most investigated targets for protection and recovery after TBI.

Inhibiting Release of Excitotoxins

Inhibiting glutamate release has been demonstrated to attenuate functional and morphological deficits after experimental TBI. Sun and Faden (3) reported that early treatment with

619C89, a sodium channel blocker that inhibits glutamate release, attenuates behavioral deficits and lessens hippocampal cell death. Riluzole (2-amino-6-trifluoromethoxy benzothiazole) has properties that include inhibition of glutamate release and is also reported to attenuate functional (4) and morphological damage (5) after TBI. Galanin, which is a neuropeptide that inhibits neurotransmitter release by opening potassium channels and closing N-type calcium channels, attenuates motor, but not cognitive deficits after TBI (6). Moreover, blocking postinjury ion fluxes with tetrodotoxin is not reported to protect against behavioral deficits (7).

Blocking Receptor Activation

Treatment with NMDA and non-NMDA receptor blockers has been shown in several models of TBI to attenuate neurological deficits. Hayes and colleagues (8) reported behavioral protection by the noncompetitive NMDA receptor antagonist phencyclidine after TBI. Studies by Faden and colleagues (9) showed behavioral protection by dextromethorphan, a noncompetitive NMDA antagonist and 3-(2-carboxypiperazin-4-yl)propyl-l-phosphonic acid (CPP), a competitive NMDA antagonist. The NMDA antagonist, MK-801, has also been reported in numerous studies to exert neuroprotection (10–13). Cortical and hippocampal damage is attenuated by both pretreatment with the NMDA antagonist CPP and the non-NMDA antagonist NBQX (14). Delayed administration (i.e., beginning 1 and 7 hours after TBI) of NBQX has been documented to prevent hippocampal damage. Remacemide hydrochloride, an NMDA receptor-associated ionophore blocker, has been reported to reduce post-traumatic cortical lesion volume but not to improve cognitive function (15). Gacyclidine, a noncompetitive NMDA receptor antagonist has been shown to attenuate neuronal death and deficits in Morris water maze (MWM) performance following frontal cortex contusion (16). Furthermore, treatment with kynurenate, an NMDA and non-NMDA antagonist, has been reported to attenuate hippocampal CA_3 neuronal loss after TBI (17). Animals treated with HU-211, a synthetic nonpsychotropic cannabinoid that acts as a noncompetitive NMDA receptor antagonist, has been reported to enhance motor function after TBI (18). The NMDA antagonist ketamine has been demonstrated to attenuate postinjury neurological (19) and cognitive deficits (20). Treatment with CP-98, 113, an NMDA receptor blocker, has been shown to attenuate motor and cognitive performance deficits (21). NPS 1506 is a noncompetitive NMDA receptor antagonist that appears less toxic than earlier agents (22) and has been reported to attenuate MWM performance and hippocampal CA_3 cell death, but not cortical lesion (22). Additionally, increasing inhibitory function through stimulation of gamma-aminobutyric acid (GABA(A)) receptors via bicuculline administration has also been reported to attenuate MWM deficits after TBI (23).

TBI-induced glutamate release can also damage tissue by activating metabotropic glutamate receptors (mGluR), which are coupled to second messenger cascades via G-proteins. Modulation of mGluRs has been shown to confer neuroprotection. Gong and colleagues (24) reported that intraventricular administration of alpha-methyl-4-carboxyphenylglycine (MCPG), an mGluR antagonist, prior to TBI attenuated motor and cognitive deficits. Administration of 2-methyl-6-(phenylethynyl)-pyridine (MTEP), an mGluR5 antagonist, has been reported to reduce lesion volume and to attenuate functional deficits after TBI (25). Administration of a group II mGluR agonist 30 minutes after TBI can improve behavioral recovery (26). Selective mGluR1 antagonists have also been reported to attenuate motor deficits and MRI-assessed lesion volume (27). The compound ZJ-43, which inhibits N-acetylaspartylglutamate (NAAG) through selective activation of presynaptic group II mGluR3, has been shown to attenuate neuronal and glial degeneration after TBI (28). PGI-02776, a newly designed di-ester pro-drug of the urea-based NAAG peptidase inhibitor ZJ-43 has been recently shown to attenuate hippocampal neuronal loss and cognitive deficits after TBI (29).

Calcium Channel Blockers

Calcium channel blockers, which reduce excessive accumulation of intracellular calcium, have been examined as possible neuroprotective agents for TBI. Postinjury administration of ziconotide (also SNX-111 and CI-1009) has been reported to attenuate motor and cognitive deficits (30). Similarly, postinjury treatment with LOE 908, a broad-spectrum inhibitor of voltage-operated cation channels and store-operated cation channels, has been demonstrated to reduce neuromotor and visuospatial memory deficits (31). Treatment with the specific N-type voltage-gated calcium channel blocker SNX-185 has been shown to attenuate functional deficits and enhance neuronal survival after TBI (32). Pharmacological blockade of calcium entry has been another important strategy to reduce postinjury excitotoxicity. Treatment with (S)-emopamil has been reported to attenuate postinjury motor deficits (33). Inhibiting polyamine-dependent calcium influx is another therapeutic target for attenuating postinjury excitotoxicity. Ifenprodil, a polyamine-site NMDA receptor antagonist, has been reported to reduce cortical morphology after TBI (34).

Oxidative Injury

Oxidative stress has been implicated in the pathology of TBI. Several agents with antioxidant properties have been evaluated in animal models of TBI. Hall and colleagues (35) re-

ported that administration of a nonglucocorticoid 21-amino-steroid U74006F (tirilazad) enhanced neurological recovery in mice. Tirilazad has also been reported to attenuate axonal injury following TBI (36). Tirilazad has not been shown to improve outcome in a randomized clinical trial, and its future development is in question (37). Clifton et al. (38) reported that pretreatment and acute posttreatment with alpha-tocopherol succinate plus polyethylene glycol attenuated motor deficits following TBI. Analogues of alpha-tocopherol have also been reported to be neuroprotective in mice following TBI (39). Administration of lidocaine has been reported to attenuate postinjury neurological and motor function, but not cognitive function (40). Deferoxamine is an iron-chelating agent that can inhibit the iron-dependent hydroxyl radical production and has been reported to improve spatial memory performance following TBI (41). Interestingly, deferoxamine did not improve functional outcome when combined with moderate hypothermia treatment (42).

Superoxide dismutase (SOD) is a metalloenzyme that catalyzes the dismutation of superoxide ion into oxygen and hydrogen peroxide. Administration of polyethylene glycol-conjugated SOD has been reported to reduce motor but not MWM deficits following TBI (43). OPC-14117, a superoxide scavenger, has been reported to attenuate tissue damage (44) and behavioral deficits (45,46) following TBI. Early treatment with LY341122, an inhibitor of lipid peroxidation and an antioxidant, has been shown to provide significant histopathological protection (47). Penicillamine is a scavenging compound that has been reported to improve motor performance in mice after TBI (48). The pineal hormone melatonin, a scavenger of free radicals, has been found to reduce contusion volume following cortical impact in rats (49). Edaravone, a novel-free radical scavenger, inhibited free radical-induced neuronal degeneration and apoptotic cell death and produced a significant increase in neuronal cell number and improvement in cognitive outcome after cortical impact injury (50). The nitrone free radical scavenger, NXY-059, initiated 30 minutes after fluid percussion brain injury reduced cortical lesion volume and significantly improved MWM performance (51). Tempol, a scavenger of peroxynitrite (PN)-derived free radicals was evaluated after a severe unilateral cortical impact injury in CF-1 mice. Administration of a single 300 mg/kg dose (i.p.) 15 minutes after TBI suppressed oxidative damage in injured cortical tissue 1 hour after injury. Furthermore, multiple doses of tempol improved motor function (52). Acute administration of the dopamine D_2 receptor agonist bromocriptine, which exhibits significant antioxidant properties, reduced TBI-induced lipid peroxidation, enhanced spatial learning in a MWM task, and increased hippocampal CA_3 neuron survival after controlled cortical impact injury (53).

Exogenous Growth Factors

Exogenous administration of several growth factors has been reported to produce beneficial effects on both cognitive performance and histological outcome measures after TBI. Sinson and colleagues have shown that nerve growth factor (NGF) attenuates cognitive dysfunction following fluid percussion brain injury (54). The same group has also reported an attenuation of cognitive deficits and cholinergic cell loss after fluid percussion injury and NGF infusion (55). Dixon et al. (56) have reported that intraventricular NGF infusion reverses the post-traumatic reduction in scopolamine-evoked ACh release and significantly improves spatial memory retention following controlled cortical impact injury. Increasing NGF protein levels by intraventricular injections of liposome/NGF cDNA complexes similarly attenuates the loss of cholinergic neuronal immunostaining in the rat septum after TBI (57).

Following fluid percussion brain injury, Frank and Ragel (58) showed a significant difference in fibroblast growth factor-2 (FGF-2) positive cells between the injured and contralateral cortex. Dietrich et al. (59) administered FGF-2 intravenously for 3 hours beginning 30 minutes after fluid percussion injury and found a 50% decrease in the total number of necrotic neurons compared to controls. Furthermore, the overall contusion lesion volume was significantly decreased. Using the same injury model, McDermott and colleagues (60) reported that postinjury FGF-2 treatment significantly attenuated post-traumatic memory dysfunction relative to vehicle-treated controls. However, no attenuation in histological damage was observed. However, in contrast to the beneficial effects reported by Dietrich et al. (59) and McDermott et al. (60) with FGF-2 treatment after fluid percussion injury, Guluma and colleagues failed to see a neurological improvement at 7 days after an injury of moderate severity in a similar same model (61). Follow-up studies using a cortical impact injury model in rats by Yan and colleagues have shown that FGF-2 administration moderately improves MWM performance compared to controls but has no effect on histological outcome (62). Yoshimura and colleagues reported that overexpression of FGF-2 increases neurogenesis in the adult mouse hippocampus after cortical impact injury and that neurogenesis is reduced in FGF-2 deficient mice (63). The authors conclude that supplementation of FGF-2 may be effective in treating TBI by simultaneously enhancing neurogenesis and reducing neurodegeneration. A recent study by Sun and colleagues showed that intraventricular administration of basic fibroblast growth factor (bFGF) (i.e., FGF-2) following TBI significantly enhanced neurogenesis and improved cognitive function (64).

Insulin-like growth factor 1 (IGF-1) is a mitogenic polypeptide structurally similar to insulin that is involved in repair and regeneration following injury to the brain. IGF-1 has been shown to be upregulated following cerebral cortical contusion via a weight drop injury model (65). A follow-up study found that the upregulation of IGF-1 mRNA levels can be blocked by NMDA receptor antagonists (66). Exogenous administration of IGF-1 has been demonstrated to improve neurological and cognitive outcome after fluid percussion brain injury in rats (67). IGF-1 has recently been evaluated in a unilateral penetration brain injury model. IGF-1 administration resulted in a significant decrease in Hsp70 and TUNEL positive cells in the peri-trauma region. The neuroprotective effects of IGF-1 treatment were not limited to the cellular level but also on behavioral outcome. Specifically, IGF-1 treated animals lost less postoperative weight and survived the trauma longer than controls (68).

Intraventricular administration of epidermal growth factor following TBI resulted in an improvement in cognitive function and a reduction in neuronal cell loss in the absence of a neurogenic response (69). Intraventricular infusion of S100B, a neurotrophic/mitogenic protein produced by astrocytes, induced neurogenesis within the hippocampus and concurrently enhanced cognitive function following experimental TBI (70). Recently, Thau-Zuchman and colleagues found that infusion of exogenous vascular endothelial growth factor (VEGF) into the lateral ventricles of mice for 7 days after TBI resulted in increased tissue sparing and greater function recovery (71).

Erythropoietin

Erythropoietin (EPO) is a glycoprotein hormone that controls erythropoiesis or red blood cell production. It has also been shown to have neuroprotective effects against various types of experimental brain injury, including TBI (72). Because the mechanism for EPO neuroprotection in TBI is not precisely known, multiple pathways are likely to be involved. EPO may have effects on the cerebral vasculature through alteration in NO production. EPO has also been shown to promote angiogenesis and increased endogenous cellular proliferation (BrdU-positive cells) in the injury boundary zone and hippocampus after TBI (73). EPO has been demonstrated in several experimental models to attenuate functional and histopathological deficits. In a weight drop closed skull model EPO treatment initiated 1 hour postinjury improved neurological, cognitive, and morphological end points (74). A daily EPO administration starting at 24 hours after injury increases markers of neurogenesis and spatial memory (75). A treatment window study examining hippocampal cell death and contusion volume supported a clinically relevant 6 hour window (72). Recently, darbepoetin alfa, an erythropoietic glycoprotein that activates the EPO receptor, has been reported to improve cerebrovascular function and attenuate histological damage after TBI (76). Clinical trials are underway to evaluate EPO therapy in TBI.

Hypothermia

During the past decade, several experimental studies have provided evidence that mild to moderate hypothermia can provide behavioral protection following TBI. Studies employing multiple models have reported that moderate hypothermia can reduce neurological deficits (77–81) and improve cognitive function (77,79,81). Reports of histological protection by moderate hypothermia have been less consistent. Some investigators have reported reductions in contusion volume (82,83), decreased cortical necrotic neurons (82), reductions in axonal injury (36), and reduced ventricular enlargement (84). However, in a rat model of severe TBI with secondary insult, moderate hypothermia for 4 hours postinjury failed to improve motor function, cognitive function, lesion volume, or hippocampal neuronal survival (85). Furthermore, moderate hypothermia was found to be detrimental in fentanyl-anesthetized rats (86). A recent study employing severe hypothermia (4°C) accomplished by infusion of 5 mL of 4°C saline over 5 minutes via the external jugular vein after TBI showed that cerebral damage, motor and proprioceptive deficits, and neuronal loss were significantly reduced in the hypothermic vs the 37°C control group

(87). Factors such as treatment window, injury severity, anesthesia, and rates of rewarming need to be further defined to optimize hypothermia treatment.

Protease Inhibitors

Both intracellular proteases (e.g., calpains) and extracellular proteases (plasminogen activator and matrix metalloproteinase) are believed to contribute to the pathophysiology of neuronal cell death (88). Treatments that target these processes have been evaluated in experimental TBI. Postinjury uncontrolled activation of calpain, a calcium-dependent neutral protease, can destroy neurons. Calpain inhibitors have been the most researched target for TBI treatment. Saatman et al. (89) reported that treatment with the calpain inhibitor AK245 attenuated motor and cognitive deficits following TBI. A follow-up study found that AK245 did not attenuate cell death (90). Treatment with calpain inhibitor 2 has been demonstrated to reduce cortical loss following TBI (91). Administration of the calpain inhibitor SJA6017 has been found to inhibit functional deficits 24-hour postinjury (92). Treatment with the nonimmunosuppressive neuroimmunophilin (NIMM) ligand V-10367 has been found to reduce calpain-mediated cytoskeletal damage (93). It has been recently demonstrated that preinjury administration of the calpain inhibitor MDL-28170 significantly reduced immunomarker of axonal injury after TBI (94). For an excellent review on the role of calpains as a therapeutic target for TBI, see Saatman et al. (95).

Inflammation

TBI can initiate several inflammatory processes that may contribute to secondary tissue damage. For instance, TBI can produce polymorphonuclear leukocyte migration into the brain that can result in neuronal damage. P-selectin blockade has been reported to reduce probe trial performance on a MWM task following TBI (96). Knoblach and Faden (97) demonstrated that anti-intracellular adhesion molecule-1 (ICAM-1) can attenuate motor deficits and neutrophil invasion after TBI. Systemic administration of a high but not a low dose of interleukin-1 receptor antagonist has been reported to attenuate neurological recovery after TBI (98). The same study observed that motor function was impaired by the high dose of interleukin-1 receptor antagonist (98). Further work by Knoblach and Faden (99) failed to find a beneficial effect of selective interleukin-1 antagonists and suggested that the post-traumatic increases in interleukin-1-beta may not contribute to subsequent neurological impairment. A recent study investigated the effects of chronic lithium (i.e., 14 days post-TBI) and showed a decrease in the loss of hemispheric tissue, cerebral edema, and hippocampal CA$_3$ cell loss. Expression of the pro-inflammatory cytokine interleukin-1β was also decreased. Furthermore, chronic lithium treatment enhanced spatial learning and memory performance (100).

Administration of anti-CD11B, a monoclonal antibody directed against the leukocyte adhesion molecules CD11B, reduced neurophil influx after TBI but did not improve function (101). Nitric oxide (NO), derived from the inducible iso-

form of NO synthase (iNOS), is an inflammatory product implicated both in secondary damage and in recovery from brain injury. Sinz et al. (102) reported that rats treated with iNOS inhibitors aminoguanidine and L-N-iminothyl-lysine exacerbated functional outcome and histological damage thereby suggesting a beneficial role for iNOS in TBI. In contrast, Lu et al. (103) found that aminoguanidine treatment improved neurobehavioral outcome. Acute administration of a selective iNOS inhibitor, 1400W, has been shown to reduce lesion volume after lateral fluid percussion injury (104). Treatment with interleukin-10 has been reported to enhance neurological recovery following fluid percussion brain injury (105). However, the administration of interleukin-10 30 minutes after experimental TBI via a controlled cortical impact was ineffective in attenuating functional and histopathological deficits with a dose that prevents neurotrophil accumulation in injured tissue (106). Cyclooxygenases (COX) play an important role in inflammatory cascades and increased expression of COX after experimental TBI has been well documented (107–110). Cernak et al. (109) found that chronic administration of the COX-2 inhibitor nimesulide improves cognitive function after TBI. Pre and postinjury treatment with DFU has been shown to attenuate functional deficits and neuronal cell death after controlled cortical impact (111). Minocycline attenuates microglia activation and thus has been studied in its role as an anti-inflammatory agent with varying success (112,113). A recent study investigated minocycline given at three time points within 24 hours post-TBI and found decreased microglial activation as well as reduced lesion volume (114). Recently, systemic delivery of etanercept, a TNF-alpha antagonist with anti-inflammatory effects, significantly was shown to improve histological and functional outcomes after TBI in rats (115). At present, anti-inflammatory treatments remain a viable strategy.

Ethanol

The neuroprotective effects of ethanol have been disputed for years. Yamakami et al. (116) demonstrated that following severe brain injury, animals pretreated with high-dose ethanol showed significantly worsened neurological deficits at 24 hours postinjury. Shapira et al. (117) reported that acute but not chronic ethanol exposure increased neurological deficit and hemorrhagic necrosis volume in rats following TBI. Janis et al. (118) reported that low-dose acute ethanol treatment could reduce MWM performance deficits. A low dose of ethanol has been found to be associated with a marked attenuation of immediate postinjury hyperglycolysis and with more normal glucose metabolism in the injury penumbra over the ensuing 3 days postinjury (119). It was further observed that the reduction in CBF typically seen within the contusion core and penumbra after TBI is less severe when ethanol is present. In contrast, in a model of multiple episodes of mild TBI, acute ethanol intoxication acute ethanol treatment was not neuroprotective in rats (120). Acute preinjury administration of ethanol has been shown to attenuate the cytokine response to injury (121). A treatment consisting of a low amount of ethanol combined with caffeine (caffeinol) has been found to be neuroprotective (122).

A recent study designed to investigate the influence of binge alcohol drinking after mild TBI in mice exposed to

7.5%, 15%, or 30% alcohol solutions for 48 consecutive hours once a week for 4 weeks found that although the no alcohol (or control) TBI mice exhibited lower memory ability in the Y-maze, higher anxiety in the elevated plus maze and lower retention in the passive avoidance test, alcohol reversed these effects at all doses. The authors suggest that alcohol drinking before mild TBI might have a protective effect on recovery from brain injury but not if consumed after the trauma (123). In contrast, another recent study showed that alcohol consumption prior to TBI is deleterious. Specifically, Katada and colleagues examined the effects of ethanol (3 g/kg ethanol intraperitoneally) pretreatment (1 hour before TBI) on brain edema, inflammatory responses, and oxidative stress in male rats. The ethanol-pretreated group showed significant cytotoxic brain edema and had a significantly decreased survival rate. Moreover, NF-kappaB and AP-1 were reduced 6 hours after contusion and COX-2 mRNA expression was increased 24 hours after contusion in the pretreated ethanol groups (124). Thus, whether alcohol ameliorates or exacerbates brain injury is still unknown.

Hormonal and Gender Influences

It has been postulated in animal studies that the effects of female hormones may play a positive role in outcome from brain injury. Roof and colleagues (125) found that the presence of circulating endogenous or synthetic progesterone had a neuroprotective effect on the reduction of cerebral edema in female rats compared to males. However, in a temporal response study, Galani and co-workers (126) found that a 4 mg/kg dose of progesterone was more effective in reducing edema after medial frontal cortex contusions when given for 5 consecutive days vs 3 days. The authors speculate that the longer duration of progesterone treatment was more effective because there are two phases of edema—one that begins within hours after trauma and another that begins several days later (128). Apparently, the longer treatment was able to effectively attenuate the later phase of edema. In a similar study from the same group, 5 days of progesterone treatment was shown to protect against necrotic damage and behavioral abnormalities (127). Progesterone has also been reported to confer protection against lipid peroxidation and to facilitate cognitive recovery and reduce secondary neuronal loss after cortical contusion in male rats (125,128). It has been reported that allopregnanolone (4, 8, or 16 mg/kg), which is a metabolite of progesterone, and progesterone (16 mg/kg) administered at 1 and 6 hours after controlled cortical impact to the prefrontal cortex and every day thereafter for 5 days resulted in less cell loss in the medio-dorsal nucleus of the thalamus and less learning and memory deficits compared with the vehicle-treated controls (129). Progesterone has also been shown to improve short-term motor recovery and attenuates edema, secondary inflammation, and cell death after aged rats after TBI (130).

Animal studies also show that estrogen treatment immediately after TBI has a protective effect in males but increases mortality and exacerbates outcome in females when assessing neurologic motor function 1 week after injury (131). Other studies (132,133) show a protective role of estrogen in maintaining cerebral blood flow, mortality, and cell death after experimental TBI. A study by Wagner and colleagues examined the effects of preinjury hormonal status and gender on neurobehavioral and cognitive performance after controlled cortical impact injury. The results showed that females performed significantly better than males on motor performance measures but were not significantly different on cognitive outcome as assessed in the MWM. Furthermore, there were no differences in performance between proestrous and nonproestrous females, suggesting that neither estrous cycle stage nor hormone level at the time of TBI have significant effects on behavioral recovery (134). These findings are supported by the results of a study in which nonovariectomized rats were subjected to a right parasagittal fluid percussion brain injury during either proestrous or nonproestrous and compared to ovariectomized female and male rats. Rats were sacrificed 3 days after TBI to assess neuropathology. The results showed that both the proestrous and nonproestrous rats had significantly smaller cortical lesions relative to males. In contrast, the ovariectomized females had contusion volumes that were significantly larger than both the proestrous and nonproestrous intact rats (135).

Dehydroepiandrosterone (DHEA) and its sulfate (DHEAS) are sex hormone precursors which have neurotrophic and/or neuroprotective activity in the central nervous system (CNS). The chronic administration of DHEAS to injured rats demonstrate that after a 7-day delay, has been reported to produce significant improvements behavioral recovery on both sensorimotor and cognitive tasks (136). DHEAS has also been shown to improve long-term cognitive and behavioral effects induced by mild TBI (137). Furthermore, the DHEA analog fluasterone has been shown to improve functional recovery after TBI (138). Taken together, these data provide evidence that endogenous circulating hormones confer histopathological and behavioral protection after TBI.

Mitochondria

Sequestration of calcium loads within the mitochondrial matrix can open the mitochondrial permeability transition pore leading to cellular oxidative and metabolic stress. Acute treatment with cyclosporin A (CsA), an inhibitor of calcium-induced mitochondrial permeability transition pore, has been reported to reduce tissue damage following TBI in rats (139–141). CsA has also been found to enhance cognitive function after TBI (142). A single dose of CsA has also been reported to blunt axonal damage following TBI (143). Continuous infusion of CsA after TBI has been found to be reduce cortical damage (141). Improved mitochondrial function and behavioral outcome has been achieved by treatment with ziconitide, a calcium channel blocker (30,144). A recent study compared the neuroprotective effects of CsA (20 mg/kg intraperitoneally) administered 15 minutes following cortical impact injury in mice. The data showed that CsA significantly attenuated the increased alpha-spectrin breakdown products observed in vehicle-treated animals and attenuated motor function impairment at 48 hours and 7 days (145). These results show that the neuroprotective mechanism of CsA involves maintenance of mitochondrial integrity (145). To determine the most efficacious therapeutic window for initiating CsA therapy after TBI, Sullivan and colleagues induced a moderate unilateral cortical impact injury in male rats and provided doses of CsA (20 mg/kg) or vehicle at 1, 3, 4, 5, 6, and 8 hours postinjury and then daily or 3 days. The data showed that CsA initiated at any of the postinjury initiation times resulted in significantly less cortical damage compared to animals receiving vehicle treatment, although earlier was better (146). These data suggest that initiating therapeutic interventions such as CsA as soon as possible following TBI provides optimal protection. For a new review of the literature supporting the safety and efficacy of cyclosporine-A in traumatic brain injury, see Lulic et al. (147).

Catecholamine Agonists

The role that catecholamines play in promoting functional recovery after TBI is well documented (148–153). Feeney and colleagues have shown that a single dose of d-amphetamine administered 24 hours after a sensorimotor cortex injury produces an immediate and enduring acceleration in beam walking recovery in rats (148) and that multiple doses of amphetamine restore binocular depth perception in cats with bilateral visual cortex ablation (154). Beneficial effects of other catecholamine agonists on functional outcome in rat and/or cat following either weight drop cortical contusion or cortical aspirations have also been reported (155). Because the administration of norepinephrine antagonists block or reinstate deficits, the noradrenergic system has been implicated in the aforementioned studies. However, as suggested by the following reports, the dopaminergic system is also involved in the rehabilitative process.

The psychostimulant methylphenidate has been reported to have pharmacological properties similar to amphetamine but without the undesirable sympathomimetic effect. A single administration followed by significant symptom relevant experience (i.e., beam walking experience) enhances recovery of motor function following sensorimotor cortex lesions (152). Moreover, daily methylphenidate treatments beginning as late as 24 hours after TBI in rats reveal significantly less spatial memory performance deficits vs saline treatment (153). The effect of daily administrations of amantadine beginning 1 day postinjury and continuing for 20 days showed that rats treated with amantadine had significantly less spatial memory performance deficits than their saline-treated counterparts (156). Biochemical studies have demonstrated that amantadine increases release of DA into extracellular pools by blocking reuptake and by facilitating the synthesis of DA (157–160). In addition to acting presynaptically, amantadine has been demonstrated to act postsynaptically to increase the density of postsynaptic DA receptors (160) or to alter their conformation (161). Evidence of a postsynaptic mechanism is clinically promising because the mechanisms of actions may not depend solely on the presence of surviving postsynaptic terminals. Because the mechanism of action of amantadine differs from other DA releasing drugs (see 162 for review), it is likely that the dopaminergic effects of amantadine are a combination of presynaptic and postsynaptic effects.

Rats receiving delayed and chronic pharmacological treatment with the dopamine D_2 receptor agonist bromocriptine exhibited both enhanced working memory and spatial acquisition in a MWM. Specifically, both injured groups exhibited significant impairments initially, but in marked

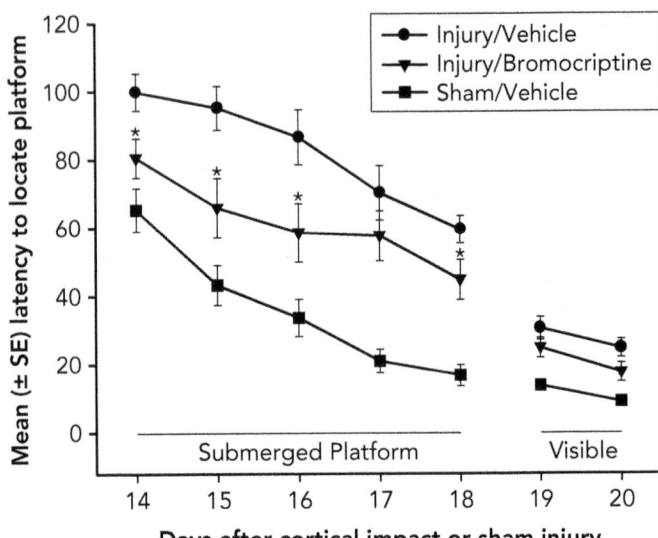

FIGURE 14-1 Mean ($\pm$ SE) latency (sec) to locate either a submerged (hidden) or raised (visible) platform in a spatial learning acquisition paradigm in the Morris water maze. The Injury/Bromocriptine group (5 mg/kg i.p., 1–20 days after cortical impact) located the hidden platform significantly quicker than the Injury/Vehicle group on the first day of training and maintained that difference at several time points throughout the testing period [p's $<$ .05]. *Significantly different from Injury/Vehicle. No differences were observed between the two CCI injured groups or the Sham/Vehicle control group in the latency to locate the visible platform [$p >$ .05]. *Reprinted from J Neurotrauma. 2002;19(4):415–425.*

contrast to the performance of the vehicle-treated group, the bromocriptine-treated animals required significantly less time to locate the platform (53) (Fig. 14-1). The dose of 5 mg/kg bromocriptine has been shown via microdialysis to increase extracellular DA levels in rats (163), suggesting that enhanced DA neurotransmission mediated the beneficial effects. However, as indicated in the "oxidative injury" section, the same dose of bromocriptine has also been reported to attenuate lipid peroxidation, suggesting that bromocriptine's antioxidant properties may also contribute to its therapeutic effects (53).

The administration of selegiline (L-deprenyl) once daily for 7 days beginning 24 hours after fluid percussion injury has been reported to improve cognitive function in the MWM and enhance neuroplasticity (164). L-deprenyl is used to enhance the action of DA by inhibiting its main catabolic enzyme in the brain, monoamine oxidase-B. Clinical studies also exist attesting to the benefits of DA augmentation following TBI (165,166).

These positive finding with delayed treatment suggests that strategies that enhance catecholamine neurotransmission during the chronic postinjury phase may be a useful adjunct in ameliorating some of the neurobehavioral sequelae following TBI in humans. Additional studies investigating this line of research are needed.

Serotonin

Investigations regarding the role of serotonergic (5-HT) responses after TBI have not been as prolific as with other neurotransmitter systems. However, several studies do exist, and they will be the topic of this section. Using a fluid percussion rat brain injury model, Busto et al. (167) reported that 5-HT levels increased from 18.85 ± 7.12 to 65.78 ± 11.36 pm/mL (mean $\pm$ SD) in the first 10 min after injury. The levels of 5-HT remained significantly higher than controls for the first 90-min sampling period. In parallel to the rise in 5-HT levels a significant 71% decrease in extracellular 5-HIAA levels was noted in the first 10 min after injury. These findings suggest that there is a rapid rise in extracellular 5-HT levels in cortical regions proximal to the injury site. Because 5-HT potentiation of excitatory amino acids has been reported in cat neocortex (168), the trauma-induced release of 5-HT might negatively impact recovery by promoting excitotoxic processes.

Serotonergic pathways originating in the raphe nuclei have extensive projections to brain areas involved in cognitive processing, and 5-HT receptor agonists and antagonists alter these processes (169,170). Of all numerous 5-HT receptors characterized thus far (5-HT_1–5-HT_7), the 5-HT_{1A} is the most widely studied. 5-HT_{1A} receptors are abundantly expressed in brain regions such as the cortex and hippocampus that play key roles in learning and memory and that are susceptible to neuronal damage induced by brain injury (171,172). Numerous studies have reported on the effects of 5-HT_{1A} receptor agonists after focal or global cerebral ischemia in both rats and mice (171–176). These studies have focused on either pre or postinjury administration of various 5-HT_{1A} receptor agonists and their potential neuroprotective effects. The general consensus is that 5-HT_{1A} receptor agonism attenuates histopathology after ischemic injury.

Since the last version of this chapter, the investigation of 5-HT_{1A} receptor agonists on neurobehavioral and cognitive recovery after TBI has flourished. In the first study assessing the role of the 5-HT_{1A} receptor agonists on recovery after brain trauma, Kline and colleagues demonstrated that a 4-hours continuous infusion of Repinotan HCL (BAY $\times$ 3702; 10 µg/kg/hours IV initiated 5 minutes after injury), a high affinity, highly selective 5-HT_{1A} receptor agonist produced a marked attenuation of TBI-induced learning and memory deficits assessed in the MWM (177). Moreover, this treatment regimen attenuated hippocampal CA_1 and CA_3 cell loss and decreased cortical lesion volume relative to vehicle-treated controls. Using the same TBI model, Kline et al. (178) have also demonstrated that the classic 5-HT_{1A} receptor agonist 8-hydroxy-2-(di-n-propylamino)tetralin (8-OH-DPAT) produces similar effects on functional and histological outcome. Briefly, in a dose response study, a single dose of 0.5 mg/kg administered intraperitoneally 15 min following cortical impact significantly attenuated water maze performance relative to the vehicle controls. Additionally, 8-OH DPAT attenuated hippocampal CA_3 cell loss (178). To elucidate whether the concomitant mild hypothermia observed in the dose response study may have mediated the benefits, a follow-up experiment was conducted. Briefly, the optimal dose from the original study was provided to 2 groups of TBI rats; one that was allowed to cool spontaneously as in the previous study and the other that was actively kept warm. The data showed that both groups (normal cooling and active warming) performed comparably in learning the location of the escape platform in the MWM, suggesting that

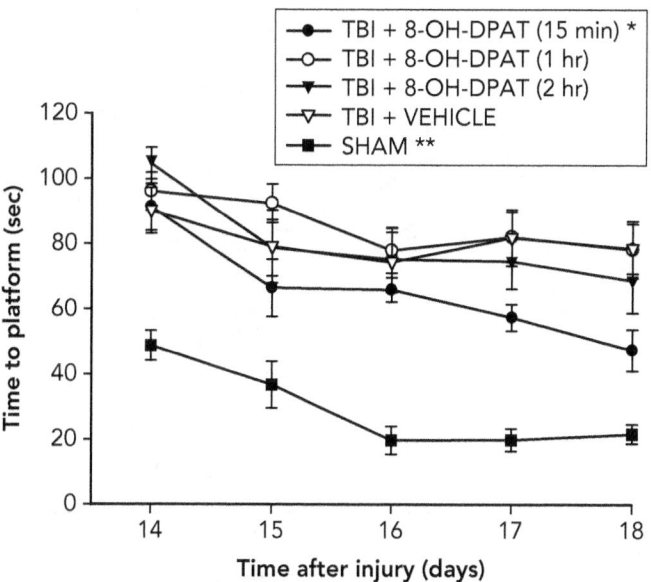

FIGURE 14-2 Mean ($\pm$ SE) time (sec) to locate escape platform in the Morris water maze on post-TBI days 14–18. $*p < .05$ vs TBI + VEHICLE, TBI + 8-OH-DPAT (1 hr), and TBI + 8-OH-DPAT (2 hr). $**p < .05$ vs all TBI groups. *Reprinted from Neurosci Lett. 2007;416(2):165–168.*

mild hypothermia did not influence the 8-OH-DPAT benefit (179). To define the therapeutic window of opportunity after a single administration of 8-OH-DPAT, a subsequent study evaluated 3 time points (i.e., 15 min, 1 hour, and 2 hours after TBI). The study showed that only the group 15 min administration group exhibited significant functional benefit (180) (Fig. 14-2), which replicated previous studies (178,179). That no benefit was observed with treatments administered at 1 and 2 hours after TBI suggests that an early and narrow critical period exists for the behavioral recovery afforded by a single 8-OH-DPAT treatment paradigm. The critical window corresponds to the well documented TBI-induced glutamate increase (9), suggesting that 8-OH-DPAT may confer neuroprotection by attenuating excitotoxicity.

Although, acute administration of 8-OH-DPAT after TBI was effective, the potential efficacy of a chronic treatment regimen was also investigated, with once daily administration of 8-OH-DPAT beginning 24 hours after TBI. The data showed that this regimen enhanced motor performance, spatial learning, and memory retention (181,182) (Fig. 14-3). These data replicated previous acute administration findings (9,178–180) and extended those results by demonstrating that the benefits could be achieved even when treatment was delayed for 24 hours, making this treatment regimen clinically feasible.

Although potential mechanisms contributing to the beneficial effects observed after a single treatment with 8-OH-DPAT in our TBI paradigm have not been reported, the results from other studies investigating 5-HT_{1A} receptor agonists suggest that it is via an attenuation of excitotoxicity. Electrophysiological studies have shown that 8-OH-DPAT, repinotan HCL, and other 5-HT_{1A} receptor agonists induce neuronal hyperpolarization by activating G-protein coupled

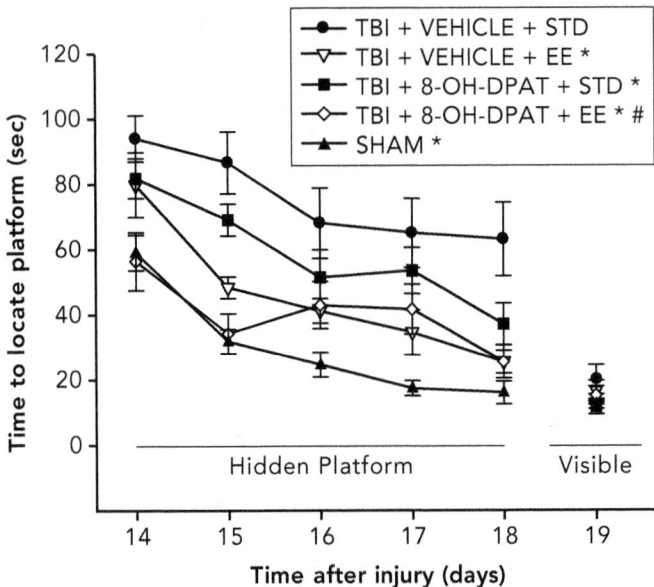

FIGURE 14-3 Mean ($\pm$ SE) time (sec) to locate either a hidden (submerged) or visible (raised) platform in a water maze. All TBI groups, except the TBI + 8-OH-DPAT + EE group, had significant difficulty with the cognitive task vs SHAM controls. However, over the subsequent 5 days of training, all groups, except the TBI + VEHICLE + STD group, became proficient at locating the escape platform. *$p < .05$ vs TBI + VEHICLE + STD. #$p < .05$ vs TBI + 8-OH-DPAT + STD. No differences were observed in locating the visible platform. Reprinted from *J Neurotrauma.* 2010;27(11):2021–2032.

inwardly rectifying K$^+$ channels (183,184) and decrease glutamate release after brain insult (171,173,174). The latter effect is likely produced by activation of presynaptic 5-HT$_{1A}$ receptors on glutamatergic terminals (185,186). 5-HT$_{1A}$ receptor activation may also contribute to neuroprotection by directly interacting with voltage-gated Na$^+$ channels to reduce Na$^+$ influx (187).

Acetylcholine

Acetylcholine (ACh) levels have been reported to change in brain and cerebral spinal fluid (CSF) following TBI. Gorman et al. (188) reported that hippocampal ACh levels (measured by microdialysis) increased significantly above control within 10 minutes after fluid percussion brain injury. Saija et al. (189,190) found that ACh turnover rate (measured by a phosphoryl [2H9]choline method) increased significantly in the brainstem at 12 minutes and was still elevated at 4 hours after moderate fluid percussion TBI in the rat. Thus, moderate TBI appears to produce a transient release of ACh and increased cholinergic neuronal activity in some brain regions for several hours after injury.

Laboratory studies have demonstrated that excessive activation of ACh muscarinic receptors contribute significantly to functional deficits associated with experimental TBI in the rat. TBI induced muscarinic receptor activation mediates excitotoxic processes by modulating ionic fluxes via altered protein kinase C activity or inositol 1,4,5-triphos-

phate associated G-protein coupled PI turnover. The role of ACh in the induction of brain injury is further strengthened by evidence indicating that blockade of muscarinic cholinergic receptors during the acute phase can reduce injury and improve outcome. For example, pretreatment (191,192) or immediate posttreatment (192) with the muscarinic receptor antagonist scopolamine has been demonstrated to significantly reduce functional motor deficits associated with TBI in the rat. Post-TBI administration of rivastigmine, an anticholinesterase drug that increases activity at both muscarinic and nicotinic receptors, has been shown to attenuate neurobehavioral and cognitive performance in mice.

In contrast, several lines of evidence indicate that experimental TBI in rats, in addition to transiently increasing ACh, also chronically decreases cholinergic neurotransmission, which may be related to disturbances in cognitive performance. Microdialysis studies at 2 weeks post-TBI have shown a reduction in the release of ACh evoked by the muscarinic autoreceptor antagonist, scopolamine (193,194). TBI can also produce increased sensitivity to disruption of spatial memory function by scopolamine that occurs concurrently with a reduction in scopolamine-evoked ACh release (195). A time-dependent loss of choline acetyltransferase (ChAT) enzymatic activity (188) and ChAT immunohistochemical staining (196,197) has also been reported after TBI. Dixon et al. (195) have reported a selective decrease in the V_{max} of choline uptake in the absence of any change in K_m after controlled cortical impact injury. However, alterations in synaptosomal choline uptake have not been reported at 1 week after closed head impact in rats (198). Ciallella and colleagues have reported chronic changes in vesicular ACh transporter (VAChT) and M2 cholinergic muscarinic receptor, two proteins involved in cholinergic neurotransmission after TBI (199). Chronic mRNA changes in VAChT and M2 have been evaluated at 4 weeks after moderate brain trauma in rats. VAChT and M2 medial septal mRNA levels evaluated by RT-PCR revealed an increase in VAChT mRNA but no significant change in M2 mRNA levels compared to sham controls (200). Changes in VAChT and M2 protein have been demonstrated to persist for up to 1 year following TBI (201). These changes may represent a compensatory response of cholinergic neurons to increase the efficiency of ACh neurotransmission chronically after TBI through differential transcriptional regulation.

Increasing levels of ACh pharmacologically can attenuate post-TBI spatial memory performance deficits. For example, increasing ACh synthesis by increasing the availability of choline using CDP-choline treatment has been reported to enhance spatial memory performance (202). Additionally, chronic post-TBI administration of BIBM 99, a selective muscarinic M2 receptor antagonist that increases ACh release by blocking presynaptic autoreceptors, has been reported to attenuate spatial memory deficits after TBI (203). Similarly, chronic post-TBI administration of MDL 26,479 (suritozole), a negative modulator at the gamma-aminobutyric acid (GABA) receptor that enhances cholinergic function, attenuates spatial memory deficits after TBI (204). Several clinical reports have described beneficial effects on memory dysfunction with the acetylcholinesterase inhibitor Aricept (donepezil) after TBI in humans (205–208). In a recent study, Fujiki and colleagues evaluated the effect of donepezil on the neurodegeneration and behavioral impairments induced by mild traumatic brain injury (mTBI). Donepezil was given orally to rats subjected to mTBI (209). The data showed that a single dose of donepezil (12 mg/kg) provided immediately after mTBI significantly attenuated hippocampal CA$_1$ neuronal death and cognitive impairment (209). Taken together, the studies described in this section suggest that therapies that attenuate the transient increase in ACh and/or alleviate the chronic decrease seen after TBI are capable of producing beneficial effects on functional outcome.

Environmental Enrichment

Environmental enrichment (EE) consists of a spacious and complex living environment with increased social interaction and novel stimuli that together promote physical and cognitive stimulation (210). Several studies in experimental models of moderate TBI (i.e., not comatose or vegetative) suggest that 3 weeks of EE exposure confer behavioral benefits. Specifically, EE facilitates learning and memory after both cortical impact (210–212) and fluid percussion brain injury (213–215) and also improves motor performance (210–212). Thus, EE may be viewed as a reasonable rodent correlate of clinical rehabilitation.

The bulk of research assessing the potential of EE to mimic rehabilitation after TBI consists of continuous exposure to the environment. However, clinical rehabilitation after brain injury consists of a limited amount of physical and occupational therapy. In practice, the length of time in therapy after TBI varies from a minimum of 1 hour up to a maximum of 8 hours per day depending on the rehabilitation setting (216–219). Thus, although the range of clinical rehabilitation may be varied, it is certainly shorter than the continuous nature of EE in the laboratory. The difference between the relatively short duration of daily clinical rehabilitation after TBI and the continuous nature of experimental EE highlights a disparity between the experimental model and the clinical environment.

To address this discrepancy, recent work has been conducted to determine the therapeutic window of EE efficacy, which will lead to further understanding of its potential contribution to clinical rehabilitation. In what is termed an abbreviated enrichment paradigm, male rats were subjected to a controlled cortical impact injury and provided 2, 4, or 6 hours of EE per day vs continuous exposure. The data showed that neither the 2-hours nor 4-hours daily EE groups benefited from the exposure as they did not differ from the standard housed animals. In marked contrast, the group receiving 6-hours of daily EE performed comparably to the continuous EE group (220). Although the translational potential to humans is not fully elucidated, this finding suggests that there may be a certain threshold of enrichment that is necessary to elicit neurobehavioral recovery within this model of TBI (220) (Fig. 14-4).

Another disparity between the clinic and the laboratory involves the time of initiation and duration of EE on neurobehavioral recovery after TBI. In the laboratory, EE is typically introduced immediately after TBI and is continued until all manipulations have been completed. Because this paradigm has consistently shown improvement on motor and cognitive performance after brain trauma (210–214), the continuous-exposure nature is inconsistent with the real

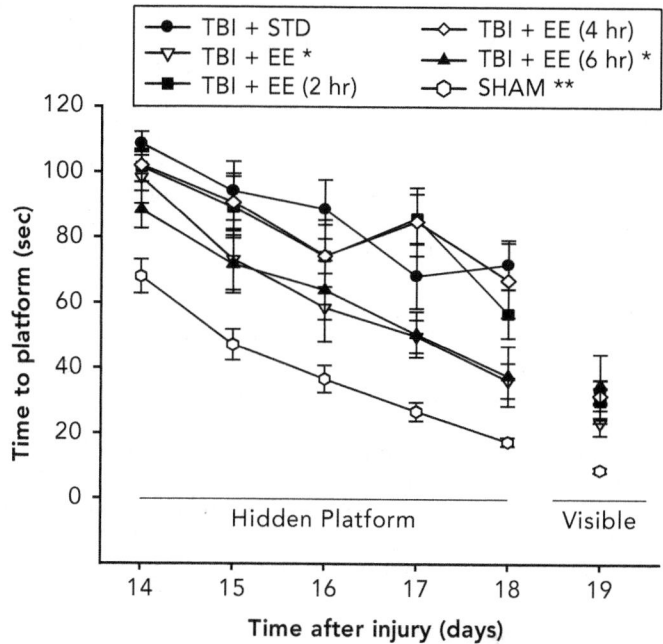

FIGURE 14-4 Mean (± S.E.M.) time (sec) to locate either a hidden (submerged) or visible (raised) platform in a water maze. *p's < .0029 vs TBI + STD, TBI + EE (2 hr), and TBI + EE (4 hr). **p < .0001 vs all TBI groups. No significant differences were revealed among the TBI groups for time to locate the visible platform, but the SHAM was able to reach it in significantly less time [p's < .0002]. Reprinted from *Neurorehabil Neural Repair.* 2011;25(4):343–350.

world where patients do not begin rehabilitation immediately after injury and also do not receive similar lengths of rehabilitation. Hence, to address this limitation, adult male rats were exposed to the EE either immediately after TBI or 1 week later and then compared their performance to standard housed rats using established motor (assessment during the first week after injury) and cognitive behavioral assessment (during the second week after injury) tasks. Motor function was facilitated in the TBI groups that received either early or continuous EE vs those receiving delayed or no EE. In contrast, cognitive performance was enhanced in the TBI groups that received continuous or delayed EE vs the early EE or standard groups. Taken together, the data suggest that EE-mediated functional improvement after TBI is contingent on task-specific neurobehavioral experience (211,221).

Potential mechanisms for the EE-mediated benefits after brain injury may include plastic changes, such as, but not limited to, increased dendritic branching and spine density, increased number of neuronal synapses and synaptic size, and greater tissue volume in the rodent cortex (222–226). EE also promotes neurogenesis, angiogenesis, and the survival of hippocampal neurons (226).

Stem Cell Therapy

Multipotential stem cells are a contemporary choice for cell therapy TBI as replacement of multiple cell types may be required for functional recovery. Several studies have demonstrated that following TBI in adult rats, the number of proliferating cells labeled with bromodeoxyuridine is significantly increased in the bilateral subventricular zone and dentate gyrus (227–230). A better understanding of these endogenous neural stem cells may lead a less invasive model of stem cell therapy. There are several promising studies in which the transplantation of various progenitor cells have improved tissue survival and functional outcome. Bone marrow stromal cells, which normally give rise to bone, cartilage, adipose tissue, and hematopoiesis-supporting cells, have been shown to differentiate in vitro and in vivo into neural-like cells. Following TBI, treatment with bone marrow stromal cells has been shown to be beneficial using intracerebral (231), intra-arterial (232), and intravenous routes of administration (233). Transplantation of the neural stem cells (clone C17.2) has been reported to survive in the injured brain, differentiate into neurons and/or glia, and attenuate motor dysfunction (234). Transplantation of embryonic stem cells has resulted in improved sensorimotor but not cognitive function after TBI (235). Lu et al. (236) found that human umbilical cord blood cells injected i.v. into TBI rats significantly reduced motor and neurological deficits compared to control groups by day 28 after the treatment. The cells were observed to preferentially enter the brain and migrate into the parenchyma and express the neuronal markers, NeuN and MAP-2, and the astrocytic marker, GFAP. These data suggest that the transplantation of progenitor cells into the brain may be a potential therapy for patients with TBI.

Nutraceuticals

Several empirical research studies have demonstrated that "natural" treatments can be effective in reducing some of the sequelae of TBI. An excellent example of a nutraceutical that has been extensively reported to reduce secondary effects of TBI and improve behavioral outcome is magnesium (Mg^{2+}). Early work has shown that the administration of Mg^{2+} 30 minutes after a fluid percussion injury in rats provides significant improvement in neurological function when compared to saline-treated rats (237). Follow-up studies from the same group have shown that Mg^{2+} therapy is also effective in decreasing cognitive and motor deficits (20), histological damage (238,239), and expression of a gene (p53) associated with the induction of cell death (240). The beneficial effects of Mg^{2+} have been observed for up to 8 months after TBI (241). Using an impact-acceleration model of severe traumatic diffuse axonal brain injury, Heath and Vink (242) have shown that intramuscular administration of $MgSO_4$ (750 µmol/kg) at 30 minutes or at 8, 12, or 24 hours after TBI significantly improves motor performance as assessed on a rotarod test vs untreated-control animals. Although the rats treated at 24 hours displayed a slower rate of recovery during the early testing period, they eventually recovered significantly beyond the vehicle-treated group by the end of the testing session, suggesting that even delayed magnesium treatment is effective after TBI (242). A more recent finding by the same group reports that $MgSO_4$ (250 µmol/kg) at 30 minutes after diffuse TBI significantly improves sensorimotor function and learning performance (243). Mg^{2+} therapy has also been shown to facilitate functional recovery and prevent subcortical atrophy after lesions of the rat sensori-

motor cortex (244). Moreover, Mg^{2+} therapy combined with riboflavin has been shown to synergistically improve functional recovery after unilateral cortical impact injury (245).

Other nutraceuticals that have been reported to positively impact the neuroprotective and/or rehabilitative process after TBI include, but are not limited to, cytidinediphosphocholine (CDP-choline), creatine, and vitamins B3 (nicotinamide), vitamin E and folic acid. CDP-choline or citicholine is a naturally occurring endogenous nucleoside and an intermediate of phosphatidylcholine synthesis. When administered as a treatment after controlled cortical impact injury (100 mg/kg, 1–18 days post-TBI), CDP-choline-treated rats performed significantly better than vehicle-treated rats on both motor and cognitive tasks (202). Also using the controlled cortical impact injury model, Baskaya et al. (246) demonstrated that intraperitoneal injections of CDP-choline (100 or 400 mg/kg twice after TBI) significantly decreased brain edema and blood brain barrier (BBB) breakdown. In a more recent study, Dempsey and colleague reported that 2 treatments of CDP-choline (200 or 400 mg/kg, immediately post-TBI and 6 hours later) after cortical impact injury significantly prevented hippocampal neuron loss, decreased cortical contusion volume, and improved neurological recovery (247). Taken together, these studies indicate that CDP-choline is an effective neuroprotective agent on secondary injuries and neurobehavioral dysfunctions that are manifested after TBI.

TBI has been observed in animals and humans to result in injury-induced glucose metabolic depression and that diets that provide an alternative fuel substrate could potentially improve cellular metabolism and recovery of function (see Chapter 12). An alternative fuel substrate under active investigation is ketones (248). Administration of a ketogenic diet has been shown to substantially reduce cortical contusion volume and attenuate functional after TBI (249,250).

Creatine, a common food supplement used by individuals as a performance enhancer, has been demonstrated to attenuate the extent of cortical damage in mice and rats by as much as 36% and 50%, respectively (251). The authors suggested that protection might have been mediated by mechanisms involving creatine-induced maintenance of mitochondrial membrane potential, decreased intramitochondrial levels of reactive oxygen species and calcium, and preservation of adenosine triphosphate levels. In a study investigating the effects of vitamin B3 (Niacin), Hoane et al. (252) reported that a 500 mg/kg dose provided 15 minutes and 24 hours after TBI produced by a cortical contusion model significantly reduced the size of the lesion and glial fibrillary acidic protein positive astrocytes compared to saline-treated rats. Furthermore, vitamin B3 treatment also significantly attenuated apoptosis and improved behavioral outcome (252). The data suggest that vitamin B3 may have therapeutic potential for the treatment of TBI. In an investigation of vitamin E or alpha-tocopherol, Inci and colleagues have demonstrated that this neutraceutical also exhibits protective effects after TBI. Specifically, guinea pigs were subjected to a TBI using a weight drop injury model and then administered 100 mg/kg of vitamin E. Lipid perixodation was measured using the thiobarbituric acid reactive substances method immediately 1 hour or 36 hours after trauma. The results indicated that alpha-tocopherol significantly suppressed the rise in lipid peroxide levels in traumatized brain tissue, suggesting that this treatment regimen has a protective effect against oxygen free radical-mediated lipid peroxidation after TBI (253). A new study has shown that vitamin E reduces MWM performance deficits after mild TBI produced by fluid percussion (254). More recently, the administration of folic acid has been shown to attenuate functional deficits in a piglet model of pediatric TBI induced by rapid axial head rotation without impact (255). Lastly, resveratrol (3, 5, 4′-trihydroxystilbene) is a plant-derived small molecule that has been recently shown to attenuate motor, cognitive, and morphological deficits (online supplemental Fig. 14-1) after TBI (256).

Antipsychotics

In addition to evaluating therapies that can potentially benefit recovery after brain trauma, it is equally important to assess agents such as antipsychotic drugs (APDs) that are currently provided to patients with TBI. APDs are frequently administered to patients with TBI to control agitated and aggressive behavior. This common practice of administering APDs continues despite a paucity of data showing their effects on functional outcome. The few studies that have investigated APDs after experimental TBI show that these drugs generally impair the recovery process and in some instances, exacerbate TBI-induced behavioral deficits. In the early 1980s, Feeney and colleagues demonstrated that a single administration of haloperidol after sensorimotor cortex lesions in adult rats markedly slowed motor recovery. Furthermore, the administration of haloperidol after the animals were recovered led to a reinstatement of the deficits (148). Similar findings have been reported by Goldstein and Bullman (257). In contrast to these studies, Kline and colleagues showed that neither a single administration of haloperidol nor the atypical APD, risperidone negatively impacted functional outcome (258). However, a significant reinstatement of motor and cognitive deficits was observed when the APDs were administered once daily for 5 days (258). Chronic administration (i.e., once daily for 3 weeks) of haloperidol and risperidone has also been shown to significantly impede recovery (259,260). These negative findings are also observed in other clinically relevant models of TBI (261–263). The findings may have significant relevance for the physician who is faced with the decision of whether to administer antipsychotics to attenuate TBI-induced aggression or agitation so that patient care can commence.

CONCLUSION

The experimental control afforded with the use of animal models of TBI has allowed for the testing of several classes of neuroprotective therapies as summarized in this chapter. Empirical studies have revealed several potential treatments that attenuate a range of neurobehavioral and morphological derangements. However, the translation of experimental neuroprotective treatments to humans has been limited. This situation may be improved by screening therapies under experimental conditions that better reproduce the clinical environment (e.g., ICU-like care, large animal models, etc.) or by conducting clinical trials that better mimic laboratory treatment administration protocols (e.g., earlier treatment windows). Animal models also serve as a useful tool to identify potentially deleterious treatments such as those reported following chronic administration of APDs.

 KEY CLINICAL POINTS

1. Excitotoxicity plays an important role in secondary neuronal injury after TBI. Experimental therapies that inhibit the release of excitotoxins, block receptor activation, or block calcium channels have been shown to be neuroprotective in several animal models.
2. The maintenance of mitochondrial integrity by agents such as cyclosporine can attenuate cellular oxidative and metabolic stress after TBI.
3. To optimize hypothermia treatment, factors such as treatment window, injury severity, anesthesia, and rates of rewarming need to be further defined.
4. Experimental studies suggest that anti-inflammatory treatments remain a viable strategy.
5. Sex hormone-base therapies show promise as a neuroprotectants and highlight the role of gender in the development of new therapies.
6. Strategies that enhance catecholamine neurotransmission during the chronic postinjury phase may be a useful adjunct in ameliorating some of the neurobehavioral sequelae following TBI in humans.
7. Regarding serotonin and TBI, the studies reviewed suggest that the administration of 5-HT$_{1A}$ receptor agonists—a pharmacotherapy novel to TBI but used routinely in treating neuropsychiatric disorders in humans—attenuate experimental TBI-induced behavioral deficits and may be an alternative and promising therapeutic approach for clinical TBI.
8. EE is a robust, noninvasive therapeutic strategy that enhances neurobehavioral recovery after experimental TBI. The studies summarized indicate that EE does not have to be initiated immediately after TBI for successful promotion of cognitive recovery. This is an important finding given that most pharmacologic and nonpharmacologic approaches require relatively early initiation for therapeutic efficacy. These studies provide a clearer understanding of the importance of initiation and duration of EE and may have important implications for clinical rehabilitation programs.
9. Antipsychotics are routinely administered after TBI to control behavioral disturbances. The studies summarized suggest that chronic administration of either haloperidol or risperidone hinder recovery in an experimental model of TBI, and hence caution should be exercised when administering these agents to human patients with TBI as similar detrimental effects may be presented.

KEY REFERENCES

1. Cherian L, Goodman JC, Robertson C. Neuroprotection with erythropoietin administration following controlled cortical impact injury in rats. *J Pharmacol Exp Ther.* 2007; 322(2):789–794.
2. Hall ED, Vaishnav RA, Mustafa AG. Antioxidant therapies for traumatic brain injury. *Neurotherapeutics.* 2010; 7(1):51–61.

3. Hoffman AN, Cheng JP, Zafonte RD, Kline AE. Administration of haloperidol and risperidone after neurobehavioral testing hinders the recovery of traumati brain injury-induced deficits. *Life Sci.* 2008;83(17–18):602–607.

4. Kline AE, Wagner AK, Westergom BP, et al. Acute treatment with the 5-HT(1A) receptor agonist 8-OH-DPAT and chronic environmental enrichment confer neurobehavioral benefit after experimental brain trauma. *Behav Brain Res.* 2007;177(2):186–194.

5. Prins M. Diet, ketones, and neurotrauma. *Epilepsia.* 2008; 49(suppl 8):111–113.

References

1. Kline AE, Dixon CE. Contemporary in vivo models of brain trauma and a comparison of injury responses. In: Miller LP, Hayes RL, eds. *Head Trauma: Basic, Preclinical and Clinical Directions.* New York, NY: John Wiley & Sons, Inc.; 2001:65–84.

2. Bittigau P, Ikonomidou C. Glutamate in neurologic diseases. *J Child Neurol.* 1997;12(8):471–485.

3. Sun FY, Faden AI. Neuroprotective effects of 619C89, a use-dependent sodium channel blocker, in rat traumatic brain injury. *Brain Res.* 1995;673(1):133–140.

4. McIntosh TK, Smith DH, Voddi M, Perri BR, Stutzmann JM. Riluzole, a novel neuroprotective agent, attenuates both neurologic motor and cognitive dysfunction following experimental brain injury in the rat. *J Neurotrauma.* 1996;13(12):767–780.

5. Stover JF, Beyer TF, Unterberg AW. Riluzole reduces brain swelling and contusion volume in rats following controlled cortical impact injury. *J Neurotrauma.* 2000;17(12):1171–1178.

6. Liu S, Lyeth BG, Hamm RJ. Protective effect of galanin on behavioral deficits in experimental traumatic brain injury. *J Neurotrauma.* 1994;11(1):73–82.

7. Di X, Lyeth BG, Hamm RJ, Bullock MR. Voltage-dependent Na + / K + ion channel blockade fails to ameliorate behavioral deficits after traumatic brain injury in the rat. *J Neurotrauma.* 1996;13(9): 497–504.

8. Hayes RL, Jenkins LW, Lyeth BG, et al. Pretreatment with phencyclidine, an N-methyl-D-aspartate antagonist, attenuates long-term behavioral deficits in the rat produced by traumatic brain injury. *J Neurotrauma.* 1988;5(4):259–274.

9. Faden AI, Demediuk P, Panter SS, Vink R. The role of excitatory amino acids and NMDA receptors in traumatic brain injury. *Science.* 1989;244(4906):798–800.

10. Mcintosh TK, Vink R, Soares H, Hayes R, Simon R. Effects of the N-methyl-D-aspartate receptor blocker MK-801 on neurologic function after experimental brain injury. *J Neurotrauma.* 1989;6(4): 247–259.

11. McIntosh TK, Vink R, Soares H, Hayes R, Simon R. Effect of non-competitive blockade of N-methyl-D-aspartate receptors on the neurochemical sequelae of experimental brain injury. *J Neurochem.* 1990;55(4):1170–1179.

12. Hamm RJ, O'Dell DM, Pike BR, Lyeth BG. Cognitive impairment following traumatic brain injury: the effect of pre- and post-injury administration of scopolamine and MK-801. *Brain Res Cogn Brain Res.* 1993;1(4):223–226.

13. Lewén A, Fredriksson A, Li GL, Olsson Y, Hillered L. Behavioural and morphological outcome of mild cortical contusion trauma of the rat brain: influence of NMDA-receptor blockade. *Acta Neurochir (Wien).* 1999;141(2):193–202.

14. Ikonomidou C, Turski L. Prevention of trauma-induced neurodegeneration in infant and adult rat brain: glutamate antagonists. *Metab Brain Dis.* 1996;11(2):125–141.

15. Smith DH, Perri BR, Raghupathi R, Saatman KE, McIntosh TK. Remacemide hydrochloride reduces cortical lesion volume following brain trauma in the rat. *Neurosci Lett.* 1997;231(3):135–138.

16. Smith JS, Fulop ZL, Levinsohn SA, Darrell RS, Stein DG. Effects of the novel NMDA receptor antagonist gacyclidine on recovery from medial frontal cortex contusion injury in rats. *Neural Plast.* 2000;7(1–2):73–91.

17. Hicks RR, Smith DH, Gennarelli TA, McIntosh T. Kynurenate is neuroprotective following experimental brain injury in the rat. *Brain Res.* 1994;655(1–2):91–96.

18. Shohami E, Novikov M, Mechoulam R. A nonpsychotropic cannabinoid, HU-211, has cerebroprotective effects after closed head injury in the rat. *J Neurotrauma.* 1993;10(2):109–119.

19. Shapira Y, Lam AM, Eng CC, Laohaprasit V, Michel M. Therapeutic time window and dose response of the beneficial effects of ketamine in experimental head injury. *Stroke.* 1994;25(8):1637–1643.

20. Smith DH, Okiyama K, Gennarelli TA, McIntosh TK. Magnesium and ketamine attenuate cognitive dysfunction following experimental brain injury. *Neurosci Lett.* 1993;157(2):211–214.

21. Okiyama K, Smith DH, White WF, McIntosh TK. Effects of the NMDA antagonist CP-98,113 on regional cerebral edema and cardiovascular, cognitive, and neurobehavioral function following experimental brain injury in the rat. *Brain Res.* 1998;792(2):291–298.

22. Leoni MJ, Chen XH, Mueller AL, Cheney J, McIntosh TK, Smith DH. NPS 1506 attenuates cognitive dysfunction and hippocampal neuron death following brain trauma in the rat. *Exp Neurol.* 2000; 166(2):442–449.

23. O'Dell DM, Gibson CJ, Wilson MS, DeFord SM, Hamm RJ. Positive and negative modulation of the GABA(A) receptor and outcome after traumatic brain injury in rats. *Brain Res.* 2000;861(2):325–332.

24. Gong QZ, Delahunty TM, Hamm RJ, Lyeth BG. Metabotropic glutamate antagonist, MCPG, treatment of traumatic brain injury in rats. *Brain Res.* 1995;700(1–2):299–302.

25. Movsesyan VA, O'Leary DM, Fan L, et al. mGluR5 antagonists 2-methyl-6-(phenylethynyl)-pyridine and (E)-2-methyl-6-(2-phenylethenyl)-pyridine reduce traumatic neuronal injury in vitro and in vivo by antagonizing N-methyl-D-aspartate receptors. *J Pharmacol Exp Ther.* 2001;296(1):41–47.

26. Allen JW, Ivanova SA, Fan L, Espey MG, Basile AS, Faden AI. Group II metabotropic glutamate receptor activation attenuates traumatic neuronal injury and improves neurological recovery after traumatic brain injury. *J Pharmacol Exp Ther.* 1999;290(1): 112–120.

27. Faden AI, O'Leary DM, Fan L, Bao W, Mullins PG, Movsesyan VA. Selective blockade of the mGluR1 receptor reduces traumatic neuronal injury in vitro and improves outcome after brain trauma. *Exp Neurol.* 2001;167(2):435–444.

28. Zhong C, Zhao X, Sarva J, Kozikowski A, Neale JH, Lyeth BG. NAAG peptidase inhibitor reduces acute neuronal degeneration and astrocyte damage following lateral fluid percussion TBI in rats. *J Neurotrauma.* 2005;22(2):266–276.

29. Feng JF, Van KC, Gurkoff GG, et al. Post-injury administration of NAAG peptidase inhibitor prodrug, PGI-02776, in experimental TBI. *Brain Res.* 2011;1395:62–73.

30. Berman RF, Verweij BH, Muizelaar JP. Neurobehavioral protection by the neuronal calcium channel blocker ziconotide in a model of traumatic diffuse brain injury in rats. *J Neurosurg.* 2000;93(5): 821–828.

31. Cheney JA, Brown AL, Bareyre FM, et al. The novel compound LOE 908 attenuates acute neuromotor dysfunction but not cognitive impairment or cortical tissue loss following traumatic brain injury in rats. *J Neurotrauma.* 2000;17(1):83–91.

32. Lee LL, Galo E, Lyeth BG, Muizelaar JP, Berman RF. Neuroprotection in the rat lateral fluid percussion model of traumatic brain injury by SNX-185, an N-type voltage-gated calcium channel blocker. *Exp Neurol.* 2004;190(1):70–78.

33. Okiyama K, Smith DH, Thomas MJ, McIntosh TK. Evaluation of a novel calcium channel blocker, (S)-emopamil, on regional cerebral edema and neurobehavioral function after experimental brain injury. *J Neurosurg.* 1992;77(4):607–615.

34. Dempsey RJ, Başkaya MK, Doğan A. Attenuation of brain edema, blood-brain barrier breakdown, and injury volume by ifenprodil, a polyamine-site N-methyl-D-aspartate receptor antagonist, after experimental traumatic brain injury in rats. *Neurosurgery.* 2000; 47(2):399–404.

35. Hall ED, Yonkers PA, McCall JM, Braughler JM. Effects of the 21-aminosteroid U74006F on experimental head injury in mice. *J Neurosurg.* 1988;68(3):456–461.

36. Marion DW, White MJ. Treatment of experimental brain injury with moderate hypothermia and 21-aminosteroids. *J Neurotrauma.* 1996;13(3):139–147.

37. Hall ED, Vaishnav RA, Mustafa AG. Antioxidant therapies for traumatic brain injury. *Neurotherapeutics.* 2010;7(1):51–61.

38. Clifton GL, Lyeth BG, Jenkins LW, Taft WC, DeLorenzo RJ, Hayes RL. Effect of D, alpha-tocopheryl succinate and polyethylene glycol on performance tests after fluid percussion brain injury. *J Neurotrauma.* 1989;6(2):71–81.

39. Grisar JM, Bolkenius FN, Petty MA, Verne J. 2,3-Dihydro-1-benzofuran-5-ols as analogues of alpha-tocopherol that inhibit in vitro and ex vivo lipid autoxidation and protect mice against central nervous system trauma. *J Med Chem.* 1995;38(3):453–458.

40. Muir JK, Lyeth BG, Hamm RJ, Ellis EF. The effect of acute cocaine or lidocaine on behavioral function following fluid percussion brain injury in rats. *J Neurotrauma.* 1995;12(1):87–97.

41. Long DA, Ghosh K, Moore AN, Dixon CE, Dash PK. Deferoxamine improves spatial memory performance following experimental brain injury in rats. *Brain Res.* 1996;717(1–2):109–117.

42. Heegaard W, Biros M, Zink J. Effect of hypothermia, dichloroacetate, and deferoxamine in the treatment for cortical edema and functional recovery after experimental cortical impact in the rat. *Acad Emerg Med.* 1997;4(1):33–39.

43. Hamm RJ, Temple MD, Pike BR, Ellis EF. The effect of postinjury administration of polyethylene glycol-conjugated superoxide dismutase (pegorgotein, Dismutec) or lidocaine on behavioral function following fluid-percussion brain injury in rats. *J Neurotrauma.* 1996;13(6):325–332.

44. Mori T, Kawamata T, Katayama Y, et al. Antioxidant, OPC-14117, attenuates edema formation, and subsequent tissue damage following cortical contusion in rats. *Acta Neurochir Suppl.* 1998;71:120–122.

45. Kawamata T, Katayama Y, Maeda T, et al. Antioxidant, OPC-14117, attenuates edema formation and behavioral deficits following cortical contusion in rats. *Acta Neurochir Suppl.* 1997;70:191–193.

46. Aoyama N, Katayama Y, Kawamata T, et al. Effects of antioxidant, OPC-14117, on secondary cellular damage and behavioral deficits following cortical contusion in the rat. *Brain Res.* 2002;934(2):117–24.

47. Wada K, Alonso OF, Busto R, et al. Early treatment with a novel inhibitor of lipid peroxidation (LY341122) improves histopathological outcome after moderate fluid percussion brain injury in rats. *Neurosurgery.* 1999;45(3):601–608.

48. Hall ED, Kupina NC, Althaus JS. Peroxynitrite scavengers for the acute treatment of traumatic brain injury. *Ann N Y Acad Sci.* 1999;890:462–468.

49. Sarrafzadeh AS, Thomale UW, Kroppenstedt SN, Unterberg AW. Neuroprotective effect of melatonin on cortical impact injury in the rat. *Acta Neurochir (Wien).* 2000;142(11):1293–1299.

50. Itoh T, Satou T, Nishida S, et al. Edaravone protects against apoptotic neuronal cell death and improves cerebral function after traumatic brain injury in rats. *Neurochem Res.* 2010;35(2):348–355.

51. Clausen F, Marklund N, Lewén A, Hillered L. The nitrone free radical scavenger NXY-059 is neuroprotective when administered after traumatic brain injury in the rat. *J Neurotrauma.* 2008;25(12):1449–1457.

52. Deng-Bryant Y, Singh IN, Carrico KM, Hall ED. Neuroprotective effects of tempol, a catalytic scavenger of peroxynitrite-derived free radicals, in a mouse traumatic brain injury model. *J Cereb Blood Flow Metab.* 2008;28(6):1114–1126.

53. Kline AE, Massucci JL, Marion DW, Dixon CE. Attenuation of working memory and spatial acquisition deficits after a delayed and chronic bromocriptine treatment regimen in rats subjected to traumatic brain injury by controlled cortical impact. *J Neurotrauma.* 2002;19(4):415–425.

54. Sinson G, Voddi M, McIntosh TK. Nerve growth factor administration attenuates cognitive but not neurobehavioral motor dysfunction of hippocampal cell loss following fluid-percussion brain injury in rats. *J Neurochem.* 1995;65(5):2209–2216.

55. Sinson G, Perri BR, Trojanowski JQ, Flamm ES, McIntosh TK. Improvement of cognitive deficits and decreased cholinergic neuronal cell loss and apoptotic cell death following neurotrophin infusion

after experimental traumatic brain injury. *J Neurosurg.* 1997;86(3):511–518.

56. Dixon CE, Flinn P, Bao J, Venya R, Hayes RL. Nerve growth factor attenuates cholinergic deficits following traumatic brain injury in rats. *Exp Neurol.* 1997;146(2):479–490.

57. Zou LL, Huang L, Hayes RL, et al. Liposome-mediated NGF gene transfection following neuronal injury: potential therapeutic applications. *Gene Ther.* 1999;6(6):994–1005.

58. Frank E, Ragel B. Cortical basic fibroblast factor expression after head injury: preliminary results. *Neurol Res.* 1995;17(2):129–131.

59. Dietrich WD, Alonso O, Busto R, Finklestein SP. Posttreatment with intravenous basic fibroblast growth factor reduces histopathological damage following fluid-percussion brain injury in rat. *J Neurotrauma.* 1996;13(6):309–316.

60. McDermott KL, Raghupathi R, Fernandez SC, et al. Delayed administration of basic fibroblast growth factor (bFGF) attenuates cognitive dysfunction following parasagittal fluid percussion brain injury in the rat. *J Neurotrauma.* 1997;14(4):191–200.

61. Guluma KZ, Saatman KE, Brown A, Raghupathi R, McIntosh TK. Sequential pharmacotherapy with magnesium chloride and basic fibroblast growth factor after fluid percussion brain injury results in less neuromotor efficacy than that achieved with magnesium alone. *J Neurotrauma.* 1999;16(4):311–321.

62. Yan HQ, Yu J, Kline AE, et al. Evaluation of combined fibroblast growth factor-2 and moderate hypothermia therapy in traumatically brain injured rats. *Brain Res.* 2000;887(1):134–143.

63. Yoshimura S, Teramoto T, Whalen MJ, et al. FGF-2 regulates neurogenesis and degeneration in the dentate gyrus after traumatic brain injury in mice. *J Clin Invest.* 2003;112(8):1202–1210.

64. Sun D, Bullock MR, McGinn MJ, et al. Basic fibroblast growth factor-enhanced neurogenesis contributes to cognitive recovery in rats following traumatic brain injury. *Exp Neurol.* 2009;216(1):56–65.

65. Sandberg Nordqvist AC, von Holst H, Holmin S, Sara VR, Bellander BM, Schalling M. Increase of insulin-like growth factor (IGF)-1, IGF binding protein-2 and -4 mRNAs following cerebral contusion. *Brain Res Mol Brain Res.* 1996;38(2):285–293.

66. Nordqvist AC, Holmin S, Nilsson M, Mathiesen T, Schalling M. MK-801 inhibits the cortical increase in IGF-1, IGFBP-2 and IGFBP-4 expression following trauma. *Neuroreport.* 1997;8(2):455–460.

67. Saatman KE, Contreras PC, Smith DH, et al. Insulin-like growth factor-1 (IGF-1) improves both neurological motor and cognitive outcome following experimental brain injury. *Exp Neurol.* 1997;147(2):418–427.

68. Kazanis I, Bozas E, Philippidis H, Stylianopoulou F. Neuroprotective effects of insulin-like factor-I (IGF-I) following a penetrating brain injury in rats. *Brain Res.* 2003;991(1–2):34–45.

69. Sun D, Bullock MR, Altememi N, et al. The effect of epidermal growth factor in the injured brain after trauma in rats. *J Neurotrauma.* 2010;27(5):923–938.

70. Kleindienst A, McGinn MJ, Harvey HB, Colello RJ, Hamm RJ, Bullock MR. Enhanced hippocampal neurogenesis by intraventricular S100B infusion is associated with improved cognitive recovery after traumatic brain injury. *J Neurotrauma.* 2005;22(6):645–655.

71. Thau-Zuchman O, Shohami E, Alexandrovich AG, Leker RR. Vascular endothelial growth factor increases neurogenesis after traumatic brain injury. *J Cereb Blood Flow Metab.* 2010;30(5):1008–1016.

72. Cherian L, Goodman JC, Robertson C. Neuroprotection with erythropoietin administration following controlled cortical impact injury in rats. *J Pharmacol Exp Ther.* 2007;322(2):789–794.

73. Ning R, Xiong Y, Mahmood A, et al. Erythropoietin promotes neurovascular remodeling and long-term functional recovery in rats following traumatic brain injury. *Brain Res.* 2011;1384:140–150.

74. Yatsiv I, Grigoriadis N, Simeonidou C, et al. Erythropoietin is neuroprotective, improves functional recovery, and reduces neuronal apoptosis and inflammation in a rodent model of experimental closed head injury. *FASEB J.* 2005;19(12):1701–1703.

75. Lu D, Mahmood A, Qu C, Goussev A, Schallert T, Chopp M. Erythropoietin enhances neurogenesis and restores spatial memory in rats after traumatic brain injury. *J Neurotrauma.* 2005;22(9):1011–1017.

76. Cherian L, Goodman JC, Robertson C. Improved cerebrovascular function and reduced histological damage with darbepoetin alfa

administration after cortical impact injury in rats. *J Pharmacol Exp Ther*. 2011;337(2):451–456.

77. Bramlett HM, Green EJ, Dietrich WD, Busto R, Globus MY, Ginsberg MD. Posttraumatic brain hypothermia provides protection from sensorimotor and cognitive behavioral deficits. *J Neurotrauma*. 1995;12(3):289–298.

78. Clifton GL, Jiang JY, Lyeth BG, Jenkins LW, Hamm RJ, Hayes RL. Marked protection by moderate hypothermia after experimental traumatic brain injury. *J Cereb Blood Flow Metab*. 1991;11(1):114–121.

79. Dixon CE, Markgraf CG, Angileri F, et al. Protective effects of moderate hypothermia on behavioral deficits but not necrotic cavitation following cortical impact injury in the rat. *J Neurotrauma*. 1998;15(2):95–103.

80. Lyeth BG, Jiang JY, Liu S. Behavioral protection by moderate hypothermia initiated after experimental traumatic brain injury. *J Neurotrauma*. 1993;10(1):57–64.

81. Markgraf CG, Clifton GL, Aguirre M, et al. Injury severity and sensitivity to treatment after controlled cortical impact in rats. *J Neurotrauma*. 2001;18(2):175–186.

82. Dietrich WD, Alonso O, Busto R, Globus MY, Ginsberg MD. Posttraumatic brain hypothermia reduces histopathological damage following concussive brain injury in the rat. *Acta Neuropathol*. 1994; 87(3):250–258.

83. Palmer AM, Marion DW, Botscheller ML, Redd EE. Therapeutic hypothermia is cytoprotective without attenuating the traumatic brain injury-induced elevations in interstitial concentrations of aspartate and glutamate. *J Neurotrauma*. 1993;10(4):363–372.

84. Bramlett HM, Dietrich WD, Green EJ, Busto R. Chronic histopathological consequences of fluid-percussion brain injury in rats: effects of post-traumatic hypothermia. *Acta Neuropathol*. 1997; 93(2):190–199.

85. Robertson CL, Clark RS, Dixon CE, et al. No long-term benefit from hypothermia after severe traumatic brain injury with secondary insult in rats. *Crit Care Med*. 2000;28(9):3218–3223.

86. Statler KD, Alexander HL, Vagni VA, et al. Moderate hypothermia may be detrimental after traumatic brain injury in fentanyl-anesthetized rats. *Crit Care Med*. 2003;31(4):1134–1139.

87. Kuo JR, Lo CJ, Chang CP, Lin HJ, Lin MT, Chio CC. Brain cooling-stimulated angiogenesis and neurogenesis attenuated traumatic brain injury in rats. *J Trauma*. 2010;69(6):1467–1472.

88. Lo EH, Wang X, Cuzner ML. Extracellular proteolysis in brain injury and inflammation: role for plasminogen activators and matrix metalloproteinases. *J Neurosci Res*. 2002;69(1):1–9.

89. Saatman KE, Murai H, Bartus RT, et al. Calpain inhibitor AK295 attenuates motor and cognitive deficits following experimental brain injury in the rat. *Proc Natl Acad Sci U S A*. 1996;93(8):3428–3433.

90. Saatman KE, Zhang C, Bartus RT, McIntosh TK. Behavioral efficacy of posttraumatic calpain inhibition is not accompanied by reduced spectrin proteolysis, cortical lesion, or apoptosis. *J Cereb Blood Flow Metab*. 2000;20(1):66–73.

91. Posmantur R, Kampfl A, Siman R, et al. A calpain inhibitor attenuates cortical cytoskeletal protein loss after experimental traumatic brain injury in the rat. *Neuroscience*. 1997;77(3):875–888.

92. Kupina NC, Nath R, Bernath EE, et al. The novel calpain inhibitor SJA6017 improves functional outcome after delayed administration in a mouse model of diffuse brain injury. *J Neurotrauma*. 2001; 18(11):1229–1240.

93. Kupina NC, Detloff MR, Dutta S, Hall ED. Neuroimmunophilin ligand V-10,367 is neuroprotective after 24-hour delayed administration in a mouse model of diffuse traumatic brain injury. *J Cereb Blood Flow Metab*. 2002;22(10):1212–1221.

94. Buki A, Farkas O, Doczi T, Povlishock JT. Preinjury administration of the calpain inhibitor MDL-28170 attenuates traumatically induced axonal injury. *J Neurotrauma*. 2003;20(3):261–268.

95. Saatman KE, Creed J, Raghupathi R. Calpain as a therapeutic target in traumatic brain injury. *Neurotherapeutics*. 2010;7(1):31–42.

96. Grady MS, Cody RF Jr, Maris DO, et al. P-selectin blockade following fluid-percussion injury: behavioral and immunochemical sequelae. *J Neurotrauma*. 1999;16(1):13–25.

97. Knoblach SM, Faden AI. Administration of either anti-intercellular adhesion molecule-1 or a nonspecific control antibody improves

recovery after traumatic brain injury in the rat. *J Neurotrauma*. 2002; 19(9):1039–1050.

98. Sanderson KL, Raghupathi R, Saatman KE, Martin D, Miller G, McIntosh TK. Interleukin-1 receptor antagonist attenuates regional neuronal cell death and cognitive dysfunction after experimental brain injury. *J Cereb Blood Flow Metab*. 1999;19(10):1118–1125.

99. Knoblach SM, Faden AI. Cortical interleukin-1 beta elevation after traumatic brain injury in the rat: no effect of two selective antagonists on motor recovery. *Neurosci Lett*. 2000;289(1):5–8.

100. Zhu ZF, Wang QG, Han BJ, William CP. Neuroprotective effect and cognitive outcome of chronic lithium on traumatic brain injury in mice. *Brain Res Bull*. 2010;83(5):272–277.

101. Weaver KD, Branch CA, Hernandez L, Miller CH, Quattrocchi KB. Effect of leukocyte-endothelial adhesion antagonism on neutrophil migration and neurologic outcome after cortical trauma. *J Trauma*. 2000;48(6):1081–1090.

102. Sinz EH, Kochanek PM, Dixon CE, et al. Inducible nitric oxide synthase is an endogenous neuroprotectant after traumatic brain injury in rats and mice. *J Clin Invest*. 1999;104(5):647–656.

103. Lu J, Moochhala S, Shirhan M, et al. Neuroprotection by aminoguanidine after lateral fluid-percussive brain injury in rats: a combined magnetic resonance imaging, histopathologic and functional study. *Neuropharmacology*. 2003;44(2):253–263.

104. Jafarian-Tehrani M, Louin G, Royo NC, et al. 1400W, a potent selective inducible NOS inhibitor, improves histopathological outcome following traumatic brain injury in rats. *Nitric Oxide*. 2005;12(2):61–69.

105. Knoblach SM, Faden AI. Interleukin-10 improves outcome and alters proinflammatory cytokine expression after experimental traumatic brain injury. *Exp Neurol*. 1998;153(1):143–151.

106. Kline AE, Bolinger BD, Kochanek PM, et al. Acute systemic administration of interleukin-10 suppresses the beneficial effects of moderate hypothermia following traumatic brain injury in rats. *Brain Res*. 2002;937(1–2):22–31.

107. Dash PK, Mach SA, Moore AN. Regional expression and role of cyclooxygenase-2 following experimental traumatic brain injury. *J Neurotrauma*. 2000;17(1):69–81.

108. Schwab JM, Seid K, Schluesener HJ. Traumatic brain injury induces prolonged accumulation of cyclooxygenase-1 expressing microglia/brain macrophages in rats. *J Neurotrauma*. 2001;18(9):881–890.

109. Cernak I, O'Connor C, Vink R. Inhibition of cyclooxygenase 2 by nimesulide improves cognitive outcome more than motor outcome following diffuse traumatic brain injury in rats. *Exp Brain Res*. 2002; 147(2):193–199.

110. Kunz T, Marklund N, Hillered L, Oliw EH. Cyclooxygenase-2, prostaglandin synthases, and prostaglandin H2 metabolism in traumatic brain injury in the rat. *J Neurotrauma*. 2002;19(9):1051–1064.

111. Gopez JJ, Yue H, Vasudevan R, et al. Cyclooxygenase-2-specific inhibitor improves functional outcomes, provides neuroprotection, and reduces inflammation in a rat model of traumatic brain injury. *Neurosurgery*. 2005;56(3):590–604.

112. Domercq M, Matute C. Neuroprotection by tetracyclines. *Trends Pharmacol Sci*. 2004;25(12):609–612.

113. Kim HS, Suh YH. Minocycline and neurodegenerative diseases. *Behav Brain Res*. 2009;196(2):168–179.

114. Homsi S, Piaggio T, Croci N, et al. Blockade of acute microglial activation by minocycline promotes neuroprotection and reduces locomotor hyperactivity after closed head injury in mice: a twelve-week follow-up study. *J Neurotrauma*. 2010;27(5):911–921.

115. Chio CC, Lin JW, Chang MW, et al. Therapeutic evaluation of etanercept in a model of traumatic brain injury. *J Neurochem*. 2010; 115(4):921–929.

116. Yamakami I, Vink R, Faden AI, Gennarelli TA, Lenkinski R, McIntosh TK. Effects of acute ethanol intoxication on experimental brain injury in the rat: neurobehavioral and phosphorus-31 nuclear magnetic resonance spectroscopy studies. *J Neurosurg*. 1995;82(5):813–821.

117. Shapira Y, Lam AM, Paez A, Artru AA, Laohaprasit V, Donato T. The influence of acute and chronic alcohol treatment on brain edema, cerebral infarct volume, and neurological outcome follow-

ing experimental head trauma in rats. *J Neurosurg Anesthesiol*. 1997; 9(2):118–127.

118. Janis LS, Hoane MR, Conde D, Fulop Z, Stein DG. Acute ethanol administration reduces the cognitive deficits associated with traumatic brain injury in rats. *J Neurotrauma*. 1998;15(2):105–115.

119. Kelly DF, Kozlowski DA, Haddad E, Echiverri A, Hovda DA, Lee SM. Ethanol reduces metabolic uncoupling following experimental head injury. *J Neurotrauma*. 2000;17(4):261–272.

120. Biros MH, Kukielka D, Sutton RL, Rockswold GL, Bergman TA. The effects of acute and chronic alcohol ingestion on outcome following multiple episodes of mild traumatic brain injury in rats. *Acad Emerg Med*. 1999;6(11):1088–1097.

121. Gottesfeld Z, Moore AN, Dash PK. Acute ethanol intake attenuates inflammatory cytokines after brain injury in rats: a possible role for corticosterone. *J Neurotrauma*. 2002;19(3):317–326.

122. Dash PK, Moore AN, Moody MR, Treadwell R, Felix JL, Clifton GL. Post-trauma administration of caffeine plus ethanol reduces contusion volume and improves working memory in rats. *J Neurotrauma*. 2004;21(11):1573–1583.

123. Baratz R, Rubovitch V, Frenk H, Pick CG. The influence of alcohol on behavioral recovery after mTBI in mice. *J Neurotrauma*. 2010; 27(3):555–563.

124. Katada R, Nishitani Y, Honmou O, Okazaki S, Houkin K, Matsumoto H. Prior ethanol injection promotes brain edema after traumatic brain injury. *J Neurotrauma*. 2009;26(11):2015–2025.

125. Roof RL, Duvdevani R, Braswell L, Stein DG. Progesterone facilitates cognitive recovery and reduces secondary neuronal loss caused by cortical contusion injury in male rats. *Exp Neurol*. 1994; 129(1):64–69.

126. Galani R, Hoffman SW, Stein DG. Effects of the duration of progesterone treatment on the resolution of cerebral edema induced by cortical contusions in rats. *Restor Neurol Neurosci*. 2001;18(4): 161–166.

127. Shear DA, Galani R, Hoffman SW, Stein DG. Progesterone protects against necrotic damage and behavioral abnormalities caused by traumatic brain injury. *Exp Neurol*. 2002;178(1):59–67.

128. Roof RL, Hoffman SW, Stein DG. Progesterone protects against lipid peroxidation following traumatic brain injury in rats. *Mol Chem Neuropathol*. 1997;31(1):1–11.

129. Djebaili M, Hoffman SW, Stein DG. Allopregnanolone and progesterone decrease cell death and cognitive deficits after a contusion of the rat pre-frontal cortex. *Neuroscience*. 2004;123(2):349–359.

130. Emerson CS, Headrick JP, Vink R. Estrogen improves biochemical and neurologic outcome following traumatic brain injury in male rats, but not in females. *Brain Res*. 1993;608(1):95–100.

131. Cutler SM, Cekic M, Miller DM, Wali B, VanLandingham JW, Stein DG. Progesterone improves acute recovery after traumatic brain injury in the aged rat. *J Neurotrauma*. 2007;24(9):1475–1486.

132. Roof RL, Hall ED. Estrogen-related gender difference in survival rate and cortical blood flow after impact-acceleration head injury in rats. *J Neurotrauma*. 2000;17(12):1155–1169.

133. Soustiel JF, Palzur E, Nevo O, Thaler I, Vlodavsky E. Neuroprotective anti-apoptosis effect of estrogens in traumatic brain injury. *J Neurotrauma*. 2005;22(3):345–352.

134. Wagner AK, Willard LA, Kline AE, et al. Evaluation of estrous cycle stage and gender on behavioral outcome after experimental traumatic brain injury. *Brain Res*. 2004;998(1):113–121.

135. Bramlett HM, Dietrich WD. Neuropathological protection after traumatic brain injury in intact female rats versus males or ovariectomized females. *J Neurotrauma*. 2001;18(9):891–900.

136. Hoffman SW, Virmani S, Simkins RM, Stein DG. The delayed administration of dehydroepiandrosterone sulfate improves recovery of function after traumatic brain injury in rats. *J Neurotrauma*. 2003; 20(9):859–870.

137. Milman A, Zohar O, Maayan R, Weizman R, Pick CG. DHEAS repeated treatment improves cognitive and behavioral deficits after mild traumatic brain injury. *Eur Neuropsychopharmacol*. 2008; 18(3):181–187.

138. Malik AS, Narayan RK, Wendling WW, et al. A novel dehydroepiandrosterone analog improves functional recovery in a rat traumatic brain injury model. *J Neurotrauma*. 2003;20(5):463–476.

139. Okonkwo DO, Büki A, Siman R, Povlishock JT. Cyclosporin A limits calcium-induced axonal damage following traumatic brain injury. *Neuroreport*. 1999;10(2):353–358.

140. Scheff SW, Sullivan PG. Cyclosporin A significantly ameliorates cortical damage following experimental traumatic brain injury in rodents. *J Neurotrauma*. 1999;16(9):783–792.

141. Sullivan PG, Rabchevsky AG, Hicks RR, Gibson TR, Fletcher-Turner A, Scheff SW. Dose-response curve and optimal dosing regimen of cyclosporin A after traumatic brain injury in rats. *Neuroscience*. 2000;101(2):289–295.

142. Alessandri B, Rice AC, Levasseur J, DeFord M, Hamm RJ, Bullock MR. Cyclosporin A improves brain tissue oxygen consumption and learning/memory performance after lateral fluid percussion injury in rats. *J Neurotrauma*. 2002;19(7):829–841.

143. Büki A, Okonkwo DO, Povlishock JT. Postinjury cyclosporin A administration limits axonal damage and disconnection in traumatic brain injury. *J Neurotrauma*. 1999;16(6):511–521.

144. Verweij BH, Muizelaar JP, Vinas FC, Peterson PL, Xiong Y, Lee CP. Improvement in mitochondrial dysfunction as a new surrogate efficiency measure for preclinical trials: dose-response and time-window profiles for administration of the calcium channel blocker Ziconotide in experimental brain injury. *J Neurosurg*. 2000;93(5): 829–834.

145. Mbye LH, Singh IN, Carrico KM, Saatman KE, Hall ED. Comparative neuroprotective effects of cyclosporin A and NIM811, a nonimmunosuppressive cyclosporin A analog, following traumatic brain injury. *J Cereb Blood Flow Metab*. 2009;29(1):87–97.

146. Sullivan PG, Sebastian AH, Hall ED. Therapeutic window analysis of the neuroprotective effects of cyclosporine A after traumatic brain injury. *J Neurotrauma*. 2011;28(2):311–318.

147. Lulic D, Burns J, Bae EC, van Loveren H, Borlongan CV. A review of laboratory and clinical data supporting the safety and efficacy of cyclosporin A in traumatic brain injury. *Neurosurgery*. 2011;68(5): 1172–1185.

148. Feeney DM, Gonzalez A, Law WA. Amphetamine, haloperidol, and experience interact to affect rate of recovery after motor cortex injury. *Science*. 1982;217(4562):855–857.

149. Goldstein LB, Davis JN. Clonidine impairs recovery of beam-walking after a sensorimotor cortex lesion in the rat. *Brain Res*. 1990;508(2):305–309.

150. Feeney DM. Pharmacologic modulation of recovery after brain injury: a reconsideration of diaschisis. *J Neuro Rehab*. 1991;5(1): 113–128.

151. Feeney DM, Weisend MP, Kline AE. Noradrenergic pharmacotherapy, intracerebral infusion and adrenal transplantation promote functional recovery after cortical damage. *J Neural Transplant Plast*. 1993;4(3):199–213.

152. Kline AE, Chen MJ, Tso-Olivas DY, Feeney DM. Methylphenidate treatment following ablation-induced hemiplegia in rat: experience during drug action alters effects on recovery of function. *Pharmacol Biochem Behav*. 1994;48(3):773–779.

153. Kline AE, Yan HQ, Bao J, Marion DW, Dixon CE. Chronic methylphenidate treatment enhances water maze performance following traumatic brain injury in rats. *Neurosci Lett*. 2000;280(3):163–166.

154. Hovda DA, Sutton RL, Feeney DM. Amphetamine-induced recovery of visual cliff performance after bilateral visual cortex ablation in cats: measurements of depth perception thresholds. *Behav Neurosci*. 1989;103(3):574–584.

155. Sutton RL, Feeney DM. α-Noradrenergic agonists and antagonists affect recovery and maintenance of beam-walking ability after sensorimotor cortex ablation in the rat. *Restor Neurol Neurosci*. 1992; 4(1):1–11.

156. Dixon CE, Kraus MF, Kline AE, et al. Amantadine improves water maze performance without affecting motor behavior following traumatic brain injury in rats. *Restor Neurol Neurosci*. 1999;14(4): 285–294.

157. Gerlak RP, Clark R, Stump JM, Vernier VG. Amantadine-dopamine interaction: possible mode of action in Parkinsonism. *Science*. 1970; 169(3941):203–204.

158. Von Voigtlander PF, Moore KE. Dopamine: release from the brain in vivo by amantadine. *Science*. 1971;174(4007):408–410.

159. Bak IJ, Hassler R, Kim JS, Kataoka K. Amantadine actions on acetyl-choline and GABA in striatum and substantia nigra of rat in relation to behavioral changes. *J Neural Transm.* 1972;33(1):45–61.

160. Gianutsos G, Chute S, Dunn JP. Pharmacological changes in dopaminergic systems induced by long-term administration of amantadine. *Eur J Pharmacol.* 1985;110(3):357–361.

161. Allen RM. Role of amantadine in the management of neuroleptic-induced extrapyramidal syndromes: overview and pharmacology. *Clin Neuropharmacol.* 1983;6(suppl 1):S64–S73.

162. Gualtieri T, Chandler M, Coons TB, Brown LT. Amantadine: a new clinical profile for traumatic brain injury. *Clin Neuropharmacol.* 1989;12(4):258–270.

163. Brannan T, Martínez-Tica J, DiRocco A, Yahr MD. Low and high dose bromocriptine have differential effects on striatal dopamine release: an in vivo study. *J Neural Transm Park Dis Dement Sect.* 1993;6(2):81–87.

164. Zhu J, Hamm RJ, Reeves TM, Povlishock JT, Phillips LL. Postinjury administration of L-deprenyl improves cognitive function and enhances neuroplasticity after traumatic brain injury. *Exp Neurol.* 2000;166(1):136–152.

165. Kraus MF, Maki PM. Effect of amantadine hydrochloride on symptoms of frontal lobe dysfunction in brain injury: case studies and review. *J Neuropsychiatry Clin Neurosci.* 1997;9(2):222–230.

166. McDowell S, Whyte J, D'Esposito M. Differential effect of a dopaminergic agonist on prefrontal function in traumatic brain injury patients. *Brain.* 1998;121(pt 6):1155–1164.

167. Busto R, Dietrich WD, Globus MY, Alonso O, Ginsberg MD. Extracellular release of serotonin following fluid-percussion brain injury in rats. *J Neurotrauma.* 1997;14(1):35–42.

168. Nedergaard S, Engberg I, Flatman JA. The modulation of excitatory amino acid responses by serotonin in the cat neocortex in vitro. *Cell Mol Neurobiol.* 1987;7(4):367–379.

169. Barnes NM, Sharp T. A review of central 5-HT receptors and their function. *Neuropharmacology.* 1999;38(8):1083–1152.

170. Meneses A. 5-HT system and cognition. *Neurosci Biobehav Rev.* 1999; 23(8):1111–1125.

171. De Vry J, Dietrich H, Glaser T, et al. BAY × 3702. *Drugs of the Future.* 1997;22:341–349.

172. De Vry J, Jentzsch KR. Discriminative stimulus properties of the 5-HT1A receptor agonist BAY × 3702 in the rat. *Eur J Pharmacol.* 1998;357(1):1–8.

173. Mauler F, Fahrig T, Horváth E, Jork R. Inhibition of evoked glutamate release by the neuroprotective 5-HT(1A) receptor agonist BAY × 3702 in vitro and in vivo. *Brain Res.* 2001;888(1):150–157.

174. Prehn JH, Welsch M, Backhauss C, et al. Effects of serotonergic drugs in experimental brain ischemia: evidence for a protective role of serotonin in cerebral ischemia. *Brain Res.* 1993;630(1–2):10–20.

175. Semkova I, Wolz P, Krieglstein J. Neuroprotective effect of 5-HT1A receptor agonist, Bay X 3702, demonstrated in vitro and in vivo. *Eur J Pharmacol.* 1998;359(2–3):251–260.

176. Torup L, Møller A, Sager TN, Diemer NH. Neuroprotective effect of 8-OH-DPAT in global cerebral ischemia assessed by stereological cell counting. *Eur J Pharmacol.* 2000;395(2):137–141.

177. Kline AE, Yu J, Horváth E, Marion DW, Dixon CE. The selective 5-HT(1A) receptor agonist repinotan HCl attenuates histopathology and spatial learning deficits following traumatic brain injury in rats. *Neuroscience.* 2001;106(3):547–555.

178. Kline AE, Yu J, Massucci JL, Zafonte RD, Dixon CE. Protective effects of the 5-HT1A receptor agonist 8-hydroxy-2-(di-n-propyl-amino)tetralin against traumatic brain injury-induced cognitive deficits and neuropathology in adult male rats. *Neurosci Lett.* 2002; 333(3):179–182.

179. Kline AE, Massucci JL, Dixon CE, Zafonte RD, Bolinger BD. The therapeutic efficacy conferred by the 5-HT(1A) receptor agonist 8-Hydroxy-2-(di-n-propylamino)tetralin (8-OH-DPAT) after experimental traumatic brain injury is not mediated by concomitant hypothermia. *J Neurotrauma.* 2004;21(2):175–185.

180. Cheng JP, Aslam HA, Hoffman AN, Zafonte RD, Kline AE. The neurobehavioral benefit conferred by a single systemic administration of 8-OH-DPAT after brain trauma is confined to a narrow therapeutic window. *Neurosci Lett.* 2007;416(2):165–168.

181. Cheng JP, Hoffman AN, Zafonte RD, Kline AE. A delayed and chronic treatment regimen with the 5-HT1A receptor agonist 8-OH-DPAT after cortical impact injury facilitates motor recovery and acquisition of spatial learning. *Behav Brain Res.* 2008;194(1): 79–85.

182. Kline AE, McAloon RL, Henderson KA, et al. Evaluation of a combined therapeutic regimen of 8-OH-DPAT and environmental enrichment after experimental traumatic brain injury. *J Neurotrauma.* 2010;27(11):2021–2032.

183. Prehn JH, Backhauss C, Karkoutly C, et al. Neuroprotective properties of 5-HT1A receptor agonists in rodent models of focal and global cerebral ischemia. *Eur J Pharmacol.* 1991;203(2):213–222.

184. Andrade R. Electrophysiology of 5-HT1A receptors in the rat hippocampus and cortex. *Drug Dev Res.* 1992;26:275–286.

185. Raiteri M, Maura G, Barzizza A. Activation of presynaptic 5-hydroxytryptamine1-like receptors on glutamatergic terminals inhibits N-methyl-D-aspartate-induced cyclic GMP production in rat cerebellar slices. *J Pharmacol Exp Ther.* 1991;257(3):1184–1188.

186. Matsuyama S, Nei K, Tanaka C. Regulation of glutamate release via NMDA and 5-HT1A receptors in guinea pig dentate gyrus. *Brain Res.* 1996;728(2):175–180.

187. Melena J, Chidlow G, Osborne NN. Blockade of voltage-sensitive Na(+) channels by the 5-HT(1A) receptor agonist 8-OH-DPAT: possible significance for neuroprotection. *Eur J Pharmacol.* 2000; 406(3):319–324.

188. Gorman LK, Fu K, Hovda DA, Murray M, Traystman RJ. Effects of traumatic brain injury on the cholinergic system in the rat. *J Neurotrauma.* 1996;13(8):457–463.

189. Saija A, Hayes RL, Lyeth BG, Dixon CE, Yamamoto T, Robinson SE. Effect of concussive head injury on central cholinergic neurons. *Brain Res.* 1988;452(1–2):303–311.

190. Saija A, Robinson SE, Lyeth BG, et al. Effect of scopolamine and traumatic brain injury on central cholinergic neurons. *J Neurotrauma.* 1988;5(2):161–170.

191. Robinson SE, Foxx SD, Posner MG, et al. The effect of M1 muscarinic blockade on behavior and physiological responses following traumatic brain injury in the rat. *Brain Res.* 1990;511(1):141–148.

192. Lyeth BG, Dixon CE, Hamm RJ, et al. Effects of anticholinergic treatment on transient behavioral suppression and physiological responses following concussive brain injury to the rat. *Brain Res.* 1988;488(1):88–97.

193. Dixon CE, Liu SJ, Jenkins LW, et al. Time course of increased vulnerability of cholinergic neurotransmission following traumatic brain injury in the rat. *Behav Brain Res.* 1995;70(2):125–131.

194. Dixon CE, Bao J, Long DA, Hayes RL. Reduced evoked release of acetylcholine in the rodent hippocampus following traumatic brain injury. *Pharmacol Biochem Behav.* 1996;53(3):579–686.

195. Dixon CE, Hamm RJ, Taft WC, Hayes RL. Increased anticholinergic sensitivity following closed skull impact and controlled cortical impact traumatic brain injury in the rat. *J Neurotrauma.* 1994;11(3): 275–287.

196. Leonard JR, Maris DO, Grady MS. Fluid percussion injury causes loss of forebrain choline acetyltransferase and nerve growth factor receptor immunoreactive cells in the rat. *J Neurotrauma.* 1994;11(4): 379–392.

197. Schmidt RH, Grady MS. Loss of forebrain cholinergic neurons following fluid-percussion injury: implications for cognitive impairment in closed head injury. *J Neurosurg.* 1995;83(3):496–502.

198. Schmidt RH, Scholten KJ, Maughan PH. Cognitive impairment and synaptosomal choline uptake in rats following impact acceleration injury. *J Neurotrauma.* 2000;17(12):1129–1139.

199. Ciallella JR, Yan HQ, Ma X, et al. Chronic effects of traumatic brain injury on hippocampal vesicular acetylcholine transporter and M2 muscarinic receptor protein in rats. *Exp Neurol.* 1998;152(1):11–19.

200. Shao L, Ciallella JR, Yan HQ, et al. Differential effects of traumatic brain injury on vesicular acetylcholine transporter and M2 muscarinic receptor mRNA and protein in rat. *J Neurotrauma.* 1999;16(7): 555–566.

201. Dixon CE, Kochanek PM, Yan HQ, et al. One-year study of spatial memory performance, brain morphology and cholinergic markers after moderate controlled cortical impact in rats. *J Neurotrauma.* 1999;16(2):109–122.

202. Dixon CE, Ma X, Marion DW. Effects of CDP-choline treatment on neurobehavioral deficits after TBI and on hippocampal and neocortical acetylcholine release. *J Neurotrauma.* 1997;14(3):161–169.

203. Pike BR, Hamm RJ. Post-injury administration of BIBN 99, a selective muscarinic M2 receptor antagonist, improves cognitive performance following traumatic brain injury in rats. *Brain Res.* 1995; 686(1):37–43.

204. O'Dell DM, Hamm RJ. Chronic postinjury administration of MDL 26,479 (Suritozole), a negative modulator at the GABAA receptor, and cognitive impairment in rats following traumatic brain injury. *J Neurosurg.* 1995;83(5):878–883.

205. Taverni JP, Seliger G, Lichtman SW. Donepezil medicated memory improvement in traumatic brain injury during post acute rehabilitation. *Brain Inj.* 1998;12(1):77–80.

206. Whelan FJ, Walker MS, Schultz SK. Donepezil in the treatment of cognitive dysfunction associated with traumatic brain injury. *Ann Clin Psychiatry.* 2000;12(3):131–135.

207. Masanic CA, Bayley MT, VanReekum R, Simard M. Open-label study of donepezil in traumatic brain injury. *Arch Phys Med Rehabil.* 2001;82(7):896–901.

208. Morey CE, Cilo M, Berry J, Cusick C. The effect of Aricept in persons with persistent memory disorder following traumatic brain injury: a pilot study. *Brain Inj.* 2003;17(9):809–815.

209. Fujiki M, Kubo T, Kamida T, et al. Neuroprotective and antiamnesic effect of donepezil, a nicotinic acetylcholine-receptor activator, on rats with concussive mild traumatic brain injury. *J Clin Neurosci.* 2008;15(7):791–796.

210. Sozda CN, Hoffman AN, Olsen AS, Cheng JP, Zafonte RD, Kline AE. Empirical comparison of typical and atypical environmental enrichment paradigms on functional and histological outcome after experimental traumatic brain injury. *J Neurotrauma.* 2010; 27(6):1047–1057.

211. Hoffman AN, Malena RR, Westergom BP, et al. Environmental enrichment-mediated functional improvement after experimental traumatic brain injury is contingent on task-specific neurobehavioral experience. *Neurosci Lett.* 2008;431(3):226–230.

212. Kline AE, Wagner AK, Westergom BP, et al. Acute treatment with the 5-HT(1A) receptor agonist 8-OH-DPAT and chronic environmental enrichment confer neurobehavioral benefit after experimental brain trauma. *Behav Brain Res.* 2007;177(2):186–194.

213. Hamm RJ, Temple MD, O'Dell DM, Pike BR, Lyeth BG. Exposure to environmental complexity promotes recovery of cognitive function after traumatic brain injury. *J Neurotrauma.* 1996;13(1):41–47.

214. Hicks RR, Zhang L, Atkinson A, Stevenon M, Veneracion M, Seroogy KB. Environmental enrichment attenuates cognitive deficits, but does not alter neurotrophin gene expression in the hippocampus following lateral fluid percussion brain injury. *Neuroscience.* 2002;112(3):631–637.

215. Passineau MJ, Green EJ, Dietrich WD. Therapeutic effects of environmental enrichment on cognitive function and tissue integrity following severe traumatic brain injury in rats. *Exp Neurol.* 2001; 168(2):373–384.

216. Blackerby WF. Intensity of rehabilitation and length of stay. *Brain Inj.* 1990;4(2):167–173.

217. Shiel A, Burn JP, Henry D, et al. The effects of increased rehabilitation therapy after brain injury: results of a prospective controlled trial. *Clin Rehabil.* 2001;15(5):501–514.

218. Vanderploeg RD, Schwab K, Walker WC, et al. Rehabilitation of traumatic brain injury in active duty military personnel and veterans: defense and Veterans Brain Injury Center randomized controlled trial of two rehabilitation approaches. *Arch Phys Med Rehabil.* 2008;89(12):2227–2238.

219. Zhu XL, Poon WS, Chan CC, Chan SS. Does intensive rehabilitation improve the functional outcome of patients with traumatic brain injury (TBI)? A randomized controlled trial. *Brain Inj.* 2007;21(7): 681–690.

220. de Witt BW, Ehrenberg KM, McAloon RL, et al. Abbreviated environmental enrichment enhances neurobehavioral recovery comparably to continuous exposure after traumatic brain injury. *Neurorehabil Neural Repair.* 2011;25(4):343–350.

221. Matter AM, Folweiler KA, Curatolo LM, Kline AE. Temporal effects of environmental enrichment-mediated functional improvement after experimental traumatic brain injury in rats. *Neurorehabil Neural Repair.* 2011;25(6):558–564.

222. Kempermann G, Kuhn HG, Gage FH. More hippocampal neurons in adult mice living in an enriched environment. *Nature.* 1997; 386(6624):493–495.

223. Leggio MG, Mandolesi L, Federico F, et al. Environmental enrichment promotes improved spatial abilities and enhanced dendritic growth in the rat. *Behav Brain Res.* 2005;163(1):78–90.

224. Olson AK, Eadie BD, Ernst C, Christie BR. Environmental enrichment and voluntary exercise massively increase neurogenesis in the adult hippocampus via dissociable pathways. *Hippocampus.* 2006;16(3):250–260.

225. Torasdotter M, Metsis M, Henriksson BG, Winblad B, Mohammed AH. Environmental enrichment results in higher levels of nerve growth factor mRNA in the rat visual cortex and hippocampus. *Behav Brain Res.* 1998;93(1–2):83–90.

226. van Praag K, Kempermann G, Gage FH. Neural consequences of environmental enrichment. *Nat Rev.* 2000;1(3):191–198.

227. Dash PK, Mach SA, Moore AN. Enhanced neurogenesis in the rodent hippocampus following traumatic brain injury. *J Neurosci Res.* 2001;63(4):313–319.

228. Kernie SG, Erwin TM, Parada LF. Brain remodeling due to neuronal and astrocytic proliferation after controlled cortical injury in mice. *J Neurosci Res.* 2001;66(3):317–326.

229. Chirumamilla S, Sun D, Bullock MR, Colello RJ. Traumatic brain injury induced cell proliferation in the adult mammalian central nervous system. *J Neurotrauma.* 2002;19(6):693–703.

230. Rice AC, Khaldi A, Harvey HB, et al. Proliferation and neuronal differentiation of mitotically active cells following traumatic brain injury. *Exp Neurol.* 2003;183(2):406–417.

231. Mahmood A, Lu D, Yi L, Chen JL, Chopp M. Intracranial bone marrow transplantation after traumatic brain injury improving functional outcome in adult rats. *J Neurosurg.* 2001;94(4):589–595.

232. Lu D, Li Y, Wang L, Chen J, Mahmood A, Chopp M. Intraarterial administration of marrow stromal cells in a rat model of traumatic brain injury. *J Neurotrauma.* 2001;18(8):813–819.

233. Lu D, Mahmood A, Wang L, Li Y, Lu M, Chopp M. Adult bone marrow stromal cells administered intravenously to rats after traumatic brain injury migrate into brain and improve neurological outcome. *Neuroreport.* 2001;12(3):559–563.

234. Riess P, Zhang C, Saatman KE, et al. Transplanted neural stem cells survive, differentiate, and improve neurological motor function after experimental traumatic brain injury. *Neurosurgery.* 2002; 51(4):1043–1052.

235. Hoane MR, Becerra GD, Shank JE, et al. Transplantation of neuronal and glial precursors dramatically improves sensorimotor function but not cognitive function in the traumatically injured brain. *J Neurotrauma.* 2004;21(2):163–174.

236. Lu D, Sanberg PR, Mahmood A, et al. Intravenous administration of human umbilical cord blood reduces neurological deficit in the rat after traumatic brain injury. *Cell Transplant.* 2002;11(3):275–281.

237. McIntosh TK, Vink R, Yamakami I, Faden AI. Magnesium protects against neurological deficit after brain injury. *Brain Res.* 1989; 482(2):252–260.

238. Bareyre FM, Saatman KE, Raghupathi R, McIntosh TK. Postinjury treatment with magnesium chloride attenuates cortical damage after traumatic brain injury in rats. *J Neurotrauma.* 2000;17(11): 1029–1039.

239. Saatman KE, Bareyre FM, Grady MS, McIntosh TK. Acute cytoskeletal alterations and cell death induced by experimental brain injury are attenuated by magnesium treatment and exacerbated by magnesium deficiency. *J Neuropathol Exp Neurol.* 2001;60(2):183–194.

240. Muir JK, Raghupathi R, Emery DL, Bareyre FM, McIntosh TK. Postinjury magnesium treatment attenuates traumatic brain injury-induced cortical induction of p53 mRNA in rats. *Exp Neurol.* 1999; 159(2):584–593.

241. Browne KD, Leoni MJ, Iwata A, Chen XH, Smith DH. Acute treatment with MgSO4 attenuates long-term hippocampal tissue loss after brain trauma in the rat. *J Neurosci Res.* 2004;77(6):878–883.

242. Heath DL, Vink R. Improved motor outcome in response to magnesium therapy received up to 24 hours after traumatic diffuse axonal brain injury in rats. *J Neurosurg.* 1999;90(3):504–509.

243. Vink R, O'Connor CA, Nimmo AJ, Heath DL. Magnesium attenuates persistent functional deficits following diffuse traumatic brain injury in rats. *Neurosci Lett.* 2003;336(1):41–44.

244. Hoane MR, Irish SL, Marks BB, Barth TM. Preoperative regimens of magnesium facilitate recovery of function and prevent subcortical atrophy following lesions of the rat sensorimotor cortex. *Brain Res Bull.* 1998;45(1):45–51.

245. Barbre AB, Hoane MR. Magnesium and riboflavin combination therapy following cortical contusion injury in the rat. *Brain Res Bull.* 2006;69(6):639–646.

246. Başkaya MK, Doğan A, Rao AM, Dempsey RJ. Neuroprotective effects of citicoline on brain edema and blood-brain barrier breakdown after traumatic brain injury. *J Neurosurg.* 2000;92(3):448–452.

247. Dempsey RJ, Raghavendra Rao VL. Cytidinediphosphocholine treatment to decrease traumatic brain injury-induced hippocampal neuronal death, cortical contusion volume, and neurological dysfunction in rats. *J Neurosurg.* 2003;98(4):867–873.

248. Prins M. Diet, ketones, and neurotrauma. *Epilepsia.* 2008;49(suppl 8):111–113.

249. Prins ML, Fujima LS, Hovda DA. Age-dependent reduction of cortical contusion volume by ketones after traumatic brain injury. *J Neurosci Res.* 2005;82(3):413–420.

250. Appelberg KS, Hovda DA, Prins ML. The effects of a ketogenic diet on behavioral outcome after controlled cortical impact injury in the juvenile and adult rat. *J Neurotrauma.* 2009;26(4):497–506.

251. Sullivan PG, Geiger JD, Mattson MP, Scheff SW. Dietary supplement creatine protects against traumatic brain injury. *Ann Neurol.* 2000;48(5):723–729.

252. Hoane MR, Akstulewicz SL, Toppen J. Treatment with vitamin B3 improves functional recovery and reduces GFAP expression following traumatic brain injury in rats. *J Neurotrauma.* 2003;20(11):1189–1199.

253. Inci S, Ozcan OE, Kilinç K. Time-level relationship for lipid peroxidation and the protective effect of alpha-tocopherol in experimental mild and severe brain injury. *Neurosurgery.* 1998;43(2):330–335.

254. Aiguo Wu, Zhe Ying, Gomez-Pinilla F. Vitamin E protects against oxidative damage and learning disability after mild traumatic brain injury in rats. *Neurorehabil Neural Repair.* 2010;24(3):290–298.

255. Naim MY, Friess S, Smith C, et al. Folic acid enhances early functional recovery in a piglet model of pediatric head injury. *Dev Neurosci.* 2010;32(5–6):466–479.

256. Singleton RH, Yan HQ, Fellows-Mayle W, Dixon CE. Resveratrol attenuates behavioral impairments and reduces cortical and hippocampal loss in a rat controlled cortical impact of traumatic brain injury. *J Neurotrauma.* 2010;27(6):1091–1099.

257. Goldstein LB, Bullman S. Differential effects of haloperidol and clozapine on motor recovery after sensorimotor cortex injury in rats. *Neurorehabil Neural Repair.* 2002;16(4):321–325.

258. Kline AE, Massucci JL, Zafonte RD, Dixon CE, DeFeo JR, Rogers EH. Differential effects of single versus multiple administrations of haloperidol and risperidone on functional outcome after experimental traumatic brain trauma. *Crit Care Med.* 2007;35(3):919–924.

259. Kline AE, Hoffman AN, Cheng JP, Zafonte RD, Massucci JL. Chronic administration of antipsychotics impede behavioral recovery after experimental traumatic brain injury. *Neurosci Lett.* 2008;448(3):263–267.

260. Hoffman AN, Cheng JP, Zafonte RD, Kline AE. Administration of haloperidol and risperidone after neurobehavioral testing hinders the recovery of traumatic brain injury-induced deficits. *Life Sci.* 2008;83(17–18):602–607.

261. Wilson MS, Gibson CJ, Hamm RJ. Haloperidol, but not olanzapine, impairs cognitive performance after traumatic brain injury in rats. *Am J Phys Med Rehabil.* 2003;82(11):871–879.

262. Hovda DA, Feeney DM. Haloperidol blocks amphetamine induced recovery of binocular depth perception after bilateral visual cortex ablation in cat. *Proc West Pharmacol Soc.* 1985;28:209–211.

263. Zhao CS, Puurunen K, Schallert T, Sivenius J, Jolkkonen J. Behavioral and histological effects of chronic antipsychotic and antidepressant drug treatment in aged rats with focal ischemic brain injury. *Behav Brain Res.* 2005;158(2):211–220.

III

NEUROIMAGING AND NEURODIAGNOSTIC TESTING

15

Structural Neuroimaging

Esther L. Yuh and Alisa D. Gean

INTRODUCTION

Neuroimaging plays a decisive role in the management of craniofacial trauma. The goals are to identify treatable injuries, assist in the prevention of secondary central nervous system (CNS) damage, and provide useful prognostic information. In particular, the findings on the initial noncontrast head computed tomography (CT) have a pivotal influence on immediate decisions regarding the need for hospitalization, intensive care unit (ICU) admission, and/or early surgical management including hematoma evacuation, the potential need for decompressive hemicraniectomy, as well as external ventricular drainage catheter and intracranial pressure (ICP) monitor placement (1–4). In addition to its role in immediate management decisions, the initial noncontrast head CT is known to carry longer-term prognostic significance following acute moderate-to-severe traumatic brain injury (TBI) (5–7).

Magnetic resonance imaging (MRI) holds great promise for both improved clinical management and outcome prediction in TBI. To date, there has been exploration of the use of both conventional MRI sequences, as well as more advanced MRI techniques including diffusion tensor imaging (DTI), magnetic resonance spectroscopy (MRS), and resting-state functional MRI (fMRI) in the diagnosis and prognosis of TBI. However, in contrast to CT, no current consensus exists on the clinical use of MRI in acute TBI. Tellingly, the question of the recommended role of MRI in clinical management of acute mild TBI was the only 1 of 4 topics that the 2008 Centers for Disease Control/American College of Emergency Physicians (CDC/ACEP) guidelines originally sought to address, but for which no recommendations could be made because of a lack of sufficient evidence (8). Unlike noncontrast CT, CT angiography (CTA), and catheter angiography, MRI in head trauma is a highly active area of research that is still in its earliest stages. As our ability to noninvasively visualize neuropathology continues to progress, and our understanding of TBI pathophysiology improves, the definitions of pathoanatomic lesions and the best methods for characterizing them using both conventional and emerging advanced MRI techniques will continue to evolve. Such advances hold promise for improved clinical care.

IMAGING MODALITIES

Radiography

Since 2002, the CDC and ACEP have indicated that skull radiographs are not routinely indicated in acute closed head injury: "Skull film radiographs are not recommended in the evaluation of mild TBI. Although the presence of a skull fracture increases the likelihood of an intracranial lesion, its sensitivity is not sufficient to be a useful screening test. Indeed, negative findings on skull films may mislead the clinician" (9). This was reconfirmed in the updated 2008 guidelines (8). For penetrating TBI, skull radiographs may assist in the 3-dimensional (3D) localization of a foreign body. In these patients, however, CT is virtually always performed. The digital CT "scout view" may serve as an adequate substitute for conventional skull radiography and may demonstrate horizontally oriented calvarial fractures that are difficult to detect on the axial CT images (Figure 15-1).

Computed Tomography

CT is currently the initial imaging modality of choice for the assessment of patients with suspected acute TBI. There are numerous reasons for this, including 24-hour availability in most hospitals; high sensitivity and specificity for acute fractures because of its exquisite delineation of bony detail, allowing for assessment not only of acute calvarial and facial fractures but also concurrent evaluation of acute cervical spine fractures; high sensitivity for acute intracranial hemorrhage (particularly for space-occupying lesions that warrant immediate neurosurgical intervention); no contraindications that would either preclude or delay imaging until screening for contraindications could be performed; and the minimal imaging time required. Indeed, standard noncontrast head CT protocols using modern (64-slice) multidetector-row CT scanners can image the entire head in approximately 1 second. This is an obvious key advantage in the setting of patients with altered mental status or claustrophobia, young children, and patients with polytrauma who require life-support or traction-stabilization devices.

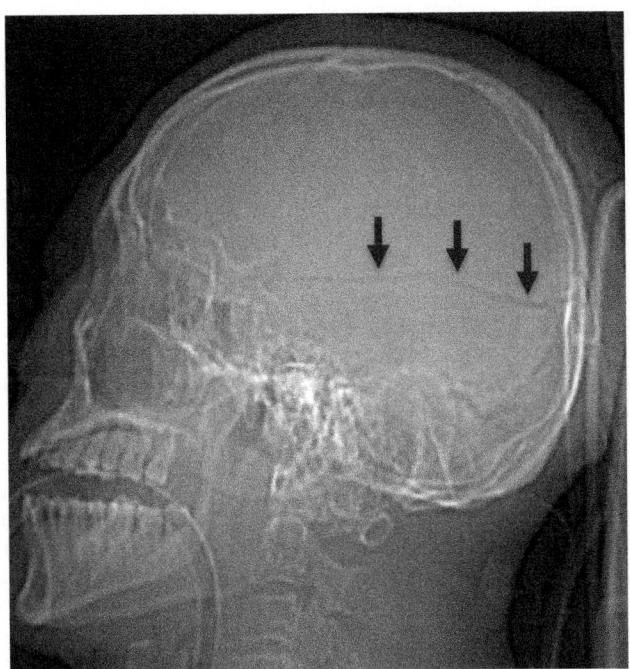

FIGURE 15–1 Horizontal skull fracture identified on the digital lateral "scout view" but missed on the axial CT images. Fractures oriented parallel to the plane of imaging acquisition can be difficult to detect without an orthogonal view. The digital scout view should always be reviewed to minimize this pitfall. It is also helpful for detecting abnormalities located outside of the CT slices (e.g., upper cervical spine and facial region).

Indications for Noncontrast Head CT in Acute Head Trauma

Currently, there is consensus that all patients with moderate-to-severe TBI (i.e., Glasgow Coma Scale [GCS] < 13) should undergo emergent imaging. The main controversy in scanning patients with TBI surrounds those with mild TBI. Each year, at least 1.7 million US civilians sustain a documented TBI, and approximately 75% of these are classified as mild TBI (10). It has been estimated that approximately 16%–21% of patients with GCS of 13–15 have acute intracranial hemor-

rhage on initial head CT (11). Borg et al. reported that 5% of patients with GCS of 15 and 30% of patients with GCS of 13 had acute intracranial hemorrhage on initial head CT (12), and only approximately 1% have intracranial findings that may require neurosurgical intervention. Many guidelines have been developed to balance clinical benefit against cost-effectiveness and radiation dose considerations. One of the most widely accepted current guidelines is the CDC/ACEP joint practice guideline (8) that includes decision rules for determining which patients with closed head injury with a GCS of 14 or 15 should undergo head CT in the emergency department (ED) (Table 15-1). These 2008 guidelines were based on an attempted synthesis of results from the best available clinical evidence at the time, including the Canadian CT Head Rule (CCHR) (13) and New Orleans Criteria (NOC) (14). Although the CDC/ACEP guidelines are accepted and widely applied by many ED physicians, there undoubtedly remains considerable variability in the practical application of these rules, partly because of the subjective nature of some of the criteria.

The noncontrast head CT protocol recommended by the Imaging Common Data Elements group established jointly by the Defense Centers of Excellence (DCOE), the National Institute of Neurological Disorders and Stroke (NINDS), the National Institute on Disability and Rehabilitation Research (NIDRR), and the Veterans Administration (VA) (15) is shown in Table 15-2. The essential features are whole-brain coverage during a series of several gantry rotations that each take place over 0.5 to 1 second, at 120–140 kVp, and 200–400 mA tube current employing the automated modern dose-modulation software now offered by all major CT vendors. Although a 1 second gantry rotation is recommended, modern CT scanners can perform a single gantry rotation in as little as 0.3 seconds, and this can be implemented for extremely agitated patients. Slice reconstruction at 2.0–3.75 mm in the axial plane using a soft-tissue algorithm is recommended for images of the brain parenchyma. An additional "bone-algorithm" series is also constructed, with slice reconstruction at 0.5–1.25 mm in axial, coronal, and sagittal planes to assess for facial and calvarial fractures. Intravenous contrast administration should not be performed without a baseline noncontrast CT exam because the contrast can both mask and mimic underlying hemorrhage. However, CTA can be performed in selected cases *after* completion of noncontrast

TABLE 15-1 Indications for Noncontrast Head CT for Closed Head Injury and Glasgow Coma Scale Score of 14 or 15

| LOSS OF CONSCIOUSNESS OR POST-TRAUMATIC AMNESIA? | |
YES	NO
Noncontrast head CT is **indicated** *for:*	*Noncontrast head CT should be* **considered** *for:*
Headache	Focal neurologic deficit
Vomiting	Vomiting
> 60 years of age	Severe headache
Drug or alcohol intoxication	> 65 years of age
Deficits in short-term memory	Physical signs of basilar skull fracture
Physical evidence of trauma above the clavicle	GCS < 15
Post-traumatic seizure	Coagulopathy
GCS < 15	Dangerous mechanism of injury (ejected from motor vehicle,
Focal neurologic deficit	pedestrian struck by motor vehicle, fall from > 3 ft or > 5 stairs)
Coagulopathy	

Abbreviations: CT, computed tomography; GCS, Glasgow Coma Scale.
Source: Jagoda et al. (8).

TABLE 15-2 Recommended Noncontrast Head CT Protocol for Acute Head Trauma

Image acquisition mode	Helical Pitch: 0.8–1:1
Gantry rotation	1 second per gantry rotation (can be decreased to 0.5 s for agitated patients)
Image acquisition parameters	120–140 kVp, 200–400 mA Dose modulation recommended to reduce dose (noise index 4–6)
Coverage and slice thickness	Whole brain coverage 2.0–3.75 mm slice thickness Slice interval = slice thickness
Slice orientation	Parallel to orbitomeatal line or hard palate

Source: Haacke et al. (15).

head CT, if significant risk factors for acute vascular injury are present, as discussed below.

Controversy remains over the necessity of repeat head CT in cases of minimal intracranial hemorrhage on the initial head CT and no neurological deterioration or new focal neurological signs. Most of the recent literature addressing this question concludes that repeat CT several hours after initial CT is unnecessary in patients with mild TBI with intracranial hemorrhage on the initial head CT and no neurological decline (16–19). Lower GCS scores and coagulopathy were the most commonly described risk factors associated with significant progression on follow-up CT leading to neurosurgical intervention (16). Nevertheless, despite the preponderance of evidence in the literature that routine scheduled follow-up CT should be performed selectively based on such factors as the (*a*) initial GCS score, (*b*) severity of initial CT findings, (*c*) serial clinical examinations, and (*d*) presence of coagulopathy, the application of these criteria in practice is highly variable, and in many institutions, follow-up CT is performed several hours after initial CT in all patients with any evidence of acute intracranial hemorrhage.

Magnetic Resonance Imaging

Because of the advantages of CT discussed earlier, MRI is virtually never the initial imaging modality performed in acute TBI. Even in children who have a greater susceptibility to radiation-induced malignancy and developmental impairment, CT remains the accepted modality of choice in acute TBI and is recommended over MRI in the current practice guidelines of the American Academy of Pediatrics (20,21). Regarding the issue of imaging time, even a fast MRI protocol for acute head trauma would require one to several minutes of image acquisition time alone, compared to 1 second or less for 16- or 64-slice CT, in which the entire brain can be imaged in a single gantry rotation that requires as little as 0.3 seconds. In addition, accessibility to unstable patients or those with other severe injuries in the smaller-bore MRI scanner is significantly limited compared to CT, and would require the use of MRI-compatible devices and equipment that may not be available.

Despite these issues, many studies have firmly established that certain conventional MRI sequences have superior *sensitivity* relative to noncontrast head CT for identification of certain acute pathoanatomic findings, including hemorrhagic traumatic axonal injury, small cortical contusions, and small extra-axial collections (22–29). Although no clear consensus exists on the current clinical role of MRI in acute TBI, it is sometimes used as a follow-up test after CT has been performed. This is particularly the case in the setting of unexplained persistent altered level of consciousness in the hospitalized patient, in suspected abusive head trauma (AHT) to assess for evidence of traumatic intracranial injuries of different ages or that were not detected on CT (Figure 15-2), and in other medicolegal settings to establish a diagnosis of TBI when CT abnormalities are absent or equivocal.

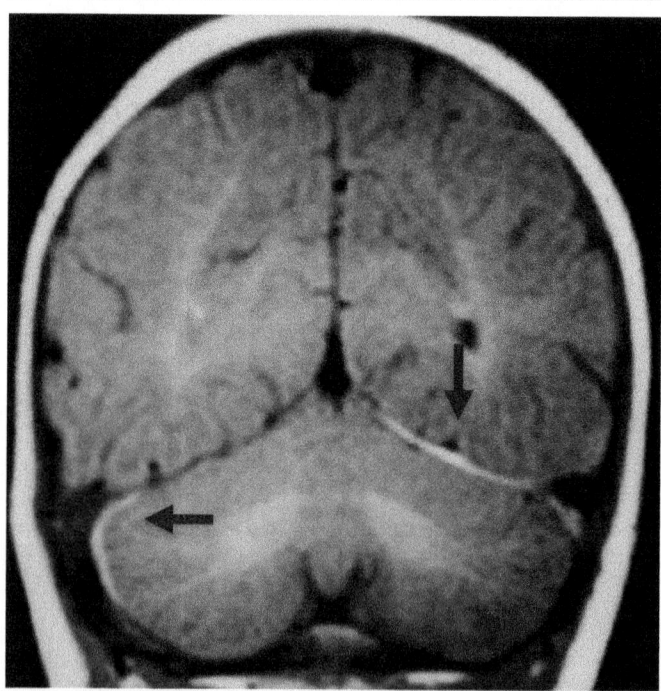

FIGURE 15–2 Abusive head trauma (AHT) identified on MRI but invisible on CT. This 2-year-old child presented with "altered mental status." Emergent noncontrast CT imaging was normal. The 4-day follow-up coronal T1-weighted MR image demonstrates subtle linear hyperintensity layering along the left tentorium and lateral to the right cerebellar hemisphere, consistent with subacute subdural hematomas (*arrows*).

Table 15-3 Brain MRI Trauma Protocol at 1.5 Tesla (Tier 1 Protocol)

SEQUENCE	2D FLAIR	GRE/ SWI	DWI	T2	3D T1	2D GRE (OPTIONAL)
Orient	Oblique axial	Oblique axial	Oblique axial	Oblique axial	Sagittal	Oblique axial
TR (ms)	9,540	50	5,400	7,000	2,000	1,110
TE (ms)	114	40	Minimum	106	3.22	26
TI (ms)	2,500					
Flip angle (degrees)	150	15	90	160	8	20
FOV (mm^2)	256 × 192	256 × 192	256 × 256	256 × 192	256 × 256	256 × 192
Matrix size	256 × 256	512 × 256	128 × 128	256 × 256	512 × 256	256 × 256
Nz/TH (mm)	32/4	64/2	32/4	32/4	120/2	32/4
Voxel size (mm)	1 × 1 × 4	0.5 × 1 × 2	2 × 2 × 4	1 × 1 × 4	0.5 × 1 × 2	1 × 1 × 4
#Acq./#DTI directions	2	1	3	1	1	1
Fat suppression	No	No	Yes	No	No	No
Phase encode direction	Right to left	Right to left	Anterior to posterior	Right to left	Anterior to posterior	Right to left
AF/CL	2/30	2/24	2/24	None	None	
BW	201	80	1,502	130	160	80
Flow Compensation	No	Yes	No	No	No	Yes
Echo train length	29		128	17		
b-value (second/mm^2)			0/1,000			
Time	2:53	5:47	2:27	2:55	8:32	3:35

Abbreviations: MRI, magnetic resonance imaging; FLAIR, fluid-attenuated inversion recovery; GRE, gradient echo; SWI, susceptibility-weighted imaging; DWI, diffusion-weighted imaging; TR, repetition time; TE, echo time; TI, inversion time; FOV, field of view; DTI, diffusion tensor imaging; AF/CL, acceleration factor and central lines for parallel imaging; BW, bandwidth.
Source: Haacke et al. (15).

In recognition of its superior *sensitivity* for focal lesions in acute TBI, protocols for MRI at 1.5 and 3.0 T consisting of conventional MRI sequences that best depict lesions in acute brain injury based on the best available current knowledge have been suggested. Examples of these are the "tiered" protocols recommended in the Imaging Common Data Elements mentioned earlier (15). The basic "Tier 1" protocol includes fluid-attenuated inversion recovery (FLAIR), gradient-echo (GRE) or susceptibility-weighted imaging (SWI), diffusion-weighted imaging (DWI), T2-weighted fast-spin-echo, and 3D T1-weighted imaging (Tables 15-3 and 15-4)

IMAGING FEATURES OF ACUTE TRAUMATIC INTRACRANIAL INJURY

Epidural Hematoma

The epidural hematoma (EDH) is located between the inner table of the skull and the outer layer of the dura mater (Figure 15-3). It classically results from a blow to the side of the head that fractures the thin squamosal temporal bone and tears a branch of the middle meningeal artery that is embedded in the inner table of the skull. The most common imaging appearance of the EDH is that of a biconvex, homogeneous, hyperdense extra-axial collection (Figure 15-4). In adults, approximately 75% of EDHs occur in the temporal region (30). A skull fracture is identified in approximately 90% of EDH cases. In pediatric patients, the EDH occurs with similar frequency in the temporal, occipital, frontal, and posterior fossa regions because the middle meningeal artery is not yet indented within the inner table and is thus less susceptible to tearing (31). A heterogeneous or "mixed-density" EDH is considered more ominous because the low density areas are believed to be caused by active extravasation

(Figure 15-5). In one recent study in pediatric patients, those with mixed-density clots presented earlier to the hospital, had poorer GCS scores at admission, exhibited larger clot volumes, had a higher incidence of active bleeding at surgery, and had increased morbidity and mortality as compared with the patients with a homogeneous EDH (32).

The EDH does not generally cross suture lines. Exceptions include the sagittal suture to which the periosteal layer of the dura is less firmly attached (Figure 15-6) (30) and in cases of sutural diastasis or skull fracture extending across a suture line (33). Thus, unlike the subdural hematoma (SDH), the EDH can cross the midline. Similarly, unlike the SDH, the EDH readily crosses the tentorium cerebelli and therefore may be seen to extend from the posterior fossa into the supratentorial space or vice versa (Figure 15-7).

Approximately 10% of EDHs are "venous" in origin, attributable to laceration of a dural venous sinus. These are most commonly the sphenoparietal sinus (Figure 15-8), transverse/sigmoid sinuses, and, less commonly, the superior sagittal sinus. Venous EDHs are considered more "benign" in nature and do not grow aggressively in the same fashion as arterial EDHs (34).

Subdural Hematoma

The SDH is located between the arachnoid and the inner layer of the dura. It usually results from tearing of cortical "bridging veins" that extend from the cortex to the dural venous sinuses but it may also result from disruption of penetrating branches of superficial cerebral arteries. On neuroimaging, the SDH most commonly appears as a crescent-shaped extra-axial collection overlying a cerebral convexity (Figures 15-9A and 15-9B). Another common manifestation is the interhemis-

TABLE 15-4 Brain MRI Trauma Protocol at 3 Tesla (Tier 1 Protocol) (15)

SEQUENCE	2D FLAIR	GRE/ SWI	DWI	3D T2	3D T1	2D GRE (OPTIONAL)
Orient	Oblique axial	Oblique axial	Oblique axial	Sagittal	Sagittal	Oblique axial
TR (ms)	9,000	30	5,000	2,500	1,950	800
TE (ms)	78	20	Minimum	359	2.26	20
TI (ms)	2500					
Flip angle (degrees)	150	15	90	Variable	8–10	15–20
FOV (mm^2)	256 × 192	256 × 192	256 × 256	256 × 256	256 × 256	256 × 192
Matrix size	256 × 256	512 × 256	128 × 128	256 × 256	256 × 256	256 × 256
Nz/TH (mm)	32/4	64/2	32/4	192/1	176/1	32/4
Voxel size (mm)	1 × 1 × 4	0.5 × 1 × 2	2 × 2 × 4	1 × 1 × 1	1 × 1 × 1	1 × 1 × 4
#Acq./#DTI directions	1	1	2	1	1	1
Fat suppression	Yes	No	Yes	No	No	No
Slice overlap	0	25%	0	0	45.5%	0
Phase encode direction	Right to left	Right to left	Anterior to posterior	Anterior to posterior	Anterior to posterior	Right to left
AF/CL	2/30	2/24	2/24	2/24	2/24	2/24
BW	250	100	1,346	751	200	180
Flow Compensation	No	Yes	No	No	No	Yes
Echo train length	15		128	141		
b-value (second/mm^2)			0/1,000			
Time	2:44	4:18	1:27	4:02	4:33	2:54

Abbreviations: MRI, magnetic resonance imaging; FLAIR, fluid-attenuated inversion recovery; GRE, gradient echo; SWI, susceptibility-weighted imaging; DWI, diffusion-weighted imaging; TR, repetition time; TE, echo time; TI, inversion time; FOV, field of view; DTI, diffusion tensor imaging; AF/CL, acceleration factor and central lines for parallel imaging; BW, bandwidth.
Source: Haacke et al. (15).

pheric SDH, which appears as a thickened "shaggy" falx cerebri (Figure 15-9C). The tentorial SDH is a third common type and is recognized as high density along the tentorium that is either bilaterally asymmetric, or symmetric bilaterally but unusually prominent (Figure 15-9D). Unlike the EDH, the SDH readily crosses suture lines but does not cross the falx cerebri or tentorium cerebelli. Also unlike the EDH, the SDH can be located at the contrecoup as well as at the coup location. In addition, there is no known consistent association between SDH and skull fracture.

Both the acute EDH and SDH most commonly appear as a uniformly hyperdense collection on CT, regardless of location. However, the SDH has several additional characteristic appearances owing to the variation in CT density of blood products over time. For example, the so-called "hyperacute" SDH that is characterized by newly extravasated blood results in heterogeneous CT density; this is analogous to the previously mentioned actively bleeding mixed-density EDH. In the case of the SDH, however, the heterogeneity may also be caused by serum extrusion during the early

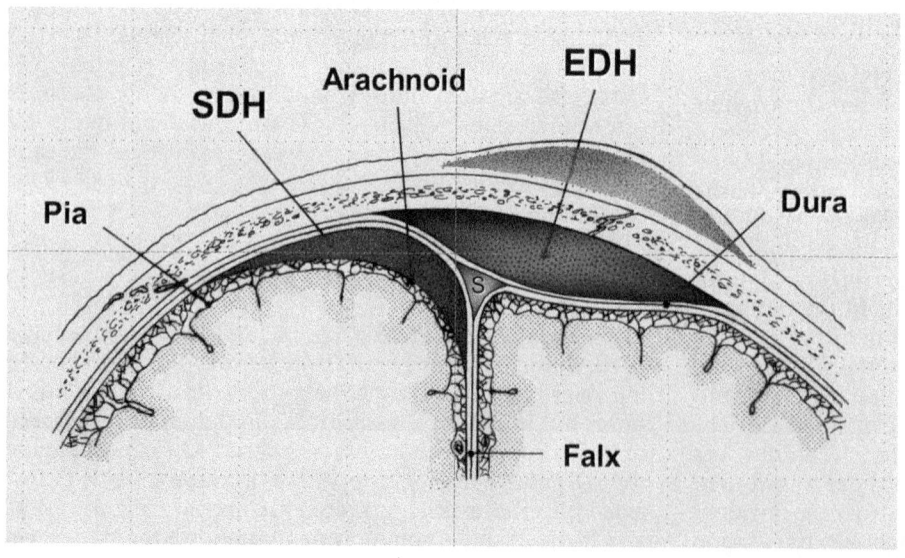

FIGURE 15–3 Diagram of the epidural hematoma (*EDH*) and the subdural hematoma (*SDH*). The EDH is located above the outer dural layer (i.e., the periosteum), and the SDH is located beneath the inner (meningeal) dural layer. The EDH does not cross sutures, with exception of the sagittal suture at the midline. The SDH does not cross the falx or the tentorium. Reprinted from Gean (30) with permission.

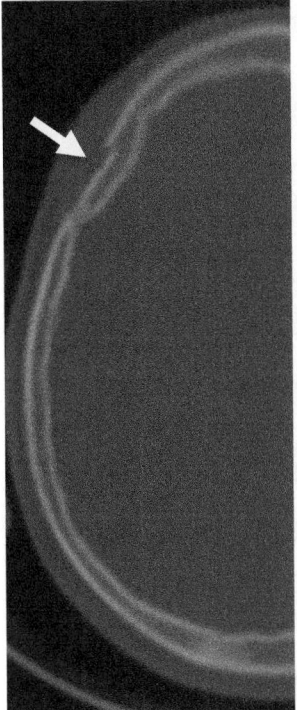
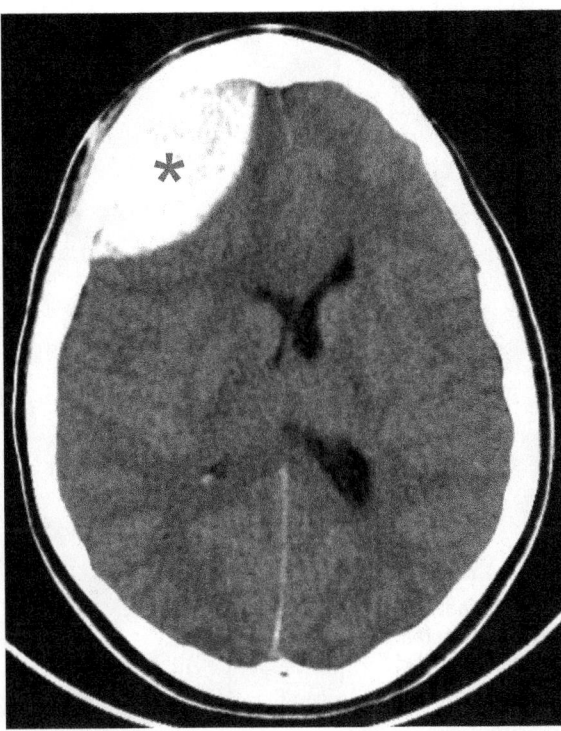

FIGURE 15–4 Acute epidural hematoma (typical). Note the well-defined biconvex homogeneous high-density extra-axial collection (*asterisk*) underlying a right frontal calvarial fracture (*arrow*). Nearly 99% of EDHs are located at the coup site, and at least 90% are associated with a skull fracture. The EDH generally does not cross suture lines; in this example, the posterior margin is limited by the right coronal suture. Also note the absence of concomitant intra-axial injury, a feature that is characteristic of the EDH in contrast to the SDH.

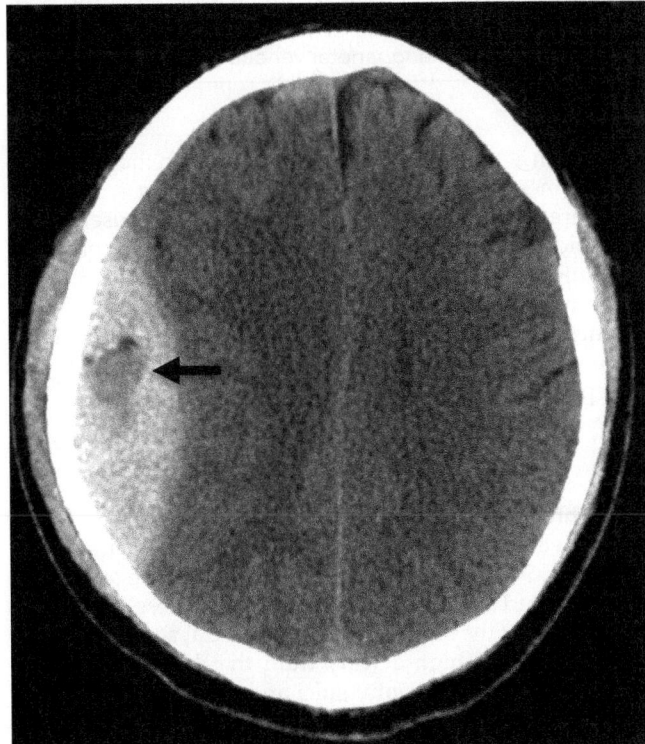

FIGURE 15–5 Acute epidural hematoma (atypical). Note the biconvex heterogeneous (i.e., mixed-density) extra-axial collection. The central area of low density likely represents a focus of active extravasation (*arrow*). Again, no underlying intra-axial injury is seen.

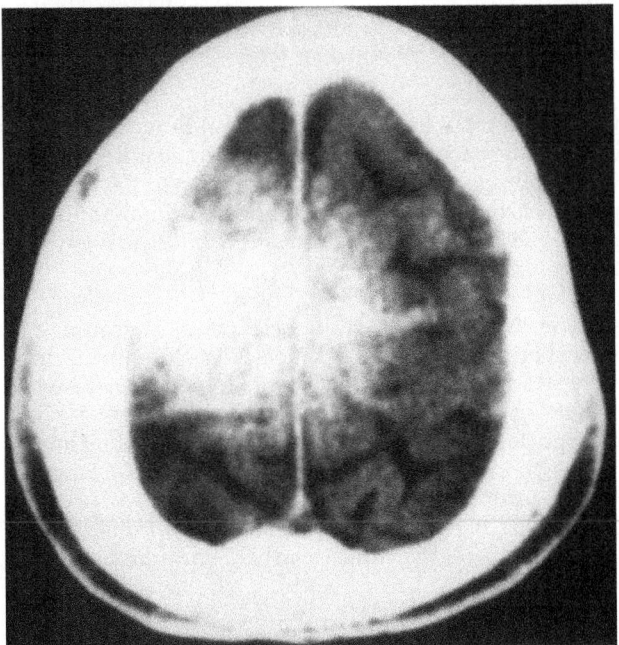

FIGURE 15–6 Acute epidural hematoma (convexity). Although the EDH usually does not cross suture lines, the high convexity EDH may cross the midline (i.e., sagittal suture) because the inner dural layer is less firmly attached to the suture in this region. Also note the more ill-defined margins of the EDH located in this region because of partial volume averaging with CSF and brain parenchyma because of the curvature of the calvarium.

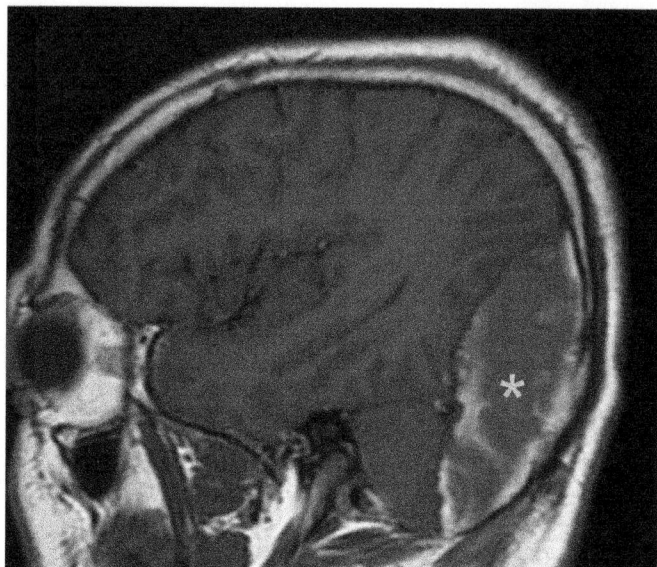

FIGURE 15–7 Subacute epidural hematoma. This 25-year-old patient presented with "rule out stroke" 1 week after a fall. The parasagittal T1-weighted image shows a large well-defined extradural lesion (*asterisk*) causing mass effect on the cerebellar hemisphere and the occipital lobes. Unlike the SDH, the EDH can directly extend from the infratentorial space to the supratentorial space. Note the peripheral areas of increased signal within the lesion that represent methemoglobin (i.e., subacute hemorrhage). The bulk of the lesion, however, is isointense to brain parenchyma and represents deoxyhemoglobin (acute hemorrhage). This EDH is most likely of venous origin.

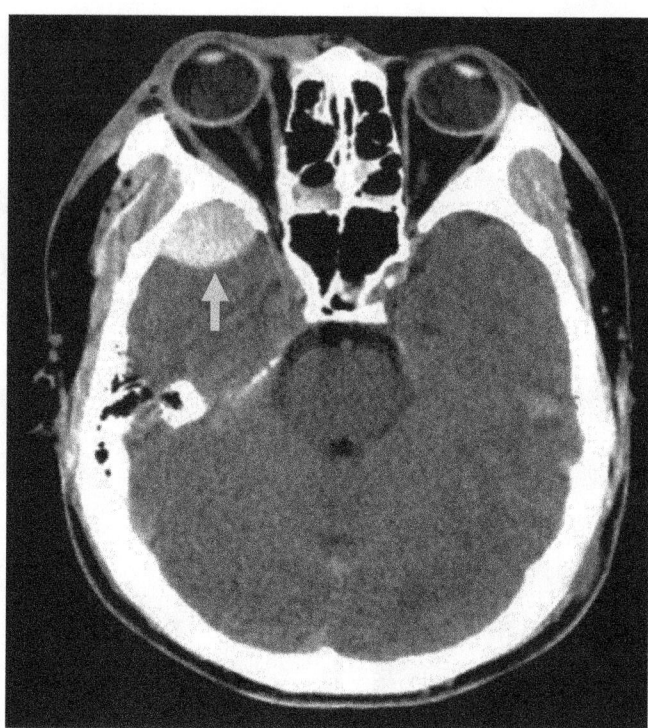

FIGURE 15–8 Acute epidural hematoma (venous). The acute venous EDH is generally attributable to laceration of a venous sinus. It is often benign in nature and rarely increases significantly in size following initial head imaging. In this example, a well-defined lentiform collection (*arrow*) is noted in the right middle cranial fossa, consistent with a venous EDH resulting from injury to the sphenoparietal venous sinus.

phase of clot retraction, or cerebrospinal fluid (CSF) within the subdural space caused by a concurrent tear in the arachnoid membrane (35). As clotting progresses, the collection typically becomes uniformly hyperdense. More than 90% of "acute" SDHs in the period from a few hours to a few days are hyperdense.

After several days, the CT density progressively decreases by an estimated 0.7 to 1.5 HU per day because of the chemical breakdown of globin molecules (36) until approximately 90% are isodense and 10% are hypodense at 3 weeks (37). During this "subacute" period between 1 and 3 weeks, approximately half of SDHs are hypodense and half are isodense to brain (Figure 15-10). As the subacute SDH evolves, it may occasionally contain a fluid–fluid level, with a dependent layering high CT-density region and a nondependent low CT-density region, rather than being uniformly isodense or hypodense.

Most chronic SDHs (> 3 weeks) are crescent-shaped, uniformly low CT-density collections with a hemosiderin-lined capillary-rich capsular membrane that enhances with contrast and demonstrates signal void on MRI sequences that have susceptibility weighting (36). However, rebleeding into a chronic SDH can result in a laminated appearance, with alternating hyperdense and hypodense layers and/or internal septations (Figure 15-11). Calcifications occur after months to years in an estimated 0.3%–2.7% of chronic SDHs (36).

In addition to the variation in appearance over time, the SDH also has variable appearances in the setting of certain systemic conditions such as anemia and coagulopathy. For

example, an acute isodense SDH can be seen in the following settings: anemia with hemoglobin concentration < 10 g/dL, admixture with CSF within the subdural space caused by an arachnoid membrane tear, and disseminated intravascular coagulation (30). Like the subacute SDH, the acute SDH in the setting of impaired coagulation can also appear as a heterogeneous collection characterized by a fluid–fluid level with a dependent layering high CT-density collection and nondependent low CT-density collection.

Subarachnoid Hemorrhage

Subarachnoid hemorrhage (SAH) results from injury to superficial vessels along the cortical surface and arachnoid membrane. SAH is therefore located between the arachnoid membrane and the pia mater, the latter being closely adherent to the surface of the brain. On noncontrast CT, acute SAH generally appears as high-density fluid that has a curvilinear morphology within cerebral sulci and cerebellar fissures or high-density fluid filling and following the outlines of the cisterns (Figure 15-12). Intraventricular hemorrhage (IVH), located within the ventricular system (usually layering dependently in the occipital horns), is observed in an estimated 1%–5% of patients with closed head injury and is attributable to retrograde reflux of SAH through the foramina of Luschka and Magendie, tearing of subependymal veins, or contiguous extension of an intraparenchymal hematoma (36). CT remains the modality of choice for detection of acute SAH and IVH

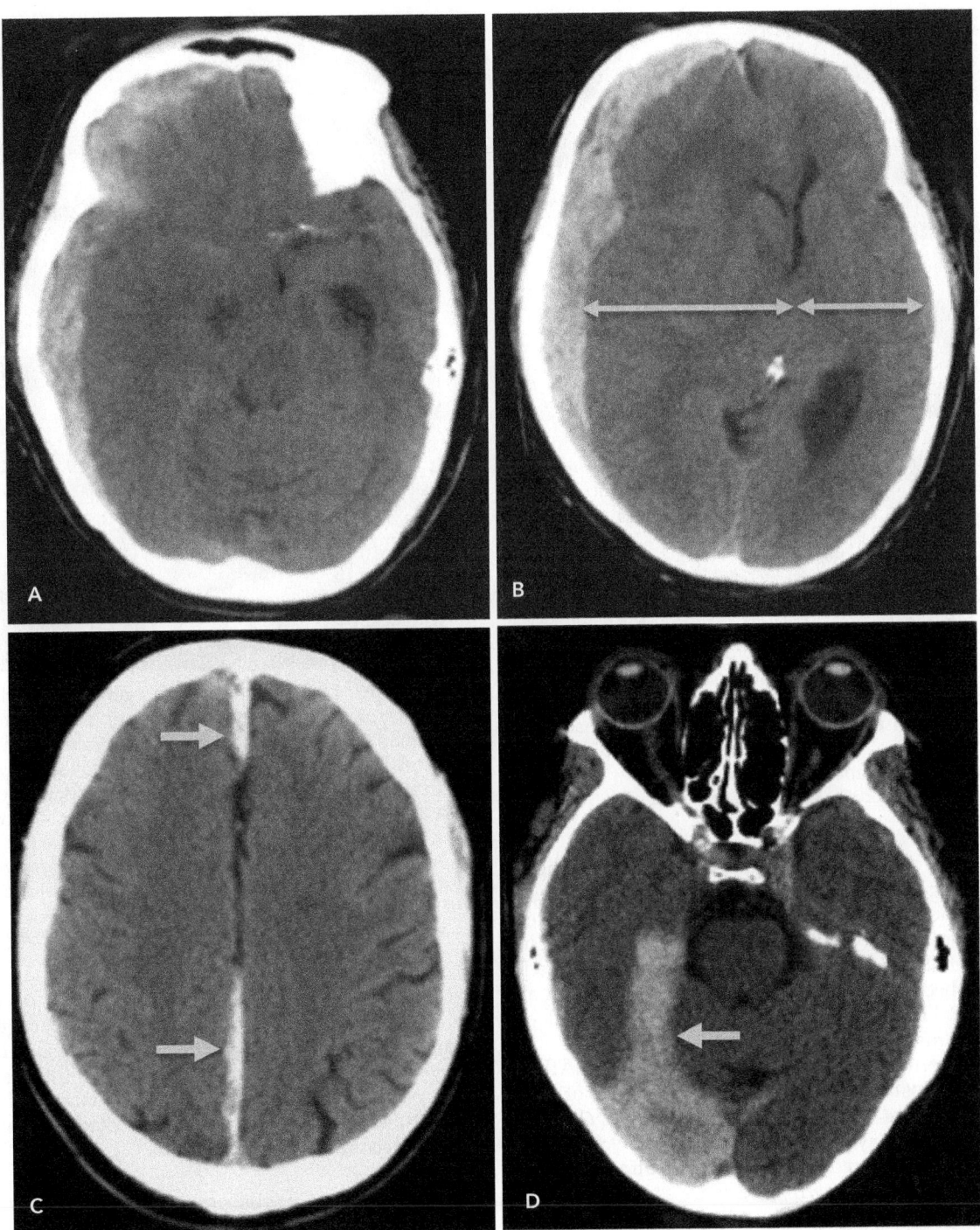

FIGURE 15–9 Acute subdural hematoma. A and B, The SDH commonly appears on imaging as a crescent-shaped extra-axial collection overlying the lateral hemisphere. Despite compression by the SDH, note how the size of the underlying hemisphere is larger than the size of the contralateral hemisphere. This asymmetry in cerebral volume may be caused by traumatic dysautoregulation (compare with Figure 15-11). C, Another common manifestation is the interhemispheric SDH, which appears as a thickened "shaggy" falx cerebri (*arrows*). D, The tentorial SDH is a third common type and is recognized as high-density layering en face along the tentorium (*arrow*). In more subtle cases, bilaterally asymmetric or symmetric high density is seen along the tentorium.

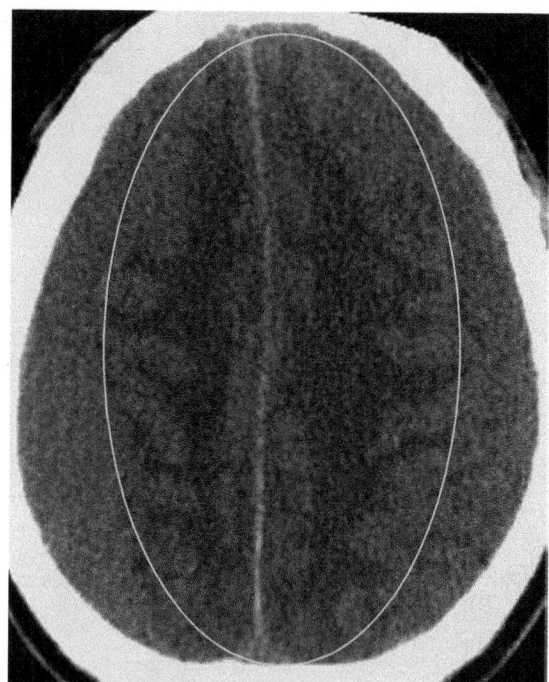

FIGURE 15–10 Subacute subdural hematoma (isodense). Note complete effacement of the cerebral sulci and white matter "buckling" because of bilateral isodense subdural collections. The compressed hemispheres are outlined by the oval. During the transition from acute to chronic SDH, an isodense phase occurs. At this stage, the SDH can be difficult to discriminate from the adjacent parenchyma.

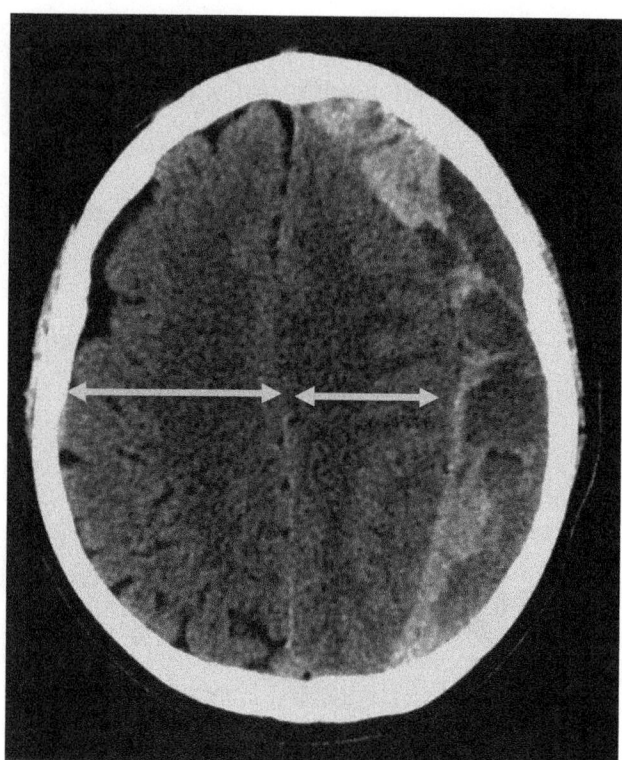

FIGURE 15–11 Chronic subdural hematoma. Although many SDHs resolve without complication, rebleeding into the collection may result in the so-called "chronic recurrent SDH" that typically appears as a heterogeneous collection with internal septations, loculations, and fluid–fluid levels. Unlike Figures 15-9A and 15-9B, the chronic SDH may be associated with minimal midline shift, that is, note how the size of the left hemisphere appears smaller than the right hemisphere (*arrows*); this may be caused by the absence of underlying parenchymal injury (e.g., dysauto-regulation).

with sensitivity depending on volume, hematocrit, and age of the hemorrhage. Although FLAIR MRI has been reported to be slightly more sensitive for acute SAH, the difference is small and does not outweigh the other advantages that CT has over MRI in the acute setting (38). Due largely to dilution with CSF, SAH becomes rapidly undetectable by CT, usually within several hours to a few days (36). Larger quantities of SAH and "tumefactive" IVH may persist much longer.

Among conventional MRI sequences, the T2 FLAIR sequence is the most sensitive for SAH (39). All types of extra-axial collections are usually evident on T2 FLAIR, although, as with CT, SAH may be visible for a relatively short time because it undergoes redistribution and dilution with CSF. FLAIR MRI has been shown to be more sensitive than CT for detection particularly of subacute and chronic SAH. Although the FLAIR sequence is the most sensitive, SAH may also be discernible on T1- or T2-weighted images as "dirty" CSF. Meningitis and carcinomatosis may mimic SAH on both MRI and noncontrast CT, although the clinical context usually prevents misinterpretation in such relatively rare cases. In addition to meningitis and carcinomatosis, oxygen therapy and magnetic field distortions because of nearby metal may also result in high signal within the CSF on FLAIR images that mimics acute SAH.

SAH and IVH carry the risk of development of chronic, communicating hydrocephalus. A recent retrospective review of 301 consecutive cases of traumatic SAH determined that 12% developed hydrocephalus. Increasing age, presence of IVH, and large quantity of SAH were associated with higher risk for hydrocephalus. Gender, admission GCS

score, location of SAH, or performance of decompressive craniectomy were not significant risk factors (40). A low-radiation-dose CT protocol, or rapid single-shot T2-weighted fast-spin-echo sequence that requires as little as 2 seconds, can be performed for follow-up evaluations of ventricular size after ventriculoperitoneal shunt placement and is particularly recommended in children.

Contusion or Hematoma

The cerebral contusion results from direct injury to the brain from direct impact at the coup and/or contrecoup sites. On CT and MRI, the contusion appears as a geographic area of patchy hemorrhage and edema within a superficial portion of the brain that is directly contiguous to the calvarium or skull base (Figure 15-13). Cerebral contusions can be very small and limited to the cortex, or more extensive and involve both cortex and underlying subcortical white matter. In this latter case, contusion may evolve into a frank intraparenchymal hematoma. The most common locations are the anterior temporal lobes (approximately 50%) followed by the frontal lobes (30%), most commonly involving the gyri recti and medial orbital gyri within the anterior cranial fossa. Parietal and occipital (13%) and cerebellar (10%) contusions are relatively less common (41).

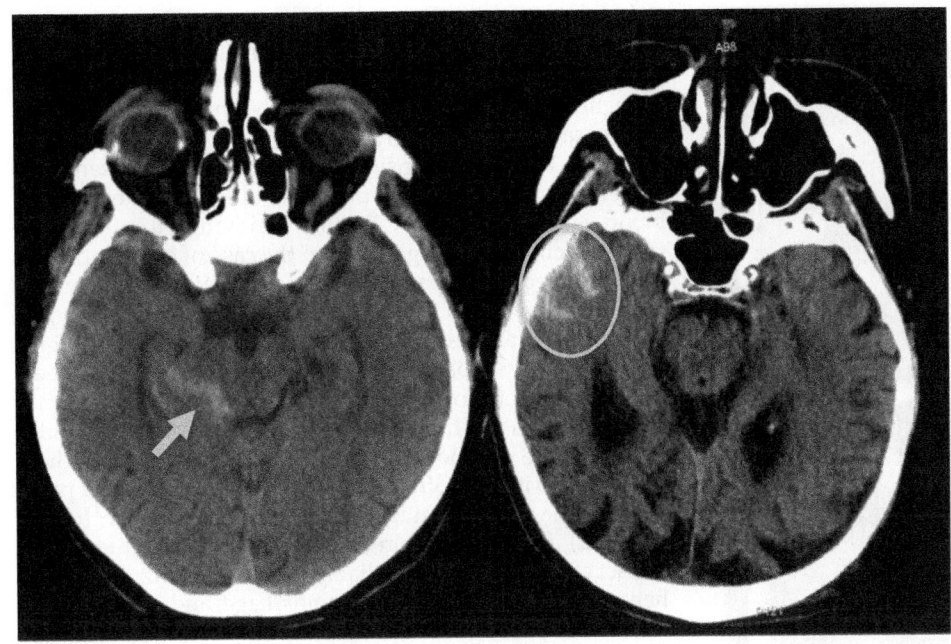

FIGURE 15–12 Acute subarachnoid hemorrhage. Traumatic SAH results from injury to superficial vessels along the brain surface and arachnoid membrane. On noncontrast CT, acute SAH generally appears as curvilinear areas of high density within cerebral sulci, cerebellar fissures, or cisterns. In this case, note the asymmetric high density within the right perimesencephalic cistern (*arrow*) and right temporal sulci (*circle*).

Brain contusions exhibit the characteristic feature of "blooming," whereby the extent of the contusion frequently expands, sometimes very dramatically, within 24 hours after injury. The blooming effect is most profound within the first several hours after injury (42). Later, in the subacute stage (1 day to several weeks after injury), the lesion demonstrates peripheral enhancement on postcontrast CT and postcontrast MRI and can thereby mimic metastatic disease, primary brain tumor, infection, abscess, cerebritis, subacute infarct, and other classic ring-enhancing lesions (Figure 15-14)

MRI is more sensitive than CT for detection of brain contusions, particularly small lesions. Sensitivities have been estimated at 98% for MRI and 56% for CT (43). 3D thin-section T1-weighted imaging is useful for detection of small cortical contusions, owing to (a) T1 shortening in methemo-globin that results in conspicuous high T1 signal that is known to typify subacute intraparenchymal hemorrhage of any etiology, including trauma and (b) thin sections made possible through 3D acquisition of these images (Figures 15-15 and 15-16). T2 FLAIR can be performed as either a 2-dimensional (2D) or a 3D sequence, and is also useful for demonstration of contusions. It is possible that 3D FLAIR—a sequence whose widespread incorporation into clinical MRI protocols is relatively recent—may perform favorably relative to 2D FLAIR because of the thin sections that are possible through this technique, just as with 3D T1-weighted imaging.

Regarding dating of intracranial hemorrhage, blood products generally progress through a series of stages, each with a characteristic constellation of CT density and T1- and

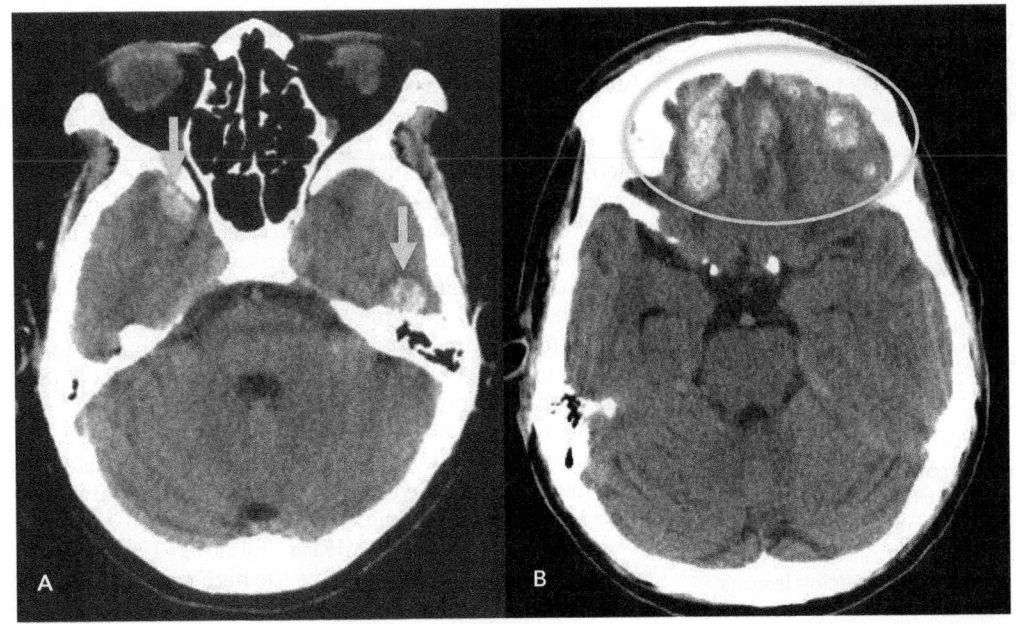

FIGURE 15–13 Hemorrhagic contusions. The cerebral contusion results from injury to the brain from impact. It occurs most commonly at the contrecoup site but is also seen at the coup site. The most common locations are (A) the anterior temporal lobes (approximately 50%) followed by (B) the orbitofrontal lobes (30%), frequently involving the gyri recti and medial orbital gyri within the anterior cranial fossa. Parietal and occipital (13%) contusions are less common, and cerebellar contusions are rare and are almost always associated with an adjacent occipital skull fracture.

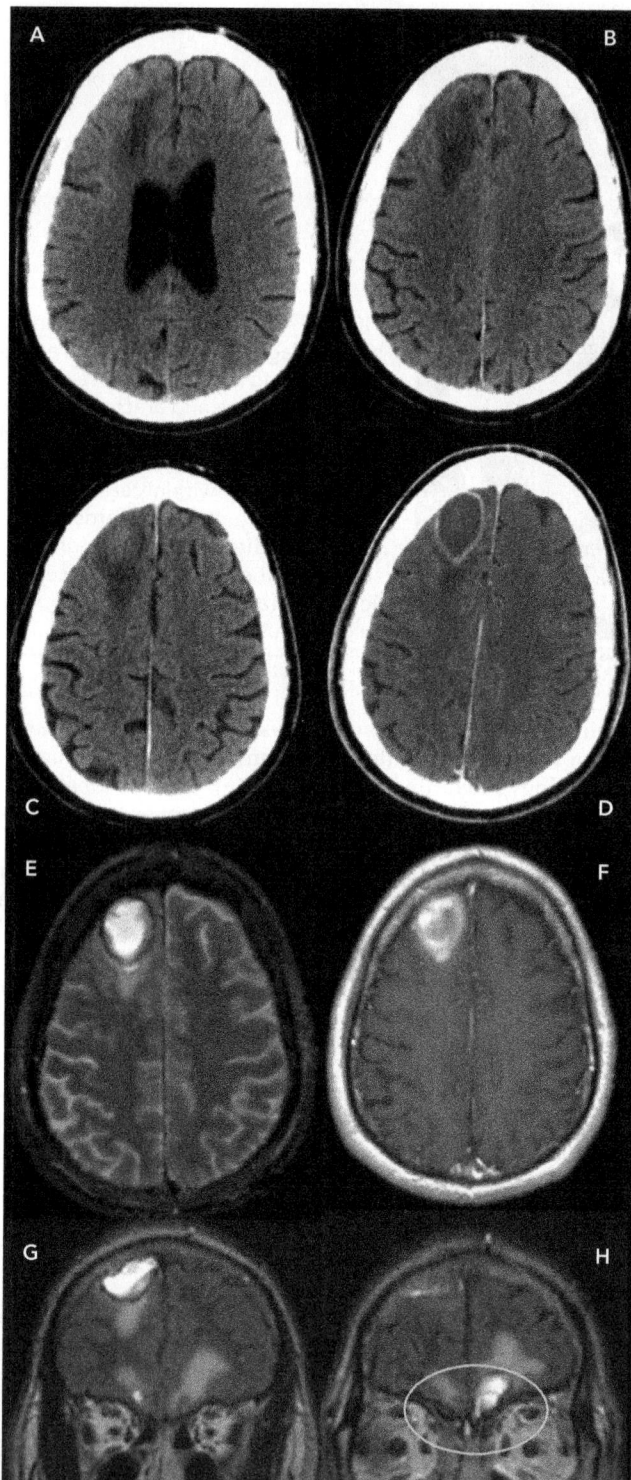

FIGURE 15-14 Subacute contusion or hematoma. In the subacute stage (approximately 48 hours to several weeks after injury), the cerebral hematoma shows surrounding vasogenic edema on (A–C) noncontrast CT and peripheral rim enhancement on (D) postcontrast CT. E, T2-weighted, (F) postcontrast T1-weighted, and (G, H) T2 FLAIR MRI images show late subacute, T1- and T2-hyperintense right frontal hematoma and smaller bilateral orbitofrontal contusions (*circle*). The peripheral rim enhancement seen with subacute hematomas can mimic metastatic disease, primary brain tumor, infection, abscess, cerebritis, subacute infarct, and other classic ring-enhancing lesions.

T2-weighted MRI signal intensities. Thus the pattern of CT density and MRI signal intensities constitutes a "signature" suggesting the approximate age of a hemorrhagic lesion or collection. Hyperacute hemorrhage (within several hours of extravasation) is generally hyperdense on CT, with low T1 and high T2 signal intensity and often a T2-hypointense peripheral rim. Extremely hyperacute, or freshly extravasated blood, is initially low in CT density, although this is uncommon in a clinical setting except in the case of coagulopathies characterized by impaired/delayed clotting. Acute hemorrhage (within hours to approximately 3 days) is also hyperdense on CT, with intermediate to low T1 and low T2 signal intensity. Early subacute hemorrhage (a few days to 1 week) is usually hyperdense on CT, with high T1 and low T2 signal; and late subacute hemorrhage (1 week to several months) is hypodense or isodense on CT with high T1 and high T2 signal intensity and often a T2-hypointense rim. Blood products in the chronic stage are hypodense on CT (unless calcified) and very low in both T1 and T2 signal intensity. These stages are more reliably observed with intra-axial hemorrhage than extra-axial hemorrhage, and can be altered in certain settings such as coagulopathy and acute-on-chronic hemorrhage. Furthermore, the rate at which blood products pass through individual stages is highly variable among individuals.

Traumatic Axonal Injury

Traumatic axonal injury (TAI), diffuse axonal injury (DAI), and shear injury are all terms that have been used to describe injuries to axons, usually within the cerebral white matter caused by shear-strain forces. Terms and definitions for the systematic description of pathoanatomic injuries in TBI recently established jointly by the DCOE, NINDS, NIDRR, and VA (15,44) recommended the use of the term "traumatic axonal injury" for 1 to 3 foci of axonal injury identified on brain imaging, and reservation of the term "diffuse axonal injury" for identification of 4 or more foci. Previously, axonal injury was thought to be generally associated with poor outcome (45). It is now known that TAI is extremely common within not only moderate and severe TBI but also in mild TBI.

Strich, (46,47) building on early classic work by Holbourn, (48) hypothesized that white matter injuries result from rotational acceleration caused by shear-strain deformation of the brain at interfaces between tissues of different density (e.g., gray/white matter). These theories were supported by postmortem observations (49,50) and experimental work on animals by Gennarelli (50). Locations in which traumatic axonal injury has been more commonly described in clinical imaging are the lobar white matter, particularly within the frontal and temporal lobes (approximately 50% of TAI detected by conventional MRI sequences), the corpus callosum (approximately 22% of lesions, with most lesions in the splenium), corona radiata (19%), internal capsule (8%, mostly within the posterior limb of the internal capsule), and dorsolateral midbrain or rostral pons (< 8%) (41). CT has very poor sensitivity for TAI, with essentially no sensitivity for nonhemorrhagic TAI and only limited sensitivity, relative to MRI, for hemorrhagic TAI (25,28).

Among conventional MRI sequences, T2*-weighted GRE and SWI are thought to have the highest sensitivity for hemorrhagic traumatic axonal injury (22,51–53). Both T2*-

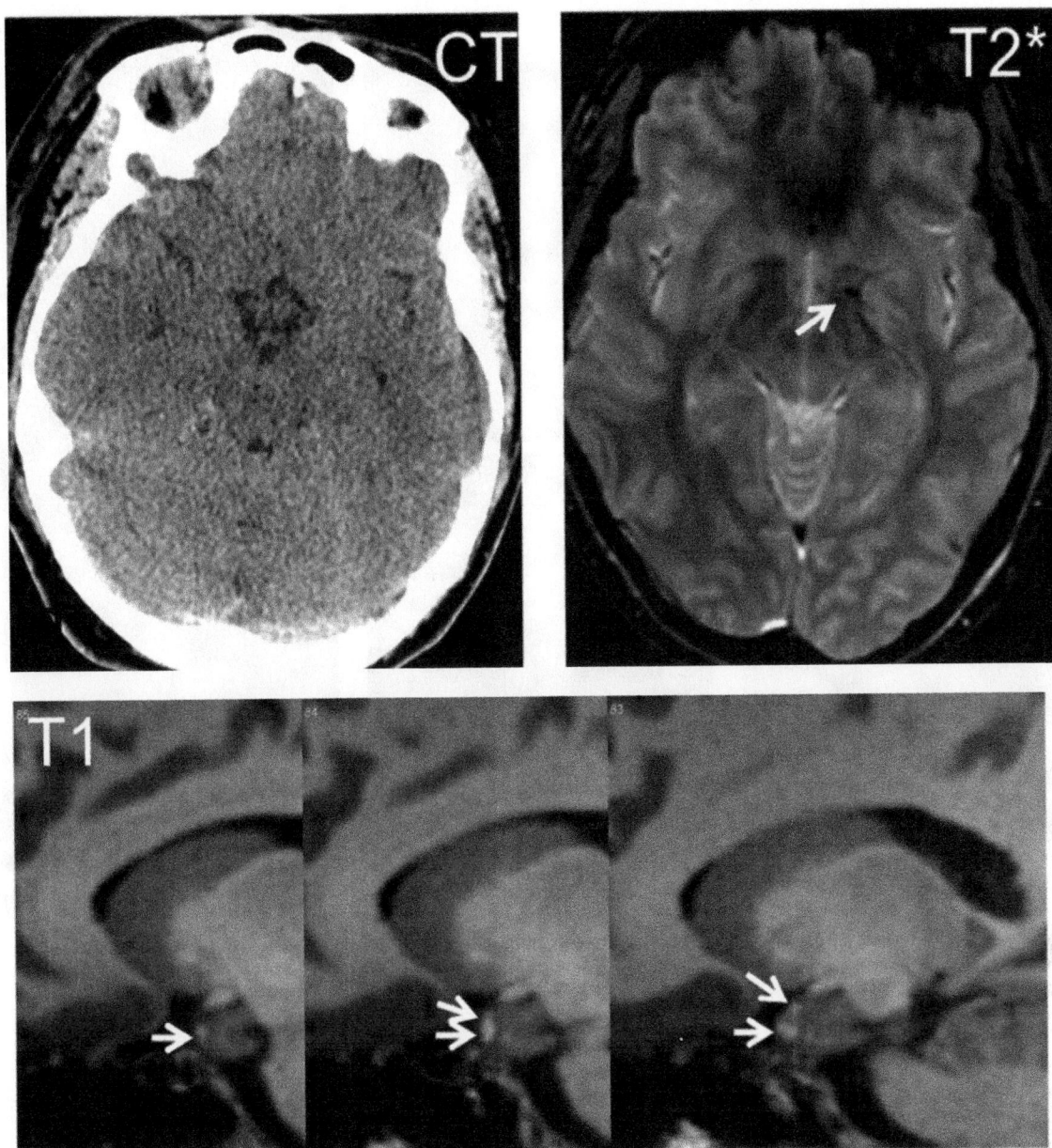

FIGURE 15–15 Hippocampal contusion. A 27-year-old woman found down near a bicycle. GCS was 12 in the field and 13 on emergency department arrival. Noncontrast head CT showed only trace subarachnoid near the vertex but no evidence of brain contusion, traumatic axonal injury, or other brain parenchymal injury. MRI within 2 weeks of injury showed a hemorrhagic contusion of the left hippocampal head, visible on T2*-weighted gradient-echo and parasagittal 3-dimensional (3D) thin-section T1-weighted images (*arrows*).

weighted GRE and SWI exploit the local magnetic field distortions resulting from paramagnetic blood products to demonstrate small foci of hemorrhagic TAI. Focal areas of signal loss on these sequences indicate the presence of small foci of acute, subacute, or chronic blood products that are often not visible on T1- or fast-spin-echo T2-weighted sequences (Figures 15-15, 15-16, 15-17, and 15-18) (27,54,55). SWI is a newer technique that has been shown to be more sensitive than T2*-weighted GRE for these hemorrhagic foci (22,51). Some knowledge of the typical geographic distribution of traumatic axonal injury may be useful in reading SWI images because blood vessels are also highly conspicuous on these images.

Itt has been estimated that less than 20% of TAI is hemorrhagic (41). Nonhemorrhagic traumatic axonal injury can sometimes be seen on FLAIR and T2-weighted images, but unless it is seen in a location that is relatively specific for TAI, it is often indistinguishable from small areas of gliosis because of chronic small vessel ischemic disease, remote infection or demyelination, or other types of injury. T2-weighted fast-spin-echo may be useful for demonstrating nonhemorrhagic TAI in the posterior fossa. In contrast to supratentorial lesions, which may be better visualized on T2 FLAIR (56), brainstem and cerebellar lesions may show up relatively poorly on T2 FLAIR sequences and are sometimes conspicuous only on T2-weighted spin-echo imaging.

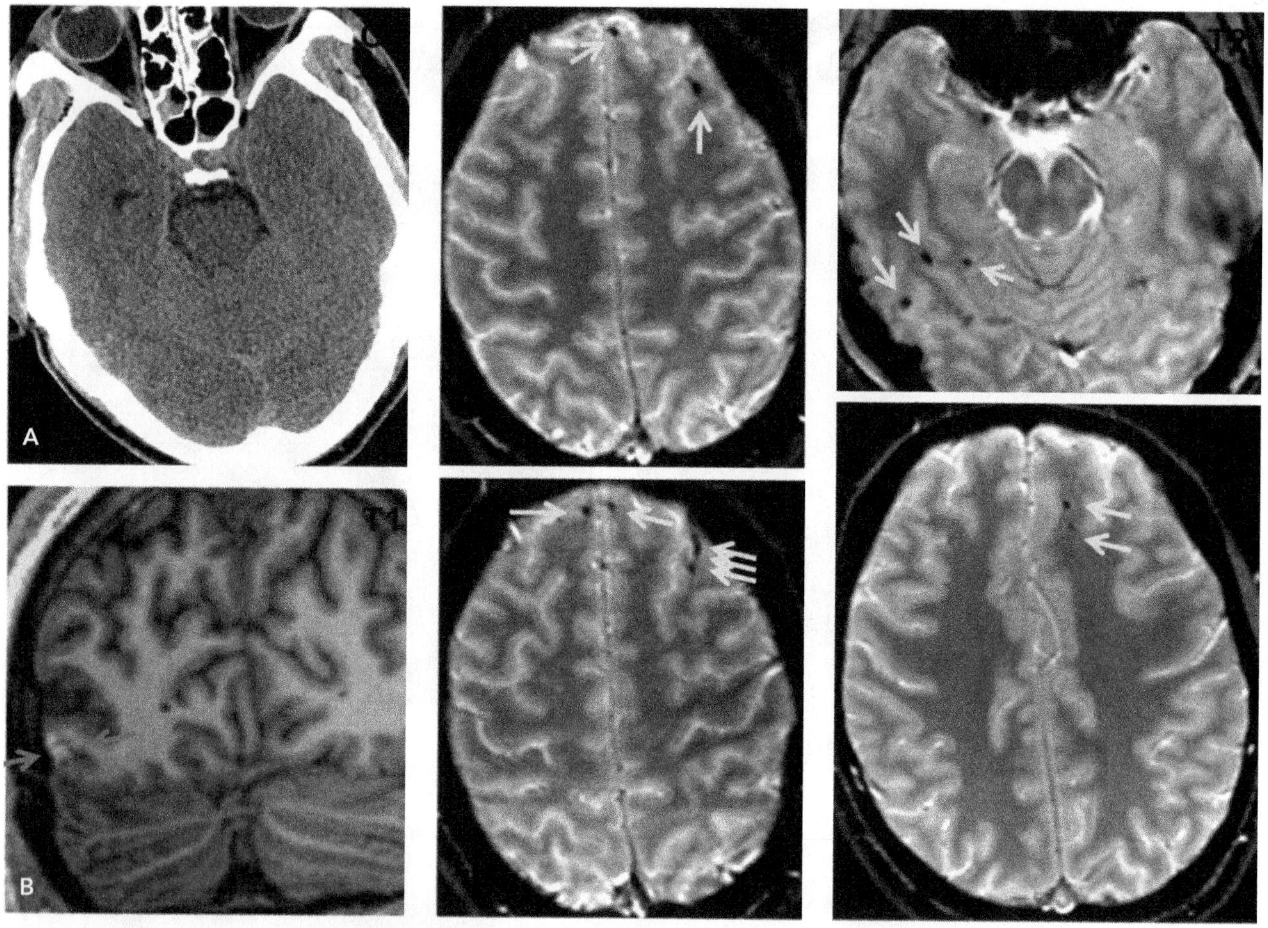

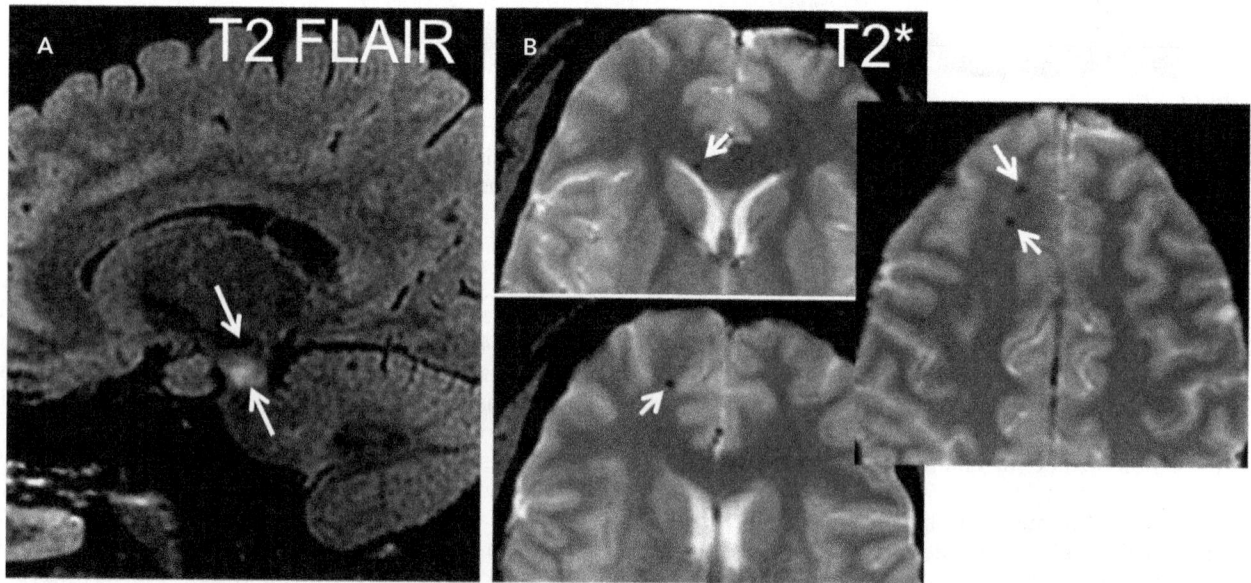

FIGURE 15–16 Greater sensitivity of MRI for brain contusion and hemorrhagic traumatic axonal injury. A, CT demonstrates subtle SAH vs hemorrhagic contusion in the posterior right temporal lobe (*arrow*). B, Coronal T1-weighted MRI more definitively demonstrates that this finding represents a hemorrhagic contusion (cortical T1 hyperintensity) (*arrows*) rather than SAH. The remaining images are from the T2*-weighted gradient-echo sequence: note innumerable foci of traumatic axonal injury not detected on CT (*arrows*).

FIGURE 15–17 Shear injury—hemorrhagic and nonhemorrhagic. A, Parasagittal 3D FLAIR demonstrates nonhemorrhagic shear injury in the midbrain (*arrows*). B, T2*-weighted gradient-echo demonstrating multiple foci of hemorrhagic shear injury. None of these injuries were visible on admission or follow-up in patient head CT exams. (FLAIR, fluid-attenuated inversion recovery.)

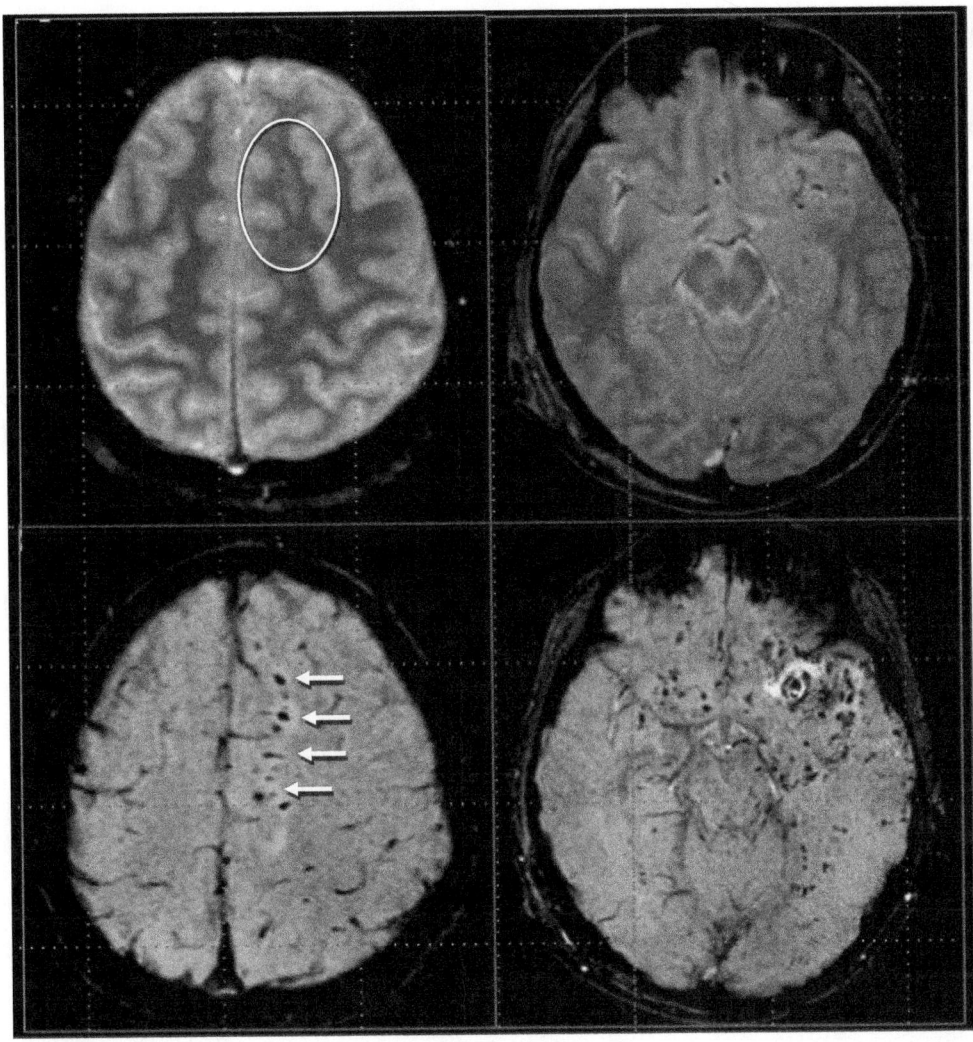

FIGURE 15–18 Diffuse axonal injury on gradient-echo (GRE) and susceptibility-weighted imaging (SWI). In the current example, the upper row images are GRE and the lower row images are SWI. Subtle asymmetric T2 hyperintensity is seen in the left centrum semiovale on the GRE sequence (*circle*). The image at the level of the midbrain is relatively unremarkable. Note the marked improvement in lesion conspicuity on the SWI sequence, evident as innumerable punctate hypointense foci representing microhemorrhages (*arrows*). The image at the level of the midbrain now demonstrates extensive bilateral hemorrhagic diffuse axonal injury (DAI). (Image courtesy of Karen A. Tong, MD, Loma Linda University Medical Center.)

DWI, which assesses the microscopic motion of water molecules in brain tissue, is complementary to T2*-weighted GRE and SWI because it can depict foci of nonhemorrhagic axonal injury that would be invisible on T2*-weighted imaging (Figure 15-19) (57,58). DWI has been described to be highly sensitive for acute TAI (59), demonstrating these lesions as foci of reduced diffusion, although the diffusion coefficient normalizes within hours to days, and is elevated in the chronic stage.

DTI represents a further advance over DWI, enabling characterization of the directionality of water diffusion in 3D space (60). Within white matter tracts with their parallel fiber bundles, water diffuses more freely along the direction of the white matter fibers than transverse to the fibers because diffusion orthogonal to the fibers is impeded by structural elements such as myelin sheaths, the axolemma, microtubules, and neurofilaments. Known as diffusion "anisotropy," this phenomenon can be quantified within white matter tracts using the DTI measure of fractional anisotropy (FA). FA is a scalar quantity that quantifies the degree of anisotropy in the diffusivity within each voxel. FA has been shown to be a quantitative metric of the microstructural integrity of white matter (58,61). Other measures include radial diffusivity (RD), the diffusivity perpendicular to the fiber bundles; and axial diffusivity (AD), the diffusivity along the

fiber bundles. Generally, one expects normal myelinated white matter to exhibit low diffusivity and high FA, and damaged white matter to demonstrate lower FA and higher diffusivity because of local decrease in longitudinally oriented microstructural elements such as the myelin sheath and axolemma.

Four major types of DTI analysis are currently in practice (62). *Histogram analysis* consists of a simple histogram of the FA values throughout the whole brain. It is easy to perform because it ignores tract-specific anatomy and instead gives a summary "gestalt" of global changes in FA throughout the brain. Studies employing histogram analysis have not shown consistent correlation with clinical measures of TBI, and may have limited use. *Region-of-interest (ROI) analysis* is likely the most common approach to date. In ROI analysis, a priori knowledge of the locations of specific white matter tracts that are known to be prone to injury in TBI is required. Manual or semiautomated segmentation of these ROIs is performed, and the DTI metrics of FA, RD, and AD are calculated. *Voxel-based analysis* comprises a variety of powerful data-driven analysis techniques in which each subject's brain is spatially warped such that its white matter tracts coincide with those of a 3D white-matter atlas. Its strength is that no a priori assumptions are made about which white matter tract are more prone to injury. Finally,

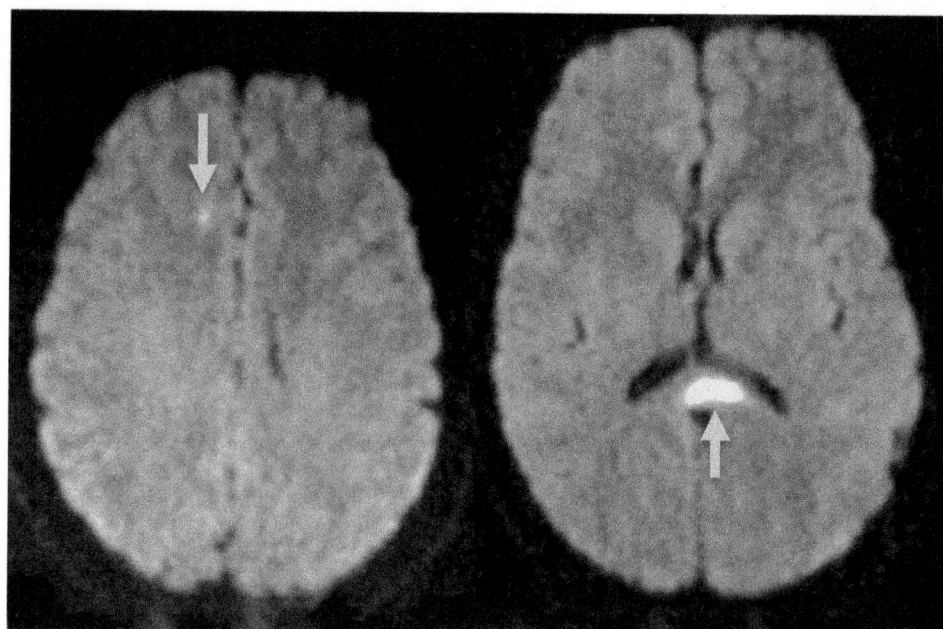

FIGURE 15–19 Acute traumatic axonal injury on diffusion-weighted imaging (DWI). DWI is complementary to T2*-weighted gradient-echo (GRE) and susceptibility-weighted imaging (SWI) because it can depict foci of nonhemorrhagic shear injury that are invisible on T2*-weighted imaging. DWI demonstrates these lesions as foci of reduced diffusion (*arrows*), although the diffusion coefficient tends to normalize within hours.

DTI tractography is a new technique that has been used to demonstrate focal discontinuity in certain white matter tracts after TBI. Tractography uses the diffusion tensor within each voxel to attempt to follow an axonal tract in 3 dimensions from voxel to voxel throughout the brain (63,64). This technique can yield captivating 3D renderings of individual white matter tracts (Figure 15-20) (65). However, most tractography in TBI reported in the literature to date is limited to case reports, to single tracts such as the corpus callosum, or to subjects with moderate or severe TBI who are likely to have significant gross abnormalities on CT and conventional MRI. In addition, tractography results are highly dependent on choices of certain user-imposed parameters such as FA threshold and deflection angle (62).

Initial studies of DTI in mild TBI using both ROI and voxel-based analysis have demonstrated in small numbers of patients that there exist group differences in FA within specific white matter tracts between patients with mild head injury and controls and/or that reduced FA values within these white matter tracts are correlated with poorer performance on neuropsychiatric tests in patients with TBI (66–69). Frontal association pathways including the anterior corona radiata, uncinate fasciculus, superior longitudinal fasciculus, and anterior corpus callosum are among the tracts most commonly identified to exhibit evidence of injury on DTI studies of mild TBI (62). Although these results are extremely promising, DTI is not currently implemented clinically in diagnosis or outcome prediction in TBI, in part because these metrics of white matter injury have not been shown to be specific for TAI rather than white matter degeneration/injury caused by other etiologies including aging. In addition, no consensus yet exists that these techniques are sufficiently powerful to provide meaningful prediction of outcome in the individual patient rather than just group differences.

From both a clinical and medicolegal perspective, neither an abnormal DTI exam nor the identification of an abnormal white matter lesion on conventional MRI sequences is specific for TBI because other disease entities can result in

both of these. Because patients with TBI tend to be younger adults, there does tend to be a lower incidence of chronic medical conditions, such as cerebrovascular disease, in a significant subset of patients with TBI. From a neuroradiologic perspective, preexisting brain lesions are rarely a complicating factor when evaluating imaging studies in children and young adults, and in the proper clinical setting, one can often assume that an abnormality identified on a young patient's imaging study is most likely caused by the trauma rather than by a preexisting nontraumatic cause. In addition, although the presence of a white matter microbleed is always suspicious for TBI, there are substantial differences in locations of microbleeds in younger patients with trauma in comparison to older patients with stroke (70). Nevertheless, because TBI is associated with alcohol and substance abuse, the severity and nature of the postinjury deficit may yet be confounded by the potential cumulative effects of repetitive brain injuries as well as by acute and chronic effects of toxic and metabolic disorders. Therefore, close clinical correlation is imperative when interpreting imaging findings.

Brain Herniation

Brain herniation is defined as displacement of a portion of the brain from its normal location to a space that it does not normally occupy. The 4 types of cerebral herniation include subfalcine herniation (sometimes referred to as "midline shift"), unilateral or bilateral descending transtentorial (i.e., "downward") herniation, uncal herniation, and external herniation. The 3 types of cerebellar herniation include ascending transtentorial (i.e., "upward") herniation, tonsillar herniation, and external herniation.

In cases of severe herniation, morbidity can result in several ways. Severe subfalcine herniation can result in infarction of part or all of the anterior cerebral artery territory from compression of its branches within the anterior interhemispheric fissure (Figure 15-21). Descending transtentorial herniation can result in compression of the ipsilateral pos-

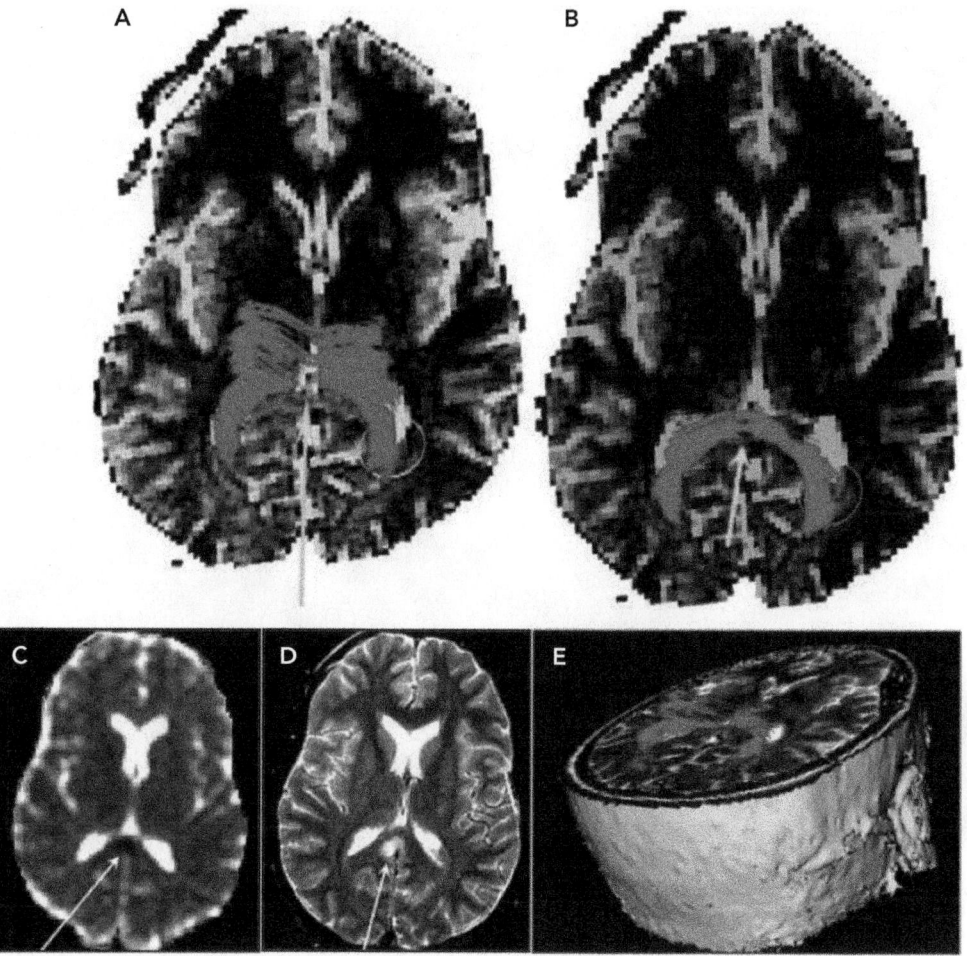

FIGURE 15–20 *See color insert.* DTI fiber tractography 3 days after TBI in a 22-year-old man with left hemialexia. Axial (A) and coronal (B) projections of DTI fiber tractography showing discontinuous fibers at the posteroinferior margin of the splenium of the corpus callosum (*green arrows*) in a 22-year-old man with left hemialexia, a functional deficit caused by disconnection of the right visual cortex from the language centers of the dominant left cerebral hemisphere. *Green circles* at the left side of the splenium of the corpus callosum in the axial (A) and coronal (B) projections show a 2-dimensional cross-section of the 3-dimensional (3D) region of interest from which diffusion tensor fiber tracking was initiated. C, Apparent diffusion coefficient (ADC) and (D) T2-weighted images of the same patient, also at 3 days after injury, demonstrate reduced diffusion and focal abnormal high T2 signal in the midline splenium, respectively. E, 3D reconstruction of the DTI fiber tractogram. Reprinted from Le (65) with permission.

terior cerebral artery (PCA) within the perimesencephalic cistern and resulting infarction within all or a portion of the PCA distribution. In rare cases, bilateral descending transtentorial herniation can result in the Duret hemorrhage (Figure 15-22). Duret hemorrhages are midbrain and pontine hemorrhages believed to be caused by either stretching and laceration of pontine perforating branches of the basilar artery, or by venous compression followed by venous infarction (71).

Cerebral ischemia and stroke may also occur when cerebral perfusion pressure, defined as the difference between mean arterial pressure and ICP, is reduced to less than the autoregulatory capacity of the brain vasculature. Normal cerebral blood flow is maintained for cerebral perfusion pressures of 50–150 mm Hg through autoregulation. When cerebral perfusion pressure is reduced to < 50 mm Hg, as in sustained increased ICP without a corresponding increase in mean arterial pressure, cerebral blood flow is reduced. This reduced flow can result in large-territory ischemia or

infarction. Increased systemic blood pressure in response to reduced cerebral perfusion pressure may result in or exacerbate existing intracranial hematomas. Reflex bradycardia may further reduce brain perfusion via a reduction in systemic blood pressure and a corresponding reduction in perfusion pressure (72).

Fast Magnetic Resonance Imaging Sequences for Patients Unable to Lie Still

Fast imaging sequences may be useful when patients, such as those with decreased levels of consciousness, are unable to lie still. Many fast imaging techniques are "single-shot 2D" techniques, meaning that a complete image of a 2D slab of the brain is obtained employing a single excitation pulse. In single-shot 2D techniques, a 2D slab of the brain is excited at once, and the complex signal that results is "decoded" by using frequency encoding in one direction, and phase encoding in the other direction, to spatially localize the signal

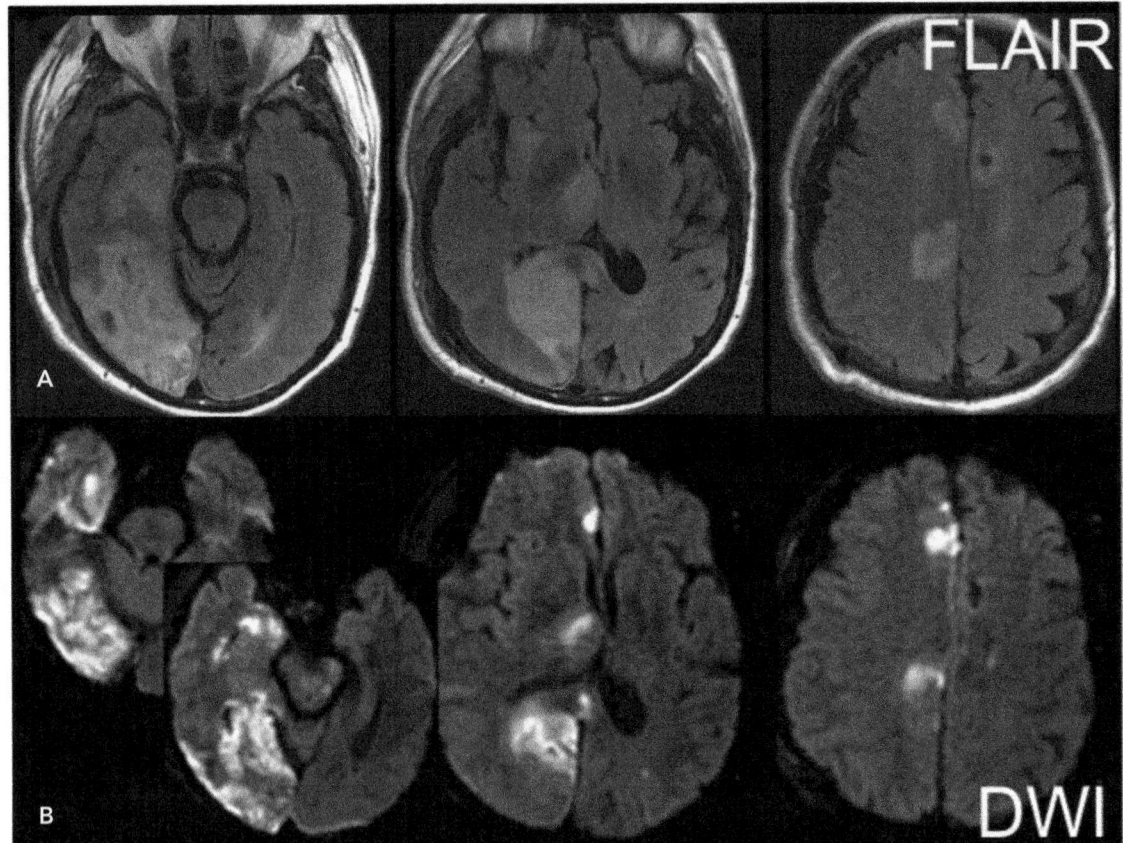

FIGURE 15–21 Post-traumatic infarction in the anterior and posterior cerebral artery territories caused by brain herniation. A, Fluid-attenuated inversion recovery (FLAIR) MR images obtained after surgical evacuation of a large right SDH demonstrates multifocal T2-hyperintense lesions. B, Diffusion-weighted imaging (DWI) shows corresponding reduced diffusion, confirming the ischemic etiology. This case illustrates that severe subfalcine herniation can result in infarction of part or all of the anterior cerebral artery territory from compression of its branches within the anterior interhemispheric fissure. Descending transtentorial herniation can result in compression of the ipsilateral posterior cerebral artery within the perimesencephalic cistern and result in infarction within all or a portion of the posterior cerebral artery distribution.

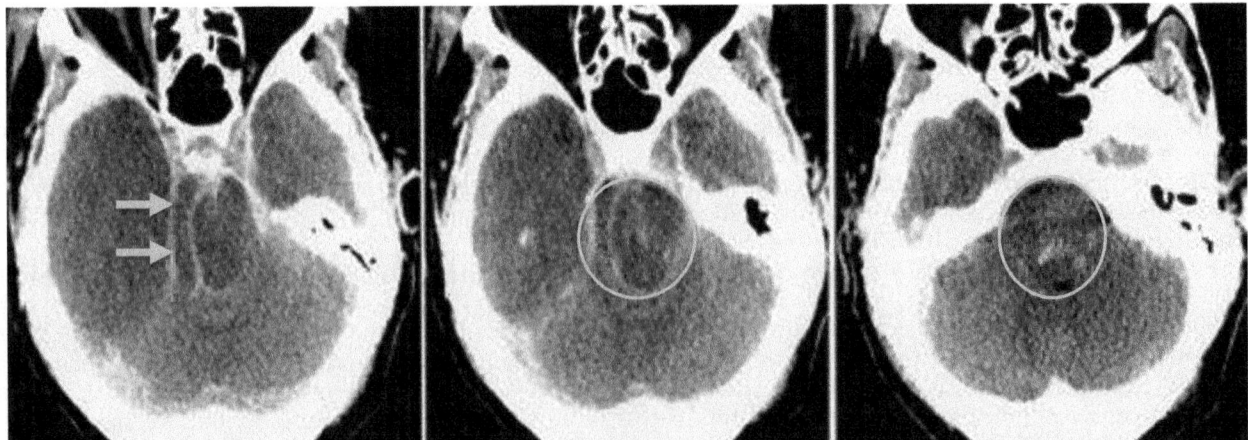

FIGURE 15–22 Duret hemorrhage. Duret hemorrhages are midbrain and/or pontine hemorrhages believed to be caused by stretching and laceration of pontine perforating branches of the basilar artery, or by venous thrombosis and infarction. It is typically seen in the setting of acute downward herniation. In this example, note complete effacement of the perimesencephalic cisterns, right medial temporal lobe downward herniation (*arrows*), deformity of the brainstem, and central pontine hemorrhage (*circles*).

coming from protons at any point within the 2D slab. Examples of single-shot 2D techniques include single-shot T2-weighted fast-spin-echo, and single-shot echo-planar diffusion-weighted imaging, which can require 2 seconds or less to acquire images of the entire brain. A rapid brain MRI protocol for acute TBI might consist of fast T1-and T2*-weighted GRE sequences, single-shot echo-planar DWI, and single-shot echo-planar T2 FLAIR.

CT ANGIOGRAPHY

Indications for CT Angiography in Acute Head Trauma

Blunt cerebrovascular injuries (BCVI) include injuries to the cervical or intracranial carotid or vertebral arteries caused by nonpenetrating trauma. The proposed mechanisms fall into several categories: stretch injuries that exceed the mechanical tolerance of the vessel wall, blunt trauma to the vessel by direct impact, and secondary trauma to a vessel (either blunt or penetrating) caused by bony fracture fragments (73).

Although no consensus exists, screening criteria have been proposed to limit radiation exposure and costs associated with CTA and conventional angiography to a subset of patients at high risk for BCVI. The Denver criteria (74) (Table 15-5A) were demonstrated to be independent predictors of BCVI in 249 patients with blunt trauma who underwent catheter angiography. Miller et al. demonstrated in a prospective study of 216 trauma patients a 29% rate of BCVI using a similar, shorter set of criteria (Table 15-5B) (75). Although several authors concur that screening for BCVI is indicated (74–79), others argue that these are unnecessary because of low yield and little bearing on clinical outcome (80,81).

Grading systems that classify the types of injuries according to morbidity rates have also been described. For example, the Denver group has proposed the Blunt Carotid and Vertebral Arterial Injury Grading scale as follows: Grade I, luminal irregularity or dissection with < 25% luminal narrowing; Grade II, dissection or intramural hematoma with ≥ 25% luminal narrowing, intraluminal thrombus, or raised

---

TABLE 15-5A Denver Screening Criteria for Blunt Cerebrovascular Injury

Signs and symptoms
Intraoral arterial hemorrhage
Cervical bruit in patient < 50 years old
Expanding cervical hematoma
Focal neurological deficit
Neurological examinations incongruous with head CT findings
Stroke on secondary head CT

Risk factors
High-energy transfer mechanism with LeFort II or III fracture
Cervical spine fracture patterns: subluxation, fractures extending into the foramen transversarium, fractures of C1–C3
Skull base fracture with carotid canal involvement
Diffuse axonal injury with Glasgow Coma Scale (GCS) score < 6
Near-hanging with anoxic brain injury

Source: Biffl et al. (74).

TABLE 15-5B Proposed "Screening Triggers" for Further Vascular Imaging to Assess for Blunt Cerebrovascular Injury

Cervical spine fracture
Neurologic exam not explained by brain imaging
Horner's syndrome
LeFort II or III fractures
Skull base fracture involving foramen lacerum
Neck soft tissue injury such as seatbelt injury or hanging

Source: Miller et al. (75).

---

intimal flap; Grade III, pseudoaneurysm; Grade IV, occlusion; Grade V, transection with free extravasation (74,76). Risk of stroke increased from 3% for Grade I injuries to 100% for Grade IV and V injuries.

CT Angiographic Features of Traumatic Intracranial or Extracranial Arterial Dissection

Traumatic arterial dissection is an injury to the vessel wall resulting in hematoma within the layers of the vessel wall. Arterial dissection is not limited to acute trauma but can also be seen spontaneously, or in vasculitides, collagen vascular diseases, and atherosclerosis. On both CTA and magnetic resonance (MR) angiography, dissection can have several appearances (73,82,83). The most classic appearance is long-segment stenosis, often with tapered edges, sometimes referred to as the "string sign." Fusiform dilatation is also a very common appearance. Abrupt occlusion is also possible, often with some tapering at the location of the occlusion rather than a blunt cutoff.

The most common extracranial location for an acute traumatic arterial dissection is the internal carotid artery, most commonly a few centimeters distal to the carotid bifurcation extending to the skull base (Figure 15-23). The vertebral artery at the C1-C2 level is also frequently affected. Symptoms include persistent neck pain, headache, or stroke. In 15% of cases of traumatic extracranial dissection, multiple locations are involved. When acute traumatic arterial dissection occurs intracranially, the most common immediate symptoms include SAH, stroke, or symptoms associated with carotid-cavernous fistula. At least 70% of acute traumatic intracranial arterial dissection occurs in an intradural vertebral artery (Figure 15-24)

THE ROLE OF NONCONTRAST HEAD CT IN ACUTE CLINICAL MANAGEMENT

In the rapid initial assessment of patients with head trauma, noncontrast CT studies play a pivotal role in determining whether hospitalization and/or early surgical management is needed. According to the most recent CDC/ACEP joint practice guidelines, patients with TBI 16 years of age older with nonpenetrating head injury, GCS of 14 or 15 on ED evaluation within 24 hours of injury, and a head CT demonstrating no acute intracranial injury may be safely discharged directly from the ED (8). However, as discussed earlier, despite the preponderance of evidence in the literature that follow-up CT may not be justified in patients with mild TBI with small amounts of intracranial hemorrhage and no neu-

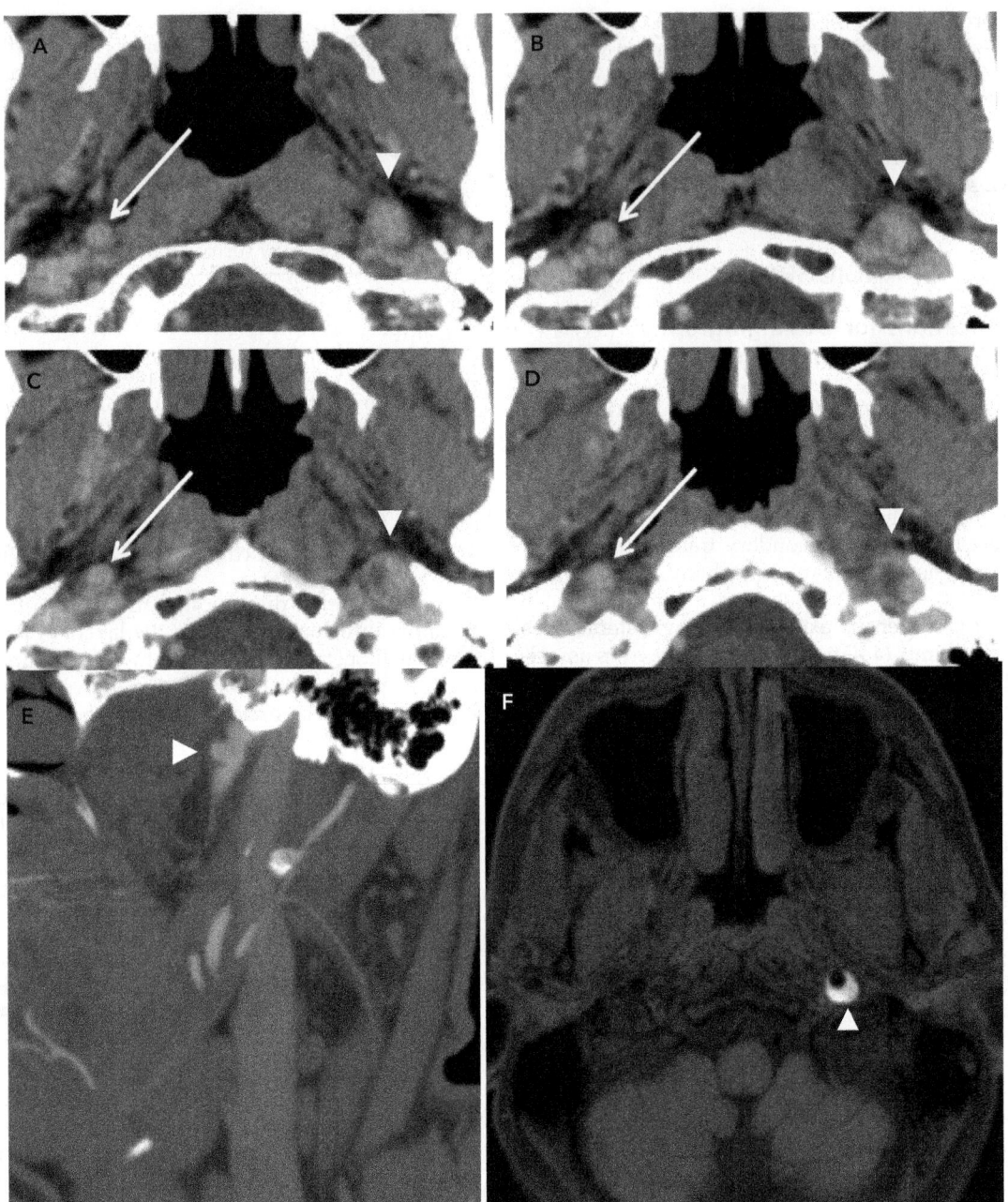

FIGURE 15–23 Internal carotid artery dissection. A–D, Axial CT angiographic images demonstrate an enlarged, ill-defined left internal carotid artery with a subtle filling defect (*arrowheads*) just below the petrous canal. Note the normal right internal carotid artery for comparison (*arrows*). E, Oblique parasagittal maximum intensity-projection (MIP) CT angiographic image shows irregular caliber of the artery (*arrow*). F, Fat-saturated axial T1-weighted MR image shows the classic intramural hyperintensity ("crescent sign") within the arterial wall.

rological decline or coagulopathy, in many institutions, all patients with evidence of acute intracranial hemorrhage on the initial CT undergo routine scheduled follow-up CT several hours after the initial CT.

ICP monitoring is indicated whenever there is a significant risk of acute intracranial hypertension. ICP monitor placement is often performed for GCS < 9 and for GCS 9–12 with an abnormal head CT (1–4). Although elevated ICP is not reliably determined by current imaging techniques, it has been shown that 60% of patients with acute closed head

injury and an admission head CT that demonstrates evidence of acute intracranial injury (intracranial hemorrhage, basal cistern effacement, midline shift) develop intracranial hypertension. In contrast, only 13% of those with normal head CT develop increased ICP. Thus, an abnormal admission head CT in patients with acute head trauma often results in invasive ICP monitor placement (84). ICP monitoring can be performed with a ventriculostomy catheter, subarachnoid screw or bolt, or with a transducer-tipped catheter that does not need to be inserted into the CSF system. Treatment of

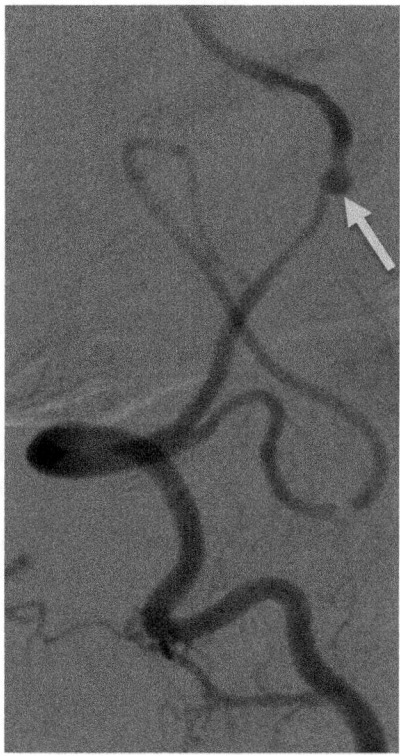

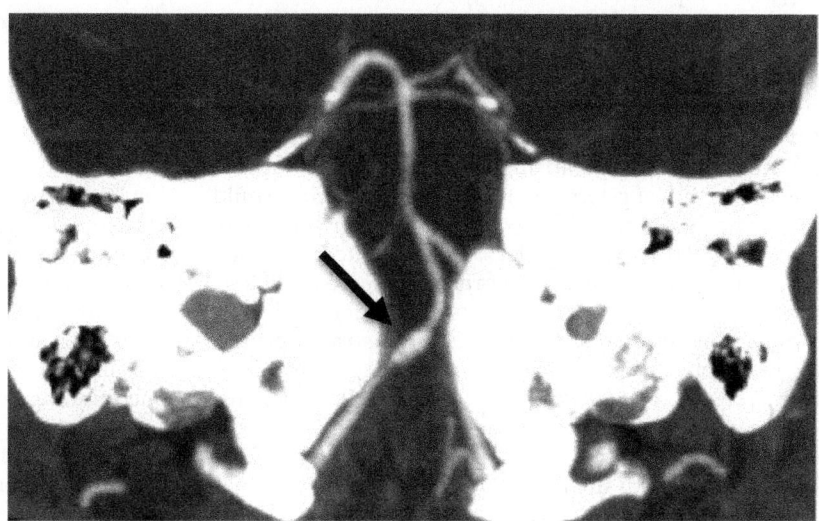

FIGURE 15–24 Vertebral artery dissection. A, Conventional catheter angiogram demonstrates abnormal caliber narrowing and irregularity of the distal right vertebral artery, consistent with an acute traumatic dissection and pseudoaneurysm (*arrow*) of the intradural right vertebral artery. B, Coronal MIP CT angiographic images in a different patient demonstrate an intradural right vertebral artery dissection (*arrow*).

acute intracranial hypertension has the following goals: (*a*) maintenance of ICP at < 20–25 mm Hg; (*b*) maintenance of cerebral perfusion pressure > 60 mm Hg; and (*c*) for patients with persistently increased ICP > 20–25 mm Hg, aggressive treatment, including hyperosmolar therapy (mannitol, hypertonic saline) or surgical intervention, is indicated (85).

Although many TBI lesions may be surgically evacuated via a craniotomy, refractory intracranial hypertension necessitates a decompressive craniectomy. The decompressive craniectomy relieves increased ICP both through evacuation of any intracranial hemorrhagic space-occupying lesions and by allowing external herniation of the brain, circumventing the Monro–Kellie doctrine (72). The decompressive craniectomy is still undergoing clinical trials to determine a consensus on its best application (86–88). It is discussed in more detail in the chapters on neurosurgical management.

CT AND MAGNETIC RESONANCE IMAGING IN OUTCOME PREDICTION

Computed Tomography

In addition to its role in immediate management decisions, the initial noncontrast head CT is known to carry longer term prognostic significance following acute TBI. The best-known head CT classification systems in acute TBI—the Marshall CT classification and more recent Rotterdam classification—are based on certain qualitative features of the admission head CT that were identified as having the greatest prognostic significance among a larger set of candidate CT features, when 6-month mortality was used as the outcome measure (5,6). These include the presence or absence of any acute traumatic intracranial abnormality (Marshall); presence or absence of significant midline shift, usually defined

as exceeding 5 mm (Marshall and Rotterdam); presence or absence and severity of basal cistern effacement (Marshall and Rotterdam); presence or absence of a large intracranial hematoma, defined as a hematoma with volume exceeding 25 cm^3 (Marshall); presence or absence of acute traumatic SAH (Rotterdam); and presence or absence of EDH (Rotterdam). The Marshall CT classification (6) divided patients with severe head trauma into 6 groups according to these head CT features and has been widely used for descriptive purposes; later, it was also used for prediction of mortality. The subsequently developed Rotterdam CT classification (5) achieved an improved discriminative value for the prediction of long-term outcome (6-month mortality) through regrouping of some CT features underlying the Marshall classification, and the addition of EDH to the model.

Just as management decisions in any clinical problem, including head trauma, are not based on imaging alone without regard to clinical information, neither is outcome prediction in head trauma based solely on a patient's head CT results. In the area of moderate-to-severe brain injury, several studies have successfully integrated clinical and imaging parameters into outcome prediction models (3,7,89). Recently, a 3-tier outcomes prediction model integrating clinical, demographic, and admission head CT features was developed by Steyerberg et al. (7) for the prediction of mortality and Glasgow Outcome Scale (GOS) score at 6 months after injury using the Internation Mission for Prognosis and Analysis of Clinical Trials in TBI (IMPACT) database. A core model based only on age, motor GCS score, and pupillary reactivity provided baseline discriminatory ability with area under the curves (AUCs) ranging from 0.66 to 0.84. Slightly higher discriminative ability with AUCs ranging from 0.71 to 0.87 could be achieved through augmentation by additional tiers of predictors, including the Marshall CT classification, hypotension, hypoxia, presence or absence of EDH, presence or absence of traumatic SAH, and serum glucose and hemoglobin on admission.

As a group, patients with mild TBI generally have a good prognosis. However, there is growing recognition that current classification schemes for mild TBI, or concussion, based on GCS and loss of consciousness/post-traumatic amnesia (LOC/PTA) duration are lacking, with small mean effect sizes in long-term impairment obscuring differences among diverse subgroups of patients with mild TBI with very different prognoses (90). It has been suggested that approximately 15% of patients with mild TBI have persistent measurable neuropsychiatric deficits at 1 year (26). Although several prior studies have demonstrated a correlation between acute intracranial hemorrhage on the admission head CT and acute, intermediate- and long-term neuropsychiatric deficits in mild TBI, a few have also shown no correlation (91), a very weak correlation (92,93), or even a better long-term outcome associated with acute intracranial hemorrhage (94). Nevertheless, the term *complicated mild* head injury is used in recognition of previous highly cited work (95) that demonstrated poorer performance on early neuropsychiatric testing, approaching levels more typical "moderate" TBI (GCS 9–12), in patients with "complicated mild" (with acute intracranial hemorrhage). Patients with "uncomplicated mild" TBI (either normal head CT or with the abnormality limited to a linear nondepressed skull fracture) performed significantly better than those with "complicated mild" TBI.

Magnetic Resonance Imaging

As discussed, many studies have demonstrated that conventional MRI techniques have superior sensitivity for identification of intracranial pathology in acute TBI (Figures 15-15 and 15-16). However, a consensus does not currently exist on the *long-term* clinical relevance of abnormal early conventional MRI findings in TBI once other routinely obtained predictive variables, such as GCS and other clinical features, and findings on the admission head CT, have been taken into account. Focal traumatic intracranial lesions on acute *conventional* brain MRI sequences have been shown to be associated with *short-term* (96,97) *but not intermediate- or long-term* dysfunction persisting for more than 3 months (26,98,99). Several prior studies have shown a correlation between focal lesions on early conventional brain MRI and intermediate- to long-term outcome in mild-to-severe (100–104) or moderate-to-severe TBI (105,106); however, in these studies there was no investigation of the *differential* predictive power of MRI, after adjusting for previously validated (5,7) predictors of long-term outcome in moderate-to-severe TBI including age, GCS, pupillary reactivity, and admission head CT features.

More advanced MRI techniques hold great promise for both characterization and outcome prediction in acute, subacute, and chronic stages of TBI (62,107–109). To date, there has been intensive investigation of DTI studies of FA changes in mild TBI, through region-of-interest, voxel-based techniques including tract-based spatial statistics, MR spectroscopy, and resting-state functional MRI (fMRI) (62,107–109). These advanced MRI techniques show great promise for outcome prediction in the area of mild TBI. Although these techniques are not currently widely implemented, largely because no consensus exists regarding their practical application to outcome prediction in the individual patient, group

differences between patients with mild brain injury and controls have already been demonstrated. It is highly likely that such emerging MRI techniques, in conjunction with statistically driven analysis of MR images, will continue to advance to the stage of routine use in not only diagnosis but also long-term management, guidance of rehabilitation therapy and/or clinical trials of therapies in TBI, and estimation of prognosis.

Another area of active research is the use of automated measurements of whole brain volume and, more recently, automated measurements of cortical volume, white matter volume, and specific subcortical gray matter structures following automated brain segmentation to diagnose and monitor diseases such as TBI, Alzheimer disease, and other neurodegenerative disorders. Many studies have demonstrated evidence that some patients with TBI demonstrate a significantly faster rate of atrophy on serial MRI, and/or that the rate of atrophy correlates with long-term outcome measures (110–113). Rate of atrophy of whole-brain volume or of individual brain structures therefore holds promise as a marker for TBI. It should be emphasized that, although such findings may support a diagnosis of TBI, the presence of brain atrophy may be seen in a variety of situations: dehydration, steroid and other medication usage, diabetes, hypertension, prior infection, alcohol use, stress, and numerous congenital medical conditions, to name just a few. More investigation is needed to determine the sensitivity and specificity of this technique over the spectrum of injury, from the mildest concussion to the severest brain injuries, and how it can be applied practically to improve diagnosis, outcome prediction, and clinical care.

CONCLUSION

Imaging will likely play an increasing and ubiquitous role in the clinical management of TBI, across the spectrum of severity from concussion to profound injury, and from the earliest time of acute management decisions and early outcome predictions, through guidance and monitoring of therapies during rehabilitation and recovery. The role of noncontrast head CT in immediate patient management—and the imaging appearance of TBI lesions on both CT and conventional brain MRI sequences—are already well established. CT angiography as a screening tool for traumatic vascular lesions in a subset of high-risk patients also has a relatively firmly established role.

Unlike noncontrast CT and CT angiography, MRI in TBI is an active area of research that is still in relatively early stages. Although CT is generally preferred in acutely injured patients, MRI is preferable to CT in subacute and chronic head injury and may also be helpful as a follow-up test in the setting of unexplained neurological deficits, in suspected abusive head trauma and in other medicolegal settings to establish a diagnosis of TBI when CT abnormalities are absent or equivocal. Finally, despite some success in the early prediction of long-term functional outcome after acute TBI, it is widely recognized that existing outcome models based on demographic and early clinical and imaging parameters still fail to satisfactorily account for the wide variability in hospital course and long-term levels of dysfunction that are observed following acute brain injury (86–88). More advanced MRI techniques, including DTI, MR spectroscopy, resting-state fMRI, and new image processing and analysis techniques such as automated brain segmentation and volumetric measurements, hold great promise for both characterization and outcome prediction in acute, subacute, and chronic stages of TBI. As our understanding of TBI pathophysiology improves, and our ability to visualize and characterize pathoanatomic lesions progresses through these new techniques, the definitions of pathoanatomic lesions and the best methods for characterizing them, and how to apply this information to clinical management, will continue to evolve.

KEY CLINICAL POINTS

1. The role of CT as the initial brain imaging modality in acute TBI is firmly established.
2. Findings on the initial noncontrast head CT are key to immediate decisions regarding the need for hospitalization, ICU admission, and/or early surgical management including both ICP monitor placement and the need for decompressive hemicraniectomy.
3. Conventional MRI sequences have superior *sensitivity* relative to noncontrast head CT for identification of certain acute pathoanatomic findings including hemorrhagic traumatic axonal injury, small cortical contusions, and small extra-axial collections.
4. Although no clear consensus exists on the current clinical role of MRI in acute TBI, it is sometimes used as a follow-up test after CT has been performed, particularly in the setting of unexplained persistent altered LOC in the hospitalized patient, in suspected abusive head trauma (AHT) to assess for evidence of traumatic intracranial injuries of different ages, and in other medicolegal settings to establish a diagnosis of TBI when CT abnormalities are absent or equivocal.
5. MRI for the characterization of both acute and remote brain injury is a highly active area of research still in relatively early stages. As our understanding of and ability to visualize pathology continue to progress, the definitions of pathoanatomic lesions and the best methods for characterizing them using both conventional and emerging advanced MRI techniques, and how to apply this information to clinical management, will continue to evolve.

KEY REFERENCES

1. Gean AD. *Imaging of Head Trauma.* New York, NY: Raven Press; 1994.
2. Gentry LR, Godersky JC, Thompson B. MR imaging of head trauma: review of the distribution and radiopathologic features of traumatic lesions. *AJR Am J Roentgenol.* 1988;150:663–672.
3. Haacke EM, Duhaime AC, Gean AD, et al. Common data elements in radiologic imaging of traumatic brain injury. *J Magn Reson Imaging.* 2010;32(3):516–543.
4. Levine B, Fujiwara E, O'Connor C, et al. In vivo characterization of traumatic brain injury neuropathology with structural and functional neuroimaging. *J Neurotrauma.* 2006;23(10):1396–1411.
5. Niogi SN, Mukherjee P. Diffusion tensor imaging of mild traumatic brain injury. *J Head Trauma Rehabil.* 2010;25: 241–255.

References

1. Guidelines for the management of severe head injury. Brain Trauma Foundation, American Association of Neurological Surgeons, Joint Section on Neurotrauma and Critical Care. *J Neurotrauma.* 1996;13(11):641–734.
2. The Brain Trauma Foundation. The American Association of Neurological Surgeons. The Joint Section on Neurotrauma and Critical Care. Resuscitation of blood pressure and oxygenation. *J Neurotrauma.* 2000;17(6–7):471–478.
3. Chestnut RM, Ghajar J, Maas AR. Guidelines for the management and prognosis of severe traumatic brain injury, Part II: early indicators of prognosis in severe traumatic brain injury. *J Neurotrauma.* 2000;17:556–627.
4. Maas AI, Stocchetti N, Bullock R. Moderate and severe traumatic brain injury in adults. *Lancet.* 2008;7:728–741.
5. Maas AI, Hukkelhoven CW, Marshall LF, Steyerberg EW. Prediction of outcome in traumatic brain injury with computed tomographic characteristics: a comparison between the computed tomographic classification and combinations of computed tomographic predictors. *Neurosurgery.* 2005;57:1173–1182.
6. Marshall LF, Eisenberg HM, Jane JA, Marshall SB, Klauber MR. A new classification of head injury based on computerized tomography. *J Neurosurgery.* 1991;75:S14–S20.
7. Steyerberg EW, Mushkudiani N, Perel P, et al. Predicting outcome after traumatic brain injury: development and international validation of prognostic scores based on admission characteristics. *PLoS Med.* 2008;5(8):e165.
8. Jagoda AS, Bazarian JJ, Bruns JJ Jr, et al; for the American College of Emergency Physicians, Centers for Disease Control and Prevention. Clinical policy: neuroimaging and decisionmaking in adult mild traumatic brain injury in the acute setting. *Ann Emerg Med.* 2008;52(6):714–748.
9. Jagoda AS, Cantrill SV, Wears RL, et al; for the American College of Emergency Physicians. Clinical policy: neuroimaging and decisionmaking in adult mild traumatic brain injury in the acute setting. *Ann Emerg Med.* 2002;40(2):231–249.
10. Centers for Disease Control and Prevention. Injury fact book. 2006. CDC Web site. http://www.cdc.gov/Injury/Publications/FactBook. Accessed July 16, 2012.
11. Iverson GL, Lovell MR, Smith S, Franzen MD. Prevalence of abnormal CT scans following mild head injury. *Brain Inj.* 2000;14: 1057–1061.
12. Borg J, Holm L, Cassidy JD, et al. Diagnostic procedures in mild traumatic brain injury: results of the WHO Collaborating Centre Task Force on mild traumatic brain injury. *J Rehabil Med.* 2004; (43)(suppl):61–75.
13. Stiell IG, Wells GA, Vandemheen K, et al. The Canadian CT Head Rule for patients with minor head injury. *Lancet.* 2001;357(9266): 1391–1396.
14. Haydel MJ, Preston CA, Mills TJ, Luber S, Blaudeau E, DeBlieux PM. Indications for computed tomography in patients with minor head injury. *N Engl J Med.* 2000;343:100–105.
15. Haacke EM, Duhaime AC, Gean AD, et al. Common data elements in radiologic imaging of traumatic brain injury. *J Magn Reson Imaging.* 2010;32:516–543.
16. Wang MC, Linnau KF, Tirschwell DL, Hollingworth W. Utility of repeat computed tomography after blunt head trauma: a systematic review. *J Trauma.* 2006;61:226–233.
17. Smith JS, Chang EF, Rosenthal G, et al. The role of early follow-up computed tomography imaging in the management of traumatic brain injury patients with intracranial hemorrhage. *J Trauma.* 2007;63(1):75–82.
18. Sifri ZC, Homnick AT, Vaynman A, et al. A prospective evaluation of the value of repeat cranial computed tomography in patients with minimal head injury and an intracranial bleed. *J Trauma.* 2006; 61(4):862–867.
19. Brown CV, Zada G, Salim A, et al. Indications for routine repeat head computed tomography (CT) stratified by severity of traumatic brain injury. *J Trauma.* 2007;62(6):1339–1345.
20. American Academy of Pediatrics. The management of minor closed head injury in children. *Pediatrics.* 1999;104(6):1407–1415.
21. Barkovich AJ, Raybaud C. *Pediatric Neuroimaging.* 5th ed. Philadelphia, PA: Lippincott Williams and Wilkins; 2012.

22. Beauchamp MH, Ditchfield M, Babl FE, et al. Detecting traumatic brain lesions in children: CT versus MRI versus susceptibility weighted imaging (SWI). *J Neurotrauma*. 2011;28(6):915–927.

23. Gentry LR, Godersky JC, Thompson B, Dunn VD. Prospective comparative study of intermediate-field MR and CT in the evaluation of closed head trauma. *AJR Am J Roentgenol*. 1988;150:673–682.

24. Jenkins A, Hadley MDM, Teasdale G, Macpherson P, Rowan JO. Brain lesions detected by magnetic resonance imaging in mild and severe head injuries. *Lancet*. 1986;328:445–446.

25. Kelly AB, Zimmerman RD, Snow RB, Gandy SE, Heier LA, Deck MD. Head trauma: comparison of MR and CT—experience in 100 patients. *AJNR Am J Neuroradiol*. 1988;9:699–708.

26. Lee H, Wintermark M, Gean AD, Ghajar J, Manley GT, Mukherjee P. Focal lesions in acute mild traumatic brain injury and neurocognitive outcome: CT versus 3T MRI. *J Neurotrauma*. 2008;25: 1049–1056.

27. Mittl RL, Grossman RI, Hiehle JF, et al. Prevalence of MR evidence of diffuse axonal injury in patients with mild head injury and normal head CT findings. *AJNR Am J Neuroradiol*. 1994;15(8): 1583–1589.

28. Orrison WW, Gentry LL, Stimac GK, Tarrel RM, Espinosa MC, Cobb LC. Blinded comparison of cranial CT and MRI in closed head injury evaluation. *AJNR Am J Neuroradiol*. 1994;15:351–356.

29. Uchino Y, Okimura Y, Tanaka M, Saeki N, Yamaura A. Computed tomography and magnetic resonance imaging of mild head injury—is it appropriate to classify patients with Glasgow Coma Scale score of 13 to 15 as "mild injury"? *Acta Neurochir (Wien)*. 2001;143:1031–1037.

30. Gean AD. *Imaging of Head Trauma*. New York, NY: Raven Press; 1994.

31. Rocchi G, Caroli E, Raco A, Salvati M, Delfini R. Traumatic epidural hematoma in children. *J Child Neurol*. 2005;20:569–571.

32. Nayil K, Ramzan A, Arif S, et al. Hypodensity of extradural hematomas in children: an ominous sign. *J Neurosurg Pediatr*. 2011;8: 417–421.

33. Huisman TA, Tschirch FT. Epidural hematoma in children: do cranial sutures act as a barrier? *J Neuroradiol*. 2009;36:93–97.

34. Gean AD, Fischbein NJ, Purcell DD, Aiken AH, Manley GT, Stiver SI. Benign anterior temporal epidural hematoma: indolent lesion with a characteristic CT imaging appearance after blunt head trauma. *Radiology*. 2010;257:212–218.

35. Reed D, Robertson WD, Graeb DA, Lapointe JS, Nugent RA, Woodhurst WB. Acute subdural hematomas: atypical CT findings. *AJNR Am J Neuroradiol*. 1986;7:417–421.

36. Parizel PM, Makkat S, Van Miert E, Van Goethem JW, van den Hauwe L, De Schepper AM. Intracranial hemorrhage: principles of CT and MRI interpretation. *Eur Radiol*. 2001;11:1770–783.

37. Lee KS, Bae WK, Doh JW, Yun IG. The computed tomographic attenuation and the age of subdural hematomas. *J Korean Med Sci*. 1997;12:353–359.

38. Yuan MK, Lai PH, Chen JY, et al. Detection of subarachnoid hemorrhage at acute and subacute/chronic stages: comparison of four magnetic resonance imaging pulse sequences and computed tomography. *J Chin Med Assoc*. 2005;68(3):131–137.

39. Noguchi K, Ogawa T, Seto H, et al. Subacute and chronic subarachnoid hemorrhage: diagnosis with fluid-attenuated inversion-recovery MR imaging. *Radiology*. 1997;203:257–262.

40. Tian HL, Xu T, Cui YH, Chen H, Zhou LF. Risk factors related to hydrocephalus after traumatic subarachnoid hemorrhage. *Surg Neurol*. 2008;69:241–246.

41. Gentry LR, Godersky JC, Thompson B. MR imaging of head trauma: review of the distribution and radiopathologic features of traumatic lesions. *AJR Am J Roentgenol*. 1988;150:663–672.

42. Yamaki T, Hirakawa K, Ueguchi T, Tenjin H, Kuboyama T, Nakagawa Y. Chronological evaluation of acute traumatic intracerebral hematoma. *Acta Neurochir (Wien)*. 1990;103:112–115.

43. Hesselink JR, Dowd CF, Healy ME, Hajek P, Baker LL, Luerssen TG. MR imaging of brain contusions: a comparative study with CT. *AJR Am J Roentgenol*. 1988;150:1133–1142.

44. Duhaime AC, Gean AD, Haacke EM, Hicks R, Wintermark M, Mukherjee P. Common data elements in radiologic imaging of traumatic brain injury. *Arch Phys Med Rehabil*. 2010;91:1661–1666.

45. Cotran RS, Kumar V, Collins T, Robbins SL. *Pathologic Basis of Disease*. 6th ed. Philadelphia, PA: Saunders; 1999.

46. Strich SJ. Shearing of nerve fibers as a cause of brain damage due to head injury, a pathological study of twenty cases. *Lancet*. 1961; 2:443–448.

47. Strich SJ. Diffuse degeneration of the cerebral white matter in severe dementia following head injury. *J Neurol Neurosurg Psychiatry*. 1956;19:163–185.

48. Holbourn AHS. Mechanics of head injuries. *Lancet*. 1943;2:438–441.

49. Adams JH, Graham DI, Murray LS, Scott G. Diffuse axonal injury due to non-missile head injury in humans: an analysis of 45 cases. *Ann Neurol*. 1982;12:557–563.

50. Adams JH, Gennarelli TA, Graham DI. Brain damage in non-missile head injury: observations in man and subhuman primates. Edinburgh, United Kingdom: Churchill Livingston; 1982.

51. Tong KA, Ashwal S, Holshouser BA, et al. Hemorrhagic shearing lesions in children and adolescents with posttraumatic diffuse axonal injury: improved detection and initial results. *Radiology*. 2003; 227:332–339.

52. Mittal S, Wu Z, Neelavalli J, Haacke EM. Susceptibility-weighted imaging: technical aspects and clinical applications, part 2. *AJNR Am J Neuroradiol*. 2009;30:232–252.

53. Li XY, Feng DF. Diffuse axonal injury: novel insights into detection and treatment. *J Clin Neurosci*. 2009;16:614–619.

54. Kuzma BB, Goodman JM. Improved identification of axonal shear injuries with gradient echo MR technique. *Surg Neurol*. 2000;53: 400–402.

55. Haacke EM, Xu Y, Cheng YC, Reichenbach JR. Susceptibility weighted imaging (SWI). *Magn Reson Med*. 2004;52(3):612–618.

56. Ashikaga R, Araki Y, Ishida O. MRI of head injury using FLAIR. *Neuroradiology*. 1997;39:239–242.

57. Liu AY, Maldjian JA, Bagley LJ, Sinson GP, Grossman RI. Traumatic brain injury: diffusion-weighted MR imaging findings. *AJNR Am J Neuroradiol*. 1999;20:1636–1641.

58. Huisman TA. Diffusion-weighted imaging: basic concept and application in cerebral stroke and head trauma. *Eur Radiol*. 2003;13: 2283–2297.

59. Schaefer PW, Huisman TAGM, Sorensen AG, Gonzalez RG, Schwamm LH. Diffusion-weighted MR imaging in closed head injury: high correlation with initial Glasgow Coma Scale score and score on Modified Ranking scale at discharge. *Radiology*. 2004;233: 58–66.

60. Pierpaoli C, Barnett A, Pajevic S, et al. Water diffusion changes in Wallerian degeneration and their dependence on white matter architecture. *Neuroimage*. 2001;13:1174–1185.

61. Arfanakis K, Haughton VM, Carew JD, Rogers BP, Dempsey RJ, Meyerand ME. Diffusion tensor MR imaging in diffuse axonal injury. *AJNR Am J Neuroradiol*. 2002;23:794–802.

62. Niogi SN, Mukherjee P. Diffusion tensor imaging of mild traumatic brain injury. *J Head Trauma Rehabil*. 2010;25:241–255.

63. Mukherjee P, Berman JI, Chung SW, Henry RG. Diffusion tensor MR imaging and fiber tractography: theoretic underpinnings. *AJNR Am J Neuroradiol*. 2008;29:632–641.

64. Mukherjee P, Chung SW, Berman JI, Hess CP, Henry RG. Diffusion tensor MR imaging and fiber tractography: technical considerations. *AJNR Am J Neuroradiol*. 2008;29:843–852.

65. Le TH, Mukherjee P, Henry RG, Berman JI, Ware M, Manley GT. Diffusion tensor imaging with three-dimensional fiber tractography of traumatic axonal shearing injury: an imaging correlate for the posterior callosal "disconnection" syndrome: case report. *Neurosurgery*. 2005;56:189.

66. Huisman TA, Schwamm LH, Schaefer PW, et al. Diffusion tensor imaging as potential biomarker of white matter injury in diffuse axonal injury. *AJNR Am J Neuroradiol*. 2004;25(3):370–376.

67. Kraus MF, Susmaras T, Caughlin BP, Walker CJ, Sweeney JA, Little DM. White matter integrity and cognition in chronic traumatic brain injury: a diffusion tensor imaging study. *Brain*. 2007;130: 2508–2519.

68. Niogi SN, Mukherjee P, Ghajar J, et al. Extent of microstructural white matter injury in postconcussive syndrome correlates with impaired cognitive reaction time: a 3T diffusion tensor imaging

study of mild traumatic brain injury. *AJNR Am J Neuroradiol*. 2008; 29:967–973.

69. Niogi SN, Mukherjee P, Ghajar J, et al. Structural dissociation of attentional control and memory in adults with and without mild traumatic brain injury. *Brain*. 2008;131:3209–3221.

70. Imaizumi T, Miyata K, Inamura S, Kohama I, Nyon KS, Nomura T. The difference in location between traumatic cerebral microbleeds and microangiopathic microbleed associated with stroke. *J Neuroimaging*. 2011;21:359–364.

71. Parizel PM, Makkat S, Jorens PG, et al. Brainstem hemorrhage in descending transtentorial herniation (Duret hemorrhage). *Intensive Care Med*. 2002;28:85–88.

72. Yuh EL, Dillon WP. Intracranial hypotension and intracranial hypertension. *Neuroimaging Clin N Am*. 2010;20:597–617.

73. Sliker CW. Blunt cerebrovascular injuries: imaging with multidetector CT angiography. *Radiographics*. 2008;28:1689–1710.

74. Biffl WL, Moore EE, Offner PJ, et al. Optimizing screening for blunt cerebrovascular injuries. *Am J Surg*. 1999;178:517–521.

75. Miller PR, Fabian TC, Croce MA, et al. Prospective screening or blunt cerebrovascular injuries. *Ann Surg*. 2002;236:386–395.

76. Biffl WL, Cothren CC, Moore EE, et al. Western Trauma Association critical decisions in trauma: screening for and treatment of blunt cerebrovascular injuries. *J Trauma*. 2009;67:1150–1153.

77. Cothren CC, Moore EE, Ray CE, et al. Screening for blunt cerebrovascular injuries is cost-effective. *Am J Surg*. 2005;190:849–854.

78. McKevitt EC, Kirkpatrick AW, Vertesi L, Granger R, Simons RK. Blunt vascular neck injuries: diagnosis and outcomes of extracranial vessel injury. *J Trauma*. 2002;53:472–476.

79. van Wessem KJ, Meijer JM, Leenen LP, van der Worp HB, Moll FL, de Borst GJ. Blunt traumatic carotid artery dissection still a pitfall? The rationale for aggressive screening. *Eur J Trauma Emerg Surg*. 2011;37(2):147–154.

80. Mayberry JC, Brown CV, Mullins RJ, Velmahos GC. Blunt carotid injury: the futility of aggressive screening and diagnosis. *Arch Surg*. 2004;139:609–613.

81. Stein DM, Boswell S, Sliker CW, Lui FY, Scalea TM. Blunt cerebrovascular injuries: does treatment always matter? *J Trauma*. 2009; 66:132–144.

82. Mascalchi M, Bianchi MC, Mangiafico S, et al. MRI and MR angiography of vertebral artery dissection. *Neuroradiology*. 1997;39: 329–340.

83. Provenzale JM, Sarikaya B. Comparison of test performance characteristics of MRI, MR angiography, and CT angiography in the diagnosis of carotid and vertebral artery dissection: a review of the medical literature. *AJR Am J Roentgenol*. 2009;193:1167–1174.

84. Rangel-Castilla L, Gopinath S, Robertson CS. Management of intracranial hypertension. *Neurol Clin*. 2008;26:521–541.

85. Juul N, Morris GF, Marshall SB, Marshall LF. Intracranial hypertension and cerebral perfusion pressure: influence on neurological deterioration and outcome in severe head injury. The Executive Committee of the International Selfotel Trial. *J Neurosurg*. 2000;92: 1–6.

86. Aarabi B, Hesdorffer DC, Ahn ES, Aresco C, Scalea TM, Eisenberg HM. Outcome following decompressive craniectomy for malignant swelling due to severe head injury. *J Neurosurg*. 2006;104(4): 469–479.

87. Cooper DJ, Rosenfeld JV, Murray LS, et al. Decompressive craniectomy in diffuse traumatic brain injury. *New Engl J Med*. 2011;364: 1493–1502.

88. Hutchinson PJ, Corteen E, Czosnyka M, et al. Decompressive craniectomy in traumatic brain injury: the randomized multicenter RESCUEicp study (www.RESCUEicp.com). *Acta Neurochir Suppl*. 2006;96:17–20.

89. Murray GD, Butcher I, McHugh GS, et al. Multivariable prognostic analysis in traumatic brain injury: results from the IMPACT study. *J Neurotrauma*. 2007;24(2):329–337.

90. Dikmen S, Machamer J, Temkin N. Mild head injury: facts and artifacts. *J Clin Exp Neuropsychol*. 2001;23:729–738.

91. McCauley SR, Boake C, Levin HS, Contant CF, Song JX. Postconcussional disorder following mild to moderate traumatic brain injury: anxiety, depression, and social support as risk factors and comorbidities. *J Clin Exp Neuropsychol*. 2001;23:792–808.

92. Jacobs B, Beems T, Stulemeijer M, et al. Outcome prediction in mild traumatic brain injury: age and clinical variables are stronger predictors than CT abnormalities. *J Neurotrauma*. 2010;27(4): 655–668.

93. Smits M, Hunink MG, van Rijssel DA. Outcome after complicated minor head injury. *AJNR Am J Neuroradiol*. 2008;29:506–513.

94. Zumstein MA, Moser M, Mottini M, et al. Long-term outcome in patients with mild traumatic brain injury: a prospective observational study. *J Trauma*. 2011;71:120–127.

95. Williams DH, Levin HS, Eisenberg HM. Mild head injury classification. *Neurosurgery*. 1990;27:422–428.

96. Kurca E, Sivak S, Kucera P. Impaired cognitive functions in mild traumatic brain injury patients with normal and pathologic magnetic resonance imaging. *Neuroradiology*. 2006;48:661–669.

97. Levin HS, Amparo E, Eisenberg HM, et al. Magnetic resonance imaging and computerized tomography in relation to the neurobehavioral sequelae of mild and moderate head injuries. *J Neurosurg*. 1987;66(5):706–713.

98. Hughes DG, Jackson A, Mason DL, Berry E, Hollis S, Yates DW. Abnormalities on magnetic resonance imaging seen acutely following mild traumatic brain injury: correlation with neuropsychological tests and delayed recovery. *Neuroradiology*. 2004;46:550–558.

99. Wilson JT, Wiedemann KD, Hadley DM, Condon B, Teasdale G, Brooks DM. Early and late magnetic resonance imaging and neuropsychological outcome after head injury. *J Neurol Neurosurg Psychiatry*. 1988;51:391–396.

100. Chastain CA, Oyoyo UE, Zipperman M, et al. Predicting outcomes of traumatic brain injury by imaging modality and injury distribution. *J Neurotrauma*. 2009;26:1183–1196.

101. Hiekkanen H, Kurki T, Brandstack N, Kairisto V, Tenovuo O. Association of injury severity, MRI-results and ApoE genotype with 1-year outcome in mainly mild TBI: a preliminary study. *Brain Inj*. 2009;23:396–402.

102. Scheid R, Preul C, Gruber O, Wiggins C, von Cramon DY. Diffuse axonal injury associated with chronic traumatic brain injury: evidence from T2*-weighted gradient-echo imaging at 3 T. *AJNR Am J Neuroradiol*. 2003;24(6):1049–1056.

103. Scheid R, Walther K, Guthke T, Preul C, von Cramon DY. Cognitive sequelae of diffuse axonal injury. *Arch Neurol*. 2006;63:418–424.

104. Sigmund GA, Tong KA, Nickerson JP, Wall CJ, Oyoyo U, Ashwal S. Multimodality comparison of neuroimaging in pediatric traumatic brain injury. *Pediatr Neurol*. 2007;36:217–226.

105. Mannion RJ, Cross J, Bradley P, et al. Mechanism-based MRI classification of traumatic brainstem injury and its relationship to outcome. *J Neurotrauma*. 2007;24:128–135.

106. van der Naalt J, Hew JM, van Zomeren AH, Sluiter WJ, Minderhous JM. Computed tomography and magnetic resonance imaging in mild to moderate head inury: early and late imaging related to outcome. *Ann Neurol*. 1999;46:70–78.

107. Kou Z, Wu Z, Tong KA, et al. The role of advanced MR imaging findings as biomarkers of traumatic brain injury. *J Head Trauma Rehabil*. 2010;25(4):267–282.

108. Levine B, Fujiwara E, O'Connor C, et al. In vivo characterization of traumatic brain injury neuropathology with structural and functional neuroimaging. *J Neurotrauma*. 2006;23(10):1396–1411.

109. Van Boven RW, Harrington GS, Hackney DB, et al. Advances in neuroimaging of traumatic brain injury and posttraumatic stress disorder. *J Rehabil Res Dev*. 2009;46(6):717–757.

110. Bigler ED, Maxwell WL. Neuroimaging and neuropathology of TBI. *NeuroRehabilitation*. 2011;28:63–74.

111. Irimia A, Chambers MC, Alger JR, et al. Comparison of acute and chronic traumatic brain injury using semi-automatic multimodal segmentation of MR volumes. *J Neurotrauma*. 2011;28(11):2287–2306.

112. Ng K, Mikulis DJ, Glazer J, et al. Magnetic resonance imaging evidence of progression of subacute brain atrophy in moderate to severe traumatic brain injury. *Arch Phys Med Rehabil*. 2008; 89(12)(suppl):S35–S44.

113. Ross DE. Review of longitudinal studies of MRI brain volumetry in patients with traumatic brain injury. *Brain Inj*. 2011;25:1271–1278.

16

Functional Neuroimaging

Joseph H. Ricker, Patricia M. Arenth, and Amy K. Wagner

INTRODUCTION

New technologies, as well as advances in existing technologies, continue to change how the brains of both healthy and injured individuals are evaluated in research and clinical settings. In combination with traditional neuromedical examination and psychometric testing, functional neuroimaging is providing a means through which additional information about brain structure, function, and recovery may be obtained. Enthusiasm for the application of functional neuroimaging can be readily appreciated, yet it must be balanced by the need for empirical evidence and a healthy level of caution.

Increasingly, clinicians are using advanced imaging techniques (e.g., single photon emission computed tomography [SPECT], positron emission tomography [PET], functional magnetic resonance imaging [FMRI]) among persons with traumatic brain injury (TBI). Clinical application of most of these techniques still remains investigational, however, within the TBI population (1). The present chapter provides an overview of several functional neuroimaging procedures and their applications in the context of TBI. This chapter will also address many limitations of these procedures, with guidelines for exercising appropriate care if they are used in clinical evaluation.

RESTING AND ACTIVATED FUNCTIONAL NEUROIMAGING

In functional neuroimaging, one can dichotomize the available techniques into 2 broad categories: "resting" or "activated" (2). Resting paradigms are those that acquire functional images during nonactivated (i.e., "static" or baseline) conditions. Resting studies, by design, have no explicit or systematic requirements of the participant other than those required to successfully acquire a technically valid image, such as having the participant lie still, minimizing head movement, and eliminating extraneous stimuli (3). Although participants do not overtly engage in any specific task, there is no systematic way to "control" random or volitional covert mental activity during the image acquisition. There have been several studies that have applied resting functional neuroimaging across multiple populations, most of which have examined chronic glucose uptake (with PET) and resting cerebral blood flow (CBF) (using PET or SPECT). These studies will be discussed later in context.

In contrast to resting paradigms, activation studies require participants to systematically receive sensory input (e.g., a visual array) or engage in an activity (e.g., motor or cognitive) to elicit changes in brain physiology that are correlated with a specific stimulus or event in time (4). These tasks are usually administered in adherence to a strict protocol, typically with some form of overt response required to provide an objective correlate of the participant's active engagement in the task. Because of the physical properties of the dependent variables examined (e.g., briefer half-lives of radioisotopes or transient changes in hemodynamic response), activation studies have much briefer time sampling windows than resting studies. Certain imaging techniques are able to depict changes over time in a somewhat continuous manner (e.g., event-related FMRI and magnetoencephalography [MEG]). With this level of experimental control, researchers are in a better position to make inferences about cerebral activity associated with the underlying cognitive process under investigation (5). Figure 16-1 presents an example.

SINGLE PHOTON EMISSION COMPUTED TOMOGRAPHY

SPECT is an approach to functional imaging that is based on the concept that regional changes in brain activity or chemistry can be measured indirectly via externally placed gamma radiation detectors (referred to as "cameras"), which detect the regional accumulations of tracer flow or receptor-binding isotopes. Although the emphasis of SPECT studies tends to be on regional cerebral blood flow (rCBF), specific neuroreceptor imaging studies are also possible with this technology (6).

The dependent variable in SPECT derives from the well-established principle of increased cerebral activity correlating with increased blood flow. That is, when neural activity in a region of the brain increases, related energy requirements also increase. Because the blood supply carries glucose and oxygen to the brain, the flow of blood to the active area increases (7). The radioisotopes themselves are absorbed into glial cells that are proximal to the active neurons, but these isotopes are not immediately excreted. Thus, the absorbed radioisotopes remain in greater concentration in the more active areas. There are also radioisotopes available that bind to specific types of receptors, for example, dopamine (6).

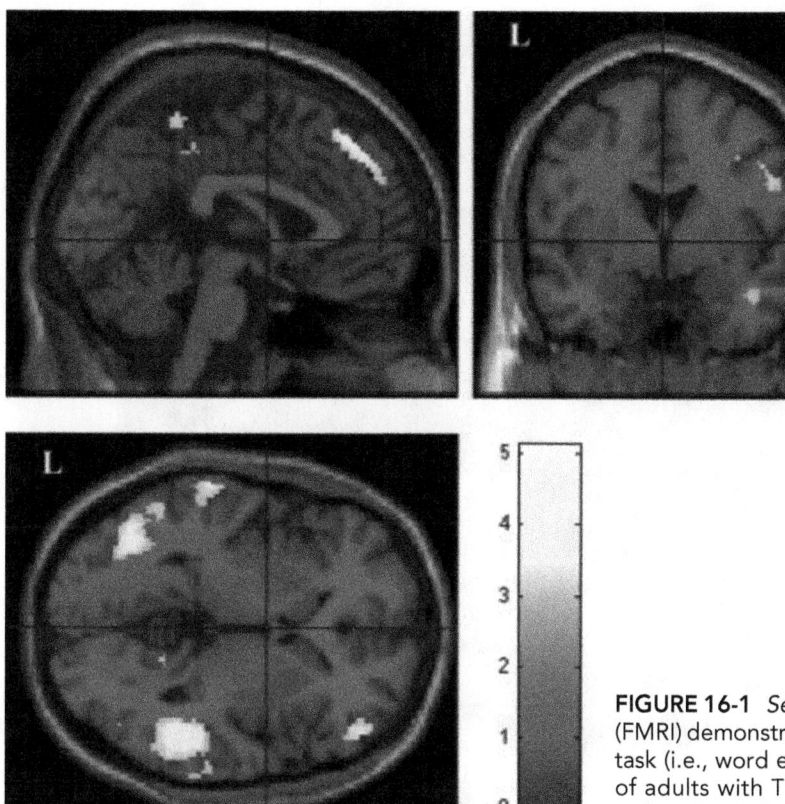

FIGURE 16-1 *See color insert.* Functional magnetic resonance imaging (FMRI) demonstrating regions of functional activation during a cognitive task (i.e., word encoding contrasted with picture encoding) in a group of adults with TBI. Adapted from Russell, Arenth, Scanlon, Kessler, Ricker (81) with permission.

Through normal radioactive decay, the isotope emits annihilated radioactive particles (i.e., photons), which are then detected by the external detectors (sometimes referred to as cameras). Computer-based reconstruction permits external representations to be derived that correlate with differences in blood flow. Compared to some of the other functional imaging techniques, there are certain advantages to SPECT (8). SPECT is more widely available than PET or FMRI. Unlike PET, the radioisotopes usually employed in SPECT can be prepared or shipped in advance, thus dispensing with the need for an on-site cyclotron and chemist.

SPECT has application in examining resting blood flow, and it has limited use in imaging a change in blood flow from one time point to another, for example, from preictal to ictal state (9). It is not appropriate, however, for use in mapping rapid changes in blood flow that occur within a single scanning session, such as encountered in most cognitive activity (6). SPECT has some potential for investigating discrete cognitive processes if multiple scanning sessions are used and explicit experimental task conditions and complex subtraction analyses that are not typically employed for clinical studies (10). SPECT is also not as diverse as other imaging techniques, such as PET, but novel ligands are under continuous development (11). Recent technologic advances have provided for multiple detector scanners, with the result being improved spatial resolution.

Regarding all assessment tools, SPECT has several sources of potential measurement error (12). Unlike other techniques (e.g., PET), SPECT requires that regional counts be normalized to an area that is presumed to be free from injury and/or physiologic abnormality, and its resolution does not yet approach that of PET imaging. This latter concern has been attenuated somewhat with the increased availability of combined SPECT/computed tomography (CT) technology (13). Color SPECT image reconstruction can produce striking images, particularly when spatially rendered into 3-dimensional (3D) "maps," but reliable and valid interpretation is best accomplished through quantitative approaches given the subjectivity and lack of standardization associated with interpreting 3D images (14). It must be emphasized, however, that although SPECT can be used quantitatively, this is not the case in most settings. Visual inspection of SPECT maps is a qualitative process and interpretation may vary across clinicians. In addition, image reconstruction is typically based on presumptions about which brain regions are "normal." Relative flow values in SPECT are often based on a region such as the thalamus or cerebellum. Although such assumptions might be valid for some populations with focal lesions (e.g., stroke), they might not be valid for populations whose involvement is more diffused (e.g., TBI). SPECT is quite sensitive to detecting regional differences in resting blood flow, but there is little specificity to the patterns that are obtained, and the results depicted in series of SPECT images can be affected by many factors including acute or chronic emotional disturbances, medications, or current substance use (15,16).

SPECT Studies of Brain Injury

Resting brain SPECT studies of individuals acquired months (or sometimes years) after moderate and severe brain trauma have demonstrated decreased CBF, primarily within prefrontal cortex (15–17), as demonstrated in Figure 16-2. In

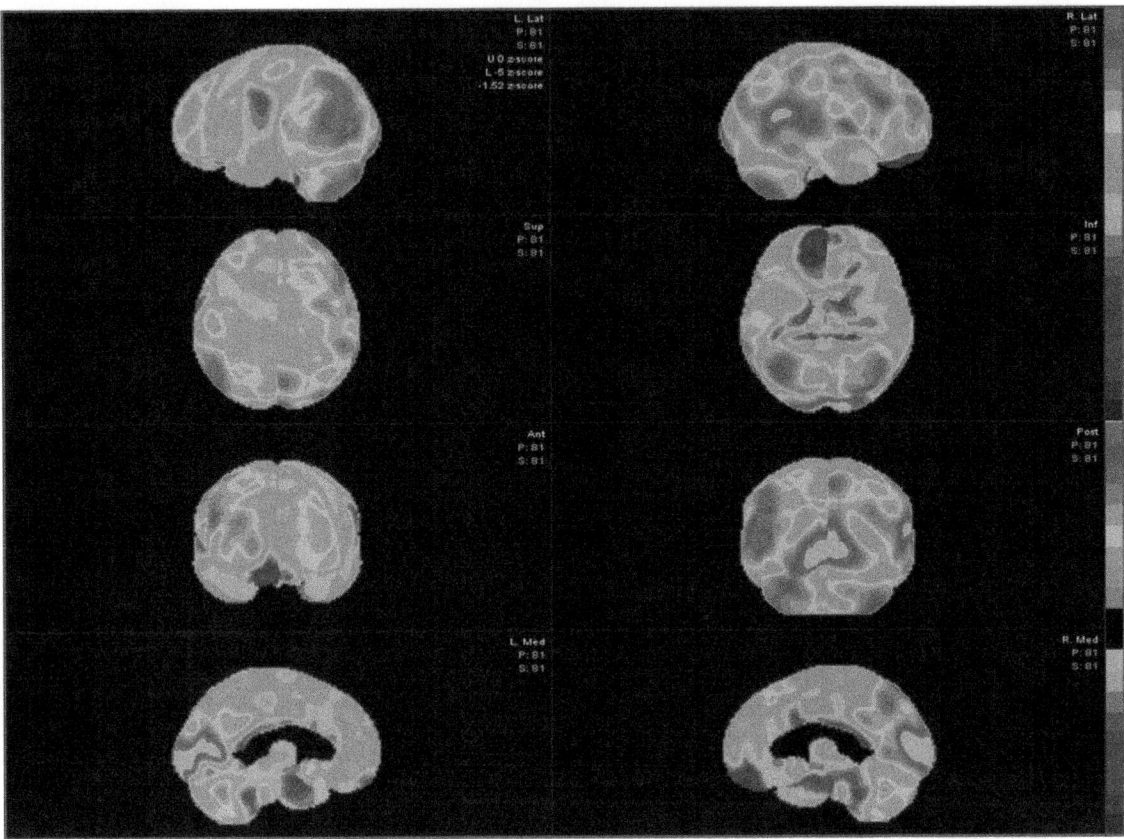

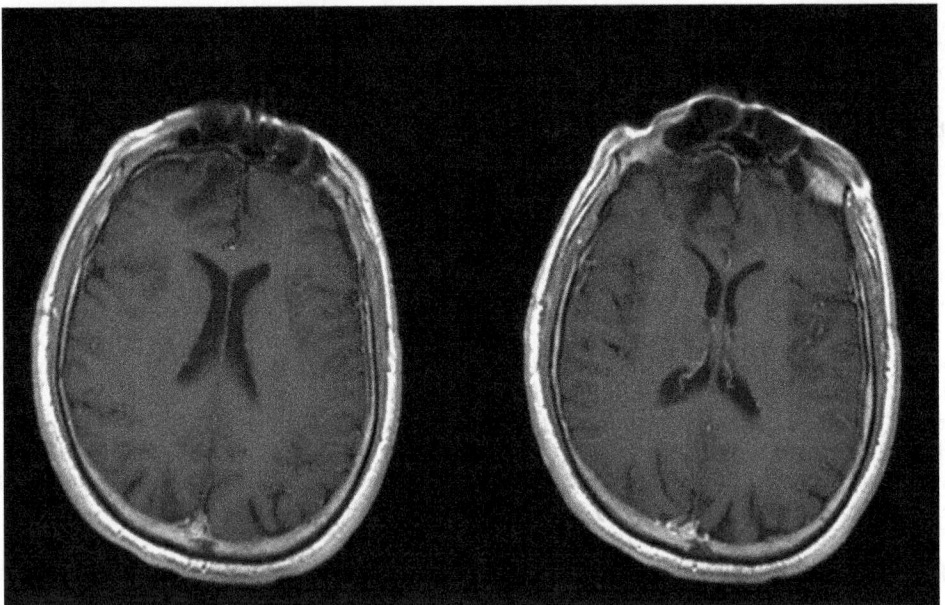

FIGURE 16-2 *See color insert.* Technetium-99m ethyl cysteinate dimer (Tc-99m-ECD) SPECT study and axial magnetic resonance imaging (MRI) slices of a man with history of motor vehicle crash and frontal lobe contusion. The SPECT surface map images show a corresponding ("purple/blue" color) deficit in the inferior right frontal lobe, consistent with an area of prior injury. This is best appreciated in column 2, in the second and fourth images downward. Image courtesy of Paul R. Jolles, MD, Department of Radiology, Virginia Commonwealth University Medical Center, Richmond, VA.

most of these studies, decreased blood flow and metabolism were generally beyond what might be expected based solely on findings from structural scans (i.e., CT and magnetic resonance imaging [MRI]). The presence of decreased resting blood flow or metabolism is not, however, in and of itself evidence of compromised or nonfunctional brain tissue (4).

Numerous investigations have demonstrated that SPECT is superior to CT and structural MRI in the detection of the presence and extent of trauma-related lesions. SPECT has been applied to mild brain injury and has demonstrated regionally decreased blood flow in the presence of normal acute CT scans, but there is much variability across individuals (i.e., no pathognomonic profile emerges). SPECT findings have also sometimes been demonstrated in cases of below average neuropsychological test scores in cases of mild brain trauma, but SPECT findings are usually not very predictive of neuropsychological test performance (18,19).

In spite of advances in technology and data analysis, the utility of SPECT in characterizing specific illness and injury states or predicting outcome remains controversial (16). Although not predictive, SPECT has some utility when correlating neuropsychological parameters with the effects of brain injury (20,21), but caution must be exercised given that SPECT findings are routinely positive in a variety of medical and neurological disorders (21–25), learning disabilities (26), as well as in substance use and emotional disorders (27–35). Some investigators have noted that when used in a *prospective* design, a negative SPECT scan is a good predictor of a favorable outcome after brain injury and that SPECT overall correlates well with the severity of the initial trauma (36). Still, there are relatively few well-controlled prospective studies of SPECT (and for that matter, PET and FMRI) being used in differential diagnosis, prognosis, and intervention (2,37). The use of normative data (8) rather than subjective impressions of SPECT images will greatly facilitate such developments.

SPECT has been shown to be of use in research studies following brain injury, but there is no particular SPECT profile that is pathognomonic or reliable for brain injury (16,37). Clinically, the literature does not support the routine use of SPECT for the evaluation of postconcussion syndrome (PCS) in specific or actually for brain injury in general. The Therapeutics and Technology Assessment Subcommittee of the American Academy of Neurology (38) has rated SPECT as an investigational procedure for the study of brain trauma. More recently in 2008, the American College of Radiology (1) continues to rate SPECT as inappropriate (a rating of 1 on a 1–9 scale, with 1 indicating *least appropriate*) in the evaluation of mild head trauma, with slightly increased appropriateness (a rating of 4 on the same scale) *"for selected cases"* of mild head trauma (across levels of injury severity) with associated neurologic or cognitive signs. In spite of the professional cautions and the present conclusions regarding the lack of scientific support for the routine use of SPECT in brain injury, SPECT appears to be used frequently in clinical and forensic contexts as a means of supporting a diagnosis of brain injury (39). With increasing evidence and appropriately designed studies, however, and greater specificity of diagnostic criteria (particularly with mild brain injury) and greater anatomic colocalization, SPECT is likely to be of

improved clinical utility in the future (40,41). SPECT has been found to be predictive of post-traumatic amnesia acutely after TBI (42) and useful in assessing the efficacy of intraventricular shunt placement after TBI (43). SPECT radioligands that label specific neurotransmitter systems or precursors are also seeing use. For example, 2-beta-carbomethoxy-3-beta-(4-fluorophenyl) tropane or CFT, a dopamine transporter-specific ligand, has been used to demonstrate nigrostriatal dysfunction after moderate and severe TBI even in the presence of a morphologically intact striatum (44).

POSITRON EMISSION TOMOGRAPHY

Like SPECT, PET is a radioisotope-based imaging technology. PET studies typically use intravenous tracers such as 18F-fluorodeoxyglucose (FDG) for the quantification of "resting" (i.e., nonactivated) regional brain metabolism (45). An exception is xenon, which is an inhaled isotope. As they are catabolized, annihilation particles are emitted and are detected by an external detector.

PET remains the "gold standard" for functional neuroimaging (46). PET has the capability of demonstrating specific biochemical or physiologic processes associated with CBF and metabolism (47). Radiolabeled ligands that target dopaminergic, serotonergic, and other receptor systems have been developed, as are genetically mediated transport markers and pathology-specific ligands (48).

PET has been widely used as a research tool since the 1970s, but requires a cyclotron to be present on site for most radioisotopes and remains a very expensive procedure. Thus, its application to persons with TBI has been minimally investigated. PET has the capability of demonstrating specific biochemical or physiologic processes associated with CBF and metabolism. As with SPECT, clinical data from PET imaging are typically portrayed visually in the form of the spatial distribution of radioisotopes projected on to actual or standardized anatomic MRI templates.

PET Studies of Brain Injury

Acute O-15 PET studies of human brain trauma have shown that significant changes in regional (but not necessarily global) hemodynamics occur, such as lower contusional and pericontusional blood flow and flow-to-volume ratios (49). There is also heterogeneity in regional glucose metabolism (50). In addition, cerebral hyperglycolysis is a pathophysiological response that occurs in response to injury-induced neurochemical cascades and can be demonstrated via FDG-PET (51,52), as illustrated in Figure 16-3.

Several studies have demonstrated PET's ability to detect brain abnormalities that are not visualized on CT or standard MRI sequences in cases of moderate and severe brain injury (2). In addition, functional imaging data exist to suggest that there can be regions of physiological dysfunction beyond the boundaries of anatomic lesions (e.g., contusions) seen with structural imaging. This has been demonstrated for many years using both FDG-PET (53) and

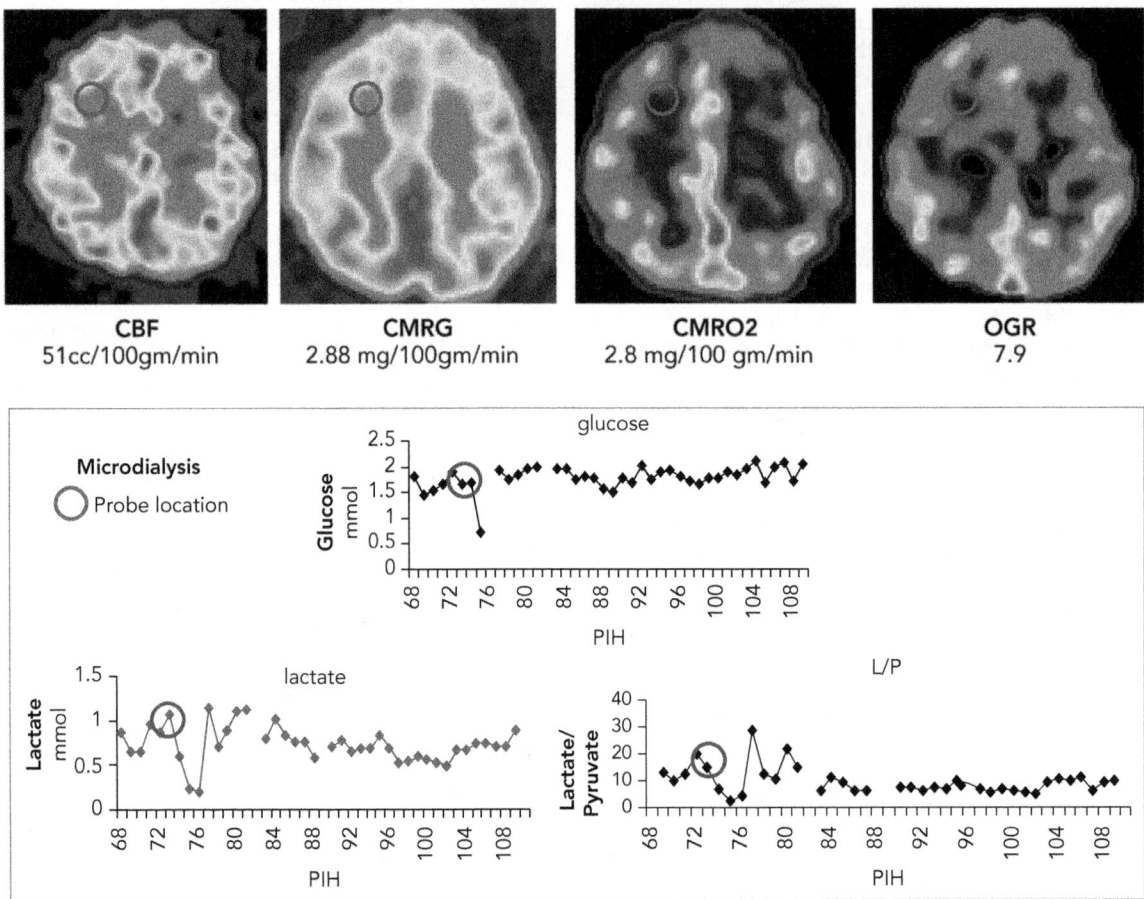

FIGURE 16-3 *See color insert.* Positron emission tomography (PET) study examining cerebral blood flow (CBF) and cerebral metabolic rate for glucose (CMRG) combined with cerebral microdialysis. The example shows elevation of the oxygen to glucose ratio in the setting of normal perfusion. This likely reflects alternative fuel use, perhaps lactate because the microdialysis lactate concentration in the extracellular compartment is low. Image courtesy of David Hovda, PhD, and Paul Vespa, MD, UCLA Brain Injury Research Center, David Geffen School of Medicine at UCLA, Los Angeles, CA.

Cobalt-55 PET (54). Such changes are seen acutely and occur more in gray matter relative to white matter, perhaps reflecting physiological diaschisis (55). Acute metabolic changes often begin to resolve within the first month following injury, regardless of injury severity, but the correlation between the extent of change in disability and the changes in brain metabolism are minimal (52).

Although PET would appear intuitively to lend itself well to the many clinical issues that emerge after brain trauma, there are surprisingly few studies that have actually attempted to directly relate functional imaging findings with cognition after TBI. In most of these studies, the findings from neuropsychological and other assessments have been obtained at times that were quite disparate from the time at which imaging occurred. For example, 1 frequently cited paper (56) described FDG-PET and neuropsychological test scores among a selected group of 9 individuals that had experienced mild head trauma. Their CT and MRI findings were negative, but PET imaging demonstrated a variety of regions of decreased FDG uptake, some (but not all) of which

corresponded to decreased cognitive testing scores. Such findings have little generalizability, however, given that subjects were specifically selected for inclusion based on their outcome criteria rather than criteria selected a priori. In addition, scanning and the neuropsychological evaluation were separated in time by an average of 11 months, thus essentially negating the reliability of any correlation between PET and cognitive findings.

In more carefully designed studies, the localized abnormal cerebral metabolic rates in frontal and temporal regions correlate with both subjective complaints and neuropsychological test results obtained during the chronic phase of recovery (57). In moderate and severe TBI, resting PET studies have demonstrated frontal hypometabolism, with related decreased performance on neuropsychological tests that are mediated by frontal lobe functioning (58). Through the use of PET, an association between post-TBI anosmia and orbitofrontal hypometabolism has been demonstrated (59). In another recent study, Ostberg and colleagues used PET to demonstrate that acetylcholinesterase activity was lower in persons with brain injury, even at more than 1-year postinjury, as compared to uninjured controls (60).

As described earlier in this chapter, activation studies are likely to be far more sensitive to the functional effects of brain injury or disease, as such paradigms introduce in vivo cognitive challenges (61). The first published PET study (62) to apply a cognitive activation paradigm with individuals that sustained brain injury demonstrated CBF changes in the left prefrontal cortex among individuals with TBI during a free recall task when compared to controls, but blood flow increases were noted in more posterior brain regions in TBI subjects during both free and cued recall. The change in allocation of neural resources during tasks with greater cognitive load may suggest increased cognitive effort among individuals with TBI (and thus greater blood flow within prefrontal cortex during task performance). During recognition tasks, both the controls and the individuals with TBI performed at comparable behavioral levels (and within normal limits), yet the individuals with TBI still demonstrated increased change in regional CBF relative to the controls. This suggests that after brain injury, individuals must exert more cognitive effort than controls to attain the same level of overt behavior. Subsequently, a different group of investigators also demonstrated comparable findings in a larger sample of individuals with TBI, again using O-15 PET and a verbal memory task (63).

FUNCTIONAL MAGNETIC RESONANCE-BASED IMAGING

Techniques based on MRI capitalize on the presence of hydrogen in all of the body's tissues. When the protons of hydrogen atoms encounter a strong magnetic field, they align in parallel to that field's direction. In MRI, radiofrequency (RF) pulses are presented at a 90° angle relative to the magnetic field. This causes roughly 1% of the hydrogen nuclei to realign and begin spinning in a different direction (a condition called "excitation"). When the RF pulse is then stopped, the nuclei return to their original alignment and spin (64). During the process of returning to previous resting status, an electromagnetic signal is emitted from nuclei. Because the body's tissues are primarily made up of water, the water content and tissue density dictate the degree of signal that is detected by the scanner and subsequently digitally reconstructed into an image (4,64).

FMRI is a variant of structural MRI. The primary difference, however, is that the dependent variable of interest in FMRI is the change in intensity of electrical signal emissions related to increases in blood flow (that are presumably caused by changes in neural activity). Although the primary goal of structural MRI is to generate high-resolution anatomic images of underlying brain structure, the goal of FMRI is to allow the investigator to make inferences about regional changes in brain activity (65).

During FMRI, specific stimuli or tasks are presented to the individual within the scanner in an attempt to elicit or increase brain activity. When neural activity increases in a brain region, there is a corresponding increase in blood flow to that region. In fact, this blood flow may increase by more than 50% (66), beyond metabolic needs. This excess of flow to the region results in a localized surplus of oxyhemoglobin relative to deoxyhemoglobin in the cerebral venous and capillary beds. Oxyhemoglobin is naturally diamagnetic, whereas deoxyhemoglobin is paramagnetic (i.e., becomes readily magnetized within a magnetic field). With increased neural activity and concomitant increased blood flow, there is a net increase in diamagnetic material (oxyhemoglobin), and a net decrease in paramagnetic material (deoxyhemoglobin). This results in an increased signal intensity that can be detected externally, and is represented as higher signal intensity on a T2 (specifically a T2* or "T2-star") weighted scan. This change in signal intensity is referred to as the blood oxygen level-dependent or "BOLD" effect (67).

As compared with other neuroimaging techniques, FMRI uses the body's natural physical responses to high-strength magnetism, thus, no exogenous radioisotopes or contrast agents are required. The anatomic and temporal resolution of FMRI is also superior to that of SPECT or PET. In addition, there are numerous activation paradigms that can be carried out in FMRI, and it allows for greater flexibility in paradigm with reference to repeatability and brevity of the overall scanning session in comparison to other techniques (2).

FMRI may also be used in conjunction with another technique, arterial spin labeling (ASL) as an alternate and noninvasive means of measuring cerebral perfusion that uses an endogenous biophysical "contrast" rather than an exogenous contrast agent. In ASL, an additional pulse sequence is transmitted, for example at the level of the carotid artery in the neck. In essence, this magnetically "labels" the protons contained within the blood's water molecules prior to reaching the brain, where they can then be detected farther up stream by the head coil (4). By then, comparing a given brain region's signal before and then after that the magnetic labeling occurs, one is able to make direct inferences about CBF and perfusion.

As with any imaging procedure, however, FMRI can be impacted by numerous variables, particularly in clinical populations such as TBI. Consideration must be made for head movement, normal high frequency noise within the scanner, morphologic brain abnormalities (e.g., frontal or temporal lobe resection secondary to trauma), claustrophobia, anxiety, boredom, or actual onset of sleep while in the scanner. As with any MR-based procedure, there are also metallic artifact and potential safety concerns that must be considered and addressed, particularly when working with high-field (e.g., 3 Tesla or beyond) MRI systems (4).

Although most contemporary MRI scanners can be adapted to perform FMRI, this technique is still investigational in most clinical populations including brain injury (1). Thus, FMRI is primarily a research tool at this time and its availability is generally limited to academic medical centers. A single FMRI session generates a large volume of data, which necessitates considerations for computer hardware, data storage, and data security. At present, FMRI protocols neither "automatically" nor "objectively" yield brain maps, nor are there normative values for FMRI scans or activity levels (65). Resulting images must therefore be carefully and skillfully reconstructed, and this reconstruction process should be considered as much of an art as science. The approach that one takes in reconstructing and displaying the data in the form of brain images data will impact the display, and potentially the interpretation, of the end product.

FMRI Studies of Brain Injury

In the first FMRI studies of individuals with TBI (68,69), the investigators examined individuals with a very recent history of mild brain injury (i.e., within the previous 30 days). The individuals with mild TBI demonstrated intact behavioral performance on a verbal working memory task, but they did show right hemisphere lateralized FMRI activation in response to increased working memory load, as compared to healthy controls. In subsequent FMRI investigations of working memory following moderate and severe TBI (70,71), increased blood flow and more widespread dispersion of cortical activation were noted during working memory tasks. This again suggests that increased cognitive effort is reflected in increased brain activation on FMRI. In a study of working memory and response inhibition, FMRI was used to demonstrate increased recruitment of cerebral resources following severe diffuse TBI, particularly during response inhibition or when task difficulty was increased (72). This greater expenditure of effort to achieve overtly normal behavioral performance has also been demonstrated in an FMRI study of simple psychomotor execution (i.e., finger tapping) among individuals with TBI examined several years after injury (73). One case study (74) has demonstrated correlations between changes in FMRI activations and improvement in cognitive status following rehabilitation of an individual with severe TBI, a compelling finding that warrants replication. Studies have also used FMRI to examine working memory in concussed athletes with cognitive symptoms (75,76) and have demonstrated findings similar to those obtained in persons with TBI sustained through other mechanisms.

In a more recent study (77), persons with severe TBI were compared to persons with orthopedic injuries using an n-back working memory task using photographs of faces as stimuli. The findings of this study were generally comparable to those of previous studies, with most group differences noted in the 1-back condition. This study only examined persons with severe TBI, however, and only up to a 2-back level of cognitive load. Thus, application of the results to other levels of TBI must be made with caution. In addition, although the stimuli used in this study were visual, faces are processed differently by the brain than other types of spatial information. As such, this paradigm did not address the specific cognitive or neural architecture of the visuospatial component of working memory. In another study, these investigators also used FMRI to examine working memory in adolescents with TBI (78), finding a disruption during the maintenance phase of working memory. To date, each of the published FMRI studies of working memory after TBI has addressed rather limited aspects of working memory processing and examined limited ranges of injury severity.

Only very recently has episodic memory, which is arguably the memory function that is most typically assessed clinically (i.e., through list recall tests), been formally studied with FMRI in persons with TBI. The first of these studies (79) involved teaching a verbal learning strategy to a group of 54 individuals with documented memory impairment after moderate or severe TBI and a matched group of controls. FMRI scanning was conducted only during the encoding phase of a verbal learning. The findings suggested that left prefrontal areas were related to strategic verbal learning. They also observed that both underactivation and overactivation in the TBI group was associated with reduced performance on memory tasks after rehabilitation, creating an inverted-U quadratic relationship between performance and activation, which was therefore predictive of outcome. The authors suggested that underactivation may represent structural injury to the gray or white matter within the region of interest or possible injury to areas projecting to that region, whereas overactivation may indicate intact and engaged cortical areas, which, despite "effortful utilization," failed to produce improvement in functional memory as tested. They subsequently conducted another study (80) of 20 participants with moderate or severe TBI and 20 healthy controls using the same behavioral and FMRI paradigm from their 2008 study. Despite baseline testing indicating significant differences in behavioral performance between groups, direct comparison of group FMRI activation across all tasks indicated no significant differences, suggesting that individuals in the TBI group activated the same general networks as healthy controls. Most recently, (81,82) both encoding and recognition of verbal and visual stimuli were examined with FMRI. Twelve adults with chronic severe, moderate, and complicated mild injuries were compared with a matched group of 12 controls. Behavioral task performance did not differentiate the groups. During neuroimaging, however, the group of individuals with TBI exhibited increased activation, as well as increased bilaterality and dispersion as compared to controls. These results were generally consistent with previous imaging and behavioral findings in TBI, but there was an additional novel finding. Persons with TBI demonstrated more subcortical activation (i.e., caudate and thalamus), whereas activations for the control group were mostly cortical. The exact nature of this finding is unknown, but there is evidence that these subcortical structures are involved in cognitive processes, and, even if not typically injured after TBI, are highly interconnected with frontal cortex through white matter tracts that are known to be susceptible to compromise after moderate and severe TBI.

Although FMRI represents a very advanced approach to brain imaging vis-à-vis cognitive functioning when compared to SPECT or PET, it has not reached a sufficient threshold of evidence for routine use at any level of injury severity after head trauma. Given the paucity of FMRI research in TBI, the American College of Radiology has not fully evaluated FMRI and continues to classify this procedure as investigational in the examination of any level brain injury.

MAGNETIC RESONANCE SPECTROSCOPY

Although not strictly a "functional" imaging procedure, magnetic resonance spectroscopy (MRS) is included within this chapter, given its capacity to characterize brain-based biomarkers and its potential relevance and application to medical rehabilitation of brain injury.

MRS is based on the same biophysical principles as MRI and FMRI. Where it differs is in the fact that it does not solely emphasize hydrogen content of water or lipids but is additionally capable of representing other endogenous biocompounds. MRS is able to detect the distinct magnetic profiles of biological markers such as creatine (Cr) or phosphocreatine (PCr), glutamate (Glu), choline-related compounds (Cho), and N-acetylaspartate (NAA), which is a product of neuronal degradation (83,84). Typically, the signal that derived from MRS is represented as a series of waveforms presented in spectra rather than as a topographic brain map. Each biomarker possesses different numbers of electrons in their nuclei. Larger numbers of electrons cause local reductions within the magnetic field, thus causing a reduction in the spectral peak. Because of this phenomenon, biomarkers can be differentially localized and quantified in space.

MRS Studies After Brain Injury

MRS is still considered to be investigational in brain injury (1), but it has been used in research. NAA is an endogenous neurochemical that can be studied with MRS and has been studied in humans (85). NAA occurs exclusively in the central nervous system. It is also only second to Glu in terms of abundance in the cerebrum. NAA is generally considered to be related to axonal repair, thus, its relationship to brain injury has received a significant amount of investigation. Animal studies have demonstrated TBI-related reductions in NAA reductions at 1 hour after injury (86). Studies of NAA in human brain injury have shown that NAA suppression can continue for several months after the initial injury (83,87,88). Another MRS index is Cho, which is comprised of indices representing levels of choline, phosphocholine, and glycerophosphocholine. It is increased when there is tissue inflammation (83). Declines in NAA accompanied by increases in Cho are seen as fairly reliable indices of the status of brain injury recovery (84). Hyperglycolysis results when Glu and other excitatory biochemical compounds are released, and levels of Glu may remain elevated for several days after injury. This may lead to neuronal overexcitation without corresponding oxygen metabolism. Hyperglycolysis can eventually result in neuronal acidosis and neuronal death. Glu has been implicated as a marker for injury severity and may also have implications for recovery. Glu has been studied in animals (89), and more recently its use has been examined in humans (90). Within the first month after injury, MRS has been shown to be useful in characterizing lactate levels in humans (91), but its predictive functional value remains to be determined. Additional markers such as myoinositol and lipid macromolecules are also under investigation in human TBI (92).

MAGNETOENCEPHALOGRAPHY AND MAGNETIC SOURCE IMAGING

In addition to electrical activity, neurons also generate minute magnetic fields that can be measured using an approach known as MEG. MEG involves the use of liquid helium that cools conducting coils to almost absolute zero. When cooled to such low temperatures, the electrical resistance of the conductor is greatly reduced, and very small changes in magnetic field can be detected (93). The miniscule mature of these fields requires significant amplification in order to be useful. Using devices known as superconducting quantum interference devices (SQUIDs), the changes in magnetic fields produced by neuronal activity can be detected. An array of conductors is situated around the head of the participant, which allows for the placement of multiple detectors (94).

The physiological basis of MEG is that of normal neuronal membrane signal conduction. The flow of electrical current within an active neuron generates a magnetic field. When a synapse becomes active, there is a current flow across the neuronal membrane. This current diffuses intracellularly and then emerges extracellularly at a fixed distance from where it began (i.e., from dendrite to synapse). This results in the opportunity for "sources" and "sinks" extracellularly. In the presence of an asymmetrically oriented neuron, the sources and sinks create dipolar electromagnetic fields that cancel one another out. The intracellular current between the region of synaptic activation and the point at which the current returns to extracellular space does not cancel out (95). This magnetic field can be recorded. Used in conjunction with localization techniques, MEG is referred to as magnetic source imaging (MSI) and may be used to construct spatial and time-course images depicting brain activity (96).

Although intuitively similar to EEG, MEG has some advantages (97). First, MEG frequencies are technically easier to record than those from EEG given that the detectors are placed in helmet for adjacent to the scalp and do not have to be individually applied (or interconnected). Second, magnetic fields are not affected by the variability in skull thickness over different regions of cortex. Third, in general, the component structure of the MEG response is actually simpler that that derived through EEG. Fourth, in contrast to all of the other modalities discussed in this chapter, MEG allows participants to be scanned in a more naturalistic, upright and seated position (see Figure 16-4). There are, of course, disadvantages to MEG. MEG is very expensive and thus not widely available. MEG also does not detect deep (e.g., subcortical) sources of activity. MEG, along with EEG, lacks the anatomic precision of other neuroimaging techniques (98).

MEG/MSI After Brain Injury

Although MEG/MSI has been used extensively in several populations, such as language disorders and autism, there have been few studies in which MES/MSI has been applied to TBI. In fact, this work has been primarily restricted to research with persons that have sustained or are suspected of having sustained mild brain injury (84). For example, in conjunction with multiple imaging modalities (including SPECT and MRI), Lewine and colleagues (99) have proposed that MEG may add useful incremental data related to persisting cognitive problems following mild head trauma. More recently, MEG/MSI has been combined with diffusion tensor imaging (DTI) in an attempt to characterize the effects of both civilian and military mild head trauma (100).

CONCLUSION

The past few years have seen even further advances in functional neuroimaging technologies and approaches to data

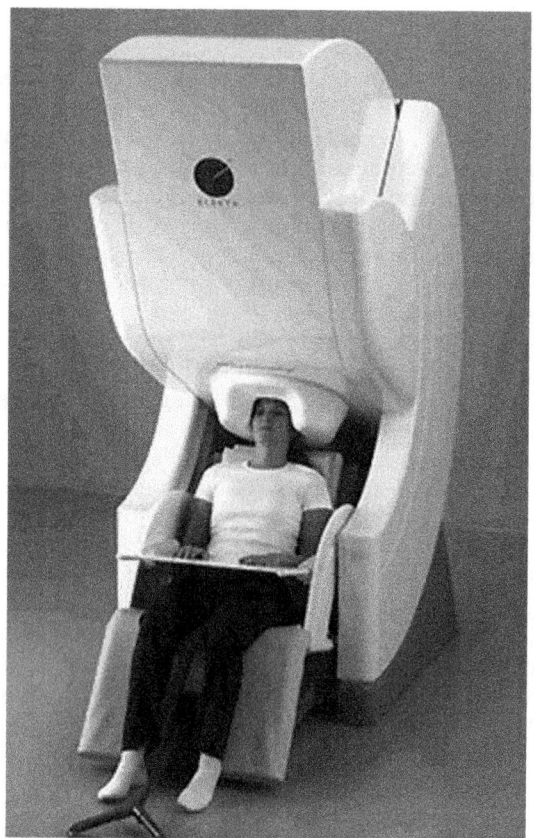

FIGURE 16-4 Magnetoencephalography (MEG) scanner. This photograph demonstrates the capability of having a participant in an upright, seated position. Image courtesy of Jeffrey David Lewine, PhD, The Mind Research Network, Albuquerque, NM.

analysis. In addition, there have been several more exploratory studies in several clinical populations, including TBI. In spite of these advances, these techniques remain investigational in most clinical applications (81,101). As with any technology, the transition from "investigational" to "routine" will neither occur overnight nor will it occur solely from the publication of a handful of case studies or small investigations drawn only from highly selected cases. It will occur after much additional, well-designed, systematic research (102).

It is also important to note that even though most of the imaging modalities discussed in this chapter are considered investigational in terms of routine clinical use in the TBI population, many imaging technologies are seeing increasing use in both the civil and criminal forensic arenas. Although a comprehensive discussion of this important topic is beyond the scope of this chapter (see recent reviews by Granacher [16] and Ricker [103]), it is important for practicing clinicians to remain cautious when presented with findings generated by novel neuroimaging technologies in the context of medicolegal cases. For example, even though essentially all functional imaging technologies remain investigational for use in persons with mild TBI or PCS, and courts are typically justifiably cautious about admitting functional imaging into evidence under *Frye* or *Daubert* challenges (104), neuroimaging will likely to see increased consideration in the forensic arena (105).

KEY REFERENCES

1. Hattori N, Huang SC, Wu HM, et al. Correlation of regional metabolic rates of glucose with Glasgow Coma Scale after traumatic brain injury. *J Nucl Med.* 2003;44(11):1709–1716.
2. McAllister TW, Saykin AJ, Flashman LA, et al. Brain activation during working memory 1 month after mild traumatic brain injury: a functional MRI study. *Neurology.* 1999;53(6):1300–1308.
3. Russell KC, Arenth PM, Scanlon JM, Kessler LJ, Ricker JH. A functional magnetic resonance imaging investigation of episodic memory after traumatic brain injury. *J Clin Exp Neuropsychol.* 2011;33(5):538–547.
4. Seo Y, Mari C, Hasegawa BH. Technological development and advances in single-photon emission computed tomography/computed tomography. *Semin Nucl Med.* 2008;38(3):177–198.
5. Strangman GE, O'Neil-Pirozzi TM, Goldstein R, et al. Prediction of memory rehabilitation outcomes in traumatic brain injury by using functional magnetic resonance imaging. *Arch Phys Med Rehabil.* 2008;89(5):974–981.

References

1. Davis PC, Drayer BP, Anderson RE, et al. Head trauma. American College of Radiology. ACR appropriateness criteria. *Radiology.* 2000;215(suppl):507–524.
2. Ricker JH. Functional neuroimaging in medical rehabilitation populations. In: DeLisa JA, Gans BM, Walsh NE, eds. *Physical Medicine and Rehabilitation: Principles and Practice.* 4th ed. Philadelphia, PA: Lippincott Williams & Wilkins; 2005:229–242.

3. Raichle ME. Functional neuroimaging: a historical and physiological perspective. In: Cabeza R, Kingstone A, eds. *Handbook of Functional Neuroimaging of Cognition.* Cambridge, MA: MIT Press; 2001: 3–26.

4. Huettel SA, Song AW, McCarthy G. *Functional Magnetic Resonance Imaging.* 2nd ed. Sunderland, MA: Sinauer Associates Inc; 2009.

5. Small SA. Neurobiological correlates of imaging. In: D'Esposito M, ed. *Functional MRI: Applications in Clinical Neurology and Psychiatry.* Boca Raton, FL: Taylor & Francis; 2006:1–8.

6. Masdeu JC, Arbizu J. Brain single photon emission computed tomography: technological aspects and clinical applications. *Semin Neurol.* 2008;28(4):423–434.

7. Ingvar DH, Risberg J. Influence of mental activity upon regional cerebral blood flow in man. A preliminary study. *Acta Neurol Scand Suppl.* 1965;14:183–186.

8. Wintermark M, Sesay M, Barbier E, et al. Comparative overview of brain perfusion imaging techniques. *J Neuroradiol.* 2005;32(5): 294–314.

9. Habert MO, Huberfeld G. Ictal single photon computed tomography and SISCOM: methods and utility [in French]. *Neurochirurgie.* 2008;54(3):226–230.

10. Ludwig C, Chicherio C, Terraneo L, Magistretti P, de Ribaupierre A, Slosman D. Functional imaging studies of cognition using 99mTc-HMPAO SPECT: empirical validation using the n-back working memory paradigm. *Eur J Nucl Med Mol Imaging.* 2008; 35(4):695–703.

11. Ogawa M, Tsukada H, Hatano K, Ouchi Y, Saji H, Magata Y. Central in vivo nicotinic acetylcholine receptor imaging agents for positron emission tomography (PET) and single photon emission computed tomography (SPECT). *Biol Pharm Bull.* 2009;32(3):337–340.

12. Sohlberg A, Watabe H, Iida H. Three-dimensional SPECT reconstruction with transmission-dependent scatter correction. *Ann Nucl Med.* 2008;22(7):549–556.

13. Seo Y, Mari C, Hasegawa BH. Technological development and advances in single-photon emission computed tomography/computed tomography. *Semin Nucl Med.* 2008;38(3):177–198.

14. Habert MO, Horn JF, Sarazin M, et al. Brain perfusion SPECT with an automated quantitative tool can identify prodromal Alzheimer's disease among patients with mild cognitive impairment. *Neurobiol Aging.* 2011;32(1):15–23.

15. Ricker JH, Zafonte RD. Functional neuroimaging and quantitative electroencephalography in adult traumatic head injury: clinical applications and interpretive cautions. *J Head Trauma Rehabil.* 2000; 15(2):859–868.

16. Granacher RP Jr. Commentary: applications of functional neuroimaging to civil litigation of mild traumatic brain injury. *J Am Acad Psychiatry Law.* 2008;36(3):323–328.

17. Ricker JH, Arenth PM. Traumatic brain injury. In: D'Esposito M, ed. *Functional MRI: Applications in Clinical Neurology and Psychiatry.* Boca Raton, FL: Taylor & Francis; 2006:197–206.

18. Hofman PA, Stapert SZ, van Kroonenburgh MJ, Jolles J, de Kruijk J, Wilmink JT. MR imaging, single-photon emission CT, and neurocognitive performance after mild traumatic brain injury. *AJNR Am J Neuroradiol.* 2001;22(3):441–449.

19. Umile EM, Plotkin RC, Sandel ME. Functional assessment of mild traumatic brain injury using SPECT and neuropsychological testing. *Brain Inj.* 1998;12(7):577–594.

20. Ichise M, Chung DG, Wang P, Wortzman G, Gray BG, Franks W. Technetium-99m-HMPAO SPECT, CT and MRI in the evaluation of patients with chronic traumatic brain injury: a correlation with neuropsychological performance. *J Nucl Med.* 1994;35(2):217–226.

21. Audenaert K, Jansen HM, Otte A, et al. Imaging of mild traumatic brain injury using 57Co and 99mTc HMPAO SPECT as compared to other diagnostic procedures. *Med Sci Monit.* 2003;9(10):MT112–MT117.

22. Dougherty DD, Rauch SL, Rosenbaum JF. *Essentials of Neuroimaging for Clinical Practice.* 1st ed. Washington, DC: American Psychiatric Publishing; 2004.

23. Garcia-Campayo J, Sanz-Carrillo C, Baringo T, Ceballos C. SPECT scan in somatization disorder patients: an exploratory study of eleven cases. *Aust N Z J Psychiatry.* 2001;35(3):359–363.

24. Mountz JM, Liu HG, Deutsch G. Neuroimaging in cerebrovascular disorders: measurement of cerebral physiology after stroke and assessment of stroke recovery. *Semin Nucl Med.* 2003;33(1):56–76.

25. Pakrasi S, O'Brien JT. Emission tomography in dementia. *Nucl Med Commun.* 2005;26(3):189–196.

26. Papanicolaou AC, Simos PG, Breier JI, et al. Brain mechanisms for reading in children with and without dyslexia: a review of studies of normal development and plasticity. *Dev Neuropsychol.* 2003; 24(2–3):593–612.

27. Haldane M, Frangou S. New insights help define the pathophysiology of bipolar affective disorder: neuroimaging and neuropathology findings. *Prog Neuropsychopharmacol Biol Psychiatry.* 2004;28(6): 943–960.

28. Kennedy SE, Zubieta JK. Neuroreceptor imaging of stress and mood disorders. *CNS Spectr.* 2004;9(4):292–301.

29. Ernst M, Kimes AS, Jazbec S. Neuroimaging and mechanisms of drug abuse: interface of molecular imaging and molecular genetics. *Neuroimaging Clin N Am.* 2003;13(4):833–849.

30. Pezawas L, Fischer G, Podreka I, et al. Opioid addiction changes cerebral blood flow symmetry. *Neuropsychobiology.* 2002;45(2): 67–73.

31. Heinz A, Goldman D, Gallinat J, Schumann G, Puls I. Pharmacogenetic insights to monoaminergic dysfunction in alcohol dependence. *Psychopharmacology (Berl).* 2004;174(4):561–570.

32. Browndyke JN, Tucker KA, Woods SP, et al. Examining the effect of cerebral perfusion abnormality magnitude on cognitive performance in recently abstinent chronic cocaine abusers. *J Neuroimaging.* 2004;14(2):162–169.

33. Modell JG, Mountz JM. Focal cerebral blood flow change during craving for alcohol measured by SPECT. *J Neuropsychiatry Clin Neurosci.* 1995;7(1):15–22.

34. Malaspina D, Harkavy-Friedman J, Corcoran C, et al. Resting neural activity distinguishes subgroups of schizophrenia patients. *Biol Psychiatry.* 2004;56(12):931–937.

35. Maron E, Kuikka JT, Ulst K, Tiihonen J, Vasar V, Shlik J. SPECT imaging of serotonin transporter binding in patients with generalized anxiety disorder. *Eur Arch Psychiatry Clin Neurosci.* 2004; 254(6):392–396.

36. Jacobs A, Put E, Ingels M, Bossuyt A. Prospective evaluation of technetium-99m-HMPAO SPECT in mild and moderate traumatic brain injury. *J Nucl Med.* 1994;35(6):942–947.

37. Herscovitch P. Functional brain imaging: basic principles and application to head trauma. In: Rizzo M, Tranel D, eds. *Head Injury and the Postconcussive Syndrome.* 1st ed. New York, NY: Churchill Livingstone; 1996:89–118.

38. Assessment of brain SPECT. Report of the Therapeutics and Technology Assessment Subcommittee of the American Academy of Neurology. *Neurology.* 1996;46(1):278–285.

39. Wortzel HS, Filley CM, Anderson CA, Oster T, Arciniegas DB. Forensic applications of cerebral single photon emission computed tomography in mild traumatic brain injury. *J Am Acad Psychiatry Law.* 2008;36(3):310–322.

40. Bonne O, Gilboa A, Louzoun Y, et al. Cerebral blood flow in chronic symptomatic mild traumatic brain injury. *Psychiatry Res.* 2003; 124(3):141–152.

41. Cihangiroglu M, Ramsey RG, Dohrmann GJ. Brain injury: analysis of imaging modalities. *Neurol Res.* 2002;24(1):7–18.

42. Lorberboym M, Lampl Y, Gerzon I, Sadeh M. Brain SPECT evaluation of amnestic ED patients after mild head trauma. *Am J Emerg Med.* 2002;20(4):310–313.

43. Mazzini L, Campini R, Angelino E, Rognone F, Pastore I, Oliveri G. Posttraumatic hydrocephalus: a clinical, neuroradiologic, and neuropsychologic assessment of long-term outcome. *Arch Phys Med Rehabil.* 2003;84(11):1637–641.

44. Donnemiller E, Brenneis C, Wissel J, et al. Impaired dopaminergic neurotransmission in patients with traumatic brain injury: a SPECT study using 123I-beta-CIT and 123I-IBZM. *Eur J Nucl Med.* 2000; 27(9):1410–1414.

45. Buckner RL, Logan JM. Functional neuroimaging methods: PET and FMRI. In: Cabeza R, Kingstone A, eds. *Handbook of Functional Neuroimaging of Cognition.* Cambridge, MA: MIT Press; 2001:27–48.

46. Chen JJ, Wieckowska M, Meyer E, Pike GB. Cerebral blood flow measurement using fMRI and PET: a cross-validation study. *Int J Biomed Imaging*. 2008;2008:516359.

47. Gulyas B, Sjoholm N. Principles of positron emission tomography. In: Hillary FG, DeLuca J, eds. *Functional Neuroimaging in Clinical Populations*. New York, NY: Guilford Press; 2007:3–30.

48. Herholz K, Carter SF, Jones M. Positron emission tomography imaging in dementia. *Br J Radiol*. 2007;80(Spec. No. 2):S160–S167.

49. Hattori N, Huang SC, Wu HM, et al. Correlation of regional metabolic rates of glucose with Glasgow Coma Scale after traumatic brain injury. *J Nucl Med*. 2003;44(11):1709–1716.

50. Hattori N, Huang SC, Wu HM, et al. Acute changes in regional cerebral (18)F-FDG kinetics in patients with traumatic brain injury. *J Nucl Med*. 2004;45(5):775–783.

51. Bergsneider M, Hovda DA, Shalmon E, et al. Cerebral hyperglycolysis following severe traumatic brain injury in humans: a positron emission tomography study. *J Neurosurg*. 1997;86(2):241–251.

52. Bergsneider M, Hovda DA, McArthur DL, et al. Metabolic recovery following human traumatic brain injury based on FDG-PET: time course and relationship to neurological disability. *J Head Trauma Rehabil*. 2001;16(2):135–148.

53. Langfitt TW, Obrist WD, Alavi A, et al. Computerized tomography, magnetic resonance imaging, and positron emission tomography in the study of brain trauma. Preliminary observations. *J Neurosurg*. 1986;64(5):760–767.

54. Jansen HM, van der Naalt J, van Zomeren AH, et al. Cobalt-55 positron emission tomography in traumatic brain injury: a pilot study. *J Neurol Neurosurg Psychiatry*. 1996;60(2):221–224.

55. Wu HM, Huang SC, Hattori N, et al. Selective metabolic reduction in gray matter acutely following human traumatic brain injury. *J Neurotrauma*. 2004;21(2):149–161.

56. Ruff RM, Crouch JA, Troster AI, et al. Selected cases of poor outcome following a minor brain trauma: comparing neuropsychological and positron emission tomography assessment. *Brain Inj*. 1994;8(4):297–308.

57. Gross H, Kling A, Henry G, Herndon C, Lavretsky H. Local cerebral glucose metabolism in patients with long-term behavioral and cognitive deficits following mild traumatic brain injury. *J Neuropsychiatry Clin Neurosci*. 1996;8(3):324–334.

58. Fontaine A, Azouvi P, Remy P, Bussel B, Samson Y. Functional anatomy of neuropsychological deficits after severe traumatic brain injury. *Neurology*. 1999;53(9):1963–1968.

59. Varney NR, Pinkston JB, Wu JC. Quantitative PET findings in patients with posttraumatic anosmia. *J Head Trauma Rehabil*. 2001;16(3):253–259.

60. Ostberg A, Virta J, Rinne JO, et al. Cholinergic dysfunction after traumatic brain injury: preliminary findings from a PET study. *Neurology*. 2011;76(12):1046–1050.

61. Baron JC. Study of functional neuro-anatomy of perception using positron emission tomography [in French]. *Rev Neurol (Paris)*. 1995;151(8–9):511–517.

62. Ricker JH, Muller RA, Zafonte RD, Black KM, Millis SR, Chugani H. Verbal recall and recognition following traumatic brain injury: a [0–15]-water positron emission tomography study. *J Clin Exp Neuropsychol*. 2001;23(2):196–206.

63. Levine B, Cabeza R, McIntosh AR, Black SE, Grady CL, Stuss DT. Functional reorganisation of memory after traumatic brain injury: a study with H(2)(15)0 positron emission tomography. *J Neurol Neurosurg Psychiatry*. 2002;73(2):173–181.

64. Springer CS, Patlak CS, Playka I, Huang W. Principles of susceptibility contrast-based functional MRI: the sign of the functional response. In: Moonen CT, Bandettini PA, eds. *Functional MRI*. Berlin, Germany: Springer-Verlag; 2000:91–102.

65. Aguirre GK. Interpretation of clinical functional neuroimaging studies. In: D'Esposito M, ed. *Functional MRI: Applications in Clinical Neurology and Psychiatry*. Boca Raton, FL: Taylor & Francis; 2006: 9–23.

66. Weisskoff RM. Basic theoretical models of BOLD signal change. In: Moonen CT, Bandettini PA, eds. *Functional MRI*. Berlin, Germany: Springer-Verlag; 2000:115–123.

67. Chen W, Ogawa S. Principles of BOLD functional MRI. In: Moonen CT, Bandettini PA, eds. *Functional MRI*. Berlin, Germany: Springer-Verlag; 2000:103–112.

68. McAllister TW, Saykin AJ, Flashman LA, et al. Brain activation during working memory 1 month after mild traumatic brain injury: a functional MRI study. *Neurology*. 1999;53(6):1300–1308.

69. McAllister TW, Sparling MB, Flashman LA, Guerin SJ, Mamourian AC, Saykin AJ. Differential working memory load effects after mild traumatic brain injury. *Neuroimage*. 2001;14(5):1004–1012.

70. Christodoulou C, DeLuca J, Ricker JH, et al. Functional magnetic resonance imaging of working memory impairment after traumatic brain injury. *J Neurol Neurosurg Psychiatry*. 2001;71(2):161–168.

71. Perlstein WM, Cole MA, Demery JA, et al. Parametric manipulation of working memory load in traumatic brain injury: behavioral and neural correlates. *J Int Neuropsychol Soc*. 2004;10(5):724–741.

72. Scheibel RS, Pearson DA, Faria LP, et al. An fMRI study of executive functioning after severe diffuse TBI. *Brain Inj*. 2003;17(11): 919–930.

73. Prigatano GP, Johnson SC, Gale SD. Neuroimaging correlates of the Halstead Finger Tapping Test several years post-traumatic brain injury. *Brain Inj*. 2004;18(7):661–669.

74. Laatsch L, Little D, Thulborn K. Changes in fMRI following cognitive rehabilitation in severe traumatic brain injruy: a case study. *Rehabil Psychol*. 2004;49:262–267.

75. Chen JK, Johnston KM, Frey S, Petrides M, Worsley K, Ptito A. Functional abnormalities in symptomatic concussed athletes: an fMRI study. *Neuroimage*. 2004;22(1):68–82.

76. Lovell MR, Pardini JE, Welling J, et al. Functional brain abnormalities are related to clinical recovery and time to return-to-play in athletes. *Neurosurgery*. 2007;61(2):352–359.

77. Newsome MR, Scheibel RS, Steinberg JL, et al. Working memory brain activation following severe traumatic brain injury. *Cortex*. 2007;43(1):95–111.

78. Newsome MR, Steinberg JL, Scheibel RS, et al. Effects of traumatic brain injury on working memory-related brain activation in adolescents. *Neuropsychology*. 2008;22(4):419–425.

79. Strangman GE, O'Neil-Pirozzi TM, Goldstein R, et al. Prediction of memory rehabilitation outcomes in traumatic brain injury by using functional magnetic resonance imaging. *Arch Phys Med Rehabil*. 2008;89(5):974–981.

80. Strangman GE, Goldstein R, O'Neil-Pirozzi TM, et al. Neurophysiological alterations during strategy-based verbal learning in traumatic brain injury. *Neurorehabil Neural Repair*. 2009;23(3): 226–236.

81. Russell KC, Arenth PM, Scanlon JM, Kessler LJ, Ricker JH. A functional magnetic resonance imaging investigation of episodic memory after traumatic brain injury. *J Clin Exp Neuropsychol*. 2011;33(5): 538–547.

82. Arenth PM, Russell KC, Scanlon JM, Kessler LJ, Ricker JH. Encoding and recognition after traumatic brain injury: neuropsychological and functional magnetic resonance imaging findings. *J Clin Exp Neuropsychol*. 2012;34(4):333–344.

83. Brooks WM, Friedman SD, Gasparovic C. Magnetic resonance spectroscopy in traumatic brain injury. *J Head Trauma Rehabil*. 2001; 16(2):149–164.

84. Hunter JV, Wilde EA, Tong KA, Holshouser BA. Emerging imaging tools for use with traumatic brain injury research. *J Neurotrauma*. 2012;29(4):654–671.

85. Alessandri B, al-Samsam R, Corwin F, Fatouros P, Young HF, Bullock RM. Acute and late changes in N-acetyl-aspartate following diffuse axonal injury in rats: an MRI spectroscopy and microdialysis study. *Neurol Res*. 2000;22(7):705–712.

86. Smith DH, Cecil KM, Meaney DF, et al. Magnetic resonance spectroscopy of diffuse brain trauma in the pig. *J Neurotrauma*. 1998; 15(9):665–674.

87. Hunter JV, Thornton RJ, Wang ZJ, et al. Late proton MR spectroscopy in children after traumatic brain injury: correlation with cognitive outcomes. *AJNR Am J Neuroradiol*. 2005;26(3):482–488.

88. Yeo RA, Phillips JP, Jung RE, Brown AJ, Campbell RC, Brooks WM. Magnetic resonance spectroscopy detects brain injury and predicts cognitive functioning in children with brain injuries. *J Neurotrauma*. 2006;23(10):1427–1435.

89. Faden AI, O'Leary DM, Fan L, Bao W, Mullins PG, Movsesyan VA. Selective blockade of the mGluR1 receptor reduces traumatic neuronal injury in vitro and improvesoOutcome after brain trauma. *Exp Neurol*. 2001;167(2):435–444.

90. Ashwal S, Holshouser B, Tong K, et al. Proton MR spectroscopy detected glutamate/glutamine is increased in children with traumatic brain injury. *J Neurotrauma*. 2004;21(11):1539–1552.

91. Hillary FG, Liu WC, Genova HM, et al. Examining lactate in severe TBI using proton magnetic resonance spectroscopy. *Brain Inj*. 2007; 21(9):981–991.

92. Panigrahy A, Nelson MD Jr, Bluml S. Magnetic resonance spectroscopy in pediatric neuroradiology: clinical and research applications. *Pediatr Radiol*. 2010;40(1):3–30.

93. King DW, Park YD, Smith JR, Wheless JW. Magnetoencephalography in neocortical epilepsy. *Adv Neurol*. 2000;84:415–423.

94. Simos PG, Papanicolaou AC, Breier JI, et al. Insights into brain function and neural plasticity using magnetic source imaging. *J Clin Neurophysiol*. 2000;17(2):143–162.

95. Tang AC, Pearlmutter BA, Malaszenko NA, Phung DB, Reeb BC. Independent components of magnetoencephalography: localization. *Neural Comput*. 2002;14(8):1827–1858.

96. Wheless JW, Castillo E, Maggio V, et al Magnetoencephalography (MEG) and magnetic source imaging (MSI). *Neurologist*. 2004;10(3): 138–153.

97. Malmivuo J. Comparison of the properties of EEG and MEG in detecting the electric activity of the brain. *Brain Topogr*. 2012;25(1):1–19.

98. Stern E, Silbersweig DA. Advances in functional neuroimaging methodology for the study of brain systems underlying human neuropsychological function and dysfunction. *J Clin Exp Neuropsychol*. 2001;23(1):3–18.

99. Lewine JD, Davis JT, Bigler ED, et al. Objective documentation of traumatic brain injury subsequent to mild head trauma: multimodal brain imaging with MEG, SPECT, and MRI. *J Head Trauma Rehabil*. 2007;22(3):141–155.

100. Huang MX, Theilmann RJ, Robb A, et al. Integrated imaging approach with MEG and DTI to detect mild traumatic brain injury in military and civilian patients. *J Neurotrauma*. 2009;26(8):1213–1226.

101. American Psychological Association Division 40. Official position of the division of clinical neuropsychology (APA Division 40) on the role of neuropsychologists in clinical use of fMri: approved by the Division 40 Executive Committee July 28, 2004. *Clin Neuropsychol*. 2004;18(3):349–351.

102. Strangman G, O'Neil-Pirozzi TM, Burke D, et al. Functional neuroimaging and cognitive rehabilitation for people with traumatic brain injury. *Am J Phys Med Rehabil*. 2005;84(1):62–75.

103. Ricker JH. Functional neuroimaging in forensic neuropsychology. In: Larrabee GJ, ed. *Forensic Neuropsychology: A Scientific Approach*. New York, NY: Oxford University Press; 2005:159–181.

104. Kaufmann P. Admissibility of expert opinions based on neuropsychological evidence. In: Larrabee G, ed. *Forensic Neuropsychology: A Scientific Approach*. 2nd ed. New York, NY: Oxford University Press; 2012:70–100.

105. Treadway MT, Buckholtz JW. On the use and misuse of genomic and neuroimaging science in forensic psychiatry: current roles and future directions. *Ch Adol Psychiatric Clin N America*. 2011;20(3): 533–546.

17

Electrophysiologic Techniques

Marine Vernet, Shahid Bashir, Syed Faaiz Enam, Hatice Kumru, and Alvaro Pascual-Leone

INTRODUCTION

Assessing the extent and functional impact of a traumatic brain injury (TBI), obtaining reliable prognostic indicators, gauging the best therapeutic interventions, and following the course of disease with reliable and objective markers is challenging. Electrophysiological techniques are relatively inexpensive, broadly deployable, repeatable, and safe methods that hold the promise of addressing some of these major clinical needs. Electrophysiological techniques can not only provide continuous and objective monitoring but can also pick up specific functional deficits and pathologies, provide a quantitative scale of severity, and be of great help in guiding rehabilitation and treatment interventions.

Electrophysiological techniques can be used to characterize the brain and central nervous system, as well as various aspects of the peripheral and autonomic nervous system. Evaluation of the peripheral and autonomic systems can be extremely important in patients after TBI because they may reflect consequences of brain injury and offer important prognostic insights. However, the focus of this chapter will be on the role of electrophysiological techniques to assess brain function with the use of electroencephalography (EEG), evoked potentials (EPs), and transcranial magnetic stimulation (TMS) in aiding the diagnosis, prognosis, and therapy of TBI.

ELECTROENCEPHALOGRAPHY

EEG measures electrical activity of the cerebral cortex through surface electrodes placed on the scalp adhering to standardized placement methods (e.g., the 10–20 International System of Electrode Placement; Figure 17-1A and 17-1B). Typical wave frequencies detected include delta (up to 4 Hz), theta (4–8 Hz), alpha (8–13 Hz), beta (13–30 Hz) and gamma (above 30 Hz). Within each frequency band, different rhythms have been indentified and ascribed to different brain/cognitive states (1). The alpha rhythm is a common starting point in the conventional analysis of a clinical EEG, is the dominant rhythm over posterior brain regions, and is attenuated with eye opening. Generally, alpha activity is thought to be related to inhibitory cortical tone and linked to thalamocortical patterns of activation. Mu rhythms are centrally located rhythms in the alpha frequency band that

are attenuated with contralateral movement of an extremity. Beta rhythms are normally activated with mental, lingual, or cognitive efforts, mostly over the frontal areas. Furthermore, many pharmacologic agents increase power in beta band activity, notably benzodiazepines, for example. Theta rhythms can be recorded intermittently over the frontocentral head regions during awake resting or while performing moderately difficult mental tasks; these are enhanced by drowsiness. Delta rhythms are considered a normal finding in the awake state in the very young and in the elderly. They are also considered normal across all ages during slow-wave sleep (1). Finally, gamma rhythms are associated with higher cognitive functions involving perception, attention, learning, and memory. These may also serve to assess the temporal dynamics of cortical networks and their interactions (2) (Table 17-1).

Abnormalities detected in EEG recordings can indicate primary cortical pathology or be the result of deeper structures modulating cortical regions erratically. In patients with TBI, EEG is one of the electrophysiological techniques often used to assess severity of brain injury and predict prognosis and outcomes (3–4). EEG analysis can be divided into conventional and quantitative methods.

Conventional EEG

Conventional EEG is the standard method for recording cortical electrical waveforms as mentioned earlier (Figure 17-1C). Although conventional EEG might have some value when assessing injury severity and depth of coma in patients with TBI (5–6), it remains a qualitative tool. Therefore, it does not provide great resolution and cannot quantify wave spectrum frequencies. This makes it impractical for long-term monitoring of patients with TBI and predicting a prognosis (6). Nevertheless, it is often used in neurocritical care for assessment and monitoring of patients with moderate-to-severe TBI (7). Conventional EEG can certainly help in the detection of epileptic activity, a common consequence of more severe TBI. However, use of conventional EEG in early evaluation of patients with mild TBI is rather limited (3).

Mild TBI

There are no clear EEG features unique to TBI of mild severity (8), and conventional EEG is not reliable in differentiat-

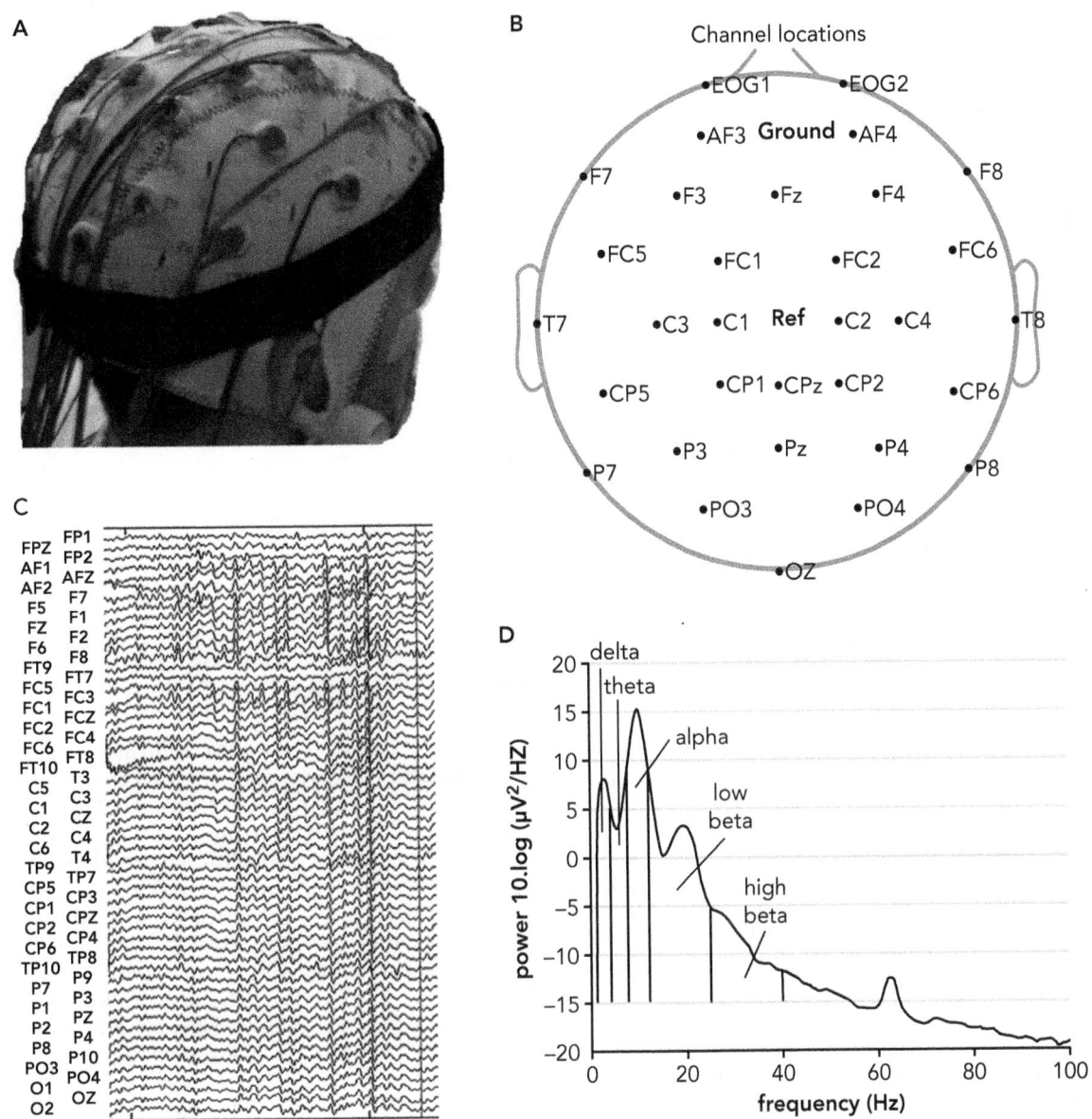

FIGURE 17-1 Electroencephalography (EEG). A, Setup of a 32 channels EEG system. B, Electrode positions on a topographical map. C, Raw recordings (conventional EEG). D, Example of the power spectrum in one channel (quantitative EEG).

ing between mild and moderate TBI either (4,9). There are studies that note an absence of any early EEG abnormalities, (10) even when a structural abnormality is present on magnetic resonance imaging (MRI) (11) or the patient clinically exhibits symptoms of TBI (12–14). However, not all studies report normal conventional EEG following mild TBI or concussion. One study, conducted in 1944 (15), involved the EEG recording of patients with industrial injuries acquired in a shipyard. Most patients, in whom EEG was measured within 15 minutes postinjury, showed little or no apparent alteration in the recording. However, certain patients who experienced the least delay between trauma and EEG recording showed diffuse slowing of EEG activity. This generally resolved within 15 minutes but for some lasted up to an hour. Within the first several hours after mild trauma, attenuated posterior alpha waves (decreased alpha fre-

quency) as well as generalized or focal slow wave activity with a preponderance of theta waves are sometimes observed (3,8,16–18). The presence of these signs may be dependent on the length of loss of consciousness (19). Further, when associated with other signs of complicated injury, these abnormalities predict a poorer prognosis (20). However, the changes are often subtle and sometimes within the range of normal findings in the general population. Even if a longer lasting abnormality is present, it often resolves completely within months after a mild TBI. Correspondence between clinical and EEG findings is relatively poor (8), and any abnormalities discovered tend to resolve during the first several months postinjury (21). In the late period postinjury, approximately 10% of the individuals tend to show mild EEG abnormalities (10). However, the etiology of these is not always clear, and they may not be indicative of brain

TABLE 17-1 Electroencephalography Rhythms and Their Significance in Healthy and TBI Populations

RHYTHMS	FREQUENCY	MAIN DISTRIBUTION	RECORDED IN HEALTHY	STANDARD EEG FINDINGS IN PATIENTS WITH TBI
Delta	< 4 Hz		Awake state in the very young and in the elderly. Across all ages during slow-wave sleep.	Increased slow waves in the delta frequency band in severe TBI.
Theta	4–8 Hz	Frontocentral	Resting or while performing moderately difficult mental tasks; enhanced by drowsiness.	Rise in slow focal or diffuse theta activity.
Alpha	8–13 Hz	Posterior	Attenuated with eye opening.	Immediate decrease in the mean frequency of alpha waves.
Mu	8–13 Hz	Central	Attenuated with contralateral movement of an extremity.	
Beta	13–30 Hz	Frontal	Mental, lingual, or cognitive efforts	
Gamma	> 30 Hz	Diffuse, central	Higher cognitive functions involving perception, attention, learning, and memory. Assess the temporal dynamics of cortical networks and their interactions	

Abbreviation: EEG, electroencephalography; TBI, traumatic brain injury.

damage. For example, a low-voltage alpha EEG pattern, months to years after a mild TBI or concussion, is indicative more of anxiety than brain injury (16).

Severe TBI

The use of EEG in severe TBI is higher than in mild TBI. EEG recordings after severe brain injury correlate well with the depth of post-traumatic coma (22–25). During initial stages of a TBI-induced coma, EEG variables such as the amplitude, frequency, and shape of wave potentials are not stable (6). Initial recordings taken within 24 hours postinjury are of less prognostic significance, however, than those from the 24- to 48- hour period (23,26). This could be caused by an interplay between both irreversible brain lesions and reversible functional disturbances. The degree of unconsciousness in patients can rapidly change, and thus continuous monitoring has been used for detecting possible signs of clinical deterioration during the first few weeks postinjury (27). Findings, during a post-traumatic coma, range from increased slow activity to amplitude suppression (28). Features typical of sleep, various sharply contoured discharges, epileptic spikes, periodic lateralized epileptiform discharges (PLEDs), and triphasic waves can also be found. However, reactivity and the typical sleep features mentioned earlier are more common among patients who show a good recovery (29).

In the late postinjury period of severe brain injuries, EEGs may show a wide variety of dysrhythmias, focal or generalized suppression, focal slowing, frontal alpha waves, and epileptiform discharges (30–31).

In summary, the use of conventional EEG in mild TBI is limited. Although there are abnormalities sometimes discovered in the EEG of patients with mild TBI, sensitivity is low, and the clinical and functional significance are uncertain. Further, any detected abnormalities may be similar to those present in the general population. Even in the late postinjury period, there is a lot of skepticism toward the significance of epileptiform EEG findings. In severe cases of TBI, however, the EEG can be more helpful and may even lend a hand in determining a prognosis for the patient.

Post-Traumatic Epilepsy

Post-traumatic epilepsy (PTE) will be covered in depth in Chapter 39 (Post-traumatic Seizures and Epilepsy) of this book. PTE is a recurrent seizure disorder that results from TBI. PTE is estimated to constitute more than 20% of cases of symptomatic epilepsy and about 5% of all cases of epilepsy. PTE must be differentiated from post-traumatic seizures (PTS), which refers to isolated seizures that occur as a sequel to brain injury either within 24 hours (immediate PTS), within 1 week (early PTS), or more than 1 week after injury (late PTS). About 20% of people who have a single late PTS never have any further seizures and should not be labeled as having PTE.

How to predict who will develop epilepsy after TBI and who will not is challenging. The onset of PTE can occur within a short time of the TBI but also months or even years later, and compared with the general population, people with TBI remain at a higher risk for epilepsy even decades after the injury. Serial EEGs may, thus, be helpful in following a patient after TBI and assessing the risk of PTE. However, this practice is not free of challenges.

The severity and type of injury certainly contribute to the risk of developing PTE, for example, penetrating injuries and those causing intracerebral hemorrhages confer a higher risk. On the other hand, development of PTE is a relatively uncommon consequence of mild TBI (32). Nonetheless, a study showed that epileptiform abnormalities assessed with magnetoencephalography (MEG) were present in 10% of the cases long after an episode of mild TBI (33). However, this statistic may not differ much from the prevalence of these abnormalities in the general population. Indeed, an earlier study (14) reported that 6 months after a mild TBI, the number of patients with epileptiform EEG abnormalities were equal to those who had sustained only a whiplash injury. However, the authors did notice that post-traumatic epileptiform abnormalities increased as time passed while other

EEG abnormalities did not. It should be noted that epileptiform activity could also be observed in healthy subjects with no history of seizures. In addition to various epileptiform variant patterns that are nonepileptic in nature (1,34,35), spontaneous interictal epileptiform discharges (IED) can be recorded in healthy volunteers (35). Overall, spontaneous IED rates appear to be higher in patients who are nonepileptic with TBI than in healthy adults (2%–12% vs 0%–6.6%), and rates for a seizure after IED detection are also higher in patients than in healthy adults (up to 14% in patients vs 2% in healthy adults).

It is, thus, difficult to predict the occurrence of PTE when based only on the recording of spontaneous IEDs, particularly after mild TBI. It is usually considered that sleep deprivation is an enhancer of epileptic discharges and seizure frequency. However, this could also be because sleep deprivation often occurs in association with physical or emotional stress and substance abuse. When controlling for these factors, sleep deprivation facilitates IEDs but does not seem to affect seizure frequency (36). However, EEGs after sleep deprivation might be a useful indicator of brain damage after TBI, and follow-up imaging studies (computer tomography [CT] or MRI) seem warranted and frequently reveal abnormalities (37).

In case of greater clinical suspicion, admission to an epilepsy monitoring unit (EMU) for prolonged video-EEG monitoring is the best way to confirm and clarify a diagnosis of epilepsy. In patients with suspected diagnosis of PTE, video-EEG monitoring can provide further diagnostic clarification and certainty in about 80% of the cases. Importantly, about 30% will be diagnosed as having psychogenic nonepileptic seizures (38). Finally, deep brain recordings might be necessary to precisely localize the epileptic focus before surgery in case of intractable epilepsy.

In summary, the development of PTE is rare after mild TBI, although higher following other more severe TBIs (particularly penetrating wounds and those with intracerebral bleeds). Symptoms can develop long time after the TBI and while EEGs can be helpful in serially assessing the relative risk; presence of epileptiform activity in the EEG does not necessarily predict the occurrence of future seizures. However, it might indicate the existence of more significant brain damage.

Quantitative EEG

With signal processing technology, EEG data can be quantified and objectively analyzed (Figure 17-1D). Computer-assisted analysis of EEG data, that is, quantitative EEG (QEEG), offers definite advantages over a trained electroencephalographer's eye in identifying the electrophysiological features of TBI (3–4). Although some studies raise questions about the overall validity and accuracy of QEEG findings (8), many discuss the reliability of use in assessing various neurological disorders (9), specifically in diagnosing and classifying the severity of TBI (4,39). Studies have determined multiple QEEG variables known as discriminant functions. Because of their low cost, speed, and objectivity, these can help in predicting functional characteristics and pathologies (40).

Thatcher et al. (4,41) showed that QEEG was very successful in distinguishing and discriminating mild TBI from controls and also from patients with more severe TBI. They were able to achieve a discriminant classification accuracy of 94.8% in 1989 amongst a population of 608 cases of mild TBI and 108 age-matched controls. In 2001, the sensitivity in discriminating between mild and severe TBI was 95.45%, and specificity was 97.44%. Thatcher et al. went on to propose "big bump theory" stating that pathological residues and/or compensation could be detectable by QEEG even years later after the original trauma. This is analogous to the big bang theory where cosmic radiation is still detected billions of years after the explosion. The study also discovered that the greatest contribution to discriminant function was actually multivariable and consisted of coherence, phase, and amplitude differences. Consensus says that QEEG of TBI cases show an immediate decrease in the mean frequency of alpha waves and a rise in slow focal or diffuse theta activity (8–9). These often later resolve within weeks and months coinciding with clinical improvement (8).

Methods of analysis of continuous EEG recording have been developed to evaluate changes in connectivity between different brain areas after TBI. EEG coherence, that is, correlation between the spectral content of 2 electrodes over time, is believed to reflect the strength of functional interactions between cortical neuraly networks; EEG phase, that is, the time lag between 2 similar activations at different locations, is believed to be linked to the speed of the connection between the 2 areas. TBI has been characterized by a decreased coherence and increased asymmetry (9). However, these coherence changes can be considered nonspecific findings and can certainly be found in pathologies other than TBI (8). Kumar et al. (42) showed that patients with mild TBI depicted normal connectivity at rest from 1 to 6 months after their concussion. These patients, however, had impaired verbal and visuospatial working memory tasks. This impairment was associated with decreased frontoparietal, frontotemporal, temporoparietal, and interhemispheric connectivity during working memory performance. Similarly, during an auditory memory activation condition, abnormal frontal connectivity measures within the low and high beta bands (coherence and phase), as well as a shift toward right temporal functioning, have been associated with auditory memory deficits in patients with TBI (43). Thus, abnormalities of functional connectivity, explored during tasks execution, might be more prominent and more sensitive than abnormalities explored during the resting state.

However, impairment in functional connectivity at rest can be revealed with more sophisticated methods. Cao and Sloubounov (44) described a method in which an independent component analysis (ICA) was run to transform multichannel EEG recordings into independent processes. A source reconstruction algorithm followed this transformation. A graph theory analysis was then performed to assess the connectivity between regions of interest (ROIs). This method was applied to athletes, selected for their high risk of concussion, up to 6 months before and 7 days after a sport-related mild TBI. TBI resulted in a decrease in the long-distance connectivity (between frontal areas and other areas of the brain) and significant increase in the short-distance connectivity (within occipital and parietal areas) at rest, which could not be observed when traditional coherence analysis was implemented.

In summary, these studies reveal how the information contained in the EEG signal is rich and can be mathemati-

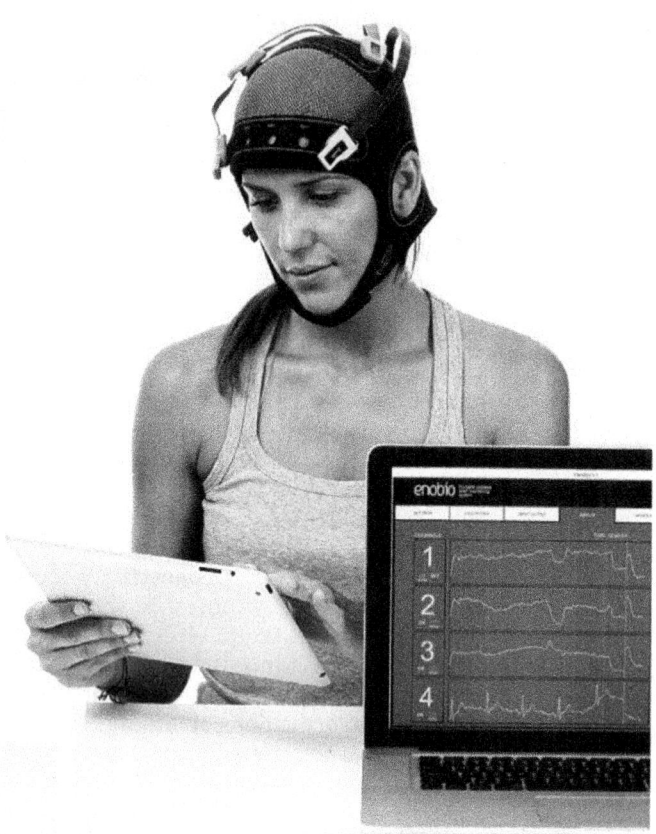

FIGURE 17–2 Setup of a wearable, modular, and wireless system of electroencephalography (EEG) recording (ENOBIO, Starlab, Barcelona, Spain).

cally processed to quantify abnormalities after severe TBI and also to reveal subtle abnormalities following mild TBI. The most consistent findings, as summarized by Thatcher (45) are (*a*) reduced power in the higher frequency bands (alpha and above), related to cortical gray matter injury; (*b*) increased slow waves in the delta frequency band in severe TBI, which are related to cerebral white matter injury; and (*c*) changes in EEG coherence and phase delays, related to gray and white matter injury, especially in frontal and temporal lobes. Novel technology that enables wearable, modular, and wireless recording of EEG (Figure 17-2) on the one hand, and the advent of more powerful, faster analysis algorithms on the other hand, promise to further increase the use of quantitative EEG in TBI.

On the Use of EEG Versus Quantitative EEG: Clinical and Forensic Considerations

In a report of the American Academy of Neurology and the American Clinical Neurophysiology Society on the assessment of digital EEG, QEEG, and EEG brain mapping published in 1997 (still holding in 2006), it was stated that QEEG remains investigational for clinical use in postconcussion syndrome resulting from mild or moderate head injury (46). This statement was criticized in later publications (e.g., 9,47–48). The superiority of visual examination over QEEG defended by the American Academy of Neurology is ques-

tioned in regard (among others) to the demonstrated subjectivity of visual examination and the large amount of publications based on QEEG. Discriminate analysis with QEEG is also challenging given the fact that frequently, the issue is not simply a differentiation between "TBI" vs "no TBI," that is, patients may have prior mental health issues, postinjury post-traumatic stress disorder (PTSD), depression, anxiety, drug abuse, alcohol, medications, and so forth. In addition, there is ongoing controversy regarding the various normative databases used for QEEG analysis. Thus, QEEG has not become fully established in the clinical realm, yet it can play a role in the medicolegal arena, where it can find some acceptance in courts and for third-party reimbursement (45). Part XIX (Medicolegal and Ethical Issues) of this book will cover in depth these forensic considerations.

EEG Biofeedback

EEG biofeedback will be covered in depth in chapter 76 (Complementary and Alternative Medicine) of this book. Here, we shall just provide some basic descriptions of the principles. EEG biofeedback offers the opportunity for EEG to go from diagnostic and prognostic applications to therapeutics. Biofeedback techniques have been used to promote improvement of cognitive functions. Biofeedback consists of measuring certain physiologic parameters from a patient and then converting them into a sensorial feedback that is provided to the patient. The feedback is positive (reward) when the desired physiological response is obtained, whereas it is negative when the undesired physiological response occurs. Thus, the patient learns to control his or her own physiological process (Figure 17-3).

When the physiological signals of interest are extracted from EEG, this technique is called EEG biofeedback, neurofeedback, or neurotherapy. The electrophysiological signals are believed to be related to different functional and mental states. The patient can hear or see an audio or visual positive feedback whenever the target parameters equal or exceed a threshold setting. The threshold is usually adjusted periodically to ensure the patient can receive the feedback over a fixed duration of time. The patient is instructed to discover the mental set or strategy to produce and maintain the positive feedback; no further instruction is given. The sessions are discontinued when the patient reaches the desired level of brain activity and/or behavioral improvement, when the neurophysiologic and/or neuropsychological outcomes remain stable, or after a fixed number of sessions.

Originally, the target electrophysiological signal in EEG biofeedback was the amplitude in a given frequency band, and the purpose was to normalize the EEG by increasing abnormally weak frequency bands and/or decreasing excessively dominant frequency bands. However, other physiological parameters can be targeted. Thornton (49) described 2 distinct categories. In addition to the absolute magnitude in a given frequency band, the activation measures are comprised of the relative magnitude (ratio of the magnitude of one band to the total magnitude of all bands), peak amplitude, peak frequency, and symmetry (peak amplitude symmetry between 2 locations in a particular bandwidth). The connection measures are mainly comprised of measures of coherence and phase.

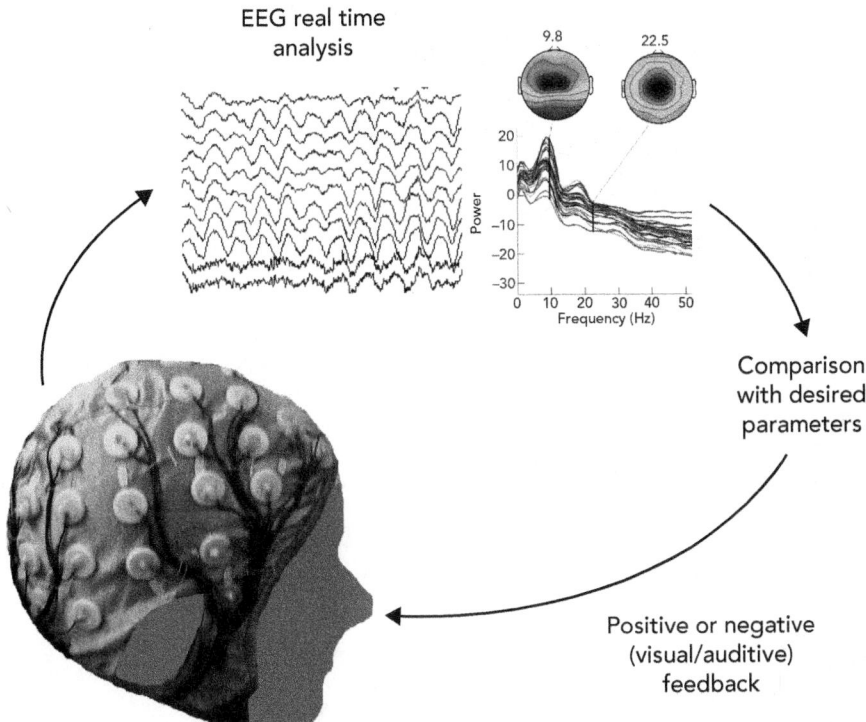

EEG real time analysis

Comparison with desired parameters

Positive or negative (visual/auditive) feedback

FIGURE 17–3 Schematic principle of electroencephalography (EEG) biofeedback.

The promise of EEG biofeedback is to promote normalization of abnormal brain activity and thus lead to behavioral and cognitive advantages. This promise is not specific to TBI, and indeed, EEG biofeedback is explored and claimed to be of benefit in a long list of diverse conditions, reaching from anxiety/mood disorders, attention deficit and hyperactivity disorders and autism, to age-related cognitive decline, and dementia. This chapter focuses on the notion that EEG biofeedback might leverage the diagnostic virtues of quantitative EEG in TBI and offer a valuable therapeutic intervention.

Two main approaches of EEG biofeedback in patients with TBI can be found in the literature. The first one relies on predefined protocols, based on previous studies revealing EEG abnormalities in patients with TBI, aiming to eliminate supposed abnormalities. The second one is based on individual deviations from normal EEG values as defined by a control group of participants or with a previously constituted database. Although most protocols train patients to control their brain activity at rest (eyes opened or eyes closed conditions), rehabilitating the EEG abnormalities while the patient is performing a task involving the target function is also possible and might increase the efficiency of EEG biofeedback.

According to the aim of the protocol, the EEG electrodes of interest can differ. By default, the vertex of the head (electrode position Cz) is generally chosen. However, in TBI, one can choose the electrode closest to the impact site of the head injury (e.g., 50) or electrodes that reveal the largest abnormalities (e.g., 51). The frequencies considered have been traditionally limited to frequencies lower than 32 Hz. Higher frequencies (high beta or gamma bands), nevertheless, may also have multiple functions in sensory and cognitive processing and are of interest for the rehabilitation of patients with TBI (52). It should be noted that different defi-

nitions of the frequency bands are given across different studies; moreover, methods of calculation of different parameters (e.g., coherence) might vary from one study to another. Thus, generalization of any results in this field requires special care.

The single-case study of Byers (50) offers an example of a protocol aiming to adjust the level of activity in predefined frequency bands. A patient who sustained a TBI 6 years earlier was trained to enhance, over the Cz location, his or her sensory motor rhythm (12–15 Hz) and in a second time his or her beta activity (15–18 Hz) while at the same time suppressing theta activity (4–7 Hz). The expected modifications of frequency were not clearly obtained; nonetheless, many symptoms of this patient were reduced during and following the EEG biofeedback training. The improvement was mainly seen in cognitive flexibility and executive functions.

An example of connectivity training at rest, to normalize coherence values toward values measured in a group of healthy subjects, can be found in the study of Walker et al. (51). Twenty-six patients with TBI with symptoms interfering with daily activities for more than 3 months, including employment, were trained to increase their reduced coherence values and to decrease any elevated coherence values. The initial training involved the use of a pair of electrodes with the most significant abnormalities. After 5 sessions, the training was dedicated to the next pair of electrodes picking up the most significant abnormalities and so on. Using a global improvement scale, based on a reduction of symptoms (e.g., headaches, memory loss or confusion) and the ability to return to work, significant improvements were noted in 88% of the patients.

The studies from Tinius and Tinius (53), Thornton (49), and Thornton and Carmody (52) exemplify EEG biofeedback training while the patient is performing cognitive training or a task involving the function to be improved. In the study of Tinius and Tinius (53), the treatment decisions for 16 patients with mild TBI followed preestablished rules based on clinical symptoms and a brain map from the Thatcher reference database. For example, if theta activity was high, the treatment aimed to decrease theta activity at Cz; if the primary symptom was pain, the target was to increase sensory motor rhythm at Cz. They postulated that it may be beneficial to use coherence training after unipolar training and that it should start with the rehabilitation of short connections before long connections. Following this methodology, patients reported a decrease in their symptoms, and there was improvement of visual and auditory sustained attention that was trained during the simultaneous cognitive tasks. For the rehabilitation of memory function in patients with TBI, Thornton (49) offered a database for normal EEG reference during 18 different tasks (obtained from subjects without neurological disorder, history of brain injury or learning problems). The EEG variables were correlated with the memory performance of 59 normal right-handed participants to determine the cortically based electrophysiological correlates of effective cognitive functioning. Then, in several multiple single-case studies (49,52), patients with TBI were trained to normalize abnormal connections (coherence and phase values), and this was associated with improvement of general cognitive abilities and memory function.

In summary, EEG biofeedback in patients with TBI is a promising field. However, it needs to be further explored. Thornton and Carmody (54) point out the heterogeneity of parameters chosen and outcomes measured in studies of EEG biofeedback in TBI. It remains to be systematically proven that (a) abnormal EEG parameters and behavioral deficits are correlated, (b) EEG biofeedback is effective in normalizing EEG, (c) EEG biofeedback is effective in improving behavior and cognition, (d) measured improved functions translate into everyday life criteria, and (e) positive changes are long lasting. Ultimately, appropriately powered, randomized, controlled trials are needed.

In this context, a few questions are worth considering. Most prominently, how soon after a TBI the EEG biofeedback should be offered remains an open question. Starting too soon may overload existing resources, whereas waiting for a longer period of time may reduce the potential benefit (50–51). Several studies point toward the absence of a link between the time since the TBI and EEG abnormalities or successful outcomes of EEG biofeedback (51,52,55). These observations contribute to the notion that the brain does not spontaneously repair the damage caused by the TBI but instead allocates different resources to accomplish the task with variable results (49).

EVOKED POTENTIALS

Following the presentation of a stimulus or multiple stimuli, an electrophysiological response from the nervous system is known as an EP. The stimuli are most frequently auditory, visual, or somatosensory, and the EPs are frequently recorded from the brain using EEG techniques. These potentials are different from conventional EEG because they are calculated from an averaged response to a presented stimulus. Such av-

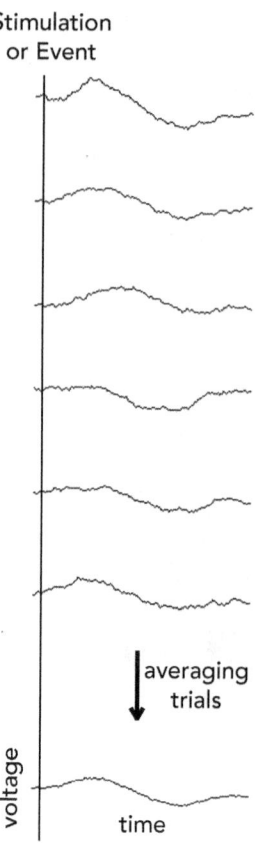

FIGURE 17–4 Principle of evoked potentials (EPs): stimulation- or event-locked averaging of several trials allows the isolation of an electroencephalography (EEG) response to stimulation (EP) or event-related potential (ERP) from background EEG activity.

eraging allows the response to the stimuli to be isolated from the background EEG activity (Figure 17-4).

Somatosensory Evoked Potential

The somatosensory EP (SEP) captures the manner in which the neural system responds to sensory input. SEPs can be elicited through electrical, tactile, vibratory, or painful stimuli applied to different body parts. However, among these different modalities, electrical stimulation is most commonly employed because of its ease of use (56). A peripheral nerve, such as the median, ulnar, or tibial nerve, is stimulated, and the EP is picked up over the scalp (Figure 17-5). A SEP is generally characterized by its amplitude and latency. Short-latency SEPs (50 ms from stimulation) are more independent from the level of consciousness than longer latencies, which generally reflect higher cognitive processes. For example, absence of the N20 component of the SEPs, the component thought to mark the arrival of the thalamic volley to the cortex, appears to be a reliable indicator of significant corticosubcortical disconnection and suggestive of poor prognosis. Overall, short-latency SEPs are considered valuable prognostic indicators for TBI (57).

Somatosensory Evoked Potentials after stimulation of Medial Nerve

Normal SEP

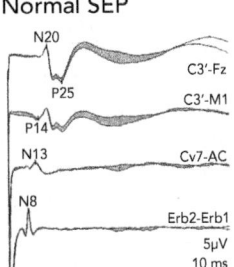

Pathological SEP from an increased central condition time

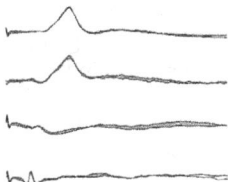

Absent cortical SEP

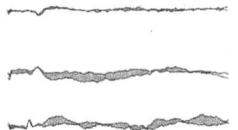

Event Related Potentials in a Oddball Paradigm

Frequent Tone

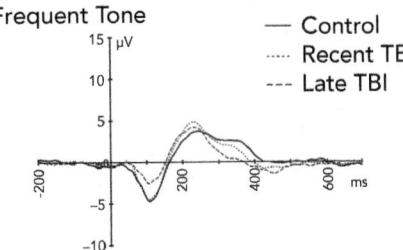

Rare Target Tone (eliciting the P3b)

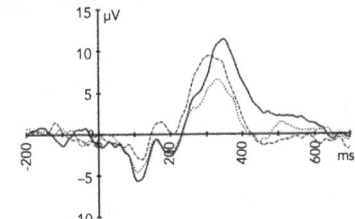

Rare Deviant Tone (eliciting the P3a)

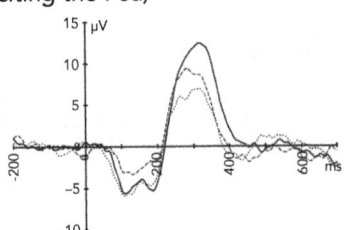

FIGURE 17–5 Illustration of somatosensory evoked potentials (SEPs) and event-related potentials (ERPs) in a traumatic brain injury (TBI) population compared to healthy controls. *Left*: SEPs. Adapted from Amantini et al. (57) with permission. *Right*: ERPs. Adapted from Thériault et al. (71) with permission.

In a consensus for the use of neurophysiologic techniques in TBI (58), short-latency EPs (including auditory and somatosensory) were found to be normal in 50% of severe TBI cases. Further, bilateral normal short-latency EPs predicted a favorable outcome in almost 80% of patients after TBI (59). However, a stronger prognostic indicator (albeit, negative) was in fact the absence of bilateral short-latency EPs (N20), and one study (57) showed a 95% predictive value of not awakening from a coma with such a recording. A systematic review of 25 studies (60) showed that SEPs are the best single overall predictor of outcome after TBI, superior to CT, EEG, Glasgow Coma Scale (GCS), and pupillary and motor responses. However, when standard clinical tests such as GCS and pupillary and motor responses are combined with SEP recordings, the predictive ability is further enhanced.

Other EP studies such as brainstem auditory evoked potential (BAEP) are limited to evaluating pharmacological effects of hearing and brainstem dysfunction after brain injury (56, 61); visual evoked potential (VEP) to disturbances in the visual cortex. One study (62) combined the use of SEPs and BAEPs but noticed that it was really only SEPs that increased the predictive value of certain clinical parameters while neither of them correlated with cognitive function at 1-year follow-up.

Because EPs provide neurophysiologic monitoring of different neural pathways (SEPs = somatosensory system, VEPs = visual system, BAEPs = auditory pathways, etc.),

and because these various pathways show limited overlap, it seems reasonable to assume that multimodal EPs may be of additive diagnostic and prognostic value. A similar argument can be made regarding multimodal EPs within a given domain, where EPs are evoked with a variety of different stimuli (e.g., SEPs can be evoked by touch, pressure, electric stimuli, etc.) because these can tap onto different receptors and be mediated by different fiber pathways. Unfortunately, despite the theoretical appeal of such considerations, the practical use of such approaches is limited. Brain imaging techniques, particularly MRI, appear to offer greater clinical use.

In summary, the use of a SEP test can be of high value when assessing patients with brain injury and can add prognostic information to the clinical assessment. Certain situations need to be considered beforehand though, such as how the use of anesthesia can decrease the amplitude of SEP recordings, to prevent false conclusions.

Event-Related Potential/P300

An event-related potential (ERP) is an EP generally influenced by higher cognitive faculties. It is a measured brain response that is the result of either internal (e.g., thoughts) or external stimuli. Similar to EPs, ERPs are typically quantitatively characterized by their amplitude and latency. An ERP is usually referred to by its polarity (positive [P] or negative [N]) and its latency in milliseconds.

A typical ERP protocol involves identifying and discriminating a specific stimulus in a larger series of stimuli (oddball paradigm). The target stimulus is generally presented 20% of the time, whereas the other stimuli (distractors) are presented 80% of the time (63). To accurately judge the brain's response to these stimuli, the experimenter must record multiple trials and then average the results. ERPs are thought to capture complex coordinated processing of widespread brain networks and appear to be a useful tool in assessing patients following brain injury because of their noninvasiveness and great temporal resolution (56).

One of the important elicited patterns of the ERP is the positive peak elicited 300 ms poststimulus (P300) (63). This response is consistently observed whether the stimulus is visual, auditory, tactile, or even olfactory. It is thought to reflect active attention, working memory, and the ability to discriminate individual stimuli among a group of other similar stimuli (64–67). Following brain injury the absence of P300 does not necessarily predict a negative outcome (68). However, another study (69) emphasized the usefulness of visual ERPs for evaluation of abnormalities following trauma. Doi et al. (69) compared 20 patients with TBI with 32 age-matched controls using a conventional oddball paradigm. They found that the P300 latency was longer in patients than in the controls. In addition, the P300 amplitudes were significantly smaller in patients than in controls but only for certain stimuli. Thus, ERPs may be a potentially useful marker for evaluating cognitive dysfunction in patients after TBI. However, detailed attention to the type of stimulus is important, and the use of ERPs at individual (rather than group) level is insufficiently studied.

Abnormalities in ERP have also been found in asymptomatic patients with TBI. For instance, a 3-tone auditory oddball paradigm revealed subclinical deficits in concussed athletes (e.g., 70–71). This paradigm consists of 3 different stimuli presented in a random order: typically a standard tone presented in 80%, a deviant target tone presented in 10%, and a deviant nontarget tone presented in 10% of the trials. Participants are instructed to press a button when they hear the target stimulus while withholding their response to both standard and deviant nontarget tones.

A P3a ERP is obtained by averaging brain responses to the rare deviant tone, whereas the P3b ERP is obtained by averaging brain responses to the rare target tone (Figure 17-5). Thus, the P3b component is analogous to the classic P300 described earlier. A P3b amplitude reduction is believed to reflect deficits in memory updating. The P3a component is thought to reflect frontal lobe function; reduced P3a amplitude and latency delays may reflect deficits in shifting of attentional resources to novel stimuli. Although concussed athletes generally show normal behavioral outcomes in the auditory (or the equivalent visual) oddball task, their P3a and/or P3b components frequently show reduced amplitude and/or an increased latency (71–73). Such abnormalities may resolve 2 years after the last multiple concussions (71), but one study showed abnormalities up to 3 decades after the last multiple concussions (70). Further studies along these lines, however, seem warranted. A reliable objective marker of brain function/dysfunction following TBI, such as this one, might provide valuable insights into the neurobiological impact of injury and the compensatory mechanisms that may render the patients asymptomatic but nevertheless render them vulnerable for long-term complications.

In summary, these ERP measures appear to represent a particularly sensitive tool to detect functional alterations unnoticed on classic neuropsychological tests. ERP-identified subclinical findings may explain the vulnerability of patients to subsequent concussions and the reported susceptibility of patients with TBI to develop long-term complications, including a progressive cognitive decline. Longitudinal studies using such measures seem to be warranted.

TRANSCRANIAL MAGNETIC STIMULATION

TMS is a noninvasive method that uses the principles of electromagnetic induction to induce currents within discrete brain regions (74,75). These currents can be of sufficient magnitude to depolarize neurons. When applied repetitively, TMS can modulate cortical excitability, decreasing or increasing it, depending on the parameters of stimulation, beyond the duration of the train of stimulation.

Following single-pulse TMS, distinct episodes of enhanced and suppressed activity can be observed. Initial induction of an excitatory postsynaptic potential is followed by a period of suppression of 100–200 ms duration. Furthermore, local and distant reentry mechanisms contribute to complex and longer lasting suppression-activation dynamics. This results in lasting neuromodulation with a complex pattern of suppression and facilitation of activity, in part related to stimulation of inhibitory and excitatory interneurons, metabotropic or metabolic processes, or even vascular responses.

TMS represents a particularly pertinent approach suitable to study the neurophysiologic effects of TBI because of its unprecedented sensitivity to central excitation/inhibition (E/I) mechanisms (76). TMS can provide additional tools to characterize severity of TBI and evaluate abnormalities in symptomatic and asymptomatic patients. Moreover, the ability to induce plasticity with TMS can provide an interventional tool to promote recovery.

Characterization of Brain Abnormalities After TBI: Single- and Paired-Pulse TMS

EP approaches can be readily adapted along with the use of TMS. TMS is applied as a controlled input to a specific brain region, and the neurophysiologic nervous system response can be recorded using electromyography (EMG) or EEG. The most commonly used EPs elicited with TMS are motor-evoked potentials (MEPs). They are produced by using TMS to target the primary motor cortex (M1) and are recorded using EMG via electrodes placed over specific target muscles. MEPs are of great interest to evaluate corticospinal integrity in patients with TBI.

Central Motor Conduction Time

Central motor conduction time (CMCT) reflects the integrity of the corticospinal tract (77). It is calculated by subtracting the peripheral conduction time (spinal cord to muscles) from the latency of MEPs evoked by TMS. CMCT has been shown to be prolonged in patients with TBI with diffuse and combined brain lesions tested 2 weeks after head trauma (78). However, CMCT was not affected in patients with TBI with minor brain concussions or focal lesions (78). Nonetheless, this absence of CMCT increase does not necessarily demonstrate an absence of impairment at the cortical level.

Resting Motor Threshold and Motor-Evoked Potentials Amplitude

Resting motor threshold (RMT) refers to the lowest TMS intensity necessary to evoke MEPs in a target muscle when single-pulse stimuli are applied to the contralateral M1. RMT reflects neuronal membrane excitability, which is highly dependent on ion channel conductivity (79–80). When TMS is applied at suprathreshold intensities, activation of excitatory interneurons results in volleys of upper motor neuron activity, which subsequently activate motor neurons in the spinal cord. The summed activity results in an MEP. Latency and peak-to-peak amplitude reflect the integrity of the corticospinal motor pathways. The MEP/M wave amplitude ratio is calculated by dividing the MEP amplitude by the maximal M wave amplitude obtained after supramaximal peripheral electrical stimulation.

RMT did not reveal any abnormality, neither in athletes with 1 to several concussions 9 months after their last concussion (81) nor in athletes with a history of sports concussions more than 30 years prior to testing (70). However, in another study, RMT was significantly increased 2 weeks after mild and moderate head injury (78). This increase was accompanied by a marked reduction in the MEP/M wave amplitude ratio. Similarly, concussed athletes evaluated sequentially between 1 and 10 days postconcussion showed a progressive increase in MEP latency and a reduction in MEP amplitude (82). The loss of the corticospinal neurons, the slowing because of demyelination or axonal disconnection, and the desynchronization of multiple descending volleys resulting in less effective temporal summation of excitatory postsynaptic potentials could explain these observations (78,82). In addition, the reduction of the MEP amplitude may also be indicative of pyramidal tract/brainstem involvement (82).

Finally, increased RMT was also found 3 months after mild-to-moderate TBI in patients with objective excessive daytime sleepiness (83). A reduced excitability of the corticospinal system during wakefulness, mimicking the hyperpolarization of the thalamocortical system in healthy subjects during sleep, might contribute to the persistent sleepiness often seen in patients with TBI.

Cortical Silent Period

When TMS is delivered over the motor cortex while the subject maintains a voluntary muscle contraction in the contralateral hand, a pause in ongoing EMG activities follows the MEP (Figure 17-6D). This pause is called the cortical silent period or contralateral silent period (CSP). The initial phase of the CSP might be related to the refractory period of the pyramidal tract neurons, whereas the latter part of the CSP has been attributed to activity of intracortical inhibitory systems of the M1 involving gamma-aminobutyric acid (GABA_B) receptors.

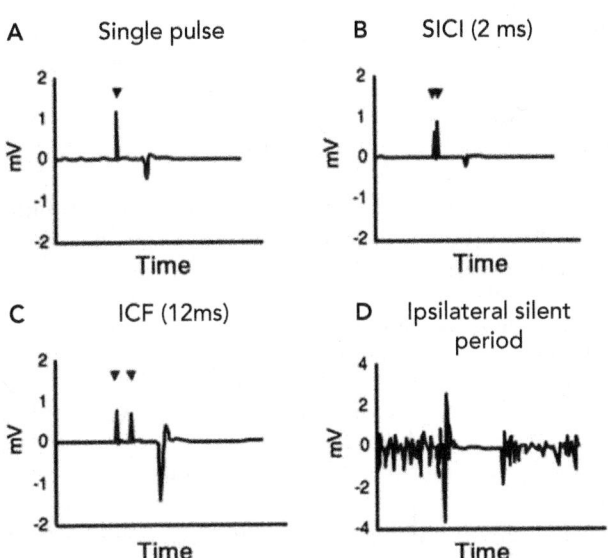

FIGURE 17–6 Examples of transcranial magnetic stimulation (TMS) paradigms. A, A single pulse of TMS over M1 evokes an MEP recorded over the contralateral first dorsal interosseous. B, Two pulses separated by 2 ms evoke an MEP of smaller amplitude, revealing short interval intracortical inhibition (SICI). C, Two pulses separated by 12 ms evoke an MEP of larger amplitude, revealing intracortical facilitation (ICF). D, A pulse applied during a voluntary contraction of the contralateral hand evokes a pause in ongoing EMG activity following the MEP. Adapted from de Beaumont et al. (81) with permission.

De Beaumont et al. (81) and Tremblay et al. (84) showed that CSP duration was prolonged in athletes who had experienced multiple concussions. Sustaining subsequent concussions exacerbates this deficit and thus provides additional support for the existence of cumulative deficit following multiple concussions; moreover, concussion severity was significantly correlated with CSP lengthening (81). Observed CSP duration lengthening in athletes with multiple concussion seemed to remain unaffected by the time elapsed since the last accident. De Beaumont et al. (70) further showed that former athletes with a history of concussion more than 30 years prior to testing also have an increased CSP duration, despite apparently normal cognitive performance and absence of neuropsychological abnormalities.

However, a previous study (78) showed no alteration of CSP duration in a similar population of patients 2 weeks after a mild TBI; only patients with moderate brain injury showed an increased CSP duration. Such discrepancy could be related to methodological aspects in relation to determination of TMS intensity (78). Alternatively, CSP prolongation could be triggered later after trauma, when acute RMT abnormalities are resolved (81).

Ipsilateral Silent Period

When TMS is applied over M1 during an ongoing tonic voluntary contraction of the muscles ipsilateral to the site of stimulation, the activity of these ipsilateral muscles can be temporarily suppressed. This ipsilateral silent period (ISP) has been attributed to transcallosal inhibition, and this method can evaluate the integrity of the corpus callosum connecting homologous motor cortices. Diffuse axonal injury, in consequence of TBI, might involve disruption of the corpus callosum, which may be uncovered as a reduction of transcallosal inhibition measured with TMS. Takeuchi et al. (85) showed that the amount of transcallosal inhibition was significantly reduced in patients with TBI several months after their concussion compared to healthy controls, and this reduction was significantly correlated with the severity of TBI as evaluated using the GCS.

Transcallosal inhibition can also be assessed by measuring the decrease in amplitude of an MEP evoked by a test pulse applied over the contralateral M1 when this test pulse is preceded by a conditioning pulse applied over the ipsilateral M1 (dual-coil paired-pulse TMS technique). This paired-pulse technique using 2 TMS coils has not yet been used in a TBI population but offers promise to further characterize possible interhemispheric and other corticocortical disconnections.

Excitatory and Inhibitory Balance

Chistyakov et al. (78) evaluated the balance between excitatory and inhibitory central mechanism by calculating the interthreshold difference (ITD) as the difference between the RMT and CSP threshold. Indeed, both RMT and CSP thresholds were significantly increased in patients who sustained mild and moderate head injury, but the increase in CSP threshold was much less pronounced than that of the MEP threshold. This resulted in a significant increase of the ITD. The increase in the ITD, accompanied by reduction of the MEP/M wave amplitude ratio, suggests dissociated impairment of inhibitory and excitatory components of the central motor control.

Alternative ways to assess excitatory and inhibitory central mechanisms is using paired-pulse TMS (ppTMS) paradigms. The ppTMS involves the application of 2 TMS stimuli of independently controllable intensity and with a variable interstimulus interval to the same cortical region. The first stimulus, thus, serves as a conditioning stimulus to the effect of the second test stimulus. Several paired-pulse paradigms have been designed to assess the short-interval intracortical inhibition (SICI; Figure 17-6B), hypothetically $GABA_A$ mediated, the long-interval intracortical inhibition (LICI), hypothetically $GABA_B$-mediated, and intracortical facilitation (ICF; Figure 17-6C), hypothetically mediated by synaptic glutamatergic transmission (80,86–88).

The studies from De Beaumont and collaborators previously cited (70,81,84) did not reveal any abnormalities in SICI or ICF in athletes with 1 or several sport concussions from 9 months to 30 years prior to testing. However, increased SICI has been found 3 months after mild-to-moderate TBI in patients with objective excessive daytime sleepiness (83). These patients also had an increased RMT. Both RMT and SICI correlated with objective measures of sleepiness. It has been suggested that the persistent sleepiness in some patients with TBI is caused by a combination of reduced excitability because of reduced hypocretin signaling (hypothalamic injury) and also injury to other sleep-wake regulating systems. Finally, LICI was enhanced in asymptomatic concussed athletes with multiple concussions that occurred more than

12 months prior to testing (84). Together with the increase in CSP duration, this result points toward the presence of specific and stable alterations of $GABA_B$ receptor activity in the M1 (84).

In summary, TMS methodology can provide useful tools to assess brain abnormalities in the acute and sustained phases of TBI of various severities. Acutely after moderate concussion, several measures point toward the loss of the corticospinal neurons, the slowing and the desynchronization of multiple descending volleys, and both excitatory and inhibitory circuits seem to be affected. This could be related to cholinergic abnormalities and excessive glutamate accumulation leading to N-methyl-D-aspartate (NMDA)-mediated excitotoxicity. Whether these deficits are also present in asymptomatic patients with mild TBI, shortly after the concussion, remains to be explored. In the long term (9 months and up to 30 years after the concussion), potential glutamatergic excitotoxicity of asymptomatic patients with mild TBI seems to resolved (normal excitability and ICF), and there is likely no deficit in $GABA_A$-mediated inhibition (normal SICI). However, an increase in CSP duration and an abnormal LICI point toward increased $GABA_B$ transmission. It has been suggested that this increase may counter preliminary excitotoxicity and prevent damage; however, it might be excessive and finally maladaptive (84). Whether similar mechanisms occur in the sustained phase of patients with more severe TBI remain to be explored.

TMS studies are of particular importance to further characterize the severity of TBI and evaluate subclinical lasting effects. They can also provide insight into the mechanisms of symptoms associated with TBI, such as sleepiness, and help to identify patients who would be suitable for treatment (83). If further developed, TMS tools could be included in the return-to-normal-life criteria. They might turn out to be useful in the prognostic concerning recovery and improve prognosis of a second TBI or the development of mild cognitive impairment or Alzheimer disease (84).

TMS Combined with EEG

The combination of brain stimulation by TMS with simultaneous EEG recording has become feasible because of the development of novel engineering solutions (89–92). The TMS-EEG integration provides real-time information on cortical reactivity and connectivity. A noninvasive input (TMS) of known spatial and temporal characteristics can be applied to study local reactivity of the brain and interactions between different brain regions with directional and precise chronometric information (Figure 17-7). TMS-EEG combination appears to be of particular interest to explore excitability of areas outside the motor cortex that are primarily affected by TBI. In addition, this methodology will allow one to assess the integrity of entire cortical circuits. Being able to study humans directly and across the lifespan is critical to translate findings from animal studies and thus identify potential biomarkers for disease and promote therapeutic monitoring. Systematic exploration of such TMS-EEG methods in TBI seems warranted and will allow the study of prefrontal, temporal, and other brain regions and distributed neural

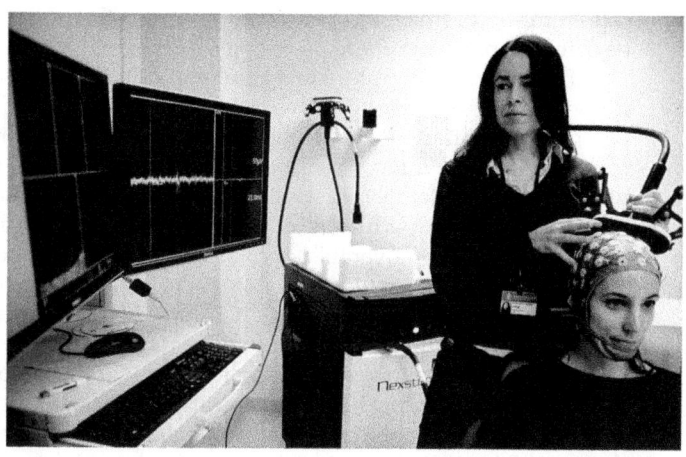
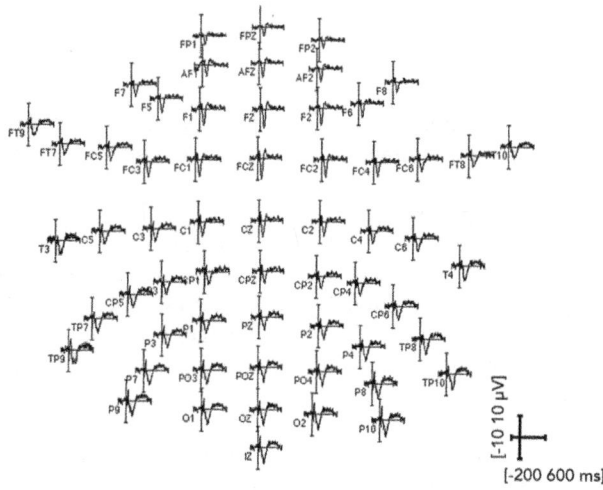

FIGURE 17–7 Transcranial magnetic stimulation (TMS) combined with electoencephalography (EEG). *Left*: a TMS-EEG system (Nexstim Oy, Helsinki, Finland). *Right*: TMS-evoked potentials for individual EEG channels.

networks that cannot be approached using TMS-EMG techniques.

Repetitive TMS

Trains of repeated TMS (rTMS) pulses can induce a lasting modification of activity in the targeted brain region, which can outlast the effects of the stimulation itself. Depending on the frequency, intensity, and the pattern of stimulation, the induced effects promote inhibition or excitation of the stimulated area. Repetitive TMS paradigms might be used to test the plasticity resources of patients at several time points after TBI of varying severities. Indeed, after a TBI, the nervous system reorganizes in response to injury. Such reorganization is restricted by existing patterns of anatomical and functional brain connectivity. The behavioral impact of such plastic reorganization is not necessarily adaptive and may prove to represent dead-end strategies that ultimately limit functional recovery and promote lasting disability. Assessment of plasticity resources at different time points after TBI might be necessary to develop differential mechanistic interventions and promote functional recovery.

In addition, rTMS can be directly used to facilitate recovery. Such rTMS approaches thus offer, similar to EEG biofeedback, the opportunity to use neurophysiologic techniques in therapeutic rather than diagnostic and prognostic applications. Pape et al. (93) performed 30 sessions (6 weeks) of an rTMS protocol in a patient with severe TBI who remained in a vegetative state for longer than 9 months. The rTMS intervention (a repetitive paired-pulse stimulation of the right dorsolateral prefrontal cortex) was designed to use potentially excitatory stimulation parameters while maximizing safety. This methodology proved to be safe, and the patient progressed clinically from a vegetative state at the time of study enrollment to a minimal conscious state by the 15th session. The patient demonstrated incremental neurobehavioral improvements simultaneously occurring with the provision of rTMS up to the 25th session. Although a mild decrease of performance occurred during the final 5 sessions, most of the neurobehavioral improvement sustained 6 weeks after rTMS withdrawal and, according to his family, up to 1 year after completion of the study. Obviously, this is a single-case study that requires cautious follow-up and demands confirmation prior to clinical adoption. Whether rTMS might promote adaptive plasticity in other patients, including patients with less severe TBI, remains to be explored. Such studies should be done with care because rTMS can induce significant side effects and complications, particularly in certain predisposed populations (94). Therefore, appropriately controlled studies are needed prior to considering the use of rTMS in clinical practice.

OTHER METHODS OF POTENTIAL INTEREST

Transcranial direct current stimulation (tDCS) is a noninvasive technique of neuromodulation, which passes low amplitude direct current (1–2 mA) through pad electrodes placed on the scalp to alter neuronal firing. Although anodal tDCS elicits prolonged increases in the cortical excitability of the underlying brain area, cathodal stimulation shows opposite effects (95–96). As with rTMS, the duration of the effects outlast the period of stimulation. The mechanisms are believed to be nonsynaptic and result from change in resting polarization of neurons. Although investigation of tDCS in patients with TBI is only starting, this technique is promising because it shows excellent safety record and has proven to be able to improve several brain functions in healthy subjects and in patient populations (for a review, see 97). Several studies conducted on the safety of tDCS have concluded that it is a painless technique for electrically stimulating the brain with almost no risk of harm. The most frequent adverse effects that have been reported include moderate fatigue (35%), mild headache (11.8%), nausea (2.9%) and temporary mild tingling sensation, itchiness, and/or redness in the area of stimulation. Overall, tDCS features a highly portable, safe, noninvasive means to modulate cortical excitability with reasonable topographic resolution and reliable experimental blinding. It can focally suppress or enhance neuronal firing following TBI and thus may offer a promising method to minimize the damage and promote functional recovery. Cathodal tDCS may be employed to suppress the acute glutamatergic hyperexcitability following TBI. In the subacute stage, when GABAergic activity is excessive and conditions the neurologic, cognitive, and functional disability, anodal tDCS may increase excitability to counter these aberrant GABAergic effects. In the chronic stage, brain stimulation coupled to rehabilitation can enhance behavioral recovery, learning of new skills, and cortical plasticity. Furthermore, tDCS can be combined, with relative ease, with other interventions with the aim of enhancing their effect. For example, tDCS can be applied during cognitive training, robot-supported arm or gait training, physical or occupational therapy, imagery, and so forth. As such, tDCS might prove to be a valuable neuromodulatory tool to promote rehabilitation and functional recovery after TBI.

Cranial electrotherapy/electrical stimulation (CES) is a technique that provides small pulses of electric current (0–4 mA) across the head, using pregelled electrodes, conductive rubber ear clips, or moistened sponges placed on the head either below or directly on the ears. This technique has primarily been investigated for the treatment of anxiety, depression, and insomnia. It is hypothesized that the outcomes of CES would be mediated by neurotransmitters. Some studies have shown effects onto QEEG. However, the mechanisms of action remain uncertain, and overall, the experimental evidence regarding clinical use is limited. In the treatment of postconcussion symptoms, CES has been shown to be useful in improving several mood measures (98), but further studies with better controlled trial designs are needed to assess its efficacy.

Transcranial pulsed ultrasound stimulation (TCPUS) is another recently developed method of potential interest for noninvasive brain stimulation (99–100). Ultrasound is a mechanical pressure wave with a frequency above the range of human hearing (> 20 kHz), capable of being transmitted over long distances through solid structures. Ultrasound can influence physiological activity through thermal and/or mechanical mechanisms. Tufail et al. (99) used a series of low-frequency ultrasound pulses (typically below 100 cycles per pulse at a frequency within one-tenths of a MHz range) repeated over time (typically hundreds of times at a frequency in the order of 1 KHz) at a low intensity (< 300 mW/cm2) to safely stimulate neural activity in the intact mouse brain. With a negligible increase of temperature, ultrasound stimulation of the motor cortex produced short bursts of activity and peripheral muscle contraction, whereas stimulation of the hippocampus triggered rhythmic bursting lasting about 3 seconds. It was suggested that the fluid-mechanical effects (*a*) modulate the resting membrane potentials of neurons, (*b*) directly modulate the kinetics of mechanically sensitive ions channels, and/or (*c*) produce ephaptic effects by altering the distribution of electric fields. The advantage of this technique over other noninvasive techniques of brain stimulation would be its spatial resolution, estimated to be of approximately 2 mm. Although this technique appears to be safe in mice, it remains to be proven as to whether it could be safely applied in other species.

Transcranial Doppler sonography (TCD) can be used in the acute assessment of cerebral ischemia following TBI (101) and may offer appealing noninvasive methods to monitor patients in the intensive care setting. A study in patients with mild-to-moderate TBI (102) showed that TCD-based measures of brain perfusion at time of hospitalization are good predictors of overall neurological outcomes. Thus, TCD might be a powerful prognostic tool in TBI. More recent advances in our understanding of TCD have lead to exciting possible therapeutic roles in TBI where clot formation may result from primary injury. One application is sonothrombolysis, a technique of focal TCD applied at diagnostic frequencies alone or in combination with standard thrombolytic therapy (tPA) (103). TCD may also have the potential to promote neuroprotection during acute TBI by increasing the local bioavailability of neuroprotective agents. TCD has been shown to transiently (i.e., hours) enhance blood–brain barrier (BBB) permeability without adverse cellular effects. The mechanism is believed to be a process of stable cavitation in which low acoustic energy causes administered microbubbles to oscillate and expand creating small eddy currents in the surrounding plasma. These currents provide shear stress on cells and large molecules to improve BBB transcellular and paracellular transport (104). Thus, TCD may increase the applicability of novel neuroprotective agents by allowing focal pharmacokinetic optimization. Finally, some studies have alluded to the potential of TCD as a direct means of neuroprotection (105). In the setting of TBI, these attributes of TCD may allow for suppression of neuronal activity in the acute energy deficient phase and facilitation in the subacute phase of active recovery, strengthening our therapeutic capacity against TBI.

Low-level laser therapy (LLLT), or photobiostimulation, is a novel method of noninvasive neural stimulation that, at specific wavelengths, can safely penetrate into the brain. LLLT is thought to promote cellular survival in times of reduced energy substrate through interactions with cytochrome c oxidase to enhance oxidative phosphorylation, improve mitochondrial function, and increases adenosine triphospate (ATP) (106,107). LLLT has been shown to accelerate wound healing, reduce neurological deficit following stroke, and improve outcome in spinal cord injury. Recently, LLLT was used for the first time in a rodent TBI model. LLLT-treated rats showed significantly reduced functional impairment and reduced lesion volume (108). Given such preclinical findings, the promising results in human stroke research (109–111), and the unique properties of LLLT, its therapeutic application in TBI seems worth exploring.

SOME LIMITATIONS OF ELECTROPHYSIOLOGICAL TECHNIQUES

Although all these techniques have proven to be helpful for TBI diagnosis, prognosis, exploration of the mechanisms, and/or rehabilitation, several concerns still need to be addressed. The reliability of most of these measures is particularly challenged by the fact that the dissociation of TBI or non-TBI is often complicated by ongoing or comorbid conditions and medications.

QEEG allows successful discrimination between mild TBI and controls of patients with more severe TBI. EPs can provide valuable prognostic information and ERPs and brain stimulation can further contribute to fine characterization of brain dysfunction in TBI. However, research is still needed to assess the impact of potential confounding factors on most of these techniques. For example, prior conditions, such as neurological or psychiatric issues, may affect the outcomes of all the previously mentioned techniques. In addition, it is difficult to disentangle neurophysiologic abnormalities as a consequence to the TBI per se from conditions that are often associated with it, such as PTSD, depression, or anxiety.

Moreover, it remains to be fully explored how medications systematically affect the normative data bases used for all the techniques described in this chapter. Among the medications relevant for TBI, anesthetics, analgesics, and antiepileptic drugs are particularly prone to modify neurophysiologic measures. Finally, often leading to a TBI event, ingestion of alcohol and toxins should be discussed prior to interpretation of EEG findings and/or application of brain stimulation. In fact, drugs and alcohol could alter brain excitability and increase the risk of adverse events associated with TMS and other stimulation techniques. Potential sleep deprivation, occurring as a consequence of TBI-related insomnia, also has to be considered in the same context. In addition, increased intracranial pressure, intracranial lesion or hematomas, and structural damage might all constitute contraindication for TMS and other brain stimulation methods because they might be aggravated by stimulation. Cranioplasty and burr holes might participate in a shunting on the induced current through skull defects, leading to poorly controlled intensity of stimulation in brain tissues. Finally, even in patients with mild TBI, where none of these complications are observed, safety studies remains to be undertaken for most brain stimulation methods.

CONCLUSION

Electrophysiological techniques are essential in the TBI care practice. They are useful for diagnosis, prognosis and monitoring, for exploration and characterization of brain deficits, and for detection of subclinical anomalies that might increase vulnerability to subsequent concussions or susceptibility to long-term complications. In addition, some of these tools can be used to guide functional recovery (e.g., EEG biofeedback, brain stimulation). Certainly, these techniques still need to be developed and improved, and for all, studies need to be done to further clarify findings and to assess the validity and safety of these methods when confounding and aggravating factors intervene.

KEY CLINICAL POINTS

1. The use of conventional EEG is limited for mild TBI. However, for more severe TBI, conventional EEG is useful for prognosis, monitoring the recovery/deterioration, detecting brain damages, or post-traumatic epilepsy.

2. QEEG allows a more objective characterization of brain abnormalities after TBI and appears sensitive to discriminate mild TBI from healthy controls and from more severe TBI. Efforts still need to be made to reconcile results from different studies and establish the full clinical use of QEEG.

3. Based on the findings of EEG anomalies, EEG biofeedback is a promising potential treatment for patients with TBI, aiming to normalize the EEG and consequently improving behavior and cognition.

4. SEPs and ERPs are useful together with other clinical assessments for prognosis of TBI, but their interpretation remains delicate. They are also sensitive tools to detect functional alterations and may help in the understanding of vulnerability to subsequent concussions as well as the susceptibility to develop long-term complications.

5. Methods of brain stimulation, such as TMS, are particularly suited to assess excitatory and inhibitory function in patients with TBI. Combined with EEG and also neuroimaging, noninvasive brain stimulation might become a particularly useful physiologic biomarker, but more work is needed.

6. Brain stimulation applied for neuromodulation (for example, repetitive TMS or tDCS) is also promising as a tool to guide functional recovery and adaptive plasticity. Safety guidelines for the TBI populations still need to be established.

KEY REFERENCES

1. De Beaumont L, Théoret H, Mongeon D, et al. Brain function decline in healthy retired athletes who sustained their last sports concussion in early adulthood. *Brain*. 2009; 132(pt 3):695–708.
2. Louise-Bender Pape T, Rosenow J, Lewis G, et al. Repetitive transcranial magnetic stimulation-associated neurobehavioral gains during coma recovery. *Brain Stimul*. 2009;2(1):22–35.
3. Robinson LR, Micklesen PJ, Tirschwell DL, Lew HL. Predictive value of somatosensory evoked potentials for awakening from coma. *Crit Care Med*. 2003;31(3):960–967.
4. Thatcher RW. Electroencephalography and mild traumatic brain injury. In: Slobounov S, Sebastianelli W, eds. *Foundations of Sport-Related Brain Injury*. New York, NY: Springer-Verlag; 2006:241–265.
5. Thornton KE, Carmody DP. Efficacy of traumatic brain injury rehabilitation: interventions of QEEG-guided biofeedback, computers, strategies, and medications. *Appl Psychophysiol Biofeedback*. 2008;33(2):101–124.

References

1. Tatum WO IV, Husain AM, Benbadis SR, Kaplan PW. Normal adult EEG and patterns of uncertain significance. *J Clin Neurophysiol*. 2006;23(3):194–207.
2. Kaiser J, Lutzenberger W. Human gamma-band activity: a window to cognitive processing. *Neuroreport*. 2005;16(3):207–211.
3. Arciniegas DB. Clinical electrophysiologic assessments and mild traumatic brain injury: state-of-the-science and implications for clinical practice. *Int J Psychophysiol*. 2011;82(1):41–52.
4. Thatcher RW, North DM, Curtin RT, et al. (2001). An EEG severity index of traumatic brain injury. *J Neuropsychiatry Clin Neurosci*. 2011;13(1):77–87.

5. Steudel WI, Kruger J. Using the spectral analysis of the EEG for prognosis of severe brain injuries in the first post-traumatic week. *Acta Neurochir Suppl (Wien)*. 1979;28(1):40–42.

6. Wallace BE, Wagner AK, Wagner EP, McDeavitt JT. A history and review of quantitative electroencephalography in traumatic brain injury. *J Head Trauma Rehabil*. 2001;16(2):165–190.

7. Abend NS, Dlugos DJ, Hahn CD, Hirsch LJ, Herman ST. Use of EEG monitoring and management of non-convulsive seizures in critically ill patients: a survey of neurologists. *Neurocrit Care*. 2010; 12(3):382–389.

8. Nuwer MR, Hovda DA, Schrader LM, Vespa PM. Routine and quantitative EEG in mild traumatic brain injury. *Clin Neurophysiol*. 2005;116(9):2001–2025.

9. Hughes JR, John ER. Conventional and quantitative electroencephalography in psychiatry. *J Neuropsychiatry Clin Neurosci*. 1999; 11(2):190–208.

10. Jacome DE, Risko M. EEG features in post-traumatic syndrome. *Clin Electroencephalogr*. 1984;15(4):214–221.

11. Voller B, Benke T, Benedetto K, Schnider P, Auff E, Aichner F. Neuropsychological, MRI and EEG findings after very mild traumatic brain injury. *Brain Inj*. 1999;13(10):821–827.

12. Denker PG, Perry GF. Postconcussion syndrome in compensation and litigation; analysis of 95 cases with electroencephalographic correlation. *Neurology*. 1954;4(12):912–918.

13. Jacome DE. EEG in whiplash: a reappraisal. *Clin Electroencephalogr*. 1987;18(1):41–45.

14. Torres F, Shapiro SK. Electroencephalograms in whiplash injury. A comparison of electroencephalographic abnormalities with those present in closed head injuries. *Arch Neurol*. 1961;5:28–35.

15. Dow RS, Ulett G, Raaf J. Electroencephalographic studies immediately following head injury. *Am J Psychiatry*. 1944;101:174–183.

16. Courjon J, Scherzer E. Traumatic disorders. In: Remond A, Magnus O, Courjon J, eds. *Handbook of Electroencephalography and Clinical Neurophysiology: Clinical EEG, IV*. Amsterdam, The Netherlands: Elsevier; 1972:1–104.

17. Fenton GW. The postconcussional syndrome reappraised. *Clin Electroencephalogr*. 1996;27(4):174–182.

18. Geets W, de Zegher F. EEG and brainstem abnormalities after cerebral concussion. Short term observations. *Acta Neurol Belg*. 1985; 85(5):277–283.

19. Geets W, Louette N. EEG and brain-stem evoked potentials in 125 recent concussions [in French]. *Rev Electroencephalogr Neurophysiol Clin*. 1983;13(3):253–258.

20. Hessen E, Nestvold K. Indicators of complicated mild TBI predict MMPI-2 scores after 23 years. *Brain Inj*. 2009;23(3):234–242.

21. Koufen H, Dichgans J. Frequency and course of posttraumatic EEG-abnormalities and their correlations with clinical symptoms: a systematic follow up study in 344 adults (author's transl) [in German]. *Fortschr Neurol Psychiatr Grenzgeb*. 1978;46(4):165–177.

22. Arfel G. Introduction to clinical and EEG studies in coma. In: Remond A, Harner R, Naquet R, eds. *Handbook of Electroencephalography and Clinical Neurophysiology: Clinical EEG, II*. Amsterdam, The Netherlands: Elsevier; 1972:5–23.

23. Bricolo A, Turella G. Electroencephalographic patterns of acute traumatic coma: diagnostic and prognostic value. *J Neurosurg Sci*. 1973;17:278–285.

24. Stone L, Keenan MA. Peripheral nerve injuries in the adult with traumatic brain injury. *Clin Orthop Relat Res*. 1988;(233):136–144.

25. Synek VM. Revised EEG coma scale in diffuse acute head injuries in adults. *Clin Exp Neurol*. 1990;27:99–111.

26. Synek VM. Prognostically important EEG coma patterns in diffuse anoxic and traumatic encephalopathies in adults. *J Clin Neurophysiol*. 1988;5(2):161–174.

27. Hakkinen VK, Kaukinen S, Heikkila H. The correlation of EEG compressed spectral array to Glasgow Coma Scale in traumatic coma patients. *Int J Clin Monit Comput*. 1988;5(2):97–101.

28. Rumpl E. Craniocerebral trauma. In: Niedermeyer E, da Silva FL, eds. *Electroencephalography*. 5th ed. Philadelphia, PA: Lippincott Williams & Wilkins; 2005:415–438.

29. Rumpl E, Prugger M, Gerstenbrand F, Hackl JM, Pallua A. Central somatosensory conduction time and short latency somatosensory evoked potentials in post-traumatic coma. *Electroencephalogr Clin Neurophysiol*. 1983;56(6):583–596.

30. Jabbari B, Vengrow MI, Salazar AM, Harper MG, Smutok MA, Amin D. Clinical and radiological correlates of EEG in the late phase of head injury: a study of 515 Vietnam veterans. *Electroencephalogr Clin Neurophysiol*. 1986;64(4):285–293.

31. Ruijs MB, Gabreels FJ, Thijssen HM. The utility of electroencephalography and cerebral computed tomography in children with mild and moderately severe closed head injuries. *Neuropediatrics*. 1994; 25(2):73–77.

32. Frey LC. Epidemiology of posttraumatic epilepsy: a critical review. *Epilepsia*. 2003;44(suppl 10):11–17.

33. Lewine JD, Davis JT, Bigler ED, et al. Objective documentation of traumatic brain injury subsequent to mild head trauma: multimodal brain imaging with MEG, SPECT, and MRI. *J Head Trauma Rehabil*. 2007;22(3):141–155.

34. Cervone RL, Blum AS. Normal variant EEG pattern. In: Blum AS, Rutkove SB, eds. *The Clinical Neurophysiology Primer*. Totowa, NJ: Humana Press; 2007:83–100.

35. So EL. Interictal epileptiform discharges in persons without a history of seizures: what do they mean? *J Clin Neurophysiol*. 2010;27(4): 229–238.

36. Malow BA. Sleep deprivation and epilepsy. *Epilepsy Curr*. 2004; 4(5):193–195.

37. Thomaides TN, Kerezoudi EP, Chaudhuri KR, Cheropoulos C. Study of EEGs following 24-hour sleep deprivation in patients with posttraumatic epilepsy. *Eur Neurol*. 1992;32(2):79–82.

38. Benbadis SR, O'Neill E, Tatum WO, Heriaud L. Outcome of prolonged video-EEG monitoring at a typical referral epilepsy center. *Epilepsia*. 2004;45(9):1150–1153.

39. Arciniegas DB, Anderson CA, Topkoff J, McAllister TW. Mild traumatic brain injury: a neuropsychiatric approach to diagnosis, evaluation, and treatment. *Neuropsychiatr Dis Treat*. 2005;1(4):311–327.

40. Leon-Carrion J, Martin-Rodriguez JF, Damas-Lopez J, Martin JM, Dominguez-Morales Mdel R. A QEEG index of level of functional dependence for people sustaining acquired brain injury: the Seville Independence Index (SINDI). *Brain Inj*. 2008;22(1):61–74.

41. Thatcher RW, Walker RA, Gerson I, Geisler FH. EEG discriminant analyses of mild head trauma. *Electroencephalogr Clin Neurophysiol*. 1989;73(2):94–106.

42. Kumar S, Rao SL, Chandramouli BA, Pillai SV. Reduction of functional brain connectivity in mild traumatic brain injury during working memory. *J Neurotrauma*. 2009;26(5):665–675.

43. Thornton K. The electrophysiological effects of a brain injury on auditory memory functioning. The QEEG correlates of impaired memory. *Arch Clin Neuropsychol*. 2003;18(4):363–378.

44. Cao C, Slobounov S. Alteration of cortical functional connectivity as a result of traumatic brain injury revealed by graph theory, ICA, and sLORETA analyses of EEG signals. *IEEE Trans Neural Syst Rehabil Eng*. 2010;18(1):11–19.

45. Thatcher RW. Electroencephalography and mild traumatic brain injury. In: Slobounov S, Sebastianelli W, eds. *Foundations of Sport-Related Brain Injury*. New York, NY: Springer-Verlag; 2006:241–265.

46. Nuwer M. Assessment of digital EEG, quantitative EEG, and EEG brain mapping: report of the American Academy of Neurology and the American Clinical Neurophysiology Society. *Neurology*. 1997;49(1):277–292.

47. Hoffman DA, Lubar JF, Thatcher RW, et al. Limitations of the American Academy of Neurology and American Clinical Neurophysiology Society paper on QEEG. *J Neuropsychiatry Clin Neurosci*. 1999;11(3):401–407.

48. Thatcher RW, Moore N, John ER, Duffy F, Hughes JR, Krieger M. QEEG and traumatic brain injury: rebuttal of the American Academy of Neurology 1997 report by the EEG and Clinical Neuroscience Society. *Clin Electroencephalogr*. 1999;30(3):94–98.

49. Thornton KE. The improvement/rehabilitation of auditory memory functioning with EEG biofeedback. *NeuroRehabilitation*. 2002; 17(1):69–80.

50. Byers AP. Neurofeedback therapy for a mild head injury. *J Neurotherapy*. 1995;1(1):22–37.

51. Walker JE, Norman CA, Weber RK. Impact of qEEG-guided coherence training for patients with a mild closed head injury. *J Neurotherapy*. 2002;6(2):31–43.

52. Thornton KE, Carmody DP. Electroencephalogram biofeedback for reading disability and traumatic brain injury. *Child Adolesc Psychiatr Clin N Am*. 2005;14(1):137–162, vii.

53. Tinius TP, Tinius KA. Changes after EEG biofeedback and cognitive retraining in adults with mild traumatic brain injury and attention deficit hyperactivity disorder. *J Neurotherapy*. 2002;4(2):27–44.

54. Thornton KE, Carmody DP. Traumatic brain injury rehabilitation: QEEG biofeedback treatment protocols. *Appl Psychophysiol Biofeedback*. 2009;34(1):59–68.

55. Thornton KE, Carmody DP. Efficacy of traumatic brain injury rehabilitation: interventions of QEEG-guided biofeedback, computers, strategies, and medications. *Appl Psychophysiol Biofeedback*. 2008; 33(2):101–124.

56. Lew HL, Lee EH, Pan SSL, Chiang JYP. Electrophysiologic assesment techniques: evoked potentials and electroencephalography. In: Zasler ND, Katz DI, Zafonte RD, eds. *Brain Injury Medicine*. New York, NY: Demos Medical Publishing; 2007:157–165.

57. Robinson LR, Micklesen PJ, Tirschwell DL, Lew HL. Predictive value of somatosensory evoked potentials for awakening from coma. *Crit Care Med*. 2003;31(3):960–967.

58. Guérit JM, Amantini A, Amodio P, et al. Consensus on the use of neurophysiological tests in the intensive care unit (ICU): electroencephalogram (EEG), evoked potentials (EP), and electroneuromyography (ENMG). *Neurophysiol Clin*. 2009;39(2):71–83.

59. Amantini A, Grippo A, Fossi S, et al. Prediction of "awakening" and outcome in prolonged acute coma from severe traumatic brain injury: evidence for validity of short latency SEPs. *Clin Neurophysiol*. 2005;116(1):229–235.

60. Carter BG, Butt W. Are somatosensory evoked potentials the best predictor of outcome after severe brain injury? A systematic review. *Intensive Care Med*. 2005;31(6):765–775.

61. Gaetz M, Bernstein DM. The current status of electrophysiologic procedures for the assessment of mild traumatic brain injury. *J Head Trauma Rehabil*. 2001;16(4):386–405.

62. Shin DY, Ehrenberg B, Whyte J, Bach J, DeLisa JA. Evoked potential assessment: utility in prognosis of chronic head injury. *Arch Phys Med Rehabil*. 1989;70(3):189–193.

63. Polich J. P300 clinical utility and control of variability. *J Clin Neurophysiol*. 1998;15(1):14–33.

64. Lew H, Chmiel R, Jerger J, Pomerantz JR, Jerger S. Electrophysiologic indices of Stroop and Garner interference reveal linguistic influences on auditory and visual processing. *J Am Acad Audiol*. 1997;8(2):104–118.

65. Polich J, Herbst KL. P300 as a clinical assay: rationale, evaluation, and findings. *Int J Psychophysiol*. 2000;38(1):3–19.

66. Polich J, Kok A. Cognitive and biological determinants of P300: an integrative review. *Biol Psychol*. 1995;41(2):103–146.

67. Viggiano MP. Event-related potentials in brain-injured patients with neuropsychological disorders: a review. *J Clin Exp Neuropsychol*. 1996;18(5):631–647.

68. Lew HL, Dikmen S, Slimp J, et al. Use of somatosensory-evoked potentials and cognitive event-related potentials in predicting outcomes of patients with severe traumatic brain injury. *Am J Phys Med Rehabil*. 2003;82(1):53–61.

69. Doi R, Morita K, Shigemori M, Tokutomi T, Maeda H. Characteristics of cognitive function in patients after traumatic brain injury assessed by visual and auditory event-related potentials. *Am J Phys Med Rehabil*. 2007;86(8):641–649.

70. De Beaumont L, Théoret H, Mongeon D, et al. Brain function decline in healthy retired athletes who sustained their last sports concussion in early adulthood. *Brain*. 2009;132(pt 3):695–708.

71. Thériault M, De Beaumont L, Gosselin N, Filipinni M, Lassonde M. Electrophysiological abnormalities in well functioning multiple concussed athletes. *Brain Inj*. 2009;23(11):899–906.

72. Gosselin N, Thériault M, Leclerc S, Montplaisir J, Lassonde M. Neurophysiological anomalies in symptomatic and asymptomatic concussed athletes. *Neurosurgery*. 2006;58(6):1151–1161; discussion 1151–1161.

73. Lavoie ME, Dupuis F, Johnston KM, Leclerc S, Lassonde M. Visual p300 effects beyond symptoms in concussed college athletes. *J Clin Exp Neuropsychol*. 2004;26(1):55–73.

74. Kobayashi M, Pascual-Leone A. Transcranial magnetic stimulation in neurology. *Lancet Neurol*. 2003;2(3):145–156.

75. Wagner T, Valero-Cabre A, Pascual-Leone A. Noninvasive human brain stimulation. *Annu Rev Biomed Eng*. 2007;9:527–565.

76. Reis J, Swayne OB, Vandermeeren Y, et al. Contribution of transcranial magnetic stimulation to the understanding of cortical mechanisms involved in motor control. *J Physiol*. 2008;586(2):325–351.

77. Rossini PM, Barker AT, Berardelli A, et al. Non-invasive electrical and magnetic stimulation of the brain, spinal cord and roots: basic principles and procedures for routine clinical application. Report of an IFCN committee. *Electroencephalogr Clin Neurophysiol*. 1994; 91(2):79–92.

78. Chistyakov AV, Soustiel JF, Hafner H, Trubnik M, Levy G, Feinsod M. Excitatory and inhibitory corticospinal responses to transcranial magnetic stimulation in patients with minor to moderate head injury. *J Neurol Neurosurg Psychiatry*. 2001;70(5):580–587.

79. Hallett M. Transcranial magnetic stimulation and the human brain. *Nature*. 2000;406(6792):147–150.

80. Ziemann U, Rothwell JC, Ridding MC. Interaction between intracortical inhibition and facilitation in human motor cortex. *J Physiol*. 1996;496(pt 3):873–881.

81. De Beaumont L, Lassonde M, Leclerc S, Théoret H. Long-term and cumulative effects of sports concussion on motor cortex inhibition. *Neurosurgery*. 2007;61(2):329–336; discussion 336–327.

82. Livingston SC, Saliba EN, Goodkin HP, Barth JT, Hertel JN, Ingersoll CD. A preliminary investigation of motor evoked potential abnormalities following sport-related concussion. *Brain Inj*. 2010; 24(6):904–913.

83. Nardone R, Bergmann J, Kunz A, et al. Cortical excitability changes in patients with sleep-wake disturbances after traumatic brain injury. *J Neurotrauma*. 2011;28(7):1165–1171.

84. Tremblay S, de Beaumont L, Lassonde M, Théoret H. Evidence for the specificity of intracortical inhibitory dysfunction in asymptomatic concussed athletes. *J Neurotrauma*. 2011;28(4):493–502.

85. Takeuchi N, Ikoma K, Chuma T, Matsuo Y. Measurement of transcallosal inhibition in traumatic brain injury by transcranial magnetic stimulation. *Brain Inj*. 2006;20(9):991–996.

86. Di Lazzaro V, Oliviero A, Profice P, et al. Muscarinic receptor blockade has differential effects on the excitability of intracortical circuits in the human motor cortex. *Exp Brain Res*. 2000;135(4): 455–461.

87. Kujirai T, Caramia MD, Rothwell JC, et al. Corticocortical inhibition in human motor cortex. *J Physiol*. 1993;471:501–519.

88. Wassermann EM. Risk and safety of repetitive transcranial magnetic stimulation: report and suggested guidelines from the International Workshop on the Safety of Repetitive Transcranial Magnetic Stimulation, June 5–7, 1996. *Electroencephalogr Clin Neurophysiol*. 1998;108(1):1–16.

89. Ives JR, Rotenberg A, Poma R, Thut G, Pascual-Leone A. Electroencephalographic recording during transcranial magnetic stimulation in humans and animals. *Clin Neurophysiol*. 2006;117 (8):1870–1875.

90. Thut G, Ives JR, Kampmann F, Pastor MA, Pascual-Leone A. A new device and protocol for combining TMS and online recordings of EEG and evoked potentials. *J Neurosci Methods*. 2005;141(2): 207–217.

91. Thut G, Northoff G, Ives JR, et al. Effects of single-pulse transcranial magnetic stimulation (TMS) on functional brain activity: a combined event-related TMS and evoked potential study. *Clin Neurophysiol*. 2003;114(11):2071–2080.

92. Virtanen J, Ruohonen J, Naatanen R, Ilmoniemi RJ. Instrumentation for the measurement of electric brain responses to transcranial magnetic stimulation. *Med Biol Eng Comput*. 1999;37(3):322–326.

93. Pape TL, Rosenow J, Lewis G, et al. Repetitive transcranial magnetic stimulation-associated neurobehavioral gains during coma recovery. *Brain Stimul*. 2009;2(1):22–35.

94. Rossi S, Hallett M, Rossini PM, Pascual-Leone A. Safety, ethical considerations, and application guidelines for the use of transcra-

nial magnetic stimulation in clinical practice and research. *Clin Neurophysiol.* 2009;120(12):2008–2039.

95. Nitsche MA, Paulus W. Excitability changes induced in the human motor cortex by weak transcranial direct current stimulation. *J Physiol.* 2000;527(pt 3):633–639.

96. Nitsche MA, Paulus W. Sustained excitability elevations induced by transcranial DC motor cortex stimulation in humans. *Neurology.* 2001;57(10):1899–1901.

97. Nitsche MA, Cohen LG, Wassermann EM, et al. Transcranial direct current stimulation: State of the art 2008. *Brain Stimul.* 2008;1(3):206–223.

98. Smith RB, Tiberi A, Marshall J. The use of cranial electrotherapy stimulation in the treatment of closed-head-injured patients. *Brain Inj.* 1994;8(4):357–361.

99. Tufail Y, Matyushov A, Baldwin N, et al. Transcranial pulsed ultrasound stimulates intact brain circuits. *Neuron.* 2010;66(5):681–694.

100. Yoo SS, Bystritsky A, Lee JH, et al. Focused ultrasound modulates region-specific brain activity. *Neuroimage.* 2011;56(3):1267–1275.

101. Vespa P. What is the optimal threshold for cerebral perfusion pressure following traumatic brain injury? *Neurosurg Focus.* 2003;15(6):E4.

102. Jaffres P, Brun J, Declety P, et al. Transcranial Doppler to detect on admission patients at risk for neurological deterioration following mild and moderate brain trauma. *Intensive Care Med.* 2005;31(6):785–790.

103. Alexandrov AV. Ultrasound enhancement of fibrinolysis. *Stroke.* 2009;40(3)(suppl):S107–S110.

104. Vykhodtseva N, McDannold N, Hynynen K. Progress and problems in the application of focused ultrasound for blood-brain barrier disruption. *Ultrasonics.* 2008;48(4):279–296.

105. Bachtold MR, Rinaldi PC, Jones JP, Reines F, Price LR. Focused ultrasound modifications of neural circuit activity in a mammalian brain. *Ultrasound Med Biol.* 1998;24(4):557–565.

106. Karu T. Primary and secondary mechanisms of action of visible to near-IR radiation on cells. *J Photochem Photobiol B.* 1999;49(1):1–17.

107. Mochizuki-Oda N, Kataoka Y, Cui Y, Yamada H, Heya M, Awazu K. Effects of near-infra-red laser irradiation on adenosine triphosphate and adenosine diphosphate contents of rat brain tissue. *Neurosci Lett.* 2002;323(3):207–210.

108. Oron A, Oron U, Chen J, et al. Low-level laser therapy applied transcranially to rats after induction of stroke significantly reduces long-term neurological deficits. *Stroke.* 2006;37(10):2620–2624.

109. Hashmi JT, Huang YY, Osmani BZ, Sharma SK, Naeser MA, Hamblin MR. Role of low-level laser therapy in neurorehabilitation. *PM R.* 2010;2(12)(suppl 2):S292–S305.

110. Lampl Y, Zivin JA, Fisher M, et al. Infrared laser therapy for ischemic stroke: a new treatment strategy: results of the Neuro-Thera Effectiveness and Safety Trial-1 (NEST-1). *Stroke.* 2007;38(6):1843–1849.

111. Zivin JA, Albers GW, Bornstein N, et al. Effectiveness and safety of transcranial laser therapy for acute ischemic stroke. *Stroke.* 2009;40(4):1359–1364.

IV

PROGNOSIS AND OUTCOME

Prognosis After Severe Traumatic Brain Injury:
A Practical, Evidence-Based Approach

Sunil Kothari and Craig DiTommaso

INTRODUCTION

It seems to be highly desirable that a physician should pay much attention to prognosis. If he is able to tell his patients when he visits them not only about their past and present symptoms but also to tell them what is going to happen, as well as to fill in the details they have omitted, he will increase his reputation as a medical practitioner and people will have no qualms in putting themselves under his care.
—*Hippocrates*

Like diagnosis and treatment, prognosis is a fundamental responsibility of all clinicians. This is especially true after a traumatic brain injury (TBI), when uncertainty about the future compounds the suffering already experienced by patients and families. Indeed, families have identified information about prognosis as one of their most important needs in the aftermath of a TBI (1–3). Unfortunately, this need often goes unmet because families report they were rarely provided adequate prognostic information (2,3,5). Physicians themselves seem to agree; a recent survey of brain injury physicians found that only 37% agreed that they currently assess prognosis accurately (6). This situation undermines the confidence that families have in their physicians and contributes to strain in the relationship between families and physicians (5).

Providing patients and families with this information can help in several ways. Knowing what the future might hold allows families to gain some cognitive control over a situation they otherwise feel powerless to affect. Moreover, there is a symbolic importance to prognosis: patients and families want to believe their condition is understood (4). Simply knowing that the clinician understands their condition can alleviate anxiety. Given the importance of prognosis for patients and families, some authors have even suggested that prognostication is an ethical *duty* for clinicians (4).

Despite its clear importance, clinicians often neglect prognosis. Some reasons for this neglect apply only to the delivery of *poor* prognoses: a lack of training in the delivery of "bad news," the emotionally demanding nature of providing a poor prognosis, a fear of extinguishing hope, and the fact that a poor prognosis highlights the limits of professional help (4). Other barriers can affect *any* act of prognosis: the belief that prognostication is arrogant or hubristic, a lack of facility in probabilistic reasoning, and the difficulty in extracting clinical guidelines from a large body of literature (4).

Because of this difficulty in developing guidelines based on the research literature, health care professionals often rely on their own clinical experiences in formulating prognoses. However, such an approach is of limited value: not only is a clinician's personal experience subject to selection bias, but it is also prone to significant cognitive distortion (7,8). Many studies have shown that a clinician's "subjective" estimation of prognoses is often far less accurate than those derived from well-designed studies (9–11).

Yet, providing prognostic information based on these studies can be difficult for TBI professionals. The literature is vast, with thousands of studies reported, all varying in focus, design, and quality. Also, most of the studies were designed or reported in a way that makes it difficult to derive *clinically* useful guidelines. Often, they report only general associations (e.g., "outcome is related to the length of coma [LOC]"). Even when these associations are quantified, it is done in a way that limits their applicability to individual cases (for instance, by using regression equations).

The purpose of this chapter is to address these obstacles and thereby derive accurate and useful guidelines from the relevant literature. It is hoped that this information will enable TBI professionals to make the most accurate prognoses possible, both to inform their own clinical decisions as well as to provide the desired information to patients and families. Of course, other reviews of this topic exist (12–28), including several, recently published, that use an evidence-based approach (29–33). The review presented here differs from the others in 1 significant way. Unlike the other reviews, the primary aim of this chapter is to present guidelines that can directly be applied to clinical practice.

This chapter is divided into 4 major sections:

- A summary of findings
- Guidelines for communicating prognostic information
- An appendix on guidelines for evaluating studies on prognosis
- An appendix describing the methodology of the literature review

The core of this chapter is contained in the next 2 sections, which summarize the findings of the evidence-based review and provide guidelines in communicating this information to patients and families. The first appendix provides

Development of Acute Care Guidelines and Effect on Outcome	Chapter 25
Neuroimaging Correlates of Functional Outcome	Chapter 19
Electrophysiologic Techniques	Chapter 17
Functional Assessment in Traumatic Brain Injury Rehabilitation	Chapter 20
Neuropsychological Assessment and Treatment Planning	Chapter 60
Conceptualizing Outcome From Mild Traumatic Brain Injury	Chapter 30
Assessment and Rehabilitative Management of Individuals With Disorders of Consciousness	Chapter 32
Pediatric Traumatic Brain Injury: Special Considerations	Chapter 34
Traumatic Brain Injury in the Elderly	Chapter 28
Returning to Work Following Traumatic Brain Injury	Chapter 81
Life Care Planning After Traumatic Brain Injury: Clinical and Forensic Issues	Chapter 86
Life Expectancy and Wellness	Chapter 21

FIGURE 18–1 Topics relevant to prognosis covered elsewhere.

a guide for evaluating future studies on prognosis. The second appendix provides a detailed description and justification for the methodology guiding this review. To maximize the usefulness of this chapter as a future reference, all the important information is summarized in the figures and tables. Therefore, after an initial reading of the entire chapter, readers can then simply refer to the tables and figures to review the essential information. This chapter does not address topics relevant to prognosis after TBI that are covered elsewhere in the textbook (see Figure 18–1).

SUMMARY OF FINDINGS

Medicine is a science of uncertainty and an art of probability.
—William Osler

Clinical Utility: The Concept of a "Threshold Value"

The primary purpose of this chapter is to provide clinicians with information that is not only evidence-based but also *practical*. The nature of the studies in this area makes this difficult for several reasons. First, many of the relevant studies do not *directly* address issues of prognosis. Instead, they often have simpler aims, such as providing a description of the possible outcomes after TBI as well as the factors associated with these outcomes. As a result, the findings are reported in such a way that only the broadest generalizations are possible (e.g., that the initial Glasgow Coma Scale [GCS] score is correlated with outcome after a TBI). Although this knowledge does represent an advance in our understanding of TBI, it does little to help clinicians who are trying to prog-

nosticate for individual patients. Even when these associations are quantified, it is in a form that is not clinically useful (e.g., as correlation coefficients).

This was a limitation even of those studies that directly addressed prognosis. For example, the relationship between a potential predictor variable and an outcome might be expressed as a path coefficient or the percentage of variance explained. Yet, both clinicians and laypeople are more used to thinking about, for instance, probabilities (e.g., "What are the chances that he will ever work again?"). Unfortunately, there is no straightforward way to translate results expressed as path coefficients, R^2, log-likelihood's, correlation matrices, and so forth, into prognoses that are meaningful to the clinician, let alone the family. For most clinicians, our knowledge begins and ends simply with the awareness that certain variables are associated with outcome (e.g., GCS, pupillary abnormalities, etc.) without knowing how to apply that information to individual cases. There were a handful of studies that actually did provide practical guidelines for clinicians (e.g., by using simple formulas, prediction trees, or scores from specially designed scales), but they did not meet the other inclusion criteria of this review.

To maximize the clinical utility of studies that did meet the inclusion criteria, the results were interpreted through the use of threshold values. These are values of a predictor variable above or below which a particular outcome was especially unlikely. For example, several studies reported that no one with a duration of post-traumatic amnesia (PTA) more than 3 months achieved a good recovery as defined by the Glasgow Outcome Scale (GOS) (Figure 18-2). Thus, 3 months would be considered a threshold value for the duration of PTA, at least in terms of excluding the possibility of a good recovery on the GOS (Figure 18-3). Conversely, several studies found that no one who had a duration of PTA of *less than* 2 months ended up severely disabled (by GOS criteria); 2 months would then be the threshold value for excluding the possibility of severe disability.

As "milestones" in a patient's recovery, threshold values can be useful to clinicians. For instance, as the length of a patient's PTA extends beyond 3 months, rehabilitation clinicians can counsel family members about realistic expectations for the future. On the other hand, if 2 months have not yet elapsed since the injury, clinicians can give hope to families even if the patient is still in PTA.

- **Dead**
- **Vegetative state** ("alive but unconscious")
- **Severe disability** ("conscious but dependent")
  - unable to live alone for more than 24 hours: the daily assistance of another person at home is essential as a result of physical and/or cognitive impairments.
- **Moderate disability** ("independent but disabled") – independent at home; able to utilize public transportation; able to work in a supported environment.
- **Good recovery** ("mild to no residual deficits")
  - capacity to resume normal occupational and social activities although there may be minor residual physical or mental deficits.

FIGURE 18–2 Glasgow Outcome Scale.

A value of a predictor variable higher or lower than which a certain outcome is especially likely or unlikely.

Example: If post-traumatic amnesia (PTA) lasts more than 3 months, a person is very unlikely to achieve a "good recovery" on the Glasgow Outcome Scale (GOS).

FIGURE 18–3 Definition of threshold value.

Outcomes studied should be relevant and meaningful to a layperson (e.g., family member) asking about prognosis.

Predictor variables should represent information easily accessible to rehabilitation clinicians and the population encountered by rehabilitation professionals.

The studies must meet minimal methodological criteria in terms of patient selection, follow-up, statistical analysis, etc.

FIGURE 18–4 General guidelines for inclusion of studies.

Studies that reported their results in a way that allowed the determination of threshold values were especially important for this review. Unfortunately, less than a third of the included studies did so. In some cases, this was because the variable in question did not turn out to have a threshold value. This occurred when, regardless of the score or value, a prognostic factor was associated with all possible outcomes. For instance, for any initial GCS value between 3 and 8, all the outcomes on the GOS are possible, so there are no threshold values for this variable. With other factors such as PTA, it does make sense to speak of threshold values. Even in these cases, however, only a minority of the studies were designed or reported so that one could determine what those threshold values actually were. The guidelines in this chapter relied heavily on these few studies because they were the ones that provided the most useful information for clinicians.

Because of the limited number of studies involved, it was important to provide independent verification of the validity of their conclusions. This was done by determining if the results were consistent with the findings of the other excluded studies. For example, excluded studies were reviewed to determine if any of them reported a significant number of cases of good recovery on the GOS when the duration of PTA extended beyond 3 months (1 of the threshold values derived from the included studies). If the excluded studies also converged on the same threshold values, one could be more certain of the validity of the original values. In fact, the results of the excluded studies were consistent with almost all the derived threshold values; the few exceptions were not clinically significant and are discussed in more detail in the following text (in the sections on individual predictor variables).

The threshold values that were chosen were those that allowed one to exclude either a good recovery on the one hand or a severe disability on the other; no attempt was made to determine similar threshold values for moderate disability. This was motivated by the belief that, for most family members, it is the GOS categories of severe disability and good recovery that are of most interest in the subacute period. Families want to know how long they can still hope for a good recovery (and may not be as concerned, during that time, about whether the alternative is moderate disability or severe disability). Conversely, it is reassuring to families to hear it is unlikely that the patient will be severely disabled (even if neither them nor the clinician knows whether the eventual outcome will be a good recovery or moderate disability).

Of course, interpreting threshold values is not unproblematic. There is a degree of statistical uncertainty for all calculated threshold values. For example, even if no one with a duration of PTA greater than 3 months had a good recovery in a particular study, such an outcome is still *statistically* possible. This statistical uncertainty can be quantified using confidence intervals (CIs). The lower end of the CI would be zero (in a study where no one had the outcome of interest), whereas the upper end would represent the largest number of people who could have had the outcome of interest. The use of CIs in this context is further explained in the second appendix.

There were also instances where 2 or more studies differed in the threshold values they identified (for instance, excluding the possibility of a good recovery after a PTA of 2 months in one study but not until a PTA of 3 months in another). As discussed subsequently, a decision was made to err on the side of conservatism in these situations by choosing the value (larger or smaller, depending on the outcome) that minimized the possibility of an inaccurately pessimistic prognosis. So, in this example, one would choose 3 months of PTA as the threshold value to avoid discounting the possibility of a good recovery in those patients whose PTA lasted between 2 and 3 months.

Brief Comment on Methodology

The inclusion criteria are summarized in Figures 18-4 and 18-5. The second appendix provides a detailed review and justification for selecting these criteria. For present purposes,

Population
1. Publication after 1983
2. Setting in North America, Western Europe, Australia, New Zealand, or Israel
3. Setting in either acute care or inpatient rehabilitation
4. Moderate and/or severe TBI (penetrating and/or closed)
5. Exclusively or primarily adult TBI

Predictors
6. Predictor variables: GCS (total), LOC PTA, age, neuroimaging (CT or MRI) and/or early neuropsychological testing

Outcomes
7. Outcomes: GOS, vocational re-entry, and/or independent living
8. Outcomes assessed at 6 months or later

Methodology
9. Sample must represent consecutive admissions (whether done prospectively or retrospectively) or a random/neutral sampling or consecutive admissions
10. Sample size > 25
11. Follow-up > 80%
12. Statistical analysis performed (or, if not, enough information provided to analyze oneself)

FIGURE 18–5 Inclusion criteria for studies.

it is noted that the review focused on studies of adults who had sustained a moderate or severe TBI (either closed or penetrating). The predictor variables represented the information most likely to be available to rehabilitation clinicians: initial GCS score, LOC, duration of PTA, age, neuroimaging findings, and results of early neuropsychological testing. The outcomes of interest (assessed at 6 months or later) were vocational reentry, return to independent living, or the classification on the GOS. The use of the GOS as the primary outcome of interest requires justification; this is provided in the second appendix.

Well over a thousand articles were reviewed, out of which only 56 studies met all the inclusion criteria: 29 using neuroimaging predictors (34–45) (46–62) (Table 18-1), 41 using clinical predictors (34,36,37,40,45,47–50,52–56,58,59, 62–85) (see Table 18-2), 2 focused on the elderly (86,87) (see Table 18-3), and 2 focused on penetrating brain injury (88,89) (see Table 18-4) (the numbers add up to more than 56 because some studies investigated more than 1 prognostic factor). No studies that used early neuropsychological testing as a predictive variable met all the inclusion criteria. More importantly, of all the studies that were included, only a quarter allowed for the determination of threshold values. In particular, 8 of the closed head injury studies reported threshold values with acceptable CIs (0%–12%): 1 for magnetic resonance imaging (MRI), 1 for LOC, 2 for length of PTA, and 4 for age. In what follows, the results of the studies are reviewed by predictor variable. The conclusions are summarized in Figure 18-6.

SYNOPSIS OF STUDIES

Magnetic Resonance Imaging

Summary

Seven studies (39,41,48,54,56,59,61) met the inclusion criteria, all using information from MRI obtained from 2–8 weeks after injury. Every study found that the depth of the lesions correlated with outcome. Specifically, they discovered that brainstem lesions were strongly associated with poor outcome. Four of the studies identified possible threshold values (39–41,48,61); they all found that good recovery on the GOS was unlikely if bilateral brainstem lesions were present. In particular, no more than 7% of patients with bilateral brainstem lesions had a good recovery in these studies. However, only 1 of the 4 studies had an acceptable CI (41). Finally, 1 study found that no one without DAI had severe disability (59).

Discussion

The advantage of conventional MRI (relative to computed tomography [CT] scanning) is that it allows for better visualization of lesions, especially those in the brainstem. As a result, MRI is ideally suited to study the centripetal model of brain injury severity (90), which claims that the stronger the forces to which the brain is subjected, the more severe the injury and the deeper the lesions. The findings of these studies (as well as others that did not meet the inclusion criteria) are consistent with this hypothesis: depth of lesion is associated with worse outcomes because it is a marker of brain injury severity.

Conclusions

If an MRI from the first 2–8 weeks after a TBI is available, the depth of the lesions is associated with worse outcome. In particular, the presence of bilateral brainstem lesions makes the possibility of a good recovery very unlikely.

Computed Tomography

Summary

Twenty-three studies (34–38,40,42–47,49–53,55–58,60,62) met the inclusion criteria; all but 2 were conducted in the acute care setting. However, even the studies from the rehabilitation setting made use of the acute care CT scan. Almost half of the studies used scales that included several different imaging variables (e.g., the Traumatic Coma Data Bank classification and the Marshall CT classification), making it difficult to isolate how individual variables contributed to outcome.

Nonetheless, certain patterns emerged. In particular, the following findings on CT were found to be correlated with worse outcome: traumatic subarachnoid hemorrhage (SAH), midline shift, cisternal compression or obliteration, subdural hematoma (SDH), and epidural hematoma (EDH). Unfortunately, clinically useful threshold effects for these variables were not found in any of the studies.

Discussion

Because the acute care CT scan (or a report) is often available to rehabilitation professionals, it would have been helpful if the CT findings yielded more definitive prognoses. Unfortunately, although it is known that certain lesions are associated with worse outcomes, the nature of the relationship is such that more specific prognoses cannot be made. Overall, all of these findings are consistent with those of the excluded studies.

Conclusions

The presence of SAH, cisternal effacement, significant midline shift, EDH, or SDH on an acute care CT scan are all associated with worse outcomes. More specific conclusions about the implications of the lesions cannot be drawn because each one individually can be associated with the full range of outcomes after TBI.

Initial Glasgow Coma Scale

Summary

Of the studies that met the inclusion criteria, 19 (45,48,50,53, 54,56,58,59,61,65,66,69,70,72,74,77,80,81) examined the relationship between the total GCS score and outcome. As mentioned earlier, studies that used only a subset of the GCS (e.g., motor score) were excluded because, although rehabilitation professionals should have access to the initial GCS score, the individual subscores are often much less available. All but 4 of the studies (48,50,61,80) found an association between lower GCS scores and worse outcomes. Although the studies measured the GCS differently (e.g., admission, post-resuscitation, highest in the first 6–24 hours, etc.), none of them discovered threshold or cutoff values for outcomes. In other words, any particular initial GCS score could potentially be associated with any outcome (although the proba-

TABLE 18–1 Neuroimaging

STUDY	POPULATION	NUMBER	OUTCOME	PREDICTOR	FINDINGS ASSOCIATED WITH WORSE OUTCOME	STATISTICS	"THRESHOLD" VALUES
Rao, 1990 (34)	Moderate and severed rehab	79	Return to work (approximately 1.5 years)	CT (acute care)	Extent of CT damage (bilateral > unilateral > normal)	Univariate	None
Fearnside, 1993 (35)	Severe; acute	315	GOS (6 months)	CT (admission)	Contusion, intracerebral hematoma and SAH	Multivariate	None
Kakarieka, 1994 (36)	Severe; acute	414	GOS (6 months)	CT (admission)	Presence of SAH	Univariate and Multivariate	None
Walder, 1995 (37)	Severe; acute	109	GOS (6 months)	CT (admission)	CT findings as characterized by Abbreviated Injury Scale and the Traumatic Coma Data Bank Classification	Univariate	None
Lobato, 1997 (38)	Severe; acute	710	GOS (6 months)	CT (admission)	CT findings as characterized by Traumatic Coma Data Bank Classification	Univariate	None
Wedekind, 1999 (39)	Severe; acute	57	GOS (> 6 months)	MRI (2 weeks)	Lesions in corpus callosum or basal ganglia or midbrain or total number of lesions	Univariate	None
Gomez, 2000 (40)	Severe; acute	810	GOS (6 months)	CT (admission)	Univariate: status of cisterns, SAH, EDH, SDH, midline shift, or contusion; multivariate: status of cisterns, SAH, EDH, and IVH	Univariate and multivariate	None
Firsching, 2001 (41)	Severe; acute	102	GOS (2 years)	MRI (8 days) Depth of lesion; (total # of lesions or corpus callosum lesions do not correlate with outcome)	Depth of lesions (total number of lesions or corpus callosum lesions do not correlate with outcome)	Univariate	No one with bilateral brainstem lesions achieved a good recovery (CI 0%–8%)
Schaan, 2001 (42)	All GCS (admitted to ICU); acute; isolated TBI	554	GOS (6 months)	CT (admission)	EDH, SDH, edema, or contusion	Multivariate	None
Vos, 2001 (43)	Severe; acute	63	GOS (6 months)	CT (admission)	CT findings as characterized by Traumatic Coma Data Bank Classification	Univariate	None

Study	Sample	N	Outcome	Imaging	Variables	Analysis	Notes
Mattioli, 2003 (44)	All GCS (admitted to ICU); acute; included GSW	605	GOS (6 months)	CT (admission)	SAH	Multivariate	None
Rovlias, 2004 (45)	Severe (isolated BI); acute	345	GOS (6 months)	CT (admission)	SAH; EDH; SDH	Multivariate	None
Hanlon, 2005 (46)	Moderate and severe; inpatient rehab	100	Return to work (12 months)	CT (admission)	SAH	Univariate	None
Hukkelhoven, 2005 (47)	Moderate and severe, acute	2269	GOS (6 months)	CT (admission)	Marshall CT classification; SAH	Univariate and multivariate	None
Carpentier, 2006 (48)	Severe, acute	40	GOS (18 months)	MRI (average 17.5 days status post trauma)	Brainstem involvement, total number of lesions	Univariate	No one with a brainstem lesion had a good recovery (CI 0%–23%)
Cremer, 2006 (49)	Severe; acute	304	GOSE (> 12 months)	CT (admission)	CT findings as characterized by Traumatic Coma Data Bank Classification	Univariate and multivariate	None
Hiler, 2006 (50)	Severe; acute	126	GOS (6 months)	CT (admission)	Marshall CT classification; lesion volume; midline shift	Univariate	None
Maas, 2007 (51)	Moderate and severe; acute	5500	GOS (6 months)	CT (admission)	Marshall CT classification; status of cisterns; EDH; SDH: midline shift; SAH	Univariate and multivariate	None
Murray, 2007 (52)	Moderate and severe; acute	8509	GOS (6 months)	CT (admission)	Marshall CT classification; status of cisterns; EDH; SDH; midline shift; SAH	Univariate and multivariate	None
Perel, 2008 (53)	Moderate and severe, acute	10,008	GOS (6 months)	CT (admission)	CT with petechial hemorrhages; cisternal obliteration; SAH; midline shift; non-evacuated hematoma	Univariate and multivariate	None
Sidaros, 2008 (54)	Severe; inpatient rehab	30	GOS (9–15 months)	MRI (5–11 weeks)	Involvement of brainstem	Univariate	None
Steyerberg, 2008 (55)	Moderate and severe; acute	8509	GOS (6 months)	CT (admission)	Marshall CT classification; status EDH; SAH	Univariate and multivariate	None

(Continued)

TABLE 18–1 Neuroimaging (*Continued*)

STUDY	POPULATION/AGE (RANGE [MEAN])	NUMBER	OUTCOME	PREDICTOR	FINDINGS ASSOCIATED WITH WORSE OUTCOME	STATISTICS	"THRESHOLD" VALUES
Lagares, 2009 (56)	Moderate and severe; acute	100	GOS (6 months)	CT (admission); MRI (15 days status post trauma)	Univariate: CT findings and DAI on MRI; multivariate: DAI in brainstem	Univariate and multivariate	None
Jacobs, 2010 (57)	Moderate and severe; acute	679	GOSE (6 months)	CT (admission)	Univariate: any cisternal compression and/or absence; multivariate: compressed and/or absent ambient cisterns and/or fourth ventricle	Univariate and multivariate	None
Nelson, 2010 (58)	Moderate and severe; acute	361	GOS (12 months)	CT (admission)	Midline shift, SAH/IVH, and cisternal compression	Univariate and multivariate	None
Skandsen, 2010 (59)	Moderate and severe, acute	106	GOSE (12 months)	MRI (4 weeks)	DAI; brainstem involvement	Univariate	No one without DAI had severe disability (CI 0%–10%)
Jacobs, 2011 (60)	Moderate and severe, acute	567	GOSE (6 months)	CT	Lesion burden; SDH; hemorrhagic contusion	Univariate and multivariate	None
Skandsen, 2011 (61)	Moderate and severe, acute	106	GOSE (12 months)	MRI (4 weeks)	Bilateral brainstem injury	Univariate and multivariate	Only 7% of patients with bilateral brainstem injury had a good recovery (CI 0%–34%)
Yeoman, 2011 (62)	Moderate and severe, acute	1,276	GOS (12 months)	CT (admission)	Marshall CT classification; SAH	Multivariate	None

Abbreviations: CI, confidence interval; CT, computed tomography; DAI, diffuse axonal injury; EDH, epidural hematoma; GOS, Glasgow Outcome Scale; GOSE, Glasgow Outcome Scale Extended; GSW, gunshot wound; ICU, intensive care unit; IVH, intraventricular hemorrhage; MRI, magnetic resonance imaging; SAH, subarachnoid hemorrhage; SDH, subdural hematoma.

TABLE 18–2 Clinical Predictors

STUDY	POPULATION/AGE (RANGE [MEAN])	NUMBER	OUTCOME	PREDICTOR	FINDINGS ASSOCIATED WITH WORSE OUTCOME	STATISTICS	"THRESHOLD" VALUES
Born, 1985 (64)	Severe; acute, 1–75 years old (23)	109	GOS (6 months)	Age	Older age	Univariate	None
Facco, 1986 (65)	Severe; acute, 15–60 years old	56	GOS (6 months)	GCS; length of coma	Lower GCS	Univariate	None
Hans, 1987 (66)	Severe; acute, 3–61 years old (23)	40	GOS (6 months)	Age; GCS	Older age; lower GCS	Univariate	None
Choi, 1988 (67)	Severe; acute (30.8 years old)	523	GOS (6 months)	Age	Older age	Multivariate	None
Tate, 1989 (68)	Severe; rehab, 15–45 years old (23.9)	100	GOS (6 years)	PTA; length of coma	Length of PTA; length of coma	Univariate	None
Narayan, 1989 (69)	Severe; acute	133	GOS (> 6 months)	Age; GCS	Older age; lower GCS	Multivariate	None
Rao, 1990 (34)	Moderate and severe; rehab, 17–66 years old (29)	79	Return to work (1 year)	PTA; age; length of coma	Older age; length of coma; (length of PTA not correlated)	Univariate	None
Levin, 1990 (70)	Severe; acute, 16–70 years old (27)	300	GOS (12 months)	GCS	Lower GCS	Univariate	None
Choi, 1991 (71)	Severe; acute (30.9 years old)	617	GOS (12 months)	Age	Older age	Multivariate	None
Marshall, 1991 (72)	Severe; acute (29.5 years old)	746	GOS (2 years)	GCS	Lower GCS	Univariate	None
Vollmer, 1991 (73)	Severe; acute, 15–80 years old	661	GOS (6 months)	Age	Older age	Univariate	No patient older than 55 years old had a good recovery (CI 0%–4%)
Bishara, 1992 (74)	Severe; acute, 15–65 years old (25.7)	93	GOS (> 6 months)	PTA; age; GCS	Length of PTA; lower GCS; (age not correlated)	Univariate and multivariate	No one had severe disability until PTA > 2 months (CI 0%–4%)
Godfrey, 1993 (75)	Severe; acute (who survived acute care), 15–61 years old (25.38)	66	Return to work (> 1 year)	PTA	Length of PTA	Univariate	None
Pennings, 1993 (76)	Severe (GCS < 5); acute, 20–92 years old	92	GOS (> 6 months)	Age	Older age	Univariate	No patient older than 60 years old had a good recovery (CI 0%–7%).

(Continued)

255

TABLE 18-2 Clinical Predictors (Continued)

STUDY	POPULATION/AGE (RANGE [MEAN])	NUMBER	OUTCOME	PREDICTOR	FINDINGS ASSOCIATED WITH WORSE OUTCOME	STATISTICS	"THRESHOLD" VALUES
Katz, 1994 (77)	Moderate and severe; rehab (with DAI), 8–89 years old	175	GOS (6 months)	PTA; age; GCS; length of coma	Univariate: length of PTA, older age, lower GCS, length of coma; Multivariate: length of PTA, older age	Univariate and multivariate	No one with length of coma > 2 weeks (CI 0%–10%) or PTA > 3 months (CI 0%–11%) had a good recovery. Only 2% of patients with a PTA < 2 months were severely disabled (CI 0.3%–9.0%). Only 5% of length of coma < 2 weeks were severely disabled (CI 2%–12%).
Kakarieka, 1994 (36)	Severe; acute, 16–70 years old (36)	414	GOS (6 months)	Age	Older age	Multivariate	None
Walder, 1995 (37)	Severe; acute, 16–78 years old (26)	109	GOS (6 months)	Age	Older age	Univariate	None
Combes, 1996 (78)	Severe; acute, (38.5 years old)	198	GOS	Age	Older age	Multivariate	None
Ellenberg, 1996 (79)	Severe; acute (that regained consciousness in acute care), 16 years old (29)	314	GOS (6 months)	PTA; age; length of coma	Length of PTA; older age; length of coma	Multivariate	None
Hawkins, 1996 (80)	Mild, moderate, but mostly severe; rehab, 17–72 years old (27)	55	Return to work; independent living	GCS	None	Multivariate	None
Hellawell, 1999 (81)	Moderate and severe; acute, 15–78 years old (39.2)	96	GOS (6 months)	PTA; GCS	Length of PTA; lower GCS	Univariate	None

Study		N	Outcome measure			Analysis	Comments
Gomez, 2000 (40)	Severe; acute, 15 to > 65 years old	810	GOS (6 months)	Age	Older age	Multivariate	Only 6% of patients older than 65 years old had a good recovery (CI 0%–14%)
Rovlias, 2004 (45)	Severe; acute (isolated BI), 16–70 years old (40)	345	GOS (6 months)	Age; GCS	Age; GCS	Multivariate	None
Formisano, 2004 (63)	Severe; rehab (coma > 15 days), 11–56 years old (26)	43 (> 1 year)	GOS coma; age	Age; length of coma	Length of coma	Univariate	None
Hawkins, 2005 (82)	Mild, moderate, and severe; inpatient rehab, 13–72 years old (35.5)	64	Return to work, independent living (12 months)	Age, GCS	Older age for return to work	Multivariate	None
Hukkelhoven, 2005 (47)	Moderate and severe; acute, 15–65 years old (32.8–40.9)	1,552–3,718	GOS (6 months)	Age	Older age	Univariate and multivariate	None
Carpentier, 2006 (48)	Severe; acute, (33 years old)	40	GOS (18 months)	GCS	Lower GCS	Univariate and multivariate	None
Cremer, 2006 (49)	Severe; acute, (41 years old)	304	GOSE (> 12 months)	Age	Older age	Univariate and multivariate	None
Hiler, 2006 (50)	Severe; acute, 14–74 years old	126	GOS (6 months)	GCS	Not significant	Univariate	None
Murray, 2007 (52)	Moderate and severe; acute, 14–70 years old	8,509	GOS (6 months)	Age	Older age	Univariate and multivariate	None
Mushkudiani, 2007 (83)	Moderate and severe; acute, 14–70 years old	8,719	GOS (6 months)	Age	Older age	Univariate and multivariate	None
Perel, 2008 (53)	Moderate and severe; acute, adults (37 years old)	10,008	GOS (6 months)	Age, GCS	Older age, lower GCS	Univariate and multivariate	None
Sherer, 2008 (84)	All GCS; inpatient rehab (28 years old)	118	Productivity (12 months)	Age, length of coma	Older age	Univariate and multivariate	None

(Continued)

TABLE 18–2 Clinical Predictors (Continued)

STUDY	POPULATION/AGE (RANGE [MEAN])	NUMBER	OUTCOME	PREDICTOR	FINDINGS ASSOCIATED WITH WORSE OUTCOME	STATISTICS	"THRESHOLD" VALUES
Sidaros, 2008 (54)	Severe; rehab, 18–65 years old (34 years old)	30	GOS (9–15 months)	PTA: age, GCS; length of coma	Length of PTA; lower GCS, length of coma	Univariate	None
Steyerberg, 2008 (55)	Moderate and severe; acute, 14–70 years old	8,509 and 6,999	GOS (6 months)	Age	Older age	Univariate and multivariate	None
Lagares, 2009 (56)	Moderate and severe; acute, 15–75 years old (33)	100	GOS (6 months)	GCS	Lower GCS on univariate analysis only	Univariate and multivariate	None
Nakase-Richardson, 2009 (85)	Moderate and severe; rehab, 16–82 years old (27 years old)	280	Employment (1 year)	PTA	Length of PTA	Univariate	Less than 10% of patients with PTA greater than 70 days were productive (CI 3%–21%)
Nelson, 2010 (58)	Moderate and severe; acute, > 15 years old	361	GOS (12 months)	Age, GCS	Older age, lower GCS	Univariate and multivariate	None
Skandsen, 2010 (59)	Moderate and severe; acute, 5–65 years old (28 years old)	106	GOSE (12 months)	GCS	Lower GCS	Univariate and multivariate	None
Skandsen, 2011 (61)	Moderate and severe; acute, 5–65 years old (28 years old)	106	GOSE (12 months)	Age, GCS	Older age	Univariate and multivariate	None
Yeoman, 2011 (62)	Moderate and severe; acute, > 16 years old (40.1 years old)	1,276	GOS (12 months)	Age	Older age	Multivariate	None

Abbreviations: BI, brain injury; CI, confidence interval; DAI, diffuse axonal injury; GCS, Glasgow Coma Scale; GOS, Glasgow Outcome Scale; GOSE, Glasgow Outcome Scale Extended; PTA, post-traumatic amnesia.

TABLE 18–3 Elderly

STUDY	POPULATION/AGE	NUMBER	OUTCOME	PREDICTOR	FINDINGS ASSOCIATED WITH WORSE OUTCOME	STATISTICS	"THRESHOLD" VALUES
Ross, 1992 (86)	All GCS; acute, age > 65 years old	195	GOS (6 months)	GCS	Lower GCS	Univariate	Only 3% of patients with an initial GCS < 8 achieved a good recovery (CI 1%–9%)
Kilaru, 1996 (87)	Severe; acute, > 65 years old	40	GOS (38 months)	GCS	Lower GCS	Multivariate	No patient with admission GCS < 8 achieved a good recovery (CI 0%–8%)

Abbreviations: CI, confidence interval; GCS, Glasgow Coma Scale; GOS, Glasgow Outcome Scale.

bility of having a good outcome decreases as the GCS score decreases).

Discussion

Although providing a general idea of the severity of the injury, the GCS by itself does not yield definitive prognoses. This is true even when the accuracy of the GCS is increased by varying the timing and content of measurement. Even the most accurate of the methods did not improve accuracy enough to allow for more specific prognoses. Also, rehabilitation professionals are often limited in which GCS score they have access to (and often don't know exactly when it was obtained). For both these reasons, it did not seem worthwhile to look more closely at the accuracy of different ways of obtaining the GCS. All of these findings are consistent with the rest of the literature (i.e., the studies that were excluded).

Conclusions

Although the initial GCS score is associated with outcome and lower GCS scores are associated with worse outcomes, one cannot draw more specific conclusions solely from the GCS score.

Length of Coma

Summary

Of the studies that met the inclusion criteria, there were 8 (34,54,63,65,68,77,79,84) that studied the relationship between the LOC and outcome. Five of the 8 defined the LOC as that period until the patient started following commands. One defined it as the time until the GCS was > 8. The other 2 studies did not specify how coma duration was measured. All but 2 (65,84) found a relationship between the duration of coma and outcome (the longer the duration of coma, the worse the outcome). In addition, 1 of the studies (77) reported its data in such a way that it was possible to determine a threshold value for excluding the possibility of a good recovery. Specifically, they found that no subject made a good recovery whose LOC exceeded 14 days (77).

Discussion

Although the duration of coma has been defined several different ways (e.g., when GCS is 9 or greater, when the eyes open, etc.), the most common method of measurement is the time to follow commands. This was also the predominant method of measurement in the rest of the literature. Therefore, the rehabilitation clinician using the LOC for prognostic

TABLE 18–4 Penetrating Missile Injury

STUDY	POPULATION	NUMBER	OUTCOME	PREDICTOR	FINDINGS ASSOCIATED WITH WORSE OUTCOME	STATISTICS	"THRESHOLD" VALUES
Grahm, 1990 (88)	All GCS; acute	100	GOS (> 6 months)	GCS; CT	Lower GCS; bilateral or transventricular injury on CT	Univariate	No patients with GCS < 8 or transventricular injury had good recovery (CI 0%–4%)
Levy, 1994 (89)	GCS 3–5; acute	190	GOS (6–12 months)	GCS; CT	Lower GCS; bilateral injury with IVH on CT	Multivariate	No patients with GCS 3–5 had a good recovery (CI 0%–2%)

CI, confidence interval; CT, computed tomography; IVH, intraventricular hemorrhage; GCS, Glasgow Coma Scale; GOS, Glasgow Outcome Scale.

GCS
  • Lower scores associated with worse outcomes
  • No threshold values

Length of Coma
  • Longer duration associated with worse outcomes
  • Threshold values:
    • Severe disability unlikely when less than 2 weeks
    • Good recovery unlikely when greater than 4 weeks

PTA
  • Longer duration associated with worse outcomes
  • Threshold values:
    • Severe disability unlikely when less than 2 months
    • Good recovery unlikely when greater than 3 months

Age
  • Older age associated with worse outcomes
  • Threshold values:
    • Good recovery unlikely when older than 65 years old

Neuroimaging
  • Certain features (e.g., depth of lesions) associated with worse outcomes
  • Threshold values:
    • Good recovery unlikely when bilateral brainstem lesions present on early MRI

FIGURE 18–6 Summary of studies of nonpenetrating TBI.

purposes should follow the same guidelines. Only 1 study (77) reported a threshold value with an acceptable CI. However, the value of 14 days they found seems too short. For instance, the Tate study (68) reported instances of a good recovery even after a month of coma. Other studies, excluded in the review, also converge on approximately 1 month as a cutoff point (beyond which the chances of a good recovery are small) (91–93). In these studies, it appears that on average, only 7%–8% of patients will make a good recovery who are not following commands beyond 1 month.

Conclusions

The longer the duration of coma (as measured by the time to follow commands), the more likely a worse outcome. In particular, a duration of coma greater than 4 weeks makes a good recovery unlikely.

Post-Traumatic Amnesia

Summary

Of the studies that met the methodological criteria, 9 (34,54, 68,74,75,77,79,81,85) investigated the relationship between the length of PTA and outcome. All but 1 found the 2 were associated (the longer the duration of PTA, the worse the outcome). Only 4 of the studies reported how they measured PTA (54,77,79,85); all of these studies relied on the Galveston Orientation and Amnesia Test (GOAT) to mark the end of PTA (i.e., a score of greater than 75 on 2 consecutive days). Three of the studies (74,77,85) reported their data in such a way that it was possible to determine threshold values for excluding the possibility of either a good recovery or a severe disability. Specifically, 1 of the studies found that no subject had an outcome of severe disability until their duration of PTA exceeded 2 months (CI 0%–3.6%) (74). Similarly, the

Katz study (77) found that only 2% of individuals with a duration of PTA less than 2 months was severely disabled (CI 0.3%–8.8%). Although these studies converged on the period during which a severe disability was unlikely, the 3 studies varied in when they were able to exclude the possibility of a good recovery. The longest reported duration of PTA before a good recovery became unlikely was 3 months (CI 0%–11%) (77).

Discussion

The duration of PTA has long been considered one of the most powerful prognostic factors available to the rehabilitation clinician (94). Besides its power, the duration of PTA has other advantages that make it especially useful. For one, the duration of PTA lends itself to the identification of threshold values. Also, many of these thresholds are crossed while the patient is in inpatient rehabilitation, allowing the rehabilitation professional an opportunity to substantively address issues of prognosis during the rehabilitation stay. In addition, because these thresholds are often reached in rehabilitation, the rehabilitation professional has much more control over the measurement of this variable.

In general, the studies that reported thresholds converge on a duration of PTA of 2–3 months when the prognosis becomes much clearer. For instance, both the Bishara (74) and Katz (77) studies agreed that the possibility of severe disability was very unlikely when the duration of PTA was less than 2 months. Also, 3 studies converged on 2–3 months as the duration of PTA before the possibility of a good recovery becomes very unlikely (74,77,85), although only the Katz study (77) had an acceptable CI.

A review of the studies on PTA that did not meet the inclusion criteria revealed findings consistent with this value. For example, one recent large study ($N = 1332$) was specifically designed to identify potential prognostic threshold values for the duration of PTA (95). They found that severe disability was unlikely when the duration of PTA was less than 40 days (85% negative predictive value) and that a good recovery was unlikely when the duration of PTA was greater than 2 months (90% positive predictive value) (95).

Conclusions

The longer the duration of PTA, the worse the outcome. In particular, it is unlikely that a person will have an outcome of severe disability if the duration of PTA is less than 2 months. Conversely, it is unlikely a person will have a good recovery when the duration of PTA extends beyond 3 months.

Age

Summary

Of the studies that met the inclusion criteria, 29 investigated the relationship between age and outcome (34,36,37,40, 45,47,49,52,53,54,55,58,61–64,66,67,69,71,73,74,76–79,82–84). All but 3 (63,74,54) found the 2 were associated (the older the patient, the worse the outcome). There were differences in whether increasing age was seen as a continuous risk factor or whether the risk increased at certain ages ("inflection points"). Four of the studies (40,73,76,77) reported threshold values of an age above which a good recovery was extremely unlikely. However, there was variability in the exact age found to represent this cutoff point. Among patients with a severe TBI, 2 studies found that no patients had a good recovery after the age of 55 (CI 0%–4.1%) (73) and 60 (CI 0%–6.9%) (76). Another study found that, although there were some patients with a good recovery after the age of 65, the probability was low (6%) (CI 2%–14%) (40).

Discussion

Age is a powerful prognostic factor. Although the risk for adults appears continuous, the prognosis worsens significantly after the age of 65. This is discussed in more detail in the next section. A review of the excluded literature is consistent with these findings.

Conclusions

Older patients have a worse outcome after a severe TBI. In particular, in patients older than 65 years, the chances of a good recovery after severe TBI are unlikely.

Special Populations: Elderly

Summary

There were 2 studies (86,87) meeting the inclusion criteria that examined prognostic factors in patients older than 65 years. Both studies found the initial GCS was associated with outcome: the lower one's GCS score, the worse the outcome. One study (87) found that no subject with an admission GCS < 8 had a good recovery at long-term follow-up (CI 0%–8.2%). This is consistent with the studies mentioned previously (73,76) that also found no subjects older than 65 years who had a good recovery after a severe TBI.

The other study on the elderly (56), however, found that a subset of those with an admission GCS < 8 did have the potential to achieve a good recovery. Specifically, they reported that those patients who regained consciousness within 72 hours had the potential to achieve a good recovery (3% in their series) (CI 0.6%–8.9%). This finding is consistent with the results of the other study mentioned previously (40) that found some patients older than 65 years who achieved a good recovery (6% in their series, with CI 2%–14%).

Discussion

The importance of TBI in the elderly is growing. This is not only because the incidence of TBI rises in the elderly but also because the percentage of the population older than 65 years is growing. Although there may be confounding factors (e.g., comorbidities), it is now clear that age is an independent risk factor in this population (96). There are many potential reasons for this, ranging from the nature of the injuries in the elderly (e.g., SDH) to changes in the brain as one ages (e.g., decreased functional reserve, less elasticity of blood vessels, etc.). These issues are discussed in more depth in the chapter on TBI in the elderly (Chapter 28). For our purposes, the main point is that a good recovery after a severe TBI in a person older than 65 years is very unlikely. The increased likelihood of poor outcomes is also found in the other severity categories. In fact, several writers have noted that, in terms of outcome, a moderate TBI in the elderly re-

sembles a severe TBI in a younger person (86,97,98). Even the outcomes of mild TBI in the elderly are much worse, with many never returning to their premorbid functional status (99).

Conclusions

In patients older than 65 years, the lower the admission GCS, the worse the outcome. In particular, older patients who have sustained a severe TBI (GCS < 8) are unlikely to achieve a good recovery.

Special Populations: Penetrating Injuries

Summary

There were 2 studies (88,89) that met the inclusion criteria which investigated prognostic factors in civilian patients with penetrating missile wounds. Both studies found the GCS was associated with outcome: the lower one's GCS score, the worse the outcome. Both studies also found that CT findings of bilateral injury or transventricular injury were associated with worse outcomes. One study (88) found that no patients who had a post-resuscitation GCS score < 8 had a good recovery at long-term follow-up (CI 0%–4.4%). The other study (89) only included patients with GCS scores of 3–5. No one in their series achieved a good recovery at long-term follow-up (CI 0%–1.6%).

Discussion

Penetrating injury differs from closed brain injuries in many ways, as discussed elsewhere in this textbook. In terms of outcome, the early mortality rate after penetrating injury is much higher than that of closed head injury (100). Among the survivors, however, there are proportionally fewer people who are left vegetative or severely disabled (100). Although many prognostic factors have been studied in penetrating injuries (100), only the GCS is readily available to rehabilitation clinicians. Unlike closed head injury, where a range of outcomes is still possible with a GCS of 3–8, in penetrating injury, it is very unlikely that patients with an initial GCS in this range will have a good recovery. These findings are consistent with those in the excluded studies; only 1 study reported any patients who achieved a good outcome with an initial GCS of 6–8 (8%) (101). However, they also found that no one achieved a good recovery with an initial GCS of 3–5.

Conclusions

In patients with a penetrating missile injury, lower GCS scores and CT findings of bilaterality or transventricular injury are associated with worse outcomes. Moreover, those patients with a post-resuscitation GCS score of 8 or less are unlikely to achieve a good recovery.

Special Populations: Moderate TBI

The focus of this chapter is on severe TBI because it is with this group of patients that the most uncertainty exists about long-term prognosis. In contrast, outcomes after moderate TBI are much clearer (12,21,102,103): more than 90% of individuals who survive a moderate TBI will achieve either a moderate disability or good recovery. This information is certainly useful for clinicians counseling family members, especially by reassuring them the odds are heavily in favor of at least independent living, if not a return to previous function.

There are certain risk factors associated with the poorer outcomes: lower GCS scores (e.g., 9 or 10), older age, and abnormalities on the CT scan (12,21,102,103). When these are present, patients are more likely to have a moderate disability (or, infrequently, even a severe disability) rather than a good recovery. This information can be used to adjust the content and tone of prognostic information provided to family members.

Although the prognosis after moderate TBI is good, it is here that the limits of the higher categories of the GOS are most obvious. Studies have shown that even individuals with a good recovery often have neurobehavioral problems that contribute significantly to the morbidity of moderate TBI (12,21). It is important to communicate this information to the family, although initially it may be in the most general of terms (e.g., "most people are able to at least live on their own after this type of brain injury, although they may have some other problems").

Neuropsychological Testing

Although early neuropsychological testing (performed within 1 month after injury or at the resolution of PTA) was originally included as a potential predictor variable, none of the studies reviewed met the methodological criteria, mainly because of limited follow-up. Still, because neuropsychological testing is so widely used in the rehabilitation setting, the findings of some of these studies (92,104–108) are reviewed here. Almost all the studies found an association between selected test results and long-term outcome, even when adjusted for demographic and injury severity variables (92). The specific tests found to be predictive varied between the studies, however, limiting the utility of the findings. Another feature of the studies that reduced their applicability was the use of statistical analyses that cannot easily be utilized in the clinical setting (e.g., correlation coefficients, principal components analysis, etc.).

Even when the findings were reported in a clinically useful way, the studies were still not helpful. This is because early neuropsychological testing, even when correlated with outcome, is not a particularly powerful predictor. In the language of the rest of the chapter, there were no threshold values that were found for neuropsychological test scores. For instance, 1 study (106) found that a normal score on 1 of 10 tests identified as predictive still had less than a 50% chance of predicting productivity at 1 year or beyond. Even an impaired score, which was a more powerful prognosticator, predicted lack of productivity in only 70% of people. The utility of testing is further diminished by the fact that only a subset of patients are able to be tested subacutely; therefore, the results of these studies are not relevant to the significant number of patients who are not testable during inpatient rehabilitation.

In fact, this distinction between those who are testable or not (rather than the test scores themselves) turns out to be the most powerful predictor in these studies and one that could potentially serve as a threshold value for prognosis. In 1 of the 2 studies that examined this relationship (106), only 6% of patients who were unable to complete any test during inpatient rehabilitation were productive at 1 year. In the other study (92), only 6% of those who were not testable at 1 month were employed a year later. In contrast, being testable was not as predictive in either study, correctly classifying only about 40%–80% of those who would be productive at 1 year. Although the inability to be tested in the subacute setting appears to be a potentially valuable prognostic variable, it does not provide significantly more information than the better supported use of LOC or duration of PTA.

Indeed, it is likely that the findings in these studies were confounded by the LOC or PTA. For instance, the first study was designed so that people were only tested when they emerged from PTA. Thus, being testable was a marker for the length of PTA. The primary reason that patients who are not testable during inpatient rehabilitation do poorly is that they have a prolonged PTA. Assuming that most patients are discharged from inpatient rehabilitation about 2–3 months after their injury, those patients who are not testable during this period must have had lengths of PTA greater than 2–3 months, which was the threshold value identified in previous studies. Similar considerations apply to the other studies (91,92). There was 1 study that did adjust for PTA duration; it found that neuropsychological test performance made a contribution to the prediction of productivity beyond that made by the duration of PTA (107). The exact improvement in predictive power made by the tests was not reported, however, and is unlikely to be clinically significant.

In conclusion, it is likely that there is an association between early neuropsychological test performance and long-term outcome. More specific conclusions cannot be made because of the methodological limitations of the studies, the lack of consensus on which tests are most important, and because, even with the most robust results, there are no threshold values for test performance. The only statement that can be made with some confidence (within the constraints of the methodological limitations already discussed) is that not being testable early on is a poor prognostic sign for a productive long-term outcome. This subject is more extensively reviewed elsewhere (108).

SUMMARY

Key Clinical Findings

The 56 studies were almost unanimous in finding that age, initial GCS score, LOC, duration of PTA, and neuroimaging findings are correlated with outcome (Figure 18-6). However, this represents information that TBI clinicians already know. Of much greater interest is the existence of threshold values for several of the variables; these allow the clinician to formulate more fine-grained prognoses in individual cases. Specifically, age, LOC, duration of PTA, and the presence of bilateral brainstem lesions all provide valuable information the clinician can use to mark milestones when either a severe disability or a good recovery are unlikely. Of course, the duration of coma and PTA are related to one another, partly because they are both markers of injury severity (as is the GCS score). Several studies have examined the relationship between these variables in a more detailed manner (77,109). These results are based on a small number of studies (less than a third of the total); however, this must be kept in mind when using this information in clinical situations. On the other hand, the fact that these results were consistent with those in the excluded studies increases confidence in the findings. In essence, the results are at least consistent with almost *all* the published literature.

There was only 1 minor exception to the general agreement between the included and excluded studies: the maximum LOC after which a good recovery is extremely unlikely. The original review found a value of 2 weeks. However, as mentioned earlier, there were several excluded studies that found a significant number of individuals with a good recovery after 2 weeks of coma. These other studies seem to converge on the value of 1 month of coma as the time after which a good recovery is very unlikely. Because of the wish to err on the side of preserving hope, 1 month of coma was adopted as the final threshold value for LOC (Figure 18-7).

Finally, the statistical uncertainty involved must be kept in mind. The upper limits of the 95% CIs for the threshold values averaged approximately 7%. This means that, on average, up to 7% of individuals could have outcomes that are considered unlikely (e.g., up to 7% of patients with a PTA greater than 3 months may have a good recovery on the GOS). This underscores the point that one should use terms such as "unlikely" or "very unlikely" rather than, for instance, "never" in talking with families. One may even want to convey the associated degree of uncertainty in quantitative terms.

Applying the Guidelines

The final guidelines are presented in Figure 18-7. They are based both on the results of the initial review as well as, for LOC, the findings of the excluded studies. There are a few final points about applying these principles. The first is to recommend the use of different sources of information at different times in the recovery process. For example, if someone older than 65 years has a severe TBI, one knows fairly early that the chances of a good recovery are low, especially if they do not regain consciousness within a few days. For those younger than the age of 65, however, one will probably need to wait until the duration of coma is known (especially when it is less than 2 weeks or greater than 4 weeks). Later,

because of its predictive power, the length of PTA should be used as the primary source of information.

This sequential use of different variables is important not only because the later variables are more powerful than the earlier ones. It is also necessary because there is not always a strong correlation between the variables (e.g., between the LOC and duration of PTA). For instance, based on clinical experience, one can have a duration of coma of less than 2 weeks (which would imply a relatively good prognosis) with a protracted PTA of greater than 2–3 months (which implies a worse prognosis). In these cases, the prognosis based on the duration of PTA should be used as the primary source of information. It is also important to keep in mind some sense of the trajectory of recovery and adjust one's predictions accordingly. In someone who is still minimally conscious at 2 months, for instance, it is extremely unlikely they will become fully conscious and clear from PTA within the following month. Thus, one does not always have to wait until the passage of a full 3 months to infer that the likelihood of a good recovery is low.

Finally, it is also important to modify one's predictions based on the presence or absence of significant focal lesions. Although it is true that almost all the studies "correct" for the presence of focal lesions (by including both those with and without such lesions), knowledge of a significant focal lesion can help with prognostication in individual cases. Someone with a left anterior lesion and significant language deficits will likely have a worse outcome than patients who have similar lengths of coma, PTA, and so forth, but who don't have the same focal lesion. On the other hand, it has been shown that patients who primarily have DAI usually do worse than those whose primary lesions are focal (77). If the predominant underlying pathology is known, clinicians can use this information to modify what they tell patients and their families. In summary, application of the principles presented here involves the sequential use of the predictor variables, modified by knowledge of the larger trajectory of recovery as well as the presence or absence of significant focal lesions.

Excursus: Prognostic Models

The approach taken in this chapter, with its emphasis on threshold values, has resulted in a focus on the prognostic value of single predictor variables in isolation from other variables. But of course, outcome after a TBI is determined by the additive and interactive effect of several different variables, only some of which are related to injury severity. For example, nonbiological premorbid factors such as education and employment are strongly correlated with outcome, especially long-term outcome (110). Theoretically, if we knew all of the factors that affect outcome (as well as their relative contribution to outcome), we would be able to make more accurate prognoses for our patients. Many studies on prognosis after TBI do attempt to model the interaction between multiple variables and their impact on outcome. These "multivariable" models (commonly referred to as prognostic models, prediction models, prediction rules, etc.) enable clinicians to use a combination of variables to estimate the probability of outcomes in patients.

Many of the studies included in our review adopt this strategy, especially more recent investigations (e.g. 47,49,52, 53,55,62,83). The prognostic models created from the studies

---

> Severe disability (according to GOS) is unlikely when
> - time to follow commands is less than 2 weeks
> - duration of PTA is less than 2 months
>
> Good recovery (according to the GOS) is unlikely when
> - Time to follow commands is longer than 1 month
> - Duration of PTA is greater than 3 months
> - Age is older than 65 years
> - MRI indicates bilateral brainstem injury

FIGURE 18–7 Summary of evidence-based guidelines for prognostication after severe TBI (see text for important qualifications).

of the 2 largest samples of patients in our review have recently been posted on the internet with the intent of aiding clinicians in prognosticating after acute TBI (111,112). After clinicians enter the patient's values for 3–10 acute care variables (e.g., GCS motor score, pupillary status, age, CT findings, serum glucose levels, etc.), the model then provides an estimate of the risk of an unfavorable outcome for that patient. These prognostic models, if they accurately predict outcome in individual patients, would seem to have significant advantages over an approach that uses threshold values for single variables. Theoretically, the predictions should be more accurate because the prognostic model accounts for more of the variables that determine outcome. In addition, prognostic models would also allow the clinician to estimate outcome at any time and not just when certain threshold values have been crossed.

Despite these apparent advantages, prognostic models have significant limitations, especially for TBI. One issue is that almost all of these models were developed in the acute care setting that may limit their applicability to patients in the rehabilitation setting. More importantly, recent systematic reviews of prognostic models in TBI have found significant problems in almost all of the models reviewed (113–115). In particular, the models were developed from small samples of patients, had poor study design, were rarely externally validated, and were not easy to use for clinicians. The issue of external validation is especially important: all models perform less well when applied to samples other than the one the model was derived from. Even TBI models that have been externally validated seem to have performance characteristics (e.g., discrimination and calibration) that would limit their usefulness in prognosticating for individual patients.

Even if these models had acceptable performance characteristics, there are other concerns. One is ease of use. Many of the models were presented in a way that made it difficult for clinicians to use in daily practice (e.g., as regression equations). Even more accessible forms of presentations (e.g., an internet based model) add an "extra step" that might limit widespread use. The issue of clinical utility arises not only for clinicians but, maybe surprisingly, also for families. In particular, it is unclear how valuable families find probabilities that are not close to either 0% or 100%. As discussed at the beginning of this chapter, it has been our experience that families are most interested in how soon it can be known that the patient won't be severely disabled or, conversely, how long they can still hope for a good recovery. The closer a probability estimate for a given outcome is to 50%, the less valuable a family seems to find the information. This is because most laypeople understand a 50% probability to mean no more than that "either (their loved one) will have the outcome or they won't," which they understandably don't find very helpful.

Thus, although an apparent advantage of prognostic models over the threshold value approach is that it allows for estimates of probabilities in the range between thresholds (e.g., between a 10% probability of a good recovery and a 90% probability of a good recovery), it is not clear how useful that information is to families. And because, as we have argued, prognostication is ultimately a *clinical* act, the clinical value of information must be judged by its relevance and value to families and patients. Of course, prognostic models

in TBI are an important source of information and have a role to play in clinical decision making. But we do not believe that they currently are any more valuable to clinicians than the threshold value approach adopted in this chapter.

COMMUNICATING PROGNOSES

Patients and their families will forgive you for wrong diagnoses, but will rarely forgive you for wrong prognoses.—David Seegal

Barriers to Communication

Formulating a prediction constitutes only part of the clinical act of prognosis; this information must then be communicated to patients and families. Clinicians' reluctance to communicate this information is just as responsible for the neglect of prognostication as is the difficulty in developing a prognosis in the first place. There are many reasons for this reluctance. Many health care professionals believe that patients and families don't want prognostic information (4). Yet, studies have shown that professionals significantly underestimate patients' and families' desire for this information (116–120). One study found that 88% of patients wanted prognostic information (121). Another study showed that, even when patients had not explicitly asked for prognostic information, they wished the clinician had discussed it with them (122).

Studies involving patients with TBI have come to similar conclusions (5). As mentioned earlier, families have identified information about the future as one of their greatest needs in the aftermath of a TBI (1–3). Of course, it is true that some patients or their families sincerely do not want prognostic information (123). It may even be true that these preferences may vary by one's ethnic or cultural group (123). Therefore, 1 of the key steps in communicating prognoses is to find out how much information the patient or the family wants.

Another reason that rehabilitation professionals may be reluctant to discuss prognosis is the fear that families will interpret any discussion of uncertainty as evidence of the clinician's lack of competence (124). There is some support for this concern; 1 study found that the presentation of probabilities in discussing possible outcomes undermined patients' confidence in their physicians (125). In addition, there is evidence that clinicians themselves are unable to tolerate uncertainty (126); this is likely to contribute to their avoidance of prognosis.

Rehabilitation professionals may also believe that communicating a poor prognosis to patients or families causes too much pain, thereby extinguishing hope that might be needed to actively engage in rehabilitation. Yet, studies in other contexts at least partially belie this concern. One study found that, although communicating a poor prognosis did result in short-term distress among cancer patients, they experienced less anxiety, more peace of mind, and better adjustment in the long-term (118). It might even be the case that not being told about a poor prognosis interferes with the grieving process by making it much more ambiguous (because one is not sure whether a loss has occurred). There is evidence this "ambiguous grief" results in more emotional distress than grief where the loss is both clear and acknowledged (127).

Finally, avoiding a discussion of prognosis can itself cause distress: the anxiety associated with uncertainty often compounds the suffering families experience. Of course, like everything else in medicine, the benefits of communication must be weighed against the risks; however, in most cases, it is probable that more is gained by open communication (4). This is not to say that minimizing distress and fostering hope are unimportant. Rather, it is to highlight the fact that the avoidance of prognosis is unlikely to achieve these goals. There are better means by which to foster hope; some of these ways will be discussed shortly.

Not only are clinicians concerned about the distress they might cause families, they themselves feel distress in communicating poor prognoses (4). Clinicians (especially physicians) might feel unprepared to deal with the emotions the patient or family might express. Also, it has been argued that conveying a poor prognosis reminds clinicians of the limits of their abilities (because they are powerless to change the outcome) and this also reduces their willingness to have these discussions. Finally, the fact remains that most clinicians (again, especially physicians) are simply not trained in "how to break bad news" (116). Their reluctance stems from not knowing *how* to proceed (compounded by their apprehension in publicly performing a skill they have not mastered).

It is hoped the guidelines presented here (summarized in Figures 18-8–18-10) will help allay some of this anxiety and improve the frequency and quality of communication of prognostic information. Several general guidelines for communicating prognostic information are presented in Figure 18-8; these guidelines will structure the discussion to follow.

Guidelines for Communicating Prognoses

Begin with the Patient and Family

Although most patients and families want prognostic information, this is not universally true. Even those who want to discuss prognosis may differ in the amount of information desired as well as how its delivery is timed. Thus, if patients or families don't explicitly ask to discuss prognosis, it is important to ask if they are interested in the information. If so, one should explore in more detail what they are interested

in (for instance, in terms of possible outcomes). It is also helpful to begin by asking the family members what they already know and what their current perceptions are. This enables the clinician to build on the knowledge they already have or, if appropriate, correct any misinformation that might distort their understanding of the information to follow. Starting with the patient or family's desires and beliefs not only ensures that the discussion addresses their need, but it also draws them into the conversation early (and thus hopefully makes it easier for them to articulate their concerns). It also gives them some sense of control in a situation where they often feel powerless.

Ensure Understanding of the Outcomes

It is important that families clearly understand the nature of the outcomes discussed. This is especially important when one is using studies that rely on the GOS. The names of the GOS categories can be confusing. In particular, the terms moderate and severe disability may imply a far worse prognosis than might actually be the case. Most families would not necessarily consider someone who can live independently and use public transportation moderately disabled, even if they can't work. Or, a person who might be independent in mobility and self-care might not be considered severely disabled, even if they were unable to live independently for cognitive reasons. Given this ambiguity, it is best to avoid the GOS

- Try to use "natural frequencies" when communicating probabilistic information (e.g., "8 out of 10 people with this type of injury will make a good recovery")
- Present information both qualitatively as well as quantitatively (e.g., "This is a very good chance of a good recovery")
- Attempt to "frame" information in both a positive and negative manner (e.g., "This is the same as saying that 2 out of 10 people with this type of injury will not make a good recovery")
- When possible, consider presenting the information visually
- Ask the person to restate, in their own words, their understanding of the information provided

FIGURE 18–9 Guidelines for the communication of quantitative information.

- Begin with the family's desire for information as well as their current beliefs.
- Ensure that the meaning and content of the outcomes are understood.
- Present quantitative information in a manner that can be understood (see Figure 18-9).
- Foster hope.
- Pay attention to the process of communication (see Figure 18-10).

FIGURE 18–8 General guidelines for communicating prognostic information.

- Find a quiet, comfortable room without interruptions
- Sit close and speak face to face
- Have the family member's support network present, if wanted
- Present the information at a pace the family can follow
- Periodically summarize the discussion to that point
- Periodically ask family members to repeat or summarize what was said
- Keep the language simple but direct without euphemism or jargon
- Allow time for questions

FIGURE 18–10 Guidelines for the communication process.

category names altogether, and simply describe concretely what the outcomes might be. It is also important to mention some of the limitations of the GOS. Families should be aware that patients who achieve a good recovery might still have significant emotional or behavioral issues. At the same time, they should also know that the category of severe disability does not automatically preclude a good quality of life. One study found that almost half of individuals classified as severely disabled by the GOS at 1 year were satisfied with their lives (and close to a third who had made a good recovery were dissatisfied with their lives) (128). Finally, it is important to stress to families that most of the studies on prognosis followed patients for only a year, on average, and that there is evidence for continued gains well beyond that time (17).

Present Statistical Information in an Understandable Manner

Prognostication is not only about the range of possible outcomes but also the likelihood of their occurring. Therefore, the ability to convey the numerical aspects of the information accurately is crucial. However, there are significant barriers to effective communication of quantitative information. The level of numerical literacy ("numeracy") in the general population is low (129). Even the understanding of the most elementary ideas of probability cannot be taken for granted. In 1 study, only half of the respondents were able to predict the results of tossing a fair coin 1,000 times. The same study found that only 16% of respondents correctly answered all 3 of a set of basic numerical questions (130). These findings have been reproduced in other studies (131).

People had the most difficulty with concepts such as relative risk (132), odds, rates (where the numerator is fixed at 1 and the denominator varies) (133), and proportions where the denominator was anything other than 10 or a 100. One common problem is that people often pay attention only to the numbers and not the form they are in. That is, they believe that the expression with the highest number must represent the highest probability, regardless of whether it is expressed as a rate, proportion, percentage, and so forth. In 1 study, subjects rated a health problem as riskier when told that it affects 1,286 out of 10,000 people compared to 1 that affects 24.14 out of 100 people (134). Other times, it is not clear why people are having difficulty. For instance, in another study, half the respondents believed that 2.6/1,000 was a larger number than 8.9/1,000 (132). Converting between proportions and percentages was particularly difficult (130,135). In summary, there is a significant chance for confusion when the likelihood of outcomes is communicated by concepts such as rates, proportions, and so forth.

However, the most common way of communicating prognostic information, both in studies and in clinical practice, is through the uses of percentages (e.g., "there is a 70% chance he will be able to go back to work"). Yet the comprehension of even such a seemingly straightforward concept as percentages cannot be taken for granted. One study that assessed the understanding of the phrase "there is a 30% chance it will rain tomorrow" found that two thirds of the subjects misinterpreted the statement (for instance, believing it meant that it will rain just 30% of the day or in 30% of the area) (136). The problem here has less to do with numbers and more with an understanding of the referent class—what the percentage is about (e.g., believing that it refers to a por-

tion of the day or the geographic area instead of the likelihood of any rainfall). Even when it seems clear to professionals what the referent class should be, patients can be confused. In 1 study where patients were told "your risk of developing breast cancer is 10%", 1 subject asked "10% of what?" (137). Besides confusion about the referent class, there are other logical or conceptual difficulties that people can have with percentages. For example, a study found that some people thought the risk of developing and dying of breast cancer was higher than the risk of simply developing breast cancer (138).

In addition to the conceptual issues, problems even arise with the numerical aspects of percentages. In looking at cumulative risks (which required addition), many subjects in 1 study ended up with totals greater than 100% (138). In another study of people who were "highly educated," 20% of the respondents were not able to state which represented the larger risk: 1%, 5%, or 10% (131). Thus, when communication about prognoses involves the use of percentages, it cannot be automatically assumed that patients or families understand this information.

The difficulty in understanding numerical information is further compounded by the quantified uncertainty associated with any prediction. That is, not only is the primary outcome itself expressed as a probability (e.g., "your son has a 70% chance of living independently . . .") but also this estimate itself is subject to uncertainty (". . . and we know this with 90% certainty"). Having to process 2 different levels of numerical uncertainty can overwhelm families and patients and, thus, ironically, end up disempowering decision making rather than enabling it (125). These expressions of uncertainty can also undermine confidence in the clinician (125) as discussed earlier.

In the end, the numbers themselves may not even be used in decision making. Several studies have found that people immediately code numbers they hear into qualitative or ordinal categories such as high, medium, or low probability or even simply "likely" or "not likely" (124,132,134). Moreover, there is evidence the categories people use were better predictors of their decision making than the actual numbers they were given (132,134). Others have found the form of the information (numerical vs qualitative) did not affect decision making (139). These findings raise the issue of whether professionals should be communicating numeric values to patients and their families in the first place, rather than using qualitative statements such as likely, unlikely, probable, and so forth.

In fact, studies have shown that about a third of people would prefer that information about the likelihood of future events be given in qualitative terms rather than numerically (140,141). The problem with qualitative information, however, is that there is a wide variation in the interpretation of the terms, both among patients as well as professionals. One study found that the range of values patients associated with the word "frequent" was 30%–90% (140). A report on the understanding of these terms by professionals finds that, for example, the range of values associated with the term "unlikely" was 0.05%–90.00% (142). A study that compared the understanding of clinicians and patients found that they differed by an order of magnitude in the numerical associations they made to the same qualitative terms (143). These findings suggest that any use of descriptive terms would need to be supplemented by numeric information, even for those patients who prefer that information be presented qualitatively.

In addition to numeric and qualitative *verbal* communication, there is evidence that graphic displays may also aid in communicating numeric information (144). However, very few studies have directly examined which format might be the most effective. One study that did investigate this question found that a row of 10 human stick figures (shaded and unshaded to represent the percentages involved) was the most easily understood graphic and preferred by most of the subjects (137). This is an area needing further study.

So far, the discussion has focused on how the quantitative content of information is presented, whether descriptively, numerically, graphically, and so forth. Yet, nonquantitative aspects of the message can also affect a person's perception of how likely an event is to occur. For example, one could state that a patient has a 10% chance of having a good outcome or a 90% chance of having a poor outcome. Almost universally, people perceived a good outcome as being more likely when presented with the "positive" statement ("10% chance of good outcome") than when presented with the "negative" statement, despite both being numerically equivalent. These findings are the result of "framing" effects, the most widely studied of which has been the "positive/negative" or "loss/gain" frame, as in the example earlier. A recent review found that, although framing effects did exist, their effect on patients' understanding was much less than that of the "innumeracy" described earlier (145). Still, the existence of framing effects has implications for how prognostic information might be communicated in TBI, as will be seen subsequently.

Although the discussion so far has primarily been about patients and families, it should be pointed out that professionals, especially physicians, often have the same problems in handling quantitative information. Studies have found that physicians are subject to positive or negative framing effects in their treatment decisions: when the same numeric data were presented in a positive frame, physicians were more likely to undertake the treatment (146). Other studies have demonstrated that the way in which the results of clinical trials are reported will affect physician prescribing practices, even when the results themselves are identical (146). For instance, physicians are more likely to prescribe medications if efficacy is presented as a relative risk reduction instead of an absolute risk reduction (147,148). Regarding the qualitative use of probability terms, there is just as much variability in physicians' understanding of these terms as is found with laypeople (142). Finally, there is widespread acknowledgement of the difficulties most physicians have in understanding other statistical concepts, including concepts used routinely in journal articles and even clinical practice (149,150).

Practical Suggestions for Presenting Statistical Information

Given the significant barriers to the communication and comprehension of numeric information, what is the best way for a professional to proceed? One solution would be to minimize the occasions in which this information would need to be presented. Clinicians could avoid these discussions during those periods of the recovery process when there are a wide range of possible outcomes. Because each of these outcomes will be associated with a different likelihood of occurring, a discussion would involve the presentation of many different probabilities, further compounding the difficulties patients and families have with quantitative information. One of the advantages of threshold values is that they minimize the cognitive demands on comprehension. To tell a family that it is extremely unlikely the patient will be severely disabled or, alternatively, that it is now extremely unlikely they will have a good recovery is comprehensible and requires minimal numeric abilities to understand. During periods before these milestones are reached, clinicians could avoid discussing the probabilities of particular outcomes and rely on more general statements such as "all we can say at this point is that there is a chance that she will be able to return to work; we will know more later as further information becomes available."

Some families, however, will request detailed information even before milestones are reached. Or, even after a threshold has been crossed, they are interested in the likelihood of a moderate disability on the one hand and either a severe disability or good recovery on the other. In these cases, there are some general principles that a TBI professional can follow to maximize the chances of comprehension (Figure 18-9). The first suggestion addresses the issue of what form the numeric information should be communicated in. As mentioned earlier, most people have significant difficulties with odds, rates, risks (especially relative risks), and so forth. Even percentages can be confusing for many people (138). The form of communicating numeric information that seems least susceptible to misunderstanding is the use of natural frequencies (136,137,150). In essence, a natural frequency describes the number of people out of an easily comprehensible set (e.g., 10 or 100) that have the outcome of interest. For instance, rather than stating "there is an 80% chance your son will have a good recovery in a year," one would say "out of 10 people like your son, 8 of them will have a good recovery in a year" (136,137,150).

As professionals, we are so used to converting 1 expression into another that we may no longer perceive the differences between these 2 formulations. There are, however, 2 important differences between using natural frequencies and using percentages. First, from a numeric point of view, people have more difficulty with percentages than they do with proportions (as long as the denominator is either 10 or 100 and is kept constant). This is not the only issue, however. To see why, compare the 2 expressions: "Your son has an 8 out of 10 chance of having a good recovery" and, "Out of 10 people like your son, 8 of them will have a good recovery." Even though both formulations use proportions, people have much less difficulty with the second formulation. This is because the second formulation specifies the referent class. By making it explicit that one is talking about people, the ambiguity that might result in questions such as "80% of what?" can be avoided. It is also relevant that the referent class refers to persons instead of outcome categories. There is increasing evidence from cognitive psychology that people are better able to handle computations if they involve persons rather than abstract concepts (136,150). This was also seen when physicians were asked to solve questions of probability involving diagnostic testing (150).

Another suggestion to improve the communication of quantitative information would be to present the information through different routes; not just numerically, as just discussed, but also qualitatively and visually. Because most studies show that people are equally divided in how they wish to receive information, it would make sense to rely on more than 1 modality. And the fact that people might have difficulty even in their preferred modality justifies presenting the information in at least 2 different ways. So, in the example cited, after the information was presented numerically, one might say, "This is a very good chance for a good recovery."

In addition, given the known effects of framing on the perception of information, one can consider framing the information both positively and negatively. One might say, "This means that 2 out of 10 people in his situation will not have a good recovery." Although framing information both positively and negatively might ensure better understanding of the actual likelihood, it could be argued that clinicians should rely mainly on positive framing so as to maximize hope (see in the following texts). Finally, as with any other medical interaction, it is helpful to ask the patient or family members to state, in their own words, their understanding of the information.

Fostering Hope

The recommendation to foster hope may seem out of place in a discussion of *techniques* for communicating prognostic information. However, hope is an important part of this process. Of course, hope is most relevant when there is uncertainty. When the eventual outcome is fairly clear (e.g., PTA duration of several days), hope is less relevant precisely because of the certainty of the outcome. In contrast, when the outcome is uncertain (and an undesired outcome is possible), hope becomes correspondingly more important. Fostering hope has many advantages. For one, it may help patients and families to mobilize their energies and resources to engage fully in rehabilitation. In addition, when the prognosis is likely to be poor, even a little hope may "cushion the landing" and allow family members more time to process and come to terms with the probability of a poor outcome. Finally, based on clinical experience, most families seem far more upset with clinicians who offered them little or no hope when the outcome turned out well than those who offered some hope when the outcome was poor.

Of course, there are risks to offering hope, most notably the fear it might prevent family members from adequately preparing for a poorer outcome than they expect. However, the standard advice to families to "hope for the best but plan for the worst" (151) should allow most families to prepare for an undesired outcome without losing hope. When the concern about lack of adequate preparation persists, the clinician can always engage the family in another conversation, trying to shift their perspective. Overall, it appears that the benefits of offering hope in prognosis outweigh the risks (at least in most situations).

It was the commitment to fostering hope that was partly responsible for the emphasis on threshold values in this chapter. For instance, the interest in the longest period of PTA before one can reasonably exclude the possibility of a good recovery was motivated by the wish to preserve justified hope as long as possible. Likewise, being able to tell family members that the chances of severe disability were unlikely if a patient emerged from PTA within a particular time frame helps to allay fears about the possibility of an especially "bad" outcome. The disadvantage of threshold values is that one has to wait until the milestones are reached before one can provide families with more precise information. One way to minimize the frustration of families during the period before a threshold value is crossed is to describe concretely what the potential outcomes are. This is much more helpful and reassuring than saying "we'll just have to wait and see what happens." Knowing what the outcomes might be gives families some sense of control (if only cognitive), while preserving hope for a favorable outcome.

Another way in which to convey hope involves framing the information in a positive way by presenting the likelihood of the favorable outcome rather than the unfavorable outcome (e.g., by saying "he has an 80% chance of a good outcome" instead of "he has a 20% chance of a poor outcome"). One could also accentuate the positive aspects of less favorable outcomes. For instance, one could point out that someone with a severe disability may still be independent in mobility and self-care. Or that there is not a strong correlation between disability category and quality of life. Or that people with TBI are usually fairly healthy. In addition, emphasizing that improvement continues beyond the first year (the end point for many of the studies discussed) is another way of providing encouragement. Even the uncertainty in the prognosis can help to foster hope; by carefully highlighting this uncertainty, one can salvage a little hope even when the prognosis is particularly poor. One could even provide a rough numerical estimation of this uncertainty based on the CIs discussed earlier (e.g., "Although it is possible that up to 5% of people in his condition could have a good recovery, it is extremely unlikely"). Finally, it is important to reassure the family they will not be abandoned and that the clinician will be available to them during the long period of recovery (if true).

Optimizing the Process

There have been several good reviews on improving the process by which this information is communicated, especially in the case of "bad news" (116–118). Some of these guidelines are summarized in Figure 18-10 and are self-explanatory.

CONCLUSION

Predictions are difficult, especially about the future.—Yogi Berra

The results of this review, as well as other recent reviews of prognostication after TBI (29–33), demonstrate that it *is* possible to prognosticate after TBI, often with a very reasonable degree of accuracy. Unfortunately, it is possible that many clinicians may not be aware of this information, given data that suggests that most physicians do not feel that they assess prognosis accurately (6). The situation might be improved if a professional organization became involved in the dissemination of this information. The process could begin with the assembly of a task force that could review the literature in order to see if they could replicate the results of this chapter. Having a group of individuals involved, rather than just 2 authors, might improve the quality of the criteria used, the scope of the literature search, as well as the classification of the studies. In addition, a larger group could expand the grading system that is used to include different levels of strength of evidence (as is common in most evidence-based reviews). Such a task force could also follow other suggestions that have recently been made about how to improve the quality of systematic reviews of studies on prognosis (152).

In addition to reviewing already existing studies, it is important that more studies be conducted in an attempt to confirm the findings of this review. However, these studies should be designed so as to build on the strengths of the current literature and to compensate for its weaknesses (in scope or design). This is crucial given how few studies formed the basis of the recommendations presented here. Most generally, it would be important for future studies to incorporate the concept of threshold values to maximize their clinical utility. Recently, there has been a promising trend toward incorporating the concept of threshold values in the design of studies on prognosis (85,95). It would also be important that studies focus on those variables that have already shown promise as being clinically useful (e.g., duration of coma or PTA) rather than those that are clearly not powerful enough to aid in clinical prognostication (such as initial GCS or CT imaging).

In addition to selecting appropriate variables, it would be important for future studies to address shortcomings in the outcome measures used previously as well as to study more relevant populations. Regarding outcome measures, given the clear limitations of the GOS, the use of supplementary outcome measures should be considered (153). The duration of follow-up should be longer as well, given what is now known about the possibility of clinically meaningful recovery that can occur a year or more after an injury (154). In terms of setting, more studies are needed that are based in inpatient rehabilitation (thus circumventing the problems that arise when attempting to extrapolate from the acute care setting to patients in rehabilitation).

Finally, it is important that studies be conducted that attempt to identify what types of prognostic information patients and families want. There have been very few studies that have explicitly addressed this issue (see the discussion in Appendix II). Yet, because prognostication is ultimately a *clinical* act (one directed at and meant to benefit patients and families), it is crucial that future studies on prognostication (as opposed to studies on outcomes more generally) be designed around the explicit needs of patients and their families. More generic guidelines on improving the quality of prognostic research are also available (155).

Another line of research involves the examination of the ability of newer technologies to improve our ability to prognosticate after TBI. These modalities include magnetic resonance spectroscopy (MRS), diffusion tensor imaging (DTI), serum biomarkers (e.g., S100B), and electrophysiological measures, amongst others (156). Although promising, these tests are still not routinely available to most clinicians. Therefore, in this chapter we have chosen to restrict ourselves to "classical" predictors of outcome after TBI. This was motivated by the wish to focus on variables that are easily accessible to rehabilitation professionals. In addition, there is a much larger body of literature available for these variables than for more recently discovered prognostic

factors. Still, rehabilitationists should be aware of these recent developments as they are likely to affect clinical practice over the next several years.

APPENDIX I: EVALUATING AN ARTICLE ON PROGNOSIS

This section discusses some general guidelines that readers can use when evaluating individual studies on prognosis; these are summarized in Figure 18-11. Interested readers are referred to more detailed discussions of these issues (157–165). In general, 3 main principles guide the critical evaluation of an article on prognosis: the *quality* of the study, its *relevance* to one's own practice, and the *utility* of the findings. A study can be methodologically sound but inapplicable to one's practice, for instance if the study population is not similar to one's own. Or the reverse can happen: the study is relevant to one's practice but, because of problems in design, one cannot rely on the study's results. Finally, a relevant and methodologically sound study may still not be helpful because the results are reported in a way that makes it difficult to apply to clinical practice.

These principles of quality, relevance, and utility guide the questions that one should ask about the various compo-

Outcomes
- Is the outcome clinically important?
- Is the outcome measure validated?
- Is the outcome measure described well enough that it can be easily applied?
- Did an appropriate amount of time elapse before the outcome was measured?

Predictor Variables
- Are the predictor variables described well enough that they can be easily applied?
- Are the predictor variables easily accessible?
- Do the predictor variables have high reliability?

Sample
- Is the population described well enough to determine if they are similar in relevant aspects to your own (including the site)?
- Was there any bias in the selection of subjects (for instance, an inception cohort vs a convenience sample)?
- Was the sample large enough?
- Was there minimal loss to follow-up?
- Were the characteristics of those who were lost to follow-up compared to those who completed the study?

Results
- Were the findings reported in a form that is useful for clinicians (e.g., absolute risk)?
- Was the precision of the estimates provided (e.g., confidence intervals)?
- Was there an evaluation of validity (replication of findings in same sample)?
- Have the findings been confirmed in other studies (reproducibility)?
- Are the findings believable on biological grounds?
- Do the findings represent an advance over already available prognostic tools?

FIGURE 18–11 Guidelines for reading an article on prognosis.

nents of the study: outcomes, predictors, sample, and results (Figure 18-11). It is also important to assess the statistical analysis performed, although this issue is only briefly addressed here. Many of the criteria listed in Figure 18-11 will be familiar: they are identical to the inclusion criteria for this review. The second appendix provides a detailed review of these criteria; therefore, they will not be discussed here. Rather, the focus will be on the new criteria listed. The following discussion is organized according to the topics mentioned earlier (outcomes, predictors, sample, results).

Outcomes

The outcomes must be of clinical relevance, one that would matter either to the clinician, the patient, or their family. Whatever outcome measure is used, it should be well described so clinicians can apply it to their own patients. The outcome should also be easy to measure in clinical practice. It should also be a measure that has either already been validated or, at least, has had some assessment of validity performed in the study itself. Finally, the outcome should be measured at an appropriate time (at least 6 months after a TBI).

Predictors

Many of the same criteria apply to the study's choice of predictor variables: they should be well described, have high reliability, and be easily accessible or easily performed by the clinician.

Sample

The sample should also be well-described, so readers can decide if the subjects are similar to their own patients. In assessing this, it is also important to keep in mind the nature of the treatments received by the study population and whether one's own patients receive similar treatments. The study should be prospective, utilizing an inception cohort, rather than retrospective (e.g., a case-control design). The sample size should also be adequate. The size of the sample not only affects the precision of the estimates (e.g., the width of the CIs) but also ensures the sample obtained is representative of the population. In addition, many of the statistical analyses performed require a sample of a certain size for the results to be valid (e.g., for multivariate analyses).

There should also be minimal loss to follow-up. Although most authors recommend the loss to follow-up should be no greater than 15%–20%, the real issue is the number of people lost to follow-up relative to the number of people with the outcome of interest. One way of evaluating this would be to examine what would happen if everyone lost to follow-up ended up in each of the outcome categories. For instance, a 15% loss to follow-up in which the outcome categories were equally likely (e.g., 50% "good" and 50% "bad") would not affect the results significantly. Even if you assume that all of those lost to follow-up either had a good outcome or a bad outcome, the percentages would shift only slightly (e.g., to 57% and 43% in either direction), not enough to affect prognostication. On the other hand, in a study in

which no one achieved a certain outcome (e.g., severe disability), a 15% loss to follow-up would be significant if all 15% were severely disabled. Finally, it would be ideal if the characteristics of those lost to follow-up were compared with those who remained in the study.

Results

The results have to be reported in a way that is clinically useful, so they can be used to formulate a prognosis for individual patients. In general, absolute risks or simple percentages are more useful than measures such as relative risk, likelihood ratios, odds, and so forth. There should also be some report of the precision of the estimate provided (e.g., the width of the CI). Ideally, there should also be some assessment of the model's validity: both by replication of the findings in the original sample as well as, more importantly, replication at other sites. Although this assessment of validity represents the ideal, it is rarely met in studies of TBI. An exception that illustrates the importance of replication was a study done in the acute care setting (166). This study applied a previously published model (167) to their own patient population. Although the model was reported to be 100% accurate in the original study, the second study found it to be only about 65% accurate in their patient population.

Finally, the results of the study should be interpreted in the larger context of the available literature. Do the findings make sense based on what is known of the pathophysiology and natural history of TBI? Have other studies confirmed the findings? Do the findings provide for more accurate prognoses than is already possible?

APPENDIX II: METHODOLOGY

Methods

Extensive literature searches (based on the inclusion criteria described subsequently) were performed on Medline, PsycINFO, and the personal database of a colleague of the author (which has more than 20,000 TBI specific articles); the search covered the period from 1983 to 2011. Over a thousand articles were retrieved and their bibliographies then reviewed for further references. All the articles were then reviewed to determine whether they met the inclusion criteria. The inclusion criteria were developed after extensive discussions with various professionals (including, for instance, neurosurgeons and biostatisticians), as well as family members and survivors. The general principles that guided the selection of the inclusion criteria are presented in Figure 18-4. The inclusion criteria themselves are listed in Figure 18-5. The sections that follow explain the rationale for the criteria chosen.

Population

Severe TBI

Because patients with severe TBI make up most of those admitted to inpatient rehabilitation, this chapter focuses on severe TBI and devotes little space to moderate TBI. This seems appropriate given the generally good outcomes in patients with moderate TBI (12) as well as the fact that patients with severe injuries are the ones for whom prognostication is often the most difficult. Studies on civilian penetrating brain injury were evaluated separately from those on closed brain injury, given the substantial differences between these 2 populations.

Subacute Period After TBI
(Acute Care and Rehabilitation)

The focus of this chapter is on prognostication during the subacute period, which was defined as the period from the initial stabilization of the patient after the injury (usually in the first week) to approximately 3 months after the injury. It was felt that this period was of most concern to rehabilitation clinicians working with TBI. Certainly, there are other periods in which the question of prognosis is relevant. Most obviously, there is a great deal of concern about prognosis in the acute setting, early after a TBI. Similarly, survivors and family members often continue to have questions about "final" recovery many months or even years after a brain injury, during the chronic phase.

In this chapter, however, the focus is on prognostication during the time that lies between these 2 periods. There are various reasons for this focus. For one, the literature on prognostication is enormous, and it would be impossible to survey all of it in a single chapter. Besides, at least regarding prognostication in the acute stage, there has already been a comprehensive evidence-based review (168). In addition, the focus in the immediate aftermath of a TBI is mostly on mortality rather than on broader outcomes. Rehabilitation professionals are less likely to be involved during the period immediately after the injury, although they often play a more important role after the patient is stabilized. Although rehabilitationists are the primary clinicians during the chronic phase (after approximately 6–12 months), the questions that arise during this period are often easier to answer because much more information is available by then.

In contrast, there is relatively little information during the subacute period, which is 1 reason why prognostication is so difficult then. At the same time, the need for prognostic information is greatest during this period. Families have often been so focused on issues of survival during the acute care stage that they are just beginning to think about the long-term implications of the injury. This is especially true after patients are admitted to inpatient rehabilitation. In many ways, then, this period represents a pivotal point after a TBI and providing information about outcomes is 1 of the clinician's most important obligations during this time (2).

The question then arose as to whether to limit the review to only those studies done in the inpatient rehabilitation setting or to also include studies done in acute care. The populations are clearly different. The primary issue is that only a subset of all patients with TBI admitted to acute care eventually goes to inpatient rehabilitation. Many patients die in the acute care setting. Of those patients that survive, some have improved to the point that they do not require inpatient rehabilitation and can be discharged with outpatient services. At the other end of the spectrum, many survivors of TBI have not made enough neurological progress to meet the criteria for admission to inpatient rehabilitation and are therefore often discharged to long-term care facilities or home. Thus, there is a concern that the acute care population would not necessarily be representative of patients seen in rehabilitation.

Despite these concerns, studies done in the acute care setting were included in this review. Because both acute care and inpatient rehabilitation usually occur during the subacute time period, it was felt that studies from both settings were needed to adequately represent this phase. Also, rehabilitation professionals often first encounter patients in the acute care setting and are often asked by other clinicians or family members about long-term prognosis early after a TBI. Additionally, despite differences between the 2 populations, the variables affecting prognosis seem to be similar; in fact, there were no appreciable differences in the findings of the studies done in the 2 settings.

The most important reason for including the acute care studies, however, is that there were only 10 studies conducted in the inpatient rehabilitation setting that met the inclusion criteria. Given the limited number of well-designed rehabilitation studies, the choice was either to include acute care studies or to liberalize the inclusion criteria so more studies based in rehabilitation could be included. It was decided that well designed studies of prognosis from the acute care setting would be more useful than methodologically weaker studies based in the rehabilitation setting.

Studies Published After 1983

Beginning in the early 1980s, changes in prehospital, neurosurgical, and ICU care have resulted in a steady decline in mortality from TBI (169–171). Whether functional outcome has also improved is less clear. There has been some concern that although mortality has declined, the survivors are disproportionately severely disabled. Recent reports don't support these fears, however, and it now appears that functional outcomes have improved along with survival (172,173). Because of these changes in care, it was decided to exclude studies published before 1984, under the assumption that the care patients received before that time differed from current care in ways that directly impact outcome. Specifically, it is assumed that studies done before the early 1980s would underestimate survival and function. Although acute medical and surgical care continued to improve after the early 1980s, most of these changes have been relatively minor compared with those of 20 years ago. The primary changes over the past 15 years have been the adoption of the new standards by an increasing number of nonacademic centers (170,173).

Setting: North America/Western Europe/
Australia/New Zealand/Israel

Although there is some documented variation in TBI care *within* the United States (as well as between the United States and Europe) (174), care in the countries listed earlier was similar enough to justify grouping them together (175). Even though care in the excluded countries may be similar to that in the countries above, there is no evidence to support this. Because variations in care are likely to affect outcomes, studies originating in countries other than those listed were excluded.

Age: Adult

Because pediatric TBI is discussed elsewhere, the studies included in this review focused exclusively or predominately on *adult* TBI. Also, because age is such a powerful predictor of outcome, also included were studies on the elderly.

Subpopulations

In general, studies that included a wide range of patients were preferred because this would most closely resemble the typical patient population seen by most rehabilitation clinicians. In addition, beyond a certain point, it becomes difficult for clinicians to use a different set of guidelines for minor variations in preinjury, injury, or postinjury factors. Some groups are so distinctive, however, that studies that focused exclusively on them were included. The most notable examples in this review were the studies on the elderly and those with civilian penetrating injuries. A few studies that focused on other subsets of the TBI population were included only if that subset made conceptual sense and was easily identifiable by a rehabilitation professional. For instance, included were studies that limited themselves to patients who regained consciousness in acute care as well as one that focused on patients with TBI who did not sustain other injuries. However, studies that focused only on those patients with, for example, traumatic SAH or a history of elevated intracranial pressure, were excluded under the assumption that this information was often not readily available and did not reflect conceptual categories that rehabilitation professionals routinely use.

Predictor Variables

The review is limited to the following predictor variables: age, initial GCS, LOC, duration of PTA, and early neuroimaging (CT and MRI). There are several reasons for focusing exclusively on these predictors. First, these variables are among the most powerful predictors of outcome available. More importantly, they represent pieces of information that are either easily available to most rehabilitation clinicians (e.g., age, initial GCS, etc.) or can be prospectively determined in the rehabilitation setting (e.g., duration of PTA). Although there are other variables that can also have a significant impact on outcome (e.g., pupillary abnormalities, hypoxia, premorbid functioning, etc.), this information is often not readily available (for instance, because of the limited availability of medical records). Thus, studies that rely on utilizing this information may not be particularly useful for rehabilitation clinicians providing subacute prognostication.

Only those studies that used the *total* GCS score were included. Although there are compelling reasons for the use of just the motor score in prognostication (176), rehabilitation clinicians do not often have access to a patient's GCS subscores. There were also many studies that combined the variables selected for this review with other variables to create a single predictive model (for instance: age, pupillary abnormalities, and GCS motor response). Although the clinical utility of these models is dependent on the *combination* of

variables (some of which are not readily available to the rehabilitation clinician), the studies making use of these models were included because they provided evidence that the variable of interest (e.g., age in the example earlier) was, after a multivariate analysis, associated with outcome.

Although neuropsychological testing during inpatient rehabilitation was originally included as a predictor of interest, none of the studies on early neuropsychological testing met the methodological criteria. Although not discussed as part of the evidence-based review, the studies that have been done are briefly reviewed in the body of the chapter.

Outcomes

Outcome Measures

One of the central issues in prognostication is to be clear about the outcome of interest. There are many outcome measures available: survival, physical impairment, ability to perform activities of daily living, cognitive and behavioral status, return to work, independent living, quality of life, and so forth (177,178). The outcome one chooses depends on the question(s) one is asking and whether these questions are being asked for research or clinical purposes. In particular, the interests of professionals (especially researchers) and families do not always coincide. For instance, there is evidence that the outcomes of most interest to family members, at least during the rehabilitation phase, have to do with broad conceptual categories such as independent living and return to work (179,180). Besides the intrinsic importance of these categories, there is a symbolic importance associated with them (181). That is, given the importance our culture places on employment and independent living, these roles come to symbolize our membership in the community at large. Even the concern with other outcomes (e.g., physical impairment, cognitive decline, etc.) is interpreted mainly by their impact on these more holistic functional categories (179,180).

Unfortunately, most studies do not use measures of these types of outcomes for several different reasons. First, these outcomes are so broad that they can include a wide range of patients within a single category. For instance, the category of severe disability in the GOS would include both a minimally conscious patient as well as someone independent in basic activities of daily living who is unable to live alone because of cognitive deficits (182). These measures are also insensitive to changes that can occur beyond the first 6 months to a year, making them less useful in studying the long-term natural history of TBI (178,183). Third, the psychometric properties of these global outcome measures often are not as good as those of more fine-grained research measures. For example, there are concerns about interobserver agreement in the clinical use of the GOS (17). Another concern with the GOS is the fact that what is documented is the rater's subjective impression of a person's abilities rather than actual outcome. For instance, the measure documents the rater's beliefs about a person's ability to work rather than actual employment (which may account for the finding that ratings on the GOS may not be as strongly correlated with measures of employment as one would expect) (177).

The broadness of categories such as return to work or independent living can obscure the underlying mechanisms that mediate the outcome. Although this is sometimes seen as an advantage of these measures (so that they "integrate" the effect of many deficits into a final outcome such as work) (184), this characteristic can also lead to the loss of valuable information. For instance, is the person unable to live independently because of executive dysfunction, impulsivity, or physical impairment? Or because of factors that have nothing to do with the brain injury (e.g., other disabling physical conditions, financial resources, family support, etc.) (27)? By collapsing these distinctions, the use of these outcome measures can obscure the underlying deficits that actually prevent people from living independently or returning to work.

There is also evidence that, at least early on, both patients and family members overestimate the contribution of certain outcomes to eventual quality of life (such as independent living) and underestimate the importance of others (such as social relationships). During the chronic phase of TBI, most studies show that emotional and behavioral issues are far more important to family members than, for instance, residence or occupational status (180,185–187). Even for patients, there is evidence the GOS categories do not correlate well with their own ratings of their quality of life (128). The broad categories of return to work, independent living, or the GOS are simply not designed to identify sequelae such as quality of life, social relationships, behavioral disturbances, and so forth.

However, although they will likely change their minds later, the fact remains that it is still these broad categories of functional outcome that families and patients are concerned with during the subacute period. To prognosticate about outcomes that are not yet relevant to them can lead to dissatisfaction and the perception that their needs for information are not being met. And because prognosis is ultimately a clinical act that tries to address the *current* needs of families and patients, their preferences have to be considered. For this reason, this review was limited to those studies that focused on return to work or independent living, either directly or through the GOS.

Despite its other limitations, the GOS actually seems to be one of the most useful measures of these sorts of outcomes. This is because the GOS utilizes outcome categories that correspond to those used by lay people, making results expressed in terms of its categories useful to clinicians. For instance, in discussing that their loved one will likely be "moderately disabled" in a year, the clinician can explain that the patient will likely be able to live independently but will have residual deficits precluding their being able to return to competitive employment. This outcome is understandable to family members because they, too, think in terms of independent living or employment.

In this respect, the GOS contrasts to measures such as the Disability Rating Scale (DRS) that either report a numerical score that has no real meaning to a layperson or is divided into categories (e.g., partial disability, moderately severe disability, etc.) that also have no clear conceptual correlates. Although it is true that information about living situation and employment can be extracted from the DRS, the data needed to do so is rarely reported in the literature (it is usually only the total score that is reported). The relatively clear meaning of the GOS categories is also an advantage relative to the results of neuropsychological testing. For most family members, a decline on a neuropsychological test is of little relevance except as it has an impact on "real-world" outcomes such as independent living.

Despite its advantages in addressing the needs of patients and families, there are still the many methodological limitations of the GOS mentioned earlier. There are newer measures that retain many of the advantages of the GOS while avoiding some of its limitations (e.g., the Community Integration Questionnaire). Unfortunately, there were no studies using these measures that also met all the other inclusion criteria. This fact reflects 1 of the primary reasons for the use of the GOS in this review. Because it is the most widely used measure in the TBI outcomes literature, including the GOS as an outcome measure significantly expanded the number of studies that could be included in this review. In fact, to exclude studies that used the GOS would have limited this review to less than a handful of studies (that met all the other criteria listed).

Outcome Measured at 6 Months or Later

For several reasons, this review is limited to studies that assess outcome no earlier than 6 months after injury. Waiting *at least* 6 months is uncontroversial given the well-known clinical observation that, for most individuals, significant improvement occurs during the first 6 months after an injury. It could be argued, however, that because recovery clearly continues after 6 months, it would be better to wait a longer period of time, for instance, at least a year. Indeed, there is growing evidence that some individuals can continue to have meaningful recovery even many years after their injury (188–190). Nonetheless, there are compelling reasons to include studies that assess outcome as early as 6 months. First, studies have shown that, despite continued improvement, it was rare for an individual's GOS category to improve after 6 months (191). More practically, if only studies that assessed outcome beyond 6 months were included, well over half of the studies would have been excluded, further limiting what is already a small evidence base.

Methodological Criteria

The methodological criteria adopted are, for the most part, self-explanatory. The review is limited to studies with consecutive admissions (or a random sample of consecutive admissions) to minimize the possibility of systemic bias (which might arise from sampling based on any other criteria). Likewise, the requirement of at least 80% follow-up minimizes the biases that might be encountered with high rates of dropout. Historically, TBI outcome studies have been characterized by high rates of loss to follow-up (one-third to one-half of the original sample); the implications of this for the validity of studies on outcome have been recently reviewed (192). Studies are only now beginning to analyze the characteristics of those lost to follow-up to see if they differed substantially from those who were included. Therefore, in the interest of having more than 1–2 studies to review, it was decided that an analysis of patients lost to follow-up would not be required of studies to be included.

The criterion specifying a minimum sample size was adopted from the American Association of Neurological Surgeons (AANS) acute care prognostication review (168). Finally, the studies were reviewed to ensure that some form of statistical analysis was performed on the data of interest. If not, the study was still included if enough information was provided for the statistical analysis to be done by a knowledgeable reader. This was an issue for some of the older studies, where the distribution of outcomes was occasionally reported only in a descriptive manner. However, there was no attempt to screen studies based on the statistical models employed. The most commonly utilized models in this area are regression models and decision trees. The features and limitations of these approaches are detailed elsewhere (193–200).

There are some potential criteria not used in this review, either because they were not applicable or because they would have greatly limited the number of studies available. Most notably, a study was included even if it did not adjust for confounding factors (because so few did so). However, those studies that performed a univariate vs a multivariate analysis (or something else to adjust for confounding factors) are noted in the tables. More importantly, the fact that the studies that did not adjust for confounds came to the same conclusions as those that did increases the confidence in the findings of the review.

Threshold Values and Confidence Intervals

It cannot be automatically inferred that a particular outcome is impossible, just because no one over or under a particular threshold value had the outcome of interest in a particular study. This is because there is always a degree of statistical uncertainty, even when the outcome of interest does not occur. For example, even if no one with a duration of PTA greater than 3 months had a good recovery in a particular study, it might still be *statistically* possible that a certain percentage of them could have achieved that outcome. This possibility can be quantified by CIs. In a study where no one had the outcome of interest, the lower end of the CI would be 0, whereas the upper end would represent the largest number of people who could statistically be expected to develop the outcome of interest. The width of this CI will depend on the sample size.

For instance, if no one out of a sample of 87 people achieved a good recovery on the GOS, the 95% CI would be approximately 0%–3%. That is, the findings are compatible (with 95% certainty) with up to 3% of that group achieving a good recovery. If, instead, no one out of a sample of only 17 people achieved a good recovery, the CI would be much wider (approximately 0%–16%). Therefore, the most that one can infer from the smaller study (with 95% certainty) is that anywhere from 0% to16% of similar people could have had the outcome of interest. It is also important to keep in mind that a study in which no one had a particular outcome is not necessarily stronger evidence for a threshold value than a study in which some subjects had the outcome. It all depends on the width of the CI. For instance, a study with a large sample (e.g., 150) that reported that 4% of subjects had a good recovery would actually have a smaller CI (1%–9%) than a study with a smaller sample (e.g., 27) in which no one achieved a good recovery (CI 0%–11%). Unfortunately, none of the studies that reported threshold values reported the associated CIs. Therefore, the author calculated the CIs for all the threshold values. However, only those threshold values with a 95% CI of no greater than 0%–12%are reported.

This figure represented a balance between the limits of tolerability of error and the wish to include as many studies as possible.

KEY CLINICAL POINTS

1. Lower **GCS** scores are associated with worse outcomes but there are no threshold values.
2. **Duration of Coma** is associated with worse outcomes
   - Severe disability is unlikely when less than 2 weeks
   - Good recovery is unlikely when greater than 4 weeks
3. **PTA** duration is associated with worse outcomes
   - Severe disability is unlikely when less than 2 months
   - Good recovery is unlikely when greater than 3 months
4. Older **age** is associated with worse outcomes
   - Good recovery is unlikely when older than 65 years old
5. Deeper lesions on **MRI** are associated with worse outcomes
   - Good recovery is unlikely when bilateral brainstem lesions are present on an early MRI

KEY REFERENCES

1. Cappa KA, Conger JC, Conger AJ. Injury severity and outcome: a meta-analysis of prospective studies on TBI outcome. *Health Psychol*. 2011;30(5):542–560.
2. Husson EC, Ribbers GM, Willemse-van Son AHP, Verhagen AP, Stam HJ. Prognosis of six-month functioning after moderate to severe traumatic brain injury: a systemic review of prospective cohort studies. *J Rehabil Med*. 2010; 42(5):425–436.
3. Kim Y. A Systematic review of factors contributing to outcomes in patients with traumatic brain injury. *J Clin Nurs*. 2011;20(11–12):1518–1532.
4. Nightingale EJ, Soo CA, Tate RL. A systematic review of early prognostic factors for return to work after traumatic brain injury. *Brain Impair*. 2006;8(2):101–142.
5. Wilmse-van Son AHP, Ribbers GM, Verhagen AP, Stam HJ. Prognostic factors of long-term functioning and productivity after traumatic brain injury: a systemic review of prospective cohort studies. *Clin Rehabil*. 2007;21(11): 1024–1037.

References

1. Consensus conference. Rehabilitation of persons with traumatic brain injury. NIH Consensus Development Panel on Rehabilitation of Persons With Traumatic Brain Injury. *JAMA*. 1999;282(10): 974–983.
2. Holland D, Shigaki CL. Educating families and caretakers of traumatically brain injured patients in the new health care environment: a three-phase model and bibliography. *Brain Inj*. 1998; 12(12)993–1009.
3. Junqué C, Bruna O, Mataró M. Information needs of the traumatic brain injury patient's family members regarding the consequences of the injury and associated perception of physical, cognitive, emotional, and quality of life changes. *Brain Inj*. 1997;11(4):251–258.
4. Christakis NA. *Death Foretold: Prophecy and Prognosis in Medical Care*. Chicago, IL: The University of Chicago Press; 1999.
5. Lefebvfre H, Levert MJ. Breaking the news of traumatic brain injury and incapacities. *Brain Inj*. 2006;20(7):711–718.

6. Perel P, Wasserberg J, Ravi RR, Shakur H, Edwards P, Roberts I. Prognosis following head injury: a survey of doctors from developing and developed countries. *J Eval Clin Pract*. 2007;13:464–465.

7. Dawes RM, Faust D, Meehl PE. Clinical versus actuarial judgment. *Science*. 1989;243(4899):1668–1674.

8. Knaus WA, Wagner DP, Lynn J. Short-term mortality predictions for critically ill hospitalized adults: science and ethics. *Science*. 1991; 254:389–393.

9. Perkins HS, Jonsen AR, Epstein WV. Providers as predictors: using outcome predictions in intensive care. *Crit Care Med*. 1986;14(2): 105–110.

10. Poses RM, Bekes C, Copare FJ, Scott WE. The answer to "What are my chances, doctor?" depends on who is asked: prognostic disagreement and inaccuracy for critically ill patients. *Crit Care Med*. 1989;17(8):827–833.

11. Chang RW, Lee B, Jacobs S, Lee B. Accuracy of decisions to withdraw therapy in critically ill patients: clinical judgment versus a computer model. *Crit Care Med*. 1989;17(11):1091–1097.

12. Van der Naalt J. Prediction of outcome in mild to moderate head injury: a review. *J Clin Exper Neuropsych*. 2001;23(6):837–851.

13. Sherer M, Madison CF, Hannay HJ. A review of outcome after moderate head injury with an introduction to life care planning. *J Head Trauma Rehabil*. 2000;15(2):767–782.

14. Levin HS. Prediction of recovery from traumatic brain injury. *J Neurotrauma*. 1995;12(5):913–922.

15. Macniven E. Factors affecting head injury rehabilitation outcome: premorbid and clinical parameters. In: Finlayson MA, Garner SH, eds. *Brain Injury Rehabilitation: Clinical Considerations*. Baltimore, MD: Williams & Wilkins; 1994:57–82.

16. Mack A, Lawrence JH. Functional prognosis in traumatic brain injury. *Phys Med & Rehab: State of the Art Reviews*. 1989;3(1):13–26.

17. Sandel ME, Labi MLC. Outcome prediction: clinical and research perspectives. *Phys Med & Rehab: State of the Art Reviews*. 1990;4(3): 409–420.

18. Jennett B. Assessment and prediction of outcome after head injury. In: Macfarlane R, Hardy DG, eds. *Outcome After Head, Neck and Spinal Trauma*. Oxford, NY: Butterworth-Heinemann; 1997:3–8.

19. Andrews BT. Prognosis in severe head injury. In: Cooper PR, Golfinos JG, eds. *Head Injury*. New York, NY: McGraw-Hill; 2000: 555–563.

20. Marion DW. Outcome from severe head injury. In: Narayan RK, Wilberger JE, Povlishock JT, eds. *Neurotrauma*. New York, NY: McGraw-Hill; 1996:767–777.

21. Stein SC. Outcome from moderate head injury. In: Narayan RK, Wilberger JE, Povlishock JT, eds. *Neurotrauma*. New York, NY: McGraw-Hill; 1996:755–765.

22. Zafonte RD, Hammond FM, Peterson J. Predicting outcome in the slow to respond traumatically brain-injured patient: acute and subacute parameters. *NeuroRehab*. 1996;6:19–32.

23. Crepeau F, Scherzer P. Predictors and indicators of work status after traumatic brain injury: a meta-analysis. *Neuropsych Rehab*. 1993;3(1):5–35.

24. Yasuda S, Wehman P, Targett P, Cifu D, West M. Return to work for persons with traumatic brain injury. *Am J Phys Med Rehabil*. 2001;80(11):852–864.

25. Goldstein FC, Levin HS. Cognitive outcome after mild and moderate traumatic brain injury in older adults. *J Clin Exper Neuropsych*. 2001;23(6):739–753.

26. Rapoport MJ, Feinstein A. outcome following traumatic brain injury in the elderly: a critical review. *Brain Inj*. 2000;14(8):749–761.

27. Wagner AK. Functional prognosis in traumatic brain injury. *Phys Med & Rehab: State of the Art Review*. 2001;15(2):245–267.

28. Shutter LA, Jallo JI, Narayan RK. Traumatic brain injury. In: Evans R, Baskin D, Yatsu F, eds. *Prognosis of Neurological Disorders*. 2nd ed. New York, NY: Oxford University Press; 2000;335–365.

29. Nightingale E, Soo C, Tate R. A systematic review of early prognostic factors for return to work after traumatic brain injury. *Brain Impair*. 2006;8(2):101–142.

30. Wilmse-van Son AHP, Ribbers GM, Verhagen AP, Stam HJ. Prognostic factors of long-term functioning and productivity after traumatic brain injury: a systemic review of prospective cohort studies. *Clin Rehab*. 2007;21:1024–1037.

31. Husson EC, Ribbers GM, Willemse-van Son AHP, Verhagen AP, Stam HJ. Prognosis of six-month functioning after moderate to severe traumatic brain injury: a systemic review of prospective cohort studies. *J Rehabil Med*. 2010;41:435–436.

32. Kim Y. A Systematic review of factors contributing to outcomes in patients with traumatic brain injury. *J Clin Nurs*. 2011;20: 1518–1532.

33. Cappa KA, Conger JC, Conger AJ. Injury severity and outcome: a meta-analysis of prospective studies on TBI outcome. *Health Psychol*. 2011;30(5):542–560.

34. Rao N, Rosenthal M, Cronin-Stubbs D, Lambert R, Barnes P, Swanson B. Return to work after rehabilitation following traumatic brain injury. *Brain Inj*. 1990;4(1):49–56.

35. Fearnside MR, Cook RJ, McDougall P, McNeil RJ. The Westmead Head Injury Project outcome in severe head injury. A comparative analysis of prehospital, clinical and CT variables. *Br J Neurosurgery*. 1993;7:267–279.

36. Kakarieka A, Braakman R, Schakel EH. Clinical significance of the finding of subarachnoid blood on CT scan after head injury. *Acta Neurochir*. 1994;129(1–2):1–5.

37. Walder AD, Yeoman PM, Turnbull A. The abbreviated injury scale as a predictor of outcome of severe head injury. *Intensive Care Med*. 1995;21(7):606–609.

38. Lobato RD, Gomez PA, Alday R, et al. Sequential computerized tomography changes and related final outcome in severe head injury patients. *Acta Neurochir* (Wien). 1997;139(5):385–391.

39. Wedekind C, Fischbach R, Pakos P, Terhaag D, Klug N. Comparative use of magnetic resonance imaging and electrophysiologic investigation for the prognosis of head injury. *J Trauma*. 1999;47(1): 44–49.

40. Gómez PA, Lobato RD, Boto GR, De la Lama A, González PJ, de la Cruz J. Age and outcome after severe head injury. *Acta Neurochair* (Wien). 2000;142(4):373–381.

41. Firsching R, Woischneck D, Klein S, et al. Classification of severe head injury based on magnetic resonance imaging. *Acta Neurochir*. 2001;143:263–271.

42. Schaan M, Jaksche H, Boszczyk B. Predictors of outcome in head injury: proposal of a new scaling system. *J Trauma*. 2002;52(4): 667–674.

43. Vos PE, Van Voskuilen AC, Beems T, et al. Evaluation of the traumatic coma data bank computed tomography classification for severe head injury. *J Neurotrauma*. 2001;18(7):649–655.

44. Mattioli C, Beretta L, Gerevini S, et al. Traumatic subarachnoid hemorrhage on the computerized tomography scan obtained at admission: a multicenter assessment of the accuracy of diagnosis and the potential impact on patient outcome. *J Neurosurg*. 2003;98: 37–42.

45. Rovlias A, Kotsou S. Classification and regression tree for prediction of outcome after severe head injury using simple clinical and laboratory variables. *J Neurotrauma*. 2004;21(7):886–893.

46. Hanlon RE, Demery JA, Kuczen C, et al. Effect of traumatic subarachnoid haemorrhage on neuropsychological profiles and vocational outcome following moderate or severe traumatic brain injury. *Brain Inj*. 2005;19(4):257–262.

47. Hukkelhoven CW, Steyerberg EW, Habbema JDF, et al. Predicting outcome after traumatic brain injury: development and validation of a prognostic score based on admission characteristics. *J Neurotrauma*. 2005;22(10):1025–1035.

48. Carpentier A, Galanaud D, Puybasset L, et al. Early morphologic and spectroscopic magnetic resonance in severe traumatic brain injuries can detect "invisible brain stem damage" and predict "vegetative states." *J Neurotrauma*. 2006;23(5):674–685.

49. Cremer OL, Moons KGM, van Dijk GW, van Balen P, Kalkman CJ. Prognosis following severe head injury: development and validation of a model for prediction of death, disability, and functional recovery. *J Trauma*. 2006;61(6):1484–1491.

50. Hiler G, Czosnyka M, Hutchingson P, et al. Predictive value of initial computerized tomography scan, intracranial pressure, and state of autoregulation in patients with traumatic brain injury. *Journal Neurosurg*. 2006;104:731–737.

51. Maas AIR, Steyerberg EW, Butcher I, et al. Prognostic value of computerized tomography scan characteristics in traumatic brain

injury: results from the IMPACT study. *J Neurotrauma*. 2007;24(2): 303–314.

52. Murray GD, Butcher I, McHuch GS, et al. Multivariable prognostic analysis in traumatic brain injury: results from the IMPACT study. *J Neurotrauma*. 2007;24(2):329–337.

53. Perel P, Arango M, Clayton T, et al. Predicting outcome after traumatic brain injury: practical prognostic models based on large cohort of international patients. *BMJ*. 2008;336:425–435.

54. Sidaros A, Engberg AW, Sidaros K, et al. Diffusion tensor imaging during recovery from severe traumatic brain injury and relation to clinical outcome: a longitudinal study. *Brain*. 2008;131:559–572.

55. Steyerberg EW, Mushkudiani N, Perel P, et al. Predicting outcome after traumatic brain injury: development and international validation of prognostic scores based on admission characteristics. *PLoS Med*. 2008;5(8):1251–1261.

56. Lagares A, Ramos A, Perez-Nunez A, et al. The role of MR imaging in assessing prognosis after severe and moderate head injury. *Acta Neurochir* (Wien). 2009;151(4):341–356.

57. Jacobs B, Beems T, van der Vliet TM, Borm GF, Vos PE. The status of the fourth ventricle and ambient cisterns predict outcome in moderate and severe traumatic brain injury. *J Neurotrauma*. 2010; 27:331–340.

58. Nelson DW, Nystron H, MacCallum RM, et al. Extended analysis of early computed tomography scans of traumatic brain injured patients and relations to outcome. *J Neurotrauma*. 2010;27:51–64.

59. Skandsen T, Kvistad KA, Solheim O, Haavde Strand I, Folvik M, Vik A. Prevalence and impact of diffuse axonal injury in patients with moderate and severe head injury: a cohort study of early magnetic resonance imaging findings and 1-year outcome. *J Neurosurg*. 2010;113:556–563.

60. Jacobs B, Beems T, van der Vliet TM, Diaz-Arrastia RR, Borm GF, Bos PE. Computed tomography and outcome in moderate and severe traumatic brain injury: hematoma volume and midline shift revisited. *J Neurotrauma*. 2011;28:203–215.

61. Skandsen T, Kvistad KA, Solheim O, Lydersen S, Haavde Strand I, Vik A. Prognostic value of magnetic resonance imaging in moderate and severe head injury: a prospective study of early MRI findings and one-year outcome. *J Neurotrauma*. 2011;28:691–699.

62. Yeoman P, Pattani H, Silcocks P, Owen V, Fuller G. Validation of the IMPACT outcome prediction score using the Nottingham head injury register dataset. *J Trauma*. 2011;71(2):387–392.

63. Formisano R, Voogt RD, Buzzi MG, et al. time interval of oral feeding recovery as a prognostic factor in severe traumatic brain injury. *Brain Inj*. 2004;18(1):103–109.

64. Born JD, Albert A, Hans P, et al. Relative prognostic value of best motor response and brain stem reflexes in patients with severe head injury. *Neurosurgery*. 1985;16(5):595–601.

65. Facco E, Zuccarello M, Pittoni G, et al. Early outcome prediction in severe head injury: comparison between children and adults. *Child's Nerv Syst*. 1986;2:67–71.

66. Hans P, Albert A, Born JD. Predicting recovery from head injury. *Brit J Hospital Med*. 1987;37(6):535–540.

67. Choi SC, Narayan RK, Anderson RL, et al. Enhanced specificity of prognosis in severe head injury. *J Neurosurg*. 1988;69:381–385.

68. Tate RL, Lulham JM, Broe GA, et al. Psychosocial outcome for the survivors of severe blunt head injury: the results from a consecutive series of 100 patients. *J Neurol & Psych*. 1989;52:1128–1134.

69. Narayan RK, Enas GG, Choi SC, et al. Practical techniques for predicting outcome in severe head injury. In: Becker DP, Gude-man SK, eds. *Textbook of Head Injury*. Philadelphia, PA: Saunders; 1989: 420–425.

70. Levin HS, Gary HE, Eisenberg HM, et al. Neurobehavioral outcome 1 year after severe head injury. *J Neurosurg*. 1990;73:699–709.

71. Choi SC, Muizelaar JP, Barnes TY, et al. Prediction tree for severely head-injured patients. *J Neurosurg*. 1991;75:251–255.

72. Marshall L F, Gautille T, Klauber MR. The outcome of severe closed head injury. *J Neurosurg*. 1991;75:S28–S36.

73. Vollmer DG, Torner JC, Jane JA, et al. Age and outcome following traumatic coma: why do older patients fare worse? *J Neurosurg*. 1991;75:S37–S49.

74. Bishara SN, Partridge FM, Godfrey HPD, et al. Post-traumatic amnesia and Glasgow Coma Scale related to outcome in survivors in a consecutive series of patients with severe closed-head injury. *Brain Inj*. 1992;6(4):373–380.

75. Godfrey HPD, Bishara SN, Partridge FM, et al. Neuropsychological impairment and return to work following severe closed head injury: implications for clinical management. *NZ Med J*. 1993;106: 301–303.

76. Pennings JL, Bachulis BL, Simons CT, et al. Survival after severe brain injury in the aged. *Arch Surg*. 1993;128:787–794.

77. Katz DI, Alexander MP. Traumatic brain injury: predicting course of recovery and outcome for patients admitted to rehabilitation. *Arch Neurol*. 1994;51:661–670.

78. Combes P, Fauvage B, Colonna M, et al. Severe head injuries: an outcome prediction and survival analysis. *Intensive Care Med*. 1996; 22:1391–1395.

79. Ellenberg JH, Levin HS, Saydjari C. Posttraumatic amnesia as a predictor of outcome after severe closed head injury. *Arch Neurol*. 1996;53:782–791.

80. Hawkins ML, Lewis FD, Medeiros RS. Serious traumatic brain injury: an evaluation of functional outcomes. *J Trauma*. 1996;41(2): 257–264.

81. Hellawell DJ, Taylor R, Pentland B. Cognitive and psychosocial outcome following moderate or severe traumatic brain injury. *Brain Inj*. 1999;13(7):489–504.

82. Hawkins ML, Lewis FD, Medeiros RS. Impact of length of stay on functional outcomes of TBI patients. *Am Surg*. 2005;71:921–929.

83. Mushkudiani NA, Engel DC, Steyerberg EW, et al. Prognostic value of demographic characteristics in traumatic brain injury: results from the IMPACT study. *J Neurotrauma*. 2007;24(2):259–269.

84. Sherer M, Yablon SA, Nakase-Richardson R, Nick TG. Effect of severity of post-traumatic confusion and its constituent symptoms on outcome after traumatic brain injury. *Arch Phys Med Rehabil*. 2008;89:42–47.

85. Nakase-Richardson R, Sepehri A, Sherer M, Yablon SA, Evans C, Mani T. Classification schema of posttraumatic amnesia duration-based injury severity relative to 1-year outcome: analysis of individuals with moderate and severe traumatic brain injury. *Arch Phys Med Rehabil*. 2009;90:17–19.

86. Ross AM, Pitts LH, Kobayashi S. Prognosticators of outcome after major head injury in the elderly. *J of Neurosci Nurs*. 1992;24(2): 88–93.

87. Kilaru S, Garb J, Emhoff T, et al. Long-term functional status and mortality of elderly patients with severe closed head injuries. *J Trauma*. 2000;142:373–381

88. Grahm TW, Williams FC Jr, Harrington T, Spetzler RF. Civilian gunshot wounds to the head: a prospective study. *Neurosurgery*. 1990;27(5):696–700.

89. Levy ML, Masri LS, Lavine S et al. Outcome prediction after penetrating craniocerebral injury in a civilian population: aggressive surgical management in patients with admission Glasgow Coma Scale scores of 3, 4, or 5. *Neurosurgery*. 1994;35(1):77–85.

90. Levin HS, Williams D, Crofford MJ, et al. Relationship of depth of brain lesions to consciousness and outcome after closed head injury. *J Neurosurg*. 1988;69:861–866.

91. Dikmen SS, Ross BL, Machamer JE. One year psychosocial outcome in head injury. *J of the Intl Neuropsych Society*. 1995;1:67–77.

92. Dikmen SS, Temkin NR, Machamer JE, Holubkov AL, Fraser RT, Winn HR. Employment following traumatic head injuries. *Arch Neurol*. 1994;51:177–179.

93. Groswasser Z, Sazbon L. Outcome in 134 patients with prolonged posttraumatic unawareness. *J Neurosurg*. 1990;72:81–84.

94. Greenwood R. Value of recording duration of post-traumatic amnesia. *Lancet*. 1997;349:1041–1042.

95. Walker WC, Ketchum JM, Marwitz JH, et al. A multicentre study on the clinical utility of post-traumatic amnesia duration in predicting global outcome after moderate-severe traumatic brain injury. *J Neurol Neurosurg Psychiatry*. 2010;81:87–89.

96. Jane JA, Francel PC. Age and outcome of head injury. In: Narayan RK, Wilberger JE, Povlishock JT, eds. *Neurotrauma*. New York, NY: McGraw-Hill; 1996:723–741.

97. Pentland B, Jones PA, Roy CW, et al. Head injury in the elderly. *Age and Aging*. 1986;15:193–202.

98. Rothweiler B, Temkin NR, Dikmen SS. Aging effect on psychosocial outcome in traumatic brain injury. *Arch Phys Med Rehabil*. 1998; 79:881–887.

99. Maurice-Williams RS. Head injuries in the elderly. *British J of Neurosurg*. 1999;13(1):5–8.

100. Pruitt BA Jr. Part 2: Prognosis in Penetrating Brain Injury. *J Trauma*. 2001;51(2, suppl):S44–S86.

101. Nagib MG, Rockswold GL, Sherman RS, Lagaard MW. Civilian gunshot wounds to the brain: prognosis and management. *Neurosurgery*. 1986;18(5):533–537.

102. Fabbri A, Servadei F, Marchesini G, Stein SC, Vandelli A. Early predictors of unfavourable outcomes in subjects with moderate head injury in the emergency department. *J Neurol Neurosurg Psychiatry*. 2008;79:567–573.

103. Compagnone C, d'Avella D, Servadei F, et al. Patients with moderate head injury: a prospective multicenter study of 315 patients. *Neurosurgery*. 2009;64(4):690–697.

104. Ip RY, Dornan J, Schentag C. Traumatic brain injury: factors predicting return to work or school. *Brain Inj*. 1995;9(5):517–532.

105. Cattelani R, Tanzi F, Lombardi F, et al. Competitive re-employment after severe traumatic brain injury: clinical, cognitive and behavioural predictive variables. *Brain Inj*. 2002;16(1):51–64.

106. Boake C, Millis SR, High WM, et al. Using early neuropsychologic testing to predict long-term productivity outcome from traumatic brain injury. *Arch Phys Med Rehabil*. 2001;82:761–768.

107. Sherer M, Sander AM, Nick TG, et al. Early Cognitive status and productivity outcome after traumatic brain injury: findings from the TBI model systems. *Arch Phys Med Rehabil*. 2002;83:183–192.

108. Sherer M, Novack TA, Sander AM, et al. Neuropsychological assessment and employment outcome after traumatic brain injury: a review. *Clin Neuropsychologist*. 2002;16(2):157–178.

109. Sherer M, Struchen MA, Yablon SA, Wang Y, Nick TG. Comparison of indices of traumatic brain injury severity: Glasgow Coma Scale, length of coma, and post-traumatic amnesia. *J Neurol Neurosurg Psychiatry*. 2008;79:678–685.

110. Novack TA, Bush BA, Meythaler JM, et al. Outcome after traumatic brain injury: pathway analysis of contributions from premorbid, injury severity, and recovery variables. *Arch Phys Med Rehabil*. 2001; 82:300–305.

111. Corticosteroid Randomisation After Significant Head Injury Investigators. CRASH Head Injury Prognostic Model. http://www.crash.lshtm.ac.uk/Risk%20calculator/index.html. Accessed February 16, 2012.

112. International Mission for Prognosis and Analysis of Clinical Trials in TBI. Prognostic Calculator. http://www.tbi-impact.org/?p=impact/calc. Accessed February 16, 2012.

113. Hukkelhoven CW, Rampen AJJ, Maas AIR, et al. Some prognostic models for traumatic brain injury were not valid. *J Clinical Epidemiol*. 2006;59:132–143.

114. Perel P, Edwards P, Wentz R, Roberts I. Systematic review of prognostic models in traumatic brain injury. *BMC Med Inform Decis Mak*. 2006;6:38.

115. Mushkudiani NA, Hukkelhoven C, Hernandez AV, et al. A systematic review finds methodological improvements necessary for prognostic models in determining traumatic brain injury outcomes. *J Clinical Epidemiol*. 2008;61(4):331–343.

116. Buckman R. *How to Break Bad News: A Guide for Healthcare Professionals*. Baltimore, MD: The Johns Hopkins University Press; 1992.

117. Ptacek JT, Eberhardt TL. Breaking bad news: a review of the literature. *JAMA*. 1996;276(6):496–502.

118. Girgis A, Sanson-Fisher RW. Breaking bad news: consensus guidelines for medical practitioners. *J of Clinical Oncology*. 1995;13(9): 2449–2456.

119. Lobb, EA, Kenny DT, Butow PN. Women's preferences for discussion of prognosis in early breast cancer. *Health Expectations*. 2001; 4:48–57.

120. Blanchard C, Labrecque M, Ruckdeschel J, et al. Information and decision-making preferences of hospitalized adult cancer patients. *Soc Sci Med*. 1988;27(11):1139–1145.

121. Butow PN, Maclean M, Dunn SM, et al. The dynamics of change: cancer patients' preferences for information, involvement and support. *Annals of Onc*. 1997;8:857–863.

122. Sanchez-Menegay C, Stalder H. Do physicians take into account patients' expectations? *J Gen Intern Med*. 1994;9:404–406.

123. Blackhall LJ, Murphy ST, Frank G, et al. Ethnicity and attitudes toward patient autonomy. *JAMA*. 1995;274(10):820–825.

124. Bottorff JL, Ratner PA, Johnson JL, et al. Communicating cancer risk information: the challenges of uncertainty. *Patient Educ Couns*. 1998;33:67–81.

125. Fong GT, Rempel LA, Hall PA. Challenges to improving health risk communication in the 21st century: a discussion. *J Natl Cancer Inst Monogr*. 1999;25:173–176.

126. Gerrity MS, DeVellis RF, Earp JA. Physicians' reactions to uncertainty in patient care. *Med Care*. 1990;28(8):724–736.

127. Boss P. *Ambiguous Loss*. Cambridge, MA: Harvard University Press; 1999.

128. Kothari S, Sander AM, Contant C, et al. The relation between level of disability and satisfaction with life in individuals with traumatic brain injury. *Arch Phys Med Rehabil*. 2001;82(10):1490.

129. Paulos JA. *Innumeracy: Mathematical Illiteracy and its Consequences*. New York. NY: Hill & Wang; 1988.

130. Schwartz LM, Woloshin S, Black WC, et al. The role of numeracy in understanding the benefit of screening mammography. *Ann Intern Med*. 1997;127(11):966–972.

131. Lipkus IM, Samsa G, Rimer BK. General performance on a numeracy scale among highly educated samples. *Med Decis Making*. 2001; 21:37–44.

132. Lloyd AJ. The extent of patients' understanding of the risk of treatments. *Qual Health Care*. 2001;10(suppl 1):i14–i18.

133. Grimes DA, Snively GR. Patients' understanding of medical risks: implications for genetic counseling. *Obstet Gynecol*. 1999;93(6): 910–914.

134. Rothman AJ, Kiviniemi MT. Treating people with information: an analysis and review of approaches to communicating health risk information. *J Natl Cancer Inst Monogr*. 1999;25:44–51.

135. Sheridan SL, Pignone MP, Lewis CL. A randomized comparison of patients' understanding of number needed to treat and other common risk reduction formats. *J Gen Intern Med*. 2003;18:884–892.

136. Gigerenzer G, Edwards A. Simple tools for understanding risks: from innumeracy to insight. *BMJ*. 2003;327:741–744.

137. Schapira MM, Nattinger AB, McHorney CA. Frequency or probability? A qualitative study of risk communication formats used in health care. *Med Decis Making*. 2001;21:459–467.

138. Weinstein ND. What does it mean to understand a risk? Evaluating risk comprehension. *J Natl Cancer Inst Monogr*. 1999;25:15–20.

139. Marteau TM. Communicating genetic risk information. *Br Med Bull*. 1999;55(2):414–428.

140. Edwards A, Elwyn G. Understanding risk and lessons for clinical risk communication about treatment preferences. *Qual Health Care*. 2001;10(suppl 1):i9–i13.

141. Mazur DJ, Hickam DH. Patients' interpretations of probability terms. *J Gen Intern Med*. 1991;6:237–240.

142. Bryant GD, Norman GR. Expressions of probability: words and numbers. *N Engl J Med*. 1980;302(7):411.

143. Paling J. Strategies to help patients understand risks. *BMJ*. 2003; 327:745–748.

144. Lipkus IM, Hollands JG. The visual communication of risk. *J Natl Cancer Inst Monogr*. 1999;25:149–63.

145. Moxey A, O'Connell D, McGettigan P, Henry D. Describing treatment effects to patients. *J Gen Intern Med*. 2003;18:948–959.

146. McGettigan P, Sly K, O'Connell D, Henry D. The effects of information framing on the practices of physicians. *J Gen Intern Med*. 1999; 14:633–642.

147. Forrow L, Taylor WC, Arnold RM. Absolutely relative: how research results are summarized can affect treatment decisions. *Am J of Med*. 1992;92:121–124.

148. Naylor CD, Chen E, Strauss B. Measured enthusiasm: does the method of reporting trial results alter perceptions of therapeutic effectiveness? *Annals of Intern Med*. 1992;117:916–921.

149. Berwick DM, Fineberg HV, Weinstein MC. When doctors meet numbers. *Amer J of Med*. 1981;71:991–998.

150. Gigerenzer G. The psychology of good judgment: frequency formats and simple algorithms. *Med Decis Making*. 1996;16:273–280.

151. Back AL, Arnold RM, Quill TE. Hope for the best, and prepare for the worst. *Ann Intern Med.* 2003;138:439–443.

152. Hayden JA, Cote P, Bombardier C. Evaluation of the quality of prognostic studies in systemic reviews. *Ann Intern Med.* 2006; 144(6):427–437.

153. Wilde EA, Whiteneck GG, Bogner J, et al. Recommendations for the use of common outcome measures in traumatic brain injury research. *Arch Phys Med Rehabil.* 2010;91:1650–1660.

154. Miller KJ, Schwab KA, Warden DL. Predictive value of an early Glasgow Outcome Scale score: 15-month score changes. *J Neurosurg.* 2005;103:239–245.

155. Hemingway H, Riley RD, Altman DG. Ten steps towards improving prognosis research. *BMJ.* 2009;340:410–414.

156. Technologies of Prognostication. *J Head Trauma Rehabil.* 2006;21(4): 293–374.

157. Wasson JH, Sox HC, Neff RK, Goldman L. Clinical prediction rules: applications and methodological standards. *New Eng J of Med.* 1985; 313(13):793–799.

158. Laupacis A, Wells G, Richardson WS, Tugwell P. Users' guides to the medical literature. V. how to use an article about prognosis. *JAMA.* 1994;272(3):234–237.

159. Wyatt JC, Altman DG. Commentary: prognostic models: clinically useful or quickly forgotten? *BMJ.* 1995;311:1539–1541.

160. Braitman LE, Davidoff F. Predicting Clinical States in Individual Patients. *Ann Intern Med.* 1996;125(5):406–412.

161. Randolph AG, Guyatt GH, Richardson WS. Prognosis in the intensive care unit: finding accurate and useful estimates for counseling patients. *Crit Care Med.* 1998;26(4):767–772.

162. Laupacis A, Sekar N, Stiell IG. Clinical prediction rules: a review and suggested modifications of methodological standards. *JAMA.* 1997;277(6):488–494.

163. Justice AC, Covinsky KE, Berlin JA. Assessing the generalizability of prognostic information. *Ann Intern Med.* 1999;130(6):515–524.

164. Simon R, Altman DG. Statistical aspects of prognostic factor studies in oncology. *Br J Cancer.* 1994;69:979–985.

165. Altman DG, Royston P. What do we mean by validating a prognostic model? *Statist Med.* 2000;19:453–473.

166. Feldman Z, Contant CF, Robertson CS, et al. Evaluation of the Leeds prognostic score for severe head injury. *Lancet.* 1991;337: 1451–1453.

167. Gibson RM, Stephenson GC. Aggressive management of severe closed head trauma: time for reappraisal. *Lancet.* 1989;369–371.

168. Chestnut RM, Ghajar J, Maas AIR, et al. Management and prognosis of severe traumatic brain injury. Part 2: early indicators of prognosis in severe traumatic brain injury. *J Neurotrauma.* 2000;17: 557–627.

169. Wilberger JE. Emergency care and initial evaluation. In: Cooper PR, Golfinos JG, eds. *Head Injury.* New York, NY: McGraw-Hill; 2000:27–40.

170. Ghajar J, Hariri RJ, Narayan RK, et al. Survey of critical care management of comatose, head-injured patients in the United States. *Crit Care Med.* 1995;23(3):560–567.

171. Jennett B. Historical perspective on head injury. In: Narayan RK, Wilberger JE, Povlishock JT, eds. *Neurotrauma.* New York, NY: McGraw-Hill; 1996:3–11.

172. Eker C, Schalen W, Asgeirsson B, et al. Reduced mortality after severe head injury will increase the demands for rehabilitation services. *Brain Inj.* 2000;14(7):605–619.

173. Bulger EM, Nathens AB, Rivara FP, et al. Management of severe head injury: institutional variations in care and effect on outcome. *Crit Care Med.* 2002; 30(8):1870–1876.

174. Hukkelhoven CWPM, Steyerberg EW, Farace E, et al. Regional differences in patient characteristics, case management, and outcomes in traumatic brain injury: experience from the Tirilazad trials. *J Neurosurg.* 2002;97:549–557.

175. Chui W. Head injuries in developing countries. In: Narayan RK, Wilberger JE, Povlishock JT, eds. *Neurotrauma.* New York, NY: McGraw-Hill; 1996.

176. Stein SC. Classification of head injury. In: Narayan RK, Wilberger JE, Povlishock JT, eds. *Neurotrauma.* New York, NY: McGraw-Hill; 1996:31–42.

177. Boake C, High WM. Functional outcome from traumatic brain injury: unidimensional or multidimensional? *Phys Med & Rehabil.* 1996;75(2):105–113.

178. Hannay HJ, Sherer M. Outcome from head injury. In: Narayan RK, Wilberger JE, Povlishock JT, eds. *Neurotrauma.* New York, NY: McGraw-Hill; 1996:723–741.

179. Evans RW, Ruff RM. Outcome and value: a perspective on rehabilitation outcomes achieved in acquired brain injury. *J Head Trauma Rehabil.* 1992;7(4):24–36.

180. Condeluci A, Ferris LL, Bogdan A. Outcome and value: the survivor perspective. *J Head Trauma Rehabil.* 1992;7(4):37–45.

181. Prigatano GP. Work, love, and play after brain injury. *Bull Menninger Clin.* 1989;53(5):414–431.

182. Jennett B, Bond M. Assessment of outcome after severe brain damage: a practical scale. *Lancet.* 1975;1:480–484.

183. Baalen BV, Odding E, Maas AIR, Ribbers GM, Bergen MP, Stam HJ. Traumatic brain injury: classification of initial severity and determination of functional outcome. *Disability & Rehabil.* 2003;25(1): 9–18.

184. Groswasser Z, Melamed S, Agranov E, Keren O. Return to work as an integrative outcome measure following traumatic brain injury. *Neuropsych Rehabil.* 1999;9(3/4):493–504.

185. Morton MV, Wehman P. Psychosocial and emotional sequelae of individuals with traumatic brain injury: a literature review and recommendations. *Brain Inj.* 1995;9(1):81–92.

186. Hoofien D, Gilboa A, Vakil E, et al. Traumatic brain injury (TBI) 10–20 years later: a comprehensive outcome study of psychiatric symptomatology, cognitive abilities and psychosocial functioning. *Brain Inj.* 2001;15(3):189–209.

187. Campbell CH. Needs of relatives and helpfulness of support groups in severe head injury. *Rehab Nursing.* 88;13(6):320–325.

188. Rappaport M, Herrero-Backe C, Rappaport ML, et al. Head injury outcome up to ten years later. *Arch Phys Med Rehabil.* 1989;70: 885–892.

189. Corrigan JD, Smith-Knapp K, Granger CV. Outcomes in the First 5 Years After Traumatic Brain Injury. *Arch Phys Med Rehabil.* 1998; 79:299–305.

190. Olver JH, Ponsford JL, Curran CA. Outcome following traumatic brain injury: s comparison between 2 and 5 years after injury. *Brain Inj.* 1996;10(11):841–848.

191. Choi SC, Barnes TY, Bullock R, Germanson TA, Marmarou A, Young HF. Temporal profile of outcomes in severe head injury. *J Neurosurg.* 1994;81:169–173.

192. Corrigan JD, Harrison-Felix C, Bogner J, Dijkers M, Sendroy-Terrill M, Whiteneck G. Systematic bias in traumatic brain injury outcome studies because of loss to follow-up. *Arch Phys Med Rehabil.* 2003;84:153–160.

193. Choi SC, Barnes TY. Predicting outcome in the head-injured patient. In: Narayan RK, Wilberger JE, Povlishock JT, eds. *Neurotrauma.* New York, NY: McGraw-Hill; 1996:779–790.

194. Concato J, Feinstein AR, Holford TR. The risk of determining risk with multivariable models. *Ann Intern Med.* 1993;118(3):201–210.

195. Harrel HE Jr, Lee KL, Matchar DB, et al. Regression models for prognostic prediction: advantages, problems, and suggested solutions. *Cancer Treat Rep.* 1985;69(10):1071–1077.

196. Hosmer DW, Taber S, Lemeshow S. The importance of assessing the fit of logistic regression models: a case study. *Am J Pub Health.* 1991;81(12):1630–1635.

197. Diamond GA. What price perfection? Calibration and discrimination of clinical prediction models. *J Clin Epidemiol.* 1992;45(1):85–89.

198. Charlson ME, Ales KL, Simon R, et al. Why predictive indexes perform less well in validation studies. *Arch Intern Med.* 1987;147: 2155–2161.

199. Andrews PJD, Sleeman DH, Statham PFX, et al. Predicting recovery in patients suffering from traumatic brain injury by using admission variables and physiological data: a comparison between decision tree analysis and logistic regression. *J Neurosurg.* 2002;97: 326–336.

200. McQuatt A, Sleeman D, Andrews PJD, et al. Discussing anomalous situations using decision trees: a head injury case study. *Methods Inf Med.* 2001;40:373–379.

Neuroimaging Correlates of Functional Outcome

Erin D. Bigler and William L. Maxwell

INTRODUCTION

How do neuroimaging findings best predict outcome once the brain has been injured? The answer is complicated. Even though many trauma-induced abnormalities can be identified by neuroimaging and such findings represent one of our best objective measures of brain injury, there are numerous neuropathological and imaging variables that have to be considered. For example, imaging—even functional imaging—represents only a particular moment in time, yet predictions of outcome typically involve statistical statements over much broader timeframes into the future, including the lifetime of the patient. Likewise, the recovery process is dynamic and ever changing particularly in the first year of injury; and neuroimaging now detects many of those dynamic brain changes. Early changes reflect the immediate effects of trauma whereas others reflect trauma-induced degeneration or changes associated with neural plasticity and adaptation. A host of injury variables apply, including the type and severity of brain injury, the brain regions most likely affected, the age at time of injury, as well as issues involving brain and cognitive reserve along with individual differences associated with neural plasticity. Because of the advent of contemporary neuroimaging, the type, degree, location, and a host of other indicators of brain imaging abnormalities have been examined in an attempt to identify neuroimaging correlates of functional outcome.

Major neuroimaging developments have occurred since the first edition of *Traumatic Brain Injury Medicine*, most importantly in automation and quantitative analyses. This same chapter in the first edition may be referred to for historical perspective on neuroimaging techniques that mostly attempted to relate clinical neuroimaging findings with outcome. Much of this past research focused on the location and size of traumatic lesions or some type of rating method that specified the amount of regional or whole brain atrophy or some region of interest (ROI) (i.e., the hippocampus), or degree of abnormalities within the white matter. Although it may still be useful for the clinician to view and rate actual neuroimaging studies as this chapter will demonstrate, several novel, elegant methods can now provide improved, statistically validated, quantitative information about brain anatomy and pathology from neuroimaging studies. The goal of these advanced imaging methods is to aid in guiding and predicting outcome from TBI as they become readily available to the clinician evaluating and treating patients with TBI (1).

Although neuroanatomists first described the major white matter pathways of the brain in the latter part of the 19th century (2,3), from a practical standpoint there were no neuroimaging methods that could efficiently demonstrate actual white matter pathways. More recently, *computed tomography (CT)* and *magnetic resonance (MR)* imaging or *MRI* of the brain allows distinction between white and gray matter, but conventional neuroimaging with these methods could only detect where macroscopic lesions occurred and not how focal or nonspecific lesions actually disrupted neural tracts until the advent of the MRI technique *diffusion tensor imaging* (DTI) (4). Now DTI methods provide a sensitive technique for examining *pathway* damage—not just where a lesion occurs—and relating this damage to outcomes (5–7). Understanding how lesions disrupt pathways provides insights into how neural networks become damaged and how this damage relates to outcome (8–10). Furthermore, the integration of DTI with other methods such as *functional MRI (fMRI)*, *magnetic resonance spectroscopy (MRS)*, and a host of quantitative MRI methods that provide volumetric, pathophysiologic, and morphologic data has considerably enhanced prediction of TBI outcomes.

Quantitative Image Analysis of Structural Scans

Automated Quantitative Image Analysis

Accurate, robust, and rapidly performed automated MR image analyses of the brain are now available (11) and have been applied to studying the effects of TBI (12). Figure 19-1A shows the standard T1 image where white matter, gray matter, and cerebrospinal fluid (CSF) can be readily differentiated. The first step in quantitative image analysis is to identify these tissue/CSF boundaries through a process referred to as *segmentation* (see Figure 19-1B). Once segmented, using common landmarks and other algorithms, the brain is parcellated and classified into numerous common anatomical divisions as shown in Figure 19-1C. All of this is done with fully automated methods that only require a volume acquisition MR scan that has been appropriately formatted.

Figure 19-2 shows some of the cortico-gyral parcellation that can be done using identified ROIs. Because these methods are fully automated, they can be performed on any scan with similar acquisition parameters required for these analyses with scan data compared to normative samples (see 13). These quantitative findings can then be used to examine neuropsychological correlates (14,15).

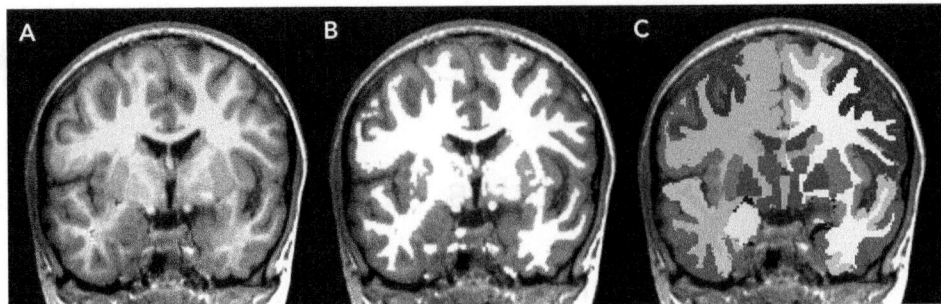

FIGURE 19–1 *See color insert.* Differences in white and gray matter are distinctly visualized in a coronal T1 MRI as shown in A. By "segmenting" the image into gray matter, white matter, and CSF as in B, all tissue types are separated into one of those 3 and then parcellated and "classified" as to region of interest. For example, for subcortical structures **light blue** identifies the caudate, **darker blue** the globus pallidus, **pink** the putamen and **dark green** the thalamus. After this type of classification, by knowing the MRI slice thickness and the number of slices where a structure is identified and classified, volumes may be calculated.

Voxel Based Morphometry

Voxel-based morphometry (VBM) capitalizes on the fact that gross cranial parenchyma is readily resolved into 3 major compartments—white matter, gray matter, and CSF. For any given brain region, the signal intensity will be defined by the predominance of a particular tissue type within a specified pixel. Right at the margin of a transition zone between white and gray matter or between parenchyma and CSF, there will be intermediate values influenced by what is referred to as partial volume effects. However, parameters and algorithms can be established, which will segment and classify brain matter based on what the greatest likelihood of tissue types may be (as described earlier) with all pixels classified on a 256 grayscale as either white matter, gray matter, or CSF. Currently, by applying techniques that standardize the individual brain image into a uniform space, such as Talairach space originally used for stereotaxic placement of electrodes (16) or what is referred to as the Montreal Neurological Institute (MNI) space (17), all brains can be placed into that standardized space where comparisons are made voxel-by-voxel per a specified region. However, it is notable that because of the inherent statistical analyses used during computer processing, some caution should be exercised in interpretation of the results obtained, which are appropriate only to comparisons across large numbers of patients or samples. VBM basically examines the "concentration" of pixel type per region. Figure 19-3 shows a VBM analysis that demonstrates where the greatest amount of gray matter loss occurs in a group of patients who experienced cortical contusions. This image will be fully discussed in the section on

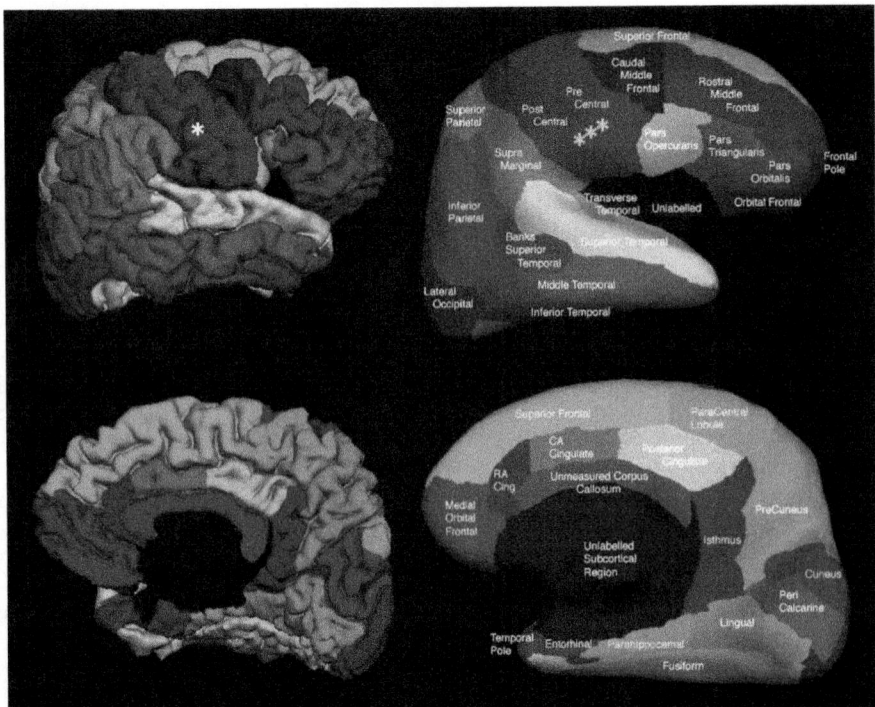

FIGURE 19–2 *See color insert.* This illustration demonstrates the cortico-gyral surface classification of major cortical anatomical regions of interest that can be identified using the automated FreeSurfer image analysis software. The left image represents the pial surface and the right image inflated cortico-gyral regions of interest. The top row depicts the lateral view of the right hemisphere while the bottom row shows the medial view of the hemisphere. The white asterisk on the image in the upper left indicates the cortex arounds the perimeter of the central sulcus that is buried within the gyri and thus not visible. In contrast, the yellow asterisks on the inflated image in the upper right indicate the cortex around the perimeter of the central sulcus that has now been inflated and is visible. From Desikan RS, Segonne F, Fischl B, et al. An automated labeling system for subdividing the human cerebral cortex on MRI scans into gyral based regions of interest. *Neuroimage.* 2006;31(3):968–980) and used with permission from Elsevier.

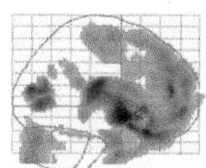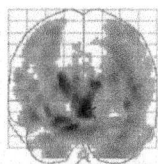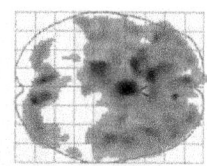

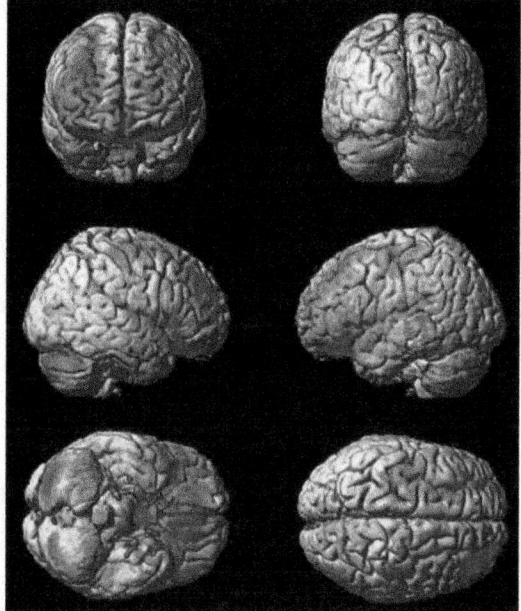

FIGURE 19–3 *See color insert*. Voxel-based morphometry depicting the location of decreased gray matter pixel intensity in patients with TBI with history of prior cortical contusion. The "glass brain" shown **at the top** depicts the "see through" appearance whereas shades of gray indicate where decreased gray matter occurred, with the darker the gray, the greater the loss of pixel density within localized voxels. Using this information, general plots are highlighted in color on a standard surface MRI reconstruction of brain surface anatomy from the anterior aspect **(top left)**, posterior aspect **(top right)**, lateral aspect **(middle)**, inferior aspect **(bottom left)** and superior aspect **(bottom right)**, where *red* depicts reduced gray matter density.

the selective frontotemporal vulnerability of brain injury, but clearly this type of VBM analysis shows the focal loss of gray matter distributed across the frontal and temporal lobes, in particular the frontal and temporal poles, the base of the frontal lobe, and the cerebellum in this group of patients with TBI.

VBM analyses also permit the statistical comparison of outcome variables with VBM differences. This is useful for group data comparisons examining regional and whole-brain differences in outcome, where the degree of whole brain white matter changes relate most with cognitive outcome following TBI (see 18,19,20).

Diffusion Tensor Imaging

Diffusion tensor images are derived from MR detected differences in water diffusion in brain parenchyma. The most common DTI metric is the measurement of *fractional anisotropy* (*FA*) where unconstrained diffusion is 0.00 and perfectly constrained diffusion in all directions is an FA value of 1.0.

Figure 19-4 provides a schematic example and this will be discussed in greater detail subsequently.

Neuroimaging and Neuropathology Correlates of Outcome in Traumatic Brain Injury

Regardless of the neuroimaging method used to detect TBI abnormalities, to understand what is being viewed as an abnormality requires a basic understanding of the neuropathology of TBI. This section relates what is viewed at the gross neuroimaging level to its underlying histopathology.

Although earlier work suggested that the human brain contains about 100 million neurons and 10 times that number of glial cells, recent work has indicated that the cellular scaling rules differ between rodents and primates. More recently, studies reviewed by Azevedo and colleagues (21), in their analysis of neurons and non-neuronal or glial cells, provide evidence that the number of neurons is smaller and that the ratio of neurons to glial cells is approximately 1:1. But there are also marked differences between different brain regions, for example, 80% of all neurons within the human brain occur within the cerebellum, 19% of all brain neurons occur in the gray matter of the cerebral cortex, and 1% within the basal ganglia, diencephalon, and brainstem (21). Azevedo et al. (21) also report that in a human male of about 50 years of age with a brain weighing 1.5 kg, there are, on average, 86.1 ± 8.1 billion NeuN-positive cells or neurons and 84.6 ± 9.8 billion NeuN negative or glia and endothelial cells. Clearly, neuroimaging is but a gross indicator of the underlying structure of the brain and, as observed in Figure 19-5 of a postmortem horizontal section of the brain or from an MRI at the level of the head of the caudate nucleus adjacent to the anterior horn of each lateral ventricle, the tissue consists of visibly discrete gray and white matter in an MRI scan but discrete pathways within the white matter are not. Myelinated axons are but a few microns in diameter and therefore within a typical MRI resolution of a cubic millimeter, what is viewed as "white matter" parenchyma is comprised of millions of axons.* Similarly, gray matter, which houses neuronal cell bodies, contains comparable numbers per cubic millimeter.

Visualization of the brain with MRI reflects its gross anatomy and can be readily appreciated in Figure 19-5. Here, the horizontal postmortem section shown is centered on the anterior genu of the corpus callosum from a healthy, typically developed young adult, who died from non-neurological and non-head injury respiratory complications of an acute infection. In addition, T1 and T2 weighted MR images oriented at approximately the same horizontal plane, but from a living individual, nicely show gross brain anatomy very similar to the postmortem section at that same level. Whether seen from the postmortem section or through conventional neuroimaging, tissue appears as a contiguous mass; however, with DTI, directionality of the fiber tracts within the white matter can also be distinguished as seen in the DTI color map in Figure 19-5. Because DTI is based on the direction of water diffusion or anisotropy, in normal myelinated axons that form the white matter tracts, the axon

---

* If one takes an axon 2.5 μm in radius and 500 μm long, then the number in a mm^3 = 101,677.68, for $r = 1.25$ then $n = 1,280,000$, for $r = 0.5$ then $n = 2,541,942$ formula is $\pi r^2 \times 500$ μm into 10^9 cu μm which is 1mm^3 of axons.

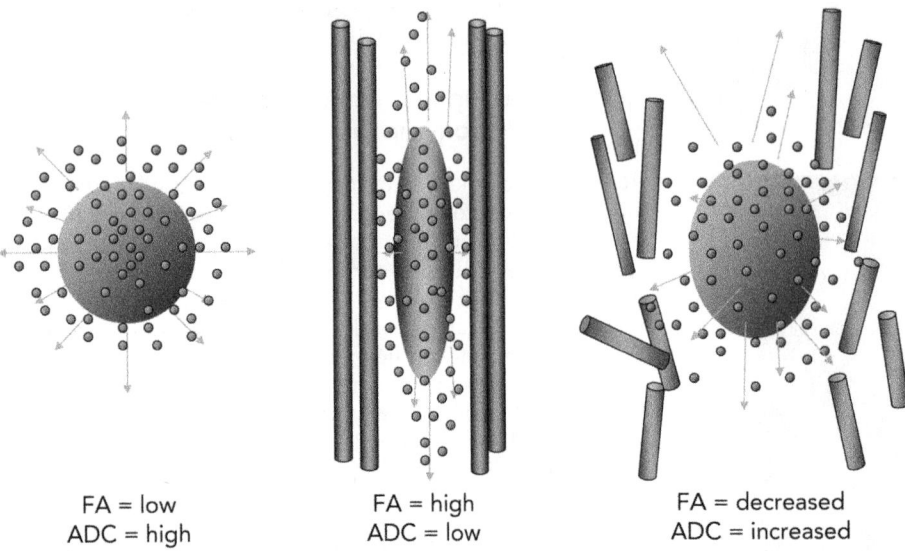

FA = low
ADC = high

FA = high
ADC = low

FA = decreased
ADC = increased

FIGURE 19–4 Diagrammatic illustration of the relationship of the DTI metrics fractional anisotropy (FA) and apparent diffusion coefficient (ADC). Illustration provided by Gerri Hanten, PhD, Baylor College of Medicine.

membrane or axolemma and myelin membranes constrain intracellular water diffusion within a common direction permitting computer-based algorithms to infer white matter tract composition based on similar water diffusion properties.

Animal studies that have integrated DTI and histology (22,23) have shown that DTI represents a sensitive tool in white matter tract identification. When the brain is viewed as a conglomeration of tracts, a much greater appreciation of the complexity and intricacy of the brain's connectivity can be obtained as shown in Figure 19-6. In this DTI image, and all others shown convention has aggregate tracts that course in the anteroposterior plane to be green, lateral or side-to-side coursing tracts are represented by warm (orange-to-red) colors, and vertically oriented tracts are blue.

Capitalizing on the physics of water diffusion (refer back to Figure 19-4), DTI not only provides a method to identify bundles of axons forming incredibly intricate neural pathways, as shown in Figure 19-6, the physics of DTI also permits measurements of the anisotropy of brain paren-

chyma. For example, normal white matter has an intermediate FA value, resulting from several factors: (*a*) intracellular water is held within the axon as well as the myelin sheath and these membranes constrain the movement of water; (*b*) the degree of myelin coating may further constrain free movement of water molecules; and/or (*c*) because of the compactness of normal, healthy neural tissue, extracellular water within tightly bundled tracts is also constrained because of the constricted configuration of axon-to-axon alignment. If there is cell loss from TBI, or a pathological disruption in the integrity of the myelin or changes in axonal membrane integrity or spacing of axons or cell bodies because some have degenerated, water molecules become freer to diffuse. DTI is a well-suited neuroimaging technique sensitive to even subtle differences in water diffusion reflecting the brain's microstructure. These DTI metrics provide a method for correlating DTI findings with neurobehavioral and neurocognitive changes, even in mild injury, and will be discussed more thoroughly later in the chapter.

Figure 19-7 shows a large focal right frontal lesion (red) in a teenager who was involved in a high-speed head-on

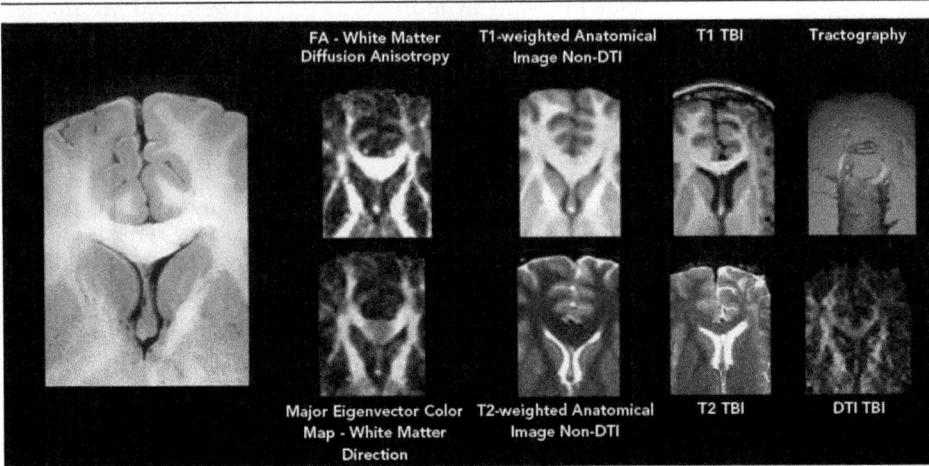

FA - White Matter Diffusion Anisotropy   T1-weighted Anatomical Image Non-DTI   T1 TBI   Tractography

Major Eigenvector Color Map - White Matter Direction   T2-weighted Anatomical Image Non-DTI   T2 TBI   DTI TBI

FIGURE 19–5 *See color insert.* The postmortem section on the left depicts the natural appearance of the brain at the time of cutting in the horizontal plane. Matched to this level are different MRI sequences showing how images differ depending on the sequence. Note in the patient with TBI (the 4 images on the **right side** of the figure) that pathology alters the basic characteristics of the MRI signal, reflecting pathological changes from the brain injury.

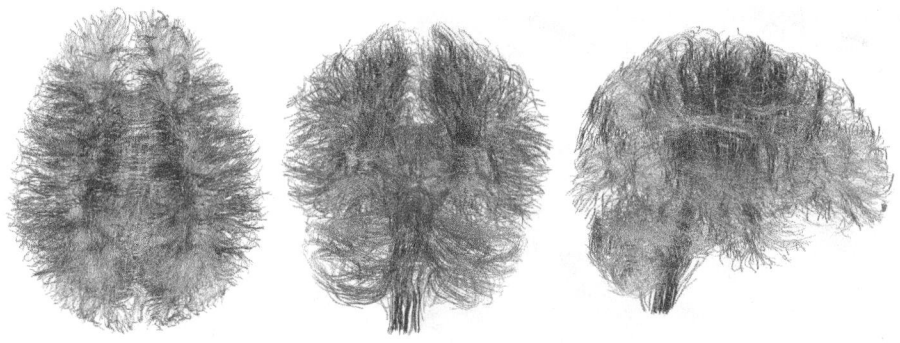

FIGURE 19-6 *See color insert.* Whole brain DTI tracts showing their orientation in 3 planes (**left** - dorsal, **middle** - frontal view, **right** - parasagittal).

and side-impact collision. This case will be used to demonstrate the major points of image analysis in predicting TBI outcome and is also the same patient with TBI shown in Figure 19-5. In addition to a blunt force head injury, this patient suffered a penetrating right inferior frontal injury from accident debris striking his head. Key points to understanding the gross pathological effects of TBI are demonstrated in the 4 conventional images (T1, T2, FLAIR and GRE) shown in Figure 19-7 as well as the 3-dimensionally reconstructed brain and DTI tractography images shown in Figure 19-8. The T1 image is often referred to as the anatomical image because of the clear definition of major brain structures and anatomical landmarks—the focal lesion in the right frontal region is readily identified because there is increased, localized CSF as a *dark* or *hypointense* signal (see

arrow). The brain is typically symmetric on either side of the vertical midline or sagittal plane and bilateral structures in typical, healthy individuals are usually symmetric. In the T1 image (bottom row in Figure 19-7) along with the anterior focal lesion, it can be seen that the anterior horn of the right lateral ventricle is dilated, compared to the left. This type of dilation reflects loss of surrounding parenchyma and passive dilation of the ventricle. Note how the anterior horn dilates in the direction of the pathology (see *arrow* in T1 image within the bottom row). In addition, there is a clear difference in the signal intensity of the residual white matter in the right frontal region surrounding the focal lesion. Even though tissue is there, the lack of normal MRI signal, particularly on the DTI, reflects loss and disorganization of white matter.

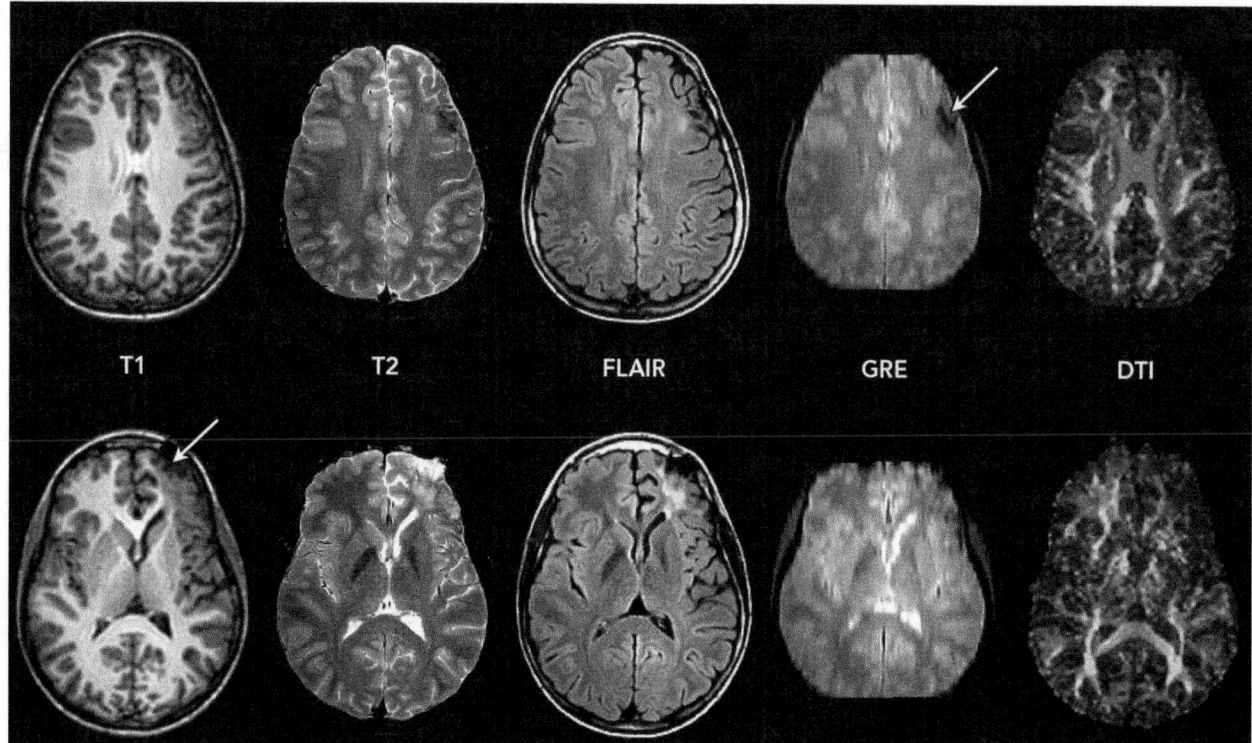

FIGURE 19-7 *See color insert.* This is the same patient originally shown in Figure 19-5 who had sustained a focal frontal injury. These horizontal images reflect different aspects of the pathology as well as sensitivity to pathological changes. To be consistent with the 3-D presentation in Figure 19-8, right is on the viewer's right. The arrow in the T1 image points to focal frontal damage and note the distinct difference between the frontal white matter, which also is different on the T2, FLAIR and DTI sequences. In the GRE sequence, the arrow points to a large hemosiderin deposit from prior hemorrhage.

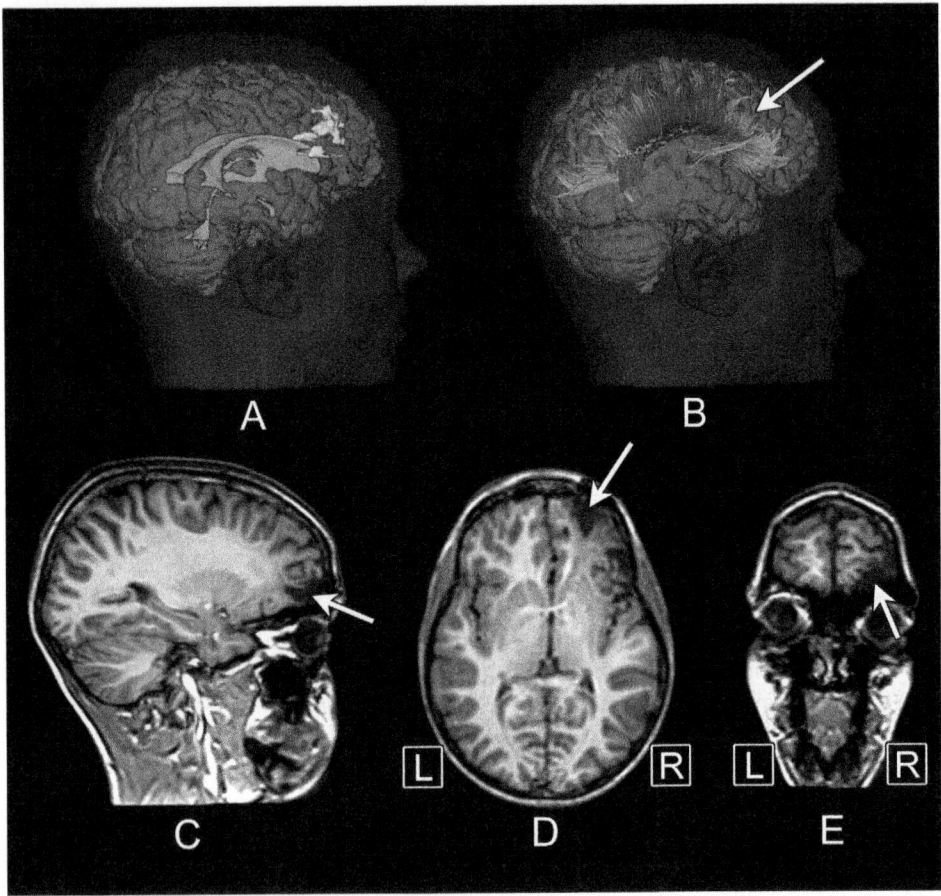

FIGURE 19–8 *See color insert.* A, 3D depiction of the focal loss of cortical gray matter (shown in *red*) compared to where focal white matter signal loss occurred (*yellow*), with the lateral ventricle shown in *aquamarine*, mostly as an internal landmark. B, Same level of posterior oblique image but now showing the tractography of the corpus callosum and the loss of fiber tracts in the frontal region. C, Sagittal view at the level of the hippocampus where the arrow points to the inferior frontal penetrating injury (*arrow*). D, Axial view of the frontal focal frontal damage (*arrow*). D, Coronal image just above the orbit depicting the location of the focal frontal injury (*arrow*). C, D, and E are not in radiological perspective because of the 3D presentation and all are T1-weighted images.

T2 image sequences (see Figure 19-7) are particularly sensitive to signal differences that highlight CSF changes, which can be readily appreciated in the bottom scan (see *arrow*). T2 is also sensitive to signal differences created by the accumulation of the blood by-product *hemosiderin* that result from prior trauma-induced hemorrhages (see **arrow** in Figure 19-7 GRE sequence). Presence of hemosiderin, as shown in Figure 19-7, reflects that trauma resulted in localized hemorrhage. In nonpenetrating, closed head injury, the presence of hemosiderin is held to be an indication of shearing action within brain parenchyma with damage to both axons and blood vessels.

The *fluid attenuated inversion recovery sequence (FLAIR)* (see Figure 19-7) is particularly sensitive to white matter changes, which are distinctly observed in this patient to be associated with damaged white matter that surrounds the focal penetrating injury and areas of encephalomalacia. The change in the white matter MR signal in the surrounding tissue suggest that the white matter projections into and out of the frontal area, where the encephalomalacia is at its apex, are damaged. Note that the FLAIR poorly defines where hemorrhage has occurred.

The DTI images provide even further information about the disruption of white matter, where the altered *directionality* of white matter pathways can now be demonstrated by the faded or less intense green in the DTI map within the right frontal pole shown in Figure 19-7. Returning to the T1 axial image shown in Figures 19-5 and 19-8, where the anterior horn of the lateral ventricle is asymmetric and dilated

on the right compared to the left, the asymmetry points to the location of greatest pathology. Medial to the anterior horn is the forceps minor, a bundle of white matter representing the anterior fibers of the corpus callosum on their way to and from the frontal lobes. DTI tractography can show these pathways in their normal and damaged state, with the normal appearance of DTI tractography shown in Figure 19-9, to be compared to the pathological appearance of corpus callosum-forceps minor tractography findings shown in Figures 19-7 and 19-8.

The discussion up to this point has been focused on the identification of structural neuroimaging findings in TBI but, obviously, what is represented in macroscopic MRI and CT findings is representation of the much more complex underlying microscopic neuroanatomy and neuropathology. How do macroscopic neuroimaging findings represent underlying neuropathology and how does all of this relate to predicting outcome?

Traumatic Brain Injury as a Diffuse Injury

Graham et al. (24) discuss TBI in the context of underlying general neuropathology, often referred to as *diffuse brain injury* or *DBI* (25,26). This is a very important concept to understand in interpreting functional outcome from brain imaging because neuroimaging methods readily detect the major features of DBI including the following: increased prominence of cortical sulci; thinning of the cortical mantle; nonspecific

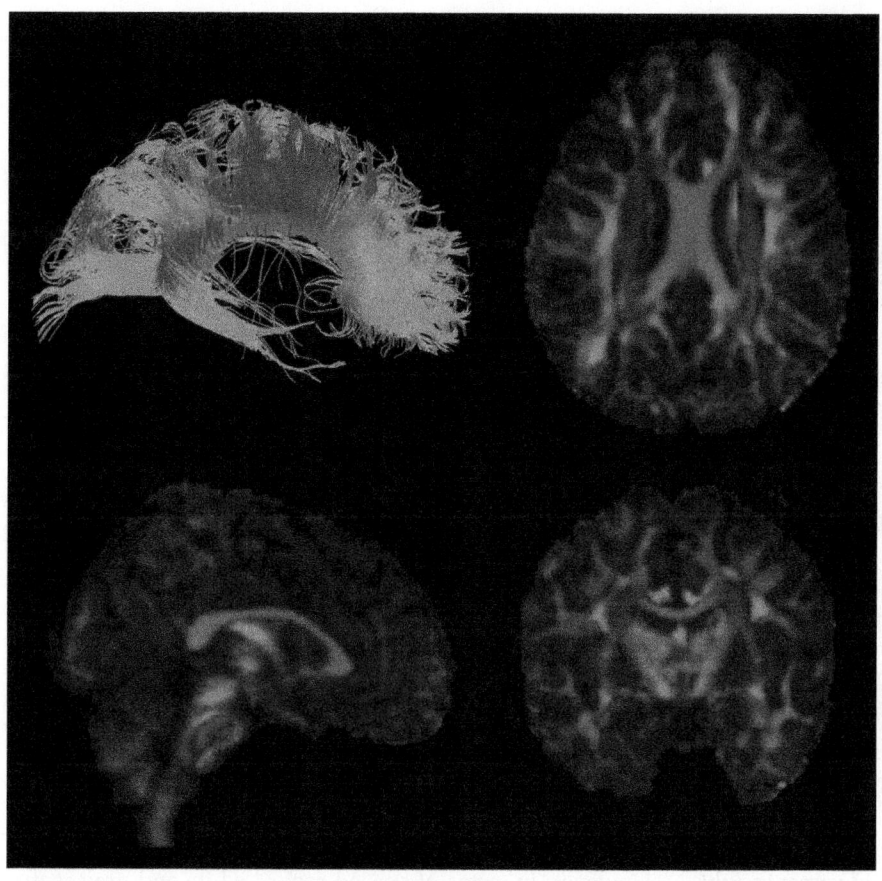

FIGURE 19–9 *See color insert.* Normal appearing DTI in 3 planes with corpus callosum tractography shown in the upper left. *Green* reflects an anteroposterior projection, *blue* vertical and *warmer colors* lateral or side-to-side projection.

reductions in gray and white matter volumes; ventricular dilation in combination with reduced overall brain volume (27); as well as where focal lesions may reside. The loss of white matter is typically disproportionate in TBI where white matter volume loss associated with the passive expansion of the ventricular system, known as hydrocephalus ex vacuo (20), occurs in proportion to the severity of injury. These ventricular changes tend to be nonspecific, except in the region of focal damage, with the non-specificity of global ventricular dilation indicating generalized volume loss of the brain following trauma and, because the ventricular system within the cerebral hemispheres is surrounded by white matter, ventricular size increases often reflect nonspecific damage to and loss of white matter. Figure 19-10 depicts these major changes in a postmortem coronal (A) section matched with an antemortem MRI (B, C, and D) as well as the surrounding changes in white matter integrity that contribute to ventricular dilation.

In the most comprehensive neuropathological study to date to address some of these issues, Maxwell and colleagues (28) examined the postmortem brains of 48 patients who had survived at least 3 months and had received Glasgow Outcome Scale (GOS) rating prior to death. At the time of brain removal, each brain was weighed and categorized by GOS severity as follows: 1,442.7 ± 105.0 g for controls, 1,329.6 ± 202.9 g for moderately disabled, 1,330.0 ± 140.7 g for severely disabled, and 1,275.0 ± 135.5 g for vegetative state patients. These observations alone nicely demonstrate that the relationship of total brain volume loss is proportional to severity of disability. Motor cortex was specifically

examined where the amount of thinning ranged from 0.50 mm in moderately disabled, 0.80 mm in severely disabled, to 1.03 mm in vegetative state patients, or up to 3 times greater than the maximum predicted change with ageing alone. In the Maxwell et al. study (28), cortical thinning was statistically greater than expected without injury, providing confidence that the changes in cortical thickness were a result of the traumatic injury. Thinning of the cortical gray matter can be assessed using MRI by measuring the thickness of the gray matter mantel, as shown in Figure 19-11 from Merkley et al. (29). In Figure 19-10, note the disproportionate thinning of frontal and temporal regions of the brain, the increased size of the ventricles, and the more discrete separation of the gyri reflecting loss of tissue with the extensive nature of the cortical thinning in patients with moderate-to-severe TBI. Figure 19-11 is from children who had sustained moderate-to-severe TBI, the majority of whom survived without major disability, yet loss of cortical thickness was extensive and did relate to changes in cognitive ability.

The diffuseness of white matter injury may be viewed in voxel-based morphometric DTI maps of the brain beginning with the acute injury as shown in Figure 19-12. For this demonstration, DTI findings in very acute yet only mild injury in patients with TBI with normal conventional imaging is used so that the perturbation of white matter is not obscured with other pathologies, such as major hemorrhage, contusion, or acute shear pathologies that commonly occur in more severe injuries. The subjects displayed in Figure 19-12 were characterized in detail in Wilde et al. (30); although all were evaluated in the emergency room and met criteria for mild

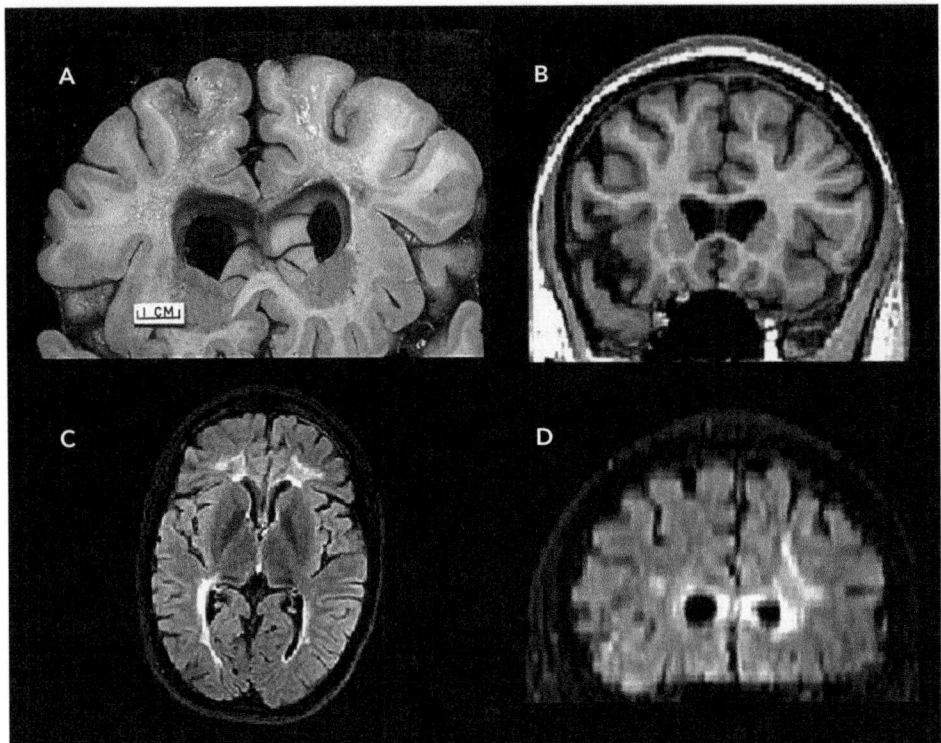

FIGURE 19-10 A, Postmortem coronal section showing ventricular dilation and loss of white matter integrity. B, MRI of a patient with TBI who sustained a severe TBI with similar type of appearance of ventricular dilation, where the FLAIR sequence shows extensive white matter signal abnormalities (C and D). From Bigler, ED & Maxwell WL. Neuroimaging and neuropathology of TBI. *NeuroRehabilitation*. 2010;28:63–74, used with permission from IOS Press.

TBI, none were hospitalized and none had any major deficit at follow-up. Nonetheless, these images provide great insight into which white matter areas of the brain were most affected and the diffuse nature of DTI white matter signal differences involving the deep white matter of the brain as already stated, but in particular, the involvement of the anterior aspect of the corpus callosum and fornix. More on the selectivity of white matter damage will be covered in subsequent sections. However, in terms of spaced foci of white and gray matter injury, the report of changes in FA within supratentorial white matter (SWM) with an increase in apparent diffusion coefficient within SWM, corpus callosum, whole brain gray matter, thalamus, and cerebellum in patients with normal appearing structural MRI scans (7) is of interest.

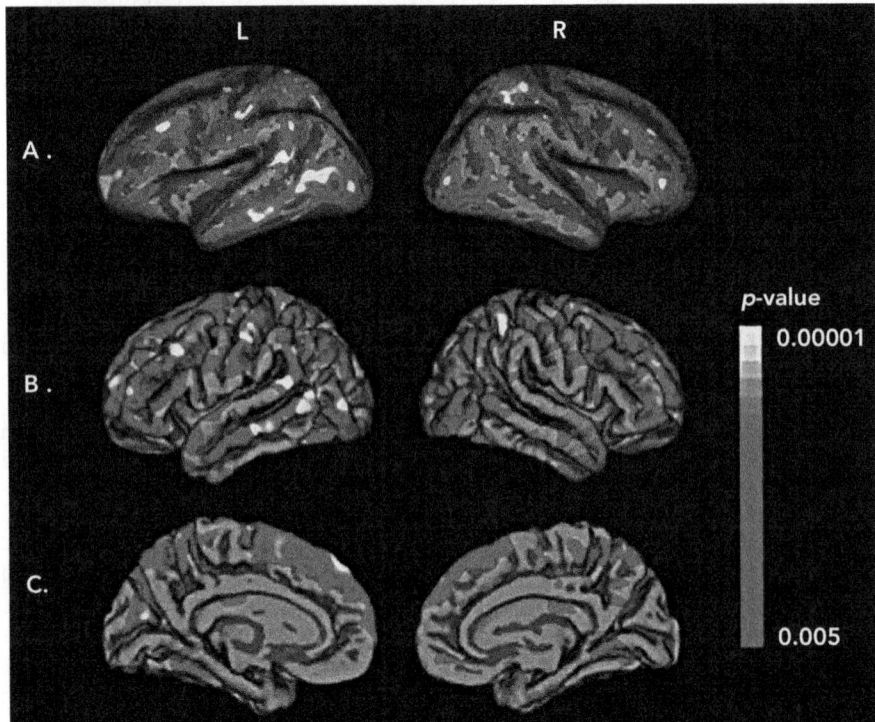

FIGURE 19-11 *See color insert.* Reduced cortical thickness in TBI in children who sustained moderate-to-severe injuries. The significance bar on the right shows that where *yellow* is present that the greatest amount of atrophic change has occurred. A, inflated brain reflecting loss even into sulcal regions. B, standard lateral surface. C, medial surface of left hemisphere in the sagittal plane. From Merkley et al. [29] used with permission from Mary Liebert Publishers.

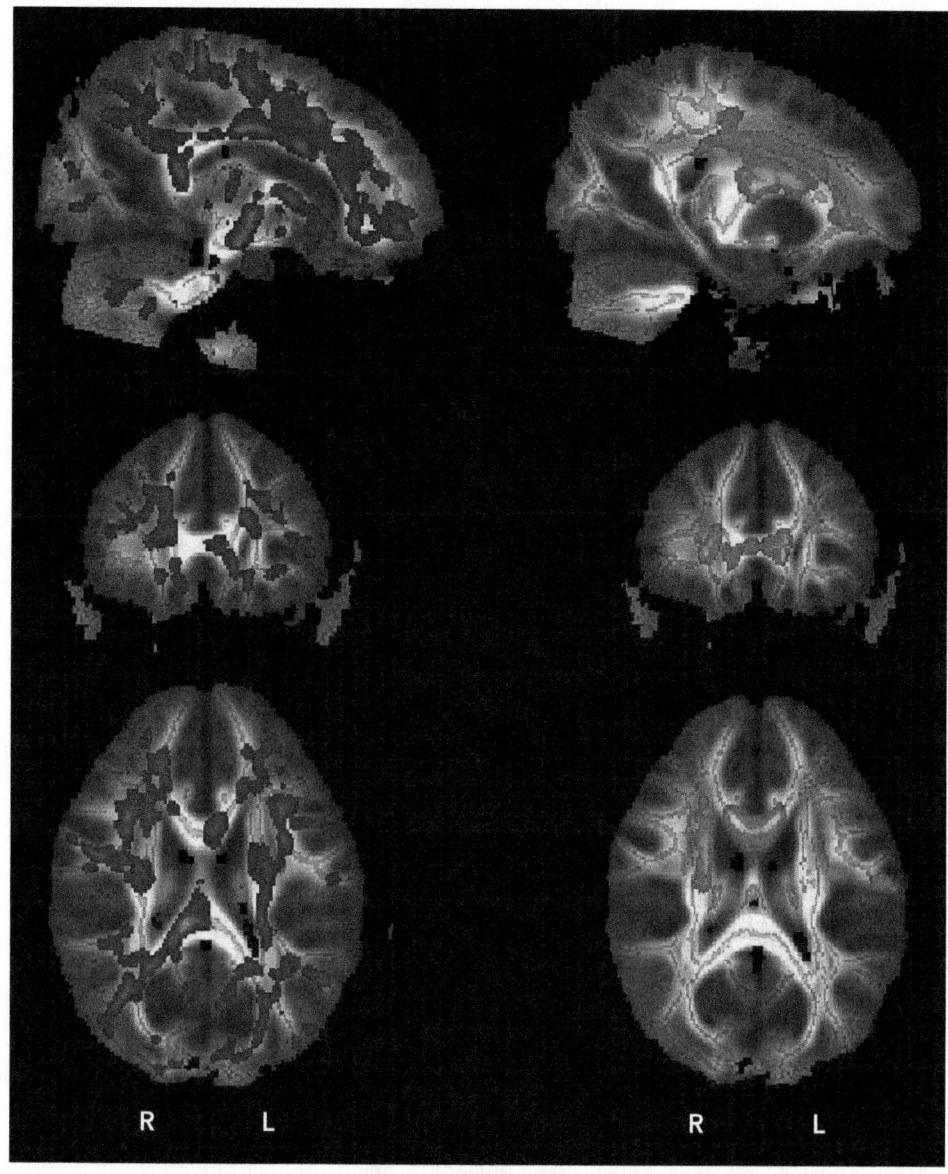

R   L

R   L

FIGURE 19–12 *See color insert.* TBSS based ADC and FA changes in acute mild TBI. Note the extensive involvement of the cingulum, corpus callosum, and fornix. Illustration courtesy of Elisabeth A. Wilde, PhD, Jill V. Hunter, MD, and Harvey S. Levin, PhD, Baylor College of Medicine.

An important overview of neuropathological changes within 85 patients who survived at least 1 month after TBI has recently been published (31). Patients were classified as to their outcome by the GOS score. Moderately disabled (MD) patients survived for a median of 4 years (1–47 years), severely disabled (SD) patients for 4 months (1 month to 14.5 years), and vegetative state (VS) patients for a median period of 9 months (5 weeks to 8.5 years) clearly demonstrating that survival is correlated with severity of injury. The absence of cortical contusions, the occurrence of diffuse axonal injury (DAI), the presence of ischemic damage within the cerebral hemispheres, ventricular enlargement (66% of SD and VS patients, about 50% of MD patients), evidence for raised intracranial pressure, and damage to the thalamus were all associated with a poorer outcome. And, importantly, when there was a combination of the aforementioned brain pathologies in TBI, the outcome was poorer (31). This is important because the patient with TBI frequently presents with several types of pathology and in this respect differs greatly from many of the current experimental models where a single

pathology is investigated. Recent MRI reports illustrate evidence for post-traumatic ongoing loss of both gray and white matter from the injured brain (32) and has led to investigation of pathology at the cellular level to increase our understanding.

As already shown in Figures 19-10 and 19-11, a general thinning of the cerebral cortex occurs in TBI related to the severity of injury. From a neuroimaging perspective, it is important to understand what neuropathological correlates are associated with changes in cortical thickness. Since this disproportionately affects the frontal lobes and because of the importance of the frontal lobes in the neurobehavioral sequelae of TBI, some detailed discussion of the underlying neuropathology that relates to changes in cortical thickness follows. As discussed earlier in relation to motor cortex, Maxwell et al. (28) reported differential thinning of cerebral cortex and loss of neurons there in patients within 3 GOS outcome groups. Figure 19-13 presents the histological findings of that study showing bar graphs for percentage changes in the thickness of cortical layers from 1 through to

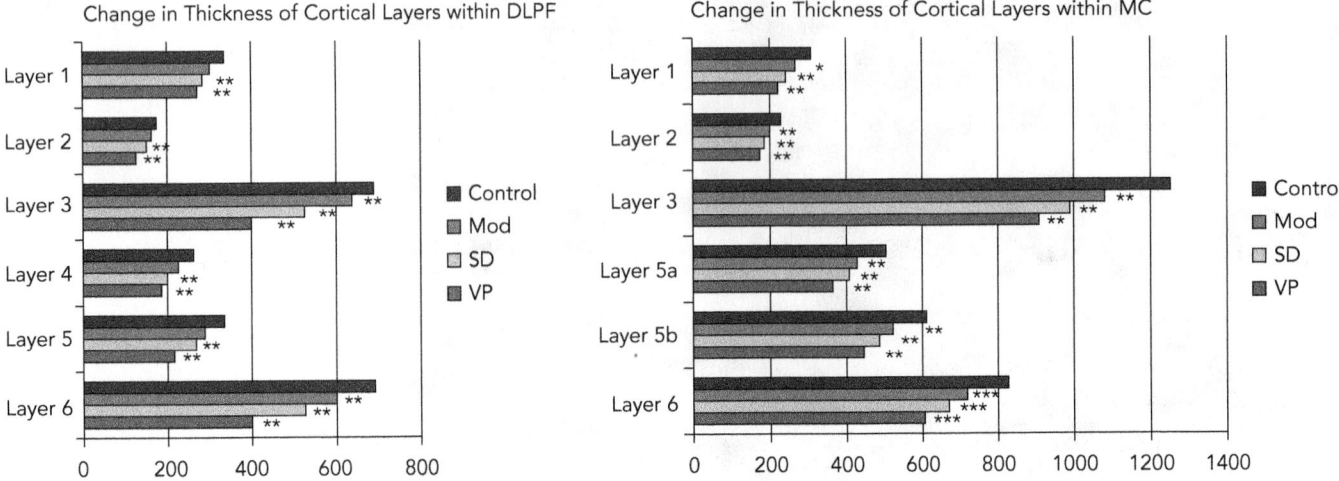

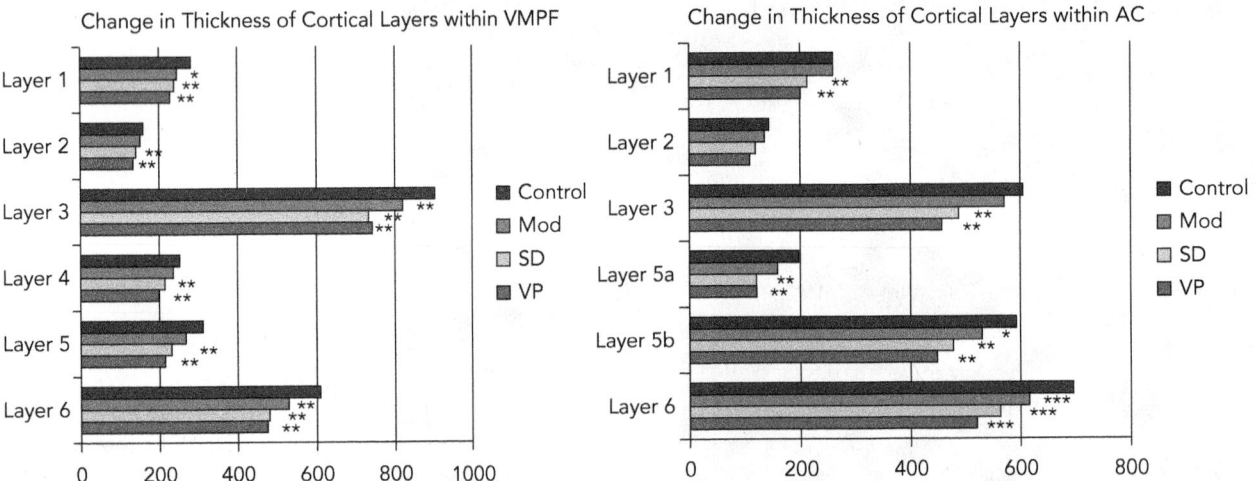

FIGURE 19–13 Histological based changes in thickness of cortical neurons. These 4 bar graphs illustrate changes in thickness of the 6 cerebral cortex layers in 4 cortical regions (medioventral prefrontal, dorsolateral prefrontal, anterior cingulated gyrus, and primary motor cortex) between control (*n* = 11), moderately disabled (*n* = 13), severely disabled (*n* = 12), and vegetative state (*n* = 12) patients from the Glasgow archive. (* indicates statistical significance from control values, Dunnett Multiple Comparisons Test. * = $p < .05$, ** = $p < .01$, *** = $p < .001$).

6 in medioventral prefrontal (VMPF), dorsolateral prefrontal (DLPF), anterior cingulate (AC) as well as motor cortex (MC) in control, moderately disabled (MoD), severely disabled (SD), and vegetative state (VS) patients who survived for a minimum of 3 months after TBI and were assessed using the Glasgow Outcome Score. It is notable that there is progressive thinning of all 6 cortical layers across MoD, SD, and VS outcome groups and that there are differences in detail between the 4 cortical areas examined. Loss from layer 1 was greater in agranular cortex (AC) being particularly marked in MC (−28%). Loss from layer 2 was greatest (−29%) within DLPF. Loss from layer 3 was greater in AC. The thickness of layer 4 was reduced across all outcome groups in VMPF, but only in MoD and SD patients from DLPF. There was loss of thickness from layer 5 across all outcome groups but loss was by 30% in VMPF compared to 36% from DLPF and 25% from AC.

Loss from layer 6 was comparable (−26%) across all 4 cortical areas in SD and VS patients. In summary, thinning

of the cerebral cortex is greater with greater severity of injury or outcome but there are differences in detail between cortical architectonic and/or functional areas. A novel finding by Maxwell et al. (28) was that cortical loss occurs by 7% within AC, 11% in prefrontal, and 14% in MC within moderately disabled patients.

Moreover, thinning of the layers of the cerebral cortex was associated with loss of neurons. Maxwell and colleagues (28) subdivided pyramidal and nonpyramidal neurons into 3 size subclasses—big, medium, and small sized cells—to test the hypotheses that cells either are reduced in size following TBI and/or secondary axotomy; that larger cells, more probably projection neurons, are more susceptible to injury and that the ratio of pyramidal to nonpyramidal cells changes on survival after TBI. Large pyramidal cells occurred in layer 3 of granular cortex and layers 3, 5a, and 5b in AC of control patients. Numbers of these cells fell significantly in MoD patients and they were totally absent in SD and VS patients. Medium and small pyramidal cells are far more numerous than large cells in controls. There was loss of between 30% and 50% of medium sized cells from VMPF in SD and 70%–80% from DLPF in VS patients. In AC the number of medium-sized pyramidal cells fell by 60%–65% in layers 5a and 5b of AC, whereas in MC the number of medium pyramidal cells did not change within layers 5a and 5b but fell in layer 6 across all outcome groups. The number of small pyramidal cells within layer 6 fell only in VS patients within granular cortex whereas there was a notable loss of cells from layer 6 across all outcome groups within AC.

Regarding nonpyramidal neurons, there was a graded loss of large and medium cells from layers 3, 5, and 6 between MoD and SD patients, to 25% of uninjured numbers in VS patients within all 4 cortical areas. The number of small nonpyramidal neurons increased in layers 3, 5, and 6 within VMPF; was unchanged within DLPF; and increased within layers 2, 3, 5a, and 5b in AC in both SD and VS patients (see 28 for greater detail). Differences in the extent of change between pyramidal and nonpyramidal cells resulted in an alteration in the proportion of the 2 groups from a value of 0.29 in granular cortex of control patients to 0.39 in VS patients. On the other hand, there was no change of proportion between pyramidal and nonpyramidal neurons within agranular cortex. In granular cortex, loss of pyramidal neurons is greater with increasing severity of outcome, whereas in AC, there is loss of both pyramidal and nonpyramidal cells such that the proportion of these does not change across outcome groups.

Efferent axons of pyramidal neurons in layers 2 and 3 extend largely to other cortical regions in the ipsilateral and contralateral hemispheres (33,34) and either form part of the cortico–cortico association inputs (35,36) via long horizontal axon collaterals from layers 3 to 6 or the transcallosal inputs between more distant regions with axons running via the underlying white matter (33). In addition, axons of pyramidal neurons in cortical layer 5 project to the striatum, brainstem, and spinal cord. Axons of large pyramidal neurons in the primary motor cortex form part of the corticospinal tract. Lastly, axons of pyramidal neurons in cortical layer 6 of the dorsal and lateral prefrontal cortices form fascicles that contribute to the corticothalamic radiation within the prefrontal white matter, the anterior corona radiata and the anterior limb of the internal capsule (37).

Afferent thalamic fibers form the thalamocortical radiation and terminate on dendrites of pyramidal neurons either within the deep part of layer 3 and layer 4 or extend up to cortical layer 1 of the prefrontal cortex. Ventromedial and dorsolateral prefrontal cortices are linked by way of association fibers to each other and, among other cortical regions, to cingulate cortex. Patients with lesions within the anterior cingulum experience psychological symptoms including apathy, inattention, change of personality, lack of distress, labile emotions, and changes in cognitive and emotional processing (38). These closely parallel reported behavioral changes in patients with TBI. MRI and DTI studies also indicate that several bundles or fascicles of myelinated fibers link the frontal cortex to other cortical regions: for example, by way of the superior longitudinal fasciculus, the uncinate fasciculus, the extreme capsule and the cingulate bundle (35,36). These fiber bundles, among others, form a major volumetric component of the prefrontal white matter.

A reduced fractional anisotropy has been reported within frontal and temporal white matter both in patients

diagnosed with postconcussion disorder (39), and with deficiencies of attention and memory (40). Quantitative evidence for loss of neurons from the overlying gray matter provides confidence that axons will have been lost from the frontotemporal white matter with survival after TBI. MRI and DTI have also provided evidence that white matter density falls within the superior longitudinal fasciculus, uncinate fasciculus, inferior longitudinal fasciculus, sagittal stratum, anterior corona radiate, and corticospinal tract after mild head injury (37,40). Furthermore, DTI provides evidence for a more widespread loss of white matter from the corpus callosum, fornix, internal and external capsules, corona radiata, superior frontal gyrus, superior longitudinal fasciculus, cingulum, sagittal strata, and parahippocampal gyrus in moderately and severely injured patients who survive either 90 days (41), 6 months (37,42), 1.0–3.0 (40) or 4.6–5.0 years (43,44) after TBI.

It has been recognized for some time that the dendritic tree of injured neurons undergoes a degenerative response following TBI. Gao and Chen (45) have greatly extended our understanding of this area using an experimental analysis after controlled cortical impact in mice. At 72 hours after injury, the density of NeuN positive neurons in injured cortex was half that in control animals, there was a marked degeneration of dendrites, a 40% reduction in the number of dendritic spines, and a 35% reduction in the number of synapses (45). In human cortex, pyramidal neurons within cortical layer 3 have dendritic trees extending into layer 1 of the cortex. With cell loss from layer 3 discussed earlier, there will clearly be a reduced number of cells contributing to the dendritic plexus that is cortical layer 1. Moreover, there is also input to cortical layer 1 from neurons within some nuclei of the thalamus and a reduced size of the thalami is a widely recognized response noted in both MRI investigations of volumetric studies of human brain after TBI and stereology of the thalami as discussed subsequently (44,46, 66). Moreover, white matter damage is frequently noted in the anterior parts of the corpus callosum and the corona radiata and it may be suggested that such damage may reflect injury both to projection neurons of prefrontal cortex and to the bilateral thalamocortical and corticothalamic radiations (46) among other tracts.

It has become appreciated that axonal injury may precipitate neuronal death as recently reported in an experimental optic nerve injury model of TBI (47). In the postacute and chronic phases of TBI, the major pathway to death of a neuron is programmed cell death (PCD) (15,47–50) of which the morphologic, most readily identified stage is the relatively short-term stage of apoptosis. But caspase-3 immunocytochemistry or TUNEL-label evidence for programmed cell death of cortical neurons has been reported in humans (51) and in numerous experimental studies. Despite the occurrence of several reports of a lack of cell death following axotomy in the experimental literature (52), it may be suggested from a small number of experimental studies (47) that the time course of PCD in models of TBI is much greater than has been appreciated earlier, and it is suggested that the study of Farkas et al. (52) examined only relatively short-term survivals. In the stretch-injury model in optic nerve, good morphological evidence for programmed cell death in retinal ganglion cells (RGC) has been reported (47) but peak numbers of degenerating cells were not obtained until 3 weeks after injury. Importantly, however, quantitative evidence in support of a continuing, low-grade loss of RGC out to 12 weeks after injury was reported (47).

Loss of pyramidal cells from layer 5 within MC (28) extend and confirm earlier reports (37) that axons within the corticospinal tract (CST) may be more susceptible to TBI. Kraus et al. (37) reported decreased FA within CST in mild TBI and a greater response at more severe levels of injury. Several studies have suggested that the long course of axons within the corticospinal tract through the brainstem into the upper spinal cord may expose those axons to physical strain during rapid movement of the head and neck during motor vehicle accidents, assaults, and falls. Loss of pyramidal cells, and in particular, large pyramidal cells from layers 5A and 5B of MC (28) supports the suggestion earlier that motor projection neurons are more susceptible to injury with a subsequent cell loss or death.

As already mentioned and previously shown in Figure 19-10, ventricular dilation is common place in TBI. In a postmortem examination of 85 individuals who survived at least a month post moderate-to-severe TBI and then died, Adams et al. (31) observed the following frequencies of gross neuropathological finding: 84% with residual indicia of a prior contusion, 68% with pathological ventricular dilation, 67% with concomitant ischemic damage with 58% meeting criteria for DAI. Ventricular enlargement is related to severity of injury, occurs in both pediatric and adult TBI (53–55) and relates to outcome (15,56). Although ventricular dilation relates to both white and gray matter degeneration, it is probable that white matter degeneration has a greater influence, in part that the largest surface areas that abut the wall of the lateral ventricle are white matter structures (32). An easy metric can be quickly calculated from either CT or MRI that reflects ventricular dilation, by dividing ventricular volume by brain volume, which provides an instantaneous correction for head size differences, allowing the ventricle-to-brain ratio (VBR) to be used by clinician as well as researcher to compare across patients with brain injury. As brain volume decreases and ventricular volume passively expands to take up the space left by trauma-induced degeneration, VBR increases as a reflection of generalized atrophy and volume loss. The VBR as a global indicator of brain pathology is associated with outcome where Tate et al. (15) have shown correlations with most major neuropsychological measures to range between 0.20 and 0.55 in predicting neuropsychological outcome when VBR is calculated at least a few weeks postinjury.

White Matter Damage

As a global indicator of white matter damage, the MRI FLAIR sequence is particularly sensitive in detecting gross pathologies as already shown in Figure 19-10. In their investigation of 106 patients with TBI with admitting GCS scores of 3–13, Skandsen et al. (57) observed that 50% of patients with moderate TBI and 90% of those with severe TBI had FLAIR-identified white matter abnormalities in lobar white matter and/or the corpus callosum, yet the presence of FLAIR-identified white matter abnormality within the cerebral hemispheres is only poorly related to outcome at 1 year postinjury whereas severity of outcome and the incidence of post-traumatic disability is associated with FLAIR-identified white matter abnormality within the brainstem (39).

Beyond the basic FLAIR detection of white matter signal hyperintensities, the DTI sequence provides an even more refined recognition of white matter changes following TBI because DTI metrics directly assess white matter diffusion

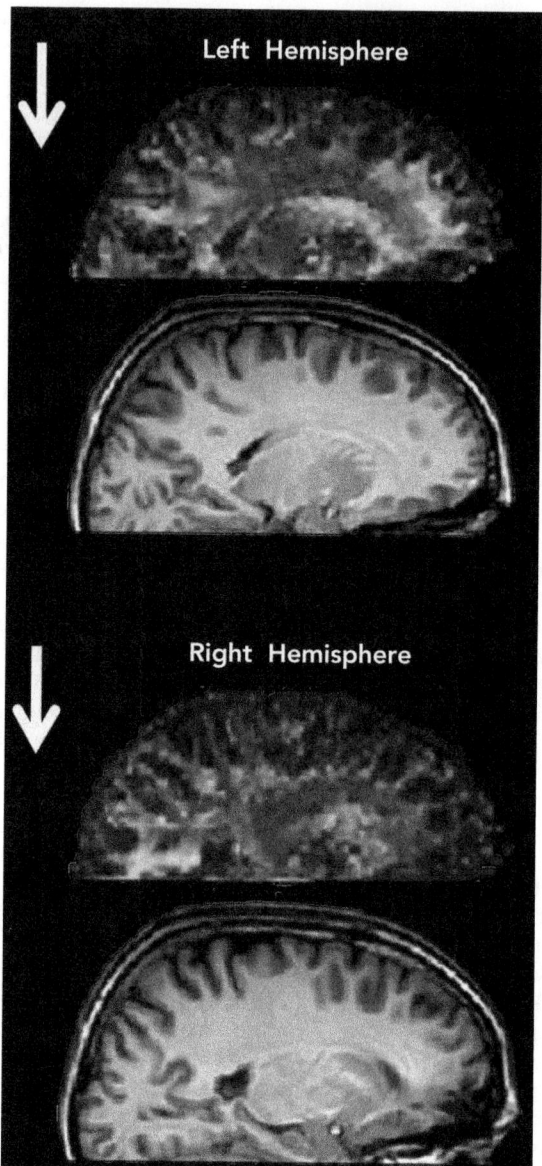

FIGURE 19–14 *See color insert.* DTI comparing the focally affected right hemisphere (bottom) with the nonfocally affected left hemisphere. Note the distinct sharpness of the DTI color maps in the more intact left hemisphere and the "fuzzier" appearance on the right, reflecting extensive disruption of white matter connectivity far beyond where the focal pathology occurred (see also Figures 19-5, 19-7, and 19-8).

characteristics, the information from which can be used to display graphic depiction of white matter disruption using DTI color maps and tractography. Based on DTI technology, axons within the corpus callosum have been shown to be particularly vulnerable to injury in TBI (22,58–60) and, to date, is the region most studied. Returning to the patient with focal frontal injury previously seen in Figures 19-5, 19-7, and 19-8, the DTI color maps of the injured brain demonstrate extensively disrupted white matter in the right frontal region compared to the left as seen in Figure 19-14. Furthermore, the DTI tractography technique graphically demonstrates the loss of aggregates of axons across the corpus callosum as also shown in Figure 19-8. Although the focal frontal traumatic injury is several centimeters from the corpus callosum per se, it nonetheless disrupts *all* of the anterior interhemispheric pathways between the region of the focal injury and the contralateral intact frontal lobe, where tractography readily demonstrates the dropout of connectivity as shown in Figures 19-7 and 19-8. In addition, the intrahemispheric pathways of the right hemisphere where the lesion disrupts all of the right superior longitudinal fasciculus is distinctly smaller and thinned out in comparison to the left. Therefore, not only is there focal damage but also the focal damage disrupts the entirety of the brain's white matter network. For example, the attentional network that connects parietal and frontal regions within the right hemisphere would be affected in the patient shown in Figure 19-14, as well as the interhemispheric tracts across both frontal lobes. So even though the focal lesion is in the right frontal lobe, the disruption of parietal input would be a distal consequence of this focal lesion.

DTI is particularly sensitive to the chronic effects of brain injury and changes within damaged white and gray matter. Using what is referred to as the *tract-based spatial statistical method* or *TBSS*, Kinnunen et al. (5) have shown the diffuse nature of white matter damage as illustrated in Figure 19-15. The TBSS method basically provides a "skeleton" through the middle of the white matter tract where normal FA values are reflected in green and abnormal values are shown in red. Where red appears indicates that a significant difference ($p < .05$) in FA has been observed corrected for multiple comparisons. Where green remains, it denotes that the changes did not reach significance after correction for multiple comparisons. Note the extensive changes in white matter in the central parts of the brain, regions that involve long tracts, and all of the corpus callosum. Note how these match the same, but a lesser degree in acute mild TBI, implicating that in some individuals with mild TBI, chronic white matter pathology develops.

Clearly, DTI provides an eloquent technique to demonstrate TBI-related pathology, but what is viewed in the DTI image is but a reflection of widespread histopathological changes that have probably taken days to months to evolve. But information at the level of individual fibers is limited in that the smallest dimension of resolution in high quality MRI/DTI machines is between 2.0 and 2.5 mm³ voxels. In addition, DTI is not able to describe the orientation of fibers where groups of fibers cross or follow different orientations (61), although progress is being made (62). The major proportion of myelinated nerve fibers within central white matter are of the order of 1.5 to 5.0 μm in diameter, for example, within the optic nerve of the adult guinea pig, 95% of the total content of nerve fibers are between 0.5 and 2.5 μm in

diameter (47). Damaged nerve fibers suffer focal disruption of the subaxolemma cytoskeleton, more frequently at nodes of Ranvier, where so called "nodal blebs" extend into the surrounding pericellular environment (see Figure 19-16). Within the nodal axolemma, sodium channels become leaky and homeostasis is lost to result in an uncontrolled influx of Na^+ and free Ca^{2+}. Release of calcium from the axoplasmic reticulum and influx of calcium allows: first, activation of neutral activated calpains and caspases which probably exacerbate axolemma damage as may be visualized using freeze-fracture techniques (Figure 19-16B and 19-1C); second, damage to mitochondria resulting in opening of the mitochondrial permeability membrane transmission pore (63); and third, loss of oxidative phosphorylation for generation of ATP with a consequent failure of ATP dependent membrane pumps and depolymerization of axonal microtubules provide a focal loss of fast axonal transport (FAT) (Figure 19-16E and 19-16F). These lead to accumulation of membranous profiles within axonal swellings large enough to be resolved by light microscopy following immunocytochemical labeling for β–amyloid precursor protein (Figure 19-16D). Axonal transport continues in the short term elsewhere in the length of the axon and continued delivery of axoplasmic components results in the region of axonal damage increasing in caliber forming axonal swellings when the axon remains in continuity.

A focal constriction then occurs at some point within the axonal swelling (Figure 19-16D), and neurofilaments of the axonal cytoskeleton become more closely spaced or compacted with a focal breakdown of the axolemma (Figure 19-16G) that may allow equilibration of calcium gradients and activation of calpains and caspases to depolymerize the remnants of the compacted neurofilaments (see Figure 19-16). The axon has then been fragmented into 2 or more fragments and the axon has undergone secondary axotomy (64). Wang et al. (65) in an analysis of axonal dieback in optic nerve after fluid percussion injury provided a detailed time course for development of axonal swellings, axotomy, and provided a novel morphological distinction between proximal and distal terminal or degeneration bulbs in mice. Wang et al. (65) reported small numbers of reactive axonal swellings at 1 hour with the occurrence of swellings some 8 μm in diameter (Figure 19-16D). Following axotomy terminal bulbs form the swollen ends of the disconnected axon. The proximal swelling or bulb remaining in continuity with the neuronal cell soma has a truncated or rod-like appearance at the distal end of the axon remnant. The distal swelling, however, expands to form a spherical terminal appendage with a diameter greater than the proximal swelling (Figure 19-16D). Ultrastructurally, the proximal swelling contains

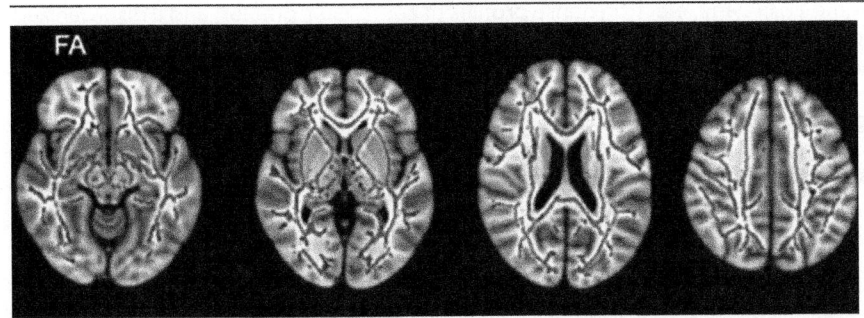

FIGURE 19–15 *See color insert.* TBSS findings of abnormal FA in TBI. *Green* indicates differences did not reach significance whereas *red* reflects definite difference. From Kinnunen et al. [5] reproduced with permission from Oxford University Press.

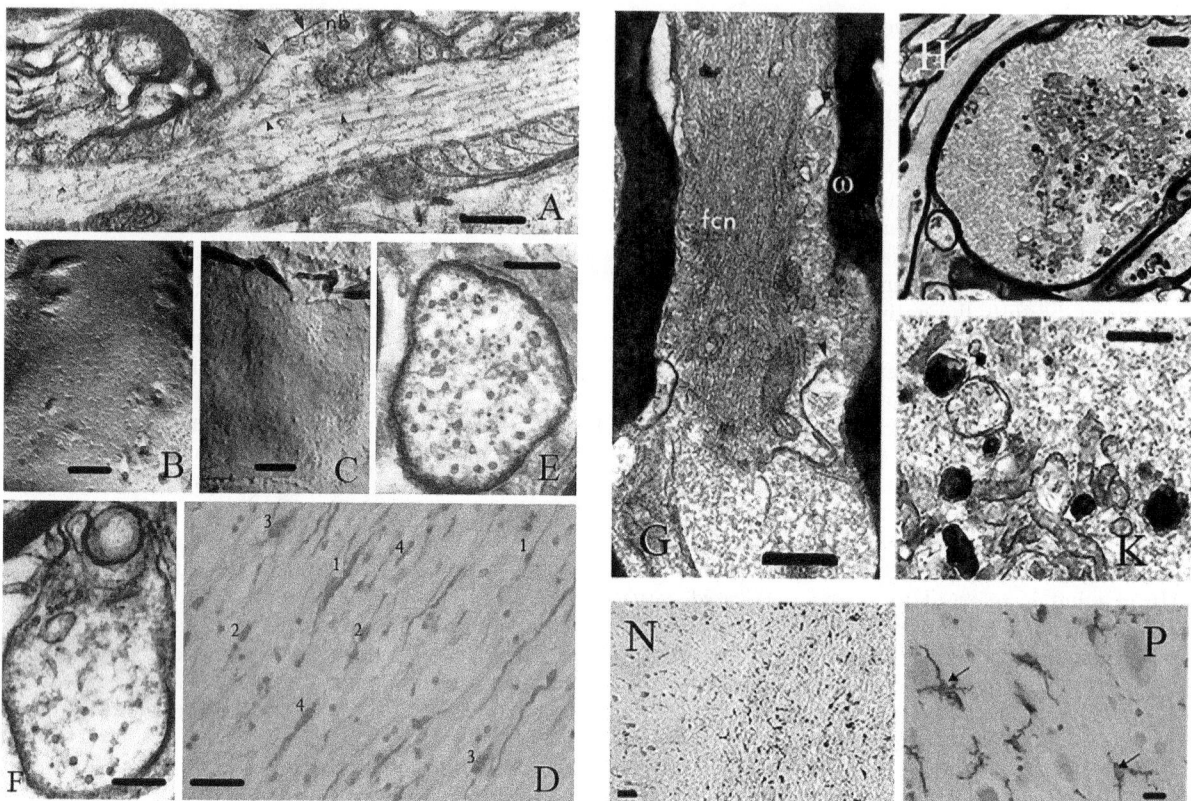

FIGURE 19–16 *See color insert.* A, A longitudinal thin section of an injured node of Ranvier at 15 minutes after stretch-injury to adult guinea pig optic nerve. A nodal bleb (*nb*) extends into the periaxonal space. This nodal bleb is limited by an intact plasmamembrane which lacks a subaxolemma density (*arrows*) and contains vesicular profiles. Axonal microtubules (*arrowheads*) extend axially but there is a suggestion of a reduced number of microtubules adjacent to the base of the nodal bleb compared to elsewhere in the axoplasm (*bar* = 0.5 μm). B and C, Freeze fracture replicas of the p-face of nodal axolemma of a control (B) and injured (C) nerve fiber. A differential number of intramembranous particles occur between the 2 replicas, which reflect changes in the structure of the membrane and numbers of ion transporters (*bar* = 300 nm). D, A field of a paraffin embedded block from the brain of a severely disabled patient 2 months after TBI. Injured or reactive axons are visualized by immunolabeling for β–amyloid precursor protein. Some axons (*1*) are in continuity and contain an axonal swelling. Others illustrate a central constriction (*2*) within the axonal swelling. Rounded swollen axonal bulbs (*3*) and truncated rod-like (*4*) bulbs occur at points of axotomy. Axons labeled (*3*) represent distal axonal swellings, (*4*) represent proximal axonal swellings (*bar* = 10 μm). E and F, Transverse thin sections of control (E) and injured (F) nodes of Ranvier. Specimen F was obtained at 15 minutes after stretch injury to optic nerve. The control specimen (E) contains many neurofilaments (*small, dark points*) and axonal microtubules (*small circular profiles*) distributed throughout the axoplasm cut in transverse section and therefore parallel to the longitudinal axis of the nerve fiber. The nodal axolemma is highlighted by the presence of the dark subaxolemma density. A nodal bleb containing membranous profiles extends toward the top of Figure 19-16F and is limited by plasmamembrane lacking subaxolemma density. There is a reduced number of widely spaced axonal neurofilaments and microtubules within the lower part of the nodal axoplasm. The decreased number of microtubules is indicative of a compromise in fast axonal transport (*bar* = 0.25 μm). G, A longitudinal thin section through a region of secondary axotomy or axonal disconnection from stretch-injured guinea pig optic nerve at 4 hours after injury. Parts of the electron dense myelin sheath are seen laterally. The upper part of the field contains a locus of compacted neurofilaments (*fcn*). These neurofilaments are absent at the bottom of the field and are replaced by a flocculent precipitate suggestive of neurofilament proteolysis. Irregular, fragmented membrane profiles occur thereby. To the left of ω occur numerous circular membrane profiles that replace a discrete axolemma and are suggestive of membrane fragmentation. Lucent, damaged mitochondria are also present (*bar* = 0.5 μm). H and K, Low magnification (H) and high magnification (K) fields of a swollen, rounded distal axonal swelling or retraction bulb at 6 days after injury. The center of the bulb contains aggregates of mitochondria, some of which (K) are lucent in structure reflecting mitochondrial damage, electron dense profiles of autophagic profiles, and a disorganized, sometimes flocculent structure of the filamentous cytoskeleton (*bar* in H = 1.0 μm and in K = 0.25 μm). N, A low power section of the corticomedullary junction in dorsolateral prefrontal cortex obtained at 8 months after TBI and immunolabeled (CR3/43 antibody) for the MHC class II marker in microglia. On the left of the field are large, pale grey unlabeled cells which are pyramidal neurons within layer 6 of the cortex. On the right is a superficial part of the white matter of subcortical tissue containing large numbers of immunolabeled microglia distributed along the length of axons. High power images (P) of microglia possessing lengthy branched cell processes indicative of a reactive state of these cells possibly suggesting removal of tissue remnants of degenerating axons.

aggregates of mitochondria with a normal appearance, axoplasmic reticulum, and a central spiral core of neurofilaments and microtubules. The distal swelling, on the contrary, is more rounded in profile; the axoplasm is relatively electron dense and contains damaged, dilated mitochondria lacking discrete cristae, aggregates of axoplasmic reticulum, and, by about a day after axotomy, groups of autophagic vesicles (65). All of this shows that what is imaged at the macroscopic DTI level of neuroimage analysis reflects the complex and multifaceted cellular pathology that underlies MRI images of the brain pathology.

In human TBI within just a few hours of injury is the common association of focal hemorrhage, probably caused by focal tissue tears, both within the posterior part of the corpus callosum and/or rostral brainstem. In addition, the occurrence of traumatic microbleeds (tMBs), defined as hemorrhagic lesions of the order of 1- to 5- mm diameter with no connection to the brain surface or the ventricular system, are frequently observed at the corticomedullary junction of frontal and temporal lobes and has increasingly been recognized by means of gradient-echo T2*-weighted (T2*-w) MRI (66), 2D and 3D gradient-recalled echo (GRE) (67), and susceptibility-weighted imaging (SWI) (68).

Deoxyhemoglobin and hematoma maturation into hemosiderin, frequently stored in macrophages, may be seen as areas of low intensity on MRI. A recent report (69) has indicated a differential distribution of microbleeds (tMBs) between patients with tMBs and after stroke. tMBs occurred in the midportion of subcortical cerebral hemispheres superior to the corpus callosum, the tectum of the midbrain, and the posterior part of the corpus callosum but were largely absent from the basal ganglia, pons, and cerebellum. Microangiopathic microbleeds (m-MB) after stroke, on the contrary, were frequent in the basal ganglia, thalamus pons and cerebellum, and the lateral parts of subcortical regions (69). It may be suggested that microbleeds increase in frequency with the age of a patient, microbleeds have a negative influence on outcome, and the distribution of tMB differs from those resulting from stroke and incipient cerebrovascular disease.

However, it is noteworthy that a considerable body of MRI literature indicates that an ongoing, low level of loss of axons within white matter may occur that is reflected in the now widely documented loss of white matter volume within cerebral hemispheres and other brain regions (32) discussed earlier. There is limited experimental literature in this area but quantitative evidence for a continued low-grade loss of myelinated nerve fibers from the optic nerve has recently been provided (47). Further investigation and quantitative analysis is required.

Strategic Loci of Traumatic Brain Injury Lesions

Since the 2007 edition of this chapter, image quantification methods have improved so significantly that TBI neuroimaging research has moved to direct examination of specific ROIs, pathways, and neural systems. The major ROIs that have yielded important insights to neuroimaging predictors of outcome are presented subsequently.

Thalamus

Maxwell et al. (70,71) in a postmortem investigation of patients who were moderately to severely disabled and vegeta-

tive following TBI demonstrated thalamic damage in the form of trauma induced neuronal degeneration, particularly notable in the dorsal medial nuclei. Both positron emission tomography (PET) (72) and DTI (73) studies have shown that the degree of thalamic abnormality during the more chronic stages of TBI correlates with increasing neuropsychological impairment in patients. Tollard et al. (74) showed that in severe TBI, the combination of DTI detected white matter abnormalities with MRS abnormalities in the thalamus assessed in the subacute timeframe (typically within a month postinjury) predicted poor outcome.

Long Tracts

Figure 19-17, from Wilde et al. (75), shows DTI tractography of the inferior occipitofrontal fasciculus, along with the cingulum bundle, and the inferior longitudinal fasciculus—several of the long tracts of the brain that can be identified with DTI (see 76). These long tracts are particularly vulnerable to injury from mechanical deformation and strain in response to blunt trauma, particularly with rotational movement (77). Given that these tracts are comprised of axons that are several centimeters in length also creates increased vulnerability to mechanical deformation (78). DTI studies examining outcome consistently show that damage within these tracts is associated with worse outcome (7,58,79–82).

DTI metrics provide objective markers of white matter integrity that can be applied to specific and individual tracts. For example, Bigler et al. (79) found robust correlations of up to 0.7 between memory function and the left inferior frontooccipital fasciculus using DTI metrics in a group of patients with moderate-to-severe TBI.

Limbic and Limbic-Associated Tracts

The fornix and cingulum bundle are the longest limbic tracts, but the mammillothalamic tract, tracts that input the hippocampus and hippocampal-amygdala pathways are all disrupted in TBI (83). All of these tracts play major roles in memory and emotional functioning, which of course, are common symptoms/problems of patients with TBI.

The tracts arising from the hippocampus that comprise the fornix have their major synaptic termination at the level of the mammillary bodies, which in turn send their input to the anterior thalamus via a short pathway, the mammillothalamic tract. Some fornix fibers also terminate in the septal nuclei. The mammillary bodies at the base of the brain are vulnerable to direct trauma (84), but probably the most common pathology involving the mammillothalamic tract are thought to result from Wallerian type degeneration (85). Although the mammillary bodies have been primarily considered to play a role mainly as a relay station, this has been reconsidered recently because the mammillary bodies also receive afferent input from other regions, most importantly from the frontal lobes and midbrain (86), leading Vann (87) to conclude that the mammillary body may have a more primary and independent role in memory (see also 88). Figure 19-18 shows an atrophied mammillary body in a case of severe TBI without focal lesion. Note also in the TBI brain there is discrete ventriculomegaly.

In a TBI study of children without focal limbic lesions, Wilde et al. (89) have shown that the frontal projections from the cingulum became thinned out. Several studies have dem-

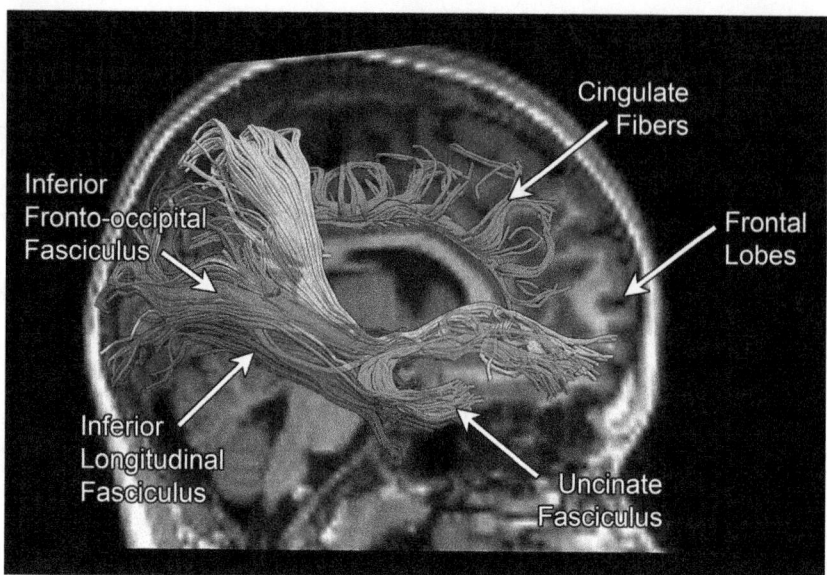

FIGURE 19–17 *See color insert.* Several major white matter tracts are depicted in this illustration.

onstrated involvement of the fornix in TBI showing altered white matter diffusion characteristics on DTI during the acute (90) as well as chronic stage (91).

The anterior commissure connects medial temporal lobe regions, in particular the amygdala across the 2 hemispheres. As shown by Wilde et al. (92) and graphically depicted in Figure 19-18, the anterior commissure is commonly affected, where DTI studies show reduced white matter tracts (93).

Although these are small tracts, they are critical ones that interconnect the two medial temporal lobes and right and left amygdala.

The uncinate fasciculus connects medial temporal lobe with the inferior frontal region, both areas vulnerable to injury (83,94). Niogi et al. (40) and Geary et al. (95) have shown that DTI relates to memory function in TBI; in addition, Johnson et al. (96) have shown that uncinate integrity predicts a

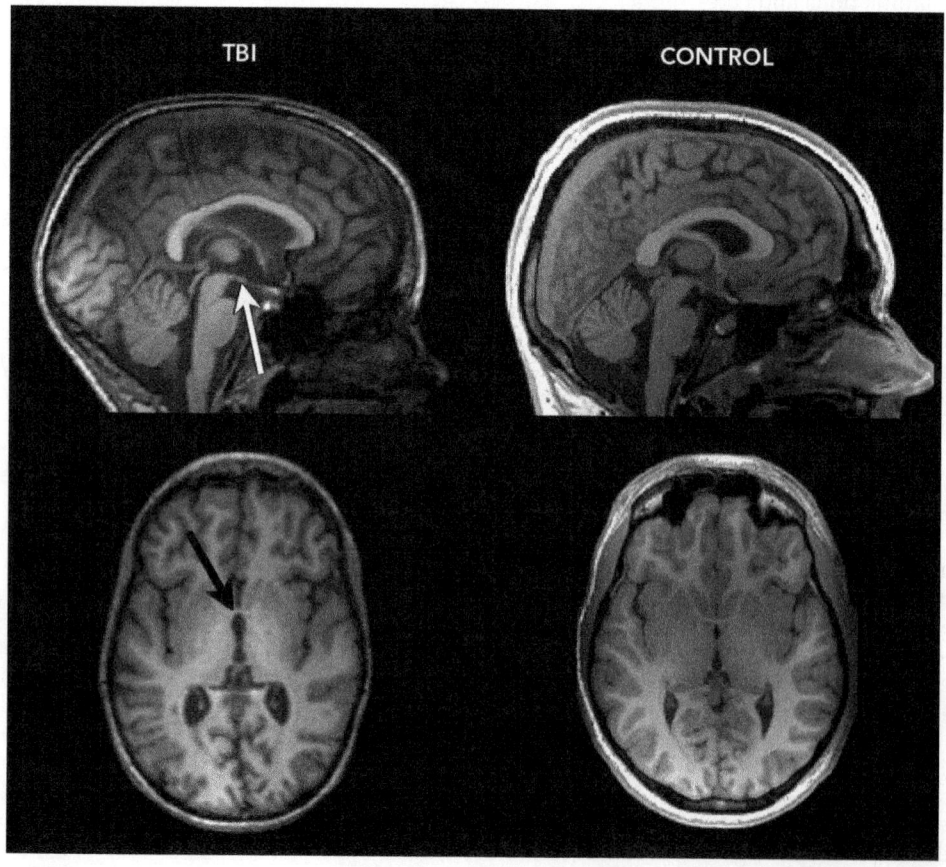

FIGURE 19–18 Mammillary atrophy in severe TBI (*white arrow*) with concomitant atrophy of the anterior commissure (*black arrow*). DTI images of these regions will also be shown.

broad spectrum of behavior deficits. Further, Smits et al. (97) have shown microstructural damage at the level of the uncinate in mild TBI.

Lesion Volume

A variety of traumatic lesions are commonplace in TBI as has been discussed in Chapter 12. Prior to methods like DTI, several studies were undertaken to categorize and localize just the lesions in attempting to predict outcome (see 93) with only limited success because lesion detection alone is only a course indicator of traumatic brain pathology (27). Nonetheless, one consistent general predictor of outcome is the size of acute lesion volume and the degree of midline shift. Jacobs et al. (98) in a large prospective study examined 605 patients demonstrating that on acute CT imaging absolute lesion volume and degree of midline shift were course predictors of outcome based on the Glasgow Outcome Scale (GOS), especially at the moderate-to-severe level of TBI. Similar findings have been reported by Chastain et al. (99). The single most consistent lesion-location predictor of poor TBI outcome is a brainstem lesion (53,57,100). As mentioned, these are but course outcome predictors since the GOS, and its more recent extension—the "extended" Glasgow Outcome Scale or GOS-E—range from dead, vegetative, severely disabled, moderately disabled, and good recovery. As such, the GOS or GOS-E do not capture more specific or subtle cognitive and behavioral deficits that accompany TBI. This is because the GOS was originally developed to allow assessment of function of the whole brain rather than to delineate focal changes.

In viewing Figure 19-19, it is straightforward to understand why larger hemorrhagic acute lesions, especially those that produce major midline shift, provide some general and global indicators of outcome. The problem comes when using neuroimaging to better predict outcome within specific neuropsychological domains such as memory, ex-

ecutive functioning, or even neuropsychiatric status. Global indicators of overall lesion volume or generalized measures of DBI, like global atrophy measures, are poor to only modest indicators of cognitive and behavioral outcome (15). Even taking in all of the nuances with lesion localization and size determination, the relationship to neuropsychological outcome has been disappointedly weak (101) to only modest at best (102).

The first issue why lesion size alone is a poor predictor of specific outcome within a cognitive domain following TBI relates to the different lesion types and their locations that occur in TBI, along with the fact that TBI often damages the brain distally to where the lesion being measured is located. Note, just in the examples given in this chapter that no 2 head injuries produce identical lesions. Furthermore, lesion boundaries differ depending on the MRI sequence and, therefore, the "size" of a lesion depends on the image sequence used. Returning to Figures 19-7 and 19-8 with the patient sustaining a focal frontal injury—the "size" of the lesion varies depending on which MRI sequence is used.

What lesion analysis alone misses is that basic measures of lesion volume are not a direct reflection of how a lesion may have disconnected pathways, both regionally within short distances of the lesion site, as well as globally. DTI methods are better suited for identifying white matter pathway disruption improving outcome predictions (5,7,103).

Given the neuroimaging technology of today, it is probably no longer useful to simply review a scan and even quantify volume of certain ROIs, as indicators of outcome. The cases presented earlier show that it is not just where a focal lesion may be, but how that lesion disrupts the network, how lesions produce focal, ipsilateral as well as contralateral, and entire network disruptions. Jirsa et al. (10) in a virtual connection model of a focal anterior cingulate lesion demonstrated an extensive disruption of the entire network of the brain, just from a singular lesion. In that TBI is comprised

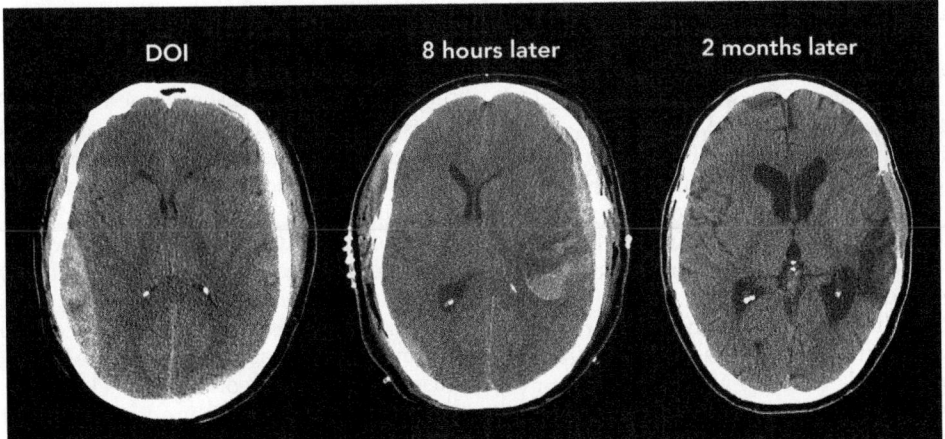

FIGURE 19–19 Day-of-injury (DOI) CT scan showing a large right hemisphere epidural hematoma and a smaller less distinct subdural **on the left**. After the right subdural was operated on, note that there was rebound bleeding and enlargement of the left subdural and occurrence of a massive intraparenchymal hemorrhage on the left, for which the patient was emergently reoperated on. Note in both the DOI and the 8-hour post-admission scans the mass effect, midline shift, and massive brain swelling. By 2 months later, global atrophy had developed along with focal encephalomalacia from the intraparenchymal hemorrhage on the left and the neurosurgical intervention.

of numerous lesion sites and potentially diffuse damage to white matter, it is no surprise that lesion analysis alone provides limited prediction of outcome because it cannot capture the complexities of the pathological issues of brain injury to predict outcome.

The limits of a singular image analysis approach compared to a multimodality approach was recently shown by Wilde et al. (75), where they compared quantitative and functional outcome measures that included ROI volume, ROI cortical thickness, DTI and fMRI activation, and neuropsychological outcome in moderate-to-severe pediatric TBI. Each neuroimaging method uniquely tapped a different aspect of pathology where no one method was superior in overall relationship to outcome. The Wilde et al. investigation demonstrated the importance of examining abnormal imaging findings across neuroimaging modalities but also how certain imaging modalities like DTI permit better detection of pathologies of disconnectivity in TBI and their relationship to a specific cognitive impairment.

Hemorrhagic Lesions

The case presented in Figure 19-5, 19-7, and 19-8 not only had diffuse white matter changes but also hemorrhagic lesions in the form of MRI-identified hemosiderin deposits. Hemorrhage is probably perivascular in the acute phase of TBI reflecting either mechanical damage to the wall of the microvessels within the brain at the time of injury or focal loss of the lining endothelium of capillaries (104). With increasing survival over 2–3 days, hemorrhage extends peripherally into juxtavascular or penumbral tissue and probably reflects incipient hypoxia/ischemia as a result of clot formation occluding or compromising perfusion through damaged vessels resulting in hypoxia and foci of ischemia. It is presently hypothesized that compromised supply of metabolites for production of ATP induce failure of membrane pumps and injury to mitochondria inducing further axons to form axonal swellings and undergo secondary axotomy. Axonal swellings and sites of axotomy increase in number over 15–18 hours and there is reactive change in capillary endothelium, astrocytes, and microglia.

It is noteworthy that damage to the capillary endothelium may result in loss of these cells and a consequent exacerbation of breakdown of the blood–brain barrier (BBB) (104,105). A progression toward a lucent or rarified lesion crossed by reactive astrocyte processes and hemosiderin containing macrophages occurs over days or a few weeks. During this phase, damaged axons fragment and their myelin sheath remnants are lost. At weeks or about 1 or possibly 2 months, active macrophages that aggregated within the lesion shortly after injury, regress to form microscopically definable groups or clumps of microglia within injured white matter and form the characteristic microglial clusters (106) within the white matter of patients who survive TBI by months or years.

Hemorrhagic lesions are common place in TBI and best detected by MR SWI sequence (107). Some forms of hemorrhagic lesions from small petechial to large hematomas were identified in 72% of patients with TBI with a GCS of 3–13 in a Scandinavian sample of 159 (57). The importance of hemorrhagic burden in predicting outcome has been shown by Babikian et al. (108) in a pediatric sample where they showed that total hemorrhagic lesion volume accounted for approximately 32% of the explained variance in predicting neuropsychological outcome. Presence of hemorrhage is probably

an important marker of TBI severity and occurrence of shear/strain injury to white matter as the volume of hemorrhage increases together with cortical contusions provide a total burden having some negative relationship to outcome (107,109). But in vivo demonstration of the number and distribution of microscopic level foci of hemorrhage, often termed petechial hemorrhages, has only recently been achieved with the realization that routine MRI techniques have been insensitive to tMBs of 5 mm or less in diameter.

The advent of SWI has allowed straightforward appreciation of microbleeds within subcortical tissues in the injured brain. It is possible, and probable, that the frequency and occurrence of tMB has been underestimated until very recently. A characterization of the cerebral distribution of tMB in a range of severities of patient outcome has not yet been published. Microvascular responses by capillary endothelium and the loss of damaged endothelium to form potential foci of breakdown of the BBB were reported in the early 1990s by Maxwell et al. (104,105) but have not until recently been an area of interest. In the light of recent developments, investigation of cerebrovascular and microvascular responses to TBI may now be a pertinent field for future investigation.

Edema and Neuroinflammation

The last point in this section on pathology is that injury to brain parenchyma produces an inflammatory response that may be acute as well as chronic (110,111). Initially, edema dominates the clinical picture as shown in Figure 19-19. Edema may congest the brain and disrupt blood flow, which may lead to cell death. The degree of initial cerebral edema coarsely relates to outcome. There are 2 mechanisms that generate edema within injured brain, vasogenic and cytotoxic edema. Vasogenic edema develops as a result of disruption of the extensive tight junctions between neighboring endothelial cells of capillaries and small vessels within the region of injury. Blood-hydrostatic pressure generated by the heart drives plasma and blood cells through gaps in the vessel wall into the perivascular space down a pressure gradient and small blood vessels may appear to be surrounded by a lucent halo or sleeve containing water, proteins, and cells that are normally excluded via the BBB.

Early work (104) following experimental lateral head acceleration in nonhuman primates reported that a short-term rise of intracranial pressure occurred followed by a reduction of both mean arterial blood pressure and cerebral perfusion pressure that, however, never dropped lower than the normal range. Formation of lucent perivascular astrocyte foot processes, endothelial microvilli, and pinocytotic vesicle development, has been related to localized inflammatory reactions in the vessel lining and probably reflects a compromise of the integrity of the BBB (112) that resolves as the BBB is reestablished. Cytotoxic edema manifests as an increase in water content inside cells resulting from an osmotic gradient. It is usually associated with failure of the ATP-dependent Na^+/K^+-pumps as a result of energy failure. In cerebral ischemia, anoxic-ischemic encephalopathy, and severe TBI blood flow to the injured brain is reduced and the delivery of O_2 and glucose falls lower than levels necessary to maintain normal cellular activity.

Mitochondrial injury prevents or compromises generation of ATP and the related transmembrane pumps fail. This leads to an abnormal content of intracellular ions and of cell osmolarity, and results in marked influx of water into cells from the extracellular space. Cytotoxic edema does not result in the brain content of water or swelling of the brain because the water moves from the extracellular to the intracellular compartments. But cytotoxic edema does compromise cellular function and depolarization of neurons, for example, may release massive amounts of neurotransmitters which are so high as to be toxic to cells within the brain. (113) But, if some degree of cerebral circulation remains or recovers, then additional water is supplied to the compromised part of the brain and vasogenic edema exacerbates the situation. Brain swelling will then result and intracranial pressure (Figure 19-19) will rise and the combination has been suggested to account for up to half of the mortality in victims of TBI. The previous discussion demonstrates the underlying complexity of the pathological changes associated with brain edema when detected in neuroimaging studies.

The Integration of Structural and Functional Imaging

The image of the brain generated by CT or MRI only represents gross brain structure. Although in the living individual, structure is never devoid of function, neither CT nor MRI structural imaging provides a direct measure of function. However, as explained in Chapter 16 on functional imaging in this book, the principles of structural imaging can be applied to obtain functional measures of the brain. As already discussed, when structural changes are detected, they merely depict where the macroscopic abnormalities are and not necessarily the totality of neural areas or systems that may be disrupted. Although at first blush this may seem straightforward, each method of brain image analysis whether assessing functional or structural relationships, probably tap unique aspects of brain function. As such, depending on the ROI, the neuroimaging method to measure the ROI and the methods to assess function or outcome findings postinjury vary. This was discussed earlier in the Wilde et al. (75) investigation which showed distinctly different outcome relationships following TBI dependent on whether the imaging metric was volume, cortical thickness, DTI, or fMRI, and which ROI examined.

These types of multimodality quantitative morphometric and neuroimaging studies are showing considerable promise in predicting TBI outcome (1,14,114). One key to this research will likely be using acute and subacute imaging findings to establish a baseline which, in turn, permit tracking pathological effects over time that may yield better predictions (74,115).

In summary, the mere presence of imaging abnormalities from trauma has only limited ability as predictors of functional outcome. What may appear straightforward (i.e., simply comparing "lesions" or counting their number to outcome) actually represents a very complex clinical question that depends on the imaging type and modality and the time postinjury. With DTI, clinical and cognitive neuroscience is moving in the direction of examining entire neural networks and brain connectivity where DTI methods hold great promise as better predictors of outcome. The capacity to use DTI to attempt to predict outcome for a particular patient is also limited by whether application of several specialized methods of MRI analysis has been undertaken and

the fact that analysis of images obtained at just 1 point after injury provides little information about the progression of neuropathology within that patient's brain. Such insight may only be obtained using sequential analysis of a series of scans during post-traumatic survival.

CONCLUSION

When first recognized in the middle of the last century, TBI was thought to represent an immediate cellular response to a single traumatic insult. Research over the last 50 years and in particular since the availability of noninvasive MRI techniques that allow examination of the living patient has generated a consensus that cellular responses within the injured brain are initiated or influenced by a range of factors that interacts with 1 or several cell types both at the initial locus of injury and extensively throughout the brain and that degenerative responses are both widespread and continue for possibly years or more after TBI. Although the initial focus of damage is to axons passing through white matter, it is now apparent that responses occur within the cell soma and the dendritic tree of a neuron. In some cases, an injured neuron may recover when injury is mild. But if injury is severe enough, the injured axon may enter the "pathological cascade" that terminates in secondary axotomy. But MRI and DTI imaging technology still lacks resolution to allow examination or identification of single injured nerve fibers. Thus the capacity to make a clinical diagnosis of mTBI in the acute or postacute phases is still not possible using just MRI techniques. However, the capacity of MRI to monitor changes in water diffusion and structural volume of white and gray matter in vivo is a considerable advance although limited to zones at which large numbers of axons or neurons have been affected.

Study of the brain of a patient with suspected TBI using only a single MRI modality is of little diagnostic value. Rather a range of different MRI techniques should be used. It is now appreciated that TBI does not only reflect injury to neurons but also injury to the microvasculature of the injured brain. MRI techniques like the SWI sequence allow resolution of microhemorrhages at the acute phase as well as detection of hemosiderin deposition in the chronic phase, important indicators that vascular injury is a component of TBI.

The spatial distribution and number of foci of structural abnormalities within the injured brain varies markedly between different patients and may, tentatively, be closely associated with possible outcomes in terms of behavioral and functional outcomes. Only a detailed appraisal of the 3-dimensional distribution of foci of injury such as reduced FA or increased diffusivity together with an appreciation of the fields of origin and termination of injured fibers combined with the volume of parenchymal damage will allow any confidence in prediction of patient outcome.

KEY CLINICAL POINTS

1. TBI disrupts white matter acutely at an initial physiological level. A structural disruption occurs thereafter that may disconnect functional cortical areas.
2. Loss of ionic homeostatis of the axolemma and associated injury to axonal mitochondria are key to the development of subsequent pathology.

3. Neuroimaging detects a pathology that arises from a complex cellular pathology across tens or hundreds of nerve fibers.
4. Contemporary research level neuroimaging methods allow resolution of foci of neuropathology at close to a microscopic level of resolution.
5. Contemporary multimodal methods of neuroimaging rather than use of a single imaging technique allows a more rigorous estimation of damage and functional impairment occurring after TBI.
6. Repeated, sequential neuroimaging assays allow increased confidence in prediction of outcomes in a patient with TBI.

KEY REFERENCES

1. Haacke EM, Duhaime AC, Gean AD, et al. Common data elements in radiologic imaging of traumatic brain injury. *J Magn Reson Imaging*. 2010;32(3):516–543.
2. Hunter JV, Wilde EA, Tong KA, Holshouser BA. Emerging imaging tools for use with traumatic brain injury research. *J Neurotrauma*. 2012;29(4):654–671.
3. Sharp DJ, Beckmann CF, Greenwood R, et al. Default mode network functional and structural connectivity after traumatic brain injury. *Brain*. 201;134:511–518.
4. Tomaiuolo F, Bivona U, Lerch, JP, et al. Memory and anatomical change in severe non missile traumatic brain injury: 1 vs. 8 years follow-up. *Brain Res Bull*. 2012;87(4–5):373–382.
5. Wang JY, Bakhadirov K, Abdi H, et al. Longitudinal changes of structural connectivity in traumatic axonal injury. *Neurology*. 2011;77(9):818–826.

ACKNOWLEDGEMENT

The assistance of Tracy Abildskov in image preparation is gratefully acknowledged.

References

1. Bigler ED, Wilde EA. Quantitative neuroimaging and the prediction of rehabilitation outcome following traumatic brain injury. *Front Hum Neurosci*. 2010;4:228.
2. Filley CM. White matter: organization and functional relevance. *Neuropsychol Rev*. 2010;20(2):158–173.
3. Filley CM. White matter: beyond focal disconnection. *Neurol Clin*. 2011;29(1):81–97, viii.
4. Gasparetto EL, Rueda Lopes FC, Domingues RC. Diffusion imaging in traumatic brain injury. *Neuroimaging Clin N Am*. 2011;21(1):115–125, viii.
5. Kinnunen KM, Greenwood R, Powell JH, et al. White matter damage and cognitive impairment after traumatic brain injury. *Brain*. 2011;134(pt 2):449–463.
6. Matsushita M, Hosoda K, Naitoh Y, Yamashita H, Kohmura E. Utility of diffusion tensor imaging in the acute stage of mild to moderate traumatic brain injury for detecting white matter lesions and predicting long-term cognitive function in adults. *J Neurosurg*. 2011;115(1):130–139.
7. Newcombe V, Chatfield D, Outtrim J, et al. Mapping traumatic axonal injury using diffusion tensor imaging: correlations with functional outcome. *PLoS One*. 2011;6(5):e19214.
8. Castellanos NP, Leyva I, Buldú JM, et al. Principles of recovery from traumatic brain injury: reorganization of functional networks. *Neuroimage*. 2011;55(3):1189–1199.
9. Hillary FG, Slocomb J, Hills EC, et al. Changes in resting connectivity during recovery from severe traumatic brain injury. *Int J Psychophysiol*. 2011;82(1):115–123.
10. Jirsa VK, Sporns O, Breakspear M, Deco G, McIntosh AR. Towards the virtual brain: network modeling of the intact and the damaged brain. *Arch Ital Biol*. 2010;148(3):189–205.
11. Friston KJ. Modalities, modes, and models in functional neuroimaging. *Science*. 2009;326(5951):399–403.
12. Bigler ED, Abildskov TJ, Wilde EA, et al. Diffuse damage in pediatric traumatic brain injury: a comparison of automated versus operator-controlled quantification methods. *Neuroimage*. 2010;50(3):1017–1026.
13. Brewer JB. Fully-automated volumetric MRI with normative ranges: translation to clinical practice. *Behav Neurol*. 2009;21(1):21–28.
14. Strangman GE, O'Neil-Pirozzi TM, Supelana C, Goldstein R, Katz DI, Glenn MB. Regional brain morphometry predicts memory rehabilitation outcome after traumatic brain injury. *Front Hum Neurosci*. 2010;4:182.
15. Tate DF, Khedraki R, Neeley ES, Ryser DK, Bigler ED. Cerebral volume loss, cognitive deficit, and neuropsychological performance: comparative measures of brain atrophy: II. Traumatic brain injury. *J Int Neuropsychol Soc*. 2011;17(2):308–316.
16. Talairach JT, Tournoux P. *Co-Planar Stereotaxic Atlas of the Human Brain: 3-Dimensional Proportional System: An Approach to Cerebral Imaging*. New York, NY: Thieme Medical Publishers; 1988.
17. Frey S, Pandya DN, Chakravarty MM, Bailey L, Petrides M, Collins DL. An MRI based average macaque monkey stereotaxic atlas and space (MNI monkey space). *Neuroimage*. 2011;55(4):1435–1442.
18. Gale SD, Prigatano GP. Deep white matter volume loss and social reintegration after traumatic brain injury in children. *J Head Trauma Rehabil*. 2010;25(1):15–22.
19. Slawik H, Salmond CH, Taylor-Tavares JV, Williams GB, Sahakian BJ, Tasker RC. Frontal cerebral vulnerability and executive deficits from raised intracranial pressure in child traumatic brain injury. *J Neurotrauma*. 2009;26(11):1891–1903.
20. Vannorsdall TD, Cascella NG, Rao V, Pearlson GD, Gordon B, Schretlen DJ. A morphometric analysis of neuroanatomic abnormalities in traumatic brain injury. *J Neuropsychiatry Clin Neurosci*. 2010;22(2):173–181.
21. Azevedo FA, Carvalho LR, Grinberg LT, et al. Equal numbers of neuronal and nonneuronal cells make the human brain an isometrically scaled-up primate brain. *J Comp Neurol*. 2009;513(5):532–541.
22. van de Looij Y, Mauconduit F, Beaumont M, et al. Diffusion tensor imaging of diffuse axonal injury in a rat brain trauma model. *NMR Biomed*. 2012;25(1):93–103.
23. Mac Donald CL, Dikranian K, Song SK, Bayly PV, Holtzman DM, Brody DL. Detection of traumatic axonal injury with diffusion tensor imaging in a mouse model of traumatic axonal injury. *Exp Neurol*. 2007;205(1):116–131.
24. Graham DI, Teasdale GT, McIntosh TK. *Trauma*. In: Graham DI Lantos LP, (Eds). *Greenfield's Neuropathology*. 7th Ed, Vol 1. London, England: Hodder Arnold Headline Group 2002.
25. Povlishock JT, Katz DI. Update of neuropathology and neurological recovery after traumatic brain injury. *J Head Trauma Rehabil*. 2005;20(1):76–94.
26. Smith DH, Meaney DF, Shull WH. Diffuse axonal injury in head trauma. *J Head Trauma Rehabil*. 2003;18(4):307–316.
27. Bigler ED. Structural imaging. In: Silver JM, McAllister TW, Yudofsky SC, eds. *Textbook of Traumatic Brain Injury*. 2nd ed. Washington, DC: American Psychiatric Publishing Inc; 2011:73–90.
28. Maxwell WL, MacKinnon MA, Stewart JE, Graham DI. Stereology of cerebral cortex after traumatic brain injury matched to the Glasgow outcome score. *Brain*. 2010;133(pt 1):139–160.
29. Merkley TL, Bigler ED, Wilde EA, McCauley SR, Hunter JV, Levin HS. Diffuse changes in cortical thickness in pediatric moderate-to-severe traumatic brain injury. *J Neurotrauma*. 2008;25(11):1343–1345.
30. Wilde EA, McCauley SR, Hunter JV, et al. Diffusion tensor imaging of acute mild traumatic brain injury in adolescents. *Neurology*. 2008;70(12):948–955.

31. Adams JH, Jennett B, Murray LS, Teasdale GM, Gennarelli TA, Graham DI. Neuropathological findings in disabled survivors of a head injury. *J Neurotrauma*. 2011;28(5):701–709.

32. Mamere AE, Saraiva LA, Matos AL, Carniero AA, Santos AC. Evaluation of delayed neuronal and axonal damage secondary to moderate and severe traumatic brain injury using quantitative MR imaging techniques. *AJNR Am J Neuroradiol*. 2009;30(5):947–952.

33. Thomson AM, Bannister AP. Interlaminar connections in the neocortex. *Cereb Cortex*. 2003;13(1):5–14.

34. Lewis DA. Structure of the human prefrontal cortex. *Am J Psychiatry*. 2004;161(8):1366.

35. Mori S, Kaufmann WE, Davatzikos C, et al. Imaging cortical association tracts in the human brain using diffusion-tensor-based axonal tracking. *Magn Reson Med*. 2002;47(2):215–223.

36. Schmahmann JD, Pandya DN, Wang R, et al. Association fibre pathways of the brain: parallel observations from diffusion spectrum imaging and autoradiography. *Brain*. 2007;130(pt 3):630–653.

37. Kraus MF, Susmaras T, Caughlin BP, Walker CJ, Sweeney JA, Little DM. White matter integrity and cognition in chronic traumatic brain injury: a diffusion tensor imaging study. *Brain*. 2007;130(pt 10):2508–2519.

38. Bush G, Luu P, Posner MI. Cognitive and emotional influences in anterior cingulate cortex. *Trends Cogn Sci*. 2000;4(6):215–222.

39. Hofman PA, Verhey FR, Wilmink JT, Rozendaal N, Jolles J. Brain lesions in patients visiting a memory clinic with postconcussional sequelae after mild to moderate brain injury. *J Neuropsychiatry Clin Neurosci*. 2002;14(2):176–184.

40. Niogi SN, Mukherjee P, Ghajar J, et al. Structural dissociation of attentional control and memory in adults with and without mild traumatic brain injury. *Brain*. 2008;131(pt 12):3209–3221.

41. Tomaiuolo F, Worsley KJ, Lerch J, et al. Changes in white matter in long-term survivors of severe non-missile traumatic brain injury: a computational analysis of magnetic resonance images. *J Neurotrauma*. 2005;22(1):76–82.

42. Kumar R, Husain M, Gupta RK, et al. Serial changes in the white matter diffusion tensor imaging metrics in moderate traumatic brain injury and correlation with neuro-cognitive function. *J Neurotrauma*. 2009;26(4):481–495.

43. Cohen BA, Inglese M, Rusinek H, Babb JS, Grossman RI, Gonen O. Proton MR spectroscopy and MRI-volumetry in mild traumatic brain injury. *AJNR Am J Neuroradiol*. 2007;28(5):907–913.

44. Fujiwara E, Schwartz ML, Gao F, Black SE, Levine B. Ventral frontal cortex functions and quantified MRI in traumatic brain injury. *Neuropsychologia*. 2008;46(2):461–474.

45. Gao X, Chen J. Mild traumatic brain injury results in extensive neuronal degeneration in the cerebral cortex. *J Neuropathol Exp Neurol*. 2011;70(3):183–191.

46. Zhang D, Snyder AZ, Fox MD, Sansbury MW, Shimony JS, Raichle ME. Intrinsic functional relations between human cerebral cortex and thalamus. *J Neurophysiol*. 2008;100(4):1740–1748.

47. Mohammed Sulaiman A, Denman N, Buchanan S, et al. Stereology and ultrastructure of chronic phase axonal and cell soma pathology in stretch-injured central nerve fibers. *J Neurotrauma*. 2011;28(3):383–400.

48. Hall ED, Sullivan PG, Gibson TR, Pavel KM, Thompson BM, Scheff SW. Spatial and temporal characteristics of neurodegeneration after controlled cortical impact in mice: more than a focal brain injury. *J Neurotrauma*. 2005;22(2):252–265.

49. Pullela R, Raber J, Pfankuch T, et al. Traumatic injury to the immature brain results in progressive neuronal loss, hyperactivity and delayed cognitive impairments. *Dev Neurosci*. 2006;28(4–5):396–409.

50. Raghupathi R. Cell death mechanisms following traumatic brain injury. *Brain Pathol*. 2004;14(2):215–222.

51. Williams S, Raghupathi R, MacKinnon MA, McIntosh TK, Saatman KE, Graham DI. In situ DNA fragmentation occurs in white matter up to 12 months after head injury in man. *Acta Neuropathol*. 2001;102(6):581–590.

52. Farkas O, Povlishock JT. Cellular and subcellular change evoked by diffuse traumatic brain injury: a complex web of change extending far beyond focal damage. *Prog Brain Res*. 2007;161:43–59.

53. Bigler ED, Ryser DK, Gandhi P, Kimball J, Wilde EA. Day-of-injury computerized tomography, rehabilitation status, and development of cerebral atrophy in persons with traumatic brain injury. *Am J Phys Med Rehabil*. 2006;85(10):793–806.

54. Ghosh A, Wilde EA, Hunter JV, et al. The relation between Glasgow Coma Scale score and later cerebral atrophy in paediatric traumatic brain injury. *Brain Inj*. 2009;23(3):228–233.

55. Wilde EA, Bigler ED, Pedroza C, Ryser DK. Post-traumatic amnesia predicts long-term cerebral atrophy in traumatic brain injury. *Brain Inj*. 2006;20(7):695–699.

56. Himanen L, Portin R, Isoniemi H, Helenius H, Kurki T, Tenovuo O. Cognitive functions in relation to MRI findings 30 years after traumatic brain injury. *Brain Inj*. 2005;19(2):93–100.

57. Skandsen T, Kvistad KA, Solheim O, Strand IH, Folvik M, Vik A. Prevalence and impact of diffuse axonal injury in patients with moderate and severe head injury: a cohort study of early magnetic resonance imaging findings and 1-year outcome. *J Neurosurg*. 2010;113(3):556–563.

58. Ljungqvist J, Nilsson D, Ljungberg M, et al. Longitudinal study of the diffusion tensor imaging properties of the corpus callosum in acute and chronic diffuse axonal injury. *Brain Inj*. 2011;25(4):370–378.

59. Matsukawa H, Shinoda M, Fujii M, et al. Genu of corpus callosum in diffuse axonal injury induces a worse 1-year outcome in patients with traumatic brain injury. *Acta Neurochir (Wien)*. 2011;153(8):1687–1693.

60. Wu TC, Wilde EA, Bigler ED, et al. Longitudinal changes in the corpus callosum following pediatric traumatic brain injury. *Dev Neurosci*. 2010;32(5–6):361–373.

61. Lazar M. Mapping brain anatomical connectivity using white matter tractography. *NMR Biomed*. 2010;23(7):821–835.

62. Tournier JD, Mori S, Leemans A. Diffusion tensor imaging and beyond. *Magn Reson Med*. 2011;65(6):1532–1556.

63. Barrientos SA, Martinez NW, Yoo S, et al. Axonal degeneration is mediated by the mitochondrial permeability transition pore. *J Neurosci*. 2011;31(3):966–978.

64. Maxwell WL, Povlishock JT, Graham DL. A mechanistic analysis of nondisruptive axonal injury: a review. *J Neurotrauma*. 1997;14(7):419–440.

65. Wang J, Hamm RJ, Povlishock JT. Traumatic axonal injury in the optic nerve: evidence for axonal swelling, disconnection, dieback, and reorganization. *J Neurotrauma*. 2011;28(7):1185–1198.

66. Scheid R, Preul C, Gruber O, Wiggins C, von Cramon DY. Diffuse axonal injury associated with chronic traumatic brain injury: evidence from T2*-weighted gradient-echo imaging at 3 T. *AJNR Am J Neuroradiol*. 2003;24(6):1049–1056.

67. Hammond KE, Lupo JM, Xu D, et al. Microbleed detection in traumatic brain injury at 3T and 7T; comparing 2D and 3D gradient-recalled echo (GRE) imaging with susceptibility-weighted imaging (SWI). *Proc Intl Soc Mag Reson Med*. 2009;17:248.

68. Park JH, Park SW, Kang SH, Nam TK, Min BK, Hwang SN. Detection of traumatic cerebral microbleeds by susceptibility-weighted image of MRI. *J Korean Neurosurg Soc*. 2009;46(4):365–369.

69. Imaizumi T, Miyata K, Inamura S, Kohama I, Nyon KS, Nomura T. The difference in location between traumatic cerebral microbleeds and microangiopathic microbleeds associated with stroke. *J Neuroimaging*. 2011;21(4):359–364.

70. Maxwell WL, MacKinnon MA, Smith DH, McIntosh TK, Graham DI. Thalamic nuclei after human blunt head injury. *J Neuropathol Exp Neurol*. 2006;65(5):478–488.

71. Maxwell WL, Pennington K, MacKinnon MA, et al. Differential responses in three thalamic nuclei in moderately disabled, severely disabled and vegetative patients after blunt head injury. *Brain*. 2004;127(pt 11):2470–2478.

72. Kawai N, Maeda Y, Kudomi N, Yamamoto Y, Nishiyama Y, Tamiya T. Focal neuronal damage in patients with neuropsychological impairment after diffuse traumatic brain injury: evaluation using ^{11}C-flumazenil positron emission tomography with statistical image analysis. *J Neurotrauma*. 2010;27(12):2131–2138.

73. Little DM, Kraus MF, Joseph J, et al. Thalamic integrity underlies executive dysfunction in traumatic brain injury. *Neurology*. 2010;74(7):558–564.

74. Tollard E, Galanaud D, Perlbarg V, et al. Experience of diffusion tensor imaging and 1H spectroscopy for outcome prediction in severe traumatic brain injury: preliminary results. *Crit Care Med.* 2009;37(4):1448–1455.

75. Wilde EA, Newsome MR, Bigler ED, et al. Brain imaging correlates of verbal working memory in children following traumatic brain injury. *Int J Psychophysiol.* 2011;82(1):86–96.

76. Catani M, Thiebaut de Schotten M. A diffusion tensor imaging tractography atlas for virtual in vivo dissections. *Cortex.* 2008;44(8):1105–1132.

77. Wright RM, Ramesh KT. An axonal strain injury criterion for traumatic brain injury. *Biomech Model Mechanobiol.* 2011;11(1–2):245–260.

78. Mao H, Guan F, Han X, Yang KH. Strain-based regional traumatic brain injury intensity in controlled cortical impact: a systematic numerical analysis. *J Neurotrauma.* 2011;28(11):2263–2276.

79. Bigler ED, McCauley SR, Wu TC, et al. The temporal stem in traumatic brain injury: preliminary findings. *Brain Imaging Behav.* 2010; 4(3–4):270–282.

80. Mayer AR, Ling J, Mannell MV, et al. A prospective diffusion tensor imaging study in mild traumatic brain injury. *Neurology.* 2010;74(8):643–650.

81. Messé A, Caplain S, Paradot G, et al. Diffusion tensor imaging and white matter lesions at the subacute stage in mild traumatic brain injury with persistent neurobehavioral impairment. *Hum Brain Mapp.* 2011;32(6):999–1011.

82. Tasker RC, Westland AG, White DK, Williams GB. Corpus callosum and inferior forebrain white matter microstructure are related to functional outcome from raised intracranial pressure in child traumatic brain injury. *Dev Neurosci.* 2010;32(5–6):374–384.

83. Bigler ED. Anterior and middle cranial fossa in traumatic brain injury: relevant neuroanatomy and neuropathology in the study of neuropsychological outcome. *Neuropsychology.* 2007;21(5):515–531.

84. Saeki N, Sunami K, Kubota M, et al. Heavily T2-weighted MR imaging of white matter tracts in the hypothalamus: normal and pathologic demonstrations. *AJNR Am J Neuroradiol.* 2001;22(8):1468–1475.

85. Ng SE, Lau TN, Hui FK, et al. MRI of the fornix and mamillary body in temporal lobe epilepsy. *Neuroradiology.* 1997;39(8):551–555.

86. L'Vovich AI. Descending pathways of the frontal lobe cortex to nuclei of the hypothalamic mamillary bodies in craniocerebral trauma in humans. *Neurosci Behav Physiol.* 2001;31(4):371–374.

87. Vann SD. Re-evaluating the role of the mammillary bodies in memory. *Neuropsychologia.* 2010;48(8):2316–2327.

88. Tsivilis D, Vann SD, Denby C, et al. A disproportionate role for the fornix and mammillary bodies in recall versus recognition memory. *Nat Neurosci.* 2008;11(7):834–842.

89. Wilde EA, Ramos MA, Yallampalli R, et al. Diffusion tensor imaging of the cingulum bundle in children after traumatic brain injury. *Dev Neuropsychol.* 2010;35(3):333–351.

90. Yallampalli R, Wilde EA, Bigler ED, et al. Acute white matter differences in the fornix following mild traumatic brain injury using diffusion tensor imaging [published online ahead of print November 17, 2010]. *J Neuroimaging.*

91. Palacios EM, Fernandez-Espejo D, Junque C, et al. Diffusion tensor imaging differences relate to memory deficits in diffuse traumatic brain injury. *BMC Neurol.* 2011;11:24.

92. Wilde EA, Bigler ED, Haider JM, et al. Vulnerability of the anterior commissure in moderate to severe pediatric traumatic brain injury. *J Child Neurol.* 2006;21(9):769–776.

93. Bigler ED. Neuroimaging correlates of functional outcome. In: Zasler ND, Katz DI, Zafonte RD, eds. *Brain Injury Medicine: Principles and Practice.* New York, NY: Demos Medical Publishing; 2007.

94. Singh M, Jeong J, Hwang D, Sungkarat W, Gruen P. Novel diffusion tensor imaging methodology to detect and quantify injured regions and affected brain pathways in traumatic brain injury. *Magn Reson Imaging.* 2010;28(1):22–40.

95. Geary EK, Kraus MF, Pliskin NH, Little DM. Verbal learning differ-

ences in chronic mild traumatic brain injury. *J Int Neuropsychol Soc.* 2010;16(3):506–516.

96. Johnson CP, Juranek J, Kramer LA, Prasad MR, Swank PR, Ewing-Cobbs L. Predicting behavioral deficits in pediatric traumatic brain injury through uncinate fasciculus integrity. *J Int Neuropsychol Soc.* 2011:1–11.

97. Smits M, Houston GC, Dippel DW, et al. Microstructural brain injury in post-concussion syndrome after minor head injury. *Neuroradiology.* 2011;53(8):553–563.

98. Jacobs B, Beems T, van der Vliet TM, Diaz-Arrastia RR, Borm GF, Vos PE. Computed tomography and outcome in moderate and severe traumatic brain injury: hematoma volume and midline shift revisited. *J Neurotrauma.* 2011;28(2):203–215.

99. Chastain CA, Oyoyo UE, Zipperman M, et al. Predicting outcomes of traumatic brain injury by imaging modality and injury distribution. *J Neurotrauma.* 2009;26(8):1183–1196.

100. Calvi MR, Beretta L, Dell'Acqua A, Anzalone N, Licini G, Gemma M. Early prognosis after severe traumatic brain injury with minor or absent computed tomography scan lesions. *J Trauma.* 2011;70(2):447–451.

101. Scheid R, von Cramon DY. Clinical findings in the chronic phase of traumatic brain injury: data from 12 years' experience in the Cognitive Neurology Outpatient Clinic at the University of Leipzig. *Dtsch Arztebl Int.* 2010;107(12):199–205.

102. Schönberger M, Ponsford J, Reutens D, Beare R, O'Sullivan R. The Relationship between age, injury severity, and MRI findings after traumatic brain injury. *J Neurotrauma.* 2009;26(12):2157–2167.

103. Perlbarg V, Puybasset L, Tollard E, Lehéricy S, Benali H, Galanaud D. Relation between brain lesion location and clinical outcome in patients with severe traumatic brain injury: a diffusion tensor imaging study using voxel-based approaches. *Hum Brain Mapp.* 2009;30(12):3924–3933.

104. Maxwell WL, Whitfield PC, Suzen B, et al. The cerebrovascular response to experimental lateral head acceleration. *Acta Neuropathol.* 1992;84(3):289–296.

105. Maxwell WL, Irvine A, Watt C, Graham DI, Adams JH, Gennarelli TA. The microvascular response to stretch injury in the adult guinea pig visual system. *J Neurotrauma.* 1991;8(4):271–279.

106. Adams JH, Doyle D, Ford I, Gennarelli TA, Graham DI, McLellan DR. Diffuse axonal injury in head injury: definition, diagnosis and grading. *Histopathology.* 1989;15(1):49–59.

107. Kou Z, Wu Z, Tong KA, et al. The role of advanced MR imaging findings as biomarkers of traumatic brain injury. *J Head Trauma Rehabil.* 2010;25(4):267–282.

108. Babikian T, Freier MC, Tong KA, et al. Susceptibility weighted imaging: neuropsychologic outcome and pediatric head injury. *Pediatr Neurol.* 2005;33(3):184–194.

109. Li XY, Feng DF. Diffuse axonal injury: novel insights into detection and treatment. *J Clin Neurosci.* 2009;16(5):614–619.

110. Gentleman SM, Leclercq PD, Moyes L, et al. Long-term intracerebral inflammatory response after traumatic brain injury. *Forensic Sci Int.* 2004;146(2–3):97–104.

111. Ramlackhansingh AF, Brooks DJ, Greenwood RJ, et al. Inflammation after trauma: Microglial activation and traumatic brain injury. *Ann Neurol.* 2011;70(3):374–383.

112. Vajtr D, Benada O, Kukacka J, et al. Correlation of ultrastructural changes of endothelial cells and astrocytes occurring during blood brain barrier damage after traumatic brain injury with biochemical markers of BBB leakage and inflammatory response. *Physiol Res.* 2009;58(2):263–268.

113. Donkin JJ, Vink R. Mechanisms of cerebral edema in traumatic brain injury: therapeutic developments. *Curr Opin Neurol.* 2010;23(3):293–299.

114. Strangman GE, O'Neil-Pirozzi TM, Goldstein R, et al. Prediction of memory rehabilitation outcomes in traumatic brain injury by using functional magnetic resonance imaging. *Arch Phys Med Rehabil.* 2008;89(5):974–981.

115. Nichol AD, Toal F, Fedi M, Cooper DJ. Early outcome prediction after severe traumatic brain injury: can multimodal magnetic resonance imaging assist in clinical prognostication for individual patients? *Crit Care Resusc.* 2011;13(1):5–8.

Functional Assessment in Traumatic Brain Injury Rehabilitation

Marcel P.J.M. Dijkers and Brian D. Greenwald

INTRODUCTION

Chronic disease and injury often result in difficulties performing day-to-day activities because of physical, cognitive, and/or emotional impairments. The process of determining the type and degree of such problems or the ability to perform normal acts, activities, and roles is typically designated as "functional assessment" (FA). This is a misnomer in that "assessment of function" or "functioning assessment" more clearly expresses the nature of this activity. Terms that overlap with FA to a considerable degree are health status assessment, disability assessment or measurement, and geriatric assessment (1,2). All of these activities aim to measure to what degree patients in their functioning deviate from "normal," where normal may refer to typical persons without disorder (either all persons or persons of the same age, gender, education, etc.) or the patient's own preinjury status.

Assessment in this context refers to quantification, where the exact position of the person on a continuum ranging from unable (complete lack of function) to very able (on a level with or even better than "average" or than preinjury) is determined and expressed in a number. This is the meaning of the term FA as commonly used in health care and rehabilitation practice and research. However, the term assessment has a second meaning, referring to evaluation or valuation: the worth or meaning attached to the (amount of) function by the person involved or by others. Although the two types of FA are strongly connected, they are not synonymous. Whereas it is generally true that the value of a particular status increases with functional ability (being able to walk fast is more valuable than being able to walk only slowly), people may differ in how they valuate one ability compared to another (talking vs. reasoning) and in how they value one specific level of an ability relative to another level (3). These interindividual differences come increasingly into play, where the issue shifts from basic human functions (e.g., grasping) to more complex ones (holding down a job). Traditional methods of FA deal exclusively with the quantification issues (which are far from simple by themselves) and not with the valuation question. However, it is becoming increasingly clear that to assess with any level of adequacy what medical care and rehabilitation "produce," issues of valuation need to be dealt with (4). In this chapter, the reasons for and some methods of capturing the subjective valuing of functional states will be discussed along with more traditional FA methodologies and measures.

THE DISABLEMENT CONTINUUM

As suggested earlier, "functioning" may cover an extremely broad area, from simple functions involving a single body system to complex activities that are dependent on multiple physical and cognitive skills and are implemented in social interactions according to established social and cultural patterns. In Figure 20-1, the World Health Organization's (WHO) International Classification of Functioning, Disability, and Health (ICF) is used as a framework to delineate various concepts and terms encountered in the FA literature.

The WHO defines *impairment* as "problems in body function or structure as a significant deviation or loss"; in spite of the word "body," impairments include deficits in psychological functions (5, p. 12). In a previous edition of the ICF, the International Classification of Impairments, Disabilities, and Handicaps (ICIDH) (6), the same term was used; the taxonomy offered, however, did not make a clear distinction between deficits of structure and deficits of function at the impairment level. An FA instrument at the impairment level often used in traumatic brain injury (TBI) care and research is the Glasgow Coma Scale (GCS) (7). Neuropsychological testing also typically results in information at the impairment level, on concentration, memory span, and so on. At the level of the person, the ICF characterizes *activity* as the "execution of a task or action by an individual"(5, p. 14); its negative aspect, *activity limitations*, is defined as "difficulties an individual may have in executing activities"(5, p. 14). The ICIDH used the term "disability" for this concept, which was defined very much like the current term "activity limitation." Within rehabilitation, the prototypical measure of activity limitations is the Functional Independence Measure (FIM) (8), but many other instruments have been used within and outside TBI rehabilitation. Finally, the person in interaction with others may have *participation restrictions*, which are defined as "problems an individual may experience in involvement in life situations" (5, p. 14); the positive counterpart is characterized as "involvement in a life situation" (5, p. 14). In the ICIDH, the term "handicap" was used for the negative aspect, which was defined in a manner quite different from the newer term. However, many of the measures

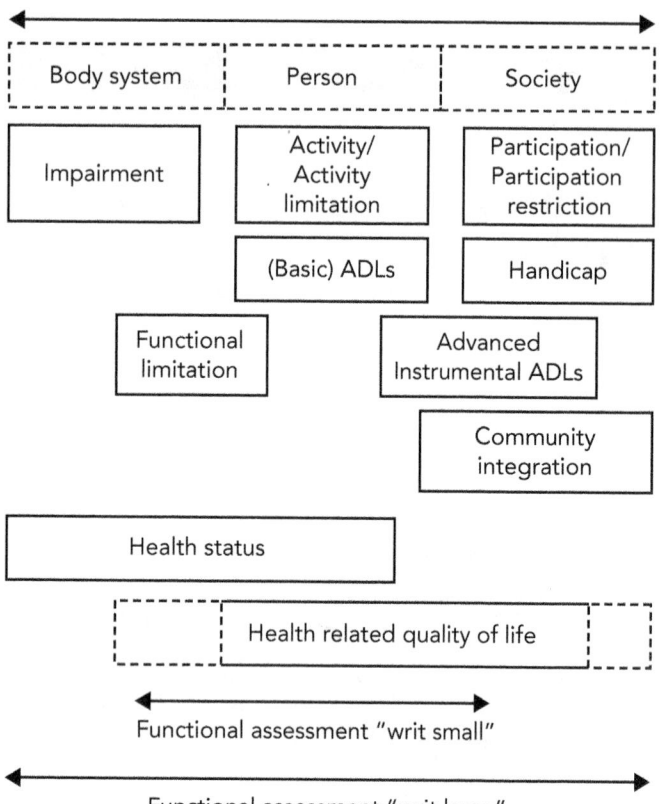

Body system	Person	Society

Impairment | Activity/ Activity limitation | Participation/ Participation restriction

(Basic) ADLs | Handicap

Functional limitation | Advanced Instrumental ADLs

Community integration

Health status

Health related quality of life

Functional assessment "writ small"

Functional assessment "writ large"

FIGURE 20-1 Aspects of functioning on a continuum from body system to societal emphasis.

developed to operationalize "handicap," such as the Craig Hospital Assessment and Reporting Technique (CHART) (9) are now used as measures of participation restrictions, including in the TBI literature.

Human functions range from simple acts, such as stretching a leg, to complicated pursuits, such as running a household, and it is difficult to define the three concepts of impairment, activity (limitation), and participation (restriction) in a clear and nonoverlapping way. The ICF offers separate concepts for the three domains of the disablement continuum, but only 2 taxonomies—one for body functions and one for activities and participation—with guidelines for users of the latter as to how the theoretical distinction might be implemented in practice using the taxonomy (10). Many measures of "functioning," such as the Disability Rating Scale (DRS) (11) overlap 2 or 3 of the concepts—intentionally or because the developers were not aware that the indicators they combined belonged to distinct conceptual classes.

FA "writ small" deals with activities/activity limitations. Rehabilitation and other specialists have developed many measures to quantify self-care, mobility, everyday communication, and other types of activities. We will try to give the readers an overview of the concepts and techniques useful in understanding and evaluating FA instruments, especially FA instruments developed for or commonly used with individuals with TBI, and in selecting them for clinical and research applications. FA "writ large" also includes measuring impairments and participation (12), and instruments that quantify the latter that are of relevance to TBI are included here.

Many terms developed prior to or outside the ICIDH/ ICF can be placed on the same disablement continuum, as shown in Figure 20-1. The core interests of rehabilitation, activities of daily living (ADLs) (sometimes designated basic ADLs), coincide with activities. Extended (instrumental, advanced) ADLs measured using, for example, the Frenchay Activities Index (FAI) (13) or the Adelaide Activities Profile (AAP) (14) are generally defined such that they straddle the activity-participation dividing line; on the other side of the continuum, functional limitations typically represent activities, such as grasping and lifting, which cross the divide between impairments and activities. Measures of functional limitations used in TBI care and research include the TEMPA(15), which assesses upper limb function. Community integration instruments, such as the CHART or, in TBI research more frequently, the Community Integration Questionnaire (CIQ) (16) or the PART (17,18) quantify aspects of instrumental activities of daily living (IADLs) and other facets of participation, with emphasis on the social interactional components.

Health status, a term used by health outcomes researchers, typically is defined and operationalized as combining elements of impairment and activity limitations, although some measures (such as the well-known Short-Form 36 [SF-36]) (19) also include indicators of participation. The SF-36 now increasingly is considered to be a measure of quality of life (QOL). QOL has been defined in a number of ways (20); most definitions and operationalizations of health-related QOL (HRQOL) overlap with activities and participation and may even include some aspects of impairment. Many disease-specific HRQOL measures include symptoms that typically are missing from activity and participation measures; however, many symptoms can be seen as impairments, which suggests that HRQOL is somehow synonymous with "disability," the term the ICF uses to represent the entire spectrum from impairments through participation restrictions.

THE STRUCTURE OF FUNCTIONAL ASSESSMENT INSTRUMENTS

At their simplest, FA measures consist of a number of separate items, each one of which refers to a narrow or broad ability or skill—for instance, lifting overhead, transferring into a bathtub, or making telephone calls. For each item, from 2 to as many as 7, different levels or categories of "ability" are distinguished, which have quantitative values from 0 (or 1) to the highest needed. The lowest category corresponds to no ability/cannot do at all/needs maximum help and the highest to independence, "normal" or even "above average." Additional metrics have been used, such as difficulty (21) and time needed (22). For measures of participation the metrics used include frequency of performing an activity (9), hours spent on an activity (23), share of activities performed (24), and others. The numbers a patient or subject receives for their performances on the constituent items typically are added together, and the total (with or without further arithmetical manipulation) reflects his or her functional status in the domain being measured. For some measures, the FIM for instance, the items all have the same number of steps and the same minimum and maximum value. The Barthel Index (BI) (25) on the other hand consists of some items with only 2 categories of ability, whereas the other items have 3 categories. Differential scoring of the categories from one item to the next can be used to express the relative weight (importance) of the constituent skills for overall functioning, as seen by the instrument's creator (25). A separate weighting step prior to addition can be used to achieve the same purpose.

The numeric values of the categories (item scale steps) represent measurement on an ordinal scale—they only indicate relative order along the able–not able (or not participating-participating) continuum, but the differences between scale steps are not equivalent in true underlying quantity, and the values chosen for them are arbitrary. As a result, adding up the scores for the items to obtain the total score is not an operation that is allowed based on the rules of mathematics. Therefore, total scores do not reflect position along a continuum that has a true 0 point and has constant distances between scale points. (These constitute the definition of a ratio scale, which is what is required for calculating means for a group or percentage improvement for a person over time). However, research has shown that if the item category values are chosen "reasonably," the sum of ordinal items corresponds quite well to values on a true ratio scale, at least for intermediate levels of the continuum of total scores (26). Rasch analysis and similar mathematical procedures based on item response theory (IRT) have been used to transform a set of scores on ordinal FA items into a score on an interval scale (9,21,26). The assumptions and mathematical manipulations underlying Rasch analysis-based FA instruments are beyond the scope of this chapter; good introductions to the technique and its application to FA may be found in Bond and Fox (27). There are several articles in the literature that explain Rasch analysis in the context of FA (28–30) and IRT more broadly (31,32).

Most FA measures used in TBI clinical services and research, such as the GCS, Disability Rating Scale (DRS), and Community Integration Questionnaire (CIQ), have never been subjected to Rasch analysis, let alone rescored based on the findings of such an analysis. They may not be unidimensional, and gains by patients from very low initial scores (e.g., a Functional Independent Measure [FIM] of 40) may be much easier to accomplish than apparently equally great increases (as expressed in score points) from medium or high starting points (e.g., an FIM of 90). As a result, one should be quite careful in interpreting FA instrument scores as applied to individuals and to groups. Especially, "percent improvement" and "change efficiency scores" should be considered as nothing but rough approximations of the mathematical precision they appear to offer. Calculation of means and all other operations (regression analysis, etc.) that require interval scales are somewhat less suspect, but the results also should be considered as approximations. Mathematical wizardry cannot make up for the basic problems created by ordinal measurement of the individual constituent skills and performances incorporated in a scale.

ISSUES IN FUNCTIONAL ASSESSMENT

Capacity and Performance

Two aspects of functioning are commonly distinguished: capacity and performance (5). *Capacity* is what people can do under optimal circumstances—well rested, encouraged to do their best—in an environment with minimal physical and other barriers. *Performance* is what they do in everyday life. People who can do self-care will not necessarily always do it for a variety of reasons. One of the most common reasons is that their environment is not accommodating or that the energy and time which a task requires preferentially are spent on other, more worthwhile, endeavors, whether that is work or watching one's favorite soap opera.

At the impairment end of the disablement continuum, measures of functional limitations tend to be capacity focused, for instance, neuropsychological testing and neurological assessment. The American Spinal Injury Association (ASIA) motor scale (33) is based on the patient's ability to contract key muscles, and the physician and patient are hardly interested in the patient's actual frequency of contracting those muscles. At the other end of the spectrum, measures of participation or community integration, without exception, quantify performance. Testing capacity is either impossible (how could one test "ability to function as a brain surgeon"?) or not of interest; actual performance is of importance as the long-term outcome of rehabilitative efforts, not potential. It is in the middle ground, the domain of activities, where a discrepancy between capacity and performance is most likely to be relevant, and performance is most modifiable with therapeutic, environmental, and other interventions.

Testing, Observation, and Reporting of Performance

Three methods are used to collect functional information. Testing involves requiring the person to perform specific tasks or skills under the direct supervision of the test administrator who times the test, assesses the amount of help from aids or aides that is needed, and so forth. This tends to occur in laboratory situations, but testing can also be done in the person's home or other setting where the activities involved typically are or should be performed (34). Depending on the degree to which the test situation approximates an optimal one, the resulting score quantifies capacity.

Most FAs of activity reported as part of inpatient or outpatient rehabilitation programs are observation based. For instance, the FIM admission and discharge scores submitted to Uniform Data System (UDS) (http://www.udsmr.org/) and eRehabData (https://web2.erehabdata.com/erehabdata/index.jsp), the 2 inpatient rehabilitation outcomes reporting systems, are based on what the patient does in the first 3 days after admission and the last 3 days before discharge. In practice, there is continuous pressure on the patients to perform at their best, especially in treatment with physical therapists (PTs) and occupational therapists (OTs), and the measure of performance turns into a measure of capacity. Automated assessment using sensors worn by the person or embedded in her environment or in tools and utensils may, in the future, offer another method of observation, but the technology still needs quite some development (35).

A third way of collecting FA information is through report by the patient or a proxy, such as a family member. These reports can involve capacity but more typically address performance. Questions are asked about how the person performs the various activities included in the FA measure in his or her daily routine, focusing on amount of assistance received or the frequency of performance. Using a standardized branching questionnaire, trained interviewers can reach a high level of inter-rater (inter-interviewer) reliability. This is how data are typically collected for follow-up assessments in the UDS and eRehabData outcomes assessment systems and in other program evaluation approaches.

All three methods have their advantages and disadvantages in terms of cost, personnel needed, required ability of the patient to cooperate with the data collection, and so on. If capacity data are of interest, testing is the preferred method; for true performance data, interviewing is the only feasible approach. Problems arise when the data obtained by 2 methods need to be linked. For instance, a typical question (clinically and in research) is whether the person manages to maintain or even improve on the skills he or she was discharged with from inpatient rehabilitation. The hospital data are typically collected using observation in an environment that tends to be more accessible than the typical residence, and with overt or covert pressure to perform one's best. The home follow-up data are normally collected using patient or proxy interview and concern performance in a different environment, in which there may be no incentive at all to use all the abilities taught in rehabilitation. If a change in functional performance is noted, is it because of the change in data collection method per se, changes in the environment, or even because of changes in the true underlying capacity, such as continued neurological recovery? This issue has hardly been studied, and we don't know enough about differences in scores from various data collection methods for assorted FA instruments to tease apart the various factors (36).

The Nature of the Items

In an IQ test, the person being tested answers multiple questions about arithmetic, similarities, and other items, which in themselves are not of interest to the test administrator. The IQ score that results is of interest because it gives an (imperfect) indication of the person's overall cognitive abilities. The focus is on the underlying trait: intelligence. In FA, however, the items most likely have intrinsic meaning to the person performing the assessment and to the individual being assessed; they reflect activities that are of importance in and of themselves, whether it is stair climbing or communicating a simple idea. That does not mean that there is no underlying construct "functional ability" that is of interest, but the underlying ability is of concern mostly because it informs on the functional items that were part of the assessment and possibly on those that were not part of it. Because the primary interest is in the functional items (tasks, activities) themselves, there always is a tendency to include in FA measures the full panoply of acts that are part of daily human routines. Maintaining a balance between feasibility (minimizing testing time required and minimally taxing the energy and interest levels of the person being measured) and inclusion of all those functional tasks that are key to living has always been a challenge for FA instrument developers. Measures that cover "all areas of life" tend to select broadly defined tasks (e.g., "dressing") and limit the number of items from 10 to 20. Instruments developed for use by specific disciplines are apt to include more narrowly defined tasks ("putting on a pullover") and include a large number; the Klein-Bell ADL scale contains 170 items to cover just 6 areas:

dressing, mobility, elimination, bathing/hygiene, eating, and emergency telephone use (37).

When the focus of FA shifts from performance of the individual key tasks to the status of broad underlying abilities ("self care," "motor strength and coordination"), the need to include each and every possible item diminishes. Traditional psychometric methods sketched in the next section can be used to show that the underlying construct can be measured with one set of items (indicators) about as well as with another set, in that the resulting total scores will have high correlations with one another. Some measures of functional limitations (the transition area between impairments and activities) do not attempt to "cover the waterfront"; they select a small number of activities that are representative of the entire universe of relevant items and use those to score, for instance, "upper extremity functioning." After all, once it is known how much difficulty a subject has picking up a can of soup and how much picking up a ream of paper, it should be fairly clear how well she would do lifting a paperback book. To what degree this same reasoning applies at the other end of the disablement spectrum, participation, is not yet known. The ICF distinguishes about 90 different aspects of "participation" in 9 chapters covering communication, mobility, domestic life, and so on. Is it necessary to obtain information on all of these to get a complete view of someone's level of participation? Or is it possible to extrapolate from 3 household tasks to all other ones and also to know quite adequately how well the person does in the domain of civic responsibilities? That depends to a large degree on whether participation is a single unidimensional construct or a large collection of disparate items that all reflect participation in some way. There presumably are key participation components that no participation FA instrument would want to omit (work, social relations with family), but the need to collect information on all others is still not known. These and other problems involved in measuring participation are discussed in greater detail in several articles (10,38–40).

The presence of a unidimensional continuum underlying functional tasks makes it possible for those whose interest is more in the patients'/clients'/subjects' status on the construct rather than their performance on each of the individual items, to use computer adaptive testing (CAT) and related techniques to administer very short sets of items matched to the individuals' ability (performance) level that produce the same quantity and quality of information as the more expansive arrays of items ("item banks") from which these sets are drawn (41–43). To date, application of CAT to FA has been more demonstration of concept than use in daily clinical and research practice.

ISSUES IN MEASUREMENT: THE METROLOGIC CHARACTERISTICS OF FUNCTIONAL ASSESSMENTS INSTRUMENTS

Whenever we measure, error creeps into the resulting score, whether it is a small error in measuring simple concrete characteristics (for instance, the area of a room) or a large error in quantifying abstract concepts, such as authoritarianism. FA is no exception, and the issue is not so much getting rid of the error (we never will be able to do that completely) but being aware of the amount of error our data contain and being attentive to what that error means for any conclusions we draw and actions we undertake based on those data. *Metrology* (the science of measuring) is a major concern in all science disciplines, and the developers and users of FA instruments have mostly relied on the methodologies for instrument development originating in psychology. "Psychometrics," as it is named, is a very technical and, for most clinicians, very boring subject, but knowledge of some of the basics is necessary for the fruitful use of FA instruments.

Traditionally, two aspects of the data resulting from measurement have had most emphasis: validity and reliability. But in clinical applications, such issues as sensitivity and practicality are increasingly getting attention. In theory, reliability is an aspect of validity, but most people tend to think of them as separate characteristics of instruments (or, more properly, of the data produced by instruments), and the techniques for quantifying validity and reliability are distinct. "Validity" refers to the question "Is this instrument measuring what we aim to measure?" If it is targeting characteristic X, do the numbers reflect X and not Y, or a little bit of X with a lot of Z mixed in? "Reliability" refers to the question "How reproducible is this measurement? If we repeated the measurement operation with the same or a similar "ruler," would we get the same result?" By definition, an instrument can be very reliable without being valid. If it is not reliable at all, it is by definition not valid. The goal we are aiming for is instruments that are both reliable (they give results that are reproducible) and valid (they measure what we set out to measure).

Over the years, a great many techniques have been developed to quantify validity and reliability, each applicable to different situations. Unfortunately, psychologists and social scientists have fallen into the habit of "inventing" new types of validity and reliability by naming them after these techniques. However, there is no such thing as test–retest reliability or construct validity. There is only one validity and one reliability of each instrument, which are estimated using different techniques, for instance, by comparing the results of testing and retesting.

Reliability

Estimating the reliability of the data produced by our measures is the easiest to understand. The estimates all are based on some form of repeat measurement. If two clinicians at the same time rate the ability of patient X on the FIM grooming item, they should come up with the same number, or else one or both are wrong (they are deficient observers), or the instructions for measurement in the FIM manual are incomplete or confusing. We can estimate the reliability of the FIM grooming data *as the item is used by these 2 clinicians* by having the 2 rate a few hundred patients and calculate how often they agree, completely or almost so. A statistical formula such as coefficient kappa (or weighted kappa) can be used to express the result. All these formulas are constructed in such a way that the result, the reliability coefficient, varies between 0.00 (no reliability whatsoever) and 1.00 (perfect reliability). "Inter-rater reliability" can be estimated based on a few raters to represent all possible raters so that we can have an idea as to how reliable this one-item FIM grooming instrument is in the hands of the average clinician.

If the same patients are rated by the same clinician twice, we similarly can calculate "intra-rater reliability," the degree to which she agrees with her own earlier ratings. There are 2 scenarios for this: either the patients' performance is videotaped, or the rater observes the patients twice. In the latter case, it is of course important that we are sure these patients have not changed in the mean time. In both instances, the clinician should "forget" about the scores she assigned the first time around, which is not that difficult if large numbers of ratings are to be made.

Functional status is a fairly broad and abstract entity (a "construct" in psychometrical parlance), and it is unlikely that a single item, such as grooming, can represent the entire construct. Typically, we select multiple items as indicators of the abstraction and combine them to adequately operationalize the theoretical definition of the construct we may have. Use of multiple indicators has another advantage; the random measurement error involved with quantifying any one item is likely offset by the random error in another item. (For that reason, the more items there are in an instrument, the more reliable it will be, because the chance of random error being eliminated is increased. Any *systematic* error will just remain, however, and practical issues come into play if instruments are too long). Because each item in an FA instrument is a repeat measurement of the construct, like the 2 raters for grooming produce repeat measurements, we can calculate the agreement between items as yet another estimate of reliability. A number of formulas to estimate "internal consistency reliability" exist, the most frequently used of which is Cronbach's coefficient alpha. "Split-half" and "parallel forms" reliability are related formulas. All of them take values between 0.00 and 1.00.

The minimal level of reliability a measure needs to have depends on the purpose to which the data are to be put. A minimum of 0.90 for situations where decisions on an individual patient need to be made (discharge Mrs. Jones or extend her stay another week?) is often quoted, whereas 0.70 or 0.80 is a typical minimum required for group applications, such as in program evaluation and research. Longer instruments tend to be more reliable, but the trend is toward the use of short forms, such as the SF-12 and the CHART-SF rather than long ones, like their parents SF-36 and CHART. With better methods of development and construction, new short instruments can offer a level of reliability approximating that of older long ones. Another development is CAT, in which only those questions that are targeted to the ability level of the person are being asked (42,43). For very simple instruments, paper-and-pencil adapted testing is possible (44,45).

Validity

Validity cannot be estimated in such a simple way as reliability can, except in one unusual situation: there is an existing instrument that we are certain is perfectly valid. In that case, we can administer the old instrument and the new one to a sample, calculate the correlation between the 2 scores, and use that correlation as the estimate of the validity of the new measure. (The issue, of course, is "If there is a perfectly good measure, why is there a need to develop a new one?" The importance of having a shorter scale may be the only acceptable reason.) Less powerful methods are used in the more common situation: there is no existing measure, or the existing ones have low validity themselves.

"Face validity" is (in the eyes of most authorities) not a form of validity determination but an answer to the question "Does the instrument 'on the face of it' measure what those completing it expect to see?" "Does a measure of X have questions about X that patients recognize as such?" Some instruments have no or little face validity but are claimed to be valid, for instance, the Minnesota Multiphasic Personality Inventory (MMPI).

The closely related term "content validity" refers to a measure covering the entire construct the developer is targeting in the eyes of experts. It is generally determined by having the experts draw up lists of necessary content for a measure of X or checking the content of the draft measure. Of course, this presumes there is a clear description (by the authors) of the concept they would like to operationalize; it makes no sense criticizing a painted portrait for lack of veracity if you don't know the person depicted. There are no standard formulas for calculating this validity aspect.

"Predictive validity" concerns the ability of a measure to predict a future state or event that is inherently linked to the characteristic being measured. A college entrance examination is said to have predictive validity if it can be used to accurately predict who will graduate in 4, 5, or 6 years. A parallel in FA would be the ability of a measure to predict who will be successfully discharged from home vs to a nursing home from a rehabilitation inpatient stay. One problem with predictive validity assessment is the fact that there are no hard and fast rules as to what should be the minimum level of success in predicting. We know that many factors affect successful independent living—the accessibility of the home, family and other support available, the person's stubbornness and willingness to run risks of falling, and so on. Does an FA instrument have adequate predictive validity if predictions based on it are correct 40% of the time? Fifty percent?

"Known group validity" is based on differences in scale scores between two groups that are known to differ in the characteristic the instrument aims to measure. The average score of persons with TBI on a measure of physical functioning should be higher than the average of persons with spinal cord injury (SCI); in case of a measure of cognitive functioning, the situation should be reversed. If the data do not parallel these expectations, quite likely, the instrument is not measuring what we think it is. Alternatively, systematic error (bias) has crept into the data. A similar problem as mentioned earlier exists for known group validity: How much of the variation in the functional status of the overall group should be explained by diagnostic category, TBI vs SCI? If every person with TBI is known to have a higher physical functioning level than every person with an SCI, things would be easy: the variation explained should be 100%, and everything lower than that would mean less than perfect validity. However, the distributions for functioning ability of the SCI and TBI groups overlap, and the variation explained by analysis of variance reflects both the difference between group means, the standard deviations around those means, and the random and systematic error in the measure we use. Stating that a good functional measure should explain between 0% and 100% of variance is not very helpful in developing or selecting an instrument.

Lastly, "construct validity" concerns the relationships between the measurement data of a (highly abstract) construct and data for other constructs. Sometimes, we have a basis in theory to predict that construct K should be strongly related to (yet not identical with) construct L and be independent of construct M. (For instance, "ADL ability is related to community integration but unrelated to political party preference"). If the data bring this out, the operationalization of K is likely to be valid (and similarly the operationalizations of L and M). If the predicted association between K and L is minimal or absent, however, we don't know if the problem is with the theory; the operationalization of K, or the measurement of L. And it is an unusual theory that specifies the exact strength of the relationship between K and L predicated on perfect measurement of the constructs involved. "Strong" or "very strong" is the best we get, and those are not very good starting points for evaluating the level of validity of the instruments involved.

The earlier discussion should make clear that the estimation of the validity of instruments always is less straightforward than the quantification of their reliability. Finding high values parallel to, for example, a 0.91 level of test–retest reliability just does not happen; validity coefficients are much lower, because all methods of validity estimation are roundabout. In practice, it is necessary to simultaneously use all possible methods of estimating validity and "patch together" evidence supporting validity based on multiple findings, which never will be ironclad. Finding encouraging levels of the various "types of" validity distinguished here, in multiple studies, with patterns of correlations that make sense based on expert knowledge, is what typically occurs. Fortunately, in the case of FA, the construct being measured is fairly concrete, and the specialists involved have extensive knowledge of the determinants, correlates, intergroup differences, and so on of various aspects of functional status, making the issue of assessing the quality of specific measures less problematic than the preceding list of issues might suggest.

"Ecological validity" does not concern validity proper but the relevance of assessment data to real-life situations outside the testing situation. For instance, the Wisconsin Card Sort Test (46) is a measure of executive functioning (the ability to plan, initiate, execute, monitor, and correct one's actions) often used by neuropsychologists to assess persons with TBI. Like all neuropsychological tests, it is administered in a quiet office after the person tested has had a good night's sleep and is still fresh, and so on. How well do the results predict the patient's ability to make breakfast for her children while testing the middle schooler on history and finishing her own makeup before leaving for work, with the TV competing for attention (47)? Testing executive functioning in situations that resemble the real world would provide data that are more "ecologically valid," but the standardization of testing might suffer. Standardization of testing has always been a keystone of psychometric methods of assessing reliability and validity of neuropsychological instruments, and of quantifying the abilities of individual patients or clients—they are capacity measures. However, standardized environments tend to be dissimilar from the settings where people perform self-care, communicate, do work, and all other things captured under the umbrella of functioning. Testing in a standardized environment almost always means in an optimal environment, and the results therefore are more indicative of capacity than of performance.

In the development of measures using Rasch analysis and IRT, reliability and validity are much intertwined issues, addressed by various parameters derived from data on samples and used to give a quantitative answer to questions such as, "Does this particular item belong in the measure?" "Do the items remaining after "misfits" are eliminated define a unidimensional scale?" "Can this scale reliably differentiate between at least three bands of people differing in ability or functioning?" "Can the instrument quantify the abilities of people at the extreme ends of the functioning spectrum (48)?"

Sensitivity

It is easy to see that if an FA "measure" has just 2 categories ("able" and "unable"), it lacks sensitivity: it cannot reflect fine distinctions in ability/performance, and it cannot be used to record minor but clinically significant changes. Sensitivity refers to the ability of an instrument to capture differences between two people or over time that are clinically relevant or small but still of importance in research. Sensitive measures allow such fine distinctions across the full extent of the range of ability of the cases to be measured. When sensitivity is discussed in relation to change, the term *responsiveness* is frequently used.

Floor effects and *ceiling effects* are one issue in sensitivity. The first terms refer to the lowest measurable level of performance on an FA instrument being higher than what is the status of the least able person to be measured. When a measure has a floor effect, all individuals who have ability equal to the lowest measurable level or lower are clumped together and given the corresponding score. Vice versa, a ceiling effect means that the highest measurable level is lower than the level of at least some of the more able patients/clients. It should be noted that very often, measures are developed for one population, in which they have no floor or ceiling effects, but then applied to another in which they do. For instance, the FIM was designed to quantify functional status of rehabilitation inpatients, and any patient who achieves the maximum score on discharge was probably an inappropriate admission. However, a few years after onset of TBI, many persons will score at the maximum of the motor FIM subscale (49,50). (It should be noted that the FIM was never designed to distinguish between people with minimal motor or cognitive deficits that do not affect day-to-day functioning, other mere mortals, and Superman; its target population is people who require and can benefit from inpatient rehabilitation. "Lack of responsiveness" often is a problem for which the instrument user is responsible, not the instrument developer.) Different instruments are needed to assess and monitor progress in this group of individuals. The measures available tend not to cover "all of functioning," such as the BI and FIM but more limited aspects—mobility only (51) or cognitive communication only (52) or even just narrative discourse (53).

The issue is similar with respect to floor effects; the functioning level of some patients is so low that the FIM and other FA instruments designed for the common rehabilitation population cannot be used to reliably assess them or monitor their progress. The JFK Coma Recovery Scale Revised (CRS-R) was developed to characterize and monitor patients functioning at Rancho Levels I–III and is a more appropriate choice for this type of patients (54). A high-quality systematic review of all measures of disorders of conscience was published recently (55).

Quantification of responsiveness is not done using formulas resulting in simple coefficients ranging from 0.0 (not responsive at all) to 1.0 (maximum responsiveness possible). All methods of quantifying responsiveness are mostly useful for comparing responsiveness of one measure with that of another, allowing one to select the most responsive one. A variety of indices are used, including effect sizes (the mean change between time 1 and time 2 divided by the standard deviation at time 1), the standardized response mean (the mean change between time 1 and time 2 divided by the standard deviation of change scores), receiver operating characteristic (ROC) analysis, and many others. Discussion of these indices is beyond the scope of this chapter; the reader is referred to the extensive literature (56–62). Reliable Change Statistics or Indices are a family of techniques developed chiefly by psychologists to determine, primarily at the level of the individual patient, from whether the amount of change resulting from treatment or other factors is beyond what might be seen as a result of measurement error (63,64).

The sensitivity of measures should be considered in relation to the population in which they are to be used. As indicated, ceiling effects may preclude the use of the FIM and other FA measures with individuals with mild TBI. However, other instruments which do not have similar range restrictions may be unsuitable for particular applications because they cannot make minor distinctions between cases or cannot capture the minor improvements rehabilitation can bring about over short or even medium time periods.

Other Metrologic Characteristics

Beyond validity, reliability, and sensitivity, there is a number of other characteristics of an FA measure that are relevant to its use in clinical, program, and research applications. Most have to do with practicality.

- Language: This is especially relevant to self-administered measures, such as the CIQ, but may also be an issue with observational and other measures. Both the required reading ability and a translation in a language the user is familiar with are of concern.
- Training required: Many observational FA instruments require the user to be trained and sometimes certified (34) to produce reliable data.
- Time and equipment required: Measures that take inordinate time on the part of the subjects or the administrator or that use special equipment may not be suitable outside research applications.
- Suitability for use with people with a disability: Self-report items developed for the population at large or for people with sensory or mobility disabilities may not be suitable for subjects/patients with TBI. The limitations that impairments may impose on the validity or use of measures are receiving increased attention (65–68).

USES OF FUNCTIONAL ASSESSMENT

The origin of FA (writ small) in medical rehabilitation lies in attempts by clinicians in the 1950s to express quantitatively the functional deficits patients had on admission to rehabilitation and determine discharge status so that there was some "proof" of the effectiveness of treatment. The forerunners of instruments such as the BI (25) were simple checklists for recording (lack of) problems with performing self-care and mobility activities (2). From these early efforts, measurement instruments of sometimes great sophistication have grown. In addition, the range of applications of these instruments has expanded tremendously so that we now can describe uses in the care of individual patients, evaluation, and development of treatment programs as a whole, reimbursement, population monitoring, and research. The type of information needed in these various applications is somewhat different, and even when the basic instrument used is the same (e.g., the FIM at this time still is the "workhorse" of medical rehabilitation and is used almost throughout all these types of applications), ideally there would be differences in scoring or other details.

Uses in Care of Individual Patients

Decisions on admissions to inpatient and outpatient programs are often based on a formal FA to see if the person has the types and degrees of deficits that the program is qualified and authorized to treat, either in general or for the person in question. The "baseline" assessment therefore often is communicated to the third-party payor, who may use it to approve program admission and allow a certain duration or intensity of treatment. The preadmission or admission assessment is frequently the basis for a prognosis, which is communicated to the patient and the payor and ideally underlies goal setting. Many programs use an FA instrument, such as the FIM to set goals, either for classes of patients or for individual patients. Software applications have been developed to assist case or care managers to make such predictions; they are based in large part on a database that contains the data on many previous patients with the same rehabilitation diagnosis, age, gender, and comorbidities.

Goal setting ideally is more individualized than the limited number of constituent items and/or outcome levels of standard instruments make available. Several methodologies have been developed to allow more or less "customized" selection and quantification of goals, which then are the basis for treatment plan development. Results can be monitored to see if goals are reached (in the time span planned) or need to be modified based on new or initially unknown complicating factors. *Goal Attainment Scaling* (GAS) is a method originally developed in the mental health arena (69) that has been applied in medical rehabilitation, mostly for research purposes, it appears (70,71). Clinical applications have been discussed more recently (72–74).

In GAS, the client and therapist together set multiple goals and, for each, determine the most likely outcome level, as well as 2 levels of lesser accomplishment and 2 of better accomplishment. For instance, for the goal mobility, the target level could be "household walker—can ambulate 50 feet without walker and without difficulty." Lower levels could reflect use of supports and/or lesser distance (scored as −1 and −2); higher levels greater distance and/or outdoors mobility (scored as +1 and +2). Each of the several goals or items (walking, bathing, doing dishes, etc.) is given an importance weight reflecting patient/client valuation. To cal-

culate the overall outcome of treatment, the outcomes for the various goals are summed after weighting by the importance factors. Thus, the GAS and derivative methods incorporate to some degree the individual valuation of functioning components, but do so only for those activities and roles that display major deficits, which have been selected for treatment, rather than for all domains of functioning. The quantification of treatment outcomes reflects success in terms of the goals set, not client functioning in terms of deviation from "normal." For that reason, these types of instruments may be more useful in clinical applications than in research on the determinants of, treatments for, and consequences of functional deficits. Appropriate use of functional measures for goal setting must take into account premorbid function, patient resources (financial assets, family, and community support), and known prognostic information. The Canadian Occupational Performance Measure (COPM) (75–78) uses a methodology very similar to GAS. A number of applications in TBI have been reported (79–81).

Treatment monitoring using an FA measure is applied in many rehabilitation programs, even if the goals have been set without patient input or without subjective a-priori weighting. Team rounds often exist of the reporting by "most responsible/knowledgeable therapies" (nursing for bladder, speech for verbal expression, etc.) of the current status of the patient on the items offered by the FA instrument used in the facility. Even if weekly or less frequent team meetings do not employ formal quantification, the status of the patient with respect to various skills and other aspects of impairment, activities, and (in outpatient programs) participation is typically discussed. Almost all rehabilitation programs quantify status on discharge because that information is needed to document program results and subsequently is used in program evaluation. Although treatment termination decisions increasingly are based on "external" criteria (e.g., a maximal length of stay [LOS] approved by a third-party payor), ideally, they are founded on either the accomplishment of goals or plateauing of the patient in terms of overall functional ability. In both instances, measurement of patient status should be performed using an instrument that has minimal error so that (lack of) change can be reliably determined.

FA information may also be used to communicate progress and outcomes of treatment to persons who are not part of the treatment team. Patients themselves, their family members, referral sources, and payors have a keen interest in the functional aspects of the patient's status, especially where it concerns activities and participation. One additional use of FA for individual cases is long-term monitoring of a patient's status. Especially in the case of progressive diseases, this type of information is important to make decisions on new treatments, changes in patient environments, and so on. In fact, this use of FA has led to a designation of functional status information as a sixth (after the standard 4 and pain) vital sign (82).

The foregoing issues suggest that the choice of an appropriate validated FA measure for the individual with TBI depends on a number of factors, including time after injury, rehabilitation setting, nature and severity of deficits, and goals of rehabilitation. When clinical improvement is seen and goals and maybe even the rehabilitation setting (inpatient acute, subacute, outpatient) are changed, the choice of the measurement tools used should be reevaluated. The use of a scale that is insensitive to the improvement that is expected or not measuring the progress toward an individual's goal should be avoided.

Uses in Program Administration

Most rehabilitation programs have as their mission statement something along the lines of improving QOL by reducing impairments and increasing activities and participation. Program evaluation aims to assess to what degree a program indeed accomplishes what it sets out to do: improve functional status of people with disablement. Basic questions are, "Do patients change for the better (program effectiveness), and if so, are resources used optimally in accomplishing this (program efficiency)?"

The choice of appropriate functional measures for the evaluation of a TBI program should be based on the span of the rehabilitation spectrum the program serves. Measures of impaired physical and cognitive functions would be appropriate for acute inpatient care, with "disorders of consciousness" scales (55) used for low-level patients. Activity measures are most appropriate for acute or subacute inpatient care; participation measures are needed to assess the effectiveness and efficiency of outpatient services in the community.

Although change in functioning between admission to and discharge from a program is common, it is unfortunately not easy to offer proof that the program deserves credit. For instance, a person with TBI may score higher on a posttest than on a pretest for a number of reasons that have nothing to do with the selection, timing, quality, and quantity of services received: natural recovery, improved test-taking ability, and many others (83). All rehabilitation programs face the same problem, and one solution that has been found is to compare outcomes between programs under the assumption that not *all* change in *all* programs can be explained by causes other than function improvement resulting from the treatment received. The "excess" change in the best programs is truly the result of interventions, the implicit claim reads. Evaluation of a program's outcomes is facilitated by creation of a minimal data set for all programs that includes patient demographics, time since injury, and measures of injury severity in addition to specific scales of functioning, selection of which depends on program type and time of follow-up (84). The UDS, in which many inpatient rehabilitation facilities in the United States participate, as well as some subacute facilities and nursing homes that offer rehabilitation, and eRehabData are 2 such data aggregators.

Comparisons between programs is fair only, of course, if their inputs (admission status) are the same; it may be much easier to bring an admit FIM score of 50 up to 100 for someone with SCI than for a patient with TBI. Thus, UDS and other aggregators produce customer reports that compare like with like, in terms of diagnostic group, comorbidities, age, and other factors that are considered relevant to chances of program success. Their focus tends to be on admission–discharge functional status change as the key indicator of effectiveness. Because the better programs may achieve a certain level of change using many fewer resources than poorly organized ones, LOS is typically used as a gross indicator of resource use. Functional status change per day

then is an indicator of program efficiency. (It may be worth repeating here that a number of assumptions that may not stand up to scrutiny, including interval-level measurement of functional status, underlie such calculations.)

There are other methods of evaluating a program's effectiveness: for example, by calculating what percentage of the patients did achieve the goals that were set at admission. It is natural that a small percentage of patients do not progress as well as anticipated, for example, because of intercurrent illness. But if a large percentage fails to reach the standardized or individualized functional goals set for them, the program is either selecting the wrong types of patients, or staff and programs are ineffective. Shifts in the program's admission policies, management, and/or processes may be needed. Unfortunately, routine program evaluation data tend to be insufficient to indicate where exactly the problem is and how it can be fixed; additional studies are needed to obtain that information.

Routine outcome data can and should be communicated to stakeholders, including current and future patients, third-party payors, and the local community. The Centers for Medicare and Medicaid Services (CMS) has started to post on its website comparative functional outcomes for nursing homes, and it is to be expected that similar "report cards," including functional FA information, will be published in the future for many other facilities that offer rehabilitation of some type.

The Commission on Accreditation of Rehabilitation Facilities (CARF) (http://www.carf.org) is a widely recognized agency that accredits organizations and programs, including TBI programs. It currently offers accreditation in 7 categories of brain injury services, including inpatient hospital rehabilitation, residential services, and home and community-based services. Accreditation is based on documenting adherence to standards as well as surveyors' evaluations. Depending on the level of care, different criteria need to be met. Ensuring patient and family education, as well as considering future rehabilitation needs, are required components of all accreditation standards. Standards for outcome measures include appropriate FA during and after treatment. Patient and family satisfaction measures also play an important role. See Chapter 6 for additional information about CARF.

FA data are also used by provider agencies in a variety of activities centering on improving program services quality. Whether they are called outcomes management, continuous quality improvement (CQI), or total quality management (TQM), they all involve considering the organization delivering services as a system, with parts and subsystems that all should be studied continuously to reduce inefficiencies, improve administrative and clinical procedures, and reduce risks and adverse events (85). FA information almost by definition plays a key role in making decisions about programs that deal with individuals with TBI. For instance, an admission-to-discharge increase in functioning less than a specified minimum could be an indicator threshold violation that triggers an in-depth investigation whether a problem ("opportunity to improve processes") exists. FA information could also function as an indicator that is collected routinely to indicate functioning of the program(s)—a vital sign for the organization.

Effective 2002, CMS has, under its prospective payment system (PPS), paid inpatient rehabilitation facilities (IRFs) fixed amounts for each patient discharged, rather than reimbursing (adjusted) charges, costs of operations, or an amount based on some other formula used in earlier years and still used by other payors. The fixed amounts are based in part on the functional status of the patient on admission, combined with diagnostic category (stroke, TBI, SCI, etc.) and age category. For functional status, a minor variation on the FIM is used, which is embedded in the IRF-Patient Assessment Instrument (IRF-PAI). The combination of diagnosis, IRF-PAI functional status score, and age defines a group whose rehabilitation requires unique resources as acknowledged in the payment amount for each case (86). (This amount is further adjusted for comorbidities ["tiers"], salary levels in the region the facility is located, etc.).

CMS is in the process of replacing the FIM, embedded in the IRF-PAI, as well as the FA instruments used in admission, periodic, and discharge assessments of nursing home residents (Minimum Data Set [MDS]) and people receiving home health (Outcome and Assessment Information Set [OASIS]) by a new FA measure, embedded in a new assessment instrument to be used with all 3 patient groups, currently known as the Continuity Assessment Record and Evaluation (CARE) tool (http://www.pacdemo.rti.org/meetingInfo.cfm?cid=caretool). The CARE tool at this time (spring 2012) is undergoing testing but will be rolled out in the near future to offer the basis for reimbursement in CMS-funded postacute care (87–89).

The National Committee on Vital and Health Statistics (NCVHS) has recommended capturing and classifying functional status information as part of routine health care transactions, so that administrative databases could be mined and used for a variety of purposes, including monitoring overall population health, health care management, public health planning, predicting costs and financial management, and policy development (90). Attempts to use computer intelligence to harvest and process such information from "free text" in medical records have been initiated (91). At the moment, only limited information on functioning is available in a systematic mode, mostly through Medicare files, on special populations: those receiving inpatient rehabilitation (IRF-PAI), nursing home residents (MDS), and people receiving home health (OASIS). The subcommittee on populations of the NCVHS, which investigated these issues, suggested that, with modifications, the ICF might be a useful taxonomic system (a "uniform code") on which to base such data collection across the continuum of care. The uniform code would not prescribe *how* to measure functional status but only specify *what* data elements need to be reported.

A German group under the guidance of Stucki and associated with the WHO has begun the development of ICF "core sets"—listings of selected impairments, activity limitations, and participation restrictions that are of particular relevance to the care and management of a particular diagnostic group. The core sets for TBI have been published (92), among many others. The ICF allows coding the severity of impairments, activity limitations, and participation restrictions (93) but offers rather primitive methods that do not operationalize measurement. Presumably, productive use of the core sets, especially in applications beyond clinical care, requires a system or systems of FA.

Uses in Research

Program evaluation typically does not address what was done for individual patients to explain changes in functional status and link those interventions to outcomes (the "black box" aspect of rehabilitation). It also does not systematically address alternative explanations for outcomes and has no hard evidence for the effectiveness of traditional or innovative treatments. This is where research comes in. Per end of April 2012, Medline contained more than 44,000 records classified under "activities of daily living," which label (MeSH term) is used to classify articles on ADLs, (chronic) limitations of activity, independent living, and self-care. FA articles are also indexed under other headings, for instance, "geriatric assessment" added another 11,000 unduplicated records. Of this total, only a small number addresses clinical application at the level of the individual (presumably less than 5%) and a slightly larger number (maybe 10%) concerns the program level uses of FA measures. Most published articles concern either the development of FA instruments, including assessing their reliability, validity, sensitivity, and practicality, or the use of FA measures to carefully compare the effects of rehabilitation treatments, describe the natural course of disablement, assess the financial and social impact of disability, and so on.

Because functioning is the central interest of rehabilitation providers and researchers and their patients/clients, it is to be expected that much of their research uses FA information as either the "independent" (predictor) variable, the "dependent" (outcome) one, or both. The same holds true with respect to TBI rehabilitation; FA measures, whether specific to individuals in this diagnostic group (CIQ, DRS) or generic (FIM) are used in a large percentage of the published research. In this literature, one also finds application of very specialized FA measures (e.g., of functional communication). It is worthwhile to remember, though, that before any use is made of the results of this research, the investigations need to be assessed in terms of the applicability of the FA instruments selected and their metrologic qualities.

SUBJECTIVE VALUATION OF FUNCTIONAL PERFORMANCE

A major criticism of most of the FA measures used in TBI clinical care, program evaluation, and research is the fact that they do not reflect the subjective view of the person involved. "Normal functioning" may be a laudable goal but not if that functioning detracts from the person's subjective QOL. Thus, the nature of the fit between functional activities and the person's values, preferences, and abilities may need to be considered and reflected in some way in FA instruments, especially in participation measures. Corrigan noted that outcomes can be defined from 3 perspectives: that of the person with TBI, that of the health care professionals treating the injury, and that of society (94). The latter 2 perspectives presumably are reflected to some degree in the FA measures commonly used. However, the point of view of the insider, the person with TBI, to date has not been investigated with the attention it deserves (39).

This case has been made most fervently by Brown and Gordon (4). They argue that in the measurement of social constructs, value judgments are involved, and the values of the insiders (here, persons with TBI) and the outsiders (persons without disability, payors, clinicians, researchers) may be different. Power imbalances occur in measurement whenever the outsider's values and preferences are incorporated into the means–ends chain leading from interventions to immediate effects to ultimate outcomes, with few, if any, mechanisms for tapping into the values and preferences of the insider. Such power imbalances are of concern because the insider's perspective can vary significantly from that of the outsider (95).

Although most instruments designed to measure aspects of "functioning" have concentrated on the "how independent" and "how much" of acts, actions, and roles, a few have explored additional dimensions. GAS and the COPM, mentioned earlier, are semistructured approaches by which rehabilitation service recipients assisted by clinicians formulate individualized goals for therapy and provide perceptions of the adequacy of their performance, their satisfaction with performance, and the importance of each goal to their lives. An importance-weighted sum of outcomes serves as the key evaluation measure. Given their open-ended nature, the GAS and COPM goals specified can reflect performance in the domains of participation and activity, and even inclusion of impairment aspects is possible. The choice of goals reflects individual valuation, as does the importance rating. A number of instruments with standardized content have included importance ratings, such as the MACTAR (96), and many instruments traditionally classified as QOL measures (97). Stineman and colleagues have used the FIM to explore preferences of patients and clinicians for performance in ADLs vis-à-vis one another (3,98). Instruments to quantify preferences for aspects of participation or satisfaction with participation have been proposed by a number of researchers (23,99,100).

Subjective measures of the type described have a number of shortcomings according to critics (39). First, they typically involve the multiplication of 2 factors: one an importance rating, the other a satisfaction rating or a desire for change indicator. The critics claim that no psychometric measurement model applies to such a procedure and that therefore, the resulting item scores and total scores have no meaning or at least cannot be considered reliable or valid. The measurement models of classical test theory underlying psychometrics and of IRT only recognize simple items, each measured on an ordinal scale as input to measurement instruments that operationalize constructs on a (pseudo) interval scale. Another criticism of individualized measures is that if individuals can determine (by exclusion or even by nomination) which particular activities should be included in a measure and with what weight, the "content" of the construct varies from person to person, and performing averaging and other statistical manipulations makes no sense. However, it may be argued that if the *content* in all instances is judged (by the instrument's user) to be relevant to the construct, there is no problem. Personal construct psychology adherents see this as a strength of the methodology, rather than a weakness (97).

SELECTION OF A FUNCTIONAL ASSESSMENT MEASURE

The selection of an FA measure for a clinical, administrative, or research application is not straightforward. A first step

always should be determining what one wants to measure; activity/activity limitation only, or aspects of impairment and participation/participation restriction in addition. Although there are a few instruments, such as the DRS, that cover (parts of) all three domains, they often do that poorly, and using 2 or 3 separate instruments may be preferable. A second question is "what aspect of functioning is of interest, capacity, or performance," and consequently, what type of administration should be selected: testing in a laboratory or other setting, observation (by a clinician, researcher, or instrument), or report by the patient or a proxy. This limits choices, and one's options might be even more restricted if the population that one deals with has particular characteristics that make application of the most common instruments impossible, for example, intubation. Yet another issue is whether one is interested on the objective facts of activity limitations and participation restrictions, or that subjective elements are (also) of interest. The resources on hand for administration of the instrument—a special laboratory, administrator training, time available of administrator and subject—typically play a major role in decisions. Lastly, metrological characteristics—reliability, validity, sensitivity, clinical use—should inform the selection; although in some situations the choice of instruments is so limited that one needs to accept a measure with less than stellar measurement characteristics.

Table 1 provides capsule descriptions of some of the better known instruments used to assess activity and participation. It refers (in the last column) to 1 book and a series of websites where descriptive and evaluative information on these and many other instruments can be found. These useful websites themselves are described in Table 2.

There is a limited number of peer-reviewed reviews of FA instruments suitable for use with individuals with TBI.(101–112). The Common Data Elements project, on which many prominent TBI clinicians and researchers cooperated, made recommendations for core and supplemental TBI outcome measures and also identified a set of "emerging" measures (113). The TBI Model Systems of Care maintain a website, COMBI (Center on Outcome Measurement in Brain Injury) (http://www.tbims.org/combi/list.html) that in Spring 2012 contained information on 34 instruments commonly used in TBI clinical services and research. For each instrument, the following are offered: the actual instrument (subject to copyright restrictions), a syllabus containing administration and scoring instructions, information on administrator training and testing required, a description of the metrologic qualities of the instrument based on the published literature, and frequently asked questions. The various sections are kept up-to-date by experts, frequently the individual(s) who created the instrument.

Just making their way into the literature are measures developed by or selected by 3 federally funded projects to make available instruments that can be used across all patients or subjects, or specifically those with TBI or other neurological disorders. The Patient Reported Outcomes Measurement Information System (PROMIS) (http://www.nihpromis.org/default), funded by the National Institutes of Health (NIH), is a system of highly reliable, valid, flexible, precise, and responsive assessment tools that measure patient-reported health status in three domains: physical, mental, and social well-being. Administration methods were

TABLE 20-1 Selected Functional Assessment Measures

INSTRUMENT NAME	DESCRIPTION	TARGET POPULATION	COMMENTS	KEY REFERENCES
Barthel Index (BI)	A 10-item measure of disability.	Adolescents/adults in inpatient rehabilitation or living in the community with significant activity limitations	The forerunner of the FIM; still used. Designed for clinician rating but often administered in questionnaire format.	EBRSR RMD StrokEngine Tate
Community Integration Measure (CIM)	A 10-item measure of the subjective aspect of participation: "experience of belonging and participating".	Community-dwelling adolescents/adults with activity limitations or participation restrictions	Completed only by the person himself or herself, using interview or self-administration.	Tate
Community Integration Questionnaire (CIQ)	A 15-item instrument used to measure community integration.	Adolescents/adults with TBI living outside institutions	Originally, the instrument of participation used in the TBI model systems. Can be self-rated or rated by a clinician or significant other.	COMBI ERABI RMD Tate
Craig Handicap Assessment and Reporting Technique (CHART, CHART-SF)	A 32-item instrument used to measure participation. The CHART-SF is a 19-item shorter version of the CHART.	Adolescents/adults with TBI living outside institutions	Modeled on the WHO ICIDH. Completed using interview with the person or a proxy or self-administration.	COMBI RMD Tate
Disability Rating Scale (DRS)	An 8-item instrument used to measure disability. DRS items address impairment, activity limitations, and participation restrictions focusing on cognitive (rather than physical) ability to perform tasks.	All individuals, from those in (near-) coma to people fully reintegrated into society	Completion is based on clinician observation and/or interview with person or proxy.	COMBI ERABI Tate
Frenchay Activities Index (FAI)	A 15-item scale to measure frequency of involvement in household chores, leisure and work, and outdoor activities.	Community dwelling adults/adolescents	Reporting by the person or a proxy is possible. Most frequently used with elderly samples.	EBRSR StrokEngine Tate
Functional Independence Measure (FIM) and Functional Assessment Measure (FAM)	The FIM is an 18-item instrument (13 motor, 5 cognitive/communicative) to measure activity limitations. The FAM is a 12-item add-on with items relevant to cognitive/communicative functioning and community living.	Inpatient rehabilitation patients (about 8 years and older) and others who have significant activity limitations. The FIM + FAM combination is targeted more to community-living individuals.	The FIM was originally developed to measure burden of care; now generally used to quantify activity limitations. Most commonly used functional limitation measure in the United States; likely will be replaced by the CareTool. Both FIM and FAM are completed on the basis of clinician observation or systematic questioning of person or proxy.	COMBI EBRSR ERABI PROQOLID RMD StrokEdge StrokEngine Tate
Functional Independence Measure for Children (WeeFIM)	The WeeFIM is a version of the FIM targeted to children with a disability.	Children between 6 months and 7 years, inclusive, with significant functional limitations	The WeeFIM contains the same items as the FIM, but scoring considers functional abilities in a developmental context. Completed based on observation or parent interview.	PROQOLID Tate

(Continued)

TABLE 20-1 Selected Functional Assessment Measures (*Continued*)

INSTRUMENT NAME	DESCRIPTION	TARGET POPULATION	COMMENTS	KEY REFERENCES
Glasgow Outcome Scale (GOS) Extended Glasgow Outcome Scale (GOS-E)	The GOS is a 1-item instrument used to characterize overall disability. The GOS-E is an extension of the GOS that has 8 disability categories rather than 5.	All individuals from those in coma to people fully reintegrated into society.	GOS and GOS-E can be completed based on observation, interview by a clinician, or standardized interview by a researcher.	COMBI ERABI Tate
Impact on Participation and Autonomy Questionnaire (IPA or IPAQ)	A measure of subjective aspects of participation, focusing on autonomy and problems. Versions with 23, 39, and 41 items have been published.	Community-dwelling adults/adolescents with activity limitations or participation restrictions	Reporting by the person only in self-administered or interview format.	Tate
Mayo Portland Adaptability Inventory (MPAI)	A 35-item instrument (version 4) that measures functioning problems (vocational, communicative, etc.) after brain injury, in abilities, adjustment, and participation.	Community dwelling adolescents/adults with a brain injury	Can be self-rated or rated by a clinician or significant other.	COMBI ERABI
Participation Objective, Participation Subjective (POPS)	A measure of participation, both objective (26 items on frequency of participation) and subjective (an additional 26 + 26 items on the importance of activities and the satisfaction with current participation).	Community-dwelling adolescents/adults with a brain injury	The subjective items can be self-rated only; the objective items may be completed by a proxy.	COMBI Tate
Reintegration to Normal Living Index (RNLI),	An 11-item measure of participation with items that focus on satisfaction.	Community-dwelling adolescents/ individuals with activity limitations or participation restrictions	Completed by self-administration or interview. A version suitable for people who use aids or aides is available.	EBRSR RMD StrokEdge StrokEngine Tate
Short-Form 36 Health Survey (SF-36)	A measure of physical and mental health status, focusing on functional health (activities and participation), with 36 items that generate 8 subscale scores and 2 component scores: physical and mental.	All institutionalized and community-dwelling adolescents and adults	The most frequently used measure of HRQOL or health status; extensive norming available. Completed by the person himself or herself only. Versions with 20 and 12 items are also available, which only generate component scores.	EBRSR RMD StrokEdge StrokEngine Tate
Sydney Psychosocial Reintegration Scale (SPRS)	A 12-item measure covering occupation, interpersonal relations, and independent living skills.	Adolescents/adults dwelling in the community	One version scores change since injury; another current competence. A set of 15 nonscored questions is used to obtain relevant information.	Tate

We have selected functional assessment instruments that are applicable in TBI, are known well enough to be part of review articles on TBI outcome measures and databases of rehabilitation outcome measures, and focus on broad aspects of activity/activity limitations and/or participation/participation restrictions. Instruments that focus on only a single aspect of function (e.g., functional communication) are omitted. However, the listing of websites and sources provided in Table 20-2 includes many resources that provide a rich listing of measures (scales, instruments) of impairments and of more narrowly defined aspects of activity and participation. The "key references" column of this table refers to these websites, with the following abbreviations: COMBI, Center for Outcome Measurement in Brain Injury; EBRSR, Evidence-based Review of Moderate to Severe Acquired Brain Injury; ERABI, Evidence-based Review of Moderate to Severe Brain Injury; PROQOLID, Patient Reported Quality of Life Research; RMD, Rehabilitation Measures Database; StrokEdge, APTA Neurology Section Outcome Measure Recommendations; StrokEngine, Canadian Stroke Network. "Tate" refers to Tate RL. *A Compendium of Tests, Scales, and Questionnaires: The Practitioner's Guide to Measuring Outcomes After Acquired Brain Impairment.* Canada, USA: Psychology Press; 2010.

TABLE 20-2 A Selection of Websites That Describe and/or Evaluate Functional Assessment Instruments

ORGANIZATION/SITE NAME AND WEB ADDRESS	SITE DESCRIPTION
APTA Neurology Section Outcome Measure Recommendations http://www.neuropt.org/go/EDGE	Recommendations for outcome measure in clinical use are categorized by practice settings: acute care hospital, inpatient rehabilitation, home health, skilled nursing facility, and outpatient, as well as by acuity level.
Canadian Stroke Network StrokEngine http://www.medicine.mcgill.ca/strokengine-assess/	Provides information about interventions and outcome measures that can be used in (stroke) rehabilitation.
Center for Outcome Measurement in Brain Injury http://www.tbims.org/combi/	Provides information about instruments used to assess individuals with brain injury. Information provided includes background, administration and scoring guidelines, training and testing materials, scale properties, references, and frequently asked questions.
Centre for Evidence-based Physiotherapy http://www.cebp.nl/	The centre searches, collects, and disseminates scientific evidence about physical therapy for health care workers, patients, and health care payers. This website also contains more than 2,500 freely available white papers.
Evidence-based Review of Moderate to Severe Acquired Brain Injury http://www.abiebr.com/module/17-assessment-outcomes-following-acquiredtraumatic-brain-injury	Provides an evidence-based review of acquired brain injury rehabilitation literature. Current literature is synthesized into a free, usable format that can be downloaded from the site. The outcome measures chapter reviews a series of TBI outcome measures.
Evidence Based Review of Stroke Rehabilitation http://www.ebrsr.com/reviews_details.php?Outcome-Measures-9	Provides in-depth reviews of literature relevant to stroke rehabilitation. The outcome measures chapter makes recommendations for rehabilitation outcomes measure selection.
Health Measurement Research Group http://www.healthmeasurement.org/	Evaluates widely used health measures in terms of their strengths and limitations.
Medical Outcomes Trust http://www.outcomes-trust.org/	Provides information on the SF-36 and various other instruments that have been approved by the Trust.
NINDS Common Data Elements http://www.commondataelements.ninds.nih.gov/#page=Default	The Common Data Elements provides a platform that allows clinical investigators to collect, analyze, and share data on such disorders as stroke, spinal cord injury, and TBI, as well as several others.
Orthopedic Scores http://www.orthopaedicscore.com/	Provides free information about instruments that can be used to assess individuals with musculoskeletal conditions. The website can also be used to calculate scores on the tests, and allows the user to print test results in diverse formats.
Patient Reported Quality of Life Research http://www.proqolid.org/	Identifies and describes patient-reported outcomes and QOL instruments. Basic information about instruments is provided free; for more detailed information, users must pay a fee.
Psychometric Laboratory for Health Sciences at Leeds University http://www.leeds.ac.uk/medicine/rehabmed/psychometric/index.htm	Several outcomes measures, generally developed using Rasch analysis, are provided and generally free.
RAND Healthcare Surveys and Tools http://www.rand.org/health/surveys_tools.html	Provides a listing of many surveys and tools produced by RAND Healthcare available without charge for noncommercial purposes.
Rehabilitation Measures Database http://www.rehabmeasures.org/rehabweb/allmeasures.aspx? PageView=Shared	Help for clinicians and researchers in identifying reliable and valid instruments used to assess patient outcomes during all phases of rehabilitation. Provides evidence-based summaries that include concise descriptions of psychometric properties, instructions for administering and scoring, as well as a representative bibliography with citations linked to PubMed abstracts.
Spinal Cord Injury Rehabilitation Evidence http://www.scireproject.com/outcome-measures	Provides a synthesis of research evidence investigating rehabilitation interventions and outcome measures in spinal cord injury.
Transport Accident Commission http://www.tac.vic.gov.au/jsp/content/Navigation Controller.do?areaID=22&tierID=2&navID= F0065BDA7F000001018056DF70ECF3D5&navLink= null&pageID=1675	The TAC clinical resources page provides information and resources useful to clinical practice, including information on outcome measures.

Modified, with permission, from the Rehabilitation Measures Database site.

developed with the situation and needs of persons with disability in mind (114). As of spring 2012, instruments were available to quantify (among others) physical function–mobility, physical function upper extremity, ability to participate in social roles and activities, satisfaction with social participation (discretionary social activities), satisfaction with social participation (social roles), and (pediatric) peer relationships. A very similar project is Neuro-QOL (http://www.Neuro-QOL.org/default.aspx), a venture funded by the National Institute of Neurological Disorders and Stroke that aims to create clinically relevant and psychometrically well-developed HRQOL (social, psychological, and mental well-being) assessment tools for adults and children with neurological disorders (115). Available tools include ability to participate in social roles and activities, lower extremity function–mobility, upper extremity function–fine motor, ADL, and communication.

While PROMIS and Neuro-QOL focus on activity (limitations) and participation (restrictions), the NIH toolbox project (http://www.nihtoolbox.org/default.aspx) is identifying or creating widely applicable instruments to quantify neurological and behavioral functions in the domains of cognition (executive function, episodic memory, working memory, processing speed, language, attention, and reading), emotion (negative affect, positive affect, stress and coping, social relationships), motor function (locomotion, balance, dexterity, strength, and endurance), and sensation (audition, olfaction, somatosensation, taste, vestibular balance) that use performance testing, where applicable. The toolbox, PROMIS, and Neuro-QOL instruments have been developed using state-of-the-art research methodology by large teams of investigators with a range of expertise and access to large samples. Because public funding supported the research and development, the resulting instruments are available free of charge.

CONCLUSION

FA refers to the quantification of functioning, specifically after onset of a major disorder, in areas ranging from body systems to societal role fulfillment, but with an emphasis on ADLs, mobility, and other skills at the person level. Because TBI, specifically moderate or severe TBI, has cognitive, emotional, and physical consequences that affect functioning, clinicians need to be familiar with FA measures for patient assessment and monitoring. Similarly, researchers investigating diagnosis of, prognosis of, and treatment of TBI need to be familiar with FA instruments.

FA instruments generally consist of a set of items (questions, subskills), which are scored and then combined using simple or advanced mathematical models to provide a total score that reflects the person's status on a continuum ranging from totally unable to normal. The relevant information can be obtained by means of observation by a clinician or researcher; report by the person or a proxy; or testing in a laboratory, clinic, or (preferably) a real-life setting. The user of FA information needs to be aware of the method of data collection, as well as the content of the FA measure. Some understanding of metrology or psychometrics (the science of measurement as it refers to human functioning) is similarly useful in understanding and using FA data, whether for individual patients/clients or for groups.

Ideally, the FA instruments used in making decisions as part of clinical or administrative management or in research are reliable, valid, sensitive to change, and otherwise appropriate for the individual(s) with whom they are used. Although most FA instruments in current usage were designed to provide objective information, the valuation by people with TBI of the roles and relationships that are part of instruments measuring functioning at the level of household, community, and society (participation measures) is an important issue; a few instruments are available to quantify the fit between participation and individual goals and preferences.

FA instruments have become more important with CMS basing payment for postacute services on functional status. To date, only functional status at admission is taken into account, but is not impossible that in the future, payment will be linked to provider performance, and functional change will be considered in reimbursing for care that has been delivered. Certainly, such change data are important in evaluating clinical programs and improving treatment approaches. With the aging of the population and more interest in comparative effectiveness research, functional status issues are only going to become more salient in clinical services, program administration, and research.

 KEY CLINICAL POINTS

In selecting a FA measure for individuals with TBI, consider the following points:

1. Does the instrument include the function(s) you want to assess at the level of impairment, activity limitation, or participation restriction?
2. Does the means of data collection and the setting of assessment correspond to the real-life situation in which functioning occurs—testing function in a different setting may yield different results (e.g., laboratory vs clinic vs community)?
3. Is the functional measure matched to the rehabilitation spectrum of clients served (e.g., inpatient vs outpatient) and their abilities?
4. If the FA measure was developed for assessing the general population, does it take into account the cognitive and emotional impairments that frequently disable persons with TBI?
5. What are the reliability, validity, and sensitivity of a candidate scale? Floor and ceiling effects as well as insensitivity to minimally important changes may limit the amount of improvement that can be measured.
6. Unless IRT or Rasch analysis was used to develop the measure, is it reasonable to assume that the instrument uses a ratio scale? An interval scale?

The same issues are relevant to the published literature using FA measures. Before accepting any conclusions, the readers have to ask themselves whether the instrument used and the way it was used were likely to generate reliable, valid, and sensitive data that can be interpreted in the manner proposed.

KEY REFERENCES

1. Dijkers MP. Issues in the conceptualization and measurement of participation: an overview. *Arch Phys Med Rehabil.* 2010;91(9)(suppl):S5–S16.
   A discussion of issues involved in measuring participation, with problems of subjective valuation of outcomes part of the expose.
2. Nichol AD, Higgins AM, Gabbe BJ, Murray LJ, Cooper DJ, Cameron PA. Measuring functional and quality of life outcomes following major head injury: common scales and checklists. *Injury.* 2011;42(3):281–287.
   This article offers a description of major FA and HRQOL measures commonly used in TBI care and research.
3. Tesio L. Functional assessment in rehabilitative medicine: principles and methods. *Eura Medicophys.* 2007;43(4):515–523.
   A nontechnical description of the principles of functional assessment, with emphasis on Rasch analysis methodology in creating measures.
4. Wilde EA, Whiteneck GG, Bogner J, et al. Recommendations for the use of common outcome measures in traumatic brain injury research. *Arch Phys Med Rehabil.* 2010;91(11):1650–1660,e17.
   This article contains recommendations by a panel of experts for TBI outcome measures that should be considered for use in any research in this area.
5. World Health Organization. *International Classification of Functioning, Disability and Health: ICF.* Geneva, OH: World Health Organization; 2001.
   This book offers a conceptual model of the disablement continuum, as well as taxonomies of body functions, body structures, activities and participation, and environmental factors.

References

1. Keith RA. Functional status and health status. *Arch Phys Med Rehabil.* 1994;75(4):478–483.
2. Crewe NM, Dijkers M. Functional assessment. In: Scherer M, Cushman L, eds. *Psychological Assessment in Medical Rehabilitation Settings.* Washington, DC: American Psychological Association; 1995:101–144.
3. Stineman MG, Wechsler B, Ross R, Maislin G. A method for measuring quality of life through subjective weighting of functional status. *Arch Phys Med Rehabil.* 2003;84(4) (suppl 2):S15–S22.
4. Brown M, Gordon WA. Empowerment in measurement: "muscle," "voice," and subjective quality of life as a gold standard. *Arch Phys Med Rehabil.* 2004;85(4)(suppl 2):S13–S20.
5. World Health Organization. *International Classification of Functioning, Disability and Health: ICF.* Geneva, OH: World Health Organization; 2001.
6. World Health Organization. *International Classification of Impairments, Disabilities and Handicaps. A Manual of Classification Relating to the Consequenses of Disease.* Geneva, OH: World Health Organization; 1980.
7. Teasdale G, Jennett B. Assessment of coma and impaired consciousness. A practical scale. *Lancet.* 1974;2(7872):81–84.
8. Keith RA, Granger CV, Hamilton BB, Sherwin FS. The functional independence measure: a new tool for rehabilitation. *Adv Clin Rehabil.* 1987;1:6–18.
9. Whiteneck GG, Charlifue SW, Gerhart KA, Overholser JD, Richardson GN. Quantifying handicap: a new measure of long-term rehabilitation outcomes. *Arch Phys Med Rehabil.* 1992;73(6):519–526.
10. Whiteneck G, Dijkers MP. Difficult to measure constructs: conceptual and methodological issues concerning participation and environmental factors. *Arch Phys Med Rehabil.* 2009;90(11 suppl):S22–S35.
11. Rappaport M, Hall KM, Hopkins K, Belleza T, Cope DN. Disability rating scale for severe head trauma: coma to community. *Arch Phys Med Rehabil.* 1982;63(3):118–123.
12. Frey W. Functional assessment in the 80s: a conceptual enigma, a technical challenge. In: Halpern A, Fuhrer M, eds. *Functional Assessment in Rehabilitation.* Baltimore, MD: Paul H. Brooks Publishing Co.; 1984:11–43.
13. Holbrook M, Skilbeck CE. An activities index for use with stroke patients. *Age Ageing.* 1983;12(2):166–170.
14. Clark MS, Bond MJ. The Adelaide activities profile: a measure of the life-style activities of elderly people. *Aging (Milano).* 1995;7(4):174–184.
15. Moseley AM, Yap MC. Interrater reliability of the TEMPA for the measurement of upper limb function in adults with traumatic brain injury. *J Head Trauma Rehabil.* 2003;18(6):526–531.
16. Willer B, Ottenbacher KJ, Coad ML. The community integration questionnaire. A comparative examination. *Am J Phys Med Rehabil.* 1994;73(2):103–111.
17. Whiteneck GG, Dijkers MP, Heinemann AW, et al. Development of the participation assessment with recombined tools-objective for use after traumatic brain injury. *Arch Phys Med Rehabil.* 2011;92(4):542–551.
18. Bogner JA, Whiteneck GG, Corrigan JD, Lai JS, Dijkers MP, Heinemann AW. Comparison of scoring methods for the participation assessment with recombined tools-objective. *Arch Phys Med Rehabil.* 2011;92(4):552–563.
19. Ware JE Jr, Sherbourne CD. The MOS 36-item short-form health survey (SF-36). I. Conceptual framework and item selection. *Med Care.* 1992;30(6):473–483.
20. Dijkers MP. Quality of life after traumatic brain injury: a review of research approaches and findings. *Arch Phys Med Rehabil.* 2004;85(4)(suppl 2):S21–S35.
21. Jette AM, Haley SM, Coster WJ, et al. Late life function and disability instrument: I. Development and evaluation of the disability component. *J Gerontol A Biol Sci Med Sci.* 2002;57(4):M209–M216.
22. Gerrity MS, Gaylord S, Williams ME. Short versions of the Timed Manual Performance Test. Development, reliability, and validity. *Med Care.* 1993;31(7):617–628.
23. Brown M, Dijkers M, Gordon WA, Ashman T, Charatz H, Cheng Z. Participation objective, participation aubjective: a measure of participation combining outsider and insider perspectives. *J Head Trauma Rehabil.* 2004;19(6):459–481.
24. Dijkers M. Measuring the long-term outcomes of traumatic brain injury: a review of the community integration questionnaire. *J Head Trauma Rehabil.* 1997;12(6):74–91.
25. Mahoney FI, Barthel DW. Functional evaluation: the Barthel Index. *Md State Med J.* 1965;14:61–65.
26. Linacre JM, Heinemann AW, Wright BD, Granger CV, Hamilton BB. The structure and stability of the Functional Independence Measure. *Arch Phys Med Rehabil.* 1994;75(2):127–132.
27. Bond TG, Fox CM. *Applying the Rasch Model. Fundamental Measurement in the Human Sciences.* Mahwah, NJ: Erlbaum; 2001.
28. Tesio L. Measuring behaviours and perceptions: Rasch analysis as a tool for rehabilitation research. *J Rehabil Med.* 2003;35(3):105–115.
29. Tesio L. Functional assessment in rehabilitative medicine: principles and methods. *Eura Medicophys.* 2007;43(4):515–523.
30. Granger CV, Carlin M, Linacre JM, et al. Rasch-derived latent trait measurement of outcomes: insightful use leads to precision case management and evidence-based practices in functional healthcare. *J Appl Meas.* 2010;11(3):230–243.
31. Coster W, Ludlow L, Mancini M. Using IRT variable maps to enrich understanding of rehabilitation data. *J Outcome Meas.* 1999;3(2):123–133.
32. Jette AM, Haley SM. Contemporary measurement techniques for rehabilitation outcomes assessment. *J Rehabil Med.* 2005;37(6):339–345.
33. Marino RJ, Barros T, Biering-Sorensen F, et al. International standards for neurological classification of spinal cord injury. *J Spinal Cord Med.* 2003;26 (suppl 1):S50–S56.

34. Park S, Fisher AG, Velozo CA. Using the assessment of motor and process skills to compare occupational performance between clinic and home settings. *Am J Occup Ther*. 1994;48(8):697–709.

35. Min CH, Ince NF, Tewfik AH. Classification of continuously executed early morning activities using wearable wireless sensors. *Conf Proc IEEE Eng Med Biol Soc*. 2008;2008:5192–5195.

36. Smith PM, Illig SB, Fiedler RC, Hamilton BB, Ottenbacher KJ. Intermodal agreement of follow-up telephone functional assessment using the Functional Independence Measure in patients with stroke. *Arch Phys Med Rehabil*. 1996;77(5):431–435.

37. Klein RM, Bell B. Self-care skills: behavioral measurement with Klein-Bell ADL scale. *Arch Phys Med Rehabil*. 1982;63(7):335–338.

38. Dijkers MP, Whiteneck G, El-Jaroudi R. Measures of social outcomes in disability research. *Arch Phys Med Rehabil*. 2000;81(12)(suppl 2):S63–S80.

39. Dijkers MP. Issues in the conceptualization and measurement of participation: an overview. *Arch Phys Med Rehabil*. 2010;91(9 suppl): S5–S16.

40. Whiteneck G, Dijkers MP. Difficult to measure constructs: conceptual and methodological issues concerning participation and environmental factors. *Arch Phys Med Rehabil*. 2009;90(11):S22–S35.

41. Webster K, Cella D, Yost K. The Functional Assessment of Chronic Illness Therapy (FACIT) measurement system: Properties, applications, and interpretation. *Health Qual Life Outcomes*. 2003;1(1):79.

42. Andres PL, Black-Schaffer RM, Ni P, Haley SM. Computer adaptive testing: a strategy for monitoring stroke rehabilitation across settings. *Top Stroke Rehabil*. 2004;11(2):33–39.

43. Dijkers MP. A computer adaptive testing simulation applied to the FIM instrument motor component. *Arch Phys Med Rehabil*. 2003; 84(3):384–393.

44. Bode RK, Heinemann AW, Semik P. Measurement properties of the Galveston Orientation and Amnesia Test (GOAT) and improvement patterns during inpatient rehabilitation. *J Head Trauma Rehabil*. 2000;15(1):637–655.

45. Cook KF, Roddey TS, Gartsman GM, Olson SL. Development and psychometric evaluation of the flexilevel scale of shoulder function. *Med Care*. 2003;41(7):823–835.

46. Vayalakkara J, Backhaus SD, Bradley JD, Simco ER, Golden CJ. Abbreviated form of the Wisconsin Card Sort test. *Int J Neurosci*. 2000;103(1–4):131–137.

47. Manchester D, Priestley N, Jackson H. The assessment of executive functions: coming out of the office. *Brain Inj*. 2004;18(11):1067–1081.

48. Hobart J, Cano S. Improving the evaluation of therapeutic interventions in multiple sclerosis: the role of new psychometric methods. *Health Technol Assess*. 2009;13(12):iii, ix–x, 1–177.

49. Hall K, Mann N, High W Jr, Wright J, Kreutzer JS, Wood D. Functional measures after traumatic brain injury: ceiling effects of FIM, FIM + FAM, DRS, and CIQ. *J Head Trauma Rehabil*. 1996;11(5):27–39.

50. Seel RT, Wright G, Wallace T, Newman S, Dennis L. The utility of the FIM + FAM for assessing traumatic brain injury day program outcomes. *J Head Trauma Rehabil*. 2007;22(5):267–277.

51. Williams G, Pallant J, Greenwood K. Further development of the High-level Mobility Assessment Tool (HiMAT). *Brain Inj*. 2010; 24(7–8):1027–1031.

52. MacDonald S, Johnson CJ. Assessment of subtle cognitive-communication deficits following acquired brain injury: a normative study of the Functional Assessment of Verbal Reasoning and Executive Strategies (FAVRES). *Brain Inj*. 2005;19(11):895–902.

53. Body R, Perkins MR. Validation of linguistic analyses in narrative discourse after traumatic brain injury. *Brain Inj*. 2004;18(7):707–724.

54. Giacino JT, Kalmar K, Whyte J. The JFK Coma Recovery Scale-Revised: Measurement characteristics and diagnostic utility. *Arch Phys Med Rehabil*. 2004;85(12):2020-2029.

55. American Congress of Rehabilitation Medicine, Brain Injury-Interdisciplinary Special Interest Group, Disorders of Consciousness Task Force, Seel RT, Sherer M, Whyte J, et al. Assessment scales for disorders of consciousness: evidence-based recommendations for clinical practice and research. *Arch Phys Med Rehabil*. 2010; 91(12):1795–1813.

56. Terwee CB, Dekker FW, Wiersinga WM, Prummel MF, Bossuyt PM. On assessing responsiveness of health-related quality of life

instruments: guidelines for instrument evaluation. *Qual Life Res*. 2003;12(4):349–362.

57. Ward MM, Marx AS, Barry NN. Identification of clinically important changes in health status using receiver operating characteristic curves. *J Clin Epidemiol*. 2000;53(3):279–284.

58. Diehr P, Chen L, Patrick D, Feng Z, Yasui Y. Reliability, effect size, and responsiveness of health status measures in the design of randomized and cluster-randomized trials. *Contemp Clin Trials*. 2005;26(1):45–58.

59. Revicki DA, Cella D, Hays RD, Sloan JA, Lenderking WR, Aaronson NK. Responsiveness and minimal important differences for patient reported outcomes. *Health Qual Life Outcomes*. 2006;4:70.

60. Revicki D, Hays RD, Cella D, Sloan J. Recommended methods for determining responsiveness and minimally important differences for patient-reported outcomes. *J Clin Epidemiol*. 2008;61(2):102–109.

61. de Vet HC, Terwee CB. The minimal detectable change should not replace the minimal important difference. *J Clin Epidemiol*. 2010; 63(7):804–805.

62. de Vet HC, Terluin B, Knol DL, et al. Three ways to quantify uncertainty in individually applied "minimally important change" values. *J Clin Epidemiol*. 2010;63(1):37–45.

63. Hinton-Bayre AD. Deriving reliable change statistics from testretest normative data: comparison of models and mathematical expressions. *Arch Clin Neuropsychol*. 2010;25(3):244–256.

64. Maassen GH, Bossema E, Brand N. Reliable change and practice effects: outcomes of various indices compared. *J Clin Exp Neuropsychol*. 2008;31(3):339–352.

65. Meyers AR, Andresen EM. Enabling our instruments: accommodation, universal design, and access to participation in research. *Arch Phys Med Rehabil*. 2000;81(12)(suppl 2):S5–S9.

66. Andresen EM. Criteria for assessing the tools of disability outcomes research. *Arch Phys Med Rehabil*. 2000;81(12)(suppl 2):S15–S20.

67. Hahn EA, Cella D. Health outcomes assessment in vulnerable populations: measurement challenges and recommendations. *Arch Phys Med Rehabil*. 2003;84(4)(suppl 2):S35–S42.

68. Johnston MV, Graves DE. Towards guidelines for evaluation of measures: an introduction with application to spinal cord injury. *J Spinal Cord Med*. 2008;31(1):13–26.

69. Kiresuk TJ, Sherman RE. Goal attainment scaling: a general method for evaluating comprehensive community mental health programs. *Community Ment Health J*. 1968:4(6): 443–453.

70. Malec JF. Goal attainment scaling in rehabilitation. *Neuropsychol Rehabil*. 1999;9(3–4):253–275.

71. Rockwood K, Joyce B, Stolee P. Use of goal attainment scaling in measuring clinically important change in cognitive rehabilitation patients. *J Clin Epidemiol*. 1997;50(5):581–588.

72. Turner-Stokes L. Goal attainment scaling (GAS) in rehabilitation: a practical guide. *Clin Rehabil*. 2009;23(4):362–370.

73. Bovend'Eerdt TJ, Botell RE, Wade DT. Writing SMART rehabilitation goals and achieving goal attainment scaling: a practical guide. *Clin Rehabil*. 2009;23(4):352–361.

74. Schlosser RW. Goal attainment scaling as a clinical measurement technique in communication disorders: a critical review. *J Commun Disord*. 2004;37(3):217–239.

75. Law M, Baptiste S, McColl M, Opzoomer A, Polatajko H, Pollock N. The Canadian occupational performance measure: an outcome measure for occupational therapy. *Can J Occup Ther*. 1990;57(2): 82–87.

76. Pollock N, Baptiste S, Law M, McColl MA, Opzoomer A, Polatajko H. Occupational performance measures: a review based on the guidelines for the client-centred practice of occupational therapy. *Can J Occup Ther*. 1990;57(2):77–81.

77. Eyssen IC, Beelen A, Dedding C, Cardol M, Dekker J. The reproducibility of the Canadian occupational performance measure. *Clin Rehabil*. 2005;19(8):888–894.

78. Dedding C, Cardol M, Eyssen IC, Dekker J, Beelen A. Validity of the Canadian occupational performance measure: a client-centred outcome measurement. *Clin Rehabil*. 2004;18(6):660–667.

79. Doig E, Fleming J, Kuipers P, Cornwell PL. Clinical utility of the combined use of the Canadian occupational performance measure and goal attainment scaling. *Am J Occup Ther*. 2010;64(6):904–914.

80. Dawson DR, Gaya A, Hunt A, Levine B, Lemsky C, Polatajko HJ. Using the cognitive orientation to occupational performance (CO-OP) with adults with executive dysfunction following traumatic brain injury. *Can J Occup Ther*. 2009;76(2):115–127.

81. Phipps S, Richardson P. Occupational therapy outcomes for clients with traumatic brain injury and stroke using the Canadian occupational performance measure. *Am J Occup Ther*. 2007;61(3):328–334.

82. Bierman AS. Functional status: the sixth vital sign. *J Gen Intern Med*. 2001;16(11):785–786.

83. Campbell DT, Stanley JC. *Experimental and Quasi-Experimental Designs for Research*. Chicago, IL: Rand McNally College Publishing Company; 1963.

84. Hall KM, Johnston MV. Outcomes evaluation in TBI rehabilitation. Part II: measurement tools for a nationwide data system. *Arch Phys Med Rehabil*. 1994;75(12, special issue):SC10–SC118.

85. Johnston MV, Eastwood E, Wilkerson DL, Anderson L, Alves A. Systematically assessing and improving the quality and outcomes of medical rehabilitation programs. In: Delisa JA, Gans BM, Walsh NE, eds. *Physical Medicine and Rehabilitation: Principles and Practice*. 4th ed. Philadelphia, PA: Lippincott Williams Wilkins; 2005:1163–1192.

86. Carter GM, Relles DA, Ridgeway GK, Rimes CM. Measuring function for Medicare inpatient rehabilitation payment. *Health Care Financ Rev*. 2003;24(3):25–44.

87. Johnston MV, Graves D, Greene M. The uniform postacute assessment tool: systematically evaluating the quality of measurement evidence. *Arch Phys Med Rehabil*. 2007;88(11):1505–1512.

88. Gage B, Stineman M, Deutsch A, et al. Perspectives on the state-of-the-science in rehabilitation medicine and its implications for Medicare postacute care policies. *Arch Phys Med Rehabil*. 2007;88(12):1737–1739.

89. Holland DE. The Medicare post-acute care payment reform initiative: impact and opportunity for case management. *Prof Case Manag*. 2008;13(1):37–42.

90. Iezzoni LI, Greenberg MS. Capturing and classifying functional status information in administrative databases. *Health Care Financ Rev*. 2003;24(3):61–76.

91. Kukafka R, Bales ME, Burkhardt A, Friedman C. Human and automated coding of rehabilitation discharge summaries according to the international classification of functioning, disability, and health. *J Am Med Inform Assoc*. 2006;13(5):508–515.

92. Bernabeu M, Laxe S, Lopez R, et al. Developing core sets for persons with traumatic brain injury based on the international classification of functioning, disability, and health. *Neurorehabil Neural Repair*. 2009;23(5):464–467.

93. Ustün TB, Chatterji S, Kostansjek N, Bickenbach J. WHO's ICF and functional status information in health records. *Health Care Financ Rev*. 2003;24(3):77–88.

94. Corrigan JD. Community integration following traumatic brain injury. *NeuroRehabilitation*. 1994;4(2):109–121.

95. Heinemann AW, Lai JS, Magasi S, et al. Measuring participation enfranchisement. *Arch Phys Med Rehabil*. 2011;92(4):564–571.

96. Tugwell P, Bombardier C, Buchanan WW, Goldsmith CH, Grace E, Hanna B. The MACTAR patient preference disability questionnaire—an individualized functional priority approach for assessing improvement in physical disability in clinical trials in rheumatoid arthritis. *J Rheumatol*. 1987;14(3):446–451.

97. Dijkers MP. Individualization in quality of life measurement: in-struments and approaches. *Arch Phys Med Rehabil*. 2003;84(4)(suppl 2):S3–S14.

98. Stineman MG, Maislin G, Nosek M, Fiedler R, Granger CV. Comparing consumer and clinician values for alternative functional states: application of a new feature trade-off consensus building tool. *Arch Phys Med Rehabil*. 1998;79(12):1522–1529.

99. Johnston MV, Goverover Y, Dijkers M. Community activities and individuals' satisfaction with them: quality of life in the first year after traumatic brain injury. *Arch Phys Med Rehabil*. 2005;86(4):735–745.

100. Cicerone KD, Mott T, Azulay J, Friel JC. Community integration and satisfaction with functioning after intensive cognitive rehabilitation for traumatic brain injury. *Arch Phys Med Rehabil*. 2004;85(6):943–950.

101. Bedell G, Coster W. Measuring participation of school-aged children with traumatic brain injuries: considerations and approaches. *J Head Trauma Rehabil*. 2008;23(4):220–229.

102. Bullock MR, Merchant RE, Choi SC, et al. Outcome measures for clinical trials in neurotrauma. *Neurosurg Focus*. 2002;13(1):ECP1.

103. Malloy P, Grace J. A review of rating scales for measuring behavior change due to frontal systems damage. *Cogn Behav Neurol*. 2005;18(1):18–27.

104. Riemsma RP, Forbes CA, Glanville JM, Eastwood AJ, Kleijnen J. General health status measures for people with cognitive impairment: learning disability and acquired brain injury. *Health Technol Assess*. 2001;5(6):1–100.

105. van Baalen B, Odding E, Maas AI, Ribbers GM, Bergen MP, Stam HJ. Traumatic brain injury: classification of initial severity and determination of functional outcome. *Disabil Rehabil*. 2003;25(1):9–18.

106. von Steinbuechel N, Richter S, Morawetz C, Riemsma R. Assessment of subjective health and health-related quality of life in persons with acquired or degenerative brain injury. *Curr Opin Neurol*. 2005;18(6):681–691.

107. Adamovich BB. Functional outcome assessment of adults with traumatic brain injury. *Semin Speech Lang*. 1998;19(3):281–290.

108. Li Wood R, Alderman N, Williams C. Assessment of neurobehavioural disability: a review of existing measures and recommendations for a comprehensive assessment tool. *Brain Inj*. 2008;22(12):905–918.

109. Nichol AD, Higgins AM, Gabbe BJ, Murray LJ, Cooper DJ, Cameron PA. Measuring functional and quality of life outcomes following major head injury: common scales and checklists. *Injury*. 2011;42(3):281–287.

110. Salter K, Foley N, Jutai J, Bayley M, Teasell R. Assessment of community integration following traumatic brain injury. *Brain Inj*. 2008;22(11):820–835.

111. Williams G, Robertson V, Greenwood K. Measuring high-level mobility after traumatic brain injury. *Am J Phys Med Rehabil*. 2004;83(12):910–920.

112. Winthrop AL. Health-related quality of life after pediatric trauma. *Curr Opin Pediatr*. 2010;22(3):346–351.

113. Wilde EA, Whiteneck GG, Bogner J, et al. Recommendations for the use of common outcome measures in traumatic brain injury research. *Arch Phys Med Rehabil*. 2010;91(11):1650–1660,e17.

114. Amtmann D, Cook KF, Johnson KL, Cella D. The PROMIS initiative: involvement of rehabilitation stakeholders in development and examples of applications in rehabilitation research. *Arch Phys Med Rehabil*. 2011;92(10)(suppl):S12–S19.

115. Cella D, Nowinski C, Peterman A, et al. The neurology quality-of-life measurement initiative. *Arch Phys Med Rehabil*. 2011;92(10)(suppl):S28–S36.

21

Life Expectancy and Wellness

Cynthia L. Harrison-Felix, Lenore A. Hawley, Allen W. Brown, and Michael J. DeVivo

INTRODUCTION

Life expectancy after major traumatic events is of interest to a wide range of audiences including those who survive the trauma, sometimes with lifelong disabilities, their family members, care providers, third-party payors, attorneys, health care planners, life-care planners, and researchers. In particular, persons who experience a traumatic brain injury (TBI) often face an increased risk of many secondary medical conditions that result in a reduction in life expectancy for those with more severe injuries.

In this chapter, we will review the current literature on life expectancy for persons with TBI compared to the general population of similar age, gender, and race. We will also review early and late causes of death, risk factors related to short- and long-term mortality, clinical implications of secondary medical complications of particular concern after TBI, recommendations for maintaining health and wellness after TBI, and medicolegal issues associated with life expectancy determination and interpretation.

TERMINOLOGY

Some terminology defined here will be helpful in understanding some of the findings from studies cited in this chapter.

- **Mortality rate** is the number of deaths per unit of time (typically 1 year) in a population, sample, or study cohort divided by the total number of individuals in the population/sample/cohort. Thus, in the following section on mortality after TBI, rates reported as percentages indicate the proportion of the study population that died during the reported time interval. Mortality rates can also reflect the probability of death that depends on the number of deaths and the midyear population for each single year of age observed during the calendar year of interest. Thus, in the following section on deaths caused by TBI, mortality rates are given such as 9 per 100,000 in 2000, which means in the year 2000, for every 100,000 persons in the population, 9 people died.
- **Person-years** are the total number of years a person is followed in a study, and then those totals are summed across all members of a study cohort. So if 1 person is in the study for 5 years and a second person is in the study for 10 years, then the total person-years for the study cohort is 15 years.
- **Life expectancy** is the average number of years of life remaining for persons who have attained a given age. Life expectancy is derived from the annual life tables published by the National Center for Health Statistics (1). Calculation of a life table is derived from the probability of death (the mortality rate), which depends on the number of deaths and the midyear population for each single year of age observed during the calendar year of interest (2). Life tables are constructed using 7 parameters: (a) the age interval (e.g., age 0–1); (b) the probability of dying during the given age interval; (c) the number of individuals surviving from the original cohort to the beginning of each successive age interval; (d) the number of individuals dying in each successive age interval out of the original total cohort; (e) the number of person-years lived by the cohort within a given age interval; (f) the total number of person-years that would be lived by the cohort after the beginning of the age interval; and (g) the life expectancy at any given age, which is derived by dividing the total person-years that would be lived above a given age by the number of person who survived to that age interval (l). Because it is the mortality rates that are the basis of calculating life expectancy, it follows that the higher the mortality rate, the shorter the life expectancy. Thus, in the following section on life expectancy, where an average life expectancy reduction is given, this indicates that on average across all ages, genders, and races, individuals with TBI will live a fewer number of years than a person in the general population of similar age, gender, and race.
- **Standardized Mortality Ratio (SMR)** is calculated as the observed number of deaths in a population or study cohort divided by the expected number of deaths in similar individuals from the general population. The expected number of deaths is calculated by assigning the U.S. mortality rate of a given year for each year postinjury for each case based on his or her gender, race, and age at each annual anniversary of injury. Once rates are assigned for each postinjury anniversary year for each case, the rates for each year are summed for each case.

Finally, the summed rate for each case is summed over all cases in a population study cohort to obtain the expected number of deaths needed to calculate the overall SMR. For example, 10 deaths are observed in the study cohort, whereas in a cohort of individuals in the general population of same or similar age, gender, and race, the expected number of deaths would be 5. Thus, the SMR would be 2.00, which indicates that individuals in the study cohort are 2 times more likely to die compared to individuals in the general population of same/similar age, gender, and race.

- **Risk factors** are characteristics or processes related to a person that can put them at greater risk of a certain outcome. For example, older age at the time of a TBI is a risk factor for earlier death after TBI.

Additional references are also included, which provide further details on statistical nomenclature and methodology used in survival studies (3–5).

MORTALITY AFTER TBI

Deaths Caused by TBI

Most of the literature on mortality after TBI focuses on the mortality rate, risk factors for death, and causes of death among individuals who have sustained a TBI and survived to some point (e.g., hospital admission or discharge), from which point they were then followed until they die, they are lost to follow-up, or until the end of the study. In contrast, a few studies have reported on death rates that are directly related to TBI. That is, TBI is considered to be 1 of the causes of death. For example, Faul et al. (6) reports that an estimated 1.7 million TBIs occur in the United States annually. Of those, 1,365,000 are seen in hospital emergency departments, 275,000 are hospitalized, and 52,000 are reported TBI-related deaths.

Early Mortality After TBI

The overwhelming majority of the literature on mortality after TBI has focused on *early* mortality, which occurs within 1 year after injury. These studies have used several different data sources, taken place in different countries, included different and overlapping years of data, varied in inclusion criteria, and tracked patients for different amounts of time postinjury. Because several of these types of studies have been published, this review will focus on those published in the past decade as being the most relevant to current knowledge. This review also attempts to group similar studies together to draw some relevant conclusions.

Several studies have specifically focused on early mortality after *severe* TBI. A number of those have focused specifically on death occurring during hospitalization (i.e., *in-hospital* mortality) (7–17). The lowest reported in-hospital mortality rates after severe TBI hover around 10%. For example, 1 study used the Pennsylvania Trauma Outcome Study database of head and neck injuries treated in trauma centers and reported a rate of 10% (17). Two studies used data from the National Trauma Data Bank and reported mortality rates of 11% (7) and 9% (included only cases with blood alcohol

level measured) (13). There are a cluster of studies that have reported higher rates closer to 30% (9,11,12,14), with the highest in-hospital mortality rate for individuals with severe TBI of 51% reported in a study using a Honolulu, Hawaii hospital trauma database (10).

Several studies have followed cases of severe TBI out to *6-months postinjury* and report rates that generally hover around 50%, which is higher than those for most in-hospital mortality rates (18–26). For example, the lowest mortality rate of 36% was reported in a study of patients admitted to a neurosurgical intensive care unit in Singapore from 1999 to 2004 (22), and the highest rate of 58% was reported in a study of patients admitted to an Argentinean Emergency Department of a level I trauma center from 2000 to 2003 (23). Finally, 1 study followed all severe TBI hospital admissions of all ages and reported a mortality rate of 29% at *1-year postinjury* (27).

Several studies have specifically focused on early mortality after *moderate-to-severe* TBI and have generally focused on *in-hospital* mortality (28–39). The rates vary depending on a number of differing inclusion criteria, from a low of 6% reported in a study using the San Diego County Trauma Registry from 1987 to 2003 (33) to a high of 38% in a study of blunt moderate to severe TBI cases ages 18 and older admitted to a level I trauma center intensive care unit between 2001 and 2004 (37). Finally, 1 study that focused only on *moderate* TBI reported a *6-months postinjury* mortality rate of 4%, using data from emergency department admissions of a general hospital in Forli, Italy between 1999 and 2005 (40).

Another group of studies have focused on all cases of TBI *admitted to trauma centers or used data from trauma registries* (37,41–48). These studies report *in-hospital* mortality rates that vary from a low of 9%, from a study using a medical center trauma database in Hawaii (41), to a high of 16%, from a study of blunt TBI admitted to a level I trauma center between 2003 and 2007 (48).

Finally, 3 *population-based* studies of early mortality after TBI have been conducted. The first used data from the Colorado TBI surveillance system from 1994 to 1998 and reported a *prehospital mortality rate* of 17% and an *in-hospital rate* of 6% (49). The second used data from the South Carolina TBI Follow-up Registry of hospital discharges from 1992 to 2003 and reported a mortality rate of 8% at 1-year postinjury, which was 7 times higher compared to the general population (50). The third was a population-based sample of hospital emergency department admissions in Hanover and Munster, Germany between 2000 and 2001, which reported a 1% mortality rate at 1-year postinjury (51).

In summary, mortality rates early on after TBI vary considerably from a low of 1% at 1-year postinjury for a population-based study of all emergency department admissions (51) to a high of 58% at 6-months postinjury reported in a study of severe TBI admitted to the emergency department of an Argentinean level I trauma center (23). It appears that mortality rates are generally higher for those with severe TBI, especially in studies that followed their cohorts to 6-months postinjury.

Later Mortality After TBI

Studies of longer term survival and mortality have tended to involve registries of military veterans (52–56), individual, or groups of hospitals (57–66); specific databases such as those of the California Department of Developmental Services (CDDS) (67–70), the Traumatic Brain Injury Model Systems (71), or the Medicare Provider Analysis and Review files (72); or population-based cohorts (73–78). Studies have followed cohorts of individuals with TBI for amounts of time ranging from 1 year posthospital discharge (77) to 60 years postinjury (56). These studies report vastly differing mortality rates depending on the cohort included and the amount of time followed (52–56,60–64,66,67,69,72,79). For example, Strauss et al. (69) reported a mortality rate of 4% up to 9 years postinjury; Pentland et al. (64) reported a mortality rate of 21% up to 20 years postinjury; McMillan et al. (63) reported a mortality rate of 40% up to 13 years postinjury; and Weiss et al. (56) reported a mortality rate of 77% up to 60 years postinjury.

Population-based studies have reported mortality rates ranging from 8% for hospitalized South Carolina cases up to 1 year posthospitalization (77); to 9% for Olmsted County, Minnesota cases up to 10 years postinjury (75); to 13% for hospitalized Colorado cases up to 8 years postinjury (78); and 13% for hospitalized Manitoba cases up to 10 years postinjury (74).

Some studies have followed individuals discharged from *inpatient rehabilitation* programs with longer follow-up periods. These studies have reported mortality rates ranging from 6% for discharges from an Australian rehabilitation hospital up to 11 years postinjury (57); to 7% for the National Institute on Disability and Rehabilitation Research-funded TBI Model System inpatient rehabilitation discharges up to 13 years postinjury (71); to 8% for discharges from a Colorado rehabilitation hospital between 1 and 41 years postinjury (59); to 20% for discharges from a Pittsburgh, Pennsylvania rehabilitation hospital up to 24 years postinjury (80); to 36% for discharges that were functionally dependent from an Australian rehabilitation hospital up to 18 years postinjury (58).

Studies *comparing mortality rates among individuals with TBI with the general population* found higher rates among those with TBI (54,57–59,67,69,71,78,80,81). For example, those studies that reported standardized mortality ratios ranged from 1.5 for discharges from a Colorado rehabilitation hospital between 1 and 41 years postinjury (59); to 2.0 for TBI Model System rehabilitation discharges up to 13 years postinjury (71); to 2.5 for hospitalized Colorado cases up to 8 years postinjury (78); to 2.77 for those receiving services from the CDDS up to 10 years postinjury (67); to 2.78 for discharges from a Pittsburgh, Pennsylvania rehabilitation hospital up to 24 years postinjury (80); to 2.9 for severe TBI trauma hospitalizations in Ontario between 1 and 9 years postinjury (81); to 13.2 for discharges that were functionally dependent from an Australian rehabilitation hospital up to 18 years postinjury (58).

In summary, mortality rates among individuals with TBI after 1 year postinjury also vary considerably from a low of 4% to a high of 77%. Studies that compare cohorts of individuals with TBI to the general population generally report a 1.5–3 times greater likelihood of death in the TBI populations.

LIFE EXPECTANCY

Although life expectancy goes hand in hand with mortality, the available literature in this area is not as plentiful, and

actual life expectancy estimates or life tables are only sparsely included (52–57,59,61,65,67–71,73,78,82). Nevertheless, 2 early studies suggest that life expectancy was reduced by 3–5 years for "highly functioning" (i.e. ambulatory) adults with TBI (55,61).

A few more recent studies have also reported specific life expectancy reductions. Harrison-Felix et al. (59) reported an average life expectancy reduction of 4 years for discharges from a Colorado rehabilitation hospital between 1 and 41 years postinjury. Ventura et al. (78) reported an average life expectancy reduction of 6 years for hospitalized Colorado cases up to 8 years postinjury. Harrison-Felix et al. (71) reported an average life expectancy reduction of 7 years for TBI Model System rehabilitation discharges up to 13 years postinjury. Finally, Brown et al. (73), in their population-based study in Olmsted County, Minnesota, reported that among individuals with moderate-to-severe TBI who survived at least to 6-months postinjury, their long-term survival was similar to that for individuals with mild TBI. They further reported that individuals with mild TBI have a small but statistically significant reduction in long-term survival (up to 17 years postinjury) compared to the general population. Further analysis by Brown et al. (83) determined for those with mild TBI that died, in no case was the cause of death either primarily or indirectly related to the head trauma. The authors commented that "though the association of mild injury with increased mortality from all causes in the short term remains worth noting, this review did not reveal any causal pattern of death other than that it was not related to the initial head trauma. A more complete analysis of this cohort, or expanding the cohort to include larger numbers of cases, may shed more light on the relationship between mild TBI and mortality" (83).

In summary, studies that have focused on long-term survival after TBI have shown that life expectancy after TBI is reduced possibly even for those with mild TBI. The average estimated life expectancy reductions in a variety of populations have been reported to be between 3 and 8 years.

CAUSES OF DEATH

Causes of Early Mortality

Few studies have detailed the specific causes of death early on after TBI; however, several attribute death primarily because of the incident causing the TBI, the TBI itself, or complications as a result of the TBI (i.e., circulatory and respiratory conditions) (12,14,32,39,46,78,84–87). For example, Sekulovic et al. (86) reported on 499 deaths occurring within 30 days of TBI based on autopsies. They reported that 59% of the deaths were caused by injury to brainstem, 12% caused by brain edema, and 7% caused by brain compression, with the next most frequent cause of death to be pneumonia (12%). In another study, Ventura et al. (78) reported that of the 504 deaths occurring in the first month after acute hospital discharge among hospitalized Colorado residents with TBI, circulatory system diseases were the most prevalent cause of death (36%), followed by "unknown" cause of death (21%), of which 86% were accompanied by TBI diagnosis codes on the death certificate. Finally, Kemp et al. (84) reported in a study of individuals with severe TBI who died during hospitalization that "of the 81 deaths attributed to a single cause, 60% died from nonsurvivable TBI or brain death, whereas the remainder died of a nonneurologic cause." They also reported that "cardiovascular and respiratory dysfunction (excluding pneumonia) contributed to mortality in 51.1% and 34.1% of patients, respectively."

Causes of Later Mortality

There have been several studies that contain varying information about the causes of death in the years following TBI. Several studies have mentioned seizures or epilepsy (59,61, 64,68,69,78,88); external causes of injury, both intentional (e.g., assaults) and unintentional (e.g., car crashes, falls) (53,59–64,69,77,78,88); and suicide (61,64,78,82,88–91). However, some studies have found both circulatory (e.g., heart disease, stroke) and respiratory (e.g., pneumonias) diseases to be more common (56,59–64,68,77,78,88). In addition, several studies have mentioned that neoplasms (e.g., lung cancer) (59,60,62–64,77,78,88) and digestive conditions (59,60,62, 63,78,88) also account for a proportion of deaths after TBI. A few studies have pointed to infections (e.g., septicemia) (61,69,78,88), neurologic conditions (e.g., Alzheimer disease) (60,78), mental/behavioral conditions (e.g., dementias), and/or drug/alcohol-related deaths (62,64,78). Finally, 2 studies have suggested that causes of death after TBI begin to mirror the patterns seen in the general population as soon as 2 (53) to 10 (56) years after injury.

A few studies have compared causes of death after TBI with the *general population* to determine if individuals with TBI are at greater risk of dying of specific causes. Selassie et al. (77) reported that individuals with TBI discharged from South Carolina hospitals and followed for a year were 36 times more likely to die of unintentional injury (note: many of these cases also indicated TBI on the death certificate suggesting the cause of death was caused by the original injury resulting in the TBI), 12 times more likely to die of cerebrovascular disease, 4 times more likely to die of heart disease, and 3 times more likely to die of cancer. Harrison-Felix et al. (88) reported that individuals discharged from the TBI Model Systems and followed up to 13 years postinjury were 37 times more likely to die of seizures, 12 times more likely to die of septicemia, 4 times more likely to die of pneumonia, and 3 times more likely to die of other respiratory conditions (excluding pneumonia), digestive conditions, and all external causes of injury/poisoning. Harrison-Felix et al. (59) reported that individuals with TBI discharged from a Colorado rehabilitation hospital and followed up to 41 years postinjury were 49 times more likely to die of aspiration pneumonia, 22 times more likely to die of seizures, 4 times more likely to die of other pneumonias, 3 times more likely to commit suicide, and 2 times more likely to die of digestive conditions. Ventura et al. (78) reported that individuals with TBI hospitalized in Colorado and followed up to 8 years postinjury were 15 times more likely to die of seizures, 5 times more likely to die of mental/behavioral disorders (includes dementia), 3 times more likely to die of nervous system conditions (includes Alzheimer disease), aspiration pneumonia, other pneumonias, septicemia, digestive conditions and assaults, and 2 times more likely to die of suicide, circulatory conditions, and unintentional injuries. Finally, McMillan et al. (63) reported that the frequency of deaths in a Scottish head injury cohort were significantly higher than

for a cohort of community controls for circulatory, respiratory, digestive, mental/behavioral, and external causes of death.

In summary, studies have implicated several different causes of death after TBI. Deaths early on after TBI appear to be mostly related to the TBI itself and/or resulting complications. Most of the deaths later on after TBI are caused by the same causes as seen in the general population, such as heart disease and cancer. What is probably the most meaningful are the later causes of death that are seen at much higher rates in individuals with TBI than in the general population, such as seizures, aspiration pneumonia, septicemia, and cerebrovascular disease. Another interesting association that has come to light is that of death after TBI caused by neurologic conditions such as Alzheimer disease, and mental/behavioral conditions such as dementia; however, the temporal association of the onset of these diseases leading to death after TBI is not clear. Finally, another topic of interest in the TBI literature of late is the risk of suicide-related death after TBI.

RISK FACTORS FOR MORTALITY

Risk Factors for Early Mortality

Studies of severe TBI that have followed individuals up to 1-year postinjury have reported several risk factors such as older age (7,9–12,17,18,20–27,85); female gender (11,18,24); Glasgow Coma Scale score (7,9,10,12,18,20–23,25,27,85); Abbreviated Injury Scale score for the head region (12,17); Injury Severity Score (7,10,17); fall-related injury (18); comorbidities (17); complications (7); hypotension (7,23,25); (systolic) blood pressure (17,21); higher blood glucose level (9,21); cerebral lactate (21); coagulopathy (15,18); platelet count (21); anemia (18); body temperature/hyperthermia (21,27); peak and admission troponin >0.3 (12); pupillary response (9,21–23,25); nonreactive unilateral and bilateral mydriasis (18); shock (18); hypoxia (18,27); intracranial pressure/hypertension (21,25,27); positive cerebrovascular pressure reactivity index (92); computed tomography (CT) findings (23); Marshall CT classification (9); Traumatic Coma Data Bank traumatic lesion categories types III, IV, V, and VI (18); subdural hematoma (18,21); subarachnoid hemorrhage (9,12,18,21); intraventricular hemorrhage (18,21); brain swelling (18); intracranial hemorrhage (21); cerebral ischemia (18); basal cisterns compressed–absent (18); midline shift (18,25); progression of neurologic insult (7); poor neurologic status (85); penetrating TBI (7,17); pedestrian-related injury (24); basilar skull fracture (12); none/low vs high EtOH (13,14,16); toxicology screen and amphetamine screen negative (10); urgent cranial surgery (18); decreased caloric intake (93); ventilation and days postinjury ventilation began (12); intubation prehospital vs in-hospital (17); ground transport mode vs other mode (17); medical care received during transport (18); level II vs level I trauma center designation (7); poor quality of care (85); and treated in lower and middle income countries vs high-income countries (19).

In addition, prehospital neuromuscular blockage (17), beta blocker therapy in patients with elevated troponin (12), and receiving care in United States compared to developing countries (43) were considered factors associated with a decreased risk of death.

Studies including individuals with *moderate-to-severe* TBI and studies of those *admitted to trauma centers* mostly focused on *in-hospital* mortality. These studies have also reported some of the same risk factors for death such as older age (33,37–39,42,43,47), Asian race (28), Glasgow Coma Scale score (28,33,39,41,42,47), Injury Severity Score (28,33,37,42), mechanism of injury (33,42), hypotension (30,33,41), heart rate(<50, 50–59, 60–69, and ≥110 vs 80–89) (34), systolic blood pressure (28), brainstem injury (39), penetrating TBI (30,35,41,42), anticoagulant use (33), pulmonary emboli diagnosis (33), hypercapnia and hypocapnia in intubated patients (32), intubation (38), pulmonary catheter use (38), mannitol use (38), the presence of a do-not-resuscitate order (38), withdrawal of therapy (38), quality of medical care (42), not having insurance (28,30), and lack of use of protective devices (41). In addition, being a perimenopausal and/or postmenopausal woman (29,31), having a higher number of surgical, medical, other specialty consultations and the number of nonneurosurgical procedures performed (38), the use of beta blockers (48), and positive EtOH (13,14) were associated with decreased risk of death.

In summary, several risk factors for death early on after TBI have been investigated and identified including those related to demographic and socioeconomic factors, injury severity, medical comorbidities and complications, mechanisms and anatomic types of injury, type and quality of care, and procedures received. The most frequently reported risk factors are older age and greater severity and/or TBI. Several studies identify several different critical medical complications such as hypotension and pupillary response. Interestingly, a couple of studies identified positive blood alcohol levels as being a protective factor after severe TBI.

Risk Factors for Later Mortality

Studies of mortality in the years after TBI report some similar and some different risk factors than those identified early on after TBI such as age (58,59,61,65,76–79,81,88), male gender (58,59,69,76,77), lower education (52), not being employed at injury (88), reduced work capacity/retirement soon after TBI (60), community-level median income of residence at injury (78), metropolitan residence at injury (78), government insurance (78), Medicare insurance (77), Glasgow Coma Scale score (59,79), Abbreviated Injury Score of the head (77,78), Injury Severity Score (81), post-traumatic amnesia (61,65), coma (53), nature of injury (hemorrhage) (79), right hemisphere injury (54), worst neurologic responsiveness (61,65), mechanism of injury (81), firearm-related injury (79), fall-related injury (78), preinjury medical history (previous brain illness, previous physical limitation) (62), preinjury characteristics (alcohol/drug abuse, social/personal problems) (80), number of cormorbidities (77,78,81), seizure/post-traumatic epilepsy (52,53,56), decreased mobility (67,69), ability to self-feed (69), level of function (57), greater disability at inpatient rehabilitation discharge (58,80,88), being in a vegetative state at inpatient rehabilitation discharge (59), longer hospitalization (59,78), received care in nontrauma center (77), earlier year of injury (59), discharge destination other than home (78,81), and suboptimal postinjury lifestyle (habitual excess alcohol use, living alone) (62).

In summary, some risk factors for death after TBI remain strong even years after injury including age, socioeconomic status, injury severity, comorbidities, certain mechanisms of injury, anatomic nature of injury, and suboptimum care. Nevertheless, some new risk factors for death emerge in the years following TBI such as seizures, suboptimum lifestyle, and level of functioning or disability.

Interestingly, early on after TBI, female gender was reported as a risk factor for death, but male gender was reported as a risk factor in the studies following individuals for many years postinjury. Another interesting point is that positive blood alcohol level was reported to be a protective factor against death early on after TBI; however, habitual excess alcohol use was reported as a risk factor for death in the later years after TBI.

WELLNESS AFTER TBI: A HOLISTIC MODEL AND RECOMMENDATIONS FOR A HEALTHY LIFESTYLE

Although individuals with TBI appear to face additional risks regarding life expectancy, every individual makes lifestyle choices that can potentially affect his or her health and life expectancy. *Health* is a state of complete physical, mental, and social well-being, encompassing more than the absence of disease (94). *Wellness* refers to being in good health and actively seeking good health (95). In 1979, Bill Hettler, MD, developed a holistic model of wellness, with the dimensions of physical, emotional, social, intellectual, spiritual, and occupational wellness displayed as sections of a hexagon (96). Numerous adaptations of Hettler's model have been developed over the years, some omitting the occupational dimension or adding other dimensions (97,98). Several of these adaptations have depicted the dimensions of wellness as interconnected sections of a wellness wheel (Figure 21-1)

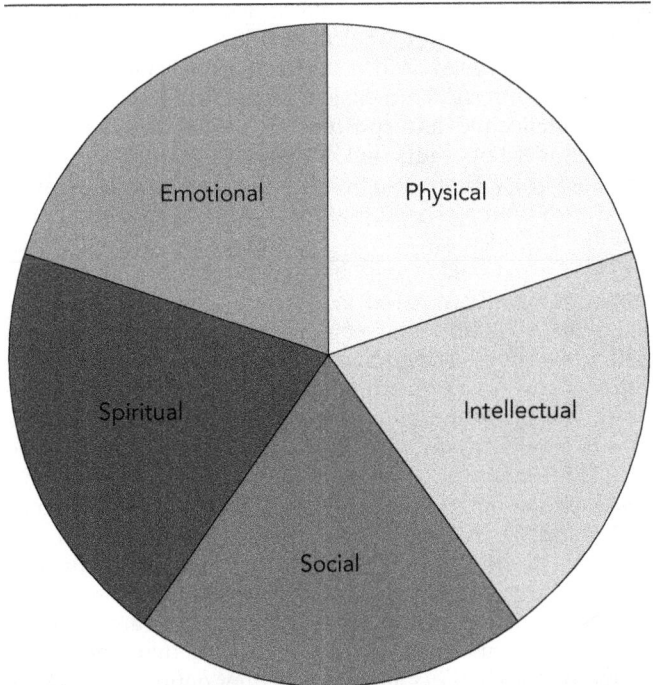

FIGURE 21-1 The wellness wheel

(99–101). A multidimensional wellness wheel lends itself to conceptualizing wellness as an integrated balanced system where the equal functioning of the parts leads to a smooth progression through life.

The wellness efforts of individuals with TBI can be facilitated by the generally accepted rehabilitation strategies of (*a*) self-assessment of one's current wellness and lifestyle and (*b*) setting relevant and realistic goals (102). Conceptualizing wellness as a holistic wellness wheel can assist in an individual's self-assessment by providing a concrete perspective of the multiple integrated dimensions of wellness. The individual can be prompted to evaluate: (*a*) What activities make up the sections of the wheel in my life? (*b*) Are there sections of my wellness wheel that need more attention? and (*c*) What lifestyle changes can I make to bring my wheel into balance? (99)

Wellness Recommendations for the General Population

Evidence-based recommendations regarding healthy lifestyle choices are available for the general population. These recommendations are applicable to individuals with TBI as well. Although individuals with TBI face additional risks, as previously cited in this chapter, they share the same most common causes of death as the general public: heart disease and cancer. Adherence to specific lifestyle behaviors has been associated with a lowered lifetime risk of heart disease and ischemic stroke (103–106). These lifestyle behaviors include maintaining a healthy weight, getting regular exercise, abstaining from smoking, and eating a high fiber, low-fat diet rich in plant-based foods. Lifestyle factors have been found to significantly affect an individual's risk of developing cancer as well (107–110). Based on the available evidence, the American Cancer Society (ACS) recommends that individuals abstain from smoking, eat a variety of healthful foods with emphasis on plant sources, adopt a physically active lifestyle, maintain a healthful weight throughout life, and limit consumption of alcohol (108).

Evidence-based information regarding recommendations for nonphysical dimensions of wellness (i.e., emotional, social, intellectual, and spiritual) also exists. *Emotional wellness* includes both reduction of stress and increased positive well-being. Psychological stress has been positively correlated with premature mortality (111), and overall emotional stability has been associated with longevity (112). Individuals who express kindness, helping behavior, and positive emotions have been found to live longer lives (113,114). *Social wellness* is defined as engaging in positive interactions with others and having a social support system (115). Social support and social integration have been positively correlated with lower mortality risk among groups with specific health conditions (i.e., cardiovascular and renal disease) (116,117). *Intellectual wellness* involves engaging in creative and stimulating mental activities (115). There is evidence that engaging in high levels of intellectual activity delays cognitive decline and may be a strong predictor of survival in the elderly (118,119).

The National Institute of Healthcare Research defines *spirituality* as the feelings and behaviors that arise from searching for what is sacred (120). Other definitions include seeking meaning or purpose in life (121). *Religion* is differentiated from spirituality in that it includes validation and support from an organization or group (120). A significant body of evidence exists supporting a positive association between religious involvement and health and longevity (120–123). Individuals who attend religious services regularly have an increased life expectancy than those who do not, even when controlling for sociodemographic and physical health factors (121).

Collectively, evidence-based recommendations for healthy lifestyle choices for *all individuals* include:

- abstain from smoking,
- maintain a healthy weight,
- engage in regular physical activity,
- eat a variety of healthful foods with an emphasis on plant sources,
- limit consumption of alcoholic beverages,
- manage stress,
- engage in intellectually stimulating activity,
- maintain positive social relationships,
- engage in altruistic behavior, and
- consider spending time in activities that search for meaning and purpose in life.

Wellness Recommendations Specific to Individuals With TBI

As noted, TBI presents additional risk factors which can affect life expectancy. Individuals with TBI also report more health-related problems than individuals of similar age without TBI (124,125). Therefore, in addition to the general recommendations outlined previously, the following wellness recommendations are provided to specifically address the needs of individuals with TBI and focus on the risk factors for death and causes of death identified in studies cited previously in this chapter. Although there is evidence to support several of these recommendations, others are included based on generally accepted clinical information in TBI rehabilitation.

- *Seek out positive support from others who have experienced TBI*. Receiving support from others who have experienced TBI has been shown to be beneficial in developing TBI knowledge, general coping skills, and the ability to cope with depression (126). Social support from peers may be gained through support groups, friendships, or peer mentoring programs.
- *Be aware of the environment*. Individuals with TBI are at greater risk of dying from assaults as well as unintentional injuries such as falls and have an increased risk of recurrent TBI (59,127–130). Those with severe TBI who resume driving have a higher risk of being involved in car accidents post-TBI (131). Individuals may be prompted to "stop and think it through" before driving (checking that directions are clear, the best route has been chosen, etc.) and before attending activities (determining if the area is safe, if there may be hazards related to balance, etc). At home, individuals who have difficulty with balance may want to remove throw rugs, keep furniture in the same position, and report changes in balance to a medical professional.

- *Use a helmet and seat belt as recommended.* As noted, individuals with TBI have been found to be at increased risk of recurrent TBI, and dying of other injuries. Therefore, such individuals may need to particularly heed general recommendations for the use of helmets in recreational activities (such as skiing, biking, etc.) and wearing seat belts in vehicles on all occasions. Seat belt use by adults is the most effective way to save lives and reduce injuries in motor vehicle accidents (132), and the use of bicycle and motorcycle helmets has been found to be highly effective in reducing head injuries in bicycle and motorcycle accidents (133,134).
- *Develop self-advocacy skills.* Advocating for oneself involves becoming aware of one's own strengths and needs, gaining knowledge about community resources, and developing the skills to communicate one's needs successfully to other people (135). Developing such awareness, knowledge, and skills have been seen as an important component of successful interventions for individuals as they seek to meet the many needs of life after TBI (126).
- *Abstain from using alcohol.* There is still much to learn about the effects of alcohol consumption by individuals with TBI. However, there are several factors that should be considered. There is an established link between excessive drinking and cognitive impairment in the general population (136). In a recent study, alcohol use post-TBI was found to have a detrimental effect on cognitive functioning (137). As mentioned, habitual alcohol consumption is a risk factor for mortality after TBI (62). Individuals who sustained a TBI in an alcohol-related event are specifically at increased risk of recurrent TBI, with even occasional intoxication leading to increased risk of recurrent injury (128). Individuals with TBI are often already grappling with cognitive impairments as well as impairments in balance and emotional regulation, and clinical observations indicate that excessive drinking may interfere with the recovery process (130, 138,139). Based on all of these factors, it is commonly suggested that individuals abstain from the use of alcohol after TBI.
- *Be aware of the signs of depression and psychiatric illness.* Depression and other psychiatric disorders are common following TBI, and individuals with TBI are at increased risk for suicide (59,91,140–142). Individuals and families should be aware of signs and symptoms of depression and suicide risk, and should be aware of available resources.
- *Follow the recommendations of a medical professional.* Individuals with TBI who are under treatment for infections or other medical conditions should remember to take all medications and attend all recommended follow-up appointments. If a special diet is prescribed, consult a physician before making any dietary changes.
- *Individuals who experience seizures should be knowledgeable about seizures, educate their family and co-workers, and follow physician's recommendations.* Individuals with TBI are at increased risk of seizures (143) and increased risk of seizure-related death (59). In general, patient education has been shown to improve health outcomes and reduce health risk factors (144,145). Patient education materials, such as publications, videos, and online educational resources, are available regarding seizure self-management (144,146). Individuals should closely follow physician recommendations regarding seizure management and medications.

Resources for Facilitating Wellness After TBI

There are several resources available to facilitate healthy lifestyle decisions following TBI. Some of these resources are accessible through the Internet and therefore are usually updated on a regular basis as new information is available. Several are listed here:

- *Cnpp.usda.gov (United States Department of Agriculture Center for Nutrition Policy and Promotion)*
  This website links scientific research to the everyday nutritional needs of Americans. It offers dietary guidelines, the food pyramid, a calorie calculator, and a food planner to help individuals reach personal goals.
- *CDC.gov (The Centers for Disease Control and Prevention)*
  This website offers information regarding physical fitness activities, physical activity planning, measurement of physical activity, nutritional information, healthy meal planning and recipes, information on weight management, as well as references and statistics.
- *Biausa.org (Brain Injury Association of America and its state affiliates)*
  This website provides information and resources regarding TBI in general, advocacy, information and support, as well as contact information for state affiliates with additional information and resources.
- *Suicidepreventionlifeline.org (National Suicide Prevention Lifeline) 1-800-273-TALK*
  This site lists suicide warning signs, crisis center locations, printable handouts, and 24-hour contact information.
- *Mentalhealthamerica.net (Mental Health America—formerly known as the National Mental Health Association)*
  This site offers information and resources regarding a wide range of mental health issues including stress management, substance abuse, specific mental health diagnoses, medication management, and advocacy.

MEDICAL/CLINICAL IMPLICATIONS

Acute Care

The goal of minimizing mortality and prolonging life expectancy after TBI is shared by federal and state governments, medical professionals, individuals with a history of TBI, their significant others, and advocates. State trauma systems have been shown to reduce all-cause trauma-related mortality by organizing services to rapidly identify injuries and safely transporting individuals to definitive care (147). Regional trauma councils within State systems promote close collaboration and interaction to solve problems unique to specific geographical areas and cultures. National and State trauma data sets provide the foundation for continuous improvement in these systems, including regular reporting of mortality and morbidity data (148,149).

Hospital-Based Care

Effective medical care after trauma requires coordinated efforts across clinical disciplines using evidence-based best practices consistently applied, which is a basic principal of trauma systems. Efficient, accurate exchanges of information between prehospital emergency providers in the field and emergency department clinicians and trauma surgeons are a continuous point of practice improvement. A process that eliminates duplicate diagnostic procedures, and their associated time and expense, facilitates an injured individual to definitive care, minimizing the risk for early mortality and/or acquiring comorbidities that may increase mortality in the postacute and chronic postinjury phases. Information about increased mortality after TBI associated with infectious causes as outlined in this chapter, such as aspiration pneumonia and sepsis, is best assimilated into a coordinated clinical trauma team by a data system that monitors their occurrence and uses a practice-based evidence method to continuously improve performance and outcome (150). Immediate provision of rehabilitation care after TBI has been shown to improve outcome and reduce hospital length of stay (151), with clinical rehabilitation services often playing a coordinating role along the continuum of care, because rehabilitation is most commonly the primary medical need for individuals soon after TBI for all degrees of injury severity. Prevention of secondary complications related to TBI and polytrauma that may affect life expectancy is a primary goal of hospital-based medical rehabilitation services (152).

Outpatient Clinical Care

As economic and other factors minimize hospital lengths of stay, and reduction in life span after TBI diminishes, comprehensive outpatient brain rehabilitation programs have become the standard of care. These multidiscipline clinical services coordinate and customize care to optimize health and minimize morbidity as individuals age with impairment-related activity limitations and restriction to participation in life roles. Clinicians with knowledge of postacute death rates and causes of death can inform patients, their families, and significant others about expected survival. Awareness of causes of death shown to be associated with TBI in the postacute period and in the long-term should lead clinicians to establish surveillance and preventative care plans that minimize this risk. Specific monitoring of epileptic, infectious, pulmonary, and cardiac conditions are important components of longitudinal medical rehabilitation care. Knowledge of conditions associated with the traumatic injury incident, such as chemical use or failure to use personal protective equipment, should prompt intervention to prevent subsequent injury (153).

Broader efforts to influence the availability and types of community-based services and advocacy can also play an important role in affecting mortality and survival after TBI. Acquired chronic health conditions related to TBI lead to increased social stressors that are associated with increased morbidity (154,155). Self and system advocacy skills are critical in the pursuit of employment, education, health insurance, social networks, and rehabilitation. Social participation, control over life events, and gaining political power have been shown to positively influence health and quality of life and affect mortality (156,157).

Medicolegal Issues in Life Expectancy Determination

A lawsuit often ensues when a TBI is caused by third-party negligence or use of faulty products. The purpose of that lawsuit is to compensate the person with TBI for the damages they have and will sustain in the future. A critical component of those damages is the future costs of medical care that result from the injury. Typically, a life-care plan is developed that identifies all the future needs of the person with TBI. Once the needs of a person with TBI have been determined, then the costs of meeting those needs must be assessed, and the present value of those future costs must be calculated. A necessary ingredient to calculating the present value of those future costs is the probability that the individual will still be alive to incur those costs when they occur (158).

There are several ways to calculate either survival probabilities over time or life expectancy given an appropriate longitudinal data set such as the TBI Model Systems database (159). Each approach has strengths and limitations, and results will be slightly different depending on the selected statistical method.

One approach would be to identify similar individuals from within the data set and apply standard life table techniques to determine long-term probabilities of survival, median survival, and life expectancy. Unfortunately, for most persons with TBI, length of follow-up in the data set will fall short of median survival. Moreover, this approach cannot adequately compensate for any trends toward improvement in survival rates over time because the estimate of median survival will of necessity be based on persons injured many years ago.

A second approach used in many studies is to calculate an expected number of deaths for the TBI population based on persons in the general population of comparable age, gender, race, and length of follow-up. The SMR is then calculated as the ratio of actual to expected deaths and is used as a multiplier for annual mortality probabilities in the general population life table. The life table is then recalculated based on the higher annual mortality probabilities associated with TBI. Separate SMR values can be calculated based on different combinations of risk factors such as age, gender, race, injury severity, and other risk factors that may be available in the data set.

The most flexible and powerful statistical approach to estimating life expectancy appears to involve the development of a logistic regression model on a person-year data set wherein each year of follow-up for each individual is treated as a separate observation. In this way, the unique effect of each risk factor on the likelihood of dying each year given survival to the start of that year can be determined (160).

An example of using these 3 different statistical methods to estimate annual probabilities of survival and life expectancy for the case of a person with spinal cord injury was provided by DeVivo (158). Life expectancy estimates were within 3% of each other depending on the selected analytic method.

Without a data set to analyze for each case, one must rely on previously published studies and try to adapt the results to account for the unique characteristics of the person with TBI for whom a life expectancy estimate is needed. Unfortunately, results of general population studies of risk factors do not readily translate to the TBI population. Risk factors that typically exert their effects later in life usually will have a reduced effect in the TBI population because a larger percentage of persons will already be deceased from some other cause before that risk factor exerts its full effect on mortality. Conversely, some general population mortality risk factors may have an increased effect in the TBI population if they exacerbate common complications following TBI. Moreover, combining risk factors identified through multiple studies will tend to overstate the total effect on life expectancy because these risk factors do not usually exert their effects in a completely independent manner as required by the statistical methods that are typically used. As a general rule, one should look for the closest match in the literature and make only minor adjustments for other factors because there are typically both positive and negative factors present, and few if any risk factors will alter life expectancy by more than 1 or 2 years.

Often, for simplicity, either the life expectancy or the median survival is used by the economist for present value calculations of lifetime costs of care. However, when these figures are used, the implicit assumption is that the person will live exactly that long, no more and no less. It is, of course, unrealistic to assume we know exactly how long anyone will live. Moreover, life-care plans often assume changing needs as a person ages. If a change in needs were expected to occur after the life expectancy was attained, then it would not contribute to the present value calculation because the person would be assumed to be dead. Nonetheless, there may be a significant chance the person will still be alive to experience those increased needs, even if that chance is less than 50%. Therefore, whenever actual annual survival probabilities are available, they should be used instead of a single estimate of life expectancy or median survival (161–163). This allows all future needs to be included in the calculation of damages whenever they are expected to occur.

When probabilities of survival over time are not available, then either the life expectancy or the median survival will be used. The choice of which to use may depend on the laws of the jurisdiction in which the case is tried. Median survival is the point at which the individual will be equally likely as not to still be alive, whereas life expectancy is the arithmetic average of remaining years of life for a group of similar persons. Because the distribution of actual survival times is almost always skewed to the left (overrepresentation of deaths at very young rather than very old age), median survival following TBI will almost always be slightly higher than life expectancy, just as it is in the general population. In other words, most people actually outlive their life expectancy. However, the difference between life expectancy and median survival is often less than 1 year, and rarely more than 2 years. Nonetheless, when it is appropriate to do so, use of the median survival will usually result in a slightly higher estimate of damages in the form of future medical expenses than would be obtained from calculations based on the life expectancy. Moreover, depending on future inflation and interest rate assumptions, as well as the needs of the individual as specified in the life-care plan, the difference in present value dollar estimates of damages based on use of the median survival or life expectancy may be substantial, and in extreme cases, could even exceed $1 million.

Although it is impossible to predict exactly how long anyone will live, an estimate of life expectancy that reflects the average experience of a similar group of individuals can be calculated. Persons with TBI and their families should not be discouraged by these reduced life expectancies. Many people with TBI will live a normal life span or more. Adhering to the wellness and healthy lifestyle recommendations described earlier in this chapter will maximize one's chances to reach or exceed their potential life expectancy.

To eliminate the uncertainty surrounding the use of life expectancy estimates in court, structured settlements should be considered whenever feasible. In this way, periodic payments can be made for as long as the person with TBI is still alive and cease as soon as the person dies. That approach guarantees that a person's needs will be met for as long as they live and that the responsible party will not overpay for potential expenses that never occur. Persons with TBI who receive a lump sum settlement should consider converting those funds to a lifetime annuity so that they will avoid the risk of running out of needed funds for their medical care in the event that they outlive their life expectancy.

KEY CLINICAL POINTS

1. Life expectancy after TBI in most samples is reduced by an average of 3–8 years when compared to those without injury.
2. Age and injury severity are the most consistently reported risk factors for death after TBI.
3. TBI and related complications are most consistently reported as causes of death in the acute period after injury.
4. Causes of death after TBI in the postacute phase are the same as for the general population (heart disease and cancer) with notable increases in death caused by seizure, infectious, and cerebrovascular diseases in multiple samples.
5. Knowledge of the literature related to life expectancy, risk factors, and causes of death after TBI is crucial in developing a life-care plan and estimating TBI-related lifetime costs of care.
6. Together with general and TBI-specific health and wellness recommendations, coordinated longitudinal medical rehabilitation care after TBI that targets known modifiable risks and causes for death for prevention should be the standard of care.

KEY REFERENCES

1. Byers T, Nestle M, McTiernan A, et al. American Cancer Society guidelines on nutrition and physical activity for cancer prevention: reducing the risk of cancer with healthy food choices and physical activity. *CA Cancer J Clin.* 2002;52(2):92–119.

2. DeVivo MJ. Estimating life expectancy for use in determining lifetime costs of care. *Top Spinal Cord Inj Rehabil.* 2002;7(4):49–58.

3. Faul M, Wald MM, Rutland-Brown W, Sullivent EE, Sattin RW. Using a cost-benefit analysis to estimate outcomes of a clinical treatment guideline: testing the Brain Trauma Foundation guidelines for the treatment of severe traumatic brain injury. *J Trauma.* 2007;63(6):1271–1278.

4. Nathens AB, Jurkovich GJ, Cummings P, Rivara FP, Maier RV. The effect of organized systems of trauma care on motor vehicle crash mortality. *JAMA.* 2000;283(15):1990–1994.

5. Pickelsimer EE, Selassie AW, Gu JK, Langlois JA. A population-based outcomes study of persons hospitalized with traumatic brain injury: operations of the South Carolina Traumatic Brain Injury Follow-up Registry. *J Head Trauma Rehabil.* 2006;21(6):491–504.

6. Salcido R, Costich JF. Recurrent traumatic brain injury. *Brain Inj.* 1992;6(3):293–298.

7. Strauss D, Shavelle R, DeVivo MJ, Day S. An analytic method for longitudinal mortality studies. *J Insur Med.* 2000;32(4):217–225.

8. Ventura T, Harrison-Felix C, Carlson N, et al. Mortality after discharge from acute care hospitalization with traumatic brain injury: a population-based study. *Arch Phys Med Rehabil.* 2010;91(1):20–29.

References

1. Kochanek K, Xu J, Murphy SAQ, Minino A, Kung H. Deaths: preliminary data for 2009. *National Vital Statistics Reports.* 2011;59(4).

2. Anderson RN. A method for constructing complete annual U.S. life tables. *Vital Health Stat 2.* 2000;(129):1–28.

3. Anderson TW. *Life Expectancy in Court: A Textbook for Doctors and Lawyers.* Vancouver, Canada: Teviot Press; 2002.

4. Rothman KJ, Greenland S, Lash TL, eds. *Modern Epidemiology.* 3rd ed. Philadelphia, PA: Lippincott Williams & Wilkins; 2008.

5. Zasler ND. Long-term survival after severe TBI: clinical and forensic aspects. *Prog Brain Res.* 2009;177:111–124.

6. Faul M, Xu L, Wald MM, Coronado VG. *Traumatic Brain Injury in the United States: Emergency Department Visits, Hospitalizations and Deaths 2002–2006.* Atlanta, GA: Centers for Disease Control and Prevention; 2010.

7. DuBose JJ, Browder T, Inaba K, Teixeira PG, Chan LS, Demetriades D. Effect of trauma center designation on outcome in patients with severe traumatic brain injury. *Arch Surg.* 2008;143(12):1213–1217.

8. Fakhry SM, Trask AL, Waller MA, Watts DD; for IRTC Neurotrauma Task Force. Management of brain-injured patients by an evidence-based medicine protocol improves outcomes and decreases hospital charges. *J Trauma.* 2004;56(3):492–500.

9. Martins ET, Linhares MN, Sousa DS, et al. Mortality in severe traumatic brain injury: a multivariated analysis of 748 Brazilian patients from Florianópolis City. *J Trauma.* 2009;67(1):85–90.

10. O'Phelan K, McArthur DL, Chang CW, Green D, Hovda DA. The impact of substance abuse on mortality in patients with severe traumatic brain injury. *J Trauma.* 2008;65(3):674–677.

11. Ottochian M, Salim A, Berry C, Chan LS, Wilson MT, Margulies DR. Severe traumatic brain injury: is there a gender difference in mortality? *Am J Surg.* 2009;197(2):155–158.

12. Salim A, Hadjizacharia P, Brown C, et al. Significance of troponin elevation after severe traumatic brain injury. *J Trauma.* 2008;64(1):46–52.

13. Salim A, Ley EJ, Cryer HG, Margulies DR, Ramicone E, Tillou A. Positive serum ethanol level and mortality in moderate to severe traumatic brain injury. *Arch Surg.* 2009;144(9):865–871.

14. Salim A, Teixeira P, Ley EJ, DuBose J, Inaba K, Margulies DR. Serum ethanol levels: predictor of survival after severe traumatic brain injury. *J Trauma.* 2009;67(4):697–703.

15. Talving P, Benfield R, Hadjizacharia P, Inaba K, Chan LS, Demetriades D. Coagulopathy in severe traumatic brain injury: a prospective study. *J Trauma.* 2009;66(1):55–62.

16. Talving P, Plurad D, Barmparas G, et al. Isolated severe traumatic brain injuries: association of blood alcohol levels with the severity of injuries and outcomes. *J Trauma.* 2010;68(2):357–362.

17. Wang HE, Peitzman AB, Cassidy LD, Adelson PD, Yealy DM. Out-of-hospital endotracheal intubation and outcome after traumatic brain injury. *Ann Emerg Med.* 2004;44(5):439–450.

18. Boto GR, Gómez PA, De la Cruz J, Lobato RD. A historical analysis of severe head injury. *Neurosurg Rev.* 2009;32(3):343–354.

19. De Silva MJ, Roberts I, Perel P, et al. Patient outcome after traumatic brain injury in high-, middle- and low-income countries: analysis of data on 8927 patients in 46 countries. *Int J Epidemiol.* 2009;38(2):452–458.

20. Gan BK, Lim JH, Ng IH. Outcome of moderate and severe traumatic brain injury amongst the elderly in Singapore. *Ann Acad Med Singapore.* 2004;33(1):63–67.

21. Lannoo E, Van Rietvelde F, Colardyn F, et al. Early predictors of mortality and morbidity after severe closed head injury. *J Neurotrauma.* 2000;17(5):403–414.

22. Ng I, Lee KK, Lim JH, Wong HB, Yan XY. Investigating gender differences in outcome following severe traumatic brain injury in a predominantly Asian population. *Br J Neurosurg.* 2006;20(2):73–78.

23. Petroni G, Quaglino M, Lujan S, et al. Early prognosis of severe traumatic brain injury in an urban Argentinean trauma center. *J Trauma.* 2010;68(3):564–570.

24. Ponsford JL, Myles PS, Cooper DJ, et al. Gender differences in outcome in patients with hypotension and severe traumatic brain injury. *Injury.* 2008;39(1):67–76.

25. Schreiber MA, Aoki N, Scott BG, Beck JR. Determinants of mortality in patients with severe blunt head injury. *Arch Surg.* 2002;137(3):285–290.

26. Tokutomi T, Miyagi T, Ogawa T, et al. Age-associated increases in poor outcomes after traumatic brain injury: a report from the Japan Neurotrauma Data Bank. *J Neurotrauma.* 2008;25(12):1407–1414.

27. Jiang JY, Gao GY, Li WP, Yu MK, Zhu C. Early indicators of prognosis in 846 cases of severe traumatic brain injury. *J Neurotrauma.* 2002;19(7):869–874.

28. Berry C, Ley EJ, Mirocha J, Salim A. Race affects mortality after moderate to severe traumatic brain injury. *J Surg Res.* 2010;163(2):303–308.

29. Berry C, Ley EJ, Tillou A, Cryer G, Margulies DR, Salim A. The effect of gender on patients with moderate to severe head injuries. *J Trauma.* 2009;67(5):950–953.

30. Bowman SM, Martin DP, Sharar SR, Zimmerman FJ. Racial disparities in outcomes of persons with moderate to severe traumatic brain injury. *Med Care.* 2007;45(7):686–690.

31. Davis DP, Douglas DJ, Smith W, et al. Traumatic brain injury outcomes in pre- and post- menopausal females versus age-matched males. *J Neurotrauma.* 2006;23(2):140–148.

32. Davis DP, Idris AH, Sise MJ, et al. Early ventilation and outcome in patients with moderate to severe traumatic brain injury. *Crit Care Med.* 2006;34(4):1202–1208.

33. Davis DP, Kene M, Vilke GM, et al. Head-injured patients who "talk and die": the San Diego perspective. *J Trauma.* 2007;62(2):277–281.

34. Ley EJ, Berry C, Mirocha J, Salim A. Mortality is reduced for heart rate 80 to 89 after traumatic brain injury. *J Surg Res.* 2010;163(1):142–145.

35. Peek-Asa C, McArthur D, Hovda D, Kraus J. Early predictors of mortality in penetrating compared with closed brain injury. *Brain Inj.* 2001;15(9):801–810.

36. Shandro JR, Rivara FP, Wang J, Jurkovich GJ, Nathens AB, MacKenzie EJ. Alcohol and risk of mortality in patients with traumatic brain injury. *J Trauma.* 2009;66(6):1584–1590.

37. Sorani MD, Lee M, Kim H, Meeker M, Manley GT. Race\ethnicity and outcome after traumatic brain injury at a single, diverse center. *J Trauma.* 2009;67(1):75–80.

38. Thompson HJ, Rivara FP, Jurkovich GJ, Wang J, Nathens AB, MacKenzie EJ. Evaluation of the effect of intensity of care on mor-

tality after traumatic brain injury. *Crit Care Med.* 2008;36(1): 282–290.

39. Utomo WK, Gabbe BJ, Simpson PM, Cameron PA. Predictors of in-hospital mortality and 6-month functional outcomes in older adults after moderate to severe traumatic brain injury. *Injury.* 2009; 40(9):973–977.

40. Fabbri A, Servadei F, Marchesini G, Stein SC, Vandelli A. Early predictors of unfavourable outcome in subjects with moderate head injury in the emergency department. *J Neurol Neurosurg Psychiatry.* 2008;79(5):567–573.

41. Chapital AD, Harrigan RC, Davis J, et al. Traumatic brain injury: outcomes from rural and urban locations over a 5-year period (Part 1). *Hawaii Med J.* 2007;66(12):318–321.

42. Demetriades D, Kuncir E, Murray J, Velmahos GC, Rhee P, Chan L. Mortality prediction of head Abbreviated Injury Score and Glasgow Coma Scale: analysis of 7,764 head injuries. *J Am Coll Surg.* 2004;199(2):216–222.

43. Harris C, DiRusso S, Sullivan T, Benzil DL. Mortality risk after head injury increases at 30 years. *J Am Coll Surg.* 2003;197(5):711–716.

44. Harris OA, Bruce CA, Reid M, et al. Examination of the management of traumatic brain injury in the developing and developed world: focus on resource utilization, protocols, and practices that alter outcome. *J Neurosurg.* 2008;109(3):433–438.

45. LeBlanc J, de Guise E, Gosselin N, Feyz M. Comparison of functional outcome following acute care in young, middle-aged and elderly patients with traumatic brain injury. *Brain Inj.* 2006;20(8): 779–790.

46. Lefering R, Paffrath T, Linker R, Bouillon B, Neugebauer EA; for Deutsche Gesellschaft für Unfallchirurgie/German Society for Trauma Surgery. Head injury and outcome—what influence do concomitant injuries have? *J Trauma.* 2008;65(5):1036–1044.

47. Mosenthal AC, Lavery RF, Addis M, et al. Isolated traumatic brain injury: age is an independent predictor of mortality and early outcome. *J Trauma.* 2002;52(5):907–911.

48. Schroeppel TJ, Fischer PE, Zarzaur BL, et al. Beta-adrenergic blockade and traumatic brain injury: protective? *J Trauma.* 2010;69(4): 776–782.

49. Gujral IB, Stallones L, Gabella BA, Keefe TJ, Chen P. Sex differences in mortality after traumatic brain injury, Colorado 1994–1998. *Brain Inj.* 2006;20(3):283–291.

50. Pickelsimer EE, Selassie AW, Gu JK, Langlois JA. A population-based outcomes study of persons hospitalized with traumatic brain injury: operations of the South Carolina Traumatic Brain Injury Follow-up Registry. *J Head Trauma Rehabil.* 2006;21(6):491–504.

51. Rickels E, von Wild K, Wenzlaff P. Head injury in Germany: a population-based prospective study on epidemiology, causes, treatment and outcome of all degrees of head-injury severity in two distinct areas. *Brain Inj.* 2010;24(12):1491–1504.

52. Corkin S, Sullivan EV, Carr FA. Prognostic factors for life expectancy after penetrating head injury. *Arch Neurol.* 1984;41(9): 975–977.

53. Rish BL, Dillon JD, Weiss GH. Mortality following penetrating craniocerebral injuries. An analysis of the deaths in the Vietnam Head Injury Registry population. *J Neurosurg.* 1983;59(5):775–780.

54. Walker AE, Blumer D. The fate of World War II veterans with posttraumatic seizures. *Arch Neurol.* 1989;46(1):23–26.

55. Walker AE, Leuchs HK, Lechtape-Grüter H, Caveness WF, Kretschman C. Life expectancy of head injured men with and without epilepsy. *Arch Neurol.* 1971;24(2):95–100.

56. Weiss GH, Caveness WF, Einsiedel-Lechtape H, McNeel ML. Life expectancy and causes of death in a group of head-injured veterans of World War I. *Arch Neurol.* 1982;39(12):741–743.

57. Baguley I, Slewa-Younan S, Lazarus R, Green A. Long-term mortality trends in patients with traumatic brain injury. *Brain Inj.* 2000; 14(6):505–512.

58. Baguley IJ, Nott MT, Slewa-Younan S. Long-term mortality trends in functionally-dependent adults following severe traumatic-brain injury. *Brain Inj.* 2008;22(12):919–925.

59. Harrison-Felix CL, Whiteneck GG, Jha A, DeVivo MJ, Hammond FM, Hart DM. Mortality over four decades after traumatic brain injury rehabilitation: a retrospective cohort study. *Arch Phys Med Rehabil.* 2009;90(9):1506–1513.

60. Himanen L, Portin R, Hämäläinen P, Hurme S, Hiekkanen H, Tenovuo O. Risk factors for reduced survival after traumatic brain injury: a 30-year follow-up study. *Brain Inj.* 2011;25(5):443–452.

61. Lewin W, Marshall TF, Roberts AH. Long-term outcome after severe head injury. *Br Med J.* 1979;2(6204):1533–1538.

62. McMillan TM, Teasdale GM. Death rate is increased for at least 7 years after head injury: a prospective study. *Brain.* 2007;130(pt 10): 2520–2527.

63. McMillan TM, Teasdale GM, Weir CJ, Stewart E. Death after head injury: the 13 year outcome of a case control study. *J Neurol Neurosurg Psychiatry.* 2011;82(8):931–935.

64. Pentland B, Hutton LS, Jones PA. Late mortality after head injury. *J Neurol Neurosurg Psychiatry.* 2005;76(3):395–400.

65. Roberts A. *Severe Accidental Head Injury: An Assessment of Long-term Prognostics.* London: Macmillan; 1979:140–179.

66. Whitnall L, McMillan TM, Murray GD, Teasdale GM. Disability in young people and adults after head injury: 5–7 year follow up of a prospective cohort study. *J Neurol Neurosurg Psychiatry.* 2006; 77(5):640–645.

67. Shavelle R, Strauss D. Comparative mortality of adults with traumatic brain injury in California, 1988–97. *J Insur Med.* 2000;32(3): 163–166.

68. Shavelle RM, Strauss D, Whyte J, Day SM, Yu YL. Long-term causes of death after traumatic brain injury. *Am J Phys Med Rehabil.* 2001; 80(7):510–516.

69. Strauss DJ, Shavelle RM, Anderson TW. Long-term survival of children and adolescents after traumatic brain injury. *Arch Phys Med Rehabil.* 1998;79(9):1095–1100.

70. Strauss DJ, Shavelle RM, Ashwal S. Life expectancy and median survival time in the permanent vegetative state. *Pediatr Neurol.* 1999;21(3):626–631.

71. Harrison-Felix C, Whiteneck G, DeVivo M, Hammond FM, Jha A. Mortality following rehabilitation in the Traumatic Brain Injury Model Systems of Care. *NeuroRehabilitation.* 2004;19(1):45–54.

72. Donohue JT, Clark DE, DeLorenzo MA. Long-term survival of Medicare patients with head injury. *J Trauma.* 2007;62(2):419–423.

73. Brown AW, Leibson CL, Malec JF, Perkins PK, Diehl NN, Larson DR. Long-term survival after traumatic brain injury: a population-based analysis. *NeuroRehabilitation.* 2004;19(1):37–43.

74. Cameron CM, Purdie DM, Kliewer EV, McClure RJ. Ten-year outcomes following traumatic brain injury: a population-based cohort. *Brain Inj.* 2008;22(6):437–449.

75. Flaada JT, Leibson CL, Mandrekar JN, et al. Relative risk of mortality after traumatic brain injury: a population-based study of the role of age and injury severity. *J Neurotrauma.* 2007;24(3):435–445.

76. Koskinen S, Alaranta H. Traumatic brain injury in Finland 1991–2005: a nationwide register study of hospitalized and fatal TBI. *Brain Inj.* 2008;22(3):205–214.

77. Selassie AW, McCarthy ML, Ferguson PL, Tian J, Langlois JA. Risk of posthospitalization mortality among persons with traumatic brain injury, South Carolina 1999–2001. *J Head Trauma Rehabil.* 2005; 20(3):257–269.

78. Ventura T, Harrison-Felix C, Carlson N, et al. Mortality after discharge from acute care hospitalization with traumatic brain injury: a population-based study. *Arch Phys Med Rehabil.* 2010;91(1):20–29.

79. Conroy C, Kraus JF. Survival after brain injury. Cause of death, length of survival, and prognostic variables in a cohort of brain-injured people. *Neuroepidemiology.* 1988;7(1):13–22.

80. Ratcliff G, Colantonio A, Escobar M, Chase S, Vernich L. Long-term survival following traumatic brain injury. *Disabil Rehabil.* 2005;27(6):305–314.

81. Colantonio A, Escobar MD, Chipman M, et al. Predictors of post-acute mortality following traumatic brain injury in a seriously injured population. *J Trauma.* 2008;64(4):876–882.

82. Teasdale TW, Engberg AW. Suicide after traumatic brain injury: a population study. *J Neurol Neurosurg Psychiatry.* 2001;71(4): 436–440.

83. Brown AW, Leibson CL, Malec JF. Letter to the editors. *NeuroRehabilitation.* 2005;20(1):67.

84. Kemp CD, Johnson JC, Riordan WP, Cotton BA. How we die: the impact of nonneurologic organ dysfunction after severe traumatic brain injury. *Am Surg.* 2008;74(9):866–872.

85. Mauritz W, Wilbacher I, Majdan M, et al. Epidemiology, treatment and outcome of patients after severe traumatic brain injury in European regions with different economic status. *Eur J Public Health.* 2008;18(6):575–580.

86. Sekulovic N, Ceramilac A. Brain injuries—causes of death, and life expectancy. *Acta Neurochir Suppl (Wien).* 1979;28(1):203–204.

87. Spiotta AM, Stiefel MF, Gracias VH, et al. Brain tissue oxygen-directed management and outcome in patients with severe traumatic brain injury. *J Neurosurg.* 2010;113(3):571–580.

88. Harrison-Felix C, Whiteneck G, Devivo MJ, Hammond FM, Jha A. Causes of death following 1 year postinjury among individuals with traumatic brain injury. *J Head Trauma Rehabil.* 2006;21(1): 22–33.

89. León-Carrión J, De Serdio-Arias ML, Cabezas FM, et al. Neurobehavioural and cognitive profile of traumatic brain injury patients at risk for depression and suicide. *Brain Inj.* 2001;15(2):175–181.

90. Silver JM, Kramer R, Greenwald S, Weissman M. The association between head injuries and psychiatric disorders: findings from the New Haven NIMH Epidemiologic Catchment Area Study. *Brain Inj.* 2001;15(11):935–945.

91. Simpson G, Tate R. Suicidality after traumatic brain injury: demographic, injury and clinical correlates. *Psychol Med.* 2002;32(4): 687–697.

92. Czosnyka M, Radolovich D, Balestreri M, et al. Gender-related differences in intracranial hypertension and outcome after traumatic brain injury. *Acta Neurochir Suppl.* 2008;102:25–28.

93. Härtl R, Gerber LM, Ni Q, Ghajar J. Effect of early nutrition on deaths due to severe traumatic brain injury. *J Neurosurg.* 2008; 109(1):50–56.

94. World Health Organization. http://who.int/about/definition. Accessed April 11, 2011.

95. Merriam-Webster Online. http://www.merriam-webster.com. Accessed April 11, 2011.

96. National Wellness Institute. http://www.nationalwellness.org. Accessed April 13, 2011.

97. Chase T. Promoting optimal health after spinal cord injury. In: Lanig I, Chase T, Butt L, Hulse K, Johnson K, eds. *A Practical Guide to Health Promotion After Spinal Cord Injury.* Gaithersburg, MD: Aspen Publishing; 1996.

98. O'Donnell MP. Definition of health promotion. *Am J Health Promot.* 1986;1(1):4–5.

99. *Healthy Choices, Healthy Lives.* Unpublished health and wellness workbook for individuals with TBI. Englewood, CO: Craig Hospital; 2011.

100. Recreational Sports. Wellness Wheel. http://oregonstate.edu/recsports/wellness-wheel. Accessed April 11, 2011.

101. Vanderbilt University. Wellness Wheel. http://www.vanderbilt.edu/wellnesscenter/wellnesswheel.html. Accessed April 11, 2011.

102. Bandura A. Health promotion from the perspective of social cognitive theory. *Psychology & Health.* 1998;13(4):623–649.

103. U.S. Department of Health & Human Services. Dietary Guidelines for Americans. http://health.gov/dietaryguidelines/. Accessed April 11, 2011.

104. Djoussé L, Driver JA, Gaziano JM. Relation between modifiable lifestyle factors and lifetime risk of heart failure. *JAMA.* 2009;302(4): 394–400.

105. Kurth T, Moore SC, Gaziano JM, et al. Healthy lifestyle and the risk of stroke in women. *Arch Intern Med.* 2006;166(13):1403–1409.

106. Stampfer MJ, Hu FB, Manson JE, Rimm EB, Willett WC. Primary prevention of coronary heart disease in women through diet and lifestyle. *N Engl J Med.* 2000;343(1):16–22.

107. Barnard RJ. Prevention of Cancer Through Lifestyle Changes. *Evid Based Complement Alternat Med.* 2004;1(3):233–239.

108. Byers T, Nestle M, McTiernan A, et al. American Cancer Society guidelines on nutrition and physical activity for cancer prevention: reducing the risk of cancer with healthy food choices and physical activity. *CA Cancer J Clin.* 2002;52(2):92–119.

109. Friedenreich CM, Courneya KS, Bryant HE. Influence of physical activity in different age and life periods on the risk of breast cancer. *Epidemiology.* 2001;12(6):604–612.

110. Ornish D, Weidner G, Fair WR, et al. Intensive lifestyle changes may affect the progression of prostate cancer. *J Urol.* 2005;174(3): 1065–1069; discussion 1069–1070.

111. Friedman HS, Tucker JS, Schwartz JE, et al. Psychosocial and behavioral predictors of longevity. The aging and death of the "termites." *Am Psychol.* 1995;50(2):69–78.

112. Terracciano A, Löckenhoff CE, Zonderman AB, Ferrucci L, Costa PT, Jr. Personality predictors of longevity: activity, emotional stability, and conscientiousness. *Psychosom Med.* 2008;70(6):621–627.

113. Danner DD, Snowdon DA, Friesen WV. Positive emotions in early life and longevity: findings from the nun study. *J Pers Soc Psychol.* 2001;80(5):804–813.

114. Post SG. Altruism, happiness, and health: it's good to be good. *Int J Behav Med.* 2005;12(2):66–77.

115. University of California–Riverside. Social Wellness. http://wellness.ucr.edu/social_wellness.html. Accessed May 11, 2011.

116. Schwarzer R, Rieckmann N. Social Support, Cardiovascular Disease and Mortality. In: Weidner G, Kopp M, Kirstenson M, eds. *Heart Disease: Environment, Stress and Gender.* Amsterdam, Netherlands: IOS Press; 2002:185–197.

117. Untas A, Thumma J, Rascle N, et al. The associations of social support and other psychosocial factors with mortality and quality of life in the dialysis outcomes and practice patterns study. *Clin J Am Soc Nephrol.* 2011;6(1):142–152.

118. Schumacher V, Martin M. Comparing age effects in normally and extremely highly educated and intellectually engaged 65–80 year-olds: potential protection from deficit through educational and intellectual activities across the lifespan. *Curr Aging Sci.* 2009;2(3): 200–204.

119. Takata Y, Ansai T, Akifusa S, Soh I, Sonoki K, Takehara T. High-level functional capacity and 4-year mortality in an 80-year-old population. *Gerontology.* 2007;53(1):46–51.

120. George LK, Ellison CG, Larson DB. Explaining the relationships between religious involvement and health. *Psychol Inq.* 2002;13(3): 190–200.

121. Williams DR, Sternthal MJ. Spirituality, religion and health: evidence and research directions. *Med J Aust.* 2007;186(10 suppl): S47–S50.

122. Miller WR, Thoresen CE. Spirituality, religion, and health. An emerging research field. *Am Psychol.* 2003;58(1):24–35.

123. Strawbridge WJ, Cohen RD, Shema SJ, Kaplan GA. Frequent attendance at religious services and mortality over 28 years. *Am J Public Health.* 1997;87(6):957–961.

124. Breed ST, Flanagan SR, Watson KR. The relationship between age and the self-report of health symptoms in persons with traumatic brain injury. *Arch Phys Med Rehabil.* 2004;85(4 suppl 2):S61–S67.

125. Hibbard MR, Uysal S, Sliwinski M, Gordon WA. Undiagnosed health issues in individuals with traumatic brain injury living in the community. *J Head Trauma Rehabil.* 1998;13(4):47–57.

126. Hibbard MR, Cantor J, Charatz H, et al. Peer support in the community: initial findings of a mentoring program for individuals with traumatic brain injury and their families. *J Head Trauma Rehabil.* 2002;17(2):112–131.

127. Annegers JF, Grabow JD, Kurland LT, Laws ER, Jr. The incidence, causes, and secular trends of head trauma in Olmsted County, Minnesota, 1935–1974. *Neurology.* 1980;30(9):912–919.

128. Jagger J, Levine JI, Jane JA, Rimel RW. Epidemiologic features of head injury in a predominantly rural population. *J Trauma.* 1984; 24(1):40–44.

129. Salcido R, Costich JF. Recurrent traumatic brain injury. *Brain Inj.* 1992;6(3):293–298.

130. Winqvist S, Luukinen H, Jokelainen J, Lehtilahti M, Näyhä S, Hillbom M. Recurrent traumatic brain injury is predicted by the index injury occurring under the influence of alcohol. *Brain Inj.* 2008; 22(10):780–785.

131. Formisano R, Bivona U, Brunelli S, Giustini M, Longo E, Taggi F. A preliminary investigation of road traffic accident rate after severe brain injury. *Brain Inj.* 2005;19(3):159–163.

132. Centers for Disease Control and Prevention. Adult Seat Belt Use in the US. http://www.cdc.gov/VitalSigns/SeatBeltUse/index.html .Accessed May 11, 2011.

133. Offner PJ, Rivara FP, Maier RV. The impact of motorcycle helmet use. *J Trauma*. 1992;32(5):636–641; discussion 641–642.

134. Thompson RS, Rivara FP, Thompson DC. A case-control study of the effectiveness of bicycle safety helmets. *N Engl J Med*. 1989; 320(21):1361–1367.

135. Hawley L. Self advocacy after brain injury. In: Hawley L, ed. *Self Advocacy for Independent Life: An Advocacy Workbook for People With Brain Injuries and Their Families*. Denver, CO: The Brain Injury Association of Colorado; 2008.

136. Williams CM, Skinner AE. The cognitive effects of alcohol abuse: a controlled study. *Br J Addict*. 1990;85(7):911–917.

137. Ponsford J, Tweedly L. The relationship between alcohol and cognitive functioning after traumatic brain injury [abstract]. *Brain Impair*. 2011;12(suppl):44.

138. Corrigan JD. Substance abuse as a mediating factor in outcome from traumatic brain injury. *Arch Phys Med Rehabil*. 1995;76(4): 302–309.

139. Sander AM, Witol AD, Kreutzer JS. Alcohol use after traumatic brain injury: concordance of patients' and relatives' reports. *Arch Phys Med Rehabil*. 1997;78(2):138–142.

140. Curran CA, Ponsford JL, Crowe S. Coping strategies and emotional outcome following traumatic brain injury: a comparison with orthopedic patients. *J Head Trauma Rehabil*. 2000;15(6):1256–1274.

141. Deb S, Lyons I, Koutzoukis C, Ali I, McCarthy G. Rate of psychiatric illness 1 year after traumatic brain injury. *Am J Psychiatry*. 1999; 156(3):374–378.

142. Jorge RE, Robinson RG, Moser D, Tateno A, Crespo-Facorro B, Arndt S. Major depression following traumatic brain injury. *Arch Gen Psychiatry*. 2004;61(1):42–50.

143. Annegers JF, Hauser WA, Coan SP, Rocca WA. A population-based study of seizures after traumatic brain injuries. *N Engl J Med*. 1998; 338(1):20–24.

144. Elliott J, Shneker B. Patient, caregiver, and health care practitioner knowledge of, beliefs about, and attitudes toward epilepsy. *Epilepsy Behav*. 2008;12(4):547–556.

145. Keulers BJ, Welters CF, Spauwen PH, Houpt P. Can face-to-face patient education be replaced by computer-based patient education? A randomised trial. *Patient Educ Couns*. 2007;67(1–2):176–182.

146. Epilepsy Foundation. Living with Epilepsy. http://www.epilepsyfoundation.org/living/. Accessed April 21, 2011.

147. Nathens AB, Jurkovich GJ, Cummings P, Rivara FP, Maier RV. The effect of organized systems of trauma care on motor vehicle crash mortality. *JAMA*. 2000;283(15):1990–1994.

148. American College of Surgeons. Trauma Programs. http://www.facs.org/trauma/ntdb/docpub.html. Accessed July 19, 2011.

149. Faul M, Wald MM, Rutland-Brown W, Sullivent EE, Sattin RW. Using a cost-benefit analysis to estimate outcomes of a clinical treatment guideline: testing the Brain Trauma Foundation guidelines for the treatment of severe traumatic brain injury. *J Trauma*. 2007;63(6):1271–1278.

150. Horn SD, Gassaway J. Practice-based evidence study design for comparative effectiveness research. *Med Care*. 2007;45(10 suppl 2): S50–S57.

151. Wagner AK, Fabio T, Zafonte RD, Goldberg G, Marion DW, Peitzman AB. Physical medicine and rehabilitation consultation: relationships with acute functional outcome, length of stay, and discharge planning after traumatic brain injury. *Am J Phys Med Rehabil*. 2003; 82(7):526–536.

152. Turner-Stokes L. Evidence for the effectiveness of multi-disciplinary rehabilitation following acquired brain injury: a synthesis of two systematic approaches. *J Rehabil Med*. 2008;40(9):691–701.

153. National Highway Traffic Safety Administration DoT. Traffic Safety Facts: Crash • Stats. Lives Saved in 2009 by Restraint Use and Minimum-Drinking-Age Laws. Recent Research and Data. September 2010. http://www-nrd.nhtsa.dot.gov/Pubs/811383 .pdf. Accessed July 19, 2011.

154. Kleinman JC, Gold M, Makuc D. Use of ambulatory medical care by the poor: another look at equity. *Med Care*. 1981;19(10):1011–1029.

155. Manton KG, Patrick CH, Johnson KW. Health differentials between blacks and whites: recent trends in mortality and morbidity. *Milbank Q*. 1987;65(suppl 1):129–199.

156. Blazer DG. Social support and mortality in an elderly community population. *Am J Epidemiol*. 1982;115(5):684–694.

157. House JS, Robbins C, Metzner HL. The association of social relationships and activities with mortality: prospective evidence from the Tecumseh Community Health Study. *Am J Epidemiol*. 1982; 116(1):123–140.

158. DeVivo M. Estimating life expectancy for use in determining lifetime costs of care. *Top Spinal Cord Inj Rehabil*. 2002;7(4):49–58.

159. Traumatic Brain Injury Model Systems National Data and Statistical Center. https://www.tbindsc.org/Default.aspx. Accessed July 22, 2011.

160. Strauss D, Shavelle R, DeVivo MJ, Day S. An analytic method for longitudinal mortality studies. *J Insur Med*. 2000;32(4):217–225.

161. Berkowitz M, Harvey C, Greene CG, Wilson SE. *The Economic Consequences of Traumatic Spinal Cord Injury*. New York: Demos Publishers; 1992:145–167.

162. DeVivo M, Whiteneck GG, Charles ED Jr. The economic impact of spinal cord injury. In: Stover S, DeLisa JA, Whiteneck GG, eds. *Spinal Cord Injury: Clinical Outcomes From the Model Systems*. Gaithersburg, MD: Aspen Publishers; 1995:234–271.

163. Cao Y, Chen Y, DeVivo MJ. Lifetime direct costs after spinal cord injury. *Top Spinal Cord Inj Rehabil*. 2011;16(4):10–16.

V

ACUTE CARE

Prehospital Assessment and Care

Holly E. Hinson and Geoffrey S. F. Ling

INTRODUCTION

To optimize clinical outcome from traumatic brain injury (TBI), rapid and efficient application of best medical practices must be instituted as soon as possible after injury. Typically, this requires initiation of care in the prehospital environment, which translates to providing care on the playing field, at the roadside, or in the battle space. Most often, it will be the emergency medical technicians who will provide this care. The goals of such providers are to stabilize the patient and then transport. Combat medics have the additional responsibility of protecting their patients, which might mean returning fire but certainly includes getting the patient to a safe location. The objective of stabilization interventions is minimizing exacerbation of TBI. The intent of transport is to rapidly get the patient to a higher echelon of care, which is a level 1 trauma center for patients with moderate-to-severe TBI, where advanced definitive care can be rendered (1).

PREHOSPITAL NEUROPHYSIOLOGY

Time is of the essence, dictating that medical care for TBI must begin prehospital. The brain can only tolerate impaired glucose and oxygen delivery for minutes at a time. Under normal conditions, the brain requires significant energy to maintain function. The body's general physiology is disproportionally committed to supporting brain metabolism. Approximately 20% of the cardiac output is devoted to meeting the needs of this single organ. Oxygen and glucose are the primary fuels of the brain. The normal healthy brain consumes glucose at a rate of about 5.5 g/100 g tissue/min or 0.31 mcM/100 g tissue/min (2). Oxygen consumption is 160 mmol/100 g/min. When the brain is injured, these rates of consumption may increase dramatically. To meet this demand, under aerobic conditions, there is a 1:36 ratio of glucose to adenosine triphosphate (ATP) generation as the product of glycolysis, which is pyruvate, can feed into the Krebs cycle of oxidative phosphorylation. If oxygen is insufficient, then anaerobic conditions will ensue. When this happens, the brain will still metabolize glucose through glycolysis, but the ratio of glucose to ATP generation falls dramatically to 1:2 ratio. Furthermore, the glycolytic product now becomes lactate. Without oxygen, pyruvate is unable to enter the Krebs cycle and thus takes the alternative path to lactate. In doing so, lactate or lactic acid accumulates, re-sulting in acidosis. The consequences of acidosis are further suppression of metabolism, cellular injury, and vasodilation.

Surprisingly for an organ with such high metabolic needs, the brain has remarkably low-stored supplies of these critical energy sources. Furthermore, it has limited capacity to produce its own energy. There is only 1 mM/kg of free glucose, 3 mM of glycogen, and almost no oxygen in the brain. At normal brain basal metabolic rate, these reserves will be consumed in for only 2 minutes (2). After injury, when demand is very high and endogenous delivery is compromised, supportive medical care needs to be instituted almost immediately, which means in the prehospital setting.

PREHOSPITAL MANAGEMENT OF MILD TBI

From a system level, medical care of mild TBI is inconsistent. Most patients do not present to medical providers and thus do not receive any advanced care. Those that do may or may not see a provider who is adequately prepared to manage this condition. The care that is provided is not standardized, and thus, the quality is highly dependent on where a patient is seen and by whom. It has been well established that creating a standard of care improves clinical outcome. The approach to sudden coronary syndrome through cardiopulmonary resuscitation (CPR) and advanced cardiac life support (ACLS) is a good example. A similar global system approach for TBI does not exist. Such as for sudden coronary syndrome, this must begin in the prehospital setting.

Clinical Signs of Mild TBI

For TBI, the first people to intervene are laypersons, such as bystanders, coaches, parents, or friends (3). Although well intentioned, very few are properly trained in TBI medical care. It is easy for them not to identify the signs and symptoms of TBI, especially mild TBI or concussion. Consequently, victims may never see a medical provider for this injury (3). There are estimates that as many as 8 million mild TBIs occur in the United States (4). The Centers for Disease Control and Prevention (CDC) reports only 1.3 million documented cases of TBI, acknowledging that more cases are not seen in an emergency department (ED) and may receive no care at all (5).

TABLE 22-1 Signs and Symptoms of Concussion

PHYSICAL	COGNITIVE	BEHAVIORAL	RED FLAGS
Headache	Poor attention	Depression	Altered consciousness
Nausea	Memory disturbance	Anxiety	Declining neurologic examination
Dizziness	Slow processing speed	Agitation	Pupillary asymmetry
Fatigue	Poor judgment	Irritability	Seizures
Blurred vision	Reduced executive function	Impulsivity	Vomiting
Sleep disturbance		Aggression	Double vision
Phonophobia			Worsening headache
Photophobia			Severe disorientation
Headache			Slurred speech
Nausea			Unsteady gait
			Weakness or loss of sensation in an extremity

TBI may be classified into 3 categories guided by initial presenting Glasgow Coma Scale (GCS)—mild, moderate, and severe (6). Mild TBI is defined by a presenting GCS of 13–15 (7). Even trained medical personnel may miss signs of mild TBI because they can be subtle. These signs and symptoms can be motor or cognitive, observed or elicited (8). Table 22-1 lists physical, cognitive, and behavioral signs of concussion plus "red flags," which might warn a provider that the victim needs more immediate medical attention. Motor signs include a patient moving slowly, exhibiting clumsiness, heading in the wrong direction, and so forth. Cognitive signs include confusion or personality changes. Retrograde amnesia may manifest as forgetting information preceding the injury such as where a person was, what the score of a game was, what they were doing, and so forth. Anterograde amnesia is the inability to remember pertinent information following an injury. Symptoms often must be elicited from the patient by direct questioning. Providers should attend to both what the patient says and how the patient answers questions. Common TBI symptoms are headache, nausea, blurry or double vision, feeling groggy or disoriented, fatigue, and photophobia or phonophobia. Answering slowly and deliberately may be related to TBI (9).

Mild TBI in the Military

In response to the significant number of patients with TBI in the war theater, in 2010, the Deputy Secretary of Defense issued the Directive Type Memorandum (DTM) 09-033, which was specific for mild TBI/concussion. A DTM is an "order" that establishes policy, assigns responsibility, and provides procedures for mild TBI. It encumbers all branches of the US military (10). In essence, it led to the creation of a TBI system of care that begins in the prehospital setting.

The motivation for beginning prehospital is mainly driven by military operational need. It is self-evident that a war fighter with TBI can be a danger to himself and to his unit. However, victims of TBI often do not recognize that they are suffering from TBI. For this reason, it considers the responsibility of unit leaders and members to refer potential victims of TBI to the medic. Thus, any war fighter who is exposed to a blast or suffers an event concerning for TBI, such as hitting one's head, will be evaluated at the site of injury by the medic. Blast exposure that necessitates evaluation is any soldier within 50 m of an explosive blast, even if inside a vehicle that may not be damaged. Recently, a blast gauge has been introduced (11). This gauge is a device worn by each war fighter, which measures pressure and acceleration (Figure 22-1). It is intended to be a dosimeter that quanti-

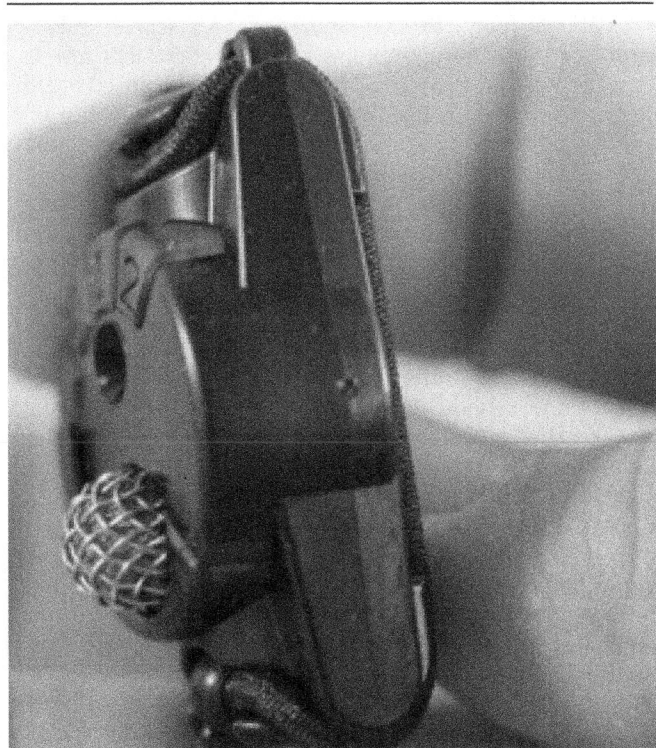

FIGURE 22-1 Defense Advance Research Projects Agency (DARPA) blast gauge. This device is worn by each war fighter and can measure pressure and acceleration. It is intended to quantify an individual's exposure to a blast. In a conversation with J. Rodgers (December 14, 2011).

fies an individual's exposure to a blast. By doing so, it will help identify which victims are at highest risk of TBI (9,12).

For mild TBI or concussion in the setting of combat, evaluation is done by the first provider using the Military Acute Concussion Evaluation (MACE), which is a standardized paper-based examination developed by the Defense and Veterans Brain Injury Center (DVBIC) (13). The MACE has 2 parts. The first is a record of the history and presenting symptoms. The second is a clinical examination using the Standardized Assessment of Concussion (SAC). SAC is a neuropsychological battery that was developed and validated for sports-related concussion (14–16). It tests orientation, immediate memory, concentration, and memory recall. An abnormal score is less than 25. If a patient is found to score less than 25, he or she is considered to have suffered a TBI. Patients who suffer mild symptoms, such as headache, but do not have abnormal SAC scores can be treated symptomatically by the medic with acetaminophen or nonsteroidal anti-inflammatory agents (12).

One significant innovation in the US military medical care system is the formation of concussion care centers. These are specific facilities dedicated to providing medical care to patients suffering from mild TBI. For the army, these are concussion care centers (CCC) and are led by occupational therapists (OTs) with battalion surgeon (physician) support. For the navy and marines, it is a concussion restoration center and is led by a sports medicine physician. For all, there are neurologists in theater available for consultation and to assume care of patients who have more serious TBI. It is interesting to note that this TBI-specific program was created by military physicians, Drs. Bell, Skipton and Nasky (personal communication, 2009), at the battlefront.

Patients found to have abnormal SAC scores or have severe or persistent symptoms concerning for TBI are referred by their medics to their military unit's advanced health care provider who is usually a physician. The provider will take a more detailed history, conduct a neurological examination, and cognitive assessment. From this, a diagnosis of mild TBI will or will not be rendered. If there is a neurological deficit, patients are sent for computed tomography (CT) scan of the head, which typically requires helicopter evacuation. If there is no deficit or the CT scan of the head is normal, then the patient is enrolled in a specific TBI care program administered at the CCC located at the patient's military base at the battle front. In this way, each patient is kept with his military unit, who is his most important support group. Although patients sleep in the CCC, they eat and socialize with their unit. Even though they remain at the front, they do not engage in military operations, such as patrol. To optimize full recovery, this is for a predetermined specified length of time, on the order of a few days. Even if they fully recover within that time, they will not be returned to full duty until the established time has elapsed.

Admission to the CCC is by the OT, who is an officer, in close coordination with the military unit's primary care provider. It is the OT who will execute each patient's specific TBI care plan. At entry, the OT performs detailed physical, neurological, and cognitive assessment. The OT is supported by an OT technician who is a noncommissioned officer (sergeant). The OT technician lives in the CCC and thus provides 24/7 supervision. Patients are seen daily by their OT. During these sessions, the patient is educated about TBI, especially

its typically self-limited course. The process is a 5-step graduated program that slowly increases physical and cognitive activity. Cognitive exercises are intellectually stimulating activities such as crossword puzzles, sudoku, and so forth but not violent video games. Cognitive testing at each step determines whether or not a patient will advance. It should be noted that the time spent in each step depends on how well the patient is recovering. Patients can complete the program within a day or may take as long as 7 days.

Military Clinical Practice Guidelines for Mild TBI

Medical management of symptoms is guided by the medical algorithms from the Department of Defense (DoD's) "DTM 09-033: Policy Guidance for Management of Concussion/Mild Traumatic Brain Injury in the Deployed Setting," as well as the Department of Veterans Affair (VA)/DoD "Clinical Practice Guidelines for Management of Concussion/Mild Traumatic Brain Injury" (10,17–19). These are evidence-based guidelines that were developed collectively by the military, veterans' administration (VA), other federal medical professionals, and civilian subject matter experts. The resulting recommendations are both pharmacologic and nonpharmacologic and the highlights of which appear in Table 22-2. The theater neurologist, who is a senior officer, is available 24/7 for consultation and is also responsible for providing continuing education to all TBI providers.

Return to full duty depends on passing a final physically strenuous exercise challenge followed by cognitive testing. If a patient has no symptoms, passes testing, and requires no medications, he or she will be returned to full duty. Patients who have persistent symptoms beyond the predetermined time are referred to the main bases at either Bagram or Kandahar, where there is an advanced TBI restoration center led by a neurologist and staffed with nurses, OT, and/or other specialty providers. At these main bases, there is also a hospital so that more advanced diagnostic modalities, including neuroimaging, and focused medical care can be

---

TABLE 22-2 Department of Veterans Affairs and Department of Defense Clinical Practice Guidelines for Management of Mild Traumatic Brain Injury/Concussion

1. There are no universal criteria for the definition of mild traumatic brain injury (mTBI), and the diagnosis is based on the characteristics of the immediate sequella following the event.

2. The symptoms associated with postconcussion syndrome (PCS) are not unique to mTBI and may appear in other conditions such as chronic pain or depression.

3. Headache is the single most common symptom associated with mTBI.

4. Most patients who have sustained a concussion/mTBI improve with no lasting sequella.

5. Early education of patients and families is the best available treatment for mTBI.

6. Patient sustaining a mTBI should return to normal activity as soon as possible, with gradual resumption of activity.

Modified from Management of Concussion/mTBI Working Group (17) with permission.

rendered. Recalcitrant cases after this are evacuated out of theater back to the United States (12).

Mild TBI in Sports

In addition to the battlefield, the sports arena is another venue in which rapid evaluation of TBI is critical. Concussion in the context of sports play is defined as "a complex pathophysiological process affecting the brain, induced by traumatic biomechanical forces" (20). The Vienna Guidelines in 2001 (21) were the first attempt to establish an international set of guidelines for sports concussion identification and management. There have been 2 revisions since, most recently in 2008 in Zurich. The Zurich Guidelines were designed to update and build on the principles outlined in previous consensus statements (20).

Evaluation of the concussion may be made prehospital by using cognitive and physical assessments. The Balance Error Scoring System (BESS) tests postural stability and may lend an objective motor parameter to the traditional cognitive domains testing in the SAC earlier (22). Conversely, the Zurich Guidelines combine both cognitive and motor assessment in a tool termed "Sport Concussion Assessment Tool 2 (SCAT2)." This 3-part assessment may be performed rapidly on the field by a layperson. Part 1 lists signs and symptoms of concussion, which overlap greatly with those listed in Table 22-1. Part 2 asks 5 questions testing the memory, including "which half is it now?" and "who scored last in this game?" Part 3 assesses balance by observing the injured player's tandem gait. If any 1 or more parts of the 3-part assessment is not normal, a concussion should be suspected. (20)

The sensitivity of testing for mild TBI increases when post-traumatic amnesia (PTA) is taken into account. PTA is defined as cognitive impairment following brain injury characterized by the difficulty in encoding and retrieving new memories, as well as other cognitive symptoms such as confusion and disorientation (23). PTA may be divided into retrograde amnesia and anterograde amnesia. Tests exist to identify the cognitive impairment. Classically, the Galveston Orientation and Amnesia Test (GOAT) was administered serially after head injury to identify PTA and track its progress. The GOAT was validated with GCS and severity of injury on head CT. The test consists of 10 items regarding orientation and memory of the injury. In an effort to simplify PTA testing, the Abbreviated Westmead PTA Scale (A-WPTAS) was developed. The scale consists of 5 orientation questions, calculation of the eye opening and motor response scores from the GCS, and 3 images to identify. If a subject is unable to correctly answer any item, the subject is instructed on the correct answer and retested after a time interval. The A-WPTAS achieved validation, and in that study, 80% of the patients with mild TBI who failed the A-WPTAS had conventional GCS of 15 (24). This observation underscores the importance of cognitive testing to reduce the rate of false negatives that an intact GCS might suggest. Duration of PTA is associated with outcome; the more lengthy the episode of PTA, the worse the prognosis (25). Historically, the Russell intervals were used to classify the length of the PTA and reflect prognosis status. More recently, the Mississippi intervals appear to be superior in classifying PTA in the sense that the model predicts productivity at 1 year postinjury and provides a more sensitive categorization of PTA values (26). Any cognitive testing to identify PTA is chal-

TABLE 22-3 Vienna Concussion Conference: Return-to-Play Recommendations

1. Removal from contest following any signs/symptoms of concussion.
2. No return to play in current game.
3. Medical evaluation following injury
   a. Rule out more serious intracranial pathology.
   b. Neuropsychological testing (considered a cornerstone of proper postinjury assessment)
4. Stepwise return to play
   a. No activity and rest until asymptomatic.
   b. Light aerobic exercise
   c. Sport-specific training
   d. Noncontact drill
   e. Full-contact drill
   f. Game play

Modified from Aubry M et al. (21) with permission.

lenging to administer in the field, given environmental distractions and need for expediency in assessment. Identification of PTA should likely be reserved for cases of mild TBI, especially when the patient has an intact GCS.

Rest is the cornerstone of therapy for concussion. This is in large part to avoid diffuse cerebral swelling, which can be a fatal consequence of repeat TBI (27). Players are advised to return to competition in a stepwise fashion in the Vienna Guidelines (Table 22-3) (21). The Zurich update outlines what type of exercise activity is permitted during the rest period (20) (Table 22-4). Practioners are also turning to computerized neuropsychological testing to aid them in determining when athletes are ready to return to play (28,29).

PREHOSPITAL MANAGEMENT OF MODERATE OR SEVERE TBI

Moderate-to-severe TBI is more easily recognized, even by laypersons. In more severe TBI, a greater degree of altered

TABLE 22-4 Graduated Return-to-Play Protocol

REHABILITATION STAGE	FUNCTIONAL EXERCISE AT EACH STAGE OF REHABILITATION
1. No activity	1. Complete physical/cognitive rest
2. Light aerobic exercise	2. Walking, swimming, or stationary bicycling, intensity < 70% MPHR
3. Sports-specific exercise	3. Skating drills in ice hockey, running drills in soccer
4. Noncontact drills	4. Progression to more complex drills
5. Full-contact practice	5. Following medical clearance, participation in normal drills
6. Return to play	6. Normal game play

Abbreviation. MPHR, maximum predicted heart rate. Modified from McCrory et al. (20).

consciousness is expected. A patient who is moderately injured will be lethargic or somnolent, whereas the patient who is severely injured will be obtunded or comatose. The astute layperson will activate 911 emergency services when faced with this type of patient.

Emergency care begins with addressing the ABCs (airway, breathing, and circulation). It is well established that hypoxemia and hypotension are associated with worse clinical outcome (30). A single episode of hypotension can double mortality risk (31). Analysis from the Traumatic Coma Database reveals that the most critical predictors of TBI outcome are hypotension, hypoxemia, and hypercapnea (31). Hypotension is systolic blood pressure (SBP) < 90 mm Hg. Hypoxemia is defined as apnea, cyanosis, or O_2 saturation < 90%. Hypercapnea is partial arterial pressure of carbon dioxide ($PaCO_2$) > 60 mm Hg. These critical predictors are independent of other predictors such as age and mechanism of injury.

Guidelines for Moderate-to-Severe TBI

The National Association of Emergency Medical Services Physicians (NAEMSP) created "Guidelines for Prehospital Management of Traumatic Brain Injury," which are summarized in Table 22-5 accompanied by each guideline's level of evidence (32). These guidelines, along with the 2007 Brain Trauma Foundation's *Guidelines for the Management of Severe Traumatic Brain Injury*, comprise the foundation of evidence-based medicine in prehospital care. Collectively, we will refer to both guidelines as prehospital clinical practice guidelines (CPGs) because of the significant overlap. Class I evidence is the strongest available, whereas class III is relatively weak evidence. The CPGs begin by recommending an artificial airway if the patient has a GCS ≤ 8 and if the patient is unable to maintain an adequate airway or suffers hypoxemia that is

not corrected by supplemental oxygen. Paralytic agents are not recommended for assisting in intubation in patients who are spontaneously breathing and able to maintain O_2 saturations > 90% on supplemental oxygen. Interestingly, there is emerging evidence that prehospital endotracheal intubation may be associated with increased mortality in moderate-to-severe TBI (33). However, this increase in mortality may be attributable to more severe injuries in the early intubation group (lower initial GCS, penetrating trauma as mechanism of injury, etc.). Prehospital providers must weigh the importance of securing an airway to maximize oxygenation, with minimizing delays in transport, hypotension, or esophageal intubation.

The CPGs also recommend monitoring for hypotension and hypoxemia (30). This can be done with automated blood pressure cuffs and pulse oximetry. End-tidal capnography can also be used if a patient is intubated. If hypoxemia is identified, it should be corrected immediately. Supplemental oxygen should be instituted as necessary to keep the O_2 saturation ≥ 90% and/or arterial partial pressure of oxygen (PaO_2) ≥ 60 mm Hg. Hyperventilation should not be performed unless there is a clear evidence of cerebral herniation, for example, posturing, asymmetric pupils, and so forth.

SBP must be maintained at ≥ 90 mm Hg. This can be achieved with intravenous (IV) fluid resuscitation with isotonic crystalloids. In the Saline vs Albumin Fluid Evaluation (SAFE) study, albumin was compared to normal saline for maintaining SBP in patients with TBI (34). It was found that 33% of the patients who received albumin died vs only 20% of the saline group. The role of hypertonic saline solutions is unclear for prehospital resuscitation in patients with TBI. There are logistical advantages to hypertonic saline when compared to isotonic fluids, but the outcome benefit has not yet been established (35). In the intensive care setting, there is increasing supportive evidence for the application of hypertonic saline solutions for treating acute cerebral herniation and increased intracranial pressure (ICP) (36–39).

TABLE 22-5 Department of Veterans Affairs Prehospital Emergency Care of Head Injury (Selected Recommendations)

RECOMMENDATION	LEVEL OF EVIDENCE
1. Patients with suspected severe TBI should be monitored in the prehospital setting for hypoxemia (< 90% SaO_2) or hypotension (< 90 mmHg SBP).	III
2. Prehospital measurement of GCS is a significant and reliable indicator of the severity of the TBI and should be used repeatedly to detect change over time.	III
3. Pupils should be assessed in the field after resuscitation and stabilization.	III
4. Patients should be maintained with normal breathing rates ($EtCO_2$ 35–40mmHg). Hyperventilation is reserved for patients showing signs of cerebral herniation.	III

$EtCO_2$, end tidal carbon dioxide; GCS, Glasgow Coma Scale; SaO_2, oxygen saturation; SBP, systolic blood pressure; TBI, traumatic brain injury. Modified from Badjatia N et al. (32) with permission.

The Glasgow Coma Scale

The GCS of a patient with TBI should be made after the ABCs are first addressed. It should be done by a trained provider and before sedatives or paralytic agents are administered. If such medications are given, then GCS assessment should be made after these drugs have worn off (32).

The GCS is a valuable prehospital clinical tool. It is used to classify, describe, and prognosticate patients with TBI. The GCS is used to differentiate a patient with moderate TBI (GCS 9–12) from the one who suffers from severe TBI (GCS ≤ 8). Perhaps the most useful application of the GCS is to describe. When field medical providers are informing the receiving hospitals of the patients they are transporting, the GCS often allows experienced clinicians to visualize the incoming patient's neurologic status and thus get a sense of the patient's condition even before they arrive. There is a prognostic value to the presenting GCS. Lower initial GCS score is correlated with poorer outcome (40). Analysis from the Traumatic Coma Database reveals that patients whose GCS score was 3 had a mortality rate of 55%, whereas those with GCS of 4–8 had only 13% mortality.

However, despite the ubiquitous nature of the GCS, it has significant limitations. The GCS is a simple tool but is unfortunately not well learned. One study demonstrated poor retention of what the GCS is, even among those providers who were all trained in Advanced Trauma Life Support (ATLS) where GCS is taught (41). This underscores the need for frequent review and practice among providers who will treat patients with TBI. There is interrater variability even in the best of circumstances. One study of emergency physicians calculating GCS on presentation to the ED found only moderate degrees of test reliability, even in this highly trained population (42). For this reason, some authors advocate simpler scoring systems to be carried out in the field (43). Controversy exists regarding the timing of the scale's calculation. GCS calculated in the field prior to resuscitation may portend a falsely poorer prognosis. A preresuscitation GCS score may allow reversible hypotension and hypoxia to negatively impact the score (44). Another complicating factor is the presence of an endotracheal airway that reduces the verbal score to 1 regardless of the orientation status of the patient in question. Preresuscitation GCS scores do not predict mortality as well as postresuscitation scores (45). Although GCS should always be calculated, it should be interpreted within the context of how it was assessed.

The Neurological Exam

The bedside neurological exam of the patient remains the best assessment method. Ideally, the neurological examination in an awake patient should include mental status, naming (for aphasia evaluation), confrontation visual fields, motor, sensory, coordination, and cranial nerve (CN) assessments. If poorly or unresponsive, then GCS, motor, sensory response to pain, and CN evaluation should be done, especially reflexes for pupillary response to light (CN III), corneal (CN V), occulovestibular (CN VIII), gag (CN IX and X), and spontaneous ventilation.

It is recognized that in the prehospital environment, a detailed neurological examination may be difficult. The CPGs recommend, at minimum, that after determining a patient's GCS, both pupils should be examined. There should be identification of any ocular trauma. Then, both left and right pupils should be assessed. Asymmetry between both eyes of > 1 mm is considered abnormal. A fixed and dilated pupil is an ominous sign that may indicate brain herniation.

Brain herniation should be suspected if there are unreactive dilated pupils, asymmetric pupils, extensor posturing or lack of movement to stimulation, or a decrease in GCS > 2 points. A "brain code" should be instituted for any actively herniating patient. The brain code consists of elevating the head of the bed to 30° angle, hyperventilating to $PaCO_2$ of 34–36 mm Hg, administering a bolus of mannitol (0.25–1.0 g/kg), and consideration of a bolus of 23.4% hypertonic saline (30 mL) (8). Hyperventilation should be considered a temporizing measure. Ventilation should be 20 times per minute with an end-tidal CO_2 goal of 30–35 mm Hg (32). There does not appear to be a role for hypothermia in the prehospital setting (46).

For moderate-to-severe TBI, military far forward providers use either the Prehospital Trauma Life Support guidelines or the Guidelines for Field Management of Combat-Related Head Trauma (47,48). These are evidence-based CPGs intended for use by medics and corpsmen on the battlefield. A unique aspect of these prehospital guidelines is that military operational demands are considered. This means that in addition to attending to the patient's medical needs, practical considerations had to be made to what a medic can reasonably do under such conditions, ensuring the physical safety of the patient and minimizing the potential that the patient could endanger the unit, for example, crying out while confused and thus give away a unit's position. Important recommendations are determining GCS and pupillary function as soon as possible, avoiding hypoxia (O_2 saturation < 90%), establishing an artificial airway for GCS $\leq$ 8, reserving hyperventilation only for active brain herniation, avoiding hypotension (SBP < 90 mm Hg), and reserving mannitol only for patients in whom intravascular volume can be maintained. Of note, no specific IV fluid is recommended. Hypertonic saline has logistical benefits and is considered an option for use. Sedation and analgesics with easily reversible pharmacologic agents is permitted for military operational considerations and transport so long as the patient can be monitored. Patients with moderate-to-severe TBI (GCS of < 13) are to be evacuated expeditiously to the nearest combat support hospital (CSH) with neurosurgical capability.

In the civilian trauma paradigm, triage of trauma patients including TBI relies on the CDC's "Guidelines for Field Triage of Injured Patients." Step 1 of triage begins with the assessment of GCS, SBP, and respiratory rate (RR). If the patient has GCS < 14, SBP < 90 mm Hg, and/or RR < 10 or > 29 breaths per minute, that patient should be transported to a dedicated trauma center. Step 2 dictates that all penetrating brain injuries should also be transported to a dedicated trauma center. The recommendations continue to describe other mechanisms and injuries that dictate higher levels of care in trauma (49).

Triage

Severity of the injury dictates the level of necessary hospital care. Patients with mild TBI (GCS of 14–15) may be evaluated in the closest ED. For more severe injuries, especially those that may require surgical intervention, a dedicated trauma center is more appropriate. Thus, patients with a GCS of 9–13 should be routed to a trauma center. For the most severe injuries, a GCS of 3–8, a level I trauma center is recommended. Such center should have several capabilities. First, access to 24-hour CT scanning. Second, access to 24-hour operating room facility. Third, prompt neurosurgical evaluation. Fourth, the center should be capable of installing an ICP monitor (50).

TECHNOLOGY

Prehospital assessment of TBI may also be aided by technology. Three technologies recently generating interest in the prehospital environment are near-infrared spectroscopy (NIRS), ultrasonography, and quantitative electroencephalography (QEEG). Although none of these techniques are new, application of these methods in the prehospital environment is novel. NIRS uses near-infrared light to measure cerebral tissue oxygenation. The light penetrates several centimeters through the skull under the probe noninvasively. The attenuation at specific wavelengths is used to determine brain tissue oxygenation saturation. The values obtained are thought to mirror cerebral venous oxygen saturation. NIRS appears to correlate with invasive brain tissue oxygenation probes in the intensive care unit (ICU) setting. Additionally, NIRS is used to detect presence of traumatic frontal hematomas (51). Limitations of NIRS include extracranial blood and ambient light contamination and location confinement to the frontal lobes (52). Additionally, there is commercial variability between systems with no accepted standardization. NIRS may be feasible during road and helicopter transport if ambient light is well shielded (53). Interventions based on the values generated by NIRS have not yet been evaluated for impact on outcomes after TBI, perhaps because thresholds for hypoxia are not well established (54).

Devices using ultrasound (U/S) are also undergoing investigation in the prehospital environment. U/S has several advantages in this arena, namely its low cost and ease of use. Transcranial Doppler (TCD) ultrasonography may be used for noninvasive measurements of cerebral autoregulation and ICP (52). However, precise quantitation, that is, millimeters of mercury discrimination, of ICP by TCD has not yet been demonstrated. Another approach to identifying elevated ICP with U/S is measurement of optic nerve sheath diameter (ONSD). Different cut points of ONSD for detection of ICP > 20 mm Hg have been used, but approximately 0.5 cm is commonly cited as both specific and sensitive (55). However, there is question whether ONSD is reliable enough to base clinical decision making on its values alone (56). At present, U/S-based technology is not a substitute for invasive ICP monitoring when the latter is available. However, optic U/S may prove to be a reasonable adjuvant in the field, although further research on feasibility is needed.

Finally, EEG after brain injury was first conducted in the 1940s and 1950s following injuries sustained by boxers and in industrial accidents. Investigators over the years noted patterns such as diffuse slowing or attenuated posterior alpha after mild TBI, although these findings are not specific to the injury sustained (57). The EEG may be abnormal even when the clinical exam is normal. Accepted EEG changes after mild TBI include slowing of the alpha frequency and increased theta (57). QEEG refers to any statistical or mathematical analysis performed on digital EEG tracings. Although many reports advocate various QEEG algorithms in diagnosis of TBI (58–61), particularly mild or concussive injury, these claims have yet to be prospectively validated.

CONCLUSION

Prehospital medical care of TBI is an important aspect of optimum care. The injured brain has only a few moments before its ability to meet its metabolic needs are exceeded. This is long before reaching definitive care. Thus, it is incumbent on the first medical provider to institute appropriate treatment. Today, CPGs that are evidence based, tailored specifically for both civilian and military first responders, are available. Similar to those used in hospital, these CPGs provide the crucial first steps in focused neurological treatment, with the intent of improving both survival and neurological outcome.

KEY CLINICAL POINTS

1. TBI is often unrecognized and thus under treated.
2. CPGs for mild, moderate, and severe TBI are now available and should be used.
3. Patients suspected of having suffered a TBI should be removed from work or play and evaluated as soon as possible by a skilled medical provider. If it is a moderate-to-severe TBI, then this should be at a level I trauma center.
4. Patients suffering from TBI should not be returned to work or play until recovery which, if mild TBI, may take days to weeks and for moderate-to-severe TBI, significantly longer.
5. Initial prehospital care begins with ABCs, with the goals of therapy being O_2 saturation $\geq$ 90% and SBP $\geq$ 90 mm Hg.
6. Neurological examination is the most valuable clinical tool available and should include cognitive assessment and GCS.
7. Prehospital providers should not administer mannitol or hyperventilation prophylactically, but reserve these treatments for evidence of cerebral herniation.
8. If there is evidence of cerebral herniation, for example, asymmetric pupils or motor posturing, then the patient's head of the bed should be elevated to 30° angle, be given mannitol (0.5–1.0 g/kg IV), and hyperventilated to $PaCO_2$ 34–36 mm Hg.
9. Hypertonic saline is an optional treatment for cerebral herniation.
10. Neuroimaging should be performed whenever a structural lesion is suspected.

KEY REFERENCES

1. Brain Trauma Foundation, American Association of Neurological Surgeons, Congress on Neurological Surgeons. Guidelines for the management of severe traumatic brain injury. *J Neurotrauma*. 2007;24(suppl 1):S1–S106.
2. Ling GSF, Marshall SA, Moore DF. Diagnosis and management of traumatic brain injury. *Continuum Lifelong Learning Neurol*. 2010;16(6):27–40.
3. Management of Concussion/mTBI Working Group. VA/DoD clinical practice guideline for management of concussion/mild traumatic brain injury. *J Rehabil Res Dev*. 2009;46(6):CP1–C68.
4. McCrory P, Meeuwisse W, Johnston K, et al. Consensus statement on concussion in sport—the 3rd international conference on concussion in sport held in Zurich, November 2008. *Phys Med Rehab*. 2009;1(5):406–420.
5. National Association of Emergency Medical Technicians. *PHTLS: Prehospital Trauma Life Support, Military Edition*. 7th ed. St. Louis, MO: Mosby Jems Elsevier; 2011:216–244.

ACKNOWLEDGMENTS

The authors express their gratitude to Ms. Eleanor Kitces and Ms. Erin Murphy for their assistance in manuscript preparation.

DISCLAIMER

The opinions expressed herein by Geoffrey S. F. Ling belong solely to him. They should not be interpreted to be those of or endorsed by the Uniformed Services University of the Health Sciences, the US Army, the Department of Defense, or any other agency of the federal government.

References

1. Brain Trauma Foundation, American Association of Neurological Surgeons, Conress on Neurological Surgeons. Guidelines for the management of severe traumatic brain injury. *J Neurotrauma.* 2007; 24(suppl1):S1–S106.
2. Posner J, Plum F. *Plum and Posner's Diagnosis of Stupor and Coma.* 4th ed. New York, NY: Oxford University Press; 2007.
3. McCrea M, Hammeke T, Olsen G, Leo P, Guskiewicz K. Unreported concussion in high school football players: implications for prevention. *Clin J Sport Med.* 2004;14(1):13–17.
4. Rimel RW, Giordani B, Barth JT, Boll TJ, Jane JA. Disability caused by minor head injury. *Neurosurgery.* 1981;9(3):221–228.
5. Faul M, Xu L, Wald MM, Coronado VG. *Traumatic Brain Injury in the United States: Emergency Department Visits, Hospitalizations, and Deaths 2002–2006.* National Center for Injury Prevention and Control. Atlanta, GA: Centers for Disease Control and Prevention; 2010.
6. Teasdale G, Jennett B. Assessment of coma and impaired consciousness. A practical scale. *Lancet.* 1974;2(7872):81–84.
7. Miller JD. Minor, moderate and severe head injury. *Neurosurg Reviews.* 1996;9(1–2):135–139.
8. Lovell M, Collins M, Bradley J. Return to play following sports-related concussion. *Clin Sports Med.* 2004;23(3):421–441.
9. Ling GSF, Marshall SA, Moore DF. Diagnosis and management of traumatic brain injury. *Continuum Lifelong Learning Neurol.* 2010; 16(6):27–40.
10. Department of Defense. *Directive-Type Memorandum (DTM) 09-033: Policy Guidance for Management of Concussion/Mild Traumatic Brain Injury in the Deployed Setting.* Washington, DC: US Department of Defense; 2010.
11. Rogers J. DARPA to field blast gauge to address TBI threat. 2011. Available at: http://www.darpa.mil/NewsEvents/Releases/2011/2011/06/09_DARPA_to_field_Blast_Gauge_to_address_TBI_threat.aspx. Accessed February 4, 2012.
12. Ling GS, Ecklund JM. Traumatic brain injury in modern war. *Curr Opin Anaesthesiol.* 2011;24(2):124–130.
13. Defense and Veterans Brain Injury Center. Military acute concussion evaluation (MACE). *DVBIC Brainwaves.* 2008;(Summer):1–2.
14. McCrea M. Standardized mental status testing on the sideline after sport-related concussion. *J Athl Train.* 2001;36(3):274–279.
15. McCrea M, Kelly JP, Kluge J, Ackley B, Randolph C. Standardized assessment of concussion in football players. *Neurology.* 1997;48(3):586–588.
16. McCrea M, Kelly JP, Randolph C, et al. Standardized assessment of concussion (SAC): on-site mental status evaluation of the athlete. *J Head Trauma Rehabil.* 1998;13(2):27–35.
17. Management of Concussion/mTBI Working Group. VA/DoD clinical practice guideline for management of concussion/mild traumatic brain injury. *J Rehabil Res Dev.* 2009;46(6):CP1–C68.
18. Defense and Veterans Brain Injury Center consensus conference on the acute management of concussion/mild traumatic brain injury (mTBI) in the deployed setting: clinical practice guidelines and recommendations; July 31–August 1, 2008; Washington, DC: Defense and Veterans Brain Injury Center; 2008:1–12.
19. Defense and Veterans Brain Injury Center consensus conference on the acute management of mild traumatic brain injury in military operational settings: clinical practice guidelines and recommendations. Washington, DC: Defense and Veterans Brain Injury Center; 2006:1–12.
20. McCrory P, Meeuwisse W, Johnston K, et al. Consensus statement on concussion in sport—the 3rd international conference on concussion in sport held in Zurich, November 2008. *Phys Med Rehab.* 2009;1(5):406–420.
21. Aubry M, Cantu R, Dvorak J, et al. Summary and agreement statement of the 1st international symposium on concussion in sport, Vienna 2001. *Clin J Sport Med.* 2002;12(1):6–11.
22. Guskiewicz KM. Postural stability assessment following concussion: one piece of the puzzle. *Clin J Sport Med.* 2001;11(3):182–189.
23. Schacter DL, Crovitz HF. Memory function after closed head injury: a review of the quantitative research. *Cortex.* 1977;13(2):150–176.
24. Meares S, Shores EA, Taylor AJ, Lammél A, Batchelor J. Validation of the abbreviated Westmead post-traumatic amnesia scale: a brief measure to identify acute cognitive impairment in mild traumatic brain injury. *Brain Inj.* 2011;25(12):1198–1205.
25. McMillan TM, Jongen EL, Greenwood RJ. Assessment of post-traumatic amnesia after severe closed head injury: retrospective or prospective? *J Neurol Neurosurg Psychiatry.* 1996;60(4):422–427.
26. Nakase-Richardson R, Sherer M, Seel RT, et al. Utility of post-traumatic amnesia in predicting 1-year productivity following traumatic brain injury: comparison of the Russell and Mississippi PTA classification intervals. *J Neurol Neurosurg Psychiatry.* 2011; 82(5):494–499.
27. McCrory P, Davis G, Makdissi M. Second impact syndrome or cerebral swelling after sporting head injury. *Curr Sports Med Rep.* 2012;11(1):21–23.
28. Collie A, Darby D, Maruff P. Computerised cognitive assessment of athletes with sports related head injury. *Br J Sports Med.* 2001; 35(5):297–302.
29. Iverson GL, Lovell MR, Collins MW. Validity of ImPACT for measuring processing speed following sports-related concussion. *J Clin Exp Neuropsychol.* 2005;27(6):683–689.
30. Bratton SL, Chestnut RM, Ghajar J, et al. Guidelines for the management of severe traumatic brain injury. I. Blood pressure and oxygenation. *J Neurotrauma.* 2007;24(suppl 1):S7–S13.
31. Chesnut RM, Marshall LF, Klauber MR, et al. The role of secondary brain injury in determining outcome from severe head injury. *J Trauma.* 1993;34(2):216–222.
32. Badjatia N, Carney N, Crocco TJ, et al. Guidelines for prehospital management of traumatic brain injury 2nd edition. *Prehosp Emerg Care.* 2008;12(suppl 1):S1–S52.
33. Bukur M, Kurtovic S, Berry C, et al. Pre-hospital intubation is associated with increased mortality after traumatic brain injury. *J Surg Res.* 2011;170(1):e117–e121.
34. Myburgh J, Cooper DJ, finfer S, et al. Saline or albumin for fluid resuscitation in patients with traumatic brain injury. *N Engl J Med.* 2007;357(9):874–884.
35. Bratton SL, Chestnut RM, Ghajar J, et al. Guidelines for the management of severe traumatic brain injury. II. Hyperosmolar therapy. *J Neurotrauma.* 2007;24(suppl 1):S14–S20.
36. Koenig MA, Bryan M, Lewin JL III, Mirski MA, Geocadin RG, Stevens RD. Reversal of transtentorial herniation with hypertonic saline. *Neurology.* 2008;70(13):1023–1029.
37. Qureshi AI, Suarez JI. Use of hypertonic saline solutions in treatment of cerebral edema and intracranial hypertension. *Crit Care Med.* 2000;28(9):3301–3313.
38. Qureshi AI, Suarez JI. More evidence supporting a "brain code" protocol for reversal of transtentorial herniation. *Neurology.* 2008; 70(13):990–991.
39. Qureshi AI, Suarez JI, Castro A, Bhardwaj A. Use of hypertonic saline/acetate infusion in treatment of cerebral edema in patients with head trauma: experience at a single center. *J Trauma.* 1999; 47(4):659–665.
40. Ono J, Yamaura A, Kubota M, Okimura Y, Isobe K. Outcome prediction in severe head injury: analyses of clinical prognostic factors. *J Clin Neurosci.* 2001;8(2):120–123.
41. Riechers RG II, Ramage A, Brown W, et al. Physician knowledge of the Glasgow Coma Scale. *J Neurotrauma.* 2005;22(11):1327–1334.
42. Gill MR, Reiley DG, Green SM. Interrater reliability of Glasgow Coma Scale scores in the emergency department. *Ann Emerg Med.* 2004;43(2):215–223.
43. Gill M, Steele R, Windemuth R, Green SM. A comparison of five simplified scales to the out-of-hospital Glasgow Coma Scale for the prediction of traumatic brain injury outcomes. *Acad Emerg Med.* 2006;13(9):968–973.

44. Marion DW, Carlier PM. Problems with initial Glasgow Coma Scale assessment caused by prehospital treatment of patients with head injuries: results of a national survey. *J Trauma*. 1994;36(1): 89–95.

45. Udekwu P, Kromhout-Schiro S, Vaslef S, Baker C, Oller D. Glasgow Coma Scale score, mortality, and functional outcome in head-injured patients. *J Trauma*. 2004;56(5):1084–1089.

46. Bukur M, Kurtovic S, Berry C, Tanios M, Ley EJ, Salim A. Prehospital hypothermia is not associated with increased survival after traumatic brain injury. *J Surg Res*. 2012;175(1):24–29.

47. Knuth T, Ling G, Moores LE, Rhee P, Tauber D, Trask A. *Guidelines for the Field Management of Combat-Related Head Trauma*. New York, NY: Brain Trauma Foundation; 2005.

48. National Association of Emergency Medical Technicians. *PHTLS: Prehospital Trauma Life Support, Military Edition*. 7th ed. St. Louis, MO: Mosby Jems Elsevier; 2011:216–244.

49. Sasser SM, Hunt RC, Faul M, et al. Guidelines for field triage of injured patients: recommendations of the national expert panel on field triage, 2011. *Morbidity and Mortality Weekly Report*. 2012; 61(RR–1):1–20.

50. Bratton SL, Chestnut RM, Ghajar J, et al. Guidelines for the management of severe traumatic brain injury. VII. Intracranial pressure monitoring technology. *J Neurotrauma*. 2007;24(suppl 1):S45–S54.

51. Gopinath SP, Robertson CS, Contant CF, Narayan RK, Grossman RG, Chance B. Early detection of delayed traumatic intracranial hematomas using near-infrared spectroscopy. *J Neurosurg*. 1995; 83(3):438–444.

52. Dagal A, Lam AM. Cerebral blood flow and the injured brain: how should we monitor and manipulate it? *Curr Opin Anaesthesiol*. 2011; 24(2):131–137.

53. Weatherall A, Skowno J, Lansdown A, Lupton T, Garner A. Feasibility of cerebral near-infrared spectroscopy monitoring in the prehospital environment. *Acta Anaesthesiol Scand*. 2012;56(2):172–177.

54. Highton D, Elwell C, Smith M. Noninvasive cerebral oximetry: is there light at the end of the tunnel? *Curr Opin Anaesthesiol*. 2010; 23(5):576–581.

55. Rajajee V, Vanaman M, Fletcher JJ, Jacobs TL. Optic nerve ultrasound for the detection of raised intracranial pressure. *Neurocrit Care*. 2011;15(3):506–515.

56. Strumwasser A, Kwan RO, Yeung L, et al. Sonographic optic nerve sheath diameter as an estimate of intracranial pressure in adult trauma. *J Surg Res*. 2011;170(2):265–271.

57. Nuwer MR, Hovda DA, Schrader LM, Vespa PM. Routine and quantitative EEG in mild traumatic brain injury. *Clin Neurophysiol*. 2005;116(9):2001–2025.

58. von Bierbrauer A, Weissenborn K, Hinrichs H, Scholz M, Künkel H. Automatic (computer-assisted) EEG analysis in comparison with visual EEG analysis in patients following minor cranio-cerebral trauma (a follow-up study) [in German]. *EEG EMG Z Elektroenzephalogr Elektromyogr Verwandte Geb*. 1992;23(3):151–157.

59. Thatcher RW, Moore N, John ER, Duffy F, Hughes JR, Krieger M. QEEG and traumatic brain injury: rebuttal of the American Academy of Neurology 1997 report by the EEG and Clinical Neuroscience Society. *Clin Electroencephalogr*. 1999;30(3):94–98.

60. Thatcher RW, North DM, Curtin RT, et al. An EEG severity index of traumatic brain injury. *J Neuropsychiatry Clin Neurosci*. 2001;13(1): 77–87.

61. Duff J. The usefulness of quantitative EEG (QEEG) and neurotherapy in the assessment and treatment of post concussion syndrome. *Clin EEG Neurosci*. 2004;35(4):198–209.

23

Critical Care

Samson Sujit Kumar Gaddam and Claudia S. Robertson

INTRODUCTION

Traumatic brain injury (TBI) includes primary brain injury (a one-time event that occurs at the time of injury, which can only be prevented) and secondary brain injury (brain edema, changes in cerebral blood flow [CBF], and secondary insults that follow the primary injury). Systematic evaluation of brain injury data over the last few decades (1,2,3) has provided us an understanding of the critical role of prehospital insults (hypotension and hypoxia), importance of intracranial hypertension, and evacuation of mass lesions, in addition to identifying various independent prognostic variables, assessment scores, and a computed tomography (CT)-based classification system. The current evidence-based management of patients with TBI involves appropriate clinical decisions for imaging, medical, and/or surgical intervention that are based on monitoring of cerebral physiological and biochemical parameters, which would help in anticipating, recognizing, and treating secondary brain injury processes. A joint committee of the Brain Trauma Foundation with the American Association of Neurological Surgeons (AANS), the Congress of Neurological Surgeons (CNS), and the AANS/CNS Joint Section on Neurotrauma and Critical Care has recently updated evidence-based guidelines for the management of severe TBI (4). These *Guidelines for the Management of Severe Traumatic Brain Injury* (3rd edition, 2007) are summarized in Tables 23-1–23-3. In this chapter, we would focus on the intensive care monitoring, treatment strategies, and controversies involved in the current management of adult patients with severe TBI.

BRAIN INJURY

Diffuse axonal injury (DAI) and focal contusion/hematoma are two characteristic pathological processes in primary brain injury and account for 56% and 42% of severe closed brain injuries respectively in the traumatic coma data bank (TCDB) series. Medical or surgical management of focal lesions depend on the clinical status of the patient (Glasgow Coma Scale [GCS] score, focal deficits, pupil response), intracranial pressure (ICP) values, and radiological characteristics (volume of hematoma, extent of midline shift, and compression of cisterns) (5–7).

The various biochemical cascades that result in secondary brain injury following the primary injury are complex, interrelated, and can have an adverse effect on the clinical outcome. The clinical manifestations of secondary brain injury involve evolution of brain edema, changes in CBF, and secondary insults because of cerebral and/or systemic causes.

Brain edema is caused by the accumulation of water in the intracellular (cytotoxic edema) or extracellular (vasogenic edema) compartments, resulting in raised ICPs and shifts of the brain within the closed calvarium. Although there are no randomized clinical trials, reduction of ICP to less than 20 mm Hg is thought to reduce mortality after severe TBI (8).

Martin et al. described the following phasic pattern of *CBF* changes following severe TBI: (a) hypoperfusion phase during the initial 24 hours characterized by low CBF and normal middle cerebral artery (MCA) flow velocity; (b) hyperemic phase between day 1 and 3 (seen in 40% of patients) with transiently increased CBF, rapidly rising MCA flow velocity with normal hemispheric index (MCA to extracranial internal carotid artery flow velocity ratio); and (c) "vasospasm" phase between day 4 and 15 with low normal CBF, high MCA flow velocity, and elevated hemispheric index (9). About one-third of the patients with severe TBI have regional or global CBF in the ischemic range (< 18 mL/100 g/min) within the first 6 hours after injury (10). Patients with a reduced CBF at any time during the first 7 days after injury have a higher mortality rate and a poor recovery in survivors (11). Hyperemia (CBF above normal values) has a variable relationship to outcome (11,12). Subarachnoid hemorrhage (SAH) is reported in 39% of patients with severe brain injury in the TCDB study.

Jones et al. reported *secondary insults* in 91% of 124 patients with TBI (13). Gopinath et al. observed poor outcome following TBI in patients with secondary insults resulting in desaturation of jugular venous blood (14). CBF is normally regulated by cerebral metabolic rate and depends on an adequate cerebral perfusion pressure (CPP) and on arterial partial pressure of carbon dioxide ($PaCO_2$). Pathophysiological processes like hypotension, hypoxia, hypocapnia, abnormal metabolism of glucose, seizures, febrile episodes, and anemia that impair cerebral energy metabolism can result in further ischemic insults in an injured brain. Therefore, monitoring of these secondary insults will be helpful in patients with TBI.

TABLE 23-1 Recommendations for Monitoring and Thresholds From *Guidelines for the Management of Severe Traumatic Brain Injury* (3rd Edition, 2007)

TOPIC	LEVEL OF RECOMMENDATION		
	I	II	III
Blood pressure and oxygenation		Monitor blood pressure and avoid hypotension (systolic blood pressure < 90 mm Hg).	Monitor oxygenation and avoid hypoxia (PaO_2 < 60 mm Hg or oxygen saturation < 90%).
Indications for ICP monitoring		Monitor ICP in all salvageable patients with a severe traumatic brain injury, GCS of 3–8 after resuscitation, and an abnormal CT scan (with hematomas, contusions, swelling, herniation, or compressed basal cisterns).	Monitor ICP in patients with severe TBI and a normal CT scan if 2 or more of the following features are noted at admission: age > 40 years, unilateral or bilateral motor posturing, or a systolic blood pressure < 90 mm Hg.
ICP monitoring technology	Ventriculostomy remains the lowest cost, most accurate monitor of ICP. It also can be recalibrated in situ (no level of recommendation assigned).		
ICP threshold		Initiate ICP treatment at an upper threshold of 20 mm Hg.	Use a combination of ICP values and clinical and CT findings to determine the need for treatment.
CPP threshold		Avoid aggressive treatment to maintain CPP > 70 mm Hg with fluids and pressors because of the increased risk of ARDS.	Avoid CPP < 50 mm Hg. Optimal CPP target lies within the 50–70 mm Hg range. Patients with intact pressure autoregulation tolerate higher CPP values. Monitoring additional parameters such as cerebral blood flow, oxygenation, or metabolism, facilitates CPP management.
Brain oxygen monitoring and threshold			Treat jugular venous saturation < 50% and brain tissue oxygen tension < 15 mm Hg. Jugular venous saturation and brain tissue oxygen measure cerebral oxygenation.

ICP, intracranial pressure; GCS, Glasgow Coma Scale; CT, computed tomography; TBI; traumatic brain injury; CPP, cerebral perfusion pressure; ARDS, acute respiratory distress syndrome.

PARAMETERS MONITORED IN A PATIENT WITH TBI

Apart from monitoring of systemic parameters (electrocardiogram [ECG], temperature, arterial blood pressure [BP], volume status, nutrition status, oxygenation, and ventilation), patients with severe brain injury should have close monitoring and treatment of ICP and cerebral perfusion. Cerebral autoregulation monitoring, when feasible, is helpful in taking clinical decisions.

Intracranial Pressure

According to the TBI guidelines, ICP should be monitored in patients with a GCS of 3–8 after resuscitation and an abnormal CT scan (Table 23-1, level II recommendation) because 50% of such patients have a risk of developing intracranial hypertension. In comatose patients with normal CT scan, ICP monitoring is recommended for patients older than 40 years, unilateral or bilateral motor posturing, or a systolic BP < 90 mm Hg (Table 23-1, level III recommendation). A severe coagulopathy is the only major contraindication to ICP monitoring.

Although various types of ICP monitoring devices are available, the ventriculostomy (with the catheter tip in the frontal horn of lateral ventricle) remains the gold standard ICP monitoring device. In addition to monitoring ICP, the ventriculostomy catheter allows therapeutic intervention through intermittent drainage of cerebrospinal fluid (CSF) and administration of intraventricular drugs. When it is difficult to canulate the ventricles, alternative devices like microsensor and fiber-optic transducers are available for implantation in brain parenchyma (15). These transducers are easy to insert (especially in patients with collapsed ventricles), provide reliable readings of ICP, and do not have a lumen to become obstructed. However, these transducers exhibit a drift over time and cannot be reset to 0 after implantation (16).

ICP monitoring is usually continued for 3–5 days or longer if needed. A secondary rise in ICP is observed in 30% of patients with intracranial hypertension, 3–10 days after injury because of the development of delayed intracerebral hematoma, cerebral vasospasm, or systemic factors such as hypoxia or hypotension (17). ICP-lowering drugs should be gradually withdrawn followed by sedatives to access the neurological status of the patient. When ICP requires little or no treatment, the ICP monitoring can be discontinued. In difficult cases, brain CT should be obtained before removal of ICP monitoring. Rarely, even patients with normal CT scan can have vasogenic ICP waves and nonconvulsive sta

TABLE 23–2 ICP Treatment Recommendations From *Guidelines for the Management of Severe Traumatic Brain Injury* (3rd Edition, 2007)

TOPIC	LEVEL OF RECOMMENDATION		
	I	II	III
Hyperosmolar therapy		Mannitol is effective for control of ICP after severe head injury at doses of 0.25–1 g/kg.	Avoid arterial hypotension. Restrict mannitol use prior to ICP monitoring to patients with signs of tentorial herniation or progressive neurological deterioration not attributable to extracranial causes.
Hyperventilation		Do not use prophylactic hyperventilation (Paco$_2$ of 25 mm Hg or less) to control ICP.	May use hyperventilation as a temporizing measure for the reduction of elevated ICP. Avoid hyperventilation during the first 24 hours after injury when cerebral blood flow is often critically reduced. If hyperventilation is used, use jugular venous oxygen saturation or brain tissue oxygen tension to monitor oxygen delivery.
Prophylactic hypothermia			Prophylactic hypothermia does not decrease mortality rate. Preliminary findings suggest that a greater decrease in mortality risk when target temperatures are maintained for 48 hours. Prophylactic hypothermia may be associated with significantly higher GOS scores.
Anesthetics, analgesics, and sedatives		Do not use prophylactic barbiturate coma to control ICP or improve outcome. High-dose barbiturate administration may control elevated ICP refractory to maximum standard medical and surgical treatment. Hemodynamic stability is essential before and during barbiturate therapy. Propofol may control ICP (does not improve outcome).	
Steroids	Steroids do not improve outcome or reduce ICP. In patients with moderate-to-severe TBI, high-dose methylprednisolone is associated with increased mortality.		

ICP, intracranial pressure; Paco$_2$, arterial partial pressure of carbon dioxide; GOS, Glasgow Outcome Scale; TBI, traumatic brain injury.

tus epilepticus, which should be considered and evaluated with an electroencephalogram (EEG) (18). Continuous digital recording of ICP helps in recording the trends in ICP and timing of ICP events with clinical events (like drop in GCS, pupil light reflex changes, ventilatory desynchronization, and nursing care such as changing position or tracheal suctioning). This helps to appropriately titrate the administration of anti-edema measures and also to time, follow-up imaging, and surgical intervention. Recent studies show that analysis of the ICP-pulse waveform (Morphological Cluster and Analysis of Intracranial Pressure-MOCAIP metrics) can be used as an indicator of global perfusion. Elevation of third peak in ICP waveform is associated with low CBF and is shown to correlate well with Xenon CBF studies (19).

Two major complications of ICP monitoring are ventriculitis and hemorrhage. Infection is reported in 1%–10% of cases and factors that predispose to ventriculitis are intraventricular hemorrhage; SAH; cranial fracture with CSF leak; craniotomy; catheter manipulation, leak, and irrigation; and duration of catheter dwelling. Prophylactic systemic antibiotics and catheter exchange do not reduce risk of infection and are not recommended. Antibiotic impregnated ventriculostomy catheters reduce the risk of infection from 9.4% to 1.3% (20). The best measures to reduce infection are usage of aseptic technique during insertion, antibiotic impregnated catheters, and minimizing the duration of monitoring. Intracerebral hemorrhage is known to occur in 1%–2% of cases with ICP monitoring.

TABLE 23–3 Recommendations for Nutrition and Prophylaxis of Complications From *Guidelines for the Management of Severe Traumatic Brain Injury* (3rd Edition, 2007)

TOPIC	LEVEL OF RECOMMENDATION		
	I	II	III
Nutrition		Provide nutrition to attain full caloric replacement by day 7 postinjury.	
Infection prophylaxis		Give periprocedural antibiotics for intubation to reduce the incidence of pneumonia (does not alter mortality or length of hospital stay).	Routine ventricular catheter exchange and systemic prophylactic antibiotics for catheter placement do not reduce infection.
		Perform early tracheostomy to reduce days of mechanical ventilation (does not alter mortality rate or incidence of pneumonia)	Early extubation in qualified patients does not increase risk of pneumonia.
Deep vein thrombosis prophylaxis			Apply graduated compression stockings or intermittent pneumatic compression stockings to reduce risk of thrombophlebitis (unless lower extremity injuries prevent their use)
Seizure prophylaxis		Prophylactic phenytoin or valproate does not prevent late post-traumatic seizures.	Prophylactic anticonvulsants decrease the incidence of early post-traumatic seizures (does not improve outcome).

Recent reports of noninvasive monitoring of ICP include techniques like measurement of tympanic membrane displacement, ultrasound "time of flight," optic sheath diameter using ultrasound or MRI, and venous ophthalmodynamometry (by measuring the intraorbital pressure required to collapse the central retinal vein) (18). Bellner, Schmidt, and Edouard have proposed equations to measure ICP based on noninvasive Transcranial Doppler (TCD) parameters (19). These studies are promising but require further validation.

ICP monitoring allows early detection and treatment of intracranial hypertension that could result in severe secondary brain injury. There are no randomized controlled trials to show the benefit or no benefit of ICP monitoring. Although ICP monitoring does have a physiological basis, aggressive ICP-driven protocols could potentially result in cardiorespiratory complications. Cremer et al. analyzed 686 patients with severe TBI admitted to 2 tertiary centers in Netherlands (one center monitored ICP and the treatment was ICP/CPP driven and the other center did not monitor ICP) and reported no difference in the survival or the functional outcome between the 2 groups (21). However, this is a retrospective study and the outcome difference could be caused by the difference in the standard of care between the 2 hospitals. Moreover, the patients who died in the first 24 hours were excluded from the study. Similarly, Shafi et al., in a retrospective analysis of National Trauma Data Bank (NTDB) cases (1994–2001) have shown a 45% reduction in survival in patients with ICP monitoring. In this study too, the patients who died in the first 48 hours were excluded from the study and the risk adjustment may not have given equivalent groups (22). However, it must be remembered that monitoring a physiological process like ICP is not a treatment and alone will not improve outcome after TBI. An effective treatment protocol must accompany the monitoring of ICP.

Cerebral Perfusion

The ideal method for monitoring of cerebral ischemia should provide continuous data both on global and regional CBF. The available methods for monitoring cerebral perfusion either directly measure CBF or indirectly estimate CBF by measuring cerebral oxygenation. Measurement of CPP, which is calculated from mean arterial pressure (MAP) minus ICP is the simplest way to measure cerebral perfusion and is a widely used method. However, in a setting of TBI, with impaired autoregulation, even with CPP values higher than 50 mm Hg, which is the normal lower limit of autoregulation, cerebral perfusion may be inadequate.

TCD ultrasonography measures flow velocity (FV), which can be used as an indicator of CBF. Increase in FV could be caused by vasospasm or hyperemia. To differentiate between the two, MCA to extracranial internal carotid artery flow velocity ratio (known as Lindegaard or hemispheric index) (23) needs to be measured. In hyperemia, velocity in both vessels will increase with no net change in the ratio, whereas in vasospasm the ratio is high because there is an increase in MCA flow velocity only. Normal hemispheric index is 1.76 ± 0.1 and values higher than 3 are suggestive of vasospasm.

Modern technology has made direct measurement of CBF more feasible in critically ill patients. Measurement of global blood flow using Kety-Schmidt technique with nitrous oxide, and both global and regional CBF with stable xenon CT imaging (using rapid diffusion of 28%–33% xenon into tissues) or perfusion CT imaging is feasible. However, these techniques measure only intermittent values and are not widely available except for research purposes. Continuous blood flow can be measured using thermal diffusion method and laser Doppler method. These methods are invasive, require placement of a probe on the surface or within the brain and provide only regional blood flow information.

The adequacy of CBF can also be measured indirectly by measuring cerebral oxygenation using jugular venous oxygen saturation ($SjvO_2$) or brain tissue oxygenation ($PbtO_2$). These methods have an advantage when compared to direct measurements of CBF in providing an indication of the relative adequacy of CBF rather than an absolute value of CBF. When CBF is low (25–30 mL/100 g/min), it can be difficult to decide whether the brain is hypoperfused or the low CBF is a response to lower cerebral metabolic requirements. Measurement of cerebral oxygenation would help make the distinction. If there is hypoperfusion, oxygen extraction will increase to compensate for the lower CBF and the $SjvO_2$ or $PbtO_2$ will be reduced. In contrast, if CBF is appropriate for the brain's metabolic requirement, then $SjvO_2$ or $PbtO_2$ will remain normal.

$SjvO_2$ monitoring can be useful in monitoring for global ischemic insults. Robertson et al. published a series of 177 patients with severe TBI and demonstrated that 39% of those patients had at least one episode of desaturation. Good recovery or moderate disability occurred in 44% of patients with no episodes of desaturation, 30% of patients with one episode, and only 15% of patients with multiple episodes of desaturation (24). Cormio et al. have reported a series of 450 patients with $SjvO_2$ monitoring; the worst outcome was noticed in patients with high $SjvO_2$ (> 75%), which occurs with severe injury because the nonviable tissue does not extract oxygen (25). In patients with brain injury, the average $SjvO_2$ is higher than normal and in a series of 116 patients with continuous $SjvO_2$; the average value was 68.1 ± 9.7 in 1,329 measurements (14). The current TBI guidelines recommend treating $SjvO_2$ < 50% (Table 23-1, level III recommendation).

Some controversy exists over optimal placement of the $SjvO_2$ catheter. Stocchetti et al. showed differences between the values of $SjvO_2$ measured from right and left jugular bulbs, suggesting incomplete mixing of jugular venous blood (26). Metz et al. compared bilateral $SjvO_2$ in 22 patients and recommended that the catheter should be placed on the dominant side in diffuse injury and on the same side when the injury is focal (27). However, if the goal is to monitor global oxygenation, it may be more logical to always monitor on the dominant side. $SjvO_2$ will not reliably identify regional ischemia and monitoring of $PbtO_2$ may have an advantage for this indication. $PbtO_2$ measures oxygenation in tissue directly surrounding the tip of the catheter so location of the catheter is very important. When placed in relatively normal brain tissue, the values closely parallel global oxygenation. When placed in more injured tissue, the $PbtO_2$ values reflect the local oxygenation and can vary substantially from global oxygenation. Normal value for $PbtO_2$ in anesthetized subjects is 20–40 mm Hg. The current TBI guidelines recommend treatment of $PbtO_2$ < 15mm Hg (Table 23-1, level III recommendation). Spiotta et al. found improvement in outcome and mortality with $PbtO_2$-guided therapy when compared to conventional ICP/CPP management in patients with severe TBI (28).

Recently, a noninvasive method (using near-infrared spectroscopy [NIRS] based on oximetry) to monitor cerebral perfusion was found useful in patients undergoing cardiopulmonary bypass surgery (29). However, in patients with TBI, NIRS has limited value because there is common occurrence of traumatic blood that confounds the oxygenation signal.

Because none of the direct or indirect methods for monitoring cerebral perfusion is ideal, a strategy combining the available technologies is often used. Imaging of cerebral perfusion, when available, is useful to understand whether areas of focal hypoperfusion exist or not. If there are no focal areas of hypoperfusion, then a technique that monitors global perfusion, such as $SjvO_2$ or a local monitor ($PbtO_2$ or CBF) placed in normal brain, is useful. When focal hypoperfusion exists, then placement of a $PbtO_2$ or CBF probe in the area of interest might provide the most useful information for management.

Cerebral Autoregulation

Cerebral autoregulation, initially described in 1964 by Lassen, is the inherent ability of the brain to maintain a constant CBF over a wide range of BPs (mean 50–150 mm Hg) by varying the diameter of arterial vessels. In TBI, the brain commonly loses the ability to autoregulate and CBF is more dependent on CPP. Autoregulation can be monitored intermittently or continuously. A hemodynamic stimulus (pharmacologic agents like phenylephrine, thigh cuff release, carotid artery compression) is applied and the resulting changes in CBF (using TCD by measuring changes in FV) are determined (30–33). An autoregulatory index (ARI) can be calculated from the change in CBF relative to the change in BP. Using spontaneous fluctuations in BP that occur in patients over time as the hemodynamic stimulus, indices like mean velocity index (Mx) and pressure reactivity index (Px) can be calculated. Both intermittent (ARI) and continuous (Px) indices are shown to correlate well with CBF studies and with clinical outcome following TBI. With an intact cerebral vascular pressure reactivity, there is a negative correlation between MAP and cerebral blood volume (and thereby ICP). In TBI, because of the loss of autoregulation, blood volume (ICP) passively follows MAP. These changes in Px can be calculated and then used to find the CPP value at which cerebral autoregulation is optimal.

Secondary Ischemic Insults

The causes of secondary ischemic insults could be cerebral causes (raised ICP, seizures) or systemic causes (hypotension, hypoxia, hypocapnia, anemia, and fever). *Raised ICP* is the most common cause of $SjvO_2$ desaturation and is discussed in the previous section. *Seizures* can dramatically increase cerebral energy requirements. If the CBF is uncoupled or marginal, ischemia can occur during the seizure. The overall risk of seizures is 2.5%–5% with all types of TBI (34). Continuous EEG is useful in patients who are sedated and paralyzed and who are a high-risk group for seizures.

Hypotension can occur in the prehospital period or during the hospital stay (intraoperatively or in the ICU). In a TCDB study, 35% of patients had a systolic BP of < 90 mm Hg on arrival in the emergency room. Many subsequent studies have shown worsening of outcome with hypotension on admission or during the hospital stay. Zafar et al. reported a bimodal distribution of mortality following moderate-to-severe TBI for the presenting systolic BP in the emergency department. Patients with emergency department systolic BP < 120 and > 140 mm Hg had higher mortality rates—2.2

times and 1.6 times respectively—when compared to patients with systolic BP between 120 and 140 mm Hg (35). Usually, an arterial catheter is used to monitor systemic BP in the ICU and the goal should be to maintain a MAP of at least 80 mm Hg so that the CPP remains at least 60 mm Hg.

Hypocapnia is the second most common cause of $SjvO_2$ desaturation (14). The beneficial effect of hyperventilation on briefly decreasing ICP comes at the expense of cerebral perfusion. If the injured brain has altered CO_2 reactivity, mild hyperventilation might constrict the blood vessels in the uninjured brain and increase regional flow to the injured and the marginally perfused brain (inverse steal response) (36). However, with more intense hyperventilation, cerebral perfusion can be globally reduced. End-tidal CO_2 ($EtcO_2$) can be used to continuously estimate $Paco_2$. In patients with brain injury without pulmonary involvement, $EtcO_2$ correlates well with $Paco_2$. In patients with pulmonary insufficiency, these values do not correlate and requires analysis of the arterial blood gases.

Hypoxia is a common cause of $SjvO_2$ desaturation. Normally, a decrease in partial pressure of arterial oxygen (PaO_2) is compensated by an increase in CBF through vasodilatation even though this results in raised ICP. Hypoxia can develop because of lung contusion, atelectasis, fat emboli, pneumonia, or acute respiratory distress syndrome (ARDS). In a study on 225 patients with TBI, hypoxia was present in 35% and increased the mortality rate from 24% to 50% (37). Pulse oximetry is a convenient way to monitor systemic oxygenation and the goal should be to maintain arterial oxygen saturation (SaO_2) $\geq$ 95%.

Anemia, if associated with significant decrease in CaO_2 (oxygen content of blood), can result in cerebral ischemia. In a normal brain, this is compensated by an increase in CBF. When the blood flow is compensated to supply oxygen, the $SjvO_2$ remains constant, but when increase in CBF is not able to compensate oxygen supply, the $SjvO_2$ decreases. Hemoglobin (Hb) content should be measured at least once daily during the early phase after injury.

Fever increases body metabolic rate by 10%–13%/°C (centigrade) and is associated with a poor neurological outcome (13). In studies using a temperature probe that is incorporated into a standard ventriculostomy ICP monitor, the intracranial temperature was 0.5°C–2°C higher than the body temperature. Therefore, measurement of rectal temperature alone could underestimate the actual brain temperature.

MANAGEMENT OF A PATIENT WITH TBI

The traditional approach to the management of patients with TBI is to control ICP using a *stair-step approach*, adding or subtracting therapies as needed. *CPP management*, advocated by Rosner et al. (38), is based on the concept of "vasodilatory cascade." According to this hypothesis, an increase in BP will break the cycle that leads to ever reducing CPP in TBI. It assumes a normal pressure autoregulation in the brain. A randomized clinical trial has compared a "CBF-targeted" strategy to a conventional "ICP-targeted" strategy in the initial management of TBI (39). The CBF-targeted treatment, where CPP was kept at least 70 mm Hg and hyperventilation was not used, reduced the incidence of secondary ischemic events by approximately 50%. However, this treatment strategy increased the incidence of ARDS by fivefold and did not

improve long-term neurological outcome. In another approach, called "*Lund therapy*"(*volume regulated*), the emphasis is on reduction of microvascular pressures to minimize edema formation in the brain by keeping physiological parameters within normal limits (Hb, PaO_2, oncotic pressure, blood volume) and avoiding factors, which favor transcapillary filtration (hypothermia, barbiturates, high CPP, CSF drainage, osmotic diuretics) (40). This approach assumes impaired autoregulation and disrupted blood–brain barrier and runs the risk of ischemia if CPP is not adequate. A final approach has been to individualize the treatment to match the underlying pathophysiology. This approach recognizes the fact that the pathophysiology of TBI evolves over time and treatment that is appropriate in the first few hours after injury may not necessarily be optimal 2–3 days after injury in the same patient. This *autoregulation-regulated therapy* aims at monitoring of cerebral autoregulation and maintenance of CPP at a value where there is optimal cerebral autoregulation and cerebral oxygenation (32,33). This approach seems to fill the gap between the CPP guided therapy and Lund therapy. These approaches are illustrated in Figure 23-1.

General Measures for Patients With TBI

General Measures

Studies have shown a reduction in ICP without a reduction in either CPP or CBF in most patients with elevation of the head end by 30° angle (41). Therefore, unless the patient is hypovolemic and head elevation results in hypotension, the reduction in ICP afforded by 30° angle of head elevation is probably advantageous.

Maintenance Measures

In choosing a sedative agent for the patient with head injury (to blunt the effect of routine nursing care), it is important to remember to avoid drugs with hypotensive side effects. A combination of morphine or fentanyl and lorazepam is frequently used. It is important to know that these drugs can alter CBF, cerebral metabolic rate of oxygen consumption ($CMRo_2$), and ICP. Propofol has the advantage of a short half-life, which allows intermittent neurological examination, but it is a potent systemic vasodilator and can cause hypotension and reduce CPP. Propofol infusion syndrome can develop in some patients.

Maintenance of fluid requirement (35 mL/kg/day of 0.9% saline) and strict estimation of fluid loses should be carefully monitored. Studies have measured that caloric expenditure after TBI averages 140% of normal resting energy expenditure, based on age, gender, and body size (42). In a retrospective study of patients with TBI, those who were not fed within 5–7 days after TBI had a twofold and fourfold increased likelihood of death, respectively (43). The average nitrogen loss for a patient with head injury is 0.2 g/kg/day (2–3 times the normal fasting nitrogen loss), which needs replacement with enteral feedings, beginning as soon after injury as possible but certainly within 72 hours. The goal should be to gradually increase the feedings and reach full caloric replacement by the end of first week (Table 23-3, level II recommendation). Enteral feedings (nasogastric/jejunal tube in acute phase or percutaneous gastrostomies in chronic phase) are preferable to parenteral feedings because gut in-

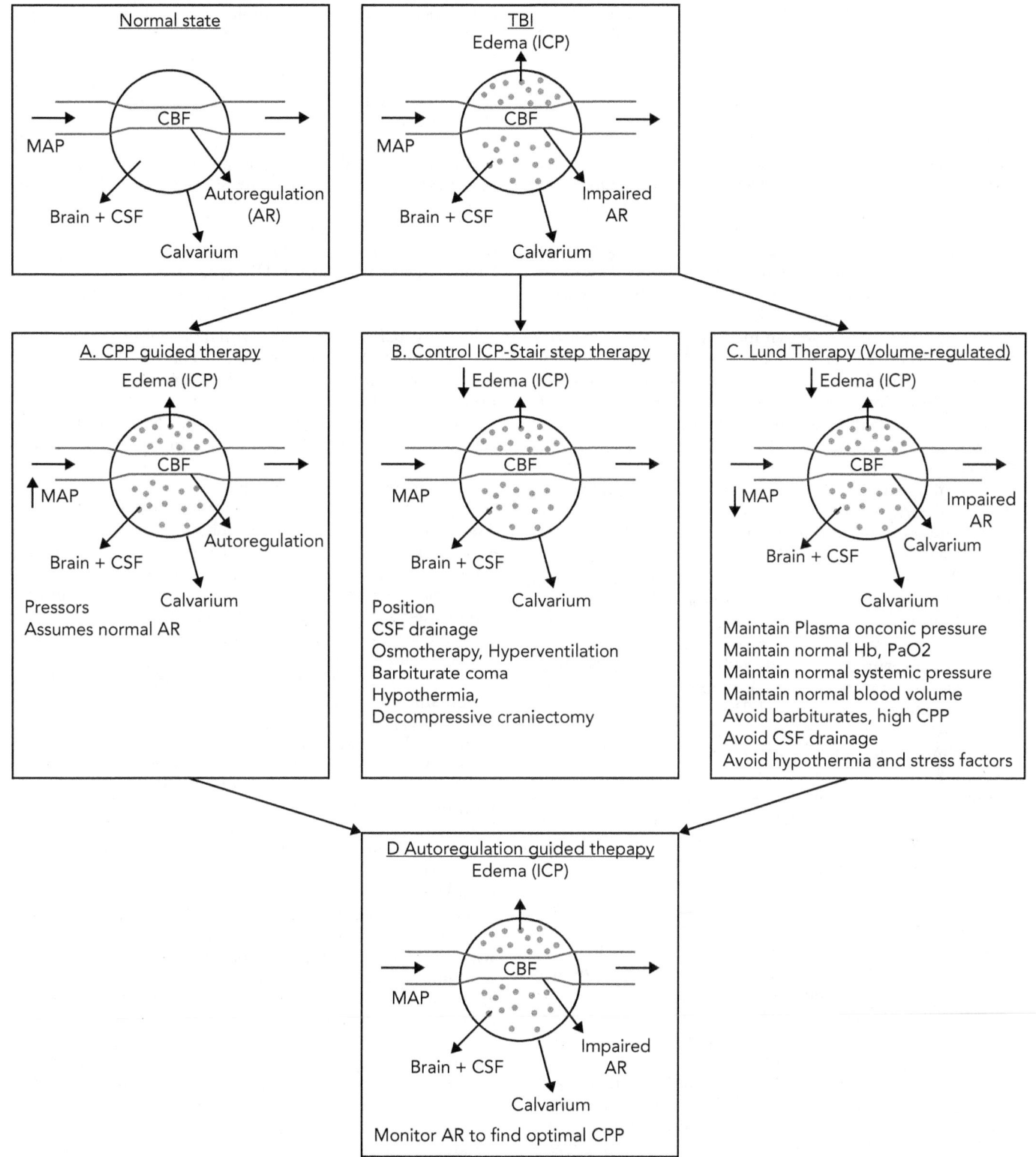

FIGURE 23-1 Approaches to management of TBI. A, The CPP-guided therapy aims at breaking the "vasodilatory cascade" by increasing MAP and assumes a normal pressure autoregulation. B, The ICP therapy aims at reducing the ICP using a stair-step approach. C, Lund therapy (volume-targeted therapy) aims at minimizing the brain edema by maintaining physiological parameters within normal limits (Hb, PaO_2, blood volume, BP, and oncotic pressure) and avoiding factors that increase edema (high CPP, barbiturates, hypothermia, and stress factors). This approach assumes an impaired pressure autoregulation. D, Autoregulation-guided therapy aims at finding a CPP at which autoregulation is optimal. This approach probably fills the gap between the CPP-guided therapy and Lund therapy.

tegrity is better maintained and probably reduces the risk of sepsis (see Chapter 54 for additional discussion of gastrointestinal dysfunction and nutritional support after brain injury).

Prophylactic Measures

The role of anticonvulsants in preventing *post-traumatic seizures* is controversial. The risk factors for late seizures after TBI are brain contusion with subdural hematoma, skull fracture, loss of consciousness, or amnesia for more than 1 day and an age of 65 years or older (see Chapter 39 for additional discussion of post-traumatic seizures). Temkin et al. reported reduction in the incidence of seizures during the first week after TBI with phenytoin in a double-blind study (44).

Some studies have shown major brain injury as a risk factor for *venous thromboembolism*. Prophylactic treatment reduces the incidence of thromboembolism from 8.98% to 2.9%. Both low-dose heparin and sequential venous compression prophylaxis are equally effective. Sequential compression devices are the class II recommendation in the third edition of the brain injury guidelines (45). Low-molecular-weight heparin may be safely started with the finding of stable hemorrhage on CT scans separated by 12–24 hours.

Following TBI, *stress ulcers* are common and are caused by increased vagal activity. Risk factors for stress ulcers are severity of TBI, burns > 25% of body surface area (BSA), respiratory failure, hypotension, sepsis, jaundice, peritonitis, coagulopathy, and hepatic failure. The use of proton pump inhibitors or sucralfate may be a better choice to treat stress ulcers in neurosurgical patients as histamine (H2) blockers and antacids can increase the risk of nosocomial pneumonia because of increase in gastric pH. There is no role for prophylactic antibiotics to prevent meningitis in TBI.

Although steroids (dexamethasone and methylprednisolone) do not improve outcome following TBI (level I recommendation), recent studies have demonstrated a neuroprotective role for progesterone and its metabolites in TBI. This neuroprotection is mediated through various mechanisms. So far, there are two phase II trials that have shown a neuroprotective effect and safety for progesterone following TBI. In the ProTECT II trial (46), 3 days IV administration of progesterone following TBI in patients with severe and moderate head injury reduced the mortality to less than half that of controls. The functional outcome at 3 months was better in the moderate head injury group compared to the control group. Similarly, Xiao et al. have demonstrated beneficial effect following intramuscular administration of progesterone for 5 days on both mortality and morbidity at 6 months following severe TBI (47). Results of subsequent clinical trails (Protect III: NCT00822900 in United States and SyNAPse: NCT01143064, multicenter, worldwide) are awaited to tell us more about the long-term effects of progesterone in TBI (48).

Intervention Measures

It is unwise to reduce *systemic BP* in patients with hypertension associated with untreated intracranial mass lesions because cerebral perfusion is maintained by the higher BP. Treatment of systemic hypertension (systolic BP > 160 mm Hg) during the postoperative course is a controversial issue. Sympathomimetic-blocking antihypertensive drugs, such as beta-blocking drugs (propanolol, esmolol, or labetalol) or centrally acting alpha receptor agonists (clonidine or alpha-methyldopa), are preferred for treating hypertension if required. Vasodilatory antihypertensive drugs, including hydralazine and nitroprusside that consistently increase ICP should be avoided.

Fever is a potent cerebral vasodilator and can raise ICP and cerebral metabolic requirements. Elevated rectal temperatures should be treated with antipyretics and/or cooling blankets.

In the TCDB studies, *hypoxia* was present in 19% of comatose patients with head injury at arrival in the emergency room. Patients with severe TBI have some type of breathing abnormality, including periodic respirations, tachypnea, and irregular breathing. Hypoxia and hypercarbia can dramatically raise ICP. Controlled ventilation helps prevent these episodes of hypoventilation (rapid changes in $Paco_2$) and intracranial hypertension and allow deeper levels of sedation to be used.

Patients with TBI have a high incidence of *pneumonia* (up to 40%), probably as a result of aspiration at the time of the injury. Antibiotic prophylaxis for ventilated patients with TBI, either cefuroxime 1,500 mg intravenous (IV) for 2 doses after intubation or ampicillin-sulbactam 3 g every 6 hours for 3 days, reduces the incidence of subsequent pneumonia (49). Other ways of minimizing the risk of ventilator-associated pneumonia include limiting the duration of intubation and mechanical ventilation, oral rather than nasal intubation, continuous aspiration of subglottic secretions, maintenance of endotracheal tube cuff pressure at least 20 cm water, nursing in semirecumbent position (30°–45° angle), emptying condensate from ventilator tubing, and not allowing condensate to contaminate the endotracheal tube.

Electrolyte abnormalities are reported in 59% of the TCDB patients (50). Syndrome of inappropriate antidiuretic hormone (ADH) secretion (SIADH) and cerebral salt-wasting are the 2 most common causes of hyponatremia in patients with brain injury. In both conditions, the urine sodium is high (> 40 mEq/L). Patients with SIADH are normovolemic or slightly volume expanded in contrast to the patients with salt-wasting syndrome who are hypovolemic. The diagnosis of SIADH also requires serum osmolarity < 280 mOsm/L and urine osmolarity greater than serum osmolarity. SIADH is treated with fluid restriction or demeclocycline. For salt-wasting syndrome, replacement of intravascular volume with normal saline is the initial treatment. Hypertonic (3%) saline may be administered slowly for patients with significant symptoms such as seizures or raised ICP.

Diabetes insipidus (DI) results in free water loss and hypovolemic hypernatremia because of inadequate ADH. DI can be treated with water replacement; however, in TBI, patients may require IV administration of aqueous desmopressin acetate (DDAVP) 2–4 µg as administration of large volumes of free water may exacerbate intracranial hypertension (see Chapter 53 for additional discussion of neuroendocrine dysfunction after brain injury).

Hyperglycemia has been associated with a poor neurological outcome after TBI. Tight control of blood glucose between 80 and 110 mg/dL has been shown to reduce morbidity and mortality rate in critically ill patients (51). However, because hypoglycemia can occur with such tight glucose control, a slightly more liberal range of 100–180 mg/dL is usually targeted during the acute recovery period following TBI.

In a TBI study of 22 patients, abnormalities of the sellar region were noticed in 80% of the patients with *hypopituitarism* compared to only 29% of those without hypopituitarism. The pituitary axis most commonly involved at 3 months post-injury is gonadotropic (32%), followed by corticotropic (19%), somatotropic (9%), and thyrotropic (8%). Adrenal insufficiency (hypotension, hypoglycemia, and hyponatremia) can be primary (from adrenal gland failure) or secondary (from pituitary or hypothalamic failure). In a study of 80 patients with moderate or severe TBI, 53% had at least transient adrenal insufficiency. Studies recommend early endocrine evaluations of all patients with moderate and severe TBI with follow-up at 3 and 12 months after injury (52).

Patients with severe TBI often have other systemic injuries (like femur fracture) that require surgical procedures. However, there is a controversy about timing of surgery for injuries that are not immediately life-threatening. McKee et al. (53) concluded that their practice of early fixation of femur fractures did not increase morbidity or mortality in patients with TBI.

Treatment of Raised Intracranial Pressure

Raised ICP that develops unexpectedly or accompanied by clinical deterioration or refractory to medical treatment requires prompt CT imaging to rule out surgical lesions. Although various studies recommend different cutoff points (ICP greater than 15, 20, or 25 mm Hg) for intervention, the current TBI guidelines recommend treating ICP that is more than 20 mm Hg (Table 23-1, level II recommendation). Sustained ICP greater than 20–25 mm Hg despite general measures as described in the previous section should be treated by specific measures that are typically added in a stepwise fashion until the ICP is controlled.

Pharmacologic Paralysis

ICP raised by agitation, posturing, or coughing should be prevented by narcotics and nondepolarizing muscle relaxants that do not alter cerebrovascular resistance although the TCDB suggests increased risk of pulmonary complications and prolonged ICU stay with this treatment. Morphine or fentanyl and lorazepam for analgesia/sedation and cisatracurium or vecuronium as a muscle relaxant, with the dose titrated by twitch response to stimulation, is a reasonable regimen. The muscle relaxants can be withheld once a day, usually before morning rounds to obtain a brief neurologic examination.

Neuromuscular blockade in patients with TBI can cause critical illness myopathy and neuropathy, which can be categorized into the following 3 general syndromes: (*a*) critical illness myopathy (common in asthmatics), (*b*) prolonged neuromuscular blockade (in patients with kidney or liver dysfunction and with aminoglycosides), and (*c*) acute polyneuropathy (in patients with sepsis and multiple organ syndrome). There is an overlap in these typical syndromes and an electromyography (EMG), a muscle and nerve biopsy, can be helpful in distinguishing weakness caused by these syndromes from the underlying brain injury. These complications can be minimized by limiting the overall use and dosage of neuromuscular blocking agents, measuring creatine phosphokinase (CPK) daily, and stopping the neuromuscular blocking agents at least once a day to observe motor response (54,55).

Hyperventilation

The relationship between hyperventilation and global CBF was examined in a series of 171 patients with head injury during the first 10 days after injury (56). Of the 1,212 CBF measurements in these patients, 132 (11%) were less than 25 mL per 100 g/min. Of the 132 low CBF values, 71 (54%) were appropriately reduced relative to the lower CMR_{O_2}, whereas 61 (46%) were associated with increased oxygen extraction and/or increased cerebral lactate production, suggesting a relative inadequacy of perfusion. The incidence of an inadequate CBF steadily increased as the $Paco_2$ decreased and was 2%, 4%, 8%, and 23% when the $Paco_2$ was greater than 30, 25–30, 20–25, and less than 20 mm Hg, respectively. Routine hyperventilation (to bring $Paco_2$ of 20–25 mm Hg) has been shown to have a detrimental effect on outcome in one randomized trial (57) and is not recommended in the current TBI guidelines (Table 23-2, level II recommendation). The authors of this study recommended using hyperventilation only in patients with intracranial hypertension rather than as a routine in all patients with brain injury.

In general, hyperventilation should not be used during the first 24-hour postinjury and used only if $Pbto_2$ or $Sjvo_2$ is monitored to be certain that ischemia is not being produced (Table 23-2, level III recommendation). In patients who have been chronically hyperventilated, abruptly returning the $Paco_2$ to normal can result in a dramatic increase in ICP. Therefore hyperventilation should be gradually withdrawn to prevent this increase in ICP (58).

Cerebrospinal Fluid Drainage

Removal of 1–2 mL of CSF through the ventriculostomy catheter in a patient with TBI can temporarily lower ICP (59). However, the effectiveness of this modality reduces when the ventricles collapse because of progressive swelling of the brain. Some advocate continuous drainage of CSF, periodically closing the ventriculostomy to measure ICP. However, if this option is chosen, ICP should be continuously monitored using some alternative method. Periodic rather than continuous measurement of ICP could allow ICP to remain elevated without treatment for a long time.

Osmotherapy

Mannitol and hypertonic saline are 2 most commonly used hyperosmolar agents for the treatment of intracranial hypertension. Mannitol administration lowers the ICP within 1–5 minutes, with a peak effect at 20–60 minutes, and lasting for 1.5–6 hours (60). Mannitol is usually given as a bolus of 0.25–1g/kg body weight (Table 23-2, level II recommendation). A bolus of 1 g/kg is required for an urgent reduction of ICP and 0.25–0.5 g/kg repeated every 2–6 hours is needed for long-term control. Serum osmolarity should be kept at less than 320 mOsm (optimal 300–320 mOsm) to avoid side effects such as hypovolemia, hyperosmolarity, and renal failure. Mannitol loses its potential after initial doses as it opens the blood–brain barrier, crosses into interstitium, draws fluid into the brain, and aggravates edema.

Hypertonic saline (3%–23.4%) reduces intracranial volume and ICP. Hypertonic saline is more effective than mannitol in reducing ICP in some studies (61,62). It has an advantage over mannitol in hypovolemic patients, where it augments intravascular volume and may increase BP in addition to decreasing ICP. It reduces ICP with concurrent durable elevations in CPP and also increases brain oxygenation levels (63). However, in severe TBI, it is not associated with improved neurologic outcome when given as a prehospital bolus to hypotensive patients (64). Hypertonic saline administration can result in adverse effects like decreased platelet aggregation, prolonged coagulation times, hypokalemia, and hyperchloremic acidosis (65).

Barbiturate Coma

Barbiturate coma, in addition to lowering ICP, decreases extracellular levels of lactate and excitatory amino acids (66–69). A randomized multicenter trial demonstrated that instituting barbiturate coma in patients with refractory intracranial hypertension resulted in a twofold greater chance of controlling the ICP (70). It is reserved for patients with ICP that is refractory to other medical measures because it can cause hypotensive complications, and also, it is difficult to examine patients during the treatment. Pentobarbital is given in a loading dose of 10 mg/kg (over 30 minutes) followed by 5 mg/kg each hour for 3 doses. The maintenance dose (1–2 mg/kg/hr) is titrated to maintain a serum level in the therapeutic range of 30–50 μg/mL or the EEG has a burst suppression pattern. These patients require monitoring of EEG and close monitoring of hemodynamics, perhaps with pulmonary wedge pressure and cardiac output (71). Barbiturates reduce ICP by probably a hemodynamic effect because the reduction in ICP is immediate. Messeter et al. have suggested that the reduction in ICP with barbiturates is closely tied to the retention of CO_2 reactivity by the brain (72,73). Barbiturate coma is reported to cause hypotension in 58%, hypokalemia in 82%, respiratory complications in 76%, infections in 55%, renal dysfunction in 47%, and hepatic dysfunction in 87% of the patients (74). In a study of barbiturate coma in patients with refractory intracranial hypertension, the most consistent cerebral effect was a reduction in $CMRO_2$ (by an average of 31%) (75). There was a significantly better outcome in patients with a good or partial ICP response to pentobarbital, with 21% of these patients having a good recovery or moderate disability at 3 months postinjury compared to 100% persistent vegetative state or death in the nonresponders. Patients with severe injuries with reduced $CMRO_2$ and patients with systemic hypotension are not likely to have a good response with barbiturates.

Hypothermia

Hypothermia has numerous potential neuroprotective roles in TBI through reductions in cerebral metabolic rate, increased ICP, cerebral edema, frequency of epileptic discharges, inflammatory response, release of glutamate, nitric oxide and free radicals, and attenuation in the opening of the blood–brain barrier (76). Hypothermia can be induced by systemic or selective methods (surface cooling, intranasal selective hypothermia, endovascular cooling, and epidural cerebral cooling). Systemic hypothermia can result in cardiovascular and pulmonary complications, infections, and thrombocytopenia. So far, use of hypothermia is limited to a level III recommendation in the guidelines for the management of TBI. Among the methods used to induce selective hypothermia, although most studies have used surface cooling, there are a couple of studies with intravascular cooling method (77). Although some studies have reported an overall beneficial effect of moderate hypothermia (32°C–33°C) in

severe TBI, in a recently concluded randomized trial (National Acute Brain Injury Study: Hypothermia II), early induction and hypothermia for 48 hours did not confirm the neuroprotective role of early hypothermia in TBI (78). The published hypothermia trials in TBI differ in the method of cooling used, target temperature used (between 31 and 35), time to achieve target temperature (3–8 hours), duration of hypothermia (24–155.3 hours), and rate of rewarming (79). In view of the conflicting results, it is important to determine the optimal hypothermia parameters and the subgroup of patients with TBI who would benefit from hypothermia. The ongoing hypothermia clinical trials may provide us a higher level of evidence for using hypothermia. A new multicenter randomized controlled trial has started recruiting patients in Europe (the Eurotherm3235 trial) and aims to study the role of titrated hypothermia for at least 48 hours in reducing ICP in TBI (80).

Decompressive Craniectomy

Decompressive craniectomy has been used to treat uncontrolled intracranial hypertension of various origins, including cerebral infarction, trauma, SAH, and spontaneous hemorrhage. Patient selection, timing of operation, type of surgery, and severity of clinical and radiologic brain injury are all factors that determine the outcome of this procedure. The effectiveness of very early decompressive craniectomy was evaluated in one randomized clinical trial (pilot study of 27 children with TBI); children treated with conventional medical management and very early decompressive craniectomy had reduced ICP, fewer episodes of raised ICP, and better functional outcome at 6 months when compared to children treated with medical treatment alone (81). Reduction in ICP and favorable outcomes following decompressive craniectomy has been reported in several case-control and case-series studies. However, a recent randomized trial (DECRA, Australia, 155 adults) concluded that in patients with diffuse TBI and intractable intracranial hypertension, bifrontotemporoparietal craniectomy decreased ICP and the length of the intensive care unit (ICU) stay but was associated with more unfavorable outcomes (82). The results of RESCUEicp trial are awaited (83).

Treatment of Cerebral Hypoperfusion

The main goal in TBI treatment is to optimize oxygen delivery to the brain, which depends on oxygen content of the blood and on CBF. Oxygen content of the blood (in mL/dL = $SaO_2 \times Hb \times 1.34 + PaO_2 \times 0.003$) can be improved by optimizing Hb concentration (at least 10 g/dL) (84) and by optimizing PaO_2 (by increasing inspiring oxygen percentage). The increase in oxygen content after Hb is 100% saturated and occurs in only small amounts (because oxygen dissolved in the blood [$PaO_2 \times 0.003$]), but even this small increase may be critical for ischemic brain tissues (85).

After TBI with impaired autoregulation, CBF is more dependent on CPP, and a higher CPP is required to maintain an adequate CBF. CPP depends on both ICP and MAP so manipulation of both parameters can influence CPP and therefore CBF. If ICP is elevated, treatment of ICP can effectively improve CBF. BP can also be manipulated to maintain a desired CPP. After ascertaining an adequate intravascular volume as assessed by a central venous catheter or a Swan-

Ganz catheter, further increase in BP to maintain CPP is achieved by adding a pressor agent.

Few studies have compared the effectiveness of various pressor agents in increasing CBF (86). Dopamine at intermediate dosage (2–6 µg/kg/min) increases CBF with a variable effect at higher and lower doses, perhaps because of direct effects of cerebral arterioles. Other pressor agents do not have a significant direct effect on either CBF or ICP. In patients with suspected vasospasm, dopamine infusion increased regional cerebral blood flow (rCBF) in more than 90% of the regions where CBF was < 25 mL per 100 g/min at baseline and also unexpectedly reduced rCBF in one-third of the nonischemic territories (87). Dopamine may not be the best agent for induced hypertension as a treatment of cerebral ischemia. The other pressor drugs such as norepinephrine or phenylephrine may have more predictable effects on CBF but can result in systemic ischemic complications.

Monitoring of cerebral autoregulation indices may help by allowing identification of an optimal CPP in individual patients with TBI. Studies have shown improvement in cerebral autoregulation with hyperventilation, acute hyperoxia, and statins (32,33,88). Further studies are required to define the clinical significance of these results.

Improved $PbtO_2$ is shown to correlate with good clinical outcome following TBI. $PbtO_2$ can be improved by increasing the oxygen percentage in the inspired air at normal atmospheric pressure (normobaric hyperoxia [NBH], 1 atmosphere absolute [ATA]) or hyperbaric oxygen. Hyperbaric oxygen therapy (HBOT) (oxygen at > 1 ATA) in experimental studies is shown to improve both $PbtO_2$ and behavioral outcome following TBI (89). Both NBH and HBOT increase the PaO_2 by increasing the amount of dissolved oxygen in plasma after 100% saturation of Hb. A recently concluded randomized prospective clinical trial using HBOT (at 1.5 ATA, 60 minutes daily for 3 days) vs normobaric oxygen therapy (NBOT) (1 ATA, 100% inspired oxygen) and standard care has shown higher $PbtO_2$ levels that correlated well with improved CBF and $CMRO_2$ and lower ICP and CSF lactate levels (90). Further studies are required to establish the optimal levels of required ATA, frequency of HBOT, duration of HBOT, and optimal levels of $PbtO_2$ that should be maintained for a good clinical outcome. The improvement that is observed in the physiological parameters with HBOT is to be correlated with clinical outcome. Apart from improved tissue oxygenation, HBOT is shown to have antiapoptotic and anti-inflammatory effects, which may contribute toward its neuroprotective effect.

Secondary Ischemic Insults: Treatment Strategies and Controversies

Hypotension
Intravascular volume, if low as assessed by a central venous pressure monitor or a Swan-Ganz catheter, should be treated with infusion of crystalloids, colloids, or blood as appropriate for the clinical situation. From the Saline vs Albumin Fluid Evaluation (SAFE) study in patients with TBI, a higher mortality rate was observed among patients with severe TBI who received 4% albumin than among those who received saline (91). Hypertonic saline allows replacement of intravascular volume with less increase in ICP than saline or dextran and is shown to have significantly better survival-to-

discharge in TBI (92). Inotropic and/or pressor agents should be used if volume replacement does not provide an adequate BP. Hypotension in adults with TBI is rarely caused by brain injury alone and blood loss from other injuries like associated spinal cord injury (hypotension and bradycardia), cardiac contusion or tamponade, and tension pneumothorax needs to be considered and treated promptly and appropriately.

Hypoxia
Hypoxia can be improved by increasing fractional inspired oxygen concentration (FiO_2). When pulmonary edema is present, addition of positive end-expiratory pressure (PEEP) may improve ventilation perfusion mismatch at a lower inspired oxygen concentration. However, PEEP can raise ICP by increasing intrathoracic pressure and central venous pressure and reduce BP by decreasing venous return to the heart. This combined effect can reduce cerebral perfusion. The effect of increasing PEEP on ICP depends on both intracranial and pulmonary compliance. In patients with normal intracranial compliance, ICP does not change because the brain is able to compensate but with decreased intracranial compliance, even small increases in cerebral venous pressure may cause dangerous increases in ICP (93). Elevating the patient's head reduces the effect of high airway pressures on ICP (94). When the lungs are poorly compliant, exposure to PEEP does not markedly increase venous pressure or ICP. Sudden removal of PEEP may precipitate a sudden increase in central blood volume and a rise in arterial BP and CPP thereby resulting in an increase in ICP (95).

Anemia
Studies correlating CBF and hematocrit demonstrate that CBF and tissue oxygen delivery increase as hematocrit and viscosity decrease until hematocrit falls to 33%. Lower than this threshold, tissue oxygen delivery decreases. In normal adults, an adequate oxygen-carrying capacity is met by a Hb concentration of at least 7g/dL (hematocrit of 21%) when the intravascular volume is normal. However, in TBI it cannot be assumed that the same hematocrit will be adequate, especially if cerebral ischemia is present. The optimal transfusion threshold in neurological critically ill patients is unknown. In patients with severe TBI and SAH with hematocrit less than 25%, red blood cell (RBC) transfusion has been shown to increase local brain tissue oxygenation in 75% of the patients (96). When cerebral ischemia is present, a hematocrit level of at least 30% may be required for maximal oxygen delivery to the brain (97).

Seizures
Seizures in a patient with brain injury should be immediately arrested using diazepam (5–10 mg IV) or lorazepam (2–3 mg IV). The action of these drugs is short-lived and requires IV administration of other antiepileptics like phenytoin to maintain antiepileptic activity. Phenytoin is administered at 25 mg/min until a loading dose of 15–20 mg/kg has been given followed by a maintenance dose of 300–400 mg/day.

Vasospasm
Hypervolemic hemodilution and induced hypertension ("Triple H" therapy) are the primary therapies of symptomatic

vasospasm after TBI. Usually, intravascular volume is expanded and monitored with a central venous or Swan-Ganz catheter. If the patient is still symptomatic after hypervolemia, a pressor agent is added; phenylephrine or norepinephrine if cardiac output is adequate or dopamine if cardiac output is inadequate, with attention to the effect of these pressor on cerebral hemodynamics as discussed earlier. Nimodipine is effective in reducing neurological complications caused by vasospasm following TBI. In blast-related injuries with vasospasm, aggressive treatment (open surgical and endovascular treatment) may improve outcome (98).

CONCLUSION

In conclusion, use of multiple strategies still remains the main stay in the management of patients with TBI. Prevention of secondary cerebral insults following TBI is crucial for favorable outcome. Intensive care monitoring, anticipation, early recognition, and treatment of cerebral insults would improve outcome. With the available experimental and clinical knowledge, we are definitely heading toward treatment based on individual patient parameters especially in optimization of autoregulation based on physiological parameters. The role of interventions like hypothermia and decompressive craniectomy are yet to be fine-tuned because they seem to benefit a particular segment of patients with TBI. The beneficial effect of HBOT on physiological parameters needs to be correlated with clinical outcome. Newer neuroprotective agents that are in various phases of trials like progesterone may further improve our understanding of pathophysiology of TBI.

KEY CLINICAL POINTS

1. Monitoring, early detection, and treatment of secondary brain injury processes are the main focus in the current management of patients with TBI.
2. Ventriculosotomy has both diagnostic and therapeutic role in the management of raised ICP. Medical management is the mainstay in controlling ICP. Role of hypothermia and decompressive craniectomy in TBI needs to be further evaluated to define the parameters and the patient groups that would benefit from these interventions.
3. Monitoring of cerebral metabolism (Pbto$_2$ along with CBF) rather than CBF alone is the ideal way to detect an evolving ischemia and treat with optimization of oxygen delivery. Role of HBOT in TBI needs further evaluation to determine its clinical benefits.
4. Role of autoregulation in management of TBI (methods of monitoring, correlation with other parameters, defining optimal range and effect on clinical outcome, and means of improving it) needs further clinical evaluation.
5. Although ICP-targeted, CPP-guided, and Lund therapies are available, current understanding of TBI is leading us toward a paradigm shift; treatment based on individual pathoanatomy and pathophysiology. Progress of genomic, proteomic, and metabolomic research in TBI may provide us an opportunity for personalized medicine in the future.
6. Newer neuroprotective agents like progesterone seem to have a beneficial role that needs further evaluation by phase III trials.

KEY REFERENCES

1. Brain Trauma Foundation, American Association of Neurological Surgeons, Congress of Neurological Surgeons. Guidelines for the management of severe traumatic brain injury. *J Neurotrauma.* 2007;24(suppl 1):S1–S106.
2. Clifton GL, Valadka A, Zygun D, et al. Very early hypothermia induction in patients with severe brain injury (the National Acute Brain Injury Study: Hypothermia II): a randomised trial. *Lancet Neurol.* 2011;10(2):131–139.
3. Cooper DJ, Rosenfeld JV, Murray L, et al. Decompressive craniectomy in diffuse traumatic brain injury. *N Engl J Med.* 2011;364(16):1493–1502.
4. Gopinath SP, Robertson CS, Contant CF, et al. Jugular venous desaturation and outcome after head injury. *J Neurol Neurosurg Psychiatry.* 1994;57(6):717–723.
5. Rockswold SB, Rockswold GL, Zaun DA, et al. A prospective, randomized clinical trial to compare the effect of hyperbaric to normobaric hyperoxia on cerebral metabolism, intracranial pressure, and oxygen toxicity in severe traumatic brain injury. *J Neurosurg.* 2010;112(5):1080–1094.
6. Spiotta AM, Stiefel MF, Gracias VH, et al. Brain tissue oxygen-directed management and outcome in patients with severe traumatic brain injury. *J Neurosurg.* 2010;113(3):571–580.
7. Steiner LA, Czosnyka M, Piechnik SK, et al. Continuous monitoring of cerebrovascular pressure reactivity allows determination of optimal cerebral perfusion pressure in patients with traumatic brain injury. *Crit Care Med.* 2002;30(4):733–738.
8. Wright DW, Kellermann AL, Hertzberg VS, et al. ProTECT: a randomized clinical trial of progesterone for acute traumatic brain injury. *Ann Emerg Med.* 2007;49(4):391–402.

References

1. Jennett B, Braakman R. Severe traumatic brain injury. *J Neurosurg.* 1990;73(3):479–480.
2. Foulkes MA, Eisenberg HM, Jane JA, Marmarou A, Marshall LF. The Traumatic Coma Data Bank: design, methods, and baseline characteristics. *J Neurosurg.* 1991;75(suppl):S8–S13.
3. Marmarou A, Lu J, Butcher I, et al. IMPACT database of traumatic brain injury: design and description. *J Neurotrauma.* 2007;24(2):239–250.
4. Brain Trauma Foundation, American Association of Neurological Surgeons, Congress of Neurological Surgeons. Guidelines for the management of severe traumatic brain injury. *J Neurotrauma.* 2007;24(suppl 1):S1–S106.
5. Bullock MR, Chesnut R, Ghajar J, et al. Surgical management of acute subdural hematomas. *Neurosurgery.* 2006;58(3)(suppl):S16–S24.
6. Bullock MR, Chesnut R, Ghajar J, et al. Surgical management of traumatic parenchymal lesions. *Neurosurgery.* 2006;58(3)(suppl):S25–S46.
7. Bullock MR, Chesnut R, Ghajar J, et al. Surgical management of acute epidural hematomas. *Neurosurgery.* 2006;58(3)(suppl):S7–S15.
8. Miller JD, Becker DP, Ward JD, Sullivan HG, Adams WE, Rosner MJ. Significance of intracranial hypertension in severe head injury. *J Neurosurg.* 1977;47(4):503–516.
9. Martin NA, Patwardhan RV, Alexander MJ, et al. Characterization of cerebral hemodynamic phases following severe head trauma: hypoperfusion, hyperemia, and vasospasm. *J Neurosurg.* 1997;87(1):9–19.
10. Bouma GJ, Muizelaar JP, Stringer WA, Choi SC, Fatouros P, Young HF. Ultra-early evaluation of regional cerebral blood flow in se-

verely head-injured patients using xenon-enhanced computerized tomography. *J Neurosurg.* 1992;77(3):360–368.

11. Robertson CS, Contant CF, Gokaslan ZL, Narayan RK, Grossman RG. Cerebral blood flow, arteriovenous oxygen difference, and outcome in head injured patients. *J Neurol Neurosurg Psychiatry.* 1992; 55(7):594–603.

12. Obrist WD, Langfitt TW, Jaggi JL, Cruz J, Gennarelli TA. Cerebral blood flow and metabolism in comatose patients with acute head injury. Relationship to intracranial hypertension. *J Neurosurg.* 1984; 61(2):241–253.

13. Jones PA, Andrews PJ, Midgley S, et al. Measuring the burden of secondary insults in head-injured patients during intensive care. *J Neurosurg Anesthesiol.* 1994;6(1):4–14.

14. Gopinath SP, Robertson CS, Contant CF, et al. Jugular venous desaturation and outcome after head injury. *J Neurol Neurosurg Psychiatry.* 1994;57(6):717–723.

15. Gopinath SP, Robertson CS, Contant CF, Narayan RK, Grossman RG. Clinical evaluation of a miniature strain-gauge transducer for monitoring intracranial pressure. *Neurosurgery.* 1995;36(6):1137–1140.

16. Czosnyka M, Czosnyka Z, Pickard JD. Laboratory testing of three intracranial pressure microtransducers: technical report. *Neurosurgery.* 1996;38(1):219–224.

17. Unterberg A, Kiening K, Schmiedek P, Lanksch W. Long-term observations of intracranial pressure after severe head injury. The phenomenon of secondary rise of intracranial pressure. *Neurosurgery.* 1993;32(1):17–23.

18. Lavinio A, Menon DK. Intracranial pressure: why we monitor it, how to monitor it, what to do with the number and what's the future? *Curr Opin Anaesthesiol.* 2011;24(2):117–123.

19. Hu X, Glenn T, Scalzo F, et al. Intracranial pressure pulse morphological features improved detection of decreased cerebral blood flow. *Physiol Meas.* 2010;31(5):679–695.

20. Zabramski JM, Whiting D, Darouiche RO, et al. Efficacy of antimicrobial-impregnated external ventricular drain catheters: a prospective, randomized, controlled trial. *J Neurosurg.* 2003;98(4):725–730.

21. Cremer OL, van Dijk GW, van Wensen E, et al. Effect of intracranial pressure monitoring and targeted intensive care on functional outcome after severe head injury. *Crit Care Med.* 2005;33(10):2207–2213.

22. Shafi S, Diaz-Arrastia R, Madden C, Gentilello L. Intracranial pressure monitoring in brain-injured patients is associated with worsening of survival. *J Trauma.* 2008;64(2):335–340.

23. Lindegaard KF, Nornes H, Bakke SJ, Sorteberg W, Nakstad P. Cerebral vasospasm diagnosis by means of angiography and blood velocity measurements. *Acta Neurochir (Wien).* 1989;100(1–2):1–224.

24. Robertson CS, Gopinath SP, Goodman JC, Contant CF, Valadka AB, Narayan RK. SjvO2 monitoring in head-injured patients. *J Neurotrauma.* 1995;12(5):891–896.

25. Cormio M, Valadka AB, Robertson CS. Elevated jugular venous oxygen saturation after severe head injury. *J Neurosurg.* 1999;90(1):9–15.

26. Stocchetti N, Paparella A, Bridelli F, Bacchi M, Piazza P, Zuccoli P. Cerebral venous oxygen saturation studied with bilateral samples in the internal jugular veins. *Neurosurgery.* 1994;34(1):38–43.

27. Metz C, Holzschuh M, Bein T, Kallenbach B, Taeger K. Jugular bulb monitoring of cerebral oxygen metabolism in severe brain injury: accuracy of unilateral measurements. *Acta Neurochir Suppl.* 1998;71:324–327.

28. Spiotta AM, Stiefel MF, Gracias VH, et al. Brain tissue oxygen-directed management and outcome in patients with severe traumatic brain injury. *J Neurosurg.* 2010;113(3):571–580.

29. Brady KM, Mytar JO, Lee JK, et al. Monitoring cerebral blood flow pressure autoregulation in pediatric patients during cardiac surgery. *Stroke.* 2010;41(9):1957–1962.

30. Czosnyka M, Brady K, Reinhard M, Smielewski P, Steiner LA. Monitoring of cerebrovascular autoregulation: facts, myths, and missing links. *Neurocrit Care.* 2009;10(3):373–386.

31. Rangel-Castilla L, Gasco J, Nauta HJ, Okonkwo DO, Robertson CS. Cerebral pressure autoregulation in traumatic brain injury. *Neurosurg Focus.* 2008;25(4):E7.

32. Rangel-Castilla L, Lara LR, Gopinath S, Swank PR, Valadka A, Robertson C. Cerebral hemodynamic effects of acute hyperoxia and

33. Steiner LA, Czosnyka M, Piechnik SK, et al. Continuous monitoring of cerebrovascular pressure reactivity allows determination of optimal cerebral perfusion pressure in patients with traumatic brain injury. *Crit Care Med.* 2002;30(4):733–738.

34. Wang HC, Chang WN, Chang HW, et al. Factors predictive of outcome in posttraumatic seizures. *J Trauma.* 2008;64(4):883–888.

35. Zafar SN, Millham FH, Chang Y, et al. Presenting blood pressure in traumatic brain njury: a bimodal distribution of death. *J Trauma.* 2011;71(5):1179–1184.

36. Stringer WA, Hasso AN, Thompson JR, Hinshaw DB, Jordan KG. Hyperventilation-induced cerebral ischemia in patients with acute brain lesions: demonstration by xenon-enhanced CT. *AJNR Am J Neuroradiol.* 1993;14(2):475–484.

37. Miller JD, Becker DP. Secondary insults to the injured brain. *J R Coll Surg Edinb.* 1982;27(5):292–298.

38. Rosner MJ, Rosner SD, Johnson AH. Cerebral perfusion pressure: management protocol and clinical results. *J Neurosurg.* 1995;83(6):949–962.

39. Robertson CS, Valadka AB, Hannay HJ, et al. Prevention of secondary ischemic insults after severe head injury. *Crit Care Med.* 1999;27(10):2086–2095.

40. Andrews PJ, Citerio G. Lund therapy—pathophysiology-based therapy or contrived over-interpretation of limited data? *Intensive Care Med.* 2006;32(10):1461–1463.

41. Feldman Z, Kanter MJ, Robertson CS, et al. Effect of head elevation on intracranial pressure, cerebral perfusion pressure, and cerebral blood flow in head-injured patients. *J Neurosurg.* 1992;76(2):207–211.

42. Clifton GL, Robertson CS, Grossman RG, Hodge S, Foltz R, Garza C. The metabolic response to severe brain injury. *J Neurosurg.* 1984;60(4):687–696.

43. Härtl R, Gerber LM, Ni Q, Ghajar J. Effect of early nutrition on deaths due to severe traumatic brain injury. *J Neurosurg.* 2008;109(1):50–56.

44. Temkin NR, Dikmen SS, Wilensky AJ, Keihm J, Chabal S, Winn HR. A randomized, double-blind study of phenytoin for the prevention of post-traumatic seizures. *N Engl J Med.* 1990;323(8):497–502.

45. Bratton SL, Chestnut RM, Ghajar J, et al. Guidelines for the management of severe traumatic brain injury. V. Deep vein thrombosis prophylaxis. *J Neurotrauma.* 2007;24(suppl 1):S32–S36.

46. Wright DW, Kellermann AL, Hertzberg VS, et al. ProTECT: a randomized clinical trial of progesterone for acute traumatic brain injury. *Ann Emerg Med.* 2007;49(4):391–402.

47. Xiao G, Wei J, Yan W, Wang W, Lu Z. Improved outcomes from the administration of progesterone for patients with acute severe traumatic brain injury: a randomized controlled trial. *Crit Care.* 2008;12(2):R61.

48. Stein DG. Is progesterone a worthy candidate as a novel therapy for traumatic brain injury? *Dialogues Clin Neurosci.* 2011;13(3):352–359.

49. Acquarolo A, Urli T, Perone G, Giannotti C, Candiani A, Latronico N. Antibiotic prophylaxis of early onset pneumonia in critically ill comatose patients. A randomized study. *Intensive Care Med.* 2005;31(4):510–516.

50. Piek J, Chesnut RM, Marshall LF, et al. Extracranial complications of severe head injury. *J Neurosurg.* 1992;77(6):901–907.

51. van den Berghe G, Wouters P, Weekers F, et al. Intensive insulin therapy in the critically ill patients. *N Engl J Med.* 2001;345(19):1359–1367.

52. Ghigo E, Masel B, Aimaretti G, et al. Consensus guidelines on screening for hypopituitarism following traumatic brain injury. *Brain Inj.* 2005;19(9):711–724.

53. McKee MD, Schemitsch EH, Vincent LO, Sullivan I, Yoo D. The effect of a femoral fracture on concomitant closed head injury in patients with multiple injuries. *J Trauma.* 1997;42(6):1041–1045.

54. Nates JL, Cooper DJ, Day B, Tuxen DV. Acute weakness syndromes in critically ill patients—a reappraisal. *Anaesth Intensive Care.* 1997;25(5):502–513.

55. Zochodne DW, Bolton CF, Wells GA, et al. Critical illness polyneuropathy. A complication of sepsis and multiorgan failure. *Brain.* 1987;110(pt 4):819–841.

hyperventilation after severe traumatic brain injury. *J Neurotrauma.* 2010;27(10):1853–1863.

56. Hayes C, Robertson CS, Narayan RK, et al. The effect of hyperventilation on cerebral blood flow in head-injured patients. American Association of Neurological Surgeons Abstracts. 1992. Abstract 1271.

57. Muizelaar JP, Marmarou A, Ward JD, et al. Adverse effects of prolonged hyperventilation in patients with severe brain injury: a randomized clinical trial. *J Neurosurg.* 1991;75(5):731–739.

58. Muizelaar JP, van der Poel HG, Li ZC, Kontos HA, Levasseur JE. Pial arteriolar vessel diameter and CO2 reactivity during prolonged hyperventilation in the rabbit. *J Neurosurg.* 1988;69(6):923–927.

59. Ghajar JB, Hariri R, Patterson RH. Improved outcome from traumatic coma using only ventricular CSF drainage for ICP control. *Adv Neurosurg.* 1993;21:173–177.

60. Knapp JM. Hyperosmolar therapy in the treatment of severe head injury in children: mannitol and hypertonic saline. *AACN Clin Issues.* 2005;16(2):199–211.

61. Battison C, Andrews PJ, Graham C, Petty T. Randomized, controlled trial on the effect of a 20% mannitol solution and a 7.5% saline/6% dextran solution on increased intracranial pressure after brain injury. *Crit Care Med.* 2005;33(1):196–202.

62. Vialet R, Albanèse J, Thomachot L, et al. Isovolume hypertonic solutes (sodium chloride or mannitol) in the treatment of refractory posttraumatic intracranial hypertension: 2 mL/kg 7.5% saline is more effective than 2 mL/kg 20% mannitol. *Crit Care Med.* 2003;31(6):1683–1687.

63. Pascual JL, Maloney-Wilensky E, Reilly PM, et al. Resuscitation of hypotensive head-injured patients: is hypertonic saline the answer? *Am Surg.* 2008;74(3):253–259.

64. Cooper DJ, Myles PS, McDermott FT, et al. Prehospital hypertonic saline resuscitation of patients with hypotension and severe traumatic brain injury: a randomized controlled trial. *JAMA.* 2004;291(11):1350–1357.

65. Doyle JA, Davis DP, Hoyt DB. The use of hypertonic saline in the treatment of traumatic brain injury. *J Trauma.* 2001;50(2):367–383.

66. Marshall LF, Smith RW, Shapiro HM. The outcome with aggressive treatment in severe head injuries. Part I: the significance of intracranial pressure monitoring. *J Neurosurg.* 1979;50(1):20–25.

67. Rea GL, Rockswold GL. Barbiturate therapy in uncontrolled intracranial hypertension. *Neurosurgery.* 1983;12(4):401–404.

68. Lee MW, Deppe SA, Sipperly ME, Barrette RR, Thompson DR. The efficacy of barbiturate coma in the management of uncontrolled intracranial hypertension following neurosurgical trauma. *J Neurotrauma.* 1994;11(3):325–331.

69. Goodman JC, Valadka AB, Gopinath SP, Cormio M, Robertson CS. Lactate and excitatory amino acids measured by microdialysis are decreased by pentobarbital coma in head-injured patients. *J Neurotrauma.* 1996;13(10):549–556.

70. Eisenberg HM, Frankowski RF, Contant CF, Marshall LF, Walker MD. High-dose barbiturate control of elevated intracranial pressure in patients with severe head injury. *J Neurosurg.* 1988;69(1):15–23.

71. Winer JW, Rosenwasser RH, Jimenez F. Electroencephalographic activity and serum and cerebrospinal fluid pentobarbital levels in determining the therapeutic end point during barbiturate coma. *Neurosurgery.* 1991;29(5):739–742.

72. Messeter K, Nordström CH, Sundbärg G, Algotsson L, Ryding E. Cerebral hemodynamics in patients with acute severe head trauma. *J Neurosurg.* 1986;64(2):231–237.

73. Nordström CH, Messeter K, Sundbärg G, Schalén W, Werner M, Ryding E. Cerebral blood flow, vasoreactivity, and oxygen consumption during barbiturate therapy in severe traumatic brain lesions. *J Neurosurg.* 1988;68(3):424–431.

74. Schalén W, Messeter K, Nordström CH. Complications and side effects during thiopentone therapy in patients with severe head injuries. *Acta Anaesthesiol Scand.* 1992;36(4):369–377.

75. Cormio M, Gopinath SP, Valadka AB, Robertson CS. Cerebral hemodynamic effects of pentobarbital coma in head injured patients. *J Neurotrauma.* 1999;16(10):927–936.

76. McIntyre LA, Fergusson DA, Hébert PC, Moher D, Hutchison JS. Prolonged therapeutic hypothermia after traumatic brain injury in adults: a systematic review. *JAMA.* 2003;289(22):2992–2999.

77. Christian E, Zada G, Sung G, Giannotta SL. A review of selective hypothermia in the management of traumatic brain injury. *Neurosurg Focus.* 2008;25(4):E9.

78. Clifton GL, Valadka A, Zygun D, et al. Very early hypothermia induction in patients with severe brain injury (the National Acute Brain Injury Study: Hypothermia II): a randomised trial. *Lancet Neurol.* 2011;10(2):131–139.

79. Faridar A, Bershad EM, Emiru T, Iaizzo PA, Suarez JI, Divani AA. Therapeutic hypothermia in stroke and traumatic brain injury. *Front Neurol.* 2011;2:80.

80. Andrews PJ, Citerio G. EUROTHERM3235Trial. *Intensive Care Med.* 2010;36(12):1990–1992.

81. Taylor A, Butt W, Rosenfeld J, et al. A randomized trial of very early decompressive craniectomy in children with traumatic brain injury and sustained intracranial hypertension. *Childs Nerv Syst.* 2001;17(3):154–162.

82. Cooper DJ, Rosenfeld JV, Murray L, et al. Decompressive craniectomy in diffuse traumatic brain injury. *N Engl J Med.* 2011;364(16):1493–1502.

83. Hutchinson PJ, Corteen E, Czosnyka M, et al. Decompressive craniectomy in traumatic brain injury: the randomized multicenter RESCUEicp study (www.RESCUEicp.com). *Acta Neurochir Suppl.* 2006;96:17–20.

84. Kee DB Jr, Wood JH. Rheology of the cerebral circulation. *Neurosurgery.* 1984;15(1):125–131.

85. Menzel M, Doppenberg EM, Zauner A, Soukup J, Reinert MM, Bullock R. Increased inspired oxygen concentration as a factor in improved brain tissue oxygenation and tissue lactate levels after severe human brain injury. *J Neurosurg.* 1999;91(1):1–10.

86. Myburgh JA, Upton RN, Grant C, Martinez A. A comparison of the effects of norepinephrine, epinephrine, and dopamine on cerebral blood flow and oxygen utilisation. *Acta Neurochir Suppl.* 1998;71:19–21.

87. Darby JM, Yonas H, Marks EC, Durham S, Snyder RW, Nemoto EM. Acute cerebral blood flow response to dopamine-induced hypertension after subarachnoid hemorrhage. *J Neurosurg.* 1994;80(5):857–864.

88. Tseng MY, Czosnyka M, Richards H, Pickard JD, Kirkpatrick PJ. Effects of acute treatment with pravastatin on cerebral vasospasm, autoregulation, and delayed ischemic deficits after aneurysmal subarachnoid hemorrhage: a phase II randomized placebo-controlled trial. *Stroke.* 2005;36(8):1627–1632.

89. Wang GH, Zhang XG, Jiang ZL, et al. Neuroprotective effects of hyperbaric oxygen treatment on traumatic brain injury in the rat. *J Neurotrauma.* 2010;27(9):1733–1743.

90. Rockswold SB, Rockswold GL, Zaun DA, et al. A prospective, randomized clinical trial to compare the effect of hyperbaric to normobaric hyperoxia on cerebral metabolism, intracranial pressure, and oxygen toxicity in severe traumatic brain injury. *J Neurosurg.* 2010;112(5):1080–1094.

91. Myburgh J, Cooper DJ, Finfer S, et al. Saline or albumin for fluid resuscitation in patients with traumatic brain injury. *N Engl J Med.* 2007;357(9):874–884.

92. Vassar MJ, Fisher RP, O'Brien PE, et al. A multicenter trial for resuscitation of injured patients with 7.5% sodium chloride. The effect of added dextran 70. The Multicenter Group for the Study of Hypertonic Saline in Trauma Patients. *Arch Surg.* 1993;128(9):1003–1013.

93. Apuzzo ML, Weiss MH, Petersons V, Small RB, Kurze T, Heiden JS. Effects of positive end expiratory pressure ventilation on intracranial pressure in man. *J Neurosurg.* 1977;46(2):227–232.

94. Frost EA. Effect of positive end-expiratory pressure on intracranial pressure and compliance in brain-injured patients. *J Neurosurg.* 1977;47(2):195–200.

95. Aidinis AJ, Lafferty J, Shapiro HM. Intracranial responses to PEEP. *Anesthesiology.* 1976;45(3):275–286.

96. Smith MJ, Stiefel MF, Magge S, et al. Packed red blood cell transfusion increases local cerebral oxygenation. *Crit Care Med.* 2005;33(5):1104–1108.

97. Pendem S, Rana S, Manno EM, Gajic O. A review of red cell transfusion in the neurological intensive care unit. *Neurocrit Care.* 2006;4(1):63–67.

98. Armonda RA, Bell RS, Vo AH, et al. Wartime traumatic cerebral vasospasm: recent review of combat casualties. *Neurosurgery.* 2006;59(6):1215–1225.

The Surgical Management of Traumatic Brain Injury

Peter S. Amenta and Jack I. Jallo

INTRODUCTION

The enormity of the problem of traumatic brain injury (TBI) cannot be underestimated, as more than 1.7 million Americans are affected annually, with many suffering fatal or permanently disabling injuries (1–4). TBI demonstrates a predilection for the young and most productive members of society, accounting for dramatically shortened life spans and a severely diminished quality of life (5,6). Within the population of young adults, TBI remains the leading cause of death and accounts for up to two-thirds of in-hospital deaths (7). For those trauma patients suffering TBI, the overall mortality is 3 times higher than in those without intracranial trauma (8). Preclinical research continues to investigate the pathophysiology of TBI; however, the limitations of animal models and complexity of the underlying cellular and biochemical processes have impeded progress in this arena. (Please refer to Chapters 10 and 11.) As a result, despite the enormous burden of this disease, medical and surgical treatment options remain limited. (Please refer to Chapter 8).

Recent trends have seen a shift toward multidisciplinary approaches to complex medical problems. The acute management of TBI is no different, with critical care specialists, neurologists, and neurosurgeons frequently involved in the comanagement of these patients (9). Neurosurgical intervention remains a key component; however, operative intervention is more frequently weighed within the context of alternative medical treatment options. Nevertheless, it remains important that an understanding of neurosurgical interventions, as well as their complications and outcomes, is held by all those invested in the care of these patients.

This chapter will discuss the diagnosis and neurosurgical management of TBI as it pertains to indications for surgery, the timing of intervention, preoperative and postoperative care, and potential complications and pitfalls of operative management. Additionally, the pathophysiology of TBI will be highlighted as it relates to mechanisms and patterns of injury.

PREOPERATIVE EVALUATION OF THE TBI PATIENT

Successful management of TBI begins in the moments immediately following the initial insult and is centered on the stabilization and resuscitation of the patient. Undoubtedly, the avoidance of prolonged periods of hypoxia and hypotension in the field limits the development of secondary injury (10). Thus, the initial evaluation of the TBI patient, as with any trauma patient, begins with the airway, breathing, and circulation (ABCs) of trauma care described in the Advanced Trauma Life Support (ATLS) protocol (11). In patients with a Glasgow Coma Scale (GCS) ≤ 8, the airway is secured via endotracheal intubation as soon as possible (12). Suspicion of elevated intracranial pressure (ICP) is treated temporarily with hyperventilation to acutely but transiently reduce the ICP until more definitive measures can be taken (13,14). The maintenance of cerebral perfusion during this time is also of the utmost importance, and fluid resuscitation must begin immediately. Ideally, patients with suspected TBI should be transferred to the nearest trauma center possessing computed tomography (CT) and neurosurgical capabilities (12).

On the arrival to the emergency department, rapid triage and preoperative planning are carried out simultaneously. The ABCs of trauma care are repeated and combined with a detailed physical exam to identify life-threatening systemic injuries. Every attempt to obtain a neurologic exam must be made; however, the use of paralytics, sedatives, and the presence of drugs and alcohol may preclude an accurate assessment of cognition and neurologic deficits. The admission GCS is routinely calculated because it has important implications in operative decision making and establishes a well-defined baseline of neurologic function (15). Blood work is drawn on admission and should include a type and cross, complete blood count (CBC) with platelet count, and partial thromboplastin time/international normalized ratio (PTT/INR). The medication profile of all potential operative candidates and those with known intracranial hemorrhage is reviewed, with special attention paid to antiplatelet agents (aspirin, clopidogrel) and anticoagulation (warfarin). These medications are reversed promptly with platelet transfusions or fresh frozen plasma/factor IX, respectively. (Please refer to Chapter 22).

In the event that the admission CT scan shows evidence of increased ICP (obliteration of the cisterns, diffuse cerebral edema) or a mass lesion resulting in herniation or brainstem compression, an ICP management protocol is initiated. Patients should be positioned with the neck in neutral position and the head of the bed elevated ≥ 30° angle to maximize venous outflow (16). Hyperventilation, as previously discussed, can temporarily decrease the ICP and consideration should be given to treatment with intravenous mannitol (1 mg/kg) or bolused hypertonic saline (15). Once an accurate neurologic exam is completed, the patient can be paralyzed and sedated.

ICP monitoring is routinely used in those patients with a GCS ≤ 8 and in those with evidence of hydrocephalus or diffuse cerebral injury without an accompanying mass lesion (13). In situations where a ventriculostomy can be accurately placed with a minimal number of passes, it is the preferred measuring device because it is both diagnostic and therapeutic.

Although beyond the scope of this chapter, the preoperative evaluation of a TBI patient should include an evaluation of salvageability and a consideration of ultimate quality of life. Such an assessment may aid in family counseling, establish realistic expectations, and avoid "heroic" measures in patients of advanced age or in those with devastating neurologic or systemic injuries. (Please refer to Chapter 18).

SURGICAL INTERVENTION AND TRAUMATIC BRAIN INJURY

As with all surgical interventions, the selection of the appropriate surgical candidate is often as important in determining the success of an intervention as is the technical skill with which the procedure is carried out. Evidence-based practice is difficult to apply to the surgical management of TBI, and there is a lack of Class I data to define the indications of operative intervention. The *Guidelines for the Surgical Management of Traumatic Brain Injury*, an extensive review of the existing TBI literature, was released in 2006 and addressed the surgical management of 5 commonly encountered traumatic injuries: acute epidural hematomas, acute subdural hematomas, traumatic intraparenchymal lesions, posterior fossa mass lesions, and depressed skull fractures (9,17). No data higher than Class III evidence was identified. As a result, the guidelines do not represent proven standards of care but are instead a comprehensive review of management options that serve as a reference for clinical decision making. Thus acquired clinical acumen and clinical suspicion must be integrated into the management algorithms for each individual patient. (Please refer to Chapter 7).

PATHOPHYSIOLOGY AND MANAGEMENT OF TRAUMATIC EXTRA-AXIAL LESIONS

Extra-axial lesions, including epidural and subdural hematomas, are commonly encountered traumatic lesions with which all medical personnel should be familiarized. Patients present with a wide spectrum of signs and symptoms and with different levels of acuity. Delayed or missed diagnoses may have catastrophic neurologic consequences, and in the presence of a neurologic deficit, these lesions are usually promptly evacuated. The following section will detail the underlying pathophysiology of epidural and subdural hematomas and review key points in their operative management.

Epidural Hematomas

Of patients presenting with a traumatic head injury, 6% are found to have an epidural hematoma (18). These lesions are commonly associated with an overlying skull fracture and are classically described as resulting from a laceration of the middle meningeal artery on the fractured bone edge (19). In these situations, the arterial source of hemorrhage, which is unlikely to tamponade, produces a continuously expanding hematoma between the periosteal layer of the dura mater and the inner table of the skull. Rarely, these lesions can develop secondary to the rupture of a dural venous sinus into the epidural space.

CT is widely available within the community and is an efficient and sensitive imaging modality for the identification of an epidural hematoma. Regardless of the source of hemorrhage, these hematomas display a characteristic appearance on standard CT. Epidural hematomas, because of their relationship with the middle meningeal artery, most commonly appear as a hyperdense extra-axial lesion in the temporoparietal region. Because of the insertion of the dura mater at the cranial sutures, these hematomas do not cross suture lines and most commonly assume a lentiform/biconvex shape.

Epidural hematomas (Figure 24-1) are associated with a relatively low incidence of underlying parenchymal injury because of the protection afforded the brain by the dura. As

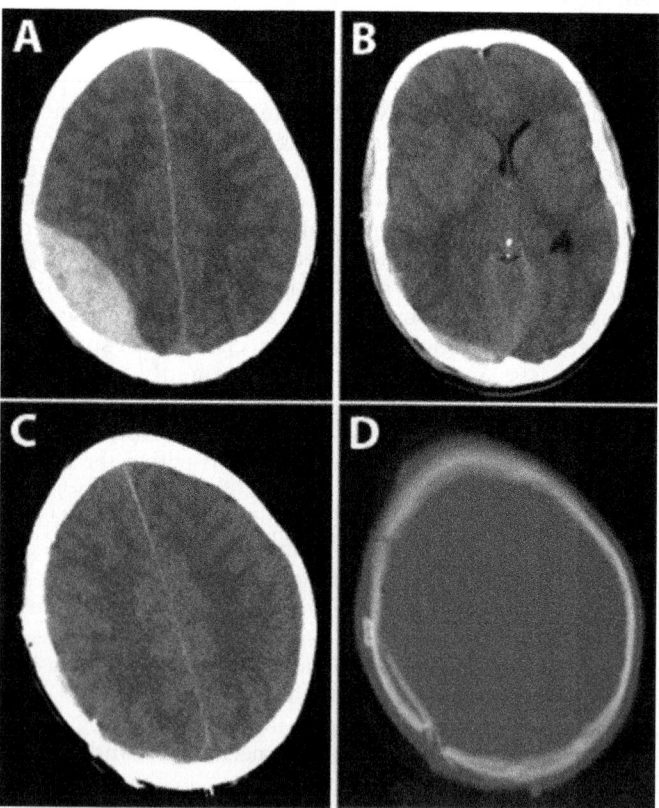

FIGURE 24-1 Epidural hematoma. A 33-year-old male presented to the emergency room with a GCS of 15 and intractable nausea and vomiting 2 hours status post falling down the stairs. CT displayed a 2.6 cm right-sided epidural hematoma (A) with 9 mm of associated right-to-left midline shift (B). The patient was taken for emergent right-sided craniotomy and hematoma evacuation (C). A drain can be seen in the epidural space on the bone windows (D). The patient was discharged home neurologically intact.

a result, isolated epidural hematomas can be associated with particularly good neurologic outcomes when diagnosed and evacuated promptly. This finding renders surgical decompression of an epidural hematoma, one of the most cost-effective of all surgical procedures in terms of quality of life and years preserved (20). Nevertheless, these lesions are also associated with rapid and devastating neurologic deterioration and have a mortality rate of 9% (18).

Prognosis is largely dependent on the neurologic exam and level of consciousness at the time of surgery. Although present in less than half of the patients undergoing operative intervention, the classic presentation is that of a "lucid interval" in the wake of a traumatic insult (21–24). These patients, as well as those with only a minimal neurologic deficit, have an extremely good prognosis. Additional variables with prognostic significance include age, time elapsed between injury and treatment, onset of immediate coma, pupillary abnormalities on exam, and postoperative ICP (25–28). Findings on CT may also be predictive of the ultimate outcome, as large hematoma volume, significant midline shift, and the presence of an intraparenchymal lesion are all associated with a worse prognosis (29).

There is currently no Class I evidence to support the indications for surgical evacuation of an epidural hematoma; however, most practitioners adhere to relatively similar standards (13). Regardless of the GCS score or neurologic examination, supratentorial epidural hematomas > 30 mL and infratentorial hematomas > 10 mL are routinely evacuated (17). CT findings of a hematoma thicker than 15 mm or midline shift greater than 5 mm are also strong indications for surgical intervention. Clinically, patients presenting with anisocoria or GCS < 9 should also be taken for emergent evacuation of the epidural hematoma (17).

Epidural hematomas are focal lesions and can be evacuated rapidly and relatively easily through a limited incision and a small craniotomy (11,17,26,30). In instances where additional intracranial lesions are present, the surgeon may opt for a larger incision and craniotomy to access multiple areas of pathology. Clot evacuation consists of a combination of suction, irrigation, and hematoma removal with cupped forceps. If there is suspicion of an underlying subdural component, the dura may be opened and the subdural space explored. Following the acquisition of meticulous hemostasis, the bone plate can usually be replaced (11).

Acute Subdural Hematomas

In patients presenting with severe closed-head injury, acute subdural hematomas, with an average mortality rate of 50%–60%, represent the most common focal intracranial lesions (18,31–33). Subdural hematomas most commonly result from the tearing of bridging veins as the mobile brain accelerates relative to the fixed skull and dura. The rupture of cortical blood vessels, dural sinuses, and intraparenchymal hematomas through the arachnoid can also result in the accumulation of blood in the subdural space. Subdural hematomas extend beyond suture lines on CT and assume a crescentic appearance. Most present as hyperdense lesions; however, up to 10% of acute subdural hematomas can appear isodense secondary to a low hemoglobin concentration (34).

In patients taking antiplatelet agents or anticoagulants, relatively mild trauma may result in an acute subdural hematoma. However, most patients with operative lesions have been subjected to significant head or neck trauma with the underlying mechanism of injury being age dependent. In the population of patients aged 18–40 years old, motor vehicle accidents are the most common causative event, whereas those aged 65 years or older are most frequently the victim of a fall (35). Unlike epidural hematomas, up to 50% of patients present with an additional intraparenchymal lesion, which may play a critical role in determining the ultimate outcome (15).

Prognosis is most heavily dependent on age, and the highest mortality rates are found in patients older than 65 years old (35). CT findings on admission are also useful in predicting outcome, with increasing hematoma thickness and midline shift associated with poorer outcomes (17). Acute subdural hematomas ≥ 18 mm in thickness or those producing ≥ 20 mm of midline shift are associated with a 50% survival rate. As shift exceeds thickness, the survival rate progressively declines. The survival rate drops to 25% when shift exceeds hematoma thickness by 5 mm and reaches 0% when there is ≥ 25 mm of shift (36).

Acute subdural hematomas (Figure 24-2) can be associated with rapid neurologic deterioration. These lesions compress adjacent structures, induce edema formation, cause an acute elevation of ICP, and eventually lead to herniation (37). Thus, rapid surgical evacuation remains the standard of care. Subdural hematoma evacuation usually requires a large craniotomy to identify sources of bleeding, address additional parenchymal lesions, and obtain adequate hemostasis. In the event that significant cerebral edema is encountered, larger craniotomies also provide additional room for the brain to swell, and the bone flap is left out in some instances (Figure 24-3).

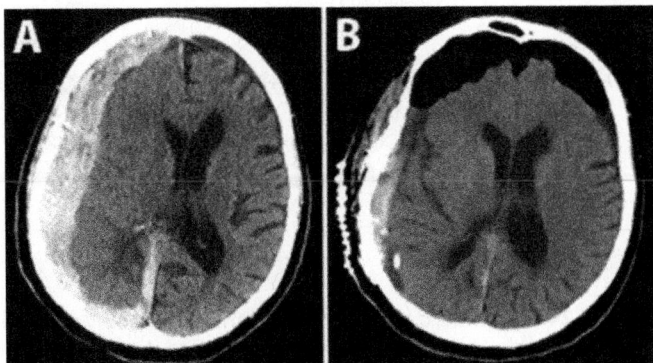

FIGURE 24-2 Acute subdural hematoma. A 79-year-old male on antiplatelet agents presented with a GCS of 8 status post fall from standing. CT demonstrated a 2.5 cm right-sided acute subdural hematoma and 6.4 mm of associated right-to-left midline shift. Following the administration of platelets, the patient was taken to the operating room for a right-sided craniotomy and hematoma evacuation. Postoperatively, the patient improved significantly and was following commands at the time of discharge.

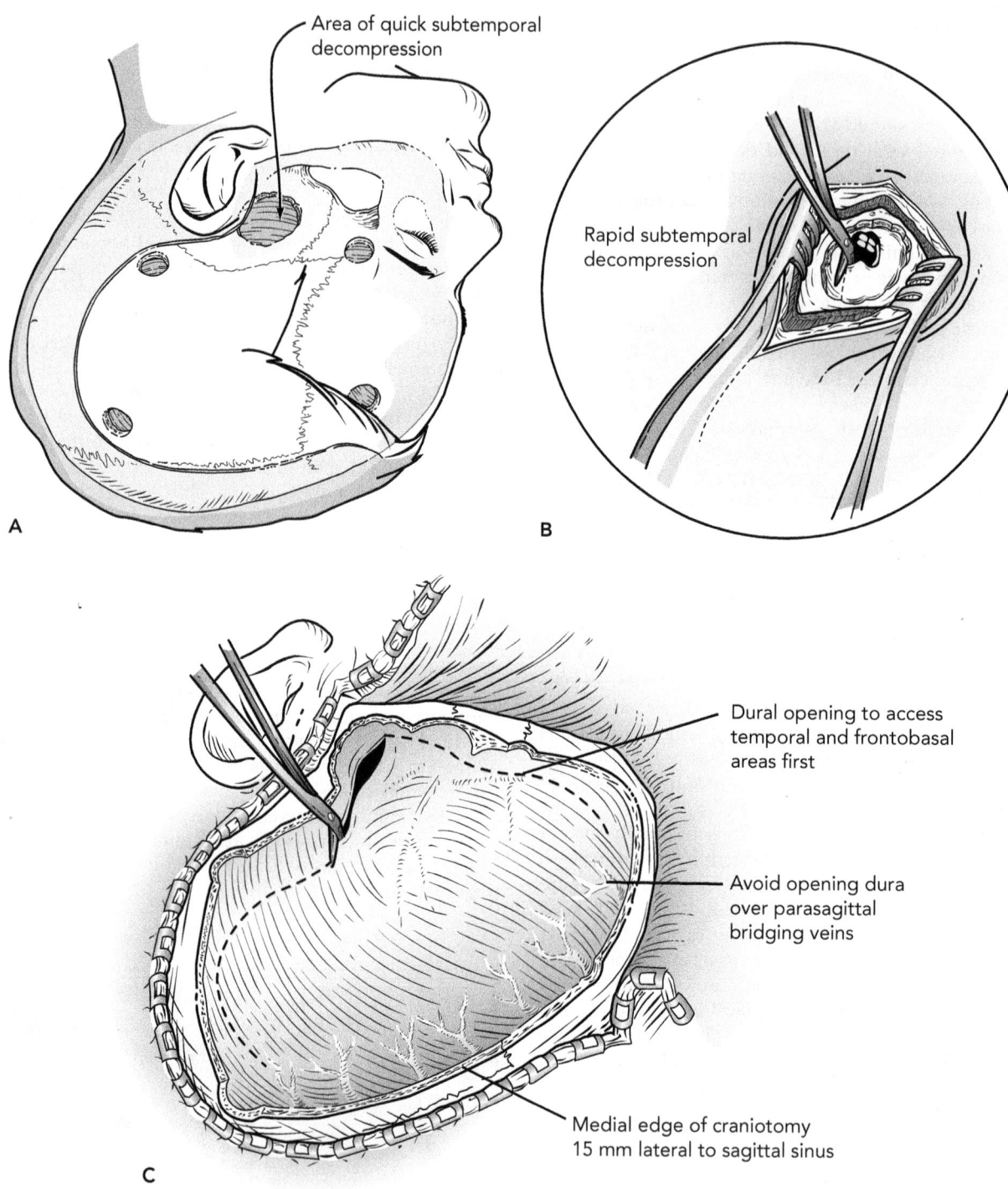

FIGURE 24-3 Standard trauma craniotomy/craniectomy and the evacuation of an acute extra-axial hematoma. A, The scalp incision and trauma flap margins are outlined for the routine evacuation of an extra-axial hematoma. B, In the event of rapid neurologic deterioration, rapid temporal decompression may be performed immediately to prevent herniation. The inferior aspect of the incision is opened, and the scalp and temporalis muscle are reflected. A small craniotomy is made over the temporal lobe, and the hematoma is evacuated prior to completing the craniotomy. C, The bone flap is removed and the dura mater is reflected to allow for subdural hematoma evacuation with cupped forceps and irrigation. Reprinted from Prabhu SS, Zauner A, Bullock MR. *Surgical Management of Traumatic Brain Injury.* 5th ed. Philadelphia, PA: Saunders; 2004.

Labels in figure:
- Area of quick subtemporal decompression
- Rapid subtemporal decompression
- Dural opening to access temporal and frontobasal areas first
- Avoid opening dura over parasagittal bridging veins
- Medial edge of craniotomy 15 mm lateral to sagittal sinus

Contusions and Intraparenchymal Hematomas

General Management Considerations

Blunt trauma to the head causes the brain to impact against the skull, leading to contusions and intracerebral hematomas in nearly all patients with severe head injury and in 25% of those with moderate injury (38–41). These lesions are classified as coup injuries when occurring directly under the site of impact and are most commonly found in the parietal and occipital lobes. Most contusions and intraparenchymal hematomas are contrecoup injuries, which occur in a region of brain opposite the side of impact. Most commonly, these lesions are found in the frontal and temporal lobes as the brain is injured while it slides over the bony irregularities of the anterior and middle cranial fossae.

When weighing the risks and benefits of medical and surgical intervention, intraparenchymal hematomas (Figure 24-4) present unique challenges in decision making (17). The lesions can often effectively be managed nonoperatively, and the hematoma will resorb in 4–6 weeks, leaving a gliotic cavity. Surgical evacuation often requires dissection of normal brain, and there is typically no clear margin between hematoma and salvageable tissue. Thus, intervention carries a significant risk of further neurologic insult.

Management decisions must take into account the neurologic examination, imaging findings, and suspicion of impending clinical deterioration. Obtaining an accurate GCS on admission is of critical importance because it establishes the baseline on which all other examinations will be compared. CT, because of its widespread availability and short acquisition time, is of particular use in the nonoperative management of these lesions. Serial CT reliably identifies progression of midline shift, loss of the cisterns, and local mass effect. Enlargement of the lesion is demonstrated on repeat imaging in 25% of cases over the first 2–3 days following the injury (42–44). ICP monitoring, which may identify a trend of rising ICP prior to clinical deterioration, is also a useful tool in the decision-making process. However, this information must be weighed against all of the existing data because a significant number of patients will exhibit delayed neurologic deterioration without an associated increase in ICP (38).

Posterior Fossa Mass Lesions and Dural Sinus Injury

Traumatic posterior fossa hemorrhages account for 3%–5% of all traumatic mass lesions and may result in devastating neurologic injury and death if not evacuated immediately. The most commonly encountered traumatic lesions of the posterior fossa are epidural hematomas, which are usually found in association with an overlying skull fracture. Eighty percent of patients will display evidence of occipital trauma, such as scalp lacerations, contusions, and open fractures. Subdural and intraparenchymal hematomas secondary to trauma are rarely encountered in the posterior fossa.

Neurologically stable patients demonstrating little or no deficit with a small posterior fossa hemorrhage and without signs of mass effect on CT may be observed and managed nonoperatively (9,17). These patients require close monitoring within intensive care units where routine serial examinations can be performed and there is ready access to CT. Subtle changes in exam must be readily identified, and a high suspicion for deterioration is necessary.

Immediate surgical evacuation is required for lesions causing midline shift, compression or obliteration of the cisterns or fourth ventricle, or obstructive hydrocephalus. Suboccipital craniectomy is the standard surgical approach for the evacuation of all traumatic posterior fossa lesions. Bony decompression should expose the pathology, allow for rapid evacuation of the hematoma, and provide adequate room for parenchymal swelling to eliminate compression of the fourth ventricle and brainstem. Posterior fossa hematomas may be associated with dural venous sinus injury, which can result in epidural, subdural, and intraparenchymal hematomas. The surgeon and the anesthesia team must anticipate the possibility of significant blood loss and recognize the need for immediate blood availability. If possible, it is helpful to identify the dominant transverse sinus with either CT venogram or angiography.

Patients with posterior fossa hematomas are at high risk for acute obstructive hydrocephalus, and the consideration of a ventriculostomy is part of the treatment algorithm. Depending on individual practitioner preference and the clinical scenario, a frontal ventriculostomy may be placed preoperatively or postoperatively. With the patient in the prone position, the occipital approach allows intraoperative placement.

NONFOCAL INTRAPARENCHYMAL LESIONS

Management of Nonfocal Intraparenchymal Lesions

Nonfocal TBI, including malignant cerebral edema, disseminated swelling, and diffuse axonal injury (DAI), lack defined margins, thereby limiting the use of surgical resection. DAI is present in up to 90% of postmortem TBI specimens and is caused by acceleration–deceleration and rotational forces applied to the parenchyma during a significant traumatic insult (45,46). These forces result in the shearing of axons

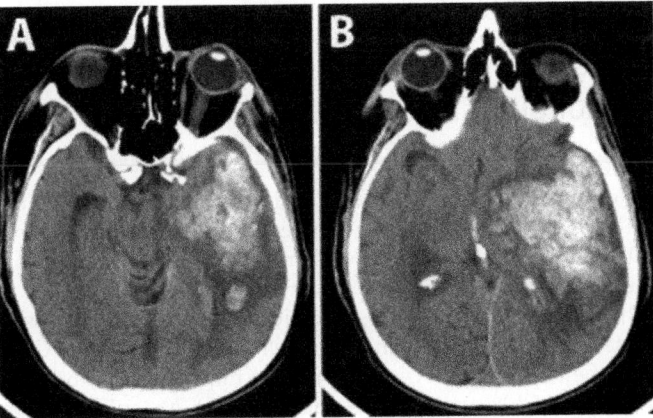

FIGURE 24-4 Traumatic intraparenchymal hematoma. A 68-year-old male on warfarin for atrial fibrillation presented with a GCS of 3 after syncopal episode and a fall down a flight of stairs. Admission CT demonstrated a 6 × 6 × 8 cm left temporoparietal intraparenchymal hematoma. The family was counseled regarding the extremely poor prognosis, and the patient expired following the withdrawal of support.

and widespread neuronal damage, most frequently seen on imaging studies in the corpus callosum and dorsal midbrain. In the absence of a focal hematoma or persistently elevated ICP, DAI is the most common cause of diminished consciousness and poor neurologic function following severe TBI (19).

The management of nonfocal TBI is founded on optimizing cerebral perfusion pressures (CPP > 60), controlling ICP (ICP < 20–25), and limiting the evolution of secondary injury (47–49). As discussed previously, upright positioning, sedation, hyperosmolar therapy, cerebrospinal fluid (CSF) drainage, and high-dose barbiturates may all be used to meet these parameters. In 10%–15% of patients with severe TBI, ICP remains elevated despite maximal medical therapy (49–51).

Persistent elevation of ICP has been demonstrated to result in substantially worse outcomes, with mortality rates ranging from 56.4%–100% in cases of medically refractory intracranial hypertension (50,52,53). In these scenarios, decompressive craniectomy has traditionally represented the definitive surgical treatment, with a significant amount of data supporting a reduction in ICP postprocedure (54–57). Clinical outcomes have been primarily investigated in retrospective analyses, a large number of which use varying measures of success. Of 50 patients with malignant cerebral edema, Aarabi et al. reported better-than-expected functional outcome following decompressive craniectomy (58). A comparison of mortality rates in 115 severe TBI patients found mortality rates of 82.4% and 40% in patients treated with pentobarbital coma or decompressive craniectomy, respectively (59). A metaanalysis, including 323 decompressive craniectomy patients, demonstrated a collective mortality rate of 22.3%, with 48.3% of patients achieving a good outcome (56–65). Despite these seemingly favorable results, the incidence of major disability and persistent vegetative state has remained stable, and the true benefit of decompressive craniectomy on outcome remains unknown (58).

The early Decompressive Craniectomy in patients with severe traumatic brain injury (DECRA) trial is a recently published prospective analysis of 155 patients with severe diffuse TBI and medically refractory ICP who were randomized to continued medical therapy or bilateral frontotemporoparietal decompressive craniectomy (66). The study found patients randomized to surgery to have improved control of ICP and a reduced length of stay in the intensive care unit. However, these patients also exhibited poorer scores on the Glasgow Outcome Scale Extended (GOSE) and a greater risk of an unfavorable outcome (vegetative state and severe disability). Multiple aspects of this study have been debated within the neurosurgical community, and the role of decompressive craniectomy remains largely undefined. The Randomized Evaluation of Surgery with Craniectomy for Uncontrollable Elevation of Intracranial Pressure (RESCUEicp), an additional ongoing prospective randomized investigation, will evaluate the Glasgow Outcome Score at the time of discharge and the GOSE at 6 months postinjury (67).

SURGICAL MANAGEMENT OF DEPRESSED SKULL FRACTURES

Linear, nondisplaced skull fractures require no surgical treatment and will heal without operative intervention.

Depressed skull fractures, which are classified as open when associated with a breach in the overlying galea, demonstrate a morbidity and mortality rate as high as 19% (68–70). These fractures are associated with infection rates of 5%–11%, and 15% of patients will develop epilepsy secondary to underlying parenchymal damage (68,70–73). For these reasons, traditional management has consisted of operative intervention for nearly all open depressed skull fractures (68,71,73). Recently, the surgical management of open depressed skull fractures has experienced an evolution due, in part, to the widespread availability of CT. In most cases, CT consistently rules out an associated hematoma, underlying dural sinus injury, and frontal sinus injury. Additionally, in the absence of gross wound contamination, routine wound care and antibiotic therapy effectively prevents infection (70). The elevation of depressed fractures has also failed to demonstrate a reduction in the incidence of epilepsy (74). Thus, in an increasingly larger number of cases, operative intervention may be avoided.

Operative management is still necessary in a subset of depressed skull fractures, and the surgical approach varies depending on the fracture location, associated injuries, and goals of intervention. Significant cosmetic deformity, grossly contaminated open fractures, fractures depressed ≥ 1 cm, and fractures associated with significant underlying hematomas or a neurologic deficit remain strong indications for surgery. Dural sinus injuries associated with depressed skull fractures also deserve consideration for operative management and present a unique number of management dilemmas. As a general rule, in the absence of mass effect on the sinus, surgical intervention is usually withheld. In cases of sinus compression, venous outflow obstruction and subsequent intracranial hypertension may lead to rapid neurologic deterioration (75). Decompression of the sinus in these situations is necessary to restore venous outflow. When associated with a hematoma, primary repair of the torn sinus may be achieved; however, irreparable lacerations require sacrifice of the sinus, thereby risking postoperative venous outflow obstruction and intracranial hypertension. Ligation of the anterior 50% of the superior sagittal sinus is usually well tolerated; however, injury to the posterior 50% is associated with mortality rates up to 24% (76).

SURGICAL MANAGEMENT OF PENETRATING BRAIN INJURY

Penetrating brain injuries arising from accidental, intentional, self-inflicted, and interpersonal traumas have an extremely poor prognosis, with mortality rates estimated as high as 94% (77). Stab and gunshot wounds (GSWs) to the head account for most of such injuries and are usually associated with homicides and suicides (78). Outcomes in GSWs to the head remain dismal, and the mortality rate for a self-inflicted GSW approximates 80% (79–81). A significant number of GSW to the head patients will die in the field, and the mortality rate of those surviving to admission approaches 60% (82). Those that survive the initial insult are at a significant risk for infection, CSF leak, and the development of epilepsy.

At present, there is no Class I data to guide the surgical management of penetrating TBI and the *Guidelines for the*

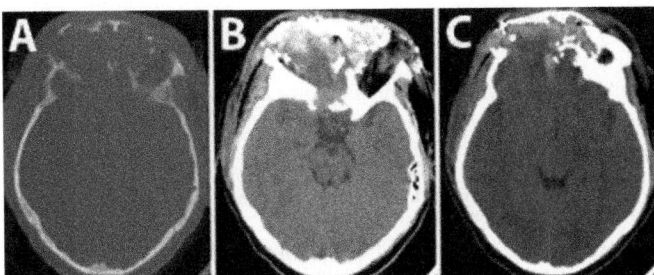

FIGURE 24-5 Gunshot wound to the head. A 28-year-old male involved in an altercation in which he was shot at close range through the orbits and anterior cranial fossa. A, CT bone windows demonstrating destruction of the orbits and anterior cranial base. B and C, Soft tissue windows showing bifrontal hematomas. The patient underwent bilateral orbital exenterations, a bicoronal craniectomy, debridement, and repair of the cranial base with a dural graft. The patient was discharged to a rehabilitation facility following commands symmetrically.

Surgical Management of Traumatic Brain Injury only establish a set of practice guidelines (83). In daily practice, there is variability in management strategies among individual practitioners. Commonalities in management stem from efforts to prevent infection and CSF leaks. Additionally, most protocols include debridement of devitalized tissue, evacuation of intracranial hematomas, acquisition of hemostasis, removal of readily accessible foreign bodies, dural repair, and revision of entrance and exit wounds to ensure scalp coverage (84,85). A watertight dural repair is of the utmost importance and often requires the use of a dural graft (9,83,84). Controversy arises when determining the extent to which contaminated bone and metal fragments should be removed from the parenchyma, with opinions ranging from minimal dissection to removal over the course of multiple interventions (86–89). Avoidance of infection is critical, and all management algorithms include broad-spectrum antibiotic therapy (Figure 24-5).

POSTOPERATIVE CARE

Postoperative care of the TBI patient is relatively standardized and adheres to the same principles regardless of the type of injury or surgical procedure. Postoperative laboratory values include a CBC, PT/INR, PTT, electrolyte panel, and serum osmolarity. Abnormalities are corrected, with special attention paid to the platelet count and coagulation panel. The likelihood of postoperative hematoma recurrence is not insignificant, and untreated coagulopathies greatly increase the risk. Unless sedation is required for the continued control of ICP, the patient should be aroused as soon as possible to accurately assess neurologic function. Persistently elevated ICP or deterioration relative to the preoperative exam requires an immediate CT to rule out new or recurrent lesions. Routine use of perioperative antibiotics is now the standard of care, and in cases of penetrating injury, the course of treatment may be extended. Surgical incisions are examined on a daily basis and evaluated for signs of infection, such as erythema, drainage, and dehiscence. In patients presenting with grossly contaminated

open wounds, suspicion for postoperative infection must be particularly high. Surgical TBI patients are at risk for seizures, and current guidelines for prophylactic treatment recommend 1 week of antiepileptic therapy (13,90–92). (Please refer to Chapter 39). Patients suffering significant head trauma are also at risk for developing delayed hydrocephalus and temporary ventriculostomy or permanent shunting may be necessary. (Please refer to Chapter 44).

Postoperative care should include an evaluation by rehabilitation medicine, physical therapy, and occupational therapy. These specialists provide insight into potential for recovery, aid in maximizing functional gains, and establish a long-term care plan. Early involvement of these practitioners facilitates a methodical transition from acute to chronic care and assists in securing disposition to an appropriate rehabilitation facility. (Please refer to Chapters 26, 59–71).

CONCLUSION

TBI remains among the most devastating of all illnesses, with a significant number of patients suffering poor functional outcomes or death. Operative management of these injuries has become increasingly integrated into a multidisciplinary approach to this complex patient population. As a result, all members of the critical care team are required to have a working understanding of the principles, goals, and complications of neurosurgical intervention.

At present, no Class I data exists to guide the management of focal and nonfocal injuries, and treatment is largely based on practice guidelines and acquired clinical acumen. Because of their focal nature, epidural and subdural hematomas readily lend themselves to surgical evacuation. Intraparenchymal hematomas and diffuse injuries may be more effectively managed, at least initially, with medical management. Decisions to observe such injuries need to be made with the understanding that neurologic decline or lesion expansion may require immediate surgical intervention. Decompressive craniectomy remains a commonly employed treatment option for medically refractory ICP; however, emerging data show that this procedure may not improve the ultimate clinical outcome. Penetrating brain injury is associated with a dismal prognosis, and there is significant variability between treatment protocols. Additional prospective randomized trials are needed to further explore treatment options for all types of TBI.

KEY CLINICAL POINTS

1. Successful management of TBI begins in the moments immediately following the initial insult and is centered on the stabilization and resuscitation of the patient.
2. In patients with a GCS ≤ 8, the airway is secured via endotracheal intubation as soon as possible (12).
3. ICP monitoring is routinely used in those patients with a GCS ≤ 8 and in those with evidence of hydrocephalus or diffuse cerebral injury without an accompanying mass lesion (13).
4. Epidural hematomas occurring in isolation can be associated with particularly good neurologic outcomes when diagnosed and evacuated promptly.

5. In patients presenting with severe closed head injury, acute subdural hematomas, with an average mortality rate of 50%–60%, represent the most common focal intracranial lesions (18,31–33).

6. Blunt trauma to the head causes the brain to impact against the skull, leading to contusions and intracerebral hematomas in nearly all patients with severe head injury and in 25% of those with moderate injury (38–41).

7. The management of nonfocal TBI is founded on optimizing (CPP > 60), controlling ICP (ICP < 20–25), and limiting the evolution of secondary injury (47–49).

8. Outcomes in GSWs to the head remain dismal, and the mortality rate for a self-inflicted GSW approximates 80% (79–81).

KEY REFERENCES

1. Aarabi B, Alden TD, Chestnut RM, et al. Guidelines for the management of penetrating brain injury. *J Trauma.* 2001;51(2)(suppl):S1–S86.

2. Bullock MR, Chesnut R, Ghajar J, et al. Guidelines for the surgical management of traumatic brain injury. *Neurosurgery.* 2006;58(3)(suppl):S1–S60.

3. Bullock R, Golek J, Blake G. Traumatic intracerebral hematoma—which patients should undergo surgical evacuation? CT scan features and ICP monitoring as a basis for decision making. *Surg Neurol.* 1989;32(3): 181–187.

4. Chestnut RM. Scientific surgical management. In: Jallo J LC, ed. *Neurotrauma and Critical Care of the Brain.* New York, NY: Thieme; 2009:255–274.

5. Jallo J, Narayan RK. Pathophysiology of head injury. In: Webb AR SM, Singer M, Suter P, eds. *Oxford Textbook of Critical Care.* Oxford: Oxford University Press; 1999.

References

1. Centers for Disease Control and Prevention. Traumatic *Brain Injury in the United States: A Report to Congress.* Atlanta, GA: Centers for Disease Control and Prevention; 1999.

2. Onyszchuk G, Al-Hafez B, He YY, Bilgen M, Berman NE, Brooks WM. A mouse model of sensorimotor controlled cortical impact: characterization using longitudinal magnetic resonance imaging, behavioral assessments and histology. *J Neurosci Methods.* 2007; 160(2):187–196.

3. McGarry LJ, Thompson D, Millham FH, et al. Outcomes and costs of acute treatment of traumatic brain injury. *J Trauma.* 2002;53(6): 1152–1159.

4. Coronado VG, Xu L, Basavaraju SV, et al. Surveillance for traumatic brain injury-related deaths—United States, 1997–2007. *MMWR Surveill Summ.* 2011;60(5):1–32.

5. Cameron P, Dziukas L, Hadj A, Clark P, Hooper S. Patterns of injury from major trauma in Victoria. *Aust N Z J Surg.* 1995;65(12): 848–852.

6. Sosin DM, Sniezek JE, Waxweiler RJ. Trends in death associated with traumatic brain injury, 1979 through 1992. Success and failure. *JAMA.* 1995;273(22):1778–1780.

7. Maas AI, Dearden M, Teasdale GM, et al. EBIC-guidelines for management of severe head injury in adults. European Brain Injury Consortium. *Acta Neurochir (Wien).* 1997;139(4):286–294.

8. Gennarelli TA, Champion HR, Sacco WJ, Copes WS, Alves WM. Mortality of patients with head injury and extracranial injury treated in trauma centers. *J Trauma.* 1989;29(9):1193–1202.

9. Chestnut RM. Scientific surgical management. In: Jallo J LC, ed. *Neurotrauma and Critical Care of the Brain.* New York, NY: Thieme; 2009:255–274.

10. Jallo J, Narayan RK. Pathophysiology of head injury. In: Webb AR, Shapiro MJ, Singer M, Suter P, eds. *Oxford Textbook of Critical Care.* Oxford: Oxford University Press; 1999.

11. Chesnut RM, Marshall LF, Klauber MR, et al. The role of secondary brain injury in determining outcome from sever head injury. *J Trauma.* 1993;34(2):216–222.

12. Badjatia N, Carney N, Crocco TJ, et al. Guidelines for prehospital management of traumatic brain injury 2nd edition. *Prehosp Emerg Care.* 2008;12(suppl 1):S1–S52.

13. Brain Trauma Foundation, American Association of Neurological Surgeons. *Management and Prognosis of Severe Traumatic Brain Injury.* New York, NY: Brain Trauma Foundation; 2000.

14. Marion DW, Firlik A, McLaughlin MR. Hyperventilation therapy for severe traumatic brain injury. *New Horiz.* 1995;3(3):439–447.

15. Narayan RK. Head trauma. In: Krantz BE, Ali J, Aprahamian C, et al, eds. *Advanced Trauma Life Support for Doctors.* Chicago, IL: American College of Surgeons; 1997:181–206.

16. Feldman Z, Kanter MJ, Robertson CS, et al. Effect of head elevation on intracranial pressure, cerebral perfusion pressure, and cerebral blood flow in the head-injured patients. *J Neurosurg.* 1992;76(2): 207–211.

17. Bullock MR, Chesnut R, Ghajar J, et al. Guidelines for the surgical management of traumatic brain injury. *Neurosurgery.* 2006;58(3) (suppl):S1–S60.

18. Marshall LF, Klauber GT, Eisenberg HM, et al. The outcome of severe closed head injury. *J Neurosurg.* 1991;75(suppl):S28–S36.

19. Adams J, Graham D. *An Introduction to Neuropathology.* Edinburgh, Scotland: Churchill Livingstone; 1994.

20. Pickard JD, Bailey S, Sanderson H, Rees M, Garfield JS. Steps towards cost-benefit analysis of regional neurosurgical care. *BMJ.* 1990;301(6753):629–635.

21. Lee EJ, Hung YC, Wang LC, Chung KC, Chen HH. Factors influencing the functional outcome of patients with acute epidural hematomas: analysis of 200 patients undergoing surgery. *J Trauma.* 1998; 45(5):946–952.

22. Cordobés F, Lobato RD, Rivas JJ, et al. Observations on 82 patients with extradural hematoma. Comparison of results before and after the advent of computerized tomography. *J Neurosurg.* 1981;54(2): 179–186.

23. Bricolo AP, Pasut LM. Extradural hematoma: toward zero mortality. A prospective study. *Neurosurgery.* 1984;14(1):8–12.

24. Jones NR, Molloy CJ, Kloeden CN, North JB, Simpson DA. Extradural haematoma: trends in outcome over 35 years. *Br J Neurosurg.* 1993;7(5):465–471.

25. Bezircioğlu H, Erşahin Y, Demirçivi F, Yurt I, Dönertaş K, Tektaş S. Nonoperative treatment of acute extradural hematomas: analysis of 80 cases. *J Trauma.* 1996;41(4):696–698.

26. Chen TY, Wong CW, Chang CN, et al. The expectant treatment of "asymptomatic" supratentorial epidural hematomas. *Neurosurgery.* 1993;32(2):176–179.

27. Bullock R, Smith RM, van Dellan JR. Nonoperative management of extradural hematoma. *Neurosurgery.* 1985;16(5):602–606.

28. Cucciniello B, Martellotta N, Nigro D, Citro E. Conservative management of extradural hematomas. *Acta Neurochir (Wien).* 1993; 120(1–2):47–52.

29. Servadei F. Prognostic factors in severely head injured adult patients with epidural haematoma's. *Acta Neurochir (Wien).* 1997;139 (4):273–278.

30. Wong CW. The CT criteria for conservative treatment—but under close clinical observation—of posterior fossa epidural haematomas. *Acta Neurochir (Wien).* 1994;126(2–4):124–127.

31. Wilberger JE Jr, Harris M, Diamond DL. Acute subdural hematoma: morbidity, mortality, and operative timing. *J Neurosurg.* 1991; 74(2):212–218.

32. Miller JD, Butterworth JF, Gudeman SK, et al. Further experience in the management of severe head injury. *J Neurosurg.* 1981;54(3): 289–299.

33. Foulkes MA, Eisenberg HM, Jane JA, Marmarou A, Marshall LF. The Traumatic Coma Data Bank: design, methods, and baseline characteristics. *J Neurosurg.* 1991;75:S8–S13.

34. Smith WP Jr, Batnitzky S, Rengachary SS. Acute isodense subdural hematomas: a problem in anemic patients. *Am J Radiol.* 1981;136(3): 543–546.

35. Howard MA III, Gross AS, Dacey RG Jr, Winn HR. Acute subdural hematomas: an age-dependent clinical entity. *J Neurosurg.* 1989; 71(6):858–863.

36. Zumkeller M, Behrmann R, Heissler HE, Dietz H. Computed tomographic criteria and survival rate for patients with acute subdural hematoma. *Neurosurgery.* 1996;39(4):708–713.

37. Gopinath SP, Cormio M, Ziegler J, Raty S, Valadka A, Robertson CS. Intraoperative jugular desaturation during surgery for traumatic intracranial hematomas. *Anesth Analg.* 1996;83(5):1014–1021.

38. Bullock R, Golek J, Blake G. Traumatic intracerebral hematoma—which patients should undergo surgical evacuation? CT scan features and ICP monitoring as a basis for decision making. *Surg Neurol.* 1989;32(3):181–187.

39. Lobato RD, Cordobes F, Rivas JJ, et al. Outcome from severe head injury related to the type of intracranial lesion. A computerized tomography study. *J Neurosurg.* 1983;59(5):762–764.

40. Nordström CH, Messeter K, Sundbärg G, Whlander S. Severe traumatic brain lesions in Sweden. Part I: aspects of management in non-neurosurgical clinics. *Brain Inj.* 1989;3(3):247–265.

41. Soloniuk D, Pitts LH, Lovely M, Bartkowski H. Traumatic intracerebral hematomas: timing of appearance and indications for operative removal. *J Trauma.* 1986;26(9):787–794.

42. Gudeman SK, Kishore PR, Miller JD, Girevendulis AK, Lipper MH, Becker DP. The genesis and significance of delayed traumatic intracerebral hematoma. *Neurosurgery.* 1979;5(3):309–313.

43. Kaufman HH, Moake JL, Olson JD, et al. Delayed and recurrent intracranial hematomas related to disseminated intravascular clotting and fibrinolysis in head injury. *Neurosurgery.* 1980;7(5):445–449.

44. Lobato RD, Gomez PA, Alday R, et al. Sequential computerized tomography changes and related final outcome in severe head injury patients. *Acta Neurochir (Wien).* 1997;139(5):385–391.

45. Adams JH, Graham DI, Gennarelli TA. Head injury in man and experimental animals: neuropathology. *Acta Neurochir Suppl (Wien).* 1983;32:15–30.

46. Gentleman SM, Roberts GW, Gennarelli TA, et al. Axonal injury: a universal consequence of fatal closed head injury? *Acta Neuropathol.* 1995;89(6):537–543.

47. Changaris DG, McGraw CP, Richardson JD, Garretson HD, Arpin EJ, Shields CB. Correlation of cerebral perfusion pressure and Glasgow Coma Scale to outcome. *J Trauma.* 1987;27(9):1007–1013.

48. Narayan RK, Kishore PR, Becker DP, et al. Intracranial pressure: to monitor or not to monitor? A review of our experience with severe head injury. *J Neurosurg.* 1982;56:650–659.

49. Eisenberg HM, Frankowski RF, Contant CF, Marshall LF, Walker MD. High-dose barbituate control of elevated intracranial pressure in patients with severe head injury. *J Neurosurg.* 1988;69(1):15–23.

50. Juul N, Morris GF, Marshall SB, Marshall LF. Intracranial hypertension and cerebral perfusion pressure: influence on neurological deterioration and outcome in severe head injury. The Executive Committee of the International Selfotel Trial. *J Neurosurg.* 2000; 92(1):1–6.

51. Marmarou A, Anderson RL, Ward JD. Impact of ICP instability and hypotension on outcome in patients with severe head trauma. *J Neurosurg (Suppl).* 1991;75:S59–S66.

52. Saul TG, Ducker TB. Effect of intracranial pressure monitoring and aggressive treatment on mortality in severe head injury. *J Neurosurg.* 1982;56(4):498–503.

53. Miller JD, Becker DP, Ward JD, Sullivan HG, Adams WE, Rosner MJ. Significance of intracranial hypertension in severe head injury. *J Neurosurg.* 1977;47(4):503–516.

54. Coplin WM, Cullen NK, Policherla PN, et al. Safety and feasibility of craniectomy with duraplasty as the initial surgical intervention for severe traumatic brain injury. *J Trauma.* 2001;50(6):1050–1059.

55. Dam Hieu P, Sizun J, Person H, Besson G. The place of decompressive surgery in the treatment of uncontrollable post-traumatic intracranial hypertension in children. *Childs Nerv Syst.* 1996;12(5): 270–275.

56. De Luca GP, Volpin L, Fornezza U, et al. The role of decompressive craniectomy in the treatment of uncontrollable post-traumatic intracranial hypertension. *Acta Neurochir Suppl.* 2000;76:401–404.

57. Guerra WK, Gaab MR, Dietz H, Mueller JU, Piek J, Fritsch MJ. Surgical decompression for traumatic brain swelling: indications and results. *J Neurosurg.* 1999;90(2):187–196.

58. Aarabi B, Hesdorffer DC, Ahn ES, Aresco C, Scalea TM, Eisenberg HM. Outcome following decompressive craniectomy for malignant swelling due to severe head injury. *J Neurosurg.* 2006;104(4): 469–479.

59. Gower DJ, Lee KS, McWhorter JM. Role of subtemporal decompression in severe closed head injury. *Neurosurgery.* 1988;23(4): 417–422.

60. Albanèse J, Leone M, Alliez JR, et al. Decompressive craniectomy for severe traumatic brain injury: evaluation of the effects at one year. *Crit Care Med.* 2003;31(10):2535–2538.

61. Gaab MR, Rittierodt M, Lorenz M, Heissler HE. Traumatic brain swelling and operative decompression: a prospective investigation. *Acta Neurochir Suppl.* 1990;51:326–328.

62. Polin RS, Shaffrey ME, Bogaev CA, et al. Decompressive bifrontal craniectomy in the treatment of severe refractory posttraumatic cerebral edema. *Neurosurgery.* 1997;41(1):84–94.

63. Schneider GH, Bardt T, Lanksch WR, Unterberg A. Decompressive craniectomy following traumatic brain injury: ICP, CPP and neurological outcome *Acta Neurochir Suppl.* 2002;81:77–79.

64. Taylor A, Butt W, Rosenfeld J, et al. A randomized trial of very early decompressive craniectomy in children with traumatic brain injury and sustained intracranial hypertension. *Childs Nerv Syst.* 2001;17(3):154–162.

65. Whitfield PC, Patel H, Hutchinson PJ, et al. Bifrontal decompressive craniectomy in the management of posttraumatic intracranial hypertension. *Br J Neurosurg.* 2001;15(6):500–507.

66. Cooper DJ, Rosenfeld JV, Murray L, et al. Decompressive craniectomy in diffuse traumatic brain injury. *N Engl J Med.* 2011;364(16): 1493–1502.

67. Hutchinson PJ, Corteen E, Czosnyka M, et al. Decompressive craniectomy in traumatic brain injury: the randomized multicenter RESCUEicp study (www.RESCUEicp.com). *Acta Neurochir Suppl.* 2006;96:17–20.

68. Braakman R. Depressed skull fracture: data, treatment, and follow-up in 225 consecutive cases. *J Neurol Neurosurg Psychiatry.* 1972; 35(3):395–402.

69. Wylen EL, Willis BK, Nanda A. Infection rate with replacement of bone fragment in compound depressed skull fractures. *Surg Neurol.* 1999;51(4):452–457.

70. van den Heever CM, van der Merwe DJ. Management of depressed skull fractures. Selective conservative management of nonmissile injuries. *J Neurosurg.* 1989;71(2):186–190.

71. Jennett B, Miller JD. Infection after depressed fracture of skull. Implications for management of nonmissile injuries *J Neurosurg.* 1972;36(3):333–339.

72. Mendelow AD, Campbell D, Tsementzis SA, et al. Prophylactic antimicrobial management of compound depressed skull fracture. *J R Coll Surg Edinb.* 1983;28(2):80–83.

73. Jennett B, Miller JD, Braakman R. Epilepsy after nonmissile depressed skull fracture. *J Neurosurg.* 1974;41(2):208–216.

74. Heary RF, Hunt CD, Krieger AJ, Schulder M, Vaid C. Nonsurgical treatment of compound depressed skull fractures. *J Trauma.* 1993; 35(3):441–447.

75. Taha JM, Crone KR, Berger TS, Becket WW, Prenger EC. Sigmoid sinus thrombosis after closed head injury in children. *Neurosurgery.* 1993;32(4):541–546.

76. Kapp JP, Gielchinsky I. Management of combat wounds of the dural venous sinuses. *Surgery.* 1972;71(6):913–917.

77. Traumatic brain injury—Colorado, Missouri, Oklahoma, and Utah, 1990–1993. *MMWR Morb Mortal Wkly Rep.* 1997;46(1):8–11.

78. Bukur M, Inaba K, Barmparas G, et al. Self-inflicted penetrating injuries at a Level I trauma center. *Injury.* 2010;42(5):474–477.

79. Suddaby L, Weir B, Forsyth C. The management of .22 caliber gunshot wounds of the brain: a review of 49 cases. *Can J Neurol Sci.* 1987;14(3):268–272.

80. Selden BS, Goodman JM, Cordell W, Rodman GH Jr, Schnitzer PG. Outcome of self-inflicted gunshot wounds of the brain. *Ann Emerg Med.* 1988;17(3):247–253.

81. Pikus HJ, Ball PA. Characteristics of cerebral gunshot injuries in the rural setting. *Neurosurg Clin N Am.* 1995;6(4):611–620.

82. Trask T, Narayan RK. Civilian penetrating head injury. In: Narayan RK, Wilberger JE, Povlishock JT, eds. *Neurotrauma.* New York, NY: McGraw Hill; 1996:869–889.

83. Aarabi B, Alden TD, Chestnut RM. Guidelines for the management of penetrating brain injury. *J Trauma.* 2001;51(2)(suppl):S1–S86.

84. Carey ME. Bullet wounds to the brain among civilians. In: Winn HR, ed. *Youmans Neurological Surgery.* Vol 4. 5th ed. Philadelphia, PA: Saunders; 2004:5223–5242.

85. Byrnes DP, Crockard HA, Gordon DS, Gleadhill CA. Penetrating craniocerebral missile injuries in the civil disturbances in Northern Ireland. *Br J Surg.* 1974;61(3):169–176.

86. Martin J, Campbell EH Jr. Early complications following penetrating wounds of the skull. *J Neurosurg.* 1946;3:58–73.

87. Aarabi B, Taghipour M, Alibaii E, Kamgarpour A. Central nervous system infections after militray missile head wounds. *Neurosurgery.* 1998;42(3):500–509.

88. Levi L, Borovich B, Guilburd JN, et al. Wartime neurosurgical experience in Lebanon, 1982–85. I: penetrating craniocerebral injuries. *Isr J Med Sci.* 1990;26(10):548–554.

89. Taha JM, Saba MI, Brown JA. Missile injuries to the brain treated by simple wound closure: results of a protocol during the Lebanese conflict. *Neurosurgery.* 1991;29:380–383.

90. Temkin NR, Haglund M, Winn HR. Post-traumatic seizures. In: Narayan R Wilberger JE, Povlishock J, eds. *Neurotrauma.* New York, NY: McGraw Hill; 1996:611–619.

91. Temkin NR, Dikmen SS, Wilensky AJ, Keihm J, Chabal S, Winn HR. A randomized, double-blind study of phenytoin for the prevention of post-traumatic seizures. *N Eng J Med.* 1990;323(8):497–502.

92. Temkin NR, Dikmen SS, Winn HR. Management of head injury. Posttraumatic seizures. *Neurosurg Clin N Am.* 1991;2(2):425–435.

Development of Acute Care Guidelines and Effect on Outcome

Jose J. Sanchez, David E. Kahn, and M. Ross Bullock

INTRODUCTION

Severe traumatic brain injury (TBI), defined by a Glasgow Coma Scale (GCS) score of 3–8, is one of the leading causes of death and disability in the United States with a massive cost to society of around $45 billion per year (1–4) (see Chapter 8 on Epidemiology and Public Health Issues). To try to reduce secondary and avoidable brain damage after severe TBI, the "Guidelines for the Management of Severe Traumatic Brain Injury" have been developed by the Brain Trauma Foundation (BTF). These guidelines are scientific-based documents that evaluate the current evidence for practice and interventions to reduce secondary brain injury and improve outcome for patients with TBI.

The BTF has drawn together different experts for the authorship of these guidelines, including emerging experts in the field that were trained under evidence-based medicine methodology. This group performed comprehensive and up-to-date electronic searches of all databases relevant to neurotrauma and human-based literature. Their data does not reflect pathomechanistic information from animal studies nor in vitro or mathematical modeling studies.

The writing group used criteria to assess the quality of the included literature that was based on the United States Preventive Services Task Force, the National Health Services Centre for Reviews and Dissemination (United Kingdom), and the Cochrane Collaboration. Independent members reviewed each selected study and classified them as class I, class II, or class III, with the aid of the neurotrauma expert panel. The literature lists and classifications were further refined by consensus discussion among the experts.

Evidence was classified into that which was derived from the strongest clinical studies of therapeutic interventions (randomized controlled trials) and was called class I evidence. Class I evidence is used to support treatment recommendations of the strongest type, reflecting a high degree of clinical certainty. Nonrandomized cohort studies, randomized controlled trials with significant design flaws, and case control studies (comparative studies with less strength) were designated as class II evidence and were used to support recommendations, reflecting a moderate degree of clinical certainty. Other sources of information, including observational studies such as case series and expert opinion (class III evidence), reflect unclear clinical certainty.

Brain injury care requires an individualized interdisciplinary approach involving prehospital and in-hospital actions, connecting personnel in emergency deparment, trauma center, critical care, and neurosurgery services. The guidelines cover prehospital phase, in-hospital management (medical and surgical), and extend through long-term care. These cover a wide range of topics including trauma systems, oxygenation and blood pressure resuscitation, intracranial pressure (ICP) monitoring, intracranial hypertension, nutrition, and pharmacological interventions for the patient with severe TBI.

There are at least 5 different sets of BTF guidelines used to manage TBI (see Table 25-1). These include prehospital management of TBI, management of severe TBI, pediatric TBI, surgical management of TBI, management of penetrating TBI, and cervical spine trauma management. There are also guidelines for the field management of combat-related head trauma. These evidence-based guidelines for military medical personnel address the assessment, treatment, triage, and transport of TBI combat casualties, particularly in the far-forward environment. The guidelines aim to improve outcomes and to reduce long-term disabilities of wounded warfighters (5) (see Chapter 33 on Military TBI: Special Considerations).

The Department of Veteran Affairs/Department of Defense (VA/DoD) clinical practice guideline for management of concussion/mild traumatic brain injury (mTBI) is an evidence-based guideline applying to adult patients (18 years or older) who are diagnosed with concussion/mTBI and complain of symptoms related to the injury. These patients were treated in VA/DoD clinical settings for their symptoms at least 7 days after the initial brain injury (6). The guideline is relevant to all health care professionals providing or directing treatment services to patients with concussion/mTBI in any VA/DoD health care settings, including both primary and specialty care. This guideline does not address management of concussion/mTBI in the acute phase (< 7 days postinjury) nor management of moderate or severe TBI.

FACTORS USED TO PREDICT OUTCOME IN SEVERE TRAUMATIC BRAIN INJURY

It still remains impossible to say with certainty what will be the future course of events for an individual suffering from

TABLE 25-1 Guidelines to Manage Severe Traumatic Brain Injury

CURRENT TBI GUIDELINES	REVIEW PROCESS	WEBSITE AND JOURNAL
Guideline of prehospital management of severe TBI, 2nd edition	1996–2005	[a]*Prehosp Emerg Care.* 2008;12(suppl 1):S1–S52.
In-hospital severe TBI guidelines		
• Management of severe head injury		*J Neurotrauma.* 1996;13:641–734.
• Management and prognosis of severe TBI, 2nd edition		*J Neurotrauma.* 2000;17(6–7):457–627.
• Guidelines for the management of severe TBI, 3rd edition	1996–2004	[a]*J Neurotrauma.* 2007;24(suppl 1):S71–S76.
• Surgical management	1975–2001	[a]*Neurosurgery.* 2006;58(3)(suppl 2):1–62.
• Management of penetrating brain injury (PBI)	1966–2000	[a]*J Trauma.* 2001;51(2):S3–S43.
Pediatric severe TBI guidelines		
• Guidelines for the acute medical management of severe TBI in infants, children, and adolescents	1966–2001	[a]*Pediatr Crit Care Med.* 2003;4(3):S1–S75.
Guidelines for the field management of combat-related head trauma	1966–2005	[a]New York, NY: Brain Trauma Foundation; 2005.
VA/DoD clinical practice guideline for management of concussion/mild TBI (mTBI)	2002–2008	[b]*J Rehabil Res Dev.* 2009;46(6):CP1–68.

[a]http://www.braintrauma.org
[b]http://www.healthquality.va.gov
Abbreviations: TBI, traumatic brain injury; VA/DoD, Deparment of Veterans Affairs/Department of Defense.

TBI. Recent research has made it possible to be much more confident about what is likely to happen and to consider prognosis in terms of probabilities rather than prophecies. With this in mind, a number of factors have been documented as important features predicting the outcome of TBI (7); these are GCS score, age, pupillary response and size, hypotension, hypoxia, hyperthermia, high ICP, and some computed tomography (CT) findings.

Glasgow Coma Scale

There is an increasing probability of poor outcome with a decreasing GCS score. When considering the use of the initial GCS score for prognosis, the 2 most important problems are the reliability of the initial measurement and its lack of precision for prediction of a good outcome if the initial GCS score is low. If the initial GCS score is reliably obtained and not tainted by prehospital medications or intubation, approximately 20% of the patients with the worst initial GCS score will survive, and 8%–10% will have a good functional survival (Glasgow Outcome Scale [GOS] 4–5) (7–11).

The GCS is fairly reliable when measured by trained medical personnel. GCS should be measured for prognostic purposes only after pulmonary and hemodynamic resuscitation and after withholding pharmacologic sedation or paralytic agents. GCS must be obtained through interaction with the patient (e.g., application of a painful stimulus for patients unable to follow commands).

Age

Age should be obtained and documented on admission. Age is not subjected to observer's measurement variability. There is strong evidence with at least 70% positive predictive value (PPV) that increasing age is a predictor of poor outcome in a stepwise manner (7,12). Age is a strong factor influencing both mortality and morbidity (13). Most literature supports children faring much better than adults who have severe

brain injury. The significant influence of age on outcome is not explained by the increased frequency of systemic complications or intracerebral hematomas with age. Increasing age is a strong independent factor for poor prognosis with a significant increase in poor outcome for patients older than age 60 (14–15). Very few patients older than age 70, who are in a prolonged coma (GCS < 9 for more than 6 hours), will recover to fully independent function Glasgow Outcome Score-Extended (GOS-E > 8) (16).

Pupillary Function

There is strong evidence, with at least a 70% PPV. that bilaterally absent pupillary light reflex is associated with poor outcome (7). Bilaterally reactive pupils correlate with a better outcome and a lower probability of transtentorial herniation (10,17,18). Pupils and pupillary light reflex should be measured by trained medical personnel after endotracheal intubation, oxygenation, and hemodynamic resuscitation. Recommendations for parameter measurement for prognosis are (a) asymmetry is a measurement difference of 1 mm or more, (b) a fixed pupil shows no response (< 1 mm) to bright light, and (c) dilated pupil has a pupillary size > 4 mm.

Systolic Blood Pressure

Systolic blood pressure (SBP) less than 90 mm Hg was found to have a 67% PPV for poor outcome and when combined with hypoxia, a 79% PPV. An early low SBP increases the probability of mortality and morbidity 15 fold. Late hypotension increases the probability 11 fold (7,11,19,20). With systemic multiple trauma, the more severe the trauma, the lower the SBP will be, forming an indirect relationship to low SBP (< 90 mm Hg). Finally, if hypotension and hypoxia are both present, there is an increased probability for a poor prognosis.

SBP and diastolic blood pressure should be measured using the most accurate system available allowed by circumstances. Monitoring by arterial line, when free of signal artifact, provides data that is both accurate and continuous and is the method of choice. Methods that do not determine the mean arterial pressure are less valuable. Blood pressures should be measured as frequently as possible. The incidence and duration of hypotension (SBP < 90 mm Hg) should be documented by direct blood pressure values.

Computed Tomography Findings

CT is the preferred imaging modality in the acute phase of head trauma (see Chapter 15 on Structural Neuroimaging). Class I and class II studies support evidence that the presence of any abnormalities on initial CT has a PPV of 77%–78% with respect to an unfavorable outcome in patients with severe brain injury, as defined by a GCS score < 9 (7). There are particular findings on head CT that confer significant prognostic value at the moment of analysis in the patient with severe TBI (21–24) (see Table 25-2 and Figure 25-1). The studies should be evaluated by a neuroradiologist or other qualified physician who are experienced in reading CT scans.

OUTCOME PREDICTION MODELS

Corticosteroid randomisation after significant head injury (CRASH) brain injury prognostic models is a practical prognostic model developed and validated for death at 14 days or severe disability 6 months after TBI. It can be used to obtain valid predictions of relevant outcomes in patients with TBI (25). The model is comprised of 10 predictors: 5 demographic and clinical variables (country, age, GCS, pupil

TABLE 25-2 Individual CT Characteristics Found to be Particularly Relevant in Terms of Prognosis/Outcome

Dural collections	SDH or EDH size expressed in millimeter
SAH	SAH should be noted in the basal cisterns or over the convexity
Intraparenchymal	Contusion: single, multiple unilateral, or bilateral Swelling (e.g., brain edema or infarction) Diffuse axonal injury (DAI)
Midline shift (MLS)	MLS should be measured at the level of the septum pellucidum; document if it is present or not. (degree expressed in millimeter)
Status of basal cisterns	Completely open Partial obliteration: cisterns visible as hypodense slits, usually in 1 hemisphere Complete obliteration: cisterns no longer visible as CSF (cerebrospinal fluid) spaces

Abbreviations: EDH, epidural hematoma; SAH, subarachnoid hemorrhage; SDH, subdural hematoma.

reactivity, and the presence of major extracranial injury) and 5 head CT scan prognosis features that include the presence of petechial hemorrhages, obliteration of the third ventricle or basal cisterns, subarachnoid bleeding, midline shift, and nonevacuated hematoma. The predictions are based on the average outcome in adult patients with a GCS < 15 within 8 hours of injury and can only support, not replace, clinical judgment.

International Mission for Prognosis and Analysis of Clinical Trials (IMPACT) in TBI (26). The investigators have developed and validated prognostic models for classification and standardized data collection of adult patients with moderate-to-severe brain injury (GCS < 13) on admission. By entering the characteristics into the calculator, the models will provide an estimate of the expected outcome at 6 months. Three models of increasing complexity (Core, Core + CT, Core + CT + Lab) are used. These models were developed and validated in collaboration with the CRASH trial collaborators on large numbers of individual patient data (the IMPACT database). The models discriminate well and are particularly suited for the purposes of classification and characterization of large patient cohorts. They provide evidence-based recommendations for improving sensitivity and efficiency of trials in TBI.

PREHOSPITAL MANAGEMENT

The prehospital care of the patient with a TBI is critical to maximizing the chances for a good outcome. It is directed toward preventing and limiting secondary brain injury while facilitating rapid transport to an appropriate facility capable of providing neurocritical care. Prehospital management includes correctly identifying the TBI, optimal treatment in the ambulance, and direct transfer to a TBI trauma center (see Chapter 22 on Emergency Care/Initial Trauma Care).

The Guidelines for Prehospital Management of Severe Traumatic Brain Injury (27) evaluated the following points that include assessment and treatment strategies, which are directed to improve the outcome of the patients with TBI: (*a*) assessment: oxygenation and blood pressure; (*b*) mental status (as measured with the GCS); (*c*) pupil examination; (*d*) maintaining airway with adequate oxygenation and ventilation; (*e*) fluid resuscitation to preserve a satisfactory perfusion; (*f*) treating cerebral herniation; and (*g*) decision making within the emergency medical services (EMS) system: dispatch, scene, transportation, and destination.

IN-HOSPITAL MANAGEMENT

A specialized trauma center with neurosurgical and neurocritical care support, which uses guideline-based standardized protocols, is advised for most optimally managed patients with TBI (see Chapter 23 on Critical Care). Once the patient is in the emergency department, treatment and diagnostic assessment is recommended according to the Advanced Trauma Life Support (ATLS) protocol. This includes ruling out other systemic trauma; stabilizing vital signs; continuous monitoring including heart rate, blood pressure, respiratory status (respiratory rate and pulse oximetry), and temperature; also a complete blood count (CBC), arterial blood gas (ABG), electrolytes, glucose, and coagulation

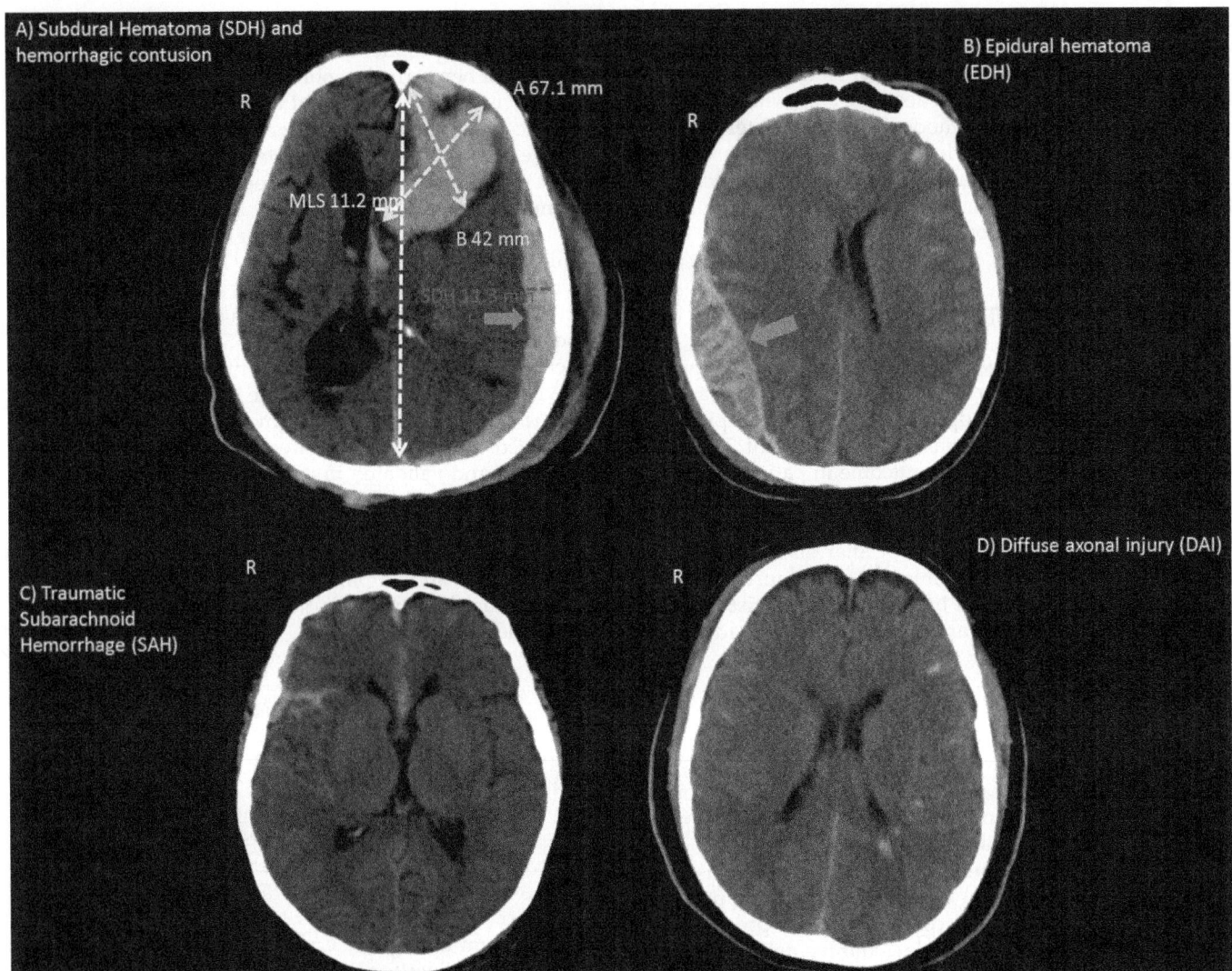

A) Subdural Hematoma (SDH) and hemorrhagic contusion

R

A 67.1 mm

MLS 11.2 mm

B 42 mm

SDH 11.5 mm

B) Epidural hematoma (EDH)

R

R

C) Traumatic Subarachnoid Hemorrhage (SAH)

R

D) Diffuse axonal injury (DAI)

FIGURE 25-1 A, Large left frontal hemorrhagic contusion and left hemispheric subdural hematoma (SDH, *arrow*). Subdural hematomas are typically crescent shape. In this case, the SDH is causing significant mass effect and causing significant left-to-right midline shift (MLS) and impending left uncal herniation, as well as suspected entrapment of the right lateral ventricle, subarachnoid, and intraventricular hemorrhages. B, CT scan demonstrating a right epidural hematoma (EDH, *red arrow*) hyperdense convex lens-shaped (lenticular) extra-axial fluid collection with mass effect and edema. C, Head CT without contrast shows subarachnoid hemorrhage predominantly overlying the right cerebral hemisphere extending to the sylvian fissure. Right frontal subdural hemorrhage measuring 3 mm in thickness, with a subdural hemorrhage along the interhemispheric fissure. D, CT scan of the brain showing diffuse axonal injury (DAI). Note small hemorrhagic lesions at the corticomedullary junction (*arrows*).

parameters should be ordered. As soon as patients are hemodynamically stable, they should be evaluated by the neurosurgical services. Initial head CT should be performed as quickly as possible (stat CT). Current guidelines recommend a head CT in all patients with TBI with a GCS < 15. Full extent of intracranial pathology may not be disclosed on initial CT. Follow-up CT scanning should be performed if there is any clinical deterioration. For "guidelines" regarding which patients to CT scan, the "Canadian CT Head Rule" was formulated (28–32). New Orleans Criteria are also recommended (33–35). In the United Kingdom, where not all patients can easily access a center with neurosurgical capabilities, the "National Institute for Health and Clinical Excellence (NICE) Guidelines" were formulated (36).

Neuromonitoring

ICP monitoring and management is central to the current guidelines of patients with severe brain injury. Increased ICP is associated with high mortality and worsened outcome. Monitoring and managing ICP should begin as soon as possible when indicated (see Table 25-3). There are 5 different devices for ICP monitoring: intraventricular devices (external ventricular drain [EVD]), parenchymal pressure transducer devices, subdural devices, subarachnoid fluid coupled devices, and epidural devices. Although the last 3 devices do not produce parenchymal damage, they are not recommended because of lack of accuracy and reliability. Clinically significant infections or hemorrhage associated with ICP are rare and should not deter the decision to monitor ICP.

TABLE 25-3 Neuromonitoring in Traumatic Brain Injury

	NEUROMONITORING	LoR
Blood pressure (BP)	BP should be monitored and hypotension (SBP < 90 mm Hg) should be avoided	Level II
Oxygenation (O$_2$) (98)	• O$_2$ should be monitored and hypoxia (PaO$_2$ < 60 mm Hg or SpO$_2$ < 90%) should be avoided	Level III
ICP monitoring Note: Clinically significant infections or hemorrhage associated with ICP devices causing patient morbidity are rare and should not prevent the decision to monitor ICP.	Indications (99): • ICP should be monitored in all salvageable patients (at least 1 reactive pupil) with a severe TBI injury (GCS score of 3–8 after resuscitation) and • an abnormal CT scan (hematomas, contusions, swelling, herniation, or compressed basal cisterns);	Level II
	Note: In case of a normal CT scan in severe TBI, ICP monitoring is indicated if 2 or more of the following features are noted at admission: 1. Age older than 40 years 2. Unilateral or bilateral motor posturing (GCS motor = 2 or 3) 3. SBP < 90 mm Hg	Level III
	Technology (100): Ventricular catheter connected to an external strain gauge transducer is the most accurate and cost-effective method for ICP. Parenchymal transducer devices are advantageous when ventricular ICP is not obtained or if there is obstruction in the fluid couple. Other ICP devices (subarachnoid, subdural, and epidural) are less accurate.	
	Thresholds (101): • Treatment should be initiated with ICP thresholds > 20 mm Hg. • A combination of ICP values, clinical, and brain CT findings should be used to determine the need for treatment.	Level II Level III
CPP = MAP − ICP (102)	• CPP target range of 50–70 mm Hg. CPP < 50 mm Hg should be avoided. • Aggressive attempts to maintain CPP > 70 mm Hg with fluids and pressors should be avoided because of the risk of ARDS. Patients with intact pressure autoregulation tolerate higher CPP values.	Level III Level II
PbtO$_2$ and SjvO2 (103)	• Jugular venous saturation (SjvO$_2$) or partial brain tissue oxygen (PbtO$_2$) monitoring measure cerebral oxygenation. SjvO$_2$ < 50% or PbtO$_2$ < 15 mm Hg are treatment thresholds.	Level III

Abbreviations: ARDS, acute respiratory distress syndrome; CPP, cerebral perfusion pressure; ICP, intracranial pressure; LoR, Level of Recommendation; MAP, mean arterial pressure; PaO$_2$, partial pressure of oxygen; SBP, systolic blood pressure; SpO$_2$, oxygen saturation.

Management of Increased Intracranial Pressure

Several approaches are used to prevent and treat elevated ICP. General protocols should be instituted as soon as possible with the goal of optimizing venous drainage. This would include raising the head of bed to 30° angle and keeping the neck in neutral position, loosening of neck braces if they are excessively tight, monitoring central venous pressure, and avoiding excessive hypervolemia. In the current guidelines, there is a documented evidence to support the use of mannitol, hyperventilation, anesthetics, analgesics, and sedatives to treat the increased ICP (see Table 25-4).

Multimodal Neuromonitoring

Current guidelines recommend multimodal neuromonitoring with jugular venous oxygen saturation (SjO$_2$) or brain tissue oxygen tension (PbrO$_2$) to ensure adequate brain oxygen delivery when hyperventilation is used to decrease the ICP through cerebral blood flow (CBF) reduction. All neurological damage from TBI does not occur at the moment of impact. Secondary brain injuries may occurs hours, days, or weeks after the primary insult. Brain tissue that is still viable is at risk for progressing to permanent cell loss (penumbra area). These delayed events are not only related to reduced cerebral perfusion pressure (CPP) or CBF. These may be associated with increased CPP or CBF (reperfusion damage), reduced brain oxygenation, metabolic disarrangement, spreading cortical depolarization (SCD), delayed neural death (apoptosis), and postischemic neural death (see Chapter 12 on Pathobiology of Secondary Brain Injury). Improved outcome results when these secondary delayed insults are prevented or respond to treatment.

To complement ICP monitoring, there are alternative technologies that are becoming available for patients with severe TBI (see Table 25-5). Some of these techniques allow for the measurement of cerebral physiology, electrical activity, and metabolic parameters with the goal of improving the detection and management of secondary brain injury. These monitoring tools provide unique information that may help to individualize severe brain injury management for patients (see Figures 25-2 and 25-3).

Seizure Prophylaxis

There is a clear risk for seizures in some types of TBI. From 4% to 90% of patients with severe TBI may develop epilepsy,

TABLE 25-4 Increased Intracranial Pressure Management of Traumatic Brain Injury

	MEDICAL MANAGEMENT OF INCREASED INTRACRANIAL PRESSURE	LoR
Hyperosmolar therapy (HO) (104)	• Mannitol is effective for control of raised ICP at doses of 0.25 g/kg to 1 g/kg body weight. Arterial hypotension (SBP < 90 mm Hg) should be avoided.	Level II
	• Restrict mannitol use prior to ICP monitoring to patients with signs of transtentorial herniation or progressive neurological deterioration not attributable to extracranial causes.	Level III
Hyperventilation (HV) PaCO$_2$ ≤25 mm Hg (105)	• HV is recommended as a temporizing measure for the reduction of elevated ICP. If HV is used, SjO$_2$ or PbtO$_2$ measurements are recommended to monitor oxygen delivery. HV should be avoided during the first 24 hours after injury when CBF is often critically reduced.	Level III
	• Prophylactic HV is NOT recommended.	Level II
Anesthetics, analgesics, and sedatives (106)	• High-dose barbiturate administration is recommended to control elevated ICP refractory to maximum standard medical and surgical treatment. Hemodynamic stability is essential before and during barbiturate therapy. Prophylactic administration of barbiturates to induce burst suppression EEG is NOT recommended. Propofol is recommended for the control of ICP but not for improvement in mortality or 6-month outcome. High-dose propofol can produce significant morbidity.	Level II
Steroids (107)	• The use of steroids is NOT recommended for reducing ICP or improving outcome.	Level I

Abbreviation: CBF, cerebral blood flow; EEG, electroencephalography; LoR, Level of Recommendation; PbtO$_2$, partial pressure of brain oxygen tissue; SBP, systolic blood pressure; SjO$_2$, jugular venous oximetry.

and brain injuries account for 20% of epilepsy. In contrast to blunt injury, patients with penetrating injury are at higher risk for late seizures and 80%–90% of patients with penetrating injury have seizures at 15 years follow-up (37). In studies that followed high-risk patients to 3 years, the incidence of early post-traumatic seizures (PTS) varied between 4% and 25%, and the incidence of late PTS varied between 9% and 42% in untreated patients (37). Certain risk factors have been identified that place patients with TBI at increased risk for developing PTS (38–39). These include the following: GCS score of 10 or less; cortical contusion; depressed skull fracture; penetrating head wound; seizure within 24 hours of injury; and subdural, epidural, and intracerebral hematoma.

PTS can have an important effect on management strategies in patients in the intensive care unit (ICU). The risks associated with multiple seizures in the acute setting include elevated ICP, release of catecholamines, hypoxia, and blood pressure changes. In addition, these patients may develop epilepsy if they survive the initial insult through the concept of *epileptogenesis*. Epileptogenesis is defined as the process by which an initial event causing a seizure transforms into spontaneous unprovoked seizures. The transformation is contingent on reorganization of the cortical electrical network secondary to deafferentation, as well as a decline in the inherent ability to modulate neuronal excitability. When neurons sustain injury after a trauma, some will undergo

TABLE 25-5 Invasive Online Multimodality Neuromonitoring in Severe Brain Injury

	TARGET	NORMAL VALUES	PROCEDURE
Jugular venous oximetry (SjO$_2$) (103)	Venous brain oxygen saturation	SjO$_2$ > 60	Retrograde cannulation of the internal jugular vein
Brain tissue oxygen tension (PbtO$_2$) (108)	Intraparenchymal oxygenation	PbtO$_2$ > 20 mmHg	Intraparenchymal oxygen electrode placement
Cerebral microdialysis (MD) (109–110)	Extracellular aerobic and anaerobic glucose metabolism and other biomarkers	Glucose (mM): 0.8–2.6 Lactate (mM): < 4 Pyruvate (μm): ≥ 120 Lactate/pyruvate ratio: < 25 Lactate/glucose ratio: < 10	Intraparenchymal microdialysis probe placement
Thermal diffusion flowmetry (TDF)	White matter regional cerebral blood flow (rCBF)	CBF 50–60 mL/100g/min	Intraparenchymal microprobe placement
Electrocorticography (ECoG) (111)	Cortical spreading depression (CSD)	Absence of CSD	ECoG strips (6 channels) placement over cortical surface after craniotomy

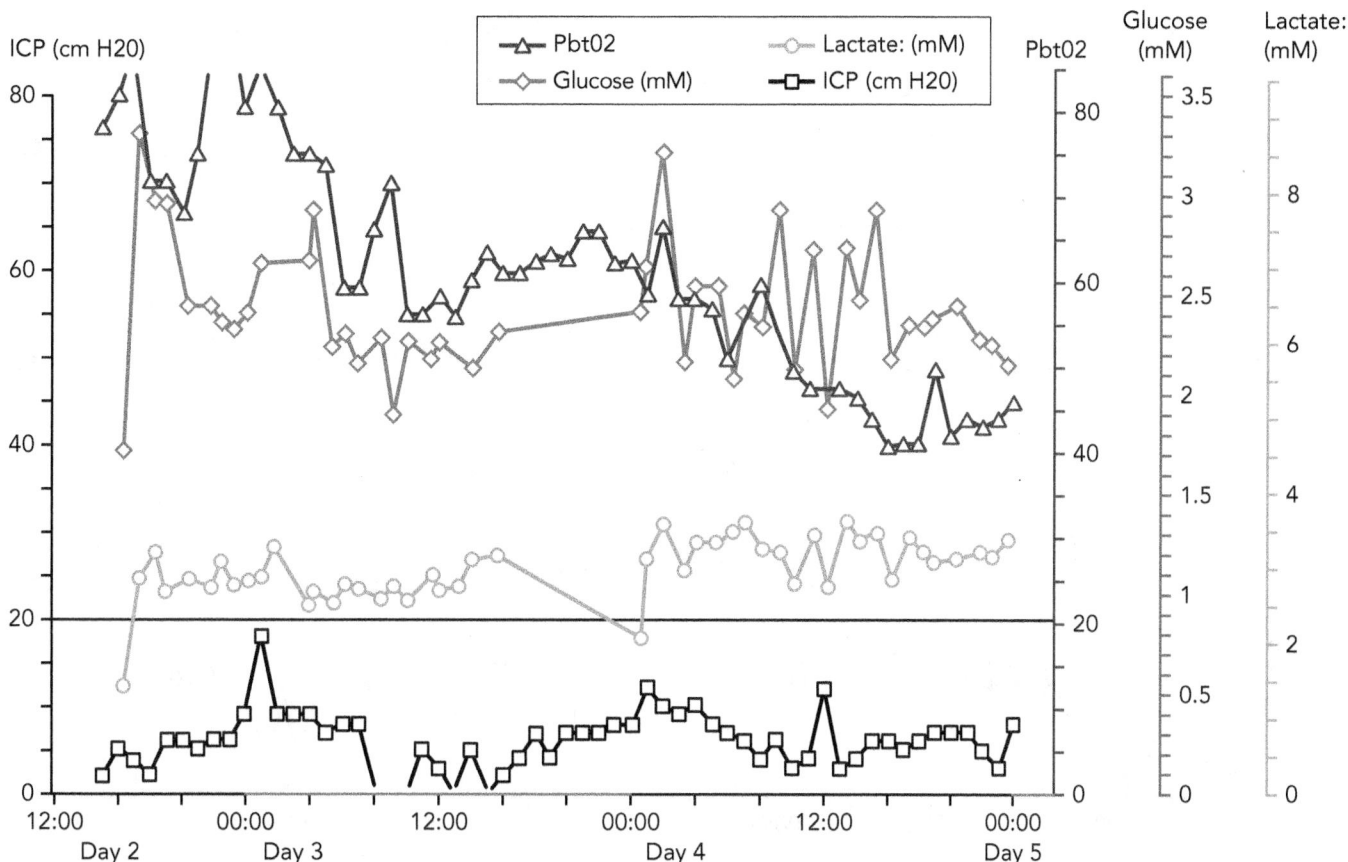

FIGURE 25-2 Multimodality neuromonitoring (intracranial pressure [ICP], cerebral perfusion pressure [CPP], partial brain tissue oxygen [PbtO$_2$], and microdialysis) from day 2 to day 5 post-emergent decompressive craniectomy because large right frontotemporal hemorrhagic contusion with right-to-left midline shift with diffuse cerebral edema and crowding of the basilar cisterns. Normal ICP (< 20 cm H$_2$O), normal PbtO$_2$ (> 20), CPP with no evidence of hypoperfusion (no represented in the graph), normal extracellular lactate (< 4 mM) but high extracellular glucose (NL [Normal Limits]: 0.8–2.6 mM) as an index of cell metabolism damage, hyperglycemia, or both. This is an 18-year-old male with severe TBI status post-motor vehicle collision with Glasgow Coma Scale (GCS) score of 3 and fixed pupils at the scene, GCS score of 4 on admission. Patient had a Glasgow Outcome Score (GOS) of 2 at discharge from hospital.

aberrant branching while others will die, triggering reactive gliosis. The pattern of astrocytic neuronal connections and synaptic efficiency are altered, leading to abnormal neocortical electrical impulses and to the generation of paroxysmal discharges. Epilepsy then develops (40). It is reasonable to consider early prophylaxis in TBI to prevent the advent of chronic epilepsy secondary to reactive gliosis. Interestingly, no studies to date have conclusively shown that treating early PTS will result in a better long-term outcome.

Long-term effects of uncontrolled seizures in TBI may include mesial temporal sclerosis and hippocampal atrophy. Vespa et al. (41) performed a study on 140 patients with moderate-to-severe TBI using continuous electroencephalogram (EEG) monitoring. Twenty-three out of 140 patients were found to be in nonconvulsive status epilepticus. Patients with seizures had greater hippocampal atrophy as compared to those without seizures. Hippocampi ipsilateral to the electrographic seizure focus demonstrated a propensity for atrophy as compared to the contralateral side (41).

Treatment decisions for PTS should be considered based on timing postinjury. By convention, 7 days is considered

the transitional point from early to late PTS. There is a level 2 evidence to support the prophylactic treatment of seizures in the first 7 days, but the prophylactic use of anticonvulsants is not recommended for preventing late PTS. Early prophylaxis has been shown to reduce the incidence of seizures in the acute setting. There is no evidence that prophylactic treatment of seizures after 7 days has any effect on mortality (42). However, recent studies have found that patients with late PTS have worse outcome. One study, performed on 508 patients with seizures within 2 years post-TBI, found that 14% had late PTS. Twenty-seven percent of these patients had died at 8–15 years postinjury, as compared to 10% of those without. Individuals with late PTS expired at a younger age (43).

Selection of antiepileptic medication must be based on the context of confounding medical risk factors. Typical anticonvulsants used in the neurocritical care setting include phenytoin, levetiracetam, and valproate (VPA). Phenytoin and VPA have been well studied in TBI. A class 2 study directed at preventing early and late PTS conducted by Temkin et al. (39) randomized 404 patients to phenytoin or pla-

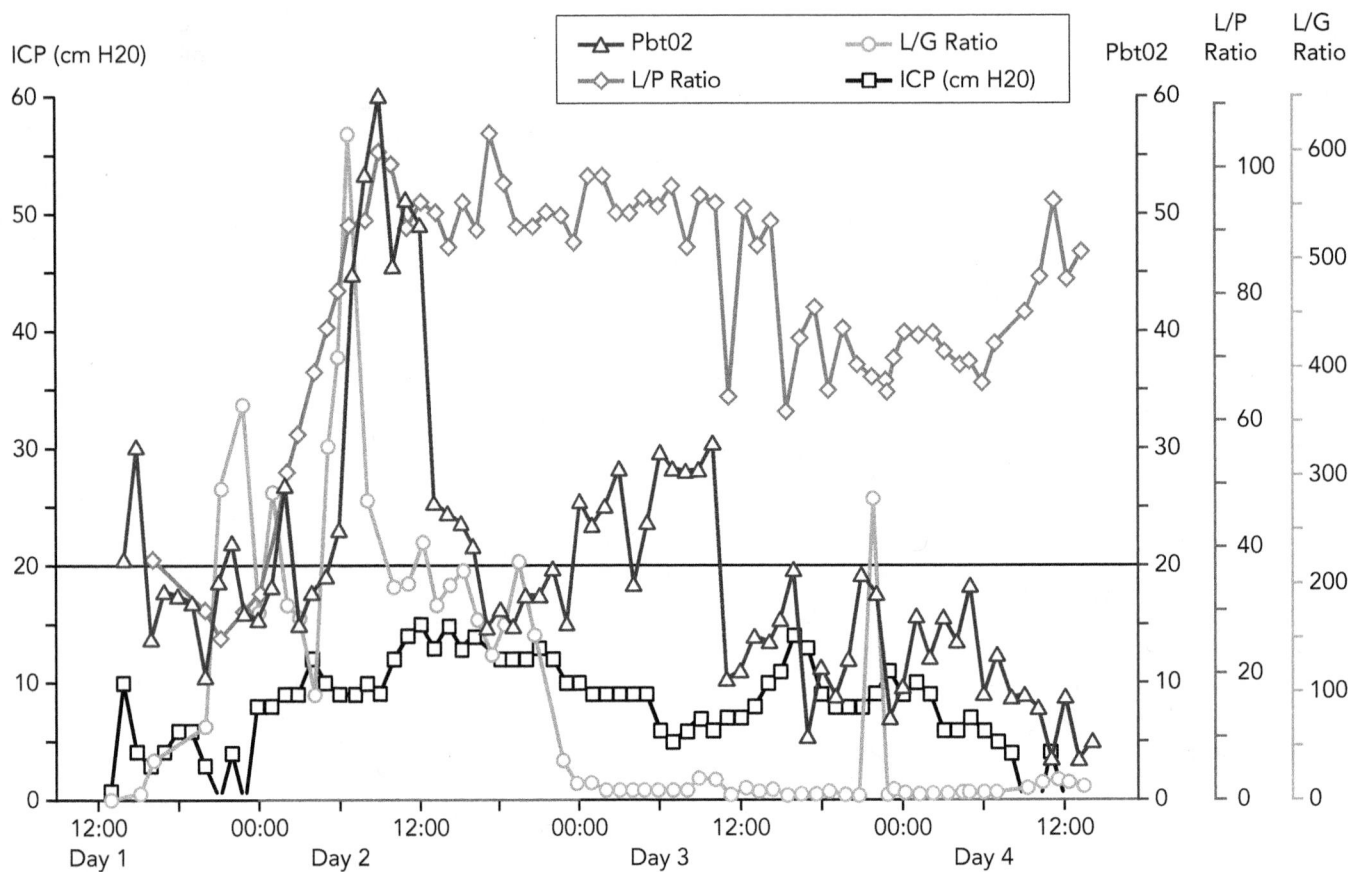

FIGURE 25-3 Multimodality neuromonitoring (ICP, CPP, PbtO$_2$, and microdialysis) from Day 1 to Day 4 post-decompressive craniectomy. Normal ICP (< 20 cm H$_2$O) and CPP with no evidence of hypoperfusion (no represented in the graph) but sustained low PbtO$_2$ (< 20) on day 3 and 4 with increased extracellular lactate and glucose. There is a predominant increasing on extracellular glucose over lactate on day 3 reflected on declines of lactate/glucose ratio representing a probable decrease on glucose anaerobic metabolism or a failure to convert glucose to lactate. This is a 21-year-old male with severe TBI status post-motor vehicle collision with a Glasgow Coma Scale (GCS) score of 5 at the scene. On day 7 postinjury, GCS decreased to 3 because of massive left brain edema with herniation syndrome requiring decompressive craniectomy. Patient had Glasgow Outcome Score (GOS) of 2 at discharge from hospital.

cebo. It revealed that phenytoin may have a favorable benefit on early PTS but little effect on late PTS (39). There was a conflicting class 3 study performed by Young et al. (44); the group concluded that phenytoin has no effect on early or late PTS. A subsequent class 2 study of 380 patients comparing VPA to phenytoin reported that VPA is noninferior to phenytoin (45).

Because of minimal hepatic metabolism and reduced risk of interactions with other medications, levetiracetam has grown in popularity for treating PTS. A recent prospective single-blinded study of 52 patients compared levetiracetam and phenytoin for seizure prophylaxis in patients with TBI or subarachnoid hemorrhage. Although a small study, patients treated with levetiracetam had the same incidence of PTS as phenytoin and experienced better long-term outcomes than those on phenytoin; the Disability Rating Scale (DRS) score was lower at 3 months, and the GCS score was higher at 6 months (46). A second study investigating levetiracetam and phenytoin in patients with TBI included 32 total patients and compared a prospective cohort of patients treated with levetiracetam to a retrospective cohort of pa-

tients treated with phenytoin. Patients treated with levetiracetam had a higher incidence of abnormal electrographic activity, but the seizure frequency was equal in both groups (47). Newer antiepileptic agents such topiramate and lacosamide are gaining popularity for treating seizures in the ICU setting, although studies supporting their efficacy are limited to case reports and small retrospective studies. More large scale studies are needed to investigate their role.

Continuous EEG monitoring in patients with TBI is commonly used as a way to detect subclinical electrographic seizures. Because patients with TBI are often comatose early in their disease course, electrographic activity provides a window into potential etiology for the patient's clinical status. For example, triphasic waves on EEG would favor a metabolic etiology as a cause of altered consciousness. A patient found to have a generalized spike and wave activity on EEG should be treated with anticonvulsant agents. Monitoring may reveal patterns of uncertain significance, including periodic lateralized epileptiform discharges (PLEDs), paroxysmal delta activity, and focal high frequency activity (48). The delayed epileptogenicity of these patterns has not yet been decisively elucidated. Also, the connection between nonconvulsive status epilepticus in TBI and increased mortality is still being studied. A small trial using microdialysis technology compared electrographic PTS to ICP measurements and lactate/pyruvate ratio. It showed that electrographic PTS are associated with increased ICP, including the percentage of time elevated, as compared with nonseizure patients with TBI. Analysis of lactate/pyruvate ratio exhibited both an episodic spike and an increase in a total period of time during the nonconvulsive seizure events compared to interictal baseline (49). PTS should be treated prophylactically for 7 days. The use of anticonvulsants after 7 days is not indicated unless clinical or electrographic seizures are present. Common anticonvulsants used in patients with TBI include phenytoin and levetiracetam, which appear to be equally efficacious on seizure treatment and mortality. Future studies should include larger scale investigation into newer antiepileptics, including topiramate and lacosamide.

Prophylactic Hypothermia

Hypothermia was first used as a treatment for TBI in the early 1800s. During the 20th century, it fell out of favor mainly because of cardiovascular and infectious side effects. Recently, the cooling has gained increased interest (50) as a possible treatment for increased ICP, fever control, and possibly seizures (51). Hypothermia has many benefits. The process provides neuroprotection via reduction of the inflammatory release of cytokines interleukin-1 beta (IL-1β) and tumor necrosis factor-alpha (TNF-α). This effect contributes to the reduction of edema formation. It has protective effects on the hippocampus (52) and decreases intracerebral O_2 consumption and CO_2 production. Hypothermia inhibits glutamatergic excitotoxicity, as well as exhibiting a reduction in cellular apoptosis. Although well studied in the animal model, beneficial effects have not translated well into human trials. In TBI, studies investigating the effect of hypothermia on outcome have been inconclusive at best.

To date, there are no positive studies pertaining to hypothermia in TBI. Investigations have suffered from a small sample size. In their notable study, Clifton et al. (53) reported no difference in mortality between hypothermia to 33° C and normothermia at their 6-month end point. "The National Acute Brain Injury Study (NABIS): Hypothermia II" induced hypothermia with target temperatures to be met at a goal of 4 hours. Patients were initially cooled to 35° C and, if they did not meet exclusion criteria, were randomized to normothermia or hypothermia to 33° C for 48 hours (53). Once again, improvement in outcome at 6 months was not demonstrated. Interestingly, patients with surgical focal TBI, such as subdural hematoma, tended to have better outcome if treated with hypothermia. No effect on outcome was found in patients with nonsurgical diffuse axonal injuries treated with hypothermia. The NABIS: Hypothermia II study was closed after only 97 patients were enrolled secondary to "futility in the interim analysis."

Despite a lack of data demonstrating improved mortality, hypothermia is very effective as a treatment for increased ICP. This efficacy is supported by more than 10 studies since 2001 (50). Interestingly, one trial, the NABIS: Hypothermia II, reported that the ICP was actually elevated in the hypothermia group, which required more medical interventions

(54). This unexpected increase in ICP occurred in relation to the rewarming phase after 48 hours likely because of rebound vasodilation. The finding raises the question of how long hypothermia can be safely and effectively applied. Increased length of time of treatment may correlate with better outcomes. Early results show that there is a lower risk of death when hypothermia is performed for more than 48 hours.

The preferred target temperature for cooling patients is being studied. Better outcomes are seen in patients with a target temperature of 32° C–33° C and 33° C–35° C. The NABIS: Hypothermia I examined the influence of different temperatures (34.8° C, 35.8° C, 36.8° C) on patient outcome in severe TBI. It reported that poor outcome was less evident in the 34.8° C and 35.8° C groups than in the 36.8° C group (53). Temperature selection has an impact on the mortality and efficacy of hypothermia. The properties of cooling that appear to be most important are minimum time to target temperature, maintaining an adequate target temperature with minimal shivering for at least 48 hours, and slow rewarming. Jiang et al. (55) investigated patients with TBI that underwent cooling for 5 days and reported better behavioral outcomes than those patients that were only cooled for 3 days. Slow rewarming must be performed to avoid potentially dangerous cellular potassium release into the blood and cardiac arrhythmias. At our institution, patients are rewarmed at a rate of 1° C every 8 hours.

Hypothermia is an exciting treatment but has yet to be proven as a decisive treatment to improve outcome. Seven randomized controlled trials concerning hypothermia in TBI failed to clearly report a significant reduction in mortality (56). However, there is a level 3 evidence that prophylactic hypothermia is not associated with reduced mortality but instead a greater decrease in "mortality risk." This is especially true when target temperatures are maintained for more than 48 hours. Prophylactic hypothermia is associated with higher GOS scores than normothermia comparison groups. There are still more questions than answers for the efficacy of hypothermia in TBI. Future studies should be informed by post hoc analysis of data from NABIS: Hypothermia II and maybe best focused on the early cooling of patient with surgical hematoma such as subdural and intracerebral contusion cases using femoral vein cooling catheter.

Infection Prophylaxis

Patients with TBI are at increased risk for infection, and early identification and treatment is a necessity. Patients in the ICU are commonly subjected to surgical interventions, prolonged intubation, invasive neuromonitoring, and prolonged bed rest. Fever control is of utmost importance, particularly in patients with prolonged ICP issues in whom fever increases ICP. Chronic systemic infections worsen ischemic brain damage. The most common causes of infection in the ICU are pneumonia and urinary tract infection; however, patients with TBI often have brain monitoring devices, craniectomies, and other invasive monitors. Consequently, the differential diagnosis for the origin of infections in patients with TBI can become complicated.

Prolonged intubation places patients at risk for nosocomial infection. There is a level 2 evidence that periprocedural antibiotics at the time of intubation should be administered to reduce pneumonia risk. Prophylactic use of antibiotics after intubation is not recommended. There is no effect on the length of stay (LOS) in the unit and mortality. It is prudent to extubate as soon as safely possible. Level 3 evidence reveals that early extubation (earlier than 1 week) improves outcome. If extubation is contraindicated, it is recommended to consider early tracheostomy, thereby reducing the number of days on mechanical ventilation and the risk of infection. A delay in extubation or tracheostomy correlates with the possible development of nosocomial pneumonia (57).

Invasive intracranial monitors may increase the risk of meningeal infection. There is a level 3 evidence stating that routine ventricular catheter exchange is not recommended because of the possibility of introducing infection and promoting hemorrhages. In addition, routine prophylactic antibiotic use for external ventricular catheter placement should not be performed. Further studies continued to support that routine catheter exchange is unnecessary. Antibiotic impregnated catheters are recommended.

Prophylactic antibiotics for the prevention of nosocomial infections are not recommended. Although patients with trauma are known to have a high rate of infection, the unnecessary use of antibiotics will allow propagation of more antibiotic-resistant gram-negative organisms (58). Prophylactic antibiotics in certain circumstances have been shown to be beneficial. This includes the use of antibiotics perioperatively for intubation (59). Patients not treated with antibiotics at the time of intubation were more likely to develop pneumonia.

Topical antibiotics applied to the mouth have been shown to reduce the risk of infections in the ICU (60). Although early tracheostomy, as defined as within 1 week post-trauma, has not been reported to reduce rates of pneumonia or mortality in most small scale studies, it is still recommended to do so when possible to avoid prolonged days in the ICU (61). Early extubation appears to be beneficial. Of course, certain criteria must be fulfilled before extubation is even considered, including an intact cough reflex and a positive leak test (62). If a patient meets criteria, early extubation does reduce the risk of infection.

In summary, there are numerous new studies that support early extubation and antibiotics prophylaxis during intubation, as well as early tracheostomies. Overuse of antibiotics may select out benign organisms and allow for the growth of more resistant ones, including *Acinetobacter* and extended spectrum β-lactamase (ESBL) organisms. The single most important aspect to infection prevention is hand washing in the ICU. Future studies should be oriented toward optimal antibiotic selection and daily measures that can be taken by doctors and nurses in the ICU to reduce the spread of infection.

Deep Vein Thrombosis Prophylaxis

Patients with TBI are at an increased risk for developing deep vein thrombosis (DVT), with an incidence reported as high as 20% (63). In moderate-to-severe TBI, the risk is up to one-third (64). Thromboprophylaxis is therefore important for outcome and can be achieved using mechanical and pharmacologic interventions. Mechanical interventions include graduated compression stockings and intermittent pneumatic compression stockings. Current pharmacologic options are low dose heparin administered subcutaneously and low molecular weight heparin (LMWH) (Lovenox). Mechanical compression devices are safer, although may, at times, not be an option if there is trauma to the legs. Heparin carries the risk of hematoma expansion and systemic bleeding, as well as heparin-induced thrombocytopenia (HIT), all of which may increase the risk of mortality.

The rates of DVT discovery depend on the mode of evaluation (Dopplers, venogram, etc.) and on the institution. In addition, most studies only include Doppler evaluation of the distal lower extremities, which are often asymptomatic. Concern arises when DVTs are found in the proximal lower extremities, pelvis, or upper limbs, which are much harder to image and which are more likely to be symptomatic and associated with pulmonary embolism.

Discovery of a pulmonary embolus in the setting of TBI can force a physician into a difficult situation. Most patients with TBI under these circumstances have some degree of intracranial blood; therefore, anticoagulation in this setting may have the unwanted side effect of hemorrhage expansion. Further complicating matters, many patients who develop DVTs and are untreated in the ICU will develop chronic venous abnormalities, causing chronic pain and swelling in long-term follow-up. Commonly, inferior vena cava (IVC) filters are placed to provide protection from further thromboembolism. It should be noted, although, that IVC filters themselves increase the risk of thrombus formation; removable IVC filters have gained popularity to thwart this effect. Patients with removable IVC filters are at risk for being lost to follow-up, and subsequently, the hardware is often not removed early.

In the TBI population, most case studies suggest that pharmacologic prophylaxis should not be initiated immediately perioperatively. Recent literature has challenged this assumption. Scuddy and colleagues (65) found no significant evidence of increased risk of TBI progression in the early thromboprophylaxis treatment group and reduced rates of DVT development over the nontreatment group. Another retrospective study on 669 patients with TBI evaluated the safety of early thromboprophylaxis, comparing the incidence of TBI progression if initiated before or after 72 hours. Once again, their results confirmed both efficacy and safety if pharmacological prophylaxis is initiated early (66). Finally, Dudley et al. (66) performed a retrospective chart review of 287 patients with TBI; prophylaxis was started within 48–72 hours of injury, without evidence of progression of intracranial bleeding.

Only class 3 studies exist to investigate the decision to use mechanical vs pharmacological prophylaxis in patients with TBI. One study, comparing enoxaparin 24 hours postoperatively to compression stockings alone in nontraumatic surgical patients, exhibited lower rates of DVT with enoxaparin (17%) than in the compression stockings group (32%) (67). There was no increased risk of bleeding between the 2 groups.

Numerous trials have reported favorable results using mechanical thromboprophylaxis. Graduated compression stockings or intermittent pneumatic compression devices should be used until patients are ambulatory. LMWH or low dose unfractionated heparin should be used in combination with mechanical devices. It should be noted that in comparison to unfractionated heparin, LMWH may have a slightly higher incidence of delayed intracranial hemorrhage.

Future studies should include a large randomized controlled trial comparing pharmacologic intervention and mechanical intervention in the prevention of DVTs in patients with TBI. An investigation should be performed to answer the question of timing of intervention in the setting of a patient with intracranial hemorrhage or traumatic subarachnoid hemorrhage. It is unknown whether the risk of hemorrhage from pharmacologic prophylaxis is increased based on mode of blood (contusion, subarachnoid hemorrhage, intracranial hemorrhage). Finally, recommendations into the use of IVC filters should be explored.

Nutrition After Traumatic Brain Injury

The importance of adequate and early nutrition on the outcome of patients with TBI cannot be overstated. In the past, it was thought that all patients in coma, regardless of etiology, had reduced metabolic requirements. In actuality, patients with TBI have a markedly increased metabolic demand. Isolated TBI yielded a mean increase of approximately 140% of the expected metabolic expenditure with variations from 120%–250% of that expected (68). In fact, patients with TBI have a metabolic requirement similar to patients with burns with 20%–40% of body area affected (69).

Timing of nutrition postinjury has been well studied. Energy requirements are at their highest within the first 2 weeks postinjury. Undernutrition during this period appears to cause worse mortality as compared to full replacement. Patients who are not fed within 5–7 days after TBI have a twofold and fourfold increased likelihood of death, respectively (70). Early refeeding may also reduce the risk of hospital-borne infection. The goal, then, is to initiate feeding as soon as possible. On average, replacement should be started no later than 24–48 hours after injury to attain full caloric goal at 7 days. Feeding should be initiated at a low rate and gradually increased to full replacement over 2–3 days.

Early refeeding may produce issues of intolerability. Patients are often given anticholinergics, paralytic agents, and opiates, which may slow gastric motility. Prokinetic agents have been investigated with mixed results. Dickerson et al. (71) investigated the use of metoclopramide as a tool to improve gastric motility in TBI. They reported that there was poor tolerability because of tachyphylaxis in the TBI population and recommend erythromycin 250 mg intravenously every 6 hours as first-line therapy or in combination with metoclopramide in this patient subset.

The recommended daily caloric intake is 50 kcal/kg/day. Most formulations contain a combination of carbohydrates, lipids, and proteins to meet this goal. Patients with TBI are at risk for losing up to 50% of administered nitrogen. Nitrogen loss in this important period may amount to 20% of the total caloric composition of daily feeding. Of note, the maximum protein content of enteral feeds for the hypermetabolic patient is 20%. These requirements can be reduced by nearly 40% via different interventions, including the use of paralysis with pancuronium bromide and barbiturate coma (72). There is evidence that branched-chain amino acids have use in septic patients, but no studies to date have been performed on patients with TBI. Glutamine supplementation, on the other hand, may improve the efficacy of intestinal villi and enhance absorption in bed-bound patients. One small study, which randomized 20 patients to placebo and early glutamine supplementation, reported improvement in length of hospital stay and infection rate in the glutamine group (73).

There is no definite advantage for choosing gastric or jejunal routes for feeding. Some evidence indicates decreased nitrogen loss in jejunal and parenteral replacement feedings. Percutaneous gastrostomy is quite common, but there is some concern over increased risk of residual formation, delayed gastric emptying, and aspiration pneumonia. Continuous feeding may achieve daily caloric intake goals better than bolus feedings, but there was no difference in clinical outcome seen between the 2 options. Jejunal feeding may have some benefit over gastric feedings. A greater percentage of patients tolerate this option over gastric feedings in the first few days because there is less risk of aspiration pneumonia. Contrary to general critical care literature, no studies yet have decisively shown increased risk of infection in patients with TBI who receive parenteral nutrition over enteral nutrition. The physician must weigh the need for early parenteral nutritional support with the risk of infection. The available studies suggest that the combination of a central line for long periods, together with parental nutrition, may worse the risk of septicemia. There have been some indications that parenteral nutrition may increase cerebral edema, but the animal studies have not transitioned into the clinical field.

Control of blood sugars in patients with TBI is important; however, the goal for glucose level is unclear. Elevated blood sugars may aggravate brain injury via various networks. A heightened stress response is precipitated causing a secondary increase in circulating catecholamines and cortisol. Elevated glucose concentrations in insulin-independent tissues (such as neurons) may contribute to secondary injury. Also, increased lactate production and brain tissue acidosis are seen with hyperglycemia. Catabolism increases by enhancing proteolysis (74). With this in mind, hyperglycemia may be associated with worse outcomes. Recently, Liu-Deryke et al. (75) demonstrated that patients with blood sugars less than 60 or more than 160 mg/dL within the first 5 days of admission had worse outcomes.

Adding electrolyte and trace element supplements to tube feeds may provide benefit. Because of the hypercatabolic and metabolic state in TBI, patients may have wide fluctuations in electrolytes including potassium, phosphorus, zinc, and magnesium. Zinc has been well studied in TBI; one study showed an improved 24-hour GCS motor score at days 15 and 21 with supplementation (76). Serum zinc concentrations are diminished because of liver sequestration and increased renal clearance (74). Magnesium may be neuroprotective because of activity at the N-methyl-D-aspartate (NMDA) receptor and modulation of cellular energy production and calcium influx. However, a single center randomized clinical trial of magnesium therapy did not show any benefit on outcome for severe TBI. Potassium and phosphorus requirements are increased in patients with TBI. One study comparing 50 patients split into trauma with TBI and trauma without TBI found that patients with TBI were more likely to develop hypokalemia and more difficult to reach a target concentration level of 4 mEq/L. Patients in the TBI group also required one-third more phosphorus supplementation than that of the non-TBI trauma group (77).

There has been some recent interest in the use of polyphenols in the setting of brain ischemia and TBI. Polyphenols are potential antioxidants found in vegetables, fruits, grains, bark, roots, tea, and wine. They may have insulin-potentiating, anti-inflammatory, anticarcinogenic, antiviral, antiulcer, and antiapoptotic properties (78). Polyphenols may be an important additive to tube feeds in the future.

Malnutrition in patients with TBI is an often underrecognized entity. Early and adequate nutrition is important for neuroprotection, as well as infection control. Feeding should be initiated within the first 24–48 hours and accelerated to goal as the patient tolerates. Care must be taken to aggressively follow electrolyte imbalances and treat accordingly. Normoglycemia is important for outcome. Additional supplements are being studied. Future studies should include target glucose goals and timing for safety of loosening those goals.

SURGICAL MANAGEMENT

Acute care guidelines for surgical management after severe TBI are based on neurologic status, usually defined by the GCS, pupils exam results, and findings on head CT criteria (see Table 25-6). In patients with indications for surgical intervention, evacuation should be performed as soon as possible because these patients can deteriorate rapidly, thus worsening their prognosis (79–83) (see Chapter 24 on Surgical Management and Procedures).

PENETRATING BRAIN INJURY

A penetrating brain injury (PBI) occurs when the dura mater is breached. PBI can be caused by high-velocity projectiles or objects of lower velocity such as bone fragments or knives from a skull fracture that are driven into the brain. Guidelines for surgical management of PBI (84) are summarized in Table 25-7 (see Figure 25-4).

IMPACT OF CURRENT GUIDELINES

TBI guidelines offer and ensure the possibility for uniformity of severe TBI care and conformity with the best standards of clinical practice, early resuscitation, rapid transport to a trauma care facility, CT scanning, and consequent prompt evacuation of significant intracranial hematomas. Guidelines are targeted to prevent and treat secondary injury.

Integration of the "Guidelines for the Management of Severe Traumatic Brain Injury" recommendations into a multidisciplinary clinical pathway for severe TBI aim to bring care to a consistently higher level of quality and thereby improving patient outcomes by the following:

1. Diminishing mortality and morbidity with improvement in functional outcome scores.
2. Decreasing the ICU and hospital LOS.

3. Reducing variability through standardization of many components of care delivery.
4. Codifying the optimal or best clinical choices suggested by the evidence to date. As a by-product of this process, the resources and costs of caring for that patient population could be substantially reduced.

Guidelines should not only be used as a roadmap to improve treatment but also as a template from which to generate high-quality research for future use providing the best milieu for the conduct of clinical trials to evaluate putative new therapies, which are being brought forth for clinical trials.

A significant improvement in patient outcomes by the implementation of the Guidelines for the Management of Severe Brain Injury has been documented. Recently, there is evidence that the use of clinical practice guidelines-based management protocol for severe TBI was independently associated with a significant reduction in hospital and ICU mortality (odds ratio = 0.45, 95% confidence interval = 0.24–0.86 and odds ratio = 0.47, 95% confidence interval = 0.23–0.96, respectively). The use of the protocol was not associated with an increase in the need for tracheostomies, mechanical ventilation duration, ICU LOS, and hospital LOS, suggesting that the improved survival was not associated with increased number of patients surviving with severe disability and that the functional status might have also improved (85).

Epidemiologic study of TBI in Australia and New Zealand that were obtained following the publication of international evidence-based guidelines in 2007 showed mortality and favorable neurologic outcomes after TBI were similar to published data before the advent of evidence-based guidelines. They suggested that a high incidence of prehospital secondary brain insults and an aging population may have contributed to these outcomes. The authors recommended strategies directed at preventive public health approaches and interventions to minimize secondary brain injuries in the prehospital period (86).

The association between implementation of clinical practice guidelines and outcome for TBI was documented by Keris et al. (87). They found that implementation of the guidelines was associated with a statistically significant decrease of hospital case fatality rate (HCFR) in patients with TBI from 3.7% during 1998–2000 to 2.6% during 2002–2004 (relative risk = 0.72, 95% confidence interval = 0.67–0.76; $P = 0.03$).

Rusnak et al. (88) analyzed the effects of guidelines-based management for severe TBI in Austria. They concluded that there is a relatively strong relation between initial resuscitation in the hospital and ICU survival and a positive influence of some of the recommendations on reduction of ICU or hospital days.

Faul et al. (89) assessed the BTF guidelines for the treatment of severe TBI using a cost–benefit analysis to estimate outcomes of a clinical treatment guideline. They determined that widespread implementation of the BTF guidelines would cost $61 million, but the substantial savings would far outweigh the cost. It was estimated that savings would amount to $262 million in annual medical costs, $43 million in annual rehabilitation costs, and $3.84 billion in lifetime

TABLE 25-6 Indications for Surgical Management in Patients With Severe Traumatic Brain Injury

SURGICAL MANAGEMENT	INDICATIONS	METHOD
Acute epidural hematoma (EDH) (79)	• An EDH $\geq$ 30 cm^3 regardless of the patient's GCS score. • Acute EDH in coma (GCS score < 9) and anisocoria. • Nonoperative management with serial head CT scanning and close neurological observation is indicated if EDH < 30 cm^3, thickness < 15 mm, MLS < 5 mm, GCS score > 8, and without focal deficit.	There are insufficient data to support 1 surgical treatment method. However, craniotomy provides a more complete evacuation of the hematoma.
Acute subdural hematoma (SDH) (80)	• An acute SDH with a thickness $\geq$ 10 mm or a MLS $\geq$ 5 mm, regardless of the patient's GCS score. • All acute SDH with GCS score < 9 should undergo intracranial pressure (ICP) monitoring. • SDH with a thickness < 10 mm or a MLS < 5 mm, GCS score < 9, should undergo surgical evacuation if the GCS decreased between the time of injury and hospital admission by 2 or more points and/or the patient presents with asymmetric or fixed and dilated pupils and/or the ICP exceeds 20 mm Hg.	Craniotomy with or without bone flap removal and duraplasty.
Traumatic parenchymal lesion (82)	• Patients with parenchymal mass lesions and signs of progressive neurological deterioration referable to the lesion, medically refractory intracranial hypertension, or signs of mass effect on CT scan. • Patients with GCS of 6–8 with frontal or temporal contusions more than 20 cm^3 in volume with MLS $\geq$ 5 mm and/or cisternal compression on CT scan. • Patients with any lesion more than 50 cm^3 in volume. • Patients with parenchymal mass lesions who do not show evidence for neurological compromise have controlled ICP, and no significant signs of mass effect on CT scan may be managed nonoperatively with intensive monitoring and serial imaging.	Craniotomy with evacuation of mass lesion for patients with focal lesions. Bifrontal decompressive craniectomy within 48 hours of injury for diffuse, medically refractory cerebral edema and increased ICP. Decompressive procedures (subtemporal decompression, temporal lobectomy, and hemispheric decompressive craniectomy) for refractory intracranial hypertension and diffuse parenchymal injury with clinical and radiographic evidence for impending transtentorial herniation.
Posterior fossa mass lesions (81)	• Patients with mass effect on CT scan or with neurological dysfunction or deterioration referable to the lesion should undergo operative intervention. Mass effect on CT scan is defined as distortion, dislocation, or obliteration of the fourth ventricle; compression or loss of visualization of the basal cisterns, or the presence of obstructive hydrocephalus. • Patients with lesions and no significant mass effect on CT scan and without signs of neurological dysfunction may be managed by close observation and serial imaging.	Suboccipital craniectomy is the predominant method reported for evacuation of posterior fossa mass lesions and is therefore recommended.
Depress cranial fracture (83)	• Patients with open (compound) cranial fractures depressed more than the thickness of the cranium should undergo early operative intervention to reduce the incidence of infection. • Patients with open (compound) depressed cranial fractures may be treated nonoperatively if there is no clinical or radiographic evidence of dural penetration, significant intracranial hematoma, depression more than 1 cm, frontal sinus involvement, gross cosmetic deformity, wound infection, pneumocephalus, or gross wound contamination. Nonoperative management of closed (simple) depressed cranial fractures is a treatment option.	Elevation and debridement is recommended as the surgical method of choice. Primary bone fragment replacement is a surgical option in the absence of wound infection at the time of surgery. All management strategies for open (compound) depressed fractures should include antibiotics.

Abbreviations: GCS, Glasgow Coma Scale; MLS, midline shift.

societal costs. The net savings were primarily because of better health outcomes and a decreased burden on lifetime social support systems. They also estimated that mortality would be reduced by 3,607 lives if the guidelines were followed in the United States.

A study for analysis of mortality from TBI was completed by Lu et al. (90). They found a progressive and significant reduction ($P < 0.05$) in severe TBI mortality from 1984 to 1996, even when adjusted for injury severity, age, and other admission prognostic parameters.

Fakhry et al. (91) studied the impact of 1995s in-hospital guideline to manage patients with severe blunt TBI from a level I trauma center over the mortality, day of LOS (in ICU and hospital), total charges, and patient outcome measured by GOS and Rancho Los Amigos Scale (RLAS). They found that from 1991–1994 to 1997–2000, ICU LOS was reduced

TABLE 25-7 Management of Penetrating Brain Injury

Neuroimaging	Plain radiographs of the head can be helpful in assessing bullet trajectory, the presence of large foreign bodies, and the presence of intracranial air. Head CT scanning is recommended. Coronal sections may be helpful in skull base or high-convexity involvement. CT angiography and/or conventional angiography should be considered when a vascular injury is suspected to identify a traumatic intracranial aneurysm (TICA) or arteriovenous fistula in patients with a penetrating brain injury (PBI) involving an orbitofacial or pterional injury, particularly in patients harboring an intracerebral hematoma.
Antibiotic prophylaxis	Use of prophylactic broad-spectrum antibiotics (usually cephalosporin) is believed to have contributed to the reduced incidence of infection in this setting.
Surgical management	Small entry wounds can be treated with simple closure in patients whose scalp are not devitalized and have no "significant" intracranial pathologic findings. Treatment of more extensive wounds with nonviable scalp, bone, or dura with more extensive debridement before primary closure or grafting to secure a watertight wound is recommended. In patients with significant fragmentation of the skull, debridement of the cranial wound with either craniectomy or craniotomy is recommended. In the presence of significant mass effect, debridement of necrotic brain tissue and safely accessible bone fragments is recommended. Evacuation of intracranial hematomas with significant mass effect is recommended. In the absence of significant mass effect, surgical debridement of the missile track in the brain is not recommended, on the basis of class III evidence that outcomes are not measurable worse in patients who do not have aggressive debridement. Routine surgical removal of fragments lodged distant from the entry site and reoperation solely to remove retained bone or missile fragments are not recommended.
Vascular complications	When a TICA or arteriovenous fistula is identified, surgical or endovascular management is recommended.
CSF leak	Surgical correction is recommended for cerebrospinal fluid (CSF) leaks that do not close spontaneously or are refractory to temporary CSF diversion. During the primary surgery, every effort should be made to close the dura and prevent CSF leaks.

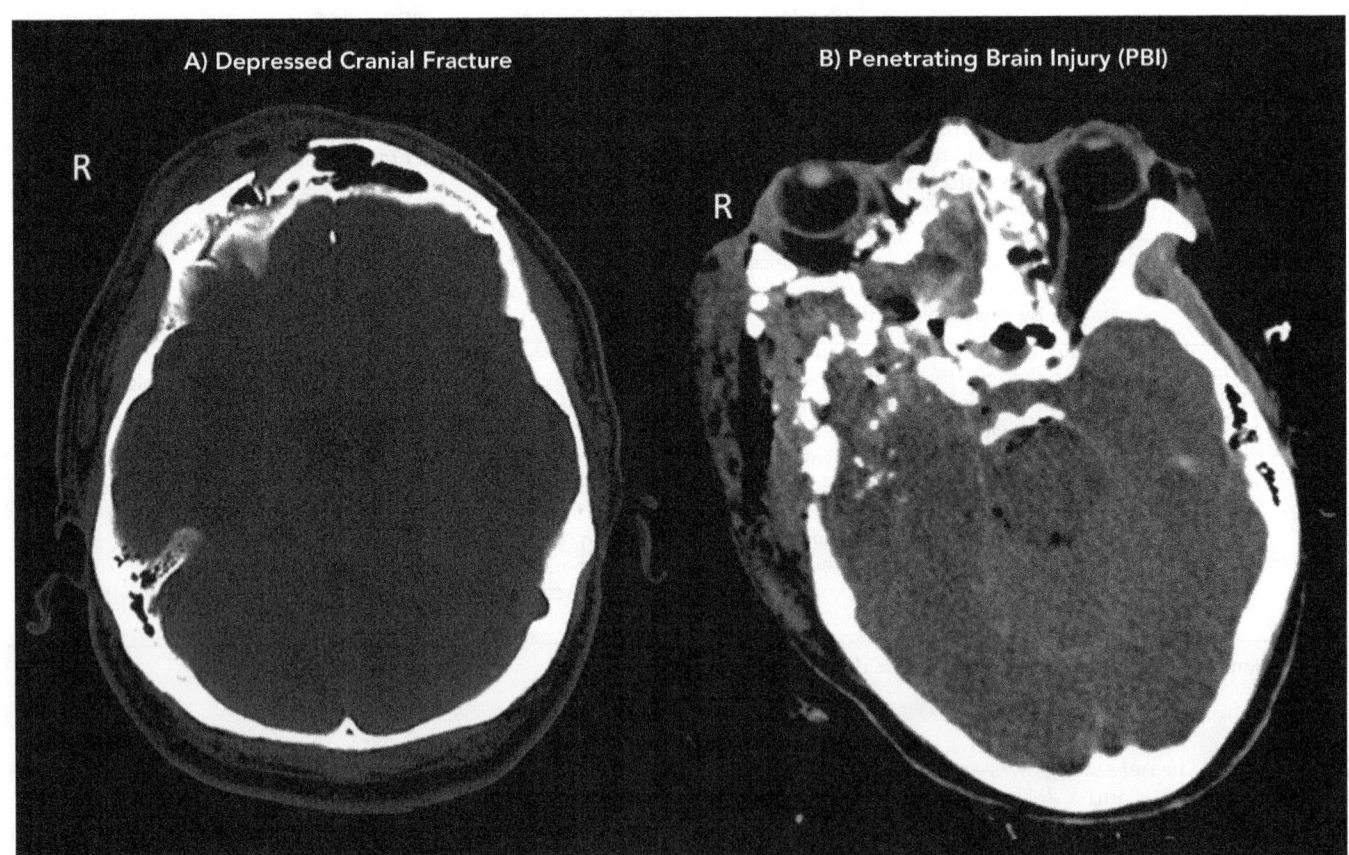

FIGURE 25-4 A, Comminuted depressed fracture of the right frontal sinus and the roof of the right orbit with adjacent small hematoma. B, Gunshot wound to the face/head with extensive soft tissue and bony destruction, multiple facial bone fractures with hemosinuses. There are bullets and/or displaced bony fragments, traumatic encephalocoele, uncal herniation, diffuse cerebral edema, pneumocephalus, subarachnoid hemorrhage, and parenchymal contusions in the right anterior temporal lobe.

by 1.8 days ($P = 0.021$), and total hospital LOS was reduced by 5.4 days ($P < 0.001$). The charge reduction (calculated in 1997 dollars) per patient for the LOS decrease was $6,577 in 1995–1996 and $8,266 in 1997–2000 ($P = 0.002$). This represents a total reduction over 6 years of $4.7 million in charges. The overall mortality rate showed a reduction of 4% from 1991–1994 to 1997–2000 (17.8% vs 13.8%), although this was significant. On the basis of the GOS score, in 1997–2000, 61.5% of the patients had either a "good recovery" or only "moderate disability" compared with 50.3% in 1995–1996 and 43.3% in 1991–1994 ($P < 0.001$). The RLAS showed a similar trend, with 56.6% of the 1997–2000 patients having appropriate responses at 10–14 days, compared with only 44% of the 1995–1996 patients and 43.9% of the 1991–1994 patients ($P = 0.004$).

Vitaz et al. (92) analyzed the development and implementation of a clinical pathway (CP) for severe TBI. They reported a significant decrease in the hospital LOS, ICU LOS, and length of ventilator support in the study group: 22.5, 16.8, and 11.5 days, respectively; compared with control group: 31, 21.2, and 14.4 days, respectively; ($P < 0.03$). They concluded that the use of this CP helped to standardize and improve patient care with fewer complications and a potential cost savings of approximately $14,000 per patient.

Palmer et al. (93) revised the impact on outcomes in a community hospital setting of using the 1995s American Association of Neurological Surgeons (AANS) TBI guidelines. They compared 2 groups of patients. Group I, the pre-TBI guidelines group consisting of 37 patients admitted between January 1994 and June 1997, was managed with an emphasis on ICP reduction. Group II, the post-TBI guidelines group consisting of 56 patients admitted between June 1997 and December 1999, was managed with an emphasis on concurrent ICP reduction, CPP enhancement, and maximization of cerebral oxygenation. They found that implementation of the guidelines increased hospital charges by more than $97,000 per patient but resulted in a 9.13 times higher odds ratio of a good outcome relative to the odds of a poor outcome or death compared with a group managed before the practice change. They concluded that the protocol resulted in an increase in resource usage, but it also resulted in statistically improved outcomes justifying the increase in expenditures.

Vukic et al. (94) retrospectively analyzed 2 groups of consecutive patients. Guidelines group was treated according to the Guidelines for the Management of Severe Brain injury with ICP monitoring. Such an approach allowed the maintenance of ICP within normal values, especially in patients with intraventricular ICP monitoring, allowing the release of cerebrospinal fluid (CSF) from the ventricular system. The "nonguidelines group" was not monitored for ICP. In this group, management consisted of the prophylactic administration of barbiturates, high-dose osmotic diuretics, and hyperventilation usually at levels below 25 mm Hg. In the guidelines group, the mortality rate was 30% compared to 44% in the nonguidelines group. Almost twice as many patients achieved a "favorable" (good recovery and moderate disability) outcome (49%) compared to the nonguidelines treated patients (25%). Furthermore, there was a 32% decrease in severe neurological disabilities in those patients in the guidelines group. They concluded that implementation of "guidelines" in the treatment of severe brain injury seems to reduce death and disability rates in patients with severe brain injury.

Evidence-based guidelines for severe TBI have been widely discussed; however, guideline adoption has tended to be slow, partial, and highly variable. Management often varies depending on the region of the country, hospital, and doctor. These variations in the treatment of patients with severe brain injury in the United States were documented in a survey published in 1995 by Ghajar et al. (95).

Because severe head trauma enlists so many providers and often involves injury to multiple body systems, it maximizes the challenges of delivering timely, consistent, and coordinated care. Management of TBI thus offers a valuable perspective on the structural problems that impede the delivery of care and the implementation of clinical guidelines.

Hesdorffer et al. (96) did a survey of 828 US trauma centers to study the implementation of guidelines for severe TBI care during 1999–2000. They found that implementation of evidence-based guidelines was infrequent. There was only 16% of full guideline compliance. Hesdorffer and Ghajar (97) published another survey in 2007, and they found that adherence to evidence-based guidelines for severe TBI has been improving dramatically. Routine ICP monitor use increased from 32.4% in 1991 and 50.8% in 2000 to 77.4% in the current survey ($P < 0.0001$). Avoidance of steroids in TBI rose from 47.8% in 1991 and 52.4% in 2000 to 86.0% in 2006 ($P < 0.0001$). Lack of guideline adherence decreased significantly from 67% in 2006 to 34.5%.

CONCLUSION

Implementation of TBI guidelines is practical and efficacious. Appropriate invasive monitoring of systemic and cerebral parameters guides therapy. Adherence to a protocol based on the BTF guidelines can result in a significant improvement on patients' outcome. In addition, guideline goal-directed therapy is economical and provides a clear pathway for physician decision making. Standardization of care in the TBI setting would also allow for more high-quality studies to be performed in multiple hospital systems, which provide care following the same guidelines.

Although much ground has been made in creating recommendations for patients with TBI, there are still more questions that need to be addressed. All neurological damage after TBI does not occur at the moment of impact. Secondary brain injuries may occur hours, days, or weeks after the primary insult and present a serious risk of viable brain tissue, leading to permanent cell loss (penumbra area). These delayed events are not simply related to increased ICP, reduced CPP, or CBF. Improved outcomes result when the penumbra is protected via guideline directed treatment, and further clarification of delayed inflammatory cascades will help to improve outcome.

New technologies, such as microdialysis and partial pressure of oxygen in brain tissue ($PbtO_2$) monitoring, are being developed to help direct management. These techniques allow for the measurement of cerebral physiologic, electrical activity, and metabolic parameters with the goal of improving the detection of secondary brain injury. New studies are necessary to evaluate such neuromonitoring technology and the effect on outcome. In addition, more specific guidelines into need and timing of prophylaxis should be explored. Alternatives to clinical scales, such as the GCS, should be considered to help accurately predict which patients will benefit from therapeutic or surgical interventions.

1. Important factors to predict outcome in severe TBI are age, GCS, pupil examination, SBP, and some particular feature on the initial head CT. The prehospital care of the patient with TBI is critical to maximizing the chances for a good outcome. Specialized neurotrauma center with neurosurgical and neurocritical care support and the use of guidelines-based standardized protocols are the most optimally management of patients with TBI.
2. ICP monitoring is the key in management of patient with severe TBI.
3. Multimodal neuromonitoring may help to individualize the management of patients with severe TBI.
4. Increased ICP should be treated with general measures to optimization of venous drainage, hyperosmolar therapy, hyperventilation, anesthetics, analgesics, and sedatives.
5. The use of steroids is NOT recommended for reducing ICP or improving outcome.
6. Prophylactic recommendations, such as starting antiepileptics, early thromboprophylaxis, early extubation, and avoiding a delay for adequate nutrition, are extremely important for outcome.
7. Patients with indications for surgical intervention and evacuation should be performed as soon as possible.

KEY REFERENCES

1. Bratton, SL, Chestnut, RM, Ghajar J, et al. Guidelines for the management of severe traumatic brain injury. XI. Anesthetics, analgesics, and sedatives. *J Neurotrauma*. 2007; 24(suppl 1):S71–S76.
2. Bullock MR, Chesnut R, Ghajar J, et al. Surgical management of acute subdural hematomas. *Neurosurgery*. 2006; 58(3)(suppl):S16–S24.
3. Carney NA, Chesnut R, Kochanek PM. Guidelines for the acute medical management of severe traumatic brain injury in infants, children, and adolescents. *Pediatr Crit Care Med*. 2003;4(3):S1–S75.
4. Chestnut RM, Ghajar J, Maas AIR, et al. Management and prognosis of severe traumatic brain injury. Part 2: early indicators of prognosis in severe traumatic brain injury. *J Neurotrauma*. 2000;17:557–627.
5. http://www.braintrauma.org
6. http://www.tbi-impact.org
7. Surgical management of penetrating brain injury. *J Trauma*. 2001;51(2)(suppl):S16–S25.

References

1. Tiesman HM, Konda S, Bell JL. The epidemiology of fatal occupational traumatic brain injury in the U.S. *Am J Prev Med*. 2011;41(1): 61–67.
2. Corrigan JD, Selassie AW, Orman JA. The epidemiology of traumatic brain injury. *J Head Trauma Rehabil*. 2010;25(2):72–80.
3. Andriessen TM, Horn J, Franschman G, et al. Epidemiology, severity classification, and outcome of moderate and severe traumatic

brain injury: a prospective multicenter study. *J Neurotrauma*. 2011; 28(10):2019–31.
4. Bruns J Jr, Hauser WA. The epidemiology of traumatic brain injury: a review. *Epilepsia*. 2003;44(suppl 10):2–10.
5. Knuth T, Letarte PB, Ling G, et al. Guidelines for the field management of combat-related head trauma. New York, NY: Brain Trauma Foundation; 2005.
6. Management of Concussion/mTBI Working Group. VA/DoD clinical practice guideline for management of concussion/mild traumatic brain injury. *J Rehabil Res Dev*. 2009;46(6):CP1–CP68.
7. Chestnut RM, Ghajar J, Maas AIR, et al. Management and prognosis of severe traumatic brain injury. Part 2: early indicators of prognosis in severe traumatic brain injury. *J Neurotrauma*. 2000;17: 557–627.
8. Fortune PM, Shann F. The motor response to stimulation predicts outcome as well as the full Glasgow Coma Scale in children with severe head injury. *Pediatr Crit Care Med*. 2010;11(3):339–342.
9. Amirjamshidi A, Abouzari M, Rashidi A. Glasgow Coma Scale on admission is correlated with postoperative Glasgow Outcome Scale in chronic subdural hematoma. *J Clin Neurosci*. 2007;14(12): 1240–1241.
10. Lieberman JD, Pasquale MD, Garcia R, Cipolle MD, Mark Li P, Wasser TE. Use of admission Glasgow Coma score, pupil size, and pupil reactivity to determine outcome for trauma patients. *J Trauma*. 2003;55(3):437–442; discussion 442–443.
11. Kamal H, Mardini A, Aly BM. Traumatic brain injury in pediatric age group; predictors of outcome in pediatric intensive care unit. *Libyan J Med*. 2007;2(2):90–94.
12. Czosnyka M, Balestreri M, Steiner L et al. Age, intracranial pressure, autoregulation, and outcome after brain trauma. *J Neurosurg*. 2005;102(3):450–454.
13. Hanif S, Abodunde O, Ali Z, Pidgeon C. Age related outcome in acute subdural haematoma following traumatic head injury. *Ir Med J*. 2009;102(8):255–257.
14. Inamasu J, Nakatsukasa M, Kuramae T, Nakagawa Y, Miyatake S, Tomiyasu K. Influence of age and anti-platelet/anti-coagulant use on the outcome of elderly patients with fall-related traumatic intracranial hemorrhage. *Neurol Med Chir (Tokyo)*. 2010;50(12):1051–1055.
15. Pompucci A, De Bonis P, Pettorini B, Petrella G, Di Chirico A, Anile C. Decompressive craniectomy for traumatic brain injury: patient age and outcome. *J Neurotrauma*. 2007;24(7):1182–1188.
16. Jacobs B, Beems T, Stulemeijer M, et al. Outcome prediction in mild traumatic brain injury: age and clinical variables are stronger predictors than CT abnormalities. *J Neurotrauma*. 2010;27(4):655–668.
17. Clusmann H, Schaller C, Schramm J. Fixed and dilated pupils after trauma, stroke, and previous intracranial surgery: management and outcome. *J Neurol Neurosurg Psychiatry*. 2001;71(2):175–181.
18. Chamoun RB, Robertson CS, Gopinath SP. Outcome in patients with blunt head trauma and a Glasgow Coma Scale score of 3 at presentation. *J Neurosurg*. 2009;111(4):683–687.
19. Coates BM, Vavilala MS, Mack CD, et al. Influence of definition and location of hypotension on outcome following severe pediatric traumatic brain injury. *Crit Care Med*. 2005;33(11):2645–2650.
20. Samant UB IV, Mack CD, Koepsell T, Rivara FP, Vavilala MS. Time of hypotension and discharge outcome in children with severe traumatic brain injury. *J Neurotrauma*. 2008;25(5):495–502.
21. Beretta L, Anzalone N, Dell'Acqua A, Calvi MR, Gemma M. Post-traumatic interpeduncular cistern hemorrhage as a marker for brainstem lesions. *J Neurotrauma*. 2010;27(3):509–514.
22. Chiewvit P, Tritakarn SO, Nanta-aree S, Suthipongchai S. Degree of midline shift from CT scan predicted outcome in patients with head injuries. *J Med Assoc Thai*. 2010;93(1):99–107.
23. Jacobs B, Beems T, van der Vliet TM, Borm GF, Vos PE. The status of the fourth ventricle and ambient cisterns predict outcome in moderate and severe traumatic brain injury. *J Neurotrauma*. 2010; 27(2):331–340.
24. Nelson DW, Nyström H, MacCallum RM, et al. Extended analysis of early computed tomography scans of traumatic brain injured patients and relations to outcome. *J Neurotrauma*. 2010;27(1):51–64.

25. Perel P, Arango M, Clayton T, et al. Predicting outcome after traumatic brain injury: practical prognostic models based on large cohort of international patients. *BMJ*. 2008;336(7641):425–429.

26. Yeoman P, Pattani H, Silcocks P, Owen V, Fuller G. Validation of the IMPACT outcome prediction score using the Nottingham Head Injury Register dataset. *J Trauma*. 2011;71(2):387–392.

27. Badjatia N, Carney N, Crocco TJ, et al. Guidelines for prehospital management of traumatic brain injury 2nd edition. *Prehosp Emerg Care*. 2008;12 (suppl 1):S1–S52.

28. Haydel MJ. The Canadian CT Head Rule. *Lancet*. 2001;358(9286): 1013–1014.

29. Maharaj I, Tosiello L. The Canadian CT Head Rule. *Lancet*. 2001; 358(9286):1013; author reply 1014.

30. Stiell IG, Lesiuk H, Wells GA, et al. Canadian CT Head Rule study for patients with minor head injury: methodology for phase II (validation and economic analysis). *Ann Emerg Med*. 2001;38(3):317–322.

31. Stiell IG, Lesiuk H, Wells GA, et al. The Canadian CT Head Rule study for patients with minor head injury: rationale, objectives, and methodology for phase I (derivation). *Ann Emerg Med*. 2001; 38(2):160–169.

32. Stiell IG, Wells GA, Vandemheen K, et al. The Canadian CT Head Rule for patients with minor head injury. *Lancet*. 2001;357(9266): 1391–1396.

33. Smits M, Dippel DW, de Haan GG, et al. External validation of the Canadian CT Head Rule and the New Orleans criteria for CT scanning in patients with minor head injury. *JAMA*. 2005;294(12): 1519–1525.

34. Stiell IG, Clement CM, Rowe BH, et al. Comparison of the Canadian CT Head Rule and the New Orleans criteria in patients with minor head injury. *JAMA*. 2005;294(12):1511–1518.

35. Edmonds M. The Canadian CT Head Rule reduced the need for CT scans more than the New Orleans criteria in minor head injury. *Evid Based Med*. 2006;11(2):61.

36. Hassan Z, Smith M, Littlewood S, et al. Head injuries: a study evaluating the impact of the NICE head injury guidelines. *Emerg Med J*. 2005;22(12):845–849.

37. Temkin NR, Dikmen SS, Winn HR. Management of head injury. Posttraumatic seizures. *Neurosurg Clin N Am*. 1991;2(2):425–435.

38. Yablon SA. Posttraumatic seizures. *Arch Phys Med Rehabil*. 1993; 74(9):983–1001.

39. Temkin NR, Dikmen SS, Wilensky AJ, Keihm J, Chabal S, Winn HR. A randomized, double-blind study of phenytoin for the prevention of post-traumatic seizures. *N Engl J Med*. 1990;323(8): 497–502.

40. Timofeev I, Bazhenov M, Avramescu S, Nita DA. Posttraumatic epilepsy: the roles of synaptic plasticity. *Neuroscientist*. 2010;16(1): 19–27.

41. Vespa PM, McArthur DL, Xu Y, et al. Nonconvulsive seizures after traumatic brain injury are associated with hippocampal atrophy. *Neurology*. 2010;75(9):792–798.

42. Bratton SL, Chestnut RM, Ghajar J, et al. Guidelines for the management of severe traumatic brain injury. XIII. Antiseizure prophylaxis. *J Neurotrauma*. 2007;24(suppl 1):S83–S86.

43. Englander J, Bushnik T, Wright JM, Jamison L, Duong TT. Mortality in late post-traumatic seizures. *J Neurotrauma*. 2009;26(9): 1471–1477.

44. Young B, Rapp RP, Norton JA, Haack D, Tibbs PA, Bean JR. Failure of prophylactically administered phenytoin to prevent late post-traumatic seizures. *J Neurosurg*. 1983;58(2):236–241.

45. Temkin NR, Dikmen SS, Anderson GD, et al. Valproate therapy for prevention of posttraumatic seizures: a randomized trial. *J Neurosurg*. 1999;91(4):593–600.

46. Szaflarski JP, Sangha KS, Lindsell CJ, Shutter LA. Prospective, randomized, single-blinded comparative trial of intravenous levetiracetam versus phenytoin for seizure prophylaxis. *Neurocrit Care*. 2010;12(2):165–172.

47. Jones KE, Puccio AM, Harshman KJ, et al. Levetiracetam versus phenytoin for seizure prophylaxis in severe traumatic brain injury. *Neurosurg Focus*. 2008;25(4):E3.

48. Ronne-Engstrom E, Winkler T. Continuous EEG monitoring in patients with traumatic brain injury reveals a high incidence of epileptiform activity. *Acta Neurol Scand*. 2006;114(1):47–53.

49. Vespa PM, Miller C, McArthur D, et al. Nonconvulsive electrographic seizures after traumatic brain injury result in a delayed, prolonged increase in intracranial pressure and metabolic crisis. *Crit Care Med*. 2007;35(12):2830–2836.

50. Jiang JY. Clinical study of mild hypothermia treatment for severe traumatic brain injury. *J Neurotrauma*. 2009;26(3):399–406.

51. Atkins CM, Truettner JS, Lotocki G, et al. Post-traumatic seizure susceptibility is attenuated by hypothermia therapy. *Eur J Neurosci*. 2010;32(11):1912–1920; doi:10.1111/j.1460-9568.2010.07467.x.

52. Feng JF, Zhang KM, Jiang JY, Gao GY, Fu X, Liang YM. Effect of therapeutic mild hypothermia on the genomics of the hippocampus after moderate traumatic brain injury in rats. *Neurosurgery*. 2010;67(3):730–742.

53. Clifton GL, Miller ER, Choi SC, et al. Lack of effect of induction of hypothermia after acute brain injury. *N Engl J Med*. 2001;344(8): 556–563.

54. Clifton GL, Valadka A, Zygun D, et al. Very early hypothermia induction in patients with severe brain injury (the National Acute Brain Injury Study: hypothermia II): a randomised trial. *Lancet Neurol*. 2011;10(2):131–139.

55. Jiang JY, Xu W, Li WP, et al. Effect of long-term mild hypothermia or short-term mild hypothermia on outcome of patients with severe traumatic brain injury. *J Cereb Blood Flow Metab*. 2006;26(6):771–776.

56. Aibiki M, Maekawa S, Yokono S. Moderate hypothermia improves imbalances of thromboxane A2 and prostaglandin I2 production after traumatic brain injury in humans. *Crit Care Med*. 2000;28(12): 3902–3906.

57. Bratton SL, Chestnut RM, Ghajar J, et al. Guidelines for the management of severe traumatic brain injury. V. Deep vein thrombosis prophylaxis. *J Neurotrauma*. 2007;24(suppl 1):S32–S36.

58. Hoth JJ, Franklin GA, Stassen NA, Girard SM, Rodriguez RJ, Rodriguez JL. Prophylactic antibiotics adversely affect nosocomial pneumonia in trauma patients. *J Trauma*. 2003;55(2):249–254.

59. Goodpasture HC, Romig DA, Voth DW. A prospective study of tracheobronchial bacterial flora in acutely brain-injured patients with and without antibiotic prophylaxis. *J Neurosurg*. 1977;47(2): 228–235.

60. Liberati A, D'Amico R, Pifferi S, Torri V, Brazzi L, Parmelli E. Antibiotic prophylaxis to reduce respiratory tract infections and mortality in adults receiving intensive care. *Cochrane Database Syst Rev*. 2009(4).

61. Sugerman HJ, Wolfe L, Pasquale MD, et al. Multicenter, randomized, prospective trial of early tracheostomy. *J Trauma*. 1997;43(5): 741–747.

62. Hsieh AH, Bishop MJ, Kubilis PS, Newell DW, Pierson DJ. Pneumonia following closed head injury. *Am Rev Respir Dis*. 1992;146(2): 290–294.

63. Kaufman HH, Satterwhite T, McConnell BJ, et al. Deep vein thrombosis and pulmonary embolism in head injured patients. *Angiology*. 1983;34(10):627–638.

64. Ekeh AP, Dominguez KM, Markert RJ, McCarthy MC. Incidence and risk factors for deep venous thrombosis after moderate and severe brain injury. *J Trauma*. 2010;68(4):912–915.

65. Scudday T, Brasel K, Webb T, et al. Safety and efficacy of prophylactic anticoagulation in patients with traumatic brain injury. *J Am Coll Surg*. 2011;213(1):148–153.

66. Dudley RR, Aziz I, Bonnici A, et al. Early venous thromboembolic event prophylaxis in traumatic brain injury with low-molecular-weight heparin: risks and benefits. *J Neurotrauma*. 2010;27(12): 2165–2172.

67. Agnelli G, Piovella F, Buoncristiani P, et al. Enoxaparin plus compression stockings compared with compression stockings alone in the prevention of venous thromboembolism after elective neurosurgery. *N Engl J Med*. 1998;339(2):80–85.

68. Deutschman CS, Konstantinides FN, Raup S, Thienprasit P, Cerra FB. Physiological and metabolic response to isolated closed-head injury. Part 1: basal metabolic state: correlations of metabolic and physiological parameters with fasting and stressed controls. *J Neurosurg*. 1986;64(1):89–98.

69. Clifton GL, Robertson CS, Grossman RG, Hodge S, Foltz R, Garza C. The metabolic response to severe head injury. *J Neurosurg*. 1984; 60(4):687–696.

70. Hartl R, Gerber LM, Ni Q, Ghajar J. Effect of early nutrition on deaths due to severe traumatic brain injury. *J Neurosurg.* 2008; 109(1):50–56.

71. Dickerson RN, Mitchell JN, Morgan LM, et al. Disparate response to metoclopramide therapy for gastric feeding intolerance in trauma patients with and without traumatic brain injury. *JPEN J Parenter Enteral Nutr.* 2009;33(6):646–655.

72. Clifton GL, Robertson CS, Choi SC. Assessment of nutritional requirements of head-injured patients. *J Neurosurg.* 1986;64(6): 895–901.

73. Falcão de Arruda IS, de Aguilar-Nascimento JE. Benefits of early enteral nutrition with glutamine and probiotics in brain injury patients. *Clin Sci (Lond).* 2004;106(3):287–292.

74. Cook AM, Peppard A, Magnuson B. Nutrition considerations in traumatic brain injury. *Nutr Clin Pract.* 2009;23(6):608–620.

75. Liu-DeRyke X, Collingridge DS, Orme J, Roller D, Zurasky J, Rhoney DH. Clinical impact of early hyperglycemia during acute phase of traumatic brain injury. *Neurocrit Care.* 2009;11(2):151–157.

76. Young B, Ott L, Kasarskis E, et al. Zinc supplementation is associated with improved neurologic recovery rate and visceral protein levels of patients with severe closed head injury. *J Neurotrauma.* 1996;13(1):25–34.

77. Lindsey KA, Brown RO, Maish GO III, Croce MA, Minard G, Dickerson RN. Influence of traumatic brain injury on potassium and phosphorus homeostasis in critically ill multiple trauma patients. *Nutrition.* 2010;26(7–8):784–790.

78. Panickar KS, Anderson RA. Role of dietary polyphenols in attenuating brain edema and cell swelling in cerebral ischemia. *Recent Pat CNS Drug Discov.* 2010;5(2):99–108.

79. Bullock MR, Chesnut R, Ghajar J, et al. Surgical management of acute epidural hematomas. *Neurosurgery.* 2006;58(3)(suppl):S7–S15; discussion Si–Siv.

80. Bullock MR, Chesnut R, Ghajar J, et al. Surgical management of acute subdural hematomas. *Neurosurgery.* 2006;58(3)(suppl): S16–S24; discussion Si–Siv.

81. Bullock MR, Chesnut R, Ghajar J, et al. Surgical management of posterior fossa mass lesions. *Neurosurgery.* 2006;58(3)(suppl): S47–S55; discussion Si–Siv.

82. Bullock MR, Chesnut R, Ghajar J, et al. Surgical management of traumatic parenchymal lesions. *Neurosurgery.* 2006;58(3)(suppl): S25–S46; discussion Si–Siv.

83. Bullock MR, Chesnut R, Ghajar J, et al. Surgical management of depressed cranial fractures. *Neurosurgery.* 2006;58(3)(suppl): S56–S60; discussion Si–Siv.

84. Surgical management of penetrating brain injury. *J Trauma.* 2001; 51(2)(suppl):S16–S25.

85. Arabi YM, Haddad S, Tamim HM, et al. Mortality reduction after implementing a clinical practice guidelines-based management protocol for severe traumatic brain injury. *J Crit Care.* 2010;25(2): 190–195.

86. Myburgh JA, Cooper DJ, Finfer SR, et al. Epidemiology and 12-month outcomes from traumatic brain injury in Australia and New Zealand. *J Trauma.* 2008;64(4):854–862.

87. Keris V, Lavendelis E, Macane I. Association between implementation of clinical practice guidelines and outcome for traumatic brain injury. *World J Surg.* 2007;31(6):1352–1355.

88. Rusnak M, Janciak I, Majdan M, Wilbacher I, Mauritz W. Severe traumatic brain injury in Austria VI: effects of guideline-based management. *Wien Klin Wochenschr.* 2007;119(1–2):64–71.

89. Faul M, Wald MM, Rutland-Brown W, Sullivent EE, Sattin RW. Using a cost-benefit analysis to estimate outcomes of a clinical treatment guideline: testing the Brain Trauma Foundation guidelines for the treatment of severe traumatic brain injury. *J Trauma.* 2007;63(6):1271–1278.

90. Lu J, Marmarou A, Choi S, Maas A, Murray G, Steyerberg EW. Mortality from traumatic brain injury. *Acta Neurochir Suppl.* 2005; 95:281–285.

91. Fakhry SM, Trask AL, Waller MA, Watts DD. Management of brain-injured patients by an evidence-based medicine protocol improves outcomes and decreases hospital charges. *J Trauma.* 2004; 56(3):492–499; discussion 499–500.

92. Vitaz TW, McIlvoy L, Raque GH, Spain D, Shields CB. Development and implementation of a clinical pathway for severe traumatic brain injury. *J Trauma.* 2001;51(2):369–375.

93. Palmer S, Bader MK, Qureshi A, et al. The impact on outcomes in a community hospital setting of using the AANS traumatic brain injury guidelines. Americans Associations for Neurologic Surgeons. *J Trauma.* 2001;50(4):657–664.

94. Vukic M, Negovetic L, Kovac D, Ghajar J, Glavic Z, Gopcevic A. The effect of implementation of guidelines for the management of severe head injury on patient treatment and outcome. *Acta Neurochir (Wien).* 1999;141(11):1203–1208.

95. Ghajar J, Hariri RJ, Narayan RK, Iacono LA, Firlik K, Patterson RH. Survey of critical care management of comatose, head-injured patients in the United States. *Crit Care Med.* 1995;23(3):560–567.

96. Hesdorffer DC, Ghajar J, Iacono L. Predictors of compliance with the evidence-based guidelines for traumatic brain injury care: a survey of United States trauma centers. *J Trauma.* 2002;52(6): 1202–1209.

97. Hesdorffer DC, Ghajar J. Marked improvement in adherence to traumatic brain injury guidelines in United States trauma centers. *J Trauma.* 2007;63(4):841–847; discussion 847–848.

98. Bratton SL, Chestnut RM, Ghajar J, et al. Guidelines for the management of severe traumatic brain injury. I. Blood pressure and oxygenation. *J Neurotrauma.* 2007;24(suppl 1):S7–S13.

99. Bratton SL, Chestnut RM, Ghajar J, et al. Guidelines for the management of severe traumatic brain injury. VI. Indications for intracranial pressure monitoring. *J Neurotrauma.* 2007;24(suppl 1):S37–S44.

100. Bratton SL, Chestnut RM, Ghajar J, et al. Guidelines for the management of severe traumatic brain injury. VII. Intracranial pressure monitoring technology. *J Neurotrauma.* 2007;24(suppl 1): S45–S54.

101. Bratton SL, Chestnut RM, Ghajar J, et al. Guidelines for the management of severe traumatic brain injury. VIII. Intracranial pressure thresholds. *J Neurotrauma.* 2007;24(suppl 1):S55–S58.

102. Bratton SL, Chestnut RM, Ghajar J, et al. Guidelines for the management of severe traumatic brain injury. IX. Cerebral perfusion thresholds. *J Neurotrauma.* 2007;24(suppl 1):S59–S64.

103. Bratton SL, Chestnut RM, Ghajar J, et al. Guidelines for the management of severe traumatic brain injury. X. Brain oxygen monitoring and thresholds. *J Neurotrauma.* 2007;24(suppl 1):S65–S70.

104. Bratton SL, Chestnut RM, Ghajar J, et al. Guidelines for the management of severe traumatic brain injury. II. Hyperosmolar therapy. *J Neurotrauma.* 2007;24(suppl 1):S14–S20.

105. Bratton SL, Chestnut RM, Ghajar J, et al. Guidelines for the management of severe traumatic brain injury. XIV. Hyperventilation. *J Neurotrauma.* 2007;24(suppl 1):S87–S90.

106. Bratton SL, Chestnut RM, Ghajar J, et al. Guidelines for the management of severe traumatic brain injury. XI. Anesthetics, analgesics, and sedatives. *J Neurotrauma.* 2007;24(suppl 1):S71–S76.

107. Bratton SL, Chestnut RM, Ghajar J, et al. Guidelines for the management of severe traumatic brain injury. XV. Steroids. *J Neurotrauma.* 2007;24(suppl 1):S91–S95.

108. Narotam PK, Morrison JF, Nathoo N. Brain tissue oxygen monitoring in traumatic brain injury and major trauma: outcome analysis of a brain tissue oxygen-directed therapy. *J Neurosurg.* 2009;111(4): 672–682.

109. Reinstrup P, Ståhl N, Mellergård P, Uski T, Ungerstedt U, Nordström CH. Intracerebral microdialysis in clinical practice: baseline values for chemical markers during wakefulness, anesthesia, and neurosurgery. *Neurosurgery.* 2000;47(3):701–709; discussion 709–710.

110. Timofeev I, Carpenter KL, Nortje J, et al. Cerebral extracellular chemistry and outcome following traumatic brain injury: a microdialysis study of 223 patients. *Brain.* 2011;134(pt 2):484–494.

111. Hartings JA, Strong AJ, Fabricius M, et al. Spreading depolarizations and late secondary insults after traumatic brain injury. *J Neurotrauma.* 2009;26(11):1857–1866.

26

Acute Rehabilitation

Cindy B. Ivanhoe, Ana Durand-Sanchez, and Eric T. Spier

INTRODUCTION

The purpose of rehabilitation in general is to allow the individual with a brain injury to progress and evolve to the best of his or her functional potential. For this to occur, the rehabilitation process should begin early and be goal directed. If one comes from the perspective that there will be recovery, to whatever degree, there are clinical considerations that will allow a greater degree of recovery and a lesser degree of avoidable complications and discomfort. Unfortunately, there are many biases and variables that affect outcome. If the treating team has a negative view of potential recovery, there may be fewer options considered for the patient. If there is a more positive perspective of what is possible, patients may be offered more opportunities to achieve goals. There is evidence that the time it takes to access rehabilitation following brain injury materially affects cost and outcome. Access within the first 6 months of injury affects rate of recovery and the degree of supervision following discharge (1). The flow of patients through the brain injury continuum of care can include the neurosurgical intensive care unit (NICU) or shock trauma unit, neurology or trauma floor, acute rehabilitation, nursing home, skilled nursing facility, long-term acute care, outpatient therapy, home health, day programs, residential rehabilitation, and residential placement (see Table 26-1. Also, see Chapter 1 for further details).

Factors that influence when and where a patient goes include a combination of medical stability, available services and facilities, insurance contracts and funding, family, and timing. In the extremely acute setting, the concerns are focused on keeping the patient alive and on stabilization. In the rehabilitation setting, the focus or goals gradually shift toward how those initial goals translate into short- and long-term function. Nonetheless, the medical issues are intimately intertwined with the "rehabilitation" issues.

TEAM APPROACH

No matter where the patient falls in the continuum of care, no one individual clinician may have all the information necessary to make well-informed prognostic and treatment decisions. A team is necessary; ideally a well-informed, communicating group of professionals who all add valuable information about the patient's plan of care. The composition of that team will vary with the level of care, institution, specialization, and location. In the acute neurosurgical setting, it will generally include the treating physicians, nurses, case manager for the facility and insurance company (at times), social worker, occupational, physical, and speech and language therapists. Neuropsychology/psychology, music therapy, art, pets, and others can be more active in the treatment program once the brain injury survivor is in the acute rehabilitation setting. Depending on each patient's situation, vision specialists, behaviorists, orthopedists, and other medical subspecialists may participate in the care.

THE ACUTE NEUROTRAUMA SETTING

There is a need and benefit to establishing a trajectory of care as early as the NICU. Risks to a patient that can derail care start at the moment of impact. In the context of moderate and severe traumatic brain injury (TBI), regardless of the nature of injury, the crisis to a patient and their entire social structure may reverberate for a lifetime. Physical and cognitive recovery, as well as psychosocial needs, can be better addressed if familiarity with a patient's injury and social structure is initiated from the start of critical care treatment.

Many of the acute medical needs such as syndrome of inappropriate antidiuretic hormone secretion (SIADH), cerebral salt wasting (CSW), elevated intracranial pressure (ICP), and other acute issues are managed mainly by the primary medical team until the patient is in an acute rehabilitation setting (see Chapter 22 and 23). In addition to medical and surgical considerations, the slope of family education about brain injury is steep and the impact of individual social situation is considerable. The goal of acute care is to keep the patient alive and minimize mortality. Morbidity-related issues such as skin breakdown, bowel and bladder management, and pain are often overlooked, and as a result, they impact outcome months or years after the date of injury. This is evidenced by the frequent need for eventual tendon lengthenings, bowel disimpactions, and pressure sore management. Early physiatric or neurorehabilitative management can limit the morbidity associated with brain injury. In the acute setting, rehabilitative goals include preparation for the next level of care and, potentially, long-term considerations. A setting where the patient is confused and medically unstable is a setting in which to evaluate and establish a plan of care, at times, addressing prognosis. Family education is an important part of rehabilitation and cannot begin too early. Families have questions about prognosis—a prognosis

TABLE 26-1 Brain Injury Rehabilitation Continuum of Care[a]

Acute hospital (ICU, ward)

Acute rehabilitation

Postacute residential

Brain injury rehabilitation day program

Outpatient individual therapy (PT, OT, ST, NP)

Home health therapy (PT, OT, ST)

Long-term acute care (LTAC)

Skilled nursing facility (SNF)

Nursing home (NH)

Abbreviations: ICU, intensive care unit; OT, occupational therapy; ST, speech therapy; NP, neuroprotective therapy.

[a]Multiple factors will affect the order, time, or necessity of any of these locations.

they often cannot imagine. All need to understand the interplay of medical, behavioral, and cognitive deficits and how they evolve. They need to understand the ins and outs of their medical coverage and how to best manage the benefits and programs available to their loved one, in the short- and long-term. The sooner this education process begins, the more manageable the situation becomes for them.

Intensive Care Unit Setting

In an intensive care unit (ICU) setting, early rehabilitative efforts should be directed towards limiting morbidity across organ systems. For the respiratory system, this will frequently mean tracheostomy and, preferably, scheduled breathing treatments because it is the unusual patient at this stage who can request a breathing treatment when feeling short of breath. The same will be true in the rehabilitation setting. Patients need to be turned regularly to prevent skin breakdown, limit contractures, and decrease abnormal postures. This may become difficult depending on the lines and cables of monitoring equipment. Bowel and bladder function and nutritional needs should be monitored and managed. From the cardiovascular standpoint, blood pressure, pulse, and autonomic storming may all be intertwined with these other physiologic functions.

Dysautonomia, also referred to as paroxysmal sympathetic hyperactivity (PSH) or paroxysmal autonomic instability with dystonia (PAID), occurs in less than one-fifth of patients, with a greater incidence among younger patients and those with lower Glasgow Coma Scale (GCS) score. Associated factors are deep lesions on cranial magnetic resonance imaging (MRI), longer ICU stays, and worse outcomes. Diencephalic-mesencephalic dysfunction or disconnection has been mentioned as a possible pathophysiologic mechanism (2) (see Chapter 11). Dysautonomia may be precipitated by constipation, urinary retention, or deep venous thrombosis (DVT) (the risks of which should be weighed against the risks of anticoagulation). See Chapter 52 for a detailed discussion of autonomic dysfunction.

The psychosocial groundwork begins in the acute ICU setting. Family members are generally the primary decision makers and are also the ones experiencing the greatest emotional trauma. They will have memories of the experience that the injured party most likely never will. Time spent educating family members early on can help them through the grieving and decision-making processes. Trust can be established, facilitating understanding and decisions later on the course of care. Ideally, families can glean information from a care provider who will potentially bridge at least parts of the continuum of care. A patient will sometimes need alternative placement prior to acute rehabilitation, and creating a plan early on may minimize patients being lost to follow-up and a cascade of undue complications.

Services, including medical, emotional, and physical, must be provided when the patient is ready, and that timing is key to recovery and to the experience of recovery. In considering medical interventions and the timing of their execution, physiatrists and neurologists familiar with neurorehabilitation can help orchestrate decisions to best facilitate recovery. Most of the recommendations are meant to help minimize future complications that interfere with care or facilitate a more independent recovery.

Gastrostomy tubes and jejunal tubes (percutaneous endoscopic gastrostomy [PEG]/percutaneous endoscopic jejunostomy [PEJ]) are often placed at the same time tracheostomies are performed. Patients may not yet have the alertness or cognition to begin swallowing evaluations. Sedating medications, impaired cognition, tracheostomy tubes, and even primitive reflexes can complicate swallowing efforts. Timing of gastrostomy tube placement should be weighed against timing of anticipated recovery and severity of injury. Having the tube placed earlier can decrease the risk of sinusitis from nasogastric tubes and may allow for earlier removal relative to the recovery (see Chapter 54).

For bladder management, a Foley catheter is best maintained while a close eye on input and output is vital. Intermittent catheterization can be done in place of using a Foley catheter, but is usually unrealistic in the acute setting. Urinary accidents and turning schedules can become difficult in patients with increased risk for skin breakdown. Condom catheters do not address the potential of underlying retention, postobstructive renal insufficiency, and bladder dysfunction. In the rehabilitation setting, the approach will change (see Chapter 50).

Skin is a carefully managed issue in most ICU settings; however, it cannot be overly stressed given the negative sequelae that can result from skin breakdown. Patients are likely to have multiple lines, surgical sites, intracranial monitors, chest tubes, and respiratory support. With a multitude of equipment and lines in place, minimizing movement and agitation is critical (3).

Frequent shifting is always best included as a standing order in patients with little or no movement; they should be shifted every 2 hours as a minimum from back, to side, and to another side (4). There are also many different trauma beds available such as rotating, beaded, and prone. Some of these create background noise and lack of support for positioning techniques and transfers but may be necessary initially depending on the other injuries sustained and staffing considerations. Unfortunately, it is not unusual for patients to transfer to a rehabilitation setting with unrecognized pressure sores, particularly in the sacral, gluteal, and occipital regions (5) (see Chapter 49).

Secondary injuries may be overlooked early in the patient's triage secondary to more pressing issues of neurosurgical considerations, major bone fractures, intra-abdominal injury, electrolytes issues, and cardiopulmonary failure. Ongoing vigilance of undetected injury may explain why a patient is not progressing with rehabilitative efforts in spite of providing appropriate interventions. Autonomic storming warrants mentioning here, as medical and physical issues may be contributing. Various treatment efforts may be worthy of trial as long as a formalized effort can be defended based on the patients' needs and underlying deficits. Pharmacologic agents often considered include beta-blockers, which may affect cognition because they can cross the blood–brain barrier, but early in rehabilitation that may be of benefit to minimize risk to the patient in a medically unstable environment (6,7). Patients in an ICU setting are limited in their mobility for many reasons including, among others, a lower level of consciousness, spasticity, and paresis. If efforts to maintain range of motion (ROM) through all joints are not continued, their mobility may be affected, secondary to rheological changes. Efforts to maintain good joint mobility not only result in better long-term outcomes (8) but can also minimize time and resources spent to reverse the lost range. Such efforts are commonly initiated in the rehabilitative setting because of contractures and muscle tightness. Some of the more common examples include loss of ankle dorsiflexion, knee flexion, and hip extension needed to ambulate. Care should also be taken in the casting or splinting of patients in positions that will preserve function, limiting contractures. Education can be done with family to initiate frequent ROM exercises with the patient to avoid a poor outcome and maximize time spent in rehabilitation. This also allows them to feel like they are involved in the patient's care.

An additional indication for neurorehabilitation monitoring in the acute care setting includes the collection of useful prognostic and treatment data. Secondary injuries such as anoxia, hypoxia, infection, and elevated ICP may be overlooked in the record but play a significant role, impacting the patient's recovery and prognosis. Such information may also be useful when the time comes for neuropsychological testing. An iatrogenic anoxic or hypoxic injury (because of hypotension or increased ICP) may exacerbate an underlying TBI but be "lost" in the record. This secondary injury may worsen outcome but may also help to explain why the course of recovery is altered. This outcome can be obviated if known to the treating team through close monitoring in the acute setting (see Chapter 23).

Pharmacologic Considerations in the Acute Hospital and Rehabilitation Setting

The neurorehabilitation approach to patient management generally takes into consideration the goals of treatment and ideally, the cognitive and behavior deficits of the individual. Neuropharmacologic management is no different. Goals should include medical stability, pain management, improved arousal, alertness and participation, decreased caregiver burden, decreased lability, improved cooperation and mood, and improved sleep. There is an array of medications that can affect an obtunded or confused patient with brain injury while still in the acute neurotrauma setting or in reha-

bilitation (see Appendix II). Although some can, and should, be removed to simplify the neuropharmacological regimen and allow improved cognition, others may still be necessary (this is further discussed in Chapters 72–74). Basic tenets of medication management acknowledge that these patients may be more susceptible to the side effects of pharmacologic interventions (9). Medications can impact recovery, complications, and the duration of time needed to recover from a confused state. Pain is a powerful distractor; analgesics should be given at the lowest dose necessary, but scheduled, because a confused patient with brain injury will not solve how long it has been since the last dose or how to ask for pain management (10). Nonsteroidal anti-inflammatories are inexpensive and useful, provided no contraindications are present. They are also not sedating. Patients may not be able to communicate their need for analgesia effectively, often presenting as agitated or uncooperative. If the need for analgesia is obvious, then the delay has been unnecessarily prolonged. Scheduling medications or using lower doses of long-acting medications can minimize side effects, discomfort, agitation, and storming. Avoid medications that have a tendency to cause extrapyramidal side-effects such as high-potency antipsychotics (such as as haloperidol and seroquel), as well as medications such as metoclopramide and phenergan (11). Some sedating medications are critical in the ICU setting to control seizures, minimize storming, and quell agitation; however, bear in mind that sedating medications prolong confusion and can thwart the rehabilitative and recovery process. Neuropharmacologic management will change frequently in the first few months of care as patients' needs change. Knowing what improvements have occurred can be difficult because of natural recovery, medical management, and/or rehabilitation interventions.

Reestablishment of sleep–wake cycles is always a safe and important place to start early in recovery. In a rehabilitative setting, time spent participating in therapy is most productive if the patient is maximally awake and rested. Medications for sleep should not be sedating during the day or leave a "hangover effect." Minimizing sedating medications during the day may also be helpful. Stimulating medications during the day can help with alertness and attention. Examples include bromocriptine, amantadine, modafinil, methylphenidate, methamphetamine, and amphetamine. Increased activity during the day can also impact the quality and quantity of sleep at night (see Chapter 43). Antidepressants such as selective serotonin reuptake inhibitors (SSRIs) and selective norepinephrine reuptake inhibitors (SNRIs) are also "activating" and can assist with behavior management. There is often a blurry line between the contributions of mood, sleep, focus, and all other neurobehavioral characteristics noted in *Brain Injury Medicine*. The tendency to add medications rather than simplify the medication regimen should be monitored. Agitation can be a manifestation of internal discomfort that should be sought out. Some examples of this include pain, confusion, fatigue, and frustration (12). Whenever possible, clinicians should be considering the short- and long-term management of their patients and how their current interventions will affect postdischarge management. For example, it is best to limit the amount of medications that will need to be administered multiple times a day because this adds a burden for caregivers and risks for those with memory issues who may not remember to take their

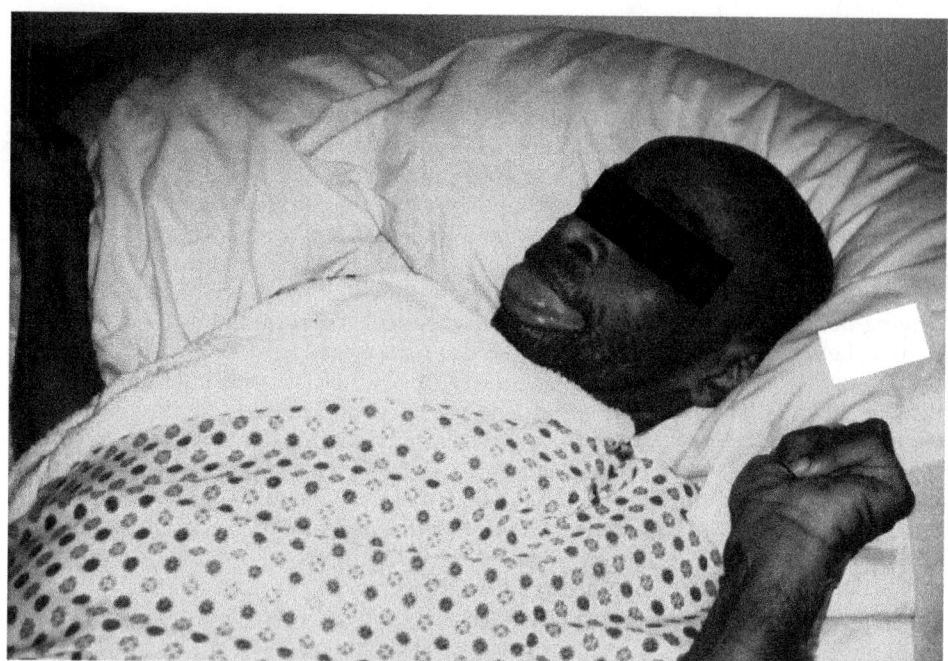

FIGURE 26-1 Acute dystonic reaction after a 2-week treatment with haloperidol for behavior in previously ambulatory patient. Reaction did not resolve after discontinuation of medication.

medications once they are out of the structured hospital setting. Long-term risks of medications should be considered, bearing in mind that this patient population is particularly susceptible to neurologic side effects. Neuroleptics, whether typical or second generation (atypical), carry a high risk of tardive movement disorders and a host of other side effects (12) (See Figure 26-1). Evidence does not bear out that second generation antipsychotics cause fewer motor side effects than the older drugs (13). Also see Chapters 72–74.

COGNITIVE–BEHAVIORAL ISSUES IN ACUTE REHABILITATION

In survivors of brain injury, behavior, cognition, and mood are all intertwined throughout the rehabilitation process and in life. Part of the art to their management is teasing out what the problems are and how to address them. Starting with regulation of pain and sleep is most practical because these have significant influence on behavior and mood. Even empirical treatment of sleep disturbances is better than having sedated, fatigued patients in the rehabilitation setting. Managing medical issues that contribute to the patient's sensation of internal discomfort is vital. Hypoxia, for example, can present with anxiety or a sense of dread. Discomfort from vaginal infections or urinary tract infections (UTIs) can lead to psychomotor agitation in a person who does not understand his or her situation or cannot express her or his needs.

The ever-evolving behavioral and cognitive changes in the patient with acute brain injury are intimately tied to his or her physical, medical, cognitive, and pharmacologic management. There are a host of potential behaviors and cognitive considerations that patients may exhibit (see Table 26-2). For example, a patient with aphasia who cannot ambulate to the bathroom may manifest what clinicians consider "agitation." The treatment for her agitation is assistance to the restroom, not restraints and antipsychotics. Brain injury care

providers need to step outside of a paradigm of judgment; to look from the perspective as the patient's advocate.

Cognitive deficits are not necessarily obvious when a patient is not speaking or interacting consistently. Once they display more behavior and more cognition, outsiders may think that the patient has actually declined, because there is more impaired behavior and impaired cognition to interpret. This can be alarming to families as well as to staff.

Ideally, behavior issues are managed behaviorally within the constraints of staffing. Possible medical causes should be assessed and addressed. Although difficult, staff dealing with patients with brain injury needs to remember that behaviors are usually more reactive than proactive at this level of care. Creating a calming or at least a less annoying environment can create a calmer patient. One-to-one supervision is ideal but expensive. Nonetheless, it can provide a less disruptive means of protecting the patient and others. A consistent caregiver can provide the patient with a sense of security and the caregiver can learn to read the patient's behavioral cues. Behavior plans are useful for the patient, family, and staff to create a consistent manner of dealing with a targeted behavior and calming all concerned. Objective measures may be of use to monitor effectiveness but they may not realistically be obtainable in a hospital setting. The realities of staffing can make behavior plans challenging because consistency is necessary across shifts and visitors. The premorbid family history and patient history are also important to consider. The patient with a possible psychiatric or substance abuse history may respond differently from a patient with a less complicated background (15).

Many considerations can contribute to resistance to participation in the rehabilitation program. The individual may not recognize their deficits, such as when anosognosia is present. Patients may not understand where they are or why, particularly when they are still in post-traumatic amnesia (PTA). Fear and anxiety may be limiting their participation, as may pain. Some patients described as "resisting" therapy

TABLE 26-2 Common Cognitive and Behavioral Considerations in the Acute Rehabilitation Setting

BEHAVIOR/MOOD/COGNITIVE DEFICIT	DEFINITION
Aggression	Hostile or violent attitudes or actions toward another.
Akathisia	Motor restlessness ranging from anxiety to inability to sit quietly or to sleep.
Anhedonia	Absence of pleasure or inability to experience it.
Anxiety	A feeling of worry, nervousness, or unease.
Apathy	Lack of emotion or feeling; lack of concern.
Aphasia	Partial or total loss of the ability to communicate. Includes 1 or a combination of verbal, written, or other types of communication.
Apraxia	Difficulty controlling fine and gross motor movement and gestures (may affect limbs or speech).
Aprosody	Lack of variations of normal speech characteristics.
Confabulation	Unconsciously attempting to fill memory gaps by fabricating information or details that one accepts as facts.
Confusion	Lack of understanding, uncertainty, disturbed orientation.
Cooperation	Willingness to assist and comply with requests.
Depression	Loss of interest or pleasure, guilt, or low self-worth with low energy. Changes in sleep, appetite, or concentration (impaired learning may appear to affect memory).
Dysthymia	A mood disorder characterized by chronic symptoms of mild to moderate depression.
Emotional lability or incontinence	Neurologic disorder characterized by involuntary episodes of crying and/or laughing or other emotional displays. Also called labile or pseudobulbar affect.
Frustration	Disappointment. Sense or state of insecurity and dissatisfaction.
Impersistence	Inability to sustain an action (usually a movement) despite understanding and trying to obey a command to repeat it.
Impulsivity	To act on impulse rather than thought.
Lack of behavior	Deficiency or absence of action, reaction, or conduct.
Lack of insight	Inability to discern or understand the nature of a situation, person, or thing.
Memory deficits	Decreased ability to retain and recall past information or experience.
Motor negativism; gegenhalten	Involuntary "resistance" to passive movement that results in movement in the opposite direction. It is related to motor apraxia.
Neglect	Decrease or absence of attention.
Perseveration	Uncontrollable repetition of a particular response: movement, thought, word, or gesture.
Poor judgment	Decreased ability to make considered decisions or come to sensible conclusions/opinions.
Poor self-awareness	The inability to acknowledge one's strengths and limitations in particular impairment and its implications (14).
Vegetative state	Characterized by the presence of sleep–wake cycles or consistent eye opening without awareness of self or the environment.

are actually displaying motor negativism or gegenhalten related to apraxia. Depression or just dysthymia are worth treating. One need not be clinically depressed or suicidal to benefit from the use of SSRIs or SNRIs. Sleep, mood, focus, behavior, and cognitive and physical endurance are interdependent. Understanding these issues is imperative to creating an environment that fosters patient participation and progress. Medications used should be those that allow improved endurance and understanding, and decrease pain without causing further cognitive impairment (16). Dopaminergics such as amantadine and bromocriptine have been suggested to help with aphasia, as have other stimulants. Supporting literature tends to involve extremely small numbers of subjects (15,17,18).

Antidepressants have been shown to improve physical recovery in poststroke patients whether depression is present or not (19). It is important to realize that patients' cognition and behavior may present as the manifestation of multiple interacting neurotransmitters, premorbid brains, personalities, social behaviors, situation, religious beliefs, hormonal dysfunction, and substance use and abuse. Time of treatment following injury is also a significant factor (12,15,20). Aside from the medical management, behavioral interventions are the foundation for dealing with patients with TBI. Ideally, environmental management should include providing a calming, nonconfrontational setting (see Chapters 62–64). Patients' reactions are generally not personal. Staff and family need to remember that inappropriate, hostile, or aggressive behaviors are more reactive than proactive, even if it is not clear what the reaction is for. The responsibility of the health care professional is to figure out the cause. The patient who is aggressive from discomfort from a cast needs the cast loosened or analgesics. Sedation does not address the underlying issue, although it may be temporarily useful. Familiar staff and caregivers can provide comfort, even if the patient is in PTA (21). The care provider learns to read the needs of the patient as the patient learns to recognize the care provider. This is often difficult to accomplish depending on staffing considerations and more responsibility has fallen on friends and family in recent years. Tracking of standardized measures such as the Galveston Orientation and Amnesia Test (GOAT), neurobehavioral measures such as the Overt Aggression Scale (OAS), as well as functional measures such as the Canadian Neurological Scale-Revised (CNS-R), in conjunction with assessments of trained staff, can help with determining prognosis and guiding medication prescription decisions. Environmental adjustments, such as net beds for fall risks, modular beds with larger mattress and walls around them, or mattresses on the floor, are less confining. Placing a belt on a patient in a wheelchair may be necessary for the patient's safety. However, there comes a point where a wheelchair should not be used as a restraining device to make up for staff shortages and/or concerns. The primary philosophical tenants of TBI neurorehabilitation are to optimize patients' function and facilitate neurorecovery. If a patient is increasingly ambulatory, it is counterintuitive to hold them back. Additionally, a mobile patient strapped to a wheelchair can become a safety hazard. Abdominal binders can be donned to prevent an agitated or confused patient from removing his or her gastrostomy tubes. Padded mittens can make it difficult to decannulate oneself.

Medication selection is ideally limited to a minimum of medications rather than layering of 1 drug on top of another. Often, weaning of medications has a strong positive impact on functional recovery. Determining what is being targeted is important: Is the problem related to decreased attention, focus, and organization, or is a mood disorder at the root of the problem? Which neurotransmitter systems might benefit from manipulation? SSRIs and SNRIs are all useful at times with alertness, interaction, and mood. Each one has its own set of potential considerations, side effects, and interactions. SSRIs have been demonstrated to help with aphasia. Aphasia can also be negatively impacted by frustration. A feeling of overstimulation or confusion can magnify frustration. In that scenario, stimulants may be of use when behavioral and environmental modifications are not enough. Although many clinicians may be fearful of placing an agitated patient on a stimulant, they can be useful in increasing attention and focus. They may also have a mild antidepressant effect. Using 1 medication for more than 1 indication is valuable both clinically and financially. An example is venlafaxine, which can be useful for mood, arousal, and neuropathic pain. Dextromethorphan hydrobromide and quinidine sulfate (DMQ or Nuedexta) is an approved combination treatment for pseudobulbar affect (PBA), also known as involuntary emotional expression disorder (IEED) (22). DMQ has been shown to markedly reduce PBA frequency and severity in multiple sclerosis and amyotrophic lateral sclerosis. DMQ's timing and indication for the brain injury population has yet to be established, but there will certainly be clinical scenarios when it may be indicated. However, it is important to realize that in TBI, disorders of affect and lability may also occur with hydrocephalus. Again, in this scenario, the treatment

is shunting; not medication. In the acute setting, patients may be changing regardless of clinical interventions and not always because of them. Neuropharmacologic, like behavioral considerations, require a larger vision of what is causing and contributing to a behavior. Interpretation of behaviors may vary with the situation and comprehension of the interpreter. Longer term management and medication selection for cognitive impairment and neuropsychiatric disturbances are also addressed in Chapters 73 and 74.

MEDICAL COMPLICATIONS IN ACUTE REHABILITATION

Goals in the acute rehabilitation setting begin with management of the medical complications that develop as a result of brain injury (see Appendix I and III). Those who transfer to this setting usually have moderate-to-severe brain injury. There is no organ system that is not affected, from the injury itself, as well as from the complications of immobility. The more severe the injury, the more imperative it becomes to manage said systems. The interplay of behavioral, cognitive, psychosocial, physical, and medical considerations must always be considered. For example, agitation may be a manifestation of pain, hypoxia, fear, discomfort, and a combination of factors. These may be reflected in the individual's behaviors, vital signs, level of cooperation, and facial expression or they may not. Ideally, health care providers must try to anticipate the needs of the individual with brain injury. On arrival to a brain injury rehabilitation setting once the basic history and physical are obtained, steps should be taken to work towards the removal of distracting tubes, decreasing pain, maximizing arousal, and improving sleep. Patients should be reoriented with small amounts of consistent information, so as not to be overwhelmed, overstimulated, and more confused. These are practical considerations that would affect the level of participation of any individual in a therapy program, with brain injury or otherwise. Once someone has sustained a brain injury, his or her level of endurance and reserve is impaired, cognitively, physically, and emotionally. Neuropharmacologically, there are some basic principles that apply. "Start low and go slow" is an expression frequently heard in the brain injury setting; it applies to starting at low doses of medications, as disruption of the blood–brain barrier can often lead to greater sensitivity to side effects. It is ideal to limit the amount of pharmacologic changes made at a time but this must be balanced with the realities of shortened lengths of stay and the need for patients to make significant progress on a weekly basis. Medications that are sedating can impair apparent recovery and interfere with the goals in the rehabilitation setting. It is also important to realize that a medication that is useful at one point in recovery might not be useful or indicated at another point. This is particularly true in the more acute setting, where patients may be changing rapidly, despite or because of their clinicians' best efforts. Targeting and measuring certain behaviors is useful but this is often not feasible. Consider the potential cost of medications and the risk of withdrawal if the patient with impaired memory or overwhelmed family members may be responsible for administration after discharge. Medications may be selected as much for their side effect profile as their primary indications. For instance, dopaminergic agents may help with movement, motor planning, attention, and alertness. They may also cause hypotension. A patient with motor apraxia, cognitive fatigue, and hypertension might reap many benefits from a dopaminergic agent. Pharmacological interventions will continue to play a key role in the acute management of acquired brain injury. Given the diversity of complications associated with brain injury, treatment often requires combinations of medications that make isolating the effect of a single intervention difficult. How pharmacology and other interventions are combined in each individual will vary with presentation, indications, and tolerance. Research into the effects of interventions within different patient groups will allow for more individualized treatment strategies resulting in improved patient outcomes (20).

Discomfort and Pain

Although pain is a consideration in multiple areas of this chapter and textbook (see Chapter 57), it warrants mentioning on its own. Just as someone may over dramatize their pain, in brain injury, one's blunted affect may not subjectively do justice to their degree of suffering (11,23). Additionally, it can be difficult to gauge pain with scales that rely on language and cognition, attention, and memory. Conversely, when someone cannot complain verbally, it is often forgotten that they may be experiencing pain. Pain can manifest as "agitation" or "aggression." For example, a patient may be attempting to get out of bed because they are lying on "road rash" or an excoriated back. They may avoid or limit their participation in therapy when an occult fracture or soft tissue injury is missed. Management in such cases is not neuroleptics or 4-point leather restraints, it is analgesia. In deference to the patient, family, and nursing staff, medications should be scheduled to prevent pain before it becomes unbearable or limiting. This allows for more consistent management and more humane care (24).

Discomfort and pain are powerful distractors. In someone who is cognitively compromised, pain management increases his or her ability to interact, focus, and participate. There is a balance to be struck between sedation and adequate pain management (see Chapters 57 and 58). In the rehabilitation setting, treating pain not only makes the patient feel better, but it can also affect all aspects of their rehabilitation experience. The treatment of pain can affect participation in therapies, rate of functional improvement, sleep, mood, and even blood pressure and pulse. It can be difficult to measure a patient's level of pain or response to treatment in the early stages of rehabilitation because patients may not be able to communicate or even comprehend their own discomfort. It is important to consider, at least the common medical issues that can be seen in this setting (see Table 26-3).

The basic premise of pharmacologic management applies: it is important to avoid sedation and cognitively impairing medications. Ideally, pain can be managed with milder medications such as nonsteroidal anti-inflammatory agents if relative contraindications are managed or monitored. Scheduling medications can limit the pattern of intermittent relief and inconsistent patient assessments.

Antidepressants and antiepileptic agents have a significant role in treating not just the affective signs and symptoms but the pain itself. Chosen appropriately, they can be used

TABLE 26-3 Common Causes of Pain and Discomfort in the Acute Rehabilitation Setting

Neuropathic pain

Complex regional pain syndrome (CRPS)

Occult fracture

Soft tissue injury (i.e., knee, ankle ligaments, shoulder)

Urinary tract infection

Vaginal yeast infection

Constipation

Spasticity

Skin lesions (road rash, pressure sores)

Headache

Visual disturbances

to treat more than 1 issue with 1 medication. For example, in a patient with a seizure disorder, perhaps the anticonvulsant chosen can target the pain as well as seizures (see Chapters 39 and 57). Venlafaxine can address neuropathic pain, mood, and, to variable degrees, arousal and cognition. It might be useful in a scenario where a patient is resistant to participating in their rehabilitation program because of their mood, coupled with pain and/or fatigue.

In cases of severe pain, opioids may be necessary, at least early on. There comes a point where concerns about addiction are secondary to the need for relief; where the ongoing pain is a greater limitation than the potential complications, short- and long-term. Occult fractures, neuropathic pain, visceral considerations, and other medical issues should be sought and addressed. It is important to understand, to the best of the treating team's ability, what the source of pain is and it's implications on the other aspects of care and function.

Respiratory

Although there is often a perception that one's transfer to the rehabilitation setting will be more easily facilitated if the patient does not have a tracheostomy, the reality is that tracheostomies allow for better airway protection, pulmonary hygiene, and, therefore, comfort and safety. Patients with TBI are at risk for aspiration, atelectasis, pneumonia, and pulmonary embolus, in conjunction with whatever potential chest traumas may have occurred. In the rehabilitation setting, the tracheostomy tube can be gradually downsized, allowing improved tolerance of a speaking valve, such as the Passy-Muir valve. Downsizing patients to a smaller tracheostomy tube without a cuff is ideal because it decreases the obstruction to swallowing and the local tissue irritation (which may cause cough). Application of the valve also allows the patient to hear their voicing often inspiring more vocalization. As secretion management and pulmonary hygiene improves, Passey-Muir valves are a good way to progress toward plugging a tracheostomy. If plugging is not tolerated or wheezing is present, albeit intermittent, the patient should undergo endotracheal endoscopy to look for granulation tissue or other causes of partial obstruction (25).

When secretion management is a significant concern that is not improving with oral motor therapy, Robinul or scopolamine may be instituted, particularly in patients who may be aspirating on their own saliva. Many patients with brain injury may experience sedation from the anticholinergic side effects of these medications. Their benefit must be weighed against that potential. If patients are receiving scheduled respiratory treatments, the risk of inspisated secretions is low. These are rarely needed long term, as patients progress with facial exercises, tongue base strengthening, positioning, and generally improved pulmonary hygiene. These medications do have anticholinergic side effects and this must be considered in light of their potential side effects on memory and bladder and bowel function.

Cardiovascular

The signs and symptoms of deconditioning and immobility include tachycardia, hypotension, hypertension, lower extremity edema, and deep venous thrombosis. These signs and symptoms can influence how the person with a brain injury feels, sleeps, participates in therapy, tolerates therapy, and even breathes. Hypotension can be managed through the usual means of applying compression stockings, perhaps an abdominal binder, managing fluid status, nutrition, anemia, and reassessing the need for medications. Some patients will be hypotensive because of medications that were started early in the course of their event which, in itself, may more acutely have caused hypertension and tachycardia. These may no longer be needed. Beta-blockers are frequently used in the acute medical setting but can often be weaned as the acute TBI is more remote. Although some may find this class useful in neurobehavioral situations, the cognitive and hypotensive side effects may be exacerbated in this population. The effect of anemia on endurance should also be factored into someone's rate of progress. Although the acute care facility may be comfortable with the patient who is asymptomatic in bed with hemoglobin of 8, the rehabilitation setting demands more. It is best to avoid the use of as needed antihypertensives that can result in rebound hypertension (e.g., clonidine). Ideally, practitioners should look at what other events or changes present before or simultaneously with the tachycardia, hypotension, or hypertension to be able to pinpoint the possible triggers.

Sleep

Sleep quality is frequently impaired in patients with brain injuries (26) (see Chapter 43). A study comparing controls and patients with brain injury found that 39% of these patients had abnormal sleep studies, 23% had obstructive sleep apnea (OSA), 3% had posttraumatic hypersomnia, 5% had narcolepsy, 7% had periodic limb movements in sleep (PLMS), and 12% had objective excessive daytime sleepiness (27). Although it is not uncommon for a brain injury program to monitor sleep–wake cycles, there are some common sense considerations to bear in mind. No matter what the diagnosis, no one is optimally awake, alert, and cooperative without adequate sleep. Also, understanding a patient's premorbid sleep patterns is important. For example, shift workers may have a particularly difficult time being awake during the day, as opposed to at night. Endocrine and electrolyte disturbances may affect sleep, as does the brain injury and ICU

experience. Other medical complications to consider include pain, hydrocephalus, infection, depression, anxiety, and seizures. Patients with TBI showed increased slow wave sleep and significantly lower levels of evening melatonin production; the latter significantly correlated with rapid eye movement (REM) sleep (26).

A distinction can be drawn between difficulty maintaining sleep and difficulty with sleep initiation. Frequently, both issues coexist and should be considered when selecting a sleep agent. Zolpidem can be helpful for sleep initiation if the patient does not have a hangover effect. Nortriptyline or the extended-release form of zolpidem may be of use when the issue is inability to sustain sleep. Trazodone is a nontricyclic antidepressant that is among the most frequently prescribed sleeping agents following TBI. It decreases sleep latency and increases total sleep time (studies done in patients with depression) (28). Other sleep medication options include ramelteon (a nonbenzodiazepine receptor-modulator option to improve sleep latency) and eszopiclone. Low-dose sedative antidepressants, such as quetiapine or olanzapine, may be used in the treatment of comorbid insomnia (29), but are not without risks of central nervous system (CNS) side effects. Additionally, if a patient is not psychotic, he or she might not need antipsychotics.

The basic neuropharmacologic principles of treating brain injury apply here. Medications that have long-term potential for side effects should be avoided, such as second-generation neuroleptics and those that cause paradoxical agitation (e.g., benzodiazepines) or a daytime hangover (30). Neurorehabilitation practitioners should attempt to help patients out of coma, not prolong it. Interruptions through the course of the night should be limited as much as possible. This can be accomplished by scheduling medication administration, toileting programs, tube feedings, and wound care so as not to be disruptive. Increasing activities during the day helps improve quality and duration of sleep at night. The same can be true of adding daytime stimulants. This may include time up in a wheelchair, which for some is still an endurance-demanding task. Limiting the amount of time the patient spends in bed during the day will gradually assist with the establishment of endurance and improved sleep cycles but must be balanced with the fatigue that accompanies brain injury. Increasing activities during the day helps improve quality and duration of sleep at night. The same can be true of adding daytime stimulants.

OSA, restless leg syndrome (RLS), and PLMS are more frequent than generally suspected (31). These can and should be considered, explored, and treated as contributing factors in patients' irritability, cognitive and physical fatigue, and mood disorders. If the suspicion is high, a trial of a dopaminergic agent such as pramipexole or ropinirole may be warranted, especially because they may help with attention and alertness. Sleep studies provide useful clinical information regarding seizure activity and movement disorders in addition to sleep. The detrimental side effects of sleep deprivation are exaggerated clinically in the setting of brain injury (27,32). These include mood and irritability, arousal, alertness, and physical and cognitive endurance.

Dysautonomia, Spasticity, and Movement Disorders

Dysautonomia, also referred to as paroxysmal sympathetic hyperactivity (PSH), paroxysmal autonomic instability with dystonia (PAID), autonomic instability, and "brain storming," is often seen in the setting of acutely severe TBI (see Chapter 52). Dysautonomia presents with posturing, hyperthermia, hypertension, tachycardia, fever, and diaphoresis. There is also a variable presentation of return of primitive reflexes. Not all acute rehabilitation facilities accept patients in this state because they tend to be more medically complex. Other factors are lack of appropriate licensure by the facility and the comfort level of the treatment team.

Aside from medications, positioning techniques help break up the abnormal muscle tone patterns, contributing to improved ROM, patient and family comfort, and stabilization of cardiovascular parameters. These techniques, taken from Bobath concepts are often best carried out in conjunction with botulinum neurotoxin injections, motor point blocks, and nerve blocks. Intrathecal baclofen (ITB) therapy has been gradually gaining favor in this clinical setting as well. Oral medications suggested in this setting include beta-blockers, morphine, valproic acid, and gabapentin (33,34). These medications may decrease posturing but may not allow as much clinical/prefunctional improvement as ITB therapy. Additionally, they are not as readily titrated and come with a host of side effects that can be counterintuitive to the process of trying to improve alertness.

Dysautonomia, like other aspects of the upper motor neuron syndrome (UMNS), can be exacerbated by infection, pain, or hydrocephalus. In other words, as with spasticity, a noxious stimulus should be sought when it increases. Dysautonomia may also increase as the person with TBI passes through the stages of neurologic recovery. Diarrhea, constipation, UTIs, and pressure sores can easily occur in the more acute setting and contribute to an increase in symptomatology. Medication selection should follow the general principles of *Brain Injury Medicine*. Dopaminergic medications, clonidine, benzodiazepines, beta-blockers, and morphine have been suggested in this setting, as has high-dose gabapentin (33). As with spasticity, contributing factors and noxious stimuli should also be assessed (35). ITB therapy has demonstrated significant utility in this setting, albeit in small studies and in clinical experiences. This can limit the need to use sedating interventions during a potentially beneficial time for rehabilitation (36–39).

Spasticity or the velocity dependent increased resistance to stretch is part of the UMNS. Therefore positive and negative signs accompany it (see Table 26-4). This is further discussed in Chapter 50.

TABLE 26-4 Upper Motor Neuron Syndrome

POSITIVE SIGNS: STEREOTYPIC BEHAVIORS (PREMORBIDLY INHIBITED)	NEGATIVE SIGNS: ABSENCE OF VOLUNTARY MOVEMENT
Athetosis	Loss of motor control
Co-contraction	Incoordination
Dystonia	Hypotonia
Hyperreflexia and clonus	Areflexia
Hypertrophy	Atrophy
Primitive reflexes	Fasciculations
Spasticity	Muscle weakness

Spasticity is often associated with clonus and some patients will come to rehabilitation with a history of "seizures," which was actually clonus noted in the acute setting. This may become a decision point for weaning yet more sedating medications. Oral medications frequently used for the treatment of spasticity include oral baclofen, diazepam, tizanidine, and dantrolene. Some physicians will try benzodiazepines or muscle relaxants (40), although the cognitive side effects are generally not worth the poor functional potential for improvement. None of these have been shown to improve function, and to variable degrees are sedating and not as well tolerated (40). They have been gradually decreasing in use in the brain injury setting, as availability of other interventions has increased. This includes the use of botulinum toxin injections and ITB therapy.

Positioning is a key part of spasticity management no matter what the setting is. If patients are allowed to assume postures created by the UMNS, they will have limited ROM, muscle endurance, and increased heterotopic ossification by the time they are ready to participate more actively in their rehabilitation. Simple techniques starting in the NICU when possible and expanded to other venues can be used to not only limit or prevent unnecessary complications but also allow ongoing progress. The more these complications are avoided, the better the outcome. Serial casting is the best option for restoring ROM (41). Occasionally, joint immobilizers and dynamic splints can also be used. They may be useful when serial casting is not available or for ongoing maintenance of ROM, but skin and nerve integrity must be monitored. It is imperative to be aware of how devices should be applied and ensure that pressure is evenly distributed to avoid injury to nerves and skin. The pain of neuropraxia or skin breakdown can be a source of increased spasticity (42). Chemodenervation with botulinum neurotoxins and neurolysis with phenol or alcohol are options that can be timed appropriately with the clinical changes and disposition in mind (40). Botulinum toxins may be injected to allow for better tolerance of devices, improved head posture, prefunctional weight bearing, bed-positioning techniques, improved speed of movement, and improved ROM (42). Neurolysis with phenol or alcohol either via nerve block or motor point block can be a useful technique to decrease muscle over activity. Nerve blocks can be temporary (i.e., diagnostic) or "permanent" and are useful adjuvants to spasticity management. Their duration of action is variable from 10 days to 28 months (43). Dosing, technique, muscle selection, and injector expertise will affect the outcome from either agent. Additionally, they are not mutually exclusive interventions. These interventions are covered in greater detail in Chapter 50.

Positioning techniques to maintain or establish proper body alignment can have a significant effect on the spread of synergistic postures. These techniques are used to break up abnormal postures such as knee extension and equinovarus. Heat, ultrasound, and cold are often tried, but their effects may not be long lived past the therapy session.

ITB therapy, although not often initiated early after TBI, has significant advantages for the management of spasticity and spastic dystonia. ITB allows for a relative ease of titration without significant sedation and cognitive impairment. Multiple joints can be affected simultaneously, particularly in the lower limbs and trunk. Dynamic changes in hypertonicity can be positively impacted. ITB therapy initiated relatively acutely is more likely than not indicative of the severity of the injury and the impact of tone on progress. Although the original approval of ITB was written for implant 1 year after brain injury, it is not wise to watch patients not progress or lose ROM and potential, waiting for an arbitrary date for intervention. Clinical judgment should be used in the context of working toward the best possible outcome for the patient.

Gastrointestinal

Dysphagia presents in approximately 33% of patients with TBI (< 60% in severe TBI). Patients develop a delay in the oral and/or pharyngeal phase of swallow. The latter is the most common cause of dysphagia and aspiration in this patient group. Patients may also present with pharyngeal weakness because of prolonged intubation. Cognitive or behavioral impairment may further affect a patient's ability to eat regular meal consistencies by mouth (44). Patients should be taught therapeutic and compensatory strategies for the swallowing disorder (45).

The Brain Trauma Foundation Guidelines recommend initiating feeding within 72 hours and reaching full caloric replacement by 1 week after injury (in moderate-to-severe TBI). The caloric target should be 100%–160% of estimated resting metabolic expenditure (although in pharmacologic coma, it may be only 80%) (46). Gastrostomy or jejunal tubes should be considered early in patients expected to have swallow difficulties for more than a few weeks. This increases meal tolerance in the acute phase of recovery, and by week 2–3 after TBI, gastric feedings are usually safe and able to meet nutritional needs (47). Although nutrition is being provided, it should be reassessed frequently with bedside or modified barium swallow (MBS) studies to advance or adjust the patient's route or diet consistency as soon as it is safe (no signs of aspiration). Once oral intake is safe, liquids may be thickened and the consistency of solid foods may be adjusted, usually starting with pureed food for the more severely affected patients. Individuals on thickened liquids are at higher risk of not meeting their fluid requirements and their hydration status should be monitored. Caloric requirements should be reassessed and adjusted to prevent malnutrition or excessive intake. Hypotonic fluids (e.g., free water) should be given as appropriate to the patient's fluid status, bearing in mind that dehydration will also affect bowel regularity. Patients receiving antibiotics may benefit from the addition of lactobacillus, decreasing the incidence of excessively loose stools and perineal excoriation. Certain nutritional supplements may be considered, for example, adding omega-3 fatty acids to the patient's diet as an adjuvant central anti-inflammatory (48).

Injury to the frontal lobes can lead to bowel incontinence or constipation via a potential impact on gastrointestinal reflexes. These include the gastrocolic reflex, parasympathetic defecation reflex, and the intrinsic myenteric reflex. Constipation can also be present because of immobility, poor hydration or diet, and as a side effect of medications. Instituting a bowel management program is important to help with issues like patients having bowel accidents during therapy sessions or becoming irritable because of constipation, distension, and elevated ammonia levels. A combination of timed bowel movements, good hydration, fiber intake, stool softeners, and suppositories can be included in the program as needed to regulate the frequency, quality, and consistency of bowel movements (47,49).

Oral thrush is a common complication after brain injury because of poor hygiene, decreased immune defense, changes in oral pH (fasting, diet modifications), and decreased transit of saliva in patients with mental status changes or dysphagia. Antifungal solutions can be swabbed, swish-and-swallowed if dysphagia allows. Oral fluconazole may be necessary but good oral hygiene must still be provided. Alternative treatments include lemon juice, lemon grass infusion, or gentian violet, used in other countries (50).

Recurrent vomiting may present secondary to the acute inflammatory process after TBI, abnormal neurotransmitter release (serotonin, dopamine, histamine), increased ICP (hydrocephalus, bleed), metabolic derangements, toxicity, side effects of medications, gastritis or esophagitis, changes in taste or smell, vertigo, dizziness, or infections (e.g., meningitis). Adequate treatment will target the cause of emesis (e.g., cerebrospinal fluid [CSF] shunt, electrolyte correction). Symptoms can be palliated with 5-HT$_3$ receptor antagonists (e.g., ondansetron) to disrupt serotonergic transmission at the brainstem structures and affect the peripheral release of serotonin from the gut (51). These should not be used to mask an underlying medical issue that may be as simple as constipation.

Intestinal colonization with *Clostridium difficile* may be present at the time of admission to rehabilitation (prevalence range 16%–66%) and may be inadvertently spread to other patients. Risk factors for *Clostridium difficile* infection include antibiotic exposure, low immune response, proton pump inhibitors (PPIs), prolonged length of stay (LOS) in a health care setting, serious underlying illness, and gastrointestinal surgery. The management of *Clostridium difficile* infection includes antibiotics, probiotics, contact precautions, and immunotherapy in some cases (52,53). Gastrostomy tubes also allow for bolus feedings, which ultimately translates into more effective bowel (and bladder) management. A daily bowel program, or one consistent with premorbid function is best because it is physiologic, minimizes impaction and the need for strong and often irritating laxatives. Impaction can present as liquid stools. Clinicians should explain to caregivers and staff that liquid stooling does not necessarily mean a bowel program is not in order. Additionally, bowel issues can lead to increased irritability, posturing, dysautonomia, and spasticity (54). Also see Chapter 54.

Genitourinary

In the rehabilitation setting, issues of bladder emptying, infection, and plans for the home setting and beyond are addressed in an effort to avoid additional neuro-urologic problems (55). Most patients with brain injury display hyperactive bladder function, urinating small amounts frequently. Urinary retention is often missed in the hospital setting because there is a tendency for families and staff to be satisfied that the patient is urinating without understanding that urinary retention can still be present. Urination may represent only overflow incontinence (55). Foley catheters are most useful when patients present to the rehabilitation setting with pressure sores or a clinical indication for strict monitoring of input and output. Agitated or confused patients will be tempted to remove them themselves. Additionally, they do not allow for bladder training.

Long-term urinary retention is associated with bladder stones, nephrolithiasis, and injury to the upper tracts as well. Polyuria may be associated with endocrine dysfunction as in cerebral salt waisting or diabetes insipidus (DI). This needs to be considered and assessed.

UTIs can present with vomiting, bowel issues, and behavioral issues. From the cognitive perspective, the discomfort of UTI is a significant and common cause of distraction and subtle decline in the rehabilitation setting. Foley catheters are rarely needed in the patient with brain injury because the majority will empty their bladders frequently (56). Anticholinergic medications may not be tolerated from the perspective of fatigue and cognition. Urodynamic studies are particularly useful when there are premorbid urologic issues, whether they were previously identified or not (55). However, the presentation will most likely improve as patients move through the recovery continuum (57). Ideally, patients can begin a timed toileting program to allow them to establish a routine. This can also limit the presence of bladder accidents in unfortunate situations, such as during gait training. When the patient can sit on a commode, even with assistance, this serves as a strong cue to the patient to void and empty. Sitting also is an opportunity to work on trunk stability and transfers. Bladder scanning or straight catheterization can be used to document post-void residual volumes (58).

Heterotopic Ossification and Myositis Ossificans

Heterotopic ossification (HO) is the formation of lamellar bone inside soft-tissue structures. Its incidence following TBI is 11%–73% (59–61) and is more common in women than men post-severe TBI; it is less common in children and elderly patients (61,62). HO often affects the hip, shoulder, elbow, and knee (60,62,63). Bone tissue formation in muscle or myositis ossificans (MO) is post-traumatic in 60%–75% of all cases and more common in adolescents and young adults (62,64,65). MO usually affects the thigh and anterior compartments of the arm (64). It has been suggested that the early presence of centrally released humoral factors following TBI stimulate osteoprogenitors within skeletal muscle (62,66–68). Prostaglandin E_2 may cause periosteal lamellar heterotopic bone formation (60). Other risk factors include tissue hypoxia, sympathetic changes, immobilization, remobilization, and spasticity (60,62,69). HO is clinically relevant in 10%–20% of cases, associated with prolonged coma, mechanical ventilation, surgically treated bone fractures, and autonomic dysregulation (70). Patients present with local heat, a palpable mass, and/or contracture. Erythrocyte sedimentation rate (ESR) may be elevated as a systemic reaction to muscle necrosis (64). Alkaline phosphatase levels may be used as a marker of HO. Complications of HO and MO include nervous or vascular entrapment, joint ankylosis, complex regional pain syndrome (CRPS), osteoporosis, infection, increased spasticity, and pressure ulcers (60,63). HO may be misperceived as accelerated bone healing or metastasis (71). A triple-phase bone scan (TPBS) is the most sensitive modality for early detection (2–4 wks) of HO and to assess its maturity. Its low specificity leads to difficulty in discriminating HO and MO from other inflammatory, traumatic, or degenerative process of the skeleton (62,72,73). Bedside ultrasound is useful to diagnose HO in severe TBI. Power Doppler aids in localization and activity of ossification (73, 74). Radiographic or computed tomography (CT) findings may not appear for 1 month; they can show the pattern of mineralization and help locate the lesion presurgically, whereas TPBS can help determine timing of excision (64). MRI is sensitive for early MO lesions but has low specificity and high cost (73).

Management of HO involves resting the affected joints in functional position during the inflammatory stage, passive ROM, and mobilization. Indomethacin and radiation therapy are appropriate for prophylaxis or early treatment, although radiation with or without excision has been associated with a risk of late sarcoma. Anti-inflammatories suppress mesenchymal cell proliferation but increase the risk of anticoagulation, dyspepsia, and delayed fracture healing. Bisphosphonates are prophylactic if initiated shortly after trauma but mineralization of the bone matrix resumes after drug discontinuation (60,72). If lesions progress (e.g., decreased ROM that impairs function, neurovascular entrapment, or impingement), surgery is indicated. Surgery is often delayed for 12–18 months, awaiting radiographic evidence of maturation and maximal neurological recovery. HO has low recurrence rates in appropriately selected patients, but small studies have suggested the rate of recurrence is not affected by its maturity and that recurrence may be more common in late resection (59,72,75). Therefore, in cases of severe pain or progressive functional limitations, earlier excision can be considered.

The Hemiplegic Shoulder

The management of the hemiplegic shoulder is a common clinical dilemma in rehabilitation. Shoulder issues can affect recovery of function and be accompanied by severe pain and immobility. Pain related to the hemiplegic shoulder can contribute to behavioral issues, distractibility, and limit progress. Impingement usually presents with pain in the shoulder or scapular area. Traumatic lesions, including traction and direct closed injuries, can be treated operatively or nonoperatively depending on the exact issue and extent. Compressive lesions (e.g., suprascapular notch impingement) have the best improvement with surgical decompression (76). This is not common in the acute rehabilitation following TBI. Peripheral nerve injuries can also accompany upper extremity fractures (77). Malpositioning of the shoulder can lead to tremendous pain and limited progress in the use of the upper limb in activities of daily living. Positioning should be monitored so that patients are not lying on the plegic side. Positioning should be performed with an eye toward potential function.

In general, neurologic injuries to the brain can create an initial weakness that, because of the anatomic characteristics of the glenohumeral joint, lead to subluxation of the humeral head and downward, lateral rotation of the scapula. Care should be taken in therapies and with passive positioning to protect the muscles, ligaments, blood vessels, nerves, and joint capsule, positioning them anatomically. As the process continues and weakness and spasticity develop, there is increased restriction and difficulty with alignment in proper posture (78). The scapula cannot glide and the cycle of pain gains momentum. This creates further pain and disability.

When attempting to get improved shoulder function and decrease pain, positioning of scapula and neck are important to avoid shoulder pain (e.g., myofascial) and contractures. It is important to maintain adequate posture whether the patient is in or out of bed. The neck should be aligned with the midline and patients may benefit from a 1–2 inch hemicylindrical pillow/support in the cervical area while supine. The shoulders can be placed in neutral position; when a patient is developing muscle hypertonicity, shoulders can be positioned in slight abduction, but internal rotation should be avoided as much as possible. Myofascial work and mobilizations should be included in the therapy program. Neck posture also impacts shoulder positioning. Botulinum toxin injections can be useful in facilitating positioning with the longer range intent of improved function. Positioning of the arm in the wheelchair should also be directed toward a healthy, "normal" position. This implies not allowing a paretic limb to dangle, positioning to decrease abnormal tone and synergy as well as elevating the hand when edema is present. Aside from the potential effects of missed upper extremity fractures and nerve injuries, the hemiplegic shoulder, no matter what stage of recovery (be it hypotonic, spastic, dystonic, or synergistic), is associated with different mechanisms leading to pain (78).

Complex Regional Pain Syndrome

Previously known as reflex sympathetic dystrophy, CRPS can be triggered by peripheral or CNS trauma, inflammation, hypoxic changes, neurogenic inflammation, and sympathetic dysregulation (79). CRPS, also addressed in Chapter 57 of this book, presents as localized autonomic dysregulation in the affected area with vasomotor and/or sudomotor changes, temperature changes, edema, color difference, sweating, and/or atrophy (80,81). Reorganization of central motor circuits with an increased activation of primary and supplementary motor area (SMA) may contribute to motor symptoms in CRPS (81). TPBS can be used as a diagnostic tool in the early stage (within 6 weeks) because it may show minimal uptake in all phases in up to 90% of patients with CRPS. However, up to 75% of patients without CRPS may show similar results. A follow-up TPBS in the range of 2–20 weeks may show moderately increased uptake for 78%, 83%, and 83%, respectively in the 3 phases of patients with CRPS, and only 16% of the patients without CRPS (80). Most of the time, the diagnosis can be made clinically.

Management consists of physical and occupational therapy and pharmacologic management, often with pulsed steroids, beta-blockers, or anticonvulsants. Sympathetic block is the interventional treatment of first choice. Stellate ganglion block in the upper extremity is diagnostic as well as therapeutic (82). This may be the most effective and timely way to treat CRPS, particularly in the acute rehabilitation setting. Radiofrequency denervation after positive diagnostic block is documented, can also be of use although tends to occur later in the course (82). It is important to note that CRPS can also be seen in the lower limb.

Fractures are occasionally missed because of the multiple trauma and changes in mental status inherent to the patient with TBI. Hypertrophic callus, MO, and HO occur frequently and can be misperceived as accelerated healing (77). These findings may be suspected when there is firm feeling at the end of ROM or a palpable bony prominence.

Neurosurgical/Neurologic Considerations

The late neurosurgical complications of TBI are covered in greater detail in Chapter 44. It is imperative that those caring for these patients in the rehabilitation setting are cognoscente of the presentations and implications of these conditions. Communicating hydrocephalus is perhaps the most common "late" neurosurgical consideration after TBI. The incidence of symptomatic post-traumatic hydrocephalus (PTH) ranges from 0.7% to 29% (83–85). However, if ventriculomegaly on CT is used to diagnose PTH, the incidence has been reported to range from 30% to 86% (86,87). Variables known to independently contribute to the development of hydrocephalus include thick subarachnoid hemorrhage (SAH), intraventricular hemorrhage, infection, or bifrontal decompression. It is important to become familiar with the radiographic appearance of hydrocephalus and subdural fluid collections and not just rely on the narrative report.

Although imaging is the usual diagnostic method, the clinical presentation is key. Although clinical presentation may be what causes the treating physician to order a scan, scans may be inconclusive. *Hydrocephalus ex-vacuo* refers to an enlargement of cerebral ventricles and subarachnoid spaces, and is usually caused by brain atrophy, post-traumatic brain injury, as well as in some psychiatric disorders. As opposed to post-traumatic hydrocephalus, this is a compensatory enlargement of the CSF spaces in response to loss of brain parenchyma. However, hydrocephalus is not solely a radiographic diagnosis. The expression, "wet, wobbly, and weird" is sometimes used to describe its clinical presentation. "Wet" refers to incontinent, "wobbly" to the ataxic and frontal gait disturbances, and "weird" to the cognitive and behavioral deficits associated with hydrocephalus. Although these are useful considerations, most patients with TBI will come to the rehabilitation unit with a variable combination of these signs and symptoms because of the nature of their brain injury (88). If a patient is progressing and declines functionally without another medical cause, certainly, hydrocephalus should be considered. It can sometimes become trickier when a patient has improved but not to the anticipated degree. The natural course of recovery from TBI includes some degree of recovery. There is still value in suspecting, monitoring, and ruling out hydrocephalus. Patients who have hydrocephalus stand a chance to improve from shunting more than their risk of a complication. The presentation of hydrocephalus can be subtle. Patients may present with abulia, emotional lability, perseveration, mutism, apraxia, or change in bladder or bowel function not related to infection. Memory and behavior may not be improving, may be improving, but not as anticipated or may demonstrate mild decline. This is representative of the influence of hydrocephalus on the frontal and temporal lobes and their projections. A behavioral example might be the patient who cannot stop picking at lint balls on a sweater (perseveration). Holding food in one's mouth or perseverating on chewing may be manifestations of hydrocephalus as well. It may also represent a deficit in initiation (i.e., to trigger a swallow). It is imperative to remember that the diagnosis of hydrocephalus is clinical and not purely radiographic. There are nonetheless certain radiographic findings that are more suggestive of hydrocephalus than cerebral atrophy alone. There is utility in comparing the degree of sulcal enlargement, which associated with atrophy, as brain tissue is lost. Ventricular shape and periventricular edema may be factors in interpretation of CT or MRI scans.

CSF tap tests are performed in some centers, taking off 30–50 ml of lumbar CSF and assessing patients for improvement (89). Often, the post-tap assessment is quite subjective. It is difficult to get useful objective measures pre- and post-tap that is sensitive to the potential changes. Gait analysis may appear reliable between 2 evaluators assuming the patient is even ambulatory (90). Quality of sleep the night before the test, family, or medical professional biases are some examples of potential confounders to the test interpretation. A positive response to a 40–50 ml tap test has a higher degree of certainty for a favorable response to shunt placement than clinical examination alone. However, this test cannot be exclusionary because of its low sensitivity (26%–61%). CSF infusion tests carry a higher sensitivity (57%–100%) to determine CSF outflow resistance and have a similar positive predictive value as CSF tap tests (75%–92%). Prolonged external lumbar drainage in excess of 300 ml is associated with high sensitivity (50%–100%) and high positive predictive value of 80%–100% (88). More assorted complex studies are possible but rarely performed (see Chapter 44). Ultimately, it is more often a matter of the referring physician's interpretation of a patient's clinical presentation and his or her relationship with the neurosurgeon.

Some studies show that unilateral decompressive craniectomy with large window diameters (≥ 15cm) has superiority over temporoparietal craniectomy of smaller diameter while lowering ICP, reducing the mortality rate, and improving cerebral compliance and neurological outcomes. However, even in the acute rehabilitation setting, one must be aware that neurosurgical complications may arise. Decompressive craniectomy may increase the incidence of delayed intracranial hematomas and subdural effusion (91,92). The effectiveness in TBI is under investigation. Concerns have been raised regarding timing, technique, patient selection, and complications. The "syndrome of the trephined" that presents after craniectomy in some patients includes headaches, apathy, hemiparesis, midbrain syndrome, tremor, gait, and cognitive functions (93). Early cranioplasty has been shown to improve those symptoms and the clinical complications seen in the acute rehabilitation setting. Currently, timing of cranioplasty varies with surgeon preference and patient characteristics (94). Overall, clinical status can improve once cranioplasties are performed, restoring the natural flow pattern.

Subdural hygromas (accumulation of serous or CSF) may occur after head trauma patients with hygromas are at higher risk for low GCS scores, midline shift < 5 mm, SAH, delayed hydrocephalus, compression of basal cisterns, and tearing of the arachnoid membrane (95).

Seizures (covered in Chapter 39) should be considered in the context of medication management, unexplained behaviors, and fluctuating cognition and movements.

Dizziness may be caused by vestibular deficits, orthostasis, and/or visual deficits. The vestibular system, oculomotor system, and the sensory-motor systems are integrated to maintain balance. Disturbances in these systems contribute to dizziness, nausea, and loss of balance. Not all patients will be physically or cognitively able to identify what they are experiencing, as with other issues following brain injury, empiric treatments can be considered. Patients may present with hearing or balance deficits, increased agitation, or vomiting related to changes in position (96) (see Chapters 46 and 47).

Visual input from enclosure beds may be overstimulating and disorienting, as may be fluorescent lights. Medications that are generally considered for dizziness include antihistamines, anticholinergics, and gamma-aminobutyric acid (GABA) agonists (see Chapters 72 and 73). Antihistamines can be profoundly sedating thus impeding progress. Meclizine, which is frequently prescribed, has both antihistaminic and anticholinergic (antimuscarinic) properties. Meclizine provides symptomatic short-term relief but limits the ability of the CNS to habituate. Anticholinergic properties increase the risk of orthostatic hypotension (97). Scopolamine patches offer the advantage of being easy to apply to combative patients although associated with anticholinergic side effects. GABA agonists such as lorazepam or diazepam are likely to prolong confusion and hamper memory. They may produce dizziness, which itself can affect memory concentration, behavior, and nutritional status. However, low doses may serve to decrease the sensation of imbalance and allow greater focus and participation.

This should be weighed against the impact of these medications. Severe vertigo associated with benign paroxysmal positional vertigo (BPPV) can be impressively managed with the Epley maneuver, which is described elsewhere in this edition (98). Vestibular derangement contributes to dizziness, nausea, and potential loss of balance. Visual- and oculomotor-related problems with convergence abnormalities may also contribute because of cranial nerve lesions or damage to eye muscles. Headache may coexist with complaints of dizziness as the individual tightens their cervical musculature to stabilize the sensation of instability and at times because of an underlying cervical dystonia.

In the acute rehabilitation setting, therapies can be designed to address visual dysfunction and fixation, cervical motion, and somatosensory deficits. A plan for longer-term follow up should also be established. Cranial nerve injuries are common in this setting and covered in Chapter 41.

Endocrine

Awareness of endocrine abnormalities following TBI has increased and is addressed in greater detail in Chapter 53. Many of the symptoms of hypopituitarism, such as fatigue, neuropsychiatric, and cognitive deficits, are often attributed to postconcussive disorder. However, various hormone deficiencies are seen in the acute phase post-TBI, including gonadotropin deficiency in up to 80% of patients, growth hormone (18%), corticotropin (16%–25%), and vasopressin (40%) (99–101). Associated risk factors include severity of injury, basilar skull fractures (especially the sphenoid), local edema or hemorrhage, systemic inflammation, and severe hypotension. Some manifestations include hypoglycemia, hyponatremia, and hypotension. Following severe TBI in children, cortisol and adrenocorticotropic hormone (ACTH) were significantly elevated on day 1 postinjury but then returned to normal by day 3. In the acute period, cortisol was low in 46% of children and ACTH in 14% (102,103). Progesterone has substantial pleiotropic properties as a neuroprotective agent in a variety of CNS injury models.

SIADH is one of the most common disturbances of sodium following TBI. Patients present with an increase in urine output, hyponatremia, and an increase in urine osmolality. SIADH is treated primarily with fluid restriction. CSW occurs less frequently than SIADH, but is another cause of hyponatremia after an injury to the brain. CSW, unlike SIADH, leads to volume depletion. Therefore, fluid restriction actually leads to a worsening of the condition. Treatment involves either hypertonic saline or oral sodium chloride, with monitoring of the clinical and laboratory response. Finally, another condition that affects sodium and urination in the brain injury population is DI. DI can be of a central etiology caused by a decrease in the secretion of antidiuretic hormone (ADH). This gives rise to polyuria and polydipsia by diminishing the patient's ability to concentrate urine.

Among long-term survivors, approximately 21%–25% still suffer from at least 1 deficiency, sometimes associated with increased disability, poor quality of life, and a greater likelihood of depression. Hypothyroidism is also a consideration on its own and when patients do not respond to antidepressants.

DISCHARGE PLANNING: FROM ACUTE TO WHERE AND WHEN

Discharge planning should begin early on in the rehabilitation process, at least in terms of presenting potential options (104). Every patient's social support and funding resources are unique, as will be their eventual deficits. These will affect everything from family ability to cope and absorb the demands of training, equipment prescriptions, medication selection, and discharge disposition. Access to ongoing therapy after discharge from inpatient rehabilitation and the need for medical follow-up are also factors in discharge planning. Patients seldom leave the acute brain injury rehabilitation setting without ongoing rehabilitation needs. Family members will need a degree of permission to remember to care for themselves as well as their loved one. Initially, there is a sense of relief that their loved one survived. The reality of what the future may bring can be unfathomable.

LOS in rehabilitation are decreasing in many health care systems across industrialized countries. In some countries, this is associated with a decrease in morbidity. In Germany, the recommended minimum LOS in neurological early rehabilitation for survivors of severe brain injury is 8 weeks (105) more than the average LOS in the United States (106). Length of rehabilitation stays are increasingly based on coding of diagnoses, functional scores, and costs of complications (107); increasingly driven by insurance constraints. A retrospective analysis of the TBI Model Systems (TBIMS) national data from 1990–2009 showed that patients admitted to in-patient rehabilitation with a Disability Rating Scale (DRS) category of moderately severe and above (score of 6.5–29.0), a median length of stay of 17 days was needed to achieve a rating of moderate disability (DRS ≤ 6). For those patients with DRS scores in the range of severe disability on admission, it took a median of 30 days to achieve a rating of moderate disability whereas patients with extremely severe disability on admission required 58 days and those in vegetative state needed 94 days to reach that level (108). Nevertheless, from 2006 to 2010, patients with TBI (not including multitrauma) in facilities subscribed to the Uniform Data System for Medical Rehabilitation (UDSMR) had a national average LOS of 17.5 days in acute rehabilitation (109). UDSMR data from 2000 to 2008 displayed consistent declines in admission and discharge functional ratings as well as in LOS. Most patients with TBI were discharged to community setting following inpatient rehabilitation, but these rates have shown a steady downward trend from 81% in 2000 to 74% in 2008, according to UDSMR data (110).

In the general population, the need for a longer LOS can be predicted by lower admission motor functional independence measure (FIM) scores and presence of comorbidities, whereas in the elderly population, women are more likely to have shorter LOS and be referred for home health (111). Patients with positive brain imaging (bilateral lesions or diffuse damage) may be less likely to be discharged home, whereas those with PTA > 1 week may be more likely to be discharged to an inpatient rehabilitation program (112). Social considerations including available services and health coverage may be factors (105). The influence of insurance plans on LOS cannot be ignored. For example, a patient may only be allowed a set amount of days for inpatient rehabilitation whether more would be beneficial or not. Although this might push the treating team to be more aggressive, it also can lead patients to be drugged inappropriately, face more complications, and push the limits of family strength and burnout. An agitated ambulatory and confused man with hydrocephalus might be discharged to home where the family members have to stop work to manage him. The goals of an inpatient rehabilitation stay are affected by the length of time a patient may be granted per their insurance policy or ability to pay. Care is often dictated more by what is a covered benefit than what is in the patient's and family's best interests, which does not necessarily result in better and quicker outcomes. The long-term socioeconomic, health, and quality of life considerations can be negatively impacted when the delivery of care is shortsighted.

GOALS, OUTCOME MEASURES, AND SOCIOECONOMIC CONSIDERATIONS

The FIM score is the most commonly used validated measure to assess a patient's progress in rehabilitation. The FIM is a standardized measure of independence in self-care, widely used and accepted in the United States and Europe. In the United States and other health care systems, LOS and therefore, reimbursement for rehabilitation, are based on ongoing improvements in functional performance as measured by improvements in serial FIM scores. "FIM efficiency" (net change in FIM score from admission to discharge, divided by LOS) has been used to "benchmark" the comparative efficiency of rehabilitation in different provider settings and in different patient populations (113,114).

In the acute brain injury rehabilitation setting, classic FIM scores have a floor effect making useful assessment of function difficult to quantify and document. FIM scores do not capture the qualitative changes necessary to move to the next level of independence. Early inpatient rehabilitation may translate into decreased long-term morbidity for the patient and family, even in individuals who remain dependent for their care needs. The use of FIM scores alone as a measure of progress may lead to failure to detect clinical gains (115). The Northwick Park Dependency Score (NPDS) and the Northwick Park Care Needs Assessment (NPCNA) are reportedly gaining favor in the United Kingdom as a measure of dependency in the more severely impaired patient population.

Brain injury rehabilitation can be cost-efficient for the most severely disabled patients with TBI, with the potential to generate substantial savings in the cost of continuing care in the community. In an English study from 2005, the initial cost of rehabilitation was £1,944/week and the weekly savings in care cost because of decreased dependency were £950/week. Over time, the proportions changed in such a way that the savings would offset the cost in 14 months (116). Many patients will go to long-term acute care hospitals or LTACHs from the acute hospital setting. This decision is often made when an acute rehabilitation program is not available or insurance benefits are limited. There are efficiencies to having a physiatrist in brain injury provide care, reducing dependency and costs of continuing care for adults with complex acquired brain injuries (115).

Family dynamics and psychosocial factors play a pivotal role in the discharge plan from the acute rehabilitation setting. It is unrealistic and unfair to patients to not acknowledge that LOS and funding sources are tightly bound. Couple that with the abrupt changes that can occur in family roles. It is not unusual to have the discharge plan affected by cultural and gender roles. In couples where the man was the primary decision maker but is now the injured survivor, it can be difficult for both the patient and the spouse to accept the change in roles. Cultures that emphasize nurturing of the infirmed may make it difficult for caregivers to allow the patient to work on acquiring new skills; to them, this may seem like tough love.

The treating inpatient rehabilitation team needs to remember that even after discharge from the hospital setting, that patient will still be progressing. What that progress looks like will be affected by what they get as inpatients, where they go following discharge, patient and family coping skills, finances, supervision needs, and many other variables that are difficult to quantify (see Chapters 20 and 25).

Goals of the inpatient stay will partially be influenced by how long that LOS can be. Constraints such as a limited number of inpatient days cannot be ignored. If someone has unlimited days based on medical necessity, those days should still be used responsibly. If someone has limited days, goals will be more directed toward family education, equipment, and medication adjustments than ongoing functional progress.

Follow-up is vital after discharge because it provides a means for persons with brain injury to continue progressing. Just because they are sent out at a particular level of function, that does not mean their improvements need to stop. Medication needs and other issues will change as patients evolve. Medications that were necessary at one point may no longer be needed. Alternatively, ongoing issues may evolve around mood, cognition, awareness, and medical complications.

Functional recovery after brain injury is tied, not only to the injury but also where services are provided, timing of services, biases, and medical advancements. Perhaps most importantly, it is tied to family, community, and social support systems. The demands financially, socially, medically, and personally can be huge (117). Even patients who have "good" outcomes will have significant changes in their role in the family and community. There will be adjustments for the rest of their lives that warrant monitoring, whether they reside in a nursing home or return to work. It is shortsighted to look at outcomes from a particular intervention in isolation of the other affected factors. Ideally, there will be an investment not just in the particular stage of a person's rehabilitation but in their lifelong outcome. Health care providers are bound by oaths to put the patient first. Insurance coverage is dictated by contracts. This imposes a potential conflict in philosophies and priorities that affects delivery of care (118).

Evidenced-based medicine (EBM) is increasingly touted as vital to provision of appropriate and cost-effective medicine. EBM has the benefits of considering the strength of evidence, not being restricted by statistical approaches alone and the goal of striving for greater scientific certainty and specificity. If used in exclusion, EBM undervalues individual preferences and differences and limits generalizability (119).

EBM does provide the medical and financial communities with useful information, although it has its limitations particularly in *Brain Injury Medicine*. It will always be difficult to factor in all the variables that make up each individual's situation. It is also difficult to control for the experience of clinicians, variable financial resources, and preinjury and postinjury condition of the affected brain. Most practice of medicine is not evidence based. Ideally, EBM is used in conjunction with logic and humanism. Hopefully, the trend will not increase in using EBM as an excuse to deny services because there is no sufficient evidence to support a given intervention. There are many studies that will never be performed because they take too long or are not financially feasible, profitable, or ethical. There are times to defend clinical decisions and remember that the practice of medicine is not just science; it is an art (120).

Rehabilitation of the patient with brain injury still, unfortunately, is often met with biases—biases regarding more than the financial benefits. Even clinicians in related fields often miss the point of interventions and do not see the potential for progress. Patients and their families may be misguided by well-meaning medical professionals who do not understand the breadth of recovery that may be achieved (see Chapter 18). Despite research on plasticity indicating otherwise, there is an inaccurate perception that recovery is complete by 12 months following the injury, when in fact recovery can continue.

CONCLUSION

Initiating the rehabilitation process early in the course of recovery not only serves to improve the experience but also the outcome. Brain injury rehabilitation can improve the medical stability of the patient, lead to judicious medication usage, and progress function. In this way, it also promotes recovery, prevents comorbidities, and allows for the education of patients and families. The prescription of appropriate equipment can make ongoing care manageable and allow for patients to continue to progress after discharge from the hospital setting. The team of medical professionals needs to serve as advocates and, in some ways, case managers of the medical, behavioral, and psychosocial factors that are variables in patients' lives. It is important to consider the variable performance and presentation from day to day but to keep perspective of the big picture. Early intervention with an integrated approach to care allows for improved understanding for families and hopefully, earlier recognition of issues that can be best managed before they grow into greater complications. Educating third-party payers and health care providers alike can be difficult, whether it is justifying an inpatient rehabilitation stay, a piece of durable medical equipment, or advocating for a ventriculoperitoneal (VP) shunt. Not all providers and services will provide the same care nor have the same outcomes. There is a wide range of patient presentations and access to care, levels of care, and provision of services at all those levels of care (104,121). The philosophy across those levels of care can be quite variable. If the treating team does not see goals, the patient will not improve.

There is an incorrect belief by some that further exacerbates the fears and stresses on family members of the injured: that recovery occurs only within the first 6 months after injury. Those involved in the long-term care of these patients know that this is only a myth. There is ongoing potential for recovery or improvement across all functional domains. If survivors are not allowed to access care, the myth becomes a reality (107,111,113,115). There is strong evidence that late rehabilitation can result in significant functional gains 5–10 years postinjury (122). Granted, it can be challenging to achieve one's full potential with the reality of limited resources (111). It can be difficult to judge the appropriate time to provide services. The costs of rehabilitation for brain injury are staggering, as are the costs of not delivering care or delivering care poorly (115,116). To provide optimal care for survivors of brain injury, the interplay of behavior, cognition, medical concerns and stability, and psychosocial factors should be considered and managed in an integrated manner. This is true from the start of acute rehabilitation through the continuum. For many survivors of brain injury, the sequelae will be lifelong (123).

In a world demanding EBM, there is limited specific data to answer many of the questions that arise. *Brain Injury Medicine* melds medical, cognitive, psychosocial, and behavioral considerations. There will often be lifelong ramifications and the ideal timing of interventions, both acutely and long-term needs to be understood. Newer interventions, including pharmacologic, stem cell use, advanced imaging, transcranial magnetic stimulation, and the assortment of therapy protocols used in this population, warrant study as we continue to advance our knowledge of treatment options and their benefits.

KEY CLINICAL POINTS

1. Medical, behavioral, cognitive, motoric, and psychosocial presentations must all be factored together holistically.
2. Medications should be used judiciously with the understanding that patients cannot plan and problem solve their own needs early on.
3. Have a high index of suspicion for hydrocephalus and subdural collections early on, even if patients are improving. Clinical findings must be given consideration.
4. Sleep disorders should be suspected and optimally managed to allow for greater progress because they affect mood, participation, cognition, and fatigue.

5. Changes in the clinical presentation have to be viewed from a fresh perspective every time (e.g., changes in behavior may reflect anything from UTI to increase in awareness to a VP shunt malfunction).
6. Think practically through the management of patients' organ systems to improve comfort, function, and potential.
7. Acute rehabilitation occurs in the beginning of the recovery process but can set the stage for optimizing longer term recovery. Neurorehabilitation practitioners are positioning patients for ongoing improvements.
8. Patients and families at this point are in crisis and cannot envision what the future looks like.

KEY REFERENCES

1. Behan LA, Phillips J, Thompson CJ, Agha A. Neuroendocrine disorders after traumatic brain injury. *J Neurol Neurosurg Psychiatry*. 2008;79(7):753–759.
2. Cuny E, Richer E, Castel JP. Dysautonomia syndrome in the acute recovery phase after traumatic brain injury: relief with intrathecal Baclofen therapy. *Brain Inj*. 2001; 15(10):917–925.
3. Flanagan SR, Elovic EP, Sandel E. Managing agitation associated with traumatic brain injury: behavioral versus pharmacologic interventions? *PM R*. 2009;1(1):76–80.
4. Masel BE, DeWitt DS. Traumatic brain injury: a disease process, not an event. *J. Neurotrauma*. 2010;27(8):1529–1540.
5. Rehabilitation of persons with traumatic brain injury. *NIH Consens Statement*. 1998;16(1):1–41.

References

1. Ashley MJ, Persel CS. Traumatic brain injury recovery rates in post acute rehabilitation: spontaneous recovery or treatment? *J Rehabil Outcomes Meas*. 1999;3(4):15–21.
2. Lv LQ, Hou LJ, Yu MK, et al. Prognostic influence and magnetic resonance imaging findings in paroxysmal sympathetic hyperactivtiy after severe traumatic brain injury. *J Neurotrauma*. 2010; 27(11):1945–1950.
3. Jastremski CA. Pressure relief bedding to prevent pressure ulcer development in critical care. *J Crit Care*. 2002;17(2):122–125.
4. Chung HT, Shu LH, Pan CC, Yang SY, Chen WI. Reducing patient pressure sore incidence in the surgical intensive care unit [in Chinese]. *Hu Li Za Zhi*. 2011;58(3)(suppl):56–63.
5. Goodrich C, March K. From ED to ICU: a focus on prevention of skin breakdown. *Crit Care Nurs Q*. 1992;15(1):1–13.
6. Huffman JC, Stern TA. Neuropsychiatric consequences of cardiovascular medications. *Dialogues Clin Neurosci*. 2007;9(1):29–45.
7. Sun H, Mao Y, Wang J, Ma Y. Effects of beta-adrenergic antagonist propranolol on spatial memory and exploratory behavior in mice. *Neurosci Lett*. 2011;498(2):133–137.
8. Lazowski DA, Ecclestone NA, Myers AM, et al. A randomized outcome evaluation of group exercise programs in long-term care institutions. *J Gerontol A Biol Sci Med Sci*. 1999;54(12):M621–M628.
9. Rehabilitation of persons with traumatic brain injury *NIH Consens Statement*. 1998;16(1):1–41.
10. Ivanhoe CB, Hartman ET. Clinical caveats on medical assessment and treatment of pain after TBI. *J Head Trauma Rehabil*. 2004;19(1): 29–39.
11. Elovic EP, Jasey NN, Eisenberg ME. The use of atypical antipsychotics after traumatic brain injury. *J Head Trauma Rehabil*. 2008; 23(2):132–135.
12. Cascade E, Kalali AH, Mehra S, Meyer JM. Real-world data on atypical antipsychotic medication side effects. *Psychiatry (Edgmont)*. 2010;7(7):9–12.

13. Peluso MJ, Lewis SW, Barnes TR, Jones PB. Extrapyramidal motor side-effects of first- and second-generation antipsychotic drugs. *Br J Psychiatry*. 2012;200:387–392.

14. Fleming J. Self-awareness. In: Stone JH, Blouin M, eds. *International Encyclopedia of Rehabilitation*. Brisbane, Australia: The University of Queensland and Princess Alexandra Hospital; 2011. http://cirrie .buffalo.edu/encyclopedia/en/article/109. Accessed August 8, 2011.

15. Flanagan SR, Elovic EP, Sandel E. Managing agitation associated with traumatic brain injury: behavioral versus pharmacologic interventions? *PM R*. 2009;1(1):76–80.

16. Barrett AM, Eslinger PJ. Amantadine for adynamic speech: possible benefit for aphasia? *Am J Phys Med Rehabil*. 2007;86(8):605–612.

17. Tanaka Y. Pharmacotherapy for aphasia. *Rinsho Shinkeigaku*. 2007; 47(11):859–861.

18. Korsukewitz C, Breitenstein C, Schomacher M, Knecht S. Present status and future possibilities of adjuvant pharmacotherapy for aphasia. *Nervenarzt*. 2006;77(4):403–415.

19. Mikami K, Jorge RE, Adams HP Jr, et al. Effect of antidepressants on the course of disability following stroke. *Am J Geriatr Psychiatry*. 2011;19(12):1007–1015.

20. Meyer MJ, Megyesi J, Meythaler J, et al. Acute management of acquired brain injury part II: an evidence-based review of pharmacologic interventions. *Brain Inj*. 2010;24(5):706–721.

21. Meyer MJ, Megyesi J, Meythaler J, et al. Acute management of acquired brain injury part I: an evidence-based review of non-pharmacological interventions. *Brain Inj*. 2010;24(5):694–705.

22. Pioro EP, Brooks BR, Cummings J, et al. Dextromethorphan plus ultra low-dose quinidine reduces pseudobulbar affect. *Ann Neurol*. 2010;68(5):693–702.

23. Lippert-Grüner M, Kuchta J, Hellmich M, Klug N. Neurobehavioural deficits after severe traumatic brain injury (TBI). *Brain Inj*. 2006;20(6):569–574.

24. Kölzsch M, Wulff I, Ellert S, et al. Deficits in pain teratment in nursing homes in Germany: A cross-sectional study [published online ahead of print December 19, 2011]. *Eur J Pain*. doi:10.1002/j.1532-2149.2011.00029.x.

25. Pelosi P, Severgnini P, Chiaranda M. An integrated approach to prevent and treat respiratory failure in brain-injured patients. *Curr Opin Crit Care*. 2005;11(1):37–42.

26. Shekleton JA, Parcell DL, Redman JR, Phipps-Nelson J, Ponsford JL, Rajaratnam SM. Sleep disturbance and melatonin levels following traumatic brain injury. *Neurology*. 2010;74(21):1732–1738.

27. Castriotta RJ, Atanasov S, Wilde MC, Masel BE, Lai JM, Kuna ST. Treatment of sleep disorders after traumatic brain injury. *J Clin Sleep Med*. 2009;5(2):137–144.

28. Flanagan SR, Greenwald B, Wieber S. Pharmacological treatment of insomnia for individuals with brain injury. *J Head Trauma Rehabil*. 2007;22(1):67–70.

29. Foral P, Dewan N, Malesker M. Insomnia: a therapeutic review for pharmacists. *Consult Pharm*. 2011;26(5):332–341.

30. Larson EB, Zollman FS. The effect of sleep medications cognitive recovery from traumatic brain injury. *J Head Trauma Rehabil*. 2010; 25(1):61–67.

31. Castriotta RJ, Wilde MC, Lai JM, Atanasov S, Masel BE, Kuna ST. Prevalence and consequences of sleep disorders in traumatic brain injury. *J Clin Sleep Med*. 2007;3(4):349–356.

32. Webster JB, Bell KR, Hussey JD, Natale TK, Lakshminarayan S. Sleep apnea in adults with traumatic brain injury: a preliminary investigation. *Arch Phys Med Rehabil*. 2001;82:316–321.

33. Srinivasan S, Lim CC, Thirugnanam U. Paroxysmal autonomic instability with dystonia. *Clin Auton Res*. 2007;17(6):378–381.

34. Baguley IJ, Heriseanu RE, Gurka JA, Nordenbo A, Cameron ID. Gabapentin in the management of dysautonomia following severe traumatic brain injury: a case series. *J Neurol Neurosurg Psychiatry*. 2007;78(5):539–541.

35. Katz RT. Management of spasticity. *Am J Phys Med Rehabil*. 1998; 67(3):108–116.

36. Turner MS. Early use of intrathecal baclofen in brain injury in pediatric patients. *Acta Neurochir Suppl*. 2003;87:81–83.

37. Cuny E. Intrathecal baclofen and traumatic brain injury. A review. *Neurochirurgie*. 2003;49(2–3, pt 2):289–292.

38. Cuny E, Richer E, Castel JP. Dysautonomia syndrome in the acute recovery phase after traumatic brain injury: relief with intrathecal Baclofen therapy. *Brain Inj*. 2001;15(10):917–925.

39. Becker R, Benes L, Sure U, Hellwig D, Bertalanffy H. Intrathecal baclofen alleviates autonomic dysfunction in severe brain injury. *J Clin Neurosci*. 2000;7(4):316–319.

40. Simpson DM, Gracies JM, Yablon SA, Barbano R, Brashear A. Botulinum neurotoxin versus tizanidine in upper limb spasticity: a placebo controlled study. *J Neurol Neurosurg Psychiatry*. 2009;80(4): 380–385.

41. Farina S, Migliorini C, Gandolfi M, et al. Combined effects of botulinum toxin and casting treatments on lower limb spasticity after stroke. *Funct Neurol*. 2008;23(2):87–91.

42. Kanellopoulos AD, Mavrogenis AF, Mitsiokapa EA, et al. Long lasting benefits following the combination of static night upper extremity splinting with botulinum toxin A injections in cerebral palsy children. *Eur J Phys Rehabil Med*. 2009;45(4):501–506.

43. Petrillo CR, Chu DS, Davis SW. Phenol block of the tibial nerve in the hemiplegic patient. *Orthopedics*. 1980;3:871–874.

44. Dray TG, Hillel AD, Miller RM. Dysphagia caused by neurologic deficits. *Otolaryngol Clin North Am*. 1998;31(3):507–524.

45. O'Gara JA. Dietary adjustments and nutritional therapy during treatment for oral-pharyngeal dysphagia. *Dysphagia*. 1990;4(4): 209–212.

46. Bratton SL, Chestnut RM, Ghajar J, et al; for Brain Trauma Foundation, American Association of Neurological Surgeons, Congress of Neurological Surgeons, Joint Section on Neurotrauma and Critical Care, AANS/CNS. Guidelines for the management of severe traumatic brain injury. XII. Nutrition. *J Neurotrauma*. 2007;24(suppl 1): S77–S82.

47. Zollman FS, ed. *Manual of Traumatic Brain Injury Management*. New York, NY: Demos Medical; 2011:187–198.

48. Pascoe MC, Crewther SG, Carey LM, Crewther DP. What you eat is what you are—a role for polyunsaturated fatty acids in neuroinflammation induced depression? *Clin Nutr*. 2011;30(4):407–415.

49. Roberts I, Yates D, Sandercock P, et al. Effect of intravenous corticosteroids on death within 14 days in 10008 adults with clinically significant head injury (MRC CRASH trial): randomised placebo-controlled trial. *Lancet*. 2004;364(9442):1321–1328.

50. Wright SC, Maree JE, Sibanyoni M. Treatment of oral thrush in HIV/AIDS patients with lemon juice and lemon grass (Cymbopogon citratus) and gentian violet. *Phytomedicine*. 2009;16(2–3):118–124.

51. Martin C, Roman V, Agay D, Fatôme M. Anti-emetic effect of ondansetron and granisetron after exposure to mixed neutron and gamma irradiation. *Radiat Res*. 1998;149(6):631–636.

52. Marciniak C, Chen D, Stein AC, Semik PE. Prevalence of Clostridium difficile colonization at admission to rehabilitation. *Arch Phys Med Rehabil*. 2006;87(8):1086–1090.

53. Hookman P, Barkin JS. Clostridium difficile associated infection, diarrhea and colitis. *World J Gastroenterol*. 2009;15(13):1554–1580.

54. Harari D, Norton C, Lockwood L, Swift C. Treatment of constipation and fecal incontinence in stroke patients: randomized controlled trial. *Stroke*. 2004;35(11):2549–2555.

55. Dorsher PT, McIntosh PM. Neurogenic bladder. *Adv Urol*. 2012; 2012:816274.

56. De Groat WC. A neurologic basis for the overactive bladder. *Urology*. 1997;50(6A)(suppl):36–52.

57. Linsenmeyer TA. Post-CVA voiding dysfunctions: clinical insights and literature review. *NeuroRehabilitation*. 2012;30(1):1–7.

58. Leary SM, Liu C, Cheesman AL, Ritter A, Thompson S, Greenwood R. Incontinence after brain injury: prevalence, outcome and multidisciplinary management on a neurological rehabilitation unit. *Clin Rehabil*. 2006;20(12):1094–1099.

59. Genêt F, Jourdan C, Schnitzler A, et al. Troublesome heterotopic ossification after central nervous system damage: a survey of 570 surgeries. *PLoS One*. 2011;6(1):e16632.

60. Cullen N, Perera J. Heterotopic ossification: pharmacologic options. *J Head Trauma Rehabil*. 2009;24(1):69–71.

61. Simonsen LL, Sonne-Holm S, Krasheninnikoff M, Engberg AW. Symptomatic heterotopic ossification after very severe traumatic brain injury in 114 patients: incidence and risk factors. *Injury*. 2007; 38(10):1146–1150.

62. Vanden Bossche L, Vanderstraeten G. Heterotopic ossification: a review. *J Rehabil Med.* 2005;37(3):129–136.

63. Cipriano CA, Pill SG, Keenan MA. Heterotopic ossification following traumatic brain injury and spinal cord injury. *J Am Acad Orthop Surg.* 2009;17(11):689–697.

64. Parikh J, Hyare H, Saifuddin A. The imaging features of post-traumatic myositis ossificans, with emphasis on MRI. *Clin Radiol.* 2002; 57(12):1058–1066.

65. Cushner FD, Morwessel RM. Myositis ossificans traumatica. *Orthop Rev.* 1992;21(11):1319–1326.

66. Cadosch D, Toffoli AM, Gautschi OP, et al. Serum after traumatic brain injury increases proliferation and supports expression of osteoblast markers in muscle cells. *J Bone Joint Surg Am.* 2010;92(3): 645–653.

67. Toffoli AM, Gautschi OP, Frey SP, Filgueira L, Zellweger R. From brain to bone: evidence for the release of osteogenic humoral factors after traumatic brain injury. *Brain Inj.* 2008;22(7–8):511–518.

68. Gautschi OP, Cadosch D, Frey SP, Skirving AP, Filgueira L, Zellweger R. Serum-mediated osteogenic effect in traumatic brain-injured patients. *ANZ J Surg.* 2009;79(6):449–455.

69. Bruno-Petrina A. Posttraumatic heterotopic ossification. Medscape Website. http://www.emedicine.com/pmr/topic112.htm. Updated July 28, 2008. Accessed April 4, 2011.

70. Van Kampen PJ, Martina JD, Vos PE, Hoedemaekers CW, Hendricks HT. Potential risk factors for developing heterotopic ossification in patients with severe traumatic brain injury. *J Head Trauma Rehabil.* 2011;26(5):384–391.

71. Shehab D, Elgazzar AH, Collier BD. Heterotopic ossification. *J Nucl Med.* 2002;43(3):346–353.

72. Mavrogenis AF, Soucacos PN, Papagelopoulos PJ. Heterotopic ossification revisited. *Orthopedics.* 2011;34(3):177. doi:10.3928/01477447-20110124-08.

73. Falsetti P, Acciai C, Palilla R, Carpinteri F, Patrizio C, Lenzi L. Bedside ultrasound in early diagnosis of neurogenic heterotopic ossification in patients with acquired brain injury. *Clin Neurol Neurosurg.* 2011;113(1):22–27.

74. Falsetti P, Acciai C, Lenzi L. Sonographic diagnosis of neurogenic heterotopic ossification in patients with severe acquired brain injury in a neurorehabilitation unit. *J Clin Ultrasound.* 2011;39(1): 12–17. doi:10.1002/jcu.20742.

75. Forsberg JA, Potter BK. Heterotopic ossification in wartime wounds. *J Surg Orthop Adv.* 2010;19(1):54–61.

76. Antoniou J, Tae SK, Williams GR, Bird S, Ramsey ML, Iannotti JP. Suprascapular neuropathy. Variability in the diagnosis, treatment, and outcome. *Clin Orthop Relat Res.* 2001;(386):131–138.

77. Kushwaha VP, Garland DG. Extremity fractures in the patient with a traumatic brain injury. *J Am Acad Orthop Surg.* 1998;6(5):298–307.

78. Gamble GE, Barberan E, Laasch HU, Bowsher D, Tyrrell PJ, Jones AK. Poststroke shoulder pain: a prospective study of the association and risk factors in 152 patients from a consecutive cohort of 205 patients presenting with stroke. *Eur J Pain.* 2002;6(6):467–474.

79. Ediz L, Hiz O, Meral I, Alpayci M. Complex regional pain syndrome: a vitamin K dependent entity? *Med Hypotheses.* 2010;75(3): 319–323.

80. Park SA, Yang CY, Kim CG, Shin YI, Oh GJ, Lee M. Patterns of three-phase bone scintigraphy according to the time course of complex regional pain syndrome type I after a stroke or traumatic brain injury. *Clin Nucl Med.* 2009;34(11):773–776.

81. Maihöfner C, Baron R, DeCol R, et al. The motor system shows adaptive changes in complex regional pain syndrome. *Brain.* 2007; 130(pt 10):2671–2687.

82. Van Eijs F, Stanton-Hicks M, Van Zundert J, et al. Evidence-based interventional pain medicine according to clinical diagnoses. 16. Complex regional pain syndrome. *Pain Pract.* 2011;11(1):70–87. doi: 10.1111/j.1533-2500.2010.00388.x.

83. Choi I, Park HK, Chang JC, Cho SJ, Choi SK, Byun BJ. Clinical factors for the development of posttraumatic hydrocephalus after decompressive craniectomy. *J Korean Neurosurg Soc.* 2008;43(5): 227–231.

84. Cardoso ER, Galbraith S. Posttraumatic hydrocephalus—a retrospective review. *Surg Neurol.* 1985;23(3):261–264.

85. Hawkins TD, Lloyd AD, Fletcher GI, Hanka R. Ventricular size following head injury: a clinico-radiological study. *Clin Radiol.* 1976;27(3):279–289.

86. Gudeman SK, Kishore PR, Becker DP, et al. Computed tomography in the evaluation of incidence and significance of post-traumatic hydrocephalus. *Radiology.* 1981;141(2):397–402.

87. Philippon J, George B, Visot A, Cophignon J. Post-operative hydrocephalus. *Neurochirurgie.* 1976;22(2):111–117.

88. Marmarou A, Bergsneider M, Klinge P, Relkin N, Black PM. The value of supplemental prognostic tests for the preoperative assessment of idiopathic normal-pressure hydrocephalus. *Neurosurgery.* 2005;57(3)(suppl):S17–S28.

89. Ishikawa M, Hashimoto M, Mori E, Kuwana N, Kazui H. The value of the cerebrospinal fluid tap test for predicting shunt effectiveness in idiopathic normal pressure hydrocephalus. *Fluids Barriers CNS.* 2012;9(1):1.

90. Virhammar J, Cesarini KG, Laurell K. The CSF tap test in normal pressure hydrocephalus: evaluation time, reliability and the influence of pain. *Eur J Neurol.* 2012;19(2):271–276.

91. Qiu W, Guo C, Shen H, et al. Effects of unilateral decompressive craniectomy on patients with unilateral acute post-traumatic brain swelling after severe traumatic brain injury. *Crit Care.* 2009;13(6): R185.

92. Timofeev I, Czosnyka M, Nortje J, et al. Effect of decompressive craniectomy on intracranial pressure and cerebrospinal compensation following traumatic brain injury. *J Neurosurg.* 2008;108(1): 66–73.

93. Dujovny M, Agner C, Aviles A. Syndrome of the trephined: theory and facts. *Crit Rev Neurosurg.* 1999;9(5):271–278.

94. Lazaridis C, Czosnyka M. Cerebral blood flow, brain tissue oxygen, and metabolic effects of decompressive craniectomy [published online ahead of print March 07, 2012]. *Neurocrit Care.*

95. Jeon SW, Choi JH, Jang TW, Moon SM, Hwang HS, Jeong JH. Risk factors associated with subdural hygroma after decompressive craniectomy in patients with traumatic brain injury: a comparative study. *J Korean Neurosurg Soc.* 2011;49(6):355–358.

96. Kroenke K, Mangelsdorff AD. Common symptoms in ambulatory care: incidence evaluation, therapy and outcome *Am J Med.* 1989; 86(3):262–266.

97. Zee DS. Vestibular adaptation. In: Herdman SJ, ed. *Vestibular Rehabilitation.* Philadelphia, PA: FA Davis Co; 1994:68–79.

98. Herdman SJ. Assessment and management of bilateral vestibular loss. In: Herdman SJ, ed. *Vestibular Rehabilitation.* Philadelphia, PA: FA Davis Co; 1994:317–330.

99. Behan LA, Phillips J, Thompson CJ, Agha A. Neuroendocrine disorders after traumatic brain injury. *J Neurol Neurosurg Psychiatry.* 2008;79(7):753–759.

100. Bavisetty S, Bavisetty S, McArthur DL, et al. Chronic hypopituitarism after traumatic brain injury: risk assessment and relationship to outcome. *Neurosurgery.* 2008;62(5):1080–1093.

101. Powner DJ, Boccalandro C. Adrenal insufficiency following traumatic brain injury in adults. *Curr Opin Crit Care.* 2008;14(2): 163–166.

102. Srinivas R, Brown SD, Chang YF, Garcia-Fillion P, Adelson PD. Endocrine function in children acutely following severe traumatic brain injury. *Childs Nerv Syst.* 2010;26(5):647–653.

103. Stein DG, Wright DW. Progesterone in the clinical treatment of acute traumatic brain injury. *Expert Opin Investig Drugs.* 2010;19(7): 847–857.

104. Cuthbert JP, Corrigan JD, Harrison-Felix C, et al. Factors that predict acute hospitalization discharge disposition for adults with moderate to severe traumatic brain injury. *Arch Phys Med Rehabil.* 2011;92(5):721–730.

105. Rollnik JD, Janosch U. Current trends in the length of stay in neurological early rehabilitation. *Dtsch Arztebl Int.* 2010;107(16):286–292.

106. Arango-Lasprilla JC, Ketchum JM, Cifu D, et al. Predictors of extended rehabilitation length of stay after traumatic brain injury. *Arch Phys Med Rehabil.* 2010;91(10):1495–1504.

107. Graham JE, Radice-Neumann DM, Reistetter TA, Hammond FM, Dijkers M, Granger CV. Influence of sex and age on inpatient rehabilitation outcomes among older adults with traumatic brain injury. *Arch Phys Med Rehabil.* 2010;91(1):43–50.

108. Ashley JG, Ashley MJ, Seneca PJ, Kreber LA. Rehabilitation length of stay following traumatic brain injury: Are patient's getting the full dose? http://www.tbi-research.org/11los.pdf. Accessed May 6, 2012.

109. Uniform Data System for Medical Rehabilitation 2011. Amherst, NY. http://www.udsmr.org. Accessed June, 2011.

110. Granger CV, Markello SJ, Graham JE, Deutsch A, Reistetter TA, Ottenbacher KJ. The uniform data system for medical rehabilitation: report of patients with traumatic brain injury discharged from rehabilitation programs in 2000–2007. *Am J Phys Med Rehabil.* 2010; 89(4):265–78.

111. Tooth L, McKenna K, Strong J, Ottenbacher K, Connell J, Cleary M. Rehabilitation outcomes for brain injured patients in Australia: functional status, length of stay and discharge destination. *Brain Inj.* 2001;15(7):613–631.

112. De Guise E, LeBlanc J, Feyz M, Lamoureux J. Predictors of outcome at discharge from acute care following traumatic brain injury. *J Head Trauma Rehabil.* 2006;21(6):527–536.

113. Granger CV, Cotter AC, Hamilton BB, Fiedler RC. Functional assessment scales: a study of persons after stroke. *Arch Phys Med Rehabil.* 1993;74(2):133–138.

114. Granger CV, Divan N, Fiedler RC. Functional assessment scales: a study of persons after traumatic brain injury. *Am J Phys Med Rehabil.* 1995;74(2):107–113.

115. Turner-Stokes L, Paul S, Williams H. Efficiency of specialist rehabilitation in reducing dependency and costs of continuing care for adults with complex acquired brain injuries. *J Neurol Neurosurg Psychiatry.* 2006;77(5):634–639.

116. Turner-Stokes L. Cost efficiency of longer-stay rehabilitation programmes: can they provide value for money? *Brain Inj.* 2007;21(10): 1015–1021.

117. Sander AM, Caroselli JS, High WM Jr, Becker C, Neese L, Scheibel R. Relationship of family functioning to progress in a post-acute rehabilitation programme following traumatic brain injury. *Brain Inj.* 2002;16(8):649–657.

118. Donovan WH. Ethics, health care and spinal cord injury: research, practiced and finance. *Spinal Cord.* 2011;49(2):162–174.

119. Malec JF. Ethical and evidence-based practice in brain injury rehabilitation. *Neuropsychol Rehabil.* 2009;19(6):790–806.

120. Sackett DL, Rosenberg WM, Gray JA, Haynes RB, Richardson WS. Evidence based medicine: what it is and what it isn't. *BMJ.* 1996; 312(7023):71–72.

121. Davis CH, Fardanesh L, Rubner D, Wanlass RL, McDonald CM. Profiles of functional recovery in fifty traumatically brain-injured patients after acute rehabilitation. *Am J Phys Med Rehabil.* 1997; 76(3):213–218.

122. Powell J, Heslin J, Greenwood R. Community based rehabilitation after severe traumatic brain injury: a randomised controlled trial. *J Neurol Neurosurg Psychiatry.* 2002;72(2):193–202.

123. Masel BE, DeWitt DS. Traumatic brain injury: a disease process, not an event. *J. Neurotrauma.* 2010;27(8):1529–1540.

124. American Society of Anesthesiologists Task Force on Acute Pain Management. Practice guidelines for acute pain management in the perioperative setting: an updated report by the american society of anesthesiologists task force on acute pain management. *Anesthesiology.* 2004;100(6):1573–1581.

125. Arnt J, Skarsfeldt T. Do novel antipsychotics have similar pharmacological characteristics? A review of evidence. *Neuropsychopharmacology.* 1998;18(2):63–101.

126. Pasero C. Assessment of sedation during opioid administration for pain management. *J Perianesth Nurs.* 2009;24(3):186–190.

127. Woods SW. Chlorpromazine equivalent doses for the newer atypical antipsychotics. *J Clin Psychiatry.* 2003;64(6):663–667.

128. Charts and tables: *Antipsychotic agents.* Lexi-Comp Inc. 1978–2012.

129. Charts and tables: *Beta-blockers.* Lexi-Comp Inc. 1978–2012.

130. Charts and tables: *Selected adverse effects.* Lexi-Comp Inc. 1978–2012.

APPENDIX I Suggested Admitting Orders: Acute Rehabilitation

Admit

Diagnoses

Condition (e.g., stable)

Activity

Vitals

Allergies

Weight-bearing precautions

Supervision/restraints/abdominal binder

DVT assessment (including vascular imaging and hose)

Fall risk

Turning schedule

Wound care

Bladder program: Remove Foley catheter if no premorbid issues with goal of timed voiding/bladder scans for post-void residuals.

Bowel program: Daily stool softener/laxative; if patient is incontinent or constipated, mini enema or suppository is scheduled. Toilet to commode when sitting, balance, and staffing allow.

Respiratory: Oxygen saturation or arterial blood gas. Nebulizer treatments should be scheduled. If patient is at a low level, he or she will need regularly scheduled treatments, tracheostomy care, and plugging.

Nutrition: Swallowing evaluation. Bolus tube feedings/diet as appropriate.

Pain medications: Should be scheduled and nonsedating whenever possible, considering half life.

Sleep: Chart sleep–wake cycles and adjust medications accordingly.

Therapy as indicated including the following: physical therapy, occupational therapy, speech and language therapy, music therapy, neuropsychology, social work, therapeutic recreation, chaplain services, and school referral.

Medications: wean unnecessary medications. Consider behaviors, nonsedating sleep aid.
Labs: CMP, CBC, TSH, Free T4 and T3, Urine analysis and culture, drug levels if appropriate.

APPENDIX II Drugs to Avoid in Acute Brain Injury Rehabilitation (124–130)

The drugs listed in the table subsequently are to be avoided in acute rehabilitation because there is evidence that the stated risks are higher than other drugs in the same class. Some medications such as doxepin, trazodone, valproic acid, or quetiapine are used because of their side-effect profile. In the drugs listed subsequently, the benefits do not usually outweigh the risks. The "+" sign indicates the most common, severe, and studied symptoms of the listed drugs. The goals of treatment must be considered.

Category	Drug	Sedation	EPS	ACH	Orth. Hyp.	Psychosis
Pain	Meperidine	+		+	+	
	Methadone	+	+	+		
Anticonvulsant	Phenytoin	+				
	Phenobarbital	+				
Antihypertensive	Clonidine			+	+	
	Propranolol	+				
	Penbutolol	+				
	Nebivolol	+				
Antipsychotic	Chlorpromazine	+			+	
	Haloperidol		+			
	Fluphenazine		+			
	Pimozide		+			
	Thiothixene		+			
	Trifluoperazine		+			
Anxiolytics	Diazepam	+				
	Alprazolam	+	Lorazepam	+		
Prokinetic/antiemetic	Metoclopramide	+	+			+
	Chlorpromazine	+			+	
	Promethazine	+	+			

Abbreviations: EPS, extrapyramidal symptoms; ACH, anticholinergic; Orth. Hyp., orthostatic hypotension.

APPENDIX III Most Common Problems and Their Treatments in the Acute Rehabilitation of Persons With Traumatic Brain Injury

Common Problem	Treatment
Awareness deficits	Environmental modifications, frequent visual and verbal cueing; patient, family, and staff education.
Balance impairments	Treat with therapy (e.g., vestibular) and medications depending on its cause.
Behavioral	Environmental modifications, staff/family education, $+/-$ pharmacologic management. See Table 26-2.
Cognitive deficits	Environmental modifications, compensatory strategies, speech therapy, pharmacologic management, minimize distractions. See Table 26-2.
Contractures	Stretching, ROM, splinting, serial casting, tone management, manipulation under anesthesia, tendon release surgery.
Decreased activities of daily living (ADL) skills and mobility	Retraining as able in therapy and by family and staff.
Deep vein thrombosis (DVT)/pulmonary embolism (PE)	Screening, high index of suspicion, mechanical/chemical prophylaxis, mobility.
Dysautonomia	Treat possible triggers (e.g., pain, wounds, infections, elevated ICP). Positioning, beta-blockers, clonidine, morphine, and antipyretics may help. Tone management and ITB therapy.
Dysphagia	Swallow evaluation. Adequate diet. Speech therapy/functional electrical stimulation (FES), Beckman exercises, family training.
Endocrine abnormalities	Treat as appropriate based on thorough screening.
Fractures	Suspect, obtain x-rays as appropriate, orthopedic consult, manage pain with scheduled analgesia.
Gait impairments	Strengthening in therapy, forced use, assistive devices, gait reeducation, tone management, tendon lengthenings.
HO/MO	Suspect, obtain x-rays as appropriate, consider bisphosphonates and indomethacin, positioning, avoid *brisk* ROM.
Hydrocephalus	Have high suspicion, follow-up scans, track physical and cognitive progress, "tap test," shunt.
Hypertension	Monitor in ward and therapies, low sodium intake, fluid intake monitoring, exercise, and medications.
Infections: UTI, pneumonia (PNA), meningitis, Candida (perineal skin, oral mucosa)	Suspect infection if patient's cognition/alertness changes, work up as appropriate, treat as needed.
Low vital capacity	Respiratory therapy consult, breathing exercises, monitor volumes for improvement, consider lung pathology.
Memory impairment	Speech therapy, neuropsychology, environmental cues, compensatory strategies, medication if source of impairment requires it (e.g., impairment because of inability to focus or maintain attention), neuropharmacologic agents.
Motor weakness	Strengthening in therapy, forced use, general neurologic facilitation/stimulation, assistive devices, adaptive equipment, durable medical equipment (DME), orthotics.
Movement disorders	Evaluate thoroughly, identify possible cause and threat with therapy, modifications for safety (e.g., during gait/handling of hot liquids), pharmacologic treatment, remove neuroleptics. Parkinsonism may mimic the stage of emergence from vegetative state if patient's cognition is not evaluated.
Neurogenic bladder	Bladder program with monitoring (timed voids), assure emptying, possible bladder studies.
Neurogenic bowel	Bowel program with monitoring and medication for upper and lower gastrointestinal (GI) functions, toilet when possible.
Orthostatic hypotension	Monitor in ward and therapies. Compression stockings and abdominal binder may help. Tilt table or stander. Medications as prescribed. Assess cardiac medications.
Pain	Scheduled and as prescribed pain meds investigate and treat cause. Monitor for CRPS.
Peripheral nerve injury	Suspect, evaluate level, consider electrodiagnostics.
Psychiatric pathologies	Decrease/limit polypharmacy, monitor and repair sleep patterns, appropriate medications, investigate pre-TBI history, consider psychiatry consultation (ideally someone familiar with TBI), psychotherapy when patient's cognition allows.
Shoulder subluxation	Strengthening $+/-$ FES, positioning program, ROM.
Sleep disorder	Sleep hygiene, environmental modifications, $+/-$ pharmacological treatment including daytime stimulants and increasing activity.
Spasticity	Therapy (stretching, desensitization, weight bearing, cold), medical management (e.g., treat infections), serial casting, splints, pharmacologic management, injections, and ITB therapy.
Speech deficits	Speech therapy $+/-$ augmentative communication devices; patient, family, and staff education.
Visual deficits	Evaluate all patients, neuro-optometry consult, visual rehabilitation, prisms/eyeglasses, family education.

Neurorehabilitation Nursing

Mary Goonan, Melinda Kahn, and Harriet Straus

INTRODUCTION

Hope for traumatic brain injury (TBI) recovery increases as medical research, therapies, and technologies advance. The bedside nurse is a critical component of the interdisciplinary team, providing the focus of round-the-clock, documented, professional care, thus giving each patient the maximum opportunity for recovery (1). Through close monitoring of and interaction with the patient, and in constant, close communication with other members of the interdisciplinary team, the nurse both puts into practice and suggests therapies and interventions and is thus a critical factor in optimal patient recovery.

This chapter will present information to nurses that will provide them with excellent patient-centered care in brain injury rehabilitation. It is the framework for assessing the rehabilitation patient, and includes the latest approaches used by rehabilitation nursing in collaboration with the interdisciplinary team.

Nurses face multiple challenges when caring for individuals with brain injury. Whether the nurse is a neophyte or has had years of practice, each patient provides new vectors for understanding the ever-changing field of brain injury and a window on the efficacy of new therapeutic approaches that meets each patient's unique presentation.

It is the responsibility of the rehabilitation nurse to understand each individual's challenges and learn from them. Facilitating the emergence of an individual who is in essence the same person they were before their brain injury but fortified, through the rehabilitation process, with strategies and strengths to deal with their changed circumstances and abilities is one of the rewards of rehabilitation nursing.

The aim of rehabilitation nursing is to help the patient be as independent as possible. If the patient is unable to do a task independently, the rehabilitation nurse facilitates the patient's direction of his or her own care. If the patient is unable to direct the care, the rehabilitation nurse teaches a family member, significant other, or caregiver to do the task.

Rehabilitation nursing, at least in the context of in-hospital care, supports the patient 24 hours per day. Each member of the interdisciplinary team contributes their disciplines' approach, as well as their individual interpretation of that disciplinary approach to give the patient the best outcomes. The nurse's job is to maintain the interdisciplinary plan of care (IPOC) and facilitate the use of the skills learned by the patient during the therapy day. Efficient and thorough communication of the IPOC to all members of the team including the patient and the family is essential to the success of the plan.

Allowing each patient time to express their needs and to accomplish therapeutic tasks is an important foundation of rehabilitation process, and enables the patient to progress steadily throughout the rehabilitation course toward discernible, meaningful goals. It is therefore important to continuously reassess the unique needs of each patient, and to communicate effectively with other members of the team to find ways to meet those needs.

Resilience, motivation, hope, and courage are hallmarks of patients who do well in rehabilitation. For those patients who lack these characteristics based on life circumstances, neurological impairment, or other factors, it is the nurses' challenge to facilitate positive attitudes and maintain motivation for functional advancement for both patients and families.

ACUTE CARE

The immediate critical care of the patient with TBI has changed dramatically over the last decade (2). Predictors of an unfavorable outcome include—but not limited to—the Glasgow Coma Scale (GCS) score after resuscitation, motor scores, and injury severity scores. Age, absence of papillary light reflex, systolic blood pressure, hypoxemia, CT findings, mechanism of injury, and glucose level all within the first 24 hours are also predictors of outcomes (3). Mastering new procedures and giving attention to infection, nutrition, prevention of pressure ulcers (especially from devices), prophylaxis for deep vein thrombosis (DVT), respiratory stability, respiratory hygiene, mouth care, removal of invasive devices, and, above all, prevention of errors are essential aspects of rehabilitation nursing. A thorough review of the initial history and physical exam tells the rehabilitation nurse how much the patient has progressed and the potential for recovery.

Rehabilitation begins in the intensive care unit and continues when the patient is on the acute care floor. The most intensive rehabilitation typically takes place in the brain injury rehabilitation unit. Following inpatient rehabilitation, the patient might go to a day rehabilitation program, residential rehabilitation program, or outpatient rehabilitation. Today, inpatient rehabilitation is only the beginning of the rehabilitation road to recovery.

Physical examination is as important for the rehabilitation nurse as it is for the acute care nurse. Changes in the skull exam such as increased ballotability or increased bulging of the area of skull removal can be a positive sign of impending neurological or neurosurgical decompensation. The lung exam monitors for pneumonia, and the abdominal exam monitors for bleeding and/or ileus. Changes in feeding tolerance may signal ileus or gastroparesis.

Abnormalities in vital signs and/or laboratory data may indicate early evidence of medical complications such as line sepsis, abscess, wound infection, skin infection, and central nervous infection. The rehabilitation nurse should monitor laboratory values, including the patient's white blood cell count, platelet count, hemoglobin levels, hematocrit levels, blood urea nitrogen levels, creatinine levels, albumin values, albumin and prealbumin levels, as well as bicarbonate values to observe trends. It is important to maintain accurate recordings of intake and output.

It is also important to watch for delayed surgical or trauma complications such as perforations, hemorrhage, thrombosis, or missed fractures in the polytrauma patient. Renal function, DVT prophylaxis, seizure medications, and sepsis are monitored. Urinary infections and constipation frequently follow trauma, and it is the responsibility of the rehabilitation nurse to observe the patient for these outcomes. Many preventable problems have negative outcomes; early notice, assessment, and implementation of changes in the plan of care are essential in preventing negative outcomes.

Rehabilitation nurses continue to monitor the patient's sensorimotor and general exam 1 to 3 times a day, monitoring for trends such as changes in cognition, behavior, sensory functions, and/or strength. The patient should be examined to determine whether they are awake, alert, and oriented as to person, place, time (A&Ox3), and event (A&Ox4). Cranial nerve impairments should be assessed and the results compared to previous exams. Pupils should be monitored for size, symmetry, and reaction to light. The assessment of cranial nerve XII should include assuring that the patient's tongue protrusion is straight and does not deviate to one side. Grip strength can also be monitored for changes in upper extremity motor function.

Any adverse clinical change may mark the onset of a medical complication such as sepsis, one of the most common sequelae to trauma (4). Nurses continue to monitor for sepsis during the rehabilitation stay. The systemic inflammatory response syndrome (SIRS) for sepsis is a heart rate greater than 90 beats per minute, respiratory rate greater than 20 respirations per minute, carbon dioxide tension ($PaCO_2$) greater than 32, temperature greater than 38°C or less than 36°C, and white blood cell count greater than 14,000 or less than 4,000 or greater than 10% (5). The rehabilitation nurse should obtain orders from the rehabilitation physician to culture all sites that may support an infection while in rehabilitation. The nurse should also know which organisms were found and treated in acute care because these organisms may now be resistant to therapy.

DVT and pulmonary embolism (PE) are serious and ever present risks for the rehabilitation patient following TBI (6,7). They can occur in acute care or after rehabilitation begins. Signs and symptoms of a DVT include pain, tenderness, warmth, discoloration, fever, and edema of the affected limb.

Symptoms of a PE may include shortness of breath, chest pain, and tachypnea. According to several studies, there is no consensus on when to start prophylaxis or which treatment to use (6,8). (See Chapter 49 for more information.)

BEHAVIORAL MANAGEMENT

Brain Injury survivors can be easily overwhelmed by overstimulation from the environment. Structured, quiet environments work well for the patient with TBI. Keeping noise, interruptions, and visitors to a minimum is helpful in decreasing the stimulation to these patients. These visitors may include well-intentioned family members. Behavior requiring intervention includes aggression, disinhibited behavior, and difficulty relating to others in the environment, all of which may cause agitation in the patient. Rehabilitation nurses proactively build therapeutic relationships with the family from the time of admission; building a trusting relationship provides a strong foundation for future interventions. Nurses and the rehabilitation team cannot promise that the patient will return to baseline. Instead, the rehabilitation nurse works with the patient and their individual challenges and therapies in the present with hope that the patient will get better in the future.

Behavioral Assessment and Planning

Mental status may vacillate from somnolent to agitated throughout the hospital stay. Behavior problems in rehabilitation are approached through working with the neuropsychologist and the interdisciplinary team to make a behavioral plan. The plan aims to modulate or extinguish some negative behaviors and encourage positive behaviors. The plan should be patient focused, parallel the patient's rehabilitation schedule, have specific goals, and include benchmarks that enable the team members working with the patient to know when the plan is successful. The major element in the success of any behavior program is consistency in following through. At the onset of each incident, the nurse needs to reintroduce herself or himself and reorient the patient to the plan as though it were new each time for the patient.

Several scales are presently in use to determine the degree, severity, and range of agitation in patients. One such scale, the Agitated Behavior Scale (ABS), uses objective scoring of 14 behaviors, and is used for ongoing assessment of agitation during the acute phase of recovery (9). Each behavior is scored 1 (absent) to 4 (severe). The total score is a measure of the level of agitation: 21–27 is mild agitation, 29–34 is moderate agitation, and greater than 35 is severe agitation (9). Scoring is done daily at predetermined intervals. Close monitoring of the ABS scores allows the team to evaluate the efficacy of the interventions and use that information to update the plan used to help the agitated patient. Accurate documentation of the ABS score and a 24-hour sleep–wake cycle provides data to the physiatrist who may adjust medications with a goal of weaning the patient from their use. Using a table for ABS documentation provides the team the ability to follow the trends in a concise format (see Table 27-1). In addition to documenting the numbers, a com-

TABLE 27-1 Agitated Behavior Scale

BEHAVIOR	TIME
Short attention span, easy distractibility, inability to concentrate	
Impulsive, impatient, low tolerance for pain or frustration	
Uncooperative, resistant to care, demanding	
Violent and/or threatening violence toward people or property	
Explosive and/or unpredictable anger	
Rocking, rubbing, moaning, or other self-stimulating behavior	
Pulling at tube restraints, etc.	
Wandering from treatment areas	
Restlessness, pacing, excessive movement	
Repetitive behaviors, motor and/or verbal	
Rapid, loud, or excessive talking	
Sudden changes of mood	
Easily initiated or excessive crying and/or laughter	
Self-abusiveness, physical and/or verbal	

Total score

1 = absent	14–20	= no agitation
2 = present to slight degree	21–27	= mild agitation
3 = present to a moderate degree	28–34	= moderate agitation
4 = present to an extreme degree	35+	= severe

TABLE 27-2 Example of Treatment Plan

0730	Lights on, open blinds, reorientation
0800	Occupational therapy—ADLs or living skills
0900	Meal
1000	Physical therapy
1030	Speech therapy
1100	Neuropsychology group or individual
1130	Quiet time
1200	Meal
1300	Occupational therapy
1330	Speech therapy
1400	Physical therapy
1430	Therapeutic recreation group or individual
1500	Quiet time
1600	Teaching group patients and families
1700	Meal
1800	Unstructured leisure time with family
1900	Medication and showers
2030	Bedtime

ADLs, activities of daily living.

ASSESSMENT TOOLS

There are numerous assessment tools that can be used for the person with TBI. They range from the Coma/Near-Coma Scale and Coma Recovery Scale-Revised to the Community Integration Scale (see Chapter 20). There are scales that assess cognition, mobility, and family coping. Some of the scales may be used once or they may be used throughout the continuum of care. Several of the more commonly used functional measures in inpatient rehabilitation include the Disability Rating Scale (DRS), the Functional Independence Measure, and the Rancho Los Amigos Scale.

The DRS shows a change in patterns of behavior, and can be used throughout, at least, the early continuum of rehabilitation health care because it has not been validated in the long-term care setting. The DRS provides concise information regarding the cognitive and functional status of a patient at a given point and allows across-time comparisons. Proper training is critical to optimize inter-rater reliability (11). The scale is composed of 8 items divided into 4 categories: arousal, cognitive ability for self-care, degree of dependence, and employability (12). The interdisciplinary team scoring indicates if a patient is progressing or not during their rehabilitation program.

The Functional Independence Measure (FIM) is a widely used scale in rehabilitation. The measure uses a 7-point scale to estimate the severity and the amount of assistance needed to complete a task or respond to a question. The point ranges from "1" (*total assistance*) to "7" (*complete independence*). Point ranges of 1 to 5 require a helper/caregiver providing care from total assistance to supervision. The FIM score provides clinicians, payers, as well as family members/caregivers with a numeric representation of the relative burden of care for that particular patient; that is, the physical level of assistance to care for that patient. The levels of dependence range from independent to fully dependent where minimal assistance is defined as when the patient is able to do 75% of the task, moderate assistance where the patient does at least 50% of the task, and maximum assistance being where the patient

ment regarding the circumstances surrounding the change of behavior and the intervention provides the team background to make changes to the behavioral program as necessary.

The rehabilitation nurse, as a member of the interdisciplinary team, uses pharmacological interventions prescribed by the neurorehabilitation or consulting physician, as well as non-pharmacological interventions and behavioral strategies planned by the team in a consistent manner. Use of restraints is presently considered somewhat controversial and its use is generally being curtailed because of the mounting evidence that it can increase agitation (10). A structured environment and training in use of de-escalation techniques are essential when dealing with the agitated patient.

Collaboration with the interdisciplinary team and frequent review of the plan facilitates timely intervention with the goal of optimizing functional outcomes (see Chapter 63 for more information). Treatment plans are altered on an individual basis. Depending on the individuals' endurance, medical stability, or behavior, they may need longer rest periods or quiet time (see Table 27-2). Suggestions for groups include cognition, aphasic, art, music, and relaxation.

is only able to do 25% of the task (13). The scoring of each of the 18 items is done collaboratively with the interdisciplinary team members. The rehabilitation nurse is essential to the scoring process because of their involvement with the patient over the 24-hour care cycle.

The Rancho Los Amigos Scale interprets the cognitive behavioral recovery process after a brain injury. The scale ranges from 1 to 10; a lower score indicates a more severe impairment of consciousness (14). The agitated patient is commonly labeled as a Rancho IV, and is the population most often medicated because of the disruptive nature of this type of behavior in the traditional rehabilitation setting (although some have argued that the drug treatments may actually be deleterious to the expedience of neurorecovery). The rehabilitation nurse collaborates with the interdisciplinary team to limit the use of medications that may impair cognition, behavior, and/or recovery. Accurate documentation of the ABS score and 24-hour sleep–wake cycle provides data to the physician, who may adjust medications with a goal of weaning the patient from their use.

Developing an individual understanding of each patient's premorbid function and age-related abilities is an important aspect of the nurse's role in the rehabilitation process and enables structuring of comprehensive interventions. These interventions take into account the patient's unique cognitive deficits and level of presentation, as does their implementation and subsequent assessments.

NUTRITION

Adequate nutritional intake is essential for the patient with TBI who has increased caloric needs in the acute recovery process. The route of nutrition can be by mouth (per os or P.O.) or enteral and less commonly parenteral (intravenously). The physician, rehabilitation nurse, speech-language pathologist, and dietitian develop a nutrition plan working together in an interdisciplinary manner.

When the patient is unable to meet their caloric needs by mouth because of aspiration, lethargy, or other impairments, then other forms of feeding must be considered. The dietitian calculates the caloric needs and determines the formula and fluids required, and percutaneous endoscopic gastrostomy tubes are placed. During the administration of tube feedings, the head of the bed must be at least 30–45° to decrease the risk of aspiration. Gastric residuals are checked before feedings and the skin around the tube site is assessed for irritation and excoriation. Medications to increase gastric motility may be administered although medications that are dopamine antagonists should ideally be avoided, particularly early in neurorecovery. Cleaning the site with soap and water are completed on a daily basis (see Chapter 54).

Dysphagia poses a serious risk of aspiration in the patient with TBI. To determine if the patient can swallow, the speech-language pathologist conducts a bedside swallow evaluation or performs a modified barium swallow in radiology. The speech-language pathologist communicates the results to the physician and the nurse who then incorporate changes into the plan of care. The speech pathologist integrates the results of the evaluation into treatment. This treatment may include trials of different solid consistencies (pure, soft, or general) as well as various liquid consistencies (honey-thick, nectar-thick, or thin liquids) or swallow strategies that increase the safety of the swallow and move the patient from enteral to oral feeding (see Chapter 66).

Swallowing strategies and interventions must often be utilized with TBI having cognitive deficits. Patients may demonstrate behaviors such as poor impulse control secondary to impulsivity, distractibility, poor attention, overstimulation, visual perceptual problems, or neglect. All the aforementioned behaviors may present with an increased risk for aspiration and poor intake. The need for 1:1 supervision in a non-distracting environment is optimal for these types of patients. Caloric intake monitoring and weekly weights are maintained for the dietitian to ensure adequate nutritional intake. Discontinuation of tube feedings is dependent on the patient's swallow abilities and/or the patient's ability to meet their caloric and fluid needs.

The speech-language pathologist may institute the Frazier Free Water Protocol after the assessment of the patient's swallow ability (15). This may be recommended for those patients on thickened liquids or those having their nutritional needs met by the use of percutaneous endoscopic gastrostomy tube. This provides the patient with the ability to increase hydration without the use of IVs. It may also increase the patient's compliance to thickened liquids as recommended by the speech-language pathologist. The protocol allows the patient to drink free water after thorough oral care. The amount of bacteria entering the lungs is decreased if the patient aspirates while drinking and the water will be absorbed. The water is allowed only between meals and no medications are to be administered with the water. Any swallow recommendations must be adhered to decrease the risk of aspiration (15) (see Chapter 66).

SLEEP

Adequate, restful, and restorative sleep is necessary for every segment of the population, but it is even more important and more elusive for those with TBIs. Nurses play an important role in facilitating sleep in their patients. The nature and scope of sleep disturbances, the impact of these disturbances on the patient, and the ways in which nurses can ensure that their patients are getting adequate sleep will be discussed in this section.

Sleep disorders are common in this population and may include sleep apnea, restless leg syndrome, periodic limb movement disorders, circadian rhythm disorders, and narcolepsy (less commonly), among others. Sleep problems may present with myriad symptoms including—but not limited to—difficulty falling asleep; inability to maintain sleep; early awakening, fitful sleep; waking not feeling refreshed; daytime hypersomnolence; among other manifestations (16,17). Brain injury, pain, affective disorders (including post-traumatic stress disorder [PTSD], anxiety disorders, and depression), daytime sleeping, boredom, environmental noise and lighting, medications, and other factors may all negatively impact sleep (see Chapter 43). Studies have shown that between 30%–70% of this population report sleep problems (16,18,19). Cohen found that the problem is more prevalent in women and older adults and states that 82% of people with a sleep disorder have difficulty initiating and maintaining sleep.

Lack of sleep can exacerbate symptoms such as pain, cognitive deficits, fatigue, or irritability (16,20). The patient with TBI already has cognitive and physical deficits, which, when compounded with a sleep disorder, can inhibit, extend, or delay the rehabilitation process. Daytime fatigue and somnolence lead to poor participation in rehabilitation and therefore directly affect patient outcomes (21,22). Therefore, observing, assessing, and facilitating the aspects of the patient with TBI are important facet of nursing care for these patients.

To promote adequate, restful sleep for the patient, a sleep history and pattern should be assessed on admission (23). The history may be from the patient, but the nurse should be aware that the patient may lack insight or the ability to communicate, and family input should also be considered and solicited. The nurse needs to listen to and document what patients say about their sleep and communicate this information to the other nurses (24). A nurse-charted 24-hour sleep–wake cycle is an important tool that serves several purposes. It provides the interdisciplinary team with information they need to determine what, if any, sleep-related problems may arise in their therapy sessions. It also provides data necessary for evaluating sleep disorder patterns and tailoring interventions based on each patient's needs.

The patient with severe brain injury may not know if they have slept well because of their lack of awareness and/or memory (25,26). Nurses should evaluate the sleep state of the patient during nightly rounds. If the patient has excessive fatigue, somnolence, or an increase in cognitive problems during the day, an evaluation of sleep patterns should be considered (27). Environment, physiology, and psychology affect sleep (28). Reid states that the hospital environment is not conducive to inducing and maintaining a good night sleep. Pain and depression also impair sleep. Nurses have the responsibility and the ability to mitigate environmental factors, to document pain and help facilitate pain management, and to bring symptoms of depression to the attention of the interdisciplinary team (17,23). Clustering of nursing care will decrease interruptions of the patient's sleep. These are ways in which the rehabilitation nurse can enhance the well-being of the patient and help them progress in their rehabilitation efforts.

Evaluation of the environment is necessary when considering the problem of sleep in the rehabilitation patient. Studies have shown that the main cause of sleep disturbance in the hospital is noise (29). Hospital staff members need to be aware of the noise in their surroundings: conversations should be quiet, swift, and timely response to equipment alarms and call bells will limit patient disturbance; and, televisions should be off. Lights at night can hinder sleep and can confuse hospitalized patients because they may not know if it is day or night; only a dim light or a night light should be left on for safety. It is also important to orient the patient by opening the window shades during the day and closing them at night. The room thermostat must be set at a temperature comfortable for each individual (28).

The patient with TBI may have pain issues and may not be able to maintain a comfortable position because of their mobility deficits. Pain management is an important aspect of sleep that should be dealt with (23). Medications need to be assessed to make sure that there are not any that interfere with sleep. Medications must also be administered when patients are awake; to avoid disturbing what may be a fragile sleep state. Constipation, urinary retention, and incontinence should also be taken into consideration. Elimination programs can be individualized to allow for sleep. Caffeine, chocolate, tea, and caffeinated soft drinks may have an effect on sleep and should not be taken within 6 hours prior to sleep (17). Alcohol, nicotine, and exercise before sleep may have an effect on their ability to fall asleep or stay asleep (17). (See Chapter 43 for more information.)

FALLS

For the population of 65 years or older, the Center for Disease Control estimates the cost of fall-related injuries to be $54.2 billion in 2020. Falls are a common occurrence in acute rehabilitation (30,31). The goal for rehabilitation is to reduce falls and the severity of injuries, and the rehabilitation nurse must focus on fall reduction and prevention of fall-related injury. Patients with TBIs have cognitive deficits and are frequently impulsive and unaware of their deficits. Their physical mobility can be limited to poor coordination and balance to flaccid limbs. Poor vision and neglect are risk factors for falls; and pharmacological interventions may further impair the person.

Initially, the individual needs to be assessed for risk factors using a standardized risk form. According to Quigley, there are 4 main factors that have a bearing on the risk for injury. The ABCs for fall risk are Age (less than 4 or greater than 85 years old, Bones (history of osteoarthritis), and Coagulation and surgery. This information should be disseminated to all of the interdisciplinary team. Safety "huddles" among the interdisciplinary staff occur throughout the day to provide interventions for safety issues.

It is necessary to educate the individual and their family about what they can do to decrease the risk of falls. The teach-back method is an effective tool in this situation. The information is taught and the person or family member describes what they heard and demonstrates the techniques (32).

When interventions are put into place to decrease the risk of falls, environmental factors should be taken into account. The patient should be assigned a bed that allows them to exit toward their strong side (31,32). A room location as close to the nurse's station as possible, furniture that does not roll or that can be locked in place, keeping personal items in reach, utilizing nonskid floor mats or nonskid socks and proper lighting, and maintaining a clutter-free floor all reduce the risk of falls (31).

Assistive devices such as walkers or wheelchairs should be available (32,33). Wheelchairs can be outfitted with alarm belts and brake extenders (31). Low beds with bed pads are now readily available at many facilities to decrease injuries, along with the use of bed alarms. Nurses should check the devices to see that they are in place and working properly. Hip protectors designed to reduce the risk of hip fractures are also valuable in preventing injuries (31). The nurse completes hourly rounds in anticipation of patient needs. Patients are assessed for pain, positioning, toileting, and environment (31). All patients should be toileted before administering a cognitively altering medication, including, but not limited, to benzodiazepines. If a fall occurs, a post-fall huddle is recommended to be attended by all interdisciplinary team members and the patient to determine the root cause and preventable measures (31,32). This procedure can assist in reducing repeat falls.

Restraints of various types continue to be used at times for patient safety although, as previously noted, there remain controversies including issues of safety secondary to risk of injury to the patient, liability concerns, and potential patient civil rights violations. The least restrictive devices should be the first to be considered for use. For fall safety, the use of an enclosure bed may make more sense relative to the aforementioned than direct use of restraints. This device allows the patient to turn and sit up in bed with the only restriction in movement being the inability to get out of bed without assistance. The roll belt is another restrictive device to use in bed, allowing the patient to roll but restricting them from getting up without assistance.

INTEGUMENATARY

Persons with TBI are at a high risk for skin breakdown because of immobility, limited range of motion, spasticity, edema, and nutritional changes. A thorough skin assessment and documentation of existing skin breakdown is essential to prevention and treatment of skin abnormalities. The rehabilitation nurse must document observable skin integrity, including, but not limited to, immobility (external splints, cast, and positioning devices), impaired nutrition, incontinence of bowel and bladder, sensory impairments, and tissue perfusion. The Braden Scale is an assessment tool that scores the risk for the patient in developing pressure ulcers. Braden looks at sensory perception, moisture, activity, mobility, nutrition, and friction (33,34). At this time, the International NPUAP-EPUAP (National Pressure Ulcer Advisory Panel-European Pressure Ulcer Advisory Panel) acknowledges that there are contributing risk factors for pressure ulcers but have not determined the significance of them.

The International NPUAP-EPUAP has collaborated to develop prevention, treatment, and classification system for pressure ulcers. Categories are associated with tissue loss caused by pressure and are not to be used for other wounds. There are 4 Categories: Category I, non-blanchable redness of intact skin; Category II, partial thickness skin loss or blister; Category III, full thickness skin loss; and Category IV, full thickness tissue loss. The United States is continuing to use the classification on unstageable and suspected deep tissue injury–depth unknown (35).

When assessing pressure ulcers, documentation includes the category, size, color, any exudate in the wound bed and surrounding skin, odor, tunneling, and evidence of granulation tissue (35). Photographs of the pressure ulcer allow a team to have a reference from baseline through the healing process. The team takes the information from the assessment to determine the plan that promotes healing. Assessment of the nutritional status of the person with a pressure ulcer is important for the healing process. The person with TBI may already have nutritional risk factors such as difficulty swallowing. A well-balanced caloric intake, hydration, and blood values need to be monitored. Prevention of pressure ulcers is not the sole responsibility of the rehabilitation nurse. The team provides significant input related to immobility and positioning. A turning and repositioning schedule is needed for those at risk. The side lying should

be at 30° angle and the head of the bed should not be at 90° angle to avoid shearing. In the bed, heel pressure is relieved either with pillows or a boot. The boot must allow a space so the heel does not rest on the bottom of the boot. The occupational and physical therapist may provide a schedule for wear time for any positioning devices. The device must be checked frequently for skin breakdown and adjusted where needed. When in the seated position, care should be taken that the individual has full range of motion. They should be upright with their feet flat on the floor or foot pedals. This seating keeps the person from sliding and shearing. Range of motion should be provided for the person with TBI on a regular schedule. The documentation of the prevention measures, including frequency, what was done, and the outcome provide the information needed to change the plan of care as needed.

It is important to have face-to-face hand off communication between shifts as well as communication with the interdisciplinary team because collaboration and communication is essential in prevention and healing of pressure ulcers. The tasks of turning, repositioning, proper hydration and nutrition, and toileting schedule should be viewed as the sole responsibility of nursing. A wound care consult is recommended for facilities that have this type of specialized expertise.

ELIMINATION

Bladder Issues

Urinary continence and retention is an important consideration in the rehabilitation of the patient with TBI. Incontinence-related problems that may arise are pressure ulcers and falls. Chua and associates found that 62% of TBI in acute rehabilitation had urinary incontinence (36) and also found that incontinence is significantly correlated with poorer outcomes and increased length of stay. Pinkowski 1996 found that poor assessment led to increase of health cost (37). Prevention of these negative outcomes requires a patient-focused approach to continence and management (38).

Several factors should be considered for the assessment. These include past and recent history of urinary continence, past medical history, physical mobility, communication, cognition, and physical exam (39,40). Urinalysis should be ordered to determine if there is any underlying cause of the incontinence (41). Determining the reasons for incontinence symptoms is important; the symptoms may stem from urge, stress, or overflow. Some patients may experience functional incontinence—an impaired ability to manage clothing openings or a mental impairment that keeps them from realizing that they need to urinate.

The rehabilitation nurse is the leader in designing an individual plan of care for the patient and is responsible for assessing, planning, implementing, and evaluating the program. Other team members provide input for successful management. The physical therapist evaluates transfer techniques and sitting balance and gait. The occupational therapist assesses for adaptive equipment for clothing management, vision, and upper extremity function as well as activities of daily living (ADLs). Determination of the patient's communication and swallowing abilities is generally under the domain of the speech therapist.

For cognitively impaired patients, a timed voiding schedule is often useful. The staff keeps a diary of the voiding pattern for 3 days. This information is used to set up a toileting program with the goal of creating continence. For the person who has some awareness, a habit training schedule is useful. If the person has increased urinary frequency, a behavior program may be established to increase the time between voids; however, urinary tract pathology including infection or stones should be ruled out. Prompted voiding may work well for the individual with some awareness but inability to consistently and fully express their needs (41). Any program that is chosen needs to be evaluated for success and plan of care changes as needed. Yates states that if the bladder programs are unsuccessful, medications could be attempted but should be used with caution (41).

To determine post-void residual (PVR), a "bladder scan" (i.e., bedside portable ultrasound of the bladder) is preferred to intermittent catheterization because it is not an invasive procedure. If there are persistent urological problems evident including excessive urination (i.e., polyuria), urgency, dysuria, nocturia, and/or hematuria, then appropriate laboratory testing may need to be recommended. On occasion, a recommendation by nursing to the physician for referral for urological work-up including potentially urodynamic studies may be indicated to further elucidate the neuro-urological status of a patient following TBI.

Bowel Issues

Changes to the brain after TBI may interfere with bowel management; often, there is a decrease in mobility and activity, dietary changes, cognitive changes, and a change in self-awareness. These changes can result in constipation, impaction, and diarrhea. Accidents during this period can also be a problem to self-esteem and skin management.

A thorough assessment including nutrition, mobility, and premorbid as well as recent history of bowel patterns is essential for care planning. Goals of the bowel program include having a predictable bowel movement to avoid accidents and facilitate evacuation. A good bowel program should assure adequate hydration and fiber with consideration of stool softener, cathartics, enemas, and/or suppository use as needed. The program should emphasize an evacuation schedule that occurs daily about an hour after eating a particular meal (i.e., breakfast) to take advantage of the normally occurring gastrocolic reflexes. As cognition and self-awareness improve, bowel continence normally follows. For diarrhea, a thorough assessment of the cause should be evaluated and acted on. Just as with urinary elimination, the interdisciplinary team is involved with the assessment and management of the patient with bowel issues (42) (see Chapter 54).

PAIN

Pain diagnosis and management in TBI is a complex and challenging situation. Many factors contribute to the problems that may be encountered in this aspect of caring for these patients. Patients with TBI present with cognitive defi-

cits and their speech and communication are often affected, which may hinder assessment of pain (43,44). Their sensory and motor functioning may also be affected, along with their perception of the pain (44). Pain may manifest in ways that are already part of the brain injury sequelae. Cognitive deficits, mood, anxiety, decreased socialization, and functional loss may all worsen if the pain is unrelieved (45,46). It is therefore imperative that pain be adequately addressed and modulated to allow for the affected individual to be able to optimally participate in their rehabilitation.

Several types of pain are addressed in the literature. Neuropathic pain is described as "pins and needles." Spasticity is the tightness or resistance to strength. Heterotopic ossification (the growth of bone in soft tissue), DVT, and headache are common sources of pain (43,44). Sherman also discusses constipations and urinary tract infections as preventable causes of discomfort that need to be addressed (44).

The TBI nurse assesses the individual for a history of premorbid pain issues, pain relief that has been tried, and the efficacy of each type of treatment. This information may need to be obtained from the family member or medical records that are available because the information from the patient may be limited and will provide the background information needed to institute an individualized pain management program.

Assessment of the individual's pain is a challenge because their communication may be compromised. In addition, cognitive impairment may cause perseveration on the pain. In spite of these issues, the best information about whether they are in pain is from the patient themselves. When taking a history, consider using assessment tools such as non-verbal scales, visual analog scales, verbal rating scales, drawing pictures of painful areas, and pain diaries. Pain assessments need to be completed on a formal tool and documented on a regular basis.

Factors that may impact pain management include attitude, belief, and culture on the part of both the patient and the nurse. Cultures that have a stoic background include Northern European and Asian, whereas Hispanic, Middle Eastern, and Mediterranean cultures are sometimes more expressive (45). Members of the medical profession, including physicians and nurses, may believe in limiting pain medication, and laws regarding the type and amount of medication that can be administered change.

Medication use should be balanced with cognitive recovery (44). Scheduled pain medication for those individuals who are unable to describe their pain or lack awareness that they have pain may be the best option (44). Behavioral strategies such as distraction or visualization may be used with the medication or alone, and having a multidisciplinary team approach will enhance the teaching and learning (47). Thermal therapies including heat- and cold-based therapies can also modulate certain types of pain.

Involving the patient and the family in the treatment plan is important to the success of the pain management program because reassessment and adjustment of the plan of care as outcomes are monitored and considered (47). Allowing the individual to have the optimum rehabilitation experience is the goal of pain treatment. Pain management is important in many aspects including helping the patient have more normalized sleep patterns. Improved sleep may facilitate daytime arousal and therapy participation, as well as, decreased anxiety. Optimally, the outcome of pain management would be that there were no associated complications to the pain condition such as falls, altered cognition or behavior, or medication related side effects (see Chapters 57 and 58).

Headache

Headaches are recognized as a common pain complaint after TBI (48,49,50). Post-traumatic headache (PTHA) is classified in the International Classification of Headache disorders as a headache that occurs 7 days after the trauma and may last less than 3 months or greater than 3 months (51) although some have questioned the clinical relevance of this classifcation. Symptoms associated with headache may include, but are not limited to, decreased cognition, anxiety, irritability, and insomnia (49,51). Headache may also aggravate TBI, as well as trauma related conditions including but not limited to cognition, behavior, PTSD, and driving skills.

Assessment of headache is generally more difficult in persons after severe TBI than in persons after mild TBI (MTBI). The person who is able to verbalize the pain and provide feedback for the treatment modality used has the most effective pain management program. The person with cognitive and communication deficits presents additional challenges when it comes to assessing pain conditions including headache. In persons after severe TBI, it is therefore even more relevant to use multiple inputs when assessing pain, including staff and family observations, patient self-report, pain scales, and/or physiological and laboratory measures (52).

The rehabilitation nurse is important in this process because they have established a relationship with the patient and family. They are able to assess for the cognitive and behavioral changes of the patient. After assessing the headache and providing the treatment, nurses must reassess to determine if the treatment plan was effective. Keeping a journal of the headaches by either the patient or the family or the nurse provides documentation of the frequency, intensity, treatment measures, and relief. The aforementioned information can be used for assessing the headache subtype(s) and to help direct treatment (see Chapter 56).

SEIZURES

Seizures are a serious potential consequence of TBI and certainly more likely to be seen with greater severity injuries including ones with dural penetration and/or prolonged periods of unconsciousness. In the acute setting, antiepileptic drugs may be used for a short time for prophylaxis. Long-term prophylaxis for seizures is no longer recommended based on current evidence-based medicine (see Chapter 39). If patients have seizures while being treated with an antiepileptic drug, it could mean that they are being inadequately treated (i.e., wrong medication, too low a serum level of the drug being used, need for more than monotherapeutic approach, etc.), that there is a new brain pathology (i.e., reaccumulation of an extra-axial clot), or an abscess formation, among other possibilities. Hypoglycemia, hypotension, and hypoxia can precede seizures and emphasizes the need for careful monitoring of vital signs.

By current standards, seizure prophylaxis is typically only continued for a week. Patients who subsequently have witnessed seizures or are deemed to likely have post-traumatic epilepsy are placed on antiepileptic medication. It may take more than one medication to control seizure activity. Laboratory values are monitored as clinically indicated to ensure therapeutic serum drug levels. The rehabilitation nurse needs to be knowledgeable regarding these and other medications and must also be aware of adverse signs related to drug side effects as well as the nuances of laboratory monitoring interpretation. The patient receiving medication such as phenytoin via a percutaneous endoscopic gastrostomy must have the tube feeding off 1 hour before and for 1 hour after receiving phenytoin for better absorption. The patient with potentially traumatic event should have their room set up appropriately in case of a seizure event including having suction set up and nasal oxygen tubing connected to wall oxygen.

If a seizure occurs, it is important to have nursing staff document as much as possible regarding the event including any noted triggers, the behavioral manifestations (eye deviation, incontinence, loss of consciousness, sensory and/or motor signs, among other possible presentations), the duration of the episode, and its aftermath including whether or not there was a post-ictal state, and/or any injuries (see Chapter 39).

Family education is essential for patients at risk for seizures. Education needs to focus on what to do in the event of a seizure, maintaining compliance with medications, education on the medication, dosage, schedule, and side effects. (See Chapter 39 for more information on seizures.)

SEXUALITY

The role of nurses regarding dealing with sexuality issues in the context of brain injury care is not clearly defined in the literature. Attention to sexual issues has the potential to help the patient with brain injury understand that he or she is still capable of experiencing and expressing sexuality and thereby work toward recovery of sexual function; however, nurses lack comprehensive training regarding this sensitive and important dimension of the patient. The nurse is in a position to observe and interact with the patient. Because the nurse also interacts with physicians, the patient's partner, and with the rehabilitation team, the nurse has the ability to communicate with others in order to facilitate this important facet of the brain injured recovery, and needs to do so in a professional manner.

Sexual dysfunction is common among patients with TBI (53). ''The loss of sexual function that often follows TBI can be devastating for the person with the injury, as well as their intimate partner'' (54). However, this is often neglected by health professionals and society in general, despite sexuality being a fundamental right of every individual (55,56).

Each individual may present with a wide range of symptoms that have a bearing on their sexuality. Physical impairments, such as paralysis or weakness, can prevent free movement or positioning. The lack of sensation can inhibit the experience. Discomfort and pain inhibit weight bearing and movement. Cognitive impairments may impact the individual's ability to concentrate and initiation may be impaired. Bowel and bladder incontinence can hinder a sexual relationship for both the individual with brain injury and the significant other. When the partner becomes the caregiver, the intimacy between the two may become strained, and impaired communication may frustrate the couple even more.

The nurse's role in addressing sexuality issues (and they may take many forms) during inpatient rehabilitation remains debated. Gan states that sexuality is not often addressed in rehabilitation (57). Sexuality for the patient with a TBI may not be a priority for the rehabilitation team because they are more concerned with functions of daily living, mobility, toileting, dressing, and nutrition. Staff may also believe that the patient is not at a level of recovery where they can make appropriate decisions about sexual intimacy.

To begin to address the sexual concerns, the permission, limited information, specific suggestions, and intensive therapy (PLISSIT) model may be used (57). The first step is to get permission to create an environment that the parties know that they can express their concerns. Limited information is shared to reduce anxiety. Specific suggestions about how the patient's concerns can be addressed are followed by intensive therapy, where the staff refers the patient to the appropriate specialist. Gan states that the goal of the intervention is to acknowledge sexuality and provide information (57). Targeted workshops are increasingly available, and every brain injury nurse should be trained to deal with the sexuality of the patient. The role of the acute rehabilitation nurse is to open the communication in this area, provide information in accordance to their knowledge base and know where to obtain the information (see Chapter 55).

ALCOHOL AND SUBSTANCE ABUSE

Much has been written about alcohol and substance abuse in relation to the TBI population and all of the literature points to the primary importance of a comprehensive assessment as key to beginning to address these problems when they are present (58,59,60). The 1997 Bombardier study reflects the readiness of the patient with TBI to change alcohol consumption habits, (61) and the Bombardier and Associates study of 2003 indicated the need for prevention programs within the first year after brain injury and before the patient begins drinking again (62). Therefore, motivational strategies implemented at the time of rehabilitation might be used with increased success to help assess and change the patient's alcohol consumption habits. Prevention efforts begin with engaging the patient in discussing how alcohol affects them and how its use will affect their recovery from the brain injury. Alcohol-dependent patients need to understand that alcohol use impacts relationships with family and friends, interferes with thinking skills, changes the balance of interactions between medications, and can promote seizures. Long-term specialized treatment programs should be recommended as follow through (62,63) (see Chapter 79).

TEAM CONFERENCES

Team conference is an important element of care for all steps in the post-TBI neurorehabilitation continuum including acute inpatient rehabilitation, sub-acute care, and all aspects of community-based rehabilitation including day and outpatient rehabilitation, as well as longer term supported care. Rehabilitation nursing should play an integral role in the team conference process as implied in the aforementioned narrative. It is pivotal for nursing to be present when discussing the plan of care because it is nursing that generally carries out the plan when other therapists are not present (at least in the context of in facility care). The nurse caring for the patient must know the plan of care to reduce miscommunication between the team and the patient and family.

Rehabilitation nursing partners with physiatry to address the medical issues of the patient with TBI. There should be adequate and ongoing communication regarding cognitive and behavioral status, neuromedical changes (particularly if potentially signaling a decline in patient status), bowel and bladder updates, nutritional/dietary follow along, fall risk assessment (along with therapy input), and reporting on integumentary status. The team meeting provides a structured opportunity for nursing to report on the aforementioned issues and further coordinate ongoing care with the team at large, as well as to modify, as necessary, the plan of care.

ROLES OF THE REHABILITATION NURSE

It is important to keep in mind that the process of rehabilitation is not limited to one setting; it is a process which starts typically in the field at the scene of the accident and moves through various phases including acute care (i.e., emergency department (ED), intensive care unit [ICU], neurosurgical step down unit), rehabilitation unit (whether or not a dedicated brain injury unit), day rehab or outpatient unit, long-term care treatment scenarios, and in the community at large. The rehabilitation nurse should use a holistic biopsychosocial approach to both evaluation and care of the person with TBI, ideally, remaining aware of the specific diagnosis and premorbid history regardless of the patient, their age, or the setting in which they practice. The expertise of the rehabilitation nurse enables them to provide a continuum of care throughout the health care system. They also work in the community through education and preventive measures.

The Association of Rehabilitation Nurses (ARN) recognizes the experienced rehabilitation nurse with advanced level of knowledge through certification and maintains a website at http://www.rehabnurse.org/. Becoming a Certified Rehabilitation Registered Nurse provides recognition of expertise and professional credibility.

The rehabilitation admission liaison nurse is an expert in the field of care coordination. They assess the physical needs, the emotional readiness, and the financial eligibility of the rehab patient, and recommend the appropriate level of care. With professional training in managed care, they negotiate cost-effective plans and serve as contacts between clients, their family, the institution, and external sources such as insurance providers. They also oversee record keeping and coordinate communication among all parties involved with rehabilitation of the patient with brain injury. It is recommended that the rehabilitation admission liaison nurse have a minimum of 2 years experience and certification in rehabilitation or a related field.

The rehabilitation staff nurse is the leader in maximizing the rehabilitation process. The experienced staff nurse works with the patient on a shift-long basis, and is therefore able to evaluate the interdisciplinary plans and communicate to the team what benefits the patient outcomes and what should be changed. In addition to being a caregiver, the staff nurse educates the patient and family and advocates for the patient because they interact with all disciplines involved in the patient's care.

The gerontological nurse specialty concentrates their practice on the population older than 65 years of age and the illness and injury that they may encounter. The pediatric specialty also recognizes the age of the population with the emphasis on the developmental theory. The nurses in both these specialties incorporate the staff nurse description and include consultation with other practitioner and research. The pain management rehabilitation nurse improves the quality of life of those affected by pain. They work with the patient to set goals and strategies for reducing pain and enable them to maximize their level of functioning. The nurse provides education for the patients, caregivers, and health care team. It is recommended that they have a minimum of 2 years experience in rehabilitation and also in acute and chronic management of pain.

The home care rehabilitation nurse is recognized as a specialty in the continuum of care from the rehabilitation facility to the home and community. They coordinate the process that has been indentified in the interdisciplinary plan of care. The nurse consults with the patient, family, and services to achieve the greatest outcomes in the community.

The advanced practice rehabilitation nurse has a graduate degree in nursing. They may function in many different roles such as a nurse practitioner, case manager, staff nurse, nurse specialist, educator, consultant, and researcher. They work in a variety of settings, from hospital rehabilitation units to community populations (64).

Regardless of the work setting, the primary function of the rehabilitation nurse is to promote the independence of the patient, to teach the family about the patient's challenges, and to carry out the interdisciplinary plan of care. Nurses should additionally advocate for the patient when medical issues arise that may hold substantive medical morbidity, be life threatening, and/or interfere with the patient's ability to participate in the rehabilitation program. The nurse should be the physician's partner in keeping the patient healthy and participatory in the rehabilitation process. Communication between the nurse and physician needs to be one of mutual respect and one in which there is trust and camaraderie but with the focus being optimization of patient outcomes. The ability to institute the plan of care to keep the patient safe is basic to the rehabilitation process. When there are barriers to the nurse communicating with the physician, then adverse outcomes are potentially increased, which is in no one's best interest, in particular, the patients'. Keeping the focus of communication on what is best for the patient will assist nurses in advocating and promoting safety in their patients with TBI. Rehabilitation nursing is the specialized approach to helping the patient reach their full potential during rehabilitation and beyond.

CONCLUSION

The rehabilitation nurse is an integral part of the treatment team as related to the care of persons following TBI, particularly as related to moderate to severe TBI cases. Along with pharmacy and the chaplains, rehabilitation nursing is the only discipline that is present round-the-clock in most care settings and as such spends the most time with the patient and the family. Nursing is often the discipline that patients feel most comfortable in confiding their fears and apprehensions to, especially on the night shift where they can be their most vulnerable. Rehabilitation nursing can make a sizable contribution to the interdisciplinary plan of care through appropriate surveillance of the myriad neuromedical, psychological, and social issues that confront patients after TBI and their families during acute, post-acute, and community reentry based care.

The roles that rehabilitation nurses play in the various settings require further research relative to working with persons following TBI to optimize nursing interventions. Additionally, this reseach should be based on nursing evidence-based-practice and medical literature. The cost benefit of specialty trained rehabilitation nursing staff in the context of care for individuals after TBI needs to be clarified to support the continued challenges and benefits of better patient surveillance relative to improving outcomes and minimizing medical and psychosocial morbidity.

KEY CLINICAL POINTS

1. Rehabilitation nurses approach the patient in a holistic manner to facilitate the best possible medical and functional outcomes.
2. Rehabilitation nurses carry out the rehabilitation plan of care over the 24-hour period, assisting the patient to use the skills learned in the other discipline therapies.
3. Rehabilitation nurses manage behavioral issues including agitation and maladaptive behaviors to facilitate the continuity of the rehabilitation process and protect the patient from self-harm.
4. Rehabilitation nurses coordinate and facilitate the quality care that is efficient and effective in bringing about the achievement of the rehabilitation plan goals.
5. Rehabilitation nurses work in an interdisciplinary manner with the patient, family, and team to facilitate the rehabilitation plan.
6. Sexuality is an important aspect of the person with TBI and is often overlooked by nurses. They must be educated and feel comfortable with the subject to meet the needs of this population.
7. Rehabilitation may begin in the earliest setting of the ICU but it continues through a potentially multistep continuum involving acute care, inpatient rehabilitation, outpatient, transitional living, long-term care, home care, and community settings—all of which may benefit from nursing involvement.
8. Rehabilitation can be a lifelong process for the person with TBI and ongoing nursing involvement can aide in optimizing functional outcomes and decreasing morbidity.

KEY REFERENCES

1. Association of Rehabilitation Nurses (ARN). http://www.rehabnurse.org/.
2. Australasian Rehabilitation Nurses' Association Inc. (ARNA). http://www.arna.com.au/
3. European Pressure Ulcer Advisory Panel and National Pressure Ulcer Advisory Panel. *Treatment of Pressure Ulcers: Quick Reference Guide*. Washington, DC: National Pressure Ulcer Advisory Panel; 2009.
4. Hoeman S. *Rehabilitation Nursing: Prevention, Intervention and Outcomes*. 4th ed. St Louis, MO: Mosby; 2007.
5. Jacelon, CJ. *The Specialty Practice of Rehabilitation Nursing: A Core Curriculum*. 6th ed. Glenview, IL: Rehabilitation Nursing Foundation of the Association Rehabilitation of the Association of Rehabilitation Nurses; 2011.

References

1. Bradley M. Brain injury: what is known? [electronic version]. Department of Neurosurgery, Hunter Holmes McGuire VAMC 145. Nursing care of the neurosurgical blast injury patient. *J Neuropsych Clin N*. (n.d.);18:141.
2. Marik P, Varon J, Trosk T. Management of head trauma. *Chest*. 2002;122(2):699–711.
3. Turgeon A. Early determination of neurological prognosis in traumatic brain injury: beyond the Glasgow Coma Scale. *Critical Care Rounds*. 2006;7(2).
4. Rivers E, Nguyen B, Havstad S, et al. Early goal-directed therapy in the treatment of severe sepsis and septic shock. *N Engl J Med*. 2001;345:1368–1377.
5. Elliot D. An evaluation of the endpoints of resuscitation. *J Am Coll Surg*. 1998;187(5):536–547.
6. Carlile MC, Yablon SA, Frol AB, Lo D, Diaz-Arrastia R. DVT management following TBI: a practice survey of the TBI model systems. *J of Head Trauma Rehabil*. 2006;21(6):483–490.
7. Reiff DA, Haricharan RN, Bullington NM, Griffin RL, McGwin G, Rue LW. Traumatic brain injury associated with the development of deep vein thrombosis independent of pharmacologic prophylaxis. *J of Trauma*. 2009;66(5):1436–1440.
8. Agency for Healthcare Research and Quality. Clinical practice guidelines. AHRQ Web site. http://www.ahrq.gov/clinic/cpgsix.htm. Accessed May 28, 2012.
9. Bogner JA, Corrigan JD, Bode RK, Heinemann AW. Rating scale analysis of the Agitated Behavior Scale. *J Head Trauma Rehabil*. 2000;15(1):656–669.
10. Motts S, Poole J, Kenrick M. Physical and chemical restraints in acute care: their potential impact on the rehabilitation of older people. *IJNP*. 2005;11(3):95–101.
11. Chin P, Finocchiaro D, Rosebrough A. *Rehabilitation Nursing Practice*. New York, NY: McGraw-Hill; 2002.
12. Rappaport M. The Disability Rating and Coma/Near-Coma scales in evaluating severe head injury. *Neuropsychol Rehabil*. 2005;15:(3–4):442–453.
13. Cournan M. Use of the functional independence measure for outcomes measurement in acute inpatient rehabilitation. *Rehabil Nurs*. 2000;36(3):111–117. http://www.rehabnurse.org/uploads/files/rnj339.pdf. Accessed May 28, 2012.
14. Rancho Los Amigos National Rehabilitation Center. Patient information: Family Guide to the Rancho levels of cognitive functioning. http://www.rancho.org/research/bi_cognition.pdf. Accessed August 8, 2006.
15. http://www.jhsmh.org/Health-Services/Rehab-Services-Frazier-Rehab/Specialties/Frazier- Water-Protocol.aspx
16. Ouellet M, Savard J, Morin CM. Insomnia following traumatic brain injury: a review. *Neurorehabil and Neural Repair*. 2004;18(4):187–198.
17. Pellatt G. Clinical skills. The nurse's role in promoting a good night's sleep for patients. *Br J Nurse*. 2007;16(10):602–605.
18. Clinchot D, Bogner J, Mysiw W, Fugate L, Corrigan J. Defining sleep disturbance after brain injury. *AM J Phys Med Rehabil*. 1998;77(4):291–295.
19. Cohen M, Olsenberg A, Snir D, Stern M, Groswasser Z. Temporally related changes of sleep complaints in traumatic brain injured patients. *J Neurol Neurosurg Psychiatr*. 1992;55(4):313–315.
20. Greenwald B, Bell K. Sleep and TBI. 2010. http://msktc.washington.edu. Accessed May 28, 2012.
21. Ouellet J, Morin C. Insomnia following traumatic brain injury: a review. *Neurorehabil and Neural Repair*. 2004;18(4):187–198.
22. Makley M, English JB, Drubach DA, Kreuz AJ, Celnik PA, Tarwater PM. Prevalence of sleep disturbance in closed head injury patients in a rehab unit. *Neurorebil Neural Repair*. 2008;22(4):341–347.
23. Nagel C, Markie M, Richards K, et al. Sleep promotion in hospitalized elders. *Med Surg Nurs*. 2003;12(5):279–289.
24. Bephag G. Clinical skills: promoting quality sleep in older people: the nursing care role. *Br J Nurs*. 2005;14(4):205–210.
25. Castriotta R, Wilde M, Lai J, Atanasov S, Masel B, Kuna S. Prevalance and consequences of sleep disorders in traumatic brain injury. *J Clin Sleep Med*. 2007;3(4):349–356.
26. Mahmood O. Neuropsycological performance and sleep disturbance following traumatic brain injury. *J Head Trauma Rehabil*. 2005;19(50):378–390.
27. Ouellet J, Cohen M, Astriotta R. Prevelence and consequences of sleep disorders in traumatic brain injury. *Clin Sleep Med*. 2007;3(4):349–356.
28. Reid E. (2001). Clinical: factors affecting how patients sleep in the environment. *Br J Nurs*. 2001;14(4):912–915.
29. Southwell M, Wistow G. Inpatient sleep disturbance: the views of staff and patients. *Nursing Times*. 1995;91(37):29–31.
30. Rabadi MH. Risk factors for falls in stroke patients during inpatient rehabilitation. *Clin Rehabil*. 2009;23(5):463.
31. Quigly PA, Bulat T, Hart-Hughes S. Stratagies to reduce risk of fall related injuries in rehabilitation nursing. *Rehabil Nurs*. 2007;32:120–121.
32. Boushon B, Nielsen G, Quigley P, Rutherford P, Taylor J, Shannon D. *Transforming Care at the Bedside How-to Guide: Reducing Patient Injuries From Falls*. Cambridge, MA: Institute for Healthcare Improvement; 2008. www.ihi.org/.../TCABHowToGuideReducingPatientInjuriesfromFalls. Accessed May 28, 2012.
33. Bergstrom N, Braden BJ, Laguzza A, Holman V. The Braden Scale for predicting pressure sore risk. *Nurs Res*. 1987;36(4):205–210.
34. Braden B, Maklebust J. Preventing pressure ulcers with the braden scale: an update on this easy to use tool that assesses a patients risk. *Am J Nurs*. 2005;105(6):70–72.
35. European Pressure Ulcer Advisory Panel and National Pressure Ulcer Advisory Panel. *Treatment of Pressure Ulcers: Quick Reference Guide*. Washington, DC: National Pressure Ulcer Advisory Panel; 2009.
36. Chua K, Chuo A, Kong K. Urinary incontinence after traumatic brain injury; incidence, outcomes and correlates. *Brain Inj*. 2003;17(6):469–478.
37. Pinkowski P. Prompted Voiding in the Long-Term Care Facility. *JWOCN*. 1996;23(2):110–114.
38. Coffey A, McCarthy G, McCormick B, Wright J, Slater P. Incontinence: assessment, diagnosis, and management in two rehabilitation units for older people. *World Evid-based Nu*. 2007;4(4):179–186.
39. Sarker PK. Management of urinary incontinence. *J Clin Pharm Ther*. 2000;25(4):251–263.
40. Williams K. Stress urinary incontinence: treatment and support. *Nursing Standard*. 2004;18(31):54–56.
41. Yates A. Identifying and managing urinary continence problems. *Practice Nurse*. 2008;36(9):31–32.
42. RehabTeamSite. Medical Problems in TBI: Bowel Program in Traumatic Brain Injury: Bowel Movements/Bowel Program TBI. http://calder.med.miami.edu/pointis/handbook.html. Accessed May 28, 2012.

43. Ivanhoe CB, Hartman ET. Clinical caveats on medical assessment and treatment of pain after TBI. *J Head Trauma Rehabil*. 2004;19(1):29–39.

44. Sherman K, Goldberg M, Bell K. Traumatic brain injury and pain. *Phys Med Rehabil Clin N Am*. 2006;17(2):473–490.

45. Horgas A, Saunjoo L. Pain Nursing Standard of Practice Protocol: Pain Management in Older Adults. http://consultgerirn.org/topics/pain/want_to_know_more. Accessed May 28, 2012.

46. Branca B, Lake AE. Psychological and neuropsycology integration in multidisplinary pain management after TBI. *J Head Trauma Rehabil*. 2004;19(1):40–57.

47. Wells N, Pasero C, McCaffery M. Improving the quality of care through pain assessment and management. In: Hughes RG, ed. *Patient Safety and Quality. An Evidence-Based Handbook for Nurses*. Rockville, MD: Agency for Healthcare Reseacrch and Quality; 2008:469–489.

48. Hoffman J, Lucas S, Dikmen S, et al. Natural history of headache after traumatic brain injury. *J of Neurotrama*. 2011;28(9):1719–1725.

49. Nicholson K, Martelli MF. The problem of pain. *J Head Trauma Rehabil*. 2004;19(1):2–9.

50. Lew HL, Lin P, Fuh J, Wang S, Clark DJ, Walker WC. Characteristics and treatment of headache after traumatic brain injury. *Am J Phys Med Rehabil*. 2006;85(7):619–627.

51. Headache Classification Subcommittee of the International Headache Society. The International Classification of Headache Disorders: 2nd edition. *Cephalalgia*. 2004;24(suppl 1):9–160.

52. Gironda R, Chait S, Walker R, Ruff R, Craine M, Scholten J. Traumatic brain injury, polytrauma and pain: challenges and treatment strategies for the polytrauma rehabilitation. *Rehabil Psyc*. 2009;54(3):247–258.

53. Kreuter M, Dahlof AG, Gudjonnson G, Sullivan M, Siosteen A. Sexual adjustment and its predictors after traumatic brain injury. *Brain Inj*. 1998;12(5):349–368.

54. Sander A. Integrating sexualtiy into traumatic brain injury rehabilitation. *Brain Injury/Professional*. 2010;7(1):9–11.

55. Kreutzer JS, Zasler ND. Psychosexual consequences of traumatic brain injury; methodology and preliminary findings. *Brain Inj*. 1989;3(2):177–120.

56. Sakellariou D. If not the disability, then what? Barriers to reclaiming sexuality following spinal cord injury. *Sex, Disabil*. 2006;24:101–111.

57. Gan C. Everything you wanted to know about sex after brain injury but were afraid to ask. http://www.brainline.org/mutimedia/presentations/Caron_Gan-R&R_slides.pdf. Accessed May 28, 2012.

58. Corrigan J, Lamb-Hart, Rust E. A programme of interventions for substance abuse following traumatic brain injury. *Brain Inj*. 1995;9:221–223.

59. Bombardier C, Rimmele C, Zintal H. The magnitude and correlates of alcohol and drug use before TBI. *Arch Phys Med Rehabil*. 2002;83:1765–1773.

60. Bogner J, Corrigan J, Mysiw J, Clinchot D, Fugate L. A comparison of substance abuse and violence in the prediction of long-term rehabilitation outcomes after traumatic brain injury. *Arch of Phys Med and Rehabil*. 2001;82(50):571–577.

61. Bombardier CH, Ehde D, Kilmer J. Readiness to change alcohol drinking habits after traumatic brain injury. *Arch Phys Med Rehabil*. 1997;78:592–596.

62. Brombardier C, Temkin N, Machamer J, Dikemen S. The natural history of drinking and alcohol related problems after brain injury. *Arch Phys Med Rehabil*. 2003;84(2):185–191.

63. Kreutzer J, Doherty K, Harris J, Zasler N. Alcohol use among persons with traumatic brain injury. *J Head Trauma Rehab*. 1990;5(3):9–30.

64. Association of Rehabilitation Nurses. Resources for role description. http://www.rehabnurse.org. Accessed May 28, 2012.

VI

SPECIAL TBI POPULATIONS

Traumatic Brain Injury in the Elderly

Jaime Levine and Steven R. Flanagan

INTRODUCTION

The elderly are the second largest age group at risk for traumatic brain injury (TBI). Current trends clearly indicate that the population of the United States is aging, which will impact TBI in 2 broad ways. First, as the population ages, more elderly will sustain a TBI. Elderly have poorer outcomes following TBI regarding mortality, functional skills, and disposition, which will clearly have a significant and growing impact in the coming decades. Second, more people with TBI will survive their injuries and will age with the short-term and long-term consequences of their injury. Imbedded in the first issue is the impact of larger numbers of older individuals will have on medicine, costs of care, and overall burden to society. Health care providers treating elderly with TBI must be familiar with the myriad of issues associated with the geriatric population, including normal age-related changes and increased medical comorbidities to ensure delivery of the best possible treatments that result in optimal outcomes. It is equally important to note that despite less optimal outcomes than their younger counterparts, elderly with TBI benefit from intense treatments, including rehabilitation, although at greater costs. The second issue, aging with a TBI, underscores the growing recognition that TBI is not an isolated event with a definitive end, but rather a chronic disease associated with increased risk of developing other diseases and shortened life expectancy. Growing constraints on health care expenditures clearly indicates the need to address this epidemic through enhanced education of health care providers of the multitude of issues impacting TBI and the elderly and innovative means to provide effective care throughout the lives of injured people. This chapter will focus on how TBI in the elderly differs from other age groups in terms of etiology, pathophysiology, outcomes, prevention, and best treatment approaches, as well as its overall impact on society and medicine.

SCOPE OF THE PROBLEM

Over the past century, average life expectancy in the industrialized countries has dramatically increased. In the United States alone, it increased from approximately 47 years in 1900 to 77 years in 2000. Accompanying the increase in life expectancy is a dramatic growth of the population of older Americans. According to the US Census Bureau, the population of individuals older than 64 years of age in 1990 was 29.6 million, which grew to 40 million in 2010. This is projected to expand to 47 million by 2015 and 88.5 million by 2050, at which time the number of people older than 64 years of age will represent 20% of the US population. The number of very old American will also increase, with 19 million people estimated to be older than 84 years old by 2050, representing 4.3% of the total population (1).

The population growth of older individuals coupled with increasing life expectancy will impact the financial, medical, and societal toll of TBI in 2 broad ways. First, the incidence of TBI is bimodal, with young adults and the elderly at increased risk for sustaining an injury. Therefore, as the population ages, a greater number of older individuals will be expected to sustain a TBI. As a group, older individuals are likely to have greater mortality and morbidity, have longer hospitalizations, and have poorer functional outcomes than their similarly injured younger counterparts. Second, as medical treatments continue to improve, combined with greater emphasis on using evidence-based practices, a greater proportion of younger individuals will survive the acute phases following injury but will face life-long disability. They will also be at increased risk for shortened life expectancy and several disabling medical conditions in addition to a poorer quality of life as they age with the consequences of TBI. This will worsen an already daunting problem because it is currently estimated that at least 1.7 million people sustain a TBI yearly in the United States, with a prevalence of 3.17 million individuals having a chronic problem related to TBI (2).

These figures likely underestimate the true burden of TBI because many individuals either do not seek medical treatment for mild injuries, whereas others with complaints of impaired cognition, altered behaviors, and multiple somatic problems resulting from a TBI are often misdiagnosed. This may be particularly true in the elderly as signs and symptoms of TBI, including mood, cognitive, and several physical changes, such as impaired balance, may be incorrectly attributed to the aging process or dementia rather than a blow to the head. The consequences of TBI are staggering and, until the recent media attention directed at the large numbers of military personnel injured in Iraq and Afghanistan and professional sports players with concussions, have been poorly understood by most health care professionals, insurers, and governmental agencies. Although many individuals post-TBI have physical problems, many people manifest only cognitive and behavioral problems, which are often either overlooked or misdiagnosed as being psychiatric in nature or simply malingering by health care providers, insurers, and others. The financial burden of TBI is enormous, including the high cost of direct health care, loss productivity of people with TBI and their families, and the inability to participate in desired societal roles. The aging population trends indicate that the health care burden of TBI will substantially grow in the coming decades and will need to be addressed in substantive and innovative ways to decrease its burden on medicine and society.

EPIDEMIOLOGY OF TBI IN THE ELDERLY

TBI is a common health problem for older individuals, with rates of TBI-related hospitalization greatest among the elderly than any other age group (3,4). This risk continues to increase in a very substantial manner after the age of 65 (5), which combined with the growing population of older people will present enormous challenges in the future. For example, the rate of subdural hemorrhage (SDH)-related hospitalizations grew by nearly 40% from 1998 to 2007, with the largest increase observed in those older than 80 years of age (6). The elderly account for more than 80,000 TBI-related emergency department visits each year in the United States (7).

The reasons accounting for increased TBI-related hospitalizations in the elderly are multiple and include their high risk of falls combined with their growing use of vitamin K antagonists and antiplatelet drugs that enhance the likelihood of intracranial hemorrhages. Similar to younger populations, severity of injury of most elderly people hospitalized with TBI is classified as mild, followed in order of frequency by moderate and severe injury (5). However, with advancing age, the percentage of elderly individuals with moderate TBI increases with a concomitant decrease in overall percentage with mild TBI (5).

Although the overall age-adjusted rate of TBI-related hospitalizations is 60.6 per 100,000, it is 155.9 per 100,000 for those 65 years and older. However, within the group aged 65 years and older, the rate increases sharply with advancing age. The TBI-related hospitalization rate is 85.1 per 100,000 for those 65–74 years old, rising to 187.4 per 100,000 for those 75–84 years of age and to a staggering 366.6 per 100,000 for those 85 years and older (5). Similar to younger groups, older men are more likely to be hospitalized than women, although the rates begin to approximate each other as people reach old age (7). As opposed to the general population where nonwhites are at increased risk for sustaining a TBI, the hospitalization rates are highest among whites for those 75 years and older. One exception is for those aged 65–74 years, where the highest rates are among American Indians/Alaskan Natives (5). Blacks have the lowest rate compared to other groups in the 65 years and older range, although blacks older than 75 years of age have the highest rate of TBI-related hospitalization among all black Americans (7).

Unlike younger individuals with TBI who sustain injuries predominantly in motor vehicle crashes, the leading cause of TBI-related hospitalizations in the elderly is an unintentional fall, with a rate of 104.9 per 100,000 (5). Advancing age within the elderly group increases the risk of a fall-related TBI. Compared to the 65–74-year-old group, the fall-related TBI hospitalization rate in the 75–84-year-old group is twice as high, which grows to 6 times the rate for those older than 85 years of age (5). Older individuals are more

likely to fall because of many reasons, including having a larger number of coexisting medical problems that predispose them to fall, such as diabetes and associated sensory and visual loss; other visual disturbances, such as glaucoma, macular degeneration, and cataracts; neurological diseases such as Parkinson disease (PD) and stroke; and other age-related problems, such as impaired balance, slow reaction times, muscle weakness, impaired cognition, polypharmacy, and postural hypotension. It has been noted that people who sustain a TBI from falling are more likely to have a greater number of medical problems than those injured in motor vehicle collisions (5). TBI and falls represent a major health risk to the elderly, with 50% of deaths from unintentional fall resulting from TBI, and 8% of nonfatal falls resulting in TBI (8). Traffic-related events, including motor vehicle crashes and pedestrian struck by moving vehicles, accounts for the second most common cause of TBI hospitalization in the elderly, with a rate of 24.2 per 100,000 (5), which is notably less than that for falls. However, elderly drivers are at significant risk for being injured in a motor vehicle collision. Although individuals aged 55 years or older constituted only 14.4% of all drivers in 1999, they accounted for 17% of all motor vehicle-related fatalities. Excluding the very youngest drivers, older drivers have the highest risk of sustaining motor vehicle crash fatalities when adjusting for total number of miles traveled (9). This problem will likely grow in the future as the percentage of drivers considered elderly is anticipated to reach 30% by 2020 and 40% by 2050 (10).

Although the rate of traffic-related injuries decreases for those individuals 85 years or older, likely because as a group, they drive less than younger people; the overall problem of elderly drivers needs to be address to decrease this burden. Older people are more likely to be at risk for traffic-related crashes and injury because of several age-related health problems. These include impairments in vision, slower reaction times, impaired cognitive skills, osteopenia, and medication use. Although older persons tend to use safety belts with greater frequency than their younger counterparts and are less likely to drink alcohol and drive, approximately 1 in 4 older adults involved in motor vehicle crashes are noncompliant with safety belt use, whereas 8% are found to have evidence of alcohol use at the time of injury (5). Other causes of TBI in the elderly are less common than falls and traffic-related incidents. For example, assaults account for only 1% of TBI in the elderly, with 17% of TBI attributed to other etiologies (7). For a more in-depth review of epidemiology pertaining to other age groups, please refer to Chapter 8.

PATHOPHYSIOLOGY

The pathophysiologic changes after TBI are common to all ages, although the elderly are at greater risk for certain findings because of normal age-related anatomical changes in the brain and premorbid conditions that require specific treatments, such as anticoagulants and antiplatelet medications that increase the risk of hemorrhaging. Focal contusions are a common example of primary injury. However, hemorrhagic conversion of bland contusions may be more likely for individuals on anticoagulants, a common medication in the elderly, requiring close monitoring for worsening neurological functioning and possibly requiring more frequent neuroimaging follow-up studies. Focal areas of ischemia are another common example of primary injury.

Older individuals are more likely to have cerebrovascular disease and therefore may be more susceptible to focal ischemic injury following trauma. Similarly, preexisting stroke or other cerebral disease may lessen restorative capability after TBI and will likely negatively impact recovery.

Extra-axial hemorrhages are common after TBI and include subarachnoid, epidural, and SDHs. Further, increasing the risk of traumatic hemorrhage, many older adults receive antiplatelet and anticoagulant therapies as part of the medical management of several premorbid conditions commonly associated with advanced age. It has been estimated that approximately 9% of older adults who sustained a TBI were taking warfarin prior to their injury, which was associated with more severe TBI and a higher rate of mortality (11).

With advancing age, the dura becomes more tightly adhered to the skull (12), and therefore, the incidence of epidural hemorrhage (EDH) in the elderly decreases. However, in association with age-related cerebral atrophy, the subdural space expands, placing the bridging veins at increased risk for shear, thereby increasing susceptibility to the development of SDHs. A large and rapidly expanding SDH manifests as acute deterioration of arousal or development of focal neurological impairments. However, an SDH may not be clinically evident during the acute stages in older adults because of the enlargement of the subdural space that naturally occurs with aging (13). An SDH may also slowly expand in the elderly as a result of abnormalities of blood vessels (14).

The combination of a larger subdural space with blood vessels abnormalities permits a larger volume of blood to accumulate over a longer period before the development of clinically significant cerebral compression, accounting for the late deterioration of neurological status commonly observed in elderly people with SDH. SDH frequently occurs in older adults after apparently trivial trauma and is often related to a fall in which there was no direct trauma to the head (15). Because symptoms related to slowly expanding hemorrhages are often not observed acutely post trauma, the diagnosis of SDH is frequently made when it appears as subacute or chronic on neuroimaging studies. Not surprisingly, many older individuals are unable to recall the traumatic event, particularly as only minimal trauma, often without a direct blow to head is required to cause an SDH. Therefore, all health care providers, including but not limited to emergency responders, primary care physicians, and rehabilitation specialists, need to be wary of elderly individuals who present with vague neurological complaints following a mild TBI or other injuries, such as orthopedic fractures that occur from falling because often it is these individuals who are just entering a period when an SDH begins to manifest clinically. Please refer to the Chapters 11 and 12 for a more detailed discussion of these topics because they pertain to the general TBI population.

ACUTE CARE MANAGEMENT

For both young and elderly persons who experience a severe TBI, a primary focus of acute care management is preventing secondary brain injury that may arise as a result of diffuse cerebral ischemia. Increased intracerebral pressure (ICP), resulting from intracranial hemorrhages or brain edema, can impede cerebral blood flow, particularly in instances of systemic hypotension. The trauma team must diligently monitor ICP and lower it if it is elevated, using such measures as evacuation of extra-axial hemorrhages, osmotic diuresis, and pharmacological induction of coma. Mean arterial pressure is also closely monitored to ensure adequate cerebral perfusion. Cerebral perfusion pressure (CPP), defined as the difference between mean arterial pressure and ICP is recommended to be maintained between 50 and 70 mm Hg (16).

However, evidence indicates that cerebral autoregulation and pressure reactivity decreases with advancing age, suggesting that the older brain is less capable of maintaining cerebrovascular reactivity post trauma and is associated with worse outcomes in elderly patients with TBI. Therefore, it has been suggested that the general recommendation for maintaining CPP between 50 and 70 mm Hg has not been adequately established for elderly patients, indicating that more studies are needed (17).

Similar to maintaining adequate perfusion, continuous assessment of systemic oxygenation is crucial to avert secondary cerebral injury. Individuals who have severe TBI may be placed on mechanical ventilation to prevent hypoxemia. Older individuals are more likely to have cardiac and pulmonary comorbidities that may make maintaining adequate oxygenation more challenging.

Rehabilitation following TBI is ideally initiated shortly after initial hospitalization, often while the elderly patient resides in an intensive care setting. The immediate goal of rehabilitation is to prevent complications associated with a prolonged period of immobilization, such as joint contracture, skin breakdown, venous stasis, and pulmonary compromise. However, older individuals have considerably more comorbidities than their younger counterparts and frequently require greater attention to several precautions during rehabilitation at this time, such as more diligent monitoring of cardiac and pulmonary status even when fairly simple interventions, such as positioning and range of motion procedures, are being performed. Once patients are permitted to be out of bed, therapists providing therapy to older individuals must be aware of potential blood pressure alterations that occur with changes in position because elderly people are prone to orthostatic hypotension and rapid changes in heart rate when sitting up in bed or in a chair. Please refer to part V for more discussions of these topics.

Inpatient Rehabilitation for the Elderly

There are various settings where TBI rehabilitation can be provided, including acute rehabilitation facilities, subacute rehabilitation facilities, home, and outpatient settings. The appropriate location depends on several factors, including the severity of injury and associated physical, cognitive, and behavioral impairments; the need for ongoing medical oversight; and time elapsed postinjury. Once an elderly person with TBI has been medically stabilized post trauma and no longer requires continual intensive care but has persistent TBI-related functional impairments, transfer to a rehabilitation setting should be considered. Acute inpatient rehabilitation ideally occurs in specialized brain injury units situated within a hospital or in a freestanding facility.

Certain admission criteria must be met before acceptance to an acute rehabilitation unit including

1. medical complexity that requires around-the-clock physician presence and specialized rehabilitative nursing expertise,

2. reasonable expectation for functional improvement and discharge to the community within a reasonable time, and
3. functional deficits requiring at least 3 hours of specialized rehabilitation treatment.

Individuals who do not meet these criteria but who cannot return to their home because of persistent TBI-related functional impairments should be considered for subacute rehabilitation, which provides less intensive medical, nursing, and rehabilitation interventions in long-term care facilities. Increasing pressure from third-party payors and government agencies has impacted admission practices for people with TBI, including the elderly. Several factors, including the trend to shorten length of rehabilitation hospitalizations accompanied by the criteria to achieve functional improvements and discharge to community settings within a reasonable time frame has forced acute inpatient rehabilitation facilities to reconsider admission of elderly patients with severe TBI-related disabilities. Older individuals, particularly those with severe TBI, have longer hospitalizations and are less likely than younger people to be discharged to their communities. Recent evidence suggests that over a span of approximately 1 decade, acute inpatient rehabilitation facilities increasingly admitted less impaired older adults with TBI, likely in response to these pressures and changing regulations (18,19).

Regardless of the setting, rehabilitation is provided in an interdisciplinary manner by a specialized team of health care providers, the patient, and his or her loved ones. The interdisciplinary model takes advantage of each member's unique knowledge and expertise while the entire team works collaboratively to address impairments that cut across multiple disciplines. The efficiency of this team model becomes extremely important in the context of mounting pressures to limit acute inpatient rehabilitation lengths of stay.

In the inpatient rehabilitation setting, a unit wide schedule is created to allow for ample rest time during the day, as well as provide opportunities for medical care and diagnostics. Elderly patients are likely to have multiple medical comorbidities necessitating more than the usual amount of diagnostic testing, medical procedures, or time-consuming medical treatments during their inpatient rehabilitation stay. It is important to schedule these tests and treatments in a manner that limit their impact on the elderly person's ability to participate in therapy. In particular, fatigue-inducing treatments, such as hemodialysis or chemotherapy, should ideally be scheduled at the end of the day after the conclusion of therapy.

It is well established that sleep architecture becomes more fragmented with aging; thus, elderly patients may require more time in which to get the same amount of sleep than their younger counterparts. For this reason, it is recommended that brain injury rehabilitation units provide both rest breaks during the day and a nighttime environment that is conducive to restful sleep. Scientific evidence supports these recommendations, indicating that providing an optimal environment and plan to ensure adequate rest and sleep for the elderly patient with TBI is a key factor in planning inpatient rehabilitation. New learning, which is often severely impaired following TBI, is essential to secure the skills necessary to achieve independence in mobility and activities of daily living. Although actual physical practice is needed to learn a specific motor skill, sleep and rest play an impor-

tant role in consolidating the memory of tasks learned throughout the day (20,21,22); this helps to induce neuronal changes that strengthen and stabilize the new skill (21). Visitors also should be advised as to the importance of scheduled rest times so that they can tailor their visits accordingly. Establishing strategic visiting hours is an easy way to help reinforce this practice. Please refer to Chapter 43 for a more detailed discussion of sleep-related problems associated with TBI.

In addition to a unit wide schedule, individual therapy schedules are tailored to the medical needs and tolerance of the older patient. For example, although all patients in an acute inpatient rehabilitation environment participate in a minimum of 3 hours of therapy daily, older patients will most likely have their needs best met with short sessions scattered throughout the day rather than in 1-hour blocks. Please refer to Chapter 26 for a more general description of TBI rehabilitation.

SENSORY ABNORMALITIES OF AGING AND THE IMPACT ON REHABILITATION

As humans age, there are some changes in sensorium, sleep, and cognition, which occur naturally that when coupled with neurological effects of TBI create a uniquely challenging scenario for rehabilitation specialists. For example, up to 60% of older adults experience some degree of presbycusis or sensorineural hearing loss by age 65 (23). Following TBI, when receptive language and cognitive processing skills are commonly impaired, it is crucial not to mistake hearing loss for another cognitive or linguistic deficit.

A limited hearing screen should be completed by a speech therapist on admission to any inpatient rehabilitation environment, and there should be a low threshold for pursuing a more in-depth audiology evaluation in any patient with meaningful deficits. Technological aids, such as hearing aids or other noise amplification devices, such as a Pocket Talkers, should be used liberally. Signage in the patient's room alerting all caregivers and visitors of the patient's hearing impaired status should be employed, coupled with good communication among team members to be sure all strategies and devices are used when appropriate to maximize communication with the patient.

On the contrary, many individuals following TBI, both young and old, may become very sensitive to noise volume and require a quiet, low-stimulus environment to succeed in rehabilitation. Excessive or high-volume noise may pose insurmountable external distraction for the individual who is already processing his or her ambient environment at a slower rate than normal, making the individual prone to agitation or "shutting down" behaviors when the level of noise or stimulus becomes too great. Although many older patients may have diminished hearing, requiring some degree of amplification assistance, they often still require an overall low-stimulus environment. It is these patients who are particularly challenging in this regard. It is important for all members of the rehabilitative team to be sensitive to all parts of this spectrum and to tailor the individual's environment accordingly, with the common goal of creating the optimum environment a given individual needs to succeed. There are also a myriad of visual changes that coincide with normal aging, including declines in extraocular muscle motion, increases in intraocular pressure, and changes in visual acuity (24), as well as a multitude of visual changes that may occur as a direct result of TBI. Any visual changes further predispose an already at-risk population for falls or other injury. Appropriate signage and internal communication should be employed to create the safest environment possible for each individual. Aside from these obvious safety implications, visual changes may prevent a patient from fully appreciating their physical environment, thus limiting the effectiveness of rehabilitative therapies if not appropriately addressed.

It is critical in designing a custom rehabilitation program to fully understand an older individual's visual status. A visual screen should be routinely completed on all new admissions to an inpatient rehabilitation setting, and further testing should be completed when appropriate. Attention should be paid to an older patient's previous visual aids, such as corrective lenses, to evaluate whether these are still appropriate or whether the TBI has induced visual changes, making these premorbid visual aids less effective or possibly dangerous. Often, a complete visual evaluation cannot be completed during the initial periods of acute rehabilitation because of cognitive and communication impairments that prevent full participation or understanding of the evaluator's instructions but should be commenced as soon as it is deemed feasible.

Addressing visual deficits and providing individualized vision rehabilitation is an important part of the inpatient rehabilitation process. Specific therapeutic exercises are taught and practiced, and individuals are encouraged to practice these techniques on their own between therapy sessions. When appropriate, strategic visual aids are used, such as patches, partial occlusion glasses, or blackout tape, depending on the specific impairments and needs of the patient. However, if they are used incorrectly, they pose a potential safety risk or serve to limit preserved vision, so all team members, including patients, loved ones, and nurses, should be trained on the correct use of these aids. Sometimes, it is appropriate to call for the expertise of a neuro-ophthalmologist to more definitively elucidate visual deficits as they relate to the specific neurological injury and to supply prognostic information, which is helpful to staff and comforting to patients and their loved ones. This is particularly important for older patients who are more likely to have other age-related visual disturbances that complicate the rehabilitation process. For a more in-depth discussion on how the visual changes associated with aging impact brain injury rehabilitation, please refer to Chapter 45 of this book.

DIAGNOSIS AND MANAGEMENT OF MEDICAL AND REHABILITATION PROBLEMS IN THE ELDERLY WITH TBI

Medical complications following TBI lengthen hospital stay and increase mortality (25). This is magnified in the older adult population because of a higher preinjury disease burden and greater susceptibility to many medical complications. Prevention, swift diagnosis, and appropriate treatment of common medical problems following TBI in the elderly should be of paramount concern to any clinician caring for this population.

Pharmacological Considerations

In the United States, 48% of community-dwelling adults aged 65 and older have arthritis; 36% have hypertension; 27% have coronary artery disease; 10% have diabetes mellitus; and 6% have had a cerebrovascular accident (26,27). In addition to medications directly targeting medical sequelae of TBI, older adults are more likely to be on several additional other medications because of the frequency of these comorbidities. Polypharmacy is a challenge for all clinicians who provide care to an elderly population, particularly following TBI because many patients become more sensitive to the effects of certain medications or more vulnerable to potential interactions.

Paralysis

Muscle weakness or complete paralysis is common following TBI, typically manifesting as hemiplegia or as more focal weakness related to traumatic neuropathy. Older patients may also have had less muscle strength preinjury because of normal age-related decreases in muscle mass or premorbid medical conditions, which will exacerbate the functional implications of the TBI-based weakness. Multiple rehabilitation therapists work to enhance motor recovery using a variety of therapeutic methods, such as neurodevelopmental techniques, therapeutic exercises targeting specific muscles or muscle groups, and electrical stimulation. Although maximizing motor recovery is an important goal, the extent of motor return varies from person to person, and learning new strategies to compensate for this loss of strength becomes a parallel goal. Therefore, various assistive devices and orthoses are introduced to enhance the function of a person with muscle weakness to optimize their level of functional independence. Proper training and education for patients and their caregivers can help ensure that these devices are used correctly because improper use can increase an individuals' fall risk and lead to devastating consequences. Please refer to Part XVI of this book for a more in-depth review of this topic.

Orthostasis

Orthostatic hypotension, which often results from periods of prolonged bed rest following trauma, is a frequent obstacle to full participation in an aggressive rehabilitation program. The combination of post-traumatic hypertension and a history of underlying hypertension, heart disease, or peripheral vascular disease often create a scenario where an elderly patient is prescribed of multiple antihypertensive agents. When combined with rapid changes in physical orientation, the inability of the cardiovascular system to quickly compensate results in orthostatic hypotension. This requires diligent monitoring of patients' cardiovascular response to exercise especially because it relates to position changes. Individualized blood pressure and heart rate parameters should be clearly established to help guide the type and intensity of interventions provided by rehabilitation therapists. The entire interdisciplinary team, including any individual interacting with the elderly patient, must be educated regarding the risk of orthostatic hypotension to ensure that a drop in blood pressure doesn't lead to a fall or other adverse event.

When orthostatic hypotension is present, drug regimens often need to be altered to permit full participation in the rehabilitation program. Additional strategies may be helpful in supporting blood pressure, such as use of abdominal binders and lower extremity pressure stockings. Other measures include slowly raising the head of the bed, followed by dangling the feet of an elderly person prior to standing them may decrease the occurrence of orthostatic hypotension. When these strategies are inadequate, pharmacological agents can be prescribed to the regimen to help maintain blood pressure.

Hydrocephalus

Hydrocephalus is among the most common treatable neurosurgical conditions following TBI, so clinicians caring for patients during the acute rehabilitation period should have a low threshold for diagnostic imaging in suspected cases. Clinical signs of hydrocephalus include worsening cognition, alterations in gait, and urinary incontinence; however, patients rarely display this classical triad of symptoms. Oftentimes, patients simply appear more tired, experience nausea or vomiting, display a change in their functional status, or cease making functional and neurological improvements when hydrocephalus develops. It is not uncommon for acute hydrocephalus to manifest initially as a decline in functional status, which is frequently first appreciated by a treating therapist. For example, a patient who required minimal assistance of 1 therapist to stand may be noticed to require moderate assistance of 2 therapists for the same maneuver. This example underscores the importance of good communication among rehabilitation team members.

Hydrocephalus following TBI often occurs as a result of traumatic subarachnoid hemorrhage or infection that scars the arachnoid inhibiting effective absorption of cerebral spinal fluid from the subarachnoid space into the general circulation. It may also develop because of the mass effect of blood product or edema compressing ventricles or causing blockage of the usual flow of cerebrospinal fluid, although this typically occurs acutely following injury and is rarely the cause of hydrocephalus that develops during acute inpatient rehabilitation.

The elderly population is already at an increased risk for developing hydrocephalus; thus, the index of suspicion must be even higher in this population. The symptoms of hydrocephalus, specifically of the normal pressure type, may be mistakenly attributed to effects of the brain injury itself because there are often overlaps in their clinical presentations. Alterations in gait, urinary problems, and confusion are not uncommon following TBI at any age but with the increased risk of hydrocephalus in the elderly population, these symptoms require special attention to arrive at a timely diagnosis. Please refer to Chapter 44 of this book for a more in-depth review of this topic.

Spasticity

Spasticity, defined as a velocity-dependent increase in resistance to passive stretch across a joint, is a commonly encountered problem following severe TBI, occurring in as many as two-thirds of patients (28). When present, it often complicates the already disabling effects of paralysis by contributing to pain and development of joint contractures and pressure sores and by making mobility, positioning, and hygiene more difficult. Spasticity is not always detrimental, however. For example, lower extremity extensor tone may enable a person to achieve greater independence with standing than they otherwise would have with a flaccid extremity.

Effective spasticity treatment requires an interdisciplinary approach and initially includes aggressive stretching by all rehabilitation team members, including family members and patients when feasible. In the elderly population, it is especially important to use nonpharmacological modalities, such as stretching, splinting, serial casting, use of neuromuscular electrical stimulation, and heat and cold modalities because, when effective, they can limit the need for pharmacological agents, all of which have the potential to interact with other pharmacological agents and cause unwanted systemic side effects.

Oral agents in the elderly must be prescribed with great caution, with careful consideration given to the possible effect of polypharmacy and diminished renal and/or hepatic function. These agents frequently have adverse effects on cognition and arousal; thus, their usefulness is limited following TBI particularly in the elderly who are typically taking many other medications and are more susceptible to the effects of medication interactions.

Spasticity that is regional, involving 1 extremity or muscle group, is effectively treated with focal delivery of antispasmodic agents. Options include selective motor point blocks with phenol or botulinum toxin injections. Continuous intrathecal delivery of baclofen through an implanted pump is sometimes offered to patients with predominantly lower extremity tone to manage their spasticity; however, special considerations must be taken into account in the elderly population. Implantation of the pump is a surgical procedure, so patients must be deemed to be at an acceptable risk for surgery, and although there are no clear guidelines on their use based on life expectancy, this treatment is not appropriate for patients with a poor prognosis. Please refer to Chapter 50 of this book for a more in-depth review of this topic.

Heterotopic ossification (HO), a common complication following TBI that limits joint range of motion and function, is routinely diagnosed using standing radiograph, computed tomography (CT), or 3-phase technetium bone scanning. Because radiographs are often insensitive to HO during the very acute phases of its development, bone scanning is typically used as the preferred diagnostic modality. There is new evidence that the use of bedside power Doppler ultrasound (DUS) is a safe, cost effective, and useful tool in the diagnosis of early HO (29,30). When diagnosing early HO in an elderly patient, DUS may be a safer modality than bone scan because it eliminates the use of contrast material, which may have harmful renal effects and avoid radiation, which is delivered with the other diagnostic tools. A more detailed review of HO is available in Chapter 51 of this book.

Cognition

Age-related cognitive changes are an expected component of normal aging, with most people experiencing a gradual decline in cognitive skills over their life span, particularly in memory. The decline is usually minor, and although may be frustrating at times, it does not impair functional abilities (31). In contrast to normal age-related changes, the term mild cognitive impairment (MCI) refers to a level of impaired cognitive function that exceeds expected changes observed in normal aging but not severe enough to meet criteria for dementia (32). The estimated prevalence of MCI in persons older than 65 years of age is significant and ranges from 10% to 20% (33–35). Preexisting MCI and dementia increase the risk of sustaining a TBI (36,37) and therefore partially accounts for the overall increased risk of sustaining a TBI later in life. Premorbid MCI or dementia is expected to complicate the rehabilitation process by slowing recovery and increasing rehabilitation lengths of stay. Moreover, cognitive changes following brain injury are important predictors of long-term functional recovery.

Understanding an elderly individual's pretrauma cognitive status is important when considering realistic goal setting and rehabilitation planning. It will influence both short-term and long-term planning, including the venue in which rehabilitation is provided (e.g., acute inpatient vs subacute), type and intensity of interventions, length of treatment, disposition after hospital discharge, distribution of financial resources, and services required if community discharge is feasible. The lack of cognitive reserve in elderly patients with MCI or dementia should be expected to both exacerbate and negatively impact the recovery of the common constellation of neurocognitive and behavioral problems that typically follow TBI, which are often the most challenging issues faced by patients and their loved ones. When post-TBI cognitive symptoms are mild, they may be similar in appearance to MCI; thus, it is often difficult to separate what aspects of cognitive impairment are caused by a preexisting condition and what may be attributable to TBI. This is made more challenging by the fact that cognitive impairment is underdiagnosed in older patients (38), so a patient's premorbid cognitive status is often unclear or misunderstood. Furthermore, older individual with mild post-TBI–related cognitive and behavioral changes may be mis-diagnosed with MCI or dementia, delaying—or worse—blocking effective rehabilitation interventions to improve function. A more detailed review of cognitive problems and treatment following TBI in other age groups can be found in part XII of this book.

Behavior/Affective

Following TBI, emotional changes are common, most often manifesting as depression and anxiety disorders. These disorders create unique challenges for the clinician because often they are difficult to diagnose and treat. Depressive disorders are the most frequent comorbid psychiatric conditions following TBI (39–41). In fact, prevalence of post-TBI depression ranges from 30% to 77% (40), which exceeds expected frequencies for community-based samples or in non-brain-injured populations of elderly adults.

Effectively recognizing and treating depression in the elderly after TBI requires both a comprehensive understanding of mood disorders in the elderly, as well as in people with TBI. Depressive disorders are among the most prevalent mental health problems in the elderly population (42), which is associated with considerable mortality (43), including an increased risk of suicide.

The process of diagnosing depression in the elderly is complicated by several factors. First, comorbid medical conditions, such as PD, may mask depressive symptoms, and yet in other circumstances, comorbid conditions, such as sleep disorders, may cause a clinical picture that mimics depression. Elderly patients with depression also often present differently than younger patients, with older individuals commonly focusing more on somatic rather than affective symptoms, making it difficult to disentangle symptoms related to a mood disorder from those of another medical condition. The elderly also tend to underreport symptoms of depression and may be less likely to admit to mood changes and feelings of sadness than their younger counterparts. Additionally, many elderly have experienced some personal loss, including illness of a spouse or death of a loved one, making it difficult for a clinician to distinguish true depression from normal grieving.

These same issues apply to elderly people with depression following TBI, which complicates recognition and treatment because many of the sequelae of the brain injury are similar to those of depression. Symptoms, such as apathy, fatigue, and cognitive slowing as well as somatic complaints, such as pain, may be erroneously attributed in their entirety to the brain injury and comorbid injuries rather than to depression. The development of depression after TBI in the elderly poses challenges for the survivor and their caregivers, including diminished quality of life, poor psychosocial functioning, and increased barriers, to successful community reentry (39,44,45) and is associated with poorer rehabilitation outcomes (46).

Multiple treatment options, which usually include a combination of medications and various psychological interventions, can be effective in treating TBI-related depression. However, careful consideration of medications is required in the elderly. Although tricyclic antidepressant medications have demonstrated efficacy in treating TBI-related depression, their associated anticholinergic effects pose possible dangers to elderly individuals who often have comorbid cardiac diseases. In general, all medications used in the elderly patient with TBI should be started at the lowest dose possible and only very gradually increased, using the "start low, go slow" approach to minimize undesirable effects.

Behavioral dysregulation following TBI in the elderly is a challenge faced by many clinicians caring for this population. Common examples of behavioral problems include restlessness, agitation, aggression, and irritability and when consistent, these often can interfere with rehabilitation participation or progress, as well as create an environment of unrest on the rehabilitation unit or at home. Behavioral problems are also quite stressful to a patient's loved ones, who require education on the topic from the rehabilitation specialist.

The first line of treatment for behavioral disturbances employs using nonpharmacological strategies and involves identification followed by mitigation of inciting causes, supportive counseling, and behavioral therapy. Some behavioral excesses, such as verbal inappropriateness, although potentially a nuisance, should be permitted as long as it is not interfering with the rehabilitation experience of other patients on the unit. When nonpharmacological treatment strategies prove ineffective, it is reasonable to trial selective medications for the management of behavioral excesses, with an additional goal of ensuring the safety and comfort of the patient and those around him or her. Considerable caution is required when prescribing psychoactive medications to the elderly because of the risk of worsening the existing TBI-related problems, such as poor balance, fatigue, and impaired cognition. Commonly used agents include atypical antipsychotics, antiepileptics, and beta-blockers, and as with other medications, it is recommended that the lowest possible dose be used initially, followed by a slow upward titration as needed. Extreme caution should be used when prescribing atypical antipsychotic agents in the elderly population because their use has been shown to increase the risk of mortality in a chronic setting by a factor of 1.7 (47). In fact, the Food and Drug Administration (FDA) has placed a black box warning on the use of atypical antipsychotic medications in this population. Beta-blockers should also be used cautiously because they have been shown to worsen memory in people with preexisting memory problems (48) and may worsen orthostatic hypotension. Finally, several drugs, including benzodiazepines and traditional neuroleptics, such as haloperidol, which may be effective in controlling undesirable behavior, have been shown to impair recovery following TBI and should therefore be avoided whenever possible (49). These medications also increase fall risk (50–52), and evidence suggests that their withdrawal decreases the frequency of fall in the elderly (53). A more detailed description of these topics pertaining to other age groups can be found in part XIV of this book.

Fatigue/Sleep Disturbance

Fatigue is among the most pervasive symptoms after TBI and occurs at a greater frequency than that in the general population (54,55). Self-reported complaints of fatigue increase with advancing age, so it is reasonable to expect that older adults are more susceptible to post–TBI-related fatigue. *Fatigue* is a frequent barrier to successful rehabilitation because it can shorten and decrease the efficiency of therapy sessions. It is important to address fatigue as part of the admission workup, monitor for signs of fatigue throughout the rehabilitation course, and employ appropriate treatments to address it both pharmacologically and through behavioral modification.

There is no universally accepted definition of fatigue, but many sources describe it as a subjective sense of overwhelming tiredness, lack of energy, and exhaustion. A general distinction is made between central and peripheral fatigue, describing the former as difficulty initiating or sustaining mental or physical tasks in the absence of motor impairments and the latter as musculoskeletal symptoms that affect mobility or the ability to perform activities of daily living. It is important to determine whether the fatigue is primary to the TBI or secondary to another condition, such as depression, pain, sleep disorders, or neuroendocrine abnormality, which have all been associated with fatigue after TBI (55).

Fatigue after TBI can be treated in several ways, including patient and caregiver education, behavioral modification, exercise, and/or pharmacological interventions. The use of neurostimulants or general wakefulness-promoting agents is a common treatment modality to accompany nonpharmacological methods or after other strategies have failed, acknowledging that evidence supporting their efficacy following TBI is lacking. Because of a higher number of comorbidities, older patients are more likely to be on several other medications; therefore, special care must be paid to avoid drug interactions and side effects when using these medications. However, several psychostimulants can be used safely in older adults when carefully attending to possible side effects and acknowledging the existence of comorbidities that may preclude their use.

Altered sleep patterns, which are commonly observed after TBI, need to be addressed regardless of age. However, the combination of age-related sleep changes and altered sleep patterns in people with TBI creates special challenges to physicians and caregivers. Treatment for post-TBI sleep disorders involves normalizing the sleep–wake cycle through behavioral, habitual, and environment strategies. Some medications may be cautiously trialed when nonpharmacological methods are insufficient; however, the avoidance of cognitive side effects, falls, and excessive sedation must be a constant concern. The goal of using medications to assist with sleep in the elderly must be to find the balance between, allowing for adequate rest at night while optimizing the patient for participation in the full therapy program on the following day.

When choosing a pharmacologic agent to assist with sleep in the elderly, it is wise to look to relatively benign medications that induce sleepiness as a side effect or to choose agents that may serve multiple functions. For example, the antidepressant agents trazodone or mirtazapine can be chosen in patients with both dysphoria and difficulty sleeping. The use of melatonin or melatonin analogues is another indirect way of normalizing sleep patterns without exposing the patient to agents that may cause unfavorable side effects, such as sedative hypnotics or benzodiazepines. For more in-depth discussions on fatigue and sleep following TBI in other age groups, please refer to Chapters 42 and 43 of this book.

CHALLENGES PRESENTED BY CURRENT HEALTH CARE REGULATIONS

Although the elderly with TBI have poorer outcomes as measured by mortality, acute hospital and rehabilitation disposition, and level of disability, most achieve significant functional recovery following acute inpatient rehabilitation. However, the improvements they realize occur over longer periods and therefore at greater costs than younger groups. Despite this, several studies have clearly demonstrated that most older individuals admitted to acute inpatient rehabilitation settings are discharged to their communities (18,19).

Interestingly, however, length of rehabilitation hospitalizations for people with TBI decreased from an average of 22.7 days in 2000 to 16.6 days in 2007. This occurred despite a notable increase in the average age for people with TBI, which increased from 47.1 to 59.1 years over the same period, with the proportion of cases for patients aged 75 years or older doubling (56).

Not surprisingly, Medicare represented the most common primary payer source for elderly people receiving inpatient rehabilitation services. The Centers for Medicare and Medicaid Services (CMS) began strict enforcement of the prospective payment system (PPS) for Medicare beneficiaries for the last decade, which provides a specific predetermined reimbursement to rehabilitation facilities based on several factors, including diagnosis and level of disability. However, because the elderly person with TBI requires longer periods of inpatient rehabilitation to realize enough functional improvement to be safely discharged to community settings as compared to younger groups, they often incur higher charges than what is reimbursed by CMS (57). Unfortunately, reimbursement to rehabilitation facilities is a main factor that determines the financial viability of providing acute inpatient rehabilitation services to the elderly. Accordingly, admission patterns of elderly people with TBI has changed over the past decade, with a greater percentage of less disabled elderly people being admitted to acute inpatient rehabilitation now than in the past, perhaps in response to pressure to control costs (19). Older patients with more severe TBI-related disabilities are therefore more likely to be discharged to less expensive alternatives than acute inpatient rehabilitation, where services are notably less intensive and outcomes less certain. Patients with TBI, both young and old, often face lifelong disability related to TBI and may incur considerable debt as resources dwindle. Older adults with TBI-related physical and cognitive impairments and their spouses are therefore often referred to elder care attorneys to assist them with protecting their resources, particularly when long-term disability is anticipated.

OUTCOMES

As mentioned previously, outcomes for older individuals are worse than their younger counterparts when controlling for injury severity. In general, older individuals with TBI are more likely to die from their injury, be more dependent on others for mobility and activity of daily living needs, and be discharged to long-term residential facilities than younger people with similarly severe injuries.

Mortality

Mortality acutely following TBI is highest among the elderly than any other age group, estimated to be approximately twice that for younger populations (58–60). The reported age at which people with TBI begin to incur higher mortality rates varies, with 1 report indicating it starts at 30 years and reaches a maximum after age 71 (61). Higher mortality occurs in the elderly across all severity levels, with age at injury an independent predictor of mortality (59), regardless of injury severity (25). Multiple reasons have been suggested for this level of mortality, most of which relate to the combination of greater comorbidities and their related treatment effects in the elderly, as well as intrinsic factors related to aging and associated impaired healing abilities. For example, older individuals are more likely to have cardiovascular disease and therefore more likely to be treated with antiplatelet drugs and vitamin K antagonists. These medications have been associated with increased mortality in elderly patients with TBI who have intracranial hemorrhages (62–66), although the degree of anticoagulation, rather than simply their use may have the greatest impact on outcomes (67). However, the medication is likely not the sole source of increased mortality because the cause of death is frequently an etiology other than expansion of an intracranial hemorrhage (62). Interestingly, others have suggested that anticoagulants may have a protective effect following hemorrhagic brain injury by reversing the hypercoaguable state induced by trauma (68,69), decreasing edema, and contusion, (70) as well as safely protecting against venous thromboembolism (71–74).

Cardiovascular diseases, which preferentially afflict older individuals, may also impair compensatory responses to hypotension and hypoxemia, resulting in further secondary injury following trauma and result in higher mortality rates. Elderly people hospitalized for TBI also have higher rates of other medical complications, likely contributing to increased mortality (59).

Another potential explanation accounting for higher mortality in the elderly is the possibility that the Glasgow Coma Scale (GCS) can underestimate injury severity in cases of SDH because of age-related increased subdural spaces, permitting greater hemorrhaging prior to developing clinical signs of cerebral compression and neurological compromise. Other injury severity measures, such as the Abbreviated Injury Severity Scale, Marshal score, or Revised Trauma Score, may provide a more accurate assessment of severity in these cases (25,75).

Functional and Disposition Outcomes

Elderly people with TBI are more likely to have poorer functional outcomes than their younger counterparts, with most studies indicating they more frequently require residential settings at the time of hospital discharge or more assistance at home when they are discharged to the community (5,76). Only slightly more than one-third of people aged 65 years or older who are hospitalized for TBI are discharged to their home with either unskilled or no assistance (5). The percentage of good recovery, as assessed by the Glasgow Outcome Scale, decreases with advancing age with an associated increase in the proportion of those deemed to have moderate and severe disability (5). These outcomes hold true even when controlling for injury severity as those elderly people with mild TBI have greater disability than their similarly injured counterparts (60,76). Poorer cognitive functioning has also been reported with advancing age post-TBI (76), which may begin as early as age 40 (77).

The reasons for poorer outcomes in the elderly are likely multifactorial. The aging central nervous system has altered responses to injury and may not be able to adequately compensate to stress. Cerebral plasticity is likely less effective in the older brain and the elderly may have impaired ability to make psychological adjustments to a traumatic event (78).

The elderly are more likely to have poorer premorbid cognitive and physical capabilities than their younger counterparts and be on more medications that impair cognitive skills.

It is important to note, however, that most studies examining functional outcomes after TBI typically assess skills at the time of hospital discharge or shortly thereafter. It is known that elderly people with TBI can experience significant recovery of function but do so at a slower pace than their younger counterparts (18,19).

Therefore, studies need to be interpreted with some caution because overall outcomes may not be as dire over the long term as some studies suggest. However, a long-term follow-up study indicates a substantial decrease in participation and increased need for assistance for cognitive-related activities as longer periods post-TBI have elapsed. The same study also indicated that age at the time of injury predicted increased complaints of fatigue and decreasing physical independence. Interestingly, however, advancing age also tended to reduce perceived environmental barriers, although injury severity was the strongest predictor for all these findings (79).

Despite overall poorer outcomes in the elderly with TBI compared to younger groups, older individuals retain considerable capacity to improve their cognitive and functional skills through intensive inpatient rehabilitation. Gains made by older people with TBI are generally only slightly less robust compared to their younger peers, although improvements occur over a longer period and therefore at a higher cost. Furthermore, most older adults who receive acute inpatient rehabilitation are able to be discharged to their communities (18,19).

PREVENTION

Falls occurring in older adults presents a significant health problem and is the leading cause of TBI in this age group. Approximately one-third of people aged 65 years or older fall each year (80–83). There are many risk factors associated with falls in the elderly, including previous falls, balance impairments, muscle weakness, visual disturbances, polypharmacy particularly with psychoactive medications, gait impairments, depression, dizziness, postural hypotension, functional limitations, incontinence, cognitive impairments, arthritis, diabetes mellitus and pain.[84]

Health care providers treating older adults are strongly recommended to routinely screen patients for falls and provide specific interventions to decrease their occurrence. More specifically, older individuals with 2 or more falls within the past 12 months or a single fall within the same time frame but with evidence of gait or balance disturbance should undergo a multidimensional fall risk assessment (see Table 28-1). Based on the findings of this assessment, specific interventions should be prescribed or recommended to mitigate the risk of falling (85).

Multiple interventions are usually recommended to decrease risk of falls and typically include a combination of exercises, correction of visual and cardiac abnormalities, environmental modifications, and reduction or elimination of psychoactive medications or other drugs contributing to postural hypotension (see Table 28-2) (85).

Elderly at risk for falls should be assessed for the need for adaptive aids, such as walking devices and shower and tub grab bars and provided training to properly use the devices. Please refer to Chapter 9 of this book for a more in-depth discussion on prevention of TBI in other age groups.

AGING WITH TBI

Older age at the time of TBI has been well established as an independent predictor of higher mortality and poorer func-

TABLE 28-1 Multifactorial Fall Assessment

1. Obtain relevant history of falls, perform physical/cognitive and functional assessment.

2. Determine multifactorial fall risk.

   a. history of falls
   b. medication use
   c. assessment of gait, balance, mobility
   d. assessment of visual acuity
   e. neurological assessment
   f. muscle strength assessment
   g. assessment of heart rate and rhythm
   h. assessment for postural hypotension
   i. assessment of feet and footwear
   j. assessment of environmental hazards

Reprinted from Panel on Prevention of Falls in Older Persons, American Geriatrics Society and British Geriatrics Society (85) with permission.

TABLE 28-2 Interventions to Reduce Fall Risk in the Elderly

1. Reduce medications, particularly psychoactive agents and drugs contributing to postural hypotension.
2. Individually tailored exercise program targeting strength, balance, endurance, and gait.
3. Management of visual disturbances, particularly correction first cataract
4. Management of postural hypotension
5. Management of heart rate and rhythm abnormalities
6. Management of foot and footwear problems
7. Modify home environment
8. Patient and family member/caregiver education

Reprinted from Panel on Prevention of Falls in Older Persons, American Geriatrics Society and British Geriatrics Society (85) with permission.

tional outcomes. However, evidence is emerging that indicates TBI should be viewed as a chronic disease that imposes increased risk of long-term health problems for those who survive the initial injury regardless of age of onset. Therefore, TBI should not simply be viewed as an isolated event similar to a fractured bone that will heal over time but rather as a chronic disease with the traumatic event representing the initiation of the disease process. In addition to direct injury to the brain, TBI has been associated with diseases of other organ systems as well as shortened life expectancy and should be viewed as disease causative or accelerative.

LIFE EXPECTANCY

Although it is well known that TBI is associated with mortality acutely after injury, it is becoming increasingly established that it is also associated with premature mortality for those who survive the acute event. Numerous studies have found significant associations between TBI and early mortality, with life expectancy reductions ranging on average from 4 to 7 years depending on several factors, such as injury severity, age at injury onset, degree of physical disability, and several psychosocial factors (86–90). Those with more severe injuries measured by either the GCS or length of unconsciousness and older age at the time of injury increase the likelihood of early mortality (87). Reported causes of premature death vary, although most commonly include seizures (89,91–96), respiratory-related problems, and infection (92,97). Other reported causes of death occurring more commonly in people with TBI include problems related to the genitourinary and digestive systems (89), accidental death (92), suicide (91,98) and cerebrovascular disease, although others have not confirmed the findings regarding the latter 2 causes (92,93,99,100). Several risk factors have also been associated with premature mortality and relate to the degree of physical disability and several psychosocial factors. More severely physically disabled individuals, as assessed by having less ability to ambulate, have a substantially higher risk of shortened life expectancy (99,101). The retrospective nature and other methodological issues inherent in studying long-term mortality following TBI makes it difficult to determine cause and effect regarding risk factors and cause of death. However, people with greater TBI-related physical disabilities are more likely to have other injury-related problems, such as dysphagia, seizures, inability to effectively clear pulmonary secretions, and neurogenic bladder that predispose to more frequent and more severe morbidities that increase the risk of mortality. Impaired mobility is also likely to negatively impact the ability to effectively participate in physical activity, which subsequently can increase the risk of cardiovascular disease (99). Substance abuse has frequently been cited as a risk factor for premature mortality post-TBI (98,101–103) with unemployment (97) and fewer years of education (87) also reported in some studies. An extensive review of literature by the Institute of Medicine (IOM) concluded that based on its evaluation, there is sufficient evidence of a causal relationship between penetrating TBI and premature mortality in survivors of the acute injury. They also concluded that there is sufficient evidence of an association between moderate or severe TBI and premature mortality in the subset of patients who are admitted into or discharged from rehabilitation centers or receive disability service (104). For a more extensive review on this topic, please refer to Chapter 21 of this book.

NEURODEGENERATIVE DISORDERS

Neurological consequences of TBI are well described and typically manifest acutely after injury. However, evidence is emerging that demonstrates an association between sustaining a TBI and developing dementia or PD many years later. Several studies examining multiple risk factors have found significant correlations with sustaining a TBI and developing senile dementia of the Alzheimer type (SDAT) many years later. One of the strongest associations was found in a long-term follow-up of veterans who served in World War II. Veterans who were hospitalized in 1944–1945 for nonpenetrating TBI were compared to veterans hospitalized during the same time for non–TBI-related illnesses 50 years later. Veterans with moderate to severe TBI as assessed by length of post-traumatic amnesia or length of unconsciousness were significantly more likely to develop SDAT than their non–TBI injured peers (36). *Mild TBI*, which was defined in this study as loss of consciousness (LOC) or amnesia lasting less than 30 minutes was not found to increase the risk for SDAT. Several other reports confirm these findings, indicating that TBI sustained earlier in life is a risk factor of developing SDAT many years later, with more severe injuries imparting a greater risk. Mild TBI, particularly without LOC, has been found to impart either a much less robust or no increase in risk (105–108). Results of other studies indicate that a history of sustaining a TBI increases the risk of earlier onset dementia (105,109), suggesting that TBI accelerates the degenerative process. Although other studies have failed to confirm these findings, indicating either only nonsignificant trends or no association, the IOM in their extensive review of the literature concluded that there is sufficient evidence of an association between moderate and severe TBI and the development of SDAT and only limited evidence of an association with SDAT if a mild TBI caused LOC (110). No evidence was found that supported an association with mild TBI without LOC. Postulated reasons accounting for this association include TBI-related injury to the blood–brain barrier that permits the passage of plasma proteins in the brain, liberation of oxygen radicals, loss of cerebral reserve tissue, enhanced development of amyloid plaques, apoptosis, and hastening of degenerative processes in people with early dementia.

A similar risk has been found with TBI and PD. Evidence supports an association between TBI that was severe enough to cause LOC and the development of PD. The association is strongest with increasingly severe TBI and lessens considerably with mild TBI with LOC. No association was found with mild TBI occurring without LOC (111–113). The association appears strongest among men (112), with other studies indicating the increased risk persists when controlling for other factors, including family history and exposure to similar environmental risks (111,113). Similar to Alzheimer's Dementia (AD), TBI may hasten the degenerative processes, leading to an earlier onset of PD (111).

Similar to their conclusions regarding SDAT, the IOM also concluded that there is an association between moderate to severe TBI and the development of PD with only limited evidence suggesting an association with mild TBI causing LOC and the development of PD (110). For a more extensive review on this topic, please refer to the chapters on neurological complications following TBI and mild TBI in this textbook.

CONCLUSION

The aging population will increase the burden of TBI as the number of people at risk for sustaining an injury will progressively increase. This will place tremendous burdens on health care systems and society, particularly given current third-party payor reimbursement practices that insufficiently cover the cost of providing adequate care to older people with TBI. The epidemiology of TBI in older people is notably different than younger populations, with older people much more likely to sustain their injury from falls as opposed to motor vehicle collisions. Older people are also at greater risk for sustaining SDHs, which unlike younger people can occur with seemingly minimal trauma and expand over long periods that delay the presentation of clinical systems and consequently its diagnosis. Older people with TBI are more likely to die from their injury compared to younger populations regardless of injury severity. The functional and disposition outcomes of older people are also less desirable because of multiple age-related factors that impact health and function. Despite this, older individuals with TBI can benefit from intensive acute inpatient rehabilitation efforts, with most of those being discharged to their communities. Successful rehabilitation of the older adult with TBI requires special attention to several age-related changes that present specific challenges to rehabilitation professionals. Finally, as people age after sustaining a TBI, it is important for health care providers to monitor them for a multitude of problems that predispose to premature mortality in addition to the development of several neurodegenerative disorders that have been associated with TBI. Additional research is needed to better define and delineate effective means of fall prevention, innovative, and cost-efficient rehabilitation strategies to improve functional outcomes for older populations, long-term impact of TBI as people age, and better means to identify and diagnose elderly with TBI.

KEY CLINICAL POINTS

1. The population in the United States is aging, with an expected growth of people aged 65 years or older expected to reach 88.5 million by 2050, representing 20% of the population. This will result in an expansion of TBI burden because older people are at increased risk for injury. Dis-

ease burden will also increase because younger people who survive their injury are at risk for long-term health problems associated with TBI.

2. Older people are more likely to sustain TBI from falls, as opposed to younger groups who are more likely to be injured in motor vehicle collisions.

3. Older people are at increased risk for SDHs, both immediate and delayed post trauma because of age-related cerebral atrophy that increased shear forces on bridging veins. Acute management of cerebral perfusion may be different in the older adult due as evidence indicates that cerebral autoregulation and pressure reactivity decreases with advancing age, suggesting that the older brain is less capable of maintaining cerebrovascular reactivity post trauma and is associated with worse outcomes in elderly patients with TBI. Therefore, it has been suggested that the general recommendation for maintaining CPP between 50 and 70 mm Hg has not been adequately established for elderly patients, indicating more studies are needed.

4. Although older individuals have worse functional and survival outcomes than their similarly injured younger counterparts, they benefit from acute inpatient rehabilitation with most of those capable of being discharged to their community. Inpatient rehabilitation programs must be tailored to meet the specific needs on an elderly population to enhance the likelihood of favorable outcomes.

5. Current reimbursement patterns for older adults with TBI insufficiently cover costs of care, which has resulted in a greater proportion of less disabled adults being admitted for inpatient care. More severely injured older adults are likely being discharged from acute care to long-term health facilities, where rehabilitation services are less intense and outcomes less certain.

6. Falls are the leading cause of TBI in the elderly, necessitating a multifactorial risk assessment and implementing a multidimensional fall-risk program tailored to the specific needs of elderly people at risk for injury.

KEY REFERENCES

1. Coronado VG, Thomas KE, Sattin RW, Johnson RL. The CDC traumatic brain injury surveillance system: characteristics of persons aged 65 years and older hospitalized with a TBI. *J Head Trauma Rehabil.* 2005;20(3):215–228.
2. Frankel JE, Marwitz JH, Cifu DX, Kreutzer JS, Englander J, Rosenthal M. A follow-up study of older adults with traumatic brain injury: taking into account decreasing length of stay. *Arch Phys Med Rehabil.* 2006;87(1):57–62.
3. *Gulf War and Health, Volume 7: Long-term Consequences of Traumatic Brain Injury.* Washington, DC: National Academies Press; 2008.
4. Jeste DV, Blazer D, Casey D, et al. ACNP white paper: update on use of antipsychotic drugs in elderly persons with dementia. *Neuropsychopharmacology.* 2008;33(5):957–970.
5. Sendroy-Terrill M, Whiteneck GG, Brooks CA. Aging with traumatic brain injury: cross-sectional follow-up of people receiving inpatient rehabilitation over more than 3 decades. *Arch Phys Med Rehabil.* 2010;91(3):489–497.

References

1. U.S. Census Bureau, Statistical Abstract of the United States: 2011. Available at http://www.census.gov/compendia/statab/2011/tables/11s0034.pdf. 2011. Accessed March 26, 2011.
2. Zaloshnja E, Miller T, Langlois JA, Selassie AW. Prevalence of long-term disability from traumatic brain injury in the civilian population of the United States, 2005. *J Head Trauma Rehabil.* 2008;23(6):394–400.
3. Adekoya N, Thurman DJ, White DD, Webb KW. Surveillance for traumatic brain injury deaths—United States, 1989–1998. *MMWR Surveill Summ.* 2002;51(10):1–14.
4. Langlois JA, Kegler SR, Butler JA, et al. Traumatic brain injury-related hospital discharges. Results from a 14-state surveillance system, 1997. *MMWR Surveill Summ.* 2003;52(4):1–20.
5. Coronado VG, Thomas KE, Sattin RW, Johnson RL. The CDC traumatic brain injury surveillance system: characteristics of persons aged 65 years and older hospitalized with a TBI. *J Head Trauma Rehabil.* 2005;20(3):215–228.
6. Frontera JA, Egorova N, Moskowitz AJ. National trend in prevalence, cost, and discharge disposition after subdural hematoma from 1998–2007. *Critical Care Medicine.* 2011;39(7):1619–1625.
7. Langlois JA, Rutland-Brown W, Thomas KE, eds. *Traumatic Brain Injury in the United States: Emergency Department Visits, Hospitalizations, and Deaths.* Atlanta, GA: National Center for Injury Prevention and Control; 2004.
8. Thomas KE, Stevens JA, Sarmiento K, Wald MM. Fall-related traumatic brain injury deaths and hospitalizations among older adults—United States, 2005. *J Safety Res.* 2008;39(3):269–272.
9. National Center for Statistics and Analysis. *Traffic Safety Facts 1998: Older Population.* Washington, DC: National Center for Statistics and Analysis, National Highway Traffic Safety Administration, US Department of Transportation; 1999. DHHS Publication No. DOT HS 808 955.
10. Ekelman BA, Mitchell SA, O'Dell-Rossi P. Driving and older adults. In: Bonder BR, ed. *Functional Performance in Older Adults.* Philadelphia, PA: Davis; 2001:448–476.
11. Lavoie A, Ratte S, Clas D, et al. Preinjury warfarin use among elderly patients with closed head injuries in a trauma center. *J Trauma.* 2004;56(4):802–807.
12. Thompson HJ, McCormick WC, Kagan SH. Traumatic brain injury in older adults: epidemiology, outcomes, and future implications. *J Am Geriatr Soc.* 2006;54(10):1590–1595.
13. Miranda LB, Braxton E, Hobbs J, Quigley MR. Chronic subdural hematoma in the elderly: not a benign disease. *J Neurosurg.* 2011;114(1):72–76.
14. Ito H, Yamamoto S, Saito K, Ikeda K, Hisada K. Quantitative estimation of hemorrhage in chronic subdural hematoma using the 51Cr erythrocyte labeling method. *J Neurosurg.* 1987;66(6):862–864.
15. Rozzelle CJ, Wofford JL, Branch CL. Predictors of hospital mortality in older patients with subdural hematoma. *J Am Geriatr Soc.* 1995;43(3):240–244.
16. Brain Trauma Foundation, American Association of Neurological Surgeons, Congress of Neurological Surgeons, Joint Section on Neurotrauma and Critical Care, et al. Guidelines for the management of severe traumatic brain injury. IX. Cerebral perfusion thresholds. *J Neurotrauma.* 2007;24(suppl 1):S59–S64.
17. Czosnyka M, Balestreri M, Steiner L, et al. Age, intracranial pressure, autoregulation, and outcome after brain trauma. *J Neurosurg.* 2005;102(3):450–454.
18. Cifu DX, Kreutzer JS, Marwitz JH, Rosenthal M, Englander J, High W. Functional outcomes of older adults with traumatic brain injury: a prospective, multicenter analysis. *Arch Phys Med Rehabil.* 1996;77(9):883–888.
19. Frankel JE, Marwitz JH, Cifu DX, Kreutzer JS, Englander J, Rosenthal M. A follow-up study of older adults with traumatic brain injury: taking into account decreasing length of stay. *Arch Phys Med Rehabil.* 2006;87(1):57–62.
20. Walker MP. A refined model of sleep and the time course of memory formation. *Behav Brain Sci.* 2005;28(1):51–104.
21. Shadmehr R, Holcomb HH. Neural correlates of motor memory consolidation. *Science.* 1997;277(5327):821–825.

22. Born J, Wagner U. Awareness in memory: being explicit about the role of sleep. *Trends Cogn Sci.* 2004;8(6):242–244.

23. Mościcki EK, Elkins EF, Baum HM, McNamara PM. Hearing loss in the elderly: an epidemiologic study of the Framingham heart study cohort. *Ear and Hearing.* 1985;6(4):184–190.

24. National Institute on Aging. Age Page: Aging and your eyes. 2009. Available at http://www.nia.nih.gov/HealthInformation/Public ations/eyes.htm. Accessed July 9, 2011.

25. Taylor MD, Tracy JK, Meyer W, Pasquale M, Napolitano LM. Trauma in the elderly: intensive care unit resource use and outcome. *J Trauma.* 2002;53(3):407–414.

26. Hoffman C, Rice D, Sung HY. Persons with chronic conditions. their prevalence and costs. *JAMA.* 1996;276(18):1473-1479.

27. Adams PF, Hendershot GE, Marano MA. Current estimates from the National Health Interview Survey, 1996. *Vital Health Stat.* 1999; 10(200).

28. Safaz I, Alaca R, Yasar E, Tok F, Yilmaz B. Medical complications, physical function and communication skills in patients with traumatic brain injury: a single centre 5-year experience. *Brain Inj.* 2008; 22(10):733–739.

29. Falsetti P, Acciai C, Lenzi L. Sonographic diagnosis of neurogenic heterotopic ossification in patients with severe acquired brain injury in a neurorehabilitation unit. *J Clin Ultrasound.* 2011;39(1): 12–17.

30. Falsetti P, Acciai C, Palilla R, Carpinteri F, Patrizio C, Lenzi L. Bedside ultrasound in early diagnosis of neurogenic heterotopic ossification in patients with acquired brain injury. *Clin Neurol Neurosurg.* 2011;113(1):22–27.

31. Petersen RC. Clinical practice. Mild cognitive impairment. *N Engl J Med.* 2011;364(23):2227–2234.

32. Petersen RC, Smith GE, Waring SC, Ivnik RJ, Tangalos EG, Kokmen E. Mild cognitive impairment: clinical characterization and outcome. *Arch Neurol.* 1999;56(3):303–308.

33. Manly JJ, Tang MX, Schupf N, Stern Y, Vonsattel JP, Mayeux R. Frequency and course of mild cognitive impairment in a multiethnic community. *Ann Neurol.* 2008;63(4):494–506.

34. Plassman BL, Langa KM, Fisher GG, et al. Prevalence of cognitive impairment without dementia in the united states. *Ann Intern Med.* 2008;148(6):427–434.

35. Busse A, Hensel A, Gühne U, Angermeyer MC, Riedel-Heller SG. Mild cognitive impairment: long-term course of four clinical subtypes. *Neurology.* 2006;67(12):2176–2185.

36. Plassman BL, Havlik RJ, Steffens DC, et al. Documented head injury in early adulthood and risk of Alzheimer's disease and other dementias. *Neurology.* 2000;55(8):1158–1166.

37. Starkstein SE, Jorge R. Dementia after traumatic brain injury. *Int Psychogeriatr.* 2005;17(suppl 1):S93–S107.

38. Garcia CA, Tweedy JR, Blass JP. Underdiagnosis of cognitive impairment in a rehabilitation setting. *J Am Geriatr Soc.* 1984;32(5): 339–342.

39. Hibbard MR, Uysal S, Kepler K, Bogdany J, Silver J. Axis I psychopathology in individuals with traumatic brain injury. *J Head Trauma Rehabil.* 1998;13(4):24–39.

40. Fann JR, Katon WJ, Uomoto JM, Esselman PC. Psychiatric disorders and functional disability in outpatients with traumatic brain injuries. *Am J Psychiatry.* 1995;152(10):1493–1499.

41. van Reekum R, Bolago I, Finlayson MA, Garner S, Links PS. Psychiatric disorders after traumatic brain injury. *Brain Inj.* 1996;10(5): 319–327.

42. Baldwin RC, Anderson D, Black S, et al. Guideline for the management of late-life depression in primary care. *Int J Geriatr Psychiatry.* 2003;18(9):829–838.

43. Lyness JM, Cox C, Curry J, Conwell Y, King DA, Caine ED. Older age and the underreporting of depressive symptoms. *J Am Geriatr Soc.* 1995;43(3):216–221.

44. Cantor JB, Ashman TA, Schwartz ME, et al. The role of self-discrepancy theory in understanding post-traumatic brain injury affective disorders: a pilot study. *J Head Trauma Rehabil.* 2005;20(6):527–543.

45. Jorge R, Robinson RG. Mood disorders following traumatic brain injury. *Int Rev Psychiatry.* 2003;15(4):317–327.

46. Fedoroff JP, Starkstein SE, Forrester AW, et al. Depression in patients with acute traumatic brain injury. *Am J Psychiatry.* 1992; 149(7):918–923.

47. Jeste DV, Blazer D, Casey D, et al. ACNP white paper: update on use of antipsychotic drugs in elderly persons with dementia. *Neuropsychopharmacology.* 2008;33(5):957–970.

48. Gliebus G, Lippa CF. The influence of beta-blockers on delayed memory function in people with cognitive impairment. *Am J Alzheimers Dis Other Demen.* 2007;22(1):57–61.

49. Goldstein LB. Common drugs may influence motor recovery after stroke. The sygen in acute stroke study investigators. *Neurology.* 1995;45(5):865–871.

50. Leipzig RM, Cumming RG, Tinetti ME. Drugs and falls in older people: a systematic review and meta-analysis: I. Psychotropic drugs. *J Am Geriatr Soc.* 1999;47(1):30–39.

51. Hartikainen S, Lönnroos E, Louhivuori K. Medication as a risk factor for falls: critical systematic review. *J Gerontol A Biol Sci Med Sci.* 2007;62(10):1172–1181.

52. Woolcott JC, Richardson KJ, Wiens MO, et al. Meta-analysis of the impact of 9 medication classes on falls in elderly persons. *Arch Intern Med.* 2009;169(21):1952–1960.

53. Salonoja M, Salminen M, Vahlberg T, Aarnio P, Kivelä SL. Withdrawal of psychotropic drugs decreases the risk of falls requiring treatment. *Arch Gerontol Geriatr.* 2011;54(1):160–167.

54. Ziino C, Ponsford J. Selective attention deficits and subjective fatigue following traumatic brain injury. *Neuropsychology.* 2006;20(3): 383–390.

55. Ouellet MC, Beaulieu-Bonneau S, Morin CM. Insomnia in patients with traumatic brain injury: frequency, characteristics, and risk factors. *J Head Trauma Rehabil.* 2006;21(3):199–212.

56. Granger CV, Markello SJ, Graham JE, Deutsch A, Reistetter TA, Ottenbacher KJ. The uniform data system for medical rehabilitation: report of patients with traumatic brain injury discharged from rehabilitation programs in 2000–2007. *Am J Phys Med Rehabil.* 2010; 89(4):265–278.

57. Hoffman JM, Doctor JN, Chan L, Whyte J, Jha A, Dikmen S. Potential impact of the new Medicare prospective payment system on reimbursement for traumatic brain injury inpatient rehabilitation. *Arch Phys Med Rehabil.* 2003;84(8):1165–1172.

58. Gan BK, Lim JH, Ng IH. Outcome of moderate and severe traumatic brain injury amongst the elderly in Singapore. *Ann Acad Med Singapore.* 2004;33(1):63–67.

59. Mosenthal AC, Lavery RF, Addis M, et al. Isolated traumatic brain injury: age is an independent predictor of mortality and early outcome. *J Trauma.* 2002;52(5):907–911.

60. Susman M, DiRusso SM, Sullivan T, et al. Traumatic brain injury in the elderly: increased mortality and worse functional outcome at discharge despite lower injury severity. *J Trauma.* 2002;53(2): 219–224.

61. Harris C, DiRusso S, Sullivan T, Benzil DL. Mortality risk after head injury increases at 30 years. *J Am Coll Surg.* 2003;197(5):711–716.

62. Ivascu FA, Howells GA, Junn FS, Bair HA, Bendick PJ, Janczyk RJ. Predictors of mortality in trauma patients with intracranial hemorrhage on preinjury aspirin or clopidogrel. *J Trauma.* 2008;65(4): 785–788.

63. Ivascu FA, Janczyk RJ, Junn FS, Bair HA, Bendick PJ, Howells GA. Treatment of trauma patients with intracranial hemorrhage on preinjury warfarin. *J Trauma.* 2006;61(2):318–321.

64. Mina AA, Knipfer JF, Park DY, Bair HA, Howells GA, Bendick PJ. Intracranial complications of preinjury anticoagulation in trauma patients with head injury. *J Trauma.* 2002;53(4):668–672.

65. Ohm C, Mina A, Howells G, Bair H, Bendick P. Effects of antiplatelet agents on outcomes for elderly patients with traumatic intracranial hemorrhage. *J Trauma.* 2005;58(3):518–522.

66. Pieracci FM, Eachempati SR, Shou J, Hydo LJ, Barie PS. Use of long-term anticoagulation is associated with traumatic intracranial hemorrhage and subsequent mortality in elderly patients hospitalized after falls: analysis of the New York State administrative database. *J Trauma.* 2007;63(3):519–524.

67. Pieracci FM, Eachempati SR, Shou J, Hydo LJ, Barie PS. Degree of anticoagulation, but not warfarin use itself, predicts adverse outcomes after traumatic brain injury in elderly trauma patients. *J Trauma.* 2007;63(3):525–530.

68. Fortuna GR, Mueller EW, James LE, Shutter LA, Butler KL. The impact of preinjury antiplatelet and anticoagulant pharmacotherapy on outcomes in elderly patients with hemorrhagic brain injury. *Surgery.* 2008;144(4):598–605.

69. Stein SC, Chen XH, Sinson GP, Smith DH. Intravascular coagulation: a major secondary insult in nonfatal traumatic brain injury. *J Neurosurg.* 2002;97(6):1373–1377.

70. Wahl F, Grosjean-Piot O, Bareyre F, Uzan A, Stutzmann JM. Enoxaparin reduces brain edema, cerebral lesions, and improves motor and cognitive impairments induced by a traumatic brain injury in rats. *J Neurotrauma.* 2000;17(11):1055–1065.

71. Norwood SH, McAuley CE, Berne JD, et al. Prospective evaluation of the safety of enoxaparin prophylaxis for venous thromboembolism in patients with intracranial hemorrhagic injuries. *Arch Surg.* 2002;137(6):696–702.

72. Norwood SH, Berne JD, Rowe SA, Villarreal DH, Ledlie JT. Early venous thromboembolism prophylaxis with enoxaparin in patients with blunt traumatic brain injury. *J Trauma.* 2008;65(5):1021–1027.

73. Kim J, Gearhart MM, Zurick A, Zuccarello M, James L, Luchette FA. Preliminary report on the safety of heparin for deep venous thrombosis prophylaxis after severe head injury. *J Trauma.* 2002; 53(1):38–43.

74. Dudley RR, Aziz I, Bonnici A, et al. Early venous thromboembolic event prophylaxis in traumatic brain injury with low-molecular-weight heparin: risks and benefits. *J Neurotrauma.* 2010;27(12): 2165–2172.

75. Rothweiler B, Temkin NR, Dikmen SS. Aging effect on psychosocial outcome in traumatic brain injury. *Arch Phys Med Rehabil.* 1998; 79(8):881–887.

76. LeBlanc J, de Guise E, Gosselin N, Feyz M. Comparison of functional outcome following acute care in young, middle-aged and elderly patients with traumatic brain injury. *Brain Inj.* 2006;20(8): 779–790.

77. Katz DI, Alexander MP. Traumatic brain injury. Predicting course of recovery and outcome for patients admitted to rehabilitation. *Arch Neurol.* 1994;51(7):661–670.

78. Vollmer DG, Torner J, Jane JA, et al. Age and outcome following traumatic coma: why do older patients fare worse? *J Neurosurg.* 1991;75:S37–S49.

79. Sendroy-Terrill M, Whiteneck GG, Brooks CA. Aging with traumatic brain injury: cross-sectional follow-up of people receiving inpatient rehabilitation over more than 3 decades. *Arch Phys Med Rehabil.* 2010;91(3):489–497.

80. Campbell AJ, Spears GF, Borrie MJ. Examination by logistic regression modelling of the variables which increase the relative risk of elderly women falling compared to elderly men. *J Clin Epidemiol.* 1990;43(12):1415–1420.

81. Tinetti ME, Speechley M, Ginter SF. Risk factors for falls among elderly persons living in the community. *N Engl J Med.* 1988; 319(26):1701–1707.

82. Nevitt MC, Cummings SR, Kidd S, Black D. Risk factors for recurrent nonsyncopal falls. A prospective study. *JAMA.* 1989;261(18): 2663–2668.

83. Centers for Disease Control and Prevention. Self-reported falls and fall-related injuries among persons aged > or = 65 years—United States, 2006. *MMWR Morb Mortal Wkly Rep.* 2008;57(9):225–229.

84. Tinetti ME, Kumar C. The patient who falls: "it's always a trade-off." *JAMA.* 2010;303(3):258–266.

85. Panel on Prevention of Falls in Older Persons, American Geriatrics Society and British Geriatrics Society. Summary of the updated American Geriatrics Society/British Geriatrics Society clinical practice guideline for prevention of falls in older persons. *J Am Geriatr Soc.* 2011;59(1):148–157.

86. Brown AW, Leibson CL, Malec JF, Perkins PK, Diehl NN, Larson DR. Long-term survival after traumatic brain injury: a population-based analysis. *Neurorehabilitation.* 2004;19(1):37–43.

87. Harrison-Felix CL, Whiteneck GG, Jha A, DeVivo MJ, Hammond FM, Hart DM. Mortality over four decades after traumatic brain injury rehabilitation: a retrospective cohort study. *Arch Phys Med Rehabil.* 2009;90(9):1506–1513.

88. Ventura T, Harrison-Felix C, Carlson N, et al. Mortality after discharge from acute care hospitalization with traumatic brain injury: a population-based study. *Arch Phys Med Rehabil.* 2010;91(1):20–29.

89. Shavelle RM, Strauss D, Whyte J, Day SM, Yu YL. Long-term causes of death after traumatic brain injury. *Am J Phys Med Rehabil.* 2001; 80(7):510–516.

90. Strauss DJ, Shavelle RM, Anderson TW. Long-term survival of children and adolescents after traumatic brain injury. *Arch Phys Med Rehabil.* 1998;79(9):1095–1100.

91. Harrison-Felix C, Whiteneck G, DeVivo MJ, Hammond FM, Jha A. Causes of death following 1 year postinjury among individuals with traumatic brain injury. *J Head Trauma Rehabil.* 2006;21(1): 22–33.

92. Lewin W, Marshall TF, Roberts AH. Long-term outcome after severe head injury. *Br Med J.* 1979;2(6204):1533–1538.

93. Rish BL, Dillon JD, Weiss GH. Mortality following penetrating craniocerebral injuries. An analysis of the deaths in the Vietnam head injury registry population. *J Neurosurg.* 1983;59(5):775–780.

94. Walker AE, Erculei F. Post-traumatic epilepsy 15 years later. *Epilepsia.* 1970;11(1):17–26.

95. Walker AE, Leuchs HK, Lechtape-Grüter H, Caveness WF, Kretschman C. Life expectancy of head injured men with and without epilepsy. *Arch Neurol.* 1971;24(2):95–100.

96. Weiss GH, Caveness WF, Einsiedel-Lechtape H, McNeel ML. Life expectancy and causes of death in a group of head-injured veterans of World War I. *Arch Neurol.* 1982;39(12):741–743.

97. Harrison-Felix C, Whiteneck G, DeVivo M, Hammond FM, Jha A. Mortality following rehabilitation in the traumatic brain injury model systems of care. *NeuroRehabilitation.* 2004;19(1):45–54.

98. Teasdale TW, Engberg AW. Suicide after traumatic brain injury: a population study. *J Neurol Neurosurg Psychiatry.* 2001;71(4): 436–440.

99. Shavelle RM, Strauss D, Whyte J, Day SM, Yu YL. Long-term causes of death after traumatic brain injury. *Am J Phys Med Rehabil.* 2001; 80(7):510–519.

100. Walker AE, Blumer D. The fate of World War II veterans with posttraumatic seizures. *Arch Neurol.* 1989;46(1):23–26.

101. McMillan TM, Teasdale GM. Death rate is increased for at least 7 years after head injury: a prospective study. *Brain.* 2007;130(pt 10): 2520–2527.

102. Ratcliff G, Colantonio A, Escobar M, Chase S, Vernich L. Long-term survival following traumatic brain injury. *Disabil Rehabil.* 2005;27(6):305–314.

103. Baguley I, Slewa-Younan S, Lazarus R, Green A. Long-term mortality trends in patients with traumatic brain injury. *Brain Inj.* 2000; 14(6):505–512.

104. Other health outcomes. In: *Gulf War and Health: Volume 7: Long-term Consequences of Traumatic Brain Iinjury.* Washington, DC: National Academies Press; 2008:333–366.

105. Schofield PW, Tang M, Marder K, et al. Alzheimer's disease after remote head injury: an incidence study. *J Neurol Neurosurg Psychiatry.* 1997;62(2):119–124.

106. Heyman A, Wilkinson WE, Stafford JA, Helms MJ, Sigmon AH, Weinberg T. Alzheimer's disease: a study of epidemiological aspects. *Ann Neurol.* 1984;15(4):335–341.

107. Guo Z, Cupples LA, Kurz A, et al. Head injury and the risk of AD in the MIRAGE study. *Neurology.* 2000;54(6):1316–1323.

108. French LR, Schuman LM, Mortimer JA, Hutton JT, Boatman RA, Christians B. A case-control study of dementia of the Alzheimer type. *Am J Epidemiol.* 1985;121(3):414–421.

109. Guskiewicz KM, Marshall SW, Bailes J, et al. Association between recurrent concussion and late-life cognitive impairment in retired professional football players. *Neurosurgery.* 2005;57(4):719–726.

110. Neurological outcomes. In: *Gulf War and Health: Volume 7: Long-term Consequences of Traumatic Brain Injury.* Washington, DC: National Academies Press; 2008:197–264.

111. Goldman SM, Tanner CM, Oakes D, Bhudhikanok GS, Gupta A, Langston JW. Head injury and Parkinson's disease risk in twins. *Ann Neurol.* 2006;60(1):65–72.

112. Bower JH, Maraganore DM, Peterson BJ, McDonnell SK, Ahlskog JE, Rocca WA. Head trauma preceding PD: a case-control study. *Neurology.* 2003;60(10):1610–1615.

113. Taylor CA, Saint-Hilaire MH, Cupples LA, et al. Environmental, medical, and family history risk factors for Parkinson's disease: a new England-based case control study. *Am J Med Genet.* 1999;88(6): 742–749.

29

Mild Traumatic Brain Injury

Grant L. Iverson, Rael T. Lange, Michael B. Gaetz, and Nathan D. Zasler

INTRODUCTION

Mild traumatic brain injuries (MTBI) are common in children, adults, and older adults. Bazarian and colleagues (1) reported that 56/100,000 people are evaluated in the emergency department each year for an *isolated* MTBI. Sosin et al. (2), based on the National Health Interview Survey in 1991, estimated that 1.5 million Americans sustain a traumatic brain injury (TBI) each year (i.e., 618/100,000), with most being mild in severity (e.g., 85%–90%). This, of course, is much higher than previous estimates based on hospital admissions because most people who sustain an MTBI are not evaluated in the emergency department or admitted to the hospital (2).

For most people, MTBIs are self-limiting and follow a predictable course. Permanent cognitive, psychological, or psychosocial problems caused by the biological effects of this injury are relatively uncommon in trauma patients and rare in athletes (see 3,4–8 for comprehensive reviews). Slow or incomplete recovery from MTBI is poorly understood despite decades of research.

The purpose of this chapter is to provide a comprehensive overview of MTBI. This chapter is divided into the following 12 sections: (*a*) definitions, (*b*) pathoanatomy and pathophysiology, (*c*) biomarkers, (*d*) neuropsychological outcome, (*e*) early intervention, (*f*) return to work, (*g*) depression, (*h*) posttraumatic stress disorder, (*i*) chronic traumatic encephalopathy, (*j*) risk for Alzheimer disease (AD), (*k*) persistent postconcussion symptoms, and (*l*) conclusions. This chapter does not provide a detailed review of concussions in sports (see Chapter 31), MTBI in children (see Chapter 34) or in the military (see Chapter 33), long-term outcome from MTBI (see Chapter 30), or neuroimaging (see Chapters 15, 16, and 19). Chapter 30 is a continuation of this topic.

DEFINITIONS

There is no universally accepted definition of MTBI. Classification is based on initial severity indicators, not outcome. The 3 primary severity indicators are duration of unconsciousness, Glasgow Coma Scale (GCS) score, and duration of posttraumatic amnesia (PTA). A definition of MTBI, provided by the World Health Organization (WHO) Collaborating Center Task Force on Mild Traumatic Brain Injury, is reprinted subsequently.

MTBI is an acute brain injury resulting from mechanical energy to the head from external physical forces. Operational criteria for clinical identification include: (*a*) 1 or more of the following: confusion or disorientation, loss of consciousness for 30 minutes or less, posttraumatic amnesia for less than 24 hours, and/or other transient neurological abnormalities such as focal signs, seizure, and intracranial lesion not requiring surgery; (*b*) Glasgow Coma Scale score of 13–15 after 30 minutes postinjury or later upon presentation for health care. These manifestations of MTBI must not be due to drugs, alcohol, medications; caused by other injuries or treatment for other injuries (e.g., systemic injuries, facial injuries, or intubation); caused by other problems (e.g., psychological trauma, language barrier or coexisting medical conditions); or caused by penetrating craniocerebral injury. (p. 115) (9)

This aforementioned definition is very similar to the definition developed by the Mild Traumatic Brain Injury Committee of the Head Injury Interdisciplinary Special Interest Group of the American Congress of Rehabilitation Medicine (10). It is also similar to the conceptual definition of MTBI offered by the Center for Disease Control (CDC) working group (11). The WHO workgroup definition has been endorsed as reasonable for use in clinical practice and research (12).

Some researchers have differentiated *complicated* from *uncomplicated* MTBI (13). A complicated MTBI is diagnosed if the person has a GCS score of 13–15 and shows an intracranial abnormality (e.g., edema, hematoma, or contusion) on a computed tomography (CT) scan. Depressed skull fractures were also considered characteristic of complicated injuries by Williams et al. (13), but fractures have been investigated separately by other researchers. The mainstream definitions of MTBI include patients with these visible structural abnormalities. Complicated MTBIs are discussed in detail in the pathoanatomy and pathophysiology and the neuropsychological outcome sections of this chapter.

PATHOANATOMY AND PATHOPHYSIOLOGY

MTBI can be characterized by limited damage to the structure of the brain and its support systems. Clinicians and researchers often emphasize that most patients with MTBI have normal structural neuroimaging studies; this is certainly true. However, a substantial minority of patients have

TABLE 29-1 Rates of Complicated Mild Traumatic Brain Injury in Adults

FIRST AUTHOR	YEAR	COUNTRY	TOTAL *N*	NUMBER SCANNED	GCS SCORES	ABNORMAL (%)
Livingston (19)	1991	United States	111	111	14–15	14
Stein (488)	1992	United States	1,538	1,538	13–15	17.2
Jeret (18)	1993	United States	712	702	15	9.4
Moran (489)	1994	United States	200	96	13–15	8.3
Borczuk (490)	1995	United States	1,448	1,448	13–15	8.2
Iverson (17)	2000	United States	912	912	13–15	15.8
Thiruppathy (491)	2004	India	381	381	13–15	38.9
Stiell (492)	2005	Canada	2,707	2,171	13–15	12.1
Stiell (492)	2005	Canada	1,822	1,822	15	8.0
Ono (493)	2007	Japan	1,064	1,064	14–15	4.7
Saboori (494)	2007	Iran	682	682	15	6.7

Abbreviation: GCS, Glasgow Coma Scale. Reprinted with permission from Iverson GL, Lange RT, Waljäs M, Liimatainen S, Dastidar P, Hartikainen KM, Soimakallio S, Öhman J. Outcome from complicated versus uncomplicated mild traumatic brain injury. *Rehabilitation Research & Practice.* 2012. Article ID 415740, 7 pages.

day-of-injury abnormalities visible on CT. Approximately 7%–20% of consecutive patients presenting to the emergency department[1] with an MTBI have bleeding, bruising, or swelling on day-of-injury CT (16–22). Borg and colleagues conducted a comprehensive review of this literature and concluded that the estimated prevalence of CT abnormalities of patients seen in the hospital was 5% for those with GCS scores of 15 and 30% or more for those with GCS scores of 13 (22). Not surprisingly, patients with *macroscopic* abnormalities on their day-of-injury CT have *microscopic* damage or dysfunction as well, as reported in both the animal and human literature. The rates of intracranial abnormalities, based on cohorts of patients who underwent acute CT scans following head trauma, are presented in Table 29-1. Patients with GCS scores of 13 or 14 are more likely to have an abnormality than patients with a GCS score of 15. Other possible reasons for differences in abnormality rates reported in the literature could relate to technology (e.g., older scanners vs newer scanners) and referral patterns for neuroimaging (i.e., more liberal vs more conservative use of imaging).

It has been reported that some patients with normal CT scans show abnormalities on magnetic resonance imaging (MRI) (23–26), single photon emission computed tomography (SPECT) (27–29), or magnetoencephalography (30). Abnormalities on positron emission tomography (29,31) and SPECT (32,33) have been observed in some patients with lingering postconcussion symptoms. In some patients with

moderate TBI, brain atrophy can be quantified on serial quantitative MRI over a several month interval (34,35). Not all studies show abnormalities on structural MRI, especially when the patient sample consists of very mild injuries (36). Most studies report structural abnormalities on MRI close to the range reported for CT (~12%–30%) in the weeks and months postinjury (30,37,38). Increased abnormality detection rates have been reported when using a scanner of greater strength (e.g., 1.5T vs 3T), when studying patients with persistent symptoms (39,40), or when using nonstandard clinical protocols. For example, a detailed MRI examination of Virchow-Robin spaces (i.e., extensions of the subpial space surrounding perforating arteries and emerging veins serving cerebral cortex—when enlarged, these have been linked to white matter injury) in uncomplicated MTBI (i.e., 23/24 with GCS of 15 and 20/24 with unremarkable MRI) revealed significant trauma-related findings (41).

Newer MRI-based techniques such as functional MRI (fMRI) and diffusion tensor imaging (DTI) have been used to study MTBI and have provided mixed results. For example, some patients with a history of MTBI who have chronic cognitive complaints do not have abnormalities on fMRI (42). However, another study described substantial increases in multiple frontotemporal areas related to verbal working memory and selective attention. These areas were statistically more activated in patients who reported more symptoms (43) (a similar pattern is found in some sport concussion studies—see Chapter 31).

DTI is an MRI technique used to examine the integrity of white matter in the brain at a microstructural level. Thermal energy causes molecules to intermingle and migrate, a process called diffusion. DTI can be used to measure both the directionality and the magnitude of water diffusion in white matter. Fractional anisotropy (FA) is a mathematical measurement used in physics to estimate diffusion at the level of a voxel, with values ranging from 0 (*isotropic*—equal in all directions) to 1 (*anisotropic*—highly directional and linear). Thus, reduced FA is believed to represent white matter that is reduced in directionality. Low FA might reflect disintegra-

---

[1] Victims of serious assault, people who fall or are struck hard enough to fracture their skull, or people in high-velocity accidents are at increased risk for intracranial abnormalities (14), and these individuals are more likely to be seen in the emergency department. Note that at least 25% of people with MTBIs seek no medical attention and 14% are seen at their doctor's office or in clinics (2). Moreover, there is a low risk for intracranial abnormalities in athletic concussions, most athletes are not taken to the hospital, and a significant percentage of athletes with minor concussions do not even report the injury to their coaches or trainers (15). Therefore, the true incidence of structural lesions in *all people* with MTBIs is likely far less than these estimates.

tive changes in white matter. As such, this technology can be used to estimate damage to white matter (see Chapter 15).

It is well established that DTI can detect microstructural white matter changes in children (44–48) and adults (49–52) who have sustained severe TBIs. Moreover, researchers have reported differences between MTBI samples and healthy control subjects on DTI acutely (i.e., 2 weeks to 3 months) (41,51,53) and chronically (i.e., 2 or more years) (54–57). Researchers have reported reduced FA and increased mean diffusivity (MD) in large white matter structures such as the centrum semiovale (54,56), internal capsule (54,56), and the corpus callosum (56,58); particularly in the splenium (53,54) and genu (51,53). However, one recent study found only a weak relation between an ICD-10 diagnosis of postconcussional disorder and DTI of the corpus callosum following uncomplicated MTBI 6–8 weeks postinjury (59). Individuals reporting chronic symptoms who were scanned 3–6 years following an MTBI had decreased FA and/or increased MD in the corpus callosum, internal capsule (39,54,56), centrum semiovale, deep cerebellar white matter (56), anterior corona radiata, uncinate fasciculus, and cingulum bundle (39) compared to healthy controls. In contrast to this pattern of results, some studies have found *increased* FA and *decreased* diffusivity in the corpus callosum in the first few days and weeks postinjury (60–62). This opposite than expected pattern is thought to be attributable to acute "cytotoxic edema associated with compressed intracellular space between corpus callosum fibers, thus restricting diffusion in a more uniform direction" (p. 953) (62).

It is important to appreciate that microstructural, as measured by DTI, white matter abnormalities are not unique to TBI. Researchers have reported that people with learning disorders (e.g., 63–65), attention deficit hyperactivity disorder (ADHD) (e.g., 66,67), substance abuse (e.g., 68–70), and depression (e.g., 71) also show abnormalities on DTI. Similarly, macroscopic white matter hyperintensities are found in (*a*) a minority of children and adults with bipolar disorder (72–74), (*b*) a minority of adults with depression (75–77) or migraines (78), and (*c*) most older adults with hypertension (79). Iverson and colleagues reported that healthy control subjects with macroscopic white matter hyperintensities also show microstructural abnormalities on DTI. Specifically, there were differences in DTI measurements of white matter integrity between control subjects with or without these incidental findings, and these measurements occurred in areas of white matter that were spatially separate from the incidental findings (80). Therefore, preexisting incidental findings (macroscopic and/or microscopic) might be present in some people who sustain MTBIs and might influence the results of research involving DTI.

Cellular Pathophysiology of MTBI

When forces are applied to the brain with sufficient magnitude, small changes in structure and function can be observed in a subset of neurons and glia. To fully understand the pathophysiology of MTBI, we must first understand how these forces differentially affect gray and white matter at cortical and subcortical levels. The first comprehensive model of TBI was proposed by Ommaya and Gennarelli (81). Their model of TBI suggested that acceleration/deceleration

forces can cause mechanical strains that occur in a "centripetal sequence." Injuries of this nature occur when the head is propelled through space and is abruptly stopped by a solid object, such as the ground, or when the head is set into motion, such as when a car is struck from behind by another car. Their theory predicted three important elements related to MTBI. First, it reinforced the principle that the *direction* of force can determine severity of injury. Second, a continuum of injury exists whereby mild, moderate, and severe brain injuries caused by acceleration (inertial)/deceleration (impact) forces are not random in magnitude but occur on a spectrum. Third, acceleration/deceleration forces alone are sufficient to cause severe TBI (head impact is not required), as supported by research in human trauma cases (82–85). The importance of acceleration/deceleration forces and their role in the pathophysiology of MTBI is evidenced by the number of methods that are being developed to measure these forces in motor vehicles (86) and in athletes (87–90) (see Chapter 10).

A review by Meaney and Smith (91) echoes some of the principles described by Ommaya and Gennarelli while adding others. The authors clearly describe two components of acceleration that occur in nearly every instance of MTBI—linear and rotational acceleration. Rotational acceleration is common during either impact or impulsive head loading. They note that because of the physical properties and complexity of the human brain, its tissue deforms more readily in response to shear forces compared with other biological tissues. Rapid head rotations generate shear forces throughout the brain, and therefore, rotational accelerations have a higher likelihood of causing shear-induced tissue damage (not to be confused with the physical "shearing" or cutting of axons—a common misconception that continues today). Lateral (coronal) plane accelerations in humans have the greatest likelihood for producing damage within the deep internal structures of the brain (91). The movement of the brain within the cranial vault may be even more complex than was originally suspected. A very interesting study that used an MRI of periodic motion showed that with consistent mild accelerations of the head inside the imaging coil, a remarkable amount of movement could be observed. Three subjects were asked to repeatedly allow the head to fall a short distance downward, when lying in the supine position. The authors showed that tethering loads may be borne by the vascular, neural, and dural elements that bind the brain to the base of the skull. These biological tethers cause the brain to compress and stretch in the anteroposterior plane followed by rotation backward and upward relative to the skull. They noted that the corpus callosum appears to follow more closely the motion of the skull than the more compliant gray matter that deforms around it, suggesting that it may be less vulnerable to movement and therefore injury compared to other brain areas (even though it is typically selected for DTI and tractography studies) (92).

When the brain moves within the cranial vault, stretching and compression can affect neuronal cell bodies, axons, and organelle as well as glial cells. Barkhoudarian et al. (93) summarized the complex neurometabolic and neurochemical cascade that can occur in neurons following stretch or compression. Briefly, they state that the first stage in this process is a disruption of the neuronal cell membrane and axon because of stretching. This allows for ion movement across the plasma membrane through previously regulated ion channels and perhaps temporary membrane defects. This in turn causes widespread release of neurotransmitters, most importantly, excitatory amino acids (EAAs) such as glutamate. Glutamate binds with the N-methyl-D-aspartate (NMDA) receptors and when activated cause further depolarization and influx of calcium ions. The resulting depolarization results in a widespread suppression of neurons, creating a condition resembling spreading depression. To restore ionic balance, ATP-dependent Na^+/K^+ pumps are activated, requiring high levels of glucose metabolism, most of which is conducted aerobically under normal conditions. Local cerebral metabolic rates for glucose are increased within the first 30 minutes followed by glucose hypometabolism several hours following the injury that can last up to 5 days in animal studies. While this is happening, oxidative metabolism is disrupted, likely from mitochondrial dysfunction, and lactate production is increased in the extracellular space (mitochondrial dysfunction will be described in detail subsequently) (93).

Axonal injury is currently thought to be the structural substrate that underlies most post-MTBI neurologic dysfunction (94) with less damage occurring at neuronal cell bodies and to the myelin itself (95). Axons of cultured human neurons have a remarkable capacity for stretch with no primary axotomy observed for strains lower than 65% of the length of the axon. In addition, axons exhibit the behavior of "delayed elasticity." In other words, stretch causes a temporary deformation of an axon that will gradually return to its original orientation and morphology (96). However, once an axon is stretched, a pathophysiologic process begins that can lead to further structural change and metabolic dysfunction (see Chapter 11).

Most studies indicate that it is acute axonal stretch and strain that causes a rapid increase in intracellular calcium. Strain on the axonal membrane causes an abnormal influx of Na^+ through mechanosensitive sodium channels, a reversal of the $Na^+ - Ca^{2+}$ exchangers, and activation of voltage-gated Ca^{2+} channels (97). This in turn causes selective proteolysis or a breakdown of Na^+ channels and progressively increasing levels of intra-axonal Ca^{2+} (98). The massive influx of Ca^{2+} leads to damage to the axonal cytoskeleton and initiates the pathophysiological process that follows.

Intracellular calcium release actually occurs during the first 1–6 seconds following axonal stretch (99) and has been linked to axonal changes such as neuritic sprouting and secondary degeneration. Stretch injury of axon bundles induces a biphasic (2-peak) increase in intracellular calcium detected by an increase in fluorescence. The initial peak increase was within 1–3 seconds of injury followed rapidly by a second peak increase that was significantly less than the first peak increase. The authors suggest that release of calcium from intracellular stores may mediate the secondary influx of calcium from extracellular locations, perhaps via capacitative or store-mediated calcium influx (99). The complexity of the process increases when considering entry of extracellular calcium into the axon. One study has shown that mild neuronal injury can result in receptor remodeling that enhances both calcium permeability and the susceptibility of these cells to secondary excitotoxic challenge (100). The basis for receptor remodeling may be altered gene expression, which has been shown to affect chromatin assembly/disassembly, nucleosome organization and assembly, organ development, developmental process, multicellular organismal development, system development, and anatomical structural development following MTBI (101).

Axons contain numerous microscopic elements including microtubules and neurofilaments. Microtubules are thick cytoskeletal fibers consisting of long polar polymers constructed of protofilaments packed in a long tubular array. They are oriented longitudinally in relation to the axon and are associated with fast axonal transport (102). Neurofilaments are essentially the "bones" or cytoskeleton of the axon and are the most abundant intracellular structural element in axons (102). When axons are stretched, excess Ca^{2+} causes damage to the axonal cytoskeleton and initiates the formation of axonal swellings. This process has been reviewed in detail (103) and will be summarized here. The pathophysiologic events that lead to secondary axotomy associated with animal models of traumatic axonal injury occur within minutes of injury. For example, at as early as 5 minutes after a moderate injury, neurofilament networks appear dense or more tightly packed and local mitochondrial abnormalities have been observed without any overt disruption of the overlying axolemma (104,105). In the hours following injury, a gradual progression of axonal pathology occurs in the absence of local hemorrhage or damage in the surrounding tissue. This pathology progresses with some axons exhibiting focal swellings and others in early stages of disconnection. Disconnection eventually progresses to resemble enlarged ball-like expansions with no continuity that can be identified between proximal and distal axonal segments, suggesting an abrupt separation of the axon cylinder (106). At this time, injured axons become distorted, appearing undulating and wavy within a highly localized region that correlated with the stretched region of the axon (107). Days later, 2 conditions are considered to be predominant (108): a degenerative response and a regenerative response (108). A human case study by Bigler (109) reported similar pathology in the frontal and temporal lobes in a patient with an MTBI who died from other causes several months postinjury.

Stretching of axons has functional and structural implications. In an animal model, stretch lower than 4 mm did not cause any morphological change in axons, a stretch of 5 mm produced changes in visual evoked potentials that were significantly different from controls, with a 6 mm stretch causing morphological change including retraction balls and axonal swellings (110). Therefore, a single acceleration/deceleration event might result in (a) no apparent change in structure or function, (b) functional or metabolic change, or (c) eventual structural change in the axon. These outcomes are dependent on the force applied to the brain.

Perhaps the most important addition to the literature relates to the fate of neurons that have been injured. It has long been assumed that axons that have been stretched to undergo subsequent axonal disconnection. When disconnection occurs close to the cell body, neuronal death ensues (e.g., 111,112) with substantial neuronal atrophy occurring with more distal lesions. New evidence suggests that axonal injury causes (a) persistent neuronal atrophy in neocortex but not neuronal death, and (b) spontaneous structural plasticity (113). In this study, the axonal swellings appeared, as expected, as early as 15 minutes following injury in layer V of the neocortex and subcortical white matter.

However, once the swelling progressed to separation, the axotomized neurons consistently underwent atrophy without evidence of cell death. Equally important was the fact that injured neurons produce an elongation of their proximal disconnection over a 28-day period, consistent with regeneration and reorganization (113). It is not known at this point whether the reorganization of axons has functional value (see Chapter 13).

There is also emerging evidence that when neurons survive, they are often structurally compromised beyond what has been described at the axon (114). Cortical impact models demonstrate that dendrites can also be affected when exposed to mild forces. Specifically, the dendrites of neurons in injured cortex swell in a manner similar to that described for axons. Over time, the amount of dendritic degeneration can be large. In one study, the volume of neuronal degeneration was substantial and was accounted for by reductions in total length of the apical dendrites and the number of dendrite branches of pyramidal cells (114). In summary, the emerging science on the pathophysiology of injured neurons is both positive and negative. It now appears to be the case that many fewer neurons die following a stretch injury that causes frank separation of the axon than previously thought, and that a regenerative attempt is made by the cell. However, it is unclear as to whether this regenerative attempt has functional value. It is also the case that surviving cells may have fewer dendrites and therefore fewer synapses, limiting their communicative potential following injury.

Neurons that have sustained a prior injury also show prolonged changes in subcellular structures such as Na^+ channels (115). Using a "tensile elongation" model of axonal stretch, a 5% strain was the minimum level of injury necessary to induce calcium influx through specific sodium channels. When axonal injury below the threshold of 5% strain was repeated 24 hours later, a significant increase in intracellular Ca^{2+} was reported equivalent to that of a strain level of single injury of 4 times the magnitude. These in vitro data suggest that mild axonal trauma induces a form of axonal sodium channelopathy that can greatly exacerbate the pathophysiologic response to subsequent injuries (115).

Neuronal survival is not only dependent on structural integrity but is also intimately linked to mitochondrial homeostasis. Mitochondria supply the central nervous system (CNS) with energy (adenosine triphosphate [ATP]), as well as regulating calcium within the cell. Mitochondria have also been linked to the pathophysiology of MTBI via either metabolic dysfunction or the release of pro-apoptotic factors such as cytochrome c (Cyt c). The proposed mechanism for mitochondrial dysfunction post-MTBI is the formation of a more permeable transition pore that may play a role in cytoskeletal alterations and axonal degeneration following acceleration brain injury (116). Another proposed impairment in mitochondrial functioning following MTBI is a reduction in ubiquitous mitochondrial creatine kinase (uMtCK), an enzyme implicated in the energetic regulation of Ca^{2+} pumps and in the maintenance of $Ca2^+$ homeostasis (117). Experimental models of MTBI have shown that mitochondrial damage occurs rapidly. Significant decrements in respiration are seen as early as 15–30 minutes postinjury, peaking within 12–24 hours and persisting for up to 14 days (118). Animal experimentation has provided evidence that depressed mitochondrial functioning might be improved by treatment with hyperbaric oxygenation (119) (see Chapter 76 for a discussion of this topic).

Metabolic change following MTBI, including that related to mitochondrial dysfunction, has been measured using magnetic resonance spectroscopy (MRS). In animal (120) and human studies (121–123), there appears to be observable changes in the vicinity of brain contusions that are related to neuronal metabolic pathophysiology (most notably with *N*-acetylaspartate [NAA], a marker of neuronal axonal viability; creatine [Cr], which reflects energy status; choline [Cho], a marker of membrane metabolism; and lactate [Lac], an indicator of ischemia). When studying the whole brain, NAA differences have been reported in patients with MTBI in the days and months following injury (124). NAA/Cr ratios in parietal white matter, Cho/Cr ratios in occipital gray matter, the NAA/Cho ratio in 4 occipital lobe regions, and all 3 ratios in temporal lobe, were shown to be significantly different in patients with MTBI (121). Cr concentrations in both white matter and the splenium have been reported to be significantly greater following MTBI and are predictive of deficits in executive functioning and increased emotional distress in these patients studied between 2 and 30 days postinjury (125). The occurrence of post-traumatic headache following MTBI was associated within reduced values of NAA/Cr in the right and left anterior regions of the frontal lobe white matter, anterior and posterior medial region of the frontal lobes, and medial region of parietal lobes. In addition, Cho/Cr increases in the posterior region of right frontal lobe white matter, anterior medial region of the frontal lobes, and medial region of the parietal lobes have been observed (126). However, thalamic NAA, Cr, and Cho levels in patients with MTBI do not statistically differ from the controls (127). In animal models of MTBI, the metabolic changes associated with a second injury are even greater than those associated with the first injury and vary relative to the interval between impacts (maximal changes were recorded when MTBIs were spaced by 3 days). In these animals, prolonging the time of sacrifice after the second MTBI up to 1 week failed to show cerebral metabolic recovery, indicating that this type of damage is difficult to reverse (128).

In addition to metabolic factors, neurotrophic factors also change following MTBI. Some neurotrophins, including brain-derived neurotrophic factor (BDNF), ciliary neurotrophic factor (CNTF), neurotrophin-3 (NT-3), neurotrophin-4 (NT-4), and β-nerve growth factor (β-NGF), have been shown to decrease as the severity of the brain injury increases (129). Others such as the insulin-like growth factor 1 (IGF-1) system (involved in growth, differentiation, and survival signaling of neurons) have been shown to increase following MTBI. IGF-1 has been implicated as a potential neuroprotective agent in brain injuries and in hypoxia–ischemia induced damage. Activation of the IGF-1R anti-apoptotic pathway by MTBI could be part of a neuroprotective and neurogenic process aimed at maintaining normal brain function following a relatively stressful event (130). This is important because animal models have shown that MTBI can cause diffuse neuronal damage and apoptosis in hippocampus (131). Tweedie et al. (132) described an interesting link between mitochondrial function and apoptosis—that mitochondria are the site for apoptotic stimuli via a biochemical cascade termed the "intrinsic pathway." Following injury, mitochondrial proteins, Cyt c and Smac/DIABLO (second mitochondria-derived activator of caspase/direct IAP-binding protein with low PI), are released into the cytoplasm. Mitochondrial Cyt c normally functions as an electron shuttle between complex III and complex IV of the respiratory chain. In contrast, cytoplasmic Cyt c associates with apoptosis activating factor-1 (Apaf-1) in the presence of deoxy-ATP or ATP and thereby forms a complex, termed an "apoptosome" (132).

It is important to recognize that neurons are not the only cells within the CNS that are affected by MTBI. The functioning of glial cells also changes and this has an impact on the functioning of the CNS as a whole. Widespread dysfunction of astrocytes can occur following MTBI (133) with most studies indicating altered homeostatic regulation (91). One of the roles played by non-injured astrocytes is clearing glutamate from the extracellular space through the high-affinity, sodium-dependent glutamate transporters, glutamate aspartate transporter (GLAST), and glutamate transporter-1 (GLT-1). In the presence of high extracellular glutamate (such as occurs during the complex neurometabolic and neurochemical cascade that occurs post-MTBI), extracellular glutamate induces a decline in GLT-1 and GLAST expression in cultured cortical astrocytes (134). This of course can be linked to a build-up of glutamate in the extracellular space that occurs in a feed-forward manner. Furthermore, astrocytes and microglia are important mediators of inflammation following MTBI. Inflammation in the CNS is driven by the activation of resident microglia, astrocytes, and infiltrating peripheral macrophages, which release a plethora of anti- and pro-inflammatory cytokines, chemokines, neurotransmitters, and reactive oxygen species. Precise regulation of inflammation is essential because mild acute inflammation usually stimulates neurogenesis; whereas the factors released by uncontrolled inflammation create an environment that is detrimental to neurogenesis (135) (see Chapter 12).

The advancements in our understanding of the pathophysiology of MTBI have allowed researchers to explore several potential treatments. Although it is acknowledged that we are not close to solving the problem, several potential mechanism are worthy of mention. For example, substances that prevent Na^+ channel remodeling or permeability that in turn lead to increased intracellular Ca^{2+} have been explored (100,136). Omega-3 fatty acid supplementation has been shown to counteract some of the challenges to mitochondrial homeostasis that occur following MTBI (117). Immediate postinjury hypothermia (32°C) for 3 hours has been shown to reduce axonal degeneration (137). Symptoms such as postinjury depression and locomotor deficits have been treated experimentally with GSK-3 inhibitors (138) and preconditioning with a low dose of NMDA (139) respectively.

Neuroscience has not only provided a new vantage point to consider the pathophysiology of injury but also given us a better understanding about which cells are vulnerable to injury. The features of cellular injury, dysfunction, and death have been described in detail in this section. It is important to appreciate that cell death is closely related to injury severity. MTBIs, especially injuries on the milder end of the spectrum, are typically characterized by cellular dysfunction that is at least somewhat reversible. Cell death is possible but emerging research points to a pattern where most cells survive stretch injury but may be compromised functionally. Very mild concussions likely produce little to

no permanent damage to cells resulting in long-term symptoms or problems whereas severe TBIs, especially those involving considerable forces, often produce widespread cellular death and dysfunction with clear functional consequences; complicated MTBIs and moderate TBIs likely fall in between. Recent science has also pointed to the importance of understanding subcellular physiology related to mitochondrial dysfunction and characteristics of ion channels. Furthermore, it is now understood that glial cells play an important role in neural signaling and are affected by MTBI.

BIOMARKERS

There is considerable interest in the role of various serum and plasma based biochemical markers for use as diagnostic and prognostic measures of TBI (140,141). Biochemical markers have the potential to serve as cost-effective measures to (a) initially screen patients in the first few hours postinjury to detect brain injury, (b) monitor the occurrence of secondary complications during recovery, and (c) predict future outcomes (142).

There are a large number of biochemical markers that have been examined by researchers over the past few decades. A discussion of all biomarkers is outside the scope of this chapter (for more information, see reviews 140,141, 143–147). Rather, 9 markers are discussed subsequently. These were selected based on their potential value for use with MTBI, and those that have received substantial attention in the literature. These include (a) S100B, (b) neuron specific enolase, (c) creatine kinase isoenzyme, (d) myelin basic protein, (e) glial fibrillary acidic protein, (f) fatty acid-binding proteins, (g) cleaved tau, (h) ubiquitin C-terminal hydrolase-L1 (UCH-L1), and (i) alpha II-spectrin breakdown products.

Prior to this discussion, it is important to appreciate that most biomarkers have been mostly studied in patients with moderate-to-severe TBI (except S100B). Few biomarkers have been studied specifically in patients with MTBI. Despite decades of research in this area, no biomarker has yet proven accurate and reliable for detecting TBI of any severity (143,146,147).

S100B

S100B is a calcium-binding protein found in high concentrations in astroglial cells. When these cells are structurally or ischemically damaged, it is believed that S100B is rapidly released into the cerebrospinal fluid (CSF) and secondarily across the blood-CSF barrier into circulation (148). S100B levels reach a concentration peak within 20 minutes (148) and are then eliminated quickly (149). S100B significantly declines within the first few hours after injury (150–153) and is estimated to have a biological half-life ranging from 30 to 113 minutes (148,149,154). Measurements of S100B can be acquired from a standard serum blood sample (155).

S100B is by far the most widely studied biomarker. Much of the literature suggests that S100B may be a useful marker for brain injury (e.g., 140,141,148,153,155–158). Researchers have reported, for example, that the concentration level of S100B is significantly higher in patients with MTBI than in controls (148,158–162). S100B levels are associated with (a) brain abnormalities detected by CT scans (148,152, 153,160,163,164); (b) prediction of poor outcome as measured by the Glasgow Outcome Scale (GOS) 1 month (165), 6 months (166), and 1 year (167) postinjury; (c) the rate of failure to return to work 1 week postinjury in patients with very mild brain injuries (168); (d) injury severity as measured by the GCS and the Coma Remission Scale (150,152,153,159, 166,169); and (e) the presence of neuropsychological deficits 2 weeks and 6 months postinjury (153). However, some researchers have reported that S100B levels are *not* associated with neuropsychological test results at 7–21 days postinjury in uncomplicated MTBI (170), or with PCS symptom reporting 1 year following MTBI (151).

Of particular interest for the diagnosis of MTBI in the acute care setting, some researchers have found that the presence of alcohol at the time of injury tends not to influence the serum concentrations of S100B in patients with MTBIs or healthy controls (156,160,161), even in injured patients with blood alcohol levels of 2.5 to 5.0 times (i.e., 250–500 mg/dl) the legal level of intoxication (148). However, not all research has supported these conclusions (162).

Despite the support for the relation between S100B levels and brain injury, there are several limitations of S100B as a diagnostic or prognostic marker for brain injury. First, S100B tends to be a *sensitive* marker for brain damage, but not a highly *specific* marker (171). Various studies have examined the clinical value of S100B levels to predict outcomes from TBI such as abnormal CT or MRI scans (148,152, 159,163,164,169,172), GOS scores (165–167), and return to work rates (168). The results from these studies are remarkably consistent with researchers reporting high to very high sensitivity (range = 0.80–1.00) and negative predictive power (NPP) (range = 0.95–1.00), moderate to high specificity (range = 0.41–0.81), but only low to moderate positive predictive power (PPP) (range = 0.21%–0.42%). In contrast to the desired results, S100B is more useful for predicting those who will *not* have certain adverse outcomes following TBI as opposed to those who *will* have adverse outcomes.

A second limitation relates to the extracranial release of S100B (151). When compared to healthy controls, higher S100B levels have been found in non-head injured trauma patients who had incurred bone fractures, soft-tissue injuries, and burns (173). Recent studies by Lange and colleagues (161,162) showed that elevated S100B levels were also found in trauma control subjects. However, S100B levels were significantly lower than groups with (a) uncomplicated MTBIs or (b) complicated MTBIs, moderate TBI, or severe TBI. Similarly, researchers examining athletes have found that the release of S100B increases after various sporting activities, compared to pre-activity levels, such as competitive boxing, jogging, running, sparring, elite basketball, ice hockey, and soccer (174–176). However, the increase in S100B was lower than in patients who have sustained an MTBI (176,177).

Neuron Specific Enolase

Neuron specific enolase (NSE) is 1 of the 5 isozymes of the glycolytic enzyme family (enolases) and is thought to be passively released into extracellular space and the bloodstream as a result of structural damage to neuronal cells (178–180). Despite its name, NSE has also been identified in "nonneuronal" locations such as neuroendocrine cells, oligodendrocytes, thrombocytes, and erythrocytres (2). NSE has a biological half-life between 20–48 hours (144,145,147) and can be detected via a blood or CSF sample (144). It is believed that levels of NSE peak within 6–12 hours after injury and then decrease during the following hours or days (144).

Studies examining the influence of injury severity on NSE levels in patients following a broad spectrum of injury severity (147) have found mixed results. Whereas some studies have found no correlation (180–182) between GCS scores and NSE levels, other studies have found significant negative correlations between GCS and NSE ($r = -0.50$ to -0.73) (150,181,183–185). In these studies, increased NSE levels were associated with lower GCS scores (and thus, increased TBI severity). Researchers have also reported no association between NSE levels and CT scan findings (183,186,187) or intracranial pressure (187,188). However, other researchers have further reported that elevated NSE are associated with (a) worse neurocognitive outcome following MTBI (150), and (b) poor neurological outcome (182), higher mortality rates (180,189), and lower GOS scores (189) following moderate-to-severe TBI. However, as a predictor of poor outcome, sensitivity, and specificity values are consistently inadequate to be considered a reliable marker (150,182,189).

Although several studies have demonstrated that NSE levels increase following moderate and/or severe TBI (150,181,183–185,189), few studies have compared NSE levels to controls or to patients following MTBI. Of the studies that have included a control or MTBI group (181,183), significantly higher NSE levels have been found following severe TBI compared to controls (181) and MTBI (181,183). However, no differences have been found between controls and MTBI (181). The one exception to this was a study by deKruijk and colleagues (158) who found slightly elevated NSE in MTBI vs healthy controls. However, there was only a small effect size noted between groups ($d = .21$). In a study by Palinka and colleagues (178), NSE increased within 48 hours of bodily trauma with or without the presence of TBI. Similarly elevated levels of NSE in the absence of TBI have also been found in patients with peripheral disorders of the CNS (i.e., polyneuropathia, myopathia) (190).

Creatine Kinase Isoenyme

Creatine kinase isoenyme BB (CK-BB) is one of three isoenzymes in the creatine kinase family: (a) muscle type, (b) heart type, and (c) brain type. In the CNS, the brain type is located in the astrocytes. CK-BB is also present in organs such as the large intestine, prostate, stomach, and bladder. However, the concentration of the enzyme in these organs is only one-third to one-fourth of that in the brain (141,145) and is found at much lower concentrations in other organs (e.g., the pancreas, uterus, liver, and spleen) (191). The biological half-life of CK-BB is estimated between 1 and 5 hours (143). It peaks rapidly within the first few hours following brain injury, and falls to normal levels within 6 hours (145,192–194).

CK-BB is one of the early serum enzyme markers examined as a biomarker for brain injury (145). Like most other biomarkers, much of the research has focused on patients following severe TBI. The results of studies examining the relation between GCS scores and CK-BB levels following TBI are mixed. Some studies have found no correlation between GCS scores and CK-BB levels (194,195), whereas other studies have found significant negative correlations between GCS and CK-BB levels (range: $r = -.63$ to $-.89$) (183,196, 197). Researchers have reported that day-of-injury CK-BB levels are not associated with 3–12 month GOS scores following severe TBI (193–195).

Increases in CK-BB levels have been found in patients following MTBI, although higher CK-BB levels are found following severe TBI (192,195,196). Despite the demonstrated increases in CK-BB following MTBI, researchers examining patients following MTBI have also found CK-BB to be a poor predictor of intracranial injury on CT scan (183,198,199). In contrast, some researchers have found elevated CK-BB levels to be a good indicator of patients that have difficulty recovering from MTBI, as indicated by neurocognitive functioning, symptom reporting, and return to pre-injury activities/work (200). Nonetheless, overall, CK-BB has not been found to have adequate sensitivity and specificity to be used as a reliable indicator of MTBI (141,197).

Myelin Basic Protein

Myelin basic protein (MBP) is a major protein component of myelin (144) and is found in growing oligodendroglial cells (the tissue consisting of glial cells that forms the myelin sheath). MBP is specific to myelin and appears to be bound to the cellular membrane on mainly central myelin. MBP can be released into CSF and serum/blood after white matter damage caused by brain injury or demyelinating diseases (141,144,145). The release of MBP is thought to occur over 2–3 days after injury and remains elevated up to 2 weeks (143,201,202).

Few studies have examined MBP for detecting TBI. In studies examining the relation between TBI severity and MBP levels, no association has been found between GCS scores and MBP levels following moderate-to-severe TBI in adults (180), or following mild-to-severe TBI in children (203). Berger and colleagues (203) found no differences in median MBP levels when comparing healthy controls with patients who had sustained either (a) isolated fractures or (b) mild-to-severe TBI. These authors did, however, find elevated MBP levels in those patients who had intracranial abnormalities versus those without. Nonetheless, the sensitivity of MBP levels to successfully identify those with intracranial abnormalities was low (44% true positives).

Thomas and colleagues (202) compared MBP values in healthy controls to patients following mild-to-severe TBI and found that those patients classified as having "good outcome" at 3 months postinjury (using the GOS) had acute MBP values that were comparable to healthy controls. However, those patients with "poor outcome" had higher acute MBP values compared to both groups. Other researchers have also found that elevated MBP levels are associated with worse GOS scores and higher mortality rates following moderate-to-severe TBI (180), and worse outcomes as measured by the GOS and GOS-E Pediatric following mild-to-severe TBI (201).

Glial Fibrillary Acidic Protein

Glial fibrillary acidic protein (GFAP) is a major protein in the cytoskeleton of astrocytes and is found only in astroglial cells

of the CNS (141,146). GFAP is released into extracellular space when cells are damaged following TBI (147,204–206). GFAP is released very soon after injury within the first few hours and begins to decrease after a few days (189). This protein is of particular interest because it is not found outside of the CNS (146) and thus may prove to be more promising marker than S100B (140,146).

To date, there are only a few studies that have examined GFAP following TBI. In a series of studies by Pelinka and colleagues (206,207) who examined patients following "CT-confirmed" TBI (presumably complicated MTBI or higher), higher GFAP levels were found in patients who died vs those who lived (206,207). GFAP appears to be unaffected by bodily injury, with normal GFAP levels reported in patients who sustained multiple bodily trauma without TBI (206). Normal GFAP levels have also been reported by other researchers in injured controls without TBI (208) and healthy controls (204). Pelinka and colleagues further reported that higher GFAP levels were also associated with increased intracranial and cerebral perfusion pressure, increased intracranial abnormality as rated by the Marshall classification, and poor outcome as measured by the GOS at 3 months postinjury (206,207). Vos and colleagues (189) also found that GFAP levels were associated with 6-month GOS scores following severe TBI.

Similarly, Nylen and colleagues (205) found that patients with an unfavorable outcome at 12 months following severe TBI (i.e., GOS < 4) had higher GFAP levels in the acute injury phase compared to those with a more favorable outcome (i.e., GOS > 3; moderate disability to good recovery).

Fatty Acid-Binding Proteins

Fatty acid-binding proteins (FABP) are small cytoplasmic, non-enzymatic proteins involved in the intracellular buffering and transport of long-chain fatty acids and regulation of gene expression (143,145). FABPs are expressed in multiple tissues including the liver, intestine, heart, muscles, and brain. FABPs are a family of 9 proteins named after the tissue in which it was first detected (209), such as heart type (H-FABP), brain type (B-FABP), and liver type (L-FABP). B-FABP is expressed exclusively in the brain (209), is released rapidly from damaged brain cells into circulation, and is thought to have a plasma half-life of 20 minutes (145).

To date, only 1 study has examined the use of FABPs to identify TBI in humans. However, this study has focused exclusively on detection of MTBI. Pelsers and colleagues (210) compared B-FABP, H-FABP, S100B, and NSE levels in 130 patients following MTBI and 14 patients undergoing electroconvulsive therapy (ECT) for depression. A sample of 92 healthy controls was used to establish reference values for elevated levels. In the MTBI group, elevated serum levels were highest for H-FABP (70%), followed by B-FABP (68%), NSE (51%), and S100B (45%). In the ECT group, elevated serum levels were low for all biomarkers (6.4% B-FABP, 16.6% H-FABP, 0.4% S100B, and NSE not reported). Pelser and colleagues concluded that B-FABP and H-FABP are more sensitive markers for MTBI than S100B or NSE. Further studies are recommended to help replicate these findings.

Cleaved Tau

Tau protein is a highly soluble microtubule-associated protein. In humans, Tau proteins constitute a family of 6 isoforms, and these proteins are found mainly in neurons (211–213). At the time of axonal injury (e.g., TBI, hypoxia), Tau is released from neurons in the CNS into extracellular space. After release, it is proteolytically cleaved at the N- and C-terminals and diffuses into the cerebrospinal fluid and plasma (213).

Researchers have found significantly increased C-Tau levels within the first 24 hours following severe TBI compared to various groups such as (*a*) healthy controls, (*b*) multiple sclerosis, (*c*) normal pressure hydrocephalus, (*d*) neurologic controls (e.g., headache, seizure, muscle weakness), and (*e*) nonneurological controls (e.g., psychiatric disorders, non-CNS trauma, renal or cardiovascular disease) (214,215). Elevated C-Tau levels have been found (214,216) to be predictive of outcome as defined by GOS scores at discharge (sen = 0.92, spec = 0.94) and 12 months postinjury (sen = 0.83, spec = 0.69); however, some researchers have failed to establish this relation using 6-month GOS scores (217). Elevated C-Tau levels have also been found to be associated with mortality (216,217), elevated intracranial pressure in the acute recovery phase (214), intracranial abnormalities on day-of-injury CT scan (213), and worse outcome defined by successful/unsuccessful discharged to the patients' home environment (217).

The relation between C-Tau levels and MTBI is less well established. Kavalci and colleagues (212) examined 88 patients following MTBI who were divided into 2 groups (CT-positive and CT-negative). Increased C-Tau was found in both groups with no differences reported between the groups. When the groups were combined, a negative correlation was found between C-Tau and GCS scores. Bazarian and colleagues (218) examined 35 patients following MTBI most of whom had no intracranial abnormalities on CT scan. There was no statistically significant correlation between C-Tau levels obtained acutely and self-reported postconcussion symptoms 3 months postinjury (218). C-Tau was a poor predictor of postconcussion symptoms (sen = 0.44, spec = 0.71, PPP = 0.64, NPP = 0.53). Of note, S100B was also not useful in this regard (sen = 0.56, spec = 0.36, PPP = 0.44, NPP = 0.33). Bulut and colleagues (219) compared 20 healthy controls to 60 patients following MTBI (25% abnormal CT). C-Tau levels were slightly higher in the MTBI group compared to controls, but this was not statistically significant. C-Tau levels did not differ between CT positive and CT negative, nor were they associated with 6 month postconcussion symptoms. There was, however, higher C-Tau levels found in patients classified as high risk for poor outcome (e.g., symptomatic, low GCS, longer loss of consciousness [LOC]/PTA, seizures) versus low risk (e.g., high GCS, no LOC/PTA, asymptomatic).

Neuroproteomics

In the past decade, a new field of biomarker technology has developed—*neuroproteomics*. Neuroproteomics is a sub-field of proteomics that is dedicated to studying the protein complexes of organs, tissues, and cells that make up the nervous system (220). The term *proteomics* refers to the study of the protein-equivalent of a genome—the proteome. There are several techniques currently available for neuroproteomic studies. However, two of the major approaches currently used in TBI biomarker research include: (*a*) protein separation mass spectrometry (MS/MS), and (*b*) high-throughput (HTP) antibody-based microarray or panel. For a comprehensive discussion of these techniques, please see (220,221).

One of the main benefits of the neuroproteomic approach is that the available technology enables the researcher to examine a large array of proteins to determine which protein might be useful (221). Using this approach, researchers have the capability of identifying unique protein biomarkers from tissues or biofluids obtained from humans or animals (222). Much of the work to date has focused on the discovery of new biomarkers undertaken largely in animals (e.g., 223–230), although human studies are increasing (e.g., 231–235). To date, a large number of candidate markers for TBI have been identified using these methods. Although researchers are working toward validating these candidate TBI markers, few studies have examined their usefulness in a clinical setting. Two biomarker markers have received some attention in this regard: UCH-L1 and αII-spectrin breakdown product.

UCH-L1 is present in almost all neurons and averages 1%–5% of total soluble brain protein (236,237). There are 3 enzymes in the UCH family: UCH-L1, UCH-L2, and UCH-L3. However, only UCH-L1 is highly enriched in the CNS (237). The primary role of these enzymes is to add or remove ubiquitin from proteins that are destined for metabolism (via the ATP-dependent proteasome pathway) (237). As such, UCH-L1 plays an important role in the removal of excessive, oxidized, or misfolded proteins (237). In a series of 3 studies by the same research group (236–238), patients who sustained a severe TBI had significantly elevated UCH-L1 compared to uninjured controls (236–238). Higher UCH-L1 levels were associated with a variety of clinical outcomes following severe TBI.

Alpha II-Spectrin Breakdown Products (αII-SBDP) are part of the cytoskeleton and are enriched in the brain. Activation of calpain or caspase, as a consequence of TBI, has been shown to cleave αII-spectrin at specific sites to generate breakdown products (221). Cleavage caused by calpain and caspase generates 4 alpha II- SBDP: 150 kDa (SBDP150), 145 kDa (SBDP145), 149 kDa (SBDP149), and 120 kDa (SBDP120) (221). Researchers (239–243) have found significantly higher levels on all SBDPs following severe TBI (i.e., SBDP280, SBDP120, SBDP150, and SBDP145) compared to controls (although there are some exceptions to this [239]), and these biomarkers have correlated with several clinical outcomes.

Most of the proof of concept work in neuroproteomics is being done in patients with severe neurotrauma. Over time, it will be extended to patients who have sustained MTBIs. At the time of writing this chapter, some work in the area of MTBI is underway.

NEUROPSYCHOLOGICAL OUTCOME

An MTBI can result in severe symptoms and problems for some people during the first 72 hours following injury. These acute symptoms and problems have been more closely and extensively examined in sports. Athletes who experience a sport-related concussion can have dramatically reduced cognitive functioning, serious balance problems, and widespread physical and neurobehavioral symptoms (e.g., headaches, dizziness, nausea, light and noise sensitivity, fatigue, hypersomnia/insomnia, irritability, and emotional dysregulation). In a meta-analysis, Broglio and Puetz reported that the acute adverse effect of sport-related concussion on objectively-measured cognition is large (Hedge's $g = -0.81$), and the adverse effect on balance ($g = -2.56$) and subjective symptoms ($g = -3.31$) are very large (244). By extension, similar symptoms and problems are likely present in adults who sustain MTBIs in daily life.

The neurocognitive outcome from uncomplicated MTBI is well documented in the literature. Injured athletes and trauma patients perform poorly on neuropsychological tests in the initial days (245–250) and up to the first month following the injury (247,251–254). Because of natural recovery, neurocognitive deficits typically are not seen in athletes after 1–3 weeks (15,245–248,255) and in trauma patients after 1–3 months (253,256,257) in prospective group studies. This has been illustrated repeatedly in reviews and meta-analyses (3,5,7,258–261).

Figure 29-1 was derived from meta-analytic reviews of the literature. It illustrates the effect of MTBI on cognitive functioning over the course of time. The adverse effects of injury on cognition are pronounced acutely and disappear by 3 months. Figure 29-2, also derived from meta-analytical reviews, illustrates the effect of MTBI on cognition relative to mental health and substance abuse problems.

This does not mean, of course, that all patients who sustain an MTBI experience a full and swift recovery of their cognitive functioning. It is possible, although this has not been demonstrated definitively and scientifically, that a small minority of people who sustain MTBIs, especially complicated MTBIs, may have some degree of permanent brain damage that is directly causing some degree of permanent impairment in cognition. However, the problem with establishing brain injury as the sole or primary cause of cognitive diminishment long after injury in any given patient is that (a) the literature suggests that this is a low prevalence condition; (b) it is well-established in medicine that low prevalence conditions can be difficult to identify accurately (they are

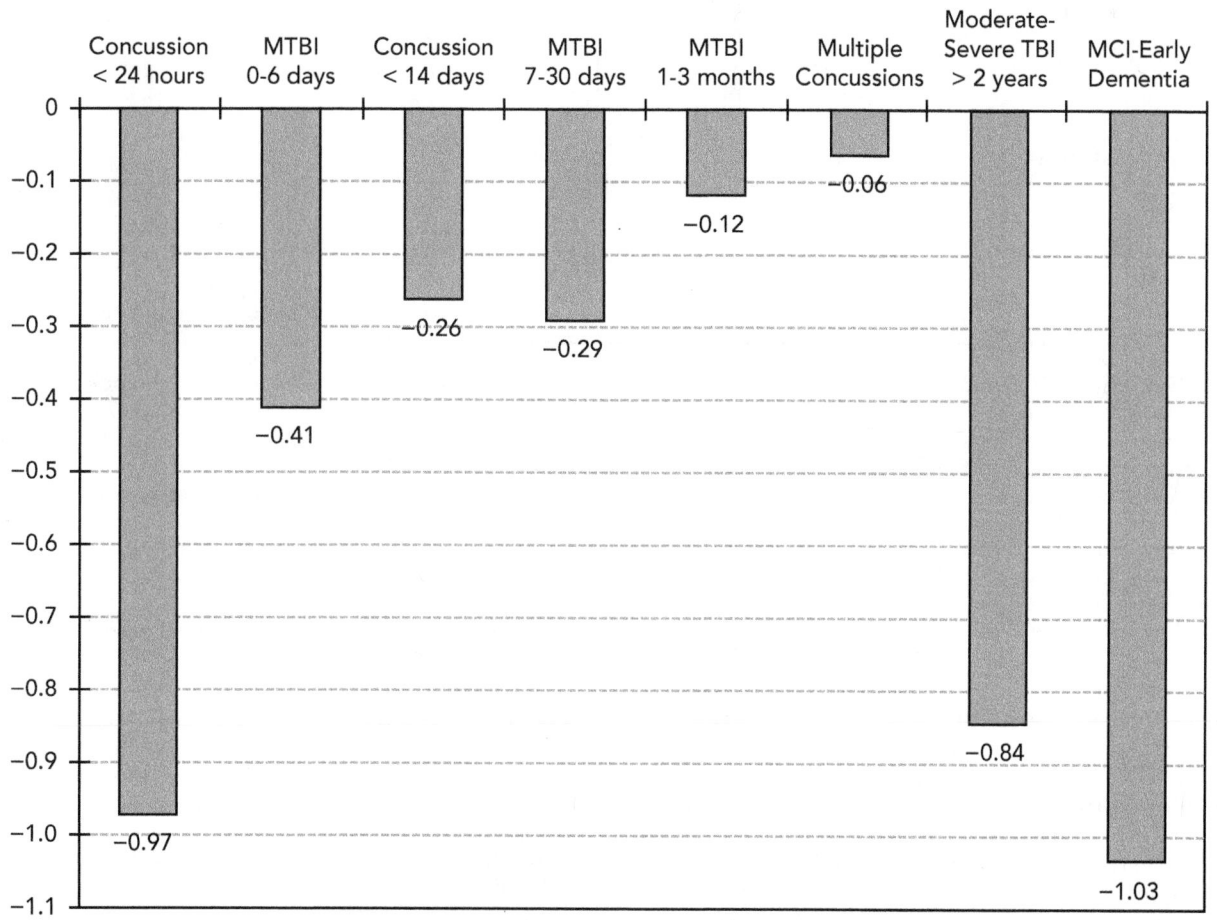

FIGURE 29-1 Meta-analytic effect sizes: adverse effects on neuropsychological functioning. Effect sizes typically are expressed in pooled, weighted standard deviation units. However, across studies, there are some minor variations in the methods of calculation. For this figure, the overall effect on cognitive or neuropsychological functioning is reported. Effect sizes < 0.3 should be considered very small and difficult to detect in individual patients because the patient and control groups largely overlap. Sport-related concussion < 24 hours from Belanger and Vanderploeg (3); concussion < 14 days from Broglio and Puetz (244); MTBI 0–6 days, 7–30 days, 1–3 months, moderate–severe > 2 years, all in Schretlen and Shapiro (7); multiple concussions (513); and mild cognitive impairment (MCI) or early dementia based on memory testing (514). Reprinted from Iverson GL. Evidence-based neuropsychological assessment in sport-related concussion. In: Webbe FM, ed, *Handbook of Sport Neuropsychology.* New York, NY: Springer Publishing Company; 2011:131-154.

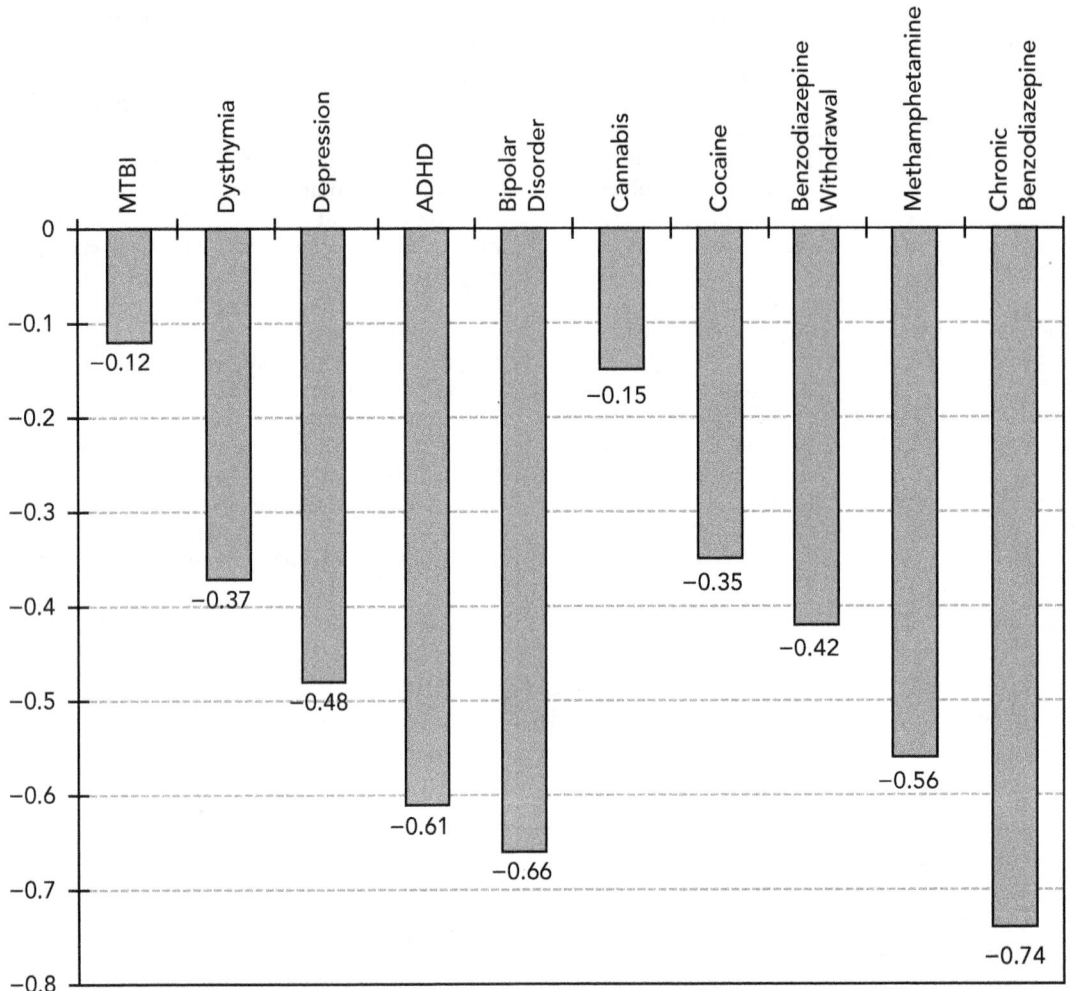

FIGURE 29-2 Effects of mild traumatic brain injury, psychiatric conditions, and substance use on neuropsychological functioning. MTBI (516), 11 studies, $N = 314$ and MTBI, $N = 308$ controls; dysthymia, depression, and bipolar disorder (517), 3 comparisons for dysthymia, 97 comparisons for depression, and 15 comparisons for bipolar disorder; ADHD (518), based on full scale IQ, 123 studies; cannabis (519), long-term regular use, 11 studies, $N = 623$ users, $N = 409$ nonuser or minimal users; cocaine (520) dependence/abuse (including some concurrent alcohol abuse), 15 studies, $N = 481$ users, $N = 586$ healthy normal controls, median (not mean) effect size reported; benzodiazepine withdrawal (521), 10 studies, long-term follow-up, 44 comparisons; chronic benzodiazepine use (522), 13 studies, $N = 384$, 61 comparisons. Adapted from Iverson GL, Lange RT. Mild traumatic brain injury. In: Schoenberg MR, Scott JG, eds, *The Black Book of Neuropsychology: A Syndrome Based Approach.* New York, NY: Springer; 2011:697–719 with kind permission from Springer+Business Media B.V.

especially prone to false positives); (*c*) numerous preexisting and comorbid developmental conditions (e.g., learning disabilities or ADHD), physical conditions, medical problems, and emotional problems are associated with cognitive problems; and (*d*) neuropsychological test results can be influenced by situational and motivational factors. As such, the identification and quantification of cognitive problems, and attributing specific causes for these problems, usually relies heavily on clinical judgment.

EARLY INTERVENTION

Most early intervention programs are designed to provide education and reassurance with the goal of helping patients better manage symptoms and more effectively return to their normal lifestyle. Several intervention protocols following

MTBI have been described in the literature (e.g., 262–264). Researchers initially reported that simple intervention programs applied within the first 3 weeks postinjury can reduce the total number and frequency of postconcussion symptoms (265) and increase return to work rates (266). The reader interested in this topic should obtain 2 systematic reviews of this literature (267,268).

The content of early intervention programs varies, ranging from, at minimum, the provision of an educational brochure containing information regarding the effects of MTBI (e.g., 269) to a more comprehensive intervention program that couples educational material with various forms of treatment (e.g., access to a multidisciplinary outpatient brain injury program; e.g., 270) and/or assessment (e.g., neuropsychological) (e.g., 271). Providing educational information is a standard component in most studies. Although the content of the educational sessions varies, these sessions typically provide information regarding common symptoms, likely time course of recovery, reassurance of recovery, and suggested coping strategies following MTBI (e.g., 272–275). The method of dissemination ranges from the distribution of written information alone (e.g., 274) to providing written educational material and a discussion of its contents with an occupational therapist or neuropsychologist (e.g., 270). Telephone delivery of the information has been shown to be effective (276).

Patients participating in intervention programs consisting of educational materials plus various additional treatments and/or assessments (e.g., neuropsychological testing, meeting with a therapist, reassurance, access to a multidisciplinary team) report fewer postconcussion symptoms at 3 months postinjury (271,274) and at 6 months postinjury (265, 272,275) compared to patients who received standard hospital treatment. However, some researchers have reported that early intervention programs using educational material alone and educational material plus access to a specialist outpatient brain injury team, did not result in reduced self-reported post-concussive symptoms in children 3 months following injury (269) and adults 6 months following injury (277). Although most research in this area points toward the usefulness of early intervention programs, our understanding of the *type* of intervention required is limited. The intervention programs evaluated in the literature to date vary considerably, ranging from economical programs (e.g., distribution of written educational materials) to much more expensive programs (e.g., multidisciplinary brain injury programs). Few studies have attempted to compare different intervention programs. In 1 of the first studies of this kind, Alves, Macciocchi and Barth (278) compared the outcome of patients provided with standard hospital treatment to 2 different intervention programs provided within the first week postinjury: (*a*) education only and (*b*) education and reassurance. They concluded that intervention assignment was not associated with the number or duration of self-reported postconcussive symptoms at 3, 6, or 12 months postinjury (although when missing data were considered differently in the analyses, education, and reassurance was associated with decreased risk of chronic symptom reporting).

Paniak and colleagues compared patients assigned to 2 different treatment methods: (*a*) single session (i.e., a brief, educational, and reassurance-oriented session) and (*b*) treatment as needed (i.e., including education, reassurance, psychological, personality, and neuropsychological testing and feedback, consultation with physical therapist, and access to multidisciplinary brain injury treatment program as needed). They concluded that the brief, educational and reassurance-oriented intervention was as effective as the more comprehensive and expensive treatment model because there was no difference between the two interventions in self-reported postconcussive symptoms at 3 months and 12 months postinjury (270,273).

The research focusing on early intervention is promising. The literature suggests that early intervention can be useful for reducing the number of individuals who experience long-term symptoms. Early intervention programs need not consist of complex multidisciplinary brain injury treatment programs, but may consist of a simple education session provided soon after injury. This is a conclusion

echoed by Borg et al. (279) in their review of interventions for people with MTBIs. The effective use of simple education-oriented programs is supported in the literature (e.g., 271,274). However, clinicians working in early intervention programs know that some people continue to report symptoms despite education, reassurance, and gradual resumption of activities. Early intervention programs certainly have limitations (267,268). Patients with significant anxiety problems, or those who swiftly develop depression, might be at risk for slower return to work and persistent symptoms. Effective treatments for people who are slow to recover or who report significant symptoms long after injury are greatly needed. Treatments for these people are discussed in detail in Chapter 30.

RETURN TO WORK

There is tremendous variability in how quickly people return to work following an MTBI, but most do so within the first month. Some, however, suffer persistent symptoms for a prolonged period which interferes with their return to work (280). For many individuals, the inability to return to work can result in economic, social, family, and interpersonal problems (281–283) (see Chapter 80).

The risk factors for delayed return to work are diverse, complex, and not well understood (284). Some researchers have reported that injury severity, as measured by duration of PTA, duration of LOC, and/or GCS scores, is associated with the time in which individuals return to pre-injury employment following TBI (e.g., 285,286–288). However, other studies have failed to support the relation between injury severity and postinjury employment status (e.g., 289–293). In general, within the spectrum of MTBI, those individuals with milder injuries (e.g., GCS = 15; no LOC) tend to have a higher return to work rate compared to those with more serious injuries (e.g., GCS = 13–14; with LOC) (e.g., 168,294,295).

The literature regarding return to work following MTBI is summarized in Table 29-2. Return to work rates range from (*a*) 22% to 84% in the first week, (*b*) 25% to 99% within the first month, (*b*) 48% to 100% 3 to 6 months postinjury, and (*c*) 46% to 100% 1 year postinjury. The variability in return to work rates may in large part be caused by methodological differences between studies. The most notable of these include (*a*) differences in definitions of return to work (e.g., return to preinjury employment vs return to meaningful activity), (*b*) variations in the definition of MTBI (e.g., inclusion of GCS = 15 only vs GCS = 13–15), (*c*) variations in the inclusion and exclusion of individuals who were unemployed or performing domestic duties prior to injury, and (*d*) the failure of some studies to take into account preinjury employment status (e.g., return to full-time vs part-time vs unemployed). For a comprehensive discussion regarding return to work following TBI, the interested reader is referred to Chapter 81.

Under most circumstances, good recovery and return to work should be anticipated following an MTBI. Health care providers should work with injured adults to address the difficulties they face with particular symptoms while they resume their normal daily activities (e.g., work or school). Unfortunately, some trauma patients transition from acute postconcussion symptoms and problems into a mild

TABLE 29-2 Summary of Return to Work Rates in the Research Literature

FIRST AUTHOR	SETTING	N	COUNTRY	TIME POSTINJURY	RTW	MTBI DEFINITION	RTW DEFINITION	PREINJURY WORK STATUS: INCLUSION/EXCLUSION CRITERIA	TYPE OF STUDY AND REFERRALS
Stranjalis (2004)	HTC	100	Greece	1 week	84.0%	GCS = 15 PTA < 15 mins LOC < 15 mins	Return to work or activities	Included = students, homemakers, retired, and unemployed.	Consecutive Prospective[a]
Wrightson (1981)	HTC	66	New Zealand	1 week	81.8%[b]	Described as "minor HI" (however, 2 patients had PTA 18–36 hours). No GCS or LOC data reported.	Return to work that is, no longer had to take days off work.	All patients in regular employment at the time of injury	Consecutive Prospective
Sadowski-Cron (2006)	HTC	176	Switzerland	1 week	22.0%	GCS = 14–15	Return to previous work or activities	No apparent exclusions based on work status	Consecutive Prospective Longitudinal
Wrightson (1981)	HTC	66	New Zealand	2 weeks	92.4%[b]	Described as minor HI (however, 2 patients had PTA 18–36 hours). No GCS or LOC data reported.	Return to work that is, no longer had to take days off work.	All patients in regular employment at the time of injury	Consecutive Prospective
Haboubi (2001)	RC	391	United Kingdom	2 weeks	44.0%	GCS = 13–15	Return to regular employment	Included those only in regular employment	Consecutive Retrospective
Dikmen (1994)	LITC	213	United States	1 month	25.0%	GCS = 13–15	Return to work irrespective of length of that employment	Excluded = students, homemakers, and retired; included = workers[c] (employed and unemployed).	Consecutive Prospective Longitudinal
Wrightson (1981)	HTC	66	New Zealand	1 month	99.0%[b]	Described as minor HI (however, 2 patients had PTA 18–36 hours). No GCS or LOC data reported.	Return to work that is, no longer had to take days off work.	All patients in regular employment at the time of injury	Consecutive Prospective
van der Naalt (1999)	HTC	43	Netherlands	1 month	39.0%	GCS = 13–14	Resumption of previous activities either partially or completely.	None	Consecutive Prospective
Stranjalis (2004)	HTC	100	Greece	1 month	99.0%	GCS = 15 PTA < 15 mins LOC < 15 mins	Return to work or activities	Included = students, homemakers, retired, and unemployed.	Consecutive Prospective
Haboubi (2001)	RC	391	United Kingdom	6 weeks	88.0%	GCS = 13–15	Return to regular employment	Included those only in regular employment	Consecutive Retrospective

Study	Setting	N	Country	Follow-up	%	Injury severity criteria	Outcome definition	Inclusion/exclusion	Design
van der Naalt (1999)	HTC	43	Netherlands	3 months	67.0%	GCS = 13–14	Resumption of previous activities either partially or completely.	None	Consecutive Prospective
Drake (2000)	NMC	121	United States	3 months	53.7%	Described as "MTBI patients" but no specific criteria provided; LOC (M = 1.4 mins, SD = 2.6 mins); PTA (M = 3 hours, SD = 1.3 hours).	Return to full military duty defined by US Navy guidelines[d]	Included if in preinjury active duty military status	Consecutive Prospective
Drake (2000)	NMC	121	United States	3 months	100.0%	Described as "MTBI patients" but no specific criteria provided; LOC (M = 1.4 mins, SD = 2.6 mins); PTA (M = 3 hours, SD = 1.3 hours).	Return to full or limited military duty defined by US Navy guidelines[d]	Included if in preinjury active duty military status	Consecutive Prospective
Sigurdardottir (2009)	LITC	40	Norway	3 months	48.0%	GCS = 13–15	Return to full-time work or study (≥ 30 hour/week)	No apparent exclusions based on work status	Consecutive Prospective Longitudinal
Sigurdardottir (2009)	LITC	40	Norway	3 months	12.0%	GCS = 13–15	Return to part-time work or study (< 30 hour/week)	No apparent exclusions based on work status	Consecutive Prospective Longitudinal
McCullaugh (2001)	TTC	20	Canada	5 months	37.5%	LOC < 20 mins PTA < 24 hours GCS = 13–14	Return to previous work or studies	Excluded = retired, unemployed because of non-TBI injury; included = employed, students, homemaker.	Consecutive Prospective
McCullaugh (2001)	TTC	37	Canada	5 months	60.0%	LOC < 20 mins PTA < 24 hours GCS = 15	Return to previous work or studies	Excluded = retired, unemployed because of non-TBI injury; included = employed, students, homemaker.	Consecutive Prospective
Kraus (2005)	HTC	201	United States	6 months	82.6%[e]	LOC < 30 mins GCS 13–15 PTA < 24 hours	No change in employment status postinjury	Preinjury work status not used to include/exclude patients.	Consecutive Prospective
Dikmen (1994)	LITC	213	United States	6 months	63.0%	GCS = 13–15	Return to work irrespective of length of that employment	Excluded = students, homemakers, and retired; included = workers[c] (employed and unemployed).	Consecutive Prospective Longitudinal

(Continued)

TABLE 29-2 Summary of Return to Work Rates in the Research Literature *(Continued)*

FIRST AUTHOR	SETTING	N	COUNTRY	TIME POSTINJURY	RTW	MTBI DEFINITION	RTW DEFINITION	PREINJURY WORK STATUS: INCLUSION/EXCLUSION CRITERIA	TYPE OF STUDY AND REFERRALS
van der Naalt (1999)	HTC	43	Netherlands	6 months	97.0%	GCS = 13–14	Resumption of previous activities either partially or completely.	None	Consecutive Prospective
Metting (2009)	HTC	76	Netherlands	6 months	78.7%	GCS = 13–15, PTA present	Return to previous work or studies	No apparent exclusions based on work status	Consecutive Prospective Selected sample (normal CT)
Metting (2009)	HTC	76	Netherlands	6 months	17.3%	GCS = 13–15, PTA present	Return to previous work or study but with lower demands or part-time	No apparent exclusions based on work status	Consecutive Prospective Selected sample (normal CT)
Metting (2009)	HTC	76	Netherlands	6 months	1.3%	GCS = 13–15, PTA present	Return to different work on significantly lower level	No apparent exclusions based on work status	Consecutive Prospective Selected sample (normal CT)
Stulemeijer (2008)	HTC	201	Netherlands	6 months	76.0%	GCS = 13–15, with or without LOC ≤ 30 mins, with or without PTA	Return to work (no longer on sick leave or no change in working status to partial or lower level employment)	No apparent exclusions based on work status	Consecutive Prospective
Benedictus (2010)	LITC	208	Netherlands	6 months	72.0%	GCS = 13–15	Return to previous work or studies	No apparent exclusions based on work status	Consecutive Prospective
Benedictus (2010)	LITC	208	Netherlands	6 months	22.0%	GCS = 13–15	Return to previous work or study but with lower demands or part-time	No apparent exclusions based on work status	Consecutive Prospective
Benedictus (2010)	LITC	208	Netherlands	6 months	4.0%	GCS = 13–15	Return to different work on significantly lower level	No apparent exclusions based on work status	Consecutive Prospective
Friedland (2001)	TTC	64	Canada	6–9 months	44.0%	Initial GCS ≥ 13 PTA ≤ 24 hours LOC ≤ 30 mins	Return to premorbid level or modified level.	Included all patients regardless of employment status.	Consecutive Prospective
Ruffolo (1999)	TTC	63	Canada	6–9 months	42.0%[f]	GCS and LOC criteria used LOC < 60 mins GCS scores obtained but not reported.	Return to premorbid employment under usual or modified[g] conditions (paid or unpaid).	All working before the accident in paid or unpaid employment (e.g., students, volunteers, homemaker)	Consecutive Prospective

Author (year)	Group	N	Country	Follow-up	%	Criteria	Outcome definition	Exclusions/Inclusions	Study design
van der Naalt (1999)	HTC	43	Netherlands	12 months	100.0%	GCS = 13–14	Resumption of previous activities either partially or completely.	None	Consecutive Prospective
Dikmen (1994)	LITC	213	United States	12 months	80.0%	GCS = 13–15	Return to work irrespective of length of that employment	Excluded = students, homemakers, and retired; included = workers[c] (employed and unemployed)	Consecutive Prospective Longitudinal
Sadowski-Cron (2006)	HTC	176	Switzerland	12 months	100.0%	GCS = 14–15	Return to previous work or activities	No apparent exclusions based on work status	Consecutive Prospective Longitudinal
Sigurdardottir (2009)	LITC	40	Norway	12 months	70.0%	GCS = 13–15	Return to full-time work/study (≥ 30 hour/week)	No apparent exclusions based on work status	Consecutive Prospective Longitudinal
Sigurdardottir (2009)	LITC	40	Norway	12 months	15.0%	GCS = 13–15	Return to part-time work/study (< 30 hour/week)	No apparent exclusions based on work status	Consecutive Prospective Longitudinal
Doctor (2005)	HTC, LITC	84	United States	12 months	46.4%	GCS = 13–15	Return to work (currently or within 7 days of assessment)	All patients in regular employment at the time of injury	Consecutive Prospective Longitudinal
Dawson (2004)	TTC	38	Canada	1 year	78.9%	GCS = 13–15	Return to productivity (i.e., paid employment and/or school)	Not described	Consecutive Prospective
van der Naalt (1999)	HTC	43	Netherlands	1 year	79.0%	GCS = 13–14	Resumed previous activities completely	None	Consecutive Prospective
Dikmen (1994)	LITC	213	United States	2 years	83.0%	GCS = 13–15	Return to work irrespective of length of that employment	Excluded = students, homemakers, and retired; included = workers[c] (employed and unemployed)	Consecutive Prospective Longitudinal
Dawson (2004)	TTC	24	Canada	4 years	79.2%	GCS = 13–15	Return to productivity (i.e., paid employment and/or school)	Not described	Consecutive Prospective
Vanderploeg (2003)	USVV	373	United States	8 years	75.1%	Described as MTBI with no reported LOC—no specific criteria presented.	Return to full-time employment	Vietnam veterans who (a) had at least 4 months of active duty, (b) served only 1 tour of duty, (c) achieved a military occupation subspecialty other than "trainee" of "duty soldier."	Consecutive Retrospective

(Continued)

449

TABLE 29-2 Summary of Return to Work Rates in the Research Literature (*Continued*)

FIRST AUTHOR	SETTING	N	COUNTRY	TIME POSTINJURY	RTW	MTBI DEFINITION	RTW DEFINITION	PREINJURY WORK STATUS: INCLUSION/EXCLUSION CRITERIA	TYPE OF STUDY AND REFERRALS
Vanderploeg (2003)	USVV	253	United States	8 years	81.8%	Described as MTBI + reported LOC—no specific criteria presented.	Return to full-time employment	Vietnam veterans who (a) had at least 4 months of active duty, (b) served only 1 tour of duty, (c) achieved a military occupation subspecialty other than "trainee" of "duty soldier."	Retrospective Random selected sample
Asikainen (1996)	HOC	118	Finland	12 years	61.9%	GCS = 13–15	Return to independent work only	No apparent exclusions based on work status	Retrospective Selected sample (patients with brain injury and postinjury problems in education and employment)
Asikainen (1996)	HOC	118	Finland	12 years	72.9%	GCS = 13–15	Return to independent work or subsidized employment or education continuing	No apparent exclusions based on work status	Retrospective Selected sample (patients with brain injury and postinjury problems in education and employment)

Abbreviations: CT, computed tomography; GCS, Glasgow Coma Scale; HI, head injury; HOC, hospital outpatient clinic; HTC, hospital trauma center; LITC, Level 1 trauma center; LOC, loss of consciousness; M, Mean; MTBI, mild traumatic brain injury; NMC, US Navel medical center; PTA, Posttraumatic amnesia; RC, Rehabilitation clinic; RTW, return to work; SD, Standard Deviation; TTC, Tertiary trauma center; USVV, US Vietnam veterans.

a Consecutive = consecutive referrals; Retrospective/Prospective = retrospective/prospective study design.

b A follow-up interview was obtained in 63 of the 66 patients 90 days postinjury regarding their condition on returning to work. Of these patients, 60% reported experiencing symptoms when they first returned to work and 46% reported that they were unable to do their work as well as usual.

c Workers were defined as individuals who defined themselves as "workers" regardless of whether they were employed or unemployed at the time of injury.

d Limited duty is a duty status within the military for individuals with ongoing medical problems; it has fewer responsibilities, some limitations, and decreased performance standards. Individuals are placed on limited duty for periods of 6 months, with the expectation of recovery and eventual return to full duty status (p. 1,106).

e It is not entirely clear whether this percentage includes individuals who were employed preinjury or also includes individuals who were retired, students, and unemployed.

f Of these patients, 12% returned to premorbid level of work and 30% returned to modified employment.

g Modified conditions was defined as "working shorter hours, performing lighter work, performing part of the job at home, or trading difficult tasks with other workers" (p. 393).

Data were derived from Asikainen, Kaste, Sarna (495); Benedictus, Spikman, van der Naalt (496); Dawson, Levine, Schwartz, Stuss (497); Dikmen, Temkin, Machamer, Holubkov, Fraser, Winn (281); Doctor, Castro, Temkin, Fraser, Machamer, Dikmen (498); Drake, Gray, Yoder, Pramuka, Llewellyn (499); Friedland, Dawson (500); Guerin, Kennepohl, Leveille, Dominique, McKerral (501); Haboubi, Long, Koshy, Ward (502); Kraus, Schaffer, Ayers, Stenehjem, Shen, Afifi (282); McCullagh, Oucherlony, Protzner, Blair, Feinstein (294); Metting, Rodiger, Stewart, Oudkerk, De Keyser, van der Naalt (503); Ruffolo, Friedland, Dawson, Colantonio, Lindsay (504); Sadowski-Cron, Schneider, Senn, Radanov, Ballinari, Zimmermann (505); Sigurdardottir, Andelic, Roe, Schanke (506); Stranjalis, Korfias, Papapetrou, et al (168); Stulemeijer, van der Werf, Borm, Vos (507); Vanderploeg, Curtiss, Duchnick, Luis (295); van der Naalt, van Zomeren, Sluiter, Minderhoud (508); Wrightson, Gronwall (283) with permission.

depression (or major depressive episode). Mental health problems can have an adverse effect on a person's ability to be effective in the workplace.

DEPRESSION

Depression following MTBI defies parsimonious explanation. In clinical psychiatry, depression is believed to arise from the cumulative impact (296–298) of genetics (299–302), adverse events in childhood (303–306), and ongoing life stressors (307–310). In neurology and neuropsychiatry, there is concern that TBIs alter brain physiology, and/or create a psychological burden, precipitating the development of depression. In fact, it is well established in the literature that people who sustain a TBI are at increased risk for developing depression (311,312), with prevalence rates varying widely (i.e., from 11% to 77%) (e.g., 313–315) (see Chapter 62). Rates of depression in the first 3 months following MTBI have ranged from 12% to 44% (316–322). A review of prevalence studies relating to depression in people following MTBI is presented in Table 29-3.

It is important to appreciate that people who suffer TBIs have higher rates of *preinjury* psychiatric disorders (314, 323–326), such as depression and substance abuse. It is established that the number of prior episodes of depression is predictive of the likelihood of developing a future episode of depression. For example, at least 60% of people who have a single episode of major depressive disorder will likely have a second episode, 70% of those who have had 2 prior episodes will likely have a third, and 90% of those who have had 3 prior episodes will likely have a fourth (*DSM-IV-TR*; p. 372; under Course; APA) (327). Therefore, patients with a history of depression, especially those with multiple prior episodes, should be at increased risk for developing depression following brain injury, bodily injury, or significant life stress. Moreover, they would be at increased risk for developing depression, at some point postinjury, yet for reasons unrelated to the injury.

It is difficult to study depression following TBI because there is some overlap in the symptoms of depression and that of moderate-to-severe brain injury (e.g., concentration problems, memory problems, irritability, amotivation/apathy, and fatigue), and there is dramatic overlap between the symptoms of depression and the "postconcussion syndrome" (328,329). Moreover, certain conditions that frequently occur in patients with MTBIs are also associated with comorbid depression (in patients without a history of MTBI). That is, people who sustain MTBIs often experience psychological traumas (e.g., in assaults or car crashes) or other bodily injuries that could lead to post-traumatic stress disorder (PTSD), other anxiety problems, chronic pain, or sleep disturbance. Anxiety problems (especially PTSD [330–333]), chronic pain (334–338), and chronic insomnia (339) are associated with depression. Chronic headaches are also associated with depression (340–343). Chronic pain can, essentially, mimic a postconcussion syndrome (344–350).

There are converging lines of evidence that provide the theoretical underpinnings for trauma-related neurobiological factors being causally related to the onset of depression. First, contusions to the frontal lobes or damage to frontal-subcortical pathways could precipitate depression. Second, microstructural disintegrative changes to white matter tracts (or more purely functional cellular changes) in the anterior

regions of the brain could explain why Chen and colleagues (351) found that concussed athletes with symptoms of depression appeared to have fMRI findings similar to what has been reported by biological psychiatry researchers in the depression literature. Finally, it is theoretically plausible that when the injured brain is recovering from a complex neurometabolic crisis, serotonin and dopamine (352) transmitter systems, especially in vulnerable individuals (e.g., genetics, adverse childhood events, and life stress), could become dysregulated and thus be a target for treatment (353–355).

Without question, depression is a heterogeneous condition. It is theoretically plausible that depression can arise (*a*) directly or indirectly from the neurobiological consequences of the brain injury, (*b*) as a psychological reaction to deficits and problems associated with having a brain injury, (*c*) as a biopsychosocial reaction to the stress of co-occurring bodily injuries and associated lifestyle changes, and/or (*d*) from a combination of these factors. Depression can also arise *de novo*, incidentally, sometime postinjury—such as in response to life stressors. It can also arise as part of a preexisting chronic relapsing and remitting condition.

Clearly, no simple theory relating to the etiology of depression following TBI will have explanatory value. From a syndromal perspective, depression is too heterogeneous. From an etiological perspective, the manifestation of depression likely represents the cumulative effect of multiple variables, not all of which are operative in any given case, such as genetics, adverse life events in childhood, mental health history, current life stress, activity restrictions and reduced exposure to positive reinforcement in daily life, general medical problems, chronic pain, insomnia, chronic headaches, a co-occurring anxiety disorder (e.g., PTSD), substance abuse, and macroscopic or microstructural damage to the brain. A theoretical model for the development of depression following MTBI is presented in Figure 29-3.

When patients report symptoms and problems many months after an injury, differential treatment often flows from differential diagnosis. Given the clear overlap between the symptoms of depression and postconcussion syndrome, some researchers have recommended treatment with antidepressants (e.g., 320,356–358) or cognitive behavior therapy (e.g., 272,359). Medications and psychotherapy would be an obvious choice, of course, if depression is simply mimicking the postconcussion syndrome. Those recommending cognitive behavior therapy have set forth a treatment protocol (360,361) that is based on CBT principles but is tailored toward the patients with chronic symptoms and belief systems relating to symptoms and brain damage (see Chapter 63).

POSTTRAUMATIC STRESS DISORDER

PTSD (327) occurs in some people who *experience intense fear, helplessness, or horror* during or immediately after experiencing or witnessing a traumatic event (except when "delayed"). Symptom onset typically occurs in the first few days (in fact the first 24 hours) in most people. The traumatic event is *persistently reexperienced* through (*a*) intrusive and distressing recollections of the event including visual images, thoughts, or perceptions; (*b*) distressing dreams (nightmares); (*c*) acting or feeling as if the traumatic event was happening again (e.g., dissociative flashbacks); (*d*) intense psychological distress when exposed to things (e.g., thoughts

TABLE 29-3 Summary of Depression Prevalence Rates in Mild Traumatic Brain Injury

FIRST AUTHOR	N	COUNTRY	POSTINJURY INTERVAL	SETTING	RATE OF DEPRESSION	MTBI DEFINITION	DEPRESSION DEFINITION	TYPE OF STUDY OR REFERRALS
Goldstein (2001)	18	United States	2 months	Acute care neurosurgery services affiliated with university hospitals	33.0%	GCS 13–15 LOC < 20 mins Normal CT or MRI	GDS > 10	Prospective Consecutive
Mooney (2001)	80	United States	Median = 25.5 weeks	Rehabilitation program, university hospital	44.0%	ACRM criteria	DSM-IV criteria	Prospective Selected sample (individuals who failed to recover as expected 3 months postinjury)
Levin (2005)	129	United States	3 months	Level I trauma center	11.6%	GCS 13–15	SCID: DSM-IV	Prospective Consecutive
McCauley (2001)	95	United States	3 months	Level I trauma center	21.4%	GCS 13–15 LOC < 20 mins Normal CT	DSM-IV Major depressive disorder criteria	Prospective Consecutive
Levin (2001)	60	United States	3 months	Level I trauma center	18.3%	GCS 13–15 LOC < 20 mins Normal CT	DSM-IV Major depressive disorder criteria	Prospective Consecutive
Ponsford (2011)	90	Australia	3 months	Trauma center	13.5%	LOC < 30 mins, PTA < 24 hrs, GCS 13–15	DSM-IV criteria	Prospective Consecutive
Hoge (2008)	118	United States	3–4 months	Military population	22.9%	Injury with LOC	DSM-IV criteria with "very difficult" impairment	Retrospective Random selection of service members
Hoge (2008)	250	United States	3–4 months	Military population	8.4%	Injury with AMS	DSM-IV criteria with very difficult impairment	Retrospective Random selection of service members
Bombardier (2010)	191	United States	12 months	Community sample	51.9%	GCS 13–15, radiological abnormality	DSM-IV criteria met at any screening call	Retrospective Consecutive

Study	N	Country	Follow-up	Setting	Prevalence	TBI definition	Depression criteria	Design
Horner (2005)	524	United States	12 months	State hospital	21.3%	Injury to the head ICD/AIS = 2[a]	"Since your injury, has a doctor told you that you had depression?"	Retrospective Random selection of TBI
Rao (2010)	43	United States	12 months	Trauma center	18.6%	LOC < 30 mins	DSM-IV criteria for mood disorder secondary to general medical condition, major depressive-like episode, or other depressive symptoms	Prospective Consecutive
Parker (1996)	33	United States	M = 20 months	Private Practice or Compensation	36.0%	Diagnosis of "whiplash" from medical records or on self description Excluded if LOC > 5 mins or presence of cerebral abnormalities.	DSM-III-R	Prospective Selected sample
Vanderploeg (2007)	254	United States	16 years	Military population	14.2%	Head injury with altered consciousness	DSM-III critieria	Retrospective

Abbreviations: ACRM, American Congress of Rehabilitation Medicine (LOC < 30 mins, initial GCS = 13–15, PTA < 24 hours); AIS, Abbreviated Injury Scale; AMS, altered mental status; CT, computed tomography; DSM-III-R, Diagnostic and Statistical Manual of Mental Disorders–3rd Edition Revised; DSM-IV, Diagnostic and Statistical Manual of Mental Disorders 4th Edition; GCS, Glasgow Coma Scale; GDS, Geriatric Depression Scale; ICD, International Classification of Diseases; LOC, loss of consciousness; MRI, magnetic resonance imaging; MTBI, mild traumatic brain injury; SCID, Structured Clinical Interview for DSM IV; TBI, traumatic brain injury.

[a] "TBI was defined as an injury to the head associated with decreased consciousness, amnesia, neurological abnormalities, skull fracture, or intracranial lesion, in accordance with the Center for Disease Control and Prevention" (p. 323). TBI severity was determined by translating ICD-9-CM codes to ICD/AIS scores using ICDMAP-90 software (p.324).

Data were derived from Bombardier, Fann, Temkin, Esselman, Barber, Dikmen (326); Goldstein, Levin, Goldman, Clark, Altonen (316); Hoge, McGurk, Thomas, Cox, Engel, Castro (509); Horner, Ferguson, Selassie, Labbate, Kniele, Corrigan (321); Levin (319); Levin, McCauley, Josic, et al (318); Mooney, Speed (317); McCauley, Boake, Levin, Contant, Song (320); Parker, Rosenblum (322); Ponsford, Cameron, Fitzgerald, Grant, Mikocka-Walus (510); Rao, Bertrand, Rosenberg, et al (511); Vanderploeg, Curtiss, Luis, Salazar (512) with permission.

453

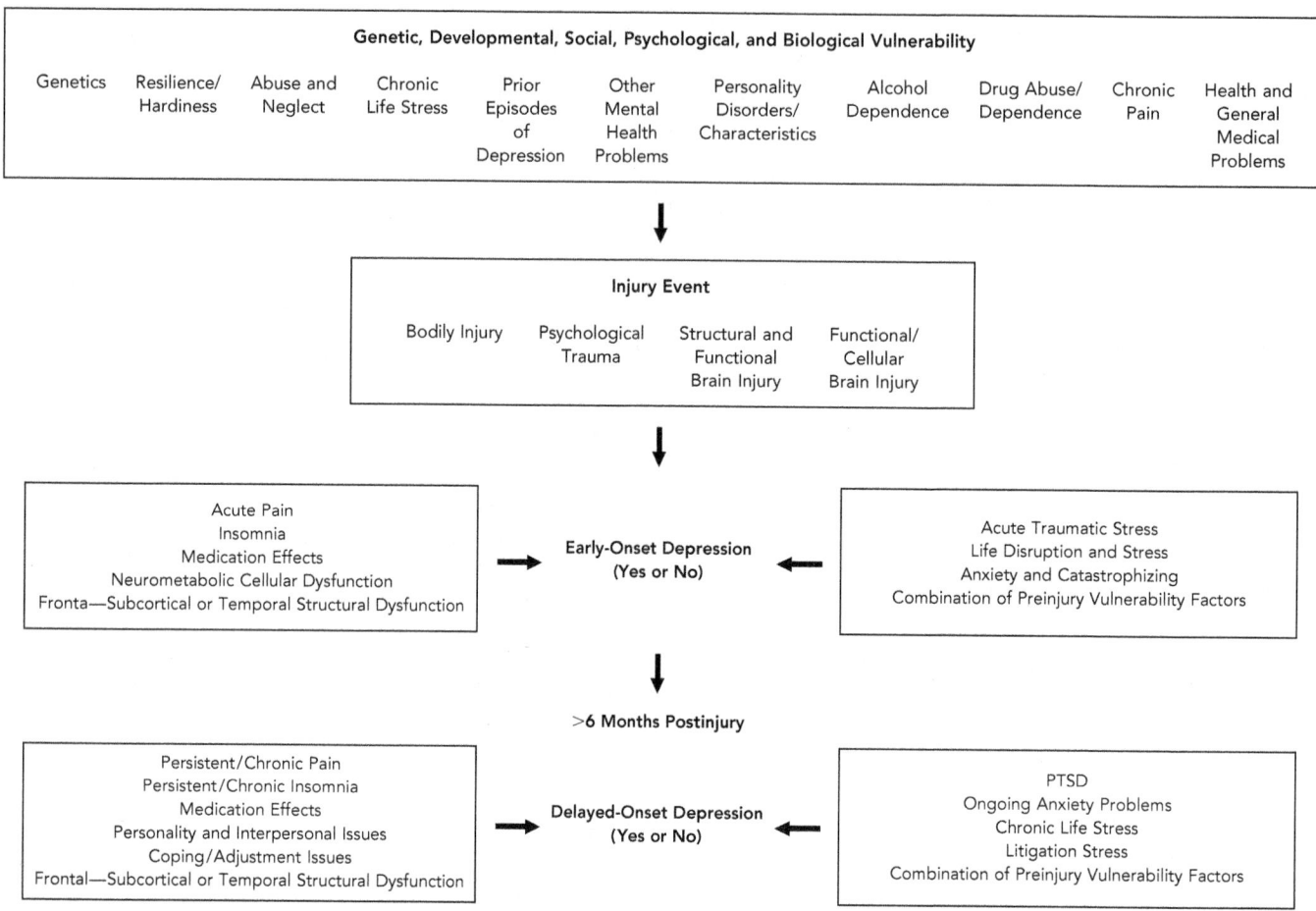

FIGURE 29-3 A theoretical model for the development of depression following mild traumatic brain injury. Copyright 2010 by Grant L. Iverson. Reprinted with permission.

or external visual reminders) that symbolize or resemble an aspect of the event; or (*e*) physiological reactivity when exposed to things that symbolize or resemble an aspect of the traumatic event. In addition to the persistent reexperiencing, there is *persistent avoidance* of things associated with the traumatic event and a numbing of general responsiveness. Examples of avoidance and numbing of responsiveness include (*a*) avoiding thoughts, feelings, or conversations associated with the event; (*b*) avoiding activities, places, or people that stimulate thoughts or memories of the event; (*c*) feeling detached or estranged from others; or (*d*) having a sense of a foreshortened future (e.g., not expecting to have a career, marriage, children, or a normal life span). In addition, the person has persistent symptoms of *increased arousal* such as (*a*) difficulty falling or staying asleep, (*b*) irritability or outbursts of anger, (*c*) difficulty concentrating, (*d*) hypervigilance, and (*e*) an exaggerated startle response.

Developing PTSD following a car accident is uncommon. Some estimates of the rate of this disorder in accident victims have been 9% (362), 12% (363), and 6.3% and 8.8% for men and women, respectively (332). Essentially, 90% of people in car accidents do not develop PTSD. For comparison, fewer than 5% of individuals develop PTSD after a natural disaster (332). In a sample of survivors of the September 11, 2001 terrorist attack on the Pentagon, 14% had PTSD 7 months after the event (364). Sexual assault is associated with

the highest incidence of PTSD, with estimates ranging from 46% to 80% (332,363).

Patients with PTSD often report the same symptoms as patients who have sustained MTBIs. For example, in a sample of 128 patients with PTSD, 89% reported irritability, 56% reported memory problems, 92% reported concentration problems, and 90% reported difficulty sleeping (330). A longstanding controversial issue relates to whether a person who sustains a TBI can develop PTSD. There are data to support the position that MTBI involving a period of dense PTA for several hours and PTSD typically are mutually exclusive (319,365–370), although researchers have put forward a compelling rationale for how, under certain circumstances, PTSD could emerge in a patient with a brain injury—especially an MTBI (371,372). The conceptual question at the heart of the debate is whether a person with no memory for a traumatic event can develop PTSD. In other words, how can you be traumatized by an event you can't remember? How can you reexperience through flashbacks, images, or dreams an event you cannot remember? Researchers suggest that the anxiety response is activated in some individuals, despite the occurrence of memory impairment, so that PTSD can be a comorbid condition with TBI (373–376). It is proposed that PTSD can develop following MTBI via several possible mechanisms, such as fear conditioning, resolution of PTA during the traumatic experience, and reconstruction of traumatic experiences (377–379) (see Chapter 61).

A well-controlled study provides additional information to better understand the relation between PTA and the development of PTSD. Gil and colleagues prospectively studied 120 accident victims who sustained an MTBI and who were hospitalized for observation immediately after their trauma. They were assessed within the first 24 hours and at 1 week, 3 months, and 6 months postinjury. At 6 months postinjury, 14% met diagnostic criteria for PTSD. Predictors of PTSD at 6 months were (*a*) PSTD symptoms, depressive symptoms, and anxiety symptoms at 1 week postinjury, (*b*) history of psychiatric disorder, and (*c*) memory for the event. Of the patients with memory for the event, 13/55 (23%) had PTSD at 6 months postinjury, compared to only 4/65 (6%) who did not have memory for the event (369). Therefore, the literature to date suggests that having no memory for the event likely protects the individual from developing PTSD—but it is still possible to develop PTSD or an anxiety disorder even when a person has no memory for the event.

Clinicians should be very cautious when diagnosing PTSD in a person who has sustained an MTBI if that person does not exhibit prominent symptoms in the initial days postinjury. The onset of symptoms in PTSD is generally rapid. For example, the onset of PTSD symptoms in the survivors of the Oklahoma City bombing was swift, with 76% reporting symptoms on the day of the event (380). For example, there were no cases of delayed onset PTSD associated with the Oklahoma City bombing (381,382) or a mass shooting incident (383,384). Delayed onset PTSD in the vast majority of studies has been considered rare (e.g., 385–387). Therefore, if delayed-onset traumatic stress symptoms appear, they might reflect a combination of (*a*) individual differences in avoidance behavior that masks other PTSD symptoms, (*b*) post-trauma stressors that exacerbate psychological distress, and/or (*c*) delayed compensation motivation (385,388). As illustrated in the study by Gil and colleagues, patients with MTBIs are likely at increased risk for developing PTSD if (*a*) they have a psychiatric history, (*b*) they have memory for the event, and (*c*) they develop major symptoms within the first 24 hours or first week postinjury (369).

CHRONIC TRAUMATIC ENCEPHALOPATHY

A detailed discussion of chronic traumatic encephalopathy (CTE) is provided in the Sport-Related Concussion chapter of this book (Chapter 31). In brief, CTE was initially described clinically and pathologically in boxers decades ago (389). In the past few years, 2 research groups have identified more specific types of neuropathology in the brains of former professional and amateur athletes who have committed suicide or died from other causes and conceptualized this neuropathology as CTE (390–393). CTE is conceptualized as a brain disease arising from cumulative, repetitive, concussive, and subconcussive blows to the head. It is considered a progressive neurodegenerative condition characterized by changes in personality, cognition, and physical functioning. Chronic psychiatric problems, substance abuse, aggression, and suicidal behavior have been linked to CTE through case studies. Omalu and colleagues (392) recently broadened the definition to include a *single* blunt force trauma to the head

as potentially causing CTE: "We define CTE as a progressive neurodegenerative syndrome caused by single, episodic, or repetitive blunt force impacts to the head and transfer of acceleration-deceleration forces to the brain" (p. 174). In a previous article, Omalu and colleagues (394) suggested that a single *severe* TBI could cause CTE, so readers should not assume that a single MTBI is the cause of CTE. Gavett et al. (391) noted that "the exact relationship between concussion and CTE is not entirely clear, although repetitive axonal perturbation may initiate a series of metabolic, ionic, membrane, and cytoskeletal disturbances, which trigger the pathologic cascade that leads to CTE in susceptible individuals" (p. 180).

To date, some researchers have made 2 broad assumptions based on these case studies. First, that the neuropathological findings (e.g., tauopathy [neurofibrillary tangles, neuropil threads, and glial tangles]; beta-amyloid deposits; and TDP-43 proteinopathy) were directly and exclusively caused by repetitive head trauma associated with playing sports. Second, that the psychiatric problems in these former athletes were caused by these specific neuropathological findings. These assumptions regarding causation might ultimately be proven to be correct or partially correct. At present, however, there are important unanswered questions. First, we do not know if patients with chronic mental health problems, drug abuse and/or alcohol abuse histories, steroid abuse histories, chronic pain conditions, diabetes, obesity, or other health conditions, singly or especially in combination, also show some of these neuropathological features. Second, we do not know if there are specific genetic risk factors for this neuropathology. Third, we do not know how to identify athletes or former athletes who are most at risk for this neuropathology. Finally, we do not know the extent to which the neuropathological features are the underlying cause of the psychiatric, substance abuse, and cognitive problems reported in the case histories of these former athletes. Much more research is needed to expand our understanding of CTE neuropathology (e.g., how common it is in people with other conditions) and clinical features (e.g., its relative contribution to psychiatric problems). Psychiatric problems and cognitive impairment often have multifactorial, not unitary, causation—this will need to be examined in future studies.

RISK FOR ALZHEIMER DISEASE

A controversial issue relating to outcome from MTBI is whether this injury increases a person's risk for the development of later-life dementia, such as AD. The most obvious risk factor for developing AD is age (especially an age-genetics interaction). Meta-analytic studies indicate that the prevalence of the disease around the world increases with age (e.g., 395–398), with the most notable rise occurring through the seventh and eighth decades of life (399). In an early meta-analysis of 22 studies, Jorm and colleagues (396) reported that the prevalence of AD doubled every 4.5 years; they reported the following prevalence rates stratified by age group: 65–69 years (1.4%), 70–74 years (2.8%), 75–79 years (5.6%), 80–84 years (11.1%), and 85 years or more (23.6%). The risk for developing the disease is low in a person's 60s and high after the age of 85 (perhaps 25%–50% of older adults); however, the incidence rates in people older than 75 years of age are more variable across studies (399).

Recent work has suggested that AD pathology is driven by genetic factors related to amyloid precursor protein (APP), not aging per se, bringing into question the long-standing adage that "age is the greatest risk factor for AD" (400).

Genetics (particularly the apolipoprotein E [APOE] gene [401–404]), singly or in combination with medical conditions and lifestyle factors, are an important risk factor for the disease. Recent reviews of the literature indicate that diabetes, hypertension, obesity, heart disease, and cerebrovascular disease are risk factors for dementia and AD (399,405). Mental health problems such as a history of depression in adulthood (406), have been associated with an increased risk for the disease—and this risk appears to be greater for men (407).

A controversial and poorly understood issue relating to outcome from MTBI is whether this injury increases a person's risk for the future development of dementia including AD. There has been considerable research interest regarding whether mild, repetitive mild, moderate, or severe TBIs increase a person's risk for developing dementia or AD. This research has been ongoing, with mixed results, for more than 25 years.

A prima facie plausible theory is that more severe forms of TBIs reduce "cognitive reserve," resulting in increased vulnerability to developing the disease (408). For example, if a severe TBI results in widespread cellular death, it seems reasonable to assume that the injured person would be more vulnerable to the adverse neurocognitive effects of natural aging, chronic medical problems, and degenerative brain disease. The relation between TBI and risk for AD is very difficult to study, from a methodological perspective. One methodology is to examine a large cross-sectional cohort of subjects with history of brain injury identified retrospectively and dementia diagnosed in the present. Another methodology is to attempt to follow patients prospectively. Over the years, using varying research designs and methodologies (including autopsy studies), some researchers have reported a statistical relation between a history of TBI (mostly moderate or severe) and a current diagnosis of AD (e.g., 409–422). However, other researchers have frequently failed to find this association (e.g., 423–431).

The animal literature has revealed evidence that some of the neuropathological features of AD arise shortly after TBI (see 432,433 for reviews), and human autopsy studies are advancing our understanding of the link between severe TBI and AD (434–438). There has been considerable interest in whether genetic factors influence the susceptibility of the human brain to injury and/or the capacity for recovery (439). If so, these genetic factors could influence the relation between TBI and the development of AD. Researchers have been most interested in the APOE allele; APOE epsilon 4 (APOEE4) reportedly is associated with worse outcome following TBI (e.g., see 440, 441 for reviews) whereas APOE epsilon 3 (APOEE3) might be neuroprotective. Thus, genetics might play an important role in the degree of permanent brain damage sustained following traumatic injury (439).

The logical extension is to study whether genetics, in combination with TBI (typically moderate or severe TBI), increase one's risk for AD. Researchers have reported mixed and contradictory findings in this area. Some researchers have reported a positive association between TBI, APOE, and dementia (e.g., 442,443), whereas other researchers have not found this relation (e.g., 413,414). Some researchers have

even reported the opposite of the "expected" relation, that TBI increases the risk for AD in those *without* the genetic characteristic (e.g., 416,434,435).

Mortimer and colleagues conducted an important meta-analytic review of the entire literature published prior to 1991 (444). They reported that TBIs were associated with a 1.82 relative risk (RR) (95% confidence interval = 1.26–2.67) for developing AD. The RR was significant for men (RR = 2.67, 95% CI = 1.64–4.41) but not for women (RR = 0.85, 95% CI = 0.43–1.70). This meta-analysis, and the individual studies reporting the connection, have slowly lead to a widespread clinical belief that TBI increases a patient's risk for AD. By extension, clinicians have assumed that an isolated *mild* TBI also increases the risk, even though most of the literature is based on moderate or severe TBIs. However, Fleminger and colleagues conducted a second meta-analytic review of the literature and reported that studies published *since 1991* did *not* reveal a statistically significant increased risk for AD (445). Fleminger and colleagues reported that if one considers the entire literature (i.e., the studies published before and after the Mortimer meta-analysis) there is an increased risk for AD associated with a history of TBI (Odds Ratio [OR] = 1.58, 95% CI = 1.21–2.06). This increased risk was significant for men (OR = 2.26, 95% CI = 1.13–4.53) but not for women (OR = 0.92, 95% CI = 0.53–1.59). Starkstein and Jorge (446) suggested that this increased risk in men and not women might simply reflect men sustaining more severe TBIs. Jellinger, in his review of the literature, concluded that the epidemiological and autopsy studies have provided evidence of an association between *severe* TBI and AD (433).

In regards to risk for AD, there are many conflicting results in this large literature spanning more than 25 years. Nonetheless, it is reasonable to conclude that patients who sustain *severe* TBIs are at a small increased risk for the future development of AD, as concluded by Starkstein and Jorge (446) and Jellinger (433). In a systematic review, Bazarian and colleagues (447) concluded that there is sufficient evidence of an association between moderate and severe TBI and AD, limited evidence of an association between MTBI with LOC and AD, and insufficient evidence to determine whether there is an association between MTBI (with no LOC) and AD.

Given that (a) many studies have failed to find an association between history of TBI (of any severity) and the disease, (b) the meta-analyses have only identified this association for men, (c) several studies have found a severity effect (i.e., risk is greater in patients with more severe brain injuries), and (d) the pathophysiology of MTBI, especially on the milder end of the spectrum of this injury, appears to be temporary and reversible, it would be a mistake to conclude, at this point, that patients with *MTBIs*, as a group, are at increased risk for AD. Several specific studies suggest that there is not a relationship between MTBI and risk for AD (e.g., 414, 418,429).

PERSISTENT POSTCONCUSSION SYMPTOMS

A minority of patients have poor long-term outcome following MTBI (448). The etiology of the so-called *persistent* postconcussion syndrome has never been agreed on (see 6,449–451 for reviews). For decades, researchers have questioned the validity of this diagnosis as a true syndrome, disorder, or disease entity (e.g., 452–457). Others have noted that the syndrome is rare in prospective studies (e.g., 278,454), and concerns regarding the role of financial compensation on symptom reporting have been expressed for many years (452,458–462). Most researchers simply suggest that the etiology is caused by the biological effects of the injury, psychological factors, psychosocial factors (broadly defined), chronic pain, or a combination of factors (463–471). Ruff and colleagues (448,451,472) have stressed a multidimensional cumulative stressor conceptualization of the persistent postconcussion syndrome. Essentially, setbacks in several aspects of a person's life (physical, emotional, cognitive, psychosocial, vocational, financial, and recreational) serve as cumulative stressors that interact with personality and premorbid physical and mental health factors, resulting in the syndrome. This model stresses the complexity of the etiology and maintenance of the syndrome.

Experienced clinicians and researchers know that it is extraordinarily difficult to disentangle the many factors that can be related to self-reported symptoms in persons who have sustained remote MTBIs (449). This is a challenging and potentially contentious diagnosis, of course, because postconcussion-like symptoms are common in healthy subjects (473–479), in patients with no history of brain injury, such as outpatients seen for psychological treatment (480), outpatients seen for minor medical problems (481), personal injury claimants (481,482), patients with PTSD (330), patients with orthopedic injuries (453), individuals with chronic pain (344,347,348,483) and patients with whiplash (484). Thus, the differential diagnosis of long-term symptoms following MTBI is very challenging. Chapter 30 in this book is devoted to conceptualizing long-term outcome from MTBI.

CONCLUSION

MTBI has been recognized as a public health problem (485–487). The pathophysiology of MTBI is predominately neurometabolic and reversible. However, as the physical forces exerted on the head and brain increase, this injury can be characterized by macroscopic damage that is visible with structural neuroimaging and cellular damage that is not visible through neuroimaging. A comprehensive overview of specific topics relating to MTBI was provided in this chapter. This chapter covered definitions, pathoanatomy and pathophysiology, biomarkers, neuropsychological outcome, early intervention, return to work, depression, PTSD, and risk for AD. The next chapter in the book provides a comprehensive discussion of how to conceptualize long-term symptoms and problems in patients who sustain this injury and a review of treatment and rehabilitation strategies. Although there is still much to learn about MTBI, we have made significant progress and further progress will clearly lead to both better diagnostic accuracy and better functional outcomes.

KEY CLINICAL POINTS

1. There is no universally accepted definition of MTBI, but the definition provided by the WHO Collaborating Center Task Force on Mild Traumatic Brain Injury is commonly used in research and clinical practice.

2. MTBIs can be characterized by damage to the structure of the brain. A minority of patients with MTBIs have visible abnormalities on CT or MRI conducted on the day-of-injury or within the first 2 weeks postinjury. For the most part, however, the pathophysiology of MTBI is neurometabolic and mostly reversible. When forces are applied to the brain with sufficient magnitude, small changes in structure and function can be observed in a subset of neurons and glia.

3. There is considerable interest in serum and plasma based biochemical markers for use as diagnostic and prognostic measures of brain injury in the first few days following MTBI. However, biomarkers have been mostly studied in moderate-severe TBI patients (except S100B). Few biomarkers have been studied specifically in MTBI patients. Despite decades of research in this area, no biomarker has yet proven accurate and reliable for detecting TBI of any severity. Algorithms involving several proteins, rather than single markers, might prove optimal diagnostically and prognostically.

4. Injured athletes and trauma patients perform poorly on neuropsychological tests in the initial days and up to the first month following the injury. Because of natural recovery, neurocognitive deficits typically are not seen in athletes after 1–3 weeks and in trauma patients after 1–3 months in prospective group studies.

5. The literature suggests that early intervention, in the form of education and reassurance, can help patients better manage symptoms and more effectively return to their normal lifestyle. Clinicians working in early intervention programs know that some people continue to report symptoms despite education, reassurance, and gradual resumption of activities. Effective treatments for people who are slow to recover or who report significant symptoms long after injury are greatly needed.

6. Depression is common following MTBI. It is theoretically plausible that depression can arise (*a*) directly or indirectly from the neurobiological consequences of the brain injury, (*b*) as a psychological reaction to deficits and problems associated with having a brain injury, (*c*) as a biopsychosocial reaction to the stress of co-occurring bodily injuries and associated lifestyle changes, and/or (*d*) from a combination of these factors. Depression can also arise *de novo*, incidentally, sometime postinjury—such as in response to life stressors. It can also arise as part of a preexisting chronic relapsing and remitting condition.

7. PTSD can occur in patients who experience an MTBI within the context of a psychologically traumatic event. Patients are at increased risk for developing PTSD if (*a*) they have a psychiatric history, (*b*) they have memory for the event (not dense PTA), and (*c*) they develop major symptoms within the first 24 hours or first week postinjury.

8. At present, the available evidence suggests that people who sustain severe TBIs are at an increased risk of AD but those who sustain MTBI are not.

KEY REFERENCES

1. Barkhoudarian G, Hovda DA, Giza CC. The molecular pathophysiology of concussive brain injury. *Clin Sports Med.* 2011;30:33–48, vii–iii.

2. Bazarian JJ, Cernak I, Noble-Haeusslein L, Potolicchio S, Temkin N. Long-term neurologic outcomes after traumatic brain injury. *J Head Trauma Rehabil*. 2009;24:439–451.

3. Ruff RM, Iverson GL, Barth JT, Bush SS, Broshek DK. Recommendations for diagnosing a mild traumatic brain injury: a National Academy of Neuropsychology education paper. *Arch Clin Neuropsychol*. 2009;24(1):3–10.

4. The Management of Concussion/mTBI Working Group. VA/DoD clinical practice guideline for management of concussion/mild traumatic brain injury (mTBI). Published April 2009. http://www.healthquality.va.gov/mtbi/concussion_mtbi_full_1_0.pdf. Accessed April 18, 2010.

References

1. Bazarian JJ, McClung J, Cheng YT, Flesher W, Schneider SM. Emergency department management of mild traumatic brain injury in the USA. *Emerg Med J*. 2005;22:473–477.

2. Sosin DM, Sniezek JE, Thurman DJ. Incidence of mild and moderate brain injury in the United States, 1991. *Brain Inj*. 1996;10:47–54.

3. Belanger HG, Vanderploeg RD. The neuropsychological impact of sports-related concussion: a meta-analysis. *J Int Neuropsychol Soc*. 2005;11:345–357.

4. Carroll LJ, Cassidy JD, Peloso PM, et al. Prognosis for mild traumatic brain injury: results of the WHO Collaborating Centre Task Force on Mild Traumatic Brain Injury. *J Rehabil Med*. 2004;84–105.

5. Belanger HG, Curtiss G, Demery JA, Lebowitz BK, Vanderploeg RD. Factors moderating neuropsychological outcomes following mild traumatic brain injury: a meta-analysis. *J Int Neuropsychol Soc*. 2005;11:215–227.

6. Iverson GL. Outcome from mild traumatic brain injury. *Curr Opin Psychiat*. 2005;18:301–317.

7. Schretlen DJ, Shapiro AM. A quantitative review of the effects of traumatic brain injury on cognitive functioning. *Int Rev Psychiatry*. 2003;15:341–349.

8. Rees PM. Contemporary issues in mild traumatic brain injury. *Arch Phys Med Rehabil*. 2003;84:1885–1894.

9. Carroll LJ, Cassidy JD, Holm L, Kraus J, Coronado VG; for WHO Collaborating Centre Task Force on Mild Traumatic Brain Injury. Methodological issues and research recommendations for mild traumatic brain injury: the WHO Collaborating Centre Task Force on Mild Traumatic Brain Injury. *J Rehabil Med*. 2004;(43)(suppl):113–125.

10. Mild Traumatic Brain Injury Committee ACoRM, Head Injury Interdisciplinary Special Interest Group. Definition of mild traumatic brain injury. *J Head Trauma Rehabil*. 1993;8:86–87.

11. National Center for Injury Prevention and Control. *Report to Congress on Mild Traumatic Brain Injury in the United States: Steps to Prevent a Serious Public Health Problem*. Atlanta, GA: Centers for Disease Control and Prevention; 2003.

12. Ruff RM, Iverson GL, Barth JT, Bush SS, Broshek DK. Recommendations for diagnosing a mild traumatic brain injury: a National Academy of Neuropsychology education paper. *Arch Clin Neuropsychol*. 2009;24(1):3–10.

13. Williams DH, Levin HS, Eisenberg HM. Mild head injury classification. *Neurosurgery*. 1990;27:422–428.

14. Vos PE, Battistin L, Birbamer G, et al; for European Federation of Neurological Societies. EFNS guideline on mild traumatic brain injury: report of an EFNS task force. *Eur J Neurol*. 2002;9(3):207–219.

15. McCrea M, Hammeke T, Olsen G, Leo P, Guskiewicz K. Unreported concussion in high school football players: implications for prevention. *Clin J Sport Med*. 2004;14:13–17.

16. French BN, Dublin AB. The value of computerized tomography in the management of 1000 consecutive head injuries. *Surg Neurol*. 1977;7:171–183.

17. Iverson GL, Lovell MR, Smith S, Franzen MD. Prevalence of abnormal CT-scans following mild head injury. *Brain Inj*. 2000;14(12):1057–1061.

18. Jeret JS, Mandell M, Anziska B, et al. Clinical predictors of abnormality disclosed by computed tomography after mild head trauma. *Neurosurgery*. 1993;32:9–16.

19. Livingston DH, Loder PA, Koziol J, Hunt CD. The use of CT scanning to triage patients requiring admission following minimal head injury. *J Trauma*. 1991;31:483–489.

20. Levin HS, Williams DH, Eisenberg HM, High WM Jr, Guinto FC Jr. Serial MRI and neurobehavioural findings after mild to moderate closed head injury. *J Neurol Neurosurg Psychiatry*. 1992;55:255–262.

21. Tellier A, Della Malva LC, Cwinn A, Grahovac S, Morrish W, Brennan-Barnes M. Mild head injury: a misnomer. *Brain Inj*. 1999;13:463–475.

22. Borg J, Holm L, Cassidy JD, et al; for WHO Collaborating Centre Task Force on Mild Traumatic Brain Injury. Diagnostic procedures in mild traumatic brain injury: results of the WHO Collaborating Centre Task Force on Mild Traumatic Brain Injury. *J Rehabil Med*. 2004:61–75.

23. Mittl RL, Grossman RI, Hiehle JF, et al. Prevalence of MR evidence of diffuse axonal injury in patients with mild head injury and normal head CT findings. *AJNR Am J Neuroradiol*. 1994;15(8):1583–1589.

24. van der Naalt J, Hew JM, van Zomeren AH, Sluiter WJ, Minderhoud JM. Computed tomography and magnetic resonance imaging in mild to moderate head injury: early and late imaging related to outcome. *Ann Neurol*. 1999;46:70–78.

25. Voller B, Auff E, Schnider P, Aichner F. To do or not to do? Magnetic resonance imaging in mild traumatic brain injury. *Brain Inj*. 2001;15:107–115.

26. Yokota H, Kurokawa A, Otsuka T, Kobayashi S, Nakazawa S. Significance of magnetic resonance imaging in acute head injury. *J Trauma*. 1991;31:351–357.

27. Lorberboym M, Lampl Y, Gerzon I, Sadeh M. Brain SPECT evaluation of amnestic ED patients after mild head trauma. *Am J Emerg Med*. 2002;20:310–313.

28. Audenaert K, Jansen HM, Otte A, et al. Imaging of mild traumatic brain injury using 57Co and 99mTc HMPAO SPECT as compared to other diagnostic procedures. *Med Sci Monit*. 2003;9:MT112–MT117.

29. Umile EM, Sandel ME, Alavi A, Terry CM, Plotkin RC. Dynamic imaging in mild traumatic brain injury: support for the theory of medial temporal vulnerability. *Arch Phys Med Rehabil*. 2002;83:1506–1513.

30. Lewine JD, Davis JT, Bigler ED, et al. Objective documentation of traumatic brain injury subsequent to mild head trauma: multimodal brain imaging with MEG, SPECT, and MRI. *J Head Trauma Rehabil*. 2007;22:141–155.

31. Chen SH, Kareken DA, Fastenau PS, Trexler LE, Hutchins GD. A study of persistent post-concussion symptoms in mild head trauma using positron emission tomography. *J Neurol Neurosurg Psychiatry*. 2003;74:326–332.

32. Abu-Judeh HH, Parker R, Singh M, et al. SPET brain perfusion imaging in mild traumatic brain injury without loss of consciousness and normal computed tomography. *Nucl Med Commun*. 1999;20:505–510.

33. Bonne O, Gilboa A, Louzoun Y, et al. Cerebral blood flow in chronic symptomatic mild traumatic brain injury. *Psychiatry Res*. 2003;124:141–152.

34. Hofman PA, Stapert SZ, van Kroonenburgh MJ, Jolles J, de Kruijk J, Wilmink JT. MR imaging, single-photon emission CT, and neurocognitive performance after mild traumatic brain injury. *AJNR Am J Neuroradiol*. 2001;22:441–449.

35. MacKenzie JD, Siddiqi F, Babb JS, et al. Brain atrophy in mild or moderate traumatic brain injury: a longitudinal quantitative analysis. *AJNR Am J Neuroradiol*. 2002;23:1509–1515.

36. Schrader H, Mickeviciene D, Gleizniene R, et al. Magnetic resonance imaging after most common form of concussion. *BMC medical imaging*. 2009;9:11.

37. Topal NB, Hakyemez B, Erdogan C, et al. MR imaging in the detection of diffuse axonal injury with mild traumatic brain injury. *Neurol Res*. 2008;30:974–978.

38. Sigurdardottir S, Andelic N, Roe C, Jerstad T, Schanke AK. Post-concussion symptoms after traumatic brain injury at 3 and 12 months post-injury: a prospective study. *Brain Inj.* 2009;23:489–497.

39. Niogi SN, Mukherjee P, Ghajar J, et al. Extent of microstructural white matter injury in postconcussive syndrome correlates with impaired cognitive reaction time: a 3T diffusion tensor imaging study of mild traumatic brain injury. *AJNR Am J Neuroradiol.* 2008; 29:967–973.

40. Datta SG, Pillai SV, Rao SL, Kovoor JM, Chandramouli BA. Post-concussion syndrome: correlation of neuropsychological deficits, structural lesions on magnetic resonance imaging and symptoms. *Neurol India.* 2009;57:594–598.

41. Inglese M, Bomsztyk E, Gonen O, Mannon LJ, Grossman RI, Rusi-nek H. Dilated perivascular spaces: hallmarks of mild traumatic brain injury. *AJNR Am J Neuroradiol.* 2005;26:719–724.

42. Perlstein WM, Cole MA, Demery JA, et al. Parametric manipulation of working memory load in traumatic brain injury: behavioral and neural correlates. *J Int Neuropsychol Soc.* 2004;10:724–741.

43. Smits M, Dippel DW, Houston GC, et al. Postconcussion syndrome after minor head injury: brain activation of working memory and attention. *Hum Brain Mapp.* 2009;30:2789–2803.

44. Feldman HM, Yeatman JD, Lee ES, Barde LH, Gaman-Bean S. Diffusion tensor imaging: a review for pediatric researchers and clinicians. *J Dev Behav Pediatr.* 2010;31:346–356.

45. Suskauer SJ, Huisman TA. Neuroimaging in pediatric traumatic brain injury: current and future predictors of functional outcome. *Dev Disabil Res Rev.* 2009;15:117–123.

46. Bosnell R, Giorgio A, Johansen-Berg H. Imaging white matter diffusion changes with development and recovery from brain injury. *Dev Neurorehabil.* 2008;11:174–186.

47. Oni MB, Wilde EA, Bigler ED, et al. Diffusion tensor imaging analysis of frontal lobes in pediatric traumatic brain injury. *J Child Neurol.* 2010;25:976–984.

48. Wilde EA, Ramos MA, Yallampalli R, et al. Diffusion tensor imaging of the cingulum bundle in children after traumatic brain injury. *Dev Neuropsychol.* 2010;35:333–351.

49. Jiang Q, Zhang ZG, Chopp M. MRI evaluation of white matter recovery after brain injury. *Stroke.* 2010;41:S112–113.

50. Kou Z, Wu Z, Tong KA, et al. The role of advanced MR imaging findings as biomarkers of traumatic brain injury. *J Head Trauma Rehabil.* 2010;25:267–282.

51. Rutgers DR, Fillard P, Paradot G, Tadie M, Lasjaunias P, Ducreux D. Diffusion tensor imaging characteristics of the corpus callosum in mild, moderate, and severe traumatic brain injury. *AJNR Am J Neuroradiol.* 2008;29:1730–1735.

52. Sidaros A, Engberg AW, Sidaros K, et al. Diffusion tensor imaging during recovery from severe traumatic brain injury and relation to clinical outcome: a longitudinal study. *Brain.* 2008;131:559–572.

53. Kumar R, Gupta RK, Husain M, et al. Comparative evaluation of corpus callosum DTI metrics in acute mild and moderate traumatic brain injury: its correlation with neuropsychometric tests. *Brain Inj.* 2009;23:675–685.

54. Inglese M, Makani S, Johnson G, et al. Diffuse axonal injury in mild traumatic brain injury: a diffusion tensor imaging study. *J Neurosurg.* 2005;103:298–303.

55. Kraus MF, Susmaras T, Caughlin BP, Walker CJ, Sweeney JA, Little DM. White matter integrity and cognition in chronic traumatic brain injury: a diffusion tensor imaging study. *Brain.* 2007;130: 2508–2519.

56. Lipton ML, Gellella E, Lo C, et al. Multifocal white matter ultra-structural abnormalities in mild traumatic brain injury with cognitive disability: a voxel-wise analysis of diffusion tensor imaging. *J Neurotrauma.* 2008;25:1335–1342.

57. Lipton ML, Gulko E, Zimmerman ME, et al. Diffusion-tensor imaging implicates prefrontal axonal injury in executive function impairment following very mild traumatic brain injury. *Radiology.* 2009;252:816–824.

58. Rutgers DR, Toulgoat F, Cazejust J, Fillard P, Lasjaunias P, Ducreux D. White matter abnormalities in mild traumatic brain injury: a diffusion tensor imaging study. *AJNR Am J Neuroradiol.* 2008;29: 514–519.

59. Lange RT, Iverson GL, Brubacher JR, Mädler B, Heran MK. Diffusion tensor imaging findings are not strongly associated with post-concussional disorder 2 months following mild traumatic brain injury. *J Head Trauma Rehabil.* 2012;27(3):188–198.

60. Mayer AR, Ling J, Mannell MV, et al. A prospective diffusion tensor imaging study in mild traumatic brain injury. *Neurology.* 2010;74: 643–650.

61. Bazarian JJ, Zhong J, Blyth B, Zhu T, Kavcic V, Peterson D. Diffusion tensor imaging detects clinically important axonal damage after mild traumatic brain injury: a pilot study. *J Neurotrauma.* 2007; 24:1447–1459.

62. Wilde EA, McCauley SR, Hunter JV, et al. Diffusion tensor imaging of acute mild traumatic brain injury in adolescents. *Neurology.* 2008; 70:948–955.

63. Carter JC, Lanham DC, Cutting LE, et al. A dual DTI approach to analyzing white matter in children with dyslexia. *Psychiatry Res.* 2009;172:215–219.

64. Rimrodt SL, Peterson DJ, Denckla MB, Kaufmann WE, Cutting LE. White matter microstructural differences linked to left perisylvian language network in children with dyslexia. *Cortex.* 2010;46: 739–749.

65. Odegard TN, Farris EA, Ring J, McColl R, Black J. Brain connectivity in non-reading impaired children and children diagnosed with developmental dyslexia. *Neuropsychologia.* 2009;47:1972–1977.

66. Konrad A, Dielentheis TF, El Masri D, et al. Disturbed structural connectivity is related to inattention and impulsivity in adult attention deficit hyperactivity disorder. *Eur J Neurosci.* 2010;31:912–919.

67. Cao Q, Sun L, Gong G, et al. The macrostructural and microstructural abnormalities of corpus callosum in children with attention deficit/hyperactivity disorder: a combined morphometric and diffusion tensor MRI study. *Brain Res.* 2010;1310:172–180.

68. Yeh PH, Simpson K, Durazzo TC, Gazdzinski S, Meyerhoff DJ. Tract-Based Spatial Statistics (TBSS) of diffusion tensor imaging data in alcohol dependence: abnormalities of the motivational neurocircuitry. *Psychiatry Res.* 2009;173:22–30.

69. Ma L, Hasan KM, Steinberg JL, et al. Diffusion tensor imaging in cocaine dependence: regional effects of cocaine on corpus callosum and effect of cocaine administration route. *Drug Alcohol Depend.* 2009;104:262–267.

70. Jacobus J, McQueeny T, Bava S, et al. White matter integrity in adolescents with histories of marijuana use and binge drinking. *Neurotoxicol Teratol.* 2009;31:349–355.

71. Dalby RB, Frandsen J, Chakravarty MM, et al. Depression severity is correlated to the integrity of white matter fiber tracts in late-onset major depression. *Psychiatry Res.* 2010;184:38–48.

72. Lyoo IK, Lee HK, Jung JH, Noam GG, Renshaw PF. White matter hyperintensities on magnetic resonance imaging of the brain in children with psychiatric disorders. *Compr Psychiatry.* 2002;43: 361–368.

73. Moore PB, Shepherd DJ, Eccleston D, et al. Cerebral white matter lesions in bipolar affective disorder: relationship to outcome. *Br J Psychiatry.* 2001;178:172–176.

74. Pillai JJ, Friedman L, Stuve TA, et al. Increased presence of white matter hyperintensities in adolescent patients with bipolar disorder. *Psychiatry Res.* 2002;114:51–56.

75. Agid R, Levin T, Gomori JM, Lerer B, Bonne O. T2-weighted image hyperintensities in major depression: focus on the basal ganglia. *Int J Neuropsychopharmacol.* 2003;6:215–224.

76. Ehrlich S, Breeze JL, Hesdorffer DC, et al. White matter hyperintensities and their association with suicidality in depressed young adults. *J Affect Disord.* 2005;86:281–287.

77. Sassi RB, Brambilla P, Nicoletti M, et al. White matter hyperintensities in bipolar and unipolar patients with relatively mild-to-moderate illness severity. *J Affect Disord.* 2003;77:237–245.

78. Cooney BS, Grossman RI, Farber RE, Goin JE, Galetta SL. Frequency of magnetic resonance imaging abnormalities in patients with migraine. *Headache.* 1996;36:616–621.

79. Greenwald BS, Kramer-Ginsberg E, Krishnan KR, et al. A controlled study of MRI signal hyperintensities in older depressed patients with and without hypertension. *J Am Geriatr Soc.* 2001;49: 1218–1225.

80. Iverson GL, Hakulinen U, Waljas M, et al. To exclude or not to exclude: white matter hyperintensities in diffusion tensor imaging research. *Brain Inj.* 2011;25:1325–1332.

81. Ommaya AK, Gennarelli TA. Cerebral concussion and traumatic unconsciousness. Correlation of experimental and clinical observations of blunt head injuries. *Brain.* 1974;97:633–654.

82. Duhaime AC, Christian CW, Rorke LB, Zimmerman RA. Nonaccidental head injury in infants—the "shaken-baby syndrome". *N Engl J Med.* 1998;338(25):1822–1829.

83. Gieron MA, Korthals JK, Riggs CD. Diffuse axonal injury without direct head trauma and with delayed onset of coma. *Pediatr Neurol.* 1998;19:382–384.

84. Henry GK, Gross HS, Herndon CA, Furst CJ. Nonimpact brain injury: neuropsychological and behavioral correlates with consideration of physiological findings. *Appl Neuropsychol.* 2000;7:65–75.

85. Varney NR, Varney RN. Some physics of automobile collisions with particular reference to brain injuries occuring without physical head trauma. *Appl Neuropsychol.* 1995;2:47–62.

86. Olvey SE, Knox T, Cohn KA. The development of a method to measure head acceleration and motion in high-impact crashes. *Neurosurgery.* 2004;54:672–677; discussion 677.

87. Crisco JJ, Chu JJ, Greenwald RM. An algorithm for estimating acceleration magnitude and impact location using multiple nonorthogonal single-axis accelerometers. *J Biomech Eng.* 2004;126:849–854.

88. Duma SM, Manoogian SJ, Bussone WR, et al. Analysis of real-time head accelerations in collegiate football players. *Clin J Sport Med.* 2005;15:3–8.

89. Pellman EJ, Viano DC, Tucker AM, Casson IR. Concussion in professional football: location and direction of helmet impacts-Part 2. *Neurosurgery.* 2003;53:1328–1341.

90. Withnall C, Shewchenko N, Gittens R, Dvorak J. Biomechanical investigation of head impacts in football. *Br J Sports Med.* 2005; 39(suppl 1):i49–i57.

91. Meaney DF, Smith DH. Biomechanics of concussion. *Clin Sports Med.* 2011;30:19–31, vii.

92. Bayly PV, Cohen TS, Leister EP, Ajo D, Leuthardt EC, Genin GM. Deformation of the human brain induced by mild acceleration. *J Neurotrauma.* 2005;22:845–856.

93. Barkhoudarian G, Hovda DA, Giza CC. The molecular pathophysiology of concussive brain injury. *Clin Sports Med.* 2011;30:33–48, vii–viii.

94. Bazarian JJ. Diagnosing mild traumatic brain injury after a concussion. *J Head Trauma Rehabil.* 2010;25:225–227.

95. Spain A, Daumas S, Lifshitz J, et al. Mild fluid percussion injury in mice produces evolving selective axonal pathology and cognitive deficits relevant to human brain injury. *J Neurotrauma.* 2010;27: 1429–1438.

96. Smith DH, Wolf JA, Lusardi TA, Lee VM, Meaney DF. High tolerance and delayed elastic response of cultured axons to dynamic stretch injury. *J Neurosci.* 1999;19:4263–4269.

97. Wolf JA, Stys PK, Lusardi T, Meaney D, Smith DH. Traumatic axonal injury induces calcium influx modulated by tetrodotoxin-sensitive sodium channels. *J Neurosci.* 2001;21:1923–1930.

98. Iwata A, Stys PK, Wolf JA, et al. Traumatic axonal injury induces proteolytic cleavage of the voltage-gated sodium channels modulated by tetrodotoxin and protease inhibitors. *J Neurosci.* 2004;24: 4605–4613.

99. Staal JA, Dickson TC, Gasperini R, Liu Y, Foa L, Vickers JC. Initial calcium release from intracellular stores followed by calcium dysregulation is linked to secondary axotomy following transient axonal stretch injury. *J Neurochem.* 2010;112:1147–1155.

100. Bell JD, Ai J, Chen Y, Baker AJ. Mild in vitro trauma induces rapid Glur2 endocytosis, robustly augments calcium permeability and enhances susceptibility to secondary excitotoxic insult in cultured Purkinje cells. *Brain.* 2007;130:2528–2542.

101. Di Pietro V, Amin D, Pernagallo S, et al. Transcriptomics of traumatic brain injury: gene expression and molecular pathways of different grades of insult in a rat organotypic hippocampal culture model. *J Neurotrauma.* 2010;27:349–359.

102. Schwartz JH. Synthesis and trafficking of neural proteins. In: Kandel ER, Schwartz JH, Jessell TM, eds. *Principles of Neural Science.* 3rd ed. New York, NY: Elsevier; 1991:49–65.

103. Gaetz M. The neurophysiology of brain injury. *Clin Neurophysiol.* 2004;115:4–18.

104. Maxwell WL, Kansagra AM, Graham DI, Adams JH, Gennarelli TA. Freeze-fracture studies of reactive myelinated nerve fibres after diffuse axonal injury. *Acta Neuropathol (Berl).* 1988;76:395–406.

105. Pettus EH, Christman CW, Giebel ML, Povlishock JT. Traumatically induced altered membrane permeability: its relationship to traumatically induced reactive axonal change. *J Neurotrauma.* 1994; 11:507–522.

106. Yaghmai A, Povlishock J. Traumatically induced reactive change as visualized through the use of monoclonal antibodies targeted to neurofilament subunits. *J Neuropathol Exp Neurol.* 1992;51:158–176.

107. Chung RS, Staal JA, McCormack GH, et al. Mild axonal stretch injury in vitro induces a progressive series of neurofilament alterations ultimately leading to delayed axotomy. *J Neurotrauma.* 2005; 22:1081–1091.

108. Povlishock JT, Becker DP. Fate of reactive axonal swellings induced by head injury. *Lab Invest.* 1985;52:540–552.

109. Bigler ED. Neuropsychological results and neuropathological findings at autopsy in a case of mild traumatic brain injury. *J Int Neuropsychol Soc.* 2004;10:794–806.

110. Bain AC, Raghupathi R, Meaney DF. Dynamic stretch correlates to both morphological abnormalities and electrophysiological impairment in a model of traumatic axonal injury. *J Neurotrauma.* 2001;18:499–511.

111. Giehl KM, Schacht CM, Yan Q, Mestres P. GDNF is a trophic factor for adult rat corticospinal neurons and promotes their long-term survival after axotomy in vivo. *Eur J Neurosci.* 1997;9:2479–2488.

112. Bonatz H, Rohrig S, Mestres P, Meyer M, Giehl KM. An axotomy model for the induction of death of rat and mouse corticospinal neurons in vivo. *J Neurosci Methods.* 2000;100:105–115.

113. Greer JE, McGinn MJ, Povlishock JT. Diffuse traumatic axonal injury in the mouse induces atrophy, c-Jun activation, and axonal outgrowth in the axotomized neuronal population. *J Neurosci.* 2011; 31:5089–5105.

114. Gao X, Chen J. Mild traumatic brain injury results in extensive neuronal degeneration in the cerebral cortex. *J Neuropathol Exp Neurol.* 2011;70:183–191.

115. Yuen TJ, Browne KD, Iwata A, Smith DH. Sodium channelopathy induced by mild axonal trauma worsens outcome after a repeat injury. *J Neurosci Res.* 2009;87:3620–3625.

116. Staal JA, Dickson TC, Chung RS, Vickers JC. Cyclosporin-A treatment attenuates delayed cytoskeletal alterations and secondary axotomy following mild axonal stretch injury. *Dev Neurobiol.* 2007; 67(14):1831–1842.

117. Wu A, Ying Z, Gomez-Pinilla F. Omega-3 fatty acids supplementation restores mechanisms that maintain brain homeostasis in traumatic brain injury. *J Neurotrauma.* 2007;24:1587–1595.

118. Gilmer LK, Roberts KN, Joy K, Sullivan PG, Scheff SW. Early mitochondrial dysfunction after cortical contusion injury. *J Neurotrauma.* 2009;26:1271–1280.

119. Daugherty WP, Levasseur JE, Sun D, Rockswold GL, Bullock MR. Effects of hyperbaric oxygen therapy on cerebral oxygenation and mitochondrial function following moderate lateral fluid-percussion injury in rats. *J Neurosurg.* 2004;101:499–504.

120. Schuhmann MU, Stiller D, Skardelly M, et al. Metabolic changes in the vicinity of brain contusions: a proton magnetic resonance spectroscopy and histology study. *J Neurotrauma.* 2003;20:725–743.

121. Govindaraju V, Gauger GE, Manley GT, Ebel A, Meeker M, Maudsley AA. Volumetric proton spectroscopic imaging of mild traumatic brain injury. *AJNR Am J Neuroradiol.* 2004;25:730–737.

122. Garnett MR, Blamire AM, Corkill RG, Cadoux-Hudson TA, Rajagopalan B, Styles P. Early proton magnetic resonance spectroscopy in normal-appearing brain correlates with outcome in patients following traumatic brain injury. *Brain.* 2000;123(pt 10):2046–2054.

123. Son BC, Park CK, Choi BG, et al. Metabolic changes in pericontusional oedematous areas in mild head injury evaluated by 1H MRS. *Acta Neurochir Suppl.* 2000;76:13–16.

124. Cohen BA, Inglese M, Rusinek H, Babb JS, Grossman RI, Gonen O. Proton MR spectroscopy and MRI-volumetry in mild traumatic brain injury. *AJNR Am J Neuroradiol.* 2007;28:907–913.

125. Gasparovic C, Yeo R, Mannell M, et al. Neurometabolite concentrations in gray and white matter in mild traumatic brain injury: an 1H-magnetic resonance spectroscopy study. *J Neurotrauma.* 2009; 26:1635–1643.

126. Sarmento E, Moreira P, Brito C, Souza J, Jevoux C, Bigal M. Proton spectroscopy in patients with post-traumatic headache attributed to mild head injury. *Headache.* 2009;49:1345–1352.

127. Kirov I, Fleysher L, Babb JS, Silver JM, Grossman RI, Gonen O. Characterizing 'mild' in traumatic brain injury with proton MR spectroscopy in the thalamus: initial findings. *Brain Inj.* 2007;21: 1147–1154.

128. Vagnozzi R, Tavazzi B, Signoretti S, et al. Temporal window of metabolic brain vulnerability to concussions: mitochondrial-related impairment—part I. *Neurosurgery.* 2007;61(2):379–389.

129. Kalish H, Phillips TM. Analysis of neurotrophins in human serum by immunoaffinity capillary electrophoresis (ICE) following traumatic head injury. *J Chromatogr B Analyt Technol Biomed Life Sci.* 2010;878:194–200.

130. Rubovitch V, Edut S, Sarfstein R, Werner H, Pick CG. The intricate involvement of the Insulin-like growth factor receptor signaling in mild traumatic brain injury in mice. *Neurobiol Dis.* 2010;38:299–303.

131. Tashlykov V, Katz Y, Volkov A, et al. Minimal traumatic brain injury induce apoptotic cell death in mice. *J Mol Neurosci.* 2009;37: 16–24.

132. Tweedie D, Milman A, Holloway HW, et al. Apoptotic and behavioral sequelae of mild brain trauma in mice. *J Neurosci Res.* 2007; 85:805–815.

133. Ekmark-Lewen S, Lewen A, Israelsson C, et al. Vimentin and GFAP responses in astrocytes after contusion trauma to the murine brain. *Restor Neurol Neurosci.* 2010;28:311–321.

134. Lehmann C, Bette S, Engele J. High extracellular glutamate modulates expression of glutamate transporters and glutamine synthetase in cultured astrocytes. *Brain Res.* 2009;1297:1–8.

135. Whitney NP, Eidem TM, Peng H, Huang Y, Zheng JC. Inflammation mediates varying effects in neurogenesis: relevance to the pathogenesis of brain injury and neurodegenerative disorders. *J Neurochem.* 2009;108:1343–1359.

136. Atalay B, Caner H, Can A, Cekinmez M. Attenuation of microtubule associated protein-2 degradation after mild head injury by mexiletine and calpain-2 inhibitor. *Br J Neurosurg.* 2007;21:281–287.

137. Ma M, Lindsell CJ, Rosenberry CM, Shaw GJ, Zemlan FP. Serum cleaved tau does not predict postconcussion syndrome after mild traumatic brain injury. *Am J Emerg Med.* 2008;26:763–768.

138. Shapira M, Licht A, Milman A, Pick CG, Shohami E, Eldar-Finkelman H. Role of glycogen synthase kinase-3beta in early depressive behavior induced by mild traumatic brain injury. *Mol Cell Neurosci.* 2007;34:571–577.

139. Costa T, Constantino LC, Mendonca BP, et al. N-methyl-D-aspartate preconditioning improves short-term motor deficits outcome after mild traumatic brain injury in mice. *J Neurosci Res.* 2010;88: 1329–1337.

140. Ingebrigtsen T, Romner B. Biochemical serum markers for brain damage: a short review with emphasis on clinical utility in mild head injury. *Restor Neurol Neurosci.* 2003;21:171–176.

141. Ingebrigtsen T, Romner B. Biochemical serum markers of traumatic brain injury. *J Trauma.* 2002;52:798–808.

142. Vos PE, Verbeek MM. Brain specific proteins in serum: do they reliably reflect brain damage? *Shock.* 2002;18:481–482.

143. Hergenroeder GW, Redell JB, Moore AN, Dash PK. Biomarkers in the clinical diagnosis and management of traumatic brain injury. *Mol Diagn Ther.* 2008;12:345–358.

144. Dash PK, Zhao J, Hergenroeder G, Moore AN. Biomarkers for the diagnosis, prognosis, and evaluation of treatment efficacy for traumatic brain injury. *Neurotherapeutics.* 2010;7(1):100–114.

145. Korfias S, Papadimitriou A, Stranjalis G, et al. Serum biochemical markers of brain injury. *Mini Rev Med Chem.* 2009;9:227–234.

146. Kobeissy FH, Sadasivan S, Oli MW, et al. Neuroproteomics and systems biology-based discovery of protein biomarkers for traumatic brain injury and clinical validation. *Proteomics Clin Appl.* 2008;2(10–11):1467–1483.

147. Kövesdi E, Lückl J, Bukovics P, et al. Update on protein biomarkers in traumatic brain injury with emphasis on clinical use in adults and pediatrics. *Acta Neurochir.* 2010;152:1–17.

148. Mussack T, Biberthaler P, Kanz KG, et al. Immediate S-100B and neuron-specific enolase plasma measurements for rapid evaluation of primary brain damage in alcohol-intoxicated, minor head-injured patients. *Shock.* 2002;18:395–400.

149. Ytrebo LM, Nedredal GI, Korvald C, et al. Renal elimination of protein S-100beta in pigs with acute encephalopathy. *Scand J Clin Lab Invest.* 2001;61(3):217–225.

150. Herrmann M, Curio N, Jost S, Wunderlich MT, Synowitz H, Wallesch CW. Protein S-100B and neuron specific enolase as early neurobiochemical markers of the severity of traumatic brain injury. *Restor Neurol Neurosci.* 1999;14:109–114.

151. Stalnacke BM, Bjornstig U, Karlsson K, Sojka P. One-year follow-up of mild traumatic brain injury: post-concussion symptoms, disabilities and life satisfaction in relation to serum levels of S-100B and neurone-specific enolase in acute phase. *J Rehabil Med.* 2005; 37:300–305.

152. Romner B, Ingebrigtsen T, Kongstad P, Borgesen SE. Traumatic brain damage: serum S-100 protein measurements related to neuroradiological findings. *J Neurotrauma.* 2000;17:641–647.

153. Herrmann M, Curio N, Jost S, et al. Release of biochemical markers of damage to neuronal and glial brain tissue is associated with short and long term neuropsychological outcome after traumatic brain injury. *J Neurol Neurosurg Psychiatry.* 2001;70(1):95–100.

154. Jönsson H, Johnsson P, Hoglund P, Alling C, Blomquist S. Elimination of S100B and renal function after cardiac surgery. *J Cardiothorac Vasc Anesth.* 2000;14(6):698–701.

155. Ingebrigtsen T, Romner B. Serial S-100 protein serum measurements related to early magnetic resonance imaging after minor head injury. Case report. *J Neurosurg.* 1996;85(5):945–948.

156. Biberthaler P, Mussack T, Wiedemann E, et al. Influence of alcohol exposure on S-100b serum levels. *Acta Neurochir Suppl.* 2000;76: 177–179.

157. Mussack T, Biberthaler P, Kanz KG, et al. Serum S-100B and interleukin-8 as predictive markers for comparative neurologic outcome analysis of patients after cardiac arrest and severe traumatic brain injury. *Crit Care Med.* 2002;30:2669–2674.

158. de Kruijk JR, Leffers P, Menheere PP, Meerhoff S, Twijnstra A. S-100B and neuron-specific enolase in serum of mild traumatic brain injury patients. A comparison with health controls. *Acta Neurol Scand.* 2001;103(3):175–179.

159. Biberthaler P, Mussack T, Wiedemann E, et al. Evaluation of S-100b as a specific marker for neuronal damage due to minor head trauma. *World J Surg.* 2001;25:93–97.

160. Biberthaler P, Mussack T, Wiedemann E, et al. Elevated serum levels of S-100B reflect the extent of brain injury in alcohol intoxicated patients after mild head trauma. *Shock.* 2001;16:97–101.

161. Lange RT, Brubacher JR, Iverson GL, Procyshyn RM, Mitrovic S. Differential effects of alcohol intoxication on S100B levels following traumatic brain injury. *J Trauma.* 2010;68:1065–1071.

162. Lange RT, Iverson GL, Brubacher JR. Clinical utility of the protein S100B to evaluate traumatic brain injury in the presence of acute alcohol intoxication. *J Head Trauma Rehabil.* 2012;27(2):123–134.

163. Castellani C, Bimbashi P, Ruttenstock E, Sacherer P, Stojakovic T, Weinberg AM. Neuroprotein s-100B—a useful parameter in paediatric patients with mild traumatic brain injury? *Acta Paediatr.* 2009; 98(10):1607–1612.

164. Muller K, Townend W, Biasca N, et al. S100B serum level predicts computed tomography findings after minor head injury. *J Trauma.* 2007;62:1452–1456.

165. Townend WJ, Guy MJ, Pani MA, Martin B, Yates DW. Head injury outcome prediction in the emergency department: a role for protein S-100B? *J Neurol Neurosurg Psychiatry.* 2002;73:542–546.

166. Žurek J, Bartlova L, Marek L, Fedora M. Serum S100B protein as a molecular marker of severity in traumatic brain injury in children. *Cesk Slov Neurol N.* 2010;1:37–44.

167. Murillo-Cabezas F, Muñoz-Sánchez MÁ, Rincón-Ferrari MD, et al. The prognostic value of the temporal course of the S100β protein in post-acute severe brain injury: a prospective and observational study. *Brain Inj.* 2010;24:609–619.

168. Stranjalis G, Korfias S, Papapetrou C, et al. Elevated serum S-100B protein as a predictor of failure to short-term return to work or activities after mild head injury. *J Neurotrauma*. 2004;21:1070–1075.

169. Ingebrigtsen T, Romner B, Marup-Jensen S, et al. The clinical value of serum S-100 protein measurements in minor head injury: a Scandinavian multicentre study. *Brain Inj*. 2000;14:1047–1055.

170. Stapert S, de Kruijk J, Houx P, Menheere P, Twijnstra A, Jolles J. S-100B concentration is not related to neurocognitive performance in the first month after mild traumatic brain injury. *Eur Neurol*. 2005;53:22–26.

171. Undén J, Romner B. A new objective method for CT triage after minor head injury—serum S100B. *Scand J Clin Lab Invest*. 2009; 69(1):13–17.

172. Ingebrigtsen T, Waterloo K, Jacobsen EA, Langbakk B, Romner B. Traumatic brain damage in minor head injury: relation of serum S-100 protein measurements to magnetic resonance imaging and neurobehavioral outcome. *Neurosurgery*. 1999;45(3):468–476.

173. Anderson RE, Hansson LO, Nilsson O, Dijlai-Merzoug R, Settergren G. High serum S100B levels for trauma patients without head injuries. *Neurosurgery*. 2001;48:1255–1260.

174. Stalnacke BM, Tegner Y, Sojka P. Playing soccer increases serum concentrations of the biochemical markers of brain damage S-100B and neuron-specific enolase in elite players: a pilot study. *Brain Inj*. 2004;18:899–909.

175. Stalnacke BM, Tegner Y, Sojka P. Playing ice hockey and basketball increases serum levels of S-100B in elite players: a pilot study. *Clin J Sport Med*. 2003;13:292–302.

176. Otto M, Holthusen S, Bahn E, et al. Boxing and running lead to a rise in serum levels of S-100B protein. *Int J Sports Med*. 2000;21: 551–555.

177. Waterloo K, Ingebrigtsen T, Romner B. Neuropsychological function in patients with increased serum levels of protein S-100 after minor head injury. *Acta Neurochir (Wien)*. 1997;139:26–32.

178. Pelinka LE, Hertz H, Mauritz W, et al. Nonspecific increase of systemic neuron-specific enolase after trauma: clinical and experimental findings. *Shock*. 2005;24(2):119–123.

179. Guzel A, Er U, Tatli M, et al. Serum neuron-specific enloase as a predictor of short-term outcome and its correlation with Glasgow Coma Scale in traumatic brain injury. *Neurosurg Rev*. 2008;31: 439–445.

180. Yamazaki Y, Yada K, Morii S, Kitahara T, Ohwada T. Diagnostic significance of serum neuron-specific enolase and myelin basic protein assay in patients with acute head injury. *Surg Neurol*. 1995; 43:267–271.

181. Ross SA, Cunningham RT, Johnston CF, Rowlands BJ. Neuron-specific enolase as an aid to outcome prediction in head injury. *Br J Neurosurg*. 1996;10:471–476.

182. McKeating EG, Andrews PJD, Mascia L. Relationship of neuron specific enolase and protein S-100 concentrations in systemic and jugular venous serum to injury severity and outcome after traumatic brain injury. *Acta Neurochir Suppl*. 1998;71:117–119.

183. Skogseid IM, Nordby HK, Urdal P, Paus E, Lilleaas F. Increased serum creatine kinase BB and neuron specific enolase following head injury indicates brain damage. *Acta Neurochir (Wien)*. 1992; 115:106–111.

184. Herrmann M, Jost S, Kutz S, et al. Temporal profile of release of neurobiochemical markers of brain damage after traumatic brain injury is associated with intracranial pathology as demonstrated in cranial computerized tomography. *J Neurotrauma*. 2000;17:113–122.

185. Ergun R, Bostanci U, Akdemir G, et al. Prognostic value of serum neuron-specific enolase levels after head injury. *Neurol Res*. 1998; 20:418–420.

186. Raabe A, Grolms C, Keller M, Döhnert J, Sorge O, Seifert V. Correlation of computed tomography findings and serum brain damage markers following severe head injury. *Acta Neurochir (Wien)*. 1998; 140:787–792.

187. Dauberschmidt R, Marangos PJ, Zinsmeyer J, Bender V, Klages G, Gross J. Severe head trauma and the changes of concentration of neuron-specific enolase in plasma and in cerebrospinal fluid. *Clin Chim Acta*. 1983;131:165–170.

188. Woertgen C, Rothoerl RD, Holzschuh M, Metz C, Brawanski A. Comparison of serial S-100 and NSE serum measurements after severe head injury. *Acta Neurochir (Wien)*. 1997;139:1161–1165.

189. Vos PE, Lamers KJB, Hendriks JCM, et al. Glial and neuronal proteins in serum predict outcome after severe traumatic brain injury. *Neurology*. 2004;62:1303–1310.

190. Finsterer J, Exner M, Rumpold H. Cerebrospinal fluid neuron-specific enolase in non-selected patients. *Scand J Clin Lab Invest*. 2004; 64:553–558.

191. Johnsson P. Markers of cerebral ischemia after cardiac surgery. *J Cardiothorac Vasc Anesth*. 1996;10(1):120–126.

192. Kaste M, Hernesniemi J, Somer H, Hillbom M, Konttinen A. Creatine kinase isoenyzmes in acute brain injury. *J Neurosurg*. 1981; 55:511–515.

193. Nordby HK, Urdal P. Creatine kinase BB in blood as index of prognosis and effect of treatment after severe head injury. *Acta Neurochir*. 1985;76:131–136.

194. Rabow L, Hedman G. CKBB-isoenzymes as a sign of cerebral injury. *Acta Neurochir Suppl*. 1979;28:108–112.

195. Cooper PR, Chalif DJ, Ramsey JF, Moore RJ. Radioimmunoassay of the brain type isoenyzme of creatine phosphokinase (CK-BB): a new diagnostic tool in the evaluation of patients with head injury. *Neurosurgery*. 1983;12:536–541.

196. Phillips JP, Jones HM, Hitchcock R, Adams N, Thompson RJ. Radioimmunoassay of serum creatine kinase BB as index of brain damage after head injury. *Br Med J*. 1980;281:777–779.

197. Bakay RAE, Ward AA. Enzymatic changes in serum and cerebrospinal fluid in neurological injury. *J Neurosurg*. 1983;58:27–37.

198. Levitt MA, Cook LAS, Simon BC, Williams V. Biochemical markers of cerebral injury in patients with minor head trauma and ethanol intoxication. *Acad Emerg Med*. 1995;2:675–680.

199. Carr ME, Masullo Ln, Brown JK, Lewis PC. Creatine kinase BB isoenyzme blood levels in trauma patients with suspected mild traumatic brain injury. *Mil Med*. 2009;174:622–625.

200. Nordby HK, Urdal P, Bjørnæs H. The prognosis of patients with concussion and increased creatine kinase BB in the cerebrospinal fluid. *Acta Neurochir*. 1984;71:205–215.

201. Berger RP, Beers SR, Richichi R, Wiesman D, Adelson PD. Serum biomarker concentrations and outcome after pediatric traumatic brain injury. *J Neurotrauma*. 2007;24:1793–1801.

202. Thomas DG, Palfreyman JW, Ratcliffe JG. Serum-myelin-basic-protein assay in diagnosis and prognosis of patients with head injury. *Lancet*. 1978;1(8056):113–115.

203. Berger RP, Adelson PD, Pierce MC, Dulani T, Cassidy LD, Kochanek PM. Serum neuron-specific enolase, S100B, and myelin basic protein concentrations after inflicted and noninflicted traumatic brain injury in children. *J Neurosurg*. 2005;103:61–68.

204. Missler U, Wiesmann M, Wittmann G, Magerkurth O, Hagenström H. Measurement of glial fibrillary acidic protein in human blood: analytic method and preliminary clinical results. *Clin Chem*. 1999;45: 138–141.

205. Nylen K, Öst M, Csajbok LZ, et al. Increased serum-GFAP in patients with severe traumatic brain injury is related to outcome. *J Neurol Sci*. 2006;240:85–91.

206. Pelinka LE, Kroepel A, Schmidhammer R, et al. Glial fibrillary acidic protein in serum after traumatic brain injury and multiple trauma. *J Trauma*. 2004;57:1006–1012.

207. Pelinka LE, Kroepel A, Leixnering M, Buchinger W, Raabe A, Redl H. GFAP versus S100B in serum after traumatic brain injury: relationship to brain damage and outcome. *J Neurotrauma*. 2004;21: 1553–1561.

208. Lumpkins KM, Bochicchio GV, Keledjian K, Simard JM, McCunn M, Scalea T. Glial fibrillary acidic protein is highly correlated with brain injury. *J Trauma*. 2008;65:778–784.

209. Glatz JF, Vusse GC. Cellular fatty acid-binding proteins: their function and physiological significance. *Prog Lipid Res*. 1996;35(3): 243–282.

210. Pelsers MM, Hanhoff T, Van der Voort D, et al. Brain- and heart-type fatty acid-binding proteins in the brain: tissue distribution and clinical utility. *Clin Chem*. 2004;50(9):1568–1575.

211. Sergeant N, Delacourte A, Buée L. Tau protein as a differential biomarker of tauopathies. *Biochim Biophys Acta.* 2005;1739(2–3): 179–197.

212. Kavalci C, Pekdemir M, Durukan P, et al. The value of serum tau protein for the diagnosis of intracranial injury in minor head trauma. *Am J Emerg Med.* 2007;25:391–395.

213. Shaw GJ, Jauch EC, Zemlan FP. Serum cleaved tau protein levels and clinical outcome in adult patients with closed head injury. *Ann Emerg Med.* 2002;39:254–257.

214. Zemlan FP, Jauch EC, Mulchahey JJ, et al. C-tau biomarker of neuronal damage in severe brain injured patients: association with elevated intracranial pressure and clinical outcome. *Brain Res.* 2002; 947:131–139.

215. Zemlan FP, Rosenberg WS, Leubbe PA, et al. Quantification of axonal damage in traumatic brain injury: affinity purification and characterization of cerebrospinal fluid tau proteins. *J Neurochem.* 1999;72:741–750.

216. Öst M, Nylen K, Csajbok LZ, et al. Initial CSF total tau correlates with 1-year outcome in patients with traumatic brain injury. *Neurology.* 2006;67:1600–1604.

217. Chatfield DA, Zemlan FP, Menon DK. Discordant temporal patterns of S100β and cleaved tau protein elevation after head injury: a pilot study. *Br J Neurosurg.* 2002;16:471–476.

218. Bazarian JJ, Zemlan FP, Mookerjee S, Stigbrand T. Serum S-100B and cleaved-tau are poor predictors of long-term outcome after mild traumatic brain injury. *Brain Inj.* 2006;20:759–765.

219. Balut M, Koksal O, Dogan S, et al. Tau protein as a serum marker of brain damage in mild traumatic brain injury: preliminary results. *Adv Ther.* 2006;23(1):12–22.

220. Alzate O. Neuroproteomics. In: Alzate O, ed. *Neuroproteomics.* Boca Raton, FL: CRC Press; 2010:1–16.

221. Wang KK, Ottens AK, Liu MC, et al. Proteomic identification of biomarkers of traumatic brain injury. *Expert Rev Proteomics.* 2005; 2(4):603–614.

222. Ottens AK, Kobeissy FH, Fuller BF, et al. Novel neuroproteomic approaches to studying traumatic brain injury. *Prog Brain Res.* 2007; 161:401–418.

223. Burgess JA, Lescuyer P, Hainard A, et al. Identification of brain cell death associated with proteins in human post-mortem cerebrospinal fluid. *J Proteome Res.* 2006;5:1674–1681.

224. Opii WO, Nukala VN, Sultana R, et al. Proteomic identification of oxidized mitochondrial proteins following experimental traumatic brain injury. *J Neurotrauma.* 2007;24:772–789.

225. Kochanek PM, Kline AE, Gao W, et al. Gel-based hippocampal proteomic analysis 2 weeks following traumatic brain injury to immature rats using controlled cortical impact. *Dev Neurosci.* 2006; 28:410–419.

226. Jenkins LW, Peters GW, Dixon CE, et al. Conventional and functional proteomics using large format two-dimensional gel electrophoresis 24 hours after controlled cortical impact in postnatal day 17 rats. *J Neurotrauma.* 2002;19:715–740.

227. Yao C, Williams AJ, Ottens AK, et al. Detection of protein biomarkers using high-throughput immunoblotting following focal ischemic or penetrating ballistic-like brain injuries in rats. *Brain Inj.* 2008;22:723–732.

228. Yao C, Williams AJ, Ottens AK, et al. P43/pro-EMAPII: a potential biomarker for discriminating traumatic versus ischemic brain injury. *J Neurotrauma.* 2009;26:1295–1305.

229. Zhang Z, Ottens AK, Sadasivan S, et al. Calpain-mediated collapsin response mediator protein-1, -2, and -4 proteolysis after neurotoxic and traumatic brain injury. *J Neurotrauma.* 2007;24:460–472.

230. Liu MC, Akinyi L, Scharf D, et al. Ubiquitin C-terminal hydrolase-L1 as a biomarker for ischemic and traumatic brain injury in rats. *Eur J Neurosci.* 2010;31:722–732.

231. Siman R, Toraskar N, Dang A, et al. A panel of neuron-enriched proteins as markers for traumatic brain injury in humans. *J Neurotrauma.* 2009;26:1867–1877.

232. Haqqani AS, Hutchison JS, Ward R, Stanimirovic DS. Protein biomarkers in serum of pediatric patients with severe traumatic brain injury identified by ICAT-LC-MS/MS. *J Neurotrauma.* 2007;24: 54–74.

233. Zhang Z, Majava V, Greffier A, Hayes RL, Kursula P, Wang KKW. Collapsin response mediator protein-2 is a calmodulin-binding protein. *Cell Mol Life Sci.* 2009;66:526–536.

234. Gao W, Chadha MS, Berger RP, et al. A gel-based proteomic comparison of human cerebrospinal fluid between inflicted and noninflicted pediatric traumatic brain injury. *J Neurotrauma.* 2007;24: 43–53.

235. Hergenroeder G, Redell JB, Moore AN, et al. Identification of serum biomarkers in brain-injured adults: potential for predicting elevated intracranial pressure. *J Neurotrauma.* 2008;25:79–93.

236. Brophy GM, Mondello S, Papa L, et al. Biokinetic analysis of ubiquitin C-terminal hydrolase-L1 (UCH-L1) in severe traumatic brain injury patient biofluids. *J Neurotrauma.* 2011;28:861–870.

237. Papa L, Akinyi L, Liu MC, et al. Ubiquitin C-terminal hydrolase is a novel biomarker in humans for severe traumatic brain injury. *Crit Care Med.* 2010;38:138–144.

238. Mondello S, Papa L, Buki A, et al. Neuronal and glial markers are differently associated with computed tomography findings and outcome *Crit Care.* 2011;15:R156.

239. Farkas O, Polgar B, Szekeres-Bartho J, Doczi T, Povlishock JT, Buki A. Spectrin breakdown products in the cerebrospinal fluid in severe head injury—preliminary observations. *Acta Neurochir (Wien).* 2005;147(8):855–861.

240. Cardali S, Maugeri R. Detection of αII-spectrin and breakdown products in humans after severe traumatic brain injury. *J Neurosurg Sci.* 2006;50:25–31.

241. Pineda JA, Lewis PC, Valadka A, et al. Clinical significance of αII-spectrin breakdown products in cerebrospinal fluid after severe traumatic brain injury. *J Neurotrauma.* 2007;24:354–366.

242. Brophy GM, Pineda JA, Papa L, et al. αII-spectrin breakdown product cerebrospinal fluid exposure metrics suggest differences in cellular injury mechanisms after severe traumatic brain injury. *J Neurotrauma.* 2009;26:471–479.

243. Mondello S, Robicsek SA, Gabrielli A, et alL. αII-spectrin breakdown products (SBDPs): diagnosis and outcome in severe traumatic brain injury patients. *J Neurotrauma.* 2010;27:1203–1213.

244. Broglio SP, Puetz TW. The effect of sport concussion on neurocognitive function, self-report symptoms and postural control : a meta-analysis. *Sports Med.* 2008;38:53–67.

245. Bleiberg J, Cernich AN, Cameron K, et al. Duration of cognitive impairment after sports concussion. *Neurosurgery.* 2004;54:1073–1080.

246. Lovell MR, Collins MW, Iverson GL, Johnston KM, Bradley JP. Grade 1 or "ding" concussions in high school athletes. *Am J Sports Med.* 2004;32:47–54.

247. Macciocchi SN, Barth JT, Alves W, Rimel RW, Jane JA. Neuropsychological functioning and recovery after mild head injury in collegiate athletes. *Neurosurgery.* 1996;39:510–514.

248. McCrea M, Guskiewicz KM, Marshall SW, et al. Acute effects and recovery time following concussion in collegiate football players: the NCAA Concussion Study. *JAMA.* 2003;290:2556–2563.

249. McCrea M, Kelly JP, Randolph C, Cisler R, Berger L. Immediate neurocognitive effects of concussion. *Neurosurgery.* 2002;50: 1032–1040.

250. Hughes DG, Jackson A, Mason DL, Berry E, Hollis S, Yates DW. Abnormalities on magnetic resonance imaging seen acutely following mild traumatic brain injury: correlation with neuropsychological tests and delayed recovery. *Neuroradiology.* 2004;46:550–558.

251. Hugenholtz H, Stuss DT, Stethem LL, Richard MT. How long does it take to recover from a mild concussion? *Neurosurgery.* 1988;22: 853–858.

252. Levin HS, Mattis S, Ruff RM, et al. Neurobehavioral outcome following minor head injury: a three-center study. *J Neurosurg.* 1987; 66:234–243.

253. Ponsford J, Willmott C, Rothwell A, et al. Factors influencing outcome following mild traumatic brain injury in adults. *J Int Neuropsychol Soc.* 2000;6:568–579.

254. Mathias JL, Beall JA, Bigler ED. Neuropsychological and information processing deficits following mild traumatic brain injury. *J Int Neuropsychol Soc.* 2004;10:286–297.

255. Pellman EJ, Lovell MR, Viano DC, Casson IR, Tucker AM. Concussion in professional football: neuropsychological testing—part 6. *Neurosurgery.* 2004;55(6):1290–1305.

256. Gentilini M, Nichelli P, Schoenhuber R, et al. Neuropsychological evaluation of mild head injury. *J Neurol Neurosurg Psychiatry.* 1985; 48:137–140.

257. Lahmeyer HW, Bellur SN. Cardiac regulation and depression. *J Psychiatry Res.* 1987;21:1–6.

258. Binder LM. A review of mild head trauma. Part II: clinical implications. *J Clin Exp Neuropsychol.* 1997;19:432–457.

259. McCrea M, Iverson GL, McAllister TW, et al. An integrated review of recovery after mild traumatic brain injury (MTBI): implications for clinical management. *Clin Neuropsychol.* 2009;23:1368–1390.

260. Rohling ML, Larrabee GJ, Millis SR. The "Miserable Minority" following mild traumatic brain injury: who are they and do meta-analyses hide them? *Clin Neuropsychol.* 2012;26(2):197–213.

261. Rohling ML, Binder LM, Demakis GJ, Larrabee GJ, Ploetz DM, Langhinrichsen-Rohling J. A meta-analysis of neuropsychological outcome after mild traumatic brain injury: re-analyses and reconsiderations of Binder et al. (1997), Frencham et al. (2005), and Pertab et al. (2009). *Clin Neuropsychol.* 2011;25:608–623.

262. Gronwall D. Rehabilitation programs for patients with mild head injury: components, problems, and evaluation. *J Head Trauma Rehabil.* 1986;1:53–62.

263. Kay T. Neuropsychological treatment of mild traumatic brain injury. *J Head Trauma Rehabil.* 1993;8:74–85.

264. Wrightson P. Management of disability and rehabilitation services after mild head injury. In: Levin HS, Eisenberg HM, Benton AL, eds. *Mild Head Injury.* New York, NY: Oxford University Press; 1989:245–256.

265. Minderhoud JM, Boelens ME, Huizenga J, Saan RJ. Treatment of minor head injuries. *Clin Neurol Neurosurg.* 1980;82:127–140.

266. Relander M, Troupp H, Af Björkesten G. Controlled trial of treatment for cerebral concussion. *Br Med J.* 1972;4(5843):777–779.

267. Al Sayegh A, Sandford D, Carson AJ. Psychological approaches to treatment of postconcussion syndrome: a systematic review. *J Neurol Neurosurg Psychiatry.* 2010;81:1128–1134.

268. Snell DL, Surgenor LJ, Hay-Smith EJ, Siegert RJ. A systematic review of psychological treatments for mild traumatic brain injury: an update on the evidence. *J Clin Exp Neuropsychol.* 2009;31:20–38.

269. Ponsford J, Willmott C, Rothwell A, et al. Cognitive and behavioral outcome following mild traumatic head injury in children. *J Head Trauma Rehabil.* 1999;14:360–372.

270. Paniak C, Toller-Lobe G, Durand A, Nagy J. A randomized trial of two treatments for mild traumatic brain injury. *Brain Inj.* 1998; 12:1011–1023.

271. Ponsford J, Willmott C, Rothwell A, et al. Impact of early intervention on outcome after mild traumatic brain injury in children. *Pediatrics.* 2001;108:1297–1303.

272. Mittenberg W, Tremont G, Zielinski RE, Fichera S, Rayls KR. Cognitive-behavioral prevention of postconcussion syndrome. *Arch Clin Neuropsychol.* 1996;11:139–145.

273. Paniak C, Toller-Lobe G, Reynolds S, Melnyk A, Nagy J. A randomized trial of two treatments for mild traumatic brain injury: 1 year follow-up. *Brain Inj.* 2000;14:219–226.

274. Ponsford J, Willmott C, Rothwell A, et al. Impact of early intervention on outcome following mild head injury in adults. *J Neurol Neurosurg Psychiatry.* 2002;73:330–332.

275. Wade DT, King NS, Wenden FJ, Crawford S, Caldwell FE. Routine follow up after head injury: a second randomised controlled trial. *J Neurol Neurosurg Psychiatry.* 1998;65(2):177–183.

276. Bell KR, Hoffman JM, Temkin NR, et al. The effect of telephone counselling on reducing post-traumatic symptoms after mild traumatic brain injury: a randomised trial. *J Neurol Neurosurg Psychiatry.* 2008;79:1275–1281.

277. Wade DT, Crawford S, Wenden FJ, King NS, Moss NE. Does routine follow up after head injury help? A randomised controlled trial. *J Neurol Neurosurg Psychiatry.* 1997;62:478–484.

278. Alves W, Macciocchi SN, Barth JT. Postconcussive symptoms after uncomplicated mild head injury. *J Head Trauma Rehabil.* 1993;8: 48–59.

279. Borg J, Holm L, Peloso PM, et al; for WHO Collaborating Centre Task Force on Mild Traumatic Brain Injury. Non-surgical intervention and cost for mild traumatic brain injury: results of the WHO Collaborating Centre Task Force on Mild Traumatic Brain Injury. *J Rehabil Med.* 2004;(43)(suppl):76–83.

280. Shames J, Treger I, Ring H, Giaquinto S. Return to work following traumatic brain injury: trends and challenges. *Disabil Rehabil.* 2007; 29:1387–1395.

281. Dikmen S, Temkin NR, Machamer JE, Holubkov AL, Fraser RT, Winn HR. Employment following traumatic head injuries. *Arch Neurol.* 1994;51:177–186.

282. Kraus J, Schaffer K, Ayers K, Stenehjem J, Shen H, Afifi AA. Physical complaints, medical service use, and social and employment changes following mild traumatic brain injury: a 6-month longitudinal study. *J Head Trauma Rehabil.* 2005;20:239–256.

283. Wrightson P, Gronwall D. Time off work and symptoms after minor head injury. *Injury.* 1981;12:445–454.

284. Andersson EE, Bedics BK, Falkmer T. Mild traumatic brain injuries: a 10-year follow-up. *J Rehabil Med.* 2011;43:323–329.

285. Cifu DX, Keyser-Marcus L, Lopez E, et al. Acute predictors of successful return to work 1 year after traumatic brain injury: a multicenter analysis. *Arch Phys Med Rehabil.* 1997;78:125–131.

286. Mazaux JM, Masson F, Levin HS, Alaoui P, Maurette P, Barat M. Long-term neuropsychological outcome and loss of social autonomy after traumatic brain injury. *Arch Phys Med Rehabil.* 1997;78: 1316–1320.

287. Ponsford JL, Olver JH, Curran C, Ng K. Prediction of employment status 2 years after traumatic brain injury. *Brain Inj.* 1995;9:11–20.

288. Stambrook M, Moore AD, Peters LC, Deviaene C, Hawryluk GA. Effects of mild, moderate and severe closed head injury on long-term vocational status. *Brain Inj.* 1990;4:183–190.

289. Franulic A, Carbonell CG, Pinto P, Sepulveda I. Psychosocial adjustment and employment outcome 2, 5 and 10 years after TBI. *Brain Inj.* 2004;18:119–129.

290. Keyser-Marcus LA, Bricout JC, Wehman P, et al. Acute predictors of return to employment after traumatic brain injury: a longitudinal follow-up. *Arch Phys Med Rehabil.* 2002;83:635–641.

291. Spikman JM, Timmerman ME, Zomeren van AH, Deelman BG. Recovery versus retest effects in attention after closed head injury. *J Clin Exp Neuropsychol.* 1999;21:585–605.

292. Ip RY, Dornan J, Schentag C. Traumatic brain injury: factors predicting return to work or school. *Brain Inj.* 1995;9:517–532.

293. Gollaher K, High W, Sherer M, et al. Prediction of employment outcome one to three years following traumatic brain injury (TBI). *Brain Inj.* 1998;12:255–263.

294. McCullagh S, Oucherlony D, Protzner A, Blair N, Feinstein A. Prediction of neuropsychiatric outcome following mild trauma brain injury: an examination of the Glasgow Coma Scale. *Brain Inj.* 2001; 15:489–497.

295. Vanderploeg RD, Curtiss G, Duchnick JJ, Luis CA. Demographic, medical, and psychiatric factors in work and marital status after mild head injury. *J Head Trauma Rehabil.* 2003;18:148–163.

296. Kendler KS, Thornton LM, Gardner CO. Genetic risk, number of previous depressive episodes, and stressful life events in predicting onset of major depression. *Am J Psychiatry.* 2001;158:582–586.

297. Kendler KS, Thornton LM, Gardner CO. Stressful life events and previous episodes in the etiology of major depression in women: an evaluation of the "kindling" hypothesis. *Am J Psychiatry.* 2000; 157:1243–1251.

298. Monroe SM, Harkness KL. Life stress, the "kindling" hypothesis, and the recurrence of depression: considerations from a life stress perspective. *Psychol Rev.* 2005;112:417–445.

299. Binder EB, Nemeroff CB. The CRF system, stress, depression and anxiety-insights from human genetic studies. *Mol Psychiatry.* 2009.

300. Hauger RL, Risbrough V, Oakley RH, Olivares-Reyes JA, Dautzenberg FM. Role of CRF receptor signaling in stress vulnerability, anxiety, and depression. *Ann N Y Acad Sci.* 2009;1179:120–143.

301. McGuffin P, Knight J, Breen G, et al. Whole genome linkage scan of recurrent depressive disorder from the depression network study. *Hum Mol Genet.* 2005;14:3337–3345.

302. Sullivan PF, Neale MC, Kendler KS. Genetic epidemiology of major depression: review and meta-analysis. *Am J Psychiatry*. 2000;157: 1552–1562.

303. Bradley RG, Binder EB, Epstein MP, et al. Influence of child abuse on adult depression: moderation by the corticotropin-releasing hormone receptor gene. *Arch Gen Psychiatry*. 2008;65:190–200.

304. Heim C, Newport DJ, Mletzko T, Miller AH, Nemeroff CB. The link between childhood trauma and depression: insights from HPA axis studies in humans. *Psychoneuroendocrinology*. 2008;33:693–710.

305. Heim C, Bradley B, Mletzko TC, et al. Effect of childhood trauma on adult depression and neuroendocrine function: sex-specific moderation by CRH receptor 1 gene. *Front Behav Neurosci*. 2009;3: 1–10.

306. Gatt JM, Nemeroff CB, Dobson-Stone C, et al. Interactions between BDNF Val66Met polymorphism and early life stress predict brain and arousal pathways to syndromal depression and anxiety. *Mol Psychiatry*. 2009;14:681–695.

307. Farmer AE, McGuffin P. Humiliation, loss and other types of life events and difficulties: a comparison of depressed subjects, healthy controls and their siblings. *Psychol Med*. 2003;33:1169–1175.

308. Friis RH, Wittchen HU, Pfister H, Lieb R. Life events and changes in the course of depression in young adults. *Eur Psychiatry*. 2002; 17:241–253.

309. Kendler KS, Hettema JM, Butera F, Gardner CO, Prescott CA. Life event dimensions of loss, humiliation, entrapment, and danger in the prediction of onsets of major depression and generalized anxiety. *Arch Gen Psychiatry*. 2003;60:789–796.

310. Kendler KS, Karkowski LM, Prescott CA. Causal relationship between stressful life events and the onset of major depression. *Am J Psychiatry*. 1999;156:837–841.

311. Kreutzer JS, Seel RT, Gourley E. The prevalence and symptom rates of depression after traumatic brain injury: a comprehensive examination. *Brain Inj*. 2001;15:563–576.

312. Seel RT, Kreutzer JS, Rosenthal M, Hammond FM, Corrigan JD, Black K. Depression after traumatic brain injury: a National Institute on Disability and Rehabilitation Research Model Systems multicenter investigation. *Arch Phys Med Rehabil*. 2003;84(2):177–184.

313. Silver JM, Kramer R, Greenwald S, Weissman M. The association between head injuries and psychiatric disorders: findings from the New Haven NIMH Epidemiologic Catchment Area Study. *Brain Inj*. 2001;15:935–945.

314. Jorge RE, Robinson RG, Starkstein SE, Arndt SV. Depression and anxiety following traumatic brain injury. *J Neuropsychiatry Clin Neurosci*. 1993;5:369–374.

315. Varney N, Martzke J, Roberts R. Major depression in patients with closed head injury. *Neuropsychology*. 1987;1:7–8.

316. Goldstein FC, Levin HS, Goldman WP, Clark AN, Altonen TK. Cognitive and neurobehavioral functioning after mild versus moderate traumatic brain injury in older adults. *J Int Neuropsychol Soc*. 2001;7:373–383.

317. Mooney G, Speed J. The association between mild traumatic brain injury and psychiatric conditions. *Brain Inj*. 2001;15:865–877.

318. Levin HS, McCauley SR, Josic CP, et al. Predicting depression following mild traumatic brain injury. *Arch Gen Psychiatry*. 2005;62: 523–528.

319. Levin HS, Brown SA, Song JX, et al. Depression and posttraumatic stress disorder at three months after mild to moderate traumatic brain injury. *J Clin Exp Neuropsychol*. 2001;23:754–769.

320. McCauley SR, Boake C, Levin HS, Contant CF, Song JX. Postconcussional disorder following mild to moderate traumatic brain injury: anxiety, depression, and social support as risk factors and comorbidities. *J Clin Exp Neuropsychol*. 2001;23:792–808.

321. Horner MD, Ferguson PL, Selassie AW, Labbate LA, Kniele K, Corrigan JD. Patterns of alcohol use 1 year after traumatic brain injury: a population-based, epidemiological study. *J Int Neuropsychol Soc*. 2005;11:322–330.

322. Parker RS, Rosenblum A. IQ loss and emotional dysfunctions after mild head injury incurred in a motor vehicle accident. *J Clin Psychol*. 1996;52:32–43.

323. Chamelian L, Feinstein A. Outcome after mild to moderate traumatic brain injury: the role of dizziness. *Arch Phys Med Rehabil*. 2004;85:1662–1666.

324. Federoff JP, Starkstein SE, Forrester AW, et al. Depression in patients with acute traumatic brain injury. *Am J Psychiatry*. 1992;149: 918–923.

325. Hibbard MR, Ashman TA, Spielman LA, Chun D, Charatz HJ, Melvin S. Relationship between depression and psychosocial functioning after traumatic brain injury. *Arch Phys Med Rehabil*. 2004; 85:S43–53.

326. Bombardier CH, Fann JR, Temkin NR, Esselman PC, Barber J, Dikmen SS. Rates of major depressive disorder and clinical outcomes following traumatic brain injury. *JAMA*. 2010;303:1938–1945.

327. American Psychiatric Association. *Diagnostic and Statistical Manual of Mental Disorders. Fourth Edition. Text Revision*. Washington, DC: American Psychiatric Association; 2000.

328. Iverson GL. Misdiagnosis of persistent postconcussion syndrome in patients with depression. *Arch Clin Neuropsychol*. 2006;21: 303–310.

329. Lange RT, Iverson GL, Rose A. Depression strongly influences postconcussion symptom reporting following mild traumatic brain injury. *J Head Trauma Rehabil*. 2011;26:127–137.

330. Foa EB, Cashman L, Jaycox L, Perry K. The validation of a self-report measure of posttraumatic stress disorder: the Posttraumatic Diagnostic Scale. *Psychol Assess*. 1997;9:445–451.

331. Franklin CL, Zimmerman M. Posttraumatic stress disorder and major depressive disorder: investigating the role of overlapping symptoms in diagnostic comorbidity. *J Nerv Ment Dis*. 2001;189: 548–551.

332. Kessler RC, Sonnega A, Bromet E, Hughes M, Nelson CB. Posttraumatic stress disorder in the National Comorbidity Survey. *Arch Gen Psychiatry*. 1995;52:1048–1060.

333. Shalev AY, Freedman S, Peri T, et al. Prospective study of posttraumatic stress disorder and depression following trauma. *Am J Psychiatry*. 1998;155:630–637.

334. Atkinson JH, Slater MA, Patterson TL, Grant I, Garfin SR. Prevalence, onset, and risk of psychiatric disorders in men with chronic low back pain: a controlled study. *Pain*. 1991;45:111–121.

335. Fishbain DA, Cutler R, Rosomoff HL, Rosomoff RS. Chronic pain-associated depression: antecedent or consequence of chronic pain? A review. *Clin J Pain*. 1997;13(2):116–137.

336. Wilson KG, Eriksson MY, D'Eon JL, Mikail SF, Emery PC. Major depression and insomnia in chronic pain. *Clin J Pain*. 2002;18:77–83.

337. Campbell LC, Clauw DJ, Keefe FJ. Persistent pain and depression: a biopsychosocial perspective. *Biol Psychiatry*. 2003;54:399–409.

338. McWilliams LA, Cox BJ, Enns MW. Mood and anxiety disorders associated with chronic pain: an examination in a nationally representative sample. *Pain*. 2003;106:127–133.

339. Ohayon MM, Lemoine P. Daytime consequences of insomnia complaints in the French general population [in French]. *Encephale*. 2004;30:222–227.

340. Hung CI, Liu CY, Fuh JL, Juang YY, Wang SJ. Comorbid migraine is associated with a negative impact on quality of life in patients with major depression. *Cephalalgia*. 2006;26:26–32.

341. Breslau N, Schultz LR, Stewart WF, Lipton RB, Lucia VC, Welch KM. Headache and major depression: is the association specific to migraine? *Neurology*. 2000;54:308–313.

342. Breslau N, Lipton RB, Stewart WF, Schultz LR, Welch KM. Comorbidity of migraine and depression: investigating potential etiology and prognosis. *Neurology*. 2003;60:1308–1312.

343. Sheftell FD, Atlas SJ. Migraine and psychiatric comorbidity: from theory and hypotheses to clinical application. *Headache*. 2002;42: 934–944.

344. Gasquoine PG. Postconcussional symptoms in chronic back pain. *Appl Neuropsychol*. 2000;7:83–89.

345. Guez M, Brannstrom R, Nyberg L, Toolanen G, Hildingsson C. Neuropsychological functioning and MMPI-2 profiles in chronic neck pain: a comparison of whiplash and non-traumatic groups. *J Clin Exp Neuropsychol*. 2005;27:151–163.

346. Haldorsen T, Waterloo K, Dahl A, Mellgren SI, Davidsen PE, Molin PK. Symptoms and cognitive dysfunction in patients with the late whiplash syndrome. *Appl Neuropsychol*. 2003;10:170–175.

347. Iverson GL, McCracken LM. 'Postconcussive' symptoms in persons with chronic pain. *Brain Inj*. 1997;11:783–790.

348. Smith-Seemiller L, Fow NR, Kant R, Franzen MD. Presence of post-concussion syndrome symptoms in patients with chronic pain vs mild traumatic brain injury. *Brain Inj.* 2003;17:199–206.

349. Jamison RN, Sbrocco T, Parris WC. The influence of problems with concentration and memory on emotional distress and daily activities in chronic pain patients. *Int J Psychiatry Med.* 1988;18:183–191.

350. Iverson GL, King RJ, Scott JG, Adams RL. Cognitive complaints in litigating patients with head injuries or chronic pain. *J Forensic Neuropsychol.* 2001;2:19–30.

351. Chen JK, Johnston KM, Petrides M, Ptito A. Neural substrates of symptoms of depression following concussion in male athletes with persisting postconcussion symptoms. *Arch Gen Psychiatry.* 2008;65:81–89.

352. Bales JW, Wagner AK, Kline AE, Dixon CE. Persistent cognitive dysfunction after traumatic brain injury: a dopamine hypothesis. *Neurosci Biobehav Rev.* 2009;33:981–1003.

353. Novack TA, Banos JH, Brunner R, Renfroe S, Meythaler JM. Impact of early administration of sertraline on depressive symptoms in the first year after traumatic brain injury. *J Neurotrauma.* 2009;26:1921–1928.

354. Rapoport MJ, Chan F, Lanctot K, Herrmann N, McCullagh S, Feinstein A. An open-label study of citalopram for major depression following traumatic brain injury. *J Psychopharmacol.* 2008;22:860–864.

355. Silver JM, McAllister TW, Arciniegas DB. Depression and cognitive complaints following mild traumatic brain injury. *Am J Psychiatry.* 2009;166:653–661.

356. Zafonte RD, Cullen N, Lexell J. Serotonin agents in the treatment of acquired brain injury. *J Head Trauma Rehabil.* 2002;17:322–334.

357. Fann JR, Uomoto JM, Katon WJ. Cognitive improvement with treatment of depression following mild traumatic brain injury. *Psychosomatics.* 2001;42:48–54.

358. Fann JR, Uomoto JM, Katon WJ. Sertraline in the treatment of major depression following mild traumatic brain injury. *J Neuropsychiatry Clin Neurosci.* 2000;12:226–232.

359. Mittenberg W, Canyock EM, Condit D, Patton C. Treatment of post-concussion syndrome following mild head injury. *J Clin Exp Neuropsychol.* 2001;23:829–836.

360. Potter S, Brown RG. Cognitive behavioural therapy and persistent post-concussional symptoms: integrating conceptual issues and practical aspects in treatment. *Neuropsychol Rehabil.* 2012;22:1–25.

361. Ferguson RJ, Mittenberg W. Cognitive-behavioral treatment of postconcussion syndrome: a therapist's manual. In: Van Hasselt VB, Hersen M, eds. *Sourcebook of Psychological Treatment Manuals for Adult Disorders.* New York, NY: Plenum; 1996:615–655.

362. Blanchard EB, Hickling EJ. *After the Crash: Psychological Assessment and Treatment of Survivors of Motor Vehicle Accidents.* Washington, DC: American Psychological Association; 1997.

363. Breslau N, Davis GC, Andreski P, Peterson E. Traumatic events and posttraumatic stress disorder in an urban population of young adults. *Arch Gen Psychiatry.* 1991;48:216–222.

364. Grieger TA, Fullerton CS, Ursano RJ. Posttraumatic stress disorder, alcohol use, and perceived safety after the terrorist attack on the pentagon. *Psychiatr Serv.* 2003;54:1380–1382.

365. Sbordone RJ, Liter JC. Mild traumatic brain injury does not produce post-traumatic stress disorder. *Brain Inj.* 1995;9:405–412.

366. Klein E, Caspi Y, Gil S. The relation between memory of the traumatic event and PTSD: evidence from studies of traumatic brain injury. *Can J Psychiatry.* 2003;48:28–33.

367. Mayou R, Bryant B, Duthie R. Psychiatric consequences of road traffic accidents. *BMJ.* 1993;307:647–651.

368. Bombardier CH, Fann JR, Temkin N, et al. Posttraumatic stress disorder symptoms during the first six months after traumatic brain injury. *J Neuropsychiatry Clin Neurosci.* 2006;18(6905):501–508.

369. Gil S, Caspi Y, Ben-Ari IZ, Koren D, Klein E. Does memory of a traumatic event increase the risk for posttraumatic stress disorder in patients with traumatic brain injury? A prospective study. *Am J Psychiatry.* 2005;162:963–969.

370. Glaesser J, Neuner F, Lutgehetmann R, Schmidt R, Elbert T. Post-traumatic Stress Disorder in patients with traumatic brain injury. *BMC Psychiatry.* 2004;4:5.

371. Bryant RA, Harvey AG. The influence of traumatic brain injury on acute stress disorder and post-traumatic stress disorder following motor vehicle accidents. *Brain Inj.* 1999;13:15–22.

372. Harvey AG, Brewin CR, Jones C, Kopelman MD. Coexistence of posttraumatic stress disorder and traumatic brain injury: towards a resolution of the paradox. *J Int Neuropsychol Soc.* 2003;9:663–676.

373. Hickling EJ, Gillen R, Blanchard EB, Buckley T, Taylor A. Traumatic brain injury and posttraumatic stress disorder: a preliminary investigation of neuropsychological test results in PTSD secondary to motor vehicle accidents. *Brain Inj.* 1998;12:265–274.

374. Mather FJ, Tate RL, Hannan TJ. Post-traumatic stress disorder in children following road traffic accidents: a comparison of those with and without mild traumatic brain injury. *Brain Inj.* 2003;17:1077–1087.

375. Harvey AG, Bryant RA. Two-year prospective evaluation of the relationship between acute stress disorder and posttraumatic stress disorder following mild traumatic brain injury. *Am J Psychiatry.* 2000;157:626–628.

376. Mayou RA, Black J, Bryant B. Unconsciousness, amnesia and psychiatric symptoms following road traffic accident injury. *Br J Psychiatry.* 2000;177:540–545.

377. Bryant RA, Marosszeky JE, Crooks J, Gurka JA. Posttraumatic stress disorder after severe traumatic brain injury. *Am J Psychiatry.* 2000;157:629–631.

378. Harvey AG, Bryant RA. Reconstructing trauma memories: a prospective study of "amnesic" trauma survivors. *J Trauma Stress.* 2001;14:277–282.

379. Bryant RA, Harvey AG. Traumatic memories and pseudomemories in posttraumatic stress disorder. *Appl Cogn Psychol.* 1998;12:81–88.

380. North CS, Nixon SJ, Shariat S, et al. Psychiatric disorders among survivors of the Oklahoma City bombing. *JAMA.* 1999;282:755–762.

381. North CS. The course of post-traumatic stress disorder after the Oklahoma City bombing. *Mil Med.* 2001;166:51–52.

382. North CS, Pfefferbaum B, Tivis L, Kawasaki A, Reddy C, Spitznagel EL. The course of posttraumatic stress disorder in a follow-up study of survivors of the Oklahoma City bombing. *Ann Clin Psychiatry.* 2004;16:209–215.

383. North CS, Smith EM, Spitznagel EL. One-year follow-up of survivors of a mass shooting. *Am J Psychiatry.* 1997;154:1696–1702.

384. North CS, McCutcheon V, Spitznagel EL, Smith EM. Three-year follow-up of survivors of a mass shooting episode. *J Urban Health.* 2002;79:383–391.

385. Buckley TC, Blanchard EB, Hickling EJ. A prospective examination of delayed onset PTSD secondary to motor vehicle accidents. *J Abnorm Psychol.* 1996;105:617–625.

386. Bryant RA, Harvey AG. Delayed-onset posttraumatic stress disorder: a prospective evaluation. *Aust N Z J Psychiatry.* 2002;36:205–209.

387. Gray MJ, Bolton EE, Litz BT. A longitudinal analysis of PTSD symptom course: delayed-onset PTSD in Somalia peacekeepers. *J Consult Clin Psychol.* 2004;72:909–913.

388. Ehlers A, Mayou RA, Bryant B. Psychological predictors of chronic posttraumatic stress disorder after motor vehicle accidents. *J Abnorm Psychol.* 1998;107:508–519.

389. McCrory P, Zazryn T, Cameron P. The evidence for chronic traumatic encephalopathy in boxing. *Sports Med.* 2007;37:467–476.

390. Stern RA, Riley DO, Daneshvar DH, Nowinski CJ, Cantu RC, McKee AC. Long-term consequences of repetitive brain trauma: chronic traumatic encephalopathy. *PM R.* 2011;3(10)(suppl 2):S460–467.

391. Gavett BE, Cantu RC, Shenton M, et al. Clinical appraisal of chronic traumatic encephalopathy: current perspectives and future directions. *Curr Opin Neurol.* 2011;24:525–531.

392. Omalu B, Bailes J, Hamilton RL, et al. Emerging histomorphologic phenotypes of chronic traumatic encephalopathy in American athletes. *Neurosurgery.* 2011;69:173–183.

393. McKee AC, Cantu RC, Nowinski CJ, et al. Chronic traumatic encephalopathy in athletes: progressive tauopathy after repetitive head injury. *J Neuropathol Exp Neurol.* 2009;68:709–735.

394. Omalu BI, Hamilton RL, Kamboh MI, DeKosky ST, Bailes J. Chronic traumatic encephalopathy (CTE) in a National Football League Player: case report and emerging medicolegal practice questions. *J Forensic Nurs.* 2010;6(1):40–46.

395. Corrada M, Brookmeyer R, Kawas C. Sources of variability in prevalence rates of Alzheimer's disease. *Int J Epidemiol.* 1995;24: 1000–1005.

396. Jorm AF, Korten AE, Henderson AS. The prevalence of dementia: a quantitative integration of the literature. *Acta Psychiatr Scand.* 1987;76:465–479.

397. Hofman A, Rocca WA, Brayne C, et al. The prevalence of dementia in Europe: a collaborative study of 1980–1990 findings. Eurodem Prevalence Research Group. *Int J Epidemiol.* 1991;20(3):736–748.

398. Rocca WA, Hofman A, Brayne C, et al. Frequency and distribution of Alzheimer's disease in Europe: a collaborative study of 1980–1990 prevalence findings. The EURODEM-Prevalence Research Group. *Ann Neurol.* 1991;30(3):381–390.

399. Reitz C, Brayne C, Mayeux R. Epidemiology of Alzheimer disease. *Nature reviews. Neurology.* 2011;7:137–152.

400. Nelson PT, Head E, Schmitt FA, et al. Alzheimer's disease is not "brain aging": neuropathological, genetic, and epidemiological human studies. *Acta Neuropathol.* 2011;121:571–587.

401. Lahiri DK. Apolipoprotein E as a target for developing new therapeutics for Alzheimer's disease based on studies from protein, RNA, and regulatory region of the gene. *J Mol Neurosci.* 2004;23: 225–233.

402. Nielsen AS, Ravid R, Kamphorst W, Jorgensen OS. Apolipoprotein E epsilon 4 in an autopsy series of various dementing disorders. *J Alzheimers Dis.* 2003;5:119–125.

403. St George-Hyslop PH, Petit A. Molecular biology and genetics of Alzheimer's disease. *C R Biol.* 2005;328(2):119–130.

404. Heininger K. A unifying hypothesis of Alzheimer's disease. III. Risk factors. *Hum Psychopharmacol.* 2000;15(1):1–70.

405. Ballard C, Gauthier S, Corbett A, Brayne C, Aarsland D, Jones E. Alzheimer's disease. *Lancet.* 2011;377:1019–1031.

406. Andersen K, Lolk A, Kragh-Sorensen P, Petersen NE, Green A. Depression and the risk of Alzheimer disease. *Epidemiology.* 2005; 16(2):233–238.

407. Dal Forno G, Palermo MT, Donohue JE, Karagiozis H, Zonderman AB, Kawas CH. Depressive symptoms, sex, and risk for Alzheimer's disease. *Ann Neurol.* 2005;57:381–387.

408. Lye TC, Shores EA. Traumatic brain injury as a risk factor for Alzheimer's disease: a review. *Neuropsychol Rev.* 2000;10:115–129.

409. Canadian Study of Health and Aging. The Canadian Study of Health and Aging: risk factors for Alzheimer's disease in Canada. *Neurology.* 1994;44(11):2073–2080.

410. van Duijn CM, Tanja TA, Haaxma R, et al. Head trauma and the risk of Alzheimer's disease. *Am J Epidemiol.* 1992;135(7):775–782.

411. Salib E, Hillier V. Head injury and the risk of Alzheimer's disease: a case control study. *Int J Geriatr Psychiatry.* 1997;12:363–368.

412. Graves AB, White KP, Koepsell TD, et al. The association between head trauma and Alzheimer's disease. *Am J Epidemiol.* 1990;131: 491–501.

413. O'Meara ES, Kukull WA, Sheppard L, et al. Head injury and risk of Alzheimer's disease by apolipoprotein E genotype. *Am J Epidemiol.* 1997;146:373–384.

414. Plassman BL, Havlik RJ, Steffens DC, et al. Documented head injury in early adulthood and risk of Alzheimer's disease and other dementias. *Neurology.* 2000;55:1158–1166.

415. Chandra V, Philipose V, Bell PA, Lazaroff A, Schoenberg BS. Case-control study of late onset "probable Alzheimer's disease". *Neurology.* 1987;37:1295–1300.

416. Guo Z, Cupples LA, Kurz A, et al. Head injury and the risk of AD in the MIRAGE study. *Neurology.* 2000;54:1316–1323.

417. Luukinen H, Viramo P, Herala M, et al. Fall-related brain injuries and the risk of dementia in elderly people: a population-based study. *Eur J Neurol.* 2005;12:86–92.

418. Luukinen H, Viramo P, Koski K, Laippala P, Kivela SL. Head injuries and cognitive decline among older adults: a population-based study. *Neurology.* 1999;52:557–562.

419. Rasmussen DX, Brandt J, Martin DB, Folstein MF. Head injury as a risk factor in Alzheimer's disease. *Brain Inj.* 1995;9:213–219.

420. Mayeux R, Ottman R, Tang MX, et al. Genetic susceptibility and head injury as risk factors for Alzheimer's disease among community-dwelling elderly persons and their first-degree relatives. *Ann Neurol.* 1993;33:494–501.

421. Schofield PW, Tang M, Marder K, et al. Alzheimer's disease after remote head injury: an incidence study. *J Neurol Neurosurg Psychiatry.* 1997;62(2):119–124.

422. Mortimer JA, French LR, Hutton JT, Schuman LM. Head injury as a risk factor for Alzheimer's disease. *Neurology.* 1985;35:264–267.

423. Amaducci LA, Fratiglioni L, Rocca WA, et al. Risk factors for clinically diagnosed Alzheimer's disease: a case-control study of an Italian population. *Neurology.* 1986;36(7):922–931.

424. Ferini-Strambi L, Smirne S, Garancini P, Pinto P, Franceschi M. Clinical and epidemiological aspects of Alzheimer's disease with presenile onset: a case control study. *Neuroepidemiology.* 1990;9: 39–49.

425. Fratiglioni L, Ahlbom A, Viitanen M, Winblad B. Risk factors for late-onset Alzheimer's disease: a population-based, case-control study. *Ann Neurol.* 1993;33:258–266.

426. Nemetz PN, Leibson C, Naessens JM, et al. Traumatic brain injury and time to onset of Alzheimer's disease: a population-based study. *Am J Epidemiol.* 1999;149:32–40.

427. Katzman R, Aronson M, Fuld P, et al. Development of dementing illnesses in an 80-year-old volunteer cohort. *Ann Neurol.* 1989;25: 317–324.

428. Li G, Shen YC, Li YT, Chen CH, Zhau YW, Silverman JM. A case-control study of Alzheimer's disease in China. *Neurology.* 1992;42: 1481–1488.

429. Mehta KM, Ott A, Kalmijn S, et al. Head trauma and risk of dementia and Alzheimer's disease: the Rotterdam Study. *Neurology.* 1999; 53(9):1959–1962.

430. Chandra V, Kokmen E, Schoenberg BS, Beard CM. Head trauma with loss of consciousness as a risk factor for Alzheimer's disease. *Neurology.* 1989;39:1576–1578.

431. Broe GA, Henderson AS, Creasey H, et al. A case-control study of Alzheimer's disease in Australia. *Neurology.* 1990;40:1698–1707.

432. Szczygielski J, Mautes A, Steudel WI, Falkai P, Bayer TA, Wirths O. Traumatic brain injury: cause or risk of Alzheimer's disease? A review of experimental studies. *J Neural Transm.* 2005;112: 1547–1564.

433. Jellinger KA. Head injury and dementia. *Curr Opin Neurol.* 2004; 17:719–723.

434. Jellinger KA, Paulus W, Wrocklage C, Litvan I. Effects of closed traumatic brain injury and genetic factors on the development of Alzheimer's disease. *Eur J Neurol.* 2001;8:707–710.

435. Jellinger KA, Paulus W, Wrocklage C, Litvan I. Traumatic brain injury as a risk factor for Alzheimer disease. Comparison of two retrospective autopsy cohorts with evaluation of ApoE genotype. *BMC Neurol.* 2001;1:3.

436. Johnson VE, Stewart W, Smith DH. Widespread tau and amyloid-Beta pathology many years after a single traumatic brain injury in humans. *Brain Pathol.* 2012;22(2):142–149.

437. Johnson VE, Stewart W, Smith DH. Traumatic brain injury and amyloid-beta pathology: a link to Alzheimer's disease? *Nat Rev Neurosci.* 2010;11:361–370.

438. Chen XH, Johnson VE, Uryu K, Trojanowski JQ, Smith DH. A lack of amyloid beta plaques despite persistent accumulation of amyloid beta in axons of long-term survivors of traumatic brain injury. *Brain Pathol.* 2009;19(2):214–223.

439. McAllister TW. Genetic factors modulating outcome after neurotrauma. *PM R.* 2010;2:S241–S252.

440. Waters RJ, Nicoll JA. Genetic influences on outcome following acute neurological insults. *Curr Opin Crit Care.* 2005;11:105–110.

441. Nathoo N, Chetty R, van Dellen JR, Barnett GH. Genetic vulnerability following traumatic brain injury: the role of apolipoprotein E. *Mol Pathol.* 2003;56:132–136.

442. Mayeux R, Ottman R, Maestre G, et al. Synergistic effects of traumatic head injury and apolipoprotein-epsilon 4 in patients with Alzheimer's disease. *Neurology.* 1995;45:555–557.

443. Koponen S, Taiminen T, Kairisto V, et al. APOE-epsilon4 predicts dementia but not other psychiatric disorders after traumatic brain injury. *Neurology.* 2004;63:749–750.

444. Mortimer JA, van Duijn CM, Chandra V, et al. Head trauma as a risk factor for Alzheimer's disease: a collaborative re-analysis of case-control studies. EURODEM Risk Factors Research Group. *Int J Epidemiol*. 1991;20(suppl 2):S28–S35.

445. Fleminger S, Oliver DL, Lovestone S, Rabe-Hesketh S, Giora A. Head injury as a risk factor for Alzheimer's disease: the evidence 10 years on; a partial replication. *J Neurol Neurosurg Psychiatry*. 2003;74(7):857–862.

446. Starkstein SE, Jorge R. Dementia after traumatic brain injury. *Int Psychogeriatr*. 2005;17(suppl 1):S93–S107.

447. Bazarian JJ, Cernak I, Noble-Haeusslein L, Potolicchio S, Temkin N. Long-term neurologic outcomes after traumatic brain injury. *J Head Trauma Rehabil*. 2009;24:439–451.

448. Ruff RM, Camenzuli L, Mueller J. Miserable minority: emotional risk factors that influence the outcome of a mild traumatic brain injury. *Brain Inj*. 1996;10:551–565.

449. Wood RL. Understanding the 'miserable minority': a diasthesis-stress paradigm for post-concussional syndrome. *Brain Inj*. 2004; 18:1135–1153.

450. Ryan LM, Warden DL. Post concussion syndrome. *Int Rev Psychiatry*. 2003;15:310–316.

451. Evered L, Ruff R, Baldo J, Isomura A. Emotional risk factors and postconcussional disorder. *Assessment*. 2003;10:420–427.

452. Cook JB. The post-concussional syndrome and factors influencing recovery after minor head injury admitted to hospital. *Scand J Rehabil Med*. 1972;4:27–30.

453. Mickeviciene D, Schrader H, Obelieniene D, et al. A controlled prospective inception cohort study on the post-concussion syndrome outside the medicolegal context. *Eur J Neurol*. 2004;11:411–419.

454. Rutherford WH, Merrett JD, McDonald JR. Symptoms at one year following concussion from minor head injuries. *Injury*. 1979;10:225–230.

455. Satz PS, Alfano MS, Light RF, et al. Persistent Post-Concussive Syndrome: a proposed methodology and literature review to determine the effects, if any, of mild head and other bodily injury. *J Clin Exp Neuropsychol*. 1999;21:620–628.

456. Mickeviciene D, Schrader H, Nestvold K, et al. A controlled historical cohort study on the post-concussion syndrome. *Eur J Neurol*. 2002;9:581–587.

457. Lees-Haley PR, Fox DD, Courtney JC. A comparison of complaints by mild brain injury claimants and other claimants describing subjective experiences immediately following their injury. *Arch Clin Neuropsychol*. 2001;16:689–695.

458. Miller H. Accident neurosis. *Br Med J*. 1961;1(5230):919–925.

459. Miller H. Accident neurosis. *Br Med J*. 1961;1(5231):992–998.

460. Reynolds S, Paniak C, Toller-Lobe G, Nagy J. A longitudinal study of compensation-seeking and return to work in a treated mild traumatic brain injury sample. *J Head Trauma Rehabil*. 2003;18:139–147.

461. Binder LM, Rohling ML. Money matters: a meta-analytic review of the effects of financial incentives on recovery after closed-head injury. *Am J Psychiatry*. 1996;153:7–10.

462. Paniak C, Reynolds S, Toller-Lobe G, Melnyk A, Nagy J, Schmidt D. A longitudinal study of the relationship between financial compensation and symptoms after treated mild traumatic brain injury. *J Clin Exp Neuropsychol*. 2002;24:187–193.

463. Binder LM. Persisting symptoms after mild head injury: a review of the postconcussive syndrome. *J Clin Exp Neuropsychol*. 1986;8:323–346.

464. Brown SJ, Fann JR, Grant I. Postconcussional disorder: time to acknowledge a common source of neurobehavioral morbidity. *J Neuropsychiatry Clin Neurosci*. 1994;6:15–22.

465. Cicerone KD, Kalmar K. Persistent postconcussion syndrome: the structure of subjective complaints after mild traumatic brain injury. *J Head Trauma Rehabil*. 1995;10:1–7.

466. Heilbronner RL. Factors associated with postconcussion syndrome: neurological, psychological, or legal? *Trial Diplomacy J*. 1993;16:161–167.

467. Youngjohn JR, Burrows L, Erdal K. Brain damage or compensation neurosis? The controversial post-concussion syndrome. *Clin Neuropsychol*. 1995;9:112–123.

468. Lishman WA. Physiogenisis and psychogenisis in the 'post-concussional syndrome'. *Br J Psychiatry*. 1986;153:460–469.

469. Mittenberg W, Strauman S. Diagnosis of mild head injury and the postconcussion syndrome. *J Head Trauma Rehabil*. 2000;15:783–791.

470. Larrabee GJ. Neuropsychological outcome, post concussion symptoms, and forensic considerations in mild closed head trauma. *Semin Clin Neuropsychiatry*. 1997;2:196–206.

471. Bijur PE, Haslum M, Golding J. Cognitive and behavioral sequelae of mild head injury in children. *Pediatrics*. 1990;86:337–344.

472. Ruff RM, Richardson AM. Mild traumatic brian injury. In: Sweet JJ, ed. *Forensic Neuropsychology: Fundamentals and Practice. Studies on Neuropsychology, Development, and Cognition*. Bristol, PA: Swets & Zeitlinger; 1999:315–338.

473. Gouvier WD, Uddo-Crane M, Brown LM. Base rates of post-concussional symptoms. *Arch Clin Neuropsychol*. 1988;3:273–278.

474. Machulda MM, Bergquist TF, Ito V, Chew S. Relationship between stress, coping, and post concussion symptoms in a healthy adult population. *Arch Clin Neuropsychol*. 1998;13:415–424.

475. Iverson GL, Lange RT. Examination of "postconcussion-like" symptoms in a healthy sample. *Appl Neuropsychol*. 2003;10:137–144.

476. Mittenberg W, DiGiulio DV, Perrin S, Bass AE. Symptoms following mild head injury: expectation as aetiology. *J Neurol Neurosurg Psychiatry*. 1992;55:200–204.

477. Trahan DE, Ross CE, Trahan SL. Relationships among postconcussional-type symptoms, depression, and anxiety in neurologically normal young adults and victims of brain injury. *Arch Clin Neuropsychol*. 2001;16:435–445.

478. Sawchyn JM, Brulot MM, Strauss E. Note on the use of the Postconcussion Syndrome Checklist. *Arch Clin Neuropsychol*. 2000;15:1–8.

479. Wong JL, Regennitter RP, Barrios F. Base rate and simulated symptoms of mild head injury among normals. *Arch Clin Neuropsychol*. 1994;9:411–425.

480. Fox DD, Lees-Haley PR, Ernest K, Dolezal-Wood S. Post-concussive symptoms: base rates and etiology in psychiatric patients. *Clin Neuropsychol*. 1995;9:89–92.

481. Lees-Haley PR, Brown RS. Neuropsychological complaint base rates of 170 personal injury claimants. *Arch Clin Neuropsychol*. 1993;8:203–209.

482. Dunn JT, Lees-Haley PR, Brown RS, Williams CW, English LT. Neurotoxic complaint base rates of personal injury claimants: implications for neuropsychological assessment. *J Clin Psychol*. 1995;51:577–584.

483. Radanov BP, Dvorak J, Valach L. Cognitive deficits in patients after soft tissue injury of the cervical spine. *Spine*. 1992;17:127–131.

484. Sullivan MJ, Hall E, Bartolacci R, Sullivan ME, Adams H. Perceived cognitive deficits, emotional distress and disability following whiplash injury. *Pain Res Manag*. 2002;7:120–126.

485. Berube J. The Traumatic Brain Injury Act Amendments of 2000. *J Head Trauma Rehabil*. 2001;16(2):210–213.

486. Center for Disease Control and Prevention. *Report to Congress on Mild Traumatic Brain Injury in the United States: Steps to Prevent a Serious Public Health Problem*. Atlanta, GA: Centers for Disease Control and Prevention; 2003.

487. National Institutes of Health. Rehabilitation of persons with traumatic brain injury. *NIH Consens Statement*. 1998;16(1):1–41.

488. Stein SC, Ross SE. Mild head injury: a plea for routine early CT scanning. *J Trauma*. 1992;33:11–13.

489. Moran SG, McCarthy MC, Uddin DE, Poelstra RJ. Predictors of positive CT scans in the trauma patient with minor head injury. *Am Surg*. 1994;60:533–536.

490. Borczuk P. Predictors of intracranial injury in patients with mild head trauma. *Ann Emerg Med*. 1995;25:731–736.

491. Thiruppathy SP, Muthukumar N. Mild head injury: revisited. *Acta Neurochir (Wien)*. 2004;146:1075–1083.

492. Stiell IG, Clement CM, Rowe BH, et al. Comparison of the Canadian CT Head Rule and the New Orleans Criteria in patients with minor head injury. *JAMA*. 2005;294:1511–1518.

493. Ono K, Wada K, Takahara T, Shirotani T. Indications for computed tomography in patients with mild head injury. *Neurol Med Chir (Tokyo)*. 2007;47:291–298.

494. Saboori M, Ahmadi J, Farajzadegan Z. Indications for brain CT scan in patients with minor head injury. *Clin Neurol Neurosurg.* 2007;109:399–405.

495. Asikainen I, Kaste M, Sarna S. Patients with traumatic brain injury referred to a rehabilitation and re-employment programme: social and professional outcome for 508 Finnish patients 5 or more years after injury. *Brain Inj.* 1996;10:883–899.

496. Benedictus MR, Spikman JM, van der Naalt J. Cognitive and behavioral impairment in traumatic brain injury related to outcome and return to work. *Arch Phys Med Rehabil.* 2010;91:1436–1441.

497. Dawson DR, Levine B, Schwartz ML, Stuss DT. Acute predictors of real-world outcomes following traumatic brain injury: a prospective study. *Brain Inj.* 2004;18:221–238.

498. Doctor JN, Castro J, Temkin NR, Fraser RT, Machamer JE, Dikmen SS. Workers' risk of unemployment after traumatic brain injury: a normed comparison. *J Int Neuropsychol Soc.* 2005;11:747–752.

499. Drake AI, Gray N, Yoder S, Pramuka M, Llewellyn M. Factors predicting return to work following mild traumatic brain injury: a discriminant analysis. *J Head Trauma Rehabil.* 2000;15:1103–1112.

500. Friedland JF, Dawson DR. Function after motor vehicle accidents: a prospective study of mild head injury and posttraumatic stress. *J Nerv Ment Dis.* 2001;189:426–434.

501. Guerin F, Kennepohl S, Leveille G, Dominique A, McKerral M. Vocational outcome indicators in atypically recovering mild TBI: a post-intervention study. *NeuroRehabilitation.* 2006;21:295–303.

502. Haboubi NH, Long J, Koshy M, Ward AB. Short-term sequelae of minor head injury (6 years experience of minor head injury clinic). *Disabil Rehabil.* 2001;23:635–638.

503. Metting Z, Rodiger LA, Stewart RE, Oudkerk M, De Keyser J, van der Naalt J. Perfusion computed tomography in the acute phase of mild head injury: regional dysfunction and prognostic value. *Ann Neurol.* 2009;66:809–816.

504. Ruffolo CF, Friedland JF, Dawson DR, Colantonio A, Lindsay PH. Mild traumatic brain injury from motor vehicle accidents: factors associated with return to work. *Arch Phys Med Rehabil.* 1999;80: 392–398.

505. Sadowski-Cron C, Schneider J, Senn P, Radanov BP, Ballinari P, Zimmermann H. Patients with mild traumatic brain injury: immediate and long-term outcome compared to intra-cranial injuries on CT scan. *Brain Inj.* 2006;20:1131–1137.

506. Sigurdardottir S, Andelic N, Roe C, Schanke AK. Cognitive recovery and predictors of functional outcome 1 year after traumatic brain injury. *J Int Neuropsychol Soc.* 2009;15:740–750.

507. Stulemeijer M, van der Werf S, Borm GF, Vos PE. Early prediction of favourable recovery 6 months after mild traumatic brain injury. *J Neurol Neurosurg Psychiatry.* 2008;79:936–942.

508. van der Naalt J, van Zomeren AH, Sluiter WJ, Minderhoud JM. One year outcome in mild to moderate head injury: the predictive value of acute injury characteristics related to complaints and return to work. *J Neurol Neurosurg Psychiatry.* 1999;66(2):207–213.

509. Hoge CW, McGurk D, Thomas JL, Cox AL, Engel CC, Castro CA. Mild traumatic brain injury in U.S. Soldiers returning from Iraq. *N Engl J Med.* 2008;358:453–463.

510. Ponsford J, Cameron P, Fitzgerald M, Grant M, Mikocka-Walus A. Long-term outcomes after uncomplicated mild traumatic brain injury: a comparison with trauma controls. *J Neurotrauma.* 2011;28: 937–946.

511. Rao V, Bertrand M, Rosenberg P, et al. Predictors of new-onset depression after mild traumatic brain injury. *J Neuropsychiatry Clin Neurosci.* 2010;22:100–104.

512. Vanderploeg RD, Curtiss G, Luis CA, Salazar AM. Long-term morbidities following self-reported mild traumatic brain injury. *J Clin Exp Neuropsychol.* 2007;29:585–598.

513. Belanger HG, Spiegel E, Vanderploeg RD. Neuropsychological performance following a history of multiple self-reported concussions: a meta-analysis. *J Int Neuropsychol Soc.* 2010;16:262–267.

514. Bäckman L, Jones S, Berger AK, Laukka EJ, Small BJ. Cognitive impairment in preclinical Alzheimer's disease: a meta-analysis. *Neuropsychology.* 2005;19:520–531.

515. Iverson GL. Evidence-based neuropsychological assessment of sport-related concussion. In: Webbe FM, ed. *Handbook of Sport Neuropsychology.* New York, NY: Springer Publishing Company; 2011: 131–154.

516. Binder LM, Rohling ML, Larrabee J. A review of mild head trauma. Part I: meta-analytic review of neuropsychological studies. *J Clin Exp Neuropsychol.* 1997;19(3):421–431.

517. Christensen H, Griffiths K, Mackinnon A, Jacomb P. A quantitative review of cognitive deficits in depression and Alzheimer-type dementia. *J Int Neuropsychol Soc.* 1997;3:631–651.

518. Frazier TW, Demaree HA, Youngstrom EA. Meta-analysis of intellectual and neuropsychological test performance in attention-deficit/hyperactivity disorder. *Neuropsychology.* 2004;18:543–555.

519. Grant I, Gonzalez R, Carey CL, Natarajan L, Wolfson T. Non-acute (residual) neurocognitive effects of cannabis use: a meta-analytic study. *J Int Neuropsychol Soc.* 2003;9:679–689.

520. Jovanovski D, Erb S, Zakzanis KK. Neurocognitive deficits in cocaine users: a quantitative review of the evidence. *J Clin Exp Neuropsychol.* 2005;27:189–204.

521. Barker MJ, Greenwood KM, Jackson M, Crowe SF. Persistence of cognitive effects after withdrawal from long-term benzodiazepine use: a meta-analysis. *Arch Clin Neuropsychol.* 2004;19:437–454.

522. Barker MJ, Greenwood KM, Jackson M, Crowe SF. Cognitive effects of long-term benzodiazepine use: a meta-analysis. *CNS Drugs.* 2004;18:37–48.

Conceptualizing Outcome From Mild Traumatic Brain Injury

Grant L. Iverson, Noah Silverberg, Rael T. Lange, and Nathan D. Zasler

INTRODUCTION

Most mainstream definitions of mild traumatic brain injury (MTBI) capture an extraordinarily broad spectrum of severity, ranging from a very mild sport-related concussion characterized by momentary confusion to a complicated MTBI following high-speed motor vehicle accident with a brief period of coma, several hours of post-traumatic amnesia, a focal brain contusion visible on day-of-injury computed tomography (CT), and multiple bodily injuries. This wide spectrum contributes to the complexity of conceptualizing outcome. Most MTBIs, especially those on the mild end of the spectrum, are expected to be self-limiting and to follow a predictable course. Permanent cognitive, psychological, or psychosocial problems are relatively uncommon in trauma patients and rare in athletes (1–5,6) (see the Chapters 30 and 31 in this book). However, some people do not recover well following MTBI (7,8). Persistent symptoms after MTBI can be associated with high levels of disability and health care service utilization (9–14).

Despite decades of research, the incidence, prevalence, etiology, natural history, and treatment of the "postconcussion syndrome" have not been well established. This has led researchers to question the validity of this diagnosis as a true syndrome or disease entity (e.g., 15,16–20). At the heart of this debate is controversy over etiology (see 4, 21, 22, and 23 for reviews). In medicine, a syndrome is traditionally defined as a group of signs and symptoms that occur together, signaling an abnormal condition. The signs and symptoms are believed to have a common cause. This is troublesome because postconcussion symptoms are nonspecific and do not occur consistently in a syndromal manner. Similar symptoms occur in healthy people and they are associated with common comorbid conditions (e.g., depression, anxiety, and chronic pain). In a proposed biopsychosocial model (see subsequently), there are numerous diverse factors that can influence how people perceive and report their symptoms and functional problems long after an MTBI.

The thesis of this chapter is that the cause of symptoms and functional problems long after an MTBI is usually multifactorial, and the only appropriate perspective when conceptualizing outcome is biopsychosocial. Poor outcome is often related to several preexisting and/or comorbid conditions, and rarely occurs without these confounding factors (13,14).

Accordingly, it cannot be assumed that when a person reports symptoms long after an MTBI that the symptoms are caused by the original brain injury or continued brain dysfunction because of this injury. A careful assessment approach is urged, in the hope that it leads to better differential diagnosis, treatment, and rehabilitation; reduced patient suffering; and overall better functional outcomes (e.g., return to work, family roles, and social and recreational pursuits).

PREVALENCE

The widely cited statistic that 15% of people who sustain an MTBI will develop a persistent postconcussion syndrome appears to have its origin largely through a misinterpretation of a prospective study completed in the mid 1970s by Rutherford and colleagues. These researchers followed consecutive hospital admissions for MTBIs and reported that 14.5% of patients had *at least one* symptom at 1-year postinjury. However, fewer than 5% had multiple (4 or more) symptoms. This latter figure is rarely cited. Although other studies reported a similar figure of about 2%–5%, some suggest that the long-term symptoms might occur in *more* than 15% of people at 1-year post MTBI (e.g., 24,25). The constellation of symptoms comprising the syndrome likely occurs in far less than 15% of patients with remote MTBIs, once 2 issues are considered that contribute to inflated incidence estimates (*a*) sample unrepresentativeness, and (*b*) liberal criteria for positive "caseness."

If *all* MTBIs are considered, the percentage of people with poor long-term outcome (e.g., significant symptoms greater than 1 year) is likely very small (i.e., clearly less than 5%). This is because the definition of concussion requires only that a person feels momentarily dazed or disoriented to meet criteria for the injury (26). Injuries at this mild end of the MTBI spectrum are common in daily life and in sports, and as a rule, do not result in symptoms that last beyond hours, days, or weeks. At least 75% of MTBI cases are not hospitalized (27) and have no contact with concussion researchers. In contrast, the Rutherford et al. study and the majority of more recent studies reported incidence rates for prospectively recruited trauma patients seen in the hospital, not athletes with MTBIs or civilians seen by their family doctors or in clinics, or those who do not present for medical attention at all. As well, researchers have reported that patients who agree to participate in prospective research on outcome from MTBI have more severe injuries than those who refuse participation (e.g., rate of CT abnormalities was 33% in participants and 6% in refusals) (28). Symptomatic patients may be more likely to remain enrolled through the follow-up period (e.g., 29). Thus, most published prospective studies began with a nonrepresentative sample and then, because of nonrandom selection and attrition (severe in some studies), the final sample is often highly nonrepresentative. Sample selection methodology may be the most influential moderator across MTBI outcome studies (3).

A second major influence on incidence estimates is the wide variability in how "symptomatic" is defined at follow-up. Some criteria are set as liberal as a single symptom (e.g., headache, fatigue, or irritability) of any frequency and severity at 1-year postinjury. Not surprisingly, studies considering various thresholds report much higher incidence rates for 1 or more symptoms compared to 3 or more symptoms (16,17, but see 25,29). If one accepts the classic definition of a syndrome as involving a *constellation* of symptoms, then having 1 or 2 symptoms would not represent a syndrome. Moreover, because most healthy people with no head or brain trauma history report 1–3 of these symptoms in their daily life (30), a cut-off within this range is probably too liberal. In addition to symptom counts, some studies include a "clinical significance" criterion, wherein only individuals whose social or occupational functioning is impacted by their symptoms are defined as having a poor outcome (e.g., 31). In the *Diagnostic and Statistical Manual of Mental Disorders, Fourth Edition (DMS-IV)* framework, this is what makes a disorder a disorder. The effect of including this criterion on incidence rates of poor outcome is not clear. Until the field arrives at a unified approach to defining poor outcome, incidence rates will continue to vary widely.

DIAGNOSTIC CRITERIA

There are 2 current sets of research criteria for the postconcussion syndrome: the International Classification of Diseases 10th edition (ICD-10) and the *DSM-IV* (32). According to the ICD-10 (33), a person must have a history of "head trauma with a loss of consciousness" preceding the onset of symptoms by a period of up to 4 weeks and have symptoms in at least 3 of 6 categories. The specific research criteria for the ICD-10 postconcussional syndrome are set out in Table 30-1. Notice that the ICD-10 criteria do not require "objective" evidence of cognitive problems (in contrast to the *DSM-IV* criteria described later). The emphasis is on subjective cognitive complaints. Therefore, a person with depression and/or anxiety, insomnia, and a preoccupation with having brain damage would meet diagnostic criteria for the syndrome. This definition implicitly assumes that symptoms reported long after an MTBI are exclusively the result of MTBI, and unfortunately does not acknowledge the need for differential diagnosis of the cause of the various symptoms after MTBI.

The *DSM-IV* included research criteria for the postconcussional disorder (see 34 for a discussion of the development and limitations of these criteria). Criterion A requires a history of head trauma causing "significant cerebral concussion." The authors provide no absolute threshold, but

TABLE 30-1 FO7.2 Postconcussional Syndrome (research criteria from the ICD-10)

The nosological status of this syndrome is uncertain, and criterion A of the introduction to this rubric is not always ascertainable. However, for those undertaking research into this condition, the following criteria are recommended:

A. The general criteria of F07 must be met.

   (The general criteria for F07, Personality and behavioral disorders due to brain disease, damage and dysfunction, are as follows: G1. Objective evidence (from physical and neurological examination and laboratory tests) and/or history of cerebral disease, damage, or dysfunction. G2. Absence of clouding of consciousness and of significant memory deficit. G3. Absence of sufficient or suggestive evidence for an alternative causation of the personality or behavior disorder that would justify its placement in section F6 (Other mental disorders due to brain damage and dysfunction and to physical disease).

B. History of head trauma with loss of consciousness, preceding the onset of symptoms by a period of up to 4 weeks (objective EEG, brain imaging, or oculonystagmographic evidence for brain damage may be lacking).

C. At least 3 of the following:

(1) Complaints of unpleasant sensations and pains, such as headache, dizziness (usually lacking the features of true vertigo), general malaise and excessive fatigue, or noise intolerance.

(2) Emotional changes, such as irritability, emotional lability, both easily provoked or exacerbated by emotional excitement or stress, or some degree of depression and/or anxiety.

(3) Subjective complaints of difficulty in concentration and in performing mental tasks, and of memory complaints, without clear objective evidence (e.g., psychological tests) of marked impairment.

(4) Insomnia.

(5) Reduced tolerance to alcohol.

(6) Preoccupation with the aforementioned symptoms and fear of permanent brain damage, to the extent of hypochondriacal overvalued ideas and adoption of a sick role.

Abbreviations: ICD-10, International Classification of Diseases 10th Edition; EEG, electroencephalography.

offer the injury severity marker examples of loss of consciousness (LOC) greater than 5 minutes, post-traumatic amnesia (PTA) greater than 12 hours, or the new onset of seizures. This definition implies, but does not explicitly state, that not at all MTBIs would meet Criterion A. Moreover, the definition implies that persistent symptoms should only follow an MTBI at the more severe end of spectrum, despite the strong evidence that MTBI severity does not predict outcome (e.g., 2,35,36,37). According to Criterion B, the individual must show objective evidence on neuropsychological testing of declines in some of his or her cognitive abilities, such as attention, concentration, learning, or memory. The person must also report 3 or more subjective symptoms from Criterion C, and these symptoms must be present for at least 3 months. The Criterion C symptoms are (a) becoming fatigued easily; (b) disordered sleep; (c) headache; (d) vertigo or dizziness; (e) irritability or aggression on little or no provocation; (f) anxiety, depression, or affective lability; (g) changes in personality (e.g., social or sexual inappropriateness); and (h) apathy or lack of spontaneity. *DSM-IV* also requires that "the disturbance causes significant impairment in social or occupational functioning and represents a significant decline from a previous level of functioning."

The most serious and obvious problem with the ICD-10 and the *DSM-IV* criteria for the syndrome is causally linking the subjective, self-reported symptoms to the original MTBI. There are also major discrepancies between them. Prevalence rates using the ICD-10 criteria are 3–6 times higher than that using the *DSM-IV* criteria (38,39), likely because the latter requires the additional (a) documentation of objective neurocognitive impairment and (b) impairment in important role functioning.

Ruff (7,40) proposed 4 modifiers for the syndrome. These modifiers are as follows: (a) postconcussional disorder with objective neuropathological features, (b) postconcussional disorder with neurocognitive features, (c) postconcussional disorder with psychopathological features, and (d) postconcussional disorder with neurocognitive and psychopathological features. The subtype with objective neuropathological features classification identifies those patients with a combination of neuropsychological deficits and abnormalities identified on neuroimaging (i.e., those with "complicated" MTBIs). The subtype with neurocognitive features is used if (a) a cluster of cognitive deficits consistent with MTBI are reliably documented on neuropsychological testing, (b) there is an absence of significant emotional overlay, and (c) there is an absence of positive neuroimaging. The subtype with psychopathological features is used when (a) persistent emotional sequelae dominate the clinical picture (e.g., acute stress reaction, depression, panic attacks), (b) neuropsychological deficits are disproportionate with the duration of LOC or PTA and absence of neuroimaging findings, and (c) symptoms tend to persist or even worsen over time. The subtype with neurocognitive and psychopathological features is used when there is a mixture of documented neurocognitive deficits and acquired emotional problems that improve over time, and there is an absence of positive neuroimaging.

CAUSES AND COMORBID CONDITIONS

A diverse range of biopsychosocial factors can influence the perception and reporting of symptoms long after an MTBI, as well as impact how the person functions in day-to-day life. These are illustrated in Figure 30-1, and described subsequently in a timeline from preinjury to postinjury (see Table 30-2 for a definition of many of these terms). Note that the preinjury, peri-injury, and early and late postinjury factors likely interact in complex ways to produce symptoms—and there are substantial individual differences in which factors are most relevant for a given person.

Preinjury

Symonds (41) famously suggested that after an MTBI, "the symptom picture depends not only on the kind of injury, but upon the kind of brain" that is injured (p. 464). By far the 2 most well researched preinjury variables are prior MTBI(s) and personality/psychological functioning. A

meta-analysis found that a history of 2 or more sport-related concussions had a trivial effect on global postinjury neuropsychological functioning and self-reported postconcussion symptoms compared to a single concussion (42). This study also reported that multiple concussions were associated with significant (small) effects for the domains of delayed memory (Cohen's $d = 0.16$) and executive functioning (Cohen's $d = 0.24$). The threshold for the number, severity, and recency of prior MTBIs that is necessary to influence outcome from a new MTBI remains uncertain. Moreover, these data are largely derived from athletes with a history of sport concussion(s); applicability to MTBIs of other mechanisms and contexts may be low. In addition to prior MTBI(s), it is certainly possible that preinjury neurological (e.g., ischemic cerebrovascular disease) or neurodevelopment problems (e.g., attention deficit hyperactivity disorder) alter outcome from MTBI in civilians, but these conditions are rarely studied.

Influential theories relating to long-term symptom reporting have highlighted the role of preinjury psychological functioning in creating vulnerability (8,43,44). In prospective studies with consecutively recruited patients with MTBI, a preinjury history of psychiatric diagnosis or treatment was related to outcome in some (45–47), but not all (48,49), patients. Samples with persistent symptoms tend to have elevated rates of preinjury psychiatric problems (14,22,46,50).

Personality characteristics influence how people respond to stressors, illness, or injury. For example, researchers have frequently reported that certain personality characteristics appear to be risk factors for major depression. People with high levels of neuroticism or negative affectivity, low self-esteem, and poor life coping skills are at increased risk for developing depression (51–55). These same personality characteristics, in addition to anger/hostility and narcissism, have been reported in studies as risk factors for posttraumatic stress disorder (PTSD) (56–59). By extension, this large literature is relevant to understanding who is at risk for developing a persistent symptoms following an MTBI.

Researchers have also investigated the personality profiles associated with long-term symptom reporting. Axis II psychopathology, particularly compulsive, histrionic, and narcissistic traits, is overrepresented (22). Kay et al. (43) elegantly described how overachievement, dependency, insecurity, grandiosity, and borderline personality traits could create vulnerability to poor outcome following MTBI. Case studies highlight the importance of these premorbid personality traits (8) (p. 562). "Type D" personality (60), characterized by negative affectivity and social inhibition, is also associated with more symptoms, lower neuropsychological performance, and symptom validity test failure after MTBI (61,62). Similar personality characteristics are associated with higher postconcussion-like symptom reporting in people without a history of concussion (63). Other studies have found more modest and nonsignificant associations between preinjury personality variables and MTBI outcome (e.g., 64). It is important to acknowledge the methodological limitations of this literature. Researchers are generally constrained to assess postinjury personality characteristics. If assessing current personality traits, they assume that such traits are invariable over time, and therefore accurately reflect preinjury personality. The alternative approach of asking patients or family members to retrospectively report personality traits is vulnerable to biases.

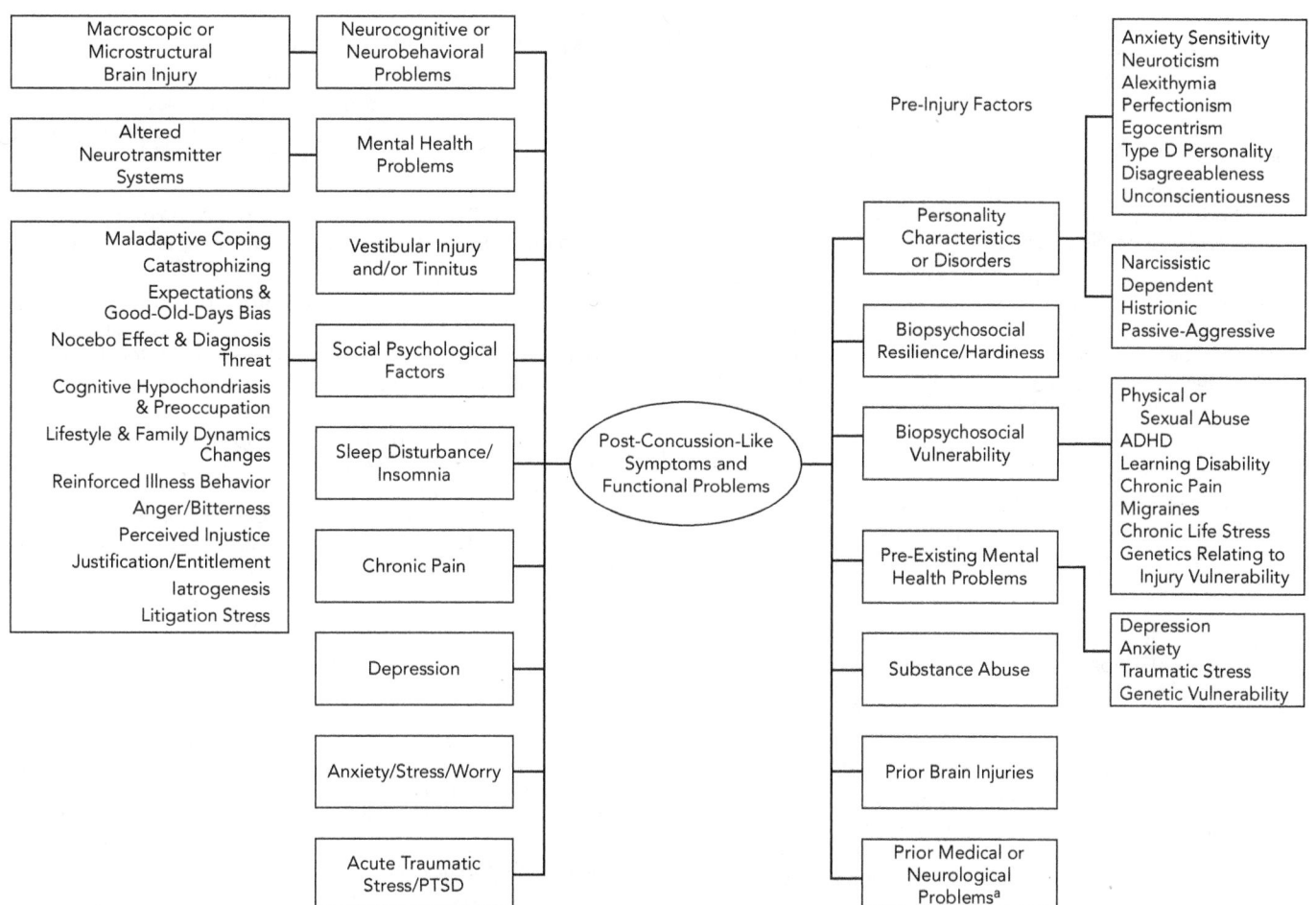

FIGURE 30–1 A biopsychosocial conceptualization of outcome from mild traumatic brain injury. Structural and/or microstructural damage to the brain is not necessary to cause or to maintain the symptoms comprising a postconcussion syndrome. Moreover, structural and/or microstructural damage, if present, is likely insufficient to causally maintain a *persistent* postconcussion syndrome. Assuming that a constellation of persistent symptoms are present (i.e., not exaggerated), there are many factors that could, singly or in combination, be the underlying cause of these symptoms. Notably, patients with chronic pain frequently report a constellation of symptoms that are postconcussion-like, and patients with depression are virtually guaranteed to report symptoms that mimic a postconcussion syndrome (in the absence of a history of head trauma). PTSD, post-traumatic stress disorder; ADHD, attention deficit hyperactivity disorder.
[a]For example, hypertension, heart disease, cardiac surgery, diabetes, thyroid problems, and small vessel ischemic disease.
Copyright © 2011, Grant L. Iverson. Used with permission.

Prior life experience may also predispose people to poor outcome from MTBI. A greater number of preinjury stressful life events are associated with depression, anxiety, and health-related quality of life after MTBI (65). In other health conditions characterized by medically unexplained symptoms, prior experience with illness (both personally and indirectly, such as observing a family member) seems to shape interpretations of symptoms and behavioral responses to them (66). This may also be true for long-term symptom reporting following MTBI.

The earlier-identified factors do not capture all aspects of preinjury functioning that contribute to individual differences in MTBI recovery. Resiliency and vulnerability are biopsychosocial concepts that confer protection against or predispose one to physical and mental health problems. They provide a broader framework for understanding preinjury risk for poor outcome. Resilience factors include positive

coping style, high self-efficacy, hardiness, positive emotions and optimism, humor, social and occupational support, genetics, serotonin transport and binding, norepinephrine biosynthesis and availability, dopaminergic brain reward systems, sympathetic nervous system regulation, neuropeptides, hypothalamic-pituitary-adrenal axis, cortisol, and other stress hormones (67–69). *Resilience,* from a psychological perspective, is an intrinsic characteristic underlying a person's ability to successfully adapt to acute stress and more chronic forms of adversity. Possible underpinnings of resilience include (a) facing fears; (b) adaptive coping; (c) optimism and positive emotions; (d) cognitive reappraisal, positive reframing, and acceptance; (e) social competence and social support; and (f) purpose in life, a moral compass, and meaning and spirituality (67).

In contrast, vulnerability can be conceptualized as a superordinate composition of individual risk factors for physi-

TABLE 30-2 Definitions of Selected Terms Used in the Biopsychosocial Model Presented in Figure 30-1.

Alexithymia: A cluster of traits characterized by difficulty identifying feelings, difficulty describing feelings to others, externally oriented thinking, and limited capacity for imaginal thinking (395).

Anxiety Sensitivity: A trait comprised of physical, psychological, and social preoccupations and concerns, is characterized by fear of anxiety-related bodily sensations.

Diagnosis Threat: This term, proposed by Suhr and Gunstad (265), was adapted from the social psychological concept of *stereotype threat* (396). Specifically, if told the reason for neuropsychological testing is because you might have problems caused by a past head trauma, a person might perform more poorly than if given a more benign explanation for the purpose of testing.

Disagreeableness: A personality trait characterized by antagonism, skepticism, and egocentrism.

Egocentrism: A personality characteristic relating to the tendency to perceive, understand, and interpret one's social interactions from a highly personalized frame of reference. This personality characteristic is related to selfishness, self-centeredness, and narcissism.

Expectation as Etiology: An expression coined by Mittenberg and colleagues (102). Following an injury, people's anticipation or expectation of certain symptoms might cause them to misattribute future normal, everyday symptoms to the remote injury—or fail to appreciate the relation between more proximal factors (e.g., life stress, poor sleep, and mild depression) and their symptoms.

Good-Old-Days Bias: This refers to the tendency to view oneself as healthier in the past and underestimate past problems. This response bias, combined with an expectation of certain symptoms following MTBI, can have a potent impact on symptom reporting.

Hardiness: A personality characteristic consisting of 3 psychological attitudes and beliefs: commitment, challenge, and control. Through commitment, a person turns events into something meaningful and important. Control refers to the belief that one can influence the course of events. Challenge refers to a belief system in which wisdom and growth are gained from difficult experiences.

Cognitive Hypochondriasis and Preoccupation: Hypochondriasis and somatic preoccupation have been recognized as dysfunctional behavior patterns for decades. They are associated with a magnified perception of bodily sensations and symptoms, fear of having serious health problems or disease, and extensive contact with health care providers. By extension, Boone (397) discussed a form of cognitive hypochondriasis that sometimes occurs in patients with poor outcome following MTBI. These patients have a fixed belief that they are significantly cognitively impaired, despite normal neuropsychological test performance, and that this impairment reflects permanent brain damage. Delis and Wetter

(398) proposed a "Cogniform Disorder," a Somatoform Disorder Subtype, characterized by pervasive and excessive cognitive symptoms and conversion-like adoption of the sick role.

Iatrogenesis: A state of ill health or adverse effect caused by medical treatment. For example, diagnosing "brain damage" as an explanation for persistent problems seen long after a mild concussion can be iatrogenic for some people.

Neuroticism: A personality trait characterized by a strong tendency to experience negative emotions such as anxiety, depression, anger, and self-consciousness. Individuals with this trait have considerable difficulty coping with stress.

Reinforced Illness Behavior: Some patients with chronic pain conditions and somatoform disorders develop entrenched reinforced illness behaviors and evolve into describing their symptoms and problems in a dramatic or exaggerated manner. That is, their behavior and interpersonal style changes over time, through environmental factors and social reinforcement, to include verbal and nonverbal illness behaviors.

Nocebo Effect: The nocebo effect is the causation of sickness by the expectations of sickness and by associated emotional states. That is, the sickness is, essentially, caused by expectation of sickness (113).

Perceived Injustice: A strongly held belief that one has been treated unfairly, disrespectfully, and/or thwarted in what one feels entitled to. Believing that one is suffering unnecessarily as a result of another's actions can underlie perceived injustice. This can be a firmly entrenched belief system that can influence the perception and reporting of symptoms, treatment adherence, and health-related behaviors.

Perfectionism: A personality characteristic characterized by an organized, disciplined, and focused striving toward perfection in behavior and activities. It can be particularly pathological when a person with high levels of neuroticism believes firmly that anything less than perfection is unacceptable.

Resilience: This is comprised of a diverse set of biological, psychological, and social factors that confer some degree of protection from physical and mental health problems. From a psychological perspective, resilience is an intrinsic characteristic underlying a person's ability to successfully adapt to acute stress and more chronic forms of adversity.

Type D Personality: This personality pattern is characterized by 2 stable personality traits: negative affectivity and social inhibition.

Unconscientiousness: A personality trait characterized by reduced self-discipline and ambition, disorganization, and a more lackadaisical approach to life.

Vulnerability: Conceptualized as a superordinate composition of individual risk factors for physical and mental health problems.

Abbreviation: MTBI, mild traumatic brain injury.
Reprinted from Silverberg ND, Iverson GL (391) with permission.

cal and mental health problems. A person's vulnerability to depression, for example, is believed to arise from the cumulative impact (70,71) of genetics (72,73), adverse events in childhood (e.g., abuse) (74), and ongoing life stressors. Obviously, there is no reason to believe that people who have sustained an MTBI would be immune to the diverse range of preinjury and co-occurring factors that contribute to both resilience and vulnerability. These preinjury factors might

influence the initial presentation, acute outcome, course, and long-term outcome from injury.

Peri-Injury

Several aspects of the injury event appear to influence outcome. Although MTBI appears to result in a characteristic neurometabolic response (75), the biomechanics of each brain trauma and resultant neuropathology are unique. Traditional severity indicators for traumatic brain injury such as the duration of LOC and PTA have repeatedly been found to poorly predict MTBI outcome (2). These severity indices may be too crude, or factors other than brain injury severity may largely account for differences in outcome. Neuroimaging findings are considered another objective marker of injury severity. Individuals with trauma-related intracranial abnormalities, considered to have a "complicated" MTBI, are intuitively at risk for worse outcome. This is discussed in more detail in Chapter 29 and in the following text.

The mechanism and context of the injury may also be important. MTBIs incurred in sport participation are associated with better outcome than those from other mechanisms, especially motor vehicle accidents (e.g., 47). There are probably several other reasons for this discrepancy. Athletes tend to be younger, in relatively good health at the time of their injury, and have more adaptive expectations (76) and incentives for recovery. As well, there is a higher probability of additional bodily injuries, potential for psychological traumatization, and access to financial compensation following car accidents. Each of these factors is associated with prolonged recovery (2,49,77–79). These and other postinjury factors are addressed subsequently.

Postinjury

A diverse set of factors influence the experience and reporting of symptoms and problems in the days, weeks, and months following an MTBI. Many of these factors are illustrated in Figure 30-1 and discussed in the sections that follow.

Pathophysiological Factors

Following the injury event, several biopsychosocial factors appear to shape the recovery trajectory. Although the neurobiological consequences of MTBI (75) are thought to resolve over the initial days and weeks in most patients with milder forms of this injury, some may be left with structural or microstructural brain damage. Initially, structural injuries (i.e., complicated MTBIs) are associated with worse neuropsychological functioning and higher incidence of comorbid vestibular injury (80–82). Studies have reported both higher (25) and lower (80) symptom reporting associated with complicated MTBIs. At follow-up, these patients often have similar affective profiles (83) and return to work rates (80) as those with uncomplicated MTBIs, but there are mixed evidence regarding whether neuropsychological performance converges in the 2 groups (83–86). Finally, there is some evidence that hemorrhagic contusions, but not other types of day-of-injury CT abnormalities, are associated with worse outcome (78).

Long white matter tracts might be particularly vulnerable (87). Modern neuroimaging techniques such as diffusion tensor imaging (DTI) and susceptibility weighted imaging (SWI) have the potential to better characterize neuropathological changes (see Chapter 15). A few studies have found group-level differences in white matter integrity between patients with persistent symptoms and matched healthy controls (88–90), but the magnitude of these effects and their correspondence with symptom severity is modest and variable. Similarly, a few studies have demonstrated functional neuroimaging differences in a subset of patients with persistent symptoms (91,92). The prevalence, specificity, and clinical relevance of neuroimaging abnormalities in patients with chronic symptoms remain poorly understood.

Leddy and colleagues (93) propose additional central and peripheral physiological mechanisms that may underlie postconcussion symptoms. Based on observations of altered physiological parameters such as increased heart rate, reduced cerebrovascular autoregulation, heightened sympathetic nervous system activity, and proinflammatory cytokine release in MTBI patients, they suggest "regulatory and autoregulatory physiologic dysfunction as a primary explanation of [postconcussion syndrome]" (p. 203). The specificity of these physiological changes to MTBI (versus a stressful event that does not involve head trauma, e.g.), their time course, and their association with symptomatic status needs to be further researched.

Psychological Factors

A variety of postinjury psychosocial factors have also been investigated. Worry, stress, and anxiety are thought to be central features of long-term symptom reporting (43,44, 94,95). Ruff and colleagues (8,22,96) presented a multidimensional cumulative stressor conceptualization of the persistent postconcussion symptom reporting. Essentially, setbacks in several aspects of a person's life (physical, emotional, cognitive, psychosocial, vocational, financial, and recreational) serve as cumulative stressors that interact with personality and premorbid physical and mental health factors, resulting in a disorder. Considerable research evidence supports the relationship between anxiety and postconcussion symptoms, which is thought to be reciprocal (e.g., 43,95,97). Measures of anxiety strongly differentiate people with and without long-term symptoms after MTBI and correlate with concurrent postconcussion symptom severity, including headaches and balance problems (13,14,47,98,99). Postconcussion symptom reporting is higher on stressful days (100) and is increased by experimentally induced stress (101).

Maladaptive health-related beliefs can contribute to anxiety and increase the risk of poor outcome. For example, Mittenberg and colleagues (102,103) proposed that expecting to have symptoms after an MTBI and misattributing bodily sensations (e.g., stress-induced sympathetic nervous system hyperarousal) to MTBI was responsible for postconcussion symptoms. Based on the key findings that (a) the number of postinjury symptoms reported by patients was the same as the number of symptoms healthy controls would *expect* to experience after a brain injury, and (b) patients with brain injuries consistently *underestimated* the normal prevalence of postconcussion-like symptoms in their retrospective accounts (i.e., their preinjury symptoms) compared with the base rate of symptoms reported by normal controls, they hypothesized that for some people the presence of symptoms following MTBI may be due to "the anticipation . . . that [postconcussion syndrome] will occur following mild head injury (p. 202)".

Following an injury, a patient may "reattribute benign emotional, physiological, and memory symptoms to their head injury" (p. 203). That is, people might "expect" to experience certain symptoms and problems, and this expectation might partially underlie symptom reporting following an injury. This mechanism may be an example of the "nocebo effect" (30), a term most associated with adverse event reporting in patients taking a placebo medication as part of a double-blinded pharmaceutical clinical trial. The nocebo effect was introduced more than 40 years ago (104,105), and research and discussion in this area is ongoing (e.g., 106, 107–112). The nocebo effect is the causation of sickness by the expectations of sickness and by associated emotional states (113). The nocebo effect may cause and/or maintain symptoms over time. There is now evidence that expecting symptoms to persist beyond a few weeks after MTBI predicts their actual persistence, that is, higher rates of symptoms months later (31,114,115). Consistent with this, persistent postconcussion symptom reporting is far less prevalent in cultures without such permanency beliefs (116–118).

Other possible maladaptive beliefs after MTBI include catastrophizing its consequences, blaming others for causing the injury, being preoccupied with injustice, and perceiving little control. The more that patients see postconcussion symptoms as interfering with their life in the first few weeks after MTBI, the more likely they are to have symptoms at follow-up, after controlling for initial symptom severity (31,114,115). Within their seminal study, Rutherford et al. (119) reported that attributing blame to an employer or impersonal organization was disproportionately common in patients with persistent symptoms. Blame attribution in acute rehabilitation is associated with later psychological functioning in moderate-to-severe traumatic brain injury (120). Perceived injustice—blaming others for unfair and irreparable losses—is associated with worse outcome from musculoskeletal injury (121), and so may also be relevant in MTBI. Finally, there is a large literature in other health conditions demonstrating that individuals who perceive that they have minimal control over their symptoms (i.e., low coping self-efficacy) have worse health outcomes (122,123).

What people think about their health condition has been well established to influence how they cope with it, which in turn influences health outcomes (123,124). Maladaptive coping behaviors, therefore, probably also contribute to long-term symptom reporting. For example, excessive rest and inactivity during the postacute period may actually worsen symptoms because of physiological deconditioning or increased depression because of limited opportunities for mastery experiences that are essential for positive mood and self-efficacy (93,125–128). At the other end of the spectrum, the cycle of "pushing through symptoms" (overexertion) and "crashing" may be even more counterproductive to recovery (115). Symptom-focused attention and related hypervigilant behaviors (e.g., keeping extremely detailed symptom diaries) may also be problematic. Hypervigilance to symptoms is also thought to mediate the nocebo effect (66,117,129), but the role of this behavior in MTBI outcome has yet to be empirically established. Avoidant coping is an important determinant of outcome in other health conditions (e.g., 123), but research of this construct in MTBI outcome to date has been minimal and mixed (48,130).

Iatrogenic Factors

How others respond to the injured person can also influence recovery. Although poorly researched, the iatrogenic potential of health professionals is widely recognized

(44,94). Certainly, incorrect diagnosis may lead to treatment that is potentially both ineffective and possibly detrimental to the patient, physically and/or psychologically. Parallel to experiences with chronic pain and whiplash-associated disorders, persons with MTBI may experience the negative ramifications of iatrogenesis in the context of overinvestigation, particularly with unproven "neurodiagnostic" techniques, inappropriate information and advice, misdiagnosis, overtreatment, and inappropriate medication prescription (the latter which may produce further impairment and/or complications) (131,132).

The tendency for medical, medical–legal, and rehabilitation professionals to diagnose "brain damage" or "diffuse axonal injury" as an explanation for persistent symptoms following an uncomplicated MTBI may, in and of itself, result in iatrogenic harm. When a person is diagnosed or misdiagnosed as having presumed permanent brain damage, it sends a strong, negative, prognostic message. It also might lead to (a) the person seeking support from Brain Injury Associations, (b) the person receiving rehabilitation services normally designated for patients with moderate to severe brain injuries and consequentially unnecessarily utilizing health care and societal resources, and (c) the failure to provide effective treatment for the person's prominent underlying problems.

Others might argue that what sometimes appears to be accidental iatrogenic illness may in fact be driven by unethical clinical practice and/or examiner secondary gain. There are tremendous financial and professional pressures in the medical–legal setting, and it is widely believed that some experts adopt rather extreme, predictable, and polarized opinions that result in routine labeling of people as having long-term problems because of permanent brain damage following a mild concussion. Better guidelines are clearly necessary to aid clinicians evaluating and treating persons with MTBI to avoid iatrogenesis.

Social and Interpersonal Factors

Family, friends, and coworkers can also act, often inadvertently, in ways that contribute to ongoing symptoms. For example, the patient may get special privileges and extra attention. The experience of being ill can then, in some ways, be rewarding for the patient. For many years, these issues have been studied in patients with chronic pain syndromes. Researchers have demonstrated that extra attention, changes in household responsibilities and routines, and the avoidance of undesirable activities all can *increase* patients' reporting of pain and disability (133–135).

It is reasonable to think that some individuals with persistent symptoms and problems following an MTBI, similar to chronic pain patients, could derive reinforcement for disability behaviors. This is sometimes referred to as a reinforced behavior pattern. In contrast, invalidating responses from others, such as minimizing the patient's symptoms, attributing their disability to being "all in your head," or advising him to "get over it" can exacerbate stress (and as a result, heightened symptoms) and/or counterproductively motivate patients to prove the validity of their condition through exaggerated illness behaviors (e.g., wearing sun glasses indoors, cancelling social plans, etc.). Note that "adoption of a sick role" is included in the ICD-10 diagnostic criteria for the syndrome (95).

Litigation-Related Factors

Many patients with chronic symptoms are involved in litigation relating to their injury, which can influence their condition in several ways. Litigation is another major source of stress. Weissman (136) described aspects of litigation stress in the quote subsequently. What is apparent from this quote is Weissman's belief that litigation produces negative effects on the plaintiff's mental state through multiple pathways, including greater susceptibility to stressors, attitude changes, motivational changes, and biases in self-reported problems.

> Involvement in litigation renders plaintiffs susceptible to stressors and to influences that may lead to increased impairment, biased reportage, and retarded recovery. Underlying personality patterns play a critical role in defining and shaping reactions to trauma, to the stress of litigation, and to treatment interventions. Protracted litigation creates conditions that promote mnemonic and attitudinal distortions, as well as conscious and unconscious motivations for secondary gain. (136) (p. 67)

Plaintiffs with acquired brain injuries or psychological problems find themselves in a very different health care environment compared to injured or emotionally distressed people not in litigation. For example, individuals other than the injured person have a vested interest in the assessment and rehabilitation of the plaintiff. As well, others have a vested interest in doubting the veracity of the patient's health problems. The effect of these vested interests can be seen in the skepticism frequently attached to diagnoses of postconcussion syndrome, PTSD, or major depressive disorder. Outside the context of litigation or disability compensation systems, these diagnoses are accepted with little skepticism. One result of these vested interests and skepticism is that plaintiffs with alleged postconcussion syndrome or psychological problems will be subjected to more intensive, frequent, and possibly hostile assessment of their health problems. There might even be pressures to avoid effective treatments and remain off work in order to illustrate the damages resulting from the cause of action.

Undoubtedly, protracted litigation can be very stressful, and a plaintiff who was once significantly injured but who has largely recovered might feel *entitled* to the compensation anticipated by his lawyer, thus feeling *justified* in his decision to significantly exaggerate his current disability. This situation may also promote disability through unconscious processes such as "cognitive dissonance" (137,138), wherein people alter their views (e.g., "I still have severe symptoms") to match their behavior (e.g., seeking compensation).

Recall Bias Factors

Postconcussion symptom reporting is also influenced by biases in self-assessment. Following an MTBI, people tend to underestimate how much they have recovered because they overestimate their preinjury well-being, a phenomenon termed the "good-old-days" bias. Researchers have reported that patients with back injuries, general trauma victims, as well as patients with MTBI, overestimate the actual degree of postinjury change that has taken place by retrospectively recalling fewer preinjury symptoms than the base rate of symptoms in healthy controls (102,137,139–144). This may

occur after negative life events other than traumatic injuries (140), and even in absence of an explicit negative event reference point (145). The tendency to recall past symptoms and functioning (e.g., work status, relationships, etc.) more favorably may be enhanced in the context of personal injury litigation (e.g., 142,144,146) and in examinees who fail effort testing in neuropsychological assessment (143).

Comorbid Conditions

There are several comorbidities that may contribute to, or even fully account for, the myriad of symptoms and problems reported by patients long after experiencing a mild injury to their head, brain, or both. In practice, it is often difficult to disentangle the many factors that can be responsible for the symptoms following a remote MTBI and/or craniocervical trauma. This is because chronic symptoms that can follow MTBI (e.g., headaches, fatigue, dizziness, irritability, poor concentration) can also be present in healthy subjects (102,147–152) and more prominently in patients with no history of brain injury, such as outpatients seen for psychological treatment (153) or minor medical problems (154), personal injury claimants (154,155), patients with PTSD (156) or depression (157), patients with orthopedic injuries (16), individuals with chronic pain (158–161), and patients with whiplash (162). Thus, differential diagnosis of persistent symptoms is very challenging but critical in the context of optimizing outcomes. It is important to note that these comorbid conditions often cooccur not just with MTBI but with each other, such as chronic pain and depression (163–167).

Cervical Injuries and Whiplash-Associated Disorders

The most common acute symptoms following whiplash are neck pain, headache, and limitation in neck range of motion (168–170). Many other symptoms have been associated with cervical injury, including visual disturbances, dizziness, auditory disturbances, balance disorders, and cognitive dysfunction (171–174). This cluster of symptoms might arise from extracranial head and neck trauma such as dislodging of otoconia (as in benign paroxysmal positional vertigo; 175, 176,177) and temporomandibular joint dysfunction (178). The cause of cognitive complaints or objective cognitive decrements in a subset of patients with whiplash is less clear; researchers suggest they might be related to damage to the brain (179), somatization (180), distraction because of pain (181), or a combination of factors.

Cranial Trauma

Head (i.e., cranial) injury can, of course, result in damage to the skull or its adjoining parts (i.e., the cranium or cranial adenexal structures). This damage might underlie some of the symptoms and problems reported acutely and postacutely in some patients (176). Skull fractures are relatively uncommon in patients who sustain MTBIs. When they occur, they may be closed, compound and depressed, or nondepressed. Longitudinal fractures are more commonly associated with conductive hearing loss because of either ossicular chain disruption or traumatic tympanic membrane tear and blood in the middle ear. Transverse temporal skull fractures often will be associated with either mixed or profound sensorineural hearing loss, hemotympanum, dizziness, and/or facial nerve injuries (182,183). The most common type of ossicular dislocation associated with temporal skull fractures is the separation of the incudostapedial joint, with or without dislocation of the body of the incus from the articulation with the malleus head (see Chapter 46).

Complaints of "dizziness" following cranial trauma and/or MTBI are common. Labyrinthine concussion can result in transient auditory and vestibular symptoms without associated skull fracture. Benign paroxysmal positional vertigo is the most common neuro-otologic problem following head trauma. Many patients demonstrate a paroxysmal positional nystagmus with rapid changes in position (184). The clinician should also consider the possibility of a post-traumatic endolymphatic hydrops (Meniere syndrome) after cranial trauma when there is ipsilateral low-frequency hearing loss, tinnitus, and a sensation of fullness in the ear.

Post-traumatic perilymphatic fistula can occur following trauma as a result of rupture of the oval and less commonly the round window with subsequent communication between the inner ear and middle ear resulting in inappropriate stimulation of labyrinthine receptors (185). Unfortunately, there is no pathognomonic or characteristic sign or test for this condition. Symptoms can include vertigo, fluctuating hearing loss (usually a late complication), tinnitus, chronic low-grade nausea, endolymphatic hydrops, abnormal cervical muscle tone (myodystonia), and persistent or exertional headache (186). Patients quite frequently complain of aural fullness (187). Patients will often complain of nonspecific balance problems worsened by sudden turning, as well as disequilibrium with perceptually complex external stimuli such as patterns and wide-field motion evidenced with escalator rides, revolving doors, and crowds (187,188). The sensation while ambulating has been described as "walking on pillows" (189). The aforementioned experiences sometimes promote a mild agoraphobia (see Chapter 47).

Olfactory and gustatory problems also can occur following injury to the cranium and/or brain (see Chapter 48). Costanzo and Zasler (190) listed the known and presumed mechanisms underlying olfactory impairment following head trauma or traumatic brain injury (TBI) as follows: (a) traumatic damage to the nasal epithelium; (b) shearing of the olfactory fila, arising from the nasal epithelium, prior to entering the olfactory bulbs, as a presumed consequence of movement of the brain relative to, and/or fracture of, the cribriform plate; and (c) contusions or edema affecting the olfactory bulb or the lateral or medial olfactory tracts. All of these mechanisms could cause impairment in the ability to detect odors. Isolated gustatory dysfunction is uncommon. Typically, peripheral injury involves the facial nerve (cranial nerve [CN] VII) because it is more prone to injury than the glossopharyngeal (CN IX) and vagus (CN X) nerves, which are also involved in mediation of taste (190).

Visual problems can occur at a peripheral level and be unrelated to a brain injury (see Chapters 45 and 47). These deficits can be caused by disorders of the vitreous, both perifoveal and foveal, commonly associated with traction on the retina with resultant subjective symptoms of floating spots (so-called "floaters") (191,192). Retinal injury, including detachment, tear, and hemorrhage (193,194), also causes visual symptoms. Approximately 20% of patients evaluated with mid-facial trauma were noted in one study to have accommodative and/or convergence insufficiency (195).

Headache and neck pain are the most common physical complaints following head trauma and MTBI (see Chapter 57). Headaches, of course, are common in the general population as well (196,197). Preexisting headaches, post-traumatic headaches, or both might largely underlie a diverse set of symptoms and problems in people who have sustained an MTBI (as well as patients with whiplash-related problems or cranial-trauma related problems). Patients with problematic headaches often have comorbid depression (198–201) or subclinical psychiatric symptoms (202–207).

Chronic Pain

Patients with chronic pain often complain of physical, cognitive, and psychological symptoms that closely resemble postconcussion-like symptoms (e.g., 158,160,180,208,209–215). For example, Iverson and McCracken (160) reported that among nonlitigating, chronic pain patients with no history of head injury, 80.6% endorsed 3 or more of the symptoms from Category C of the postconcussional disorder research criteria in the DSM-IV (32). Patients who sustain MTBIs in falls or motor vehicle accidents frequently have a comorbid chronic pain problem. Uomoto and Esselman (216) reported that 95% of patients with MTBIs reported the presence of at least 1 chronic pain symptom 24 months postinjury (e.g., headaches, neck/shoulder pain, or back pain). Pain is associated with postconcussion symptom reporting in individuals with and without a recent MTBI (46). In summary, because chronic pain often accompanies MTBI and influences postconcussion symptom reporting, attributing symptoms to brain injury in patients with comorbid chronic pain is problematic (see Chapters 57 and 58).

Mood and Anxiety Disorders

Depression is common following TBIs of all severities (217, 218), as well as in conditions that are often comorbid with MTBI such as chronic pain (163,165,166,219), chronic headaches (201,220–222), PTSD (156,223–225), and substance abuse problems (226–230). The cause(s) of depression following MTBI are not well understood. It is theoretically plausible that depression can arise (a) directly or indirectly from the neurobiological consequences of the MTBI; (b) as a psychological reaction to deficits and problems associated with having an MTBI; (c) as a comorbid condition with an anxiety disorder such as PTSD, chronic pain, and/or insomnia; or (d) a combination of these factors. Of course, depression can also arise de novo, incidentally, sometime postinjury—such as in response to life stressors that are unrelated or peripherally related to the original injury. It can also arise as part of a preexisting chronic relapsing and remitting condition.

Depression has a very large effect on postconcussion-like symptom reporting (63,150,157,231,232). For example, in patients with depression who do not have a history of head trauma, approximately 90% met self-report symptom criteria for ICD-10 postconcussional syndrome when defined liberally (i.e., symptoms endorsed as "mild" were included), and more than 50% met these criteria when defined conservatively (i.e., all symptoms had to be reported as "moderate–severe") (232). This is not surprising because the symptoms associated with depression have considerable overlap with the symptoms comprising the postconcussion syndrome. The diagnostic criteria for major depression include the following symptoms: (a) diminished ability to think or concentrate, (b) indecisiveness, (c) fatigue or loss of energy, and (d) sleep problems (*DSM-IV*; 32) (p. 327). In addition, major depression often is associated with irritability, excessive worry over one's health, and headaches (32) (p. 323). Even when this confound is minimized by identifying cases with depression on the basis of nonoverlapping features (e.g., sadness, guilt, worthlessness, suicidality), a substantial effect of depression on postconcussion-like symptom reporting remains (157).

Comorbid depression further complicates differential diagnosis because perceived cognitive impairment is a *cardinal feature* of depression (233). Depression can also be associated with objective impairment on neuropsychological testing (234–236). There are no published studies showing that the cognitive effects of depression can be reliably differentiated from the cognitive effects of an MTBI. Therefore, it is extremely difficult to determine if a person's low neuropsychological test scores are attributable to depression, a remote MTBI, or both.

Another challenging differential diagnosis is PTSD. Traumatic stress co-occurs with MTBI in 33%–39% of military personnel and 12%–27% of civilian trauma patients (237,238). Traumatic stress may be more common in patients with MTBI compared to those with moderate-to-severe TBI, perhaps because the former are less likely to have extensive amnesia for the traumatic event (239–241). Patients with PTSD (and no MTBI) often report the same symptoms as patients who have sustained MTBIs. For example, in a sample of 128 patients with PTSD, 89% reported irritability, 56% reported memory problems, 92% reported concentration problems, and 90% reported difficulty sleeping (156). Therefore, it is easy to misdiagnose PTSD as a postconcussion syndrome and vice versa. Several studies have reported that PTSD largely explained the relationship between MTBI and postconcussion-like symptom reporting (242,243) or had an additive effect on symptom reporting (239,244).

It is unclear whether anxiety disorders other than PTSD are more common after MTBI. The small literature in this area contains significant discrepancies (245). For example, of patients with MTBI referred to a rehabilitation program for poor outcome, 2% had a preinjury anxiety disorder and 24% had a current anxiety disorder (246). Patients with MTBI from a prospective cohort of consecutive trauma admissions had a similar rate of current anxiety disorder (18%), but this proportion did not differ from the preinjury period or from a non-MTBI trauma control group (46). Regardless, given the symptom overlap between the postconcussion syndrome and all anxiety disorders, they should be considered in the differential diagnosis.

Substance-Related Disorders and Medications

Alcohol and drug use might also contribute to symptom reporting. Analgesics for post-traumatic headache, including over-the-counter acetaminophen, caffeine, and/or opiates can actually perpetuate headaches if used too frequently (e.g., medication overuse headache) (247). Gabapentin and anticonvulsant medications such as topiramate and valproic acid are also sometimes prescribed for post-traumatic headache (248); several of these medications have well-documented cognitive side effects. Benzodiazepines, used to treat anxiety and/or insomnia, can cause or aggravate fatigue and, with prolonged regular use, they may be depressogenic

and cause or aggravate cognitive impairment (249,250). Excessive use of caffeine and over-the-counter agents such as guarana and gotu kola can cause or aggravate irritability. Illicit drug use of marijuana, cocaine, and other agents may cause both cognitive and behavioral changes, some of which may confound interpretation of patient complaints regarding postconcussive symptoms. Lastly, alcohol abuse may cause behavioral disinhibition and other behavioral dysregulations, as well as impede cognitive function. Early on after injury, it may also theoretically impede neurorecovery through GABAergic mechanisms (251) (see Chapter 79).

ASSESSMENT

Eliciting self-reported symptoms is the cornerstone of assessment. Subjective symptoms are necessary for a diagnosis under both the ICD-10 and *DSM-IV* frameworks, and sufficient for the ICD-10. There are several standardized postconcussion symptom checklists and questionnaires (e.g., 252). Such measures can help to quantify severity and track change over time. Because reporting postconcussion-like symptoms is normal to some extent, it can also be helpful to compare obtained scores to normative standards for healthy adults and adults with mental health problems, chronic pain, or both. Concerns have been raised, however, that post-concussion symptom endorsement rates are markedly higher when elicited by a standardized rating scale vs an interview (253,254). For example, worker's compensation patients with MTBI often endorse having moderate to severe symptoms on a questionnaire after not mentioning the symptom in a clinical interview, even when domain prompts (e.g., "... any problems with your thinking?") are provided (254).

A thorough history taking can enrich case conceptualization, providing context for symptom reporting. Although many of the preinjury resilience and vulnerability factors outlined earlier cannot be directly measured, proxy indicators of preinjury functioning can be probed in a clinical interview. A history of low academic achievement, childhood abuse, unemployment, alcohol and drug use, legal problems, relationship dysfunction, family mental health history, and psychiatric treatment may be gross indicators of preinjury neurobiological and psychological vulnerability. Inquiring about an examinee's prior experience with injury, illness, and other major stressors can shed light on his or her resiliency, self-efficacy, and coping styles. The clinician should also listen for idealized language in an examinee's description of their preinjury life. Insistence on having a "photographic" memory, "perfect" marriage, sleeping "like a rock" every night, never feeling irritable, or never feeling tired, for example, is suggestive of a good-old-days bias.

Neuropsychological Assessment

Neuropsychological assessment can be helpful for documenting a person's current functioning, determining whether or not a person has measurable cognitive deficits, and planning treatment and rehabilitation services. However, requiring impaired performance on objective cognitive testing to define poor outcome from MTBI, such as in the *DSM-IV* diagnostic framework, is fraught with challenges. Meta-analyses have documented that the acute neuropsychological effects of

MTBI are substantial (255,256). After 3 months, however, MTBI effects disappear in unselected (prospective) samples (256,257). Neuropsychological deficits remain large or even increase in samples of patients who are in litigation or presenting to clinic (3). Studies comparing patients with persistent symptoms to matched healthy controls, orthopedic injury controls, recovered MTBI patients, or normative data have yielded mixed findings regarding whether persistent symptom reporting is associated with detectable neuropsychological impairment (13,14,258–262). It is possible, although unproven (257), that these group-level analyses may aggregate a small subgroup with persistent cognitive deficits and the majority who made a complete recovery (263). However, the long-term neuropsychological impairment after MTBI might be too uncommon and too subtle to reliably identify in most individual patients without excessive false positive diagnostic errors (256).

Clearly, not all patients with multiple persisting symptoms after MTBI produce impaired scores on neuropsychological testing. In those who do, some have preexisting factors that can result in lower neuropsychological test results, such as innate intelligence, attention deficit hyperactivity disorder, learning disabilities, or substance abuse. Test results obtained from patients long after an MTBI can also be adversely affected by situational factors (e.g., serious test anxiety or lapses in attention), social psychological factors (264,265), and comorbid clinical conditions such as pain (266), depression (234,235,267–278), and poor effort (279, 280). Finally, having a few low test scores in a comprehensive neuropsychological test battery is common in healthy children, adults, and older adults (281), and so is not necessarily abnormal.

Effort and Validity Testing

Symptom exaggeration and below-capacity performance on neuropsychological testing represent a major assessment challenge. When answering interview questions or responding to questionnaire items, examinees may fabricate symptoms, overstate their severity, or misattribute actual symptoms to the compensable event. On testing, they may underperform, intentionally choose wrong answers, slow their responding, or use other strategies to appear more impaired than they actually are. When an examinee deliberately engages in these behaviors to influence the outcome of the assessment for financial gain, they are considered to be malingering. The base rates of malingering following MTBI may be among the highest seen in neuropsychological practice (282). They are particularly high in the context of disability evaluations and personal injury litigation.

It is important to point out that malingering (*a*) is not an all-or-none phenomenon, that is, it occurs along a continuum; (*b*) does not rule out having legitimate signs and/or symptoms—an examinee with genuine problems attributable to an MTBI and/or a comorbid condition could also malinger; and (*c*) is not the only explanation for symptom exaggeration and below-capacity performance. A determination of malingering requires an inference about the examinee's intent. Several other motivations can underlie symptom exaggeration and below-capacity performance, including a "cry for help" (a euphemism implying that the person has serious problems and is desperately seeking recognition of, and attention for, these problems), dramatizing personality style, or a deep-seated psychological need to be perceived as sick and disabled (as in factitious disorder). The occurrence of effort test failures in outpatient rehabilitation and other settings outside of a medicolegal context (e.g., 283) supports the notion that malingering is not the only cause of symptom exaggeration and below-capacity performance.

Diagnosis Threat

Another challenge to the validity of neuropsychological assessment is "diagnosis threat." Suhr and Gunstad (265) hypothesized that the well-documented social-psychological phenomenon "stereotype threat," wherein an individual's performance on a particular task can be negatively affected by the threat of an inferior and/or negative stereotype (e.g., men are superior to women in mathematics), might be relevant in MTBI. They predicted that in people with MTBI, "calling attention to a personal history of head injury and its potential effects on cognition might lead to worse cognitive performance than that seen in individuals with similar head injury history, but who do not have attention called to either the head injury history or the possible consequences of head injury" (p. 450). Their experimental manipulation to create "diagnosis threat" in undergraduate students with a history of MTBI resulted in substantially lower performance on selected neuropsychological measures. It remains unclear whether increased anxiety, reduced effort, or other factors mediate the diagnosis threat effect (264,284).

Neuroimaging

Structural neuroimaging with CT is primarily used to screen for neurosurgical intervention needs shortly after an MTBI. In patients with severe persisting symptoms, it may also be used to rule out other neurological conditions that could explain a worsening course, but CT is insensitive to MTBI neuropathology (285). High-resolution magnetic resonance imaging (MRI) techniques including T1, T2, FLAIR, and SWI are also frequently used in patients with long-term symptoms following an MTBI. They can reveal white matter abnormalities from shear injury and/or hemosiderin deposits. The sensitivity of traditional MRI has not been documented in large prospective studies. Its specificity is another consideration, because incidental white matter hypertensities are fairly common in healthy people (286,287) (especially older than the age of 55 years) (288). Experimental techniques such as DTI are sometimes used in clinical settings. However, the diagnostic accuracy associated with cut-off points on quantitative measures (e.g., fractional anisotropy in DTI) is typically unknown, limiting their utility in clinical assessment. Functional neuroimaging techniques such as functional MRI, single photon emission CT (SPECT), and magnetic resonance spectroscopy can sometimes detect abnormalities in patients with acute MTBI who do not have visible structural lesions (289). An abnormal neuroimaging finding is not necessary for diagnosing someone with long-term symptoms attributable to an MTBI, and is probably not sufficient to fully account for these residual symptoms. On the other hand, the available technology is not adequate to rule out neurobiological contributions to a patient's clinical presentation if their neuroimaging is "normal."

Evaluating for Comorbidities

Assessment of patients with chronic postconcussion symptoms is incomplete without evaluating for comorbid conditions. Reports of dizziness and balance problems are suspicious of traumatic vestibular injury. Vestibular disorders often resolve quickly without treatment, but when this does not happen, there is often a lengthy delay in treatment referrals (290). Neurodiagnostic evaluation of the dizzy patient might include bedside vestibular tests, audiologic testing, a platform fistula test, electronystagmography with calorics, rotary chair testing, and/or posturography (177,291). There are a number of other objective assessment tools for vestibular dysfunction (see 292 for a recent review), several of which may only be available at a specialty vestibular rehabilitation clinic. The role of psychological factors in exacerbating dizziness and slowing recovery must also be considered (293).

Tinnitus may be a major source of distress and disability (294), so this should also be reviewed as part of a comprehensive evaluation. Chronic tinnitus has stress-inducing effects, it is associated with depression and anxiety, and tinnitus-related psychological distress is worse in individuals who have certain personality characteristics, such as type D personality and anxiety sensitivity (295).

Characterization of headache type (e.g., migraine vs tension-type presentations), medication use patterns, and lifestyle factors (e.g., missed meals, inadequate hydration) can help guide headache treatment. Medical conditions that can contribute to sleep and fatigue problems (e.g., sleep apnea) should also be ruled out.

Assessing for psychiatric comorbidity is also essential (see Chapter 61). MTBI outcome research suggests that a psychodiagnostic interview should, at minimum, cover mood, anxiety, and substance use disorders. Standardized multidimensional self-report tools with embedded validity can also be helpful to identify underreporting or overreporting response styles and to characterize personality traits that color the clinical picture. Well-validated psychopathology screening measures can be administered as part of routine care at concussion clinics to help identify individuals who require referral for psychiatric/psychological assessment (see Chapter 59).

"Postconcussion Syndrome" in Patients With MTBIs Other Clinical Groups, and Controls

It is well established and understood that postconcussion-like symptoms are nonspecific. For example, headaches, fatigue, sleep problems, irritability, and having difficulty concentrating are common in daily life, and extremely common in patients with medical or psychiatric problems. Rates of *individual* symptom reporting, such as headaches and irritability, in patients with MTBIs and other clinical groups have been presented in table form in a previous article (4). In Table 30-3, we present rates of *clusters* of symptoms across groups. By carefully studying articles relating to symptom reporting, we can determine how often people with MTBIs, assessed at different times, report clusters of symptoms and compare those rates to patients with other diagnoses and healthy controls. Careful study of this table reveals several themes, as listed subsequently.

1. Rates of multiple symptom reporting 3 or more months following MTBI vary widely, from 7.8% (296) to 91% (14) across studies.
2. Symptom reporting can be related to nonspecific effects of trauma vs MTBI. This was illustrated in 2 studies by Meares and colleagues (46,297) who reported that 43%–50% of trauma control subjects (without head injury), evaluated within approximately 1 week of injury, report multiple postconcussion-like symptoms compared to 40%–43% of patients with MTBIs.
3. Studies using questionnaires to elicit symptoms usually have higher rates of symptom endorsement than studies relying on interviewing (254).
4. How symptoms are conceptualized on a questionnaire dramatically alters rates of endorsement. For example, many questionnaires use Likert scales—so symptoms can be counted as present if they are endorsed as "mild or greater" or "moderate or greater." Simply requiring a "mild" experience of irritability, for example, greatly increases the prevalence of individual symptom endorsement. This was illustrated dramatically in a study by Iverson and Lange (149) in which healthy, uninjured community control subjects—free of mental health problems—completed a postconcussion questionnaire. Most healthy controls (72.1%) met ICD-10 symptom criteria for the postconcussional syndrome when symptoms endorsed as mild or greater were counted, and 13.9% met criteria when symptoms endorsed as moderate or greater were counted.
5. Patients with depression (63,157,232) or chronic pain (158,160), in the absence of head trauma, report very high levels of postconcussion-like symptoms. A substantial minority of healthy control subjects also endorse high levels of symptoms (63,142,149,298,299).

In conclusion, high levels of symptom reporting are common following MTBI. The cause of these symptoms might be multifactorial. Symptoms can be related to the pathophysiology of the MTBI, psychological factors, and/or a diverse range of biopsychosocial factors illustrated in Figure 30-1. In most cases of patients who present with a heavy symptom burden long after injury, identifying a single or predominant cause for the symptoms will be difficult unless the person clearly has a significant comorbid condition such as depression. A significant problem with depression or anxiety, combined with chronic pain, virtually guarantees high levels of symptom reporting regardless of a person's history of head trauma.

PROGNOSIS

Several prospective studies have noted that symptom reporting is stable or modestly increases/decreases from 3 months to 1 year after MTBI (16,29,300–304). Compared to full samples of consecutive MTBI cases, the trajectory of recovery appears to plateau earlier and improve less in the subgroup with persistent symptoms (37,99,300). The few studies that followed patients beyond 1 year note that symptom remission in this subgroup is uncommon, even after litigation settlement (305,306). To the extent that research participants who are retained at follow-up tend to be more symptomatic, these estimates are overly pessimistic.

TABLE 30-3 Rates of "Postconcussion Syndrome" in Patients With Mild Traumatic Brain Injuries, Depression, Trauma Controls Subjects, and Healthy Controls.

FIRST AUTHOR (YEAR)	COUNTRY	SAMPLE SIZE	SAMPLE CHARACTERISTICS	RECRUITMENT SETTING	TIME POSTINJURY (IF APPLICABLE)	RATE OF PCS	PCS DEFINITION
Dischinger (2009)	United States	180	Mild TBI	Level 1 Trauma Center	3–10 days	84.2%	4 or more symptoms
Meares (2008)	Australia	90	Mild TBI	Level 1 Trauma Center	Average 4.9 days	43.3%	3 or more symptoms from ICD-10 PCS symptom criteria
Meares (2011)	Australia	62	Mild TBI	Level 1 Trauma Center	Average 4.9 days	40.3%	3 or more symptoms from ICD-10 PCS symptom criteria
Kashluba (2006)	Canada	110	Mild TBI	Emergency department	1 month	72.7%	5 or more symptoms
Dikmen (2010)	United States	603	Mild-severe TBI	Level 1 Trauma Center	1 month	74.0%	3 or more symptoms
Rutherford (1977)	United Kingdom	145	Mild TBI	Emergency department	6 weeks	24.8%	5 or more symptoms
Lange (2011a)	Canada	60	Mild TBI	Level 1 Trauma Center	6–8 weeks	81.7%	ICD-10 Criteria, symptoms mild or greater
Lange (2011a)	Canada	60	Mild TBI	Level 1 Trauma Center	6–8 weeks	35.0%	ICD-10 Criteria, symptoms moderate or greater
Lange (2011b)	Canada	37	Mild TBI (no depression)	Outpatient clinic	51.8 ± 61.1 days	83.8%	ICD-10 Criteria, symptoms mild or greater
Lange (2011b)	Canada	23	Mild TBI + Depression	Outpatient clinic	51.8 ± 61.1 days	100.0%	ICD-10 Criteria, symptoms mild or greater
Lange (2011b)	Canada	37	Mild TBI (no depression)	Outpatient clinic	51.8 ± 61.1 days	48.6%	ICD-10 Criteria, symptoms moderate or greater
Lange (2011b)	Canada	23	Mild TBI + Depression	Outpatient clinic	51.8 ± 61.1 days	95.7%	ICD-10 Criteria, symptoms moderate or greater
Lange (2010a)	Canada	86	Mild TBI	Outpatient clinic	1.8 ± 1.7 months	94.2%	3 or more symptoms
Lange (2010a)	Canada	86	Mild TBI	Outpatient clinic	1.8 ± 1.7 months	82.6%	5 or more symptoms
Yang (2009)	Taiwan	180	Mild TBI	Inpatient clinic	2 months	9.0%	ICD-10 Criteria
Lange (2010b)	Canada	63	Mild TBI—failed effort testing	Outpatient clinic	2 ± 1 months	93.3%	5 or more symptoms
Lange (2010b)	Canada	63	Mild TBI—passed effort testing	Outpatient clinic	2 ± 1 months	66.0%	5 or more symptoms
Iverson (2010)	Canada	61	Mild TBI	Outpatient clinic	2.3 ± 1.6 months	91.8%	4 or more symptoms (questionnaire)
Iverson (2010)	Canada	61	Mild TBI	Outpatient clinic	2.3 ± 1.6 months	44.4%	4 or more symptoms (semi-structured interview)
Rimel (1982)	United States	424	Mild TBI	Hospital	3 months	5.0%	2 or more symptoms
Alves (1993)	United States	360	Mild TBI	Emergency department	3 months	7.2%	4 or more symptoms
Dischinger (2009)	United States	110	Mild TBI	Level 1 Trauma Center	3 months	41.4%	4 or more symptoms

Study	Country	N	TBI Severity	Setting	Time Post-Injury	%	Criteria
Kraus (2009)	United States	687	Mild TBI	Emergency department	3 months	32.1%	3 or more symptoms
McCauley (2001)	United States	95	Mild TBI	Emergency department, inpatient clinic	3 months	28.4%[a]	DSM-IV Criteria (structured interview)
McCauley (2005)	United States	340	Mild TBI	Level 1 Trauma Center	3 months	17.3%	DSM-IV Criteria (structured interview)
McCauley (2005)	United States	340	Mild TBI	Level 1 Trauma Center	3 months	53.8%	ICD-10 Criteria (structured interview)
Roe (2009)	Norway	52	Mild TBI	Neurosurgical department	3 months	55.8%	ICD-10 Criteria
Ingebrigtsen (1998)	Norway, Sweden	113	Mild TBI	Neurosurgical department	3 months	40.0%	ICD-9 Criteria, symptoms mild or greater
Sigurdardottir (2009)	Norway	115	Mild–severe TBI	Level 1 Trauma Center	3 months	27.8%	ICD-10 Criteria, symptoms moderate or greater
Meares (2011)	Australia	62	Mild TBI	Level 1 Trauma Center	Average 106.2 days	47.5%	3 or more symptoms from ICD-10 PCS symptom criteria
Schneiderman (2008)	United States	275	Mild TBI	Survey of military sample	5 months or greater	35.0%	3 or more symptoms
Ma (2008)	United States	41	Mild TBI	Level 1 Trauma Center	20 ± 6 weeks	53.7%	3 or more symptoms (scored 2 or higher)
McCauley (2008)	United States	139	Mild TBI	Level 1 Trauma Center	6 months	14.4%	DSM-IV Criteria (structured interview)
McCauley (2008)	United States	139	Mild TBI	Level 1 Trauma Center	6 months	44.6%	ICD-10 Criteria (structured interview)
McCauley (2008)	United States	46	Mild TBI with compensation	Level 1 Trauma Center	6 months	28.3%	DSM-IV Criteria (structured interview)
McCauley (2008)	United States	90	Mild TBI without compensation	Level 1 Trauma Center	6 months	7.8%	DSM-IV Criteria (structured interview)
McCauley (2008)	United States	46	Mild TBI with compensation	Level 1 Trauma Center	6 months	60.9%	ICD-10 Criteria (structured interview)
McCauley (2008)	United States	90	Mild TBI without compensation	Level 1 Trauma Center	6 months	37.8%	ICD-10 Criteria (structured interview)
Roe (2009)	Norway	52	Mild TBI	Neurosurgical department	6 months	42.3%	ICD-10 Criteria
Rutherford (1979)	United Kingdom	131	Mild TBI	Emergency department	12 months	4.6%	4 or more symptoms
Alves (1993)	United States	189	Mild TBI	Emergency department	12 months	5.8%	4 or more symptoms
Watson (1995)	United Kingdom	25	Mild TBI	Emergency department	12 months	28.0%	3 or more symptoms
Roe (2009)	Norway	52	Mild TBI	Neurosurgical department	12 months	46.2%	ICD-10 Criteria
Mickeviciene (2004)	Lithuania	192	Mild TBI	Hospital	12 months	78.0%	ICD-9 Criteria
Sigurdardottir (2009)	Norway	115	Mild–severe TBI	Level 1 Trauma Center	12 months	23.6%	ICD-10 Criteria, symptoms moderate or greater

(Continued)

TABLE 30-3 Rates of "Postconcussion Syndrome" in Patients With Mild Traumatic Brain Injuries, Depression, Trauma Controls Subjects, and Healthy Controls. (Continued)

FIRST AUTHOR (YEAR)	COUNTRY	SAMPLE SIZE	SAMPLE CHARACTERISTICS	RECRUITMENT SETTING	TIME POSTINJURY (IF APPLICABLE)	RATE OF PCS	PCS DEFINITION
Dikmen (2010)	United States	603	Mild–severe TBI	Level 1 Trauma Center	12 months	53.0%	3 or more symptoms
Smith-Seemiller (2003)	United States	32	Mild TBI	Outpatient clinic	12.3 ± 15.5 months	81.3%	DSM-IV Criteria
Mooney (2005)	United States	67	Mild TBI	Outpatient clinic	Average 15 months	91.0%	3 or more symptoms (rated 4 or higher out of 5)
Edna (1987)	Norway	485	Mild–severe TBI	Surgical department	3–5 years	22.0%	3 or more symptoms
Sterr (2006)	United Kingdom	38	Mild TBI	Community	Average ~7 years	28.9%	3 or more symptoms (rated 3 or higher)
Dean (2012)	United States	106	Mild TBI	Community	Average ~8 years	31.0%	3 or more symptoms
Smith-Seemiller (2003)	United States	63	Chronic pain	Outpatient clinic	38.6 ± 38.0 months	82.5%	DSM-IV Criteria
Iverson (1997)	Canada	170	Chronic pain	Outpatient clinic	79.7 ± 92.5 months	39.0%	DSM-IV Criteria
Garden (2010)	Australia	24	Depression	Community	N/A	96.0%	ICD-10 Criteria
Garden (2010)	Australia	24	Depression	Community	N/A	83.0%	ICD-10 Criteria, symptoms moderate or greater
Iverson (2006)	Canada	64	Depression	Inpatient/outpatient clinic	N/A	53.1%	DSM-IV Criteria, symptoms moderate or greater
Iverson (2006)	Canada	64	Depression	Inpatient/outpatient clinic	N/A	57.8%	ICD-10 Criteria, symptoms moderate or greater
Lange (2011b)	Canada	58	Depression	Outpatient clinic	N/A	82.8%	ICD-10 Criteria, symptoms moderate or greater
Iverson (2006)	Canada	64	Depression	Inpatient/outpatient clinic	N/A	85.9%	DSM-IV Criteria, symptoms mild or greater
Iverson (2006)	Canada	64	Depression	Inpatient/outpatient clinic	N/A	89.1%	ICD-10 Criteria, symptoms mild or greater
Lange (2011b)	Canada	58	Depression	Outpatient clinic	N/A	96.6%	ICD-10 Criteria, symptoms mild or greater
Meares (2008)	Australia	85	Injured controls	Level 1 Trauma Center	Average 4.9 days	43.5%	ICD-10 Criteria
Meares (2011)	Australia	58	Injured controls	Level 1 Trauma Center	Average 4.9 days	50.0%	3 or more symptoms from ICD-10 PCS symptom criteria
Dikmen (2010)	United States	119	Injured controls	Level 1 Trauma Center	1 month	53.0%	3 or more symptoms
Lange (2011a)	Canada	34	Injured controls	Level 1 Trauma Center	6–8 weeks	52.9%	ICD-10 Criteria, symptoms mild or greater
Lange (2011a)	Canada	34	Injured controls	Level 1 Trauma Center	6–8 weeks	11.8%	ICD-10 Criteria, symptoms moderate or greater
Kraus (2009)	United States	1318	Injured controls	Emergency department	3 months	18.9%	3 or more symptoms

Study	Country	N	Controls	Setting	Time	%	Criteria
McCauley (2001)	United States	85	Injured controls	Emergency department, inpatient clinic	3 months	15.3%	DSM-IV Criteria (structured interview)
Meares (2011)	Australia	58	Injured controls	Level 1 Trauma Center	Average 106.2 days	48.3%	3 or more symptoms from ICD-10 PCS symptom criteria
Mickeviciene (2004)	Lithuania	215	Injured controls	Hospital	12 months	47.0%	ICD-9 Criteria
Dikmen (2010)	United States	119	Injured controls	Level 1 Trauma Center	12 months	24.0%	3 or more symptoms
Garden (2010)	Australia	96	Healthy controls	Community	N/A	60.0%	ICD-10 Criteria
Garden (2010)	Australia	96	Healthy controls	Community	N/A	29.0%	ICD-10 Criteria, symptoms moderate or greater
Sterr (2006)	United Kingdom	38	Healthy controls	Community	N/A	0.0%	3 or more symptoms (rated 3 or higher)
Lange (2010a)	Canada	117	Healthy controls	Community	N/A	47.5%	3 or more symptoms
Lange (2010a)	Canada	117	Healthy controls	Community	N/A	29.9%	5 or more symptoms
Lange (2011b)	Canada	72	Healthy controls	Community	N/A	13.9%	ICD-10 Criteria, symptoms mild or greater
Lange (2011b)	Canada	72	Healthy controls	Community	N/A	1.4%	ICD-10 Criteria, symptoms moderate or greater
Iverson (2003)	Canada	104	Healthy controls	Community	N/A	12.5%	ICD-10 Criteria, symptoms moderate or greater
Iverson (2003)	Canada	104	Healthy controls	Community	N/A	14.6%	DSM-IV Criteria, symptoms moderate or greater
Dean (2012)	USA	244	Healthy and injured controls	Community	N/A	34.0%	3 or more symptoms
Kashluba (2006)	Canada	118	Healthy controls	Community	N/A	39.0%	5 or more symptoms
Iverson (2003)	Canada	104	Healthy controls	Community	N/A	72.1%	ICD-10 Criteria, symptoms mild or greater
Iverson (2003)	Canada	104	Healthy controls	Community	N/A	79.6%	DSM-IV Criteria, symptoms mild or greater

Abbreviations: MTBI, mild traumatic brain injury; ICD-10, International Classification of Diseases 10th Edition; DSM-IV, Diagnostic and Statistical Manual of Mental Disorders 4th Edition.

The focus of this table was studies published in the past 10 years. We included only a few studies from previous decades for comparison. Data were derived from Alves, Macciocchi, Barth (29); Dean, O'Neill, Sterr (298); Dikmen, Machamer, Fann, Temkin (25); Dischinger, Ryb, Kufera, Auman (399); Edna, Cappelen (400); Garden, Sullivan (63); Ingebrigtsen, Waterloo, Marup-Jensen, Attner, Romner (401); Iverson (232); Iverson, Brooks, Ashton, Lange (253); Iverson, Lange (149); Iverson, McCracken (160); Kashluba, Casey, Paniak (299); Kraus et al. (402); Lange, Iverson, Rose (142); Lange, Iverson, Brooks, Ashton Rennison (279); Lange, Iverson, Brubacher, Madler, Heran (90); Lange, Iverson, Rose (157); Ma, Lindsell, Rosenberry, Shaw, Zemlan (403); McCauley et al. (39); McCauley et al. (404); McCauley, Boak, Levin, Contant, Song (405); Meares et al. (297); Mickeviciene et al. (16); Mooney, Speed, Sheppard (14); Rimel, Giordani, Barth, Jane (296); Roe, Sveen, Alvsaker, Bautz-Holter (302); Rutherford (119); Rutherford, Merrett, McDonald (17); Schneiderman, Braver, Kang (406); Sigurdardottir, Andelic, Roe, Jerstad, Schanke (303); Smith-Seemiller, Fow, Kant, Franzen (158); Sterr, Herron, Hayward, Montaldi (36); Watson et al. (407); Yang, Hua, Tu, Huang (408) with permission.

[a]Note that there was a typographical error in the original article and the percentage reported was not accurate.

The group data described earlier suggests a stable course in the subgroup with persistent symptoms but might aggregate patients with variable recovery patterns. When individual patient trajectories are tracked, there are similar numbers who recover or deteriorate over the first year (15%–30% of each) (46,302). Distinct patterns of recovery have been identified in children following MTBI (307), further suggesting that individual differences are substantial. Finally, in a given patient, there may be waxing and waning of the symptoms over time (100,308), possibly caused by situational and mental health factors. In summary, the available evidence suggests that the course of symptom reporting is fairly stable from 3 to 12 months in the average patient, although recovery trends are probably variable between and within individual patients. The long-term prognosis for the subgroup who remain symptomatic (i.e., after 1 year) may be poor but has not been well studied.

TREATMENT

Effective treatments for people who are slow to recover or who report significant symptoms long after injury are greatly needed. Most intervention research has focused on *prevention* by delivering early education and reassurance (see 309,310) (see also Chapter 29 in this book). In this section, we review treatment studies that recruited patients with MTBI who are symptomatic at 3 or more months following injury.

Cognitive Rehabilitation

Cognitive rehabilitation has been the subject of at least 6 clinical trials (310,311). These interventions primarily target attention, memory, and other cognitive problems with therapist and/or computer-assisted remediation training. A recent systematic review described their efficacy as "inconclusive" (p. 28) because of methodological problems such as practice effects on outcome measures and lack of demonstrated transfer of cognitive process training to everyday functioning (310). Because of the considerable intensity and duration of these interventions, their cost-effectiveness was also questioned.

Psychological Treatment

Several authors have described how cognitive-behavioral therapy (CBT) can be tailored to patients with postconcussion symptoms (312,313). The efficacy of this treatment modality has been the subject of some empirical investigation. Miller and Mittenberg (314) delivered a manualized 12-session CBT program to a small (*n* = 4) case series of patients with MTBIs. Treatment components included graded resumption of activities, collaborative reexamination of symptom attribution, and relaxation training. Average symptom severity declined following treatment. In an unpublished study, Leonard and Tucker (315) found qualified support for a group-based intervention with a similar protocol. Tiersky et al. (316) included CBT in their holistic intervention, but the treatment benefits owing to the CBT component are unclear. Because not one randomized controlled trial of

CBT as a stand-alone treatment for persistent postconcussion symptoms has been published to date, its empirical status remains tentative. The support for using CBT comes from the broader literature on treating depression, anxiety, chronic pain, and sleep problems. If tinnitus-related psychological distress appears to be a prominent part of a person's clinical presentation, CBT might reduce this distress and associated disability (317).

Another psychological therapy that holds promise in treating people who report symptoms and functional problems long after an MTBI, especially those with associated comorbidities such as chronic pain, depression, anxiety, insomnia, and substance abuse, is Acceptance and Commitment Therapy (ACT) (318). ACT is a principles-driven treatment designed to help people behave and think in more flexible and adaptive ways. Psychological flexibility is fostered through 6 core processes of change, including acceptance, defusion, mindfulness, self-as-context, values, and committed action (see 319 for an in-depth discussion). Employing such therapeutic strategies as mindfulness and acceptance, ACT focuses on the role experiential avoidance plays in exacerbating and maintaining psychological problems. The primary goal of ACT is not symptom reduction; it is to live more adaptively and effectively, consistent with one's core values.

Researchers have reported that ACT is effective for several conditions relevant to poor outcome following MTBI, including chronic pain (320–325), depression (326), tinnitus (327), work-related stress and burnout (328–330), diagnosis acceptance (331), generalized social anxiety disorder (332), comorbid substance abuse and PTSD (333), and comorbid depression and alcohol use disorders (334). ACT has been heralded as a good fit for people with long-term problems following MTBI (30,335) because of its application to these other conditions. However, we are not aware of any completed trials evaluating this intervention in patients with chronic problems following MTBI. Using a more focused mindfulness-based intervention, a small (*n* = 10) pre–post design trial in "mild/moderate TBI" with dropouts serving as controls found improvement on psychological measures after a group-based program that involved meditation practice and discussion to foster acceptance (336,337).

Self-management is an intervention approach designed to engender coping self-efficacy, promote health behavior change, and support valued living with a chronic health condition (338). It has been extensively researched in various chronic health conditions, such as diabetes, arthritis, chronic pain, and depression (see Newman et al. and Nolte et al. for reviews) (338,339). As with mindfulness-based therapies, the goal is not to eliminate symptoms but to function better with symptoms. It is also based on the assumption that, similar to patients with chronic tinnitus and pain conditions, unwillingness to accept symptoms and relentlessly pursuing a cure for them may be counterproductive (340,341). As such, this treatment may be appropriate for patients who remain symptomatic for a year or more following MTBI. A retrospective case series with pre–post assessments found large gains with goal attainment in a sample of acquired brain injury patients (~85% with MTBIs) (342).

Exercise as Treatment

There is considerable interest in using exercise as an adjunct treatment for people who have sustained a TBI (343–345).

Converging lines of diverse medical and scientific evidence support the use of exercise as a core component of treatment for children and adults who have poor outcome from MTBI. Exercise facilitates molecular markers of neuroplasticity and promotes neurogenesis in both the healthy and the injured brain (346–352). Exercise is associated with changes in neurotransmitter systems (353,354) and can be an effective adjunctive treatment for depression (355–362) and anxiety (363–368) in adults. Exercise in older adults is associated with improved cognitive functioning (369). Exercise is associated with higher ratings of self-esteem (370), and it has beneficial effects on sleep quality (371). Most directly, there is preliminary evidence that exercise as treatment is associated with reduced symptom reporting in children (372) and adults (308) who are slow to recover from MTBI.

Leddy et al. (308) conducted a phase I (safety) trial of exercise as treatment. Participants meeting eligibility criteria (n = 12; 50% athletes) were still symptomatic at rest, seen 6–52 weeks postinjury, were free of comorbid psychiatric disorder and orthopedic injury, and were not litigating. They completed a treadmill exercise at a heart rate that was lower than their individualized threshold for symptom exacerbation 5–6 days per week for an average of 5 weeks. Leddy et al. (308) reported no adverse events and very large effect sizes for postconcussion symptom improvement, as well as positive functional outcomes (return to work and sport). Further study of subthreshold exercise appears warranted in patients who are slow to recover, especially with less rigorously screened samples to establish external validity.

Alternative and Complementary Treatments

Few alternative and complementary treatments have been studied in patients with long-term problems following MTBI. Chapman et al. (373) conducted a randomized double-blinded placebo-controlled trial of homeopathy in patients with MTBIs. Homeopathic medicines were matched to participants' presenting symptoms according to a systematic algorithm. This treatment was associated with improved symptoms and daily functioning. Although it is already being commercially marketed, there is limited research on the use of hyperbaric oxygen therapy for patients with chronic symptoms following MTBI. Supplementing evidence from a few published case studies, a recent pre–post design case series reported improved symptoms, cognitive performance, and SPECT findings (374). Adverse effects were common but reversible and led to study withdrawal in only 1 out of 16 participants. A multisite double-blind randomized sham controlled trial of this intervention is in progress (clinicaltrials.gov identifier: NCT01220713).

Targeted Symptomatic Treatment

A now widely recommended approach for treatment of patients who are slow to recover or who report chronic problems following MTBI is to focus on specific symptoms (e.g., headache) or comorbid conditions (e.g., mood, anxiety, or vestibular disorders) with a variety of pharmaceutical, psychological, and physiological interventions. Psychological treatments are effective for reducing symptoms and improving functioning in patients with depression (375,376),

depression with comorbid medical problems (377,378), generalized anxiety disorder (379), social anxiety disorder (380), and PTSD (381). Psychological and behavioral treatments can also be effective for improving sleep and reducing psychological distress in people with insomnia (382) and chronic tinnitus (317). It is important to aggressively treat chronic pain, and it is often helpful to focus treatment and rehabilitation services on cooccurring chronic pain and anxiety (383). Vestibular rehabilitation appears effective for dizziness and balance disorders after MTBI (289,384). The interested reader is referred to the Veteran Affairs/Department of Defense (VA/DoD) Clinical Practice Guideline for Management of Concussion/Mild Traumatic Brain Injury (385) or the recently released Ontario Neurotrauma Foundation Mild Traumatic Brain Injury and Persistent Symptoms Guidelines (386) for more thorough evidence-based recommendations derived from this literature. The VA/DoD Clinical Practice Guideline (385) recommends a variety of symptomatic treatments such as antidepressants, mood-stabilizing anticonvulsants, sleep hygiene education, regularly scheduled aerobic exercise, and referral for psychological treatment.

The Ontario Guidelines (386) propose that when taking a symptom-based approach to treatment, the clinician should (*a*) address symptoms in hierarchical manner, starting with those that are most likely to respond to targeted treatment and result in functional improvement (which they identify as mood symptoms, sleep disturbance, and headache); and (*b*) given the scarcity of clinical trials involving patients with long-term symptoms and problems after MTBI, the clinician should be guided by extrapolation from the best available evidence for treating these problems outside of an MTBI context. For example, post-traumatic headache should be treated according to the class of headache its characteristics most closely resemble (e.g., tension-type or migraine; see also 388 and Chapter 57). Similarly, CBT could be used for chronic fatigue following MTBI because it has been found to be helpful in chronic fatigue syndrome (388,389).

CONCLUSION

Following MTBI, there is no doubt that most people experience a constellation of symptoms such as headaches, dizziness, fatigue, balance problems, sleep disturbance, difficulty thinking (e.g., concentration or memory), and/or emotional changes (e.g., irritability). As a rule, these symptoms are at their worst in the first few hours to days postinjury and tend to get progressively better thereafter. A minority of people does not follow this trajectory but rather continue to have symptoms months to years later. There is no universally agreed upon cause or diagnostic criteria for this outcome—it is often simply conceptualized as a postconcussion syndrome. However, for patients with chronic symptoms, it is usually not possible to know what, precisely, is causing their symptoms. This is because patients with depression, anxiety, PTSD, chronic pain, chronic insomnia, tinnitus with associated psychological distress, vestibular problems combined with anxiety, and/or major life stressors will report a diverse number of postconcussion-like symptoms. Therefore, it is parsimonious but inaccurate to assume that persistent symptoms are the direct and/or indirect consequence of an injury to the brain. A wide range of biopsychosocial factors influence symptom reporting and disability. A mild injury to the

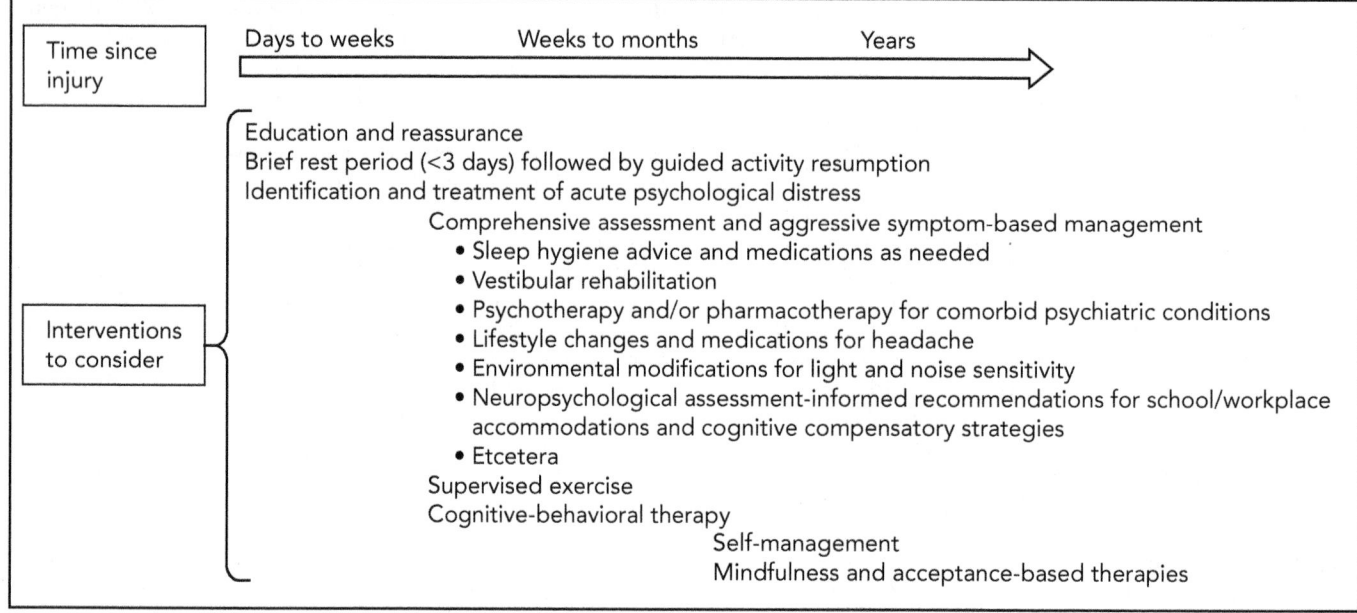

FIGURE 30–2 Sequenced care model for mild traumatic brain injury.

brain is not necessary, and usually not sufficient, to cause a constellation of long-term symptoms and problems.

For the minority of patients with chronic long-lasting symptoms, spontaneous recovery is likely uncommon. However, chronic symptoms following MTBI are *treatable* in some patients. Treatment planning flows from a differential diagnostic process that considers diverse biopsychosocial factors and comorbid conditions. Based on available evidence, a sequenced care model is recommended. This model is illustrated in Figure 30-2. Attempting secondary prevention soon after MTBI may be optimal. For patients with significant symptoms at 3–12 months postinjury, medical symptom management, CBT, and/or graded exercise may be most effective, although the evidence base is currently weak. If remission is still not achieved after 1 or more years, intervention approaches that move the focus from eliminating symptoms to enhancing quality of life (e.g., acceptance and commitment therapy or self-management) may be pursued. The antiquated notion of a binary distinction between "organic and psychological" etiologies is a barrier to effective treatment. It is hoped that researchers will increasingly turn their attention away from debating etiology to designing and testing interventions that aim to reduce patients' suffering and improve their daily functioning.

Designing interventions requires a thorough understanding of specific treatment targets. This is needed at 2 phases. First, many questions remain about how acute postconcussion symptoms evolve into chronic disability (390). For example, practitioners and researchers need to go beyond recognizing that psychosocial factors contribute to the development of chronic symptoms and more clearly specify which maladaptive beliefs, coping behaviors, and environmental reinforcers are at play. With improved characterization of the modifiable risk factors involved in this process, health care professionals involved as treaters could identify at-risk patients and design early intervention programs to mitigate this risk. Research is also needed in the chronic stage. Conceptualizing long-term symptoms and problems following MTBI as a chronic health condition such

as chronic pain, chronic fatigue syndrome, and chronic tinnitus would facilitate linkage to the relatively abundant research into these conditions. Several variables have been identified in these related chronic conditions that moderate the relationship between symptoms and disability. Acceptance—willingness to experience symptoms and engage in activities regardless of symptoms—is one example (391–393). Interventions that aim to weaken the link between symptoms and disability have most promise. Finally, although the subgroup with poor outcome from MTBI is often characterized as the "miserable minority" (44), a positive psychology research agenda may identify resiliency and other factors that facilitate post-traumatic (or adversarial) growth, which is possible even after moderate-to-severe TBI (394).

 KEY CLINICAL POINTS

1. Most people recover from an MTBI within days, weeks, or months. Having multiple persistent symptoms is uncommon when considering the entire unselected population of people who sustain this injury (i.e., including those who seek no medical attention and those with sport-related concussions).

2. Patients who are highly symptomatic at 3 months postinjury, on average, remain so at 1 or more years postinjury, although individual recovery trajectories probably vary.

3. It cannot be assumed that when a person reports symptoms many months or years after an MTBI that the symptoms are caused by brain damage. The cause of symptoms and functional problems long after an MTBI is likely multifactorial, usually related to several preexisting and/or comorbid conditions, and rarely occurs without these confounding factors.

4. Comprehensive assessment leads to better differential diagnosis, treatment, and rehabilitation. The primary focus of clinical assessment should be on differential diagnosis

of treatable comorbid conditions such as insomnia, depression, PTSD, vestibular disorders, chronic pain, and substance use disorders. A diverse range of social psychological factors can magnify postconcussion-like symptoms, and many of these factors might be modifiable through treatment.

5. Targeted symptomatic treatment, relying largely on extrapolated evidence from related and comorbid conditions (e.g., insomnia, headaches, depression, and anxiety), is the cornerstone of clinical management in the first year postinjury.

6. Potentially effective behavioral treatments for "chronic postconcussion syndrome" include CBT, supervised exercise, self-management, and mindfulness-based therapies.

KEY REFERENCES

1. King NS. Post-concussion syndrome: clarity amid the controversy? *Br J Psychiatry*. 2003;183:276–278.
2. Meares S, Shores EA, Taylor AJ, et al. The prospective course of postconcussion syndrome: the role of mild traumatic brain injury. *Neuropsychology*. 2011;25(4):454–465.
3. Ontario Neurotrauma Foundation. *Guidelines for Mild Traumatic Brain Injury and Persistent Symptoms*. Ontario Neurotrauma Foooundation; 2011. http://www.onf.org/documents/Guidelines%20for%20Mild%20Traumatic%20Brain%20Injury%20and%20Persistent%20Symptoms.pdf. Accessed November 4, 2011.
4. Ruff RM. Mild traumatic brain injury and neural recovery: rethinking the debate. *NeuroRehabilitation*. 2011;28(3):167–180.

References

1. Belanger HG, Vanderploeg RD. The neuropsychological impact of sports-related concussion: a meta-analysis. *J Int Neuropsychol Soc*. 2005;11:345–357.
2. Carroll LJ, Cassidy JD, Peloso PM, et al. Prognosis for mild traumatic brain injury: results of the WHO Collaborating Centre Task Force on Mild Traumatic Brain Injury. *J Rehabil Med*. 2004;(suppl 43):84–105.
3. Belanger HG, Curtiss G, Demery JA, Lebowitz BK, Vanderploeg RD. Factors moderating neuropsychological outcomes following mild traumatic brain injury: a meta-analysis. *J Int Neuropsychol Soc*. 2005;11:215–227.
4. Iverson GL. Outcome from mild traumatic brain injury. *Curr Opin Psychiat*. 2005;18:301–317.
5. Schretlen DJ, Shapiro AM. A quantitative review of the effects of traumatic brain injury on cognitive functioning. *Int Rev Psychiatry*. 2003;15:341–349.
6. Rees PM. Contemporary issues in mild traumatic brain injury. *Arch Phys Med Rehabil*. 2003;84:1885–1894.
7. Ruff R. Two decades of advances in understanding of mild traumatic brain injury. *J Head Trauma Rehabil*. 2005;20:5–18.
8. Ruff RM, Camenzuli L, Mueller J. Miserable minority: emotional risk factors that influence the outcome of a mild traumatic brain injury. *Brain Inj*. 1996;10:551–565.
9. Vanderploeg RD, Curtiss G, Duchnick JJ, Luis CA. Demographic, medical, and psychiatric factors in work and marital status after mild head injury. *J Head Trauma Rehabil*. 2003;18:148–163.
10. Wrightson P, Gronwall D. Time off work and symptoms after minor head injury. *Injury*. 1981;12:445–454.
11. Kraus J, Schaffer K, Ayers K, Stenehjem J, Shen H, Afifi AA. Physical complaints, medical service use, and social and employment

12. Drake AI, Gray N, Yoder S, Pramuka M, Llewellyn M. Factors predicting return to work following mild traumatic brain injury: a discriminant analysis. *J Head Trauma Rehabil*. 2000;15:1103–1112.
13. King NS, Kirwilliam S. Permanent post-concussion symptoms after mild head injury. *Brain Inj*. 2011;25:462–470.
14. Mooney G, Speed J, Sheppard S. Factors related to recovery after mild traumatic brain injury. *Brain Inj*. 2005;19:975–987.
15. Cook JB. The post-concussional syndrome and factors influencing recovery after minor head injury admitted to hospital. *Scand J Rehabil Med*. 1972;4:27–30.
16. Mickeviciene D, Schrader H, Obelieniene D, et al. A controlled prospective inception cohort study on the post-concussion syndrome outside the medicolegal context. *Eur J Neurol*. 2004;11:411–419.
17. Rutherford WH, Merrett JD, McDonald JR. Symptoms at one year following concussion from minor head injuries. *Injury*. 1979;10:225–230.
18. Satz PS, Alfano MS, Light RF, et al. Persistent post-concussive syndrome: a proposed methodology and literature review to determine the effects, if any, of mild head and other bodily injury. *J Clin Exp Neuropsychol*. 1999;21:620–628.
19. Mickeviciene D, Schrader H, Nestvold K, et al. A controlled historical cohort study on the post-concussion syndrome. *Eur J Neurol*. 2002;9:581–587.
20. Lees-Haley PR, Fox DD, Courtney JC. A comparison of complaints by mild brain injury claimants and other claimants describing subjective experiences immediately following their injury. *Arch Clin Neuropsychol*. 2001;16:689–695.
21. Ryan LM, Warden DL. Post concussion syndrome. *Int Rev Psychiatry*. 2003;15:310–316.
22. Evered L, Ruff R, Baldo J, Isomura A. Emotional risk factors and postconcussional disorder. *Assessment*. 2003;10:420–427.
23. Evans RW. Persistent post-traumatic headache, postconcussion syndrome, and whiplash injuries: the evidence for a non-traumatic basis with an historical review. *Headache*. 2010;50(4):716–724.
24. Stalnacke BM, Bjornstig U, Karlsson K, Sojka P. One-year follow-up of mild traumatic brain injury: post-concussion symptoms, disabilities and life satisfaction in relation to serum levels of S-100B and neurone-specific enolase in acute phase. *J Rehabil Med*. 2005;37(5):300–305.
25. Dikmen S, Machamer J, Fann JR, Temkin NR. Rates of symptom reporting following traumatic brain injury. *J Int Neuropsychol Soc*. 2010;16:401–411.
26. Holm L, Cassidy JD, Carroll LJ, Borg J. Summary of the WHO Collaborating Centre for Neurotrauma Task Force on Mild Traumatic Brain Injury. *J Rehabil Med*. 2005;37:137–141.
27. Cassidy JD, Carroll LJ, Peloso PM, et al. Incidence, risk factors and prevention of mild traumatic brain injury: results of the WHO Collaborating Centre Task Force on Mild Traumatic Brain Injury. *J Rehabil Med*. 2004;(suppl 43):28–60.
28. McCullagh S, Feinstein A. Outcome after mild traumatic brain injury: an examination of recruitment bias. *J Neurol Neurosurg Psychiatry*. 2003;74:39–43.
29. Alves W, Macciocchi SN, Barth JT. Postconcussive symptoms after uncomplicated mild head injury. *J Head Trauma Rehabil*. 1993;8:48–59.
30. Iverson GL, Zasler ND, Lange RT. Post-Concussive disorder. In: Zasler ND, Katz HT, Zafonte RD, eds. *Brain Injury Medicine: Principles and Practice*. New York, NY: Demos Medical Publishing; 2007:373–405.
31. Snell DL, Siegert RJ, Hay-Smith EJ, Surgenor LJ. Factor structure of the brief COPE in people with mild traumatic brain injury. *J Head Trauma Rehabil*. 2011;26(6):468–477.
32. American Psychiatric Association. *Diagnostic and Statistical Manual of Mental Disorders*. 4th ed. Washington, DC: American Psychiatric Association; 1994.
33. World Health Organization. *International Statistical Classification of Diseases and Related Health Problems*. 10th ed. Geneva, Switzerland: World Health Organization; 1992.

34. Ruff RM, Grant I. Postconcussional disorder: background to the *DSM-IV* and future considerations. In: Varney NR, Roberts RJ, eds. *The Evaluation and Treatment of Mild Traumatic Brain Injury.* Mahwah, NJ: Lawrence Erlbaum Associates Inc; 1999:315–325.

35. Ruff RM, Jurica P. In search of a unified definition for mild traumatic brain injury. *Brain Inj.* 1999;13:943–952.

36. Sterr A, Herron KA, Hayward C, Montaldi D. Are mild head injuries as mild as we think? Neurobehavioral concomitants of chronic post-concussion syndrome. *BMC Neurol.* 2006;6:7.

37. Kashluba S, Paniak C, Casey JE. Persistent symptoms associated with factors identified by the WHO Task Force on Mild Traumatic Brain Injury. *Clin Neuropsychol.* 2008;22:195–208.

38. Boake C, McCauley SR, Levin HS, et al. Diagnostic criteria for postconcussional syndrome after mild to moderate traumatic brain injury. *J Neuropsychiatry Clin Neurosci.* 2005;17:350–356.

39. McCauley SR, Boake C, Pedroza C, et al. Postconcussional disorder: are the DSM-IV criteria an improvement over the ICD-10? *J Nerv Ment Dis.* 2005;193:540–550.

40. Ruff RM. Mild traumatic brain injury and neural recovery: rethinking the debate. *NeuroRehabilitation.* 2011;28:167–180.

41. Symonds CP. The assessment of symptoms following head injury. *Guys Hospital Gazette.* 1937;51:461–468.

42. Belanger HG, Spiegel E, Vanderploeg RD. Neuropsychological performance following a history of multiple self-reported concussions: a meta-analysis. *J Int Neuropsychol Soc.* 2010;16:262–267.

43. Kay T, Newman B, Cavallo M, Ezrachi O, Resnick M. Toward a neuropsychological model of functional disability after mild traumatic brain injury. *Neuropsychology.* 1992;6:371–384.

44. Wood RL. Understanding the 'miserable minority': a diathesis-stress paradigm for post-concussional syndrome. *Brain Inj.* 2004; 18(11):1135–1153.

45. Luis CA, Vanderploeg RD, Curtiss G. Predictors of postconcussion symptom complex in community dwelling male veterans. *J Int Neuropsychol Soc.* 2003;9:1001–1015.

46. Meares S, Shores EA, Taylor AJ, et al. The prospective course of postconcussion syndrome: the role of mild traumatic brain injury. *Neuropsychology.* 2011;25:454–465.

47. Ponsford J, Willmott C, Rothwell A, et al. Factors influencing outcome following mild traumatic brain injury in adults. *J Int Neuropsychol Soc.* 2000;6:568–579.

48. Snell DL, Siegert RJ, Hay-Smith EJ, Surgenor LJ. Associations between illness perceptions, coping styles and outcome after mild traumatic brain injury: preliminary results from a cohort study. *Brain Inj.* 2011;25:1126–1138.

49. Stulemeijer M, van der Werf S, Borm GF, Vos PE. Early prediction of favourable recovery 6 months after mild traumatic brain injury. *J Neurol Neurosurg Psychiatry.* 2008;79:936–942.

50. Greiffenstein FM, Baker JW. Comparison of premorbid and postinjury mmpi-2 profiles in late postconcussion claimants. *Clin Neuropsychol.* 2001;15:162–170.

51. Kendler KS, Neale MC, Kessler RC, Heath AC, Eaves LJ. A longitudinal twin study of personality and major depression in women. *Arch Gen Psychiatry.* 1993;50:853–862.

52. Ormel J, Oldehinkel AJ, Vollebergh W. Vulnerability before, during, and after a major depressive episode: a 3-wave population-based study. *Arch Gen Psychiatry.* 2004;61:990–996.

53. Maier W, Lichtermann D, Minges J, Heun R. Personality traits in subjects at risk for unipolar major depression: a family study perspective. *J Affect Disord.* 1992;24:153–163.

54. Van Os J, Jones PB. Early risk factors and adult person—environment relationships in affective disorder. *Psychol Med.* 1999;29: 1055–1067.

55. Hirschfeld RM, Klerman GL, Clayton PJ, Keller MB. Personality and depression. Empirical findings. *Arch Gen Psychiatry.* 1983;40: 993–998.

56. Bachar E, Hadar H, Shalev AY. Narcissistic vulnerability and the development of PTSD: a prospective study. *J Nerv Ment Dis.* 2005; 193:762–765.

57. Heinrichs M, Wagner D, Schoch W, Soravia LM, Hellhammer DH, Ehlert U. Predicting posttraumatic stress symptoms from pretraumatic risk factors: a 2-year prospective follow-up study in firefighters. *Am J Psychiatry.* 2005;162:2276–2286.

58. Brewin CR, Andrews B, Valentine JD. Meta-analysis of risk factors for posttraumatic stress disorder in trauma-exposed adults. *J Consult Clin Psychol.* 2000;68:748–766.

59. McNally RJ. Psychological mechanisms in acute response to trauma. *Biol Psychiatry.* 2003;53:779–788.

60. Mols F, Denollet J. Type D personality among noncardiovascular patient populations: a systematic review. *Gen Hosp Psychiatry.* 2010; 32:66–72.

61. Stulemeijer M, Vos PE, Bleijenberg G, van der Werf SP. Cognitive complaints after mild traumatic brain injury: things are not always what they seem. *J Psychosom Res.* 2007;63:637–645.

62. Stulemeijer M, Andriessen TM, Brauer JM, Vos PE, Van Der Werf S. Cognitive performance after mild traumatic brain injury: the impact of poor effort on test results and its relation to distress, personality and litigation. *Brain Inj.* 2007;21:309–318.

63. Garden N, Sullivan KA. An examination of the base rates of postconcussion symptoms: the influence of demographics and depression. *Appl Neuropsychol.* 2010;17:1–7.

64. Rush BK, Malec JF, Moessner AM, Brown AW. Preinjury personality traits and the prediction of early neurobehavioral symptoms following mild traumatic brain injury. *Rehabil Psychol.* 2004;49: 275–281.

65. van Veldhoven LM, Sander AM, Struchen MA, et al. Predictive ability of preinjury stressful life events and post-traumatic stress symptoms for outcomes following mild traumatic brain injury: analysis in a prospective emergency room sample. *J Neurol Neurosurg Psychiatry.* 2011;82:782–787.

66. Brown RJ. Psychological mechanisms of medically unexplained symptoms: an integrative conceptual model. *Psychol Bull.* 2004;130: 793–812.

67. Feder A, Nestler EJ, Charney DS. Psychobiology and molecular genetics of resilience. *Nat Rev Neurosci.* 2009;10:446–457.

68. Hoge EA, Austin ED, Pollack MH. Resilience: research evidence and conceptual considerations for posttraumatic stress disorder. *Depress Anxiety.* 2007;24:139–152.

69. Southwick SM, Vythilingam M, Charney DS. The psychobiology of depression and resilience to stress: implications for prevention and treatment. *Annu Rev Clin Psychol.* 2005;1:255–291.

70. Kendler KS, Thornton LM, Gardner CO. Genetic risk, number of previous depressive episodes, and stressful life events in predicting onset of major depression. *Am J Psychiatry.* 2001;158:582–586.

71. Monroe SM, Harkness KL. Life stress, the "kindling" hypothesis, and the recurrence of depression: considerations from a life stress perspective. *Psychol Rev.* 2005;112:417–445.

72. Binder EB, Nemeroff CB. The CRF system, stress, depression and anxiety-insights from human genetic studies. *Mol Psychiatry.* 2010; 15(6):574–588.

73. Sullivan PF, Neale MC, Kendler KS. Genetic epidemiology of major depression: review and meta-analysis. *Am J Psychiatry.* 2000;157: 1552–1562.

74. Heim C, Newport DJ, Mletzko T, Miller AH, Nemeroff CB. The link between childhood trauma and depression: insights from HPA axis studies in humans. *Psychoneuroendocrinology.* 2008;33:693–710.

75. McCrea M, Iverson GL, McAllister TW, et al. An integrated review of recovery after mild traumatic brain injury (MTBI): implications for clinical management. *Clin Neuropsychol.* 2009;23:1368–1390.

76. van Wilgen CP, Kaptein AA, Brink MS. Illness perceptions and mood states are associated with injury-related outcomes in athletes. *Disabil Rehabil.* 2010;32:1576–1585.

77. Bryant RA, Harvey AG. Relationship between acute stress disorder and posttraumatic stress disorder following mild traumatic brain injury. *Am J Psychiatry.* 1998;155:625–629.

78. Jacobs B, Beems T, Stulemeijer M, et al. Outcome prediction in mild traumatic brain injury: age and clinical variables are stronger predictors than CT abnormalities. *J Neurotrauma.* 2010;27:655–668.

79. Stulemeijer M, van der Werf SP, Jacobs B, et al. Impact of additional extracranial injuries on outcome after mild traumatic brain injury. *J Neurotrauma.* 2006;23:1561–1569.

80. de Guise E, Lepage JF, Tinawi S, et al. Comprehensive clinical picture of patients with complicated vs uncomplicated mild traumatic brain injury. *Clin Neuropsychol.* 2010;24:1113–1130.

81. Iverson GL. Complicated vs uncomplicated mild traumatic brain injury: acute neuropsychological outcome. *Brain Inj.* 2006;20: 1335–1344.

82. Lange RT, Iverson GL, Franzen MD. Neuropsychological functioning following complicated vs. uncomplicated mild traumatic brain injury. *Brain Inj.* 2009;23:83–91.

83. Borgaro SR, Prigatano GP, Kwasnica C, Rexer JL. Cognitive and affective sequelae in complicated and uncomplicated mild traumatic brain injury. *Brain Inj.* 2003;17:189–198.

84. Kurca E, Sivak S, Kucera P. Impaired cognitive functions in mild traumatic brain injury patients with normal and pathologic magnetic resonance imaging. *Neuroradiology.* 2006;48:661–669.

85. Sadowski-Cron C, Schneider J, Senn P, Radanov BP, Ballinari P, Zimmermann H. Patients with mild traumatic brain injury: immediate and long-term outcome compared to intra-cranial injuries on CT scan. *Brain Inj.* 2006;20:1131–1137.

86. Hughes DG, Jackson A, Mason DL, Berry E, Hollis S, Yates DW. Abnormalities on magnetic resonance imaging seen acutely following mild traumatic brain injury: correlation with neuropsychological tests and delayed recovery. *Neuroradiology.* 2004;46:550–558.

87. Bigler ED. Neuropsychology and clinical neuroscience of persistent post-concussive syndrome. *J Int Neuropsychol Soc.* 2008;14:1–22.

88. Lo C, Shifteh K, Gold T, Bello JA, Lipton ML. Diffusion tensor imaging abnormalities in patients with mild traumatic brain injury and neurocognitive impairment. *J ComputAssist Tomogr.* 2009;33(2):293–297.

89. Smits M, Houston GC, Dippel DW, et al. Microstructural brain injury in post-concussion syndrome after minor head injury. *Neuroradiology.* 2011;53:553–563.

90. Lange RT, Iverson GL, Brubacher JR, Mädler B, Heran MK. Diffusion tensor imaging findings are not strongly associated with postconcussional disorder 2 months following mild traumatic brain injury [published online ahead of print June 2, 2011]. *J Head Trauma Rehabil.*

91. Chen SH, Kareken DA, Fastenau PS, Trexler LE, Hutchins GD. A study of persistent post-concussion symptoms in mild head trauma using positron emission tomography. *J Neurol Neurosurg Psychiatry.* 2003;74:326–332.

92. Kant R, SmithSeemiller L, Isaac G, Duffy J. Tc-HMPAO SPECT in persistent postconcussion syndrome after mild head injury: comparison with MRI/CT. *Brain Inj.* 1997;11:115–124.

93. Leddy JJ, Kozlowski K, Fung M, Pendergast DR, Willer B. Regulatory and autoregulatory physiological dysfunction as a primary characteristic of post concussion syndrome: implications for treatment. *NeuroRehabilitation.* 2007;22:199–205.

94. Lishman WA. Physiogenesis and psychogenesis in the 'post-concussional syndrome'. *Br J Psychiatry.* 1988;153:460–469.

95. World Health Organization. *The ICD-10 Classification of Mental and Behavioural Disorders: Clinical Descriptions and Diagnostic Guidelines.* Geneva, Switzerland: World Health Organization; 1992.

96. Ruff RM, Richardson AM. Mild traumatic brian injury. In: Sweet JJ, ed. *Forensic Neuropsychology: Fundamentals and Practice. Studies on Neuropsychology, Development, and Cognition.* Bristol, PA: Swets & Zeitlinger; 1999:315–338.

97. Bay E, de-Leon MB. Chronic stress and fatigue-related quality of life after mild to moderate traumatic brain injury. *J Head Trauma Rehabil.* 2011;26:355–363.

98. Cooper DB, Kennedy JE, Cullen MA, Critchfield E, Amador RR, Bowles AO. Association between combat stress and post-concussive symptom reporting in OEF/OIF service members with mild traumatic brain injuries. *Brain Inj.* 2011;25:1–7.

99. Snell DL, Siegert RJ, Hay-Smith EJ, Surgenor LJ. An examination of the factor structure of the Revised Illness Perception Questionnaire modified for adults with mild traumatic brain injury. *Brain Inj.* 2010;24:1595–1605.

100. Gouvier WD, Cubic B, Jones G, Brantley P, Cutlip Q. Postconcussion symptoms and daily stress in normal and head-injured college populations. *Arch Clin Neuropsychol.* 1992;7:193–211.

101. Hanna-Pladdy B, Berry ZM, Bennett T, Phillips HL, Gouvier WD. Stress as a diagnostic challenge for postconcussive symptoms: sequelae of mild traumatic brain injury or physiological stress response. *Clin Neuropsychol.* 2001;15:289–304.

102. Mittenberg W, DiGiulio DV, Perrin S, Bass AE. Symptoms following mild head injury: expectation as aetiology. *J Neurol Neurosurg Psychiatry.* 1992;55:200–204.

103. Mittenberg W, Tremont G, Zielinski RE, Fichera S, Rayls KR. Cognitive-behavioral prevention of postconcussion syndrome. *Arch Clin Neuropsychol.* 1996;11:139–145.

104. Kennedy WP. The nocebo reaction. *Med Exp Int J Exp Med.* 1961;95:203–205.

105. Luparello T, Lyons HA, Bleecker ER, McFadden ER Jr. Influences of suggestion on airway reactivity in asthmatic subjects. *Psychosom Med.* 1968;30:819–825.

106. Bootzin RR, Bailey ET. Understanding placebo, nocebo, and iatrogenic treatment effects. *J Clin Psychol.* 2005;61:871–880.

107. Lancman ME, Asconape JJ, Craven WJ, Howard G, Penry JK. Predictive value of induction of psychogenic seizures by suggestion. *Ann Neurol.* 1994;35:359–361.

108. Schweiger A, Parducci A. Nocebo: the psychologic induction of pain. *Pavlov J Biol Sci.* 1981;16:140–143.

109. Benedetti F, Pollo A, Lopiano L, Lanotte M, Vighetti S, Rainero I. Conscious expectation and unconscious conditioning in analgesic, motor, and hormonal placebo/nocebo responses. *J Neurosci.* 2003;23:4315–4323.

110. Benson H. The nocebo effect: history and physiology. *Prev Med.* 1997;26:612–615.

111. Evans RW, Rogers MP. Headaches and the nocebo effect. *J Head Face Pain.* 2003;43:1113–1115.

112. Speigel H. Nocebo: the power of suggestibility. *Prev Med.* 1997;26:616–621.

113. Hahn RA. The nocebo phenomenon: concept, evidence, and implications for public health. *Prev Med.* 1997;26:607–611.

114. Whittaker R, Kemp S, House A. Illness perceptions and outcome in mild head injury: a longitudinal study. *J Neurol Neurosurg Psychiatry.* 2007;78:644–646.

115. Hou R, Moss-Morris R, Peveler R, Mogg K, Bradley BP, Belli A. When a minor head injury results in enduring symptoms: a prospective investigation of risk factors for postconcussional syndrome after mild traumatic brain injury. *J Neurol Neurosurg Psychiatry.* 2012;83:217–223.

116. Ferrari R, Obelieniene D, Russell AS, Darlington P, Gervais R, Green P. Symptom expectation after minor head injury. A comparative study between Canada and Lithuania. *Clin Neurol Neurosurg.* 2001;103:184–190.

117. Ferrari R, Russell AS. Why blame is a factor in recovery from whiplash injury. *Med Hypotheses.* 2001;56:372–375.

118. Spinos P, Sakellaropoulos G, Georgiopoulos M, et al. Postconcussion syndrome after mild traumatic brain injury in Western Greece. *J Trauma.* 2010;69:789–794.

119. Rutherford WH. Sequelae of concussion caused by minor head injuries. *Lancet.* 1977;1:1–4.

120. Hart T, Hanks R, Bogner JA, Millis S, Esselman P. Blame attribution intentional and unintentional traumatic brain injury: longitudinal changes and impact on subjective well-being. *Rehabil Psychol.* 2007;52:152–161.

121. Sullivan MJ, Adams H, Horan S, Maher D, Boland D, Gross R. The role of perceived injustice in the experience of chronic pain and disability: scale development and validation. *J Occup Rehabil.* 2008;18:249–261.

122. Hagger MS, Orbell S. A meta-analytic review of the common-sense model of illness representations. *Psychol Health.* 2003;18:141–184.

123. Roesch SC, Weiner B. A meta-analytic review of coping with illness: do causal attributions matter? *J Psychosom Res.* 2001;50:205–219.

124. Leventhal H, Brissette I, Leventhal EA. The common-sense model of self-regulation of health and illness. In: Cameron LD, Leventhal H, eds. *The Self-Regulation of Health and Illness Behaviour.* New York, NY: Routledge; 2003.

125. McLean SA, Clauw DJ. Predicting chronic symptoms after an acute "stressor"—lessons learned from 3 medical conditions. *Med Hypotheses.* 2004;63:653–658.

126. Nijs J, Paul L, Wallman K. Chronic fatigue syndrome: an approach combining self-management with graded exercise to avoid exacerbations. *J Rehabil Med.* 2008;40:241–247.

127. Veale D. Behavioural activation for depression. *Adv Psychiatr Treat.* 2008;14:29–36.

128. Willer B, Leddy JJ. Management of concussion and post-concussion syndrome. *Curr Treat Options Neurol.* 2006;8:415–426.

129. Barsky AJ, Saintfort R, Rogers MP, Borus JF. Nonspecific medication side effects and the nocebo phenomenon. *J Am Med Assoc.* 2002;287:622–627.

130. Woodrome SE, Yeates KO, Taylor HG, et al. Coping strategies as a predictor of post-concussive symptoms in children with mild traumatic brain injury versus mild orthopedic injury. *J Int Neuropsychol Soc.* 2011;17:317–326.

131. Kouyanou K, Pither CE, Rabe-Hesketh S, Wessely S. A comparative study of iatrogenesis, medication abuse, and psychiatric morbidity in chronic pain patients with and without medically explained symptoms. *Pain.* 1998;76:417–426.

132. Cote P, Soklaridis S. Does early management of whiplash-associated disorders assist or impede recovery? *Spine.* 2011;36(suppl 25): S275–S279.

133. Flor H, Kerns RD, Turk DC. The role of spouse reinforcement, perceived pain, and activity levels of chronic pain patients. *J Psychosom Res.* 1987;31:251–259.

134. Wooley SC, Blackwell B, Winget C. A learning theory model of chronic illness behavior: theory, treatment, and research. *Psychosom Med.* 1978;40:379–401.

135. Jolliffe CD, Nicholas MK. Verbally reinforcing pain reports: an experimental test of the operant model of chronic pain. *Pain.* 2004; 107:167–175.

136. Weissman HN. Distortions and deceptions in self presentation: effects of protracted litigation on personal injury cases. *Behav Sci Law.* 1990;8:67–74.

137. Gunstad J, Suhr JA. Cognitive factors in postconcussion syndrome symptom report. *Arch Clin Neuropsychol.* 2004;19:391–405.

138. Festinger LA. *A Theory of Cognitive Dissonance.* Stanford, CA: Stanford University Press; 1957.

139. Davis CH. Self-perception in mild traumatic brain injury. *Am J Phys Med Rehabil.* 2002;81:609–621.

140. Gunstad J, Suhr JA. "Expectation as etiology" versus "the good old days": postconcussion syndrome symptom reporting in athletes, headache sufferers, and depressed individuals. *J Int Neuropsychol Soc.* 2001;7:323–333.

141. Hilsabeck RC, Gouvier WD, Bolter JF. Reconstructive memory bias in recall of neuropsychological symptomatology. *J Clin Exp Neuropsychol.* 1998;20:328–338.

142. Lange RT, Iverson GL, Rose A. Post-concussion symptom reporting and the "good-old-days" bias following mild traumatic brain injury. *Arch Clin Neuropsychol.* 2010;25:442–450.

143. Iverson GL, Lange RT, Brooks BL, Rennison VL. "Good old days" bias following mild traumatic brain injury. *Clin Neuropsychol.* 2010; 24:17–37.

144. Lees-Haley PR, Williams CW, Zasler ND, Marguilies S, English LT, Stevens KB. Response bias in plaintiffs' histories. *Brain Inj.* 1997;11:791–799.

145. Panayiotou A, Crowe S, Jackson M. An analogue study of the psychological and psychosocial processes associated with postconcussion symptoms. *Aust Psychol.* 2011:1–9.

146. Lees-Haley PR, Williams CW, English LT. Response bias in self-reported history of plaintiffs compared with nonlitigating patients. *Psychol Rep.* 1996;79:811–818.

147. Gouvier WD, Uddo-Crane M, Brown LM. Base rates of postconcussional symptoms. *Arch Clin Neuropsychol.* 1988;3:273–278.

148. Machulda MM, Bergquist TF, Ito V, Chew S. Relationship between stress, coping, and post concussion symptoms in a healthy adult population. *Arch Clin Neuropsychol.* 1998;13:415–424.

149. Iverson GL, Lange RT. Examination of "postconcussion-like" symptoms in a healthy sample. *Appl Neuropsychol.* 2003;10:137–144.

150. Trahan DE, Ross CE, Trahan SL. Relationships among postconcussional-type symptoms, depression, and anxiety in neurologically normal young adults and victims of brain injury. *Arch Clin Neuropsychol.* 2001;16:435–445.

151. Sawchyn JM, Brulot MM, Strauss E. Note on the use of the Postconcussion Syndrome Checklist. *Arch Clin Neuropsychol.* 2000;15:1–8.

152. Wong JL, Regennitter RP, Barrios F. Base rate and simulated symptoms of mild head injury among normals. *Arch Clin Neuropsychol.* 1994;9:411–425.

153. Fox DD, Lees-Haley PR, Ernest K, Dolezal-Wood S. Post-concussive symptoms: base rates and etiology in psychiatric patients. *Clin Neuropsychol.* 1995;9:89–92.

154. Lees-Haley PR, Brown RS. Neuropsychological complaint base rates of 170 personal injury claimants. *Arch Clin Neuropsychol.* 1993; 8:203–209.

155. Dunn JT, Lees-Haley PR, Brown RS, Williams CW, English LT. Neurotoxic complaint base rates of personal injury claimants: implications for neuropsychological assessment. *J Clin Psychol.* 1995; 51:577–584.

156. Foa EB, Cashman L, Jaycox L, Perry K. The validation of a self-report measure of posttraumatic stress disorder: the Posttraumatic Diagnostic Scale. *Psychol Assess.* 1997;9:445–451.

157. Lange RT, Iverson GL, Rose A. Depression strongly influences postconcussion symptom reporting following mild traumatic brain injury. *J Head Trauma Rehabil.* 2011;26:127–137.

158. Smith-Seemiller L, Fow NR, Kant R, Franzen MD. Presence of postconcussion syndrome symptoms in patients with chronic pain vs mild traumatic brain injury. *Brain Inj.* 2003;17:199–206.

159. Radanov BP, Dvorak J, Valach L. Cognitive deficits in patients after soft tissue injury of the cervical spine. *Spine.* 1992;17:127–131.

160. Iverson GL, McCracken LM. 'Postconcussive' symptoms in persons with chronic pain. *Brain Inj.* 1997;11:783–790.

161. Gasquoine PG. Postconcussional symptoms in chronic back pain. *Appl Neuropsychol.* 2000;7:83–89.

162. Sullivan MJ, Hall E, Bartolacci R, Sullivan ME, Adams H. Perceived cognitive deficits, emotional distress and disability following whiplash injury. *Pain Res Manag.* 2002;7:120–126.

163. Atkinson JH, Slater MA, Patterson TL, Grant I, Garfin SR. Prevalence, onset, and risk of psychiatric disorders in men with chronic low back pain: a controlled study. *Pain.* 1991;45:111–121.

164. Fishbain DA, Cutler R, Rosomoff HL, Rosomoff RS. Chronic pain-associated depression: antecedent or consequence of chronic pain? A review. *Clin J Pain.* 1997;13:116–137.

165. Wilson KG, Eriksson MY, D'Eon JL, Mikail SF, Emery PC. Major depression and insomnia in chronic pain. *Clin J Pain.* 2002;18:77–83.

166. Campbell LC, Clauw DJ, Keefe FJ. Persistent pain and depression: a biopsychosocial perspective. *Biol Psychiatry.* 2003;54:399–409.

167. McWilliams LA, Cox BJ, Enns MW. Mood and anxiety disorders associated with chronic pain: an examination in a nationally representative sample. *Pain.* 2003;106:127–133.

168. Balla JI. Headache and cervical disorders: report to the motor accidents board of Victoria on whiplash injuries. In: Hopkins A, ed. *Headache, Problems in Diagnosis and Management.* London, United Kingdom: Saunders; 1988:256–269.

169. Pearce JM. Whiplash injury: a reappraisal. *J Neurol Neurosurg Psychiatry.* 1989;52:1329–1331.

170. Hildingsson C, Toolanen G. Outcome after soft-tissue injury of the cervical spine. A prospective study of 93 car-accident victims. *Acta Orthop Scand.* 1990;61:357–359.

171. Tollison CD, Satterthwaite, eds. Painful cervical trauma: diagnosis and rehabilitation treatment of neuromusculoskeletal injuries. Baltimore, MD: Williams & Wilkins; 1992.

172. Croft AC. Soft tissue injuries: long- and short-term effects. In: Foreman SM, Croft AC, eds. *Whiplash Injuries: The Cervical Acceleration/Deceleration Syndrome.* 3rd ed. Philidelphia, PA: Lippincott Williams & Wilkins; 2002:335–428.

173. Zasler ND. Post-traumatic sensory disorders in TBI. In: Arciniegas DB, Zasler ND, Vanderploeg R, Jaffee MS, eds. *Clinical Manual for the Management of Adults With Traumatic Brain Injury.* Washington, DC: American Psychiatric Publishing Inc. In press.

174. Zasler ND. Confounding factors in postconcussive disorders. In: Zollman FS, ed. *Manual of Traumatic Brain Injury Management.* New York, NY: Demos Medical Publishing; 2011:125–131.

175. Marzo SJ, Leonetti JP, Raffin MJ, Letarte P. Diagnosis and management of post-traumatic vertigo. *Laryngoscope.* 2004;114:1720–1723.

176. Zasler ND. Neuromedical diagnosis and management of post-concussive disorders. In: Horn L, Zasler ND, eds. *Medical Rehabilitation of Traumatic Brain Injury.* Philadelphia, PA: Hanley & Belfus Inc; 1996:133–170.

177. Ernst A, Basta D, Seidl RO, Todt I, Scherer H, Clarke A. Management of posttraumatic vertigo. *Otolaryngol Head Neck Surg.* 2005; 132:554–558.

178. Boniver R. Temporomandibular joint dysfunction in whiplash injuries: association with tinnitus and vertigo. *Int Tinnitus J.* 2002;8: 129–131.

179. Kischka U, Ettlin T, Heim S, Schmid G. Cerebral symptoms following whiplash injury. *Eur Neurol.* 1991;31:136–140.

180. Guez M, Brannstrom R, Nyberg L, Toolanen G, Hildingsson C. Neuropsychological functioning and MMPI-2 profiles in chronic neck pain: a comparison of whiplash and non-traumatic groups. *J Clin Exp Neuropsychol.* 2005;27:151–163.

181. Antepohl W, Kiviloog L, Andersson J, Gerdle B. Cognitive impairment in patients with chronic whiplash-associated disorder—a matched control study. *NeuroRehabilitation.* 2003;18:307–315.

182. Healy GB. Hearing loss and vertigo secondary to head injury. *N Engl J Med.* 1982;306:1029–1031.

183. Williams GH, Giordano AM. Temporal bone trauma. In: Becker DP, Gudeman SK, eds. *Textbook of Head Injury.* Philadelphia, PA: W. B. Saunders; 1989:367–377.

184. Zasler ND, Ochs AL. Oculovestibular dysfunction in symptomatic mild traumatic brain injury. *Arch Phys Med Rehabil.* 1992;73:963.

185. Maitland CG. Perilymphatic fistula. *Curr Neurol Neurosci Rep.* 2001; 1:486–491.

186. Black FO, Lilly DJ, Peterka RJ, Shupert C, Hemenway WG, Pesznecker SC. The dynamic posturographic pressure test for the presumptive diagnosis of perilymph fistulas. *Neurol Clin.* 1990;8: 361–374.

187. Bourgeois B, Ferron C, Bordure P, Beauvillain de Montreuil C, Legent F. Exploratory tympanotomy for suspected traumatic perilymphatic fistula [in French]. *Ann Otolaryngol Chir Cervicofac.* 2005; 122(4):181–186.

188. Grimm RJ, Hemenway WG, Lebray PR, Black FO. The perilymph fistula syndrome defined in mild head trauma. *Acta Otolaryngol Suppl.* 1989;464:1–40.

189. Brandt T. *Vertigo: its multisensory syndromes.* New York, NY: Springer-Verlag; 1991.

190. Costanzo RM, Zasler ND. Epidemiology and pathophysiology of olfactory and gustatory dysfunction in head trauma. *J Head Trauma Rehabil.* 1992;7:15–24.

191. Daily L. Whiplash injury as one cause of the foveolar splinter and macular wisps. *Arch Ophthalmol.* 1979;97:360.

192. Cytowic R, Stump DA, Larned DC. Closed head trauma: cognitive, somatic and ophthalmic sequellae in nonhospitalized patients. In: Whitaker HA, ed. *Neuropsychological Studies of Nonfocal Brain Damage.* New York, NY: Springer-Verlag; 1988:226–264.

193. Carter JE, McCormick AQ. Whiplash shaking syndrome: retinal hemorrhages and computerized axial tomography of the brain. *Child Abuse Negl.* 1983;7:279–286.

194. Kowal L. Ophthalmic manifestations of head injury. *Aust N Z J Ophthalmol.* 1992;20:35–40.

195. al-Qurainy IA. Convergence insufficiency and failure of accommodation following midfacial trauma. *Br J Oral Maxillofac Surg.* 1995; 33:71–75.

196. Rasmussen BK. Epidemiology of headache. *Cephalalgia.* 2001;21: 774–777.

197. Rasmussen BK, Jensen R, Schroll M, Olesen J. Epidemiology of headache in a general population—a prevalence study. *J Clin Epidemiol.* 1991;44:1147–1157.

198. Pine DS, Cohen P, Brook J. The association between major depression and headache: results of a longitudinal epidemiologic study in youth. *J Child Adolesc Psychopharmacol.* 1996;6:153–164.

199. Mitsikostas DD, Thomas AM. Comorbidity of headache and depressive disorders. *Cephalalgia.* 1999;19:211–217.

200. Zwart JA, Dyb G, Hagen K, et al. Depression and anxiety disorders associated with headache frequency. The Nord-Trøndelag Health Study. *Eur J Neurol.* 2003;10:147–152.

201. Breslau N, Lipton RB, Stewart WF, Schultz LR, Welch KM. Comorbidity of migraine and depression: investigating potential etiology and prognosis. *Neurology.* 2003;60:1308–1312.

202. Magnusson JE, Becker WJ. Migraine frequency and intensity: relationship with disability and psychological factors. *Headache.* 2003; 43:1049–1059.

203. Wacogne C, Lacoste JP, Guillibert E, Hugues FC, Le Jeunne C. Stress, anxiety, depression and migraine. *Cephalalgia.* 2003;23: 451–455.

204. Kowacs F, Socal MP, Ziomkowski SC, et al. Symptoms of depression and anxiety, and screening for mental disorders in migrainous patients. *Cephalalgia.* 2003;23:79–89.

205. Venable VL, Carlson CR, Wilson J. The role of anger and depression in recurrent headache. *Headache.* 2001;41:21–30.

206. Lipton RB, Hamelsky SW, Kolodner KB, Steiner TJ, Stewart WF. Migraine, quality of life, and depression: a population-based case-control study. *Neurology.* 2000;55:629–635.

207. Holroyd KA, Stensland M, Lipchik GL, Hill KR, O'Donnell FS, Cordingley G. Psychosocial correlates and impact of chronic tension-type headaches. *Headache.* 2000;40:3–16.

208. Parmelee PA, Smith B, Katz IR. Pain complaints and cognitive status among elderly institution residents. *J Am Geriatr Soc.* 1993;41: 517–522.

209. Haldorsen T, Waterloo K, Dahl A, Mellgren SI, Davidsen PE, Molin PK. Symptoms and cognitive dysfunction in patients with the late whiplash syndrome. *Appl Neuropsychol.* 2003;10:170–175.

210. Jamison RN, Sbrocco T, Parris WC. The influence of problems with concentration and memory on emotional distress and daily activities in chronic pain patients. *Int J Psychiatry Med.* 1988;18:183–191.

211. McCracken LM, Iverson GL. Predicting complaints of impaired cognitive functioning in patients with chronic pain. *J Pain Symptom Manage.* 2001;21:392–396.

212. Muñoz M, Esteve R. Reports of memory functioning by patients with chronic pain. *Clin J Pain.* 2005;21:287–291.

213. Roth RS, Geisser ME, Theisen-Goodvich M, Dixon PJ. Cognitive complaints are associated with depression, fatigue, female sex, and pain catastrophizing in patients with chronic pain. *Arch Phys Med Rehabil.* 2005;86:1147–1154.

214. Schnurr RF, MacDonald MR. Memory complaints in chronic pain. *Clin J Pain.* 1995;11:103–111.

215. Iverson GL, King RJ, Scott JG, Adams RL. Cognitive complaints in litigating patients with head injuries or chronic pain. *J Forensic Neuropsychol.* 2001;2:19–30.

216. Uomoto JM, Esselman PC. Traumatic brain injury and chronic pain: differential types and rates by head injury severity. *Arch Phys Med Rehabil.* 1993;74:61–64.

217. Kreutzer JS, Seel RT, Gourley E. The prevalence and symptom rates of depression after traumatic brain injury: a comprehensive examination. *Brain Inj.* 2001;15:563–576.

218. Seel RT, Kreutzer JS, Rosenthal M, Hammond FM, Corrigan JD, Black K. Depression after traumatic brain injury: a National Institute on Disability and Rehabilitation Research Model Systems multicenter investigation. *Arch Phys Med Rehabil.* 2003;84:177–184.

219. Ericsson M, Poston WS, Linder J, Taylor JE, Haddock CK, Foreyt JP. Depression predicts disability in long-term chronic pain patients. *Disabil Rehabil.* 2002;24:334–340.

220. Hung CI, Liu CY, Fuh JL, Juang YY, Wang SJ. Comorbid migraine is associated with a negative impact on quality of life in patients with major depression. *Cephalalgia.* 2006;26:26–32.

221. Breslau N, Schultz LR, Stewart WF, Lipton RB, Lucia VC, Welch KM. Headache and major depression: is the association specific to migraine? *Neurology.* 2000;54:308–313.

222. Sheftell FD, Atlas SJ. Migraine and psychiatric comorbidity: from theory and hypotheses to clinical application. *Headache.* 2002;42: 934–944.

223. Franklin CL, Zimmerman M. Posttraumatic stress disorder and major depressive disorder: investigating the role of overlapping symptoms in diagnostic comorbidity. *J Nerv Ment Dis.* 2001;189: 548–551.

224. Kessler RC, Sonnega A, Bromet E, Hughes M, Nelson CB. Posttraumatic stress disorder in the National Comorbidity Survey. *Arch Gen Psychiatry.* 1995;52:1048–1060.

225. Shalev AY, Freedman S, Peri T, et al. Prospective study of posttraumatic stress disorder and depression following trauma. *Am J Psychiatry.* 1998;155:630–637.

226. Nunes EV, Levin FR. Treatment of depression in patients with alcohol or other drug dependence: a meta-analysis. *JAMA.* 2004; 291:1887–1896.

227. Grothues J, Bischof G, Reinhardt S, et al. Intention to change drinking behaviour in general practice patients with problematic drinking and comorbid depression or anxiety. *Alcohol Alcohol.* 2005;40: 394–400.

228. Frisher M, Crome I, Macleod J, Millson D, Croft P. Substance misuse and psychiatric illness: prospective observational study using the general practice research database. *J Epidemiol Community Health.* 2005;59:847–850.

229. Grant BF, Stinson FS, Dawson DA, et al. Prevalence and co-occurrence of substance use disorders and independent mood and anxiety disorders: results from the National Epidemiologic Survey on Alcohol and Related Conditions. *Arch Gen Psychiatry.* 2004;61: 807–816.

230. Brady KT, Verduin ML. Pharmacotherapy of comorbid mood, anxiety, and substance use disorders. *Subst Use Misuse.* 2005;40(13–14): 2021–2041, 2043–2048.

231. Suhr JA, Gunstad J. Postconcussive symptom report: the relative influence of head injury and depression. *J Clin Exp Neuropsychol.* 2002;24:981–993.

232. Iverson GL. Misdiagnosis of the persistent postconcussion syndrome in patients with depression. *Arch Clin Neuropsychol.* 2006; 21:303–310.

233. American Psychiatric Association. *Diagnostic and Statistical Manual of Mental Disorders.* 4th ed. Text Rev. Washington, DC: American Psychiatric Association; 2000.

234. Austin MP, Mitchell P, Wilhelm K, et al. Cognitive function in depression: a distinct pattern of frontal impairment in melancholia? *Psychol Med.* 1999;29:73–85.

235. Zakzanis KK, Leach L, Kaplan E. On the nature and pattern of neurocognitive function in major depressive disorder. *Neuropsychiatry Neuropsychol Behav Neurol.* 1998;11:111–119.

236. McDermott LM, Ebmeier KP. A meta-analysis of depression severity and cognitive function. *J Affect Disord.* 2009;119:1–8.

237. Carlson KF, Kehle SM, Meis LA, et al. Prevalence, assessment, and treatment of mild traumatic brain injury and posttraumatic stress disorder: a systematic review of the evidence. *J Head Trauma Rehabil.* 2011;26:103–115.

238. Hoffman JM, Dikmen S, Temkin N, Bell KR. Development of posttraumatic stress disorder after mild traumatic brain injury. *Arch Phys Med Rehabil.* 2012;93:287–292.

239. Jamora CW, Young A, Ruff RM. Comparison of subjective cognitive complaints with neuropsychological tests in individuals with mild vs more severe traumatic brain injuries. *Brain Inj.* 2012;26: 36–47.

240. Bryant RA, Creamer M, O'Donnell M, Silove D, Clark CR, McFarlane AC. Post-traumatic amnesia and the nature of post-traumatic stress disorder after mild traumatic brain injury. *J Int Neuropsychol Soc.* 2009;15:862–867.

241. Gil S, Caspi Y, Ben-Ari IZ, Koren D, Klein E. Does memory of a traumatic event increase the risk for posttraumatic stress disorder in patients with traumatic brain injury? A prospective study. *Am J Psychiatry.* 2005;162:963–969.

242. Hoge CW, McGurk D, Thomas JL, Cox AL, Engel CC, Castro CA. Mild traumatic brain injury in U.S. Soldiers returning from Iraq. *N Engl J Med.* 2008;358:453–463.

243. Belanger HG, Kretzmer T, Vanderploeg RD, French LM. Symptom complaints following combat-related traumatic brain injury: relationship to traumatic brain injury severity and posttraumatic stress disorder. *J Int Neuropsychol Soc.* 2010;16:194–199.

244. Brenner LA, Ivins BJ, Schwab K, et al. Traumatic brain injury, posttraumatic stress disorder, and postconcussive symptom reporting among troops returning from iraq. *J Head Trauma Rehabil.* 2010;25: 307–312.

245. Moore EL, Terryberry-Spohr L, Hope DA. Mild traumatic brain injury and anxiety sequelae: a review of the literature. *Brain Inj.* 2006;20:117–132.

246. Mooney G, Speed J. The association between mild traumatic brain injury and psychiatric conditions. *Brain Inj.* 2001;15:865–877.

247. Gladstone J. From psychoneurosis to ICHD-2: an overview of the state of the art in post-traumatic headache. *Headache.* 2009;49: 1097–1111.

248. Patil VK, St Andre JR, Crisan E, et al. Prevalence and treatment of headaches in veterans with mild traumatic brain injury. *Headache.* 2011;51:1112–1121.

249. Barker MJ, Greenwood KM, Jackson M, Crowe SF. Persistence of cognitive effects after withdrawal from long-term benzodiazepine use: a meta-analysis. *Arch Clin Neuropsychol.* 2004;19:437–454.

250. Barker MJ, Greenwood KM, Jackson M, Crowe SF. An evaluation of persisting cognitive effects after withdrawal from long-term benzodiazepine use. *J Int Neuropsychol Soc.* 2005;11:281–289.

251. Zasler ND. Update on pharmacology. Neuromedical aspects of alcohol use following traumatic brain injury. *J Head Trauma Rehabil.* 1991;6:78–80.

252. Alla S, Sullivan SJ, Hale L, McCrory P. Self-report scales/checklists for the measurement of concussion symptoms: a systematic review. *Br J Sports Med.* 2009;(43, suppl 1):i3–i12.

253. Nolin P, Villemure R, Heroux L. Determining long-term symptoms following mild traumatic brain injury: method of interview affects self-report. *Brain Inj.* 2006;20:1147–1154.

254. Iverson GL, Brooks BL, Ashton VL, Lange RT. Interview vs. questionnaire symptom reporting in people with post-concussion syndrome. *J Head Trauma Rehabil.* 2010;25:25–30.

255. Dikmen SS, Corrigan JD, Levin HS, Machamer J, Stiers W, Weisskopf MG. Cognitive outcome following traumatic brain injury. *J Head Trauma Rehabil.* 2009;24:430–438.

256. Rohling ML, Binder LM, Demakis GJ, Larrabee GJ, Ploetz DM, Langhinrichsen-Rohling J. A meta-analysis of neuropsychological outcome after mild traumatic brain injury: re-analyses and reconsiderations of Binder et al. (1997), Frencham et al. (2005), and Pertab et al. (2009). *Clin Neuropsychol.* 2011;25:608–623.

257. Rohling ML, Larrabee GJ, Millis SR. The "miserable minority" following mild traumatic brain injury: who are they and do meta-analyses hide them? *Clin Neuropsychol.* 2012;26(2):197–213.

258. Vanderploeg RD, Curtiss G, Belanger HG. Long-term neuropsychological outcomes following mild traumatic brain injury. *J Int Neuropsychol Soc.* 2005;11:228–236.

259. Geary EK, Kraus MF, Pliskin NH, Little DM. Verbal learning differences in chronic mild traumatic brain injury. *J Int Neuropsychol Soc.* 2010;16:506–516.

260. Heitger MH, Jones RD, Macleod AD, Snell DL, Frampton CM, Anderson TJ. Impaired eye movements in post-concussion syndrome indicate suboptimal brain function beyond the influence of depression, malingering or intellectual ability. *Brain.* 2009;132:2850–2870.

261. Konrad C, Geburek AJ, Rist F, et al. Long-term cognitive and emotional consequences of mild traumatic brain injury. *Psychol Med.* 2010:1–15.

262. Ettenhofer ML, Abeles N. The significance of mild traumatic brain injury to cognition and self-reported symptoms in long-term recovery from injury. *J Clin Exp Neuropsychol.* 2009;31:363–372.

263. Iverson GL. Mild traumatic brain injury meta-analyses can obscure individual differences. *Brain Inj.* 2010;24:1246–1255.

264. Suhr JA, Gunstad J. Further exploration of the effect of "diagnosis threat" on cognitive performance in individuals with mild head injury. *J Int Neuropsychol Soc.* 2005;11:23–29.

265. Suhr JA, Gunstad J. "Diagnosis Threat": the effect of negative expectations on cognitive performance in head injury. *J Clin Exp Neuropsychol.* 2002;24:448–457.

266. Hart RP, Martelli MF, Zasler ND. Chronic pain and neuropsychological functioning. *Neuropsychol Rev.* 2000;10:131–149.

267. Benoit G, Fortin L, Lemelin S, Laplante L, Thomas J, Everett J. Selective attention in major depression: clinical retardation and cognitive inhibition. *Can J Psychol.* 1992;46:41–52.

268. Ellis HC. Focused attention and depressive deficits in memory. *J Exp Psychol Gen.* 1991;120:310–312.

269. Lemelin S, Baruch P, Vincent A, Everett J, Vincent P. Distractibility and processing resource deficit in major depression. Evidence for two deficient attentional processing models. *J Nerv Ment Dis.* 1997; 185:542–548.

270. Ilsley JE, Moffoot AP, O'Carroll RE. An analysis of memory dysfunction in major depression. *J Affect Disord.* 1995;35:1–9.

271. Sternberg DE, Jarvik ME. Memory functions in depression. *Arch Gen Psychiatry.* 1976;33:219–224.

272. Weingartner H, Cohen RM, Murphy DL, Martello J, Gerdt C. Cognitive processes in depression. *Arch Gen Psychiatry.* 1981;38:42–47.

273. Wolfe J, Granholm E, Butters N, Saunders E, Janowsky D. Verbal memory deficits associated with major affective disorders: a comparison of unipolar and bipolar patients. *J Affect Disord.* 1987;13: 83–92.

274. Degl'Innocenti A, Agren H, Backman L. Executive deficits in major depression. *Acta Psychiatr Scand.* 1998;97:182–188.

275. Channon S. Executive dysfunction in depression: the Wisconsin Card Sorting Test. *J Affect Disord.* 1996;39:107–114.

276. Channon S, Green PS. Executive function in depression: the role of performance strategies in aiding depressed and non-depressed participants. *J Neurol Neurosurg Psychiatry.* 1999;66:162–171.

277. Merriam EP, Thase ME, Haas GL, Keshavan MS, Sweeney JA. Prefrontal cortical dysfunction in depression determined by Wisconsin Card Sorting Test performance. *Am J Psychiatry.* 1999;156:780–782.

278. Rajkowska G, Miguel-Hidalgo JJ, Wei J, et al. Morphometric evidence for neuronal and glial prefrontal cell pathology in major depression. *Biol Psychiatry.* 1999;45:1085–1098.

279. Lange RT, Iverson GL, Brooks BL, Ashton Rennison VL. Influence of poor effort on self-reported symptoms and neurocognitive test performance following mild traumatic brain injury. *J Clin Exp Neuropsychol.* 2010;32:961–972.

280. Green P, Rohling ML, Lees-Haley PR, Allen LM III. Effort has a greater effect on test scores than severe brain injury in compensation claimants. *Brain Inj.* 2001;15:1045–1060.

281. Binder LM, Iverson GL, Brooks BL. To err is human: "abnormal" neuropsychological scores and variability are common in healthy adults. *Arch Clin Neuropsychol.* 2009;24:31–46.

282. Mittenberg W, Patton C, Canyock EM, Condit DC. Base rates of malingering and symptom exaggeration. *J Clin Exp Neuropsychol.* 2002;24:1094–1102.

283. Locke DE, Smigielski JS, Powell MR, Stevens SR. Effort issues in post-acute outpatient acquired brain injury rehabilitation seekers. *NeuroRehabilitation.* 2008;23:273–281.

284. Ozen LJ, Fernandes MA. Effects of "diagnosis threat" on cognitive and affective functioning long after mild head injury. *J Int Neuropsychol Soc.* 2011;17:219–229.

285. Bigler E. Neuroimaging in mild traumatic brain injury. *Psychol Inj Law.* 2010;3:36–49.

286. Wen W, Sachdev PS, Li JJ, Chen X, Anstey KJ. White matter hyperintensities in the forties: their prevalence and topography in an epidemiological sample aged 44–48. *Hum Brain Mapp.* 2009;30:1155–1167.

287. Hopkins RO, Beck CJ, Burnett DL, Weaver LK, Victoroff J, Bigler ED. Prevalence of white matter hyperintensities in a young healthy population. *J Neuroimaging.* 2006;16:243–251.

288. Ylikoski A, Erkinjuntti T, Raininko R, Sarna S, Sulkava R, Tilvis R. White matter hyperintensities on MRI in the neurologically nondiseased elderly. Analysis of cohorts of consecutive subjects aged 55 to 85 years living at home. *Stroke.* 1995;26:1171–1177.

289. Belanger HG, Vanderploeg RD, Curtiss G, Warden DL. Recent neuroimaging techniques in mild traumatic brain injury. *J Neuropsychiatry Clin Neurosci.* 2007;19:5–20.

290. Alsalaheen BA, Mucha A, Morris LO, et al. Vestibular rehabilitation for dizziness and balance disorders after concussion. *J Neurol Phys Ther.* 2010;34:87–93.

291. Rubin W. How do we use state of the art vestibular testing to diagnose and treat the dizzy patient? An overview of vestibular testing and balance system integration. *Neurol Clin.* 1990;8:225–234.

292. Slattery EL, Sinks BC, Goebel JA. Vestibular tests for rehabilitation: applications and interpretation. *NeuroRehabilitation.* 2011;29:143–151.

293. Yardley L, Redfern MS. Psychological factors influencing recovery from balance disorders. *J Anxiety Disord.* 2001;15:107–119.

294. Andersson G, Westin V. Understanding tinnitus distress: introducing the concepts of moderators and mediators. *Int J Audiol.* 2008;(47, suppl 2):S106–S111.

295. Malouff JM, Schutte NS, Zucker LA. Tinnitus-related distress: a review of recent findings. *Curr Psychiatry Rep.* 2011;13:31–36.

296. Rimel RW, Giordani B, Barth JT, Jane JA. Moderate head injury: completing the clinical spectrum of brain trauma. *Neurosurgery.* 1982;11:344–351.

297. Meares S, Shores EA, Taylor AJ, et al. Mild traumatic brain injury does not predict acute postconcussion syndrome. *J Neurol Neurosurg Psychiatry.* 2008;79:300–306.

298. Dean PJA, O'Neill D, Sterr A. Post-concussion syndrome: prevalence after mild traumatic brain injury in comparison with sample without head injury. *Brain Inj.* 2012;26:14–26.

299. Kashluba S, Casey JE, Paniak C. Evaluating the utility of ICD-10 diagnostic criteria for postconcussion syndrome following mild traumatic brain injury. *J Int Neuropsychol Soc.* 2006;12:111–118.

300. McLean SA, Kirsch NL, Tan-Schriner CU, et al. Health status, not head injury, predicts concussion symptoms after minor injury. *Am J Emerg Med.* 2009;27:182–190.

301. Norrie J, Heitger M, Leathem J, Anderson T, Jones R, Flett R. Mild traumatic brain injury and fatigue: a prospective longitudinal study. *Brain Inj.* 2010;24:1528–1538.

302. Roe C, Sveen U, Alvsaker K, Bautz-Holter E. Post-concussion symptoms after mild traumatic brain injury: influence of demographic factors and injury severity in a 1-year cohort study. *Disabil Rehabil.* 2009;31:1235–1243.

303. Sigurdardottir S, Andelic N, Roe C, Jerstad T, Schanke AK. Postconcussion symptoms after traumatic brain injury at 3 and 12 months post-injury: a prospective study. *Brain Inj.* 2009;23:489–497.

304. van der Naalt J, van Zomeren AH, Sluiter WJ, Minderhoud JM. One year outcome in mild to moderate head injury: the predictive value of acute injury characteristics related to complaints and return to work. *J Neurol Neurosurg Psychiatry.* 1999;66:207–213.

305. Fee CR, Rutherford WH. A study of the effect of legal settlement on post-concussion symptoms. *Arch Emerg Med.* 1988;5:12–17.

306. Packard RC. Posttraumatic headache: permanency and relationship to legal settlement. *Headache.* 1992;32:496–500.

307. Yeates KO, Taylor HG, Rusin J, et al. Longitudinal trajectories of postconcussive symptoms in children with mild traumatic brain injuries and their relationship to acute clinical status. *Pediatrics.* 2009;123:735–743.

308. Leddy JJ, Kozlowski K, Donnelly JP, Pendergast DR, Epstein LH, Willer B. A preliminary study of subsymptom threshold exercise training for refractory post-concussion syndrome. *Clin J Sport Med.* 2010;20:21–27.

309. Al Sayegh A, Sandford D, Carson AJ. Psychological approaches to treatment of postconcussion syndrome: a systematic review. *J Neurol Neurosurg Psychiatry.* 2010;81:1128–1134.

310. Snell DL, Surgenor LJ, Hay-Smith EJ, Siegert RJ. A systematic review of psychological treatments for mild traumatic brain injury: an update on the evidence. *J Clin Exp Neuropsychol.* 2009;31:20–38.

311. Comper P, Bisschop SM, Carnide N, Tricco A. A systematic review of treatments for mild traumatic brain injury. *Brain Inj.* 2005;19:863–880.

312. Potter S, Brown RG. Cognitive behavioural therapy and persistent post-concussional symptoms: integrating conceptual issues and practical aspects in treatment. *Neuropsychol Rehabil.* 2012;22:1–25.

313. Ferguson RJ, Mittenberg W. Cognitive-behavioral treatment of postconcussion symdrome: a therapist's manual. In: Van Hasselt VB, Hersen M, eds. *Sourcebook of Psychological Treatment Manuals for Adult Disorders.* New York, NY: Plenum; 1996:615–655.

314. Miller LJ, Mittenberg W. Brief cognitive behavioral interventions in mild traumatic brain injury. *Appl Neuropsychol.* 1998;5:172–183.

315. Leonard KN, Tucker DM. Group-based cognitive-behavioral therapy for persistent postconcussion syndrome: a controlled treatment outcome study. Poster presented at: International Neuropsychological Society Meeting; 2004 February; Baltimore, MD.

316. Tiersky LA, Anselmi V, Johnston MV, et al. A trial of neuropsychologic rehabilitation in mild-spectrum traumatic brain injury. *Arch Phys Med Rehabil.* 2005;86:1565–1574.

317. Hesser H, Weise C, Westin VZ, Andersson G. A systematic review and meta-analysis of randomized controlled trials of cognitive-behavioral therapy for tinnitus distress. *Clin Psychol Rev.* 2011;31:545–553.

318. Hayes SC, Strosahl K, Wilson KG. *Acceptance and commitment therapy: an experiential approach to behavior change.* New York, NY: Guilford Press; 1999.

319. Strosahl KD, Hayes SC, Wilson KG, Gifford EV. An ACT primer: core therapy processes, intervention strategies, and therapist competences. In: Hayes SC, Strosahl KD, eds. *A Practical Guide to Acceptance and Commitment Therapy.* New York, NY: Springer Publishing; 2004:31–58.

320. Dahl J, Wilson KG, Nilsson A. Acceptance and commitment therapy and the treatment of persons at risk for long-term disability resulting from stress and pain symptoms: a preliminary randomized trial. *Behav Ther*. 2004;35:785–802.

321. Gutierrez O, Luciano C, Fink BC. Comparison between an acceptance-based and a cognitive-control-based protocol for coping with pain. *Behav Ther*. 2004;35:767–784.

322. Johnston M, Foster M, Shennan J, Starkey NJ, Johnson A. The effectiveness of an Acceptance and Commitment Therapy self-help intervention for chronic pain. *Clin J Pain*. 2010;26:393–402.

323. McCracken LM, Vowles KE, Eccleston C. Acceptance-based treatment for persons with complex, long standing chronic pain: a preliminary analysis of treatment outcome in comparison to a waiting phase. *Behav Res Ther*. 2005;43:1335–1346.

324. Vowels KE, Loebach-Wetherell J, Sorrell JT. Targeting acceptance, mindfulness, and values based action in chronic pain: findings of two preliminary trials of an outpatient group-based intervention. *Cogn Behav Pract*. 2008;16:49–58.

325. Wicksell RK, Melin L, Lekander M, Olsson GL. Evaluating the effectiveness of exposure and acceptance strategies to improve functioning and quality of life in longstanding pediatric pain—a randomized controlled trial. *Pain*. 2009;141:248–257.

326. Forman EM, Herbert JD, Moitra E, Yeomans PD, Geller PA. A randomized controlled effectiveness trial of acceptance and commitment therapy and cognitive therapy for anxiety and depression. *Behav Modif*. 2007;31:772–799.

327. Hesser H, Westin V, Hayes SC, Andersson G. Clients' in-session acceptance and cognitive defusion behaviors in acceptance-based treatment of tinnitus distress. *Behav Res Ther*. 2009;47:523–528.

328. Bond FW, Bunce D. Mediators of change in emotion-focused and problem-focused worksite stress management interventions. *J Occup Health Psychol*. 2000;5:156–163.

329. Bond FW, Bunce D. The role of acceptance and job control in mental health, job satisfaction, and work performance. *J Appl Psychol*. 2003;88:1057–1067.

330. Hayes SC, Bissett R, Roget N, et al. The impact of acceptance and commitment training on stigmatizing attitudes and professional burnout of substance abuse counselors. *Behav Ther*. 2004;35:821–836.

331. Blackledge JT, Hayes SC. Using acceptance and commitment training in the support of parents of children diagnosed with autism. *Child Fam Behav Ther*. 2006;28:1–18.

332. Dalrymple KL, Herbert JD. Acceptance and commitment therapy for generalized social anxiety disorder: a pilot study. *Behav Modif*. 2007;31:543–568.

333. Batten SV, Hayes SC. Acceptance and commitment therapy in the treatment of comorbid substance abuse and post-traumatic stress disorder: a case study. *Clin Case Stud*. 2005;4:246–262.

334. Petersen CL, Zettle RD. Treating inpatients with comorbid depression and alcohol use disorders: a comparison of acceptance and commitment therapy and treatment as usual. *Psychol Rec*. 2009;59:521–536.

335. Kangas M, McDonald S. Is it time to act? The potential of acceptance and commitment therapy for psychological problems following acquired brain injury. *Neuropsychol Rehabil*. 2011;21:250–276.

336. Bedard M, Felteau M, Mazmanian D, et al. Pilot evaluation of a mindfulness-based intervention to improve quality of life among individuals who sustained traumatic brain injuries. *Disabil Rehabil*. 2003;25:722–731.

337. Bedard M, Felteau M, Gibbons C, et al. A mindfulness-based intervention to improve quality of life among individuals who sustained traumatic brain injuries: one-year follow-up. *J Cogn Rehabil*. 2005:8–13.

338. Newman S, Steed L, Mulligan K. Self-management interventions for chronic illness. *Lancet*. 2004;364:1523–1537.

339. Nolte S, Elsworth GR, Sinclair AJ, Osborne RH. The extent and breadth of benefits from participating in chronic disease self-management courses: a national patient-reported outcomes survey. *Patient Educ Couns*. 2007;65:351–360.

340. McCracken LM. Learning to live with the pain: acceptance of pain predicts adjustment in persons with chronic pain. *Pain*. 1998;74:21–27.

341. Budd RJ, Pugh R. Tinnitus coping style and its relationship to tinnitus severity and emotional distress. *J Psychosom Res*. 1996;41:327–335.

342. Kendrick D, Silverberg ND, Miller WC, Moffat J. Acquired brain injury self-management program: a pilot evaluation. In press.

343. Mossberg KA, Amonette WE, Masel BE. Endurance training and cardiorespiratory conditioning after traumatic brain injury. *J Head Trauma Rehabil*. 2010;25:173–183.

344. Devine JM, Zafonte RD. Physical exercise and cognitive recovery in acquired brain injury: a review of the literature. *PM R*. 2009;1:560–575.

345. Lojovich JM. The relationship between aerobic exercise and cognition: is movement medicinal? *J Head Trauma Rehabil*. 2010;25:184–192.

346. Michelini LC, Stern JE. Exercise-induced neuronal plasticity in central autonomic networks: role in cardiovascular control. *Exp Physiol*. 2009;94:947–960.

347. Neeper SA, Gomez-Pinilla F, Choi J, Cotman C. Exercise and brain neurotrophins. *Nature*. 1995;373:109.

348. van Praag H. Neurogenesis and exercise: past and future directions. *Neuromolecular Med*. 2008;10:128–140.

349. Griesbach GS, Sutton RL, Hovda DA, Ying Z, Gomez-Pinilla F. Controlled contusion injury alters molecular systems associated with cognitive performance. *J Neurosci Res*. 2009;87:795–805.

350. Griesbach GS, Hovda DA, Molteni R, Wu A, Gomez-Pinilla F. Voluntary exercise following traumatic brain injury: brain-derived neurotrophic factor upregulation and recovery of function. *Neuroscience*. 2004;125:129–139.

351. Griesbach GS, Gomez-Pinilla F, Hovda DA. Time window for voluntary exercise-induced increases in hippocampal neuroplasticity molecules after traumatic brain injury is severity dependent. *J Neurotrauma*. 2007;24:1161–1171.

352. Griesbach GS, Hovda DA, Gomez-Pinilla F, Sutton RL. Voluntary exercise or amphetamine treatment, but not the combination, increases hippocampal brain-derived neurotrophic factor and synapsin I following cortical contusion injury in rats. *Neuroscience*. 2008;154:530–540.

353. Molteni R, Ying Z, Gomez-Pinilla F. Differential effects of acute and chronic exercise on plasticity-related genes in the rat hippocampus revealed by microarray. *Eur J Neurosci*. 2002;16:1107–1116.

354. Chaouloff F. Physical exercise and brain monoamines: a review. *Acta Physiologica Scandinavia*. 1989;137:1–13.

355. Penninx BW, Rejeski WJ, Pandya J, et al. Exercise and depressive symptoms: a comparison of aerobic and resistance exercise effects on emotional and physical function in older persons with high and low depressive symptomatology. *J Gerontol B Psychol Sci Soc Sci*. 2002;57:P124–P132.

356. Dunn AL, Trivedi MH, Kampert JB, Clark CG, Chambliss HO. Exercise treatment for depression: efficacy and dose response. *Am J Prev Med*. 2005;28:1–8.

357. Mead GE, Morley W, Campbell P, Greig CA, McMurdo M, Lawlor DA. Exercise for depression. *Cochrane Database Syst Rev*. 2008:CD004366.

358. Babyak M, Blumenthal JA, Herman S, et al. Exercise treatment for major depression: maintenance of therapeutic benefit at 10 months. *Psychosom Med*. 2000;62:633–638.

359. Lawlor DA, Hopker SW. The effectiveness of exercise as an intervention in the management of depression: systematic review and meta-regression analysis of randomised controlled trials. *BMJ*. 2001;322:763–767.

360. Daley A. Exercise and depression: a review of reviews. *J Clin Psychol Med Set*. 2008;15:140–147.

361. Mead GE, Morley W, Campbell P, Greig CA, McMurdo M, Lawlor DA. Exercise for depression. *Cochrane Database Syst Rev*. 2009:CD004366.

362. Rethorst CD, Wipfli BM, Landers DM. The antidepressive effects of exercise: a meta-analysis of randomized trials. *Sports Med*. 2009;39:491–511.

363. Wang C, Bannuru R, Ramel J, Kupelnick B, Scott T, Schmid CH. Tai Chi on psychological well-being: systematic review and meta-analysis. *BMC Complement Altern Med*. 2010;10:23.

364. Herring MP, O'Connor PJ, Dishman RK. The effect of exercise training on anxiety symptoms among patients: a systematic review. *Arch Intern Med*. 2010;170:321–331.

365. Greenwood BN, Fleshner M. Exercise, learned helplessness, and the stress-resistant brain. *Neuromolecular Med*. 2008;10:81–98.

366. Barbour KA, Edenfield TM, Blumenthal JA. Exercise as a treatment for depression and other psychiatric disorders: a review. *J Cardiopulm Rehabil Prev*. 2007;27:359–367.

367. Merom D, Phongsavan P, Wagner R, et al. Promoting walking as an adjunct intervention to group cognitive behavioral therapy for anxiety disorders—a pilot group randomized trial. *J Anxiety Disord*. 2008;22:959–968.

368. Smits JA, Berry AC, Rosenfield D, Powers MB, Behar E, Otto MW. Reducing anxiety sensitivity with exercise. *Depress Anxiety*. 2008; 25:689–699.

369. Smith PJ, Blumenthal JA, Hoffman BM, et al. Aerobic exercise and neurocognitive performance: a meta-analytic review of randomized controlled trials. *Psychosom Med*. 2010;72:239–252.

370. Ekeland E, Heian F, Hagen KB, Abbott J, Nordheim L. Exercise to improve self-esteem in children and young people. *Cochrane Database Syst Rev*. 2004:CD003683.

371. Youngstedt SD. Effects of exercise on sleep. *Clin Sports Med*. 2005; 24:355–365, xi.

372. Gagnon I, Galli C, Friedman D, Grilli L, Iverson GL. Active rehabilitation for children who are slow to recover following sport-related concussion. *Brain Inj*. 2009;23:956–964.

373. Chapman EH, Weintraub RJ, Milburn MA, Pirozzi TO, Woo E. Homeopathic treatment of mild traumatic brain injury: a randomized, double-blind, placebo-controlled clinical trial. *J Head Trauma Rehabil*. 1999;14:521–542.

374. Harch PG, Andrews SR, Fogarty EF, et al. A phase I study of low-pressure hyperbaric oxygen therapy for blast-induced postconcussion syndrome and post-traumatic stress disorder. *J Neurotrauma*. 2012;29:168–185.

375. Bortolotti B, Menchetti M, Bellini F, Montaguti MB, Berardi D. Psychological interventions for major depression in primary care: a meta-analytic review of randomized controlled trials. *Gen Hosp Psychiatry*. 2008;30:293–302.

376. Ekers D, Richards D, Gilbody S. A meta-analysis of randomized trials of behavioural treatment of depression. *Psychol Med*. 2008; 38:611–623.

377. van Straten A, Geraedts A, Verdonck-de Leeuw I, Andersson G, Cuijpers P. Psychological treatment of depressive symptoms in patients with medical disorders: a meta-analysis. *J Psychosom Res*. 2010;69(1):23–32.

378. Beltman MW, Voshaar RC, Speckens AE. Cognitive-behavioural therapy for depression in people with a somatic disease: meta-analysis of randomised controlled trials. *Br J Psychiatry*. 2010;197: 11–19.

379. Hunot V, Churchill R, Silva de Lima M, Teixeira V. Psychological therapies for generalised anxiety disorder. *Cochrane Database Syst Rev*. 2007:CD001848.

380. Acarturk C, Cuijpers P, van Straten A, de Graaf R. Psychological treatment of social anxiety disorder: a meta-analysis. *Psychol Med*. 2009;39:241–254.

381. Bisson J, Andrew M. Psychological treatment of post-traumatic stress disorder (PTSD). *Cochrane Database Syst Rev*. 2007;3:CD003388.

382. Zeitzer JM, Hubbard J, Litsch S, Luzon A, Friedman L, O'Hara R. Sleep disorders in the context of traumatic brain injury. *State of the Art (SOTA)*. Arlington, VA: Department of Veterans Affairs; 2008.

383. Asmundson GJ, Katz J. Understanding the co-occurrence of anxiety disorders and chronic pain: state-of-the-art. *Depress Anxiety*. 2009; 26:888–901.

384. Gottshall K. Vestibular rehabilitation after mild traumatic brain injury with vestibular pathology. *NeuroRehabilitation*. 2011;29: 167–171.

385. The Management of Concussion/mTBI Working Group. *VA/DoD Clinical Practice Guideline for Management of Concussion/Mild Traumatic Brain Injury (mTBI)*. Washington, DC: Department of Veterans Affairs and Department of Defense; 2009.

386. Ontario Neurotrauma Foundation. *Guidelines for mild traumatic brain injury and persistent symptoms*. Ontario Neurotrauma Foundation; 2011.

387. Zasler ND. Pharmacotherapy and posttraumatic cephalalgia. *J Head Trauma Rehabil*. 2011;26:397–399.

388. Malouff JM, Thorsteinsson EB, Rooke SE, Bhullar N, Schutte NS. Efficacy of cognitive behavioral therapy for chronic fatigue syndrome: a meta-analysis. *Clin Psychol Rev*. 2008;28:736–745.

389. Price JR, Mitchell E, Tidy E, Hunot V. Cognitive behaviour therapy for chronic fatigue syndrome in adults. *Cochrane Database Syst Rev*. 2008;(3):CD001027.

390. Silverberg ND, Iverson GL. Etiology of the post-concussion syndrome: physiogenesis and psychogenesis revisited. *NeuroRehabilitation*. 2011;29(4):317–329.

391. Van Damme S, Crombez G, Van Houdenhove B, Mariman A, Michielsen W. Well-being in patients with chronic fatigue syndrome: the role of acceptance. *J Psychosom Res*. 2006;61:595–599.

392. Westin V, Hayes SC, Andersson G. Is it the sound or your relationship to it? The role of acceptance in predicting tinnitus impact. *Behav Res Ther*. 2008;46:1259–1265.

393. McCracken LM, Eccleston C. Coping or acceptance: what to do about chronic pain? *Pain*. 2003;105:197–204.

394. Powell T, Ekin-Wood A, Collin C. Post-traumatic growth after head injury: a long-term follow-up. *Brain Inj*. 2007;21:31–38.

395. Nemiah JC, Freyberger H, Sifneos PE. Alexithymia: a view of the psychosomatic process. In: Hill OW, ed. *Modern Trends Psychosomatic Medicine*. Vol. 2. London, United Kingdom: Butterworths; 1976:26–34.

396. Steele CM, Aronson J. Stereotype threat and the intellectual test performance of African Americans. *J Pers Soc Psychol*. 1995;69: 797–811.

397. Boone KB. Fixed belief in cognitive dysfunction despite normal neuropsychological scores: neurocognitive hypochondriasis? *Clin Neuropsychol*. 2009;23:1016–1036.

398. Delis DC, Wetter SR. Cogniform disorder and cogniform condition: proposed diagnoses for excessive cognitive symptoms. *Arch Clin Neuropsychol*. 2007;22:589–604.

399. Dischinger PC, Ryb GE, Kufera JA, Auman KM. Early predictors of postconcussive syndrome in a population of trauma patients with mild traumatic brain injury. *J Trauma*. 2009;66(2):289–297.

400. Edna TH, Cappelen J. Late post-concussional symptoms in traumatic head injury. An analysis of frequency and risk factors. *Acta Neurochir* (Wien). 1987;86(1–2):12–17.

401. Ingebrigtsen T, Waterloo K, Marup-Jensen S, Attner E, Romner B. Quantification of post-concussion symptoms 3 months after minor head injury in 100 consecutive patients. *J Neurol*. 1998;245:609–612.

402. Kraus J, Hsu P, Schaffer K, et al. Preinjury factors and 3-month outcomes following emergency department diagnosis of mild traumatic brain injury. *J Head Trauma Rehabil*. 2009;24:344–354.

403. Ma M, Lindsell CJ, Rosenberry CM, Shaw GJ, Zemlan FP. Serum cleaved tau does not predict postconcussion syndrome after mild traumatic brain injury. *Am J Emerg Med*. 2008;26:763–768.

404. McCauley SR, Boake C, Pedroza C, et al. Correlates of persistent postconcussional disorder: DSM-IV criteria versus ICD-10. *J Clin Exp Neuropsychol*. 2008;30:360–379.

405. McCauley SR, Boake C, Levin HS, Contant CF, Song JX. Postconcussional disorder following mild to moderate traumatic brain injury: anxiety, depression, and social support as risk factors and comorbidities. *J Clin Exp Neuropsychol*. 2001;23:792–808.

406. Schneiderman AI, Braver ER, Kang HK. Understanding sequelae of injury mechanisms and mild traumatic brain injury incurred during the conflicts in Iraq and Afghanistan: persistent postconcussive symptoms and posttraumatic stress disorder. *Am J Epidemiol*. 2008;167:1446–1452.

407. Watson MR, Fenton GW, McClelland RJ, Lumsden J, Headley M, Rutherford WH. The post-concussional state: neurophysiological aspects. *Br J Psychiatry*. 1995;167:514–521.

408. Yang CC, Hua MS, Tu YK, Huang SJ. Early clinical characteristics of patients with persistent post-concussion symptoms: a prospective study. *Brain Inj*. 2009;23(4):299–306.

Sport-Related Concussion

Michael W. Collins, Grant L. Iverson, Michael B. Gaetz,
William P. Meehan III, and Mark R. Lovell

INTRODUCTION

Concussions are common in sports (1–3). Moreover, these injuries might be more prevalent than initially thought because some concussions go unrecognized (4). Injuries without loss of consciousness (LOC) occur most frequently; in fact, approximately 90% of concussions in sport occur without LOC (5–8). Because most concussions lack the dramatic on-field nature of those with LOC, they can be more difficult to detect and might be underdiagnosed (9). There is a mature body of literature illustrating that concussions cause acute adverse changes in subjectively experienced symptoms, balance, and neuropsychological test performance (6,7,9–20). The importance of accurate diagnosis, management, and return-to-play decisions extends from the elite ranks of professional athletes to the child athlete. This chapter, designed to be a comprehensive overview, is divided into the following 8 sections: (a) definition of concussion, (b) pathophysiology, (c) injury severity markers (signs), (d) symptoms, (e) balance, (f) cognition, (g) multiple concussions, (h) concussive convulsions, (i) chronic traumatic encephalopathy, (j) structural and functional neuroimaging, (k) recovery time and return-to-play decision making, (l) prevention, and (m) conclusions.

DEFINITION OF CONCUSSION

In 2001, 2004, and 2008, International Symposia on Concussion in Sport were held and concussion experts from around the world met to discuss specific issues related to the injury. One outcome of these symposia was the adoption of a definition of concussion. The current definition of concussion is reprinted in the following text.

> Concussion is defined as a complex pathophysiological process affecting the brain, induced by traumatic biomechanical forces. Several common features that incorporate clinical, pathological, and biomechanical injury constructs that may be utilized in defining the nature of a concussive head injury include
> 1. Concussion may be caused either by a direct blow to the head, face, neck, or elsewhere on the body with an "impulsive" force transmitted to the head.

> 2. Concussion typically results in the rapid onset of short-lived impairment of neurologic function that resolves spontaneously.
> 3. Concussion may result in neuropathological changes, but the acute clinical symptoms largely reflect a functional disturbance rather than a structural injury.
> 4. Concussion results in a graded set of clinical symptoms that may or may not involve loss of consciousness. Resolution of the clinical and cognitive symptoms typically follows a sequential course; however, it is important to note that in a small percentage of cases, however, post-concussive symptoms may be prolonged.
> 5. No abnormality on standard structural neuroimaging studies is seen in concussion. (21).

PATHOPHYSIOLOGY

The pathoanatomy and pathophysiology of mild traumatic brain injury (MTBI) is reviewed in detail in the MTBI chapter in this book. As described in that chapter, brain injuries produced by acceleration/deceleration forces occur along a continuum of severity dependent on the mechanical forces that caused them (22,23). Concussion in athletes is typically produced by acceleration/deceleration forces (e.g., helmet-to-helmet contact in North American football or helmet-to-ice contact in ice hockey). In athletics, all traumatic accelerations of the head involve both linear (translational) and rotational components (24). Although it is possible that both linear and rotational accelerations can result in concussive brain injury, rotational forces appear to be a more significant etiological factor (22,25,26). Concussion can be considered an injury at the mild end of the MTBI continuum with LOC (when it occurs) and post-traumatic amnesia being considerably briefer in duration. Further, Giza and Hovda (27) describe the complex interwoven cellular and vascular changes that occur following concussion as a multilayered neurometabolic cascade. The primary mechanisms include ionic shifts, abnormal energy metabolism, diminished cerebral blood flow (CBF), and impaired neurotransmission. A brief summary of this process, derived from several sources (27,28), is provided in the following text.

Stretching of an axon results in an indiscriminate release of neurotransmitters and uncontrolled ionic fluxes. When ionic gradients are disrupted, cells respond by activating ion pumps in an attempt to restore the normal membrane potential. Pump activation increases glucose use. This contributes to dramatic increases in the local cerebral metabolic rate for glucose. This hypermetabolism occurs in tandem with mildly decreased CBF, which contributes to the disparity between glucose supply and demand. There also appears to be impaired oxidative metabolism and diminished mitochondrial function, resulting in the overuse of anaerobic energy pathways and elevated lactate as a by-product. Moreover, intracellular magnesium levels appear to decrease significantly and remain depressed for several days following injury. This is important because magnesium is essential for the generation of adenosine triphosphate (ATP; energy production). Magnesium is also essential for the initiation of protein synthesis and the maintenance of the cellular membrane potential. A sustained initial influx of Ca^{2+} can result in mitochondrial accumulations of this ion contributing to metabolic dysfunction and energy failure. High intracellular Ca^{2+} levels, combined with stretch injury, can initiate an irreversible process of destruction of microtubules within axons.

Fortunately, the brain undergoes a dynamic restorative process in the initial days to weeks following a concussion. From a commonsense perspective, the ionic shifts, abnormal energy metabolism, diminished CBF, and impaired neurotransmission believed to be associated with concussions in sports, reinforces the importance of immediate rest, both physically and cognitively, following injury. Although not fully established scientifically, it seems reasonable to assume that vigorous exercise, intensive academic work, or blows to the head or body could exacerbate the pathophysiology described earlier.

INJURY SEVERITY MARKERS (SIGNS)

Appropriate acute care and management of the concussed athlete begins with a detailed and accurate assessment of the severity of the injury. As with any serious injury, the first priority is always to evaluate the athlete's level of consciousness, airway, breathing, and circulation. The designated medical first responder should be prepared with an emergency action plan in the event that the evacuation of a critically head- or neck-injured athlete is necessary. This plan should be familiar to all staff, be well delineated, and frequently rehearsed.

Loss of Consciousness

On ruling out more severe injury via neurological and clinical examination, the acute evaluation continues with the assessment of concussion. At the outset, the first responder should establish whether an LOC has occurred. By definition, LOC represents a state of brief coma in which the eyes are typically closed completely or partially, and the athlete is unresponsive to external stimuli. The definitive presence of LOC is difficult to determine, especially because some athletes may report "blacking out," which may actually be a visual disturbance rather than a frank LOC or could be related to impaired memory formation (i.e., post-traumatic amnesia). Regardless, LOC is relatively uncommon and re-

portedly occurs in fewer than 10% of concussive injuries in most (5–8) but not all (17) studies. Moreover, prolonged LOC (> 1–2 minutes) in sport-related concussion occurs much less frequently. Athletes with LOC are typically unresponsive for only a brief period of time, sometimes only 1–2 seconds. This makes LOC difficult to identify because first responders typically initiate care beyond this time window.

Research on the relation between LOC and outcome is mixed. Large scale studies with patients with trauma have not revealed a definitive relation between brief LOC and neuropsychological outcome (e.g., 29,30). Some researchers examining athletes with concussions have reported an association between LOC and immediate or short-term outcome (e.g., 17,31,32), whereas others have not (e.g., 14,33). One factor that might help to explain different research results has to do with the nature and severity of the sample being studied. Generally speaking, LOC that takes place within the context of sports is most often very brief (seconds), and LOC that extends beyond a minute of 2 is relatively rare. Yeates and his colleagues (34) found that a sample of children with LOC and other severity markers following MTBI were more likely to have higher levels of postconcussive symptoms in comparison to an orthopedic control group and to a group with less severe injuries. However, this sample was drawn from children who had been evaluated in an emergency department setting, which may represent an inherently different group than concussed athletes injured in sports settings. Lau and colleagues reported that LOC within the athletic environment was not a significant predictor of persistent postconcussive difficulties (35).

Confusion

A more common form of mental status change following concussion involves confusion and amnesia. *Confusion* (i.e., disorientation), by definition, represents impaired awareness and orientation to surroundings, although memory systems are not necessarily directly affected. An athlete with postinjury confusion will typically appear stunned, dazed, or "glassy eyed" on the sideline or playing field. Confusion is sometimes manifested in athletes who do not remove themselves from play in the form of difficulty with appropriate play calling, failure to correctly execute their positional assignment during play, or difficulty in communicating game information to teammates or coaches. Teammates are often the first to recognize that an athlete has been injured when the athlete shows these behaviors and has difficulty maintaining the flow of the game. On the sidelines, confused athletes may answer questions slowly, may inappropriately ask, "What is going on?" or "What happened?" and may repeat themselves during evaluation. Some may be temporarily disoriented to time or place and even, very rarely, to people they know well (e.g., not knowing coaches or teammates). To assess the presence of confusion, first responders can ask the athlete simple questions such as the name of the opposing team or what period or half is it. A standard set of orientation questions are included in the second edition of the Sideline Concussion Assessment Tool (SCAT2).

Amnesia

Amnesia is emerging as perhaps the most important sign to carefully assess following concussion (after more serious injuries have been ruled out). Amnesia, because of concussion, may present as retrograde amnesia (difficulty with memory for events prior to the injury) or post-traumatic/anterograde amnesia (difficulty with memory for events following the injury). Athletes who present with 1 or both types of amnesia may initially have difficulty recalling large spans of time before the injury, after the injury, or both. These larger periods of amnesia typically shrink as the injury becomes less acute. The presence and duration of amnesia, disorientation, or mental status disturbance has been associated with immediate outcome or slower recovery (17,32,33,36,37) in many but not all studies (e.g., 14).

Post-traumatic amnesia and anterograde amnesia are synonymous terms that represent the duration of time between the head trauma (e.g., an ice hockey player's face striking the protective glass as the result of a hit from behind) and the point at which the athlete reports a return of normal continuous memory functioning (e.g., remembering the athletic trainer asking the athlete orientation questions in the locker room).

At times, especially during a sideline assessment, confusion and post-traumatic amnesia may be difficult to disentangle. It is important to remember that confusion is not necessarily associated with a loss of memory, whereas amnesia is only present with a loss of memory. This memory loss may span only a few seconds or minutes. It sometimes can span several hours but rarely exceeds a day. A practitioner may be unable to differentiate confusion and amnesia until the athlete's confusion has resolved—the point when memories surrounding the injury can actually be discussed. Once the athlete is more lucid, the practitioner may gain additional insight into any existing post-traumatic amnesia by asking the athlete to recall the events that occurred immediately following the trauma (e.g., rising from the ground, walking/skating to sideline, memory for any part of the game played or observed after the injury, memory for the score of the contest, memory of the ride home, etc.). *Post-traumatic amnesia* is inferred by failure to remember events following the injury.

Retrograde amnesia is defined as the inability to recall events before the injury event. Medical personnel may ask for the athlete's memory of the actual injury (e.g., seeing a linebacker charge toward him with his helmet down, then falling backward and striking the back of his head to the ground). Then, additional questions can probe events that are increasingly remote from the injury (e.g., what was done for pregame warm-up, the coach's pregame instructions, and the score at the end of the first quarter). The duration of retrograde amnesia will typically "shrink" over time. As recovery occurs, the period of retrograde amnesia may shrink from several minutes to a few seconds (in rare cases, an athlete will have retrograde amnesia for hours or days). The presence and duration of retrograde amnesia has been associated with worse initial presentation and with slower recovery (31–33,36).

SYMPTOMS

The initial signs and symptoms of concussion vary from athlete to athlete. A summary of on-field signs and symptoms

TABLE 31-1 University of Pittsburgh Medical Center's Sideline Concussion Card: Signs and Symptoms of Concussion

SIGNS/BEHAVIORS OBSERVED BY STAFF	SYMPTOMS REPORTED BY ATHLETE
Loss of consciousness	Feeling "foggy" or groggy
Forgets events prior to play (retrograde)	Change in sleep pattern (appears later)
Forgets events after hit (post-traumatic)	Feeling fatigued
Appears to be dazed or stunned	Headache
Is confused about assignment	Nausea
Forgets plays	Balance problems or dizziness
Is unsure of game, score, or opponent	Double or fuzzy/blurry vision
Moves clumsily	Sensitivity to light or noise
Answers questions slowly	Feeling sluggish or slowed down
Shows behavior or personality change	Concentration or memory problems

of concussion is presented in Table 31-1. It is important to note that an athlete may present with as few as 1 symptom or potentially a constellation of symptoms.

Headaches and dizziness are the most commonly reported symptoms of injury (5,38). Moreover, headaches lasting more than 3 hours postinjury (31), those present at 7 days postinjury (37), or those that are migraine-like (39) have been associated with slower recovery. However, the absence of headache does not rule out a concussion, highlighting the importance of a thorough assessment of all symptoms. Assessment of postconcussion headache may be complicated by the presence of musculoskeletal headaches and other preexisting headache syndromes (e.g., migraine disorder or frequent stress headaches) or headache because of focal head, but not brain, trauma.

Most frequently, a "concussion headache" is a uniquely described sensation of pressure in the skull that may be localized to 1 region of the head or may be generalized in nature. In some athletes (particularly athletes with a history of migraine), the headache may take the form of a vascular headache; it may be unilateral, and it is often described as throbbing or pulsating. The headache may develop in the minutes or even hours following injury. Therefore, it is important to question the potentially concussed athlete regarding the development of symptoms beyond the first few minutes after injury. Postconcussion headache is often worsened with physical or cognitive exertion. Thus, if the athlete complains of worsening headache during exertional testing or returns to play, postconcussion headache should be suspected and conservative management is indicated. Moreover, it is common for student athletes to exhibit worsening headaches while attending school and engaging in cognitive activities, such as reading, math class, and taking notes during the days, weeks, and sometimes months following injury. Although headache immediately following a concussion usually does not constitute a medical emergency, a severe or progressively worsening headache, particularly when accompanied by vomiting or declining mental status, may signal a life-threatening situation, such as an epidural or subdural hematoma. This should prompt immediate transport to the hospital and imaging of the brain.

In addition to headaches, many other symptoms may emerge in the days following concussion. An athlete may report increased fatigue, feeling "a step slow," or feeling "sluggish." Fatigue is especially prominent in the days following injury, and this symptom may be as notable as headache. Some athletes will experience blurred vision, changes in peripheral vision, or other visual disturbance. Athletes may report cognitive changes, including problems with attention, concentration, short-term memory, learning, and multitasking. These symptoms sometimes become more noticeable after the athlete has returned to school or work. Emotional and psychological symptoms are also reported by some athletes in the initial days postinjury. For those who are slow to recover, these symptoms sometimes become prominent. Most often, athletes will report increased irritability or having a "shorter fuse." However, symptoms of anxiety and depression might also occur.

Monitoring Symptoms

Symptom rating scales are helpful for monitoring recovery from concussion. The Post-Concussion Scale is well suited for this purpose (40–42). This 22-item test is based on a 7-point Likert scale with 0 and 6 reflecting the anchor points. Athletes report symptoms based on the severity of each symptom that day. This scale, in slightly modified forms, has been used by the National Football League (NFL) (40) and the National Hockey League (NHL) (43,44). It has been used as an outcome measure in numerous published studies (e.g., 36,37,45–47). The internal consistency of the scale ranges from 0.88 to 0.94 in high school and college students, and 0.92 to 0.93 in concussed athletes (48). Normative data for the scale are based on 1,391 young males and 355 young females (48).

The Concussion Symptom Inventory (CSI; 49) is a new 12-item scale. It was developed using samples of more than 16,000 uninjured athletes and more than 600 concussed athletes. Although it can be derived from the Post-Concussion Scale and the SCAT2, the CSI combines balance problems/dizziness into a single symptom. Therefore, clinicians could sum and average the 2 symptoms to compute the CSI total score. The SCAT2, a new on-field assessment test that includes symptom ratings, balance testing, and cognitive screening (21), is now being widely used in clinical settings. At present, however, there are no normative or psychometric data for the symptom scale within the SCAT2. If normative scores are desired, the clinician using the SCAT2 could calculate the CSI total score and compare it to scores derived from healthy and concussed athletes.

BALANCE

Concussions can have an adverse effect on balance during the early stages of recovery; thus, balance testing can be used to track recovery (6,14,19,20). Early studies into the effects of concussion on balance used electronic pressure transducers placed under athletes' feet to measure postural sway (50). Later, the Sensory Organization Test has been used to assess postural sway after injury (14,51,52). For the Sensory Organization Test, athletes are asked to remain as motionless as possible. Postural sway of the center of gravity is assessed while the support surface, the visual surround, or both are tilted (14). These studies have revealed an increase in postural sway after sport-related concussion that persists for several days after injury (50).

Because force plates, associated software, and the expertise to use them are not widely available, more practical means of measuring postural stability were developed and validated using posturography (14,53). The most well known is the Balance Error Scoring System (BESS; 6,14,20,54).

The BESS is a rapid, relatively easy-to-administer, and inexpensive measure of static balance and postural stability. A combination of 3 stances (narrow double leg stance, single leg stance, and tandem stance) and footing surfaces (firm surface/floor or medium density foam) are used for the test. Each stance is held, with hands on hips and eyes closed, for 20 seconds. "Error" points are given for specific behaviors, including opening eyes, lifting hands off hips, or stepping, stumbling, or falling (6,14,20,54).

The BESS was included as an outcome measure in a large-scale National Collegiate Athletic Association (NCAA) football study (6). BESS error scores in concussed players changed from baseline on average by 5.7 points when measured on the sideline, immediately following injury. At 1 day postinjury, their average BESS score was only 2.7 points above baseline performance. BESS performance returned to preseason baseline levels (average 12 errors) by 3–7 days postinjury for most athletes. These modest changes in BESS performance and rapid recovery of static balance have been reported in other studies with athletes (14,19,20).

A modified version of the BESS (M-BESS), using the 3 stances on a hard surface only, has been included in the SCAT2 and recommended for widespread use in sports (21). At present, only limited research is available to guide its clinical use. Iverson and Gaetz (55) examined M-BESS performance in 36 amateur athletes before and after a heavy exertion exercise protocol. Women outperformed men before and after the exercise protocol. There were no significant differences between pre- or post-exercise balance scores for men or women. Therefore, in that study, M-BESS performance was different for men and women—but it was minimally affected by aerobic exercise. Unfortunately, large-scale normative data and data for estimating reliable change are not available for the M-BESS. Iverson (56) provided preliminary normative data for the M-BESS across the adult lifespan (age 20–69). However, high school and university athletes were not included in this sample. Preliminary normative data for the M-BESS, based on relatively small samples of university athletes, are provided in Table 31-2. As seen in the interquartile ranges (IQR), scores from 0–5 are broadly normal for the young men, and scores from 0–2 are broadly normal for young women. The information presented in the table shows that interpretation of M-BESS scores is not straightforward, and it would be helpful to gather normative data on much larger samples.

COGNITION

There is a mature body of evidence indicating that some athletes who sustain concussions experience cognitive defi-

TABLE 31-2 Preliminary Normative Reference Values for the SCAT2 M-BESS

AGE	N	MEAN	MEDIAN	SD	ABOVE AVERAGE	BROADLY NORMAL	BELOW AVERAGE	POOR	VERY POOR
University men	47	2.7	2.0	3.2	—	0–5	6–8	9–11	12+
University women	58	1.5	1.0	1.6	—	0–2	3	4–7	8+
Adults: 20–29	65	2.7	2.0	2.5	0	1–4	5–6	7–10	11+
Men: 20–29	26	2.5	2.0	2.5	0	1–4	5–6	7–10	11+
Women: 20–29	39	2.8	2.0	2.4	0	1–4	5–6	7–10	11+

The maximum score for each trial was truncated at 10 points. These classification ranges correspond to the following percentile ranks: very poor = < 2nd percentile; poor = 2nd–9th percentile; below average = 10th–24th percentile; broadly normal = 25th–75th percentile. Approximately 15% of the community adult sample obtained a score of zero. The 105 university students (47 men and 58 women) were amateur athletes from sports teams. The 65 adults between the ages of 20 and 29 were taking part in a comprehensive preventive health screen at a private multidisciplinary health care center. They did not have significant medical, neurologic, or lower extremity problems that might have an adverse effect on balance. The differences amongst the subgroups are very subtle. The distributions are skewed, so the classification ranges are more accurate for referencing a person's performance than using the mean and standard deviation (SD) to compute a z-score. Abbreviation: N, total sample size; M-BESS, modified version of the Balance Error Scoring System; SCAT2, Sideline Concussion Assessment Tool 2.

cits that can be detected with traditional and computerized tests (e.g., 6,7,9,14–16,33,36,47,57,58–70). Based on group data, researchers have reported that athletes usually recover within 2 weeks (6,7,17,47,71,72). When analyzing individual cases, however, some athletes take longer to recover, and their slower recovery can be obscured in group analyses (63,73). Moreover, Lovell and colleagues reported much longer recovery times in a sample of athletes (i.e., several weeks) and noted that those athletes with the greatest functional activation on functional magnetic resonance imaging (fMRI) in the first week postinjury took the longest to recover (74).

There is some evidence that there are important differences in recovery time relating to age and level of play; for example, professional football players appear to recover faster than high school athletes (75). Results from a 6-year, prospective NFL concussion study have been published in a series of articles (32,38,72,76–80). A total of 887 concussions were recorded in 650 players during the study period. The time taken to return to play was as follows: (a) day of injury = 56%, (b) 1–6 days = 35.9%, (c) 7–14 days = 6.5%, and (d) more than 14 days = 1.6% (32). Those athletes who returned to play in the same game had fewer and briefer signs and symptoms of concussion, and they did not appear to have significantly increased risk for a second injury either in the same game or during the season (80).

A subset of concussed NFL players underwent baseline paper-and-pencil neuropsychological evaluations and then completed a second evaluation (N = 95) within a few days following their concussion (M = 1.4 days, SD = 1.3) (76). The players did not show a single statistically significant decrement on any paper-and-pencil neuropsychological test when seen in the first few days postinjury. These results are inconsistent with studies in both collegiate and high school athletes, where neurocognitive decrements are more pronounced. The NFL study relied on a relatively small sample of concussed athletes, and baseline test results were not available for the entire sample, so postinjury performance was compared to normative rather than to individual baseline values. These results also might reflect a selection bias (NFL athletes return to play earlier, perhaps because of genetics/biological hardiness) or that age/developmental factors or being a professional athlete may play a role in recovery from concussion.

In a NCAA prospective cohort study (6), 1,631 football players from 15 colleges completed preseason baseline testing during the 3-year study. Players with concussions (n = 94) and noninjured controls (n = 56) underwent assessment of symptoms, cognitive functioning via the measurement of paper-and-pencil neuropsychological tests, and postural stability immediately, 3 hours, and 1, 2, 3, 5, 7, and 90 days after injury. Concussed athletes' balance problems resolved within 3–5 days, self-reported postconcussion symptoms gradually resolved by day 7, and paper-and-pencil neurocognitive functioning improved within 5–7 days. By 7 days postinjury, 91% of athletes appeared to be functionally recovered.

Collins and colleagues conducted a 3-year, prospective, naturalistic, cohort study of high school football players (65). Outcome measures included measurement of symptoms, as well as computerized neurocognitive assessment. Participants were 2, 141 high school athletes from Western Pennsylvania. During this 3-year study, athletes were carefully followed clinically, until they were cleared to return to competition. The recovery rates for athletes with no prior history of injury, compared to those with 1 or more previous concussions, are presented in Figure 31-1.

The high school football players, as illustrated in Figure 31-1, took considerably longer to recover than university (6) or professional (32,72,75) football players. The reasons for slower recovery following multiple concussions are not known but could be related to a number of factors, including neurodevelopmental differences in response to concussion-related neuropathophysiology, genetics, and injury resilience. Moreover, young athletes who are more susceptible to concussions, or who are slow to recover, might not advance to higher levels of play. Thus, the more rapid recovery time in college and professional athletes could, in part, reflect a selection bias.

Neuropsychological Assessment in Concussion Management Programs

Over the past 2 decades, neuropsychologists have led scientific and clinical initiatives aimed at identifying the symptoms and problems associated with concussions, monitoring recovery, and facilitating return to school and sports. This

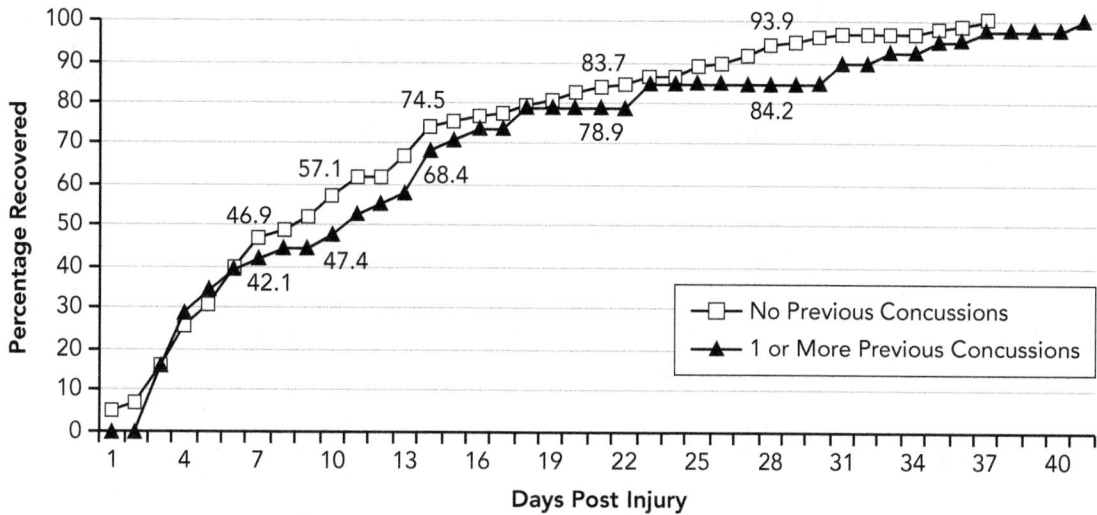

FIGURE 31–1 Recovery times for concussed high school football players (N = 134) *Note*: These recovery curves were calculated based on a reanalysis of data from Collins et al. (65). The sample size was 134 concussed high school football players. Recovery curves for those with no previous concussions vs one or more previous injuries are presented. The percentages of athletes deemed recovered at 7, 10, 14, 21, and 28 days are noted.

has resulted in evidence-based approaches to the clinical assessment and management of concussion in athletes. The Vienna Summary and Agreement Statement referred to neuropsychological testing as the "cornerstone" of a concussion management program (81). The Prague Summary and Agreement Statement (82) emphasized that neuropsychological testing was most appropriate for athletes who are slow to recover (e.g., more than 10 days). A National Academy of Neuropsychology Position Statement recommended the use of neuropsychological testing to monitor recovery from concussion (83). The Zurich Consensus Statement noted that neuropsychological testing was an important component of a more comprehensive assessment that also included subjective symptoms and balance (21), and neurocognitive testing was recommended for athletes who are slow to recover.

Neuropsychologists get involved at 2 points in time: preseason and/or postinjury. Many athletic teams now use preseason neuropsychological testing. The preseason testing provides a benchmark for each player to help gauge recovery should the player get concussed during the season. Several computerized packages are available for preseason testing, including ImPACT, AxonSports (previously known as Cogsport), and the HeadMinder Concussion Resolution Index (13,15,36,63,64,66,69,84). In the United States, ImPACT appears to be the most commonly used (85). Often, however, neuropsychologists become involved only after an athlete has been injured. The clinical goal is to determine if the athlete has subjectively experienced symptoms and/or neuropsychological impairments. Assessment procedures typically include an interview with the athlete, postconcussion self-report questionnaires, administering neuropsychological tests, and possibly balance testing. The clinician, in cooperation with the family physician, might set out specific recommendations for return to play, provide advice about any potential for establishing short-term accommodations in school and/or work, and give information to the athlete on

recovery following more serious concussions or persisting injuries.

MULTIPLE CONCUSSIONS

There is a concern that athletes who sustain more than 1 concussion will be at increased risk for long-term changes to brain structure and/or function, slower recovery, and increased risk of future injuries. The concerns stem in part from the well-publicized cases of athletes in sports such as American football, ice hockey, and especially combatants in sports such as boxing who have been reported to have significant functional impairments after retirement, as well as structural changes to their brain at autopsy.

Athletes who may be at the greatest risk for the effects of multiple concussive and subconcussive impacts are participants in combat sport, such as boxing. Few would debate that a *career* in boxing can result in changes to the structure and function of the brain (86–91) (a discussion of chronic traumatic encephalopathy [CTE] in boxers follows this section). However, this may not be the case with amateur boxers and noncombat sport participants. For example, professional boxing differs from amateur boxing in a number of ways: amateur boxers are typically not the elite in their weight class, they use headgear and larger gloves, and they have fewer rounds per fight. Taken as a whole, studies on amateur boxers have offered mixed results regarding changes in brain structure and function (e.g., 92,93–96). In a longitudinal study, Porter (97) observed no statistical change in a group of 19 amateur boxers over a period of 9 years using neuropsychological testing compared to nonboxing athletic controls.

The literature on subconcussive blows to the head in other sports is also mixed. Some studies reported neuropsychological decrements (16) or temporary adverse effects immediately following repeatedly heading a soccer ball during practice (98). A greater number of studies showed that heading the soccer ball, tournament boxing, helmet impacts in American football, or springboard diving generally result in no statistically significant neuropsychological (99–105) or balance effects (106).

Based on the combat sport literature alone, there appears to be the potential for a continuum of lingering or cumulative structural and/or functional changes to the brain following repeated exposure to multiple subconcussive events or concussions. In contact sports such as American football, ice hockey, and rugby, there appears to be some support for the effects of multiple concussions as well, although more research is needed in this regard. Researchers have reported that a history of 3 or more concussions is associated with changes in cognitive neurophysiology (107,108), subjective symptoms (46,107,109), worse neuropsychological test performance (e.g., 46), and long-term cognitive decrements (110). Although not demarcating 3 concussions specifically, 2 recent studies have shown a positive relationship between concussion history and worse neuropsychological performance (105,109). However, not all studies have shown neuropsychological group differences with a history of 3 or more concussions (111,112). Similarly, NFL athletes with a history of 3 or more concussions did not perform more poorly on neuropsychological testing than those with fewer than 3 (72). However, high school and university athletes who experienced 3 or more concussions revealed small but measurable group effects (45,107,113) and increased risk for future concussions (114,115).

The research evidence for group differences following 2 or fewer concussions is expectedly less conclusive. Regarding possible long-term effects, some researchers have reported significant findings (9,116), others have not (107), and others reported equivocal results (e.g., 117). In a large-scale study that examined jockeys with 2 or more concussions (20/27 jockeys had listed 2 concussions or did not specify), individuals with multiple concussions vs history of a single concussion performed more poorly on the Stroop Color-Word and Trails 2 tests. It should be noted that jockeys in the study who were multiply concussed did not differ from those who were never concussed on the Stroop test, making logical conclusions difficult to draw.

Another important functional change linked to multiple concussions is slowed recovery time. Studies have shown that athletes who sustained multiple concussions may have slowed recovery time (114,118) and may have greater acute changes in memory performance (46). Very few studies have measured the effects of 2 concussions within a season compared to a preinjury baseline. Slobounov et al. (119) reported a differential rate of recovery for the complexity of the electroencephalogram (EEG), indicating a better functional outcome after the first compared to the second concussion.

Another concern related to a history of multiple concussions is that the risk of sustaining a future concussion may be dependent on concussion history. It has been reported that athletes who sustain a concussion are at statistically increased risk for sustaining another concussion (120, 121). The reasons for this are unclear but could relate to style of play, position, genetics, or lowering a biological susceptibility threshold.

In summary, *most* studies on multiple concussions indicate that group differences exist in the structure and/or functioning of the brain that increase with exposures in a cumulative response manner. What is not clear at this time is whether all athletes respond in a similar way to multiple impacts and concussions, or whether a small number of athletes are largely responsible for these group effects. Furthermore, inherent methodological difficulties occur in studying lingering effects of concussions, and such studies usually have not always taken into account the timing of prior injuries, management (or lack thereof) of these injuries, developmental differences, or the potential inaccuracy and self-report nature of these data. More research must be completed studying multiply concussed athletes prospectively using a within subject methodologies (e.g., 119) if statements about cumulative effects in multiply concussed athletes are to be accurately made.

Second Impact Syndrome

Second impact syndrome is conceptualized as an *extraordinarily rare* cascade of events, in which an athlete experiences a catastrophic brain injury following a seemingly mild concussion. The second impact syndrome, as a true clinical entity, has been questioned (122–124). In fact, in a recent review of the literature, McCrory and colleagues stated that "the scientific evidence to support this concept is nonexistent" (124, p. 21). It has been noted in the literature that diffuse cerebral swelling is a rare and catastrophic consequence of a *single* seemingly mild brain injury—creating a conceptual problem for the assumption that the small number of cases really represent second impact syndrome. In theory, however, sustaining a second brain injury during a period of increased vulnerability with unresolved metabolic dysfunction has been linked to second impact syndrome. The pathophysiological basis for second impact syndrome is thought to be cerebrovascular congestion or a loss of cerebrovascular autoregulation leading to considerable brain swelling and edema (125,126). It has been reported that relatively few athletes, approximately 35 or more in the years between 1980 and 1993, have succumbed to this syndrome (125) (18 cases identified in another literature review; 127). When it occurs, morbidity is 100%, and mortality is reported to occur in up to 50% of cases (125). To date, most cases of second impact syndrome have been reported in children (e.g., 128) or adolescents (129,130).

Animal modeling has indicated that a single MTBI revealed transient and minimal impairment on a composite neuroscore test and minimal breach of the blood–brain barrier. If a second mild injury was inflicted within 24 hours of the first injury, a marked breakdown of the blood–brain barrier occurred leading to swelling and edema (131). This change in blood–brain barrier integrity following a second concussive injury occurring shortly after the first could be a possible mechanism for the rapid swelling and edema formation that occurs in humans.

A concern that affects all injured athletes (as opposed to a tiny percentage that could experience second impact syndrome) is the possibility of magnified pathophysiology attributable to overlapping injuries. For example, there is evidence in the animal literature that there is a temporal window of vulnerability in which a second injury results in magnified cognitive and behavioral deficits and greater levels of traumatic axonal injury (131–133). Specifically, mice that are reinjured during this "temporal window" have worse behavioral and neurophysiological outcome than mice that are reinjured after the temporal window. These animal studies support the idea that athletes should not be returned to contact sports during the *acute recovery stage* from concussion.

CONCUSSIVE CONVULSIONS

Some sport-related concussions occasionally are associated with a "concussive convulsion" (134–137). Using video analysis from Australian rules football matches, McCrory and Berkovic describe these in detail. Concussive convulsions occur when an athlete is unconscious after sustaining a blow to the head. Beginning within 2 seconds of impact, these convulsions involve a period of initial tonicity of the upper extremities, classically in a "bear-hug" position. The tonic phase then progresses to a bilateral myoclonic phase. Concussive convulsions are brief in duration, typically lasting less than 30 seconds; the longest reported concussive convulsion lasted 150 seconds (135,136). Some authors estimate the occurrence of convulsions at 1 in every 70 concussions, although they are careful to point out, this is a "crude" estimation (134).Concussive convulsions are not thought to be epileptic in nature (134,136–139), although this opinion is not universal (140). Concussive convulsions themselves require no specific management; they resolve spontaneously. They do not appear to be associated with prolonged recovery, and they are not associated with an increased risk of future epilepsy (134,136,137).

CHRONIC TRAUMATIC ENCEPHALOPATHY

CTE was historically described as a progressive neurodegenerative syndrome occurring in boxers who had a significant history in the sport. Martland (141) was the first to describe the syndrome known as "punch drunk" that characterized many of the cognitive-behavioral changes attributed to the pathophysiology of CTE. Parker (142) was among the first to use the term *traumatic encephalopathy* and described early signs and symptoms such as ataxia and confusion, postcareer signs such as dysarthria, deafness, "physical slowing up," and mental deterioration, finally leading to a neurological syndrome that in severe cases resulted in mental or physical helplessness. The often cited classic study by Corsellis et al. (143) described a characteristic pattern of brain injury in boxers: a fenestrated or a cavum septum pellucidum, scarring to cerebellar tonsils and other cerebral areas, neuronal loss in substantia nigra and locus coeruleus, ventricular enlargement, thinning of the corpus callosum, and neurofibrillary tangles in cerebral cortex and temporal lobe. Roberts (144) randomly sampled 250 retired boxers and showed severe CTE pathophysiology in 5% of boxers and demonstrable lesions in 17%.

The modern era of CTE study is different from the historical reports in several ways. First, the more recent cases have been "autopsy confirmed" (e.g., 145). Second, most of the athletes were not boxers (e.g., American football, ice hockey, and professional wrestling). These case reports have generated a significant amount of attention within the media, advisory boards for the professional sports leagues, and within the amateur levels of sport perhaps because CTE

was reported to have been connected to, or *caused*, the death of these athletes (146).

The pathophysiologic hallmark of these cases is the development of regionally specific tau-immunoreactive neurofibrillary pathology of neurofibrillary tangles, astrocytic tangles, neuropil, and neurites observed in subcortical (e.g., hippocampus, entorhinal cortex, amygdala, as well as throughout the diencephalon and brainstem) and cortical areas (e.g., insular, temporal, dorsolateral parietal, inferior occipital, and dorsolateral frontal cortices) (147). A possible mechanism for tau deposition is linked to the stretch of axons that occurs with traumatic axonal injury. Gavett et al. (148) reported that the stretching of axons results in alterations in axonal membrane permeability, calcium influx, and caspase and calpain release. Caspases and calpains may in turn trigger tau abnormalities (e.g., misfolding, truncation, aggregation), as well as dissolution of microtubules and neurofilaments (148). The neurofibrillary tangles often have a perivascular distribution and are preferentially located in cortical layers II and the upper third of layer III (147). A second characteristic feature of CTE is β-amyloid (Aβ) deposition. Aβ deposits are found in 40%–45% of individuals with CTE, in contrast to the extensive Aβ deposits that characterize nearly all cases of Alzheimer disease (148). At present, the pathogenesis of CTE is unknown, but Blaylock and Maroon (149) reported that the accumulation of hyperphosphorylated tau proteins might be related, in large part, to an interaction between proinflammatory cytokines and glutamate receptors.

Of the total number of autopsy confirmed cases of CTE described by McKee et al., most were professional boxers (147). Of the more recently described nonboxers, 5 were football players, with 1 soccer, professional wrestling, and ice hockey case also described (e.g., 145,147,150,151). A perceived increase in public interest accompanied the reports of CTE in the nonboxing athletes, perhaps because they participated in more mainstream sports that a significant percentage of North Americans participate in during childhood and recreationally as adults.

The more recent autopsy confirmed case reports provided detailed descriptions of the neuropathology as well as some description of the life circumstances of these athletes and, furthermore, created a causal link between them—this has resulted in criticism. The primary criticisms have been that the neuropathological findings were not consistent with the CTE literature on boxers and that adequate clinical case histories were not provided. Importantly, the case reports attributed the *entirety* of the gross and microscopic pathology to neurotrauma while ignoring other possible contributing factors (152). This is problematic, as later acknowledged by the primary research group studying CTE, in part because of the highly selective and unique case histories of these athletes (153). This and other issues require further discussion and consideration.

For example, steroid use was common in athletes who played specific positions in these sports—roles that required power over speed and agility. One of the athletes described died with elevated levels of exogenous testosterone in his system. Another was suspended by the NFL for contravening the performance enhancement policies. Therefore, another possible hypothesis is that chronic steroid use caused or significantly contributed to the pathophysiology, the psychiatric problems, or both that has been solely attributed to repetitive trauma.

Chronic anabolic steroid use can result in psychiatric problems that resemble those attributed to CTE in football, hockey, and wrestling. For example, anabolic-androgenic steroid (AAS) abuse has been reported to result in aggressiveness, anxiety, and depression linked to functional change in monoamine and peptidergic systems (154). AAS-induced hypogonadism may require normalization of neuroendocrine function that can include antidepressant treatments and reversal of dependence via mechanisms shared with classical addictive drugs (155).

Another possible factor contributing to the psychiatric problems reported in the autopsy-confirmed cases of CTE is chronic pain—a common problem faced by athletes in contact sport. Chronic pain is associated with depression, drug and alcohol abuse, and suicide in some people (156). Chronic pain can also lead to dependence on prescription medication. For example, on his death, one of the described cases of CTE had detectable levels of hydrocodone in his system. Therefore, mental health and substance abuse problems, solely attributed to CTE, could also be related to chronic pain.

Unfortunately, there are no detailed autopsy cases for patients with chronic pain, drug and alcohol abuse, psychiatric illness, and/or steroid abuse without significant neurotrauma. Hopefully, this work will be done in the near future. In addition, some of the autopsy-confirmed cases had cardiovascular disease, a history of nonsport-related brain injury, and had in some cases survived 1 or more suicide attempts (including repetitive poisoning). Autopsy work in patients with hypertension, insulin resistance, diabetes, and cardiovascular disease also would be helpful. When considering all of these factors, the statement that "CTE is the only known neurodegenerative dementia with a specific identifiable cause; in this case, head trauma" (148, p. 184) is not scientifically supported at this time.

Much remains unknown about the neuropathophysiology and putative psychiatric manifestations of CTE, including whether it is triggered by repetitive concussions or perhaps repetitive subconcussive blows, whether all people who experience multiple blows to the head are at risk for CTE, or whether or not there are certain predisposing conditions (e.g., genetic and environmental factors) that make some people vulnerable. Moreover, no research, to date, has studied other potential causal or moderating variables that could be responsible for tau and Aβ deposition. Furthermore, most of these cases are not typical of retired athletes from sports such as football and ice hockey. They can be considered to be at an extreme of a continuum for retired athletes in these sports based on their early and complicated deaths alone. It may one day prove correct that neurotrauma is the primary cause for the pattern of neuropathological and the psychiatric problems reported in these cases. However, research on CTE must be done in a more systematic and generalizable way if definitive links to CTE pathophysiology, psychiatric problems, and neurotrauma are to be made.

STRUCTURAL AND FUNCTIONAL NEUROIMAGING

Given that concussion is largely a functional as opposed to a structural injury, techniques such as computed tomography

(CT) or standard clinical magnetic resonance imaging (MRI) are almost always normal following a single concussion. Nonetheless, these techniques are useful for ruling out other pathology (e.g., intracranial bleed, swelling, or skull fracture) that occasionally occur in sports-related head and brain injuries (157). Athletes who are most likely to show abnormalities on structural neuroimaging are boxers. This is not particularly surprising because historically, brain damage sustained when boxing could be seen with the naked eye at autopsy (143). Studies of professional boxers, active and retired, have revealed the greatest number of CT abnormalities estimated to be between 25%–50% (89,158–160). In these boxers, a cavum septum pellucidum was considered a CT sign of traumatic encephalopathy (161). CT abnormalities were correlated with the number of bouts fought (162) and were estimated to be less frequently observed in amateur boxers (between 0% and 20% had abnormalities) (94,163, 164). This pattern is not unique to boxing; however, Sortland and Tysvaer (165) reported that approximately 33% of a sample of retired Norwegian international soccer players had widening of the lateral ventricles suggesting some form of generalized cerebral atrophy. MRI studies on boxers show a similar pattern of results as those using CT with the exception that MRI was able to detect subdural hematoma, white matter changes, and focal contusion not detected using CT (89,166,167). In 1 study, 42/49 (86%) of retired professional boxers had normal clinical MRIs with small numbers showing chronic hemorrhage, cavum septum pellicidum, and injury to white matter (168). Another study reported smaller pituitary volumes in 8 retired boxers with growth hormone deficiency compared to 9 retired boxers with normal growth hormone levels (169). MRI studies on young or amateur boxers typically show no change as a result of participation in their sport (94,167,170,171).

Diffusion Tensor Imaging

Diffusion tensor imaging (DTI) is an MRI technique used to examine the integrity of white matter in the brain at a microstructural level (as opposed to the macrostructural level examined by traditional MRI scans). Thermal energy causes molecules to intermingle and migrate, a process called *diffusion*. DTI can be used to measure both the directionality and the magnitude of water diffusion in white matter. *Fractional anisotropy* (FA) is a mathematical measurement used in physics to estimate diffusion at the level of a voxel, with values ranging from 0 ("isotropic" equal in all directions) to 1 ("anisotropic" highly directional and linear). Thus, reduced FA is believed to represent white matter that is reduced in directionality. Low FA might reflect disintegrative changes in white matter. As such, this technology can be used to estimate damage to white matter. Pulsipher et al. (172) note that DTI can also provide important information regarding grey matter integrity, particularly as it relates to gliosis and necrosis, which may be indicators of brain injury from concussion (172). Two studies on professional boxers reported small but significant differences from a control group in corpus callosum, internal capsule, basal nuclei structures, cerebral peduncles, and longitudinal fasciculi (168,173). Zhang et al. (174) compared 15 concussed athletes to 15 controls and found no significant changes in FA or in number of fibers between groups, but small but significant differences in apparent diffusion coefficient (ADC) at both left and right dorsolateral prefrontal cortex (174). Others have reported increased mean diffusivity in a group of varsity level athletes who continued to present with symptoms for at least 1 month, with a pattern that more closely resembled that of the boxers (e.g., longitudinal fasciculi, internal capsule, and thalamic radiations with no difference in FA reported) (175). Henry and colleagues (176) compared 18 concussed athletes to 10 control subjects at 1–6 days and 6 months postinjury. They reported significant differences in white matter in the corpus callosum and the corticospinal tract. Bazarian and colleagues (177) imaged a small group of football and hockey players before and after the season. It was estimated that these players experienced between 26 and 289 subconcussive head blows. Pre-post season changes in white matter were observed in several athletes.

Positron Emission Tomography and Single Photon Emission Computerized Tomography

Cerebrovascular dynamics have also been studied in boxers using positron emission tomography (PET) and single photon emission computerized tomography (SPECT). Two SPECT studies reported "perfusion abnormalities" in samples of active boxers compared to nonboxing controls (92,178). However, these studies did not clearly indicate whether the abnormalities were perfusion increases, decreases, or both, or what the physiological basis of the abnormalities was. PET studies of regional cerebral blood flow (rCBF) in boxers have described hypometabolism in professional boxers especially in frontocentral regions (179). For example, in a sample of boxers with recent history of poor competitive performance or knockout, Provenzano et al. (180) reported significant levels of hypometabolism in bilateral frontal lobes, parietal, occipital lobes bilaterally, posterior cingulate gyrus, and cerebellum compared to nonboxing controls (180). In summary, there is some evidence that hypoperfusion/hypometabolism is present in samples of professional boxers with a history of poor competitive performance. There is not sufficient evidence at this time to suggest that this is a pattern of pathophysiology expected in all boxers, especially amateurs, those with fewer bouts, or those with good performance.

Functional Magnetic Resonance Imaging

The past few years have witnessed a significant increase in the research literature using blood oxygen level dependent (BOLD) activity. BOLD signals measure changes in the state of oxygenation of hemoglobin (and thus signal intensity), and it is, therefore, assumed that brain regions associated with these changes represent the neural substrates of the task performed (172). BOLD activity has been used to assess the functional changes that can occur following concussion. Two primary patterns emerge from the BOLD literature: (*a*) overactivation or recruitment of adjacent areas (e.g., 181,182) or (*b*) underactivation or recruitment of adjacent brain regions; both associated with increased symptom reporting and injury. Brain regions such as medial, frontal, and right temporoparietal gyri may be overactive in athletes with prolonged recovery times (74). Parietal, dorsolateral prefrontal,

hippocampal, and visual cortex have been reported to be overactivated during spatial memory tasks in symptomatic athletes (174,183). Similarly, frontal and parietal areas have been reported to be overactive in highly symptomatic concussed athletes during a working memory task (184). These findings have been generally explained as consistent with recruitment of brain regions beyond those normally expected.

On the other hand, some studies report reductions in activity in brain regions such as the frontal lobe during working memory tasks in symptomatic athletes (181,185), including those with depressive symptomology (186). Others have described a reduction in a posterior parietal circuit during a working memory task (74). Functional interhemispheric connectivity was shown to be reduced in primary visual cortex hippocampus, parahippocampal and perirhinal cortex, and dorsolateral prefrontal cortex at rest, as well as following an exercise stress test and recovery (187). Therefore, the data do not, at this point, support a convergent pattern of results for the BOLD methodology. Differences in experimental design and subject characteristics may account for the different patterns of results—more research is needed.

Magnetic Resonance Spectroscopy

Magnetic resonance spectroscopy (MRS) is a noninvasive technique that measures the presence of neurometabolites in tissue such as N-acetylaspartate (NAA; found in mitochondria and felt to be a marker of neuronal integrity), creatine (Cr; involves cellular energy metabolism), or choline (a marker of neuronal damage and membrane turnover) (172). Animal models of concussion show that a group of rats that sustained a second injury 3 days following a first had decreased neurometabolite expression that was prolonged when compared to a group of rats that experienced a second brain injury 5 days after the first (188). In humans, a similar pattern was observed, whereby 3 of 13 patients had a second concussive injury within 15 days of the first. Compared to the other 10 subjects, the 3 subjects who sustained repeat concussions had a similar decrease of the NAA-to-Cr ratio at 3 days; however, they continued to worsen until 15 days and had a prolonged metabolic recovery compared to the single concussion subjects (188). Brain regions that exhibit significant metabolic disruption in acutely concussed athletes include depressed levels of NAA in the dorsolateral prefrontal cortex and primary motor cortex (189).

Electroencephalogram and Evoked Potentials

The past few years have seen a substantial increase in the number and quality of studies using the EEG (and related techniques such as event-related potentials or ERPs) for detecting group differences related to concussion history. Historically, standard clinical EEG assessments revealed abnormalities associated with several years of involvement in boxing and soccer in some people (e.g., 190,191,192). Amplitude reductions were reported in recently concussed athletes during standard paradigms (193) or those that involved balance paradigms (194). More recently, EEG studies have shown left/right power asymmetry and decreased left/right hemisphere coherence in concussed athletes compared their preinjury baselines and to matched controls (195). The EEG has also been coupled with complex nonlinear mathematical techniques that help to examine change in the underlying spatial and temporal characteristics associated with concussion. For example, Slobounov et al. (119) reported a significant reduction in Shannon entropy transformed EEG at occipital, temporal, and parietal locations in 21 athletes who had sustained a concussion compared to a preinjury baseline. Furthermore, this effect was most pronounced after a second concussion. The same analytical tool was used to show that the peak EEG frequency and EEG nonstationarity (a measure of complexity in the EEG) were both decreased in 30 athletes 30 days following concussion compared to age and sex matched controls (196). A shift to slower EEG frequencies has also been reported during sleep in athletes recovering from concussion (197).

In addition to the EEG, cognitive ERPs have been used to describe changes in brain function associated with concussion. The ERP most often used to describe electrophysiological change related to concussion is the *N2/P3 or P300 response*, a series of averaged EEG responses time locked to a stimulus, with positive or negative peaks associated with different cognitive processes. P3 amplitude is considered to index allocation of attention (198,199), whereas latency is related to stimulus evaluation and categorization time (200), transfer of information to consciousness and memory systems (199), and stimulus saliency (201).

Early studies on small numbers of boxers did not report consistent change in auditory N2/P3 latencies or amplitudes (95,202). However, recent studies indicate increased auditory N2/P3 latency and/or decreased amplitude between symptomatic athletes compared to asymptomatic recently concussed athletes and controls (203,204) and in former university level athletes between the ages of 50 and 65 who sustained their last sports concussion during early adulthood (205).

Visual N2/P3 studies have been shown to be sensitive to changes associated with concussion for over a decade (206). Researchers have reported significant reductions in visual P3 amplitude in concussed compared to recently concussed but asymptomatic athletes and never concussed athletes (207,208) and in athletes with 1 or more concussions compared to 0 (209). Longer visual P3 latencies were correlated with self-reported attention and memory deficits in athletes with 3 or more concussions (107). A recent study that used a nonstandard working memory paradigm did not find changes in visual N2 or P3 responses but did report that athletes with 3 or more concussions exhibited significantly attenuated late component response amplitudes when contrasted with athletes with 2 or fewer concussions (108).

Averaged brain responses associated with movement and balance are important to consider given the unique demands of the athlete. These techniques have been used to distinguish motor responses variations between concussed and nonconcussed groups of athletes (194,210). Magnetic excitation of motor cortex can be used to elicit motor evoked potentials (MEP) in the extremities. De Beaumont et al. (211) showed that the length of the quiescent period following MEP generation until the onset of ongoing EMG activity was prolonged when compared to that of normal control participants and was correlated with concussion severity. A similar difference was reported between former university level athletes between the ages of 50 and 65 compared to age and sex matched athletes with no concussion history (205). Magnetic stimulation of motor cortex has also been used to elicit difference in MEP latency in concussed vs nonconcussed athletes on day 1 vs day 10 postinjury (212).

In summary, the electrophysiological studies to date have enough consistency to no longer be considered purely experimental and preliminary. Numerous studies have revealed differences in brain function for groups of male and female athletes who are active or retired, symptomatic and asymptomatic, with fewer vs greater number of concussions, and in multiple sensory and motor systems. As Broglio et al. (104) stated, these studies suggest that concussed individuals do not allocate the same level of cognitive resources toward their environment and are less capable of initiating and monitoring their actions compared to athletes with no history of injury. Furthermore, these techniques are sensitive to the number of concussions sustained and the time since injury. Future studies should focus on how to improve the clinical use of these techniques, so that they can be used to manage individual cases rather than to simply show group differences.

Exercise and Cerebrovascular Dynamics

Finally, newly developed exercise-based return-to-play protocols that use standardized cycle ergometry (213) or treadmill tests (214) afford the opportunity to study the cerebrovascular dynamics associated with central nervous system functioning at rest and following various stressors. Len and Neary (215) explain that there is a differential age-related pattern that occurs following traumatic brain injury (TBI) and MTBI. In pediatric studies, CBF increased following MTBI on the day of the injury in younger subjects (< 30 years old) and was then followed by a subsequent decrease in the following days, whereas in adults (> 30 years old) there is typically a decrease in CBF (215). In addition, variables of interest related to MTBI include cerebral perfusion pressure (CPP), cerebrovascular reactivity, and cerebral oxygenation (215). Recent studies report that middle cerebral arterial (MCA) velocity may be lower following concussion in athletes during a hyperventilation and breath-holding paradigms (215). However, another recent study showed an increase in MCA flow velocity to the pathological level with decreased venous reactivity to hypercapnia reflecting impairment to the regulation of venous tone (216). Cerebrovascular dynamics are important to understand because of the relation between the nervous system and the vascular system. This relation becomes even more important and potentially more complex when studying injured children and adults. To understand injury and recovery in a neuron completely, we must also understand the cerebrovascular changes that co-occur following a concussion—a hypofunctional cerebrovascular system might negatively impact recovery in the nervous system.

RECOVERY TIME AND RETURN-TO-PLAY DECISION MAKING

Although significant individual variability exists in recovery from concussion, most group studies have indicated that a single concussion typically resolves in less than 2 weeks for most athletes (6,7,17,36,47,71,72). As noted earlier, however, studies of individual outcome reveal a minority of athletes who take longer to recover. Moreover, clinicians specializing in this injury are aware of a cohort of patients that may have chronic and persistent symptoms. Current clinical experience and research has suggested that proper management of concussion should lead to a good prognosis in most cases. Returning an athlete to contact sport participation prior to recovery increases the risk for overlapping injuries. Thus, the most important step a practitioner can take toward a positive prognosis is proper assessment and management of concussion in the acute and follow-up stages of injury.

Importantly, new and evolving research has focused on the ability to predict which concussed athletes will suffer prolonged recoveries, lasting more than a few weeks. Such data are important to begin to delineate a risk profile that may suggest more complicated recovery, and, perhaps, a cohort of patients that may be at greater risk of postconcussion syndrome. In a series of studies, Lau et al. showed that male football players who had symptoms persisting for more than 10 days were more likely to have problems with visual memory and processing speed, as measured by computerized neurocognitive testing, and were more likely to have a higher Post-Concussion Symptom Scale (PCSS) score acutely after injury than their peers who recovered within 10 days (217). Similarly, those patients whose symptoms were predominantly migrainous in nature, had decreases in reaction time postinjury, or had difficulties with either visual or verbal memory postinjury, were more likely to suffer concussion lasting longer than 14 days than their peers (218). By combining computerized neurocognitive outcomes with symptom clusters, they developed an algorithm that might help clinicians predict which patients are likely to suffer protracted recoveries after sport-related concussions. Studies assessing the ability of individual symptoms to predict recovering show some promising results. Iverson et al. showed that athletes who reported subjective fogginess after injury were more likely to have symptoms lasting beyond 1 week postinjury (45).

In addition to acute predictors, athlete's activities after injury and during recovery may effect recovery times. Preliminary evidence suggests that mild amounts of subsymptom threshold exercise after sport-related concussion may be safe (219), whereas high levels of physical and cognitive exertion may delay recovery and negatively impact cognitive function (220).

Return-to-Play Criteria

It is recommended that an athlete satisfy 3 conditions before returning to play. These conditions are described in the following:

1. Asymptomatic status at rest

    Before progressing to any significant level of physical exertion, the athlete should report being asymptomatic at rest for at least 24 hours. Again, in the case of a student athlete, it is critically important to closely monitor symptoms during their regular academic and general life activities. If the athlete's report of asymptomatic status is suspected to be false, a careful discussion of the impor-

tance of reporting all symptoms should be undertaken. If there are others who present for evaluation with the athlete (e.g., parents, athletic trainers, or teammates), asking these third party informants about the athlete's previous or current symptom complaints might be helpful.

2. Asymptomatic status with physical and cognitive exertion

    Once an athlete is asymptomatic at rest and with school-based activities, he or she can begin a graduated return to physical exertion prior to contact participation because postconcussion difficulties might evolve with the increased metabolic demands of physical activity. The Vienna, Prague, and Zurich statements encourage a graduated protocol (81,82). Briefly, the protocol involves an athlete successfully moving through the following exertional steps in 24-hour periods: (a) light aerobic exercise (walking, stationary biking), (b) sport-specific training (ice-skating in hockey, running in soccer—typically moderately exertional), and (c) noncontact training drills (usually heavily exertional). Although the focus has, to date, been on physical activity, the athlete should also be able to complete normal school work without eliciting or exacerbating symptoms. If the athlete's previously resolved postconcussion symptoms return at any point during the graded return to physical exertion or activities of school, the athlete should return to the previous exertion level at which he or she was last asymptomatic.

3. Intact neurocognitive function (either compared to baseline or normative data)

    Neurocognitive recovery can be considered achieved when the athlete's performance either returns to baseline levels or, in the absence of baseline, is consistent with premorbid estimates of functioning when the test data are compared to normative values (clinicians should use test batteries that have good quality and representative norms).

    Preseason or baseline neuropsychological assessment can be helpful for comparing postinjury functioning to "normal" functioning for the injured athlete. Some practitioners prefer to complete serial follow-up using computerized neuropsychological testing. The first test is often performed while the athlete remains symptomatic, then completed again once the athlete is asymptomatic to gauge progress and ensure a return to baseline or premorbid expectations of cognitive functioning. In the case of a protracted recovery from concussion, interim tests may also be completed to help in preparing academic accommodations for student athletes (221).

    Once the athlete is symptom free at rest and with physical/cognitive exertion, as well as within expected levels on cognitive testing (if available), he or she may return to full-contact training, then to competition. Again, if any symptoms emerge with return-to-contact participation, the athlete should return to noncontact physical exertion or perhaps complete rest depending on the severity of symptoms that return.

    It is possible that some athletes will score uncharacteristically high in their preseason baseline assessments. After recovering from a sport-related concussion, such athletes' neurocognitive scores may regress to the mean. In other words, despite fully recovering from their concussions, they may not reachieve their previously, un-

TABLE 31-3 Factors to Consider for Decisions Regarding Discontinuing an Athlete's Season

- Number of lifetime concussions
- Duration of symptoms
- Severity of symptoms
- Duration of neurocognitive deficits
- Severity of neurocognitive deficits
- Decreasing force required to produce injury
- Life goals (professional vs recreational athletes)
- Prolonged losses of consciousness or periods of post-traumatic amnesia
- Ongoing cognitive/emotional issues that may complicate diagnosis
- Time of year/season

characteristically high baseline levels of performance. Thus, there may be circumstances where athletes can be safely cleared to return to play without reachieving their baseline values. These situations are, however, rare and should be approached cautiously.

Discontinuation for the Season and Retirement From Sport Decisions

It is inherently difficult to determine when an athlete should discontinue participation in, or retire from, contact sports. This represents a very challenging issue for even the most senior clinician. To the greatest extent possible, this should be a personal choice. Clinicians are encouraged to respect autonomy and freedom of choice. However, the athlete and his or her family, coach, athletic trainer, and physician need good information on which they can make informed decisions. In Table 31-3, we present some factors to consider regarding decisions to discontinue an athlete's season or consider retiring from contact sports.

Echemendia and Cantu (222) indicated that there are 2 main changes that should raise concern about retirement from contact sports. The first change relates to the *duration* of postconcussion symptoms. These symptoms typically resolve within a few days or weeks. However, a progressively increasing period of symptom duration, especially in those who have sustained multiple concussions, is an obvious concern. The second change to consider is the *force* required to produce a concussion. Blows that produce concussion usually strike the head. However, there is anecdotal evidence that some athletes with a history of multiple injuries become more susceptible to a concussion from blows to other parts of the body. Possible changes in the athlete's susceptibility to concussions could be an impetus for discussions about retirement.

PREVENTION

Thoughtful rule and policy changes are the primary way to reduce the number of concussions in specific sports. At present, there is no proven way to prevent this injury. However, there may be ways athletes can reduce their risk of sustaining a concussion. Studies in American football and ice hockey show that most concussions occur when athletes sustain blows that they do not anticipate (79,223). When athletes anticipate a blow, they instinctively contract their muscles. This muscle contraction may result in less acceleration of the brain after impact, thereby reducing the chance of concussive injury. Thus, by learning to constantly be aware of what is taking place around them, athletes may reduce their risk of injury.

The musculature of the neck and shoulders attach the skull to the remainder of the body. These muscles act as a restraint to acceleration of the head after impact. Stronger muscles are more effective at reducing acceleration after impact (25). Thus, strengthening of the neck and posterior shoulder muscles might reduce the risk of injury in some athletes.

It should be noted that helmets were originally designed to prevent skull fractures and severe brain injuries. All participants in sports that mandate the use of helmets should wear an undamaged, properly fitted helmet. However, helmets have not been shown to prevent concussions (224,225). Similarly, mouth guards were originally designed to prevent dental injury. They are effective at preventing dental injury, as well as facial bone fracture. Therefore, all persons participating in sports where mouth guard use is recommended should wear a properly fitting mouth guard. However, mouth guards have not been shown to reduce the risk of concussion (224–226).

CONCLUSION

This chapter was intended to be a comprehensive overview of concussion in sport, dealing with topics such as definitions, on-field/sideline presentation, pathophysiology, structural and functional imaging, neuropsychological outcome, cumulative effects, and return-to-play decision making. The pathophysiology of concussion may include ionic shifts, abnormal energy metabolism, diminished CBF, and impaired neurotransmission. Fortunately, the brain undergoes a dynamic restorative process in the initial days to weeks following a concussion. From a commonsense perspective, the ionic shifts, abnormal energy metabolism, diminished CBF, and impaired neurotransmission believed to be associated with concussions in sports, reinforce the importance of immediate rest following injury until multisystemic homeostasis can be regained.

Many athletes with concussions have neurocognitive decrements as measured by traditional paper-and-pencil and computerized neuropsychological tests in the initial hours, days, and occasionally weeks postinjury. In terms of group data, it has become a fairly robust finding that athletes tend to recover in terms of perceived symptoms and neuropsychological test performance within 2–14 days. However, individual variability exists in recovery rates, especially in high school athletes, and the duration of symptoms can persist well beyond 2 weeks postinjury. In fact, at 4 weeks postinjury, 84% of high school football players with a prior history of concussion and 94% of those experiencing their first concussion were deemed recovered based on symptoms and neurocognitive testing (see Figure 31-1).

Researchers have reported that 3 or more concussions in high school and university athletes are associated with measurable effects in some people and increased risk for future concussions. The literature on the long-term effects of 1 or 2 previous concussions is mixed. In general, there is insufficient evidence at this time to conclude that 1–2 previous concussions results in adverse long-term effects in the average athlete.

Ideally, athletes should satisfy 3 conditions before returning to play. The athlete should be asymptomatic at rest, with full academic activity, and during noncontact exertion. Once asymptomatic at rest, the athlete is then progressed through increasing noncontact physical exertion, until he or she has demonstrated asymptomatic status with heavy noncontact physical exertion and noncontact sport-specific training. In addition, the athlete should demonstrate recovery of neurocognitive function exhibited by his or her performance on a neuropsychological testing battery (if available).

There remain several substantial deficiencies in the overall body of knowledge regarding concussion that require further investigation. First, one of the leading theories regarding the molecular pathophysiological basis of concussion (227) relies on data gathered using the fluid percussion model of injury (228–236). As has been pointed out by other investigators (237–239), the fluid percussion mechanism of injury may be distinct from the rotational acceleration experienced by athletes who sustain sport-related concussions, whether the same molecular events occur after rotational acceleration needs to be investigated. Second, there is no definitive diagnostic test for concussion. Investigation should continue into the use of neuroimaging studies, biomarkers, EEG modalities, and other techniques to assist in diagnosing the injury and monitoring recovery. Third, there is no effective treatment for concussive brain injury (240,241). Future investigations should focus on treatments that directly target the underlying neurobiology of this injury. Finally, the ability to predict duration of recovery would allow patients, as well as other parties affected by concussion, such as employers, clinicians, coaches, and teammates, to plan accordingly. Thus, future studies should attempt to discern risk factors for prolonged recovery.

Contemporary models of care have recognized the complexity of the recovery process following concussion and are beginning to consider the unique contribution of factors, such as the athlete's age, developmental history, and past injury status in determining outcome. This recognition of the interplay between multiple variables is leading to the development of a more sophisticated understanding of the recovery process; we anticipate that this will continue in the near future. Given the current trend towards research-based models of clinical care, we anticipate that concussion management will continue to grow and develop as our capacity for completing large-scale clinical research projects increases, and we are able to meld this information with other advances in the neurosciences, such as structural and functional neuroimaging, as well as cerebrovascular and electrophysiological techniques.

KEY CLINICAL POINTS

1. A sport-related concussion, by definition, is a MTBI.
2. Concussion cannot be visualized by standard structural neuroimaging modalities (e.g., CT or MRI).

3. Athletes who sustain sport-related concussions should be removed from play and reduce physical and cognitive exertion during the recovery process.
4. A comprehensive concussion care program will assess symptoms, neurocognitive functioning, and balance.
5. Neurocognitive assessments are sensitive to detecting cognitive deficits associated with sport-related concussions, and they are useful for monitoring recovery.
6. Athletes should not be returned to play until they are symptom free with both physical and cognitive exertion, and cognitive functioning has returned to baseline levels or estimates of premorbid functioning.

KEY REFERENCES

1. Barkhoudarian G, Hovda DA, Giza CC. The molecular pathophysiology of concussive brain injury. *Clin J Sport Med*. 2011;30(1):33–48.
2. Iverson GL. Evidence-based neuropsychological assessment of sport-related concussion. In: Webbe FM, ed. *Handbook of Sport Neuropsychology*. New York, NY: Springer Publishing; 2011: 131–154.
3. McCrea M, Guskiewicz KM, Marshall SW, et al. Acute effects and recovery time following concussion in collegiate football players: the NCAA Concussion Study. *JAMA*. 2003;290(19):2556–2563.
4. McCrory P, Meeuwisse W, Johnston K, et al. Consensus statement on concussion in sport: the 3rd International Conference on Concussion in Sport held in Zurich, November 2008. *Br J Sports Med*. 2009;43(suppl 1):i76–i90.

References

1. Koh JO, Cassidy JD, Watkinson EJ. Incidence of concussion in contact sports: a systematic review of the evidence. *Brain Inj*. 2003; 17(10):901–917.
2. Delaney JS. Head injuries presenting to emergency departments in the United States from 1990 to 1999 for ice hockey, soccer, and football. *Clin J Sport Med*. 2004;14(2):80–87.
3. Powell JW, Barber-Foss KD. Traumatic brain injury in high school athletes. *JAMA*. 1999;282(10):958–963.
4. McCrea M, Hammeke T, Olsen G, Leo P, Guskiewicz K. Unreported concussion in high school football players: implications for prevention. *Clin J Sport Med*. 2004;14(1):13–17.
5. Guskiewicz KM, Weaver NL, Padua DA, Garrett WE Jr. Epidemiology of concussion in collegiate and high school football players. *Am J Sports Med*. 2000;28(5):643–650.
6. McCrea M, Guskiewicz KM, Marshall SW, et al. Acute effects and recovery time following concussion in collegiate football players: the NCAA Concussion Study. *JAMA*. 2003;290(19):2556–2563.
7. Macciocchi SN, Barth JT, Alves W, Rimel RW, Jane JA. Neuropsychological functioning and recovery after mild head injury in collegiate athletes. *Neurosurgery*. 1996;39(3):510–514.
8. Meehan WP III, d'Hemecourt P, Comstock RD. High school concussions in the 2008–2009 academic year: mechanism, symptoms, and management. *Am J Sports Med*. 2010;38(12):2405–2409.
9. Collins MW, Grindel SH, Lovell MR, et al. Relationship between concussion and neuropsychological performance in college football players. *JAMA*. 1999;282(10):964–970.
10. Barr WB, McCrea M. Sensitivity and specificity of standardized neurocognitive testing immediately following sports concussion. *J Int Neuropsychol Soc*. 2001;7(6):693–702.
11. Delaney JS, Lacroix VJ, Gagne C, Antoniou J. Concussions among university football and soccer players: a pilot study. *Clin J Sport Med*. 2001;11(4):234–240.

12. Erlanger D, Feldman D, Kutner K, et al. Development and validation of a web-based neuropsychological test protocol for sports-related return-to-play decision-making. *Arch Clin Neuropsychol.* 2003;18(3):293–316.

13. Erlanger D, Saliba E, Barth J, Almquist J, Webright W, Freeman J. Monitoring resolution of postconcussion symptoms in athletes: preliminary results of a web-based neuropsychological test protocol. *J Athl Train.* 2001;36(3):280–287.

14. Guskiewicz KM, Ross SE, Marshall SW. Postural stability and neuropsychological deficits after concussion in collegiate athletes. *J Athl Train.* 2001;36(3):263–273.

15. Makdissi M, Collie A, Maruff P, et al. Computerised cognitive assessment of concussed Australian Rules footballers. *Br J Sports Med.* 2001;35(5):354–360.

16. Matser JT, Kessels AG, Lezak MD, Troost J. A dose-response relation of headers and concussions with cognitive impairment in professional soccer players. *J Clin Exp Neuropsychol.* 2001;23(6):770–774.

17. McCrea M, Kelly JP, Randolph C, Cisler R, Berger L. Immediate neurocognitive effects of concussion. *Neurosurgery.* 2002;50(5):1032–1040.

18. Warden DL, Bleiberg J, Cameron KL, et al. Persistent prolongation of simple reaction time in sports concussion. *Neurology.* 2001;57(3):524–526.

19. Peterson CL, Ferrara MS, Mrazik M, Piland S, Elliott R. Evaluation of neuropsychological domain scores and postural stability following cerebral concussion in sports. *Clin J Sport Med.* 2003;13(4):230–237.

20. Riemann BL, Guskiewicz KM. Effects of mild head injury on postural stability as measured through clinical balance testing. *J Athl Train.* 2000;35(1):19–25.

21. McCrory P, Johnston K, Meeuwisse W, Aubry M, Cantu R, Dvorak J, Graf-Baumann T, Kelly J, Lovell M, Schamasch P. Summary and agreement statement of the 2nd international conference on concussion in sport, Prague 2004. *British Journal of Sports Medicine,* 2005; 39(4):196–204.

22. Ommaya AK, Gennarelli TA. Cerebral concussion and traumatic unconsciousness. Correlation of experimental and clinical observations of blunt head injuries. *Brain.* 1974;97(4):633–654.

23. Gaetz M. The neurophysiology of brain injury. *Clin Neurophysiol.* 2004;115(1):4–18.

24. Elson LM, Ward CC. Mechanisms and pathophysiology of mild head injury. *Semin Neurol.* 1994;14(1):8–18.

25. Viano DC, Casson IR, Pellman EJ. Concussion in professional football: biomechanics of the struck player—part 14. *Neurosurgery.* 2007;61:313–327; discussion 327–318.

26. McCaffrey MA, Mihalik JP, Crowell DH, Shields EW, Guskiewicz KM. Measurement of head impacts in collegiate football players: clinical measures of concussion after high- and low-magnitude impacts. *Neurosurgery.* 2007;61:1236–1243; discussion 1243.

27. Giza CC, Hovda DA. The pathophysiology of traumatic brain injury. In: Lovell MR, Echemendia RJ, Barth JT, Collins MW, eds. *Traumatic Brain Injury in Sports.* Lisse, The Netherlands: Swets & Zeitlinger; 2004:45–70.

28. Iverson GL. Outcome from mild traumatic brain injury. *Curr Opin Psychiat.* 2005;18(3):301–317.

29. Iverson GL, Lovell MR, Smith SS. Does brief loss of consciousness affect cognitive functioning after mild head injury? *Arch Clin Neuropsychol.* 2000;15(7):643–648.

30. Lovell MR, Iverson GL, Collins MW, McKeag D, Maroon JC. Does loss of consciousness predict neuropsychological decrements after concussion? *Clin J Sport Med.* 1999;9(4):193–198.

31. Asplund CA, McKeag DB, Olsen CH. Sport-related concussion: factors associated with prolonged return to play. *Clin J Sport Med.* 2004;14(6):339–343.

32. Pellman EJ, Viano DC, Casson IR, Arfken C, Powell J. Concussion in professional football: injuries involving 7 or more days out—part 5. *Neurosurgery.* 2004;55:1100–1119.

33. Collins MW, Iverson GL, Lovell MR, McKeag DB, Norwig J, Maroon J. On-field predictors of neuropsychological and symptom deficit following sports-related concussion. *Clin J Sport Med.* 2003; 13(4):222–229.

34. Yeates KO, Taylor HG, Rusin J, et al. Longitudinal trajectories of postconcussive symptoms in children with mild traumatic brain injuries and their relationship to acute clinical status. *Pediatrics.* 2009;123(3):735–743.

35. Lau BC, Kontos AP, Collins MW, Mucha A, Lovell MR. Which on-field signs/symptoms predict protracted recovery from sport-related concussion among high school football players? *Am J Sports Med.* 2011;39(11):2311–2318.

36. Lovell MR, Collins MW, Iverson GL, et al. Recovery from mild concussion in high school athletes. *J Neurosurg.* 2003;98(2):296–301.

37. Collins MW, Field M, Lovell MR, et al. Relationship between postconcussion headache and neuropsychological test performance in high school athletes. *Am J Sports Med.* 2003;31(2):168–173.

38. Pellman EJ, Powell JW, Viano DC, et al. Concussion in professional football: epidemiological features of game injuries and review of the literature—part 3. *Neurosurgery.* 2004;54(1):81–94; discussion 94–96.

39. Mihalik JP, Stump JE, Collins MW, Lovell MR, Field M, Maroon JC. Posttraumatic migraine characteristics in athletes following sports-related concussion. *J Neurosurg.* 2005;102 (5):850–855.

40. Lovell MR. Evaluation of the professional athlete. In: New Developments in Sports-Related Concussion Conference; July 16–18, 2004; Pittsburgh, Philadelphia.

41. Lovell MR. Evaluation of the professional athlete. In: Bailes JE, Lovell MR, Maroon JC, eds. *Sports-Related Concussion.* St. Louis, MO: Quality Medical Publishing; 1999:200–214.

42. Lovell MR, Collins MW. Neuropsychological assessment of the college football player. *J Head Trauma Rehabil.* 1998;13:9–26.

43. Lovell MR, Echemendia RJ, Burke CJ. Traumatic brain injury in professional hockey. In: Lovell MR, Echemendia RJ, Barth J, Collins MW, eds. *Traumatic Brain Injury in Sports: An International Neuropsychological Perspective.* Netherlands: Swets & Zeitlinger; 2004:221–231.

44. Lovell MR, Burke CJ. The NHL concussion program. In: Cantu R, ed. *Neurologic Athletic Head and Spine Injury.* Phildelphia, PA: WB Saunders; 2002:32–45.

45. Iverson GL, Gaetz M, Lovell MR, Collins MW. Relation between subjective fogginess and neuropsychological testing following concussion. *J Int Neuropsychol Soc.* 2004;10(6):904–906.

46. Iverson GL, Gaetz M, Lovell MR, Collins MW. Cumulative effects of concussion in amateur athletes. *Brain Inj.* 2004;18(5):433–443.

47. Lovell MR, Collins MW, Iverson GL, Johnston KM, Bradley JP. Grade 1 or "ding" concussions in high school athletes. *Am J Sports Med.* 2004;32:47–54.

48. Lovell MR, Iverson GL, Collins MW, et al. Measurement of symptoms following sports-related concussion: reliability and normative data for the post-concussion scale. *Appl Neuropsychol.* 2006; 13(3):166–174.

49. Randolph C, Millis S, Barr WB, et al. Concussion symptom inventory: an empirically derived scale for monitoring resolution of symptoms following sport-related concussion. *Arch Clin Neuropsychol.* 2009;24(3):219–229.

50. Guskiewicz KM, Perrin DH, Gansneder BM. Effect of mild head injury on postural stability in athletes. *J Athl Train.* 1996;31(4):300–306.

51. Sosnoff JJ, Broglio SP, Shin S, Ferrara MS. Previous mild traumatic brain injury and postural-control dynamics. *J Athl Train.* 2011;46(1):85–91.

52. Guskiewicz KM. Balance assessment in the management of sport-related concussion. *Clin Sports Med.* 2011;30(1):89–102, ix.

53. Reimann BL, Guskiewicz KM, Sheilds E. Relationship between clinical and forceplate measures of postural stability. *J Sport Rehabil.* 1999;8:71–82.

54. Guskiewicz KM. Postural stability assessment following concussion: one piece of the puzzle. *Clin J Sport Med.* 2001;11(3):182–189.

55. Iverson GL, Gaetz M. Effects of standardized aerobic exercise on balance in non-injured athletes: implications for concussion management. *Br J Sports Med.* 2009;43:i101.

56. Iverson GL. Evidence-based neuropsychological assessment of sport-related concussion. In: Webbe FM, ed. *Handbook of Sport Neuropsychology.* New York, NY: Springer Publishing; 2011:131–154.

57. Iverson GL, Gaetz M, Lovell MR, Collins MW. Relation between fogginess and outcome following concussion. *Arch Clin Neuropsychol.* 2002;17:769–770.

58. Iverson GL, Lovell MR, Collins MW. Interpreting change on ImPACT following sport concussion. *Clin Neuropsychol.* 2003;17(4):460–467.

59. Fazio VC, Lovell MR, Pardini JE, Collins MW. The relation between post concussion symptoms and neurocognitive performance in concussed athletes. *NeuroRehabilitation.* 2007;22(3):207–216.

60. Iverson G. Predicting slow recovery from sport-related concussion: the new simple-complex distinction. *Clin J Sport Med.* 2007;17(1):31–37.

61. Covassin T, Schatz P, Swanik CB. Sex differences in neuropsychological function and post-concussion symptoms of concussed collegiate athletes. *Neurosurgery.* 2007;61(2):345–350; discussion 350–341.

62. McClincy MP, Lovell MR, Pardini J, Collins MW, Spore MK. Recovery from sports concussion in high school and collegiate athletes. *Brain Inj.* 2006;20(1):33–39.

63. Iverson GL, Brooks BL, Collins MW, Lovell MR. Tracking neuropsychological recovery following concussion in sport. *Brain Inj.* 2006;20(3):245–252.

64. Van Kampen DA, Lovell MR, Pardini JE, Collins MW, Fu FH. The "value added" of neurocognitive testing after sports-related concussion. *Am J Sports Med.* 2006;34(10):1630–1635.

65. Collins M, Lovell MR, Iverson GL, Ide T, Maroon J. Examining concussion rates and return to play in high school football players wearing newer helmet technology: a three year prospective cohort study. *Neurosurgery.* 2006;58(2):275–286.

66. Broglio SP, Macciocchi SN, Ferrara MS. Sensitivity of the concussion assessment battery. *Neurosurgery.* 2007;60(6):1050–1057; discussion 1057–1058.

67. Sosnoff JJ, Broglio SP, Hillman CH, Ferrara MS. Concussion does not impact intraindividual response time variability. *Neuropsychology.* 2007;21(6):796–802.

68. Broshek DK, Kaushik T, Freeman JR, Erlanger D, Webbe F, Barth JT. Sex differences in outcome following sports-related concussion. *J Neurosurg.* 2005;102(5):856–863.

69. Erlanger D, Kaushik T, Cantu R, et al. Symptom-based assessment of the severity of a concussion. *J Neurosurg.* 2003;98(3):477–484.

70. Collie A, Makdissi M, Maruff P, Bennell K, McCrory P. Cognition in the days following concussion: comparison of symptomatic versus asymptomatic athletes. *J Neurol Neurosurg Psychiatry.* 2006;77(2):241–245.

71. Bleiberg J, Cernich AN, Cameron K, et al. Duration of cognitive impairment after sports concussion. *Neurosurgery.* 2004;54(6):1073–1078; discussion 1078–1080.

72. Pellman EJ, Lovell MR, Viano DC, Casson IR, Tucker AM. Concussion in professional football: neuropsychological testing—part 6. *Neurosurgery.* 2004;55(6):1290–1303.

73. Iverson GL. Mild traumatic brain injury meta-analyses can obscure individual differences. *Brain Inj.* 2010;24(10):1246–1255.

74. Lovell MR, Pardini JE, Welling J, et al. Functional brain abnormalities are related to clinical recovery and time to return-to-play in athletes. *Neurosurgery.* 2007;61(2):352–359; discussion 359–360.

75. Pellman EJ, Lovell MR, Viano DC, Casson IR. Concussion in professional football: recovery of NFL and high school athletes assessed by computerized neuropsychological testing—part 12. *Neurosurgery.* 2006;58(2):263–274; discussion 263–274.

76. Pellman EJ, Viano DC, Casson IR, et al. Concussion in professional football: repeat injuries—part 4. *Neurosurgery.* 2004;55:860–873; discussion 873–876.

77. Pellman EJ. Background on the National Football League's research on concussion in professional football. *Neurosurgery.* 2003;53(4):797–798.

78. Pellman EJ, Viano DC, Tucker AM, Casson IR; for the Committee on Mild Traumatic Brain Injury, National Football League. Concussion in professional football: location and direction of helmet impacts—part 2. *Neurosurgery.* 2003;53(6):1328–1340; discussion 1340–1341.

79. Pellman EJ, Viano DC, Tucker AM, Casson IR, Waeckerle JF. Concussion in professional football: reconstruction of game impacts and injuries. *Neurosurgery.* 2003;53(4):799–812; discussion 812–814.

80. Pellman EJ, Viano DC, Casson IR, Arfken C, Feuer H. Concussion in professional football: players returning to the same game—part 7. *Neurosurgery.* 2005;56(1):79–90.

81. Aubry M, Cantu R, Dvorak J, et al. Summary and agreement statement of the First International Conference on Concussion in Sport, Vienna 2001. Recommendations for the improvement of safety and health of athletes who may suffer concussive injuries. *Br J Sports Med.* 2002;36(1):6–10.

82. McCrory P, Johnston K, Meeuwisse W, et al. Summary and agreement statement of the 2nd International Conference on Concussion in Sport, Prague 2004. *Br J Sports Med.* 2005;39(4):196–204.

83. Moser RS, Iverson GL, Echemendia RJ, et al. Neuropsychological evaluation in the diagnosis and management of sports-related concussion. *Arch Clin Neuropsychol.* 2007;22(8):909–916.

84. Collie A, Maruff P, McStephen M, Darby DG. Psychometric issues associated with computerised neuropsychological assessment of concussed athletes. *Br J Sports Med.* 2003;37(6):556–559.

85. Meehan WP III, d'Hemecourt P, Collins CL, Taylor AM, Comstock RD. Computerized neurocognitive testing for the management of sport-related concussions. *Pediatrics.* 2012;129(1):38–44.

86. Zhang L, Ravdin LD, Relkin N, et al. Increased diffusion in the brain of professional boxers: a preclinical sign of traumatic brain injury? *AJNR Am J Neuroradiol.* 2003;24(1):52–57.

87. Rabadi MH, Jordan BD. The cumulative effect of repetitive concussion in sports. *Clin J Sport Med.* 2001;11(3):194–198.

88. Dale GE, Leigh PN, Luthert P, Anderton BH, Roberts GW. Neurofibrillary tangles in dementia pugilistica are ubiquitinated. *J Neurol Neurosurg Psychiatry.* 1991;54(2):116–118.

89. Jordan BD, Zimmerman RD. Computed tomography and magnetic resonance imaging comparisons in boxers. *JAMA.* 1990;263(12):1670–1674.

90. Roberts GW, Allsop D, Bruton C. The occult aftermath of boxing. *J Neurol Neurosurg Psychiatry.* 1990;53(5):373–378.

91. Miele VJ, Carson L, Carr A, Bailes JE. Acute on chronic subdural hematoma in a female boxer: a case report. *Med Sci Sports Exerc.* 2004;36(11):1852–1855.

92. Kemp PM, Houston AS, Macleod MA, Pethybridge RJ. Cerebral perfusion and psychometric testing in military amateur boxers and controls. *J Neurol Neurosurg Psychiatry.* 1995;59(4):368–374.

93. Haglund Y, Edman G, Murelius O, Oreland L, Sachs C. Does Swedish amateur boxing lead to chronic brain damage? 1. A retrospective medical, neurological and personality trait study. *Acta Neurol Scand.* 1990;82(4):245–252.

94. Haglund Y, Bergstrand G. Does Swedish amateur boxing lead to chronic brain damage? 2. A retrospective study with CT and MRI. *Acta Neurol Scand.* 1990;82(5):297–302.

95. Murelius O, Haglund Y. Does Swedish amateur boxing lead to chronic brain damage? 4. A retrospective neuropsychological study. *Acta Neurol Scand.* 1991;83(1):9–13.

96. Haglund Y, Persson HE. Does Swedish amateur boxing lead to chronic brain damage? 3. A retrospective clinical neurophysiological study. *Acta Neurol Scand.* 1990;82(6):353–360.

97. Porter MD. A 9-year controlled prospective neuropsychologic assessment of amateur boxing. *Clin J Sport Med.* 2003;13(6):339–352.

98. Schmitt DM, Hertel J, Evans TA, Olmsted LC, Putukian M. Effect of an acute bout of soccer heading on postural control and self-reported concussion symptoms. *Int J Sports Med.* 2004;25(5):326–331.

99. Moriarity J, Collie A, Olson D, et al. A prospective controlled study of cognitive function during an amateur boxing tournament. *Neurology.* 2004;62(9):1497–1502.

100. Putukian M, Echemendia RJ, Mackin S. The acute neuropsychological effects of heading in soccer: a pilot study. *Clin J Sport Med.* 2000;10(2):104–109.

101. Zillmer EA. The neuropsychology of repeated 1- and 3-meter springboard diving among college athletes. *Appl Neuropsychol.* 2003;10(1):23–30.

102. Rutherford A, Stephens R, Potter D. The neuropsychology of heading and head trauma in Association Football (soccer): a review. *Neuropsychol Rev.* 2003;13(3):153–179.

103. Straume-Naesheim TM, Andersen TE, Dvorak J, Bahr R. Effects of heading exposure and previous concussions on neuropsychological performance among Norwegian elite footballers. *Br J Sports Med*. 2005;39(suppl 1):i70–i77.

104. Broglio SP, Eckner JT, Surma T, Kutcher JS. Post-concussion cognitive declines and symptomatology are not related to concussion biomechanics in high school football players. *J Neurotrauma*. 2011; 28(10):2061–2068.

105. Stephens R, Rutherford A, Potter D, Fernie G. Neuropsychological consequence of soccer play in adolescent U.K. school team soccer players. *J Neuropsychiatry Clin Neurosci*. 2010;22(3):295–303.

106. Mangus BC, Wallmann HW, Ledford M. Analysis of postural stability in collegiate soccer players before and after an acute bout of heading multiple soccer balls. *Sports Biomech*. 2004;3(2):209–220.

107. Gaetz M, Goodman D, Weinberg H. Electrophysiological evidence for the cumulative effects of concussion. *Brain Inj*. 2000;14(12): 1077–1088.

108. Theriault M, De Beaumont L, Tremblay S, Lassonde M, Jolicoeur P. Cumulative effects of concussions in athletes revealed by electrophysiological abnormalities on visual working memory. *J Clin Exp Neuropsychol*. 2011;33(1):30–41.

109. Thornton AE, Cox DN, Whitfield K, Fouladi RT. Cumulative concussion exposure in rugby players: neurocognitive and symptomatic outcomes. *J Clin Exp Neuropsychol*. 2008;30(4):398–409.

110. Guskiewicz KM, Marshall SW, Bailes J, et al. Association between recurrent concussion and late-life cognitive impairment in retired professional football players. *Neurosurgery*. 2005;57(4):719–726; discussion 719–726.

111. Broglio SP, Ferrara MS, Piland SG, Anderson RB, Collie A. Concussion history is not a predictor of computerised neurocognitive performance. *Br J Sports Med*. 2006;40(9):802–805; discussion 802–805.

112. Collie A, McCrory P, Makdissi M. Does history of concussion affect current cognitive status? *Br J Sports Med*. 2006;40(6):550–551.

113. Collins MW, Lovell MR, Iverson GL, Cantu RC, Maroon JC, Field M. Cumulative effects of concussion in high school athletes. *Neurosurgery*. 2002;51(5):1175–1179; discussion 1180–1181.

114. Guskiewicz KM, McCrea M, Marshall SW, et al. Cumulative effects associated with recurrent concussion in collegiate football players: the NCAA Concussion Study. *JAMA*. 2003;290(19):2549–2555.

115. Zemper ED. Two-year prospective study of relative risk of a second cerebral concussion. *Am J Phys Med Rehabil*. 2003;82(9):653–659.

116. Moser RS, Schatz P, Jordan BD. Prolonged effects of concussion in high school athletes. *Neurosurgery*. 2005;57(2):300–306; discussion 300–306.

117. Moser RS, Schatz P. Enduring effects of concussion in youth athletes. *Arch Clin Neuropsychol*. 2002;17(1):91–100.

118. Covassin T, Stearne D, Elbin R. Concussion history and postconcussion neurocognitive performance and symptoms in collegiate athletes. *J Athl Train*. 2008;43(2):119–124.

119. Slobounov S, Cao C, Sebastianelli W. Differential effect of first versus second concussive episodes on wavelet information quality of EEG. *Clin Neurophysiol*. 2009;120(5):862–867.

120. Delaney JS, Lacroix VJ, Leclerc S, Johnston KM. Concussions during the 1997 Canadian Football League season. *Clin J Sport Med*. 2000;10(1):9–14.

121. Gerberich SG, Priest JD, Boen JR, Straub CP, Maxwell RE. Concussion incidences and severity in secondary school varsity football players. *Am J Public Health*. 1983;73(12):1370–1375.

122. McCrory P. Does second impact syndrome exist? *Clin J Sport Med*. 2001;11(3):144–149.

123. McCrory P, Berkovic SF. Second impact syndrome. *Neurology*. 1998; 50(3):677–683.

124. McCrory P, Davis G, Makdissi M. Second impact syndrome or cerebral swelling after sporting head injury. *Curr Sports Med Rep*. 2012;11(1):21–23.

125. Cantu RC. Second-impact syndrome. *Clin Sports Med*. 1998;17(1): 37–44.

126. Kelly JP, Rosenberg JH. Diagnosis and management of concussion in sports. *Neurology*. 1997;48(3):575–580.

127. Mori T, Katayama Y, Kawamata T. Acute hemispheric swelling associated with thin subdural hematomas: pathophysiology of repetitive head injury in sports. *Acta Neurochir Suppl*. 2006;96:40–43.

128. Bruce DA, Alavi A, Bilaniuk L, Dolinskas C, Obrist W, Uzzell B. Diffuse cerebral swelling following head injuries in children: the syndrome of "malignant brain edema." *J Neurosurg*. 1981;54(2): 170–178.

129. Kelly JP, Nichols JS, Filley CM, Lillehei KO, Rubinstein D, Kleinschmidt-DeMasters BK. Concussion in sports. Guidelines for the prevention of catastrophic outcome. *JAMA*. 1991;266(20): 2867–2869.

130. McQuillen JB, McQuillen EN, Morrow P. Trauma, sport, and malignant cerebral edema. *Am J Forensic Med Pathol*. 1988;9(1):12–15.

131. Laurer HL, Bareyre FM, Lee VM, et al. Mild head injury increasing the brain's vulnerability to a second concussive impact. *J Neurosurg*. 2001;95(5):859–870.

132. Vagnozzi R, Tavazzi B, Signoretti S, et al. Temporal window of metabolic brain vulnerability to concussions: mitochondrial-related impairment—part I. *Neurosurgery*. 2007;61(2):379–388.

133. Longhi L, Saatman KE, Fujimoto S, et al. Temporal window of vulnerability to repetitive experimental concussive brain injury. *Neurosurgery*. 2005;56(2):364–374; discussion 364–374.

134. McCrory PR, Berkovic SF. Concussive convulsions. Incidence in sport and treatment recommendations. *Sports Med*. 1998;25(2):131–136.

135. McCrory PR, Berkovic SF. Video analysis of acute motor and convulsive manifestations in sport-related concussion. *Neurology*. 2000; 54(7):1488–1491.

136. McCrory PR, Bladin PF, Berkovic SF. Retrospective study of concussive convulsions in elite Australian rules and rugby league footballers: phenomenology, aetiology, and outcome. *BMJ*. 1997; 314(7075):171–174.

137. Chadwick D. Not everything that jerks is epilepsy. *Br J Sports Med*. 1997;31(3):173.

138. Stephenson J. Concussive convulsions. Editorial perpetuated myths about convulsive syncope. *BMJ*. 1997;314(7089):1283.

139. Gordon AG. Early seizures after closed head injury. *Can J Neurol Sci*. 1997;24(4):359–360.

140. Sander JW, O'Donoghue MF. Epilepsy: getting the diagnosis right. *BMJ*. 1997;314(7075):158–159.

141. Martland HS. Punch drunk. *JAMA*. 1928;19:1103–1107.

142. Parker HL. Traumatic encephalopathy ("Punch Drunk") of professional pugilists. *J Neurol Psychopathol*. 1934;15(57):20–28.

143. Corsellis JA, Bruton CJ, Freeman-Browne D. The aftermath of boxing. *Psychol Med*. 1973;3(3):270–303.

144. Roberts A. *Brain Damage in Boxers: A Study of Prevalence of Traumatic Encephalopathy Among Ex-professional Boxers*. London, UK: Pitman Medical & Scientific Publishing; 1969.

145. Omalu BI, DeKosky ST, Minster RL, Kamboh MI, Hamilton RL, Wecht CH. Chronic traumatic encephalopathy in a National Football League player. *Neurosurgery*. 2005;57(1):128–134; discussion 128–134.

146. Cantu RC. Chronic traumatic encephalopathy in the National Football League. *Neurosurgery*. 2007;61(2):223–225.

147. McKee AC, Cantu RC, Nowinski CJ, et al. Chronic traumatic encephalopathy in athletes: progressive tauopathy after repetitive head injury. *J Neuropathol Exp Neurol*. 2009;68(7):709–735.

148. Gavett BE, Stern RA, McKee AC. Chronic traumatic encephalopathy: a potential late effect of sport-related concussive and subconcussive head trauma. *Clin Sports Med*. 2011;30(1):179–188, xi.

149. Blaylock RL, Maroon J. Immunoexcitotoxicity as a central mechanism in chronic traumatic encephalopathy—a unifying hypothesis. *Surg Neurol Int*. 2011;2:107.

150. Omalu BI, DeKosky ST, Hamilton RL, et al. Chronic traumatic encephalopathy in a National Football League player: part II. *Neurosurgery*. 2006;59(5):1086–1092; discussion 1092–1083.

151. Omalu BI, Fitzsimmons RP, Hammers J, Bailes J. Chronic traumatic encephalopathy in a professional American wrestler. *J Forensic Nurs*. 2010;6(3):130–136.

152. Casson IR, Pellman EJ, Viano DC. Chronic traumatic encephalopathy in a National Football League player. *Neurosurgery*. 2006;58(5): E1003.

153. Stern RA, Riley DO, Daneshvar DH, Nowinski CJ, Cantu RC, McKee AC. Long-term consequences of repetitive brain trauma: chronic traumatic encephalopathy. *PM R*. 2011;3(10)(suppl 2): S460–S467.

154. Hallberg M. Impact of anabolic androgenic steroids on neuropeptide systems. *Mini Rev Med Chem.* 2011;11(5):399–408.

155. Kanayama G, Brower KJ, Wood RI, Hudson JI, Pope HG Jr. Treatment of anabolic-androgenic steroid dependence: emerging evidence and its implications. *Drug Alcohol Depend.* 2010;109(1–3):6–13.

156. Cheatle MD. Depression, chronic pain, and suicide by overdose: on the edge. *Pain Med.* 2011;12(suppl 2):S43–S48.

157. Miele VJ, Bailes JE, Cantu RC, Rabb CH. Subdural hematomas in boxing: the spectrum of consequences. *Neurosurg Focus.* 2006;21(4):E10.

158. Casson IR, Sham R, Campbell EA, Tarlau M, Didomenico A. Neurological and CT evaluation of knocked-out boxers. *J Neurol Neurosurg Psychiatry.* 1982;45(2):170–174.

159. Casson IR, Siegel O, Sham R, Campbell EA, Tarlau M, DiDomenico A. Brain damage in modern boxers. *JAMA.* 1984;251(20):2663–2667.

160. Jordan BD, Jahre C, Hauser WA, et al. CT of 338 active professional boxers. *Radiology.* 1992;185(2):509–512.

161. Bogdanoff B, Natter HM. Incidence of cavum septum pellucidum in adults: a sign of boxer's encephalopathy. *Neurology.* 1989;39(7):991–992.

162. Ross RJ, Cole M, Thompson JS, Kim KH. Boxers—computed tomography, EEG, and neurological evaluation. *JAMA.* 1983;249(2):211–213.

163. McLatchie G, Brooks N, Galbraith S, et al. Clinical neurological examination, neuropsychology, electroencephalography and computed tomographic head scanning in active amateur boxers. *J Neurol Neurosurg Psychiatry.* 1987;50(1):96–99.

164. Sironi VA, Scotti G, Ravagnati L, Franzini A, Marossero F. CT-scan and EEG findings in professional pugilists: early detection of cerebral atrophy in young boxers. *J Neurosurg Sci.* 1982;26(3):165–168.

165. Sortland O, Tysvaer AT. Brain damage in former association football players. An evaluation by cerebral computed tomography. *Neuroradiology.* 1989;31(1):44–48.

166. Autti T, Sipilä L, Autti H, Salonen O. Brain lesions in players of contact sports. *Lancet.* 1997;349(9059):1144.

167. Loosemore M, Knowles CH, Whyte GP. Amateur boxing and risk of chronic traumatic brain injury: systematic review of observational studies. *BMJ.* 2007;335(7624):809.

168. Zhang L, Heier LA, Zimmerman RD, Jordan B, Ulug AM. Diffusion anisotropy changes in the brains of professional boxers. *AJNR Am J Neuroradiol.* 2006;27(9):2000–2004.

169. Tanriverdi F, Unluhizarci K, Kocyigit I, et al. Brief communication: pituitary volume and function in competing and retired male boxers. *Ann Int Med.* 2008;148(11):827–831.

170. Levin HS, Lippold SC, Goldman A, et al. Neurobehavioral functioning and magnetic resonance imaging findings in young boxers. *J Neurosurg.* 1987;67(5):657–667.

171. Jordan BD, Zimmerman RD. Magnetic resonance imaging in amateur boxers. *Arch Neurol.* 1988;45(11):1207–1208.

172. Pulsipher DT, Campbell RA, Thoma R, King JH. A critical review of neuroimaging applications in sports concussion. *Curr Sports Med Rep.* 2011;10(1):14–20.

173. Chappell MH, Uluğ AM, Zhang L, et al. Distribution of microstructural damage in the brains of professional boxers: a diffusion MRI study. *J Magn Reson Imaging.* 2006;24(3):537–542.

174. Zhang K, Johnson B, Pennell D, Ray W, Sebastianelli W, Slobounov S. Are functional deficits in concussed individuals consistent with white matter structural alterations: combined FMRI & DTI study. *Exp Brain Res.* 2010;204(1):57–70.

175. Cubon VA, Putukian M, Boyer C, Dettwiler A. A diffusion tensor imaging study on the white matter skeleton in individuals with sports-related concussion. *J Neurotrauma.* 2011;28(2):189–201.

176. Henry LC, Tremblay J, Tremblay S, et al. Acute and chronic changes in diffusivity measures after sports concussion. *J Neurotrauma.* 2011;28(10):2049–2059.

177. Bazarian JJ, Zhu T, Blyth B, Borrino A, Zhong J. Subject-specific changes in brain white matter on diffusion tensor imaging after sports-related concussion. *Magn Reson Imaging.* 2012;30(2):171–180.

178. Houston AS, Kemp PM, Macleod MA, Francis JR, Colohan HA, Matthews HP. Use of significance image to determine patterns of cortical blood flow abnormality in pathological and at-risk groups. *J Nucl Med.* 1998;39(3):425–430.

179. Rodriguez G, Vitali P, Nobili F. Long-term effects of boxing and judo-choking techniques on brain function. *Ital J Neurol Sci.* 1998;19(6):367–372.

180. Provenzano FA, Jordan B, Tikofsky RS, Saxena C, Van Heertum RL, Ichise M. F-18 FDG PET imaging of chronic traumatic brain injury in boxers: a statistical parametric analysis. *Nucl Med Commun.* 2010;31(11):952–957.

181. Chen JK, Johnston KM, Frey S, Petrides M, Worsley K, Ptito A. Functional abnormalities in symptomatic concussed athletes: an fMRI study. *Neuroimage.* 2004;22(1):68–82.

182. Jantzen KJ, Anderson B, Steinberg FL, Kelso JA. A prospective functional MR imaging study of mild traumatic brain injury in college football players. *AJNR Am J Neuroradiol.* 2004;25(5):738–745.

183. Slobounov SM, Zhang K, Pennell D, Ray W, Johnson B, Sebastianelli W. Functional abnormalities in normally appearing athletes following mild traumatic brain injury: a functional MRI study. *Exp Brain Res.* 2010;202(2):341–354.

184. Pardini JE, Pardini DA, Becker JT, et al. Postconcussive symptoms are associated with compensatory cortical recruitment during a working memory task. *Neurosurgery.* 2010;67(4):1020–1027; discussion 1027–1028.

185. Chen JK, Johnston KM, Collie A, McCrory P, Ptito A. A validation of the post concussion symptom scale in the assessment of complex concussion using cognitive testing and functional MRI. *J Neurol Neurosurg Psychiatry.* 2007;78(11):1231–1238.

186. Chen JK, Johnston KM, Petrides M, Ptito A. Neural substrates of symptoms of depression following concussion in male athletes with persisting postconcussion symptoms. *Arch Gen Psychiatry.* 2008;65(1):81–89.

187. Slobounov SM, Gay M, Zhang K, et al. Alteration of brain functional network at rest and in response to YMCA physical stress test in concussed athletes: RsFMRI study. *Neuroimage.* 2011;55(4):1716–1727.

188. Vagnozzi R, Signoretti S, Tavazzi B, et al. Temporal window of metabolic brain vulnerability to concussion: a pilot 1H-magnetic resonance spectroscopic study in concussed athletes—part III. *Neurosurgery.* 2008;62(6):1286–1295; discussion 1295–1286.

189. Henry LC, Tremblay S, Boulanger Y, Ellemberg D, Lassonde M. Neurometabolic changes in the acute phase after sports concussions correlate with symptom severity. *J Neurotrauma.* 2010;27(1):65–76.

190. Kaplan HA, Browder J. Observations on the clinical and brain wave patterns of professional boxers. *J Am Med Assoc.* 1954;156(12):1138–1144.

191. Kröss R, Ohler K, Barolin GS. Effect of heading in soccer on the head—a quantifying EEG study of soccer players. *EEG EMG Z Elektroenzephalogr Elektromyogr Verwandte Geb.* 1983;14(4):209–212.

192. Tysvaer AT, Storli OV. Soccer injuries to the brain. A neurologic and electroencephalographic study of active football players. *Am J Sports Med.* 1989;17(4):573–578.

193. Thompson J, Sebastianelli W, Slobounov S. EEG and postural correlates of mild traumatic brain injury in athletes. *Neurosci Lett.* 2005;377(3):158–163.

194. Slobounov S, Sebastianelli W, Simon R. Neurophysiological and behavioral concomitants of mild brain injury in collegiate athletes. *Clin Neurophysiol.* 2002;113(2):185–193.

195. McCrea M, Prichep L, Powell MR, Chabot R, Barr WB. Acute effects and recovery after sport-related concussion: a neurocognitive and quantitative brain electrical activity study. *J Head Trauma Rehabil.* 2010;25(4):283–292.

196. Cao C, Slobounov S. Application of a novel measure of EEG nonstationarity as "Shannon- entropy of the peak frequency shifting" for detecting residual abnormalities in concussed individuals. *Clin Neurophysiol.* 2011;122(7):1314–1321.

197. Gosselin N, Lassonde M, Petit D, et al. Sleep following sport-related concussions. *Sleep Med.* 2009;10(1):35–46.

198. Duncan-Johnson CC, Donchin E. On quantifying surprise: the variation of event-related potentials with subjective probability. *Psychophysiol.* 1977;14(5):456–467.

199. Picton TW. The P300 wave of the human event-related potential. *J Clin Neurophysiol.* 1992;9(4):456–479.

200. Kutas M, McCarthy G, Donchin E. Augmenting mental chronometry: the P300 as a measure of stimulus evaluation time. *Science.* 1977;197(4305):792–795.

201. Polich J. Attention, probability, and task demands as determinants of P300 latency from auditory stimuli. *Electroencephalogr Clin Neurophysiol.* 1986;63(3):251–259.

202. Breton F, Pincemaille Y, Tarriere C, Renault B. Event-related potential assessment of attention and the orienting reaction in boxers before and after a fight. *Biol Psychol.* 1991;31(1):57–71.

203. Gosselin N, Thériault M, Leclerc S, Montplaisir J, Lassonde M. Neurophysiological anomalies in symptomatic and asymptomatic concussed athletes. *Neurosurgery.* 2006;58(6):1151–1161; discussion 1151–1161.

204. Thériault M, De Beaumont L, Gosselin N, Filipinni M, Lassonde M. Electrophysiological abnormalities in well functioning multiple concussed athletes. *Brain Inj.* 2009;23(11):899–906.

205. De Beaumont L, Théoret H, Mongeon D, et al. Brain function decline in healthy retired athletes who sustained their last sports concussion in early adulthood. *Brain.* 2009;132(pt 3):695–708.

206. Gaetz M, Bernstein DM. The current status of electrophysiologic procedures for the assessment of mild traumatic brain injury. *J Head Trauma Rehabil.* 2001;16(4):386–405.

207. Dupuis F, Johnston KM, Lavoie ME, Lepore F, Lassonde M. Concussion in athletes produce brain dysfunction as revealed by event-related potentials. *NeuroReport.* 2000;11(18):4087–4092.

208. Lavoie ME, Dupuis F, Johnston KM, Leclerc S, Lassonde M. Visual p300 effects beyond symptoms in concussed college athletes. *J Clin Exp Neuropsychol.* 2004;26(1):55–73.

209. Broglio SP, Pontifex MB, O'Connor P, Hillman CH. The persistent effects of concussion on neuroelectric indices of attention. *J Neurotrauma.* 2009;26(9):1463–1470.

210. Slobounov S, Sebastianelli W, Moss R. Alteration of posture-related cortical potentials in mild traumatic brain injury. *Neurosci Lett.* 2005;383(3):251–255.

211. De Beaumont L, Brisson B, Lassonde M, Jolicoeur P. Long-term electrophysiological changes in athletes with a history of multiple concussions. *Brain Inj.* 2007;21(6):631–644.

212. Livingston SC, Saliba EN, Goodkin HP, Barth JT, Hertel JN, Ingersoll CD. A preliminary investigation of motor evoked potential abnormalities following sport-related concussion. *Brain Inj.* 2010; 24(6):904–913.

213. Gaetz M, Iverson GL. Sex differences in self-reported symptoms following aerobic exercise in non-injured athletes: implications for concussion management programs. *Br J Sports Med.* 2009;43(7): 508–513.

214. Leddy JJ, Baker JG, Kozlowski K, Bisson L, Willer B. Reliability of a graded exercise test for assessing recovery from concussion. *Clin J Sport Med.* 2011;21(2):89–94.

215. Len TK, Neary JP. Cerebrovascular pathophysiology following mild traumatic brain injury. *Clin Physiol Funct Imaging.* 2011;31(12): 85–93.

216. Dicheskul ML, Kulikov VP. Arterial and venous brain reactivity in the acute period of cerebral concussion. *Neurosci Behav Physiol.* 2011;41:64–67.

217. Lau B, Lovell MR, Collins MW, Pardini J. Neurocognitive and symptom predictors of recovery in high school athletes. *Clin J Sport Med.* 2009;19(3):216–221.

218. Lau BC, Collins MW, Lovell MR. Sensitivity and specificity of subacute computerized neurocognitive testing and symptom evaluation in predicting outcomes after sports-related concussion. *Am J Sports Med.* 2011;39(6):1209–1216.

219. Leddy JJ, Kozlowski K, Donnelly JP, Pendergast DR, Epstein LH, Willer B. A preliminary study of subsymptom threshold exercise training for refractory post-concussion syndrome. *Clin J Sport Med.* 2010;20(1):21–27.

220. Majerske CW, Mihalik JP, Ren D, et al. Concussion in sports: postconcussive activity levels, symptoms, and neurocognitive performance. *J Athl Train.* 2008;43(3):265–274.

221. McGrath N. Supporting the student-athlete's return to the classroom after a sport-related concussion. *J Athl Train.* 2010;45(5):492–498.

222. Echemendia RJ, Cantu RC. Return to play following sports-related mild traumatic brain injury: the role for neuropsychology. *Appl Neuropsychol.* 2003;10(1):48–55.

223. Mihalik JP, Blackburn JT, Greenwald RM, Cantu RC, Marshall SW, Guskiewicz KM. Collision type and player anticipation affect head impact severity among youth ice hockey players. *Pediatrics.* 2010; 125(6):e1394–e1401.

224. Daneshvar DH, Baugh CM, Nowinski CJ, McKee AC, Stern RA, Cantu RC. Helmets and mouth guards: the role of personal equipment in preventing sport-related concussions. *Clin Sports Med.* 2011;30:145–163, x.

225. Benson BW, Hamilton GM, Meeuwisse WH, McCrory P, Dvorak J. Is protective equipment useful in preventing concussion? A systematic review of the literature. *Br J Sports Med.* 2009;43(suppl 1): i56–i67.

226. Blignaut JB, Carstens IL, Lombard CJ. Injuries sustained in rugby by wearers and non-wearers of mouthguards. *Br J Sports Med.* 1987; 21(2):5–7.

227. Giza CC, Hovda DA. The neurometabolic cascade of concussion. *J Athl Train.* 2001;36(3):228–235.

228. Fineman I, Giza CC, Nahed BV, Lee SM, Hovda DA. Inhibition of neocortical plasticity during development by a moderate concussive brain injury. *J Neurotrauma.* 2000;17(9):739–749.

229. Fineman I, Hovda DA, Smith M, Yoshino A, Becker DP. Concussive brain injury is associated with a prolonged accumulation of calcium: a 45Ca autoradiographic study. *Brain Res.* 1993;624(1–2): 94–102.

230. Ginsberg MD, Zhao W, Alonso OF, Loor-Estades JY, Dietrich WD, Busto R. Uncoupling of local cerebral glucose metabolism and blood flow after acute fluid-percussion injury in rats. *Am J Physiol.* 1997;272(6, pt 2):H2859–H2868.

231. Katayama Y, Becker DP, Tamura T, Hovda DA. Massive increases in extracellular potassium and the indiscriminate release of glutamate following concussive brain injury. *J Neurosurg.* 1990;73(6): 889–900.

232. Osteen CL, Moore AH, Prins ML, Hovda DA. Age-dependency of 45calcium accumulation following lateral fluid percussion: acute and delayed patterns. *J Neurotrauma.* 2001;18(2):141–162.

233. Pettus EH, Christman CW, Giebel ML, Povlishock JT. Traumatically induced altered membrane permeability: its relationship to traumatically induced reactive axonal change. *J Neurotrauma.* 1994; 11(5):507–522.

234. Sunami K, Nakamura T, Ozawa Y, Kubota M, Namba H, Yamaura A. Hypermetabolic state following experimental head injury. *Neurosurg Rev.* 1989;12(suppl 1):400–411.

235. Yamakami I, McIntosh TK. Effects of traumatic brain injury on regional cerebral blood flow in rats as measured with radiolabeled microspheres. *J Cereb Blood Flow Metab.* 1989;9(1):117–124.

236. Yoshino A, Hovda DA, Kawamata T, Katayama Y, Becker DP. Dynamic changes in local cerebral glucose utilization following cerebral conclusion in rats: evidence of a hyper- and subsequent hypometabolic state. *Brain Res.* 1991;561(1):106–119.

237. Denny-Brown D, Russell W. Experimental cerebral concussion. *Brain.* 1941;64:93–164.

238. Kane MJ, Angoa-Pérez M, Briggs DI, Viano DC, Kreipke CW, Kuhn DM. A mouse model of human repetitive mild traumatic brain injury. *J Neurosci Methods.* 2012;203(1):41–49.

239. Prins ML, Hales A, Reger M, Giza CC, Hovda DA. Repeat traumatic brain injury in the juvenile rat is associated with increased axonal injury and cognitive impairments. *Dev Neurosci.* 2010;32(5–6): 510–518.

240. Chew E, Zafonte RD. Pharmacological management of neurobehavioral disorders following traumatic brain injury—a state-of-the-art review. *J Rehabil Res Dev.* 2009;46(6):851–879.

241. Meehan WP III. Medical therapies for concussion. *Clin Sports Med.* 2011;30(1):115–124, ix.

Assessment and Rehabilitative Management of Individuals With Disorders of Consciousness

Joseph T. Giacino, Douglas I. Katz, Kent Garber, and Nicholas Schiff

The pace of progress in understanding and managing disorders of consciousness (DOC) after acquired brain injury continues to evolve at a rapid rate. American and European initiatives to establish practice guidelines for assessment, prognosis, and rehabilitation of individuals in coma, the vegetative state (VS), and the minimally conscious state (MCS) (1–4) have been completed, and specialized behavioral, electrophysiologic, and neuroimaging procedures developed. These are perhaps the two most important drivers behind the dramatic expansion of clinical and scientific knowledge of the continuum of consciousness. This chapter will update and critique the major developments in this area that have influenced the clinical management of DOC over the last 5 years. Following a review of the diagnostic criteria associated with coma, VS, and MCS, the chapter presents pathophysiologic findings from structural and functional neuroimaging studies of patients with severely altered consciousness, outlines the diagnostic and prognostic utility of behavioral assessment procedures developed specifically for this population, and reviews the effectiveness of treatment interventions designed to facilitate recovery of cognition. General recommendations for clinical management of the conditions discussed are also provided.

DEFINITIONS AND DIAGNOSTIC CRITERIA

Professional organizations in the United States and Europe have established consensus-based behavioral criteria to improve differential diagnostic precision among DOC. In the United States, diagnostic guidelines have been published by the American Academy of Neurology (AAN) for VS (1) and by the Aspen Neurobehavioral Workgroup for MCS (4). Internationally, guidelines have been developed in the United Kingdom (5), France (6), and Australia (7). Despite the availability of practice guidelines to aid diagnostic assessment, estimates of misdiagnosis among patients with DOC range from 15%–43% (8–11). These figures are startling and possibly unrivaled by other neurologic conditions. In a study published in 2009 by Belgian and US researchers (11), the investigators hypothesized that diagnostic accuracy among DOC would be higher now, relative to when error rates were first released in the 1990s. The basis for this hypothesis was that MCS was not operationally defined until 2002, well after the original studies were published. Using a standardized

assessment instrument, the Coma Recovery Scale- Revised (12) as the "gold standard," the authors found that 41% of the diagnoses established by team consensus were incorrect, 89% of which were in the false-negative direction (i.e., conscious but believed to be unconscious). This rate is roughly equivalent to the rates reported before the criteria for MCS were published. The authors suggested that the examiners' reliance on unstructured bedside observations, rather than on standardized test administration and scoring procedures, was most likely the strongest contributor to the high rate of misdiagnosis.

Many factors have been implicated as causes of diagnostic error in DOC, including patient, examiner, and environmental influences (13); however, diagnostic precision is also hindered by the wide array of terms that have been proposed to characterize states of altered consciousness, many of which have not been operationalized (see Table 32-1). Among these the most controversial is the vegetative state, which has been viewed as pejorative in view of its similarity to the word vegetable. This has led to occasional efforts to abandon the term VS (14), most recently a proposal by the European Task Force on Disorders of Consciousness to adopt "unresponsive wakefulness" in place of VS (15). The task force also felt that VS conflates consciousness and behavioral responsiveness. Nonetheless, the term VS remains deeply ingrained in medical terminology, registries, and diagnostic coding systems.

The following section summarizes the neuropathologic characteristics and distinguishing behavioral features of three major DOC: coma, VS, and MCS.

Coma

Coma is a state of pathologic unconsciousness in which the eyes remain closed and the patient cannot be aroused (16). It is most often the result of severe, diffuse bihemispheric lesions of the cortex or underlying white matter; bilateral thalamic damage; or paramedian tegmental lesions. The clinical criteria for diagnosing coma were described by Plum and Posner in 1982 (16) and remain well accepted. The defining feature of coma is the complete loss of spontaneous or stimulus-induced arousal. The eyes remain continuously closed despite the application of noxious stimuli and there are no sleep/wake cycles on electroencephalography (EEG). On ex-

TABLE 32-1 Terms Used to Refer to Disorders of Consciousness

Akinetic mutism	Minimally responsive state
Apallic syndrome	Permanent vegetative state
Coma	Persistent vegetative state
Coma vigil	Post coma unawareness
Cognitive death	Prolonged coma
Decerebrate state	Prolonged posttraumatic
Low level	unconsciousness
Minimally conscious state	Vegetative state
Unresponsive wakefulness	Wakeful unconsciousness

amination, there is no evidence of purposeful motor activity, no response to command, and no indication of receptive or expressive language ability. Coma is a self-limiting state that typically resolves within 2–4 weeks in those who survive the initial injury.

Vegetative State

The vegetative state has been mired in controversy since it was first introduced by Jennett and Plum (17) more than 25 years ago. The term itself is controversial because it is considered to be pejorative by the lay public and because clinicians have not been able to agree on the prognostic parameters associated with this diagnosis. Despite the ongoing dissatisfaction with this term, it is deeply embedded in the scientific literature, diagnostic coding systems, and surveillance registries and has not been supplanted by proposed alternatives.

VS is a condition in which awareness of self and environment is presumed to be absent and there is an inability to interact with others, although the capacity for spontaneous or stimulus-induced arousal is preserved (18). VS typically follows a period of coma but may also arise from developmental malformations or may represent the culmination of progressive degenerative or metabolic disorders. The neuropathologic substrate is usually determined by the cause of injury. Diffuse axonal injury is the most common finding in posttraumatic VS. Vascular causes of VS are often associated with paramedial thalamic damage, and diffuse laminar cortical necrosis is frequently noted following anoxic brain injury.

The diagnosis of VS is made when spontaneous eye opening has reemerged (signaling recovery of the reticular activating system) and there is no discernible evidence of

- sustained or reproducible purposeful behavioral responses to visual, auditory, tactile, or noxious stimuli or
- language comprehension or expression.

The AAN recommends that the term *persistent VS* (PVS) be used to describe VS when it persists for 1 month following either traumatic or nontraumatic brain injury (1). In view of the high rate of recovery of consciousness that occurs between 3 and 12 months postinjury in individuals who remain in VS longer than 1 month (19,20), the Aspen Neurobehavioral Workgroup recommended that the term *PVS* be abandoned in favor of accompanying the diagnosis of "VS" with a description of the injury and the length of time since onset,

as both of these factors provide prognostic information (14). The current AAN practice guideline also recommends that the term *permanent VS* be applied 3 months after nontraumatic brain injury and after 12 months following traumatic injury, implying that further recovery of consciousness is highly improbable after these time points. New evidence from recently published outcome studies extending out to 5 years postinjury suggests that a substantial minority of patients who remain in VS for longer than 1 month recover consciousness and continue to demonstrate meaningful functional recovery after 12 months. These findings are discussed in some detail in the subsequent section on *Prognosis*.

Minimally Conscious State

MCS is a condition of severely altered consciousness in which there is minimal but definite behavioral evidence of self or environmental awareness (4). MCS usually represents a transitional state reflecting improvement in consciousness from coma or VS, or progressive decline as in neurodegenerative disease (e.g., Alzheimer disease). The pathophysiology, natural history, long-term outcome, and attendant ethical issues associated with MCS have received considerable attention over the last 5 years. A search of core clinical journals included on PubMed revealed more than 100 publications on MCS since this condition was defined in 2002. This represents a tenfold increase since the first edition of *Brain Injury Medicine* was published.

Jennett and colleagues conducted a postmortem analysis to investigate the neuropathologic substrate of posttraumatic MCS (21).The authors found that the typical lesion profile consists of grade 2 or 3 diffuse axonal injury with multifocal cortical contusions, sometimes accompanied by thalamic involvement. In comparison to patients diagnosed with VS, thalamic lesions were notably less prevalent in MCS (50%) relative to VS (80%). Based on these findings, MCS appears to be characterized by greater sparing of corticothalamic connections, which may account for why patients in MCS retain some capacity for cognitive processing.

The diagnosis of MCS is based on clearly discernible *and* reproducible evidence of one or more of the following behaviors:

- Simple command following.
- Intelligible verbalization.
- Recognizable verbal or gestural "yes/no" responses (without regard to accuracy).
- Movements or emotional responses that are triggered by relevant environmental stimuli and cannot be attributed to reflexive activity. Examples of the fourth criterion include (*a*) smiling or crying following exposure to emotional (e.g., family photographs) but not neutral stimuli (e.g., photographs of objects), (*b*) vocalizations or gestures that occur in direct response to specific linguistic prompts, (*c*) accurate reaching toward objects placed within the immediate visual field, (*d*) manipulation of objects placed in the hand, and (*e*) sustained visual fixation or pursuit eye movements.

In making the diagnosis of MCS, it is important to consider the frequency and complexity of the behavior observed. When there is evidence of rudimentary cognition only (e.g., visual tracking), the diagnosis of MCS requires serial reassessment. At the opposite end of the MCS spectrum, patients who demonstrate consistent evidence of complex cognitively mediated behavior (e.g., command following) fall at the upper limit of MCS.

Some patients in MCS infrequently initiate volitional behavior and often fail to respond to environmental prompts, but on occasion, exhibit behaviors that infer complex cognitive processing (e.g., follow countermanding or go-no go commands, verbalize at sentence level). These individuals tend to show marked fluctuations in behavioral responsiveness across examinations. Responses to a series of yes/no questions may be consistent and reliable on one examination, but inconsistent or inaccurate on a follow-up conducted 24 hours later. It is unclear whether patients who infrequently engage in complex responses should be included in the MCS category because it is difficult to determine whether the low rate of behavioral responsiveness is primarily due to underarousal, sensory impairment, motor dysfunction, or loss of drive.

Emergence From Minimally Conscious State

Emergence from MCS is signaled by the recovery of interactive communication or functional object use. These behaviors were selected as exit criteria for two reasons. First, both are dependent on widely distributed cortical connectivity to engage and sustain the actions required. Second, these behaviors permit meaningful environmental interaction and basic restoration of personal autonomy. In keeping with the conceptual underpinnings of MCS, emergence from MCS requires *reliable* and *consistent* evidence of either communication or object use. Communication may occur through verbal responses, gestural means, or augmentative devices. "Functional object use" requires discrimination among items presented (e.g., comb brought to head and toothbrush to mouth). Aphasia and apraxia must be ruled out as contributing or causative factors in patients who don't meet the criteria for reliable communication ability or functional object use.

The criteria for emergence from MCS have received increased scrutiny and calls for review. Nakase-Richardson and others tested the appropriateness of the "functional communication" criterion in a cohort of patients whom they defined as "responsive" but unable to communicate on admission to rehabilitation (22). This definition served as a proxy for emergence from MCS. The sample was subdivided into "confused" and "nonconfused" subgroups, based on *Diagnostic and Statistical Manual of Mental Disorders, Fourth Edition* (*DSM-IV*) criteria for delirium, and four "simple" yes/no questions were serially administered over the course of the rehabilitation stay. Results indicated that 59% of yes/no responses were inconsistent in the nonconfused group, prompting the investigators to suggest that the existing criteria for emergence from MCS may be too difficult. Although methodologic issues in the study design (e.g., compatibility of proxy and actual definitions of "emergence," difficulty level of yes/no questions) limit the direct applicability of the findings, this study raises an important question that deserves further analysis.

The last 10 years have witnessed movement toward achieving universally agreed upon terminology for DOC. As of this writing, a jointly sponsored systematic review of diagnostic, prognostic, and treatment evidence pertinent to patients with DOC has been launched by the AAN, Ameri-

can Congress of Rehabilitation Medicine, and TBI Model Systems. This effort is expected to provide new guidelines for clinical practice. This is an essential first step toward assuring diagnostic accuracy, prognostic precision, and well-informed treatment decisions.

PATHOPHYSIOLOGY AND NEUROIMAGING

Neuropathology of Vegetative State and Minimally Conscious State

Traumatic and nontraumatic VS have distinct and identifiable pathologies. Adams et al. (23) studied 49 patients remaining in VS for at least 1 month until death and found that nontraumatic injuries included severe bilateral thalamic damage in all instances and, in the majority of cases, were associated with diffuse cortical damage. In contrast, traumatic etiologies associated with VS showed grade 2 and 3 diffuse axonal injuries and severe thalamic degeneration in the majority of patients who survived for 3 months before death. These pathological studies confirm the intuition that the chronic vegetative state is characterized by overwhelming cerebral damage. An important conclusion that is often overlooked is that the most consistent and severe pathologies arising from both types of injuries are in subcortical structures, particularly the thalamus. The cerebral cortex is generally spared in traumatic VS, with only about 10% of patients showing diffuse ischemic neocortical injury patterns; brainstem damage is uncommon in chronic VS patients emphasizing that VS is primarily a disorder of cerebral integration at the thalamocortical level.

No comprehensive study has evaluated specific anatomic pathologies associated with MCS. Jennett and colleagues (21) reported 65 autopsies of patients with traumatic brain injury leading either to VS or severe disability and found wide variation in underlying neuroanatomical substrates. This study included 12 patients with histories consistent with MCS at the time of death. Of note, two of the MCS patients demonstrated only focal brain injures, without DAI or focal thalamic infarction (a consistent finding in approximately half of the severely disabled patients). Further work to determine the pathological correlates of MCS is required.

Functional Neuroimaging Studies

Characterization of Resting Brain Activity and Response to Passively Presented Stimuli

Several brain imaging techniques are now providing important insight into the mechanisms of neurological DOC. Functional MRI (fMRI) and functional positron emission tomography (15O-PET) studies respectively correlate changes in blood oxygen level and cerebral blood flow with neuronal activation. Both techniques have been employed to characterize the resting brain activity across patients with DOC (24). Precise correlational studies of single-unit and multiunit neuronal recordings from brain regions simultaneously studied using fMRI techniques indicate that fMRI signal activations are tightly correlated with neuronal population activity (25). These findings support the use of both fMRI and 15O-PET activations as a proxy for neuronal activation per se. Brain metabolism can also be quantified in neuroimaging studies using fluorodeoxyglucose positron emission tomography (FDG-PET) imaging, a measure of cerebral glucose metabolic rates. FDG-PET studies in patients with Parkinson disease have correlated regional glucose metabolism with neuronal firing rates in cerebral structures (26). Direct measurements of cerebral metabolism and neuronal activity demonstrate a rough equivalence of metabolic rate and mean firing rate of population of neurons (27). Combined with traditional structural magnetic resonance imaging (MRI) and EEG (or magnetoencephalography [MEG] recordings obtained from measurements of the brain magnetic field), these techniques offer an integrative view of the damaged brain.

The clinical judgment of unconsciousness in chronic VS was first supported in imaging studies by FDG-PET studies that revealed overall cerebral metabolism to be reduced by 50% or more below normal levels in VS patients (1,28–30). FDG-PET studies have also identified novel evidence of the modular organization of brain systems in patients who retained small islands of cerebral metabolic activity that correlated with clinically identified behavioral fragments (31,32).

Resting state fMRI studies have identified evidence that a midline frontoparietal "default mode" state activation may correlate with level of brain function indexed by clinical examination (33–35). Compared to VS patients, MCS patients show intermediate expression pattern of the "default mode" pattern with a higher functional connectivity of the posterior cingulate/precuneus area as compared to unresponsive patients (35). Similar findings have been obtained using FDG-PET measurements (36).

Several studies have employed 15O-PET imaging techniques to evaluate responses to sensory VS patients. Laureys and colleagues have identified a marked loss of distributed network processing in the vegetative state (37–39). In their studies, elementary auditory and somatosensory stimuli were presented to PVS patients and normal control subjects and compared to baseline resting conditions in 15O-PET subtraction paradigms; in VS, patients demonstrated a loss of brain activations outside of primary sensory cortices for both types of stimuli. Cortical regions identified as "hierarchically higher order" multimodal association areas active in the normal control subjects did not activate in the VS patients; these findings are consistent with evidence of early sensory processing in VS patients as measured by evoked potential studies and add important additional information about the integrity of cerebral information processing in PVS. Menon and colleagues (40) described a 26-year-old woman in a PVS 4 months following an attack of acute disseminated encephalomyelitis that functionally impaired both cortical and subcortical (brainstem and thalamic) structures. Right occipital-temporal regions in this patient demonstrated selective activation of the right fusiform gyrus and extrastriate visual association areas with visual stimulation. These results were obtained in response to presentation of familiar faces and scrambled images. No other evidence of cortical processing was reported but the patient became increasingly responsive at 6 months and minimally expressive at 8 months into the course of her illness. Menon et al. interpreted this activity measured at 4 months as indicating a recovery of minimal awareness. However, such selective identification of relatively complex information processing may not alone index recovery of cognitive function or even potential for recovery (31,41).

Compared to findings in patients in VS, functional neuroimaging studies obtained from those in MCS have consistently showed a higher level of functional segregation (i.e.,

more widespread activation) and functional integration (i.e., more functional long-range connectivity with frontoparietal "awareness" networks) for both auditory (42,43) and noxious processing (44). Responses to emotionally relevant stimuli have also been elicited in some MCS patients (45).

Measurement of Active Response Using Neuroimaging: Command Following and Communication Paradigms

Although several neuroimaging studies have found group differences in resting patterns of brain activity or response to passively presented stimuli comparing patients in VS and MCS patients, such approaches have not shown features that provide unambiguous information to establish or contravene a clinical diagnosis. The first such demonstration of the use of neuroimaging for diagnostic assessment was carried out by Owen et al. (46), who employed fMRI in a patient diagnosed with traumatic VS. The patient was asked to imagine playing tennis and activated the supplementary motor area of the brain, consistent with response profiles of normal subjects. Similarly, when asked to imagine moving around in her house, she produced an expected activation within the same parahippocampal area seen in controls. The same paradigm was further extended by Monti et al. (47) to establish evidence of fMRI-based communication in a single subject who had appear to fulfill VS criteria for 5 years prior to the assessment. Subsequent to the Owen et al. study, other investigators have used motor imagery (48,49) and activation of the expressive language Broca region (50) to show fMRI evidence of command following in subjects fulfilling MCS and VS criteria. Bardin et al. have importantly demonstrated two subjects for whom fMRI-based command following did not lead to communication using this, with a test–retest confirmation of this dissociation (49).

Complementing these fMRI approaches are methods using electrophysiological assessments, a considerably less expensive and portable technology. Goldfine and colleagues (51) developed a quantitative EEG methodology and evaluated subjects studied by Bardin et al. (49) in fMRI. EEG evidence for command following demonstrated similar variations in linking behavioral evaluations to directly measured brain signal evaluations of command following seen in this study (Figure 32-1). Schnakers and coworkers demonstrated that some MCS patients increased the amplitude of the "P3" potential when instructed to count a target name (52). Both steady-state and event-related EEG paradigms are likely to find continued use in the assessment of VS and MCS.

CLINICAL ASSESSMENT

Prior to the last decade, procedures for evaluating individuals with DOC were largely limited to the Glasgow Coma Scale (GCS) (53), MRI, and EEG studies. These procedures continue to be useful during the acute stage of recovery but represent relatively gross indicators of cerebral dysfunction. Specialized behavioral and neuroradiologic protocols have been developed in an attempt to provide a more specific means of monitoring recovery across the subacute and postacute periods and to improve outcome prediction.

Bedside Examination

There are no standardized evaluation procedures for the clinical bedside examination of patients with impaired con-

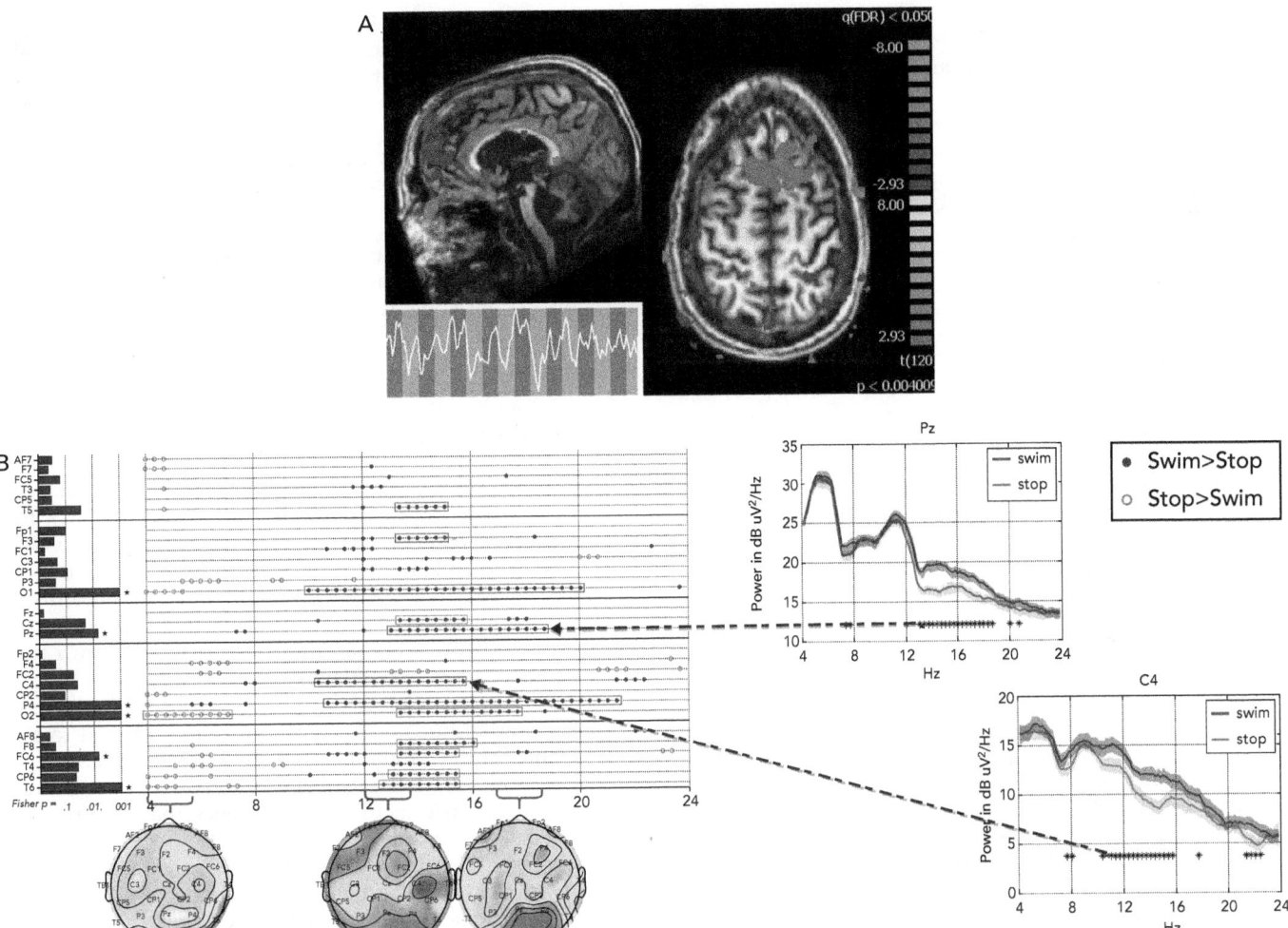

FIGURE 32-1 *See color insert.* Multimodal fMRI and EEG evidence of covert command-following in a patient who failed to demonstrate bedside evidence of command-following. *Panel A* shows selective activation of the supplementary motor area in response to the command to 'imagine swimming.' *Panel B* shows a concomitant increase in EEG power over primary motor and parietal cortices during the active command condition. Modified from *Brain.* 2011;134(pt 3):769–782.

sciousness. Most clinicians rely on systematic evaluations of arousal and behavioral responses to various forms of stimulation. Nevertheless, frequent errors in diagnosis occur, (9,10) either because of a misinterpretation of responses or examinations that are inadequate to detect minimal, inconsistent responsiveness.

The bedside neurological examination of patients with impaired consciousness should focus on two general areas: assessment of the integrity of the central nervous system, particularly brainstem pathways (e.g., pupillary responses, ocular movements, oculovestibular reflexes, breathing patterns), and the presence of higher level cortical functions (e.g., purposeful, voluntary behaviors). The examiner's task is to systematically elicit and distinguish behaviors that are reflexive or automatic, reliant on spinal or subcortical pathways, or isolated cortical-subcortical networks from those that are mediated by integrated cortical activity and represent some level or awareness or purposeful intent.

Cognitive awareness or conscious intent may be difficult to interpret when responses are extremely inconsistent or simple. There is an inverse relationship between the dimensions of *complexity* and *consistency* when judging whether particular behaviors imply consciousness. When a behavior is more complex, such as a verbalization, fewer instances of the response are sufficient to demonstrate consciousness. When a behavior is less complex, such as a finger movement, more frequent occurrences are necessary to establish a link to stimulus awareness or conscious intention. For this reason, single bedside examinations are often inadequate to conclusively establish level of unconsciousness. Repeated assessments and use of standardized evaluations (see later) may be necessary for diagnostic accuracy. Table 32-2 presents a systematic approach to the neurological examination of patients with impaired consciousness.

There are several common problems that can lead to inaccurate diagnosis of consciousness in patients with impaired consciousness. These include

- attributing purposeful intent for responses that are reflexive or generalized to any form of stimulation;
- inadequate evaluation to detect conscious behavior—for example, insufficient sampling time, inadequate arousal, inappropriate choice of stimuli;

TABLE 32-2 A Systematic Approach to the Examination of Patients With Impaired Consciousness Includes the Following Steps

1. Brainstem integrity and other subcortical evaluation
   - Pupillary response, blink reflex to visual threat
   - Ocular movements, gaze deviations
   - Oculovestibular reflexes (oculocephalic ["doll's eyes"] maneuvers, calorics)
   - Corneal response
   - Gag reflex
   - Breathing pattern
   - Decerebrate postures
   - Other posturing, reflexes, and tone

2. Cortical functioning
   a. Observation of spontaneous activity
      - Purposeful, complex movements (involving cortically mediated isolated motor control) vs posturing (decorticate or decerebrate) or reflex or stereotyped, patterned (subcortically mediated) movements
      - Spontaneous vocalizations or verbalizations
      - Eye movements (signs of fixation or tracking vs nonspecific roving or no movement)

   b. Responses to stimulation or environment
      - Tracking or fixation to stimuli (try salient stimuli such as familiar pictures, faces, mirror)
      - Verbal stimulation (e.g., patient's name, commands, social greetings):
        Begin with simple commands sampling a variety of areas under different neural control, favoring those areas of potentially preserved movement.
        - Eye commands—e.g., "look up," "blink twice"
        - Limb commands—e.g., "make a fist," "show two fingers," "raise your arm"
        - Oral commands—e.g., "open mouth," "stick out tongue"
        - Axial or whole body commands—e.g., "turn your head," "lean forward"
        - Ask patient to "stop moving" or "hold still" to distinguish from spontaneous repetitive movements.
      - Noxious stimulation
        - Look for localization or purposeful defensive maneuvers vs reflexive or generalized, stereotyped movements or facial expressions.
      - Response in contingent relationship to environment or other stimuli
        - Look for intentional reach for or manipulation of objects on or around the patient (e.g., pulling at tubes, clothing, items placed in the hand)
        - Look for changes in facial expression contingent on stimuli such as familiar voices, particular conversation, pictures, music, etc.
        - Look for attempts at purposeful mobility in bed, chair, and even ambulation
        - Gestural behaviors indicating intentive communication (e.g., yes/no signals)
      - Confounding factors affecting arousal (e.g., centrally acting medications, concurrent illness, subclinical seizures, undetected pain)
      - The potential influence of aphasia, apraxia, and other higher cortical disorders that may affect the ability to respond to commands

- overconsideration or underconsideration of family or other's observations of purposeful behavior (i.e., failure to recognize that family may be first to observe signs of consciousness or to overattribute purposeful intent); and
- simple, cortically mediated behaviors of uncertain cognitive significance—for example, simple isolated limb movements.

The examiner should use strategies to account for some of these confounds and maximize the chance of detecting signs of conscious behavior. The clinician should:

1. *Assure optimal arousal.* There should be an adequate warm-up period, with verbal and tactile stimulation to promote wakefulness. Deep pressure stimulation is often effective. Positioning is important and patients are usually more wakeful sitting up. The time of day, the patient's sleep-wake cycles, and fatigue from activities preceding the neurological examination all have to be considered. Sedating medications should be avoided, and treatable medical conditions should be addressed.

2. *Assure optimal environmental conditions.* Avoid distractions, provide adequate lighting, remove physical restrictions to movement, and position stimuli to the patient's best advantage.

3. *Consider stimulus duration and rate.* Use a long enough presentation time and interstimulus interval to allow time for the patient to respond and to minimize perseveration. Recognize that as the interval between stimulus and response increases, the chance that a spurious response is mistakenly attributed to a stimulus also increases. Watch for signs of response fatigue.

4. *Avoid unnecessary complexity in command following trials.* Use simple declarative language, one request at a time.

5. *Consider the patient's motor repertoire in choosing commands.* Use commands that incorporate motor responses that appear to be within the patient's capabilities, such as spontaneously observed movements.

6. *Distinguish purposeful from reflexive behavior.* When attempting to elicit movements to command, avoid responses that may represent common reflexive behaviors—for example, squeeze hands, blink eyes.

7. *Evaluate a variety of potential responses and employ a range of different stimuli.* Attempt to elicit responses to a few different types of command—for example, a limb command and an eye command. Look for other forms of purposeful behavior—for example, manipulation of an object placed in the patient's hand, social handshake, purposeful resistance to unpleasant stimulation.

8. *Assess for signs of pain.* Untreated pain can constrain behavioral response repertoires and thus confound the assessment of level of consciousness. Consider using the recently developed Nociception Coma Scale to help detect and manage pain in noncommunicative patients in VS or MCS (54).

9. *Assure adequate examination time and perform serial reassessments.* Quick bedside evaluations such as typical morning rounds are often not adequate in detecting responses in patients with DOC. Repeated reassessments are necessary to establish response consistency, validity of examination findings, and accuracy of the diagnosis.

10. *Pay attention to observations of others.* Families, nurses, and therapists who are more familiar or spend more time with the patient often observe behaviors associated with

consciousness before they are observed by the physician. The physician's assessment should incorporate these observations.

Standardized Rating Scales

Neurorehabilitation specialists have long recognized the need for reliable assessment instruments that can detect subtle but potentially important clinical findings to guide diagnostic and prognostic assessment. A wide variety of standardized neurobehavioral assessment scales have been circulated over the last 20 years and have become an important component of the clinician's tool box. Although most instruments that have entered the clinical mainstream (55–60) have obvious face validity and provide a comprehensive overview of neurobehavioral functions, other important psychometric characteristics including diagnostic and prognostic utility have not been well studied.

In response to the dearth of information available about the psychometric strength of standardized assessment measures designed for this population, the Disorders of Consciousness Task Force of the American Congress of Rehabilitation Medicine completed a systematic review of 13 behavioral assessment scales for DOC (61). The results of this review yielded insufficient evidence to support the use of any of these measures for use in differential diagnosis or outcome prediction. The lack of support for these indications was directly attributable to the failure to employ appropriate masking procedures to mitigate the risk of examiner bias. The task force reviewed all scales to determine standardization procedures, content validity, interrater and test–retest reliability, internal consistency, criterion/construct validity, diagnostic and prognostic validity, and user characteristics. One scale, the Coma Recovery Scale-Revised (CRS-R) (12), was recommended by the task force with "minor reservations" for use in individuals with DOC. The CRS-R was also recently selected as the measure of choice for assessment of recovery of consciousness in traumatic brain injury (TBI) research by the Traumatic Brain Injury Common Data Elements (CDE) Outcomes Workgroup, cosponsored by the National Institute of Neurological Disorders and Stroke (NINDS), Defense Centers of Excellence for Psychological Health and Traumatic Brain Injury, US Department of Veterans Affairs, and the National Institute on Disability and Rehabilitation Research (62).

The CRS-R is composed of six subscales addressing auditory, visual, motor, oromotor/verbal, communication, and arousal functions. Subscale items are hierarchically arranged, corresponding to brainstem, subcortical, and cortically mediated functions. Administration and scoring guidelines are manualized and the scale is intended for use by medical and allied health professionals. The scale is well represented in the scientific literature and has been used to investigate diagnostic accuracy (12,63), the relationship between behavioral and neurophysiologic markers of consciousness (64–66), outcome prediction (67,68), and treatment effectiveness (69,70). Additional information is available on the NINDS TBI CDE website (http://www.commondataelements.ninds.nih.gov/TBI.aspx).

Individualized Behavioral Assessment

The rigorous attention to methodologic consistency afforded by standardized measures does not allow case-specific ques-

tions to be addressed. For example, standardized procedures may not be able to differentiate between random movement and low-frequency movement to command because the investigational technique is fixed and the number of observations restricted. For example, finger movement that occurs on two of four trials immediately after the command to "move your fingers" raises the possibility of verbal comprehension. However, if finger movement fails to occur during the next 20 trials administered, the probability that the two earlier responses represented evidence of verbal comprehension is diminished. Conversely, a patient may move his or her fingers following command on 10 consecutive trials but, if the same finger movement precedes the command or persists well after the last command is administered, it is less likely that this response is an indication of verbal comprehension. To address this problem, DiPasquale and Whyte (71) developed an approach termed, "Individualized Quantitative Behavioral Assessment (IQBA)." IQBA applies principles of single subject research design to assess the cognitive and behavioral capacities of individuals with marked limitations in responsiveness. In this technique, clinical questions are individually tailored, stimuli and response criteria are operationally defined, and behavioral frequencies are analyzed statistically to determine whether the behavior of interest exceeds the rate predicted by chance. This approach has been successfully employed to investigate command following, visual function, communication ability, emotional responses, and drug efficacy (72).

Standardized and individualized procedures should be viewed as complementary as they serve different purposes. Standardized methods are designed to provide a broad overview of the integrity of sensory, motor, and cognitive processes. When viewed in toto, these findings can help establish diagnosis, prognosis, and lesion locus and may inform the optimal approach to treatment. The inherent flexibility offered by the individualized approach provides an opportunity to control case-specific influences on behavior, which contribute to diagnostic inaccuracy and erroneous judgments concerning consciousness.

TREATMENT INTERVENTIONS AND EFFECTIVENESS

The primary goal in treating individuals with DOC is to restore basic functional competence. The degree to which this goal can be achieved is dependent on multiple factors including arousal level, sensorimotor functions, communication ability, initiation and drive mechanisms, and executive control processes. Treatment strategies, therefore, are usually designed to improve or augment one or more of these areas. Unfortunately, no treatment has definitively been shown to alter the natural course of recovery from coma, VS, or MCS. This may be due, in part, to the lack of prospective, randomized controlled trials (RCTs). RCTs represent the gold standard for testing treatment effectiveness but are particularly difficult to organize because they require large sample sizes, tight control over exposure to related treatments, and an extended period of follow-up. Not surprisingly, most of the published research on treatment efficacy consists of uncontrolled case studies and case series. For a discussion of the ethical issues surrounding the treatment of patients with brain injury, including those with DOC, see the chapter by Fins et al.

Types of Treatment

Interventions available for individuals with DOC can be grouped into three broad categories: sensory stimulation, physical rehabilitation, and neuromodulation. Treatments that rely on *sensory stimulation (SS)* provide systematic exposure to a variety of environmental stimuli. The intent of SS is to improve arousal level and increase the frequency of purposeful behavior. Treatment interventions focus on systematically exposing the patient to unimodal (e.g., music therapy) or multimodal stimuli of varying intensity and duration. *Physical rehabilitation* strategies employ traditional rehabilitation techniques to promote physical health and prevent secondary complications. Interventions such as range of motion exercises, positioning schedules, bowel and bladder training, splinting, and casting for spasticity management fall within this category. *Neuromodulation* protocols are designed to promote recovery by directly altering the neurophysiologic substrate presumed to be responsible for mediating consciousness. Pharmacologic interventions, deep brain stimulation, and noninvasive brain stimulation techniques (i.e., repetitive magnetic stimulation) represent examples of neuromodulatory approaches. Table 32-3 provides an overview of the treatments described previously.

Treatment Efficacy

Treatment decisions should be guided by the strength of empirical evidence available for a particular intervention. As a direct consequence of the lack of prospective RCTs, most existing treatment efficacy studies have significant methodologic limitations that limit their interpretability and clinical application.

Research methods are often flawed and results are difficult to compare across studies. Diagnostic criteria are nonuniform, subject characteristics are inadequately reported, outcome measures are psychometrically weak or too insensitive to detect prognostically important changes over time, and there is significant variation in the frequency and duration of the treatments employed. Consequently, the existing base of evidence is insufficient to support empirically derived clinical practice guidelines. The interested reader is referred to the AAN Clinical Practice Guideline Process Manual available at http://www.aan.com/globals/axon/assets/3749.pdf for further information about evidence classification and corresponding recommendations for clinical practice. The following is a brief summary of the results of systematic reviews and representative studies from each treatment category.

Sensory Stimulation

Studies investigating the effectiveness of SS comprise primarily class III and IV evidence (96), such as case studies and retrospective data analyses (73–75,77,97,98). No class I prospective, RCTs have been completed. Prior systematic reviews (99,100) have demonstrated significant methodologic weaknesses including infrequent use of masking, inadequate subject and treatment descriptions, and insufficient information concerning the equivalence of the treatment and comparison groups. One class II RCT carried out by Johnson, Roethig-Johnston, and Richards (76) provided multimodal SS to 14 patients in coma or VS within 24 hours of injury. Biochemical and physiologic markers were monitored before

and after SS. On average, the treatment group received SS for 8 days and the placebo group was treated for 4 days. The authors reported that there was a significant stimulation effect noted between groups at 6 days postinjury on only one of six biochemical markers. No difference was noted in biochemical or physiologic measures between survivors and deceased subjects.

In view of the dearth of methodologically sound studies involving SS, definitive conclusions regarding the effectiveness of this type of intervention cannot be drawn. It is incumbent on clinicians to clearly elucidate to family members the high degree of clinical uncertainty associated with this form of treatment. To date, there have not been any published reports of harm associated with the use of SS.

Physical Management

Despite the universal acceptance and widespread use of physical management strategies employed to facilitate recovery of consciousness and function, no prospective RCTs have been conducted to date. Leong (78) completed an evidence-based review of the efficacy of traditional physical therapy interventions including prolonged muscle stretch, passive range of motion exercises, and serial casting as applied to pediatric patients in VS and MCS. Of the 17 studies identified, including three RCTs and three randomized crossover studies, none specifically enrolled patients in VS or MCS. Among those reviewed, many had methodologic weaknesses prompting the author to conclude that the available evidence for the effectiveness of treatments for spasticity and reduced range of motion was inconclusive.

Mackay et al. (79) completed a retrospective study to assess the effectiveness of an organized inpatient rehabilitation protocol on length of stay and cognitive outcome. Retrospective chart reviews were completed on 38 individuals with severe TBI (initial GCS of 3 to 8) consecutively discharged from an inpatient rehabilitation facility. Seventeen individuals received an aggressive, formal program of multidisciplinary rehabilitation during the acute hospitalization. Treatment methods were not specifically described but were designed to promote physical recovery and prevent complications. The 21 remaining individuals did not receive any formal rehabilitative treatment. There were no statistically significant differences between the two groups on injury severity, brainstem reflexes, associated injuries, or level of function on admission. Outcome data indicated that duration of coma and length of rehabilitation were approximately 66% shorter, discharge ratings on the Levels of Cognitive Functioning Scale (LCFS) (101) were significantly higher, and the percentage of home discharges was greater in the group that received the structured rehabilitation program. The generalizability of these findings is limited because they are based on a retrospective chart review and treatment interventions were unspecified.

Timmons et al. (80) evaluated the degree of functional improvement noted in 47 patients who received interventions designed to promote health maintenance. All patients were admitted to rehabilitation at LCFS levels II to III within 6 months of injury. Because none of the patients reportedly showed functional communication, all were presumably in VS or MCS. Treatment consisted of interventions aimed at improving "physiologic integrity" and preventing complications. Procedures were administered by nursing staff and included hygiene procedures, positioning protocols, range

TABLE 32-3 Overview of Treatment Interventions Used in Disorders of Consciousness

TYPE OF INTERVENTION	RATIONALE	METHOD	INTENDED OUTCOME	EFFICACY STUDIES
Sensory Stimulation				
Structured sensory stimulation	Information processing efficiency is dependent on proper calibration of stimulus intensity and response to threshold	Administration of multimodal sensory stimuli (e.g., auditory, visual, tactile, olfactory) titrated to existing sensory thresholds	Improve breadth and reliability of behavioral response repertoire	Hall et al. (73) Pierce et al. (74) Wood et al. (75) Johnson et al. (76) Formisano et al. (77)
Physical Rehabilitation				
Health maintenance and physical reconditioning maximize the likelihood and rate of recovery of spared neurologic functions	Implementation of range of motion exercises, positioning protocols, bowel/bladder schedules, skin care regimens, etc.	Prevention of aspiration, contractures, decubiti, malnourishment, heterotopic ossification, infection	Leong (78) Mackay et al. (79) Timmons et al. (80) Tanhehco and Kaplan (81)	
Neuromodulation				
Pharmacologic: Dopaminergic	Increasing dopamine release or blocking dopamine reuptake may potentiate damaged neurotransmitter systems responsible for mediating attention and intention	Administration of dopaminergic, agonist medications	Improve arousal (i.e., wakefulness), alertness (i.e., vigilance), and intention (i.e., behavioral initiation)	Martin and Whyte (82) Powell et al. (83) Passler and Riggs (84) Meythaler et al. (85) Schnakers et al. (69) Whyte et al. (86) Patrick et al. (87)
Pharmacologic: GABAergic	Modulation of spinal cord circuits or neural networks may mediate cortical structures involved in consciousness	Administration of GABAergic agonist medications orally or intrathecally	Improve arousal	Clauss and Nel (88) Brefel-Courbon et al. (89) Whyte and Myers (90) Sarà et al. (91)
Deep brain stimulation	Electrophysiologic stimulation of the thalamus or brainstem reticular system produces physiologic and behavioral changes associated with arousal	Chronic electrical stimulation of mesodiencephalic structures	Amelioration of arousal and/or cognitive deficits (e.g., neglect, memory disturbance) associated with disruption of thalamocortical circuits	Kanno et al. (92) Tsubokawa et al. (93) Yamamoto and Katayama (94) Schiff et al. (70)
Noninvasive brain stimulation	Electrophysiologic stimulation of the brain cortex or subcortical structures induces physiologic and behavioral changes associated with arousal	Administration of repetitive transcranial magnetic stimulation (rTMS)	Improvement of awareness of self and surroundings and amelioration of arousal and/or cognitive defects	Louise-Bender Pape et al. (95)

of movement, pulmonary care, and multisensory stimulation. By 12 months postinjury, 83% of the level III patients demonstrated functional improvement as compared to 31% of level II patients. Overall, 44% of the sample had regained functional communication, mobility, or were able to use an upper extremity to perform activities of daily living. The authors suggested that amount of treatment influenced outcome as patients who did not improve received fewer hours of treatment than those who did (15 vs 25 hours per week).

This relationship did not appear to be related to length of time postinjury; however, the authors did not consider spontaneous recovery as a possible cause of the improvements noted.

Two additional case study reports describe functional improvement following introduction of physical management strategies. Tanhehco and Kaplan (81) reported significant improvements in communication and self-care abilities in a 31-year-old woman with a 6-year history of eyes-closed coma resulting from a motor vehicle accident. The patient was admitted from a nursing home for inpatient rehabilitation after family members reportedly observed eye opening, accurate head nods, and occasional verbalizations. On admission, the patient was severely contracted with multiple decubiti, speech intelligibility was 10%–25%, and communication was compromised by vocal cord paralysis and limb contractures. Range of motion, stretching, serial casting, and surgical releases were performed to facilitate motor function while breath control and single syllable vocabulary exercises were implemented to increase communication ability. An exercise regimen was begun to increase strength and endurance. After approximately 6 months of treatment, the patient was discharged home. By 14 months, she was able to self-feed and groom with setup and could dress and transfer with moderate assistance. She was able to communicate bowel and bladder needs and rarely experienced incontinence. The decubiti healed and active range of movement improved enough to allow her to use her right upper extremity for pointing. This case is of interest given the late reemergence of consciousness and degree of functional recovery that occurred after physically based rehabilitation strategies were initiated at 6 years postinjury.

Neuromodulation

Neuromodulatory approaches to treatment of DOC seek to normalize the neurophysiologic disturbances that accompany severe brain injury. Although pharmacologic intervention is the most widely used form of neuromodulation, invasive and noninvasive brain stimulation techniques are receiving increasing attention as a means of modulating brain activity to improve functional capacity in this patient population.

Pharmacologic Interventions

Drug therapy has been used to improve arousal, promote behavioral initiation and persistence, stimulate speech, and reduce agitation in patients with DOC. The "workhorse" agents used in rehabilitation of individuals with disturbances in consciousness have historically included dopamine agonists such as methylphenidate (82), levodopa (102,103), bromocriptine (83,84), and amantadine (85,87). More recent investigations have focused on GABA agonists (e.g., zolpidem and baclofen) (88–91,104–107) and apomorphine (108).

There is some evidence that dopamine agonists are effective for improving arousal (i.e., wakefulness) and basic attentional functions (109). Significant improvements in behavioral initiation and response persistence have been noted following administration of bromocriptine (83,84) and amantadine (69,85–87). Recovery of spontaneous speech (110) and increases in verbal fluency (83) have also been tied to the use of bromocriptine in individuals diagnosed with MCS.

As with other therapies, data on the efficacy of pharmacologic intervention comes largely from case reports, case series, and a small number of cohort studies. There are few controlled medication trials in patients with DOC. Meythaler and colleagues (85) conducted a prospective, single-center randomized, controlled trial of amantadine hydrochloride (100 mg, bid) or placebo in 35 patients who were 1–6 weeks postinjury and had Disability Rating Scale (DRS) scores between 15 and 22. A crossover design was used in which half the group received amantadine first, followed by placebo,

whereas the other half received placebo first, followed by amantadine. Results indicated that cognitive and functional improvement was more rapid during the on-drug phase, regardless of whether subjects received AH or placebo first. At 3- and 6-month follow-up, there was no significant difference in DRS scores between treatment groups. Two important methodologic problems challenge the authors' conclusions, however. The group that received amantadine first was less severely disabled prior to treatment than the placebo group and may have achieved more favorable outcomes independent of treatment. Second, because a crossover design was used early in the course of recovery, the group that received amantadine first had improved substantially at the point of crossover, limiting their opportunity to improve to the same extent as the comparison group during the second phase of treatment. By the time the group treated with amantadine first reached crossover, the range of possible improvement on the DRS had narrowed from 15 points (during the active drug phase) to 5 points (during the placebo phase).

Patrick et al. (87) completed a randomized, double-blind study comparing the effectiveness of amantadine versus pramipexole, another dopamine agonist, in improving mental status in a group of 10 children who scored less than or equal to level III on the Rancho Los Amigos Scale at least 1 month after traumatic brain injury. The subjects, ranging in age from 8 to 21, were randomly assigned to either amantadine or pramipexole and were treated with escalating doses of the assigned drug for the first 4 weeks of the 8-week trial. They were then weaned from the drug for 2 weeks and monitored for the final 2 weeks. Performance on the DRS, Coma-Near Coma Scale (C-NCS), and Western Neurosensory Stimulation Profile was measured prior to, during, and after medication exposure. Significant improvements were seen on all three scales for both groups during the medication phase, with no further improvements during weaning. No between-group difference was observed in degree of improvement between amantadine and pramipexole. This study did not include a placebo arm, and many of the subjects were less than 2 months postinjury, raising the possibility that spontaneous improvement accounted for the improvements noted.

The effectiveness of several other dopaminergic agents has been explored in single and multiple case studies, few of which have incorporated robust controls. Passler and Riggs (84) investigated bromocriptine (2.5 mg, bid) in improving functional outcome in a series of five patients in VS. Bromocriptine was used in association with multidisciplinary rehabilitation interventions. The authors reported that physical and cognitive recovery at 12 months postinjury was greater in the bromocriptine-treated patients, relative to a group of historical controls. The strength of this study is limited by the small sample size, questionable comparability of the historical control group, and failure to adequately address the influence of spontaneous recovery on outcome. It should be noted that a number of studies have reported adverse behavioral and cognitive side effects associated with the use of dopaminergic agents, including agitation, perseveration (111), and exacerbation of neglect (112).

Fridman and colleagues (108) investigated the dopamine agonist apomorphine as a therapy for patients in VS or MCS. The study consisted of eight patients (VS = 6; MCS = 2) ranging in age from 22 to 41, all of whom were between 1 and 4 months post severe TBI. Apomorphine was administered with a continuous subcutaneous infusion pump 12–16 hours a day. Outcomes were measured with the Coma-Near Coma Scale and DRS. Prior to apomorphine administration, no patients demonstrated response to command. The authors reported that all patients recovered command following between 1 and 62 days after initiation of the medication and C-NCS scores fell to 0 after 1 year. These improvements were maintained after discontinuation of treatment. These findings cannot be confidently attributed to the study drug because all patients were well within the window for spontaneous recovery after severe TBI.

GABA agonists have received growing attention as a potential treatment for patients with DOC (88–91,104–107). Two particular GABA agonists—zolpidem, a selective omega-1 GABA agonist, and baclofen, a GABA-B receptor agonist—have been studied. In the most robust study conducted to date, Whyte and Myers (90) used a placebo-controlled, double-blind, crossover design to study the effects of zolpidem in 15 patients who were in VS or MCS for at least 1 month following traumatic or nontraumatic brain injury. All participants had a DRS score greater than 11 and lacked consistent command following and functional communication at enrollment. Zolpidem (10 mg administered through a feeding tube) or placebo was administered in blinded order on two different occasions, separated by 1–7 days. On each assessment day, CRS-R scores were recorded every hour for 5 hours following drug or placebo administration. Of the 15 patients enrolled in the study, one patient, who had been in a traumatic vegetative state for more than 4 years, transiently emerged from VS to MCS after administration of zolpidem and not placebo. The remaining fourteen patients did not show a significant difference in response. Additional published case reports describing the effects of zolpidem have shown conflicting results (104,106).

Intrathecal baclofen (ITB) has also been reported to promote recovery of consciousness in patients in VS and MCS (91,107). ITB has traditionally been used to treat muscle spasticity by promoting inhibitory GABAergic transmission. Unfortunately, existing published reports do not clearly characterize subjects' baseline functional status, making conclusive statements difficult. Sarà and colleagues (91) administered ITB to five patients who were in VS for 6–12 months following traumatic or nontraumatic brain injury. The patients were followed on the CRS-R for 6 months to assess changes in consciousness. Increases in sustained eye opening were documented in all five patients within the first 4 weeks, and variable improvements in alertness, visual pursuit, and verbal abilities were seen over the 6-month follow-up, as indicated by scores on the CRS-R. Sarà hypothesized that ITB may improve alertness and consciousness either by modulating spinal circuits or by entering the brain through cerebral spinal fluid. However, given the limited size of this sample and the paucity of data to establish a mechanistic link between baclofen and alterations in consciousness, these results require confirmation in a controlled trial.

Invasive and Noninvasive Brain Stimulation Approaches

In 2005, a study of the effectiveness of amantadine hydrochloride, funded by the National Institute on Disability and Rehabilitation Research, was launched. The primary aims of this study, the largest multicenter randomized controlled trial conducted to date in patients with DOC (i.e., eight rehabilitation centers in the United States and three in Europe), were to determine if functional improvement is

significantly more favorable on the DRS after 4 weeks of treatment with amantadine relative to placebo, and whether amantadine-induced improvements persist following drug washout (116). There were 184 patients with TBI, ages 16 to 65, in VS or MCS between 4 and 16 weeks post-injury enrolled and randomized to receive either amantadine, (staring does 200mg, increase up to 400mg/day weeks 3 and 4 if < 2 points change on DRS) or placebo for 4 weeks. Recovery was assessed with the DRS at weekly intervals before and during the 4 weeks of treatment and for 2 weeks after completion of treatment. CRS-R scores were measured at baseline, week 4 at treatment completion and week 6 after the 2 week washout period to characterize the quality of clinical changes. The amantadine treatment and placebo groups were well-matched on demographic characteristics and had equivalent baseline DRS and CRS-R scores. During the 4-week treatment period, the rate of recovery was significantly faster in the amantadine treatment group than in the placebo group, as measured by DRS scores (P = 0.007). The pace of recovery was faster in patients receiving amantadine whether in a vegetative state or in a minimally conscious state at the time of enrollment or whether enrolled earlier (28-70 days) or later (71-112 days) after injury. The rate of improvement in the amantadine group slowed significantly with respect to the placebo group (P = 0.02) during the 2 weeks after treatment but the functional gains of the amantadine treatment were maintained after treatment. There were no significant differences in the incidence of adverse events. A greater proportion of the group receiving amantadine recovered key behavioral benchmarks, including consistent command following, accurate response to yes/no questions, functional object use, and intelligible verbalization, as indicated by scores on the CRS-R. After 4 weeks of treatment only 18% of the amantadine group remained in a VS compared to 31% in the placebo group. The results support that amantadine is effective and safe in promoting more rapid functional recovery of clinically significant, functionally meaningful behaviors in patients with prolonged DOC after TBI. Additional study is required to determine if the benefit of amantadine is limited to a temporary improvement in rate of recovery or whether it promotes better outcome over the long-term.

Brain stimulation procedures include deep brain stimulation (DBS) of the thalamus and spinal cord and repetitive transcranial magnetic stimulation (rTMS) of the cortex. In DBS, electrical pulses are delivered through electrodes implanted in the spinal cord, brainstem, or thalamic structures in an effort to stimulate neurons within those structures. This technique is derived from experimental findings in animals showing behavioral and EEG arousal responses in response to stimulation of the reticular system (113).

A series of Japanese studies beginning in the 1980s have reported on the effects of DBS in patients diagnosed with VS. Kanno and colleagues (92) observed improvements in eye opening, emotional expressiveness, verbal command following, and communication ability in three of the four patients treated during the course of the trial. Tsubokawa and others (93) applied DBS to the mesencephalic reticular formation and nonspecific thalamic nuclei in eight patients (TBI = 4, vascular = 3, anoxia = 1) reportedly in VS for more than 6 months and recorded increases in arousal, vocalization, and movement of the extremities, coinciding with desynchronization of the EEG and marked increases in regional cerebral blood flow and metabolic markers. Yamamoto and Katayama (94) tracked 26 patients, including five in MCS, exposed to DBS between 3 and 6 months postinjury for 10 years from the time of initial exposure. In 19 of the 21 VS cases and in all of the MCS cases, DBS was administered to the thalamic central median-parafascicular complex. In the two remaining VS cases, DBS was administered to the mesencephalic reticular formation. The investigators reported that all five MCS patients showed improvements in communication and four were no longer confined to bed. Of the VS patients, all 21 reportedly showed increased arousal responses immediately after stimulation, with 8 of 21 emerging from VS, based on reemergence of command following or discernible gestural communication. Kanno and colleagues (114) reviewed the results of studies employing spinal cord stimulation completed over a 20-year period (n = 214) in patients who were reported to be in a persistent vegetative state. The spinal cord stimulator was implanted at the C2-C4 level and programmed to apply regular daytime stimulation in 15-minute on/15-minute off waves. The investigators reported improvements in orientation to self or surroundings in 109 patients as measured on an assessment scale devised by the authors.

It is important to note that all of the DBS studies described previously were compromised by significant methodologic flaws limiting their clinical applicability. Crude assessment and outcome measures were employed across studies, making it difficult to determine the accuracy of the patients' diagnoses as well as the nature and extent of the changes reported. Because some patients were early in the recovery course and important treatment controls were lacking, spontaneous recovery cannot be excluded to explain the improvements noted.

In 2000, Schiff, Rezai, and Plum (115) proposed a circuit model of DBS that identified carefully selected thalamic targets tied to downstream cortical fields. In this approach, specific subdivisions of the intralaminar nuclei of the thalamus were targeted for stimulation to facilitate activation of downregulated but still viable cortical areas responsible for mediating critical executive functions. This protocol was specifically developed for use with patients in MCS as this subgroup has greater potential to harness the effects of DBS through spared thalamocortical and corticocortical pathways.

In 2007, Schiff and coworkers (70) published the results of a 6-month, double-blind alternating crossover case study of a patient who had remained in MCS for more than 6 years following traumatic brain injury. DBS was applied bilaterally to the central thalamus, and stimulation was alternated on and off in 30-day periods for 6 months. The investigators found that DBS was associated with significant improvements in arousal, communication, and motor ability, as measured by scores on the CRS-R. These findings, although limited to a single case, demonstrated "proof of principle" that DBS can promote meaningful behavioral improvement well after the typical period of spontaneous recovery following TBI.

A single case study has been published to date describing the results of noninvasive brain stimulation techniques. Louise-Bender Pape (95) administered repetitive transcranial magnetic stimulation, or rTMS, to a 26-year-old patient who was in VS for 287 days following a traumatic brain injury. In rTMS, rapidly changing magnetic fields are used to induce electrophysiologic changes in specific areas of the brain.

Stimulation was applied over the right dorsolateral prefrontal cortex for a total of 30 sessions, 5 days a week, over 6 weeks. The authors reported that the patient began to verbalize single words and answer yes/no questions using an eyes-open/eyes-closed paradigm, and scores on the Disorders of Consciousness Scale (DOCS) showed a trend toward significance over time. The absence of treatment controls limits the interpretability of this study as the treatment was conducted within the window of spontaneous recovery.

There is a clear need for additional clinical trials of interventions designed to speed the pace of recovery from severe brain injury and improve functional outcome. Because relatively few rehabilitation centers offer services for patients with DOC, this can only be accomplished through multicenter collaborative studies.

PROGNOSIS

Prognosis for patients with DOC has been analyzed with respect to three main outcome areas: mortality, recovery of consciousness, and functional recovery. Outcome of VS and MCS are considered below but outcome information concerning MCS is more limited because it has more recently been operationally defined. It is not known if some patients who were labeled VS in outcome studies performed before 2002, when MCS diagnostic criteria were published, included some patients who would be diagnosed as MCS in more recent studies.

Mortality

According to the Multi-Society Task Force report in 1994, mortality is relatively high for patients in VS at least 1 month (82% at 3 years, and 95% at 5 years). Younger patients have a greater chance for survival (117). In a recent study of 51 patients admitted to an intensive care unit (ICU) who were either at a VS or MCS level after TBI or nontraumatic brain injury (non-TBI) at 1 year postinjury, mortality was 75% for 12 patients in VS and 35.9% for 36 patients in MCS followed for 5 years postinjury.

As would be expected, mortality rates are somewhat lower for patients with DOC who survive to rehabilitation admission. In a recent study of 50 patients admitted to rehabilitation who were in VS after TBI or non-TBI at 6 months postinjury, mortality was 42% at a mean follow-up of 25.7 months after onset (118). Mortality was 8% at a mean of 2.1 years postdischarge for a series 337 patients who were not following commands (based on DRS scores) on admission to 16 rehabilitation centers of the NIDRR TBI Model Systems Program (119). The lower mortality in this study compared to the previously noted study is predictable because the sample includes patients with DOC of shorter duration than 6 months.

Recovery of Consciousness

In 1994, the Multi-Society Task Force on PVS (18) analyzed all available reports on outcome of VS and summarized prognosis for recovery of consciousness (120). They used the term *persistent* vegetative state (PVS) to define those who remain unconscious for at least a month. The report included data on 434 adults and 106 children with TBI, and 169 adults and 45 children with non-TBI—primarily anoxic brain injury and stroke. Prognosis for recovery was substan-

TABLE 32-4 Prognosis and Functional Outcome According to the Glasgow Outcome Scale at 1 Year After Prolonged Unconsciousness in Adults With Traumatic Brain Injury (TBI) or Nontraumatic Brain Injury (Non-TBI)

TBI	NON-TBI
Unconscious at least 1 month:	
Death 33%	53%
VS 15%	32%
SD 28%	11%
MD 17%	3%
GR 7%	1%
Unconscious at least 3 months:	
Death 35%	46%
VS 30%	47%
SD 19%	6%
MD/GR 16%	1%
Unconscious at least 6 months:	
Death 32%	28%
VS 52%	72%
SD 12%	0%
MD/GR 4%	0%

VS, vegetative state; SD, severe disability; MD, moderate disability; GR, good recovery. From *N Engl J Med.* 1994;330(21):1499–1508.

tially better for victims of TBI than those with non-TBI. Of adults with traumatic brain injury who were unconscious at least 1 month, 33% recovered consciousness by 3 months postinjury, 46% by 6 months, and 52% by 1 year. Approximately 35% of patients with TBI who were still unconsciousness at 3 months regained consciousness by 1 year; if still unconscious for 6 months, 16% regained consciousness by 1 year. Of those adults with non-TBI unconscious for 1 month, only 11% recovered consciousness by 3 months and 15% by 6 months. No person with non-TBI regained consciousness after 6 months postinjury.

Prognosis in children was only slightly more favorable. For those children with TBI who were unconscious at 1 month, 51% regained consciousness by 6 months and up to 62% of children with TBI recovered consciousness at 1 year after injury. After non-TBI, recovery of consciousness occurred mainly within the first 3 months (11%), but a very small percentage (2%) regained consciousness between 6 and 12 months. Table 32-4 shows a summary of these outcome data.

The task force concluded that prognosis for recovery of consciousness was very poor 12 months after traumatic injuries and 3 months after non-TBI for both adults and children. They suggested the term *permanent vegetative state* for patients who were still unconscious beyond these intervals after injury. The Royal College of Physicians in the United Kingdom recommended deferring the diagnosis of permanent VS for at least 6 months in patients with non-TBI; however, this was based on consensus opinion. Although unlikely, the chance of recovering consciousness is not absolutely lost. There are several reports of later recovery of consciousness (18,121). Childs and Mercer (121) pointed out that there is insufficient evidence in the task force study or any other studies to predict the incidence of late improvement. In fact, using the limited number of cases followed beyond 12 months in the task force report, they recalculated

that the incidence of regaining consciousness after 12 months in that limited series of patients was 14%. Late recovery from VS is supported by a subsequent report of 50 patients with TBI and non-TBI (hemorrhagic stroke or anoxic brain injury) who were in VS for at least 6 months and followed for a mean of 25.7 months after injury (118). At latest follow-up, 42% of the sample died, 24% recovered to an MCS level, and 20% recovered to at least an MCS level after 12 months postinjury. It is noteworthy that of the 10 patients who recovered beyond a VS level after 12 months, four were patients with non-TBI (three with anoxia and one with hemorrhagic stroke). Six of these patients went on to emerge from MCS to a higher level of consciousness (four with TBI, two with non-TBI), all remaining at a severe to extremely severe level on the DRS (122) at latest follow-up. In another report that included 12 patients in VS at 1 year postinjury (2 with TBI and 10 with non-TBI) that were part of long-term follow-up of patients with DOC, none regained consciousness at 5 years postinjury (123). In the same study, patients in MCS at 1 year postinjury fared better. Of the 36 of 39 patients who were followed for 5 years, 14 died, 9 remained in MCS, and 13 emerged from MCS, remaining at the severe disability level on the Glasgow Outcome Scale (123). Among the 337 patients with DOC admitted to the NIDRR Model Systems centers, 8 patients regained the capacity to follow commands after 1 year postinjury (119). All of these reports of late recoveries suggest that the time frames designated by the Multi-Society Task Force for permanence should be reconsidered or that the term *permanent* should be avoided as a diagnostic label. The issue of life expectancy, key to life care planning, and medicolegal decision making after severe TBI is discussed in the chapter by Harrison-Felix et al.

Functional Outcome

The Multi-Society Task Force report described functional outcome using the Glasgow Outcome Scale. By 12 months postinjury, more than one-half of the patients were *severely disabled*, nearly one-third were *moderately disabled*, and a little more than an eighth achieved a *good recovery* level. Functional outcome was worse after nontraumatic injury; nearly three-quarters of those who regained consciousness were severely disabled at 12 months. Outcome for children was somewhat better at 12 months: one-half were severely disabled, whereas most of the remainder achieved a good recovery. Older adults (older than 40 years old) tended toward a worse functional outcome, rarely improving beyond the level of severe disability.

Functional outcome appears to be substantially better and faster for patients in MCS than those in VS when evaluated at a similar time postinjury. In a small series of patients with impaired consciousness followed for 4 months, Rappaport et al. (57) reported improvement in 25% of a small group of patients with impaired consciousness noting that only those in MCS (referred to as "near-coma") improved; none in VS improved in the follow-up period. Figure 32-2 depicts the results of a study conducted by Giacino and Kalmar (67) that investigated functional outcome on the DRS (122) across the first year postinjury in patients diagnosed with VS (n = 55) or MCS (n = 49). The VS and MCS groups were stratified further according to etiology: TBI = 70, non-TBI = 34. Although both diagnostic groups presented with similar levels of disability at 1 month postinjury, outcome was signifi-

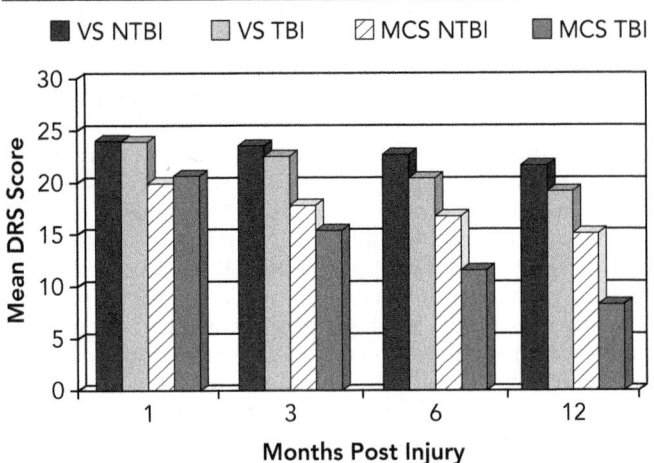

FIGURE 32-2 Comparison of mean DRS outcome scores between patients diagnosed with the vegetative and minimally conscious states at 1, 3, 6, and 12 months post-injury. From *J Head Trauma Rehabil.* 1997;12(4):42. Copyright 1997 by Aspen Publishers, Inc. Reprinted with permission.

cantly more favorable by 12 months in the MCS group, particularly after TBI. The differences in outcome became progressively more apparent at 3, 6, and 12 months postinjury. The probability of a more favorable outcome (moderate or no disability) by 1 year was much greater for the MCS group (38%) than the VS group (2%) and only occurred in those patients with TBI.

Lammi and colleagues (124) followed 18 patients in traumatic MCS for 2–5 years after discharge from an inpatient brain injury rehabilitation program located in Australia. The authors found that 15% of their sample had partial disability or less at follow-up, whereas 20% fell in the extremely severe to vegetative category. In comparison, Giacino and Kalmar reported that 23% of their sample had no more than partial disability at 12 months, with 17% classified as extremely severe to vegetative. In both samples, the most common outcome was moderate disability, which occurred in approximately 50% of patients. Of particular importance, Lammi et al. also noted that 50% of their sample had regained independence in activities of daily living.

In a consecutive series of 36 patients admitted to rehabilitation in VS (n = 11) or MCS (n = 25) after TBI (n = 22) or non-TBI (n = 14) and followed for 1–4 years postinjury, Katz et al. found that 72% emerged from MCS and 58% recovered further, clearing from the posttraumatic confusional state and amnesia (CS/PTA) (124,125). Patients admitted in VS took significantly longer than those admitted in MCS to emerge from MCS (mean 16.4 weeks for VS; 7.4 weeks for MCS) and to emerge from CS/PTA (mean 30.1 weeks for VS; 11.5 weeks for MCS). Patients who failed to clear CS/PTA at latest follow-up were either patients with non-TBI or those with VS lasting more than 8 weeks. Of those followed over 1 year, nearly half achieved household independence, 22% returned to work or school, 17% at or near preinjury levels.

A recent larger series of patients admitted to rehabilitation with a DOC at the NIDRR Model Systems centers and followed up to 5 years also demonstrated a substantial proportion of patients with more favorable functional outcome. Of the 396 patients, 68% regained consciousness and 23%

cleared CS/PTA, 21% were capable of living without in-house supervision, and 20% were employable based on DRS criteria.

All of these studies suggest a clear separation between MCS and VS in course of recovery and eventual functional outcome. Patients with TBI have better outcomes and a more prolonged trajectory of recovery than those with non-TBI. In those followed a year or more postinjury, a substantial proportion achieve household independence and some level of employability. These studies also show ongoing improvements in DRS scores that extend 2 years or more postinjury (119,125).

Outcome Prediction

Although the Multi-Society Task Force analysis and other studies have provided some general guidelines and probabilities for outcome after prolonged DOC, outcome prediction for individuals with prolonged unconsciousness is difficult at best. There have been a few studies that reported prediction models for patient with DOC. A multicenter study by Whyte and colleagues of 124 patients with severely impaired consciousness (VS or MCS) of 1 month or more after TBI examined a number of demographic, injury severity, functional, and neuroimaging variables to predict short-term outcome. Of all the variables tested, the best predictors in the outcome models for both recovery of consciousness (time to follow commands) and functional outcome at 4 months postinjury were time from injury to initial rehabilitation evaluation, initial functional level on the DRS, and the rate of early functional recovery on the DRS over the first 2 weeks (86). The same group evaluated short-term outcome at 13 weeks postinjury on the DRS and time to follow commands for a larger cohort of patients with DOC of 1 month or more that included non-TBI patients in addition to the previously reported TBI group (126). The prediction models included similar variables including time from injury to initial rehabilitation evaluation and initial functional level on the DRS for 13-week outcome on the DRS. Faster early rates of recovery on the DRS and initial DRS score were best variables in the model for predicting time to follow commands. Etiology, TBI versus non-TBI, was a significant variable in the model predicting for functional recovery on the DRS at 6 weeks but only approached significance in predicting DRS at 13 weeks. For longer term outcome, Katz et al. found that the functional independence measure (FIM) score at inpatient rehabilitation facility discharge along with age or duration of MCS along with age were best predictors of DRS scores at 1–4 years postinjury in the outcome models of 36 patients admitted to rehabilitation in VS or MCS after TBI or non-TBI (125). It was noteworthy in that study that the duration of time for injury to resolution of MCS was a significant predictor of the duration of CS/PTA after emergence from MCS, accounting for 57% of the variance.

A study by Fischer and others (123) demonstrated that if the cognitive-evoked potential was present in patients with prolonged coma, the patient did not remain in a vegetative state. In that study, the best predictors for regaining wakefulness, although not necessarily consciousness, after coma of various etiologies were the presence of a pupilary reflex, followed by the presence of late auditory-evoked potentials (N100) and middle latency–evoked potentials. A recent study demonstrated that the presence of increased complexity as reflected in nonlinear EEG parameters, referred to as approximate entropy, predicted survival and recovery from VS to MCS or higher levels of consciousness in a group of 38 patients in VS (127).

Structural neuroimaging (CT and MRI) has not been very helpful in prognosticating outcome of impaired unconsciousness but there are some correlates with worse outcome. Kamplf and colleagues (128) found that location of brain lesions after trauma was a better predictor of recovery from prolonged unconsciousness than GCS scores, age, and papillary abnormalities. Patients who did not recover consciousness by 12 months had a significantly higher frequency of corpus callosum, corona radiata, and dorsolateral brainstem lesions than those that did regain consciousness. These locations are not specific for unconsciousness but are correlates of more severe grades of diffuse axonal injury (129).

Functional MRI may have more value in predicting outcome in patients with impaired consciousness. In a group of 41 patients in VS or MCS after TBI or non-TBI, 2–122 months postinjury, fMRI activity indicating higher levels of auditory processing of sound and speech (from no response, to sound processing alone, to speech processing, to semantic processing) was predictive of better outcome on the CRS-R 6 months after the imaging (65). Assessments using combinations of newer structural imaging techniques, such as diffusion tensor imaging or arterial spin labeling (130); various functional imaging protocols; and electrophysiologic technologies offer promise to improve outcome prediction in the future. For further discussion of prognosis and outcomes in patients with impaired consciousness, see Outcome Prediction section of this text.

RECOMMENDATIONS FOR A RATIONAL APPROACH TO CLINICAL MANAGEMENT

In the absence of empirically established standards of care for clinical management of individuals with DOC, clinicians should adhere to a core set of basic tenets to guide evaluation and treatment of patients with DOC. In that spirit, the following recommendations are proposed, not as a prescriptive mandate, but rather, as a self-study reference for brain injury rehabilitation programs that offer services to this population.

Assessment Strategies

Carefully defined *admissions criteria* should be developed for patients with DOC seeking entry into an inpatient rehabilitation facility. This population has unique needs that may not be easily accommodated by traditional rehabilitative interventions. Specialized training is essential for staff members responsible for providing assessment and treatment services as few academic training programs directly address the care of patients with DOC. Diagnosis, cause of injury, length of time postonset, degree of medical stability, age, level of disability, and adequacy of support system are factors that should be considered in admission decisions as each may influence outcome. Creation of a local database is useful for monitoring these variables and may help identify admission and discharge trends, gauge program effectiveness, and facilitate longitudinal research.

A *comprehensive neuromedical workup* should be obtained on admission. This should include a complete review of the history, comprehensive physical examination, neurologic assessment, neuroimaging studies (if recent scans are una-

vailable), nutritional assessment, and review of current medications. Undetected or coexisting medical conditions such as posttraumatic epilepsy, hydrocephalus, late subdural hematoma, neuroendocrine dysfunction, nutritional deficiency, occult infection, and drug toxicity must be excluded as potential causes of underarousal and underresponsiveness (4).

A *well-defined assessment protocol* should be developed to monitor changes in neurologic, cognitive, physical, and functional status. Standardized measures of neurobehavioral responsiveness (55–58,60) and functional disability (122) should be used and supplemented with individualized assessment techniques (71) as needed. When conducting medication trials, treatment objectives should be operationally defined and objective measures employed to track progress. In most cases, patients should be serially reevaluated across the course of rehabilitation to detect fluctuations in level of responsiveness. Assessment frequency should be determined by the patient's rate of change. When possible, telephone follow-up should be conducted at 12 months to ascertain level of function and determine if additional assessment and treatment needs have surfaced since discharge.

There are no universally accepted criteria for determining when rehabilitative treatment should be discontinued. It is incumbent on individual programs to determine local decision-making criteria to assure consistency across patients. There are four clinical factors that should be considered in the decision to discontinue treatment (99). The first two, cause of injury and length of time post-onset, represent important determinants of outcome, particularly when they are used in combination. As discussed earlier, the probability of recovering from VS after 3 months is significantly higher following traumatic versus nontraumatic brain injury (18,67, 124). Current level of neurobehavioral responsiveness is a third factor that should be taken into account as there is compelling evidence that patients who retain at least partial awareness of self and environment experience more favorable outcomes (67,124,125). Response profiles dominated by reflexive brainstem activity offer little opportunity to promote higher order cognitive processing given the loss of cortical connectivity. The fourth factor, rate of recovery, is perhaps the most important variable. Prior studies suggest that evidence of ongoing change is a favorable predictor of functional outcome, even in patients who have not yet regained signs of consciousness (55,86). The specific weight that should be assigned to each factor has not yet been elucidated. Additional research is needed before algorithms can be developed to guide treatment discontinuation decisions.

Treatment Strategies

Physical management interventions (e.g., range of motion, positioning, hygiene) should be considered a standard component of the rehabilitation regimen of patients with DOC. Although it is unknown whether these interventions can facilitate the pace or degree of neurophysiologic recovery, there are strong rational indications for their use and little evidence that they are ineffective or unsafe. Steps should be taken to ensure that comfort is maintained and pain alleviated, particularly when intrusive medical and rehabilitative procedures are performed. Other interventions such as sensory stimulation and medication trials should be considered treatment *options* and should be construed as supplementary to the basic rehabilitative strategies described previously.

Special emphasis should be placed on using behavioral and pharmacologic strategies to promote arousal and facilitate neurogenic drive. Preserved cognitive function may be masked by deficiencies in these areas. Alternative or augmentative communication systems should be implemented in individuals diagnosed with MCS because sensory and neuromuscular impairments often accompany disturbances in consciousness (9,10). Assisted communication systems should not be incorporated into long-term care plans until there has been an adequate period of assessment in which response consistency and reliability have been demonstrated.

Finally, a formal protocol for providing family/surrogate education and training should be developed. An explicit mechanism for allowing ongoing communication between caretakers and the rehabilitation team across the span of treatment is a prerequisite for effective treatment. At a minimum, family conferences should be held shortly after admission and prior to discharge. The initial conference should include discussion of the preliminary assessment findings, particularly those that pertain to functional capacity and prognosis for further recovery. The treatment objectives recommended by the clinical team should be presented and integrated with the goals stipulated by the caretakers. Specific treatment methods should be outlined and accompanied by information regarding the efficacy of the proposed interventions and the anticipated outcome in each targeted area. A second meeting should be held prior to discharge to confirm or modify the initial diagnostic and prognostic impressions, to clarify recommendations for clinical management, and to establish a plan for follow-up assessment as indicated.

CONCLUSION

DOCs are among the most clinically daunting and scientifically challenging conditions in medicine. This is not surprising when one considers the fact that "consciousness" itself has not been adequately defined. Nonetheless, the last decade has been witness to remarkable neuroscientific discoveries and game-changing advances in technology. Terminology and diagnostic criteria have been carefully vetted but require further refinement to reduce diagnostic error. Functional neuroimaging has provided particularly exciting insights into the mechanisms underlying neurological deficits associated with DOC, although these efforts have yet to yield sufficiently robust findings to justify incorporation into clinical practice. A multimodal approach, combining information garnered from bedside examination and functional neuroimaging/electrophysiologic studies, is likely to become the norm. Current options for the treatment of DOC include sensory stimulation, physical rehabilitation, pharmacology, and invasive or noninvasive brain stimulation; however, existing evidence for effectiveness is inconclusive for most interventions due to weaknesses in methodology. Although outcome prediction remains challenging at the level of the individual patient, recent research demonstrates that meaningful recovery occurs after 12 months in a substantial minority of persons with prolonged DOC.

Future research should be directed toward (a) clarifying the natural history of recovery from VS and MCS, (b) identifying predictors of recovery of consciousness and function,

(c) elucidating the pathophysiology underlying specific DOC, (d) developing treatments capable of altering outcome in patients with DOC, and (e) tracking outcomes beyond 12 months postinjury. To accomplish these goals, it will be necessary to establish collaborative partnerships across rehabilitation centers and across disciplines. In the current health care climate, few rehabilitation centers can recruit patient samples large enough to carry out adequately powered clinical trials. In addition, most centers do not have ready access to neuroscientists, biophysicists, neurosurgeons, neurologists, and bioethicists, all of whom contribute uniquely to the study of patients with DOC.

KEY CLINICAL POINTS

1. Despite the existence of well-accepted diagnostic criteria for coma, VS, and MCS, rates of misdiagnosis have consistently remained at 30%–40%.

2. Functional neuroimaging studies have greatly improved our understanding of the neurophysiologic substrate underlying DOC. Residual cortical connectivity and the integrity of the default monitoring network appear to be linked to level of consciousness.

3. Although the availability of standardized neurobehavioral assessment procedures has improved the reliability and validity of bedside examination, recent evidence suggests high variability in the psychometric and clinical strength of specific measures.

4. There are currently no empirically based guidelines to govern the selection of pharmacologic, physical, behavioral, or electrophysiologic treatment interventions that are currently in clinical use. Two multicenter, randomized, controlled drug trials, one involving amantadine and the other zolpidem, are nearing completion and are expected to yield robust evidence for or against effectiveness.

5. Outcome studies suggest a clear separation between MCS and VS in course of recovery and eventual functional outcome. Additionally, patients with TBI have better outcomes and a more prolonged trajectory of recovery than those with nontraumatic injuries. Recently completed long-term outcome studies show ongoing functional improvements in both diagnostic subgroups that extend 2 years or more postinjury.

KEY REFERENCES

1. Nakase-Richardson R, Whyte J, Giacino JT, et al. Longitudinal outcome of patients with disordered consciousness in the NIDRR TBI Model Systems Programs. *J Neurotrauma.* 2012;29(1):59–65.

2. Newcombe VF, Williams GB, Scoffings D, et al. Aetiological differences in neuroanatomy of the vegetative state: insights from diffusion tensor imaging and functional implications. *J Neurol Neurosurg Psychiatry.* 2010;81(5):552–561.

3. Schnakers C, Vanhaudenhuyse A, Giacino J, et al. Diagnostic accuracy of the vegetative and minimally conscious

state: clinical consensus versus standardized neurobehavioral assessment. *BMC Neurol.* 2009;9:35.
4. Seel RT, Sherer M, Whyte J, et al. Assessment scales for disorders of consciousness: evidence-based recommendations for clinical practice and research. *Arch Phys Med Rehabil.* 2010;91(12):1795–1813.
5. Whyte J, Katz D, Long D, et al. Predictors of outcome in prolonged posttraumatic disorders of consciousness and assessment of medication effects: a multicenter study. *Arch Phys Med Rehabil.* 2005;86(3):453–462.

ACKNOWLEDGMENTS

The authors wish to thank Maria Brandao and Sara Midwood for their invaluable administrative and technical support in preparing this manuscript.

References

1. Practice parameters: assessment and management of patients in the persistent vegetative state (summary statement). The Quality Standards Subcommittee of the American Academy of Neurology. *Neurology.* 1995;45(5):1015–1018.
2. Recommendations for use of uniform nomenclature pertinent to patients with severe alterations in consciousness. American Congress of Rehabilitation Medicine. *Arch Phys Med Rehabil.* 1995;76(2): 205–209.
3. Andrews K. International Working Party on the Management of the Vegetative State: summary report. *Brain Inj.* 1996;10(11): 797–806.
4. Giacino JT, Ashwal S, Childs N, et al. The minimally conscious state: definition and diagnostic criteria. *Neurology.* 2002;58(3): 349–353.
5. The permanent vegetative state. Review by a working group convened by the Royal College of Physicians and endorsed by the Conference of Medical Royal Colleges and their faculties of the United Kingdom. *J R Coll Physicians London.* 1996;30(2):119–121.
6. French Society of Physical Medical and Rehabilitation. Adult head trauma in physical medicine and rehabilitation: coma vigil. Paper presented at: Consensus Conference; 2001; Bordeaux, France.
7. National Health and Medical Research Council. Post-coma unresponsiveness (vegetative state): a clinical framework for diagnosis. Canberra, Australia: Author; 2003.
8. Schnakers C, Vanhaudenhuyse A, Giacino J, et al. Diagnostic accuracy of the vegetative and minimally conscious state: clinical consensus versus standardized neurobehavioral assessment. *BMC Neurol.* 2009;9:35.
9. Andrews K, Murphy L, Munday R, Littlewood C. Misdiagnosis of the vegetative state: retrospective study in a rehabilitation unit. *BMJ.* 1996;313(7048):13–16.
10. Childs NL, Mercer WN, Childs HW. Accuracy of diagnosis of persistent vegetative state. *Neurology.* 1993;43(8):1465–1467.
11. Tresch DD, Sims FM, Duthie EH, Goldstein MD, Lane PS. Clinical characteristics of patients in the persistent vegetative state. *Arch Intern Med.* 1991;151(5):930–932.
12. Giacino JT, Kalmar K, Whyte J. The JFK Coma Recovery Scale-Revised: measurement characteristics and diagnostic utility. *Arch Phys Med Rehabil.* 2004;85(12):2020–2029.
13. Giacino JT, Schnakers C, Rodriguez-Moreno D, Kalmar K, Schiff N, Hirsch J. Behavioral assessment in patients with disorders of consciousness: gold standard or fool's gold? *Prog Brain Res.* 2009; 177:33–48.
14. Giacino JT, Zasler ND, Katz DI, Kelly JP, Rosenberg JH, Filley CM. Development of practice guidelines for assessment and management of the vegetative and minimally conscious states. *J Head Trauma Rehabil.* 1997;12(4):79–89.
15. Laureys S, Celesia GG, Cohadon F, et al; European Task Force on Disorders of Consciousness. Unresponsive wakefulness syndrome:

16. a new name for the vegetative state or apallic syndrome. *BMC Med.* 2010;8:68.
16. Plum F, Posner JB. *The Diagnosis of Stupor and Coma.* 3rd ed. Philadelphia, PA: F.A. Davis; 1982.
17. Jennett B, Plum F. Persistent vegetative state after brain damage. A syndrome in search of a name. *Lancet.* 1972;1(7753):734–737.
18. Medical aspects of the persistent vegetative state (1). The Multi-Society Task Force on PVS. *N Engl J Med.* 1994;330(21):1499–1508.
19. Choi SC, Barnes TY, Bullock R, Germanson TA, Marmarou A, Young HF. Temporal profile of outcomes in severe head injury. *J Neurosurg.* 1994;81(2):169–73.
20. Dubroja I, Valent S, Miklić P, Kesak D. Outcome of post-traumatic unawareness persisting for more than a month. *J Neurol Neurosurg Psychiatry.* 1995;58(4):465–466.
21. Jennett B, Adams JH, Murray LS, Graham DI. Neuropathology in vegetative and severely disabled patients after head injury. *Neurology.* 2001;56(4):486–490.
22. Nakase-Richardson R, Yablon SA, Sherer M, Evans CC, Nick TG. Serial yes/no reliability after traumatic brain injury: implications regarding the operational criteria for emergence from the minimally conscious state. *J Neurol Neurosurg Psychiatry.* 2008;79(2): 216–218.
23. Adams JH, Graham DI, Jennett B. The neuropathology of the vegetative state after an acute brain insult. *Brain.* 2000;123(pt 7): 1327–1338.
24. Laureys S, Owen AM, Schiff ND. Brain function in coma, vegetative state, and related disorders. *Lancet Neurol.* 2004;3(9):537–546.
25. Logothetis NK. The neural basis of the blood-oxygen-level-dependent functional magnetic resonance imaging signal. *Philos Trans R Soc Lond B Biol Sci.* 2002;357(1424):1003–1037.
26. Eidelberg D, Moeller JR, Kazumata K, et al. Metabolic correlates of pallidal neuronal activity in Parkinson's disease. *Brain.* 1997; 120(pt 8):1315–1324.
27. Smith AJ, Blumenfeld H, Behar KL, Rothman DL, Shulman RG, Hyder F. Cerebral energetics and spiking frequency: the neurophysiological basis of fMRI. *Proc Natl Acad Sci U S A.* 2002;99(16): 10765–10770.
28. Levy DE, Sidtis JJ, Rottenberg DA, et al. Differences in cerebral blood flow and glucose utilization in vegetative versus locked-in patients. *Ann Neurol.* 1987;22(6):673–682.
29. DeVolder AG, Goffinet AM, Bol A, Michel C, de Barsy T, Laterre C. Brain glucose metabolism in postanoxic syndrome. Positron emission tomographic study. *Arch Neurol.* 1990;47(2):197–204.
30. Rudolf J, Ghaemi M, Ghaemi M, Haupt WF, Szelies B, Heiss WD. Cerebral glucose metabolism in acute and persistent vegetative state. *J Neurosurg Anesthesiol.* 1999;11(1):17–24.
31. Schiff N, Ribary U, Plum F, Llinás R. Words without mind. *J Cogn Neurosci.* 1999;11(6):650–656.
32. Schiff ND, Ribary U, Moreno DR, et al. Residual cerebral activity and behavioural fragments can remain in the persistently vegetative brain. *Brain.* 2002;125(pt 6):1210–1234.
33. Soddu A, Boly M, Nir Y, et al. Reaching across the abyss: recent advances in functional magnetic resonance imaging and their potential relevance to disorders of consciousness. *Prog Brain Res.* 2009; 177:261–274.
34. Vanhaudenhuyse A, Demertzi A, Schabus M, et al. Two distinct neuronal networks mediate the awareness of enviroment and of self. *J Cogn Neurosci.* 2011;23(3):570–578.
35. Vanhaudenhuyse A, Noirhomme Q, Tshibanda LJ, et al. Default network connectivity reflects the level of consciousness in noncommunicative brain-damaged patients. *Brain.* 2010;133(pt 1): 161–171.
36. Phillips CL, Bruno M, Maquet P, et al. "Relevance vector machine" consciousness classifier applied to cerebral metabolism of vegetative and locked-in patients. *Neuroimage.* 2011;56(2):797–808.
37. Laureys S, Goldman S, Phillips C, et al. Impaired effective cortical connectivity in vegetative state: preliminary investigation using PET. *Neuroimage.* 1999;9(4):377–382.
38. Laureys S, Faymonville ME, Degueldre C, et al. Auditory processing in the vegetative state. *Brain.* 2000;123(pt 8):1589–1601.

39. Laureys S, Faymonville ME, Peigneux P, et al. Cortical processing of noxious somatosensory stimuli in the persistent vegetative state. *Neuroimage.* 2002;17(2):732–741.

40. Menon DK, Owen AM, Williams EJ, et al. Cortical processing in persistent vegetative state: Wolfson Brain Imaging Center Team. *Lancet.* 1998;352(9153):200.

41. Schiff ND, Plum F. Cortical function in the persistent vegetative state. *Trends Cogn Sci.* 1999;3(2):43–44.

42. Boly M, Faymonville ME, Peigneux P, et al. Auditory processing in severely brain injured patients: differences between the minimally conscious state and the persistent vegetative state. *Arch Neurol.* 2004;61(2):233–238.

43. Schiff ND, Rodriguez-Moreno D, Kamal A, et al. fMRI reveals large-scale network activation in minimally conscious patients. *Neurology.* 2005;64(3):514–523.

44. Boly M, Faymonville ME, Schnakers C, et al. Perception of pain in the minimally conscious state with PET activation: an observational study. *Lancet Neurol.* 2008;7(11):1013–1020.

45. Bekinschtein T, Leiguarda R, Armony J, et al. Emotion processing in the minimally conscious state. *J Neurol Neurosurg Psychiatry.* 2004;75(5):788.

46. Owen AM, Coleman MR, Boly M, Davis MH, Laureys S, Pickard JD. Detecting awareness in the vegetative state. *Science.* 2006; 313(5792):1402.

47. Monti MM, Vanhaudenhuyse A, Coleman MR, et al. Willful modulation of brain activity in disorders of consciousness. *N Engl J Med.* 2010;362(7):579–589.

48. Bekinschtein TA, Manes FF, Villarreal M, Owen AM, Della-Maggiore V. Functional imaging reveals movement preparatory activity in the vegetative state. *Front Hum Neurosci.* 2011;27(5):5.

49. Bardin JC, Fins JJ, Katz DI, et al. Dissociations between behavioural and functional magnetic resonance imaging-based evaluations of cognitive function after brain injury. *Brain.* 2011;134(pt 3):769–782.

50. Rodriguez-Moreno D, Schiff ND, Giacino J, Kalmar K, Hirsch J. A network approach to assessing cognition in disorders of consciousness. *Neurology.* 2010;75(21):1871–1878.

51. Goldfine AM, Victor JD, Conte MM, Bardin JC, Schiff ND. Determination of awareness in patients with severe brain injury using EEG power spectral analysis. *Clin Neurophysiol.* 2011;122(11):2157–2168.

52. Schnakers C, Perrin F, Schabus M, et al. Voluntary brain processing in disorders of consciousness. *Neurology.* 2008;71(20):1614–1620.

53. Jennett B, Teasdale G. Aspects of coma after severe head injury. *Lancet.* 1977;1(8017):878–881.

54. Schnakers C, Chatelle C, Vanhaudenhuyse A, et al. The Nociception Coma Scale: a new tool to assess nociception in disorders of consciousness. *Pain.* 2010;148(2):215–219.

55. Giacino JT, Kezmarsky MA, DeLuca J, Cicerone KD. Monitoring rate of recovery to predict outcome in minimally responsive patients. *Arch Phys Med Rehabil.* 1991;72(11):897–901.

56. Ansell BJ, Keenan JE. The Western Neuro Sensory Stimulation Profile: a tool for assessing slow-to-recover head-injured patients. *Arch Phys Med Rehabil.* 1989;70(2):104–108.

57. Rappaport M, Dougherty AM, Kelting DL. Evaluation of coma and vegetative states. *Arch Phys Med Rehabil.* 1992;73(7):628–634.

58. Gill-Thwaites H, Munday R. The Sensory Modality Assessment Rehabilitation Technique (SMART): a valid and reliable assessment for the vegetative and minimally conscious state patient. *Brain Injury.* 2004;18(12):1255–1269.

59. Horn S, Watson M, Wilson BA, McLellan DL. The development of new techniques in the assessment and monitoring of recovery from severe head injury: a preliminary report and case history. *Brain Inj.* 1992;6(4):321–325.

60. O'Dell MW, Jasin P, Lyons N, Stivers M, Meszaro F. Standardized assessment instruments for minimally-responsive, brain-injured patients. *NeuroRehabil.* 1996;6:45–55.

61. Seel RT, Sherer M, Whyte J, et al. Assessment scales for disorders of consciousness: evidence-based recommendations for clinical practice and research. *Arch Phys Med Rehabil.* 2010;91(12):1795–1813.

62. Wilde EA, Whiteneck GG, Bogner J, et al. Recommendations for use of common outcome measures in traumatic brain injury research. *Arch Phys Med Rehabil.* 2010;91(11):1650–1660.

63. Schnakers C, Majerus S, Giacino J, et al. A French validation study of the Coma Recovery Scale-Revised (CRS-R). *Brain Inj.* 2008;22(10):786–792.

64. Smart CM, Giacino JT, Cullen T, et al. A case of locked-in syndrome complicated by central deafness. *Nat Clin Pract Neurol.* 2008;4(8):448–453.

65. Coleman MR, Davis MH, Rodd JM, et al. Towards the routine use of brain imaging to aid the clinical diagnosis of disorders of consciousness. *Brain.* 2009;132(pt 9):2541–2552.

66. Newcombe VF, Williams GB, Scoffings D, et al. Aetiological differences in neuroanatomy of the vegetative state: insights from diffusion tensor imaging and functional implications. *J Neurol Neurosurg Psychiatry.* 2010;81(5):552–561.

67. Giacino JT, Kalmar K. The vegetative and minimally conscious states: a comparison of clinical features and functional outcome. *J Head Trauma Rehabil.* 1997;12(4):36–51.

68. Vanhaudenhuyse A, Schnakers C, Brédart S, Laureys S. Assessment of visual pursuit in post-comatose states: use a mirror. *J Neurol Neurosurg Psychiatry.* 2008;79(2):223.

69. Schnakers C, Hustinx R, Vandewalle G, et al. Measuring the effect of amantadine in chronic anoxic minimally conscious state. *J Neurol Neurosurg Psychiatry.* 2008;79(2):225–227.

70. Schiff ND, Giacino JT, Kalmar K, et al. Behavioural improvements with thalamic stimulation after severe traumatic brain injury. *Nature.* 2007;448(7153):600–603.

71. DiPasquale MC, Whyte J. The use of quantitative data in treatment planning for minimally conscious patients. *J Head Trauma Rehabil.* 1996;11(6):9–17.

72. Whyte J, Laborde A, DiPasquale MC. Assessment and treatment of the vegetative and minimally conscious patient. In: Rosenthal M, Griffith E, Kreutzer J, Pentland B, eds. *Rehabilitation of the Adult and Child with Traumatic Brain Injury.* 3rd ed. Philadelphia, PA: F.A. Davis; 1999:435.

73. Hall ME, MacDonald S, Young GC. The effectiveness of directed multisensory stimulation versus non-directed stimulation in comatose CHI patients: pilot study of a single subject design. *Brain Inj.* 1992;6(5):435–445.

74. Pierce JP, Lyle DM, Quine S, Evans NJ, Morris J, Fearnside MR. The effectiveness of coma arousal intervention. *Brain Inj.* 1990;4(2):191–197.

75. Wood RL, Winkowski TB, Miller JL, Tierney L, Goldman L. Evaluating sensory regulation as a method to improve awareness in patients with altered states of consciousness: a pilot study. *Brain Inj.* 1992;6(5):411–418.

76. Johnson DA, Roethig-Johnston K, Richards D. Biochemical and physiological parameters of recovery in acute severe head injury: responses to multisensory stimulation. *Brain Inj.* 1993;7(6):491–499.

77. Formisano R, Vinicola V, Penta F, Matteis M, Brunelli S, Weckel JW. Active music therapy in the rehabilitation of severe brain injured patients during coma recovery. *Ann Ist Super Sanita.* 2001;37(4):627–630.

78. Leong B. The vegetative and minimally conscious states in children: spasticity, muscle contracture and issues for physiotherapy treatment. *Brain Inj.* 2002;16(3):217–230.

79. Mackay LE, Bernstein BA, Chapman PE, Morgan AS, Milazzo LS. Early intervention in severe head injury: long-term benefits of a formalized program. *Arch Phys Med Rehabil.* 1992;73(7):635–641.

80. Timmons M, Gasquoine L, Scibak JW. Functional changes with rehabilitation of very severe traumatic brain injury survivors. *J Head Trauma Rehabil.* 1987;2(3):64–67.

81. Tanhehco J, Kaplan PE. Physical and surgical examination of patient after 6-year coma. *Arch Phys Med Rehabil.* 1982;63(1):36–38.

82. Martin RT, Whyte J. The effects of methylphenidate on command following and yes/no communication in persons with severe disorders of consciousness: a meta-analysis of n-of-1 studies. *Am J Phys Med Rehabil.* 2007;86(8):613–620.

83. Powell JH, al-Adawi S, Morgan J, Greenwood RJ. Motivational deficits after brain injury: effects of bromocriptine in 11 patients. *J Neurol Neurosurg Psychiatry.* 1996;60(4):416–421.

84. Passler MA, Riggs RV. Positive outcomes in traumatic brain injury-vegetative state: patients treated with bromocriptine. *Arch Phys Med Rehabil.* 2001;82(3):311–315.

85. Meythaler JM, Brunner RC, Johnson A, Novack TA. Amantadine to improve neurorecovery in traumatic brain injury-associated diffuse axonal injury: a pilot double-blind randomized trial. *J Head Trauma Rehabil.* 2002;17(4):300–313.

86. Whyte J, Katz D, Long D, et al. Predictors of outcome in prolonged posttraumatic disorders of consciousness and assessment of medication effects: a multicenter study. *Arch Phys Med Rehabil.* 2005; 86(3):453–462.

87. Patrick PD, Blackman JA, Mabry JL, Buck ML, Gurka MJ, Conaway MR. Dopamine agonist therapy in low-response children following traumatic brain injury. *J Child Neurol.* 2006;21(10):879–885.

88. Clauss R, Nel W. Drug induced arousal from the permanent vegetative state. *NeuroRehabilitation.* 2006;21(1):23–28.

89. Brefel-Courbon C, Payoux P, Ory F, et al. Clinical and imaging evidence of zolpidem effect in hypoxic encephalopathy. *Ann Neurol.* 2007;62(1):102–105.

90. Whyte J, Myers R. Incidence of clinically significant responses to zolpidem among patients with disorders of consciousness: a preliminary placebo controlled trial. *Am J Phys Med Rehabil.* 2009;88(5): 410–418.

91. Sarà M, Pistoia F, Mura E, Onorati P, Govoni S. Intrathecal baclofen in patients with persistent vegetative state: 2 hypotheses. *Arch Phys Med Rehabil.* 2009;90(7):1245–1249.

92. Kanno T, Kamei Y, Yokoyama T, Jain VK. Neurostimulation for patients in vegetative status. *Pacing Clin Electrophysiol.* 1987;10(1 pt 2):207–208.

93. Tsubokawa T, Yamamoto T, Katayama Y, Hirayama T, Maejima S, Moriya T. Deep-brain stimulation in a persistent vegetative state: follow-up results and criteria for selection of candidates. *Brain Inj.* 1990;4(4):315–327.

94. Yamamoto T, Katayama Y. Deep brain stimulation therapy for the vegetative state. *Neuropsychol Rehabil.* 2005;15(3–4):406–413.

95. Louise-Bender Pape T, Rosenow J, Lewis G, et al. Repetitive transcranial magnetic stimulation-associated neurobehavioral gains during coma recovery. *Brain Stimul.* 2009;2(1):22–35.

96. Woolf SH. Practice guidelines, a new reality in medicine. II. Methods of developing guidelines. *Arch Intern Med.* 1992;152(5):946–952.

97. Wilson SL, Powell GE, Elliott K, Thwaites H. Sensory stimulation in prolonged coma: four single case studies. *Brain Inj.* 1991;4(5): 393–400.

98. Wilson SL, Powell GE, Brock D, Thwaites H. Vegetative state and responses to sensory stimulation: an analysis of 24 cases. *Brain Inj.* 1996;10(11):807–818.

99. Giacino JT. Sensory stimulation: theoretical perspectives and the evidence for effectiveness. *NeuroRehabil.* 1996;6(1):69–78.

100. Lombardi F, Taricco M, De Tanti A, Telaro E, Liberati A. Sensory stimulation for brain injured individuals in coma or vegetative state. *Cochrane Database Syst Rev.* 2002;(2):CD001427.

101. Hagen C, Malkmus D, Durham P. Levels of cognitive function. In: *Rehabilitation of the Head-Injured Adult: Comprehensive Physical Management.* Downey, CA: Professional Staff Association of Rancho Los Amigos Hospital; 1979.

102. Matsuda W, Komatsu Y, Yanaka K, Matsumura A. Levodopa treatment for patients in persistent vegetative or minimally conscious states. *Neuropsychol Rehabil.* 2005;15(3–4):414–427.

103. Koeda T, Takeshita K. A case report of remarkable improvement of motor disturbances with L-dopa in a patient with post-diffuse axonal injury. *Brain Dev.* 1998;20(2):124–126.

104. Shames JL, Ring H. Transient reversal of anoxic brain injury-related minimally conscious state after zolpidem administration: a case report. *Arch Phys Med Rehabil.* 2008;89(2):386–388.

105. Cohen SI, Duong TT. Increased arousal in a patient with anoxic brain injury after administration of zolpidem. *Am J Phys Med Rehabil.* 2008;87(3):229–231.

106. Singh R, McDonald C, Dawson K, et al. Zolpidem in a minimally conscious state. *Brain Inj.* 2008;22(1):103–106.

107. Taira T. Intrathecal administration of GABA agonists in the vegetative state. *Prog Brain Res.* 2009;177:317–328.

108. Fridman EA, Krimchansky BZ, Bonetto M, et al. Continuous subcu-

taneous apomorphine for severe disorders of consciousness after traumatic brain injury. *Brain Inj.* 2010;24(4):636–641.

109. Whyte J. Neurologic disorders of attention and arousal: assessment and treatment. *Arch Phys Med Rehabil.* 1992;73(11):1094–1103.

110. Ross ED, Stewart, RM. Akinetic mutism from hypothalamic damage: successful treatment with dopamine agonists. *Neurology.* 1981; 31(11):1435–1439.

111. Giacino JT, Rodriguez M, Cicerone KD. Exacerbation of frontal release behaviors with use of amantadine following traumatic brain injury [abstract]. *Arch Phys Med Rehabil.* 1992;73:975.

112. Barrett AM, Crucian GP, Schwartz RL, Heilman KM. Adverse effect of dopamine agonist therapy in a patient with motor-intentional neglect. *Arch Phys Med Rehabil.* 1999;80(5):600–603.

113. Moruzzi G, Magoun HW. Brain stem reticular formation and activation of the EEG. *Electroencephalogr Clin Neurophysiol.* 1949;1(4): 455–473.

114. Kanno T, Morita I, Yamaguchi S, et al. Dorsal column stimulation in persistent vegetative state. *Neuromodulation.* 2009;12(1):33–38.

115. Schiff ND, Rezai AR, Plum F. A neuromodulation strategy for rational therapy of complex brain injury states. *Neurol Res.* 2000;22(3): 267–272.

116. Giacino JT, Whyte J, Bagiella E, Kalmar K, Childs N, Khademi A, Eifert B, Long D, Katz DI, Cho S, Yablon SA, Luther M, Hammond FM, Nordenbo A, Novak A, Mercer W, Maurer-Karattup P, Sherer M. Placebo-Controlled Trial of Amantadine for Severe Traumatic Brain Injury. *N Engl J Med.* 2012;366:819–826.

117. Strauss DJ, Shavelle RM, Ashwal A. Life expectancy and median survival time in the permanent vegetative state. *Pediatr Neurol.* 1999;21(3):626–631.

118. Estraneo A, Moretta P, Loreto V, Lanzillo B, Santoro L, Trojano L. Late recovery after traumatic, anoxic, or hemorrhagic long-lasting vegetative state. *Neurology.* 2010;75(3):239–245.

119. Nakase-Richardson R, Whyte J, Giacino JT, et al. Longitudinal outcome of patients with disordered consciousness in the NIDRR TBI Model Systems Programs. *J Neurotrauma.* 2011;29(1):59–65.

120. Jennett B, Bond M. Assessment of outcome after severe brain damage: a practical scale. *Lancet.* 1975;1(7905):480–484.

121. Childs NL, Mercer WN. Brief report: late improvement in consciousness after post-traumatic vegetative state. *N Engl J Med.* 1996; 334(1):24–25.

122. Rappaport M, Hall KM, Hopkins K, Belleza T, Cope DN. Disability rating scale for severe head trauma: coma to community. *Arch Phys Med Rehabil.* 1982;63(3):118–123.

123. Fischer C, Luauté J, Adeleine P, Morlet D. Predictive value of sensory and cognitive evoked potentials for awakening from coma. *Neurology.* 2004;63(4):669–673.

124. Lammi MH, Smith VH, Tate RL, Taylor CM. The minimally conscious state and recovery potential: a follow-up study 2 to 5 years after traumatic brain injury. *Arch Phys Med Rehabil.* 2005;86(4): 746–754.

125. Katz DI, Polyak M, Coughlan D, Nichols M, Roche A. Natural history of recovery from brain injury after prolonged disorders of consciousness: outcome of patients admitted to inpatient rehabilitation with 1–4 year follow-up. *Prog Brain Res.* 2009;177:73–88.

126. Whyte J, Gosseries O, Chervoneva I, et al. Predictors of short-term outcome in brain-injured patients with disorders of consciousness. *Prog Brain Res.* 2009;177:63–72.

127. Sarà M, Pistoia F, Pasqualetti P, Sebastiano F, Onorati P, Rossini PM. Functional isolation within the cerebral cortex in the vegetative state: a nonlinear method to predict clinical outcomes. *Neurorehabil Neural Repair.* 2011;25(1):35–42.

128. Kampfl A, Schmutzhard E, Franz G, et al. Prediction of recovery from post-traumatic vegetative state with cerebral magnetic-resonance imaging. *Lancet.* 1998;351(9118):1763–1767.

129. Adams JH, Doyle D, Ford I, Gennarelli TA, Graham DI, McLellan DR. Diffuse axonal injury in head injury: definition, diagnosis and grading. *Histopathology.* 1989;15(1):49–59.

130. Liu AA, Voss HU, Dyke JP, Heier LA, Schiff ND. Arterial spin labeling and altered cerebral blood flow patterns in the minimally conscious state. *Neurology.* 2011;77(16):1518–1523.

Military Traumatic Brain Injury: Special Considerations

Kimberly S. Meyer, Michael S. Jaffee, and Jamie Grimes

INTRODUCTION

Traumatic brain injury (TBI) is one of the hallmark injuries stemming from the current conflicts in Afghanistan (Operation Enduring Freedom [OEF]) and Iraq (Operation Iraqi Freedom [OIF]). TBI ranges in severity from mild to severe or penetrating. Combat-related TBI is most often mild in nature (see also Chapter 29, MTBI). Concussion or mild TBI (MTBI) may be overlooked in those without external evidence of trauma. In contrast, it may also be underrecognized in patients with polytrauma with more significant or life-threatening injuries (1). Since the initiation of military surveillance efforts in 2009, 229,108 service members have been diagnosed with TBI (2). More than 82% of these injuries are categorized as mild or concussive injury (Figure 33-1)(2,3).

The context of military TBI requires additional considerations, including mechanism(s) of injury, a population-centered approach to screening, complicating comorbidities of other physical injuries and psychological stress reactions, and return-to-duty considerations.

VARIANCES BETWEEN CIVILIAN AND COMBAT-RELATED TRAUMATIC BRAIN INJURY

In the United States, civilian TBI is largely attributable to blunt trauma, with falls and motor vehicle collisions comprising most acceleration–deceleration type injuries (4) (see Chapter 10, Biomechanics). Rarely is the general population affected by blast injury; the most notable in recent US history occurring in the Oklahoma City bombing, where 56% of survivors sustained injuries to the head (5). Because of civil unrest, civilians in countries such as Gaza/Israel, Libya, Sudan, and others are at higher risk for blast-related injury (6). However, combat-related brain injury is frequently associated with blast injury and in many cases, a combination of blast and blunt trauma.

Although most civilian injuries occur during relatively homeostatic conditions, combatants are likely to be under some degree of physiologic stress at the time of injury. Temperature extremes, dehydration, fatigue, chronic cortisol elevations, and other factors may impact tolerance from otherwise minor injuries (7). It is unclear the impact factors such as these have on symptom reporting and recovery after TBI.

Because of the nature of war, combatants are also under variable degrees of psychological stress at the time of injury. Resilience training is aimed at minimizing the effects of psychological stress on overall function and recovery from injury. Although fear and anxiety can precede injury, acute stress reaction and post-traumatic stress disorder (PTSD) may follow, especially in those sustaining TBI (8,9). These psychological comorbidities can provide a diagnostic challenge given the overlap of symptoms between TBI and PTSD. In addition, the presence of comorbidities may complicate TBI management. Brenner et al. (10) recently demonstrated that patients who had both TBI and PTSD reported more symptoms than patients who had TBI without PTSD or patients who had PTSD without TBI.

Another factor complicating the evaluation and management of combat-related TBI is that it may coexist in the setting of other injuries or polytrauma. In cases of life- or limb-threatening injuries such as amputations or burns, concussion may not be immediately identified. This situation requires coordination of TBI rehabilitation and care with that of other associated injuries.

MECHANISMS OF INJURY

Blast is thought to cause bodily injury by 4 main mechanisms. Primary injury is generally postulated to result directly from rapid pressure changes caused by the blast wave and most commonly affects organs with air-fluid interfaces (11,12). Recent research has led to additional theories that further explain the pathophysiology of primary blast injury and how the energy is transmitted to the brain. Some findings have suggested that the effects of a blast are transmitted to the brain via great vessels in the thorax (13). Advanced computer modeling of the blast-brain interface has suggested that the transmission is more direct through orifices in the cranium, such as the eyes and ears (14). Experimental primary brain injury results in abnormalities in the corpus callosum, hippocampus, cerebellum, brainstem, and axonal tracts (11,15,16). More recently, animal models have indicated that injury may also be attributed to electromagnetic changes following the blast (17).

Other mechanisms of blast-related injury involve a more direct physical force. Secondary injury occurs when debris set in motion by kinetic energy from the blast strikes the body, usually causing localized trauma. Tertiary injury re-

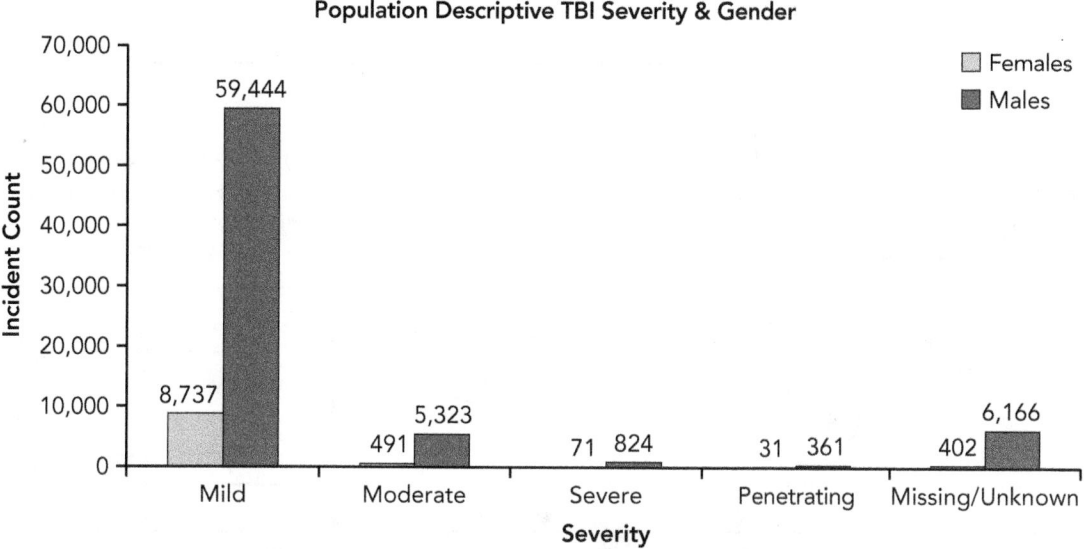

FIGURE 33–1 Traumatic brain injury severity and gender distribution.

sults when the body is displaced, striking a surface that can cause injury. Finally, quaternary injury results from other mechanisms, including toxic inhalation, radiation, and other similar factors (12,18,19).

Injury may result from 1 or more blast-related mechanisms. In addition, blast injury may cooccur with blunt trauma, commonly referred to as "blast +" mechanism. Passengers in a vehicle struck by an improvised explosive device (IED), which came to an abrupt halt in the crater formed by the explosion, would be at risk for "blast+" mechanism of injury. Those subjected to blast injury are more likely to sustain injuries to other body systems, including the extremities and the spine (3).

Current protective gear largely protects the head from penetrating injury. However, exposed areas of the face may allow shrapnel and other objects entry to the cranial vault, leading to penetrating TBI. Penetrating TBI is generally quickly recognized and treated. Prevention of penetrating injury is of high importance because this injury pattern carries a higher risk for long-term complications, including seizures (see also Chapter 39, Post-Traumatic Seizures and Epilepsy) (20). Some evidence suggests that shielding of the thorax (15) and face/head (21) may lessen intracranial effects of blast. In evaluating different helmet types, helmets with a face shield appeared to impede stress waves through the face, thereby reducing impact on the brain (21).

SYMPTOMS ASSOCIATED WITH BLAST BRAIN INJURY (VARIANCE FROM BLUNT INJURY)

Symptoms following blast-induced TBI are similar to those seen following blunt trauma. However, mounting evidence suggests etiologic differences in these symptoms, which may impact treatment planning.

Headache

Headache is one of the most prevalent postconcussive symptoms in soldiers returning from Iraq who screened positive for MTBI (22,23), as well as other postconcussive patients (24) (see also Chapter 56, Post-Traumatic Cephalgia). Blunt trauma is commonly associated with tension-type headaches. However, this headache phenotype is less common following blast injury. Instead, headaches following blast injury are described more often as migrainous (vascular) in nature. (25) Consideration of headache type should influence management, potentially affecting outcome (Figure 33-2). Initial management of post-traumatic headaches may lead to the development of overuse or rebound headaches, which can further complicate care. Post-traumatic headaches may be difficult to treat, although small studies show benefit from medications, such as propranolol and amitriptyline (26,27). Given the forces associated with blast injury, cervicogenic headaches could be anticipated. However, this headache phenotype has not been as well described in combat veterans.

Visual Dysfunction

Currently, a large percentage of patients treated at the Veterans Affairs Polytrauma Rehabilitation or network centers sustained blast-related injuries. More than 80% of these patients had associated moderate or severe TBI (28). In the TBI population, subjective visual complaints are common and may be nonspecific, such as blurry vision (29). Oculomotor dysfunction is more common in concussive injury than previously thought (30) (see also Chapter 45, Evaluating and Treating Visual Dysfunction). Saccadic abnormalities and difficulties with pursuit were found to be twice as high in those with blast injury compared to a nonblast group with visual complaints (28). Other manifestations include convergence and accommodation insufficiency (28,29). This suggests that appropriate screening is warranted in those with any visual complaints.

Vestibular and Hearing Difficulties

Blast injury contributes to vestibular dysfunction, manifested as dizziness or imbalance that is associated with TBI

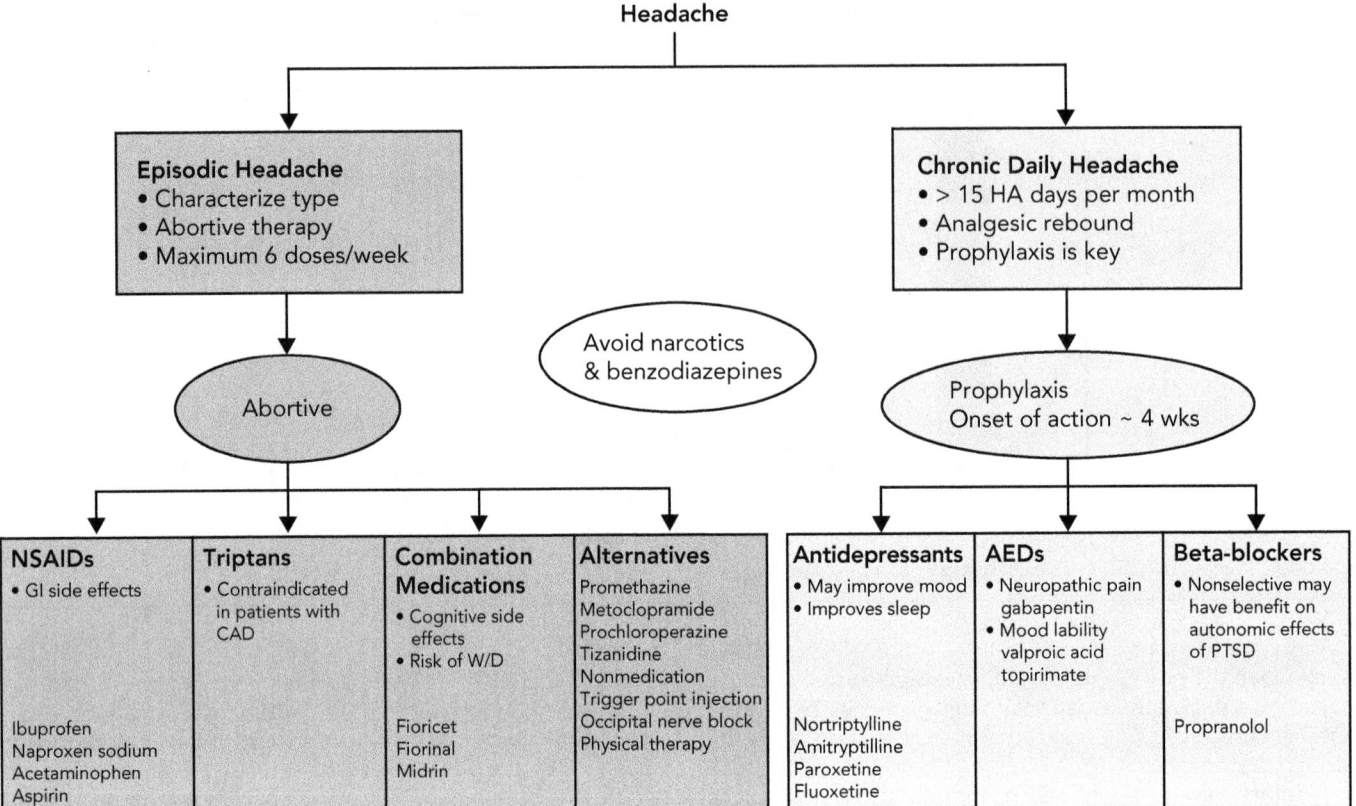

FIGURE 33–2 Considerations in headache management. AEDs, antiepileptic drugs; CAD, coronary artery disease; GI, gastrointestinal; HA, headache; NSAIDs, nonsteroidal anti-inflammatory drugs; PTSD, post-traumatic stress disorder; W/D, withdrawal. From Defense and Veterans Brain Injury Center, 2008, with permission.

(see also Chapter 47, Balance and Dizziness). Dynamic posturography has shown differences in lag times between blast and blunt brain injury (31). This may explain the variance in outcomes following vestibular rehabilitation in the 2 populations. Based on objective testing, dizziness can be characterized as post-traumatic migraine associated dizziness, positional vertigo, or spatial disorientation (32). Depending on etiology, canalith repositioning or vestibular rehabilitation are routinely used therapies. Medications such as meclizine and valium are used only in dizziness that causes significant impairments in activity because they may aggravate other TBI-related symptoms and impair recovery of central habituation (33).

Hearing dysfunction following TBI also appears to vary by mechanism of injury (see also Chapter 46, Audiologic Impairment). Lew et al. (34) report hearing loss in 62% and tinnitus in 38% in blast-related TBI compared to 44% and 18% respectively in a similar nonblast sample. Pure sensorineural hearing loss occurred most frequently followed by mixed type loss.

Sleep Disturbances

There has been a known association between sleep complaints and TBI (see also Chapter 42, Fatigue, and Chapter 43, Sleep-Wake Disturbances). Understanding this association becomes even more of a challenge in the military population because of the known preinjury status, which includes a de-

creased total sleep time in this population, especially in the deployed environment. Various studies have illustrated a premorbid total sleep time of from 5.6 to 6.5 hours (35,36,37).

There are a variety of factors that may contribute to premorbid sleep deprivation including military culture, environmental factors, a high prevalence of delayed circadian phase that is described in the same age population of a large percentage of service members, and poor sleep hygiene (38). Chronic sleep deprivation is known to be associated with decreased cognitive performance. This may be a confounding factor when assessing postinjury cognitive performance, as well as complaints of insomnia following a concussion/MTBI. There are emerging thoughts that quality and quantity of sleep prior to an injury may be a factor of resiliency affecting recovery.

The complaint of excessive daytime somnolence is the most common sleep complaint following TBI. Rates are reported as high as 50%. This is followed by the complaint of insomnia, which has been reported at 33% (39). Insomnia has been more commonly reported with MTBI than it has with severe injuries. Evaluation of these subjective complaints can be challenging in the military population. Other injuries and pain medications can affect the results of evaluations such as polysomnography and multiple sleep latency testing. In addition, the high prevalence of TBI injuries with psychological comorbidities, such as traumatic stress conditions, is another confounder in that most of the comorbid psychological conditions are associated with sleep disruptions.

It has been described that sleep disruption can further exacerbate and contribute to a variety of postconcussive symptoms to include post-traumatic headaches and affect the recovery process. Some studies have demonstrated that insomnia can interfere with the pain inhibitory control center (40). Furthermore, the pain itself may further exacerbate and contribute to insomnia with both factors mediating the other (41).

A study of active duty personnel confirmed previous findings that insomnia is associated with a higher probability of headache following a concussion/MTBI (42). The results of this study indicated that insomnia increased probability of endorsement of a headache following MTBI, whereas increases in headache severity were associated with loss of consciousness (LOC), PTSD symptoms, and slowed reaction time (43).

To further complicate these relationships, there have been several recent reports of associating PTSD with obstructive sleep apnea (OSA) in veterans. A predilection for such a primary sleep disorder can significantly complicate analyses and attribution of sleep complaints to TBI (43). A recent analysis suggested that the younger active duty population had an increased risk for OSA independent of whether or not an individual had PTSD (44). These relationships require further investigation.

Severe injuries have been reported to be an etiology for a hypersomnolence syndrome. Severity of symptoms has been reported as correlating with severity of injury, and 25% may have persistent symptoms at 1 year following the injury (45). A proposed pathophysiology for this phenomenon postulates that there may be associated injury to posterolateral hypothalamus that typically produces the wake-promoting hypocretin-1 hormone. Low cerebrospinal fluid (CSF) levels of hypocretin-1 have been reported in 95% moderate-to-severe TBI (46).

Management of sleep issues in military concussion begins with a clinical assessment that identifies which sleep issues are present. Diagnostic polysomnography is primarily used when there is a suspicion for a comorbid sleep breathing disorder, such as OSA. Insomnia is primarily targeted with cognitive-behavioral techniques, such as stimulus control or sleep restriction. These therapies are aimed at increasing homeostatic drive for sleep and reduction of fragmented sleep (47). There is not as much evidence for these techniques in the TBI population but there has been a report of effectiveness (48). Department of Defense/Veterans Affairs (DoD/VA) guidelines (49) recommend short-term adjunctive pharmacotherapy with zolpidem (maximum duration of 10 days), trazodone, or amitriptyline to promote adequate sleep. When using hypnotic agents in a TBI population, it is important to consider possible adverse effects on cognition and neuroplasticity. For this reason, benzodiazepines are discouraged (50). Hypersomnolence not secondary to insomnia can be managed with wake-promoting agents (modafinil, armodafinil) and other stimulants. Sleep-disordered breathing can be addressed with the appropriate positive airway pressure modality such as continued positive airway pressure (CPAP) for OSA. Issues of circadian rhythm disorders can be addressed with phototherapy and melatonin, using the same standardized recommendations as in the non-TBI population. It should be noted that medications initiated for other conditions, such as pain, may have an adverse effect on daytime somnolence and insomnia. Evaluating the evolution and response of sleep complaints should be a regular component of the clinical follow-up in this population.

TBI AND PTSD SYMPTOM OVERLAP

As previously stated, PTSD frequently co-occurs with combat-related TBI. Some have investigated the association between TBI and PTSD, finding that PTSD is more commonly seen in those with less severe TBI and shorter durations of alterations in consciousness (51,52). Others report that those with other visible physical injuries may be less likely to develop PTSD (53). The cause of persistent postconcussive symptoms is likely multifactorial, but the presence of coexisting psychiatric conditions, such as PTSD, may be implicated (54,55,56,57).

In a survey of soldiers returning from Iraq with self-reported symptoms of MTBI or PTSD, Hoge et al. found that symptoms such as memory problems, balance problems, irritability, ringing in the ears, fainting spells, fatigue, and sleep problems were prevalent in both TBI and PTSD populations (58). In this sample, only headache was found to be more associated with MTBI. Another study looking at remote injury, found that headaches, memory problems, sleep problems, and fainting were associated with MTBI even after controlling for PTSD (59). Symptoms of both disorders can be clustered into the more general categories of physical, cognitive, or emotional. In general, physical symptoms such as headache, dizziness, and visual deficits are considered to be a result of MTBI, whereas symptoms such as reexperiencing, nightmares and hypervigilance are more likely associated with PTSD (see also Chapter 64, Psychological Issues and Amelioration of Emotional and Behavioral Problems).

Symptoms in the cognitive cluster may be seen with both conditions. Neuropsychological testing of the subjective complaints of memory may facilitate identification of specific areas of difficulty (see Chapter 60, Neuropsychological Assessment and Treatment Plans). Additionally, neuropsychological testing may help substantiate a dual diagnosis. Nelson et al. demonstrated that processing speeds and executive functioning were significantly more impaired in those diagnosed with TBI and PTSD compared to those with TBI alone (60). Specific impairments can be managed with appropriate intervention or compensatory techniques. For example, deficits in attention, processing speeds, and executive function may be perceived as memory problems, yet each requires a different approach to treatment. Cognitive strategy training, using group therapy to practice compensatory strategies, may be a useful approach to minor cognitive dysfunction (61). A multidimensional approach has been suggested as the most appropriate way to capture all symptom clusters to fully delineate areas of dysfunction (62).

SEVERE AND PENETRATING TBI

Severe and penetrating TBI comprise only a small percentage of combat-related TBI (2). As in the civilian TBI population, this cohort requires intensive resources. Recent studies have shown that blast-related severe or penetrating TBI are at higher risk for vascular injury or complications compared

TABLE 33-1 Indications for Vascular Imaging in Blast-Related Brain Injury

INDICATIONS FOR VASCULAR IMAGING IN BLAST-RELATED BRAIN INJURY
• Penetrating head injury
• Nonpenetrating blast brain injury with Glasgow Coma Scale (GCS) score ≤ 8
• Transcranial Doppler (TCD) evidence of vasospasm
• Spontaneous decrease in brain tissue oxygenation (pBO₂) or cerebral blood flow (CBF) in otherwise stable patient

Reprinted from Bell et al. (63) with permission.

to blunt brain injury of similar severity. Pathologies such as traumatic aneurysm, dissections, and vascular fistulae are found in this population (63). In those with traumatic intracranial aneurysms, almost half developed vasospasm (63). The duration of vasospasm has been shown to average 14 days, although it may continue up to 30 days (64). Factors associated with the development of vasospasm include the presence of pseudoaneurysm, number of lobes injured, and degree of hemorrhage. As in aneurysmal subarachnoid hemorrhage, the presence of vasospasm is associated with higher mortality. However, advances in endovascular management (angioplasty, stenting, coiling) have contributed to improved long-term outcomes (64). These findings have led to aggressive screening for vascular injury in this subpopulation. Indications for using digital subtraction angiography are listed in Table 33-1 (63). The use of computed tomography angiography (CTA) can be considered in the evaluation of vascular structures of the head and neck, although visualization of the vessels may be impaired in the presence of retained foreign bodies.

Decompressive craniectomy is considered controversial in the civilian trauma population (see also Chapter 24, Surgical Management and Procedures). However, this is a widely used modality in the management of severe and penetrating combat-related TBI (65). Despite presenting with lower admission Glasgow Coma Scale (GCS) scores, 60% of those undergoing bilateral or bicompartmental craniectomy in-theater achieved independent living by 2-year follow-up (66). Patients with systemic infections or cerebrovascular injury were less likely to make a full recovery. Because of wound contamination, sterilization, or processing difficulties, autologous skull reconstruction is often not feasible. Alloplastic grafts are viable solutions for skull reconstructions in this population. Infection, requiring graft removal occurred in 5%, whereas other complications including extraaxial fluid collections, seizures, and contour abnormalities were commonly seen (67).

Coagulopathy remains a concern in patients with severe/penetrating TBI. A study evaluating all combat casualties revealed that those injured by blast presented with higher degrees of coagulopathy compared to those with non-blast mechanisms (68). In addition, these patients presented with more tachycardia and greater base deficits. A similar study compared isolated TBI resulting from combat injury to non-TBI patients. Those with more severe TBI (lower GCS score) had a higher admission International Normalized Ratio (INR) (69). Aggressive correction of elevated INR is critical to minimize the expansion of intracranial hemorrhage.

DIAGNOSTIC TESTING

As with MTBI resulting from blunt trauma, traditional imaging (computed tomography [CT] and magnetic resonance imaging [MRI]) following blast-related MTBI is often void of pathologic findings. Studies using more sophisticated imaging techniques indicate that structural lesions may be present following blast brain injury (see also Part III, Neuroimaging and Neurodiagnostic Testing). Diffusion tensor imaging (DTI) has demonstrated differences in fractional anisotropy among blast and blunt patients with TBI. In some cases, DTI illustrates disruptions in white matter fiber tracts following blast brain injury (70,71,72). Other investigators have shown that in comparing DTI patterns of TBI with a blast component compared to TBI without blast, the injuries associated with blast demonstrated a more diffuse pattern of injury on DTI. In patients with persistent symptoms, functional MRI (fMRI) has shown abnormalities in the basal ganglia and dorsolateral prefrontal cortex (73). It should be noted that many patients with combat-related TBI may not be candidates for MRI or advanced MRI modalities such as DTI or fMRI because of safety concerns of associated shrapnel or retained metallic fragments. Investigators for one of the combat TBI DTI studies were only able to enroll 15% of patients evaluated for this reason (71). Other diagnostic modalities including electroencephalogram (EEG) and fluorodeoxyglucose positron emission tomography (FDG-PET) have demonstrated defects in similar locations (16). To date, these modalities are limited to academic and research applications; however, they are helping to elucidate important pathophysiological information.

EVALUATION AND MANAGEMENT OF COMBAT-RELATED TBI

In-Theater Evaluation

Existing military TBI protocols require medical evaluation as soon as tactically possible following blast exposure. Previous practice guidelines relied on a service member to endorse and report symptoms following an injury to medical personnel. Given that these injuries often had no outward or external manifestation, combined with the high motivation to remain on full duty, it was believed that many symptoms were underreported in theater. To better address this situation, recent policy changes developed in collaboration with US military medical and tactical command now mandate screening for any service member involved in an incident with high risk of exposure to blast or TBI regardless of whether or not they endorse symptoms. This mandatory screening is intended to identify service members with injury who may fail to self-report symptoms to avoid removal from combat activities (74). During this evaluation, the Military Acute Concussion Evaluation (MACE) is used to screen for concussion. Developed in 2006 by the Defense and Veterans Brain Injury Center (DVBIC), in conjunction with authors of the Standardized Assessment of Concussion (SAC) (75), this screener has been adopted by other North American Treaty Organization (NATO) forces, including Great Britain, Canada, and Belgium. This tool captures history of the traumatic event—the critical component required for diagnosing concussion, a brief cognitive exam, and presence of symptoms. The MACE has been shown to be most sensitive within 12 hours of injury (76). Another example of the motivation of service members to not be removed from duty is the fact that many had memorized the initial version of the MACE to artificially improve their performance. To address this, additional versions of the MACE were developed, and different versions are used in the postinjury evaluation and in the return-to-duty evaluation. Given the limited resources that are available in some combat settings, management algorithms suggest criteria for imaging and initial management. Treatment follows a primary care model of rest, acute symptom management, especially headache and sleep in conjunction with education, which highlights the expectation of recovery (77). Once symptoms resolve, exertional testing is performed to ensure that symptoms do not return when the body is stressed. This procedure involves a brief period of aerobic activity followed by reevaluation for physical and cognitive symptoms. Return-to-duty determinations may be further informed following administration of a computerized neurocognitive test with results compared to performance on a baseline assessment done prior to deployment. Those who have sustained multiple concussions are required to undergo more detailed evaluation prior to returning to unrestricted duty. In cases with persistent symptoms, management may also involve combat stress evaluations, as conditions such as PTSD are known to occur at higher rates in patients with TBI (9,78). The current system includes in-theater concussion care centers for those patients who do not completely recover within a few days. These centers offer up to several weeks of focused therapy for those service members who needed a longer recovery time. These centers have reported a favorable return-to-duty rate and are thought to reduce the number of service members requiring evacuation from theater. Failure to resolve or control symptoms within a few weeks may result in evacuation for more esoteric evaluations (79).

Stateside Evaluation

Stateside evaluation of TBI may occur during the subacute phase, although chronic injury, either inadequately resolved or previously undiagnosed, is more common (80). Screening occurs on redeployment through Post-Deployment Health Assessment (PDHA). This DoD postdeployment screening has been done with questions adapted from the validated Brief TBI Screen (BTBIS), which has been supported by the Institute of Medicine (IOM). It should be noted that this form of screening is intended to identify those service members who need further clinical evaluation and is not considered diagnostic in the absence of further clinical correlation and evaluation. In one brigade combat team, 23% sustained a clinician-confirmed TBI (28). Although 33% of the sample reported postconcussive symptoms immediately following the injury, only 7.5% reported persistent symptoms on return to the states (23). In newly diagnosed TBI, the primary care

model of evaluation and management is instituted. Those with refractory or complicated symptom clusters are referred to designated TBI centers within the Military Health System (MHS). These centers offer sophisticated neurologic, vestibular, ophthalmologic, and neuropsychological care (81).

Service members may transition to care within the VA medical system for a variety of reasons. On entry into this system, those serving in OEF or OIF undergo TBI screening in an effort to ascertain injury, alterations of consciousness, and past/present symptoms. This screening is done with the VA TBI Clinical Reminder, which is also an adaptation of the BTBIS. Similar to the DoD postdeployment screening program, this VA screening is intended to identify those veterans who are in need of further evaluation and in the absence of further clinical correlation is not considered diagnostic. This assessment includes a clinical interview and any appropriate specialty evaluations, such as neuropsychological testing and neuroimaging, which help to delineate complaints. A challenge for any system attempting to identify an injury months to years after the incident is determining the attribution of current symptoms to a prior injury. The VA has the additional challenge of disability implications that may be a contributing factor to some patients' subjective reports. The VA has reported that of all the patients identified by their entry TBI screen, approximately 15% are found to have current symptoms that are attributable to a prior TBI.

A joint DoD/VA workgroup developed evidence-based guidelines for the evaluation and management of concussion (49). These guidelines recommend a functional assessment (Table 33-2), in addition to providing recommendations for diagnostic evaluation and symptom management strategies. Generally, this is accomplished at local VA primary care facilities, although those service members and veterans with TBI and polytrauma may receive advanced rehabilitation care at 1 of the 5 VA polytrauma centers.

Service members or veterans with lingering symptoms are frequently treated within VA medical system, although some receive care through the MHS or in civilian settings. Concerns regarding exaggeration of symptom reporting related to both TBI and PTSD are evident across all treatment settings. Studies looking at the effects of different measures of effort testing and validity testing have shown variable results. It has been suggested that some of the disparity between self-report and objective testing of symptoms may be based on the patients' overestimation of premorbid function (82). One study revealed that when a group of patients were instructed they were to undergo neuropsychological testing based on their MTBI history, the group had significantly worse performance than a second group who was not told that testing was related to previous TBI (83).

The Minnesota Multiphasic Personality Inventory II (MMPI-2) was used to evaluate groups of compensation-seeking vs noncompensation-seeking veterans (84). Significant differences in subscale scoring were found between the 2 groups. Another study using the MMPI-2 profiles of a group of US Army soldiers and veterans diagnosed with concussion, demonstrated that participants with comorbid PTSD or ongoing disability claims had elevated scores in certain subscales (96). This would suggest that the MMPI-2 may be a useful tool in evaluating veterans with concussion and PTSD.

TABLE 33-2 Functional Assessment

Work	Have there been any changes in productivity?
	Is there an increase in tardiness, loss of motivation, or loss of interest?
	Has the patient been more forgetful, easily distracted?
School	Have there been changes in grades?
	Have there been changes in relationships with friends?
	Has there been a recent onset or increase in acting-out behaviors?
	Has there been a recent increase in disciplinary actions?
	Has there been increased social withdrawal?
	Has there been a change in effort required to complete assignments?
Family relationships	Have there been negative changes in relationship with significant others?
	Is the patient irritable or easily angered by family members?
	Has there been a withdrawal of interest in or time spent with family?
	Has there been any violence within the family?
Housing	Does the patient have adequate housing?
	Are there appropriate utilities and services?
	Is the housing situation stable?
Legal	Are there outstanding warrants, restraining orders, or disciplinary actions?
	Is the person regularly engaging in, or at risk to be involved in, illegal activity?
	Is the patient on probation or parole?
	Is the patient seeking litigation for compensation?
	Is there family advocacy/Department of Social Services (DSS) involvement?
Financial	Is there a stable source of income?
	Are there significant outstanding or past-due debts, alimony, child support?
	Has the patient filed for bankruptcy?
	Does the patient have access to health care and/or insurance?
Unit/community involvement	Does the patient need to be put on profile, MEB, or limited duty?
	Is the patient functional and contributing in the unit environment?
	Is there active/satisfying involvement in a community?

Reprinted from The Management of Concussion/mTBI Working Group. *VA/DoD clinical practice guideline. For management of concussion/mTBI*. 2009. Available at: http://www.healthquality.va.gov/mtbi/concussion_mtbi_full_1_0.pdf. Accessed August 25, 2011.

SCREENING CONSIDERATIONS IN THE MILITARY POPULATION

There have been some suggestions that motivation and effort may affect the results of concussion screening. There has been confusion in the medical literature regarding DoD screening for TBI. Many articles indicate that results of a positive screen are equivalent to a confirmed diagnosis of TBI. This is not an accurate representation. Screening identifies those who need a clinical evaluation to determine if they

had a TBI or concussion. Official DoD screening includes a requirement that an individual have symptoms at the time of screening. The emphasis is identifying those who need further evaluation.

The timing of screens also appears to be a factor in symptom reporting. In the official in-theater survey of US Army soldiers, the reported incidence of concussion was 11.2% (36). Currently, in-theater screening is conducted using the MACE, which incorporates key history, a brief exam, and a cognitive screen adapted from the validated SAC. As stated, the desire for return to duty led service members to memorize the initial version of the MACE, which led to increased versions and more controlled release of the instrument. The motivation to deny symptoms was also a reason that the new guidelines were implemented requiring event-based mandatory screening regardless of whether a service member may be endorsing symptoms.

There have been some misunderstandings by the media that the DoD is using computerized neurocognitive assessment testing as a screen for TBI and concussion. These instruments are not used as a diagnostic screen. Current policy defines their role as informing a return-to-duty determination after a clinical diagnosis of concussion or TBI has been made. Results are compared to the individual's predeployment baseline to help inform this decision. Currently, the DoD is using the Automated Neuropsychological Assessment Metrics (ANAM) for this purpose. An objective head-to-head evaluation of available computerized instruments is in progress to determine which program best meets the needs of the military. One limitation of the ANAM as identified by DVBIC and other subject matter experts has been its lack of an effort scale. However, the officer responsible for the program described unpublished data that indicated that less than 5% of deployed service members score below cutoff indicative of poor effort (97).

At the conclusion of a deployment, service members have been screened with the PDHA that incorporates an adaptation of the validated BTBIS. Data from the Defense Medical Surveillance Center has consistently averaged 4.5%. These results indicate that most service members who sustained a concussion have recovered before the end of their tour. This is consistent with the known natural history of concussion recovery.

Results are different in surveys conducted retrospectively long after our service members have returned home. The incidence of in-theater concussion was reported by the Research and Development (RAND) Corporation as 19% based on a retrospective telephone survey (85). There was no clinical correlation of these self-reports. These results are similar to those reported by the VA, where screening of all OIF/OEF veterans entering their system yielded positive results of 18.5%. It should be noted that after these, veterans received clinical correlation with evaluations and diagnostic testing.

CURRENT RESEARCH EFFORTS

A challenging aspect of military TBI is understanding the multiple dimensions of blast injury and if this mechanism is clinically different than other mechanisms of injury. To better determine the role of blast as a mechanism of injury, 75 experts were gathered from the DoD, the Department of Transportation, the Department of Veterans Affairs, academia, and industry from 5 countries in May 2009 to evaluate evidence from past and ongoing blast research at the International State-of-the-Science Meeting on Non-Impact, Blast-Induced Mild Traumatic Brain Injury (87). Based on the information reviewed, including published studies and newly acquired data, the meeting determined that there was evidence that blast-induced mild trauma to the brain does occur (Table 33-3). Investigators continue to evaluate the different components of blast injury. In addition to the shock wave, other mechanisms such as thermal, electromagnetic, and kinetic factors are now thought to contribute to injury (17,86). Some initial clinical data did not readily illustrate such a difference. Belanger et al. (86) evaluated performance of these 2 populations on neuropsychological testing and did not find any difference on neuropsychological testing between these 2 populations when matched for severity of injury. An understanding of the clinical correlation of blast injury continues to evolve.

There has been a great deal of investigation of identifying a clinically valid and reliable biomarker that may help identify service members with TBI. Biomarkers previously studied include lactate dehydrogenase (LDH), glial fibrillary acid protein (GFAP), neuron specific enolase (NSE), and S-100β (88). Although some have shown promise in preclinical trials, they appear to lack either the necessary sensitivity or brain specificity to be of clinical use. More recently, a number of new candidate biomarkers have been discovered. The emerging data suggest ubiquitin carboxy-terminal hydrolase L1 (UCH-L1), microtubule-associated protein 2 (MAP2), tau proteins, and the spectrin protein breakdown products (SBDPs) are possibilities for effective biomarkers (89).

There continue to be studies of the efficacy of cognitive rehabilitation in improving the deficits seen in combat-related TBI. Areas of investigation include what techniques of cognitive rehabilitation are most effective and whether cognitive rehabilitation may be effective in speeding recovery in MTBI. In addition, there are long-term epidemiological initiatives to better understand potential long-term sequelae and complications of military TBI. It is anticipated that the use of common data elements, developed jointly between the DoD, National Institute of Health (NIH), and academia

---

TABLE 33-3 Differences in Blunt and Blast-Related Brain Injury

---

Statistically significant differences in diffusion tensor imaging-based fractional anisotropy between service members with documented MTBI associated with blast and service members with impact-only MTBI

Statistically significant differences in event-related potentials between blast and nonblast exposures in human studies

Preliminary evidence of disturbed phase synchrony following blast exposure

Differences in functional magnetic resonance imaging (fMRI) between Breacher instructors and students (statistically significant fMRI results, nonstatistically significant neurocognitive results

Alterations in inflammatory markers in animal studies.

Abbreviation: MTBI, mild traumatic brain injury. Reprinted from International State-of-the-Science Meeting on Non-Impact, Blast-Induced Mild Traumatic Brain Injury (87) with permission.

---

will assist in such determinations (74). Preliminary plans have been discussed to establish a military brain bank to determine if a pattern of neuropathology exists, similar to the recently described chronic traumatic encephalopathy noted in athletes who sustained multiple concussions.

Clinically, there are efforts to develop assessment techniques that can facilitate return-to-duty determinations rapidly in a field hospital or clinic setting. These assessments may include evaluation of vestibular function, evaluation of nystagmus, neurocognitive assessment tests to include visuospatial reaction time, or combinations of the aforementioned.

Clinical practice guidelines continue to be developed and revised as more data becomes available. There have been efforts to develop practice guidance for patients who have significant symptoms from both TBI, as well as psychological stress.

DEVELOPMENTS ON THE HORIZON

Initiatives aimed at identifying service members who may have been exposed to a blast or head injury are focusing on the use of blast dosimeters or helmet-mounted accelerometers. Proteomic and genomic studies are in progress, which may lead to the identification of innate factors of vulnerability and resiliency that may better correlate duty assignments based on risk of injury.

More data may emerge regarding use of neuroprotection, both following injury and as a primary preventive measure. The role of progesterone as a neuroprotective agent is being evaluated by the NIH for civilian injuries but is yet to be evaluated in military injuries. A recent IOM (90) report identifies nutritional interventions as a possible means of promoting metabolic recovery following injury.

Technology continues to emerge, which facilitates the identification and rehabilitation of those with TBI. Virtual reality and the use of telemedicine are used for remote monitoring and assessment. A goal is the eventual development of a portable handheld point-of-care detection tool. There have been preliminary initiatives considering the emerging role of nanotechnology in the design of protective equipment. More experience is being gained in the use of electrical stimulation technology from the use of deep brain stimulators for severe injuries to the possible use of transcranial magnetic stimulation incorporated into rehabilitation.

INTERNATIONAL COMBAT-RELATED TBI FINDINGS

Several NATO countries have ongoing research related to blast injury as a result of their military involvement in Iraq and Afghanistan. However, availability of formal findings remains limited at this point.

TBI rates in British forces appear lower than that of the United States. Rona et al. (91,92) reported that this variance is likely related to duration of deployment as US troops are deployed twice as long as the Royal Army and Marines. Dutch researchers evaluated the relationship between certain glucocorticoid receptor components and the subsequent development of PTSD in military personnel (93). It appears that those with high predeployment numbers of glucocorticoid receptors and low messenger RNA (mRNA) expression of receptor gene FKBP5 were at greater risk of PTSD symptom reporting, although MTBI was not considered in analysis. MACE results and long-term outcomes are under investigation in a group of medically evacuated Dutch personnel who sustained blast brain injury, but results are not yet available.

In a Canadian study, students and instructors at an explosive forced entry training program underwent medical evaluations 1 day prior to blast exposure and 10 days following the blast. Most of the instructors and half of the students reported prior head injury. Results indicate that most subjects had baseline deficits in postural stability, which did not change significantly after blast exposure (94). Blast exposure prior to this training program was not specified in the current study. Another study of Canadian troops found that those who screened positive for MTBI were more likely to report poor health than those who screened negative for MTBI (95).

CONCLUSION

Most combat-related TBI is mild or concussive in nature and most often result from blast injury. Early intervention facilitates recovery and return to duty in this special population. Later screening identifies those individuals with persistent symptoms that require further evaluation and management. Refractory symptoms may be attributable to other conditions: pain, depression, anxiety-type disorders, multiple concussions, and less commonly, secondary gain. Mounting evidence suggests that there may be subtle differences in the pathophysiology of brain injury itself, as well as related posttraumatic sequelae between blast and blunt TBI.

Advances in military TBI have been caused by innovative partnerships between the DoD, Department of Veterans Affairs, academia, and industry from many countries. Care is being further optimized through important NATO collaborative efforts. The experience and lessons learned from the military regarding TBI pathophysiology, blast injury, as well as management in the context of comorbidities, such as polytrauma or PTSD, are helping to further both military and civilian TBI care.

KEY CLINICAL POINTS

1. Blast exposure may result in TBI via several different mechanisms, but military TBI most commonly results from a combination of blast and blunt trauma.
2. TBI and PTSD may coexist in patients with combat-related TBI, thereby complicating management.
3. Advanced imaging modalities including fMRI and DTI sequences may be useful in understanding neuropathology associated with blast-related TBI.
4. Headache phenotypes vary between blast and blunt injury and should be considered in developing treatment plan.
5. Visual dysfunction is common following TBI, and screening should be considered in those with vague or persistent TBI symptoms.
6. The emphasis of DoD screening is to identify those in need of further evaluation and symptom management.
7. Penetrating injury is associated with the development of vascular injuries, such as dissections and pseudoaneurysms.

8. Decompressive craniectomy is a viable treatment option in the management of combat-related severe or penetrating TBI.

KEY REFERENCES

1. Kennedy JE, Leal FO, Lewis JD, Cullen MA, Amador RR. Posttraumatic stress symptoms in OIF/OEF service members with blast-related and non–blast-related mild TBI. *NeuroRehabilitation.* 2010;26(3):223–231.
2. Kocsis JD, Tessler A. Pathology of blast-related brain injury. *J Rehabil Res Dev.* 2009;46(6):667–672.
3. Meyer KS, Marion DW, Coronel H, Jaffee MS. Combat-related traumatic brain injury and its implications to military healthcare. *Psychiatr Clin North Am.* 2010;33(4):783–796.

E-BOOK SUGGESTIONS

1. The Management of Concussion/mTBI Working Group. *VA/DoD clinical practice guideline. For management of concussion/mTBI.* 2009. Available at: http://www.healthquality.va.gov/mtbi/concussion_mtbi_full_1_0.pdf. Accessed May 20, 2012.
2. Department of Veterans Affairs. Veterans health initiative study guide to help health providers care for veteran patients who've suffered traumatic brain injuries. 2010. Available at: http://www.publichealth.va.gov/docs/vhi/traumatic-brain-injury-vhi.pdf. Accessed. May 20, 2012

References

1. Scott SG, Belanger HG, Vanderploeg RD, Massengale J, Scholten J. Mechanism-of-injury approach to evaluating patients with blast-related polytrauma. *J AM Osteopath Assoc.* 2006;106(5) 265–70.
2. Defense and Veterans Brain Injury Center. TBI numbers. Available at: http://www.dvbic.org/TBI-Numbers/aspx. Accessed January 5, 2012.
3. MacGregor AJ, Dougherty AL, Galarneau MR. Injury-specific correlates of combat-related traumatic brain injury in Operation Iraqi Freedom. *J Head Trauma Rehabil.* 2001;26(4): 312–318.
4. Centers for disease Control and Prevention, National Center for Injury Prevention and Control. Traumatic brain injury in the United States: Emergency department visits, hospitalization and deaths, 2002–2006. 2010. Available at: http://www.cdc.gov/traumaticbraininjury/pdf/tbi_blue_book_externalcause.pdf. Accessed September 9, 2011.
5. Walilko T, North C, Young LA, et al. Head injury as a PTSD predictor among Oklahoma City bombing survivors. [Erratum appears in *J Trauma.* 2010;69(1):242]. *J Trauma.* 2009;67(6):1311–1319.
6. Zarocostas J. Use of bombs in populated areas is having a devastating effect on civilians, say reports. *BMJ.* 2011;342:d2161.
7. Mountain SJ, Tharion WJ. Hypohydration and muscular fatigue of the thumb alter median nerve somatosensory evoked potentials. *Appl Physiol Nutr Metab.* 2010;35(4): 456–463.
8. Elder GA, Mitsis EM, Ahlers ST, Cristian A. Blast-induced mild traumatic brain injury. *Psychiatr Clin North Am.* 2010;33(4):757–781.
9. Kennedy JE, Leal FO, Lewis JD, Cullen MA, Amador RR. Posttraumatic stress symptoms in OIF/OEF service members with blast-related and non–blast-related mild TBI. *NeuroRehabilitation.* 2010; 26(3):223–231.
10. Brenner LA, Ivins BJ, Schwab K, et al. Traumatic brain injury, posttraumatic stress disorder, and postconcussive symptom reporting among troops returning from Iraq. *J Head Trauma Rehabil.* 2010; 25(5):307–312.

11. Park E, Gottlieb JJ, Cheung B, Shek PN, Baker AJ. A model of low-level primary blast brain trauma results in cytoskeletal proteolysis and chronic functional impairment in the absence of lung barotrauma. *J Neurotrauma.* 2011;28(3):343–357.

12. Plurad DS. Blast injury. *Mil Med.* 2011;176(3):276–282.

13. Cernak I, Savic VJ, Ignjatovic D, Jevtic M. Blast injury from explosive munitions. *J Trauma.* 1999;47(1):96–103.

14. Moore DM, Jérusalem A, Nyein M, Noels L, Jaffee MS, Radovitzky RA. Computational biology—modeling of primary blast effects on the central nervous system. *Neuroimage.* 2009;(47)(suppl 2): T10–T20.

15. Koliatsos VE, Cernak I, Xu L, et al. A mouse model of blast injury to brain: Initial pathological, neuropathological, and behavioral characterization. *J Neuropathol Exp Neurol.* 2011;70(5):399–416.

16. Peskind ER, Petrie EC, Cross DJ, et al. Cerebrocerebellar hypometabolism associated with repetitive blast exposure mild traumatic brain injury in 12 Iraq war veterans with persistent post-concussive symptoms. *Neuroimage;* 2011;(54)(suppl 1): S76–S82.

17. Lee KY, Nyein MK, Moore DF, et al. Blast-induced electromagnetic fields in the brain from bone piezoelectricity. *Neuroimage.* 2011; (54)(suppl 1):S30–S36.

18. Born CT. Blast trauma: the fourth weapon of mass destruction. *Scand J Surg.* 2005;94(4):279–285.

19. Kocsis JD, Tessler A. Pathology of blast-related brain injury. *J Rehabil Res Dev.* 2009;46(6):667–672.

20. Raymont V, Salazar AM, Lipsky R, Goldman D, Tasick G, Grafman J. Correlates of posttraumatic epilepsy 35 years following combat brain injury. *Neurology.* 2010;75(3):224–229.

21. Nyein MK, Jason AM, Yu L, et al. In silico investigation of intracranial blast mitigation with relevance to military traumatic brain injury. *Proc Natl Acad Sci U S A.* 2010;107(48):20703–20708.

22. Kozminski M. Combat-related posttraumatic headache: diagnosis, mechanisms of injury, & challenges to treatment. *J Am Osteopath Assoc.* 2010;110(9):514–519.

23. Terrio H, Brenner LA, Ivins BJ, et al. Traumatic brain injury screening: preliminary findings in a US Army Brigade Combat Team. *J Head Trauma Rehabil.* 2009;24(1):14–23.

24. Lew HL, Lin PH, Fuh JL, Wang SJ, Clark DJ, Walker WC. Characteristics and treatment of headache after traumatic brain injury: a focused review. *Am J Phys Med Rehabil.* 2006;85(7):619–627.

25. Vargas BB. Posttraumatic headache in combat headache soldiers and civilians: what factors influence the expression of tension-type versus migraine? *Curr Pain Headache Rep.* 2009;13(6):470.

26. Janculjak D, Fingler M, Bras M, Heċimoviċ I, Splavski B, Vukoviċ V. Efficiency of pharmacological treatment of chronic post-traumatic headaches [in Croatian]. *Acta Med Croatica.* 2008;62(2):151–155.

27. Weiss HD, Stern BJ, Goldberg J. Post-traumatic migraine: chronic migraine precipitated by minor head or neck trauma. *Headache.* 1991;31(7):451–456.

28. Braham KD, Wilgenburg HM, Kirby J, Ingalla S, Cheng CY, Goodrich GL. Visual impairment and dysfunction in combat-injured servicemembers with traumatic brain injury. *Optom Vis Sci.* 2009;86(7): 817–825.

29. Kelts EA. Traumatic brain injury and visual dysfunction: a limited overview. *NeuroRehabilitation.* 2010;27(3):223–229.

30. Ciuffreda KJ, Kapoor N. Oculomotor dysfunctions, their remediation, and reading-related problems in mild traumatic brain injury. *J Behav Optom.* 2007;18(3):72–77.

31. Hoffer ME, Donaldson C, Gotshall KR, Balaban C, Balough BJ. Blunt and blast head trauma: different entities. *Int Tinnitus J.* 2009; 15(2):115–118.

32. Hoffer ME, Gottshall KR, Moore R, Balough BJ, Wester D. Characterizing and treating dizziness after mild head trauma. *Otol Neurotol.* 2004;25(2):135–138.

33. Donaldson, CJ, Hoffer ME, Balough BJ, Gotshall KR. Prognostic assessments of medical therapy and vestibular testing in post-traumatic migraine-associated dizziness patients. *Otolaryngol Head Neck Surg.* 2010;143(6):820–825.

34. Lew HL, Jerger JF, Guillory SB, Henry JA. Auditory dysfunction in traumatic brain injury. *J Rehabil Res Dev.* 2007;44(7):921–928

35. Peterson AL, Goodie JL, Satterfield WA, Brim WL. Sleep disturbance during military deployment. *Mil Med.* 173(3);230–235.

36. Mental Health Advisory Team V. *Operation Iraqi Freedom, 2006–2008.* Available at: http://www.armymedicine.army.mil/ reports/mhat/mhat_v/MHAT_V_OIFandOEF-Redacted.pdf. Accessed January 5, 2012.

37. Seelig AD, Jacobson IG, Smith B, et al. Sleep patterns before, during, and after deployment to Iraq and Afghanistan. *Sleep.* 2010; 33(12):1615–1622.

38. Luxton DD, Greenburg D, Ryan J, Niven A, Wheeler G, Mysliwec V. Prevalence and impact of short sleep duration in deployed OIF soldiers. *Sleep.* 2010;34(9):1189–1195.

39. Fichtenberg NL, Zafonte RD, Putnam S, Mann NR, Millard AE. Insomnia in a post-acute brain injury. *Brain Inj.* 2002;16:197–206.

40. Lautenbacher S, Kundermann B, Krieg JC. Sleep deprivation and pain perception. *Sleep Med Rev.* 2006;10:357–369.

41. Smith MT, Haythornthwaite JA. How do sleep disturbance and chronic pain inter-relate? Insights from the longitudinal and cognitive-behavioral clinical trials literature. *Sleep Med Rev.* 2004;8(2): 119–132.

42. Chaput G, Giguère JF, Chauny JM, Denis R, Lavigne G. Relationship among subjective sleep complaints, headaches, and mood alterations following a mild traumatic brain injury. *Sleep Med.* 2009; 10(7):713–716.

43. Bryan CJ, Hernandez AM. Predictors of post-traumatic headache severity among deployed military personnel. *Headache.* 2011;51(6): 945–953.

44. Capaldi VF II, Guerrero ML, Killgore WD. Sleep disruptions among returning combat veterans from Iraq and Afghanistan. *Mil Med.* 2011;176(8):879–888

45. Watson NF, Dikmen S, Machamer J, Doherty M, Temkin N. Hypersomnia following traumatic brain injury. *J Clin Sleep Medicine.* 2007; 3(4):363–368.

46. Baumann CR, Stocker R, Imhof HG, et al. Hypocretin-1 (orexin A) deficiency in acute traumatic brain injury. *Neurology.* 2005;65(1): 147–149.

47. Zeitzer JM, Friedman L, O'Hara R. Insomnia in the context of traumatic brain injury. *J Rehabil Res Dev.* 2009;46(6):827–836

48. Ouellet MC, Beaulieu-Bonneau S, Morin CM. Insomnia in patients with traumatic brain injury: frequency, characteristics, and risk factors. *J Head Trauma Rehabil.* 2006;21(3):199–212.

49. VA/DoD TBI Workgroup. *Clinical practice guideline: Management of concussion/mTBI.* 2009. Available at: http://www.healthquality .va.gov/mtbi/concussion_mtbi_full_1_0.pdf. Accessed August 25, 2011.

50. Larson EB, Zollman FS. The effect of sleep medications on cognitive recovery from traumatic brain injury. *J Head Trauma Rehabil.* 2010; 25(1):61–67.

51. Bryant R. Post traumatic stress disorder versus traumatic brain injury. *Dialogues Clin Neurosci.* 2009;13(3):251–262.

52. Zatzick DF, Rivara FP, Jurkovich GJ, et al. Multisite investigation of traumatic brain injuries, posttraumatic stress disorder, and self-reported health and cognitive impairments. *Arch Gen Psychiatry.* 2010;67(12):1291–1300.

53. Kennedy JE, Cullen MA, Amador RR, Huey JC, Leal FO. Symptoms in military service members after blast mTBI with and without associated injuries. *NeuroRehabilitation.* 2010;26(3):191–197.

54. Brenner LA, Ivins BJ, Schwab K, et al. Traumatic brain injury, posttraumatic stress disorder, and postconcussive symptom reporting among troops returning from Iraq. *J Head Trauma Rehabil.* 2010; 25(5):307–312.

55. Cooper DB, Kennedy JE, Cullen MA, Critchfield E, Amador RR, Bowles AO. Association between combat-stress and and postconcussive symptom reporting in OEF/OIF service members with mild traumatic brain injury. *Brain Inj.* 2011;5(1):1–7.

56. Lew HL, Otis JD, Tun C, Kerns RD, Clark ME, Cifu DX. Prevalence of chronic pain, posttraumatic stress disorder, and persistent postconcussive symptoms in OIF/OEF veterans: a polytrauma clinical triad. *J Head Trauma Rehabil.* 2008;46(6):697–702.

57. Polusny MA, Kehle SM, Nelson NW, Erbes CR, Arbisi PA, Thuras P. Longitudinal effects of mild traumatic brain injury and posttraumatic stress disorder comorbidity on postdeployment outcomes in national guard soldiers deployed to Iraq. *Archives Gen Psych.* 2011; 68(1):79–89.

58. Hoge CW, McGurk D, Thomas JL, Cox AL, Engel CC, Castro CA.

Mild traumatic brain injury in U.S. Soldiers returning from Iraq. *New Eng J Med.* 2008;358(5):453–463.

59. Vanderploeg RD, Belanger HD, Curtiss G. Mild traumatic brain injury and post-traumatic stress disorder and their associations with health symptoms. *Arch Phys Med Rehabil.* 2009;90(7): 1084–1093.

60. Nelson LA, Yoash-Gantz RE, Pickett TC, Campbell TA. Relationship between processing speed and executive functioning performance among OEF/OIF veterans: implications for postdeployment rehabilitation. *J Head Trauma Rehabil.* 2009;24(1):32–40.

61. Huckans M, Pavawalla S, Demadura T, et al. A pilot study examining effects of group based Cognitive Strategy Training treatment on self-reported cognitive problems, psychiatric symptoms, functioning, and compensatory strategy use in OIF/OEF combat veterans with persistent mild cognitive disorder and history of traumatic brain injury. *J Rehab Res Dev.* 2010;47(1):43–60.

62. Halbauer JD, Ashford JW, Zeitzer JM, Adamson MM, Lew HL, Yesavage JA. Neuropsychiatric diagnosis and management of chronic sequelae of war-related mild to moderate traumatic brain injury. *J Rehabil Res Devel.* 2009;46(6):757–796.

63. Bell RS, Ecker RD, Severson MA III, Wanebo JE, Crandall B, Armonda RA. The evolution of the treatment of traumatic cerebrovascular injury during wartime. *Neurosurg Focus.* 2010;28(5):E5.

64. Armonda RA, Bell RS, Vo AH, et al. Wartime traumatic cerebral vasospasm: recent review of combat casualties. *Neurosurgery.* 2006; 59(6):1215–1225.

65. Bell RS, Mossop CM, Dirks MS, et al. Early decompressive craniectomy for severe penetrating and closed head injury during wartime. *Neurosurgical Focus.* 2010;28(5):E1.

66. Ecker RD, Mulligan LP, Dirks M, et al. Outcomes of 33 patients from the wars in Iraq and Afghanistan undergoing bilateral or bicompartmental craniectomy. *J Neurosurgery.* 2011;115(1):124–129.

67. Kumar AR, Bradley JP, Harshberger R, et al. Warfare-related craniectomy defect reconstruction: early success using custom implant alloplast implants. *Plast Reconstr Surg.* 2011;127(3):1279–1287.

68. Simmons JW, White CE, Ritchie JD, Hardin MO, Dubick MA, Blackbourne LH. Mechanism of injury affects acute coagulopathy of trauma in combat casualties. *J Trauma.* 2011;71(1)(suppl): S74–S77.

69. Cap AP, Spinella PC. Severity of head injury is associated with increased risk of coagulopathy in combat casualties. *J Trauma.* 2011; 71(1)(suppl):S78–S81.

70. Levin HS, Wilde E, Troyanskaya M, et al. Diffusion tensor imaging of mild to moderate blast-related traumatic brain injury and its sequelae. *J Neurotrauma.* 2010;27(4):683–694.

71. Mac Donald CL, Johnson AM, Cooper D, et al. Detection of blast-related traumatic brain injury in U.S. military personnel. *N Engl J Med.* 2011;364(22):2091–2100.

72. Matthews SC, Strigo IA, Simmons AN, O'Connell RM, Reinhardt LE, Moseley SA. A multimodal imaging study in U.S. veterans of Operations Iraqi and Enduring Freedom with and without major depression after blast-related concussion. *Neuroimage.* 2001;(54) (suppl 1):S69–S75.

73. Gosselin N, Bottari C, Chen JK, et al. Electrophysiology and functional MRI in post-acute mild traumatic brain injury. *J Neurotrauma.* 2011;28(3):329–341.

74. Marion DW, Curley KC, Schwab K, Hicks RR; for mTBI Diagnostics Workgroup. Proceedings of the military mTBI Diagnostics Workshop, St. Pete Beach, August 2010. *J Neurotrauma.* 2011;28(4): 517–526.

75. McCrea M, Kelly J, Randolph C, et al. Standardized assessment of concussion (SAC): on-site mental status evaluation of the athlete. *J head Trauma Rehab.* 1998;13(2):27–35.

76. Coldren RL, Kelly MP, Parish RV, Dretsch M, Russell ML. Evaluation of the Military Acute Concussion Evaluation for use in combat operations more than 12 hours after injury. *Mil Med.* 2010;175(7): 477–481.

77. Ponsford J, Willmott C, Rothwell A, et al. Impact of early intervention on outcome following mild head injury in adults. *J Neurol Neurosurg Psychiatry.* 2002;73(3):330–332.

78. Rosenfeld JV, Ford NL. Bomb blast, mild traumatic brain injury and psychiatric morbidity: a review. *Injury.* 2010;41(5):437–443.

79. Jaffee MS, Helmick KM, Girard PD, Meyer KS, Dinegar K, George K. Acute clinical care and care coordination for traumatic brain injury within Department of Defense. *J Rehabil Res Dev.* 2009;46(6): 655–666.

80. Drake AI, Meyer KS, Cessante LM, et al. Routine TBI screening following combat deployments. *NeuroRehabilitation.* 2010;26(3): 183–189.

81. Meyer KS, Marion DW, Coronel H, Jaffee MS. Combat-related traumatic brain injury and its implications to military healthcare. *Psychiatr Clin North Am.* 2010;33(4):783–796.

82. Iverson GL, Lange RT, Brooks BL, Rennison VL. "Good old days" bias following mild traumatic brain injury. *Clin Neuropsychol.* 2010; 24(1):17–37.

83. Suhr JA, Gunstad J. Further exploration of the effect of "diagnosis threat" on cognitive performance in individuals with mild head injury. *J Int Neuropsychol Soc.* 2005;11(1):23–29.

84. Tolin DF, Steenkamp MM, Marx BP, Litz BT. Detecting symptom exaggeration in combat veterans using the MMPI-2 symptom validity scales: a mixed group validation. *Psychol Assess.* 2010;22(4): 729–736.

85. Adamson DM, Burnam MA, Burns RM, et al. *Invisible wounds of war: Psychological and cognitive injuries, their consequences, and services to assist recovery, Santa Monica, Calif: RAND Corporation, MG-720-CCF, 2008.* Available at: http://www.rand.org/pubs/monographs/. Accessed December 20, 2011.

86. Belanger HG, Kretzmer T, Yoash-Gantz R, Pickett T, Tupler LA. Cognitive sequelae of blast-related versus other mechanisms of brain trauma. *J Int Neuropsychol Soc.* 2009;15(1):1–8.

87. International State-of-the-Science on Non-Impact, Blast-Induced Mild Traumatic Brain Injury. Available at: http://www.dvbic .org/images/pdfs/Summary-of-Meeting-Proceedings–Non-Impact,-Blast.aspx. Acccessed August 25, 2011.

88. Vos PE, Jacobs B, Andriessen TM, et al. GFAP and S100B are biomarkers of traumatic brain injury: an observational cohort study. *Neurology.* 2010;75(20):1786–1793.

89. Mondello S, Papa L, Buki A, et al. Neuronal and glial markers are differently associated with computed tomography findings and outcome in patients with severe traumatic brain injury: a case control study. *Crit Care.* 2011;15(3):R156.

90. Erdman J, Oria M, Pillsbury L. *Nutrition and Traumatic Brain Injury: Improving Acute and Subacute Health Outcomes in Military Personnel.* Institute of Medicine; 2011.

91. Rona RJ, Jones M, Fear NT, Sundin J, Hull L, Wessley S. Frequency of mild traumatic brain injury in Iraq and Afghanistan: are we measuring incidence or prevalence? *J Head Trauma Rehabil.* 2012; 27(1):75–82.

92. Rona RJ, Jones M, Fear NT, et al. Mild traumatic brain injury in UK military personnel returning from Afghanistan and Iraq: cohort and cross-sectional analyses. *J Head Trauma Rehabil.* 2012;27(1): 33–44.

93. Van Zuiden M, Geuze E, Willemen HL, et al. Glucocorticoid receptor pathway components predict posttraumatic stress disorder symptom development: a prospective study. *Biol Psychiatry.* 2011; 71(4):309–316.

94. Baker AJ, Topolovec-Vranic J, Michalak A, et al. Controlled blast exposure during forced explosive entry training and mild traumtic brain injury. *J Trauma.* 2011;71(5)(suppl 1):S472–S477.

95. Nelson C, St Syr K, Weisser M, Gifford S, Gallimore J, Morningstar A. Knowledge gained from the Brief Traumatic Brain Injury Screen—implications for treating Canadian military personnel. *Mil Med.* 2011;176(2):156–160.

96. Nelson NW, Hoetzle JB, McGuire KA, et al. Self-report of psychological function among OEF/OIF personnel who also report combat-related concussion. *Clin Neuropsychol.* 2011;25(5):716–740.

97. Bryan C, Hernandez A. Magnitudes of decline on ANAM subtest scores relative to predeployment baseline performance among service members evaluated for traumatic brain injury in Iraq. *J Head Trauma Rehab.* 2012;27(12):45–54.

VII

PEDIATRIC TBI

Pediatric Traumatic Brain Injury: Special Considerations

Brad G. Kurowski, Linda Michaud, Lynn Babcock, and Tara Rhine

INTRODUCTION

Because of ongoing brain development in children, the effects of traumatic brain injury (TBI) differ in children compared to adults, and the evaluation and management of TBI in children needs to include special considerations. This chapter will address these special considerations in children with TBI from an epidemiologic, pathophysiologic, assessment, and management perspective. This chapter will supplement other chapters in the text and provide a perspective on the current framework for the care of children with TBI.

EPIDEMIOLOGY

TBI is the most common cause of morbidity and mortality in children. In children aged 0–14 years, 473,947 emergency department (ED) visits, 35,136 hospitalizations, and 2,174 deaths occur annually in the United States (1). The rate of TBI is highest in children aged 0–4 years (1,256 per 100,000) and older adolescents aged 15–19 years (757 per 100,000) (1). In children aged 0–14 years, 50.2% of TBI are caused by falls, 24.8% are caused by being struck by/against an object (e.g., colliding with a moving or stationary object), and 6.8% are caused by motor vehicle accidents. The rate of fall related TBI is highest among children aged 0–4 years (839 per 100,000) and the rate of motor vehicle accident related TBI is highest among children aged 15–19 years (195 per 100,000). Boys are more likely to sustain a TBI than girls. Boys aged 0–4 years having the highest injury rate (1,357 per 100,000); however, girls aged 0–4 years have the second highest injury rate (1,150 per 100,000).

TBI in children is also associated with large economic and societals costs. In the year 2006, it was estimated that pediatric TBI-associated hospital charges were approximately $2.56 billion annually in the United States (2). Additionally, in the year 2000, pediatric TBIs resulted in an estimated $60 billion direct and indirect medical cost in the United States (3).

PATHOPHYSIOLOGY

The brain of a child differs from the adult brain regarding anatomy, biomechanics, and physiology; therefore, a child's brain likely responds differently to brain injury than an adult's brain (see Chapters 10–13). Children have increased brain water content, less myelination, increased cerebral metabolic rate, increased blood flow, greater number of synapses, and different skull elasticity compared to an adult (4–8). The degree of primary injury, including contusions and shear injury, is likely influenced by these factors. Secondary injury is similar to that encountered in adult TBI and occurs because of complications after the initial injury. Secondary injury factors typically include hypotension, hypoxia, seizure activity, infarction, and edema. One of the primary goals after the initial injury is to minimize these complications. Control of cerebral perfusion pressure and intracranial pressure (ICP) after pediatric TBI is important during the initial management to improve mortality and morbidity (9–11). Additionally, it was previously thought that recovery from brain injury during childhood was more favorable than brain injury in adulthood because a developing brain was more flexible and had the ability to reorganize. However, recent research is finding that very early insults are associated with poorer outcomes compared to lesions that occur later in childhood (12).

GRADING OF INJURY SEVERITY

Glasgow Coma Scale

The Glasgow Coma Scale (GCS) is a validated clinical tool created to assist with evaluating level of consciousness using 3 scores assigned based on motor response, verbal response, and eye opening response (13). The issue with using the GCS in infants, young children, and children with neurodevelopmental delay is that the score requires a specific level of cognitive ability in order to be an appropriate assessment tool. Multiple modifications of the GCS and additional coma scales have been created and validated, although there is often inconsistent use within hospitals secondary to health care providers' preferences, comfort level, and knowledge of pediatric coma scales (14–19). It has been found that when comparing these scales, the interobserver agreement was highest for the Pediatric GCS (Table 34-1) (14). This validated scale (19) is recommended for use in infants and children by the American Heart Association's Pediatric Advanced Life Support guidelines (20).

TABLE 34-1 Pediatric Glasgow Coma Scale

EYE OPENING		VERBAL RESPONSE		MOTOR RESPONSE	
Spontaneous	4	Oriented to sound or visual stimuli, interacts	5	Normal spontaneous movement	6
To verbal or touch stimuli	3	Cries but consolable	4	Withdraws to touch	5
To painful stimuli	2	Inconsistently consolable, moaning	3	Withdraws to pain	4
None	1	Inconsolable, agitated	2	Flexion to pain	3
		None	1	Extension to pain	2
				None	1

When assigning a GCS score to a patient, one must remember to account for confounders that complicate the score, such as medications that could decrease arousal, endotracheal intubation, or facial trauma causing eye swelling. Classically, if a patient is intubated, their GCS verbal component's score will be assigned as a "1-T" (1 point assigned for verbal, plus a "T" for tube). Research has found that a Grimace Score (Table 34-2) has good interobserver reliability and could replace the verbal component in intubated children given that facial expression is an important part of both verbal and nonverbal communication that begins early on in life (18). Finally, if a patient's eyes are swollen shut secondary to trauma, then the GCS eye component's score should be assigned a "1-C" (1 point for eye opening, plus a "C" for closed). If there are multiple confounders and scoring becomes complicated, studies have found that the motor component is the most important score of the three and it is comparable to the total GCS score (17).

The critical GCS score is the score cutoff that has been found to best predict a patient's outcome. The critical GCS score has been set at "8" for adult TBIs (21); however, multiple studies have shown that a critical GCS score of "5" is more strongly correlated with the outcome of pediatric TBI. In children with GCS scores of 3–5, about 11% subsequently die and the vast remainder goes on to develop severe disabilities. Pediatric patients with TBI and a GCS score >5, without deterioration within the first 24 hours after injury, usually have good outcomes (21–26). However, when predicting outcomes other clinical variables such as the presence of a hypoxic-ischemic event, head computed tomography (CT) findings, and pupillary response must also be considered.

Post-Traumatic Amnesia

The Children's Orientation and Amnesia Test (COAT) was developed to assess post-traumatic amnesia (PTA) in children and adolescents from ages 3 to 15 years (27). The COAT assesses general orientation to person and place, temporal orientation, and memory (immediate, short-term, and remote). The temporal orientation items cannot be used reliably in children younger than 8 years. Serial COAT scores provide an objective monitor of cognitive improvement in early post-TBI recovery in children and adolescents. Deferral of neuropsychological evaluation until COAT scores improve to the average range, that is, after resolution of PTA, ensures neuropsychological test scores that are more representative of post-traumatic abilities (27). Duration of PTA has been associated with severity of injury and with outcome post-TBI, with shorter durations reflecting lesser injury severity and better outcomes. Time to follow commands postinjury, however, may be a better predictor of outcome than PTA in children (28).

Duration of Unconsciousness

Duration of unconsciousness is used to rate brain injury severity similar in adults and children. In children, less than 15–30 minutes of unconsciousness is commonly categorized as mild TBI, 15 minutes to 24 hours of unconsciousness as moderated TBI, 1–90 days of unconsciousness as severe TBI, and greater than 90 days of unconsciousness as profound TBI (29).

MILD TRAUMATIC BRAIN INJURY

Acute Assessment and Management

In the acute setting, initial assessment for children with milder injury (see Chapters 29 and 31), such as those with GCS 13–15, is focused on symptom management and select-

TABLE 34-2 Grimace vs Verbal Score

VERBAL RESPONSE		GRIMACE RESPONSE	
Oriented to sound or visual stimuli, interacts	5	Normal spontaneous facial movement	5
Cries but consolable	4	Less than usual spontaneous facial changes	4
Inconsistently consolable, moaning	3	Vigorous grimace to pain	3
Inconsolable, agitated	2	Mild grimace or change in facial expression to pain	2
None	1	No facial response to pain	1
Intubated	1-T		

ing those children who are in need of imaging to detect possible intracranial injury. Currently, cranial CTs are performed in about 50% of these children who present to EDs in the United States. For this mild cohort, the incidence of intracranial injury such as subdural, epidural, or intracerebral hematomas in mild TBI is between 3% and 7% among children and between 4% and 48% in children less than 2 years of age (30–34). Although imaging every child would reduce the risk of missing some of the intracranial injuries, this approach is neither feasible nor practical, and may even be risky. Early exposure to radiation, increased length of stay in the ED, and risks of sedations are potential complications of this approach. Recently, several prospective studies have identified a group of historical and physical findings that can predict those children who are at low risk of intracranial injury, thus negating the need for cranial CT (33,35,36). Key variables in rules include GCS <15, the presence of vomiting, headache, loss of consciousness, scalp hematoma, signs of skull fracture, signs of basilar skull fracture, and the mechanism of injury. Perhaps in the best designed and largest (more than 50,000 children) study to date, a multicenter pediatric emergency medicine network (PECARN) derived and validated prediction rule for younger and older children had near perfect negative predictive values with very narrow 95% confidence intervals (33). Although these rules can identify children at low risk of intracranial injury with a high degree of sensitivity, potentially decreasing cranial CT rates by approximately 25%, they have been slow to be integrated into clinical practice (33,37).

Management of mild TBI is directed at minimizing the individual symptoms. Aside from the pharmacologic treatment of headaches, usually with over-the-counter nonsteroidal anti-inflammatory agents such as acetaminophen or ibuprofen, rest and reduction of activity levels is generally recommended. However, there is little evidence for these recommendations. In one of the only and best designed pediatric mild TBI treatment studies to date, Ponsford and colleagues (38) compared the relative efficacy of an informational booklet outlining common symptoms of mild TBI and strategies for addressing them relative to usual care in 119 children with mild TBI. At 3 months postinjury, individuals who did not receive the booklet had higher levels of behavioral symptoms and stress, suggesting that the information provided reduced anxiety, thereby resulting in fewer behavioral consequences. In an effort to increase recognition and to ensure adequate basic treatment of the mild TBI and possible sequelae, the Centers for Disease Control and Prevention (CDC) recently sponsored the development of Acute Concussion Evaluation (ACE) and the ACE–Emergency Department version (Assessment and Care Plan). These plans delineate general instructions for practitioners to better identify concussions, provide patients with information on concussion symptoms, provide instructions for gradual return to cognitive or physical activities, and can be used for children ages 5 years and up (39).

Outcome

Mild TBI accounts for more than 90% of TBIs that occur in children in the United States (40) and clinically significant deficits long-term (> 1 year) after mild injuries are rare (41); however, a significant percentage of individuals may develop persistent symptoms. Mild TBI can result in a constellation of physical, cognitive, emotional, and/or sleep-related symptoms that may last from several minutes to days, weeks, months, or even longer in some cases (42). The resultant sequelae are commonly referred to as postconcussion syndrome (PCS) (see Chapter 29) and can lead to impairment of physical, psychological, and academic functioning. Prospective follow-up data suggest that about 60% of children with mild TBI meet criteria for PCS 1 month after injury and about 10% continue to meet criteria for PCS 3 months after injury (43–46). Headaches (30%–58%), fatigue (19%–78%), and dizziness (17%) are the predominant physical symptoms following mild TBI (43,44,47–49). Evidence regarding persistent consequences of mild TBI in children is equivocal. Although there are some reports of increased hyperactivity (50), visual defects (51,52), and reading impairments (51) following mild TBI in children, a recent systematic review (53) found that most studies did not demonstrate long-term cognitive or behavioral deficits attributable to the brain injury. In the largest longitudinal prospective study of recovery from mild TBI in children published to date, significant impairments in memory, psychomotor speed, and language were found up to 1 year following injury; however, similar differences were also found in the cohort of children with other injuries, but not with noninjured children (54). In youth, the presence of headaches (47) and dizziness (55) immediately after mild TBI has been shown to predict the development of PCS and protracted recovery, respectively. Interestingly, an association between loss of consciousness at the time of injury and the development of PCS or cognitive deficits has not been demonstrated (47,53). In addition to factors associated with the injury itself, premorbid personal and social factors have been shown to be equally, if not more, important determinants of outcomes following mild TBI (56,57). Personal characteristics such as age (58,59), gender (60), prior head injury (43,61), premorbid cognitive ability (62), preexisting learning disabilities (43,63), comorbid conditions (64,65), and coping skills (66) may influence the persistence of symptoms. Other environmental factors, including socioeconomic status and family functioning, may also affect postinjury trajectory (60,67–70).

Sequelae of the injury may also affect school attendance and performance. Although the acute injury usually results in 2–3 days out of school, children who develop PCS miss an average of 8 days of school (47). Returning to school without provisions for reduced cognitive workloads can aggravate symptoms and further delay recovery. As such, all children with mild TBI and concomitant PCS would benefit from a few global informal modifications such as reduced workloads, shortened school days, and postponed testing in the first few days/weeks after the injury to assist with the transition back to school (71,72).

MODERATE AND SEVERE TRAUMATIC BRAIN INJURY

Acute Assessment and Management

Regardless of severity, the goal of initial management is to prevent or ameliorate secondary injury by maintaining adequate aeration, ventilation, and circulation (73). For children with moderate and severe injury (GCS 3–12), more aggressive management is often necessary. Stabilization of the cervical spine is also necessary because of high incidence of comorbidity (74). Early and rapid transfer to a pediatric trauma center should be considered for these children. Airway support is often required and rapid sequence intubation is indicated in children with a GCS <8, significant hypoxemia, inadequate ventilation, inability to control or protect the airway, or hemodynamic instability. The goal is to provide adequate oxygenation to the brain and normalize partial pressure of carbon dioxide (PcO_2) to prevent adjunctive vasoconstriction. Maintenance of adequate perfusion, usually through the intravascular administration of isotonic solutions, is necessary to avoid hypotension to maintain adequate cerebral perfusion pressure. At the present time, maintenance of euthermia is recommended because worse outcomes have been associated with hyperthermia (75). Furthermore, the effect of induced moderate hypothermia on neurologic outcomes for children with moderate/severe TBI remains controversial, especially in light of a recent multi-center study that did not improve neurologic outcomes (75). Cranial CTs have a pivotal role in the immediate assessment and subsequent management of children with signs of moderate/severe TBI and can detect structural anomalies such as fractures, subdural, epidural, or brain parenchymal hematomas, subarachnoid hemorrhage, brain swelling, edema, and mass effects. Pediatric specific grading systems (76) such as the Marshall classification (77) or Rotterdam classification (78) are used to report findings in a structured/universal format.

The remainder of the management for children with moderate and severe injury is primarily dependent on presenting signs and symptoms (79). Most children will be in need of analgesia and sedation. Ideal agents are ones that do not raise intracranial pressure, such as midazolam or lorazepam, fentanyl, or propofol. If a child is acutely having seizures, pharmacologic control is necessary with intravenous benzodiazepine such as lorazepam or diazepam. Prophylactic use of longer acting antiseizure medicines such as fosphenytoin/phenytoin or levetiracetam to prevent the incidence of post-traumatic seizures may decrease further seizures for the first week following injury; however, longer term use is controversial and needs further study.

For acute signs of increasing ICP and acute brain herniation—such as third nerve palsy, diminished pupillary responses, fixation and dilation of pupils, rising systemic blood pressure or ICP, and decreasing heart rate—immediate aggressive intervention is needed. Simple measures should be initially performed, such as elevating head of bed to 30° to decrease venous obstruction and mild hyperventilation (PcO_2 30–35 mm Hg) to cause vasoconstriction. Depending on severity, initiation of hyperosmolar therapy with agents such as mannitol or hypertonic saline to acutely decrease the interstitial volume should be considered. The recommended dose of mannitol is 0.5 mg/kg of 20% solution to raise serum osmolality to 320 mOsm/L. Complications may include hypovolemia and electrolyte disturbances. Hypertonic saline can also reduce ICP (80,81). It may be advantageous to use mannitol in that it has less osmotic diuresis and it may better control a sustained uniform reduction in ICP (82); however, it may cause reversible renal insufficiency and trigger central pontine myelinosis that can be associated with

rapid changes in serum sodium, yet this has not been seen in clinical trials (80). Optimal dosing has not been clearly established; however, 3% saline at 2–6 mL/kg boluses over 5–10 minutes is commonly used to raise serum osmolality to 360 mOsm/L. Because intracranial hypertension is associated with poor neurologic outcomes, ICP monitoring is recommended for children with GCS <8. Age stratified norms for ICP have not been established, yet the consensus is to keep ICP less than 20 mm Hg. In addition to positioning, mild hyperventilation, and administration of osmotic agents, other therapies such as paralysis and barbiturate therapy, as well as decompressive craniectomy if needed, can be used to control ICP (79).

Other potential therapeutic agents primarily targeting secondary mechanisms of brain injury, including antioxidants, free radical scavengers, ion channel blockers, N-methyl-d-aspartate (NMDA) antagonists, gamma-aminobutyric acid (GABA) agonists, and other neuroprotectants including progesterone that can protect neurons from the sequelae of ischemia and hypoxia immediately postinjury either have not been tested or proven effective in children.

Outcomes

Mortality rate for severe TBI in children ranges from 30% to 59% (40,83–85). Age less than 2 years, GCS of 5 or less, accidental hypothermia, hyperglycemia, and coagulation disorders were found to be independent predictors of mortality (83). Multiple risk factors have also been associated with increased morbidity after TBI in children, including abnormal oculocephalic and light reflexes, posturing, GCS <7, need for ventilator support, longer duration of coma, age of injury lower than 2 years, hypotension, hyperglycemia, increased intracranial pressure with cerebral perfusion pressure lower than 50 mm Hg, development of post-traumatic amnesia, and physical abuse as the cause of injury (9–11, 86–89). Facco et al. specifically found that the combined evaluation of oculocephalic reflex and need for ventilation provided the best prognostic information in children (86). Children may often survive longer in a minimally conscious or vegetative state than adults with TBI (see Chapter 32) and are more likely to regain consciousness after a prolonged period of unconsciousness. In a study of 60 children with, primarily, TBI who were unconscious for 90 days or greater, 8 died, 13 remained in a persistent vegetative state (PVS), and 39 regained consciousness (90). Children who remain in a PVS have the highest risk of mortality (90,91). Factors most predictive of disability after severe TBI are GCS motor responses 72 hours after injury and level of oxygenation in the ED (85). Indices most predictive of early and 1-year neurobehavioral and functional measures in children are days to 75% age-adjusted performance on the COAT, number of days to GCS score of 15, and initial GCS score (92). Additionally, 1 study found that children 6 years and older had better cognitive and motor outcomes and less brain atrophy outcomes than younger children (93). In summary, the mortality rate is slightly lower in children with severe TBI compared to adults; however, younger age at injury is associated with worse functional outcomes in general.

Rehabilitation

The goals of rehabilitation for children with brain injuries include maximizing developmentally appropriate and age-appropriate function and participation by addressing seven domains: general management; family-centered care; cognitive-communication speech, language, and swallowing; gross and fine motor skills; neuropsychological, social, and behavior; school reentry; and community integration (94). School entry or reentry is a major concern unique to post-TBI rehabilitation of youth. TBI can have a major impact on vocational development and the achievement of economic independence, with significant implications because of injury occurring in childhood and adolescence, when the individual's entire potentially productive life lies ahead. A child's TBI often places stressors on the entire family, including on siblings. In addition to physical, occupational, speech-language, and recreational therapists, psychologists, social workers, and vocational counselors, children additionally benefit from interventions by child life therapists and educators to address all of the aforementioned domains of function as needed.

Pediatric inpatient rehabilitation units and units with higher volumes of children with TBI are more likely to have adequate specialized equipment, a classroom, a medical director who is pediatric subspecialty trained, and more than 75% of therapists with pediatric training (95). Whether outcomes post-TBI in youth are improved in association with such variations in the structure and organization of pediatric rehabilitation remains to be demonstrated. Efforts to use common outcome measures in pediatric TBI research should facilitate better evaluation of comparative effectiveness of components of rehabilitation care addressing the affected domains of function leading to more efficient clinical research and ultimately improved care (96).

Sub-Acute and Chronic Medical and Rehabilitative Issues

Autonomic Dysfunction

Autonomic dysfunction or paroxysmal sympathetic hyperactivity (PSH)after TBI is characterized similarly in adults and children by increased heart rate, respiratory rate, temperature, blood pressure, sweating, and muscle overactivity (see Chapter 52). The exact incidence of PSH in children after TBI has not been well elucidated. However, 1 study found 14.1% of children who had been unconscious for 24 hours or more after an acquired brain injury developed PSH (97). This is similar to reported rates of 9.3%–33% in adult TBI (98,99). PSH is associated with an increased duration of unconsciousness, worse cognitive and motor outcomes, and mortality in children with TBI (97). Treatment for PSH in children most commonly includes propranolol (100,101); however, there have been reports of successful management of PSH in children with bromocriptine (102) and intrathecal baclofen (103).

Post-Traumatic Epilepsy

Seizure susceptibility differs between the adult (also see Chapter 39) and child brain because the immature and developing brain primarily favors neuronal excitability (104). Age is a primary factor in the development of seizures (104,105). The incidence of post-traumatic seizures after pediatric TBI ranges from 9.6% to 68% for early (<7days) seizures (104, 106–109) and from 1% to 20% for late (> 7 days) seizures (108–110). Most seizures are immediate (< 24 hours) after pediatric TBI (104,106–108). Children younger than 3 years of age with severe injury (GCS of 3–8), cerebral edema, or a depressed skull fracture have an increased risk of early post-traumatic seizures (111). Additionally, compared to adults, children with severe TBI need longer follow-up because they are at increased risk of developing seizures late (> 10–15 years) after injury (112,113). Family history of epilepsy is also associated with the development of post-traumatic seizures after mild (Relative Risk = 5.75) and severe (Relative Risk = 10.09) TBI in children and young adults (113).

Prophylactic use of phenytoin for early post-traumatic seizures after pediatric TBI may be considered for high-risk individuals; however, prophylactic use of phenytoin to prevent late post-traumatic seizures is not recommended (114). Antiepileptic drugs (AED) commonly used include phenytoin (115); however, various other AEDs are also used in clinical practice. Early seizures increase the risk of development of late seizures (110). AEDs are typically initiated for treatment of late post-traumatic epilepsy. A trial off AEDs is typically considered after a seizure free period of 2 years while on medications (116–118).

Post-Traumatic Hydrocephalus

As with adult TBI, ventriculomegaly can be seen after pediatric TBI, especially severe TBI (119). Differentiating post-traumatic hydrocephalus and cerebral atrophy as causes of ventriculomegaly is important. Ventricular enlargement is common (29%–72%) after severe pediatric TBI (120), but true hydrocephalus is relatively uncommon (1%–9%) (120,121). Signs of hydrocephalus on CT scan commonly include distended appearance of the frontal horns of the lateral ventricles, enlargement of the temporal horns and third ventricles, normal or absent sulci, enlargement of the basal cisterns and fourth ventricle, and the presence of periventricular hypodensity (120,122,123). Cerebral atrophy is characterized by diffuse ventriculomegaly in the presence of prominent sulci and absence of periventricular lucency (120,123). Clinical signs of hydrocephalus can include irritability or depressed mental status, seizures, increase tone, and functional decline. Definitive treatment for post-traumatic hydrocephalus is often shunt placement that may lead to neurologic improvement (120,124).

Neuroendocrine Dysfunction

Endocrine dysfunction after pediatric TBI most commonly includes hypothalamic-pituitary axis dysregulation. This is similar to adult TBI (see Chapter 53); however, surveillance for endocrine dysfunction after pediatric TBI is especially important because growth and physical and neurocognitive development can be significantly affected by hormone abnormalities (125–129). Endocrine dysfunctions that occur in the first days after moderate to severe TBI in childhood is similar to changes that occur after other critical illnesses (125,128). Longer term sequelae of neuroendocrine dysfunction are beginning to be explored. In a prospectively followed cohort of children with moderate to severe TBI, the incidence of endocrine dysfunction was 15% at 1 month, 75% at 6 months, and 29% at 12 months. At 12 months postinjury,

14% had precocious puberty, 9% had hypothyroidism, and 5% had growth hormone deficiency (130). Systematic screening for neuroendocrine dysfunction should be performed after moderate to severe pediatric TBI (127). Endocrine dysfunction may present months or years postinjury; therefore, monitoring for symptoms long-term postinjury is important. Additionally, neuroendocrine dysfunction has been associated with mild TBI in adolescence and screening should also be considered based on symptoms in this population (131). Timely management of endocrine dysfunction after pediatric TBI will help to facilitate normal growth and development (126).

Respiratory Dysfunction

Children with the more severe brain injuries are commonly intubated and many—especially those with severe injury with GCS ≤8—require tracheostomy for management of central respiratory problems and control of oral and pulmonary secretions. Tracheostomy is believed to be associated with higher morbidity in children with TBI, in whom the size of the airway is smaller than in adults (132). Complications of tracheostomy in pediatric patients with TBI include aspiration pneumonia, tracheal granuloma formation, vocal cord paralysis or other phonation dysfunction, tracheal stenosis, glottic or subglottic stenosis, tracheomalacia, tube obstruction, and unintentional decannulation (132–135). Ongoing surveillance and preventive maintenance can be helpful in decreasing the incidence and adverse outcomes of some of these complications. However, surgical intervention may be indicated for airway reconstruction in some children.

Gastrointestinal

Most children with severe brain injuries sustain associated injuries to other body systems, commonly abdominal (85). Even without concurrent gastrointestinal (GI) injury, children with severe TBI are at risk for GI complications (see Chapter 54). These include predisposition to develop upper GI bleeding (136), for which the use of histamine H_2 antagonists is common practice, especially while nasogastric feeding tubes remain in place. Gastroesophageal reflux is common after pediatric TBI and is typically managed medically, although for some children fundoplication is warranted. Ischemic injury and medications may result in elevations in liver enzymes, generally transiently. Increases in pancreatic enzymes are also common in children after severe TBI. Delayed increases are associated with intracranial hypertension and intracranial hemorrhage, suggesting a possible interaction between the brain and GI system, with the implication that disturbances in cerebral hemodynamics may lead to pancreatic dysfunction (137). Early recognition is crucial for institution of therapies in some cases (parenteral nutrition, bowel rest, jejunostomy tube feeding).

Genitourinary

Following TBI in children and adolescents, micturition disturbances have not been a topic of focused research. In one study of urinary disturbances following TBI, children as young as 9 years of age were included; however, results were not analyzed separately for children and adults (138). Findings in this study indicate that patients with moderate or severe brain injuries may commonly have asymptomatic urodynamic abnormalities and that these abnormalities are

associated with the presence of motor deficits and are likely generalizable to the pediatric population based on clinical experience. A useful guide to prediction of normal bladder capacity for age that can aid in recognition of abnormal voiding patterns in children with TBI is as follows: normal bladder capacity (ounces) equals age (years) plus 2 (139). This simple formula may be used until the age of 14 years, when the 16-ounce (480 mL) bladder capacity is that of an adult. Postvoid residual volumes should be kept lower than 10% of bladder capacity for age to avoid complications such as urinary tract infections. The possibility of medication-related urinary retention must be kept in mind, in particular for those children undergoing acute rehabilitation. Post-TBI voiding abnormalities in adults has a good prognosis to resolve (140) and, based on clinical experience, this is likely applicable to children as well.

Heterotopic Ossification

The incidence of neurogenic heterotopic ossification (HO) seems lower in children (10%–15%) than in adults after TBI (see Chapter 49) (141–143). Clinical presentation is similar in children in comparison to adults, with warmth and swelling, pain, and/or restricted mobility, occurring on average of 4 months post-trauma, with a range from 3 weeks to 20 months post-TBI (141). The hip, knee, shoulder, and elbow are the most commonly involved sites (142). Risk factors in youth with severe TBI include age after the first decade and greater length of coma (142). Post-TBI HO can occur in the preschool years and develop after the child is no longer in coma (141). Management of HO includes range of motion exercises. Disodium etidronate therapy in youth may result in a rachitic syndrome and alternate treatments should be considered (144). Salicylates have been suggested to have a useful role in children with severe TBI in prophylaxis and postsurgical management (143). Surgical excision, when indicated, is generally deferred for at least 1 year (141).

Venous Thromboembolism

Deep vein thrombosis (DVT) and pulmonary embolism have been reported to occur rarely in children with TBI (145–146). Although the incidence of DVT in the pediatric trauma population is lower than that in adults and thus may not warrant routine prophylaxis, exceptions might be indicated for those likely to remain immobile for an extended period, require prolonged rehabilitation, have venous manipulations, or present with clinical symptoms (147). There is growing evidence that venous thromboembolism (VTE) is not as rare as previously thought after major trauma in pediatric patients (148). Risk factors for VTE in a population of 58,716 pediatric trauma-related discharges across 19 states in the United States in which the rate of VTE was 0.77 per 1,000 discharges (compared with an overall VTE rate of 6 per 1,000 discharges for 534,487 adult trauma patients in the same study) included increased age within the pediatric age range (relative risk 6.1 for age 10–15 years in comparison to children < 5 years), TBI, greater severity of injury, and craniotomy; venous catheters posed the greatest risk, with a rate of 28.6 of 1,000 discharges (149). Lack of available evidence has precluded definitive recommendations regarding prophylaxis for VTE in the pediatric TBI population to date (149).

Cognitive

Attention problems after pediatric TBI (see Chapters 59–61) are relatively common and referred to as secondary attention deficit hyperactivity disorder (SADHD). In school-age children, SADHD ranges from 14.5% to 21% in the first 24 months postinjury (150–152). Divided and sustained attention are most commonly affected (153–155), which has implications for return to school-based actives that require adequate divided and sustained attention for success. Severe TBI in children is more frequently associated with attention problems postinjury than mild or moderate TBI (150,155); however, preinjury psychosocial adversity and preinjury attention problems are associated with a greater risk of developing SADHD (150). Attention problems are also often comorbid with intellectual and adaptive function deficits, personality change, and new-onset disruptive behavior problems postinjury (150–156). Attention problems may persist for years postinjury, especially after severe TBI (157). Neurostimulant medications may be used to manage attention problems after pediatric TBI (151), but large trials specific to pediatric TBI are lacking.

Memory problems also commonly occur after pediatric TBI. School-aged children with TBI demonstrate poor encoding and acquisition of new verbal memories compared to age-matched controls, suggesting that the nature of learning and memory problems after pediatric TBI is related to working memory impairment (158). Prospective memory deficits typically worsen with increasing cognitive demand in children and adolescents after TBI and children younger at the time of injury tend to perform worse than adolescents (159). Memory difficulties often lead to school difficulties in children. Catroppa and Anderson found that severe TBI, poorer verbal memory indices, and poorer preinjury academic abilities predict greater academic difficulties in up to 24 months postinjury in children ages 8–12 years (160). Additionally, children who sustain a brain injury before age 2 years are at risk of developing global cognitive and adaptive behavior problems up to 2 years postinjury, indicating the importance of monitoring long-term after an early childhood TBI (161). Executive functioning involves multiple constructs, including attention, memory, organization, planning, and problem solving and it is often impaired after pediatric TBI. It is estimated that 18%–38% of children with TBI have significant executive dysfunction during the first year after injury (162). Executive dysfunction can persist long-term postinjury, with dysfunction being most pronounced after severe TBI (163).

Behavioral

Behavioral problems commonly occur after pediatric TBI (also see Chapters 62–64). Increased behavior problems have been reported 6 and 12 months and 4 years postinjury in children who sustained a TBI between age 6 and 12 years (164). The 36% of individuals with severe TBI and 22% of individuals with moderate TBI were found to have persistent long-term behavior problems compared to 10% of a reference group (164). Severe TBI in children who sustained an early injury (ages 3–7 years) is also associated with long-term externalizing behavior problems and executive function problems (165). Psychosocial environment is associated with behavioral problems after injury; social disadvantage is associated with increased behavioral problems both short- and long-term after moderate and severe TBI (69). Preinjury and postinjury family dysfunction, personal or family history of a psychiatric disorder, lower socioeconomic status, and severe TBI are also associated with an increased risk of developing behavioral or psychiatric problems postinjury, including personality syndromes, major depression, attention deficit disorder, oppositional defiant disorder, anxiety disorders, post-traumatic stress disorder, obsessive compulsive disorder, and adjustment disorder (166,167). Preinjury conduct disorder is associated with a greater risk of postinjury conduct disorder; however, an 8% new-onset incidence of oppositional defiant disorder and 9% new-onset incidence of conduct disorder 1 year post-TBI have been reported (168). Personality changes measured using the Neuropsychiatric Rating Schedule (NPRS) occurred in 13% (6–12 months) and in 12% (12–24 months) after TBI in children between ages 5 and 14 years (169). Personality changes 6–12 months postinjury were associated with lesions in the superior frontal gyrus whereas personality changes 12–24 months postinjury were associated with lesions in the frontal white matter (169).

Language

Children with TBI may demonstrate a range of deficits in speech and language function (also see Chapter 65). Recovery of speech, reflecting motor function, is often earlier and more complete than recovery of higher level receptive and expressive language abilities. Communication disorders following pediatric TBI may be expressive, receptive, or mixed, and may impact recovery of already-developed written and/or oral skills, as well as the development of further skills higher than the premorbid level. Dysarthria and dysphasia are common expressive speech and language problems seen in children with TBI. Receptive language impairments commonly involve auditory-perceptual problems. The type and extent of language deficits in children depend on numerous factors, including age at the time of injury and premorbid language development as well as the location, type, and severity of injury (170).

Problems in language are often associated with impairments in cognition and social skills. Severe TBI early in childhood results in increased risk for persisting deficits in higher level discourse abilities, that is, impairments in the pragmatics of language use (171). Childhood TBI may disrupt the ability to abstract the central meaning or "gist" from connected language (172). Even subtle language processing deficits may adversely affect academic performance as well as communication and social interaction (173). Predictors of language and literacy skills at 2 years post-TBI in school-aged children have been identified to include age at injury, preinjury communication skills, and socioeconomic status, as well as vocabulary (173). Intervention by a speech-language pathologist is directed at improving the speech and/or language disorder as well as the associated cognitive and social impairments.

Motor

The site(s) of brain injury determines the type of motor dysfunction that follows pediatric TBI (also see Chapters 49–51). Spasticity, rigidity, ataxia/tremor, weakness, and deficits in balance and coordination are common motor abnormalities. Associated injuries sustained at the time of TBI, such as fractures of the spine or extremities, as in adults, may be associated with concurrent spinal cord injury and/or peripheral nerve injury, including brachial or lumbosacral plexopathies. Functional deficits associated with these impairments may include deficits in developmentally appropriate and age-appropriate mobility, including ambulation and self-care skills, as well as the ability to fully participate in higher level sports and recreational activities.

Physical and occupational therapy are commonly indicated to assist the child in maximizing independence in age-appropriate motor function. Exercises and activities should include an individualized home program after acute inpatient rehabilitation to increase strength, balance, and coordination; reduce spasticity; and prevent contractures and deformities. Orthoses and adaptive equipment for gait and mobility may be needed and the child will need to be monitored for fit and function with growth.

Useful medications to treat spasticity and rigidity include those that are used to treat spasticity in adults after TBI: in particular, baclofen (Lioresal), dantrolene (Dantrium), tizanidine (Zanaflex), and diazepam (Valium). Baclofen can be administered intrathecally as well as orally. As with adults with TBI, management of spasticity may also include nerve blocks, such as with botulinum toxin A or phenol. The effects of Botox last for several months, but repeated injections are required if spasticity persists. Intramuscular injections of botulinum toxin A have demonstrated effectiveness in reducing localized spasticity in children. Serial casting may be used post-Botox for prolonged stretching in some cases of spasticity associated with muscle shortening.

Orthopedic surgery may be required in some chronic situations. Spasticity and weakness may result in an imbalance of forces surrounding joints. Over a prolonged period in the growing child, when asymmetries of muscle tone and strength occur, muscle growth may not keep pace with bone growth and the result can be fixed deformities of the extremities and spine. Long-term contractures or deformities may need to be managed with tendon lengthening or release, osteotomies, or spine stabilization.

Sensory

Vision and hearing can both be affected by TBI in children (also see Chapters 45 and 46). Diplopia may result from cranial nerve involvement (174). Nystagmus, caused by injury to the areas of the brain controlling eye movements, also occurs among children with severe TBI. Less commonly, a crush injury (e.g., blunt object) may injure the globe or a missile injury (e.g., gunshot) may damage the visual pathway; both types of injury may cause irreversible damage. Injury affecting the visual pathway may result in cuts in the visual fields. Retinal hemorrhage is strongly associated with abusive head trauma (175). Finally, a TBI accompanied by severe brain swelling in a child can result in cortical blindness. Cortical blindness involves a visual cortical abnormality; partial or complete recovery can occur. Visual–perceptual and visual–motor deficits can compromise eye–hand coordination and fine motor function. Consultation with pediatric ophthalmology should be obtained for evaluation of children with TBI with any behaviors suggestive of visual impairment.

Hearing loss after TBI (also see Chapter 46) most commonly results from a fracture of the temporal bone and is usually unilateral. Transverse fractures can affect the cochlea and result in sensorineural hearing loss. The more common longitudinal fractures tend to involve the middle ear structures and are associated with conductive hearing loss. Audiologic assessment should be conducted following temporal bone fractures in children because of the frequency with which hearing loss occurs. Deafness is uncommon because involvement is usually unilateral and resolution is frequent (176). Even a mild hearing loss, however, should be identified and corrected with amplification, if indicated, so that the child can benefit maximally from his or her educational environment.

Often underrecognized in children with TBI are abnormalities in smell and/or taste (see Chapter 48) resulting from injuries to cranial nerves I and/or VII. These may be associated with decreases in appetite leading to feeding problems. Inability to appreciate body odor and maintain appropriate hygiene may lead to further social challenges in teens with dysosmia and TBI.

Neuropharmacology

Neuropharmacology in pediatric TBI has not been extensively studied (177). Several specific studies of neuropharmacology in pediatric TBI are highlighted here whereas neuropharmacology for TBI in general is covered in depth elsewhere (see Chapter 72).

Dopamine-enhancing medications are some of the best studied medications to date in pediatric TBI. A retrospective review of various dopamine agonists suggested an association between dopamine-enhancing medications and acceleration of recovery for some children in a low response state (178). A retrospective case-control study specific to amantadine use in pediatric TBI found an improvement in Ranchos Los Amigos level in the amantadine group compared to the control group (179). In a pilot randomized, double-blind, placebo-controlled crossover trial, amantadine facilitated recovery of consciousness in pediatric acquired brain injury (180). These studies suggest that amantadine may be effective in pediatric TBI associated with low response states.

Several other medications specific to pediatric TBI have been evaluated; however, many of the agents commonly used in pediatric TBI are "off label" (177). The extrapolation of medications used in adult TBI to children should be done judiciously. A child's response to medications is likely different than an adult's response. Future research is needed in the use of neuropharmacology in the management of pediatric TBI (see reference 177 for a review of the current state of neuropharmacology in pediatric TBI).

SPECIAL CIRCUMSTANCES

Non-Accidental Trauma

The mechanism of inflicted TBI in young children is most frequently shaking, often associated with impact (181). Incidence is about 17 per 100,000 in children younger than 2 years of age, with highest occurrence in the first year of life (182). The angular deceleration of the brain because of shaking-impact can lead to subdural hematomas, which may be accompanied by contact injuries including skull fractures and brain contusions (181). Secondary injury may include cerebral swelling, which can result in loss of gray–white matter differentiation, predictive of worse recovery. Concurrent injuries on physical exam and radiographs may include retinal hemorrhages, long bone fractures of varying ages, and skin lesions in unusual locations (183). The history provided is often inaccurate, inconsistent with the injuries sustained, and may be implausible and evolve over time. Mortality is 11%–33% (181). Although outcomes are variable in survivors, ranging from apparent absence of functional deficits to persisting physical and cognitive deficits across the spectrum of severity, outcomes overall are worse than those following nonintentional trauma when severity of injury is considered (184). About two-thirds with subdural hematomas have neurological deficits affecting function. Neurobehavioral deficits after injuries sustained in early childhood may not be appreciated until higher level functions mediated by area(s) of the injured brain mature, often not until the child is in elementary school. Thus, follow-up for inflicted TBI should be long-term. Challenges to long-term follow-up in this population of children with brain injury include psychosocial factors that may be associated with the need to place these children with caregivers who are not their parents—sometimes with multiple caregivers—as well as with strict legal and confidentiality restrictions (185).

Anoxic Injury

Severe, anoxic brain injury in children is often associated with poorer cognitive and motor outcomes compared to severe, nonhypoxic TBI in children (90,186). A comparison of severe hypoxic brain injury and nonhypoxic TBI leading to PVS in children and adolescents showed that individuals with hypoxic brain injury were less likely to emerge from PVS (186). Hypoxic injury was also associated with a higher incidence and frequency of seizures and more pneumonia, GI, and HO complications (186). In general, hypoxic injuries are associated with worse overall outcomes and complications than nonhypoxic brain injuries in children.

PREVENTION

Falls account for most TBIs in children that are seen in the ED. Other etiologies include sports-related injuries, assault, and motor vehicle injuries, the latter being the leading cause of TBI-related deaths (1). Whether a patient sustains a mild or severe TBI, this type of injury cannot only result in a large financial burden, but more importantly, long-term clinical effects. It is important to do what is possible to best prevent accidents that cause TBI (see Chapter 9), especially in the vulnerable pediatric population.

Motor vehicle accidents are the leading cause of death among children in the United States (187). However, with proper seating placement of the child within the car and usage of age- and size-appropriate car seats or booster seats, almost one-third of these deaths can be prevented, and injuries can be reduced by more than half (188–191). Across age groups, safety restraints have been found to substantially decrease the risk for motor vehicle associated TBI (192). The American Academy of Pediatrics Committee on Injury, Violence, and Poison Prevention published a policy statement in 2011 providing 5 evidence-based recommendations regarding car restraints to optimize safety for children from birth to adolescence: (a) rear-facing car safety seats for most

infants up to 2 years of age and 40 lb, (b) forward-facing car safety seats for most children through 4 years of age and 80 lb, (c) belt-positioning booster seats for most children through 8 years of age and 4 feet 9 inches, (d) lap-and-shoulder seat belts for all children who have outgrown booster seats, (e) all children younger than 13 years to ride in the rear seat of vehicles (193).

Special considerations include premature infants and children with special health care needs. To ensure that preterm infants are transported safely, the proper selection and use of car seats or car beds are necessary. Although rear-facing car seats provide the best protection for an infant, a car bed may be indicated for infants who manifest apnea, bradycardia, and/or low oxygen saturation when placed in a semireclined position in a car seat (194). Regarding children with special health care needs, rear-facing seats may be indicated in children with higher ages and weights if they have low muscle tone, poor head control, or who are at risk for airway obstruction. Specialized medical seats or standard seats with rolled towels can provide improved support (195).

It is important to establish safety guidelines, but implementation is the key. There is strong evidence that passing legislation, safety seat distribution, educational programs, and enforcement campaigns are all effective in increasing child safety seat use (196). Additionally, it is essential to not only use child safety seats, but also to educate on how to use them properly. Child restraint systems have been found to be secured incorrectly up to 72% of the time, which could increase a child's risk of injury during a crash (191).

As children grow older and become more mobile, parents and guardians must begin child-proofing their home environments in order to prevent TBI. Falls account for most TBIs in young children and are the most common home injury in the United States (197), including falling down stairs, falling off of playground equipment, and falling out of windows (198). Much effort is being put toward educating parents on how to prevent household falls by using tools such as stair gates, window locks, window stops that allow only a 4 inch opening, and discontinuing the use of baby walkers; all measures which have been shown to decrease the risk for falls when properly implemented (199). Furthermore, when placed in conjunction with enforced legislation, injury prevention tools, such as window guards, have been shown to reduce fall injuries by up to 96% (200). Regarding play areas, thus far the only intervention proven to reduce the risk of TBI is to ensure that 12 inches of soft surface materials, such as sand or wood chips, are used for the playground instead of asphalt or dirt (201).

Bicycling accounts for tens of thousands of pediatric ED visits each year. Helmets, when worn properly, have been shown to reduce head injuries by almost 70%, although there is no federal law that legally mandates their use and their reported usage is low. In certain states, there are laws on helmet use based on age, although many times this does not extend to include skates, skateboards, scooters, or all-terrain vehicles that can also put children at risk (201,202). Other recreational sports in organized leagues such as baseball, football, hockey, and lacrosse require helmets, although mild TBI continues to be an issue in these young athletes, as well as in semicontact sports such as basketball and soccer (203,204). Additionally, it has been reported that snow skiing and snowboarding can be high-risk activities for TBI, helmet use, although not a mandated law, significantly reduces the risk for serious head and neck trauma and is strongly recommended for all ages (205).

CONCLUSION

TBI is the most common cause of mortality and morbidity in children. TBI in children leads to large medical and societal costs, especially because injury occurs at such a young age. Sequelae of pediatric TBI often parallel problems seen after adult TBI; however, ongoing brain development must be considered in the context of injury. Younger age at injury is often associated with poorer outcomes. Assessment and management protocols used in adults with TBI may not apply to children and future research needs to be performed to elucidate many of these factors.

FUTURE DIRECTIONS

Biomarkers

Differences in children in terms of mechanism of injury, anatomy, and physiology may result in different biomarker expression patterns than adults, thus extrapolation of findings from adult TBI studies to children must be approached with caution. Biomarkers that have been studied in children include S100B, neuron specific enolase, myelin basic protein, cleaved-tau, creatine kinase BB, glial fibrillary acidic protein, neurofilament heavy chain, alpha II-spectrin breakdown products, and most recently ubiquitin C-terminal hydrolase-L1. Most of the published work on biomarkers in children has been small studies with a single focus on their ability to predict abnormal CT scan, injury severity, or outcomes. To date, there is not one ideal candidate biomarker that has been identified. Age-dependent variations in the permeability of the blood–brain barrier, cell development, and cell stability complicate the study of biomarkers in children. S100B, a calcium-binding protein highly expressed in astroglial cells in the brain, is the best studied marker at this time. In children, studies have found that there is an association between higher levels and poorer outcomes (206–208), yet there are conflicting reports about the usefulness of this marker in children with mild TBI (209–211). The search for the ideal biomarker continues.

Imaging

The sensitivity and specificity of various forms of magnetic resonance (MR) for brain injury is superior to CT, particularly for detection of diffuse axonal injury (DAI) (see Chapters 15–17). For children, the principal advantage is the absence of radiation; yet long imaging times may necessitate sedation, which is a key limiting factor. Perhaps one of the most promising MR techniques is diffusion tensor imaging (DTI) for the detection of DAI in children. Most DTI studies have involved children following moderate/severe TBI in the chronic phases of recovery and have reported decreased fractional anisotropy (FA) and increased apparent diffusion coefficient (ADC) (212–217). These findings have been attributed to diffuse degenerative changes, including Wallerian degeneration, axonal collapse, and myelin degeneration (213,216,218–220). In some studies, changes in DTI metrics

correlated with initial clinical severity as well as functional outcomes (212,213,217,221). As for mild TBI, pilot work in adolescents during the acute phase by Wilde (222) and Levin (223) showed an increased FA and decreased or no changes in ADC in the corpus callosum and cingulum as compared to controls, indicative of transient cytotoxic edema. Another promising technique, susceptibility-weighted imaging, may be much more sensitive than traditional T2-weighted gradient-echo sequences in detecting the number, size, volume, and distribution of hemorrhagic lesions in DAI following moderate/severe TBI in children (224–226). In addition, number and size of lesions detected correlated with neuropsychological outcomes in these cohorts.

There is very limited data about the use of other imaging techniques—including magnetization transfer imaging and arterial spin tag labeling—in children with TBI. Electrophysiological techniques such as magnetoencephalography (MEG) and magnetic source imaging (MSI) also have limited data in children with TBI, yet there may be a role for these techniques in understanding postconcussion symptoms in mild TBI. Further research is needed to clarify the role of any of the earlier mentioned techniques in the care of children with TBI.

Genetics

The association of genetics with survival and recovery after TBI is beginning to be explored. However, genetics studies specific to pediatric TBI are limited. Overall, the studies to date have focused primarily on the apolipoprotein E (APOE) alleles and the results have been mixed. In predominantly severe injury, Brichtová and Kozák found that children with the APOE e4 allele were more likely to have severe clinical symptomatology and unfavorable outcome compared to other alleles (227). Additionally, Lo et al. demonstrated that different APOE alleles potentially affect cerebral ischemic tolerance, but that the APOE e4 allele was associated with poor outcomes in general (228). Alternatively, Quinn et al. found no association between the APOE e4 allele and posttraumatic brain swelling postmortem (229). In 1 study of mild TBI in children, the APOE e4 allele was not consistently related to outcomes after mild TBI (230). Further work needs to be done to better elucidate the association of genetics with outcomes after TBI in children.

KEY CLINICAL POINTS

1. Pediatric TBI is the most common cause of morbidity and mortality in children.
2. TBI in children leads to large economic and societal costs.
3. TBI in childhood affects normal brain growth and development. Injury at a younger age is not necessarily associated with better outcomes, and may be associated with poorer outcomes.
4. Neuroendocrine dysfunction can lead to problems with normal growth and development; monitoring for long-term clinical signs and symptoms is important.
5. Post-traumatic early seizures are common but do not correlate with late seizures.
6. In general, anoxic brain injury outcomes are worse than traumatic brain injury in children.

7. The neuropharmacology related to pediatric TBI needs to be better elucidated; medications used in adult TBI may have different effects in children.

8. CT scan decision criteria can reduce unnecessary scans in children with milder injuries.

9. Proper use of car seats and helmets when appropriate are important for primary prevention of TBI in children.

10. The role of advanced imaging, biomarkers, and genetics in pediatric TBI needs to be better elucidated.

KEY REFERENCES

1. Centers for Disease Control and Prevention. Injury Prevention & Control: Traumatic Brain Injury. http://www.cdc.gov/TraumaticBrainInjury/

2. Faul M, Xu L, Wald MM, Coronado VG. *Traumatic Brain Injury in the United States: Emergency Department Visits, Hospitalizations and Deaths 2002–2006.* Atlanta, GA: Centers for Disease Control and Prevention, National Center for Injury Prevention and Control; 2010.

3. Kuppermann N, Holmes JF, Dayan PS, et al. Identification of children at very low risk of clinically-important brain injuries after head trauma: a prospective cohort study. *Lancet.* 2009;374(9696):1160–1170.

4. McDonald CM, Jaffe KM, Fay GC, et al. Comparison of indices of traumatic brain injury severity as predictors of neurobehavioral outcome in children. *Arch Phys Med Rehabil.* Mar 1994;75(3):328–337.

5. Pangilinan PH, Giacoletti-Argento A, Shellhaas R, Hurvitz EA, Hornyak JE. Neuropharmacology in pediatric brain injury: a review. *PM R.* 2010;2(12):1127–1140.

References

1. Faul M, Xu L, Wald MM, Coronado VG. *Traumatic Brain Injury in the United States: Emergency Department Visits, Hospitalizations and Deaths 2002–2006.* Centers for Disease Control and Prevention, National Center for Injury Prevention and Control; 2010.

2. Shi J, Xiang H, Wheeler K, et al. Costs, mortality likelihood and outcomes of hospitalized US children with traumatic brain injuries. *Brain Inj.* 2009;23(7):602–611.

3. Finkelstein E, Corso PS, Miller TR. *The Incidence and Economic Burden of Injuries in the United States.* New York, NY: Oxford University Press; 2006.

4. Chugani HT. Positron emission tomography: principles and applications in pediatrics. *Mead Johnson Symp Perinat Dev Med.* 1987;(25):15–18.

5. Prins ML, Hovda DA. Developing experimental models to address traumatic brain injury in children. *J Neurotrauma.* 2003;20(2):123–137.

6. Thibault KL, Margulies SS. Age-dependent material properties of the porcine cerebrum: effect on pediatric inertial head injury criteria. *J Biomech.* 1998;31(12):1119–1126.

7. Zwienenberg M, Muizelaar JP. Cerebral perfusion and blood flow in neurotrauma. *Neurol Res.* 2001;23(2–3):167–174.

8. Guskiewicz KM, Valovich McLeod TC. Pediatric sports-related concussion. *PM R.* 2011;3(4):353–364.

9. Hackbarth RM, Rzeszutko KM, Sturm G, Donders J, Kuldanek AS, Sanfilippo DJ. Survival and functional outcome in pediatric traumatic brain injury: a retrospective review and analysis of predictive factors. *Crit Care Med.* 2002;30(7):1630–1635.

10. Carter BG, Butt W, Taylor A. ICP and CPP: excellent predictors of long term outcome in severely brain injured children. *Childs Nerv Syst.* 2008;24(2):245–251.

11. Downard C, Hulka F, Mullins RJ, et al. Relationship of cerebral perfusion pressure and survival in pediatric brain-injured patients. *J Trauma.* 2000;49(4):654–659.

12. Anderson V, Jacobs R, Spencer-Smith M, et al. Does early age at brain insult predict worse outcome? Neuropsychological implications. *J Pediatr Psychol.* 2010;35(7):716–727.

13. Teasdale G, Jennett B. Assessment of coma and impaired consciousness. A practical scale. *Lancet.* 1974;2(7872):81–84.

14. Simpson DA, Cockington RA, Hanieh A, Raftos J, Reilly PL. Head injuries in infants and young children: the value of the Paediatric Coma Scale. Review of literature and report on a study. *Childs Nerv Syst.* 1991;7(4):183–190.

15. Browne GJ, Cocks AJ, McCaskill ME. Current trends in the management of major paediatric trauma. *Emerg Med (Fremantle).* 2001;13(4):418–425.

16. Hahn YS, Chyung C, Barthel MJ, Bailes J, Flannery AM, McLone DG. Head injuries in children under 36 months of age. Demography and outcome. *Childs Nerv Syst.* 1988;4(1):34–40.

17. Van de Voorde P, Sabbe M, Rizopoulos D, et al; for PENTA study group. Assessing the level of consciousness in children: a plea for the Glasgow Coma Motor subscore. *Resuscitation.* 2008;76(2):175–179.

18. Tatman A, Warren A, Williams A, Powell JE, Whitehouse W. Development of a modified paediatric coma scale in intensive care clinical practice. *Arch Dis Child.* 1997;77(6):519–521.

19. Holmes JF, Palchak MJ, MacFarlane T, Kuppermann N. Performance of the pediatric glasgow coma scale in children with blunt head trauma. *Acad Emerg Med.* 2005;12(9):814–819.

20. Ralson M, Hazinski MF, Zaritsky AL, Schexnayder SM, Kleinman ME. *Pediatric Advanced Life Support Provider Manual.* Dallas, TX: American Heart Association; 2006.

21. Chung CY, Chen CL, Cheng PT, See LC, Tang SF, Wong AM. Critical score of Glasgow Coma Scale for pediatric traumatic brain injury. *Pediatr Neurol.* 2006;34(5):379–387.

22. Wagstyl J, Sutcliffe AJ, Alpar EK. Early prediction of outcome following head injury in children. *J Pediatr Surg.* 1987;22(2):127–129.

23. Bruce DA, Schut L, Bruno LA, Wood JH, Sutton LN. Outcome following severe head injuries in children. *J Neurosurg.* 1978;48(5):679–688.

24. Lieh-Lai MW, Theodorou AA, Sarnaik AP, Meert KL, Moylan PM, Canady AI. Limitations of the Glasgow Coma Scale in predicting outcome in children with traumatic brain injury. *J Pediatr.* 1992;120(2, pt 1):195–199.

25. Grewal M, Sutcliffe AJ. Early prediction of outcome following head injury in children: an assessment of the value of Glasgow Coma Scale score trend and abnormal plantar and pupillary light reflexes. *J Pediatr Surg.* 1991;26(10):1161–1163.

26. Ducrocq SC, Meyer PG, Orliaguet GA, et al. Epidemiology and early predictive factors of mortality and outcome in children with traumatic severe brain injury: experience of a French pediatric trauma center. *Pediatr Crit Care Med.* 2006;7(5):461–467.

27. Ewing-Cobbs L, Levin HS, Fletcher JM, Miner ME, Eisenberg HM. The Children's Orientation and Amnesia Test: relationship to severity of acute head injury and to recovery of memory. *Neurosurgery.* 1990;27(5):683–691.

28. Suskauer SJ, Slomine BS, Inscore AB, Lewelt AJ, Kirk JW, Salorio CF. Injury severity variables as predictors of WeeFIM scores in pediatric TBI: time to follow commands is best. *J Pediatr Rehabil Med.* 2009;2(4):297–307.

29. Krach LE, Gormley ME, Ward M. Traumatic Brain Injury. In Alexander MA, Matthews D, eds. *Pediatric Rehabilitaiton: Principles and Practice.* 4th ed. New York, NY: Demos Medical; 2010:231–260.

30. Quayle KS, Jaffe DM, Kuppermann N, et al. Diagnostic testing for acute head injury in children: when are head computed tomography and skull radiographs indicated? *Pediatrics.* 1997;99(5):E11.

31. Schunk JE, Rodgerson JD, Woodward GA. The utility of head computed tomographic scanning in pediatric patients with normal neurologic examination in the emergency department. *Pediatr Emerg Care.* 1996;12(3):160–165.

32. Dietrich AM, Bowman MJ, Ginn-Pease ME, Kosnik E, King DR. Pediatric head injuries: can clinical factors reliably predict an ab-

normality on computed tomography? *Ann Emerg Med.* 1993;22(10): 1535–1540.

33. Kuppermann N, Holmes JF, Dayan PS, et al; for Pediatric Emergency Care Applied Research Network. Identification of children at very low risk of clinically-important brain injuries after head trauma: a prospective cohort study. *Lancet.* 2009;374(9696):1160–1170.

34. Schutzman SA, Barnes P, Duhaime AC, et al. Evaluation and management of children younger than two years old with apparently minor head trauma: proposed guidelines. *Pediatrics.* 2001;107(5): 983–993.

35. Dunning J, Daly JP, Lomas JP, Lecky F, Batchelor J, Mackway-Jones K; for Children's head injury algorithm for the prediction of important clinical events study group. Derivation of the children's head injury algorithm for the prediction of important clinical events decision rule for head injury in children. *Arch Dis Child.* 2006;91(11):885–891.

36. Osmond MH, Klassen TP, Wells GA, et al.; for Pediatric Emergency Research Canada (PERC) Head Injury Study Group. CATCH: a clinical decision rule for the use of computed tomography in children with minor head injury. *CMAJ.* 2010;182(4):341–348.

37. Stiell IG, Bennett C. Implementation of clinical decision rules in the emergency department. *Acad Emerg Med.* 2007;14(11):955–959.

38. Ponsford J, Willmott C, Rothwell A, et al. Impact of early intervention on outcome after mild traumatic brain injury in children. *Pediatrics.* 2001;108(6):1297–1303.

39. Gioia GA, Collins M, Isquith PK. Improving identification and diagnosis of mild traumatic brain injury with evidence: psychometric support for the acute concussion evaluation. *J Head Trauma Rehabil.* 2008;23(4):230–242.

40. Kraus JF, Fife D, Conroy C. Pediatric brain injuries: the nature, clinical course, and early outcomes in a defined United States' population. *Pediatrics.* 1987;79(4):501–507.

41. Fay GC, Jaffe KM, Polissar NL, et al. Mild pediatric traumatic brain injury: a cohort study. *Arch Phys Med Rehabil.* 1993;74(9):895–901.

42. National Center for Injury Prevention and Control. *Report to Congress on Mild Traumatic Brain Injury in the United States: Steps to Prevent a Serious Public Health Problem.* Atlanta, GA: Centers for Disease Control and Prevention; 2003.

43. Ponsford J, Willmott C, Rothwell A, et al. Cognitive and behavioral outcome following mild traumatic head injury in children. *J Head Trauma Rehabil.* 1999;14(4):360–372.

44. Barlow KM, Crawford S, Stevenson A, Sandhu SS, Belanger F, Dewey D. Epidemiology of postconcussion syndrome in pediatric mild traumatic brain injury. *Pediatrics.* 2010;126(2):e374–e381.

45. Sroufe NS, Fuller DS, West BT, Singal BM, Warschausky SA, Maio RF. Postconcussive symptoms and neurocognitive function after mild traumatic brain injury in children. *Pediatrics.* 2010;125(6): e1331–e1339.

46. Babcock Cimpello L, Bazarian JJ, Fisher S. *Acute Predictors of Poor Outcomes in Children with Mild Traumatic Brain Injury 2009.* Rochester, NY: MPH Thesis (in process).

47. Babcock Cimpello L, Byczkowski TL, Bazarian JJ. Acute Predictors of Post-Concussion Syndrome. *Academic Emergency Medicine.* 2011; 18:S4–S249.

48. Mittenberg W, Wittner MS, Miller LJ. Postconcussion syndrome occurs in children. *Neuropsychology.* 1997;11(3):447–452.

49. Yeates KO, Luria J, Bartkowski H, Rusin J, Martin L, Bigler ED. Postconcussive symptoms in children with mild closed head injuries. *J Head Trauma Rehabil.* 1999;14(4):337–350.

50. Bijur PE, Haslum M, Golding J. Cognitive and behavioral sequelae of mild head injury in children. *Pediatrics.* 1990;86(3):337–344.

51. Wrightson P, McGinn V, Gronwall D. Mild head injury in preschool children: evidence that it can be associated with a persisting cognitive defect. *J Neurol Neurosurg Psychiatry.* 1995;59(4):375–380.

52. Brosseau-Lachaine O, Gagnon I, Forget R, Faubert J. Mild traumatic brain injury induces prolonged visual processing deficits in children. *Brain Inj.* 2008;22(9):657–668.

53. Carroll LJ, Cassidy JD, Peloso PM, et al.; for WHO Collaborating Centre Task Force on Mild Traumatic Brain Injury. Prognosis for mild traumatic brain injury: results of the WHO Collaborating Centre Task Force on Mild Traumatic Brain Injury. *J Rehabil Med.* 2004(suppl 43):84–105.

54. Babikian T, Satz P, Zaucha K, Light R, Lewis RS, Asarnow RF. The UCLA longitudinal study of neurocognitive outcomes following mild pediatric traumatic brain injury. *J Int Neuropsychol Soc.* 2011; 17(5):886–895.

55. Lau BC, Kontos AP, Collins MW, Mucha A, Lovell MR. Which on-field signs/symptoms predict protracted recovery from sport-related concussion among high school football players? *Am J Sports Med.* 2011;39(11):2311–2318.

56. Bijur PE, Haslum M, Golding J. Cognitive outcomes of multiple mild head injuries in children. *J Dev Behav Pediatr.* 1996;17(3): 143–148.

57. Greenspan AI, MacKenzie EJ. Functional outcome after pediatric head injury. *Pediatrics.* 1994;94(4, pt 1):425–432.

58. McClincy MP, Lovell MR, Pardini J, Collins MW, Spore MK. Recovery from sports concussion in high school and collegiate athletes. *Brain Inj.* 2006;20(1):33–39.

59. Gioia G, Collins M. CDC-RFA-CE-08-006: Feasibility of Acute Concussion Management in the Emergency Department. Centers for Disease Control and Prevention; 2008.

60. Yeates KO, Taylor HG, Rusin J, et al. Premorbid child and family functioning as predictors of post-concussive symptoms in children with mild traumatic brain injuries [published online ahead of print May 27, 2011]. *Int J Dev Neurosci.*

61. Collins MW, Lovell MR, Iverson GL, Cantu RC, Maroon JC, Field M. Cumulative effects of concussion in high school athletes. *Neurosurgery.* 2002;51(5):1175–1181.

62. Fay TB, Yeates KO, Taylor HG, et al. Cognitive reserve as a moderator of postconcussive symptoms in children with complicated and uncomplicated mild traumatic brain injury. *J Int Neuropsychol Soc.* 2010;16(1):94–105.

63. Massagli TL, Jaffe KM. Pediatric traumatic brain injury: prognosis and rehabilitation. *Pediatr Ann.* 1994;23(1):29–30, 33–36.

64. Mihalik JP, Stump JE, Collins MW, Lovell MR, Field M, Maroon JC. Posttraumatic migraine characteristics in athletes following sports-related concussion. *J Neurosurg.* 2005;102(5):850–855.

65. Luis CA, Mittenberg W. Mood and anxiety disorders following pediatric traumatic brain injury: a prospective study. *J Clin Exp Neuropsychol.* 2002;24(3):270–279.

66. Woodrome SE, Yeates KO, Taylor HG, et al. Coping strategies as a predictor of post-concussive symptoms in children with mild traumatic brain injury versus mild orthopedic injury. *J Int Neuropsychol Soc.* 2011;17(2):317–326.

67. Taylor HG, Dietrich A, Nuss K, et al. Post-concussive symptoms in children with mild traumatic brain injury. *Neuropsychology.* 2010; 24(2):148–159.

68. Yeates KO, Taylor HG, Walz NC, Stancin T, Wade SL. The family environment as a moderator of psychosocial outcomes following traumatic brain injury in young children. *Neuropsychology.* 2010; 24(3):345–356.

69. Taylor HG, Yeates KO, Wade SL, Drotar D, Stancin T, Minich N. A prospective study of short- and long-term outcomes after traumatic brain injury in children: behavior and achievement. *Neuropsychology.* 2002;16(1):15–27.

70. Yeates KO, Taylor HG. Predicting premorbid neuropsychological functioning following pediatric traumatic brain injury. *J Clin Exp Neuropsychol.* 1997;19(6):825–837.

71. Glang A, Ylvisaker M, Stein M, Ehlhardt L, Todis B, Tyler J. Validated instructional practices: application to students with traumatic brain injury. *J Head Trauma Rehabil.* 2008;23(4):243–251.

72. Ylvisaker M, Feeney TJ. Traumatic brain injury in adolescence: assessment and reintegration. *Semin Speech Lang.* 1995;16(1):32–45.

73. American Association for the Surgery of Trauma, Child Neurology Society, International Society for Pediatric Neurosurgery, et al. Guidelines for the acute medical management of severe traumatic brain injury in infants, children, and adolescents. *J Trauma.* 2003; 54(suppl 6):S235–S310.

74. Leonard JC, Kuppermann N, Olsen C, et al.; for Pediatric Emergency Care Applied Research Network. Factors associated with cervical spine injury in children after blunt trauma. *Ann Emerg Med.* 2011;58(2):145–155.

75. Hutchison JS, Ward RE, Lacroix J, et al.; for Hypothermia Pediatric Head Injury Trial Investigators and the Canadian Critical Care Trials Group. Hypothermia therapy after traumatic brain injury in children. *N Engl J Med.* 2008;358(23):2447–2456.

76. Duhaime AC, Holshouser B, Hunter JV, Tong K. Common data elements for neuroimaging of traumatic brain injury: pediatric considerations [published online ahead of print November 2, 2011]. *J Neurotrauma.*

77. Marshall LF, Marshall SB, Klauber MR, et al. The diagnosis of head injury requires a classification based on computed axial tomography. *J Neurotrauma.* 1992;9(suppl 1):S287–S292.

78. Maas AI, Hukkelhoven CW, Marshall LF, Steyerberg EW. Prediction of outcome in traumatic brain injury with computed tomographic characteristics: a comparison between the computed tomographic classification and combinations of computed tomographic predictors. *Neurosurgery.* 2005;57(6):1173–1182.

79. Adelson PD, Bratton SL, Carney NA, et al. Guidelines for the acute medical management of severe traumatic brain injury in infants, children, and adolescents. Chapter 3. Prehospital airway management. *Pediatr Crit Care Med.* 2003;4(suppl 3):S9–S11.

80. Khanna S, Davis D, Peterson B, et al. Use of hypertonic saline in the treatment of severe refractory posttraumatic intracranial hypertension in pediatric traumatic brain injury. *Crit Care Med.* 2000; 28(4):1144–1151.

81. Knapp JM. Hyperosmolar therapy in the treatment of severe head injury in children: mannitol and hypertonic saline. *AACN Clin Issues.* 2005;16(2):199–211.

82. Mirski AM, Denchev ID, Schnitzer SM, Hanley FD. Comparison between hypertonic saline and mannitol in the reduction of elevated intracranial pressure in a rodent model of acute cerebral injury. *J Neurosurg Anesthesiol.* 2000;12(4):334–344.

83. Tude Melo JR, Di Rocco F, Blanot S, et al. Mortality in children with severe head trauma: predictive factors and proposal for a new predictive scale. *Neurosurgery.* 2010;67(6):1542–1547.

84. Berger MS, Pitts LH, Lovely M, Edwards MS, Bartkowski HM. Outcome from severe head injury in children and adolescents. *J Neurosurg.* 1985;62(2):194–199.

85. Michaud LJ, Rivara FP, Grady MS, Reay DT. Predictors of survival and severity of disability after severe brain injury in children. *Neurosurgery.* 1992;31(2):254–264.

86. Facco E, Zuccarello M, Pittoni G, et al. Early outcome prediction in severe head injury: comparison between children and adults. *Childs Nerv Syst.* 1986;2(2):67–71.

87. Kieslich M, Marquardt G, Galow G, Lorenz R, Jacobit G. Neurological and mental outcome after severe head injury in childhood: a long-term follow-up of 318 children. *Disabil Rehabil.* 2001;23(15): 665–669.

88. Vavilala MS, Bowen A, Lam AM, et al. Blood pressure and outcome after severe pediatric traumatic brain injury. *J Trauma.* 2003;55(6): 1039–1044.

89. Cochran A, Scaife ER, Hansen KW, Downey EC. Hyperglycemia and outcomes from pediatric traumatic brain injury. *J Trauma.* 2003; 55(6):1035–1038.

90. Kriel RL, Krach LE, Jones-Saete C. Outcome of children with prolonged unconsciousness and vegetative states. *Pediatr Neurol.* 1993; 9(5):362–368.

91. Fields AI, Coble DH, Pollack MM, Cuerdon TT, Kaufman J. Outcomes of children in a persistent vegetative state. *Crit Care Med.* 1993;21(12):1890–1894.

92. McDonald CM, Jaffe KM, Fay GC, et al. Comparison of indices of traumatic brain injury severity as predictors of neurobehavioral outcome in children. *Arch Phys Med Rehabil.* 1994;75(3):328–337.

93. Kriel RL, Krach LE, Panser LA. Closed head injury: comparison of children younger and older than 6 years of age. *Pediatr Neurol.* 1989;5(5):296–300.

94. Rivara FP ES, Mangione-Smith R, MacKenzie EJ, Jaffe KM; and The National Expert Panel for the Development of Pediatric Rehabilitation Quality of Care Indicators. Quality of care indicators for the rehabilitation of children with traumatic brain injury. *Arch Phys Med Rehabil.* In press.

95. Zumsteg JM ES, Jaffe KM, Mangione-Smith R, Mackenzie EJ, Rivara FP; and the National Expert Panel for the Development of Pediatric Rehabilitatiion Quality of Care Indicators. Quality of care indicators for the structure and organization of inpatient rehabilitation care of childen with traumatic brain injury. *Arch Phys Med Rehabil.* In press.

96. McCauley SR, Wilde EA, Anderson VA, et al. Recommendations for the use of common outcome measures in pediatric traumatic brain injury research [published online ahead of print August 24, 2011]. *J Neurotrauma.*

97. Krach LE, Kriel RL, Morris WF, Warhol BL, Luxenberg MG. Central autonomic dysfunction following acquired brain injury in children. *Neurorehabil Neural Repair.* 1997;11:41–45.

98. Baguley IJ, Heriseanu RE, Felmingham KL, Cameron ID. Dysautonomia and heart rate variability following severe traumatic brain injury. *Brain Inj.* 2006;20(4):437–444.

99. Baguley IJ, Slewa-Younan S, Heriseanu RE, Nott MT, Mudaliar Y, Nayyar V. The incidence of dysautonomia and its relationship with autonomic arousal following traumatic brain injury. *Brain Inj.* 2007; 21(11):1175–1181.

100. Pranzatelli MR, Pavlakis SG, Gould RJ, De Vivo DC. Hypothalamic-midbrain dysregulation syndrome: hypertension, hyperthermia, hyperventilation, and decerebration. *J Child Neurol.* 1991;6(2): 115–122.

101. Meythaler JM, Stinson AM, III. Fever of central origin in traumatic brain injury controlled with propranolol. *Arch Phys Med Rehabil.* 1994;75(7):816–818.

102. Russo RN, O'Flaherty S. Bromocriptine for the management of autonomic dysfunction after severe traumatic brain injury. *J Paediatr Child Health.* 2000;36(3):283–285.

103. Turner MS. Early use of intrathecal baclofen in brain injury in pediatric patients. *Acta Neurochir Suppl.* 2003;87:81–83.

104. Statler KD. Pediatric posttraumatic seizures: epidemiology, putative mechanisms of epileptogenesis and promising investigational progress. *Dev Neurosci.* 2006;28(4–5):354–363.

105. Asikainen I, Kaste M, Sarna S. Early and late posttraumatic seizures in traumatic brain injury rehabilitation patients: brain injury factors causing late seizures and influence of seizures on long-term outcome. *Epilepsia.* 1999;40(5):584–589.

106. Chiaretti A, De Benedictis R, Polidori G, Piastra M, Iannelli A, Di Rocco C. Early post-traumatic seizures in children with head injury. *Childs Nerv Syst.* 2000;16(12):862–866.

107. Hahn YS, Fuchs S, Flannery AM, Barthel MJ, McLone DG. Factors influencing posttraumatic seizures in children. *Neurosurgery.* 1988; 22(5):864–867.

108. Ratan SK, Kulshreshtha R, Pandey RM. Predictors of posttraumatic convulsions in head-injured children. *Pediatr Neurosurg.* 1999;30(3): 127–131.

109. Barlow KM, Spowart JJ, Minns RA. Early posttraumatic seizures in non-accidental head injury: relation to outcome. *Dev Med Child Neurol.* 2000;42(9):591–594.

110. Appleton RE, Demellweek C. Post-traumatic epilepsy in children requiring inpatient rehabilitation following head injury. *J Neurol Neurosurg Psychiatry.* 2002;72(5):669–672.

111. Ateş O, Ondül S, Onal C, et al. Post-traumatic early epilepsy in pediatric age group with emphasis on influential factors. *Childs Nerv Syst.* 2006;22(3):279–284.

112. Manaka S, Takahashi H, Sano K. The difference between children and adults in the onset of post-traumatic epilepsy. *Folia Psychiatr Neurol Jpn.* 1981;35(3):301–304.

113. Christensen J, Pedersen MG, Pedersen CB, Sidenius P, Olsen J, Vestergaard M. Long-term risk of epilepsy after traumatic brain injury in children and young adults: a population-based cohort study. *Lancet.* 2009;373(9669):1105–1110.

114. Adelson PD, Bratton SL, Carney NA, et al. Guidelines for the acute medical management of severe traumatic brain injury in infants, children, and adolescents. Chapter 19. The role of anti-seizure prophylaxis following severe pediatric traumatic brain injury. *Pediatr Crit Care Med.* 2003;4(suppl 3):S72–S75.

115. Hunt EA. Phenytoin in traumatic brain injury. *Arch Dis Child.* 2002; 86(1):62–63.

116. Kim CT, Moberg-Wolff E, Trovato M, Kim H, Murphy N. Pediatric rehabilitation: 1. Common medical conditions in children with disabilities. *PM R.* 2010;2(3):S3–S11.

117. Randomised study of antiepileptic drug withdrawal in patients in remission. Medical Research Council Antiepileptic Drug Withdrawal Study Group. *Lancet*. 1991;337(8751):1175–1180.

118. Shinnar S, Vining EP, Mellits ED, et al. Discontinuing antiepileptic medication in children with epilepsy after two years without seizures. A prospective study. *N Engl J Med*. 1985;313(16):976–980.

119. Kriel RL, Krach LE, Sheehan M. Pediatric closed head injury: outcome following prolonged unconsciousness. *Arch Phys Med Rehabil*. 1988;69(9):678–681.

120. Silver BV, Chinarian J. Neurologic improvement following shunt placement for post-traumatic hydrocephalus in a child. *Pediatr Rehabil*. 1997;1(2):123–126.

121. Massimi L, Paternoster G, Fasano T, Di Rocco C. On the changing epidemiology of hydrocephalus. *Child Nerv Syst*. 2009;25(7):795–800.

122. Gudeman SK, Kishore PR, Becker DP, et al. Computed tomography in the evaluation of incidence and significance of post-traumatic hydrocephalus. *Radiology*. 1981;141(2):397–402.

123. Kishore PR, Lipper MH, Miller JD, Girevendulis AK, Becker DP, Vines FS. Post-traumatic hydrocephalus in patients with severe head injury. *Neuroradiology*. 1978;16:261–265.

124. Licata C, Cristofori L, Gambin R, Vivenza C, Turazzi S. Post-traumatic hydrocephalus. *J Neurosurg Sci*. 2001;45(3):141–149.

125. Acerini CL, Tasker RC. Traumatic brain injury induced hypothalamic-pituitary dysfunction: a paediatric perspective. *Pituitary*. 2007;10(4):373–380.

126. Pinyerd B. 2010 update: consequences of hypothalamic-pituitary dysfunction following traumatic brain injury in children. *J Pediatr Nurs*. 2010;25(3):231–233.

127. Schneider HJ, Corneli G, Kreitschman-Andermahr I, et al. Traumatic brain injury and hypopituitarism in children and adolescents: is the problem under-estimated? *Pediatr Endocrinol Rev*. 2007; 4(3):205–209.

128. Acerini CL, Tasker RC. Endocrine sequelae of traumatic brain injury in childhood. *Horm Res*. 2007;68(suppl 5):14–17.

129. Acerini CL, Tasker RC. Neuroendocrine consequences of traumatic brain injury. *J Pediatr Endocrinol Metab*. 2008;21(7):611–619.

130. Kaulfers AM, Backeljauw PF, Reifschneider K, et al. Endocrine dysfunction following traumatic brain injury in children. *J Pediatr*. 2010;157(6):894–899.

131. Ives JC, Alderman M, Stred SE. Hypopituitarism after multiple concussions: a retrospective case study in an adolescent male. *J Athl Train*. 2007;42(3):431–439.

132. Citta-Pietrolungo TJ, Alexander MA, Cook SP, Padman R. Complications of tracheostomy and decannulation in pediatric and young patients with traumatic brain injury. *Arch Phys Med Rehabil*. 1993; 74(9):905–909.

133. Carr MM, Poje CP, Kingston L, Kielma D, Heard C. Complications in pediatric tracheostomies. *Laryngoscope*. 2001;111(11, pt 1):1925–1928.

134. Woo P, Kelly G, Kirshner P. Airway complications in the head injured. *Laryngoscope*. 1989;99(7, pt 1):725–731.

135. Nowak P, Cohn AM, Guidice MA. Airway complications in patients with closed-head injuries. *Am J Otolaryngol*. 1987;8(2):91–96.

136. Cochran EB, Phelps SJ, Tolley EA, Stidham GL. Prevalence of, and risk factors for, upper gastrointestinal tract bleeding in critically ill pediatric patients. *Crit Care Med*. 1992;20(11):1519–1523.

137. de Toledo JS, Adelson PD, Watson RS, et al. Relationship between increases in pancreatic enzymes and cerebral events in children after traumatic brain injury. *Neurocrit Care*. 2009;11(3):322–329.

138. Moiyadi AV, Devi BI, Nair KP. Urinary disturbances following traumatic brain injury: clinical and urodynamic evaluation. *NeuroRehabilitation*. 2007;22(2):93–98.

139. Berger RM, Maizels M, Moran GC, Conway JJ, Firlit CF. Bladder capacity (ounces) equals age (years) plus 2 predicts normal bladder capacity and aids in diagnosis of abnormal voiding patterns. *J Urol*. 1983;129(2):347–349.

140. Singhania P, Andankar MG, Pathak HR. Urodynamic evaluation of urinary disturbances following traumatic brain injury. *Urol Int*. 2010;84(1):89–93.

141. Kluger G, Kochs A, Holthausen H. Heterotopic ossification in childhood and adolescence. *J Child Neurol*. 2000;15(6):406–413.

142. Hurvitz EA, Mandac BR, Davidoff G, Johnson JH, Nelson VS. Risk factors for heterotopic ossification in children and adolescents with severe traumatic brain injury. *Arch Phys Med Rehabil*. 1992;73(5):459–462.

143. Mital MA, Garber JE, Stinson JT. Ectopic bone formation in children and adolescents with head injuries: its management. *J Pediatr Orthop*. 1987;7(1):83–90.

144. Silverman SL, Hurvitz EA, Nelson VS, Chiodo A. Rachitic syndrome after disodium etidronate therapy in an adolescent. *Arch Phys Med Rehabil*. 1994;75(1):118–120.

145. Radecki RT, Gaebler-Spira D. Deep vein thrombosis in the disabled pediatric population. *Arch Phys Med Rehabil*. 1994;75(3):248–250.

146. Sobus KM, Cawley MF, Alexander MA. Pulmonary embolism in the traumatic brain injured adolescent: report of two cases. *Arch Phys Med Rehabil*. 1994;75(3):362–364.

147. Grandas OH, Klar M, Goldman MH, Filston HC. Deep venous thrombosis in the pediatric trauma population: an unusual event: report of three cases. *Am Surg*. 2000;66(3):273–276.

148. Mayer MP, Suskauer SJ, Houtrow A, Watanabe T. Venous thromboembolism prophylaxis in the pediatric population. *PM R*. 2011; 3(6):578–585.

149. Vavilala MS, Nathens AB, Jurkovich GJ, Mackenzie E, Rivara FP. Risk factors for venous thromboembolism in pediatric trauma. *J Trauma*. 2002;52(5):922–927.

150. Max JE, Schachar RJ, Levin HS, et al. Predictors of secondary attention-deficit/hyperactivity disorder in children and adolescents 6 to 24 months after traumatic brain injury. *J Am Acad Child Adolesc Psychiatry*. 2005;44(10):1041–1049.

151. Levin H, Hanten G, Max J, et al. Symptoms of attention-deficit/hyperactivity disorder following traumatic brain injury in children. *J Dev Behav Pediatr*. 2007;28(2):108–118.

152. Max JE, Schachar RJ, Levin HS, et al. Predictors of attention-deficit/hyperactivity disorder within 6 months after pediatric traumatic brain injury. *J Am Acad Child Adolesc Psychiatry*. 2005;44(10):1032–1040.

153. Ginstfeldt T, Emanuelson I. An overview of attention deficits after paediatric traumatic brain injury. *Brain Inj*. 2010;24(10):1123–1134.

154. Anderson V, Anderson D, Anderson P. Comparing attentional skills in children with acquired and developmental central nervous system disorders. *J Int Neuropsychol Soc*. 2006;12(4):519–531.

155. Catroppa C, Anderson V. A prospective study of the recovery of attention from acute to 2 years following pediatric traumatic brain injury. *J Int Neuropsychol Soc*. 2005;11(1):84–98.

156. Max JE, Lansing AE, Koele SL, et al. Attention deficit hyperactivity disorder in children and adolescents following traumatic brain injury. *Dev Neuropsychol*. 2004;25(1–2):159–177.

157. Catroppa C, Anderson VA, Morse SA, Haritou F, Rosenfeld JV. Children's attentional skills 5 years post-TBI. *J Pediatr Psychol*. 2007; 32(3):354–369.

158. Mandalis A, Kinsella G, Ong B, Anderson V. Working memory and new learning following pediatric traumatic brain injury. *Dev Neuropsychol*. 2007;32(2):683–701.

159. Ward H, Shum D, McKinlay L, Baker S, Wallace G. Prospective memory and pediatric traumatic brain injury: effects of cognitive demand. *Child Neuropsychol*. 2007;13(3):219–239.

160. Catroppa C, Anderson V. Recovery in memory function, and its relationship to academic success, at 24 months following pediatric TBI. *Child Neuropsychol*. 2007;13(3):240–261.

161. Keenan HT, Hooper SR, Wetherington CE, Nocera M, Runyan DK. Neurodevelopmental consequences of early traumatic brain injury in 3-year-old children. *Pediatrics*. 2007;119(3):e616–e623.

162. Sesma H, Slomine B, Ding R, McCarthy M. Executive functioning in the first year after pediatric traumatic brain injury. *Pediatrics*. 2008;121(6):E1686–E1695.

163. Nadebaum C, Anderson V, Catroppa C. Executive function outcomes following traumatic brain injury in young children: a five year follow-up. *Dev Neuropsychol*. 2007;32(2):703–728.

164. Schwartz L, Taylor HG, Drotar D, Yeates KO, Wade SL, Stancin T. Long-term behavior problems following pediatric traumatic brain injury: prevalence, predictors, and correlates. *J Pediatr Psychol*. 2003;28(4):251–263.

165. Chapman LA, Wade SL, Walz NC, Taylor HG, Stancin T, Yeates KO. Clinically significant behavior problems during the initial 18 months following early childhood traumatic brain injury. *Rehabil Psychol.* 2010;55(1):48–57.

166. Max JE, Smith WL Jr, Sato Y, et al. Traumatic brain injury in children and adolescents: psychiatric disorders in the first three months. *J Am Acad Child Adolesc Psychiatry.* 1997;36(1):94–102.

167. Max JE, Lindgren SD, Robin DA, et al. Traumatic brain injury in children and adolescents: psychiatric disorders in the second three months. *J Nerv Ment Dis.* 1997;185(6):394–401.

168. Gerring JP, Grados MA, Slomine B, et al. Disruptive behaviour disorders and disruptive symptoms after severe paediatric traumatic brain injury. *Brain Inj.* 2009;23(12):944–955.

169. Max JE, Levin HS, Schachar RJ, et al. Predictors of personality change due to traumatic brain injury in children and adolescents six to twenty-four months after injury. *J Neuropsychiatry Clin Neurosci.* 2006;18(1):21–32.

170. Sullivan JR, Riccio CA. Language functioning and deficits following pediatric traumatic brain injury. *Appl Neuropsychol.* 2010;17(2):93–98.

171. Chapman SB, Sparks G, Levin HS, et al. Discourse macrolevel processing after severe pediatric traumatic brain injury. *Dev Neuropsychol.* 2004;25(1–2):37–60.

172. Chapman SB, Gamino JF, Cook LG, Hanten G, Li X, Levin HS. Impaired discourse gist and working memory in children after brain injury. *Brain Lang.* 2006;97(2):178–188.

173. Catroppa C, Anderson V. Recovery and predictors of language skills two years following pediatric traumatic brain injury. *Brain Lang.* 2004;88(1):68–78.

174. Kapoor N, Ciuffreda KJ. Vision disturbances following traumatic brain injury. *Curr Treat Options Neurol.* 2002;4(4):271–280.

175. Levin AV. Retinal hemorrhage in abusive head trauma. *Pediatrics.* 2010;126(5):961–970.

176. Roizen NJ. Etiology of hearing loss in children. Nongenetic causes. *Pediatr Clin North Am.* 1999;46(1):49–64, x.

177. Pangilinan PH, Giacoletti-Argento A, Shellhaas R, Hurvitz EA, Hornyak JE. Neuropharmacology in pediatric brain injury: a review. *PM R.* 2010;2(12):1127–1140.

178. Patrick PD, Buck ML, Conaway MR, Blackman JA. The use of dopamine enhancing medications with children in low response states following brain injury. *Brain Inj.* 2003;17(6):497–506.

179. Green L, Hornyak J, Hurvitz E. Amantadine in pediatric patients with traumatic brain injury: a retrospective, case-controlled study. *Am J Phys Med Rehabil.* 2004;83(12):893–897.

180. McMahon M, Vargus-Adams J, Michaud L, Bean J. Effects of amantadine in children with impaired consciousness caused by acquired brain injury: a pilot study. *Am J Phys Med Rehabil.* 2009;88(7):525–532.

181. Chiesa A, Duhaime AC. Abusive head trauma. *Pediatr Clin North Am.* 2009;56(2):317–331.

182. Keenan HT, Runyan DK, Marshall SW, Nocera MA, Merten DF, Sinal SH. A population-based study of inflicted traumatic brain injury in young children. *JAMA.* 2003;290(5):621–626.

183. Reece RM, Nicholson, CE. Inflicted Childhood Neurotrauma. *American Academy of Pediatrics.* 2003.

184. Hymel KP, Makoroff KL, Laskey AL, Conaway MR, Blackman JA. Mechanisms, clinical presentations, injuries, and outcomes from inflicted versus noninflicted head trauma during infancy: results of a prospective, multicentered, comparative study. *Pediatrics.* 2007;119(5):922–929.

185. Duhaime AC, Christian C, Moss E, Seidl T. Long-term outcome in infants with the shaking-impact syndrome. *Pediatr Neurosurg.* 1996;24(6):292–298.

186. Heindl UT, Laub MC. Outcome of persistent vegetative state following hypoxic or traumatic brain injury in children and adolescents. *Neuropediatrics.* 1996;27(2):94–100.

187. Centers for Disease Control and Prevention. Web-based Injury Statistics Query and Reporting System. 2010.

188. National Highway Traffic Safety Administration. *Traffic Safety Facts 2008: Children.* Washington, DC: National Highway Traffic Safety Administration; 2008.

189. Arbogast KB, Durbin DR, Cornejo RA, Kallan MJ, Winston FK. An evaluation of the effectiveness of forward facing child restraint systems. *Accid Anal Prev.* 2004;36(4):585–589.

190. Zaloshnja E, Miller TR, Hendrie D. Effectiveness of child safety seats vs safety belts for children aged 2 to 3 years. *Arch Pediatr Adolesc Med.* 2007;161(1):65–68.

191. Elliott MR, Kallan MJ, Durbin DR, Winston FK. Effectiveness of child safety seats vs seat belts in reducing risk for death in children in passenger vehicle crashes. *Arch Pediatr Adolesc Med.* 2006;160(6):617–621.

192. Muszynski CA, Yoganandan N, Pintar FA, Gennarelli TA. Risk of pediatric head injury after motor vehicle accidents. *J Neurosurg.* 2005;102(suppl 4):374–379.

193. Committee on Injury, Violence, and Poison Prevention, Durbin DR. Child passenger safety. *Pediatrics.* 2011;127(4):788–793.

194. Bull MJ, Engle WA. Safe transportation of preterm and low birth weight infants at hospital discharge. *Pediatrics.* 2009;123(5):1424–1429.

195. Bull M, Agran P, Laraque D, et al. American Academy of Pediatrics. Committee on Injury and Poison Prevention. Transporting children with special health care needs. *Pediatrics.* 1999;104(4, pt 1):988–992.

196. Arbogast KB, Jermakian JS, Kallan MJ, Durbin DR. Effectiveness of belt positioning booster seats: an updated assessment. *Pediatrics.* 2009;124(5):1281–1286.

197. Kendrick D, Watson MC, Mulvaney CA, et al. Preventing childhood falls at home: meta-analysis and meta-regression. *Am J Prev Med.* 2008;35(4):370–379.

198. National SAFE KIDS Campaign. *Falls Fact Sheet.* Washington, DC: National SAFE KIDS Campaign; 2004.

199. Britton JW. Kids can't fly: preventing fall injuries in children. *WMJ.* 2005;104(1):33–36.

200. Pressley JC, Barlow B. Child and adolescent injury as a result of falls from buildings and structures. *Inj Prev.* 2005;11(5):267–273.

201. Werner P. Playground injuries and voluntary product standards for home and public playgrounds. *Pediatrics.* 1982;69(1):18–20.

202. All-terrain vehicle injury prevention: two-, three-, and four-wheeled unlicensed motor vehicles. *Pediatrics.* 2000;105(6):1352–1354.

203. Halstead ME, Walter KD. American Academy of Pediatrics. Clinical report—sport-related concussion in children and adolescents. *Pediatrics.* 2010;126(3):597–615.

204. Gessel LM, Fields SK, Collins CL, Dick RW, Comstock RD. Concussions among United States high school and collegiate athletes. *J Athl Train.* 2007;42(4):495–503.

205. Russell K, Christie J, Hagel BE. The effect of helmets on the risk of head and neck injuries among skiers and snowboarders: a meta-analysis. *CMAJ.* 2010;182(4):333–340.

206. Berger RP. The use of serum biomarkers to predict outcome after traumatic brain injury in adults and children. *J Head Trauma Rehabil.* 2006;21(4):315–333.

207. Berger RP, Beers SR, Richichi R, Wiesman D, Adelson PD. Serum biomarker concentrations and outcome after pediatric traumatic brain injury. *J Neurotrauma.* 2007;24(12):1793–1801.

208. Wiesmann M, Steinmeier E, Magerkurth O, Linn J, Gottmann D, Missler U. Outcome prediction in traumatic brain injury: comparison of neurological status, CT findings, and blood levels of S100B and GFAP. *Acta Neurol Scand.* 2010;121(3):178–185.

209. Herrmann M, Curio N, Jost S, Wunderlich MT, Synowitz H, Wallesch CW. Protein S-100B and neuron specific enolase as early neurobiochemical markers of the severity of traumatic brain injury. *Restor Neurol Neurosci.* 1999;14(2–3):109–114.

210. Herrmann M, Jost S, Kutz S, et al. Temporal profile of release of neurobiochemical markers of brain damage after traumatic brain injury is associated with intracranial pathology as demonstrated in cranial computerized tomography. *J Neurotrauma.* 2000;17(2):113–122.

211. Townend W, Ingebrigtsen T. Head injury outcome prediction: a role for protein S-100B? *Injury.* 2006;37(12):1098–1108.

212. Levin HS, Wilde EA, Chu Z, et al. Diffusion tensor imaging in relation to cognitive and functional outcome of traumatic brain injury in children. *J Head Trauma Rehabil.* 2008;23(4):197–208.

213. Wilde EA, Chu Z, Bigler ED, et al. Diffusion tensor imaging in the corpus callosum in children after moderate to severe traumatic brain injury. *J Neurotrauma.* 2006;23(10):1412–1426.

214. Rutgers DR, Fillard P, Paradot G, Tadié M, Lasjaunias P, Ducreux D. Diffusion tensor imaging characteristics of the corpus callosum in mild, moderate, and severe traumatic brain injury. *AJNR Am J Neuroradiol.* 2008;29(9):1730–1735.

215. Xu J, Rasmussen IA, Lagopoulos J, Håberg A. Diffuse axonal injury in severe traumatic brain injury visualized using high-resolution diffusion tensor imaging. *J Neurotrauma.* 2007;24(5):753–765.

216. Benson RR, Meda SA, Vasudevan S, et al. Global white matter analysis of diffusion tensor images is predictive of injury severity in traumatic brain injury. *J Neurotrauma.* 2007;24(3):446–459.

217. Yuan W, Holland SK, Schmithorst VJ, et al. Diffusion tensor MR imaging reveals persistent white matter alteration after traumatic brain injury experienced during early childhood. *AJNR Am J Neuroradiol.* 2007;28(10):1919–1925.

218. Arfanakis K, Haughton VM, Carew JD, Rogers BP, Dempsey RJ, Meyerand ME. Diffusion tensor MR imaging in diffuse axonal injury. *AJNR Am J Neuroradiol.* 2002;23(5):794–802.

219. Inglese M, Makani S, Johnson G, et al. Diffuse axonal injury in mild traumatic brain injury: a diffusion tensor imaging study. *J Neurosurg.* 2005;103(2):298–303.

220. Newcombe VF, Williams GB, Nortje J, et al. Analysis of acute traumatic axonal injury using diffusion tensor imaging. *Br J Neurosurg.* 2007;21(4):340–348.

221. Kraus MF, Susmaras T, Caughlin BP, Walker CJ, Sweeney JA, Little DM. White matter integrity and cognition in chronic traumatic brain injury: a diffusion tensor imaging study. *Brain.* 2007;130(pt 10):2508–2519.

222. Wilde EA, McCauley SR, Hunter JV, et al. Diffusion tensor imaging of acute mild traumatic brain injury in adolescents. *Neurology.* 2008; 70(12):948–955.

223. Wu T, Wilde EA, Bigler ED, et al. Evaluating the relationship between memory functioning and cingulum bundles in acute mild traumatic brain injury using diffusion tensor imaging. *J Neurotrauma.* 2010;27(2):303–307.

224. Tong KA, Ashwal S, Holshouser BA, et al. Diffuse axonal injury in children: clinical correlation with hemorrhagic lesions. *Ann Neurol.* 2004;56(1):36–50.

225. Tong KA, Ashwal S, Holshouser BA, et al. Hemorrhagic shearing lesions in children and adolescents with posttraumatic diffuse axonal injury: improved detection and initial results. *Radiology.* 2003;227(2):332–339.

226. Babikian T, Freier MC, Tong KA, et al. Susceptibility weighted imaging: neuropsychologic outcome and pediatric head injury. *Pediatr Neurol.* 2005;33(3):184–194.

227. Brichtová E, Kozák L. Apolipoprotein E genotype and traumatic brain injury in children—association with neurological outcome. *Childs Nerv Syst.* 2008;24(3):349–356.

228. Lo TY, Jones PA, Chambers IR, et al. Modulating effect of apolipoprotein E polymorphisms on secondary brain insult and outcome after childhood brain trauma. *Childs Nerv Syst.* 2009;25(1):47–54.

229. Quinn TJ, Smith C, Murray L, Stewart J, Nicoll JA, Graham DI. There is no evidence of an association in children and teenagers between the apolipoprotein E epsilon4 allele and post-traumatic brain swelling. *Neuropathol Appl Neurobiol.* 2004;30(6):569–575.

230. Moran LM, Taylor HG, Ganesalingam K, et al. Apolipoprotein E4 as a predictor of outcomes in pediatric mild traumatic brain injury. *J Neurotrauma.* 2009;26(9):1489–1495.

Pediatric Neurocritical Care: Special Considerations

Kristin Guilliams, Andranik Madikians, Jose Pineda, and Christopher C. Giza

INTRODUCTION

Traumatic brain injury (TBI) is the most common cause of morbidity and mortality in pediatrics, with nearly 500,000 emergency department visits annually for children younger than age 14 (http://www.cdc.gov). Of these, some 29,000 are hospitalized and 3,000 die. Although most cases of TBI fall into the mild-to-moderate range, which is usually defined as a Glasgow Coma Score between 9 and 15, the primary focus of this chapter will be on severe TBI, as defined by a Glasgow Coma Score of ≤ 8, and often includes a period of care in the intensive care unit (ICU). Research specific to pediatric TBI of all levels has rapidly grown over the past 2 decades including at least 2 large, international randomized clinical trials. Intervention and management to optimize outcomes begin before the patient arrives in the hospital and continues well past their discharge (Figure 35-1). There is a mantra in pediatrics that "kids are not little adults." This is well borne out in TBI characteristics, acute management, and long-term recovery.

DISTINCTIONS OF THE IMMATURE BRAIN

Biomechanics

The developing brain has distinct vulnerabilities to traumatic injury. As the brain develops across age groups, it has different unique properties and susceptibilities. Mechanism of injury also varies with age: children younger than the age of 4 are more likely to have TBI from a fall or an assault, whereas the 15–19-year-old population is more likely to have a motor vehicle accident as the primary cause of their injury (1). These multiple sources of injury challenge our ability to classify pediatric TBI into a single category.

Velocity, 3-dimensional (3D) angular acceleration, and impact force all contribute to the biomechanics of injury in any head trauma, but there are differences in these forces between accidental and nonaccidental (or abusive) trauma (2). Duhaime et al. (3) found that in infants diagnosed with "shaken baby syndrome," 63% had evidence of blunt trauma, such as a hematoma or skull fracture, in addition to the intracranial findings associated with forceful shaking. All infants who died had evidence of blunt trauma. They also determined through infant modeling that although shaking

alone could generate forces with peak tangential accelerations of 9.29 G, shaking associated with the impact of a skull against a surface generated cranial peak accelerations nearly 50 times greater. High angular acceleration and velocity of impact correlate with intracranial hemorrhage and white matter injury (2). The unique proportion of an infant's head weight to total body weight and general head to body ratio also create biomechanical forces on the brain not commonly seen in TBI in other age groups. The exact tension, compression, and bending properties of an infant neck are currently not well known (2), but the neck may be hyperextended in the young infant, leading to brainstem and cervical cord injury (4,5). Unilateral or bilateral hematomas in the third through fifth cervical spinal nerve roots, which innervate the diaphragm, frequently occur in children with suspected neck hyperextension (6). The head-to-body proportions also influence the directional forces to which the young brain may be subjected. Infant models demonstrate in falls less than 1 m that axial, but not coronal, rotation of the skull occurs on occipital impact. This is important because Gennarelli et al. (7) demonstrated through primate models that those who sustained injury with coronal rotation experienced unconsciousness for more than 6 hours and had diffuse axonal injury (DAI), whereas only approximately half of the animals with axial rotation injury experienced prolonged unconsciousness or DAI.

The newborn skull consists of thin, partially calcified bony tissue plates joined together at the sutures by periosteal and endosteal membranes (8). Unlike adult sutures, infant sutures do not have the enhanced ability to absorb energy, and thus are unable to function as "shock absorbers" to help protect the brain as adult sutures do. (8) The lack of shock absorption, along with high rates of acceleration, may contribute to the formation of acute subdural hematomas in TBI. Based on animal models and clinical observation, impact does not need to occur to induce subdural hematomas because enough acceleration force may be generated with non-impact trauma to tear the bridging veins (9). For reasons that have not yet been determined, the young brain is also more susceptible to a specific pattern of tissue loss noted by computed tomography (CT) hypodensity, affecting the entire supratentorial hemisphere in association with the acute subdural hematomas. This may be present at initial evaluation or may develop over several days and has been termed "big black brain" (10).

injury → Pre-hospital	Trauma Bay	PICU	Medical Floor	Inpatient Rehabilitation	Home & School environments
• Avoid secondary insults: hypotension, hypoxia, hyper-ventilation • Treat clinical signs of herniation	• Avoid secondary insults: hypoxia, hypotension, hyper-ventilation • Treat clinical/radio-logical signs of herniation • To OR for treatment of intracranial hematomas if indicated	• Avoid secondary insults: intracranial hypertension, hypotension, low cerebral perfusion pressure, hypoxia, hyperventilation, low brain tissue oxygen tension, fever, seizures, hyponatremia, severe anemia, severe hyperglycemia	• Physical, occupational, cognitive therapy • Address other comorbid or secondary medical problems, i.e. headaches, depression, seizures	• Aggressive physical, occupational, and cognitive therapy	• Outpatient rehabilitation therapy • Formal testing to determine learning needs • Integrative therapy and education plan • Education of teachers and peers

FIGURE 35-1 Traumatic brain injury continuum of therapy. *OR*, operating room; *PICU*, pediatric intensive care unit.

Cerebral Blood Flow and Metabolism

The developing brain also differs from the adult brain in its physiologic properties. Cerebral blood flow (CBF) and CBF velocity vary based on age (11–14). Quantitative perfusion CT measured age-dependent changes in regional CBF of 40 mL/100 g/min in the first 6 months, which then increases to approximately 130 mL/100 g/min between 2 and 4 years before stabilizing at about 50 mL/100 g/min, which is consistent with other published estimates (15). In addition to absolute CBF varying by age, CBF velocity is also age dependent. As measured by transcranial Doppler (TCD) of the middle cerebral artery (MCA), healthy newborns have a CBF velocity of approximately 24 cm/s, which slowly increases to a peak at age 6–9 years of approximately 97 cm/s, and then settles out to the average adult velocity of approximately 50 cm/s. Across the age ranges, girls tend to have higher flow velocities than boys (16–18). Historically, it was originally thought that TBI in children induced hyperemia and edema when pediatric TBI CBFs were compared to adult and late teen normal values (19,20). Later, it was found that CBF was naturally higher in younger kids. Zwienenberg and Muizelaar (12) republished the Japanese data on age-dependent CBF changes in 80 normal children that Suzuki (21) had published in *Nagoya Medical Journal*, which is not widely available. These findings provided age-matched control data for pediatric TBI and changed the impression of the incidence of true hyperemia (12).

The age-dependent fluctuations in CBF are consistent with neurometabolic coupling because cerebral metabolism of glucose also varies by age. Metabolism is initially lower at birth, increasing to a peak around 3–4 years of age, where it sustains its elevated rate until about 9 years of age, after which it declines to its adult rate (22,23). The extent to which TBI disrupts the natural coupling of CBF to metabolism has signifi-

cant implications for both acute management and long-term recovery. After TBI, there are 3 phases of change noted in CBF (24): (a) Poor perfusion and ischemia, which usually occurs within the first 6–12 hours, followed by (b) hyperemia with "luxury perfusion" and increased intracranial pressure (ICP), and finally, (c) poor perfusion and possibly vasospasm. CBF is an important predictor of outcome because it appears that the initial increase in CBF, presumably to supply increased metabolic demands, is a necessary step for functional recovery (25,26). Supranormal elevations of CBF, however, and excessive elevations of ICP lead to poor outcomes. This may be caused by impaired cerebral autoregulation and uncoupling between CBF and metabolism.

Cerebral autoregulation (AR) is a homeostatic mechanism by which cerebral arteries and arterioles constrict to increase resistance in response to increases in mean arterial pressure (MAP) or increased cerebral perfusion pressure (CPP) or conversely dilate in response to lower MAP or CPP. Maintenance of cerebral AR is an important protective factor after TBI. AR maintains normal CBF when blood pressure changes, which in turn has important implications for intracranial blood volume and consequently ICP (Figure 35-2). Younger age appears to be a risk factor for impaired AR (27). If AR is impaired, CBF, cerebral blood volume, and ICP may vary passively with blood pressure fluctuations, which may lead to increased secondary insults or unintended consequences with therapeutic interventions (28,29). Alternatively, disrupted AR may make the brain more susceptible to hypoperfusion during periods of low or even normal CPP. AR disruption in children can occur in up to 40% of cases of moderate-to-severe TBI, may be unilateral or bilateral, and may range from mild impairment to complete absence of AR (16,30). Partial pressure of carbon dioxide ($PaCO_2$) is a potent vasodilator and influences both CBF and AR. Data from healthy, anesthetized children suggest that children

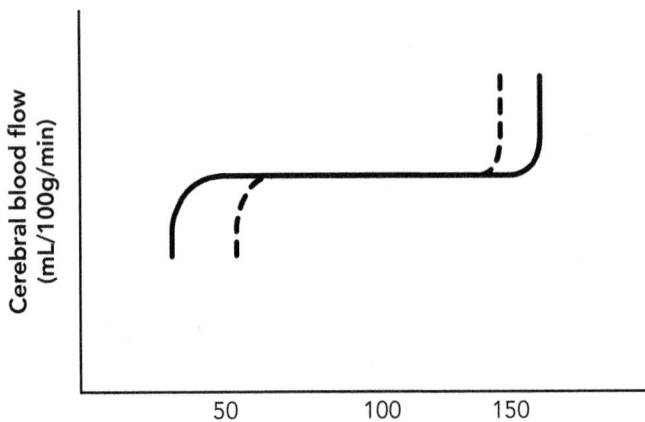

FIGURE 35-2 Cerebral autoregulation maintains a steady blood flow over a wide range of blood pressures. Dotted line depicts abnormal autoregulation.

have more vasoreactivity to fluctuations in CO_2 than adults (31). Reactivity to CO_2 may be transiently impaired in pediatric TBI (16) and, although not routinely monitored at bedside, poor vasoreactivity correlates with poor outcome (25,26,32). Brain CO_2 vasoreactivity has important implications for a patient's response to hyperventilation: Under conditions of hyperemia (excessive CBF), the benefit of hyperventilation may be decreased ICP because of decreased cerebral blood volume (33). However, in patients with brain injury, hyperventilation may cause brain ischemia, and hyperemia in children with TBI is not common (12,34). Intact AR does not provide immunity from deleterious vascular response to TBI: Patients with intact blood pressure AR but reduced intracranial compliance may experience "Cushing vasodilator cascade," where decreased MAP leads to vasodilatation, which in turn may cause increased cerebral blood volume, which elevates ICP, causing decreased CPP and leading to further vasodilatation (16). The initial treatment steps in such patients should be directed toward normalizing the MAP.

Cerebral metabolism is also closely linked with CBF. Most current knowledge of molecular metabolism after TBI comes from animal models, particularly rats. Young rats provide a workable model for juvenile TBI because they, like humans, have postnatal brain maturation, including cellular proliferation and migration, apoptosis, pruning, synaptogenesis, and myelination (35). In these animal models, and presumably in humans as well, after TBI there is an initial increase in glucose metabolism followed by a dip. In young rats, the period of decreased glucose metabolic rate was much shorter than that observed in adult rats (3 days vs 10 days) (36). This may have important implications because children have higher baseline glucose metabolism rates, and local glucose metabolism rates have been proposed as surrogate markers of synaptogenesis and plasticity (35).

Although glucose is the primary substrate for cerebral metabolism, ketones also play an important role and may have neuroprotective properties for TBI, particularly in the developing brain. Children adapt more rapidly to ketone metabolism, and after a 24-hour period of fasting, ketone

levels in children are inversely proportional to age (37). In animal models of developmental TBI, postinjury ketones decrease lesion volume and improve behavioral outcome (38–40). This may be caused by several mechanisms, including increased expression of monocarboxylate transporter 2, which allows for increased ketone transport across the blood–brain barrier, making it available to the neuron for use as an energy substrate (41). Although the ketogenic diet has not been used clinically for TBI, it is employed to control intractable childhood epilepsy, and thus, it may be a therapy more readily translatable from the bench to the bedside.

The immature brain is exquisitely sensitive to excitotoxicity of TBI. In TBI, there is excessive release of potassium and glutamate (42). Glutamate is an important neurotransmitter for proper synaptic pruning, but excessive glutamate activation may lead to intracellular calcium overload, production of free radicals, lipid peroxidation, and cell death (43). After TBI during the developmental period, animal models suggest a downregulation of N-methyl-d-aspartate (NMDA) receptors in hippocampus lasting for 2–4 days. This is in contrast to adult animals, in which alterations of hippocampal NMDA receptor subunits are less prominent (44,45). Impairment of NMDA-mediated neurotransmission after injury may impair long-term potentiation and plasticity (46,47). Importantly, administration of NMDA antagonists is neuroprotective in adult rodents after TBI but worsens injury, particularly secondary apoptotic damage, in immature animal models (48).

The metabolite adenosine also plays a role in the pathology of TBI. In humans, it is elevated regardless of age, mechanism of injury, or GCS score, although significantly higher levels are found in children with a GCS of ≤ 4 (49). Adenosine may be a "retaliatory metabolite" because it may decrease excitatory amino acids, improve CBF, inhibit platelet aggregation, and reduce free radicals and oxidative damage. Adenosine decreases glutamate release via A_1 binding. It may also mediate vasodilatation via A_2 binding, although A_2 binding inhibits A_1 binding, thus counteracting the inhibition of glutamate release (49). Finally, the inhibitory neurotransmitter gamma-aminobutyric acid (GABA) may actually be excitotoxic in the neonatal brain (50,51). In addition to direct excitotoxicity acutely, secondary downregulation of GABA receptors and, thus, reduction of GABA binding during key time points in brain maturation may impair plasticity (52).

Plasticity

Plasticity is "a change in a structure in response to an external force and the maintenance of that shape after removal of the force" (53). The developing brain is intrinsically plastic as it learns and adapts to a variety of experiences. This adds a layer of complexity to recovery and outcome measurements in pediatric TBI, however, as the baseline measurement of recovery changes as expectations of development and skills change throughout childhood. The Kennard Principle of "younger is better" was founded on observation that focal sensorimotor cortex lesions sustained during development had better recovery than lesions sustained in adulthood (44). This was the mantra of fierce optimism for pediatric brain injuries for decades, but more recent data may suggest otherwise (54,55). The principle of "growing into the lesion" postulates that if a particular function is not normally well developed at the time of injury, then such a deficit may not necessarily be observed until a later developmental stage. For example, a 3-month-old may sustain TBI and appear to recover over a few weeks to a developmental level similar to other noninjured 4-month-olds; however, injury to speech centers may not become apparent until well after the child's first birthday. Recovery may also be tenuous because disruption of neurotransmission, such as a decrease or blockade of NMDA receptors, may cause recrudescence of symptoms (56). The plasticity that contributes to the spontaneous recovery from TBI may come at the cost of experience-dependent plasticity. Animal models of pediatric TBI demonstrate that in absence of clinical neurological deficits or neuronal loss, environment induced increases in learning, and cortical thickness were impaired in those animals who sustained early life TBI compared to noninjured animals (57). These theories have not been tested in children with TBI, however. Finally, the plasticity of the developing brain may not always be beneficial. "Bad plasticity" may lead to the abnormal reorganization of damaged networks, leading to ongoing injury as the brain develops (44). This may be the root of post-traumatic epilepsy.

CLINICAL MANAGEMENT OF SEVERE TRAUMATIC BRAIN INJURY

The primary goals of clinical management of TBI are to mitigate secondary injury and prevent secondary insult. Secondary injury generally refers to pathophysiological processes, such as mitochondrial dysfunction, caspase activation, or cytoskeletal damage, which follow as a consequence of the primary traumatic injury. Secondary insult is a direct insult to the brain, such as hypotension or hypoxia, which occurs after the primary traumatic event and has the potential to increase or exacerbate the primary injury. In 2003, the "Guidelines for the Acute Medical Management of Severe Traumatic Brain Injury of Infants, Children, and Adolescents" were published by the Brain Trauma Foundation, based on relevant evidence-based knowledge available at the time. This was primarily in response to the publication of "Guidelines for the Management of (Adult) Severe Traumatic Brain Injury" (58,59) and the recognition that "children are not little adults." An updated version was published in 2012, with a few significant changes from new clinical evidence that were incorporated into the guidelines (60). The following sections in this chapter reflect contemporary management of severe TBI in children. The management principles are consistent with the Brain Trauma Foundation guidelines and relevant published literature.

Basic Physiologic Parameters

Blood Pressure

Systolic blood pressure (SBP) should be kept above 90 mm Hg or fifth percentile for age (70 mmHg + [2 × age in years]) (61). Although the fifth percentile for age is commonly used as the lower threshold for SBP, at least 1 study reports 75th percentile for age as the threshold associated with poor outcome (62). Blood pressure is a key component of total CPP (MAP − ICP = CPP). Children with severe TBI who presented to emergency room (ER) with hypotension had a 61% mortality rate, compared to 22% in the absence of hypoten-

sion. When children were hypotensive and hypoxic, mortality rate rose to 85% (63). Early hypotension in pediatric TBI has also been associated with prolonged length of stay and worse outcome at 3 months postinjury (64). Mild hypertension should not be aggressively treated, however, as hypertension up to 30 mm Hg above age corrected normal values has been correlated with lower mortality rates (65), and children may have a 5% increase in odds of survival for every 1 mm Hg increase in SBP (24). However, children with disrupted blood pressure AR may experience increases in ICP as blood pressure increases. Advanced neuromonitoring techniques such as brain tissue oxygen tension (PbtO$_2$) monitoring may be helpful under these complex hemodynamic circumstances, but experience in children with TBI is limited.

Intracranial Pressure

ICP should be kept below 20 mm Hg because this has been associated with improved outcomes (60,66,67). Smaller children may benefit from a lower threshold than 20 mm Hg for ICP intervention, but ICP thresholds for children younger than 2 years of age have not been well established (68). Extremely elevated ICP (>40 mm Hg) has been associated with high mortality rates (69,70). ICP monitoring is recommended for all patients with severe TBI (GCS of 8 or less) with abnormalities on the admission computed tomography (CT) scan, including children younger than 1 year of age because an open fontanel does not preclude the need for ICP monitoring. ICP monitoring may be done with an external strain gauge transducer, a catheter tip pressure transducer device, or a ventriculostomy catheter (60,71). The ventriculostomy catheter has the advantage of also allowing for simultaneous cerebrospinal fluid (CSF) drainage.

Cerebral Perfusion Pressure

CPP is calculated as MAP − ICP and should be maintained at least greater than 40 mm Hg. There may be a continuous threshold ranging from 40–60 mm Hg based on age (60,72), but this requires further study. The goal of maintaining adequate CPP is to adequately perfuse and prevent secondary ischemic injury throughout the brain. CPP below 40 mm Hg has been associated with significantly higher rates of mortality and unfavorable outcomes (60,66,68,73). As CPP drops below the lower limit of AR, blood vessels become maximally dilated, oxygen extraction increases, and CBF can no longer respond to increased metabolic demand. As vessels further dilate to attempt to compensate, they may collapse, leading to irreversible ischemia (74).

Control of Intracranial Pressure—First Tier

Maintaining adequate CPP requires aggressive intervention to control both blood pressure and ICP. Blood pressure is primarily supported by volume resuscitation and inotropic/vasopressor support. ICP management has a greater array of options and levels of evidence behind practices. The "Guidelines for the Acute Medical Management of Severe Traumatic Brain Injury of Infants, Children, and Adolescents" relating to ICP management provide level I–III recommendations for several aspects in the care of children with severe TBI (60). In this chapter, we follow a tiered approach to sequential implementation of ICP directed therapies that is consistent with the recommendations and additional published literature.

Maintain Head of Bed at 30 Degrees

Basic maneuvers may assist in venous drainage and lowering ICP with minimal risk. Midline head positioning prevents kinking of the jugular veins. Tight cervical collars may also limit venous drainage. Elevating the head of the bed by flexing the patient at the hip (not the abdomen) promotes drainage from the cranial vault. If the patient is hypotensive, however, the benefits of head elevation may be outweighed by the potential risk of exacerbating hypoperfusion and ischemia.

Sedation and Analgesics

Sedation may be helpful in lowering ICP by controlling pain, facilitating mechanical ventilation, preventing shivering, decreasing seizure activity, as well as alleviating long-term psychological trauma (60). Noxious or stressful stimuli may increase ICP (75) or increase the cerebral metabolic rate for oxygen (60). Commonly used sedatives and analgesics include midazolam, fentanyl, and morphine. Barbiturates are discussed separately under second tier therapies.

Midazolam and fentanyl are often used either separately or in conjunction for sedation in the pediatric ICU, despite a lack of evidence for their specific use in pediatric TBI. Fentanyl and midazolam are reported as sedative agents in several studies of pediatric TBI management (73,76,77), and many studies report a generic "sedation" in the management section. No pediatric TBI studies have looked specifically at midazolam or fentanyl use, although several studies in adults included an age range down to 17. There is one report of midazolam in adults with TBI (with teenage inclusion) showing no effect on lowering and even possibly increasing ICP (78). One report in the literature of fentanyl use in a child is limited to an elevated ICP after fentanyl administration (79). Diazepam is effective in providing sedation in adults with relatively minimal effects on blood pressure of CBF (80).

Ketamine has historically been discouraged from use in TBI because of concerns of increased ICP (81–83). However, when used in conjunction with an anesthestic, it does not always have the same effect on ICP (84) and may, in fact, decrease ICP in patients with TBI (85). Comparison studies demonstrate ketamine in conjunction with midazolam to be as effective as fentanyl (or sufentanil) (86,87) and midazolam in controlling ICP.

Propofol is sometimes used in adult TBI, but with reports of increased incidence of propofol syndrome and cardiac arrest. In the pediatric TBI population, propofol may be effective in controlling ICP (88). However, propofol is not recommended for continuous sedation in critically ill children because of safety warnings from the Food and Drug Administration.

As stated in the first edition of the guidelines,

> [An] ideal sedative for patients with severe TBI is one that is rapid in onset and offset, is easily titrated to effect, has a well-defined metabolism (preferably independent of end-organ function), neither accumulates nor has active metabolites, exhibits anticonvulsant actions, has no adverse cardiovascular or immune action, and lacks drug–drug interactions while preserving the neurologic examination. (89)

Unfortunately, such a drug does not currently exist, thus leaving the choice of these agents largely in the hands of the treating physician.

Drain Cerebrospinal Fluid

If the ICP remains elevated after proper patient positioning and sedation, the guidelines recommend CSF drainage if a ventriculostomy is already in place (level III recommendation) (60).

Neuromuscular Blockade

The guidelines recommend consideration of neuromuscular blockade for persistently elevated ICP, although no specific trials have examined its effect on pediatric ICP. There may be potential benefits contributing to ICP control, including reduction in airway and intrathoracic pressure leading to improved cerebral venous outflow, reduction in shivering, posturing, or breathing against the ventilator and decrease in metabolic demands (60,90). One retrospective analysis of adult TBI found that early, routine use of neuromuscular blockade did not have any added benefit on ICP control or outcome and added to ICU length of stay and risk of pneumonia (91).

Osmotic Therapy

Mannitol and hypertonic saline (HTS) are both forms of hyperosmolar therapy that may be effective in controlling ICP. Mannitol had early acceptance and establishment in clinical protocols of controlling ICP, and thus has had limited clinical trials. Typical dosing is 1 g/kg of body weight (60). Mannitol reduces ICP by osmotic effect (92) and decreases blood viscosity, which contributes to decreased blood vessel diameter (93,94). Potential adverse effects of mannitol include renal failure (95) and hypovolemia (96). Adult literature supports not exceeding an upper limit of 320 mOsm/L in serum osmolality during mannitol administration because there is an increased risk of acute tubular necrosis and renal failure above 320 mOsm/L (58). However, it is important to note that evidence supporting this cutoff is limited. HTS therapy in the pediatric population is typically 3% sodium chloride at a rate of 0.1–1.0 mL/kg/hr used in a sliding scale manner to keep ICP <20 mm Hg (60). However, adult practice may use HTS of up to 23.4% (97). A slightly higher serum osmolality of up to 360 mOsm/L may be tolerated during HTS therapy (60,98,99). A double-blind crossover study comparing normal saline (0.9%) to HTS (3%) in children with severe TBI found that HTS lowered ICP and reduced the number of other interventions required (100). A recent meta-analysis of mannitol vs HTS in adult TBI found that HTS had a small but potentially clinically significant advantage over mannitol for controlling ICP (101). With insufficient evidence to support or refute mannitol use in children, however, the choice between mannitol and HTS is left to the treating physician.

Control of Intracranial Pressure—Second Tier

Second tier therapies may be employed when ICP is refractory to the previously discussed measures. These therapies have been shown in some studies to lower ICP, but adequate evidence comparing them to other therapies is lacking to establish a relative risk/benefit ratio.

Hyperventilation
Aggressive hyperventilation may be necessary for discrete, short time intervals to counteract impending herniation or acute neurologic deterioration, but mild, prophylactic, or chronic hyperventilation should be avoided (33,60,102). Hyperventilation induces hypocapnia leading to cerebral vasoconstriction and a reduction in CBF, which may cause both local and global secondary ischemic injury (34,60,102). There is little evidence of hyperemia in children with severe TBI, therefore minimal benefit for CBF reduction, even if CPP is transiently improved (60,103). A retrospective study found that when controlling for initial GCS score, injury severity score, $PaCO_2$, and year of admission, increased episodes of hypocarbia were associated with increased mortality. Children with 3 or more documented episodes of hypocarbia had an odds ratio for mortality of 3.93 compared to children without hypocarbia (104).

Decompressive Craniectomy
Decompressive craniectomy has potential benefit for children with severe TBI and medically refractory intracranial hypertension (60) (Figure 35-3). Taylor et al. (105) reported lowered ICP and improved 6-month outcomes of children receiving early bitemporal craniectomy. Although this was a pilot study, it had a significant influence on the 2006 *Cochrane Database System Review*, in support to consider decompressive craniectomy for children with refractory elevated ICP secondary to TBI (106). (Please refer to "Beyond the Guidelines" section of this article for further discussion of decompressive craniectomy.)

Barbiturates
High-dose barbiturate therapy may be considered in patients with salvageable brain tissue and refractory ICP elevation who are hemodynamically stable, although no studies have examined whether or not barbiturates improve outcome or survival in children (60). Barbiturates are theorized to lower ICP by suppression of metabolism and alteration of vascular tone and may also provide neuroprotective effects of inhibition of lipid peroxidation and membrane stabilization (107). Barbiturates lower cardiac index and systemic vascular resistance and are frequently associated with increased use of pressors (108). It is prudent to have electroencephalography (EEG) and invasive blood pressure monitoring in place prior to initiating barbiturate therapy. There have been no trials comparing effectiveness or associated adverse events with ICP control among specific barbiturates.

Moderate Hypothermia
Extrapolation from adult data led to the recommendation of avoidance of hyperthermia and consideration of moderate hypothermia (<32–34°C) in children in the first version of the guidelines (109). Fever is independently associated with worse outcome in neurologic injury (110), including pediatric TBI (111). In the updated Brain Trauma Foundation Guidelines, moderate hypothermia is listed as an option to consider in the treatment of ICP. This option should be exercised with caution because a pediatric randomized controlled clinical trial reported no benefit and potential risk associated with the use of hypothermia in children with TBI (112). At the time of this publication, a second clinical trial of hypothermia in pediatric TBI had been closed because of futility, and the results of an additional trial were pending publication. The take-home message from these studies was that short (<24 hour) duration hypothermia with rapid rewarming did not improve outcomes, at least in part to rebound elevations in ICP. Longer hypothermia (more than 48 hours) with gradual passive rewarming appeared to be beneficial in an early publication (113). Currently, it is the authors' recommendation to pursue strict maintenance of normothermia. However, if moderate hypothermia is used for any reason, it should be used for a minimum duration of 48 hours and rewarming should occur at a rate of no more than 0.5°C/hr (60).

Nutrition
The 2012 guideline update addressed the concern of providing optimal nutrition to children with severe TBI; however, only one study met inclusion criteria. Briassoulis et al. (114) performed a randomized controlled trial comparing the use of standard enteral formula to an immune-enhancing diet, which included greater amounts of protein, fat, and selected vitamins and minerals, in children with severe TBI. There was no significant difference between the 2 groups in survival, length of stay, or length of mechanical ventilation

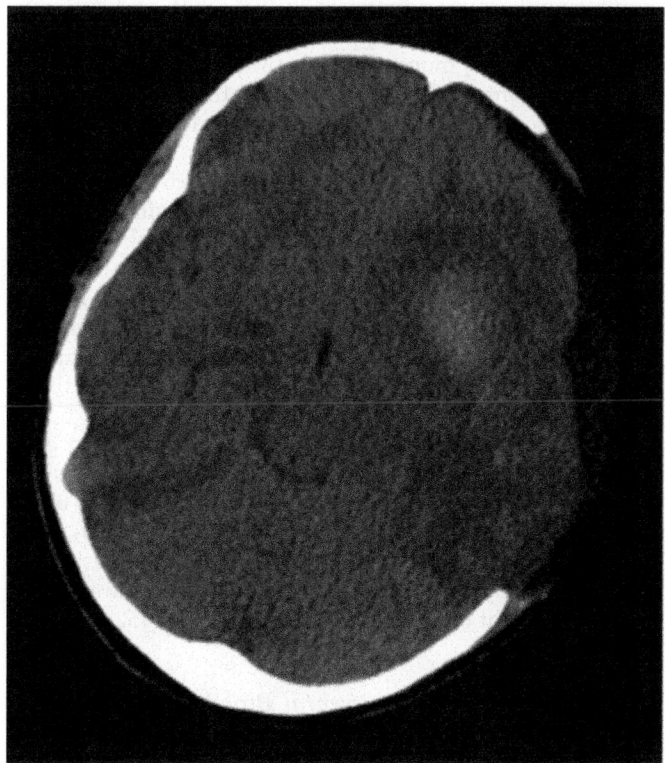

FIGURE 35-3 Typical appearance of CT scan following decompressive craniectomy where the edematous hemisphere may visibly protrude through the bony defect.

(114). At this time, there is insufficient evidence to recommend manner of nutritional support (i.e., total parenteral nutrition vs enteral feeds) or specific formulas or supplements. The guidelines do recommend that all children be on full nutritional support of some manner by day 7 post-TBI (60).

Adjunctive Therapies

Glucose Control

A delicate balance must be achieved in maintaining glucose control. Hyperglycemia of >300 mg/dL (16.6 mmol/L) was associated with 100% mortality rate in one study of pediatric TBI (115), and >200 mg/dL (11.1 mmol/L) was associated with poor outcome in another study (116). In animal models, hyperglycemia causes a significant increase in extracellular glutamate levels in the hippocampus and cortex and greater histologic injury (117). However, the brain has increased demands for glycolysis after injury (118), and, in adults, tight systemic glucose control of keeping the glucose below 120 mg/dL (6.7 mmol/L) has been associated with increased incidence of cerebral hypoglycemia, elevated lactate/pyruvate ratios, and increased glutamate release, sometimes collectively deemed a "brain energy crisis," (119,120) and may lead to increased mortality (121).

Hyperbaric Oxygen

With the observation that hypoxia and secondary ischemia contribute significantly to TBI morbidity and mortality, hyperbaric oxygen has been proposed as an adjunctive therapy. A *Cochrane Database System Review* found that although hyperbaric oxygen may reduce mortality, it does not improve overall outcomes for patients with TBI (122). A recent prospective, randomized trial in adults (123) comparing hyperbaric oxygen to normobaric hyperoxia found both groups to be associated with lower lactate levels and the hyperbaric group to have lower ICP values over the 3 days following treatment. ICP reduction was not observed in the normobaric oxygen group. Although several small studies with self-recognized flaws purport the benefit of hyperbaric oxygen therapy for long-term neuropsychological and/or physiologic improvement in patients with brain injury (124,125), there is a paucity of evidence to support its use. Lack of supportive evidence has not stopped direct-to-consumer marketing as a potential therapy, however. Hyperbaric oxygen used in children for other neurologic conditions, such as cerebral palsy and autism, has been associated with a significant risk of inducing or exacerbating seizures (126) without evidence of efficacy (127,128).

Hyperoxia

Even normobaric hyperoxia has little to no evidence to support its use. In adults with TBI, hyperoxia with ventilation of 100% oxygen did not change cerebral metabolic rate for oxygen ($CMRO_2$) when measured directly by positron emission tomography (129). Preclinical work in an animal model of cardiac arrest demonstrated increased oxidative stress and cell death after hyperoxic resuscitation compared to normoxic resuscitation (130). Further studies particularly regarding the potential long-term outcome in the pediatric population are needed.

Potential Upcoming Therapies

Other therapies currently in the pipeline for treatment of TBI in pediatrics and adults include progesterone (131,132), cyclosporine (133), erythropoietin (134), and an acetylcholinesterase inhibitor (135).

BEYOND THE GUIDELINES

Physiological Neuromonitoring in the Intensive Care Unit

Continuous Electroencephalography

The use of continuous EEG monitoring in the pediatric intensive care unit (PICU) has grown substantially over the past decade, although limited data exist currently for its specific use in pediatric TBI. A retrospective analysis found that 12% of children with moderate-to-severe TBI developed early post-traumatic seizures, both convulsive and nonconvulsive. Of these children, 68% developed seizures within 12 hours postinjury. Independent risk factors for seizures included age <2 years, GCS of ≤ 8, and nonaccidental trauma (136). In adults, nonconvulsive seizures in the TBI population have been associated with episodic elevations of ICP and metabolic crises consisting of marked increases in the lactate/pyruvate ratio . Prospective continuous EEG monitoring found nonconvulsive seizures occurring in 22% of moderate-to-severe adult patients with TBI (137).

Brain Tissue Oxygen Monitoring

$PbtO_2$ monitoring may play an important role in monitoring patients with TBI, complementing ICP and other physiologic monitoring, because adherence to ICP, CPP, and systemic monitoring may not be adequate to prevent brain tissue hypoxia (138). $PbtO_2$ monitoring was added to the guidelines for management of adult TBI in 2007 (60,139). $PbtO_2$ monitoring and intervening for $PbtO_2$ lower than 20 mm Hg has been associated with decreased mortality and improved 6-month outcomes in both adults and children (140–142). Conversely, low $PbtO_2$ has been associated with poor outcomes (143–145). There is insufficient data available to make recommendations for absolute critical $PbtO_2$ thresholds in children. Based on available literature, the authors recommend 20 mm Hg as the lower limit to initiate intervention (Table 35-1). Precisely what $PbtO_2$ is monitoring is not firmly established, largely because the physiology of oxygen distribution between cerebral microvasculature and brain tissue is not yet well understood, but it may be considered as a measure of a combination of factors that affect perfusion, diffusion, and consumptive characteristics of oxygen in brain tissue. Partial pressure of oxygen (PaO_2), CBF, $PaCO_2$, ICP, CPP, hemoglobin level, and tissue barriers to diffusion all may influence $PbtO_2$, although none of these parameters alone has a tight correlation with PbtO2 (146–152).

Noninvasive Cerebral Blood Flow

Measuring CBF directly may be beneficial in pediatric TBI because it influences ICP and CPP, and normal cerebral AR may be impaired. Current methods of measuring CBF include the use of Xenon (Xe)-133 (153), brain tissue oxygen reactivity (154), laser-Doppler flowmetry (although this has

TABLE 35-1 Steps to Respond to Low PbtO₂

ASSESSMENT	POTENTIAL INTERVENTION
Check monitor placement.	Confirm no new pathology interfering with monitor probe.
Assess for adequate ventilatory support.	Adjust ventilation tomaintain adequate oxygenation (increase FiO₂, increase PEEP).
Review MAP, volume status.	Consider NS bolus and/or pressor support.
Assess for metabolic changes in demand.	Review vitals signs and patient.
	Treat possible pain, seizures, shivering, or fever.
Check hemoglobin.	Transfuse if hemoglobin <7 g/dL.

Abbreviations: FiO₂, fraction of inspired oxygen; MAP, mean arterial pressure; NS, normal saline; PbtO₂, partial pressure of oxygen in brain tissue; PEEP, positive end expiratory pressure.

not been used in children) (29), and transcranial Doppler (TCD) (155). TCD monitoring has the advantages of being noninvasive, quick, and easy to use. The MCA is the most commonly insonated. Changes in TCD-MCA flow velocity parallel changes in CBF with age (29). In adults, the pulsatility index can calculate the cerebrovascular resistance and estimate ICP (156), but the use of TCD in children is more controversial. Figaji et al. (157) did not find TCD to be a reliable indicator of ICP, but Melo et al. (158) found high sensitivity and negative predictive value of the diastolic velocity and pulsatility index measurements for predicting ICP when used early in resuscitation. Philip et al. (159) found a wide variation in CBF velocity in children with CPP >40 mm Hg, but a low MCA flow velocity (<2 SD for age) is associated with a poor 6-month Glasgow Outcome Score (GOS) (160). More research and multicenter trials are needed, particularly with this user-dependent technology.

Role of Surgical Intervention

As noted before, a primary goal of TBI management is prevention of secondary insults. One of the most important parameters to control is ICP. The goal of therapy is to medically and surgically manage ICP, and, as a result, the CPP (106). Performance of craniotomies for evacuation of focal mass lesions plays a pivotal role in the surgical management of patients with TBI (161–163). Although not a standard of care, surgically placed pressure monitoring devices remain a focal adjuvant in management of patients with moderate-to-severe TBI.

Intracranial Pressure Monitoring

Ventriculostomy was the original form of ICP monitoring (164) and remains a commonly used method. A ventricular catheter is surgically placed via a burr hole into the lateral ventricle, and the ICP is measured via a transducer. The main advantage of this system is that it allows for both pressure waveform analysis and therapeutic drainage of CSF as needed. One caveat to this method is that air cannot enter the system because it will cause an air lock and may render unreliable measurements. The most commonly used system today is the intraparenchymal microsensor. The microsensor is extremely dependable (165), but its inability to drain CSF is a major shortcoming.

Decompressive Craniectomy

Pediatric patients with severe TBI may be more prone than adults to develop diffuse, severe cerebral edema in the ab-

sence of large mass lesions (20,166), which, in turn, may make their ICP management more difficult. The current guidelines for management of pediatric TBI list decompressive craniectomy as a level III recommendation for patients who are showing signs of neurologic deterioration or herniation or are developing intracranial hypertension refractory to medical management during the early stages of their treatment (60) (Figure 35-3). Decompressive craniectomy has more typically been used after medical management has failed to control ICP and maintain adequate cerebral perfusion pressure, although in some centers there has been a move toward earlier surgical decompression.

Although most of the large studies/series of decompressive craniectomy have been done in adults for either hemispheric stroke or TBI, there are some pediatric studies that support the role of early decompressive craniectomy for severe TBI (105). In a randomized, prospective study of approximately 30 pediatric patients, it was reported that early decompressive craniectomy after severe TBI improved global outcome at 6 months. The median time to surgery was 19 hours, and ICP tended to be lower in the decompressed patients. Although this was a pilot study, nevertheless it is the only randomized, controlled, prospective study done in pediatric population. Most recently, a large randomized multicenter study of decompressive craniectomy in adults (n = 155) concluded that early bilateral decompressive craniectomy significantly decreased elevated ICP and shortened the duration of the ICU stay; however, it did not improve outcome but actually was associated with poorer 6-month scores on the extended GOS (167).

There is no clear guidance on the surgical technique to craniectomies. The bone removals could be small or substantial; the procedure could be unilateral or bilateral; the dura could be left intact or opened (105,106,167,168). The location of the decompression could also be variable, such as subtemporal, bifrontal, and temporoparietal decompressions (105,167,169).

Decompressive craniectomy is a valuable tool in managing increased ICP but is not without risks. Large skull defects may change CSF dynamics (170) and lead to the development of hydrocephalus (167). Decompressive craniectomies often create subdural and/or subgaleal CSF collections on the ipsilateral side of the surgical procedure (167,171), and there are also case reports of external brain tamponade with accumulation of subgaleal fluid collection thought to result from leakage of CSF through the dural repair across a pressure gradient (172). The injured brain herniates externally postprocedure, putting it at risk for direct trauma, interruption of the surface blood vessels, and epidural hematomas (171). As cerebral edema improves and the externally herniated brain recedes back into the calvarium, the brain is again at risk for "paradoxical" herniation. Paradoxical herniation may result from a combination of atmospheric pressure and gravitational forces and is more common in patients with acute CSF drainage, such as a lumbar puncture or ventriculoperitoneal shunt placement. Other possible complications of a decompressive craniectomy include surgical wound infections and poor wound healing, which occur in the setting of a protracted hospital stay, often with imperfect nutrition, exposure to nosocomial bacteria, and the presence of invasive monitoring devices.

Overall, decompressive craniectomy remains part of the arsenal to manage elevated ICP associated with severe diffuse TBI in children, although data remain unclear as to how effective this intervention is at improving long-term outcomes. It is likely that TBI pathology, timing of surgery, and age of subjects are all important considerations in determining the use of surgical decompression.

Role of Hypothermia

Induced hypothermia is a level III recommendation in the "Guidelines for the Acute Medical Management of Severe Traumatic Brain Injury of Infants, Children, and Adolescents" (60). The theories behind hypothermia's benefit are multifactorial, including slowing cerebral metabolic rate, reducing excitotoxicity, diminishing postinjury inflammation, and in general, mitigating secondary injury. Minimization of secondary injury in patients with TBI plays a pivotal role in having a successful final outcome. A complex chain of events unfolds at the cellular level immediately after injury and may continue for several days post initial injury. This sequence of events is what many consider to be the secondary injury (175–177). Some of the described mechanisms of secondary injury after TBI include ischemia and reperfusion (178,179), local or generalized swelling of the brain as a result of cytotoxic edema, disruption of the blood–brain barrier, development of hyperemia and venous congestion, and formation of local hematomas with exposure of neural tissue to toxic blood products (179–181). In clinical and animal studies, hypothermia has been shown to affect multiple secondary injury cascades, exerting beneficial effects by attenuating calpain-mediated proteolysis, decreasing metabolic demands, improving mitochondrial function, lessening post-traumatic epileptic activity, and reducing edema formation by stabilizing the permeability of the blood–brain barrier (175–177,182–184).

There are multiple studies pointing to improved outcomes using induced hypothermia in neonates with mild-to-moderate perinatal asphyxia. With moderate hypothermia (33–35°C), the side effects appear to be modest and global developmental outcomes improved (185–188). The use of hypothermia in pediatric patients with TBI remains a controversial subject. Earlier smaller studies suggested the use of hypothermia was both safe and showed promise of benefit (181,189,190). However, a major randomized, multicenter trial of 225 children with severe TBI showed that 24 hours of moderate hypothermia did not improve neurological outcome and may actually increase mortality (112). This is concordant with the lack of benefit seen in a large, randomized

hypothermia trial for severe adult TBI (191), although some caveats remain (see "Moderate Hypothermia" section discussed previously). Studies of therapeutic hypothermia have uncovered many challenges in these types of investigations, including standardization of TBI management protocols, determination of optimal windows for intervention, appropriate stratification of patients, and reduction of intercenter variability.

Advanced Neuroimaging

Advanced neuroimaging is now being used to expand our ability to better manage and prognosticate TBI in the pediatric population (192). The availability of the current technology also helps with better understanding of nonaccidental head injury in this patient population (193–196). After a central nervous system injury, neuroimaging plays an important role in identifying acute and chronic implications of such trauma and is a critical guide to management (196,197). (Please also refer to Chapter 15 for more discussion on structural neuroimaging.)

Computed Tomography

CT is an ideal method for evaluating an acute TBI. It is readily available, relatively quick, and easy to perform. These characteristics are paramount to its use for guiding emergent medical or surgical interventions. One of the advantages of CT scanning is its ability to evaluate both the skull and the brain. CT has also been used to differentiate nonaccidental head trauma from accidental injury (194). More recently, it has been suggested that a combination of CT and magnetic resonance imaging (MRI) may provide a more comprehensive picture of the complexity of TBI, with each modality providing valuable data for patient care (194,198). Despite the quality images provided by the CT in a speedy fashion, it remains limited in identifying only the most obvious injuries in an acute setting. Axonal and ischemic injuries may not be fully appreciated using CT. Ionized radiation is also a significant concern when multiple CT scans are being conducted, so this modality might not be the best way to conduct longitudinal studies (195). This may also limit the use of CT scanning in low-risk situations, such as mild TBI (199,200).

Magnetic Resonance Imaging

MRI is a much more sensitive modality of investigating TBI than CT because it can identify more intricate findings, such as axonal injuries, microhemorrhages, and ischemia (201). Advanced MRI techniques are particularly valuable in further evaluation and management of TBI, including susceptibility-weighted imaging (SWI), magnetic resonance spectroscopy (MRS), diffusion-weighted imaging (DWI), and diffusion tensor imaging (DTI) (194) (Figure 35-4).

SWI can be performed on conventional MRI scanners as the technology uses paramagnetic properties of blood products such as deoxyhemoglobin and methemoglobin to detect injuries (202,203). Because it uses the paramagnetic properties of blood, SWI is a much more sensitive modality than conventional MRI in detecting small hemorrhagic lesions associated with axonal injuries (193,204). This ability to detect diffuse axonal injury allows for better understand-

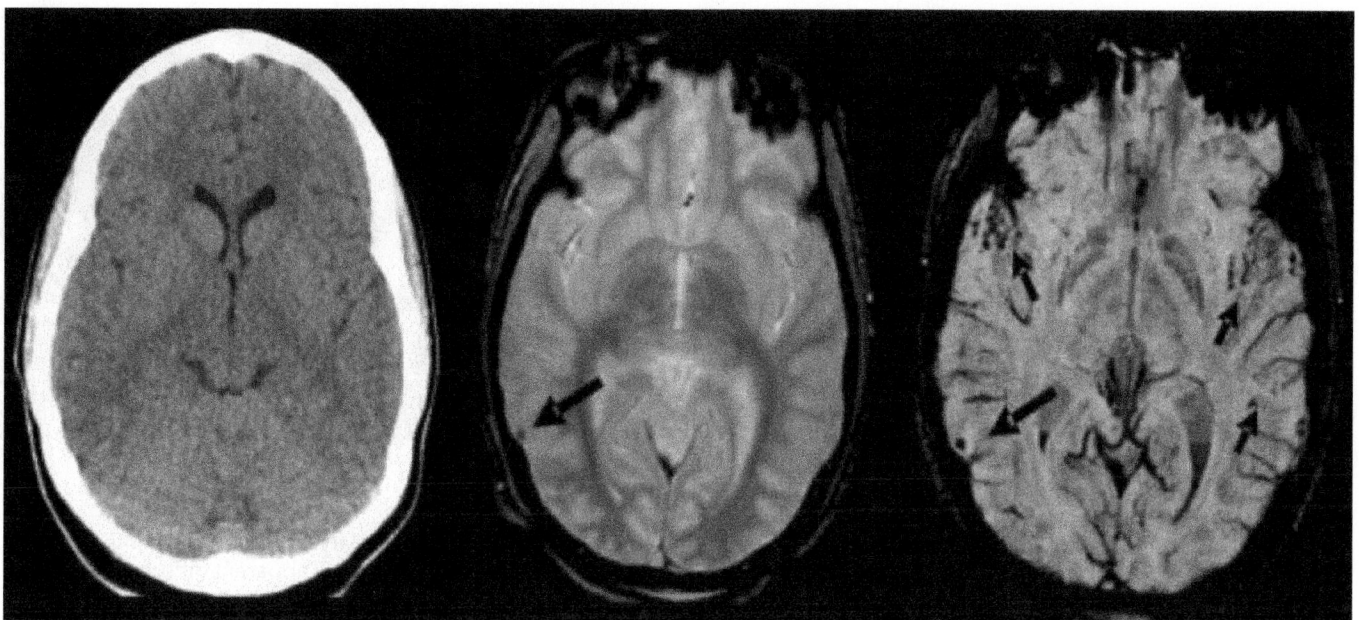

FIGURE 35-4 Comparison of different imaging modalities, demonstrating the increased sensitivity of susceptibility-weighted imaging (*SWI*) to detect microhemorrhages indicative of diffuse axonal injury. *GRE*, gradient echo. Reprinted from Tong (205) with permission.

ing of number, volume, and location of the hemorrhagic lesions, which, in turn can help prognosticate long-term neurologic outcome (205,206).

MRS offers a noninvasive mode of assessing neurochemical changes after brain injury. One of the major neurometabolites measured by MRS is *N*-acetylaspartate (NAA). NAA is a neuronal marker found to be decreased as a result of neuronal loss and dysfunction. Other measures include (*a*) creatinine, a marker of brain energy metabolism; (*b*) choline, which may represent cell turnover; and (*c*) lactate, a marker for anaerobic glycolysis. Disturbances in the balance of these neurochemicals have been shown to be predictive of cognitive and behavioral outcomes after pediatric TBI (192). MRS has also been shown to help in distinguishing global vs focal injuries in nonaccidental trauma (194) and be predictive of long-term prognosis in this population (207).

DWI is a neuroimaging method that uses differences in the rate of water molecule diffusion to distinguish injured vs normal brain tissue. This modality often detects ischemic injury before it is seen on the conventional MRI (208,209) (Figure 35-5). It is known that abusive head trauma is often associated with hypoxic ischemic insults, and therefore, DWI could help understand the extent of injury much earlier (198,210). In this setting, DWI may provide additional information regarding long-term prognosis (210,211).

DTI has similarities with DWI with the added advantage of measuring the directionality of water diffusion, which then serves as a surrogate marker for structural anatomy of white matter fiber tracts in the brain (Figure 35-6). The rate and direction of water molecule diffusion may be categorized as anisotropic (where the diffusion is restricted in its direction, such as parallel to the fiber tracks) (212) or isotropic (where there is no restriction to the direction of water diffusion, such as in CSF) (195). DTI applies a diffusion gradient along multiple anatomical directions: this then allows representation of the amount of anisotropic diffusion through calculation of fractional anisotropy (FA). DTI has been used successfully in the evaluation of developing nervous system, especially maturation of the white matter and has been shown to be a sensitive tool in evaluation of early white matter injury. In the setting of TBI, abnormalities in FA are interpreted as the result of disruption of axonal microstructure (193). DTI has also begun to be used to prognosticate TBI in multiple stages and degree of injury (213,214). Correlations between DTI, MRS, and neurocognitive performance have been proven significant in the recovery from moderate-to-severe pediatric TBI (215).

Neurocritical Care Issues for Mild to Moderate Traumatic Brain Injury

Mild Traumatic Brain Injury

Although many studies and guidelines focus on severe TBI (GCS ≤ 8), many children present for medical attention with mild (GCS of 14–15) or moderate (GCS of 9–13) TBI. Whether or not a GCS of 13 should be classified as a mild or moderate category has recently been debated in both adult and pediatric literature (216,217), but for the purposes of this chapter, we will classify it in the moderate category. One of the challenges of less severe head injury is determining which children are safe to follow in the outpatient setting, and which children require admission to minimize secondary insults and injuries. More than 170,000 children annually visited emergency departments in the United States for sports-related TBIs. Of these, almost 160,000 were treated and released home, presumably with a diagnosis of mild or moderate TBI (218). As discussed earlier, CT has limitations and is not reasonable to perform in all children. Kuppermann et al. (199) validated a prediction rule for determining which

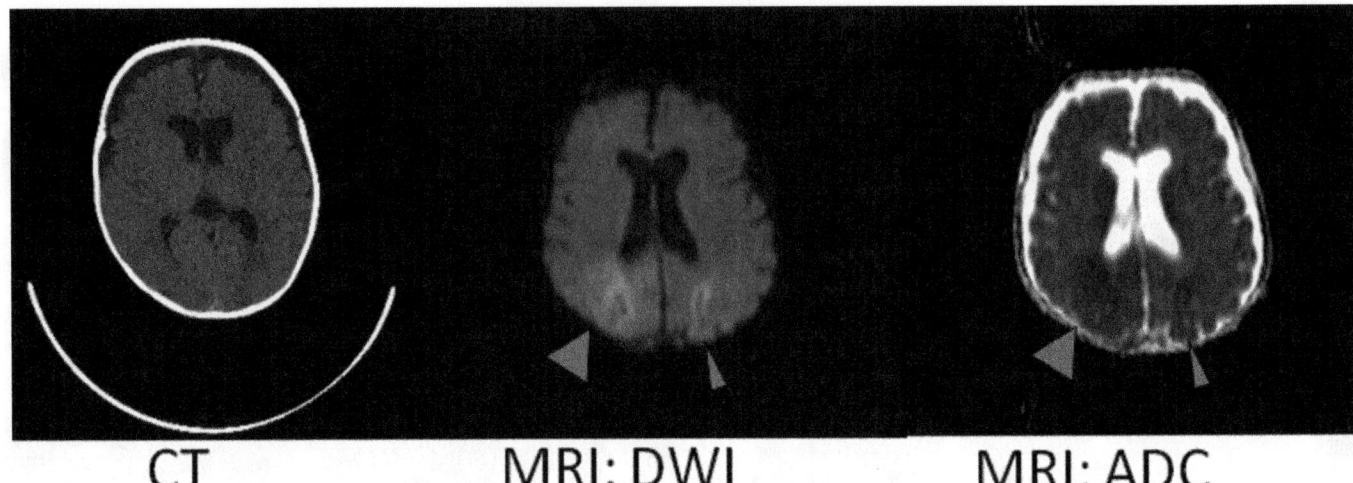

FIGURE 35-5 Comparison of different imaging modalities, demonstrating the increased sensitivity of diffusion-weighted imaging (DWI and ADC) to detect areas of restricted diffusion (*arrowheads*) indicative of ischemic injury. *ADC*, apparent diffusion coefficient.

children presenting with mild TBI ultimately had clinically important TBI (ciTBI), as defined by that which resulted in death from TBI, neurosurgery, intubation >24 hours, or hospital admission for 2 or more nights. If children younger than 2 years old had a normal mental status on exam, no scalp hematoma except frontal, loss of consciousness (LOC) for 0–5 seconds, nonsevere injury mechanism, no palpable skull fracture, and were acting normally according to parents, this had a 100% negative predictive value and sensitivity for a ciTBI. If children aged 2 years or older had a normal mental status, no LOC, no vomiting, nonsevere injury mechanism, no signs of basilar skull fracture, and no severe headache, this had a 99.95% negative predictive value with 96.8% sensitivity. Children who meet all of the aforementioned criteria do not require a CT and may be observed only. Children who fall into an intermediate status, that is, normal mental status and no sign of skull fracture, but are vomiting, with LOC, severe headache, or a severe mechanism of injury may either have a CT or observation alone depending on other factors, such as physician experience, multiple vs isolated findings, worsening symptoms during observation, or parental preference. A follow-up study (219) found that children in the intermediate category who are observed to determine whether or not a CT was necessary had equal incidences of ciTBI (~0.9%) as with children who did not have an observation period but had significantly fewer head CTs performed. Further studies are needed before an appropriate interval of observation can be specifically recommended. Whether the observation occurs in the inpatient hospital setting or the outpatient general pediatrician's or pediatric neurologist's office depends on other factors, such as resource availability and social situations, will vary from patient to patient. It is important for health care providers to help prevent secondary injury specifically by emphasizing avoiding high-risk behaviors during which a second TBI may occur in the days to weeks immediately after a mild TBI. The Center for Disease Control and Prevention has published several resources for patients and health care provid-

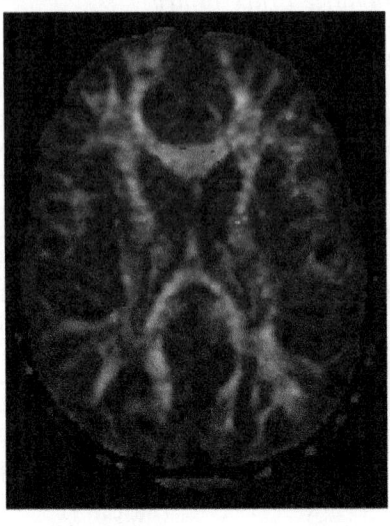
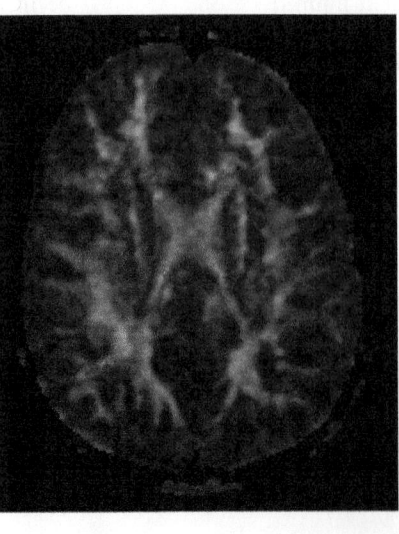

FIGURE 35-6 *See color insert.* Colored image of diffusion tensor map of adolescent after mild traumatic brain injury (TBI). *Red* indicates fibers crossing left–right, *green fibers* are front–back, and *blue fibers* are up–down (into the plane of the image slice).

ers on mild TBI (http://www.cdc.gov/concussion/index.html). (Please also refer to Chapters 29 and 31 for a more detailed discussion of mild TBI and sports-related concussions, respectively.)

Moderate Traumatic Brain Injury

Moderate TBI is a gray zone because it is sometimes cohorted with mild TBI (223) or, more frequently, with severe TBI (27,30,136) when included in study populations. Although there are no published consensus guidelines on the management of moderate pediatric TBI, the same principles of severe TBI management apply. It is the authors' experience that most patients with moderate TBIs are admitted to the ICU for close neurological monitoring and to have rapid intervention available if secondary neurological deterioration (SND) is detected. There is not currently a model to predict which patients will experience SND, although some researchers are investigating the use of TCD in adults to help predict SND (221,222). Patients should have urgent imaging, either CT or MRI, to look for lesions requiring neurosurgical intervention and to better characterize the extent of the injury. Principles of acute management of moderate TBI are similar to those discussed earlier for severe TBI, and both groups benefit from early resuscitative efforts (223). Although the studies have focused on the severe TBI population, patients with moderate TBI should also maintain adequate CPP, avoid hypotension and hypoxia, provide adequate pain control, maintain normothermia, and control seizures. Close monitoring is central to ICU management of patients with moderate TBI, so that clinical deterioration or signs of increased ICP can be detected early and timely escalation of therapy may be implemented.

It is important to note that many children with mild or moderate TBI may be victims of abusive head trauma (AHT), particularly children younger than 2 years old. It is important that the evaluation for TBI in this young population also includes a fundoscopic exam to look for retinal hemorrhages and a thorough skin exam to look for subtle bruising, swelling, or burn marks. It is reasonable to obtain a skeletal survey to look for other occult fractures or signs of injury. Children who are suspected to be victims of AHT may be admitted for a multidisciplinary team investigation regardless of the stability of the patient (224).

BRIDGING THE GAP FROM ACUTE CARE TO RECOVERY

Effects of Sedation and Anticonvulsants

When considering long-term outcomes, there is increasing concern about the chronic effects of acutely administered sedative and anticonvulsant agents in the immature brain. Although it is recognized that the use of these medications is often essential to the proper management of the critically ill patient, there is substantial and growing evidence that the use of these agents may have significant developmental consequences. Preclinical data in immature rodent models indicates that even brief or single dose administration of many types of sedation or anticonvulsants results in substantial apoptotic cell death (225,226) and later cognitive/learning impairments (227). These effects may represent underlying vulnerabilities of the developing brain. For example, the young brain naturally undergoes discrete periods of increased apoptosis as well as higher baseline levels of apoptosis than are seen in the mature brain (228,229). Developing neurons require physiological activation to promote neurite outgrowth, synaptic strengthening, and expression of neurotrophic factors. Both sedatives and anticonvulsants interfere with normal neurotransmission, and thus reduce neural activation, potentially interfering with ongoing developmental processes. Interestingly, in one comparative preclinical study, the newer anticonvulsants topiramate and levetiracetam did not show dose-dependent increases in apoptosis (Table 35-2) (225).

From a clinical perspective, it has long been known that anticonvulsants and sedatives can interfere in cognitive processes, particularly in children. Often, it is difficult to isolate the cause of cognitive impairment in children with acute neurological injury exposed to these pharmacological agents because the underlying cerebral insult may also interfere with learning and development. However, there are some clinical studies that support the animal data. In a study of phenobarbital prophylaxis for febrile seizures, after 2 years of treatment the phenobarbital group scored 8.4 IQ points lower than the placebo group. Six months after discontinuation of phenobarbital, the treated group's mean IQ remained 5.2 points lower than the controls. This study is important because children with febrile seizures do not typically have higher rates of cognitive impairment than normal children. The authors conclude that phenobarbital depressed cognition and this side effect outweighed any benefit of febrile seizure prevention (230).

More recently a population-based retrospective birth cohort study was conducted looking at the risk of developing a learning disability as related to anesthetic exposure early in life (231). Of 5,357 children, 593 received general anesthesia at less than 4 years of age. There was a dose-dependent increased risk for subsequent development of learning disability based on either the number of anesthetic exposures or a longer cumulative duration of anesthesia. A single anesthetic exposure resulted in no increased risk of learning disability; however, children exposed to anesthetics 2, 3, or more times show increased risk of learning disability (hazard ratio 1.59 and 2.60 respectively). The authors did attempt to control for comorbidities and found no major differences between the anesthesia and no anesthesia groups regarding Apgar scores or peripartum complications with the exception that mothers of children exposed to anesthesia had a slightly higher rate of peripartum hemorrhage and prolonged labor. When stratified by the American Society of Anesthesiologists physical status (ASA PS) classification and excluding those with the most severe comorbidities (ASA PS class III or greater), the findings were similar. This study concluded that early exposure to anesthesia was a significant risk for development of learning disability in children; however, it was not possible from these data to ascertain whether a learning disability was related directly to the anesthesia, or anesthesia was simply a marker for some other as yet unidentified risk factor. A follow-up study showed multiple anesthetic exposure was associated with a higher risk of learning disability, use of an individualized education plan for speech and language, and lower cognitive testing scores, even when controlling for burden of illness (232).

TABLE 35-2 Effects of Drugs on the Developing Rodent Brain

DRUG AND DOSING	CELL DEATH	BEHAVIORAL CHANGE	REFERENCE
Ethanol	+ + +		Ikonomidou, 2000
Levetiracetam	0		Kaindl, 2006
N₂0, midazolam, isoflurane	+ + +	↓ Memory ↓ LTP	Jetorovic-Todorovic, 2003
Phenytoin	+ + +		Bittigau, 2002; Kaindl, 2006
Phenobarbital	+ + +		Bittigau, 2002; Kaindl, 2006
Sulthiame	+ + + +		Kaindl, 2006
Topiramate	+/−		Kaindl, 2006
Valproate	+ + + +		Bittigau, 2002; Kaindl, 2006

Abbreviations: LTP, long term potentiation, an electrophysiological correlate of learning; N₂O, nitrous oxide.

Although these preclinical and clinical studies should not preclude the appropriate use of sedation or anticonvulsants in the pediatric critical care setting, they do caution against indiscriminate use of these agents in situations where their administration may not be essential. There may be benefit from minimizing exposure by using the lowest effective dose and/or the shortest duration for these pharmacologic agents. For example, continuous cerebral monitoring such as EEG may allow more judicious use of these drugs, and thus limit exposure to those individuals who require anticonvulsants.

Timing and Type of Rehabilitative Therapy in the Intensive Care Unit

The primary goal of critical care is not simply to ensure survival of a patient with significant brain injury but specifically to support the individual through severe acute illness and ultimately to return them to optimal function and quality of life. The challenge is perhaps even greater in children and adolescents, who must not only recover to their premorbid baseline but also reassume their normal developmental trajectory (50). Thus, the parameters with which rehabilitative therapies are introduced to the child recovering from a significant brain injury are extremely relevant, even in the ICU.

In the setting of acute neural injury, it is known that additional excitatory stimulation may exacerbate the initial damage and potentially worsen outcome. An example of this would be acute prolonged post-traumatic seizures; in adults, prolonged subclinical seizures have been associated with later hippocampal atrophy and worse global cognitive function (233). Following TBI, superimposed excitotoxic injury such as that caused by hypotension or hypoxia is the strongest treatable factor in determining TBI outcome (234).

Preclinical data provides further background to our understanding of these complex timing issues. Following an acute sensorimotor cortex lesion, forced overuse of the paretic limb (i.e., the limb controlled by the damaged cortex) can result in a larger histological lesion. If, however, the forced overuse is delayed for 1 week after the injury, there is no worsening of the lesion size, and functional recovery is improved (235,236). It is well known that voluntary wheel running or rearing in enriched environment (EE) can result in enhanced cognition and up regulation of proplasticity molecular pathways. After lateral fluid percussion injury in adult rats, immediate exposure to voluntary exercise (in the form of access to a running wheel) fails to increase neuro-

trophic factors such as brain-derived neurotrophic factor (BDNF) and actually results in greater cognitive impairment. If running wheel access is delayed for 1 week or longer after injury, the beneficial effects of exercise on plasticity markers and cognition are reinstated (237,238). Furthermore, the duration of the post-TBI period of vulnerability appears to be proportional to the severity of the initial injury (239).

Uninjured rats typically show both morphological (increased cortical thickness, increased dendritic arborization, etc.) and behavioral (improved spatial memory, enhanced rate of learning) benefits from EE rearing (240). In a paradigm of EE rearing following experimental developmental TBI, injured rat pups did not show overt cognitive impairment when reared in a normal environment. However, they failed to respond to EE rearing, showing no increase in cortical thickness, no expanded dendritic arbors, and no cognitive superiority in young adulthood (57,41,242). This period of unresponsiveness to experience-dependent plasticity coincided with a window of impaired glutamatergic neurotransmission (46).

These clinical and preclinical data would suggest that overstimulation of the injured brain in the hyperacute or acute phase may be deleterious. Thus, rehabilitation protocols that include very aggressive stimulation should be monitored carefully for both beneficial and detrimental effects. The challenge regarding initiation of rehabilitation lies in determining when any individual patient may be physiologically ready for therapies designed to promote neural activation without the potential risk of overstimulation.

Another practical consideration is that once a patient is recovering in the acute care setting, there is often a delay or lack of continuity in the transition to rehabilitation. These challenges are generally occurring in the subacute state, theoretically beyond the window of vulnerability discussed earlier. In this stage of injury recovery there appears to be clinical benefit from a rapid and smooth transition from the ICU to rehabilitation. In adults with stroke or severe TBI, observational studies of relatively early intervention showed improved functional outcomes; however, these studies often were retrospective in nature or lacked a prospective control group (243,244). This made it difficult to ascertain what time window was actually optimal for the best functional outcome. Interestingly, a retrospective pediatric TBI registry study showed a negative relationship between delay in transition from ICU to rehabilitation and the degree of functional recovery, with longer delays associated with smaller functional benefits and a lower "efficiency" of rehabilitation (245) and other studies in pediatric TBI support this (246).

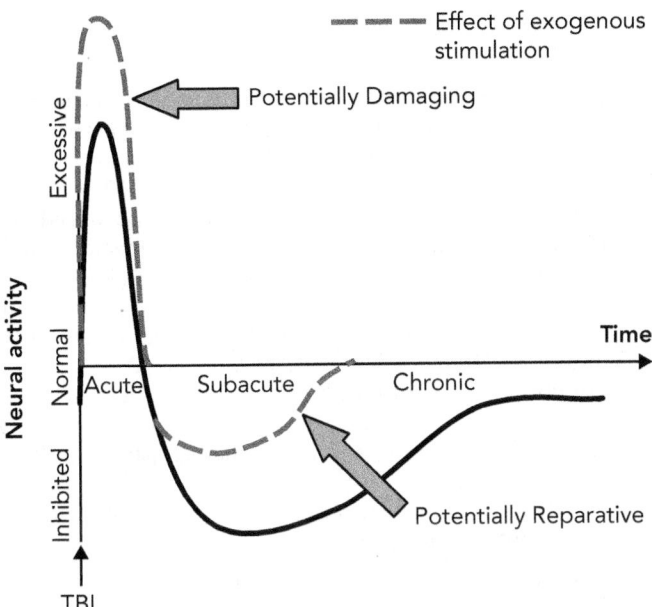

FIGURE 35-7 Model for excitatory neural activity after traumatic brain injury (TBI). Exogenous stimulation in the acute phase may result in excessive and potentially injurious activity. Exogenous stimulation at the right time may facilitate more rapid recovery. Late stimulation may or may not be as effective.

These seemingly conflicting results can actually fit into a unified model that relates to timing of rehabilitation (Figure 35-7). Very early stimulation of the acutely injured brain is subject to a physiological risk of overactivating metabolically vulnerable cells and potentially worsening injury. This biological response need to be kept in mind, although in most cases, acutely injured patients are not subjected to vigorous active therapy. There may next be a period of relative quiescence during which vulnerability is uncertain but when neurons may be incapable of normal activation—this time period represents a window of time where external therapy is less effective but also may be a period for potential therapeutic trials. Once the patient has stabilized medically and neurologically, and certainly when the intensity of the patient's acute care is being drawn down, prompt and seamless transition from ICU care to rehabilitative therapy is preferable to delaying these interventions.

Connecting Acute Data to Long-term Outcomes

One of the greatest challenges in pediatric neurocritical care is determining the long-term effects of specific characteristics of the initial traumatic injury, as well as the consequences of the many therapeutic interventions conducted in the acute phase. Very elegant, longitudinal studies of chronic neurocognitive outcomes have been conducted, but the relevant acute variables may be limited to injury severity (as determined by the Glasgow Coma Score), mechanism of injury, and/or gross neuroimaging abnormalities (54,247,248). These studies often originate in the fields of neurorehabilitation or neuropsychology. Conversely, studies looking at very particular management issues in the critical care phase may

include detailed physiological variables such as hourly measures of CPP or ICP, serum biomarkers, or invasive cerebral monitoring (PbtO$_2$), with relatively blunt long-term outcomes, such as global scales or even dichotomized good–bad outcomes (68,143,160). This perspective generally comes from those in critical care or neurosurgery.

Clearly, there is a severity-dependent effect on many global and more detailed cognitive and behavioral outcomes. In addition, some treatable parameters of the acute injury are highly relevant, such as the prevention of secondary hypoxic or hypotensive injury (234); in fact, more detailed acute studies have begun to delineate age-specific measures that take into consideration both absolute values and temporal duration of physiological abnormalities (72,249, 250). One goal of these approaches is to ultimately have prognostic use at the level of the individual patient.

Other acute parameters that may reflect on long-term functional outcomes include accurate diagnosis of early post-traumatic seizures; concomitant use of anesthetics, anticonvulsants, and other medications; and specific clinicopathological characterization of the initial TBI. For example, a Glasgow Coma Score of 5 may be caused by diffuse cerebral edema, epidural hematoma, cerebral contusion with subarachnoid hemorrhage, or diffuse axonal injury, each having a different prognosis and potentially leading to distinct long-term outcomes.

Linking acute measures of cerebral physiology and critical care management with chronic developmental outcomes remains a worthy goal and is particularly difficult and yet also particularly relevant in the pediatric population, where recovery is superimposed on normal developmental trajectories. The concept of measuring longitudinal outcome from pediatric TBI arises from the nature of impairments seen after these injuries (50,251). Often, it is not possible to detect subtle deficits after TBI in infants and young children, and these impairments may only become overt as maturational milestones are achieved (or missed). There is still some controversy as to whether the trajectory of recovery is fundamentally altered by pediatric TBI, with some studies showing stabilization and then age-appropriate advances in development (54), whereas other analyses indicate that slopes of development and recovery rates are different based on injury severity, with divergence over time after severe pediatric TBI (251).

Combining data from different centers/studies is often yet another challenge. Even when the data point in question is theoretically the same (i.e. initial Glasgow Coma Score), differences in how this is recorded may preclude easy compilation of data from different research groups (GCS in the field, postresuscitation GCS, highest GCS in the first 6 hours or 24 hours, etc.). A major effort in adult TBI was faced with these challenges (252,253). In an effort to promote consistent and accurate data collection for TBI (and other neurological diagnoses), the National Institute of Neurological Diseases and Stroke (NINDS) has embarked on a Common Data Elements (CDEs) initiative with the goal of achieving some uniformity in data collection for a given diagnosis (254). In this effort, data is classified as "core," "supplemental," and "emerging," with specific recommendations as to how the data should be collected and recorded (255,256). As part of this effort, several pediatric working groups have developed amendments to the originally published CDEs to incorporate data elements that have specific relevance for those working in children and adolescents. These CDEs and their associated tools are available at http://www.commondataelements.ninds.nih.gov. Pediatric amendments have been published for demographics and acute clinical assessment (257), neuroimaging (258), and outcomes (259).

CONCLUSION

TBI is a major public health problem, particularly in the pediatric population. Advances in neurocritical care are leading to lower mortality rates, and it is important that with increased survival come improved functional outcomes. Acute management of severe pediatric TBI has various levels of recommendations as outlined in evidence-based guidelines published in 2003 and updated in 2012. Since the initial publication of these guidelines, advances in neuro-ICU monitoring and neuroimaging have moved clinical practice forward in our ability to delineate the underlying characteristics of individual brain injuries and to monitor and treat the pathophysiology as it evolves over time.

Furthermore, the realm of neurocritical care for pediatric TBI is no longer limited to the ICU. Better understanding the long-term effects of powerful neuroactive drugs administered in the ICU will help to target these double-edge therapies to individuals most likely to benefit. Careful consideration of the timing and intensity of rehabilitative efforts, and smooth transition from the ICU to the neurorehab unit, promise to improve recovery after these often devastating injuries. Most importantly, the comprehensive linkage of acute care physiological variables and treatment with long-term neurocognitive and developmental outcomes is essential to move the area of severe pediatric TBI care to the next level. Prevention campaigns aim at reducing the incidence of TBI, striking at the root of the problem. Through establishment of multidisciplinary neurocritical care teams, with close follow-up between acute care and rehabilitation, the possibilities are great for developing and successfully implementing novel therapies and management strategies.

KEY CLINICAL POINTS

1. Biomechanical properties of the infant (i.e., less calcified skull, large head/body ratio) and common mechanisms of injury (i.e., forceful shaking and direct head impact of nonaccidental trauma) render the young brain vulnerable to injury.
2. Neurometabolism and CBF vary by age; injury and intervention at different time points along the developmental spectrum may have different consequences.
3. Careful attention to bedside management of blood pressure, ICP, and $PbtO_2$ can prevent secondary injury and improve long-term outcomes.
4. Advanced neuroimaging can provide detailed information about the extent of the injury and may help prognosticate recovery.
5. One of the greatest challenges in predicting and following outcome in pediatric TBI is superposing recovery on normally expected developmental trajectory.

KEY REFERENCES

1. Adelson PD, Pineda J, Bell MJ, et al. Common data elements for pediatric traumatic brain injury: recommendations from the working group on demographics and clinical assessment. *J Neurotrauma.* 2012;29(4):639–653.
2. Ashwal S, Holshouser BA, Tong KA. Use of advanced neuroimaging techniques in the evaluation of pediatric traumatic brain injury. *Dev Neurosci.* 2006;28(4–5):309–326.
3. Babikian T, Asarnow R. Neurocognitive outcomes and recovery after pediatric TBI: meta-analytic review of the literature. *Neuropsychology.* 2009;23(3):283–296.
4. Duhaime AC, Gennarelli TA, Thibault LE, Bruce DA, Margulies SS, Wiser R. The shaken baby syndrome. A clinical, pathological, and biomechanical study. *J Neurosurg.* 1987;66(3):409–415.
5. Giza CC, Kolb B, Harris NG, Asarnow RF, Prins ML. Hitting a moving target: basic mechanisms of recovery from acquired developmental brain injury. *Dev Neurorehabil.* 2009;12(5):255–268.

Reference

1. Kraus JF, Rock A, Hemyari P. Brain injuries among infants, children, adolescents, and young adults. *Am J Dis Child.* 1990;144(6):684–691.
2. Coats B, Margulies SS. Potential for head injuries in infants from low-height falls. *J Neurosurg Pediatr.* 2008;2(5):321–330.
3. Duhaime AC, Gennarelli TA, Thibault LE, Bruce DA, Margulies SS, Wiser R. The shaken baby syndrome. A clinical, pathological, and biomechanical study. *J Neurosurg.* 1987;66(3):409–415.
4. Shannon P, Becker L. Mechanisms of brain injury in infantile child abuse. *Lancet.* 2001;358(9283):686–687.
5. Brennan LK, Rubin D, Christian CW, Duhaime AC, Mirchandani HG, Rorke-Adams LB. Neck injuries in young pediatric homicide victims. *J Neurosurg Pediatr.* 2009;3(3):232–239.
6. Matshes EW, Evans RM, Pinckard JK, Joseph JT, Lew EO. Shaken infants die of neck trauma, not of brain trauma. *Acad For Path.* 2011;1(1):82–91.
7. Gennarelli TA, Thibault LE, Adams JH, Graham DI, Thompson CJ, Marcincin RP. Diffuse axonal injury and traumatic coma in the primate. *Ann Neurol.* 1982;12(6):564–574.
8. Margulies SS, Thibault KL. Infant skull and suture properties: measurements and implications for mechanisms of pediatric brain injury. *J Biomech Eng.* 2000;122(4):364–371.
9. Gennarelli TA, Thibault LE. Biomechanics of acute subdural hematoma. *J Trauma.* 1982;22(8):680–686.
10. Duhaime AC, Durham S. Traumatic brain injury in infants: the phenomenon of subdural hemorrhage with hemispheric hypodensity ("Big Black Brain"). *Prog Brain Res.* 2007;161:293–302.
11. Kennedy C, Sokoloff L. An adaptation of the nitrous oxide method to the study of the cerebral circulation in children; normal values for cerebral blood flow and cerebral metabolic rate in childhood. *J Clin Invest.* 1957;36(7):1130–1137.
12. Zwienenberg M, Muizelaar JP. Severe pediatric head injury: the role of hyperemia revisited. *J Neurotrauma.* 1999;16(10):937–943.
13. Kehrer M, Schoning M. A longitudinal study of cerebral blood flow over the first 30 months. *Pediatr Res.* 2009;66(5):560–564.
14. Takahashi T, Shirane R, Sato S, Yoshimoto T. Developmental changes of cerebral blood flow and oxygen metabolism in children. *AJNR Am J Neuroradiol.* 1999;20(5):917–922.
15. Wintermark M, Lepori D, Cotting J, et al. Brain perfusion in children: evolution with age assessed by quantitative perfusion computed tomography. *Pediatrics.* 2004;113(6):1642–1652.
16. Udomphorn Y, Armstead WM, Vavilala MS. Cerebral blood flow and autoregulation after pediatric traumatic brain injury. *Pediatr Neurol.* 2008;38(4):225–234.

17. Tontisirin N, Muangman SL, Suz P, et al. Early childhood gender differences in anterior and posterior cerebral blood flow velocity and autoregulation. *Pediatrics*. 2007;119(3):e610–e615.

18. Vavilala MS, Kincaid MS, Muangman SL, Suz P, Rozet I, Lam AM. Gender differences in cerebral blood flow velocity and autoregulation between the anterior and posterior circulations in healthy children. *Pediatr Res*. 2005;58(3):574–578.

19. Bruce DA, Alavi A, Bilaniuk L, Dolinskas C, Obrist W, Uzzell B. Diffuse cerebral swelling following head injuries in children: the syndrome of "malignant brain edema." *J Neurosurg*. 1981;54(2):170–178.

20. Aldrich EF, Eisenberg HM, Saydjari C, et al. Diffuse brain swelling in severely head-injured children. A report from the NIH Traumatic Coma Data Bank. *J Neurosurg*. 1992;76(3):450–454.

21. Suzuki K. The changes of regional cerebral blood flow with advancing age in normal children. *Nagoya Med J*. 1990;34:159–170.

22. Chugani HT, Phelps ME, Mazziotta JC. Positron emission tomography study of human brain functional development. *Ann Neurol*. 1987;22(4):487–497.

23. Chugani HT, Phelps ME. Maturational changes in cerebral function in infants determined by 18FDG positron emission tomography. *Science*. 1986;231(4740):840–843.

24. White JR, Farukhi Z, Bull C, et al. Predictors of outcome in severely head-injured children. *Crit Care Med*. 2001;29(3):534–540.

25. Kelly DF, Martin NA, Kordestani R, et al. Cerebral blood flow as a predictor of outcome following traumatic brain injury. *J Neurosurg*. 1997;86(4):633–641.

26. Adelson PD, Clyde B, Kochanek PM, Wisniewski SR, Marion DW, Yonas H. Cerebrovascular response in infants and young children following severe traumatic brain injury: a preliminary report. *Pediatr Neurosurg*. 1997;26(4):200–207.

27. Freeman SS, Udomphorn Y, Armstead WM, Fisk DM, Vavilala MS. Young age as a risk factor for impaired cerebral autoregulation after moderate-to-severe pediatric traumatic brain injury. *Anesthesiology*. 2008;108(4):588–595.

28. Bouma GJ, Muizelaar JP, Bandoh K, Marmarou A. Blood pressure and intracranial pressure-volume dynamics in severe head injury: relationship with cerebral blood flow. *J Neurosurg*. 1992;77(1):15–19.

29. Figaji AA. Practical aspects of bedside cerebral hemodynamics monitoring in pediatric TBI. *Childs Nerv Syst*. 2010;26(4):431–439.

30. Vavilala MS, Tontisirin N, Udomphorn Y, et al. Hemispheric differences in cerebral autoregulation in children with moderate and severe traumatic brain injury. *Neurocrit Care*. 2008;9(1):45–54.

31. Karsli C, Luginbuehl I, Farrar M, Bissonnette B. Cerebrovascular carbon dioxide reactivity in children anaesthetized with propofol. *Paediatr Anaesth*. 2003;13(1):26–31.

32. Vavilala MS, Muangman S, Tontisirin N, et al. Impaired cerebral autoregulation and 6-month outcome in children with severe traumatic brain injury: preliminary findings. *Dev Neurosci*. 2006;28(4–5):348–353.

33. Muizelaar JP, Marmarou A, Ward JD, et al. Adverse effects of prolonged hyperventilation in patients with severe head injury: a randomized clinical trial. *J Neurosurg*. 1991;75(5):731–739.

34. Stringer WA, Hasso AN, Thompson JR, Hinshaw DB, Jordan KG. Hyperventilation-induced cerebral ischemia in patients with acute brain lesions: demonstration by xenon-enhanced CT. *AJNR Am J Neuroradiol*. 1993;14(2):475–484.

35. Babikian T, Prins ML, Cai Y, et al. Molecular and physiological responses to juvenile traumatic brain injury: focus on growth and metabolism. *Dev Neurosci*. 2010;32(5–6):431–441.

36. Thomas S, Prins ML, Samii M, Hovda DA: Cerebral metabolic response to traumatic brain injury sustained early in development: a 2-deoxy-D-glucose autoradiographic study. *J Neurotrauma*. 2000; 17(8):649–665.

37. Saudubray JM, Marsac C, Limal JM, et al. Variation in plasma ketone bodies during a 24-hour fast in normal and in hypoglycemic children: relationship to age. *J Pediatr*. 1981;98(6):904–908.

38. Prins ML, Fujima LS, Hovda DA. Age-dependent reduction of cortical contusion volume by ketones after traumatic brain injury. *J Neurosci Res*. 2005;82(3):413–420.

39. Prins ML. Cerebral metabolic adaptation and ketone metabolism after brain injury. *J Cereb Blood Flow Metab*. 2008;28(1):1–16.

40. Appelberg KS, Hovda DA, Prins ML. The effects of a ketogenic diet on behavioral outcome after controlled cortical impact injury in the juvenile and adult rat. *J Neurotrauma*. 2009;26(4):497–506.

41. Prins ML, Giza CC. Induction of monocarboxylate transporter 2 expression and ketone transport following traumatic brain injury in juvenile and adult rats. *Dev Neurosci*. 2006;28(4–5):447–456.

42. Katayama Y, Becker DP, Tamura T, Hovda DA. Massive increases in extracellular potassium and the indiscriminate release of glutamate following concussive brain injury. *J Neurosurg*. 1990;73(6):889–900.

43. Choi DW. Excitotoxic cell death. *J Neurobiol*. 1992;23(9):1261–1276.

44. Giza CC, Prins ML. Is being plastic fantastic? Mechanisms of altered plasticity after developmental traumatic brain injury. *Dev Neurosci*. 2006;28(4–5):364–379.

45. Kumar A, Zou L, Yuan X, Long Y, Yang K. N-methyl-D-aspartate receptors: transient loss of NR1/NR2A/NR2B subunits after traumatic brain injury in a rodent model. *J Neurosci Res*. 2002;67(6):781–786.

46. Giza CC, Maria NS, Hovda DA. N-methyl-D-aspartate receptor subunit changes after traumatic injury to the developing brain. *J Neurotrauma*. 2006;23(6):950–961.

47. D'Ambrosio R, Maris DO, Grady MS, Winn HR, Janigro D. Selective loss of hippocampal long-term potentiation, but not depression, following fluid percussion injury. *Brain Res*. 1998;786(1–2):64–79.

48. Pohl D, Bittigau P, Ishimaru MJ, et al. N-methyl-D-aspartate antagonists and apoptotic cell death triggered by head trauma in developing rat brain. *Proc Natl Acad Sci U S A*. 1999;96(5):2508–2513.

49. Robertson CL, Bell MJ, Kochanek PM, et al. Increased adenosine in cerebrospinal fluid after severe traumatic brain injury in infants and children: association with severity of injury and excitotoxicity. *Crit Care Med*. 2001;29(12):2287–2293.

50. Giza CC, Kolb B, Harris NG, Asarnow RF, Prins ML. Hitting a moving target: basic mechanisms of recovery from acquired developmental brain injury. *Dev Neurorehabil*. 2009;12(5):255–268.

51. Ben-Ari Y. Excitatory actions of gaba during development: the nature of the nurture. *Nat Rev Neurosci*. 2002;3(9):728–739.

52. Hensch TK, Fagiolini M, Mataga N, Stryker MP, Baekkeskov S, Kash SF. Local GABA circuit control of experience-dependent plasticity in developing visual cortex. *Science*. 1998;282(5393):1504–1508.

53. Berlucchi G, Buchtel HA. Neuronal plasticity: historical roots and evolution of meaning. *Exp Brain Res*. 2009;192(3):307–319.

54. Anderson V, Spencer-Smith M, Leventer R, et al. Childhood brain insult: can age at insult help us predict outcome? *Brain*. 2009;132(pt 1):45–56.

55. Anderson V, Catroppa C, Morse S, Haritou F, Rosenfeld J. Functional plasticity or vulnerability after early brain injury? *Pediatrics*. 2005;116(6):1374–1382.

56. Felt BT, Schallert T, Shao J, Liu Y, Li X, Barks JD. Early appearance of functional deficits after neonatal excitotoxic and hypoxic-ischemic injury: fragile recovery after development and role of the NMDA receptor. *Dev Neurosci*. 2002;24(5):418–425.

57. Fineman I, Giza CC, Nahed BV, Lee SM, Hovda DA. Inhibition of neocortical plasticity during development by a moderate concussive brain injury. *J Neurotrauma*. 2000;17(9):739–749.

58. The Brain Trauma Foundation, The American Association of Neurological Surgeons, The Joint Section on Neurotrauma and Critical Care. Use of mannitol. *J Neurotrauma*. 2000;17(6–7):521–525.

59. Adelson PD, Bratton SL, Carney NA, et al. Guidelines for the acute medical management of severe traumatic brain injury in infants, children, and adolescents. Chapter 1: introduction. *Pediatr Crit Care Med*. 2003;4(3)(suppl):S2–S4.

60. Kochanek PM, Carney N, Adelson PD, et al. Guidelines for the acute medical management of severe traumatic brain injury in infants, children, and adolescents—second edition. *Pediatr Crit Care Med*. 2012;13(suppl 1):S1–S82.

61. Adelson PD, Bratton SL, Carney NA, et al. Guidelines for the acute medical management of severe traumatic brain injury in infants, children, and adolescents. Chapter 4. Resuscitation of blood pressure and oxygenation and prehospital brain-specific therapies for

the severe pediatric traumatic brain injury patient. *Pediatr Crit Care Med.* 2003;4(3)(suppl):S12–S18.

62. Vavilala MS, Bowen A, Lam AM, et al. Blood pressure and outcome after severe pediatric traumatic brain injury. *J Trauma.* 2003;55(6): 1039–1044.

63. Pigula FA, Wald SL, Shackford SR, Vane DW. The effect of hypotension and hypoxia on children with severe head injuries. *J Pediatr Surg.* 1993;28(3):310–314; discussion 315–316.

64. Kokoska ER, Smith GS, Pittman T, Weber TR. Early hypotension worsens neurological outcome in pediatric patients with moderately severe head trauma. *J Pediatr Surg.* 1998;33(2):333–338.

65. Luerssen TG, Klauber MR, Marshall LF. Outcome from head injury related to patient's age. A longitudinal prospective study of adult and pediatric head injury. *J Neurosurg.* 1988;68(3):409–416.

66. Downard C, Hulka F, Mullins RJ, et al. Relationship of cerebral perfusion pressure and survival in pediatric brain-injured patients. *J Trauma.* 2000;49(4):654–658; discussion 658–659.

67. Michaud LJ, Rivara FP, Grady MS, Reay DT. Predictors of survival and severity of disability after severe brain injury in children. *Neurosurgery.* 1992;31(2):254–264.

68. Mehta A, Kochanek PM, Tyler-Kabara E, et al. Relationship of intracranial pressure and cerebral perfusion pressure with outcome in young children after severe traumatic brain injury. *Dev Neurosci.* 2010;32(5–6):413–419.

69. Pfenninger J, Kaiser G, Lutschg J, Sutter M. Treatment and outcome of the severely head injured child. *Intensive Care Med.* 1983;9(1): 13–16.

70. Esparza J, M-Portillo J, Sarabia M, Yuste JA, Roger R, Lamas E. Outcome in children with severe head injuries. *Childs Nerv Syst.* 1985;1(2):109–114.

71. Adelson PD, Bratton SL, Carney NA, et al. Guidelines for the acute medical management of severe traumatic brain injury in infants, children, and adolescents. Chapter 7. Intracranial pressure monitoring technology. *Pediatr Crit Care Med.* 2003;4(3)(suppl):S28–S30.

72. Chambers IR, Stobbart L, Jones PA, et al. Age-related differences in intracranial pressure and cerebral perfusion pressure in the first 6 hours of monitoring after children's head injury: association with outcome. *Childs Nerv Syst.* 2005;21(3):195–199.

73. Elias-Jones AC, Punt JA, Turnbull AE, Jaspan T. Management and outcome of severe head injuries in the Trent region 1985–1990. *Arch Dis Child.* 1992;67(12):1430–1435.

74. Chambers IR, Kirkham FJ. What is the optimal cerebral perfusion pressure in children suffering from traumatic coma? *Neurosurg Focus.* 2003;15(6):E3.

75. Kerr ME, Weber BB, Sereika SM, Darby J, Marion DW, Orndoff PA. Effect of endotracheal suctioning on cerebral oxygenation in traumatic brain-injured patients. *Crit Care Med.* 1999.27(12): 2776–2781.

76. Wahlstrom MR, Olivecrona M, Koskinen LO, Rydenhag B, Naredi S. Severe traumatic brain injury in pediatric patients: treatment and outcome using an intracranial pressure targeted therapy—the Lund concept. *Intensive Care Med.* 2005–31(6):832–839.

77. Stiefel MF, Udoetuk JD, Storm PB, et al. Brain tissue oxygen monitoring in pediatric patients with severe traumatic brain injury. *J Neurosurg.* 2006;105(4)(suppl):281–286.

78. Papazian L, Albanese J, Thirion X, Perrin G, Durbec O, Martin C. Effect of bolus doses of midazolam on intracranial pressure and cerebral perfusion pressure in patients with severe head injury. *Br J Anaesth.* 1993;71(2):267–271.

79. Tobias JD. Increased intracranial pressure after fentanyl administration in a child with closed head trauma. *Pediatr Emerg Care.* 1994; 10(2):89–90.

80. Cotev S, Shalit MN. Effects on diazepam on cerebral blood flow and oxygen uptake after head injury. *Anesthesiology.* 1975;43(1): 117–122.

81. Ben Yehuda Y, Watemberg N. Ketamine increases opening cerebrospinal pressure in children undergoing lumbar puncture. *J Child Neurol.* 2006;21(6):441–443.

82. Sari A, Okuda Y, Takeshita H. The effect of ketamine on cerebrospinal fluid pressure. *Anesth Analg.* 1972;51(4):560–565.

83. Gardner AE, Dannemiller FJ, Dean D. Intracranial cerebrospinal fluid pressure in man during ketamine anesthesia. *Anesth Analg.* 1972;51(5):741–745.

84. Mayberg TS, Lam AM, Matta BF, Domino KB, Winn HR. Ketamine does not increase cerebral blood flow velocity or intracranial pressure during isoflurane/nitrous oxide anesthesia in patients undergoing craniotomy. *Anesth Analg.* 1995;81(1):84–89.

85. Albanese J, Arnaud S, Rey M, Thomachot L, Alliez B, Martin C. Ketamine decreases intracranial pressure and electroencephalographic activity in traumatic brain injury patients during propofol sedation. *Anesthesiology.* 1997;87(6):1328–1334.

86. Bourgoin A, Albanese J, Wereszczynski N, Charbit M, Vialet R, Martin C. Safety of sedation with ketamine in severe head injury patients: comparison with sufentanil. *Crit Care Med.* 2003;31(3): 711–717.

87. Kolenda H, Gremmelt A, Rading S, Braun U, Markakis E. Ketamine for analgosedative therapy in intensive care treatment of head-injured patients. *Acta Neurochir (Wien).* 1996;138(10):1193–1199.

88. Spitzfaden AC, Jimenez DF, Tobias JD. Propofol for sedation and control of intracranial pressure in children. *Pediatr Neurosurg.* 1999; 31(4):194–200.

89. Adelson PD, Bratton SL, Carney NA, et al. Guidelines for the acute medical management of severe traumatic brain injury in infants, children, and adolescents. Chapter 9. Use of sedation and neuromuscular blockade in the treatment of severe pediatric traumatic brain injury. *Pediatr Crit Care Med.* 2003;4(3)(suppl):S34–S37.

90. Vernon DD, Witte MK. Effect of neuromuscular blockade on oxygen consumption and energy expenditure in sedated, mechanically ventilated children. *Crit Care Med.* 2000;28(5):1569–1571.

91. Hsiang JK, Chesnut RM, Crisp CB, Klauber MR, Blunt BA, Marshall LF. Early, routine paralysis for intracranial pressure control in severe head injury: is it necessary? *Crit Care Med.* 1994;22(9): 1471–1476.

92. Bouma GJ, Muizelaar JP. Cerebral blood flow, cerebral blood volume, and cerebrovascular reactivity after severe head injury. *J Neurotrauma.* 1992;9(suppl 1):S333–S348.

93. Muizelaar JP, Lutz HA III, Becker DP. Effect of mannitol on ICP and CBF and correlation with pressure autoregulation in severely head-injured patients. *J Neurosurg.* 1984;61(4):700–706.

94. Muizelaar JP, Wei EP, Kontos HA, Becker DP. Cerebral blood flow is regulated by changes in blood pressure and in blood viscosity alike. *Stroke.* 1986;17(1):44–48.

95. Tsai SF, Shu KH. Mannitol-induced acute renal failure. *Clin Nephrol.* 2010;74(1):70–73.

96. Diringer MN, Zazulia AR. Osmotic therapy: fact and fiction. *Neurocrit Care.* 2004.1(2):219–233.

97. Paredes-Andrade E, Solid CA, Rockswold SB, Odland RM, Rockswold GL. Hypertonic saline reduces intracranial hypertension in the presence of high serum and cerebrospinal fluid osmolalities [published online ahead of print July 2, 2011]. *Neurocrit Care.*

98. Khanna S, Davis D, Peterson B, et al. Use of hypertonic saline in the treatment of severe refractory posttraumatic intracranial hypertension in pediatric traumatic brain injury. *Crit Care Med.* 2000; 28(4):1144–1151.

99. Peterson B, Khanna S, Fisher B, Marshall L. Prolonged hypernatremia controls elevated intracranial pressure in head-injured pediatric patients. *Crit Care Med.* 2000;28(4):1136–1143.

100. Fisher B, Thomas D, Peterson B Hypertonic saline lowers raised intracranial pressure in children after head trauma. *J Neurosurg Anesthesiol.* 1992;4(1):4–10.

101. Kamel H, Navi BB, Nakagawa K, Hemphill JC III, Ko NU. Hypertonic saline versus mannitol for the treatment of elevated intracranial pressure: a meta-analysis of randomized clinical trials. *Crit Care Med.* 2011;39(3):554–559.

102. Adelson PD, Bratton SL, Carney NA, et al. Guidelines for the acute medical management of severe traumatic brain injury in infants, children, and adolescents. Chapter 12. Use of hyperventilation in the acute management of severe pediatric traumatic brain injury. *Pediatr Crit Care Med.* 2003;4(3)(suppl):S45–S48.

103. Skippen P, Seear M, Poskitt K, et al. Effect of hyperventilation on regional cerebral blood flow in head-injured children. *Crit Care Med.* 1997;25(8):1402–1409.

104. Curry R, Hollingworth W, Ellenbogen RG, Vavilala MS. Incidence of hypo- and hypercarbia in severe traumatic brain injury before and after 2003 pediatric guidelines. *Pediatr Crit Care Med*. 2008;9(2): 141–146.

105. Taylor A, Butt W, Rosenfeld J, et al. A randomized trial of very early decompressive craniectomy in children with traumatic brain injury and sustained intracranial hypertension. *Childs Nerv Syst*. 2001;17(3):154–162.

106. Sahuquillo J, Arikan F. Decompressive craniectomy for the treatment of refractory high intracranial pressure in traumatic brain injury. *Cochrane Database Syst Rev*. 2006;(1):CD003983.

107. Piatt JH Jr, Schiff SJ. High dose barbiturate therapy in neurosurgery and intensive care. *Neurosurgery*. 1984;15(3):427–444.

108. Kasoff SS, Lansen TA, Holder D, Filippo JS. Aggressive physiologic monitoring of pediatric head trauma patients with elevated intracranial pressure. *Pediatr Neurosci*. 1988;14(5):241–249.

109. Adelson PD, Bratton SL, Carney NA, et al. Guidelines for the acute medical management of severe traumatic brain injury in infants, children, and adolescents. Chapter 14. The role of temperature control following severe pediatric traumatic brain injury. *Pediatr Crit Care Med*. 2003;4(3)(suppl):S53–S55.

110. Greer DM, Funk SE, Reaven NL, Ouzounelli M, Uman GC. Impact of fever on outcome in patients with stroke and neurologic injury: a comprehensive meta-analysis. *Stroke*. 2008;39(11):3029–3035.

111. Natale JE, Joseph JG, Helfaer MA, Shaffner DH. Early hyperthermia after traumatic brain injury in children: risk factors, influence on length of stay, and effect on short-term neurologic status. *Crit Care Med*. 2000;28(7):2608–2615.

112. Hutchison JS, Ward RE, Lacroix J, et al. Hypothermia therapy after traumatic brain injury in children. *N Engl J Med*. 2008;358(23): 2447–2456.

113. Adelson PD, Ragheb J, Kanev P, et al. Phase II clinical trial of moderate hypothermia after severe traumatic brain injury in children. *Neurosurgery*. 2005;56(4):740–754; discussion 740–754.

114. Briassoulis G, Filippou O, Kanariou M, Papassotiriou I, Hatzis T. Temporal nutritional and inflammatory changes in children with severe head injury fed a regular or an immune-enhancing diet: a randomized, controlled trial. *Pediatr Crit Care Med*. 2006;7(1):56–62.

115. Cochran A, Scaife ER, Hansen KW, Downey EC. Hyperglycemia and outcomes from pediatric traumatic brain injury. *J Trauma*. 2003; 55(6):1035–1038.

116. De Salles AA, Muizelaar JP, Young HF. Hyperglycemia, cerebrospinal fluid lactic acidosis, and cerebral blood flow in severely head-injured patients. *Neurosurgery*. 1987;21(1):45–50.

117. Li PA, Shuaib A, Miyashita H, He QP, Siesjo BK, Warner DS. Hyperglycemia enhances extracellular glutamate accumulation in rats subjected to forebrain ischemia. *Stroke*. 2000;31(1):183–192.

118. Bergsneider M, Hovda DA, Shalmon E, et al. Cerebral hyperglycolysis following severe traumatic brain injury in humans: a positron emission tomography study. *J Neurosurg*. 1997;86(2):241–251.

119. Oddo M, Schmidt JM, Carrera E, et al. Impact of tight glycemic control on cerebral glucose metabolism after severe brain injury: a microdialysis study. *Crit Care Med*. 2008;36(12):3233–3238.

120. Vespa P, Boonyaputthikul R, McArthur DL, et al. Intensive insulin therapy reduces microdialysis glucose values without altering glucose utilization or improving the lactate/pyruvate ratio after traumatic brain injury. *Crit Care Med*. 2006;34(3):850–856.

121. Meier R, Bechir M, Ludwig S, et al. Differential temporal profile of lowered blood glucose levels (3.5 to 6.5 mmol/l versus 5 to 8 mmol/l) in patients with severe traumatic brain injury. *Crit Care*. 2008;12(4):R98.

122. Bennett MH, Trytko B, Jonker B. Hyperbaric oxygen therapy for the adjunctive treatment of traumatic brain injury. *Cochrane Database Syst Rev*. 2004;(4):CD004609.

123. Rockswold SB, Rockswold GL, Zaun DA, et al. A prospective, randomized clinical trial to compare the effect of hyperbaric to normobaric hyperoxia on cerebral metabolism, intracranial pressure, and oxygen toxicity in severe traumatic brain injury. *J Neurosurg*. 2010; 112(5):1080–1094.

124. Golden Z, Golden CJ, Neubauer RA. Improving neuropsychological function after chronic brain injury with hyperbaric oxygen. *Disabil Rehabil*. 2006;28(22):1379–1386.

125. Stoller KP. Quantification of neurocognitive changes before, during, and after hyperbaric oxygen therapy in a case of fetal alcohol syndrome. *Pediatrics*. 2005;116(4):e586–e591.

126. McDonagh MS, Morgan D, Carson S, Russman BS. Systematic review of hyperbaric oxygen therapy for cerebral palsy: the state of the evidence. *Dev Med Child Neurol*. 2007;49(12):942–947.

127. Jepson B, Granpeesheh D, Tarbox J, et al. Controlled evaluation of the effects of hyperbaric oxygen therapy on the behavior of 16 children with autism spectrum disorders. *J Autism Dev Disord*. 2011; 41(5):575–588.

128. Collet JP, Vanasse M, Marois P, et al. Hyperbaric oxygen for children with cerebral palsy: a randomised multicentre trial. HBO-CP Research Group. *Lancet*. 2001;357(9256):582–586.

129. Diringer MN, Aiyagari V, Zazulia AR, Videen TO, Powers WJ. Effect of hyperoxia on cerebral metabolic rate for oxygen measured using positron emission tomography in patients with acute severe head injury. *J Neurosurg*. 2007;106(4):526–529.

130. Vereczki V, Martin E, Rosenthal RE, Hof PR, Hoffman GE, Fiskum G. Normoxic resuscitation after cardiac arrest protects against hippocampal oxidative stress, metabolic dysfunction, and neuronal death. *J Cereb Blood Flow Metab*. 2006;26(6):821–835.

131. Sayeed I, Stein DG. Progesterone as a neuroprotective factor in traumatic and ischemic brain injury. *Prog Brain Res*. 2009;175: 219–237.

132. Wright DW, Kellermann AL, Hertzberg VS, et al. ProTECT: a randomized clinical trial of progesterone for acute traumatic brain injury. *Ann Emerg Med*. 2007;49(4):391–402.

133. Hatton J, Rosbolt B, Empey P, Kryscio R, Young B. Dosing and safety of cyclosporine in patients with severe brain injury. *J Neurosurg*. 2008;109(4):699–707.

134. Mammis A, McIntosh TK, Maniker AH. Erythropoietin as a neuroprotective agent in traumatic brain injury Review. *Surg Neurol*. 2009;71(5):527–531; discussion 531.

135. Stein DG. Progesterone in the treatment of acute traumatic brain injury: a clinical perspective and update. *Neuroscience*. 2011;191: 101–106.

136. Liesemer K, Bratton SL, Zebrack CM, Brockmeyer D, Statler KD. Early posttraumatic seizures in moderate-to-severe pediatric traumatic brain injury: rates, risk factors, and clinical features. *J Neurotrauma*. 2011;28(5):755–762.

137. Vespa PM, Miller C, McArthur D, et al. Nonconvulsive electrographic seizures after traumatic brain injury result in a delayed, prolonged increase in intracranial pressure and metabolic crisis. *Crit Care Med*. 2007;35(12):2830–2836.

138. Figaji AA, Fieggen AG, Argent AC, Leroux PD, Peter JC. Does adherence to treatment targets in children with severe traumatic brain injury avoid brain hypoxia? A brain tissue oxygenation study. *Neurosurgery*. 2008;63(1):83–91; discussion 91–82.

139. Bratton SL, Chestnut RM, Ghajar J, et al. Guidelines for the management of severe traumatic brain injury. X. Brain oxygen monitoring and thresholds. *J Neurotrauma*. 2007;24(suppl 1):65S–70S.

140. Stiefel MF, Spiotta A, Gracias VH, et al. Reduced mortality rate in patients with severe traumatic brain injury treated with brain tissue oxygen monitoring. *J Neurosurg*. 2005;103(5):805–811.

141. Narotam PK, Morrison JF, Nathoo N. Brain tissue oxygen monitoring in traumatic brain injury and major trauma: outcome analysis of a brain tissue oxygen-directed therapy. *J Neurosurg*. 2009;111(4): 672–682.

142. Spiotta AM, Stiefel MF, Gracias VH, et al. Brain tissue oxygen-directed management and outcome in patients with severe traumatic brain injury. *J Neurosurg*. 2010;113(3):571–580.

143. Figaji AA, Zwane E, Thompson C, et al. Brain tissue oxygen tension monitoring in pediatric severe traumatic brain injury. Part 1: relationship with outcome. *Childs Nerv Syst*. 2009;25(10):1325–1333.

144. Maloney-Wilensky E, Gracias V, Itkin A, et al. Brain tissue oxygen and outcome after severe traumatic brain injury: a systematic review. *Crit Care Med*. 2009;37(6):2057–2063.

145. Narotam PK, Burjonrappa SC, Raynor SC, Rao M, Taylon C. Cerebral oxygenation in major pediatric trauma: its relevance to trauma severity and outcome. *J Pediatr Surg*. 2006;41(3):505–513.

146. Rohlwink UK, Figaji AA. Methods of monitoring brain oxygenation. *Childs Nerv Syst*. 2010;26(4):453–464.

147. Maloney-Wilensky E, Le Roux P. The physiology behind direct brain oxygen monitors and practical aspects of their use. *Childs Nerv Syst.* 2010;26(4):419–430.

148. Figaji AA, Zwane E, Thompson C, et al. Brain tissue oxygen tension monitoring in pediatric severe traumatic brain injury. Part 2: relationship with clinical, physiological, and treatment factors. *Childs Nerv Syst.* 2009;25(10):1335–1343.

149. Smith MJ, Stiefel MF, Magge S, et al. Packed red blood cell transfusion increases local cerebral oxygenation. *Crit Care Med.* 2005;33(5):1104–1108.

150. Figaji AA, Zwane E, Kogels M, et al. The effect of blood transfusion on brain oxygenation in children with severe traumatic brain injury. *Pediatr Crit Care Med.* 2010;11(3):325–331.

151. Figaji AA, Zwane E, Fieggen AG, et al. Pressure autoregulation, intracranial pressure, and brain tissue oxygenation in children with severe traumatic brain injury. *J Neurosurg Pediatr.* 2009;4(5):420–428.

152. Figaji AA, Zwane E, Graham Fieggen A, Argent AC, Le Roux PD, Peter JC. The effect of increased inspired fraction of oxygen on brain tissue oxygen tension in children with severe traumatic brain injury. *Neurocrit Care.* 2010;12(3):430–437.

153. Muizelaar JP, Marmarou A, DeSalles AA, et al. Cerebral blood flow and metabolism in severely head-injured children. Part 1: relationship with GCS score, outcome, ICP, and PVI. *J Neurosurg.* 1989;71(1):63–71.

154. Jaeger M, Schuhmann MU, Soehle M, Meixensberger J. Continuous assessment of cerebrovascular autoregulation after traumatic brain injury using brain tissue oxygen pressure reactivity. *Crit Care Med.* 2006;34(6):1783–1788.

155. Steiner LA, Coles JP, Johnston AJ, et al. Assessment of cerebrovascular autoregulation in head-injured patients: a validation study. *Stroke.* 2003;34(10):2404–2409.

156. Bellner J, Romner B, Reinstrup P, Kristiansson KA, Ryding E, Brandt L. Transcranial Doppler sonography pulsatility index (PI) reflects intracranial pressure (ICP). *Surg Neurol.* 2004;62(1):45–51; discussion 51.

157. Figaji AA, Zwane E, Fieggen AG, Siesjo P, Peter JC. Transcranial Doppler pulsatility index is not a reliable indicator of intracranial pressure in children with severe traumatic brain injury. *Surg Neurol.* 2009;72(4):389–394.

158. Melo JR, Di Rocco F, Blanot S, et al. Transcranial Doppler can predict intracranial hypertension in children with severe traumatic brain injuries. *Childs Nerv Syst.* 2011;27(6):979–984.

159. Philip S, Chaiwat O, Udomphorn Y, et al. Variation in cerebral blood flow velocity with cerebral perfusion pressure >40 mm Hg in 42 children with severe traumatic brain injury. *Crit Care Med.* 2009;37(11):2973–2978.

160. Chaiwat O, Sharma D, Udomphorn Y, Armstead WM, Vavilala MS. Cerebral hemodynamic predictors of poor 6-month Glasgow Outcome Score in severe pediatric traumatic brain injury. *J Neurotrauma.* 2009;26(5):657–663.

161. Bullock MR, Chesnut R, Ghajar J, et al. Surgical management of traumatic parenchymal lesions. *Neurosurgery.* 2006;58(3)(suppl):S25–46; discussion Si–Siv.

162. Bullock MR, Chesnut R, Ghajar J, et al. Surgical management of acute epidural hematomas. *Neurosurgery.* 2006;58(3)(suppl):S7–S15; discussion Si–Siv.

163. Bullock MR, Chesnut R, Ghajar J, et al. Surgical management of acute subdural hematomas. *Neurosurgery.* 2006;58(3)(suppl):S16–S24; discussion Si–Siv.

164. Wiegand C, Richards P. Measurement of intracranial pressure in children: a critical review of current methods. *Dev Med Child Neurol.* 2007;49(12):935–941.

165. Gelabert-Gonzalez M, Ginesta-Galan V, Sernamito-Garcia R, Allut AG, Bandin-Dieguez J, Rumbo RM. The Camino intracranial pressure device in clinical practice. Assessment in a 1000 cases. *Acta Neurochir (Wien).* 2006;148(4):435–441.

166. Lang DA, Teasdale GM, Macpherson P, Lawrence A. Diffuse brain swelling after head injury: more often malignant in adults than children? *J Neurosurg.* 1994;80(4):675–680.

167. Cooper DJ, Rosenfeld JV, Murray L, et al. Decompressive craniectomy in diffuse traumatic brain injury. *N Engl J Med.* 2011;364(16):1493–1502.

168. Munch E, Horn P, Schurer L, Piepgras A, Paul T, Schmiedek P. Management of severe traumatic brain injury by decompressive craniectomy. *Neurosurgery.* 2000;47(2):315–322; discussion 322–313.

169. Ruf B, Heckmann M, Schroth I, et al. Early decompressive craniectomy and duraplasty for refractory intracranial hypertension in children: results of a pilot study. *Crit Care.* 2003;7(6):R133–R138.

170. Fodstad H, Love JA, Ekstedt J, Friden H, Liliequist B. Effect of cranioplasty on cerebrospinal fluid hydrodynamics in patients with the syndrome of the trephined. *Acta Neurochir (Wien).* 1984;70(1–2):21–30.

171. Aarabi B, Hesdorffer DC, Ahn ES, Aresco C, Scalea TM, Eisenberg HM. Outcome following decompressive craniectomy for malignant swelling due to severe head injury. *J Neurosurg.* 2006;104(4):469–479.

172. Akins PT, Guppy KH. Sinking skin flaps, paradoxical herniation, and external brain tamponade: a review of decompressive craniectomy management. *Neurocrit Care.* 2008;9(2):269–276.

173. Oyelese AA, Steinberg GK, Huhn SL, Wijman CA. Paradoxical cerebral herniation secondary to lumbar puncture after decompressive craniectomy for a large space-occupying hemispheric stroke: case report. *Neurosurgery.* 2005;57(3):E594; discussion E594.

174. Fields JD, Lansberg MG, Skirboll SL, Kurien PA, Wijman CA. "Paradoxical" transtentorial herniation due to CSF drainage in the presence of a hemicraniectomy. *Neurology.* 2006;67(8):1513–1514.

175. Small DL, Morley P, Buchan AM. Biology of ischemic cerebral cell death. *Prog Cardiovasc Dis.* 1999;42(3):185–207.

176. Ghajar J. Traumatic brain injury. *Lancet.* 2000;356(9233):923–929.

177. Oku K, Kuboyama K, Safar P, et al. Cerebral and systemic arteriovenous oxygen monitoring after cardiac arrest. Inadequate cerebral oxygen delivery. *Resuscitation.* 1994;27(2):141–152.

178. Graham DI, Ford I, Adams JH, et al. Fatal head injury in children. *J Clin Pathol.* 1989;42(1):18–22.

179. Adams JH, Graham DI, Murray LS, Scott G. Diffuse axonal injury due to nonmissile head injury in humans: an analysis of 45 cases. *Ann Neurol.* 1982;12(6):557–563.

180. Muizelaar JP, Ward JD, Marmarou A, Newlon PG, Wachi A. Cerebral blood flow and metabolism in severely head-injured children. Part 2: autoregulation. *J Neurosurg.* 1989;71(1):72–76.

181. Polderman KH. Induced hypothermia and fever control for prevention and treatment of neurological injuries. *Lancet.* 2008;371(9628):1955–1969.

182. Auer RN. Nonpharmacologic (physiologic) neuroprotection in the treatment of brain ischemia. *Ann N Y Acad Sci.* 2001;939:271–282.

183. Karkar KM, Garcia PA, Bateman LM, Smyth MD, Barbaro NM, Berger M. Focal cooling suppresses spontaneous epileptiform activity without changing the cortical motor threshold. *Epilepsia.* 2002;43(8):932–935.

184. Maeda T, Hashizume K, Tanaka T. Effect of hypothermia on kainic acid-induced limbic seizures: an electroencephalographic and 14C-deoxyglucose autoradiographic study. *Brain Res.* 1999;818(2):228–235.

185. Eicher DJ, Wagner CL, Katikaneni LP, et al. Moderate hypothermia in neonatal encephalopathy: efficacy outcomes. *Pediatr Neurol.* 2005;32(1):11–17.

186. Eicher DJ, Wagner CL, Katikaneni LP, et al. Moderate hypothermia in neonatal encephalopathy: safety outcomes. *Pediatr Neurol.* 2005;32(1):18–24.

187. Gluckman PD, Wyatt JS, Azzopardi D, et al. Selective head cooling with mild systemic hypothermia after neonatal encephalopathy: multicentre randomised trial. *Lancet.* 2005;365(9460):663–670.

188. Shankaran S, Laptook AR, Ehrenkranz RA, et al. Whole-body hypothermia for neonates with hypoxic-ischemic encephalopathy. *N Engl J Med.* 2005;353(15):1574–1584.

189. Hutchison J, Ward R, Lacroix J, et al. Hypothermia pediatric head injury trial: the value of a pretrial clinical evaluation phase. *Dev Neurosci.* 2006;28(4–5):291–301.

190. Adelson PD. Hypothermia following pediatric traumatic brain injury. *J Neurotrauma.* 2009;26(3):429–436.

191. Clifton GL, Miller ER, Choi SC, et al. Lack of effect of induction of hypothermia after acute brain injury. *N Engl J Med*. 2001;344(8): 556–563.

192. Babikian T, Freier MC, Ashwal S, Riggs ML, Burley T, Holshouser BA. MR spectroscopy: predicting long-term neuropsychological outcome following pediatric TBI. *J Magn Reson Imaging*. 2006;24(4): 801–811.

193. Ashwal S, Holshouser BA, Tong KA. Use of advanced neuroimaging techniques in the evaluation of pediatric traumatic brain injury. *Dev Neurosci*. 2006;28(4–5):309–326.

194. Ashwal S, Wycliffe ND, Holshouser BA. Advanced neuroimaging in children with nonaccidental trauma. *Dev Neurosci*. 2010;32(5–6): 343–360.

195. Suskauer SJ, Huisman TA. Neuroimaging in pediatric traumatic brain injury: current and future predictors of functional outcome. *Dev Disabil Res Rev*. 2009;15(2):117–123.

196. Lee B, Newberg A. Neuroimaging in traumatic brain imaging. *NeuroRx*. 2005;2(2):372–383.

197. Ewing-Cobbs L, Prasad M, Kramer L, et al. Acute neuroradiologic findings in young children with inflicted or noninflicted traumatic brain injury. *Childs Nerv Syst*. 2000;16(1):25–33; discussion 34.

198. Kemp AM, Rajaram S, Mann M, et al. What neuroimaging should be performed in children in whom inflicted brain injury (iBI) is suspected? A systematic review. *Clin Radiol*. 2009;64(5):473–483.

199. Kuppermann N, Holmes JF, Dayan PS, et al. Identification of children at very low risk of clinically-important brain injuries after head trauma: a prospective cohort study. *Lancet*. 2009;374(9696): 1160–1170.

200. Hall EJ, Brenner DJ. Cancer risks from diagnostic radiology. *Br J Radiol*. 2008;81(965):362–378.

201. Gentry LR, Godersky JC, Thompson B, Dunn VD. Prospective comparative study of intermediate-field MR and CT in the evaluation of closed head trauma. *AJR Am J Roentgenol*. 1988;150(3):673–682.

202. Reichenbach JR, Venkatesan R, Schillinger DJ, Kido DK, Haacke EM. Small vessels in the human brain: MR venography with deoxyhemoglobin as an intrinsic contrast agent. *Radiology*. 1997;204(1): 272–277.

203. Sehgal V, Delproposto Z, Haacke EM, et al. Clinical applications of neuroimaging with susceptibility-weighted imaging. *J Magn Reson Imaging*. 2005;22(4):439–450.

204. Ashwal S, Babikian T, Gardner-Nichols J, Freier MC, Tong KA, Holshouser BA. Susceptibility-weighted imaging and proton magnetic resonance spectroscopy in assessment of outcome after pediatric traumatic brain injury. *Arch Phys Med Rehabil*. 2006;87(12)(suppl 2): S50–S58.

205. Tong KA, Ashwal S, Holshouser BA, et al. Diffuse axonal injury in children: clinical correlation with hemorrhagic lesions. *Ann Neurol*. 2004;56(1):36–50.

206. Tong KA, Ashwal S, Holshouser BA, et al. Hemorrhagic shearing lesions in children and adolescents with posttraumatic diffuse axonal injury: improved detection and initial results. *Radiology*. 2003; 227(2):332–339.

207. Aaen GS, Holshouser BA, Sheridan C, et al. Magnetic resonance spectroscopy predicts outcomes for children with nonaccidental trauma. *Pediatrics*. 2010;125(2):295–303.

208. Huisman TA, Sorensen AG, Hergan K, Gonzalez RG, Schaefer PW. Diffusion-weighted imaging for the evaluation of diffuse axonal injury in closed head injury. *J Comput Assist Tomogr*. 2003;27(1): 5–11.

209. Suh DY, Davis PC, Hopkins KL, Fajman NN, Mapstone TB. Nonaccidental pediatric head injury: diffusion-weighted imaging findings. *Neurosurgery*. 2001;49(2):309–318; discussion 318–320.

210. Zimmerman RA, Bilaniuk LT, Farina L. Nonaccidental brain trauma in infants: diffusion imaging, contributions to understanding the injury process. *J Neuroradiol*. 2007;34(2):109–114.

211. Ichord RN, Naim M, Pollock AN, Nance ML, Margulies SS, Christian CW. Hypoxic-ischemic injury complicates inflicted and accidental traumatic brain injury in young children: the role of diffusion-weighted imaging. *J Neurotrauma*. 2007;24(1):106–118.

212. Klingberg T, Vaidya CJ, Gabrieli JD, Moseley ME, Hedehus M. Myelination and organization of the frontal white matter in children: a diffusion tensor MRI study. *Neuroreport*. 1999;10(13): 2817–2821.

213. Lipton ML, Gulko E, Zimmerman ME, et al. Diffusion-tensor imaging implicates prefrontal axonal injury in executive function impairment following very mild traumatic brain injury. *Radiology*. 2009;252(3):816–824.

214. Lo C, Shifteh K, Gold T, Bello JA, Lipton ML. Diffusion tensor imaging abnormalities in patients with mild traumatic brain injury and neurocognitive impairment. *J Comput Assist Tomogr*. 2009; 33(2):293–297.

215. Babikian T, Marion SD, Copeland S, et al. Metabolic levels in the corpus callosum and their structural and behavioral correlates after moderate to severe pediatric TBI. *J Neurotrauma*. 2010;27(3): 473–481.

216. Mena JH, Sanchez AI, Rubiano AM, et al. Effect of the modified Glasgow Coma Scale score criteria for mild traumatic brain injury on mortality prediction: comparing classic and modified Glasgow Coma Scale score model scores of 13. *J Trauma*. 2011;71(5): 1185–1192; discussion 1193.

217. Melo JR, Lemos-Junior LP, Reis RC, et al. Do children with Glasgow 13/14 could be identified as mild traumatic brain injury? *Arq Neuropsiquiatr*. 2010;68(3):381–384.

218. Centers for Disease Control and Prevention. Nonfatal traumatic brain injuries related to sports and recreation activities among persons aged ≤19 years—United States, 2001–2009. *MMWR Morb Mortal Wkly Rep*. 2011;60(39):1337–1342.

219. Nigrovic LE, Lee LK, Hoyle J, et al. Prevalence of clinically important traumatic brain injuries in children with minor blunt head trauma and isolated severe injury mechanisms. *Arch Pediatr Adolesc Med*. 2012;66(4):356–361.

220. Schiehser DM, Delis DC, Filoteo JV, et al. Are self-reported symptoms of executive dysfunction associated with objective executive function performance following mild to moderate traumatic brain injury? *J Clin Exp Neuropsychol*. 2011;33(6):704–714.

221. Bouzat P, Francony G, Declety P, et al. Transcranial Doppler to screen on admission patients with mild to moderate traumatic brain injury. *Neurosurgery*. 2011;68(6):1603–1609; discussion 1609–1610.

222. Jaffres P, Brun J, Declety P, et al. Transcranial Doppler to detect on admission patients at risk for neurological deterioration following mild and moderate brain trauma. *Intensive Care Med*. 2005;31(6): 785–790.

223. Zebrack M, Dandoy C, Hansen K, Scaife E, Mann NC, Bratton SL. Early resuscitation of children with moderate-to-severe traumatic brain injury. *Pediatrics*. 2009;124(1):56–64.

224. Herman BE, Makoroff KL, Corneli HM. Abusive head trauma. *Pediatr Emerg Care*. 2011;27(1):65–69.

225. Kaindl AM, Asimiadou S, Manthey D, Hagen MV, Turski L, Ikonomidou C. Antiepileptic drugs and the developing brain. *Cellr Mol Life Sci*. 2006;63(4):399–413.

226. Olney JW, Young C, Wozniak DF, Jevtovic-Todorovic V, Ikonomidou C. Do pediatric drugs cause developing neurons to commit suicide? *Trends Pharmacol Sci*. 2004;25(3):135–139.

227. Jevtovic-Todorovic V, Hartman RE, Izumi Y, et al. Early exposure to common anesthetic agents causes widespread neurodegeneration in the developing rat brain and persistent learning deficits. *J Neurosci*. 2003;23(3):876–882.

228. Buss RR, Sun W, Oppenheim RW. Adaptive roles of programmed cell death during nervous system development. *Annu Rev Neurosci*. 2006;29:1–35.

229. Kim WR, Sun W. Programmed cell death during postnatal development of the rodent nervous system. *Dev Growth Differ*. 2011;53(2): 225–235.

230. Farwell JR, Lee YJ, Hirtz DG, Sulzbacher SI, Ellenberg JH, Nelson KB. Phenobarbital for febrile seizures—effects on intelligence and on seizure recurrence. *N Engl J Med*. 1990;322(6):364–369.

231. Wilder RT, Flick RP, Sprung J, et al. Early exposure to anesthesia and learning disabilities in a population-based birth cohort. *Anesthesiology*. 2009;110(4):796–804.

232. Flick RP, Katusic SK, Colligan RC, et al. Cognitive and behavioral outcomes after early exposure to anesthesia and surgery. *Pediatrics*. 2011;128(5):e1053–e1061.

233. Vespa PM, McArthur DL, Xu Y, et al. Nonconvulsive seizures after traumatic brain injury are associated with hippocampal atrophy. *Neurology*. 2010;75(9):792–798.

234. Chesnut RM, Marshall LF, Klauber MR, et al. The role of secondary brain injury in determining outcome from severe head injury. *J Trauma*. 1993;34(2):216–222.

235. Humm JL, Kozlowski DA, James DC, Gotts JE, Schallert T. Use-dependent exacerbation of brain damage occurs during an early post-lesion vulnerable period. *Brain Res*. 1998;783(2):286–292.

236. Kozlowski DA, James DC, Schallert T. Use-dependent exaggeration of neuronal injury after unilateral sensorimotor cortex lesions. *J Neurosci*. 1996;16(15):4776–4786.

237. Griesbach GS, Gomez-Pinilla F, Hovda DA. The upregulation of plasticity-related proteins following TBI is disrupted with acute voluntary exercise. *Brain Res*. 2004;1016(2):154–162.

238. Griesbach GS, Hovda DA, Molteni R, Wu A, Gomez-Pinilla F. Voluntary exercise following traumatic brain injury: brain-derived neurotrophic factor upregulation and recovery of function. *Neuroscience*. 2004;125(1):129–139.

239. Griesbach GS, Gomez-Pinilla F, Hovda DA. Time window for voluntary exercise-induced increases in hippocampal neuroplasticity molecules after traumatic brain injury is severity dependent. *J Neurotrauma*. 2007;24(7):1161–1171.

240. Rosenzweig MR, Bennett EL. Psychobiology of plasticity: effects of training and experience on brain and behavior. *Behav Brain Res*. 1996;78(1):57–65.

241. Giza CC, Griesbach GS, Hovda DA. Experience-dependent behavioral plasticity is disturbed following traumatic injury to the immature brain. *Behav Brain Res*. 2005;157(1):11–22.

242. Ip EY, Giza CC, Griesbach GS, Hovda DA. Effects of enriched environment and fluid percussion injury on dendritic arborization within the cerebral cortex of the developing rat. *J Neurotrauma*. 2002;19(5):573–585.

243. Choi JH, Jakob M, Stapf C, Marshall RS, Hartmann A, Mast H. Multimodal early rehabilitation and predictors of outcome in survivors of severe traumatic brain injury. *J Trauma*. 2008;65(5):1028–1035.

244. Hu MH, Hsu SS, Yip PK, Jeng JS, Wang YH. Early and intensive rehabilitation predicts good functional outcomes in patients admitted to the stroke intensive care unit. *Disabil Rehabil*. 2010;32(15):1251–1259.

245. Tepas JJ III, Leaphart CL, Pieper P, et al. The effect of delay in rehabilitation on outcome of severe traumatic brain injury. *J Pediatr Surg*. 2009;44(2):368–372.

246. Melchers P, Maluck A, Suhr L, Scholten S, Lehmkuhl G. An early onset rehabilitation program for children and adolescents after traumatic brain injury (TBI): methods and first results. *Restor Neurol Neurosci*. 1999;14(2–3):153–160.

247. Taylor HG, Yeates KO, Wade SL, Drotar D, Stancin T, Minich N. A prospective study of short- and long-term outcomes after traumatic brain injury in children: behavior and achievement. *Neuropsychology*. 2002;16(1):15–27.

248. Levin HS, Hanten G, Chang CC, et al. Working memory after traumatic brain injury in children. *Ann Neurol*. 2002;52(1):82–88.

249. Chambers IR, Jones PA, Lo TY, et al. Critical thresholds of intracranial pressure and cerebral perfusion pressure related to age in paediatric head injury. *J Neurol Neurosurg Psychiatry*. 2006;77(2):234–240.

250. Brady KM, Shaffner DH, Lee JK, et al. Continuous monitoring of cerebrovascular pressure reactivity after traumatic brain injury in children. *Pediatrics*. 2009;124(6):e1205–e1212.

251. Babikian T, Asarnow R. Neurocognitive outcomes and recovery after pediatric TBI: meta-analytic review of the literature. *Neuropsychology*. 2009;23(3):283–296.

252. Maas AI, Marmarou A, Murray GD, Teasdale SG, Steyerberg EW. Prognosis and clinical trial design in traumatic brain injury: the IMPACT study. *J Neurotrauma*. 2007;24(2):232–238.

253. Maas AI: Standardisation of data collection in traumatic brain injury: key to the future? *Crit Care*. 2009;13(6):1016.

254. Thurmond VA, Hicks R, Gleason T, et al. Advancing integrated research in psychological health and traumatic brain injury: common data elements. *Arch Phys Med Rehabil*. 2010;91(11):1633–1636.

255. Maas AI, Harrison-Felix CL, Menon D, et al. Common data elements for traumatic brain injury: recommendations from the interagency working group on demographics and clinical assessment. *Arch Phys Med Rehabil*. 2010;91(11):1641–1649.

256. Miller G. Neuroscience. New guidelines aim to improve studies of traumatic brain injury. *Science*. 2010;328(5976):297.

258. Duhaime AC, Holshouser B, Hunter JV, Tong K. Common data elements for neuroimaging of traumatic brain injury: pediatric considerations. *J Neurotrauma*. 2012;29(4):629–633.

259. McCauley SR, Wilde EA, Anderson VA, et al. Recommendations for the use of common outcome measures in pediatric traumatic brain injury research. *J Neurotrauma*. 2012;29(4):678–705.

Pediatric Neuropsychological Issues and Cognitive Rehabilitation

Bradford Ross and Peter Patrick

INTRODUCTION

Although pediatric brain injury presents some commonalities with brain injury in general, the nature of the developing child introduces unique challenges to pediatric neuropsychologists. In this chapter on pediatric neuropsychological issues, the importance of understanding the developing brain and its impact on assessment and treatment will be explored. This chapter will describe common sequelae after brain injury, as well as review neuropsychological assessment and treatment approaches to acquired neurocognitive and psychosocial deficits.

Pediatric Neuropsychology

Pediatric clinical neuropsychology is the branch of clinical psychology that attempts to describe, explain, and predict behavior based on knowledge and application of neurobiological models of brain functioning and brain-behavior relationships. Pediatric neuropsychology is the subspecialty that dedicates its research and clinical application to neurodevelopmental models that apply to the growing brain of children and adolescents. Pediatric neuropsychologists assess the neurocognitive, neurobehavioral, psychosocial, and adaptive behavioral functioning of the children and adolescents through formal assessment, behavioral observations, and family and school reports. A neuropsychological profile is obtained that identify relative strengths and weaknesses that are used to assess ongoing development and develop interventions and recommendations to address areas of weakness in the home, community, and academic settings.

The pediatric neuropsychologist knows that brain changes do not occur in isolation. Bernstein (1) provides a very useful heuristic model for the neuropsychologist to understand and study the interface between brain development and environmental/cultural influences. The author begins with the premise, "Brain is the necessary—albeit not sufficient—substrate for behavior." That even within an injured brain, the behaviors we see are not just only the expression of the limits of the injury but also the product of the complementary contribution of preserved intact systems as they struggle without the holistic contribution of a complete working brain. Our understanding of brain performance is always the result of the brain attempting to do the best it can. The resulting behavior is always an interaction between those systems preserved and those diminished or absent.

Bernstein turns her attention next to context. The author notes that "neither the structure nor the development of the brain is independent of the context in which it operates." Neuroscience and developmental biology have supported the complementary relationship between brain structural development, organization, and the shaping influences of the surrounding context. Bernstein encourages us to appreciate that the phrase "contextual variables" be broadly appreciated and explored when attempting to describe, explain, and predict behaviors. She continues by encouraging that assessment of brain-behavior relationships should explore the influence of context, including the observing evaluator and clinician. Her second guiding principle states, "Brain does not operate in isolation."

Finally, Bernstein offers that development cannot be separated from the context in which the brain operates. Guiding principle 3 states, "The child is a developing organism." The author encourages us to realize that the parent discipline to neuropsychology "is not adult neuropsychology" but that of developmental neuroscience, developmental psychology, and the like. Development is the collective history of the child's evolving brain and environment including the child's "elaboration" of behaviors over time. It is the "systemic circle" of interactions between brain, context, and development that clarifies the risks and benefits to the child, which may lead to recommendations for change or continuation of the present behavior repertoire needed to prosper and foster further growth. It is this "child-world system" that is the object of observation, evaluation, description, and explanation.

NEUROPSYCHOLOGICAL SEQUELAE OF PEDIATRIC BRAIN INJURY

Although each brain injury is unique, there are conditions that frequently occur. These neuropsychological sequelae are in the areas of cognitive and psychosocial issues. The changes summarized subsequently are outlined in more detail by Harris, Mishkin, and Ross (2).

Cognitive changes are common in students after brain injury; can affect school and social functioning; and include reduced attention and concentration, communication skills, rate of processing information, mental organization, memory, and executive functioning. Visuoperceptual and visuomotor impairments can occur that can affect visual recognition, visual scanning, visual construction and handwriting, and visual analysis and problem solving. Executive impairments can affect self-regulation and self-monitoring of behavior, initiation, inhibition, planning and organization, task completion, working memory, and higher order problem solving. As indicated in the section on brain development, because of the late development of frontal lobe connections, executive functioning skills are one of the last areas to mature in neuropsychological development. Refer to Chapter 59 for further discussion of cognitive impairments after brain injury.

Behavior and personality changes after brain injury can be newly acquired or an exacerbation of previous behavior and personality traits. These changes can occur across all severity levels. These changes not only can be a direct result of brain damage, such as in frontal lobe and temporal damage but also the result of adjustment difficulties to newly acquired areas of weakness as described earlier and how these changes in functioning impact peer, family, and community relationships. Peers often do not know how to react to changes in behavior, cognitive, and possible physical changes. Cognitive and perceptual changes impact social learning as much if not more than the impact on more traditional academic learning. Slowness in processing can lead to difficulty in following social conversation, which can affect relationships. The inability to pick up on social cues can occur after frontal and parietal damage. A child who cannot read nonverbal cues, such as facial expressions or tone of voice, is at risk for causing strained social interactions. Adolescents can have a particularly hard time adjusting to a change in self and learning because their self-identification is so important at that stage. Adolescents can end up feeling isolated because family and peers do not understand the difficulties in adjusting to the acquired areas of weakness. Refer to Chapter 62 for further discussion of emotional and behavioral sequelae of brain injury.

A child's job is learning, and the work setting is at school. The previously described cognitive and psychosocial changes can directly impact academic functioning. Although children with learning disabilities can also experience difficulty in school, not only there are similarities in the brain injury population but also differences when compared with other learning disabilities. Both groups of children can have reduced attention, concentration and memory, difficulties in problem solving, slowed processing, weak organizational skills, low frustration tolerance, and poor social judgment. Differences in the students with brain injury are greater variability in performance, wider gaps in abilities, more pronounced memory deficits, more difficulty in new learning with intact old learning, adjusting to changes in cognition and self, altered psychosocial relationships, reduced self-control, and lack of insight (2). Refer to Chapter 37 for discussion of educational issues and school reentry.

The limitations described previously can be seen immediately or can be expressed over time because of the process of "growing into an injury," where development "unmasks" an injury that may be asymptomatic earlier in life. For example, a child at age 2 is not expected to have executive skills such as regulation of behavior, but a child in elementary school would be expected to have behavior control. Therefore, frontal lobe damage resulting in executive skills limitations may not be as readily apparent until the child is older.

NEUROPSYCHOLOGICAL ASSESSMENT IN PEDIATRIC BRAIN INJURY

Neuropsychological assessment is used to understand the brain-behavior relationship of the child. A neuropsychological evaluation assists in a better understanding of pediatric functioning in areas such as attention, concentration, memory, intellectual functioning, academic functioning, verbal abilities and language, visuoperceptual abilities, executive functioning, fine motor skills, and social-emotional status. The initial evaluation after brain injury can serve as a baseline in which to measure progress during the recovery process and the efficacy of treatment. The goal is to ascertain a neuropsychological profile of relative strength and weaknesses that can be used to develop a plan for appropriate interventions.

A pediatric neuropsychological assessment differs from an adult assessment not only in the selection of instruments but also in the fact that the pediatric brain is undergoing development as outlined earlier in this chapter. Developmental factors may make an assessment less generalizable over time, unlike the older person who has more static underlying systems. Also, lack of development of basic/fundamental skills, depending on age, can interact with the injury itself requiring a careful differentiation between evaluation results due to brain injury and those due to lack of early skill achievement.

Miller (3) outlined 3 goals of neuropsychological assessment. First, determine the nature of the underlying problem through obtaining a neuropsychological profile. Second, understand the nature of the brain injury or dysfunction, the resulting neurocognitive deficit, and its impact on the individual. Although the neuropsychological assessment can identify areas of weaknesses, it is also important to identify areas of relative strengths. These relative strengths can then be used to develop compensatory strategies for the areas of weaknesses, which have not yet been remediated or cannot be remediated. For example, a child after a brain injury that resulted in decreased verbal abilities may use visual learning styles to compensate and aid in acquiring new information. The opposite would be true for a child with acquired visual reasoning weaknesses. The results of the neuropsychological evaluation show a child's relative strengths and weakness and can be used to develop treatment recommendations or remediation or compensatory strategies. The results can help to determine a child's ability to carry out a certain tasks (such as ability to return to school). Lastly, assessments may be used to measure change in functioning because a child's brain develops over time, resulting in modification of a rehabilitation program or recommendations over time. In summary, pediatric neuropsychological assessment is closely tied to the changing development of psychological skills and abilities that inherently serve as the back drop to understanding the nature of the underlying problem, understanding the nature of the brain injury, and measuring the change in functioning.

The Role of the Family in Neuropsychological Assessment

In all likelihood, the neuropsychologist did not know the child prior to brain injury. Therefore, it is important to obtain a history of the child through parent interview and report from the family. Premorbid relative strengths and weaknesses in cognitive and social-emotional areas are obtained, which aid in the interpretation of evaluation results. It is helpful when parents are completing scales and inventories to note which items are a change in functioning since the brain injury.

Estimation of Premorbid Ability and Academic Functioning

The results of neuropsychological assessment in children with brain injuries need to be compared to premorbid functioning to determine what changes have occurred after the brain injury. Yet, unless a child was a classified student or had prior neuropsychological condition, it is unlikely that there is a previous neuropsychological or psychological testing available for review. Grade reports, school records, parents and sibling intellectual and educational history, and standardized academic testing provide an estimate of premorbid status. Other estimates of premorbid status can be derived from vocabulary level unless specific language areas of the brain were damaged.

Early Assessment of Brain Injury

The Ranchos Los Amigos Scale (4) is often used to assess a patient's state in the early stages of cognitive recovery ranging from a patient in a low-level state showing no response to a state of purposeful and appropriate with modified independence. The scale has been modified for infants and preschoolers (5). The children's version assesses functioning through the child's ability to interact with the environment in the case of infants and orientation to self and surroundings for the preschool age and older.

Additionally, coma scales have been developed for use in assessing lower level patients such as the JFK Coma Recovery Scale (6), which is a standardized instrument for grading level of neurobehavioral responsiveness following severe brain injury in patients at Rancho Levels II–IV. It assesses levels of responsiveness that are (*a*) generalized; (*b*) localized; (*c*) emergent; or (*d*) cognitively-mediated in the areas of arousal/attention, auditory function, visual function, motor function, oromotor/verbal ability, and communication. Although this scale was developed for the adult population, it has also been used in the pediatric population.

Post-traumatic amnesia (PTA) is the inability to store new memories after a brain trauma. Severity of injury and persistence of cognitive impairments are related to the length of PTA (7). The Children's Orientation and Amnesia Test (COAT) (8) (aged 3–15) and the Galveston Orientation and Amnesia Test (GOAT) (9) (aged 15 and older) are widely used measures of orientation of PTA.

After a patient is oriented and PTA has resolved, more formal neuropsychological assessment can occur. A full neuropsychological evaluation can be lengthy, and in early stages of recovery, neurofatigue can affect performance making it difficult for the child to tolerate such a lengthy examination. Therefore, neuropsychological screening may be better suited for the patient. *Ross Information Processing Assessment—Primary* (10) (aged 5–12) and *Pediatric Test of Brain Injury (PTBI)* (11) (aged 6–16) are examples of screening tools for the pediatric population that are relatively short but yield valuable information about a child's cognitive, attention, and memory. A neuropsychologist can also devise his or her own screening battery test by selecting abbreviated versions of longer tests or selecting subtests within given measure.

Once the child has sufficient stamina to endure a more lengthy battery test, a more complete evaluation can be conducted. For a very detailed overview of the various measures available for the neuropsychologist, the reader is recommended to read section III: "Pediatric Neuropsychological Assessment" in Davis' *Handbook of Pediatric Neuropsychology* (12).

Infant and Toddler

Neuropsychological assessment for children younger than the preschool age consists mainly of developmental measures that are often composed of series of typical tasks or ways that a child interacts within the environment (13–16).

Intellectual Functioning and Cognitive Abilities

For preschoolers and older, tests of intellectual functioning (17–20) and cognitive abilities (21,22) assess a combination of verbal, visual, attention, memory, and processing speed. Although tests of intellectual functioning can yield an overall IQ in brain injury, there can be significant variation among individual scores or indices that can make the IQ less meaningful as a description of overall functioning. It can be more helpful to look at individual subscores and subscales.

Verbal Abilities

The tests of cognitive abilities described earlier include verbal assessments of word definition vocabulary and word knowledge. In addition, there are verbal tests of confrontational naming (picture naming vocabulary) (23) and receptive vocabulary (24). The latter does not require verbalization but allows the child to point to the answer, which is helpful when working with children who have disorders such as expressive aphasia. Word fluency or generation is assessed through a combination of phonemic fluency (generating words beginning with target letters or sounds) or categorical fluency (25,26).

Visual and Visual Motor Abilities

The assessment of visual problem solving includes puzzle-type tasks where the child is shown a finished patterned design and given either 2- or 3-dimensional pieces that are to be put together to reproduce the design (17–20,26).

Nonmotor visual problem solving is assessed through matrix reasoning, which measures nonverbal abstract reasoning, inductive, and spatial reasoning (17,19,21).

Geometric design copy can be one of the components of neuropsychological batteries (26) or as stand-alone tests (27,28). In addition to assessing a child's accuracy in reproducing a design, the neuropsychologist also assesses the child's organizational approach to design through qualitative observation or through standardized scoring. Does the child approach the design copy in a piecemeal approach where individual details were at times fairly accurate but were not organized or integrated with respect to one another? Or did the child appreciate the part-to-whole relationship, which simplified copying the figure?

Tests of intellectual functioning and cognitive abilities and neuropsychological batteries have tasks that require fine motor manipulation of puzzle-type pieces, which can be qualitatively observed and test visual processing speed on time measures of visual scanning and copying. Raw motor speed and fine motor manipulation are assessed unilaterally with dominant and nondominant hands (26,29–32) and the ability to use both hands in tandem (33). The neuropsychologist assesses lateralization of motor functioning in addition to speed, which is especially important when the motor strip on one of the brain hemispheres has been damaged.

Attention and Concentration

Auditory and visual attention can be assessed in the areas of sustained, divided, alternating attention and concentration. Attention can be assessed through clinician behavioral observations, parents, teachers, and self-reports and through formalized tests of attention and concentration, which can be stand alone or within a battery of tests. Although a child's memory and learning can appear average during formal testing, it should be noted that a student's performance in a small office setting with the examiner directly across the table and with a few distractions is different than performance in a school classroom or at home, which have more distractions and emphasizes the need for parents' and teacher's report and classroom observation when possible.

Memory and Learning

Tests of memory and learning include those instruments that cover both auditory and visual immediate and delayed memory (34–36). In addition, there are tests that target specific types of memory such as list learning over a series of trials, which allow the neuropsychologist to examine a child's learning curve (37,38). Pure tests of visual memory without verbal mediation are difficult when memorizing images of everyday objects. To prevent verbal mediation tests, some tests use complex ambiguous designs and a recognition format to measure visual learning and memory (39).

Executive Functioning

Assessment of executive functioning in the child's typical environment occurs through parents, teacher, and self-

report on measures that assess everyday functioning including behavior regulation such as the ability to inhibit responses, transition, self-monitor of behavior and emotional control, and metacognition including working memory, planning, and organization—the ability to complete tasks (40). Formal assessment of executive functioning can occur with inventories that assess planning and higher order problem solving and the ability to shift sets, profit from feedback, and learn from mistakes (32,33,41).

Behavior and Social-Emotional Functioning

Although behavioral observations in the office setting are of value, a child one-on-one with a neuropsychologist in a nondistracting setting is different than behavioral and social-emotional functioning in the child's everyday world. Parents, teacher, and self-report of home and community functioning are critical in understanding the child's typical everyday functioning. Behavioral and social-emotional inventories assess the areas of attention, hyperactivity, conduct, anxiety, depression, atypical behaviors, social skills, aggression, attitude toward school, relations with parents and teachers, and self-esteem (42–44). Such inventories provide valuable information that cannot be obtained in the office. For children with acquired brain injuries (ABIs), it is important for the parents, teacher, and the child to indicate which behaviors represent changes since the brain injury. Obtaining a social-emotional and behavioral profile will aid in developing treatment recommendations for supportive psychotherapeutic and psychiatric intervention for the child to reintegrate into the community and can aid the school psychologist in providing supportive services in the school.

In addition to standardized assessment, behavioral observation in the child's everyday environment is also useful. The ability to pay attention is different to one-on-one in the office setting compared to a child who is in a busy home or in a classroom with 25 children. Behavioral observation and feedback from teachers concerning classroom behavior and from parents concerning behavior and functioning at home add to the overall assessment of neuropsychological functioning.

Adaptive Behavior

Adaptive behaviors are those behaviors that give one the ability to adapt to the environmental demands to allow successful growth and development. These skills develop over time into adulthood and include activities of daily living, communication, socialization, and moving within one's environment (45). Changes in cognitive, psychosocial, and motor skills are brain injury that can impact adaptive behavior. Adaptive behaviors can be assessed through reports from the home and school settings by parents and teachers (46–48). Refer to Chapter 60 for further discussion of neuropsychological assessment in brain injury.

Table 36-1 presents a list of assessments and inventories and age ranges that are commonly used in neuropsychological evaluation of children and adolescents with ABIs.

TABLE 36-1 Assessments and Inventories Used in Neuropsychological Assessment

DOMAINS	EVALUATION INSTRUMENTS AND AGE RANGES
Estimation of premorbid ability and academic functioning	Wechsler Individual Achievement Test (WIAT-III) (49) (aged 4 and older) Woodcock-Johnson Tests of Achievement (WJ-III) (50) (aged 2 and older)
Neuropsychological test batteries	Halstead-Reitan Test Battery for Young & Older Children (32,33) (aged 5 and older) Kaufmann Assessment Battery for Children (K-ABC) (22) (aged 3–18) NEuroPSYchological Assessment (NEPSY-II) (26) (aged 3–17) Luria-Nebraska Neuropsychological Test Battery (29) (aged 15 and older)
Cognitive abilities	Stanford-Binet Intelligence Scales (SB5) (17) (aged 2 and older) Wechsler Preschool and Primary Scales of Intelligence (WPPSI-III) (18) (aged 2 years 6 months to 7 years 3 months) Wechsler Individual Scales of Intelligence (WISC-IV) (19) (aged 6–16) Wechsler Adult Intelligence Scales (WAIS-IV) (20) (aged 16 and older) Woodcock-Johnson Tests of Cognitive Abilities (21) (aged 2 and older) Kaufman Assessment Battery for Children (K-ABC) (22) (aged 3–18)
Verbal abilities	Boston Naming Test (23) (5 and older) Peabody Picture Vocabulary Test (PPVT-4) (24) (aged 2 years 6 months and older)
Memory and learning	Children's Memory Scale (CMS) (34) (aged 5–16) Tests of Memory and Learning (TOMAL-2) (35) (aged 5 and older) Wide Range Assessment of Memory and Learning (WRAML2) (36) (aged 5 and older) California Verbal Learning Test (CVLT –C and CVLT-II) (37,38) (aged 5 and older) Continuous Visual Memory Test (CVMT) (39) (aged 7 and older)
Attention and concentration	Conners' Continuous Performance Test-II (CPT-II) (51) (aged 4 and older) Test of Everyday Attention for Children (TEA–Ch) (52) (aged 6 and older) Test of Everyday Attention (TEA) (53) (aged 6 and older)
Visual construction	Beery-Buktenica Developmental Test of Visual-Motor Integration (VMI) (27) (aged 2 and older) Rey Complex Figure Test and Recognition Trial (RCFT) (28) (aged 6 and older)
Executive functioning	Behavior Rating Inventory of Executive Functioning (BRIEF) (40) (aged 8 and older) Delis-Kaplan Executive Functioning System (D-KEFS) (25) (aged 8 and older) Wisconsin Card Sorting Test (41) (aged 6 and older) Halstead-Reitan Neuropsychological Test Battery (18,19) (aged 5 and older)
Behavior and social-emotional functioning	Behavior Assessment System for Children (BASC2) (42) (aged 2 and older) Child Behavior Checklist (43) (aged 1 year 6 months and older) Conners' 3rd Edition Manual (44) (aged 6 and older)
Adaptive behavior	Scales of Independent Behavior-Revised (SIB-R) (46) (infancy and older) Vineland Adaptive Behavior Scales (II) (47) (birth and older) Adaptive Behavior Assessment System (ABAS-II) (48) (birth and older)
Fine motor skills	Grooved Pegboard (30) (aged 5 and older) Purdue Pegboard (33) (aged 5 and older)
Developmental	Bayley Scales of Infant and Toddler Development (13) (birth–3 years old) Mullen Scales of Early Learning (14) (birth–68 months) Battelle Developmental Inventory (15) (birth–7 years old) Differential Ability Scales (16) (aged 2 years 6 months to 17 years)

Assessment of Motivation and Effort

Neuropsychological groups such as the American Academy of Clinical Neuropsychology (AACN) have supported the assessment of motivation, effort, and response bias in their guidelines for neuropsychological assessment (54). The way a child answers test questions can be influenced by brain development, response bias, motivation, or malingering. Response bias, the tendency to answer questions such as true or false and yes or no, can also occur when the questions are unclear, especially in the younger child whose cognitive skills are not as developed. Therefore, the age and cognitive level of the child are important when examining responses. Studies have suggested that younger preschoolers exhibit a "yes" bias because of the underdeveloped cognitive abilities, whereas older preschoolers exhibit a response bias because of other factors (55). Courtney et al. (56) found that because the executive functioning are not fully developed, response bias and maintenance of effort appears to be significantly related to age and reading ability level, and the use of these tests in children younger than 11 years old is questionable. The conscious or unconscious tendency to answer questions in a socially desirable light can also affect self-report of behaviors. Some tests such as the Behavior Assessment System for Children (BASC2) have built-in scales to detect possible "faking good" (to be seen in a favorable light) or "faking bad" (a cry for help or possible malingering) (57).

Malingering or faking bad on neuropsychological tests had been discussed in the adult literature (58) in the area of forensics and is beginning to be more frequently discussed in the pediatric neuropsychology literature (59,60). Performing with less than full effort can be the result of consciously or unconsciously wanting to skew the results in a negative direction. The goal could be monetary gain as in the case of litigation, to obtain extra assistance and accommodations such as extra time on standardized tests in educational settings, or a child may not want to be in the testing situation. Behavioral observations and interview can assess behaviors such as test avoidance and variable cooperation and motivation.

Although there are formal tests to assess effort, many are normed on the adult population (61–63). There are fewer assessments that have been used in both the adult and pediatric populations. The *Test of Memory Malingering (TOMM)* (64) is one such instrument that has been used in the pediatric population aged 5 and older (65,66). The individual is shown 50 drawings one at a time and then asked to select the drawing they have seen before from a pair of drawings. The advantage of the *TOMM* is that it requires no reading that lends itself in work with younger children. Although the use of measures developed for adults in a pediatric population is a legitimate concern, Kirk et al. (65) found that 96% of a large clinic-referred pediatric population was able to pass the adult cutoff point on the *TOMM*, and Constantinou et al. (66) found a 98% accuracy rate. Donders (67) showed on the *TOMM* that 90% of children aged 6–8 years old met the adult criteria for sufficient effort. MacAllister et al. (68) in work with children and adolescents aged 6–17 years old with epilepsy found that the passing rate was 90% and was not related to age.

Other measures used in both adults and children with at least a second grade reading skills is the Word Memory Test (WMT) (69) and Computerized Assessment of Response Bias (CARB) (70,71).

Although formal tests of effort are available, the neuropsychologist can also use tests that are already a part of the neuropsychological battery, even though they were not developed specifically to be tests of effort. An example is the *Peabody Picture Vocabulary Test (PPVT-4)*. This test of receptive vocabulary presents a page with 4 picture scenes. The examinee is orally presented with a word that matches 1 of the 4 picture scenes. By chance, performance would be at 25%. Similar tests that are multiple choice in format can be used in a similar way to determine effort. A child who consistently scores below statistical cutoffs (and certainly below chance) on these measures should be suspected for suboptimal effort, and the resultant implication is that the remainder of the formal testing may be of questionable validity. Refer to Chapter 85 for further discussion of response bias in evaluations.

NEUROPSYCHOLOGICAL TREATMENTS AND INTERVENTIONS

Cognitive Remediation

Traditionally, the role of neuropsychology has been focused on evaluation and assessments. However, with time, neuropsychology has become more involved in the treatment of

neuropsychological disorders. This includes treatment of neurocognitive and neurobehavioral disturbances as well as comorbid mental health difficulties. The types of interventions have ranged from remedial/instructional treatments to neurocognitive/perceptual disorders and memory retraining to psychotherapeutic treatment of emotional motivational disorders as well as treatment of social pragmatic disorders. In addition, the venue of treatment has expanded from the classic psychotherapeutic setting to remedial and computerized retraining activities to social pragmatic training in the natural environment. Many target specific syndromes and needs. Probably, some of the best known have focused on memory and cognitive retraining, as well as dysexecutive disorders and "frontal lobe" syndrome. Each of these efforts grew out of a need to restore and improve neuropsychological functioning and to add to the armamentarium of treatments needed to recover from ABIs. Some of the treatment demands arose from the family and survivors themselves as they got beyond the acute medical recovery needs of traditional therapies. Other treatments arose from clinical and investigational inquiry into neuropsychological systems and functions

The history of neuropsychological treatment for traumatic brain injury (TBI) developed through the well-known work of Diller and Ben-Yishay (72), Ben-Yishay and Gold (73), and others who strove to systematize the remedial process. They addressed individual tasks (e.g., attention, scanning) as well as addressing complex behavioral disturbances. Much of the history remained focus on young adults and adults while efforts to assist children mainly developed through special education, speech and language, (74) and eventually psychology (75). There is a little literature or research on systematized programs for children, especially the very young.

Cognitive retraining, which had its origins with survivors of the 2 World Wars, was more robustly developed in the late 1970s for use with acute and postacute TBIs (76). According to Trexler (77), "Cognitive rehabilitation can, therefore, be viewed as a battery of interventive strategies designed to ameliorate circumscribed aspects (cognitive) of the consequences of brain injury." These strategies are based on learning and relearning principles and are applied by a number of individuals with varied professional backgrounds, including speech/language, special education, occupational therapy, and psychology.

Models of Cognitive Remediation

Attempts to learn or restore cognitive skills emerged from several efforts of help to children, and multiple models of approach have been described. Teeter (78) reviews several paradigms of intervention, stating that "to view remediation as one approach or another is to 'oversimplify' the complexity of intervention." There is a need to be aware and address the neurocognitive, behavioral/emotional, and psychosocial factors in developing and maintaining skills for daily living. The author points out that although single neuropsychological components are important, treating single elements of habilitation/remediation may be too limiting. Horton and Puente's review (79) points out that although "behavioral interventions have been helpful for disorders resulting from brain injury and learning disability," behavior treatments should be a part of a program of care. When used in combination with other interventions, behavioral therapies are complement neurocognitive treatments.

Interventions with a psychosocial component have also been recommended. Teeter (78) points out that those psychosocial factors are "bidirectional" with cognitive functioning. She points out that psychosocial factors affect cognitive functioning, and alterations in cognitive function impact psychosocial skills. Social discourse skills, pragmatic communication, and social reasoning all have an impact on peer relationships, social collaboration, and family interactions.

Some remedial approaches are more closely "linked" to the assessment process than others. Teeter (78) presented a "multistage neuropsychological model" that begins with "behavioral interventions" based on initial observations and assessment. According to the author, if initial efforts do not result in functional changes, then the addition of neurocognitive/psychosocial interventions are introduced. Teeter's 1995 work (80) yields an 8-step progression set up such as a treatment algorithm: stage 1, problem identification; stage 2, behavioral-based intervention; stage 3, cognitive child study; stage 4, cognitive-based intervention; stage 5, neuropsychological assessment; stage 6, integrated neuropsychological intervention; stage 7, neurological and neuroradiological assessment; and stage 8, medical-neurological rehabilitation. Models by Rourke, Fish, and Strang (81); Reitan (82); and Levine (83) also closely relate the assessment process with interventions.

Probably, the most complex demands are those programs that require integration of methods to address cognitive, academic, and psychosocial challenges. Along with specific interventions for cognitive limitations, this approach includes treating interpersonal skills required through coaching, modeling, and corrective feedback as well as rehearsal training. According to the literature, this works best when multiple resources are incorporated into the routine academic milieu when possible, which include use of peer supports allowing for normalization of experiences (84). Multiple strategies have been offered that include self-management training (85), attention training (86), home-based extension of activities (87), and "peer tutoring" (88).

One model of note is the neurodevelopmental model offered by Kade and Fletcher-Janzen (89). Frequently used in treatment of children with TBI, the authors compare and contrast this more active/adaptive model with the standard neuropsychological intervention. Relying on assessment of age-appropriate skills and knowledge of the severity and stage of injury recovery, the authors emphasize the use of multidisciplinary team with strong family involvement. This model coordinates multiple modalities of treatment that address, as mentioned, the cognitive, behavioral/emotional, and psychosocial factors addressed in other models. Using a paradigm similar to Dillard and Ben-Yishay (72), Kade and Fletcher-Janzen (89) promote progress through several stages. These stages begin with the progress in the child's active *engagement* in treatment, through growing awareness of needs and deficits through mastery of skills, use, and *control* of the use of skills onto *acceptance* and emergence of a repaired identity.

Overall, neuropsychological rehabilitation is an instructional intervention that is targeted at modification, compensation, and/or remediation of neuropsychological systems, which broadly include cognitive, perceptual, and learning subroutines. At times, the intervention is focused on selected subroutines, whereas at other times, there is an intervention looking at the more integrated macroroutines such as executive function, pragmatic communication, and social discourse skills.

In a 1998 National Institutes of Health (NIH) Consensus Development Conference on Rehabilitation of Persons With Traumatic Brain Injury, Prigatano (90) begins by stating, "Cognitive rehabilitation aims to directly remediating an impairment of brain function remains controversial"; however, citing Ben Yishay and Dillard (72), the authors caution that a definitive conclusion would be "premature." The authors collectively point out that "the brain learns and even an injured brain still learns." The rules of application for such relearning are not readily known. For example, are they the same as initial learning? What differences may be noticed on the pace, rate, and volume of learning with an injured brain? It is imperative to study how and under what conditions learning and relearning best takes place following brain injury.

Literature Review of Cognitive Remediation for Children/Adolescents

When considering cognitive remediation treatments, the developmental variability in the pediatric population is not uniformly addressed with one review. The evidence-based practice of treatment for the older adolescent is probably more consistent with findings from the adult population, whereas the child and very young poses different results. The 2005 review of Cicerone et al. (91) is a repeat review and update from the author's 2000 publication and does yield additional class I findings and recommendations. The older adolescent would benefit from the literature that supports the following findings. For further discussion of cognitive rehabilitation in brain injury refer to Chapter 61.

To date, there are 3 comprehensive reviews of the neuropsychological care of the younger child. These are Slomine and Locascio's (92), Laatsch's (93), and Limond and Leeke's (94). However, there remains an absence of literature on a preschool age child with ABI as well as a general lack of information about how cognitive remediation is applied to the infant with cognitive injuries. The preschool child currently receives "early intervention" services, and these services are akin to "special education services" familiar to most school systems. In the area of cognitive recovery for this youngest group of children, there are no currently available clinical investigations found in the literature.

Slomine and Locascio's (92) review presents in the spirit of Cicerone and colleagues' review (91) that focuses on evidence-based findings for the application of cognitive remediation techniques with children who suffered from brain injury. This follows and builds on the 2 other reviewers all of which share several common conclusions. Collectively, the reviewers conclude that there is a general lack of controlled randomized studies (class I evidence) of treatment interventions, and there is no generalized conclusion for efficacy of treatments, but individual small sample studies (randomized and matched group level of evidence) do exist for some very specific areas of treatment. Also, each review details the research and methodological difficulties in gaining class I and class II research that hinders advancement of the evidence-based findings. However, similar to Cicerone and colleagues' review (91), Slomine and Locascio (92) like others do believe that the literature does yield focused recommendations on practice guidelines and practice options. They both stated most assuredly that the research, because of their efficacy, should continue. The major reviews yielded the following results.

Attention

Attention is known to be a multicomponent process with many subroutines represented differently throughout the neuroaxis. Manley et al. (95) using structural equation modeling was able to isolate and identify these subroutines within a clinical model of attention. Typically, subsets included focused, sustained, selective, alternating, and divided attention. Clinical and daily demands usually mobilize 1 or more of these subroutines at any given task. Efforts to remediate these subroutines have been a center of focus for various diagnostic groups, including ABIs, attention deficit hyperactivity disorder (ADHD), and even "functional "psychiatric disorders (e.g., schizophrenia). According to Limond and Leeke (94), attention-training strategies can be grouped under 4 headings: (a) attention processing training (APT), (b) the use of self-management strategies and environmental modifications, (c) external aids to help track and organize material, and (d) psychosocial supports to address emotional and social factors that impact attention. Most therapeutic attempts have combined features of these 4 approaches. The study of these categories has not yielded uniform levels of evidence, but a few studies have yielded findings that support guidelines or recommendations. Both adult (81) and pediatric literatures (82) recommend a practice guideline for attention retraining.

Slomine and Locascio (92) report on 3 randomized controlled trials with a total of 230 children with diagnosis ranging from ABI (n = 38), radiation after tumor resection (n = 31), and children with " central nervous system (CNS) disease" (n = 161). The overall sample age ranged from 6 years to 22 years of age. From these studies, interventions included cognitive rehabilitation program (CRP) (n = 192) and an "attention training program" (n = 38)—these were the children with ABI. Range of intervention was between 17 and 20 weeks in 2 studies, whereas the other study did not indicate length of treatment (these were the 31 children who are having radiation). The children with ABI group received a daily 30-minute sessions of "attention training," the other 2 studies' frequency of treatment was not mentioned. All studies reported "improvement." The sample of children who underwent radiation therapy reported improved performance on measures of attention, but there were no measures for generalization or follow-up. The sample of children with ABI reportedly improved on measures of sustained and selective attention and again on generalization measures or follow-up measures. The largest sample of children with "CNS disease" reported significant increase in academic achievement, with some measures indicating improved generalization and improvement on follow-up for the clinical sample in the study. However, in contrast, a study by Butler et al. (96) did not find significant changes on measures of focus attention, vigilance, working memory, or memory recall when comparing the clinical and comparison group sample.

The APT appears to be the most referenced intervention. Based on Sohlberg et al. (97), the APT approach is designed to strengthen multidimensional aspects of attentional processes. APT is described as "a cognitive rehabilitation program designed to remediate attention deficits in individuals with brain injury." The APT materials consist of a group of hierarchically organized tasks that exercise different components of attention commonly impaired after brain injury including sustained, selective, alternating, and divided attention. The program tasks place increasing demands on complex attentional control and working memory systems. The new APT-3 (98) published in 2010 is mostly used in adults, but the children's literature does also indicate its use in studies.

The other approach used in the class II studies is the Cognitive Remediation Program (CRP). According to Butler et al. (96), the evaluation of the CRP approach consists of 20 weekly sessions for 2 hours over 4–5 months. The CRP has 3 interdependent components: (a) hierarchically graded massed practice, (b) strategy acquisition, and (c) cognitive-behavioral interventions. These components are not orthogonal. As part of the CRP participants, also, completed a modified version of the APT cognitive rehabilitation program. The intervention for the clinical trial described here was identical to the CRP approach as described previously by Butler et al. (96). An interesting element of this approach was the inclusion of APT protocol with specific focus on attention training. The main components of CRP include (a) APT; (b) a variant of metacognitive strategies to address preparedness, task approach, on-task behaviors, and generalization; and (c) cognitive-behavior interventions to reduce distractibility. The "cognitive-behavior intervention" segment also includes "self-coaching" as well as mnemonics. Although studies report statistically significant changes following CRP participation, it remains difficult to assess multicomponent interventions and to determine which components were effective and which components did not reach efficacy. What elements of the CRP that produced the changes in measures of attention have not been explicitly reported. There are no indications of what are the necessary and sufficient factors of CRP that produced the change in attention and other outcomes. Also, currently, there is no literature on what type of injury profile constitutes "a responder" to either CRP or APT. Changes at a class II level have been reported, but more exact understanding of what changes APT or CRP produced in what type of injured child is not currently available.

Memory

Memory, another multicomponent process with representation throughout the neural axis and across the cortical mantel, is understood to be the acquisition/retention of information that can be systematically stored and retrieved for problem solving. Heuristic models of memory have variously divided up these subroutines according to function (short term, long term) or types of information processed (semantic, episodic). However, most models point out common subroutines of encoding, storage, and retrieval.

Reestablishing memory after injury has proven difficult and if successful results from a combination of remedial intervention and compensatory strategies. The adult literature indicates that restoration of memory skills is very much dependent on the degree of impairment or severity of injury (94,99). Consequently, there is a recommendation to use remedial intervention for "mild memory disturbances." In contrast, Cicerone (99) went on to recommend that compensatory aides, such as external memory supports, electrical devices, and so forth, should be a practice guideline.

However, in children, the level of evidence consists of 1 investigation of class II findings (100). Although this study covered children at 9 years of age to older adolescents at 17 years of age, it does use a randomized trial. The authors citing work from the Amsterdam Memory and Retraining Program reported improve delayed memory and attention, but there was no follow-up measures and no measures of generalization.

Although most of the remaining support for memory training is case-series or single-case study, the investigation of Brett and Laatsch (101) (class III) used a multicomponent approach with teenagers 14–18 years old (N = 10) and measured outcomes in (a) alertness, attenton, concentration; (b) perception and memory; and (c) executive processes. Using the learning asymptote as the outcome measure or when the learning curve "leveled off," the authors reported "significantly increased memory scores," mostly because of improved verbal memory. However, as mentioned earlier, multifactorial interventions are difficult to assess because of the problem of noting which elements contributed to test scores and performance. Here again, the study by Brett and Laatsch (101) did not have follow-up measures or measures of generalization.

As with the adult literature (91,99), there is evidence that compensatory strategies and aides do reportedly help children as well. A study by Wilson et al. (102) can be cited that studied the 8–17 years age range. This study used class II evidence with a randomized, crossover design of 12 children using a 7-week training period. Wilson et al. reported that 80% of the sample of 9 children reported "significant gains in reporting target accuracy after training with pagers." Here again, there was no follow-up and no measure of generalization.

In general, the effort to retrain memory disorders does not find robust support as a primary intervention. Instead, the literature supports retraining in mild memory cases and the use of compensatory aides with more severe cases.

Medical approaches to cognitive rehabilitation have also been investigated. Refer to Chapter 73 for discussion of pharmacotherapy of cognitive impairment.

Neurobehavioral and Executive Functions

Alteration in complex behaviors and changes in self-directing skills (e.g., goal setting, self control) has been identified as some of the most challenging and most difficult problems after brain injury (103). These challenges require the mobilization of mental health, neuropsychiatric, and behavior neurology resources. In 2006, the National Institute of Neurological Disorders working group published a paper on "Cognitive Rehabilitation Interventions for Executive Function: Moving from Bench to Bedside in Patients With Traumatic Brain Injury" (104). The group outlined 4 currently identified subroutines all of which come under the umbrella concept of "executive function." First, they identify an "exec-

utive cognitive function" that correlates with activities of the dorsolateral prefrontal cortex and its associated hippocampal relationships and interconnection with various cortical zones. Next, they propose a "behavioral self-regulatory function," which is associated with the orbitofrontal cortex and associated limbic interconnections. Then, the authors identify an "activation regulation function," which provides the initiation, persistence, and follow through for goal attainment. Lastly, they describe a "metacognitive process" associated with frontal poles of the cortex and how this subroutine is important in social cognition, self-awareness, personality, autonoetic consciousness, and self-assessment. The working group proposes that when examining executive functions, each subroutine may require its own assessment instrument, and recognizing each of these functions may not currently have means for standardized assessment. Furthermore, when assessing treatment options and interventions, each subroutine may require their own outcome measures and monitoring. Consequently, understanding, measuring, and studying changes in executive function may be somewhat limited by the current state of assessment tools, outcome measures, and research design. In addition, the authors' comments are directed toward the state of the adult and do not address the complexity of the neurodevelopmental distribution of such tasks in the growing brain or the related examination and outcome measures of these various subroutines in the young and very young.

Malone and Slomine's (105) review of executive functioning points out that the adult literature, ala Cicerone, has yielded 1 practice guideline for problem-solving training using goal management training (GMT) (106). Although both Malone and Slomine wrote the importance "to teach problem solving during everyday activities in the real world," writing large scale class I evidence do not exist. However, there are a number of single-subject (SS) design interventions in the current literature at a class III level of evidence. It is important to point out that although SS designs cannot provide evidence of guideline or recommendations at a population level, SS when applied in a "particular-to-particular" situation may inform clinical decision making at the level of the individual. Ylvisaker et al. (107) outline the criteria provided by Horner et al. (108), wherein SS may be considered sufficient evidence for clinical decision making if it (a) meets acceptable methodological criteria and published in peer-reviewed journals, (b) are conducted by at least 3 different researchers across at least 3 different geographical regions, and (c) include at least 20 participants. Slomine and Locascio (92) identified 6 SS design interventions for executive functioning worth mentioning. Two studies, 1 with a 16-year-old adolescent (109) and another with 3 children 6–10 years of age (110) focused on the use of direct instructional techniques to teach self-monitoring. In both studies, authors reported improvement in "targeted instructional areas." Both studies also reported a modest measure/report of generalization and continuation of effects on follow-up. Suzman et al. (111) in another SS design also reported success with a problem-solving training program that focused on self-instruction, self-regulation, metacognition, and attribution training. Suzman an colleagues' study of 5 children 6–11 years old reported improvement on computer-based task as well as improvement on neuropsychological measures. There was no report of continuation effect.

Studies by Selznic and Savage (112) also looked at the importance of teaching children self-monitoring techniques after brain injury. Using SS with multiple baseline comparisons, they instructed 3 adolescents in self-monitoring skills. All 3 subjects elevated on task behavior from 44%–84% at baseline to 100%. Using multiple techniques, no self-monitoring condition was associated with the change alone. First, this study pointed out that on-task behavior can be enhanced by teaching self-monitoring and that there is a relationship between this skill and academic performance that also improved. The effect was maintained when the intervention was withdrawn, with the authors speculating that "on-task" behaviors may establish their own reinforcements.

Feeney and Ylvisaker (113,114) looked at a younger sample of 4 children 6 and 7 years of age (some of the youngest subjects mentioned in the literature). The report reduced "target behavior" aggression and disinhibited behaviors with increased "quantity of work completed" using cognitive-behavioral strategies and graphic organizers. Here, generalization is reported "anecdotally" with good report of continuation response 1 year and beyond.

A set of problems closely related to alteration in executive behaviors are the emotional/behavior problems. These are clusters of symptoms also associated with frontolimbic disruption and/or ventralfronto/frontolimbic disconnections. Two clusters are frequently mentioned. First is the "pseudopsychopathic" type with an array of symptoms including disinhibition, impulsiveness, lability, reduced anger control, perseveration, acting out poor social judgment, and poor learning. The second is a "pseudodepressed" presentation with poor initiation, persistence and follow through, apathy/lethargy, lack of animation or emotional concern, and reduced spontaneity of behavior. The latter group has been associated with the lack of activation-regulation function reviewed earlier.

In 2007, Ylvisaker et al. (107) provided a comprehensive review of behavior intervention strategies that not only reviews the literature but also compare 2 important theoretical approaches to care. The authors compared the approach based on applied behavior analysis (ABA)/contingency management procedures (CMP) with positive behavior interventions and supports (PBIS). See Table 36-1 of the original review to compare these differing approaches. ABA is based on the understanding that through changes in positive or negative contingency (reward) schedules, the child can learn to increase or decrease a discrete behavior. PBIS is more focused on changing macrolifestyle routines and interactions, rather than focused/specific behaviors (ABA/CMP). PBIS rely on antecedent conditioning or the staging of cues, directives that guide positive behavior, and can guide retention of successful behaviors. The PBIS approach also occurs in natural settings with collaboration among family members, staff, and the individual to effect change rather than sole reliance on professional/technician intervention. In contrast to reinforcement schedules and token economies, PBIS uses more external/environmental and internal/cognitive sets structuring in meaningful settings, also including meaningful individuals/relationships that teach positive communication styles to support changes in behavior and emotional management.

Ylvisaker and Turkstra et al. pointed out that both children and adults tend to display more problematic externalizing behaviors post-brain injury than internalizing problems. The exception being that the younger the child (injury prior to 6 years of age) demonstrate more internalizing problems. It is not clear if this is because of injury alone or a combination effects including age expectations and so forth. Citing a paper by Winkler (115), the review by Ylvisaker, Turkstra, and Coehlo focused on loss of emotional control (LEC) with such symptoms as irritability, aggression, and disinhibition. The authors related these symptoms to some identified neural networks such as orbitofrontal structures, anterior temporal lobe, and limbic structures as they relate to dysfunction of contextual analysis, processing of social information, and processing of pragmatic communication skills. In particular, the authors point out that externalizing behaviors, unlike other cognitive consquences of brain injury, may worsen over time with some evidence provided that children's LEC may worsen with age. The review goes on to indicate that the worsening of emotional control may be a product of interactions between academic demands, social support networks, and brain injury.

In a review of the literature as of the 2007 publication, there was 1 class I randomized control trial with children. This was a work of Wade et al. (116), which was an experimental group of 16 and 16 controls with an average age of 11 years old. The investigators used a family intervention format with emphasis on antecedent staging, cognitive supports, positive communication patterns (PBIS) over a 6-month period of care. Training for parents was done both in the clinic and at home using various rating scales (Child Behavior Checklist, Brief Symptom Inventory, and so forth). There was a reported reduction in the injured child's symptoms for internalizing behaviors (depression, anxiety, withdrawal), improved parent-child relationships, and improved knowledge base with no effect on parent's sense of distress. This study is consistent with 2 earlier studies by Braga et al. (117) and Ponsfeld et al. (118) that also used more of a family intervention format with psychoeducational supports and parent training to effect cognitive, emotional, and behavioral changes. Braga and colleagues' study compared "direct clinician-delivered" with "indirect family-supported" rehabilitation. The parents received training on how to deliver cognitive interventions "within the context of everyday routines of the child's life at home." Both the experimental and control groups demonstrated improvements; however, "only the children in the family-supported interventing group demonstrated statistically significant and clinically important improvements." Both the Braga et al. and Ponsford et al. studies used family training to implement PBIS principles of antecedent staging/conditioning, as well as emphasis on positive communications.

Overall, the Ylvisaker and Turkstra review (107) provided many important conclusions that not only informs clinical decision making but also leads the way for further research and investigation. In their section "Clinical Themes Emerging . . . ," they point out the following: (a) children/adolescents benefit from facilitating knowledge to understanding communication competence that support successful interpersonal interactions, (b) context-sensitive training that are personally important is beneficial, (c) practicing personally important social interactions in a more natural setting is important, (d) using coaching of interaction so that they are successful helps navigate "potentially problematic interactions," (e) situational training that supports improving social perceptiveness is also important, as well as (f) learning to monitor personal stress during social interactions, with (g) person-centered goal setting is more meaningful and explicit. Also, the lesson is not lost in translation, and finally, (h) counseling focused on restoring social interaction strategies that are positive also contributes to a "personally compelling sense of self."

Psychotherapy

An area of considerable importance is the use of psychotherapy to support, guide, and teach the child or adolescent recovering from brain injury. However, this area of work is not currently well researched in children. Brown et al. (119) found that 25% of those children with TBI who premorbidly had no known prior abnormality exhibited definite psychological and psychiatric disorders 1 year after their injury, and another 25% showed milder emotional and behavioral problems. The rate rose to 50% in children who had some prior psychological abnormality, with the rest displaying mild emotional and behavioral problems.

Following brain injury, children and adolescents often have difficulty interpreting nonverbal cues and emotions that impact social interactions. Children with brain injuries need to understand their injury, accept changes in functioning and acquired areas of weakness, and learn ways to compensate (120).

Frequently, comprehensive programs dedicated to neuropsychological recovery include a counseling or psychotherapeutic component. Such interventions may be individual attention or through group therapy format. As early as the hallmark program by Ben Yishay and Diller (72,73), there has been emphasis on themes of psychological recovery. In the New York University (NYU) program, there has been a focus on understanding, appreciating, and applying new found personal knowledge or perspective following brain injury. The "holistic" approach as it is described followed a neuropsychological paradigm as compared to biomedical paradigms of the day. This more dynamic approach was a patient-family centered approach that was health promoting vs a deficit reduction model focus. This approach used an integrated team including the use of psychotherapeutic themes. The emphasis on "cognitive adjustment" to brain injury was viewed as a progression through various phases and themes of recovery. The program began with a focus on *engagement*, which could be the most confrontational stage with emphasizing basic goal setting and involvement in recovery. This was followed by the stage of *awareness*. This stage actively confronted the patients' unawareness of their own circumstances and the consequences of the injury in their life. Next came the *mastery* stage "where the patient is in the process of mastering compensatory techniques for the deficits identified by the interdisciplinary team." Mastery is followed by the *control* stage. The *control* stage is a critical phase for stabilizing living skills with increasingly less structure/supervision outside of the hospital or residential setting. The stage of *acceptance* follows, which works on internalizing needed skills for living with an expressed understanding and appreciation of the changes that have occurred and how the patient will live with these changes over time. The final stage is *identity*. This is the last

step in clinical adjustment with emphasis on gaining age-appropriate cognitive/perceptual abilities including patient's knowledge of changes to self. Successful completion of this stage is demonstrated through appropriate understanding of events surrounding the injury, the residual deficits, and the mastery and control of compensatory strategies. The eventual outcome is skill development, personal insight, and appreciation of the new combination of things that represent the "self."

Prigatano and Naar-King (121) described the importance in a pediatric brain injury population of an integrated team approach, approaching rehabilitation in a holistic way. Luria (122) and Prigatano (123,124) focused on neuropsychological rehabilitation. They refer to training and learning exercises that attempt to restore higher integrative skills and/or teaching patients to compensate for residual disturbances that impact personal and interpersonal life. These activities are employed with both adults and children. According to these authors, neuropsychological rehabilitation with adults and older adolescents is to help them deal with the problem of "lost normality" by working to return to a productive lifestyle and find ways of maintaining mutually satisfying interpersonal relationships (i.e., work and love). For parents, the treatment is to help them both deal with the problem of the child and stop those factors that keep the child from "not developing normally." This requires considerable effort at helping the child and parents realistically adjust to whatever permanent changes may be imposed by brain injury, without having children lose their "individuality." That is, in adults, adolescents, and children, the goal is to help them improve in their higher cerebral functioning and adjust to those to unalterable changes, but to do so in a manner that still allows them to be true to who they are. The goal is more than adjusting to society.

Psychotherapeutic referral remains a popular resource for behavior management, coping, and adjustment as well as classic themes of anxiety and mood management. It was Prigatano (123) who focused early on the "catastrophic response." Although there is little literature addressing psychotherapy to children, especially the very young, in most practices today, you can expect community-based, hospital-based, and school-based mental health services being involved in the process of recovery, especially when confronting late effects. Much of the present literature is most applicable to the adolescent, especially the older adolescent. In contrast, there exists little of any literature on psychotherapeutic intervention in prepubertal children or the very young. Most of this literature for children is, rightfully, now addressed to family types of interventions, psychoeducational assistance, and school-based guidance/behavior interventions.

A brief review is presented herein of the existing state of counseling and psychotherapeutic interventions that will mostly apply to adolescent and the older adolescent in particular. Prigatano's 2010 paper (124) presented perspective for all. He focused on the need to address the consequences of lost "higher order brain disturbances" and the impact on interpersonal exchange and relationships. Although both the child and adult suffer the loss of "normalcy," the child/adolescent confronts "not developing normally." The developmental challenges will affect family members and child alike. While retaining the goal of developing individuality, the family/child must cope to adjustment, which will require considerable resources, attention, and effort to adequately address. In a very pointed and profound manner, Prigatano goes on to conclude that although recovery for adult and child alike must address attempts to regain/gain higher mental skills that were lost, it also must include the ability to adjust to permanent changes in skills in a manner that is "true to who they are." The goal is not only to adjust to society and environmental demands but also to adjust and cope with who they are now.

Jean Elbaum (125) in her chapter "Counseling Individuals Post Acquired Brain Injury" pointed out the unique challenges. When counseling children/adolescent, there is a special need to understand how knowledge of neurocognitive/neuroaffective disorders interact with a person's ability to cope, adjust, and regain a meaningful role in life. Mateer et al. (126) reemphasized the importance of including emotional reintegration into a comprehensive treatment program and holistic approach to programming.

Neuropsychological impairments of self-assessment, self-awareness, limitations of reflective thought, and lack of personal problem solving because of cognitive perceptual limitations may hinder the individual from full participation in traditional counseling sessions. In preparation to more traditional therapies, a precounseling series of treatments may be necessary to prepare full participation. Prigatano and Schacter (127) early on addressed the lack of insight, perspective taking, and adequate personal problem solving because of lack of "self awareness," the ability to accurately think, and reason about the topic of "me." Sherer (128) reported that as the number of lesions on neuroradiographic findings increase, the increasing likelihood that the subroutines needed for "self-awareness" are affected, and the lack of personal awareness increases. Evans et al. (129) reported that when the lack of self-awareness is addressed earlier in recovery, counseling outcomes improve. In part, this is caused by the fundamental importance of self-awareness in gaining insight and having appropriate self-perspective. Earlier work by Crosson et al. (130) pointed out that the restoration of insight can be a progressive process that moves from the factual understanding (cognitive elements) of events and circumstances to the integration with emotional consequences (perceptual elements). Crosson et al. outlined levels of awareness beginning with (a) intellectual awareness, wherein the individual can report, understand the factual changes in them after injury, and describe these changes; (b) emergent awareness is the product of the individual's ability to understand and report the emotional significances of these changes in skill, role, and life events; and (c) anticipatory awareness, the point at which the individual can use the knowledge of facts and understanding of emotional consequences to foresee and predict the impact on future.

Also related to a successful recovery, one must address mood and emotional management difficulties. Changes in mood and emotional life are caused by a combination of neuroemotional changes as well as psychological confrontation with change. In particular, late-onset changes in mood, frustration, and anger management are particularly challenging. In some ways, it is after the discharge from the hospital and with repeated confrontation with loss of function and confrontations with everyday demands that the individual will demonstrate depression, frustration, and anger

management problems (131). Scicutella (132) pointed out that factors associated with depression are (a) lesion location (left greater than right), (b) poor social functioning, and (c) preexisting history of mood disorder. Scicutella goes on to differentiate mood disturbance from both neurologically based "apathy," noted by its amotivational elements in the absence of endorsement of mood disturbance. Also, Scicutella mentioned the differences between mood disturbance and pseudobulbar emotion—a state of pathological laughing or crying, which has different lesion localization (disruption to cerebro-ponto-cerebellar pathway or disruption in pyramidal tracts between brainstem nuclei mediating laughing, crying with facial expression, and respiration) and is characterized by incongruity of emotional expression, circumstance, or personal experience. The latter, pseudobulbar affect, is much less seen in the younger person. In a 2006 article by Bagueley et al. (133), the author offered that there are multiple contributing factors to anger management problems. The author listed difficulty with communications that lead to frustration because of no conventional outlet for expression of anger without "acting out." In addition, there may exist post-traumatic stress disorder characteristics that reduced resilience and disrupted sleep, as well as neurobiological limitations undermining complex neuropsychological skills. For those individuals in acute stage of rehabilitation, Bagueley et al. emphasized the importance that disorientation to time and place play an important role in episodes of anger. In part, the individual has periods of delirium that affected the ability to cope, adjust, and express one's self-effectively. Bagueley et al. (133) goes on to mention the importance of preinjury characteristics that play an important role in anger management, especially preexisting emotional/behavior problems along with drug abuse history.

Anger management problems have received much attention after brain injury because of their disruptive nature in the home and community. Separated from suicidal ideation or acts, the child/adolescent is more easily frustrated and more likely to act out the frustration in verbal or physical aggression. Because of the nature of this problem, medication strategies have been explored aggressively. Bagueley et al. cited that in a sample of 228 patients at a 5-year follow-up, 25% presented difficulties with anger management. The author stated that the factors most predictive of anger difficulties were comorbid depression, traumatic complaints, low self-satisfaction, and younger age at time of injury.

Treatment of the complex conditions has not been systematically studied as to the best type of therapy, for whom, and at what point in recovery. Instead, the literature addresses the practical demands of daily clinical responsibility to respond and empirically intervene. Cognitive-behavioral therapy has been applied with clinical report of improvement (134). Giles and Manchester (135) presented 2 approaches to addressing the "disorders" following brain injury. They listed operant neurobehavioral approach (ONA) and relational neurobehavioral approach (RNA). Both approaches are based in ABA, and as Giles and Manchester (135) reported, both addressed situational elements that triggered irritation/anger, provided a positive non-aversive engagement teaching social norms (ONA), and increased attention to therapeutic relationship opportunities to learn interpersonal skills (RNA). A review in 2009 by

Slifer and Amari (136) provided focus more specifically to children and adolescents after TBI. Again, reviewing the history of ABA as it relates to addressing disinhibition, irritability, restlessness, distractibility, and aggression, the authors pointed out the long history of ABA with ABIs. The authors support the successes of ABA across diagnostic groups, age span, injury severity, and stage of recovery. The article emphasized the need for direct observation of the child's presenting problem and assessment of environmental "triggers." As the the case in ABA, the authors pointed out the need to manage antecedent conditions for success and that situational staging plays an important role. Differential rewarding systems are also considered important elements of shaping positive and functional behaviors. The authors went on to point out the need for well-trained experienced professionals to engage the child who are able to monitor target behaviors for needed updates and modifications as the child changes. The authors concluded by stating the need for well-structured, repetitive clinical trial assessment of ABA approaches in the brain injury population and endorse SS as well as multicentered large randomized controlled trials.

Within a psychotherapeutic model emphasizing skill sets, Elbaum (125) offered the COP anachronym: C, communicate needs/irritations; O, identify outlets of expression and distress; P, preparation. Prigatano and Schacter (127) offered guiding principles for counseling and psychotherapeutic intervention as well: (*a*) work within the individual's subject experience, (*b*) address disorders of awareness, (*c*) consider preinjury characteristics, and (*d*) understand between cognition and personality. Prigatano and Schacter concluded that "focus on the present, but with a sophisticated understanding of how the past may have contributed to problem behavior."

Parent-child interaction therapy (PCIT) (137) that uses a combination of behavior therapy, play therapy, and parent training has been used in children with brain injury to teach more effective discipline techniques and improve the parent-child relationship, reducing negative behaviors and parental stress (138).

Refer to Chapters 66 and 67 for further information about behavior modification amelioration of emotional and behavioral problems and Chapter 74 for pharmacotherapy of neuropsychiatric disturbances.)

Family and Caregiver Support

The care of a child with significant brain injury can cause significant stress on the family. Tips for the caregiver have been developed (139). Parent and sibling support groups are present in many states and can be found through state brain injury association and affiliations. It is important for parents to take care of themselves, which means maintaining enough sleep and eat to maintain their strength. Although parents want to put full effort in the recovery process, it is important to delegate responsibilities such as assigning someone to stay with their loved one when they are not there or to oversee household responsibilities and child care. Having a designated person assigned to contact family and friends with updates on patient status can ease stress. It can be helpful when talking with medical staff to have someone with the family member to provide another set of ears for clarification

or to write the information down to review at a later time. A voice recorder may also be useful. Maintaining a journal of medical updates or a record of thoughts and feelings can become a valuable reference in the future. Parents should remember that they are part of a medical or school team and serve as their child's advocate. Parents should allow themselves to grieve and express emotions. Refer to Chapter 38 on "Family Assessment and Intervention" for further information in working with families of children with brain injuries.

CONCLUSION

Pediatric neuropsychology assessment and treatment is a subspecialty in the area of brain injury rehabilitation. A key component is that a child's brain continues to change and develop through early adulthood. Therefore, it is imperative for a child with a brain injury to be assess by clinicians who understand the developing brain. Neuropsychological sequelae of pediatric brain injury include physical, cognitive, visuoperceptual, visuomotor, behavior, and psychosocial issues. Assessing the child can begin at early stages of recovery in low-level patients through behavioral observations or standardized screening. More formalized neuropsychological assessment assesses the brains ability to receive information from the environment and express behaviors.

Neuropsychological assessment covers the domains of verbal and visual intellectual functioning, attention, concentration, memory and learning for new information, recall of previously learned information, academic functioning, higher order executive skills, processing speed, visuomotor functioning, adaptive behavior, and psychosocial functioning. Tests of effort in children should be a part of an evaluation to assess response bias, possible malingering, or variable motivation in the assessment process. Information is obtained through standardized assessment, behavioral observations, and key to understanding how the child is functioning in their typical environment, input from parents, teachers, and the children themselves.

With a neuropsychological profile established, strengths and weaknesses can be determined and a treatment plan developed. Cognitive and psychotherapeutic intervention is unevenly supported in the area of brain injury, especially in the pediatric population, and further research in the area of efficacy of these interventions is needed.

KEY CLINICAL POINTS

1. The parent discipline for pediatric neuropsychology is not adult neuropsychology but that of developmental neurosciences.
2. Brain context development should serve as the overriding model for pediatric clinical neuropsychology evaluation, research, instruction, and intervention.
3. Neuropsychological sequelae of pediatric brain injury include physical, cognitive, visuoperceptual, visuomotor, behavior, and psychosocial issues.
4. Neuropsychological assessment of pediatric brain injury should be sensitive to the developmental level of the

child, current level of current functioning, and include a combination of standardized instruments and behavioral observations from family and community.

5. The area of effort testing is a fairly new area in pediatric neuropsychology and should be further studied.

6. Cognitive and psychotherapeutic intervention is unevenly supported in the literature, and among developmental levels, clinician, investigator, and instructor must be familiar with the findings within each developmental level and within each mental subroutine being addressed. The efficacy of cognitive and psychotherapeutic intervention should be addressed in future research.

7. Compare and contrast ABA and PBIS as 2 differing and essential models for understanding neuropsychological remediation.

8. There is an important and essential need for cognitive and neuropsychological intervention effectiveness with the very young who sustain an ABI prior to preschool.

KEY REFERENCES

1. Davis A. *Handbook of Pediatric Neuropsychology*. New York, NY: Springer Publishing; 2011:191–434.
2. Laatsch HD, Harrington D, Hotz G, et al. An evidence-based review of cognitive and behavioral rehabilitation treatment studies in children with acquired brain injury. *J Head Trauma Rehabil*. 2007;22(4):248–256.
3. Limond J, Leeke R. Practitioner review: cognitive rehabilitation for children with acquired brain injury. *J Child Psychol Psychiatry*. 2005;46(4):339–352.
4. Slomine B, Locascio G. Cognitive rehabilitation for children with acquired brain injury. *Dev Disabil Res Rev*. 2009; 15(2):133–143.
5. Ylvisaker M, Turkstra L, Coehlo C, et al. Behavioural interventions for children and adults with behaviour disorders after TBI: a systematic review of the evidence. *Brain Inj*. 2007;21(8):769–805.

References

1. Bernstein JH. Developmental neuropsychological assessment. In: Yeates KO, Taylor HG, Ris MD, eds. *Pediatric Neuropsychology, Research, Theory, and Practice*. 2000;405–438.
2. Harris J, Mishkin L, Ross B. Consequences of brain injury. In: Brain Injury Association of New Jersey, Inc, eds. *Brain Injury: A Guide for Educators*. North Brunswick, NJ: Brain Injury Association of New Jersey, Inc; 2010;10–12.
3. Miller E. Some basic principles of neuropsychological assessment. In: Crawford JR, Parker DM, McKinlay WM, eds. *A Handbook of Neuropsychological Assessment*. Hove, United Kingdom: Laurence Erlbaum Associates; 1992:7–20.
4. Hagen C. *The Ranchos Levels of Cognitive Functioning*. Encinitas, CA: Ranchos Los Amigos Medical Center; 1998.
5. Brink JD, Imbus C, Woo-Sam J. Physical recovery after severe closed head trauma in children and adolescents. *J Pediatr*. 1980; 97(5): 721–727
6. Giacino, J, Kalmar K. *The JFK Coma Recovery Scale-Revised*. Edison, NJ: The Center for Outcome Measurement in Brain Injury; 2006.
7. McDonald CM, Jaffe KM, Fay GC, et al. Comparison of indices of traumatic brain injury severity as predictors of neurobehavioral outcomes in children. *Arch Phys Med Rehab*. 1994;75(3):328–337.
8. Ewing-Cobbs L, Levin HS, Fletcher JM, Miner ME, Eisenberg HM. The children's orientation and amnesia test: relationship to severity of acute head injury and to recovery of memory. *Neurosurgery*. 1990;27(5):683–691.
9. Levin H, O'Donell V, Grossman R. The Galveston orientation and amnesia test. A practical scale to assess cognition after head injury. *J Nerv Ment Dis*. 1979;167(11):675–684.
10. Ross-Swain D. *Ross Information Processing Assessment—Primary*. Austin, TX: Pro-Ed Inc; 1999.
11. Holz G, Helm-Estabrooks N, Wolf Nelson N, Plante N. *Pediatric Test of Brain Injury (PTBI)*. Baltimore, MD: Brookes Publishing; 2010.
12. Davis A. *Handbook of Pediatric Neuropsychology*. New York, NY: Springer Publishing; 2011:191–434.
13. Bayley N. *Bayley Scales of Infant and Toddler Development*. 3rd ed. San Antonio, TX: Pearson; 2006.
14. Mullen EM. *Mullen Scales of Early Learning*. Circle Pines, MN: American Guidance Service Publishing; 1984.
15. Newborg J. *Batelle Developmental Inventory*. 2nd ed. Itasca, IL: Riverside Publishing; 2005.
16. Elliot C. *Differential Ability Scales*. San Antonio, TX: National Computer System, Pearson; 2007.
17. Roid G. *Stanford-Binet Intelligence Scales*. 5th ed. Itasca, IL: Riverside Publishing; 2003.
18. Wechsler D. *Wechsler Preschool and Primary Scales of Intelligence*. 3rd ed. San Antonio, TX: Pearson; 2002.
19. Wechsler D. *Wechsler Intelligence Scales for Children*. 4th ed. San Antonio, TX: Pearson; 2003.
20. Wechsler D. *Wechsler Adult Intelligence Scales*. 4th ed. San Antonio, TX: Pearson; 2009.
21. Woodcock R, McGrew K, Mather N. *Woodcock–Johnson Tests of Cognitive Abilities*. 3rd ed. Itasca, IL: Riverside Publishing; 2001.
22. Kaufmann A, Kaufmann N. *Kaufmann Assessment Battery for Children*. 2nd ed. Circle Pines, MN: American Guidance Service Publishing; 2004.
23. Kaplan E, Goodglass H, Weintraub S. *Boston Naming Test*. 2nd ed. Austin, TX: Pro-Ed; 2001.
24. Dunn L, Dunn D. *Peabody Picture Vocabulary Test (PPVT4)*. San Antonio, TX: National Computer System, Pearson; 2007.
25. Delis D, Kaplan E, Kramer JH. *Delis-Kaplan Executive Functioning System (D-KEFS)*. San Antonio, TX: National Computer System, Pearson; 2001.
26. Korkman M, Kirk U, Kemp S. *NEPSY-II. A Developmental Neuropsychological Assessment*. San Antonio, TX: Psychological Corporation; 2007.
27. Beery K, Beery N. *Beery-Buktenica Developmental Test of Visual–Motor Integration: Administration, Scoring, and Teaching Manual*. 5th ed. San Antonio, TX: National Computer System, Pearson; 2004.
28. Meyers J, Meyers K. *Rey Complex Figure Test and Recognition Trial*. Lutz, FL: PAR Inc; 1995.
29. Golden CJ, Purisch, AD, Hammeke TA. *Luria-Nebraska Neuropsychological Battery: Forms I and II Manual*. Los Angeles, CA: Western Psychological Services; 1985.
30. Trites R. *Neuropsychological Test Manual*. Ontario, Canada: Royal Ottawa Hospital; 1977.
31. Reitan R. *Reitan-Indiana Test Battery for Young Children (RITB-C)*. Tuscon, AZ: Reitan Neuropsychology Laboratory; 1969.
32. Reitan R, Davison L. *Halstead-Reitan Neuropsychological Test Battery for Older Children (HRNB-C)*. Tuscon, AZ: Reitan Neuropsychology Laboratory; 1974.
33. Tiffin J. *Purdue Pegboard Examiners Manual*. Rosemount, IL: London House; 1968.
34. Cohen M. *Manual for the Children's Memory Scale*. San Antonio, TX: The Psychological Corporation; 1997.
35. Reynolds C, Voress J. *Test of Memory and Learning (TOMAL2)*. 2nd ed. North Tonawanda, NY: Multi-Health Systems; 2011.
36. Sheslow D, Adams W. *Wide Range Assessment of Memory and Learning (WRAML2)*. 2nd ed. Lutz, FL: Psychological Assessment Resources; 2003

37. Delis D, Kramer J, Kaplan E, Ober B. *California Verbal Learning Test (CVLT-II)*. San Antonio, TX: National Computer System, Pearson; 2000.

38. Delis D, Kramer J, Kaplan E, Ober B. *California Verbal Learning Test (CVLT-C)*. San Antonio, TX: National Computer System, Pearson; 1994.

39. Trahan D, Larrabee G. *Continuous Visual Memory Test (CVMT)*. San Antonio, TX: National Computer System; 1988.

40. Gioia G, Isquith S, Guy S, Kenworthy L. *Behavior Rating Inventory of Executive Functioning (BRIEF)*. Lutz, FL: Psychological Assessment Resources; 2000.

41. Heaton R, Chelune G, Talley J, Kay G, Curtiss G. *Wisconsin Card Sorting Test*. Lutz, FL: Psychological Assessment Resources; 1993.

42. Reynolds C, Kamphaus R. *The Behavior Assessment System for Children*. 2nd ed. Circle Pines, MN: American Guidance Service Publishing; 2004.

43. Achenbach T. *Child Behavior Checklist*. Burlington, VT: Achenbach of System Empirically Based Assessment, University of Vermont; 2001.

44. Conners K. *Conners 3rd Edition Manual*. North Tonawanda, NY: Multi-Health Systems; 2008.

45. Reva K, Bardos A. Assessing adaptive skills in a pediatric population. In: Davis A, ed. *Handbook of Pediatric Neuropsychology*. New York, NY: Springer Publishing; 2011:245–250.

46. Bruininks R, Woodcock R, Weatherman R, Hill B. *Scales of Independent Behavior*. Rev ed. Chicago, IL: Riverside Publishing; 1996.

47. Sparrow S, Cicchetti D, Balla D. *Vineland Adaptive Behavior Scales*. 2nd ed. San Antonio, TX: Pearson; 2005.

48. Harrison P, Oakland T. *Adaptive Behavior Assessment System (ABAS-II)*. San Antonio, TX: National Computer System, Pearson; 2003.

49. Wechsler D. *Wechsler Individual Achievement Tests—Third Edition (WIAT—III)*. San Antonio, TX: Pearson; 2005.

50. Woodcock R, McGrew K, Mather N. *Woodcock-Johnson Tests of Achievement*. 3rd ed. Itasca, IL: Riverside Publishing; 2001.

51. Conners K, Multi-Health System Staff, eds. *Conners' Continuous Performance Test—II*. North Tonawanda, NY: Multi-Health System; 2000.

52. Manly T, Robertson IH, Anderson V, Nimmo-Smith I. *Test of Everyday Attention for Children (TEA-Ch)*. San Antonio, TX: Pearson; 1998.

53. Robertson I, Ward T, Ridgeway V, Nimmo-Smith I. *Test of Everyday Attention (TEA)*. San Antonio, TX: National Computer System, Pearson; 1994.

54. American Academy of Clinical Neuropsychology. American Academy of Clinical Neuropsychology (AACN) practice guidelines for neuropsychological assessment and consultation. *Clin Neuropsychol.* 2007;21(2):209–231.

55. Okanda M, Itakura S. Do young and old preschoolers exhibit response bias due to different mechanisms? Investigating children's response time. *J Exp Child Psychol.* 2007;110(3):453–460.

56. Courtney JC, Dinkins JP, Allen LM III, Kuroski K. Age related effects in children taking computerized assessment of response bias and word memory test. *Child Neuropsychol.* 2003;9(2):109–116.

57. Merrill KW. Response bias and error variance. In: Merrel KW, eds. *Behavioral, Social, and Emotional Assessment of Children and Adolescents*. New York, NY: Larwrence Erlbaum Associates, Inc; 2003: 172–173.

58. Lezak MD. Testing for functional complaints. In: Lezak MD, Howieson DB, Loring DW, eds. *Neuropsychological Assessment*. 4th ed. New York, NY: Oxford University Press; 2004:792–806.

59. Kirkwood MW, Kirk JW, Blaha RZ, Wilson P. Noncredible effort during pediatric neuropsychological exam: a case series and literature review. *Child Neuropsychol.* 2010;16(6):604–618.

60. Slick DJ, Tan JE, Sherman EM, Strauss E. Malingering and related conditions in pediatric populations. In: David AS, ed. *Handbook of Pediatric Neuropsychology*. New York, NY: Oxford University Press; 2010:457–470.

61. Rogers RR. *Structured Interview of Reported Symptoms (SIRS-2)*. 2nd ed. Lutz, FL: Psychological Assessment Resources; 2010.

62. Smith GP. *Structured Inventory of Malingered Symptomatology (SIMS)*. Lutz, FL: Psychological Assessment Resources; 2003.

63. Miller HA. *Miller Forensic Assessment of Symptoms Test (M-FAST)*. Lutz, FL: Psychological Assessment Resources; 2001.

64. Tombaugh TN. *TOMM: Test of Memory Malingering*. Ontario, Canada: Multi-Health Ssystems; 1996.

65. Kirk JW, Harris B, Hutaff-Lee CF, Koelemay SW, Dinkins JP, Kirkwood MW. Performance on the test of memory malingering (TOMM) among a large clinic-referred pediatric sample. *Child Neuropsychol.* 2011;17(3):242–254.

66. Constantinou M, McCaffrey RJ. Using the TOMM for evaluating children's effort to perform optimally on neuropsychological measures. *Child Neuropsychol.* 2003;9(2):81–90.

67. Donders J. Performance on the test of memory malingering in a mixed pediatric sample. *Child Neuropsychol.* 2005;11(2):221–227.

68. MacAllister WS, Nakhutina L, Bender HA, Karantzoulis S, Carlson C. Assessing effort during neuropsychological evaluation with the TOMM in children and adolescents with epilepsy. *Child Neuropsychol.* 2009;15(6):521–531.

69. Green P. *Green's Word Memory Test for Windows: User's Manual*. Edmonton, Canada: Green's Publishing; 2003.

70. Allen LM III, Conder RL, Green P, Cox DR. *CARB '97: Manual for the Computerized Assessment of Response Bias*. Durham, NC: CogniSyst; 1997.

71. Allen LM III, Green P. Severe TBI Sample Performance on CARB and the WMT. (Supplement for the Computerized Assessment of Response Bias, Word Memory Test, and Memory Complaints Inventory). Durham, NC: CogniSyst; 1999.

72. Diller L, Ben-Yishay Y. Outcomes and evidence in neuropsychological rehabilitation in closed head injury. In: Levin J, Grafman HS, Eisenberg HM, eds. *Neurobehavioral Recovery From Head Injury*. New York, NY: Oxford University Press; 1987:146–165.

73. Ben-Yishay Y, Gold J. Therapeutic milieu approach to neuropsychological rehabilitation. In: Wood R, ed. *Neuro-behavioral Sequelae of Traumatic Brain Injury*. Hillsdale NJ: Erlbaum; 1990: 194–215

74. Ylvisaker M, Szekeres S, Haarbauer-Krupa J. Cognitive rehabilitation: organization, memory, and language. In: Ylvisaker M, ed. *Traumatic Brain Injury Rehabilitation: Children and Adolescents*. Boston, MA: Butterworth–Heinemann; 1998:181–220.

75. Diller L, Gordon WA. Interventions for cognitive deficits in brain-injured adults. *J Consult Clinical Psychol.* 1981;49(6):822–834.

76. Diller L, Gordon WA. Rehabilitation and clinical neuropsychology. In: Fiskov S, Bolls TJ, eds. *Handbood of Clinical Neuropsychology*. New York, NY: Wiley; 1981:702–733.

77. Trexler L. *Cognitive Rehabilitation: Conceptualization and Intervention*. New York, NY: Plenum Press; 1982.

78. Teeter PA. Neurocognitive interventions for childhood and adolescent disorders: a transactional model. In: Reynolds CR, Fletcher-Janzen E, eds. *Handbook of Clinical Child Neuropsychology*. 3rd ed. New York, NY: Springer Publishing; 2009:427–458.

79. Horton AM, Puente AE. Behavioral neuropsychology in children. In: Obrzut JE, Hynd GW, eds. *Child neuropsychology: Theory and Research. Clinical practice*. Vol 2. Orlando, FL: Academic Press; 1986: 299–316.

80. Teeter PA, Semrud-Clikeman M. Integrating neurobiological, psychosocial, and behavioral paradigms: a transactional model for the study of ADHD. *Arch Clin Neuropsychol.* 1995;10(5):433–461

81. Rourke B, Fisk J, Strang J. *The Neuropsychological Assessment of children: A Treatment-Oriented Approach*. New York, NY: Guildford Press; 1986.

82. Reitan R. *REHABIT—Reitan Evalution of Hemispheric Abilities and Brain Improvement Training*. Tucson, AZ: Neuropsychology Laboratory and University of Arizona; 1980.

83. Levin L. *Educational Care*. Cambridge, MA: Educators Publishing Service; 1994.

84. Vaughn S, McIntosh R, Hogan A. Why social skills training doesn't work: an alternative model. In: Scruggs TE, Wong BYL, eds. *Intervention Research in Learning Disabilties*. Berlin, Germany: Springer-Verlag; 1990:263–278.

85. Lloyd J, Landrum TJ. Self recording of attending to task: treament components and generalization of effects. In: Scruggs TE, Wong BYL, eds. *Intervention Research in Learning Disabilities*. Berlin, Germany: Springer-Verlag; 1990:235–262.

86. Heins E, Lloyd J, Hallahan D. Cued and noncued self-recording to task. *Behav Modif*. 1986;10(2):235–254.

87. Semrud-Clikeman M. *Attention Training for Children With Attentional-Hyperactive Problems*. San Francisco, CA: American Educational Research Association; 1995.

88. Greenwood C, Maheady L, Carta J. Peer tutoring programs in the regular education classroom. In: Stoner G, Shinn M, Walker H, eds. *Interventions for Achievement and Behavior Problems*. Silver Springs, MD: National Association of School Psychologists; 1991:179–200.

89. Kade H, Fletcher-Janzen E. Brain injury rehabilitation of children and youth: neurodevelopmental perspective. In: Reynolds C, Fletcher-Janzen E, eds. *Handbook of Clinical Child Neuropsychology*. New York, NY: Springer Publishing; 2009:459–504.

90. Prigatano G. Cognitive rehabitation: an impairment-oriented approach embedded in a holistic perspective. In: *NIH Consensus Development Conference on Rehabilitation of Persons With Traumatic Brain Injury*. Washington, DC: 1998;36–39.

91. Cicerone K, Dahlberg C, Malec J, et al. Evidence-based cognitive rehabilitation: updated review of the literature from 1998 through 2002. *Arch Phys Med Rehabil*. 2005;86(8):1681–1692

92. Slomine B, Locascio G. Cognitive rehabilitation for children with acquired brain injury. *Dev Disabil Res Rev*. 2009;15(2):133–143.

93. Laatsch HD, Harrington D, Hotz G, et al. An evidence-based review of cognitive and behavioral rehabilitation treatment studies in children with acquired brain injury. *J Head Trauma Rehabil*. 2007; 22(4):248–256.

94. Limond J, Leeke R. Practitioner review: cognitive rehabilitation for children with acquired brain injury. *J Child Psychol Psychiatry*. 2005; 46(4):339–352.

95. Manley T, Anderson V, Nimmo-Smith I, Turner A, Watson P, Robertson I. The differential assessment of children's attention: the Test of Everyday Attention for Children (TEA-Ch) normative sample and ADHD performance. *J Child Psychol Psychiatry*. 2002;42(8): 1065–1081.

96. Butler R, Copeland DR, Fairclough DL, et al. A multicenter, randomized clinical trial of a cogntive remediation program for childhood survivors of a pediatric malignancy. *J Consult Clin Psychol*. 2008;76(3):367–378.

97. Sohlberg MM, McLaughlin K, Pavese A, Heidrich A, Posner M. Evaluation of attention process training in persons with acquired brain injury. *J Clin Exp Neuropsychol*. 2000;22(5):656–676.

98. Sohlberg MM, Mateer C. *Attention Process Training APT-3: A Direct Attention Training Program for Persons With Acquired Brain Injury*. Youngsville, NC: Lash & Associates Publishing; 2010.

99. Cicerone K. What is cognitive rehabilitation? Panel II. Development of Cognitive Rehabilitation Therapy for TBI. In: Institute of Medicine, JFK—Johnson Rehabilitation Institute Conference Proceedings; February 7, 2011.

100. Hooft IV, Andersson K, Bergman B, Sejersen T, Von Wendt L, Bartfai A. Beneficial effect from a cognitive training programme on children with acquired brain injuries demonstrated in a controlled study. *Brain Inj*. 2005;19(7):511–518.

101. Brett AW, Laatsch L. Cognitive rehabilitation therapy of bain injured children in a public high school setting. *Pediatr Rehabil*. 1998; 2(1):27–31.

102. Wilson BA, Emslie HC, Quirk K, Evans JJ. Reducing everyday memory and planning problems by means of a paging system: a randomized control crossover study. *J Neurol Neurosurg Psychiatry*. 2001;70(4):477–482.

103. Levin H. Cognitive rehabilitation: unproved but promising. *Arch Neurol*. 1990;47(2): 223–224.

104. Cicerone K, Levin H, Malec J, Stuss D, Whyte J. Cognitive rehabilitation intervention for executive function: moving from bench to bedside in patients with traumatic brain injury. *J Cogn Neurosci*. 2006;18(7):1212–1222.

105. Malone E, Slomine B. Managing dysexecutive disorder. In: Hunter S, Donders J, eds. *Pediatric Neuropsychological Intervention*. New York, NY: Cambridge Press; 2011:287–313.

106. Levine B, Robertson IH, Clare L, et al. Rehabilitation of executive functioning: an experimental-clinical validation of goal management training. *J Int Neuropsychol Soc*. 2000;6(3):299–312.

107. Ylvisaker M, Turkstra L, Coehlo C, et al. Behavioural interventions for children and adults with behaviour disorders after TBI: a systematic review of the evidence. *Brain Inj*. 2007;21(8):769–805.

108. Horner RD, Carr EG, Halle J, McGee G, Odom S, Wolery M. The use of single-subject research to identify evidence-based practice in special education. *Excep Chil*. 2005;71:165–180.

109. Glang A, Singer G, Cooley E, Tish N. Tailoring direct instruction techniques for use with elementary students with traumatic brain injury. *J Head Trauma Rehabil*. 1992;7(4):93–108.

110. Glang A, Ylvisaker M, Stein M, Ehlhardt L, Todis B, Tyler J. Validated instructional practices: application to students with traumatic brain injury. *J Head Trauma Rehabil*. 2008;23(4):243–251.

111. Suzman KB, Morris RD, Morris MK, Milan MA. Cognitive-behavioral remediation of problem solving deficits in children with acquired brain injury. *J Behav Ther Exp Psychiatry*. 1997;28(3):203–212.

112. Selznick L, Savage R. Using self-monitoring procedures to increase on-task behaviors with three adolescent boys with brain injury. *Behav Intervent*. 2000;15:243–260.

113. Feeney T, Ylvisaker M. Context sensitive cognitive-behavioural supports for young children with TBI: a replication study. *Brain Inj*. 2006;20(96):629–645.

114. Feeney T, Ylvisaker M. Context-sensitive behavioral supports for young children with TBI: short-term effects and long-term outcomes. *J Head Trauma Rehabil*. 2003;18(1):33–51.

115. Winkler D, Unsworth C, Sloan S. Factors that lead to successful community integration following severe traumatic brain injury. *J Head Trauma Rehabil*. 2006;21(1):8–21.

116. Wade SL, Michaud L, Brown TM. Putting the pieces together: preliminary efficacy of a family problem-solving intervention for children with traumatic brain injury. *J Head Trauma Rehabil*. 2006;21(1): 57–67.

117. Braga LW, Da Paz AC, Ylvisaker M. Direct clinician-delivered versus indirect family-supported rehabilitation of children with traumatic brain injury: a randomized controlled trial. *Brain Inj*. 2004; 19(10):819–831.

118. Ponsford J, Willmott C, Rothwell A, et al. Impact of early intervention on outcome after mild traumatic brain injury in children. *Pediatrics*. 2001;108(6):1297–1303.

119. Brown G, Chadwick O, Shaffer D, Rutter M, Traub M. A prospective study of children with head injuries: III. Psychiatric sequelae. *Psychol Med*. 1981;11(1):63–78.

120. Thurneck DA, Warner PJ, Cobb HC. Children and adolescents with disabilities and health care needs: Implications for intervention. In: Thompson PH, Brown D, eds. *Counseling and Psychotherapy With Children and Adolescents Theory and Practice for School and Clinical Settings*. 4th ed. Hoboken, NJ: John Wiley & Sons; 2007:419–454.

121. Prigatano G, Naar-King S. Neuropsychological rehabilitation of school-age children: an integrated team approach to individualized interventions. In: Hunter S, Donders J, eds. *Pediatric Neuropsychological Intervention*. New York, NY: Cambridge University Press; 2007:465–476.

122. Luria AR. *Restoration of Function After Brain Injury*. Oxford, NY: Pergamon Press; 1963.

123. Prigatano G. *Principles of Neuropsychological Rehabilitation*. New York, NY: Oxford University Press; 1999.

124. Prigatano G. Neuropsychological rehabilitation. In: Weiner IB, Craighead WE, eds. *Corsini Encyclopedia of Psychology*. Vol 2. 4th ed. Hoboken, NJ: Wiley; 2010:1082–1084.

125. Elbaum J. Counseling individuals post acquired brain injury: consideration and objectives. In: Elbaum J, Benson DM, eds. *Acquired Brain Injury. An Integrative Neuro-rehabilitation Approach*. New York, NY: Springer Publishing; 2007:259–273.

126. Mateer CA, Sira CS, O'Connell ME. Putting Humpty Dumpty together again: the importance of integrating cognitive and emotional interventions. *J Head Trauma Rehabil.* 2005;20(1):62–75.

127. Prigatano G, Schacter D. *Awareness of Deficits After Brain Injury.* New York, NY: Oxford University Press; 1991.

128. Sherer M. Rehabilitation of impaired awareness. In: High WM Jr, Sander AM, Struchen MA, Hart KA, eds. *Rehabilitation of Traumatic Brain Injury.* New York, NY: Oxford University Press; 2005.

129. Evans CC, Sherer M, Nick TG, Nakase-Richardson R, Yablon SA. Early impaired self-awareness, depression, and subjective well-being following traumatic brain injury. *J Head Trauma Rehabil.* 2005; 20(6):488–500.

130. Crosson BP, Barco BP, Velozo C, et al. Awareness and compensation in post acute head injury rehabilitation. *J Head Trauma Rehabil.* 1989;4(3):46–54.

131. Alderfer B, Arciniegas D, Silver J. Treatment of depression following traumatic brain injury. *J Head Trauma Rehabil.* 2005;20(6): 544–562.

132. Scicutella A. Neuropsychiatry of traumatic brain injury. In: Elbaum J, ed. *Counseling Individuals Post Acquired Brain Injury.* New York, NY: Springer Publishing; 2007:81–120.

133. Bagueley IJ, Cooper J, Felmingham K. Aggressive behavior following traumatic brain injury: how common is common? *J Head Trauma Rehabil.* 2006;21(1):45–56.

134. Medd J, Tate RL. Evaluation of an anger management therapy program following acquired brain injury: a preliminary study. *Neuropsychol Rehabil.* 2000;10:185–201.

135. Giles GM, Manchester D. Two Approaches to disorder after traumatic brain injury. *J Head Trauma Rehabil.* 2006;21(2):168–178.

136. Slifer KJ, Amari A. Behavior management for children and adolescents with acquired brain injury. *Dev Disabil Res Rev.* 2009;15(2): 144–151.

137. Eyberg C, Boggs SR, Algina J. Parent–child interaction therapy: a psychosocial model for the treatment of young children with conduct problem behavior and their families. *Psychopharmacol Bull.* 1995;l31(1):83–91.

138. Cohen M, Heaton SC, Ginn N, Eyberg SM. Parent–child interaction therapy as a family-oriented approach to behavioral management following pediatric traumatic brain injury: a case report. *J Pediatric Psychol.* 2012;37(3):251–261.

139. Brain Injury Alliance of New Jersey. *Tips for the Caregiver.* North Brunswick, NJ: Brain Injury Alliance of New Jersey, Inc; date unkown.

Educational Issues and School Reentry for Students With Traumatic Brain Injury

Ann Glang, Debbie Ettel, Janet Siantz Tyler, and Bonnie Todis

INTRODUCTION

Each year, approximately 40% of traumatic brain injuries (TBIs) in the United States occur in the pediatric population (ages 0–19 years) (1). The Centers for Disease Control (CDC) estimates that more than 60,000 children and adolescents are hospitalized annually in the United States after sustaining moderate-to-severe brain injuries from motor vehicle crashes, falls, sports, and physical abuse; an additional 631,146 children are seen in hospital emergency departments and released (1). In all, nearly 145,000 children aged 0–19 years are currently living with long-lasting, significant alterations in social, behavioral, physical, and cognitive functioning following a TBI (2).

Reduced federal funding and managed care have resulted in shorter inpatient rehabilitation stays for patients, fewer services dedicated to families, and lack of access to ongoing rehabilitative services (3,4). Increasingly, children with mild-to-moderate TBI are released from treatment with no plans for long-term rehabilitation support. The result is that children who may have intense physical and/or cognitive needs return home to families who are largely responsible for supporting them through the rehabilitation process with little or no support from medical or community-based agencies (5,6). As a function of shortened hospital stays and the chronic problems arising from pediatric TBI, the primary service provider for children and adolescents has become the school. This chapter will describe the challenges students with TBI present to schools and strategies schools can use to address them.

OVERVIEW OF IMPACT OF TBI ON SCHOOL PERFORMANCE

Predicting the impact of a pediatric TBI on school performance is difficult, in part because no 2 injuries are alike, and also because the same etiological factor can cause diverse outcomes depending on the child and the context. Researchers (7) suggest that several variables influence student outcomes, including (a) the child's age at injury (8), (b) the severity of the TBI (9), (c) premorbid behavioral and learning status (10,11), (d) history of previous injury (12–15), and (e) postinjury pain or stress (16,17).

Academic Achievement, Executive Dysfunction, and Social Behavior Problems

Although the impact of pediatric TBI on a child's school performance is unique and dynamic, some general characteristics typify the course of impact and recovery (7). The most reported TBI sequelae related to school performance are (a) a progressive lag in academic achievement (18–21), (b) executive dysfunction, and (c) social and behavioral problems (22–24).

Academic Achievement

Most children make academic gains postinjury, but for students with moderate to severe injury, the rate of academic achievement gains tends to slow progressively over time, and the effects are long-term (18,25,26). Researchers (27) found that children with moderate TBI showed impaired academic skills both postacutely and chronically, whereas those with severe TBI showed greater impairment with only partial recovery in certain areas over time. One critical factor in children's lag in academic achievement was cognitive deficit as a result of brain injury.

In young children with TBI, recovery of cognitive skills across time may show no improvement (28) or may actually decline (29), demonstrating a failure to develop age-appropriate cognitive skills at typical rates. These cognitive deficits can be parsed into components of executive dysfunction, memory problems, diminished attention and impulse control, and information processing problems, all areas critical to learning and school success (30–32). Notably, some effects are immediate, and some sequelae may not become apparent until the child returns to the school environment or much later, when the demands for competence in reasoning, executive functioning, self-regulation, and social skills increase (33,34). Because TBI cognitive sequelae are diverse and dynamic, educator awareness is critical to providing students with appropriate monitoring and support as needs and issues change, sometimes dramatically, over time.

Executive Dysfunction

Disruptions in executive function (EF), characterized by skills in attentional control, planning, goal setting, problem solving, cognitive flexibility, and abstract reasoning, can occur as a result of direct damage to frontal regions or from disruption of connections among these and other brain regions. Because EF orchestrates so many domains of cognition, emotion, and behavior, the functional results of executive dysfunction are multidimensional and debilitating (35–37).

At the root of many of the academic, social emotional, and behavioral issues that can follow a TBI are problems with self-regulation, the internal control functions that direct and organize all nonreflexive or nonautomatic behavior, including social, cognitive, and linguistic behavior (38). The same regulatory deficits that underlie learning problems (e.g., trouble focusing on classroom work, irritability, and impulsiveness) can also negatively affect social-emotional behavior and interpersonal relationships with peers and adults (39–42). For example, self-regulation skills required in a school setting include keeping hands and feet to oneself, taking turns in a conversation, and maintaining an emotional state appropriate to the school context. Neural systems that regulate these behaviors might be compromised, making both appropriate academic behavior and interpersonal behavior challenging for students.

In a school setting, deficits in EF can manifest as impulsiveness, poor social judgment, disorganization, social disinhibition, weakly regulated attention, slowed processing, ineffective planning, and reduced initiation (31,33). Because of difficulty with organization and attention, educators might observe students having problems managing their assignments, gathering materials, starting on tasks, or staying on task. In addition, some students struggle with transitions from one class to the next, and they might have difficulty sequencing multistep procedures or recalling assignments. Thus, executive dysfunction in the classroom presents myriad challenges for students with TBI.

After TBI, students may perform poorly on tasks of sustained, selective, and shifting attention (43). A student may have difficulty concentrating for extended periods, performing 2 tasks simultaneously (such as listening while taking notes), or completing 1 task and switching attention to a new task. Lack of attentional flexibility can also result in diminished problem solving skills. For example, a student who loses a pencil might not be able to generate problem-solving ideas for replacing it. Both initiation skills and attentional flexibility are needed to keep the lack of a pencil from being an insurmountable barrier to work completion. For children with mild injury, inattention and behavior challenges are the most frequently reported problems (44).

The speed with which students process information may change dramatically after a TBI (43). Students may take longer to respond to teacher questions or instructions, or they may need longer to complete tasks or process teacher directions. This greater response latency can be misinterpreted as refusal to respond or begin work. Students should be allowed adequate time to process and comprehend assignments (45). Language production and processing can also be impaired, resulting in problems in word finding, language fluency, receptive language comprehension, reading comprehension, and writing skills.

TBI often results in memory problems (sensory, working, and/or long-term memory; retrograde and anterior grade amnesia) that can negatively affect the assimilation of new material or skills (46–48). It has been found (49) that among young children, skills emerging at the time of brain injury were more vulnerable to disruption than skills already learned. Previously learned skills might be intact or compromised, and difficulties with working memory can negatively affect the child's ability to learn new material. Educators might notice uneven academic performance, with some lower level skills missing while more sophisticated skills remain intact, making appropriate instruction more challenging.

Social Behavioral Problems

Social dysfunction might be the most debilitating of all the TBI sequelae, affecting not only functional aspects of daily living but also quality of life (50). Unfortunately, much of the research focus has been on the effect of TBI on physical and cognitive domains, and social-emotional skills have not received as much attention. Children with an early brain injury (especially before 2 years of age) are at risk of significant social impairment (50). Social and emotional problems can become increasingly apparent during the transition from childhood to adolescence, when expectations for the use of appropriate social skills increase (51–53). Students with TBI might display disruptive behavior, emotional distress, poor conduct, and problems with empathy, moral reasoning, and peer relationships (35). Addressing potential social behavior deficits is just as critical to successful school functioning as addressing academic and cognitive skills—perhaps more so (54–56).

Sometimes overlooked is the emotional grief, sadness, or anger resulting from loss of preinjury abilities or identity. Even years after their injury, adults who sustained a childhood TBI report differences in self-concept postinjury, with the current self viewed more negatively than the preinjury self, and development of new identity as an ongoing process (57). Unfortunately, counseling or therapeutic support addressing post-traumatic stress or grief is often lacking for students with TBI. Grief and recovery from emotional trauma, especially when combined with poor impulse control, can lead to unpredictable emotional outbursts, irritability, labile affect, and depression. Educators might observe social withdrawal behaviors, poor adaptive behaviors, or apparent egocentrism as a result (58,59). The combination of these deficits can also result in problems with delinquency if not identified and addressed with appropriate intervention and support. High rates of incarceration among people with TBI have been noted (60).

A commonly noticed area of concern is lack of self-awareness, particularly of students' own skill deficits. For example, a student might express an emotional response inappropriate for a given situation (e.g., laughing when discussing a serious topic) and remain unaware of the inappropriateness of the action despite negative reactions from peers. These deficits in insight can cause misperceptions or distortions of social cues and interactions, affecting how the student relates to others or interprets their intentions and behaviors, resulting in confusion, misunderstanding, and conflict. Peers may be frustrated with the student if he or she misses important social cues, fails to regulate behaviors such as talking out of turn, or denies postinjury deficits and rejects support offered. Ironically, some research (58) has found awareness of the discrepancy between the preinjury and current (postinjury) self negatively correlated with self-esteem and positively correlated with depression; that is, lack of self-awareness is associated with 1 set of problems, whereas increased awareness has its own array of psychological costs (61).

Other functional areas pertinent to school performance include perceptual skill deficits and physical impairment. Sensorimotor changes can occur, resulting in increased sensitivity to environmental stimuli such as hypersensitivity to light and sound or diminished ability to screen out background sounds. For example, students who once had no difficulty copying notes from a blackboard might find the task coordination difficult because of visual–motor changes (62,63). Classrooms are highly stimulating environments—visually, aurally, and kinesthetically—that can overtax the cognitive abilities of a student in recovery from a brain injury. A student with poor impulse control might react inappropriately to such stimuli.

Educators also need to be aware that students can experience extreme fatigue (64), especially early in the postacute recovery phase when ordinary tasks might require greater mental exertion by the student because of difficulty in processing, organizing, initiating, and maintaining academic engagement. The student's physical stamina might be compromised, requiring increased rest or shortened school days or class periods to address fatigue and support the recovery process. In addition to fatigue, the student might have sustained other physical injuries that can adversely affect school performance. Furthermore, anticonvulsant or other medications may be prescribed prophylactically to reduce the likelihood of seizures or address behavioral or attentional concerns. Educators should be made aware of the intended and unintended effects of any such prescriptions on student behavior, attention, mood, and learning (65).

Mediating and Moderating Factors

Several factors have been found to mediate and moderate the effects of TBI on school performance. The most commonly noted factors include (a) age at injury, (b) severity of injury, and (c) family environment.

Age at Injury
It was previously thought that the developing brain was more resilient to trauma because of neuroplasticity, the flexibility of the young brain to reorganize or reassign tasks from one functional area to another area (66,67). Newer evidence has shown that early injury is associated with poorer outcomes than later injury (29,49,68). As young children with TBI develop, behavioral and cognitive problems might continue to emerge (51,69).

Other specific outcomes associated with early injury include deficits in executive functioning, expressive language, attention, academic achievement, and social skills, and less recovery of cognitive skills compared with children injured later (18,29,68,70–73). Longitudinal studies have shown that early age at injury negatively impacts outcomes in likelihood of postsecondary education enrollment, employment, and independent living. Early age at injury and severe injury were associated with employment in primarily entry level or low-skilled jobs, fewer hours worked per week, and lower pay for both males and females (29,68).

Injury Severity
In young children with TBI, severity of injury also predicted postacute effects on cognitive and school readiness skills, including memory, spatial reasoning, and EF. More severe TBI predicted more negative outcomes (74–78). However, some studies found mixed results of the impact of injury severity on outcomes, with severity of injury becoming less predictive of outcomes 1 year postinjury (79). A severe injury at an early age has been associated with the poorest long-term outcomes, including cognitive skill recovery (24,68,80).

Family Environment
Particularly in relation to social and behavioral outcomes, family environmental characteristics—such as socioeconomic status (SES), overall family functioning, and parenting behavior—can significantly affect student educational performance (26,32,55,81–84). Premorbid child and family functioning have been linked to outcomes; children with prior psychiatric disorders and families already struggling are more likely to manifest negative postinjury psychosocial effects (80,85–90). Negative social outcomes from TBI are exacerbated by postinjury family environments that are lower SES, lacking resources, and have poorer family functioning (55). Other researchers (84) reported a "double hazard" effect in which family socioeconomic disadvantage combined with severe injury to lead to the poorest long-term outcomes. Although family variables can moderate psychosocial outcomes for children with TBI (especially behavioral adjustment and social competencies), this moderating influence can wane with time among children with severe TBI (74,91).

Specific parenting behaviors have also been associated with children's outcomes after TBI. It was found (74) that high levels of permissive or authoritarian parenting were associated with increased behavior problems in children with TBI, particularly for those with severe injury. Poorer outcomes associated with these parenting styles are in contrast to those from *authoritative* parenting, characterized by parental warmth, clear boundaries and expectations, consistent rule application, and active parental monitoring. Authoritative parenting was associated with better psychosocial outcomes (74). In general, strong family social support and cohesion was predictive of students' better adaptive functioning, social competence, and global functioning postinjury (26,82). Other family variables believed to interact with factors predicting recovery include family expectations, stress and functioning (32,92–94), and genetic vulnerability (95,96). These factors interact with each other to mediate effects, but all predictors also directly affect all outcomes (74).

Outcomes by Age Group

Preschool-Aged Children
Young children (birth to age 5) who experience a TBI are at greater risk for deficits in expressive language, attention, and academic achievement than children who are injured at later ages (18,29,63,68,71,74,97). An early injury affects a developing brain that has not yet formed critical features necessary for mature function, potentially interrupting or hindering the developmental process. Some suggest that poorer outcomes in children injured early in life might be caused by the developing brain's greater susceptibility to diffuse brain

insult, resultant abnormalities in neurogenesis, or resultant difficulties in acquiring new skills postinjury (18,70,71,98,99). Some researchers (70) have stressed the link between early developmental level and TBI; those injured very young demonstrate persistent deficits in academic skills (reading, decoding, comprehension, spelling, and arithmetic). Difficulties in global cognitive function, adaptive behavior, EF, and nonverbal abilities have been observed as well (74,97). Others (74) have found that preschool-aged children with TBI had weaknesses in nonverbal abilities and EF and recommended the use of memory cues and direct instruction teaching methods—structured curricula, multiple presentations, and many opportunities for students to practice new skills.

Children injured when young might present no immediately observable deficits; however, such children should be monitored for the potential emergence of latent TBI sequelae that might appear as task and setting demands increase. For example, behavior difficulties after early injury may not be apparent until the child attends elementary school, when expectations for self-regulation, control of attention, and task complexity rise appreciably (100).

School-Aged Youth

Issues for school-aged youth with TBI (grades K–12) become heightened as the task and setting demands of school progressively increase. Some (88) have found that children who sustained moderate-to-severe TBI during their school years were likely to need special assistance in school at 1 year postinjury. Others (101) reported that reading skills are often compromised by TBI, and still others have found greater academic deficits in arithmetic, possibly because of arithmetic's necessary component skills in attention, memory, and executive functioning (102). Students are expected to become more independent learners, demonstrate self-regulatory skills (staying on task, completing work, keeping hands to self, answering when called on), and master increasingly complex skills and more abstract concepts. For the school-aged child with TBI, these can all present challenges in the school setting. In addition to the academic expectations, the child's social focus shifts from family to peers, where interpersonal social skills take on increasing importance and begin to include communication, negotiation, reciprocal interaction, and social participation (54,56,103). In summary, educators need to be aware that school-aged youth with TBI might be challenged by the increasing cognitive, academic, and behavioral demands in the school setting and by the increasing importance and complexity of their developing social relations with peers.

Post-High School Outcomes

A growing body of research indicates that for many students with TBI, post-high school outcomes are poor (68,104–106). The second National Longitudinal Transition Study (108) found that fewer than half of students with TBI who had been out of school a year or more had a paid job outside the home. Young adults (ages 18 years or older) with TBI who received special education were employed and enrolled in postsecondary education at lower rates than peers in the general population (107).

Furthermore, rates of engagement in employment and postsecondary training and education remain low through-

out early adulthood. In a recent longitudinal study of post-high school outcomes (68), the highest rate of enrollment in postsecondary education was 34% at age 21. Enrollment decreased with being male, earlier age at injury, and lower SES (68). A key finding was that although few students injured before age 14 enrolled in postsecondary education, students who sustained a TBI during adolescence attempted to pursue their preinjury college plans, often with negative results. Unable to meet academic, social, and independent living demands, many study participants struggled for several years before leaving college without degrees. A few were able to set new goals, discover helpful strategies, and eventually complete 2- or 4-year degree programs (106). Participants in the same study also experienced challenges in the area of employment, working fewer hours for lower wages than their nondisabled peers. None of the student participants worked more than 30 hours per week, and wages averaged slightly above minimum wage. At age 25, most still worked at entry level or low-skilled jobs as their nondisabled peers were moving up to higher paid, skilled, and professional positions (108). Earlier age at injury and more severe injury were associated with fewer hours worked per week and lower pay (68).

In a qualitative study with the same study sample, receipt of postsecondary transition services (in which individuals were linked with support agencies and disability services) was associated with completion of postsecondary programs (106). Focus on the modifiable variables that affect postsecondary outcomes is important for improving the lives of students with TBI.

MODIFIABLE FACTORS IN TBI OUTCOMES

In addition to child- and family-centered factors, a range of other external or environmental variables affect outcomes among children with brain injury. Challenging as it can be to address these factors, they hold promise for improving outcomes for students with TBI because they can be modified through improved training and changes in policy and practice.

Lack of Educator Awareness

Effective educational practices implemented by trained educators can contribute to successful school outcomes for children and youth with TBI (106). However, many teachers receive little or no training in childhood TBI (119,110). In a recent survey of educators working with students with TBI, 92% reported having no training in the academic effects of TBI (111). Furthermore, a recent analysis of university textbooks revealed that TBI is rarely discussed in current special education texts and is virtually absent from the general education texts reviewed (112). The lack of information about TBI for educators leads to a continued lack of awareness about the school-related implications of TBI and absence of strategies for addressing them. This lack of awareness leads to a perception among school personnel that TBI is a "low-incidence disability," which in turn contributes to the under-identification of children with TBI for special education.

Underidentification and Misidentification

The most recent special education census data suggest that there continues to be a significant discrepancy between the incidence of TBI and the identification of children with TBI for special education services (113). Approximately 145,000 children live with persistent disability following TBI (2). However, according to the most recent figures from the US Department of Education, the total number of students receiving special education services under the TBI category is 23,509 (114). This rate is likely an underestimate, given that 60,000 children are hospitalized each year for TBI (1). Rates of identification for special education are higher for students with severe TBI, problem behavior, poor academic performance, and socioeconomic disadvantage (88,115–118). Of particular concern, given the changing needs of children as they grow older and school demands increase, is that special education identification rarely occurs after the first year post-injury (118). Although it is likely that some children with TBI receive services under different disability labels (e.g., speech-language, physical disability, or "other") (118–120), it is unclear whether such services meet the cognitive and behavioral needs of students with TBI. Because most children with TBI rely on schools rather than medical settings for rehabilitation services, the underidentification and misidentification of children with TBI presents a significant obstacle to the provision of effective services.

Lack of Hospital–School Communication

There continues to be a weak link between the hospitals that treat children for TBI and the schools who educate them—in terms of both their respective understanding of one another's worlds and their mutual communication and coordination efforts (121,122). Between April 1994 and January 1999, the National Pediatric Trauma Registry tracked children ages 5–19 who were hospitalized with TBI in participating trauma centers and children's hospitals across the United States and who were discharged to their homes following treatment. Of this group, 13.2% had documented cognitive impairments resulting from their brain injury at the time of discharge, and 11.6% had behavioral impairments; yet less than 1% of these children were recommended by medical staff for referral to special education (121). A critical modifiable factor contributing to identification of students with TBI for formal services is communication and linkage between hospitals and schools. Although informing educators that a student has a TBI does not guarantee that appropriate services will follow, *not* being informed by hospital personnel or parents decreases the likelihood that educational services will be tailored to the student's specific needs (122).

Parent–Educator Relationships

A critical factor that influences school outcomes for children with TBI is the degree of collaboration between the child's parents and educators (123). When parents and educators have trouble working in partnership, conflicts arise, and the student's education suffers (124–126). Unfortunately, parent–professional relationships can easily become adversarial because of the many stressors both families and school staff face in designing educational programs for students with TBI. From the school's perspective, families often have unrealistic expectations and/or are unable to support the school's efforts (127). Parents, on the other hand, often retain preinjury expectations about academic achievement and perceive school staff as having low expectations that do not change, even as the child's school performance improves (127). Furthermore, because prior to the injury, most children with TBI progressed typically through school, parents are often unfamiliar with the provisions of the Individuals with Disabilities Education Act and their role and rights in the educational process.

EFFECTIVE EDUCATIONAL PRACTICES

Because of the physical, cognitive, academic, and psychosocial sequelae of TBI, students may require special education services, special assistance, or accommodations on returning to school, with many students continuing to require such services throughout their education. From the hospital-to-school transition to the post-high school transition to community-based services, training, and employment, the hub of the support system for students with TBI and their families is the school.

Coordinated Hospital-to-School Transition

One of the most critical points in a child's rehabilitation process is at the transition from hospital to school. It is at this point that the child can most easily gain access to formal services through communication between hospital and school staff (122). Recommendations regarding school reentry planning include having school personnel observe the student in the hospital, attend hospital predischarge meetings, and obtain information from the hospital before the child's school reentry (128–130). Although it may be difficult under managed care for hospital staff to fully participate in the transition process, the hospital–school communication link should begin early in the child's hospital stay, so that protocols are in place for hospital staff to alert school staff to those students with brain injuries, even those with mild injury (131,132). Referral is also needed for students who were already receiving special education services at the time of their injury (e.g., for a learning disability or a behavior disorder), as moderate-to-severe TBI can cause significant additional cognitive impairment in children with preexisting learning difficulties, and programming modifications are often needed after injury (133).

The Individuals with Disabilities Education Improvement Act of 2004 (IDEA) (134), provides guidelines for referral, evaluation, eligibility determination, parent involvement in decision-making, individual education plans, and delivery of specially designed instruction and related services.

Given the eligibility requirements of IDEA, and the current underidentification of students with TBI, TBI researchers and advocates are exploring ways to assure that all students with TBI who need special education services are able to access them. Recent research has demonstrated that in addition to severity of injury, the provision of hospital–school transition services is strongly related to being identified for formal services (either via individual education plan [IEP] or 504 plan) (128). Although hospital-to-school transition support emerged in this study as a strong predictor of being identified for formal special education services, only half (50.9%) of students in this study received any form of transition information or guidance from the hospital. Stated briefly, informing educators that a student has TBI does not guarantee that appropriate services will follow, but *not* being informed by hospital personnel or parents decreases the likelihood that educational services will be tailored to a student's specific needs.

Two promising practices are currently being evaluated and could improve identification processes at the state level. The School Transition Re-entry Program (STEP) is a systematic notification system designed to increase effective transition from hospital to school (135). Essential elements of this model are (*a*) hospital staff obtain a release from parents and notify an identified contact at the state Department of Education (DOE) about the child, (*b*) DOE notifies a regional transition facilitator that a child who has been treated for TBI is returning to school in that region, and (*c*) the transition facilitator contacts the child's school and family to offer resources and support. Preliminary analyses suggest that among students who do not receive hospital rehabilitation services, students receiving STEP services—systematic transition from hospital to school—are identified significantly more often for special education than those who do not receive systematic transition. Furthermore, students in the STEP group received more services, and their parents reported significantly greater satisfaction with the school and found a greater number of school staff helpful compared with parents of students in the control group (135). Thus, the STEP intervention appears to provide the essential link from hospital to school previously available only to students receiving rehabilitation services.

A second promising approach systematically tracks and supports students with mild TBIs as they transition back to school athletic and academic activities. The Reduce, Educate, Accommodate and Pace (REAP) model is a systematic notification system to increase effective concussion management from emergency department to school (www.youthsportsmed.com). A person at the emergency department obtains a release from the family and provides the REAP manual of concussion management. That person then faxes the release and an information form to an identified contact at a centralized site. The centralized site contacts a point person at the child's school within 48 hours. The point person then coordinates concussion management within the school until the child recovers, tracking and monitoring for latent concerns. Concussion management may also include providing information on physical and academic accommodations and other ways educators can reduce the cognitive, emotional, and physical load on students recovering from mild TBI.

These are 2 models of systematic communication between hospitals and schools. Central to both models is the presence of school-based professionals trained in TBI who can ensure the student receives the support necessary to succeed in school.

Special Education Law

When the provision of special education in public schools became federal law in 1975 (136), guaranteeing all students a "free and appropriate public education," no specific category for TBI was included. TBI was not introduced as a separate disability category until 1991 in IDEA. Before that time, students with TBI were identified for special education as "other health impaired" or under a specific learning disability. Some students received services under Section 504 of the Rehabilitation Act of 1973, and others were not served through either mechanism (122). Given the long-term effects of underidentifying students with TBI for special education services (137–139), accurate and appropriate assessment is critical to identify and address students' needs for educational support (119,140).

Referral Process

Parents, teachers, therapists, medical personnel, or others can begin the process of evaluating the child's educational needs by making a referral to the school's support services team or administrator. The team—made up of teachers, specialists, administrators, and others—is charged with evaluating the child's educational needs in all areas of suspected disability and determining whether the student meets eligibility criteria (as a child with a disability) to receive special education services. Each category of disability has specific eligibility criteria in the law.

Eligibility for Special Education Services

To determine whether a child is eligible for services, an evaluation based on the guidelines specific to the area of suspected disability must be conducted. The evaluation requirements for TBI are outlined in Table 37-1.

Issues in Assessment and Instruction of Students With TBI

Because of the diversity within the population of students with TBI, there is no *one* TBI assessment; each assessment must be tailored to the student's unique and changing needs. Several general principles and strategies, however, are recommended to guide educators (34,131,138,142,143). First, accurate interpretation of assessment results requires an understanding of the potential effects of TBI on students' learning and response patterns. For example, students' performance may be uneven across academic domains. They might show relatively strong performance on material mastered preinjury, although evidence of new learning could be lacking. Also, because content and skill gaps could be present throughout the range of skills, examiners might need to suspend typical basal and ceiling rules of standardized measures to more accurately capture student performance.

Second, the potential for both skill recovery and skill deterioration over time makes ongoing formative assessment and frequent monitoring especially important for students with TBI (144,145). Educators should rely on ecologically valid sources of information, such as parent and teacher behavior scales and interviews, curriculum-based assessment, and permanent product evaluation, and they should choose methods closely tied to instruction and intervention (138,146). In addition to being more relevant to instruction, these measures are more sensitive to small changes in student performance and could prove more beneficial to

TABLE 37-1 IDEA Criteria for Special Education Eligibility Under Traumatic Brain Injury

	IDEA CRITERIA FOR ELIGIBILITY UNDER TRAUMATIC BRAIN INJURY
Definition of TBI	An acquired injury to the brain caused by an external physical force resulting in total or partial functional disability or psychosocial impairment, or both, that adversely affects a child's educational performance. The term applies to open or closed head injuries resulting in impairments in one or more areas, such as cognition; language; memory; attention; reasoning; abstract thinking; judgment; problem-solving; sensory, perceptual, and motor abilities; psychosocial behavior; physical functions; information processing; and speech. The term does not apply to brain injuries that are congenital or degenerative, or to brain injuries induced by birth trauma.

Evaluation must include	(a) A medical or health assessment statement indicating that an event may have resulted in a TBI.
	(b) A comprehensive psychological assessment, using a battery of instruments to identify deficits associated with TBI, administered by a licensed school psychologist or the state Board of Psychological Examiners or others having training and experience to administer and interpret tests in the battery.
	(c) Other assessments, *as needed*, such as motor, communication, and psychosocial assessments
	  (A) Other information related to the child's suspected disability, including preinjury performance and a current measure of adaptive ability.
	  (B) Observation in the classroom and at least 1 other setting.
	  (C) Other additional assessments needed to determine the effect of the suspected disability on the child's educational performance for his/her age group.
	  (D) Other assessments needed to identify the child's educational needs.

Conditions must be met	(a) Must have an acquired brain injury caused by external physical force
	(b) Condition is permanent or expected to last for more than 60 calendar days
	(c) Injury results in an impairment in 1 or more areas:
	  (A) Communication
	  (B) Behavior
	  (C) Cognition, memory, attention, abstract thinking, judgment, problem-solving, reasoning, and/or information processing
	  (D) Sensory, perceptual, motor, and/or physical abilities

The evaluation must determine	(a) The child's disability has an adverse effect on the child's educational performance (b) The child needs special education services as a result of the disability
Definition of TBI excludes	Brain injuries that are congenital, degenerative, or induced by birth trauma

From idea.ed.gov (141).

student progress than norm-based measures standardized on noninjured student populations.

Third, schools could consider bringing neuropsychological experts into the planning process by including independent neuropsychologists in the assessment of and planning for students. The neuropsychologist's expertise in the clinical and neuropsychological aspects of functioning after TBI combined with the school psychologists' familiarity with academic assessment, instruction, and contextual issues within the school setting makes for a comprehensive assessment team (146,147). Also, building the capacity of existing staff by offering further neuropsychological training for school psychologists and others and improving in-service for staff to include basic information on the cognitive, academic, and behavioral profiles of students with TBI can increase the capacity of the broader school community (rather than a few select individuals) to support these students' unique needs across contexts.

Fourth, contextual assessment is a good framework for assessing the student with TBI in the educational setting (138,148). Contextual assessment, also referred to as ecological assessment (149), stresses the importance of multisource, multidimensional assessment, gathering relevant informa-

tion about the child's strengths and needs including (*a*) observations within the school setting; (*b*) parent interviews; (*c*) review of medical records; (*d*) file review of preinjury performance; (*e*) interviews with medical personnel, including rehabilitation teachers and home instruction staff; (*f*) behavior rating scales and checklists; (*g*) motor, sensory, and physical assessments as needed; (*h*) standardized and curriculum-based performance measures; and (*i*) adaptive behavior (146,147,150). Adaptive behaviors or activities of daily living are not routinely assessed in the school setting apart from evaluations for students with serious developmental delay. For students with TBI, the activities of daily living (e.g., independent skills in walking, talking, getting dressed, going to school, going to work, preparing a meal, cleaning the house, and adapting to the demands of one's environment) might be compromised by injury and need to be addressed.

Comprehensive Assessment

Within the student's school, home, and community, functional domains to be assessed include cognition, language, memory and concentration, sensory recognition and percep-

TABLE 37-2 Tests Commonly Used With Students With Traumatic Brain Injury

DOMAIN	TEST
Cognition	• Cognitive Assessment System (152) • Comprehensive Test of Nonverbal Intelligence, 2nd ed. (153) • Differential Abilities Scale, 2nd ed. (154) • Kaufman Assessment Battery for Children, 2nd ed. (155) • Stanford-Binet Intelligence Scales, 5th ed. (156) • Wechsler Preschool and Primary Scale of Intelligence, 3rd ed. (157) • Wechsler Abbreviated Scale of Intelligence (WASI) (158) • Wechsler Intelligence Scale for Children, 4th ed. (159) • Woodcock Johnson, 3rd ed.; Tests of Cognitive Abilities (160)
Neurospsychological	• Children's Category Test (161) • Functional Independence Measure (FIM) (162) • ImPACT (Immediate Postconcussion Assessment and Cognitive Testing) (163) • NEPSY-II, 2nd ed. (164) • Repeatable Battery for the Assessment of Neuropsychological Status (RBANS) (165)
Memory	Children's Memory Scale (166) Continuous Performance Test-II (167) Logical Memory I and II (168) Wechsler Memory Scale–IV (169) Wide Range Assessment of Memory and Learning 2 (WRMAL2) (170)
Executive function	Behavior Rating Inventory of Executive Function (BRIEF) (171) Delis-Kaplan Executive Function System (172) Executive Control Battery (173) Stroop Color and Word Test (174) Trail Making Test—Part B (175) Wisconsin Card Sorting Test (176)
Attention/concentration	Delayed Gratification Task (177) Digit Span (Forward and Reversed) (Wechsler scales) (178)
Language/verbal learning	Boston Naming Test (179) Children's Auditory Verbal Learning Test (180) Multilingual Aphasia Examination (181) Token Test—Short Form (182)
Visual perception	Developmental Test of Visual Perception, 2nd ed. (183) Test of Visual Perceptual Skills (184)
Academic-general	Kaufman Tests of Educational Achievement, 2nd ed. (185) Peabody Individual Achievement Test-III (186) Wechsler Individual Achievement Test, 3rd ed. (187) Woodcock Johnson, 3rd ed.; Tests of Academic Achievement (188)
Academic-targeted	Key Math Diagnostic Test (189) Woodcock Reading Mastery Tests, 3rd ed. (190)
Behavior	Child Behavior Checklist (ASEBA Preschool and School Age) (191)
Social behavior	Behavior Assessment System for Children, 2nd ed. (BASC-II) (192) School Social Behavior Rating Scale (SSBR) (193)
Adaptive behavior	Adaptive Behavior Assessment System, 2nd ed. (ABAS-II) (194) Scales of Independent Behavior-Revised (SIB-R) (195) Vineland Adaptive Behavior Scales, 2nd ed. (VABS-II) (196)
Motor skills	Grooved Pegboard (197)

tion, academic achievement, behavior, and personality. In addition to input from parents and educators, a neuropsychologist, school psychologist, or other certified specialist may use individually-administered tests to assess the student's skills in the aforementioned domains. Two recent reviews (146,151) provide examples of the neuropsychological and psychoeducational tests used in schools (Table 37-2).

These batteries or more narrowly focused tests should be used, when necessary, to target specific areas of suspected

disability or concern in conjunction with observation, behavior checklists, curriculum-based measurement, and other context-based measures as described earlier. Many of the aforementioned tests require standardized administration, including timed tasks, specific cut-off points, and scripted instructions for items in order to provide scorable results based on testing norms. However, students with brain injury often require additional time to process information, and would be penalized for slow or partial responses on such standardized measures. If the goal of the assessment is to compare the student's performance with typically developing peers, then measures should be administered as directed. If, however, the goal is to gather information about the student's ability to perform given appropriate accommodations and modifications (additional time on tests), then the efficacy of various accommodations could be tested during the assessment.

Special Test Considerations

Prior to assessment, examiners should be familiar with strategies to address potential problems confronting many students with TBI. These include cognitive and physical fatigue (198–199), attention deficits (200), memory problems (201), delayed processing and response time, low motivation or apathy (202), and impulse control deficits. For example, a test requiring extended focus and engagement may be broken into subtests administered at separate times to minimize cognitive fatigue. Attention problems may be managed more effectively in a quiet setting with few distractions (hallway noise, clocks, alarms, people entering and leaving the room), and may require more frequent and consistent reinforcement of student effort with age-appropriate positive contingencies (203). For tests that are untimed, examiners should allow the student sufficient time to respond to questions. Potential problems with motivation could be addressed prior to testing by asking parents or teachers to identify things that are reinforcing to the student (202,204). If the test is nonstandardized (or administered in a nonstandard way) students with short-term memory deficits may benefit from precorrections (reminders of the expected response type) before each response set. Examiner awareness of the challenges often associated with TBI can help build therapeutic rapport with the student so that a valid sample of performance is obtained during testing.

Individual Education Plan Development

Once a student is found eligible for special education services, the team (including parents) develops the student's IEP that describes the type and amount of specially designed instruction, the settings in which instruction takes place, and any accommodations or related services the student needs to benefit from school. Related services could include instruction from a speech-language pathologist, a behavioral plan for the classroom, and/or participation in a social skills group. The IEP written for a child with TBI will require procedures that vary from traditional IEP development in several ways (205). Because of the underlying medical cause of the disability, the initial IEP requires a joint venture among the health care facility, the school, and the family. Information from a variety of sources and disciplines outside the school system needs to be translated and used to determine the child's current levels of functioning. Rapidly changing needs will require the child's IEP review to be conducted more frequently than required by law (e.g., every 3–4 months initially).

Related Services

Ideally, students returning to school following a TBI have access to a variety of concomitant outpatient services with therapists specially trained to serve pediatric and adolescent TBI populations. Unfortunately, although access to such services is sometimes available in large urban settings (if the child has the appropriate insurance or qualifies for government assistance), in reality there is generally a lack of such services for most children in the school setting (206,207).

A variety of supportive services that may be required to assist the child to benefit from special education are also available through IDEA. These related services can include physical therapy, occupational therapy, speech-language therapy, audiology services, psychological services, recreation therapy, counseling services, social work services, school health services, parent counseling and training, and transportation.

As a child with TBI transitions from the hospital/rehabilitation setting back to school, questions often arise as to funding sources for related services, as there is no clear demarcation between rehabilitation services and those services that are a necessary part of the child's education. According to IDEA, children are entitled to receive "related services" deemed "educationally relevant." How individual districts interpret educational relevance is often open to debate. For example, a school district might argue that physical therapy to increase the head control of a student who is severely injured is rehabilitation therapy; others could argue that it is educationally relevant therapy because increasing head control might allow the student to use a head switch to access a computer in the school setting. In many cases, as students with TBI transition from the medical or rehabilitation setting to school, they receive a combination of educationally based therapy at school and outpatient medical therapy that is paid for by their insurance providers or Medicaid.

Special Education Placements and Settings

Although IDEA requires that students with disabilities, including TBI be educated in the least restrictive environment (LRE) "to the maximum extent possible," a full continuum of options regarding where children can receive services is available. This can include general education classes, special education classes (e.g., resource rooms, self-contained classes), special education schools, hospitals, public or private institutions, and instruction at home. There are many factors to consider in making a decision about the LRE decision and there are no standardized procedures to follow (208–210). However, IEP teams can use both case law and guidelines put forward by researchers who have examined LRE placement policy to inform their decision-making (e.g., Cheatham et al. [211]; Rozalski and Stewart [212]). In general, the child's team, based on considerations of the child's unique needs and the LRE in which those needs can be addressed, makes placement decisions. Frequent progress monitoring of student performance is helpful in guiding changes and adaptations in support provided, which might include changes in instructional setting and content.

For example, a school team may decide that a student returning to school with moderate deficits in memory, processing speed, and verbal comprehension following a TBI may best be served in the general education classroom with support from the special education teacher delivered within the child's own classroom. In another case, a school team may determine that the most appropriate placement for a student with severe language and learning problems as a result of a TBI is a self-contained classroom in the student's home school. There the student can receive more needed one-on-one learning time, yet still participate with general education peers in daily activities such as lunch, recess, art, and music class. In keeping with the intent of the law, it is unusual for a school team to recommend a placement such as a special day school or residential placement. These options are costly and are not available in many areas. Moreover, with school systems currently serving a number of students who have severe or profound disabilities as a result of various conditions, the medical needs of the child with TBI should not be a hindrance to an education in the LRE. In some cases, a residential placement or special school may be necessary if a school district is unable to provide supports that allow the student to benefit from the educational program. In the end, the child's IEP team, including medical and rehabilitation providers who have treated the student, must consider the specific needs of the student, the quality and type of resources available within the school district, and the legal mandate to place the child in the LRE to makes recommendations about school placement.

Specially Designed Instruction

Regardless of the setting, the term *special education* involves "specially designed instruction," which IDEA defines as instruction that "adapts the content, methodology, or delivery of instruction to address the unique needs of the child that result from the child's disability" [34 CFR §300.39(b)(3)]. The purpose of the specially designed instruction is to ensure

the child gains access to the general curriculum so that he or she can meet the educational standard that applies to all children within the jurisdiction of the public agency (school district or state). Although there is very little empirical evidence of the effectiveness of interventions to promote positive educational outcomes for children and youth following a TBI (213,214), a number of promising practices can be identified from research with children with other disability labels (131,144). Because children with TBI share commonalities with children with other disabilities, this research can provide guidance for educators working with students with TBI.

Perhaps the most critical factor in educating students with TBI is ensuring high levels of accuracy in their academic work; there is a strong correlation between maintaining high rates of learner success and increased acquisition and retention of newly learned information (215–217). The provision of guided practice (218–221) and cumulative review (222) address inefficient and inconsistent learning characteristics of students with TBI. Students with TBI also benefit from using well-rehearsed instructional routines or strategies. Instructional routines consist of a set of steps applicable across a range of examples (e.g., consistent sequence of steps for solving math story problems) (218,221,223). Brisk instructional pacing, appropriately adjusted to the student's response rate, can increase the acquisition rate of new material (224). Providing systematic corrective feedback (225,226) is important for students with learning and memory problems after TBI (216,227,228); immediate, nonjudgmental feedback

---

TABLE 37-3 Evidence-Based Instructional Practices and Strategies

INSTRUCTIONAL STRATEGY	DESCRIPTION	TBI CHARACTERISTIC
Appropriate pacing	Delivering material in small increments and requiring responses at a rate consistent with a student's processing speed increases acquisition of new material	• Fluctuating attention • Decreased speed of processing
High rates of success	Acquisition and retention of new information tends to increase with high rates of success	• Memory impairment • High rates of failure
Task analysis	Careful organization of learning tasks, including systematic sequencing of teaching targets	• Organizational impairment • Inefficient learning
Sufficient practice and review (including cumulative review)	Acquisition and retention of new information is increased with frequent review	• Inefficient learning • Inconsistency
Corrective feedback	Learning is enhanced when errors are followed by nonjudgmental corrective feedback	• Inefficient feedback loops • Implicit learning of errors
Teaching to mastery	Learning is enhanced with mastery at the acquisition phase	• Possibility of gaps in the knowledge base
Facilitation of generalization	Generalizable strategies and general case teaching (wide range of examples and settings) increases generalization	• Frequent failure of transfer • Concrete thinking and learning
Ongoing assessment	Adjustment of teaching based on ongoing assessment of students' progress facilitates learning	• Inconsistency • Unpredictable recovery

From Ylvisaker et al. (132).

is critical to improving accuracy when the task is presented again. Table 37-3 presents a summary of research-based instructional strategies that address cognitive characteristics common to many students with TBI.

In addition to the evidence supporting specific instructional strategies, there is substantial research on the efficacy of metacognitive interventions in promoting student success (217,218). Designed to facilitate a strategic approach to difficult academic tasks, metacognitive strategies are procedures that students can use to improve their performance across a variety of academic tasks. Strategies can be task specific or more general. For example, a self-regulatory self-talk strategy like "I need to check my work" is generally applicable to a wide variety of academic tasks. Using a graphic organizer for writing a story is an example of a metacognitive strategy that is task-specific.

Educational Accommodations

Educational accommodations allow students with disabilities to access the same curriculum as their peers through changes in teaching methods and/or materials. For example, a student with memory problems may require multisensory presentations or a child with vision deficits may require large print books to be able to work towards the same goals as their classmates in the general education classroom. Children returning to a general education setting following TBI will more than likely require multiple accommodations. Table 37-4 presents examples of educational accommoda-

tions that address cognitive and physical characteristics common to many students with TBI. These accommodations can be successfully employed in general education settings or in the context of special education environments. Accommodations such as these minimize the student's deficits and allow him or her to remain in a less restrictive school environment.

Behavioral and Social Support Strategies

Individual education plans for students with TBI often include social and behavioral goals, as difficulties with EF, including impulse control and control of attention, are common sequelae of TBI (22,24,203). Addressing behavioral challenges is often difficult and time intensive for school staff, however, appropriate school and social behavior is critical to student success (229). There is a large research base on strategies to support students with behavioral issues including Functional Behavior Assessment; monitored trials of accommodations and modifications, for example, modified schedule, preferential seating, and so forth; small group instruction; and individual behavioral interventions (230). Collaboration with district or outside agency specialists such as vocational rehabilitation counselors, transition specialists, therapists, and so forth, may also be useful (146). Table 37-5 includes validated approaches to behavioral and social intervention.

504 Eligibility

Although TBI often affects learning, not all students with TBI need, or are eligible for, assistance under IDEA. Some

TABLE 37-4 Educational Accommodations

COMMON DEFICITS FOLLOWING TBI	CLASSROOM EXAMPLES	POSSIBLE ACCOMMODATIONS
Fatigue	Student struggles to stay alert in class; physical exhaustion impacts student's learning	Modified school day; schedule most taxing courses early in day; rest breaks
Attention/concentration	Student is unable to sustain or maintain focus to complete task or activities; is easily distracted; if interrupted cannot go back and pick up where he or she left off	Reduce distractions in student's work area; divide work into smaller sections; use verbal or nonverbal cueing system to remind student to pay attention
Memory	Student has difficulty remembering instructions; is able to read assigned chapter, but cannot recall what was read; does well on daily assignment, but poorly on tests	Provide written instructions for student; shorten reading passages; frequently repeat and summarize information; link new information to student's relevant prior knowledge
Organization	Student is often late to class; comes to class without necessary materials; does not automatically carry out the class schedule; does not remember what class is next; leaves out steps in a project or when solving a complex problem	Assign person to review schedule at start of school day and organize materials for each class; use color-coded materials for each class (book, notebook, supplies); provide written schedule of daily routine and give reinforcement for referring to schedule; provide written checklist for complex tasks
Processing speed	When called on in class, student does not respond right away, gives appearance of not attending or knowing the answer; has difficulty carrying out multi-step directions; performs poorly on timed tests	Give student advanced notice he or she is going to be called on; allow extra time for the student to respond when answering; supply written set of directions; provide extended time on assignments and tests
Visual–motor	Student has difficulty copying problems from the blackboard; decreased motor speed makes keeping up with taking lecture notes impossible; visual field deficit causes student to ignore information presented on right side	Assign someone to take notes for student during lectures; provide copy of problems on blackboard; allow for alternatives to paper-pencil writing (oral responses, computer); provide preferential seating to maximize visual field

TABLE 37-5 Integrated Approaches to Behavioral and Social Intervention

APPROACH	DESCRIPTION	TBI CHARACTERISTIC
Self-awareness/attribution training	Facilitation of students' understanding of their role in learning; validated for students with learning difficulties (231)	• Decreased self-awareness • Denial of deficits
Cognitive behavior modification	Facilitation of self-control of behavior; validated with adolescents with ADHD and aggressive behavior (232)	• Weak self-regulation related to frontal lobe injury • Disinhibited and potentially aggressive behavior
Positive, antecedent-focused behavior supports	Approach to behavior management that focuses primarily on the antecedents of behavior (in a broad sense); validated in developmental disabilities and with some TBI subpopulations (233,234)	• Impulsive behavior • Inefficient learning from consequences • History of failure • Defiant behavior • Initiation impairment • Working memory impairment
Circle of friends	A set of procedures designed to support students' social life and ongoing social development; validated in developmental disabilities and TBI (235,236)	• Frequent loss of friends • Social isolation • Weak social skills

Abbreviations: ADHD, attention deficit hyperactivity disorder. From Ylvisaker et al. (132).

students are able to participate in the general education program with supports and accommodations provided through a Section 504 plan (237). This civil rights act protects individuals from discrimination based on their disability, ensuring individuals' equal rights to participate in and have access to program benefits and services, including public education. The definitions of disability in this law are broader and more inclusive than those in IDEA; an individual with a disability is someone with a physical or mental impairment that substantially limits 1 or more major life activities, such as caring for oneself, walking, seeing, hearing, speaking, breathing, working, performing manual tasks, and learning (238). The Rehabilitation Act Section 504 is a civil rights law that applies to *all* settings, not just public school, so it continues to protect individuals from discrimination after high school graduation. A written 504 plan might include accommodations to address physical, cognitive, or behavioral needs, including, for example, a reduced schedule to compensate for fatigue, a note taker for fine motor difficulties, or increased time to complete tests and assignments to compensate for processing delays.

Transition Planning or Services

Under IDEA, transition services are mandated for all students with disabilities beginning at age 16 (141). The law specifies that each student have an IEP to facilitate movement from school to post-school life, that the plan take into account the student's abilities, preferences, and interests, and include measurable postsecondary goals (239). The plan must include instruction, services, experiences, development of objectives for employment and adult living, and acquisition of living and vocational skills. The National Secondary Training and Technical Assistance Center (NSTTAC) recommends that transition plans incorporate the following evidence-based practices: (*a*) transition planning focused on post-school goals and self-determination; (*b*) help coordinating postsecondary plans with adult agencies; (*c*) instruction in academic, vocational, independent living, and per-

sonal–social content areas; (*d*) support for completing high school; and (*e*) paid job training while in the program and help securing employment or entering postsecondary training on leaving the program (240).

Building Capacity of Educators: Recommendations for Teacher Training

There continues to be a lack of awareness of the impact of TBI on school performance (112). Numerous resources exist for educators who want to learn more about childhood TBI (e.g., http://cokidswithbraininjury.com/, http://www.la-publishing.com, http://www.projectlearnet.org/, http://www.brainlinekids.org/). Further, with the increased awareness of the impact of concussion on young learners and the need for schools to address these students' needs, a variety of new resources have been developed (e.g., http://brain101.orcasinc.com/, http://www.cdc.gov/concussion/HeadsUp/schools.html).

The challenge remains that many teachers leave their university training programs with little or no training in TBI (241–243). Training for general education teachers in working with students with TBI is minimal (109,110,244), and most special education teacher preparation programs offer training in strategies designed to support students with higher incidence disabilities (e.g., Specific Learning Disability and attention-deficit/hyperactivity disorder) (245).

More comprehensive teacher training efforts in TBI have focused on training educators who are currently working in schools (137,138). The past 30 years of research on professional development for educators points to a number of critical components for effectiveness regardless of the particular subject or method being taught. To have an impact on students, training and support for educators must

- require teachers to practice new skills in the school environment (246–250);
- provide access to sufficient organizational supports (251);

- include information about the causes, incidence, treatment, outcomes, and challenges of TBI;
- include a variety of evidence-based strategies (252,253);
- include consultation on implementation of new skills in the instructional setting (e.g., Bowen [254]; Fuchs and Fuchs [255]; Gersten et al. [256]; Sailors and Price [257]); and
- be of sufficient duration (e.g., 7–8 sessions) to produce long-term sustained use of new strategies in the instructional setting (250,258,259).

There are currently 2 teacher training models that incorporate these features in use with educators serving students with TBI: the TBI Consulting Team model (137) and Brain-STARS (260–262). Although these models show promise, both lack evidence of impact on child outcome, which is the standard for evaluating the effectiveness of professional development models (263–265).

CONCLUSION

Although hospitals treat children and adolescents with TBI in their initial course of recovery, it is ultimately the school system that serves as the long-term provider of services for this population. Because TBI has significant and on-going effects on academic, cognitive, and psychosocial functioning, in 1991 TBI was added to the list of disabilities that qualify students for special education services under IDEA, and thus students, if identified, can receive an array of supports to address individual needs. However, despite the fact that the foundation for providing appropriate service to students with TBI exists in special education law, students with TBI continue to experience significant challenges in school and as a group experience poor post-secondary outcomes.

For students with TBI, school performance is most often affected by executive dysfunction, social behavioral problems, and a progressive lag in academic achievement. Several factors have been found to mediate and moderate the effect of TBI on school performance. Early injury is associated with poorer outcomes than later injury, and generally more severe TBI is associated with more negative outcomes. Family environmental characteristics, such as SES, overall family functioning, and parenting behavior can also significantly affect student educational performance. In addition to child- and family-centered factors, a range of environmental variables negatively affect student outcomes. For example, the lack of training in TBI for educators, as well as ineffective hospital–school communication, has led to underidentification of children with TBI for special education. Adversarial parent–educator relationships have often hampered the design of educational programs for students with TBI.

Like other students with disabilities, students with TBI need and deserve to be promptly and accurately identified so they can be appropriately served by educators who are knowledgeable about the challenges they experience and who can implement effective instructional and behavioral strategies. Because most parents of students with TBI will have had no prior experience with special education, school systems should provide information and link parents with skilled advocates. Linking students with TBI and their families to community-based resources—throughout their school years but especially at transition from high school—should be a high priority for the IEP team.

These improvements in service delivery will involve systemic changes. Well-developed preservice and in-service training programs for school personnel will help educators accurately identify students with TBI, implement effective educational practices, develop strategies for collaborating with parents, and link students to appropriate community-based supports as they leave high school. Well-established hospital–school linkages with school reentry protocols will help to increase identification rates and ensure smooth transitions back to school. Significantly improving outcomes for students with TBI will require comprehensive research efforts that examine these and other efficacious interventions and bringing these interventions into broader use through a coordinated process of development, training, technical assistance, and dissemination.

KEY CLINICAL POINTS

1. Reduced hospital stays have resulted in children with significant needs returning to school with little or no support from medical or community-based agencies; the primary service provider for children and adolescents has become the school.
2. For students with moderate to severe injury, the rate of academic achievement gains tends to slow progressively over time, and the effects are long-term. Changes in social behavior affect not only functional aspects of daily living but also quality of life.
3. A growing body of research indicates that post-high school outcomes for many students with TBI are poor.
4. Effective instructional and behavioral support strategies implemented by trained educators can help mitigate the academic and behavioral challenges associated with childhood TBI.
5. Instructional methodologies that have proven effective with learners with different disability labels but similar functional challenges can be used effectively with students with TBI.
6. Improved identification of students with TBI for special education services could lead to more effective provision of educational and social/behavioral support strategies tailored to students' specific needs.
7. To lead to positive student outcomes, training and support for educators must include training in evidence-based interventions, supervised practice in both the training site and classroom, and continued mentoring, feedback, and consultation in the classroom.

KEY REFERENCES

1. Babikian T, Asarnow R. Neurocognitive outcomes and recovery after pediatric TBI: meta-analytic review of the literature. *Neuropsychology.* 2009;23(3):283–296.
2. Taylor HG, Swartwout MD, Yeates KO, Walz NC, Stancin T, Wade SL. Traumatic brain injury in young children: postacute effects on cognitive and school readiness skills. *J Int Neuropsychol Soc.* 2008;14(5):734–745.
3. Todis B, Glang A, Bullis M, Ettel D, Hood D. Longitudinal investigation of the post-high school transition experi-

ences of adolescents with traumatic brain injury. *J Head Trauma Rehabil.* 2011;26(2):138–149.

4. Yeates KO, Anderson V. Childhood traumatic brain injury, executive functions, and social outcomes: toward an integrative model for research and clinical practice. In: Anderson V, Jacobs R, Anderson PJ, eds. *Executive Functions and the Frontal Lobes: A Lifespan Perspective.* Philadelphia, PA: Taylor & Francis; 2008:243–267.

5. Ylvisaker M, Todis B, Glang A, et al. Educating students with TBI: themes and recommendations. *J Head Trauma Rehabil.* 2001;16(1):76–93.

RECOMMENDED WEBSITES

http://www.cbirt.org
http://www.projectlearnet.org
http://www.cokidswithbraininjury.com

References

1. Faul M, Xu L, Wald MM, Coronado VG. *Traumatic Brain Injury in the United States: Emergency Department Visits, Hospitalizations and Deaths 2002–2006.* Atlanta, GA: Centers for Disease Control and Prevention; 2010.

2. Zaloshnja E, Miller T, Langlois JA, Selassie AW. Prevalence of long-term disability from traumatic brain injury in the civilian population of the United States, 2005. *J Head Trauma Rehabil.* 2008;23(6):394–400.

3. Hosack K, Rocchio C. Serving families of persons with severe brain injury in an era of managed care. *J Head Trauma Rehabil.* 1995;10(2):57.

4. Shigaki C, Hagglund K, Clark M, Conforti K. Access to health care services among people with rehabilitation needs receiving Medicaid. *Rehabil Psychol.* 2002;47(2):204–218.

5. Conoley J, Sheridan S. Pediatric traumatic brain injury: challenges and interventions for families. *J Learn Disabil.* 1996;29(6):662–669.

6. Batavia A, DeJong G, Eckenhoff EA, Materson RS. After the Americans with Disabilities Act: the role of the rehabilitation community. *Arch Phys Med Rehabil.* 1990;71(12):1014–1015.

7. Kirkwood MW, Yeates KO, Taylor HG, Randolph C, McCrea M, Anderson VA. Management of pediatric mild traumatic brain injury: a neuropsychological review from injury through recovery. *Clin Neuropsychol.* 2008;22(5):769–800.

8. McKinlay A, Dalrymple-Alford JC, Horwood LJ, Fergusson DM. Long term psychosocial outcomes after mild head injury in early childhood. *J Neurol Neurosurg Psychiatry.* 2002;73(3):281–288.

9. Hessen E, Nestvold K, Sundet K. Neuropsychological function in a group of patients 25 years after sustaining minor head injuries as children and adolescents. *Scand J Psychol.* 2006;47(4):245–251.

10. Brown G, Chadwick O, Shaffer D, Rutter M, Traub M. A prospective study of children with head injuries: III. Psychiatric sequelae. *Psychol Med.* 1981;11(1):63–78.

11. Massagli TL, Fann JR, Burington BE, Jaffe KM, Katon WJ, Thompson RS. Psychiatric illness after mild traumatic brain injury in children. *Arch Phys Med Rehabil.* 2004;85:1428–1434.

12. Collins MW, Lovell MR, Iverson GL, Cantu RC, Maroon JC, Field M. Cumulative effects of concussion in high school athletes. *Neurosurgery.* 2002;51:1175–1179.

13. Guskiewicz KM, Marshall SW, Bailes J, et al. Association between recurrent concussion and late-life cognitive impairment in retired professional football players. *Neurosurgery.* 2005;57:719–726.

14. Ponsford J, Willmott C, Rothwell A, et al. Cognitive and behavioral outcome following mild traumatic head injury in children. *J Head Trauma Rehabil.* 1999;14(4):360–372.

15. Swaine BR, Tremblay C, Platt RW, Grimard G, Zhang X, Pless IB. Previous head injury is a risk factor for subsequent head injury in children: a longitudinal cohort study. *Pediatrics.* 2007;119(4):749–758.

16. Luis CA, Mittenberg W. Mood and anxiety disorders following pediatric traumatic brain injury: a prospective study. *J Clin Exp Neuropsychol.* 2002;24(3):270–279.

17. Smith-Seemiller L, Fow NR, Kant R, Franzen MD. Presence of post-concussion syndrome symptoms in patients with chronic pain vs. mild traumatic brain injury. *Brain Inj.* 2003;17(3):199–206.

18. Ewing-Cobbs L, Prasad MR, Landry SH, Kramer L, DeLeon R. Executive functions following traumatic brain injury in young children: a preliminary analysis. *Dev Neuropsychol.* 2004;26(1):487–512.

19. Yeates KO, Anderson V. Childhood traumatic brain injury, executive functions, and social outcomes: toward an integrative model for research and clinical practice. In: Anderson V, Jacobs R, Anderson PJ, eds. *Executive Functions and the Frontal Lobes: A Lifespan Perspective.* Philadelphia, PA: Taylor & Francis; 2008:243–267.

20. Cattelani R, Lombardi F, Brianti R, Mazzucchi A. Traumatic brain injury in childhood: intellectual, behavioural, and social outcome into adulthood. *Brain Inj.* 1998;12(4):283–296.

21. Klonoff H, Clark C, Klonoff PS. Long-term outcome of head injuries: a 23 year follow up study of children with head injuries. *J Neurol Neurosurg Psychiatry.* 1993;56(4):410–415.

22. Chapman LA, Wade SL, Walz NC, Taylor HG, Stancin T, Yeates KO. Clinically significant behavior problems during the initial 18 months following early childhood traumatic brain injury. *Rehabil Psychol.* 2010;55(1):48–57.

23. Babikian T, Asarnow R. Neurocognitive outcomes and recovery after pediatric TBI: Meta-analytic review of the literature. *Neuropsychology.* 2009;23(3):283–296.

24. Catroppa C, Anderson VA, Morse SA, Haritou F, Rosenfeld JV. Outcome and predictors of functional recovery 5 years following pediatric traumatic brain injury (TBI). *J Pediatr Psychol.* 2008;33(7):707–718.

25. Asikainen I, Kaste M, Sarna S. Patients with traumatic brain injury referred to a rehabilitation and re-employment programme: social and professional outcome for 508 Finnish patients 5 or more years after injury. *Brain Inj.* 1996;10(12):883–899.

26. Yeates KO, Taylor HG, Wade SL, Drotar D, Stancin T, Minich N. A prospective study of short- and long-term neuropsychological outcomes after traumatic brain injury in children. *Neuropsychology.* 2002;16(4):514–523.

27. Vu J, Babikian T, Asarnow RF. Academic and language outcomes in children after traumatic brain injury: a meta-analysis. *Except Child.* 2011;77(3):263–281.

28. Ewing-Cobbs L, Barnes MA, Fletcher JM. Early brain injury in children: development and reorganization of cognitive function. *Dev Neuropsychol.* 2003;24(2–3):669–704.

29. Anderson V, Catroppa C, Morse S, Haritou F, Rosenfeld J. Functional plasticity or vulnerability after early brain injury? *Pediatrics.* 2005;116(6):1374–1382.

30. Tonks J, Yates P, Williams WH, Frampton I, Slater A. Peer-relationship difficulties in children with brain injuries: comparisons with children in mental health services and healthy controls. *Neuropsychol Rehabil.* 2010;20(6):922–935.

31. Sohlberg MM, Mateer C. *Cognitive Rehabilitation: An Integrated Neuropsychological Approach.* New York, NY: Guilford Publication; 2001.

32. Anderson VA, Anderson P, Northam E, Jacobs R, Catroppa C. Development of executive functions through late childhood and adolescence in an Australian sample. *Dev Neuropsychol.* 2001;20(1):385–406.

33. Sohlberg M, Ness B. Practical Strategies for Serving Students with TBI in the Schools. Paper presented at: Brain Injury Association of Oregon; October 5–6, 2007; Portland, OR.

34. Harvey VS. Best practices in teaching study skills. In: Thomas A, Grimes J, eds. *Best Practices in School Psychology IV.* Vol 1. Bethesda, MD: National Association of School Psychologists; 2002:831–845.

35. Anderson V, Catroppa C. Recovery of executive skills following paediatric traumatic brain injury (TBI): a 2 year follow-up. *Brain Inj.* 2005;19(6):459–470.

36. Cicerone K, Levin H, Malec J, Stuss D, Whyte J. Cognitive rehabilitation interventions for executive function: moving from bench to bedside in patients with traumatic brain injury. *J Cogn Neurosci.* 2006;18(7):1212–1222.

37. Gioia GA, Kenworthy L, Isquith PK. Executive function in the real world: BRIEF lessons from Mark Ylvisaker. *J Head Trauma Rehabil.* 2010;25(6):433–439.

38. Ylvisaker M, Szekeres SF, Feeney T. Cognitive rehabilitation: executive functions. In: Ylvisaker M, ed. *Traumatic Brain Injury Rehabilitation: Children and Adolescents.* Rev. ed. Newton, MA: Butterworth-Heinemann; 1998:221–269.

39. Ylvisaker M, Feeney T. Executive functions, self-regulation, and learned optimism in paediatric rehabilitation: a review and implications for intervention. *Pediatr Rehabil.* 2002;5(2):51–70.

40. Eslinger PJ, Biddle KR. Adolescent neuropsychological development after early right prefrontal cortex damage. *Dev Neuropsychol.* 2000;18(3):297–329.

41. Anderson SW, Damasio H, Tranel D, Damasio AR. Long-term sequelae of prefrontal cortex damage acquired in early childhood. *Dev Neuropsychol.* 2000;18(3):281–296.

42. Morgan AB, Lilienfeld SO. A meta-analytic review of the relation between antisocial behavior and neuropsychological measures of executive function. *Clin Psychol Rev.* 2000;20(1):113–136.

43. Catroppa C, Anderson V, Godfrey C, Rosenfeld JV. Attentional skills 10 years post-paediatric traumatic brain injury (TBI). *Brain Inj.* 2011;25(9):858–869.

44. McKinlay A, Grace RC, Horwood LJ, Fergusson DM, MacFarlane MR. Long-term behavioural outcomes of pre-school mild traumatic brain injury. *Child Care Health Dev.* 2010;36(1):22–30.

45. The University of the State of New York. *Traumatic Brain Injury: A Guidebook for Educators.* Albany, NY: The State Education Department, Office of Special Education Services; 1997. http://www.rojectlearnet.org/for teachers.html. Accessed July 27, 2011.

46. Conklin H, Salorio C, Slomine B. Working memory performance following paediatric traumatic brain injury. *Brain Inj.* 2008;22(11):847–857.

47. Begali V, ed. *Head Injury in Children and Adolescents: A Resource and Review for School and Allied Professionals.* 2nd ed. Brandon, VT: Clinical Psychology; 1992.

48. Bulgren JA, Schumaker JB. Teaching practices that optimize curriculum access. In: Deshler DD, Schumaker JB, eds. *Teaching Adolescents with Disabilities: Accessing the General Education Curriculum.* Thousand Oaks, CA: Corwin Press; 2006:79–120.

49. Anderson V, Jacobs R, Spencer-Smith M, et al. Does early age at brain insult predict worse outcome? Neuropsychological implications. *J Pediatr Psychol.* 2010;35(7):716–727.

50. Greenham M, Spencer-Smith MM, Anderson PJ, Coleman L, Anderson VA. Social functioning in children with brain insult. *Front Hum Neurosci.* 2010;4:22.

51. Tonks J, Slater A, Frampton I, Wall SE, Yates P, Williams WH. The development of emotion and empathy skills after childhood brain injury. *Dev Med Child Neurol.* 2009;51(1):8–16.

52. Turkstra LS. Should my shirt be tucked in or left out? The communication context of adolescence. *Aphasiology.* 2000;14(4):349–364.

53. Turkstra L, McDonald S, DePompei R. Social information processing in adolescents: data from normally-developing adolescents and preliminary data from their peers with traumatic brain injury. *J Head Trauma Rehabil.* 2001;16(5):469–483.

54. Ylvisaker M, Feeney T. Pediatric brain injury: social, behavioral, and communication disability. *Phys Med Rehabil Clin N Am.* 2007;18(1):133–44, vii.

55. Yeates KO, Swift E, Taylor HG, et al. Short- and long-term social outcomes following pediatric traumatic brain injury. *J Int Neuropsychol Soc.* 2004;10(3):412–426.

56. Yeates KO, Bigler ED, Dennis M, et al. Social outcomes in childhood brain disorder: a heuristic integration of social neuroscience and developmental psychology. *Psychol Bull.* 2007;133(3):535–556.

57. Muenchberger H, Kendall E, Neal R. Identity transition following traumatic brain injury: a dynamic process of contraction, expansion and tentative balance. *Brain Inj.* 2008;22(12):979–992.

58. Carroll E, Coetzer R. Identity, grief and self-awareness after traumatic brain injury. *Neuropsychol Rehabil.* 2011;21(3):289–305.

59. Charles N, Butera-Prinzi F. Acquired brain injury: reconstructing meaning following traumatic grief. *Grief Matters: Australian J Grief Bereavement.* 2008;11(2):64–69.

60. Langlois J, Rutland-Brown W, Wald M. The epidemiology and impact of traumatic brain injury: a brief overview. *J Head Trauma Rehabil.* 2006;21(5):375–378.

61. Landau J, Hissett J. Mild traumatic brain injury: impact on identity and ambiguous loss in the family. *Fam Syst Health.* 2008;26(1):69–85.

62. Nance ML, Polk-Williams A, Collins MW, Weibe DJ. Neurocognitive evaluation of mild traumatic brain injury in the hospitalized pediatric population. *Ann Surg.* 2009;249(5):859–863.

63. Anderson V, Catroppa C, Morse S, Haritou F, Rosenfeld JV. Intellectual outcome from preschool traumatic brain injury: a 5-year prospective, longitudinal study. *Pediatrics.* 2009;124(6):e1064–e1071.

64. Ashman TA, Cantor JB, Gordon WA, et al. Objective measurement of fatigue following traumatic brain injury. *J Head Trauma Rehabil.* 2008;23(1):33–40.

65. Cernich AN, Kurtz SM, Mordecai KL, Ryan PB. Cognitive rehabilitation in traumatic brain injury. *Curr Treat Options Neurol.* 2010;12(5):412–423.

66. Thickbroom GW, Mastaglia FL. Plasticity in neurological disorders and challenges for noninvasive brain stimulation (NBS). *J Neuroeng Rehabil.* 2009;6:4.

67. Lane SJ, Schaaf RC. Examining the neuroscience evidence for sensory-driven neuroplasticity: implications for sensory-based occupational therapy for children and adolescents. *Am J Occup Ther.* 2010;64(3):375–390.

68. Todis B, Glang A, Bullis M, Ettel D, Hood D. Longitudinal investigation of the post-high school transition experiences of adolescents with traumatic brain injury. *J Head Trauma Rehabil.* 2011;26(2):138–149.

69. Savage RC, Urbanczyk B. Growing up with a brain injury. *The Perspectives Network.* 1995;V-3.

70. Barnes MA, Dennis M, Wilkinson M. Reading after closed head injury in childhood: effects on accuracy, fluency, and comprehension. *Develop Neuropsychol.* 1999;15:1–24.

71. Ewing-Cobbs L, Fletcher JM, Levin HS, Francis DJ, Davidson K, Miner ME. Longitudinal neuropsychological outcome in infants and preschoolers with traumatic brain injury. *J Int Neuropsychol Soc.* 1997;3(6):581–591.

72. Catroppa C, Anderson V. Intervention approaches for executive dysfunction following brain injury in childhood. In: Anderson V, Jacobs R, Anderson PJ, eds. *Executive Functions and the Frontal Lobes: A Lifespan Perspective.* Philadelphia, PA: Taylor & Francis; 2008:439–469.

73. Ewing-Cobbs L, Prasad MR, Swank P, et al. Arrested development and disrupted callosal microstructure following pediatric traumatic brain injury: relation to neurobehavioral outcomes. *Neuroimage.* 2008;42(2):1305–1315.

74. Taylor HG, Swartwout MD, Yeates KO, Walz NC, Stancin T, Wade SL. Traumatic brain injury in young children: postacute effects on cognitive and school readiness skills. *J Int Neuropsychol Soc.* 2008;14(5):734–745.

75. Anderson VA, Catroppa C, Dudgeon P, Morse SA, Haritou F, Rosenfeld JV. Understanding predictors of functional recovery and outcome 30 months following early childhood head injury. *Neuropsychology.* 2006;20(1):42–57.

76. Fletcher JM, Ewing-Cobbs L, Francis DJ, Levin HS. Variability in outcomes after traumatic brain injury in children: a developmental perspective. In: Broman SH, Michel ME, eds. *Traumatic Head Injury in Children.* New York, NY: Oxford University Press; 1995:3–21.

77. Schwartz L, Taylor HG, Drotar D, Yeates KO, Wade SL, Stancin T. Long-term behavior problems following pediatric traumatic brain injury: prevalence, predictors, and correlates. *J Pediatr Psychol.* 2003;28(4):251–263.

78. Taylor HG, Yeates KO, Wade SL, Drotar D, Stancin T, Burant C. Bidirectional child-family influences on outcomes of traumatic brain injury in children. *J Int Neuropsychol Soc.* 2001;7(6):755–767.

79. Novack TA, Alderson AL, Bush BA, Meythaler JM, Canupp K. Cognitive and functional recovery at 6 and 12 months post-TBI. *Brain Inj.* 2000;14(11):987–996.

80. Anderson V, Catroppa C, Morse S, Haritou F, Rosenfeld J. Recovery of intellectual ability following traumatic brain injury in childhood: impact of injury severity and age at injury. *Pediatr Neurosurg.* 2000;32:282–290.

81. Donders J, Nesbit-Greene K. Predictors of neuropsychological test performance after pediatric traumatic brain injury. *Assessment.* 2004;11(4):275–284.

82. Rivara JB, Jaffe KM, Fay GC, et al. Family functioning and injury severity as predictors of child functioning one year following traumatic brain injury. *Arch Phys Med Rehabil.* 1993;74(10):1047–1055.

83. Rivara JB, Jaffe KM, Polissar NL, et al. Family functioning and children's academic performance and behavior problems in the year following traumatic brain injury. *Arch Phys Med Rehabil.* 1994; 75(4):369–379.

84. Taylor HG, Drotar D, Wade S, Yeates KO, Stancin T, Klein S. Recovery from traumatic brain injury in children: the importance of the family. In: Broman S, Michel ME, eds. *Traumatic Head Injury in Children.* New York, NY: Oxford University Press; 1995:188–216.

85. Catroppa C, Anderson V. Recovery of educational skills following paediatric traumatic brain injury. *Pediatr Rehabil.* 1999;3(4):167–175.

86. Fletcher JM, Ewing-Cobbs L, Miner ME, Levin HS, Eisenberg HM. Behavioral changes after closed head injury in children. *J Consult Clin Psychol.* 1990;58(1):93–98.

87. Goldstrohm SL, Arffa S. Preschool children with mild to moderate traumatic brain injury: an exploration of immediate and post-acute morbidity. *Arch Clin Neuropsychol.* 2005;20(6):675–695.

88. Kinsella GJ, Prior M, Sawyer M, et al. Predictors and indicators of academic outcome in children 2 years following traumatic brain injury. *J Int Neuropsychol Soc.* 1997;3(6):608–616.

89. Max JE, Castillo CS, Robin DA, et al. Predictors of family functioning after traumatic brain injury in children and adolescents. *J Am Acad Child Adolesc Psychiatry.* 1998;37(1):83–90.

90. Max JE, Koele SL, Castillo CC, et al. Personality change disorder in children and adolescents following traumatic brain injury. [Erratum appears in *J Int Neuropsychol Soc.* 2000;6(7):854]. *J Int Neuropsychol Soc.* 2000;6(3):279–289.

91. Yeates KO, Taylor HG, Walz NC, Stancin T, Wade SL. The family environment as a moderator of psychosocial outcomes following traumatic brain injury in young children. *Neuropsychology.* 2010; 24(3):345–356.

92. Hawley CA, Ward AB, Magnay AR, Long J. Parental stress and burden following traumatic brain injury amongst children and adolescents. *Brain Inj.* 2003;17(1):1–23.

93. Nacajauskaite O, Endziniene M, Jureniene K, Schrader H. The validity of post-concussion syndrome in children: a controlled historical cohort study. *Brain Dev.* 2006;28(8):507–514.

94. Testa JA, Malec JF, Moessner AM, Brown AW. Predicting family functioning after TBI: impact of neurobehavioral factors. *J Head Trauma Rehabil.* 2006;21:236–247.

95. Nathoo N, Chetty R, van Dellen JR, Barnett GH. Genetic vulnerability following traumatic brain injury: the role of apolipoprotein E. *Mol Pathol.* 2003;56:132–136.

96. Teasdale GM, Murray GD, Nicoll JA. The association between APOE epsilon4, age and outcome after head injury: a prospective cohort study. *Brain.* 2005;128(11):2556–2561.

97. Keenan HT, Hooper SR, Wetherington CE, Nocera M, Runyan DK. Neurodevelopmental consequences of early traumatic brain injury in 3-year-old children. *Pediatrics.* 2007;119(3):e616–e623.

98. Wetherington C, Hooper S. Preschool traumatic brain injury: a review for the early childhood special educator. *Exceptionality.* 2006; 14(3):155–170.

99. Anderson V, Moore C. Age at injury as a predictor of outcome following pediatric head injury. *Child Neuropsychol.* 1995;1:187–202.

100. Wetherington CE, Hooper SR, Keenan HT, Nocera M, Runyan D. Parent ratings of behavioral functioning after traumatic brain injury in very young children. *J Pediatr Psychol.* 2010;35(6):662–671.

101. Hawley CA, Ward AB, Magnay AR, Mychalkiw W. Return to school after brain injury. *Arch Dis Child.* 2004;89(2):136–142.

102. Walz NC, Cecil KM, Wade SL, Michaud LJ. Late proton magnetic resonance spectroscopy following traumatic brain injury during early childhood: relationship with neurobehavioral outcomes. *J Neurotrauma.* 2008;25(2):94–103.

103. Muscara F, Catroppa C, Eren S, Anderson V. The impact of injury severity on long-term social outcome following paediatric traumatic brain injury. *Neuropsychol Rehabil.* 2009;19(4):541–561.

104. Koskiniemi M, Kyykkä T, Nybo T, Jarho L. Long-term outcome after severe brain injury in preschoolers is worse than expected. *Arch Pediatr Adolesc Med.* 1995;149(3);249–254.

105. Nybo T, Sainio M, Muller K. Stability of vocational outcome in adulthood after moderate to severe preschool brain injury. *J Int Neuropsychol Soc.* 2004;10(5):719–723.

106. Todis B, Glang A. Redefining success: results of a qualitative study of postsecondary transition outcomes for youth with traumatic brain injury. *J Head Trauma Rehabil.* 2008;23(4):252–263.

107. US Department of Education. 2004. National Longitudinal Transition Study 2 (NLTS-2) Web site. http://www.nlts2.org/index.html. Accessed August 1, 2011.

108. US Bureau of Labor Statistics. 2006. *Current Population Survey* (Employed persons by detailed occupation, sex, and age, Annual Average). http://www.bls.gov/cps/home.htm#data. Accessed August 1, 2011.

109. Chapman JK. Traumatic brain injury: a regional study of rural special and general education preparation experiences. *Rural Spec Educ Q.* 2000;19(2):3–14.

110. Chapman JK. Traumatic brain injury: a five state study of special and general education preparation experiences. *Physical Disabilities: Education and Related Services.* 2005;21(1):17–34.

111. Glang A, Dise-Lewis J, Tyler J. Identification and appropriate service delivery for children who have TBI in schools. *J Head Trauma Rehabil.* 2006;21(5):411–412.

112. Bersani H, Glang A. What is taught about TBI: an analysis of TBI content in 54 teacher preparation textbooks. In press.

113. Langlois JA, Rutland-Brown W, Thomas KE. The incidence of traumatic brain injury among children in the United States: differences by race. *J Head Trauma Rehabil.* 2005;20(3):229–238.

114. US Department of Education. *Twenty-Ninth Annual Report to Congress on the Implementation of the Individuals with Disabilities Education Act.* Vol 2. Washington DC: US Department of Education; 2007: Table 1–9.

115. Donders J. Academic placement after traumatic brain injury. *J School Psychol.* 1994;32:53–65.

116. Ewing-Cobbs L, Fletcher JM, Levin HS, Iovino I, Miner ME. Academic achievement and academic placement following traumatic brain injury in children and adolescents: a two-year longitudinal study. *J Clin Exp Neuropsychol.* 1998;20(6):769–781.

117. Miller LJ, Donders J. Prediction of educational outcome after pediatric traumatic brain injury. *Rehabil Psychol.* 2003;48(4):237–241.

118. Taylor HG, Yeates KO, Wade SL, Drotar D, Stancin T, Montpetite M. Long-term educational interventions after traumatic brain injury in children. *Rehabil Psychol.* 2003;48(4):227–236.

119. Cantor JB, Gordon WA, Schwartz ME, Charatz HJ, Ashman TA, Abramowitz S. Child and parent responses to a brain injury screening questionnaire. *Arch Phys Med Rehabil.* 2004;85(4)(suppl 2): S54–S60.

120. McCaleb KN. The relationship between brain injury and the provision of school services. *Physical Disabilities: Education and Related Services.* 2006;25(1):61–76.

121. DiScala C, Osberg JS, Savage RC. Children hospitalized for traumatic brain injury: Transitions to post-acute care. *J Head Trauma Rehabil.* 1997;12(2):1–10.

122. Glang A, Todis B, Thomas C, Hood D, Bedell G, Cockrell J. Return to school following childhood TBI: who gets services? *NeuroRehabilitation.* 2008;23(6):477–486.

123. Sharp NL, Bye RA, Llewellyn GM, Cusick A. Fitting back in: adolescents returning to school after severe acquired brain injury. *Disabil Rehabil.* 2006;28(12):767–778.

124. Darling RB. Parent-professional interaction: the roots of misunderstanding. In: Seligman M, ed. *The Family With a Handicapped Child: Understanding and Treatment.* Orlando, FL: Grune & Stratton; 1983: 175–202.

125. Turnbull AP, Turnbull HR. *Families, Professionals, and Exceptionality: A Special Partnership.* Columbus, Ohio: Charles E Merrill; 1986.

126. Walker BR. Creating effective educational programs through parent-professional partnerships. In: Glang A, Singer GHS, Todis B, eds. *Students With Acquired Brain Injury: The School's Response.* Baltimore, MD: Paul H Brookes; 1996:295–322.

127. Todis B, Glang A, Fabry M. Family, school, child: qualitative study of the school experiences for students with ABI. In: Glang A, Singer GHS, Todis B, eds. *Students With Acquired Brain Injury: The School's Response.* Baltimore, MD: Paul H Brookes; 1996:33–72.

128. Ylvisaker M, Hartwick P, Stevens MB. School reentry following head injury: managing the transition from hospital to school. *J Head Trauma Rehabil.* 1991;6(1):10–22.

129. Savage RC. Identification, classification, and placement issues for students with traumatic brain injuries. *J Head Trauma Rehabil.* 1991; 6(1):1–9.

130. Mira MP, Tyler JS. Students with traumatic brain injury: making the transition from hospital to school. *Focus on Exceptional Children.* 1991;23(5):1–12.

131. Ylvisaker M, Todis B, Glang A, et al. Educating students with TBI: themes and recommendations. *J Head Trauma Rehabil.* 2001;16(1): 76–93.

132. Ylvisaker M, Feeney T, Mullins K. School reentry following mild traumatic brain injury: a proposed hospital-to-school protocol. *J Head Trauma Rehabil.* 1995;10(6):42–49.

133. Donders J, Strom D. The effect of traumatic brain injury on children with learning disability. *Pediatr Rehabil.* 1997;1(3):179–184.

134. Individuals with Disabilities Education Improvement Act of 2004. Pub L No. 108-446, 118 Stat 2647 (2004).

135. Glang A, Todis B, Ettel D. *Empirically-based interventions to improve cognitive, behavioral, and academic outcomes following pediatric TBI.* Federal Interagency Conference on TBI. Washington, DC; 2011.

136. The Education for All Handicapped Children Act (PL 94-142), 20 USC §1401 et seq. (1975).

137. Glang A, Tyler J, Pearson S, Todis B, Morvant M. Improving educational services for students with TBI through statewide consulting teams. *NeuroRehabilitation.* 2004;19(3):219–231.

138. Glang A, Todis B, Sublette P, Brown BE, Vaccaro M. Professional development in TBI for educators: the importance of context. *J Head Trauma Rehabil.* 2010;25(6):426–432.

139. Savage RC, DePompei R, Tyler J, Lash M. Paediatric traumatic brain injury: a review of pertinent issues. *Pediatr Rehabil.* 2005;8: 92–103.

140. Dettmer JL, Daunhauer L, Detmar-Hanna D, Sample PL. Putting brain injury on the radar: exploratory reliability and validity analyses of the Screening Tool for Identification of Acquired Brain Injury in School-Aged Children. *J Head Trauma Rehabil.* 2007;22(6): 339–349.

141. Individuals with Disabilities Education Act of 1990, 20 USC §1400 et seq. (1990). http:// idea.ed.gov. Accessed August 2, 2011.

142. Hibbard M, Gordon W, Martin T, Rashkin B, Brown M. *Students with Traumatic Brain Injury: Identification, Assessment, and Classroom Accommodations.* New York, NY: Research and Training Center on Community Integration of Individuals with Traumatic Brain Injury; 2001.

143. Bohmann J. Traumatic brain injury and teens: information for school administrators. *Principal Leadership.* 2007:12–15.

144. Glang A, Ylvisaker M, Stein M, Ehlhardt L, Todis B, Tyler J. Validated instructional practices: application to students with TBI. *J Head Trauma Rehabil.* 2008;23(4):243–251.

145. Arroyos-Jurado EC, Savage TA. Intervention strategies for serving students with traumatic brain injury. *Interv Sch Clin.* 2008;43: 252–254.

146. Cleary M, Scott A. Developments in clinical neuropsychology: implications for school psychological services. *J School Health.* 2010; 81:1–7.

147. Miller DC. *Essentials of School Neuropsychological Assessment.* Hoboken, NJ: John Wiley & Sons Inc; 2007:351–354.

148. Telzrow CF. Role of the school in serving children with learning disabilities. *Semin Neurol.* 1991;11(1):50–56.

149. Merrell KW. *Behavioral, social, and emotional assessment of children and adolescents.* 2nd ed. Mahwah, NJ: Lawrence Erlbaum; 2003: 52–53.

150. Hale JB, Fiorello CA. *School Neuropsychology: A Practitioner's Handbook.* New York, NY: Guilford Press; 2004.

151. Fiorello CA, Hale JB, Decker SL, Coleman S. Neuropsychology in school psychology. In: Garcia-Vazquez E, Crespi TD, Riccio CA, eds. *Handbook of Education, Training and Supervision of School Psychologists in School and Community.* Vol 1. New York, NY: Taylor & Francis; 2009:213–232.

152. Naglieri JA, Das JP. *Cognitive Assessment System.* Itasca, IL: Riverside Publishing; 1997.

153. Hammill DD, Pearson NA, Wiederholt JL. *Comprehensive Test of Nonverbal Intelligence.* 2nd ed. Rolling Meadows, IL: Riverside Publishing; 2009.

154. Elliott CD. *Differential Ability Scales.* 2nd ed. San Antonio, TX: Harcourt Assessment; 2007.

155. Kaufman AS, Kaufman NL. *Kaufman Assessment Battery for Children.* 2nd ed. Circle Pines, MN: AGS Publishing; 2004.

156. Roid GH. *Stanford-Binet Intelligence Scales.* 5th ed. Itasca, IL: Riverside Publishing. 2003.

157. Wechsler D. *Wechsler Primary and Preschool Scale of Intelligence (WPPSI-III).* 3rd ed. San Antonio, TX: Harcourt Assessment; 2002.

158. Wechsler D. *Wechsler Abbreviated Scale of Intelligence (WASI).* San Antonio, TX: Harcourt Assessment; 1999.

159. Wechsler D. *The Wechsler Intelligence Scale for Children.* 4th ed. London, United Kingdom: Pearson Assessment; 2004.

160. Woodcock RW, Mather N, McGrew KS. *Woodcock-Johnson III Tests of Cognitive Abilities Examiner's Manual.* Itasca, IL: Riverside Publishing; 2001.

161. Boll T. *Children's Category Test.* San Antonio, TX: Pearson; 1993.

162. Functional Independence Measure (FIM). *Uniform Data System for Medical Rehabilitation.* Buffalo, NY: University of Buffalo; 1996.

163. Lovell M, Maroon J. *ImPACT: Immediate Post-Concussion Assessment and Cognitive Testing.* Pittsburgh, PA: NeuroHealth Systems; 2000.

164. Korkman M, Kirk U, Kemp S. *NEPSY-II.* 2nd ed. San Antonio TX: Pearson, Psychological Corporation; 2007.

165. Randolph C. *Repeatable Battery for the Assessment of Neuropsychological Status (RBANS).* San Antonio, TX: Pearson, Psychological Corporation; 1998.

166. Cohen M. *Children's Memory Scale.* San Antonio, TX: Pearson, Psychological Corporation; 1997.

167. Conners CK, Staff MHS. *Conners' Continuous Performance Test II: Computer Program for Windows Technical Guide and Software Manual.* North Tonawanda, NY: Multi-Health Systems; 2000.

168. Wechsler D. *Logical Memory I and II subtests of Wechsler Memory Scale.* 4th ed. San Antonio, TX: Psychological Corporation; 2009.

169. Wechsler D. *Wechsler Memory Scale.* 4th ed. San Antonio, TX: Pearson; 2009.

170. Sheslow D, Adams W. *Wide Range Assessment of Memory and Learning 2 (WRMAL2).* Wilmington, DE: Wide Range; 2003.

171. Gioia GA, Isquith PK, Guy SC, Kenworthy L. *Behavior Rating Inventory of Executive Function.* Odessa, FL: Psychological Assessment Resources, Inc.; 2000.

172. Delis DC, Kaplan E, Kramer JH. *Delis-Kaplan Executive Function System.* San Antonio, TX: Pearson, Psychological Corporation; 2001.

173. Goldberg E, Podell K, Bilder R, Jaeger J. *Executive Control Battery (ECB).* Melbourne, Australia: Psych Press; 2000.

174. Stroop JR. Studies of interference in serial verbal reactions. *J Exp Psychol.* 1935;18:643–662.

175. Army Individual Test Battery. *Manual of directions and scoring. (Trail Making Test-part B).* Washington, DC: War Department, Adjutant General's Office; 1944.

176. Grant DA, Berg EA. *Wisconsin Card Sorting Test.* Los Angeles, CA: Western Psychological Services; 1948.

177. Mischel W, Ebbesen EB, Zeiss AR. Cognitive and attentional mechanisms in delay of gratification. *J Pers Soc Psychol.* 1972;21(2): 204–218.

178. Wechsler D. *Digit Span (Forward and Reversed) Subtests of The Wechsler Intelligence Scale for Children.* 4th ed. London, United Kingdom: Pearson Assessment; 2004.

179. Kohn SE, Goodglass H, Werintraub S. *The Boston Naming Test.* Philadelphia, PA: Lea & Febiger; 1983.

180. Talley JL. *Children's Auditory Verbal Learning Test-2 (CAVLT-2):* Odessa, FL: Psychological Assessment Resources; 1993.

181. Benton AL, Hamsher K, Sivan AB. *Multilingual Aphasia Examination (MAE).* 3rd ed. Odessa, FL: Psychological Assessment Resources; 1994.

182. Spellacy FJ, Spreen O. A short form of the token test. *Cortex.* 1969; 5:390–397.

183. Hammill DD, Pearson NA, Voress JK. *Developmental Test of Visual Perception.* 2nd ed. Austin, TX: PRO-ED;1993.

184. Gardner MF. *Test of Visual Perceptual Skills (non-motor).* Rev ed. San Francisco, CA: Psychological and Educational Publications; 1996.

185. Kaufman AS, Kaufman NL. *Kaufman Test of Educational Achievement*. 2nd ed. Circle Pines, MN: AGS Publishing; 2004.

186. Markwardt FC. *Peabody Individual Achievement Test*. Rev ed. Circle Pines, MN: American Guidance Service; 1989.

187. Wechsler D. *Wechsler Individual Achievement Test*. 3rd ed. San Antonio, TX: Pearson, SAGE Publications Inc; 2009.

188. Woodcock RW, McGrew KS, Mather N. *Woodcock Johnson Tests of Academic Achievement*. 3rd ed. Itasca, IL: Riverside; 2007.

189. Connolly AJ. *KeyMath-3 diagnostic assessment: Manual forms A and B*. Minneapolis, MN: Pearson; 2007.

190. Woodcock RW. *Woodcock Reading Mastery Tests*. 3rd ed. San Antonio, TX: Pearson, Psychological Corporation; 2011

191. Achenbach TM, Rescorla LA. *Manual for the ASEBA school-age forms and profiles: an integrated system of multinformant assessment*. Burlington, VT: University of Vermont, Research Center for Children, Youth and Families; 2001.

192. Reynolds CR, Kamphaus RW. *Behavior Assessment System for Children (BASC-II)*. 2nd ed. San Antonio, TX: PsychCorp; 2004.

193. Merrell KW. *School Social Behavior Scales*. 2nd ed. Eugene, OR: Assessment-Intervention Resources; 2002.

194. Harrison P, Oakland T. *Adaptive Behavior Assessment System (ABAS-II)*. 2nd ed. San Antonio, TX: Pearson, Psychological Corporation; 2003.

195. Bruininks RH, Woodcock RV, Weatherman RF, Hill BK. *Scales of Independent Behavior (SIB-R)*. Rev ed. Itasca, IL: Riverside Publishing; 1984.

196. Sparrow SS, Cicchetti DV, Balla DA. *Vineland Adaptive Behavior Scales (VABS-II)*. 2nd ed. San Antonio, TX: Pearson, Psychological Corporation; 2005.

197. Tiffin J. *Purdue Grooved Pegboard*. Chicago, IL: Research Associates; 1968.

198. Dikmen SS, Corrigan J, Levin HS, Machamer J, Stiers W, Weisskopf MG. Cognitive outcome following traumatic brain injury. *J Head Trauma Rehabil*. 2009;24(6):430–438.

199. Johansson B, Berglund P, Ronnback L. Mental fatigue and impaired information processing after mild and moderate traumatic brain injury. *Brain Inj*. 2009;23(13–14):1027–1040.

200. Himanen L, Portin R, Tenovuo O, et al. Attention and depressive symptoms in chronic phase after traumatic brain injury. *Brain Inj*. 2009;23(3):220–227.

201. Kinsella G, Prior M, Sawyer M, et al. Neuropsychological deficit and academic performance in children and adolescents following traumatic brain injury. *J Pediatr Psychol*. 1995;20:753–767.

202. Lane-Brown A, Tate R. Interventions for apathy after traumatic brain injury. *Cochrane Database Syst Rev*. 2009;(2):CD006341. http://www.thecochranelibrary.com. Accessed August 10, 2011.

203. Feeney TJ, Ylvisaker M. Context-sensitive cognitive-behavioral supports for young children with TBI: a second replication study. *J Positive Behav Interv*. 2008;10(2):115–128.

204. Alderman N, Wood RL, Williams C. The development of the St Andrew's-Swansea Neurobehavioural Outcome Scale: validity and reliability of a new measure of neurobehavioural disability and social handicap. *Brain Inj*. 2011;25(1):83–100.

205. Tyler JS, Savage RC. Students with traumatic brain injury. In: Obiakor FE, Utley CA, Rotatori AF, eds. *Advances in Special Education: Psychology of Effective Education for Learners with Exceptionalities*. Boston, MA: JAI Press; 2003:299–323.

206. Johnstone B, Nossaman LD, Schopp LH, Holmquist L, Rupright SJ. Distribution of services and supports for people with traumatic brain injury in rural and urban Missouri. *J Rural Health*. 2002;18(1):109–117.

207. Sample PL, Tomter H, Johns N. The left hand does not know what the right hand is doing": rural and urban cultures of care for persons with traumatic brain injuries. *Subst Use Misuse*. 2007;42(4):705–727.

208. Champagne JF. Decisions in sequence: how to make decisions in least restrictive environments. *EdLaw Briefing Paper*. 1993;9 & 10;1–16.

209. Kluth P, Villa RA, Thousand JS. "Our school doesn't offer inclusion" and other legal blunders. *Educ Leadership*. 2002;59(4):24–27.

210. Sharp GK, Pitasky VM. *The Current Legal Status of Inclusion. Individuals With Disability Law Report*. Special Report No. 29, LPR Publications. 2002.

211. Cheatham GA, Hart JE, Malian I, McDonald J. Six Things to Never Say or Hear During an IEP Meeting. *Teaching Exceptional Children*. 2012;44(3):50-57.

212. Rozalski MAJ. How to determine the least restrictive environment for students with disabilities. *Exceptionality*. 2010;18(3):151–163. doi:10.1080/09362835.2010.491991.

213. Laatsch L, Harrington D, Hotz G, et al. An evidence-based review of cognitive and behavioral rehabilitation treatment studies in children with acquired brain injury. *J Head Trauma Rehabil*. 2007;22:248–256.

214. Limond J, Leeke R. Practitioner review: cognitive rehabilitation for children with acquired brain injury. *J Child Psychol Psychiatry*. 2005;46(4):339–352.

215. Gersten RM, White WA, Falco R, Carnine D. Teaching basic discriminations to handicapped and non-handicapped individuals through a dynamic presentation of instructional stimuli. *Anal Interv Dev Disabil*. 1982;2(4):305–317.

216. Sohlberg MM, Ehlhardt L, Kennedy M. Instructional techniques in cognitive rehabilitation: a preliminary report. *SeminSpeech Lang*. 2005;26:268–279.

217. Weeks M, Gaylord-Ross R. Task difficulty and aberrant behavior in severely handicapped students. *J Appl Behav Anal*. 1981;86(4):449.

218. Carnine DW, Silbert J, Kameenui EJ. *Direct Instruction Reading*. 2nd ed. Columbus, Ohio: Merrill; 1990.

219. Englert CS. Effective direct instruction practices in special education settings. *Remedial Spec Educ*. 1984;5(2):38–47.

220. Kryzanowski J, Carnine DW. The effects of massed versus spaced formats in teaching sound-symbol correspondences to young children. *J Reading Behav*. 1980;12(3):225.

221. Paine SC, Carnine DW, White WA, Walters G. Effects of fading teacher presentation structure (covertization) on acquisition and maintenance or arithmetic problem-solving skills. *Educ Treat Chil*. 1982;5(2):93–107.

222. Rosenshine B, Stevens R. Teaching functions. In: Wittrock MC, ed. *Handbook of Research on Teaching*. 3rd ed. New York, NY: Macmillan; 1986:376–391.

223. Stein M, Kinder D, Silbert J, Carnine DW. *Designing Effective Mathematics Instruction: A Direct Instruction Approach*. Columbus, Ohio: Pearson-Merrill Prentice Hall; 2006.

224. Carnine DW. Effects of two teacher-presentation rates on offtask behavior, answering correctly, and participation. *J Appl Behav Anal*. 1976;9(2):199–206.

225. Carnine D. Relationships between stimulus variation and the formation of misconceptions. *J Educ Res*. 1980;74(2):106–110.

226. Gersten RM, Carnine DW, Williams PB. Measuring implementation of a structured educational model in an urban school district: an observational approach. *Educ Eval Policy Anal*. 1982;4(1):67–79.

227. Baddeley A, Wilson BA. When implicit learning fails: amnesia and the problem of error elimination. *Neuropsychologia*. 1994;32:53–68.

228. Wilson BA, Baddeley AD, Evans J, Shiel A. Errorless learning in the rehabilitation of memory-impaired people. *Neuropsychol Rehabil*. 1994;4:307–326.

229. Hawley CA. Behavior and school performance after brain injury. *Brain Inj*. 2004;18:645–659.

230. Ylvisaker M, Turkstra LS, Coelho C, et al. Behavioural interventions for Children and adults with behavior disorders after TBI: a systematic Review of the evidence. *Brain Injury*. 2007;21(8):769–805.

231. Borkowski JG, Chan KS, Muthukrishna N. A process-oriented model of metacognition: links between motivation and executive functioning. In: Schraw G, ed. *Issues in the Measurement of Metacognition*. Lincoln, NE: University of Nebraska Press; 2000:1–41.

232. Robinson TR, Smith SW, Miller MD, Brownell MT. Cognitive behavior modification of hyperactivity impulsivity and aggression: a meta-analysis of school-based studies. *Educ Psychol*. 1999:91:195–203.

233. Carr EG, Homer RH, Turnbull AP, et al. *Positive Behavior Support for People with Developmental Disabilities: A Research Synthesis*. Washington, DC: American Association of Mental Retardation; 1999.

234. Feeney TJ, Ylvisaker M. Choice and routine: antecedent behavioral interventions for adolescents with severe traumatic brain injury. *J Head Trauma Rehabil.* 1995;10(3):67–86.

235. Forest M, Lusthaus E. Promoting educational equality for all students: circles and maps. In: Stainback S, Stainback W, Forest M, eds. *Educating all Students in the Mainstream of Regular Education.* Baltimore, MD: Paul H. Brookes Publishing; 1989.

236. Glang A, Singer GHS, Todis B, eds. *Students With Acquired Brain Injury: The School's Response.* Baltimore, MD: Paul H Brookes; 1996.

237. Rehabilitation Act, 29 USC §794 (1973).

238. United States Department of Health and Human Services/Office for Civil Rights. USDHHS Web site. http://www.hhs.gov/ocr/civilrights/resources/laws/index.html. Accessed July 20, 2011.

239. Savage RC. The great leap forward: transitioning into the adult world. *Preventing School Failure.* 2005;49(4):43–52.

240. National Secondary Training and Technical Assistance Center (NSTTAC). Evidence-based secondary transition practices. NSTTAC Web site. http://www.nsttac.org/ebp/evidence_based_practices.aspx.Accessed August 1, 2011.

241. Farmer JE, Johnson-Gerard M. Misconceptions about traumatic brain injury among educators and rehabilitation staff: a comparative study. *Rehabil Psychol.* 1997;42(4):273–286.

242. Funk P, Bryde S, Doelling J, Hough D. Serving students with traumatic brain injury: a study of educators' knowledge level and personnel preparation needs in Missouri. *Physical Disabilities: Education and Related Services.* 1996;15:49–64.

243. Tyler J. Preparing educators to serve children with ABI. In: Glang A, Singer G, Todis B, eds. *Students with Acquired Brain Injury: The school's response.* Baltimore, MD: Paul H. Brookes Publishing. 1997:323–341.

244. Blosser JL, DePompei R. Preparing education professionals for meeting the needs of students with traumatic brain injury. *J Head Trauma Rehabil.* 1991;6(1):73–82.

245. Turnbull HR, Turnbull AP, Shank M, Smith S. *Exceptional Lives: Special Education in Today's Schools.* 4th ed. Upper Saddle River, NJ: Merrill-Prentice Hall; 2004.

246. Borko H. Professional development and teacher learning: mapping the terrain. *Educ Res.* 2004;33(8):3–15.

247. Darling-Hammond L, Richardson N. Teacher learning: what matters? *Educ Leadersh.* 2009;66(5):46–53.

248. Grossman P, Wineburg S, Woolworth S. Toward a theory of teacher community. *Teach Coll Rec.* 2001;103(6):942.

249. Little JW. Locating learning in teachers' communities of practice: opening up problems of analysis in records of everyday work. *Teach Teach Educ.* 2002;18(8):917.

250. Yoon KS, Duncan T, Lee SW-Y, Scarloss B, Shapley KL. *Reviewing the Evidence on How Teacher Professional Development Affects Student Achievement* (Issues & Answers. REL 2007-No. 033). Washington,

DC: US Department of Southwest; 2007. http://ies.ed.gov/ncee/edlabs. Accessed August 11, 2011.

251. Fixsen DL, Naoom SF, Blase KA, Friedman RM, Wallace F. *Implementation Research: A Synthesis of the Literature.* Tampa, FL: University of South Florida, Louis de la Parte Florida Mental Health Institute, The National Implementation Research Network; 2005.

252. Jones HA, Chronis-Tuscano A. Efficacy of teacher in-service training for attention-deficit/hyperactivity disorder. *Psychol Sch.* 2008;45(10):918–929.

253. Lerman DC, Tetreault A, Hovanetz A, Strobel M, Garro J. Further evaluation of a brief, intensive teacher-training model. *J Appl Behav Anal.* 2008;41(2):243–248.

254. Bowen JM. Classroom interventions for students with traumatic brain injuries. *Preventing School Failure.* 2005;49(4):34–41.

255. Fuchs LS, Fuchs D. Effects of expert system consultation within curriculum-based measurement, using a reading maze. *Except Child.* 1992;58(5):436–450.

256. Gersten R, Chard DJ, Jayanthi M, Baker SK, Morphy P, Flojo J. Mathematics instruction for students with learning disabilities: a meta-analysis of instructional components. *Rev Educ Res.* 2009;79(3):1202–1242.

257. Sailors M, Price LR. Professional development that supports the teaching of cognitive reading strategy instruction. *Elem Sch J.* 2010;110(3):301–322.

258. Benedict E, Horner R, Squires J. Assessment and implementation of behavior support in preschools. *Topics Early Child Spec Educ.* 2007;27(3):174–192.

259. Noell GH, Witt JC, Gilbertson DN, Ranier DD, Freeland JT. Increasing teacher intervention implementation in general education settings through consultation and performance feedback. *Sch Psychol Q.* 1997;12(1):77–88.

260. Davis AS. Review of brainSTARS—brain injury: strategies for teams and reeducation for students. *J Sch Psychol.* 2004;42(1):87–92.

261. Dise-Lewis JE, CalveryME, LewisHC. *BrainSTARS:Brain Injury—Strategies for Team and Re-education for Students.* Wake Forest, NC: Lash and Associates Publishing and Educational Services; 2006.

262. Dise-Lewis JE, Lewis HC, Reichardt CS. BrainSTARS: pilot data on a team-based intervention program for students who have acquired brain injury. *J Head Trauma Rehabil.* 2009;24(3):166–177.

263. Carpenter TP, Fennema E, Peterson PL, Chiang C-P, Loef M. Using knowledge of children's mathematics thinking in classroom teaching: an experimental study. *Am Educ Res J.* 1989;26(4):499–531.

264. McCutchen D, Abbott RD, Green LB, et al. Beginning literacy: links among teacher knowledge, teacher practice, and student learning. *J Learn Disabil.* 2002;35(1):69.

265. Odom SL. The tie that binds: evidence-based practice, implementation science, and outcomes for children. *Topics Early Child Spec Educ.* 2009;29(1):53–61.

Family Assessment and Intervention

Caron Gan, Roberta DePompei, and Marilyn Lash

INTRODUCTION

When a brain injury occurs to a child/adolescent, the focus is often placed on the child and the delivery of acute care. Although this stage of adaptation to injury is important, parents often state that they had no idea how their lives would continually change over time. In a series of family focus groups, DePompei (1) reported themes that emerged throughout the 6 different family groups. Theme One: Loss of friends and extended family support. One family stated, "Everyone was there for us when our daughter was pulled from the water. Her story was in all the newspapers and on TV, claiming it a miracle she survived. But where are they now to see what it really means to live with a brain injury?" Theme Two: Significant time and effort are required to reinvent a family's daily functioning and routines. A mom reported, "It's just a new and different normal day for our family. Each day we experience the new person our child is becoming." Theme Three: Community members often misunderstand the child who exhibits learning and social behaviors and require unacceptable levels of efforts to educate or inform them. A dad stated, "Our son looks fine but he is unable to concentrate, memory problems continue, and he gets angry easily. The teachers just do not understand." These families also reported that there is little emphasis placed on anything other than the medical condition of their child; there needs to be a broader focus from the time of the injury forward to address the full multidimensional impact of childhood trauma.

This chapter is based on the authors' premise that the family is central to the lifelong living issues that accompany a child's brain injury from several important perspectives. First, family systems change. Caring for a child with a brain injury is a long-term process and families become the critical support system. Second, families who function as the critical support system are themselves in need of help as they learn how to adapt to the medical, social, behavioral, and educational challenges over time. Although it is widely acknowledged that families are instrumental in the outcomes of rehabilitation and community integration for their child, there is a serious dearth of community, emotional, and day-to-day instrumental support available for them (2,3). Whereas long-term support of children with brain injury and their families has been advocated in the literature (2,4), this is impractical given limited health care and professional resources. It is therefore essential to find ways of strengthening families to help sustain optimal coping and functioning over the life course.

To help achieve this goal, it is critical to dispel the traditional notion that professionals are the only experts. In the social model of disability (5), the question "who is the expert" is raised and requires self-analysis by all who live within the broader social network of individuals with disabilities. Holland (6) similarly challenged the traditional assumption that "professional" is synonymous with "expert." She indicated that there are 3 experts to be considered within any family interaction: (*a*) the professional who has technical knowledge and the ability to acquire resources that can be made available to clients, (*b*) the person who lives *in* the disorder, and (*c*) those family members who live *with* the disorder. Working with families therefore indicates that interactions are dynamic and include at least 3 experts—the professional, the person with the disability, and those whose lives are affected by the person with the disability.

Holland states:

> This expanded concept became clear to me even before the advent of the social model of disability. As a beginning clinician, I often found myself smugly amused when parents would comment about their child, "He never acts like that at home."
>
> "Humm," I would think—"It's amazing what sort of blinders parents wear, particularly if experts aren't around." And then I had children. The first time I heard myself utter, "He isn't like this at home," I recognized my limitations as an expert. I learned that as clinicians, we could claim only 1 of the 2 or 3 places at the expert's table (6).

Thus, this chapter is based on 2 premises: first, that professionals have an essential but not exclusive role in the ongoing treatment process; and second, that families can be resilient and healthy supports for their child after a brain injury. This chapter supports this notion by: (*a*) reexamining the literature on families of children and youth with brain injury, (*b*) presenting a resilience-based family systems framework for clinical assessment and intervention, and (*c*) proposing a multicomponent approach to family intervention.

An *acquired brain injury* (ABI) is defined as a trauma to the brain that occurs after birth, is not related to a congenital disorder, and is not a chronic deteriorating condition. This definition can apply to children and youth, as well as adults. It generally includes external causes caused by trauma (i.e., motor vehicle collision, fall, assault, sports injury) as well as internal causes (i.e., tumor, encephalitis, meningitis, stroke, anoxia, etc). With children and youth, an injury to the brain can interrupt and delay ongoing brain development and maturation and the subsequent achievement of developmental milestones. For this reason, some children with ABI may become developmentally disabled and may be eligible for services within the developmental disability community; however, this varies greatly across and within states, provinces, and countries.

THE MEDICAL MODEL: A FAMILY SYSTEMS-ILLNESS PERSPECTIVE

The medical model of diagnosis and treatment has been the primary paradigm underlying rehabilitation programs. This traditional medical model has 4 major components:

1. There is an identified patient—in this case the child or youth with ABI.
2. There is an expert (usually the professional) who provides a diagnosis and a plan for treatment.
3. There is a period where treatment is provided by the expert.
4. The expert determines when treatment is successful or ineffective and recommends discharge based on that determination.

Rolland's Family Systems-Illness Model (7) extends the medical model beyond the lens of deficits and pathology. Rolland suggests that several condition specific factors such as onset of the injury, family and illness life cycles, and belief systems including culture and ethnicity, interact with family development to influence family, school, and community relationships. Instead of the professional being the expert, the family is viewed as a resource. Disability is viewed from a more holistic, interactive, and normative perspective. Rolland's inclusive perspective supports Masel's (8) assertion that persons with ABI have a potential for numerous medical conditions to emerge over time. Masel further suggests that ABI be considered a chronic disease and treated as such.

Repositioning Acquired Brain Injury in Children and Youth in Research and Practice

To date, there has been a preponderance of research on family distress and burden after ABI in children (9–12). Stress and burden among families have often been identified with the following concerns: child's behavioral adjustment and future potential (10,12), increased marital stress and deteriorating family functioning (11,12), sibling stress and negativity (13–15), uncertainty about the nature of the injury and uneven trajectory of ability to recover or adapt after the ABI, and continued need for monitoring and advocacy by parents after the ABI (15–17). All these issues can contribute to instability and unbalance the delicate interactions and supports of the family system. Although there are many families who experience burden and distress, there is growing indication that other families are successfully reacting and adjusting to the demands of their child's challenges (18). From the

authors' clinical experience, many families have demonstrated a resilience that outweighs any burden. Yet, there is an overwhelming dearth of literature on families that cope well and that emerge strengthened after ABI. The need for additional research on protective factors in the child's environment has been recently advocated in the literature (19).

To help us reposition ABI among children and youth using a strength-based focus, we draw on the growing body of research on resilience, which has found considerable application in the childhood disability literature (20–22). This literature supports a shift away from the deficit or pathology approach to a competency-based and family resilience framework. *Resilience* is defined as "the ability to withstand and rebound from disruptive life challenges, strengthened and more resourceful" (20). According to Rolland and Walsh (20), resilience is not about innate hardiness, invulnerability, or simply bouncing back. "It rather involves struggling well, effectively working through and learning from adversity and integrating the experience into the fabric of individual and shared lives."

Walsh (22) identifies key processes in family resilience: belief systems, organizational patterns, and communication patterns. Families who demonstrate resilient belief systems are able to normalize their suffering and distress in the context of families facing similar predicaments. They also approach their adversity as a shared challenge so that they can find new meaning and maintain a positive outlook as a family unit. Organizational patterns of resilient families are flexible, mutually supportive, and respectful of individual needs, differences, and boundaries. Communication processes of resilient families involve clear messages, open emotional expression, and collaborative problem solving. This resilience approach fundamentally alters the traditional medical model of viewing children and families as damaged and in need of fixing to seeing them as challenged with potential for healing and growth in all members. This resiliency perspective explains why the same adversity may result in different outcomes, with some families emerging strengthened and more resourceful, whereas others become devastated and deteriorate.

Repositioning Grief and Loss Issues

Linear models of psychosocial adjustment have been published extensively in the literature and are based on a series of sequential phases. The landmark work of Kubler-Ross in the early 1970s described 5 stages that terminally ill individuals and their families experience, namely denial, anger, bargaining, depression, and acceptance. This model has been widely applied to the grieving process of families and survivors of brain injury (23). However, research has not examined this model's relevance for children and youth with ABI.

Lezak's work in the 1980s focused specifically on reactions of family members during in-patient rehabilitation with 6 stages identified: helping families observe the patient accurately amidst denial, families becoming more receptive to incomplete recovery, families pulling back as coping mechanisms develop, families seeing the person as different than before the injury, families actively mourning despite the person's survival, and emotional detachment to preserve the family (24). However, Lezak's model was developed during a time when in-patient adult rehabilitation stays were much longer than those now available under managed care and insurance caps. Again, this model does not address the unique aspects of grief and mourning for families with a child who has ABI.

A more recent linear 6-step adjustment model with time frames is used by the Academy of Certified Brain Injury Specialists (25). This model includes shock, hope, and denial (1–3 mos.); recognition of severity, helplessness, and frustration (3–9 months); expectations vs impairments: seeking information (6–24 months); realism sets in: exhaustion, bereavement (10–24 months); profound sadness, grieving, mourning, loss of personality (12–24 months); and understanding, acceptance, attention to family unit (2–3 years). Again, this model is adult oriented and does not account for emerging latent effects of brain trauma among children and youth and the changing impact on parental grief and adjustment over time. Because rehabilitation services are more limited for children, many families provide care at home even for those with more severe injuries (26). The impact of becoming the child's primary caregiver on the family's stress and coping skills has not been well studied.

As linear models of psychosocial adjustment are not well suited for families of children and youth with ABI; the episodic loss model of grieving developed by Williams is proposed instead (27). The episodic loss reaction is activated during transitional points or developmental milestones that remind the family of their losses such as birthdays, transition to high school, graduation, or the anniversary date of the injury. In this type of loss, closure is impossible and has been coined by Boss as ambiguous loss (28). According to Boss (28), there are 2 types of ambiguous loss situations. The first one occurs when there is physical absence and psychological presence, such as when a loved one is physically missing. In the second type, there is physical presence but psychological absence, such as with brain injury. In this second type of ambiguous loss, the person you care about is psychologically, emotionally, or cognitively absent. This is reflected in a key theme from a recent qualitative study of parents' experiences following their child's brain injury, "grieving for the child I knew" (29). Parents expressed sorrow for the child they once knew. This type of loss experienced by families often goes unrecognized and unacknowledged by friends and family, especially because the individual with the brain injury is still physically present, yet different in personality. Normalization of these episodic and ambiguous loss reactions is needed to foster resilience and to prepare families for these recurring events over the course of the child's life.

A RESILIENCE-BASED FAMILY SYSTEMS FRAMEWORK FOR ASSESSMENT AND INTERVENTION

Although the need for a family systems framework after ABI has been widely espoused (15,30–32), a systemic review by Boschen and colleagues (33) indicated a paucity of family system interventions in both pediatric and adult populations. The family system perspective indicates that it is inadequate to simply intervene with the primary caregiver or the individual with the ABI. Healthy family functioning depends on the functioning of each individual within the system, their interactions with one another, and their influence on the overall functioning of the unit.

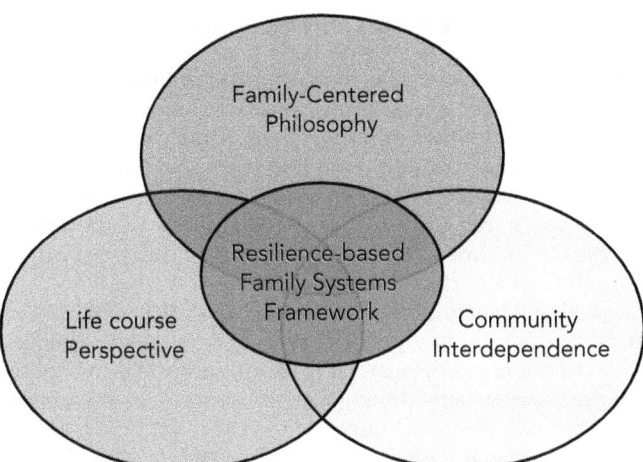

FIGURE 38-1 Resilience-based family systems framework.

In this section, a resilience lens is incorporated into the family systems framework. A resilience-based family systems framework is grounded in the recognition that ongoing crises and persistent challenges impact the whole family after ABI. This framework offers a nonpathologizing approach that reduces vulnerabilities and fosters coping and mastery of family system challenges over the life course. The resilience-based family systems framework is comprised of three components: (*a*) family-centered philosophy, (*b*) life course perspective, and (*c*) community interdependence (see Figure 38-1). Each of these components is addressed subsequently.

Family-Centered Service

Families are considered the most important influence on the child's development, recovery and overall adjustment and is the underlying principle for family-centered service (FCS), which has been widely embraced in the field of childhood chronic illness and disability (34). Similar to the Holland concept, FCS is about mutual respect, information sharing, participation, and collaborative partnerships with clients and families. It emphasizes that clients, families, and health care providers are (*a*) partners in health care; (*b*) that care must be comprehensive; and (*c*) that it must be tailored to family and client strengths, needs, priorities, and values. FCS has been associated with increased client and family satisfaction, adherence to treatment recommendations, and improved client outcomes (35–37). Despite general recognition of the benefits of FCS, service providers often find it difficult to translate these principles into action, particularly within the constraints of time and resources available (38). Moreover, there may be educational barriers as many rehabilitation professionals have not been trained in FCS and may lack the skills for collaboration and forming professional–family partnerships (39). Readers are referred to the Institute for Family-Centered Care, which provides leadership and training in advancing the practice of FCS for hospitals and health care systems (Web link: http://www.familycenteredcare.org).

Life Course Perspective

When a child sustains a brain injury, the family has to adapt to the "new" child whose needs, skills, challenges, and identity may have changed (40). They also face the complex process of the child's reintegration and transition back into the home, school, and community. Ongoing assistance is essential for their transitions because the needs of the child changes over time and as the child and family progress through their life cycle.

Unlike brain injury in an adult, an ABI in childhood occurs amidst ongoing physical and cognitive development. As the brains of children and adolescents are still developing well into young adulthood, their recovery patterns differ from those of adults. Children with ABI often "grow into" their disabilities because the latent brain injury-related challenges may not become readily apparent until the child enters adolescence (41–43). The stage of normal adolescence also coincides with increased risk-taking behavior, opposition to authority, impulsivity, and emotional reactivity, all of which create added confusion for parents because these are also common characteristics of ABI. As adolescents with ABI assert their natural desire for greater autonomy, independence, and acceptance by peers, parents struggle with the delicate balancing act of how much to let go vs how much protection and support are needed. Families also need guidance for forming appropriate developmental expectations of the adolescent who has an ABI for attainment of life skills as adulthood approaches.

This life course perspective takes into account the developmental transitions and the changing dynamics and priorities that emerge over the course of the life of both the child and family. Each transition challenges the family to readjust and reorganize. It is essential for families to learn how to pace themselves to avoid burnout, normalize relationships with other family members, sustain intrafamilial and extrafamilial relationships, and support the growing autonomy of the adolescent with ABI during the process of transitioning into adulthood.

Community Interdependence

The medical, educational, and community living aspects of service provision have traditionally been described as a continuum of care. This traditional continuum begins with the delivery of emergency medical services to the injured child and transportation to an acute hospital where trauma and medical teams provide specialized medical interventions. When stabilized, most children are discharged directly home in the care of parents; however, those more seriously injured may be transferred to an in-patient rehabilitation program for intensive rehabilitation treatment. As the child returns home and enters school and the community, parents become the ongoing caregivers and coordinators of outpatient programs, continuing rehabilitation services and educational programs.

According to DePompei and Tyler (44), the continuum of care is insufficient to explain the complexity of school, family, and community services and supports after ABI in children and youth. An alternative concept is found in Condeluci's model of community interdependence (45–47). The interdependence concept suggests that there must be an interconnection or interrelationship among 2 or more entities. The circle of community interdependence is not a linear model as suggested by the continuum of care but a circular concept that begins and ends in the community. In this concept, the beginning point is not emergency medical service. The injury or illness begins in the community where the child or youth is a living contributing member. Treatment of the child's brain injury then engages experts in medicine, education, community, and the family who collaborate with the same goal: to return the child to the community. Because this concept is based on a circle, any point on the circle may be the beginning point of care.

The circle of interdependence requires service providers to assume responsibility for the entire circle of care regardless of the primary work environment. Thus, those who work in the medical community provide treatment with consideration of the eventual return of this child to the community; those who work in educational and life-long living community agencies receive the child or youth with an appreciation of the complex and unique medical and behavioral aspects that will affect learning and community living. All professionals work in tandem with families to achieve successful community participation and access to resources. The circle of interdependence accounts for all aspects of service equally within the community. This concept is supported heavily in the literature (45–50).

RESILIENCE-BASED CLINICAL FAMILY SYSTEM ASSESSMENT

Over the past 2 decades, there has been increasing interest in measures of family functioning after brain injury. In 2 recent reviews (51,52), a critical analysis of caregiver and family measures was conducted. Based on this review, only the studies by Gan and colleagues (53,54) employed a family systems framework, with the unit of analysis being the interactions of the family as a whole rather than an individual member. It should be noted that most empirical measures have been standardized using samples of English-speaking, white, middle-class, 2-parent families who are not under stress and may not be suitable for a more diverse sample of families (51). Furthermore, families of children with chronic health conditions may score in "unhealthy" or "dysfunctional" ranges using norms and cut-offs developed in the general population; however, these patterns of functioning may actually be adaptive within these families (51). It is therefore important to go beyond any one-norm-fits-all model of family assessment. A multimodal resilience-based approach to family system assessment is proposed, incorporating both quantitative (see Table 38-1) as well as qualitative methods (see Appendix I).

Table 38-1 includes selected family assessment measures, including measures of family functioning, measures used in the childhood disability field, and measures of FCS—all with reported reliability and validity. Appendix I offers a practical guideline for resilience-based clinical family system assessment that includes the perspectives of 3 experts: child/youth with ABI, family, and professionals. This partnership approach helps to identify the family system challenges after ABI and the resources and competencies that facilitate optimal coping and adaptation. Moreover, this framework is more suited to families from diverse ethnocult-

TABLE 38-1 Family Assessment Measures

GENERAL FAMILY FUNCTIONING MEASURES

MEASURE	CONSTRUCTS MEASURED	FORMAT	COMMENTS
Family Assessment Device (FAD) (75)	Family functioning (i.e., problem solving, communication, role changes, behavioral control)	Self-report: family members 4-point Likert 60 items	• Most widely used measure of ABI family outcomes (both adult and pediatric populations) • Designed for individuals 12 years and older
Family Assessment Measure-III (FAM-III) (76)	Family system functioning (i.e., communication, problem solving, role changes)	Self-report: family members 4-point Likert 50-item general scale	• Clinical utility in measuring family system functioning with a variety of clinical populations including ABI • Designed for individuals 10 years and older • Brief 15-item version available
Family Adaptability and Cohesion Evaluation Scales-IV (FACES-IV) (77)	Family adaptability and cohesion	Self-report by family members 5-point Likert 42 items	• Earlier version, FACES II used in ABI family outcome studies • Designed for individuals 12 years and older • Discriminates between "healthy" and "unhealthy" families

MEASURES USED IN CHILDHOOD DISABILITY LITERATURE

MEASURE	CONSTRUCTS MEASURED	FORMAT	COMMENTS
Family Burden of Injury Interview (FBII) (78)	Injury-related stress and burden for families, including child adjustment, relationship with spouse and extended family, impact on siblings	Parent interview yes/no with stress rating 0 (*not at all*) to 5 (*extremely stressful*)	• Widely used in pediatric ABI family outcome studies • Designed for use with parents of school-aged children with ABI • Has shown sensitivity to change over time
Impact on Family Scale (IOF) (79)	Impact of child chronic illness on family, including strain, financial burden, and mastery/coping	Parent self-report 4-point Likert 33 items	• Used with parents of children with a variety of chronic health conditions, including children with ABI • Includes 6 sibling-related items
Coping Health Inventory for Parents (CHIP) (80)	Parent coping responses to managing life with a child with chronic illness or disability	Parent self-report 4-point Likert 45 items	• Applicable to the ABI population given its wide use in childhood chronic illness (i.e., epilepsy, autism, cystic fibrosis, multiple disabilities) • Allows for comparisons of mothers' and fathers' coping patterns

COPING MEASURE

MEASURE	CONSTRUCTS MEASURED	FORMAT	COMMENTS
Family Crisis Oriented Personal Evaluation Scales (F-COPES) (81)	Family coping patterns: problem solving and behavioral strategies used to manage difficult situations	Self-report: parents and youth 5-point Likert 30 items	• Used in studies of families of adults with ABI; families of children with learning, developmental, cognitive and/or physical disabilities; families of at-risk youth

MEASURES OF FAMILY-CENTERED SERVICE IN PEDIATRIC REHABILITATION

MEASURE	CONSTRUCTS MEASURED	FORMAT	COMMENTS
Measure of Processes of Care (MPOC) (82)	Parental perception of family-centered service (i.e., partnerships, coordinated and respectful care)	Parent self-report 7-point rating 56 item	• Demonstrated utility in assessing parents' perspectives of family-centered service in rehabilitation settings including ABI • Brief 20-item version available (MPOC-20)
Giving Youth a Voice (GYV) (83)	Youths' perceptions of client and family-centeredness of services (i.e., respect, information sharing, teen-centered service).	Self-report: youth (ages 13–19) 7-point rating 56 items	• Demonstrated utility in assessing the level of client and family-centeredness of services from the perspective of youth with chronic illness and disabilities including ABI • Brief 20-item version available (GYV-20)

ural backgrounds as assessment considers their values, priorities, belief systems, and unique coping resources.

MENU OF FAMILY SUPPORTS AFTER ACQUIRED BRAIN INJURY IN CHILDREN AND YOUTHS

In a recent qualitative study of family caregivers' support needs after brain injury, a need for family access to a variety of modalities of support over the life course was identified by caregivers, professionals, and researchers. Identified needs included psychosocial and instrumental support, peer support, professional counseling and therapy, financial planning, and respite (55). Cole (56) has also proposed family intervention guidelines for ABIs in children and adolescents. These include (*a*) selection of developmentally appropriate interventions, (*b*) matching the intervention to the family, (*c*) advocacy, (*d*) injury education, (*e*) focus on family realignment, (*f*) appropriate adjustment of the child's environment, and (*g*) skills training for the family and child. Consistent with these guidelines and the study findings of Gan and colleagues (55), Figure 38-2 acknowledges the multiple needs of families after ABI in children and youth and the menu of supports needed throughout the life course.

Education About Acquired Brain Injury in Children and Adolescents

Families face the formidable challenge of focusing on both the present and the future because ABI has both an immediate and developmental impact on the child, depending on the age of onset. ABI also impacts each member of the family differently. Educational interventions help families reduce their fears, normalize their experiences, and prepare them for future developmental transitions. In the acute care stage,

families face the crisis of threatened loss of their child. With the child's survival, they reorganize around the crisis and focus on their child's recovery. At this stage, it is critical for families to have written information about ABI, the natural course of recovery, and expectations for the child's return home. Because the stress of hospitalization often makes it difficult for families to comprehend and absorb information, education needs to be provided in both verbal and written formats and at multiple times. After hospital discharge, it is helpful to review this information once families have had some experience living with their child's brain injury. As the child "grows into" the disability, families need further education to help them understand the developmental impact of ABI, the developing brain, and the effects of brain injury on social, behavioral, and academic functioning. As the child approaches adolescence, additional educational intervention is needed because families often struggle with differentiating between the sequelae of ABI and the changes caused by adolescence.

It is important that educational materials be presented in layman's terms and in different formats depending on the family's preferences, needs, and priorities. Some prefer written modalities (i.e., pamphlets, handouts, booklets), whereas others want information presented verbally (i.e., workshops, lectures). Some welcome group formats, whereas others prefer more personalized one-on-one discussion. The family, child, or youth with ABI, as well as siblings, also need access to age-appropriate information about brain injury. Educating uninjured siblings about brain injury has been found to be important in promoting favorable behavioral outcome (57). Web-based resources, such as specific brain injury Web sites are increasingly popular. Some of these include sites in the United States (Web link: http://www.brainline.org/landing_pages/features/blkids.html), Australia (Web link: http://www.braininjurycentre.com.au/aus/index.php?option=com_content&view=frontpage&Itemid=1), United Kingdom (Web link: http://www.childbraininjurytrust.org.uk/index.html), and educational sites for children and youth (Web link: http://faculty.washington.edu/chudler/neurok.html).

Peer Support

When parents learn that their child has an ABI, they begin a journey that is often filled with different and conflicting emotions, difficult choices, stress, anxiety, and uncertainty. At the same time, they enter an arena of complex and often unfamiliar service systems. Feelings of isolation and aloneness are universal among parents, especially at the time of diagnosis; therefore, it is critical for them to have access to peer support from the outset. This may include one-on-one support and parent groups, both in the hospital system and in the community. At this early stage, it is important to link families with local brain injury associations as caregivers have consistently noted the value of peer supports. Knowing they are not alone and that other people are coping with similar issues provides families with encouragement and hope.

In addition to ABI support groups, families can also benefit from joining groups that are not disability specific because parents often face similar challenges regardless of their child's disability. A good starting place for parents to

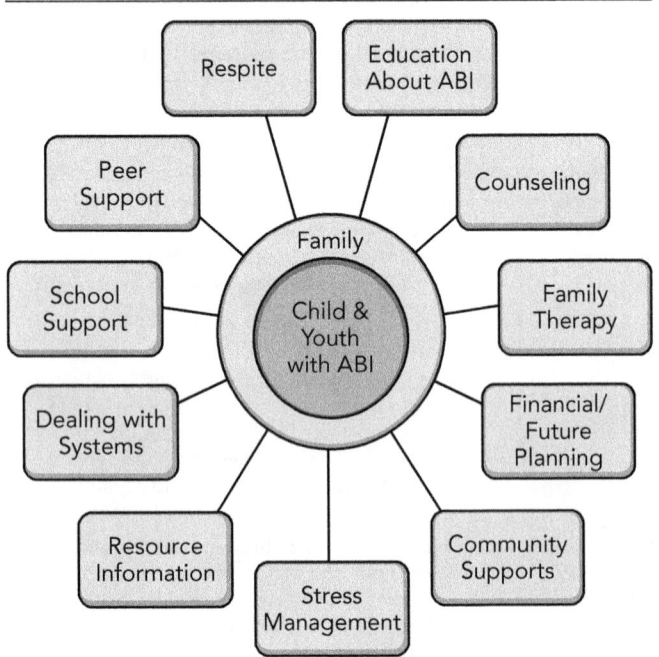

FIGURE 38-2 Menu of family supports after ABI in children and adolescents.

identify state resources in the United States is the National Dissemination Center for Children with Disabilities (NIC HCY) (Web link: http://www.nichcy.org). NICHCY offers fact sheets on specific disabilities, including traumatic brain injury. The fact sheets define the disability, describe its characteristics, offer tips for parents and teachers, and offer links to additional disability organizations.

Peer-mentoring programs are additional resources where trained peer mentors or facilitators—survivor-to-survivor and caregiver-to-caregiver—are matched to provide support through the internet, in person, or by phone. As an example, the Family-to-Family Link Up Program in Australia benefits families through brief, time-limited contacts with a trained facilitator (58). Multiple family groups have also been validated as an effective intervention for improving family functioning after brain injury (59). With the rise in technology, Web-based supports are becoming increasingly popular, especially for those who live in rural communities. Regardless of the mode of peer support, resiliencies are enhanced through building social support and contact with other families dealing with similar challenges.

Community Linkages

Access to community resources and supportive relationships outside the family are key protective factors contributing to resilience. This includes access to financial resources, respite services, legal services, school supports, recreational/social programs, camps, volunteering, work, independent living, or services for future planning. These resources are critical for providing financial security, practical assistance, social support, and a basic sense of connectedness through social support networks (60). Case management can be very helpful as families negotiate the complexities of legal, medical, rehabilitation, and insurance systems.

Family Counseling and Skills Training

Resilience is promoted by normalizing the challenges that families face after an ABI and by offering useful guidelines for coping in the present and in the future. Families need concrete and practical information for expectations, the recovery process, methods of assistance, strategies for coping with new roles, and information about community and professional supports (55,61). Families require help to balance the needs of the child with ABI with the needs of the rest of the family. Helping families maintain normalcy in family routines and activities is essential so the child's brain injury does not become the central focus of family life.

Family intervention is needed not just in the early stages of rehabilitation but also at critical developmental transitions or as salient issues arise, such as during adolescence or during transition to adulthood. During periods of stability, periodic booster sessions or "psychosocial checkups" (20) can be beneficial to reinforce strategies and maintain gains that families have made. Maintaining family organizational patterns, supporting healthy boundaries, and fostering open communication are key factors in fostering family resilience.

Counseling for siblings can help them understand not only the changes in their brother or sister caused by the ABI but their reactions and emotions as well. The sibling relationship is altered by ABI; siblings face feelings of loss and disruption in family roles and dynamics. Just as parents struggle to cope with the emotional impact of the trauma, siblings also struggle to find effective ways of coping. Far too often, their needs are overlooked, even though studies have consistently noted how their lives are profoundly affected (14). Supporting generational boundaries is essential so that the sibling does not take on a parentified role within the family. Involvement of siblings in individual, group, and family counseling sessions provides a forum to acknowledge and legitimize their needs for information, education, and support. Siblings who feel supported are more likely to have better behavioral outcome (57). Like the child or adolescent with ABI, siblings' needs also change over time and the importance of including them in "psychosocial checkups" (20) is underscored.

Families also benefit from skills training in problem solving, stress management, positive parenting, and strategies for dealing with ABI-related behavioral, cognitive, and emotional changes in the child (55,62,63). As proposed by Walsh (22), fostering collaborative problem solving can help families become more resilient. This also entails taking a proactive stance and helping families deal with anticipated challenges, such as dealing with the developmental changes of adolescence and preparing for adulthood.

Dealing with sexuality issues is an example of proactive intervention, yet this is seldom addressed with children and youth with ABI. Adolescence is a particularly challenging phase for families as this coincides with teenagers' emerging interest in sex. They live in a society where they are surrounded by sexual messages, and some of the messages they see and hear can be confusing. Parents play an important role in providing accurate information and promoting positive aspects of sexuality, yet they may not view this as a priority given the array of issues that they have to grapple with.

Parents will need help in understanding how an ABI can affect emerging sexuality and how to support their child/adolescent in a proactive way. For example, there may be physical changes such as mobility issues or sensorimotor problems, which can have a devastating effect on self-image. Early or delayed onset of puberty can also be disturbing for a young person who is not prepared for these changes. Preparing parents for these unexpected physical changes is important to normalizing family response to these issues.

From a behavioral perspective, there may be increased risk-taking behavior caused by problems with poor judgment, disinhibition, or impulsive behaviors. Risk of unplanned pregnancy, sexually transmitted infections, sexual assault, or exploitation are concerns often expressed by parents. The child or adolescent may need firm and clear guidelines around what is acceptable behavior and what is not. They may also need help differentiating between safe vs unsafe behaviors and healthy vs unhealthy relationships.

Social skills deficits and communication impairments can make it difficult for teenagers to establish or maintain friendships. Changes in body image, fitting in with peers, and reduced self-esteem can affect one's confidence and comfort in forming new relationships. Meeting people, carrying a conversation, learning to date, and learning appropriate boundaries are some of the social skills that may need to be taught.

To safely negotiate the stage of adolescence, youth need to be supported in finding positive and healthy ways to express their sexuality. They need to know who they can talk to about sexuality. They need to know what to do to avoid unwanted pregnancy, sexual diseases, loss of friendship, exploitaton, or trouble with the law. It is important for clinicians to be proactive by initiating discussions, acknowledging the importance of this topic, and providing opportunities for dialogue with children, youth, and their families. Readers are referred to this podcast on sexuality in teenagers with brain injury (Web link: www.holland bloorview.ca/programsandservices/rehabcomplexcare/br aininjurysexuality.php).

Family Therapy

Research on family therapy outcomes suggest that client and family factors account for the greatest variance in outcomes, not the skills or expertise of the therapist (64). A resilience-based model of family therapy after ABI therefore supports best outcomes because it amplifies family strengths and resources, enhances communication, facilitates problem solving, focuses on successes, encourages mutual family collaboration, and focuses on future possibilities.

The therapeutic approach used by clinicians also needs to consider the developmental aspects of working with children and adolescents. Engaging teenagers is challenging as the adolescent survivor will often resist or refuse active counseling because of developmental issues, which prioritize peer identification and increasing independence (65). Brief solution-focused therapy (BSFT) approaches have been found to be helpful in engaging children and youth with a variety of challenges (66). BSFT is client driven, collaborative, and focuses on strengths and successes vs failures and problems. Because BSFT orients toward the future, promotes competence, and fosters hope, it is very compatible with a resilience framework.

In addition to face-to-face interventions, Web-based interventions for families of children and adolescents with ABI have also been developed (62,63,67). There is evidence that Web-based programs are effective in reducing the number of parent–adolescent conflicts and improving behavior in adolescents with severe TBI (68). Web-based interventions may be particularly useful for families in more remote areas or where travel and time are barriers to participation.

Families may also present with complex issues that preceded the child's injury, have been compounded by the injury, or are independent of the injury. Current or preexisting issues of domestic abuse, marital breakdown, addictions, complicated grief, emotional trauma, or mental health concerns are examples of challenges that may warrant additional referrals to a family therapist, ideally one who is knowledgeable about brain injury. Because very few family therapists have expertise in ABI, collaboration between the brain injury specialists and the family therapist is essential.

Respite Care

The fundamental concept underlying respite care is to provide families with temporary relief by giving them a break from the ongoing demands of caregiving. Every parent needs some time off and away from their children to recharge; however, for most families of children with special needs or disabilities, relying on the neighborhood sitter is simply not an option. Respite services can range from something as informal as someone coming into the home to care for or watch a child, to a community outing with a respite worker, a residential option for overnight, or a respite camp for several weeks. Access to respite services varies widely both across and within Canada and the United States. Some programs are funded by state or provincial funds or community organizations, some have partial insurance coverage, and others are private pay. Finding qualified respite workers is another challenge that directly affects a parent's level of confidence and comfort for leaving the child in another person's care, whether it be at home or in a more formal program (69).

Advocacy

Parents can be effective advocates for their child in settings as diverse as medical, educational, social, and community programs. Advocacy can be viewed broadly as a strategy for educating others about the sequelae of ABI, ensuring that services and programs best fit the child's needs, and developing partnerships with professionals. The essential characteristics of an effective parent advocate are assertiveness, collaboration, and negotiation. Parental advocacy is essential for overcoming barriers of limited knowledge about brain injury, attitudinal biases and stereotypes, and inadequate funding for services (70).

Parents and Educators as Partners

Few parents know what to expect as their child returns home from the hospital or rehabilitation program. As their child enters or returns to school, new questions arise. "How will the brain injury affect his or her ability to learn? Will my child need special help in school? Why has his or her behavior changed? Why does it take his or her so much longer to do his or her homework? Will the teachers know what a brain injury is? Will they know how to help my child in school? How will his or her friends react?"

Many parents are alarmed and discouraged when they hear that "your child is the first student we have had with a brain injury." This comment not only worries them but raises many questions about the ability of teachers and school staff to recognize the impact of the ABI on their child's ability to learn and function in school. Learning about the laws and regulations for special education services and the language of Identification, Placement, and Review Committee (IPRC), individualized education program (IEP), or 504 plans thrusts many parents into an unfamiliar and bureaucratic service system.

Many schools consider ABI to be a low-incidence population when compared to other developmental disabilities despite the fact that it is the leading cause of death and disability among children (71). School is the setting where the child will spend more time and access more resources than any other arena. Yet the National Pediatric Trauma Registry found that less than 2% of children discharged home from a trauma center were referred to special educational services within the local school system (49). This means that the critical transition from hospital to home to school falls largely to parents at a critical time when they need more support and information. Thus, it is critical for educators and parents to work as partners to jointly address the educational needs of the child and student. There are fundamental skills used by professional case managers that have been adapted for families to use with school systems. They are (*a*) assessment or "how has the brain injury affected my child," (*b*) information gathering or "what do I need to know," (*c*) referral or "when do I need to get a specialist involved," (*d*) service coordination or "how do I pull this all together," (*e*) advocacy or "how can I help others understand what my child needs," and (*f*) evaluation or "how do I know if this is working?" Research has demonstrated that by using these skills, parents can be more effective negotiators, coordinators, and advocates for educational services for their child after a brain injury (72).

A SPECIAL NOTE ON FOSTER FAMILIES

Child abuse and assault are major causes of injury to children in the youngest and oldest age groups. According to the national Pediatric Trauma Registry, more than 1 in 5 children younger than 1 year of age were victims of child abuse and more than 1 in 10 in the 15–19-year age range were victims of assault. Despite the presence of multiple traumas in many of these children who were admitted to participating trauma centers, the mean length of stay for the youngest group was only 4.7 days and increased to a mean of 7 days for the older group. Children injured because of abuse or assault have very different discharge patterns than other age groups. Foster care is identified as the discharge disposition for 38.6% of children younger than the age of 1 year with 1–3 impairments; for 32.9% of children with 4 or more impairments. In both categories, a higher percentage of children younger than 1 year of age are discharged from trauma centers to foster care than to rehabilitation programs (26).

Foster families are largely unrecognized in the research literature, yet are the primary caregivers for these vulnerable young children. They often have limited access to the child's medical and developmental history, yet are the primary coordinators of services in the community. Furthermore, the person who inflicted the abuse is most often a family member or significant other, which increases the complexity of the dynamics for the biological family. Criminal charges and incarceration of a family member are common and further complicate family dynamics.

BRAIN INJURY FAMILY INTERVENTION FOR ADOLESCENTS

The Brain Injury Family Intervention for Adolescents (BIFI-A) is a community-based family system intervention for adolescents with brain injury and their families (73). BIFI-A is a 12-session protocol that encompasses education, skill building, and emotional support (see Table 38-2). Three key theoretical components underlie BIFI-A: family systems theory, cognitive behavioral therapy, and BSFT. Family members are provided with education about brain injury and its impact on the family, information about adolescent development, and how brain injury affects the developmental process. Through family discussion, supportive interventions are incorporated to address issues around grief, emotional expression, coping with loss and change, and supporting one another around the losses. These are considered core family tasks for healthy adaptation to loss (74).

BIFI-A is also designed to foster skill building around goal setting, stress management, and problem solving, which are key features of family hardiness (60). Families are provided with tools to support successful school transitions and to prepare for adulthood. Because BIFI-A is an interactive program that is designed to engage all members of the family system including siblings, families gain relational resilience by pulling together as a functional family unit.

TABLE 38-2 Brain Injury Family Intervention for Adolescents (BIFI-A) Curriculum

SESSION	TOPICS
1	Assessment
2	What happens after brain injury
3	Brain injury happens to the whole family
4	Being a teen and achieving independence
5	Emotional and physical recovery are different things
6	Coping with loss and change
7	Managing intense emotions
8	Managing stress and taking care of self
9	Setting SMART goals and tracking progress
10	Learning patience and solving problems
11	School, transitions, and preparing for adulthood
12	Wrap-up—celebrating successes and accomplishments

Web link: http://informahealthcare.com/doi/abs/10.3109/0269905100 3692142.

CONCLUSION

The focus of this chapter has been on family coping and resilience after ABI in children and youth. In contrast to the medical model and traditional rehabilitation approaches to family intervention after adult ABI, a resilience-based family systems framework has been introduced. Key highlights of this framework include the following:

1. Viewing families as resilient vs burdened—a strength-based approach underscores families' adaptive resources and changes the focus from deficits and pathology to how families can be strengthened to master adversity (20).
2. Family-centered approach—the child/adolescent with the ABI, the family, and the professional all work together in partnership to identify the resources and competencies that facilitate optimal coping and adaptation.
3. The circle of community interdependence—all service providers assume responsibility for the entire circle of care, regardless of primary work environment.

4. The life course perspective—helps families take a proactive approach as they prepare for the unique developmental challenges of ABI in children and youth.

Using this framework as a guideline, clinicians can help families become more resilient by focusing on their strengths and resources vs dysfunction. Reframing the family's distress as a normal response to an abnormal condition can help depathologize families so that they can maintain a positive outlook to sustain them over the long term. Clinicians are encouraged to focus on the emotional adjustment of all members, the strength of their relationships, and the resources within the family unit. Adopting a family systems perspective is crucial in order to help family members reorganize and adapt to the unique challenges arising from the child's brain injury. Clinicians can also offer practical guidelines and skill training around effective communication and collaborative problem solving, key processes in family resilience. Facilitating access to community resources and fostering supportive relationships outside the family are also important protective factors that contribute to resilience.

This chapter encourages professionals to focus on providing family support that develops resilience and enhances independence. Means for understanding family functioning from a positive perspective are supported with guidelines for resilience-based family system assessment and best practice suggestions. However, it is noted that many of these approaches are not yet confirmed with empirical data.

Because limited knowledge is available about family adaptation after ABI in children and youth, there is a clear need for research to understand resiliency and healthy adaptation in these families. Instead of studying dysfunctional families and the burden and distress associated with ABI, we need to learn about well-functioning families and what enables them to pull together and succeed. As proposed by Walsh (60), "We have much to learn from resilient families to inform our interventions with distressed families." We need to learn about the many pathways to family resilience so we can enable families to rebound from their experience with the strength and coping resources to sustain them over their life course.

KEY CLINICAL POINTS

1. The family is central to the lifelong living issues that accompany a child's brain injury.
2. As the entire family system is affected when a child or adolescent sustains an ABI, it is essential to provide intervention to the entire system and its individual members.
3. Families can be resourceful and resilient despite the challenges of having a child or adolescent with ABI.
4. Clinicians can help families become more resilient by focusing on their strengths and resources vs dysfunction. A resilience-based family systems framework for assessment and intervention is proposed.
5. Recovery patterns of children and youth with ABI differ from adults because their brains are still developing into adulthood. Hence, a life course perspective is essential to take into account the developmental transitions and changing dynamics that emerge over the course of life of the child and family.

6. There is benefit to incorporating principles of FCS and forming collaborative partnerships with clients and families.
7. A model of community interdependence is proposed, encompassing experts in medicine, education, community, and the family who work in tandem with one another to return the child to the community.
8. Families need access to a variety of modalities of support over the life course, including education about ABI, peer support, community linkages, family counseling and skills training, family therapy, respite, and advocacy. Parents and educators need to work in partnership to facilitate the child's successful return to school.
9. A practical guideline for resilience-based clinical family assessment is provided to identify family strengths and resources that foster resilience in families.
10. More research is needed on resilience and healthy family adaptation after ABI in children and adolescents.

KEY REFERENCES

1. Condeluci A. *The Essence of Interdependence: Building Community for Everyone.* Youngsville, NC: Lash & Associates Publishing/Training Inc; 2008.
2. Gan C, Gargaro J, Brandys C, Gerber G, Boschen K. Family caregivers' support needs after brain injury: a synthesis of perspectives from caregivers, programs, and researchers. *NeuroRehabilitation.* 2010;27(1):5–18.
3. Gan C, Gargaro J, Kreutzer J, Boschen KA, Wright FV. Development and preliminary evaluation of a structured family system intervention for adolescents with brain injury and their families. *Brain Inj.* 2010;24(4):651–663.
4. Rolland JS, Walsh F. Facilitating family resilience with childhood illness and disability. *Curr Opin Pediatr.* 2006; 18(5):527–538.
5. Walsh F. *Strengthening Family Resilience.* 2nd ed. New York, NY: Guilford Press; 2006.

References

1. Gillette Y, DePompei R. The potential of electronic organizers as a tool in the cognitive rehabilitation of young people. *Neurorehabilitation.* 2004;19(3):233–243.
2. Anderson V, Catroppa C. Advances in postacute rehabilitation after childhood-acquired brain injury: a focus on cognitive, behavioral, and social domains. *Am J Phys Med Rehabil.* 2006;85(9):767–778.
3. Sherk Consulting Group. *Provincial review of services for children and youth living with the effects of an acquired brain injury: Provincial report.* ON: Pediatric Sub-Committee of the Provincial Acquired Brain Injury Advisory Committee (PABIAC); 1999.
4. Chevignard MP, Brooks N, Truelle JL. Community integration following severe childhood traumatic brain injury. *Curr Opin Neurol.* 2010;23(6):695–700.
5. Barnes C, Mercer G, Shakespeare T. *Exploring Disability: A Sociological Introduction.* Cambridge, United Kingdom: Polity; 1999.
6. Holland AL. *Counseling in Communication Disorders: A Wellness Perspective.* San Diego, CA: Plural Publishers; 2007.
7. Rolland JS. *Families, Illness and Disability: An Interactive Treatment Model.* New York, NY: Basic Books; 1994.
8. Masel BE, DeWitt DS. Traumatic brain injury: a disease process, not an event. *J Neurotrauma.* 2010;27(8):1529–1540.
9. Aitken M, McCarthy M, Slomine B, et al. Family burden after traumatic brain injury in children. *Pediatrics.* 2009;123(1):199–206.
10. Anderson VA, Catroppa C, Haritou F, Morse S, Rosenfeld JV. Identifying factors contributing to child and family outcome 30 months

after traumatic brain injury in children. *J Neurol Neurosurg Psychiatry.* 2005;76(3):401–408.

11. Taylor HG, Yeates KO, Wade SL, Drotar D, Stancin T, Burant C. Bidirectional child–family influences on outcomes of traumatic brain injury in children. *J Int Neuropsychol Soc.* 2001;7(6):755–767.

12. Rivara JM, Jaffe KM, Polissar NL, Fay GC, Liao S, Martin KM. Predictors of family functioning and change 3 years after traumatic brain injury in children. *Arch Phys Med Rehabil.* 1996;77(8):754–764.

13. McMahon M, Noll R, Michaud L, Johnson JC. Sibling adjustment to pediatric traumatic brain injury: a case-controlled pilot study. *J Head Trauma Rehabil.* 2001;16(6):587–594.

14. Sambuco M, Brooks N, Lah S. Paediatric traumatic brain injury: a review of siblings' outcome. *Brain Inj.* 2008;22(1):7–17.

15. Savage RC, Depompei R, Tyler J, Lash M. Paediatric traumatic brain injury: a review of pertinent issues. *Pediatr Rehabil.* 2005;8(2):92–103.

16. Savage RC, Pearson S, McDonald H, Potoczny-Gray A, Marchese N. After hospital: working with schools and families to support the long term needs of children with brain injuries. *NeuroRehabilitation.* 2001;16:49–58.

17. Blosser J, DePompei R. *Pediatric Traumatic Brain Injury: Proactive Intervention.* 2nd ed. Clifton Park, NY: Delmar; 2003.

18. Wade S, Walz C. Family, school, and community: their role in the rehabilitation of children. In: Frank RG, Rosenthal M, Caplan B, eds. *Handbook of Rehabilitation Psychology.* 2nd ed. Washington, DC: American Psychological Association Books; 2010:345–354.

19. Gerring JP, Wade S. The essential role of psychosocial risk and protective factors in pediatric traumatic brain injury research. *J Neurotrauma.* 2012;29(4):621–628.

20. Rolland JS, Walsh F. Facilitating family resilience with childhood illness and disability. *Curr Opin Pediatr.* 2006;18(5):527–538.

21. Spina S, Ziviani J, Nixon J. Children, brain injury and the resiliency model of family adaptation. *Brain Impair.* 2005;6(1):33–44.

22. Walsh F. *Strengthening Family Resilience.* 2nd ed. New York, NY: Guilford Press; 2006.

23. Kubler-Ross E. *On Death and Dying.* London, United Kingdom: Routledge; 1973.

24. Lezak MD. Psychological implications of traumatic brain damage for the patient's family. *Rehabil Psycho.* 1986;31(4):241–250.

25. Russell D. Brain injury: a family perspective. In: *The Essential Brain Injury Guide.* 4th ed. Alexandria, VA: Brain Injury Association of America; 2007.

26. DiScala C, Savage RC. Epidemiology of children with TBI requiring hospitalization. *Brain Inj Source.* 2003;6(3):8–13.

27. Williams J. Family reaction to head injury. In: Williams JT, Kay T, eds. *Head Injury: A Family Matter.* 1991:81–99.

28. Boss P. *Ambiguous Loss: Learning to Live With Unresolved Grief.* Cambridge, MA: Harvard University Press; 1999.

29. Roscigno C, Swanson K. Parents' experiences following children's moderate to severe traumatic brain injury: a clash of cultures. *Qual Health Res.* 2011;21(10):1413–1426.

30. Kay T, Cavallo MM. The family system: impact, assessment, and intervention. In: Hales RE, Silver JM, Yudofsky SC, eds. Neuropsychiatry of Traumatic Brain Injury. Washington, DC: American Psychiatric Press; 1994:533–567.

31. Larøi F. The family systems approach to treating families of persons with brain injury: a potential collaboration between family therapist and brain injury professional. *Brain Inj.* 2003;17(2):175–187.

32. Maitz EA, Sachs PR. Treating families of individuals with traumatic brain injury from a family systems perspective. *J Head Trauma Rehabil.* 1995;10(2):1–11.

33. Boschen K, Gargaro J, Gan C, Gerber G, Brandys C. Family interventions after acquired brain injury and other chronic conditions: a critical appraisal of the quality of the evidence. *NeuroRehabilitation.* 2007;22(1):19–41.

34. Conoley JC, Sheridan SM. Pediatric traumatic brain injury: challenges and interventions for families. *J Learn Disabil.* 2005;29(6):662–669.

35. King S, Kertoy M, King G, Rosenbaum P, Hurley P, Law M. *Perceptions About Family-Centered Service Delivery for Children With Disabil-*

ities. Hamilton, ON: McMaster University, *CanChild* Centre for Childhood Disability Research; 2000.

36. King G, King S, Rosenbaum P. *Interpersonal Aspects of Caregiving and Client Satisfaction, Adherence and Stress: A Review of the Medical and Rehabilitation Literature.* Hamilton, ON: McMaster University, Neurodevelopmental Clinical Research Unit; 1994.

37. Law M, Hanna S, King G, et al. *Factors Affecting Family-Centered Service Delivery for Children with Disabilities.* Hamilton, ON: McMaster University, *CanChild* Centre for Childhood Disability Research; 2001.

38. Wilkins S, Pollock N, Rochon S, Law M. Implementing client-centred practice: why is it so difficult to do? *Can J Occup Ther.* 2001; 68(2):70–79.

39. Sohlberg MM, McLaughlin KA, Todis B, Larsen J, Glang A. What does it take to collaborate with families affected by brain injury? A preliminary model. *J Head Trauma Rehabil.* 2001;16(5):498–511.

40. Lash M. Family-centered case management: preparing parents to become service coordinators for children with ABI. In: Singer GHS, Glang A, Williams J, eds. *Children With ABI: Educating and Supporting Families.* Baltimore, MD: Paul H. Brookes Pub.; 1996.

41. Anderson V, Catroppa C, Morse S, Haritou F, Rosenfeld JV. Intellectual outcome from preschool traumatic brain injury: a 5-year prospective, longitudinal study. *Pediatrics.* 2009;124(6):e1064–e1071.

42. Ewing-Cobbs L, Prasad MR, Kramer L, et al. Late intellectual and academic outcomes following traumatic brain injury sustained during early childhood. *J Neurosurg Nurs.* 2006;105(4)(suppl):287–296.

43. Taylor H, Alden J. Age-related differences in outcomes following childhood brain insults: an introduction and overview. *J Int Neuropsychol Soc.* 1997;3(6):555–567.

44. Depompei R, Tyler J. Children and adolescents: practical strategies for school participation and transition. In: Ashey M, ed. *Traumatic Brain Injury: Rehabilitation, Treatment, and Case Management.* 3rd ed. Boca Raton, FL: CRC Press; 2010.

45. Condeluci A. *Together Is Better.* Wake Forest, NC: Lash and Associates Publishing/Training Inc; 2008.

46. Condeluci A. *The Essence of Interdependence.* Wake Forest, NC: Lash and Associates Publishing/Training Inc.; 2008.

47. Condeluci A. Opening the Doors to Community. Wake Forest, NC: Lash and Associates Publishing/Training Inc; 2002.

48. Bedell GM, Dumas HM. Social participation of children and youth with acquired brain injuries discharged from inpatient rehabilitation: a follow-up study. *Brain Inj.* 2004;18(1):65–82.

49. DiScala C. *National Pediatric Trauma Registry Biannual Report.* Boston, MA: Research and Training Center, Tufts University School of Medicine; 2001.

50. Depompei R, Blosser JL. Managing transitions for education. In: Rosenthal M, Griffith ER, Kreutzer J, et al., eds. *Rehabilitation of the Adult and Child With Traumatic Brain Injury.* 3rd ed. Philadelphia, PA: F.A. Davis; 1999:393–404.

51. Alderfer MA, Fiese BH, Gold JL, et al. Evidence-based assessment in pediatric psychology: family measures. *J Pediatr Psychol.* 2008; 33(9):1046–1061.

52. Thompson H. A critical analysis of measures of caregiver and family functioning following traumatic brain injury. *J Neurosci Nurs.* 2009;41(3):148–158.

53. Gan C, Schuller R. Family system outcome following acquired brain injury: clinical and research perspectives. *Brain Inj.* 2002; 16(4):311–322.

54. Gan C, Campbell K, Gemeinhardt M, McFadden GT. Predictors of family system functioning after brain injury. *Brain Inj.* 2006;20(6):587–600.

55. Gan C, Gargaro J, Brandys C, Gerber G, Boschen K. Family caregivers' support needs after brain injury: a synthesis of perspectives from caregivers, programs, and researchers. *NeuroRehabilitation.* 2010;27(1):5–18.

56. Cole WR, Paulos SK, Cole CA, Tankard C. A review of family intervention guidelines for pediatric acquired brain injuries. *Dev Disabil Res Rev.* 2009;15(2):159–166.

57. Sambuco M, Brookes N, Catroppa C, Lah S. Predictors of long-term sibling behavioral outcome and self-esteem following pediat-

ric traumatic brain injury. *J Head Trauma Rehabil.* 2011. Epub ahead of print.

58. Butera-Prinzi F, Charles N, Heine K, Rutherford B, Lattin D. Family-to-family link up program: a community-based initiative supporting families caring for someone with an acquired brain injury. *NeuroRehabilitation.* 2010;27(1):31–47.

59. Charles N, Butera-Prinzi F, Perlesz A. Families living with acquired brain injury: a multiple family group experience. *NeuroRehabilitation.* 2007;22(1):61–76.

60. Walsh F. The concept of family resilience: crisis and challenge. *Fam Process.* 1996;35(3):261–281.

61. Armstrong K, Kerns KA. The assessment of parent needs following paediatric traumatic brain injury. *Pediatr Rehabil.* 2002;5(3):149–160.

62. Wade SL, Wolfe C, Brown TM, Pestian JP. Putting the pieces together: preliminary efficacy of a web-based family intervention for children with traumatic brain injury. *J Pediatr Psychol.* 2005;30(5):437–442.

63. Wade S, Walz N, Carey J, Williams KM. Brief report: description of feasibility and satisfaction findings from an innovative online family problem-solving intervention for adolescents following traumatic brain injury. *J Pediatr Psychol.* 2009;34(5):517–522.

64. Duncan BL, Miller SD. *The Heroic Client: Doing Client-Directed, Outcome-Informed Therapy.* 1st ed. San Francisco, CA: Jossey-Bass; 2000.

65. Anderson VA, Catroppa C. Advances in postacute rehabilitation after childhood-acquired brain injury: a focus on cognitive, behavioral, and social domains. *Am J Phys Med Rehabil.* 2006;85(9):767–778.

66. Selekman M. *Solution-Focused Therapy With Children. Harnessing Family Strengths for Systemic Change.* New York, NY: The Guillford Press; 1997.

67. Wade SL, Carey J, Wolfe CR. An online family intervention to reduce parental distress following pediatric brain injury. *J Consult Clin Psychol.* 2006;74(3):445–454.

68. Wade SL, Walz N, Carey J, et al. Effect on behavior problems of teen online problem-solving for adolescent traumatic brain injury. *Pediatrics.* 2011;128(4):e947–e953.

69. Baskin A, Fawcett H. *More Than a Mom: Living a Full and Balanced Life When Your Child Has Special Needs.* 1st ed. Bethesda, MD: Woodbine House; 2006.

70. Lash M, Depompei R. The right to know: educating families when a child has a brain injury. *Brain Inj Source.* 2003;20–24.

71. Kimes K, Lash M, Savage RC. *Students With Brain Injury: Challenges for Identification, Learning and Behavior in the Classroom.* Wake Forest, NC: Lash and Associates Publishing/Training, Inc; 2008.

72. Lash M. Families and educators: creating partnerships for students with brain injuries. In: Savage RC, Wolcott G, eds. *An Educators Manual: What Educators Need to Know About Students With Brain Injuries.* Washington, DC: Brain Injury Association, Inc; 1995:40–48.

73. Gan C, Gargaro J, Kreutzer J, Boschen KA, Wright FV. Development and preliminary evaluation of a structured family system intervention for adolescents with brain injury and their families. *Brain Inj.* 2010;24(4):651–663.

74. Walsh F, McGoldrick M. Loss and the family: a systemic perspective. In: Walsh F, McGoldrick M, eds. *Living Beyond Loss: Death in the Family.* New York, NY: W.W. Norton; 1991.

75. Epstein N, Baldwin L, Bishop D. *The McMaster Family Assessment Device. J Marital Fam Ther.* 1983;9(2):171–180.

76. Skinner H, Steinhauer P, Sitarenios G. Family Assessment Measure (FAM) and process model of family functioning. *J Fam Ther.* 2000;22(2):190–210.

77. Olson D. FACES IV and the Circumplex Model: validation study. *J Marital Fam Ther.* 2011;37(1):64–80.

78. Burgess ES, Drotar D, Taylor HG, Wade S, Stancin T, Yeates KO. The family burden of injury interview: reliability and validity studies. *J Head Trauma Rehabil.* 1999;14(4):394–405.

79. Stein RE, Jessop DJ. The impact on family scale revisited: further psychometric data. *J Dev Behav Pediatr.* 2003;24(1):9–16.

80. McCubbin HI, McCubbin MA, Nevin R, et al. Coping Health Inventory for Parents (CHIP). In: McCubbin HI, Thompson AI, McCubbin MA, eds. *Family Assessment: Resiliency, Coping and Adaptation—Inventories for Research and Practice.* Madison, WI: University of Wisconsin System; 1981:407–453.

81. McCubbin HI, Olson D, Larsen A. Family Crisis Oriented Personal Evaluation Scales (F-COPES). In: McCubbin HI, Thompson AI, McCubbin MA, eds. *Family Assessment: Resiliency, Coping and Adaptation—Inventories for Research and Practice.* Madison, WI: University of Wisconsin System; 1981:455–508.

82. King S, Rosenbaum P, King G. *The Measure of Processes of Care (MPOC): A Means to Assess Family-Centered Behaviours of Health Care Providers.* Hamilton, ON: McMaster University, Neurodevelopmental Clinical Research Unit; 1995.

83. Gan C, Campbell K, Snider A, Snider A, Cohen S, Hubbard J. Giving Youth a Voice (GYV): a measure of youths' perceptions of the client-centredness of rehabilitation services. *Can J Occup Ther.* 2008;75(2):96–104.

APPENDIX I Guidelines for Resilience-Based Family System Assessment

Child/Youth System

Academic, social, and developmental history—are there previous concerns and how has the child/family dealt with these challenges? Child's understanding of the injury and beliefs regarding the injury

- What ABI-related changes have been noticed by the child?
- What has the child been told about the ABI?
- What does having a brain injury mean for the child?
- How does having a brain injury affect how the child feels about himself or herself?

Effects of ABI on current functioning

- School functioning—what are the challenges, have the special needs been identified, what is working, where is the child succeeding, who are the resources and supports?
- Peer relations—who are the friends, how did the child cultivate these friendships, what activities do they enjoy together?
- Family functioning—who best understands the child, who does he or she go to for support, who provides comfort and advice?
- Emotional and behavioral functioning—what helps the child deal with stress and intense emotions, what coping strategies work, how does he or she maintain calm in the face of stress?

Protective factors

- Social environment, including family, school, and peer relations—what hobbies, activities, and programs does the child enjoy, what special interests or talents does the child have, what is he or she good at, in what situations does the child excel?
- Health—what does the child do to optimize his or her health, nutrition, sleep, and physical fitness?
- Psychological factors, belief systems, and temperament—what personality traits are endearing and sources of strength, how does the child rebound from difficult situations, what are the 3 things that the child is most proud of?

What are the child's goals, wishes, and hopes—for now and for the future?

- How have these changed since the injury?
- How similar/divergent are the parents' vision vs the child's vision of the future?

Family System

Family/social history

- What are the family history and relationship patterns?
- Are there any illness patterns including mental health history?
- What previous losses and significant life events have occurred?
- What culture does the family identify with and what is their immigration history?
- What other stressors have piled up over time?
- What are their coping resources and patterns of resilience based on the earlier discussion?

Family's understanding of the injury

- Information and education—what has been provided, what has helped, what other information is needed to help with current situation and to prepare for the next stage?
- Beliefs regarding the injury—what does having a child with ABI mean for the family, how does it affect their outreach to the community, are there cultural beliefs around what it means to have an ABI and help seeking practices?

Changes in the family system

- Family life cycle and normative transitions—what is the stage of family life, what associated stresses and transitions can be expected, what can the family do to prepare for these?
- Relationship and role changes—what is the family doing to reorganize around the changes, how do members acknowledge their losses with one another, what normalizing activities do the family share and enjoy with one another, how does the family make decisions and brain storm together to find solutions to their problems?
- Parental/marital subsystem and caregiver coping—how are parents supporting one another, how is leadership negotiated and shared, how are decisions made, what helpful caregiver coping strategies are being used?
- Sibling subsystem coping—how are sibling relationships maintained, what shared activities are enjoyed, how is balance between family/peer life maintained, what new meanings and life perspectives have evolved for siblings?
- Financial resources and financial impact of ABI—how is the family reorganizing, what supports have been accessed, what other supports might be available?
- What other concurrent stressors and unexpected events are affecting the family?

(Continued)

APPENDIX I Guidelines for Resilience-based Family System Assessment *(Continued)*

Family System

Protective factors

- Family strengths, extended family supports—what 3 things are the family most proud of, who can they lean on in times of need, how can other friends and relatives help?
- Belief systems including cultural belief systems that help to make meaning of the brain injury event—how do these beliefs foster hope and optimism for the future?
- Community networks—what are the social supports, ethnocultural resources, work-related supports, and economic resources that help?
- Spiritual resources—what is the role of prayer, faith, and spirituality in fostering strength, hope, and social support?

Expectations regarding treatment

- What is important for the family (both short-term and long-term), when are things working at their best, what are the possibilities?
- What is the family's identified needs, goals, priorities, and wishes—for now and for the future?

Professional System

- Injury related information—what are the details and circumstances regarding the injury? How long has it been since the injury? When was the child diagnosed?
- What is the rehabilitation history, including previous assessments, specialists, and treatments? What has worked (make special effort to highlight the successes and strengths when reviewing assessment and treatment reports)?
- School system—what information has been provided to the school, how is the school working together with the student and parents in identifying educational goals and preparing the individualized education program (IEP), what are the strengths and needs of the student as identified in the IEP, what modifications and accommodations are helpful for the student, how are parents and students involved in transition planning?
- Has there been involvement with the child welfare system? What resources were available?
- Social support system—what has worked, which resources have been helpful, what additional resources might be anticipated given the child's/family's developmental stage, what does the family need to help plan for the future?
- Rehabilitation needs—what are the priorities based on child's and family's identified needs, goals, and wishes; what other supports would help to facilitate transition planning?
- Litigation supports (as appropriate)—is the child/family involved in litigation? How is this impacting adjustment?

VIII

NEUROLOGICAL DISORDERS

Post-Traumatic Seizures and Epilepsy

Stuart A. Yablon and Alan R. Towne

INTRODUCTION

Traumatic brain injuries (TBIs) remain a leading cause of neurologic disability and death in the population of the United States and westernized nations. An estimated 1.7 million people each year sustain a TBI, including 52,000 deaths and 275,000 hospitalizations with the remaining 80% treated and released from emergency departments (1). Among the survivors of TBI, a sizable number remain with important medical and neurological sequelae, including seizures and epilepsy.

The relationship between TBI and subsequent development of post-traumatic seizures (PTS) including incidence, risk factors for initial occurrence, recurrence, and management comprises the central themes of this review. Issues pertinent to diagnostic and therapeutic management of PTS in patient with TBI are emphasized.

CLASSIFICATION AND CLINICAL PRESENTATIONS

It is useful to review terms employed in the discussion of PTS disorders. These are defined in "Practice Parameter: Antiepileptic Drug Treatment of Post-traumatic Seizures" by the Brain Injury Special Interest Group of the American Academy of Physical Medicine and Rehabilitation (2) and "Standards for Epidemiologic Studies and Surveillance of Epilepsy" by the International League Against Epilepsy (ILAE) (3). An *epileptic seizure* is a clinical manifestation presumed to result from an abnormal and excessive discharge of a set of neurons in the brain. The clinical manifestation consists of sudden and transitory abnormal phenomena, which may include alterations of consciousness, motor, sensory, autonomic, or psychic events, perceived by the patient or an observer (3). *Epilepsy* is a condition characterized by recurrent (2 or more) epileptic seizures, unprovoked by any immediate identified cause (3).

Post-traumatic epilepsy (PTE) is a disorder characterized by recurrent late seizure episodes not attributable to another obvious cause in patients with TBI (2). PTS denote single or recurrent seizures occurring after TBI (2) and are commonly classified into early (< 1 week after TBI) and late (> 1 week after TBI). Classification of early seizures as those occurring within the first 7 days after TBI has sparked some controversy (4), particularly regarding long-term antiepileptic drug (AED) treatment decisions. There is little data to suggest that seizures that occur at day 8 or 14 have recurrence characteristics that justify classification as late seizures, and underlying mechanisms of seizure appearance are more likely to reflect acute pathophysiologic processes rather than those of chronic epilepsy. In practice, the terms PTE and PTS tend to be used interchangeably, although only recurrent late seizures represent PTE.

The exclusion of "other obvious causes" is especially relevant to this patient population. Seizures occurring among patients with TBI may be the result of precipitants unrelated to mechanisms currently linked with post-traumatic epileptogenesis. *Seizure precipitants* have been defined as any endogenous or exogenous factor that promotes the occurrence of epileptic seizures (5). Examples of seizure precipitants among patients with TBI include hydrocephalus (6), sepsis (7), hypoxia (8), metabolic abnormalities (9), and mass-occupying lesions, including hemorrhage (10,11). Among patients with epilepsy, more than 60% cite precipitants among recurrent seizures that they experience (5).

Drugs (12,13) including alcohol (14,15), prescribed psychotropic agents (13,16–21), and recreational/illicit drugs (12,22) warrant particular scrutiny as seizure precipitants among patients with TBI. In one study, for example, 19% of patients with severe TBI developed seizures attributed to tricyclic antidepressants (21). Antidepressants other than tricyclic agents are also implicated with seizure occurrence, including immediate (20) and sustained-release formulations of bupropion (16). Although selective serotonin reuptake inhibitors (SSRIs) are considered to have lower proconvulsant activity than other common antidepressants (23–25), several uncontrolled case studies of patients with epilepsy and depression have reported that SSRI administration increased seizure frequency (26,27). However, SSRIs appear to be relatively safe and are the drug of choice for patients with comorbid epilepsy and depression (28). Certain antipsychotic drugs including newer atypical antipsychotic agents, particularly clozapine, may induce electroencephalography (EEG) abnormalities and seizures (17). Antibiotics, particularly imipenem (29) and quinolone agents (30), have been associated with seizures. Seizure risk is generally elevated among patients who are critically ill (31), and proper dose adjustment for renal clearance may mitigate much of the risk attributed to antibiotic administration (31,32). Bromocriptine and amantadine, dopamine receptor agonists used to treat impaired arousal after TBI, have been implicated as seizure precipitants (33), although this association presently appears to be largely anecdotal. Recreational/illicit stimulants with well-known seizure-inducing properties include cocaine; however, few are probably aware that caffeine at high doses may also induce epileptic seizures (34). Amphetamine and related drugs rarely induce epileptic seizures at therapeutic doses (34). Moreover, methylphenidate and dextroamphetamine do not appear to be associated with increased seizure risk among patients with TBI (33,35). Opioid analgesics, especially meperidine, have been implicated in lowering seizure threshold (36). Seizures have been reported with tramadol monotherapy both at recommended and high doses. The coadministration of antidepressants with tramadol appears to heighten the seizure risk in some cases (37).

Seizures and epilepsy are classified according to their clinical and electroencephalographic characteristics, as developed by the Commission on Classification and Terminology of the International League Against Epilepsy (38,39). This classification is currently undergoing revisions; however, seizures can be divided into 2 categories based primarily on pattern of onset (Table 39-1). These include focal seizures and generalized seizures (40). Generalized seizures denote those

---

TABLE 39-1 Simplified Clinical Classification of Seizure Types

I. FOCAL SEIZURES

A. Focal seizures without impairment of consciousness
Consciousness is not impaired during these focal seizures. The patient can respond appropriately to questions and commands and can remember events occurring during the seizure. The principal types are the following:

1. *Motor seizures*, which are characterized by localized stiffening or jerking of the face or extremity on the same side of the body.
2. *Somatosensory or special sensory seizures*, which can include any sensory modality including smell, taste (often unpleasant—e.g., a metallic sensation), vision (such as flashing lights), hearing, or touch (such as paresthesias and electrical sensations).
3. *Autonomic seizures*, which are relatively common and may include changes in visceral sensation (e.g., in abdomen or chest) and change in heart or breathing rates.
4. *Psychic seizures* in which patients report feelings of fear, depression, or anxiety, or altered perceptions of time such as *déjà vu* and *jamais vu*.

B. Focal seizures with impairment of consciousness
Formerly called complex partial seizures, these seizures are characterized by impairment of consciousness. Frequently, the patient has automatisms, characterized by automatic movements such as lip smacking, picking at bed sheets, grunting, or more complex acts. Complex partial seizures (CPS) usually last no longer than 3 min, with postictal confusion lasting 15 min or less. They may begin as focal seizures without impairment of consciousness (e.g., focal motor, focal sensory) and progress to impairment of consciousness, or there may be impairment of consciousness at the onset.

C. Focal onset evolving to a bilateral convulsive seizure (e.g., tonic, clonic, tonic-clonic)
Focal seizures can evolve to a bilateral or convulsive seizure. Patients may describe an aura, which is a focal seizure preceding loss of consciousness. Patients may also experience a focal seizure with impairment of consciousness before evolution to a convulsive seizure.

II. GENERALIZED SEIZURES (SEIZURES WITHOUT FOCAL ONSET)—THE MAJOR TYPES ARE ABSENCE, MYOCLONIC, ATONIC, TONIC, AND TONIC-CLONIC

A. Absence seizures
Absence seizures are usually classified as either typical absence (previously known as *petit mal*) or atypical absence.

1. *Typical absence seizures* are characterized by abrupt onset of impairment of awareness and responsiveness lasting 3–20 sec. Return to awareness is immediate after the seizure ends. There is no warning before the seizure and no postictal confusion. The patient may report automatisms such as eye blinking and lip smacking. The electroencephalography (EEG) is important in making a diagnosis in this type of seizure and demonstrates a generalized 3-Hz spike-and-wave discharge.
2. *Atypical absence seizures* are usually seen in children with cognitive impairment as opposed to typical absence. They may be associated with atonic and tonic seizures. The EEG usually shows a generalized, slow, spike-and-wave complex (i.e., < 2.5 Hz).

B. Myoclonic seizures
Myoclonic seizures are characterized by very brief bilateral synchronous jerks. Consciousness is usually not impaired unless there are successive myoclonic seizures. EEG generally demonstrates a polyspike-and-slow-wave discharge.

C. Atonic seizures
Atonic seizures are characterized by a sudden loss of postural tone with impairment of consciousness. These seizures rarely last more than 1 min and generally last less than 5 sec.

D. Tonic seizures
Tonic seizures are characterized by flexion or extension of both the upper and lower extremities. They generally last from 5–20 sec and are common in patients with other neurologic abnormalities.

E. Tonic-clonic seizures
Primary generalized tonic-clonic seizures are not preceded by an aura and are characterized by an initial tonic phase of stiffening followed by a clonic phase of jerking of the extremities. The seizure lasts about from 30 sec to 2 min.
It may be difficult to differentiate a primary generalized tonic-clonic seizure from a secondarily generalized seizure.

Adapted from Waterhouse and Towne (36) and Berg et al. (40) with permission.

that are bilaterally symmetrical in origin without apparent focal onset (38). The most commonly recognized example is the generalized tonic-clonic (GTC) seizure or generalized convulsive seizure. Generalized onset seizures or focal onset seizures with secondary generalization are reported in approximately half of the patients with PTS (41) and appear more frequently in patients with nonpenetrating TBI (42) and among children (43).

Focal seizures originate in a localized area of 1 cerebral hemisphere. Focal seizures are further classified according to whether consciousness is maintained, commonly known as simple partial seizures (SPS), or impaired (complex partial seizures [CPS]). In the revised classification, these terms are being replaced by more descriptive terms of focal seizures associated with alteration of consciousness for CPS and focal seizures (motor, sensory, psychic, and other seizures) without alteration of consciousness for SPS. Characteristics of both vary depending on the location of the seizure activity within the brain. Twelve percent of focal seizures with alteration of consciousness in the general population may be attributable to TBI (44). Focal-onset seizures are observed in slightly more than half of all patients with PTS and appear more frequently in adults (4) and patients with early seizures (4,42,45), focal lesions on (computed tomography) CT (46), penetrating TBI (PTBI) (42,47), and nonpenetrating TBI of greater severity (46). Studies that incorporate video electroencephalography (VEEG) are more likely to detect subtle clinical signs that may indicate focal-onset PTS (48,49).

Psychogenic nonepileptic seizures (PNES), often called *pseudoseizures* or *psychogenic seizures*, are terms used for episodic behavioral events, which superficially resemble epileptic attacks but are not associated with paroxysmal activity within the brain (50). PNES must be differentiated from other nonepileptic events such as syncopal episodes and cardiac events. PNES are common in neurologic settings (51) and may coexist with epileptic seizures in patients with epilepsy (51,52). The differentiation between nonepileptic and epileptic seizures cannot be made on the basis of clinical characteristics alone. EEG monitoring (particularly with video) (52) is often helpful in establishing a diagnosis. Postictal prolactin (PRL) measurement (53) may provide additional diagnostic information if significant elevations are observed, suggesting that an epileptic seizure has occurred within 1 hour (54). The use of this test to discriminate between epileptic seizures and PNES has been questioned, however, as a subset of patients with VEEG-documented; PNES have also been reported to experience an increase in PRL, particularly if the sample is obtained within 10–20 min of a suspected PNES (54). Although recognized to occur among patients with TBI, relatively few studies address post-traumatic PNES. Hudak et al. reported that one-third of patients with moderate-to-severe TBI undergoing VEEG for diagnosis of epilepsy were found to have PNES (48). When nondiagnostic VEEG studies were excluded, patients with nonepileptic seizures (NES) comprised 40% of the TBI sample (48). Barry et al. (55) described the characteristics of 16 patients thought to have PTS, who actually had PNES, as confirmed on VEEG monitoring. Patients with PNES were characterized by injuries of much milder severity, although the disability associated with the PNES was pronounced. The patients usually had manifestations of other conversion disorders as well and psychiatric histories that predate the TBI (55). In a study comparing veterans and civilians admitted to the epilepsy monitoring unit (EMU), PNES was identified in 25% of veterans and 26% of civilians. Fifty-eight percent of veterans with PNES were thought to have seizures related to TBI. In the veteran group, PNES was the single most common discharge diagnosis and more common than the discharge diagnosis of epilepsy. Post-traumatic stress disorder (PTSD) has also been shown to be a significant risk factor for developing PNES (56).

Epilepsy and seizures can be characterized by their underlying etiology and fall under 3 categories: genetic, structural/metabolic, and unknown (40). Genetic epilepsy is the direct result of a known or presumed genetic defect. Previously, genetic epilepsies were known as *idiopathic*. Structural/metabolic epilepsies, also known as *symptomatic epilepsies*, are considered to be the consequence of a known or suspected disorder of the central nervous system, such as TBI, stroke, and infection (3,39). Recurrent late PTS or PTE is a common and important type of structural epilepsy (3), accounting for 20% of all lesional epilepsies in the general population (57). Structural/metabolic epilepsies comprise syndromes of great individual variability based mainly on seizure type and anatomic localization. The third etiology is "unknown" designating that the nature of the underlying cause in not yet known. Previously, the term for this type of epilepsy was "cryptogenic."

MANIFESTATIONS OF POST-TRAUMATIC SEIZURES AND EPILEPSY

Seizures may present with various manifestations, including cognitive, behavioral, and affective changes that may not be attributed to an underlying epileptic disorder (58,59). Patients with severe TBI may exhibit cognitive, behavioral, and affective sequelae that potentially confound attribution of episodic behavioral changes to an underlying epileptic disorder (48). The varied semiology of seizures that originate in the frontal or temporal lobes and their associated ictal or postictal alteration of consciousness justify their consideration in the differential diagnosis of any patient with TBI with episodic (especially stereotypic) changes in mental status. Given the propensity of TBI contusion localization to the frontal and temporal lobes (60,61), it is not surprising that these regions are the most frequent sites of origin for VEEG-verified partial-onset PTE (48). Presumed or pathologically confirmed PTS foci, however, have been described in all major lobes of the brain (48,61–64).

Patients with frontal lobe epilepsy may exhibit complex, semipurposeful motor automatisms such as kicking, screaming, and thrashing episodes (59). Frontal lobe interictal and postictal manifestations also include cognitive or affective symptoms, such as confusion, anger, hostility, and hallucinations (65,66). Complex partial seizures of temporal lobe origin may also present with emotional symptoms such as fear or panic, followed by periods of postictal confusion and amnesia (39). Seizure-related aggression, however, is rare (67,68). It is usually associated with postictal confusion, particularly while the patient is being restrained (68,69). Conversely, reports of aggression are more frequent among patients who are epileptic, particularly with younger age, male gender, psychopathology, and prior brain injury (70), but aggression episodes are typically unrelated to seizure type, frequency, or age of onset (71). Conventional interictal scalp EEG is of limited diagnostic assistance in such cases. Electrographic manifestations of seizure activity in the orbitofrontal and medial temporal regions of the brain may be difficult to recognize and can be misleading (59) by showing no abnormality (39) at all. Table 39-2 shows the characteristics of focal-onset epilepsies based on the involved lobe of the brain (39,66,72–78).

Ictal Versus Postictal Focal Neurological Deficits

The presence of focal motor, sensory, or language deficit of new onset should alert the clinician to the possibility of a recent unwitnessed PTS. Todd's paralysis or postictal paresis (PP) is defined as a transient focal deficit that may follow a focal (9) or tonic-clonic seizure (79). It is a recognized postictal manifestation of PTS (80). These do not reflect permanent structural damage but rather represent transient *postictal* disruption of function that typically resolves within 24–48 hours (9). In one VEEG study, PP was found in 13.4% of patients and was always unilateral and contralateral to the seizure focus. The duration of the PP ranged from 11 seconds to 22 minutes (81). PP should be differentiated from ictal paralysis, a "negative" *ictal* epileptic manifestation. (82)

Unclassified Phenomena (Not Considered to be Post-Traumatic Seizures)

Transient behavioral changes, reminiscent of focal seizures with impairment of consciousness (83–85), have been noted among patients with TBI without concurrent seizures. In most reports, patients manifest interictal discharges on EEG, without the hypersynchronous EEG activity and stereotyped behaviors, which characterize partial seizures and localization-related epilepsies (84,85). When described among patients with TBI, these are usually reported among individuals with mild injury severity (84,85). In these reports, many patients respond favorably to AEDs such as carbamazepine (CBZ) (86).

The resemblance of the behaviors to some focal seizures of temporal or frontal lobe origin and favorable response to AEDs tends to confuse clinical diagnosis. At present, the description of these behavioral abnormalities should not be considered diagnostic for epileptic seizures, although further EEG studies may be indicated to fully elucidate the etiology.

EPIDEMIOLOGY OF POST-TRAUMATIC SEIZURES

TBIs are an important cause of epilepsy, accounting for 20% of structural epilepsy observed in the general population and 5% of all epilepsy (57). TBI is the leading cause of epilepsy in young adults (86). Many studies addressing the relationship between TBI and epilepsy derive from observations of veterans sustaining PTBI in battle (47,87–99). Studies in civilian settings (4,41,43,46,100–130) generally appeared later and reflect a larger patient population with nonpenetrating TBI, as opposed to PTBI. The observed results vary, reflecting differences in inclusion and exclusion criteria, methods for evaluation and description of seizure phenomena, attention to confounding variables, duration of follow-up, and patient

population studied (131). Nevertheless, these studies provide useful information regarding the incidence, risk factors, and natural history of PTS/PTE.

In summary, the overall incidence of late seizures in hospitalized patients following nonpenetrating TBI is approximately 4%–7%, varying with the injury and patient characteristics (4,103). Late seizures are observed less frequently among children (43,103,123). The incidence of PTS among patients with nonpenetrating TBI observed in the rehabilitation setting appears substantially higher than that reported in other civilian settings (104,108,109,114,119,126, 128,132) approximately 17%. This is probably a reflection of the increased severity of injury and concurrence of multiple risk factors encountered among inpatients in these settings (104,114). In contrast, the incidence of seizures among adults after mild TBI is slightly greater than that observed in the general population (102,103). PTS will be observed in approximately 35%–65% of patients with PTBI (47,88,91,92, 114). Discussion regarding the influence of specific risk factors on the incidence of PTS follows later in this chapter.

The incidence of early seizures is approximately 5% (4,133) among all patients with nonpenetrating TBI and is higher in young children (4,42,43,104,106), among whom the incidence is approximately 10% (43,104). However, continuous EEG monitoring of patients with severe TBI in the intensive care unit suggests that the incidence of early convulsive and nonconvulsive PTS may be considerably higher than initially believed at approximately 22% (49). Immediate seizures, which make up 50%–80% of early post-traumatic seizures (EPTS) (4,42,93,123,134), are particularly frequent among children with severe TBI (43,103). EPTS are occasionally observed among children with mild TBI (4,43) but are comparatively much less frequent among adults with mild TBI. Early seizures among these adults warrant investigation for an underlying intracranial hemorrhage. In a study of > 4,000 adults with mild TBI, an intracranial hemorrhage was found in almost half of the patients with EPTS (124).

Late seizures are observed less frequently among children (43,105,125) than adults.

NATURAL HISTORY OF POST-TRAUMATIC SEIZURES AND EPILEPSY

Onset

Approximately one-half to two-thirds of patients who suffer from PTS will experience seizure onset within the first 12 months and 75%–80% by the end of the second year following injury (41,46,47,92,96,97,110). After 5 years, adults with mild TBI do not appear to have a significantly increased risk relative to the general population (102); however, patients with moderate or severe TBI and PTBI will remain at increased risk after this postinjury duration (42,46,47,102).

Recurrence

It is increasingly evident that seizure recurrence is a critical factor in determination of subsequent disability and quality of life (QOL) (135,136). Greater seizure frequency significantly correlates with lower employment rates, which in one study ranged from 57% among patients who are seizure free

TABLE 39-2 Characteristics of Focal Onset Epilepsies

SITE OF ORIGIN	MANIFESTATIONS
Frontal	**Features:** Features strongly suggestive of frontal lobe epilepsies include (a) generally short seizures, (b) impairment of consciousness often with minimal/no postictal confusion, (c) rapid secondary generalization, (d) prominent tonic/postural motor manifestations, (e) complex gestural automatisms at onset (frequent), (f) falling with bilateral discharge (frequent), and (g) seizures often occurring several times a day and frequently during sleep.
Cingulate	**Features:** Seizures with impairment of consciousness associated with complex gestural automatisms at onset, autonomic signs (common), changes in mood and affect (common), and psychic/emotional auras including fear and anger (frequent).
Orbitofrontal	**Features:** Alteration of consciousness with initial sudden, complex, bizarre motor and gestural automatisms that may be bilateral and mixed with staring, olfactory hallucinations/illusions, and autonomic signs; psychoemotional auras are rare.
Dorsolateral	**Features:** Tonic (common) or clonic (less common) with versive eye and head movements and speech arrest. *Dorsolateral premotor cortex*—onset usually without aura, with tonic head/neck/eye movement or "pseudo-absence" (very brief lapse of consciousness < 10 sec duration); *prefrontal/frontopolar*—psychic auras, visual illusions, or initial loss of consciousness followed by head and eye movements.
Motor cortex	**Features:** Focal motor (most common) with manifestations reflecting the side and topography of the area involved: *Lower prerolandic area*—speech arrest, vocalization or dysphasia, contralateral tonic-clonic movements of the face, or swallowing. Generalization is frequent. *Rolandic area*—focal motor without "march" (Jacksonian seizures), particularly beginning in contralateral upper extremity. *Paracentral lobule*—tonic movements of the ipsilateral foot and contralateral leg, postictal paralysis (frequent).
Supplementary motor cortex	**Features:** Postural, focal tonic seizures, with vocalization, speech arrest, and fencing postures; usually no aura; may have autonomic symptoms.
Temporal	**Features:** Features strongly suggestive of temporal lobe epilepsies include (a) focal seizures typically characterized by autonomic and/or psychic symptoms and certain sensory phenomena (e.g., olfactory and auditory), epigastric, often rising, sensation (most common); (b) focal seizures with impairment of consciousness with onset of motor arrest or stare followed by oroalimentary automatism (often); other automatisms frequently follow. Aura is common. Seizure duration typically > 1 min, with postictal confusion/amnesia and gradual recovery (common); and (c) interictal scalp EEG with no abnormality, slight or marked asymmetry of background activity, focal slowing or temporal spikes, sharp waves, not always confined to the temporal region. Ictal scalp EEG onset may not precisely correlate with clinical onset.
Mesiobasa / limbic	**Features:** Focal seizures with visceromotor and behavioral symptoms, including rising epigastric discomfort, nausea, marked autonomic signs, and other symptoms, including belching, pallor, fullness/flushing of the face, respiratory changes, pupillary dilatation, fear, panic, and olfactory and gustatory hallucinations. Auditory symptoms do not occur. Interictal scalp EEG may be normal.
Lateral	**Features:** Focal seizures with auditory hallucinations or illusions or dreamy states, visual misperceptions, or language disorders (dominant hemisphere). May progress to CPS with propagation to mesial temporal or extratemporal structures. The scalp EEG may show unilateral, bilateral, midtemporal, or posterior temporal spikes.
Occipital	**Features:** Usually visual manifestations, appearing in the visual field contralateral to the discharge (unless generalization occurs). Nonvisual symptoms have been reported but most often reflect spread to other lobes. *Positive phenomena:* Visual hallucinations (most common), including sparks and flashes. Visual illusions have been reported but probably reflect nondominant parietal lobe involvement. *Negative phenomena:* Ictal amaurosis, fleeting scotoma, and hemianopsia (well recognized but less common).
Parietal	**Features:** Predominantly sensory with many characteristics, also some rotatory or postural motor phenomena may occur. *Positive phenomena:* Most common: (tingling, electric shock-like sensations, desire/sensation of movement in body part) usually involving hand, arm, and/or face contralateral to seizure focus. Less common: intra-abdominal sensation of sinking/nausea, particularly with inferior and lateral parietal lobe involvement. Rare: pain and visual phenomena occurring as formed hallucinations. *Negative phenomena:* numbness (common), disturbance in body image (a feeling that a body part is absent; asomatognosia [loss of awareness of a part or a half of the body, particularly with nondominant hemisphere involvement]), severe vertigo or spatial disorientation (inferior parietal lobe), receptive or conductive languages disturbances (dominant parietal lobe), and lateralized genital sensation (paracentral parietal lobe).
Insula	**Features:** Throat/laryngeal discomfort, paresthesias on contralateral (typical) side of the body, dysarthria/aphonia, and hypersalivation.

Abbreviations. CPS, complex partial seaizure; EEG, electroencephalography.

for 3 months to 30% in patients with daily seizures. As seizure frequency increased, health care costs increased and measures of QOL declined (135).

Limited data exist regarding PTS recurrence. Earlier studies reported that about one-half of patients will experience a single PTS without recurrence (111,123) and another quarter will suffer a total of 2–3 seizures (123). These reports addressed recurrence following early seizures. Recent studies addressing late post-traumatic seizure (LPTS) recurrence, however, suggests a more ominous prognosis (137,138). Semah et al. (138) investigated the relationship between prognosis for seizure recurrence and the etiology of epilepsy. Among 50 patients with remote symptomatic (lesional) epilepsy with history or radiographic evidence of TBI, only 30% of those with partial epilepsy experienced seizure-free durations of more than 1 year without recurrence (138). Haltiner and colleagues (137) followed 63 adults with moderate or severe TBI who developed LPTS during the course of participation in a randomized, placebo-controlled study of the effectiveness of phenytoin (PHT) prophylaxis for prevention of LPTS (139). The cumulative incidence of recurrent late seizures was 86% by 2 years. However, 52% experienced at least 5 late seizures, and 37% had 10 or more late seizures within 2 years of the first late seizure (137).

Pohlmann-Eden (41) published results of a PTE study population derived from a tertiary referral epilepsy clinic. Fifty-seven patients with PTE were compared with 50 age- and sex-matched control patients with severe TBI. Of all PTE patients, 35% became seizure free (no seizures within the last 3 years) and 3.5% without any treatment. Twenty-one percent experienced more than 1 seizure per week. The most important risk factors for poor seizure control were missile injuries, "combined seizure patterns," high seizure frequency, AED noncompliance, and alcohol abuse (41).

In summary, recent evidence suggests that although patients with EPTS will experience a late seizure in 20%–30% of cases, seizure onset after the first week is associated with a much higher likelihood of a seizure recurrence (97,137). Seizure frequency within the first year after injury may be predictive of future recurrence, particularly with PTBI (47). Persistent PTS may be more common in focal seizures and less common in generalized seizures (47,138). Immediate post-traumatic seizures (IPTS) are generally believed to carry no or little increased risk of recurrence (4, 140). On the other hand, between one-fifth to one-third of patients with LPTS will experience frequent recurrences, apparently refractory to conventional AED therapy (41,132,137). Some of these patients may be helped with surgical intervention (62,63,143). TBI neuroimaging characteristics may be of value in predicting the appearance (114) and intractability (142) of PTE. Finally, few studies explicitly address rates of PTE remission, that is, disappearance of seizures (143). Early studies that are derived mostly from PTBI populations describe remission rates that range from 25%–40%. Higher overall remission rates are reported in studies conducted after the development of effective AEDs (143).

Complications and Consequences of Post-Traumatic Seizures

Potentially significant complications accompany seizures in patient with TBI. Indeed, occurrence or recurrence of seizures is an important cause of nonelective rehospitalization (144) and death (145) among patients with severe TBI. Among patients with newly diagnosed (146) or chronic structural epilepsy, persistent seizures are associated with increased mortality, particularly among individuals with status epilepticus (SE) or generalized convulsions (147). Several studies have examined the sequelae of PTS (148–151). An appreciation of these potential consequences is useful when evaluating risk-benefit relationships for decisions regarding AED therapy.

Cognitive and Behavioral Function

As introduced earlier, manifestations of PTS include cognitive and behavioral dysfunction. Evidence of cognitive impairment may occur or persist during the interictal state, when the patient who is epileptic is not actively manifesting seizures (152–154). Similarly, persistent behavioral abnormalities and a significantly higher incidence of psychiatric-related hospitalizations have been noted among patients with PTS when compared with nonepileptic controls with PTBI (155). Mazzini et al. (126) found that disinhibited behavior, irritability, and aggressive behavior were significantly more frequent and severe among rehabilitation in patients with PTE when compared with patients with TBI without seizures.

Influence on Neurological Recovery

Animal studies suggest the existence of a complex relationship between PTS and neurological recovery (156). Specifically, depending on the severity of the seizure induced and time of presentation, seizures may inhibit, improve, or not affect functional recovery. In studies conducted with rodents, if "mild" subclinical kindled seizures occur early after brain damage, no delay is noted in somatosensory recovery. This suggests that brief, infrequent PTS occurring during the early post-traumatic period did not adversely affect functional recovery. However, if more severe and widespread seizures are kindled within a 6-day critical period after a brain lesion, a permanent impairment of functional recovery results. When these same seizures occur after this critical period, recovery of function proceeds unimpeded. It is important to note that contrasting results have been found using models of brain injury other than kindling models (156).

Outcome

Recurrent PTS may exert an adverse impact on functional status among adults (157) and children (106) with TBI, independent of that attributable to the severity of injury. Among patients with PTBI in the Vietnam Head Injury Study, PTS was 1 of the 7 impairments that independently and cumulatively predicted employment status (157). PTS and increasing brain volume loss have been noted to exert independent and profound effects on cognitive performance among patients with restricted frontal lobe lesions because of PTBI (158).

However, studies among patients with nonpenetrating TBI less clearly discriminate the influence of seizures on functional prognosis (104,105) and cognition (159) from those injury. Haltiner, et al. (160) examined the relationship of LPTS to neuropsychological performance and aspects of psychosocial functioning. Although patients with LPTS demonstrated greater impairment than those without seizures, after adjusting for injury severity, there were no significant differences in outcome at 1 year as a function of seizures. The authors concluded that poorer outcomes encountered among patients with PTS at 1-year postinjury reflect the severity of injury and not the effects of LPTS *per se*. Asikainen et al. noted that patients with PTS had poorer outcome as measured by the Glasgow Outcome Scale (GOS), a gross global outcome measure, but no significant differences in employment outcome when compared with patients who are nonepileptic with TBI (105). Mazzini et al. (126) also found that PTS correlated with significantly poorer outcome, as measured by the GOS, disability rating scale, functional independence measure, and subscales of the neurobehavioral rating scale at 1 year after severe TBI. In contrast, early seizures appear to have little influence on outcome (133,161).

Status Epilepticus

SE is the most clinically significant manifestation of PTS and carries the greatest risk of adverse outcome. The Working Group on Status Epilepticus (162) defines SE as more than 30 minutes of (*a*) continuous seizure activity or (*b*) 2 or more sequential seizures without full recovery of consciousness between seizures (162). More recent publications define SE as seizures that persist for shorter durations (163,164) based on estimates of the duration necessary to cause injury to CNS neurons (164). Because the duration of most seizures is generally no longer than 3 minutes, it is felt that treatment for SE should be instituted after 5–10 minutes of continuous seizure activity (165). SE needs to be distinguished from other terms describing multiple seizure episodes, including serial seizures and acute repetitive seizures. Serial seizures are 2 or more seizures occurring over a relatively brief period (i.e., minutes to many hours) but with patient regaining consciousness between the seizures (164). Acute repetitive seizures are clusters of seizures that appear to increase in frequency or severity over a short time. Acute repetitive seizures may become SE, but the frequency of this occurrence is unclear (166).

Clinical manifestations of SE vary and may include clinically obvious tonic-clonic movements or small amplitude twitching movements of the eyes, face, or extremities (164). Some patients have no observable repetitive motor activity, and the detection of SE requires EEG. One study employing continuous EEG monitoring suggests that early nonconvulsive SE may not be rare, occurring perhaps in as many as 6% of patients with severe TBI despite "therapeutic" levels of AED prophylaxis (49). Moreover, SE among patients early after TBI is associated with a very high mortality risk (49). Fortunately, *convulsive* SE remains an infrequent manifestation of PTS (123).

Additionally, SE is usually attributable to another cause, such as AED withdrawal; acute systemic or neurologic injury, such as anoxic encephalopathy or stroke (167); sepsis; metabolic derangements; or a combination of these conditions (7). SE is more likely to be encountered as a PTS manifestation in children (168). Deaths associated with SE are usually attributable to the disorder that precipitated it, comorbidities, and the age of the patient (169–171).

Mortality

Mortality among patients with PTS remains consistently elevated in most reports (148,150,151,172). However, the contribution of PTS to this increased mortality is unclear. Walker and Blumer (150) noted that men with PTS have a death rate somewhat exceeding that of comparable normal men. However, information supplied by relatives suggested that causes of death were not specific for men with TBI and seemed to reflect those found in elderly people (150). In another related series of studies, deaths among patients with PTBI and PTS appeared because of the sequelae of injury and unrelated to seizures. These patients approached the actuarial mortality norm for their peers after only 3 years (134,149).

Sudden unexpected death in epilepsy (SUDEP) accounts for 18% of all deaths among patients treated in major epilepsy centers (173). *SUDEP* can be defined as a sudden unexpected death in people with epilepsy occurring in the absence of an obvious medical cause (174). Walczak and colleagues (173) noted that occurrence of tonic-clonic seizures, treatment with more than 2 AEDs, and full-scale IQ of less than 70 are independent risk factors for SUDEP. Tonic-clonic seizure frequency may be a risk factor but only in women. The presence of cerebral structural lesions was not found to be a risk factor for SUDEP (173), and this phenomenon has not been described among patients with PTE.

In summary, sequelae associated with isolated LPTS are comparable to those found in any seizure. Isolated or infrequent late seizure episodes are generally associated with relatively little risk. Increasing frequency and severity of seizure disorders, including status epilepticus, carry greater associated risks of increased morbidity or mortality and worsened cognitive and functional prognosis.

POST-TRAUMATIC EPILEPTOGENESIS

Epileptogenesis

Epileptogenesis refers to the dynamic process underlying the appearance and natural history of epilepsy (10). For decades, physicians treating patients with TBI have sought to prevent the appearance of PTS by interrupting the process of the development of seizures through the prophylactic administration of AEDs. However, the pathophysiologic mechanisms involved in acquired epileptogenesis are not well understood, although they clearly involve multiple pathways at the molecular and cellular level as well as changes in neural networks that result in the appearance of spontaneous seizures (175). This limited understanding of the pathophysiology of acquired epileptogenesis has probably influenced the failures encountered with clinical trials of AED prophylaxis (176), which will be discussed later in this chapter. Propelled by insights into the molecular genetics of epilepsy (177), the topic of acquired epileptogenesis is attracting increasing scientific investigation.

Aside from careful observations derived from clinical, electrographic, and neuroimaging studies among human subjects (178), much of what is known or postulated regarding acquired epileptogenesis has been derived from studying pathological specimens from surgical patients with epilepsy as well as a large number of animal models of epilepsy (175, 178–181). These animal epilepsy models simulate human epilepsy and provide a system for studying mechanisms that account for the characteristics of acquired epilepsy in humans (175). Such characteristics include the presence of a "latent" period between time of injury and recurrent seizure onset (178), as demonstrated in the kindling model of epilepsy or the propensity for seizure occurrence with specific characteristics of TBI (182), as found in patients with hemorrhagic contusions and modeled in the ferric chloride model. Indeed, the presence of an unambiguous stimulus (TBI) for later appearance of epilepsy in patients with clearly identified risk factors has prompted great interest in PTE and epileptogenesis as an archetypal model for remote symptomatic epilepsy (183). The development of relevant animal models is important because selection of AEDs for development for marketing worldwide are primarily based on results of preclinical animal model studies (176,184). Several of these models suggest that some AEDs have antiepileptogenic potential (175). The theoretical and clinical implications of such models in the treatment of epilepsy, including PTE and epileptogenesis, have been reviewed elsewhere (156,175,178,182,184,185). In the discussion that follows, animal models of epilepsy with historic relevance to post-traumatic epileptogenesis are followed by a review of more recent studies addressing this issue.

Ferric Chloride Model

Initially described by Willmore in 1978, the iron or ferric chloride model is the first considered to reflect mechanisms responsible for PTE in humans. Specifically, it is felt to model pathophysiologic processes resulting from a cortical contusion/focal neocortical injury. It is of theoretical interest because cortical deposits of hemosiderin may be important in the development of recurrent PTS (176). Patients with cerebral injuries characterized by contact of blood and cortical tissue manifest an increased incidence of PTS (187). Contusion or cortical laceration causes extravasation of red blood cells, with hemolysis and deposition of hemoglobin. Willmore demonstrated that recurrent focal epileptiform discharges could result from cortical injection of ferrous or ferric chloride (186). It is felt that the iron salts and hemoglobin in neural tissue may contribute to epileptogenesis by initiating lipid peroxidation, damaging cell membranes, and inhibiting neuronal Na-K ATPase (sodium-potassium adenosine triphosphatase) (182).

Kindling Models

The kindling model of epilepsy is arguably the most recognized animal model of epileptogenesis (180,188). When initially described (189), brief trains of weak electrical stimulation were applied to susceptible areas of rodent brains until a seizure was observed. When continued over a prolonged period of time, progressively less stimulation was required to induce the seizures and spontaneous seizures eventually appeared. Once established, this enhanced sensitivity to electrical stimulation appears to be permanent for the life of the animal. Here, epileptogenesis is triggered by the kindling paradigm. The relevance of kindling to remote symptomatic epilepsy derives from the hypothesis that other stimuli, such as subclinical seizures or structural brain lesions, may trigger epileptogenesis (190).

Agents that retard or abort the kindling process are considered "antiepileptogenic," whereas those that merely suppress or block seizures in fully "kindled" animals are "anticonvulsant." Such studies have demonstrated that PHT (191) and CBZ (192,193) have anticonvulsant effects but lack antiepileptogenic action. By contrast, studies that examined the effects of gamma-aminobutyric acid (GABA)ergic drugs, including valproic acid (VPA), diazepam (DZP), and phenobarbital (PB), on kindling have shown that they demonstrate antiepileptogenic properties (175,191,194,195). Among the newer AEDs, tiagabine (TGB) and levetiracetam (LEV) show antiepileptogenic action (175) in kindling models. In contrast, topiramate (TPM) (175) and lamotrigine (LTG) show limited antiepileptogenic activity in kindling (196–198) and rodent SE models (199). Retardation of kindled seizures appears to outlast the period of exposure to antiepileptogenic drugs, suggesting that they were not simply masking seizure expression.

Several notable limitations exist with the kindling model. For example, the original kindling studies were performed on rats. Subsequently, this phenomenon was demonstrated in rabbits, cats, and later in genetically seizure-predisposed primates (191). Because neuroanatomical structural differences between species imply functional differences, it is not surprising that animal kindling models demonstrate significant phylogenetic variability in expression (200). Further, despite the efficacy of some compounds on the kindling model, none of them has had an indisputable antiepileptogenic action in animal models with spontaneous seizures (183) or in humans (175). Also, no disease-modifying effects have been described (199). Thus, the extent of this model's relevance to investigations of human PTE is considered controversial (188).

Fluid-Percussion Injury Model of Post-Traumatic Epilepsy

In 2004, D'Ambrosio and colleagues described the results of a series of experiments that demonstrate, perhaps for the first time, a reproduction of PTE induced by a single episode of lateral fluid-percussion injury (201), a clinically relevant model of nonpenetrating TBI (202). Prior studies of experimental TBI (including those incorporating fluid-percussion experimental injury) (203) describe acute seizures (204) and hippocampal hyperexcitability to electrical stimulation (203, 205) or exposure to proconvulsant agents (206). However, spontaneous chronic seizures, the hallmark of epilepsy, have not been described (201). Moreover, although neocortical epileptic foci commonly develop in humans following TBI (62), changes in neocortical excitability have not been studied in rat models of nonpenetrating TBI, which have focused on the hippocampus (201). To date, investigation of neocortical pathophysiology in PTE has been limited to 2 approaches: the first involves studying neocortical islands isolated by undercuts from the surrounding gray matter, and the second involves chronic neocortical implantation of ferrous chloride (186,201). Both models bear limited resemblance to the human post-traumatic condition; however, they lack its unique focal and diffuse mechanical and hemorrhagic components (201). These limitations, in turn, potentially influence the relevance of these models to mechanisms of human post-traumatic epileptogenesis and subsequent therapies that can be translated to human PTE (201).

The study's main findings demonstrate that a single episode of fluid-percussion injury is sufficient to cause PTE in the rat. The characteristics of PTE appeared comparable to those of human PTE because seizure manifestations emerged after a latent period and were partial in onset after a focal injury. Moreover, epileptiform activity is first detected in the neocortex at the site of injury, which electrophysiologic studies demonstrate is chronically hyperexcitable after fluid-percussion injury. Finally, postmortem pathological examination reveals that intense glial reactivity is observed at the site of injury. Animal studies suggest that seizure activity after TBI may worsen histopathological damage after fluid-percussion brain injury and exaggerate the primary insult. These findings emphasize the need to control seizures after TBI to limit further damage to the brain (207). In summary, the clinical, electrophysiological, and structural changes of severe lateral fluid-percussion injury appear to parallel changes seen after neocortical injury in human PTE (202).

Synaptic Plasticity

During recent years, a large (and increasing) number of studies demonstrate the ability of the brain to adapt to injury with changes in functional and structural reorganization (205,208,209). These reorganizational changes, termed plasticity, may serve as an adaptive role in development and recovery (210,211) or a maladaptive role when they contribute to disorders such as epilepsy (211–214). Pathological studies of TBI reveal that compensatory collateral axonal sprouting occurs following brain injury (215) and may be a mechanism of importance in functional neurological recovery (209,216). Under certain circumstances, however, collateral sprouting may give rise to the development of seizure foci (217) or the spread of epilepsy from a primary focus to synaptically related brain regions (214). Additional excitatory synaptic contacts on cell somata could produce a marked increase in cell excitability, particularly if the new excitatory synapses replaced inhibitory ones (217). If the induced alterations in connectivity increase excitability, neural pathways could become progressively susceptible to epileptic events and may contribute to the subsequent development of seizures (218).

Although sprouting and subsequent formation of new synaptic connections have been proposed as post-traumatic epileptogenic mechanisms, they are not likely to be the only pathways to neuronal hyperexcitability (185). Postinjury development of neuronal hyperexcitability may be the result of 3 general types of plastic change: (a) alterations in intrinsic membrane properties, (b) changes in synaptic connectivity, and (c) modifications of receptors and receptor subunits (185,219). Direct axonal injury may render surviving neurons more excitable through alterations in intrinsic membrane properties. Loss of afferents can induce sprouting of axons, leading to hyperexcitability by increasing recurrent cortical pathways (185). One approach that has been proposed to mitigate "maladaptive plasticity" involves the use of local pharmacological agents to either prevent hyperpolarization or increase depolarizing influences (220).

If the aforementioned models are important mechanisms common to both "adaptive plasticity" after TBI and "maladaptive plasticity" in PTS, potentially significant implications follow. Specifically, AEDs whose potential effects are exerted by preventing the development of compensatory excitatory neural pathways, that is, a seizure focus, may concurrently retard neurological recovery through a similar mechanism of action (221). Moreover, because PTS occur among a minority of all patients with TBI, including severe TBI, AED therapy broadly directed against subclinical seizure activity among all patients with TBI during recovery may be more detrimental to neurological and functional outcome than either seizures alone or initiation of AED therapy after seizure onset.

EXPLOSIVE BLAST NEUROTRAUMA

TBI is considered the "signature injury" of the wars in Iraq and Afghanistan. Improvements in body armor and the ability to quickly evacuate wounded soldiers from the battlefield results in a high survival rate, even for those who suffer from TBI. Many of the casualties are injured by an explosive blast, usually secondary to an improvised explosive device (IED). In Operation Enduring Freedom (OEF) and Operation Iraqi Freedom (OIF), it has been estimated that blast injuries account for more than 60% of combat injuries. Blast TBI (bTBI) may also be associated with secondary, tertiary, and quaternary blast effects that may also contribute to a patient's presentation. The precise mechanisms of primary bTBI remain unknown, and the current understanding is incomplete (222). The incidence of seizures in this population is unknown and is currently the subject of ongoing research between the Department of Veterans Affairs and the Department of Defense.

MANAGEMENT OF POST-TRAUMATIC SEIZURES & EPILEPSY: PREVENTION, PROPHYLAXIS AND PRACTICE GUIDELINES

The term *prophylaxis* has been defined as "specific measures taken to prevent disease in an individual . . ." (223). In the context of PTS, the term applies to AED treatment administered to patients who have not manifested seizures. Several justifications can be proposed for prophylaxis of PTS. First, AEDs might prevent PTS at a time when they potentially pose the greatest risk of secondary injury, such as seizure-induced elevations in intracranial pressure (224). Second, seizure prevention may help avoid loss of employment, loss of driving privileges, or accidental injury (224). Third, there may exist concern over the medicolegal implications of negligent treatment if PTS appears. Finally, there exists the possibility that administration of AEDs may alter or arrest epileptogenesis. Thus far, however, animal and human studies fail to provide evidence that AED therapy prevents the development of the PTS focus (175) or alters the course of seizure recurrence aside from suppression of the seizure focus (184).

Identification of the "High-Risk" Patient

Methods have been proposed to improve identification of those patients at risk for PTS development; therefore, they are mostly to gain from its prevention or potential recurrence. These include assessment of the clinical characteristics

TABLE 39-3 Risk Factors for Late Post-Traumatic Seizures

RISK FACTOR	REFERENCE
Patient characteristics	
Age	43,103,105,123
Alcohol use	93,116,118,122,231
Family history	4,93,117,225
APOE allele	229
Injury characteristics	
Bone/metal fragments	47,88,96
Depressed skull fracture	4,43,94,130
Focal contusions/injury	46,100,112,114,116,232
Focal neurological deficits	4,46,47
Lesion location	46,93,158,233
Dural penetration	47,58,93,114,233
Intracranial hemorrhage	43,114,118,126,232,233
Injury severity	4,47,93,97,102,103
	126,233
Focal hypoperfusion	126
Other	
Early post-traumatic seizures	4,47,114,116,233

Abbreviation. ALOE, alipoprotein E.

of the patient, the injury, as well as information yielded by neuroimaging and electrophysiologic assessment techniques (Table 39-3).

Patient Characteristics

Age, history of alcohol abuse, and family history represent the patient characteristics most frequently cited as factors influencing subsequent seizure risk. Patients with histories of alcohol abuse, particularly chronic alcoholism, demonstrate an increased risk of early (133) and late seizure development (93,116,118,122,123,125,225,226) and recurrence (41) following TBI. Few data exist regarding PTS risk associated with low levels of alcohol use, either before or after TBI. Patient age appears to exert a strong influence on PTS risk (43,103,105,123). Children demonstrate markedly lower risk for LPTS and considerably higher risk for IPTS and EPTS when compared with adult patients with comparable injury severity. Some studies suggest that age at onset of injury (63) or seizures (227) may influence susceptibility to seizures later in life. Some authors note a modestly increased incidence of PTS among patients with nonpenetrating TBI and a family history of seizures (4,93,117,225). This has not been consistently observed (47,98,228), suggesting that the influence of a family history of seizures appears weak when compared to the effects of extensive cerebral trauma (47). However, Diaz-Arrastia and colleagues noted that the inheritance of the apolipoprotein E (APOE) allele was significantly associated with development of late seizures but not poorer outcome after moderate and severe TBI (229). If such findings are replicated, genetic influence may ultimately be shown to have an important role in post-traumatic epileptogenesis. The identification of specific biomarkers for PTE has been limited but remains a particularly important area for future research (230).

Injury Characteristics

Certain injury characteristics demonstrate an increased likelihood of resulting in recurrent, late PTS. Virtually uniform agreement exists regarding observations of markedly increased seizure risk among patients with PTBI (41,47,88,90–93,97). Blood appears to demonstrate an extremely irritating effect on cortical neurons, as demonstrated by increased seizure incidence among patients with TBI and intracranial bleeding (4,41,43,47,103,113,117,118,122,125,232,233) particularly with subdural hematoma (114,233). Increased extent of PTBI (47,92,172) and severity of nonpenetrating TBI (41, 43,91,101,127,129), as evidenced by prolonged duration of post-traumatic amnesia (4,41,93,103,113,115,128), prolonged duration to follow commands (233), lower Glasgow Coma Scale (GCS) scores (4,102,103,233), or impairment of consciousness (115,118,125,128) are prominently associated with increased seizure risk.

General agreement exists regarding observations of increased PTS risk in patients with TBI characterized by focal neurologic deficits (4,41,47,91,95,97,109,110,118,125), depressed skull fractures (4,93,94,113,130), cerebral contusions (46,100,101,105,110,111,116,232), and retained bone or metal fragments (88,89,93,97). Lesion location may affect incidence (46,93,95–101,158,233,234), type (63), and possible frequency (234) and treatment response (62) of PTS. The concurrent presence of multiple risk factors is consistently associated with increased seizure risk (4,91,118,123,125).

Late PTS rarely occur after mild TBI (102). Among adults, trivial blows to the head almost never result in seizures but may occur in the presence of preexisting (235) or concurrent (124) brain lesions. In a recent multicenter study, 8% of patients with GCS scores in the mild range (12–14) developed late PTS within 24 months; all had CT scan evidence of contusion or intracranial hemorrhage (114). Despite their rarity, PTS and even recurrent PTS *do* occur after mild TBI, but their presence in the adult patient should prompt an investigation for a precipitating cause, such as an intracranial mass lesion. Moreover, frequent LPTS after mild TBI should also prompt careful evaluation for NES (55).

Electroencephalography

The use of the interictal EEG as an objective predictor of subsequent PTS appears limited (116,127,236,237). It is frequently abnormal in patients with TBI, both with and without PTS (46,232,238,239), reflecting the severity of brain damage sustained (46,237). Sleep-deprivation activation procedures similarly do not appear to differentiate between patients with and without PTS (240). The rare change of focal slow-wave activity to focal spike discharges, particularly during the first month postinjury (101), or persistence of focal spike or sharp wave discharges may be suggestive of increased seizure risk (122,236,239). However, such discharges may be observed on the EEG of patients who are nonepileptic (232,241). Conversely, a normal EEG may precede PTS onset (236–238,242), although this finding is more frequently associated with a favorable prognosis (122,232). EEG findings should be evaluated in context with other clinical risk factors when assessing the likelihood of PTS onset.

The EEG provides valuable information in focus localization, seizure persistence, and severity prognostication once PTS have been observed (89,236,243). In addition, the EEG may identify the presence of nonconvulsive seizures among patients with impaired consciousness, particularly early after severe TBI (49). The use of the EEG in predicting

PTS recurrence following a seizure-free period has not been established.

In the neurorehabilitation setting, EEG is potentially helpful when considering the continuation of AED therapy in patients with a history of EPTS.

Antiepileptic Drug Prophylaxis: Clinical Trials and Guidelines

Encouraged by animal studies suggesting that anticonvulsants may prevent the development of epileptic foci in animals, several studies have been published addressing the efficacy of AED prophylaxis in TBI. These studies have been extensively reviewed elsewhere (244), and their relevant findings and conclusions are summarized here. These clinical trials and literature reviews have also served as basis for practice management guidelines addressing AED prophylaxis of early and late seizures (2,245).

Retrospective studies and nonrandomized open trials involving human subjects appeared first in the scientific literature (92,116,122,134,246–251) with generally favorable results (247–251). Decidedly unimpressive results were observed among prospective investigations (125,141,226,232, 252–256) of chronic prophylaxis for late PTS. Indeed, published randomized, controlled prospective investigations almost uniformly fail to substantiate evidence of efficacy for CBZ (232), PHT (139,252,253,255,256), PB (125), or VPA prophylaxis (254) of late PTS. In 4 of these trials, the incidence of PTS was actually higher among the PHT-treated groups (139,252,255). Meta-analyses of these trials indicate that AED prophylaxis is not accompanied by a reduction in LPTS (175, 253,257–259), mortality, or neurological disability (257,259).

In contrast, AED prophylaxis consistently reduces the incidence of early PTS (139,226,232,260). As in some of the studies cited previously, however, there is no clinical evidence that AED prophylaxis of early seizures reduces the occurrence of LPTS or has any effect on death or neurological disability (259). Most published trials lack sufficient numbers of patients with PTBI to conclude whether AED prophylaxis exerts a favorable or adverse influence on seizure incidence in this high-risk subset of patients with TBI (261).

Although disappointing, treatment failure among trials conducted, thus far, should not imply that future trials are similarly destined to fail. Different approaches are currently under investigation (262). These include (*a*) the use of available AEDs that have not been previously studied for prophylaxis of PTE, such as $MgSO_4$; (*b*) different timing of administration (e.g., < 12-hour postinjury) with presently available AEDs (262); and (*c*) development and investigation of future AEDs, preferably with demonstrated efficacy in a relevant animal model of human PTE.

Four medical societies that have published guidelines pertinent to AED prophylaxis of PTS include the Brain Injury Special Interest Group of the American Academy of Physical Medicine and Rehabilitation (BI-SIG) (2), the American Academy of Neurology (AAN) (263), the Brain Trauma Foundation (BTF; in conjunction with the Joint Section on Neurotrauma and Critical Care) (245), and the Penetrating TBI Committee (261). The guidelines of the BI-SIG, AAN, and BTF are all very similar and primarily address nonpenetrating TBI in adults (2,263). The guidelines of the Penetrating TBI Committee specifically address prophylaxis with penetrating TBI and conclude that AED prophylaxis for LPTS appears unjustified (261).

MANAGEMENT OF POST-TRAUMATIC SEIZURES AND EPILEPSY

It is beyond the practical scope of this review to critically examine the breadth of literature pertinent to the treatment of all patients with epilepsy, and the reader is referred to textbooks that serve this role (264,265). Nevertheless, treatment issues that are particularly germane to patients with TBI and recurrent PTS will be briefly reviewed. In the discussion that follows, the authors' clinical experience will be incorporated into the literature review extrapolated from other epileptic populations when addressing symptomatic management of patients with PTS/PTE.

Diagnosis

An initial step in the management of suspected seizures is establishing whether or not a seizure disorder indeed exists (58). In light of the social, economic, and medical implications that accompany the diagnosis of an epileptic disorder, errors need to be avoided. In many cases, a diagnosis can be reliably made from clinical observations of seizure phenomena, particularly those noted by experienced staff in the hospital setting. Classification of the observed seizures is similarly important because categorization can have significant prognostic and therapeutic implications.

There are situations, however, where the diverse or subtle clinical presentations of PTS complicate diagnosis. As noted earlier, epileptic manifestations (particularly those of CPS) may not be recognized in patients with significant cognitive and behavioral dysfunction. Alternatively, nonepileptic phenomena such as PNES, myoclonus, or syncopal episodes may be mistaken for PTS. Clinical observations alone may thus be insufficient to render or rule out a diagnosis of PTS, prompting the use of other diagnostic options (48).

The EEG is the single most informative laboratory test for the diagnosis of epileptic disorders (266–268) and should be obtained in any patient with suspected PTS. The EEG may assist in assessing the likelihood of an underlying epileptic condition when correlated with the clinical diagnosis (269) or in localization of the seizure focus (266). Although interictal epileptiform activity is apparent in only approximately 50% of single awake recordings in adults with epilepsy, this proportion rises to approximately 80%–85% if sleep is included. Two recordings obtained while the patient is awake will demonstrate epileptiform activity in 85% of individuals with epilepsy, and this rises to 92% of persons within 4 recordings (266). In patients who manifest only generalized seizures, interictal discharges are bilateral, symmetrical, and synchronous, generally of greatest amplitude over the frontal regions but sometimes located posteriorly. In patients with partial seizures, discharge topography will more or less closely correspond to that of the focus from which seizures arise. These focal interictal discharges may spread, producing secondarily generalized spike-and-slow-wave activity. If the generalization is rapid, the focal onset may be difficult to detect (266).

There exist limitations in the diagnostic sensitivity of the standard interictal EEG, however, and absence of EEG abnormalities does not exclude the presence of a seizure disorder (266). Postictal PRL measurement may be useful in some of these patients because significant elevations in serum PRL levels reliably occur within 20–40 minutes following GTC seizures (271) and many CPS (270). PRL elevations are typically not observed after SPS (271), CPS of frontal lobe origin (272), or after 30 minutes in most patients with NES (53,54,271). Significant PRL elevation occurring after a possible PTS episode may help confirm clinical suspicion of an underlying epileptic disorder (273). Given the significant diurnal variation in serum PRL levels, however, it is often prudent to obtain a baseline value for comparison, drawn at the same time of day as the postictal specimen within a few days.

When initial standard evaluations fail to resolve the clinical diagnosis, long-term EEG monitoring techniques including ambulatory EEG monitoring (274,275) and/or inpatient VEEG telemetry (266,276) are effective and clinically valuable (48). Ambulatory EEG monitoring offers an intermediate-level option for recording while the patient conducts normal activities at home, work, or school (8,274,275). It is most useful for investigating the patient in a natural environment; for example, to test the claim that a patient has seizures at home that are not observed in the hospital (266). A patient or observer log is maintained to identify the times and descriptions of behavioral episodes suspected of representing seizure activity (8). Ambulatory monitoring has been transformed by the recent development of recorders using solid-state memory or removable miniature digital discs (266). Ambulatory monitoring is usually performed without simultaneous video registration, however, and thus EEG telemetry with video monitoring provides the best opportunity to obtain an artifact-free ictal EEG while observing and evaluating associated clinical behavior (276). Concurrent computerized automatic seizure detection often identifies important events, particularly at night, which are not reported by the patient or nursing staff. Definitive diagnosis requires recorded examples of all seizure types experienced by the patient (266). Conversely, an absence of discharges during prolonged monitoring, particularly in a patient with frequent seizures, may serve to cast a doubt on the diagnosis of epilepsy (266).

Hudak et al. described the use of prolonged VEEG monitoring in the clinical management of paroxysmal behaviors in TBI survivors (48). In this retrospective record review, 127 patients with a documented history of moderate-to-severe brain injury preceding onset of frequent disabling paroxysmal behaviors were evaluated in an EMU for management of medically intractable epilepsy. VEEG monitoring was conducted for an average of 4.6 days. AED administration was suspended during the assessment period. Monitoring was successful in establishing a diagnosis in 82% of the cases referred. Sixty-two percent of the evaluated patients had focal seizures, 6% had generalized seizures, and 33% had psychogenic NES. The authors concluded that VEEG is a useful procedure in the evaluation of TBI survivors with paroxysmal behaviors suggestive of epilepsy and that the yield of diagnoses that may alter treatment is substantial (48).

Treatment and Selection of the Antiepileptic Drug

Although broad agreement exists regarding the appropriateness of AED treatment among patients who manifest 2 or more seizures, considerable debate remains concerning the benefits of treatment in reducing recurrence risk following a first seizure (277,278). Overall, about 33% of patients with a first unprovoked seizure can be expected to have a second within the subsequent 3–5 years. This risk varies considerably, however, depending on clinical characteristics of the patient (278). Increased risk is observed among patients with remote lesional (symptomatic) epilepsy (278,280,281). Approximately 44%–48% of patients with a first remote lesional seizure will experience a second seizure in the next 3–5 years (277,280). Of the patients with a second seizure, almost 87% will experience a third seizure at 5 years (278). Seizures occurring immediately following an acute precipitant or injury to the brain carries a lower risk of recurrence than a late seizure (282).

Treatment after first seizure has been advocated, although few randomized clinical trials have been conducted to establish the efficacy of this practice. One randomized multicenter clinical trial concluded that treatment of the first seizure with AEDs leads to a significant reduction of relapse risk. The authors added, however, that the decision to start treatment in patient with a first seizure must balance that patient's risk of relapse, the benefits of avoiding the consequences of a second seizure, and the risk of AED toxicity (283).

Once a decision has been reached that pharmacological treatment of a patient with PTS is indicated, a primary goal is to attain control of seizures with 1 medication (8,284). The decision of which specific agent to use will reflect the type of PTS, the route and frequency of drug administration, and the anticipated adverse effects and comorbities. Among patients with structural or lesional epilepsy (284), including patients with TBI who manifest seizures of focal onset, extended release of CBZ remains a commonly preferred drug (244,284,285). Patients with tonic-clonic seizures of generalized, secondarily generalized, or multifocal onset respond well to VPA (284–286). CBZ (286) and PHT (286,287) are also effective anticonvulsants for GTC seizures. Although generally effective for seizure control of tonic-clonic seizures (8,287), the use of PB is severely limited by prominent adverse effects on cognition and behavior (288) and is rarely used in current practice (289).

Neurologists and physiatrists increasingly employ newer "second generation" AEDs in symptomatic management of selected patients with PTE. Unfortunately, there currently exists little scientific data, specific to PTE, which support (or refute) the benefits of this practice. A recent review of the effectiveness and safety of antiepileptic medications in patients with epilepsy compared the newer vs the older AEDs. There was no significant difference in efficacy when the newer AEDs were compared to PHT, CBZ, or VPA .The older AEDs had more adverse events but did not lead to a higher rate of withdrawal (290).

Two previous expert consensus panels address the use of the newer AEDs as initial monotherapy (284,291), including patients with symptomatic localization-related epilepsy (SLRE) and symptomatic generalized epilepsy (SGE) (284). The Quality Standards and the Therapeutics and Technology

Assessment Subcommittees of the AAN published a practice parameter summarizing an evidence-based assessment regarding the efficacy, tolerability, and safety of 7 new AEDs in the management of new onset partial or generalized epilepsy, including gabapentin (GBP), LTG, TPM, TGB, oxcarbazepine (OXC), LEV, and zonisamide (ZNS) (291). They found evidence that GBP, LTG, TPM, and OXC are effective as immunotherapy in newly diagnosed adolescents and adults with either partial or mixed seizure disorders but not generalized epilepsy syndromes. No specific guidelines were provided regarding AED use in remote symptomatic epilepsy or PTE (291). Karceski et al. employed an "expert consensus method" to survey epilepsy specialists (284) regarding AED preference in specific clinical scenarios. The survey revealed a preference for CBZ as the initial AED for management of symptomatic epilepsies. Besides CBZ, PHT, OXC, and LTG were also cited as initial first-line agents for SLRE manifested by SPS or CPS. For management of SLRE with secondarily generalized seizures, PHT, OXC, LTG, and VPA were identified as initial first-line AEDs (284). A limitation of this consensus statement (284) is that it does not address the place of ZNS or LEV in the clinical armamentarium because these agents were not in wide use at the time the survey data were obtained. Table 39-4 summarizes the characteristics of commonly used AEDs in the long-term management of PTE.

Adverse Effects of Antiepileptic Drug Therapy

AEDs that are commonly employed in the treatment of PTS may be associated with significant idiosyncratic and dose-related adverse drug reactions (291–293), requiring their discontinuation or substitution in as many as 20%–30% of patients (294,295). These include hematologic, dermatologic, hepatic, neurologic, endocrinology, urologic, and teratogenicity adverse effects (291,296,297). Transient or persistent leukopenia and thrombocytopenia may be observed in patients taking PHT and CBZ, although idiosyncratic aplastic anemia is extremely rare. Rashes are occasionally encountered with many AEDs and severe dermatologic reactions are more rarely noted with LTG and PHT (291,292). Hirsutism and gingival hyperplasia may be problematic in patients treated with PHT (292). Weight gain has been associated with VPA and GBP treatment, and weight loss reported with ZNS and TPM (286,291). Mild and transient elevations of hepatic enzymes, up to 2–3 times normal in some cases, are reported to occur in patients receiving PHT, CBZ, and VPA (299). Frequent and rigorous routine laboratory monitoring regimens, however, aside from baseline determination of hematologic and hepatic function or closer observation of noted abnormalities, are unjustified for most AEDs (with the notable exception of felbamate [FBM]). These typically do not provide meaningful protection from rare and potentially life-threatening manifestations (299,300). Appropriate counseling for the patient, family, and/or caregivers regarding potential complications and symptoms that might herald an adverse event is far more useful and important (300).

Cognitive effects of AEDs warrant particular attention in the patient with TBI. Newer AEDs demonstrate superior cognitive adverse effect profiles and tolerability when compared with older agents (301–303). In contrast, older AEDs, particularly PB, PHT, and CBZ, significantly impair memory

performance in double-blind crossover trials among healthy adults (304). Patients with severe TBI already have significant cognitive impairment. AEDs may exert independent and additional adverse cognitive effects on the patient with TBI who is receiving chronic therapy (305). Among patients with severe TBI participating in the landmark prophylaxis trial of Temkin et al. (138), a significantly greater proportion (78%) of individuals treated with PHT demonstrated cognitive impairment sufficient to preclude testing at 1-month postinjury. This was observed in only 47% of corresponding patients treated with placebo (305).

Among older established AEDs, most studies demonstrate no comparative advantage in cognitive adverse effect profile between CBZ, PHT, or VPA, although few include subjects with TBI (306–309). Smith (309) found no significant difference on cognitive testing results among patients randomized to withdrawal from PHT and CBZ prophylaxis. Only 13 of the 82 studied patients sustained severe TBI, however, with the remainder receiving prophylaxis following craniotomy or mild/moderate TBI. There remains considerable evidence suggesting that PHT provides a relatively unfavorable cognitive side effect profile among patients with severe TBI (305,306). Patients randomized to receive 6 months of VPA for prophylaxis of LPTS following severe TBI demonstrated no evidence of adverse cognitive effects when compared with those receiving 1 week of PHT (306). In contrast, an earlier study among comparably patients who are injured receiving PHT prophylaxis yielded unequivocal evidence of cognitive impairment among patients treated with AED (306).

Although attention regarding adverse drug effects frequently focuses on observable phenomena, such as lethargy, the influence of AED therapy on the course of postinjury neurologic recovery also warrants consideration (310). Specifically, certain drugs, including AEDs, clearly impair recovery after brain injury in laboratory animals (311–313). Schallert et al. (313) demonstrated that DZP administered to rats within 12 hours of neocortical damage delayed recovery indefinitely, whereas delayed administration of DZP resulted in only transient reinstatement of neurologic deficit (313). Brailowsky observed that PHT increased the severity of cannula-induced cortical hemiplegia in rats, although motor impairment was not seen when administered to the animals after their hemiplegic syndrome had cleared (311). These findings suggest that AED administration with DZP or PHT during certain critical periods following brain injury may exert a deleterious effect on subsequent neurologic recovery.

In summary, dose-related and idiosyncratic adverse effects occur among a substantial subset of treated patients, particularly with older AEDs. Cognitive adverse effects may be particularly problematic, particularly with the older established agents, impacting on long-term tolerability. The cited studies serve as a reminder that decisions regarding chronic AED treatment and particularly prophylaxis cannot be considered solely on the merits of effectiveness in seizure prevention. Rather, consideration must also be given to potentially significant adverse effects and toxicities of the AED regimen.

Antiepileptic Drug Substitution

Neurosurgeons and neurologists have preferred PHT for prophylaxis (314,315) and symptomatic AED treatment primar-

TABLE 39-4 Antiepileptic Drugs Used for Treatment of Seizures in Adults

DRUG	PRIMARY ROUTE OF ELIMINATION/ MECHANISM OF ACTION	ADVANTAGES/ DISADVANTAGES	POTENTIAL ADVERSE EFFECTS	IDIOSYNCRATIC REACTIONS	REPRESENTATIVE MAINTENANCE DOSE
Carbamazepine	Hepatic/blocks voltage- dependent sodium channels	Inexpensive	Dizziness, diplopia, ataxia, drowsiness	Rash, blood dyscrasia, SIADH, hepatic failure	400–800 mg twice a day except for XR (once daily)
Phenobarbital	Hepatic/enhances GABA	Inexpensive	Sedation, drowsiness, cognitive impairment	Hypersensitivity reactions, seizure exacerbation	90 mg once a day
Phenytoin	Hepatic/blocks voltage-dependent sodium channels	Inexpensive	Ataxia, gingival hyperplasia, hirsutism, lymphadenopathy	Rash, hepatotoxicity, SJS, blood dyscrasias, aplastic anemia,	300 mg once a day
Valproate	Hepatic/blocks voltage-dependent sodium channels, enhance GABA release, decrease T-type calcium currents	Broad spectrum	Tremor, nausea, ataxia, somnolence	Rash, blood dyscrasias, pancreatitis, SJS, thrombocytopenia, hepatotoxicity	750–1500 mg daily in divided doses except for ER (once daily)
Felbamate	Hepatic/blocks NMDA, augments GABA	Broad spectrum	Anorexia, nausea, weight loss, insomnia	SJS, hepatic failure, rash, aplastic anemia	400 mg 3 times daily
Lamotrigine	Hepatic/blocks voltage- dependent sodium channels, other mechanisms not fully understood	Broad spectrum	Rash, tremor, dizziness, nausea, headache	Rash, hepatotoxicity, SJS, blood dyscrasias,	75–150 mg twice daily
Oxcarbazepine	Hepatic/blocks voltage-dependent sodium channels	Better tolerated than carbamazepine/ expensive	Dizziness, diplopia, nausea, somnolence, hyponatremia	Hypersensitivity reactions, blood dyscrasias, SJS, TEN	600 mg twice daily
Tiagabine	Hepatic/enhances GABA	Clearly defined mechanism of action; no significant drug interactions.	Confusion. dizziness, sedation,	Rash, paresthesias, SE	32–56 mg daily in 3 divided doses
Levetiracetam	Hepatic and renal/ unknown	No significant drug interactions; broad spectrum.	Agitation, psychosis, somnolence, dizziness, incoordination	Hepatic failure	500–1500mg twice daily
Zonisamide	Hepatic and renal/ blocks voltage-dependent sodium and T-type channels	Broad spectrum, can be given once daily.	Dizziness, ataxia, weight loss, somnolence, agitation, impaired concentration	Aplastic anemia, nephrolithiasis, rash, SJS, cross-allergy to sulfonamides	200–600 mg daily (can be given once or twice a day)
Topiramate	Renal/blocks voltage-dependent sodium channels, enhances GABA, antagonizes NMDA-glutamate receptor, inhibits carbonic anhydrase	Broad spectrum	Cognitive impairment, dizziness, ataxia, tremor, fatigue, anorexia, weight loss, sedation, paresthesias	Nephrolithiasis, narrow-angle glaucoma, metabolic acidosis, hyperthermia, maculopathy	100–300 twice daily

(Continued)

TABLE 39-4 Antiepileptic Drugs Used for Treatment of Seizures in Adults (*Continued*)

DRUG	PRIMARY ROUTE OF ELIMINATION/ MECHANISM OF ACTION	ADVANTAGES/ DISADVANTAGES	POTENTIAL ADVERSE EFFECTS	IDIOSYNCRATIC REACTIONS	REPRESENTATIVE MAINTENANCE DOSE
Gabapentin	Renal/binds to the auxiliary alpha-2/ delta subunit of a voltage-dependent calcium channel.	No significant interactions with other AEDs.	Dizziness, fatigue, somnolence, peripheral edema	Neutropenia, renal failure, SJS, pancreatitis, hepatitis	300–800 mg 3 times daily
Lacosamide	Renal/enhances slow inactivation of voltage-dependent sodium channels	No significant interactions with other AEDs.	Drowsiness, dizziness, ataxia, cognitive, difficulties, nausea	PR interval prolongation, hypersensitivity reactions	100–200 mg twice daily
Ezogabine/ retigabine	Renal/opens KCNQ2/3 voltage-gated potassium channels	Novel mechanism of action; minimal drug actions with other AEDs; recently approved by FDA	Dizziness, somnolence, fatigue, confusional state, unknown potential AEs because it is a new AED	Urinary retention, psychiatric symptoms, QT prolongation	300–1200 mg daily in 3 divided doses
Vigabatrin	Renal/irreversible inhibitor of GABA transaminase that raises the concentration of GABA	Physicians need to be registered to prescribe; frequent visual field testing required.	Fatigue, weight gain, dizziness, depression	Irreversible visual field deficits, MRI abnormalities	1000–1500 mg twice daily
Pregablin	Renal/inhibition of neuronal excitability modulates release of glutamate, noradrenaline, and calcium currents	No significant interactions with other AEDs.	Dizziness, somnolence, confusion, ataxia	Hypersensitivity reactions, myoclonus	300–600 mg daily in divided doses

Abbreviations. AEs, antiepileptics; AEDs, antiepileptic drugs; FDA, Food and Drug Administration; GABA, gamma-aminobutyric acid; MRI, magnetic resonance imaging; NMDA, N-methyl-D-aspartate; PR, pulse rate; SE, status epilepticus; SIADH, syndrome of inappropriate diuretic hormone; SJS, Stevens-Johnson syndrome; TEN, toxic epidermal necrolysis. Adapted from UpToDate and package inserts.

ily because of its availability in parenteral forms that can be administered in the acute setting where seizures are more likely to occur. Since the publication of prophylaxis guidelines (2,263,245), however, we have observed a clear trend toward less frequent use of AED prophylaxis. In addition, among patients receiving symptomatic AED treatment, PB use is rare with PHT remaining the most commonly observed AED used in acute care settings for initial symptomatic management. These patients are commonly maintained on the chosen AED until a satisfactory seizure-free duration has passed. AED substitution has previously been usually reserved for failure of seizure control or the manifestation of significant drug reactions (8). As mentioned earlier, selection of a newer AED as initial monotherapy is likely to improve tolerability, particularly with cognitive adverse effects, while maintaining comparable efficacy. For similar reasons, many neurorehabilitation specialists consider substitution of PHT monotherapy for other less cognitively impairing medications, such as LTG, as clinical circumstances allow.

When substituting an AED for another drug, clinically effective levels of the latter AED should be attained prior to discontinuation of the former drug (8). Among the newer AEDs, serum levels are not commonly obtained, although these are available at reference laboratories. Once appropriate and effective doses of the new drug are achieved, a gradual taper of the former drug ensues. At one time, CBZ was the most common AED employed for substitution instead of PHT in our center. More recently, however, we use LTG as slow add-on therapy (usually added to PHT), followed by gradual withdrawal of PHT after maintenance of seizure control and effective doses of LTG (approximately 4–500mg/ day). Our preference for LTG derives from a clearly favorable cognitive adverse effect profile, particularly when compared with either PHT or CBZ (316). Among patients requiring more rapid additional seizure control, LTG is not a therapeutic option because of the increased danger of serious rash or Stevens-Johnson syndrome (317) associated with rapid dose increases. Instead, we employ VPA because it is effective for both generalized and partial seizures (286), it demonstrates generally favorable tolerability among patients with TBI (306), and it is available in parenteral and once-daily oral formulations. VPA may also be a practical choice among patients with PTE that are also demonstrating post-traumatic mood lability and irritability. We are aware of colleagues that favor LEV as a preferred AED for substitution among patients with TBI, citing its ability to be rapidly titrated to effective dose range (318) as well as its tolerability. However, anecdotal reports of a lack of persistent antiepileptic effect and documented psychiatric adverse effects (319) may limit the use of this agent in some patients.

Duration of Antiepileptic Drug Therapy

No clinical studies specifically address the duration of AED therapy for patients with recurrent LPTS. In general, it is reasonable to consider AED withdrawal from patients with epilepsy after a 2-year period free of seizures (321). Reported rates of relapse vary considerably and reflect the type of seizure disorder being treated (8). The risk of seizure recurrence under a policy of slow AED withdrawal is still substantial when compared with a policy of continued treatment, particularly during the first year of withdrawal (322). Increased risk of recurrence has been reported among patients with a history of more frequent seizures, treatment with more than one AED, a history of GTC seizures (322), and abnormal or epileptiform discharges on prewithdrawal EEGs (321,323). Among patients for whom the risk of relapse after discontinuation appears low, the psychosocial benefits of discontinuation may be considerable (324). There is no consensus regarding the ideal period over which AEDs should be withdrawn in patients with recurrent seizures, although conservative recommendations advise a period of 12 months (8,325). Other authors consider seizure freedom after patients have gone without seizures for a period equal to 3 times the preinterval interseizure interval. Although, in certain cases, it may be necessary to wait up to 6 times this interval to confirm seizure freedom (326). Worsening of seizures following PHT (327,328) or CBZ (328) discontinuation is believed to reflect the loss of therapeutic drug effect rather than a withdrawal phenomenon. In contrast, withdrawal exacerbation of seizures is prominent, especially with rapid tapering, for barbiturates (329) and benzodiazepines (330) and does not indicate that the drug was necessary for maintenance of seizure control (8).

Surgical Treatment of Post-Traumatic Seizures

Recent studies are providing valuable insight into the natural course of history regarding PTS recurrence (137). These studies identify a subset of patients remaining refractory to treatment even with multiple AEDs. The definition of "refractory" is debatable, and there is evidence that adding a second or third AED may facilitate seizure remission in about one-fifth of patients that remain with seizures while taking a single AED (330). Nevertheless, for those patients who continue to experience frequent seizures despite various AED monotherapy or polytherapy combinations, early surgical treatment options should be considered (331).

Surgical Resection of Epileptic Focus
Advances in neuroimaging technology, coupled with results of recent landmark studies, have prompted a dramatic shift toward surgical treatment for certain types of medically refractory epilepsy (240,332). There is now growing sentiment among epilepsy specialists that surgical treatment for refrac-

tory epilepsy is seriously underused (332,333). In the first randomized study comparing surgical and medical treatment for temporal lobe epilepsy, 58% of surgically treated patients were free of disabling seizures at 1 year vs only 8% of those assigned to receive medical treatment (334). Significant improvements in outcome were observed in measures of QOL as well as a trend with respect to social functioning (334). The Multicenter Study of Epilepsy Surgery similarly reported that resective surgery significantly reduced seizure recurrence after medial temporal (77% in 1-year remission) and neocortical resection (56% in 1-year remission) (335). In light of such findings, the AAN, in association with the American Epilepsy Society and the American Association of Neurological Surgeons, published a practice parameter supporting the benefits of anteromesial temporal lobe resection for disabling CPS. It further recommended referral of patients with these seizures to an epilepsy surgery center (332).

Surgical Excision of the Post-Traumatic Seizure Focus
Surgical excision of the seizure focus also provides an important treatment option for carefully selected patients with refractory PTE. Favorable responses including seizure freedom have been described among selected patients with PTE treated with resective surgery (62,141,336). Patients with unilateral post-traumatic frontal lesions who undergo complete resection of perilesional encephalomalacia/gliosis and adjacent electrophysiologically abnormal tissue respond particularly well to surgery (337,338). The cumulative experience described in published studies, however, also highlight the challenges accompanying accurate identification of the seizure focus in patients with severe TBI who often demonstrate bilateral and multifocal injury (62,63). Marks et al. described 25 patients with PTE treated in their tertiary epilepsy center; 21 of whom were treated surgically. Seventeen of these patients were felt to have mesial temporal lobe epilepsy, and another 8 patients were judged to have neocortical epilepsy. Of the 21 patients treated with surgery, only 9 (43%) had favorable outcomes, characteristically those with well-circumscribed hippocampal or neocortical focal lesions (63). Schuh and associates (339) reported on 102 patients who underwent anterior temporal lobectomy. A history of TBI, alone or in combination with other factors, was significantly correlated with continued seizures after surgery (339).

Vagus Nerve Stimulation
Vagus nerve stimulation (VNS) is an alternative to pharmacologic treatment of seizures in patients who have failed conventional pharmacotherapy, either because of lack of efficacy or adverse effects (340). The mechanism of action of VNS is not yet clear (341).

VNS is approved by the Food and Drug Administration (FDA) for adjunctive treatment of intractable partial seizures in patients above 12 years old. Based on controlled, randomized trials, approximately 30% of these patients can be expected to have at least a 50% decrease in overall seizure frequency (342,343). Many patients with VNS continue to need AEDs for maximum seizure control. However, medications can usually be reduced resulting in less adverse effects. Efficacy in LPTS has not been specifically studied. Persistence of benefits has been demonstrated (344). Although this technique is indeed invasive, no intracranial surgery is required, and surgical morbidity and mortality are limited. Adverse effects include hoarseness, cough, and dysesthetic sensations in the throat (343).

Although numbers of patients treated with this technique are limited compared to AED therapy, in 1999, the American Academy of Neurology Therapeutics and Technology Subcommittee classified VNS as safe and effective for intractable partial seizures based on sufficient class I evidence (345). At present, VNS is considered to be an appropriate therapy for patients with medically refractory epileptic seizures who are not optimal candidates for resective epilepsy surgery (340).

A potential advantage to the use of VNS in the context of LPTS is the relative absence of cognitive adverse effects. However, the role of this technology in the treatment of epilepsy in the context of TBI remains to be delineated.

Consultation and Referral

Guidelines for the appropriate level of primary and specialty care of patients with seizures, including recommendations for referral to specialty centers, have been published (346). In summary, the first step for individuals experiencing an initial seizure or seizures is to consult their primary care physician in their own community. The primary physician may then choose to begin a treatment program or refer the individual to a general neurologist for consultation. In any case, if seizures continue to occur after 3 months, a referral to a general neurologist is indicated. When the seizures are controlled, many patients appropriately return to the care of their primary physicians, with follow-up to the neurologist as needed. If seizure control is not achieved at the end of the first year of treatment, referral to a center that offers comprehensive diagnostic and treatment services to patients with intractable seizures is indicated (339).

CONCLUSION

Epilepsy is the nation's fourth most common neurological disorder after migraine, stroke, and Alzheimer disease. An estimated 2.2 million Americans have epilepsy, with approximately 150, 000 new cases diagnosed in the United States each year. Approximately 1 in 26 people will develop epilepsy at some point in their lives (347). TBI is an acknowledged and preventable cause of seizures and is responsible for 20% of lesional/structural causes of epilepsy and 5% of all epilepsy. In light of the evidence previously discussed, one possible management approach for LPTS is presented. Patients with acute TBI who are transferred to the neurorehabilitation hospital setting receiving an AED for prophylaxis and without reported early seizures are gradually tapered from AEDs early in their hospital course. As mentioned earlier, routine chronic AED prophylaxis of LPTS is unjustified, and with few exceptions no AED therapy is provided unless

---

[1] Exceptions to this general rule include (a) history of episodes suggestive of EPTS, especially SE; (b) anticipated intracranial surgical procedure within the next 7–14 days; (c) EEG findings consistent with epileptiform activity and/or electrographic seizures; (d) concurrent serious medical or neurological complications, such as sepsis or hydrocephalus awaiting shunt placement; and (e) patient history of severe alcohol or substance abuse with poor family/caregiver support. (Our experience has found that the number of this latter group of patients have probably experienced undiagnosed seizures or epilepsy prior to their most recent TBI.)

late seizures are reported (2,263). AED prophylaxis withdrawal in the hospital setting facilitates monitoring for the potentially varied manifestations of seizures. Because seizures tend to occur in the earlier postinjury period, this also helps ensure the presence of trained personnel should a seizure be observed during or after AED withdrawal. Marked improvements in the cognitive status of patients frequently coincide with termination of AED prophylaxis.

If a possible LPTS is observed, either during the patient's hospitalization or after discharge, a search for an identifiable seizure precipitant takes place and includes a neuroimaging study of the brain. If no obvious correctable seizure precipitant is identified, establishment of a diagnosis of seizure disorder ideally precedes initiation of AED therapy. Clinical description of the episode alone, provided by a family member or other witnesses, may be sufficiently convincing to initiate AED therapy. The patient and family are given instructions for keeping a "seizure logbook," and more frequent follow-up visits are often warranted. If a LPTS has been documented, selection of an AED for symptomatic seizure management is initiated. AED selection is influenced by the (a) patient's cognitive and behavioral status, (b) type/manifestation of the seizure (e.g., GTC, SE vs SPS lip twitching), (c) perceived need for rapid achievement of a therapeutic dose, and (d) whether or not the patient has already been started on PHT or another AED in the emergency department. If the patient is receiving PHT and seizures are well controlled, an alternative AED is usually substituted at the earliest suitable point to minimize adverse side effects, particularly cognitive impairment.

For most physicians caring for patients with TBI in the rehabilitation setting, the issue of whether to institute prophylaxis of EPTS is usually moot. Nevertheless, postinjury prophylaxis of EPTS with PHT, FPT, or LEV may be justified in patients with severe TBI belonging to high-risk groups. The patient is at their highest risk for seizure development at a time when they can least afford to endure complications from a seizure. Prophylaxis may be continued for approximately 1 week if seizures are not observed and then tapered gradually. Again, this should take place in a setting in which close observation can be provided. The risks incurred with such a short duration of treatment currently appear minimal and acceptable.

Insufficient data exist to definitively guide AED therapy among patients whose only manifestation of a seizure disorder is EPTS. Most published reports exclude these patients from further study, thereby losing valuable information regarding the influence of continued AED therapy on LPTS recurrence risk. Issues to consider include onset (day 1 vs day 7 or later), severity (particularly SE), recurrence frequency, and clinical risk factors for recurrence. Factors favoring continuation of AED therapy would include later time of seizure onset, documented episodes of SE, persistent epileptiform activity or electrographic seizures on EEG, multiple seizure episodes throughout the first week of injury, and the presence of multiple risk factors suggestive of high risk for LPTS occurrence, such as PTBI. In contrast, it may be reasonable to consider a monitored withdrawal of AED therapy in selected patients with isolated EPTS, particularly those with IPTS. Most patients with nonpenetrating TBI and isolated EPTS will tolerate discontinuation of AED therapy without seizure recurrence (132,348).

Major themes involving the symptomatic management of patients with PTS have been discussed earlier and will not be repeated here. Still, important research questions remain and involve a broad range of topics pertinent to the diagnosis and treatment of epileptic disorders. Investigation must be directed toward identifying laboratory models that reflect human response to prevention of an initial or recurrent PTS. Further study is needed to clarify the natural history of PTS, the prognostic implications of single or isolated seizures, and the effect of AED therapy on recurrence risk. Future studies should address the comparative use and adverse effects of symptomatic seizure treatment, including surgery, *on adult and pediatric subjects with TBI*, and explore the potential effects of these therapies on neurologic recovery and functional outcome.

Finally, assessment of each patient's risk and suitability for treatment must be made on an individual basis, guidelines, or algorithms notwithstanding. Even with the publication of guidelines (2,263,245,261) addressing the issue of AED prophylaxis, discussion of issues related to PTS with the patient and family members is useful and important. Moreover, the clinician should be aware of the prevailing regional standards of care regarding symptomatic management. Lastly, in instances where questionable or repeated seizures occur, using the assistance of neurological and neurosurgical consultants with specific interest in the unique management issues of this patient population can be invaluable.

ACKNOWLEDGMENTS

We would like to acknowledge funding support provided through the Wilson Research Foundation, Jackson, Mississippi; the National Institute on Disability and Rehabilitation Research (grants H133A020514 and H133A980035); and the Epilepsy Centers of Excellence, Department of Veteran's Affairs.

KEY CLINICAL POINTS

1. PTE is a disorder characterized by recurrent late seizure episodes not attributable to another obvious cause in patients with TBI.
2. There is no standard treatment of PTS, and management needs to be tailored to the individual patient regarding medication selection and possible surgical intervention.
3. Psychogenic nonepileptic seizures are common in patients with TBI and may coexist with epileptic seizures in patients with epilepsy.
4. Prolonged EEG monitoring (particularly with video) is often helpful in establishing a diagnosis, especially when the history or routine EEG fails to clearly define the ictal focus.
5. TBIs are an important cause of epilepsy, accounting for 20% of symptomatic structural epilepsy observed in the general population and 5% of all epilepsy.
6. TBI is the leading cause of epilepsy in young adults.
7. The overall incidence of late seizures in hospitalized patients following nonpenetrating TBI is approximately 4%–7%; PTS will be observed in approximately 35%–65% of patients with penetrating TBI.

8. Approximately one-half to two-thirds of patients who suffer from PTS will experience seizure onset within the first 12 months and 75%–80% by the end of the second year following injury.
9. Because the duration of most seizures is generally no longer than 3 minutes, it is felt that treatment for SE should be instituted after 5–10 minutes of continuous seizure activity.
10. The EEG is the single most informative laboratory test for the diagnosis of epilepsy and should be obtained in any patient with suspected PTS.

KEY REFERENCES

1. Engel J Jr, Pedley TA, eds. Epilepsy: A Comprehensive Textbook. 2nd ed. Philadelphia, PA: Lippincott Williams & Wilkins; 2007.
2. Institute of Medicine. *Epilepsy Across the Spectrum: Promoting Health and Understanding.* Washington, DC: The National Academies Press; 2012.
3. Panayiotopoulos CP. *Atlas of Epilepsies.* London, United Kingdom: Springer Verlag; 2010.
4. Pellock JM, Dodson WE, Bourgeois BF, eds. *Pediatric Epilepsy: Diagnosis and Therapy.* New York, NY: Demos Medical Publishing; 2007.
5. Wyllie E, ed. *The Treatment of Epilepsy: Principles and Practice.* 5th ed. Philadelphia, PA: Lippincott Williams & Wilkins; 2011.

References

1. Faul M, Xu L, Wald MM, Coronado VG. *Traumatic Brain Injury in the United States: Emergency Department Visits, Hospitalizations, and Deaths.* Atlanta, GA: Centers for Disease Control and Prevention, National Center for Injury Prevention and Control; 2010.
2. Brain Injury Special Interest Group of the American Academy of Physical Medicine and Rehabilitation. Practice parameter: antiepileptic drug treatment of post-traumatic seizures. *Arch Phys Med Rehabil.* 1998;79:594–597.
3. ILAE Epidemiology Commission Report. Standards for epidemiologic studies and surveillance of epilepsy. *Epilepsia.* 2011;52(suppl 7):2–26.
4. Chang BS, Lowenstein DH; Quality Standards Subcommittee of the American Academy of Neurology. Practice parameter: antiepileptic drug prophylaxis in severe traumatic brain injury: report of the Quality Standards Subcommittee of the American Academy of Neurology. *Neurology.* 2003;60:10–16.
5. Frucht MM, Quigg M, Schwaner C, Fountain NB. Distribution of seizure precipitants among epilepsy syndromes. *Epilepsia.* 2000;41: 1534–1539.
6. Mazzini L, Campini R, Angelino E, Rognone F, Pastore I, Oliveri G. Post-traumatic hydrocephalus: a clinical, neuroradiologic, neuropsychologic assessment of long-term outcome. *Arch Phys Med Rehabil.* 2003;84:1637–1641.
7. Delanty N, French JA, Labar DR, Pedley TA, Rowan AJ. Status epilepticus arising *de novo* in hospitalized patients: an analysis of 41 patients. *Seizure.* 2001;10:116–119.
8. Engel J Jr, ed. *Seizures and Epilepsy.* Philadelphia, PA: FA Davis; 1990.
9. Messing RO, Simon RP. Seizures as a manifestation of systemic disease. *Neurol Clin.* 1986;4:563–584.
10. Hasan D, Schonck RSM, Avezaat CJJ, Tanghe HLJ, van Gijn J, van der Lugt PJM. Epileptic seizures after subarachnoid hemorrhage. *Ann Neurol.* 1993;33:286–291.
11. Jamjoon AB, Kane N, Sanderman D, Cummins B. Epilepsy related to traumatic extradural hematomas. *BMJ.* 1991;302:448.

12. Neiman J, Haapaniemi HM, Hillbom M. Neurological complications of drug abuse: pathophysiological mechanisms. *Eur J Neurol.* 2000;7:595–606.

13. Messing RO, Closson RG, Simon RP. Drug-induced seizures: a 10-year experience. *Neurology.* 1984;34:1582–1586.

14. Hauser A, Ng SKC, Brust JCM. Alcohol, seizures, and epilepsy. *Epilepsia.* 1988;29(suppl 2):S66–S78.

15. Hillbom ME. Occurrence of cerebral seizures provoked by alcohol abuse. *Epilepsia.* 1980;21:459–466.

16. Bergmann F, Bleich S, Wischer S, Paulus W. Seizure and cardiac arrest during bupropion SR treatment. *J Clin Psychopharmacol.* 2002; 22:630–631.

17. Centorrino F, Price BH, Tuttle M, et al. EEG abnormalities during treatment with typical and atypical antipsychotics. *Am J Psychiatry.* 2002;159:109–115.

18. Gross A, Devinsky O, Westbrook LE, Wharton AH, Alper K. Psychotropic medication use in patients with epilepsy: effect on seizure frequency. *J Neuropsych Clin Neurosci.* 2000;12:458–464.

19. Hedges DW, Jeppson KG. New-onset seizure associated with quetiapine and olanzapine. *Ann Pharmacother.* 2002;36:437–439.

20. Johnston JA, Lineberry CG, Ascher JA, et al. A 102-center prospective study of seizure in association with bupropion. *J Clin Psychiatry.* 1991;52:450–456.

21. Wroblewski BA, McColgan K, Smith K, Whyte J, Singer WD. The incidence of seizures during tricyclic antidepressant drug treatment in a brain-injured population. *J Clin Psychopharmacol.* 1990; 10:124–128.

22. Smith PEM, McBride A. Illicit drugs and seizures. *Seizure.*1999;8: 441–443.

23. Favale E, Audenino D, Cocito L, Albano C. The anticonvulsant effect of citalopram as an indirect evidence of serotonergic impairment in human epileptogenesis. *Seizure.* 2003;12:316–318.

24. Hernandez EJ, Williams PA, Dudek FE. Effects of fluoxetine and TFMPP on spontaneous seizures in rats with pilocarpine-induced epilepsy. *Epilepsia.* 2002;43:1337–1345.

25. Spigset O. Adverse reactions of selective serotonin reuptake inhibitors: reports from a spontaneous reporting system. *Drug Saf.* 1999; 20:277–287.

26. Hargrave R, Martinez D, Bernstein AJ. Fluoxetine-induced seizures. *Psychosomatics.* 1992;33:236–239.

27. Prasher VP. Seizures associated with fluoxetine therapy. *Seizure.* 1993;2:315–317.

28. Barry J, Huynh N. Psychotropic drug use in patients with epilepsy and developmental disabilities. In: Devinsky O, Westbrook LE, eds. *Epilepsy and Developmental Disabilities.* Boston, MA: Butterworth-Heinemann; 2001:205–217.

29. Calandra G, Lydick E, Carrigan J, Weiss L, Guess H. Factors predisposing to seizures in seriously ill infected patients receiving antibiotics: experience with imipenem/cilastin. *Am J Med.* 1988;84: 911–918.

30. Tattevin P, Messiaen T, Pras V, Ronco P, Biour M. Confusion and general seizures following ciprofloxacin administration. *Nephrol Dial Transplant.* 1998;13:2712–2713.

31. Koppel BS, Hauser WA, Politis C, van Duin D, Daras M. Seizures in the critically ill: the role of imipenem. *Epilepsia.* 2001;42:1590–1593.

32. Pestotnik SL, Classen DC, Evans RS, Stevens LE, Burke JP. Prospective surveillance of imipenem/cilastin use and associated seizures using a hospital information system. *Ann Pharmacother.* 1993;27: 497–501.

33. Wroblewski B. Epileptic potential of stimulants, dopaminergics, and antidepressants. *J Head Trauma Rehabil.* 1992;7(3):109–111.

34. Zagnoni PG, Albano C. Psychostimulants and epilepsy. *Epilepsia.* 2002;43(suppl 2):28–31.

35. Wroblewski BA, Leary JM, Phelan AM, Whyte J, Manning K. Methylphenidate and seizure frequency in brain injured patients with seizure disorders. *J Clin Psychiatry.* 1992;53:86–89.

36. Waterhouse E, Towne A. Seizures in the elderly: nuances in presentation and treatment. *Cleve Clin J Med.* 2005;72(suppl 3):S26–S37.

37. Sansone R, Sansone L. Tramadol: seizures, serotonin syndrome and coadministered antidepressants. *Psychiatry (Edgmont).* 1999; 6(4):17–21.

38. Commission on Classification and Terminology of the International League Against Epilepsy. Proposal for revised clinical and electroencephalographic classification of epileptic seizures. *Epilepsia.* 1981;22:489–501.

39. Commission on Classification and Terminology of the International League Against Epilepsy. Proposal for revised classification of epilepsies and epileptic syndromes. *Epilepsia.* 1989;30:389–399.

40. Berg A, Berkovic S, Brodie M, et al. Revised terminology and concepts for organization of seizures and epilepsies: report of the ILAE Commission on Classification and Terminology, 2005–2009. *Epilepsia.* 2010;51(4):676–685.

41. Pohlmann-Eden B, Bruckmeir I. Predictors and dynamics of post-traumatic epilepsy. *Acta Neurol Scand.* 1997;95:257–262.

42. Pagni CA. Post-traumatic epilepsy. Incidence and prophylaxis. *Acta Neurochir Suppl (Wien).* 1990;50:38–47.

43. Hahn YS, Fuchs S, Flannery AM, Barthe MJ, McClone DG. Factors influencing post-traumatic seizures in children. *Neurosurgery.* 1988; 22:864–867.

44. Rocca WA, Sharbrough FW, Hauser WA, Annegers JF, Schoenberg BS. Risk factors for complex partial seizures: a population based case-control study. *Ann Neurol.* 1987;21:22–31.

45. Locke GE, Molaie M, Biggers S, Leonard E. Risk factors for post-traumatic epilepsy [abstract]. *Epilepsia.* 1991;32(suppl 3):S104–S105.

46. Da Silva AM, Nunes B, Vaz AR, Mendonça D. Post-traumatic epilepsy in civilians: clinical and electroencephalographic studies. *Acta Neurochir Suppl (Wien).* 1992;55:56–63.

47. Salazar AM, Jabbari B, Vance SC, Grafman J, Amin D, Dillon JD. Epilepsy after penetrating head injury: I. Clinical correlates. *Neurology.* 1985;35:1406–1414.

48. Hudak AM, Trivedi K, Harper CR, et al. Evaluation of seizure-like episodes in survivors of moderate and severe traumatic brain injury. *J Head Trauma Rehabil.* 2004;19:290–295.

49. Vespa PM, Nuwer MR, Nenov V, et al. Increased incidence and impact of nonconvulsive and convulsive seizures after traumatic brain injury as detected by continuous electroencephalographic monitoring. *J Neurosurg.* 1999;91:750–760.

50. Holmes GL, Sackellares JC, McKiernan J, Ragland M, Dreifuss FE. Evaluation of childhood pseudoseizures using EEG telemetry and video tape monitoring. *J Pediatrics.* 1980;97:554–558.

51. Betts T. Pseudoseizures: seizures that are not epilepsy. *Lancet.* 1990; 336:163–164.

52. Leis AA. Psychogenic seizures. *The Neurologist.* 1996;2:141–149.

53. Pritchard PB III, Wannamaker BB, Sagel J, Daniel CM. Serum prolactin and cortisol levels in evaluation of pseudoepileptic seizures. *Ann Neurol.* 1985;18:87–89.

54. Willert C, Spitzer C, Kusserow S, Runge U. Serum neuron-specific enolase, prolactin, and creatine kinase after epileptic and psychogenic non-epileptic seizures. *Acta Neurol Scand.* 2004;109: 318–323.

55. Barry E, Krumholz A, Bergey GK, Chatha H, Alemayehu S, Grattan L. Nonepileptic post-traumatic seizures. *Epilepsia.* 1998;39:427–431.

56. Salinsky M, Spencer D, Boudreau E, et al. Psychogenic nonepileptic seizures in US veterans. *Neurology.* 2011;77:945.

57. Hauser WA, Annegers JF, Kurland LT. Prevalence of epilepsy in Rochester, Minnesota: 1940–1980. *Epilepsia* 1991;32: 429–445.

58. Broglin D, Delgado-Escueta AV, Walsh GO, Bancaud J, Chauvel P. Clinical approach to the patient with seizures and epilepsies of frontal origin. *Adv Neurol.* 1992;57:59–88.

59. Williamson PD, Spencer SS. Clinical and EEG features of complex partial seizures of extratemporal origin. *Epilepsia.* 1986;27(suppl 2): S46–S63.

60. Hardman JM. The pathology of traumatic brain injuries. *Adv Neurology.* 1979;22:15–50.

61. Payan H, Toga M, Berard-Badier M. The pathology of post-traumatic epilepsies. *Epilepsia.* 1970;11:81–94.

62. Diaz-Arrastia R, Agostini MA, Frol AB, et al. Neurophysiologic and neuroradiologic features of intractable epilepsy after traumatic brain injury in adults. *Arch Neurol.* 2000;57:1611–1616.

63. Marks DA, Kim J, Spencer DD, Spencer SS. Seizure localization following head injury in patients with uncontrolled epilepsy. *Neurology.* 1995;45:2051–2057.

64. Oller L, Fossas P, Sanchez ME, Russi A. Versive seizures of probable occipital origin in a case of post-traumatic epilepsy. *Eur Neurol.* 1985;24(5):355–399.

65. Adachi N, Onuma T, Nishiwaki S, et al. Inter-ictal and post-ictal psychoses in frontal lobe epilepsy: a retrospective comparison with psychoses in temporal lobe epilepsy. *Seizure.* 2000;9:328–335.

66. Delgado-Escueta AV, Swartz BE, Walsh GO, Chauvel P, Bancaud J, Broglin D. Frontal lobe seizures and epilepsies in neurobehavioral disorders. *Adv Neurol.* 1991;55:317–340.

67. Engel J Jr. Neurobiology of behavior: anatomic and physiological implications related to epilepsy. *Epilepsia.* 1986;27(suppl 2):S3–S13.

68. Treiman DM. Psychobiology of ictal aggression. In: Smith D, Treiman D, Trimble M, eds. *Advances in Neurology.* Vol. 55. New York, NY: Raven Press; 1991:341–356.

69. Devinsky O, Luciano D. Psychic phenomena in partial seizures. *Semin Neurol.* 1991;11:100–109.

70. Mendez MF. Post ictal violence and epilepsy. *Psychosomatics.* 1998;39:478–480.

71. Bogdanovic MD, Mead SH, Duncan JS. Aggressive behaviour at a residential epilepsy centre. *Seizure.* 2000;9:58–64.

72. Kotagal P, Arunkumar GS. Lateral frontal lobe seizures. *Epilepsia.* 1998;39(suppl 4):S62–S68.

73. Kotagal P, Arunkumar G, Hammel J, Mascha E. Complex partial seizures of frontal lobe onset statistical analysis of ictal semiology. *Seizure.* 2003;12:268–281.

74. Wieser H-G. Ictal manifestations of temporal lobe epilepsy. *Adv Neurol.* 1991;55:301–315.

75. Quesney LF. Clinical and EEG features of complex partial seizures of temporal lobe origin. *Epilepsia.* 1986;27(suppl 2):S27–S45.

76. Kuzniecky R. Symptomatic occipital lobe epilepsy. *Epilepsia.* 1998;39(suppl 4):S24–S31.

77. Kutsy RL. Focal extra temporal epilepsy: clinical features, EEG patterns, and approach. *J Neurol Sci.* 1999;166:1–15.

78. Isnard J, Guénot M, Sindou M, Maugiére F. Clinical manifestations of insular lobe seizures: a stereo-electroencephalographic study. *Epilepsia.* 2004;45:1079–1090.

79. Rolak LA, Rutecki P, Ashizawa T, Harati Y. Clinical features of Todd's post-epileptic paralysis. *J Neurol Neurosurg Psychiatry.* 1992;55:63–64.

80. Efron R. Post-epileptic paralysis: theoretical critique and report of a case. *Brain.* 1961;84:381–394.

81. Gallmetzer P, Leutmezer F, Serles W, Assem-Hilger E, Spatt J, Baumgartner C. Postictal paresis in focal epilepsies—incidence, duration, and causes: a video-EEG monitoring study. *Neurology.* 2004;62:2160–2164.

82. Iriarte J, Urrestarazu E, Artieda J, et al. Ictal paralysis mimicking Todd's phenomenon. *Neurology.* 2002;59:464–466.

83. Roberts RJ, Gorman LL, Lee GP, et al. The phenomenology of multiple partial seizure-like symptoms without stereotyped spells: an epilepsy spectrum disorder? *Epilepsy Res.* 1992;13:167–177.

84. Varney NR, Hines ME, Bailey C, Roberts RJ. Neuropsychiatric correlates of theta bursts in patients with closed head injury. *Brain Inj.* 1992;6:499–508.

85. Verduyn WH, Hilt J, Roberts MA, Roberts RJ. Multiple partial seizure-like symptoms following "minor" closed head injury. *Brain Inj.* 1992;6:245–260.

86. Annegers JF. The epidemiology of epilepsy. In: Wyllie E, ed. *The Treatment of Epilepsy: Principles and Practice.* 2nd ed. Baltimore, MD: Williams & Wilkins; 1996: 165–172.

87. Ameen AA. Penetrating craniocerebral injuries: observations in the Iraqi-Iranian war. *Milit Med.* 1987;152:76–79.

88. Ascroft PB. Traumatic epilepsy after gunshot wounds of the head. *Br Med J.* 1941;1:739–744.

89. Askenasy JJM. Association of intracerebral bone fragments and epilepsy in missile head injuries. *Acta Neurol Scand.* 1989;79:47–52.

90. Brandvold B, Levi L, Feinsod M, George ED. Penetrating craniocerebral injuries in the Israeli involvement in the Lebanese conflict, 1982–1985. Analysis of a less aggressive surgical approach. *J Neurosurg.* 1990;72:15–21.

91. Caveness WF, Liss HR. Incidence of post-traumatic epilepsy. *Epilepsia.* 1961;2:123–129.

92. Caveness WF, Meirowsky AM, Rish BL, et al. The nature of post-traumatic epilepsy. *J Neurosurg.* 1979;50:545–553.

93. Evans JH. Post-traumatic epilepsy. *Neurology.* 1962;12:665–674.

94. Phillips G. Traumatic epilepsy after closed head injury. *J Neurol Neurosurg Psychiatry.* 1954;17:1–10.

95. Russell WR, Whitty CWM. Studies in traumatic epilepsy: I. Factors influencing the incidence of epilepsy after brain wounds. *J Neurol Neurosurg Psychiatry.* 1952;15:93–98.

96. Walker AE, Jablon S. A follow-up of head injured men of World War II. *J Neurosurg.* 1959;16:600–610.

97. Walker AE, Jablon S. *A Follow-up Study of Head Wounds in World War II. (Veterans Administration Medical Monograph).* Washington, DC: U.S. Government Printing Office; 1961.

98. Watson CW. Incidence of epilepsy following cranial cerebral injury. II. Three year follow-up study. *AMA Arch Neurol Psychiatry.* 1952:68:831–834.

99. Whitty CWM. Early traumatic epilepsy. *Brain.* 1947;70:416–439.

100. Eide PK, Tysnes OB. Early and late outcome in head injury patients with radiological evidence of brain damage. *Acta Neurol Scand.* 1992;86:194–198.

101. Angeleri F, Majkowski J, Cacchio G, et al. Post-traumatic epilepsy risk factors: one-year prospective study after head injury. *Epilepsia.* 1999;40:1222–1230.

102. Annegers JF, Hauser WA, Coan SP, Rocca WA. A population-based study of seizures after traumatic brain injuries. *N Engl J Med.* 1998; 338:20–24.

103. Annegers JF, Grabow JD, Broover RV, Laws ER, Elveback LR, Kurland LT. Seizures after head trauma: a population study. *Neurology.* 1980;30:683–689.

104. Armstrong KK, Saghal V, Block R, Armstrong KJ, Heinemann A. Rehabilitation outcomes in patients with post-traumatic epilepsy. *Arch Phys Med Rehabil.* 1990;71:156–160.

105. Asikainen I, Kaste M, Sarna S. Early and late post-traumatic seizures in traumatic brain injury rehabilitation patients: brain injury factors causing late seizures and influence of seizures on long-term outcome. *Epilepsia.* 1999;40:584–589.

106. Barlow KM, Spowart JJ, Minns RA. Early post-traumatic seizures in non-accidental head injury: relation to outcome. *Dev Med Child Neurol.* 2000;42:591–594.

107. Black P, Shepard RH, Walker AE. Outcome of head trauma: age and post-traumatic seizures. *Ciba Found Symp.* 1975;34:215–219.

108. Bontke CF, Lehmkuhl LD, Englander J, et al. Medical complications and associated injuries of patients treated in TBI Model System programs. *J Head Trauma Rehabil.* 1993;8:34–46.

109. Cohen M, Groswasser Z. Epilepsy in traumatic brain-injured patients [abstract]. *Epilepsia.* 1991;32(suppl 1):S55.

110. Da Silva AM, Vaz AR, Ribeiro I, Melo AR, Nunes B, Correia M. Controversies in post-traumatic epilepsy. *Acta Neurochir Suppl (Wien).* 1990;50:48–51.

111. De Santis A, Cappricci E, Granata G. Early post-traumatic seizures in adults. *J Neurosurg Sci.* 1979;23:207–210.

112. De Santis A, Sganzerla E, Spagnoli D, Bello L, Tiberio F. Risk factors for late post-traumatic epilepsy. *Acta Neurochir Suppl (Wien).* 1992; 55:64–67.

113. Desai BT, Whitman S, Coonley-Hoganson R, Coleman TE, Gabriel G, Dell J. Seizures and civilian head injuries. *Epilepsia.* 1983;24: 289–296.

114. Englander J, Bushnik T, Duong TT, et al. Analyzing risk factors for late post-traumatic seizures: a prospective, multicenter investigation. *Arch Phys Med Rehabil.* 2003;84:365–373.

115. Guidice MA, Berchou RC. Post-traumatic epilepsy following head injury. *Brain Inj.* 1987;1:61–64.

116. Heikinnen ER, Ronty HS, Tolonen U, Pyhtinen J. Development of post-traumatic epilepsy. *Stereotact Funct Neurosurg.* 1990;54–55: 25–33.

117. Hendrick E, Harris L. Post-traumatic epilepsy in children. *J Trauma.* 1968;8:547–555.

118. Japan Follow-up Group for Post-traumatic Epilepsy. The factors influencing post-traumatic epilepsy; multicentric cooperative study. *No Shinkei Geka.* 1991;19:1151–1159.

119. Kalisky Z, Morrison DP, Meyers CA, Von Laufen AV. Medical problems encountered during rehabilitation of patients with head injury. *Arch Phys Med Rehabil.* 1985;66:25–29.

120. Kollevold T. Immediate and early cerebral seizures after head injuries, part I. *J Oslo City Hosp.* 1976;26:99–114.

121. Kollevold T. Immediate and early cerebral seizures after head injuries, part II. *J Oslo City Hosp.* 1977;27:89–99.

122. Kollevold T. Immediate and early cerebral seizures after head injuries, part III. *J Oslo City Hosp.* 1978;28:78–86.

123. Kollevold T. Immediate and early cerebral seizures after head injuries, part IV. *J Oslo City Hosp.* 1979;29:35–47.

124. Lee S-T, Lui T-N. Early seizures after mild closed head injury. *J Neurosurg.* 1992;76:435–439.

125. Manaka S, Japan Follow-Up Research Group of Post-traumatic Epilepsy. Cooperative prospective study on post-traumatic epilepsy risk factors and the effect of prophylactic anticonvulsant. *Jpn J Psychiatry Neurol.* 1992;46:311–315.

126. Mazzini L, Cossa FM, Angelino E, Campini R, Pastore I, Monaco F. Neuroradiologic and neuropsychological assessment of long-term outcome. *Epilepsia.* 2003;44:569–574.

127. Paillas JE, Paillas N, Bureau M. Post-traumatic epilepsy. Introduction and clinical observations. *Epilepsia.* 1970;11:5–16.

128. Sazbon L, Groswasser Z. Outcome in 134 patients with prolonged post-traumatic unawareness. Part 1: parameters determining late recovery of consciousness. *J Neurosurg.* 1990;72:75–80.

129. Thomsen IV. Late outcome of very severe blunt head trauma: a 10–15 year second follow-up. *J Neurol Neurosurg Psychiatry.* 1984; 47:260–268.

130. Wiederholt WC, Melton LJ III, Annegers JF, Grabow JD, Laws ER Jr, Ilstrup DM. Short-term outcomes of skull fracture: a population-based study of survival and neurologic complications. *Neurology.* 1989;39:96–100.

131. Deymeer F, Leviton A. Post-traumatic seizures: an assessment of the epidemiologic literature. *Cent Nerv Syst Trauma.* 1985;2:33–43.

132. Ng WK, Yablon SA, Dostrow VG. Risk of late post-traumatic seizure recurrence after withdrawal of antiepileptic drug therapy [abstract]. *Arch Phys Med Rehabil.* 2000;81:1266–1267.

133. Wiedemayer H, Triesch K, Schafer H, Stolke D. Early seizures following non-penetrating traumatic brain injury in adults: risk factors and clinical significance. *Brain Inj.* 2002;16:323–330.

134. Rish B, Caveness W. Relation of prophylactic medication to the occurrence of early seizures following craniocerebral trauma. *J Neurosurg.* 1973;38:155–158.

135. Van Hout B, Gagnon D, Souétre E, et al. Relationship between seizure frequency and costs and quality of life of outpatients with partial epilepsy in France, Germany, and the United Kingdom. *Epilepsia.* 1997;38:1221–1226.

136. Baker GA, Nashef L, van Hout BA. Current issues in the management of epilepsy: the impact of frequent seizures on cost of illness, quality of life, and mortality. *Epilepsia.* 1997;38(suppl 1):S1–S8.

137. Haltiner AM, Temkin NR, Dikmen SS. Risk of seizure recurrence after the first late post-traumatic seizure. *Arch Phys Med Rehabil.* 1997;78:835–840.

138. Semah F, Picot M-C, Adam C, et al. Is the underlying cause of epilepsy a major prognostic factor for recurrence? *Neurology.* 1998; 1256–1262.

139. Temkin NR, Dikmen SS, Wilensky AJ, Keihm J, Chabal S, Winn HR. A randomized, double-blind study of phenytoin for the prevention of post-traumatic seizures. *N Engl J Med.* 1990;323:497–502.

140. McCrory PR, Bladin PF, Berkovic SF. Retrospective study of concussive convulsions in elite Australian rules and rugby league footballers: phenomenology, aetiology, and outcome. *BMJ.* 1997;314: 171–174.

141. Jabbari B, Prokhorenko O, Khajavi K, Mena H. Intractable epilepsy and mild brain injury: incidence, pathology and surgical outcome. *Brain Inj.* 2002;16:463–467.

142. Kumar J, Gupta RK, Husain M, et al. Mgnetization transfer MR imaging in patients with post-traumatic epilepsy. *AJNR Am J Neuroradiol.* 2003;23:218–224.

143. Frey LC. Epidemiology of post-traumatic epilepsy: a critical review. *Epilepsia.* 2003;44(suppl 10):11–17.

144. Cifu DX, Kreutzer JS, Marwitz JH, et al. Etiology and incidence of rehospitalization after traumatic brain injury: a multicenter analysis. *Arch Phys Med Rehabil.* 1999;80:85–90.

145. Shavelle RM, Strauss D, Whyte J, Day SM, Yu YL. Long-term causes of death after traumatic brain injury. *Am J Phys Med Rehabil.* 2001; 80:510–516.

146. Lindsten H, Nystrom L, Forsgren L. Mortality risk in an adult cohort with a newly diagnosed unprovoked epileptic seizure: a population-based study. *Epilepsia.* 2000;41:1469–1473.

147. Strauss DJ, Day SM, Shavelle RM, Wu YW. Remote symptomatic epilepsy. Does seizure severity increase mortality? *Neurology.* 2003; 60:395–399.

148. Corkin S, Sullivan EV, Carr FA. Prognostic factors for life expectancy after head injury. *Arch Neurol.* 1984;41:975–977.

149. Rish BL, Dillon JD, Weiss GH. Mortality following penetrating craniocerebral injuries. *J Neurosurg.* 1983;59:775–780.

150. Walker AE, Blumer D. The fate of World War II veterans with post-traumatic seizures. *Arch Neurol.* 1989;46:23–26.

151. Weiss GH, Caveness WF, Eisiedel-Lechtape H, McNeel M. Life expectancy and causes of death in a group of head-injured veterans of World War I. *Arch Neurol.* 1982;39:741–743.

152. Aarts JHP, Binnie CD, Smit AM, Wilkins AJ. Selective cognitive impairment during focal and generalized epileptiform EEG activity. *Brain.* 1984;107:293–308.

153. Aldenkamp AP. Effect of seizures and epileptiform discharges on cognitive function. *Epilepsia.* 1997;38(suppl 1):S52–S55.

154. Binnie CD, Marston D. Cognitive correlates of interictal discharges. *Epilepsia.* 1992;33(suppl 6):S11–S17.

155. Swanson SJ, Rao SM, Grafman J, Salazar AM, Kraft J. The relationship between seizure subtype and interictal personality. Results from the Vietnam Head Injury Study. *Brain.* 1995;118:91–103.

156. Hernandez TD, Naritoku DK. Seizures, epilepsy, and functional recovery after traumatic brain injury: a reappraisal. *Neurology.* 1997;48:803–806.

157. Schwab K, Grafman J, Salazar AM, Kraft J. Residual impairments and work status 15 years after penetrating head injury: report from the Vietnam Head Injury Study. *Neurology.* 1993;43:95–103.

158. Grafman J, Jonas B, Salazar A. Epilepsy following penetrating head injury to the frontal lobes. In: Chauvel P, Delgado-Escueta AV, eds. *Advances in Neurology.* Vol 57. New York, NY: Raven Press; 1992: 369–378.

159. Dikmen S, Reitan RM. Neuropsychological performance in post-traumatic epilepsy. *Epilepsia.* 1978;19:177–183.

160. Haltiner AM, Temkin NR, Winn HR, Dikmen SS. The impact of post-traumatic seizures on 1-year neuropsychological and psychosocial outcome of head injury. *J Int Neuropsychol Soc.* 1996;2: 494–504.

161. Lee S-T, Lui T-N, Wong C-W, Yeh Y-S, Tzaan W-C. Early seizures after moderate closed head injury. *Acta Neurochir (Wien).* 1995;137: 151–154.

162. Working Group on Status Epilepticus. Treatment of convulsive status epilepticus. Recommendations of the Epilepsy Foundation of America's Working Group on status epilepticus. *JAMA.* 1993; 270:854–859.

163. Waterhouse EJ. Status epilepticus. *Curr Treat Options Neurol.* 2002; 4:309–317.

164. Lowenstein DH, Alldredge BK. Status epilepticus. *N Engl J Med.* 1998;338:970–976.

165. Lowenstein DH, Bleck T, MacDonald RL. It's time to revise the definition of status epilepticus. *Epilepsia.* 1999;40:120–122.

166. Vining E. Gaining a perspective on childhood seizures. *N Engl J Med.* 1998;338:1916–1918.

167. Leppik IE. Status epilepticus. *Neurol Clin.* 1986;4:633–643.

168. Kennedy CR, Freeman JM. Post-traumatic seizures and post-traumatic epilepsy in children. *J Head Trauma Rehabil.* 1986;1(4): 66–73.

169. Hauser WA. Status epilepticus: epidemiologic considerations. *Neurology.* 1990;40(suppl 2):9–13.

170. Leppik I. Status epilepticus: the next decade. *Neurology.* 1990; 40(suppl 2):4–9.

171. Towne AR, Pellock JM, Ko D, DeLorenzo RJ. Determinants of mortality in status epilepticus. *Epilepsia.* 1994;35(1):27–34.

172. Walker AE, Erculei F. Post-traumatic epilepsy 15 years later. *Epilepsia.* 1970;11:17–26.

173. Walczak TS, Leppik IE, D'Amelio M, et al. Incidence and risk factors in sudden unexpected death in epilepsy: a prospective cohort study. *Neurology.* 2001;56:519–525.

174. Nashef L, So E, Ryvlin P, Tomson T. Unifying the definitions of sudden unexpected death in epilepsy. *Epilepsia.* 2012;53(2):227–233.

175. Temkin NR, Jarell AD, Anderson GD. Antiepileptogenic agents: how close are we? *Drugs.* 2001;61:1045–1055.

176. Stables JP, Bertram EH, White HS, et al. Models for epilepsy and epileptogenesis: report from the NIH Workshop, Bethesda, Maryland. *Epilepsia.* 2002;43:1410–1420.

177. Chang BS, Lowenstein DH. Epilepsy. *N Engl J Med.* 2003;349:1257–1266.

178. Herman ST. Epilepsy after brain insult: targeting epileptogenesis. *Neurology.* 2002;59(9)(suppl 5):S21–S26.

179. Pitkänen A. Drug-mediated neuroprotection and antiepileptogenesis. *Neurology.* 2002;59:S27–S33.

180. Sato M, Racine RJ, McIntyre DC. Kindling: basic mechanisms and clinical validity. *Electroenceph Clin Neurophysiol.* 1990;76:459–472.

181. Willmore LJ. Post-traumatic epilepsy: cellular mechanisms and implications for treatment. *Epilepsia.* 1990;31(suppl 3):S67–S73.

182. White HS. Animal models of epilepsy. *Neurology.* 2002;59:S7–S14.

183. LöscherW. Animal models of epilepsy for the development of antiepileptogenic and disease-modifying drugs. A comparison of the pharmacology of kindling and post-status epilepticus models of temporal lobe epilepsy. *Epilepsy Res.* 2002;50:105–123.

184. Schmidt D, Rogawski MA. New strategies for the identification of drugs to prevent the development or progression of epilepsy. *Epilepsy Res.* 2002;50:71–78.

185. Jacobs KM, Graber KD, Kharazia VN, Parada I, Prince DA. Postlesional epilepsy: the ultimate brain plasticity. *Epilepsia.* 2000;41(suppl 6):S153–S161.

186. Willmore LJ, Sypert GW, Munson JB. Recurrent seizures induced by cortical iron injection: a model of post-traumatic epilepsy. *Ann Neurol.* 1978;4:329–336.

187. D'Alessandro R, Ferrara R, Benassi G, Lenzi PL, Sabattini L. Computed tomographic scans in post-traumatic epilepsy. *Arch Neurol.* 1988;45:42–43.

188. Goldensohn ES. The relevance of secondary epileptogenesis to the treatment of epilepsy: kindling and the mirror focus. *Epilepsia.* 1984;25(suppl 2):S156–S173.

189. Goddard BV. Development of epileptic seizures through brain stimulation at low intensity. *Nature.* 1967;214:1020–1021.

190. Cavalheiro EA, Leite JP, Bortolotto ZA, Turski WA, Ikonomidou C, Turski L. Long-term effects of pilocarpine in rats: structural damage of the brain triggers kindling and spontaneous recurrent seizures. *Epilepsia.* 1991;32:778–782.

191. Schmutz M, Klebs K, Baltzer V. Inhibition or enhancement of kindling evolution by antiepileptics. *J Neural Transm.* 1988;72:245–257.

192. Albertson TE, Joy RM, Stark LG. Carbamazepine: a pharmacological study in the kindling model of epilepsy. *Neuropharmacology.* 1984;23:1117–1123.

193. Wada JA, Sato M, Wake A, Green JR, Troupin AS. Prophylactic effects of phenytoin, phenobarbital, and carbamazepine examined in kindling cat preparations. *Arch Neurol.* 1976;33:426–434.

194. Silver JM, Shin C, McNamara JO. Antiepileptogenic effects of conventional anticonvulsants in the kindling model of epilepsy. *Ann Neurol.* 1991;29:356–363.

195. Wada JA. Pharmacological prophylaxis in the kindling modelof epilepsy. *Arch Neurol.* 1977;34:389–395.

196. Postma T, Krupp E, Li X-L, Post RM, Weiss SRB. Lamotrigine treatment during amygdala-kindled seizure development fails to inhibit seizures and diminishes subsequent anticonvulsant efficacy. *Epilepsy.* 2000;41:1514–1521.

197. Stratton S, Large CH, Cox B, Davies G, Hagan RM. Effect of lamotrigine and levetiracetam on seizure development in a rat amygdala kindling model. *Epilepsy Res.* 2003;53:95–106.

198. Otsuki K, Morimoto K, Sato K, Yamada N, Kuroda S. Effects of lamotrigine and conventional antiepileptic drugs on amygdala-and hippocampal-kindled seizures in rats. *Epilepsy Res.* 1998;31:101–112.

199. Nissinen J, Large CH, Stratton SC, Pitkänen A. Effect of lamotrigine treatment on epileptogenesis: an experimental study in rat. *Epilepsy Res.* 2004;58:119–132.

200. Wada JA. Erosion of kindled epileptogenesis and kindling-induced long-term seizure suppressive effect in primates. In: Wada JA, ed. *Kindling 4.* New York, NY: Plenum Press; 1990: 383–385.

201. D'Ambrosio R, Fairbanks JP, Fender JS, Born DE, Doyle DL, Miller JW. Post-traumatic epilepsy following fluid percussion injury in the rat. *Brain.* 2004;127:304–314.

202. Laurer HL, McIntosh T. Experimental models of brain trauma. *Curr Opin Neurol.* 1999;12:715–721.

203. Santhakumar V, Ratzliff AD, Jeng J, Toth Z, Soltesz I. Long-term hyperexcitability in the hippocampus after experimental head trauma. *Ann Neurol.* 2001;50:708–717.

204. Nilsson P, Ronne-Engström E, Flink R, Ungerstedt U, Carlson H, Hillered L. Epileptic seizure activity in the acute phase following cortical impact trauma in rat. *Brain Res.* 1994;637:227–232.

205. Lowenstein DH, Thomas MJ, Smith DH, McIntosh TK. Selective vulnerability of dentate hilar neurons following traumatic brain injury: a potential mechanistic link between head trauma and disorders of the hippocampus. *J Neurosci.* 1992;12:4846–4853.

206. Golarai G, Greenwood AC, Feeney DM, Connor JA. Physiological and structural evidence for hippocampal involvement in persistent seizure susceptibility after traumatic brain injury. *J Neurosci.* 2001;21:8523–8537.

207. Bao Y, Bramlett H, Atkins C, et al. Post-traumatic seizures exacerbate histopathological damage after fluid-percussion brain injury. *J Neurotrauma.* 2011;28:35–42.

208. Levin HS. Neuroplasticity following non-penetrating traumatic brain injury. *Brain Inj.* 2003;8:665–674.

209. Seitz RJ, Huang Y, Knorr U, Tellman L, Herzog H, Freund HJ. Large-scale plasticity of the human motor cortex. *Neuroreport.* 1995; 6:742–744.

210. Albensi B, Janigro D. Traumatic brain injury and its effects on synaptic plasticity. *Brain Inj.* 2003;17:653–656.

211. Schwartzkroin PA. Mechanisms of brain plasticity: from normal brain function to pathology. *Int Rev Neurobiol.* 2001;45:1–15.

212. Salin P, Tseng GF, Hoffman S, Parada I, Prince DA. Axonal sprouting in layer V pyramidal neurons of chronically injured cerebral cortex. *J Neurosci.* 1995;15:8234–8245.

213. Sankar R, Shin D, Liu H, Wasterlain C, Mazarati A. Epileptogenesis during development: injury, circuit recruitment, and plasticity. *Epilepsia.* 2002;43(suppl 5):47–53.

214. Teyler TJ, Morgan SL, Russell RN, Woodside BL. Synapticplasticity and secondary epileptogenesis. *Int Rev Neurobiol.* 2001;45:253–267.

215. Tsukahara N. Synaptic plasticity in the mammalian central nervous system. *Annu Rev Neurosci.* 1981;4:351–379.

216. Gage RH, Bjorklund A, Stenevi U. Reinnervation of the partially deafferented hippocampus by compensatory collateral sprouting from spared cholinergic and noradrenergic afferents. *Brain Res.* 1983;268:27–37.

217. Prince DA, Connors BW. Mechanisms of epileptogenesis in cortical structures. *Ann Neurol.* 1984;16(suppl):S59–S64.

218. Sutula T, Xiao-Xian H, Cavazos J, Scott G. Synaptic reorganization in the hippocampus induced by abnormal functional activity. *Science.* 1988;239:1147–1150.

219. Coulter DA. Epilepsy-associated plasticity in gamma-aminobutyric acid receptor expression, function, and inhibitory synaptic properties. *Int Rev Neurobiol.* 2001;45:237–252.

220. Timofeev I, Bazhenov M, Avramescu S, Nita D. Posttraumatic epilepsy: the roles of synaptic plasticity. *Neuroscientist.* 2010;16:19–27.

221. Montanez S, Kline AE, Gasser TA, Hernandez TD. Phenobarbital administration directed against kindled seizures delays functional recovery following brain insult. *Brain Res.* 2000;860:29–40.

222. Ling G, Bandak F, Armonda R, Grant G, Ecklund J. Explosive blast neurotrauma. *J Neurotrauma.* 2009;26:815–825.

223. *International Dictionary of Medicine and Biology.* New York, NY: John Wiley & Sons, Inc.; 1986.

224. Deutschmann CS, Haines SJ. Anticonvulsant prophylaxis in neurological surgery. *Neurosurgery.* 1985;17:510–517.

225. Caveness WF. Onset and cessation of fits following craniocerebral trauma. *J Neurosurg.* 1963;20:570–583.

226. Pechadre JC, Lauxerois M, Colnet G, et al. Prevention de L'epilepsie post-traumatique tardive par phenytoine dans les traumatismes craniens graves. Suivi durant 2 ans. *Presse Med.* 1991;20:841–845.

227. Koh S, Storey TW, Santos TC, Mian QY, Cole AJ. Early-life seizures in rats increase susceptibility to seizure-induced brain injury in adulthood. *Neurology.* 1999;53:915–921.

228. Schaumann BA, Anneger JF, Johnson SB, Moore KJ, Lubozynski MF, Salinsky MC. Family history of seizures in post-traumatic and alcohol-associated seizure disorders. *Epilepsia.* 1994;35:48–52.

229. Diaz-Arrastia R, Gong Y, Fair S, et al. Increased risk of late post-traumatic seizures associated with inheritance of APOE epsilon4 allele. *Arch Neurol.* 2003;60:818–822.

230. Lowenstein D. Epilepsy after head injury: an overview. *Epilepsia.* 2009;50(suppl 2):4–9.

231. Hauser WA, Tabaddor K, Factor PR, Finer C. Seizures and head injury in an urban community. *Neurology (Cleveland).* 1984;34: 746–751.

232. Glötzner FL, Haubitz I, Miltner F, Kapp G, Pflughaupt KW. Epilepsy prophylaxis with carbamazepine in severe brain injuries. *Neurochirurgia.* 1983;26:66–79.

233. Temkin NR. Risk factors for post-traumatic seizures. *Epilepsia.* 2003; 44(suppl 10):18–20.

234. Salazar AM, Amin D, Vance SC, Grafman J, Schlesselman S, Buck D. Epilepsy after penetrating head injury: effects of lesion location. In: Wolf P, Dam M, Janz D, Dreifuss FE, eds. *Advances in Epilepsy.* Vol 16. New York, NY: Raven Press; 1987:753–757.

235. Clear D, Chadwick DW. Seizures provoked by blows to the head. *Epilepsia.* 2000;41:243–244.

236. Courjon J. A longitudinal electro-clinical study of 80 cases of post-traumatic epilepsy observed from the time of the original trauma. *Epilepsia.* 1970;11:29–36.

237. Jennett B, van de Sande. EEG prediction of post-traumatic epilepsy. *Epilepsia* 1975;16:251–256.

238. Blackwood D, McQueen JK, Harris P, et al. A clinical trial of phenytoin prophylaxis of epilepsy following head injury: preliminary report. In: Dam M, Gram L, Penry JK, eds. *Advances in Epileptology: XIIth Epilepsy International Symposium.* New York, NY: Raven Press; 1981:521–525.

239. Scherzer E, Wessely P. EEG in post-traumatic epilepsy. *Eur Neurol.* 1978;17:38–42.

240. Thomaides TN, Kerezoudi EP, Chaudhuri KR, Cheropoulos C. Study of EEGs following 24-hour sleep deprivation in patients with post-traumatic epilepsy. *Eur Neurol.* 1992;32:79–82.

241. Zivin L, Ajmone-Marsan C. Incidence and prognostic significance of "epileptiform" activity in the EEG of non-epileptic subjects. *Brain.* 1968;91:751–758.

242. Reisner T, Zeiler K, Wessely P. The value of CT and EEG in cases of post-traumatic epilepsy. *J Neurol.* 1979;221:93–100.

243. Jabbari B, Vengrow MI, Salazar AM, Harper MG, Smutok MA, Amin D. Clinical and radiological correlates of EEG in the late phase of head injury: a study of 515 Vietnam veterans. *Electroenceph Clin Neurophysiol.* 1986;64:285–293.

244. Yablon SA. Post-traumatic seizures. *Arch Phys Med Rehabil.* 1993; 74:983–1001.

245. Bullock R, Chestnut RM, Clifton GL, et al. Role of antiseizure prophylaxis following head injury. *J Neurotrauma.* 2000;17:49–53.

246. Murri L, Arrigo A, Bonuccelli U, Rossi G, Parenti G. Phenobarbital in the prophylaxis of late post-traumatic seizures. *Ital J Neurol Sci.* 1992;13:755–760.

247. Murri L, Parenti G, Bonnucelli. Phenobarbital prophylaxis of post-traumatic epilepsy. *Ital J Neurol Sci.* 1980;1:225–230.

248. Price DJ. The efficiency of sodium valproate as the only anticonvulsant administered to neurosurgical patients. In: Parsonage MJ, Caldwell ADS, eds. *The Place of Sodium Valproate in the Treatment of Epilepsy.* London, United Kingdom: Academic Press;1980:23–34.

249. Servit Z, Musil F. Prophylactic treatment of post-traumatic epilepsy: results of a long-term follow-up in Czechoslovakia. *Epilepsia.* 1981;22:315–320.

250. Wohns RNW, Wyler AR. Prophylactic phentoin in severe head injuries. *J Neurosurg.* 1979;57:507–509.

251. Young B, Rapp R, Brooks W, Madauss W, Norton JA. Post-traumatic epilepsy prophylaxis. *Epilepsia.* 1979;20:671–681.

252. McQueen JK, Blackwood DHR, Harris P, Kalbag RM, Johnson AL. Low risk of late post-traumatic seizures following severe head injury: implications for clinical trials of prophylaxis. *J Neurol Neurosurg Psychiatry.* 1983;46:899–904.

253. Temkin NR, Dikmen SS, Winn HR. Post-traumatic seizures. *Neurosurg Clin.* 1991;2:425–435.

254. Temkin NR, Dikmen SS, Anderson GD, et al. Valproate therapy for prevention of post-traumatic seizures: a randomized trial. *J Neurosurg.* 1999;91:593–600.

255. Young B, Rapp RP, Norton JA, Haack D, Tibbs PA, Bean JR. Failure of prophylactically administered phenytoin to prevent late post-traumatic seizures. *J Neurosurg.* 1983;58:236–241.

256. Young B, Rapp RP, Norton JA, Haack D, Walsh JW. Failure of prophylactically administered phenytoin to prevent post-traumatic seizures in children. *Child's Brain.* 1983;10:185–192.

257. Beghi E. Overview of studies to prevent post-traumatic epilepsy. *Epilepsia.* 2003;44(suppl 10):21–26.

258. Schierhout G, Roberts I. Anti-epileptic drugs for preventing seizures following acute traumatic brain injury. *Cochrane Database Syst Rev.* 2001;(4):CD000173.

259. Schierhout G, Roberts I. Prophylactic antiepileptic agents after head injury: a systematic review. *J Neurol Neurosurg Psychiatry.* 1998;64:108–112.

260. Young B, Rapp RP, Norton JA, Haack D, Tibbs PA, Bean JR. Failure of prophylactically administered phenytoin to prevent early post-traumatic seizures. *J Neurosurg.* 1983;58:231–235.

261. Antiseizure prophylaxis for penetrating brain injury. *J Trauma.* 2001;51(2)(suppl):S41–S43.

262. Benardo LS. Prevention of epilepsy after head trauma: do we need new drugs or a new approach? *Epilepsia.* 2003;44(suppl 10):27–33.

263. Chang BS, Lowenstein DH; Quality Standards Subcommittee of the American Academy of Neurology. Practice parameter: antiepileptic drug prophylaxis in severe traumatic brain injury: report of the Quality Standards Subcommittee of the American Academy of Neurology. *Neurology.* 2003;60:10–16.

264. Engel J Jr, Pedley TA, eds. *Epilepsy: A Comprehensive Textbook.* 2nd ed. Philadelphia, PA: Lippincott Williams & Wilkins; 2007.

265. Wyllie E, ed. *The Treatment of Epilepsy: Principles and Practice.* 5th ed. Philadelphia, PA: Lippincott Williams & Wilkins; 2011.

266. Binnie CD, Stefan H. Modern electroencephalography: its role in epilepsy management. *Clin Neurophys.* 1999;110:1671–1697.

267. Blume WT. Current trends in electroencephalography. *Curr Opin Neurol.* 2001;14:193–197.

268. Chadwick D. Diagnosis of epilepsy. *Lancet.* 1990;336:291–295.

269. Van Donselaar CA, Schimsheimer RJ, Geerts AT, Declerck AC. Value of the electroencephalogram in adult patients with untreated idiopathic first seizures. *Arch Neurol.* 1992;49:231–237.

270. Dana-Haeri J, Trimble MR, Oxley J. Prolactin and gonadotropin change following generalized and partial seizures. *J Neurol Neurosurg Psychiatry.* 1983;46:331–335.

271. Laxer KD, Mullooly JP, Howell B. Prolactin changes after seizures classified by EEG monitoring. *Neurology.* 1985;35:31–35.

272. Meierkord H, Shorvon S, Lightman S, Trimble MB. Comparison of the effects of frontal and temporal lobe seizures on prolactin levels. *Arch Neurol.* 1992;49:225–230.

273. Hammond FM, Yablon SA, Bontke CA. Potential role of serum prolactin measurement in the diagnosis of late post-traumatic seizures. A case report. *Am J Phys Med Rehabil.* 1996;75:304–306.

274. Ebersole JS, Leroy RF. An evaluation of ambulatory, casette EEG monitoring: II. Detection of interictal abnormalities. *Neurology.* 1983;33:8–18.

275. Ebersole JS, Leroy RF. Evaluation of ambulatory casette EEG monitoring: III. Diagnostic accuracy compared to intensive inpatient EEG monitoring. *Neurology.* 1983;33:853–860.

276. American Academy of Neurology, Therapeutics and Technology Assessment Subcommittee. Assessment: intensive EEG/video monitoring for epilepsy. *Neurology.* 1989;39:1101–1102.

277. Hauser WA. Should people be treated after a first seizure? *Arch Neurol.* 1986;1287–1288.

278. Treiman DM. Current treatment strategies in selected situations in epilepsy. *Epilepsia.* 1993;34(suppl 5):S17–S23.

279. Hauser WA, Rich SS, Lee JRJ, Anneger JF, Anderson VE. Risk of recurrent seizures after two unprovoked seizures. *N Engl J Med.* 1998;338:429–434.

280. Hauser WA, Rich SS, Annegers JF, Anderson VE. Seizure recurrence after a 1st unprovoked seizure: an extended follow-up. *Neurology*. 1990;40:1163–1170.

281. Lindsten H, Stenlund H, Forsgren L. Seizure recurrence in adults after a newly diagnosed unprovoked epileptic seizure. *Acta Neurol Scand*. 2001;104:202–207.

282. Hart YM, Sander JWAS, Johnson AL, Shorvon SD. National General Practice Study of Epilepsy: recurrence after a first seizure. *Lancet*. 1990;336:1271–1274.

283. First Seizure Trial Group. Randomized clinical trial on the efficacy of antiepileptic drugs in reducing the risk of relapse after a first unprovoked tonic-clonic seizure. *Neurology*. 1993;43:478–483.

284. Karceski S, Morrell M, Carpenter D. The expert consensus guideline series: treatment of epilepsy. *Epilepsy Behav*. 2001;2:A1–A50.

285. Pellock JM. Who should receive prophylactic antiepileptic drug following head injury? *Brain Inj*. 1989;3:107–108.

286. Mattson RH, Cramer JA, Collins JF, Department of Veterans Affairs Epilepsy Cooperative Study No. 264 Group. A comparison of valproate with carbamazepine for the treatment of complex partial seizures and secondarily generalized tonic-clonic seizures in adults. *N Engl J Med*. 1992;327:765–771.

287. Mattson RH, Cramer JA, Collins JF, et al. Comparison of carbamazepine, phenobarbital, phenytoin, and primidone in partial and secondarily generalized tonic-clonic seizures. *N Eng J Med*. 1985;313: 145–151.

288. Farwell JR, Lee YJ, Hirtz DG, Sulzbacher SI, Ellenberg JH, Nelson KB. Phenobarbital for febrile seizures-effects on intelligence and on seizure recurrence. *N Engl J Med*. 1990;322:364–369.

289. Feely M. Drug treatment of epilepsy. *BMJ*. 1999;318:106–109.

290. Talati R, Scholle JM, Phung OJ, et al. Effectiveness and safety of antiepileptic medications in patients with epilepsy. Comparative Effectiveness Review No. 40. (Prepared by the University of Connecticut/Hartford Hospital Evidence-based Practice Centerunder Contract No. 20-2007-10067-I.) AHRQ Publication No. 11(12)-EHC082-EF. Rockville, MD: Agency for Healthcare Research and Quality. http://www.effectivehealthcare.ahrq.gov/reports/final.cfm.

291. French JA, Kanner AM, Bautista J, et al. Efficacy and tolerability of the new antiepileptic drugs I: treatment of new onset epilepsy: report of the Therapeutics and Technology Assessment Subcommittee and Quality Standards Subcommittee of the American Academy of Neurology and the American Epilepsy Society. *Neurology*. 2004;62:1252–1260.

292. Collaborative Group for Epidemiology of Epilepsy. Adverse reactions to antiepileptic drugs: a follow-up study of 355 patients with chronic antiepileptic drug treatment. *Epilepsia*. 1988;29:787–793.

293. Collaborative Group for Epidemiology of Epilepsy. Adverse reactions to antiepileptic drugs: a multicenter survey of clinical practice. *Epilepsia*. 1986;27:323–330.

294. Homan RW, Miller B, Veterans Administration Epilepsy Cooperative Study Group. Causes of treatment failure with epileptic drugs vary over time. *Neurology*. 1987;37:1620–1623.

295. Smith DB, Mattson RH, Cramer JA, et al. Results of a nationwide Veterans Administration cooperative study comparing the efficacy and toxicity of carbamazepine, phenobarbital, phenytoin, and primidone. *Epilepsia*. 1987;28(suppl 3):S50–S58.

296. Meythaler JM, Yablon SA. Antiepileptic drugs. *Phys Med Rehabil Clin N Am*. 1999;10:275–300.

297. Scolnik D, Nulman I, Rovet J, et al. Neurodevelopment of children exposed in utero to phenytoin and carbamazepine monotherapy. *JAMA*. 1994;271:767–770.

298. Porter RJ, Kelley KR. Antiepileptic drugs and mild liver function elevation. *JAMA*. 1985;253:1791–1792.

299. Camfield C, Camfield P, Smith E, Tibbles JAR. Asymptomatic children with epilepsy: little benefit from screening for anticonvulsant-induced liver, blood, or renal damage. *Neurology*. 1986;36:838–841.

300. Pellock JM, Willmore LJ. A rational guide to routine blood monitoring in patients receiving antiepileptic drugs. *Neurology*. 1991;41: 961–964.

301. Brodie MJ, Richen A, Yuen AWC, for the UK Lamotrigine/Carbamazepine Monotherapy Trial Group. Double-blind comparison of lamotrigine and carbamazepine in newly diagnosed epilepsy. *Lancet*. 1995;345:476–479.

302. Gilliam F, Vazquez B, Sackellares JC, et al. An active-control trial of lamotrigine monotherapy for partial seizures. *Neurology*. 1998; 51:1018–1025.

303. Steiner TJ, Dellaportas CI, Findley LJ. Lamotrigine monotherapy in newly diagnosed untreated epilepsy. *Epilepsia*. 1999;40:601–607.

304. Meador KJ, Loring DW, Abney OL, et al. Effects of carbamazepine and phenytoin on EEG and memory in healthy adults. *Epilepsia*. 1993;34:153–157.

305. Dikmen SS, Temkin NR, Miller B, Machamer J, Winn HR. Neurobehavioral effects of phenytoin prophylaxis of post-traumatic seizures. *JAMA*. 1991;265:1271–1277.

306. Dikmen SS, Machamer JE, Winn HR, Anderson GD, Temkin NR. Neuropsychological effects of valproate in traumatic brain injury: a randomized trial. *Neurology*. 2000;54:895–902.

307. Massagli TL. Neurobehavioral effects of phenytoin, carbamazepine, and valproic acid: implications for use in traumatic brain injury. *Arch Phys Med Rehabil*. 1991;72:219–226.

308. Kirschner KL, Sahgal V, Armstrong KJ, Bloch R. A comparative study of the cognitive effects of phenytoin and carbamazepine in patients with blunt head injury. *J Neuro Rehab*. 1991;5:169–174.

309. Smith KR Jr, Goulding PM, Wilderman D, Goldfader PR, Holterman-Hommes P, Wei F. Neurobehavioral effects of phenytoin and carbamazepine in patients recovering from trauma: a comparative study. *Arch Neurol*. 1994;51:653–660.

310. Goldstein LB. Prescribing of potentially harmful drugs to patients admitted to hospital after head injury. *J Neurol Neurosurg Psychiatry*. 1995;58:753–755.

311. Brailowsky S, Knight RT, Efron R. Phenytoin increases the severity of cortical hemiplegia in rats. *Brain Res*. 1986;376:71–77.

312. Feeney DM, Gonzalez A, Law WA. Amphetamine, haloperidol, and experience interact to affect rate of recovery after motor cortex injury. *Science*. 1982;217:855–857.

313. Schallert T, Hernandez TD, Barth TM. Recovery of function after brain damage: severe and chronic disruption by diazepam. *Brain Res*. 1986;379:104–111.

314. Dauch WA, Schutze M, Guttinger M, Bauer BL. Post-traumatic seizure prevention—results of a survey of 127 neurosurgery clinics. *Zentralbl Neurochir*. 1996;57:190–195.

315. Rapport RL II, Penry JK. A survey of attitudes toward the pharmacological prophylaxis of post-traumatic epilepsy. *J Neurosurg*. 1973; 38:159–166.

316. Gillham R, Kane K, Bryant-Comstock L, Brodie MJ. A double-blind comparison of lamotrigine and carbamazepine in newly-diagnosed epilepsy with health-related quality of life as an outcome measure. *Seizure*. 2000;9:375–379.

317. Messenheimer JA. Rash in adult and pediatric patients treated with lamotrigine. *Can J Neurol Sci*. 1998;25:S14–S18.

318. LaRoche SM, Helmers SL. The new antiepileptic drugs: clinical applications. *JAMA*. 2004;291:615–620.

319. White JR, Walczak TS, Leppik IE, et al. Discontinuation of levetiracetam because of behavioral side effects: a case-control study. *Neurology*. 2003;61:1218–1221.

320. Callaghan N, Garrett A, Goggin T. Withdrawal of anticonvulsant drugs in patients free of seizures for two years: a prospective study. *N Engl J Med*. 1988;318:942–946.

321. Medical Research Council Antiepileptic Withdrawal Study Group. Randomised study of antiepileptic drug withdrawal in patients in remission. *Lancet*. 1991;337:1175–1180.

322. Gherpelli JLD, Kok F, dal Forno S, Elkis LC, Lefevre BHW, Diament AJ. Discontinuing medication in epileptic children: a study of risk factors related to recurrence. *Epilepsia*. 1992;33:681–686.

323. Jacoby A, Johnson A, Chadwick D, Medical Research Council Antiepileptic Drug Withdrawal Study Group. Psychosocial outcomes of antiepileptic drug discontinuation. *Epilepsia*. 1992;33:1123–1131.

324. Schmidt D. Withdrawal of antiepileptic drugs. In: Wolf P, Dam M, Janz D, Dreifuss FE, eds. *Advances in Epilepsy*. Vol 16. New York, NY: Raven Press; 1987:373–377.

325. Westover B, Cormier J, Bianchi M, et al. Revising the "rule of three" for inferring seizure freedom. *Epilepsia*. 2012;53(2):368–376.

326. Bromfield EB, Dambrosia J, Devinsky O, Nice FJ, Theodore WH. Phenytoin withdrawal and seizure frequency. *Neurology.* 1989;39: 905–909.

327. Marks DA, Katz A, Scheyer R, Spencer SS. Clinical and electrographic effects of acute anticonvulsant withdrawal in epileptic patients. *Neurology.* 1991;41:508–512.

328. Theodore WH, Porter RJ, Raubertas RF. Seizures during barbiturate withdrawal: relation to blood level. *Ann Neurol.* 1987;22: 644–647.

329. Vining EPG. Use of barbiturates and benzodiazepines in treatment of epilepsy. *Neurol Clin.* 1986;4:617–632.

330. Stephen LJ, Brodie MJ. Seizure freedom with more than one antiepileptic drug. *Seizure.* 2002;11:349–352.

331. Diaz-Arrastia R, Agostini MA, Van Ness PC. Evolving treament epilepsy. *JAMA.* 2002;287:2917–2920.

332. Engel J Jr, Wiebe S, French J, et al. Practice parameter: temporal lobe and localized neo-cortical resections for epilepsy. *Neurology.* 2003;60:538–547.

333. Engel J Jr. Finally, a randomized, controlled trial of epilepsy surgery. *N Engl J Med.* 2001;345:165–167.

334. Wiebe S, Blume WT, Girvin JP, Eliasziw M; Effectiveness and Efficiency of Surgery for Temporal Lobe Epilepsy Study Group. A randomized, controlled trial of surgery for temporal-lobe epilepsy. *N Engl J Med.* 2001;345;311–318.

335. Spencer SS, Bert AT, Vickrey BG, et al. Initial outcomes in the multicenter study of epilepsy surgery. *Neurology.* 2003;61:1680–1685.

336. Doyle WK, Devinsky O, Perrine K, Pacia S, Vasquez B, Luciano D. Surgical management of post-traumatic epilepsy who underwent surgical management. *Epilepsia.* 1996;37(suppl 5):185.

337. Hosking PG. Surgery for frontal lobe epilepsy. *Seizure.* 2003;12: 160–166.

338. Kazemi NJ, So EL, Mosewich RK, et al. Resection of frontal encephalomalacias for intractable epilepsy: outcome and prognostic factors. *Epilepsia.* 1997;38:670–677.

339. Schuh LA, Henry TR, Fromes G, Blaivas M, Ross DA, Drury I. Influence of head trauma on outcome following anterior temporal lobectomy. *Arch Neurol.* 1998;55:1325–1328.

340. Salinsky MC. Vagus nerve stimulation as treatment for epileptic seizures. *Curr Treat Options Neurol.* 2003;5:110–120.

341. Vonck K, Van Laere K, Dedeurwaerdere S, Caemaert J, De Reuck J, Boon P. The mechanism of action of vagus nerve stimulation for refractory epilepsy: the current status. *J Clin Neurophysiol.* 2001;18: 394–401.

342. Handforth A, De Giorgio CM, Schachter S, et al. Vagus nerve stimulation therapy for partial-onset seizures: a randomized active-control trial. *Neurology.* 1998;51:48–55.

343. The Vagus Nerve Stimulation Study Group. A randomized controlled trial of chronic vagus nerve stimulation for treatment of medically intractable seizures. *Neurology.* 1995;45:224–230.

344. Morris GL, Mueller WM. Long-term treatment with vagus nerve stimulation in patients with refractory epilepsy. The Vagus Nerve Stimulation Study Group E01–E05. *Neurology.* 1999;53: 1731–1735.

345. Fisher RS, Handforth A. Reassessment: vagus nerve stimulation for epilepsy: a report of the Therapeutics and Technology Assessment Subcommittee of the American Academy of Neurology. *Neurology.* 1999;53:666–669.

346. National Association of Epilepsy Centers. Patient referral to specialty epilepsy care. *Epilepsia.* 1990;31(suppl 1):S10–S11.

347. Institute of Medicine. *Epilepsy Across the Spectrum: Promoting Health and Understanding.* Washington, DC: The National Academic Press; 2012.

348. McCarthy AD, Barletta AP, Lux WE, Bleiberg J. Withdrawal of anticonvulsants in a head injury rehabilitation setting [abstract]. *Arch Phys Med Rehabil.* 1991;72:818.

Movement Disorders After Traumatic Brain Injury

Joachim K. Krauss and Joseph Jankovic

INTRODUCTION

Movement disorders after traumatic brain injury appear to occur less frequently than in the past, but, unfortunately, war-related injuries continue to contribute to severe disability in young and otherwise healthy individuals. Trauma to the central and peripheral nervous system is an important etiologic factor in a variety of movement disorders. Although it is widely accepted that traumatic brain injury may result in both transient and persistent movement disorders (1,2), their occurrence after peripheral injury still has not become generally appreciated (3–6). Kinetic tremors and dystonia are the best investigated post-traumatic movement disorders after severe brain injury (7–9), but many other types of hypokinetic and hyperkinetic movement disorders have been reported as sequelae of injury to the central nervous system. The manifestation of movement disorders after moderate or mild brain injury has been less well documented. The association between brain injury and Parkinson disease (PD) is the subject of ongoing research (10,11). Trauma, as a cause for the development of movement disorders, has multifaceted implications regarding not only medical and psychological but also legal aspects (12–14). In some cases of post-traumatic movement disorders, a definite cause-and-effect relationship is difficult to establish. This is partly caused by associated cirumstances including not only medicolegal factors but also because the appearance of movement disorders may be delayed and cause-and-effect relationships may not be recognized.

Reviews on post-traumatic movement disorders have concentrated more on phenomenological aspects and medical treatment options (1,2,15) and less on neurorehabilitation and neurosurgical options (16). Contemporary functional stereotactic surgery may provide long-term symptomatic and functional benefits in many patients with movement disorders who do not benefit sufficiently from medical treatment (17,18). Radiofrequency lesioning of the thalamus and pallidum was the method of choice for years for patients with disabling tremor or parkinsonism and levodopa-induced dyskinesias, but in patients with diffuse axonal injury (DAI), ablative procedures, particularly when performed bilaterally, have been frequently associated with complications such as increased dysarthria or gait disturbance. Deep brain stimulation (DBS) nowadays has become the procedure of choice in such patients. In this chapter, we update the current understanding of the role of central trauma in the development of movement disorders, their diagnosis, and treatment including neurosurgical options.

MOVEMENT DISORDERS AND BRAIN INJURY

Phenomenologic Classification of Movement Disorders

Movement disorders in the following context are understood as phenomenological entities manifested either by slowness and poverty of movement (i.e., hypokinesia); by excessive, abnormal involuntary movements (i.e., hyperkinesia); or by other signs and symptoms that cannot easily be grouped under these 2 categories. Note that the term movement disorder is not synonymous with *motor disorder* covering also paresis, spasticity, and ataxia, which will not be discussed in this chapter. Also, the hypertonic postures seen in comatose patients with chronic decorticate and decerebrate rigidity after severe head injury will not be the subject of this review. Most frequently, movement disorders are associated with dysfunction of the thalamus or the basal ganglia and their circuitry. Therefore, such disorders have also been summarized as *extrapyramidal disorders* previously. This term, however, is not considered useful anymore because the arbitrary concept of a pyramidal vs an extrapyramidal motor system does not adequately reflect the complexity of the organization of the motor system. In the past few years, much progress has been made in the understanding of the functional neuroanatomy, the neurochemistry, and the neurophysiology of the basal ganglia and their circuitry. In particular, recordings of local field potentials have provided new insights (19–21). These advances have had an extraordinary impact on new pharmacological treatments and the reevaluation of surgical approaches.

Many different classifications of movement disorders exist. The International Classification of Diseases Tenth Revison: Neurological Adaptation, a result of collaboration between the World Health Organization and the Movement Disorder Society provided a classification that serves as a basis for international communication, research, and education (22). *Tremor* has been defined as a rhythmic, oscillatory movement, and it can be further divided according to the position, posture, or motor activity necessary to make it manifest (23). *Rest tremor* is seen when the body part is in complete repose. Maintenance of a posture such as holding the arms outstretched reveals *postural tremor*, whereas moving the body part from one position to another (e.g., the finger-to-nose maneuver) brings on *kinetic tremor* (termed *intention tremor* when tremor occurs only shortly before the goal of the movement is reached). *Dystonia* is characterized by involuntary, sustained, patterned muscle contractions of opposing muscles resulting in repetitive twisting movements or abnormal postures (24). Dystonic movement disorders often are misdiagnosed or they are not even recognized because the full spectrum of phenomenology has not been appreciated. Dystonia may be accompanied by tremor or rapid jerking movements. It may be present at rest, but it is usually exacerbated or elicited by voluntary activity (action dystonia). According to its distribution, dystonia can be classified as focal, segmental, generalized, or as hemidystonia. The term *athetosis* is used when phasic writhing dystonic movements of the extremities prevail in patients with secondary generalized dystonia. In *chorea*, rapid unpredictable movements spreading from one muscle group to the other prevail, predominantly affecting the distal limbs. *Ballism* has been defined as continuous, nonpatterned, purposeless movements involving chiefly proximal portions of limbs (25). It usually presents as hemiballism and is related most frequently to lesions of the contralateral subthalamic nucleus. Experimental data suggest that chorea and ballism are parts of a continuum of movement disorders (26). Ballism, thus, can be considered a form of forceful, flinging, high-amplitude, coarse chorea. *Tics* are usually rapid jerklike movements or involuntarily produced sounds and words occurring out of a background of normal activity. Both motor and vocal tics may be categorized as simple or complex. Tics are differentiated from other movement disorders also regarding their particular features such as the presence of premonitory feelings or sensations, variability, temporary suppressibility, and distractibility. *Myoclonus* is defined as a sudden, brief, shocklike involuntary movement that may be caused by both active muscle contraction (positive myoclonus) and inhibition of ongoing muscle activity (negative myoclonus). *Hyperekplexia* is characterized by exaggerated startle responses to sudden unexpected stimuli. *Stereotypy* is an involuntary, patterned, repetitive, continuous, coordinated, purposeless, or ritualistic movement, posture, or utterance that may either be simple or complex, such as self-caressing. *Akathisia* refers to a sense of restlessness and the feeling of a need to move. *Paroxysmal dyskinesias* occur intermittently with bouts of sudden-onset, short-lived involuntary movements that may be dystonic or choreic. *Parkinsonism* is characterized by a combination of bradykinesia, rigidity, rest tremor, and postural instability. *Bradykinesia*—slowness of movement—is the clinical hallmark of hypokinetic movement disorders.

Epidemiology of Movement Disorders Related to Brain Injury

Most post-traumatic movement disorders are caused by severe brain injury. There are only few epidemiologic studies that have investigated the relative incidence of post-traumatic movement disorders. These studies yielded a wide variability ranging from 13% to 66% of patients who suffered severe brain injury (27–31). In a study on severe pediatric brain injury in Poland "extrapyramidal syndromes" were described in 18 out of 100 (18%) children (30). In another study from Japan, 33 of 57 (58%) patients who were in a

persistent vegetative state secondary to severe brain injury in motor vehicle accidents had "involuntary movements" (29). In this group, palatal myoclonus and dystonia were observed most frequently. In another study of severe pediatric closed head injury, 4 out of 31 children were described to develop a "basal ganglia syndrome" (27). Exceedingly high rates of post-traumatic tremors were found in a questionnaire-based survey, screening children with severe head injury for the presence of "significant tremor" (28). Tremors were reported in 66% of the responders to the survey (131 of 199 children). Taking into account that tremors might not have been present in cases that did not return the questionnaires the frequency of tremor in this pediatric population still was as high as at least 45%. We have analyzed the frequency of post-traumatic movement disorders in survivors of severe head injury who were admitted to a multidisciplinary trauma unit over a period of 5 years (30). This study included 398 consecutively admitted patients with a Glasgow Coma Score (GCS) of 8 or less. Follow-up was available on 221 of the 264 survivors. Overall, post-traumatic movement disorders were found in 22.6% (50 of 221 patients); they were only transient in 10.4% (23 of 50 patients) but were still present at the time of the investigation at a mean follow-up of 3.9 years in 12.2% (27 of 50 patients) (Table 40-1). Tremors were the most frequent movement disorders. Only in 5.4% of all patients, however, were the movement disorders considered disabling. The presence of generalized edema on the CT scan at admission was significantly associated with the occurrence of movement disorders. Similar associations were detected for focal cerebral lesions but not for subdural or epidural hematomas.

The absolute number of severe head injuries has decreased in most industrialized countries during the last decades. Also, the management of head injury has improved considerably. In particular, decompressive craniectomy has become a routine procedure nowadays (32). It is still unclear

TABLE 40-1 Frequency of Movement Disorders Secondary to Severe Brain Injury

	TRANSIENT	PERSISTENT
Low frequency intention tremor (2.5–4 Hz)	1.4%	0.9%
Postural/kinetic tremor (2.5–4 Hz)	—	3.2%
Postural/intention tremor (> 4 Hz)	4.1%	3.6%
Unclassified tremor	4.5%	1.4%
Focal dystonia	0.5%	1.8%
Hemidystonia	—	0.9%
Hemidystonia + contralateral focal Dystonia	—	0.9%
Hemidystonia + cervical dystonia	—	0.5%
Stereotypies	—	0.9%
Myoclonus	—	0.5%
Parkinsonism	—	0.9%
Paroxysmal hypnogenic Dyskinesias	—	0.5%
Hyperekplexia (exaggerated startle)	—	0.5%

The percentages refer to a cohort of 221 patients (GCS between 3 and 8 at the time of trauma) with long-term follow-up at a mean of 3.9 years. Several patients had more than one movement disorder. Reprinted from Krauss, Tränkle, Kopp (30) with permission.

whether and how these factors translated into a lower frequency and a difference in the severity of movement disorders secondary to craniocerebral injury. Different movement disorders may co-occur in a patient subsequent to severe head injury. In the study on the frequency of post-traumatic movement disorders in survivors of severe head injury mentioned previously, 50 patients had a total of 59 phenomenologically distinct movement disorders (30). Treating one component with medication or surgery will not necessarily have an impact on the other. Furthermore, the coexistence of spastic hemiparesis or quadriparesis is observed frequently. In the individual patient, it may be difficult to distinguish dystonia from accompanying spasticity. It is pivotal to appreciate coexisting neurologic deficits in these patients in order to determine whether or not surgical treatment directed specifically to the movement disorder will make an impact in the patient's overall functional disability.

Systematic study of the frequency of post-traumatic movement disorders after moderate or mild brain injury is sparse. Such associations have been documented, however, by numerous anecdotal case reports or case series. In a survey of 519 patients who suffered head injury with a GCS between 9 and 15 on admission to the hospital, 158 patients were available for a detailed follow-up study (33). In 16 of these 158 patients (10.1%) we diagnosed a post-traumatic movement disorder. Overall, movement disorders were transient in 7.6% (12 patients) and persisted only in a minority of 2.6% (4 patients). Regarding possible bias by selection of the sample group, the frequency of post-traumatic movement disorders could be even lower. Movement disorders that occurred in this series are listed in Table 40-2. Postural or intention tremor phenomenologically similar to enhanced physiologic or essential tremor was the most frequent finding. Movement disorders were not disabling and did not require medical therapy in any instance in this series. Patients suffering from "minor" brain injury, that is those with a GCS of 15, developed movement disorders less frequently than those with a GCS ranging from 9 to 14—the difference being statistically significant.

General Pathomechanisms in Movement Disorders After Brain Injury

Movement disorders after trauma often have a delayed onset, sometimes up to months or years postinjury. In exceptional cases, a delay of more than 20 years has been reported (34). In most patients with movement disorders secondary to severe brain injury, structural or functional lesions will be seen with contemporary imaging techniques. The pathomechanisms resulting in a post-traumatic movement disorder are only partially understood. It is likely that both primary and secondary lesions are responsible for their development. Primary damage involves focal contusions particularly to the basal ganglia and their pathways, DAI with preferential lesions of the superior cerebellar peduncles and ischemia or hemorrhage caused by injury of penetrating arteries associated with rotational forces of the trauma (35,36). Secondary damage caused by hypoxia, hypotension, and increased intracranial pressure may also contribute to the extent of the lesion and the subsequent development of movement disorders. Sequential imaging analyses of the lesions that result in post-traumatic movement disorders have only rarely been performed (37). Figure 40-1 shows serial CT scans and the development of a thalamic lesion causing focal dystonia. Other factors that might be involved in the pathophysiology of post-traumatic movement disorders include the release of toxic cytokines, other neurotoxins, oxidative stress associated with the deposition of hemosiderin and iron facilitating the production of free radicals and other metabolic effects (38–41). The sequelae of mechanical injury have been studied also at cellular and molecular levels (42–44). Genetic factors may influence the rate and extent of recovery after severe brain injury (45,46). The balance between neurodegeneration and restorative neuroplasticity may determine whether a lesion results in permanent damage or in subsequent recovery (47,48). Restorative processes themselves, however, could also contribute to the development of a post-traumatic movement disorder. Neuroplastic phenomena including aberrant sprouting, ephaptic transmission, and alterations of neurotransmitter sensitivity could be responsible for the delay of onset of movement disorders (49).

DIAGNOSIS OF POSTTRAUMATIC MOVEMENT DISORDERS

Tremor

The most common post-traumatic movement disorder is tremor. High-amplitude postural and kinetic tremors that may interfere with any motor function are the most disabling tremors (50,51). Often, the tremor is present during the whole range of a movement and increases in amplitude toward reaching the goal. The frequency of these coarse tremors, in general, ranges between 2.5 and 4 Hz and the amplitudes can be larger than 10 cm. The rhythmic oscillatory movements may be interrupted by irregular jerking movements leading to a "myoclonic" appearance (52) and may even resemble "hemiballistic" movements (53). Tremor may be present also at rest. A recent electromyographic study revealed a mixed pattern of synchronous and alternating types of contractions (54). Slow post-traumatic tremors have been categorized as "midbrain," "rubral" or "Holmes" tremors, or "myorhythmias" (23,50,55,56). In a series of 35 patients with severe post-traumatic tremor, the kinetic component of the tremor was the most prominent feature (57). Bilateral tremor was evident in 10 patients. Commonly, post-traumatic tremor affects predominantly or exclusively the upper extremity. Persistent post-traumatic kinetic tremors are usually secondary to severe closed head injury (57,58).

TABLE 40-2 Frequency of Movement Disorders Secondary to Moderate or Mild Brain Injury

	TRANSIENT	PERSISTENT
Postural/intention tremor (> 4 Hz)	8.2%	1.3%
Hyperekplexia (exaggerated startle)	–	0.6%
cervical myoclonic twitches	–	0.6%

The percentages refer to a cohort of 158 patients (GCS between 9 and 15 at the time of trauma) with long-term follow-up at a mean of 5.2 years. One patient had both a transient and a persistent movement disorder. Reprinted from Krauss, Tränkle, Kopp (33) with permission.

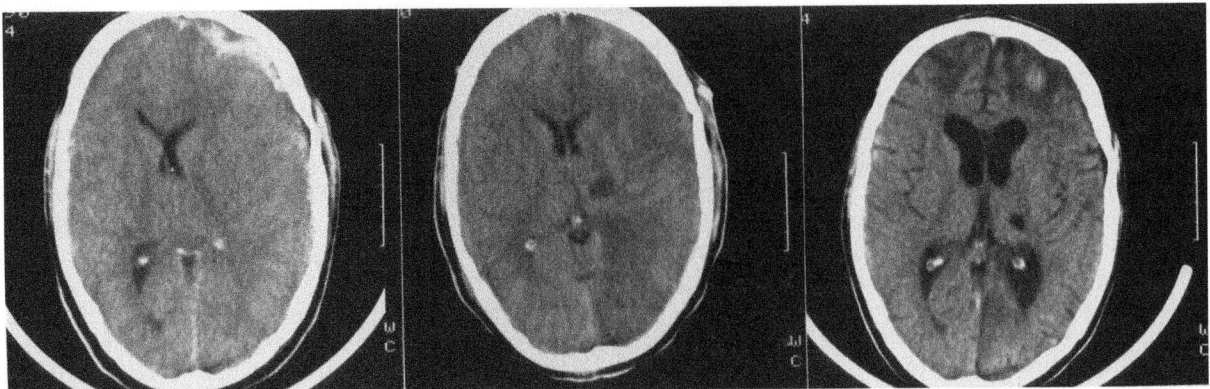

FIGURE 40-1 Serial CT scans of a patient who sustained severe head injury at age 23 and suffered from post-traumatic dystonia of his right hand showing the development of a left thalamic lesion thought to be responsible for his focal dystonia. The scan obtained immediately after head injury shows a left frontal subdural hematoma and generalized brain edema **(left)**; there is less midline shift 10 days after trauma, but a hypodense lesion in the left thalamus is now visible **(middle)**; five weeks later, the thalamic lesion is clearly demarcated **(right)**. Reprinted from Krauss, Mohadjer, Nobbe, Mundinger (57) with permission.

The most frequent cause is automobile accident with a history of deceleration trauma of the car driver. Kinetic tremors have also been described to occur in pedestrians who were strucked by cars and suffered closed head injury. The mean age at trauma was 11 years with a range from 3 to 29 years in one series (57). Most patients are comatose for weeks and often exhibit transient apallic syndromes or akinetic mutism during recovery. The delay between the trauma and the manifestation of the tremor is variable, ranging from 4 weeks up to a year. Commonly, the tremors are associated with ataxia of the affected limb. Tremor almost never is an isolated symptom. Psychological/cognitive alterations were found in 91% of patients, dysarthria in 86%, oculomotor nerve deficits in 69%, truncal ataxia in 91%, and residual hemiparesis or tetraparesis in 91% at a mean of 7 years after brain injury (57).

The history of deceleration trauma and the associated clinical findings indicate that most patients with post-traumatic tremor suffer DAI. This is also supported by neuroradiological findings. In a series of 19 patients with post-traumatic kinetic tremor, there was evidence of DAI in 18 patients according to late-phase magnetic resonance (MR) studies revealing corpus callosal atrophy, ventriculomegaly, subcortical lesions, and brainstem lesions (59). Lesions of the dentatothalamic pathways were found in 22 out of 25 instances (59). Lesions affecting the predecussational course of the dentatothalamic pathway will result in ipsilateral tremor (Figure 40-2), whereas postdecussational lesions are responsible for contralateral tremor (Figure 40-3). Two of 3 patients with an accompanying parkinsonian-like rest tremor had lesions involving the substantia nigra (Figure 40-4). Tremor at rest may be present in patients with lesions of the dentatothalamic pathways without any evidence of contralateral nigrostriatal lesions. Traumatic lesions of the red nucleus and adjacent 3rd nerve nucleus may cause ipsilateral ptosis and limitation of ocular adduction and contralateral postural and rest tremor (Benedikt or Claude syndrome) (60). Isolated cases of thalamic lesions have been reported to cause tremor. In both, cerebellar and thalamic tremors the crescendo appearance with goal-directed movements may be the result of amplification of the tremor in reverberating circuits secondary to impaired thalamic relay. The patho-

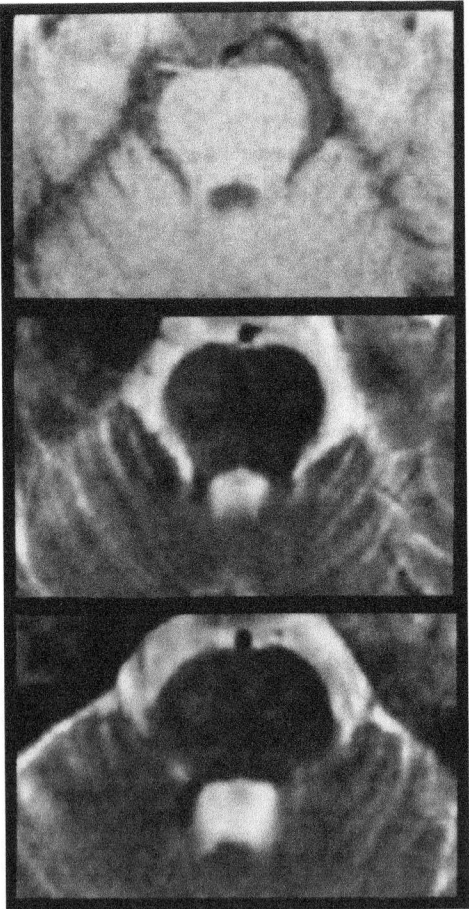

FIGURE 40-2 Axial MR imaging studies at 2.0 T in a 27-year-old man with right-sided postural and kinetic tremor 22 years after a traffic accident. T1-weighted images **(upper)** show a small *ipsilateral* hypointense signal alteration of the right brachium conjunctivum adjacent to the fourth ventricle—that is predecussational. Heavily T2-weighted rapid acquisition relaxation enhanced (RARE) images demonstrate a corresponding apparently larger hypointense lesion **(middle and lower)**. Reprinted from Krauss, Wakhloo, Nobbe, Tränkle, Mundinger, Seeger (59) with permission.

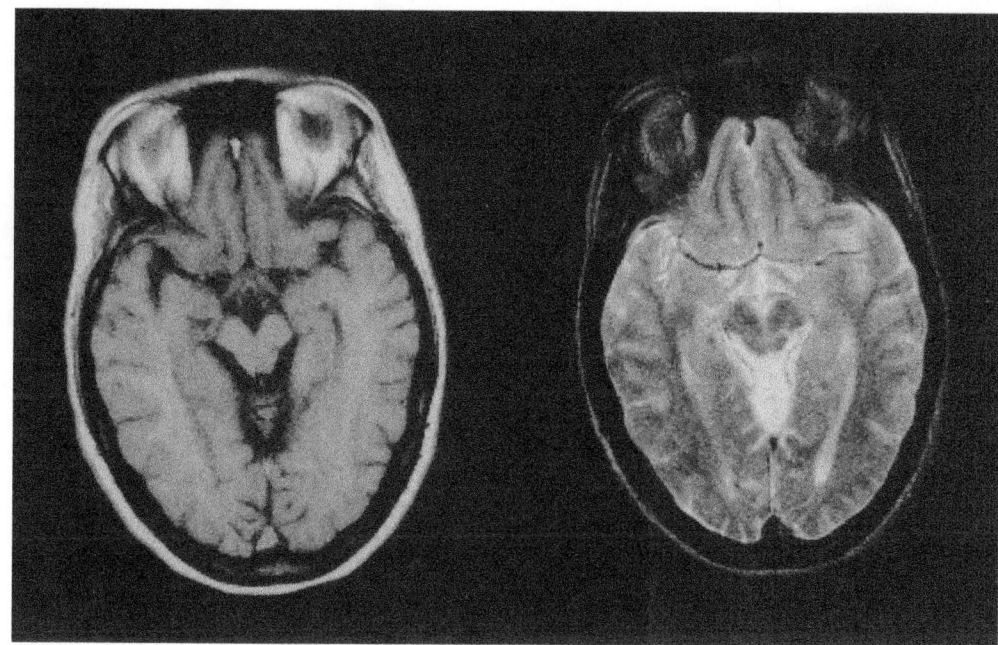

FIGURE 40-3 MR imaging studies at 1.0 T in a 30-year-old woman with right-sided postural and kinetic tremor 12 years after having sustained severe head injury. The axial scans reveal a small *contralateral* postdecussational lesion not extending to the substantia nigra. Reprinted from Krauss, Wakhloo, Nobbe, Tränkle, Mundinger, Seeger (59) with permission.

physiologic mechanisms how lesions of the dentatothalamic pathways result in the delayed appearance of tremor have not been fully elucidated (61). It is well known that such lesions trigger both orthograde and retrograde fiber degeneration. MR spectroscopic techniques suggest transsynaptic changes in the development of post-traumatic tremor (62). Transsynaptic neuronal degeneration could also involve the inferior olives, although palatal myoclonus, a well-known symptom in olivary degeneration, is not commonly observed in post-traumatic tremor. Finally, the disinhibition of thalamic rhythmic network oscillations and modifications of long-loop reflexes could be relevant. Marked decrease in

18F-dopa uptake in the contralateral striatum without significant changes in the D2-specific binding was found in patients with post-traumatic midbrain tremor who improved with levodopa therapy (63). In another patient with post-traumatic tremor who had a complete contralateral loss of the nigrostriatal pathway after midbrain injury as shown by missing [123I]FP-CIT uptake in the contralateral striatum, it was thought that concurrent lesioning of the subthalamic nucleus had prevented the occurrence of parkinsonism (64).

Traumatic neck injury may cause cervical radiculopathy, which may be associated with a postural tremor in the ipsilateral arm (65).

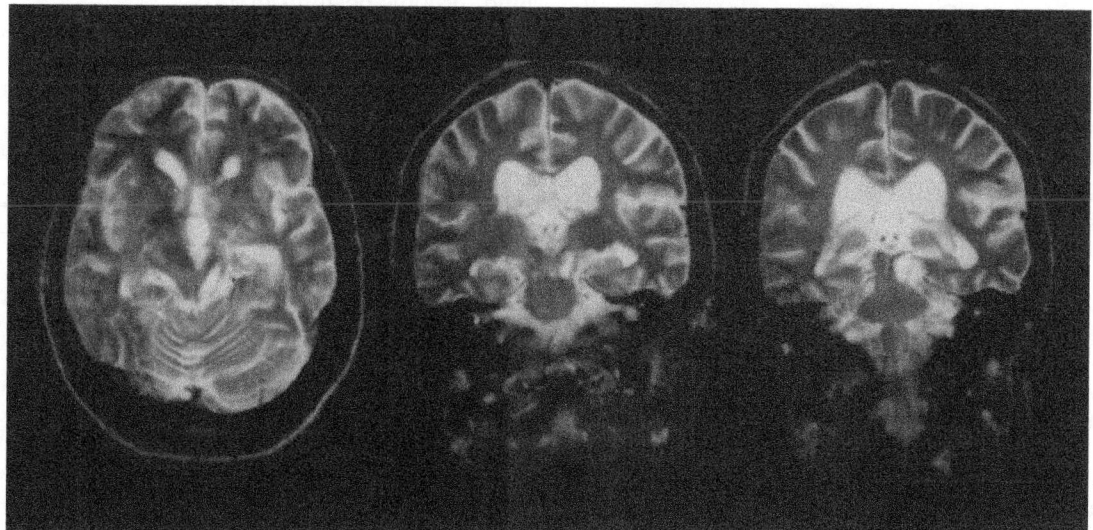

FIGURE 40-4 MR imaging studies at 2.0 T in a 37-year-old man with right-sided parkinsonian tremor at rest, postural and kinetic tremor 33 years after severe head injury. The axial **(left)** and coronal **(middle and right)** scans show a *contralateral* postdecussational lesion extending into the substantia nigra. Reprinted from Krauss, Wakhloo, Nobbe, Tränkle, Mundinger, Seeger (59) with permission.

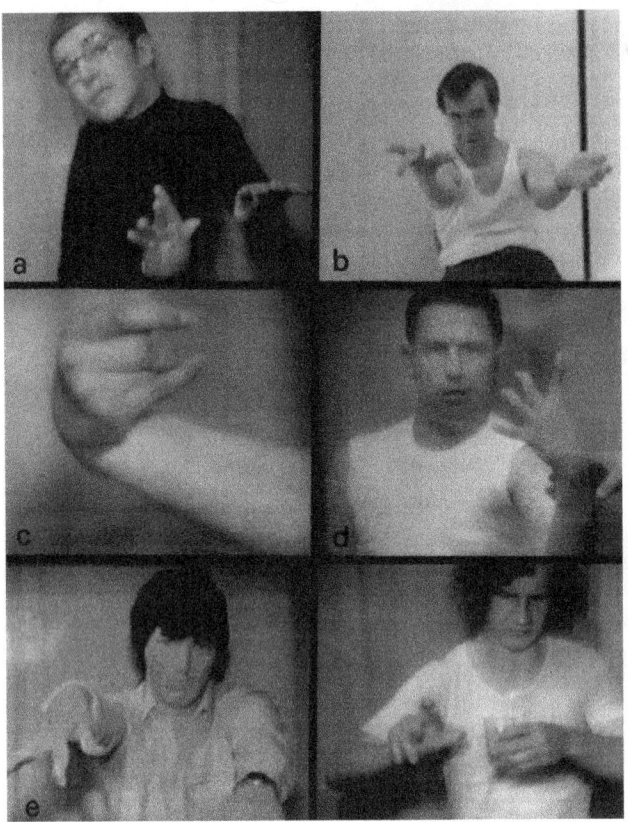

FIGURE 40-5 Clinical presentation of patients with post-traumatic dystonia. **A**, patient with right-sided hemidystonia and cervical dystonia before thalamotomy. **B**, same patient at long-term follow-up after left-sided thalamotomy. **C**, dystonic posture of right hand. **D**, left-sided dystonia with superimposed athetotic movements. **E**, right-sided hemidystonia. **F**, typical increase of dystonia on intended movement. Reprinted from Krauss, Mohadjer, Braus, Wakhloo, Nobbe, Mundinger (8) with permission.

Dystonia

Hemidystonia is the most typical presentation of post-traumatic dystonia (8,9,66–69) (Figure 40-5). In patient series with symptomatic hemidystonia from different etiologies, head injury accounted for 7% to 9% of the cases (70,71). Rare manifestations of craniocerebral trauma include cervical dystonia, segmental axial dystonia, and spasmodic dysphonia (7,72,73). Dystonic overactivity of plantar flexor and foot inversion muscles can be a major predisposing factor to ankle contracture, in particular after severe brain injury (74).

The presence of the DYT1 mutation does not seem to increase the risk of secondary dystonia, and the latter is not associated with the DYT1 mutation (75). The DYT1 mutation is found more frequently among dystonic patients with Ashkenazi Jewish origin, and it is characterized by a 3 base-pair deletion in a gene coding for an ATP-binding protein termed torsinA. In a recent case-control study, there was no association between a history of head trauma and the development of primary cranial dystonia (76).

Several patients with post-traumatic hemidystonia were described over the decades since the first report by Austregesilio in 1928 (77). Nevertheless, post-traumatic dystonia still is probably underreported. There is a predominance of men that, however, most likely reflects the male preponderance among patients suffering craniocerebral trauma. Age at the time of trauma varies but almost all patients with only few exceptions were in their infancy or adolescence. It is possible that the delay of onset of dystonia after static brain lesions is associated with the age at trauma. Patients with hemidystonia secondary to brain damage before the age of 7 years had a longer latency between the lesion and the manifestation of dystonia than adults who suffered structural cerebral damage (49). Most patients suffer severe brain injury but occasional cases of hemidystonia and cervical dystonia were reported after moderate or mild head injury (78). Post-traumatic hemidystonia frequently is preceded by or associated with ipsilateral hemiparesis. The delay between trauma and appearance of hemidystonia is variable and may be as short as one day but may take as long as 6 years (49,71,79). In a series of patients with post-traumatic hemidystonia, the mean latency between injury and the onset of dystonia was 20 months (8). The natural history of hemidystonia seems to be initial progression with spread over months to years followed by eventual stabilization (80).

Post-traumatic dystonia is associated most frequently with basal ganglia or thalamic lesions. Pathoanatomical correlations are similar to those reported for other causes of secondary dystonia (70,71,80). Figure 40-6 illustrates typical early MR imaging findings in a 19-year-old patient who later developed right hemidystonia. In one series, 7 of 8 patients with post-traumatic hemidystonia had lesions involving the contralateral caudate or putamen (8) (Figure 40-7). Cases of pallidal lesions resulting in dystonia are rare (81,82) (Figure 40-8). Occasionally, hemidystonia or focal dystonia, in particular hand dystonia, is associated with thalamic lesions (37). In some instances also, pontomesencephalic lesions mainly concerning the dorsolateral tegmentum were found to be associated with the occurrence of dystonia after severe traumatic brain injury (8,83) (Figure 40-9). Patients with post-traumatic kinetic tremor caused by mesencephalic lesions or by lesions of the superior cerebellar peduncles may also have mild dystonic postures (57).

Primary as well as secondary factors are likely to contribute to the basal ganglia lesions in post-traumatic dystonia. Some of the caudatoputaminal lesions in post-traumatic hemidystonia correspond to vascular territorries, in particular to the anterior (and more rarely posterior) group of the lateral lenticulostriate branches of the middle cerebral artery. Stretch of these vessels by rotating forces may either result in hemorrhage or in ischemia secondary to lesions of the intima (84). This mechanism is probably also responsible for the fact that in patients with dystonia caused by brain injury as compared to patients with other secondary dystonia, caudotoputaminal lesions are much more frequent than thalamic lesions (70). In general, the prognosis of traumatic basal ganglia hematoma is poor. In a series of 34 patients, only 6 (16%) made a favorable recovery (35). Rarely, blunt or penetrating carotid artery injuries have been described to result in ischemic cerebral lesions with subsequent development of dystonia (85,86). Secondary damage to the basal ganglia is also possible. Many patients with post-traumatic dystonia were reported to have hematoma contralateral to the hemidystonia as well. Hypoxia is known to result in damage following "topistic" patterns, that is, damage of specific nuclei

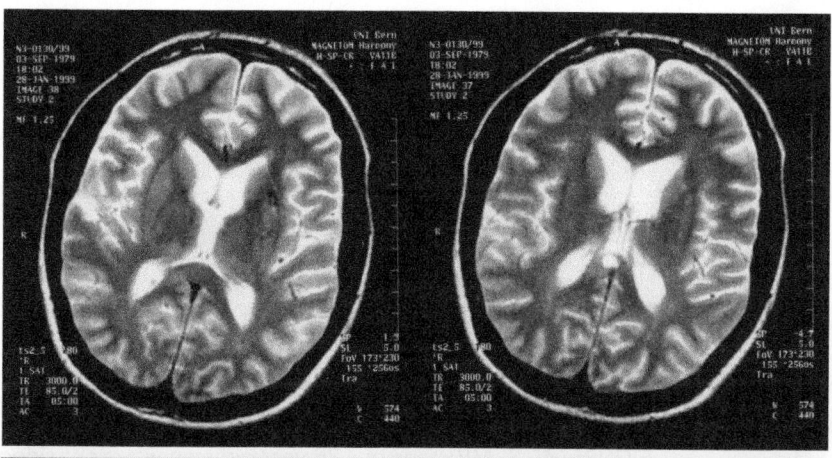

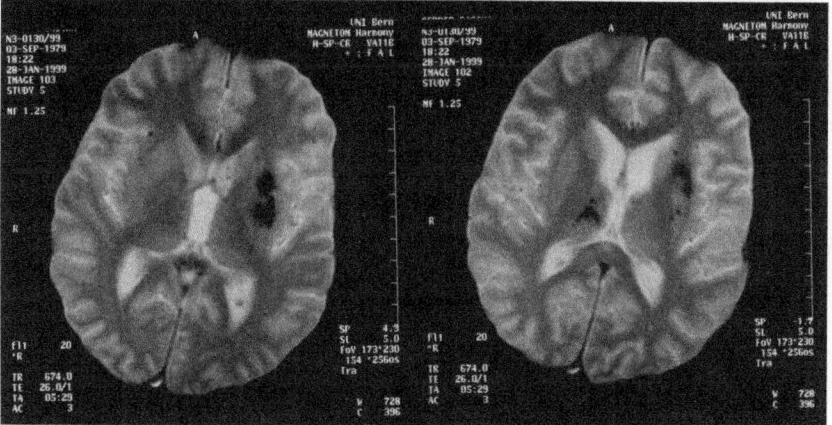

FIGURE 40-6 MR imaging studies of a 19-year-old man 2 months after suffering severe closed head injury with an initial GCS of 4. Later on, right hemidystonia and cervical dystonia developed. **Upper row**: Axial Turbospin-Echo 3000/85 scans show poorly defined lesions of the left putamen. **Lower row**: Axial T2 FLASH 674/26 sequences that are more susceptible to hemosiderin better demonstrate the extent of the hypointense lesions in the putamen and reveal other small lesions in addition. Reprinted from Krauss, Jankovic (16) with permission.

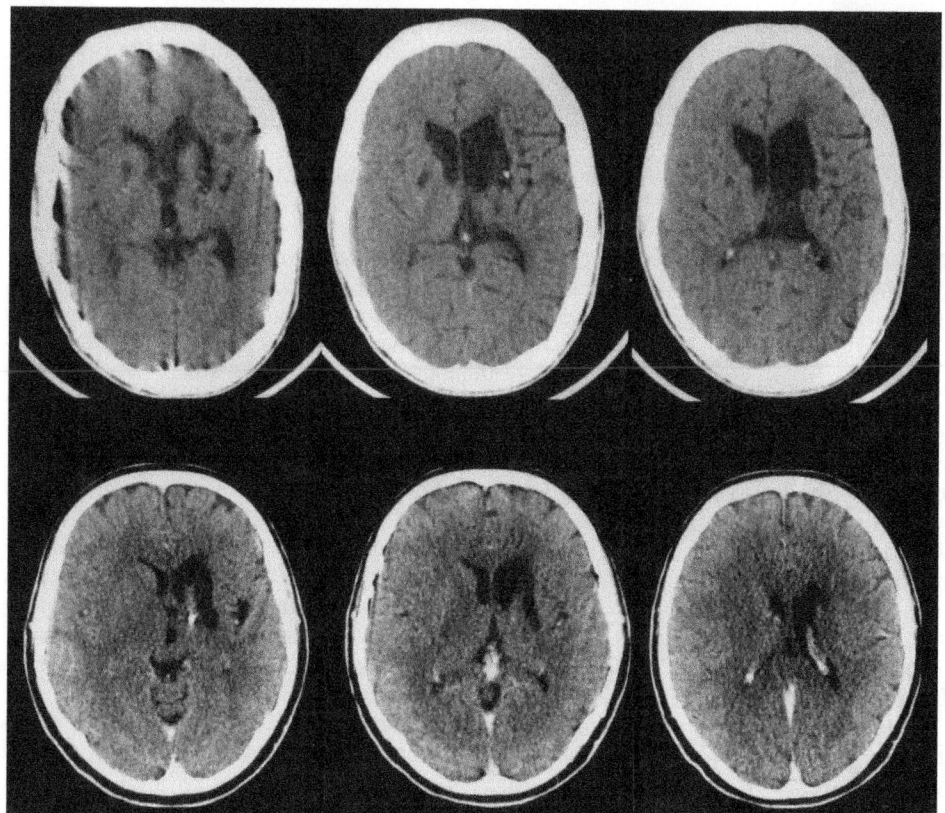

FIGURE 40-7 CT scans of a 21-year-old man who sustained a severe closed head injury at age 7 and subsequently developed *bilateral* hemidystonia. On the left side, there is a lesion of the caudate, anterior internal capsule and putamen corresponding to supply of lateral lenticulostriate branches of middle cerebral artery and small lesions of the ventrolateral thalamus; on the right side, there is a lesion of anterior putamen **(upper)**. CT scans showing a caudatoputaminal lesion in a 50-year old woman who sustained a moderate brain injury at age 9 and who developed contralateral hemidystonia 4 years thereafter **(lower)**. Reprinted from Krauss, Mohadjer, Braus, Wakhloo, Nobbe, Mundinger (8) with permission.

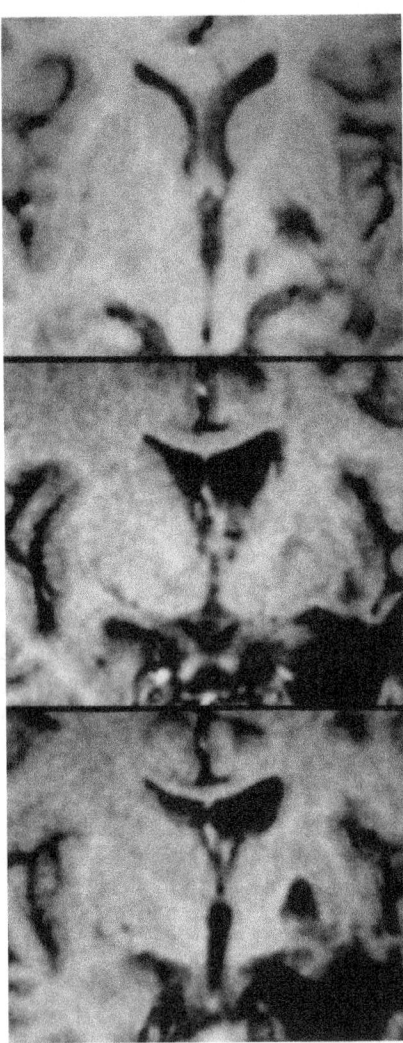

FIGURE 40-8 MR imaging studies in a 32-year-old man with post-traumatic hemidystonia after severe head injury at age 7 years. The axial scan through the lower part of the basal ganglia **(upper)** shows the post-traumatic pallidal lesion extending to the posterior putamen and a small lesion in the subthalamic region after stereotactic surgery, which provided partial relief of the hemidystonia for more than 16 years. The coronal scans **(middle and lower)** more clearly show the additional lesion to the putamen. Reprinted from Krauss, Mohadjer, Braus, Wakhloo, Nobbe, Mundinger (8) with permission.

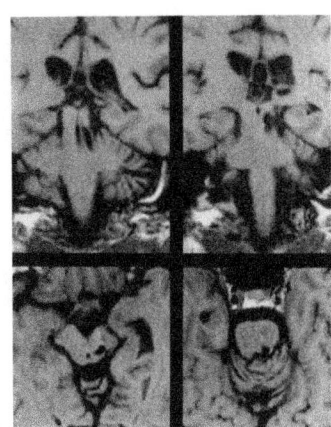

FIGURE 40-9 MR scans of a 28-year-old man with right-sided hemidystonia and cervical dystonia. The coronal images show a longish pontomesencephalic tegmental lesion on the left side **(upper row)**. The axial scans demonstrate more clearly the lesion also affecting the dentatothalamic pathway thought to be responsible for the additional tremor in this case **(lower row)**. Reprinted from Krauss, Mohadjer, Braus, Wakhloo, Nobbe, Mundinger (8) with permission.

or to neuronal subpopulations such as selective striatal vulnerability, for example (87).

Deranged function of both the direct and the indirect striatopallidal pathways is thought to underlie the development of dystonia. Regional cerebral blood flow studies in acquired hemidystonia secondary to basal ganglia or thalamic lesions have shown frontal overactivity on movement indicating that dystonia ultimately is caused by thalamo-frontal disinhibition secondary to disruption of the normal inhibitory control by the basal ganglia (88). It is puzzling that isolated lesions of the globus pallidus internus in healthy people can result in dystonia, but lesioning or stimulation of the same structure in dystonic people can alleviate dystonia. This observation, nevertheless, emphasizes that disturbed pallidal discharge and subsequent deranged pallidothalamic output is responsible for secondary dystonia (89).

It has been noted that dystonic movement disorders may also be seen in patients with brain injury because of a variety of etiologies during their stay in the intensive care unit (90). Most frequently, cervical or oromandibular dystonia has been described within this context. Typically, this type of dystonia is not related to lesions in the basal ganglia. Although only limited follow-up information has been available for these patients, it appears that dystonia improves over time and may actually resolve (90).

Ballism and Chorea

Overall, ballism is a rare movement disorder. There have been occasional descriptions of hemiballism and hemichorea secondary to craniocerebral trauma (25,81,91–93). Although some reports appear to describe true hemiballism, the categorization of the movement disorder remains somewhat unclear in other instances (53,94). Often, the term "violent" movement disorder has been wrongly used to assign the diagnosis of hemiballism in patients with large amplitude hyperkinesia including tremors with superimposed irregular myoclonic jerks. Post-traumatic hemiballism is associated with severe closed head injury. Hemorrhage to the subthalamic nucleus may result in hemiballism as early as one day after brain injury (93). It may also occur with a delay of weeks or months when patients recover from coma. Histopathological examination revealed subthalamic nucleus atrophy in a patient with a traumatic pallidal lesion who developed hemiballism at 2 years postinjury (81). In another patient with post-traumatic hemiballism, no structural abnormalities were found with conventional imaging studies but single photon emission computed tomography (SPECT) revealed a subthalamic lesion (95).

Choreatic movement disorders may be caused by epidural or subdural hematomas in the rare case (96). Chronic subdural hematomas may present with contralateral, ipsilateral, or bilateral choreatic or choreoathetotic movements (97–99).

Paroxysmal Autonomic Instability With Dystonia

The syndrome of paroxysmal autonomic instability with dystonia (PAID) has been outlined only recently by Blackman and colleagues (100). It is characterized by intermittent marked agitation, diaphoresis, hyperthermia, hypertension, tachycardia, tachypnea, and muscular hypertonia with extensor posturing. Observed most frequently in adolescents or young adults after traumatic brain injury (100,101), it is thought to be associated with dysfunction of autonomic centers in the diencephalon involving sympathoexcitatory mechanisms. Involvement of both dopaminergic and GABAergic transmission has been assumed. The syndrome has been labeled in the past with a variety of terms such as *brainstem attacks, neurostorming, acute midbrain syndrome, hyperpyrexia associated with sustained muscle contractions*, etc. The muscular hypertonia has been designated most often as *rigidity* or as *decerebrate posturing*. Differential diagnoses include *neuroleptic malignant syndrome, malignant hyperthermia, diencephalic seizures, autonomic dysreflexia*, and *central fever*. In some patients who present with an *arc de cercle* posture, the movement disorder was classified also as catatonia (102). Whether or not the muscular hypertension seen in this syndrome should be labeled as dystonia or not remains open to debate.

Paroxysmal Dyskinesias

The pathophysiology of paroxysmal dyskinesias remains unclear. It has been assumed that they present a certain type of subcortical epilepsy or reflex epilepsy. They are also thought to be associated with dysfunction of sensory processing at the level of the basal ganglia or the thalamus. There have been several reports on paroxysmal dyskinesias secondary to brain injury (103–110). Imaging findings have been inconclusive. In single cases, putaminal lesions were found (103). Positron emission tomographic scan studies showed abnormal metabolism in the contralateral basal ganglia during an attack of paroxsymal post-traumatic hemidystonia (107).

Tics and Tourettism

Adult-onset disorders with both motor tics and vocalizations secondary to a known cause have been referred to as "tourettism" to contrast it with the more common idiopathic Tourette's syndrome (111). Post-traumatic tics and tourettism following head trauma have been described in few patients (112–118). Because tics are relatively common, the coincidental occurrence of tics after head trauma must always deserve special consideration. A causative role of trauma is favored in patients with evidence of other post-traumatic sequelae and a negative history of motor tics prior to head injury. A history of well documented trauma to the head is mandatory. The older age at onset of patients with post-traumatic tourettism is notable, in contrast to Tourette syndrome. We studied the characteristics in 6 patients with tics secondary to craniocerebral trauma (113). All patients were male and the mean age at the time of the trauma was 28 years. Craniocerebral injury was moderate or mild in 5 patients, and neuroimaging studies did not reveal basal ganglia lesions. In another patient who had tics and marked obsessive-compulsive behavior secondary to severe brain injury, extensive periventricular and subcortical leukencephalopathy was detected by MR imaging studies (113) (Figure 40-10). Preexisting tics may exacerbate after head injury (15).

Other Posttraumatic Hyperkinesias

Various other hyperkinetic movement disorders, often in the frame of case reports, were reported after craniocerebral trauma including instances of myoclonus, opsoclonus, palatal myoclonus, stereotypies, akathisia, and galloping tongue (119–127).

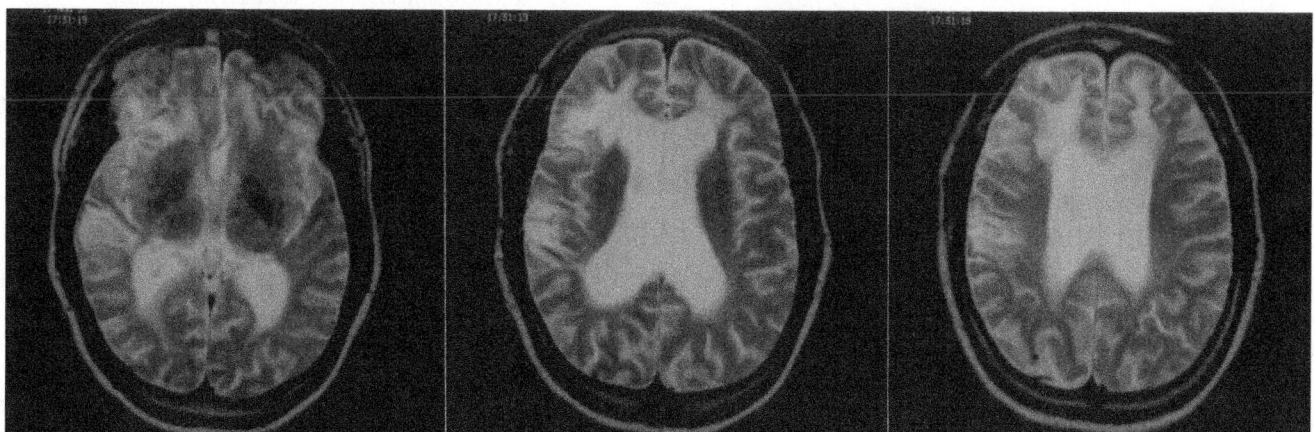

FIGURE 40-10 MR imaging studies of a 33-year-old man with post-traumatic tics and obsessive-compulsive behavior 12 years after he sustained a series of two severe head injuries. There is panventricular dilatation, cortical atrophy, and extensive periventricular and subcortical leukencephalopathy, particularly of the frontal and the right temporoparietal white matter. There are no focal basal ganglia lesions. Reprinted from Jankovic, Kwak (111) with permission.

Post-Traumatic Parkinsonism and Parkinson Disease

Parkinsonism After Single Head Injury

Although the concept of post-traumatic parkinsonism was well accepted in the first part of the 20th century, review of cases in the literature raises doubts that most are truly examples of parkinsonism resulting from trauma (128,129). The causal relationship in most cases has been largely speculative and the interpretation complicated by medicolegal issues. In some cases, the initial injury actually seemed to have resulted from—rather than caused—motor impairment. Post-traumatic parkinsonism, in general, is not caused by a single (130,131) but multiple, repeated closed head injuries. Occasionally, parkinsonism has been described to be associated with lesions of the substantia nigra (132,133). Direct lesions to the substantia nigra have been reported secondary to injuries by knives, screwdrivers, shell splinters, or gunshots and usually present with hemiparkinsonism (134–136). The parkinsonian syndrome is dominated by akinetic-rigid symptoms. Other movement disorders and pyramidal dysfunction may be present. We have studied a young man who suffered acute flexion-extension injury playing American football, followed by 3-week coma attributed to bilateral hemisphere hemorrhage, who is left with residual, levodopa-responsive parkinsonism, without any evidence of damage to the substantia nigra on imaging studies. Interestingly, in a patient who developed hemiparkinsonism after severe head injury but who did not have a structural lesion of the substantia nigra, brain parenchyma sonography revealed normal echogenicity of the substantia nigra as opposed to patients with PD (137).

There have been several reports of parkinsonism secondary to chronic subdural hematoma (138). Parkinsonian symptoms become evident within weeks after trivial head injury. The clinical picture is dominated by hypomimia, bradykinesia, and tremor. Other neurological signs and symptoms are usually present, although some instances of pure parkinsonism have been described (138,139). Diagnostic evaluations appear to be delayed and initial misinterpretations are common. Favorable outcome is achieved in most instances after drainage of the hematoma with complete or almost complete remission of parkinsonism. Chronic subdural hematomas may also cause deterioration of preexisting parkinsonian syndromes (138). Also, acute subdural hematomas, when associated with brainstem compression and reduced fluorodopa uptake in the contralateral putamen can induce a hemiparkinsonian syndrome (140).

Parkinsonism After Repeated Head Injury

Boxing is the most frequent cause for parkinsonism associated with repeated head trauma (141–145). Obvious tremors, bradykinesia, and hypophonia in Muhammed Ali has helped to draw the public attention to this problem. Although cumulative brain injury occurs also in other professional sports (146), only exceptional instances of parkinsonism have been reported (145,147,148). "Pugilistic" parkinsonism (PP) or "punch-drunk" syndrome is a chronic encephalopathy that results from the cumulative effects of subclinical concussions secondary to rotational acceleration traumas by direct blows to the head. Usually, PP appears with a delay of several years after ending an active boxing career (149). The frequency of PP has been estimated to range between 20% and 50% of professional boxers. The severity of PP correlates with the length of the boxing career and the number of bouts (150). Clinically, a variable spectrum of signs and symptoms can be present including behavioral changes, dementia, and corticospinal and cerebellar symptoms. Another frequent finding is marked dysarthria or hypophonia. In contrast to post-traumatic parkinsonism secondary to a single severe head injury, tremor at rest is a relatively frequent feature of PP. The diagnosis of chronic traumatic brain injury in patients with a history of boxing has been classified by Jordan as *improbable*, *possible*, and *probable* (combination of dementia, cerebellar dysfunction, pyramidal tract, and "extrapyramidal" symtoms) (151).

In addition to extensive nigral damage, dysfunction of striatal dopaminergic terminals has been suggested. Proton MR spectroscopy studies have demonstrated a significant reduction in the concentration of N-acetylaspartate in the lenticular nuclei of PP patients as compared to controls and PD patients (152). PET studies showed uniform nigrostriatal involvement but relative sparing of caudate function in PP (145). Neuropathological studies have revealed depigmentation of the substantia nigra but an absence of Lewy bodies, the histological hallmark for PD. A recent study showed extensive tau-immunorective neurofibrillary tangles, and spindle-shaped and threadlike neurites throughout the brain (147). Also deposition of beta amyloid was frequent.

Although the number of fatalities has decreased steadily over the years because of preventive measures in the ring, it remains to be seen whether this will ultimately result, also, in a decrease of PP among boxers (153). There has been controversy regarding the development of chronic encephalopathy in amateur boxing. Most studies do not show clinical evidence of chronic encephalopathy (154). In one study, finger-tapping performance was worse in some amateur boxers as compared to other athletes (155). It has been shown that high-exposure professional boxers with an apolipoprotein epsilon 4 allele have significantly greater scores on a scale measuring chronic encephalopathy than those without the allele (156). Thus, genetic susceptibility to the effects of repeated head trauma is likely.

Parkinson Disease and Head Trauma

In his original *Essay on the Shaking Palsy*, James Parkinson suggested that the disease that now bears his name might result from trauma to the medulla. Head trauma, as a possible risk factor for PD, has been the subject of controversy for years (10,11,157–160). It has been shown that head trauma sustained in motor vehicle accidents can exacerbate parkinsonism transiently in patients with PD, however, without resulting in increased persistent disability or acceleration of the clinical course of the disease (161). Several studies have found a higher frequency of head injury in patients with PD (162,163).

Usually, the history of head trauma dates back to 20 or 30 years prior to onset of PD and, therefore, any cause-and-effect relationship is difficult to establish. Regarding head injury and other possible environmental factors, it has been suggested that PD might be the consequence of clinically silent exposure in early or middle life with symptoms becoming manifest only later when there is a further decline of dopaminergic neurons with advancing age. Some studies suggested that susceptibility to trauma is more important than the severity of trauma itself. Several studies that have shown a positive association between head injury and trauma suffer from methodological flaws. The major problem with retrospective case control studies is recall bias. Unfortunately, there is a paucity of cohort studies that might be better suited to answer the inherent questions. One cohort study did not detect a significant increase in standardized morbidity ratios for PD in adults with head injury (164). However, this study had a 30% probability of not detecting a hypothetical twofold relative risk. In a case-control study, participants who experienced a mild head trauma with only amnesia had no increased risk for PD; however, participants who had a mild head trauma with loss of consciousness or a more severe trauma had a much higher odds ratio (11). Because head trauma, overall, was considered rather a relatively rare event, the population attributable risk was estimated to be at 5%.

A recent case-control study in 93 twin pairs discordant for PD showed that prior head injury with amnesia or loss of consciousness resulted in a significantly increased risk for PD (165). Risk increased further with a subsequent head injury whereas duration of unconsciousness was not associated with increased risk of parkinsonism. Nationwide population-based studies from Denmark, however, yielded different findings. Although a history of severe head injury did not appear to increase the risk of PD more than a decade after trauma (166), there was an increased frequency of hospital contacts for head injury during the months of onset of PD, which was thought rather a consequence of the evolving movement disorder than its cause (167).

TREATMENT OF POST-TRAUMATIC MOVEMENT DISORDERS

Rehabilitation of patients with post-traumatic movement disorders must consider both associated neurological and psychosocial dysfunction resulting from brain injury and the specific movement disorders. The physical disability of patients with severe kinetic tremors can be extreme because they are neither able to reach or to manage an object when the syndrome is fully expressed. Their disabilities should be treated according to the standard principles of rehabilitation care. It is important to anticipate and prevent potential obstacles for reintegration, to identify and offer strategies to man-

age present disabilities, and to develop adaptive and coping skills to achieve more independance. Physical therapy is helpful to prevent contractures in the most severely affected cases with dystonia.

Tremor After Severe Brain Injury

Medical Treatment

It is difficult to predict the prognosis of post-traumatic tremor in the initial period after its manifestation. It may lessen or resolve spontaneously within 1 year after its onset. Most patients, however, have persistent violent shaking movements. Post-traumatic tremor, then, is notoriously difficult to treat. Only few patients have been reported to respond favorably to medical treatment. Drugs reported to improve post-traumatic tremor include glutethimide, isoniazid, L-tryptophan, propranolol, benzodiazepines, carbamazepine, levodopa/carbidopa, and anticholinergics (62, 168–170). Botulinum toxin injections may be helpful to relieve the tremor temporarily but the high dosages administered to both proximal and distal arm muscles limit the usefulness of this treatment (171).

Surgical Treatment

The largest surgical experience for post-traumatic tremor comes from ablative functional stereotactic surgery with radiofrequency lesioning in the ventrolateral thalamus and the subthalamic region, which can effectively abate post-traumatic tremor (53,57,172–189) (Figure 40-11). The data of a total of 128 patients who underwent ablative stereotactic surgery as documented in the literature are shown in Table 40-3. Persistent improvement on long-term follow-up has been observed in 88% of patients with the tremor being absent or markedly reduced in 65% in one study (57). Tremor at rest usually is completely abolished but the most striking improvement is the reduction of postural and kinetic tremor. Also, valuable gain in functional disability has been achieved. Functional improvement was more striking in patients who had severe incapacitating tremor but comparatively less other neurological or mental deficits. There is a marked risk for adverse effects, however, in this vulnerable group of patients. Immediate postoperative side effects have been reported to occur in 50%–90% of patients and persistent side effects are being observed in up to 63%. Most frequently,

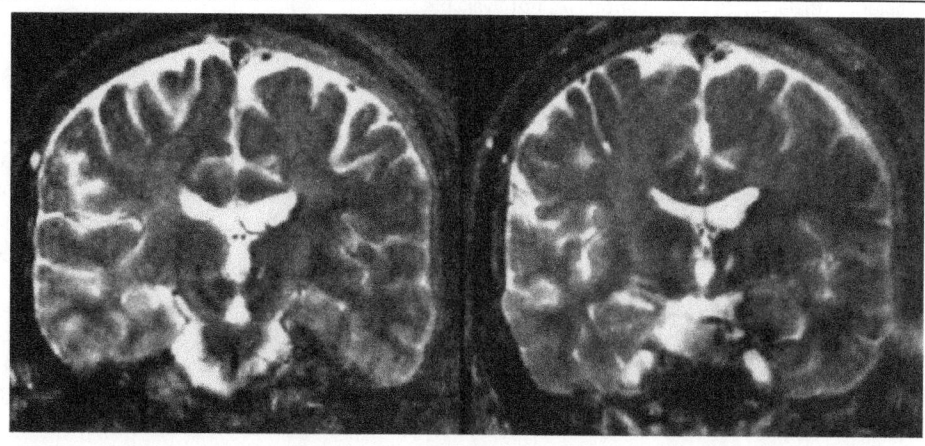

FIGURE 40-11 MR imaging studies obtained 3 years after combined ablative stereotactic surgery in the ventrolateral thalamus and zona incerta for treatment of post-traumatic tremor of the right arm. The coronal scans demonstrate the location of the small left stereotactic lesion and its topography in relation to adjacent nuclei. Reprinted from Krauss, Mohadjer, Nobbe, Mundinger (57) with permission.

TABLE 40-3 Functional Stereotactic Surgery for Post-Traumatic Tremor: Lesioning Procedures

AUTHOR(S) AND YEAR	TARGET	CASES	IMMEDIATE IMPROVEMENT	LONG-TERM FOLLOW-UP	LAST FOLLOW-UP, MEAN YEARS (RANGE)	SYMPTOMATIC IMPROVEMENT (%)	FUNCTIONAL IMPROVEMENT (%)	PERSISTENT SIDE EFFECTS
Cooper, 1960	VL	2	2	1	1.3	1/1	1/1	NA
Spiegel et al., 1963	STR	1	1	1	NA	0/1	NA	NA
Fox and Kurtzke, 1966	VL	1	1	1	0.5	1/1	1/1	0/1
Samra et al, 1970	VL	5	5	NA	NA	5/5 (100)	NA	NA
Van Manen, 1974[a]	VL	2	2	2	7	1/2	NA	1/2
Eiras and Garcìa, 1980	GP, Vop	1	1	1	2.5	1/1	1/1	0/1
Andrew et al., 1982	VL	8	8	NA	NA	8/8 (100)	8/8 (100)	5/8 (63)
Kandel, 1982[a]	VL, STR, GP	10	NA	NA	NA	NA	NA	NA
Niizuma et al., 1982[a]	Vim, Sub-Vim	3	3	NA	NA	NA	NA	NA
Ohye et al., 1982	Vim	8	8	NA	NA	NA	NA	1/8 (13)
Hirai et al., 1983	VL	5	4	NA	NA	NA	NA	0/5
Bullard and Nashold, 1984	VL	7	7	7	1.5 (0.2–3.0)	7/7 (100)	6/7 (86)	3/7 (43)
Bullard and Nashold, 1988[b]	VL	10	10	8	1.3 (0.2–3.0)	8/8 (100)	7/8 (90)	4/8 (50)
Iwadate et al, 1989	VL	3	2	NA	NA	2/3 (66)	NA	NA
Richardson, 1989	VL	1	1	NA	NA	1/1	NA	NA
Goldman and Kelly, 1992	VL	4	4	4	3 (1.4–4.5)	3/4 (75)	3/4 (75)	0/4 (0)
Marks, 1993	Vim	7	6	NA	NA	6/7 (86)	NA	1/7 (14)
Taira et al., 1993	Vop, Vim	3	1	NA	3	2/3 (66)	0.5	1/3 (33)
Krauss et al., 1994	VL, Zi	35	35	32	10.5 (0.5–24.0)	28/32 (88)	26/29 (90)	12/32 (38)
Jankovic et al., 1995	Vim	6	6	6	4	6/6 (100)	3/6 (50)	3/6 (50)
Shahzadi et al., 1995[a]	Vim	11	11	NA	NA	NA	NA	6/11 (55)
Louis et al., 1996	VL	2	2	2	0.3 and 4	2/2	NA	NA
Total		128	113/118 (96%)	68 (53%)		81/92 (88%)	56/65 (86%)	38/103 (37%)

GP, globus pallidus; STR, subthalamic region; Vim, (nucleus) ventralis intermedius (thalami); VL, ventrolateral thalamus; Vop, (nucleus) ventro-oralis posterior (thalami); Zi, zona incerta; NA, not available.
[a] Series with tremors of different etiologies, usually cerebellar-type tremors. Specific data for post-traumatic tremor not always available.
[b] The series of Bullard & Nashold from 1988 includes the patients in the series from 1984.
Reprinted from Krauss, Jankovic (16) with permission.

such side effects consist chiefly of aggravation of preoperative symptoms such as dysarthria or gait disturbance. There is a trend for patients with left-sided surgery to present more frequently with increased dysarthria than patients who have right-sided procedures. Surprisingly, single patients may benefit from marked amelioration of their dysarthria after radiofrequency lesioning (57). On long-term follow-up, it has been observed that there may be an increase in dystonic postures despite improvement of tremor, or new dystonic symptoms may become manifest. It is unclear whether this is related to the surgical procedure or whether this may present delayed-onset dystonia (49). The high frequency of side effects is remarkably different from that observed after thalamotomy for other types of tremor, for example, essential tremor. The size of the lesions necessary to control severe kinetic tremors has been debated. It has been stated that larger lesions should be made in such cases to achieve long-term relief (183). On the other hand, regarding the propensity of these patients for postoperative morbidity, small lesions in the basal ventrolateral thalamus and the subthalamic region involving the zona incerta might be more advantageous. Gamma knife Vim thalamotomy has been reported also to result in modest improvement in post-traumatic tremor (190) but delayed effects of radiation may limit this procedure.

There is still relatively little experience with thalamic DBS for treatment of post-traumatic tremor (191–197). Similar to other kinetic tremors caused by stroke or multiple sclerosis (198), DBS has been found to be less effective than in parkinsonian tremor or essential tremor. Occasionally, thalamic DBS was described as completely ineffective (195). In other instances, however, patients achieved variable symptomatic and functional benefit. Some patients may need relatively high voltage to control tremor (197). It appears that DBS may be less effective in control of tremor but is associated with fewer side effects than radiofrequency lesioning in this special group of patients. Long-term follow-up data is very limited. There have been divergent opinions what should be considered the ideal thalamic target for DBS to treat proximal kinetic tremors. Nguyen et al. suggested that proximal contacts in the Vim would be most beneficial (194), whereas others think that stimulation of a target located more anteriorly is important (196). Kitagawa et al. demonstrated that stimulation of the subthalamic area can be effective in patients with proximal tremors (199). Electrodes placed in the zona incerta were most effective to control contralateral tremor. We recommend waiting at least 1 year after onset of post-traumatic tremor before surgery is considered. Still, further studies are clearly necessary to establish the role of DBS in post-traumatic tremor. We prefer DBS over thalamotomy in these patients regarding the high occurrence of side effects, presently.

A new technique that received more attention only recently is stimulation via multiple electrodes either within the same target or different targets (200). It has been shown that combined stimulation of both the thalamic Vim and Voa region may yield additional benefit in selected cases with post-traumatic tremor (201). In another patient, the kinetic component was well controlled by thalamic DBS but additional subthalamic DBS was required for suppression of the resting tremor (202).

Tremor After Moderate and Mild Brain Injury

The postural and intention tremors that may occur after mild and moderate head injury usually do not require therapy and subside spontaneously (33). In some patients, tremor persists and head tremor can also develop. In those cases, medical therapy with clonazepam, propranolol or primidone, or botulinum toxin injections may provide relief (203,204).

Dystonia

Medical Treatment

In patients with post-traumatic dystonia, spontaneous remission is unusual, although some improvement can be seen particularly in patients with thalamic lesions. Medical treatment is usually ineffective. Occasionally, there is a mild response to anticholinergic drugs. Botulinum toxin injections are the treatment of first choice in patients with post-traumatic torticollis and other focal dystonias (24,171).

Surgical Treatment

The prognosis is favorable in the rare cases of dystonia related to subdural hematoma after drainage of the hematoma (205–207). Functional stereotactic surgery is a treatment option in patients with disabling hemidystonia or segmental dystonia (8,208). Targets include ventrolateral thalamus, the subthalamic region, the pulvinar, and the globus pallidus internus. Improvement of dystonia in the early postoperative period has been described in most instances. Experience with long-term follow-up, however, is limited (Figure 40-9). At a mean follow-up of 18 years after thalamic radiofrequency lesioning, 3 of 6 patients with post-traumatic hemidystonia still benefited from some improvement of their hemidystonia (8). Since several years, the pallidum has been the preferred target for treatment of dystonia (209). In contrast to thalamotomy, it was observed that the improvement after pallidotomy may be delayed by several weeks or months. It is still unclear at this time whether thalamic or pallidal targets should be preferred in patients with secondary dystonia (210). In a series of patients with various forms of dystonia, the response to pallidal surgery for dystonia was dependent on etiology (211). Patients with secondary dystonia who had extensive structural cerebral lesions had no improvement after pallidal surgery, whereas patients with primary dystonia, particularly those with DYT1 dystonia, had striking benefit and patients with secondary dystonia without structural lesions had mild benefit. Villemure and colleagues reported on 2 dystonia patients with secondary dystonia who did not improve with pallidal surgery but benefited with thalamic targets (212). In another study, however, no difference in outcome between pallidal and thalamic targets was seen in patients with secondary dystonia (213). Overall, patients with secondary dystonia experience more modest improvement as compared to patients with primary dystonia regardless of the target used. The response of post-traumatic dystonia to pallidotomy appears to be difficult to predict. We did not observe improvement of post-traumatic hemidystonia after pallidotomy in a young patient despite his imaging studies did not show structural brain lesions. In contrast, bilateral pallidotomy was reported to result in marked improvement in a patient with generalized post-traumatic dystonia (214).

DBS has been used in only few patients with hemidystonia secondary to craniocerebral trauma. Again, treatment response is not consistent. Marked improvement of dystonic movements and postures has been described in a 16-year-old boy with a thalamic lesion who underwent stimulation of the ventroposterolateral thalamus over 8 months (215). We have followed a patient for 10 years who continues to show consistent improvement of post-traumatic dystonia of the left arm with stimulation of the contralateral globus pallidus internus (216,217) (Figure 40-12). Chronic intrathecal baclofen administered via implanted pumps may provide useful improvement in patients with more generalized dystonia or accompanying spasticity (218–220).

Ballism and Chorea

In contrast to vascular hemiballism, post-traumatic hemiballism seems to be more persistent with fewer tendencies for spontaneous improvement. Patients who do not respond adequately to conservative treatment such as tetrabenazine, a monoamine depleting drug, can benefit from functional ste-

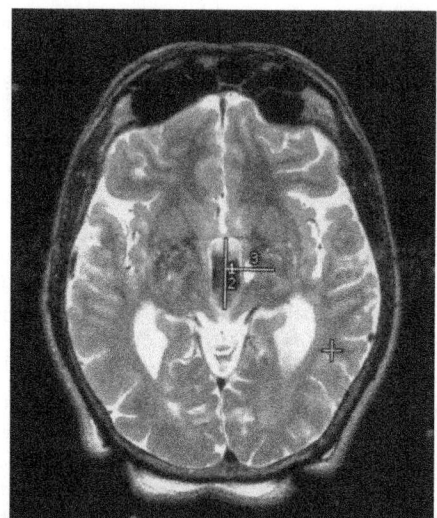

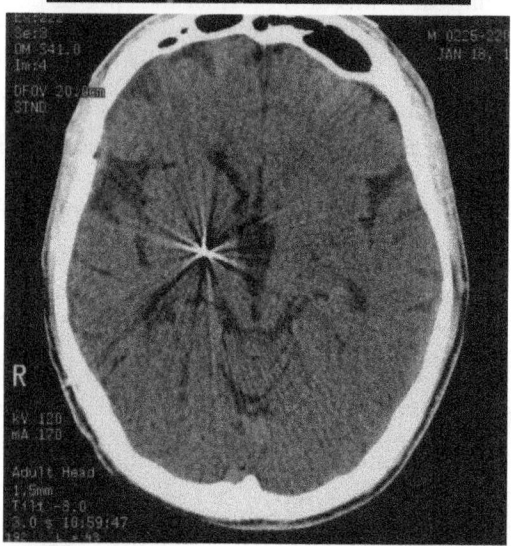

FIGURE 40-12 A, Stereotactic T2-weighted axial MR scan of a 24-year-old man who sustained severe closed head injury at age 15 and who subsequently developed left-sided low-frequency tremor and hemidystonia. The tremor was successfully relieved by a right-sided thalamotomy; hemidystonia, however, increased over the years. This MR image was used for target calculation to implant an electrode in the posteroventral lateral globus pallidus internus (sides are reversed). **B,** Axial CT scan 4 years later demonstrating the position of the electrode in the pallidal target providing relief of dystonic posture and phasic movements and dystonia-associated pain. Reprinted from Loher, Hasdemir, Burgunder, Krauss (216) with permission.

reotactic surgery (221,222). Because of the rarity of post-traumatic hemiballism, however, experience is very limited. Targets in the contralateral pallidum or thalamus are useful.

In chorea or choreoathetosis associated with chronic subdural hematoma, the prognosis usually is favorable after drainage of the hematoma (99).

Paroxysmal Dyskinesias

Post-traumatic paroxysmal dyskinesias often respond favorably to anticonvulsive medication—in particular kinesigenic dyskinesias (110). Thalamic stimulation has been shown to be beneficial in a patient with paroxysmal nonkinesigenic dyskinesia (223).

Post-Traumatic Parkinsonism

Patients with substantia nigra lesions may benefit from levodopa therapy (133). Medical treatment of post-traumatic parkinsonism, in general, is similar to that for idiopathic PD (224). There are only limited data available for the specific outcome of functional stereotactic surgery in patients with parkinsonism secondary to brain injury. Combined subthalamic nucleus and thalamic Vim DBS was applied successfully in a young man who sustained post-traumatic hemiparkinsonism and kinetic tremor secondary to an acute traumatic subdural hematoma (225).

CONCLUSION

Traumatic brain injury can result in a variety of movement disorders. The mediation of the effects of trauma and the pathophysiology of the development of post-traumatic movement disorders require further study. Proper identification of such movement disorders is pivotal for rehabilitation. Functional stereotactic neurosurgery should be considered in patients with disabling movement disorders refractory to medical treatment.

KEY CLINICAL POINTS

1. Post-traumatic movement disorders may occur in about 20% of survivors of severe brain injury.
2. They may be persistent in about half of these patients.
3. Kinetic, cerebellar outflow, tremor is the most frequent post-traumatic movement disorder.
4. Post-traumatic movement disorders persist only in a minority of patients with mild or moderate brain injury (up to 3%).
5. Overall, the frequency and occurrence of post-traumatic movement disorders seems to decline, which may be secondary to improved treatment of brain injury.
6. Kinetic tremors are most frequently associated with DAI involving the upper brainstem or the superior cerebellar peduncles.
7. Hemidystonia is the most frequent manifestation of post-traumatic dystonia and is often associated with basal ganglia lesions.
8. There is still controversy whether or not head injury is a risk factor for the manifestation of PD, although repeated head traumay may lead to PP.
9. Peripheral trauma to the nerve roots or nerves may be associated with tremor or focal dystonia, with occasional spread.
10. DBS has replaced radiofrequency lesioning for the surgical treatment of post-traumatic movement disorders.
11. Stimulation with multiple electrodes within the same target or in different targets is an evolving technique that is also applied to post-traumatic movement disorders.

KEY REFERENCES

1. Jordan BD. Chronic traumatic brain injury associated with boxing. *Semin Neurol.* 2000;20(2):179–185.
2. Krauss JK, Jankovic J. Head injury and posttraumatic movement disorders. *Neurosurgery.* 2002;50(5):927–940.
3. Krauss JK, Tränkle R, Kopp KH. Post-traumatic movement disorders in survivors of severe head injury. *Neurology.* 1996;47(6):1488–1492.
4. Krauss JK, Mohadjer M, Nobbe F, Mundinger F. The treatment of posttraumatic tremor by stereotactic surgery. Symptomatic and functional outcome in a series of 35 patients. *J Neurosurg.* 1994;80(5):810–819.
5. McKee AC, Cantu RC, Nowinski CJ, et al. Chronic traumatic encephalopathy in athletes: progressive tauopathy after repetitive head injury. *J Neuropathol Exp Neurol.* 2009; 68(7):709–735.

References

1. Jankovic J. Post-traumatic movement disorders: central and peripheral mechanisms. *Neurology.* 1994;44(11):2006–2014.
2. Goetz CG, Pappert EJ. Trauma and movement disorders. *Neurol Clin.* 1992;10(4):907–919.
3. Jankovic J. Can peripheral trauma induce dystonia and other movement disorders? Yes! *Mov Disord.* 2001;16(1):7–12.
4. Weiner WJ. Can peripheral trauma induce dystonia? No! *Mov Disord.* 2001;16(1):13–22.
5. Jankovic J. Peripherally induced movement disorders. *Neurol Clin.* 2009;27(3):821–832.
6. van Rooijen DE, Geraedts EJ, Marinus J, Jankovic J, van Hilten JJ. Peripheral trauma and movement disorders: a systematic review of reported cases. *J Neurol Neurosurg Psychiatry.* 2011;82(8):892–898.
7. Curran TG, Lang AE. Trauma and tremor. In: Findley LJ, Koller WC, eds. *Handbook of Tremor Disorders.* New York, NY: Marcel Dekker; 1995: 411–428.
8. Krauss JK, Mohadjer M, Braus DF, Wakhloo AK, Nobbe F, Mundinger F. Dystonia following head trauma: a report of nine patients and review of the literature. *Mov Disord.* 1992;7(3):263–272.
9. Lee MS, Rinne JO, Ceballos-Baumann A, Thompson PD, Marsden CD. Dystonia after head trauma. *Neurology.* 1994;44(8):1374–1378.
10. Ben-Shlomo Y. How far are we in understanding the cause of Parkinson's disease? *J Neurol Neurosurg Psychiatry.* 1996;61(1):4–16.
11. Bower JH, Maraganore DM, Peterson BJ, McDonnell SK, Ahlskog JE, Rocca WA. Head trauma preceding PD: a case-control study. *Neurology.* 2003;60(10):1610–1615.
12. Hawley JS, Weiner WJ. Psychogenic dystonia and peripheral trauma. *Neurology.* 2011;77(5):496–502.
13. Monday K, Jankovic J. Psychogenic myoclonus. *Neurology.* 1993; 43(2):349–352.
14. Scarano VR, Jankovic J. Post-traumatic movement disorders: effect of the legal system on outcome. *J Forensic Sci.* 1998;43(2):334–339.
15. Koller WC, Wong GF, Lang A. Posttraumatic movement disorders: a review. *Mov Disord.* 1989;4(1):20–36.
16. Krauss JK, Jankovic J. Head injury and posttraumatic movement disorders. *Neurosurgery.* 2002;50:927–940.
17. Krauss JK, Jankovic J, Grossman RG, eds. *Surgery for Parkinson's disease and movement disorders.* Lippincott Williams & Wilkins; 2001.
18. Wichmann T, Delong MR. Deep-brain stimulation for Basal Ganglia Disorders. *Basal Ganglia.* 2011;1(2):65–77.
19. Kühn AA, Tsui A, Aziz T, et al. Pathological synchronisation in the subthalamic nucleus of patients with Parkinson's disease relates to both bradykinesia and rigidity. *Exp Neurol.* 2009;215(2):380–387.
20. Kühn AA, Brücke C, Schneider GH, et al. Increased beta activity in dystonia patients after drug-induced dopamine deficiency. *Exp Neurol.* 2008;214(1):140–143.
21. Sharott A, Grosse P, Kühn AA, et al. Is the synchronization between pallidal and muscle activity in primary dystonia due to peripheral afferance or a motor drive? *Brain.* 2008;131(pt 2):473–484.
22. Jankovic J. International Classification of Diseases, tenth revision: neurological adaptation (ICD-10 NA): extrapyramidal and movement disorders. *Mov Disord.* 1995;10(5):533–540.
23. Deuschl G, Bain P, Brin M. Consensus statement of the Movement Disorder Society on Tremor. Ad Hoc Scientific Committee. *Mov Disord.* 1998;13(suppl 3):2–23.
24. Jankovic J, Fahn S. Dystonic disorders. In: Jankovic J, Tolosa E, eds. *Parkinson's Disease and Movement Disorders.* 4th ed. Philadelphia, PA: Lippincott Williams & Wilkins; 2002:331–357.
25. Krauss JK, Borremans JJ, Nobbe F, Mundinger F. Ballism not related to vascular disease: a report of 16 patients and review of the literature. *Parkinsonism Relat Disord.* 1996;2(1):35–45.
26. Dewey RB Jr, Jankovic J. Hemiballism-hemichorea. Clinical and pharmacologic findings in 21 patients. *Arch Neurol.* 1989;46(8): 862–867.
27. Costeff H, Groswasser Z, Goldstein R. Long-term follow-up review of 31 children with severe closed head trauma. *J Neurosurg.* 1990; 73(5):684–687.
28. Johnson SL, Hall DM. Post-traumatic tremor in head injured children. *Arch Dis Child.* 1992;67(2):227–228.
29. Kono M, Oka N, Horie T, et al. Involuntary movements after severe head injury. In: Proceedings of the Xth International Congress of Neurological Surgery; October 17–22, 1993; Acapulco, Mexico. Abstract.
30. Krauss JK, Tränkle R, Kopp KH. Post-traumatic movement disorders in survivors of severe head injury. *Neurology.* 1996;47(6): 1488–1492.
31. Szelozyńska K, Znamirowski R. Zespól pozapiramidowy w pourazowych niedowl adach pol owiczych u dzieci [Extrapyramidal syndrome in post-traumatic hemiparesis in children]. *Neurol Neurochir Pol.* 1974;8(2):167–170.
32. Eberle BM, Schnüringer B, Inaba K, Gruen JP, Demetriades D, Belzberg H. Decompressive craniectomy: surgical control of traumatic intracranial hypertension may improve outcome. *Injury.* 2010; 41(9):894–898.
33. Krauss JK, Tränkle R, Kopp KH. Posttraumatic movement disorders after moderate or mild head injury. *Mov Disord.* 1997;12(3): 428–431.
34. Krack P, Deuschl G, Kaps M, Warnke P, Schneider S, Traupe H. Delayed onset of "rubral tremor" 23 years after brainstem trauma. *Mov Disord.* 1994;9(2):240–242.
35. Boto GR, Lobato RD, Rivas JJ, Gomez PA, de la Lama A, Lagares A. Basal ganglia hematomas in severely head injured patients: clinicoradiological analysis of 37 cases. *J Neurosurg.* 2001;94(2):224–232.
36. Kampfl A, Franz G, Aichner F, et al. The persistent vegetative state after closed head injury: clinical and magnetic resonance imaging findings in 42 patients. *J Neurosurg.* 1998;88(5):809–816.
37. Tränkle R, Krauss JK. Posttraumatische fokale Dystonie nach kontralateraler Thalamusläsion. *Nervenarzt.* 1997;68(6):521–524.
38. Baker AJ, Moulton RJ, MacMillan VH, Shedden PM. Excitatory amino acids in cerebrospinal fluid following traumatic brain injury in humans. *J Neurosurg.* 1993;79(3):369–372.
39. Bullock R, Zauner A, Woodward JJ, et al. Factors affecting excitatory amino acid release following severe human head injury. *J Neurosurg.* 1998;89(4):507–518.
40. Halliwell B. Oxidants and the central nervous system: some fundamental questions. Is oxidant damage relevant to Parkinson's disease, Alzheimer's disease, traumatic injury or stroke? *Acta Neurol Scand Suppl.* 1989;126:23–33.
41. Muizelaar JP, Marmarou A, Young HF, et al. Improving the outcome of severe head injury with the oxygen radical scavenger polyethylene glycol-conjugated superoxide dismutase: a phase II trial. *J Neurosurg.* 1993;78(3):375–382.
42. Bullock MR, Lyeth BG, Muizelaar JP. Current status of neuroprotection trials for traumatic brain injury: lessons from animal models and clinical studies. *Neurosurgery.* 1999;45(2):207–220.
43. Hodge CJ Jr, Boakye M. Biological plasticity: the future of science in neurosurgery. *Neurosurgery.* 2001;48(1):2–16.

44. Andriessen TM, Jacobs B, Vos PE. Clinical characteristics and pathophysiological mechanisms of focal and diffuse traumatic brain injury. *J Cell Mol Med.* 2010;14(10):2381–2392.

45. Teasdale GM, Graham DI. Craniocerebral trauma: protection and retrieval of the neuronal population after injury. *Neurosurgery.* 1998;43(4):723–738.

46. Teasdale GM, Nicoll JA, Murray G, Fiddes M. Association of apolipoprotein E polymorphism with outcome after head injury. *Lancet.* 1997;350(9084):1069–1071.

47. Boyeson MG, Jones JL, Harmon RL. Sparing of motor function after cortical injury. A new perspective on underlying mechanisms. *Arch Neurol.* 1994;51(4):405–414.

48. Carr LJ, Harrison LM, Evans AL, Stephens JA. Patterns of central motor reorganization in hemiplegic cerebral palsy. *Brain.* 1993;116(pt 5):1223–1247.

49. Scott BL, Jankovic J. Delayed-onset progressive movement disorders after static brain lesions. *Neurology.* 1996;46(1):68–74.

50. Kremer M, Russell WR, Smyth GE. A mid-brain syndrome following head injury. *J Neurol Neurosurg Psychiatry.* 1947;10(2):49–60.

51. Samie MR, Selhorst JB, Koller WC. Post-traumatic midbrain tremors. *Neurology.* 1990;40(1):62–66.

52. Obeso JA, Narbona J. Post-traumatic tremor and myoclonic jerking. *J Neurol Neurosurg Psychiatry.* 1993;46(8):788.

53. Bullard DE, Nashold BS Jr. Stereotaxic thalamotomy for treatment of posttraumatic movement disorders. *J Neurosurg.* 1984;61(2):316–321.

54. Netravathi M, Pal PK, Ravishankar S, Indira Devi B. Electrophysiological evaluation of tremors secondary to space occupying lesions and trauma: correlation with nature and sites of lesions. *Parkinsonism Relat Disord.* 2010;16(1):36–41.

55. Friedman JH. "Rubral" tremor induced by a neuroleptic drug. *Mov Disord.* 1992;7(3):281–282.

56. Masucci EF, Kurtzke JF, Saini N. Myorhythmia: a widespread movement disorder. Clinicopathological correlations. *Brain.* 1984;107(pt 1):53–79.

57. Krauss JK, Mohadjer M, Nobbe F, Mundinger F. The treatment of posttraumatic tremor by stereotactic surgery. Symptomatic and functional outcome in a series of 35 patients. *J Neurosurg.* 1994;80(5):810–819.

58. Louis ED, Lynch T, Ford B, Greene P, Bressman SB, Fahn S. Delayed-onset cerebellar syndrome. *Arch Neurol.* 1996;53(5):450–454.

59. Krauss JK, Wakhloo AK, Nobbe F, Tränkle R, Mundinger F, Seeger W. Lesion of dentatothalamic pathways in severe post-traumatic tremor. *Neurol Res.* 1995;17(6):409–416.

60. Seo SW, Heo JH, Lee KY, et al. Localization of Claude's syndrome. *Neurology.* 2001;57(12):2304–2307.

61. Elble RJ. Animal models of action tremor. *Mov Disord.* 1998;13(suppl 3):35–39.

62. Newmark J, Richards TL. Delayed unilateral post-traumatic tremor: localization studies using single-proton computed tomographic and magnetic resonance spectroscopy techniques. *Mil Med.* 1999;164(1):59–64.

63. Remy P, de Recondo A, Defer G, et al. Peduncular 'rubral' tremor and dopaminergic denervation: a PET study. *Neurology.* 1995;45(3, pt 1):472–477.

64. Zijlmans J, Booij J, Valk J, Lees A, Horstink M. Posttraumatic tremor without parkinsonism in a patient with complete contralateral loss of the nigrostriatal pathway. *Mov Disord.* 2002;17(5):1086–1088.

65. Hashimoto T, Sato H, Shindo M, Hayashi R, Ikeda S. Peripheral mechanisms in tremor after traumatic neck injury. *J Neurol Neurosurg Psychiatry.* 2002;73(5):585–587.

66. Burke RE, Fahn S, Gold AP. Delayed-onset dystonia in patients with "static" encephalopathy. *J Neurol Neurosurg Psychiatry.* 1980;43(9):789–797.

67. Mauro AJ, Fahn S, Russman B. Hemidystonia following "minor" head trauma. *Trans Am Neurol Assoc.* 1980;105:229–231.

68. Messimy R, Diebler C, Metzger J. Dystonie de torsion du membre superieur gauche probablement consecutive a un traumatisme cranien. *Rev Neurol* (Paris). 1977;133(3):199–206.

69. Wijemanne S, Jankovic J. Hemidystonia-hemiatrophy syndrome. *Mov Disord.* 2009;24(4):583–589.

70. Marsden CD, Obeso JA, Zarranz JJ, Lang AE. The anatomical basis of sympomatic hemidystonia. *Brain.* 1985;108(pt 2):463–483.

71. Pettigrew LC, Jankovic J. Hemidystonia: a report of 22 patients and a review of the literature. *J Neurol Neurosurg Psychiatry.* 1985;48(7):650–657.

72. Jabbari B, Paul J, Scherokman B, Van Dam B. Posttraumatic segmental axial dystonia. *Mov Disord.* 1992;7(1):78–81.

73. Lee MS, Lee SB, Kim WC. Spasmodic dysphonia associated with a left ventrolateral putaminal lesion. *Neurology.* 1996;47(3):827–828.

74. Singer BJ, Jegasothy GM, Singer KP, Allison GT, Dunne JW. Incidence of ankle contracture after moderate to severe acquired brain injury. *Arch Phys Med Rehabil.* 2004;85(9):1465–1469.

75. Bressman SB, de Leon D, Raymond D, et al. Secondary dystonia and the DYT1 gene. *Neurology.* 1997;48(6):1571–1577.

76. Martino D, Defazio G, Abbruzzese G, et al. Head trauma in primary cranial dystonias: a multicentre case-control study. *J Neurol Neurosurg Psychiatry.* 2007;78(3):260–263.

77. Austregesilo A, Marques A. Dystonies. *Rev Neurol.* 1928;2:562–575.

78. Brett EM, Hoare RD. Progressive hemi-dystonia due to focal basal ganglia lesion after mild head trauma. *J Neurol Neurosurg Psychiatry.* 1981;44(5):460.

79. Silver JK, Lux WE. Early onset dystonia following traumatic brain injury. *Arch Phys Med Rehabil.* 1994;75(8):885–888.

80. Chuang C, Fahn S, Frucht SJ. The natural history and treatment of acquired hemidystonia: report of 33 cases and review of the literature. *J Neurol Neurosurg Psychiatry.* 2002;72(1):59–67.

81. King RB, Fuller C, Collins GH. Delayed onset of hemidystonia and hemiballismus following head injury: a clinicopathological correlation. *J Neurosurg.* 2001;94(2):309–314.

82. Münchau A, Mathen D, Cox T, Quinn NP, Marsden CD, Bhatia KP. Unilateral lesions of the globus pallidus: report of four patients presenting with focal or segmental dystonia. *J Neurol Neurosurg Psychiatry.* 2000;69(4):494–498.

83. Loher TJ, Krauss JK. Dystonia associated with pontomesencephalic lesions. *Mov Disord.* 2009;24(2):157–167.

84. Maki Y, Akimoto H, Enomoto T. Injuries of basal ganglia following head trauma in children. *Child's Brain.* 1980;7(3):113–123.

85. Andrew J, Fowler CJ, Harrison MJ, Kendall BE. Post-traumatic tremor due to vascular injury and its treatment by stereotactic thalamotomy. *J Neurol Neurosurg Psychiatry.* 1982;45(6):560–562.

86. Krauss JK, Jankovic J. Hemidystonia secondary to carotid artery gunshot injury. *Childs Nerv Syst.* 1997;13(5):285–288.

87. Hawker K, Lang AE. Hypoxic-ischemic damage of the basal ganglia. Case reports and a review of the literature. *Mov Disord.* 1990;5(3):219–224.

88. Ceballos-Baumann AO, Passingham RE, Marsden CD, Brooks DJ. Motor reorganization in aquired hemidystonia. *Ann Neurol.* 1995;37(6):746–757.

89. Sanghera MK, Grossman RG, Kalhorn CG, Hamilton WJ, Ondo WG, Jankovic J. Basal ganglia neuronal discharge in primary and secondary dystonia in patients undergoing pallidotomy. *Neurosurgery.* 2003;52(6):1358–1373.

90. Lo SE, Rosengart AJ, Novakovic RL, et al. Identification and treatment of cervical and oromandibular dystonia in acutely brain-injured patients. *Neurocrit Care.* 2005;3(2):139–145.

91. Levesque MF, Markham C, Nakasato N. MR-guided ventral intermediate thalamotomy for posttraumatic hemiballismus. *Stereotact Funct Neurosurg.* 1992;58(1–4):88.

92. Naddeo M, Bioliho P, Zappi D. L'hemiballisme post-traumatique. *Neurochirurgie.* 1983;29(4):285–287.

93. Kim HJ, Lee DH, Park JH. Posttraumatic hemiballism with focal discrete hemorrhage in contralateral subthalamic nucleus. *Parkinsonism Relat Disord.* 2008;14(3):259–261.

94. Bullard DE, Nashold BS Jr. Posttraumatic movement disorders. In: Lunsford LD, ed. *Modern Stereotactic Neurosurgery.* Boston, MA: Martinus Nijhoff; 1988:341–352.

95. Kant R, Zeiler D. Hemiballismus following closed head injury. *Brain Inj.* 1996;10(2):155–158.

96. Adler JR, Winston KR. Chorea as a manifestation of epidural hematoma. Case report. *J Neurosurg.* 1984;60(4):856–857.

97. Kotagal S, Shutter E, Horenstein S. Chorea as a manifestation of bilateral subdural hematoma in an elderly man. *Arch Neurol.* 1981;38(3):195.

98. Yoshikawa M, Yamamoto M, Shibata K, et al. Hemichorea associated with ipsilateral chronic subdural hematoma—case report. *Neurol Med Chir* (Tokyo). 1992;32(10):769–772.

99. Young VE, Pickett G, Richardson PL, Leach P. Choreathetoid movement as an unusual presentation of subdural haematoma. *Acta Neurochir* (Wien). 2008;150(7):733–735.

100. Blackman JA, Patrick PD, Buck ML, Rust RS Jr. Paroxysmal autonomic instability with dystonia after brain injury. *Arch Neurol.* 2004;61(3):321–328.

101. Baguley IJ, Heriseanu RE, Cameron ID, Nott MT, Slewa-Younan S. A critical review of the pathophysiology of dysautonomia following traumatic brain injury. *Neurocrit Care.* 2008;8(2):293–300.

102. Diesing TS, Wijdicks EF. Arc de cercle and dysautonomia from anoxic injury. *Mov Disord.* 2006;21(6):868–869.

103. Biary N, Singh B, Bahou Y, al Deeb SM, Sharif H. Posttraumatic paroxysmal nocturnal hemidystonia. *Mov Disord.* 1994;9(1):98–99.

104. Chandra V, Spunt AL, Rusinowitz MS. Treatment of post-traumatic choreo-athetosis with sodium valproate. *J Neurol Neurosurg Psychiatry.* 1983;46(10):963.

105. Demirkiran M, Jankovic J. Paroxysmal dyskinesias: clinical features and classification. *Ann Neurol.* 1995;38(4):571–579.

106. Drake ME Jr, Jackson RD, Miller CA. Paroxysmal choreoathetosis after head injury. *J Neurol Neurosurg Psychiatry.* 1986;49(7):837–838.

107. Perlmutter JS, Raichle ME. Pure hemidystonia with basal ganglion abnormalities on positron emission tomography. *Ann Neurol.* 1984;15(3):228–233.

108. Richardson JC, Howes JL, Celinski MJ, Allman RG. Kinesigenic choreoathetosis due to brain injury. *Can J Neurol Sci.* 1987;14(4):626–628.

109. Robin JJ. Paroxysmal choreoathetosis following head injury. *Ann Neurol.* 1977;2(5):447–448.

110. Blakeley J, Jankovic J. Secondary paroxysmal dyskinesias. *Mov Disord.* 2002;17(4):726–734.

111. Jankovic J, Kwak C. Tics in other neurological disorders. In: Kurlan R, ed. *Handbook of Tourette's Syndrome and Related Tic and Behavioral Disorders.* New York, NY: Marcel Dekker; 2004.

112. Fahn S. A case of post-traumatic tic syndrome. In: Chase TN, Friedhoff AJ, eds. *Gilles de la Tourette Syndrome.* New York, NY: Raven Press; 1982:349–350.

113. Krauss JK, Jankovic J. Tics secondary to craniocerebral trauma. *Mov Disord.* 1997;12(5):776–782.

114. Siemers E, Pascuzzi R. Posttraumatic tic disorder. *Mov Disord.* 1990;5(2):183.

115. Singer C, Sanchez-Ramos J, Weiner WJ. A case of post-traumatic tic disorder. *Mov Disord.* 1989;4(4):342–344.

116. Majumdar A, Appleton RE. Delayed and severe but transient Tourette syndrome after head injury. *Pediatr Neurol.* 2002;27(4):314–317.

117. Kwak CH, Jankovic J. Tourettism and dystonia after subcortical stroke. *Mov Disord.* 2002;17(4):821–825.

118. Ranjan N, Nair KP, Romanoski C, Singh R, Venketswara G. Tics after traumatic brain injury. *Brain Inj.* 2011;25(6):629–633.

119. Deuschl G, Mischke G, Schenck E, Schulte-Mönting J, Lücking CH. Symptomatic and essential rhythmic palatal myoclonus. *Brain.* 1990;113(pt 6):1645–1672.

120. Hallett M, Chadwick D, Marsden CD. Cortical reflex myoclonus. *Neurology.* 1979;29(8):1107–1125.

121. Keane JR. Galloping tongue: post-traumatic, episodic, rhythmic movements. *Neurology.* 1984;34(2):251–252.

122. Obeso JA, Artieda J, Rothwell JC, Day B, Thompson P, Marsden CD. The treatment of severe action myoclonus. *Brain.* 1989;112(pt 3):765–777.

123. Starosta-Rubinstein S, Bjork RJ, Snyder BD, Tulloch JW. Posttraumatic intention myoclonus. *Surg Neurol.* 1983;20(2):131–132.

124. Stewart JT. Akathisia following traumatic brain injury: treatment with bromocriptine. *J Neurol Neurosurg Psychiatry.* 1989;52(10):1200–1201.

125. Troupin AS, Kamm RF. Lingual myoclonus. Case report and review. *Dis Nerv Syst.* 1974;35(8):378–380.

126. Turazzi S, Alexandre A, Bricolo A, Rizzuto N. Opsoclonus and palatal myoclonus during prolonged post-traumatic coma. A clinico-pathologic study. *Eur Neurol.* 1977;15(5):257–263.

127. Desai A, Nierenberg DW, Duhaime AC. Akathisia after mild traumatic head injury. *J Neurosurg Pediatr.* 2010;5(5):460–464.

128. Grimberg L. Paralysis agitans and trauma. *J Nerv Ment Dis.* 1934;79:14–42.

129. Lindenberg R. Die Schädigungsmechanismen der Substantia nigra bei Hirntraumen und das Problem des posttraumatischen Parkinsonismus. *Dtsch Z Nervenheilkd.* 1964;185:637–663.

130. Doder M, Jahanshahi M, Turjanski N, Moseley IF, Lees AJ. Parkinson's syndrome after closed head injury: a single case report. *J Neurol Neurosurg Psychiatry.* 1999;66(3):380–385.

131. Giroud M, Vincent MC, Thierry A, Binnert D, Marin A, Dumas R. Parkinsonian syndrome caused by traumatic hematomas in the basal ganglia [in French]. *Neurochirurgie.* 1988;34(1):61–63.

132. Bhatt M, Desai J, Mankodi A, Elias M, Wadia N. Posttraumatic akinetic-rigid syndrome resembling Parkinson's disease: a report on three patients. *Mov Disord.* 2000;15(2):313–317.

133. Nayernouri T. Posttraumatic parkinsonism. *Surg Neurol.* 1985;24(3):263–264.

134. Krauss JK, Trankle R, Raabe A. Tremor and dystonia after penetrating diencephalic-mesencephalic trauma. *Parkinsonism Relat Disord.* 1997;3(2):117–119.

135. de Morsier. Parkinsonisme consecutife a une lesion traumatique du nojau rouge et du locus niger. *Psychiatr Neurol* (Basel). 1960;139:60–84.

136. Rondot P, Bathien N, de Recondo J, et al. Dystonia-parkinsonism syndrome resulting from a bullet injury in the midbrain. *J Neurol Neurosurg Psychiatry.* 1994;57(5):658.

137. Kivi A, Trottenberg T, Kupsch A, Plotkin M, Felix R, Niehaus L. Levodopa-responsive posttraumatic parkinsonism is not associated with changes of echogenicity of the substantia nigra. *Mov Disord.* 2005;20(2):258–260.

138. Wiest RG, Burgunder JM, Krauss JK. Chronic subdural haematomas and Parkinsonian syndromes. *Acta Neurochir* (Wien). 1999;141(7):753–758.

139. Peppard RF, Byrne E, Nye D. Chronic subdural haematomas presenting with Parkinsonian signs. *Clin Exp Neurol.* 1986;22:19–23.

140. Turjanski N, Pentland B, Lees AJ, Brooks DJ. Parkinsonism associated with acute intracranial hematomas: an [18F]dopa positron-emission tomography study. *Mov Disord.* 1997;12(6):1035–1038.

141. Friedman JH. Progressive parkinsonism in boxers. *South Med J.* 1989;82(5):543–546.

142. Mawdsley C, Ferguson FR. Neurological disease in boxers. *Lancet.* 1963;2(7312):799–801.

143. Roberts AH. *Brain Damage in Boxers: A Study of the Prevalence of Traumatic Encephalopathy among Ex-Professional Boxers.* London, UK: Pitman Medical & Scientific Publishing Co, Ltd; 1969.

144. Roberts GW, Allsop D, Bruton C. The occult aftermath of boxing. *J Neurol Neurosurg Psychiatry.* 1990;53(5):373–378.

145. Turjanski N, Lees AJ, Brooks DJ. Dopaminergic function in patients with posttraumatic parkinsonism: an 18F-dopa PET study. *Neurology.* 1997;49(1):183–189.

146. Bailes JE, Cantu RC. Head injury in athletes. *Neurosurgery.* 2001;48(1):26–45.

147. McKee AC, Cantu RC, Nowinski CJ, et al. Chronic traumatic encephalopathy in athletes: progressive tauopathy after repetitive head injury. *J Neuropathol Exp Neurol.* 2009;68(7):709–735.

148. Lolekha P, Phanthumchinda K, Bhidayasiri R. Prevalance and risk factors of Parkinson's disease in retired Thai traditional boxers. *Mov Disord.* 2010;25(12):1895–1901.

149. Corsellis JA, Brierley JB. Observations on the pathology of insidious dementia following head injury. *J Ment Sci.* 1959;105:714–720.

150. Lampert PW, Hardman JM. Morphological changes in brains of boxers. *JAMA.* 1984;251(20):2676–2679.

151. Jordan BD. Chronic traumatic brain injury associated with boxing. *Semin Neurol.* 2000;20(2):179–185.

152. Davie CA, Pirtosek Z, Barker GJ, Kingsley DP, Miller PH, Lees AJ. Magnetic resonance spectroscopic study of parkinsonism related to boxing. *J Neurol Neurosurg Psychiatry.* 1995;58(6):688–691.

153. Ryan AJ. Intracranial injuries resulting from boxing. *Clin Sports Med.* 1998;17(1):155–168.

154. Butler RJ, Forsythe WI, Beverly DW, Adams LM. A prospective controlled investigation of the cognitive effects of amateur boxing. *J Neurol Neurosurg Psychiatry.* 1993;56(10):1055–1061.

155. Haglund Y, Eriksson E. Does amateur boxing lead to chronic brain damage? A review of some recent investigations. *Am J Sports Med.* 1993;21(1):97–109.

156. Jordan BD, Relkin NR, Ravdin LD, Jacobs AR, Bennett A, Gandy S. Apolipoprotein E epsilon4 associated with chronic traumatic brain injury in boxing. *JAMA.* 1997;278(2):136–140.

157. Factor SA, Weiner WJ. Prior history of head trauma in Parkinson's disease. *Mov Disord.* 1991;6(3):225–229.

158. Hubble JP, Cao T, Hassanein RE, Neuberger JS, Koller WC. Risk factors for Parkinson's disease. *Neurology.* 1993;43(9):1693–1697.

159. Stern MB. Head trauma as a risk factor for Parkinson's disease. *Mov Disord.* 1991;6(2):95–97.

160. Ward CD, Duvoisin RC, Ince SE, Nutt JD, Eldridge R, Calne DB. Parkinson's disease in 65 pairs of twins and in a set of quadruplets. *Neurology.* 1983;33(7):815–824.

161. Goetz CG, Stebbins GT. Effects of head trauma from motor vehicle accidents on Parkinson's disease. *Ann Neurol.* 1991;29(2):191–193.

162. Godwin-Austen RB, Lee PN, Marmot MG, Stern GM. Smoking and Parkinson's disease. *J Neurol Neurosurg Psychiatry.* 1982;45(7):577–581.

163. Tanner CM, Chen B, Wang WZ, et al. Environmental factors in the etiology of Parkinson's disease. *Can J Neurol Sci.* 1987;14(3)(suppl):419–423.

164. Williams DB, Annegers JF, Kokmen E, O'Brien PC, Kurland LT. Brain injury and neurologic sequelae: a cohort study of dementia, parkinsonism, and amyotrophic lateral sclerosis. *Neurology.* 1991;41(10):1554–1557.

165. Goldman SM, Tanner CM, Oakes D, Bhudhikanok GS, Gupta A, Langston JW. Head injury and Parkinson's disease risk in twins. *Ann Neurol.* 2006;60(1):65–72.

166. Spangenberg S, Hannerz H, Tüchsen F, Mikkelsen KL. A nationwide population study of severe head injury and Parkinson's disease. *Parkinsonism Relat Disord.* 2009;15(1):12–14.

167. Rugbjerg K, Ritz B, Korbo L, Martinussen N, Olsen JH. Risk of Parkinson's disease after hospital contact for head injury: population based case-control study. *BMJ.* 2008;337:a2494.

168. Ellison PH. Propranolol for severe post-head injury action tremor. *Neurology.* 1978;28(2):197–199.

169. Harmon RL, Long DF, Shirtz J. Treatment of post-traumatic midbrain resting-kinetic tremor with combined levodopa/carbidopa and carbamazepine. *Brain Inj.* 1991;5(2):213–218.

170. Jacob PC, Pratap Chand R. Posttraumatic rubral tremor responsive to clonazepam. *Mov Disord.* 1998;13(6):977–978.

171. Jankovic J, Brin MF. Therapeutic uses of botulinum toxin. *N Engl J Med.* 1991;324(17):1186–1194.

172. Andrew J, Fowler CJ, Harrison MJ. Tremor after head injury and its treatment by stereotaxic surgery. *J Neurol Neurosurg Psychiatry.* 1982;45(9):815–819.

173. Cooper IS. Neurosurgical alleviation of intention tremor of multiple sclerosis and cerebellar disease. *N Engl J Med.* 1960;263:441–444.

174. Eiras J, García Cosamalón J. Síndrome mioclónico posttraumático. Efectividad de las lesiones talámicas sobre las mioclonías de acción. *Arch Neurobiol* (Madr.) 1980;43(1):17–28.

175. Fox JL, Kurtzke JF. Trauma-induced intention tremor relieved by stereotaxic thalamotomy. *Arch Neurol.* 1966;15(3):247–251.

176. Goldman MS, Kelly PJ. Symptomatic and functional outcome of stereotactic ventralis lateralis thalamotomy for intention tremor. *J Neurosurg.* 1992;77(2):223–229.

177. Hirai T, Miyazaki M, Nakajima H, Shibazaki T, Ohye C. The correlation between tremor characteristics and the predicted volume of effective lesions in stereotaxic nucleus ventralis intermedius thalamotomy. *Brain.* 1983;106(pt 4):1001–1018.

178. Iwadate Y, Saeki N, Namba H, Odaki M, Oka N, Yamaura A. Post-traumatic intention tremor—clinical features and CT findings. *Neurosurg Rev.* 1989;12(suppl 1):500–507.

179. Jankovic J, Cardoso F, Grossman RG, Hamilton WJ. Outcome after stereotactic thalamotomy for parkinsonian, essential, and other types of tremor. *Neurosurgery.* 1995;37(4):680–687.

180. Kandel EI. Treatment of hemihyperkinesias by stereotactic operations on basal ganglia. *Appl Neurophysiol.* 1982;45(3):225–229.

181. Marks PV. Stereotactic surgery for post-traumatic cerebellar syndrome: an analysis of seven cases. *Stereotact Funct Neurosurg.* 1993;60(4):157–167.

182. Niizuma H, Kwak R, Ohyama H, et al. Stereotactic thalamotomy for postapoplectic and posttraumatic involuntary movements. *Appl Neurophysiol.* 1982;45(3):295–298.

183. Ohye C, Hirai T, Miyazaki M, Shibazaki T, Nakajima H. Vim thalamotomy for the treatment of various kinds of tremor. *Apl Neurophysiol.* 1982;45(3):275–280.

184. Richardson RR. Rehabilitative neurosurgery: posttraumatic syndromes. *Stereotact Funct Neurosurg.* 1989;53(2):105–112.

185. Samra K, Waltz JM, Riklan M, Koslow M, Cooper IS. Relief of intention tremor by thalamic surgery. *J Neurol Neurosurg Psychiatry.* 1970;33(1):7–15.

186. Shahzadi S, Tasker RR, Lozano A. Thalamotomy for essential and cerebellar tremor. *Stereotact Funct Neurosurg.* 1995;65(1–4):11–17.

187. Spiegel EA, Wycis HT, Szekely EG, Adams DJ, Flanagan M, Baird HW III. Campotomy in various extrapyramidal disorders. *J Neurosurg.* 1963;20:871–884.

188. Taira T, Speelman JD, Bosch DA. Trajectory angle in stereotactic thalamotomy. *Stereotact Funct Neurosurg.* 1993;61(1):24–31.

189. van Manen J. Stereotaxic operations in cases of hereditary and intention tremor. *Acta Neurochirur* (Wien). 1974;(suppl 21):49–55.

190. Young RF, Jacques S, Mark R, et al. Gamma knife thalamotomy for treatment of tremor: long-term results. *J Neurosurg.* 2000;93(suppl 3):128–135.

191. Andy OJ. Thalamic stimulation for control of movement disorders. *Appl Neurophysiol.* 1983;46(1–4):107–111.

192. Benabid AL, Pollak P, Gao D, et al. Chronic electrical stimulation of the ventralis intermedius nucleus of the thalamus as a treatment of movement disorders. *J Neurosurg.* 1996;84(2):203–214.

193. Broggi G, Brock S, Franzini A, Geminiani G. A case of posttraumatic tremor treated by chronic stimulation of the thalamus. *Mov Disord.* 1993;8(2):206–208.

194. Nguyen JP, Degos JD. Thalamic stimulation and proximal tremor. A specific target in the nucleus ventrointermedius thalami. *Arch Neurol.* 1993;50(5):498–500.

195. Standhart H, Pinter MM, Volc D, Alesch F. Chronic eletrical stimulation of the nucleus ventralis intermedius of the thalamus for the treatment of tremor. *Mov Disord.* 1998;13(suppl 3):141.

196. Vesper J, Funk T, Kern BC, et al. Thalamic deep brain stimulation: present state of the art. *Neurosurg Q.* 2000;10(4):252–260.

197. Umemura A, Samadani U, Jaggi JL, Hurtig HI, Baltuch GH. Thalamic deep brain stimulation for posttraumatic action tremor. *Clin Neurol Neurosurg.* 2004;106(4):280–283.

198. Krauss JK, Simpson RK Jr, Ondo WG, Pohle T, Burgunder JM, Jankovic J. Concepts and methods in chronic thalamic stimulation for treatment of tremor: technique and application. *Neurosurgery.* 2001;48(3):535–543.

199. Kitagawa M, Murata J, Kikuchi S, et al. Deep brain stimulation of subthalamic area for severe proximal tremor. *Neurology.* 2000;55(1):114–116.

200. Voges J, Krauss JK. Neurological and technical aspects of deep brain stimulation [in German]. *Nervenarzt.* 2010;81(6):702–710.

201. Foote KD, Seignourel P, Fernandez HH, et al. Dual electrode thalamic deep brain stimulation for the treatment of posttraumatic and multiple sclerosis tremor. *Neurosurgery.* 2006;58(4)(suppl 2):ONS-280–286.

202. Romanelli P, Brontë-Stewart H, Courtney T, Heit G. Possible necessity for deep brain stimulation of both the ventralis intermedius and subthalamic nuclei to resolve Holmes tremor. Case Report. *J Neurosurg.* 2003;99(3):566–571.

203. Biary N, Cleeves L, Findley L, Koller W. Post-traumatic tremor. *Neurology.* 1989;39(1):103–106.

204. Jankovic J, Schwartz K. Botulinum toxin treatment of tremors. *Neurology.* 1991;41(8):1185–1188.

205. Dressler D, Schönle PW. Bilateral limb dystonia due to chronic subdural hematoma. *Eur Neurol.* 1990;30(4):211–213.

206. Eaton JM. Hemidystonia due to subdural hematoma. *Neurology.* 1988;38(3):507.

207. Nobbe FA, Krauss JK. Subdural hematoma as a cause of contralateral dystonia. *Clin Neurol Neurosurg.* 1997;99(1):37–39.

208. Cardoso F, Jankovic J, Grossman RG, Hamilton WJ. Outcome after stereotactic thalamotomy for dystonia and hemiballismus. *Neurosurgery.* 1995;36(3):501–508.

209. Ondo WG, Desaloms JM, Jankovic J, Grossman RG. Pallidotomy for generalized dystonia. *Mov Disord.* 1998;13(4):693–698.

210. Ondo WG, Krauss JK. Surgical therapies for dystonia. In: Brin MF, Comella C, Jankovic J, eds. *Dystonia: Etiology, Clinical Features, and Treatment.* Philadelphia, PA: Lippincott Williams & Wilkins; 2004: 125–147.

211. Alkhani A, Khan F, Lang AE, Hutchison WD, Dostrovsky J. The response to pallidal surgery for dystonia is dependent on the etiology. *Neurosurgery.* 2000;47:504.

212. Villemure JG, Vingerhoets F, Temperli P, Pollo C, Ghika J. Dystonia: pallidal or thalamic target. *Acta Neurochir* (Wien). 2000;142: 1194.

213. Yoshor D, Hamilton WJ, Ondo W, Jankovic J, Grossman RG. Comparison of thalamotomy and pallidotomy for the treatment of dystonia. *Neurosurgery.* 2001;48(4):818–826.

214. Teive H, Sa D, Grande CV, Fustes OJH, Antoniuk A, Werneck LC. Bilateral simultaneous globus pallidus internus pallidotomy for generalized posttraumatic dystonia. *Mov Disord.* 1998;13(suppl 2):33.

215. Sellal F, Hirsch E, Barth P, Blond S, Marescaux C. A case of symptomatic hemidystonia improved by ventroposterolateral thalamic electrostimulation. *Mov Disord.* 1993;8(4):515–518.

216. Loher TJ, Hasdemir MG, Burgunder JM, Krauss JK. Long-term follow-up study of chronic globus pallidus internus stimulation for posttraumatic hemidystonia. *J Neurosurg.* 2000;92(3):457–460.

217. Loher TJ, Capelle HH, Kaelin-Lang A, et al. Deep brain stimulation for dystonia: outcome at long-term follow-up. *J Neurol.* 2008;255(6): 881–884.

218. Meythaler JM, Guin-Renfroe S, Grabb P, Hadley MN. Long-term continuously infused intrathecal baclofen for spastic-dystonic hypertonia in traumatic brain injury: 1-year experience. *Arch Phys Med Rehabil.* 1999;80(1):13–19.

219. Penn RD, Gianino JM, York MM. Intrathecal baclofen for motor disorders. *Mov Disord.* 1995;10(5):675–677.

220. Hou JG, Ondo W, Jankovic J. Intrathecal baclofen for dystonia. *Mov Disord.* 2001;16(6):1201–1202.

221. Krauss JK, Mundinger F. Functional stereotactic surgery for hemiballism. *J Neurosurg.* 1996;85(2):278–286.

222. Jankovic J. Treatment of hyperkinetic movement disorders. *Lancet Neurol.* 2009;8(9):844–856.

223. Loher TJ, Krauss JK, Burgunder JM, Taub E, Siegfried J. Chronic thalamic stimulation for treatment of dystonic paroxysmal nonkinesigenic dyskinesia. *Neurology.* 2001;56(2):268–270.

224. Jankovic J. Therapeutic strategies in Parkinson's disease. In: Jankovic J, Tolosa E, eds. *Parkinson's Disease & Movement Disorders.* 4th ed. Philadelphia, PA: Lippincott Williams & Wilkins; 2002:116–151.

225. Reese R, Herzog J, Falk D, et al. Successful deep brain stimulation in a case of posttraumatic tremor and hemiparkinsonism. *Mov Disord.* 2011;26(10):1954–1955.

Cranial Nerve Disorders

Flora M. Hammond and Todd Masel

INTRODUCTION

Cranial nerves provide motor and sensory innervation to the head, neck, viscera, glands, and vasculature and are termed such owing to the fact that they emerge from the cranium. Injury to the cranial nerves is common with traumatic brain injury (TBI) and has even been shown to occur in TBI so mild as to be associated with a Glasgow Coma Scale (GCS) score of 14–15 and no initial findings on CT imaging of the head (42). In this chapter, the anatomy, pathway, function, injury incidence, mechanism of injury, examination, treatment, and prognosis will be discussed for each of the cranial nerves. Introductory information about cranial nerves and their injury is briefly reviewed before discussing each nerve individually.

The true incidence of cranial nerve injuries is difficult to estimate. The olfactory nerve (cranial nerve I) is reported to be the most often injured, followed next in frequency by the facial and vestibulocochlear nerves, less commonly the optic and oculomotor nerves, and rarely the trigeminal and lower cranial nerves (1). Cranial nerve palsies may occur with TBI for several reasons, including acceleration-deceleration, shearing forces, skull fracture, intracranial hemorrhage, intracranial mass lesion, uncal herniation, infarct, or vascular occlusion. These circumstances may cause insults to the nerves through such mechanisms as compression, traction, transection, or ischemia. Central injury may occur from brainstem or cerebral damage; peripheral injury results from fracture or local injury. Cranial nerves are particularly at risk for injury as they traverse over bony protuberances and through bony canals or by direct injury from basilar skull fracture. The cranial nerves most susceptible to injury because of fracture are olfactory, optic, oculomotor, trochlear, facial, auditory, and trigeminal (first two branches). The site of cranial fractures should indicate to the clinician the possibility of cranial nerve injury.

Injury to the cranial nerves may result in significant consequences to the individual with TBI, which may be further compounded by the deficits caused by cortical injury. Resulting impairments in sensation (sight, hearing, smell, taste) and motor function (facial expression, mastication, swallowing, speech) may impact such things as appetite, safety, interpersonal communication, and cosmesis.

Cranial nerves originate from the brainstem (see Figure 41-1), and thus, abnormality in these nerves may serve as a reflection of injury severity. For example, pupillary, oculo-vestiluar, and oculocaloric reflexes have been shown to be strong prognostic indicators of mortality (2–6) and persistent cognitive disability (7).

Diagnosis is generally based on physical examination. Table 41-1 lists the examination tests and supplies for each cranial nerve. In the presence of altered consciousness, examination may be difficult and incomplete. Thus, as one recovers from TBI, those aspects of the examination that were previously not possible will need to be performed. A good cranial nerve examination can help identify cranial nerve impairment. Electromyography and nerve conduction studies may aid the clinician in lesion localization and prognostication. A range of treatment approaches exist for cranial nerve deficits. In fact, it has been shown that surgical decompression can significantly increase the chance of recovery in these patients (43). In many cases, measures should be instituted to avoid secondary injury. In addition to this chapter, further information about cranial nerve (CN) injury, prognosis and treatment may be found in Chapters 45 (Evaluating and Treating Visual Function), 46 (Audiological Impairment), 47 (Balance and Dizziness), 48 (Smell and Taste), and 66 (Evaluation and Treatment of Swallowing Problems).

OLFACTORY NERVE (CRANIAL NERVE I)

Cranial nerve I provides the special sensory function of smell. The central axons of the bipolar olfactory neurons pass through the cribiform plate of the ethmoid bone, synapsing in the olfactory bulbs to relay sensations of smell to the brain. From here, projections travel to the entorhinal cortex, hypothalamus, and the dorsal medial thalamic nucleus and then to the orbitofrontal cortex. Of note, the olfactory system is the only sensory pathway that does not project to the thalamus before making its connections in the cortex (44).

Cranial nerve I lesions may result in alteration of smell. Olfactory nerve injury may also alter the sense of taste because flavor perception results from a combination of smell, taste, and stored memories. Altered smell and taste may impact safety, appetite/weight control, confusion, behavior, daily activities, avocational and vocational pursuits. Table 41-2 summarizes several terms used to describe the nature and extent of the altered olfactory sensation.

As many as 2 million people in the United States experience some type of olfactory dysfunction, causes of which include head trauma, upper respiratory infections, tumors

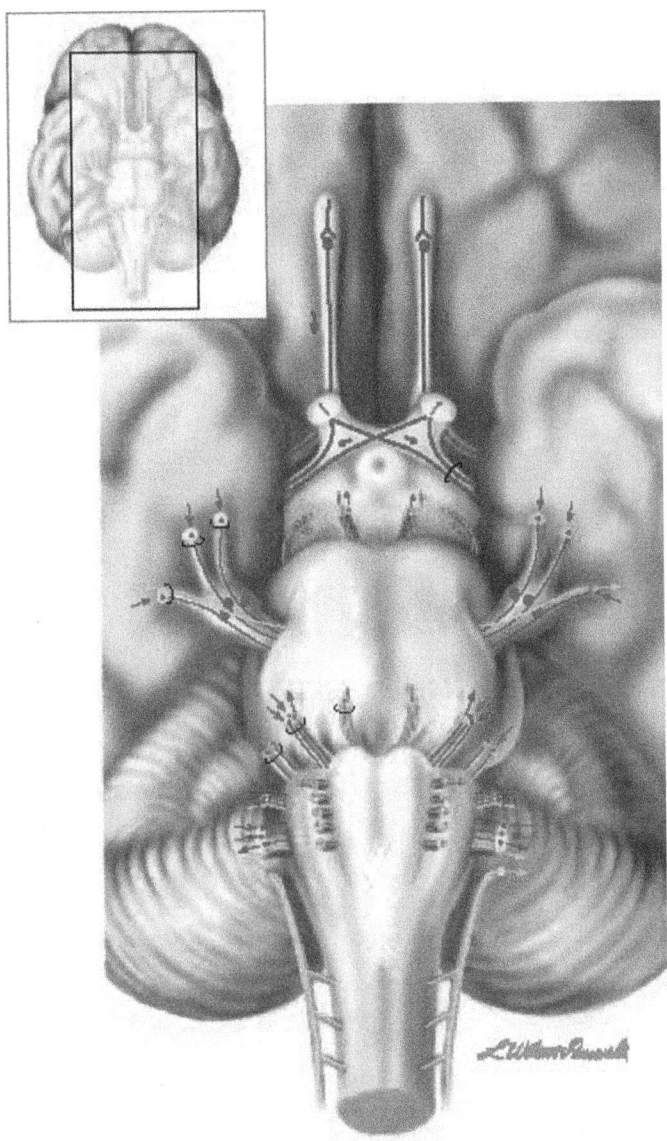

FIGURE 41-1 *See color insert.* Basal view cranial nerves exiting the brain and brainstem. The components of the cranial nerves are indicated by color aqua = general sensory; purple = visceral sensory; green = special sensory; pink = somatic motor; yellow = branchia motor; blue = visceral motor.

the olfactory bulb. There should be a high index of suspicion for olfactory nerve injury in the following cases: cerebral spinal fluid (CSF) rhinorrhea, frontal and occipital blows, frontal vault fractures. It is reported that 40% of those with CSF rhinorrhea after TBI experience anosmia.

Cranial nerve I injury may occur from damage to the olfactory nerves in the nasal mucosa, damage to the nerves as they cross the cribriform plate, or intracranial lesions affecting the olfactory bulbs. The olfactory filaments are particularly vulnerable to injury, as they may be sheared during the rotation of the brain or injured by cribriform plate fractures. The olfactory bulbs may be compressed by hemorrhage, edema, contusion, or abrasion by the cribriform plate. Olfactory structures may also be injured during craniotomies involving the anterior cranial base or from subarachnoid hemorrhage, which may disrupt the fine fibers of the olfactory nerve. Delayed onset olfactory nerve dysfunction may be the consequence of scarring or gliosis of the tissues in the cribriform plate. Other causes of olfactory sensory abnormality should also be considered such as nasal obstruction, injury to the nasal passages, acute viral respiratory infections, rhinitis sicca, allergic sinusitis, chronic polyposis, depression, medications, and seizures. Partial complex epilepsy with a mesial temporal focus classically includes an aura of foul-smelling odors that occur before seizure onset. Olfactory hallucinations from uncinate fits do not imply actual olfactory nerve involvement. Paranasal sinus endoscopy may lead to violation of the cribriform plate with associated olfactory nerve injury and also potential infectious complications.

Report of impaired smell may be the first signal of olfactory nerve injury. Because olfactory nerve function is not often evaluated in an emergency situation, the dysfunction may not be detected until weeks after the injury when the patient complains of changes in taste or smell. To examine cranial nerve I function, first, evaluate the patency of both nasal passages. Then, determine if the person can detect odor in each nostril by testing with a familiar substance and an empty bottle. Stimulants such as organic solvents, camphor, peppermint, or ammonia should be avoided as they may also stimulate cranial nerve V (13). Next, smell discrimination can be tested with the patient choosing between a series of common odors such as coffee, lemon, and soap. Providing choices is a helpful way of limiting the influence of word-finding problems on testing. Several different scratch and sniff cards are available to make testing more convenient. The University of Pennsylvania Smell Identification Test (UPSIT) is one useful tool, consisting of 40 items that evaluate olfactory and trigeminal nerve function in the nasal cavity. Central hyposmia may manifest as abnormalities in odor recognition rather than odor detection.

Ethmoid tomography may be used to determine if a basal skull fracture is present. Positron emission tomography (PET) and functional MRI are promising modalities to assist in making the diagnosis of different types of hyposmia (central vs peripheral), as well as in delineation of the role of limbic structures as sites of odor recognition, memory, and integration of multisensory inputs. Thorough evaluation of patients who have anosmia includes imaging of the anterior cranial structures. Patients experiencing parosmia should be evaluated for seizure activity on electroencephalography.

of the anterior cranial fossa, and exposure to toxic chemicals or infections. It is difficult to estimate the true incidence of olfactory nerve injury in association with TBI because of the inability to examine cranial nerve I function in the unresponsive patient, and the inconsistent medical attention sought after mild TBI. Olfactory nerve injury is reported to occur in 7% of all patients with TBI (8–11). The incidence is higher following moderate and severe TBI than mild TBI. Costanzo and Becker (12) report 19.4% with moderate TBI and 24.5% with severe TBI. Injury to the olfactory nerve is the only cranial nerve commonly associated with mild TBI. This is because the fine nerve filaments of the olfactory nerve are particularly at risk for injury, even in mild TBI, as the fibers run through the cribriform plate of the ethmoid bone to reach

TABLE 41-1 Cranial Nerve Function and Examination

NERVE	FUNCTION	TEST	SUPPLIES
Olfactory (I)	Smell	Evaluate patency of the nasal passages. Then, determine if the person can detect familiar, nonnoxious smells with eyes closed. Giving the person choices may help overcome word finding problems.	Odors or smelling card
Optic (II)	Visual acuity; visual fields	Have patient identify number of fingers held in visual fields and read up-close and far-away	Snellen visual acuity card
Oculomotor (III)	Pupillary reaction; lid retraction; and eye movement	Shine light in each eye to assess pupil reaction; note lid function; test eye movement for upward, downward, and medial gaze	Penlight
Trochlear (IV)	Intorsion and downward eye movement	Have patient follow finger to move eye downward	
Trigeminal (V)	Facial sensation; corneal sensation; chewing function	Test facial sensation for all 3 divisions; test corneal reflex; hold mouth open against resistance; clench teeth	
Abducens (VI)	Lateral eye movement	Have patient move eyes from side to side	
Facial (VII)	Facial motor function; lid closure; taste sensation (anterior)	Lateral gaze smile, wrinkle forehead, wink, puff cheeks, close eye tight, identify tastes with anterior tongue	
Acoustic (VIII)	Hearing; balance	Test hearing; assess for nystagmus; finger to nose and heel to knee; Dix-Hallpike; vestibulo-ocular reflex; Rhomberg; Sharpened Rhomberg; Fucada Stepping Test; Caloric Stimulation Test	
Glossopharyngeal (IX)	Swallowing; voice	Say "ah"; swallow; test gag reflex	Tongue depressor
Vagus (X)	Gag reflex	Tested above via gag reflex	Tongue depressor
Spinal (XI)	Neck strength	Resist head rotation, shoulder shrugs	
Hypoglossal (XII)	Tongue movement and strength	Stick out tongue; resist tongue movement with tongue depressor	Tongue depressor

Unfortunately, there are no established effective treatments for this condition (1), whereas nontraumatic causes and seizure may be amenable to treatment. Early recovery may occur caused by resolution of edema or pressure; whereas later recovery is attributable to neurofibril regrowth and central adaptation (14). Many regain the sense of smell within 2 years, but for some, this remains a permanent problem. Costanzo and Becker (12) observed 33% recovery, 27% worsening, and 40% no change. When recovery occurs, it is usually noticed within the first 6 months and complete by 12 months postinjury (13). However, late recoveries up to 5 years have been reported (8). Although it is a generally annoying development, parosmia may be the first evidence of functional return. For safety purposes, individuals with altered olfactory sensation should be aware of potential risks associated with the lack of smell (e.g., inability to detect dangers such as smoke, spoiled foods, toxins) and reminded to install smoke alarms on all floors of their home.

TABLE 41-2 Types of Olfactory Dysfunction

TERM	DEFINITION
Dysnosmia	impaired sense of smell
Anosmia	complete loss of smell
Hyposmia	partial loss of smell
Parosmia	sensation of smell in the absence of stimulus
Cacosmia	awareness of a disagreeable or unusually offensive order that does not exist; may be part of an aura prior to seizure onset

OPTIC NERVE (CRANIAL NERVE II)

The optic nerve, a fiber tract of the brain containing 1 million axons, provides the special sense of sight. This nerve receives its input from the rods and cones (first order neurons) which pass the signal to the ganglion cell layer of the retina (secondary sensory neurons). The long axons of the ganglion cells penetrate the lamina cribrosa as the optic nerve, which passes posteriorly through the optic canal. At the optic chiasm, where fibers from the nasal halves of the retina cross, the optic tract is formed, containing fibers from the ipsilateral halves of the retina. The optic tract continues posteriorly to the lateral geniculate bodies, where a third synaptic relay occurs. At this point, a small number of axons leave the optic tract and project to the pretectal midbrain to form the afferent loop of the Edinger–Westphal nucleus. From the lateral geniculate body, the optic tract continues posteriorly as the optic radiations, which project to the occipital lobe. Throughout their projection to the occipital lobe, the neurons maintain a highly topographic orientation of the retinal image.

Optic nerve injury occurs in up to 5% of individuals with TBI (9). Optic nerve palsy may occur with injury to the globe, causing damage to the intraorbital portion of the nerve within the optic canal (15). In the orbit, the nerve is redundant and cushioned by fat. It is, therefore, not liable to indirect injury. However, the nerve is strongly tethered to bone intermittently throughout the canal. It is, therefore, subject to shearing forces as the brain and orbital contents are free to move, while the nerve is not (16). Injury to the optic nerve occurs most frequently in the intracanalicular portion of the nerve (17). Injury to the intracranial portion is less common.

Injury to the optic nerve typically occurs in 1 of 2 ways: (*a*) primary lesions causing hemorrhages in the nerve, dura and sheath spaces, tears in the nerve or chiasm, and, rarely, contusion necrosis; or (*b*) secondary lesions from circulatory events subsequent to the initial injury causing edematous swelling of the nerve, necrosis from circulatory failure or local compression, and infarction related to vascular obstruction. Because the optic nerve is a direct extension of the brain, any injury to the optic nerve axons, which do not regenerate, is permanent.

Immediate monocular blindness occurs frequently in optic nerve injuries, especially in the intracanalicular portion of the nerve. Monocular blindness may be partial, and the extent of partial blindness should be documented immediately and followed closely for deterioration. The treatment of traumatic optic neuropathy is controversial. Although some studies have shown that steroids and/or optic canal decompression to be of benefit (18–20), other studies have shown that irrespective of timing postinjury, neither treatment improved visual outcome (21,22). Complete monocular blindness with preservation of normal pupillary reflexes is usually a sign of malingering or other types of functional (nonorganic) disorders.

Visual field defects are caused by injury to the optic nerve or its tracts posterior to the bulbar portion. These defects are quadrantanopias or hemianopsias of varying degrees. When such defects are due to causes other than direct pressure from a mass lesion, surgical intervention is rarely helpful. Some visual field deficits may be helped by special optics that allows the individual to "see" in the affected field (15,23). Careful evaluation by a neuro-opthalmologist or neuro-optometrist is warranted, and training in the use of such lenses is often necessary. Visual training may improve the visual spatial disorders for those with visual neglect (24). It is also important for the clinician to recognize nonphysiologic visual field deficits.

Non–nerve-related injury may also affect visual function. Trauma to the cornea may cause visual blurring and scotomata. Visual blurring may be caused by vitreous tears, traumatically induced cataracts, retinal hemorrhage, or retinal detachment. Injury to the cornea or contents of the anterior chamber (including the lens) may cause monocular diplopia (25). If eyeglasses are of no benefit, surgery may be necessary to correct blurring caused by either corneal or lens problems. Visual blurring also may be caused by Torsion syndrome (intrabulbar hemorrhage). The hemorrhage may resorb spontaneously over time or may require surgical removal for complete restoration of vision. The potential presence of occipital seizures should also be considered (26).

Examination includes testing visual acuity, visual fields, pupillary reactivity, and direct visualization by ophthalmoscope. These tests are reviewed briefly:

Pupillary Reactivity to Light. Light is shown into each eye and pupillary constriction (or lack of response) observed. It is also helpful to test for an afferent pupillary defect using the swing eye-to-eye test. If there is an afferent lesion involving the optic nerve, light shone into the affected eye fails to produce a response in either eye (contrast that with an efferent defect as described with cranial nerve III injury).

Vision Acuity. This can be performed by testing the ability to read a visual acuity card or newsprint. Unfortunately, this is often unable to be performed in individuals who are minimally responsive, confused, or aphasic. Saccadic responses to optokinetic stimuli may be checked to provide evidence of residual visual acuity function. The presence of an accommodation reflex can also provide evidence of visual fixation. Visual-evoked potentials may also help establish the integrity of the optic nerve and its cortical pathways.

Visual Fields. This entails asking the person to count fingers or identify a small object along the periphery of the vision. Each eye should be tested separately. Confrontation using a red-colored object is preferred. Evidence of visual inattention may be detected using a test of double, simultaneous extinction by presenting the test stimulus to bilateral visual fields at the same time. Tangent screen testing can provide visual field maps of deficits. Deficits may not be detected if the person is not able to fixate.

Direct Visualization by Ophthalmoscope. This may be helpful in identifying papilloedema (a hallmark of increased intracranial pressure), anterior chamber hemorrhage, and retinal detachment.

Visual Evoked Response (VER) may be considered to evaluate the integrity of the visual system from the eye to the occipital cortex.

OCULOMOTOR NERVE (CRANIAL NERVE III)

The oculomotor nerve provides somatic motor and visceral motor functions. The nucleus of the oculomotor nerve arises in the paramedian midbrain ventral to the aqueduct of Sylvius near the superior colliculus. Mainly uncrossed fibers course anteriorly through the red nucleus and inner side of the substantia nigra, emerging on the medial side of the cerebral peduncles near the pontomedullary junction at the midline, penetrating the dura at the cavernous sinus. It travels along the lateral wall of the cavernous sinus, adjacent to the trochlear nerve, and superior to the abducens. Parasympathetic fibers from the Edinger–Westphal nucleus, which lies superior and dorsal to the oculomotor nucleus, course in close proximity to the oculomotor nerve through the cavernous sinus. The oculomotor nerve emerges through the superior orbital fissure to innervate the internal, superior and inferior rectus muscles, inferior oblique muscle, and levator palpebrae muscle. The parasympathetic nerve fibers that travel with the oculomotor nerve innervate the sphincter muscle of the iris and to the ciliary muscle, which controls the shape of the lens during accommodation.

A palsy of this nerve can be caused by brain disorders (such as a head injury, tumor, or an aneurysm in an artery supplying the brain) or by diabetes. Injury may occur along its course: at the orbit, cavernous sinus, or an intracranial locus. This nerve is often injured at the point it exits through the dura, or from compression caused by uncal herniation due to increased intracranial pressure.

Isolated oculomotor nerve palsies due solely to TBI are not unusual, occurring in 17% of individuals in one study (27). Another study showed that persons with complete oculomotor palsy have a high incidence of traumatic subarachnoid hemorrhage (71%) or skull fractures (57%) (28). An orbital blowout fracture may produce clinical findings suggesting an oculomotor palsy; however, the simultaneous finding of infraorbital numbness argues against the diagnosis of an oculomotor nerve palsy (8).

Oculomotor nerve palsy causes a characteristic clinical picture: Divergent strabismus, because the eye is turned out by the intact lateral rectus muscle and slightly depressed by the intact superior oblique muscle. The eye may only be moved laterally. The affected eye turns outward when the unaffected eye looks straight ahead, producing double vision. The affected eye can move only to the middle when looking inward and cannot look upward and downward. There is ptosis of the eyelid, absent accommodation and in cases of complete palsy, a dilated and fixed ipsilateral pupil.

Assessment involves tracking an object in the 6 cardinal positions, convergence on near targets, pursuit movements, saccades, pupillary reaction, and eyelid elevation. Clinical testing of oculomotor function in the conscious patient is not difficult. The examiner observes difficulty in moving the eye inward or upward and downward, with preserved outward movement suggesting third nerve dysfunction (often with pupillary dilatation and ptosis).

In the unconscious patient, oculomotor testing is not possible, and thus, information is gathered during the performance of such tests as the doll's eye maneuver and pupillary light reflex. Such tests must be performed serially, especially in the acutely injured patient, to ensure that an expanding lesion, uncal herniation, and/or hemorrhage are not overlooked. A fixed and dilated pupil serves as a warning sign of herniation because of the nerves location medial to the temporal lobe at the edge of the tentorium. Dilation and fixation of both pupils indicates deep coma and possibly brain death.

Each eye is tested separately for pupillary reaction to light. With an efferent defect involving cranial nerve III, light shone into either eye fails to produce a response in the affected eye while light shone in the affected eye produces constriction of the opposite pupil. Pupillary dilation on one side is a characteristic of cranial nerve III palsy, and is commonly accompanied by ptosis and lateral eye deviation (due to unopposed abducen's function). The swinging flashlight test (moving light rapidly from one eye to the next) may be helpful. The normal response to this test is constriction in the illuminated eye. A Marcus Gunn sign is present when there is dilation of the pupil of the abnormal eye after light is shone briefly into it.

The diagnosis is based on the results of neurologic examination as described earlier. Assessment of cause starts with computed tomography (CT) or magnetic resonance imaging (MRI). A spinal tap (lumbar puncture) is performed only if hemorrhage is supected and CT does not detect blood. Cerebral angiography is performed when a hemorrhage caused by an aneurysm is suspected or when the pupil is affected but no head injury has occurred.

Return of function may begin within 2–3 months of injury but generally remains incomplete. The chances for complete recovery are poor (28), with 40% reported to experience complete recovery (25). However, the majority fortunately experience functional recovery, which generally occurs within 6–12 months of injury.

Occlusive therapy (patching) will resolve the diplopia while the patch is on but produces no long-term effects. Pleoptics (ocular exercises) also have not been proven to be very effective (29). Strabismus surgery should not be undertaken until maximum visual acuity has been restored. Surgery should be delayed 6–9 months postinjury, as one-third of patients will recover spontaneously (30). The procedure is empirical and consistent results cannot be guaranteed. Nevertheless, one large study showed successful alignment in 81% of adults who underwent strabismus surgery (31). This correction only improves the cosmetic deformity, however, and does nothing to improve the underlying cause.

TROCHLEAR NERVE (CRANIAL NERVE IV)

The trochlear nerve is the smallest of all the cranial nerves. It is somatic motor and innervates only 1 muscle, the superior oblique muscle. The trochlear nucleus is located in the lower midbrain and projects dorsally to cross the midline and is the only cranial nerve that decussates. It eventually emerges from the dorsal aspect of the midbrain immediately caudal to the inferior colliculus. The trochlear nerve then traverses the lateral aspect of the cavernous sinus and enters the orbit through superior orbital fissure to innervate the *contralateral* superior oblique muscle. Injury of the trochlear nerve may result from trauma, ischemia, infarction, hemorrhage, aneurysm, cavernous sinus thrombosis, inflammation, meningitis, or tumor. TBI is the most common cause. The trochlear nerve is particularly liable to traumatic injury in that it has the longest course of any cranial nerve within the skull. Trochlear nerve injury is reported to occur in 0.2%–1.4% of individuals with TBI (25).

Usually, the diagnosis is suspected in a person who, after a head injury, complains of vertical diplopia and cannot turn the affected eye inward and downward. The affected eye is typically observed to be rotated outward. The individual may also have a compensatory head tilt away from the affected side. In this position, unaffected muscles are employed and the vertical diplopia can often be eliminated. The double vision is commonly precipitated when walking down stairs.

What causes the vertical diplopia? With the superior oblique muscle paralyzed on one side, the antagonist inferior oblique extorts and slightly elevates the involved eye. Consequently, the visual fields are projected to different areas of the right and left retinae resulting in the perception of 2 different images.

The superior oblique muscle performs 2 major functions: intorsion and downward gaze. Intorsion is difficult to detect on examination. Watching for movement of the conjuctival vessel may prove useful in this effort. Downward gaze is easier to detect. Thus, cranial nerve IV is generally tested by having the person adduct the involved eye and attempt to gaze downward. Individuals with trochlear nerve palsy are unable to look downward when the eye is adducted. Adduction of the eye prior to testing downward gaze is important because movement of the superior oblique muscle depends on the starting position of the eye.

Further examination may be pursued with CT scan or MRI imaging. Treatment depends on the cause of the palsy. Eye exercises may help. Sometimes surgery is necessary to eliminate double vision.

TRIGEMINAL NERVE (CRANIAL NERVE V)

The trigeminal nerve provides general sensory and branchial motor modalities. The nerve arises from the ventrolateral pons with a large sensory and small motor root. The 2 roots extend forward to the tip of the petrous bone, where the sensory portion merges with the gasserian (semilunar) ganglion and then forms the 3 divisions of the trigeminal nerve. The motor portion travels along the inferior aspect of the ganglion and becomes part of the mandibular division.

The motor fibers exit through the foramen ovale to innervate the muscles of mastication: the masseter, temporalis, and medial and lateral pterygoid muscles. The fibers also innervate several smaller muscles: the tensor tympani and tensor veli palatini via the otic ganglion, and the mylohyoid and anterior belly of the digastric via the mylohyoid nerve.

The ophthalmic division (V-1) exits through the cavernous sinus and then the superior orbital fissure to supply sensation from the forehead, conjunctiva and cornea, as well as the mucosa of the nose, frontal, sphenoid and ethmoid sinuses, and the lacrimal duct. The maxillary division (V-2) also travels through the cavernous sinus and exits the foramen rotundum to supply sensation from the skin of the midface, the mucosa of the anterior nasopharynx, the upper portion of the hard and soft palate, the gums of the upper jaw and the upper teeth. The sensory portion of the mandibular division (V-3) supplies sensation from the lower face, the mucosa of the lower jaw, floor of the mouth, lower teeth and gum. It supplies general sensation (but not taste) from the anterior two-thirds of the tongue.

The incidence of trigeminal nerve injury from TBI is 1.4%–2% (8). The supraorbital nerve, from V-1 and the infraorbital nerve, from V-2 can be injured exiting the skull as the result of direct trauma such as blow-out fractures of the orbit. Such injuries tend to occur in motor vehicle accidents, unprotected falls, golfing and baseball injures. The peripheral branches may also be injured by a superficial blow to the face. Numbness typically follows the distribution of the nerve.

The roots and/or the gasserian ganglion may be damaged in transverse skull fractures (32) but are rare in blunt head trauma (8). Penetrating wounds involving the gasserian ganglion are also rare but may cause severe dysesthesias and trigeminal neuralgia-type pain.

Clinical testing of the trigeminal nerve involves testing of all 3 divisions for sensation along all of the peripheral pathways. The examiner should look for sensory sparing at the angle of the jaw which is supplied by the upper cervical roots. Testing of corneal sensation involves a crossed reflex, and involves a motor response from the facial nerve. Thus, touching 1 cornea lightly with a wisp of cotton normally evokes a prompt closure of both eyelids. The masseters are

among the most powerful muscles in the body, and subtle weakness may be difficult to detect. Pterygoid weakness is easier to detect, and the examiner may note jaw deviation toward the affected muscles on jaw opening.

Decreased corneal sensation may lead to corneal abrasions and drying as indicated by marked scleral injection. Treatment includes frequent eye irrigation and use of a lubricating gel with patching of the affected eye, especially at night. If irritation continues, lateral or complete tarsorrhaphy becomes the treatment of choice to avoid corneal ulceration and the development of corneal opacities.

Although injuries to the gasserian ganglion causing dysesthetic pain are rare, as with any peripheral nerve, stretch injuries tend to damage the nerves at fixed attachments at points of sharp angulation (8). Patients with trigeminal injuries may therefore complain of dysesthesias and symptoms of trigeminal neuralgia. Patients may respond to various anticonvulsants including: carbamazepine, gabapentin, lamotrigine, zonisamide, oxcarbazepine, and levetiracetam (33). Nerve block, neurectomy, and decompressive surgery may also be of benefit.

ABDUCENS NERVE (CRANIAL NERVE VI)

The abducens nerve is somatic motor. The nerve originates at the abducens nucleus in the pons; exits the ventral pons near the midline at the pontomedullary junction; pierces the dura lateral to the dorsum sellae of the sphenoid bone; continues forward between the dura and the petrous temporal bone; takes a deep right angle turn; traverses the cavernous sinus and enters the orbit through superior orbital fissure to innervate the lateral rectus muscle. Within the cavernous sinus cranial nerve VI is situated lateral to the internal carotid artery and medial to cranial nerves III, IV, V_1, and V_2. The cranial nerves III, IV, V_1, and V_2 travel through the dural wall, whereas cranial nerve VI does not travel through the dura but is free within the cavernous sinus. Cranial nerve VI palsies are the most commonly reported ocular motor palsies, owing to its long intracranial course (34). This nerve has the longest intracranial course of all the cranial nerves.

Abducens nerve palsy may result from TBI, tumor, diabetes, hypertension, multiple sclerosis, meningitis, blockage of an artery supplying the nerve, aneurysm, surgery, increased pressure within the skull, orbit fractures, hydrocephalus/shunt malfunction. Due to the long course which the abducens nerve travels along the clivus and over the sharp ridge of the petrous temporal bone, it is especially vulnerable to downward traction injury resulting from increased intracranial pressure, and an abducens palsy (unilateral or bilateral) can therefore serve as an early indicator of increased intracranial pressure resulting from a variety of causes (45). Injury to the abducens nerve in association with TBI is reported to occur in 0.4%–4.1% (25).

Cranial nerve VI is often associated with injury to other cranial nerves depending on where, along its course, the abducens nerve is injured. Injury at the abducens nucleus is invariably associated with ipsilateral facial nerve palsy as fascicles of fascial nerve loops around the 6-nerve nucleus. Cranial nerves III, IV, V_1, and V_2 may also be damaged when the injury occurs within the cavernous sinus due to their close proximity. When injured as the nerve passes through the superior orbital fissure, cranial nerves III, IV, and V_1 may be affected as they also pass through the fissure.

The lateral rectus muscle serves to move the eye laterally away from the midline (abduction). The affected eye cannot fully turn outward and may be turned inward when the person looks straight ahead. Double vision results when the person looks toward the side of the affected eye. Coordinated movements of the medial and lateral rectus muscles are required for horizontal movements. If both eyes cannot align on the same target, the visual fields will be projected to different areas of the right and left retinae, resulting in the perception of 2 images.

These individuals have an esotropia that is worsened by lateral gaze, and will often turn their heads laterally toward the paretic side to compensate. To test the abducens nerve function specifically, the patient is instructed to move the eyes through the full extent of the horizontal plane while the examiner looks for deficiency in lateral gaze.

Abducens nerve palsy is usually easy to identify, but the cause is less obvious. In the case of TBI, the cause is often apparent but not necessarily the location of the nerve injury. Injury to the nucleus of the nerve causes complete lack of ipsilateral gaze; injury to the nerve after it comes off the brainstem results in inability to look to the side. Depending on the history and presentation, further work up may be needed. CT scan or MRI may be warranted to exclude tumors. A spinal tap (lumbar puncture) may be useful if meningitis is suspected.

Treatment depends on the cause of the palsy. When the cause is treated, the palsy usually resolves. Abducens nerve palsy following TBI generally resolves over time.

FACIAL NERVE (CRANIAL NERVE VII)

Four modalities are carried by the facial nerve: general sensory (tactile sensation to parts of the external ear, auditory canal, and external tympanic membrane), special sensory (taste sensation to anterior two-thirds of the tongue), branchial motor (muscles of facial expression), and visceral motor (lacrimal glands and mucous membranes of mouth and nose; submandibular and sublingual salivary glands). The sensory components originate in the geniculate ganglion, the branchial motor in the main motor nucleus (pons), and the visceral motor in the superior salivatory nucleus (pons). The facial nerve exits the lower pons laterally and passes through the internal auditory meatus into the middle ear (where the chorda tympani branch arises to carry taste fibers); then enters the facial canal and exits the cranium through the stylomastoid foramen. In the parotid gland, the facial nerve divides into its terminal branches.

The main function of each of the 2 seventh cranial nerves is ipsilateral facial movement including forehead wrinkle, eyelid closure, and movement of half of the face. A message is sent from the motor strip of the cerebral cortex crossing over to stimulate the contralateral cranial nerve VII.

Injury to the facial nerve is the second most common, one-third as common as olfactory nerve palsy (1). Facial nerve injury most commonly occurs within its passage through the temporal bone, although it may occur at any point (13). Facial nerve injury caused by TBI is most commonly peripheral, in association with temporal bone fractures. Temporal bone fractures are most commonly longitudinal accounting for 90% of all temporal bone fractures (14). Transverse fractures of the petrous bone result in immediate and complete cranial nerve VII paralysis in 30%–50% of cases due to tearing of the nerve (13,14). The facial nerve and vestibulocochlear nerve (cranial nerve VIII) course through the petrous bone in close proximity, and thus transverse petrous bone fractures may injure one or both of these nerves. Fractures near the internal auditory meatus usually involve both nerves resulting in ipsilateral facial weakness (i.e., the forehead musculature is involved as well as the face), ageusia in the anterior two-thirds of the tongue, and ipsilateral deafness. Temporal bone fractures further along its course may result in ipsilateral facial weakness (1).

Longitudinal fracture may result in a delay of cranial nerve VII paralysis from 2 to 3 days and up to 2 weeks. Delayed facial weakness, especially in patients with hemotympanum, is indicative of facial nerve swelling in the facial canal. In this setting, corticosteroids should be initiated, otolaryngology consulted, and facial nerve decompression considered (1). The nerve is usually intact and typically recovers within 6–8 weeks (13,14).

Facial nerve palsy may occur from injury anywhere along its course from the cortex to the innervation site. Forehead wrinkle is the one clinical feature that can differentiate the cause of facial weakness. Owing to the bilateral innervation of the upper face by the two cerebral hemispheres, upper motor neuron lesions (lesions above the level of the motor nucleus of cranial nerve VII) only cause contralateral paralysis of the face below the eyes. This occurs because the part of the nucleus that innervates the frontalis and orbicularis muscles continues to receive input from the ipsilateral hemisphere, allowing these muscles to continue functioning. On the other hand, lower motor neuron VII lesions (damage to the facial nucleus or its axons along its course after leaving the nucleus) cause ipsilateral paralysis of the entire face on one side with flattening of the forehead and inability to close the eye. Pontine lesions involving the facial nucleus cause complete ipsilateral facial paralysis along with contralateral hemiparesis (resulting from damage to the descending corticospinal fibers from the motor cortex before crossing over in the medulla), and are often accompanied by lateral rectus muscle paralysis (due to proximity of abducens nucleus to the facial nucleus).

Lesions within the fallopian canal may be localized to 1 of the 3 major segments (mastoid, tympanic, and labyrinthine) based on the presentation. Loss of taste on the ipsilateral anterior two-thirds of the tongue indicates damage of the mastoid segment (which branches into the chorda tympani). Injury to the tympanic segment which serves the stapedius muscle to dampen sound waves may cause hyperacusis (sounds appear excessively loud) and loss of the stapedius reflex, as well as loss of ipsilateral taste. Impaired ipsilateral tear production (in addition to the earlier findings) indicates damage to the labyrinthine segment from which the greater superficial petrosal nerve originates.

Comprehensive examination of the facial nerve involves testing the 5 main functions of this nerve: facial expression, taste, external ear sensation, stapedius muscle function and lacrimal and salivary gland function. First, facial expression in conversation should be observed, followed by requesting performance of specific facial actions: wrinkle forehead by raising eyebrows (frontalis), close eyes tightly (orbicularis oris), press lips firmly together (buccinator and orbicularis oris), smile, and clench jaw (platysma). An enlarged palpebral fissure may be a subtle sign of facial nerve injury. Taste may be tested by using a cotton swab moistened in a sugary or salty solution. The cotton is applied to one side of the protruded tongue, taste identified, cotton applied to other side to test for side-to-side differences; mouth rinsed with water; test repeated with the other solution. This test may be facilitated by using prewritten choices of sweet, sour, bitter, salty to which the person may point. Pain and light touch sensation is tested at the small strip of skin supplied by the facial nerve at the posteriomedial surface of the auricle, although abnormality is rarely detectable. Stapedius muscle function may be tested by having the person compare the loudness of sudden clapping behind each ear. Lacrimal and salivatory function may be assessed by asking about dry eyes, dry mouth, and need for drinking water to swallow food. Lacrimal function may be formally tested using the Schirmer test which a 5 mm by 25 mm piece of filter paper is inserted into the lower conjunctival sac for 5 minutes with less than 10 mm moisture indicating abnormal function. Because of the close proximity to cranial nerve VIII, balance and hearing should also be assessed when cranial nerve VII is found to be damaged.

Electromyography and nerve conduction studies may be helpful in providing prognostic information. Brain imaging may be warranted to aid in distinguishing between central and peripheral lesions. In cases of complete facial nerve disruption, surgical techniques may be helpful such as microsurgical cranial nerve XII crossover to the cranial nerve VII. Nerve-muscle pedicle grafts from the contralateral side may offer more rapid return of nerve function without compromising neck function (35).

Misguided nerve regeneration of the salivary and lacrimal fibers may result in "crocodile tears" (tearing instead of salivation on eating).

Inadequate lid closure may result in drying of the cornea (exposure keratitis). The problem may be further compounded by accompanying loss of corneal sensation (trigeminal nerve) (13). A topical lubricant should be used frequently to protect the eye from dryness. Additional protection may be provided by taping the lid closed with eye pad, although this is not fool proof. In severe cases, tarsorrhaphy (operation to close eye lid) may be required for protection. Surgical implantation of weights (typically gold or platinum) in the eyelid is another technique that is used.

VESTIBULOCOCHLEAR NERVE (CRANIAL NERVE VIII)

Cranial nerve VIII provides special sensory functions of hearing and equilibrium/balance. Disorders of the VIII nerve may result in vertigo, tinnitus, and/or deafness. The vestibular nerve originates at the vestibular ganglion and the cochlear nerve at the spiral ganglion. In the internal auditory meatus the vestibular and cochlear nerves join and enter the brainstem at the cerebellopontine angle. Because the vestibulocochlear nerve is actually 2 distinct nerves that course together in close proximity through the internal auditory meatus and across the cerebellopontine angle, these 2 nerves are usually injured simultaneously. Once synapsing at their nuclei the nerves take different courses, and thus, are less likely to both be injured as they run more proximally. The vestibular nuclei project through the thalamus to the somato-

sensory cortex providing conscious awareness of head position and balance. The cochlear nerve is represented bilaterally via fibers from the ventral cochlear nuclei.

Trauma may cause sensory and conductive types of hearing loss. *Sensory hearing loss* is caused by disruption of the transmission of auditory pathway impulses. Projections from the cochlea run bilaterally. Thus, unilateral central nervous system (CNS) injury alone should not cause hearing loss. *Conductive hearing loss* results from disruption of sound transmission from damage to the tympanic membrane, ossicles, or cochlea. Hearing loss associated with TBI is more commonly sensorineural than conductive (36). Sensorineural hearing loss is reported to occur with TBI at an incidence of 85% and 71% in the absence of temporal bone fracture (36).

Vestibulocochlear nerve injury is common with temporal bone fractures. Of all temporal bone fractures, 80%–90% are longitudinal and 10%–20% transverse (13). The type of temporal bone fracture, transverse or longitudinal, provides a clue as to the injury and type of hearing loss that might result. *Transverse fractures*, which tend to result from frontal or occipital blow, have been reported to result in sensorineural hearing loss in 100% of cases (37). Such injury is thought not to be amenable to surgery (13). On the other hand, *longitudinal fractures* (which occur from temporal or parietal forces) tend to result in conductive hearing loss or mixed conductive and sensorineural hearing loss (37). The incidence of sensorineural or mixed hearing loss in association with longitudinal fracture is 88%. Conductive hearing loss associated with temporal bone fractures occurs because of either ossicular chain disruption or tympanic membrane tear (13). Spontaneous recovery is reported in 80% of patients with conductive hearing loss occurring with temporal bone fractures (38). When conductive hearing loss fails to recover spontaneously, surgery should be considered. Surgical repair is associated with excellent results for all types of conductive hearing loss (37). Disruption at the incudostapedial joint occurs in 82% of cases, fracture of the stapedial arch in 30%, and malleus fracture in 11% (39). In 75% of cases of ossicular chain disruption, the posterior auditory wall is also fractured (13). Although conductive hearing loss is more common with longitudinal fractures, sensorineural or mixed hearing loss may also occur with this type of injury.

Patient examination and hospital record review may reveal important findings often associated with cranial nerve VIII injury by looking for evidence of battle's sign, mastoid fracture, otorrhea, bleeding from the ear, and hemotympanum. Hemorrhage from the ear is a common sign of longitudinal temporal bone fracture. Visualization of the tempanic membrane can be helpful to reveal tears. Cranial nerve VIII is tested through testing eye movements, postural responses, and hearing. These assessments and how they guide lesion localization are discussed in brief detail later.

Vestibular dysfunction may manifest clinically with vertigo, nystagmus, and/or ataxia. Vertigo, the sensation of the room spinning, is a specific symptom of vestibular dysfunction. When the eyes are open, patients see the environment move; and when the eyes closed, patients feel like they are turning or whirling in space. Abnormalities in vestibular testing can be associated with lesions in the vestibular apparatus of the inner ear, the vestibular portion of cranial nerve VIII, the vestibular nuclei in the brainstem, the cerebellum, or pathways in the brainstem (such as the medial longitudinal fasciculus) that connect the vestibular and oculomotor systems. It is through observations of nystagmus and responses to provocative tests that a clinician can narrow down the origin of the problem. Thus, nystagmus elicited with extraocular movement testing, cold water caloric response testing, Dix-Hallpike maneuver, or a rotating chair test (Bárány Test) are key diagnostic tests in the diagnosis of vestibular pathway injury. Accompanying signs and symptoms may also provide clues to distinguish peripheral and vestibular lesions. Peripheral vestibular lesions may be accompanied by ipsilateral hearing loss and tinnitus; whereas central lesions may be associated with motor and sensory disturbances of the limbs, dysarthria, dysphagia or diplopia, indicating additional cranial nerve injuries.

Nystagmus

Nystagmus is the movement of the eye in response to stimulation of the vestibular labyrinth, retro-cochlear pathways, or central vestibulo-ocular pathways. To test for nystagmus, the patient is asked to follow the examiner's finger with the eyes while the examiner's finger moves through horizontal and vertical gaze. There are 2 components to nystagmus: slow and fast. The slow component is caused by vestibular stimulation and is mediated through the 3-neuron arc from the semicircular canals to the extraocular muscles. The fast component returns eyes to the resting position and requires a functioning cerebral cortex. As a result, the fast component will not be present in coma or under general anesthesia. If nystagmus is present, record the directions of the fast-phase and slow-down phases. Nystagmus is described clinically in terms of the direction of the *fast corrective* phase, not the direction of gaze. Nystagmus is a particularly important finding because it is generally not as performance dependent as balance and coordination tests. Electronystagmography (ENG) may be used to quantify the nystagmus and provide information on the suppressive potential of visual fixation. However, ENG is not required for the diagnosis and may be considerably uncomfortable for the patient to endure.

Vertigo

The vertigo presentation and the type of nystagmus present are important as they can help differentiate central (CNS) from peripheral (vestibular) origin. These characteristic features are described here. *Peripheral vertigo*, commonly presenting with vertigo and emesis, is usually characterized by horizontal nystagmus with a rotary component. The fast component points away from the affected side. Duration of peripheral nystagmus is generally minutes to weeks. Some of the causes of peripheral vertigo include: benign positional vertigo, labyrinthitis, vestibular neuronitis, motion sickness, Meniere disease, peripheral vestibulopathy, acoustic neuroma, and perilymphatic fistula. *Central vertigo* may have more insidious onset and produce mild symptoms. Central nystagmus can occur in any direction, and dissociation of movements between the eyes is possible. In central nystagmus, there is no relation between the direction of the nystagmus and the location of the lesion. In general, the following types of nystagmus are central in origin: vertical nystagmus, active nystagmus without vertigo, direction changing/uni-positional nystagmus, gaze paretic nystagmus, nystagmus with disconjugate eye movement, and failure of fixed suppression. Vertical nystagmus is always central in location. Central nystagmus is generally longer in duration and may be present for years. Some of the processes that present with central vertigo are dysfunction of the vestibular portion of cranial nerve VIII, upper and lower brainstem lesions, basilar artery migraines, vertebrobasilar ischemia or infarctions, multiple sclerosis, acute cerebellar lesions (hemorrhage or infarction), cerebellopontine tumors, seizures, and spinocerebellar degeneration. Metabolic causes of vertigo may be appropriate to consider which include drug toxicity, hypoglycemia, and hypothyroidism. The response to provocative tests, as described subsequently, may also help provide such distinction. Most causes of dizziness can be determined by a complete patient history and physical examination including some of the observations described here.

Nylen-Bárány or Dix-Hallpike Positional Testing

This test can help distinguish peripheral from central causes of vertigo. The patient sits on the examining table, rotates the head 45° angle with one ear down, and the examiner supports the patient's head as the patient lays back with the head extending over the edge of the table. The patient is asked to keep their eyes open and report any sensations of vertigo, while the examiner looks for nystagmus. The maneuver is then performed with the opposite ear down. The position change causes maximal stimulation of the posterior semicircular canal of the ear that is down and of the anterior semicircular canal of the ear that is up. With *peripheral lesions*, there is usually a few second delay in the onset of nystagmus and vertigo, which then fades away within approximately 1 minute. The nystagmus is horizontal or rotatory and does not change directions (just as with peripheral nystagmus described in the previous paragraph). If the same maneuver is repeated, there is often adaptation, so that the nystagmus and vertigo are briefer and less intense each time. In *central lesions*, the nystagmus and vertigo generally begin immediately and do not adapt. Nystagmus that persists while in this position but is not present while sitting is indicative of a central vestibular lesion.

Vestibulo-Ocular Reflex (VOR)

This is a simple test that can be performed at the bedside and is used to determine whether or not the vertigo is vestibular in origin. Through the VOR, rapid movement of the head produces an equal and opposite movement of the eyes. This test would only be preformed when there is no suspicion of spinal column instability. The patient fixates on a target while the physician quickly moves the patient's head approximately 15°. When the VOR is intact, the eyes will remain focused immediately on the target after the head is thrust. If the patient must make corrective eye movement to see the target, the VOR is decreased. Corrective eye movements (saccade) with left and right head thrust indicate vestibular dysfunction on the left and right sides, respectively.

Head-Shaking Nystagmus

This is nystagmus that appears after vigorous horizontal head shaking for about 15 seconds, at a frequency of approximately 2 Hz. Head-shaking nystagmus occurs when there are differences in the peripheral vestibular input reaching the central velocity storage mechanism of the brainstem. Thus, a positive head-shake test is suggestive of a peripheral lesion.

Walking With Sudden Turns Test

This test produces veering toward the side of cerebellar or labyrinthine disease. To perform this test, the patient should pivot on given points on the floor.

Fucada Stepping Test

This test is performed by asking the patient to march *in place* with eyes closed for 50 steps at normal walking speed. The examiner makes note of distance and angle of displacement from starting to final standing point, angle of rotation, body sway, changes in head position relative to the body, position of the arms in horizontal or vertical directions. The final standing position is regarded as abnormal if there is more than 30° angle of body rotation or more than 50 cm of displacement from the starting point. Individuals with unilateral vestibular pathology often turn excessively. The test is not specific to vestibular dysfunction but may provide a supportive finding taking other findings into account.

Caloric Stimulation Testing

For individuals in a low neurologic functioning state, assessment of the vestibular system through the aforementioned tests is not possible. In such patients, caloric stimulation testing may be particularly helpful for this purpose. This test is performed with the head of the bed placed at 30° angle to have the horizontal semicircular canal in a vertical plane. The external auditory canal is then irrigated with 30°C water over 30 minutes while direction of eye deviation and nystagmus are observed. With the intact vestibular system, the eyes tonically deviate to the side of cold irrigation, and then after an approximate 20 second latent period is followed by nystagmus to the opposite side that generally lasts 1.5–2 minutes. The procedure is repeated using 44°C water. With warm water irrigation the nystagmus is normally to the side of the irrigation. The normal nystagmus response to caloric testing follows the mnemonic COWS (Cold Opposite Warm Same). When there is dysfunction in the vestibular pathway, this response may be reduced or absent.

Hearing loss can be caused by lesions in the acoustic and mechanical elements of the ear, the neural elements of the cochlea or the acoustic nerve (cranial nerve VIII). There are 3 general types of deafness: conductive, sensorineural, and central. Conductive hearing loss results from a defect in the mechanism by which sound is transformed and conducted to the cochlea as occurs with disorders of the external or middle ear. Sensorineural hearing loss results from disease of the cochlea or of the cochlear division of the eighth cranial nerve. Central hearing loss is caused by lesions of the cochlear nuclei and their connections with the primary receptive areas for hearing in the temporal lobes.

After the hearing pathways enter the brainstem, they cross over at multiple levels and ascend bilaterally to the thalamus and auditory cortex. Therefore, clinically significant unilateral hearing loss is invariably caused by peripheral neural or mechanical lesions, whereas the bilaterality of the CNS connections prevents unilateral central injury from causing significant hearing loss.

Hearing may be assessed at the bedside by seeing if the patient can hear the examiner's fingers rubbed together outside of the auditory canal. Similarly, the patient may be asked to cover one ear while the examiner whispers in the other ear and has the patient repeat what is heard. Testing on the 2 sides is compared. If hearing impairment is detected the cause may be localized and differentiated as sensorineural or conductive using the Rinne and Weber tests.

Rinne Test

For the Rinne test, a 512 Hz tuning fork is placed over the mastoid process (bone conduction) until the patient indicates that the ringing sound is no longer heard, and then the tuning fork is placed a few centimeters from the external auditory canal (air conduction). In this second position of air conduction, sound is normally conducted through the external and middle ear to the cochlea. Normally, the tone is heard better by air conduction, and thus, with normal hearing, the ringing should be heard again in the second position. Not being able to hear the sound again by air conduction implies conductive hearing loss. That is, the problem is in the external or middle ear. With conductive hearing loss, bone conduction is heard as it bypasses problems in the external or middle ear. Rinne test findings in sensorineural hearing loss are the same as with normal hearing; air conduction is greater than bone conduction in both ears, except hearing is decreased in the affected ear.

Weber Test

The Weber test is performed by placing the tuning fork over the middle of the forehead transmitting sound via bone to the cochlea and bypassing the middle ear mechanism. Normally, the sound is heard equally on both sides. In sensorineural hearing loss, the ringing is not as loud on the affected side, while in conductive hearing loss, the ringing is heard louder on the affected side. You can replicate this increase in sound on the side of conduction block by covering and uncovering one ear with the cup of your hand while humming.

Formal audiometry may be helpful to detect and quantify hearing loss, differentiate sensorineural from conductive loss, and guide treatment decisions. In the lower neurologic functioning individual with TBI, brainstem auditory evoked potentials can be used to test the intactness of the auditory pathway. This may be particularly important in helping guide therapy towards more visual stimuli in trying to elicit reactions. CT of the temporal bones may be indicated to assess for skull fracture in the region of the auditory canal.

Treatment of cranial nerve VIII injuries can best be discussed in terms of the two main problems of vestibular and hearing impairment. Hearing loss and vestibular dysfunction may pose significant obstacles to the patient and treatment team in rehabilitation and community integration that should be considered in the rehabilitation program. Treatment of vestibular dysfunction is based on the vestibular system's capacity to habituate to stimuli (13). To decrease the vestibular sensitivity, labyrinthine exercises are used that incorporate equilibrium and righting reflexes (40). Referral to a physical therapists knowledgeable in the diagnosis and treatment of dizziness related to TBI can be a valuable component in the management of this disorder. Medications commonly used for vestibular problems (such as meclazine or dimenhydrinate) are generally not helpful and are discouraged due to potential sedation, cognitive side effects, and prevention of central adaptation (13).

Significant unilateral hearing loss may be improved using a CROS (contralateral routing of signal) type hearing aid which transfers sound to the intact ear (13). Surgical correction is an important consideration for conductive hearing loss that fails to recover spontaneously. For the management of tinnitus, masking sound devices and biofeedback have both been successful in some cases (13) and may be worth consideration.

GLOSSOPHARYNGEAL NERVE (CRANIAL NERVE IX)

The glossopharyngeal nerve serves general, visceral, and special sensory functions, as well as branchial and visceral motor functions. This nerve exits from the jugular foramen in close proximity to the last 3 cranial nerves; therefore, lesions, especially traumatic ones, tend to affect some or all of those nerves. The glossopharyngeal nerve provides general cutaneous function and taste to the posterior one-third of the tongue, and sensation to the soft palate, pharynx, faucil tonsils, tragus of the ear and nasopharynx. Its tympanic branch supplies sensation to the tympanic membrane, eustachian tube, and mastoid area. Chemo and baroreceptors are also carried by the glossopharyngeal nerve from the carotid body and carotid sinus. Its motor fibers innervate the stylopharyngeus muscle and, along with the vagus nerve, the pharyngeal constrictor muscles. Parasympathetic secretory and vasodilatory fibers innervate the parotid gland.

The incidence of glossopharyngeal dysfunction following trauma is 0.5%–1.6% (8). Symptoms include loss of taste over the posterior one-third of the tongue, deviation of the uvula toward the contralateral side, decreased salivation, and slight dysphagia. Examination includes testing oropharyngeal sensation and gag reflex. Loss of sensation to the posterior palate with a subsequent absent gag reflex may place the patient at risk for aspiration. Treatment for an isolated glossopharyngeal nerve injury is symptomatic, because the symptoms are usually minimal. However, injury to the glossopharyngeal nerve usually involves the vagus as well, and thus, may result in severe laryngeal and pharyngeal dysfunction. Treatment of such injuries is covered subsequently.

VAGUS (CRANIAL NERVE X)

The vagus nerve arises from the lateral medulla, leaving the skull through the jugular foramen with the glossopharyngeal and accessory nerves. It contains motor, sensory, and parasympathetic fibers. The vagus nerve supplies motor fibers to all the striated muscles of the pharynx and soft palate except the tensor veli palatini and stylopharyngeus. Through the superior and recurrent laryngeal nerves, the vagus sup-

plies all of the striated muscles of the larynx. Parasympathetic motor fibers supply the smooth muscle of the trachea, bronchi, esophagus, and gastrointestinal tract, and cause gastrin release from the antral mucosa. It also sends inhibitory fibers to the heart muscle, slowing the heart rate, and reducing the amplitude of the heartbeat. Sensory fibers innervate the pharyngeal plexus, larynx, and thoracoabdominal viscera.

The incidence of vagal involvement in TBI is 0.05%–0.16% (8), usually as the result of blunt trauma associated with occipital condyle fractures. Bilateral vagal disruption is fatal.

To examine vagus nerve function, palate elevation and gag reflex are tested. Injury to the vagus nerve, especially the superior and recurrent laryngeal nerves, may result in paralysis of the palate with loss of the gag reflex, dysphagia, aphonia, or hypophonia due to unilateral paralysis of the vocal fold. Alternative feeding techniques should be identified for those at risk for aspiration. Pharyngeal exercises may improve dysarthria in individuals with mild dysfunction (40). Glottic incompetence can be treated by procedures that augment vocal cord bulk such as the injection of Teflon, Gelfoam, or fat. More aggressive surgical procedures such as thyroplasty and arytenoids adduction have been reported beneficial to those with high vagal lesions (41).

SPINAL ACCESSORY (CRANIAL NERVE XI)

The spinal accessory nerve is a pure motor nerve with 2 parts. The cranial part (accessory vagal nerve) arises from the medulla, exits the skull via the jugular foramen, and in conjunction with the vagus nerve, supplies all the intrinsic muscles of the larynx except the cricothyroid. The spinal part (accessory spinal nerve) arises from anterior horn cells of the first through sixth cervical cord segments. The fibers form a trunk that ascends and enters the foramen magnum, where it joins the accessory vagal nerve before exiting the jugular foramen. After joining with the vagus nerve, the fibers split off to descend in the neck to supply the sternocleidomastoid muscle and the upper half of the trapezius.

Trauma, especially from missiles, is the most common cause of spinal accessory nerve dysfunction. Symptoms include the inability to turn the head to the opposite side and ipsilateral shoulder drooping resulting in shoulder dysfunction and pain.

Examination includes testing trapezius function on shoulder shrug, sternocleidomastoid on contralateral head turning, and flaring of the scapula. Aggressive physical therapy should be initiated as soon as possible. Surgical repair of the accessory nerve after sectioning may be possible in some individuals.

HYPOGLOSSAL (CRANIAL NERVE XII)

The hypoglossal nerve serves somatic motor function. It emerges from the medulla and leaves the skull via the hypoglossal canal. It innervates the ipsilateral intrinsic tongue musculature as well as the hyoglossus, styloglossus, genioglossus, and geniohyoid muscles. It is responsible for tongue protrusion to the opposite side.

Injury to the hypoglossal nerve causes dysarthria and dysphagia. Injury to the hypoglossal nerve alone most often occurs with penetrating wounds to the neck and submental region. Ipsilateral atrophy and tongue fasciculations are noted on examination. On protrusion, the tongue deviates toward the lesion by the unopposed, contralateral muscles. With a supranuclear (central) lesion, however, the tongue will deviate opposite the lesion due to contralateral innervation of the brainstem. Examination of hypoglossal nerve function involves noting tongue protrusion. The tongue deviates to the side of the lesion. The presence of dysphagia may indicate the need for swallowing precautions and oral-motor exercises. Exercises for the treatment of dysarthria may help to improve tongue coordination and strength. Treatment of hypoglossal nerve injuries caused by penetrating wounds is surgical, and the nerve tends to recover quite well.

COMMONLY MISSED CRANIAL NERVE INJURIES

Although all cranial nerve injuries can be detected by a sufficiently thorough neurological exam, some cranial nerve injuries are more apt to be detected than others. Because even the most rudimentary neurological exam often includes testing of pupillary reaction to light and because vision problems tend to not go unnoticed by the patient, optic nerve injury is less likely to be missed than many other cranial nerve injuries. Hypoglossal nerve function and sensory function of the trigeminal nerve are also among the most likely cranial nerve functions to be tested, and therefore injuries to those functions are less likely to be missed. Although extraocular movements are commonly tested, injuries to these nerves can be missed if careful attention is not paid to the subtle differences between these nerves that have overlapping functions. For example, because downward eye movement is carried out by both the superior oblique muscle, which is innervated by the trochlear nerve, and the inferior rectus muscle, which is innervated by the oculomotor nerve, the observation of intact downward eye movement after a traumatic brain injury does not necessarily signify that both the superior oblique and the inferior rectus are still innervated, and therefore denervation of either one of these muscles can be missed (and keep in mind that the intact function of some of the oculomotor-innervated muscles does not necessarily guarantee intact function of all of them, because different branches of the nerve can be selectively injured). Therefore, in the case of intact downward eye movement, the only way to truly exclude denervation of both the superior oblique and the inferior rectus is to pay special attention to the functions that distinguish them. Olfactory nerve injury is also likely to be missed initially, due to the simple fact that olfactory sensation is a very commonly overlooked component of the cranial nerve exam, particularly in acute settings such as the emergency room after a trauma. Taste sensation is also commonly overlooked in those situations, and these injuries to the nerve branches involved in taste are also likely to missed initially. In addition, the fact that taste sensation is conveyed by more than 1 cranial nerve and makes injury to 1 of these nerves an easy target for being missed clinically, as evidenced by the fact that patients presenting with Bell Palsy often have taste impairment that has gone unnoticed by the patient and is detected for the first time during careful examination testing different regions of the tongue separately. The underlying theme, therefore, is that although some cranial nerve injuries are commonly missed, this can usually be successfully avoided by performing a very diligent, detailed, and informed cranial nerve examination.

ABERRANT REINNERVATION

After a cranial nerve injury, reinnervation of denervated structures often takes place. This reinnervation can sometimes be aberrant, however, resulting in a phenomenon known as synkinesis, which refers to a unique state of abnormal interactions between nerves and innervated structures. Perhaps the most well-known example is the syndrome of "crocodile tears," which occurs after facial nerve injury, and is characterized by an abnormal relationship between the salivary glands and lacrimal glands that causes the patient to lacrimate while eating. Other examples of synkinesis include aberrant reinnervation of the lateral rectus by the trigeminal nerve (resulting in eye abduction while chewing), as well as a host of aberrant interactions between various extraocular nerves and muscles.

CONCLUSION

Cranial nerve injuries are a common complication of TBI and can significantly impact a patient's quality of life both from a functional standpoint and a cosmetic standpoint. Although much is known about the mechanisms and clinical sequelae of cranial nerve injuries in TBI, one area of knowledge that seems to be lacking in this area is that of treatment. Although surgical treatment is sometimes used for certain injuries involving cranial nerves III, IV, VII, VIII, X, and XI, many of these surgical techniques do not confer consistent results, and many of them result in incomplete treatment such as strabismus surgery for cranial nerve III injury, which has cosmetic benefits but does not repair function. Therefore, an important direction for future research would be to develop newer, more efficacious surgical techniques for restoring cranial nerve function after TBI, and surgical techniques should be developed cranial nerve injuries than what is currently available. In addition, newer nonsurgical methods of cranial nerve injury treatment should be explored. Biofeedback is sometimes used for cranial nerve VIII injuries, and eye exercises are sometimes used for injuries involving the extraocular nerves, so perhaps similar principles can be applied to develop nonsurgical treatments for other cranial nerve injuries. Research aimed at developing a more extensive arsenal for treatment of cranial nerve injuries may significantly improve the quality of life for patients with TBI.

KEY CLINICAL POINTS

1. Cranial nerves provide motor and sensory innervation to the head, neck, viscera, glands, and vasculature and are termed such owing to the fact that they emerge from the cranium.
2. Cranial nerve injury is common with traumatic brain injury (TBI) and can even be seen in cases when the TBI is mild (42).
3. The olfactory nerve (cranial nerve I) is reported to be the most often injured, followed next in frequency by the facial and vestibulocochlear nerves, less commonly the optic and oculomotor nerves, and rarely the trigeminal and lower cranial nerves (1).

4. Cranial nerve palsies may occur with TBI for several reasons, including acceleration–deceleration, shearing forces, skull fracture, intracranial hemorrhage, intracranial mass lesion, uncal herniation, infarct, or vascular occlusion.

5. Cranial nerves are particularly at risk for injury as they traverse over bony protuberances and through bony canals or by direct injury from basilar skull fracture.

6. Injury to the cranial nerves may result in significant consequences to the individual with TBI, which may be further compounded by the deficits caused by cortical injury.

7. In patients with TBI, it is essential to identify any cranial nerve injuries using physical examination and ancillary tests, so that these deficits may be addressed, thereby optimizing clinical outcome and quality of life.

KEY REFERENCES

1. Summary: http://rad.usuhs.mil/cranial_nerves/timrad.html
2. Summary and exam: http://library.med.utah.edu/neurologicexam/html/cranialnerve_anatomy.html#02
3. Video of cranial nerve exam:http://www.sports-anatomy-research.com/clinical-examination-tutorials
4. Wilson-Pauwels L, Akesson EJ, Stewart PA, Spacey SD, eds. *Cranial Nerves in Health and Disease.* 2nd ed. Hamilton, ON: B.C. Decker Inc; 2002.

References

1. Weiner WJ, Goetz CG, eds. *Neurology for the Non-neurologist.* 2nd ed. Philadelphia, PA: JB Lippencott Company; 1989.
2. Zafonte RD, Hammond FM, Peterson J. Predicting outcome in the slow to respond traumatically brain-injured patient: acute and subacute parameters. *NeuroRehab.* 1996;6(1):19–32.
3. Braakman R, Jennett WB, Minderhoud JM. Prognosis of posttraumatic vegetative state. *Acta Neurochir (Wein).* 1988;95(1–2):49–52.
4. Levati A, Farina ML, Vecchi G, Rossanda M, Marrubini MB. Prognosis of severe head injuries. *J Neurosurg.* 1982;57(6):779–783.
5. Narayan RK, Greenberg RP, Miller JD, et al. Improved confidence of outcome prediction in severe head injury. A comparative analysis of the clinical examination, multimodality evoked potentials, CT scanning, and intracranial pressure. *J Neurosurg.* 1981;54(6):751–62.
6. Braakman R, Gelpke GJ, Habbema JD, Maas AI, Minderhoud JM. Systematic selection of prognostic features in patients with severe head injury. *Neurosurgery.* 1980;6(4):362–370.
7. Alexandre A, Colombo F, Nertempi P, Benedetti A. Cognitive outcome and early indices of severity of head injury. *J Neurosurg.* 1983; 59(5):751–761.
8. Keane JR, Baloh RW. Posttraumatic cranial neuropathies. *Neurol Clin.* 1992;10(4):849–867.
9. Rovit RL, Murali R. Injuries to the cranial nerves. In: Cooper PR, ed. *Head Injury.* 3rd ed. Baltimore, MD: Lippincott Williams & Wilkins; 1993.
10. Jennett B, Teasdale G, eds. *Management of Head Injuries.* Philadelphia, PA: F.A. Davis Company; 1981:272–278.
11. Sumner D. On testing the sense of smell. *Lancet.* 1962;2(7262): 895–897.
12. Costanzo RM, Becker DFP. Sense of smell and taste disorders in head injury and neurosurgery patients. In: Meiselman HL, Rivlin RS, eds. *Clinical Management of Taste and Smell.* New York, NY: Macmillan Publishing Co; 1986:565–578.
13. Berrol S. *Cranial nerve dysfunction: physical medicine and rehabilitation: state of the art review.* Vol. 3. Philadelphia, PA: Hanley & Belfus, Inc; 1989:85–93.
14. Horn LJ, Zasler ND, eds. Sensory-perceptual disorders after traumatic brain injury. In: Thomas MD, Zasler ND, eds. *Medical Rehabilitation of Traumatic Brain Injury.* Philadelphia, PA: Hanley & Belfus, Inc; 1996:499–514.
15. Padula WV. Neuro-optometric rehabilitation for persons with a TBI or CVA. *J Optom Vis Devel.* 1992;23:4–8.
16. Glaser RA. *Neuro-opthalmology.* Baltimore, MD: Harper and Row; 1978:126.
17. Canavero S. Dynamic reverberation. A unified mechanism for central and phantom pain. *Med Hypotheses.* 1994;42(3):203–207.
18. Awerbuch GI, Sandyk R. Mexiletine for thalamic pain syndrome. *Int J Neurosci.* 1990;55(2–4):129–133.
19. Spoor TC, McHenry JG. Management of traumatic optic neuropathy. *J Craniomaxillofac Trauma.* 1996;2(1):14–26.
20. Li KK, Teknos TN, Lai A, Lauretano A, Terrell J, Joseph MP. Extracranial optic nerve decompression: a 10-year review of 92 patients. *J Craniofac Surg.* 1999;10(5):454–459.
21. Levin LA, Beck RW, Joseph MP, Seiff S, Kraker R. The treatment of traumatic optic neuropathy: the International Optic Nerve Trauma Study. *Ophthalmology.* 1999;106(7):1268–1277.
22. Steinsapir KD. Traumatic optic neuropathy. *Curr Opin Ophthalmol.* 1999;10(5):340–342.
23. Padula WV, Shapiro JB. Head injury and the post-trauma vision syndrome. *Review.* 1993;24:153–158.
24. Kerkhoff G. Rehabilitation of visuospatial cognition and visual exploration in neglect: a cross-over study. *Restor Neurol Neurosci.* 1998; 12(1):27–40.
25. Keane JR. Neuro-ophthalmic signs and symptoms of hysteria. *Neurology.* 1982;32(7):757–762.
26. Obyan A, Zafonte R, Hammond F. Occipital status epilepticus: an unusual cause of post-traumatic blindness. *Arch Phys Med Rehabil.* 1995;76(11):1085.
27. Sabates NR, Gonce MA, Farris BK. Neuro-ophthalmological findings in closed head trauma. *J Clin Neuroophthalmol.* 1991;11(4):273–277.
28. Tokuno T, Nakazawa K, Yoshida S, et al. Primary oculomotor nerve palsy due to head injury: analysis of 10 cases [in Japanese]. *No Shinkei Geka.* 1995;23(6):497–501.
29. Vaughn D, Asbury T. *General Ophthalmology.* Los Altos, CA; Lange Medical Publications; 1974:182.
30. Lagrèze WA. Neuro-ophthalmology of trauma. *Curr Opin Ophthalmol.* 1998;9(6):33–39.
31. Beauchamp GR, Black BC, Coats DK, et al. The management of strabismus in adults—I. Clinical characteristics and treatment. *J AAPOS.* 2003;7(4):233–240.
32. Dacey RG, Jane JA. Craniocerebral trauma. In: Baker AB, Baker IH, eds. *Clinical Neurology.* Rev ed. Philadelphia, PA: Harper and Row; 1987:1–61.
33. Backonja MM. Use of anticonvulsants for treatment of neuropathic pain. *Neurology.* 2002;59(5)(suppl 2):S14–S17.
34. *Rosen's Emergency Medicine: Concepts and Clinical Practice.* 4th ed. Mosby-Year Book, Inc;1998:1278.
35. Kay PP, Kinney SE, Levine H, Tucker HM. Rehabilitation of facial paralysis in children. *Arch Otolaryngol.* 1983;109(10):642–647.
36. Podoshin L, Fradis M. Hearing loss after head injury. *Arch Otolaryngol.* 1975;10(1):15–18.
37. Sismanis A. Post-concussive neuro-otological disorders. *Phys Med Rehab: State of the Art Reviews.* 1992;6(1):79–88.
38. Tos M. Prognosis of hearing loss in temporal bone fractures. *J Laryngol Otol.* 1971;85(11):1147–1159.
39. Hough JV. Restoration of hearing loss after head trauma. *Ann Otol Rhinol Laryngol.* 1969;78(2):210–226.
40. Tangeman PT, Wheeler J. Inner ear concussion syndrome: vestibular implications and physical therapy treatment. *Top Acute Care Rehabil.* 1986;1:72–73.
41. Yorkston KM, Beukelman DR, Strand EA, Bell KR. *Management of Motor Speech Disorders.* 2nd ed. Austin, TX: Pro-ed, Inc; 1999.
42. Coello AF, Canals AG, Gonzalez JM, Martín JJ. Cranial nerve injury after minor head trauma. *J Neurosurg.* 2010;113(3):547–555.
43. Jin H, Wang S, Hou L, et al. Clinical treatment of traumatic brain injury complicated by cranial nerve injury. *Injury.* 2010;41(9):918–923.
44. Souayah N. *Specialty Board Review: Neurology.* 2nd ed. McGraw Hill; 2010:22.
45. Blumenfield H. *Neuroanatomy through Clinical Cases.* Sinauer Associates, Inc; 2002:540.

Fatigue: Assessment and Treatment

Michael Henrie and Elie P. Elovic

INTRODUCTION

Fatigue is a commonly reported symptom following traumatic brain injury (TBI), yet it is both poorly understood and challenging to treat. The word symptom is used in contradistinction to diagnosis because fatigue in general and specifically in TBI is problematic to define and operationalize. Because TBI is a descriptive term for a heterogeneous collection of injuries to the brain that can result in physical, behavioral, cognitive, or emotional dysfunction, it has been particularly vexing to determine the origin of and how to best characterize post-traumatic fatigue (PTF). As a result, the determination of its incidence has been problematic. Some past attempts to quantify its incidence in TBI have placed the range between 21% and 73 % (1–3). There has been some criticism of these numbers as the reporting was based on reporting on the presence or absence of fatigue. More recently, a study was performed by Englander et al. (4) who reported a rate of between one-third and one-half when using more formalized metrics, including the Fatigue Severity Scale (FSS) and the Multidimensional Assessment of Fatigue (MDAF). PTF affects not only an individual's emotional well-being but may potentially also affect functional recovery from brain injury. Kreutzer et al. (5) reported an incidence of 46% among persons in an outpatient TBI clinic and suggested that further information needs to be gathered regarding prognostication and the efficacy of treatment alternatives. Although the overall burden of fatigue in this population is not precisely known, probably secondary to its multifaceted nature, individuals with TBI clearly suffer from fatigue with resultant diminished functioning in multiple spheres of cognition, quality of life, and activities of daily living (ADLs). This functional limitation is especially problematic because one must be able to sustain purposeful, goal-directed mental effort to function independently. Classically, clinicians who attended to persons with TBI often possessed few diagnostic and/or therapeutic resources to offer accurate assessment and treatment. Recently, however, several new and sophisticated neuroimaging tools and techniques have helped to begin unraveling the underlying pathophysiology of PTF and should soon reveal more about diagnosis and treatment. The following discussion will review the available knowledge concerning fatigue in the TBI population. Our intent is to simultaneously educate and increase readers' interest and understanding of fatigue; to promote research in this critical area, leading to productive, multidisciplinary efforts addressing the problem of fatigue;

and to facilitate the development of treatment protocols through the identification of possible fatigue-generating mechanisms. Meanwhile, the state of the art approach to managing PTF is offered.

For the following discussion, TBI will be defined using the well-established definition advanced by the TBI Model Systems Task Force: "damage to brain tissue caused by an external mechanical force, as evidenced by loss of consciousness, post-traumatic amnesia, skull fracture, or objective neurological findings that can be reasonably attributed to TBI on physical examination or mental status examination" (6).

DEFINITION

Prior to embarking on a further discussion of PTF, a working definition should be developed. It is important to recognize that no universally accepted definition or broad consensus on a conceptual framework of fatigue exists. Nevertheless, discussions in the fatigue literature make a distinction between central fatigue, which results from dysfunction of supratentorial structures involved in mentation, vs peripheral fatigue, which is of a more purely physical, metabolic, or muscular origin. Clearly, it is the central type that is of greatest interest regarding those with isolated TBI. Beyond this dichotomy, the debate over PTF or fatigue in general has moved beyond the idea of fatigue as a unitary concept and toward a belief that fatigue is multifaceted (7–9), with components likely arising from distinct mechanisms and brain networks (10). Additionally, fatigue must be differentiated from excessive daytime sleepiness (EDS). The latter is common following TBI (11) and remains a separate but related construct. This differentiation can be difficult because fatigue and EDS often coexist.

Lezak's reductionist, "fatigue needs no definition" (12), may be the battle cry of the lumpers in this debate; however, such a pronouncement does little to advance our understanding of this phenomenon and for the development of effective treatment strategies. On the other end of the spectrum, Chauduri and Behan (13) carefully define PTF as ". . . the failure to initiate and/or sustain attentional tasks and physical activities requiring self-motivation (as opposed to external stimulation) . . ." and they lay out an elegant clinico-anatomic, pathophysiological explication of why fatigue follows acquired brain injury. Clinical experience echoes their definition in that fatigue impacts on cognitive function (14,15), quality of life, well-being (16), return to work (17), and the ability to perform ADLs.

Historically, various surrogates, markers, synonyms, and clinical imitators of fatigue have been pursued in the literature, leading the casual reader astray from a purer characterization of the fatigue that follows TBI. Yet, almost paradoxically, as the research on the essence of fatigue becomes more focused, the less singular a phenomenon it appears to be. Thus, even as one measures, correlates, and localizes the fundamental components of fatigue, the syndrome or symptom cannot merely be appreciated in isolation. Rather, fatigue must be appreciated in its full context, across various domains and with the understanding that the fatigue experience is not static or constant. Ultimately, the clinical picture of PTF that emerges is colored and textured by a multitude of primary, secondary, and even tertiary factors that reliably engender the principle aspects of fatigue for persons with TBI. The current discussion hopes to elucidate the most likely generators of PTF and critique the current literature, as well as propose an operational definition based on the most appropriate measurement tools for its assessment.

EPIDEMIOLOGY

Currently employed methods of surveillance for disease burden because of TBI do not collect information beyond that of the total number of emergency department visits and the total number of hospitalizations. Moreover, most TBI's are deemed mild and the Centers for Disease Control and Prevention has labeled this variant the "silent epidemic" because many such cases never receive medical attention. Consequently, the magnitude of the problem of fatigue among all TBI survivors or that subset who are "permanently disabled" is not directly known. Disappointingly, even databases developed through the comprehensive TBI Model Systems are simply silent with respect to surveillance of PTF or its consequences. Thus, TBI stands as a persistent public health burden that, despite primary prevention successes, will likely continue to grow because of the increasing sophistication and effectiveness of contemporary emergency care further resulting in a growing prevalence of TBI-associated problems, such as fatigue. In most studies, PTF is evaluated predominantly by self-report—in other words, subjectively. Several investigators over the last several decades have attempted to identify the incidence or prevalence of fatigue in the TBI population, but these studies have not always been adequately controlled for such common confounds as anxiety and depression. Lezak (12) identified fatigue as one of the "subtle" sequelae of brain damage, along with distractibility and perplexity, and compared the incidence of fatigue between those patients seen in consultation, (i.e., relatively briefly), with those enrolled in detailed, longitudinal research protocols. Forty-two percent of 50 subjects reported fatigue if examined once and 60% if examined more often. Among the group in research studies ($n = 46$) the reporting of fatigue reached an astounding 98%. This study exposes how a methodological flaw can seriously compromise the estimated incidence of PTF. The marked discrepancy suggests that thoroughness of assessment is essential and that without such an approach, patients are at risk for having their fatigue go unrecognized, especially as TBI severity in-

creases and with it, cognitive dysfunction such as memory and self-awareness.

Middleboe et al. (1) analyzed a cohort of 51 patients with mild TBI and noted that 21% reported fatigue 1 year postinjury. Olver et al. (3) studied fatigue over a longer follow-up period, his group followed 254 patients who had been hospitalized for their TBI at 2 years, and 103 patients at 5 years. Most of these patients had suffered a severe injury as reflected by a mean Glasgow Coma Scale score of 5.1. Fatigue was reported by 68% at 2 years, and 73% at 5 years. Masson et al. (18) studied a group of 231 adults 5 years after injury. The sample was stratified with respect to TBI severity and in addition, a lower limb injury cohort was used for comparison. Among the 4 groups, 30.6% of limb injured, 35.1% of mild TBI, 32.4% of moderate TBI, and 57.7% of severe TBI subjects endorsed fatigue suggesting an association between severity of brain injury and fatigue incidence. Hillier et al. (2) examined a cohort of 67, primarily of people with severe brain injury and noted a fatigue self-report rate of 37% 5 years post-TBI. This number may be artificially low in light of the under self-reporting noted by Lezak especially because the overwhelming majority of patients in this study were severely injured (73%) and likely to have disabling cognitive impairments. Kreutzer et al. (5) examined the epidemiology of depression in a cohort of 722 TBI outpatients on an average 2.5 years after injury and with a mean duration of unconsciousness of 10 days. The self-report of fatigue in this severely injured group was 46%, and fatigue was the most frequently reported problem. Norrie et al (19) studied 263 patients with mild TBI at 1 week, 3 months, and 6 months postinjury. The prevalence of fatigue was 68%, 38%, and 34%, respectively. In this study, the prevalence decreased the first 3 months then stabilized. Early fatigue and depression were predictors of late fatigue. Unfortunately, patients were not studied beyond 6 months. However, Bushnik et al. (20) studied a cohort of patients with TBI at 1 and 2 years postinjury. There was no significant change in the amount of patients reporting fatigue at 1 year (16%–32%) and 2 years (21%–34%).

From epidemiological studies that were based on self-report, PTF ranges from 2% to 98% (21). What remains unclear from these reports is how fatigue impacts mentation and on function. Limited formal neuropsychological evidence exists to elucidate the effect of PTF on cognitive performance. Additionally, the natural history of fatigue remains unclear, as well as the associations between fatigue and a multitude of TBI-specific factors, such as length of coma, duration of post-traumatic amnesia, and mechanism of injury. Finally, it is still unclear how the incidence and magnitude of fatigue interrelate, affect, and are affected by other common TBI sequelae.

ASSESSMENT

To date, there is no single measurement instrument that has been validated to study PTF. Nevertheless, it is important to continue assessing the impact of PTF. Efforts at the assessment of PTF have been complicated by its multifaceted nature, and many measures that are commonly used rely on subjective reporting. To date, several scales have been used

TABLE 42-1 Metrics Used to Measure Fatigue

METRIC	KEY FEATURES
Visual Analogue Scale	Ease of administration
Epworth Sleepiness Scale	Measures daytime sleepiness rather than fatigue
Fatigue Severity Scale (FSS)	Score is an average of 9 items, each rated 1–7 Measures impact of scale, not actual fatigue
Fatigue Impact Scale	40-item questionnaire More intensive evaluation of fatigue's impact on life function than FSS Takes longer to administer
Barrow Neurologic Institute Fatigue Scale	Designed for use early in the injury
Modified Fatigue Impact Scale (FIS)	Modification from FIS Primarily designed for use in MS

Abbreviation: MS, multiple sclerosis.

to evaluate fatigue in TBI (7) (see Table 42-1). The FSS (9), Fatigue Impact Scale (FIS) (15), the Modified Fatigue Impact Scale (MFIS), the Barrow Neurologic Institute Fatigue Scale (BNI), and the Cause of Fatigue Questionnaire (COF). The FSS (9) is assessed by having participants rate 9 different questions rating one's fatigue from 1 (*low*) to 7 (*high*). The FSS is the average of these 9 values. The FIS (15) is a 40-item questionnaire that the person rates from 0 (*no problems*) to 4 (*severe problems*). These items are grouped into 3 separate functional categories: physical, cognitive, and psychosocial. The MFIS is a 21-item derivative of the FIS that is more commonly used in the multiple sclerosis (MS) population. The BNI (22) assesses people with brain injury in early stages of recovery by asking them to describe their difficulty on 10 fatigue-related items using a 0–7 scale.

In an effort to delineate both subjective and objective assessment of fatigue, Lachapelle and Finlayson (23) evaluated 30 subjects with TBI with a mean of 44.3 months after injury and compared them to an age and gender matched healthy control group. The study purported to parse fatigue into objective and subjective components; the paradigm for objective fatigue measurement was a continuous thumb-pressing task. Over time, normal and TBI groups demonstrated a decline in the number of repetitions per unit of time; however, the difference was statistically insignificant. The subjective evaluation of fatigue was quantified by the visual analogue, the FSS, and FIS scales. Despite the statistical parity on the objective measure, patients with TBI demonstrated significantly greater subjective fatigue scores on the FSS and FIS vs normal controls. Likewise, Walker et al. (21) looked at the measures of quadriceps strength and physical endurance to test those complaining of PTF vs normal and found no statistical difference. Researchers trying to characterize peripheral fatigue recognize the significant impact on challenging physical actions facing those with brain trauma, such as mobility, ADLs, and sustaining endurance for a given task. Brain trauma often involves lesions of central pathways governing simple and complex motor function,

for instance, resulting in hemiplegia, spasticity, ataxia, or the upper motor neuron syndrome with various well-known positive and negative signs and static and dynamic disturbances. Given the working definition of peripheral fatigue as "any reduction of maximal force output" (24), it is easily appreciated how impaired motor and sensory (modulation) centers translate into increased energy demands and reduced efficiency of ambulation, for example, quickly resulting in a fatigued individual. Thus, although some effort has been made to distinguish central from peripheral fatigue in theory, there remains such overlap that no specific study targeting this distinction has yet been published.

Therefore, the tools currently available allow only for crude assessment, leaving the clinician sliding either way on a slippery slope because even purely peripheral fatigue must necessarily be perceived by and processed within the context of the central nervous system (CNS). It should, thus, not be surprising that so frequent a dichotomy exists between what is measured and what is perceived.

General Medical Workup in the Fatigued Patient

Neurogenic fatigue related to TBI is a diagnosis of exclusion, and other causes should be investigated. The differential diagnosis is broad and outlined in Table 42-2. A systematic approach to evaluation guided primarily by clinical history is appropriate. The history should attempt to characterize the patient's fatigue, evaluating the onset and duration of symptoms and how physical activity, cognitive activity, and rest impacts symptoms. Fatigue must be differentiated from apathy and boredom. Although boredom and fatigue may present in a similar fashion, boredom generally responds to changes in activity or environment. Fatigue must also be differentiated from sleepiness, with the latter typically responding to the appropriate application of rest. Risk factors associated with fatigue should be identified. A detailed review of medications should also be undertaken as many medications, including those commonly used in TBI rehab, can cause fatigue (see Table 42-3). Additionally, a psychiatric screening and a detailed review of quality and quantity of sleep should be performed. The physical examination can assist in ruling out specific causes of fatigue. Examination begins with assessing the general appearance. The examination of individual body systems should be guided by the history. In the absence of history and physical examination findings, laboratory analysis is not usually helpful. However, initial testing should probably include erythrocyte sedimentation rate (ESR), complete blood count, chemistry panel, liver panel, and fasting blood glucose. Additional testing should depend on the clinical evaluation. If hypopituitarism is suspected, measurement of the basal anterior pituitary hormones should be obtained. The presence of risk factors of an infectious etiology should prompt additional testing (i.e., human immunodeficiency virus [HIV], hepatitis serology, Epstein Barr, etc.). Signs and symptoms of cardiopulmonary disease, autoimmune disease, and malignancy should also be considered and further evaluated if necessary. Finally, Table 42-4 is a brief description of some of the more commonly seen causes for fatigue and recommended items for evaluation.

TABLE 42-2 Differential Diagnosis of Fatigue[a]

Cardiopulmonary	**Heart failure**
	Acute myocardial ischemia
	Atrial fibrillation
	COPD
	Obstructive sleep apnea
Metabolic	**Anemia**
	Iron deficiency without anemia
	Vitamin D deficiency
Endocrine	**Diabetes mellitus**
	Hypothyroidism and hyperthyroidism
	Hypopituitarism
	Addison disease
Neurologic	**Stroke**
	Restless leg syndrome
	Multiple sclerosis
	Parkinson disease
Psychiatric	**Depression**
	Alcohol dependence
	Drug dependency
Infectious	Epstein Barr virus
	HIV
	Tuberculosis
	Toxoplasmosis
	Cytomegalovirus
	Lyme disease
	Brucellosis
Gastrointestinal	Celiac disease
	Primary biliary cirrhosis
Neoplastic	Myelodysplastic syndrome
	Chronic myeloid leukemia
	Non-Hodgkin lymphoma
	Hodgkin lymphoma
	Other malignancy
Other	**Primary insomnia**
	Medication-induced fatigue
	Chronic renal disease
	Fibromyalgia
	Systemic lupus erythematosus
	Chronic fatigue syndrome

Abbreviation: COPD, chronic obstructive pulmonary disease; HIV, human immunodeficiency virus.
[a]Common diagnoses are in bold.

TABLE 42-3 Common Medications Associated With Fatigue

MEDICATIONS FREQUENTLY ASSOCIATED WITH FATIGUE	MEDICATIONS COMMONLY USED IN TBI REHABILITATION
Antiepileptics	Levetiracetam, carbamazepine, valproate
Antihistamines	
Antipsychotics, typical and atypical	Olanzapine, quetiapine, clozapine
Corticosteroids	
Antiarrhythmics	Propranolol, verapamil
Antidepressants	SSRIs, trazadone, tricyclic antidepressants
Antiemetics	Phenergan, zofran

Abbreviation: SSRIs, selective serotonin reuptake inhibitors.

known pathophysiological mechanisms. For instance, TBI may include focal or diffuse, hemorrhagic or nonhemorrhagic, coup and contrecoup, contusional, and compressive (epidural and subdural), as well as numerous secondary and clinically superimposed causes of CNS tissue damage. Because natural traumatic forces never injure the brain in exactly the same way, the various neural circuits that support optimal cognition are differentially impaired. This leads to different degrees of cognitive dysfunction from individual to individual, further permutated by the occurrence of damage within the context of each brain's unique set of premorbid strengths and weaknesses. From a strictly statistical standpoint, the generally fatigued brain may yield a potentially infinite number of specific patterns of underperformance.

The multiple structures subserving arousal are known collectively as the ascending reticular activating system (ARAS) (Figure 42-1), emanating from the brainstem and represented in each of its 3 divisions by the following nuclei:

Medulla: raphe and reticularis ventralis (serotonergic)
Pons: parabrachialis (cholinergic), locus ceruleus (noradrenergic), reticularis pontis oralis and caudalis, and the gigantocellularis

TABLE 42-4 Medical Workup for Common Etiologies of Fatigue

Iatrogenic	Medication review
Depression	History
	Depression inventory
Cardiovascular	History, EKG, echo, stress testing, cardiac catheterization
Endocrine	History and laboratory analysis for hormonal evaluations (74)
Neurologic	History, neurological examination, imaging
Infectious	Organism specific, CBC, ESR, chest xray
Insomnia	ESS, sleep diary, overnight pulse oximetry, sleep study

Abbreviations: EKG, electrocardiography; CBC, complete blood count; ESR, erythrocyte sedimentation rate; ESS, Epworth Sleepiness Scale.

MECHANISMS

The biological "substrate" of fatigue in normal individuals is not known. Furthermore, the study of PTF is made more difficult by the fact that, in our clinical experience, this symptom does not occur in isolation but rather is part of a broader array of signs and symptoms postinjury. Functional neuroimaging reflects yet another level of inquiry into the morphology of the fatigued brain, attempting to correlate anatomy with task-specific activity.

Anatomical

Given the heterogeneity and variety of lesions from TBI, a discussion of the source of fatigue should begin with a consideration of the underlying neuroanatomy associated with

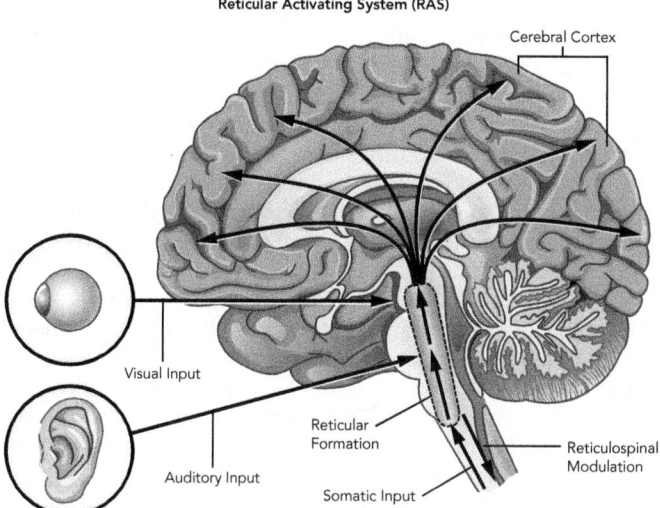

Reticular Activating System (RAS)

FIGURE 42-1 The reticular activating system regulates sleep/wake cycles and is composed of several neuronal pathways connecting the brainstem to the cortex.

Midbrain: pedunculopontine tegmental (PPT) and laterodorsal tegmental (LDT) nucleus (cholinergic); raphe (serotonergic) and ventral tegmental area (VTA) (dopaminergic).

The outputs from these structures coalesce into 2 pathways: the ventral and dorsal pathways of the reticular activating system (RAS). The ventral pathway terminates in the subthalamus and posterior hypothalamus, which in turn send histaminergic fibers to a broad array of cortical end points. In addition, the ventral pathway contains a projection via the medial forebrain bundle (MFB) to the septal nucleus and basal forebrain, which in turn send a broad array of cholinergic fibers to the cortex. The dorsal pathway projects to the interlaminar nucleus of the thalamus from which, in turn, glutaminergic tracts emerge to project across a variety of cortical and striatocortical end points (25).

The ARAS is a fundamental structure maintaining arousal as a prelude to alertness and bilateral injures in the brainstem nuclei that result in loss of consciousness (26). This system, however, is a part of a larger and more complex system, which maintains sensory attention and tonic arousal. When there is sufficient diffuse damage (DAI) to tracts or pathways mediating general arousal, immediate unconsciousness continues over a period of variable duration depending on the extent of damage (see Chapter 11). Therefore, a frequent and major component of TBI is injury of the axonal connections leading to a disruption in the neuroanatomical structures maintaining arousal. DAI thus results in insufficient amounts of neurotransmitters normally released by more caudal structures reaching their targets, yielding an unstable platform from which to launch desired cognitive processes and behaviors, including fundamental elements subserving cognition, such as attention and processing speed. Moreover, as mentioned by Arciniegas and Silver (27), damage to white matter results in inefficient and slowed information processing.

Basal Ganglia

In their review article, the investigators Chauduri and Behan (13) offer the hypothesis that the basal ganglia (BG) are the neuroanatomical site at which fatigue is generated following neurological injury. Specifically, they identify the disruption of 2 "loops": the striatocortical fibers and the striato-thalamo-cortical fibers as the mechanism responsible for central fatigue. Such critical pathways have been carefully delineated over the last 2 decades and now reveal influential and tight connections between the striatum of BG and a key component of limbic signaling: the archistriatum or amygdala. The limbic system clearly provides a route by which unconscious, spontaneous, emotionally driven motivational forces may exert influence on the motor system, thereby altering the chances that goal-directed behaviors get initiated and sustained.

In bilateral BG damage, a lack of drive, initiation, and motivation is often encountered. This is termed *abulia* when severe. When mild, it may be misinterpreted or overlooked altogether and is usually identified as mere apathy by rehabilitation team members. A dopaminergic pathway called the mesencephalofrontal activating system (MFAS) projects from the VTA of the midbrain to frontal regions, especially cingulate gyrus and drives internal states toward motivated behavior. Thus, under normal circumstances, initiation and sequential performance of a task require an internally driven mechanism integrated at the level of the BG to prepare the emotive, motor, and sensory apparatus responsible for the next and subsequent set of responses. Disruption of these algorithms of the sequential task processing mechanism would have the effect of not only delaying initiation but also preventing the seamless, well-timed execution of the target task (13).

Although direct support for their theory is lacking, if it is placed within the context of the ARAS as the "substrate" for maintaining alertness, then fatigue may represent a decrease in this normal state of alertness. How this occurs is not known; however, Whyte et al. (28) have demonstrated how difficulty sustaining arousal and attention post-TBI affects cognition. They compared a cohort of 26 patients with TBI with normal controls using a visual vigilance task. The results revealed "severe TBI does result in difficulties maintaining stable performance over time in an attention-demanding task, independent of specific distracting events." Although there was no formal assessment of fatigue in the TBI cohort in this study, the authors hypothesize that this inability to sustain performance reflects declining arousal or increasingly frequent lapses of attention. In a separate paper, Whyte drew a distinction between the tonic and phasic arousal. The former term is used to describe baseline alertness and wakefulness, whereas the latter refers to the arousal that is demonstrated in response to stimuli or as demanded by a distinct task. This runs parallel to the concept of the ARAS as not only mediating tonic activation and arousal but also playing an important role in the ability to phasically turn on cortical tissue in an efficient manner to perform on demand.

This concept is also reflected by Heilman and Valenstein's (29) assertion that "brain regions . . . are essentially silent unless and until activated by release of the appropriate transmitter . . ." Thus, PTF may be conceptualized as an inability not only to activate but also to efficiently sustain and recruit cortical tissue subserving cognitive tasks.

Riese et al. (30) attempted to study the impact of central (mental) fatigue on cognition. These investigators studied 8 young severely injured patients with TBI for more than 9 months postinjury. All of the patients studied had suffered not only severe but also diffuse injury, and in fact, 1 inclusion criterion was "no documented focal lesions." Fatigue was not assessed via self-report. Rather, the authors assessed the ability to sustain workload via a "continuous dynamic divided attention task." The study findings revealed no difference between control and TBI subject groups in terms of the effect of "task load" on performance, but an increased amount of mental effort was required among the TBI cohort for maintaining the task. The finding of increased mental effort among the TBI cohort was corroborated through both subjective and physiological indicators of distress. The relationship between subjective fatigue and selective attention deficits in patients with TBI has been investigated by Ziino and Ponsford (31). They studied 46 patients with mild to severe TBI and 46 controls. Their metrics included Visual Analogue Scale-Fatigue (VAS-F), FSS, COF, and attentional measures, including subtests from the Test of Everyday Attention and the Complex Selective Attention Task. TBI participants reported greater levels of subjective fatigue; they also performed more slowly and reported more errors on attentional tasks. The findings suggested a relationship between subjective fatigue and impairment with tasks that require higher attentional processes. In another study, Ziino and Ponsford (32) examined the relationship between vigilance and subjective fatigue. Forty-six participants with TBI and 46 controls completed the VAS-F and a selective attention task before and after a vigilance task. Their findings suggested that the increased psychophysiologic costs expended on patients with TBI were associated with increased subjective fatigue. Johansson et al. (33) assessed patients with TBI for subjective fatigue, information processing speed, working memory, and attention. They concluded that a relationship was present between information processing speed and subjective mental fatigue. Belmont et al. (34) studied 27 patients with subacute and chronic TBI. Subjective fatigue levels were measured (FSS and VAS-F) in the TBI and control group before and after a long duration selective attention task. Participants also rated their perceived degree of mental effort. The TBI group exhibited significant correlations between decreased performance on attention tasks, mental effort, and increased subjective fatigue.

The presumed increase in mental effort needed to overcome impaired attention, and processing speed has been referred to as the "coping hypothesis" (7). Although these studies do not conclusively define a relationship between post-TBI cognitive impairments and increased central fatigue, they certainly add support to the "coping hypothesis." It is certainly conceivable that this increased effort may contribute to perceived fatigue.

Two functional magnetic resonance imaging (fMRI) studies may offer 1 possible explanation for the findings noted in the studies discussed earlier. The first study by Christodoulou et al. (35) examined the differences in cortical activation in 7 controls vs 9 TBI subjects while performing the modified paced auditory serial addition task (mPASAT), a progressively more difficult computation task commonly used to assess working memory. Impairments in working memory among TBI subjects resulted not surprisingly in a higher incidence of error on the mPASAT test but interest-ingly, fMRI scanning further revealed a more regionally dispersed and more lateralized pattern of cerebral activation. Kohl et al. (36) used fMRI to assess cognitive fatigue in 11 patients with moderate or severe TBI and matched them to 11 "healthy" controls. The activity performed was a modified Symbol Digit Modalities Test. They found that patients with TBI exhibited increased activity, whereas controls exhibited decreased activity in several regions, including the BG, anterior cingulate gyrus, middle frontal gyrus, and superior parietal cortex.

This increased level of cortical activation for a given task likely reflects not only inefficiency in "phasic" recruitment of cortical assets but also suggests that the inefficiency results in increased metabolic demands as visualized on the fMRI images. The increased amount of cortex required per task in TBI vs normal controls is accompanied by the perception of greater mental effort as well.

Therefore, informed speculation leads the clinician to identify motor coordination centers (BG), executive and motor planning areas (frontal circuits), and internal motivational apparatus (hypothalamus and related limbic structures) as the main arbiters of fatigue-associated behavior. When 1 or more of these systems is affected, individuals routinely fail to complete the execution of incremental or serial tasks that demand sustained motivation and attention.

Functional

In seeking an all-inclusive, unifying theory of the mechanism of PTF, the contribution of several clinically encountered factors cannot be ignored. Clinicians will certainly recognize the recurring theme of 1 symptom or system dysfunction reflexively exacerbating another component of the index disease. For example, mood disturbances will impact on sleep/wake cycles which, when disturbed, tend to amplify mood disorders. Pain (frequently encountered with comorbid multicervical or craniocervical trauma) puts the individual at higher risk for mood and sleep disturbance, and conversely, those with dysfunctional mood or sleep are more apt to experience magnified pain (37–39). It is easy to appreciate how these interactions pose a mounting burden that cumulatively impedes optimal cognitive function. Perhaps, at its simplest mechanistic level, PTF represents and reflects the final common pathway's *product* of neural processing, impaired by some combination of primary damage and secondary or tertiary factors impeding cohesive, efficient, and coordinated cognitive output.

OTHER COMPONENTS OF TRAUMATIC BRAIN INJURY-RELATED FATIGUE

In addition to primary neurological injury, there are many other factors that can impact both the functional and subjective reporting of fatigue in populations other than TBI. Because they are also found in TBI, such factors can also likely impact PTF. The following sections discuss these issues.

Psychology/Psychiatry

Depression commonly manifests as disturbances in sleep and appetite, decreased concentration, loss of interest, fatigue, and suicidal behaviors—all of which may often be found following TBI. At least two-thirds of those studied describe fatigue, low energy, or listlessness making this one of the most common somatic complaints of depression (40,41). Kreutzer et al. (5) and Seel and Kreutzer (42) also found fatigue to be the most common symptom endorsed by depressed individuals with TBI, and Englander et al. (4) found depression to be a predictor of higher FSS scores with a robust correlation to PTF in patients with TBI. However, another study failed to show a correlation between depression and post-TBI fatigue (34). Although, statistically, depression predicts fatigue and fatigue predicts depression in the general population, this distinction can be difficult to make in people with TBI, and there is a need for further investigation.

The neurobiological dysfunction in depression consistently involves 5-hydroxytryptamine (HT) and norepinephrine (NE) systems and the limbic-hypothalamic-pituitary-adrenal (LHPA) axis (43), again demonstrating tremendous overlap with impairments following TBI (see endocrinology section later). Many attentional and cognitive deficits seen in depression are thought to be mediated by the prefrontal cortex, which receives significant NE and 5-HT input (44). Functional neuroimaging studies have elucidated frontal corticolimbic pathways critical to modulation of depression and anxiety (45,46). Given the frequency with which frontal damage occurs in TBI, one should expect that psychological dysfunction with its additive burden on cognition, especially with what is known about how these internally distracting disease states would interfere with cognition in those without TBI. A more detailed discussion of treatment of neuropsychiatric disorders can be found in Chapter 74 of this book.

Biochemical

TBI results in a cascade of events that includes biochemical and cellular derangements. The ability to make sense of these changes is limited by the complexity of neurochemical processing in the brain. At the biochemical level, it is well known that amino acid levels are altered by TBI. Aquilani et al. (47) noted that levels of tyrosine and essential amino acids are decreased after TBI and that there is a persistent decline even on discharge from acute rehabilitation. Two especially important amino acids for CNS function are tyrosine, a precursor to brain catecholamines, and tryptophan, an essential amino acid and precursor to serotonin. The neurotransmitter serotonin has been implicated in fatigue. The relationship between TBI disruptions in neurochemistry and the sensation of fatigue is suggested by Dwyer and Browning (48) who noted that m-chlorophenylpiperazine (m-CPP), a 5-HT$_{1A}$ agonist, induces fatigue in an animal model and that exercise training over a prolonged period diminished the response to this agent. Blomstrand (49) concluded that exercise-related fatigue in the CNS was correlated to 5-HT because elevated levels impaired performance, whereas decreased levels improved running in an animal model. One known mechanism of tryptophan regulation provides further support for its role in central fatigue, namely that, through competitive binding for CNS transport proteins, branched-chain amino acids (BCAA) have an inverse relationship with tryptophan levels. During exercise, the ratio of tryptophan to BCAA increases and, as shown by Blomstrand and colleagues (50), giving BCAA reduces perceived exer-

tion and mental fatigue and improves cognitive performance after exercise.

Agents commonly used in the clinical treatment of fatigue, such as the psychostimulants methylphenidate (MP), dextroamphetamine (DAA), pemoline, and amantadine act via the dopamine neurotransmitter, whereas those currently used to treat depression elevate levels of 5-HT. Additional neurotransmitters to consider include histamine, which has an arousing effect on the CNS and histaminergic fibers, project diffusely to cortex as discussed earlier with respect to the ARAS. Clinically, pharmaceuticals with an antihistaminergic mechanism of action induce sedation and fatigue. The agent modafinil acts, through one of its known mechanisms, as a histamine agonist. The ARAS is known to use cholinergic, histaminergic, glutaminergic, and serotoninergic neurotransmission (25).

Endocrine

In non-TBI populations, with endocrine abnormalities, especially anterior pituitary dysfunction, a wide variety of symptoms including fatigue are reported (51–53). Of course, no one hormonal abnormality is correlated exclusively with fatigue, and there are numerous other symptoms that are manifested as a result. However in other populations, the association between endocrine dysfunction and fatigue has been particularly well documented regarding thyroid, growth hormone (GH), and cortisol deficiencies. Deficiencies in GH has been associated with decreased bone mineral densities (54), aerobic capacity, muscle strength, lower quality of life, and cognitive impairments, in addition to increased fatigue (55,56).

Treating these deficits has been shown to be helpful in other populations. In particular, treatment of GH insufficiency has been shown to increase lean body mass and reduce body fat (57), increase exercise tolerance (58), improve quadriceps strength (59), increase energy and mood (60), increase activity and alertness (61), and an individual's sense of well-being and quality of life (62).

The importance of this issue is of course dependent on the overall incidence of endocrine dysfunction associated with TBI. It has been known for nearly 100 years that injury may produce endocrine dysfunction but until recently was considered a relatively rare event (63). In 1942, Escamilla and Lisser (64) reported an incidence of only 0.7% (4 of 595 TBI subjects) manifesting endocrine dysfunction, whereas in 1985 and 1986 respectively, Kalisky et al. (65) reported an incidence of only 4%, and Edwards and Clark (66) reported a small percentage of TBI cases that were associated with hypopituitarism. However, they did say that the low number reported in the past was possibly related to mortality and with the improvement noted in intensive care, they may now be more prevalent. More recently, the magnitude of the problem has become evident. Benvenga et al. (67) documented 367 cases of head trauma associated with hypopituitarism. Among these patients, 15% were not diagnosed with pituitary dysfunction until more than 5 years after injury.

In the past few years, post-traumatic endocrine dysfunction has been studied in a prospective manner. As a result of this work, the scientific and medical communities are becoming more aware of the issue of post-traumatic endocrinopathy. Kelly et al. (68) reported that 8 of 22 individuals with TBI had endocrine abnormalities when they underwent provocative testing. Lieberman et al. (63) studied 70 patients with TBI in a postacute brain injury program and identified endocrine abnormalities in 59% of subjects: growth hormone deficiency (GHD) in 14%, hypothyroidism in 21%, and low morning basal cortisol in 45%. Bushnik et al. (69) studied 64 individuals at least 1 year post-TBI. They found the prevalence of at least 1 neuroendocrine abnormality in more than 90% of patients studied, and 79% had severe GHD. Englander and colleagues (4) studied 119 patients and found moderate or severe GHD in 65%, adrenal insufficiency in 64%, central hypothyroidism in 12%, and testosterone deficiency in 15% of men.

Most studies in TBI, however, only addressed the presence of endocrine abnormalities. The relationship between endocrine abnormalities and fatigue in the individual with TBI is an area that remains under investigation. In pilot work, Elovic et al. (70) have demonstrated an inverse relationship between fatigue and insulin-like growth factor 1 (IGF-1) in persons with TBI. Similar results were reported in a follow-up study (71) where IGF-1 levels were noted to be inversely related to subjective fatigue. IGF-1 is commonly used as a screening measure for GHD because of their correlation. In the study by Bushnik et al. (69), the relationship between self-reported fatigue level and neuroendocrine function was explored. A trend in association between adrenal insufficiency and increased levels of fatigue was noted, but none was identified between fatigue, hypothyroidism, and low testosterone . Interestingly, there was a significant association between higher peak GH levels following dynamic stimulation and higher FSS scores, suggesting that the degree of GHD may not correlate with fatigue in persons with TBI. This study was limited by a small sample size, the possibility of selection bias, the fact that adrenal function was not ideally measured, and they did not consider many of the nonendocrine causes of fatigue that may combine with pituitary dysfunction and mask endocrine related causes of fatigue. Nevertheless, the results warrant consideration. On the other hand, Kelly et al. (72) studied quality of life changes associated with GHD in patients with TBI. They found that GH-deficient patients had reduced quality of life in the domain of limitation because of low energy and fatigue. On the other hand, a study published in 2010 disputes the idea of the relationship between GHD and cognitive sequelae after TBI (73). The issue of treatment of endocrine dysfunction and cognition will be discussed in the treatment section later in this chapter. Although the body of literature is growing, there are still few studies looking at the relationship between endocrine abnormality and PTF in the TBI population. It is clear that neuroendocrine abnormalities are common post-TBI, and Ghigo et al. (74), in their 2005 consensus statement, recommended systematic screening for hypopituitarism in all patients with TBI. Other hormones that have also been linked to fatigue after TBI include thyroid, the gonadotropic hormones, and cortisol (74). However, at this point in time, the literature regarding hypopituitarism and PTF remains conflicted. Future research will need to better define the relationship between endocrinopathy and PTF to outline the potential for effective treatment. A more detailed discussion of this area can be found in Chapter 65 of this book.

Sleep

In general, disturbances of sleep may be characterized as insomnia (deficient sleep initiation or maintenance), hypersomnia (excessive sleep or what is referred to as EDS), and altered sleep–wake cycles (circadian pattern disarray). Sleep disturbances following TBI range in frequency from 36% to 70% (75,76). Several key CNS loci regulate sleep patterns, including brainstem, basal forebrain, and hypothalamic nuclei—all areas commonly disrupted in brain trauma. Serotonin and acetylcholine are the 2 common substances involved. The comprehensive study of post-traumatic sleep disorders is complicated by the frequently encountered comorbidities of depression, anxiety, substance abuse, chronic pain, and medication use, all of which independently exert negative influences on normal sleep. Also not to be overlooked is whether one may implicate a prior (perhaps undiagnosed) sleep disorder as the proximate cause of the brain injury itself. As an example, falling asleep while driving is not uncommon, especially in persons with sleep apnea.

Controversy exists over whether severity of TBI is directly correlated with increased prevalence of insomnia and sleep disturbance. Clinchot et al. (77) and Fictenberg et al. (78) showed an inverse relationship, and Cohen et al. (79) noted increased prevalence with increasing TBI severity. Some researchers have postulated that the reason for this counterintuitive finding lies in the fact that the people with severe brain injury likely underreport, and those with milder injury are more aware of their problems and therefore are more likely to report or perhaps overly attribute their fatigue to poor sleep. More recently, Verma et al. (80) looked at the more objective data that can be collected with polysomnography and the multiple sleep latency test. Their work noted that there was a relationship between severity of TBI and some, but not all, of the measures of sleep disorder. In particular, more severe TBI was associated with a higher percentage of stage I sleep, number of awakenings per night, and the night spent awake each night. The objective data collected by Verma's group was relatively immune from the potential bias of subjective reporting.

Baumann et al. (81) assessed sleep disturbances in 65 patients with TBI 6 months postinjury. They found new onset sleep–wake disturbances following TBI in 47 (72%) of patients. Subjective EDS was reported in 18 (28%) of patients, and objective EDS was documented in 16 (25%) of patients. Eleven (17%) reported fatigue; 14 (22%) reported post-traumatic hypersomnolence; and 3 (5%) reported insomnia. In 28 (43%) of patients, a specific cause of sleep–wake disturbances other than TBI could not be identified. Clinchot et al. (77) examined 100 patients with TBI during inpatient rehabilitation and followed up with them 1 year later. These authors reported that 50% of TBI subjects complained of difficulty sleeping. Of this subgroup, 64% admitted waking up too early, 25% experienced increased sleep time, and 45% reported difficulty falling asleep. In this same cohort of 100 patients, 63% reported significant problems with fatigue. Interestingly, 80% of those admitting to sleeping difficulty also admitted to fatigue as a problem. Kemf et al. (82) studied sleep–wake disturbances in 51 patients 3 years after TBI. They found sleep–wake disturbances in 34 (67%) of patients.

Fourteen (27%) reported hypersomnia; 6 (12%) reported EDS; 18 (35%) reported fatigue; and 5 (10%) reported insomnia. Cohen et al. (79) have pointed to a temporally differentiated sleep disruption pattern whereby difficulty initiating or maintaining sleep tends to occur soon after TBI, and EDS tends to occur more often over the months and years following TBI. Controversy also exists over whether TBI may cause a secondary narcolepsy (see Chapter 43).

Several varieties of disturbed sleep–wake cycles are seen—the delayed, advanced, and disorganized types—with very little literature available specific to the TBI population. Schreiber et al. (83) described sleep–wake disturbance in 15 persons with mild TBI and without history of apnea syndrome, neurological, or psychiatric illness. Using polysomnography and actigraphy (activity detection device), more than half were found to have delayed phase and the rest disorganized type.

Thus, the population of people with brain injury experience disruption in normal sleep physiology. Specific abnormalities discovered include reductions in rapid eye movement (REM) sleep, sleep spindles, vertex sharp waves, and K complexes. These electroencephalographic findings point to an overall decrease in total sleep time, a disappearance of the deeper stages of sleep, as well as more frequent awakening (84). Conversely, it has been also found that as cognition improves, so too does REM sleep architecture. There also appears to be an association between cognition and sleep architecture among patients with TBI across time so that as the former improves, so too does the latter (85). In addition, it has been well described in the normal, non–TBI-injured population, that as sleep time declines and sleep quality worsens, there is a decline in cognitive performance, as well as an increase in fatigue (85).

Overall, although sleep disturbance after TBI is common, there is little work directly relating this disturbance with fatigue. However, it is likely that the relationship between sleep and fatigue observed in other populations applies to persons with TBI. Although these findings are perhaps predictable, unfortunately even in the normal population, the mechanism whereby sleep reduces the self-perception of fatigue and enhances cognitive performance is not known.

MANAGEMENT OF POST-TRAUMATIC FATIGUE

As is the case for most medical conditions in general and neurological conditions in particular, complete cure remains elusive. Nevertheless, it remains critical to start on the road to cure by addressing the fundamentals, relying on the interdisciplinary treatment team when available. Routine performance of a home exercise program not only optimizes cardiovascular health and physical well-being but secondarily enhances important emotional and immune system functioning, which may play important roles in the fatigue experience. Classic rehabilitation practice includes instructing the fatigued individual in compensatory strategies to conserve "energy" and can be tailored to one's specific functional requirements as they intersect with the particular areas of cognitive functional deficit. The instruction may be as simple as the admonition to pace oneself. Psychoeduca-

tion frequently comprises teaching the person with PTF (and involved caregiver)—how the clinical sequelae of focal and diffuse injuries alter the brain's ability to successfully perform certain tasks that consistently engender fatigue. Therefore, clients may learn how to prioritize activities to meet the goals of daily functioning. When efforts fall short, personal expectations may need to be reconciled with actual abilities and performance (see later discussion). Attempts should be made to counsel those with PTF about dietary habits, with the goal of both weight reduction (given the frequency of post-TBI weight gain) and energy efficiency. At a minimum, obtaining a sleep history should lead to counseling about basic sleep hygiene (see Chapter 43). When appropriate, more in-depth investigation with polysomnography may reveal a treatable sleep disorder at the root of PTF. As alluded to in the endocrine section, serum hormonal screening may reveal a remediable imbalance, although too few studies exist to predict how much success may be expected from a neuropharmacoendocrinologic intervention.

Formal psychiatric care or psychological counseling may be needed to minimize the influence of psychological distress on cognition and fatigue behavior through treatment of anxiety and depressive states. Pharmacological management by a professional knowledgeable in TBI leads to the best choice aimed at neutralizing internally distracting states while often parsimoniously addressing other sequelae of TBI, such as headache, irritability, perseveration, and sleep disturbance. Practically, our bias is to use the most activating of antidepressants, such as fluoxetine, bupropion (whose putative dopaminergic action may also address abulic features), venlafaxine at higher doses (more noradrenergic), protriptyline, and duloxetine, which has with a novel mechanism of selective noradrenergic and serotonergic reuptake inhibition.

Once modifiable factors have been addressed and conservative measures fail, the first practical pharmacological approach to PTF is to substitute for or eliminate those agents that cause fatigue itself or potentiate any of the common components of PTF. One of the most common obstacles to optimizing efficient cognitive function is the often inappropriately prolonged use of anticonvulsants (86–88) (see Chapter 39). If post-traumatic epilepsy exists, the least sedating and cognitively debilitating choice of drug must be pursued. Some literature even suggests that some anticonvulsants, lamotrigine and levetiracetam, may even be stimulatory. Commonly used gastric promotility, antispasticity, psychoactive, and antihypertensive agents may also hamper optimal cognitive and behavioral (e.g., motivational) function (89).

Regarding clinical use of drugs targeting fatigue, most of the information and experience comes from their use for sequelae other than PTF and from the treatment of fatigue in other disease states. Thus, amantadine has been used sometimes with dramatic effect in TBI to improve various facets of the fatigue experience (e.g., arousal, abulia) and long ago showed efficacy in treating the fatigue associated with MS (9,90). Numerous papers have reported on the use of MP, DAA, and amantadine to treat cognitive deficits secondary to brain injury and fatigue in other populations. Brietbart and associates (91) demonstrated the benefit of MP and pemoline in HIV-related fatigue, whereas Wagner and

Rabkin (92) reported a similar benefit of DAA. Emonson and Vanderbeek (93) reported that DAA was also useful for flight crews flying during Desert Shield.

The "classic" stimulants enjoy widespread use in TBI but few, if any, well designed and powered studies have specifically named PTF as the dependent variable despite the intuitive connection. Until such studies become available, dosing remains mostly symptomatic, aimed at improving function and quality of life. Short-acting MP and DAA, dosed in accordance with their relatively short half-lives, to coincide with therapy sessions or periods of important activity are currently used. Long-acting preparations clearly have many advantages, but cost remains a major drawback. Although these drugs (including pemoline) enhance catecholaminergic activity in general, a newer agent atomexitine is noradrenergic selective. With this class of stimulant drugs, clinicians should heed the typical cautions (although not seen clinically to a significant degree) (94) and monitor blood pressure and heart rate at a minimum.

The novel wake-promoting agent modafinil is known to less likely cause psychomotor agitation than the classic stimulants, reflecting animal studies showing activation of more subcortical, particularly hypothalamic regions. Originally approved for the treatment of narcolepsy and, more recently, for shift work sleep disorder and undertreated sleep apnea, it does not activate dopaminergic pathways but seems to exert at least part of its action through histaminergic stimulation. Modafinil has been reported to be useful in various populations with neurological disorder, including stroke, MS, depression, Parkinson disease, and schizophrenia (95). It has also been shown to reduce the fatigue associated with cancer (96) and narcolepsy (97). However, Kaiser et al. (98) in a prospective, double-blind, randomized, placebo-controlled pilot study assessed 20 patients with who had fatigue, EDS, or both. Their results showed a significant improvement in EDS in the treatment group compared to placebo; however, there was no impact on PTF. Although the numbers are small, this study provides class 1 evidence that modafinil does not improve PTF when compared to a placebo. Jha et al. (99), in a double-blind, randomized, placebo-controlled crossover trial also compared modafinil to placebo in 53 patients with TBI with PTF. They did not see a clear beneficial effect of modafinil in the treatment of PTF at 4 weeks or 10 weeks but did note Epworth Sleepiness Scale (ESS) improvement but only at week 4. Armodafinil, the R-isomer of modafinil has recently received Food and Drugs Administration (FDA) approval for treatment of EDS related to obstructive sleep apnea, narcolepsy, and shift worker disorder. Despite a similar half-life, armodafinil sustains higher plasma concentrations later in the day than modafinil. This may provide a better clinical response than modafinil; however, to date, the efficacy of a higher concentration of medication has not been established by head-to-head trials.

Hormone replacement is another modality of treatment that is currently being evaluated. The one that is most commonly discussed at this time is GH replacement. Bhagia and colleagues (100) reported a case report where GH replacement was used in a woman with mild TBI and GHD. They noted no significant improvement in neuropsychological testing and did not have significant improvements in strength, oxygen consumption, and ventilator equivalents. Although fatigue was not assessed, the previously discussed parameters suggest that it may have responded to this intervention. Tanriverdi et al. (101) reported on 2 retired boxers with history of TBI who responded to GH replacement with improvements in lipid profiles, body composition, and quality of life. Two other studies (102,103) reported significant cognitive improvements with GH administration. Further work is needed to delineate the relationship between fatigue, and these parameters thought they are suggestive of potential use in the treatment of fatigue.

Although modafinil together with atomexitine have the distinct advantage of being less scheduled, making prescription refills possible, and theoretically reducing the risk of medication abuse, which is of particular concern in TBI, it remains unclear whether treatment with stimulant medications actively ameliorates dysfunction at the level of the supposed fatigue generator, at the behavioral or output level, at the perceptual level, or simply mitigates one to several of the secondary inputs to the ultimate fatigue experience. Given this lack of hard data, the therapeutic relationship may be enhanced through the suggestion that rational trials of complementary or alternative remedies may, so long as they are not patently harmful, be beneficial. Examples in this category include piracetam (a non–FDA-approved nootropic widely used outside of but obtainable from certain compounding pharmacies in the United States), acupuncture, and various herbal preparations.

Chapter 76 in this book is dedicated to the pharmacological properties of herbal medication, and the readers are referred to that section for an in-depth discussion of the material. However, these agents are becoming more widely used by the medical community (104) and are being recommended for the treatment of fatigue (105).

Ginkgo biloba (106) has been suggested as a treatment for many different conditions in numerous populations with suggested doses ranging from 120 to 240 mg/day. Some evidence of its efficacy in the treatment of chronic fatigue syndrome has been demonstrated (107). Ginseng is a complex alternative medication that consists of many compounds and has been suggested to exert its effect through activity on nitric oxide (108). Work by Scholey and colleagues (109) demonstrated that American-produced ginseng was effective in the enhancement of working memory. Acetyl-L-carnitine in doses of 1,500 mg twice a day has been suggested to be beneficial in energy issues and cognitive function post-TBI (110). In animal studies, it has been shown to be active in the cholinergic system (111), as well as having a neuroprotective effect on brain cells (112). Citicoline or cytidine diphosphate-choline (CDP-choline), which readily crosses the blood–brain barrier, dissociates to the acetylcholine precursor choline (110). It has a demonstrated neuroprotective effect and has been widely used in Europe and Asia in the treatment of patients with stroke and TBI. A study by León-Carrión and colleagues (113) demonstrated an improvement in both attention and vigilance, with suggested dosing ranging from 1 to 3 g/day (110). A recent review article (114) states the need for further clinical trials but that there is a potential for treatment efficacy in TBI.

CONCLUSION

The cause of PTF has not been demonstrated to uniquely follow from damage to one particular anatomic locus. The works of Christodoulou et al. (35) and Kohl et al. (36) suggest that neuroimaging may, at sometime in the future, be better able to correlate deficits in function with morphology. In addition, as neuropharmacological interventions improve and the potential to target medications to specific abnormalities becomes more developed, better treatment outcomes may be obtained. The potential for the use of imaging modalities to select pharmacologic interventions and to predict effectiveness is an exciting prospect. In addition, improved management of endocrine abnormalities, cognitive deficits, mood, and sleep disorders may also lead to improved treatment outcomes. Finally, the potential promise of hormone replacement should be more fully explored as the works of High et al. (102) and Bhagia et al. (100) suggest and warrant further research efforts.

Additional efforts to establish the relationship between fatigue and well-known TBI-related deficits particularly arousal, attention, vigilance, and memory will be critical. The future holds tremendous promise in uncovering the mechanisms of fatigue generation after TBI through a combination of neuroimaging, pharmaceutical interventions, and traditional neuropsychological test batteries.

Finally, individuals with TBI have numerous medical issues that differentiate them from other patients who have fatigue. Improvements in the treatment of spasticity, endocrine abnormality, sleep disturbance, and mood disorder are just some of the areas where better medical management may make a substantial difference in the nebulous area of the treatment of fatigue associated with TBI.

KEY CLINICAL POINTS

1. Fatigue is commonly found after TBI even with mild injury and normally decreases with time
2. When treating fatigue, it is important to use a relevant metric either subjective or objective.
3. TBI-related fatigue is often a diagnosis of exclusion and can be a symptom of 1 or more other medical conditions
4. Although often related, daytime sleepiness is distinct from fatigue.
5. Fatigue's etiology is multifactorial and can be a result of inefficient cognitive processing, affect or attentional, or biochemical to name some of the most commonly discussed etiologies.
6. Fatigue may be a result of a medication side effect, and many of the medications commonly used to treat the sequelae of TBI can cause or exacerbate fatigue.
7. Anterior pituitary dysfunction has been proposed as a potential source of fatigue, especially GH. High et al. (102) suggested beneficial effects from GH replacement, but more research is required for a definitive answer.
8. Nonpharmacologic management of fatigue should always be considered in the treatment of fatigue and include dietary modification, weight loss, and activity modification focusing on energy conservation.
9. Pharmacologic treatment often includes the use of stimulants (e.g., MP).

10. A recent well-designed, double-blinded, placebo-controlled trial of modafinil for the treatment of post-TBI fatigue shows that the agent was effective for daytime sleepiness but not fatigue.

KEY REFERENCES

1. Arciniegas DB, Silver JM. Psychopharmacology. In: Silver JM, McAllister TW, Yudofsky SC, eds. *Textbook of Traumatic Brain Injury*. Arlington, VA: American Psychiatric Publishing; 2011:553–570.
2. Belmont A, Agar N, Hugeron C, Gallais B, Azouvi P. Fatigue and traumatic brain injury. *Ann Readapt Med Phys*. 2006;49(6):283–288.
3. British Medical Journal. Assessment of Fatigue Monograph. Available at http://bestpractice.bmj.com/bestpractice/monograph/571.html. Accessed November 1, 2011.
4. Bushnik T, Englander J, Wright J. The experience of fatigue in the first 2 years after moderate-to-severe traumatic brain injury: a preliminary report. *J Head Trauma Rehabil*. 2008;23(1):17–24.
5. Eisenberg DM, Davis RB, Ettner SL, et al. Trends in alternative medicine use in the United States, 1990–1997: results of a follow-up national survey. *JAMA*. 1998;280(18):1569–1575.
6. Fosnocht KM, Ende J. Approach to the adult patient with fatigue. *UpToDate*. Available http://www.uptodate.com/contents/approach-to-the-adult-patient-with-fatigue. Accessed November 1, 2011.
7. Ghigo E, Masel B, Aimaretti G, et al. Consensus guidelines on screening for hypopituitarism following traumatic brain injury. *Brain Inj*. 2005;19(9):711–724.
8. Goldstein LB. Rehabilitation and recovery after stroke. *Curr Treat Options Neurol*. 2000;2(4):319–328.
9. High WM Jr, Briones-Galang M, Clark JA, et al. Effect of growth hormone replacement therapy on cognition after traumatic brain injury. *J Neurotrauma*. 2010;27(9):1565–1575.

References

1. Middleboe T, Andersen HS, Birket-Smith M, Friis ML. Minor head injury: impact on general health after 1 year. A prospective follow-up study. *Acta Neurol Scand*. 1992;85(1):5–9.
2. Hillier SL, Sharpe MH, Metzer J. Outcomes 5 years post-traumatic brain injury (with further reference to neurophysical impairment and disability). *Brain Inj*. 1997;11(9):661–675.
3. Olver JH, Ponsford JL, Curran CA. Outcome following traumatic brain injury: a comparison between 2 and 5 years after injury. *Brain Inj*. 1996;10(11):841–848.
4. Englander J, Bushnik T, Oggins J, Katznelson L. Fatigue after traumatic brain injury: association with neuroendocrine, sleep, depression and other factors. *Brain Inj*. 2010;24(12):1379–1388.
5. Kreutzer JS, Seel RT, Gourley E. The prevalence and symptom rates of depression after traumatic brain injury: a comprehensive examination. *Brain Inj*. 2001;15(7):563–576.
6. Harrison-Felix C, Zafonte R, Mann N, Dijkers M, Englander J, Kreutzer J. Brain injury as a result of violence: preliminary findings from the traumatic brain injury model systems. *Arch Phys Med Rehabil*. 1998;79(7):730–737.
7. Belmont A, Agar N, Hugeron C, Gallais B, Azouvi P. Fatigue and traumatic brain injury. *Ann Readapt Med Phys*. 2006;49(6):283–288.
8. Brassington JC, Marsh NV. Neuropsychological aspects of multiple sclerosis. *Neuropsychol Rev*. 1998;8(2):43–77.

9. Krupp LB, Elkins LE. Fatigue and declines in cognitive functioning in multiple sclerosis. *Neurology*. 2000;55(7):934–939.

10. Iriarte J, Subirá ML, Castro P. Modalities of fatigue in multiple sclerosis: correlation with clinical and biological factors. *Mult Scler*. 2000;6(2):124–130.

11. Watson NF, Dikmen S, Machamer J, Doherty M, Temkin N. Hypersomnia following traumatic brain injury. *J Clin Sleep Med*. 2007;3(4):363–368.

12. Lezak MD. *Neuropsychological Assessment*. New York, NY: Oxford University Press; 1995.

13. Chaudhuri A, Behan PO. Fatigue and basal ganglia. *J Neurol Sci*. 2000;179(S 1–2):34–42.

14. Deluca J. *Fatigue as a Window to the Brain*. Cambridge, MA: MIT Press; 2005.

15. Bushnik T, Englander J, Wright J. Patterns of fatigue and its correlates over the first 2 years after traumatic brain injury. *J Head Trauma Rehabil*. 2008;23(1):25–32.

16. Cantor JB, Ashman T, Gordon W, et al. Fatigue after traumatic brain injury and its impact on participation and quality of life. *J Head Trauma Rehabil*. 2008;23(1):41–51.

17. McCrimmon S, Oddy M. Return to work following moderate-to-severe traumatic brain injury. *Brain Inj*. 2006;20(10):1037–1046.

18. Masson F, Maurette P, Salmi LR, et al. Prevalence of impairments 5 years after a head injury, and their relationship with disabilities and outcome. *Brain Inj*. 1996;10(7):487–497.

19. Norrie J, Heitger M, Leathem J, Anderson T, Jones R, Flett R. Mild traumatic brain injury and fatigue: a prospective longitudinal study. *Brain Inj*. 2010;24(13–14):1528–1538.

20. Bushnik T, Englander J, Wright J. The experience of fatigue in the first 2 years after moderate-to-severe traumatic brain injury: a preliminary report. *J Head Trauma Rehabil*. 2008;23(1):17–24.

21. Walker GC, Cardenas DD, Guthrie MR, McLean A Jr, Brooke MM. Fatigue and depression in brain-injured patients correlated with quadriceps strength and endurance. *Arch Phys Med Rehabil*. 1991;72(7):469–472.

22. Borgaro SR, Gierok S, Caples H, Kwasnica C. Fatigue after brain injury: initial reliability study of the BNI Fatigue Scale. *Brain Inj*. 2004;18(7):685–690.

23. LaChapelle DL, Finlayson MA. An evaluation of subjective and objective measures of fatigue in patients with brain injury and healthy controls. *Brain Inj*. 1998;12(8):649–659.

24. Krupp LB, Pollina DA. Mechanisms and management of fatigue in progressive neurological disorders. *Curr Opin Neurol*. 1996;9(6):456–460.

25. Carpenter MB. *Core Text of Neuroanatomy*. 3rd ed. Baltimore, MD: Williams & Williams; 1985.

26. Plum F, Posner JB. *The Diagnosis of Stupor and Coma*. Philadelphia, PA: F.A. Davis; 1980.

27. Arciniegas DB, Silver JM. Psychopharmacology. In: Silver JM, McAllister TW, Yudofsky SC, eds. *Textbook of Traumatic Brain Injury*. Arlington, VA: American Psychiatric Publishing; 2011:553–570.

28. Whyte J, Polansky M, Fleming M, Coslett HB, Cavallucci C. Sustained arousal and attention after traumatic brain injury. *Neuropsychologia*. 1995;33(7):797–813.

29. Heilman KM, Valenstein E. *Clinical Neuropsychology*. 4th ed. Oxford: Oxford University Press; 2003.

30. Riese H, Hoedemaeker M, Brouwer WH, Mulder LJM, Cremer R, Veldman JBP. Mental fatigue after very severe closed head injury: sustained performance, mental effort, and distress at two levels of workload in a driving simulator. *Neuropsychol Rehabil*. 1999;9:189–205.

31. Ziino C, Ponsford J. Selective attention deficits and subjective fatigue following traumatic brain injury. *Neuropsychology*. 2006;20(3):383–390.

32. Ziino C, Ponsford J. Vigilance and fatigue following traumatic brain injury. *J Int Neuropsychol Soc*. 2006;12(1):100–110.

33. Johansson B, Berglund P, Rönnbäck L. Mental fatigue and impaired information processing after mild and moderate traumatic brain injury. *Brain Inj*. 2009;23(13–14):1027–1040.

34. Belmont A, Agar N, Azouvi P. Subjective fatigue, mental effort, and attention deficits after severe traumatic brain injury. *Neurorehabil Neural Repair*. 2009;23(9):939–944.

35. Christodoulou C, Deluca J, Ricker JH, et al. Functional magnetic resonance imaging of working memory impairment after traumatic brain injury. *J Neurol Neurosurg Psychiatry*. 2001;71(2):161–168.

36. Kohl AD, Wylie GR, Genova HM, Hillary FG, Deluca J. The neural correlates of cognitive fatigue in traumatic brain injury using functional MRI. *Brain Inj*. 2009;23(5):420–432.

37. Covington EC. Depression and chronic fatigue in the patient with chronic pain. *Prim Care*. 1991;18(2):341–358.

38. Manu P, Matthews DA, Lane TJ, et al. Depression among patients with a chief complaint of chronic fatigue. *J Affect Disord*. 1989;17(2):165–172.

39. Wessely S, Powell R. Fatigue syndromes: a comparison of chronic "postviral" fatigue with neuromuscular and affective disorders. *J Neurol Neurosurg Psychiatry*. 1989;52(8):940–948.

40. Tylee A. Depression in the community: physician and patient perspective. *J Clin Psychiatry*. 1999;60(suppl 7):12–16.

41. Maurice-Tison S, Verdoux H, Gay B, Perez P, Salamon R, Bourgeois ML. How to improve recognition and diagnosis of depressive syndromes using international diagnostic criteria. *Br J Gen Pract*. 1998;48(430):1245–1246.

42. Seel RT, Kreutzer JS. Depression assessment after traumatic brain injury: an empirically based classification method. *Arch Phys Med Rehabil*. 2003;84(11):1621–1628.

43. Holsboer F. Implications of altered limbic-hypothalamic-pituitary-adrenocortical (LHPA)-function for neurobiology of depression. *Acta Psychiatr Scand Suppl*. 1988;341:72–111.

44. Drevets WC. Functional anatomical abnormalities in limbic and prefrontal cortical structures in major depression. *Prog Brain Res*. 2000;126:413–431.

45. Liotti M, Mayberg HS, Brannan SK, McGinnis S, Jerabek P, Fox PT. Differential limbic—cortical correlates of sadness and anxiety in healthy subjects: implications for affective disorders. *Biol Psychiatry*. 2000;48(1):30–42.

46. Brody AL, Barsom MW, Bota RG, Saxena S. Prefrontal-subcortical and limbic circuit mediation of major depressive disorder. *Semin Clin Neuropsychiatry*. 2001;6(2):102–112.

47. Aquilani R, Iadarola P, Boschi F, Pistarini C, Arcidiaco P, Contardi A. Reduced plasma levels of tyrosine, precursor of brain catecholamines, and of essential amino acids in patients with severe traumatic brain injury after rehabilitation. *Arch Phys Med Rehabil*. 2003;84(9):1258–1265.

48. Dwyer D, Browning J. Endurance training in Wistar rats decreases receptor sensitivity to a serotonin agonist. *Acta Physiol Scand*. 2000;170(3):211–216.

49. Blomstrand E. Amino acids and central fatigue. *Amino Acids*. 2001;20(1):25–34.

50. Blomstrand E, Hassmén P, Newsholme EA. Effect of branched-chain amino acid supplementation on mental performance. *Acta Physiol Scand*. 1991;143(2):225–226.

51. Elovic EP. Anterior pituitary dysfunction after traumatic brain injury, Part I. *J Head Trauma Rehabil*. 2003;18(6):541–543.

52. Elovic EP, Glenn MB. Anterior pituitary dysfunction after traumatic brain injury, part II. *J Head Trauma Rehabil*. 2004;19(2):184–187.

53. Larsen PR, Kronenberg HM, Melmed S, Polonsky KS. *Williams Textbook of Endocrinology*. Philadelphia, PA: Saunders; 2003.

54. Colào A, Di Somma C, Pivonello R, et al. Bone loss is correlated to the severity of growth hormone deficiency in adult patients with hypopituitarism. *J Clin Endocrinol Metab*. 1999;84(6):1919–1924.

55. Deijen JB, de Boer H, Blok GJ, van der Veen EA. Cognitive impairments and mood disturbances in growth hormone deficient men. *Psychoneuroendocrinology*. 1996;21(3):313–322.

56. Simpson H, Savine R, Sönksen P, et al. Growth hormone replacement therapy for adults: into the new millennium. *Growth Horm IGF Res*. 2002;12(1):1–33.

57. Newman CB, Kleinberg DL. Adult growth hormone deficiency. *Endocrinologist*. 1998;8:178–186.

58. Jørgensen JO, Thuesen L, Müller J, Ovesen P, Skakkebaek NE, Christiansen JS. Three years of growth hormone treatment in growth hormone-deficient adults: near normalization of body composition and physical performance. *Eur J Endocrinol.* 1994;130(3):224–228.

59. Johansson JO, Landin K, Johannsson G, Tengborn L, Bengtsson BA. Long-term treatment with growth hormone decreases plasminogen activator inhibitor-1 and tissue plasminogen activator in growth hormone-deficient adults. *Thromb Haemost.* 1996;76(3):422–428.

60. Gibney J, Wallace JD, Spinks T, et al. The effects of 10 years of recombinant human growth hormone (GH) in adult GH-deficient patients. *J Clin Endocrinol Metab.* 1999;84(8):2596–2602.

61. Burman P, Broman JE, Hetta J, et al. Quality of life in adults with growth hormone (GH) deficiency: response to treatment with recombinant human GH in a placebo-controlled 21-month trial. *J Clin Endocrinol Metab.* 1995;80(12):3585–3590.

62. Carroll PV, Christ ER, Bengtsson BA, et al. Growth hormone deficiency in adulthood and the effects of growth hormone replacement: a review. Growth Hormone Research Society Scientific Committee. *J Clin Endocrinol Metab.* 1998;83(2):382–395.

63. Lieberman SA, Oberoi AL, Gilkison CR, Masel BE, Urban RJ. Prevalence of neuroendocrine dysfunction in patients recovering from traumatic brain injury. *J Clin Endocrinol Metab.* 2001;86(6):2752–2756.

64. Escamilla RF, Lisser H. Simmonds disease. *J Clin Endocrin.* 1942;2:65–96.

65. Kalisky Z, Morrison DP, Meyers CA, Von Laufen A. Medical problems encountered during rehabilitation of patients with head injury. *Arch Phys Med Rehabil.* 1985;66(1):25–29.

66. Edwards OM, Clark JD. Post-traumatic hypopituitarism. Six cases and a review of the literature. *Medicine (Baltimore).* 1986;65(5):281–290.

67. Benvenga S, Campenní A, Ruggeri RM, Trimarchi F. Clinical review 113: hypopituitarism secondary to head trauma. *J Clin Endocrinol Metab.* 2000;85(4):1353–1361.

68. Kelly DF, Gonzalo IT, Cohan P, Berman N, Swerdloff R, Wang C. Hypopituitarism following traumatic brain injury and aneurysmal subarachnoid hemorrhage: a preliminary report. *J Neurosurg.* 2000;93(5):743–752.

69. Bushnik T, Englander J, Katznelson L. Fatigue after TBI: association with neuroendocrine abnormalities. *Brain Inj.* 2007;21(6):559–566.

70. Elovic E, Doppalapudi HS, Miller M, et al. Endocrine abnormalities and fatigue after traumatic brain injury [abstract]. *J Head Trauma Rehab.* 2006;21(5):426–427.

71. Lequerica A, Elovic E, Naqvi A, Sheffield-Moore M. The relationship between fatigue, sleep disorders, and endocrine abnormalities following traumatic brain injury. 39th Annual Meeting of the International Neuropsychological Society 2011. Abstract

72. Kelly DF, McArthur DL, Levin H, et al. Neurobehavioral and quality of life changes associated with growth hormone insufficiency after complicated mild, moderate, or severe traumatic brain injury. *J Neurotrauma.* 2006;23(6):928–942.

73. Pavlovic D, Pekic S, Stojanovic M, et al. Chronic cognitive sequelae after traumatic brain injury are not related to growth hormone deficiency in adults. *Eur J Neurol.* 2010;17(5):696–702.

74. Ghigo E, Masel B, Aimaretti G, et al. Consensus guidelines on screening for hypopituitarism following traumatic brain injury. *Brain Inj.* 2005;19(9):711–724.

75. McLean A Jr, Dikmen S, Temkin N, Wyler AR, Gale JL. Psychosocial functioning at 1 month after head injury. *Neurosurgery.* 1984;14(4):393–399.

76. Keshavan MS, Channabasavanna SM, Reddy GN. Post-traumatic psychiatric disturbances: patterns and predictors of outcome. *Br J Psychiatry.* 1981;138:157–160.

77. Clinchot DM, Bogner J, Mysiw WJ, Fugate L, Corrigan J. Defining sleep disturbance after brain injury. *Am J Phys Med Rehabil.* 1998;77(4):291–295.

78. Fictenberg NL, Putnam SH, Mann NR, Zafonte RD, Millard AE. Insomnia screening in postacute traumatic brain injury: utility and validity of the Pittsburgh Sleep Quality Index. *Am J Phys Med Rehabil.* 2001;80(5):339–345.

79. Cohen M, Oksenberg A, Snir D, Stern MJ, Groswasser Z. Temporally related changes of sleep complaints in traumatic brain injured patients. *J Neurol Neurosurg Psychiatry.* 1992;55(4):313–315.

80. Verma A, Anand V, Verma NP. Sleep disorders in chronic traumatic brain injury. *J Clin Sleep Med.* 2007;3(4):357–362.

81. Baumann CR, Werth E, Stocker R, Ludwig S, Bassetti CL. Sleep–wake disturbances 6 months after traumatic brain injury: a prospective study. *Brain.* 2007;130:1873–1883.

82. Kempf J, Werth E, Kaiser PR, Bassetti CL, Baumann CR. Sleep–wake disturbances 3 years after traumatic brain injury. *J Neurol Neurosurg Psychiatry.* 2010;81(12):1402–1405.

83. Schreiber S, Klag E, Gross Y, Segman RH, Pick CG. Beneficial effect of risperidone on sleep disturbance and psychosis following traumatic brain injury. *Int Clin Psychopharmacol.* 1998;13(6):273–275.

84. Busek P, Faber J. The influence of traumatic brain lesion on sleep architecture. *Sb Lek.* 2000;101(3):233–239.

85. Ron S, Algom D, Hary D, Cohen M. Time-related changes in the distribution of sleep stages in brain injured patients. *Electroencephalogr Clin Neurophysiol.* 1980;48(4):432–441.

86. Temkin NR, Dikmen SS, Wilensky AJ, Keihm J, Chabal S, Winn HR. A randomized, double-blind study of phenytoin for the prevention of post-traumatic seizures. *N Engl J Med.* 1990;323(8):497–502.

87. Practice parameter: antiepileptic drug treatment of posttraumatic seizures. Brain Injury Special Interest Group of the American Academy of Physical Medicine and Rehabilitation. *Arch Phys Med Rehabil.* 1998;79(5):594–597.

88. Chang BS, Lowenstein DH; for Quality Standards Subcommittee of the American Academy of Neurology. Practice parameter: antiepileptic drug prophylaxis in severe traumatic brain injury: report of the Quality Standards Subcommittee of the American Academy of Neurology. *Neurology.* 2003;60(1):10–16.

89. Goldstein LB. Rehabilitation and recovery after stroke. *Curr Treat Options Neurol.* 2000;2(4):319–328.

90. Cohen RA, Fisher M. Amantadine treatment of fatigue associated with multiple sclerosis. *Arch Neurol.* 1989;46(6):676–680.

91. Breitbart W, Rosenfeld B, Kaim M, Funesti-Esch J. A randomized, double-blind, placebo-controlled trial of psychostimulants for the treatment of fatigue in ambulatory patients with human immunodeficiency virus disease. *Arch Intern Med.* 2001;161(3):411–420.

92. Wagner GJ, Rabkin R. Effects of dextroamphetamine on depression and fatigue in men with HIV: a double-blind, placebo-controlled trial. *J Clin Psychiatry.* 2000;61(6):436–440.

93. Emonson DL, Vanderbeek RD. The use of amphetamines in U.S. Air Force tactical operations during Desert Shield and Storm. *Aviat Space Environ Med.* 1995;66(3):260–263.

94. Burke DT, Glenn MB, Vesali F, et al. Effects of methylphenidate on heart rate and blood pressure among inpatients with acquired brain injury. *Am J Phys Med Rehabil.* 2003;82(7):493–497.

95. Rammohan KW, Rosenberg JH, Lynn DJ, Blumenfeld AM, Pollak CP, Nagaraja HN. Efficacy and safety of modafinil (Provigil) for the treatment of fatigue in multiple sclerosis: a two centre phase 2 study. *J Neurol Neurosurg Psychiatry.* 2002;72(2):179–183.

96. Cooper MR, Bird HM, Steinberg M. Efficacy and safety of modafinil in the treatment of cancer-related fatigue. *Ann Pharmacother.* 2009;43(4):721–725.

97. Mitler MM, Harsh J, Hirshkowitz M, Guilleminault C. Long-term efficacy and safety of modafinil (PROVIGIL((R))) for the treatment of excessive daytime sleepiness associated with narcolepsy. *Sleep Med.* 2000;1(3):231–243.

98. Kaiser PR, Valko PO, Werth E, et al. Modafinil ameliorates excessive daytime sleepiness after traumatic brain injury. *Neurology.* 2010;75(20):1780–1785.

99. Jha A, Weintraub A, Allshouse A, et al. A randomized trial of modafinil for the treatment of fatigue and excessive daytime sleepiness in individuals with chronic traumatic brain injury. *J Head Trauma Rehab.* 2008;23(1):52–63.

100. Bhagia V, Gilkison C, Fitts RH, et al. Effect of recombinant growth hormone replacement in a growth hormone deficient subject

recovering from mild traumatic brain injury: a case report. *Brain Inj.* 2010;24(3):560–567.

101. Tanriverdi F, Unluhizarci K, Karaca Z, Casanueva FF, Kelestimur F. Hypopituitarism due to sports related head trauma and the effects of growth hormone replacement in retired amateur boxers. *Pituitary.* 2010;13(2):111–114.

102. High WM Jr, Briones-Galang M, Clark JA, et al. Effect of growth hormone replacement therapy on cognition after traumatic brain injury. *J Neurotrauma.* 2010;27(9):1565–1575.

103. Reimunde P, Quintana A, Castañón B, et al. Effects of growth hormone (GH) replacement and cognitive rehabilitation in patients with cognitive disorders after traumatic brain injury. *Brain Inj.* 2011;25(1):65–73.

104. Eisenberg DM, Davis RB, Ettner SL, et al. Trends in alternative medicine use in the United States, 1990–1997: results of a follow-up national survey. *JAMA.* 1998;280(18):1569–1575.

105. Diamond BJ, Shiflett SC, Feiwel N, et al. Ginkgo biloba extract: mechanisms and clinical indications. *Arch Phys Med Rehabil.* 2000; 81(5):668–678.

106. Elovic EP, Zafonte RD. Ginkgo biloba: applications in traumatic brain injury. J Head Trauma Rehabil. 2001;16(6):603–607.

107. Logan AC, Wong C. Chronic fatigue syndrome: oxidative stress and dietary modifications. *Altern Med Rev.* 2001;6(5):450–459.

108. Gillis CN. Panax ginseng pharmacology: a nitric oxide link? *Biochem Pharmacol.* 1997;54(1):1–8.

109. Scholey A, Ossoukhova A, Owen L, et al. Effects of American ginseng (Panax quinquefolius) on neurocognitive function: an acute, randomised, double-blind, placebo-controlled, crossover study. *Psychopharmacology (Berl).* 2010;212(3):345–356.

110. Brown RB, Gerbarg PL. Alternative treatments. In: Silver JM, McAllister TW, Yudofsky SC, eds. *Textbook of Traumatic Brain Injury.* Washington, DC: American Psychiatric Press; 2005:679–696.

111. Pettegrew JW, Levine J, McClure RJ. Acetyl-L-carnitine physical-chemical, metabolic, and therapeutic properties: relevance for its mode of action in Alzheimer's disease and geriatric depression. *Mol Psychiatry.* 2000;5(6):616–632.

112. Calvani M, Arrigoni-Martelli E. Attenuation by acetyl-L-carnitine of neurological damage and biochemical derangement following brain ischemia and reperfusion. *Int J Tissue React.* 1999;21(1):1–6.

113. León-Carrión J, Dominguez-Roldán JM, Murillo-Cabezas F, del Rosario Dominguez- Morales M, Muñoz-Sanchez MA. The role of citicholine in neuropsychological training after traumatic brain injury. *NeuroRehabilitation.* 2000;14(1):33–40.

114. Arenth PM, Russell KC, Ricker JH, Zafonte RD. CDP-choline as a biological supplement during neurorecovery: a focused review. *PMR.* 2011;3(6)(suppl 1):S123–S131.

43

Sleep-Wake Disturbances

Marie-Christine Ouellet, Simon Beaulieu-Bonneau, and Charles M. Morin

INTRODUCTION

Sleep-wake disturbances and alterations in daytime functioning are common following a traumatic brain injury (TBI). Persons having sustained TBI often complain of unrefreshing or fragmented sleep, and reports of fatigue and daytime sleepiness are also widespread. The past few decades have seen an emergence of scientific literature corroborating these subjective complaints by showing that abnormalities are present in the architecture of sleep in this population and that sleep-wake disorders are more prevalent following TBI than in the general population. Sleep-wake disturbances are present across the whole spectrum of injury severity (1) and can arise early after the injury (2) as reported during hospitalization or inpatient rehabilitation (3,4). Studies conducted several years after the injury with persons who have reintegrated into the community also indicate high levels of sleep-wake disturbances. A large spectrum of sleep disorders is observed, such as insomnia, excessive daytime sleepiness, sleep apnea, hypersomnia, and disruptions of circadian rhythms (5,6).

Following TBI, sleep-wake disorders emerge in a complex context where a large range of neurophysiological, psychological, behavioral, and environmental factors are at play. Recently, clinicians and researchers have been calling for increased attention to sleep-wake problems, which may be often overlooked in the context of other seemingly more pressing physical, cognitive, or functional issues during rehabilitation. Disorders of sleep and waking can potentially accentuate other functional consequences of TBI, for example, by exacerbating headaches, heightening irritability, or decreasing one's capacity to concentrate on a given task. Evidence is emerging that post-TBI sleep disturbances impact negatively on mood, social participation, and cognition (7–10). Despite this recent surge of interest, our comprehension of the etiology and evolution of sleep-wake disorders after TBI is still fragmentary, and the most appropriate evaluation and treatment methods still need to be identified.

This chapter provides a review of normal sleep and circadian rhythms, recent scientific findings relative to alterations in sleep following TBI, and the main clinical features of the common sleep-wake disorders seen in this population. The chapter concludes with suggested guidelines for assessment and treatment, based on the data available to date, albeit still somewhat limited.

BRIEF OVERVIEW OF THE ROLES AND NATURE OF SLEEP

Although sleep is as necessary as light, food, and water, its specific roles and functions are still not completely understood. Crucial to the development and maturation of the brain during the neonatal period as well as during childhood and adolescence (11,12), sleep in adults is thought to have a restorative function for the organism, allowing the replenishment of physical energy, repair of organic tissues, and modulation of psychological functions (13–15). Sleep regulates immune function by fostering an adaptive immune response (16). It also acts as a modulator of endocrine function, in particular the secretion of growth hormone and inhibition of cortisol, which are both critical in neural recovery (17–19). Sleep also has been shown to promote neural plasticity and memory processing, including encoding, consolidation, and retrieval (20,21). Sleep is thus thought to play an essential role in the recovery from illness and injury, but the specific processes by which it influences neurological recovery after TBI remain unclear (19,22).

Sleep is a complex amalgam of physiological and behavioral processes (23). It can be objectively studied using a technique called polysomnography (PSG), which combines the measurement of brain activity, eye movements, and muscle tone. Using PSG, 2 types of sleep states can be distinguished: nonrapid eye movement (NREM) sleep and rapid eye movement (REM) sleep. The different brain activity patterns detected during NREM sleep are usually subdivided into 4 distinct stages (stages 1, 2, 3, and 4) (24), although recently, the American Academy of Sleep Medicine has suggested that stages 3 and 4 should be combined (now called N3) (25). The onset of sleep in normal adults is through NREM sleep. During NREM sleep, the brain progressively becomes less responsive to stimuli in the environment; mental activity is fragmented, and the body can move. From a state of drowsiness, the individual usually first enters stage 1 where the alpha rhythm is attenuated and replaced by low amplitude, mixed frequency waves. Stage 1 is of short duration (1–7 minutes) and is a state of light sleep that can be easily discontinued. The person then progresses to deeper stages. Stage 2 (lasting 10–25 minutes in the first sleep cycle) is characterized by low amplitude, mixed frequency waves, and the presence of sleep spindles and K complexes. In stage 2, a more intense stimulus is needed to provoke arousal. For most people, stage 2 corresponds to the phenomenological experience of falling asleep. Next, the person enters deeper sleep with stages 3 and 4 (or N3), which last 20–40 minutes in the first sleep cycle. Stages 3 and 4 are often referred to as "delta" or "slow-wave sleep" because of the presence of slow waves of high amplitude called delta waves. After reaching stages 3 and 4, the electroencephalography (EEG) pattern usually reverses through stage 2 and then transitions to the first REM sleep period. REM sleep (which is also called paradoxical sleep) is defined by brain activation, muscle atonia, and episodic bursts of rapid eye movements. This is also the state where the most vivid dreams occur.

These NREM/REM cycles are repeated 4–5 times during any given night and follow an organized sequence where slow wave or deep sleep is more prominent in the first third of the night, and REM sleep periods are more prominent in the last part of the night or early morning hours. Adults with normal sleep patterns spend approximately 25% of their sleep time in REM sleep and 75% in NREM sleep. NREM stage 1 represents about 5%, stage 2 about 45%–60%, stages 3–4 between 5% and 20%, and REM sleep represents 15%–35% of total sleep time.

Sleep is regulated by circadian and homeostatic factors. Internal biological clocks located in the hypothalamus control the alternation between different states while interacting closely with time cues in environment called *zeitgebers*. For sleeping functions, the most important of these environmental cues is the light–dark cycle, but other extrinsic cues include social interactions, work schedules, and meal times. Daily variations in core body temperature, which are also controlled by circadian factors, are closely tied to sleep-wake patterns. Because of homeostatic factors, the time to fall asleep (sleep onset latency) is inversely related to the duration of the previous period of wakefulness. Prolonged sleep deprivation is thus associated with an increased drive to sleep. On recovery of sleep deprivation, there is a rebound effect producing shorter sleep onset latency, increased total sleep time, and a larger proportion of deep sleep.

ALTERATIONS OF SLEEP AFTER TBI

Macrostructure of Sleep

The first objective studies of sleep in the TBI population examined EEG patterns in comatose patients and found that sleep stages were difficult to distinguish in the acute phase (26–28). Furthermore, the absence of spontaneous sleep patterns in the EEG was found to be associated with a poorer prognosis, such as vegetative state or death, and the presence of recognizable sleep patterns in the EEG was associated with better prognoses and improved cognitive recovery (28–30).

When examining the macrostructure of sleep using PSG (describing the proportion of time spent in each stage of sleep and shifts between different sleep stages and awakenings), there are now a good number of studies indicating that TBI affects sleep continuity. Findings of increased time spent awake, more frequent awakenings, or decreased sleep efficiency have been reported across the TBI severity continuum and at different time points following injury (6,31–37). These results thus corroborate the frequent subjective reports of poor sleep quality in this population.

Increases in the percentage of stage 1(6,35,38) and stage 2 sleep (6,38,39) have been reported by several teams. Some

authors have suggested that this increase in light sleep reflects processes resembling those seen in normal aging where older adults have increased proportions of stages 1 and 2 sleep and decreased proportions of slow-wave (or deep) sleep (32,39). It has also been suggested that an increase in light sleep could be linked to the subjective complaints of difficulty falling asleep or fragmented or unrefreshing sleep (35), complaints which are not always corroborated by objective PSG measures of sleep onset latency or awakenings.

Most studies do not report alterations in slow-wave sleep following TBI. However, Parcell and colleagues (36) recently did note a significant increase in slow-wave sleep in a sample of 10 persons with moderate-to-severe TBI compared with 10 age- and sex-matched controls. In this study, time since injury ranged from 2 months to 3 years. These authors suggest that diffuse injuries may alter homeostatic processes of sleep following TBI or that this increase in slow-wave sleep is a marker of neural reorganization and plasticity following TBI.

An early study by Ron and collaborators (28) found that survivors of severe TBI evaluated 1–6 months after the injury had significantly decreased REM sleep percentage. George and Landau-Ferey (32) later corroborated this finding in a study of 16 young adults with severe TBI but also noted that these REM-sleep alterations had normalized by 12 months. Using a normal age- and sex-matched control group, Parcell's team (36) also found abnormalities in REM sleep in a small sample of severe TBI survivors. Reduced proportions of REM sleep have also been reported in mild TBI (39). In a larger but more heterogeneous sample of 60 patients with post-TBI sleep complaints evaluated 3 months–2 years postinjury, work by Verma's team (6) showed that 24% had reduced REM sleep percentage. Thus, it seems that REM sleep is vulnerable, particularly in the first 6 months postinjury and possibly more so in persons with severe TBI. This vulnerability persists in certain individuals for unclear reasons.

REM sleep latency is the time taken before an individual enters the first REM stage during a sleep period. Several teams have found shorter REM sleep latencies in TBI samples (6,35,37). Some authors have suggested that this finding resembles sleep characteristics found in patients with depression (35) or patients with narcolepsy—a disorder characterized by severe daytime sleepiness (described later). This hypothesis in line with several studies, which have found narcoleptic-like activity following TBI because of the observation of the onset of REM periods during daytime naps (referred to as sleep-onset REM periods [SOREMPs]) (6, 39,40).

Microstructure of Sleep

Beyond the more macroscopic features of sleep architecture, PSG measures can also yield rich information about the microstructure of sleep via spectral analysis, an approach that quantifies the sleep EEG by decomposing the EEG signals into its constituting frequency components (delta and alpha band wave activities, for example). A few studies have examined the microstructure of sleep following TBI. All were conducted following mild injuries. Parsons et al. (41) examined the microstructure of sleep of 8 adolescents within 72 hours, 6 and 12 weeks following minor TBI. Their results indicate increased delta, theta, and alpha waveforms within 72 hours postinjury, which all normalized by the subsequent follow-ups. Theta activity was found to intrude into the first REM cycle at 6 weeks postinjury. The increases in alpha waveforms were the last to return to normal. The most significant changes were seen in non-REM sleep. In a more recent study of 9 individuals with mild TBI studied much later after the injury, on average of 30 months, Williams and coworkers (37) did not reveal significant differences in the microstructure of sleep in the TBI sample when compared to a normal control group, except in the beta frequency band. However, they did find greater variability in the patients with mild TBI for sigma, theta, and delta power during sleep onset.

Gosselin and colleagues (42) studied athletes with concussions (1–11 months postinjury) and compared them with healthy individuals. They found that mild TBI increased delta activity and decreased alpha activity during wakefulness. They hypothesized that these intrusions of sleep EEG in the waking state may be the result of a slower dissipation of sleep inertia (the transitional state of lowered arousal or performance occurring immediately after awakening) in the TBI group, thus possibly explaining feelings of fatigue and

impairments in daytime functioning in this group. Recently, Rao and collaborators (43) studied the power spectra of 7 persons acutely following mild TBI. Compared to controls, they found abnormalities in several power bands in both NREM and REM periods. They suggested that because mild TBI is difficult to diagnose, alterations in the microstructure of sleep could become an objective indicator of brain injury.

NATURE AND PREVALENCE OF SLEEP-WAKE DISORDERS FOLLOWING TBI

In addition to alterations in the macrostructure and microstructure of sleep following TBI, specific sleep disturbances and disorders have been described in this population, the most frequent being insomnia, excessive daytime sleepiness, sleep-disordered breathing, narcolepsy, and circadian rhythm dysregulation. Table 43-1 provides a definition of the most

TABLE 43-1 Brief Definition of Sleep Disorders Most Frequently Reported Following TBI

Insomnia

Main feature	Dissatisfaction with the quality or quantity of sleep.
Common symptoms	Subjective complaints of difficulty falling asleep, difficulty maintaining sleep (with frequent awakenings and/or difficulty returning to sleep after awakenings), early morning awakenings (with insufficient sleep duration) and/or nonrestorative sleep.
Additional criteria	To be considered as an insomnia disorder, symptoms have to be present at least 3 nights/week, last more than 1 or 6 months (depending on the nosology being used), and cause significant distress or impairment in daytime functioning.

Sleep-related breathing disorders

Main feature	Altered respiration during sleep.
Main subtypes	Obstructive sleep apnea (OSA): breathing alteration associated with complete (apnea) or partial (hypopnea) obstruction of the upper airway during sleep. Central apnea: breathing alteration associated with temporary loss of ventilatory effort.
Common symptoms	Daytime sleepiness, frequent awakenings to restart breathing, restless and nonrestorative sleep, snoring.
Additional criteria	Presence of at least 5 polysomnography-documented apneas or hypopneas per hour of sleep.

Narcolepsy

Main feature	Rare disorder characterized by recurrent unplanned daytime napping or sleep episodes.
Common symptoms	Tetrad of classic symptoms (that are not always all present): daytime sleepiness, cataplexy (i.e., episodic loss of muscle function), hypnagogic hallucinations (i.e. dream-like experiences while falling asleep, dozing or awakening), and sleep paralysis (i.e., transitory, inability to talk, or move upon awakening).

Post-traumatic hypersomnia

Main feature	Hypersomnia because of medical condition (TBI) when other primary sleep disorders have been ruled out.
Common symptoms	Excessive daytime sleepiness, increased sleep duration.

Circadian rhythm sleep disorders

Main feature	Mismatch between one's sleep-wake rhythm and the 24-hour environment. In addition to the sleep-wake cycle, melatonin secretion and body temperature rhythms can be disrupted.
Main subtypes	Delayed sleep phase disorder: prolonged delay in the sleep-wake episodes relative to conventional times. Advanced sleep phase disorder: advance in the sleep-wake episodes relative to conventional times. Irregular sleep-wake rhythm: high day-to-day variability in sleep onset and offset.
Common symptoms	Sleep disturbances when trying to conform with conventional times (inability to fall asleep or remain asleep); normal sleep quality and duration when choosing the preferred schedule.

Useful references: *Diagnostic and Statistical Manual of Mental Disorders*, 4th ed., text revision (49); *The International Classification of Sleep Disorders*, 2nd ed. (57); *The International Classification of Diseases*, 10th ed. (157).

commonly reported sleep disorders after TBI. Other sleep disorders such as restless leg syndrome, periodic leg movements, or parasomnias (e.g., sleep terrors, somnambulism, bruxism) are seldom associated with TBI but can nonetheless be present as in any other population. Sleep-wake disorders are not mutually exclusive and can influence each other if present comorbidly.

Insomnia

Insomnia, characterized by difficulty falling asleep, staying asleep, or unrefreshing sleep, is highly prevalent in the general population with approximately 9% suffering from a clinically significant insomnia syndrome (44). Insomnia is more frequent among women and is associated with poorer physical or mental health, as well as pain and perceived stress (45). In the TBI population, self-reported symptom rates of insomnia vary greatly with most studies reporting numbers between 30% and 60% (46,47). A recent review compiling data from 23 studies, including civilian and military samples, suggest an average of about 40% (47). These studies are, however, very heterogeneous in terms of definitions of insomnia, assessment methods, and factors such as injury severity and time since injury (few studies assessing insomnia beyond the first year postinjury). Fichtenberg's team (48) was the first to use the standardized criteria of the *Diagnostic and Statistical Manual of Mental Disorders, Fourth Edition, Text Revision* (DSM-IV-TR) (49). These researchers consecutively recruited 50 patients admitted to a rehabilitation hospital for mild-to-severe TBI and evaluated them at 4 months postinjury. They found that 30% presented with all the diagnostic criteria for an insomnia syndrome. In a subsequent study of 452 patients with mild-to-severe TBI surveyed much later postaccident (on average 8 years postaccident), Ouellet and colleagues (8) used a combination of the *International Classification of Diseases, Tenth Revision* (ICD-10) and DSM-IV-TR criteria and found a very similar result with 29.4% of the sample fulfilling the diagnostic criteria for an insomnia syndrome. An additional 20.8% suffered from insomnia symptoms without meeting all clinical criteria. For those who did meet all criteria, insomnia appeared a few weeks to a few months after the injury, was present on an average of 5.7 nights per week and was rated as being of moderate-to-severe intensity according to the Insomnia Severity Index (50). Of importance, 60% were not receiving any treatment for their insomnia, despite the fact that it had been present for an average of 6.2 years. Taken together with the results of studies conducted in the first months or year postinjury, these results suggest that insomnia is a highly chronic and undertreated condition in many individuals with TBI. Table 43-2 presents key considerations on the etiology, assessment, and treatment of insomnia following TBI.

Even though the presence of post-TBI insomnia does not seem related to time since injury, injury severity does seem to be a modulating factor. Indeed, several studies indicate that insomnia complaints are more frequent in milder injuries (8,36,51–55) possibly because TBI survivors with mild TBI are more aware of their limitations and are therefore more distressed by their sleep disturbance. Other factors frequently found to be associated with the presence of insomnia following TBI include pain, depressive symptoms, and fatigue (5,8,52,53).

Excessive Daytime Sleepiness (or Hypersomnia or Hypersomnolence)

Excessive daytime sleepiness (EDS) is a tendency to fall asleep or an incapacity to maintain a desired level of alertness during the day. Variations exist in the literature as to the definition of EDS: Some researchers or clinicians define it as sleeping more than usual (e.g., at least 2 hours more); others define it as a tendency to fall asleep during activities or at inappropriate times and places. EDS can be a symptom of a specific sleep disorder such as sleep apnea or narcolepsy or can present independently as a subjective complaint (referred to as subjective EDS) or as an objectively measurable problem (referred to as objective EDS) (56). Subjective EDS is often defined as exceeding a cut-off score on the Epworth Sleepiness Scale (57) (described later in the Evaluation section). To objectify EDS, however, PSG measures are needed, such as the Multiple Sleep Latency Test (MSLT) or the Maintenance of Wakefulness Test (MWT) (see Evaluation section subsequently for descriptions).

Persistent daytime fatigue, which is one of the most common problems following TBI, is often confused with EDS (a separate chapter is in fact dedicated to fatigue in this book; see Chapter 42, Fatigue: Assessment and Treatment). Fatigue is a subjective state defined as a feeling of weariness and a difficulty to sustain an activity because of depleted energy. It is considered very difficult to measure objectively following TBI (58,59). Sleepiness, however, is a physiological propensity or need for sleep, measurable with PSG and characterized by reduced alertness, drowsiness, and objective signs, such as yawning and eyelids drooping (60). It is imperative to differentiate these 2 problems because they are evaluated and managed in different ways. Fatigue can be a consequence of poor sleep or of daytime sleepiness, yet, in most cases, it is a problem probably independent of sleep-wake disturbances and may be present in the absence of sleepiness (59,61).

Following TBI, various studies have yielded rates of subjective reports of EDS between 14% and 55% (5,6,51, 62–65). As for insomnia, these studies vary greatly in terms of definition of EDS, assessment methods, time since injury, and injury severity. Subjective EDS is not always corroborated by objective PSG measures, however. For example, Verma's team (6) noted that in a subset of patients with elevated scores on the Epworth Sleepiness Scale (> 11), 53% fulfilled the criterion for objective EDS (defined as a mean sleep onset latency of <5 minutes on the MSLT). In a study of head-neck trauma, Guilleminault and coworkers (66) noted that only 28% of patients with a complaint of sleepiness had confirmed objective EDS. In the general population, it has also often been shown that subjective measures of sleepiness (e.g., with the Epworth Sleepiness Scale) is not well correlated with objective measures of sleepiness, thereby suggesting that these are different problems. This is perhaps even more true in the TBI population because post-TBI fatigue may often be confounded with sleepiness. In samples presenting with a larger spectrum of sleep complaints, recent studies suggest that about 11%–25% of patients with TBI exceed the criterion for objective EDS (9,65). Table 43-3 pre-

TABLE 43-2 Insomnia Following TBI: A Summary of Etiological Factors and Key Considerations for Assessment and Treatment

Etiological factors

- Neuropathological processes. Damage to brain structures involved in sleep regulation (e.g., brainstem, reticular formation) through primary or secondary lesions (e.g., contusions, hemorrhages, increased intracranial pressure, abnormal neurotransmitter, protein or hormonal secretion patterns).
- Medication. Therapeutic or side effects of pharmacological agents routinely prescribed after TBI (e.g., psychostimulants, corticosteroids, anticonvulsants, antidepressants).
- Pain. Pain associated to TBI and related injuries, leading to prolonged sleep onset latency and fragmented and nonrestorative nighttime sleep.
- Psychological factors. Emotional adjustments to newly acquired cognitive and physical limitations, inability to return to premorbid functioning (e.g., working/studying, driving), problems in interpersonal relationships and litigation issues, causing increased cognitive and emotional arousal at bedtime or during the night. Development of full-blown anxiety or mood disorders interfering with sleep.
- Environmental factors. Hospital and rehabilitation settings contributing to sleep problems because of variety and frequency of diagnostic or therapeutic procedures, noise, light, bed discomfort, and general lack of *zeitgebers*.
- Life habits. Difficulty implementing a sleep-wake routine (e.g., irregular bedtime and arising time) because of lifestyle changes and compensatory strategies to cope with fatigue and sleepiness (e.g., increased time spent in bed, frequent daytime napping, use of stimulants).

Assessment considerations

- Clinical interview. Gathering information on current and premorbid sleep-wake patterns with questions on the nature, severity, duration, and evolution of insomnia; typical sleep-wake schedule; daytime functioning; fatigue; and sleep-related behaviors and cognitions. Assessment of potential comorbid psychopathology and use of prescribed and over-the-counter medication, caffeine, energy drinks, alcohol, and drugs are essential.
- Subjective measures. Daily sleep diary to monitor sleep patterns, duration, and quality, and nature, severity, and frequency of

insomnia symptoms. Insomnia Severity Index (125) or Pittsburgh Sleep Quality Index (119) to assess nature and severity of insomnia symptoms, ideally completed both by individual with TBI and a significant other, especially when severe cognitive deficits impact self-awareness of symptoms.

- Objective measures. Insomnia diagnosis and treatment planning do not require polysomnography, unless other sleep disorders have to be ruled out.

Treatment considerations

- Pharmacological treatment. Data on the safety and efficacy of pharmacological agents for insomnia following TBI is scarce, leading most clinicians to rely on evidence obtained in nonrehabilitation patients to choose hypnotic medications with the best therapeutic efficacy and least side effects (e.g., nonbenzodiazepine sedative hypnotics or z-drugs such as zolpidem, zaleplon, zopiclone, and eszopiclone). Caution is warranted when prescribing benzodiazepines (because of side effects, impacts on sleep architecture, risk of dependence) and drugs with anticholinergic effects, such as tricyclic antidepressants and diphenhydramine (because of effects on memory, attention, and seizure threshold).
- Psychological interventions. Cognitive-behavior therapy is the treatment of choice for primary insomnia and has also shown promising outcome in individuals with TBI. Typical treatment components include structured restriction of time in bed (curtailing time spent in bed to the actual time spent sleeping), stimulus control procedures (regulating sleep-wake schedule and curtailing sleep-incompatible behaviors, such as excessive napping and using the bed and bedroom for other activities than sleep), relaxation techniques (alleviating anxiety and arousal with deep breathing, positive imagery, progressive muscle relaxation or meditation), cognitive therapy (identifying, challenging, and modifying dysfunctional cognitions, such as misconceptions about insomnia causes and consequences, unrealistic expectations about sleep, and perception of lack of control over sleep), sleep hygiene recommendations (fostering healthy sleep-promoting lifestyle habits), and fatigue management strategies (monitoring and scheduling activities and rest times and optimizing the environment).

---

sents key considerations on the etiology, assessment, and treatment of EDS following TBI.

There is little research pointing to the correlates or risk factors of post-TBI EDS. Parcell and colleagues (64) reported that a higher level of subjective EDS was associated with higher levels of anxiety and with increased napping during the day. Some studies have suggested that more severe injuries are associated with increased frequency or severity of sleepiness (64,65), but others have not found such a relationship (5,9). It is also unclear whether time since injury influences the severity or evolution of EDS. EDS is often described as a persistent symptom following TBI, and some authors have suggested that its prevalence may increase with time (62,63). If it was present before the accident, EDS may even have been a causal factor for the TBI.

Narcolepsy

Narcolepsy is an uncommon sleep disorder characterized by the presence of EDS, recurrent daytime naps, cataplexy (i.e.,

sudden loss of muscle tone), hypnagogic hallucinations (i.e., vivid perceptual experiences during sleep onset), and sleep paralysis (i.e., inability to move during sleep onset or awakening). Although most narcolepsy cases are idiopathic and have a strong genetic basis, the disorder can develop secondary to various conditions, including TBI. The prevalence of this disorder following TBI remains unclear, but results are emerging pointing to narcoleptic-like activity in some patients (6,39,40). A narcolepsy diagnosis should be confirmed by nocturnal PSG to rule out other sleep disorders, followed by a MSLT that demonstrates a mean sleep latency of less than 5 minutes and during which at least 2 sleep onset REM periods (SOREMPs) are identified (67). Again, in the study by Verma and coworkers (6), narcolepsy was diagnosed in 32% of patients who underwent MSLT because of subjective reports of sleepiness. A paper reviewing 22 published cases of post-traumatic narcolepsy (68) concluded that the clinical presentation of this condition is not uniform after TBI. Symptom onset varies from a few hours to 18 months post-TBI and appears to be unrelated to the severity of injury, loss of

TABLE 43-3 Excessive Daytime Sleepiness (EDS) following TBI: A Summary of Etiological Factors and Key Considerations for Assessment and Treatment

Etiological factors
- Underlying sleep disorders. EDS is a core feature of several sleep disorders that may either have been present prior to the injury or develop post-TBI (e.g., obstructive sleep apnea, central apnea, narcolepsy, circadian rhythm sleep disorders).
- Neuropathological processes. Damage to brain structures involved in the regulation of the sleep-wake cycle (e.g., brainstem, hypothalamus); changes in hypothalamic function, especially disruption of the hypocretin-orexin neurotransmitting system (which has also been documented in idiopathic narcolepsy); and neuroelectrical changes causing cortical hypoexcitability.
- Genetic factors. Apolipoprotein E (APOE) genotype and its ε4 allele, known to be associated with obstructive sleep apnea.
- Medication. Side effects of pharmacological agents routinely prescribed after TBI (e.g., hypnotics, analgesics, anticonvulsants, antidepressants, muscle relaxants).
- Psychological factors. Comorbid psychopathology, especially mood disorders (e.g., major depression, dysthymia) and substance abuse disorders, can cause or significantly worsen EDS.

Assessment considerations
- Clinical interview. Collecting information (ideally from patient and collateral informant) on the frequency, duration, severity, context, and physiological manifestations of daytime sleepiness; premorbid sleep history; nighttime sleep pattern, quality, and duration; daytime napping; common symptoms of specific sleep disorders associated with EDS (e.g., presence of snoring, breathing interruptions, cataplexy); presence of comorbid psychiatric and medical conditions; and use of medication and other substances.
- Subjective measures. Epworth Sleepiness Scale (57) to assess general level of sleepiness within the last month and Stanford Sleepiness Scale (122) to assess sleepiness at the present time, ideally completed both by individual with TBI and a significant other especially when severe cognitive deficits impact self-awareness of symptoms and difficulties.
- Objective measures. Polysomnography is the gold standard for objective assessment of EDS and underlying sleep disorders. Daytime tests: Multiple Sleep Latency Test (125) (instruction: falling asleep as quickly as possible; useful for diagnostic purposes), Maintenance of Wakefulness Test (125) (instruction: remaining awake as long as possible; useful to determine capacity to remain awake during the day in the absence of external stimulations).

Treatment considerations
- Pharmacological treatment. Data on the safety and efficacy of pharmacological agents for insomnia following TBI is scarce. The use of stimulants, especially modafinil and methylphenidate, to increase alertness in patients with TBI has been documented in a few studies with mixed results.
- Nonpharmacological treatment. Very limited evidence regarding the applicability of typical treatment options (e.g., continuous positive airway pressure for obstructive sleep apnea) in the context of TBI, despite special issues potentially interfering with efficacy and compliance (e.g., motor limitations, cognitive deficits, neuropsychiatric symptoms).

consciousness, or to neuroimaging findings. The presenting symptom can be EDS, cataplexy, or both. The progressive nature of the disorder seems to be more consistent across patients.

Disordered Breathing During Sleep

In sleep-related breathing disorders, respiration is pathologically altered during sleep. Sleep apnea syndromes are part of this broader category and can be divided into 2 types: obstructive sleep apnea (OSA), which is the most common, and central apnea. OSA is characterized by episodes of complete or partial upper airway obstruction presenting during sleep (67). Persons with OSA will frequently snore loudly and complain of restless sleep, daytime sleepiness, and headaches in the morning. Central apnea is characterized by intermittent loss of ventilator effort. The diagnosis of a sleep apnea syndrome usually necessitates an evaluation in a sleep laboratory where at least 5 episodes of apnea (cessation of airflow for at least 10 seconds) or hypopnea (partial obstruction of airflow) per hour must be documented (apnea/hypopnea index [AHI] ≥ 5) (67,69). Guilleminault and collaborators (66,70) found that 30%–40% of TBI survivors who complain of daytime sleepiness suffer from a sleep-related breathing disorder. A study by Webster et al. (71) reported that 30% of a sample studied on an average of 35 days after TBI had an abnormal AHI (≥ 5 events per hour), and 11% had a severely abnormal AHI (≥ 10). Another study conducted in patients further along after their accident (38 ± 60 months)

found that 6% had a severely abnormal AHI (72). In a more recent investigation of 60 patients complaining of poor sleep who were 3–24 months postinjury, 30% presented a severely abnormal AHI,(6), and in 74% of these case, the respiratory events were obstructive in nature.

Post-Traumatic Hypersomnia

According to the *International Classification of Sleep Disorders, Second Edition* (67), when subjective complaints of EDS are present almost daily following TBI, a diagnosis of post-traumatic hypersomnia can be made (part of the broader diagnostic category of hypersomnia because of a medical condition). However, all other sleep disorders causing EDS (e.g., sleep apnea, narcolepsy) need to have been ruled out. Furthermore, there must be no premorbid history of daytime sleepiness or other sleep-wake problems. It has been suggested that a large proportion of patients with TBI fit into this diagnostic category, possibly 10%–30% (9,65,72–74). Post-traumatic hypersomnia may encompass a constellation of symptoms including sleepiness, fatigue, headaches, and cognitive impairment (65).

Circadian Rhythm Sleep Disorders

Circadian rhythm sleep disorders (CRSD) are defined by a mismatch between the person's sleep-wake timing schedule and the 24-hour environment, which brings about significant functional impairments (e.g., difficulty staying awake during the day). Melatonin secretion and body temperature,

TABLE 43-4 Circadian Rhythm Sleep Disorders Following TBI: A Summary of Etiological Factors and Key Considerations for Assessment and Treatment

Etiological factors
- Neuropathological processes. Damage to brain structures involved in the regulation of the sleep-wake cycle (e.g., suprachiasmatic nucleus of the hypothalamus).
- Psychological factors. Presence of comorbid psychopathology (e.g., mood or anxiety disorders).
- Life habits. Changes in daily routines, or lack thereof, associated to the inability to return to work or other social participation roles. Irregular sleep-wake patterns may have been present prior to the injury and may also be associated with secondary gains post-TBI.

Assessment considerations
- Clinical interview. Gathering information on preinjury and postinjury sleep-wake patterns, including questions about usual and preferred bedtime and arising time, variability of sleep schedule, sleep quality and quantity, daytime napping, presence and fluctuations of daytime sleepiness and fatigue symptoms, presence of common symptoms of other sleep, psychiatric and medical disorders, and use of medication and other substances.
- Subjective measures. Morningness-Eveningness Questionnaire (120) to determine preferences in sleep-wake schedules (e.g., morning type, evening type). Sleep diary or Sleep Timing Questionnaire (121) to monitor habitual sleep schedule, quantity, and quality.
- Objective measures. Actigraphy to monitor variations in sleep-wake schedule and associated nighttime and daytime sleep.

Treatment considerations
- Pharmacological treatment. Very limited data available. Melatonin has been suggested to be effective for post-TBI delayed sleep phase disorder. Sedatives and hypnotics have also been tried.
- Nonpharmacological treatment. Chronotherapy (i.e., gradually and systematically shifting bedtime and arising time toward desired schedule), bright light therapy, or a combination of both appear to be promising options but still need further scientific evidence.

which also follow circadian rhythms, can thus also be altered in CRSD. There are a few published cases of CRSD following TBI (75–78). Most of these individuals displayed a delayed sleep phase syndrome, that is, their sleep-wake schedules were delayed, usually by more than 2 hours, in comparison with socially accepted sleep-wake timing norms. Delayed sleep phase actually often can be confused with insomnia because individuals complain of being unable to fall asleep at a conventional time (79). Using actigraphy (wrist-worn devices used to objectively measure sleep-wake schedules, described later in the Evaluation section), Ayalon et al. (80) reported data on 15 persons diagnosed with CRSD after having sustained mild TBI. Eight of these individuals had a delayed sleep phase syndrome, and 7 had high day-to-day variability in their sleep onset and awakening times. These authors also found delayed melatonin and body temperature rhythms in the TBI sample compared to controls. Table 43-4 presents key considerations on the etiology, assessment, and treatment of CRSD following TBI. Additional research is warranted to obtain valid data on the prevalence and nature of CRSD after TBI because most of the published accounts are case studies.

ETIOLOGY OF POST-TBI SLEEP-WAKE DISTURBANCES

The causes of sleep-wake disturbances following TBI remain poorly understood. Many authors have hypothesized that TBI causes damage to specific structures or systems involved in the regulation of the sleep-wake cycle, thus leading to structural and/or neurochemical dysfunction in areas important for coordinating sleep. Environmental and psychological causes have also been put forward and should not be overlooked.

Pathophysiological Factors

Structural Damage
Many authors have posited that any primary or secondary damage to areas of the brain regulating the sleep-wake cycle (e.g., suprachiasmatic nuclei of the hypothalamus, reticular activating system, pontine nuclei) can be sufficient to cause dysregulation in sleep-wake functions (81–84). Early studies involving experimentally provoked brain injury in animals revealed that forces of the impact seem to converge in the brainstem and reticular formation, thereby rendering the mesencephalic and diencephalic structures more vulnerable to damage after head trauma (85–88). It has also been suggested that TBI induces changes in intracranial pressure control during sleep. Intracranial pressure is normally higher during sleep compared to waking hours. Some authors have suggested that this augmentation could be exaggerated following TBI, thus potentially affecting sleep quality (81,89). Intracranial pressure can also cause compression or reduced perfusion to certain regions important for sleep-wake regulation, for example, the hypothalamus (40). In addition, structural damage to other parts of the body can have the potential to influence sleep following TBI, for example, orofacial fractures, which can cause breathing disorders such as sleep apnea (66).

Neurochemical Alterations
In 1981, George et al. (33) hypothesized that TBI might bring on a phenomenon akin to the premature aging of brain stem structures through a decrease in catecholamines. Alterations in the secretion of growth hormone and prolactin have also been reported after TBI (84). Recent findings indicate that alterations in hypothalamic function are probably also important factors. Indeed, Baumann's team has been seminal in showing that in the acute phase following the accident (40,65,90,91), TBI survivors have significantly decreased secretion of hypocretin-1 (92), a hypothalamic neuropeptide involved in sleep-wake regulation that is usually reduced in patients with narcolepsy. These researchers found that hypocretin-1 deficiency was present in 95% of 31 patients with moderate-to-severe TBI (90) acutely after the injury. This decrease seems more pronounced during the acute phase following trauma and in cases of greater TBI severity. Because reduced hypocretin levels have also been shown in

idiopathic narcolepsy (93), this specific abnormality may play a specific role in the onset of post-TBI EDS. Findings supporting the hypothesis of narcoleptic-like activity after TBI also include an abnormally shortened latency to REM sleep found in some patients (6,35,37), as well as reports of sleep onset REM periods in subsets of patients with TBI during daytime PSG-recorded sleep (6,39,65,66).

Reduced secretion of melatonin has also been reported recently, both in the acute (94) and chronic (95) phase after the injury. Diurnal variations in melatonin have also been found to correlate with the Glasgow Coma Score with patients with more severe injuries showing more abnormalities in melatonin secretion patterns (94).

Neuroelectric Alterations

It has been suggested that, following mild TBI, subsets of individuals present with spontaneous cortical hyperarousability (i.e., significantly more cortical arousals compared to controls) or with spontaneous cortical hypoarousability (i.e., significantly less cortical arousals compared to controls) (96). Recently, Nardone and coworkers (97) used transcranial magnetic stimulation (TMS) to study changes in the excitability of the cerebral cortex in 11 TBI survivors with EDS. They found that resting motor threshold was higher and that short latency intracortical inhibition was more pronounced in patients with objective EDS than in control subjects. These authors suggested that the observed hypoexcitability seen in TBI reflects the dysregulation in the excitatory hypocretin/orexin neurotransmitter system.

Genetic Factors

The apolipoprotein E (APOE) genotype and its ε4 allele are known to be linked to OSA (98). In the TBI population, it has been associated with more adverse outcomes such as mortality, vegetative state, and disability. Some authors have suggested that it could also be linked to sleep disorders but this hypothesis needs to be investigated further (99). Sundström and coworkers (100) recently found that fatigue was more pronounced for persons having sustained mild TBI and who were carriers of the APOE ε4 allele.

Pain

Pain has been associated with sleep disturbance following TBI, especially insomnia, because it can cause significant arousal at sleep onset, during sleep, as well as during nighttime awakenings (8,51). According to a recent systematic review (101), 57.8% of TBI survivors suffer from chronic headaches, and other types of pain are also extremely common. In a study of 202 individuals with mild-to-severe TBI, Beetar and colleagues (51) found that 60%–80% of TBI survivors endured pain and that those who suffered pain also had more complaints of insomnia. In fact, the presence of pain increased by twofold the likelihood of suffering from insomnia, particularly maintenance insomnia (difficulty staying asleep). Pain can cause a phenomenon known as alpha-delta sleep (102), in which frequent intrusions of wakefulness are observed during NREM sleep. These microarousals can cause awakenings, or feelings of unrefreshing sleep, thereby increasing fatigue, depression, and exacerbating pain the next day.

Medications

Different drugs used in the treatment of TBI such as corticosteroids, sedatives, analgesics, anticonvulsants, myorelaxants, and antidepressants can modify sleep architecture by influencing sleep quality and quantity or causing daytime sleepiness or fatigue (103,104). For example, antidepressants are known to alter sleep architecture: Some increase REM sleep latency (105–107), others decrease stage 1 sleep (108, 109), more energizing ones (e.g., selective serotonin reuptake inhibitors) can also delay sleep onset. Anticonvulsant medication, such as carbamazepine, can also have impacts on REM sleep (110). Inadequate timing in the administration of different pharmacological agents may in itself cause sleep-wake problems (103,111). To avoid a decrease in daytime alertness and other related undesirable consequences, a careful evaluation and monitoring of the potential side effects and interactions of medications is thus warranted.

Environmental and Psychosocial Factors

Environmental Factors

In an investigation of patients hospitalized for acquired brain injury, Cohen et al. (62) found that 82% reported having problems initiating or maintaining sleep, and 36% of these considered the hospital environment to be an important causal factor of these problems. In the acute phase following the accident, circadian rhythms can be desynchronized because of the absence of *zeitgebers* (e.g., light–dark cycles, meal times, social routines) in the intensive care unit or hospitalization setting. Frequent interventions, administration of sedative or pain medication, pain itself, anxiety, or loneliness linked to hospitalization, noise, lack of routines, bright lights are all potential environmental factors, which can alter sleep quality or quantity (94,112). Studies examining sleep of patients treated in the intensive care unit have indeed found evidence of longer sleep onset latencies, frequent arousals during sleep, and significant decreases or even eradication of deep- or slow-wave sleep and REM sleep (82,112). When reintegrating in the community, individuals can again experience environmental disruptions to their sleep-wake patterns, for example, when adjusting to a new living and sleeping environment or in the absence of regular sleep-wake routines (e.g., fixed arising time, regular meal times, regular bedtime routine and timing).

Psychosocial Stressors and Comorbid Psychopathology

Major psychosocial stressors often accompany the recuperation process following TBI as individuals strive to adjust to new cognitive or physical limitations and attempt to reintegrate their social and familial roles. These stressors can trigger anxiety, rumination, or somatized tension, which in turn are known to increase cognitive or emotional arousal when trying to fall asleep or during awakenings (113). Insomnia, hypersomnia, or daytime sleepiness could also be caused or exacerbated by comorbid psychopathology, in particular depression and anxiety, which are very prevalent after TBI. Insomnia is often a feature of major depression and generalized anxiety disorder, the 2 most frequent psychiatric disorders in the TBI population (114,115). Major depression, dysthymia, and substance abuse can also cause or worsen hypersomnia or EDS (116). Persons suffering from post-traumatic stress disorder (PTSD) can also have nightmares (8), but these have not been a frequently reported cause of sleep disorder in the available literature.

Behavioral Factors

Life habits such as irregular sleep-wake schedules, caffeine consumption (e.g., energy drinks, coffee, and colas), use of alcohol and drugs can all have effects on sleep-wake patterns. To counteract fatigue, persons with TBI may engage in rest-seeking behaviors, such as inactivity, frequent nap taking, or excessive time in bed. These habits could actually contribute to sleep-wake disturbances by affecting the structure of nighttime sleep (46). Furthermore, the lack of a routine associated to the inability to return to work can lead to maladaptive shifts in bedtime and arising time. In addition, secondary gain (i.e., advantages) can reinforce sleep disturbances following TBI, for example, when family members take over unwanted roles or provide desired attention.

IMPACTS OF SLEEP DISTURBANCES FOLLOWING TBI

There is still limited data on the impacts of sleep-wake disturbances following TBI. Objective studies are needed to evaluate the interaction between sleep alterations and functional recovery at the physical, cognitive, or emotional levels.

Impacts on Rehabilitation and Daily Activities

In a naturalistic study of 135 adults receiving community-based rehabilitation services many years following severe TBI, Worthington and Melia (7) asked rehabilitation staff to evaluate the nature and impact of sleep and arousal disturbances on the delivery of rehabilitation treatments. They found that 47.4% of participants had some sign of disturbed sleep or arousal. In 65.6% of these cases, sleep and arousal issues disrupted rehabilitation interventions and daily activities (e.g., being unable to stay awake during an activity, missing appointments or opportunities because of late awakening time). In a study of 452 TBI survivors (mild to severe) on an average 8 years of postinjury, Ouellet and colleagues (8) collected the patients' perspective about the impacts of insomnia. Among those fulfilling the criteria for an insomnia syndrome, 60% reported that insomnia significantly affected their mood; 69% that it interfered with their mental abilities (e.g., attention, concentration, memory); 57 % reported impacts on their social, leisure, or productive activities; and 46% felt that insomnia had affected past or present rehabilitation activities (e.g., physical therapy, occupational therapy).

Impacts on Psychopathology and Pain

Studies of sleep-wake patterns following TBI have systematically found a link between sleep disorders and psychiatric disturbance, particularly anxiety and depression following TBI (5,8,63). Frieboes et al. (84) hypothesized that the nighttime hormonal changes, which may take place following TBI, resemble those seen in depression. Rao's team (4) noted that the presence of insomnia in the acute period following TBI (within 3 months) was related to the appearance of anxiety as evaluated with the structured clinical interview for *DSM-IV-TR*. Kempf and colleagues (5) also recently noted that both insomnia and impaired vigilance during the day were linked to the presence of depressive and anxious symptoms. Chaput and coworkers (2) reviewed the charts of 443 patients with mild TBI at 10 days and 6 weeks postaccident and found that persons with subjective complaints of sleep disturbance were 3 times more likely to have headaches during the first 6 weeks postinjury. Furthermore, depression and irritability were also more frequent when sleep disturbances were present. These authors thus suggest that sleep disturbance may play a role in establishing the chronicity of other types of symptoms, such as pain and mood alterations.

Potential Impacts on Cognition

Despite the potential of sleep-wake disturbances to exacerbate cognitive deficits, very few studies have yet closely examined the impact of alterations in sleep on cognition after TBI.

In the first few days following TBI, decreased sleep efficiency has been suspected to negatively affect memory return after TBI (83). Recently, Bloomfield and colleagues (117) compared performances on an objective measure of sustained attention between good and poor sleepers identified within a sample of mainly moderate-to-severe TBI. They found that individuals suffering from insomnia were significantly more likely to make errors of commission on the task, reflecting poorer sustained attention. Although more depressive symptoms were observed in the poor sleeper group, further analyses suggested that poorer performance on the attention task was more likely to be attributable to sleep disturbance rather than to depression.

TBI survivors suffering from daytime sleepiness have been found to have slower average reaction times and more lapses in a vigilance measure, compared to nonsleepy counterparts (73). In the general population, sleep apnea is well known to be associated with cognitive impairments, particularly in the attentional domain (118). Only one study has investigated the impact of the presence of sleep-related breathing disorders on several neuropsychological measures (10). Results indicated that patients with TBI with OSA performed significantly worse than patients without OSA on measures of sustained attention and episodic memory. Both groups were comparable on motor, visual construction, and other attention measures. The inverse relationship between TBI severity and frequency of sleep complaints probably complicates the relationship between sleep and cognition following TBI. Indeed, Mahmood et al. (54) found that better executive functioning and speed of processing were in fact associated with more sleep disturbances. This result may be explained by the tendency of individuals with milder injuries to report more sleep disturbance than those with more severe injuries. Further research is thus warranted to tease out the specific effects of sleep alterations on cognition following TBI, for example, how alterations in REM sleep may affect memory consolidation and learning.

EVALUATING SLEEP-WAKE PROBLEMS FOLLOWING TBI

Given the high prevalence of complaints of poor sleep and sleepiness in patients with TBI and the potential impact of these difficulties on daytime functioning, quality of life, and mental and physical health, individuals with TBI should be systematically investigated for the presence of underlying, concomitant sleep disorders. To obtain a complete picture of the patient's experience, we recommend using various tools (e.g., clinical interview, objective measures, self-reported measures) and sources of information. Ideally, information obtained from the patient should be validated with a reliable informant, especially if the patient has important cognitive limitations and impaired self-awareness, which might preclude the use of certain self-report tools. Castriotta and coworkers (73) suggest that patients with TBI should preferably undergo PSG followed by a MSLT for the detection of sleep disorders and sleepiness. Some disorders (e.g., sleep apnea, periodic leg movements, or narcolepsy) necessitate PSG measures (nocturnal and/or diurnal) to confirm the diagnosis. However, access to PSG, which requires highly specialized facilities and equipment, is often limited. Further, agitation and confusion may preclude the use of PSG in certain patients. Fortunately, other tools can be used to assess sleep-wake disorders, premorbid history, and contributing factors.

Clinical Interviews

A detailed interview with the patient, ideally complemented by information obtained from a significant other who lives with the patient, is important to document the perceived quality of sleep and potential subjective complaints. It is essential to document premorbid sleep history to evaluate whether nondiagnosed sleep disorders provoking EDS (e.g., apnea) may have been present before the injury (9,73) or even have caused the accident leading to TBI. In addition, clinicians must have a clear portrait of the medications taken, interactions between medications, and of the presence of other medical conditions (e.g., possibly causing pain) or psychiatric disorders (e.g., depression, anxiety, substance abuse). This is especially important in the TBI population given the high occurrence of comorbidity and polypharmacy.

Ideally, the clinical interview should cover (*a*) the sleep-wake schedule (initial bedtime and final arising time); (*b*) estimates of sleep-onset latency, number and duration of awakenings, total sleep time; (*c*) the nature of the sleep-wake complaint (problems falling asleep, staying asleep, early morning awakening, daytime sleepiness, unusual experiences during sleep); (*d*) daytime consequences (e.g., mood disturbances, fatigue, sleepiness, social discomfort, and cognitive impairment); (*e*) the natural history of the sleep problem (onset, duration, and evolution); (*f*) environmental factors (e.g., noise, light, room temperature, mattress comfort); (*g*) medication use; (*h*) sleep hygiene factors (e.g., meal times, caffeine, nicotine, alcohol, exercise); (*i*) napping habits; (*j*) snoring, breathing interruptions; (*k*) unusual events at

sleep onset or during the night (e.g., cataplexy, hypnagogic hallucinations, paralysis, sleep terrors); (*l*) the presence of limb movements; (*m*) the patient's medical history (e.g., pain, anemia, hyperthyroidism); and (*n*) elements of a functional analysis, including antecedents, consequences, secondary gain, and precipitating and perpetuating factors.

In Table 43-5 we propose an interview canvas adapted for TBI, which is based on the *Insomnia Interview Schedule* (23), a semistructured interview, which was developed by Morin and has been used in previous studies of insomnia and TBI (13,20). Although it was initially designed for the evaluation of insomnia, this interview can also be used as a source of information regarding other sleep-wake disturbances.

Self-Report Questionnaires

A wide variety of self-reported questionnaires exists evaluating various aspects of sleep and sleepiness. In the following section, we present the tools most commonly used and potentially helpful in the TBI population.

Sleep Quality Measures

The *Pittsburgh Sleep Quality Index* (119) evaluates sleep quality and disturbances over a 1-month time interval. It provides information on subjective sleep quality, sleep latency, sleep duration, habitual sleep efficiency, sleep disturbances, use of sleep promoting medication, and daytime dysfunction. A total score, ranging from 0 to 21, can be obtained and a score higher than 5 suggests poor sleep quality.

The *Insomnia Severity Index* (113) is a short questionnaire assessing the severity of difficulties with sleep onset, maintenance and early awakening, satisfaction with sleep, interference of sleep disturbance in daily functioning, and how noticeable and distressing the sleep-related impairment is. The total score ranges from 0 to 28 with scores from 0 to 7 indicating no clinically significant insomnia, scores from 8 to 14 pointing to subthreshold insomnia, scores from 15 to 21 suggesting clinical insomnia of moderate severity, and scores from 22 to 28 indicating of severe clinical insomnia.

Circadian Preferences

The *Morningness-Eveningness Questionnaire* (MEQ) (120) can be used to determine preferences in engaging in activities in the morning or evening (e.g., going to bed and rising early vs late). Higher scores indicate more morning tendencies and lower scores indicate more evening tendencies. Because it relies on hypothetical situations, the MEQ can be influenced by cognitive limitations, especially with patients with severe TBI. The *Sleep Timing Questionnaire* (121) can be an alternative.

Daytime Sleepiness

The *Epworth Sleepiness Scale* (58) is commonly used to evaluate sleepiness. It includes 8 daytime situations for which the respondent has to rate the probability to doze off or fall asleep. Some authors have suggested that this scale may not be the best measure to assess sleepiness in moderate-to-severe TBI because of the accompanying cognitive and self-

TABLE 43-5 Clinical Interview Canvas. *TBI*, traumatic brain injury. Adapted from Morin (113) with permission.

INTERVIEW SECTION	GOALS	SAMPLE QUESTIONS
History of sleep-wake disturbance	■ Obtain the patients perceptions of sleep quality and quantity. ■ Verify if sleep problems were present before the injury. ■ Get a sense of the causes, nature, and evolution of the sleep-wake disturbances.	■ Do you presently have problems with your sleep or difficulty staying awake during the day? ■ Can you give me some examples? ■ Has your sleep quality or quantity changed since your injury? How so? ■ How long have you had this sleep problem (specify if before/after TBI)? ■ Were there any stressful life events related to its onset? ■ Was the onset gradual or sudden? ■ What has been the course of your sleep problems since its onset (e.g., persistent, episodic, seasonal, etc.?)
Typical nighttime sleep patterns	■ Screen for insomnia. ■ Evaluate the timing and variability of the sleep-wake schedule.	■ What is your usual bedtime? ■ At what time is your last awakening in the morning (without falling back asleep)? ■ What is your usual arising time? ■ Is your sleep schedule stable? If not, how does it vary? ■ Do you have trouble falling asleep? ■ On a typical night (past month), how long does it take you to fall asleep after you go to bed and turn the lights off? ■ In the past month, how many nights per week did you take at least 30 minutes to fall asleep? ■ Do you have trouble staying asleep in the middle of the night? ■ What wakes you up at night? (e.g., pain, noise, snoring, breathing interruption, movements) ■ On a typical night (past month), how many times do you wake up in the middle of the night? ■ Are your awakenings linked to a particular cause such as noise, pain, or worrying? ■ On a typical night (past month), how long do you spend awake in the middle of the night (total for all awakenings)? ■ In the past month, how many nights per week did you spend at least 30 minutes awake in the middle of the night (total for all awakenings)? ■ Do you have trouble waking up earlier than desired in the morning? ■ In the past month, how many nights per week did you wake up at least 30 minutes before your desired time (total for all awakenings)? ■ In the past month, how many nights per week did you have an impression of nonrefreshing sleep despite adequate sleep duration? ■ How many hours of sleep do you usually get?
Screening for various symptoms	■ Screen for signs and symptoms of sleep-related breathing disorders (e.g. obstructive sleep apnea, central sleep apnea), circadian rhythm sleep disorders (e.g., delayed or advance sleep-phase syndrome), parasomnias (e.g., sleepwalking, sleep terrors, nightmares, bruxism), and sleep-related movement disorders (e.g., periodic limb movement disorder, restless legs syndrome).	■ Have you or your spouse ever noticed one of the following, and if so, how often on a typical week would you say you experience these symptoms? - Loud snoring. - Gasping, choking, breathing interruptions, or holding your breath while sleeping? - Urge to move your legs or inability to keep your legs still? - Leg cramps while sleeping? - Twitches or jerks in your legs or arms while sleeping? - Inability to move while in bed? - Grinding your teeth while sleeping? - Confusion or strange sensory experiences when falling asleep or waking up? - Recurrent nightmares or disturbing dreams? Are these related to the accident?
Daytime sleepiness and impacts of sleep-wake disturbances on daytime functioning	■ Screen for hypersomnias of central origin (e.g., narcolepsy, hypersomnia because of medical condition). ■ Evaluate perceived impacts of sleep-wake disturbances on other spheres of functioning. ■ Screen for excessive napping and excessive worrying about sleep.	■ How often do you take intentional naps during the day? ■ Do you usually fall asleep when you try to take a nap? For how long? ■ Do you have any trouble staying awake during the day? ■ If so, in what circumstances (e.g., reading, watching TV, eating, talking, driving)? ■ How often do you fall asleep during the day without intending to do so? ■ Do your sleep problems cause or exacerbate any problems in the daytime such as - Fatigue, tiredness, or lack of energy? - Difficulty with concentration, attention, or memory? - Lack of motivation or initiative? - Physical symptoms such as headaches, muscle tension, or upset stomach? - Worries or concerns about sleep and/or the consequences of your sleep problems?
Life habits, medication and substance use	■ Screen for unhealthy habits, which may contribute directly to the disturbance (e.g., exercising close to bedtime, nicotine, caffeine, alcohol, drugs, medications), ■ Screen for medications, which may impact on sleep because of inadequate type, dosage, or timing of administration,	■ What strategies do you use to cope with your sleep problem or to stay awake during the day? ■ How many times per week do you exercise? When do you typically exercise? ■ How many caffeinated beverages do you drink per day? (e.g., coffee, energy drinks), ■ Do you smoke? (amount and timing) ■ Do you take any drugs or alcohol to help you sleep or function better during the day? ■ Besides the ones used to improve sleep or daytime alertness, do you take any other prescribed or over-the-counter medication? (if so, specify name of medication, dosage, and frequency of days/use [number of days/nights per week])
Treatment	■ Explore current use of pharmacological agents or substances for sleep. ■ Explore other treatments attempted in the past (e.g., relaxation, light therapy, etc.)	■ In the past month, have you used any prescribed or over-the-counter medication to improve your sleep or your daytime alertness? (if so, specify name of medication, dosage, and frequency of use [number of days/nights per week]) ■ In the past month, have you used any other substance to improve your sleep or your daytime alertness (e.g., alcohol, drugs, energy drinks, caffeine)? (if so, specify name of medication, amount, frequency of use [number of days/nights per week]) ■ Have you received treatment in the past for your sleep problems (other than medication)?
Comorbidity	■ Screen for comorbid psychopathology or medical problems that may contribute to the sleep problem.	■ In the past 6 months, have you been particularly nervous or anxious or worried? ■ In the past month, have you been down or depressed? ■ When was your last physical exam? ■ Do you have any medical problems currently? If so, what are they?

awareness impairments (42,63). The *Stanford Sleepiness Scale* (122) can also be used to measure state sleepiness. The patient rates how sleepy he or she is at the present moment using a 1–7 rating.

Sleep Diary

A simple sleep diary can be used to identify factors, which may affect sleep-wake patterns, and to monitor changes in sleep before, during, and after any given treatment (see Figure 43-1 for an example). It is a precious tool to obtain the patient's perception of sleep quantity and quality and impacts on daytime functioning. The information gathered from the sleep diary is also invaluable to decide on pertinent treatment recommendations (e.g., changes in sleep hygiene and sleep-wake schedules) and to assess changes following treatment (113). Patients are typically asked to record bedtime and arising times, estimate how long they took to fall asleep (sleep onset latency), as well as the number and duration of awakenings. They can also use the diary to document naps and the use of medications, alcohol, caffeine, and other substances. A period of at least 2 consecutive weeks of com-

pleted sleep diaries is usually recommended to get a good overview of sleep patterns and internight variability (23).

Polysomnography

Nighttime Polysomnography

Nighttime PSG is the standard tool for measurement of sleep disturbances, such as OSA, central sleep apnea, upper airway resistance syndrome, nocturnal seizures, and periodic limb movements (69). However, objective evidence of insomnia with PSG is not necessary to pose a diagnosis. PSG usually involves at least a 1-night study of an individual's sleep in a specialized laboratory with trained technicians who code the PSG data into different sleep stages according to standardized criteria. PSG includes a standard montage of EEG (brain activity), electrooculographic (EOG; eye movements), and electromyographic (EMG; muscle movements) recordings. Additional measures can be included (e.g., heart rate, airflow, blood oxygenation, muscle movements) and monitored through devices such as electrocardiograms, thoracic and abdominal straps, nasal sensors of airflow, electrodes on leg muscles (anterior tibialis), and oxymeters (usually

		Example	Date ___ /	Date ___ /	Date ___ /	Date ___ /	Date ___ /	Date ___ /	Date ___ /
		Tuesday 25/03							
	Evening questions (before going to bed)								
A.	In general today, I felt. . .choose a number from the scale) 0 1 2 3 4 5 6 7 8 9 10 0: I was not tired at all. 10: I felt extremely tired.	4							
B.	In general today, I. . . (choose a number from the scale) 0 1 2 3 4 5 6 7 8 9 10 0: I did not accomplish anything at all. 10: I took full advantage of my day.	7							
	Morning questions (after getting up)								
1.	Yesterday, I napped from __ to __. (Note the times of all naps) Did you fall asleep during this nap (YES/NO)?	1:50–2 :30 (Yes)							
2.	Yesterday, I took __ mg of medication and/or __ oz of alcohol as a sleeping aid.	Ativan 1 mg							
3.	Last night, I went to bed at ____. I turned the lights off at ____.	10:45 pm 11:15 pm							
4.	After turning the lights off, I fell asleep in ____ minutes.	40 min							
5.	My sleep was interrupted ____ times. (Specify number of nighttime awakenings)	2							
6.	Each time, my sleep was interrupted for ____ minutes. (Specify duration of each awakening)	5 45							
7.	Last night, I got out of bed ____ times. (Specify number of times you got out of bed)	3							
8.	This morning, I woke up at ____. (Note time of last awakening without falling back asleep afterwards)	6:15 am							
9.	This morning, I got out of bed at ____.	7:00 am							

FIGURE 43–1 Sleep diary. Adapted from Morin (113) with permission.

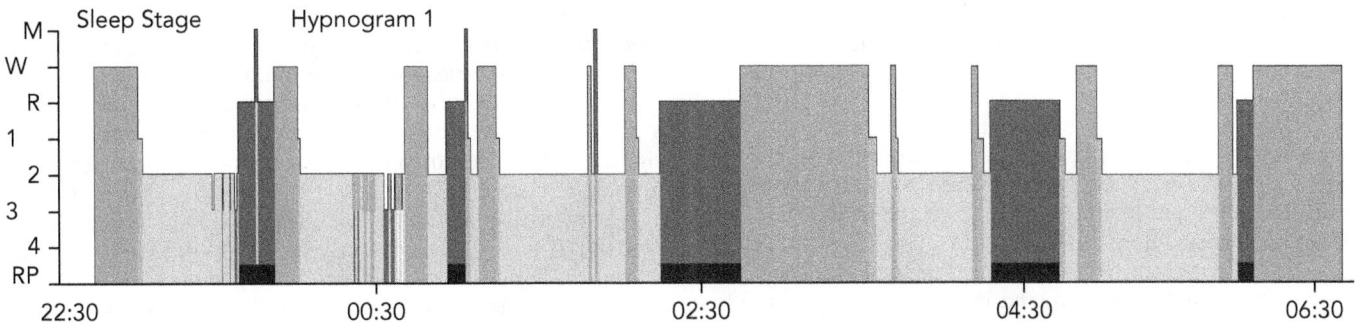

FIGURE 43-2 Example of a hypnogram showing multiple periods of wakefulness during the night. *M*, movement; *W*, wakefulness; *R*, rapid eye movement (REM) sleep; *1*, stage 1; *2*, stage 2; *3*, stage 3; *4*, stage 4; *RP*, REM period. From Beaulieu-Bonneau and Morin, unpublished data.

placed on the finger tip) (123). PSG yields comprehensive information on sleep continuity, such as exact sleep onset latency, time spent awake after sleep onset, total time slept, sleep efficiency, and time spent in different sleep stages, which can be represented graphically with a hypnogram (see Figure 43-2 for an example). Ambulatory PSG devices have also been developed to measure sleep in the patient's home. They allow the measurement of sleep parameters in a more naturalistic environment.

Multiple Sleep Latency Test

To evaluate EDS, daytime PSG recordings are used. The MSLT is a well-validated objective measure of daytime sleepiness. It is a useful tool to quantify daytime sleepiness and differentiate pathological sleep abnormalities from subjective complaints of sleepiness and post-TBI fatigue (103). The MSLT consists of providing the subject with 4 or 5 nap opportunities of 20 minutes each spaced at 2-hour intervals. Excessive sleepiness is generally defined as a mean sleep onset latency of less than 5 minutes on average during these nap opportunities. To diagnose narcolepsy, for example, patients must fall asleep in less than 5–10 minutes and present with at least 2 sleep onset REM periods (SOREMPs) across nap opportunities (127).

Maintenance of Wakefulness Test

The MWT is an alternative test for sleepiness where subjects are instructed to stay awake during 40-minute periods. As in the MSLT, mean sleep onset latency for all nap opportunities is measured. Falling asleep in less than 5 minutes during the nap opportunities is also the criterion for EDS in this test. This test is less useful to diagnose narcolepsy but may be particularly relevant in the TBI population because it measures one's aptitude to stay awake, information which may be importantly linked to variations in daytime vigilance or fluctuations in cognitive function (125,126).

Actigraphy

An actigraph represents a lower cost alternative to PSG. It is a small watch-like device worn on a limb (usually at the wrist) that continuously records data regarding patient motor activity over several days (127). The data from the

actigraph allows the objective estimation of sleep-wake parameters based on the presence or absence of motor activity detected in the limb. This technology has been used for several years in sleep research and has been successfully employed in populations where PSG is more difficult to use, such as persons with dementia and children. Moreover, actigraphy has been shown to be promising to study circadian rhythm disorders in patients with acquired brain injury and apathy (128). Recently, Zollman and collaborators (129) used actigraphy with 5 TBI survivors with motor impairment or cognitive and behavioral disturbances (e.g., agitation, impulsivity). These authors express caution as to the use of actigraphy in this population because of problems such as spasticity, paresis, impulsivity, and agitation. They offer guidelines for use of actigraphy in patients with TBI , for example placing the device on the least affected limb when motor impairments are present, and using actigraphy only with patients with a Rancho Los Amigos cognitive Level of II or above.

EVIDENCE BASE FOR TREATMENT OF POST-TBI SLEEP DISTURBANCES

Still limited research has been conducted to date on different treatment options for post-TBI sleep-wake disturbances. Given their high prevalence, however, it is crucial to verify that treatments are as safe, effective, and well tolerated in TBI survivors, who typically present with particularities (e.g., motor limitations, cognitive deficits, neuropsychiatric symptoms, self-awareness impairments), which complicate therapeutic interventions (e.g., drug interactions, fatigue because of treatments exacerbating other problems).

Pharmacological Treatment Options

Few studies have evaluated the safety and efficacy of different medications to treat sleep-wake disturbances in the TBI population. Most clinicians thus need to choose pharmacological agents while relying on the evidence gathered in nonneurological populations. There is also little data regarding issues of adherence to sleep medications in the TBI populations. In the light of various factors such as memory problems, lack of initiative, difficulties with organization, impulsivity, or substance use, research is warranted to describe TBI survivors' sleep medication consumption habits (e.g., timing, regularity) and respect of therapeutic guidelines (e.g., avoiding alcohol).

Benzodiazepines

In animal studies of brain damage, the use of benzodiazepines has been associated with impaired neurological recovery in the acute phase after an impact to the head (130,131). Hence, several authors have called for caution when using these drugs in patients with TBI. Based on their clinical experience, Flanagan, Greenwald, and Wieber (132) suggested to avoid benzodiazepines following TBI because they negatively influence normal sleep architecture, present a potential for abuse, and because of their deleterious effects such as dizziness, impaired memory, and altered psychomotor skills. They also do not recommend the use of drugs, which have anticholinergic effects (e.g., tricyclic antidepressants, diphenhydramine), because of their possible deleterious effects on memory and attention and their potential to lower the seizure threshold. Recently, Worthington et al. (7) found that 34% of a sample of moderate-to-severe TBI survivors who were on an average of 9 years postinjury were using benzodiazepines and other hypnotic drugs. Of importance, they observed that in all of the cases they studied, the period of use of the prescribed hypnotics exceeded the guidelines recommended in the United Kingdom.

Nonbenzodiazepines

In nonneurologically impaired populations, the newer nonbenzodiazepine sedative agents (e.g., zolpidem, zaleplon, zopiclone, and eszopiclone) have been shown to have fewer adverse effects, a lower risk for tolerance and withdrawal effects, and to produce fewer daytime effects on cognition. Very few data are available, however, concerning the efficacy and safety of these agents specifically following TBI. In one study of patients with stroke and brain injury reporting symptoms of insomnia during rehabilitation, Li Pi Shan and colleagues (133) compared lorazepam (a benzodiazepine hypnotic) and zopiclone (a nonbenzodiazepine hypnotic) administered for 1 week. They found no difference between the 2 drugs in reported sleep duration or sleep continuity. However, they did not measure whether these agents were effective in reducing insomnia symptoms from pre- to post-treatment. Flanagan and his collaborators (132) have advocated in favor of the use of nonbenzodiazepine agents over benzodiazepines, yet in a recent paper, Larson and Zollmann (134) issued a warning that we still have insufficient data to make conclusions about the safety of nonbezodiazepines, especially given that both acute and residual effects on cognition have been noted in normal healthy volunteers with the administration of these drugs. These authors underline the fact that these drugs are known to have distinctive effects in different patient populations, especially those with cognitive impairment.

Neurostimulants

A few studies have described results on the administration of neurostimulants (i.e., modafinil, methylphenidate) for the treatment of sleepiness specifically following TBI. One case study (135) suggested benefits of methylphenidate with a patient who had developed narcolepsy after TBI. The patient was asymptomatic after 6 months of treatment. In a larger study of 30 patients with TBI, Lee and coworkers (136) found that daytime alertness was improved by methylphenidate but not by sertraline, an antidepressant. However, according to a retrospective study, methylphenidate does not seem to significantly reduce the number of hours slept during night-time or daytime (137).

Modafinil is known to be effective in alleviating sleepiness in patients with narcolepsy, sufferers of OSA, and shift workers (138). A first randomized controlled trial conducted by Jha and colleagues (139) on 51 mild-to-severe TBI survivors found that modafinil did not provide significant benefits over placebo for sleepiness and fatigue symptoms. In addition, these authors found that modafinil administration was more frequently associated with insomnia as an adverse effect. Castriotta's team (126) also reported mitigated success (2 out of 5 patients) of modafinil in a subgroup of 5 patients with TBI, with post-traumatic hypersomnia, and narcolepsy. Recently, however, Kaiser and collaborators (140) reported positive effects of modafinil in a pilot prospective, double-blind, randomized study of 20 patients reporting post-TBI fatigue and/or EDS. Compared to placebo-treated patients, subjective EDS (as measured by the Epworth Sleepiness Scale) was significantly reduced, as well as objective sleepiness measures obtained with the MWT. Similarly to Jha and colleagues' results, however, fatigue was not improved by modafinil, further underscoring the independence of these 2 phenomena in TBI. No significant side effects were reported with modafinil in this study.

Melatonin

There is still very little data describing the effectiveness of melatonin to treat sleep-wake disturbances following TBI. Nagtegaal and colleagues (76) reported the case of a 15-year-old girl with a circadian disorder, specifically a delayed sleep phase disorder (her sleep-wake cycle was delayed almost 12 hours), who was successfully treated with melatonin. Kemp and colleagues (141) conducted a preliminary trial with 7 patients complaining of insomnia symptoms (problems initiating or maintaining sleep), who were a mean of 3-year postinjury. They compared melatonin to amitriptyline and found that the use of amitriptyline was associated with improvements in sleep duration and reduced sleep onset latency, whereas the use of melatonin was accompanied with improved daytime alertness.

Other Unstudied Pharmacological Options

Limited data are available to document the efficacy of natural products (e.g., Valerian, St. John's wort) in the treatment of primary sleep disturbances, yet alone sleep disorders in the context of TBI. Futhermore, if they are not regulated by the Food and Drug Administration, there is little information available to the consumer about the different substances used to make up these products. Caution is thus indicated.

Nonpharmacological Treatment Options

Cognitive and Behavioral Interventions for Insomnia

Cognitive-behavioral therapies (CBTs) are now established as a treatment of choice for either primary insomnia (insomnia unrelated to other medical conditions) or insomnia comorbid with medical or psychiatric conditions because they are as effective as pharmacotherapy in the short term and even more effective in the longer term (142–144). The main goal of these treatments is to act on factors perpetuating insomnia, such as unhealthy sleep hygiene, maladaptive sleep habits, autonomic and cognitive arousal, and dysfunctional beliefs and attitudes about sleep.

Ouellet and Morin (145,146) made simple adaptations to the original treatment protocol of CBT developed by Morin (113) (e.g., use of simplified material, repetition, involvement of a significant other) and studied its efficacy in a series of 12 cases of mild-to-severe TBI survivors suffering from insomnia (146). With this treatment protocol, they obtained success rates comparable to those found in the primary insomnia or insomnia secondary to medical disorders literature with statistically and clinically significant improvements in 73% of participants up to 3 months posttreatment.

CBT for insomnia usually involves the following components: *Stimulus control*, which consists in a set of instructions aimed at reassociating the bed, bedroom, and bedtime stimuli with sleep rather than with frustration, anxiety, or tension (147); *sleep restriction* (or restriction of time in bed), which consists in limiting the time spent in bed to the actual total time spent sleeping as assessed by daily sleep logs (148); *cognitive therapy for insomnia*, which is designed to identify, challenge, and alter a set of dysfunctional beliefs and attitudes about sleep (113); and *sleep hygiene education*, which is aimed at educating about the impact of certain lifestyle factors (e.g., diet, drug use, exercise) and the influence of different environmental factors (e.g., light, noise, temperature) on sleep (149). Ouellet and Morin (146) also proposed a *fatigue management* component aimed at recognizing and managing fatigue more effectively and at revising dysfunctional attitudes about fatigue and rest.

Naps

Although napping may be recommended by some clinicians to counteract the effects of fatigue or daytime sleepiness following TBI, the positive and negative impacts of nap taking have not yet been scientifically studied in the TBI population. Post-TBI fatigue can lead to frequent nap and rest taking. Obviously, the need for daytime sleep is increased in the acute phase following the accident, but the continuation of nap taking in the chronic phases following TBI may eventually become problematic. Indeed, on an average of 8 years postaccident, Ouellet and Morin (59) found that 56% of TBI survivors took naps between 3 and 7 times a week. Although daytime naps are known to be beneficial to maintain arousal and enhance performance and learning, they can also cause sleep inertia and negatively impact the next nocturnal sleep episode, particularly if they are too long, are taken too late during the day, and contain more slow-wave sleep (150). The need for a nap must thus be evaluated depending on the time since the injury and the severity of daytime sleepiness (and not fatigue). The timing and length of naps should also be revised carefully. Ideally naps should be shorter than 30 minutes and be taken before 3:00 PM (113).

Continuous Positive Airway Pressure for Sleep Apnea

A typical treatment of OSA is a device delivering continuous positive airway pressure (CPAP) (151). This device is worn over the nose (sometimes also the mouth) and prevents soft tissues in the upper airway from collapsing during sleep by providing a constant pressure throughout the respiratory cycle. The efficacy, safety, and acceptability of this device have not yet been studied specifically in the TBI population. In 13 patients with TBI with OSA, Castriotta et al. (126) reported dramatic improvements in the AHI after 3 months of CPAP treatment, but unfortunately, these changes were not accompanied by improvements in daytime sleepiness as measured either subjectively with the Epworth Sleepiness Scale or objectively with the MSLT. It did, however, increase the amount of REM sleep. More research is thus needed to confirm that CPAP is as efficacious after TBI as in other populations.

Acupuncture

Recently, Zollman and colleagues (152) have proposed that acupuncture holds promise to treat post-TBI insomnia because it is effective in other populations and has few adverse effects. They conducted a pilot study with 24 adult TBI survivors reporting chronic insomnia symptoms, who were randomized to either acupuncture treatment or a treatment-as-usual control condition. They found that the patients treated with acupuncture who were taking sleep medication were able to taper off this usage. Groups did not differ on total sleep time, but patients treated with acupuncture had a significantly higher perceived sleep quality and also showed improvement in cognitive function as measured with the Paced Auditory Serial Addition Test and the Repeatable Battery for the Assessment of Neuropsychological Status.

Chronotherapy and Phototherapy (Bright Light Therapy)

Chronotherapy aims at gradually and systematically shifting bedtime and arising time toward a more desirable sleep-wake schedule. Compliance to recommendations is, however, often difficult with chronotherapy, thus potentially compromising the success of the intervention. Quinto and coworkers (78) reported on an unsuccessful attempt to treat a delayed sleep phase syndrome with chronotherapy in a 48-year-old car accident survivor. In addition to chronotherapy, bright light therapy could be considered as a treatment option. It consists of exposing a person to a source of bright light (typically 10,000 lux) for a period of usually about 2 hours/day. The timing of the light exposure (e.g. early vs later in the day) depends on the characteristics of the patient's sleep-wake patterns. Published data on the efficacy of bright light therapy is still lacking, yet research efforts by Ponsford's team (unpublished data) are currently underway in Australia (particularly with blue light therapy) and could hold promise for the amelioration of sleepiness and post-TBI fatigue.

Other Unstudied Nonpharmacological Options

To our knowledge, relaxation therapies have not yet been investigated in the treatment of post-TBI sleep disturbances. The use of cranial electrotherapy stimulation has been suggested for insomnia in non-TBI populations (153) or for the treatment of mild TBI or head-injury related mood changes

(154,155), but still, very limited evidence exists regarding the safety or efficacy of this treatment option (156).

CONCLUSION

Despite recent scientific advances in documenting alterations in sleep-wake patterns and sleep-wake disorders following TBI, much research is still needed to provide the best guidelines for appropriate evaluation and treatment of these often overlooked, yet significant problems. In particular, there is a need to study how sleep-wake problems impact other domains of functioning (e.g., cognitive functioning, mood, quality of life, return to work). Furthermore, the interactions with psychiatric comorbidities and with prescribed medications still need to be better understood.

KEY CLINICAL POINTS

1. Sleep-wake disturbances are prevalent after TBI and should not be overlooked.
2. Poor sleep quality, insufficient sleep quantity, and EDS are among the most common symptoms. A thorough assessment is necessary to confirm the presence of a sleep disorder, such as insomnia, sleep apnea, narcolepsy, or CRSD.
3. Daytime sleepiness should be differentiated from fatigue. Sleepiness arises from a physiological drive to sleep and implies normal variations or abnormal disruptions of the sleep-wake cycle. Fatigue is a subjective state of depleted energy and is not necessarily linked to sleep.
4. Assessment of sleep-wake disturbances should include a clinical interview with the TBI survivor and an informant, as well as subjective measures (questionnaires). If the presence of specific sleep disorders, such as sleep apnea or narcolepsy is suspected, nighttime and/or daytime PSG may be necessary.
5. Both premorbid and current sleep patterns should be considered because symptoms may have been already present prior to the injury.
6. Data on the efficacy and safety of pharmacological treatment options for sleep-wake disturbances following TBI is scarce. Therefore, medication should be prescribed cautiously, medication interactions and psychiatric/medical comorbidities should be taken into consideration, and therapeutic and side effects should be monitored closely.
7. CBT, which is the treatment of choice for primary insomnia, has been shown to be effective to treat insomnia after TBI. Several other nonpharmacological options can be considered but need to be studied further in this population.

KEY REFERENCES

1. American Academy of Sleep Medicine. Practice guidelines for different sleep disorders. Available at: http://www.aasmnet.org/practiceguidelines.aspx. Accessed May 16, 2012.
2. Baumann CR, Werth E, Stocker R, Ludwig S, Bassetti CL. Sleep-wake disturbances 6 months after traumatic brain injury: a prospective study. *Brain*. 2007;130(pt 7):1873–1883.
3. Castriotta RJ, Murthy JN. Sleep disorders in patients with traumatic brain injury: a review. *CNS Drugs*. 2011;25(3):175–185.
4. Kryger MH, Roth T, Dement WC. *Principles and Practice of Sleep Medicine*. 4th ed. Philadelphia, PA: Elsevier Saunders; 2005.
5. Orff HJ, Ayalon L, Drummond SP. Traumatic brain injury and sleep disturbance: a review of current research. *J Head Trauma Rehabil*. 2009;24(3):155–165.

References

1. Wiseman-Hakes C, Colantonio A, Gargaro J. Sleep and wake disorders following traumatic brain injury: a systematic review of the literature. *Crit Rev Phys Rehabil Med*. 2009;21(3–4):317–374.
2. Chaput G, Giguere JF, Chauny JM, Denis R, Lavigne G. Relationship among subjective sleep complaints, headaches, and mood alterations following a mild traumatic brain injury. *Sleep Med*. 2009;10(7):713–716.
3. Makley MJ, English JB, Drubach DA, Kreuz AJ, Celnik PA, Tarwater PM. Prevalence of sleep disturbance in closed head injury patients in a rehabilitation unit. *Neurorehabil Neural Repair*. 2008;22(4):341–347.
4. Rao V, Spiro J, Vaishnavi S, et al. Prevalence and types of sleep disturbances acutely after traumatic brain injury. *Brain Inj*. 2008;22(5):381–386.
5. Kempf J, Werth E, Kaiser PR, Bassetti CL, Baumann CR. Sleep-wake disturbances 3 years after traumatic brain injury. *J Neurol Neurosurg Psychiatry*. 2010;81(12):1402–1405.
6. Verma A, Anand V, Verma NP. Sleep disorders in chronic traumatic brain injury. *J Clin Sleep Med*. 2007;3(4):357–362.
7. Worthington AD, Melia Y. Rehabilitation is compromised by arousal and sleep disorders: results of a survey of rehabilitation centres. *Brain Inj*. 2006;20(3):327–332.
8. Ouellet M, Beaulieu-Bonneau S, Morin C. Insomnia in patients with traumatic brain injury: frequency, characteristics, and risk factors. *J Head Trauma Rehabil*. 2006;21(3):199–212.
9. Castriotta RJ, Wilde MC, Lai JM, Atanasov S, Masel BE, Kuna ST. Prevalence and consequences of sleep disorders in traumatic brain injury. *J Clin Sleep Med*. 2007;3(4):349–356.
10. Wilde MC, Castriotta RJ, Lai JM, Atanasov S, Masel BE, Kuna ST. Cognitive impairment in patients with traumatic brain injury and obstructive sleep apnea. *Arch Phys Med Rehabil*. 2007;88(10):1284–1288.
11. Marks GA, Shaffery JP, Oksenberg A, Speciale SG, Roffwarg HP. A functional role for REM sleep in brain maturation. *Behav Brain Res*. 1995;69(1–2):1–11.
12. Jenni OG, Borbely AA, Achermann P. Development of the nocturnal sleep electroencephalogram in human infants. *Am J Physiol Regul Integr Comp Physiol*. 2004;286(3):R528–R538.
13. Adam K. Sleep as a restorative process and a theory to explain why. *Prog Brain Res*. 1980;53:289–305.
14. Benington JH, Heller HC. Restoration of brain energy metabolism as the function of sleep. *Progr Neurobiol*. 1995;45(4):347–360.
15. Horne J. Human slow wave sleep: a review and appraisal of recent findings, with implications for sleep functions, and psychiatric illness. *Experientia*. 1992;48(10):941–954.
16. Lange T, Dimitrov S, Born J. Effects of sleep and circadian rhythm on the human immune system. *Ann N Y Acad Sci*. 2010;1193:48–59.
17. Van Cauter E, Plat L, Copinschi G. Interrelations between sleep and the somatotropic axis. *Sleep*. 1998;21(6):553–566.
18. Van Cauter E, Leproult R, Plat L. Age-related changes in slow wave sleep and REM sleep and relationship with growth hormone and cortisol levels in healthy men. *JAMA*. 2000;284(7):861–868.
19. Friese RS. Sleep and recovery from critical illness and injury: a review of theory, current practice, and future directions. *Crit Care Med*. 2008;36(3):697–705.
20. Born J, Rasch B, Gais S. Sleep to remember. *Neuroscientist*. 2006;12(5):410–424.
21. Walker MP, Stickgold R. Sleep, memory, and plasticity. *Annu Rev Psychol*. 2006;57:139–166.

22. Valenza MC, Rodenstein DO, Fernandez-de-las-Penas C. Consideration of sleep dysfunction in rehabilitation. *J Bodyw Mov Ther.* 2011; 15(3):262–267.

23. Carskadon MA, Dement WC. Normal human sleep : An overview. In: Kryger TR, Dement WC, eds. *Principles and Practice of Sleep Medicine.* 3rd ed. Philadelphia, PA: WB Saunders; 2000:15–25.

24. Rechtschaffen A, Kales A. *A Manual of Standardized Terminology, Techniques, and Scoring System for Sleep Stages of Human Subjects.* Washington, DC: US Public Health Service; 1968.

25. Iber C, Ancoli-Israel S, Chesson A, Quan S. *The AASM Manual for the Scoring of Sleep and Associated Events.* Westchester, IL: American Academy of Sleep Medicine; 2007.

26. Evans BM, Bartlett JR. Prediction of outcome in severe head injury based on recognition of sleep related activity in the polygraphic electroencephalogram. *J Neurol Neurosurg Psychiatry.* 1995;59(1): 17–25.

27. Laffont F. Les insomnies organiques. In: Billiard M, ed. *Le Sommeil Normal et Pathologique: Troubles du Sommeil et de L'éveil.* 2nd ed. Paris, France: Masson; 1998:178–188.

28. Ron S, Algom D, Hary D, Cohen M. Time-related changes in the distribution of sleep stages in brain injured patients. *Electroencephalogr Clinl Neurophysiol.* 1980;48(4):432–441.

29. Bergamasco B, Bergamini L, Doriguzzi T, Fabiani D. EEG sleep patterns as a prognostic criterion in post-traumatic coma. *Electroencephalogr Clinic Neurophysiol.* 1968;24(4):374–377.

30. Bricolo A, Gentilomo A, Rosadini G, Rossi GF. Long-lasting post-traumatic unconsciousness. A study based on nocturnal EEG and polygraphic recording. *Acta Neurol Scand.* 1968;44(4):513–532.

31. Prigatano GP, Stahl ML, Orr WC, Zeiner HK. Sleep and dreaming disturbances in closed head injury patients. *J Neurol Neurosurg Psychiatry.* 1982;45(1):78–80.

32. George B, Landau-Ferey J. Twelve months' follow-up by night sleep EEG after recovery from severe head trauma. *Neurochirurgia (Stuttg).* 1986;29(2):45–47.

33. George B, Landau-Ferey J, Benoit O, Dondey M, Cophignon J. Night sleep disorders during recovery of severe head injuries. *Neurochirurgie.* 1981;27(1):35–38.

34. Kaufman Y, Tzischinsky O, Epstein R, Etzioni A, Lavie P, Pillar G. Long-term sleep disturbances in adolescents after minor head injury. *Pediatr Neurol.* 2001;24(2):129–134.

35. Ouellet MC, Morin CM. Subjective and objective measures of insomnia in the context of traumatic brain injury: a preliminary study. *Sleep Med.* 2006;7(6):486–497.

36. Parcell DL, Ponsford JL, Redman JR, Rajaratnam SM. Poor sleep quality and changes in objectively recorded sleep after traumatic brain injury: a preliminary study. *Arch Phys Med Rehabil.* 2008;89(5): 843–850.

37. Williams BR, Lazic SE, Ogilvie RD. Polysomnographic and quantitative EEG analysis of subjects with long-term insomnia complaints associated with mild traumatic brain injury. *Clin Neurophysiol.* 2008;119(2):429–438.

38. Lenard HG, Pennigstorff H. Alterations in the sleep patterns of infants and young children following acute head injuries. *Acta Paediatr Scand.* 1970;59(5):565–571.

39. Schreiber S, Barkai G, Gur-Hartman T, et al. Long-lasting sleep patterns of adult patients with minor traumatic brain injury (mTBI) and non-mTBI subjects. *Sleep Med.* 2008;9(5):481–487.

40. Baumann CR, Bassetti CL, Valko PO, et al. Loss of hypocretin (orexin) neurons with traumatic brain injury. *Ann Neurol.* 2009;66(4): 555–559.

41. Parsons LC, Crosby LJ, Perlis M, Britt T, Jones P. Longitudinal sleep EEG power spectral analysis studies in adolescents with minor head injury. *J Neurotrauma.* 1997;14(8):549–559.

42. Gosselin N, Lassonde M, Petit D, et al. Sleep following sport-related concussions. *Sleep Med.* 2009;10(1):35–46.

43. Rao V, Bergey A, Hill H, Efron D, McCann U. Sleep disturbance after mild traumatic brain injury: indicator of injury? *J Neuropsychiatry Clin Neurosci.* 2011;23(2):201–205.

44. Morin CM, LeBlanc M, Daley M, Gregoire JP, Merette C. Epidemiology of insomnia: prevalence, self-help treatments, consultations, and determinants of help-seeking behaviors. *Sleep Med.* 2006; 7(2):123–130.

45. LeBlanc M, Beaulieu-Bonneau S, Merette C, Savard J, Ivers H, Morin CM. Psychological and health-related quality of life factors associated with insomnia in a population-based sample. *J Psychosom Res.* 2007;63(2):157–166.

46. Ouellet MC, Savard J, Morin CM. Insomnia following traumatic brain injury: a review. *Neurorehabil Neural Repair.* 2004;18(4): 187–198.

47. Zeitzer JM, Friedman L, O'Hara R. Insomnia in the context of traumatic brain injury. *J Rehabil Res Dev.* 2009;46(6):827–836.

48. Fichtenberg NL, Zafonte RD, Putnam S, Mann NR, Millard AE. Insomnia in a post-acute brain injury sample. *Brain Inj.* 2002;16(3): 197–206.

49. American Psychiatric Association. *Diagnostic and Statistical Manual of Mental Disorders.* 4th ed., text rev. Washington, DC: American Psychiatric Association; 2000.

50. Bastien CH, Vallieres A, Morin CM. Validation of the Insomnia Severity Index as an outcome measure for insomnia research. *Sleep Med.* 2001;2(4):297–307.

51. Beetar JT, Guilmette TJ, Sparadeo FR. Sleep and pain complaints in symptomatic traumatic brain injury and neurologic populations. *Arch of Phys Med Rehabil.* 1996;77(12):1298–1302.

52. Clinchot DM, Bogner J, Mysiw WJ, Fugate L, Corrigan J. Defining sleep disturbance after brain injury. *Am J Phys Med Rehabil.* 1998; 77(4):291–295.

53. Fichtenberg NL, Millis SR, Mann NR, Zafonte RD, Millard AE. Factors associated with insomnia among post-acute traumatic brain injury survivors. *Brain Inj.* 2000;14(7):659–667.

54. Mahmood O, Rapport LJ, Hanks RA, Fichtenberg NL. Neuropsychological performance and sleep disturbance following traumatic brain injury. *J Head Trauma Rehabil.* 2004;19(5):378–390.

55. Mayou R, Bryant B, Ehlers A. Prediction of psychological outcomes one year after a motor vehicle accident. *Am J Psychiatry.* 2001;158(8): 1231–1238.

56. American Academy of Sleep Medicine. *The International Classification of Sleep Disorders.* 2nd ed. Westchester, IL: American Academy of Sleep Medicine; 2005.

57. Johns MW. A new method for measuring daytime sleepiness: the Epworth sleepiness scale. *Sleep.* 1991;14(6):540–545.

58. Elovic E, Dobrovic N, Fellus J. Fatigue after traumatic brain injury. In: DeLuca J, ed. *Fatigue as a Window to the Brain.* London, England: MIT Press; 2005:89–105.

59. Ouellet MC, Morin C. Fatigue following traumatic brain injury: frequency, characteristics, and associated factors. *Rehabil Psychol.* 2006;51(2):140–149.

60. Pigeon WR, Sateia MJ, Ferguson RJ. Distinguishing between excessive daytime sleepiness and fatigue: toward improved detection and treatment. *J Psychosom Res.* 2003;54(1):61–69.

61. Cantor JB, Ashman T, Gordon W, et al. Fatigue after traumatic brain injury and its impact on participation and quality of life. *J Head Trauma Rehabil.* 2008;23(1):41–51.

62. Cohen M, Oksenberg A, Snir D, Stern MJ, Groswasser Z. Temporally related changes of sleep complaints in traumatic brain injured patients. *J Neurol Neurosurg Psychiatry.* 1992;55(4):313–315.

63. Parcell DL, Ponsford JL, Rajaratnam SM, Redman JR. Self-reported changes to nighttime sleep after traumatic brain injury. *Arch Phys Med Rehabil.* 2006;87(2):278–285.

64. Watson NF, Dikmen S, Machamer J, Doherty M, Temkin N. Hypersomnia following traumatic brain injury. *J Clin Sleep Med.* 2007; 3(4):363–368.

65. Baumann CR, Werth E, Stocker R, Ludwig S, Bassetti CL. Sleep-wake disturbances 6 months after traumatic brain injury: a prospective study. *Brain.* 2007;130(pt 7):1873–1883.

66. Guilleminault C, Yuen KM, Gulevich MG, Karadeniz D, Leger D, Philip P. Hypersomnia after head-neck trauma: a medicolegal dilemma. *Neurology.* 2000;54(3):653–659.

67. American Academy of Sleep Medicine. *The International Classification of Sleep Disorders.* 2nd ed. Westchester, IL: American Academy of Sleep Medicine; 2005.

68. Ebrahim IO, Peacock KW, Williams AJ. Post-traumatic narcolepsy—two case reports and a mini review. *J Clin Sleep Med.* 2005; 1(2):153–156.

69. Kushida CA, Littner MR, Morgenthaler T, et al. Practice parameters for the indications for polysomnography and related procedures: an update for 2005. *Sleep.* 2005;28(4):499–521.

70. Guilleminault C, Faull KF, Miles L, van den Hoed J. Posttraumatic excessive daytime sleepiness: a review of 20 patients. *Neurology.* 1983;33(12):1584–1589.

71. Webster JB, Bell KR, Hussey JD, Natale TK, Lakshminarayan S. Sleep apnea in adults with traumatic brain injury: a preliminary investigation. *Arch Phys Med Rehabil.* 2001;82(3):316–321.

72. Masel BE, Scheibel RS, Kimbark T, Kuna ST. Excessive daytime sleepiness in adults with brain injuries. *Arch Phys Med Rehabil.* 2001; 82(11):1526–1532.

73. Castriotta RJ, Lai JM. Sleep disorders associated with traumatic brain injury. *Arch Phys Med Rehabil.* 2001;82(10):1403–1406.

74. Kemp S, Agostinis A, House A, Coughlan AK. Analgesia and other causes of amnesia that mimic post-traumatic amnesia: a cohort study. *J Neuropsychol.* 2010;4(pt 2):231–236.

75. Boivin DB, Caliyurt O, James FO, Chalk C. Association between delayed sleep phase and hypernyctohemeral syndromes: a case study. *Sleep.* 2004;27(3):417–421.

76. Nagtegaal JE, Kerkhof GA, Smits MG, Swart AC, van der Meer YG. Traumatic brain injury-associated delayed sleep phase syndrome. *Funct Neurol.* 1997;12(6):345–348.

77. Patten SB, Lauderdale WM. Delayed sleep phase disorder after traumatic brain injury. *J Am Acad Child Adolesc Psychiatry.* 1992; 31(1):100–102.

78. Quinto C, Gellido C, Chokroverty S, Masdeu J. Posttraumatic delayed sleep phase syndrome. *Neurology.* 2000;54(1):250–252.

79. Orff HJ, Ayalon L, Drummond SP. Traumatic brain injury and sleep disturbance: a review of current research. *J Head Trauma Rehabil.* 2009;24(3):155–165.

80. Ayalon L, Borodkin K, Dishon L, Kanety H, Dagan Y. Circadian rhythm sleep disorders following mild traumatic brain injury. *Neurology.* 2007;68(14):1136–1140.

81. Mahowald MW. Sleep in traumatic brain injury and other acquired CNS conditions. In: Culebras A, ed. *Sleep Disorders and Neurological Disease.* New York, NY: Dekker; 2000:365–385.

82. Gabor JY, Cooper AB, Hanly PJ. Sleep disruption in the intensive care unit. *Curr Opin Crit Care.* 2001;7(1):21–27.

83. Makley MJ, Johnson-Greene L, Tarwater PM, et al. Return of memory and sleep efficiency following moderate to severe closed head injury. *Neurorehabil Neural Repair.* 2009;23(4):320–326.

84. Frieboes RM, Muller U, Murck H, von Cramon DY, Holsboer F, Steiger A. Nocturnal hormone secretion and the sleep EEG in patients several months after traumatic brain injury. *J Neuropsychiatry Clin Neurosci.* 1999;11(3):354–360.

85. Foltz EL, Jenkner FL, Ward AA Jr. Experimental cerebral concussion. *J Neurosurg.* 1953;10(4):342–352.

86. Foltz EL, Schmidt RP. The role of the reticular formation in the coma of head injury. *J Neurosurg.* 1956;13(2):145–154.

87. Denny-Brown D, Russell WR. Experimental cerebral concussion. *J Physiol.* 1940;99(1):153.

88. Ward AA Jr. Physiological basis of concussion. *J Neurosurg.* 1958; 15(2):129–134.

89. Cooper R, Hulme A. Changes of the EEG, intracranial pressure and other variables during sleep in patients with intracranial lesions. *Electroencephalogr Clin Neurophysiol.* 1969;27(1):12–21.

90. Baumann CR, Stocker R, Imhof HG, et al. Hypocretin-1 (orexin A) deficiency in acute traumatic brain injury. *Neurology.* 2005;65(1): 147–149.

91. Fronczek R, Baumann CR, Lammers GJ, Bassetti CL, Overeem S. Hypocretin/orexin disturbances in neurological disorders. *Sleep Med Rev.* 2009;13(1):9–22.

92. Baumann CR, Bassetti CL. Hypocretins (orexins): clinical impact of the discovery of a neurotransmitter. *Sleep Med Rev.* 2005;9(4): 253–268.

93. Dauvilliers Y, Baumann CR, Carlander B, et al. CSF hypocretin-1 levels in narcolepsy, Kleine-Levin syndrome, and other hypersomnias and neurological conditions. *J Neurol Neurosurger Psychiatry.* 2003;74(12):1667–1673.

94. Paparrigopoulos T, Melissaki A, Tsekou H, et al. Melatonin secretion after head injury: a pilot study. *Brain Inj.* 2006;20(8):873–878.

95. Shekleton JA, Parcell DL, Redman JR, Phipps-Nelson J, Ponsford JL, Rajaratnam SM. Sleep disturbance and melatonin levels following traumatic brain injury. *Neurology.* 2010;74(21):1732–1738.

96. Keller-Wossidlo H, Suter N. Polysomnography in patients with mild traumatic brain injury and excessive daytime somnolence. *J Sleep Res.* 2004;13(suppl 1):389.

97. Nardone R, Bergmann J, Kunz A, et al. Cortical excitability changes in patients with sleep-wake disturbances after traumatic brain injury. *J Neurotrauma.* 2011;28(7);1165–1171.

98. Gottlieb DJ, DeStefano AL, Foley DJ, et al. APOE epsilon4 is associated with obstructive sleep apnea/hypopnea: the Sleep Heart Health Study. *Neurology.* 2004;63(4):664–668.

99. O'Hara R, Luzon A, Hubbard J, Zeitzer JM. Sleep apnea, apolipoprotein epsilon 4 allele, and TBI: mechanism for cognitive dysfunction and development of dementia. *J Rehabil Res Dev.* 2009;46(6): 837–850.

100. Sundström A, Nilsson LG, Cruts M, Adolfsson R, Van Broeckhoven C, Nyberg L. Fatigue before and after mild traumatic brain injury: pre-post-injury comparisons in relation to Apolipoprotein E. *Brain Inj.* 2007;21(10):1049–1054.

101. Nampiaparampil D. Prevalence of chronic pain after traumatic brain injury: a systematic review. *JAMA.* 2008;300(6):711–719.

102. Moldofsky H. Sleep and fibrositis syndrome. *Rheum Dis Clin North Am.* 1989;15(1):91–103.

103. Mahowald M, Mahowald M. Sleep disorders. In: Rizzo M, Tranel D, eds. *Head Injury and Postconcussive Syndrome.* New York, NY: Churchill Livingstone; 1996:285–304.

104. Pagel JF. Medications and their effects on sleep. *Prim Care.* 2005; 32(2):491–509.

105. Mouret J, Lemoine P, Minuit MP, Benkelfat C, Renardet M. Effects of trazodone on the sleep of depressed subjects—a polygraphic study. *Psychopharmacology (Berl).* 1988;95 (suppl):S37–S43.

106. Hubain PP, Castro P, Mesters P, De Maertelaer V, Mendlewicz J. Alprazolam and amitriptyline in the treatment of major depressive disorder: a double-blind clinical and sleep EEG study. *J Affect Disord.* 1990;18(1):67–73.

107. Ott GE, Rao U, Lin KM, Gertsik L, Poland RE. Effect of treatment with bupropion on EEG sleep: relationship to antidepressant response. *Int J Neuropsychopharmacol.* 2004;7(3):275–281.

108. Yamadera H, Nakamura S, Suzuki H, Endo S. Effects of trazodone hydrochloride and imipramine on polysomnography in healthy subjects. *Psychiatry Clin Neurosci.* 1998;52(4):439–443.

109. Kaynak H, Kaynak D, Gozukirmizi E, Guilleminault C. The effects of trazodone on sleep in patients treated with stimulant antidepressants. *Sleep Med.* 2004;5(1):15–20.

110. Zafonte R, Mann N, Fichtenberg N. Sleep disturbance in traumatic brain injury: pharmacologic options. *Neurorehabilitation.* 1996;7(3): 189–196.

111. Kowatch RA. Sleep and head injury. *Psychiatr Med.* 1989;7(1):37–41.

112. Friese RS, Diaz-Arrastia R, McBride D, Frankel H, Gentilello LM. Quantity and quality of sleep in the surgical intensive care unit: are our patients sleeping? *J Trauma.* 2007;63(6):1210–1214.

113. Morin C. *Insomnia:Psychological Assessment and Management.* New York, NY: Guilford Press; 1993.

114. Ashman TA, Spielman LA, Hibbard MR, Silver JM, Chandna T, Gordon WA. Psychiatric challenges in the first 6 years after traumatic brain injury: cross-sequential analyses of Axis I disorders. *Arch Phys Med Rehabil.* 2004;85(4)(suppl 2):S36–S42.

115. Fann JR, Leonetti A, Jaffe K, Katon WJ, Cummings P, Thompson RS. Psychiatric illness and subsequent traumatic brain injury: a case control study. *J Neurol Neurosurg Psychiatry.* 2002;72(5):615–620.

116. Krahn LE. Psychiatric disorders associated with disturbed sleep. *Semin Neurol.* 2005;25(1):90–96.

117. Bloomfield IL, Espie CA, Evans JJ. Do sleep difficulties exacerbate deficits in sustained attention following traumatic brain injury? *J Int Neuropsychol Soc.* 2009;16(1):17–25.

118. Aloia MS, Arnedt JT, Davis JD, Riggs RL, Byrd D. Neuropsychological sequelae of obstructive sleep apnea-hypopnea syndrome: a critical review. *J Int Neuropsychol Soc.* 2004;10(5):772–785.

119. Buysse DJ, Reynolds CF III, Monk TH, Berman SR, Kupfer DJ. The Pittsburgh Sleep Quality Index: a new instrument for psychiatric practice and research. *Psychiatry Res.* 1989;28(2):193–213.

120. Horne JA, Ostberg O. A self-assessment questionnaire to determine morningness-eveningness in human circadian rhythms. *Int J Chronobiol.* 1976;4(2):97–110.

121. Monk TH, Buysse DJ, Kennedy KS, Pods JM, DeGrazia JM, Miewald JM. Measuring sleep habits without using a diary: the sleep timing questionnaire. *Sleep.* 2003;26(2):208–212.

122. Hoddes E, Zarcone V, Smythe H, Phillips R, Dement WC. Quantification of sleepiness: a new approach. *Psychophysiology.* 1973;10(4):431–436.

123. Besset A. Polysomnography. In: Billiard M, ed. *Sleep: Physiology, Investigations and Medicine.* New York, NY: Plenum Publishers; 2003:127–138.

124. Littner MR, Kushida C, Wise M, et al. Practice parameters for clinical use of the multiple sleep latency test and the maintenance of wakefulness test. *Sleep.* 2005;28(1):113–121.

125. Arand D, Bonnet M, Hurwitz T, Mitler M, Rosa R, Sangal RB. The clinical use of the MSLT and MWT. *Sleep.* 2005;28(1):123–144.

126. Castriotta RJ, Atanasov S, Wilde MC, Masel BE, Lai JM, Kuna ST. Treatment of sleep disorders after traumatic brain injury. *J Clin Sleep Med.* 2009;5(2):137–144.

127. Ancoli-Israel S, Ayalon L. Diagnosis and treatment of sleep disorders in older adults. *Am J Geriatr Psychiatry.* 2006;14(2):95–103.

128. Muller U, Czymmek J, Thöne-Otto A, Von Cramon DY. Reduced daytime activity in patients with acquired brain damage and apathy: a study with ambulatory actigraphy. *Brain Inj.* 2006;20(2):157–160.

129. Zollman FS, Cyborski C, Duraski SA. Actigraphy for assessment of sleep in traumatic brain injury: case series, review of the literature and proposed criteria for use. *Brain Inj.* 2010;24(5):748–754.

130. Goldstein LB. Prescribing of potentially harmful drugs to patients admitted to hospital after head injury. *J Neurol Neurosurg Psychiatry.* 1995;58(6):753–755.

131. Schallert T, Hernandez TD, Barth TM. Recovery of function after brain damage: severe and chronic disruption by diazepam. *Brain Res.* 1986;379(1):104–111.

132. Flanagan SR, Greenwald B, Wieber S. Pharmacological treatment of insomnia for individuals with brain injury. *J Head Trauma Rehabil.* 2007;22(1):67–70.

133. Li Pi Shan RS, Ashworth NL. Comparison of lorazepam and zopiclone for insomnia in patients with stroke and brain injury: a randomized, crossover, double-blinded trial. *Am J Phys Med Rehabil.* 2004;83(6):421–427.

134. Larson EB, Zollman FS. The effect of sleep medications on cognitive recovery from traumatic brain injury. *J Head Trauma Rehabil.* 2010;25(1):61–67.

135. Francisco GE, Ivanhoe CB. Successful treatment of post-traumatic narcolepsy with methylphenidate: a case report. *Am J Phys Med Rehabil.* 1996;75(1):63–65.

136. Lee H, Kim SW, Kim JM, Shin IS, Yang SJ, Yoon JS. Comparing effects of methylphenidate, sertraline and placebo on neuropsychiatric sequelae in patients with traumatic brain injury. *Hum Psychopharmacol.* 2005;20(2):97–104.

137. Al-Adawi S, Burke DT, Dorvlo AS. The effect of methylphenidate on the sleep-wake cycle of brain-injured patients undergoing rehabilitation. *Sleep Med.* 2006;7(3):287–291.

138. Kumar R. Approved and investigational uses of modafinil: an evidence-based review. *Drugs.* 2008;68(13):1803–1839.

139. Jha A, Weintraub A, Allshouse A, et al. A randomized trial of modafinil for the treatment of fatigue and excessive daytime sleepiness in individuals with chronic traumatic brain injury. *J Head Trauma Rehabil.* 2008;23(1):52–63.

140. Kaiser PR, Valko PO, Werth E, et al. Modafinil ameliorates excessive daytime sleepiness after traumatic brain injury. *Neurology.* 2010;75(20):1780–1785.

141. Kemp S, Biswas R, Neumann V, Coughlan A. The value of melatonin for sleep disorders occurring post-head injury: a pilot RCT. *Brain Inj.* 2004;18(9):911–919.

142. Murtagh D, Greenwood K. Identifying effective psychological treatments for insomnia: a meta-analysis. *J Consult Clin Psychol.* 1994;63:79–89.

143. Morin CM, Bootzin RR, Buysse DJ, Edinger JD, Espie CA, Lichstein KL. Psychological and behavioral treatment of insomnia:update of the recent evidence (1998–2004). *Sleep.* 2006;29(11):1398–1414.

144. Morin CM, Culbert JP, Schwartz SM. Nonpharmacological interventions for insomnia: a meta-analysis of treatment efficacy. *Am J Psychiatry.* 1994;151(8):1172–1180.

145. Ouellet MC, Morin CM. Cognitive behavioral therapy for insomnia associated with traumatic brain injury: a single-case study. *Arch Phys Med Rehabil.* 2004;85(8):1298–1302.

146. Ouellet MC, Morin CM. Efficacy of cognitive-behavioral therapy for insomnia associated with traumatic brain injury: a singlecase experimental design. *Arch Phys Med Rehabil.* 2007;88(12):1581–1592.

147. Bootzin RR, Epstein D, Wood JM. Stimulus control instructions. In: Hauri PJ, ed. *Case Studies in Insomnia.* New York, NY: Plenum Publishers; 1991:19–28.

148. Spielman AJ, Saskin P, Thorpy MJ. Treatment of chronic insomnia by restriction of time in bed. *Sleep.* 1987;10(1):45–56.

149. Hauri PJ. *Case Studies in Insomnia.* New York, NY: Plenum Press; 1991.

150. Dhand R, Sohal H. Good sleep, bad sleep! The role of daytime naps in healthy adults. *Curr Opin Pulm Med.* 2006;12(6):379–382.

151. Kushida CA, Littner MR, Hirshkowitz M, et al; for American Academy of Sleep Medicine. Practice parameters for the use of continuous and bilevel positive airway pressure devices to treat adult patients with sleep-related breathing disorders. *Sleep.* 2006;29(3):375–380.

152. Zollman FS, Larson EB, Wasek-Throm LK, Cyborski CM, Bode RK. Acupuncture for treatment of insomnia in patients with traumatic brain injury: a pilot intervention study. *J Head Trauma Rehabil.* 2012;27(2):135–142.

153. Kirsch DL, Gilula MF. CES in the treatment of insomnia: a review and meta-analysis. *Pract Pain Manage.* 2007;7(7):28–39.

154. Kirsch DL. CES for mild traumatic brain injury. *Pract Pain Manage.* 2008;8(6):70–77.

155. Smith RB, Tiberi A, Marshall J. The use of cranial electrotherapy stimulation in the treatment of closed-head-injured patients. *Brain Inj.* 1994;8(4):357–361.

156. Klawansky S, Yeung A, Berkey C, Shah N, Phan H, Chalmers TC. Meta-analysis of randomized controlled trials of cranial electrostimulation. Efficacy in treating selected psychological and physiological conditions. *J Nerv Ment Dis.* 1995;183(7):478–484.

157. World Health Organization. *The International Classification of Diseases.* 10th ed. Geneva, Switzerland: World Health Organization; 1992.

Diagnosis and Management of Late Intracranial Complications of Traumatic Brain Injury

David F. Long

INTRODUCTION

Purpose and Overview

Purpose

Although many patients show excellent progress during rehabilitation from traumatic brain injury (TBI), intracranial complications occur frequently and can result in an adverse outcome. In many instances, prompt and accurate diagnosis of these complications can either be lifesaving or can dramatically improve the extent of recovery which takes place.

Overview

Complications addressed in this chapter include central nervous system (CNS) infections and the conditions predisposing to them, hydrocephalus and shunt management, and late post-traumatic vascular and mass lesions.

Specific Chapter Sections

Infection and Risk of Infection

The potential risk of serious CNS infection changes the management of some patients even before an infection occurs. Topics discussed in this section include compound depressed skull fractures, penetrating injuries, basilar skull fractures, cerebrospinal fistulae, and pneumocephalus. CNS infections themselves are then discussed including meningitis, brain abscess, and subdural empyema. Because specific management options, especially antibiotic selection, are frequently subject to change, the general approach to diagnosis and management is emphasized in this section. The section on craniectomy and cranioplasty has also been revised considerably in view of both the increasing use of craniectomy and changing approach to cranioplasty.

Hydrocephalus and Shunts

Hydrocephalus is probably the most difficult common complication to diagnose and manage during the rehabilitation of patients with TBI. Not only it is a challenge to identify which patients will benefit from a shunt, but also management often becomes even more complicated after shunting. To optimally manage these patients, physicians need to understand the different types of shunts and their physiology, as well as common shunt complications. Programmable shunts and other recent innovations are now routinely available and offer an opportunity for intervention to improve outcome during rehabilitation without requiring further surgery.

Vascular and Late Mass Lesions

Although vascular lesions such as post-traumatic aneurysm and carotid cavernous fistula are relatively uncommon, physicians treating patients with TBI need to be aware of these complications to recognize and treat them promptly when they do occur. Finally, late mass lesions such as chronic subdural hematoma and hygroma, late presenting epidural hematoma, and delayed post-traumatic intracerebral hemorrhage are discussed.

CONDITIONS INVOLVING RISK OF INFECTION

Skull Fractures and Penetrating Injuries

Depressed Skull Fractures

Depressed skull fractures are best seen on tangential skull radiographs, and if the fragment is depressed below the inner table of the skull by more than the thickness of the skull, it is usually elevated surgically both for appearance and in the hope of preventing epilepsy (1). Compound depressed skull fractures are distinguished from simple depressed skull fractures by the presence of an overlying open wound or laceration and account for 85% of depressed skull fractures (1). Because of the high risk of having intracranial infection, including subdural empyema and brain abscess, compound depressed skull fractures are debrided either acutely or once cerebral perfusion pressure stabilizes (2). Prophylactic antibiotics are also often administered (3–5).

Penetrating Injuries

Gunshot wounds confer a high risk for infection, and post-traumatic brain abscess is the most common after missile injury for several reasons: (a) the bullet is retained inside the skull in about 70% of civilian gunshot wounds and becomes a nidus for infection, (b) retained bone fragments are an even greater problem increasing the risk of infection by a factor of 10 (6), and (c) focal necrosis of tissue in the path of the bullet is also believed to be crucial in the possible development of brain abscess. For these reasons, surgical debridement has been emphasized, and antibiotic prophylaxis is routinely employed by almost 90% of neurosurgeons (7).

Basilar Skull Fractures

The base of the skull is comprised of 5 bones: the sphenoid, ethmoid (including cribriform plate), frontal, temporal (petrous and squamous), and occipital bones (1). Clues to likely basilar skull fracture include cerebrospinal fluid (CSF) leaks, pneumocephalus, hemotympanum, Battle sign (ecchymosis in the mastoid region), hearing impairment, peripheral facial nerve weakness, periorbital ecchymosis, fracture of the frontal sinus, and anosmia (8). Because the dura is closely adherent to the bones of the skull base, basilar fractures are frequently associated with dural tears; the resultant fistulous connection between the brain and sinuses or ear provides a possible route of entry for infection. Antibiotic prophylaxis after basilar skull fracture has been controversial. A recent meta-analysis of 12 studies with a total of 1,241 patients with basilar skull fracture did not find a statistically significant decrease in meningitis in patients treated with antibiotic prophylaxis (9).

Cerebrospinal Fluid Fistula

Cerebrospinal Fluid Rhinorrhea

CSF rhinorrhea is a definite indication of a fistulous tract from the intracranial compartment through the dura and skull base. It is therefore important to determine whether CSF rhinorrhea is present in patients with brain injury. CSF rhinorrhea is typically a watery discharge with a salty taste, which does not cause nasal excoriation or stiffen bed linen (10). It may be unilateral, may increase with leaning over or prone positioning, and may be associated with a dull, constant, or orthostatic headache from low intracranial pressure (ICP) (10,11). Differential diagnosis includes vasomotor rhinitis, which is typically bilateral with sneezing and lacrimation, and pseudo-CSF rhinorrhea after surgery in the region of the pericarotid sympathetic plexus (12), with nasal stuffiness and hypersecretion, facial flushing, and absent ipsilateral lacrimation.

Glucose strips or tape are notoriously unreliable for the diagnosis of CSF rhinorrhea with false-positive rates as high as 75% (13). The definitive test is the beta-2 transferrin assay, which is sensitive and specific for CSF (14). Beta-2 transferrin is not normally found in serum, tears, saliva, or nasal secretions. A different test called the beta-trace protein test measures the amount of prostaglandin D synthase, which is much more concentrated in CSF than in serum or nasal secretions and has also been used in screening and in postoperative confirmation of fistula closure (15).

Common fistula sites causing CSF rhinorrhea include the ethmoid/cribriform plate region, posterior frontal sinus, roof of the orbit, and sphenoid sinus regions. When rhinorrhea is unilateral, it accurately predicts the site of the dural tear and fracture in 95% of cases. However, only one-half of patients with bilateral rhinorrhea have bilateral dural tears (1). Fractures are particularly common into the ethmoidal air cells just lateral and posterior to the cribriform plate

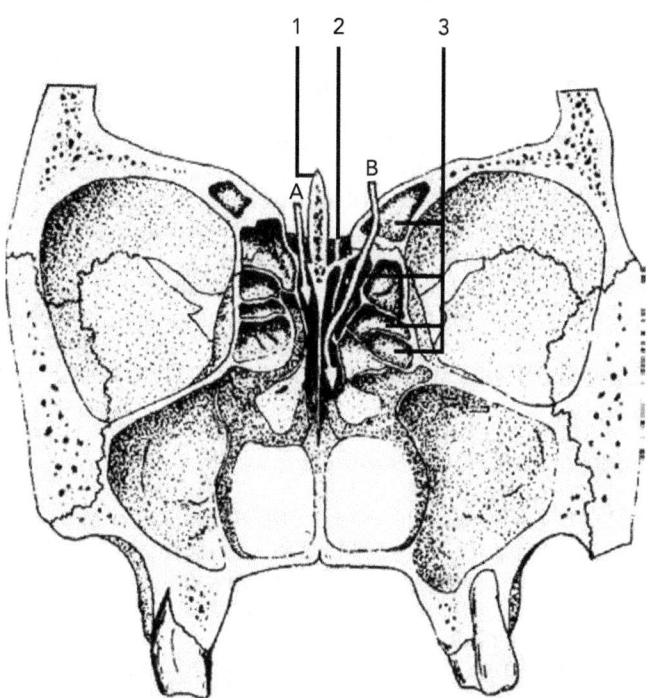

FIGURE 44-1 *A*, Fracture in cribriform plate. *B*, Fracture through ethmoidal cells, which is the more usual type. (*1*) crista galli, (*2*) cribriform plate, (*3*) ethmoidal cells. Reprinted from MacGee (10) with permission.

(Figure 44-1) (10), and injury in this area is characteristically associated with anosmia (1). Ethmoid/cribriform plate fistulas sometimes close spontaneously, whereas dural tears of the posterior wall of the frontal sinus do not tend to heal and typically require surgery (10). Frontal sinus fracture can be associated with anesthesia of the supraorbital nerves, subconjunctival ecchymosis, palpable depression over the frontal sinus region, and air in the orbit. A leak into the sphenoid sinus is particularly likely to cause profuse rhinorrhea (16).

Several diagnostic techniques are used to localize the site of a CSF leak. Radioisotope cisternography, with radioisotope injected into the CSF and measured in pledgets placed in the nose can be useful for lateralization of a slow or intermittent leak (17). Sometimes, magnetic resonance imaging (MRI) techniques using images with heavy T2 weighting may highlight CSF sufficiently to show the leak (17,18). Computed tomography (CT) cisternography, with CT scan after injection of a contrast dye, is effective in patients with an active CSF leak but may fail to visualize intermittent leaks. Intrathecal fluorescein with endoscopic visualization has been reported as a very effective means of precisely identifying slow leaks, especially as part of an endoscopic surgical repair procedure (17–19).

Cerebrospinal Fluid Fistula and Meningitis Risk

CSF rhinorrhea implies a tenfold increase in the risk of subsequent meningitis (20). CSF rhinorrhea resolves within a week in 85% of cases (21). However, if the underlying fistula persists, there is now strong evidence of a very high (30%–40% or more) risk of late meningitis (8,17,18,22); sometimes these cases have been described years later. In one study of 44 patients with meningitis, more than one-half of the episodes occurred more than a year after injury (8). Rhinorrhea has also presented years after the original trauma in multiple cases (22–25). Coughing, sneezing, hard work, or inverted posture may facilitate opening of the leak. In a recent study of 23 patients with late post-traumatic fistula, meningitis occurred 1.3 times per case, and 12–15 months typically elapsed between presentation and surgery (19). Such late occurrences of meningitis and CSF rhinorrhea underscore the importance of taking an aggressive approach to ensure closure of dural tears acutely and of considering a possible fistula when patients with a prior TBI present with meningitis.

CT or MRI may show evidence of encephalocele (brain protrusion through a skull defect) without clinical signs of basal fracture or CSF leak. In some late presenting cases, brain tissue has been trapped in the dural defect, apparently making a temporary seal but preventing dural closure (23). In cases presenting years after the injury, the cerebral plug may become inadequate with brain atrophy or change in cerebral compliance.

Endoscopic extracranial techniques can now repair 90% of fistulae without requiring craniotomy (17). This avoids additional brain trauma and often preserves sense of smell, which is typically lost with intracranial repair. Large defects or those associated with mass lesions may still require craniotomy. Lumbar drainage has often been used postoperatively after definitive dural repair, but it is not usually recommended as a sole treatment (21,22,26).

Although prophylactic antibiotic use in patients with CSF rhinorrhea remains highly controversial, there is more support for prophylaxis in patients with rhinorrhea than in patients with basilar skull fracture alone (1,9,10,20,27,28). One meta-analysis study found a statistically significant benefit by pooling studies, which showed a similar trend but individually lacked sufficient numbers to achieve statistical significance (27), whereas another meta-analysis came to the opposite conclusion (9).

Cerebrospinal Fluid Otorrhea

Otorrhea occurs when petrous temporal bone fracture and dural tear are combined with tympanic membrane tear. The exact incidence of temporal bone fracture is uncertain because as many as 60% of these fractures may be missed with routine CT imaging (29). However, they are believed to constitute over one-third of basilar skull fractures (29). Otorrhea has been estimated to occur in approximately 7% of all patients with basilar skull fractures (30) or approximately 20%–25% of those with temporal bone fractures (1). Petrous temporal bone fractures are divided into longitudinal and transverse types. Both types are associated with otorrhea. Longitudinal fractures run in the anteroposterior direction and are 5 times more common. Longitudinal fractures are often associated with torn tympanic membrane, ossicular disruption, and delayed transient impairment of the facial nerve. Transverse fractures run at right angles to the petrous axis and are associated with injury to the inner ear and eighth nerve and immediate lasting injury to the facial nerve. Unlike CSF rhinorrhea, CSF otorrhea almost always resolves spontaneously in less than a week (1,23). In the few cases that

persist, the reported rate of cessation after a single surgical procedure is 98% (1).

Pneumocephalus

Pneumocephalus is defined as the presence of gas within the cranial cavity. In TBI, this is usually air, with the exception of gas being produced in a brain abscess by anaerobic infection. Air may be present in any of the intracranial compartments, but frontal, subdural, or intracerebral air was most common in a study of 295 patients (31). Pneumocephalus occurs in 15% of patients with a fistula (22), and concurrent rhinorrhea is reported in 30%–50% (31).

Two major mechanisms for post-traumatic pneumocephalus have been proposed: the inverted bottle mechanism and the ball-valve mechanism. Relatively early pneumocephalus in patients with rhinorrrhea or otorrhea is consistent with the inverted bottle mechanism. It is similar to what happens when one drinks or pours from a bottle; as CSF escapes from the cranium, eventually, air must enter to allow more CSF to exit. On the other hand, in the ball-valve mechanism, air is forced into the cranium with pressure as by a cough or a sneeze, and then cannot exit because the meninges or cerebral tissue tamponades the leak. The delayed build up of intracranial air from this recurrent one-way valve mechanism fits the peak incidence of pneumocephalus at 1–3 months postinjury.

The term "tension pneumocephalus" is used when intracranial air acts as a mass lesion, compressing the underlying brain and causing headache, motor paresis, meningeal signs, and even psychosis. Sometimes this type of picture is seen postoperatively, such as after evacuation of a subdural hematoma (Figure 44-2).

Tension pneumocephalus has been described to present with severe, progressive, unilateral headache as much as 4 years after original brain injury (32). Although this late presentation is not common, it underscores the importance of considering this diagnosis in the comprehensive assessment of the patient with post-traumatic headache.

Intracranial air is considered a potential risk for airplane travel in view of the possible expansion and development of tension pneumocephalus at high altitude (33). It is not, however, an absolute contraindication, and other factors also need to be considered in decisions of transport (34).

One bedside finding, the "bruit hydroaerique" (31), or cranial succession splash, is pathognomonic for pneumocephalus. It is heard by auscultation of the head during head movement and is sometimes also described subjectively by the patient. Although reported in only 7% of patients with pneumocephalus, it is likely that many examiners have not looked for it.

Definitive treatment for pneumocephalus entails repair of the underlying dural tear and fistula. In some obtunded patients with tension pneumocephalus, the air collection is tapped via a burr hole as an initial temporizing measure (31).

INFECTIOUS COMPLICATIONS

Meningitis

Presentation and Approach to Management

Trauma to the head is the most common cause of meningitis in adults (35). The classical symptoms of meningitis are well

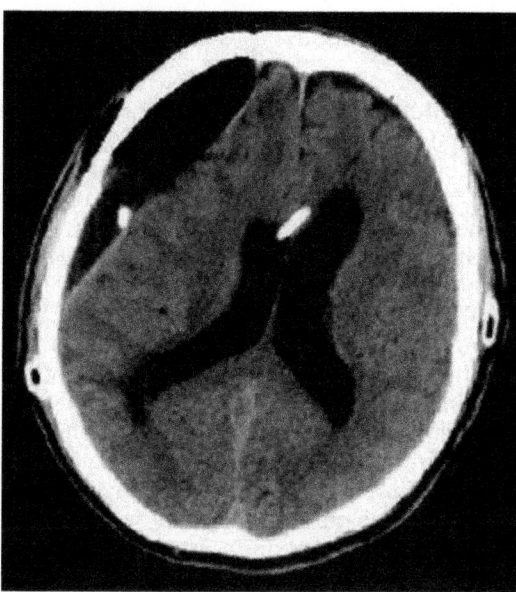

FIGURE 44–2 CT scan showing sizeable right-sided extra-axial pneumocephalus. Patient initially had TBI with subdural hematoma, later hydrocephalus, and recurrent right subdural hygroma treated with ventriculoperitoneal shunt and shunt into subdural space on right, followed by subsequent postoperative development of pneumocephalus. In this film, some fluid is seen inferiorly in the subdural space surrounding the catheter, in addition to the air superiorly. Catheter is also seen entering the right lateral ventricle. Despite the mild mass effect seen, both the subdural air and fluid eventually resolved from this point with conservative management

known, including headache, fever, stiff neck, and confusion. However, typical features may be lacking in 20% of patients, particularly the very young, the very old, and the immunosuppressed (36). Focal signs are typically absent in meningitis, and their presence warrants obtaining a CT scan to rule out abscess, empyema, or other mass lesion. Lumbar puncture characteristically reveals CSF pleocytosis (predominantly polymorphonuclear cells) with lowered glucose (less than one-third the blood glucose in three-fourths of patients). Identification of the causative organism in the CSF generally guides specific antibiotic selection along with general principles such as the ability of the antibiotic to cross the blood–brain barrier, effectiveness in purulent fluid, and ability to exert a bactericidal effect (37). Because of the changing development of drug-resistant strains, availability of newer antibiotics, and the need for treatment to be tailored to the specifics of each case, only some broad guidelines are offered here, and the readers are advised to check updated resources for best management of each case.

Common Organisms and Management

Streptococcus pneumoniae is by far the most common causative organism causing post-traumatic meningitis accounting for more than 80% of some studies (35). Adult meningitis during the first few days after a nonpenetrating injury is almost always pneumococcal. Whereas penicillin was previously the mainstay of treatment for these pneumococci, with the emergence of resistant strains, the use of third generation

cephalosporins (such as cefotaxime, ceftazidime, or ceftriaxone) is now often suggested, sometimes accompanied by vancomycin and rifampin (37). Haemophilis influenza is important in young children, and third generation cephalosporins have also been advocated (37). Patients with penetrating injuries are more likely to have *Staphylococcus aureus* or gram-negative meningitis (20). *S. aureus* can be treated with nafcillin or oxacillin, or vancomycin for resistant organisms. Postoperative meningitis after neurosurgery is most often from a gram-negative organism (38). Gram-negative infections usually present later, necessitating broader spectrum coverage in late presenting meningitis. Shunt-related infections warrant special mention because they often are indolent clinically and usually caused by *Staphylococcus epidermidis*. Shunt removal is generally necessitated along with vancomycin intravenously or even intrathecally for refractory cases (see "Hydrocephalus" section for further discussion) (37). Broad-spectrum coverage of post-traumatic meningitis with a combination of agents, such as vancomycin plus ceftazidime, can sometimes be instituted when diagnostic results from CSF are not available (37).

Subdural Empyema

Risk Factors and Presentation

Subdural empyema is said to be most common in males younger than age 20 and more often secondary to paranasal or ear infections than trauma (20). Post-traumatic subdural empyema is frequently secondary to septic compound skull fracture, comprising 77% of one study of 53 cases of post-traumatic subdural empyema (39). Presentation is typically acute and fulminant with fever, headache, and obtundation (20). Periorbital swelling (40) or tenderness over the sinuses or mastoid may provide additional clues. Focal signs and seizures are common (36).

With the increasing frequency of craniectomy in the acute management of TBI, the diagnosis of subdural empyema after cranioplasty has become an increasing problem (41). Because many of these patients are more medically complex, may have had recent antibiotic treatment for pneumonia or other infection, and have disorders of consciousness or severe cognitive impairments, the presentation may be more insidious and diagnosis be more difficult.

Evaluation and Management

Nonspecific laboratory clues can include elevated white blood count (WBC), elevated C reactive protein, and elevated Westergren sedimentation rate. CT scans show an extra-axial collection with medial membrane enhancement (41). MRI scans typically shows low signal on Tl-weighted imaging and high signal on T2-weighted imaging (42). Diffusion-weighted MRI imaging can be used to differentiate subdural empyema from chronic subdural hematoma or hygroma. Subdural empyema tends to be hyperintense on diffusion-weighted imaging and has low apparent diffusion coefficient (ADC) maps, both the opposite of findings with chronic hematoma or hygroma (41). Lumbar puncture is contraindicated in suspected subdural empyema. Multiple organisms are usually present at surgery, including *Streptococci*. When only 1 organism is cultured, it is most often *Staphylococcus*. In addition to appropriate antibiotics, either burr hole drainage or craniotomy is recommended (40). Although success has frequently been reported with burr holes (40), large size, midline shift, parafalcine or posterior fossa location, and loculation have been identified as factors favoring craniotomy (43). Of course, cranioplasty flaps need to be removed when infection develops under them.

Brain Abscess

Risk Factors and Clinical Presentation

Trauma is a less common cause of brain abscess compared with spread from sinusitis, middle ear infection, or hematogenous spread from pulmonary or dental infection. In fact, only approximately 10% of brain abscesses are secondary to TBI or neurosurgical procedure. Among patients with TBI, brain abscess is 3 times as likely after gunshot wounds and 8 times as likely with wound complications, such as hematomas, fluid collections, wound infection, and cerebrospinal fistula (44,45). Classically, the presentation of brain abscess peaks at about 2–3 weeks after injury, but the mean time of presentation was actually more than 3 months postinjury in one study of 36 patients (46). Presentation is frequently with signs of increased ICP rather than with acute febrile illness. In one study, headache was present in 90% of the patients and vomiting in 65%, whereas as many as 50% of patients are afebrile at presentation (47). Focal signs occur in 50%–75%, with changes in mental status notable in one-half of the patients and seizures in one-third (45). Table 44-1 contrasts key features of meningitis, subdural empyema, and brain abscess.

Abscess Stages and Imaging

Stages of abscess formation have been recognized pathologically and correlated with CT and MRI scan findings (45).

Early on the term cerebritis is used because of the presence of inflammatory cells in a perivascular location. CT scan at this stage shows low density with little enhancement, which may be solid. MRI during cerebritis is more sensitive (36) and shows uniform signal with indistinct margins (47). Later in cerebritis, both the necrotic center and surrounding edema may reach maximal size, fibroblasts and macrophages are found at the periphery, and CT scan may show a thin rim of enhancement and increasing edema. Next, a capsule of collagen and reticulin begins to develop; this forms more slowly on the ventricular side of the abscess. CT scan now shows a ring-enhancing capsule (less medially) and a low-density center. MRI scan shows the capsule as low signal on T2-weighted images (47). Diffusion-weighted MRI has been effective in distinguishing brain abscess from other mass lesions, such as brain tumors. On diffusion-weighted MRI, the central core of a brain abscess is hyperintense, whereas tumors such as glioblastoma or metastasis are typically hypointense centrally (48). Diffusion-weighted MRI also has been used to track response to treatment (49).

Organisms and Treatment

Most brain abscesses are polymicrobial and include anaerobes. Gas on CT scan may help in early differentiation from tumor and suggests anaerobic organisms. Staphylococci are found in about 10% of brain abscesses and are more frequent after trauma (45). Lumbar puncture is contraindicated in brain abscess and usually not diagnostically helpful if performed inadvertently. Therefore, choice of antibiotic reflects the anticipated polymicrobial etiology supplemented by information from aspiration of the abscess. For example, in the absence of specific culture information, a combination of a third generation cephalosporin, nafcillin or vancomycin for Staphylococcus, and metronidazole for anaerobes might be used. Given the presence of anaerobes in many brain ab-

TABLE 44-1 Different Types of Intracranial Infection

	RISK FACTORS	CLINICAL PRESENTATION	FEVER	HIGH WBC	MRI SCANS	LP
Meningitis	Basal fractures	Acute headache, stiff neck, mental state	Yes	Yes	Meningeal enhance	Yes
Subdural empyema	Penetrating wounds, depressed fractures, sinus fracture, ear infection, cranioplasty	Acute or subacute periorbital swelling, sinus tenderness, increased ICP, focal signs, seizures	Yes	Yes	Extra-axial, medial rim enhance, hyperintense DWI	No[a]
Brain abscess	Penetrating, depressed fractures, sinus fracture, ear infection, hematogenous	Subacute, progressive, increased ICP, focal signs	50%	No	Intra-axial ring enhance (late) capsule low T2 signal	No[a]
Shunt infection	Recent shunt shunt revision	Indolent malaise	Low grade	No	Nondiagnostic	No[b]

Abbreviations: WBC, white blood count; LP, lumbar puncture; ICP, intracranial pressure; DWI, diffusion-weighted imaging.
[a]Contraindicated
[b]Diagnose with shunt tap

scesses, the recent report of adjunctive use of hyperbaric oxygen therapy in a small number of cases of brain abscess is of interest (50).

As an abscess heals, the capsule becomes more isodense on serial CT scans. Steroids are frequently used effectively in brain abscess to decrease edema but may delay encapsulation of the abscess and make monitoring of response to therapy more difficult. Surgical management of brain abscess includes excision or CT-guided stereotactic aspiration (51). Indications to the stereotactic approach include surgically inaccessible location, cerebritis stage, or poor neurologic or general medical condition. Excision is useful for removal of foreign material and necessary for posterior fossa lesions. Adverse prognostic factors in brain abscess include young or old age, large deep abscess, coma, or rupture into the ventricular system. Mortality from brain abscess in Vietnam was 54%, and survival was worse with gram-negative organisms. However, good recovery can occur, and 30% or less of survivors are reported to have significant residual hemiparesis.

CRANIECTOMY AND CRANIOPLASTY

Craniectomy and Cranioplasty

Syndrome of the Trephined

Craniectomy (skull flap left out) is currently performed acutely in many patients with TBI in the context of managing increased ICP, hemorrhages, or penetrating or contaminated wounds. Traditionally, cranioplasty (replacement of bone flap or prosthesis) was often delayed 6 months or longer to minimize the risks of infection or complication (16,52), and the procedure was considered more cosmetic and protective rather than therapeutic. However, it now appears that some patients with chronic craniectomy may develop the "syndrome of the trephined" (53), a syndrome where the craniectomy flap becomes markedly sunken, with associated neurologic impairments. When this occurs, performance of cranioplasty can be associated with improvements in many neurologic symptoms and deficits including headaches, apathy, hemiparesis (54), midbrain syndrome with eye movement disorder (55), tremor, ataxia, and cognitive impairment (53). The syndrome of the trephined is particularly likely to occur in patients with concurrent shunts for hydrocephalus (56) because fluid is drained internally from the ventricular system predisposing to an ingoing skull flap.

In those patients where marked clinical improvement occurs with cranioplasty, the improvement has correlated with cerebral blood flow improvements of up to 30%, as well as improved distribution of flow. This has now also been confirmed with MR perfusion imaging (57). Based on measurements of transcranial cerebral oximetry and of ratios of phosphocreatine to inorganic phosphate (sensitive to rate of oxygen depletion), it has been suggested that cranioplasty induces more energy efficient mitochondrial function (53).

Recently, there has also been increased concern about craniectomy changing brain compliance and playing a role in inducing hydrocephalus (53,56–60). Hydrocephalus is particularly likely to occur when the superior margin of the craniectomy flap is within 25 mm of the midline (59). As a result of concerns about developing hydrocephalus or syndrome of the trephined, there has been considerable recent interest in performing cranioplasty much earlier, such as within the first month or even during the initial acute care hospitalization (58).

Cranioplasty is not a procedure to be taken lightly, however, because the risk of significant complications has been reported to be as high as 34%, including infection, hemorrhage, and brain swelling; and up to 25% of patients may require reoperation (61). Although some studies have suggested comparable complication rates with early and late cranioplasty (58), the best timing of cranioplasty continues to be a matter of much debate and also dependent on the specific features of each individual case.

Cranioplasty Alternatives

Cranioplasty can be performed with the patient's own bone flap, which can be frozen or stored in the patient's abdomen (62). Alternatively, computerized techniques can be used to generate a custom-made cranioplasty prosthesis; multiple materials can be used (63), but lowest rates of postoperative infection are reported with titanium or titanium mesh (64,65). For patients with shunts and depressed skull flaps, it has been suggested to clip the shunt or turn up the setting of a programmable shunt temporarily to reexpand the brain prior to cranioplasty to minimize dead space at the time of surgery (66).

HYDROCEPHALUS

Overview

Definition

Hydrocephalus is defined as "an active distention of the ventricular system of the brain related to inadequate passage of CSF from its point of production within the ventricular system to its point of absorption into the systemic circulation" (67).

Importance After Traumatic Brain Injury

Hydrocephalus is the most common treatable neurosurgical complication during rehabilitation of TBI (68), and its treatment can sometimes have a dramatic impact on rehabilitation and outcome. One recent study estimated an incidence of post-traumatic hydrocephalus at 45% in patients with severe TBI (69). However, differentiation of dynamic hydrocephalus from central atrophy or ex vacuo ventricular dilation remains problematic. This is especially true because ventriculomegaly is also known to be a marker of severe diffuse axonal injury (70). Practical management after a shunt includes prevention and treatment of other complications such as overdrainage and subdural hematoma, and the introduction of programmable shunts now offers additional opportunity for the physician to intervene medically during rehabilitation.

Types and Variants

Hydrocephalus is divided into communicating and noncommunicating types (67,68). In communicating hydrocephalus, the different portions of the ventricular system are interconnected, and fluid may exit the ventricular system freely to the cisterns and subarachnoid space, whereas in noncommunicating (obstructive) hydrocephalus, CSF flow is obstructed either between the ventricles or in exiting the ventricular system.

Post-traumatic hydrocephalus is communicating in most cases, and enlargement characteristically involves all components of the ventricular system. Blood products, protein, or fibrosis typically interfere with the circulation of CSF and its absorption into the bloodstream through the arachnoid granulations (67).

When only selected portions of the ventricular system are enlarged, noncommunicating hydrocephalus should be considered. For example, large lateral and third ventricles with a small fourth ventricle in a patient with a large head circumference is generally attributable to aqueductal stenosis—a congenital condition which may become decompensated by TBI. Lumbar puncture is contraindicated in these patients. Endoscopic third ventriculostomy can effectively bypass the aqueductal obstruction without requiring a shunt in some cases (71). The procedure involves placing a hole in the floor of the third ventricle creating a connection with the adjacent cistern.

Focal ventricular enlargement frequently occurs on an atrophic or porencephalic basis in brain areas that have sustained known damage. Less often, trapping of an isolated portion of the ventricular system may produce focal enlargement with signs of increased ICP or focal deficits (72,73). Occasional cases of multiloculated hydrocephalus are encountered usually secondary to meningitis, ventriculitis, or intraventricular hemorrhage (74). The multiple irregular intraventricular septations of the enlarged ventricular system can be effectively treated with fenestration by intraventricular endoscopy (74–76).

Pathophysiology of Chronic Communicating Hydrocephalus Including Normal Pressure Hydrocephalus

Pascal Law
Pascal law of hydraulic systems states that $F = P \times A$, where F is the force against the ventricular wall, P is the intraventricular pressure, and A is the area of the ventricular wall (77). This formula implies that when the area of the ventricular wall is large, a substantial expanding force may be generated from within the ventricle without the necessity of high pressure. For example, if a certain degree of ventricular enlargement initially results from increased pressure, ongoing enlargement may take place, even though pressures are no longer elevated (78).

Decreased Parenchymal Pressure and Compliance
Rather than the absolute intraventricular pressure, the difference between the intraventricular pressure and that of the surrounding tissue determines ventricular size (77,79). This concept may be understood more clearly by considering that the size of a balloon is determined not only by the pressure inside the balloon but also by the pressure of the air inside relative to the air outside the balloon. Changes in the viscoelastic properties of brain parenchyma with related decrease in parenchymal pressure, therefore, probably contribute significantly to the development of hydrocephalus because it is the difference between CSF pressure and intraparenchymal pressure that determines ventricular size (80). A gradient of reduced blood flow has been documented in the periventricular white matter of patients with normal pressure hydrocephalus (NPH), as well as altered blood flow autoregulation, which likely contributes to watershed ischemia (81). Damage to myelin and axons has also been described when hydrocephalus is long standing (82). These factors are probably among those that contribute to the decreased elasticity or compliance of the brain parenchyma, which is felt to be important in the development of NPH.

Pulsatile Cerebrospinal Fluid Flow
Disturbances of pulsatile CSF flow may be more important than blockage of CSF absorption in causing chronic communicating hydrocephalus (83). According to the Monro-Kellie doctrine, the volume of the intracranial contents including brain, blood, and CSF is constant (84). This means that arterial blood inflow during systole is accompanied by both outflow of venous blood and shifting of CSF into the spinal compartment (84). Furthermore, CSF movement is not a simple, unidirectional flow but complex, and the basal cisterns probably play an important role in dynamic compliance. When intracranial compliance is decreased, restricted arterial pulsation and increased pulse pressure in brain capillaries have been postulated to play a causative role in chronic hydrocephalus (85).

Clinical Presentation of Hydrocephalus

Risk Factors
Intracranial hemorrhage, especially subarachnoid or intraventricular hemorrhage, meningitis, and craniectomy are all risk factors for the subsequent development of hydrocephalus (58,59,68).

Acute Hydrocephalus
Early postinjury acute hydrocephalus can present with symptoms of increased ICP including headache, nausea, vomiting, and lethargy or decreasing mental status. Associated signs can include a tense bulging craniectomy flap, papilledema, and Cushing triad of hypertension, bradycardia, and hypoventilation.

Normal Pressure Hydrocephalus
NPH is well known to present with the clinical triad of dementia, gait ataxia, and urinary incontinence. Of the 3, gait impairment is the most important diagnostically and most likely to respond to shunting. The classic gait disturbance has a shuffling, short stepping, "magnetic" quality with difficulty in lifting the feet and is characteristic of frontal or subcortical rather than cerebellar dysfunction (86,87). Reduced cadence, reduced step height, and loss of counter rotation have been described (87). The cognitive difficulties in NPH are apt to include long latency responses, decreased attention, and poor initiation rather than deficits such as aphasia or agnosia. In patients with TBI, the presentation of hydrocephalus is not limited to the classic triad of NPH and should be considered in any patient who worsens or fails to

progress adequately. A pretectal syndrome (88) or akinetic mutism is additional clinical syndromes that should particularly raise suspicion for hydrocephalus.

Computed Tomography and Magnetic Resonance Imaging

Ventriculomegaly

CT and MRI scans have been invaluable in providing information about ventriculomegaly, and multiple methods have been devised for measuring ventricular size, calculating ventricle to brain ratios, and assessing shunt function (89–93). However, ventricular size alone has not been a reliable predictor of whether a patient has shunt-responsive hydrocephalus rather than cerebral atrophy (94). In fact, ventriculomegaly has been reported in as many as 72% of patients with severe TBI (95), and it is now recognized that the extent of ventriculomegaly can be correlated with severity of diffuse axonal injury and outcome, complicating assessment for hydrocephalus in patients already known to have severe TBI (70,96,97). Ventricular configurations favoring dynamic hydrocephalus include enlargement of temporal horns, convex shape of the frontal horns, widening of the frontal horn radius, and frontal horn location closer to midline narrowing the "ventricular angle" (72).

Sulcal Absence and Periventricular Lucency

Ex vacuo ventricular dilatation or cerebral atrophy typically involves sulcal prominence. Small or absent sulci on a CT scan in combination with ventriculomegaly are predictors of a good response to shunting, although the presence of sulci does not preclude a positive response (94). Patients with hydrocephalus often do show decreased sulcal prominence in the high convexity region, even if other fissures and sulci are more prominent—a so-called "tight high convexity" sign (98). Periventricular lucency has been a valuable predictor of a good response to shunting, especially when lucencies have been seen in multiple periventricular locations (see Figure 44-3) (94,99). In hydrocephalus, fluid seeps across the ependymal lining of the ventricle and causes interstitial edema. This transependymal fluid is seen as lucency on CT and as smooth increased T2 signal on MRI. Contusion, infarction, or demyelination in the periventricular white matter can be difficult to distinguish from transependymal fluid but are usually more irregular and asymmetric (100).

Additional Magnetic Resonance Imaging Findings

Patients with hydrocephalus may have more rapid than normal CSF flow through the Sylvian aqueduct because of decreased compliance of the ventricular wall of the third ventricle during systole (72,101,102). This can be detected on MRI as decreased signal or "flow void" in the aqueduct in patients with hydrocephalus.

A series of linear measurements on MRI, essentially reflecting size and configuration of the third ventricle, can be used to distinguish obstructive hydrocephalus from atrophy, but the effectiveness of this approach in chronic communicating hydrocephalus in TBI has not been assessed (103).

Single Photon Emission Computed Tomography Scans

Only limited information is available about the use of single photon emission computed tomography (SPECT) scans in diagnosing hydrocephalus. Subcortical low flow attributed to hydrocephalus improved after shunting in 10 of 11 clinically responding patients in one study and temporal lobe hypoperfusion improved in another small study (104).

Invasive Testing

Cisternography

Radioisotope cisternography does not improve the diagnostic accuracy of combined clinical and CT assessment. Cisternography-based predictions were the same in 43% of patients, better in 24%, and worse in 33% (105).

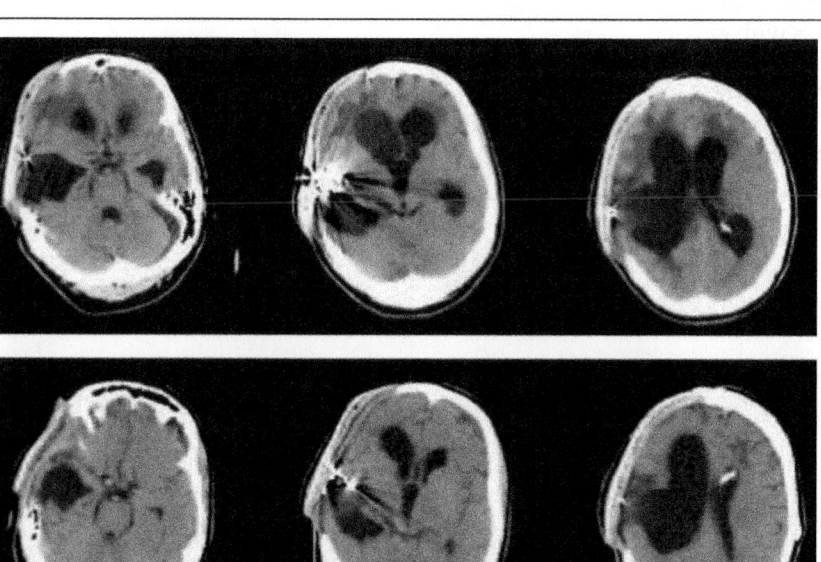

FIGURE 44–3 Hydrocephalus preshunting and postshunting. In the preshunt scans (*top*), note marked periventricular lucency in the white matter consistent with transependymal fluid in addition to ventricular enlargement. There is also artifact from aneurysm clip and right hemispheric encephalomalacia, maximal in the right temporal lobe. Postshunt scans show persisting encephalomalacia of the right hemisphere including the right lateral ventricle and right temporal horn. Shunt is now seen entering the left lateral ventricle, which has now normalized (including left temporal horn), and periventricular lucency has largely resolved. Surprisingly, a cerebrospinal fluid (CSF) tap test (see discussion) has actually been negative in this patient, but after performance of ventriculoperitoneal shunt, there was nonetheless marked clinical improvement.

Lumbar Infusion Studies

Infusion of fluid via a lumbar or ventricular catheter with measurement of drainage at designated pressures allows calculation of the outflow resistance—a measure of the difficulty of CSF absorption (94). If the outflow resistance is low, significant volumes of CSF can be readily absorbed, and a shunt is not likely to help. On the other hand, increased outflow resistance means that CSF is not readily absorbed. It is related to decreased compliance of the system and is predictive of a positive response to shunting (94,106–110). Of interest, ventricular size does not correlate well with either outflow resistance or response to shunting (84,106). Infusion studies have relatively low risk compared with the long-term morbidity of a shunt (107,108). Despite their reported value and frequent use in Europe, these studies are infrequently performed in many US hospitals.

Cerebrospinal Fluid Tap Test

A lumbar puncture with the removal of 50 mL of CSF has been advocated as a CSF tap test (99,103,111–116). If the patient shows an improvement in neurologic status after lumbar puncture, the test is viewed as positive. However, a lack of response does not preclude response to a shunt because shunting produces more sustained ventricular decompression (67,86). Therefore, the CSF tap test is most useful to identify patients who otherwise might not be shunted; a strong candidate would be shunted even in the face of a negative tap test. Combining lumbar infusion testing and CSF tap test (114) or combining serial MRI or SPECT scanning with CSF tap tests may improve yield (115).

Lumbar Catheter Drainage Trial

A more prolonged CSF drainage trial with a lumbar catheter for 3–5 days has been shown to have both greater sensitivity and predictive value of shunt success than a simple tap test alone and is increasingly used in specialized centers for the diagnosis of NPH (111,112). In ambulatory patients with gait dysfunction, quantitative and video gait assessments before and after lumbar drainage can be used. Identification of a positive clinical response to drainage is more problematic in severely impaired TBI, such as those with disorders of consciousness.

Approach to Shunt Decision Making

Establishing the Diagnosis and Therapeutic Expectations

Table 44-2 reviews multiple considerations relevant to identifying dynamic hydrocephalus. The combination of the clinical course and findings, CT and MRI appearance, and in some cases of CSF tap test or lumbar infusion testing may help establish the diagnosis. Patients with TBI are likely to show only a partial response to shunting because deficits from hydrocephalus are superimposed on deficits from the original TBI. This should be clearly explained to family members before pursuing shunting to prevent or minimize any unrealistic expectations. However, given the potential significant benefit to patient outcome, an aggressive approach to identification and treatment of hydrocephalus is warranted for the patient with severe TBI.

Treatment

Treatment Without a Shunt

The definitive treatment of hydrocephalus is surgical, usually the placement of a shunt. Treatment with carbonic anhydrase inhibitors, such as acetazolamide or furosemide (116), or with serial lumbar punctures is only a temporizing measure. Similarly, external ventricular drainage may be used on a temporary basis, particularly for obstructive mass effect or when excessive blood products are likely to clog a shunt, but conversion to a shunt is needed for treatment of persisting hydrocephalus. Third ventriculostomy, where a connection is endoscopically created between the floor of the third ventricle and the underlying cistern, is the one exception of a definitive treatment for hydrocephalus not requiring placement of a shunt. It is most commonly used to treat aqueductal stenosis (117), where the procedure can bypass the obstruction at the Sylvian aqueduct. More recently, there has been renewed interest in the procedure for other forms of hydrocephalus as well, mainly because of the potential to improve intracranial compliance without diverting fluid from the CSF compartment (118).

Shunt Types

Ventriculoperitoneal shunts are used most commonly for post-traumatic hydrocephalus, but ventriculoatrial, ventriculopleural, and lumboperitoneal shunts are useful in certain

---

TABLE 44-2 Hydrocephalus vs Atrophy

	DYNAMIC HYDROCEPHALUS	EX VACUO/ATROPHY
History	SAH, IVH, meningitis, craniectomy	DAI, anoxia
Clinical	NPH triad (gait, incontinence, MSE), akinetic mute, Parinaud decline	C/W injury severity/location
CT/MRI	Ventricles enlarged and convex, prominent third ventricle and temporal horns, sulci decreased at high convexity, periventricular transependymal fluid	Diffuse ventriculomegaly, porencephalic tissue loss, increased sulci
Lumbar drainage	Improvement, especially gait	Lack of improvement

Abbreviations: SAH, subarachnoid hemorrhage; IVH, intraventricular hemorrhage; DAI, diffuse axonal injury; CT, computerized tomography; MRI, magnetic resonance imaging; NPH, normal pressure hydrocephalus; MSE, mental status exam; C/W, consistent with.

circumstances. Ventriculoatrial shunts are used more frequently in children with obstructive hydrocephalus. Occasionally, ventriculopleural shunts may be substituted in cases with abdominal infection, very high CSF protein, or rarely to drain very low pressure hydrocephalus to the negative pressure of the pleural space (119). Ventriculopleural shunts characteristically cause a small pleural effusion that disappears with shunt malfunction. Pleural shunts are avoided in younger children because of the likelihood of symptomatic hydrothorax with a smaller pleural cavity (75). Lumboperitoneal shunts are not commonly seen but can be used for communicating but not obstructive forms of hydrocephalus. Lumboperitoneal shunts have also been used for pseudotumor cerebri when ventriculoperitoneal shunt placement may be difficult because of small ventricular size. Placement of a lumboperitoneal shunt often obliterates the basal cisterns on CT scan of the head, and the return of previously obliterated cisterns is a reliable indicator of shunt malfunction (120). Although usually asymptomatic, cerebellar tonsillar herniation (iatrogenic Chiari malformation) has been described in as many as 70% of patients with lumboperitoneal shunts (121).

Shunt Valves and Components

The basic components of a ventriculoperitoneal shunt are the ventricular catheter, valve, and distal tubing. Almost all shunt systems have some type of one-way valve to allow forward flow down the shunt when the pressure gradient exceeds a threshold range and to prevent back flow from the peritoneum. Therapy staff often ask whether a shunt contraindicates inverted position; because of the one-way valve, this is not a problem. Basic valve types include slit valves, cruciate valves, mitre valves, diaphragm valves, and ball/spring valves (122–124); detailed diagrams on a variety of different past and present valve systems and components are available (122).

Reservoirs or flushing chambers are added to many shunt systems. They allow manual pumping of the shunt and potential access to sample CSF or to inject into the shunt system. If the chamber is proximal to all valves, compressing it after first compressing the distal tubing sends fluid back into the ventricle. If the chamber is between or after valves, compression will push fluid only in the forward direction. It is important to know the specifics of a shunt system before injecting into it because some shunt components may be damaged by needle perforations (125). Most modern shunts, however, have a portion that can be injected without damage.

Shunt valves are also specified by the approximate pressure necessary for opening and forwarding CSF flow and are commonly divided into low, medium, and high pressure valves (122,123). Such valve settings are approximate and function differently depending on the compliance of the ventricular system (126). In general, because of Pascal law (F = P × A), larger ventricles require a lower pressure for adequate decompression. When patients do not respond to a shunt, conversion to a shunt of lower pressure occasionally results in clinical improvement (128). Because of the obvious undesirability of reoperation to place a valve with a different pressure, programmable valves have been developed, which allow changing the effective opening pressure of the valve noninvasively at the bedside with an external magnet (see further discussion in the following texts).

Shunt Complications

Frequency of Shunt Complications

The overall incidence of shunt complications is high. Shunt complications include shunt failure, infection, seizures, subdural hematoma, and overdrainage. In 356 adult patients over an 18-year interval, the incidence of revision was 29% (129). In a study of 1,179 patients shunted for hydrocephalus (only 312 patients older than age of 5), the probability of shunt malfunction after 12 years was 81% (130).

Shunt Failure

Shunt failure may present with irritability, confusion, lethargy, and headache unrelieved by position change. However, shunt failure may also present in a more fulminant manner than the original hydrocephalus, requiring prompt treatment (131). Proximal occlusion of the ventricular catheter is the most common source of blockage, usually accounting for at least 30% of cases of shunt dysfunction (131). Ventricular overdrainage may predispose to proximal occlusion by abutting the catheter tip against the ventricular wall (130). Distal shunt obstruction can be caused by encystment and loculation of the peritoneal contents around the distal catheter tip (72,75). Abdominal pain, palpable pseudocyst, and ultrasound or abdominal CT may establish the diagnosis. Disconnections of shunt components have accounted for as much as 15% of shunt revisions and often are shown by a shunt series of plain radiographs (132).

Bedside palpation of the shunt sometimes gives a clue to shunt malfunction; excessive resistance to digital compression of the shunt chamber suggests possible distal occlusion, whereas inadequate refill suggests proximal occlusion. Unfortunately, palpation was neither sensitive nor reliable for determining shunt malfunction in a consecutive study of 200 patients (133). CT scans are helpful in demonstrating interval increase in ventricular size in many cases of shunt malfunction.

Definitive information about shunt blockage can be obtained by performing a shuntogram, where a needle is inserted into the safely perforable portion of the shunt, a pressure recording is done, and the progression of isotope or contrast is followed down the catheter and into the peritoneum (134,135). With distal obstruction, pressure may be elevated with rapid ventricular filling but lack of distal flow. With proximal occlusion, the distal catheter fills but pressure is low with slow disappearance of tracer and lack of ventricular filling (135).

Shunt Infection

Shunt infection has been described in 7%–29% of cases. Most infections are acquired at the time of surgery, and 70% present within the first 2 months (136). *S. epidermidis* is most common, accounting for approximately one-half of infections, followed by *S. aureus* and gram-negative organisms (137). Presentation is typically insidious with low-grade fever, malaise, irritability, and nausea; meningeal irritation is usually not present (137,138). Erythema over the shunt site, however, is a highly specific sign (136–138).

Diagnosis should be established by performing a shunt tap not by doing a lumbar puncture. Tapping the shunt leads to accurate diagnosis in 95% of cases, whereas lumbar puncture is positive in only 7%–26% of cases (136). Diagnosis is based on culture results because CSF protein and glucose may be normal, and cell count may not be much greater with shunt infection than with shunt alone.

Treatment needs to be individualized to the clinical situation, but in general, the highest overall response rate (96%) has been reported with shunt removal or externalization combined with antibiotics (136). *S. epidermidis* is the most common organism causing shunt infection and sometimes can be difficult to eradicate; intravenous vancomycin, intrathecal vancomycin, or a regimen of both vancomycin and rifampin are sometimes used (139).

Seizures

The prevalence of seizures after shunting has ranged from 5% to 48%, but in patients with post-traumatic hydrocephalus, seizures may also result from the original TBI.

Overdrainage

Overdrainage by shunts is a major clinical problem, causing acute and chronic clinical symptoms and fostering both proximal shunt obstruction and development of postoperative subdural collections. It has been the driving force behind the development of antisiphon devices, programmable valves, and gravitational shunts (140–147). Intraventricular pressure normally becomes slightly subatmospheric when we stand. However, after placement of a shunt, orthostatic intraventricular pressure becomes markedly low (124), reflecting the additional negative hydrostatic pressure from the distal tubing (Figure 44-4). This may cause excessive siphoning of CSF and a low-pressure syndrome of orthostatic headache, dizziness, nausea and vomiting, lethargy, and diplopia (131,140–142). Some patients with chronically overdraining shunts develop the slit-ventricle syndrome (131,140,141). Such patients develop severe nonpostural headaches in the face of persistently small ventricles. Slight increase in ventricular size at the time of clinical symptoms and sluggish shunt refill suggest intermittent proximal shunt malfunction with ventricular collapse against the catheter. Such symptoms develop at an average of 4.5 years after shunting and are analogous to pseudotumor cerebri in the tendency toward elevated pressures with small stiff ventricles (140,141).

Chronic Subdural Hematoma

Chronic subdural hematomas and hygromas are recognized complications of shunting, occurring in 4.5%–28% of patients and are particularly likely when ventricles are extremely large preoperatively. Normally, intracranial pulsatile flow and upright posture both shift CSF within the cranium and to the lumbar region but CSF remains within the CSF compartment; however, with shunting, CSF exits to the peritoneum, and this can result in an underfilled CSF compartment (84,118). Because the volume in the cranium is fixed, a loss of fluid in the ventricular compartment may result in creation of increased potential subdural space leading to development of subdural hygroma and hematoma (142,143). Furthermore, with upright posture, low intraventricular pressures caused by standing are thought to predispose to tearing and leakage from bridging veins. The occurrence of subdural hematoma may require tying off the shunt or turning up the valve pressure setting if the patient has a programmable valve (see subsequent texts) (86,143). Not all subdural collections are clinically significant; with MRI, even very small fluid collections can be imaged (72). Postshunt meningeal fibrosis, with collagenous material in

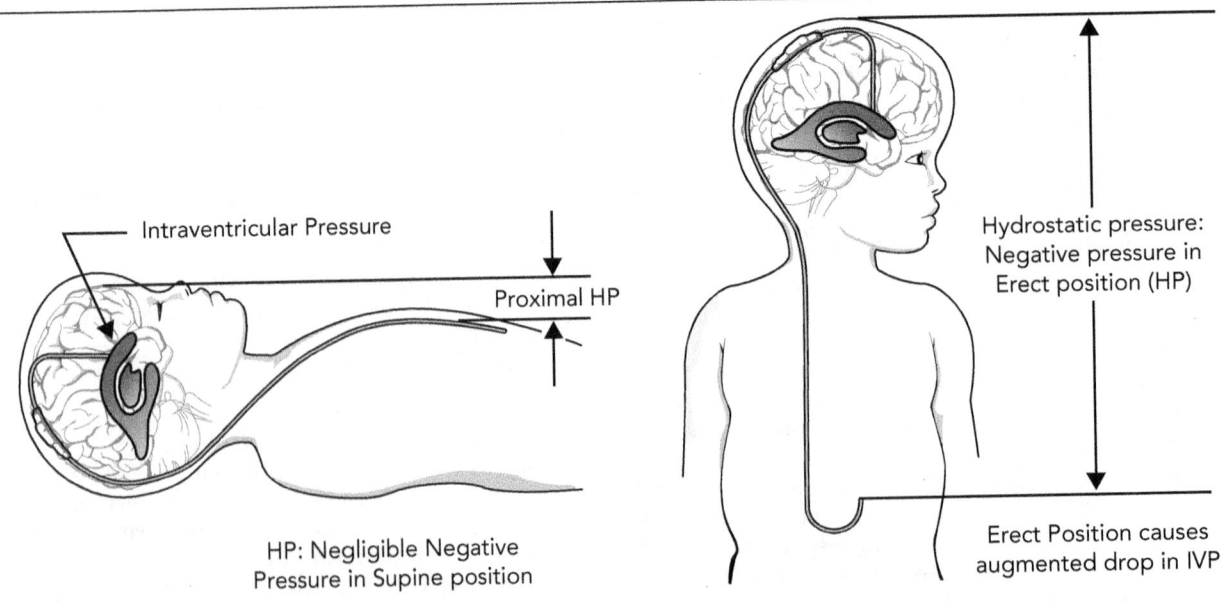

Supine Position   **Erect Position**

FIGURE 44-4 Positional changes in hydrostatic pressure (HP). IVP, intraventricular pressure.

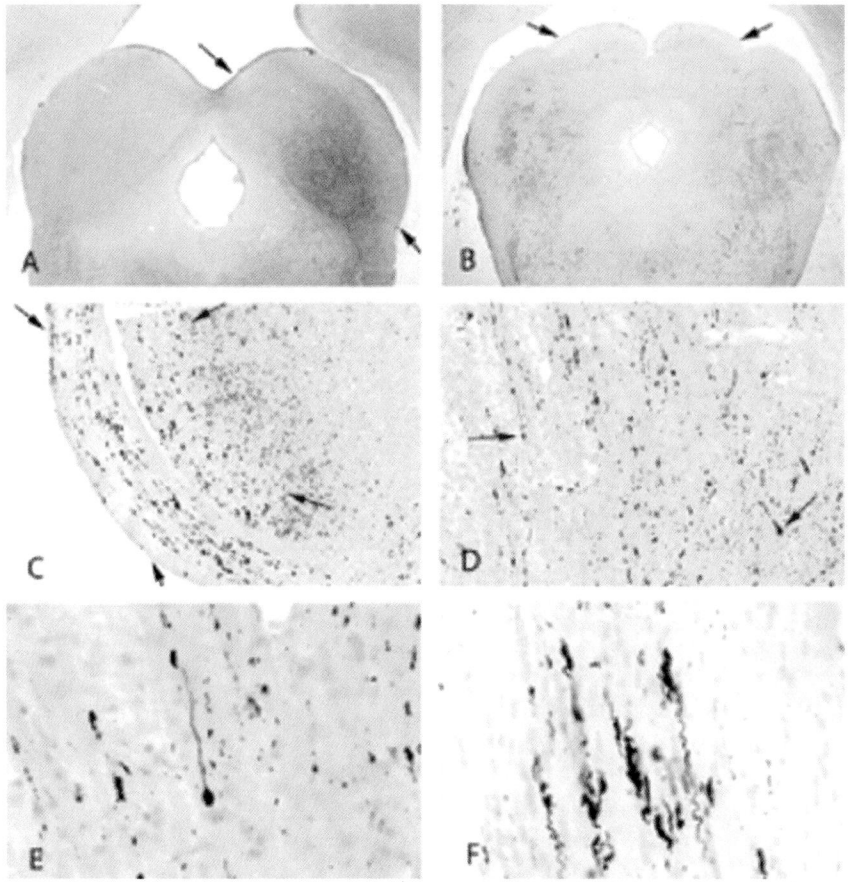

FIGURE 12–8

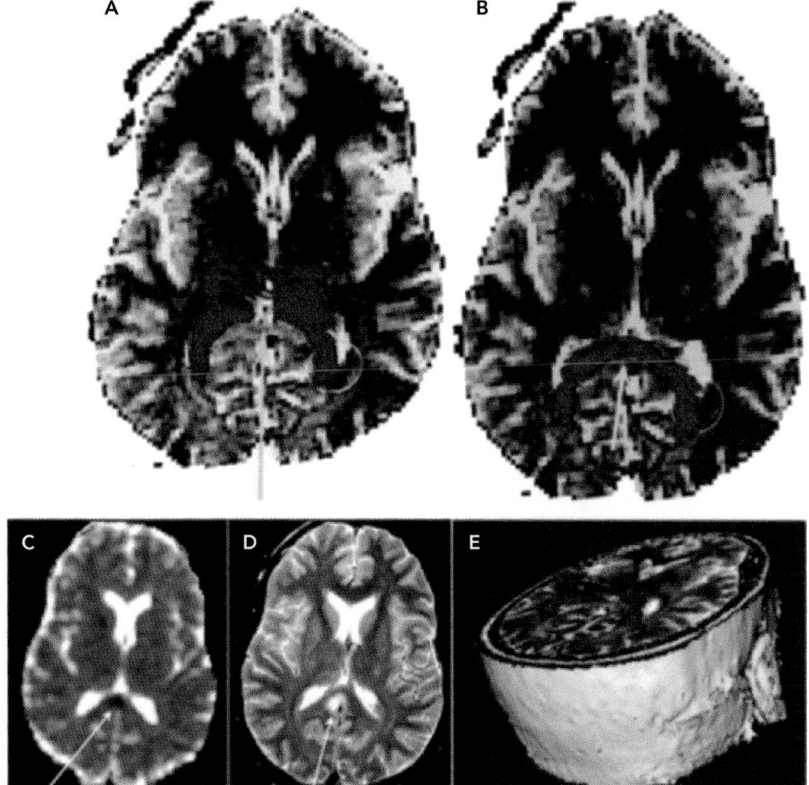

FIGURE 15–20

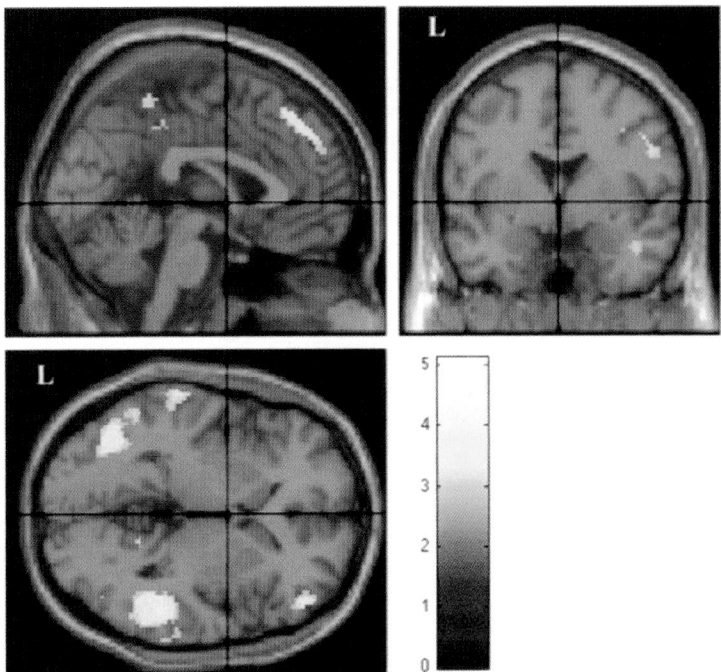

FIGURE 16-1

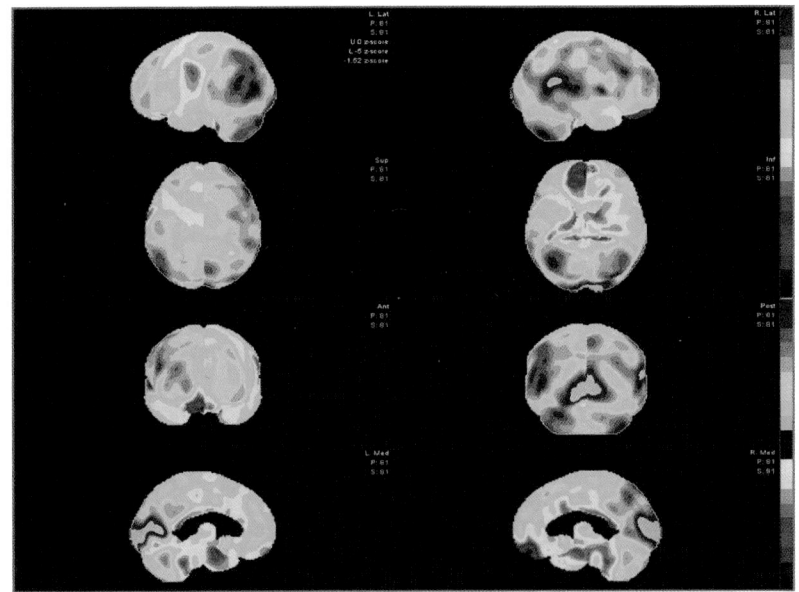

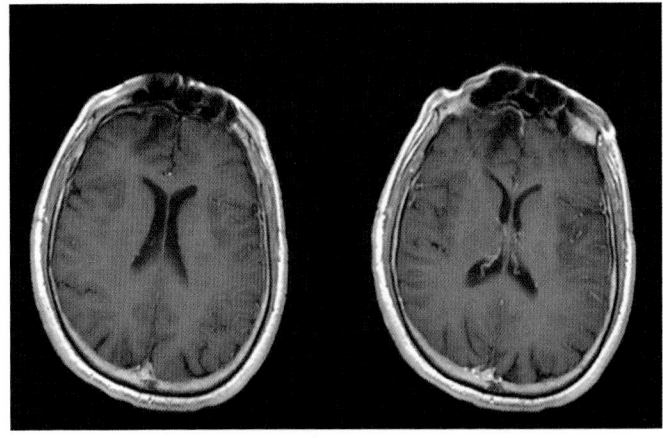

FIGURE 16-2

PET with simultaneous microdialysis
Elevated Oxygen/Glucose Ratio indicating alternative fuel consumption

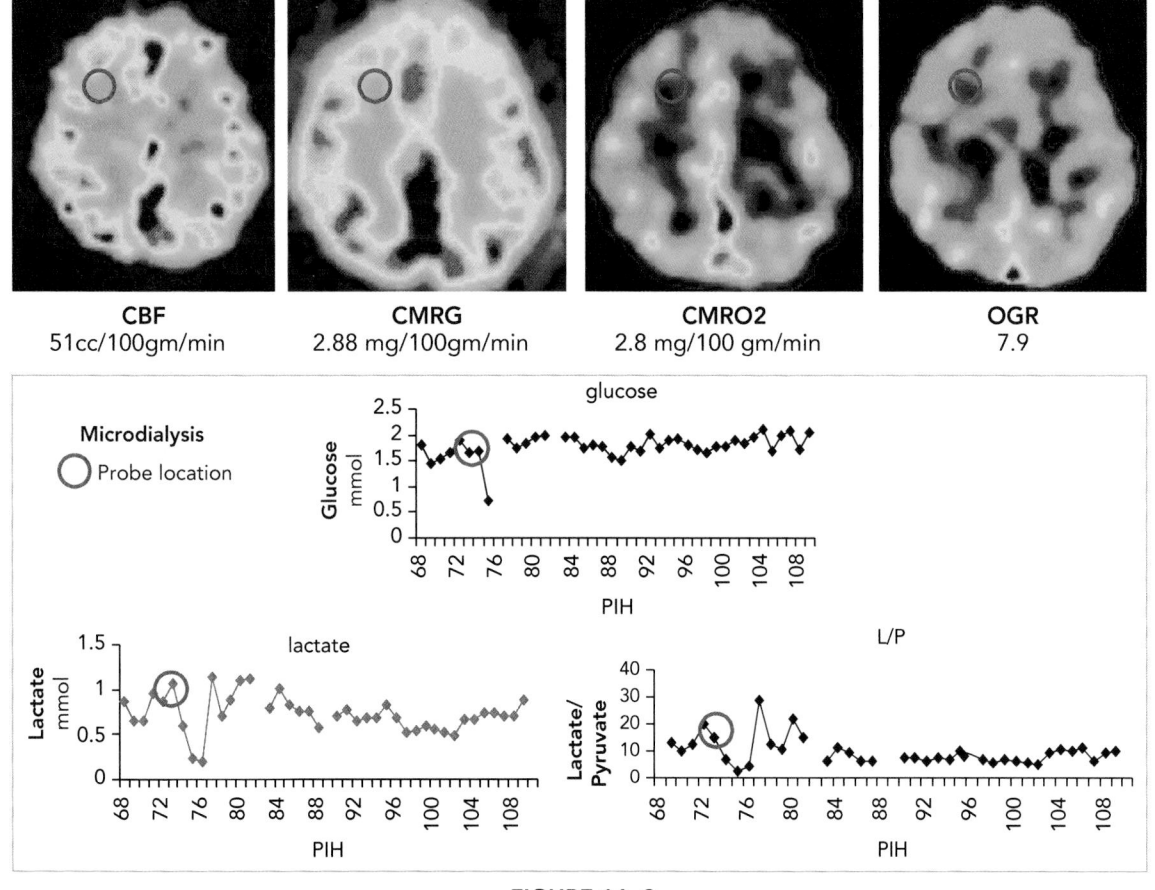

CBF	**CMRG**	**CMRO2**	**OGR**
51cc/100gm/min	2.88 mg/100gm/min	2.8 mg/100 gm/min	7.9

Microdialysis
◯ Probe location

FIGURE 16–3

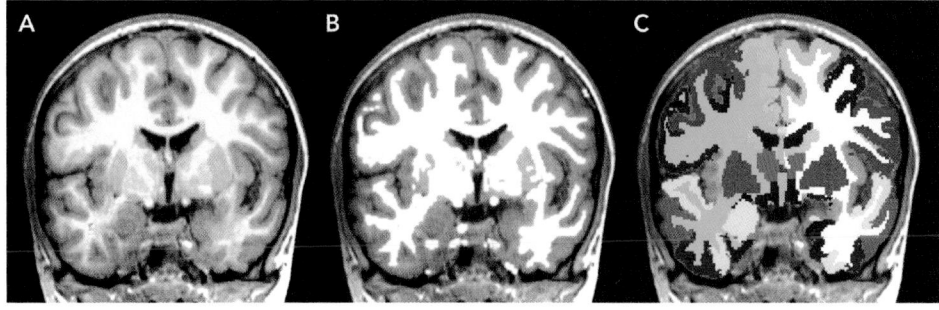

FIGURE 19–1

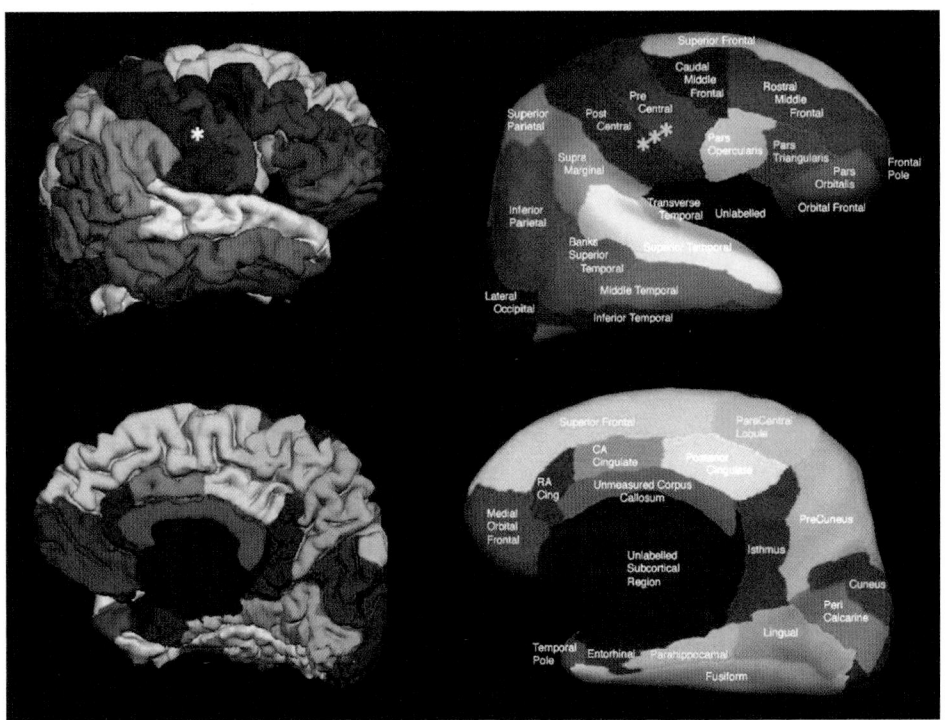

FIGURE 19–2

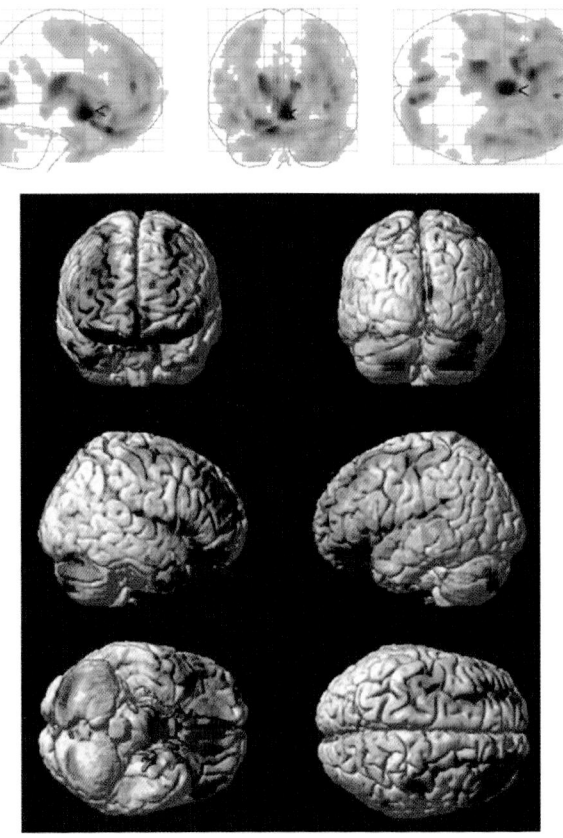

FIGURE 19–3

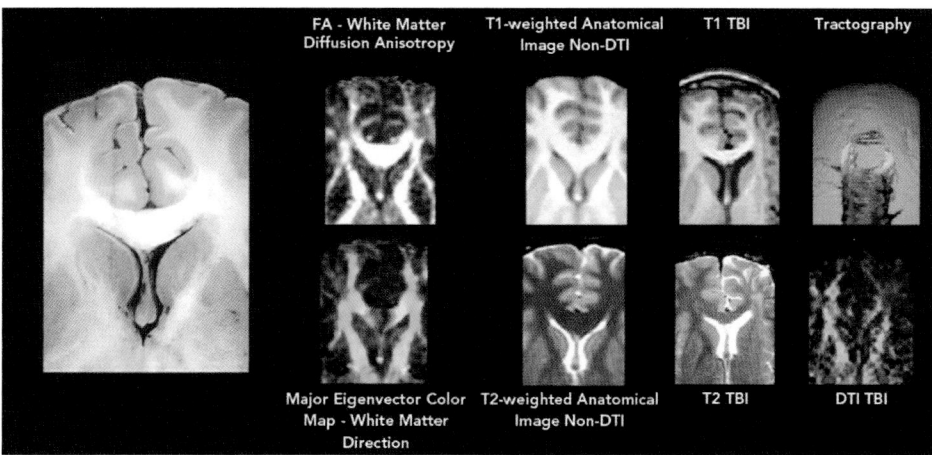

FA - White Matter Diffusion Anisotropy   T1-weighted Anatomical Image Non-DTI   T1 TBI   Tractography

Major Eigenvector Color Map - White Matter Direction   T2-weighted Anatomical Image Non-DTI   T2 TBI   DTI TBI

FIGURE 19–5

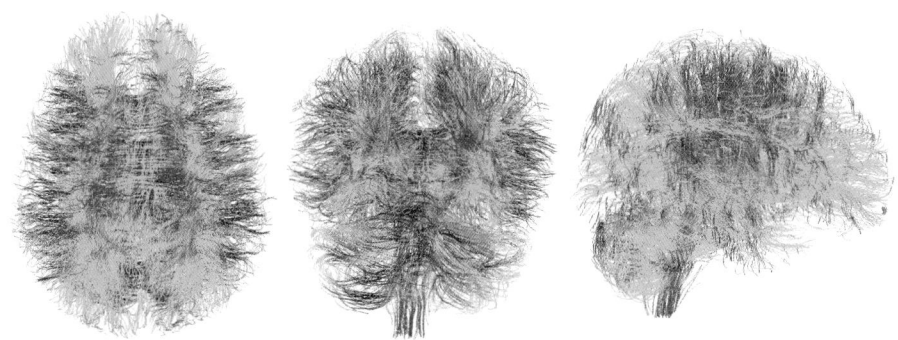

FIGURE 19–6

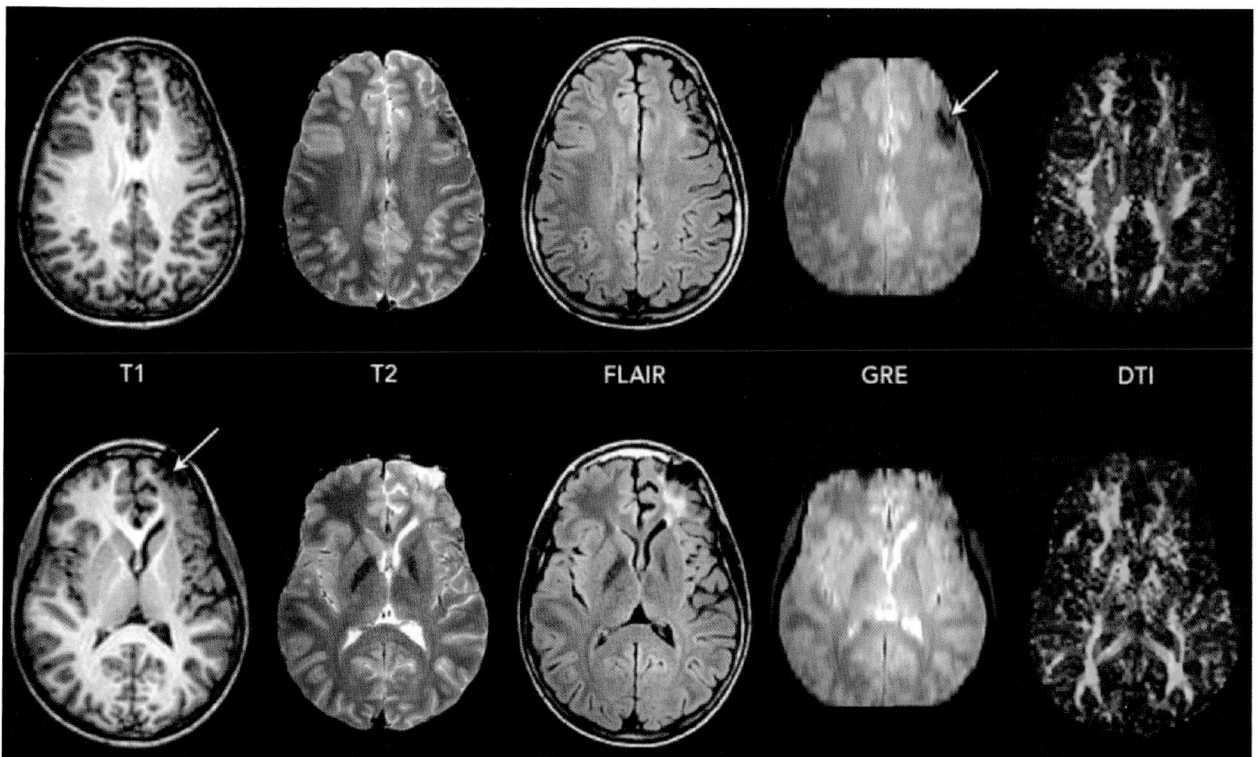

T1   T2   FLAIR   GRE   DTI

FIGURE 19–7

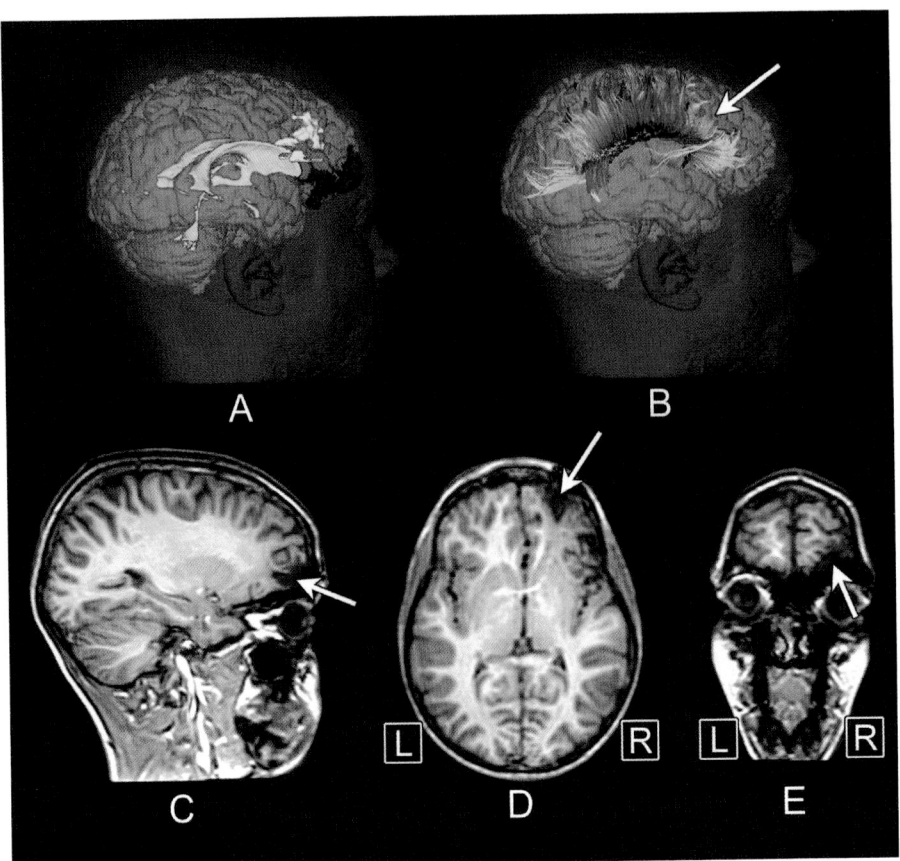

FIGURE 19–8

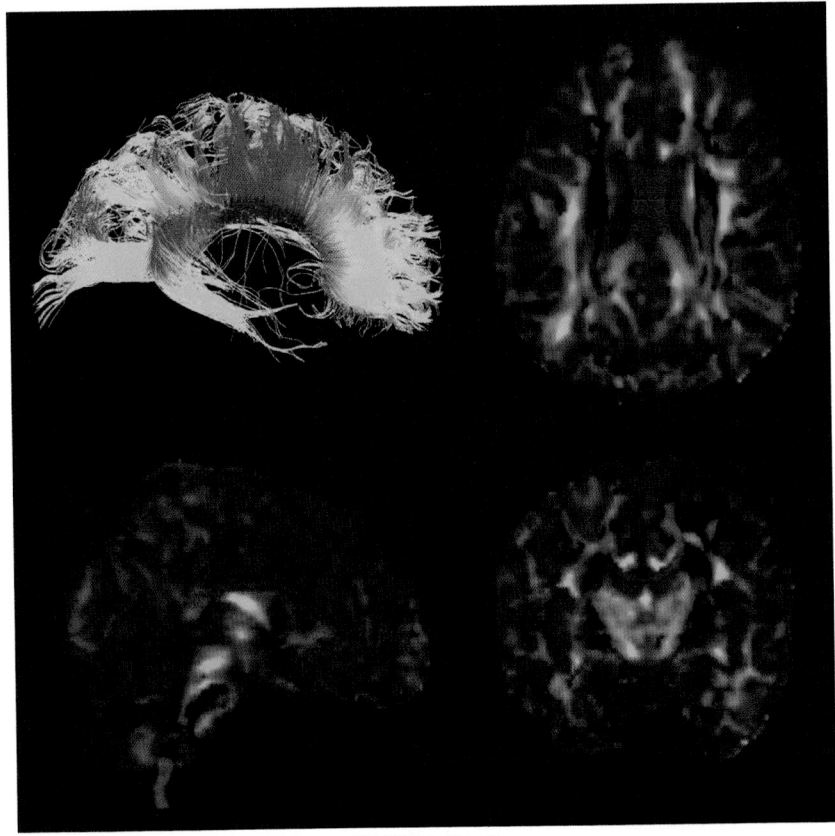

FIGURE 19–9

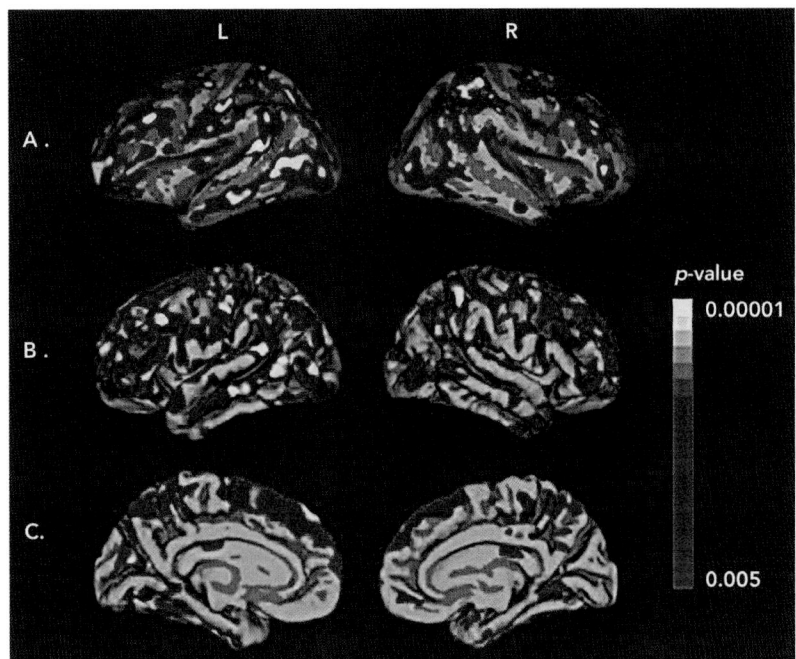

FIGURE 19-11

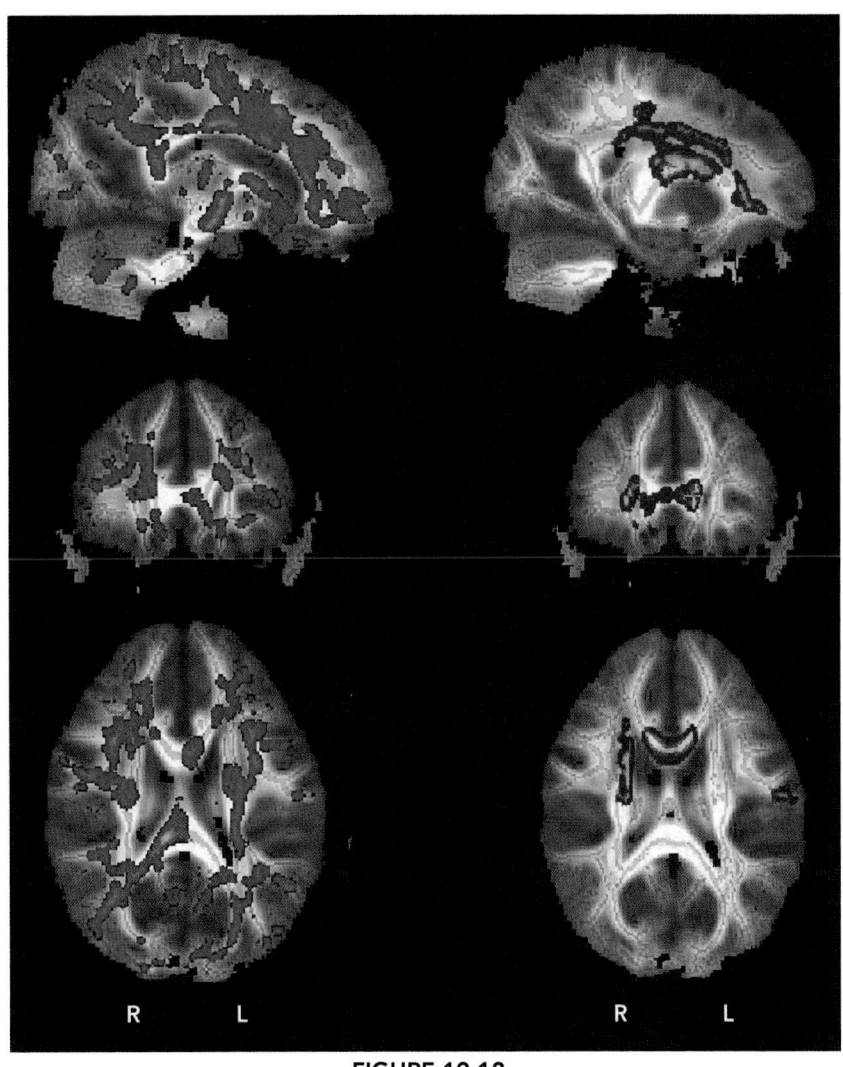

FIGURE 19-12

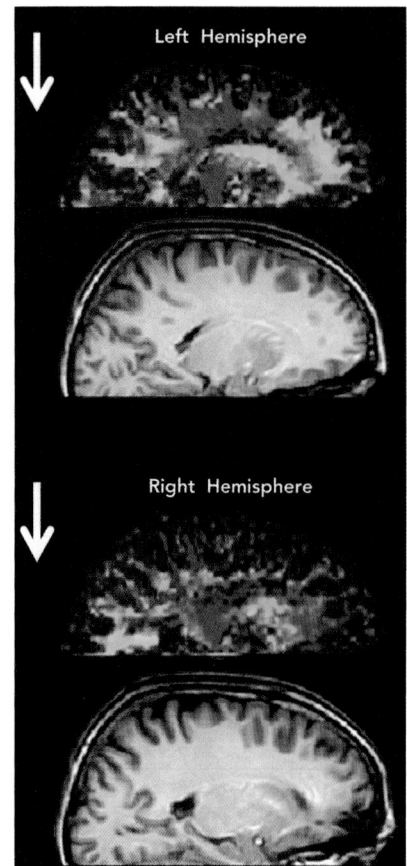

Left Hemisphere

Right Hemisphere

FIGURE 19–14

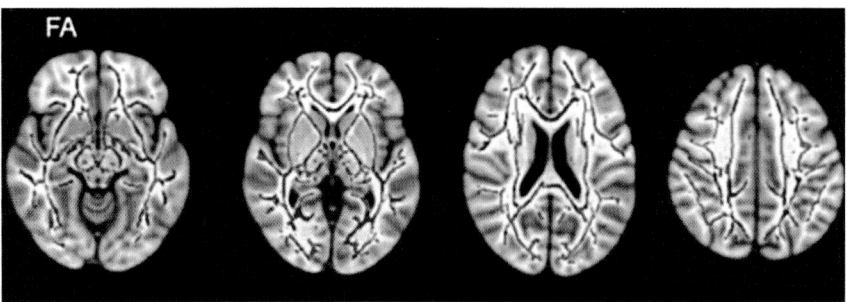

FA

FIGURE 19–15

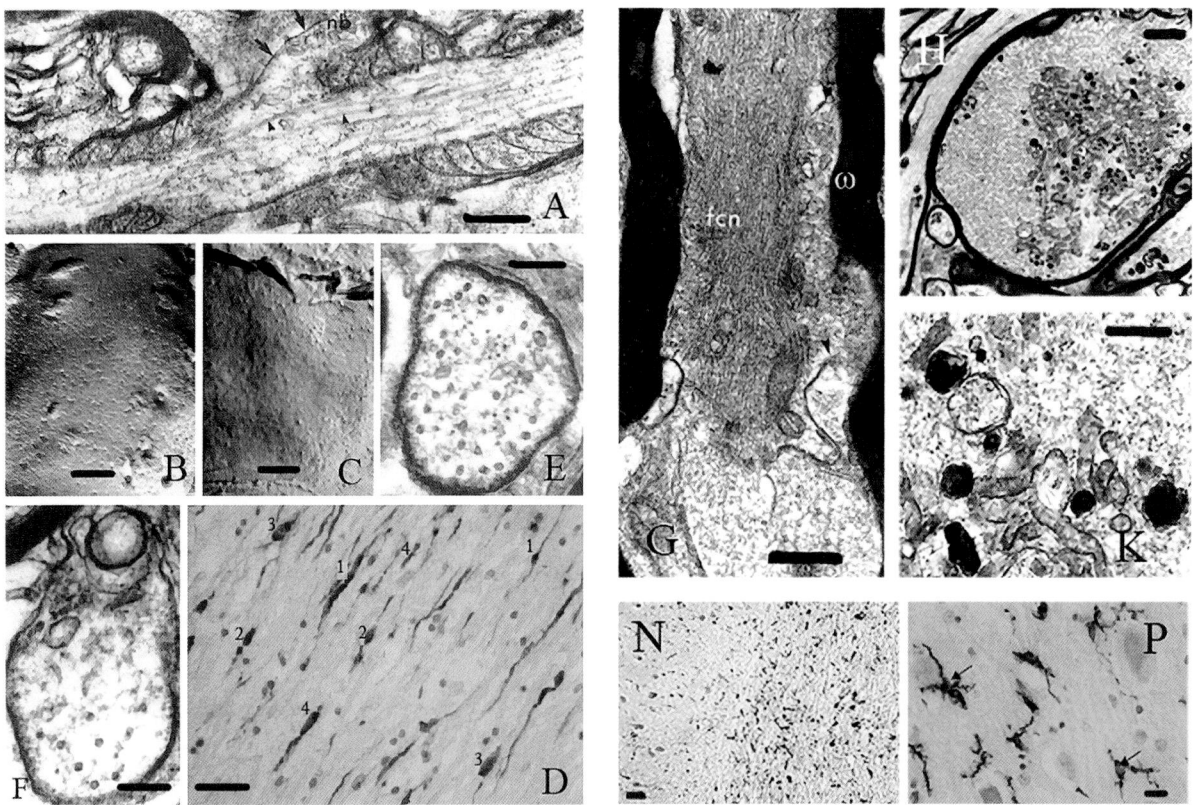

FIGURE 19–16

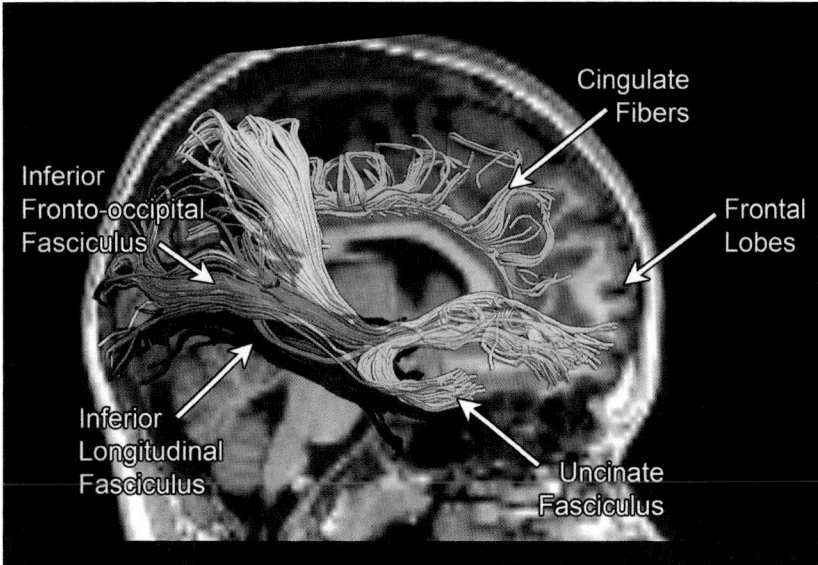

FIGURE 19–17

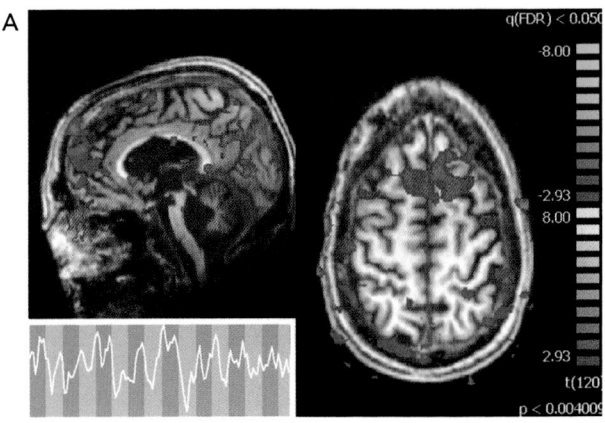

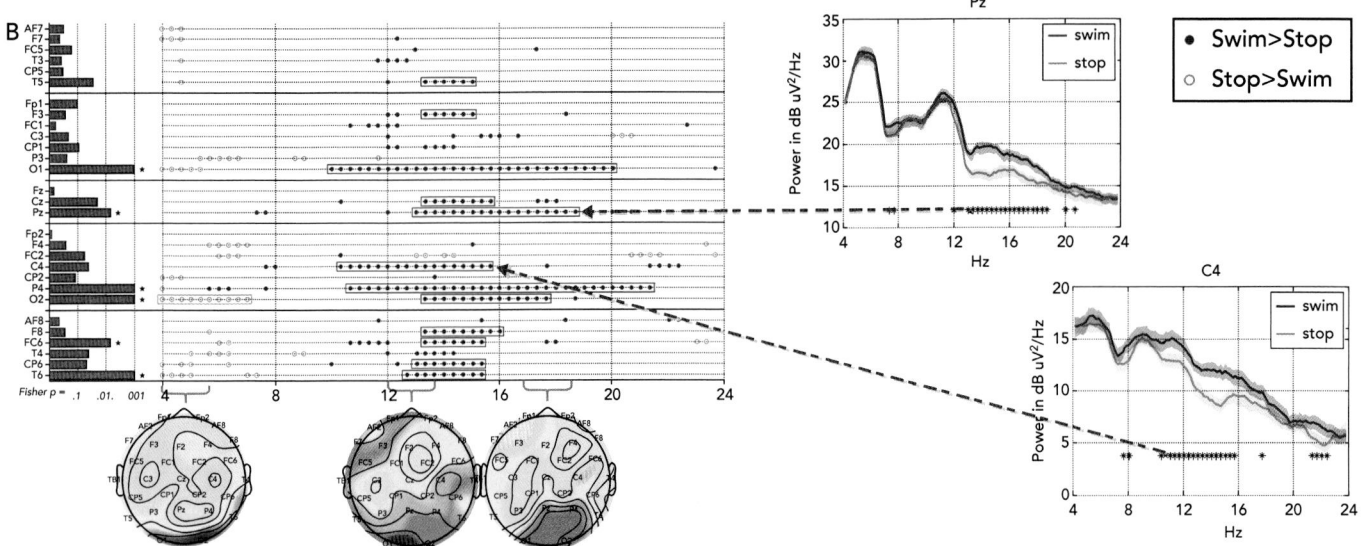

FIGURE 32–1

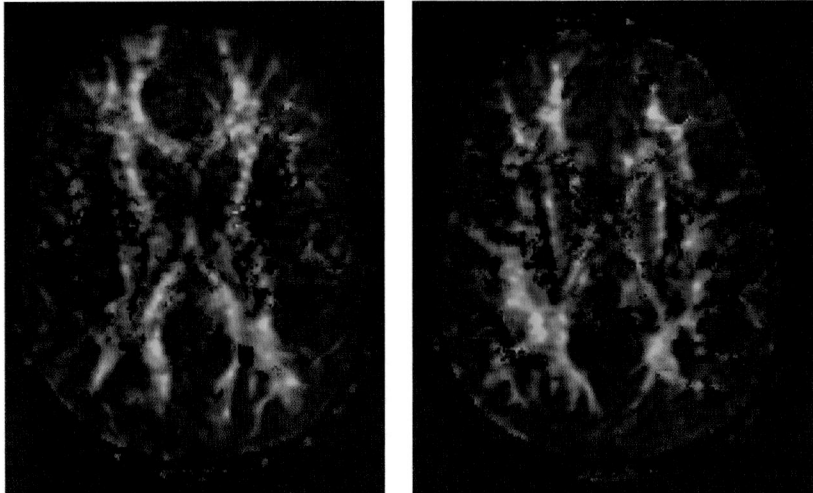

FIGURE 35–6

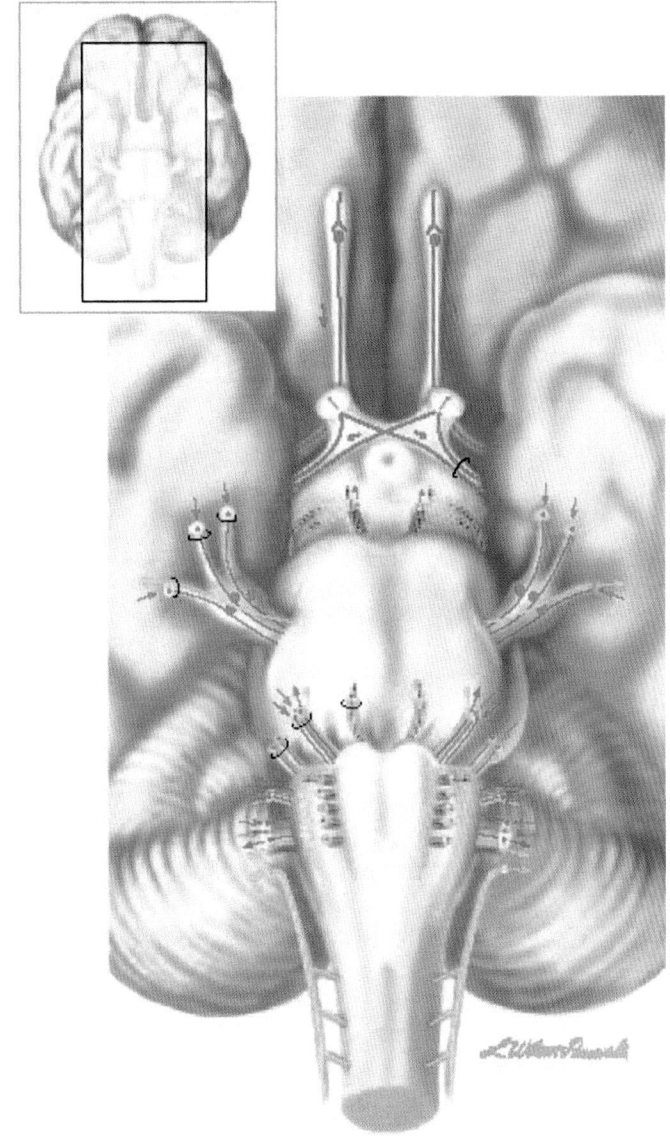

FIGURE 41–1

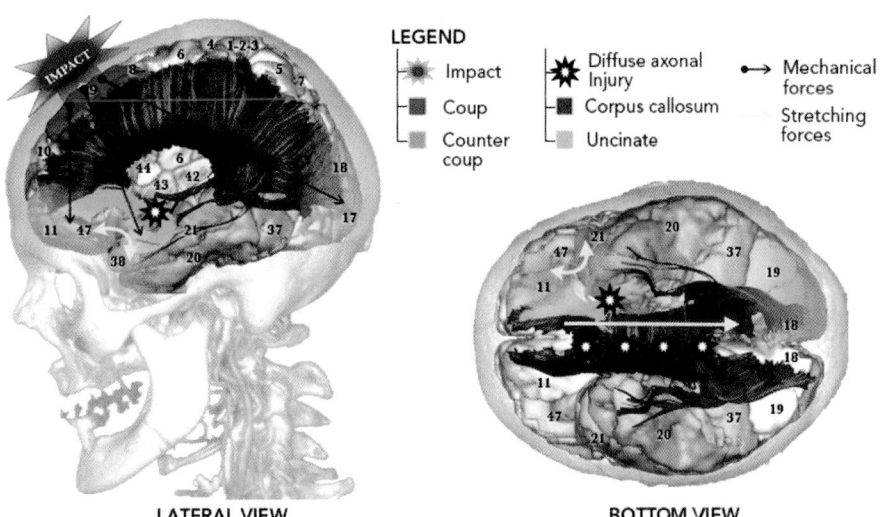

LATERAL VIEW

BOTTOM VIEW

FIGURE 59–1

ORBITOFRONTAL PARALIMBIC DIVISION

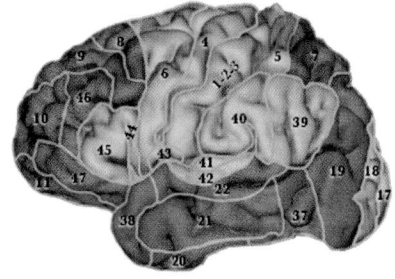

LATERAL ORBITOFRONTAL FIBERS

TEMPORAL FIBERS
- amygdala
- temporal pole (38)
- inferior temporal cortex (20)
- uncus (36)

MEDIAL ORBITOFRONTAL FIBERS

24, 32, 33, 36, 21, 22, 11, 47

Phylogeny and cytoarchitectonic
Paleocortical
granule cell

Anatomy
Amygdala, anterior parahippocampal, insula, temporal pole, subcallosal cingulate

Functions
Implicit processing, visceral integration, visual features analysis, appetite drives, social awareness, mood

FIGURE 59–2

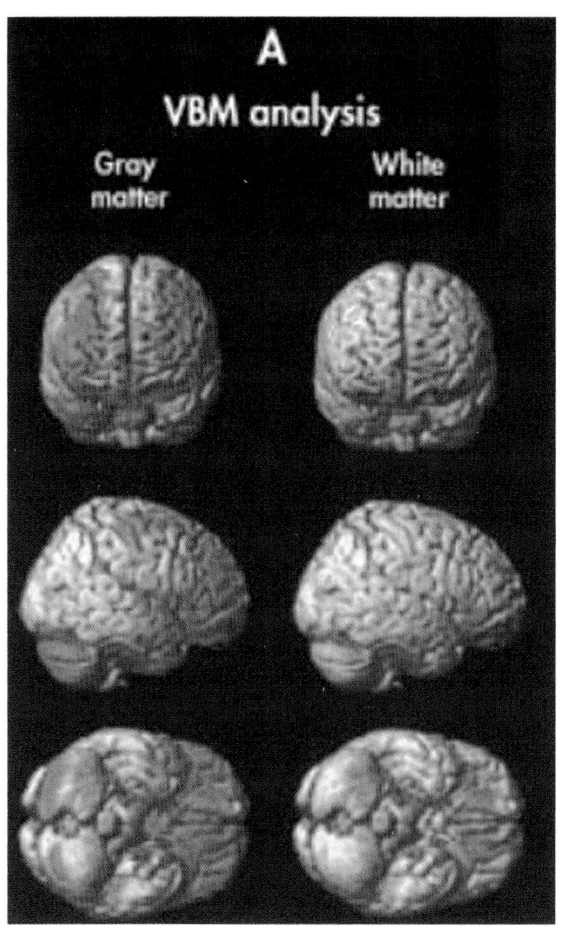

FIGURE 62–1

the subdural space, is distinguished from subdural fluid by its dramatic enhancement with gadolinium (72).

Programmable Valves, Antisiphon Devices, and Gravitational Valves

Programmable Valves

Programmable valves that can have their opening pressure changed at the bedside by use of an external magnet are now in routine use (147–153). These allow the valves to be adjusted at bedside without requiring a further surgical procedure. Valve opening pressure can be decreased for poor clinical response of hydrocephalus or increased for headaches, subdurals, or other indications of overdrainage. Programmable valves have been demonstrated to be cost-effective compared with nonadjustable ones (149). Four different programmable valve systems are currently available (68,152); each will be described briefly subsequently. One problem encountered with programmable valves has been inadvertent valve resetting by MRI scan, external magnets, valve filliping, and transcranial magnetic stimulation (68,147,152–154). MRI scans are not contraindicated with programmable valves but settings need to be checked before and after MRI scan. For some of the programmable valves, an x-ray is needed to confirm valve setting (152).

Codman Programmable Valves

The Codman Hakim was the first programmable valve released in the United States and has been tested in multiple clinical trials (147–152). It has 18 settings at 10 mm increments from 30 to 200 mm H$_2$O. The manufacturer recommends not increasing or decreasing settings by more than 30 mm at one time. Programming is with an electromagnet, which must be carefully centered and oriented over the valve mechanism in order that the proper valve setting is achieved. In cases where the shunt mechanism is difficult to palpate because of scar tissue, fluoroscopy, or use of an opaque marker (BB) on a preliminary x-ray view may confirm precise location of the active valve mechanism. MRI can reset the valve and the setting can only be determined by x-ray. Reading the setting on x-ray requires that the x-ray beam be precisely perpendicular to the valve mechanism; otherwise, it may be very difficult to see the valve setting. The x-ray beam should pass thru the shunt valve before going through the skull, which will orient the marker on the right, and the valve setting can then be determined by the location of a notch out of the opaque circle (see Figure 44-5). More recently, Codman has released the Certas valve, with 8 settings including virtual off, and designed to be more resistant to inadvertent shunt readjustment by MRI, although it is still advised to check settings after MRI.

Medtronic PS Medical Strata Valve

This valve has 5 settings, from 0.5 to 2.5 corresponding to opening pressures from 15 to 170 mm H$_2$O (152). MRI can reset the valve. The valve setting can be read at bedside without x-ray and also can be easily confirmed by x-ray (see Figure 44-6). Adjustments of the opening pressure are done with simple magnet and bedside tools.

Sophysa Programmable Valves

The Sophy valve was released in Europe even before the Codman Hakim valve was released in the United States. More recently, Sophysa has also released a Polaris valve with a locking mechanism intended to make reprogramming by MRI less likely to occur; it has 5 positions, which can be read on x-ray (152).

Aesculap-Miethke proGAV Programmable Shunt

This system combines a programmable valve in a series with a gravitational valve (which will be described in the following texts) (152,155). The valve has a brake to prevent inadvertent settings change, such as by MRI, and valve setting can be read at bedside without requiring x-ray. The device has been shown safe and reliable in a recent multicenter study (155). One complaint has been that releasing the brake requires some local pressure on the head, deemed uncomfortable by some patients.

Antisiphon Devices

Problems related to overdrainage have led to the development of several special shunt components. Antisiphon devices have been developed with diaphragms that close to counteract negative standing hydrostatic pressures with some success (124,144,145). Several valves have been designed to assist with CSF overdrainage. The delta valve is similar to an antisiphon device in combination with a standard valve but engineered to minimize the area of the valve diaphragm responsive to pressure effects of fluid in the distal tubing (146). The Orbis-Sigma valve is a flow regulated valve, with variable resistance and 3 stages of flow. It initially functions like a standard low-pressure valve but shows increased resistance with larger flow rates; it also has a decreased resistance safety valve to deal with higher pressures.

Gravitational Shunts

Overdrainage of shunts has been particularly problematic because of the negative intraventricular pressures generated in the upright position by the column of fluid in the distal shunt tubing and the related siphon effects. To address this problem in a specific manner, gravitational shunts are designed with a higher opening pressure in the upright position than supine. The one used most extensively has been the Miethke dual-switch valve (156,157). This is actually 2 valves in 1, ingeniously designed so that the lower pressure valve opens in the supine position but is mechanically closed off by a ball in the vertical position, forcing flow through the higher pressure half of the valve when upright. A related invention is the Shunt Assistant valve (157,158), in which a tantalum sphere compresses a sealing ball to substantially increase the opening pressure of the valve system when the patient is upright (see Figure 44-7). The Aesculap proGAV system combines a valve of this type in series with a programmable valve (155), and the Shunt Assistant valve has also been successfully used in combination with the Codman Hakim programmable shunt. Good clinical response of hydrocephalus with low incidence of overdrainage and only mild decrease in ventricular size on scan has been reported with both these systems (155–158).

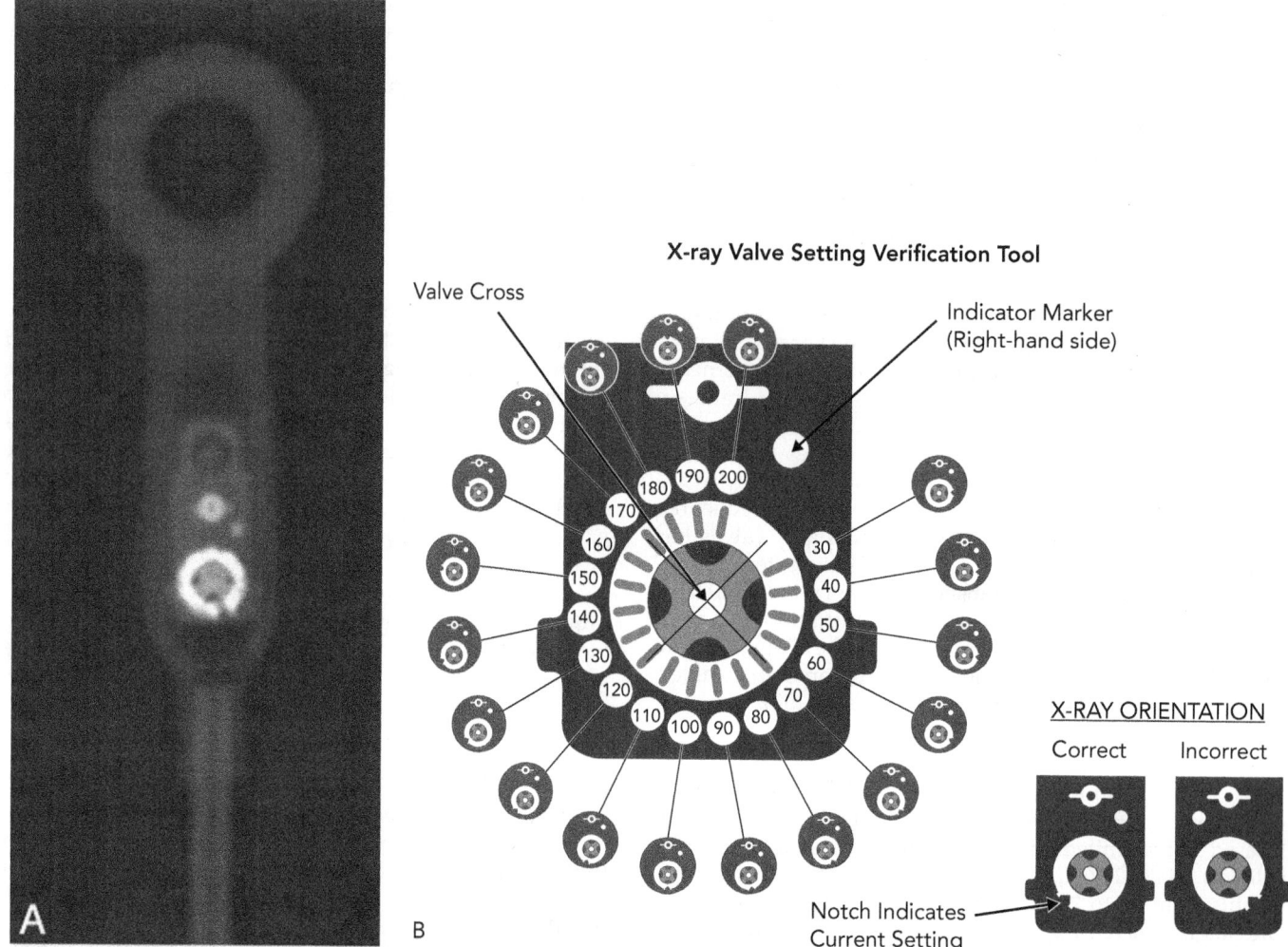

FIGURE 44-5 X-ray verification setting of Codman Hakim programmable valve. A, valve set at 80. B, different pressure settings and corresponding x-ray notch locations. Pictures at far right show that x-ray film must be shot, so that marker is on the right (achieved by x-ray beam perpendicular thru shunt, then skull, then x-ray plate). The picture marked as correct shows a shunt setting of 120.

VASCULAR COMPLICATIONS

Traumatic Aneurysm

Intracranial Traumatic Aneurysms

Traumatic intracranial aneurysms are rare; they comprise less than 1% of all intracranial aneurysms (159–161) and are more common after missile injuries than closed head injury. In missile injuries, direct contact of missile or bone fragments with the artery is common, whereas in blunt injuries, up to 40% of cases do not have associated fracture (161). Traumatic aneurysms can be classified as true, false, mixed, or dissecting types, but false aneurysms are the most common (162–164). In true aneurysms, the adventitial wall is preserved, whereas in false aneurysms, all elements of the vascular wall are disrupted, and blood is contained only by the surrounding arachnoid, hematoma, or brain parenchyma. Mixed aneurysms have a combination of true and false elements. In dissecting aneurysms, blood channels within the vessel wall, effectively narrowing or occluding the vessel itself.

Common clinical presentations of traumatic intracranial aneurysms include seizures, focal neurological deficits, altered consciousness, and severe persistent headache (159,161). Traumatic intracranial aneurysms are highly unstable and prone to rupture (162,163); in fact, although the time interval from injury to rupture varies from days to years, 90% bleed within 3 weeks of injury (160,163). The most common locations for traumatic aneurysms are the distal middle cerebral branches, distal anterior cerebral artery, and proximal carotid and vertebral arteries (161). Traumatic petrous and cavernous carotid aneurysms are often associated with basilar skull fracture, whereas supraclinoid carotid aneurysms are sometimes associated with orbital or anterior clinoid process fractures (161). Epistaxis, pharyngeal mass, and delayed cranial nerve palsy have also been described with aneurysms near the skull base (161,165). In such cases, MRI with contrast, especially combined with perfusion-weighted imaging or magnetic resonance angiography (MRA) may be a useful screening tool and identify aneurysms that might not show on noncontrast CT or MRI (161). Delayed subarachnoid hemorrhage or intracerebral hemor-

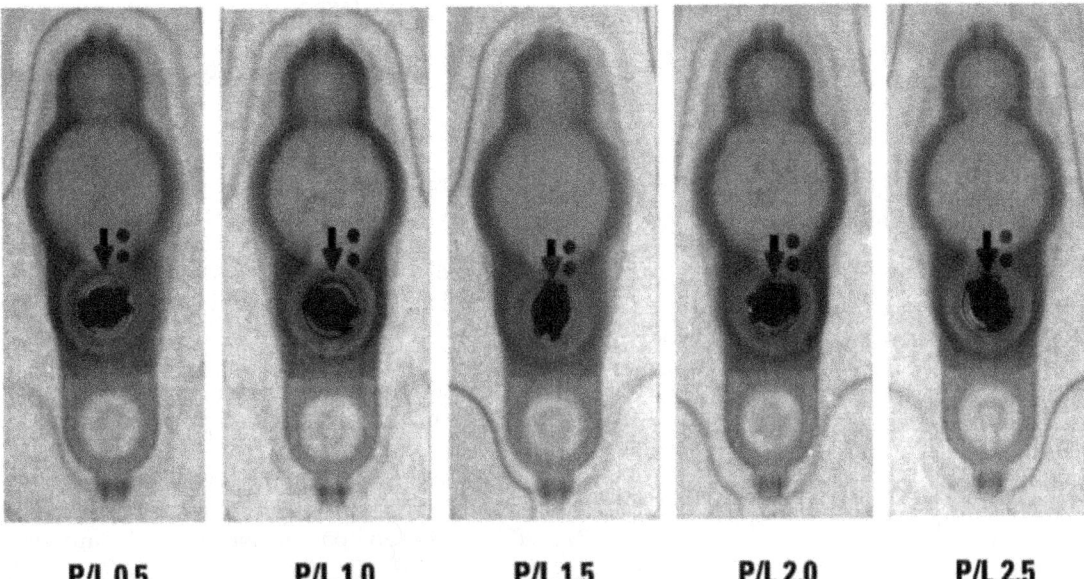

| P/L 0.5 | P/L 1.0 | P/L 1.5 | P/L 2.0 | P/L 2.5 |

FIGURE 44–6 Medtronic PS Medical Strata valve. Fluoroscopic appearance of valve mechanism for each of its 5 settings. P/L, performance level.

rhage should raise suspicion for traumatic aneurysm. Angiography remains the definitive test for aneurysm diagnosis.

Treatment of traumatic intracranial aneurysms can be problematic because they are typically false aneurysms and therefore cannot be clipped (162–164). Because the parent vessel often must be sacrificed, extracranial to intracranial distal revascularization procedures are sometimes performed at the time of definitive treatment (161). Endovascular approaches have often been useful, including detachable balloons, detachable coils to occlude the parent vessel, or stents to exclude the aneurysm from the circulation while maintaining the patency of the parent vessel (161).

Cervical Arterial Trauma Including Dissection

Traumatic injury to the cervical internal carotid or vertebral arteries may be seen after penetrating injuries or after hyperextension and flexion neck injuries, as in motor vehicle accidents. Many patients with blunt injuries show little or no overt external neck trauma (161). The incidence of injury to the carotid artery in patients with TBI has been estimated at 0.5% (161). When carotid injury occurs, mortality is esti-

mated at 20%–40%, and neurologic deficits are seen in 80% of survivors. Presentation is typically that of infarction in the distribution of the involved vessel, either secondary to thrombosis, embolism, or dissection. For example, after carotid artery trauma, hemiparesis and hemisensory loss occur, but onset of these symptoms exceeds 10 hours from initial injury in half of cases and is sometimes delayed for up to 48 hours (161). Acute headache can be a very important clue to the early diagnosis of arterial dissection, occurring in 60% of cases of carotid dissection and slightly less often with vertebral artery dissection where the headache tends to be occipital (166). Other important clues to possible cervical carotid injury include mandibular fracture, neck pain, pulsatile tinnitus, visual changes, lower cranial nerve palsies, and ipsilateral Horner syndrome (161). Revascularization or direct repair is sometimes attempted for carotid dissection but only if it can be done within 4 hours of onset in a conscious patient (162). Otherwise, management is medical, with consideration of antiplatelet or anticoagulation therapy depending on clinical course and associated injuries. Anticoagulation with heparin or warfarin (Coumadin) has been the

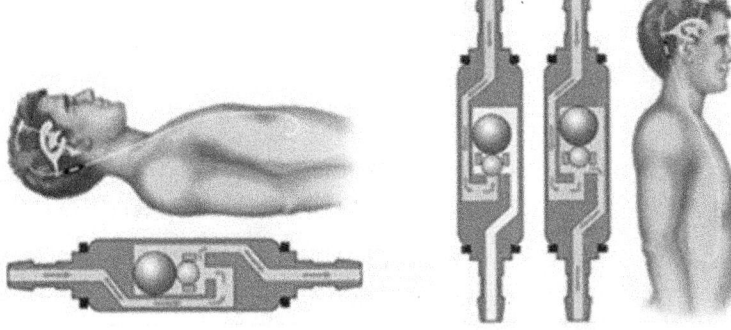

FIGURE 44–7 Shunt assistant valve A, supine flow occurs readily thru the valve. B, upright flow must additionally push up the 2 balls, effectively increasing the opening pressure of the valve. This type of gravitational valve is combined with a programmable valve in the Aesculap proGAV system.

traditional management when not contraindicated but lacks a strong evidence base (166).

Carotid Cavernous Fistula

Types

The cavernous sinus is anatomically unique in that a large artery passes through a large venous space. For this reason, a tear in the arterial wall alone can create an arteriovenous fistula without any additional venous anomaly (167–169). Thus, traumatic carotid cavernous fistulas are typically direct fistulas from the internal carotid artery with fast flow and high pressure (type A). They contrast with spontaneous carotid cavernous fistulas (types B, C, and D), which typically receive dural blood supply and therefore have low pressure or slow flow (167,168).

Presentation

Delayed visual loss or impairment raises concern for possible development of carotid cavernous fistula. In fact, 43.5% are diagnosed over 1 month after trauma (170). Additional presenting signs of carotid cavernous fistula include supraorbital bruit, exophthalmos, orbital congestion, oculomotor palsies, and trigeminal nerve involvement (167,170,171). Pulsatile tinnitus may result from arteriovenous fistulas or from altered jugular venous flow (173–176). Prevention of further visual loss is a priority in these patients.

Treatment

Although spontaneous low-flow carotid cavernous fistulas sometimes close spontaneously or with manual decompression, this is uncommon in post-traumatic high-flow fistulas (177,178). The definitive treatment of traumatic carotid cavernous fistula has become the endovascular placement of detachable balloons or coils (177–180). Successful fistula closure was accomplished by the detachable balloon technique in 92 of 95 cases of traumatic carotid cavernous fistula, with preservation of the internal carotid artery in more than 70% of cases (168).

LATE INTRACRANIAL MASS LESIONS

Subdural Hematoma and Hygroma

Differences Between Acute and Chronic Subdural Hematoma

Subdural hematoma is the most common late presenting mass lesion. Although acute, subacute (3–20 days), and chronic (3 weeks or more) subdural hematomas are distinguished by time of detection after injury, it is important to recognize that chronic subdural hematoma has a different pathophysiologic process than acute subdural hematoma and not simply an older blood clot (181–185). As a result, differences are also seen in the epidemiology, clinical presentation, prognosis, and treatment techniques (73,182,184) (Table 44-3). The incidence of chronic subdural hematoma peaks in the 7th and 8th decades, and only 60%–65% of patients have known TBI (184,186). Male predominance (70%–90%) and parietal location (91%) are some characteristics (181,184). Headaches are a cardinal symptom (184,187), sometimes following a symptom-free interval. Three major clinical presentations include hemiparesis (40%), personality or intellectual change (30%), and signs of increased ICP, including papilledema (20%) (181). In contrast with acute subdural hematoma, seizures are relatively uncommon with chronic subdural hematoma (4%–7%), and ongoing anticonvulsant prophylaxis is not routinely required (188), although some authorities have recommended it in the immediate postoperative period (187). Transient episodes of aphasia or sensorimotor disturbances have also been described with chronic subdural hematomas, mimicking either transient ischemic attacks or seizures and resolving after the immediate postoperative period following surgical drainage (189,190).

Scan Findings in Subdural Hematoma

CT scans characteristically show decreased density in chronic subdural hematoma. However, the isodense appearance characteristic of subacute subdural hematoma may last longer than 1 month in some instances (191). In questionable cases, contrast enhancement helps to identify isodense subdural collections (192). In other cases, a layer of isodensity or increased

TABLE 44-3 Differences Between Acute and Chronic Subdural Hematoma

FEATURE	ACUTE SUBDURAL HEMATOMA	CHRONIC SUBDURAL HEMATOMA
Age peak	30–49 years	60–70 years
Known TBI	Virtually all	60%–65%
Clinical presentation	Acute mental status change, focal signs, seizures, increased intracranial pressure	Personality or chronic mental status change, headache, hemiparesis, increased intracranial pressure
Composition	Blood clot	Fluid, membrane
Pathophysiology	Venous bleeding especially from torn bridging veins	Initial subdural hygroma or initial venous bleeding, inflammatory process with leaky macrocapillaries, disordered hemostatic mechanism
Treatment	Craniotomy	Burr holes, twist drill craniostomy, or craniotomy

density is seen below a hypodense layer; this sedimentation level likely reflects interval rebleeding (192,193).

Compared with CT scan density, the factors determining signal intensity on MRI are much more complex. Subacute subdural hematoma is seen as a hyperintense collection on Tl-weighted images, largely because of the presence of methemoglobin. Chronic subdural hematoma presents with more variable signal intensity on Tl-weighted images but consistently shows increased signal intensity on T2-weighted images (29,187,194,195). In addition, fluid collections that are homogeneous on CT sometimes show hypointense septations and mixed intensities on MRI. In some instances, a sedimentation level of a hyperintense (fluid) upper layer and hypointense (more cellular) lower layer is seen. Such findings are consistent with the conceptualization of subdural hematoma as an ongoing process with interval rebleeding rather than a static collection of blood. As described subsequently, an outer membrane is a characteristic in chronic subdural collections; this membrane enhances significantly with gadolinium on Tl-weighted imaging in many cases (29).

Pathology of Chronic Subdural Hematoma

On pathologic examination, the fluid of chronic subdural hematoma shows a range of color and appearance, including brown-black, dark red, amber-brown, and almost clear and watery (184,194). Coagulated masses of blood and fibrin are sometimes present. A thicker outer membrane attached to the dura and thinner inner membrane bordering on the arachnoid are characteristics (184). Enlarged ectatic capillaries, often called giant capillaries or sinusoids, are prominent on the outer membrane and associated with inflammatory cells, fibroblasts, and hemosiderin-laden macrophages (184). With age, the outer membrane also may become calcified.

Subdural Hygroma

Subdural hygroma has been described as a subdural collection of CSF, often with a modified composition (196). The distinction between subdural hygroma and chronic subdural hematoma has often been unclear in the literature, partly because subdural fluid composition varies, sometimes exhibiting xanthochromia or containing blood products. Also, the term *hygroma* has sometimes been used to describe low-density extra-axial collections on CT scan without mass effect (196), even when identification of cortical veins lateral to the collection on MRI might more correctly identify it as subarachnoid fluid associated with atrophy (29). It has been proposed that a tear in the arachnoid may acutely allow CSF into the subdural space, and rare surgical documentation of this process has been provided (196). More often, the development of subdural hygroma may be more gradual, and in these cases, subdural hygroma formation requires separation of the dura arachnoid interface and sufficient potential subdural space (143,197–199). Low ICP (such as orthostatic negative pressures with a shunt), an underfilled CSF compartment, and atrophy are factors in creating sufficient subdural space (84,118,142,143). Many patients have a slight cranial asymmetry in the occipital region, with 1 side flatter than the other. In the supine position the cranium tends to turn slightly to the flattened side, and subdural hygromas tend to form frontally to the opposite side or bilaterally in patients with a more symmetrical cranium (143,197). The

time course of hygroma development, enlargement, and, in most instances, resolution can be plotted.

Pathophysiology of Chronic Subdural Hematoma

Recent work has significantly clarified our understanding of the relationship between subdural hygroma and chronic subdural hematoma and the pathophysiology of their development. Chronic subdural hematomas occasionally develop from acute subdural hematomas, but more often, chronic subdural hematomas develop from subdural hygromas (143). When hygromas do not resolve, a neomembrane forms from the dural border cells, followed by leakage of blood from the fragile giant capillaries in the outer membrane induced by the inflammatory process (182,200,201). A disordered local hemostatic mechanism has been identified in fluid from chronic subdural hematoma (182,183), with both excessive activation of the clotting system and the fibrinolytic system. Chronic subdural collections can sometimes show increasing density on CT scans for a period of weeks to months (143). The size of a chronic subdural collection may resolve spontaneously if absorption exceeds rebleeding, or alternatively, the collection may continue to enlarge (143).

Approach to Chronic Subdural Management

Management of the patient with chronic subdural hygroma or chronic subdural hematoma is largely a matter of clinical judgment. Conservative management can be employed in patients with smaller collections, less mass effect, stable neurologic exam, and more fragile general medical condition. Serial scanning in 2–4 weeks, or sooner if clinical worsening, and early neurosurgical consultation are advised. In a recent survey, about half of neurosurgeons favored steroid use in conservatively managed patients (202).

Surgery for Chronic Subdural Hematoma

Burr holes are the first-line treatments for chronic subdural hematoma (181,184,202–204). Occasionally, the presence of sizable clots or loculation may necessitate craniotomy, as is commonly done for acute subdural hematoma (182,205). Surgical removal of a certain critical mass of fluid containing degradation products from the subdural space may be important in interrupting the vicious cycle of disordered hemostasis and facilitating the recovery from chronic subdural hematoma (182,183). Successful surgery, therefore, may reduce the residual volume to a degree that allows further resorption rather than fully removing the blood clot. In fact, persisting subdural fluid was described postoperatively in 78% of patients but had returned to normal by 40 days postoperatively in 27 of 32 cases. Therefore, it has been suggested that reoperation should be avoided until at least 3 weeks postoperatively unless marked clinical deterioration occurs (208). Neurosurgical opinions vary on the use of a drain but most reserve these for refractory cases (202). The overall prognosis from chronic subdural hematoma is much more favorable than the prognosis for acute subdural hematoma (184). Patients with even severe neurologic deficits preoperatively may have successful outcomes (181).

Epidural Hematoma

Presentation

Although epidural hematoma is usually considered the most acute post-traumatic mass lesion, it presents more than 5 days after injury in 10% of cases (209) and may present as late as the second or third week after injury (210). Although epidural hematoma most often presents in the temporal fossa (57%–83% of cases) because of injury to the middle meningeal artery, delayed presentation is more common with extratemporal location, especially frontal or posterior fossa lesions (209,211). Clouding or decreased level of consciousness is considered the most important sign of epidural hematoma (209). Onset is slowest with frontal lesions, and symptoms may be vague. Unilateral exophthalmos is an unusual sign that has been described with subfrontal epidural hematoma (211).

Posterior Fossa Epidural Hematoma

Posterior fossa epidural hematomas are unique among epidural hematomas in that they are of venous rather than arterial in origin. An occipital bone fracture is seen in 84.2% of cases and characteristically crosses the venous sinus causing this venous bleeding (212). The venous origin helps explain why a slower clinical presentation may occur. A lucid interval is common, and progressive decrease in the level of consciousness is a characteristic. Battle sign is often seen, and neck stiffness, occipital headache, and vomiting may be prominent. Symptoms and signs of increased ICP as well as brainstem, cranial nerve, and cerebellar dysfunction are common (212,213). Posterior fossa epidurals are not common; they are seen in only 0.3% of patients with TBI (212). However, they have the highest mortality rate (209) and are notoriously difficult to diagnose (211).

Intracerebral Hemorrhage

Delayed traumatic intracerebral hemorrhage is defined as an intracerebral hematoma that is not visualized on initial CT but is seen on a follow-up study. It occurs in 5.6%–7.4% of patients with severe TBI (214). Time of onset is typically about 24 hours after original injury (214), and 80% of cases occur within 48 hours of injury (187). Cardinal signs of delayed traumatic intracerebral hemorrhage include decreased level of consciousness, focal signs, or seizures (215). Factors postulated to play a role in the pathogenesis include dysregulation of blood flow, coagulation disorders, and removal of tamponade effect by evacuation of another mass lesion, such as an epidural or subdural hematoma. Outcome is worse with temporal lobe location, which shows an increased incidence of herniation (216).

CONCLUSION

Late intracranial complications continue to be extremely important concerns during the rehabilitation of TBI and warrant particular consideration when patients do not progress as anticipated. Best timing for cranioplasty and accurate identification of which patients will benefit from shunts are ongoing challenges for additional research. Further technological advances in shunt technology may help with their effectiveness and safety. Interventional approaches without craniotomy are advancing the management of vascular complications.

KEY CLINICAL POINTS

1. Cerebrospinal fistulas require careful identification and definitive treatment because of the late risk of meningitis. CSF can be identified in nasal secretions by assay for beta-2 transferrin, which is present in CSF but not in blood or nasal secretions.

2. Subdural empyema, although classically a fulminant infection, can present more insidiously after cranioplasty. MRI with diffusion-weighted imaging can help distinguish subdural empyema (hyperintense) from subdural hygroma or hematoma.

3. Cranioplasty is now often performed much earlier than in the past. This reflects the increasing frequency of craniectomy acutely, as well as increasing concern about developing either hydrocephalus or the syndrome of the trephined. Patients with this syndrome may show significant clinical improvement when cranioplasty is performed.

4. Dynamic hydrocephalus can be extremely difficult to differentiate from atrophy with ex vacuo ventricular dilation in patients with TBI. History (hemorrhage, infection, craniectomy), exam findings (NPH triad, akinetic mutism, or Parinaud syndrome), clinical course (worsening or nonprogressive), scan findings (ventriculomegaly, transependymal fluid, tight high convexity), and sometimes even lumbar drainage (showing positive clinical response) may help with identification of patients likely to respond to a shunt.

5. Shunt infections are frequently indolent, most often caused by *S. epidermidis* and are best diagnosed by tapping the shunt (not by lumbar puncture).

6. Programmable shunts are now in routine use and can be adjusted in rehabilitation, including decreasing the opening pressure for poor clinical response and increasing it for headache, subdural hematoma, or overdrainage. MRI scans can reset programmable shunts, and shunt settings need to be rechecked after MRI in some instances requiring careful x-ray to read the setting. Specifics of Codman Hakim, Medtronic PS Medical Strata, Sophy valve, and Aesculap proGAV shunts are discussed and referenced.

7. Traumatic aneurysms and carotid cavernous fistulas are relatively rare but need to be considered, especially with late hemorrhage, visual loss, new neurologic deficits, cranial nerve involvement, or sudden severe headache. Endovascular management with coils and balloons can be very effective when these problems are identified.

8. Chronic subdural hematoma is not just an older acute subdural hematoma, it has a very different clinical profile—patient demographics, pathophysiology, clinical presentation, and approach to treatment.

KEY REFERENCES

1. Dujovny M, Agner C, Aviles A. Syndrome of the trephined: theory and facts. *Crit Rev Neurosurg.* 1999;9(5):271–278.

2. Lollis SS, Mamourian AC, Vaccaro TJ, Duhaime AC. Programmable CSF shunt valves: radiographic identification and interpretation. *AJNR Am J Neuroradiol.* 2010;31(7):1343–1346.

3. Long DF. Hydrocephalus. In: Zollman FS, ed. *Manual of Traumatic Brain Injury Management.* New York, NY: Demos Medical Publishing; 2011:303–308.

4. Marmarou A, Bergsneider M, Klinge P, Relkin N, Black PM. The value of supplemental prognostic tests for the preoperative assessment of idiopathic normal-pressure hydrocephalus. *Neurosurgery.* 2005;57(3)(suppl):S17–S28; discussion ii–v.

5. Swift AC, Foy P. Advances in the management of CSF rhinorrhoea. *Hosp Med.* 2002;63(1):28–32.

References

1. Cooper PR. Skull fracture and traumatic cerebrospinal fluid fistulas. In: Cooper PR, ed. *Head Injury.* 3rd ed. Baltimore, MD: Williams & Wilkins; 1993:115–136.

2. Curry DJ, Frim DM. Delayed repair of open depressed skull fracture. *Pediatr Neurosurg.* 1999;31(6):294–297.

3. Ali B, Ghosh A. Antibiotics in compound depressed skull fractures. *Emerg Med J.* 2002;19(6):552–553.

4. Dunn LT, Foy PM. Anticonvulsant and antibiotic prophylaxis in head injury. *Ann R Coll Surg Engl.* 1994;76(3):147–149.

5. Al-Haddad SA, Kirollos R. A 5-year study of the outcome of surgically treated depressed skull fractures. *Ann R Coll Surg Engl.* 2002;84(3):196–200.

6. Roy R, Cooper PR. Penetrating injuries of the skull and brain. In: Braakman R, ed. *Handbook of Clinical Neurology.* Amsterdam, The Netherlands: Elsevier; 1990:299–315.

7. Kaufman HH. Care and variations in the care of patients with gunshot wounds to the brain. *Neurosurg Clin N Am.* 1995;6(4):727–739.

8. Laun A. Traumatic cerebrospinal fluid fistulas in the anterior and middle cranial fossae. *Acta Neurochir (Wien).* 1982;60(3–4):215–222.

9. Villalobos T, Arango C, Kubilis P, Rathore M. Antibiotic prophylaxis after basilar skull fractures: a meta-analysis. *Clin Infect Dis.* 1998;27(2):364–369.

10. MacGee E. Cerebrospinal fluid fistula. In: Vinken PJ, Bruyn GW, eds. *The Handbook of Clinical Neurology.* Amsterdam, The Netherlands: Elsevier; 1976:183–199.

11. Frederiks JAM. Post-traumatic CSF hypotension. In: Vinken PJ, Bruyn GW, eds. *Handbook of Clinical Neurology.* New York, NY: Elsevier; 1976:255–259.

12. Cusimano MD, Sekhar LN. Pseudo-cerebrospinal fluid rhinorrhea. *J Neurosurg.* 1994;80(1):26–30.

13. Wakhloo AK, van Velthoven V, Schumacher M, Krauss JK. Evaluation of MR imaging, digital subtraction cisternography, and CT cisternography in diagnosing CSF fistula. *Acta Neurochir (Wien).* 1991;111(3–4):119–127.

14. Ryall RG, Peacock MK, Simpson DA. Usefulness of beta 2-transferrin assay in the detection of cerebrospinal fluid leaks following head injury. *J Neurosurg.* 1992;77(5):737–739.

15. Meco C, Arrer E, Oberascher G. Efficacy of cerebrospinal fluid fistula repair: sensitive quality control using the beta-trace protein test. *Am J Rhinol.* 2007;21(6):729–736.

16. Miller JD. Infection after head injury. In: Vinken PJ, Bruyn GW, eds. *Handbook of Clinical Neurology.* Amsterdam, The Netherlands: Elsevier; 1976:215–230.

17. Schlosser RJ, Bolger WE. Nasal cerebrospinal fluid leaks. *J Otolaryngol.* 2002;31(suppl 1):S28–S37.

18. Swift AC, Foy P. Advances in the management of CSF rhinorrhoea. *Hosp Med.* 2002;63(1):28–32.

19. Giannetti AV, de Morais Silva Santiago AP, Becker HM, Guimarães RE. Comparative study between primary spontaneous cerebrospinal fluid fistula and late traumatic fistula. *Otolaryngol Head Neck Surg.* 2011;144(3):463–468.

20. Tunkel AR, Scheld WM. Acute infectious complications of head trauma. In: Braakman R, ed. *Handbook of Clinical Neurology.* Amsterdam, The Netherlands: Elsevier; 1990:317–326.

21. Shapiro SA, Scully T. Closed continuous drainage of cerebrospinal fluid via a lumbar subarachnoid catheter for treatment or prevention of cranial/spinal cerebrospinal fluid fistula. *Neurosurgery.* 1992;30(2):241–245.

22. Probst C. Neurosurgical treatment of traumatic frontobasal CSF fistulae in 300 patients (1967–1989). *Acta Neurochir (Wien).* 1990;106(1–2):37–47.

23. Okada J, Tsuda T, Takasugi S, Nishida K, Tóth Z, Matsumoto K. Unusually late onset of cerebrospinal fluid rhinorrhea after head trauma. *Surg Neurol.* 1991;35(3):213–217.

24. Sindou M, Guyotat-Pelissou I, Chidiac A, Goutelle A. Transcutaneous pressure adjustable valve for the treatment of hydrocephalus and arachnoid cysts in adults. Experiences with 75 cases. *Acta Neurochir (Wien).* 1993;121(3–4):135–139.

25. Salca HC, Danaila L. Onset of uncomplicated cerebrospinal fluid fistula 27 years after head injury: case report. *Surg Neurol.* 1997;47(2):132–133.

26. McCormack B, Cooper PR, Persky M, Rothstein S. Extracranial repair of cerebrospinal fluid fistulas: technique and results in 37 patients. *Neurosurgery.* 1990;27(3):412–417.

27. Brodie HA. Prophylactic antibiotics for posttraumatic cerebrospinal fluid fistulae. A meta-analysis. *Arch Otolaryngol Head Neck Surg.* 1997;123(7):749–752.

28. Friedman JA, Ebersold MJ, Quast LM. Post-traumatic cerebrospinal fluid leakage. *World J Surg.* 2001;25(8):1062–1066.

29. Gean AD. *Imaging of Head Trauma.* New York, NY: Raven Press; 1994.

30. Jennett B, Teasdale G. *Management of Head Injuries.* Philadelphia, PA: FA Davis; 1982..

31. Markham JW. Pneumocephalus. In: Vinken PJ, Bruyn GW, eds. *Handbook of Clinical Neurology.* New York, NY: Elsevier; 1976:201–213.

32. Zasler ND. Posttraumatic tension pneumocephalus. *J Head Trauma Rehabil.* 1999;14(1):81–4.

33. Seth R, Mir S, Dhir JS, Cheeseman C, Singh J. Fitness to fly post craniotomy—a survey of medical advice from long-haul airline carriers. *Br J Neurosurg.* 2009;23(2):184–187.

34. Donovan DJ, Iskandar JI, Dunn CJ, King JA. Aeromedical evacuation of patients with pneumocephalus: outcomes in 21 cases. *Aviat Space Environ Med.* 2008;79(1):30–35.

35. Hand WL, Sanford JP. Posttraumatic bacterial meningitis. *Ann Intern Med.* 1970;72(6):869–874.

36. Anderson M. Management of cerebral infection. *J Neurol Neurosurg Psychiatry.* 1993;56(12):1243–1258.

37. Chowdhury MH, Tunkel AR. Antibacterial agents in infections of the central nervous system. *Infect Dis Clin North Am.* 2000;14(2):391–408.

38. Srinivas D, Veena Kumari HB, Somanna S, Bhagavatula I, Anandappa CB. The incidence of postoperative meningitis in neurosurgery: an institutional experience. *Neurol India.* 2011;59(2):195–198.

39. Nathoo N, Nadvi SS, Van Dellen JR. Traumatic cranial empyemas: a review of 55 patients. *Br J Neurosurg.* 2000;14(4):326–330.

40. Bok AP, Peter JC. Subdural empyema: burr holes or craniotomy? A retrospective computerized tomography-era analysis of treatment in 90 cases. *J Neurosurg.* 1993;78(4):574–578.

41. Tamaki T, Eguchi T, Sakamoto M, Teramoto A. Use of diffusion-weighted magnetic resonance imaging in empyema after cranioplasty. *Br J Neurosurg.* 2004;18(1):40–44.

42. Feuerman T, Wackym PA, Gade GF, Dubrow T. Craniotomy improves outcome in subdural empyema. *Surg Neurol.* 1989;32(2):105–110.

43. Pathak A, Sharma BS, Mathuriya SN, Khosla VK, Khandelwal N, Kak VK. Controversies in the management of subdural empyema.

A study of 41 cases with review of literature. *Acta Neurochir (Wien).* 1990;102(1–2):25–32.

44. Clark WC, Muhlbauer MS, Lowrey R, Hartman M, Ray MW, Watridge CB. Complications of intracranial pressure monitoring in trauma patients. *Neurosurgery.* 1989;25(1):20–24.

45. Malavi A, Dinubile MJ. Brain abscess. In: Harris AA, ed. *Handbook of Clinical Neurology.* Amsterdam, The Netherlands: Elsevier; 1988: 143–166.

46. Patir R, Sood S, Bhatia R. Post-traumatic brain abscess: experience of 36 patients. *Br J Neurosurg.* 1995;9(1):29–35.

47. Yang SY, Zhao CS. Review of 140 patients with brain abscess. *Surg Neurol.* 1993;39(4):290–296.

48. Guzman R, Barth A, Lövblad KO, et al. Use of diffusion-weighted magnetic resonance imaging in differentiating purulent brain processes from cystic brain tumors. *J Neurosurg.* 2002;97(5):1101–1107.

49. Fanning NF, Laffan EE, Shroff MM. Serial diffusion-weighted MRI correlates with clinical course and treatment response in children with intracranial pus collections. *Pediatr Radiol.* 2006;36(1):26–37.

50. Kurschel S, Mohia A, Weigl V, Eder HG. Hyperbaric oxygen therapy for the treatment of brain abscess in children. *Childs Nerv Syst.* 2006;22(1):38–42.

51. Stapleton SR, Bell BA, Uttley D. Stereotactic aspiration of brain abscesses: is this the treatment of choice? *Acta Neurochir (Wien).* 1993;121(1–2):15–19.

52. Rish BL, Dillon JD, Meirowksy AM, et al. Cranioplasty: a review of 1030 cases of penetrating head injury. *Neurosurgery.* 1979;4(5): 381–385.

53. Dujovny M, Agner C, Aviles A. Syndrome of the trephined: theory and facts. *Crit Rev Neurosurg.* 1999;9(5):271–278.

54. Muramatsu H, Nathan RD, Shimura T, Teramoto A. Recovery of stroke hemiplegia through neurosurgical intervention in the chronic stage. *Neurorehabilitation.* 2000;15(3):157–166.

55. Gottlob I, Simonsz-Tòth B, Heilbronner R. Midbrain syndrome with eye movement disorder: dramatic improvement after cranioplasty. *Strabismus.* 2002;10(4):271–277.

56. Czosnyka M, Copeman J, Czosnyka Z, McConnell R, Dickinson C, Pickard JD. Post-traumatic hydrocephalus: influence of craniectomy on the CSF circulation. *J Neurol Neurosurg Psychiatry.* 2000; 68(2):246–248.

57. Kemmling A, Duning T, Lemcke L, et al. Case report of MR perfusion imaging in sinking skin flap syndrome: growing evidence for hemodynamic impairment. *BMC Neurol.* 2010;10:80.

58. Beauchamp KM, Kashuk J, Moore EE, et al. Cranioplasty after postinjury decompressive craniectomy: is timing of the essence? *J Trauma.* 2010;69(2):270–274.

59. De Bonis P, Pompucci A, Mangiola A, Rigante L, Anile C. Posttraumatic hydrocephalus after decompressive craniectomy: an underestimated risk factor. *J Neurotrauma.* 2010;27(11):1965–1970.

60. Waziri A, Fusco D, Mayer SA, McKhann GM, Connolly ES Jr. Postoperative hydrocephalus in patients undergoing decompressive hemicraniectomy for ischemic or hemorrhagic stroke *Neurosurgery.* 2007;61(3):489–493.

61. Gooch MR, Gin GE, Kenning TJ, German JW. Complications of cranioplasty following decompressive craniectomy: analysis of 62 cases. *Neurosurg Focus.* 2009;26(6):E9.

62. Flannery T, McConnell RS. Cranioplasty: why throw the bone flap out? *Br J Neurosurg.* 2001;15(6):518–520.

63. Spetzger U, Vougioukas V, Schipper J. Materials and techniques for osseous skull reconstruction. *Minim Invasive Ther Allied Technol.* 2010;19(2):110–121.

64. Matsuno A, Tanaka H, Iwamuro H, et al. Analyses of the factors influencing bone graft infection after delayed cranioplasty. *Acta Neurochir (Wien).* 2006;48(5):535–540

65. Cabraja M, Klein M, Lehmann TN. Long term results following titanium cranioplasty of large skull defects. *Neurosurg Focus.* 2009; 26(6): E10

66. Li G, Wen L, Zhan RY, Shen F, Yang XF, Fu WM. Cranioplasty for patients developing large cranial defects combined with post-traumatic hydrocephalus after head trauma. *Brain Inj.* 2008; 22(4)333–337.

67. Rekate HL. A contemporary definition and classification of hydrocephalus. *Semin Pediatr Neurol.* 2009;16(1):9–15.

68. Long DF. Hydrocephalus. In: Zollman FS, ed. *Manual of Traumatic Brain Injury Management.* New York, NY: Demos Medical Publishing; 2011:303–308.

69. Mazzini L, Campini R, Angelino E, Rognone F, Pastore I, Oliveri G. Posttraumatic hydrocephalus: a clinical, neuroradiologic, and neuropsychologic assessment of long-term outcome. *Arch Phys Med Rehabil.* 2003;84(11):1637–1641.

70. Bigler ED. Neurological correlates of functional outcome. In: Zasler ND, Katz DI, Zafonte RD, eds. *Brain Injury Medicine: Principals and Practice.* New York, NY: Demos Medical Publishing; 2007:201–224.

71. Nishiyama K, Mori H, Tanaka R. Changes in cerebrospinal fluid hydrodynamics following endoscopic third ventriculostomy for shunt-dependent noncommunicating hydrocephalus. *J Neurosurg.* 2003;98(5):1027–1031.

72. Barkovich AJ, Edwards MS. Applications of neuroimaging in hydrocephalus. *Pediatr Neurosurg.* 1992;18(2):65–83.

73. Boyar B, Ildan F, Begdatoglu H, Cetinalp E, Karadayi A. Unilateral hydrocephalus resulting from occlusion of foramen of Monro: a new procedure in the treatment: stereotactic fenestration of the septum pellucidum. *Surg Neurol.* 1993;39(2):110–114.

74. Nida T Y, Haines SJ. Multiloculated hydrocephalus: craniotomy and fenestration of intraventricular septations. *J Neurosurg.* 1993; 78(1):70–76.

75. Epstein F. How to keep shunts functioning or ''the impossible dream.'' *Clin Neurosurg.* 1985;32:608–631.

76. Nowoslawska E, Polis L, Kaniewska D, et al. Effectiveness of neuroendoscopic procedures in the treatment of complex compartmentalized hydrocephalus in children. *Child's Nerv Syst.* 2003;19(9): 659–665.

77. Zander E, Foroglou G. Posttraumatic hydrocephalus. In: Vinken PJ, Bruyn GW, eds. *Handbook of Clinical Neurology.* New York, NY: Elsevier; 1976:231–253.

78. Friedland RP. ''Normal''-pressure hydrocephalus and the saga of the treatable dementias. *JAMA.* 1989;262(18):2577–2581.

79. Conner ES, Foley L, Black PM. Experimental normal-pressure hydrocephalus is accompanied by increased transmantle pressure. *J Neurosurg.* 1984;61(2):322–327.

80. Hakim CA, Hakim R, Hakim S. Normal-pressure hydrocephalus. *Neurosurg Clin N Am.* 2001;12(4):761–773.

81. Momjian S, Owler BK, Czosnyka Z, Czosnyka M, Pena A, Pickard JD. Pattern of white matter regional cerebral blood flow and autoregulation in normal pressure hydrocephalus. *Brain.* 2004;127(pt 5): 965–972.

82. Del Bigio MR. Pathophysiologic consequences of hydrocephalus. *Neurosurg Clin NA.* 2001;12(4):639–660.

83. Scott RM, Madsen JR. Shunt technology: contemporary concepts and prospects. *Clin Neurosurg.* 2002;5(14):256–267.

84. Bergsneider M. Evolving concepts of cerebrospinal fluid physiology. *Neurosurg Clin N Am.* 2001;12(4):631–638.

85. Greitz D. Radiological assessment of hydrocephalus: new theories and implications for therapy. *Neurosurg Rev.* 2004;27(3):145–165.

86. Sudarsky L, Simon S. Gait disorder in late life hydrocephalus. *Arch Neurol.* 1987;44(3):263–267.

87. Relkin N, Marmarou A, Klinge P, Bergschneider M, Black PM. Diagnosing idiopathic normal-pressure hydrocephalus. *Neurosurgery.* 2005;57(3)(suppl):S4–S16.

88. Keane JR. The pretectal syndrome: 206 patients. *Neurology.* 1990; 40(4):684–690.

89. Pakkenberg B, Boesen J, Albeck M, Gjerris F. Unbiased and efficient estimation of total ventricular volume of the brain obtained from CT-scans by a stereological method. *Neuroradiology.* 1989;31(5): 413–417.

90. Hamano K, Iwasaki N, Takeya T, Takita H. A comparative study of linear measurement of the brain and three-dimensional measurement of brain volume using CT scans. *Pediatr Radiol.* 1993;23(3): 165–168.

91. O'Hayon BB, Drake JM, Ossip MG, Tuli S, Clarke M. Frontal and occipital horn ratio: a linear estimate of ventricular size for multiple imaging modalities in pediatric hydrocephalus. *Pediatr Neurosurg.* 1998;29(5):245–249.

92. Mesiwala AH, Avellino AM, Ellenbogen RG. The diagonal ventricular dimension: a method for predicting shunt malfunction on the

basis of changes in ventricular size. *Neurosurgery.* 2002;50(6): 1246–1252.

93. Jamous M, Sood S, Kumar R, Ham S. Frontal and occipital horn width ratio for the evaluation of small and asymmetrical ventricles. *Pediatr Neurosurg.* 2003;39(1):17–21.

94. Børgesen SE, Gjerris F. The predictive value of conductance to out-flow of CSF in normal pressure hydrocephalus. *Brain.* 1982;105(pt 1):65–86.

95. Levin HS, Meyers CA, Grossman RG, Sarwar M. Ventricular en-largement after closed head injury. *Arch Neurol.* 1981;38(10): 623–629.

96. Bigler ED, Kurth SA, Blatter D, Abildskov T. Day-of-injury CT as an index to pre-injury brain morphology: degree of post-injury degenerative changes identified by CT and MR neuroimaging. *Brain Injury.* 1993;7(2):125–134.

97. Blatter DD, Bigler ED, Gale SD, et al. MR-based brain and cerebro-spinal fluid measurement after traumatic brain injury: correlation with neuropsychological outcome. *AJNR Am J Neuroradiol.* 1997; 18(1):1–10.

98. Ishikawa M, Oowaki H, Matsumoto A, Suzuki T, Furuse M, Nis-hida N. Clinical significance of cerebrospinal fluid tap test and magnetic resonance imaging/computed tomography findings of tight high convexity in patients with possible idiopathic normal pressure hydrocephalus. *Neurol Med Chir (Tokyo).* 2010;50(2): 119–123; discussion 123.

99. Poca MA, Mataró M, Del Mar Matarín M, Arikan F, Junqué C, Sahuquillo J. Is the placement of shunts in patients with idiopathic normal-pressure hydrocephalus worth the risk? Results of a study based on continuous monitoring of intracranial pressure. *J Neuro-surg.* 2004;100(5):855–866.

100. Gerard G, Weisberg LA. Magnetic resonance imaging in adult white matter disorders and hydrocephalus. *Semin Neurol.* 1986;6(1): 17–23.

101. Bradley WG Jr. Diagnostic tools in hydrocephalus. *Neurosurg Clin N Am.* 2001;12(4):661–684.

102. Stollman AL, George AE, Pinto RS, de Leon MJ. Periventricular high signal lesions and signal void on magnetic resonance imaging in hydrocephalus. Diagnostic and prognostic significance. *Acta Ra-diol Suppl.* 1986;369:388–391.

103. Segev Y, Metser U, Beni-Adani L, Elran C, Reider-Grosswasser I, Constantini, S. Morphometric study of midsagittal MR imaging plane in cases of hydrocephalus and atrophy and in normal brains. *AJNR Am J Neuroradiol.* 2001;22(9):1674–1679.

104. Waldemar G, Schmidt JF, Delecluse F, Andersen AR, Gjerris F, Paulson OB. High resolution SPECT with [99m Tc]-d, I-HMPAO in normal pressure hydrocephalus before and after shunt operation. *J Neurol Neurosurg Psychiat.* 1993;56(6):655–664.

105. Vanneste J, Augustijn P, Davies GA, Dirven C, Tan WF. Normal-pressure hydrocephalus: is cisternography still useful in selecting patients for a shunt? *Arch Neurol.* 1992;49(4):366–370.

106. Børgesen SE, Gjerris F. Relationships between intracranial pres-sure, ventricular size, and resistance to CSF outflow. *J Neurosurg.* 1987;67(4):535–539.

107. Marmarou A, Foda MA, Bandoh K, et al. Posttraumatic ventriculo-megaly: hydrocephalus or atrophy? A new approach for diagnosis using CSF dynamics. *J Neurosurg.* 1996;85(6):1026–1035.

108. Morgan MK, Johnston IH, Spittaler PJ. A ventricular infusion tech-nique for the evaluation of treated and untreated hydrocephalus. *Neurosurgery.* 1991;29(6):832–836.

109. Sahuquillo J, Rubio E, Codina A, et al. Reappraisal of the intracra-nial pressure and cerebrospinal fluid dynamics in patients with so-called "normal pressure hydrocephalus" syndrome. *Acta Neurochir (Wien).* 1991;112(1–2):50–61.

110. Tans JT, Poortvliet DC. Relationship between compliance and resis-tance to outflow of CSF in adult hydrocephalus. *J Neurosurg.* 1989; 71(1):59–62.

111. McGirt MJ, Woodworth G, Coon AL, Thomas G, Williams MA, Rigamonti D. Diagnosis, treatment, and analysis of long-term out-comes in idiopathic normal-pressure hydrocephalus. *Neurosurgery.* 2005;57(4):699–705.

112. Marmarou A, Bergsneider M, Klinge P, Relkin N, Black PM. The value of supplemental prognostic tests for the preoperative assess-ment of idiopathic normal-pressure hydrocephalus. *Neurosurgery.* 2005;57(3)(suppl):S17–S28; discussion ii–v.

113. Meier U, Miethke C. Predictors of outcome in patients with normal-pressure hydrocephalus. *J Clin Neurosci.* 2003;10(4):453–459.

114. Kahlon B, Sundbärg G, Rehncrona S. Comparison between the lumbar infusion and CSF tap tests to predict outcome after shunt surgery in suspected normal pressure hydrocephalus. *J Neurol Neu-rosurg Psychiatry.* 2002;73(6):721–726.

115. Hertel F, Walter C, Schmitt M, et al. Is a combination of Tc-SPECT or perfusion weighted magnetic resonance imaging with spinal tap test helpful in the diagnosis of normal pressure hydrocephalus? *J Neurol Neurosurg Psychiatry.* 2003;74(4):479–484.

116. Gilmore HE. Medical treatment of hydrocephalus. In: Scott RM, ed. *Hydrocephalus.* Baltimore, MD. Williams & Wilkins; 1990:37–46.

117. Oi S, Shimoda M, Shibata M, et al. Pathophysiology of long-stand-ing overt ventriculomegaly in adults. *J Neurosurg.* 2000;92(6): 933–940.

118. de Jong DA, Delwel EJ, Avezaat CJ. Hydrostatic and hydrody-namic considerations in shunted normal pressure hydrocephalus. *Acta Neurochir (Wien).* 2000;142(3):241–247.

119. Owler BK, Jacobson EE, Johnston IH. Low pressure hydrocephalus: issues of diagnosis and treatment in five cases. *Br J Neurosurg.* 2001; 15(4):353–359.

120. Chuang S, Hochhauser L, Fitz C, et al. Lumbo-peritoneal shunt malfunction. A new, simple and reliable CT sign. *Acta Radiol Suppl.* 1986;369:645–648.

121. Chumas PD, Armstrong DC, Drake JM, et al. Tonsillar herniation: the rule rather than the exception after lumboperitoneal shunting in the pediatric population. *J Neurosurg.* 1993;78(4):568–573.

122. Drake JM, Sainte-Rose C. *The Shunt Book.* Cambridge, MA: Black-well Scientific; 1995:228.

123. Post EM. Currently available shunt systems: a review. *Neurosur-gery.* 1985;16(2):257–260.

124. Portnoy HD, Schulte RR, Fox JL, Croissant PD, Tripp L. Anti-siphon and reversible occlusion valves for shunting in hydrocepha-lus and preventing post-shunt subdural hematomas. *J Neurosurg.* 1973;38(6):729–738.

125. Shurtleff DB. Characteristics of the various CSF shunt systems. *Clin Pediatr (Phila).* 1978;17(2):154–160.

126. Watts C, Keith HD. Testing the hydrocephalus shunt valve. *Childs Brain.* 1983;10(4):217–228.

127. Cook SW, Bergsneider M. Why valve opening pressure plays a relatively minor role in the postural ICP response to ventricular shunts in normal pressure hydrocephalus: modeling and implica-tions. *Acta Neurochir Suppl.* 2002;81:15–17.

128. Seliger, GM, Katz DI, Seliger M, Ditullio M Jr. Late improvement in closed head injury with a low-pressure valve shunt. *Brain Inj.* 1992;6(1):71–73.

129. Puca A, Anile C, Maira G, Rossi G. Cerebrospinal fluid shunting for hydrocephalus in the adult: factors related to shunt revision. *Neurosurgery.* 1991;29(6):822–826.

130. Sainte-Rose C, Piatt JH, Renier D, et al. Mechanical complications in shunts. *Pediatr Neurosurg.* 1991–1992;17(1):2–9.

131. Rekate HL. Shunt revision: complications and their prevention. *Pediatr Neurosurg.* 1991–1992;17(3):155–162.

132. Aldrich EF, Harmann P. Disconnection as a cause of ventriculoperi-toneal shunt malfunction in multicomponent shunt systems. *Pedi-atr Neurosurg.* 1990–1991;16(6):309–311.

133. Piatt JH Jr. Physical examination of patients with cerebrospinal fluid shunts: is there useful information in pumping the shunt? *Pediatrics.* 1992;89(3):470–473.

134. Hayden PW, Rudd TG, Shurtleff DB. Combined pressure-radionu-clide evaluation of suspected cerebrospinal fluid shunt malfunc-tion: a seven year clinical experience. *Pediatrics.* 1980;66(5):679–684.

135. Uvebrant P, Sixt R, Bjure J, Roos A. Evaluation of cerebrospinal fluid shunt function in hydrocephalic children using 99mTc-DTPA. *Childs Nerv Syst.* 1992;8(2):76–80.

136. Klein DM. The treatment of shunt infections. In: Scott RM, ed. *Hydrocephalus.* Baltimore, MD: Williams & Wilkins; 1990:87–98.

137. Schoenbaum SC, Gardner P, Shillito J. Infections of cerebrospinal fluid shunts: epidemiology, clinical manifestations, and therapy. *J Infect Dis.* 1975;13(1):543–552.

138. Quintaliani R, Cooper BW. Central nervous system infections due to staphylococci. In: Harris AA, ed. *Handbook of Clinical Neurology.* Amsterdam, The Netherlands: Elsevier; 1988:71–76.

139. Chapman PH, Borges LF. Shunt infections: prevention and treatment. *Clin Neurosurg.* 1985;32:652–664.

140. Foltz EL. Hydrocephalus: slit ventricles, shunt obstructions, and third ventricle shunts: a clinical study. *Surg Neurol.* 1993;40(2):119–124.

141. Wisoff JH, Epstein FJ. Diagnosis and treatment of the slit ventricle syndrome. In: Scott RM, ed. *Hydrocephalus.* Baltimore, MD: Williams & Wilkins; 1990:79–86.

142. Kelley GR, Johnson PL. Sinking brain syndrome: craniotomy can precipitate brainstem herniation in CSF hypovolemia. *Neurology.* 2004;62(1):157.

143. Lee KS. Natural history of chronic subdural haematoma. *Brain Inj.* 2004;18(4):351–358.

144. Foltz EL, Blanks J, Meyer R. Shunted hydrocephalus: normal upright ICP by CSF gravity-flow control. A clinical study in young adults. *Surg Neurol.* 1993;39(3):210–217.

145. Chapman PH, Cosman ER, Arnold MA. The relationship between ventricular fluid pressure and body position in normal subjects and subjects with shunts: a telemetric study. *Neurosurgery.* 1990;26(2):181–189.

146. Watson DA. The delta valve: a physiologic shunt system. *Childs Nerv Syst.* 1994;10(4):224–230.

147. Zemack G, Romner B. Seven years of clinical experience with the programmable Codman Hakim valve: a retrospective study of 583 patients. *J Neurosurg.* 2000;92(6):941–948.

148. Kay AD, Fisher AJ, O'Kane C, et al. A clinical audit of the Hakim programmable valve in patients with complex hydrocephalus. *Br J Neurosurg.* 2000;14(6):535–542.

149. Zemack G, Romner B. Do adjustable shunt valves pressure our budget? A retrospective analysis of 541 implanted Codman Hakim programmable valves. *Br J Neurosurg.* 2001;15(3):221–227.

150. Muramatsu H, Koike K, Teramoto A. Ventriculoperitoneal shunt dysfunction during rehabilitation: prevalence and countermeasures. *Am J Phys Med Rehabil.* 2002;81(8):571–578.

151. Pollack IF, Albright AL, Adelson PD. A randomized controlled study of a programmable shunt valve versus a conventional valve for patients with hydrocephalus. Hakim–Medos investigator group. *Neurosurgery.* 1999;45(6):1399–1408.

152. Lollis SS, Mamourian AC, Vaccaro TJ, Duhaime AC. Programmable CSF shunt valves: radiographic identification and interpretation. *AJNR Am J Neuroradiol.* 2010;31(7):1343–1346.

153. Miwa K, Kondo H, Sakai N. Pressure changes observed in Codman–Medos programmable valves following magnetic exposure and filliping. *Child's Nerv Syst.* 2001;17(3):150–153.

154. Lefranc M, Ko JY, Peltier J, et al. Effect of transcranial magnetic stimulation on four types of pressure-programmable valves. *Acta Neurochir (Wien).* 2010;152(4):689–697

155. Sprung C, Schlosser HG, Lemcke J, et al. The adjustable proGAV shunt: a prospective safety and reliability multicenter study. *Neurosurgery.* 2010;66(3):465–474

156. Meier U, Kiefer M, Sprung C. Evaluation of the Miethke dual-switch valve in patients with normal pressure hydrocephalus. *Surg Neurol.* 2004;61(2):119–127; discussion 127–128.

157. Kiefer M, Eymann R, Meier U. Five Years experience with gravitational shunts in chronic hydrocephalus of adults. *Acta Neurochir (Wien).* 2002;144(8):755–767.

158. Tokoro K, Suzuki S, Chiba Y, Tsuda M. Shunt assistant valve: bench test investigations and clinical performance. *Childs Nerv Syst.* 2002;18(9–10):492–499.

159. Tureyen K. Traumatic intracranial aneurysm after blunt trauma. *Br J Neurosurg.* 2001;15(5)429–431.

160. Kumar M, Kitchen ND. Infective and traumatic aneurysms. *Neurosurg Clin N Am.* 1998;9(3):577–586.

161. Burke JP, Marion DW. Cerebral revascularization in trauma and carotid occlusion. *Neurosurg Clin N Am.* 2001;12(3):595–611.

162. Batjer HH, Giller CA, Kopitnik TA, et al. Intracranial and cervical vascular injuries. In: Cooper PR, ed. *Head Injury.* 3rd ed. Baltimore, MD: Williams and Wilkins; 1993:373–404.

163. Salazar Flores J, Vaquero J, Garcia Sola R, et al. Traumatic false aneurysms of the middle meningeal artery. *Neurosurgery.* 1986;18(2):200–203.

164. Wortzman D, Tucker WS, Gershater R. Traumatic aneurysm in the posterior fossa. *Surg Neurol.* 1980;13(5):329–332.

165. Matricali B. Internal carotid artery aneurysms. In: Samii M, Brihaye J, eds. *Traumatology of the Skull Base.* New York, NY: Springer Verlag; 1983:196–200.

166. Rothrock JF. Headaches due to vascular disorders. *Neurol Clin.* 2004;22(1):21–37.

167. Bonafe A, Maneife C. Traumatic carotid-cavernous sinus fistulas. In: Braakman R, ed. *Handbook of Clinical Neurology.* Amsterdam, The Netherlands: Elsevier; 1990:345–366.

168. Debrun GM, Viñuela F, Fox AJ, Davis KR, Ahn AS. Indications for treatment and classification of 132 carotid-cavernous fistulas. *Neurosurgery.* 1988;22(2):285–289.

169. Phatouros CC, Meyers PM, Dowd CF, Halbach VV, Malek AM, Higashida RT. Carotid artery cavernous fistulas. *Neurosurg Clin N Am.* 2000;11(1):67–84.

170. Dubov WE, Bach JR. Delayed presentation of carotid-cavernous sinus fistula in a patient with traumatic brain injury. *Am J Phys Med Rehabil.* 1991;70(4):178–180.

171. Miyachi S, Negoro M, Handa T, Sugita K. Dural carotid cavernous sinus fistula presenting as isolated oculomotor nerve palsy. *Surg Neurol.* 1993;39(2):105–109.

172. Koehler PJ, Blaauw G. Late posttraumatic nonvascular pulsating eye. *Acta Neurochir (Wien).* 1992;116(1):62–64.

173. Buckwalter JA, Sasaki CT, Virapongse C, Kier EL, Bauman N. Pulsatile tinnitus arising from jugular megabulb deformity: a treatment rationale. *Laryngoscope.* 1983;93(12):1534–1539.

174. Hentzer E. Objective tinnitus of the vascular type. A follow-up study. *Acta Otolaryngol.* 1968;66(4):273–281.

175. Rouillard R, Leclerc J, Savary P. Pulsatile tinnitus: adehiscent jugular vein. *Laryngoscope.* 1985;95(2):188–189.

176. Vallis RC, Martin FW. Extracranial arteriovenous malformation presenting as objective tinnitus. *J Laryngol Otol.* 1984;98(11):1139–1142.

177. Luo CB, Teng MM, Chang FC, Shen MH, Guo WY, Chang CY. Bilateral traumatic carotid-cavernous fistulae: strategies for endovascular treatment. *Acta Neurochir (Wien).* 2007;149(7):675–680.

178. Higashida RT, Hieshima GB, Halbach VV, Bentson JR, Goto K. Closure of carotid cavernous sinus fistulae by external compression of the carotid artery and jugular vein. *Acta Radiol Suppl.* 1986;369:580–583.

179. Batjer HH, Purdy PD, Neiman M, Samson DS. Subtemporal transdural use of detachable balloons for traumatic carotid-cavernous fistulas. *Neurosurgery.* 1988;22(2):290–296.

180. Brosnahan D, McFadzean RM, Teasdale E. Neuro-ophthalmic features of carotid cavernous fistulas and their treatment by endoarterial balloon embolization. *J Neurol Neurosurg Psychiatry.* 1992;55(7):553–556.

181. Cameron MM. Chronic subdural hematoma: a review of 114 cases. *J Neurol Neurosurg Psychiatry.* 1978;41(9):834–839.

182. Drapkin AJ. Chronic subdural hematoma: pathophysiological basis for treatment. *Br J Neurosurg.* 1991;5(5):467–473.

183. Kawakami Y, Chikama M, Tamiya T, Shimamura Y. Coagulation and fibrinolysis in chronic subdural hematoma. *Neurosurgery.* 1989;25(1):25–29.

184. Loew F, Kivelitz R. Chronic subdural hematomas. In: Vinken PJ, Bruyn GW, eds. *Handbook of Clinical Neurology.* New York, NY: Elsevier; 1976:297–327.

185. Stone JL, Rifai MH, Sugar O, et al. Subdural hematomas. I. Acute subdural hematoma: progress in definition, clinical pathology, and therapy. *Surg Neurol.* 1983;19(3):216–231.

186. Feldman RG, Pincus JH, McEntee WJ, et al. Cerebrovascular accident or subdural fluid collection? *Arch Intern Med.* 1963;112:204–214.

187. Cooper PR. Posttraumatic intracranial mass lesions. In: Cooper PR, ed. *Head Injury.* 3rd ed. Baltimore, MD: Williams & Wilkins; 1993:275–330.

188. Rubin G, Rappaport ZH. Epilepsy in chronic subdural haematoma. *Acta Neurochir (Wien).* 1993;123(1–2):39–42.

189. Kaminski HJ, Hlavin ML, Likavec MJ, Schmidley JW. Transient neurologic deficit caused by chronic subdural hematoma. *Am J Med.* 1992;92(6):698–700.

190. Rahimi AR, Poorkay M. Subdural hematomas and isolated transient aphasia. *J Am Med Dir Assoc.* 2000;1(3):129–131.

191. Kim KS, Hemmati M, Weinberg PE. Computed tomography in isodense subdural hematoma. *Radiology.* 1978;128(1):71–74.

192. Tsai FY, Huprich JE. Further experience with contrast-enhanced CT in head trauma. *Neuroradiology.* 1978;16:314–317.

193. Kao MCK. Sedimentation level in chronic subdural hematoma visible on computerized tomography. *J Neurosurg.* 1983;58(2):246–251.

194. Hosoda K, Tamaki N, Masumura M, et al. Magnetic resonance images of chronic subdural hematomas. *J Neurosurg.* 1987;67:677–683.

195. Vezina G. Assessment of the nature and age of subdural collections in nonaccidental head injury with CT and MRI. *Pediatr Radiol.* 2009;39(6):586–590.

196. St. John JN, Dila C. Traumatic subdural hygroma in adults. *Neurosurgery.* 1981;9(6):621–626.

197. Lee KS, Bae WK, Yoon SM, Doh JW, Bae HG, Yun IG. Location of the traumatic subdural hygroma: role of gravity and cranial morphology. *Brain Inj.* 2000;14(4):355–361.

198. Lee KS, Bae WK, Doh JW, Bae HG, Yun IG. Origin of chronic subdural hematoma and relation to traumatic subdural lesions. *Brain Inj.* 1998;12(11):901–910.

199. Lee KS, Bae WK, Bae HG, Yun, IG. The fate of traumatic subdural hygroma in serial computed tomographic scans. *J Korean Med Sci.* 2000;15(5):560–568.

200. Yamashima T, Yamamoto S, Friede RL. The role of endothelial gap junctions in the enlargement of chronic subdural hematomas. *J Neurosurg.* 1983;59(2):298–303.

201. Yamoshima T, Yamamoto S. How do vessels proliferate in the capsule of a chronic subdural hematoma? *Neurosurgery.* 1984;15(5):672–678.

202. Santarius T, Lawton R, Kirkpatrick PJ, Hutchinson PJ. The management of primary chronic subdural hematoma: a questionnaire survey of practice in the United Kingdom and the Republic of Ireland. *Br J Neurosurg.* 2008;22(4):529–534

203. Weigel R, Schmiedek P, Krauss JK. Outcome of contemporary surgery for chronic subdural hematoma: evidence based review. *J Neurol Neurosurg Psychiatry.* 2003;74(7):937–943.

204. Frati A, Salvati M, Mainiero F, et al. Inflammation markers and risk factors for recurrence in 35 patients with a posttraumatic chronic subdural hematoma: a prospective study. *J Neurosurg.* 2004;100(1):24–32.

205. Mohamed EE. Management of chronic subdural haematoma. *Br J Neurosurg.* 1991;5(5):525–526.

206. Ram Z, Hadani M, Sahar A, Spiegelmann R. Continuous irrigation-drainage of the subdural space for the treatment of chronic subdural haematoma. A prospective clinical trail. *Acta Neurochir (Wien).* 1993;120(1–2):40–43.

207. Robinson RG. Chronic subdural hematoma: surgical management in 133 patients. *J Neurosurg.* 1984;61(2):263–268.

208. Markwalder TM, Steinsiepe KF, Rohner M, Reichenbach W, Markwalder H. The course of chronic subdural hematomas after burr-hole craniostomy and closed-system drainage. *J Neurosurg.* 1981;55(3):390–396.

209. Jamieson KG, Yelland JDN. Extradural hematoma. *J Neurosurg.* 1968;29(1):13–23.

210. Illingworth R, Shawdon H. Conservative management of intracranial extradural haematoma presenting late. *J Neurol Neurosurg Psychiatry.* 1983;46(6):558–560.

211. Hirsh LF. Chronic epidural hematomas. *Neurosurgery.* 1980;6:508–512.

212. Hooper RS. Extradural hemorrhages of the posterior fossa. *Br J Surg.* 1954;42(171):19–26.

213. Roda JM, Giménez D, Pérez-Higueras A, Blázquez MG, Pérez-Alvarez M. Posterior fossa epidural hematomas: a review and synthesis. *Surg Neurol.* 1983;19(5):419–424.

214. Mertol T, Guner M, Acar U, Atabay H, Kirisoglu U. Delayed traumatic intracerebral hematoma. *Br J Neurosurg.* 1991;5(5):491–498.

215. Cooper PR. Delayed traumatic intracerebral hemorrhage. *Neurosurg Clin N Am.* 1992;3(3):659–665.

216. Andrews BT, Chiles BW III, Olsen WL, Pitts LH. The effect of intracerebral hematoma location on the risk of brain-stem compression and on clinical outcome. *J Neurosurg.* 1988;69(4):518–522.

IX

SPECIAL SENSES

Evaluating and Treating Visual Dysfunction

William V. Padula, Eric Singman, Vincent Vicci, Raquel Munitz,
and W. Michael Magrun

INTRODUCTION

Visual dysfunction after brain injury (BI) is common (1). Epidemiological studies of vision problems relating to BI demonstrate that any part of the visual process can be affected. A wide variety of symptoms related to vision have been reported (2–4), including headaches, diplopia, vertigo, eye fatigue, focusing difficulty, movement of print when reading, difficulty with tracking, sensitivity to light, reduction in scope of field of vision, reduced color perception, reduced contrast sensitivity, reduced reading speed, difficulty with depth perception, spatial disorientation, altered sense of midline, difficulty with posture and balance, delayed reaction time, and impaired visual memory.

Recent studies of Veterans Affairs (VA) polytrauma facilities have indicated that more than 74% of all inpatients with BI receiving medical treatment have reported visual complaints (3). Oculomotor, binocular, perceptual, and reading problems were among the most common visual deficits identified in service members with traumatic brain injury (TBI). Visual field defects are also common following a BI (5). One study showed that 38% of the subjects displayed a visual field defect of which the most common were compression of peripheral fields and homonymous hemianopsia. Binocular dysfunction is prevalent following a BI (6,7) and relates to many of the visual symptoms. Notably, these studies indicate that most patients with BI present with normal ocular examinations.

Visual sensory deficits can be caused by damage to the striate cortex of the occipital lobe (the primary visual cortex), as well as other cortical regions. The impact of a BI on overall sensory function can be profound but simultaneously subtle so that patients may have difficulty verbalizing their complaints. Mechanisms for treating sensory deficits require awareness and recognition of the varied problems facing patients by the rehabilitation team.

The ability of vision to guide motor function is often compromised following a BI. New evidence has emerged demonstrating that neuromotor function also contributes to spatial awareness and a normal egocentric concept of visual midline (4).The influence of a visual field defect, such as homonymous hemianopsia, will also affect the perception of visual midline, as well as posture and balance. Dysfunctional visual processing may contribute to strabismus following TBI.

It has long been proposed that vision is a bimodal process (8), where detailed visual information and information pertaining to motion in the visual periphery are channeled separately. Our understanding of bimodal processing of vision has become clinically relevant because this may help better explain how damage to the cortical and subcortical mechanisms organizing vision and the integration of sensorimotor information lead to visual dysfunction in patients with TBI. Specifically, binocular dysfunctions are the characteristics of the visual processing imbalance, and this has been termed Post-Trauma Vision Syndrome (PTVS). The visuospatial dysfunction caused by mismatch in visual processing in association with sensorimotor systems has led to recognition of Visual Midline Shift Syndrome (VMSS) affecting balance and posture. The use of this bimodal visual process enables the practitioner and therapist to establish a common model of visual processing that will be effective in understanding and diagnosing visual dysfunction affecting cognitive perceptual difficulties, as well as balance, posture, and mobility difficulties.

NEUROANATOMY OF THE AFFERENT VISUAL PATHWAYS: A BIMODAL PROCESS

Vision in humans can be considered a bimodal process whereby highly detailed or focal information about an object of regard is integrated with ambient information about the subject's surroundings (8). This bimodal processing begins in the human retina and is carried forth through the afferent and efferent visual pathways. This section will describe the anatomic relationships underlying the focal and ambient processing of afferent visual information.

Retina

Light is projected onto the retina by the optical apparatus of the eye (the cornea and lens), and the retina then transforms this energy into bioelectrical signals that are transmitted not only to the thalamus but also to other parts of the brain, including the midbrain (see later discussion). The light is most focused on the fovea, which is in the center of the area known as the macula. In this region, the density of photoreceptors (rod and cone cells) and retinal ganglion cells,

cells extending axons through the optic nerve to the brain, is greatest. The retinal cells create a map of the visual field, and this retinotopic mapping remains preserved throughout the different visual pathways in the brain. The cone cells, the photoreceptors that allow us to perceive color, are concentrated in the macula and function with higher spatial frequencies. Furthermore, photoreceptors (rod cells) allow us to perceive motion, as well as brightness in shades of gray, and are more responsive to low spatial frequency wavelengths. These are more predominant in the peripheral retina, although they are totally absent from the fovea.

The demographics of retinal cells permit the initiation of bimodal processing of vision. The central 10° angle of fixation are analyzed in extremely high detail by cones and small retinal ganglion cells (P-cells, where "P" stands for *parvo*, meaning "small" in Greek), whereas the remaining peripheral visual field is detected by rods, some cones, and larger retinal ganglion cells (M-cells, where "M" stands for *magno*, meaning "big" in Greek) best able to evaluate motion and changes in illumination. The P-cells initiate a channel of input to the 4 outermost layers of the thalamic lateral geniculate nucleus (LGN), that is, the parvocellular layers. The M-cells create a channel to the inner 2 LGN layers, that is, the magnocellular layers. Between these layers, thalamic konio cells (or K-cells) receive input from retinal ganglion cells excited specifically by blue-sensitive cones (rather than by green-sensitive or red-sensitive cones). The koniocellular pathway is believed to be the most important in providing information about color of the object of regard (9) and is therefore an adjunct to the mode of visual processing related to fine detail rather than motion detection. However, it is interesting to note that the blue cones are not located within the fovea but rather surround it. In addition, they represent only about 2% of all the cones in the retina. Furthermore, they are more sensitive to low levels of illumination intensity than red-green cones and are stimulated by light in the blue end of the visible spectrum, like the rods. Finally, some recent data have suggested that the koniocellular pathway may indeed contribute to motion detection (10). In primates, the K-cells form 3 layers of cells in the lateral geniculate: the middle, dorsal, and ventral layers. The ventral layer of the lateral geniculate functions in close association with the superior colliculus (SC). Anatomically, the koniocellular pathway may represent a transition between the parvocellular and magnocellular pathways and might ultimately be found to support both modes of visual processing or even represent a third mode of visual processing that must be considered when treating injuries to the visual pathways.

Retino-Collicular Projection

The SC of the midbrain (or optic tectum) is a critical center for coordinating eye movements with movement of the body and head, enabling us to have an awareness of our surroundings and find and fixate on an object of regard, even when we become aware of the object through auditory rather than visual cues. The SC is able to do this because it receives information from many parts of the brain, including the retina, visual cortex, auditory centers of the midbrain (inferior colliculus), spinal cord, and the cerebellum. Here, visual spatial information becomes related to posture, movement, and orientation to positional space (11). In turn, the SC projects

to the LGN, the thalamic pulvinar nucleus (which in turn projects to the visual cortex), the spinal cord, and brainstem nuclei controlling eye movements (12).

As with the LGN, the visual world is mapped retinotopically onto the SC. Furthermore, color and brightness stimuli arrive from the retina in separate channels and terminate in distinct collicular layers. However, it is believed that the cerebral cortex is the main driver of SC-initiated eye movements. Although the SC is known to be able to initiate rapid, yoked eye movements called saccades, studies suggest that the SC is also very important in the maintenance of fixation, smooth visual pursuits, head turns, and arm-reaching movements toward an object of interest and binocularity. Clearly, the SC is a vital adjunct for the ambient processing of visual information.

Geniculo-Cortical Projections

The LGN is the main relay center between the retina and the visual cortex, projecting predominantly in the area known as V1 or the striate cortex. The magnocellular, parvocellular, and koniocellular channels remain segregated during this projection and innervate cells in differing layers of V1 while maintaining the retinotopic map.

It should be recognized that the LGN is probably much more than a relay station for afferent visual information traveling from the eye to the brain (13). Recent studies have shown that the LGN may be very important as an early gate-keeper in the control of visual attention and awareness (14). Furthermore, the koniocellular pathway projects directly to area V5 (also called MT for middle temporal), a region of the extra-striate visual cortex involved in motion detection (15). This projection might account for the ability of some patients with severe damage to V1 and subsequent cortical blindness to demonstrate the ability to unconsciously detect motion in their visual fields (16). Finally, the LGN receives direct inputs from other parts of the visual pathways, including the visual cortex and the SC. Although the central image from the macula occupies the major portion of our cortical attention and concentration for perception and cognitive processing, how we organize and process visual information is not a simple phenomenon. It seems reasonable to suggest that the LGN may be important in helping coordinate visual information from the focal and ambient modes of visual processing.

It has also been demonstrated that 20% of the peripheral retinal nerve fibers relay information through axons to the thalamus or midbrain for spatial matching with kinesthetic, proprioceptive, and vestibular information being received from other sensorimotor systems. This may help organize spatial information involved in sensorimotor experiences affecting posture, movement, and balance. The occipital cortex is probably intimately involved in this processing as well. The visual cortex is divided into primary or striated visual cortex (V1) and extrastriate or accessory visual cortices (V2, V3, V4, and V5). Current theories of vision assume that visual information from V1 is distributed anteriorly through V2 via either a ventral stream (to V4) or dorsal stream (to V5) (17), maintaining the segregation of focal processing (i.e., detail) and ambient processing (i.e., motion detection), respectively. However, recent research strongly suggests that although there is channeling of information from V1 outward, there is magnocellular and parvocellular information reaching both V4 and V5, suggesting that the ventral and dorsal stream concept may require some modification (18).

NEUROANATOMY OF THE EFFERENT VISUAL PATHWAYS: EXTRAOCULAR MUSCLES

Each eye is controlled by 6 extraocular muscles (EOMs) capable, when working in concert, of rotating the globe in any direction. The EOMs are the medial, lateral, superior and inferior rectus muscles, and the superior and inferior oblique muscles. The orbital anatomy has been found to be far more complex than previously imagined (19,20). Functional magnetic resonance imaging or fMRI (21), high-resolution MRI (22), and histological studies (e.g., see 29) have confirmed the existence of fascial pulleys within the orbit (21), and it is the location of these pulleys that determine the functional origins of the EOMs, rather than the site of muscle attachment to the globe or orbit. In addition, EOMs have been shown to be bilaminate structures with global and orbital leaves, each with different types of muscle fibers (e.g., slow and fast twitch), different arborizations of nerve fiber innervations, and disparate vascular supplies (23).

The orbital anatomy permits the globe's significant range and speed of rotation. The bilaminate construction of the EOMs and the different composition of muscle fibers in each layer provide the globe with the ability to not only sustain tonic fixation but also rapidly shift gaze and cease eye movement at will. The range, speed, and accuracy of eye motion frequently decreases after TBI (24), and this reduction often leads to complaints of intermittent or constant diplopia.

Cortical Control of Ocular Motility

Extraocular motility is required for a subject to gaze on or smoothly pursue a visual target and also to rapidly refixate to an either novel target or a target that moves too rapidly to pursue smoothly. Supranuclear input, that is, input to the extraocular motor nuclei from the cerebrum and cerebellum may be divided into either visually guided or nonvisually guided movements. The pathways controlling smooth pursuit have not been identified completely in humans.

During visually guided pursuit eye movements, there is retinal image slip detected in the retino-geniculo-striate cortex pathway (likely via the magnocellular pathway, i.e., the pathway subserving ambient visual processing) and transmitted thereon to the extrastriate visual areas. The extrastriate areas (including the V5 and posterior parietal cortex [PPC]) share bidirectional transmission with the frontal eye fields (FEFs), a portion of the motor cortex. The motor cortex in turn distributes its fibers via the internal capsule to the pons and from there to the cerebellum. The cerebellar input is directed to the nuclei of the cranial nerves controlling eye movement (25).

It is believed that executive control of visually guided eye movements, that is, initiation/motivation to seek a target of interest and inhibition to avoid distraction from that target, may begin within the premotor cortex of the frontal lobes (26). However, there may be even more preliminary steps to this process. There may be a preconscious step or series of steps, whereby the ambient visual process organizes the motor fields and delivers a spatial domain from which visual information will be mapped for support of fixations, pursuits, saccades, convergence (adduction), and divergence (abduction). This preconscious ambient process would use movement, parallax, and contrast to initiate first the release of attention from one target of interest so as to permit attention to a novel fixation point. Feed-forward input of ambient processing, perhaps from the visual cortices to the FEFs, may be the true initiator of saccadic movement. Once initiated, the direction of movement becomes a complex dynamic process between the ambient and focal processes or the balance between spatial and detail information. This dynamic process involves feed-forward of spatial information and frontal lobe feedback and conscious directional/correctional information.

It has been shown that multiple regions in the frontal lobe are organized retinotopically, that is, with maps of visual space, thereby enabling the eyes to reorient to a novel object of regard. In humans, it has been established with certainty that there are at least 2 retinotopic mappings, that is, the FEF and supplementary eye fields (SEF) (27). Whereas the FEFs seem to be active during the anticipation of eye movement, the SEF may be important in inhibiting movement (28).

Studies have shown that both the FEFs and PPC are important for visual target detection, although the PPC but not the FEFs appear to be dependent on the response required by the task. In other words, the FEFs may guide visual searching while the PPC helps turn that search into manual action (29). Further, the PPC appears to actively monitor visual information to maintain conjugacy of eye movements (30).

Notably, the FEFs receive retinal input not only from the retino-geniculo-cortical pathway described earlier but also from a more direct retino-pulvino-cortical pathway (31). Studies on patients with pulvinar lesions have shown that they are more easily affected by visual distractions (32).

Visually guided refixation eye movements (i.e., saccades) can be initiated voluntarily or as a response to sensory stimuli (33). Studies have suggested that prior to a voluntary saccade, there is an anticipatory remapping of the visual image, perhaps occurring in the visual cortex, from the presaccadic state to the expected postsaccadic position (34), thereby promoting stability of the visual image. Voluntary saccades require not only an anticipated novel target of attention but also a planned disengagement from a salient stimulus, a process that may require separate cortical effort (35). Patients with TBI have demonstrated difficulty in this regard (36). Notably, reactive saccades may parallel other subconscious reflexes during which the stimulus reaches consciousness coincident with or even after the reflex has been initiated and the reflex arc is transmitted independently of prefrontal cortex (37). The clinical relevance of diplopia related to bimodal processing is that it may not be enough to consider treatment solely regarding the dysfunction of the oculomotor system and related neurology. If there is an ambient or spatial visual dysfunction, treatment of the visual process as an afferent sensory model incorporating surgical alignment of the eyes and/or with compensating prisms may not be successful. An understanding of the bimodal visual process will lead the clinician to recognize the potential of PTVS (see below) as an underlying condition that degrades the effort of treatment and rehabilitation.

Brainstem Control of Ocular Motility

Nonvisually initiated eye movements are mostly provided by infranuclear input to the EOM nuclei. These movements can be initiated from auditory stimuli, as well as by changes in head position. Both of these stimuli are detected by structures in the inner ear (the cochlea and semicircular canals, respectively) and transmitted to the brain by the vestibulocochlear (8th cranial) nerve. The vestibulo-ocular reflexes maintain steady gaze when the head moves and are probably subserved by relatively direct connections from the semicircular canals to the brainstem vestibular nuclei in the medulla and then onto the nuclei of the cranial nerves supplying the EOMs, that is, pontine abducens (6th cranial), midbrain trochlear (4th cranial), and oculomotor (3rd cranial) nerves. It is likely that auditory neural inputs stimulating nonvisually guided eye movements converge on the SC (i.e., optic tectum).

The SC is a midbrain structure that receives direct retinal input visuotopically. It also receives direct and indirect input from the FEFs, somatosensory, visual and auditory cortices, and cerebellum. The SC distributes information to the pulvinar and lateral geniculate nuclei and also shares bidirectional transmission with the pontine gaze centers (see later discussion) and cerebellum. The SC is probably involved in initiating saccades and supporting smooth pursuit and tonic gaze. In addition, through inhibitory activity, possibly via a projection through the pulvinar to the visual association cortex, the SC may help suppress the sensation of image blur during small eye movements (38).

Once fixation is established, steady gaze is needed to evaluate that target. Tonic gaze is supported by horizontal and vertical gaze centers. The horizontal gaze center is located within the 6th cranial nerve nucleus of the pons, and the vertical gaze center is in the rostral midbrain. These centers coordinate their activity through a fiber tract called the medial longitudinal fasciculus (MLF). The gaze centers and MLF are bilateral structures that communicate across the midline either through various crossover tracts, such as the posterior commissure and the MLF decussation. During steady gaze, tonic input to the horizontal and vertical gaze centers is respectively provided by nuclei located at the pontomedullary junction (nucleus prepositus hypoglossi or NPH) and midbrain (interstitial nucleus of Cajal). In addition, the cerebellum provides critically important input to gaze control. The cerebellum serves to integrate head position, body position, and eye position and has been shown to modulate the speed of eye movements (39). Just as the ability to fixate is critical to performance, so is the release of fixation. Clinically, persons with BI often demonstrate difficulty releasing from the intended point of fixation. In terms of the model of bimodal visual processing, this "focal binding" occurs when the preconscious component of the ambient or spatial visual process is dysfunctional. Normally, much of the visual function is preconscious because of the organization of the ambient visual process. However, in PTVS (see below), vision becomes oriented to conscious control of ocular movement in an environment that lacks a disas-

sociation between detail and spatial domain. To picture what this loss of ambient organization would be like for a patient, one can imagine the experience of driving at night in a snowstorm using high beams: all that can be seen are flakes of snow coming at the driver, and the driver must struggle to find the road. In other words, for patients with PTVS, movement in the environment is chaotic because there is a loss of spatial reference.

Fusion: The Result and Driver of Ocular Motility

The 2 eyes in humans are symmetrically placed in the face, highly mobile, forward facing, and each possessing visual fields spanning approximately 160° angle horizontally and 135° angle vertically (40). These attributes permit a significant overlap of the 2 visual fields of approximately 120° angle horizontally. However, because the pupils (in adults) are approximately 6 cm apart, each eye will receive a different perspective of a common object of regard. It is the process of fusion provided by the visual cortex (and perhaps even to some extent by the thalamic LGN) (41) that permits the 2 disparate ocular views to be transformed into a single stereoscopic perception.

The range of image disparity within which the 2 eyes can fuse stereoscopically can be measured in the clinic by challenging the subject with prismatic dislocation of either visual field. This measurement is referred to as fusional amplitudes. Normally, vertical fusional amplitudes are much smaller than horizontal fusional amplitudes, divergence amplitudes are less than convergence amplitudes, amplitudes for distance vision are less than for near vision.

How the brain creates the perception of fusion and stereopsis (depth perception) has been the subject of intense interest. Much of the perception of depth is created with monocular cues, the same cues frequently employed by artists to give a sense of dimensionality in paintings. Binocularity adds finedepth perception to the gross sense of depth provided by monocular cues; studies of visual cortical activity employing fMRI have demonstrated that humans can reliably differentiate image disparities of less than 1/60° angle (42). Binocular vision cues are provided in part by kinesthetic feedback received from the converging eyes (i.e., the more the eyes converge to view a target, the closer that target is perceived to be) (43), as well as perceived disparity in space of the images focused on the retinas (discussed later).

Although the cortical representation of eye position has not been fully elucidated, it has been shown using fMRI techniques that eye muscle proprioception in humans is represented bilaterally in the somatosensory cortex and the motor cortex (44).

Electrophysiologic (45) and fMRI (46) techniques have been used to demonstrate that widespread regions of the visual cortex are highly responsive to binocularly disparate stimuli; these regions are likely to also be involved in stereoscopic vision. Further, it is likely that the focal and ambient (i.e., bimodal) visual processing discussed earlier in this chapter is critical for stereopsis. The foveas of the 2 eyes are normally in correspondence and contribute heavily to the focal pathway. The reduced acuity supported by the peripheral retina is probably a significant benefit in that this lack of clarity may be required to permit the brain to adjust to rapid changes in viewing direction and distance without the subject perceiving a loss of depth perception, that is, ambient vision. It has been proposed that the parvocellular pathway stream is involved in processing disparate images allowing for depth perception, whereas the magnocellular stream processed disparities that drive vergences (47). Further, it has been reported that image disparity cues are processed differently in the central and peripheral retinas of macaques (48), providing additional support for the importance of the bimodal visual processing in the perception of stereopsis.

PHYSIOLOGY OF THE RELATIONSHIP BETWEEN VISION AND POSTURE

Efficient sensorimotor function requires an awareness of time and space made possible by internal mapping of inputs from vision, vestibular, somatosensory, and motor pathways (49,50). The information from each of these systems is continuously integrated to effect coordinated movements and proper balance. The visual process is highly dependent on the vestibular and somatosensory system (51,52). This is alternatively referred to as the visual-vestibular-cervical triad (53,54). According to systems theory (49), coordinated neck musculature action for posture is present at approximately 2 months of age and remains a critical component of sensory processing. This is followed by consecutive mappings of the visual, somatosensory, and vestibular systems to the neck musculature and it leads to activation of the upper thoracic spine, thereby allowing the visual system to orient to a stable base of support. Specifically, this provides the opportunity for ambient processes to organize and match to somatosensory and vestibular information (54). Without this supporting postural framework, skilled motor control is inefficient and deteriorates (55). Inefficiency and deterioration in motor control can be observed in individuals who have BI precisely because they have lost the ability to accurately match neural systems.

Research has shown that feed-forward activation of the neck muscles is necessary to achieve stability for the visual and vestibular systems, as well as ensuring stabilization of the cervical spine (56). It has also been shown that a reciprocal relationship exists, in that the visual process is important for organizing head–trunk relationships (57). Specifically, it appears that visual information stabilizes posture by reducing the variability of the head's position in space and the position of the center of mass within the support surface defined by the feet.

Assessment must take into account the inseparable relationships between posture, movement, and vision (58,59). BI causes alteration of the alignment of body segments (58,59). Clinically, this may be observed by abnormal postural tone, imbalances in weight bearing, and disruption of stability-mobility factors necessary for coordinated function. As a result, the neuropostural base is compromised, and in the presence of visual dysfunction, an inefficient matching of the visual-vestibular-somatosensory triad results. In turn, the inefficient righting, balance, and equilibrium responses cannot refine automatic postural adjustments, leading to poor quality movements that further deteriorate with continuous attempts.

Following a BI, the compromise of the ambient process affects the musculoskeletal organization. Although the mechanism is unclear, it has been suggested that the abnormal proprioceptive integration is associated, perhaps causally, with a disruption of the normal relationship of the 2 modes of visual processing leading to VMSS (60).

Postural analysis is needed to guide therapeutic interventions. Normalized alignment, particular in the vertical plane, allows the ambient and focal visual processes to relate normally (58,60). Therefore, the quality of the movement response is directly related to the quality of the starting posture. Any activation of movement from a misaligned starting position will result in compensatory and abnormal motor responses, thus exacerbating the mismatch of neural systems (57,60).

The photos shown subsequently illustrate the importance of proper alignment and positioning. As stated by Sherrington, "Posture follows movement like a shadow."

An attribute of normal central nervous system (CNS) function is the calibrating and recalibrating of responses to enable the "feel" of a movement to be perceived anticipatorily to the actual completion of the movement. This occurs preconsciously as the ambient visual process enables the matching of visual and postural cures

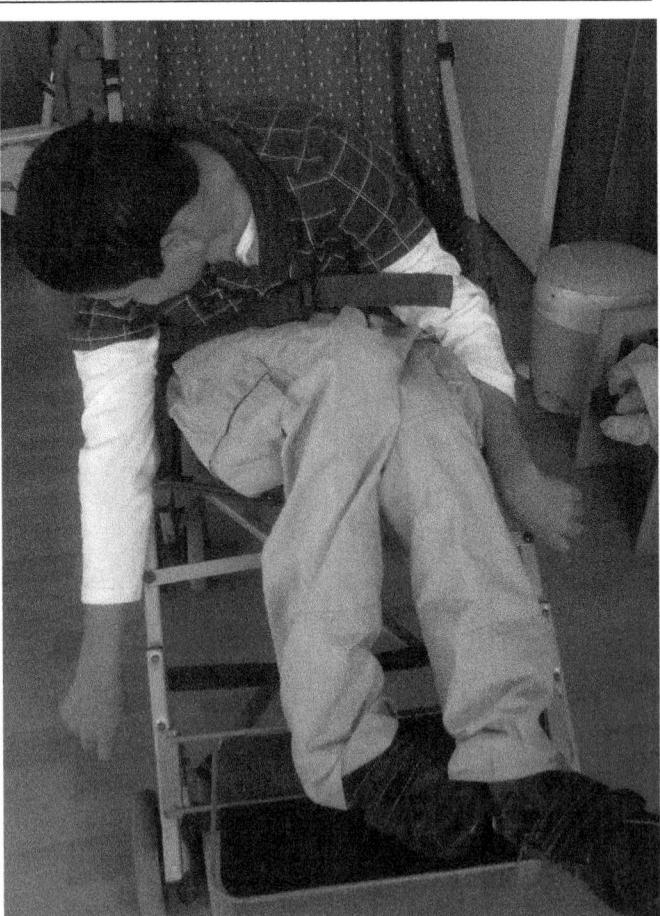

FIGURE 45-1 Child lacking stable trunk, which interferes with head position, thereby affecting visual development and function.

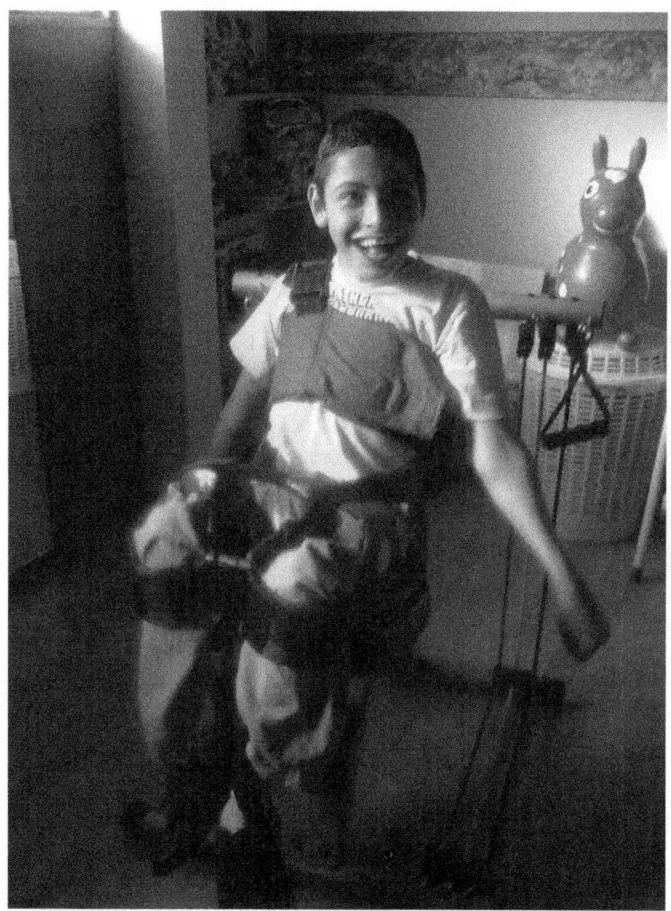

FIGURE 45-2 Child with supported trunk position enables an erect posturing of the head and providing support for visual process and spatial function.

Individuals affected by head trauma frequently have corresponding soft tissue injuries that affect muscular function (59). Depending on the extent of the injury, there can be corresponding muscle paresis, joint misalignment, and mobility restrictions. Therapeutic efforts should normalize the interactions of the visual-vestibular-sensory triad (60). In turn, this helps to reestablish a patient's neuropostural base and improve the patient's awareness of the body's relationship to itself, gravity, and time-space factors (see Chapter 68). Intervention may include the use of prisms to counter visual-sensory mismatch. In addition, physical manipulation may be employed to release tissue restrictions, mobilize joint restrictions, and reestablish biomechanical kinesiological relationships of the musculoskeletal system. Taken together, these therapeutic approaches recouple vision and posture.

Visual intervention without physical handling to organize the musculoskeletal processes could result in reinforcing abnormal motor compensations. Conversely, physical handling to increase joint range, release tissue restrictions, and increase muscle function will not be as successful if the visual imbalance is not treated. This is because the abnormal visual process will continue to enforce abnormal postural reactions.

Rehabilitative visual intervention should begin with analysis of postural misalignments and structural shifts in relationship to the bimodal process and the sensorimotor system. Once the individual is in the most erect posture against gravity that can be sustained with or without external aid, visual-motor rehabilitation should include body movement components as part of the response.

For example, efforts to encourage a patient's visual pursuits to cross the midline or improve the efficiency of the patient's saccades must incorporate rotational neck and trunk movements (4). As improvements are achieved, the head and neck can then be disassociated from the training so as to provide a stable platform for further enhancement of ocular motility. Likewise, the components of body extension

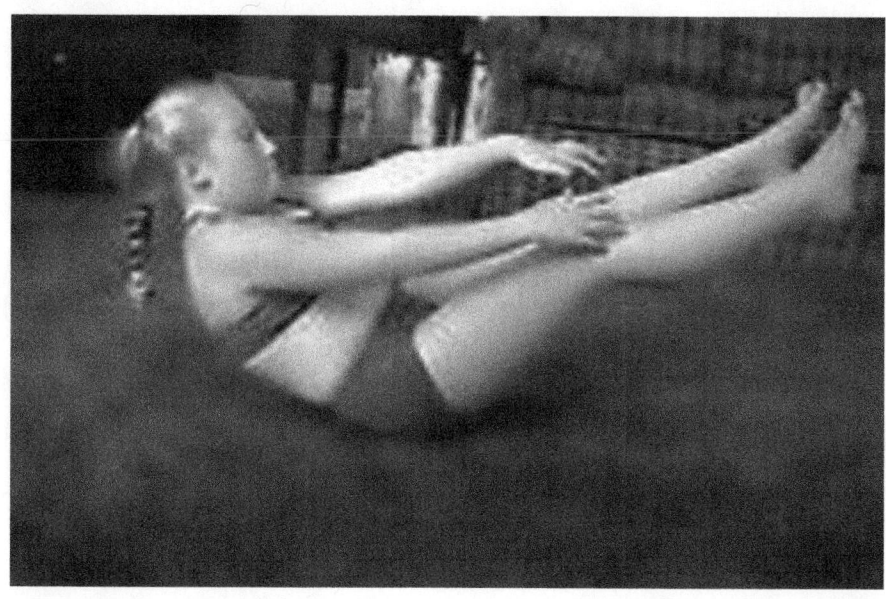

FIGURE 45-3 Attempt to assume a supine flexion posture with poor head/neck organization. The neck does not activate to allow the head to align properly over the shoulders.

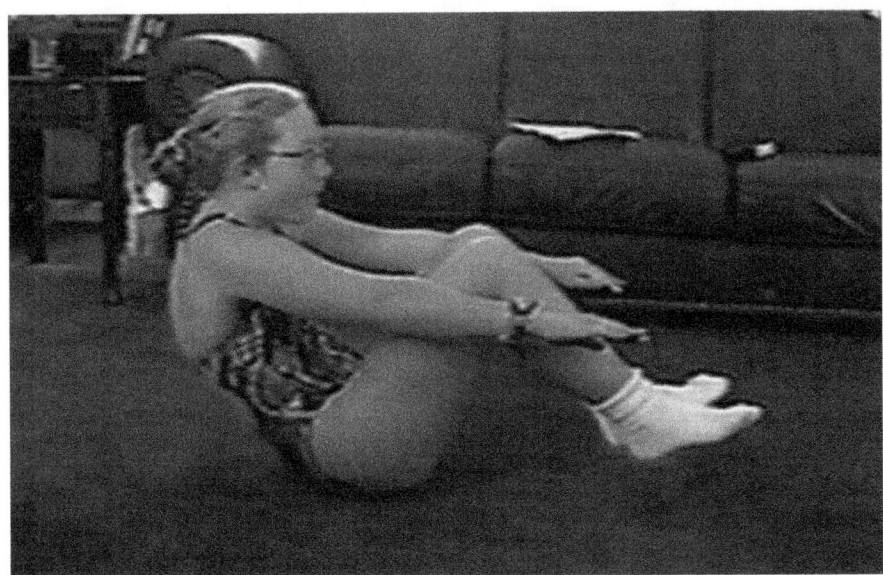

FIGURE 45-4 After several months of physical handling to align and organize the head/neck/shoulder girdle and vision intervention through prism lenses, the attempt to assume supine flexion becomes efficient and organized.

and flexion should be incorporated to assist in convergence and divergence.

Early in development, the organization of the basic movement components yields refinement of movement against gravity (61), leading to neck extension (2 months) and organization of ocular alignment and a shift from near viewing to far. The practice of lifting the head to reach visually into space permits the relationship to be established between extension–flexion and eye movements to orient vision spatially to shift orientation from near to far.

Graded flexion and extension components of movement are often inefficient in individuals with BI and children with neuromotor disorders, thereby affecting the relationship of vision to posture (62).

An inability to dynamically control postural adaptations leads to extreme compensatory stability postures. For example, hyperextension of the head and neck in prone position will ultimately lead to an intermittent or constant collapse in flexion. In either case, vision will be overemphasized in the inferior and/or superior visual fields. These abnormal vision and postural relationships will reinforce each other and inhibit a return to normal function.

Mismatch of visual-postural relationships interfere with normal development. For example, elevating an object so that a child can visually interact reinforces hyperextension of the child's posture in association with coordination between the eyes, head, and neck. This leads to a compensatory postural stability that reinforces the overuse of specific fields of vision, thus creating abnormal visual adaptation and inhibits the development of efficient postural adaptation.

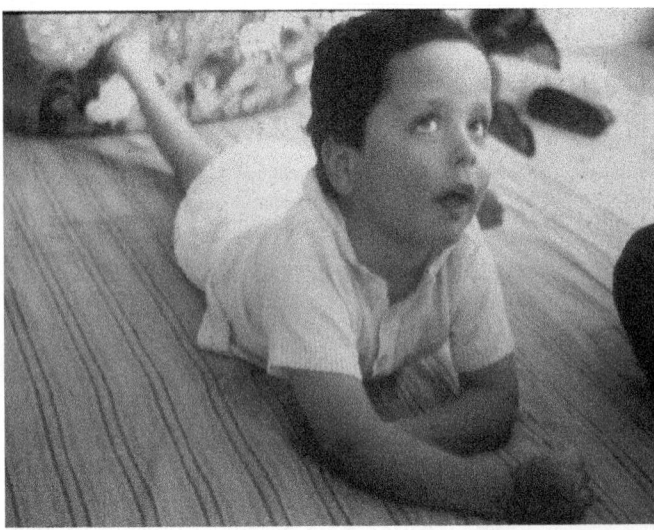

FIGURE 45-5 The child props in prone with hyperextension of the neck and trunk with capital extension of the head. This posture is not dynamic, and there is limited visual-motor adaptation.

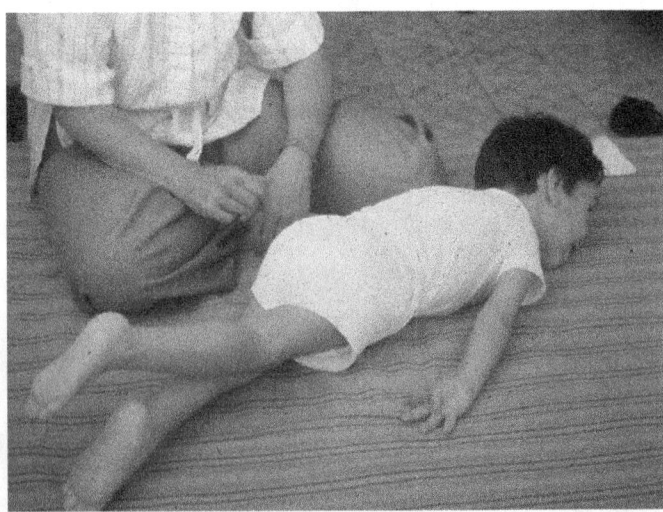

FIGURE 45-6 The child collapses into the surface, unable to posturally maintain normal prone extension. This posture severely limits visual experience. Abnormal postural control leads to the development of abnormal or inefficient visual-motor development.

Disorganization between bimodal visual processing in the superior and inferior visual fields will directly influence both the development for a child, as well as the postural organization for an adult following a BI.

VISUAL PROCESSING DYSFUNCTION FOLLOWING BRAIN INJURY

Post-Trauma Vision Syndrome

PTVS encompasses several vision complaints (see Table 45-1), including diplopia, the perception that print appears to move, difficulty shifting gaze, difficulty focusing, difficulty adapting to new visual environments, and intolerance to glare (4). Diplopia is specifically a result of binocular dysfunction, and neuro-ophthalmic examination may demonstrate strabismus, convergence insufficiency, and divergence excess. Notably, patients may adopt abnormal postures to compensate for vision dysfunction and reduce the sense of diplopia, particularly when the diplopia depends on a particular direction of gaze. These patients can develop muscle spasm or even contractures. Postconcussive diplopia that varies with direction of gaze is often attributable to cranial nerve palsy. However, the mechanism for the cause of the binocular dysfunctions related to abnormal vergences appears to stem from more complex trauma affecting bimodal visual processing. In studies employing visual evoked potential (VEP) researchers demonstrated that reduction in amplitude and an increase in latency were evident (63–65). Padula et al. (63) found a statistically significant correlation regarding VEP changes when comparing patients with TBI experiencing symptoms of binocular dysfunction and normal subjects. They also demonstrated an increase in amplitude following treatment with base-in prism and binasal occlusion for the experimental group of subjects, whereas intervention caused a decrease in amplitude for those in the control group. The clinical significance from this data indicates that some binocular symptoms following a BI are caused by visual processing dysfunction at multiple levels of the cortex and midbrain (8,14,63–65). Therefore, the binocular conditions of convergence insufficiency, accommodative insufficiency, deficiencies of pursuit tracking, and saccadic eye movements according to this percept become characteristics of the visual processing dysfunction rather than specific diagnoses requiring separate therapeutic interventions. The greater implications of this research are that

by treating the cause of the visual processing problem (PTVS), the characteristics will be diminished or resolved. This will be discussed later in this chapter in greater depth.

As mentioned earlier, spatially matched information between the ambient visual-motor and sensorimotor processes is directed to the occipital cortical areas involved in binocular integration (i.e., stereoptic fusion) of the disparate retinal images. This supports the idea that a reduction in ambient visual processing leads to reduced fusion capabilities.

The predominance of focal over ambient visual processing may also cause a patient to fixate on unnecessarily fine details while simultaneously impairing the ability of the patient to appropriately perceive visual context, anticipate visual changes, release fixation, and refixate on novel stimuli. Notably, all of these deficits in eye teaming have been reported after TBI (66–68).

It must be emphasized that patients demonstrating PTVS will often have excellent visual acuity and normal ocular examinations. Therefore, familiarity with PTVS is critical for ensuring that patients are evaluated by the appropriate specialists, rather than being relegated to years of undertreatment or unnecessary treatment from misdiagnosed psychological impairment.

Ocular Misalignment

Misalignment of the eyes as a result of a visual processing dysfunction is common. When this occurs, a patient loses the ability to fuse and could report diplopia (double vision) and visual confusion. *Diplopia* is the perception of seeing 2 identical images located in differing positions in space and is believed to occur when images from a single object of regard fall on noncorresponding regions of the 2 retinas. Visual confusion is the perception of disparate images overlapping each other and occurs when two dissimilar images fall on the two respective foveas and compete for visual attention. Children under the age of 8–10 years have sufficient cortical plasticity to suppress the input from one eye, thereby eliminating or significantly reducing diplopia and confusion. The cost of this plasticity, however, may be the development of amblyopia and concomitant reduction of visual acuity in the suppressed eye. Adults with acquired strabismus demonstrate less plasticity. However, they often demonstrate the ability to ignore the input from 1 eye. Notably, there is evidence that this ability may indeed be true suppression (69) rather than simple neglect.

Double vision after TBI can be caused by a visual processing dysfunction, direct damage to the EOMs and/or architecture of the orbit, to the nervous tissue subserving coordinated eye movements or, from reduced alertness, concentration or effort to maintain fusion. In addition, patients may report the perception of double vision from monocular factors, such as reduction in accommodative amplitude (70), cataract, and macular hole (71). Brain trauma can also be associated with epiphenomena that lead to nervous tissue damage, including ischemia, hypoxia, abnormal cerebrospinal fluid (CSF) pressure (either too high from hydrocephalus or too low from CSF leak) (72), toxic metabolic changes, edema, and secondary structural changes, such as aneurysm or progression of Chiari malformation (a condition in which low-lying cerebellar tonsils advance further downward, compressing brainstem structures) (73,74).

TABLE 45-1 Characteristics and Symptoms of Post-Trauma Vision Syndrome

COMMON CHARACTERISTICS	COMMON SYMPTOMS
Exotropia/exophoria	Diplopia
Accommodative insufficiency	Blurred near vision
Convergence insufficiency	Perceived movement of print or stationary objects
Oculomotor dysfunction	Asthenopia
Increased myopia	Headaches
Low blink rate	Photophobia

Damage to the cranial nerves innervating the EOMs probably stems from compression at the dural entry points (where the nerves enter openings in the skull extending into the orbit) or at locations where the nerve is in close approximation to bone (75,76). It is at these locations that a subdural hematoma can compress the nerve against bone, or that the tethered nerve can be stretched against resistance, or where an accelerating brain can create an impact against the nerve. Cranial nerve palsy affecting the extraocular musculature usually has a stereotypical presentation with noncomitant strabismus, that is, a strabismus that worsens as the eye attempts to move into the field of primary action of the denervated muscle. When multiple cranial nerves are affected, it can be more difficult to differentiate nerve damage from damage to nuclear structures or supranuclear tissue (77,78).

Subtle nerve damage can be difficult to diagnosis because patients may describe visual discomfort without mentioning diplopia specifically. In addition, there can be considerable discrepancy between objectively measured strabismus and a patient's subjective complaints (79).

Complaints of intermittent and/or mild diplopia after BI require proactive investigation. Patients may be found to demonstrate a reduction in the ability to converge at near (convergence insufficiency) (80), to visually pursue moving targets (deficiency of pursuits) (81), or to generate normal saccades (saccadic insufficiency) (24). These problems can often be ameliorated with neurorehabilitative therapy but unfortunately are probably underdiagnosed (82,83). Therapy for frank diplopia that does not resolve spontaneously will usually include a combination of therapies, including the prescription of spectacle-mounted prism, surgical realignment of the EOMs, and/or chemical penalization of relatively overactive muscles with agents such as botulinum toxin.

Hallucinations

Visual phenomena following a TBI are diverse and include visual hallucinations, such as flashing lights, palinopsia, variations in homonymous field defects, and scintillating scotomas. Some of these phenomena may be aura from the migraine syndromes that often follow concussion (84). However, some patients with TBI specifically describe the experience of movement of the visual field that may or may not accompany body, head, or eye movements. These symptoms are features of the PTVS and are amenable to neuro-optometric rehabilitation. Unfortunately, because visual hallucinations can also accompany temporal or occipital lobe disorders, patients might be offered psychiatric medication unnecessarily, or a patient might be accused of malingering if the PTVS is not recognized as a possible etiology. At present, there is no anatomic data that explain the visual hallucinations associated with PTVS.

Visual-Vestibular Integration Dysfunction

Coordinated movement involves a complex interaction between sensory afferents from the visual system, somatosensory system, and the vestibular system. In particular, the semicircular canals and utricle/saccule respond to rotational and linear/gravitational information and is transmitted via the vestibulocochlear nerve through the ascending and descending axon branches of the brainstem vestibular nuclei. Visual stimuli enhance and can even override vestibular input. The vestibulo-ocular reflex (which maintains foveal fixation during head movements), the vestibulospinal pathways (which are responsible for postural control under static and dynamic circumstances), and the vestibulocerebellar pathways (allowing for modulation of motor output via the flocculonodular lobe of the cerebellum) are all integrated at this level of the brainstem.

Diplopia, dizziness, vertigo (a sense of spinning), and imbalance are the most common symptoms accompanying dysfunction of integration of visual and vestibular input. A complete medical history with careful analysis of the visual process and vestibular system is necessary for diagnosis and prognosis. Too often, functional vestibular rehabilitation for vertigo and dizziness is began before the relationship to visual processing problems is determined. Less than the age of 50, TBI is the most common cause of dizziness and vertigo from a direct head trauma or whiplash.

The differential diagnosis for dizziness without vestibular dysfunction is wide and can include PTVS, hyperventilation, dehydration, cerebral ischemia (e.g., from orthostatic hypotension, vasovagal syndrome, arteriosclerosis, and arterial insufficiency), osteoarthritis, and other CNS disorders, including vestibular neuritis (acute labyrinthitis), benign paroxysmal positional vertigo (BPPV), nucleoreticular vestibular syndrome, Meniere disease, perilymphatic hypertension, and perilymphatic fistula.

Vertigo and dizziness are associated with PTVS and may be secondary to damage or compromise to the ambient visual processes. Notably, the treatment of PTVS, which entails efforts to improve coordination of vestibular, kinesthetic, proprioceptive inputs as well as the visual bimodal process, has been shown to lessen the patient's sense of dizziness, supporting the connection between abnormal visual processing and vestibular symptoms.

Visual Midline Shift Syndrome

The sense of postural orientation develops during infancy and establishes our balance, awareness of our spatial orientation, and locomotive abilities. The vestibular, visual, and kinesthetic senses provide the input to our balance centers that enable us to make smooth, coordinated, and planned movements. It is the ambient visual process that helps us establish an egocentric visual midline necessary for postural stability and orientation (85).

Research has documented that in patients developing a hemiparesis following a stroke, a shift in perception of egocenter (visual midline) can occur and is related to shift in weight bearing (86,87). This phenomenon has also been demonstrated in patients with TBI accompanied by hemiplegia or homonymous visual field defects. These patients often demonstrate a tendency to lean or walk toward on or the other side, and studies on these patients have reported that the egocentric visual midline can indeed shift (88). In addition, these patients demonstrate a reduced ability to determine egocentric straight ahead and a neglect of visual space (89). The shift in perceived egocenter, or VMSS, may be demonstrated by passing an object in front of a patient's face and asking them to report when the object appears to be directly in front of their nose. Patients with visual field loss may perceive the target as being front center when in fact it is on the side of the body opposite the loss of visual field. The asymmetric weight bearing and abnormal posture associated with VMSS interferes with many aspects of physical rehabilitation. Further, the shifting of perceived visual midline may reinforce the neglect of visual space.

In terms of visual processing, it may be that the VMSS is caused by a unilateral compression and contemporaneous expansion of ambient vision. The shift can occur anteroposteriorly or laterally but will usually be opposite the affected side. Notably, VMSS can also occur in patients who do not develop hemianopsia.

CLINICAL EXAMINATION

The neuromotor assessment can be performed to evaluate the role of the visual process in establishing concepts of visual midline, and how it affects posture, balance, and movement. This assessment can also help guide further diagnostic studies. The examiner should carefully review the medical and rehabilitative records, as well as establish a history based on visual and spatial dysfunction. This history will enable the provider to differentiate current symptoms from premorbid conditions. It is also important to reconstruct the event causing the BI to assess injury and lesions relative to inertial force and impact.

The neuro-optometric assessment will include a careful study of the patient's refractive state. This often reveals accommodative defects known to occur after BI. An oculomotor evaluation will also be performed to determine cranial nerve function. The most common result of lesions of the cranial nerve following a TBI is third nerve palsy. A third nerve palsy is associated with exotropia as well as ptosis and mydriasis of the pupil on the affected side with complete compromise. In most cases, the effect is incomplete causing variations from decompensated exophoria to intermittent exotropia. Diplopia depends on visual fatigue and chronic development of suppression. Vertical palsies resulting from damage to the fourth cranial nerve will produce hyperphoria and hypertropia, cyclotorsional strabismus, as well as decompensation in specific gaze direction and head tilt. Sixth cranial nerve palsy interferes with abduction of the related eye, causing esotropia.

A variety of binocular function tests are available to evaluate fusional mechanisms. In patients with strabismus or phorias (tendency of the eyes to deviate when fusion is prevented), these tests will elicit either diplopia or suppression. The ability with which a patient can retain fusion is a good indicator of the health of their eye teaming.

It is important to evaluate higher order binocular functions as well. For example, the visual midline test for VMSS is extremely useful. However, prior to offering this test, the examiner must first observe the patient in a seated position, as well as during ambulation, to evaluate for any tendency to drift to 1 side and/or lean forward or backward during ambulation. Lateral shift of the visual midline will often cause a lean or drift during ambulation. An anterior shift can cause a lean or flexion forward. In more severe cases of the anterior shift of visual midline, toe walking will develop in an attempt to compensate for the imbalance. A posterior shift of visual midline will cause an extension posture and tendency to lean backward after retropulsion.

In addition to the neuromotor assessment, there are several psychophysical evaluations that should be offered in the

clinical setting. Indeed, the basis of the clinical exam is the assessment of visual acuity. Visual acuity specifically tests the health of the macular pathways. Acuities should be assessed monocularly and binocularly. Usually, this testing is performed at 20 ft (6 m) and 14 in (40 cm), although this distance can be adapted to patients with visual impairment. A variety of acuity testing systems are available to provide objective measurements regardless of whether a patient is verbal or even able to cooperate well with testing.

During visual acuity testing, important clues of pathology can be sought by an experienced examiner who might notice that a patient demonstrates a head tilt or abnormal posture, asymmetry of near and distance acuity, neglect of portions of the test materials, and differences in monocular and binocular acuity. A reduction in visual acuity will usually stem from pathology affecting the eye or optic nerve. However, patients with BI may show evidence of reduced contrast sensitivity despite enjoying a normal eye examination (85).

Once visual acuity has been evaluated, it is very useful to offer visual field assessment to patients with TBI; this can help localize damage affecting the afferent visual pathways. Each eye has a visual field that spans approximately 135° angle at the horizon, and the right and left visual fields overlap frontally by approximately 120° angle at the horizon.

Homonymous visual field defects refer to losses on the same side of the 2 visual fields, whereas a *heteronymous defect* refers to losses affecting opposite sides of the 2 visual fields, either bitemporally or binasally. Because of the anatomy of the visual system, it is possible for a patient to lose a quarter of their visual field (i.e., a quadrantanopsia). The degree to which the field loss in the 2 eyes is symmetric (i.e., congruous) is a hint to the location of the etiologic lesion in the visual pathways.

It should be noted that there is a condition known as visual field neglect in which a patient appears to have functional loss of peripheral vision despite normal perimetric testing. Patients ignore information seen in either the left or right hemifields. Like true visual field loss, visuospatial neglect may manifest as a complete loss of visual perception on the side affected or as a relative loss where less is perceived in the neglected field, particularly when there are competing stimuli in the opposite hemifields of the 2 eyes.

An experienced examiner will usually detect most significant visual field losses by employing confrontational testing. However, more precise and sensitive visual field testing is available using manual and automated perimetry. Notably, patients with PTVS are more prone to fatigue of attention, delayed response time, and intolerance to glare, both of which tend to degrade their ability to participate with formal perimetry. For this reason, Goldmann perimetry, which encourages interaction between the examiner and the patient, may be more appropriate for evaluating patients with neurological impairments. Furthermore, Goldmann perimetry involved the presentation of kinetic stimuli, which may be more useful for patients with BI (90).

Visual field defects stemming from lesions posterior to the optic chiasm will always cause a homonymous hemianopsia with varying degrees of congruity. Temporal lobe lesions can cause an incongruous superior quadrantanopsia. Parietal lobe lesions can cause inferior field defects and can be associated with a patient's lack of awareness of the field loss. When patients with parietal lobe lesions are presented with simultaneous stimuli on either side of midline, the extinction phenomenon can be demonstrated during which patients will deny seeing the stimulus on the side of the impaired visual field. Notably, moving targets do not elicit extinction.

Occipital lobe lesions are characterized mostly by their congruous nature. These field defects can encompass the entire hemifield of either eye. Some patients with occipital lobe lesions demonstrate Riddoch phenomenon, the inability to detect stationary objects presented to the impaired visual field while retaining the ability to detect motion in that field. The neurologic basis for this phenomenon is not well understood. One could propose that stationary targets could fail to sufficiently stimulate a damaged ambient visual pathway, allowing a patient to overfocalize on some other stimulus and ignore the test object. On the other hand, a moving target would stimulate the ambient system sufficiently to engage a patient's consciousness.

There is currently no treatment to truly increase visual field loss in patients with BI. However, there are reports that patients can be trained in such a way as to reduce the functional effect of the defect. Yoked spectacle-mounted prisms have been shown to help patients develop a better sense of awareness of their surroundings, allowing them to negotiate obstacles more effectively. This therapy can be helpful with patient affected by true visual field loss (91) or visuospatial neglect (92). Patients can also receive training in adaptive search strategies (93, 94) during which they are taught to scan into the area of visual field loss. Automated systems to teach patients these strategies have become more widely available and are receiving greater attention (95).

The assessment of patients with TBI would not be complete without an evaluation of motion perception. Motion perception depends on higher cortical processing of visual information. Motion perception is tested by presenting various types of stimuli (usually images of dots, sinusoidal strips, or bars projected onto a screen) and recording the responses to questions concerning direction, orientation, and speed of perceived movement. Deficiencies of motion perception, or akinetopsia, have been reported in patients with damaged lateral parieto-occipital structures (96).

DIAGNOSTIC EVALUATIONS

Visual Evoked Potential

The VEP, also called visual evoked response or VER, is an electrical response created by the visual pathways and recorded by electrodes on the scalp (see Chapter 17). The amplitude of the response is usually less than 20 μV, and the response latencies are measured within 250–300 ms. To evoke these responses, subjects are presented with lights. These lights can be altered with respect to size, pattern, frequency of flicker, brightness, color, and location within the visual field(s) depending on which portion of the visual pathway is being evaluated. The latency of the VEP is a more reliable metric and has clinical application with respect to acuity and focalization. The amplitude of VEP under binocular assessment may have more relevance to ambient spatial relationships, especially when left- and right-sided responses are compared.

The recording device is programmed to average the VER, thereby improving the signal-to-noise ratio of the recordings. This permits the VER to be more easily discernible from background bioelectric activity despite their relatively low amplitudes.

The graphical report from a VEP recording usually shows a waveform with negative and positive deflections of potential. These deflections occur within well-documented limits of amplitude and latency for normal patients aged 18–60 years; young children and the elderly will require separate norms (97).

There are several strategies employed during VEP testing, including the flash VEP, pattern VEP, and multifocal VEP. These tests can help localize areas of damage to the visual pathways, even in patients who are suboptimally cooperative (98–100).

The stimulus for the flash VEP is a brief flash of light subtending 20° angle of visual field and presented at a rate of 1 Hz (1 flash/second) (97). The flash VEP is particularly helpful when working with uncooperative patients, such as children or patients with significant TBI. It can be used to determine whether the visual pathways are grossly intact; this is particularly important for patients reporting no-light-perception (NLP) vision. The flash VEP is also helpful in ascertaining the function of surgically implanted prosthetic visual devices (101). The flash VEP can be presented through goggles mounted with light-emitting diodes (LEDs); these stimuli are sufficient to elicit responses even through a closed eyelid.

The pattern VEP uses a checkerboard of white and black squares as the stimulus. The black and white squares are rapidly reversed during the stimulus presentation, allowing the overall luminance to stay constant while preventing habituation in the responding retinal cells. Pattern VEP is most useful when multiple trials using different sized checks are offered to cooperative patients, as well as from enabling more reliable estimates of speed and amplitude of visual pathway transmissions; comparison of responses to these trials can even help estimate a subject's visual acuity (98). Abnormalities in the brain can alter the pattern VEP results. For instance, TBI may desynchronize visual responses generated by different parts of the brain (65) and deform the pattern VEP waveform (102).

There are several variations of the pattern VEP. For example, the checkerboard can be moved, or the squares can be increased in size to simulate motion, permitting a "motion-onset" VEP. Further, the patterns can be colored in many ways. These tests allow evaluations that discriminate between the different vision processing streams, that is, pattern, motion, and color. The sweep VEP uses vertical bars rather than checks, and these bars can be alternated or narrowed to help obtain a rough measure of visual acuity. VEPs can also be measured using multichannel devices; much like an electrocardiogram (EKG), the use of multiple channels can help further localize areas of dysfunction in the brain.

Multifocal VEP allows the examiner to stimulate the subject's visual field at discrete points. This technique, as well as a more generalized variant called hemifield VEP, permits exploration of damage to more finely localized portions of the retina and optic nerve, as well as the retrochiasmal visual pathways (99).

VEP is an important tool in the evaluation of patients with brain injury. Perhaps the most important use we have for the VEP is to confirm or refute the presence of damage to the visual pathways when there is discord between the subjective findings and other objective findings. Electrophysiologic studies are often more sensitive than readily available imaging studies, and therefore can often detect damage to smaller areas of the brain than can imaging. For example, a VEP will often be abnormal in patients with traumatic optic neuropathy prior to the onset of physical findings, such as optic atrophy. In addition, physical conditions that heal relatively well may never be demonstrable on imaging studies, such as the computed tomography (CT) scan. Depending on the placement of the recording electrodes and the number of channels monitored, the VEP can help localize damage to the visual pathways as being pre- or postchiasmal. Interestingly, VEPs can appear normal in patients with cortical blindness (100), and this is believed to occur when more anterior visual cortex (i.e., association areas) are damaged. VEP can detect hemifield losses in patients who might not otherwise be able to cooperate with automated visual field testing (103). It can demonstrate reduction in stereovision (104), the presence of the PTVS (63), and it can detect higher level visual processing errors, such as discrimination of textures segregated by orientation or motion (105). These conditions can occur after TBI, yet can only be evaluated otherwise by subjective means.

Although VEPs do not generate waveforms that are absolutely diagnostic for any particular condition, they can often help support a diagnosis. The VEP becomes an even more powerful tool when employed synergistically with other testing modalities, such as fMRI, electroretinogram (ERG), and electroencephalogram (EEG).

Electroretinogram

The ERG is a recording of the bioelectric activity that occurs in the retina and retinal pigment epithelium (RPE) during photostimulation. The recording electrodes are usually attached to either corneal contact lenses or strips of foil tucked into the bulbar conjunctiva after the subject receives topical anesthesia. The subject's pupils are chemically dilated, and testing occurs after the subject is adapted to dark . The stimulus can be adjusted to distinguish between the activity of the rod and cone photoreceptors and retinal ganglion cells to measure the sensitivity of the photoreceptors; evaluate the ability of the photoreceptors to adjust to differing levels of illumination and to follow stimuli of varying presentation rates. The main responses during ERG testing are displayed in units of microvolts and occur within a latency of 100 ms. The 3 main strategies for testing ERG are full field (or ganzfeld), pattern, and multifocal.

There are several strategies employed with ERG, including the full-field ERG, the pattern ERG (PERG), and the multifocal ERG (mfERG). These tests can help evaluate the health of the different retinal layers and also identify isolated regional damage in the retina that might not be obvious on clinical examination (106–110).

Neither the full-field ERG nor the mfERG receive significant contributions from retinal ganglion cell activity, whereas the PERG is almost completely dependent on the ganglion cell response. Further, it has been reported that the full-field ERG is unchanged in patients with mild TBI (mTBI) (111). Taken together, these results suggest that the different ERG modalities used in combination with other tests, such as VEP and perimetry, could be very helpful in localizing visual loss to the retinal photoreceptors, macular ganglion cells, or optic nerve. Recognizing that visual complaints are very common in patients with TBI (3,112), it is clear that ERG should have a prominent role in diagnostic efforts. Some important conditions for which occult retinal damage has been identified with ERG include *commotio retinae* (a disruption of the photo-

receptor layer after blunt ocular trauma) (113), laser injury (114), photostress (115), and external beam radiation (116). At present, although no studies have been published specifically exploring ERG changes seen after blast injury, this area is currently being explored in both humans (117) and animals (118).

Electrooculogram

The electrooculogram (EOG) indirectly measures the bioelectric activity of the RPE during varying illuminations and during eye movement (119). There is an electric potential created across the RPE that decreases during dark adaptation and then rises during light adaptation. As a subject's eyes move back and forth horizontally, the potential recorded at electrodes placed at the nasal and lateral canthi rises and falls in a wavelike pattern. These waveforms are recorded during scotopic and photopic conditions and peak and trough potentials can be identified.

An important metric derived from EOG testing is called the Arden ratio. It is calculated as the quotient of the peak potential during illumination and the trough potential during dark adaptation. Measurement of the Arden ratio can help differentiate certain diseases of the RPE, such as Best disease, an autosomal dominant inherited condition (120), or damage to the RPE from toxicity, such as might occur from retained metal foreign bodies (121) or from chronic use drugs, such as hydroxychloroquine (122), vigabatrin (123), lamotrigine (124), interferon alpha (125), and desferrioxamine (126).

The EOG tracing is very sensitive to eye movements and can detect global directional changes of only 2° angle, as well as eye blinking. For this reason, good patient cooperation is required when exploring RPE function. However, this same sensitivity allows the EOG to create excellent recordings of oculomotor amplitude, speed, and accuracy. EOG has therefore proven useful in the evaluation of patients with ocular motility abnormalities, such as acquired nystagmus (127) or abnormal saccades (128).

EOG testing has been offered to patients with BI. Patients exposed to blast injury could be assessed for evidence of RPE dysfunction caused by a retained metal foreign body in the eye. In addition, EOG can detect and document abnormalities in positional-induced nystagmus exhibited by patients with post-traumatic vertigo (129) and abnormal saccades and pursuits found in patients with whiplash injuries (130).

Electro and Video Nystagmography

The visual pathways are intimately connected with the vestibular pathways; together, these pathways help us maintain a sense of balance and inform us of our position in space relative to the pull of gravity. The vestibular pathways project directly and indirectly to the oculomotor systems of the brain, thereby aligning the 2 eyes in the horizontal, vertical, and torsional axes and assisting in the control of rapid eye refixation (saccades).

Nystagmography is the study of eye movements associated with saccades, pursuits, and fixation using electrophysiologic and/or infrared video recording technology. Although nystagmography records eye position, the results are evaluated with the intent of exploring dizziness and balance disorders secondary to vestibular dysfunction. For this reason, otolaryngologists and physiatrists, rather than eye care providers, usually offer nystagmography.

During nystagmography, the examiner attempts to stimulate a patient's vestibular activity either by changing the patient's head position through voluntary or passive movements or by calorically stimulating the patient's semicircular canals through irrigation of the ear canal with hot or cold water (131). Electronystagmography (ENG) depends on the same corneo-retinal potential evaluated during electro-oculography.

Videonystagmography (VNG) employs infrared recording sensors built into masks or goggles, as well as digital image processing software to evaluate eye movements. Although ENG and VNG can complement each other because of the different advantages each technique offers, VNG appears to be supplanting ENG (132).

Vestibular system injury is common in patients with TBI (133) and has been a particular challenge for patients exposed to blast (134,135). Abnormal vestibular activity can result from damage to the vestibulo-cerebellar pathways (136), as well as to the vestibular organs, delicate bony structures of the inner ear (137). Patients with even mild TBI were found to demonstrate delayed or hypometric saccades and slowed pursuits (138). Spontaneous nystagmus can also occur after cerebellar concussion (139). Although a thorough history and clinical evaluation can often detect vestibular injury, nystagmography can help differentiate central or peripheral damage and may help identify the affected side when injury is unilateral.

Imaging Studies

Static imaging techniques of cranial anatomy are critical for the initial evaluation of the patient affected by BI (see Chapter 15). CT scan reliably and rapidly detects cranial fractures, hematoma, and intracranial hemorrhage. MRI provides an excellent follow-up study for assessing damage to the brain and tracking whether that damage will lead to a loss of nervous tissue. In addition, our understanding of the mapping of the visual world onto many brain regions often permits correlation of the anatomic findings on static CT/MRI with pathologic findings demonstrated in the clinic, such as visual field defects, strabismus, pupillary abnormalities, nystagmus, and hypometric eye movements. Furthermore, angiographic techniques can complement routine CT/MRI; CT and MRI angiography are useful adjuncts to explore posttraumatic disease of the circulatory system of the brain, such as aneurysm, arterial dissection, and arteriovenous fistula.

Advances in technology have enabled the study of brain physiology through novel applications of imaging methodologies. These methodologies permit relatively rapid, minimally invasive high-resolution evaluations of brain function and dysfunction and are often more sensitive than conventional CT and MRI (see Chapter 16). Clinical useful techniques for evaluating brain physiology include fMRI, positron emission tomography (PET), single photon emission computed tomography (SPECT), magnetoencephalography (MEG) and diffusion tensor imaging (DTI). Because these imaging methods have been discussed in detail in other sections of this book, we will briefly review their use in the diagnosis and rehabilitation of visual disturbances after BI.

fMRI studies of patients with BI have demonstrated abnormal prefrontal cortex activity (140), abnormal frontal cortex connectivity (141), and abnormal interhemispheric connectivity in the primary visual cortex (142). PET scan studies of patients demonstrating chronic postconcussion syndrome after exposure to blast injury have described subnormal glucose metabolism in visually important portions of the brain, such as the cerebellum and temporal lobes of the cerebral cortex (143). MEG activity was shown to be abnormal in most patients with mTBI; evaluated and demonstrated associations between abnormal activities in the temporal, parietal, and frontal lobes; and dysfunction in memory, visual attention, and executive tasks, respectively (144). A separate study integrating MEG and DTI further confirmed that the abnormal MEG signals arise from gray matter deafferented by the injured white matter tracts (145).

The newer imaging modalities are being explored for their potential to predict outcomes (see Chapter 19), follow the progress of patients, explore those patients for whom complaints are disproportionate to results seen on routine CT and MRI scans, evaluate whether therapeutic interventions can aid in recovery after BI, and advance the science of neuroplasticity after BI. For example, fMRI has demonstrated that patients with cortical blindness undergoing vision restoration training were found to have small increases in receptive field size in the brain, possibly accounting for the small improvements some patients demonstrate with this therapy (146). In addition, a SPECT study of patients with brain damage suggested that the drug zolpidem, a sedative hypnotic, improves outcomes (147), and a MEG study demonstrated how auditory stimulation with music or speech enhances recovery of sensory processing after stroke (148).

VISION REHABILITATION

Prisms

Prisms are lenses that bend light in such a way that the object of regard appears to be shifted from its actual position. They are extremely useful for bringing objects into the view of an eye that cannot move to look in the direction of an object of interest. Prisms are also used clinically to help reestablish balance of ambient and focal visual relationships causing visual dysfunction or in a compensatory manner to offset the effects of a binocular imbalance.

In binocular dysfunction, the use of prism can reduce symptoms and perhaps even hasten recovery. When a patient has a unilateral strabismus, a prism can shift the perception of the visual world for the affected eye so that the patient perceives the 2 eyes as being aligned. This greatly enhances the ability to fuse. Prisms can also be used over both eyes. In cases of convergence insufficiency, the prisms can be placed so that the eyes need not converge. Binocular prisms are also employed to improve spatial imbalance caused by ambient and focal dysfunction (see PTVS and VMSS). In this case, yoked prisms (i.e., prisms which have the same orientation over either eye) are prescribed so that the visual perception of the world is completely shifted for the viewer. Finally, bilateral prisms can be placed on portions of each spectacle lens to improve a patient's awareness of visual information that would fall within a hemifield scotoma. This is referred to as an enhanced sector prism system.

The experienced clinician will recognize that individuals who have a VMSS, as well as a homonymous hemianopsia, will often have difficulty adapting to and succeeding with an enhanced sector prism system because the midline reinforces the spatial neglect. Therefore, treatment with yoked prisms for VMSS is necessary prior to or in conjunction with an enhanced sector prism system. Rehabilitation with yoked prisms to treat VMSS will directly affect field neglect, as well as VMSS. Training can then be established to use the enhanced sector prism systems (149). In other cases of visual loss, including trauma with constricted visual fields, single or multiple prisms are used mounted laterally on each lens (149).

Sector prism systems used to increase a patient's peripheral awareness can be made out of Fresnel press-on prisms. Several reports confirm that the press-on sectoral prisms improve simultaneous awareness and greater obstacle avoidance (150–152), and this should decrease risk of further injury. However, because of the poor optical quality of the press-on Fresnel prisms, sometimes patients experience a decrease in acuity or have problems with reflections or distortions, which negatively affect the patient's acceptance and success. Gottlieb et al.(153) found that press-on prisms might occasionally decrease a patient's tendency to scan into their field of neglect because of the reduced clarity, and this would limit rehabilitative efforts. However, most patients who use enhanced sector prism appreciate an increased awareness of peripheral vision.

Patching

Patching has frequently been used to eliminate diplopia. Although effective, patching renders the patient monocular vision. The chief problems of monocular vision are loss of stereopsis, reduction of peripheral visual field, and VMSS (152). Monocular vision reduces the field of vision by approximately 25%, decreases visual acuity (caused by lack of binocular summation), and impairs spatial orientation. Monocular vs binocular individuals will have a disadvantage in visual-motor skills, exteroception for form and color, and appreciation of the dynamic relationship of the body to the environment needed to facilitate control of manipulation, reaching, and balance. Problems arising from acquired monocular vision will manifest as difficulties in eye-hand coordination, negotiating obstacles, climbing or descending stairs and street curbs, ambulating, driving, and engaging in sports. In the case of diplopia following TBI, a standard recommendation in acute care facilities and rehabilitation hospitals is to patch 1 eye. As discussed previously in the section about VMSS, this will cause and/or reinforce a shift in concept of visual midline affecting posture and balance, as well as having an adverse affect on physical/occupational therapy.

Patching can be performed but should be done with respect to the ambient visual process. A central occlusion patch can be placed on the deviating eye. In this way, diplopia will be eliminated when the person looks directly at something, but the peripheral field of the deviating eye is visible. This allows the ambient visual process of both eyes to begin to match information with other sensorimotor systems. This will support visual midline concept for posture, balance, and ambulation.

Another method involves use of a partial and selective occlusion. The spot patch is a procedure that eliminates diplopia without compromising peripheral vision (154). It is a small round or oval patch made of adhesive tape, blurring film, or other filters. It is placed on the lens of glasses and directly in the line of sight of 1 eye. The diameter is generally about 1 cm but will vary based on the degree of strabismus. Final size and placement is determined by evaluating different sizes and shapes to arrive at the smallest one, which effectively eliminates the diplopia. By eliminating diplopia through central occlusion, the ambient process becomes more effective and supportive. The spot patch is indicated in cases of intractable diplopia where other methods of treatment are either not viable, have failed, or are contraindicated. Central occlusion is effective if the diplopia is constant and the patient exhibits relief and improved general function as a result of eliminating the diplopia.

Determining size, shape, and placement of a central occlusion patch requires measuring the diplopic field, determining limitation of ocular motility, and measuring the angle of strabismic deviation.

Vision Therapy

Vision therapy (also referred to as vision training or orthoptics) is a clinical approach to treat a variety of visual disorders, including certain strabismic conditions. The practice of vision therapy uses a variety of nonsurgical procedures. By first evaluating the bimodal processing of vision, the physician will establish a plan of treatment designed to affect balance between the focal and ambient visual processes, as well as the ability to match information with sensorimotor systems. The goal is to improve the visual processes affecting binocularity, spatial organization, balance, movement, and reaction speed, as well as lessen dizziness, diplopia, and abnormal postures.

Vision therapy will typically require multiple treatment sessions conducted under optometric supervision. Vision therapy techniques employ lenses, prisms, computers, biofeedback, stereoscopic devices, balancing exercises, and eye-hand coordination exercises. Table 45-2 provides an orientation for approaches of treatment for visual processing disorders.

Electrophysiologic Instruments

VEP may be helpful in documenting improvement and perhaps even offering prognostic insight for certain conditions, such as PTVS (63), cortical visual impairment (155), traumatic optic neuropathy (156) and postconcussion visual cognition, and sensory processing (157). However, more studies are needed to explore the use of VEP in the rehabilitative process.

The ERG has already been used to follow a patient undergoing restorative vision rehabilitation with surgically implanted optic nerve prosthesis (101). Another avenue of research that may benefit from electroretinographic evaluation is the effort to explain hypersensitivity to light after BI. It has been reported using non-ERG techniques that this common finding has been associated with elevated dark adaptation thresholds (119) and elevated critical flicker frequency (158) metrics that ERG testing explores thoroughly.

TABLE 45-2 Options for Treatment Including Prisms, Patching, and Vision Therapy

CONDITION	PRISMS	PATCHING	VISION THERAPY
Post Trauma Vision Syndrome (PTVS)	Base-in prisms or asymmetrical yoked prisms		(after treatment for PTVS if needed)
Visual Midline Shift Syndrome (VMSS)	Yoked prisms or asymmetrical yoked prisms		Physical/occupational therapy Neuro-visual postural therapy
Amblyopia		Patch 2 hours/day	Vision therapy
Diplopia	Compensating prisms or asymmetrical yoked prisms	Central occlusion patch	Vision therapy, botox to selected EOMs, and surgical reorienting of EOMs

Abbreviation: EOMs, extraocular muscles.

The EOG has been used to follow patients during the rehabilitative year after BI (130,159) and will likely remain a research and clinical tool of interest as the different manifestations of head injury are explored. However, a particularly exciting variation on the use of EOG in rehabilitation therapy takes advantage of the exquisitely sensitive eye motion-detection technology afforded by the EOG recording. Computer interfaces employing EOG recorders are being developed that assist patients in communicating with and controlling their environment using voluntary globe movements (160,161). Although EOG recording technology has not yet been employed to assist patients in using their blink to control activity, other devices have been developed to allow this (162). Perhaps EOG technology may prove helpful toward blink-driven rehabilitation in the future.

Studies employing ENG (163) and VNG measurements (164) provided objective evidence of the documented clinical improvements patients can hope to achieve when undergoing vestibular rehabilitation for dizziness and balance disorders. Nystagmography is also an important study to consider offering patients who are not improving during vestibular rehabilitation efforts and may help identify undetected injury.

Surgical Intervention

Diplopia can result from interrupted neuromuscular connections, as well as derangement of craniofacial anatomy. Surgical relocation of EOMs can weaken or strengthen underactive or (relatively) overactive muscles, and botulinum toxin injection can also be employed to weaken a relatively overacting muscle. These techniques, as well as oculoplastic reconstruction, can often reorient the 2 eyes so that a patient can enjoy stereo fusion, at least in primary gaze.

Damage to the globe itself is often reparable. The natural crystalline lens can be replaced with an artificial prosthesis. Detached retinas can be reattached using passive means such as gas bubbles or silicon oil in the eye or buckles attached to the sclera, as well as active means of reinforcing the retina to the globe, such as with the use of laser. Corneas can be replaced with natural full- or partial-thickness grafts, and eyes with irreparable surface damage are candidates for implantable lenses, such as the Boston Keratoprosthesis (165). Eyelids that do fail to close can be reanimated with small inserted springs or even with nerve redirection (166). As

might be expected, surgical therapy to the eye carries a risk of morbidity and complications, and therefore, noninvasive therapies are preferred when possible.

Reduced vision and visual field can result from injury to the optic nerve and central visual pathways, respectively. Novel surgical therapies, including prosthetic retinal, optic nerve, and cortical implants, that is, implanted microarrays of stimulators transmitting optical images, are currently under investigation (167).

CONCLUSION

Rehabilitation of a person with a TBI requires a team approach with members representing the spectrum of health care applying modern brain science and technology. Until recently, if a person displays visual dysfunction in the way of binocular, spatial perception, and/or perceptual motor dysfunction, rehabilitation treatment was limited to patching of the deviating eye causing diplopia or primarily hospital-based occupational and physical therapy.

BI affects the entire patient, and there is no aspect of the patient's life that should be overlooked if a patient is to recover fully (see Chapters 38 and 81). Recent advances in diagnostic tests and the understanding of the visual experience have demonstrated a need to ensure that rehabilitative care is integrated and that rehabilitative teams communicate well so that efforts are not counterproductive.

The contribution of vision rehabilitation after BI continues to grow. Novel optical, medical, and surgical techniques are available to improve visual acuity, awareness of visual field, stereoscopic vision, posture, visual reaction time and visual stamina, and attentiveness. An important component of the vision rehabilitation effort is the neuro-optometric rehabilitation optometrist, who brings a burgeoning expertise of visuospatial motor disorders and therapy.

It is our belief that research efforts on behalf of patients affected by TBI should be aimed at exploring the anatomic and physiologic changes causing visual dysfunction. In addition, therapies that promote neuroprotection, neurorecovery (see Chapter 14) and neuroplasticity (see Chapter 13) should receive particular attention, especially as the tools needed to assess these therapies become more widely available. In addition, further research is needed to demonstrate that visuospatial distortion affecting posture and balance can be quantified through measurement of shifts in weight bearing and that rehabilitative approaches incorporating yoked prisms can predict normalizing postural orientation.

KEY CLINICAL POINTS

Although non-ocular vision problems are extremely common after BI, they are often underdiagnosed and undertreated. The following key points represent blending the current state-of-the-art methods for ocular evaluation and neurologic analysis with an understanding of functional organization of vision processing. This amalgam is applied toward an improved model of clinical rehabilitation.

1. Vision is a bimodal process involving ambient and focal pathways. Visual problems after BI can often be presented in terms of an imbalance between these 2 mechanisms of processing.
2. Novel uses of standard physiologic tests (VEP, ERG, EOG) and new imaging modalities (fMRI, DTI, MEG) are expanding our ability to identify damage caused by BI and correlate the symptoms with neuroanatomy.
3. PTVS is a visual processing dysfunction caused by a disassociation between the focal and the ambient processes. Specifically, there is overfocalization on detail (focal binding) and reduction of spatial visual processes.
4. VMSS is a visual processing dysfunction caused by a mismatch of information between the ambient visual process and the sensorimotor system affecting postural control, balance, movement, and spatial orientation.
5. Treatment of the visual processing dysfunction producing PTVS and VMSS employs prisms. This therapy will often reduce symptoms, improve binocular dysfunction, and positively affect balance, posture, and spatial orientation. Combining prisms with physical therapy, occupational therapy, and vestibular therapy maximizes potentials for patient outcome. This highlights the need for an interdisciplinary team to treat BI.
6. Neuro-optometric rehabilitation, a burgeoning discipline distinct from traditional vision therapy and low vision rehabilitation, approaches the visual processing disorders of PTVS and VMSS by attempting to restore the normal interaction of visuomotor and visuoperceptual processes. Neuro-optometric assessment together with traditional neuro-ophthalmologic evaluation offers a means to more completely assess the patient for visual dysfunction and to initiate visual rehabilitation.

KEY REFERENCES

1. Defense and Veterans' Brain Injury Center. Available at: http://www.dvbic.org/Research.aspx. Accessed 2010.
2. Department of Defense/Veterans Administration Vision Center of Excellence. Available at: http://vce.health.mil/resources.aspx. Accessed 2010.
3. Miller NR, Newman NJ, Biousse V, et al, eds. *Walsh and Hoyt's Clinical Neuro-Ophthalmology*. Philadelphia, PA: Lippincott Williams & Wilkins; 2005.
4. Neuro-Optometric Rehabilitation Association. Available at: http://www.nora.cc/. Accessed 2011.
5. Padula WV, Argyris S. Post-trauma vision syndrome and visual midline shift syndrome. *NeuroRehabilitation*. 1996; 6:165–171.

ACKNOWLEDGMENTS

We would like to express our appreciation to Amy Frey, MA for her contributions in support of this chapter.

References

1. Risdall JE, Menon DK. Traumatic brain injury. *Philos Trans R Soc Lond B Biol Sci*. 2011;366(1562):241–250.
2. Sabates NR, Gonce MA, Farris BK. Neuro-ophthalmological findings in closed head trauma. *J Clin Neuroophthalmol*. 1991;11(4): 273–277.
3. Cockerham GC, Goodrich GL, Weichel ED, et al. Eye and visual function in traumatic brain injury. *J Rehabil Res Dev*. 2009;46(6): 811–818.
4. Padula W. *Neuro-Optometric Rehabilitation*. Santa Ana, CA: Optometric Extension Program Publishers; 2000.
5. Suchoff IB, Kapoor N, Ciuffreda KJ, Rutner D, Han E, Craig S. The frequency of occurrence, types, and characteristics of visual field defects in acquired brain injury: a retrospective analysis. *Optometry*. 2008;79(5):259–265.
6. Ciuffreda KJ, Kapoor N, Rutner D, Suchoff IB, Han ME, Craig S. Occurrence of oculomotor dysfunctions in acquired brain injury: a retrospective analysis. *Optometry*. 2007;78(4):155–161.
7. Jin H, Wang S, Hou L, et al. Clinical treatment of traumatic brain injury complicated by cranial nerve injury. *Injury*. 2010;41(9): 918–923.
8. Post RB, Leibowitz HW. Two modes of processing visual information: implications for assessing visual impairment. *Am J Optom Physiol Opt*. 1986;63(2):94–96.
9. Roy S, Jayakumar J, Martin PR, et al. Segregation of short-wavelength-sensitive (S) cone signals in the macaque dorsal lateral geniculate nucleus. *Eur J Neurosci*. 2009;30(8):1517–1526.
10. Ruppertsberg AI, Wuerger SM, Bertamini M. When S-cones contribute to chromatic global motion processing. *Vis Neurosci*. 2007; 24(1):1–8.
11. Rolfs M, Ohl S. Visual suppression in the superior colliculus around the time of microsaccades. *J Neurophysiol*. 2011;105(1):1–3.
12. McDowell JE, Dyckman KA, Austin BP, Clementz BA. Neurophysiology and neuroanatomy of reflexive and volitional saccades: evidence from studies of humans. *Brain Cogn*. 2008;68(3):255–270.
13. Sherman SM. The thalamus is more than just a relay. *Curr Opin Neurobiol*. 2007;17(4):417–422.
14. Saalmann YB, Kastner S. Gain control in the visual thalamus during perception and cognition. *Curr Opin Neurobiol*. 2009;19(4):408–414.
15. Sincich LC, Park KF, Wohlgemuth MJ, Horton JC. Bypassing V1: a direct geniculate input to area MT. *Nat Neurosci*. 2004;7(10): 1123–1128.
16. Vakalopoulos C. A theory of blindsight—the anatomy of the unconscious: a proposal for the koniocellular projections and intralaminar thalamus. *Med Hypotheses*. 2005;65(6):1183–1190.
17. Brown JM. Visual streams and shifting attention. *Prog Brain Res*. 2009;176:47–63.
18. Sincich LC, Jocson CM, Horton JC. V1 interpatch projections to v2 thick stripes and pale stripes. *J Neurosci*. 2010;30(20):6963–6974.
19. Demer JL. Mechanics of the orbita. *Dev Ophthalmol*. 2007;40: 132–157.
20. Miller JM. Functional anatomy of normal human rectus muscles. *Vision Res*. 1989;29(2):223–240.
21. Clark RA, Miller JM, Demer JL. Location and stability of rectus muscle pulleys. Muscle paths as a function of gaze. *Invest Ophthalmol Vis Sci*. 1997;38(1):227–240.
22. Demer JL. The orbital pulley system: a revolution in concepts of orbital anatomy. *Ann N Y Acad Sci*. 2002;956:17–32.
23. Demer JL. Gillies Lecture: ocular motility in a time of paradigm shift. *Clin Experiment Ophthalmol*. 2006;34(9):822–826.
24. Kraus MF, Little DM, Donnell AJ, Reilly JL, Simonian N, Sweeney JA. Oculomotor function in chronic traumatic brain injury. *Cogn Behav Neurol*. 2007;20(3):170–178.

25. Leigh RJ, Zee DS. *The neurology of eye movements*. Available at: http://www.loc.gov/catdir/enhancements/fy0637/2005022301-d.html. Accessed 2006.

26. Xu GQ, Lan Y, Huang DF, et al. Visuospatial attention deficit in patients with local brain lesions. *Brain Res*. 2010;1322:153–159.

27. Amiez C, Petrides M. Anatomical organization of the eye fields in the human and non-human primate frontal cortex. *Prog Neurobiol*. 2009;89(2):220–230.

28. Boy F, Husain M, Singh KD, Sumner P. Supplementary motor area activations in unconscious inhibition of voluntary action. *Exp Brain Res*. 2010;206(4):441–448.

29. Muggleton NG, Kalla R, Juan CH, Walsh V. Dissociating the contributions of human frontal eye fields and posterior parietal cortex to visual search. *J Neurophysiol*. 2011;105(6):2891–2896.

30. Vernet M, Yang Q, Kapoula Z. Guiding binocular saccades during reading: a TMS study of the PPC. *Front Hum Neurosci*. 2011;5:14.

31. Leh SE, Chakravarty MM, Ptito A. The connectivity of the human pulvinar: a diffusion tensor imaging tractography study. *Int J Biomed Imaging*. 2008;2008:789539.

32. Van Ettinger-Veenstra HM, Huijbers W, Gutteling TP, Vink M, Kenemans JL, Neggers SF. fMRI-guided TMS on cortical eye fields: the frontal but not intraparietal eye fields regulate the coupling between visuospatial attention and eye movements. *J Neurophysiol*. 2009;102(6):3469–3480.

33. Chen LL, Tehovnik EJ. Cortical control of eye and head movements: integration of movements and percepts. *Eur J Neurosci*. 2007; 25(5):1253–1264.

34. Biber U, Ilg UJ. Visual stability and the motion aftereffect: a psychophysical study revealing spatial updating. *PLoS One*. 2011;6(1): e16265.

35. Born S, Kerzel D, Theeuwes J. Evidence for a dissociation between the control of oculomotor capture and disengagement. *Exp Brain Res*. 2011;208(4):621–631.

36. DeHaan A, Halterman C, Langan J, et al. Cancelling planned actions following mild traumatic brain injury. *Neuropsychologia*. 2007; 45(2):406–411.

37. Cotti J, Panouilleres M, Munoz DP, Vercher JL, Pélisson D, Guillaume A. Adaptation of reactive and voluntary saccades: different patterns of adaptation revealed in the antisaccade task. *J Physiol*. 2009;587(pt 1):127–138.

38. Berman RA, Wurtz RH. Signals conveyed in the pulvinar pathway from superior colliculus to cortical area MT. *J Neurosci*. 2011;31(2): 373–384.

39. Walker MF, Tian J, Shan X, Tamargo RJ, Ying H, Zee DS. The cerebellar nodulus/uvula integrates otolith signals for the translational vestibulo-ocular reflex. *PLoS One*. 2010;5(11):e13981.

40. Dagnelie G. *Visual Prosthetics: Physiology, Bioengineering, Rehabilitation*. New York, NY: Springer; 2011.

41. Wunderlich K, Schneider KA, Kastner S. Neural correlates of binocular rivalry in the human lateral geniculate nucleus. *Nat Neurosci*. 2005;8(11):1595–1602.

42. Backus BT, Fleet DJ, Parker AJ, Heeger DJ. Human cortical activity correlates with stereoscopic depth perception. *J Neurophysiol*. 2001; 86(4):2054–2068.

43. Trotter Y, Celebrini S, Beaux JC, Grandjean B, Imbert M. Long-term dysfunctions of neural stereoscopic mechanisms after unilateral extraocular muscle proprioceptive deafferentation. *J Neurophysiol*. 1993;69(5):1513–1529.

44. Balslev D, Albert NB, Miall C. Eye muscle proprioception is represented bilaterally in the sensorimotor cortex. *Hum Brain Mapp*. 2011;32(4):624–631.

45. Cottereau BR, McKee SP, Ales JM, Norcia AM. Disparity-tuned population responses from human visual cortex. *J Neurosci*. 2011; 31(3):954–965.

46. Minini L, Parker AJ, Bridge H. Neural modulation by binocular disparity greatest in human dorsal visual stream. *J Neurophysiol*. 2010;104(1):169–178.

47. Erkelens CJ. Organisation of signals involved in binocular perception and vergence control. *Vision Res*. 2001;41(25–26):3497–3503.

48. Durand JB, Celebrini S, Trotter Y. Neural bases of stereopsis across visual field of the alert macaque monkey. *Cereb Cortex*. 2007;17(6): 1260–1273.

49. Magrun W. *Integrating Neural Systems: improving Performance in Children With Learning Disabilities*. Las Cruces, NM: Clinician's View; 2006.

50. Moore J. *The Neuroanatomy of the Visual System*. Las Cruces, NM: Clinician's View; 2001.

51. Shumway-Cook A, Woollcott M. *Motor Control Theory and Practical Applications*. Baltimore, MD: Williams & Wilkins; 1995.

52. Gahery Y, Massion J. Coordination between posture and movement. *Trends Neuroscience*. 1981;4:199–202.

53. Falla D, Rainoldi A, Merletti R, Jull G. Spatio-temporal evaluation of neck muscle activation during postural perturbations in healthy subjects. *J Electromyogr Kinesiol*. 2004;14(4):463–474.

54. Buchanan JJ, Horak FB. Emergence of postural patterns as a function of vision and translation frequency. *J Neurophysiol*. 1999;81(5): 2325–2339.

55. Bobath B. *Abnormal Postural Reflex Activity Caused by Brain Damage*. 3rd ed. London, UK: Heinnemann Medical Books; 1987.

56. Schlageter K, Gray B, Hall K, Shaw R, Sammet R. Incidence and treatment of visual dysfunction in traumatic brain injury. *Brain Inj*. 1993;7(5):439–448.

57. Crutchfield C, Barnes MR. *Motor Control and Motor Learning in Rehabilitation*. Atlanta, GA: Stokesville Publishing; 1993.

58. Magrun W. Evaluating quality in motor behavior. In: Padula WV, ed. *Neuro-Optometric Rehabilitation*. Santa Ana, CA: Optometric Extension Program Foundation; 2000.

59. Nelson C. *Head Trauma and Related Tissue Trauma*. Las Cruces, NM: Clinician's View; 2008.

60. Nelson C, Senesa C. Management of clinical problems of children with CP. In: Umphred D, ed. *Neurological Rehabilitation*. Philadelphia, PA: Mosby-Elsevier; 2007:357–385.

61. Benabib R, Nelson CA. Efficiency in visual skills and postural control: a dynamic interaction. *Occupational Therapy Practice*. 1993: 57–68.

62. Nelson C. *Improving Movement and Postural Control in Children With Neuromotor Dysfunction*. Las Cruces, NM: Clinician's View; 2002.

63. Padula WV, Argyris S, Ray J. Visual evoked potentials (VEP) evaluating treatment for post-trauma vision syndrome (PTVS) in patients with traumatic brain injuries (TBI). *Brain Inj*. 1994;8(2): 125–133.

64. Rappaport M, Herrero-Backe C, Winterfield K, et al. Visual evoked potential pattern abnormalities and disability in severe traumatically brain injured patients. *J Head Trauma*. 1989;4(2):45–52.

65. Sarno S, Erasmus LP, Lippert G, Frey M, Lipp B, Schlaegel W. Electrophysiological correlates of visual impairments after traumatic brain injury. *Vision Res*. 2000;40(21):3029–3038.

66. Thiagarajan P, Ciuffreda KJ, Ludlam DP. Vergence dysfunction in mild traumatic brain injury (mTBI): a review. *Ophthalmic Physiol Opt*. 2011;31(5): 456–468.

67. Suh M, Kolster R, Sarkar R, McCandliss B, Ghajar J; for Cognitive and Neurobiological Research Consortium. Deficits in predictive smooth pursuit after mild traumatic brain injury. *Neurosci Lett*. 2006;401(1–2):108–113.

68. Suh M, Basu S, Kolster R, Sarkar R, McCandliss B, Ghajar J. Increased oculomotor deficits during target blanking as an indicator of mild traumatic brain injury. *Neurosci Lett*. 2006;410(3):203–207.

69. Wright KW, Fox BE, Eriksen KJ. PVEP evidence of true suppression in adult onset strabismus. *J Pediatr Ophthalmol Strabismus*. 1990; 27(4):196–201.

70. Green W, Ciuffreda KJ, Thiagarajan P, Szymanowicz D, Ludlam DP, Kapoor N. Accommodation in mild traumatic brain injury. *J Rehabil Res Dev*. 2010;47(3):183–99.

71. Rossi T, Boccassini B, Esposito L, et al. The pathogenesis of retinal damage in blunt eye trauma: finite element modeling. *Invest Ophthalmol Vis Sci*. 2011;52(7):3994–4002.

72. Schievink WI. Spontaneous spinal cerebrospinal fluid leaks. *Cephalalgia*. 2008;28(12):1345–1356.

73. Wan MJ, Nomura H, Tator CH. Conversion to symptomatic Chiari I malformation after minor head or neck trauma. *Neurosurgery*. 2008;63(4):748–53.

74. Pilon A, Rhee P, Newman T, Messner L. Bilateral abducens palsies and facial weakness as initial manifestations of a Chiari 1 malformation. *Optom Vis Sci*. 2007;84(10):936–940.

75. Janssen K, Wojciechowski M, Poot S, De Keyser K, Ceulemans B. Isolated abducens nerve palsy after closed head trauma: a pediatric case report. *Pediatr Emerg Care.* 2008;24(9):621–623.

76. Sam B, Ozveren MF, Akdemir I, et al. The mechanism of injury of the abducens nerve in severe head trauma: a postmortem study. *Forensic Sci Int.* 2004;140(1):25–32.

77. Sharpe JA, Kumar S, Sundaram AN. Ocular torsion and vertical misalignment. *Curr Opin Neurol.* 2011;24(1):18–24.

78. Brodsky MC, Donahue SP, Vaphiades M, Brandt T. Skew deviation revisited. *Surv Ophthalmol.* 2006;51(2):105–128.

79. Kushner BJ, Hariharan L. Observations about objective and subjective ocular torsion. *Ophthalmology.* 2009;116(10):2001–2010.

80. Bodack MI. Pediatric acquired brain injury. *Optometry.* 2010;81(10):516–527.

81. Caeyenberghs K, van Roon D, van Aken K, De Cock P. Static and dynamic visuomotor task performance in children with acquired brain injury: predictive control deficits under increased temporal pressure. *J Head Trauma Rehabil.* 2009;24(5):363–373.

82. Scheiman M, Gwiazda J, Li T. Non-surgical interventions for convergence insufficiency. *Cochrane Database Syst Rev.* 2011;(3):CD006768.

83. Ciuffreda KJ, Han Y, Kapoor N, Ficarra AP. Oculomotor rehabilitation for reading in acquired brain injury. *NeuroRehabilitation.* 2006;21(1):9–21.

84. Erickson JC. Treatment outcomes of chronic post-traumatic headaches after mild head trauma in US soldiers: an observational study. *Headache.* 2011;51(6):932–944.

85. Padula W, Argyris S. Post-trauma vision syndrome and visual midline shift syndrome. *NeuroRehab.* 1996;6:165–171.

86. Padula WV, Nelson CA, Benabib R, Yilmaz T, Krevisky S. Modifying postural adaptation following a CVA through prismatic shift of visuo-spatial egocenter. *Brain Inj.* 2009;23(6):566–576.

87. Padula W, Munitz R, Magrun M. eds. *Neuro-Visual Processing: An Integrated Model of Rehabilitation.* Santa Ana, CA: Optometric Extension Program Foundation Press; 2012.

88. Zoltan B. Visual, visual perceptual and perceptual-motor deficits in brain injured adults. *Traumatic Brain Injury.* 1992;3:337–355.

89. Saj A., Honoré J, Richard C, Bernati T, Rousseaux M. Hemianopia and neglect influence on straight-ahead perception. *Eur Neurol.* 2010;64(5):297–303.

90. Leys M, Verriest G, de Bie S. Results of manual and automated perimetry in the postconcussive patient. In: Proceedings of the VIII International Perimetry Society Meeting; 1988; Vancouver, Canada.

91. O'Neill EC, Connell PP, O'Connor JC, Brady J, Reid I, Logan P. Prism therapy and visual rehabilitation in homonymous visual field loss. *Optom Vis Sci.* 2011;88(2):263–268.

92. Fortis P, Maravita A, Gallucci M, et al. Rehabilitating patients with left spatial neglect by prism exposure during a visuomotor activity. *Neuropsychology.* 2010;24(6):681–697.

93. Machner B, Sprenger A, Sander T, et al. Visual search disorders in acute and chronic homonymous hemianopia: lesion effects and adaptive strategies. *Ann N Y Acad Sci.* 2009;1164:419–426.

94. Kerkhoff G, Oppenländer K, Finke K, Bublak P. Therapy for cerebral visual perception disturbances (in German). *Nervenarzt.* 2007;78(4):457–469.

95. George S, Hayes A, Chen C, Crotty M. The effect of static scanning and mobility training on mobility in people with hemianopia after stroke: a randomized controlled trial comparing standardized versus non-standardized treatment protocols. *BMC Neurol.* 2011;11:87.

96. Barton JJ. Disorders of higher visual processing. *Handb Clin Neurol.* 2011;102:223–261.

97. Odom JV, Bach M, Brigell M, et al. ISCEV standard for clinical visual evoked potentials (2009 update). *Doc Ophthalmol.* 2010;120(1):111–119.

98. Hajipour S, Shamsollahi MB, Abootalebi V. Visual acuity classification using single trial visual evoked potentials. *Conf Proc IEEE Eng Med Biol Soc.* 2009;2009:982–985.

99. Heckenlively JR, Arden GB, eds. *Principles and Practice of Clinical Electrophysiology of Vision.* 2nd ed. Cambridge, MA: MIT Press; 2006.

100. Wygnanski-Jaffe T, Panton CM, Buncic JR, Westall CA. Paradoxical robust visual evoked potentials in young patients with cortical blindness. *Doc Ophthalmol.* 2009;119(2):101–107.

101. Brelén ME, Vince V, Gérard B, Veraart C, Delbeke J. Measurement of evoked potentials after electrical stimulation of the human optic nerve. *Invest Ophthalmol Vis Sci.* 2010;51(10):5351–5355.

102. Sannita WG, Carozzo S, Fioretto M, Garbarino S, Martinoli C. Abnormal waveform of the human pattern VEP: contribution from gamma oscillatory components. *Invest Ophthalmol Vis Sci.* 2007;48(10):4534–4541.

103. Yukawa E, Matsuura T, Kim YJ, Taketani F, Hara Y. Usefulness of multifocal VEP in a child requiring perimetry. *Pediatr Neurol.* 2008;38(5):360–362.

104. Johansson B, Jakobsson P. Fourier-analysed steady-state VEPs in pre-school children with and without normal binocularity. *Doc Ophthalmol.* 2006;112(1):13–22.

105. Lachapelle J, McKerra M, Jauffret C, Bach M. Temporal resolution of orientation-defined texture segregation: a VEP study. *Doc Ophthalmol.* 2008;117(2):155–162.

106. Marmor M, Fulton AB, Holder GE, Miyake Y, Brigell M, Bach M; for International Society for Clinical Electrophysiology of Vision. ISCEV Standard for full-field clinical electroretinography (2008 update). *Doc Ophthalmol.* 2009;118(1):69–77.

107. Miura G, Wang MH, Ivers KM, Frishman LJ. Retinal pathway origins of the pattern ERG of the mouse. *Exp Eye Res.* 2009;89(1):49–62.

108. Holder G, Brigell MG, Hawlina M, Meigen T, Vaegan, Bach M; for International Society for Clinical Electrophysiolog of Vision. ISCEV standard for clinical pattern electroretinography—2007 update. *Doc Ophthalmol.* 2007;114(3):111–116.

109. Hood D, Bach M, Brigell M, et al. ISCEV guidelines for clinical multifocal electroretinography (2007 edition). *Doc Ophthalmol.* 2008;116(1):1–11.

110. Hood D, Odel JG, Chen CS, Winn BJ. The multifocal electroretinogram. *J Neuroophthalmol.* 2003;23(3):225–235.

111. Freed S, Hellerstein LF. Visual electrodiagnostic findings in mild traumatic brain injury. *Brain Inj.* 1997;11(1):25–36.

112. Dougherty A, MacGregor AJ, Han PP, Heltemes KJ, Galarneau MR. Visual dysfunction following blast-related traumatic brain injury from the battlefield. *Brain Inj.* 2011;25(1):8–13.

113. Noia Lda C, Berezovsky A, Freitas D, Sacai PY, Salomão SR. Clinical and electroretinographic profile of commotio retinae (in Portuguese). *Arq Bras Oftalmol.* 2006;69(6):895–906.

114. Link B, Michelson G, Horn FK, Jünemann A. Accidental focal laser injury—a correlation of electrophysiology, perimetry and clinical findings. *Doc Ophthalmol.* 2008;117(1):69–72.

115. Tanito M, Kaidzu S, Anderson RE. Protective effects of soft acrylic yellow filter against blue light-induced retinal damage in rats. *Exp Eye Res.* 2006;83(6):1493–1504.

116. Mizota A, Tanaka M, Kubota M, et al. Dose-response effect of charged carbon beam on normal rat retina assessed by electroretinography. *Int J Radiat Oncol Biol Phys.* 2010;78(5):1532–1540.

117. Smith D. Clinical update: the wounds of war. Brain injury and vision loss from blast trauma. In: *EyeNet Magazine.* American Academy of Ophthalmology; 2008.

118. Harper M, et al. Visual system damage in a rodent model of blast-*induced* traumatic brain injury. Poster presented at: 3rd Annual Midwest Eye Research Symposium: 2010; University of Iowa.

119. Du T, Ciuffreda KJ, Kapoor N. Elevated dark adaptation thresholds in traumatic brain injury. *Brain Inj.* 2005;19(13):1125–1138.

120. Schatz P, Bitner H, Sander B, et al. Evaluation of macular structure and function by OCT and electrophysiology in patients with vitelliform macular dystrophy due to mutations in BEST1. *Invest Ophthalmol Vis Sci.* 2010;51(9):4754–4765.

121. Good P, Gross K. Electrophysiology and metallosis: support for an oxidative (free radical) mechanism in the human eye. *Ophthalmologica.* 1988;196(4):204–209.

122. Rigaudière F, Ingster-Moati I, Hache JC, et al. Up-dated ophthalmological screening and follow-up management for long-term antimalarial treatment (in French). *J Fr Ophtalmol.* 2004;27(2):191–199.

123. Rigolet M, Baulac M, Nordmann JP. Electrophysiological monitoring of epileptic patients treated with Vigabatrin. *J Fr Ophtalmol.* 2005;28(6):535–541.

124. Arndt CF, Husson J, Derambure P, Hache JC, Arnaud B, Defoort-Dhellemmes S. Retinal electrophysiological results in patients receiving lamotrigine monotherapy. *Epilepsia.* 2005;46(7):1055–1060.

125. Crochet M, Ingster-Moati I, Even G, Dupuy P. Retinopathy caused by interferon alpha associated with ribavirin therapy and the importance of the electro-oculogram: a case report. *J Fr Ophtalmol.* 2004;27(3):257–262.

126. Hidajat R, McLay JL, Goode DH, Spearing RL. EOG as a monitor of desferrioxamine retinal toxicity. *Doc Ophthalmol.* 2004;109(3):273–278.

127. Starck M, Albrecht H, Pöllmann W, Dieterich M, Straube A. Acquired pendular nystagmus in multiple sclerosis: an examiner-blind cross-over treatment study of memantine and gabapentin. *J Neurol.* 2010;257(3):322–327.

128. Mosimann U, Müri RM, Burn DJ, Felblinger J, O'Brien JT, McKeith IG. Saccadic eye movement changes in Parkinson's disease dementia and dementia with Lewy bodies. *Brain.* 2005;128(pt 6):1267–1276.

129. Jackson L, Morgan B, Fletcher JC Jr, Krueger WW. Anterior canal benign paroxysmal positional vertigo: an underappreciated entity. *Otol Neurotol.* 2007;28(2):218–222.

130. Prushansky T, Dvir Z, Pevzner E, Gordon CR. Electro-oculographic measures in patients with chronic whiplash and healthy subjects: a comparative study. *J Neurol Neurosurg Psychiatry.* 2004;75(11):1642–1644.

131. Lang EE, McConn Walsh R. Vestibular function testing. *Ir J Med Sci.* 2010;179(2):173–178.

132. Gananca MM, Caovilla HH, Gananca FF. Electronystagmography versus videonystagmography. *Braz J Otorhinolaryngol.* 2010;76(3):399–403.

133. Ernst A, Basta D, Seidl RO, Todt I, Scherer H, Clarke A. Management of posttraumatic vertigo. *Otolaryngol Head Neck Surg.* 2005;132(4):554–558.

134. Fausti SA, Wilmington DJ, Gallun FJ, Myers PJ, Henry JA. Auditory and vestibular dysfunction associated with blast-related traumatic brain injury. *J Rehabil Res Dev.* 2009;46(6):797–810.

135. Scherer MR, Shelhamer MJ, Schubert MC. Characterizing high-velocity angular vestibulo-ocular reflex function in service members post-blast exposure. *Exp Brain Res.* 2011;208(3):399–410.

136. Corrales CE, Monfared A, Jackler RK. Facial and vestibulocochlear nerve avulsion at the fundus of the internal auditory canal in a child without a temporal bone fracture. *Otol Neurotol.* 2010;31(9):1508–1510.

137. Adil EA, Choudhary AK, Moser KW, Ghossaini SN. Vestibular pneumolabyrinth: why assessment with temporal bone computed tomography utilizing dynamic focal spot mode is important for the diagnosis. *Emerg Radiol.* 2011;18(1):43–45.

138. Heitger MH, Jones RD, Macleod AD, Snell DL, Frampton CM, Anderson TJ. Impaired eye movements in post-concussion syndrome indiate suboptimal brain function beyond the influence of depression, malingering or intellectual ability. *Brain.* 2009;132(pt 10):2850–2870.

139. Fumeya H, Hideshima H. Cerebellar concussion—three case reports. *Neurol Med Chir (Tokyo).* 1994;34(9):612–615.

140. Mayer AR, Mannell MV, Ling J, Gasparovic C, Yeo RA. Functional connectivity in mild traumatic brain injury. *Hum Brain Mapp.* 2011;32(11):1825–1835.

141. Slobounov SM, Gay M, Zhang K, et al. Alteration of brain functional network at rest and in response to Y MCA physical stress in concussed athletes: RsFMRI study. *Neuroimage.* 2011;55(4):1716–1727.

142. Matthews S, Simmons A, Strigo I. The effects of loss versus alteration of consciousness on inhibition-related brain activity among individuals with a history of blast-related concussion. *Psychiatry Res.* 2011;191(1):76–79.

143. Peskind ER, Petrie EC, Cross DJ, et al. Cerebrocerebellar hypometabolism associated with repetitive blast exposure mild traumatic brain injury in 12 Iraq war veterans with persistent post-concussive symptoms. *Neuroimage.* 2011;54(suppl 1):S76–S82.

144. Lewine JD, Davis JT, Bigler ED, et al. Objective documentation of traumatic brain injury subsequent to mild head trauma: multimodal brain imaging with MEG, SPECT, and MRI. *J Head Trauma Rehabil.* 2007;22(3):141–155.

145. Huang MX, Theilmann RJ, Robb A, et al. Integrated imaging approach with MEG and DTI to detect mild traumatic brain injury in military and civilian patients. *J Neurotrauma.* 2009;26(8):1213–1226.

146. Raemaekers M, Bergsma DP, van Wezel RJ, van der Wildt GJ, van den Berg AV. Effects of vision restoration training on early visual cortex in patients with cerebral blindness investigated with functional magnetic resonance imaging. *J Neurophysiol.* 2011;105(2):872–882.

147. Nyakale N, Clauss RP, Nel W, Sathekge M. Clinical and brain SPECT scan response to zolpidem in patients after brain damage. *Arzneimittelforschung.* 2010;60(4):177–181.

148. Särkämö T, Pihko E, Laitinen S, et al. Music and speech listening enhance the recovery of early sensory processing after stroke. *J Cogn Neurosci.* 2010;22(12):2716–2727.

149. Gottlieb DD, Fuhr A, Hatch WV, Wright KD. Neuro-optometric facilitation of vision recovery after acquired brain injury. *Neuro Rehabilitation.* 1998;11(3)197–199.

150. Lee AG, Perez AM. Improving awareness of peripheral visual field using sectoral prism. *J Am Optom Assoc.* 1999;70(10):624–628.

151. Peli E. Field expansion of homonymous hemianopsia by optically induced peripheral exotropia. *Optom Vis Sci.* 2000;77(9):453–464.

152. Park W. Post-trauma vision syndrome: prescribing prism for the brain injury patient. *Primary Care Optometry News.* 1998:31–32.

153. Gottlieb D, Allen CH, Eikenberry J, et al. Living with vision loss—independence, driving, and low vision solutions. Atlanta, GA: St. Barthelemy Press, Ltd.; 1996.

154. Politzer TA. Case studies of a new approach using partial and selective occlusion for the clinical treatment of diplopia. *Neuro Rehab.* 1996;6:213–217.

155. Watson T, Orel-Bixler D, Haegerstrom-Portnoy G. Early visual-evoked potential acuity and future behavioral acuity in cortical visual impairment. *Optom Vis Sci.* 2010;87(2):80–86.

156. Bhattacharjee H, Bhattacharjee K, Jain L, et al. Indirect optic nerve injury in two-wheeler riders in northeast India. *Indian J Ophthalmol.* 2008;56(6):475–480.

157. Folmer RL, Billings CJ, Diedesch-Rouse AC, Gallun FJ, Lew HL. Electrophysiological assessments of cognition and sensory processing in TBI: applications for diagnosis, prognosis and rehabilitation. *Int J Psychophysiol.* 2011;82(1):4–15.

158. Chang TT, Ciuffreda KJ, Kapoor N. Critical flicker frequency and related symptoms in mild traumatic brain injury. *Brain Inj.* 2007;21(10):1055–1062.

159. Kongsted A, Jørgensen LV, Leboeuf-Yde C, Qerama E, Korsholm L, Bendix T. Are altered smooth pursuit eye movements related to chronic pain and disability following whiplash injuries? A prospective trial with one-year follow-up. *Clin Rehabil.* 2008;22(5):469–479.

160. Usakli AB, Gurkan S, Aloise F, Vecchiato G, Babiloni F. A hybrid platform based on EOG and EEG signals to restore communication for patients afflicted with progressive motor neuron diseases. *Conf Proc IEEE Eng Med Biol Soc.* 2009;2009:543–546.

161. Barea R, Boquete L, Mazo M, López E. *System for assisted mobility using eye movements based on electrooculography.* IEEE Trans Neural Syst Rehabil Eng. 2002;10(4):209–218.

162. Tota A, Lancioni GE, Singh NN, O'Reilly MF, Sigafoos J, Oliva D. Evaluating the applicability of optic microswitches for eyelid responses in students with profound multiple disabilities. *Disabil Rehabil Assist Technol.* 2005;1(4):217–223.

163. Rzewnicki I, Rogowski M. Vestibular rehabilitation of vertigo and dizziness (in Polish). *Pol Merkur Lekarski.* 2008;24(141):244–246.

164. Patatas OH, Gananca CF, Gananca FF. Quality of life of individuals submitted to vestibular rehabilitation. *Braz J Otorhinolaryngol.* 2009;75(3):387–394.

165. Pujari S, Siddique SS, Dohlman CH, Chodosh J. The Boston keratoprosthesis type II: the Massachusetts Eye and Ear Infirmary experience. *Cornea.* 2011;30(12):1298–1303.

166. Chan JY, Byrne PJ. Management of facial paralysis in the 21st century. *Facial Plast Surg.* 2011;27(4):346–357.

167. Guenther T, Lovell NH, Suaning GJ. Bionic vision: system architectures—a review. *Expert Rev Med Devices.* 2012;9(1):33–48.

Audiologic Impairment

Daniel H. Coelho and Michael Hoffer

INTRODUCTION

Traumatic brain injury (TBI) is the leading cause of death and disability in the Unites States, with an estimated incidence of 1.4 million persons each year (1,2). Given the severity of the force required to cause TBI, many patients will have concurrent trauma to the auditory pathway (3). Large series suggest that 48%–74% of individuals who suffer head trauma will display some type of hearing loss (4,5). Despite the protection of the middle and inner ear afforded by its location deep within the temporal bone, different kinds of injuries can affect hearing in different ways. Civilian populations are susceptible to blunt, penetrating, baro-, electric, acoustic, and thermal injury, which all result in different patterns of auditory dysfunction. Many of these classes of injury can result from one traumatic event. Within military populations, blast and acoustic trauma are frequent sequela of modern warfare. One-quarter of all injuries among marines during Operation Iraqi Freedom through 2004 sustained auditory injury—the most common single injury type (6). Auditory dysfunction is the most prevalent service-connected disability for US military personnel, with compensation topping more than $1 billion annually (7). This number can only be expected to grow because traumatic sensorineural hearing loss (SNHL) is often progressive with time.

Unfortunately, many patients who sustain massive cranial injury do not survive to report subjective hearing loss. For the patients that do survive, the clinician must always maintain a high index of suspicion for otologic and neurotologic dysfunction, irrespective of etiology. Failure to identify and treat even mild injury to the auditory system can result in a significant detriment to quality of life.

ANATOMY AND PHYSIOLOGY

Damage to the auditory system can occur in many forms, and soft tissue damage and neurologic dysfunction may occur independently. However, because of the important role in sound conduction and hearing that each of the structures of the ear provide, most injuries are likely to result in some degree of hearing loss. Before engaging in detailed discussion of the mechanisms of traumatic hearing loss, review of the normal anatomy and physiology of hearing is warranted.

Developmentally and functionally, the anatomy of the human ear can be divided into the external ear (including the pinna and external auditory canal), the middle ear (including the tympanic membrane (TM), the middle ear cavity, and the ossicular chain), and the inner ear (including the cochlea, vestibular organs, facial nerve, and supporting structures). The inner ear contains the most sensitive neurosensory portions of the auditory system, and is encased completely by the otic capsule of the temporal bone—the hardest bone in the human body.

Sound is a form of mechanical energy. Vibrations from a source cause small oscillations of air molecules that in turn vibrate adjacent air molecules. As sound propagates away from its source, the wave of pressure is characterized by frequency (pitch) and intensity (volume). Sound waves travel fastest in solids, slower in liquids, and slowest in air. Therefore, because the cochlea is a fluid-filled structure, land dwelling animals adapted to offset the volume decrease caused by the energy dissipated going from air to liquid. This has been achieved in multiple ways. Large pinna function as sound collectors increase gain by approximately 20 dB. The large surface area of the ear drum compared to the small surface area of the stapes (14:1) increases vibrational amplitude. Furthermore, lever action between the incus and malleus results in an additional 1.3:1 gain. Overall, the gain achieved from the middle ear is more than 30 dB. These mechanical force amplifiers are able to overcome the energy lost from the air/fluid impedance mismatch. The fluid wave travels within the cochlea and vibrates the organ of Corti. The organ of Corti includes approximately 20,000 auditory nerve receptors, each with its own hair cell. The shearing of the hair cells results in depolarization of the auditory nerve, leading to signal transmission to the spiral ganglion, cochlear nucleus within the brainstem, through the thalamus, and ultimately to the auditory cortex. The reception and transmission of sound is part of a highly specialized sensory system that allows for the human ear to hear frequencies ranging from 20 Hz to 20,000 Hz with an intensities ranging more than a 100,000-fold difference in energy (120 dB).

Although the ear is able to withstand massive forces, certain injuries are significant enough to damage the delicate structures within temporal bone and brain. Depending on where in the pathway of sound the insult occurs, different types and severities of hearing loss can occur. Conductive hearing loss (CHL) occurs when physical or mechanical obstruction of the external or middle ears prevents the transmission of energy to the inner ear. This results in a decrease in the volume of sounds presented to the patient, but rarely affects the clarity of the sounds received. SNHL occurs when damage to the structures of the inner ear interferes with either the conversion of mechanical energy to neural energy or directly by neural injury. Patients with SNHL also have a decrease in the volume of sounds perceived, but when severe enough, the clarity of sound signal can deteriorate. CHL and SNHL can occur independently, but when both types of injury are present, it is called mixed hearing loss.

For centuries, the main focus of conventional hearing loss has been on the peripheral auditory system—those mechanisms of hearing housed in the ear. However, over time, great strides in neuroscience have revealed critical portions of the hearing pathways within the brainstem, midbrain, and cerebral cortex. When damage occurs to this central auditory system, as is frequently seen in TBI, the injury can go undiagnosed because such injury is unfamiliar to many in the hearing health field traditionally trained only in disorders of the peripheral auditory system.

EVALUATION

Unfortunately, otologic damage (both audiologic and vestibular) are overlooked in patients with significant head trauma. Moreover, patients with TBI can be misdiagnosed as unresponsive or underresponsive when hearing loss is present (8). A thorough understanding of the diagnosis and management of auditory dysfunction is critical to the comprehensive care of the patient with trauma.

For patients with multitrauma, examination for signs or symptoms of audiologic dysfunction is secondary to the ABCs of emergency resuscitation. Once airway and neurologic stabilization has occurred, attention can be then focused on potential otologic trauma. As with any injury, proper evaluation begins with a thorough history. Understanding of the situation in which the trauma occurred is crucial toward predicting and managing the injuries sustained. The mechanism of injury, strength, distance, duration, and volume of exposure are all key variables. Patients must be questioned regarding symptoms suggestive of otologic injury, including hearing loss, tinnitus, vertigo, aural fullness, pain, or otorrhea.

The physical exam begins with careful inspection of the auricle, mastoid, and facial structures. Periorbital ecchymosis (raccoon eye) and ecchymosis overlying the mastoid (Battle's sign) are indicative of skull base fractures—heightening clinical suspicion of possible otologic damage. Otoscopic examination, ideally under the microscope, assesses the auricle, external auditory canal, tympanic membrane, and, frequently, the ossicles. Debris and blood should be carefully removed from the external auditory canal, and squamous debris should be removed from the middle ear to prevent possible cholesteatoma ingrowth. Clear drainage from the ear canal or middle ear may signify cerebrospinal fluid (CSF) leak. Pneumatic otoscopy can help distinguish fluid in the middle ear, perforations, or malleus fractures. Nystagmus and vertigo with pneumatic otoscopy may indicate violation of the inner ear, resulting in a perilymph fistula. The Weber and Rinne tuning fork tests provide a gross assessment of hearing, and can help lateralize pathology and distinguish conductive hearing loss from SNHL. Finally, weakness of cranial nerves, especially facial function may indicate significant injury to the temporal bone.

A variety of audiologic testing can be performed to localize, characterize, and quantify hearing loss. Both air and bone conducting pure-tone audiometry can determine the type of hearing loss (CHL, SNHL, or mixed) as well as degree of loss across a range of frequencies. Speech discrimination scores test clarity and can therefore provide insight toward

potential cochlear damage. However, the aforementioned tests may not be sufficient for all patients. Patients with trauma who have sustained significant soft tissue damage to the mastoid, auricle, or auditory canal may not be able to wear the headphones or inserts necessary to perform this test. Furthermore, because tone and speech audiometry require subjective responses, results of behavioral response audiometry in those individuals with varying levels of consciousness may not be reliable. For these patients, objective measures of hearing must be used. Impedance testing, including tympanometry and acoustic reflexes, can give valuable information about the tympanic membrane, ossicles, and central auditory pathway through the brainstem. Otoacoustic emissions (OAE), auditory brainstem response (ABR, also known as brainstem electric response (BSER) or brainstem evoked response (BAER)), auditory steady-state response testing (ASSR) can be used.

For patients who have sustained significant head trauma, several radiologic imaging techniques have likely been obtained prior to seeing an otolaryngologist. Although general head imaging (computed tomography [CT], magnetic resonance imaging [MRI]) can be helpful in determining the extent of cranial or intracranial injuries likely to signify concurrent auditory damage, not all patients with subjective hearing loss require radiologic assessment. In the absence of CSF otorrhea or rhinorrhea, facial paresis or paralysis, or loss of consciousness, additional imaging may not necessarily change the plan of care and would therefore be considered an inefficient use of resources. However, for the previously listed symptoms, high-resolution computed tomography (HRCT) of the temporal bone with thin cuts (3 mm or less) can prove to be a very useful diagnostic tool. Because most of the structures of hearing are encased within the boney otic capsule of the petrous temporal bone, CT is the preferred modality over MRI, which is better for soft tissue involvement.

EXTERNAL EAR

Damage to pinna and external auditory canal can result from any mechanism of injury, including blunt, blast, burn, and penetrating injuries. This results in lacerations, abrasions, contusions, hematomas, thermal damage, and even avulsions. These injuries alone may prevent the transmission of sound to the middle ear and often result in conductive hearing loss. However, in more severe injuries, a high suspicion of inner ear damage and possible SNHL must be entertained. For burn victims, it is important to note that several intravenous antibiotics used to treat or prevent secondary infection can be ototoxic, leading to severe cochlear and/or vestibular damage.

External ear injuries are managed like other soft tissue injuries, however, with significant soft tissue loss or cartilage exposure, the remnant auricle can be buried in a postauricular pocket. Once the damaged auricle is revascularized, it can be lifted from the pocket and either grafted or allowed to epithelialize secondarily.

TYMPANIC MEMBRANE AND MIDDLE EAR

Tympanic Membrane Perforation

The tympanic membrane is exquisitely sensitive to variations in pressure. When impulse or extreme continuous noise exceeds the compliance of the membrane (usually by medial displacement), injury occurs. This may result in conditions ranging from microscopic intratympanic hemorrhage to tympanic laceration to total perforation. For blast injuries, the vector of the concussive wave affects TM trauma. Perforations may be unilateral or bilateral, small, total, single, or multiple. Lateral-to-medial forces subject greater damage than anteroposterior forces, and those to the side of the head vs those in front of the patient have a greater risk for TM injury.

Children and adults are prone to traumatic TM injury, but children are more likely to have penetrating injuries, often unintentionally self-inflicted by a foreign body (9). Additionally, younger men who are more likely to engage in high-risk activities are more susceptible to TM perforations. The true incidence is unknown, but reports vary widely, ranging from 1.4 to 8.6 per 100,000 population (10). In 1979, Griffin reported 0.6% of all patients seen in his general otolaryngology practice sustained traumatic TM perforations (11). Blast injury puts the tympanic membrane at particular risk, with reports of TM involvement reaching up to 79% (12). Recent studies have demonstrated up to a 50% perforation rate in adults exposed to 5 psi (approximately 185 dB) depending on noise spectra and duration (13,14). For perspective, explosives used in Operation Iraqi Freedom/Operation Enduring Freedom produce pressures in excess of 60 psi (7). When compared with adults, children exposed to blasts tend to have lower rates of perforations, likely because of increased compliance of their tympanic membranes (15). Although common in blast injuries, damage to the inner ear and resultant SNHL is likely minimized by the dispersion of energy to the tympanic membrane and ossicles (16).

Tympanic membrane rupture is an extremely important indicator of the force sustained by the patient, and may give important clues as the likelihood of other life-threatening injuries. The presence of a TM perforation may indicate concussive injury, though the converse is not true—absence of a TM perforation does not ensure that TBI hasn't occurred. So important is tympanic membrane status in determining the likelihood of life-threatening injury; assessment of the TM is included in the algorithm for the initial evaluation of blast-injury patients. Once basic life support and immediate treatment of life-threatening penetrating or blunt injuries are performed, TM perforation can be used to triage those at highest risk for late primary blast internal injuries. When the TM is intact, serious primary blast injuries can be conditionally excluded in the absence of other indicators such as dyspnea, respiratory distress, or abdominal pain. When the TM is ruptured, even in the absence of other injuries at initial evaluation, a period of observation is critical to evaluate for delayed pulmonary or visceral damage.

Damage to the tympanic membrane and the consequences on hearing have been well-known for hundreds of years. In 1640, Banzer attempted repair of ruptured TM using pieces of pig bladder stretched across an ivory tube. Since then, great advances in the diagnosis and treatment of TM perforations have allowed for today's highly successful management of these injuries. In the acute setting, when external auditory canal blood or debris obscures visualization of the entire tympanic membrane, further management should be deferred until it can be suctioned and cleaned under a microscope by an otolaryngologist. Depending on the extent of perforation, management plans differ. Most small to moderate sized perforations will spontaneously resolve (15,17,18). Perforations with inverted flaps may require realignment in the office to promote healing and prevent cholesteatoma, although perforations typically resolve within 3 months following injury. Seamon et al. reported a 12% incidence of cholesteatoma (secondary acquired) in 110 Vietnam War veterans with traumatic TM perforations (19). More recently, Kronenberg reported a 7.5% incidence of cholesteatoma observed in 210 ears of Israeli soldiers with TM perforations (13). Surgical intervention (myringoplasty, tympanoplasty) is indicated when the perforation fails to close after close observation, however, the ideal timing of the procedure remains controversial (13,20,21).

Hemotympanum

Hemotympanum, which refers to either blood in the middle ear space or hemorrhage of the tympanic membrane itself, can occur following almost any kind of trauma, although it is most likely to occur following blunt and barotrauma. Occasionally, hemotympanum can occur as the sole manifestation of otologic trauma, although depending on the force of trauma sustained, a high index of suspicion for concomitant injury should be entertained. It can also occur following surgical intervention, acute otitis media, spontaneously from coagulopathies, or result from retrograde flow of blood up the Eustachian tube during epistaxis. Patients will subjectively complain of aural fullness and hearing loss. Otoscopic examination will show dark red or purple middle ear fluid behind an intact eardrum that is nonmobile to pneumotoscopy. Tuning forks confirm conductive hearing loss, and tympanogram will show a noncompliant or flat ("type B") membrane. Management consists of observation and reassurance that the hemotympanum will ultimately liquefy and reabsorb in the middle ear mucosa. If the hemotympanum persists past 6 weeks, the blood should be liquefied sufficiently to allow myringotomy and aspiration in the office. Generally, obtaining an audiogram is deferred until the hemotympanum has resolved. Conductive hearing loss once the middle ear space is clear may indicate ossicular disruption.

Ossicular Disruption

Disruption of the ossicles most frequently occurs following blunt trauma. Depending on the vector and severity of cranial injury, reported incidence has reached up to 80% (22,23). Hasso and Ledington reported up to 50% association of temporal bone fractures and ossicular disolation (24). Brodie and Thompson report 21% of all patients with documented hearing loss after temporal bone fracture had conductive hearing loss (25). The incidence following blast injury is much lower. Wolf reported a 5.7% rate of conductive hearing loss in 210 exposed ears (26). Ossicular disruption following any type of injury may also be considered a protective mechanism. Without an intact ossicular chain, the huge forces sustained during trauma are transmitted fully to the inner ear, resulting in significant and nonreversible SNHL.

The incus is the most commonly involved ossicle. This is because the malleus and stapes have more support structures to keep them in place. In addition, the blood supply to the long process of the incus is susceptible to disruption—leading to avascular necrosis. For both these reasons, the incudostapedial joint in the area is most likely involved in traumatic ossicular disruption. Other injuries, including incudomalleolar and mid-ossicular fractures or displacements occur. Delayed fixation of a dislocated malleus to the epitympanum can also cause conductive hearing loss years after injury.

Because physical exam will likely show a normal tympanic membrane and middle ear space (once possible hemotympanum is resolved), audiologic workup is crucial. Tuning forks can grossly establish a conductive hearing loss, whereas a proper audiogram will quantify the extent of loss. Different degrees of loss in different frequencies can help indicate which parts of the ossicular chain may be involved. In addition, impedance tests including tympanograms and acoustic reflex patterns can give clues whether the ossicular chain is intact, fixed, or dislocated. HRCT of the temporal bone can be helpful in determining the nature of the ossicular injury, although may not be necessary for diagnosis or for preoperative planning. Although HRCT images taken at the time of injury can support your presumptive diagnosis, only direct operative microscopic visualization will afford the detail necessary to determine how to reconstruct.

Management of ossicular injuries is controversial. Many patients can simply be observed over time as fibrosis and scarring of the remnant ossicular chain may ultimately allow for significant—if incomplete—transmission of sound from the tympanic membrane to the inner ear. For those patients with persistent CHL who undergo surgical repair, a host of reconstruction options exists, including repositioning and reshaping ossicular or cartilaginous autografts, interposing artificial prostheses, and/or medial repositioning of the tympanic membrane. In the hands of a qualified otologic surgeon, results are generally very good, with repair of conductive hearing loss within 10 dB of maximal potential gain.

INNER EAR

Sensorineural Hearing Loss

There are 2 main classes of closely related traumatic sensorineural (or nerve) hearing loss—acoustic (noise) and blast. These causative etiologies are not limited to the military and can affect civilians as well, especially those who work in heavy industry or certain construction jobs. Although it may be convenient to lump acoustic trauma and blast trauma as the same etiology, they are actually different from each other as we will see in the next 2 sections. Acoustic trauma is noise-induced damage to the hearing apparatus, whereas blast injury is pressure-induced damage to the hearing apparatus as well as the brain.

Acoustic Trauma Hearing Loss (Noise-Induced Hearing Loss)

There are 2 general types of acoustic trauma to the ear as follows: continuous noise (noise that produces damage over time) and impulse noise (noise that is loud enough to produce damage with a single exposure). Although continuous noise does technically represent a traumatic etiology, it is a very slow damage over time and, therefore, beyond the scope of this chapter. Impulse noise is very much an immediate traumatic etiology. Work by several groups has demonstrated that hair cell damage and death are observed after impulse noise and the resultant hearing loss is thought secondary to this hair cell loss (27–29). The mechanisms whereby noise produces hair cell damage are not fully eluci-

dated, but there are likely 2 causes of hair cell damage associated with impulse noise (30). Impulse noise can actually sheer cells away from their supporting membrane destroying not only the hair cells but other inner ear structures as well. In addition, cells can succumb to apoptosis (31). Apoptosis (programmed cell death) results after a cascade of chemical changes within the cell. Cells can protect themselves against this cascade to a certain extent but, when overwhelmed, apoptotic cell death ensues. The prevention of the induction of apoptosis as well as strengthening of the cells' own defenses are the focuses of many of the novel pharmaceutical approaches to treating/ameliorating noise induced hearing loss.

Because damage is largely limited to the inner ear, impulse noise creates a SNHL. The degree of the SNHL can be difficult to determine because, often times, impulse noise occurs in individuals who work in noisy environments and might already have some component of continuous noise damage. A recent hearing test from just before the incident, if available, would be the best guide. As far as predicting how much hearing loss will occur from an impulse of a given decibel (dB) intensity, which is also difficult because it depends on a host of factors that can largely be broken down into 2 categories—mechanical and biological. Mechanical factors that affect the amount of hearing loss include the use (or non-use) of hearing protection at the time of the impulse and the level of protection afforded by this protection (based both on the type and the fit), the distance from the impulse, and the environment in which the impulse occurs. Biologic factors include individual susceptibility, genetic factors, and degree of previous hearing loss. This last factor is controversial because conventional wisdom suggested that an ear with previous damage from continuous noise is more likely to suffer even more damage from an impulse noise. However, others believe that previous noise exposure "hardens" the ear and, therefore, reduces the impact of the impulse noise (32).

There has been some emphasis on studying the rates of hearing loss from continuous noise in both military and nonmilitary populations, but the incidence of noise damage from impulse has been less well characterized. Part of the issue involves the denominator in 2 ways. First, it is difficult to determine the actual numbers of impulses loud enough to produce sudden hearing loss in any given population so that a percentage of affected exposed compared to unexposed cannot be accurately determined. Secondly, if the number of impulses in a military or civilian setting is increased, the amount of hearing loss might increase, simply as a factor of the total number of exposures so population incidence figures may not be accurate as well. There has been some work calculating the percentage of individuals with hearing loss secondary to impulse from war. A British study of individuals who were machine gunners in a short military operation showed a 20% incidence of hearing loss as compared to no hearing loss in the control group. This study was imperfect for assessing the effect of a single impulse because even though the machine gun fire was short-duration, it was more than a single incidence (33). Lew's group found nearly the same incidence (21%–22.7%) of hearing loss from US troops returning from Southwest Asia (Iraq and Afghanistan) who had not been exposed to blast (34). Again, this data is confounded becauset individuals may have never been exposed to even a single impulse or had many exposures over the 6–12 months of deployment. It is definitely true that in the almost decade long war on terror, the incidence of hearing loss disability claims has skyrocketed at Veterans Affairs Hospitals. Of course, there are several factors accounting for this and many of the patients did not suffer a single impulse noise. Tinnitus is a common complaint but even harder to quantify. Estimates vary from 20% to 60% of individuals returning from an overseas deployment as having tinnitus. However, it is difficult to know how many of these individuals (given previous noise exposure in the military) had tinnitus before they deployed and how many developed the tinnitus on deployment over time vs from a single event. Moreover, tinnitus is a subjective complaint, and the level as well as the frequency can be difficult to fully characterize.

Blast-Related Hearing Loss

As noted previously, blast has a different effect on the ears than noise. In blast injury, the damage done to the ear is caused by the pressure wave and not by the actual intensity of the noise. Most blasts produce a Friedlander-shaped pressure wave in which there is large positive pressure followed by a negative pressure. Theoretically, it is the actual positive or negative pressure that causes damage. Also, in contradistinction to noise, blast affects other areas of the brain beyond just the cochlea. These other areas of the brain may be involved in the process of hearing and damage to these areas may produce hearing disorders even in the presence of a normal hearing end organ. Despite an increasing understanding of the damage patterns caused by blast exposure, there is still a very incomplete understanding of the mechanism whereby blast produces damage within the brain, let alone the ear itself. However, there is little doubt about the impact of blast on hearing and balance. Hoffer's lab examined 3 groups of individuals with blast exposure—acute (within the first 72 hours of exposure), subacute (7–30 days after exposure), and chronic (more than 30 days after exposure). Most, but not all of these individuals, had a single blast exposure. This lab demonstrated that hearing loss rose from 33% of those seen acutely to almost half of those seen chronically (35). It is critical to note that these percentages are percentages of those individuals with any complaints at all and does not include the individuals exposed to blast who do not report complaints. It is possible that many of these individuals do indeed have a hearing loss from blast that they either ignore or that later gets assigned as being secondary to continuous noise. Moreover, despite increasing awareness of the dangers of multiple blast exposures, little is known about the impact of multiple blast exposures on hearing. In a simple questionnaire survey, one-third of individuals who were exposed to at least 1 blast complain of hearing loss after returning from that deployment (34). It is important to note that even 20% of those without a blast exposure complain of hearing loss after a deployment; so it is difficult to determine what contribution the blast exposure had to this 33% hearing loss rate. This is particularly true because those with blast exposure are more likely to be in more noise intensive jobs than those without blast exposure, and this increased noise alone could account for the increased percentage of hearing loss.

Unlike with noise, blast damage is not limited to SNHL and tinnitus alone. The pressure of a blast wave can produce conductive hearing loss from damage to the ear drum or ossicles. Depending on the extent of the damage and what

is actually damaged, this hearing loss may self-correct or may require surgical intervention. In addition, blast-injury patients suffer from an unusually high level of central auditory process abnormalities (CAPD) (32). At the current time, we are only just beginning to understand the impact of CAPD in this group of individuals. Likely, CAPD occurs secondary to blast damage in other areas of the brain. Similarly, tinnitus suffered by blast-exposed individuals can be different from tinnitus seen after noise. Certainly, individuals with blast and hearing loss suffer from tinnitus that is likely cochlear in origin. However, there are a significant number of individuals with blast exposure that suffer tinnitus without coincident hearing loss. A Finnish study examined the impact of a blast event at a shopping mall and found that although two-thirds of the patients had tinnitus, only 41% had both tinnitus and hearing loss (36).

There is an additional area in which blast-induced hearing disorders differ significantly from impulse noise. That is, that these disorders worsen over time. As can be seen from our group's study, the hearing loss rate increased from one-third to almost one-half of the individuals over time (35). It also appears that there is an increase in CAPD over time, but it is difficult to determine if this is indeed new symptoms or simply symptoms that are not diagnosed acutely. Our group and others have postulated an increased frequency of post-traumatic endolymphatic hydrops. This disorder, which often occurs approximately 1 year after the event, would produce a worsening of hearing loss, tinnitus, and aural pressure along with vertigo. It has been postulated that blast can produce a post-traumatic hydrops whereas there is little evidence that noise can do the same.

Treatment of Sensorineural Hearing Loss

As with all forms of trauma, the best management comes from prevention. For civilian populations, this includes protective equipment such as bicycle helmets, seatbelts, airbags, and so forth. In the military, despite advances in hearing protection devices, they are not always worn for a variety of reason. Usually, those in a battlefield or industrial setting complains that conventional hearing protection prevents their ability to communicate with those around them, which may be vital to their job performance or lives (in combat). Moreover, impulse noise can come unexpectedly when hearing protection would not normally be in use. Finally, the hearing protection may not fully protect the ear against the noise if the noise is loud enough or if the protection is not properly fitted. The same mechanical solution of hearing protection may not prevent blast-induced damage because the pressure wave may affect the inner ear right through the skull. There are several companies looking at products that can be worn on the body or over the head and absorb pressure before it penetrates into the cranium or body cavities. Unfortunately, there are no other treatments available to rescue, reverse, or prevent these hearing disorders.

For acute SNHL, treatment varies significantly. A small percentage of SNHL (usually caused by noise) will improve over the first 3–7 days. Almost any hearing loss present after 10 days is generally permanent. Nevertheless, we recommend aggressive medical therapy early on. Our treatment regimen consists of oral steroids (60 mg orally every 9 AM × 7–10 days) accompanied by intratympanic steroid injection (0.3 mL of 10 mg/mL dexamethasone) injected into the ear for 3 injections spaced 2 weeks apart. Because there is little level 1 evidence supporting this regimen, the oral and the intratympanic dosage and steroid used as well as the frequency of the injections will vary by provider. Some have also advocated *N*-acetyl cysteine (Mucomyst) in the same dosage as used for Tylenol overdose in all cases of noise-induced hearing loss. There has been a great deal of work on pharmaceutical solutions for traumatic hearing loss. A detailed examination of this work is beyond the scope of this chapter but suffice it to say that none of these treatments has yet to be proven beneficial in human subjects for hearing loss or tinnitus.

For those in whom hearing loss persists, treatment is primarily provided by amplification. Some hearing losses are not bad enough to require hearing aids but may require help in certain situations (over the phone, in a classroom, etc.). A variety of assistive listening devices (ALDs) are available for this population. For those that require more assistance, hearing aids (largely digital)—either worn in the ear, partially in the ear, or behind the ear—are extremely effective in improving environmental and speech perception. Ultimately, most hearing aids are simply amplifiers that improve volume, but not clarity. In cases of severe auditory damage, loss of hair cell modulation leads to a decrease in speech discrimination, such that conventional hearing aids are unable to provide serviceable benefit. For those patients, a variety of newly developed implantable auditory technologies (osseointegrated bone vibrating devices, middle ear implants, or cochlear implants) can provide significant improvement in hearing that, only recently, was considered untreatable.

Temporal Bone Fractures

Up to 30% of head injuries involve a fracture of the cranial base, and nearly 1 in 5 patients with skull fractures will involve the temporal bone (37–40). These fractures most commonly result from motor vehicle collisions, followed in incidence by falls, blunt assault, and penetrating gunshots. Damage to structures of the temporal bone can include hearing loss (CHL, SNHL, and mixed), facial nerve paresis or paralysis, labyrinthine concussion, tinnitus, benign paroxysmal positional vertigo, CSF leak, perilymph fistula, post-traumatic endolymphatic hydrops, cholesteatoma, meningocele/encephalocele, and late otogenic meningitis (25,37,39,41–46). Associated injuries to adjacent structures, although less common, can occur and include palsies of other cranial nerves, especially the abducens (VI), glossopharyngeal (IX), vagus (X), and spinal accessory (XI). These patients also can sustain critical intracranial injuries including subarachnoid hemorrhage, subdural hemorrhage, epidural hematoma, brain contusion, and cerebral edema (38). In a series of 115 with facial paralysis secondary to temporal bone fracture, 33% presented with a Glasgow Coma Scale (GCS) score of <7 (44). In Alvi et al., the authors report 44% of all patients required open neurosurgical intervention, including 86% of those who had 2 or more intracranial injuries. Forty-nine percent showed mental status changes and 7% had limb paralysis. Mortality related to the neurologic sequela in patients with temporal bone fracture population is as high as 10%, with up to 16% of patients requiring institutional care beyond initial in-hospital acute management (38). Cervical spine injury is twofold to sixfold higher in patients with temporal bone fractures vs those without (47).

Historically, temporal bone fractures have been classified as "longitudinal" or "transverse", with the later addition of terms "oblique" and "mixed." However, more recently changing patterns of injury and better understanding of clinical course have led to terms "otic capsule-sparing" and "otic capsule-violating" as better predictors of outcome. Those that are "otic capsule-violating" are more likely to result in significant SNHL, tinnitus, and vestibular disturbance. Overall, approximately 24% of patients will have a subjective complaint of hearing loss (25). Hearing loss in patients with temporal bone fractures may be immediate or delayed, temporary or permanent, or progressive.

Other Post-Traumatic Inner Ear Auditory Conditions

SNHL can also occur after severe temporal trauma in the absence of fracture. Microfractures of the otic capsule and intracochlear hemorrhage have been identified on postmortem histopathologic analsysis, which may explain the condition known as "cochlear concussion" (48). Cochlear concussion can cause temporary or permanent SNHL.

A rare delayed hearing loss can occur in the contralateral ear months to years after the initial trauma. This condition, known as sympathetic hearing loss, has reported rate of occurrence ranging from 1% to 11% (43). Such hearing loss is believed to be associated with the exposure of the privileged inner ear antigens to the general immune system, resulting in an autoimmune attack on the contralateral ear.

Perilymph fistula (PLF) occurs when fractures of the otic capsule causes egress of perilymph from the inner ear. Patients with PLF typically appear more ill than patients with other otologic conditions, and the symptoms of postural instability, headache, tinnitus, cognitive dysfunction, nausea, hearing loss, visual disturbances, and aural fullness can be extremely disabling. Diagnosis can be difficult given that many of the symptoms are shared with other inner ear and brain damage conditions. Because there is no "gold standard" test for diagnosing these patients, history and physical assessment is critical, especially with a history of trauma. Many patients have a diurnal pattern of symptoms that begins innocuously in the morning, but worsen throughout the day. Over time, PLF symptoms tend to be persistent, insidious, and progressive in nature rather than episodic, although periods of exacerbation can occur. Fluctuating, progressively deteriorating hearing loss as well as the failure of vestibular symptoms to resolve should raise the suspicion of PLF. When hearing is not affected, management is conservative with strict bed rest and head elevation. In cases with hearing loss, treatment is urgent operative exploration with patching of the oval and round windows.

One extremely rare condition that can lead to profound hearing loss is post-traumatic cochlear nerve avulsion. This has been reported following blunt trauma, likely a result of medial displacement of the pons and cerebellum away from the fixed entry point of the cochlear nerve within the temporal bone (49). Patients who sustain the forces required to cause such an avulsion are unlikely to survive. For those who do survive, careful radiographic evaluation, including fast imaging employing steady-state acquisition (FIESTA) or constructive interference on steady state (CISS) sequences on MRI can help determine the integrity of the cochlear nerve. To restore ipsilateral hearing, an auditory brainstem implant (ABI) may be the most viable option because cochlear implantation would clearly provide no benefit (50).

Post-traumatic pulsatile tinnitus is a rare but extremely serious condition that can worsen over months to years following initial injury. This symptom can be the result of skull base fracture–associated aneurysm (both venous and arterial) formation or from arteriovenous fistula formation. In cases of caroticocavernous fistula, presenting symptoms and signs will also include diplopia, chemosis, proptosis, headache, elevated intraocular pressure, 3rd and 6th cranial nerve palsies, exophthalmia, and extrabulbar loops. If this condition is expected, urgent ophthalmological referral is necessary. Angiography and endovascular treatment is the gold standard for both diagnosis and management.

CENTRAL AUDITORY SYSTEM DAMAGE

As mentioned earlier, the main focus of today's conventional hearing evaluation is on peripheral auditory pathology. However, we are becoming increasingly aware of the important role that the central auditory pathway plays in post-traumatic hearing loss—particularly in patients with TBI. In head trauma, most notably in primary and secondary blast injury, there are significant changes that the brain suffers injury. The movement of the brain within the skull results in hemorrhage and edema (51). In addition, angular forces exerted on axons can result in shearing, swelling, or disconnection of both axons and blood vessels (52).

The brainstem is responsible for providing sensitivity to both frequency and temporal structure of auditory stimuli. The cochlear nucleus is tonotopically organized and plays a vital role in the relative pitch and harmonic relationships of auditory stimuli. It is also within the brainstem and, in particular, at the medial longitudinal fasciculus, where auditory fibers cross the midline, allowing for processing of very subtle intra-aural timing differences. Under normal conditions, this binaural signal allows for the ability to localize sounds. Damage to this area will interfere with the highly sensitive mechanisms that allow for sound localization and lateralization. In addition, loss of binaural processing will interfere with the brain's normal ability to distinguish among multiple sound sources, and therefore organize sound meaningfully (53). Clinically, patients with brainstem injury may complain of difficulty hearing only in the setting of additional background noise. The impact of such real-world dysfunction can be severe, although testing of these abilities is rarely performed.

Less is known about thalamic and cortical injury. Taber reported that the auditory cortex in the temporal lobe is among the most commonly affected regions in neurotrauma (52). In rare cases of bilateral damage to the primary auditory cortex (the superior temporal gyrus), a condition known as "cortical deafness" can occur. This presents as immediate and persistent inability to respond to any auditory stimuli. Other additional auditory cortical processing deficits can interfere selectively with receptive speech, expressive speech, environmental sounds, and even music. The clinical realities of this condition are devastating, and unfortunately most of the traditional rehabilitative and restorative modalities used in the management of peripheral auditory dysfunction cannot be employed.

The clinical manifestation of central auditory damage can be subtle and often overlooked. Damage affects auditory processing and interferes with localization, hearing in background noise, and perception of different temporal speech patterns. These are not routinely tested as part of the audio-

metric battery, and many patients may be relatively asymptomatic within the quiet and controlled confines of doctors or audiologists offices. Hearing screens and basic behavioral audiometry may be completed. Again, a high index of suspicion for central auditory dysfunction must be entertained. In addition to the electrophysiologic tests discussed earlier, the audiologist and neuropsychologist should include special tests of temporal processing and patterning tests, dichotic speech tests, monaural low-redundancy speech tests, binaural interaction tests, and others in order to better evaluate for post-traumatic CAPD. Fausti recommends standardized and validated questionnaires that can be used to assess the impact of hearing loss, tinnitus, and/or dizziness in all patients with TBI (7). Any information concerning pre-injury function can be extremely helpful. In addition, modifications of existing protocols may be necessary for patients with cognitive impairment and/or potential CAPD.

Current treatment of CAPD, based on anecdotal rather than scientific evidence, largely consists of 2 components—generalized management and auditory training. Generalized management includes environmental strategies (amplification by hearing aids or frequency modulation [FM] systems) and behavioral compensation techniques. Auditory training, which seeks to take advantage of neural plasticity, can help to alter the encoding of sound and timing of brainstem responses. It should begin as soon as possible after injury. Additional phonological awareness and discrimination training, speech reading, prosody training, and other auditory exercises can improve interhemispheric transfer of information via cross-modality activies (7). When successful, patients can "relearn" speech and environmental sounds that were lost after injury.

Although this is an area of recent and promising research, our understanding of the central auditory system is minimal, and the therapeutic options we can offer our patients is limited. Animal studies have revealed much about the central auditory system, and we can extrapolate the findings for certain conditions (54–56). Nonetheless, the damage and its effects to the central auditory system have not been systemically studied in humans. Even more complicated is how attention and behavioral processing contribute to central auditory dysfunction. As Fausti recently stated, "The diagnosis, rehabilitation, and prevention of central auditory system damage is currently in its infancy, with only the barest indications of the directions in which it should be headed" (7).

TINNITUS AND HYPERACUSIS

Subjective tinnitus, defined as sounds perceived by the patient in the absence of external auditory stimulation, is an extremely common problem in the general population as well as in patients with trauma. Objective tinnitus, which stems from aberrant or altered blood flow within the neck and skull base as well as from myoclonus, is very rare and will not be reviewed in this chapter. Some patients may report a low volume of tinnitus that they find extremely distressing, even crippling, whereas other patients may report very loud tinnitus that is not bothersome to them at all.

Multiple hypotheses have been proposed regarding the etiology of tinnitus, yet no common mechanism has been proven. Theories include damaged inner ear hair cells resulting in unregulated discharge and overstimulation of the auditory nerve, hyperactive auditory nerve fibers, or lack of suppression of peripheral nerve activity from cortical control (57,58). Most patients with any kind of auditory damage, including those with post-traumatic dysfunction, will complain of some degree of tinnitus. However, many post-traumatic patients will complain of tinnitus despite any evidence of auditory dysfunction. Although the exact pathophysiology of tinnitus following trauma has yet to be fully elucidated, we now understand that tinnitus can and frequently does occur even in the absence of objective auditory damage. Neurologic, infectious, metabolic, musculoskeletal, and psychogenic disorders are all associated with tinnitus and are systems frequently involved in trauma victims. One must also consider the potential role of iatrogenic pharmacologic causes including salicylates, nonsteroidal anti-inflammatory drugs (NSAIDs), aminoglycoside antibiotics, loop diuretics, some chemotherapy drugs, opioids, and other medications frequently used in the care of patients with trauma (59,60).

In the post-traumatic population with tinnitus, central processes within the brain are intimately involved in the perception of tinnitus. Causality and contribution of various neurologic and psychologic conditions are certain, but the exact interaction is unknown. Many post-traumatic patients, even those without head trauma, will suffer from depression, anxiety, fibromyalgia, and post-traumatic stress disorder (PTSD)—to name a few. All which have been clearly associated with tinnitus (57,61). Folmer reported 34% of 436 patients with tinnitus had a history of depression (61). He showed depression correlated with tinnitus severity, but not with reported loudness, suggesting a strong psychological component of the disease. Fagelson reviewed 300 patients enrolled in the Veterans Affairs Medical Center Tinnitus Clinic and found a 34% incidence of PTSD. Patients with PTSD had worse tinnitus severity, suddenness of onset, sound intolerance, and sound-triggered exacerbation of tinnitus compared to patients without PTSD. He provides an excellent review of the several neural mechanisms linked to both tinnitus and PTSD—to which the reader is referred (62). Ultimately, better understanding of PTSD and indeed any one of the neuropsychological conditions that modulate tinnitus may facilitate the treatment and management strategies.

As with hearing loss, evaluation of the patient with tinnitus begins with a thorough history. Patterns of onset following trauma can vary, with some patients complaining immediately of tinnitus (with or without hearing loss). It can also occur weeks to months later once the acute stress of the trauma subsides, or if progressive hearing loss occurs. Tinnitus can take on different frequencies, timbres, intensities, and duration, pattern, and can have varying aggravating or alleviating conditions. Symptoms do not necessarily correlate with the mechanism or severity of auditory injury. Patients with tinnitus have widely differing needs regarding their symptoms. For many patients, the tinnitus is so mild that they never seek medical care. For the remainder of tinnitus patients, a well designed and efficient protocol should be in place to provide patient relief. Moreover, mild tinnitus can often be managed by simple reassurance that it, particularly that associated with sudden audiologic injury, is likely to improve. Although the improvement can take months to years, patients are frequently encouraged by the positive prognosis.

The management of tinnitus can be extremely challenging. If there is an identified underlying pathology, clearly addressing that pathology is the initial treatment of choice. If this does not work then there are several options. There is little Level 1 evidence to suggest that any option is necessarily superior to the others, although several studies are ongoing. Therapy generally breaks down into medical therapy, device therapy, cognitive-based therapy, and magnetic stimulation. Medical therapy uses a variety of medicines from antianxiety medications to some of the new sleeping medicines. For the most part, these medicines are used to treat associated anxiety or inability to sleep because of the tinnitus rather than the tinnitus itself. Device therapy refers to a range of devices from hearing aids (usually because of an associated hearing loss) to tinnitus-masking devices. Some individuals do profit from these therapies, but in most cases, the relief does not extend once the device is out of the ear. There are some emerging new device technologies using customized acoustical stimuli (63). The Neuromonics device is one such acoustical stimulus. This device uses a novel acoustical signal pattern in an attempt to provide stimuli to acoustical regions "deprived by hearing loss." The success of this particular device varies between 50% and 70% but might be increased by determining a specific group of patients in whom to apply this technology (64).

Early data also indicates that these devices may outperform traditional masking type devices by providing some residual disinhibition (control while the device is not on). More work needs to be done on the use of these devices, especially because more become approved and available. There is some novel work examining cochlear implants for tinnitus. This work is to date experimental but has shown some promising results (65,66). A great deal of recent emphasis has been placed on cognitive-based therapy such as tinnitus retraining therapy. These therapies are usually biofeedback/counseling therapy. They have been found to be effective in a subset of patients. There has been increased interest in combining this therapy with sound therapy, and some evidence is emerging that the combination is the most beneficial (67). Tinnitus retraining therapy (TRT) is a form of habituation therapy that uses a combination of counseling and noise to allow individuals to end the negative reaction to the tinnitus precept and eventually to end the tinnitus. TRT is becoming increasingly popular and available, and early studies suggest that patients do experience significant improvement with this therapy. The most aggressive therapy for tinnitus is magnetic stimulation. Transcranial magnetic stimulation (TMS) uses a stimulus placed on the skull. Outcomes have been mixed with some patients showing a significant response and others showing no response. The average response exceeds placebo in some studies but not in other studies (68,69). Magnetic stimulation has been extended to intracranial use. This technique does involve doing an awake craniotomy. There is some early work in this area documenting sustained response to this therapy but more work is needed in this area (70).

Rarely, some post-traumatic patients will suffer from hyperacusis. The term hyperacusis, however, does not imply suprathreshold sensitivity to sound. Neither does it relate to the auditory recruitment phenomenon—in which cochlear outer hair cell loss results in abnormally increased perceived loudness with increasing sound intensity (71). Rather, hyperacusis refers to phenomenon where sound levels considered comfortable by most listeners are perceived as unbearably uncomfortable. Similar conditions include phonophobia (fear of sound) and misophobia (dislike of sound). Little epidemiologic data exist regarding hyperacusis, and extensive literature review found no research performed specifically on post-traumatic hyperacusis. Like tinnitus, hyperacusis is centrally modulated, and the systems that are frequently affected by trauma (both neurologic and psychological) play important roles in the altered perception of sound. Conditions that are frequently comorbid with head trauma have also been associated with hyperascusis—including PTSD, migraine, and depression (72). Both tinnitus and hyperacusis are hypothesized to occur secondary to abnormal neural gain—for tinnitus, it is gain in the absence of sound and for hyperacusis, it is gain in the presence of sound. Therefore, strategies to treat hyperacusis have invoked methods used in the treatment of tinnitus. For many patients who suffer from hyperacusis, the first reaction is to use earplugs to prevent sound perception. However, because sound deprivation is thought to increase central gain, such methods are not recommended (just as most patients with tinnitus will complain that the noises are louder in quiet environments). Unfortunately, other than this and other anecdotal methods, no evidence of any quality exists to support any one method over another in the effective treatment of hyperacusis.

CONCLUSION

Damage to the auditory system is common following head trauma. Patients can present with overt or subtle signs and symptoms of hearing loss. All clinicians involved in the care of patients with trauma should have a high index of suspicion for concurrent auditory damage, especially for blast victims. A wide variety of diagnostic tools are available to help distinguish the location and severity of injury. Although great strides have been made in the understanding and treatment of peripheral auditory dysfunction, much is still to be learned for the management of central auditory dysfunction, tinnitus, and hyperacusis. Although patients with cranial injury frequently have other more pressing injuries in the acute setting, failure to identify and treat auditory trauma can lead to significant and lasting consequences.

KEY CLINICAL POINTS

1. Damage to the auditory system is common following trauma, and the clinician should have a high index of suspicion for hearing loss.
2. Many diagnostic tools can be helpful in defining the location, type, and severity of hearing loss. With the proper diagnosis, proper treatment can be initiated.
3. Hearing loss can be divided into conductive (CHL), sensorineural (SNHL), mixed, and central types.
4. Depending on the type of injury, treatment of auditory dysfunction can be supportive, medical, surgical, behavioral, or a combination of each.
5. Although central auditory dysfunction, tinnitus, and hyperacusis are fairly common following trauma, understanding of central auditory pathophysiology and effective treatment modalities remains limited.

KEY REFERENCES

1. Brodie HA, Thompson TC. Management of complications from 820 temporal bone fractures. *Am J Otol*. 1997;18(2): 188–197.

2. DePalma RG, Burris DG, Champion HR, Hodgson MJ. Blast injuries. *N Engl J Med*. 2005;352(13):1335–1342.
3. Fagelson MA. The association between tinnitus and post-traumatic stress disorder. *Am J Audiol*. 2007;16:107–117.
4. Fausti SA, Wilmington DJ, Gallun FJ, Myers PJ, Henry JA. Auditory and vestibular dysfunction associated with blast-related traumatic brain injury. *J Rehabil Res Dev*. 2009;46(6):797–810.
5. Lew HL, Jerger JF, Guillory SB, Henry JA. Auditory dysfunction in traumatic brain injury. *J Rehabil Res Dev*. 2007; 44(7):921–928.

DISCLAIMER

The views expressed in this article are those of the author(s) and do not necessarily reflect the official policy or position of the Department of the Navy, Department of Defense, or the U.S. Government.

References

1. Centers for Disease Control and Prevention. Incidence rates of hospitalization related to traumatic brain injury—12 states, 2002. *MMWR Morb Mortal Wkly Rep*. 2006;55(8):201–204.
2. Lew HL, Poole JH, Guillory SB, Salerno RM, Leskin G, Sigford B. Persistent problems after traumatic brain injury: the need for long-term follow-up and coordinated care. *J Rehabil Res Dev*. 2006;43(2): vii–x.
3. Lew HL, Jerger JF, Guillory SB, Henry JA. Auditory dysfunction in traumatic brain injury. *J Rehabil Res Dev*. 2007;44(7):921–928.
4. Zimmerman WD, Ganzel TM, Windmill IM, Nazar GB, Phillips M. Peripheral hearing loss following head trauma in children. *Laryngoscope*. 1993;103(1, pt 1):87–91.
5. Bergemalm PO. Progressive hearing loss after closed head injury: a predictable outcome? *Acta Otolaryngol*. 2003;123(7):836–845.
6. Gondusky JS, Reiter MP. Protecting military convoys in Iraq: an examination of battle injuries sustained by a mechanized battalion during Operation Iraqi Freedom II. *Mil Med*. 2005;170(6):546–549.
7. Fausti SA, Wilmington DJ, Gallun FJ, Myers PJ, Henry JA. Auditory and vestibular dysfunction associated with blast-related traumatic brain injury. *J Rehabil Res Dev*. 2009;46(6):797–810.
8. Chandler D. Blast-related ear injury in current U.S. military operations. *Asha Leader*. 2006;11:8–9,21.
9. Robbins JM, Mentz HA, Blair PA. Traumatic perforations of the tympanic membrane. *J La State Med Soc*. 1987;139(6):13–15.
10. Kristensen S. Spontaneous healing of traumatic tympanic membrane perforations in man: a century of experience. *J Laryngol Otol*. 1992;106(12):1037–1050.
11. Griffin WL Jr. A retrospective study of traumatic tympanic membrane perforations in a clinical practice. *Laryngoscope*. 1979;89(2, pt 1):261–282.
12. Lucić M. Therapy of middle ear injuries caused by explosive devices [in Serbian]. *Vojnosanit Pregl*. 1995;52(3):221–224.
13. Kronenberg J, Ben-Shoshan J, Modan M, Leventon G. Blast injury and cholesteatoma. *Am J Otol*. 1988;9(2):127–130.
14. Zajtchuk JT. Otolaryngic health service support in the airland battle. *Ann Otol Rhinol Laryngol Suppl*. 1989;140:5–8.
15. Kerr AG, Byrne JE. Concussive effects of bomb blast on the ear. *J Laryngol Otol*. 1975;89(2):131–143.
16. Helling ER. Otologic blast injuries due to the Kenya embassy bombing. *Mil Med*. 2004;169(11):872–876.
17. Garth RJ. Blast injury of the auditory system: a review of the mechanisms and pathology. *J Laryngol Otol*. 1994;108(11):925–929.
18. Pahor AL. The ENT problems following the Birmingham bombings. *J Laryngol Otol*. 1981;95(4):399–406.
19. Seaman RW, Newell RC. Another etiology of middle ear cholesteatoma. *Arch Otolaryngol*. 1971;94(4):440–442.

20. Sprem N, Branica S, Dawidowsky K. Tympanoplasty after war blast lesions of the eardrum: retrospective study. *Croat Med J.* 2001;42(6): 642–645.

21. Gapany-Gapanavicius B, Brama I, Chisin R. Early repair of blast ruptures of the tympanic membrane. *J Laryngol Otol.* 1977;91: 565–573.

22. Tos M. Prognosis of hearing loss in temporal bone fractures. *J Laryngol Otol.* 1971;85:1147–1159.

23. Podoshin L, Fradis M. Hearing loss after head injury. *Arch Otolaryngol.* 1975;101(1):15–18.

24. Hasso AN, Ledington JA. Traumatic injuries of the temporal bone. *Otolaryngol Clin North Am.* 1988;21(2):295–316.

25. Brodie HA, Thompson TC. Management of complications from 820 temporal bone fractures. *Am J Otol.* 1997;18(2):188–197.

26. Wolf M, Kronenberg J, Ben-Shoshan J, Roth Y. Blast injury of the ear. *Mil Med.* 1991;156(12):651–653.

27. Coleman JK, Littlesunday C, Jackson R, Meyer T. AM-111 protects against permanent hearing loss from impulse noise trauma. *Hear Res.* 2007;226(1–2):70–78.

28. Xiong M, Lai H, He Q, Wang J. Astragaloside IV attenuates impulse noise-induced trauma in guinea pig. *Acta Otolaryngol.* 2011;131(8): 809–816.

29. Bohne BA, Harding GW, Lee SC. Death pathways in noise-damaged outer hair cells. *Hear Res.* 2007;223(1–2):61–70.

30. Abrashkin KA, Izumikawa M, Miyazawa T, et al. The fate of outer hair cells after acoustic or ototoxic insults. *Hear Res.* 2006;218(1–2): 20–29.

31. Hu BH, Henderson D, Nicotera TM. Involvement of apoptosis in progression of cochlear lesion following exposure to intense noise. *Hear Res.* 2002;166(1–2):62–71.

32. Canlon B. Protection against noise trauma by sound conditioning. *Ear Nose Throat J.* 1997;76(4):248–5.

33. Anderson J. An audiometric survey of Royal Artillery gun crews following "Operation Corporate". *J R Army Med Corps.* 1984;130(2): 100–108.

34. Lew HL, Pogoda TK, Baker E, et al. Prevalence of dual sensory impairment and its association with traumatic brain injury and blast exposure in OEF/OIF veterans. *Journal of Head Trauma Rehabilitation.* 2011;26(6):489–496.

35. Hoffer ME, Balaban C, Gottshall K, Balough BJ, Maddox MR, Penta JR. Blast exposure: vestibular consequences and associated characteristics. *Otol Neurotol.* 2010;31(2):232–236.

36. Mrena R, Pääkkönen R, Bäck L, Pirvola U, Ylikoski J. Otologic consequences of blast exposure: a Finnish case study of a shopping mall bomb explosion. *Acta Otolaryngol.* 2004;124(8):946–952.

37. Cannon CR, Jahrsdoerfer RA. Temporal bone fractures. Review of 90 cases. *Arch Otolaryngol.* 1983;109(5):285–288.

38. Alvi A, Bereliani A IV. Trauma to the temporal bone: diagnosis and management of complications. *J Craniomaxillofac Trauma.* 1996;2(3): 36–48.

39. Dahiya R, Keller JD, Litofsky NS, Bankey PE, Bonassar LJ, Megerian CA. Temporal bone fractures: otic capsule sparing versus otic capsule violating clinical and radiographic considerations. *J Trauma.* 1999;47(6):1079–1083.

40. Nosan DK, Benecke JE Jr, Murr AH. Current perspective on temporal bone trauma. *Otolaryngol Head Neck Surg.* 1997;117(1):67–71.

41. Lyos AT, Marsh MA, Jenkins HA, Coker NJ. Progressive hearing loss after transverse temporal bone fracture. *Arch Otolaryngol Head Neck Surg.* 1995;121(7):795–799.

42. Shea JJ Jr, Ge X, Orchik DJ. Traumatic endolymphatic hydrops. *Am J Otol.* 1995;16(2):235–240.

43. ten Cate WJ, Bachor E. Autoimmune-mediated sympathetic hearing loss: a case report. *Otol Neurotol.* 2005;26(2):161–165.

44. Darrouzet V, Duclos JY, Liguoro D, Truilhe Y, De Bonfils C, Bebear JP. Management of facial paralysis resulting from temporal bone fractures: our experience in 115 cases. *Otolaryngol Head Neck Surg.* 2001;125(1):77–84.

45. Sudhoff H, Linthicum FH Jr. Temporal bone fracture and latent meningitis: temporal bone histopathology study of the month. *Otol Neurotol.* 2003;24(3):521–522.

46. Majmundar K, Shaw T, Sismanis A. Traumatic cholesteatoma presenting as a brain abscess: a case report. *Otol Neurotol.* 2005;26:65–67.

47. Diaz JJ Jr, Gillman C, Morris JA Jr, May AK, Carrillo YM, Guy J. Are five-view plain films of the cervical spine unreliable? A prospective evaluation in blunt trauma patients with altered mental status. *J Trauma.* 2003;55(4):658–663.

48. Ohlrogge M, Francis HW. Temporal bone fracture. *Otol Neurotol.* 2004;25(2):195–196.

49. Corrales CE, Monfared A, Jackler RK. Facial and vestibulocochlear nerve avulsion at the fundus of the internal auditory canal in a child without a temporal bone fracture. *Otol Neurotol.* 2010;31(9): 1508–1510.

50. Colletti V, Carner M, Miorelli V, Colletti L, Guida M, Fiorino F. Auditory brainstem implant in posttraumatic cochlear nerve avulsion. *Audiol Neurootol.* 2004;9(4):247–255.

51. DePalma RG, Burris DG, Champion HR, Hodgson MJ. Blast injuries. *N Engl J Med.* 2005;352(13):1335–1342.

52. Taber KH, Warden DL, Hurley RA. Blast-related traumatic brain injury: what is known? *J Neuropsychiatry Clin Neurosci.* 2006;18(2): 141–145.

53. Darwin CJ. Listening to speech in the presence of other sounds. *Philos Trans R Soc Lond B Biol Sci.* 2008;363(1493):1011–1021.

54. Joris PX, Schreiner CE, Rees A. Neural processing of amplitude-modulated sounds. *Physiol Rev.* 2004;84(2):541–577.

55. Kaas JH, Hackett TA. Subdivisions of auditory cortex and processing streams in primates. *Proc Natl Acad Sci U S A.* 2000;97(22): 11793–11799.

56. Mickey BJ, Middlebrooks JC. Representation of auditory space by cortical neurons in awake cats. *J Neurosci.* 2003;23(25):8649–8663.

57. Crummer RW, Hassan GA. Diagnostic approach to tinnitus. *Am Fam Physician.* 2004;69(1):120–126.

58. Fortune DS, Haynes DS, Hall JW III. Tinnitus. Current evaluation and management. *Med Clin North Am.* 1999;83(1):153–162, x.

59. Lockwood AH, Salvi RJ, Burkard RF. Tinnitus. *N Engl J Med.* 2002; 347(12):904–910.

60. Guitton MJ, Caston J, Ruel J, Johnson RM, Pujol R, Puel JL. Salicylate induces tinnitus through activation of cochlear NMDA receptors. *J Neurosci.* 2003;23(9):3944–3952.

61. Folmer RL, Griest SE, Meikle MB, Martin WH. Tinnitus severity, loudness, and depression. *Otolaryngol Head Neck Surg.* 1999;121(1): 48–51.

62. Fagelson MA. The association between tinnitus and posttraumatic stress disorder. *Am J Audiol.* 2007;16(2):107–117.

63. Jang DW, Johnson E, Chandrasekhar SS. Neuromonics™ tinnitus treatment: preliminary experience in a private practice setting. *Laryngoscope.* 2010;120(suppl 4):S208.

64. Goddard JC, Berliner K, Luxford WM. Recent experience with the neuromonics tinnitus treatment. *Int Tinnitus J.* 2009;15(2):168–173.

65. Van de Heyning P, Vermeire K, Diebl M, Nopp P, Anderson I, De Ridder D. Incapacitating unilateral tinnitus in single-sided deafness treated by cochlear implantation. *Ann Otol Rhinol Laryngol.* 2008; 117(9):645–652.

66. Amoodi HA, Mick PT, Shipp DB, et al. The effects of unilateral cochlear implantation on the tinnitus handicap inventory and the influence on quality of life. *Laryngoscope.* 2011;121(7):1536–1540.

67. Bauer CA, Brozoski TJ. Effect of tinnitus retraining therapy on the loudness and annoyance of tinnitus: a controlled trial. *Ear Hear.* 2011;32(2):145–155.

68. Piccirillo JF, Garcia KS, Nicklaus J, et al. Low-frequency repetitive transcranial magnetic stimulation to the temporoparietal junction for tinnitus. *Arch Otolaryngol Head Neck Surg.* 2011;137(3):221–228.

69. Vanneste S, Plazier M, Van de Heyning P, De Ridder D. Repetitive transcranial magnetic stimulation frequency dependent tinnitus improvement by double cone coil prefrontal stimulation. *J Neurol Neurosurg Psychiatry.* 2011;82(10):1160–1164.

70. Seidman MD, Ridder DD, Elisevich K, et al. Direct electrical stimulation of Heschl's gyrus for tinnitus treatment. *Laryngoscope.* 2008; 118(3):491–500.

71. Tyler RS, Conrad-Armes D. The determination of tinnitus loudness considering the effects of recruitment. *J Speech Hear Res.* 1983;26(1): 59–72.

72. Baguley DM. Hyperacusis. *J R Soc Med.* 2003;96(12):582–585.

Balance and Dizziness

Neil T. Shepard, Jaynee A. Handelsman, and Richard A. Clendaniel

INTRODUCTION

Although a large number of different etiologies can be the cause for complaints of dizziness (representing a wide variety of specific symptoms) and imbalance, traumatic brain injury (TBI) ranks among those of significant complexity and difficult to rehabilitate. Patients diagnosed with TBI often present with dizziness complaints in the midst of a wide variety of other symptoms, as is evidenced by the diversity of discussion in this chapter. Experience in treating this group of patients for imbalance and other dizziness complaints shows that the time course of recovery is significantly longer than patients with similar damage to the peripheral or central balance system, yet for reasons other than TBI. To date—as a group—those with TBI diagnoses do poorer overall in treatment formats of vestibular and balance rehabilitation therapy than other groups with peripheral vestibular injuries, not of a brain injury origin.

For reference, it will be useful to start with a brief overview of the elements of the balance system and its normal functioning.

No single structure subserves balance function. Rather, the system consists of multiple sensory inputs from the vestibular end-organs, the visual system, and the somatosensory or proprioceptive systems. The input information is then integrated at the level of the brain stem and cerebellum with significant influence from the cerebral cortex, including the frontal, parietal, and occipital lobes. The integrated input information results in various stereotypic responses for eye movement, postural control, and perception of movement and orientation in space. For those desiring more detailed information about the normal functioning of the balance system, see the references listed (1–9).

Central Vestibular Compensation Process

The vestibular system is the only special sensory system in which unilateral loss of function can seriously threaten the long-term survival or well-being of an organism. In humans, injury to the central or peripheral system may result in considerable disability. Fortunately, most disease processes involving the vestibular labyrinth are self-limited, and spontaneous functional recovery can be expected. This is caused by the remarkable ability of the central nervous system (CNS) to recover after a labyrinthine injury, a process known as vestibular compensation. Failure to recover from a peripheral labyrinthine insult may be caused by ongoing fluctuating condition in the vestibular end- organ itself or to failure of central vestibular compensation. Being alert to this critical distinction and its clinical implications is crucial for successful management of the dizzy patient (10,11).

SOURCES OF BALANCE AND DIZZINESS COMPLAINTS AFTER A TBI EVENT

Combinations of specific disorders resulting from a head injury can occur, but for the purposes of this discussion, the most common entities will be considered individually. For all of the disorders of the peripheral or central systems, the temporal course of the symptoms (length of spells or events if symptoms are not continuous), and the nature of the symptom onset being spontaneous or provoked by head or visual motion and whether hearing loss is involved with the symptoms are the key features of the history. The history, as with other patients complaining of dizziness or unsteadiness, is the single most important evaluation tool for the investigation of the cause of the complaints. For each of the encapsulated description disorders below these features will be reported.

Disorders of Peripheral Vestibular Origin

Posttraumatic injury to the peripheral vestibular system can occur in isolation or in association with a hearing loss. In cases where clear indications for peripheral vestibular involvement is lacking—but suspected—the presence of a documented postinjury hearing loss adds significantly to the argument for peripheral vestibular dysfunction.

Benign Paroxysmal Positional Vertigo

This is considered one of the most common causes for complaints of dizziness (vertigo) and imbalance, and the most common source for dizziness post head trauma. It is characterized by brief spells (typically < minute) of vertigo, falling or lightheadedness provoked by a movement of the head. In the most common form of this disorder, the provocative movements are in the saggital plane. The provoked symptoms are very frequently accompanied by complaints of general unsteadiness during daily routines. The character of the disorder is to have it resolve spontaneously and then recur.

The length of time for symptoms can vary from as short as a single day to greater than 1 year. Resolution length is equally as large as a variance. This is a disorder of the inner ear where the semicircular canals, which are not sensitive to the pull of gravity, have an altered mechanics that make them sensitive to gravity. This occurs secondary to suspected displacement of crystal structures from the otoliths into the semicircular canal system. Hearing loss is not a typical feature associated with this disorder, but certainly could occur given head trauma as the precipitating source. Treatments are highly successful and typically consist of head maneuvers referred to as "canalith repositioning procedures" during which the crystal structures are repositioned out of the involved canal (see the following texts) (12–17).

Labyrinthine Concussion

This disorder is characterized by hearing loss and vertigo—both of sudden onset following a head trauma. The symptoms typically improve over days and, in many cases, some recovery of hearing may occur. Usually, the symptoms of continuous vertigo resolve into being present only when provoked by head movements in any direction. It is thought that the violent movement of the fluids and tissues within the inner ear can cause tearing of tissues and/or set up a series of events where, metabolically, the cells undergo deterioration and death. This condition occurs in the absence of a documented fracture of the temporal bone (18). Secondary to the typical long-term symptoms of head movement provoked brief spells (seconds to minutes <5), these patients are good candidates for management with vestibular and balance rehabilitation therapy. Suppressive medication is many times needed at the initiation of this condition to control the sudden onset of vertigo and associated neurovegetative symptoms (19,20).

A long-term consequence of damage to the vestibular labyrinth, independent of the etiology, is the development of spontaneous spells of vertigo lasting from minutes to hours. In some cases, these can be associated with fluctuant or progressive hearing loss in a format classic for Ménière disease. However, this is considered a secondary Ménière resulting from the previous trauma. When it takes the form of only the spells of vertigo without associated auditory symptoms, the older term is that of posttraumatic endolymphatic hydrops. If the symptoms involve only the spontaneous events, vestibular and balance rehabilitation therapy is typically not applicable, and the treatment options are the same as those used in cases of Ménière of idiopathic origin (21).

Temporal Bone Fractures

Both blunt and penetrating trauma to the temporal bone can lead to damage to the ear or the eighth nerve complex. These injuries may result in a conductive hearing loss secondary to trauma to the external and/or middle ears, or a sensorineural hearing loss secondary to labyrinthine or eighth nerve trauma. Vertigo and subsequent imbalance may occur as an isolated symptom, or may be associated with a sensorineural hearing loss (18,19). Penetrating trauma is a less common cause of temporal bone injury, with etiologic agents for this form of injury ranging from bullets and knives to pencils and cotton swabs.

Temporal bone fractures elicited by blunt trauma have classically been defined by the relationship of the axis of the fracture line to the long axis of the temporal bone. Thus, longitudinal fractures course along the external auditory canal, through the tegmen of the middle ear, and then pass anterior to the labyrinth to terminate in one of the foramina (lacerum or spinosum).

Transverse fractures run perpendicular to the long axis of the temporal bone, traversing the petrous bone between the foramen magnum and the foramen spinosum or lacerum, typically disrupting either the bony labyrinth or internal auditory canal. More recent data indicate that most temporal bone fractures possess properties of both longitudinal and transverse fractures, and are thus classified as mixed or oblique fractures. Projectiles may involve any or all components of the temporal bone, depending on their trajectory. More benign penetrating objects (e.g., pencils, cotton swabs) may elicit neurovestibular symptoms by disrupting the interface between the stapes and the labyrinth, creating a perilymph fistula (see the following texts).

The hallmark of a labyrinthine injury secondary to blunt or penetrating trauma is the presence of vertigo and hearing loss. In cases of brain injury, in which the patient has been comatose for a period of time, the symptom of vertigo may be supplanted by the complaint of imbalance. Fractures that approximate a longitudinal course do not cause a direct disruption of the inner ear or the eighth nerve. However, patients may suffer both sensorineural hearing loss and vertigo secondary to what has been referred to as a *labyrinthine concussion* (see in previous texts). In contrast, fractures that traverse the otic capsule or internal auditory canal will cause profound hearing loss and vertigo.

No specific treatment exits for blunt or penetrating inner ear trauma. Vestibular suppressants can be used for acute vertigo control, if not otherwise contraindicated by the patient's overall medical status. Hearing aid amplification may be useful in patients with partial sensorineural hearing loss, and vestibular rehabilitation therapy is indicated in those patients with a slow recovery from their vestibular loss. Benign paroxysmal positional vertigo (BPPV) is a common sequela of head injury and is in fact, the most common form of posttraumatic vertigo. Any patient complaining of vertigo after a head trauma should have a Dix–Hallpike maneuver performed in the office (see Fig. 47-1). If the diagnosis of BPPV is confirmed, then a canalith repositioning maneuver (see Fig. 47-2) should be performed.

Perilymphatic Fistula

A perilymph fistula (PLF) of the round or oval windows occurs when the boundary between the middle and inner ear has been violated, allowing egress of perilymph and inner ear dysfunction. The topic of PLF remains controversial, particularly with respect to the spontaneous variety (22).

The development of a PLF caused by disruption of the oval (or less commonly, round) window secondary to external trauma is the most common cause for this disorder. This trauma may be iatrogenic (e.g., poststapes surgery) or secondary to blunt or penetrating trauma. Barotrauma and acoustic trauma have been proposed to create fistula via the transmission of rapid pressure changes to the round and oval windows (so called "implosive trauma") (23–25).

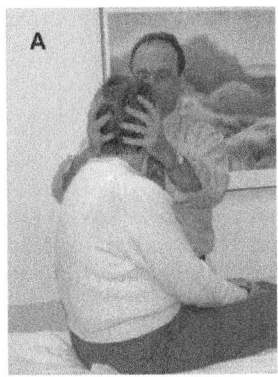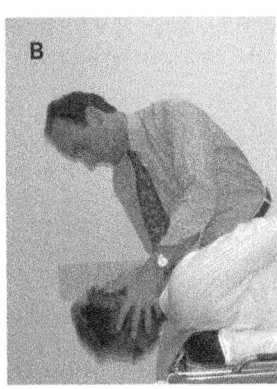

FIGURE 47-1 The left Dix–Hallpike Test. A, The patient sits with legs extended on the table and cervical spine rotated 45° to the left. The examiner places his hands on either side of the patient's head with his right forearm behind the patient's left shoulder. B, The patient is quickly brought into supine and the cervical spine extended approximately 10°. The examiner observes the patient for nystagmus and other symptoms.

A form of PLF that is thought to be a developmental defect that causes thinning or absence of bone over the superior semicircular canal is a confirmed source for PLF. In this case, the abnormal communication is between the perilymphatic space and the middle cranial fossa. In cases where the dura acts to seal the deficit or the bone is very thin but

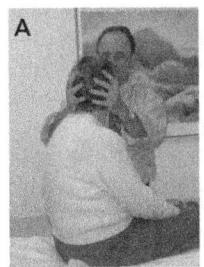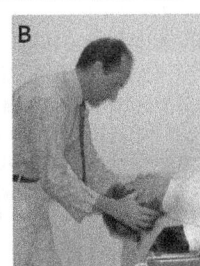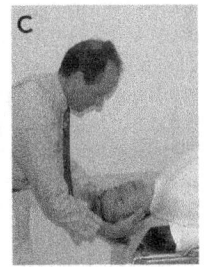
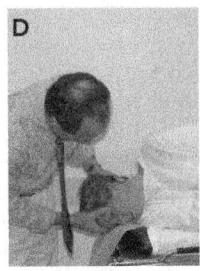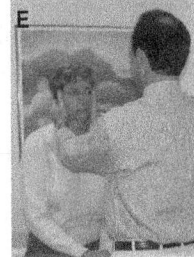

FIGURE 47-2 The Canalith Repositioning Maneuver for left-sided BPPV. A, The starting position is identical to the initial position in the Dix–Hallpike test, with the cervical spine rotated 45° to the left. B, The patient is brought into supine and the cervical spine is extended approximately 10° (45° of left cervical rotation is maintained). C, The cervical spine is rotated 90° to the right to end up in a 45° rotation to the right. D, The patient is rotated onto their right side, maintaining the cervical rotation to the right. The cervical spine is brought out of extension, and is laterally flexed to the right. E, The patient is brought into sitting position. As the patient rises from right side lying to sitting position, the cervical rotation to the right is maintained.

not absent, a simple head strike or whiplash injury can bring the defect to a clinically recognizable status (26).

A wide gamut of symptomatology has been ascribed to the PLF. Currently, most otologists would consider the diagnosis of a fistula when a patient presents with a sudden sensorineural hearing loss associated with tinnitus and vertigo, occurring immediately subsequent to a traumatic insult. Fluctuations in hearing may support the diagnosis if they appear provoked by pressure fluctuations or straining. The exception to this is the superior canal dehiscence where the clinical features are more distinct including a conductive hearing loss that is not of middle ear origin, autophony (abnormal perception of body sounds), loud sound, and straining induced dizziness (26).

Despite intense effort, no valid and accurate diagnostic test for PLF exists. Most authorities agree that the only manner in which the presence of a PLF can be confirmed is by direct observation of the leakage (27,28). Based on recent results, it would appear that the most accurate way of performing this exploration is by using endoscopes passed through a myringotomy incision (28,29). The superior canal dehiscence has a more well-defined set of specific test and clinical markers, including the use of high resolution CT with reconstructed images at 0.2–0.4 mm thickness together with Vestibular Evoked Myogenic Potentials (VEMP) (30).

Central Nervous System Causes for Balance and Dizziness

There are multiple sources of injury and secondary disorders to head trauma that can originate in the CNS and manifest in symptoms of balance and dizziness. Both posttraumatic seizures and posttraumatic stress syndrome or anxiety disorders can be direct causes for complaints of symptoms ranging from vertigo to vague lightheadedness and imbalance. Mechanisms, investigation, and treatment for these entities are considered elsewhere in this text and will not be repeated herein. It is important to realize that there can be dramatic effects of psychological disorders that develop with long term disorders and are expressed in the complaints of dizziness (31–33).

Direct trauma to the brain stem and/or cerebellum will result in complaints of imbalance with standing and walking and occasional complaints of true vertigo. The pathophysiology of injuries of this nature is addressed in another chapter in this text. The nature of the signs and symptoms will vary depending on the location of the lesion with in the CNS (34). Lesions within the brain stem and cerebellum have typical ocularmotor abnormalities that can be recognized during the office or laboratory examinations of these patients. Given that these are typically stationary lesions, vestibular and balance rehabilitation therapy will comprise a major portion of the treatment plan. These are usually not spontaneous events of symptoms but are more likely to be continuous sensations of disorientation and imbalance with gait (35).

Posttraumatic migraine headaches, as with nontraumatic migraines, can have dizziness as an aura for the migraine event. This can occur with or without the pain phase of the migraine event. When the events of dizziness are not temporally related to actual headaches, this entity can be quite difficult to diagnose because it has to be a diagnosis of exclusion. Symptoms from migraine-associated dizziness can be spontaneous spells of true vertigo to vague complaints of increased sensitivity to motion sickness. Recognition of this is typically accomplished by having a history that the headaches being experienced meet the criteria for migraine, or pretrauma the patient had a migraine history. Once diagnosed, these are treated by direct treatment of the headaches (36,37). In some cases, the patient can be assisted with the use of vestibular and balance therapy as long as there is simultaneous focused treatment on the underlying migraine disorder.

In addition to the aforementioned descriptions of the direct effects of the CNS lesions producing symptoms of dizziness and imbalance, all of those can have an indirect effect as well. In patients with combined peripheral and central lesions, the presence of the central lesion in the brain stem and/or cerebellum may not be causing direct symptoms of dizziness or imbalance, but could cause disruptions in the natural central system compensation process. This would have the effect of slowing or preventing the compensation process from reducing the symptoms from the peripheral vestibular insult. This disruption in the compensation process can also occur from psychological difficulties, migraines, or seizure disorders. In these instances, direct treatment for the other disorders would be necessary in order to allow for as full a compensation process as possible.

Post-TBI can rarely result in the development of other possible causes for dizziness of a nonvertiginous or vertigo form. Development of epilepsy can rarely take on a complaint of dizziness before or during an epileptic event. These patients may complain of event of vertigo lasting typically less than 15 minutes in association with other seizure behavior. It would be rare for myofacial pain to be a direct cause of dizziness, but pain causing a restriction in head movement on the body can be a source for difficulty with imbalance. This same mechanism of restriction of head movement on the torso is felt to be the common manner in which cervical soft tissue injuries can be a source for unsteadiness (called cervical vertigo). It would be extremely rare for cervical region injuries to be a source for true vertigo symptoms. Lastly, the medications needed in some of the patients with TBI can cause mild unsteadiness or exacerbate the effects of direct vestibular system injuries primarily by stalling the compensation process. A team approach is needed to develop an approach that allows for judicious use of the needed medications without over medicating along with the use of dominantly vestibular and balance rehabilitation at the same time to promote compensation.

In situations such as BPPV or development of secondary Ménière, the symptoms of the dizziness will likely come and go. BPPV is a disorder with high recurrence rate for which the approach to treatment is to teach the patient to manage recurrence—we do not talk about curing BPPV. For Ménière, the treatment approach would be that for idiopathic Ménière syndrome with use of medication, therapy, and, when needed, surgery all managed by a neurotologist. For most other dizziness provoked by head and/or brain injury, the issue of remission and recurrence would typically not be a problem.

Sports and Blast Injuries

More recently, especially with the military action over the last decade, much attention has been given to sport and blast injuries, both of which can produce either peripheral or central vestibular system insults.

Sports Induced Traumatic Brain Injury

Physicians who treat athletes are frequently faced with making a decision about when an athlete is ready to return to play following a cerebral concussion, yet there are no clear protocols for evaluating patients or for determining readiness to play (38). Although neuropsychological testing and sideline assessment tools have been developed, there is lack of agreement about the use of available metrics.

Evaluating postural stability has been suggested as a valid way of assessing the impact of TBI on athletes. In an ongoing study comparing athletes with mild brain injury to control subjects, the data suggest that subjects tend to have sensory integration problems and decreased postural stability for approximately 3 days after which they gradually recover to normal performance to about 10 days postinjury (38). Previous studies have investigated the relationship between symptom severity, neuropsychological test results, and postural stability, and have not found any relationship between symptom severity and the other two measures. Although each is important to the evaluation of an athlete with TBI, postural control testing may provide a unique perspective on the assessment of readiness to play.

Blast Injuries

Blast exposure is the most common cause of injury in modern warfare, and the primary injury results from a shock wave that is propagated through tissue resulting in a global compression and then decompression of the contents of the skull (39). That same blast exposure may also result in trauma to the sensory structures of the middle and inner ear because of a peak positive pressurization followed by extreme negative pressure (40). Damage to the vestibular nerve or other components of the vestibular pathway is also possible (41). When comparing active duty military personnel who suffered TBI because of purely blast injuries vs those whose injuries were a result of purely blunt head trauma, it is apparent that blast exposure results in a higher prevalence of hearing loss and cognitive impairment, and that unilateral vestibular loss is more common with blunt trauma. Postural control problems are also more prevalent following blast injury (39). Common findings in patients following blast exposure are posttraumatic migraine associated dizziness or migraine headache coupled with a balance disorder and anxiety. Also prevalent are cognitive complaints such as short-term memory deficits or mental processing problems, and it is apparent that the prevalence of central auditory processing problems and posttraumatic stress disorder (PTSD) increase over time (42). Whereas blunt trauma results in localized axonal damage, blast exposure results in global brain injury that gets worse over time. Recovery for these patients (compensation for vestibular loss) may be complicated by visual field deficits and lower limb loss in polytrauma (41). Because of the difference in performance between patients suffering from blast exposure and those with blunt trauma, clinicians cannot use the wealth of information that has been obtained about blunt head injury to predict the pathologies that are associate with blast exposure or to know how best to treat them (40).

Blast exposure frequently results in multiple traumatic injuries, in which case, ear and balance problems may be overlooked. As a result, a comprehensive multidisciplinary approach to evaluation of patients with TBI is essential (41). It is important that nonvestibular causes of dizziness such as postural hypotension, cervical vertigo, and visual impairment are ruled out (43). Additionally, because self-report of symptoms and determining whether PTSD is present will likely underestimate the extent of TBI following blast exposure, vestibular testing is important to understanding the magnitude of the disorder (42).

OVERVIEW OF ASSESSMENT TOOLS AND THEIR USE IN DIAGNOSIS AND TREATMENT

Even though a head trauma with or without TBI may be the precipitating event that results in complaints of imbalance and dizziness, one must proceed in the evaluation of those complaints in a systematic manner to uncover the source of the symptoms. Therefore, the evaluation is not different from what would be performed for a patient presenting without a known antecedent event. In considering the evaluation of the patient with complaints of vertigo, lightheadedness, imbalance, or combinations of these descriptors, one must look beyond just the peripheral and central vestibular system with its oculomotor connections. The various pathways involved in postural control—only part of which have direct or indirect vestibular input—should be kept in mind during an evaluation.

The evaluation of the dizzy patient should proceed being guided by what information is needed to make initial and subsequent management decisions. When various tests are reviewed and correlated with high-level activities of daily living, virtually no significant relationships exist for the chronic dizzy patient. Tests considered extent and site-of-lesion studies, electronystagmography (ENG) and videonystagmography (VNG), rotational chair, and specific protocols in postural control assessment (3,4), give results that are unable to be used to predict symptom type, magnitude, or the level of disability of an individual patient. Conversely, patient complaints cannot be used to predict the outcomes of these tests (44–47). In a limited manner, more functionally oriented evaluation tools—computerized dynamic posturography (CDP), dynamic visual acuity testing (48)—provide for some correlation between results, patient symptoms, and functional limitations. Add to the testing specific or general health inventories like the Dizziness Handicap Inventory (44) and predictive assessment of disability is improved but remains significantly limited. It is hypothesized that the reason for this dichotomy in test results vs functional disability and symptom complaints is the inability of the tests to adequately characterize the status of the central vestibular compensation process (5,10,11).

The following discussion will be a very brief overview of the major elements available for assessment. A recent comprehensive summary of the evaluation of the dizzy patient and detailed descriptions are found elsewhere for the interested reader (3,4).

Neurotologic History

Given the various tools for assessment, the history is the single most important factor in determining the course of management. The differentiation between the various peripheral vestibular disorders that can result from a head injury is particularly dependent on historical information and the conclusions that the physician draws from the interview. Most vestibular disorders cannot be distinguished from one another simply by vestibular testing or other diagnostic interventions. Failure to properly discriminate these disorders on historical grounds may lead to improper management. In addition, balance function study results are best interpreted in light of a proper clinical history (4).

Office Examination

A variety of test procedures may be used in the office setting to assess the balance-disorder patient. These, like the laboratory studies, assist in the identification of the extent and site of the lesion. These straightforward clinical tests are essential variations of the related laboratory studies, but have less ability to quantify the outcomes. The theoretical basis behind many of these tests is well-founded in the physiological considerations discussed earlier and in the references provided. Because of the subjective nature of these tools, the validity and reliability of these tests are reduced compared to the formal laboratory studies (9).

Laboratory Studies

Electronystagmography or Videonystagmography
Traditional ENG, using electrodes placed around the eyes or VNG with infrared video techniques for eye movement recordings, is a process that estimates the position of the eye as a function of time. Because the primary purpose of the vestibular apparatus is to control eye movements, the movements of the eyes may be used to examine the activity of the peripheral vestibular end-organs and their central vestibulo-ocular pathways. The ENG or VNG evaluation is a series of subtests performed to assess portions of the peripheral and central vestibular systems. It is important to understand that peripheral vestibular system assessment with ENG or VNG is significantly limited, typically reflecting function of the horizontal semicircular canal with restricted information from vertical canals and otolith organs.

Rotary Chair
Rotary chair testing has been used to expand the evaluation of the peripheral vestibular system. As with the ENG or VNG findings, the rotational chair evaluation can assist in site-of-lesion determination, counseling the patient, and confirmation of clinical suspicion of diagnosis and lesion site, but is not likely to significantly alter or impact on the course of patient management, excepting the bilateral peripheral weakness patient.

Otolith Organ Assessment
There are currently 3 methods that are used to provide for this assessment. Two of the techniques are the Vestibular Evoked Myogenic Potential (VEMP) test. The purpose of the VEMP is to provide information regarding the eighth nerve and otolith organ function and to potentially separate superior from inferior vestibular nerve and likewise utricular

from saccular involvement. Like the caloric test, one benefit of the VEMP is that it provides ear specific information. There are 2 types of VEMP responses: the cervical VEMP (cVEMP) (dominantly saccular) and the ocular VEMP (oVEMP) (felt to be mediated via the utricle). The third test is that of unilateral centrifugation, a test performed with rotary chair equipment. With unilateral centrifugation, the chair is translated laterally, which projects the vertical axis of rotation through the peripheral vestibular organ on the right or the left. The purpose of the test is to allow for a dynamic evaluation of each utricular organ individually by applying a horizontal force to 1 utricle at a time.

Postural Control Assessment

Just as all patients that are being evaluated in the laboratory need tests for peripheral and central vestibulo-ocular pathway involvement, they also require some assessment of postural control ability. There are several different general approaches to formal postural control testing, each with specific technical equipment requirements and goals for the testing (5,49). Three principle testing protocols are used in patient evaluation, the Sensory Organization Test (SOT), the Motor Control Test (MCT), and the Postural Evoked Responses (PER). These allow for assessment ranging from strictly functional (not site-of-lesion) with the SOT to site and limited pathology specific results with PER. Because of the functional assessment using SOT, postural control assessment is useful in the development and monitoring of vestibular and balance rehabilitation management option discussed subsequently.

OVERVIEW OF TREATMENT OPTIONS

The options for management of the dizzy and balance-disordered patient fall into the major categories of medication, surgery, dietary changes, and vestibular and balance rehabilitation therapy (VBRT), or combinations of these techniques (5). In general, it will be the rare patient with dizziness secondary to head injury that is going to be managed with medication alone. The most common use of medications in this arena would be short-term or "as needed" use of vestibular suppressant medications for acute symptom control at the onset or with recurrent spontaneous events of vertigo lasting for hours. Other than migraine and psychological disorders, there is little call for use of chronic medication. Of the medications most commonly used for vestibular suppression, the primary classes are those of antihistamines (Meclizine and Promethazine), anticholinergics (Scopolamine), phenothiazine (Prochlorperazine), and benzodiazepines (Diazepam, Lorazepam, and Clonazepam). There are other classes and other specific medications within these listed drug classes that have been used for the control of acute vertigo and the vegetative symptoms that accompany the sensation of vertigo. It is important to remember that use of these medications should be on a short-term basis and only "as needed" when possible. These classes of medications have an effect that can significantly slow the natural compensation process and the effectiveness of VBRT (17).

Surgical intervention for this group of patients is used even less frequent than medication. The patients for whom surgery may be considered are those discussed earlier, asso-

ciated with temporal-bone injuries and perilymphatic fistulas. The treatment option that would be the most common is VBRT.

The major feature that drives an initial decision about the use of medication or surgery vs VBRT is the evidence that the peripheral or central vestibular lesion is unstable (varying over time), as opposed to an uncompensated stable lesion. This distinction comes dominantly from the patient's presenting symptoms. Therefore, the patient should be asked to describe the progression of symptoms over time, along with the nature and duration of typical spells. Specifically, one wishes to know if the symptoms are continuous or occur in discrete episodes. If the symptoms are episodic, it is extremely important to distinguish whether they are spontaneous or motion-provoked. If the symptoms are brief and predictably produced by head movements or body position changes, the patient most likely has a stable lesion, but has not yet completed CNS compensation. Those who describe these symptoms sometimes also note a chronic underlying sense of disequilibrium or lightheadedness. The chronic symptoms may be quite troublesome, but any intense vertigo should be primarily motion-provoked. These patients are suitable candidates for vestibular rehabilitation. It is important to point out that historical information is essential in deciding who might benefit from rehabilitation therapy.

If the episodic spells described by the patient are longer periods of intense vertigo that occur spontaneously and without warning, this is probably a progressive or unstable peripheral dysfunction. One must also suspect a progressive lesion if the vertigo is accompanied by fluctuating or progressive sensorineural hearing loss. Such patients are managed with medical therapy, and if this fails, they constitute the best candidates for surgical intervention. Such patients are not candidates for vestibular rehabilitation, except as an adjunctive modality. For the chronic patient, including those with known brain trauma event, the primary effort is to determine why they have not had the natural central compensation process run to completion.

When dealing with the group of patient with TBI, VBRT is many times used as 1 component of a comprehensive TBI rehabilitation program involving physical, occupational, speech, and cognitive therapy aspects.

VESTIBULAR AND BALANCE REHABILITATION THERAPY PROGRAMS

As indicated earlier, VBRT is the most frequently used management option for patients with balance and dizziness complaints from brain injury, or other causes. Therefore, the remainder of this chapter will be a discussion of this technique.

Because TBI can lead to damage of the vestibular system from peripheral to central structures, as well as cause other CNS damage, the types of exercises used to treat the dizziness and imbalance can be quite comprehensive.

The use of exercise for the treatment of individuals with vestibular dysfunction is not new. In the 1940s, Sir Terrence Cawthorne, an otolaryngologist, and FS Cooksey, a physiotherapist, devised a series of exercises for the treatment of individuals with unilateral vestibular paresis and postconcussion syndrome (50–52). Cawthorne and Cooksey realized that head movements often provoked an individual's symptoms of dizziness. They also observed that patients who were active recovered faster and hypothesized that head movements must be important in the recovery of function. The exercises used in a VBRT program generally fall under 4 different categories: exercises to promote habituation, exercises to promote adaptation, exercises to promote substitution, and exercises designed to treat BPPV.

Habituation exercises, like those described initially by Cawthorne and Cooksey, are based on the principle that repeated exposure to a noxious or provocative stimulus (in this case movements) will lead to a reduction in the body's response to that stimulus.

The exercises to induce adaptation of the vestibular system, although similar to the approaches mentioned earlier, reflect our increased knowledge of the function and adaptation of the vestibular system. Adaptation exercises are designed to promote long-term (plastic) changes in the neuronal response of the vestibular system to a given head movement, with the goals of decreasing retinal slip, improving postural stability, and decreasing symptoms. These exercises are typically used in individuals with an uncompensated unilateral vestibular loss. The treatment approach for individuals with unilateral vestibular hypofunction differs in both theory and practice from the approach for individuals with bilateral vestibular loss. For individuals with bilateral vestibular loss, exercises to promote the substitution of alternative strategies for gaze stability and postural control are appropriate.

Finally, the exercises to treat BPPV are based on the hypothesis that there are crystalline structures, which are consistent with degenerating otoconia from the otolithic membrane (53). BPPV can occur in conjunction unilateral vestibular loss, central vestibular disorders, and in some cases with bilateral vestibular loss. Consequently, the treatment of BPPV is often combined with other exercise approaches to treat the identified problems.

Who Is an Appropriate Candidate for Vestibular Rehabilitation?

Generally, individuals with stable vestibular function and symptoms provoked by head motion (either self-motion or motion in the environment) or environmental situations (e.g., absence of visual cues, altered somatosensory cues) will benefit from vestibular rehabilitation. Individuals with vestibular function that fluctuates—as in Ménière disease—or those who have true spontaneous episodic bouts of dizziness, typically will not benefit from vestibular rehabilitation.

Treatment of Individuals With Benign Paroxysmal Positional Vertigo

BPPV can affect any of the 3 semicircular canals, although the most commonly encountered presentation is that of posterior canal BPPV (54). In addition, the BPPV is thought to be caused by 1 of 2 mechanisms: cupulolithiasis (55) or canalithiasis (56,57). In canalithiasis, the otoconia are mobile in the long arm of the semicircular canal; in cupulolithiasis, the otoconia are adherent to the cupula. The effect, in both cases, is to make the involved canal sensitive to the pull of gravity. The presentation of the 2 types of BPPV differs, as do the treatments for each condition. The methods used to determine the involved canal and the nature of the BPPV as well as a comprehensive review of the various treatment tech-

niques are beyond the scope of this chapter. The treatment for the most common form of BPPV associated with the posterior canal is shown in Figure 47-2, the other modifications for treatment of posterior canal and the other canal is likewise beyond the scope of this chapter. The interested reader is referred to the following articles for review (13,58–63).

Treatment of Gaze Instability

One of the primary functions of the vestibular system is to generate compensatory eye movements to a given head movement—the vestibulo-ocular reflex (VOR). The VOR, when functioning appropriately, allows the individual to maintain the object of interest on the fovea, thereby preserving visual clarity. If the vestibular system is not functioning appropriately, the eye movements generated in response to head movement will not be sufficient to keep the object of interest on the fovea. The resulting movement of the image on the retina, retinal slip, will lead to a degradation of visual acuity. In individuals with remaining vestibular function (e.g., those with a unilateral vestibular deficit), the exercises are designed to foster adaptation of the remaining vestibular signals to generate the appropriate eye movement responses. For those individuals without vestibular function (e.g., those with bilateral vestibular loss), there is no remaining vestibular signal to adapt. Consequently, the exercises for these individuals are designed to promote the use of alternative strategies to promote gaze stability during head movements. The 2 general exercise approaches and the rationale behind the exercises will be explained separately.

Exercises to Enhance Vestibular Adaptation
The rehabilitation of individuals with unilateral peripheral vestibular hypofunction (UVH) or loss is based on the plasticity inherent within the vestibular system. The ability of the vestibular system to modify its behavior during development, as well as in disease states, has been well documented (for a review, see review by du Lac and colleagues) (64). In the case of an insufficient VOR caused by vestibular hypofunction, the vestibular system will not generate sufficient eye movements in response to head movements. This will cause the visual image to move across the retina. This retinal slip in the presence of head movements appears to be an effective stimulus for inducing adaptation of the VOR (65). For patients with remaining vestibular function, the exercises used in the treatment of gaze stability deficits are designed to generate these error signals and thereby foster adaptation of the vestibular system (66). The goals of this aspect of the rehabilitation program are to (a) improve visual acuity during head movements, (b) improve visual-vestibular interactions during head movements, and (c) decrease the individual's sensitivity to head movements.

As a consequence of the error signal produced by the exercises, performance of the exercise is frequently associated with symptoms of dizziness or nausea. The patient must be aware that provocation of their symptoms is a necessary part of the rehabilitation process. If there is no symptom provocation with the exercises, then the patient is not challenging the vestibular system and adaptation will not occur. The first exercise to address the gaze instability issue is often called ×1 (times one) viewing because the eye velocity must

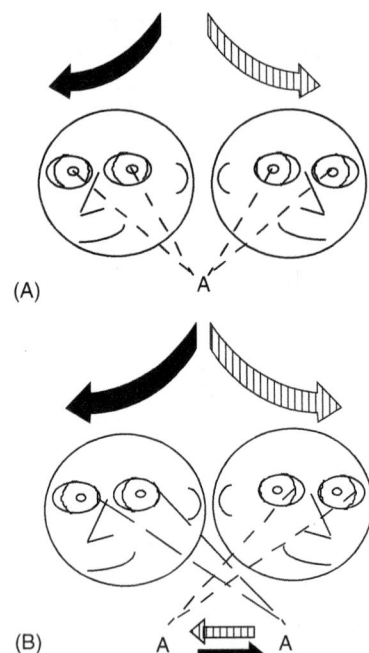

FIGURE 47-3 Exercises to induce adaptation of the vestibulo-ocular reflex. A, ×1 viewing exercise. The patient views a stationary target—which should be a letter, number, or word (in this case, the letter A)—while he turns his head back and forth. The speed of the rotation is increased to the point where faster movements would induce oscillopsia. Both horizontal and vertical rotations are performed. B, ×2 viewing exercise. The patient views a target that moves in the opposite direction of the head movement while he turns his head back and forth. As with the ×1 viewing exercise, the target should be a letter, number, or word (in this case, the letter A). The speed of the rotation is increased to the point where faster movements would induce oscillopsia. Both horizontal and vertical head rotations and target movements are performed.

equal the inverse of the head velocity to maintain visual fixation (Fig. 47-3A). To perform the exercise, the patient fixates on a visual target (a small letter or number) located on a plain visual background, approximately 3 ft away. The patient then rotates his or her head, maintaining fixation on the visual target throughout the head rotation. The image should remain in focus and stable in space. The amount of head rotation should be approximately 30°–45° to either side of the midline. Head rotation, both horizontal and vertical, should be performed as rapidly as the individual can tolerate, with the restriction that the visual target must remain in focus and stationary. The duration should be progressed gradually to avoid severe exacerbation of the symptoms or provocation of cervical pain. As the individual improves, the velocity of head rotation can be increased. Altering the postural demands or the visual conditions will vary the stimulus context. The progression in postural demands occurs over the course of several weeks. On any given day, the patient will perform the ×1 viewing exercise under only 1 postural condition.

Because adaptation of the vestibular system is context specific (67), the context of the visual stimulus should vary to reflect the different visual conditions that an individual normally encounters. The influence of the optokinetic system

(parafoveal visual stimuli) on gaze stability can be incorporated into the exercise program by placing the visual target within a "full-field" visual stimulus such as a checkerboard. When the visual target is at the same depth as the full-field visual stimulus, then the optokinetic system will assist the VOR in generating the appropriate compensatory eye movements. If the visual target is in front of the full-field visual stimulus, then the optokinetic system will actually generate anticompensatory eye movements because the visual world behind the object of interest appears to move in the same direction as the head movement. Because both of these stimulus conditions are encountered in normal activities, both conditions are incorporated into the rehabilitation program.

When the object of interest is near, the translation of the eyes relative to the visual target is greater than when the target is at a distance. The neural circuitry controlling the VOR normally takes target distance into account when generating the compensatory eye movements. Therefore the ×1 viewing exercises are also performed with larger visual targets at a distance (8–15 ft). Again, these exercises are performed in standing, with the feet positioned to challenge postural stability. The head is rotated as quickly as possible for 2 minutes, with the restriction that the visual target must remain in focus and stationary.

Gaze stability during head movements requires not only normal functioning of the VOR, but also interaction with other visual systems, such as the smooth pursuit system. To encourage this interaction, the ×1 viewing exercise is modified. The individual is again challenged to maintain clear and stable vision during head movements; however, rather than use a stationary target, the individual holds the target and moves it in the direction opposite to the head movement (Fig. 47-3B). If the target moves at the same speed as the head but in the opposite direction, then the eyes have to move at twice the head velocity to maintain clear vision. Consequently, this exercise is often referred to as ×2 (times two) viewing. This exercise can be performed in sitting, if necessary, and progressed to standing with a progressively decreasing base of support. The exercise can be performed with both a simple visual target as well as a target located in a complex visual background.

Exercises to Foster the Substitution of Alternative Strategies for Gaze Stability

Bilateral vestibular hypofunction (BVH) may result in major or complete loss of bilateral vestibular function. Therefore, the exercises are designed to enhance the remaining function of the vestibular system and to foster substitution for the loss of vestibular function with alternative strategies to maintain gaze stability (66). In the absence of vestibular signals, these individuals must use cervical inputs and knowledge of upcoming head movements (preplanning) to generate the compensatory eye movements (see Table 47-1).

The cervico-ocular reflex (COR) normally contributes less than 15% to the generation of compensatory eye movements for low frequency head rotations (66). Following bilateral vestibular loss, the COR can account for up to 25% of the compensatory eye movements for both low- and high-frequency head rotations (68). The ×1 viewing exercise described in the previous section can be used to increase the gain of the COR and to enhance the remaining function of the VOR. Generally, these exercises will be conducted at lower

TABLE 47-1 Exercises to Promote Alternative Strategies for Gaze Stability

1. ×1 viewing exercises

2. Active eye–head movements between 2 targets:

   Horizontal targets: Look directly at one target being sure that your head is also lined up with the target. Look at the other target with your eyes and then turn your head to the target. Be sure to keep the target in focus during the head movement. Repeat in the opposite direction.

   Vary the speed of the head movement, but always keep the targets in focus.

   Note: Place the 2 targets close enough together that when you are looking directly at one, you can see the other with your peripheral vision. Practice for 2–5 minutes, resting if necessary. This exercise can also be performed with 2 vertically placed targets.

3. Visualization of imaginary targets:

   Look at a target directly in front of you. Close your eyes and turn your head slightly, imagining that you are still looking directly at the target. Open your eyes and check to see if you have been able to keep your eyes on the target. Repeat in the opposite direction. Be as accurate as possible.

   Vary the speed and the amount (stopping point) of head rotation.

   Practice for 2–5 minutes, resting if necessary.

   Note: This exercise can be performed actively or passively while looking at a near target (within 2 ft) or at a distant target (across the room); it can also be performed vertically.

velocities than in individuals with unilateral vestibular hypofunction. When these exercises are performed actively, the CNS can also use foreknowledge of the upcoming movement to generate a compensatory eye movement. If performed passively, then the preplanning information is lost and the eye movements must be generated by the COR.

Another exercise that may improve the response of the COR, but uses the CNS's knowledge of upcoming movements, is the visualization of a remembered target location during head rotation. In this exercise, the patient fixates a visual target, closes his eyes, and rotates his head in one direction. While turning his head, the patient attempts to keep his eyes on the target location. When the patient stops the head rotation, he opens his eyes and looks at the visual target. If his gaze is accurate, he will be looking directly at the target. If his compensatory eye movements are insufficient, his eyes will have moved with his head and he will have to make a corrective saccade to view the target. This exercise should be performed with both horizontal and vertical head movements. The visual target should be placed at different eccentric positions and different distances relative to the patient. The degree and speed of the rotation should be varied to force the patient to attend to all sensory cues.

Difficult tasks for individuals with BVH are gaze shifts that require both eye and head movements. Normally, this task is accomplished by a patterned response. Initially, there is a saccade that is directed toward the object of interest. A head movement toward the target begins shortly after the saccade. Although both the eye and the head are moving toward the target, the VOR must be suppressed. When the

eye reaches the desired location, the head is typically still turning. At this point, the VOR must be used to keep the eyes on target during the remaining head movement. For patients with BVH, this head movement would cause the eyes to move beyond the intended object of interest and visual acuity would diminish. Individuals with BVH typically adopt 1 of 2 strategies to minimize this visual disturbance (68). One strategy is to make a hypometric saccade and allow the head movement to carry the eyes onto the object of interest. A second approach is to make an accurate initial saccade, followed by a corrective backward saccade that is triggered by the head movement. Both of these strategies will minimize the amount of time that the visual image is not on the fovea. We do not attempt to teach one strategy or the other. We simply have the patient perform an activity that will encourage adoption of one of these strategies.

Treatment of Motion Sensitivity

Symptom provocation caused by either head movements or visual motion is a common finding in individuals with vestibular dysfunction, and these findings are very common in individuals with dizziness secondary to TBI. Patients with sensitivity to head movements will describe increased symptoms associated with either head movements in general or rather specific movements. Patients with visual motion sensitivity will note increased symptoms when they are in busy visual environments such as crowds, department or grocery stores, or in traffic. The determination of head motion or visual motion sensitivity can often be made through the patient interview. One method of determining head motion sensitivity is through a series of rapid positioning maneuvers designed to elicit symptoms (69). These movements incorporate horizontal, vertical, and diagonal head movements with the head in different orientations relative to gravity. The symptom severity and duration in each of these movements is noted and used to determine a "motion sensitivity quotient." The results of this test can be used to identify patterns of motion that provoke symptoms and to track changes in the patient's motion sensitivity. The general approach to the treatment of motion sensitivity is that of habituation, defined here as the long-term reduction of the response to a noxious stimulus (specific movement), brought about by repeated exposure to the provocative stimulus (70).

Exercises to Decrease Head Motion Sensitivity

The ×1 viewing exercises, since they involve head movements, can be used as a habituation exercise. So in some individuals with head motion sensitivity, who have normal visual acuity during head movements, performance of the ×1 viewing exercise can lead to a reduction in their symptoms. For other individuals, however, performing the ×1 viewing exercise may be too symptom-provoking, or may not reduce all of their symptoms. In these cases, habituation exercises may be used to reduce the motion sensitivity. These exercises are generally of greater amplitude and velocity than the ×1 viewing exercises. However, the amplitude and velocity of the head movement is adjusted to the patient's condition. The exercises are designed to provoke symptoms, but following completion of each exercise session, the symptoms should return to baseline levels within 15–30 minutes.

TABLE 47-2 Exercises to Decrease Motion Sensitivity

1. While sitting, turn your head quickly from right to left 5 times. Look in the direction you are turning. Wait for your symptoms to subside. Repeat 3 times.

2. While sitting, alternate looking up at the ceiling and down at the floor quickly 5 times. Look in the direction you are moving your head. Wait for your symptoms to subside. Repeat 3 times.

3. Sit on the edge of your bed. Turn your head about 45° to the left. Now quickly lie on your right side. Wait for any symptoms to pass. Keeping your head turned, quickly sit up. Again, wait for the symptoms to pass. Now turn your head approximately 45° to the right. Quickly lie on your left side. Wait for the symptoms to pass. Quickly sit upright. Wait for the symptoms to pass. Repeat 5 times.

4. Lie on your back. Quickly roll to the right side. Wait for symptoms to pass. Return to your back. Quickly roll to the left side. Wait for symptoms to pass. Return to your back. Repeat 5 times.

5. While sitting in a chair, bend your head forward about halfway toward your knees. Now quickly sit upright. Wait for the symptoms to pass. Repeat 5 times. (Note: this can be done tipping the head to the right or left knee instead of straight down if that movement is more provocative.)

6. Stand in a corner with your back to the wall. Now make a quick turn so that you are facing the wall. Stop and wait for symptoms to pass. Now make a turn in the opposite direction so that your back is again facing the wall. Repeat 5 times.

The selection of the exercises and movement patterns may be based on either the patient's description of provocative movements or on the results of the motion sensitivity examination. Examples of these exercises are presented in Table 47-2.

Exercises to Decrease Visual Motion Sensitivity

Several previously described exercises can be used to try and decrease visual motion sensitivity. Performance of the ×1 viewing exercise with the visual target located in front of a complex visual background can be used as an effective exercise to decrease visual motion sensitivity. As noted earlier, this exercise will induce movement of the visual background in an anticompensatory fashion relative to the head movement. The habituation exercises described earlier (particularly the horizontal and vertical head movement exercises), if performed with eyes open, facing a visual scene with lots of color and contrast, can also be used as an exercise to decrease the visual motion sensitivity. If the combination of visual motion and head motion is too symptom-provoking, then another exercise, which does not involve head movement, may be used. In this case, the patient performs a visual following task, with the object of interest located in front of a busy visual background. The exercise is similar to the ×1 viewing exercise; however, the patient keeps their head still and moves the visual target from side to side (or up and down).

Another approach to this problem is to immerse patients in the environments that provoke their symptoms. Patients are encouraged to walk through grocery stores, department stores, shopping malls, or crowds (provided these environ-ments provoke symptoms). They can grade the intensity of the exercise in several ways. One is they can control their exposure by limiting the time they are in the particular environment. They can often adjust the intensity of the visual motion by selecting different times of the day to perform this exercise. Early in the morning, there are generally fewer people in the stores than later in the day or evening. Because their symptoms decrease, they are encouraged to walk for longer periods and at times when the stores are more crowded.

Treatment of Postural Instability

Another function of the vestibular system is to help maintain postural stability, or postural control. Postural control is defined as the ability to maintain the center of gravity over the base of support within a given sensory environment. Postural control requires the ability to perceive sensory information (somatosensory, visual, and vestibular), to centrally weight and select the appropriate sensory information, and to generate a suitable motor response to maintain stability. The selection of the appropriate motor response is based on the available sensory information, biomechanical constraints, environmental contexts, and prior experience. Vestibular, visual, and somatosensory cues are all used to detect movement of the body and to trigger appropriate postural responses. If the vestibular system is not functioning appropriately, then the individual will have difficulty maintaining their balance when visual or somatosensory cues are altered or absent (e.g., at night, walking on uneven or compliant surfaces). In individuals with remaining vestibular function (e.g., those with a unilateral vestibular deficit), the exercises are designed to foster adaptation of the remaining vestibular signals to generate the appropriate postural responses. Unlike the VOR, the signal used for modification of the vestibulospinal reflexes (VSR) is not known. Presumably, a similar visual-somatosensory-vestibular error signal is needed (71). Exercises used in the treatment of UVH are designed to generate these error signals and thereby foster adaptation of the vestibular system (66). For those individuals without vestibular function (e.g., those with bilateral vestibular loss) there is no remaining vestibular signal to adapt. Consequently, the exercises for these individuals are designed to promote the use of alternative strategies to promote postural stability.

Exercises to Improve Static and Dynamic Postural Stability in Patients With Remaining Vestibular Function

Exercises to promote static and dynamic postural stability in various sensory environments involve the manipulation of visual, vestibular, and somatosensory cues to force the individual to use vestibular cues for postural stability (see Table 47-3). Single, progressing to multiple, sensory modalities are manipulated to increase the difficulty of the postural control task. Varied sensory conditions may include (a) somatosensory changes (firm, conforming, level, uneven, and moving surfaces), (b) visual changes (eyes open with foveal, full field, or moving visual stimuli, or eyes closed), and (c) vestibular changes (different head orientations and head

TABLE 47-3 Exercises to Improve Static and Dynamic Postural Stability

The purpose of these exercises is to develop strategies for performing daily activities even when deprived of visual, somatosensory, or normal vestibular inputs. The activities are designed to help you develop confidence and establish functional limits. On all of these exercises, precautions should be taken to prevent *falls*.

1. Stand with your feet shoulder-width apart with both hands helping you keep your balance by touching a wall (or countertop). Take your hands off the wall for longer and longer periods while keeping your balance. Try moving your feet closer together. Practice for 5 minutes.

2. Stand with your feet shoulder-width apart with eyes open looking straight ahead at a target on the wall. Progressively narrow your base of support (move your feet 1 in at a time) from feet apart, to feet together, to a semi-heel-to-toe position, to heel-to-toe (one foot in front of the other), to heel-to-toe onto to on "tip-toes."

    Do the exercises first with arms outstretched, then with arms close to your body, and then with arms folded across your chest.

    Hold each position for 15 seconds, and then move to the next most difficult position.

3. Repeat exercise #2 with head bent forward 30° and then bent back 30°.

4. Repeat exercise #2 with eyes closed, at first intermittently and then continuously, while making an effort to mentally visualize your surroundings.

5. Repeat exercise #2 and/or #4 while standing on a foam pillow.

6. Stand with your feet in a comfortable distance apart and eyes open. Now sway forward and backward so that weight shifts from your toes to your heels. Make sure there is no jack-knifing at the hips. Practice this for a minute or so. Now stop and close your eyes and stand as still and steady as possible. To progress this activity: practice the swaying activity with eyes closed, practice with narrow base of support, and practice on compliant surfaces.

7. Walk close to a wall with your hand available for balancing. Walk with a narrower base of support. Finally, walk heel-to-toe. Do this with eyes open or closed. Practice for 2 minutes.

8. Walk close to a wall and turn your head to the right and left as you walk. Try to focus on different objects as you walk. Gradually turn your head further and faster. Practice for 2 minutes.

9. Practice turning around while you walk. At first, turn in a large circle but gradually make smaller and smaller turns. Be sure to turn in both directions.

10. Take five steps and turn around to the right (180°) and keep walking. Take five more steps, turn left (180°) and keep walking. Repeat five times, rest, and repeat the entire sequence.

11. Walk outside on an uneven surface or walk inside on a compliant surface.

12. Climb up your stairs without using your arms. Practice for 2 minutes.

13. Practice walking in a grocery store. To make it more difficult: try to walk without a grocery cart, go when there are few people there, then when it is crowded, and increase the number of aisles you walk through.

14. Practice walking in a shopping mall: first when it is not crowded, then when it is crowded, but walk with the flow of the crowd, and then when it is crowded, but walk against the flow of the crowd.

15. Participate in golf, tennis, dance, racquetball, etc.

    The following balance exercises are performed at home with a partner:

    While standing, kick a ball between you.

    Practice batting a NERF ball.

    Play a game of catch. Progress in the following manner:

    Start with just an easy game keeping the ball in the midline.

    Then throw to either side.

    Take a step to the side to catch the ball. Your partner should let you know to which side he will be throwing the ball.

    To further progress, throw randomly from one side to another.

    Catch the ball without taking a step as the ball is thrown to either side.

    All of the activities listed can be performed on a compliant surface.

rotation). The exercises are also progressed from static to dynamic activities.

Exercises for improving dynamic postural stability involve progressively more difficult head and trunk movements while moving through space. Initially, the individual works on simple weight shifting activities, holding the end-range position for 3–5 seconds, and independent ambulation. The progression from assisted to independent ambulation is usually very rapid. Providing there are no underlying orthopedic or other neurological problems, the patients are generally able to walk independently within several days of the initiation of ambulation. Typically, these individuals avoid head rotation during ambulation and assume a wide base of support while walking. Once they are able to walk independently, low-frequency, small amplitude head rotations with concurrent gaze shifts are incorporated into the exercise program. To avoid excessive symptom

provocation and marked gait ataxia, the individual performs the head rotation–gaze shift every fifth step. This may be performed with both horizontal and vertical head movements. This exercise forces the individual to adapt to the head rotations and prevents them from using visual fixation for postural stability. As recovery proceeds, the amplitude and peak velocity of the head rotation can be increased. To decrease the base of support, the patients walk with a progressively narrower base of support, ultimately walking heel-to-toe (tandem gait). Patients can also walk with the head tilted in either the frontal or sagittal planes to alter the otolith inputs. Patients are also encouraged to walk outdoors, which poses 2 distinct sensorimotor challenges. One, the support surface will change, which necessitates rapid postural adjustments. Two, visual cues for postural stability are at a greater distance than those indoors. This change in visual cues often causes increased disequilibrium because the normal degree of postural sway results in smaller movements of visual images across the retina. This is an analogous situation to the normal experience of height vertigo.

The exercises described previously challenge an individual's ability to move linearly. Another set of exercises is designed to rehabilitate the ability to rotate. This exercise involves walking approximately 10 ft and turning around 180°. This is then repeated with rotation in the opposite direction. As the individual's balance improves, the radius of the turn is gradually decreased. This exercise can ultimately be performed with an abrupt rotation, or standing pivot. This exercise can also be performed with the eyes closed. A further extension of the exercise for the advanced stages of the rehabilitation process is rapid rotation combined with higher velocity linear movements. Examples include dance steps or shifting from a forehand to backhand in any of the racquet sports.

One of the final exercises used in the rehabilitation of dynamic postural stability is an obstacle course, where the individual walks over various surfaces, rotates, side-steps, and goes through a series of position changes (sit to stand, bending over, reaching, etc.). Lastly, individuals are encouraged to resume their normal activities, especially those activities that involve postural changes and head movements, such as dancing, racquet sports, and golf.

Exercises to Improve Static and Dynamic Postural Stability in Patients Without Vestibular Function

The exercises to improve static and dynamic postural stability are similar to the exercises described for patients with remaining vestibular function (Table 47-2). Unlike the individuals with compensated unilateral vestibular lesions, those with bilateral vestibular hypofunction will have varying degrees of difficulty maintaining their balance when both visual and somatosensory cues are perturbed. Consequently, the exercises may need to be modified to allow the use of 1 sensory cue or to decrease the task complexity by widening the base of support.

Individuals with BVH tend to initially rely solely on visual cues but gradually use somatosensory cues for postural stability (72). If the examination of the patient reveals that they are not using somatosensory cues for postural stability, then the standing balance exercises can be performed with the eyes closed. Eye closure may need to be intermittent at first but is progressed until the patient can perform the exercise for 30 seconds. It is often helpful in the beginning stages of this exercise to have the individuals visualize their surroundings when their eyes are closed. In addition, active weight shifting with eyes closed increases somatosensory awareness and awareness of the supporting surface.

The role of cervical input in the maintenance of postural stability is questionable. Bles et al. (73) reported that static cervical positions did not contribute to postural stability in BVH. In light of these findings, the static postural exercises performed with head tilts may challenge the balance system by changing the visual frame of reference. The role of dynamic cervical input is not known at this time. Individuals with BVH have difficulty maintaining balance with head rotation during ambulation. This degradation of balance may be caused by the loss of a stable visual frame of reference. However, their ability to walk and turn their head does improve with practice.

Patients with BVH also tend to walk with a wide base of support. Having these patients walk with a decreased step width, ultimately ambulating heel-to-toe, can challenge their dynamic postural stability. Changes in direction, as described for the patients with UVH, are also a challenge for the individual with BVH. An obstacle course or functional tasks that require positional changes, movement, and changing visual or somatosensory cues are also beneficial by forcing the patient to adapt to changing environmental conditions and to shift between the available sensory cues.

Exercise Guidelines for Individuals With Traumatic Brain Injury

Confounding orthopedic and neurological factors often complicates treatment of vestibular deficits in patients with TBI. The exercise programs described earlier will provoke the patient's symptoms. The exercises, if conducted appropriately, will generate an error signal in the CNS, which is thought to provoke symptoms of vertigo, dizziness, or disequilibrium. Depending on the individual's symptoms, cognitive level, and degree of agitation, the symptom provocation may not be tolerated well. In those individuals with marked dizziness, motion sensitivity, and agitation, the ×1 viewing exercises may simply provoke too many symptoms. In these cases, it is recommended that the initial course of vestibular rehabilitation be simple habituation exercises—performed to tolerance. Once the habituation exercises have decreased the motion sensitivity, then ×1 viewing exercises, if needed, may be initiated.

As the patient's status improves and their agitation decreases, the intensity of the exercises (either habituation or adaptation exercises) can be increased. With this increase, patients are told to expect greater symptom provocation and that provocation of their symptoms is actually beneficial to their recovery. A general guideline is that symptoms may be provoked for 15–30 minutes following the exercises. If the increased symptoms persist longer, the speed, duration, or context of the stimulus should be reduced. If the exercises are performed in a manner that does not challenge the system or provoke the symptoms, then the error signal will not be generated. Consequently, there will be no stimulus for adaptation. Similarly, the use of CNS depressants (such as meclizine or benzodiazepines) to treat the symptoms of vertigo and disequilibrium are thought to retard the adaptation process.

Vestibular and Balance Rehabilitation Therapy Outcomes

At this point, there have been no comprehensive studies examining vestibular and balance rehabilitation therapy outcomes in patients with TBI. There are, however, numerous studies that have demonstrated the efficacy of VBRT programs in different populations of patients with vestibular disorders (74–77). Herdman and colleagues (74) demonstrated that, following acoustic neuroma resection, patients that underwent vestibular adaptation exercises demonstrated improvements in disequilibrium, ataxia, and static postural stability as compared to individuals that had undergone a sham exercise program. Horak and colleagues (78) reported that individuals with chronic vestibular dysfunction treated with vestibular rehabilitation exercises developed improved motion sensitivity measures and static postural stability measures when compared to similar individuals treated with either condition exercises or vestibular suppressant medication. Similar results have been shown in patients with bilateral vestibular loss (76). Shepard and colleagues (75) reported that patients that underwent a customized VBRT program had greater improvements than those that received a generic VBRT program. Are the exercises always effective? No, but reports suggest that the exercise approach is successful in reducing symptoms and improving function up to 85% of the time (75,79).

CONCLUSION

Dizziness remains one of the most common long-term sequela of TBI and although recognition of mechanisms and treatments for direct peripheral vestibular involvement are appreciated, there remains significant lack of understanding regarding why rehabilitation of these peripheral disorders require a protracted time course. Additionally, those without any evidence of direct peripheral involvement yet consistent complaints of dizziness after TBI with no findings of peripheral or central involvement continue to be an enigma. The direction of future research will need to further investigate diagnostic tools for elements of the peripheral vestibular system that to date are difficult to assess but may well participate in subtle symptoms after TBI especially when there is additional central system involvement suspected. Further work into the impact of psychological effects in the production of dizziness symptoms and improved avenues for vestibular and balance rehabilitation techniques, with or without medication, provides very fertile areas for future clinical research activities.

KEY CLINICAL POINTS

1. No single structure subserves balance function. Rather, the system consists of multiple sensory inputs from the vestibular end-organs, the visual system, and the somatosensory/proprioceptive systems. The input information is then integrated at the level of the brain stem and cerebellum with significant influence from the cerebral cortex, including the frontal, parietal, and occipital lobes.
2. The vestibular system is the only special sensory system in which unilateral loss of function can seriously threaten the long-term survival or well-being of an organism. In humans, injury to the central or peripheral system may result in considerable disability. Fortunately, most disease processes involving the vestibular labyrinth are self-limited, and spontaneous functional recovery can be expected. This is caused by the remarkable ability of the CNS to recover after a labyrinthine injury, a process known as vestibular compensation.
3. Benign paroxysmal positional vertigo—This is considered one of the most common causes for complaints of dizziness (vertigo) and imbalance, and the most common source for dizziness post head trauma.
4. It is important to realize that there can be dramatic effects of psychological disorders that develop with long term

disorders and are expressed in the complaints of dizziness.
5. Even though a head trauma with or without TBI may be the precipitating event that results in complaints of imbalance and dizziness, one must proceed in the evaluation of those complaints in a systematic manner to uncover the source of the symptoms. Therefore, the evaluation is not different from what would be performed for a patient presenting without a known antecedent event.
6. Given the various tools for assessment, the history is the single most important factor in determining the course of management.
7. The major feature that drives an initial decision regarding the use of medication or surgery vs VBRT is the evidence that the peripheral or central vestibular lesion is unstable (varying over time), as opposed to an uncompensated stable lesion. This distinction comes dominantly from the patient's presenting symptoms.

KEY REFERENCES

1. Eggers DZ, Zee DS. *Vertigo andIimbalance: Clinical Neurophysiology of the Vestibular System*. New York, NY: Elsevier; 2010.
2. Herdman SJ. *Vestibular Rehabilitation*. 3rd ed. Philadelphia, PA: FA Davis Co; 2007.
3. Jacobson GP, Shepard NT. *Balance Function Assessment and Management*. San Diego, CA: Plural; 2008.
4. Minor LB. Labyrinthine fistulae: pathobiology and management. *Curr Opin Otolaryngol Head Neck Surg*. 2003; 11(5):310–346.
5. Staab JP. Diagnosis and treatment of phychologic symptoms and psychiatric disorders in patients with dizziness and imbalance. In: Shepard NT, Solomon D, eds. *The Otolaryngologic Clinics of North America*. Philadelphia, PA: WB Saunders Co; 2000;33 (3):617–636.

References

1. Baloh RW, Honrubia V. *Clinical Neurophysiology of the Vestibular System*. 2nd ed. Philadelphia, PA: FA Davis Company; 1990.
2. Leigh RJ, Zee DS, eds. *The Neurology of Eye Movements*. 4th ed. Philadelphia, PA: FA Davis Company; 2006.
3. Jacobson GP, Shepard NT. *Balance Function Assessment and Management*. San Diego, CA: Plural; 2008.
4. Eggers SD, Zee DS. *Vertigo and Imbalance: Clinical Neurophysiology of the Vestibular System: Handbook of Clinical Neurophysiology*. New York, NY: Elsevier; 2010.
5. Shepard NT, Telian SA. *Practical Management of the Balance Disorder Patient*. Singular Publishing Group, Inc; 1996.
6. Allum JH, Shepard NT. An overview of the clinical use of dynamic posturography in the differential diagnosis of balance disorders. *J of Vestib Res*. 1999;9(4):223–252.
7. Woollacott MH, Shumway-Cook A, eds. *Development of Posture and Gait Across the Life Span*. Columbia, SC: University of South Carolina Press; 1989.
8. Bronstein AM, Brandt T, Woolacott M. *Clinical Disorders of Balance, Posture and Gait*. London, UK: Oxford University Press & Arnold; 1996.
9. Shepard NT, Solomon D. Practical issues in the management of the dizzy and balance disorder patient. In: Shepard NT, Solomon D, eds. *The Otolaryngologic Clinics of North America*. Philadelphia, PA:WB Saunders Co; 2000;33(3).
10. Curthoys IS, Halmagyi GM. Vestibular compensation: clinical changes in vestibular function with time after unilateral vestibular

loss. In: Herdman SJ, ed. *Vestibular Rehabilitation*. 3rd ed. Philadelphia, PA: FA Davis Co; 2007:76–97.

11. Zee DS. Vestibular adaptation. In: Herdman SJ, ed. *Vestibular Rehabilitation*. 3rd ed. Philadelphia, PA: FA Davis Co; 2007:19–31.

12. Brandt T, Daroff RB. Physical therapy for benign paroxysmal positional vertigo. *Arch Otolaryngol*. 1980;106(8):484–485.

13. Epley JM. The canalith repositioning procedure: for treatment of benign paroxysmal positional vertigo. *Otolaryngol Head Neck Surg*. 1992;107(3):399–404.

14. Brandt T, Steddin S. Current view of the mechanism of benign paroxysmal positioning vertigo: cupulolithiasis or canalolithiasis? *J Vestib Res*. 1993;3(4):373–382.

15. Brandt T. Benign paroxysmal positioning vertigo. *Adv Otorhinolaryngol*. 1999;55:169–194.

16. Herdman SJ, Tusa RJ, Zee DS, Proctor LR, Mattox DE. Single treatment approaches to benign paroxysmal positional vertigo. *Arch Otolaryngol Head Neck Surg*. 1993;119(4):450–454.

17. Herdman SJ. *Vestibular Rehabilitation*. 3rd ed. Philadelphia, PA: FA Davis Co; 2007.

18. Hasso AN, Ledington JA: Traumatic injuries of the temporal bone. *Otolaryngol Clin North Am*. 1988;21(2):295–316.

19. Cannon CR, Jahrsdoerfer RA. Temporal bone fractures. Review of 90 cases. *Arch Otolaryngol*. 1983;109(5):285–288.

20. Schuknecht HF. *Pathology of the Ear*. Cambridge, NY: Harvard University Press; 1974:295–298.

21. Ruckenstein MJ. Vertigo and dysequilibrium with associated hearing loss. In: Shepard NT, Solomon D, eds. *The Otolaryngologic Clinics of North America*. Philadelphia, PA: WB Saunders Co; 2000:33(3): 535–562.

22. Phelps PD. Congenital cerebrospinal fluid fistulae of the petrous temporal bone. *Clin Otolaryngol Allied Sci*. 1986;11(2):79–92.

23. Goodhill V. Sudden deafness and round window rupture. *Laryngoscope*. 1971;81(9):1462–1474.

24. Friedland DR, Wackym PA. A critical appraisal of spontaneous perilymphatic fistulas of the inner ear. *Am J Otol*. 1999;20(2): 261–279.

25. Hughes GB, Barna BP, Kinney SE, Calabrese LH, Nalepa NL. Predictive value of laboratory tests in "autoimmune" inner ear disease: preliminary report. *Laryngoscope*. 1986;96(5):502–505.

26. Minor LB. Labyrinthine fistulae: pathobiology and management. *Curr Opin Otolaryngol Head Neck Surg*. 2003;11(5):340–346.

27. Buchman CA, Luxford WM, Hirsch BE, Fucci MJ, Kelly RH. Beta-2 transferrin assay in the identification of perilymph. *Am J Otol*. 1999;20(2):174–178.

28. Poe DS, Bottrill ID. Comparison of endoscopic and surgical explorations for perilymphatic fistulas. *Am J Otol*. 1994;15(6):735–738.

29. Poe DS, Rebeiz EE, Pankratov MM. Evaluation of perilymphatic fistulas by middle ear endoscopy. *Am J Otol*. 1992;13(6):529–533.

30. Zhou G, Gopen Q, Poe DS. Clinical and diagnostic characterization of canal dehiscence syndrome: a great otologic mimicker. *Otol Neurotol*. 2007;28(7):920–926.

31. Staab JP. Diagnosis and treatment of psychologic symptoms and psychiatric disorders in patients with dizziness and imbalance. *Otolaryngol Clin North Am*. 2000;33(3):617–636.

32. Tusa RJ. Psychological problems and the dizzy patient. In: Herdman SJ, ed. *Vestibular Rehabilitation*. 3rd ed. Philadelphia, PA: FA Davis Co; 2000:316–330.

33. Yardley L. Overview of psychologic effects of chronic dizziness and balance disorders. *Otolaryngol Clin North Am*. 2000:33(3): 603–616.

34. Brandt T, Dietrich M. Assessment and management of central vestibular disorders. In: Herdman SJ, ed. *Vestibular Rehabilitation*. 3rd ed. Philadelphia, PA: FA Davis Co; 2000:264–297.

35. Schumway-Cook A. Vestibular rehabilitation of the patient with traumatic brain injury. In: Herdman SJ, ed. *Vestibular Rehabilitation*. 3rd ed. Philadelphia, PA: FA Davis Co; 2000:476–493.

36. Tusa RJ. Diagnosis and management of neuro-otological disorders due to migraine. In: Herdman SJ, ed. *Vestibular Rehabilitation*. 3rd ed. Philadelphia, PA: FA Davis Co; 2000:298–315.

37. Neuhauser H Leopold M, von Brevern M, Arnold G, Lempert G. The interrelations of migraine, vertigo, and migrainous vertigo. *Neurology*. 2001;56(4):436–441.

38. Guskiewicz KM. Postural stability assessment following concussion: one piece of the puzzle. *Clin J Sport Med*. 2001;11(3):182–189.

39. Hoffer ME, Balaban C. Traumatic brain injury and blast exposures: auditory and vestibular pathology. In: Moller AR, Langguth B, De Ridder D, Kleinjung T, eds. *Textbook of Tinnitus*. New York, NY: Springer Science and Business Media, LLC; 2011.

40. Aikin FW, Murnane OD. Head injury and blast exposure: vestibular consequences. *Otolaryngol Clin North Am*. 2011;44(2):323–334.

41. Fausti SA, Wilmington DJ, Gallun FJ, Myers PJ, Henry JA. Auditory and vestibular dysfunction associated with blast-related traumatic brain injury. *J Rehabil Res Dev*. 2009;46(6):797–810.

42. Hoffer ME, Balaban C, Gottshall K, Balough BJ, Maddox MR, Penta JR. Blast Exposure: vestibular consequences and associated characteristics. *Otol Neurotol*. 2010;31(2):232–236.

43. Myers PJ, Wilmington DJ, Gallun FJ, Henry JA, Fausti SA. Hearing impairment and traumatic brain injury among soldiers: special considerations for the audiologist. *Seminars in Hearing Journal*. 2009; 30(1):5–27.

44. Jacobson GP, Newman CW. The development of the dizziness handicap inventory. *Arch Otolaryngol Head Neck Surg*. 1990;116(4): 424–427.

45. Jacobson GP, Newman CW, Hunter Left, Balzer G. Balance function test correlates of the dizziness handicap inventory. *J Am Acad Audiol*. 1991;2(5):253–260.

46. Robertson DD, Ireland DJ. Dizziness Handicap Inventory correlates of computerized dynamic Posturography. *J Otolaryngol*. 1995; 24(2):118–124.

47. Shepard NT. Management of the patient with chronic complaints of dizziness: an overview of laboratory studies. Clackamas, OR: NeuroCom; 2003.

48. Herdman SJ, Tusa RJ, Blatt P, Suzuki A, Venuto PJ, Roberts D. Computerized dynamic visual acuity test in the assessment of vestibular deficits. *Am J Otol*. 1998;19(6):790–796.

49. Shepard NT, Janky K. Background and technique of computerized dynamic posturography. In: Jacobson GP, Shepard NT, eds. *Balance Function Assessment and Management*. San Diego, CA: Plural; 2008: 339–357.

50. Cawthorne T. The physiological basis for head exercises. *J Chart Soc Physiother*. 1944:106–107.

51. Hecker HC, Haug CO, Herndon JW. Treatment of the vertiginous patient using Cawthorne's vestibular exercises. *Laryngoscope*. 1974; 84(11):2065–2072.

52. McCabe BF. Labyrinthine exercises in the treatment of diseases characterized by vertigo: their physiologic basis and methodology. *Laryngoscope*. 1970;80(9):1429–1433.

53. Welling DB, Parnes LS, O'Brien B, Bakaletz LO, Brackmann DE, Hinojosa R. Particulate matter in the posterior semicircular canal. *Laryngoscope*. 1997;107(1):90–94.

54. Korres S, Balatsouras DG, Kaberos A, Economou C, Kandiloros D, Ferekidis E. Occurrence of semicircular canal involvement in benign paroxysmal positional vertigo. *Otol Neurotol*. 2002;23(6): 926–932.

55. Schuknecht HF. Cupulolithiasis. *Arch Otolaryngol*. 1969;90(6): 765–778.

56. Parnes LS, McClure JA. Free-floating endolymph particles: a new operative finding during posterior semicircular canal occlusion. *Laryngoscope*. 1992;102(9):988–992.

57. Moriarty B, Rutka J, Hawke M. The incidence and distribution of cupular deposits in the labyrinth. *Laryngoscope*. 1992;102(1):56–59.

58. Herdman SJ, Tusa RJ, Zee DS, Proctor LR, Mattox DE. Single treatment approaches to benign paroxysmal positional vertigo. *Arch Otolaryngol Head Neck Surg*. 1993;119:450–454.

59. Parnes LS, Agrawal SK, Atlas J. Diagnosis and management of benign paroxysmal positional vertigo (BPPV). *CMAJ*. 2003;169(7): 681–693.

60. Dix M, Hallpike C. The pathology, symptomatology, and diagnosis of certain common disorders of the vestibular systems. *Ann Otol Rhinol Laryngol*. 1952;61(4):987-1016.

61. Parnes LS, Price-Jones RG. Particle repositioning maneuver for benign paroxysmal positional vertigo. *Ann Otol Rhinol Laryngol*. 1993; 102(5):325–331.

62. Wolf JS, Boyev KP, Manokey BJ, Mattox DE. Success of the modified Epley maneuver in treating benign paroxysmal positional vertigo. *Laryngoscope.* 1999;109(6):900–903.

63. Epley JM. Positional vertigo related to semicircular canalithiasis. *Otolaryngol Head Neck Surg.* 1995;112(1):154–161.

64. du Lac S, Raymond JL, Sejnowski TJ, Lisberger SG. Learning and memory in the vestibulo-ocular reflex. *Ann Rev Neurosci.* 1995;18: 409–441.

65. Gauthier GM, Robinson DA. Adaptation of the human vestibuloocular reflex to magnifying lenses. *Brain Res.* 1975;92(2):331–335.

66. Herdman SJ. Exercise strategies for vestibular disorders. *Ear Nose Throat J.* 1989;68(12):961–964.

67. Shelhamer M, Robinson DA, Tan HS. Context-specific adaptation of the gain of the vestibulo-ocular reflex in humans. *J Vestib Res.* 1992;2(1):89–96.

68. Kasai T, Zee DS. Eye-head coordination in labyrinthine-defective human beings. *Brain Res.* 1978;144(1):123–141.

69. Smith-Wheelock M, Shepard NT, Telian SA. Physical therapy program for vestibular rehabilitation. *Am J Otol.* 1991;12(3):218–225.

70. Norré ME, De Weerdt W. Treatment of vertigo based on habituation. 1. Physio-pathological basis. *J Laryngol Otol.* 1980;94(7): 689–696.

71. Gonshor A, Jones GM. Postural adaptation to prolonged optical reversal of vision in man. *Brain Res.* 1980;192(1):239–248.

72. Bles W, Vianney de Jong JM, de Wit G. Compensation for labyrinthine defects examined by the use of a tilting room. *Acta Otolaryngol.* 1983;95(5–6):576–579.

73. Bles W, de Jong JM, Rasmussens JJ. Postural and oculomotor signs in labyrinthine-defective subjects. *Acta Otolaryngol Suppl.* 1984;406: 101–104.

74. Herdman SJ, Clendaniel RA, Mattox DE, Holliday MJ, Niparko JK. Vestibular adaptation exercises and recovery: acute stage after acoustic neuroma resection. *Otolaryngol Head Neck Surg.* 1995; 113(1):77–87.

75. Shepard NT, Telian SA. Programmatic vestibular rehabilitation. *Otolaryngol Head Neck Surg.* 1995;112(1):173–182.

76. Krebs DE, Gill-Body KM, Riley PO, Parker SW. Double-blind, placebo-controlled trial of rehabilitation for bilateral vestibular hypofunction: preliminary report. *Otolaryngol Head Neck Surg.* 1993; 109(4):735–741.

77. Yardley L, Beech S, Zander L, Evans T, Weinman J. A randomized controlled trial of exercise therapy for dizziness and vertigo in primary care. *Br J Gen Pract.* 1998;48(429):1136–1140.

78. Horak FB, Jones-Rycewicz C, Black FO, Shumway-Cook A. Effects of vestibular rehabilitation on dizziness and imbalance. *Otolaryngol Head Neck Surg.* 1992;106(2):175–180.

79. Krebs DE, Gill-Body KM, Parker SW, Ramirez JV, Wernick-Robinson M. Vestibular rehabilitation: useful but not universally so. *Otolaryngol Head Neck Surg.* 2003;128(2):240–250.

48

Smell and Taste

Richard M. Costanzo, Evan R. Reiter, and Joshua C. Yelverton

INTRODUCTION

Smell and taste disturbances are common sequelae of head trauma (1). We use our senses of smell and taste every day to prepare and taste foods, appreciate perfumes and flowers, detect noxious and hazardous vapors, maintain personal hygiene, and in our social and intimate interactions with others. Loss of these senses thus greatly affects one's ability to perform several activities of daily living (ADL), can have a negative impact on quality of life (QOL), and has been associated with an increased risk of depression (2). For these reasons, as well as their relative frequency following head trauma, alterations in the senses of smell and taste may have a significant impact on rehabilitation and QOL outcomes. An understanding of the pathophysiology, evaluation, management strategies, and prognosis of posttraumatic disturbances of smell and taste is essential to the physician managing patients after head trauma.

Incidence

The first reported cases of posttraumatic smell and taste dysfunction were presented in the late 19th century. A case reported in the *London Hospital Report* in 1864 (3) described a 50-year-old man who was knocked off his horse sustaining a brain concussion and complete loss of his sense of smell. Ogle, in 1870, reported on a patient with loss of taste following head trauma, but thought that the ageusia was secondary to an inability to "discriminate aromas and flavors" (4). The incidence of olfactory dysfunction following head trauma reported in the literature (5–12) varies widely and likely reflects differences in the severity of injury as well as methods used to assess loss of function (13–15). In 1991, Costanzo and Zasler reviewed estimates from several published studies and found that anosmia occurred in 25%–30% of patients with severe head injuries, 15%–19% of those with moderate injuries, and 0%–16% of those with mild injuries (16). Other studies employing objective methods for testing olfactory function have reported similar correlations between the degree of olfactory loss and the degree of head injury (17–20). Costanzo and Becker evaluated the incidence of olfactory disturbances in 592 patients with head injuries from a variety of mechanisms (Table 48-1), finding that injuries resulting in olfactory or gustatory dysfunction occurred more frequently in the young adult male population between the

ages of 15 and 24 years, and occurred most commonly from motor vehicle accidents (21).

In the older adult population, falls and assaults were more common causes of chemosensory dysfunction, particularly when the falls resulted in strikes to the occiput (23). Gustatory dysfunction following head trauma is seen less frequently than olfactory dysfunction, occurring in approximately 0.5% of cases, although the incidence increases to 5%–7% in patients with documented loss of olfactory function (23).

ANATOMY AND PHYSIOLOGY OF SMELL AND TASTE

Smell (Olfaction)

The olfactory system proper is the primary and most sensitive system for detection and identification of odors. The peripheral elements of the olfactory system are found in approximately 22 cm^2 of pseudostratified columnar epithelium in the superior nasal cavity, located below the cribriform plate of the ethmoid and along the superior septum and the middle and superior turbinates (24). The first of these peripheral elements are the bipolar olfactory receptor cells, of which there are approximately 6 million in the human nose (24,5). Olfactory receptor cells have several unique features. First, they are continuously being regenerated from basal cells located within the olfactory neuroepithelium throughout one's life span and following injury. This remarkable regenerative capacity allows the basal cells to differentiate into neurons, grow back to the olfactory bulb, and even reestablish functional connections to higher centers (26–30). Second, each olfactory bipolar receptor cell acts as both a sensory receptor cell and a first-order neuron with direct projection into the brain, unique among sensory systems(24). Lastly, each receptor cell expresses a single odorant receptor gene derived from a single allele. There are approximately 1,000 distinct types of odorant receptor genes within the vertebrate olfactory system, a discovery that garnered Drs. Linda Buck and Richard Axel the 2004 Nobel Prize in Physiology (31). The survival importance of olfaction is underscored by the finding that these genes comprise roughly 3%–5% of all expressed genes of the mammalian genome. Although a single olfactory receptor cell expresses only 1 odorant receptor gene, each cell can respond to more than

TABLE 48-1 Olfactory Impairment in Moderate to Severe Head Injury by Accident Type

ACCIDENT TYPE (N = 592)	OCCURRENCE	MEAN AGE (Y)	OLFACTORY IMPAIRMENT
Motor vehicle	51.5%	27	23.6%
Domestic falls	14.5%	44	26.6%
Cycle or bicycle	10.1%	23	22.5%
Pedestrian	9.2%	32	13.5%
Assault	6.8%	39	22.7%
Other	7.6%	35	16.0%

Reprinted from Reiter ER, Dinardo LJ, Costanzo RM (22) with permission from Elsevier.

1 odorant. It is the central integration of inputs from the entire olfactory neuroepithelium in response to a complex odor, the so-called "spatial coding" of the stimulus, which leads to the unique odor perception associated with each stimulus (32).

Along with the bipolar receptor cells, there are several other cell types that comprise the olfactory neuroepithelium. The sustentacular cells, or supporting cells, along with the acinar and ductal cells of Bowman's glands, produce the mucus found coating the neuroepthilium (24). These cells serve a vital function in olfactory transduction; as for transduction to take place, odorants must pass from the gaseous phase within the nasal cavity to the aqueous phase within the mucus coating the olfactory neuroepithelium (25). Odorants diffuse through the mucus layer to reach the bipolar receptor cell cilia where the odorant receptors are located. Odorant binding to a specific receptor then triggers action potentials within the receptor cells (25,33). For this reason, alterations in nasal mucus quantity or viscosity may affect olfactory function. The horizontal and globose basal cells located near the basement membrane are responsible for the regenerative

capacity of the olfactory neuroepithelium. These basal cells give rise to new olfactory receptor cells as well as sustentacular cells. Last are the microvillar cells, which have no known role in olfaction.

The axons of the bipolar receptor cells group together to form olfactory nerve bundles, or fila, which course from the olfactory neuroepithelium through the cribriform plate of the ethmoid bone to form the first and outermost concentric layer of the olfactory bulb. Groupings of approximately 50, these olfactory fila make up cranial nerve (CN) I. Within the next deeper layer of the bulb, axons converge and synapse onto dendrites of second-order neurons (mitral and tufted cells) forming oval-like structures called glomeruli. Within the glomerular layer, axons from the different odorant receptor subtypes converge onto individual glomeruli and establish a special mapping of odorant information within the olfactory bulb. With normal aging, the number of glomeruli declines (34), corresponding to the gradual decrease in olfactory function often seen in the elderly (35).

Upon leaving the olfactory bulb via the olfactory tract, the axons of the mitral and tufted cells synapse in areas of the primary olfactory cortex (Figure 48-1). The primary olfactory cortex is composed of the olfactory tubercle, the pyriform cortex, the amygdala, the periamygdaloid complex, and the entorhinal cortex.

The secondary olfactory cortex is located in the orbitofrontal region of the brain. Connections between the primary and secondary olfactory cortices occur via the mediodorsal nucleus of the thalamus. The olfactory system is somewhat unique among sensory systems in that it also has components that travel directly to other cortical regions without traveling through the thalamus (24,25), including entorhinal cortex projections to the hippocampus and hypothalamus (36).

Each of these areas has a unique role in central processing of odor perception. The pyriform cortex is associated with learning and odor memory, and with integration of

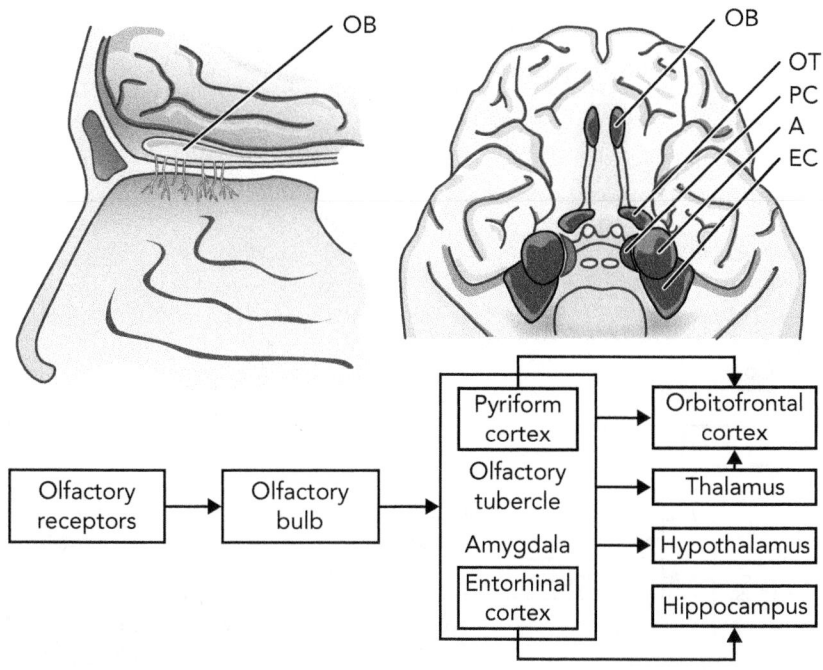

FIGURE 48-1 Diagram illustrating the major components and pathways of the olfactory system. OB, olfactory bulb; OT, olfactory tubercle; PC, pyriform cortex; A, amygdala; EC, entorhinal cortex.

olfactory, visual, and gustatory inputs (37). The amygdala responds to the intensity of emotionally significant odors. The caudal oribitofrontal cortex is associated with odor detection, whereas the rostral oribitofrontal cortex is associated with working memory, associative learning, and both short-term and long-term odor recognition. The medial orbitofrontal and ventromedial prefontal cortices are activated by pleasant odors, whereas the lateral orbitofrontal and inferior prefontal cortices are activated by unpleasant odors (25,37).

In addition to the olfactory system, which generates specific odor perceptions, the trigeminal system also plays an important role in the detection of chemical stimuli. Somatosensory fibers of CN V innervate the entire nasal cavity and respond to tactile, temperature, and pain stimuli, which may also serve to trigger reflexive responses within the nasal cavity and beyond, including mucus production, mucosal congestion, cessation of inhalation, and sneezing (24). Because of its deeper, more protected course, and bilateral innervation, CN V is more resistant to injury that the olfactory nerves and its function thus commonly spared even in cases of severe head injury. As such, patients' subjective inability to detect even strong noxious stimuli that are known trigeminal stimulants such as ammonia, is often a clue to malingering.

Taste (Gustation)

Taste is a specialized chemical sense typically described as capable of detecting 5 distinct qualities: salty, sweet, bitter, sour, and umami (the taste evoked by monosodium glutamate). Taste buds are distributed throughout the oral cavity and to a lesser degree in the oropharynx, but are concentrated on the tongue. In humans, taste is a highly redundant sensory system with bilateral innervation carried to the taste buds of the oral cavity and oropharynx via 3 CNs, the facial (CN VII), glossopharyngeal (CN IX), and vagus (CN X) nerves bilaterally. Thus, with 6 CNs carrying taste fibers, it

is rare that even a patient with severe head trauma will present with gustatory dysfunction. In addition, as with odor detection, the somatosensory fibers of the lingual nerve (CN V) respond to tactile, temperature, and pain stimuli, which also assist with detection of oral chemical stimuli (Figure 48-2).

The glossopharyngeal nerve provides chemosensory information from the posterior third of the tongue and the pharynx through its lingual branches (38). These branches travel deep to the tonsillar fossa to the inferior petrosal ganglion located within the parapharyngeal space medial to the internal and external carotid arteries. These fibers enter the skull base via the jugular foramen, where the superior petrosal ganglion is found. After exiting the jugular foramen anterior to the rest of the foramen contents, fibers travel 10–20 mm through the cerebellopontine angle (CPA) before entering the medulla, where they terminate in the nucleus solitarius.

The chorda tympani branch of the facial nerve carries taste sensory fibers to the anterior two-thirds of the tongue. Within the tongue, the chorda tympani fibers travel with the lingual nerve, a branch of the third division of the trigeminal nerve. Taste fibers of CN VII and somatosensory fibers of CN V course together from the undersurface of the tongue. These fibers then enter the infratemporal fossa where they split, with the chorda tympani fibers entering the petrous portion of the temporal bone via the petrotympanic fissure, and the remaining fibers passing through the foramen ovale as the lingual nerve to enter the middle cranial fossa. The chorda tympani then courses through the middle ear, running between the malleus and incus before entering a bony canal just medial to the posterior portion of the ear drum. After leaving the middle ear, the nerve travels through the mastoid with the facial nerve until it reaches the geniculate ganglion. At this point, the taste fibers leave the geniculate ganglion as the nervus intermedius, and pass via the internal auditory canal and cerebellopontine angle to enter the pons, terminating in the upper portion of the nucleus solitarius.

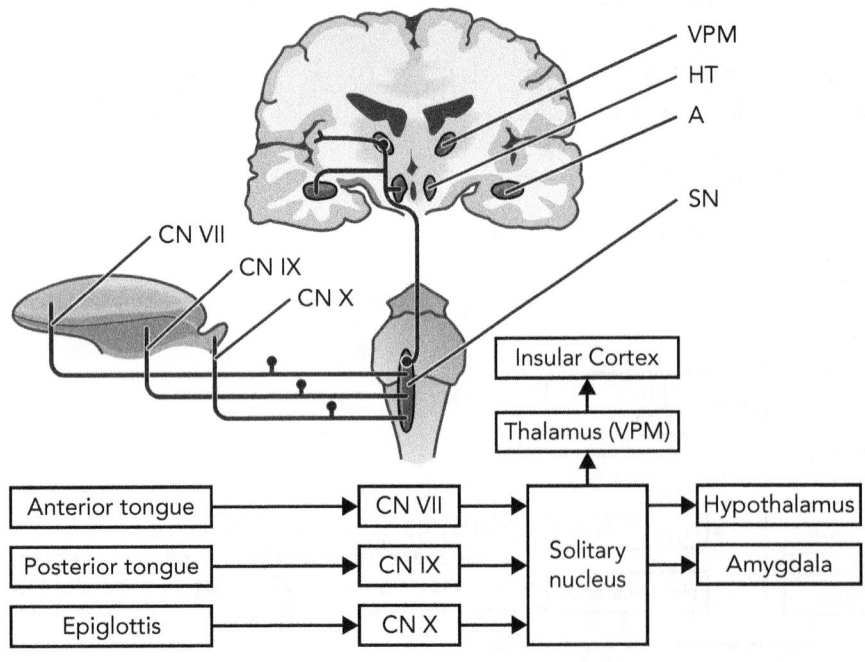

FIGURE 48-2 Diagram illustrating the major components and pathways of the gustatory system. CN VII, facial nerve; CN IX, glossopharyngeal nerve; CN X, vagus nerve; SN, solitary nucleus; VPM, ventral posteromedial thalamus; HT, hypothalamus; A, amygdala.

The vagus nerve has a limited contribution to taste. The superior laryngeal nerve carries somatosensory and some taste innervation from the laryngeal surface of the epiglottis. After leaving the larynx via the thyrohyoid membrane, the nerve passes medial to the carotid artery to join the main trunk of the vagus nerve. These fibers travel to the superior petrosal ganglion at the jugular foramen, and then course to the nucleus solitarius where they join fibers from CNs VII and IX.

After peripheral taste fibers carried by CNs VII, IX, and X terminate in their respective rostral to caudal regions of the nucleus solitarius in the medulla, higher projections are sent to the most medial small-celled division of the ventroposteromedial nucleus of the thalamus. This area is immediately adjacent to the neurons of somatosensation of the tongue and oral cavity (38). In addition, there are also direct projections from the nucleus solitarius to the hypothalamus and amygdala that do not pass through the thalamus. Thalamic taste pathways project to cortical regions in the anterodorsal insula and frontal cortex in an ipsilateral distribution (39).

MECHANISMS OF TRAUMATIC SMELL AND TASTE DYSFUNCTION

Olfactory (Smell) Dysfunction

Olfactory transduction requires a patent nasal airway and intact nasal mucosa with an appropriate mucus coating in addition to intact neural pathways from the nasal cavity up to the higher cortical processing centers. Olfactory dysfunction may occur in the patient suffering head injury by any or all of the following mechanisms causing disruption of critical components of the olfactory system: (*a*) disruption of the sinonasal tract, (*b*) shearing of the olfactory nerves at the level of the cribriform plate, and (*c*) focal trauma to the olfactory bulb and cortex (Figure 48-3). In addition, either preexisting or treatment-related etiologies of olfactory

dysfunction may also exist, such that these should also be considered in the patient with head injury, and are thus reviewed briefly here.

Sinonasal Tract Disruption

Sinonasal tract disruption is most commonly associated with nasal bone or midface fractures. Distortion of the normal sinonasal tract anatomy can result in airflow disruption leading to a conductive smell loss, essentially preventing odorants from reaching the olfactory neuroepithelium. In a study examining smell and taste disturbances after maxillofacial injuries, it was found that nasozygomatic LeFort fractures, fronto-orbital fractures, and pure LeFort fractures have a higher incidence of alterations of the sense of smell than more isolated nasal bone, nasoorbitoethmoid, or frontal bone fractures (40). Although it seems logical that more extensive factures would be more likely to cause significant obstruction of the nasal airway, the study did not examine the precise mechanism of olfactory dysfunction. Thus, it is also likely that more extensive fractures are associated with higher likelihood of disruption of other segments of the olfactory pathways.

In addition to bony fractures, soft tissue injuries within the nasal cavity may also distort sinonasal anatomy and function, resulting in olfactory dysfunction. This may occur from obstruction of nasal airflow by mucosal or septal hematoma or edema, or scar formation either from the traumatic injury itself or nasal life support tubes used in resuscitation and treatment (41). Further, rhinosinusitis resulting from sinus ostial obstruction from bony or soft tissue injuries to the sinonasal tract may subsequently lead to inflammatory changes in the nasal mucosa causing limitation of airflow or alterations in nasal mucus quantity or viscosity, which may also affect olfaction.

Although it is rare that such nasal issues arising after head injury will cause complete anosmia, either hyposmia or dysosmia may occur. Because such conductive olfactory losses are those most amenable to medical or surgical treat-

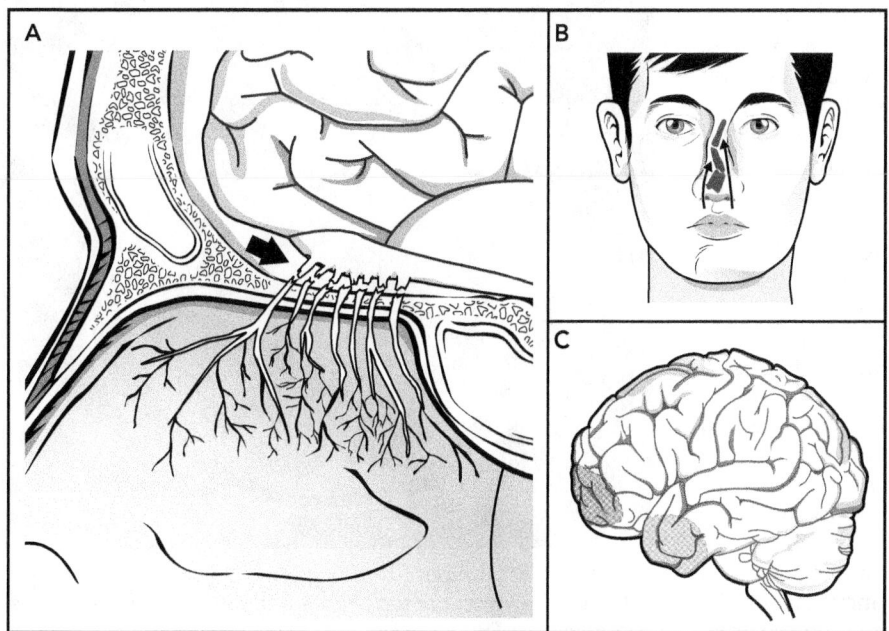

FIGURE 48-3 Diagram illustrating mechanisms of injury associated with impaired olfactory function. A, Injury to the olfactory nerves; B, Disruption of the sinonasal tract; C, Injury to olfactory centers in the brain. Reprinted from Costanzo RM, Zasler ND with permission.

ment, it is important that such potential etiologies are not overlooked.

Olfactory Nerve Injury

The sensory axons of the bipolar olfactory receptor cells course through the many foramina of the cribriform plate at the roof of the nasal cavity to enter the olfactory bulbs. It is at this site that they are particularly prone to injury. Head trauma resulting in either a fracture of the bone in the ethmoid roof–cribriform plate region, or alternately a rapid shift in position of the brain relative to the skull base, as may occur with abrupt deceleration experienced in motor vehicle accidents, can easily result in stretching or shearing of the fragile neurofilaments (Figure 48-3A). This latter mechanism of injury is caused by the fact that the olfactory bulb and brain are mobile within the calvarium, whereas the bone of the nasal cavity and cribriform plate from which the olfactory receptor axons originate is not. This type of injury most commonly results in a complete bilateral anosmia or severe hyposmia because the olfactory fibers can be severed from the olfactory bulbs, or otherwise severely stretched resulting in subsequent axonal degeneration (20). Classically, such shearing injuries are more common following mechanisms of injury that result in generation of posteroanterior coup and contrecoup forces that result in significant impact of the brain, mobile within the cerebrospinal fluid (CSF) contained by the meninges, against the skull base (7,20,22,42). This mechanism of injury may be seen with high-velocity mechanisms such as motor vehicle accidents, or even in the elderly patient suffering a ground level fall, falling backward and striking the occiput.

Central Lesions

Olfactory dysfunction may also occur following head trauma resulting in injuries to central components of the olfactory system. This may include significant cerebral edema, hemorrhage, or hematoma occurring anywhere from the olfactory bulbs to the cortical processing centers of the frontal and temporal lobes. In 1985, Levin et al. (43) suggested that damage to these regions could result in dysfunction of olfactory recognition, but not complete anosmia. Then in 1996, Yousem et al. (44) elaborated on the extensive and bilateral cortical projections of the olfactory pathways, providing the rationale for the low likelihood of complete anosmia following cortical injuries. The olfactory bulbs themselves are precariously situated beneath the mobile inferior portion of the cerebral hemispheres, sitting atop the fixed cribriform plate of the ethmoid bone, where they may be susceptible to compressive forces and possibly secondary ischemic insults. Costanzo and Zasler reported that injury to the olfactory bulbs can occur even in the absence of involvement of other brain regions, suggesting an increased susceptibility of this structure to injury, potentially by these mechanisms (45).

The olfactory cortices of the fronto-orbital and temporal lobes are some of the cortical regions most likely to sustain hemorrhage or contusion in traumatic head injuries. This is likely attributable to the anatomy of these regions. The sphenoid wings are in contact with the anterior borders of both temporal lobes, whereas the anterior clinoid process of the sphenoid is immediately anterior to the uncus bilaterally. Because the primary olfactory cortex is located on the ante-

romedial portion of the uncus and the olfactory tract passes on the lateral surface of the cerebral hemisphere, any violent forward movement of the brain against the skull base, as would occur with extreme deceleration such as when the head strikes a fixed immobile object, may cause injury to the olfactory cortex (46). Similarly, the location of the orbitofrontal cortex, abutting the posterior surface of the frontal bone, places it at risk of injury with such forces. Although it is intuitive that a blow to the frontal skull or facial region may result in such injuries, the same may also occur with blows to the occiput from a so called coup–contrecoup forces. In this case, with a blow to the posterior head such as may occur with a backward ground level fall, the occipital lobes are forced posteriorly against the cranium, potentially resulting in injuries to that region. Secondarily, the recoil of the elastic and compressible brain subsequently leads to rapid anterior displacement, thus forcing the forward brain regions such as the frontal lobes and anterior horns of the temporal lobes against the adjacent portions of the calvarium (Figure 48-4).

Nontraumatic Causes of Olfactory Dysfunction

The health care professional caring for patients after head injury with olfactory or gustatory dysfunction must also consider the possibility of preexisting or treatment-induced causes of olfactory dysfunction. Thus, a broad differential diagnosis must be considered even when evaluating the patient with significant head injury, where traumatic injury to the olfactory pathways is presumed. In some cases, the possibility of a preexisting deficit may be difficult to identify because the patient may have previously been unaware of the deficit, or in some cases, posttraumatic cognitive dysfunction may prevent recollection of having had such a

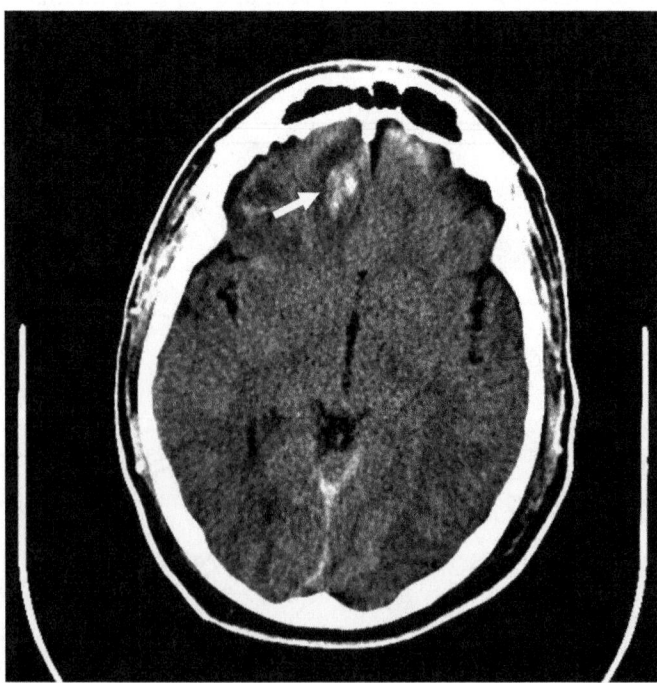

FIGURE 48-4 Computed tomography (CT) scan showing right-sided orbitofrontal contusion in a patient with unilateral anosmia following TBI.

deficit (12). Conductive smell losses may occur from inflammatory disorders such as rhinosinusitis, allergic rhinitis, or nasal polyposis, iatrogenic causes such as scarring from sinus or neurosurgical procedures or nasal tube placement as used for acute trauma resuscitation, or a wide variety of benign and malignant sinonasal neoplasms (47). Sensorineural smell loss has an even broader differential diagnosis. Common causes include aging, dementia, and other neurodegenerative disorders, virally mediated injury following upper respiratory tract infection, previous head trauma, medications including anticonvulsants often prescribed in patients with head injuries, toxic exposures, or congenitally absent sense of smell.

Gustatory (Taste) Dysfunction

Ageusia caused by traumatic injuries is uncommon, reported in only 0.4%–0.5% of traumatic head injuries (48). This may be attributable to the redundant nature and protected course of the innervation of the sensory structures of the oral cavity and pharynx, and the widely distributed cortical projections involved in gustation. As with traumatic disturbances of olfaction, traumatic disturbances of gustation may be categorized into 3 broad mechanisms: (*a*) injuries to the tongue and sensory structures; (*b*) injuries of CNs VII, IX, or X; and (*c*) injuries to cortical processing centers (22,48).

Injuries to the Tongue

Damage to the tongue itself is quite common in the patients suffering trauma to the head. This can result from direct penetration from displaced maxillomandibular fractures, self-inflicted bite or crush wounds, or foreign body penetration (48). However, the tongue is a resilient organ because of its extensive vascularization and ability for epithelial regeneration. Often, changes in taste will resolve as mucosal injuries heal and edema resolves. In addition, it is unusual for such injuries to be extensive enough to compromise taste function of all regions of the tongue, and thus, complete loss of taste from such injuries is unlikely. Despite its resilience, significant tongue injury may occasionally result in permanent alteration in gustation (22).

Injuries to Cranial Nerves V, VII, IX, or X

Maxillofacial fractures have been shown to cause gustatory dysfunction. In 1976, Obrebowski et al. reported a 0.9% incidence of asymmetrical gustatory loss following midface fractures (49). The mechanism of injury in these patients was unclear, but because of the nature of injuries sustained, it was thought to be secondary to CN damage.

CN VII is the most likely of the gustatory nerves to be injured following the head trauma because of its long anatomical course from the tongue to the brain (38,48). Longitudinal fractures of the temporal bone, representing 70%–90% of such fractures, have been found to have a 10%–20% incidence of facial nerve injury. Transverse fractures of the temporal bone are less common, but carry a 50% incidence of facial nerve damage (50). Temporal bone fractures most often result in damage to CN VII at the level of the geniculate ganglion. In addition, the chorda tympani branch is particularly vulnerable as it crosses the middle ear space, passing between the ossicles and along the medial surface of the tympanic membrane. The characteristic course of longitudinal fractures of the temporal bone extends through the external auditory canal and tympanic membrane, thus potentially causing injury to the chorda tympani at this location.

Taste fibers to the posterior third of the tongue are carried by CNs IX and X. Because of the course these nerves take to the brain via deep spaces of the neck and the wide jugular foramen, traumatic injury of these nerves is rare (22,48). Also, because of the redundant taste innervation of the tongue, patients with unilateral CN IX and X injuries will rarely complain of taste dysfunction, but more commonly will report hoarseness or dysphagia because of deficits in vocal fold mobility (CN X) or laryngopharyngeal sensation (CN IX and X) (22).

Cortical Lesions

Gustatory dysfunction caused by brain lesions following traumatic brain injury (TBI) is still an area of debate. Some of the controversy is caused by current limitations in our understanding of the interconnections between and functions of the various cortical regions involved in taste perception. This is further complicated by limitations in techniques used for objective measurement of gustatory function. It has been found that temporal and frontal lobe injuries often result in bilateral taste dysfunction (51). Unilateral pontine or rostral insular cortex lesions have been found to cause ipsilateral taste loss (38,52,53). Injuries to the ventral posteromedial thalamic nucleus have been implicated in the posttraumatic anosmia–ageusia syndrome (54). However, further research into the gustatory pathways, improved testing techniques, and potentially new imaging techniques and modalities may be required to better delineate the relationships between such traumatic central lesions and gustatory deficits.

Nontraumatic Causes of Gustatory Dysfunction

As with olfactory deficits, when considering the etiology of taste deficits in patients following head injury, the possibility of either preexisting or treatment-related causes of gustatory dysfunction must not be overlooked. In particular, many medications may alter taste perceptions either from their effect on saliva production, or their excretion into the saliva, often leading to unpleasant taste sensations, or dysgeusias. The proper saliva milieu is critical for the dissolution of ingested foods to be able to reach the taste buds. This is illustrated by the extreme example of Sjögren syndrome, an autoimmune disorder in which circulating autoantibodies initiate a brisk inflammatory response in all salivary gland tissue, ultimately leading to severe xerostomia and secondary dysgeusia or even ageusia. Although the effect of medications on saliva production would not be expected to be severe enough to cause ageusia, either hypogeusia or dysgeusia may occur. Infections of the middle ear, resulting in inflammation of the chorda tympani branch of the facial nerve, may alter transmission of gustatory information from the anterior regions of the tongue. Neoplasms located in the oral cavity, pharynx, or skull base, either affecting the taste bud containing mucosa or CNs V, VII, IX, or X, may also lead to deficits in taste function.

Lastly, one of the more common causes of subjective alteration in taste sensation is olfactory dysfunction, which occurs far more commonly following head injury than gustatory dysfunction. Although in the physiologic sense, taste refers to the basic perceptions elicited by the taste buds, one's overall perception of food is more appropriately termed *flavor*. Flavor is a more complex sensation incorporating both olfactory and gustatory perceptions simultaneously. As a result, many patients presenting with complaints of taste alterations are actually experiencing deficits of flavor perception secondary to olfactory dysfunction (55,56). It is estimated that approximately 80% of a meal's flavor perception comes from olfaction, either orthonasal, in which odorants from foods pass through the nose anteriorly to reach the olfactory neuroepithelium, or retronasal, in which odorants pass posteriorly from the oral cavity through the nasopharynx to reach the nasal cavity (38,47,57). Retronasal olfactory perceptions occur simultaneously with taste perceptions as masticated foods within the oral cavity dissolve in saliva to reach the taste buds, whereas odorants are also released, which passes to the nasopharynx and nasal cavity. As such, any complaint of taste dysfunction should also prompt thorough investigation for olfactory dysfunction.

CLINICAL PRESENTATION AND HISTORY

In patients suffering head trauma, the presence of gustatory or olfactory disturbances may not be realized until days, weeks, or even months after the traumatic event. In the period immediately after the event, attention to other potentially life threatening injuries understandably takes precedence for the health care team, such that chemosensory deficits may not even be considered initially. In some cases, altered mental status may reduce the patient's awareness of such deficits until alterations in eating behavior or lack of awareness of strong odor stimuli may be noted by family members or caregivers. Delayed resumption of oral feeding, either caused by mental status changes or traumatic injuries to the larynx, pharynx, or lower CNs, may also contribute to lack of awareness of such deficits.

To begin exploring a suspected disturbance in smell or taste, the nature of the deficit should be characterized. Is this a complete loss of smell (anosmia) or taste (ageusia), or a reduction of sensitivity (hyposmia or hypogeusia, respectively)? Qualitative distortions of olfactory perceptions are referred to as *dysosmias*, and of taste perceptions as dysgeusias. In some cases, distortions may lead to unpleasant or even foul smell (cacosmia) or taste (cacogeusia) perceptions with previously pleasant stimuli. Some may also report phantom smell or less commonly phantom taste perceptions in the absence of real stimuli, so-called "phantom" sensations (Table 48-2).

The laterality of the deficit should be explored, although this is generally hard for most patients to realize, even in the unusual setting of a completely unilateral loss. The onset and time course of the deficit should be analyzed because a traumatic injury to sensory pathways would be expected to lead to an immediate deficit. However, as noted earlier, many patients will not remember or will not have gained awareness of the sensory dysfunction in the time immediately following their traumatic event, and thus will not be able to elucidate the timing of onset. In addition, immediately following the injury, the patient is likely to have undergone multiple treatments that might affect taste or smell.

TABLE 48-2 Terms of Smell and Taste Dysfunction

DYSFUNCTION	SMELL TERM	TASTE TERM
Total inability to sense	Ansomia	Ageusia
Decreased ability to sense	Hyposmia	Hypogeusia
Altered perception	Dysosmia	Dysgeusia
Perception in the absence of a stimulus	Phantosmia	Phantgeusia
Distorted perception with stimulus	Parosmia or troposmia	Parageusia
Unpleasant or foul sensation	Cacosmia	Cacogeusia

This includes administration of multiple medications (20,48, 58), placement of oral and nasal life support tubes, and surgical treatment including maxillofacial and neurosurgical procedures. A thorough review of the medical record is thus crucial in the assessment of patients presenting with smell and taste dysfunction, but even more so in the patient with head injury. Any indication of previous nasal or sinus disease, viral infection, chemotherapy treatment, and head and neck radiation should be noted, and all medications administered should be reviewed. The history should seek to elucidate possible mechanisms of injury. This should include a detailed account of the patient's preinjury sensory function. The interviewer should inquire about any previous sensory deficits, even those that may have been only transient, and potential causes of such deficits. A history of chronic rhinosinusitis, previous maxillofacial trauma or surgery, neurosurgical procedures, upper respiratory infection-related losses, head and neck irradiation, systemic disease, or medication use may all suggest a potential preexisting sensory impairment.

Next, events surrounding the traumatic injury should be discussed with the patient, or ascertained from the medical record. In particular, some characteristics of the traumatic event, or postinjury findings may predict the likelihood of posttraumatic sensory dysfunction. Swann et al. (59) reported that patients with posttraumatic amnesia (PTA) of greater than 5 minutes duration had a significantly higher likelihood of olfactory dysfunction than those with PTA of less than 5 minutes, with an odds ratio of 9.6. Similarly, Green et al. reported that patients experiencing 10 days or more of PTA were 6 times more likely to demonstrate impairment on smell testing than those experiencing no PTA (46). Several studies have demonstrated a correlation between anosmia and injury severity (10,16,46,55). Callahan and Hinkebein (10) found that the severity of brain injury correlated not only with the severity of olfactory dysfunction, but also with the likelihood of the patient being unaware of their olfactory deficit. Green et al. (46) found that patients with more severe injury (Glasgow Coma Scale [GCS] <13) were 10–12 times more likely to have olfactory deficits than those with less severe injuries (GCS >13). The location of head strike in traumatic injuries may also be predictive for occurrence of olfactory deficits. Zusho (7) reported that the direction of external force most often resulting in anosmia was posterior-to-anterior. Doty et al. (55) subsequently found a slightly higher incidence of anosmia following occipital (39.3%) vs frontal (36.3%) head strikes.

Another clinical finding shown to correlate with olfactory dysfunction is the presence of CSF rhinorhea (60,61). The thin bone of the ethmoid roof, including the cribriform plate, is susceptible to fracture, which may lead to CSF leakage from this area. Fracture in this area suggests transmission of significant traumatic forces to this region, also placing the delicate olfactory nerve fibers at risk of injury. The patient should thus be asked about the presence of clear watery drainage from the nose, or alternately a salty taste in the mouth. Patients with disorders of smell and taste following head injury are also at high risk of executive function impairment (12,46,62–65). Roberts and Simcox reported that 52% of pediatric patients in their study with anosmia were also found to have executive dysfunction (63). They further reported that children suffering TBIs with a compromised sense of smell were 3 times more likely to manifest daily problems in self-regulation of behavior as were children with similar injuries but with intact smell. Sigurdardottir et al. (64) found that patients with olfactory dysfunction exhibited poor performance on verbal fluency tests and marked decision-making deficits at 3 months postinjury. Callahan and Hinkebein (12) reported that patients with anosmia were more likely to have deficits in complex attention, new learning and memory, problem solving, and awareness of olfactory deficit. Although these associations may simply be related to the overall increased severity of the injuries sustained, this may also be caused by the proximity of the olfactory nerves at their most susceptible point—at the cribriform plate, olfactory bulbs, and cortical processing centers to the frontal lobe regions—critical in such executive functions. As such, it has been suggested that a psychosocial history and evaluation be considered for all patients with olfactory loss (66). Lastly, associations have been reported between posttraumatic anosmia and hearing loss (41%), tinnitus (22.6%), disequilibrium (14.2%), and visual disturbances (2.8%) (7).

After a detailed history is obtained from the patient, an extensive review of the trauma record from the emergency department and inpatient record should be performed. The examiner should look for descriptions of any facial or head lacerations or ecchymosis, epistaxis, CSF leak, and CN deficits. Any brain or maxillofacial imaging obtained in the initial trauma evaluation or subsequent work-up should be obtained and reviewed. If possible, both the radiologist's report and the images themselves should be reviewed, paying special attention to the anterior skull base and orbitofrontal lobes, where subtle changes may be missed when scans are initially interpreted while looking primarily for life-threatening intracranial injuries. Any operative reports from neurosurgical or maxillofacial reconstructive procedures should be reviewed for descriptions of locations of injury as well as details of the procedure performed, in particular proximity to olfactory or gustatory pathway elements. Records from other treating physicians should be obtained and reviewed for documentation of complaints of olfactory or gustatory dysfunction.

Attention should be given to correlation between the patient's medical record and their provided history, specifically previous complaints or denials of sensory disturbance. Inconsistencies may suggest malingering, particularly in patients potentially seeking legal action. It should be noted that complete ageusia is rare even following severe head injury because of the redundant innervation, and thus patients with this complaint should be suspected for possible malingering. In all patients, but particularly in such cases of suspected malingering, objective assessment of sensory function is imperative.

PHYSICAL EXAMINATION

The examination of the patient with posttraumatic olfactory or gustatory dysfunction should begin with close inspection of the head, taking note of indications of focal head trauma such as lacerations, ecchymosis, edema, or tenderness. Any of the these findings, especially in the frontal or occipital regions, may suggest a potential coup–contrecoup type injury that may result in injury to the olfactory nerve fibers or contusion of the orbitofrontal cortex. Battle's sign (ecchymosis over the mastoid process) or periorbital ecchymosis are suggestive of basilar skull fractures. Telecanthus (increased intercanthal distance) is a classic finding in patients who have suffered nasooribitoethmoid fractures. These fractures commonly result in direct damage to the cribriform plate, and are also indicative of transmission of significant force to the midface and frontal region, which can alternately lead to shearing or stretching of the olfactory fibers. The maxillofacial skeleton—in particular the orbital rims and nasal bones—should be palpated to assess for step-offs resulting from fractures with bony displacement.

Next, attention should be turned to the ears. Otoscopic examination may reveal lacerations or bony step-offs in the external auditory canal, hemotympanum, ossicular dislocation, or tympanic membrane rupture, all findings suggestive of temporal bone fracture. Fracture lines passing through the middle ear space may result in damage to the fragile chorda tympani nerve, leading to gustatory deficits. Alternately, fractures affecting the more proximal segments of the facial nerve, prior to the take off of the chorda tympani branch may result in gustatory complaints, and are also associated with ipsilateral facial weakness. In cases of facial paralysis, clinical testing of functions mediated by other facial nerve branches such as Shirmer test for lacrimation (greater superficial petrosal branch), gustatory testing of the anterior two-thirds of the tongue (chorda tympani branch), and audiometric impedance testing of stapedial reflex (stapedial branch) may be used to localize the site of lesion along the intratemporal course of the facial nerve.

Attention is then turned to the nose. Beyond inspection for fractures as mentioned earlier, the external nose should be evaluated for posttraumatic or preexisting structural issues that might affect nasal airflow and, thus, olfaction. This includes significant deformity of the bony or cartilaginous skeleton of the external nose, or static or dynamic collapse of the nasal sidewall that may limit airflow and thus odorant access to the superior nasal cavity. Initial examination may be performed with a nasal speculum or otoscope to allow visualization of the anterior nasal cavity. Improved access to the nasal cavity may be afforded by application of a topical decongestant such as 0.25% phenylephrine or 0.025% oxymetazoline, either as a spray or on cotton balls or pledgets inserted into the nose. The septum should be evaluated for significant deformity or deviation (either preexisting or traumatic), mucosal laceration, edema, or ecchymosis. Similarly, the inferior turbinates should be inspected for mucosal injury or deformity that might obstruct nasal airflow. In addition, indirect evidence of sinonasal injury is provided by the presence of blood, clot, or CSF within the nasal cavity.

Nasal endoscopy is critical in the assessment of patients with olfactory or gustatory complaints because it provides the only means whereby the entire nasal cavity can be inspected. Endoscopy should ideally be performed twice—both before and after the application of topical decongestants—to determine the degree of reversible mucosal edema. Either a flexible fiber-optic nasopharyngoscope or a rigid nasal endoscope may be used. As with any examination, the endoscopic examination should be systematic, including inspection of the inferior, middle, and superior meatus as well as the nasopharynx. Rhinosinusitis, either preexisting or secondary to indwelling nasal tubes used in acute resuscitation or subsequent enteral feeding following major trauma, may be suggested by the presence of purulent drainage emanating from the middle or superior meatus. Although the associate mucosal edema may cause hyposmia, more commonly, patients may report dysosmia because of the purulence. Other specific abnormalities that should be noted if present are septal hematoma, septal deviation, turbinate enlargement or deformities, neoplasms, or polyposis, any of which can hinder odorant access to the olfactory neuroepithelium in the superior nasal cavity and thus contribute to the subjective sensory deficit. As the superior nasal cavity and olfactory cleft is approached, the narrow dimensions may necessitate use of a smaller endoscope (as commonly used for pediatric endoscopy) or gentle lateralization of the middle turbinate with an instrument or the endoscope itself. The olfactory cleft should be inspected for evidence of injury, such as mucosal edema, lacerations, ecchymosis, or CSF leak.

Next, the oral cavity is examined. The mucosal surfaces should be inspected for adequacy and quality of saliva. Wharton and Stenson ducts on each side should be visualized during massage of the submandibular and parotid glands, respectively, to verify flow of clear saliva because alteration in the salivary milieu of the oral cavity may result in taste dysfunction. Edema, ecchymosis, or penetrating injuries of the tongue, floor of mouth, or even externally in the submandibular or submental triangles of the neck may be indicative of lingual nerve injury. The dorsal and ventral surfaces of the tongue should be evaluated for atrophy, edema, hematoma, or laceration. Tongue sensation (carried by CN V) and mobility (provided by CN XII) should be evaluated. The state of dentition should be noted because poor dentition or malfitting dental appliances can result in taste problems. Palate elevation and gag reflex should also be tested to verify integrity of CNs IX and X.

SMELL AND TASTE TESTING

Olfactory Function Testing

All patients reporting olfactory or gustatory deficits following head trauma should undergo olfactory testing to confirm the presence of and quantify the degree of loss. As discussed earlier, because of the impact of olfactory input on taste—or more appropriately flavor perception—many patients presenting with a complaint of only taste loss may actually have an olfactory deficit alone, underscoring the need for olfactory assessment in these individuals. Unfortunately, there is no single accepted standard test of olfactory function, and several validated test methods are in common use for the objective assessment of olfactory function. These differ by functions tested—either odorant detection or odorant identification and ease or manner of administration—with differences in cost, time of testing, and potential for self-administration. These factors should be considered before selecting the test used in any clinical application. Some of the commonly used testing methods are discussed subsequently.

The University of Pennsylvania Smell Identification Test (UPSIT) (67,68) is a 40-item self-administered test that uses 4 booklets, each containing 10 "scratch and sniff" microencapsulated odorants. For each scratch and sniff odorant, 4 possible odors are provided as possible answers, and the subject is required to select 1 of the 4 choices for each item (the so-called "forced-choice" technique). The number of stimuli correctly identified yields a score ranging from 0 to 40 correct answers. Normal olfaction is a score of 34–40 correct for males and 35–40 for females. From these scores, the degree of olfactory dysfunction is classified into 6 categories: normosmia, mild hyposmia, moderate hyposmia, severe hyposmia, anosmia, and malingering. The forced-choice technique allows for detection of possible malingering. Because a patient with complete anosmia taking random guesses would be expected to achieve a score of approximately 10 (25% correct) on the test, malingering is considered if a patient scores in the 0–5 range. This would suggest correct identification of odors, with intentional selection of the incorrect responses in an effort to achieve a poor score. There are multiple forms of the UPSIT including the full 40-item version, and more compact and less expensive screening versions such as the 3-item Pocket Smell Test and the 12-item Brief Smell Identification Test, which may be more conducive to rapid screening in the emergency room or most outpatient clinical settings.

The Alberta Smell Test (69,70) is another test of odorant identification that uses scented markers containing food-grade essences such as lemon, orange, and mint as stimuli. The scented markers are presented to each side of the nose, whereas the opposite side is occluded using gentle pressure by the patient. The patient is asked to identify the odors from a list of possible options. The test is scored using the number of correct responses out of 10 for each nostril. This test does not categorize the level of dysfunction, but it does allow for testing of laterality. The test has been devised primarily for use as a screening tool because it is easily reusable and inexpensive. The test developers suggest that abnormal results should then be verified with a more comprehensive test technique such as the UPSIT (67), or a test that includes odor detection and threshold testing (71).

The University of Connecticut Chemosensory Clinical Research Center test assesses a patient's ability to both detect and identify odors (14,71). This test measures detection threshold by using nine serial dilutions of butanol in nanopure-deionized water. Each concentration is presented along with an odorless water control in a double-blind, forced-choice paradigm. Detection threshold is defined as the dilution at which the butanol bottle is correctly identified in 4 consecutive trials. If the water bottle is incorrectly selected in more than one trial, the next higher concentration is tested. This test also allows for the detection of malingering. Using the forced-choice technique, a complete anosmic taking random guesses would be expected to correctly identify the butanol bottle in 50% of trials. Thus, if a patient consistently scores lower than 50, and in particular when the subject chooses the water bottle in four out of four choices, the suspicion for malingering is high. The odor identification portion of the test consists of assessing the subject's ability to recognize 7 common olfactory stimuli (baby powder, chocolate, soap, peanut butter, cinnamon, coffee, and mothballs) and 3 trigeminal stimuli (ammonia, wintergreen, and Vicks VapoRub). Ten jars, each containing 1 of the 10 odorants, are presented sequentially to each side of the nose independently, with the opposite side occluded, and the patient asked to identify the smell from a list of choices. The olfactory stimulants are used in the assessment of olfactory function, whereas the trigeminal stimulants are used in the assessment of trigeminal function, and, moreover, to assist in the detection of malingering. The latter is based on the extreme rarity of complete and bilateral loss of trigeminal sensation, such that if the subject indicates they are unable to detect even the trigeminal stimulants, malingering is suspected. The odor threshold and odor identification scores for each side of the nose are scored independently and then added together to obtain a composite olfactory function score for that side.

In Japan, two commonly used olfactory testing methods are T&T olfactometry (19) and the Alinamin test (72). T&T olfactometry uses a test kit that includes 5 odorants: β-phenyl ethyl alcohol, cyclotene, isovaleric acid, γ-undecalactone, and skatole (rose, burning, sweat, fruit, and vegetable chips, respectively). Each odorant is presented at multiple concentrations that are used to determine both detection and recognition thresholds. The detection threshold is defined as the lowest concentration detectable by the subject, whereas the recognition threshold is defined as the lowest concentration at which the odor can be identified. The Alinamin test is an intravenous test involving the injection of a thiol-type derivative of vitamin B_1, which results in a garlic-like smell sensation when injected (72). The median vein of the left arm is injected with 10 mg of Alinamin solution at a constant rate for 20 seconds. The latency (time from injection to the detection of smell) and the duration (time from detection to the disappearance of the smell) of the smell perception are measured. Normal latency is 7–8 seconds, and normal duration is 1–2 minutes. The Alinamin test can also be used when malingering is suspected because test subjects are typically unaware of the normal latency and duration times and would be unable to differentiate between the injection of alinamin or a saline control.

Gustatory Function Testing

Clinical tests commonly used for the sense of taste involve either spatial testing techniques, which attempt to test isolated segments of the tongue independently by selective application of test substances for localization of neural deficits, or whole mouth testing techniques. Techniques involve either application of a small aliquot of tastant in solution (73–75), a flavored wafer (76), or a tasting tablet (77) to the tongue, with the patient then asked to detect or identify the taste (sweet, salty, bitter, or sour). Electrogustometry is a method used to evaluate taste nerve function, which has been used in a few clinical studies, but more commonly as

a research tool (78). Small amounts of current are applied to different regions of the tongue to activate the underlying taste nerves and determine threshold levels for generating a taste sensation.

Another indirect method of assessing taste function and more specifically evaluating for gustatory nerve deficits following traumatic injury was described in 1990 by Miller and Reedy (79). In this method, the tongue is stained with methylene blue and examined with microscopy in vivo. Taste buds with intact innervation stain blue, whereas those with loss of innervation do not stain. In cases of dysgeusia or phantom taste sensations, the abolition or diminution of such aberrant taste sensations by application of local anesthetics to the tongue provides an indication of a peripheral etiology, either at the taste bud or peripheral gustatory nerve level (80).

NEUROIMAGING

The complexity of the skull base and CN anatomy, as well as the need to rule out central nervous system pathology have placed high-resolution computed tomography (CT) and magnetic resonance imaging (MRI) in the forefront as the imaging modalities of choice in the evaluation of patients with smell and taste dysfunction. Although plain film imaging may still be used, albeit infrequently, as a screening tool in cases of suspected craniofacial bony trauma, their inability to adequately image the neuroanatomy, intricacies of the ethmoid roof and cribriform fossa, and relevant soft tissue structures of the oral cavity severely limits their utility in the evaluation of patients with posttraumatic olfactory or gustatory dysfunction. Most often, high-resolution CT scanning is the imaging modality of choice for its ability to delineate both bony and soft tissue structures and injuries. However, for some indications, MRI may provide additional diagnostic sensitivity, in particular with subtle brain injuries.

For optimal assessment of the maxillofacial region including the cribriform fossa, CT is performed using high-resolution thin-cut (1 mm or less) protocols in both the axial and coronal planes without contrast. Because direct coronal imaging requires the patient to lay prone with the head extended, patients with cervical spine injuries may be limited to axial plane imaging only, with coronal images then obtained by computer reconstruction. CT is sensitive for detecting abnormalities of the nasal cavities that may result in airflow obstruction, sinusitis, or fractures of the cribriform plate, the latter, in particular, being best detected with coronal plane imaging. In patients with taste dysfunction, CT of the temporal bones may identify fractures in the proximity of the facial nerve as it travels through the fallopian canal, whereas injury to the chorda tympani may be suggested by dislocation of the ossicles or the presence of fractures extending through the middle ear space (81). In addition, CT is capable of detecting skull base fractures in the vicinity of the jugular foramen that might pose risk of injury to the glossopharyngeal or vagus nerves. Brain imaging with CT may detect areas of brain hemorrhage or edema in the proximity of higher pathways and central processing centers for olfaction and gustation. Use of intravenous contrast may further increase sensitivity for detection of these abnormalities.

MRI has limited ability to assess bony structures, but may provide enhanced ability to evaluate and detect abnormalities of soft tissue structures, in particular, within the brain parenchyma. It allows for superior visualization of cerebral hemorrhage, infarct, or contusion compared with CT. MRI is particularly useful in evaluating structures near the skull base such as the olfactory bulbs and inferior frontal lobes, where beam-hardening artifacts and partial volume effects limit sensitivity of CT imaging (44). Yousem et al. (44), compared MRI findings within the olfactory pathways with objective olfactory test results, finding that 88% of anosmic patients had injuries of the olfactory bulbs and tracts, 60% within the subfrontal region, and 32% within the temporal lobes.

Other imaging modalities have also been explored for detection and localization of specific neural deficits in patients with posttraumatic olfactory deficits. A study using single-photon emission computed tomography (SPECT) revealed hypoperfusion in the frontal, left parietal, and left temporal lobes corresponding to posttraumatic anosmia (82). Application of positron-emission tomography (PET) revealed hypometabolism in the orbitofrontal cortex and the medial prefrontal cortex in patients with posttraumatic anosmia (83). Recently, PET has shown some utility in the evaluation of olfactory dysfunction in elderly patients suffering from Alzheimer or Parkinson disease (84). Because further research is directed toward application of existing imaging modalities to the assessment of olfactory dysfunction, and new modalities are developed, our ability to localize the site of posttraumatic olfactory dysfunction and correlate with subjective complaints and objective test findings will improve.

TREATMENT AND PROGNOSIS

As reviewed earlier, chemosensory dysfunction may arise following traumatic injuries either as a direct result of the trauma or alternately as a sequela of treatment for the traumatic injuries, either medical or surgical. Because in most cases, there are no active treatments available for neural injuries of the olfactory or gustatory pathways, patient evaluation should attempt to identify any existing reversible etiologies such as medication effects, nasal obstruction, or sinusitis, which might be amenable to treatment. Airflow limitation caused by direct trauma to the sinonasal region leading to mucosal edema or hematoma may be ameliorated by treatment with nasal corticosteroid sprays often commonly used in the management of nasal allergy or sinusitis (85,86). Bony abnormalities such as significant septal deviation or displaced middle turbinate may be corrected surgically to relieve symptomatic nasal obstruction, which may also improve olfactory function. Patients developing chronic rhinosinusitis refractory to medical therapy from fractures or scarring from nasal life support tubes causing sinus ostial obstruction or from mucosal injuries may benefit from functional endoscopic sinus surgery to relieve infection, reduce sinonasal inflammation, and secondarily improve olfaction (87). As a patient's general medical status allows, medications contributing to nasal mucosal drying or xerostomia should be discontinued for their possible effects on olfaction or gustation. Similarly, patients with dysgeusias taking medications known for such side effects should, where possible, be given a month-long holiday from

such medications, one at a time, in an effort to identify and discontinue the offending agent.

Although there are currently no specific treatments available for chemosensory deficits caused by neuronal injury, spontaneous recovery may occur. In particular, the unique regenerative capacity of the olfactory neuroepithelium has been shown to allow recovery because of regeneration of the olfactory nerves following traumatic injuries (88–90). Costanzo and Becker reported that 33% of all patients with moderate to severe head injuries with olfactory deficits showed some improvement in olfaction, whereas 27% worsened (21). However, the likelihood of experiencing any recovery of olfaction diminished with time after injury, such that if recovery had not occurred within 6 months to 1 year following injury, it was unlikely (21). Similarly, Doty et al. (55) found that 36% of patients with olfactory dysfunction following trauma improved, 45% had no change, and 18% worsened over several years. Considerable research efforts have been directed at fostering the intrinsic regenerative process of the olfactory nerve fibers following traumatic injuries. Costanzo and Kobayashi found in a murine model that the subcutaneous injection of dexamethasone for 5 days following olfactory neuron injury reduced the amount of scar tissue formation and aided in the neural reinnervation of the olfactory bulb (90). Ikeda et al. reported that 4 out of 17 (24%) anosmic patients showed slight recovery of their olfactory function following systemic or intranasal topical administration of corticosteroids (86). Others have suggested the use of zinc sulfate to improve recovery from posttraumatic olfactory deficits (91). Kern and his colleagues found that intraperitoneal injections of minocycline in a mouse model inhibited the death of olfactory neurons and suggested its use in the management of peripheral olfactory loss (92). More recent work has sought to identify alternative methods of restoring olfactory function in cases of anosmia. Recent studies have found that the olfactory epithelium can be transplanted into different regions of the brain and still retain cell characteristics of normal olfactory epithelium (93–96). This raises the possibility of olfactory tissue grafting as a potential method for the restoration of smell to anosmic patients. However, application of such techniques to human subjects is still some time off.

In most instances, no specific treatment exists for posttraumatic ageusia, however, spontaneous recovery occurs more frequently than from posttraumatic anosmia (3,23, 97,98). Improvement or resolution of taste loss usually occurs over several months after the injury. It has also been found that individual taste qualities may be affected differently (99). The ability to taste bitterness (mediated by the glossopharyngeal nerve) has been found to be particularly susceptible to traumatic insults (100). However, sweet taste perception, mediated primarily by the facial nerve, seems to recover more quickly flowing traumatic insults than bitter taste perception. Specific mechanisms of recovery remain unclear, although possibilities include (a) resolution of cortical contusion or intraparenchymal bleed; (b) recovery of neurapraxic injury to taste fibers of the chorda tympani, lingual, or glossopharyngeal nerves; (c) restoration of normal salivary flow; or (d) resolution of edema of the tongue or floor of the mouth. It should be noted that disruption of taste fibers to one side of the tongue usually does not lead to a perceived disruption in taste (101). It is for this reason that surgical decompression or repair of an isolated lingual or hypoglossal nerve injury is seldom indicated.

PATIENT MANAGEMENT AND REHABILITATION

Although in most cases, there are no specific medical treatments available, the practitioner treating the patient with posttraumatic smell and taste dysfunction may provide support and counseling, which may be quite invaluable to a patient already burdened with numerous other physical and neuropsychiatric sequelae of their traumatic injuries (102). The American Medical Association impairment rating system suggests a "1%–5% impairment of the whole person" in those with bilateral loss of smell and taste, whereas unilateral losses preclude any level of impairment rating (103). However, this does not necessarily represent the functional disability associated with such losses, which may vary widely between patients depending on the role of smell and taste in each individual's daily life. In particular, the evaluating professional must consider the patient's vocational status and other avocational pursuits to determine each patient's true functional disability. Patients in olfaction- or gustation-dependent occupations such as firefighters, chemists, plumbers, cooks, cosmeticians, and florists may be impaired significantly in their job performance by a posttraumatic loss. A previous study found a significant negative correlation between the presence of anosmia and successful vocational reintegration. Appropriate job analysis is required prior to making final recommendations regarding whether or not a given patient should attempt reentry into their previous vocation. Employee and employer education may be critical, as might job or workplace modifications to increase patient safety.

There are many other potential adverse effects of smell or taste loss affecting daily activities and QOL, including safety, appetite and nutrition, hygiene, homemaking, child care, and hobbies. A retrospective survey of patients undergoing evaluation for olfactory dysfunction found the most commonly cited activities impaired by olfactory loss were detection of spoiled foods (75%), detection of gas leaks (61%), eating (53%), detection of smoke (50%), cooking (49%), buying fresh food (36%), and using perfume or cologne (33%).

Personal safety considerations should also be explored because patients commonly report the inability to detect smoke, gas leaks, spoiled foods, or chemical vapors, which certainly places patients and those they care for in potential danger (104). Patients should thus be advised to ensure proper installation and maintenance of smoke and carbon monoxide detectors, as well as the routine monitoring of gas appliances. Perishable foods should all be dated when purchased because patients will often not be able to smell or taste spoiled foods. Precautions should be exercised in the use and storage of noxious substances used in household cleaning and gardening.

From a cooking and nutrition standpoint, there are many challenges to be overcome in this patient population. Patients with olfactory or gustatory dysfunction will experience alterations in the taste of foods, which may lead to decreased enjoyment of foods, or even alteration in appetite and food aversions. The latter may occur with dysgeusias or dysosmias, who may avoid foods that trigger unpleasant flavor perceptions. To the extreme, patients with severe taste distortions, ageusia, or anosmia may experience significant loss of appetite even leading to malnutrition. Further, some patients with anosmia seeking to compensate for loss of flavor perception by appealing to their intact taste function may adopt compensatory food items that may be very salty, sweet, or crunchy (105,106). This may pose problems for hypertensive patients because of excess salt ingestion, or diabetic patients because of excess sugar ingestion. Patients may be able to overcome loss of olfactory input in flavor perception by use of spices or "hot" seasonings to heighten stimulation of other preserved taste modalities or by stimulating CN V thus restoring some enjoyment to their meals. Physicians may suggest rehabilitative interventions such as menu planning, dietary consultation, and techniques to enhance meal enjoyment with more visual cues and texture qualities. In preparing meals, the patient should be counseled to follow recipes verbatim and not to rely on taste or smell, which may be distorted.

In addition, patients with olfactory losses may have problems with personal hygiene, child care, and pet care. Anosmic patients may not be able to detect their own body odor, the body odor of others, or the smell of colognes or perfumes. A schedule should be established for hygiene tasks such as washing clothes and bathing. Appropriate use of body fragrances can be encouraged by training the person to measure out specified quantities of fragrances. Child care issues are multiple and require education regarding timely diaper changes, hygiene timing, and food preparation. Pet care should include scheduled litter box and animal pen inspections.

Beyond the potential for direct impairment in performance of myriad daily activities, chemosensory dysfunction may have significant impact on QOL. One seldom considers what it would be like not to be able to smell spring flowers or coffee in the morning, to enjoy the specific scents of one's children or spouse, or taste one's favorite meal. Studies have shown reduced QOL in patients who have impaired olfaction (21,107) and a significant relationship between olfactory disturbances and clinical depression or other psychological effects (8,108). In Miwa et al.'s study (2) of patients with impaired olfaction from a variety of causes, only 50% reported being either very or somewhat satisfied with life, whereas 34% reported being either very or somewhat dissatisfied with life. Thus, patient counseling not only for compensatory strategies but also for reassurance and validation of their perceived concerns are important in helping patients cope with the psychological burden of their loss. By helping patients understand that they have a medical condition experienced by others, the physician may help to allay patients' fears or frustrations.

MEDICOLEGAL CONSIDERATIONS

Assessment of olfaction and gustation in the patients sustaining head injuries may be an important factor in medicolegal matters involving personal injury litigation. Because subjective reports or simple bedside testing may be unreliable in objectively documenting loss of chemosensory function and identifying malingerers, special protocols for sensory testing should be employed to validate or refute patient complaints (109,110). In any legal case, a complete and thorough evaluation, including neurological, otolaryngological, and radiological examinations, should be performed to support or refute any patient claims of chemosensory deficits. Unfortunately, in most cases, in particular where objective evidence of a deficit is present following a traumatic event, there are rarely pretraumatic event objective test results available to confirm the presence of normal function prior to the injury under consideration. For this reason, the history should include a thorough investigation, including a review of any preinjury medical records, for previous complaints of and other possible causes of preexisting olfactory or gustatory dysfunction. In addition, thorough examination of the oral cavity, oropharynx, and endoscopic examination of the nasal cavities should be performed to assess for evidence of previous injuries or surgical procedures that may potentially have caused pre-traumatic deficits.

KEY CLINICAL POINTS

1. Olfactory impairment may occur following traumatic head injuries because of disruption of the sinonasal passages, olfactory nerves injury, and/or damage to olfactory brain regions.
2. Although loss of taste function following traumatic head injury is relatively rare compared to loss of smell function, many patients with olfactory losses also experience altered taste perception because of the interplay of these 2 sensory modalities.
3. Evaluation including thorough history with exploration for possible causes of pretraumatic sensory disturbances and mechanism of traumatic injury, physical examination with nasal endoscopy, and neuroimaging may help to identify the mechanism of dysfunction and suggest possible treatments.
4. A variety of tests of olfactory and gustatory function are available, which may be used in settings ranging from the emergency department, physician's office, or specialty smell and taste centers to document the severity of the deficit, and if needed identify malingers.
5. With most posttraumatic olfactory deficits being neurally mediated, specific treatments do not exist, however, spontaneous improvement occurs in about one-third of cases, and may be seen up to 18 months after the time of injury.
6. Patient counseling should focus on avoidance of risks and health hazards associated with chemosensory disturbances, along with compensatory strategies for maintenance of safety and QOL.

KEY REFERENCES

1. Costanzo RM, DiNardo LJ, Reiter ER. Head injury and olfaction. In: Doty RL, ed. *Handbook of Olfaction and Gustation*. 2nd ed. New York, NY: Marcel Dekker, Inc.; 2003: 629–638.
2. Doty RL, Bromley SM, Panganiban WD. Olfactory function and dysfunction. In: Bailey BJ, Johnson JT, Newlands SD, eds. *Head & Neck Surgery—Otolaryngology*. Vol 1. 4th

ed. Philadelphia, PA: Lippincott Williams & Wilkins; 2006:289–305.
3. Santos DV, Reiter ER, DiNardo LJ, Costanzo RM. Hazardous events associated with impaired olfactory function. *Arch Otolaryngol Head Neck Surg.* 2004;130(3):317–319.
4. Sumner D. Distubance of the senses of smell and taste after head injuries. In: Vinken PJ, Bruyn GW, eds. *Handbook of Clinical Neurology*. Amsterdam, The Netherlands: North-Holland Publishing Co.; 1975:1–25.
5. Zasler ND, Costanzo RM. Smell and taste dysfunction. In: *Journal of Head Trauma Rehabilitation*. Frederick, MD: Aspen Publishers; 1992.

Electronic Resources

ACHEMS (The Association for Chemoreception Sciences)
  http://www.achems.org
Anosmia Foundation
  http://www.anosmiafoundation.com/
NIDCD (National Institute on Deafness and Other Communication Disorders)
  http://www.nidcd.nih.gov/health/smelltaste/
MedLine Plus—The National Institutes of Health's website for patients, family and friends
  http://www.nlm.nih.gov/medlineplus/ency/article/003052.htm

References

1. Zasler ND, Costanzo RM. Smell and taste dysfunction. In: *Journal of Head Trauma Rehabilitation*. Frederick, MD: Aspen Publishers; 1992.
2. Miwa T, Furukawa M, Tsukatani T, Costanzo RM, DiNardo LJ, Reiter ER. Impact of olfactory impairment on quality of life and disability. *Arch Otolaryngol Head Neck Surg.* 2001;127(5):497–503.
3. Jackson JH. Illustrations of diseases of the nervous system. *London Hospital Report.* 1864;1:470–471.
4. Ogle W. Anosmia, or cases illustrating the physiology and pathology of the sense of smell. *Med Chir Trans.* 1870;53:263–290.
5. Leigh AD. Defects in smell after head injury. *Lancet.* 1943;1:38–40.
6. Mifka P. Post-traumatische anosmie [The traumatically caused loss of smell]. *Wien Med Wochenschr.* 1964;114:793–796.
7. Zusho H. Posttraumatic anosmia. *Arch Otolaryngol.* 1982;108(2): 90–92.
8. Costanzo RM, Heywood PG, Ward JD, Young HF. Neurosurgical applications of clinical olfactory assessment. *N Y Acad Sci.* 1987; 510:242–244.
9. Ogawa T, Rutka J. Olfactory dysfunction in head injured workers. *Acta Otolaryngol Suppl.* 1999;119(suppl 540):50–57.
10. Callahan CD, Hinkebein JH. Assessment of anosmia after traumatic brain injury: performance characteristics of the University of Pennsylvania Smell Identification Test. *J Head Trauma Rehabil.* 2002;17(3):251–256.
11. Kraus W, Fife D, Ramstein K, Conroy C, Cox P. The relationship of family income to the incidence, external causes, and outcomes of serious brain injury, San Diego County, California. *Am J Public Health.* 1986;76(11):1345–1347.
12. Callahan CD, Hinkebein J. Neuropsychological significance of anosmia following traumatic brain injury. *J Head Trauma Rehabil.* 1999; 14(6):581–587.
13. Takagi SF. A standardized olfactometer in Japan. A review over ten years. *Ann NY Acad Sci.* 1987;510:113–118.
14. Cain WS, Gent J, Catalanotto FA, Goodspeed RB. Clinical evaluation of olfaction. *Am J Otolaryngol.* 1983;4(4):252–256.
15. Doty RL, Shaman P, Dann M. Development of the University of Pennsylvania Smell Identification Test: a standardized microencapsulated test of olfactory function. *Physiol Behav.* 1984;32(3): 489–502.

16. Costanzo RM, Zasler ND. Head trauma. In: Getchell TV, Doty RL, Bartoshuk LM, Snow JB Jr, eds. *Smell and Taste in Health and Disease.* New York, NY: Raven Press; 1991:711–730.

17. Cain WS. Testing olfaction in a clinical setting. *Ear Nose Throat J.* 1989;68(4):316, 322–328.

18. Ikeda K, Tabata K, Oshima T, Nishikawa H, Hidaka H, Takasaka T. Unilateral examination of olfactory threshold using the Jet Stream Olfactometer. *Auris Nasus Larynx.* 1999;26(4):435–439.

19. Kondo H, Matsuda T, Hashiba M, Baba S. A study of the relationship between the T&T olfactometer and the University of Pennsylvania Smell Identification Test in a Japanese population. *Am J Rhinol.* 1998;12(5):353–358.

20. Costanzo RM, DiNardo LJ, Reiter ER. Head injury and olfaction. In: Doty RL, ed. *Handbook of Olfaction and Gustation.* 2nd ed. New York, NY: Marcel Dekker, Inc.; 2003:629–638.

21. Costanzo RM, Becker DP. Smell and taste disorders in head injury and neurosurgery patients. In: Meiselman HL, Rivlin RS, eds. *Clinical Measurements of Taste and Smell.* New York, NY: MacMillan Publishing Company; 1986:565–578.

22. Reiter ER, DiNardo LJ, Costanzo RM. Effects of head injury on olfaction and taste. *Otolaryngol Clin North Am.* 2004;37(6):1167–1184.

23. Sumner D. Post-traumatic ageusia. *Brain.* 1967;90(1):187–202.

24. Doty RL, Bromley SM, Panganiban WD. Olfactory function and dysfunction. In: Bailey BJ, Johnson JT, Newlands SD, eds. *Head & Neck Surgery—Otolarnygology.* Vol 1. 4th ed. Philadelphia, PA: Lippincott Williams & Wilkins; 2006;289–305.

25. Doty RL. The olfactory system and its disorders. *Semin Neurol.* 2009;29(1):74–81.

26. Yee KK, Costanzo RM. Changes in odor quality discrimination following recovery from olfactory nerve transection. *Chem Senses.* 1998;23(5):513–519.

27. Costanzo RM, Graziadei PP. A quantitative analysis of changes in the olfactory epithelium following bulbectomy in hamster. *J Comp Neurol.* 1983;215(4):370–381.

28. Costanzo RM. Rewiring the olfactory bulb: changes in odor maps following recovery from nerve transection. *Chem Senses.* 2000;25(2):199–205.

29. Costanzo RM. Neural regeneration and functional reconnection following olfactory nerve transection in hamster. *Brain Res.* 1985; 361(1–2):258–266.

30. Schwob JE. Neural regeneration and the peripheral olfactory system. *Anat Rec.* 2002;269(1):33–49.

31. Buck L, Axel R. A novel multigene family may encode odorant receptors: a molecular basis for odor recognition. *Cell.* 1991;65(1):175–187.

32. Johnson BA, Leon M. Chemotopic odorant coding in a mammalian olfactory system. *J Comp Neurol.* 2007;503(1):1–34.

33. Pevsner J, Hou V, Snowman AM, Snyder SH. Odorant-binding protein. Characterization of ligand binding. *J Biol Chem.* 1990; 265(11):6118–6125.

34. Smith CG. Age incidence of atrophy of olfactory nerves in man. A contribution to the study of the process of ageing. *J Comp Neurol.* 1942;77(3):589–594.

35. Doty RL, Shaman P, Applebaum SL, Giberson R, Siksorski L, Rosenberg L. Smell identification ability: changes with age. *Science.* 1984;226(4681):1441–1443.

36. Brunjes PC, Illig KR, Meyer EA. A field guide to the anterior olfactory nucleus (cortex). *Brain Res Brain Res Rev.* 2005;50(2):305–335.

37. Gottfried JA, Deichmann R, Winston JS, Dolan RJ. Functional heterogeneity in human olfactory cortex: an event-related functional magnetic resonance imaging study. *J Neurosci.* 2002;22(24):10819–10828.

38. Kveton JF, Bartoshuk LM. Taste. In: Bailey BJ, Johnson JT, Newlands SD, eds. *Head & Neck Surgery—Otolaryngology.* 4th ed. Philadelphia, PA: Lippincott Williams & Wilkins; 2006;567–578.

39. Pritchard TC, Macaluso DA, Eslinger PJ. Taste perception in patients with insular cortex lesions. *Behav Neurosci.* 1999;113(4):663–671.

40. Renzi G, Carboni A, Gasparini G, Perugini M, Becelli R. Taste and olfactory disturbances after upper and middle third facial fractures: a preliminary study. *Ann Plast Surg.* 2002;48(4):355–358.

41. Costanzo RM, DiNardo LJ, Zasler ND. Head injury and olfaction. In: Doty RL, ed. *Handbook of Olfaction and Gustation.* New York, NY: Marcel Dekker, Inc.; 1995:493–502.

42. Sumner D. Disturbance of the senses of smell and taste after head injuries. In: Vinken PJ, Bruyn GW, eds. *Handbook of Clinical Neurology.* Vol. 24. Amsterdam: North-Holland Publishing Co.; 1975:1–25.

43. Levin HS, High WM, Eisenberg HM. Impairment of olfactory recognition after closed head injury. *Brain.* 1985;108(pt 3):579–591.

44. Yousem DM, Geckle RJ, Bilker WB, McKeown DA, Doty RL. Posttraumatic olfactory dysfunction: MR and clinical evaluation. *AJNR Am J Neuroradiol.* 1996;17(6):1171–1179.

45. Costanzo RM, Zasler ND. Epidemiology and pathophysiology of olfactory and gustatory dysfunction in head trauma. *J Head Trauma Rehabil.* 1992;7(1):15–24.

46. Green P, Rohling ML, Iverson GL, Gervais RO. Relationships between olfactory discrimination and head injury severity. *Brain Inj.* 2003;17(6):479–496.

47. Wrobel BB, Leopold DA. Clinical assessment of patients with smell and taste disorders. *Otolaryngol Clin North Am.* 2004;37(6):1127–1142.

48. Costanzo RM, DiNardo LJ, Reiter ER. Head injury and taste. In: Doty RL, ed. *Handbook of Olfaction and Gustation.* 2nd ed. New York, NY: Marcel Dekker, Inc.; 2003;959–966.

49. Obrebowski A, Pruszewicz A, Barańczakowa Z, Flieger S. Early and delayed changes in the olfactory and gustatory function following maxillofacial fractures [in Polish]. *Otolaryngol Pol.* 1976; 30(4):391–398.

50. Sofferman PA. Facial nerve injury and decompression. In: Nadol JB, Schuknecht HF, eds. *Surgery of the Ear and Temporal Bone.* New York, NY: Raven Press; 1993;329–344.

51. Auerbach SH. The pathophysiology of traumatic brain injury. In: Horn LJ, Cope DN, eds. *Traumatic Brain Injury: State of the Art Reviews in Physical Medicine and Rehabilitation.* Philadelphia, PA: Hanley and Belfus; 1989.

52. Rousseaux M, Muller P, Gahide I, Mottin Y, Romon M. Disorders of smell, taste, and food intake in a patient with a dorsomedial thalamic infarct. *Stroke.* 1996;27(12):2328–2330.

53. Sunada I, Akano Y, Yamamoto S, Tashiro T. Pontine haemorrhage causing disturbance of taste. *Neuroradiology.* 1995;37(8):659.

54. Herberhold C, Westhofen M. On the central-nervous localization of the anosmia-ageusia-syndrome (author's transl) [in German]. *Laryngol Rhinol Otol (Stuttg).* 1980;59(9):570–574.

55. Doty RL, Yousem DM, Pham LT, Kreshak AA, Geckle R, Lee WW. Olfactory dysfunction in patients with head trauma. *Arch Neurol.* 1997;54(9):1131–1140.

56. Deems DA, Doty RL, Settle RG, et al. Smell and taste disorders, a study of 750 patients from the University of Pennsylvania Smell and Taste Center. *Arch Otolaryngol Head Neck Surg.* 1991;117(5):519–528.

57. Pierce J, Halpern BP. Orthonasal and retronasal odorant identification based upon vapor phase input from common substances. *Chem Senses.* 1996;21(5):529–543.

58. Schiffman SS, Zervakis J, Suggs MS, Shaio E, Sattely-Miller EA. Effect of medications on taste: example of amitriptyline HCl. *Physiol Behav.* 1999;66(2):183–191.

59. Swann IJ, Bauza-Rodriguez B, Currans R, Riley J, Shukla V. The significance of post-traumatic amnesia as a risk factor in the development of olfactory dysfunction following head injury. *Emerg Med J.* 2006;23(8):618–621.

60. Nakayama H, Ishikawa T, Yamashita S, et al. CSF leakage and anosmia in aneurysm clipping of anterior communicating artery by basal interhemispheric approach [in Japanese]. *No Shinkei Geka.* 2011;39(3):263–268.

61. Jin H, Wang S, Hou L, et al. Clinical treatment of traumatic brain injury complicated by cranial nerve injury. *Injury.* 2010;41(9):918–923.

62. Varney NR. Prognostic significance of anosmia in patients with closed-head trauma. *J Clin Exp Neuropsychol.* 1988;10(2):250–254.

63. Roberts MA, Simcox AF. Assessing olfaction following pediatric traumatic brain injury. *Appl Neuropsychol.* 1996;3(2):86–88.

64. Sigurdardottir S, Jerstad T, Andelic N, Roe C, Schanke AK. Olfactory dysfunction, gambling task performance and intracranial lesions after traumatic brain injury. *Neuropsychology.* 2010;24(4):504–513.

65. Martzke JS, Swan CS, Varney NR. Posttraumatic anosmia and orbital frontal damage: neuropsychological and neuropsychiatric correlates. *Neuropsychology.* 1991;5(3):213–225.

66. Mott AE, Leopold DA. Disorders in taste and smell. *Med Clin North Am.* 1991;75(6):1321–1353.

67. Doty RL, Shaman P, Kimmelman CP, Dann MS. University of Pennsylvania Smell Identification Test: a rapid quantitative olfactory function test for the clinic. *Laryngoscope.* 1984;94(2, pt 1):176–178.

68. Doty RL, Agrawal U. The shelf life of the University of Pennsylvania Smell Identification Test (UPSIT). *Laryngoscope.* 1989;99(4):402–404.

69. Fortin A, Lefebvre MB, Ptito M. Traumatic brain injury and olfactory deficits: the tale of two smell tests! *Brain Inj.* 2010;24(1):27–33.

70. Green P, Iverson GL. Effects of injury severity and cognitive exaggeration on olfactory deficits in head injury compensation claims. *NeuroRehabilitation.* 2001;16(4):237–243.

71. Cain WS, Gent JF, Goodspeed RB, Leonard G. Evaluation of olfactory dysfunction in the Connecticut Chemosensory Clinical Research Center. *Laryngoscope.* 1988;98(1):83–88.

72. Furukawa M, Kamide M, Miwa T, Umeda R. Significance of intravenous olfaction test using thiamine propyldisulfide (Alinamin) in olfactometry. *Auris Nasus Larynx.* 1988;15(1):25–31.

73. Bartoshuk L. Clinical evaluation of the sense of taste. *Ear Nose Throat J.* 1989;68(4):331–337.

74. Yamauchi Y, Endo S, Sakai F, Yoshimura I. [Whole mouth gustatory test (Part 1)—basic considerations and principal component analysis]. *Nippon Jibiinkoka Gakkai Kaiho.* 1995;98(1):119–129.

75. Yamauchi Y, Endo S, Sakai F, Yoshimura I. A new whole-mouth gustatory test procedure. 1. Thresholds and principal components analysis in healthy men and women. *Acta Otolaryngol Suppl.* 2002;(546):39–48.

76. Hummel T, Erras A, Kobal G. A test for the screening of taste function. *Rhinology.* 1997;35(4):146–148.

77. Ahne G, Erras A, Hummel T, Kobal G. Assessment of gustatory function by means of tasting tablets. *Laryngoscope.* 2000;110(8):1396–1401.

78. Frank ME, Smith DV. Electrogustometry: a simple way to test taste. In: Getchell TV, Doty RL, Bartoshuk LM, Snow JB, II, eds. *Smell and Taste in Health and Disease.* New York, NY: Raven Press; 1991:503–514.

79. Miller IJ Jr, Reedy FE Jr. Variations in human taste bud density and taste intensity perception. *Physiol Behav.* 1990;47(6):1213–1219.

80. Formaker BK, Mott AE, Frank ME. The effects of topical anesthesia on oral burning in burning mouth syndrome. *Ann N Y Acad Sci.* 1998;855:776–780.

81. Darrouzet V, Duclos JY, Liguoro D, Truilhe Y, De Bonfils C, Bebear JP. Management of facial paralysis resulting from temporal bone fractures: our experience in 115 cases. *Otolaryngol Head Neck Surg.* 2001;125(1):77–84.

82. Atighechi S, Salari H, Baradarantar MH, Jafari R, Karimi G, Mirjali M. A comparative study of brain perfusion single-photon emission computed tomography and magnetic resonance imaging in patients with post-traumatic anosmia. *Am J Rhinol Allergy.* 2009;23(4):409–412.

83. Varney NR, Pinkston JB, Wu JC. Quantitative PET findings in patients with posttraumatic anosmia. *J Head Trauma Rehabil.* 2001;16(3):253–259.

84. Wong KK, Muller ML, Kuwabara H, Studenski SA, Bohnen NI. Olfactory loss and nigrostriatal dopaminergic denervation in the elderly. *Neurosci Lett.* 2010;484(3):163–167.

85. Fujii M, Fukazawa K, Takayasu S, Sakagami M. Olfactory dysfunction in patients with head trauma. *Auris Nasus Larynx.* 2002;29(1):35–40.

86. Ikeda K, Sakurada T, Takasaka T, Okitsu T, Yoshida S. Anosmia following head trauma: preliminary study of steroid treatment. *Tohoku J Exp Med.* 1995;177(4):343–351.

87. Delank KW, Stoll W. Olfactory function after functional endoscopic sinus surgery for chronic sinusitis. *Rhinology.* 1998;36(1):15–19.

88. Schwob JE, Costanzo RM. Regeneration of the olfactory epithelium. In: Smith DV, Firestein S, Beauchamp GK, eds. *Olfaction and Taste.* San Diego, CA: Academic Press; 2008:591–612.

89. Monti Graziadei GA, Karlan MS, Bernstein JJ, Graziadei PP. Reinnervation of the olfactory bulb after section of the olfactory nerve in monkey (Saimiri sciureus). *Brain Res.* 1980;189(2):343–354.

90. Kobayashi M, Costanzo RM. Regeneration of the olfactory nerves following mild and severe injury and efficacy of steroid treatment [abstract]. *International Union of Physiological Sciences, 36th World Congress.* 2009.

91. Aiba T, Sugiura M, Mori J, et al. Effect of zinc sulfate on sensorineural olfactory disorder. *Acta Otolaryngol Suppl.* 1998;538:202–204.

92. Kern RC, Conley DB, Haines GK III, Robinson AM. Treatment of olfactory dysfunction, II: studies with minocycline. *Laryngoscope.* 2004;114(12):2200–2204.

93. Yagi S, Costanzo RM. Grafting the olfactory epithelium to the olfactory bulb. *Am J Rhinol Allergy.* 2009;23(3):239–243.

94. Chen X, Fang H, Schwob JE. Multipotency of purified, transplanted globose basal cells in olfactory epithelium. *J Comp Neurol.* 2004;469(4):457–474.

95. Holbrook EH, DiNardo LJ, Costanzo RM. Survival of olfactory epithelial grafts in the brain [abstract]. Holbrook EH, DiNardo LJ, Costanzo RM. *Virginia Society of Otolaryngology-Head and Neck Surgery.* 2001.

96. Monti Graziadei AG, Graziadei PP. Experimental studies on the olfactory marker protein. V. Olfactory marker protein in the olfactory neurons transplanted within the olfactory bulb. *Brain Res.* 1989;484(1–2):157–167.

97. Rotch TM. A case of traumatic anosmia and ageusia, with partial loss of hearing and sight. *Bost Med Surg J.* 1878;99:130–132.

98. Szmeja Z, Pruszewicz A, Tokarz F, Zwoździak W, Obrebowski A. Value of otoneurologic examinations in the certification of late results of craniocerebral injuries [in Polish]. *Patol Pol.* 1974;25(3):469–473.

99. Semeria C. Le alterazioni della sensibilita olfattiva e gustative consecutive a traumi cranici [Changes in olfactory and gustatory sensitivity caused by cranial nerves]. *Minerva Otorhinolaring.* 1957;7(3):111–115.

100. Henkin RI, Schechter PJ, Hoye R, Mattern CFT. Idiopathic hypogeusia with dysgeusia, hyposmia, and dysosmia. A new syndrome. *JAMA.* 1971;217(4):434–440.

101. Saito T, Manabe Y, Shibamori Y, et al. Long-term follow-up results of electrogustometry and subjective taste disorder after middle ear surgery. *Laryngoscope.* 2001;111(11, pt 1):2064–2070.

102. Zasler ND, McNeney R, Heywood PG. Rehabilitative management of olfactory and gustatory dysfunction following brain injury. *J Head Trauma Rehabil.* 1992;7(1):66–75.

103. Rondinelli RD, Genovese E, Brigham CR. *Guides to the Evaluation of Permanent Impairment.* 6th ed. Chicago, IL: American Medical Association; 2008.

104. Santos DV, Reiter ER, DiNardo LJ, Costanzo RM. Hazardous events associated with impaired olfactory function. *Arch Otolaryngol Head Neck Surg.* 2004;130(3):317–319.

105. Mattes RD, Cowart BJ. Dietary assessment of patients with chemosensory disorders. *J Am Diet Assoc.* 1994;94(1):50–56.

106. Duffy VB, Ferris AM. Nutritional management of patients with chemosensory disturbances. *Ear Nose Throat J.* 1989;68(5):395–397.

107. Temmel AF, Quint C, Schickinger-Fischer B, Klimek L, Stoller E, Hummel T. Characteristics of olfactory disorders in relation to major causes of olfactory loss. *Arch Otolaryngol Head Neck Surg.* 2002;128(6):635–641.

108. Toller SV. Assessing the impact of anosmia: review of a questionnaire's findings. *Chem Senses.* 1999;24(6):705–712.

109. Doty RL, McKeown DA, Lee WW, Shaman P. A study of the test-retest reliability of ten olfactory tests. *Chem Senses.* 1995;20(6):645–656.

110. Heywood PG, Costanzo RM. Identifying normosmics: a comparison of two populations. *Am J Otolaryngol.* 1986;7(3):194–199.

X

MOTOR AND MUSCULOSKELETAL PROBLEMS

Complications Associated With Immobility

Kathleen R. Bell and Christian N. Shenouda

INTRODUCTION

Immobilization of the human body has long been known to affect physiology in ways detrimental to normal function, even in the time of Hippocrates (1). Despite this knowledge, prolonged bed rest was used for many years in the treatment of medical disorders. However, studies emanating from the manned space program since the 1960s defining the effects of a gravity-free environment have clarified many of these effects in healthy humans. Most of the studies performed on animals, however, rely on hind limb suspension models of immobilization, and many studies on humans rely on the head-down tilt position in bed to mimic microgravity. None of these conditions precisely reproduces the conditions of prolonged bed rest in a medical situation. Nonetheless, general principles regarding the effect of inactivity on the body can be derived from these experiments. As an additional complicating factor for persons with traumatic brain injury (TBI), immobilization may be prolonged and worsened by several disorders stemming from the brain injury itself such as posturing, spasticity, dysautonomia, endocrine abnormalities, and other body system injuries. Thus, the importance of prevention and prompt management of these disorders is highlighted in addition to early mobilization of the patient with TBI. It should be noted that many of the conditions discussed in this chapter may be associated with other types of acquired brain injury as well (2).

Prolonged bed rest results in reduced function in multiple body systems simultaneously. For example, deconditioning is a diagnosis in its own right (3). Deconditioning results from reduced functional capacity of both the musculoskeletal and cardiovascular systems; changes to one system are unlikely to be significant without accompanying decrements in the other system. The effects of deconditioning can be studied in young, healthy experimental subjects, eliminating the effects of pathology. The effects of mobilization and exercise on this group emphasizes the importance of early mobilization for those with illness or injury (3).

This chapter seeks to address those general aspects of immobility that may be seen in any situation where prolonged bed rest occurs and to discuss the impact of TBI on related causal factors and treatment (Table 49-1). There are very few studies that actually examine the specific effects of immobility on persons recovering from TBI (or any other illness or injury) so associations and recommendations are made derived from literature on healthy individuals or those with other disorders.

EFFECTS OF IMMOBILITY ON THE PERSON WITH TRAUMATIC BRAIN INJURY

Musculoskeletal System

Significant changes occur in the musculoskeletal system in the first 4–6 weeks of immobilization affecting all components of the system, including up to 40% loss of muscle strength, decrements in bone density, and shortening of collagen-containing tissues. These changes are the results of a lack of the usual weight-bearing forces acting in the vertical position and the decrease in muscular contraction especially in the postural muscles (4). Although these types of changes occur in even healthy young people, the effects are magnified in populations such as the elderly with baseline alterations in muscle strength and bone density. One concern is whether persons subjected to prolonged periods of bed rest will be at higher risk of osteoporosis as they age if stores are not recovered (4). Persons with TBI are likely to be more profoundly affected as well because of associated conditions.

Bone Density Loss

Bone is constantly undergoing alteration and remodeling during normal activities. The activity of osteoclasts that reabsorb mineralized bone matrix and osteoblasts, which are responsible for the synthesis and mineralization of bone is governed by mechanical stresses and systemic stimuli. Participants in the regulation of bone density include mechanical stresses, hormones, growth factors, and cytokines. In addition to osteoclasts and osteoblasts, chondroprogenitor cells may become either chondrocytes covering the joint surface of bone or growth plate chondrocytes that are the basis for metaphyseal bone formation. These cells form bone modeling units (BMUs) whose activity is altered by physical activity or immobility, nutrition, aging, and illness (5). Specifically, skeletal muscle activity at least partially regulates bone density maintenance via growth factors (e.g., IGF-1) even during periods of disuse (6). There is increasing evidence of neural control of bone growth that is mediated by neurotransmitters and neuropeptides. In particular, the sympathetic nervous system (SNS) influences bone mass through β-adrenergic receptors in bone. SNS activity is altered by

TABLE 49-1 A Summary of the Effects of Immobility on Organ Systems With Associated TBI-Related Physiological Stressors

ORGAN SYSTEMS	POSSIBLE EFFECTS	TBI-RELATED DISORDERS
Musculoskeletal	Muscle weakness, osteopenia, muscle, and joint contracture	Spasticity and other movement related disorders, paresis, heterotopic ossification, associated trauma
Respiratory	Atelectasis, low lung volumes, hypoventilation, pooling of secretions, pneumonia	Tracheostomy, impaired cough and swallow mechanisms
Cardiovascular	Deconditioning, postural hypotension, resting tachycardia	Autonomic instability, hyperhidrosis, paresis, fluid and metabolic disorders
Hematological	Decreased red blood cell mass, thrombogenesis	Deep venous thrombosis
Dermatological	Pressure ulcers, poor wound healing	Paresis, catabolism, dysphagia
Neurological/psychological	Sensory deprivation, balance disorder	Special senses disturbances, cognitive impairment, vertigo
Metabolic/neuroendocrine	Volume contraction, hypercalcemia	Sodium disorders, hyperhidrosis, hormonal imbalance
Gastrointestinal	Constipation, decreased absorption, reflux	Dysphagia and impaired cognition requiring enteral feeding, stress ulcers
Urological	Urinary stasis, urinary tract infection	Urinary incontinence

both mobility and potentially by brain injury, resulting in neurogenic osteoporosis (7).

Chronic illness or prolonged recovery from trauma such as that seen in TBI is most likely associated with the growth hormone/IGF-1 axis, along with impaired thyroid and gonadal function (5,8). Immobilization, specifically, is associated with a moderate decrease in bone resorption but an even larger decrease in mineralization of bone matrix (9,10). A negative calcium balance occurs within a week of bed rest and 20 weeks of bed rest in healthy young men results in a 60% increase in urinary calcium. Fecal calcium loss also occurs in conjunction with reduced intestinal absorption (4). There are decrements on bone mineral density in the lumbar spine, femoral neck, tibia, and calcaneus but not the radius noted in young men on 4 months of bed rest (11). There are no significant changes in serum parathyroid hormone or in serum 1,25-dihydroxyvitamin D during bed rest in healthy men, but persons with spinal cord injury have been shown to have decreased levels of both (12). In persons with TBI, an additional factor to consider in factoring the degree of bone loss is the frequent presence of hemiplegia or other patterns of paralysis. Data from persons recovering from stroke and other neurologic disorders offer some insight although not directly applicable to the population with brain injury because of the differences in average age and degree of paralysis and immobility. Bone loss early after stroke appears to be primarily caused by increased bone resorption, whereas later bone loss is more clearly related to the degree of paresis and vitamin D levels (13). The 1,25-dihyroxyvitamin D production appears to be inhibited (14). Nearly all fractures after falls occur on the hemiparetic side in stroke patients (15). Bone mineral density was significantly lower in both femurs in stroke patients who were nonambulatory after stroke. The difference in bone loss, only on the hemiparetic side, between the nonambulatory and ambulatory patients was also significant. Most of the loss occurred within the first 7 months after stroke (16). Bone density loss is even more striking after spinal cord injury in the limbs; however, vertebral bone density is not significantly compromised because of continued weightbearing in the seated position (17).

Recovery of bone mineral density after loss is quite slow for longer periods of immobilization. Although dogs recover to baseline after 12 weeks of immobilization, for longer periods of immobility, bone did not recover even after 7 months (18). Calcaneal bone density deficits have been noted in astronauts even 5 years after space flight (4,19). There are few studies of reversing or minimizing bone loss after neurologic insults. Vitamin D and calcium supplementation have been demonstrated to be helpful in preventing fracture in elderly patients but caution should be used after stroke in the presence of hypercalcemia (20,21). Etidronate, which inhibits bone resorption and has been studied in spinal cord injury and stroke, may be effective in preventing bone resorption (22,23). Recently, many other bisphosphonates have been introduced to prevent osteoporosis, which offer benefits of weekly or monthly dosing. Although clenbuterol, a β_2-agonist, had been tested to prevent muscle and bone loss in rats with increased bone mass initially reported, later studies have shown (24) negative effects on trabecular bone architecture and increased muscle mass predisposing fractures (25).

Muscle Weakness and Atrophy

There is no doubt that muscle strength and size are affected after prolonged bed rest. As might be predicted, the weightbearing muscles of the lower limb are affected to a greater degree than the muscles of the arm (26). There are even more local differences in the degree of muscle atrophy. The knee extensors lose more mass than do the knee flexors (27). There are several possible mechanisms that result in muscle weakness and atrophy that are further discussed subsequently. Prolonged bed rest is noted to cause selective atrophy in lumbar musculature, including the multifidi, erector spinae, quadrati lumborum, and psoas muscles as well as changes in disc volumes (28).

Protein Breakdown

By the fifth day of bed rest, there is a significant increase in the urinary excretion of nitrogen, peaking in the second week of bed rest. This reflects protein degradation and an early marker of muscle atrophy (29–31). The cross-sectional area of muscles is reduced 7%–14% in 4–6 weeks of immobilization, especially in muscles responsible for resisting gravity such as the knee extensors (32,33). Lower limb muscles are affected more than upper limb muscles.

Decreased Protein Synthesis

Shortly after a limb is immobilized, decreases in total RNA and protein synthesis can be seen in muscles (34). Some alterations in pretranslational and translational mechanisms for protein production begin within 6 hours of immobilization, reflected in decreased alpha-actin and cytochrome c protein synthesis and decreased cytochrome c mRNA in rats (30,35–37).

Regrowth after inactivity-induced atrophy involves several mechanisms including (a) increased protein synthesis, (b) continued elevations of protein degradation, (c) increased proliferation of muscle precursor cells, (d) and increases in myonuclear number (myonuclei per 100 myofibers) (30). Unfortunately, muscle regrowth after atrophy is not always complete, especially in the elderly (38,39).

Disruption of Antioxidants in Skeletal Muscle

In pathological conditions such as post-trauma catabolism, other mechanisms may be at play in the volume of muscle loss during bed rest and immobilization. Typically, antioxidant protein and scavenger protection protect skeletal muscle against oxidative stress. However, during hind limb unloading in rats, there has been demonstrated large shifts in superoxide dismutase activity with impaired antioxidant activity (decreased catalase, glutathione peroxidase, and nonenzymatic antioxidant scavenging capacity) (40–42). This disruption of protection can result in muscle fiber damage and loss that, when combined with a state of protein loss after severe trauma, is accelerated.

There is disagreement between animal and human experiments on which muscle fibers appear to be most affected by this loss of volume induced by immobilization. Generally, in animals, slow-twitch fibers are predominantly affected. In humans, however, fast-twitch fibers appear to be most affected. It is possible that this may be somewhat misleading because the relative sizes of slow- and fast-twitch muscle are different in rats and humans (4).

There is some evidence that some of the muscle atrophy and loss of oxidative capacity can be prevented by isometric exercise during the period of immobilization (43,44). Isometric exercises appear to be more effective in slow tonic muscles like the soleus as compared to the fast-twitch muscles such as the gastrocnemius (43). In addition to its effects on bone density, clenbuterol also appears to reduce muscle degeneration in dystrophic or denervated muscle (25). There is some evidence that oral creatine supplementation enhances the muscle hypertrophy response to exercise after a period of immobilization (45).

Not unexpectedly, these findings suggesting protein breakdown and a loss of muscle mass would lead one to predict an accompanying decrease in muscle strength. Microgravity studies have demonstrated that 30 days of bed rest will result in an 18%–20% decrease in knee extensor strength (46,47).

Endurance is also decreased after prolonged immobility. Decrements up to 17% are noted in torque production in limbs unloaded for 4 weeks; this does not recover to baseline even after 7 weeks of recovery (48). These findings may be caused by changes in muscle oxidative enzymes as well as decreased oxygen delivery to muscle after disuse (4). In vivo studies have revealed that mitochondrial uncoupling may be a mechanism for muscle weakness and poor endurance with those who are sedentary, especially increasing with age (49).

Part of the loss of muscle strength observed after prolonged bed rest is the result of decreased efficiency in motor neuron recruitment. Although electromyographic activity is reduced by half in muscles that are shortened, there does not appear to be a relationship between the electrical activation of muscle and the relative decrease in muscle mass (50). However, there is evidence for reduced motor neuron activation after immobilization and a subsequent need for increased neuronal activation to produce the same degree of muscle force output (51–53). These neuromuscular inefficiencies can be totally reversed with training after the cessation of bed rest (52). This data also supports early movement and weightbearing, as much of the muscle loss seen in the first 2 weeks of bed rest can be easily restored.

Joint Contractures

Changes in connective tissue and muscle during immobilization of a limb can ultimately result in contracture formation. Common to all forms of contracture is the loss of passive range of motion in the affected joint. Studies have demonstrated reductions in both the length and diameter of muscle fibers and in muscle extensibility (54–56). Additionally, there is an increase in intramuscular connective tissue and reduced capillary density in muscle (57,58). In addition to these muscle changes, there is a significant increase in endomysial and perimysial connective tissue. More fibers are deposited perpendicularly to the adjacent muscle fibers. The network of collagen fibers become indistinguishable from each other (59).

Patients with TBI have an assortment of risk factors associated with their injuries that may contribute to the formation of joint contractures. Spasticity and rigidity may be extremely difficult to control in the acute stages of TBI. In examining the patient with TBI for contractures, it is important to assess the contribution of dynamic (spasticity dependent) aspects of joint movement limitation. It may be useful to perform a peripheral nerve block for this purpose (please see Chapter 50 for further information). With severe TBI, postural control, especially of the axial skeleton, may lead to contractures of the neck and spine that are challenging to address. Weakness and prolonged maintenance of any posture will also contribute to joint contracture. Other general risk factors include age, edema, and diabetes mellitus. Reported incidence of ankle plantar flexion contractures in persons with acute moderate-to-severe TBI has ranged from 16% to 76%, depending on the definition of contracture (60,61).

Prevention of joint contracture depends on the maintenance of proper joint position with the use of splints, adequate treatment of spasticity, and active and passive range of motion exercises to the joint several times daily. Standing is the optimal method of maintaining ankle range of motion, and prone lying is very helpful to prevent hip flexion contractures. Serial casting is one option to treat mild-to-moderate equinovarus deformities of the ankle and contractures of the upper limb (62,63). Short changing intervals of 1–4 days were more effective than intervals of 5–7 days in restoring range of motion (63). (see Chapter 51 on Neuro-orthopedics for further information).

Heterotopic Ossification
Ectopic bone formation is a common feature of nervous system injury as well as fractures and burns. The pathophysiology remains unclear; local changes in capillary permeability and hormonal influences on mesenchymal stem cells have been noted to induce osteoblast formation (64). The incidence in the population with TBI has been estimated between 11% and 76% (65,66). Common locations include hips, knees, shoulder, and elbows, all of which can present with restricted range of motion, pain, and swelling. If suspected, elevated alkaline phosphatase may help with diagnosis, but triple-phase bone scan is the most definitive. Nonsteroidal anti-inflammatory agents and bisphosphonates are used to prevent progression, and surgical intervention is usually reserved for 12–18 months (67). New data suggest that earlier surgical intervention within 1 year resulted in improved functional outcomes with no increase in recurrence rates (68,69). Potential complications of ectopic bone formation include pain, nerve entrapment, limited range of motion, and increased spasticity. Safaz and colleagues examined patients with TBI over a 5-year period and noted significantly lowered ambulation levels in those with heterotopic ossification (70). (Please see Chapter 51 on Neuro-orthopedics for further information).

Respiratory System

Many patients with severe TBI have tracheostomies for assisted ventilation and respiratory toilet in the acute stages. In addition, impaired alertness will result in a decreased drive for deep inspiration. Therefore, patients with TBI are already at risk for pulmonary complications during their rehabilitation. Prolonged bed rest adds to that risk. Simulated weightlessness with a head-down tilt in healthy individuals demonstrates that the functional residual capacity of the lungs falls by 33% during this period with insignificant changes in lung tissue volume. Diffusing capacity decreases gradually to 4%–5% lower than baseline values. Pulmonary blood flow also decreases by 16% (71). All of these changes result in higher risk for atelectasis and pulmonary infection. Treatment consists of early mobilization of the patient and aggressive pulmonary toilet with suction and the use of equipment such as the in-exsufflator to assist in the management of secretions.

Pneumonia is a common nosocomial infection in the population with brain injury. In stroke literature, pneumonia is responsible for a threefold increase in death (72). Impaired cough/swallow mechanism, low lung volumes, and ventilator usage place those with acute TBI at particular risk of pneumonia. It is estimated that the population with TBI is four times more likely to die of respiratory complications as compared to the general public (73). At 1-year after injury, patients with TBI are 49 times more likely to die from aspiration pneumonia compared to matched individuals from the general population (74), underscoring the importance of swallow evaluation in the acute setting.

Cardiovascular System

Research on cardiovascular effects of immobility is drawn both from microgravity experiments during space flight and from experiments using a head-down tilt position to mimic weightlessness. Obviously, these studies seek to maximize the effects of bed rest. Normal positioning of patients in bed after TBI will mitigate the severity of cardiovascular effects.

Reduction of Cardiopulmonary Functional Capacity and Postural Hypotension
Functional efficiency of the heart depends on both intravascular volume (hydrostatic forces) and coordinated filling and emptying of the ventricles (hydrodynamic forces). Normally, arterial pressures and certain levels of intravascular volume interact to maintain adequate body and cerebral perfusion in the face of gravity. However, when the body is placed horizontally for a prolonged period, about a liter of fluid is relocated from the legs to the chest area. Initially, this increases diastolic filling and increases the stroke volume of each cardiac contraction (i.e., the Frank-Starling mechanism). However, baroreceptor responses eventually result in a diuresis and loss of plasma volume within 24–48 hours (75). When a normal upright position is resumed, there is a sudden decrease in both ventricular filling and stroke volume that results in orthostatic symptoms (76). Cardiovascular baroreflex responses become attenuated without the challenges of baroreceptor unloading that comes from upright standing (77). Other factors may include disordered sympathetic activation in combination with hypovolemia and diminished baroreceptor reflexes (78). Particularly interesting in the context of TBI is the involvement of brain autonomic nuclei such as the paraventricular nucleus of the hypothalamus that includes basal and reflex control of the SNS vasopressin and oxytocin release and secretion of corticotrophin-releasing factor (79).

Other changes in cardiac function have been noted. After immobilization, the maximal oxygen uptake ($\dot{V}o_{2max}$) is reduced and the heart rate is increased in response to submaximal exercise (80). This equates to a loss in aerobic capacity of 0.9% per day over 30 days of bed rest (3). The heart rate during prolonged bed rest is higher for the same oxygen requirement (81) (see Figure 49-1). Part of this is related to the fluid changes noted previously; these effects are much less during supine submaximal exercise (80). The heart rate is probably increased because of increased beta-adrenergic receptor sensitivity (81).

Simple replacement of volume does not abolish the orthostatic response (82). It appears that there are some alterations to the ventricles themselves during a period of prolonged bed rest leaving them less distensible (83). This appears to be an effect on cardiac muscle similar to the loss of muscle volume seen in skeletal muscle during prolonged immobilization (76). Actual muscle contractile properties seem to be preserved (84). The effects on stroke volume and cardiac output after prolonged bed rest will persist for at least a month (84). These effects are partially masked by

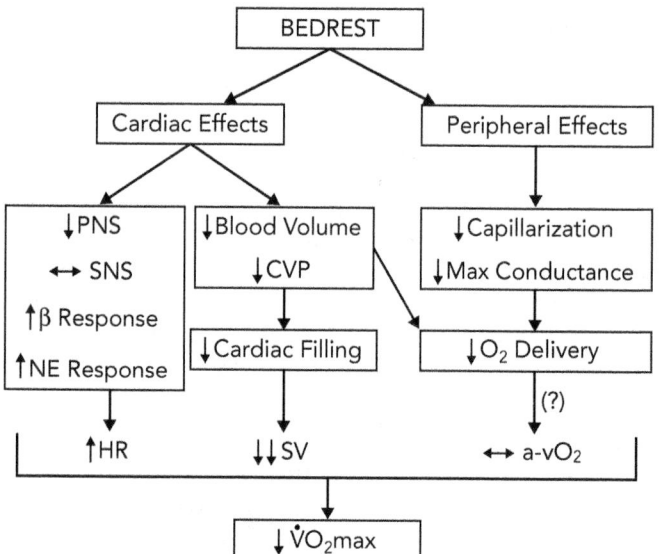

FIGURE 49-1 Model of cardiovascular mechanisms controlling maximal oxygen uptake during bed rest. Reprinted from Convertino (81) with permission.

an increase in peripheral volume and retention of sodium and, at least initially, an increase in sympathetic nerve activity (85).

Hematological System

Deconditioning causes a reduction in red blood cell mass by 5%–25% that may compromise blood oxygen-carrying capacity. However, the hematocrit generally remains stable during bed rest. Therefore, the effect of reduced blood cell mass is still unclear (81). As noted elsewhere in this chapter, there is a significant decrease in resting blood flow to the leg muscles and a reduction in capillarization. This is correlated with fatigability in calf muscles (81,86,87). Reversing these effects requires not only the upright position and adequate fluid volume but also the exercise that induces arterial baroreceptor loading (77). In animals, daily standing for only 1 hour per day prevented depression of myocardial contractility (88).

Thrombogenesis

Thromboembolic disease is a well-described risk in the setting of immobilization. In the patient with brain injury, this risk remains present with significant complicating factors for diagnosis and treatment. Often after significant trauma, each of the factors of Virchow triad (stasis, endothelial damage, and hypercoagulable state) is present on admission to the emergency department. In the patient with TBI, one sequelae of the injury may be hemiparesis, which contributes to stasis in a more discrete and prolonged manner. Patients with TBI may also present with bleeding in the subdural or subarachnoid space, limiting the choice of treatment modalities. The patient with TBI may also be impulsive and have considerable fall risk, which may limit pharmacologic prophylaxis and treatment options. Identification and treatment of venous

thromboembolism is therefore of increased complexity but of great necessity in the population with TBI (89).

Initial traumatic injury inherently carries with it risk for hypercoagulability when multiple organ systems are involved and bleeding present at one or more sites. When bleeding occurs, the body initiates the coagulation cascade, a response that may be prolonged when blood remains present acting as a nidus for continued production of coagulation factors. With TBI, bleeding may occur at any site in the body because of concomitant trauma but is of particular concern intracranially. The patient may require prolonged monitoring to ensure resorption or neurosurgical intervention to reduce mass effect because of bleeding, contributing to further stasis. A functional limitation of TBI may be hemiparesis or bilateral weakness, which may persist following the acute period of immobility after trauma. Thrombi are noted to occur most frequently in the paralyzed limb of hemiparetic patients and more likely to occur in the proximal segment of the limb, placing them at higher risk for propagation (90). In a similar setting, deep vein thrombosis (DVT) risk has been found to be comparable following brain tumor surgery as in the orthopedic hip replacement population (91). The patient with TBI is also likely to have suffered endothelial damage with the initial inciting injury.

Identification of thromboembolism may be suspected clinically by the presence of a warm, edematous, and painful limb. Unfortunately, the affected limb often exhibits no signs at all of thrombophlebitis; therefore, physical exam is unreliable for venous thrombosis diagnosis (92). The venous duplex exam is the mainstay of diagnosis. Testing carries high accuracy, is noninvasive, and often readily available at the bedside (93). If pulmonary embolism (PE) is suspected by clinical findings of decreased oxygen saturation, tachypnea, and pleuritic chest pain, studies to assist in diagnosis for PE should be employed as well as the previously mentioned venous duplex to identify potential source of the embolus. The D-dimer assay, spiral computed tomography (CT), and ventilation-perfusion studies are all well-accepted means to assist in diagnosis of PE. In the patient with TBI, there are noted limitations to the use of these means of diagnosis. Following trauma, it is anticipated that D-dimer levels will be unspecifically high and therefore are noncontributory to assisting in diagnosis. Using D-dimer levels has not been shown to be useful in predicting DVT after acute TBI (94). However, a low D-dimer may assist to rule out a PE if this be the goal. A ventilation-perfusion scan may be limited by any other concomitant pulmonary conditions such as pneumonia, secretions, or atelectasis. The spiral CT is the most readily available tool for reliable diagnosis, albeit at a higher initial cost.

Treatment for identified thromboembolism is primarily pharmacologic by using unfractionated or regular heparin. Heparin acts initially by enhancing antithrombin III activity. In high doses, heparin also acts to inhibit prothrombin and platelet aggregation. This constitutes its efficacy in meeting the key treatment goals for PE and thromboembolism by inducing a hypocoagulable state and decreased potential for clot propagation (92). However, the patient with TBI may have comorbidities limiting the use of anticoagulation in his pharmacologic regimen. Anticoagulation with heparin prophylaxis has been noted to be safe in patients with intracranial bleeds who had stable or improved head imaging at

24 hours (95). Early anticoagulation resulted in a statically significant lower rate of thromboembolism. A 2010 observational study examined screening, prophylaxis, and treatment in patients with TBI in the rehabilitation setting (96). No definitive proof of prevention of venous thromboembolism was observed in those treated with propyhylactic medications. For those individuals who are not candidates for anticoagulation, the use of retrievable inferior vena cava filters provide an alternative to disrupt the clot pathway to decrease risk of PE. These filters are generally used in patients in whom recurrent PE has occurred despite treatment with anticoagulants or those in whom anticoagulant therapy is contraindicated (97). A review of case series has indicated that these filters are successfully removed in 91% of cases; 9% of filters could not be removed because of large trapped thrombus (98). It is important to note that these filters are associated with a twofold increase in the incidence of recurrent DVT. If it is safe to anticoagulate a patient, they should remain on therapeutic anticoagulation even with a filter in place for the recommended length of time (99).

Integumentary System

Pressure ulcers are a well-known complication of bed rest, particularly when complicated by paresis of any kind. Pressure ulcers are associated with increased mortality, morbidity, length of stay, and cost of treatment (100,101). Although pressure ulcer in patients with TBI have not been specifically examined, immobility and decreased body weight are both independent risk factors for the development of pressure sores (102). After acute TBI, inadequate tissue perfusion because of unrelieved pressure at bony prominences is chiefly responsible for the development of pressure ulcers (103,104). Pressure wounds heal best when kept moist with occlusive dressings. Other methods used to improve healing have included serial casting in patients with spasticity; the casts are thought to reduce friction associated with repetitive movements. Prevention of pressure ulcers should be a priority with turning at least every 2 hours. Pressure-mapping studies show continued pressure at the skin-surface interface even with turning by experienced nursing staff (105). Risk reduction strategies at the organizational level with interventions such as specialty mattresses are of particular interest in facilities with high-risk patients. (Please see Chapter 27 on Neurorehabilitation Nursing.)

Neurological System

Effects of Bed Rest on Cognitive and Psychiatric Function

Confinement to bed has been associated with several undesirable psychological and cognitive effects. Much of the data has come from studies on healthy young men as part of the space program research projects. These studies have used a 6° angle head-down tilt that more closely reproduces microgravity conditions than normal bed rest. Nonetheless, these studies have some application to medically driven bed rest. These studies have noted enhanced levels of depression and emotional distress. In addition, impairments in overall cognitive capabilities have been noted as well with self-reported confusion and depressed scores on cognitive testing (106,107).

An additional area that may be affected by prolonged immobilization in bed is sleep. Chronic insomnia can be perpetuated by increased time spent in bed (108). Studies on elderly hospitalized patients on bed rest in poorly lit rooms show that patients report poor sleep quality and that phase shifts for sleep are noted (109). Individuals with TBI are noted to have both problems with nighttime sleep pathology and daytime somnolence. Patients with brain injuries as well as those critically ill patients are noted to have poor sleep with altered sleep architecture, increased sleep latency, and poor sleep quality (110). (Please see Chapter 43 on Sleep Disturbance for further information.)

Balance Dysfunction and Incoordination

Neuromuscular changes associated with inefficient recruitment of motor neurons may be partly responsible for the findings of increased postural sway, gait changes, and impaired kinesthetic sense after prolonged space travel (4,111,112). These changes in response to immobilization and bed rest may occur at multiple levels of the nervous system (113). For instance, it has been demonstrated that training can enlarge the size of the cortical area involved in the task. Conversely, it appears that there are reduced cortical responses after immobilization of a joint that are proportional to the length of time of immobilization. The amplitude of motor-evoked potentials decreases after joint splinting during motor imagery tasks but not motor activation tasks (114). Other changes have been noted in the motor strategies used to perform a static muscle contraction after immobilization; some people were noted to produce a bursting pattern with reduced electromyogram (EMG) amplitude in contrast to the preimmobilization pattern of progressive increase in the amplitude of EMG activity (115,116). The organization of neurons to provide maximal voluntary contraction appears to be diminished after 6 weeks of immobilization of a limb; peak force produced voluntarily during a maximum contraction was lower than that produced by electrical stimulation (117). Although the specific effects of immobilization on sensory inputs on control of movement have not been studied, there is evidence that sensory feedback such as vibration can evoke a cross-training effect and increase the power production capability of muscles (52,118). Peripheral nerve fibers can also be affected. In animal models, the axon diameter of large myelinated nerve fibers has been shown to decrease proportionally to the length of immobilization (119). (Please see Chapter 47 on Balance and Dizziness for more information.)

Endocrine and Metabolic System

There is scant literature that directly addresses the influence of bed rest on the endocrine system or metabolism after TBI. A few points, however, may be interesting to review with an emphasis on how these factors may be affected by conditions after TBI such as hyperhidrosis resulting in volume loss and intrinsic damage to the pituitary–adrenal axis. Growth hormone resistance has been observed in chronic illness and/or malnutrition resulting from resistance at the hepatic growth hormone receptor leading to impaired hepatic IGF-1 generation and decreased growth hormone bioactivity. Growth hormone and thyroid hormone have synergistic actions and potentiate the effects of each other on normal skeletal growth while acting on osteoblasts to stimulate bone remodeling. Involvement of growth hormone/IGF-1 and thyroid hormones can result in decreased skeletal growth, low bone mass, and low serum concentration of osteocalcin (4). Prolonged immobilization can be seen as a physiological stress and, as such, has been associated with elevated corticosterone levels and decreased plasma adrenocorticotropic hormone (ACTH) levels (120). There is also noted glucose intolerance because of resistance to endogenous insulin, which is ameliorated after mobilization (121). (Please see Chapter 53 on Neuroendocrine Dysfunction for more information.)

Hypercalcemia has been noted to be a particular problem in young adolescents who are immobilized for prolonged periods, particularly after spinal cord injury. However, there has been noted suppression of the parathyroid—1,25—dihydroxyvitamin D axis resulting in calcium loss as well as increased serum phosphorus and an elevated phosphorus renal threshold (122). Additionally, losses of magnesium in both feces and urine during immobilization in rats has been observed, resulting in a negative magnesium balance despite replacement (123). Nitrogen loss has been studied for many years; urinary nitrogen excretion peaks in the second week of bed rest at 20%–43% higher than baseline values (29).

Volume-regulating systems are affected by head-down bed rest (HDBR) and likely, by extension but to a lesser degree, to bed rest. Sodium and chloride are excreted as volume is lost—reflected by weight loss. Potassium excretion is delayed but then is elevated for the duration of HDBR experiments. An elevation in plasma renin activity accompanies these changes as well as a decrease in autonomic responses, with a shift toward sympathetic control (124). A high-sodium diet does not seem to stabilize this loss of plasma volume (125).

Gastrointestinal System

Constipation and Abnormal Absorption

Intestinal absorption, in general, is decreased during the period of bed rest (4). This can be particularly acute for patients with TBI who already have severe nutritional challenges, leading to heightened malabsorption (126). More specifically, calcium absorption decreases from 31% to 24% of dietary intake over 17 weeks of bed rest (127). However, bone resorption accounts for a large proportion of the hypercalcuria seen after prolonged bed rest. Constipation may result from altered central input into the enteric nervous system (128). Medications that slow gastrointestinal motility are frequently used in the acute hospital setting; untreated constipation can progress to obstruction. A bowel regime consisting of fiber supplementation and rectal suppositories is recommended. (Please see Chapter 54 on Gastrointestinal and Nutritional Issues for more information.)

Gastroesophageal Reflux

After severe TBI, there are many issues that interfere with normal ingestion and digestion of food. Both neurologically and cognitively based dysphagia predispose the patient to aspiration and almost always result in the use of parenteral feeding via a gastric or jejunal feeding tube. One study of all patients admitted to a hospital via the emergency department found that those on bed rest or who received nonsteroidal anti-inflammatory drugs had increased risk of refluxlike symptoms (129). Patients with prolonged nasogastric tube feeding have demonstrated increased rates of esophageal damage (129).

Stress Ulcers

The population with brain injury are particularly prone to gastric ulcerations. This was first noted by Harvey Cushing and detailed in 1932 (130). These gastric ulcerations occur in the setting of increased intracranial pressure and, if suspected, need close monitoring for perforation. Proton pump inhibitors are now a mainstay of treatment in the acute setting and help reduce the risk of gastritis and ulcer formation associated with glucocorticoids.

Urologic System

Urinary Incontinence

Urinary incontinence may occur in those with TBI for several reasons: cognitive impairment, damage to micturition centers, peripheral nerve damage, or even bladder trauma. Recent studies have shown 62% of patients with TBI have urinary incontinence in the acute setting (131). It is also noted that urinary incontinence is associated with poorer functional outcomes in the population with TBI and likely present more challenges to community living.

Urinary Stasis and Infection

The recumbent position is associated with a reduced urinary flow rate and, although the difference in postvoid residuals did not reach the level of significance, there was a trend toward higher volumes in recumbent voiding (132). In conjunction with urinary stasis, alterations of urine composition because of dehydration predispose the immobilized patient to calcium-containing renal stones (133). Urinary tract infections are common in the acute setting and occur more frequently with indwelling catheters. After the indwelling catheter is removed, postvoiding residual measurements are recommended to ensure that the patient is adequately emptying the bladder.

PREVENTION OF COMPLICATIONS

In general, it can be said that any mobilization is beneficial in ameliorating the effects of prolonged bed rest. From the limited work done on the effects of exercise during prolonged bed rest, it is apparent that both isotonic and isokinetic exercises help to maintain cardiac functional capacity (peak $\dot{V}O_2$) and help to preserve the red cell volume and positive body water balance. However, these 2 types of exercise had varying effects on quality of sleep and mental concentration (isotonic exercise surprisingly seemed to impair both) and had no effect on orthostatic tolerance when the experimental subjects were remobilized (134).

Remobilization after prolonged bed rest of the elderly patient with TBI should be done cautiously because the effects on bone density will be magnified in this population. Exercise directed at the weight-bearing trunk and lower limbs should be approached in a graduated basis. Although there are studies showing some efficacy of electrical stimulation to prevent immobility-associated atrophy in specific limb regions, this modality has limited use in persons who are at risk for generalized atrophy (135,136).

Adequate hydration and nutrition are extremely important in maintaining bone, skin, and muscle integrity during rehabilitation after TBI, especially during bed rest. Hydration is often difficult to maintain in patients with spasticity and dysautonomia. Range of motion and good positioning of the limbs, trunk, and head are essential in preventing contractures and preserving the ability of the patient to use neurological recovery effectively at a later date.

CONCLUSION

The field of TBI rehabilitation has limited data on those with chronic care needs and how best to intercede and maximize function. Specifically, there are few well-powered controlled studies to provide a strong rationale for specific rehabilitation measures in patients with TBI with prolonged immobilization. This being said, individuals are noted to have functional improvements years after their original injury when effectively mobilized. In this chapter, research from various fields including orthopedics, neurosurgery, endocrinology, and other areas has been presented, but there are many areas with little specific information about the interaction of TBI with outcome. For instance, there are no guidelines regarding the timing of intervention for surgical treatment of heterotopic ossification and outcome and the use of anticoagulation in the setting of intracerebral hemorrhage. How does early mobilization and exercise affect long-term cognitive outcome and what type of mobilization is most efficient and productive? Do certain types of mobilization impact the quality and extent of motor return after TBI? Can exercise be an effective treatment for depression and anxiety after TBI? Although the heterogeneity of TBI can be a challenge to the researcher, there are very practical questions of clinical management to be answered as well as mapping the influence of specific areas of brain injury on the comorbidities associated with immobilization.

KEY CLINICAL POINTS

1. In caring for an individual with a brain injury, the clinician must monitor for complications of immobility, which could negatively affect function later in recovery.
2. Changes in the musculoskeletal system can be profound with changes seen in bone and muscle. Bone pathology includes decreased density as well as heterotopic ossification. Muscles show weakness and atrophy because of a variety of factors, including decreased protein synthesis and increased protein breakdown. Joint contractures and reduced endurance are also commonly seen and frequently exacerbated by spasticity and paresis.
3. Impaired cough and swallow mechanisms, low lung volumes, and ventilator use predispose these patients to pneumonia and prolonged ventilator use.
4. Immobilized individuals are particularly susceptible to venous thromboembolism. Prophylactic anticoagulation using unfractionated heparin is recommended to start

after 24 hours in those with stable or improved head CT findings.
5. Persons with TBI have numerous risk factors for pressure ulcers when on bed rest. Prevention should include good nutrition, frequent turning, and staff education.
6. Immobility predisposes to constipation and a bowel regime should be instituted to provide daily bowel movements. Similarly, urinary stasis contributes to renal stones and urinary tract infections.
7. Cardiovascular function is affected by prolonged bed rest and can result in tachycardia, hypotension, and deconditioning with reduced cardiac output.

KEY REFERENCES

1. Belavý DL, Armbrecht G, Richardson CA, Felsenberg D, Hides JA. Muscle atrophy and changes in spinal morphology: is the lumbar spine vulnerable after prolonged bedrest? *Spine.* 2011;36(2):137–145.
2. Bloomfield SA. Changes in musculoskeletal structure and function with prolonged bed rest. *Med Sci Sports Exerc.* 1997;29(2):197–206.
3. Carlile M, Nicewander D, Yablon SA, et al. Prophylaxis for venous thromboembolism during rehabilitation for traumatic brain injury: a multicenter observational study. *J Trauma.* 2010;68(4):916–923.
4. Harrison-Felix C, Whiteneck G, Jha A, DeVivo MJ, Hammond FM, Hart DM. Mortality over four decades after traumatic brain injury rehabilitation: a retrospective cohort study. *Arch Phys Med Rehabil.* 2009;90(9):1506–1513.
5. Safaz I, Alaca R, Yasar E, Tok F, Yilmaz B. Medical complications, physical function and communication skills in patients with traumatic brain injury: a single centre 5-year experience. *Brain Inj.* 2008;22(10):733–739.

References

1. Chadwick J, Mann WN, eds. *The Medical Works of Hippocrates.* Oxford, United Kingdom: Blackwell; 1950.
2. Kumar S, Selim MH, Caplan LR. Medical complications after stroke. *Lancet Neurol.* 2010;9(1):105–118.
3. Convertino VA, Bloomfield SA, Greenleaf JE. An overview of the issues: physiological effects of bed rest and restricted physical activity. *Med Sci Sports Exerc.* 1997;29(2):187–90.
4. Bloomfield SA. Changes in musculoskeletal structure and function with prolonged bed rest. *Med Sci Sports Exerc.* 1997;29(2):197–206.
5. Daci E, van Cromphaut S, Bouillon R. Mechanisms influencing bone metabolism in chronic illness. *Horm Res.* 2002;58(suppl 1): 44–51.
6. Alzghoul MB, Gerrard D, Watkins BA, Hannon K. Ectopic expression of IGF-I and Shh by skeletal muscle inhibits disuse-mediated skeletal muscle atrophy and bone osteopenia in vivo. *Faseb J.* 2004; 18(1):221–3.
7. Qin W, Bauman WA, Cardozo CP. Evolving concepts in neurogenic osteoporosis. *Curr Osteoporos Rep.* 2010;8(4):212–218.
8. Zdanowicz MM, Teichberg S. Effects of insulin-like growth factor-1/binding protein-3 complex on muscle atrophy in rats. *Exp Biol Med (Maywood).* 2003;228(8):891–897.
9. Schneider VS, Hulley SB, Donaldson CL, et al. Prevention of bone mineral changes induced by bed rest: modification by static compression, simulated weight bearing, combined supplementation of oral calcium and phosphate, calcitonin injections, oscillating compression, the oral diphosphonate disodium etidronate, and lower body negative pressure (Final Report). San Francisco, CA:

Public Health Hospital NASA CR-141453; 1974. Report No. NTIS No. N75-13331/1st.

10. Vico L, Chappard D, Alexandre C, et al. Effects of a 120 day period of bed-rest on bone mass and bone cell activities in man: attempts at countermeasure. *Bone Miner.* 1987;2(5):383–394.

11. LeBlanc A, Schneider VS, Evans HJ, Engelbretson DA, Krebs JM. Bone mineral loss and recovery after 17 weeks of bed rest. *J Bone Miner Res.* 1990;5(8):843–850.

12. Bloomfield SA, Girten BE, Weisbrode SE. Effects of vigorous exercise training and beta-agonist administration on bone response to hindlimb suspension. *J Appl Physiol.* 1997;83(1):172–178.

13. Sato Y, Kuno H, Kaji M, Ohshima Y, Asoh T, Oizumi K. Increased bone resorption during the first year after stroke. *Stroke.* 1998;29(7):1373–1377.

14. Sato Y, Oizumi K, Kuno H, Kaji M. Effect of immobilization upon renal synthesis of 1,25-dihydroxyvitamin D in disabled elderly stroke patients. *Bone.* 1999;24(3):271–275.

15. Chiu KY, Pun WK, Luk KD, Chow SP. A prospective study on hip fractures in patients with previous cerebrovascular accidents. *Injury.* 1992;23(5):297–299.

16. Jørgensen L, Jacobsen BK, Wilsgaard T, Magnus JH. Walking after stroke: does it matter? Changes in bone mineral density within the first 12 months after stroke. A longitudinal study. *Osteoporos Int.* 2000;11(5):381–387.

17. Biering-Sørensen F, Bohr HH, Schaadt OP. Longitudinal study of bone mineral content in the lumbar spine, the forearm and the lower extremities after spinal cord injury. *Eur J Clin Invest.* 1990; 20(3):330–335.

18. Jaworski ZF, Uhthoff HK. Reversibility of nontraumatic disuse osteoporosis during its active phase. *Bone.* 1986;7(6):431–439.

19. Tilton FE, Degioanni JJ, Schneider VS. Long-term follow-up of Skylab bone demineralization. *Aviat Space Environ Med.* 1980;51(11):1209–1213.

20. Dawson-Hughes B, Harris SS, Krall EA, Dallal GE. Effect of calcium and vitamin D supplementation on bone density in men and women 65 years of age or older. *N Engl J Med.* 1997;337(10):670–676.

21. Tilyard MW, Spears GF, Thomson J, Dovey S. Treatment of postmenopausal osteoporosis with calcitriol or calcium. *N Engl J Med.* 1992;326(6):357–362.

22. Storm T, Steiniche T, Thamsborg G, Melsen F. Changes in bone histomorphometry after long-term treatment with intermittent, cyclic etidronate for postmenopausal osteoporosis. *J Bone Miner Res.* 1993;8(2):199–208.

23. Grigoriev AI, Morukov BV, Oganov VS, Rakhmanov AS, Buravkova LB. Effect of exercise and bisphosphonate on mineral balance and bone density during 360 day antiorthostatic hypokinesia. *J Bone Miner Res.* 1992;7(suppl. 2):S449–S455.

24. Zeman RJ, Hirschman A, Hirschman ML, Guo G, Etlinger JD. Clenbuterol, a beta 2-receptor agonist, reduces net bone loss in denervated hindlimbs. *Am J Physiol.* 1991;261(2, pt 1):E285–E289.

25. Bonnet N, Brunet-Imbault B, Arlettaz A, et al. Alteration of trabecular bone under chronic beta2 agonists treatment. *Med Sci Sports Exerc.* 2005;37(9):1493–1501.

26. LeBlanc AD, Schneider VS, Evans HJ, Pientok C, Rowe R, Spector E. Regional changes in muscle mass following 17 weeks of bed rest. *J Appl Physiol.* 1992;73(5):2172–2178.

27. Miles MP, Clarkson PM, Bean M, Ambach K, Mulroy J, Vincent K. Muscle function at the wrist following 9 d of immobilization and suspension. *Med Sci Sports Exerc.* 1994;26(5):615–623.

28. Belavý DL, Armbrecht G, Richardson CA, Felsenberg D, Hides JA. Muscle atrophy and changes in spinal morphology: is the lumbar spine vulnerable after prolonged bed-rest? *Spine.* 2011;36(2):137–145.

29. Deitrick JE, Whedon GD, Shorr E. Effects of immobilization upon various metabolic and physiologic functions of normal men. *Am J Med.* 1948;4:3–36.

30. Goldspink DF, Morton AJ, Loughna P, Goldspink G. The effect of hypokinesia and hypodynamia on protein turnover and the growth of four skeletal muscles of the rat. *Pflugers Arch.* 1986;407(3):333–340.

31. Thomason DB, Booth FW. Influence of performance on gene expression in skeletal muscle: effects of forced inactivity. *Adv Myochem.* 1989;2:79–82.

32. Berg HE, Dudley GA, Häggmark T, Ohlsén H, Tesch PA. Effects of lower limb unloading on skeletal muscle mass and function in humans. *J Appl Physiol.* 1991;70(4):1882–1885.

33. Hather BM, Adams GR, Tesch PA, Dudley GA. Skeletal muscle responses to lower limb suspension in humans. *J Appl Physiol.* 1992; 72(4):1493–1498.

34. Machida S, Booth FW. Regrowth of skeletal muscle atrophied from inactivity. *Med Sci Sports Exerc.* 2004;36(1):52–59.

35. Morrison PR, Muller GW, Booth FW. Actin synthesis rate and mRNA level increase during early recovery of atrophied muscle. *Am J Physiol.* 1987;253(2, pt 1):C205–C209.

36. Morrison PR, Montgomery JA, Wong TS, Booth FW. Cytochrome c protein-synthesis rates and mRNA contents during atrophy and recovery in skeletal muscle. *Biochem J.* 1987;241(1):257–263.

37. Watson PA, Stein JP, Booth FW. Changes in actin synthesis and alpha-actin-mRNA content in rat muscle during immobilization. *Am J Physiol.* 1984;247(1, pt 1):C39–C44.

38. Chakravarthy MV, Davis BS, Booth FW. IGF-I restores satellite cell proliferative potential in immobilized old skeletal muscle. *J Appl Physiol.* 2000;89(4):1365–1379.

39. Zarzhevsky N, Menashe O, Carmeli E, Stein H, Reznick AZ. Capacity for recovery and possible mechanisms in immobilization atrophy of young and old animals. *Ann N Y Acad Sci.* 2001;928:212–225.

40. Girten B, Oloff C, Plato P, Eveland E, Merola AJ, Kazarian L. Skeletal muscle antioxidant enzyme levels in rats after simulated weightlessness, exercise and dobutamine. *Physiologist.* 1989;32(1)(suppl):S59–S60.

41. Lawler JM, Song W, Demaree SR. Hindlimb unloading increases oxidative stress and disrupts antioxidant capacity in skeletal muscle. *Free Radic Biol Med.* 2003;35(1):9–16.

42. Kondo H, Nakagaki I, Sasaki S, Hori S, Itokawa Y. Mechanism of oxidative stress in skeletal muscle atrophied by immobilization. *Am J Physiol.* 1993;265(6, pt 1):E839–E844.

43. Hurst JE, Fitts RH. Hindlimb unloading-induced muscle atrophy and loss of function: protective effect of isometric exercise. *J Appl Physiol.* 2003;95(4):1405–1417.

44. Motobe M, Murase N, Osada T, et al. Noninvasive monitoring of deterioration in skeletal muscle function with forearm cast immobilization and the prevention of deterioration. *Dyn Med.* 2004;3(1):2.

45. Hespel P, Op't Eijnde B, Van Leemputte M, et al. Oral creatine supplementation facilitates the rehabilitation of disuse atrophy and alters the expression of muscle myogenic factors in humans. *J Physiol.* 2001;536(pt 2):625–633.

46. Dudley GA, Duvoisin MR, Convertino VA, Buchanan P. Alterations of the in vivo torque–velocity relationship of human skeletal muscle following 30 days exposure to simulated microgravity. *Aviat Space Environ Med.* 1989;60(7):659–663.

47. Adams GR, Caiozzo VJ, Baldwin KM. Skeletal muscle unweighting: spaceflight and ground-based models. *J Appl Physiol.* 2003;95(6):2185–2201.

48. Tesch PA, Berg HE, Häggmark T, Ohlsén H, Dudley GA. Muscle strength and endurance following lowerlimb suspension in man. *Physiologist.* 1991;34(1)(suppl):S104–S106.

49. Conley KE, Jubrias SA, Amara CE, Marcinek DJ. Mitochondrial dysfunction: impact on exercise performance and cellular aging. *Exerc Sport Sci Rev.* 2007;35(2):43–49.

50. Fournier M, Roy RR, Perham H, Simard CP, Edgerton VR. Is limb immobilization a model of muscle disuse? *Exp Neurol.* 1983;80(1):147–156.

51. Kozlovskaia IB, Grigor'eva LS, Gevlich GI. Comparative analysis of effect of weightlessness and its models on velocity–strength properties and tonus of human skeletal muscles [in Russian]. *Kosm Biol Aviakosm Med.* 1984;18(6):22–26.

52. Sale DG, McComas AJ, MacDougall JD, Upton AR. Neuromuscular adaptation in human thenar muscles following strength training and immobilization. *J Appl Physiol.* 1982;53(2):419–424.

53. Deschenes MR, Britt AA, Chandler WC. A comparison of the effects of unloading in young adult and aged skeletal muscle. *Med Sci Sports Exerc.* 2001;33(9):1477–83.

54. Tabary JC, Tabary C, Tardieu C, Tardieu G, Goldspink G. Physiological and structural changes in the cat's soleus muscle due to immobilization at different lengths by plaster casts. *J Physiol*. 1972;224(1):231–244.

55. Williams PE, Goldspink G. Changes in sarcomere length and physiological properties in immobilized muscle. *J Anat*. 1978;127(pt 3):459–468.

56. Kannus P, Jozsa L, Kvist M, Lehto M, Järvinen M. The effect of immobilization on myotendinous junction: an ultrastructural, histochemical and immunohistochemical study. *Acta Physiol Scand*. 1992;144(3):387–394.

57. Booth FW. Regrowth of atrophied skeletal muscle in adult rats after ending immobilization. *J Appl Physiol*. 1978;44(2):225–230.

58. Kvist M, Hurme T, Kannus P, et al. Vascular density at the myotendinous junction of the rat gastrocnemius muscle after immobilization and remobilization. *Am J Sports Med*. 1995;23(3):359–364.

59. Järvinen TA, Józsa L, Kannus P, Järvinen TL, Järvinen M. Organization and distribution of intramuscular connective tissue in normal and immobilized skeletal muscles. An immunohistochemical, polarization and scanning electron microscopic study. *J Muscle Res Cell Motil*. 2002;23(3):245–254.

60. Yarkony GM, Sahgal V. Contractures. A major complication of craniocerebral trauma. *Clin Orthop Relat Res*. 1987(219):93–96.

61. Singer BJ, Jegasothy GM, Singer KP, Allison GT, Dunne JW. Incidence of ankle contracture after moderate to severe acquired brain injury. *Arch Phys Med Rehabil*. 2004;85(9):1465–1469.

62. Singer BJ, Jegasothy GM, Singer KP, Allison GT. Evaluation of serial casting to correct equinovarus deformity of the ankle after acquired brain injury in adults. *Arch Phys Med Rehabil*. 2003;84(4):483–491.

63. Pohl M, Rückriem S, Mehrholz J, Ritschel C, Strik H, Pause MR. Effectiveness of serial casting in patients with severe cerebral spasticity: a comparison study. *Arch Phys Med Rehabil*. 2002;83(6):784–790.

64. Pape HC, Marsh S, Morley JR, Krettek C, Giannoudis PV. Current concepts in the development of heterotopic ossification. *J Bone Joint Surg Br*. 2004;86(6):783–787.

65. Garland DE, Blum CE, Waters RL. Periarticular heterotopic ossification in head-injured adults. Incidence and location. *J Bone Joint Surg Am*. 1980;62(7):1143–1146.

66. Sazbon L, Najenson T, Tartakovsky M, Becker E, Grosswasser Z. Widespread periarticular new-bone formation in long-term comatose patients. *J Bone Joint Surg Br*. 1981;63-B(1):120–125.

67. Mavrogenis AF, Soucacos PN, Papagelopoulos PJ. Heterotopic ossification revisited. *Orthopedics*. 2011;34(3):177.

68. Genêt F, Jourdan C, Schnitzler A, et al. Troublesome heterotopic ossification after central nervous system damage: a survey of 570 surgeries. *PLoS On*. 2011;6(1):e16632.

69. Beingessner DM, Patterson SD, King GJ. Early excision of heterotopic bone in the forearm. *J Hand Surg Am*. 2000;25(3):483–488.

70. Safaz I, Alaca R, Yasar E, Tok F, Yilmaz B. Medical complications, physical function and communication skills in patients with traumatic brain injury: a single centre 5-year experience. *Brain Inj*. 2008;22(10):733–739.

71. Schulz H, Hillebrecht A, Karemaker JM, et al. Cardiopulmonary function during 10 days of head-down tilt bedrest. *Acta Physiol Scand Suppl*. 1992;604:23–32.

72. Katzan IL, Cebul RD, Husak SH, Dawson NV, Baker DW. The effect of pneumonia on mortality among patients hospitalized for acute stroke. *Neurology*. 2003;60(4):620–625.

73. Harrison-Felix C, Whiteneck G, Devivo MJ, Hammond FM, Jha A. Causes of death following 1 year postinjury among individuals with traumatic brain injury. *J Head Trauma Rehabil*. 2006;21(1):22–33.

74. Harrison-Felix CL, Whiteneck GG, Jha A, DeVivo MJ, Hammond FM, Hart DM. Mortality over four decades after traumatic brain injury rehabilitation: a retrospective cohort study. *Arch Phys Med Rehabil*. 2009;90(9):1506–1513.

75. Perhonen MA, Zuckerman JH, Levine BD. Deterioration of left ventricular chamber performance after bed rest: "cardiovascular deconditioning" or hypovolemia? *Circulation*. 2001;103(14):1851–1857.

76. Levine BD, Zuckerman JH, Pawelczyk JA. Cardiac atrophy after bed-rest deconditioning: a nonneural mechanism for orthostatic intolerance. *Circulation*. 1997;96(2):517–525.

77. Convertino VA. Effects of exercise and inactivity on intravascular volume and cardiovascular control mechanisms. *Acta Astronaut*. 1992;27:123–129.

78. Kamiya A, Michikami D, Fu Q, et al. Pathophysiology of orthostatic hypotension after bed rest: paradoxical sympathetic withdrawal. *Am J Physiol Heart Circ Physiol*. 2003;285(3):H1158–H1167.

79. Mueller PJ, Cunningham JT, Patel KP, Hasser EM. Proposed role of the paraventricular nucleus in cardiovascular deconditioning. *Acta Physiol Scand*. 2003;177(1):27–35.

80. Convertino V, Hung J, Goldwater D, DeBusk FR. Cardiovascular responses to exercise in middle-aged men after 10 days of bed rest. *Circulation*. 1982;65(1):134–140.

81. Convertino VA. Cardiovascular consequences of bed rest: effect on maximal oxygen uptake. *Med Sci Sports Exerc*. 1997;29(2):191–196.

82. Gaffney FA, Buckey JC, Lane LD, et al. The effects of a 10-day period of head-down tilt on the cardiovascular responses to intravenous saline loading. *Acta Physiol Scand Suppl*. 1992;604:121–130.

83. Saltin B, Blomqvist G, Mitchell JH, Johnson RL Jr, Wildenthal K, Chapman CB. Response to exercise after bed rest and after training. *Circulation*. 1968;38(5)(suppl):VII1–V78.

84. Sundblad P, Spaak J, Linnarsson D. Cardiovascular responses to upright and supine exercise in humans after 6 weeks of head-down tilt (-6 degrees). *Eur J Appl Physiol*. 2000;83(4–5):303–309.

85. Johansen LB, Gharib C, Allevard AM, et al. Haematocrit, plasma volume and noradrenaline in humans during simulated weightlessness for 42 days. *Clin Physiol*. 1997;17:203–210.

86. Convertino VA, Doerr DF, Mathes KL, Stein SL, Buchanan P. Changes in volume, muscle compartment, and compliance of the lower extremities in man following 30 days of exposure to simulated microgravity. *Aviat Space Environ Med*. 1989;60(7):653–658.

87. Greenleaf JE, Kozlowski S. Physiological consequences of reduced physical activity during bed rest. *Exerc Sport Sci Rev*. 1982;10:84–119.

88. Sun B, Yu ZB, Zhang LF. Daily 1 h standing can prevent depression of myocardial contractility in simulated weightless rats [in Chinese]. *Space Med Med Eng (Beijing)*. 2001;14(6):405–409.

89. Yablon SA, Rock WA Jr, Nick TG, Sherer M, McGrath CM, Goodson KH. Deep vein thrombosis: prevalence and risk factors in rehabilitation admissions with brain injury. *Neurology*. 2004;63(3):485–491.

90. Turpie AG. Prophylaxis of venous thromboembolism in stroke patients. *Semin Thromb Hemost*. 1997;23(2):155–157.

91. Carman TL, Kanner AA, Barnett GH, Deitcher SR. Prevention of thromboembolism after neurosurgery for brain and spinal tumors. *South Med J*. 2003;96(1):17–22.

92. Rogers FB. Venous thromboembolism in trauma patients. *Surg Clin North Am*. 1995;75(2):279–291.

93. Hamilton MG, Hull RD, Pineo GF. Venous thromboembolism in neurosurgery and neurology patients: a review. *Neurosurgery*. 1994;34(2):280–296.

94. Meythaler JM, Fisher WS, Rue LW, Johnson A, Davis L, Brunner RC. Screening for venous thromboembolism in traumatic brain injury: limitations of D-dimer assay. *Arch Phys Med Rehabil*. 2003;84(2):285–290.

95. Scudday T, Brasel K, Webb T, et al. Safety and efficacy of prophylactic anticoagulation in patients with traumatic brain injury. *J Am Coll Surg*. 2011;213(1):148–153.

96. Carlile M, Nicewander D, Yablon SA, et al. Prophylaxis for venous thromboembolism during rehabilitation for traumatic brain injury: a multicenter observational study. *J Trauma*. 2010;68(4):916–923.

97. Stein PD, Kayali F, Olson RE. Twenty-one-year trends in the use of inferior vena cava filters. *Arch Intern Med*. 2004;164(14):1541–1545.

98. Stein PD, Alnas M, Skaf E, et al. Outcome and complications of retrievable inferior vena cava filters. *Am J Cardiol*. 2004;94(8):1090–1093.

99. Streiff MB. Vena caval filters: a review for intensive care specialists. *J Intensive Care Med*. 2003;18(2):59–79.

100. Allman RM, Laprade CA, Noel LB, et al. Pressure sores among hospitalized patients. *Ann Intern Med*. 1986;105(3):337–342.

101. Allman RM, Goode PS, Burst N, Bartolucci AA, Thomas DR. Pressure ulcers, hospital complications, and disease severity: impact on hospital costs and length of stay. *Adv Wound Care.* 1999;12(1): 22–30.

102. Allman RM, Goode PS, Patrick MM, Burst N, Bartolucci AA. Pressure ulcer risk factors among hospitalized patients with activity limitation. *JAMA.* 1995;273(11):865–870.

103. Wywialowski EF. Tissue perfusion as a key underlying concept of pressure ulcer development and treatment. *J Vasc Nurs.* 1999;17(1): 12–16.

104. Curry K, Casady L. The relationship between extended periods of immobility and decubitus ulcer formation in the acutely spinal cord-injured individual. *J Neurosci Nurs.* 1992;24(4):185–189.

105. Peterson MJ, Schwab W, van Oostrom JH, Gravenstein N, Caruso LJ. Effects of turning on skin-bed interface in healthy adults. *J Adv Nurs.* 2010;66(7):1556–1564.

106. Ishizaki Y, Ishizaki T, Fukuoka H, et al. Changes in mood status and neurotic levels during a 20-day bed rest. *Acta Astronaut.* 2002; 50(7):453–459.

107. Gouvier WD, Pinkston JB, Lovejoy JC, et al. Neuropsychological and emotional changes during simulated microgravity: effects of triiodothyronine alendronate, and testosterone. *Arch Clin Neuropsychol.* 2004;19(2):153–163.

108. Spielman AJ, Saskin P, Thorpy MJ. Treatment of chronic insomnia by restriction of time in bed. *Sleep.* 1987;10(1):45–56.

109. Monk TH, Buysse DJ, Billy BD, Kennedy KS, Kupfer DJ. The effects on human sleep and circadian rhythms of 17 days of continuous bedrest in the absence of daylight. *Sleep.* 1997;20(10):858–864.

110. Kamdar BB, Needham DM, Collop NA. Sleep deprivation in critical illness: its role in physical and psychological recovery. *J Intensive Care Med.* 2012;27(2):97–111.

111. Chekirda IF, Bogdashevskiy RB, Yeremin AV, Kolosov IA. Coordination structure of walking of Soyuz-9 crew members before and after flight. *Kosm Biol Med.* 1971;5:48–52.

112. Purakhin IuN, Kakurin LI, Georgievskiŭ VS, Petukhov BN, Mikhaĭlov VM. Vertical posture regulation following flight in "Soiuz-6"–"Soiuz-8" spaceships and 120-day hypokinesia [in Russian]. *Kosm Biol Med.* 1972;6(6):47–53.

113. Duchateau J, Enoka RM. Neural adaptations with chronic activity patterns in able-bodied humans. *Am J Phys Med Rehabil.* 2002; 81(11)(suppl):S17–S27.

114. Kaneko F, Murakami T, Onari K, Kurumadani H, Kawaguchi K. Decreased cortical excitability during motor imagery after disuse of an upper limb in humans. *Clin Neurophysiol.* 2003;114(12): 2397–2403.

115. Semmler JG, Kutzscher DV, Enoka RM. Gender differences in the fatigability of human skeletal muscle. *J Neurophysiol.* 1999;82(6): 3590–3593.

116. Semmler JG, Kutzscher DV, Enoka RM. Limb immobilization alters muscle activation patterns during a fatiguing isometric contraction. *Muscle Nerve.* 2000;23(9):1381–1392.

117. Duchateau J, Hainaut K. Electrical and mechanical changes in immobilized human muscle. *J Appl Physiol.* 1987;62(6):2168–2173.

118. Bosco C, Cardinale M, Tsarpela O. Influence of vibration on mechanical power and electromyogram activity in human arm flexor muscles. *Eur J Appl Physiol Occup Physiol.* 1999;79(4):306–311.

119. Malathi S, Batmanabane M. Effects of varying periods of immobilization of a limb on the morphology of a peripheral nerve. *Acta Morphol Neerl Scand.* 1983;21(3):185–198.

120. Hauger RL, Millan MA, Lorang M, Harwood JP, Aguilera G. Corticotropin-releasing factor receptors and pituitary adrenal responses during immobilization stress. *Endocrinology.* 1988;123(1):396–405.

121. Myllynen P, Koivisto VA, Nikkilä EA. Glucose intolerance and insulin resistance accompany immobilization. *Acta Med Scand.* 1987;222(1):75–81.

122. Mechanick JI, Brett EM. Endocrine and metabolic issues in the management of the chronically critically ill patient. *Crit Care Clin.* 2002; 18(3):619–641, viii.

123. Zorbas YG, Yaroshenko YY, Kuznetsov NK, Verentsov GE. Daily magnesium supplementation effect on magnesium deficiency in rats during prolonged restriction of motor activity. *Metabolism.* 1998;47(8):903–907.

124. Grenon SM, Sheynberg N, Hurwitz S, et al. Renal, endocrine, and cardiovascular responses to bed rest in male subjects on a constant diet. *J Investig Med.* 2004;52(2):117–128.

125. Williams WJ, Schneider SM, Gretebeck RJ, Lane HW, Stuart CA, Whitson PA. Effect of dietary sodium on fluid/electrolyte regulation during bed rest. *Aviat Space Environ Med.* 2003;74(1):37–46.

126. Charrueau CL, Belabed L, Besson V, Chaumeil JC, Cynober L, Moinard C. Metabolic response and nutritional support in traumatic brain injury: evidence for resistance to renutrition. *J Neurotrauma.* 2009;26(11):1911–1920.

127. LeBlanc A, Schneider V, Spector E, et al. Calcium absorption, endogenous excretion, and endocrine changes during and after long-term bed rest. *Bone.* 1995;16(4)(suppl):301S–304S.

128. Altaf MA, Sood MR. The nervous system and gastrointestinal function. *Dev Disabil Res Rev.* 2008;14(2):87–95.

129. Newton M, Kamm MA, Quigley T, Burnham WR. Symptomatic gastroesophageal reflux in acutely hospitalized patients. *Dig Dis Sci.* 1999;44(1):140–148.

130. Cushing H. Peptic ulcer and the interbrain. *Surg Gynec Obst.* 1932; 55:1–34.

131. Chua K, Chuo A, Kong KH. Urinary incontinence after traumatic brain injury: incidence, outcomes and correlates. *Brain Inj.* 2003; 17(6):469–478.

132. Riehmann M, Bayer WH, Drinka PJ, et al. Position-related changes in voiding dynamics in men. *Urology.* 1998;52(4):625–630.

133. Hwang TI, Hill K, Schneider V, Pak CY. Effect of prolonged bedrest on the propensity for renal stone formation. *J Clin Endocrinol Metab.* 1988;66(1):109–112.

134. Greenleaf JE. Intensive exercise training during bed rest attenuates deconditioning. *Med Sci Sports Exerc.* 1997;29(2):207–215.

135. Petrofsky JS. Electrical stimulation: neurophysiological basis and application. *Basic Appl Myol.* 2004;14:205–213.

136. Qin L, Appell HJ, Chan KM, Maffulli N. Electrical stimulation prevents immobilization atrophy in skeletal muscle of rabbits. *Arch Phys Med Rehabil.* 1997;78(5):512–517.

Managing Upper Motoneuron Muscle Overactivity

Nathaniel H. Mayer and Alberto Esquenazi

INTRODUCTION

Lesions that impair corticospinal tract function are called *upper motoneuron* (UMN) lesions (1,2). Since the days of Hughlings Jackson, clinicians have classified UMN signs as positive or negative. Negative signs signify impairment of voluntary motor behaviors (e.g., force production, dexterity, selective movement control). In a general sense, negative signs of voluntary movement can be described as *phenomena of underactivity*. In contrast, involuntary positive signs, (e.g., spasticity, flexor spasms, associated reactions) signify *phenomena of involuntary overactivity*.

"Spasticity" has frequently been used as a catchall term for all positive signs but, as Lance's classical definition indicates, spasticity is only one of many different positive signs seen in the UMN syndrome (UMNS) (3). Different signs with different pathophysiologies invite different treatments. What all positive signs have in common is that they are generated by involuntary muscle overactivity. Therefore, in this chapter, "muscle overactivity" is preferred as a catchall term rather than spasticity because muscle overactivity captures the feature of excessive muscle contraction underlying all positive signs, many of which do not have "spastic" (stretch related) features as their source (4).

Many studies have suggested that UMN muscles become stiff and develop contracture (fixed shortening) after they have been subjected to prolonged overactivity (5–7). Some have argued that changes in the rheologic (viscous, elastic, and plastic) properties of muscle are often more dysfunctional for the patient than the positive and negative signs of neurological origin (8). This perspective is agreeable to us namely problems seen in the UMNS result from interactions between impaired voluntary control of movement (negative signs), involuntary muscle overactivity (positive signs), and rheologic stiffness and contracture of muscle. In addition to positive and negative signs, changes in the rheologic properties of muscle and other soft tissues are a third contributor to disability in UMNS. Moreover, Herman (5) has shown that the degree of muscle overactivity can be influenced by the stiffness characteristics of muscle itself. He studied the triceps surae of 220 patients who are hemiplegic and found that reduced tissue extensibility was associated with reduced tonic stretch reflex activity for patients with contracture. Increased resistance to passive stretch was in large measure because of changes in the physical stiffness of the triceps surae muscle for these patients. It is well known that patients with calf muscle contracture typically have gait difficulties.

From a therapeutic perspective, treatment of contracture is very different from treatment of negative signs of muscle underactivity and positive signs of muscle overactivity.

POSITIVE SIGNS

1. Spasticity

Spasticity is a term linked with stretch reflexes (9), and we do not use it to mean flexor spasms generated by flexor reflex afferent activity or associated reactions. Co-contraction of antagonist muscles is generated by volitional effort (see discussion later) and, the combination term "spastic co-contraction," implies that stretch-induced activity is superimposed on volitionally generated co-contraction. It has a specific meaning regarding stretch reflexes, but it has also been confusingly used as a catchall term for other positive signs such as flexor spasms, co-contraction, and associated reactions that are not connected with stretch reflexes. Whatever else clinicians bundle with the term spasticity, it has classically meant an increase in excitability of skeletal muscle stretch reflexes. Both phasic and tonic stretch reflexes are found in many, if not most, patients with an UMN lesion (10). Clinically, the defining characteristic of spasticity is excessive resistance of muscle to being passively stretched. It is the nature of that resistance to increase as the examiner increases the velocity of stretch (11); slow stretch usually offers little resistance, but faster stretches elicit more and more resistance. Sherrington's seminal studies (12,13) of the cat's myotatic stretch reflex provided strong physiological underpinnings for later clinical descriptions of spasticity. Stretch reflex behavior is aptly described by Nathan (9):

> Spasticity is a condition in which the stretch reflexes that are normally latent become obvious. The tendon reflexes have a lowered threshold to tap, the response of the tapped muscle is increased, and usually muscles besides the tapped one respond; tonic stretch reflexes are affected in the same way (pp. 13-14).

The brief tendon tap blow resembles an engineering impulse function. Its quick jerk response helps classify it as a phasic reflex, meaning short duration phasic response. In contrast, passive muscle stretch of longer duration induces more sustained tension and reflects underlying stretch reflex activity of the tonic (sustained) type. Tonic stretch reflexes have a lowered threshold and an increased response to stretch. Resistance perceived by an examiner stretching a group of muscles across a joint is elevated in the spastic state and it varies with velocity. If a large enough resistance to stretch develops suddenly during passive movement, continuous passive stretch performed by an examiner may be interrupted momentarily, giving rise to a "spastic catch" sensation. Clonus may also develop under such circumstances.

Physiologically, afferent signals generated by stretch of the muscle spindle are transmitted to the central nervous system by group Ia and group II afferents. Spindle afferent activity, however, is not increased in patients who are spastic (14). Rather, the central excitatory state of the spinal cord appears to be elevated (15,16). A number of theories of spasticity are linked to the concept of signal "mishandling" at the level of the spinal cord. Delwaide (17) points out that the normal mechanism of presynaptic inhibition in the spinal cord is altered for patients with hyperreflexia. Group Ia afferent activity from the muscle spindle is normally adjusted at a premotoneuron level depending on supraspinal facilitation and preceding group Ia discharges. In spasticity, according to Delwaide, the interneuron responsible for presynaptic inhibition becomes less active because of a reduction of supraspinal facilitation influences. Accordingly, the stretch reflex of the patient with hyperreflexia is no longer subjective to tonic inhibitory control by the mechanism of presynaptic inhibition. Instead, proprioceptive signals are able to access alpha motoneurons directly and elicit spastic behavior in corresponding muscles. A change in the excitability of the spinal cord was also the basis of the hypothesis of Veale, Rees, and Mark (18) who pointed to abnormality in the Renshaw system. *Renshaw cells*, small interneurons in the ventromedial horn of the cord, are monosynaptically excited by recurrent collaterals from nearby motoneurons. Renshaw cell axons form inhibitory synapses on nearby motoneurons and produce indirect disinhibition of motoneurons by their action on inhibitory interneurons. Veale, Rees, and Mark postulated that impaired supraspinal regulation of the Renshaw system produced disinhibition of motoneurons, leading to clinical spasticity. Along similar lines, Jankowska et al. (19) proposed that a specific interneuronal system in the spinal cord mishandled group II afferent activity from the muscle spindle. Therefore, what is common to the aforementioned theories is an enhanced central excitatory state.

After a UMN lesion, a net loss of inhibition impairs descending control over motoneurons and interneurons. The result is disordered regulation of segmental spinal reflexes including stretch reflexes.

Lance (20) characterized spasticity as an increase in velocity-dependent *tonic* stretch reflexes with exaggerated tendon jerks. Generally, the term "phasic" implies time varying. "Tonic" has a time invariant quality. However, the literature's use of the terms phasic and tonic can be confusing because some authors refer to an input stimulus as either phasic or tonic, whereas others characterize the output response as either phasic or tonic. In Lance's consensus definition, *tonic stretch reflexes* referred to the output response of a muscle group that was stretched at different velocities of stretch. "Exaggerated tendon jerks" were examples of phasic stretch reflexes. In routine practice at the bedside, the 2 ways of assessing phasic and tonic stretch reflexes are tendon taps and passive stretch of a muscle group at different rates of stretch. As the rate of muscle stretch increases, resistance of the muscle group being stretched also increases. From an electromyographic (EMG) perspective, tonic stretch reflex activity also increases as the rate of stretch increases. Figure 50-1 illustrates stretch reflex EMG activity in a patient with traumatic brain injury (TBI) undergoing different rates of passive stretch by an examiner. The figure shows that different muscles respond differently to the same input (stretch). Differential muscle responses raise the possibility of differential treatment.

Stretch reflex activity in antagonist muscles can be triggered during voluntary concentric contraction of agonists. Many patients move slowly; consequently, the velocity of antagonist stretch is low, and spastic activity is negligible. Nevertheless, spasticity of antagonist muscles can be triggered during voluntary movement, but it can be confused with the phenomenon of co-contraction. Co-contraction is characterized by *simultaneous* activation of agonist and antagonist muscles during voluntary effort (21). In contrast with co-contraction, the onset of spasticity is *not simultaneous* with the onset of movement because spasticity depends on muscle stretch, and no muscle stretch occurs until at least some motion has developed. Simultaneous activation of agonists and antagonists is more easily inferred on EMG recordings than on clinical examination (see Figure 50-2).

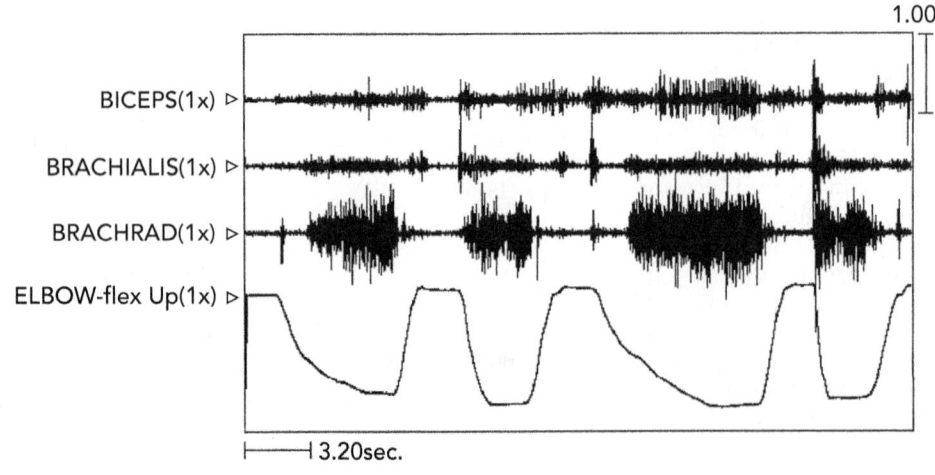

FIGURE 50–1 Passive stretch of elbow flexors performed by an examiner at different rates of stretch in a patient with traumatic brain injury (TBI) and upper motoneuron overactivity (UMN). As the velocity of stretch increases, more electromyography (EMG) is generated. Note, however, that different muscles respond differently to the same input. BRACHRAD, brachioradialis.

Voluntary Alternating Motion of Elbow

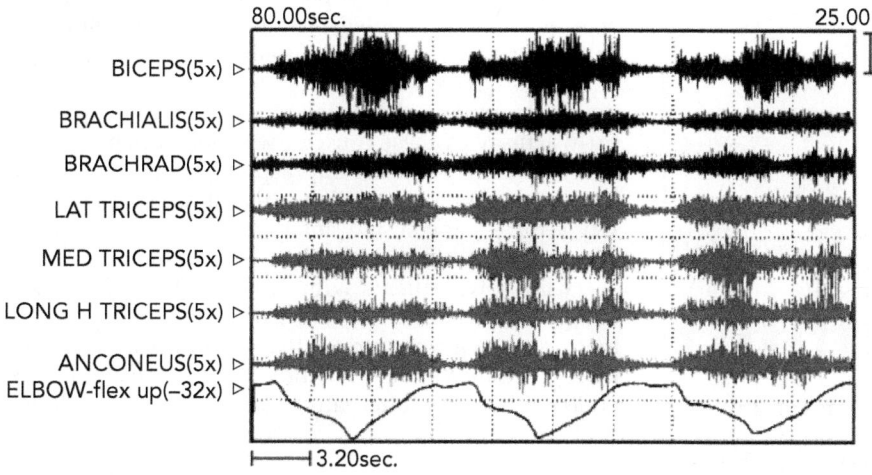

FIGURE 50–2 Co-contraction of elbow flexors and extensors during voluntary alternating movements at the elbow. The patient complained of fatigue and she felt as if she were "fighting herself" when she made these movements. BRACHRAD, brachioradialis; LAT, lateral; MED, medial.

2. Clonus

Clonus is a low frequency rhythmic oscillation in 1 or more limb segments (Figure 50-3). Clonus may be triggered by rapid stretch and hold of a muscle group. It may also be induced by a patient who inadvertently stretches a muscle group during limb positioning (e.g., planting the foot on a wheelchair pedal). Clonus may be triggered during voluntary movement. EMG of clonus reveals a short duration electrical activity at typical frequencies of 6–8 Hz. In Figure 50-4, a patient with hemiparesis secondary to gunshot wound of the brain was asked to extend his elbow.

Bursts of EMG activity alternating between medial triceps and brachioradialis are seen. Spread of activity to extensor carpi radialis and first dorsal interosseous (DI) is also seen. Clonus does not have to be alternating. Clonus can be sustained or unsustained, and it can be stopped by repositioning muscles to shorter lengths. Clonus is usually associated with other hyperexcitable phasic stretch reflexes. In

addition to rapid stretch, various cutaneous stimuli, especially cold or noxious stimuli, may give rise to ipsilateral or even contralateral clonus (22). Clonus may represent auto-oscillation of a hyperexcitable stretch reflex loop (23). Rack et al. (24) felt that the frequency of clonus was determined by peripheral parameters such as load rather than central mechanisms. On the other hand, Dimitrijevic et al. (25) felt that a central oscillator was operating to produce clonus. Therapeutically, a drug such as dantrolene sodium is often effective in reducing low-frequency, low-tension phenomena such as clonus.

3. Co-contraction

Co-contraction may be described as the activation of antagonist muscles during voluntary activation of agonists. Humphrey and Reed (26) indicated that co-contraction can be activated and deactivated at a cortical level and that it relates

ELBOW ALTERNATIONS: 2.5 yrs post TBI

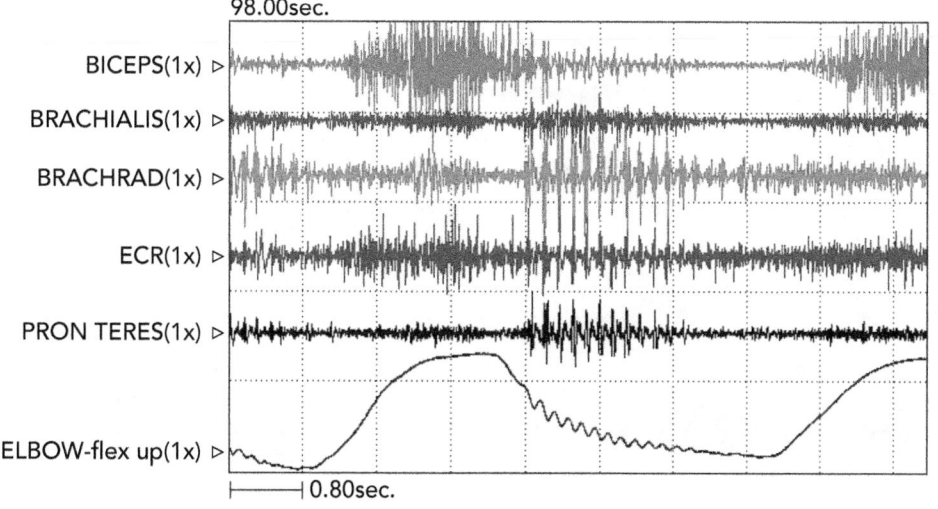

FIGURE 50–3 Illustration of clonus during extension phase of voluntary alternating movements of the elbow Clonus is a low frequency rhythmic oscillation, approximately 6–8 Hz, in one or more limb segments. This patient illustrates clonic bursts of electromyography (EMG) in brachioradialis, extensor carpi radialis (ECR), and pronator teres. The displacement trace reveals clonic oscillations of the elbow "sitting atop" the extension phase of the movement. BRACHRAD, brachioradialis.

EXTENSION PHASE, ELBOW ALTERNATIONS

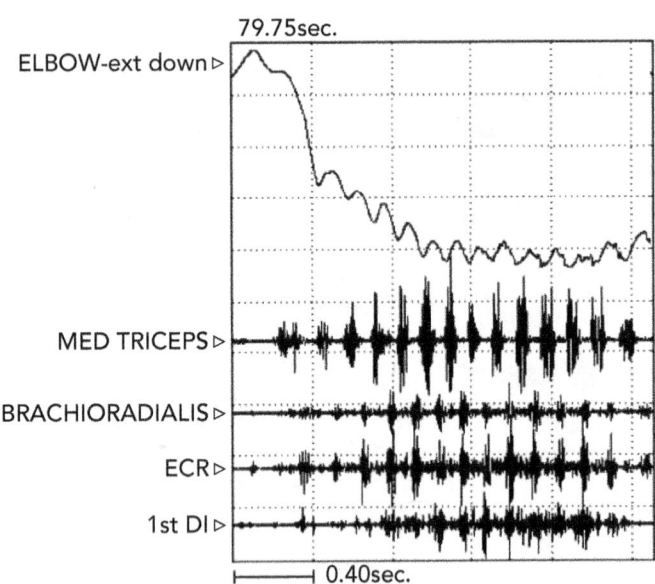

FIGURE 50-4 A patient with hemiparesis (gunshot wound of the brain) extends his elbow. Alternating bursts of clonic EMG activity are seen between medial triceps and brachioradialis. Spread of activity to distal muscles (e.g., first dorsal interosseous [DI]) is also observed. MED, medial.

to the switching mechanism of reciprocal inhibition whose circuitry is in the cord. Pathological co-contraction may represent an impairment of supraspinal control of reciprocal inhibition. Abnormalities of group Ia reciprocal inhibition have been reported in patients with UMN (27–29). Co-contraction may occur during isometric effort so that it is not necessarily related to muscle stretch. Figure 50-5 illustrates co-contraction during forward reach by an adult with UMNS. Simultaneous activation of flexors and extensors of the elbow is observed in the record. The movement trace reveals a slow, nonsmooth extension trajectory. Although co-

contraction can be a normal mechanism that provides joint stability, in this case, the patient's elbow flexors appear to be exerting an unwanted restraining action. Clinically, the patient struggled to extend his elbow as part of a reach pattern. Figure 50-5 reveals that brachioradialis and biceps activity occurred at the onset of movement, indicating that early activity in these muscles was not stretch induced but was likely linked to the supraspinal reach "command." A key feature of co-contraction is that it occurs during voluntary effort—agonist and antagonist muscles receiving signals that are activated simultaneously (30).

Clinically, patients with co-contraction of agonist and antagonist muscles make slow, effortful movements. Movement is often asymmetrical, that is, slower in one direction more than another. For example, when an examiner asks a patient to perform alternating movements at the elbow, co-contraction of flexors during extension phase will prolong extension phase and lead to obvious asymmetry of extension movement time and, often, movement amplitude. We typically test for antagonist restraint by asking the patient to perform voluntary "back" and "forth" movements about a joint for the full available range. Normally, alternating back and forth movements are symmetrical in time and amplitude. Patients with restraining co-contraction, however, exhibit temporal and spatial asymmetries. Therapeutically, co-contracting antagonist muscles may respond to a weakening strategy (e.g., chemodenervation, tendon lengthenings). Among central muscle relaxants, only tizanidine (TZD) has been described as having a potential effect on group Ia reciprocal inhibition (31).

4. Flexor and Extensor Spasms

According to Lance (32), a characteristic feature of UMNS is the release of flexor reflex afferents. The flexor reflex, a polysynaptic reflex that results in flexor muscle contraction, is elicited by afferent stimuli collectively known as flexor reflex afferents. Among others, these afferents include exteroceptive cutaneous receptors responding to touch, temperature, and pressure; nociceptors responding to painful

Reaching Forward with Left Upper Limb

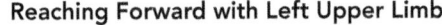

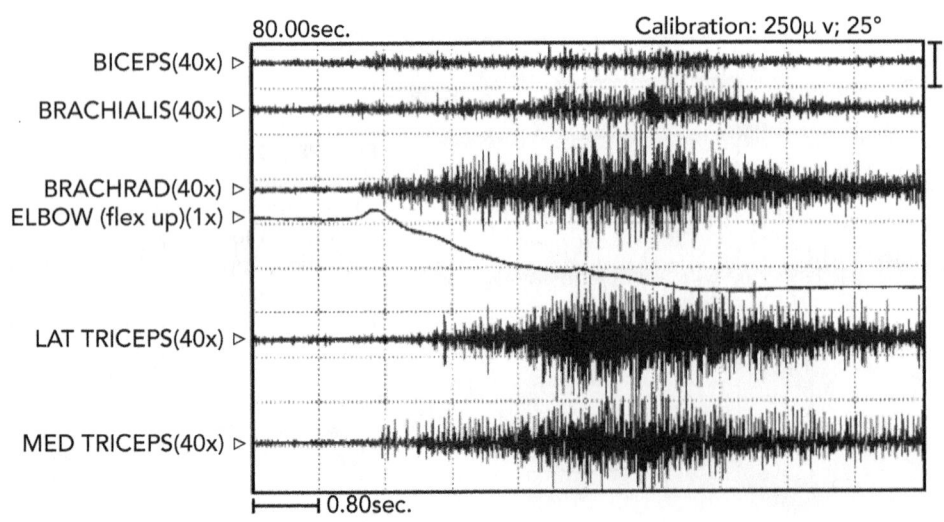

FIGURE 50-5 Co-contraction during forward reach by an adult with upper motoneuron syndrome (UMNS). Simultaneous activation of flexors and extensors of the elbow is observed in the record. The movement trace reveals a slow, nonsmooth extension trajectory (flexors restrain extensors). BRACHRAD, brachioradialis; LAT, lateral; MED, medial.

stimuli; secondary endings from muscle spindles (group II afferents); and free nerve endings scattered ubiquitously over muscles that generate slowly conducting afferent activity along group III and IV axons. The polysynaptic flexor reflex has a long latency (more than twice that of a monosynaptic tendon jerk) due both to slow afferent conduction into the cord and to central delay. In the cord, flexor reflex afferent activity travels up and down, synapsing in the internuncial pool—a system of spinal interneurons that is influenced by inputs coming from peripheral as well as central sources, including the brainstem. Compared to segmental stretch reflexes, the time course of polysynaptic flexor reflexes is slower, and unlike segmental stretch reflexes, flexor reflexes represent coordinated activity of motoneuron pools spanning many segments, resulting in muscle contraction across several joints, sometimes bilaterally. By typically recruiting flexor muscles across several joints, the flexor reflex is an example of an interjoint reflex that has tissue protective value such as enabling quick withdrawal from a noxious stimulus. Extensor reflexes are also polysynaptic and interjoint in nature and may aid upright bodily support functions. Flexor and extensor reflexes may play a role as core substrate for more complex coordinated patterns, such as locomotor stepping generators.

After UMNS, particularly after spinal cord lesions, release of inhibitory descending influences augments the flexor reflex clinically. When patient complaints are traced to flexor and extensor spasms, it is likely that these spasms represent disinhibited flexor and extensor reflexes. Flexor and extensor spasms occur in response to a variety of overt stimuli or they may occur "spontaneously," the latter placed in quotes because spasms are also triggered by covert stimuli such as a full bladder, a stool distended bowel, a tight diaper, a wheelchair restraint compressing the groin, or unappreciated skin ischemia from sitting in one position too long.

Clinically, flexor reflexes can range from the familiar Babinski sign to a mass flexor reflex characterized by intense, often painful interjoint flexion. Patients may call it a muscle spasm, but a history will reveal that they mean whole limb involvement rather than focal spasm of a single muscle group. In UMN lesions, the threshold of the flexor reflex is reduced, the intensity of muscle contraction for the same stimulus input is increased, and interjoint components of the reflex are often expanded (i.e., more muscles and more joints are recruited). Drugs such as baclofen and diazepam can inhibit polysynaptic activity in the cord, reducing frequency and intensity of flexor spasms. In TBI, these drugs may sedate (baclofen and diazepam) or affect memory (diazepam). Excessive flexor withdrawal on ground contact can impair stance phase of gait. Excessive flexion during swing can mimic steppage gait and impair limb advancement.

5. "Spastic Dystonia"

The term "spastic dystonia" originated from Denny-Brown (33). He examined postural reactions of monkeys after cerebral cortex ablations. Lesions were independent of, or in addition to, damage to the pyramidal tract. When the bodies of animals with cortical ablations were held in different positions, their limbs developed fixed positions or postures. For all postures, any attempt by the examiner to pull the limb away from its fixed position was met with an increasing resistance of spring-like quality. The limb would "fly" back to

its original posture when released. Denny-Brown called this fixed attitude *dystonia*, a term that meant the posture was being maintained by *active muscle contraction*. The continuous nature of muscle contraction that maintained cortical dystonia was present without the monkey making movements elsewhere. The dystonia did not depend on afferent input from the limb because it persisted even after the relevant dorsal roots were cut. Moreover, EMG recordings of dystonic monkey muscles revealed sustained (tonic) activity, and Denny-Brown thought that dystonia of this kind represented release of motor mechanisms that had direct access to alpha motoneurons. What seems clear, therefore, is that these dystonic postures were mediated efferently from above and had nothing to do with spinal reflex activity. However, what is not clear to us is the exact meaning of the term spastic dystonia. Denny-Brown himself pointed out that there were dystonic monkeys without spastic features. Nevertheless, dystonia may have stretch sensitive (spastic) features and it was necessary to recognize such a combination as spastic dystonia. Many clinicians seem to use the term spastic dystonia when they see a patient with UMN with fixed limb postures in the absence of obvious stretch or voluntary effort. By just looking, however, it is not always clear that a fixed posture is being generated by tonic muscle contraction. A net balance of force created by passive tissue stiffness alone may be sufficient to maintain limb posture. Contracture can also hold a limb in fixed position as will joint fusions and heterotopic ossification (HO). EMG recording "at rest" is helpful in demonstrating spastic dystonia. Spastic dystonia is primarily caused by an abnormal pattern of supraspinal descending drive, characterized by an inability to relax muscles despite efforts to do so. Gracies et al. (34) state that spastic dystonia is sensitive to the degree of tonic or sustained stretch imposed on the dystonic muscle. For example, Figures 50-6 and Figure 50-7 illustrate a patient with right hemiparesis secondary to gunshot wound of the brain who was asked to stand quietly at rest. EMG recordings of biceps and brachioradialis reveal tonic activity in biceps and occasional activity in brachioradialis. The flexed posture of the elbow was persistent, and the patient was not making a voluntary effort to hold the position. Passive stretch revealed spastic resistance, and the patient had tendon hyperreflexia as well. One might describe this patient as having spastic dystonia—a persistent posture driven by active contraction of the biceps (at a minimum) in the absence of phasic stretch or voluntary effort. In Denny-Brown's sense of mechanism for the behavior, continuous biceps contraction is mediated efferently from supraspinal sources driving alpha motoneurons. This is not so easy to prove, yet its assertion has therapeutic implications. For example, central agents such as diazepam and baclofen, known to suppress spinal reflex activity, would not be expected to be useful in treating spastic dystonia. Focal chemodenervation/neurolysis with botulinum toxin, phenol, or dantrolene, a direct skeletal muscle relaxant, would seem to have a better therapeutic rationale.

6. Associated Reactions

UMN associated reactions were first described by Walshe (35) in 1923 as released postural reactions deprived of voluntary control. "Synkinesis" is a term used by Bourbonnais (36) more recently. An associated reaction refers to involuntary activity in 1 limb that is associated with a voluntary move-

REST

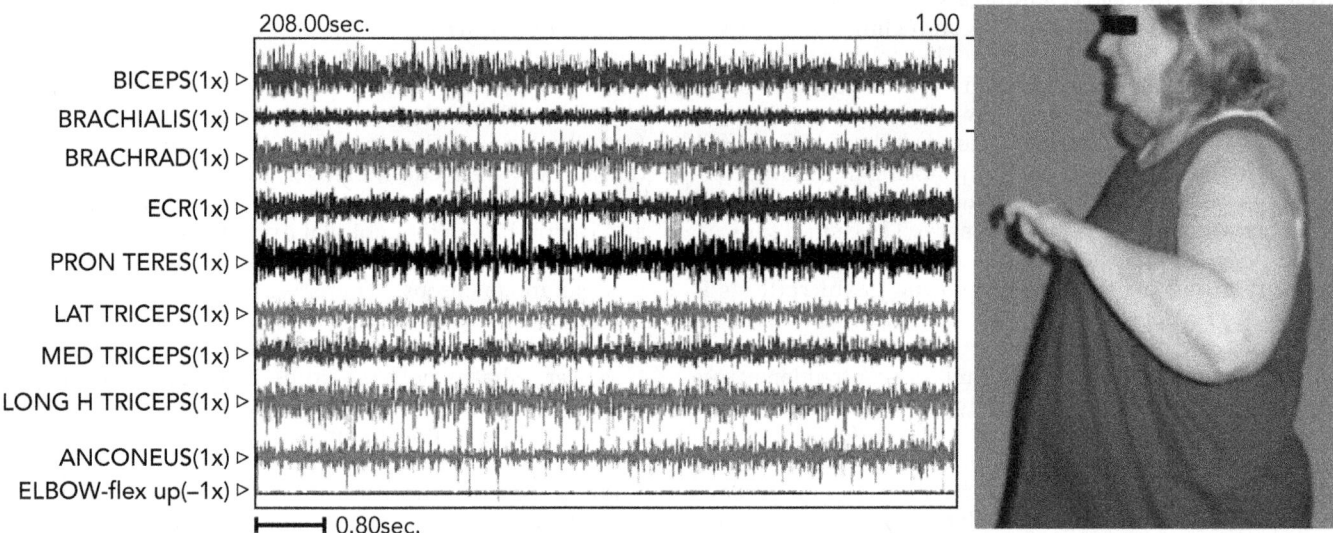

FIGURE 50–6 Spastic dystonia. This patient with an upper motoneuron syndrome and left hemiparesis was asked to stand quietly "at rest." The flexed posture of the elbow was persistent, and the patient readily acknowledged that she was not making any voluntary effort to hold this position. Persistent elbow flexion was her chief complaint. An electromyographic (EMG) record during "rest" revealed persistent activity in many muscles about the elbow and forearm. BRACHRAD, brachioradialis; ECR, extensor carpi radialis; H, head; LAT, lateral; MED, medial;

ment effort made in other limbs. Associated reactions may be caused by disinhibited spread of voluntary motor activity into the limb affected by a UMN lesion. Figure 50-8 shows a patient with left hemiparesis (brain gunshot wound) attempting to readjust his sitting position by pushing down on the wheelchair's armrest. The patient was unable to use the left upper extremity in this task because voluntary control was severely impaired. Dynamic EMG of elbow musculature during this activity revealed high EMG recruitment in flexor and extensor muscles about the elbow (Figure 50-9). Despite elbow extensor activity, the photograph reveals *flexed* elbow posturing, indicating that a net balance of muscle forces about the elbow favored flexion. The intensity of an associated reaction may depend on how much voluntary effort is made by the patient elsewhere. Dewald and Rymer (37) thought that impaired descending supraspinal com-

mands generated associated reactions. They hypothesized that unaffected bulbospinal motor pathways may have taken over the role of damaged UMN tracts during the transmission of descending voluntary commands.

Making the assumption that associated reactions are supraspinal in origin, modification by oral agents such as baclofen and diazepam would not be expected. Depending on the intensity of muscle contraction evoked in an associated reaction, dantrolene sodium, an inhibitor of muscle contraction, may be potentially useful therapeutically. TZD has known effects at spinal levels; however, it may also act supraspinally by influencing activity in descending coeruleospinal pathways. However, reports of depressed neuronal activity in the locus coeruleus by alpha-2 adrenergic agonist drugs have emphasized their impact on cord mediated reflexes such as flexor reflexes but not on supraspi-

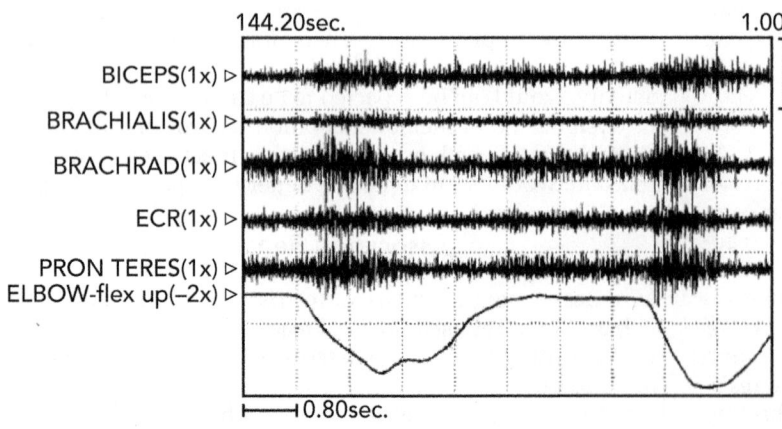

FIGURE 50–7 Passive stretch of the elbow flexors of the patient in Figure 50-6 revealed that her dystonic activity was stretch sensitive. According to Denny-Brown (33), the dystonic phenomenon (activity at rest) is of supraspinal origin and is mediated efferently, not afferently. However, the presence of stretch sensitivity suggests that some patients may also have a component of spasticity. ECR, extensor carpi radialis; PRON, pronator.

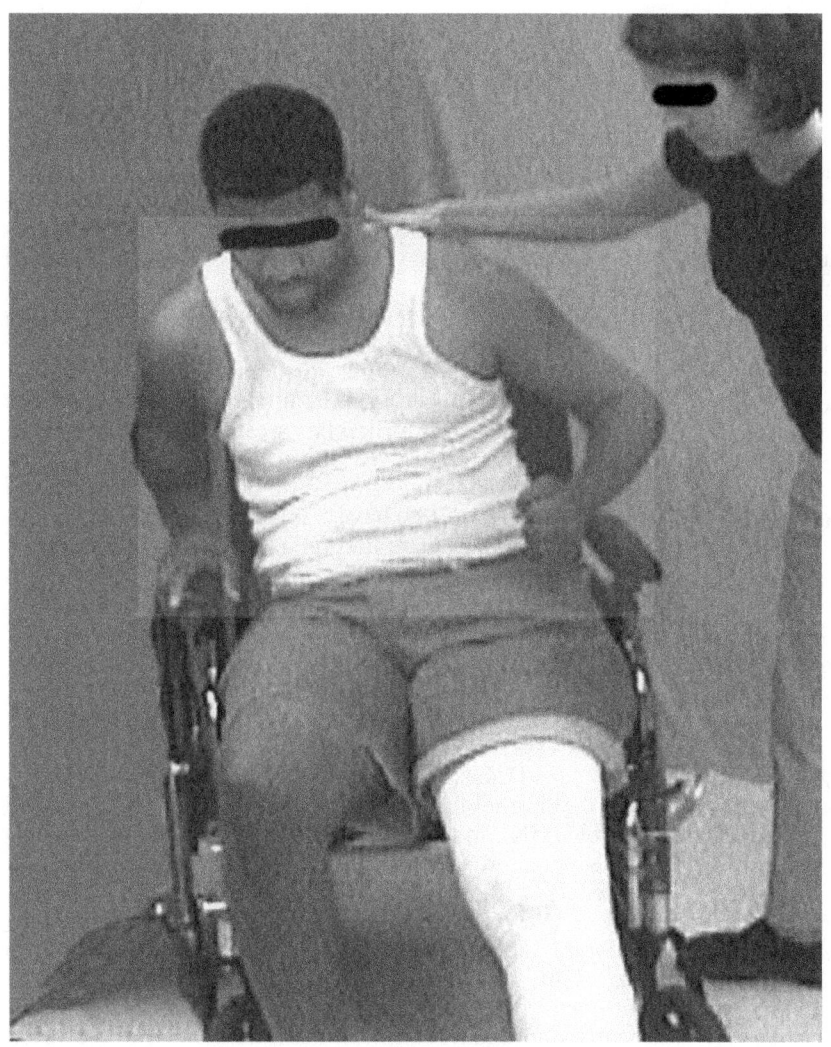

FIGURE 50–8 An "associated reaction" refers to involuntary activity in one limb that is associated with a voluntary movement effort made in other limbs. This figure illustrates an associated reaction in the left arm of a patient with left hemiparesis (gunshot wound of brain) who is readjusting his sitting position in the wheelchair by volitionally pushing down on the armrest with his right arm. The patient was unable to use the left upper extremity in this task because voluntary motor control was severely impaired on the left.

GSW L hemi: Adjusting Self with Right Arm by Pushing Down on Arm Rest of Wheelchair

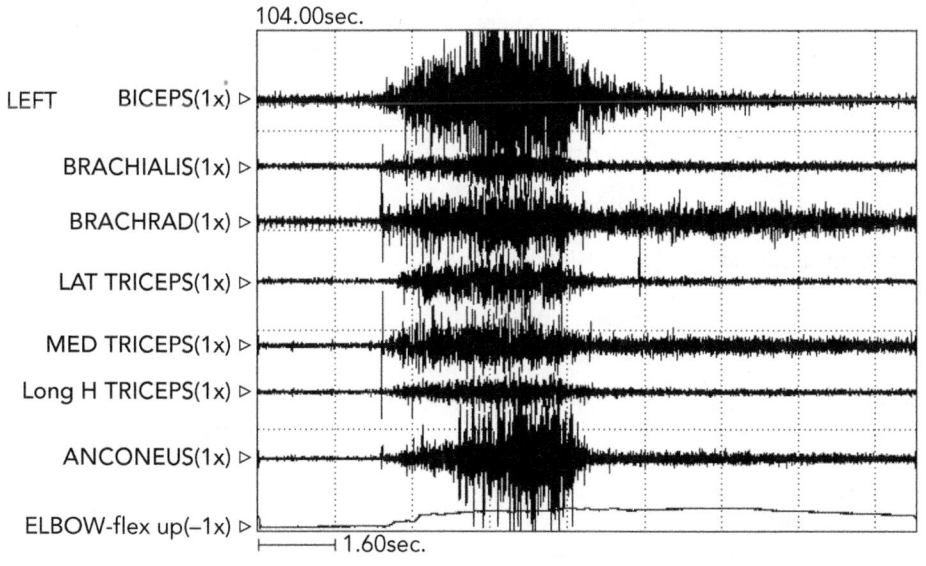

FIGURE 50–9 Dynamic electromyography (EMG) study of elbow musculature in the patient of Figure 50-8 was performed during the same maneuver of readjusting position in the wheelchair. Findings revealed high EMG recruitment for flexor and extensor muscles about the elbow. Despite elbow extensor EMG activity, the photograph in Figure 50-8 reveals *flexed* elbow posturing indicating that, despite extensor muscle contraction, a net balance of muscle forces about the elbow favored flexion posturing. The intensity of a limb's associated reaction may depend on the magnitude of voluntary effort made by the patient elsewhere. L, left; H, head; GSW, gunshot wound.

nally mediated behaviors, such as associated reactions (38). The authors are not aware of reports regarding TZD and associated reactions in man.

Although clinician's seem to be more aware of the spasticity than other positive signs of UMN, its impact may be less than advertised when one reflects on how often patients and caregivers actually stretch spastic muscles at rates that would elicit intense spastic responses. We commonly see patients and caregivers performing limb manipulations at slow rates of stretch to minimize rate-sensitive spastic resistance. In addition, what frequently passes for spastic resistance may, in large measure, reflect an increase in static stiffness because of intrinsic changes in the physical properties of muscle. On the other hand, the frequent development of associated reactions in the form of released postural reactions may be unavoidable because voluntary movement efforts made by "good" limbs occur throughout the day. High-intensity voluntary efforts required during transfers, gait, and activities of daily living (ADLs) might be expected to provide many opportunities for generating associated reactions. For patients with UMN, it is conceivable that the everyday potential for generating UMN-associated reactions may contribute more than the phenomenon of spasticity toward the development of muscle stiffness and contracture. More studies along this line would help.

7. Muscle Stiffness and Contracture

Muscle contracture refers to physical shortening of muscle length, and it is often accompanied by shortening of other soft tissues such as fascia, nerves, blood vessels, and skin. Muscle *contracture*, an invariant physical state of fixed shortening, should not be confused with muscle *contraction*, a dynamic state of internal shortening produced by sliding action of actin and myosin filaments within a muscle fiber. Contracture development is promoted by a number of processes that start with an acute UMN lesion: (*a*) paresis impairs cycles of shortening and lengthening of agonist and antagonist muscles promoted by everyday muscle usage; (*b*) gravity generates positional effects on jointed limb segments; (*c*) positional effects are created by a net balance of static rheologic forces across joints; and (*d*) as preferential muscle overactivity develops in specific muscle groups, a net balance of dynamic contractile forces promotes postures leading to contracture. Contracture implies that even if one blocked all muscle *contraction* by local or general anesthesia, physical shortening of muscle would still remain. Because central muscle relaxants such as TZD and baclofen, peripheral agents such as dantrolene, or chemodenervation/neurolytic agents such as botulinum toxin or phenol affect dynamic muscle contraction only, a clinical picture dominated by contracture will not respond to these types of interventions. Physical and surgical methods are necessary to undo contracture.

After a UMN lesion, paralyzed muscles immobilized for long periods in a shortened position became shortened and stiffer. When muscle overactivity develops in these shortened muscles, tension is generated at shorter lengths. A lack of voluntary contraction in the antagonists of these shortened muscles prevents their natural reextension, leading to a continuation of the process of stiffness and fixation. In the upper limb, for example, muscles that typically shorten include shoulder adductors or internal rotators, elbow flexors,

forearm pronators, wrist, finger, and thumb flexors and thumb adductors. Familiar UMN patterns of deformity develop in both the upper and lower limbs (Table 50-1) (Figures 50-10 and 50-11). The position of a given joint results from a net balance of static and dynamic muscle forces acting across 1 or more joints.

Literature support for this idea comes from many studies. Herman (5) described changes in the rheologic properties of spastic muscles in a large number of patients who are hemoplegic. Patients with contracture often had *reduced* reflex activity, yet resistance to passive stretch was high because of increased tissue stiffness. His study indicated that a description of muscle tone must necessarily consider the complex interaction between rheologic and reflex properties of muscle because stretch reflex properties may be influenced by alterations in the physical properties of muscle. Along similar lines, Dietz et al. (6) (stroke, cerebral palsy) and Thilmann et al. (39) have argued that hypertonia might not be related to exaggerated reflexes but rather to changes in soft tissues. Hufschmidt and Mauritz (40) proposed that abnormal cross-bridge connections in antagonist muscles could contribute to resistance to passive movement and that these changes would very likely occur in muscles subjected to prolonged positioning. Akeson et al. (41) demonstrated that immobility in animals led to stiffness associated with water loss and collagen deposition. Gossman et al. (42), Herbert (43), and Carey and Burghardt (44) described the various ways that immobility imposed on a patient by the negative signs of UMN can result in contracture. Other animal studies have suggested that when muscles are immobilized in a shortened position, some sarcomeres are lost and others become shorter and stiffer (Tabary et al. [45]; Williams and Goldspink [46]; Witzmann, Kim, and Fitts [47]). Soft tissues other than muscle become less compliant in chronically shortened positions. It is for this reason that a severe contracture undergoing surgical manipulation is not corrected more than half the lost range for fear of snapping nerves and occluding blood vessels. These soft tissues will require gradual stretching techniques postoperatively to achieve reversal of the second half of lost range. Skin contracture requiring special surgical intervention is also seen.

Human biopsy studies of contractured muscle have shown decreased fiber lengths for patients with cerebral palsy (48). Shorter than normal muscle fiber lengths have fewer sarcomeres in series. When muscle fibers with fewer

---

TABLE 50-1 Common Patterns of Upper Motoneuron Dysfunction

UPPER LIMB	LOWER LIMB
Adducted/internally rotated Shoulder	Flexed hip
	Scissoring thigh(s)
Flexed elbow	Stiff knee
Pronated forearm	Flexed knee
Bent wrist	Equinovarus foot with curl or claw toes
Clenched fist	Valgus foot
Thumb-in-palm	
Intrinsic plus hand	Hitchhiker hyperextended great toe

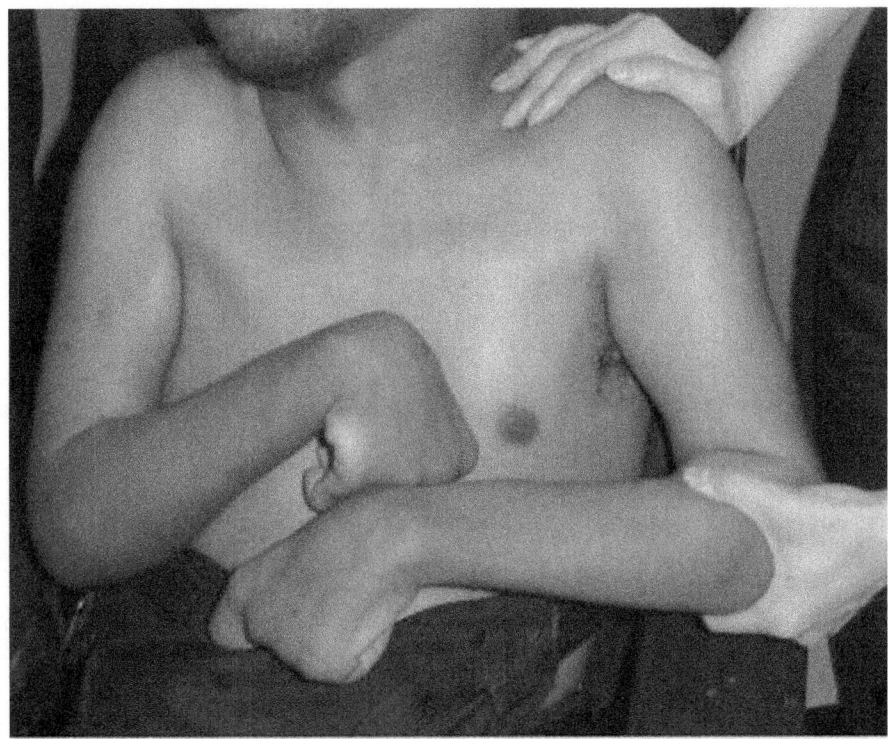

FIGURE 50–10 A familiar upper motoneuron (UMN) pattern of upper limb deformity: adducted/internally rotated shoulder, flexed elbow, pronated forearm, bent wrist, clenched fist, and thumb-in-palm. The position of a given joint results from a net balance of static and dynamic muscle forces acting across one or more joints that are promoted by a variety of UMN phenomena that are triggered frequently, likely every day (e.g., spasticity, co-contraction, flexor and extensor spasms, associated reactions).

sarcomeres are stretched during normal concentric movement, stretched sarcomeres become longer, more so than normal muscle fibers. During stretch, these longer sarcomeres are thought to be the main reason that many patients with cerebral palsy have excessive passive tension in their muscles. Similar processes might conceivably account for elevated passive tension in adults with UMN lesions. In contrast, Friden and Lieber (49) found that single fibers taken from spastic subjects with cerebral palsy developed passive tension at significantly shorter sarcomere lengths than fibers taken from subjects without spasticity. Muscle fibers were almost twice as stiff as controls, and resting sarcomere

lengths were shorter. Friden and Lieber found that force borne by spastic fibers was similar to normal fibers, even though the cross-sectional area of spastic fibers was less by two-thirds. When such spastic fibers were passively stretched, greater stress resulted. Their study suggested that sarcomeres in cerebral palsy do not have to be stretched beyond normal lengths to develop excessive passive tension. From this perspective, their study challenges the assumption that tendon lengthening or stretching exercises that aim to allow a muscle to relax at normal sarcomere lengths will lessen passive tension to normal levels. Their study challenges the current theoretical framework, suggesting that as muscle-

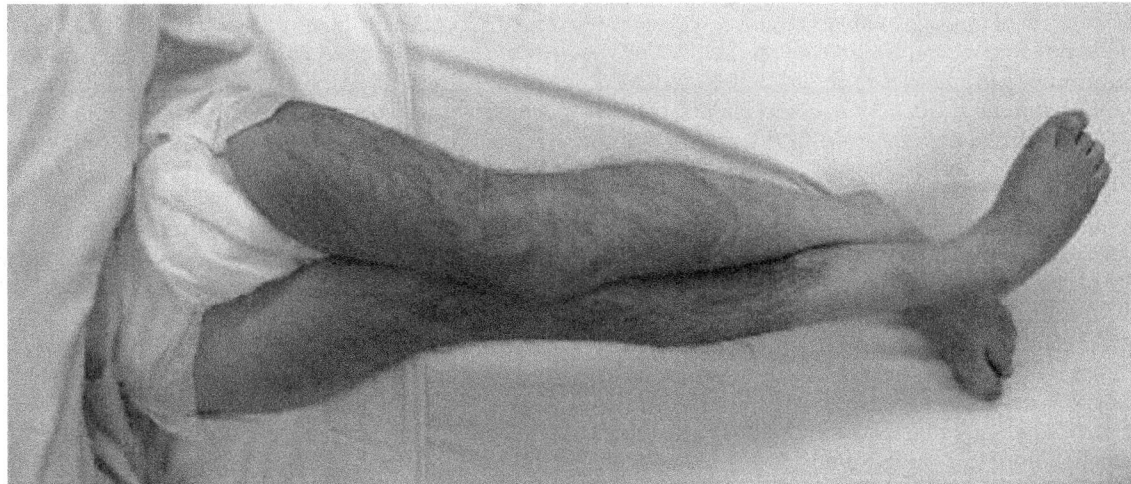

FIGURE 50–11 A familiar upper motoneuron (UMN) pattern of lower limb deformity: flexed hip, adducted (scissoring thighs); flexed knee; stiff knee; and equinovarus foot

tendon length is adjusted appropriately, sarcomeres will operate over a more normal range of lengths, with a reduction in passive tension and an increase in dynamic force potential. Their study of chronic spastic muscle fibers (during childhood development) points to a process of considerable structural remodeling of muscle components that may not be easily reversed by current surgical or physical manipulations.

GENERAL COMMENTS ON THE APPROACH TO EVALUATION

Clinical Aspects of Evaluation

In broad terms, evaluation of muscle overactivity focuses on 3 issues: (a) identifying the clinical pattern of motor dysfunction, (b) identifying the patient's ability to control muscles involved in the clinical pattern, and (c) identifying the role of muscle stiffness and contracture as it relates to functional problems. In Table 50-1, we identify 14 common patterns of motor dysfunction, organized by joint or limb segment, which are typically found in patients with TBI and UMN lesions. For each pattern, a number of muscles may be involved in motor dysfunction.

Evaluation focuses on the characteristics of these muscles in terms of their voluntary or selective control, type of muscle overactivity, rheologic stiffness, and contracture. Does the patient have voluntary control over a given muscle? What is the nature of a muscle's overactivity? (e.g., Is the muscle spastic? Does the muscle co-contract? Is it dystonic? Is it part of an associated reaction? Does the muscle have increased stiffness when slowly stretched? Is contracture present?). Two or more muscles cross each axis of most limb joints, and each muscle can vary in its UMN characteristics. Because each muscle may contribute to movement of the joint it crosses, information about each muscle's contribution is useful to assess. We often use dynamic EMG to identify the characteristics of muscle overactivity and voluntary control during upper and lower limb movements (see discussion later). We use anesthetic nerve blocks to identify properties of stiffness and contracture in particular muscle groups.

Technology Evaluation

Laboratory measurement of upper and lower extremity motion is a cornerstone of modern analysis of muscle overactivity. Gait and movement analysis is capable of measuring specific contributions of muscles to movement by means of multichannel (dynamic) EMG. EMG activity is linked to simultaneous recordings of joint motion (kinematics) and ground reaction forces (kinetics). Force platforms installed flush with a walkway enable measurement of ground reaction forces during walking and standing, permitting weight bearing and force vector analysis. By means of computer-processed optoelectronic marker systems, 3-dimensional quantitative motion data may be obtained to provide information regarding range, direction, velocity, and acceleration of limb movement during a variety of functional tasks. Clinical interpretations are enhanced by slow motion, stop-action video that provides clearer visualization of walking, reaching, and other motor behaviors. Kinetic forces, kinematics, and dynamic EMG information obtained from patients performing movement tasks allows for more in-depth interpretation of voluntary and involuntary motor behaviors. Similar measurements of passive movement responses combined with prediagnostic and postdiagnostic nerve block data allow for clinical interpretation of tone and contracture. Especially after TBI, it is clear that clinical examination alone is often insufficient to identify voluntary and involuntary characteristics of movements impaired by a UMN lesion. Combined with clinical information, laboratory measurements often provide the critical degree of detail necessary to formulate practical plans regarding treatment of complicated cases.

Considerations Related to Time Course of Motor Recovery

Evaluation and treatment will also depend on a clinician's expectations for motor recovery. Neurological recovery may be divided into 2 periods: an early period during which motor recovery may be expected and a late period when neurological motor recovery has ended. In our experience, neurological UMN recovery after head injury tapers significantly 6 months after injury. Functional recovery is a different story. Even if many years have elapsed after a head injury, altering movements and postures by interventions aimed at specific muscles can produce adaptive functional results. For example, a patient who cannot ambulate because his or her base of support is severely compromised by equinovarus deformity in stance phase may regain ambulation function through neuro-orthopedic interventions that improve the base of support by rebalancing muscles crossing the ankle joint (see Chapter 51 on Neuro-orthopedics by Hosalkar et al.). Functional recovery may occur at any time after head injury provided that the patient has sufficient motor control to take advantage of changes that can be wrought in biomechanical conditions, conservatively or neuro-orthopedically.

Clinical Commentary on Treatment Perspectives

Patients with severe disability after TBI were not considered candidates for rehabilitation, and those with lesser disability who were admitted to a rehabilitation center were given physical rehabilitation based on approaches used for patients with stroke and spinal cord injury. Before 1980, limited emphasis was given to cognitive, behavioral, and psychosocial aspects of TBI. However, the pendulum shifted in the next several decades as professionals began to recognize that families were more vulnerable to the burdensome effects of impaired behavior and cognition than they were to the consequences of physical impairment (50). With a relative reduction in emphasis on physical rehabilitation, treatment of muscle overactivity was approached less aggressively. Drugs used in spinal cord injury and multiple sclerosis such as diazepam, baclofen, and dantrolene were looked on cautiously because of their sedating, fatiguing, and weakening side effects. Nonphysician staff who typically dealt with cognitive and behavioral issues generally thought that surgery was an aggressive choice of last resort and many nonsurgical physicians thought so too, especially because the experience of local surgeons with an interest in neurological problems varied greatly. For their part, surgeons often focused on reducing severe contracture and deformity rather than increasing functional performance. They were also not well acquainted with cognitive and behavioral issues that might affect their preoperative decisions and postoperative care.

We believe that good conservative and surgical methods are available for improving function of patients with muscle overactivity. Psychosocial considerations and time course of motor recovery are important considerations during the planning process. Most importantly, our approach emphasizes a joint-by-joint analysis of muscles that are involved in generating positive and negative signs of UMN—a diffuse pathology that can be highly variable. When TBI produces an upper motoneuron syndrome, the degree of voluntary function that remains is highly variable across muscles and limb segments and must be assessed focally. Distinctions are made between factors that reflect poor production and regulation of movement from those that reflect different forms of muscle overactivity and rheologic tissue factors. These distinctions are based not only on physical examination, but also on technology-based evaluations that provide a sound basis for both conservative and surgical management.

Patterns of Upper Motoneuron Motor Dysfunction

In time, muscle overactivity leads to a net balance of contractile and rheologic forces across joints, resulting in clinically familiar maladaptive postural patterns. Common UMN patterns of motor dysfunction are outlined in Table 50-1. We now expand their description, assessment, and treatment subsequently. The following section elaborates on the description, assessment, and enteral and chemoneurolytic treatments of these maladaptive postural patterns. (Corresponding surgical interventions may be found in Chapter 51 on Neuro-orthopedics by Hosalkar et al.).

The Adducted, Internally Rotated, Flexion Restricted Shoulder

Description, Functional Consequences, and Penalties

Signs and Symptoms: The shoulder is adducted and internally rotated; passive stretching of tight adductors may be painful; some patients have hyperextension as their main problem.

Passive Function: Axillary redness, maceration, and skin breakdown may be present; access to axilla for washing is restricted and problematic for caregivers and patients.

Active Function: Some shoulder adductors are also extensors so impaired voluntary flexion, abduction, and rotation of the shoulder can make whole limb actions such as reaching, pushing, stabilizing, and otherwise placing the hand in space problematic; difficulty raising the arm and placing the hand behind and on top of the head is common.

Differential Diagnosis and Diagnostic Workup

Muscles that may contribute: Restricted abduction and/or external rotation: pectoralis major (PM), teres major (TM), latissimus dorsi (LD), anterior deltoid (AD), subscapularis (SC); restricted flexion or active hyperextension: long head of triceps (LHT), TM, LD, posterior deltoid (PD). Taut tendons of PM, TM, and LD are palpable in the axilla; resistance to passive abduction, external rotation, and extension of shoulder is typically high and may be painful. Restricted motion from capsular tightness needs to be distinguished from muscle hypertonia; examine passive in-ternal and external rotation with humerus at side of thorax and with humerus abducted.

Single voluntary movements: When passive exceeds active range for abduction, abductor weakness or adductor overactivity are considered; when passive exceeds active flexion range, flexor weakness or extensor overactivity are considered; when passive exceeds active external rotation range, external rotator weakness or internal rotator overactivity are considered.

Alternating (to and fro) movements: If voluntary abduction is slower than adduction, voluntary flexion is slower than extension, voluntary external rotation is slower than flexion, then weakness of abductors, flexors, external rotators, and/or overactivity of adductors, extensors, and internal rotators may be present. With so many muscles potentially weak or overactive, dynamic EMG helps supplement clinical examination.

Radiographs should be obtained to rule out restricted motion caused by HO. Local anesthetic blocks may clarify sources of restriction (muscles overactivity, contracture): motor point (MP) blocks for PM, TM, LHT AD, PD; thoraco-dorsal nerve block for LD; access to SC is difficult.

Findings and Treatment Options

Unmasked voluntary shoulder flexion and/or abduction and/or external rotation after diagnostic blocks improve prospects for placing the hand in space, especially for reaching. Consider chemodenervation with botulinum toxin and/or neurolysis with phenol. Use of phenol for large muscles (e.g., LD, PM) offsets the need to use large doses of botulinum toxin in such muscles, thereby preserving the use of toxin for many smaller, more distal muscles; PM, TM, LHT, AD, PD are amenable to both chemodenervation and neurolysis. Limited change in range of motion after local anesthetic block suggests muscle contracture and/or capsular tightness. Drugs for pain and blocks for overactivity may help an aggressive range of motion program for focal contracture.

The Flexed Elbow Deformity

Description, Functional Consequences, and Penalties

Signs and Symptoms: Elbow "riding up" during standing and walking; fist and fingers may contact throat or face; pain may be present on passive stretching.

Passive Function: Reddened, macerated elbow crease, and skin breakdown; caregiver has difficulty with dressing and bathing; flexed elbow, often with abducted shoulder, may affect balance during gait.

Active Function: Restrained elbow extension during forward reaching; bringing objects to and from the body is impaired.

Differential Diagnosis and Diagnostic Workup

Muscles contributing to this deformity may include biceps, brachialis, brachioradialis, and pronator teres (PT). Even extensor carpi radialis (ECR) can provide an elbow flexor force when wrist is held fixed in flexion distally. Resting postures: elbow is flexed, forearm more often pronated than supinated; ECR and PT may contribute when wrist is flexed, forearm pronated; an acutely flexed elbow can lead to stretch injury of the ulnar nerve. Very slow passive stretch establishes the available range of motion and the likely presence of contracture (Figure 50-12). Changing the velocity of stretch from slow to fast helps identify presence of spasticity. Ashworth Scale can provide an ordinal score for hypertonia: take the joint through its fully available passive extension in about 1 second. Brachioradialis and biceps reflex contractions, when present, are easily observed. It is much more difficult to ascertain the contribution of the brachialis for which dynamic EMG study is useful.

When "single" joint voluntary extension movements fall short of the available passive range of motion, flexor overactivity is likely, but extensor weakness and changes in physical stiffness of flexors must be considered. When patient is able to do alternating voluntary movements of flexion and extension, timing and amplitude asymmetries can be identified. When extension movements are visibly longer in duration than flexion movements, overactivity of flexors is likely, but extensor weakness and flexor stiffness may be factors. Amplitude asymmetries have similar implications. In addition, contracture may be present. An effort to move the limb as a whole as in reaching for an object or pushing a door may exhibit flexor or extensor synergy (pattern overlay), either partly or fully. Pattern overlay, a centrally generated phenomenon, is less amenable to relief by peripheral interventions.

Radiographs are obtained when bony block and HO is suspected. Musculocutaneous nerve block in the axillary region can help differentiate role of muscle overactivity vs contracture of biceps and brachialis. A separate MP block of brachioradialis is required to determine its role. Flexor blocks may unmask voluntary extension.

Findings and Treatment Options

If range of motion improves completely after nerve blocks, muscle overactivity without contracture is a likely cause of the posturing. Partial improvement in range or no improvement suggests contracture. Serial casting may be considered, preceded by local anesthetic block or phenol block if a dynamic component has been established by maneuvers described earlier.

An x-ray positive for HO establishes a mechanical block as the likely source of motion impairment. Underlying motor control in the patient with HO may be established using dynamic EMG (even if motion is not present) because the patient with good motor control can produce alternating voluntary recruitment patterns in flexors and extensors, respectively. In the early period of recovery, serial casting, phenol blocks of musculocutaneous nerve, and MP of brachioradialis may be considered. Botulinum toxin is useful for biceps, brachioradialis, brachialis, and PT. Treating elbow musculature should be accompanied by treatment of shoulder, wrist, and finger muscles, as necessary. The limb should be thought of as a whole.

The Pronated Forearm

Description, Functional Consequences, and Penalties

Signs and Symptoms: Forearm is pronated excessively at all times; passive stretching may be painful.

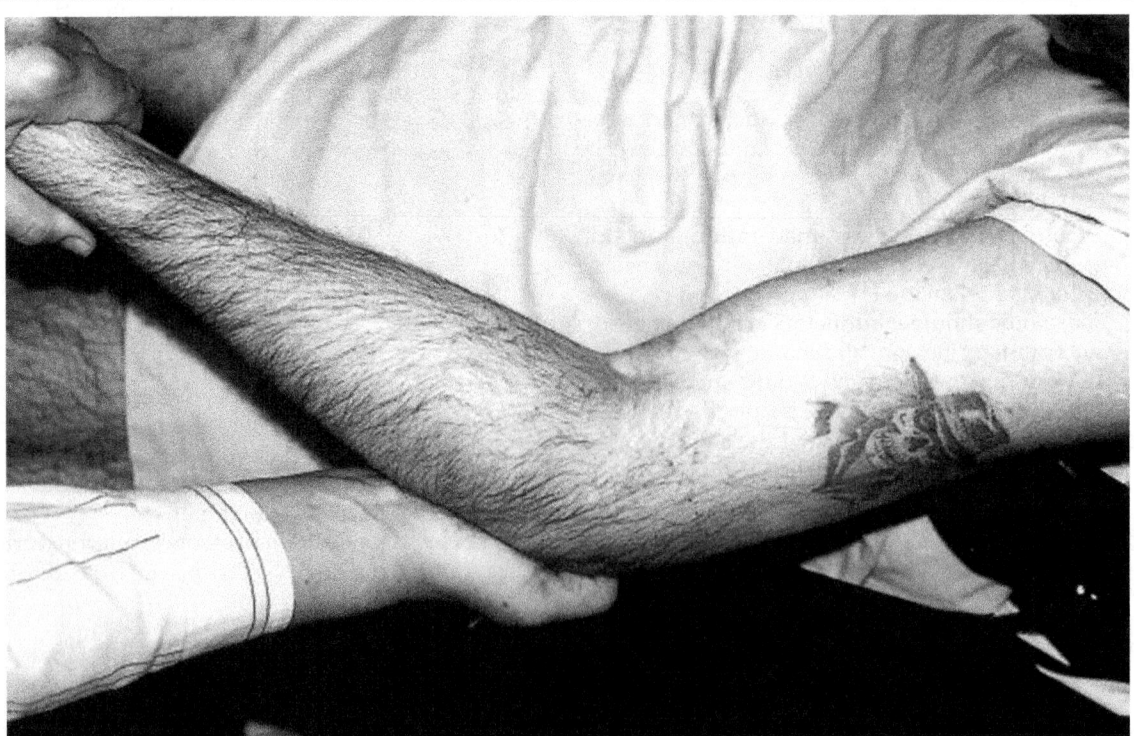

FIGURE 50–12 Example of an elbow flexion contracture. Very slow passive stretch establishes the available range of motion and the likely presence of contracture (fixed shortening). Contracture is a physical phenomenon and requires physical methods of treatment, such as aggressive stretching, serial casting, or surgical lengthening.

Passive Function: It may be difficult to passively supinate palm for washing and fingernail clipping because of tight pronators.

Active Function: Impaired voluntary underhand reaching; patient has difficulty orienting hand to objects.

Differential Diagnosis and Diagnostic Workup

Muscles that may contribute: PT and pronator quadratus (PQ). Resting posture: forearm is pronated; elbow typically flexed by flexor muscles including PT. Very slow passive stretch establishes the available range of motion and the likely presence of pronator contracture. Because PT crosses the axis of rotation of the elbow, an extended elbow may increase tension in PT. Stretching the pronators by passive supination at different velocities helps identify presence of spasticity. Tension in PT is clinically palpable, but PQ is not palpable. Dynamic EMG is useful (Figure 50-13).

When voluntary supination movement falls short of the available passive range, pronator overactivity is likely, but supinator weakness and changes in physical stiffness of pronators must be considered. When a patient is able to do alternating voluntary pronation and supination movements, timing and amplitude asymmetries can be identified. When supination movements are visibly longer in duration than pronation movements, overactivity of pronators is likely, but supinator weakness and pronator stiffness may be factors. Amplitude asymmetries may also suggest pronator contracture.

Radiographs are obtained to rule out bony block, especially if forearm fractures have occurred. MP blocks of PT and PQ (through the interosseous membrane) can be performed to distinguish between intense muscle overactivity and contracture, but it is not usual to do so. Dynamic EMG helps identify patterns of weakness in supinators and overactivity in pronators.

Findings and Treatment Options

When dynamic EMG suggests overactivity in PT and/or PQ and contracture is mild or absent, consider chemodenervation with botulinum toxin. When contracture is present, chemodenervation combined with serial casting can be used but casts must go above the elbow and include the wrist to be effective. When neurological recovery is no longer expected, consider surgical lengthening of PT and PQ.

The Flexed Wrist Deformity

Description, Functional Consequences, and Penalties

Signs and Symptoms: The wrist is flexed excessively; passive stretching may be painful; pressure in carpal tunnel may lead to carpal tunnel syndrome.

Passive Function: Redness and possible skin breakdown in wrist increase; flexed wrist may create difficulty for caregivers during dressing.

Active Function: Impaired wrist extension during reaching; ulnar deviation may be present.

Differential Diagnosis and Diagnostic Workup

Muscles that may contribute: flexor carpi radialis (FCR), palmaris longus (PL), flexor carpi ulnaris (FCU), flexor digitorum sublimis and profundus, extensor carpi ulnaris (ECU) (consider when ulnar deviation is present), weak wrist extensors. Wrist range is examined with elbow extended to maximize flexor stretch (and simulate what would occur during a full reach). Because extrinsic finger flexors as well as wrist flexors can provide stretch-activated flexion forces across the wrist, their respective contributions are sorted out by passive extension of the wrist with fingers held flexed by the examiner and with fingers held extended.

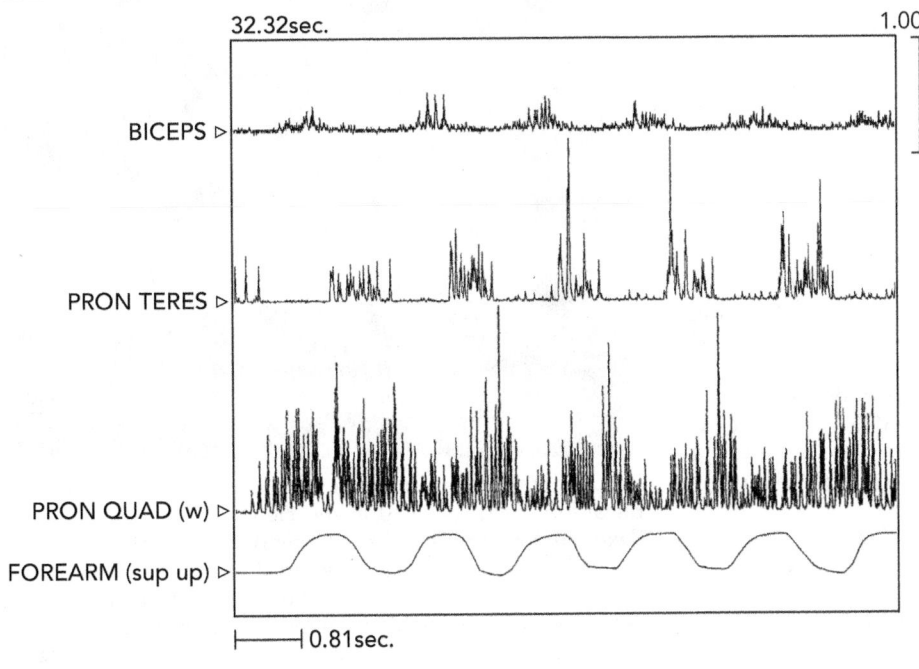

32.32sec.   1.00

BICEPS ▷

PRON TERES ▷

PRON QUAD (w) ▷

FOREARM (sup up) ▷

├──┤ 0.81sec.

FIGURE 50–13 Dynamic electromyography (EMG) study of pronation/supination of the forearm. This patient with traumatic brain injuty (TBI) complained of difficult reaching underhand. The record shows good reciprocal innervation of biceps and pronator teres. When biceps is active as a forearm supinator, pronator teres is inactive. When pronator teres is active as a forearm pronator, biceps is inactive. The same cannot be said of pronator quadratus, which is active during pronation *as well as* supination. These findings are consistent with co-contraction phenomenon in pronator quadratus but not pronator teres. Treatment implication: focal chemodenervation or surgery should be aimed at pronator quadratus, not pronator teres. PRON, pronator.

Passive stretch: bowstringing of FCR is common, PL often involved as is FCU; resistance to stretch is enhanced by holding elbow in maximum available extension; passive abduction with wrist in neutral reveals stretch activity in ulnar deviators (FCU and ECU); when resistance to passive extension of the wrist is enhanced by simultaneous finger extension, extrinsic finger flexor spasticity also contributes to the wrist flexion deformity.

Dynamic EMG is helpful in identifying whether wrist flexor overactivity and/or wrist extensor underactivity is present during reaching, and whether overactivity is present in superficial or deep finger flexors or in both. When selective voluntary extension of the wrist falls short of the available passive range of motion, flexor overactivity is likely but extensor weakness and physical stiffness of flexors may be factors. When a patient is able to do alternating voluntary flexion and extension, timing and amplitude asymmetries can be identified. When extension movements are visibly longer in duration than flexion movements, overactivity of flexors is likely, but extensor weakness and flexor stiffness may be factors. Amplitude asymmetries have similar implications. In addition, contracture may limit extension amplitude. MP block of FCU and/or ECU can help sort their contributions to ulnar deviation.

Findings and Treatment Options

Consider chemodenervation with botulinum toxin for overactive wrist flexors and finger flexors without significant contracture. When contracture and overactivity both limit range, chemodenervation and serial casting are considered. We use an approximate 2-week delay before cast application to allow chemodenervation to take hold. Alternatively, proximal median nerve infiltration with local anesthetic can block not only most of the major wrist flexors, but also most of the extrinsic finger flexors. Proximal ulnar nerve block can be added, if needed. When additional neurological recovery is not expected, consider surgical tendon lengthenings and carpal tunnel release as indicated.

The Clenched Fist Deformity

Description, Functional Consequences, and Penalties

Signs and Symptoms: Fingers are clenched into the palm, wrist most often flexed, but some patients have an extended wrist that will exacerbate finger flexion by tenodesis. Malodor and maceration are common; skin breakdown occurs when fingernails dig into the palm.

Passive Function: Washing and maintaining a dry, clean palm; donning splints and gloves; and filing and painting fingernails all pose problems for patients with a clenched fist and for caregivers (Figure 50-14).

Active Function: Impaired finger extension occurs during reaching; individual fingers or groups of fingers may flex; flexed index and long fingers impair object acquisition through the web space on radial side of hand (Figure 50-15).

Differential Diagnosis and Diagnostic Workup

Muscles that may contribute: Flexor digitorum sublimis (FDS), flexor digitorum profundus (FDP): intrinsic overactivity

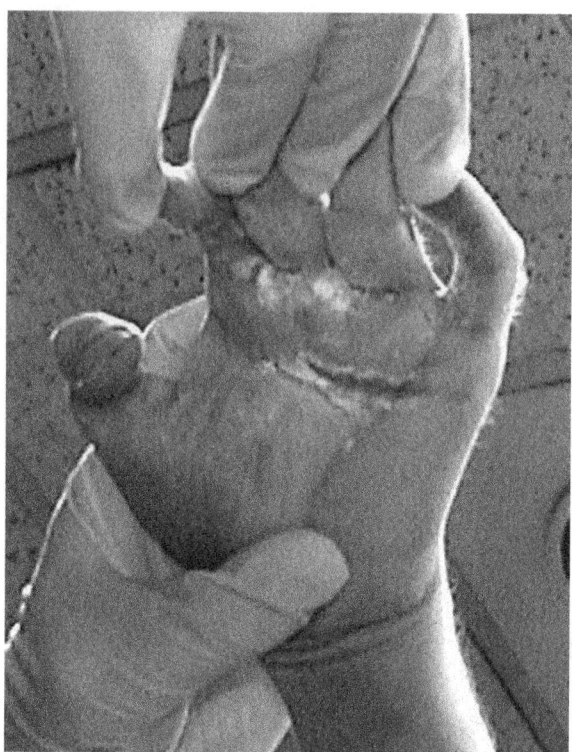

FIGURE 50–14 An example of passive dysfunction of the hand reflected by poor cleanliness and hygiene of the hand. A clenched fist reduces access to the palm for cleaning and leads to moisture retention, malodor, and tissue maceration.

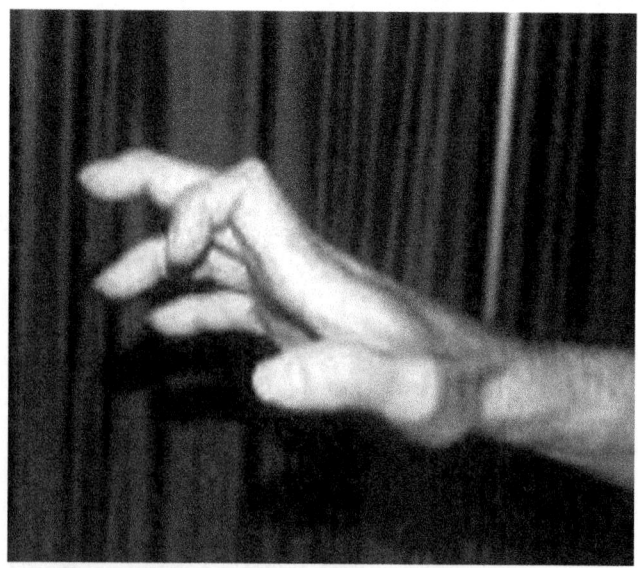

FIGURE 50–15 This photo reveals that individual fingers can be differentially involved in the clenched fist deformity. The flexed index finger and flexed thumb of this patient narrowed the web space opening on the radial side and limited the size of objects that could be acquired by the hand. Focal chemodenervation applied solely to the muscle slip of flexor digitorum of the index finger and to flexor pollicis longus is indicated.

may be masked by strength of extrinsics; weakness of extensor digitorum communis (EDC).

Resting position: When FDP is overactive, fingernails are not easily seen as they dig into the palm; when FDS but not FDP is involved, the distal interphalangeal joint (DIP) is extended; the fingernails are visible; and the proximal interphalangeal joint (PIP) is flexed.

Passive stretch: We examine fingers with elbow relatively flexed and wrist in neutral (when possible) so as not to be fighting overly tight wrist flexors; finger flexor tension is reduced by flexing the wrist, and this allows assessment of intrinsic musculature (interossei and lumbricales) as well as finger joints for contracture. Although many examine the group of extrinsic finger flexors as a whole, we prefer to examine FDS and FDP for each finger individually, keeping in mind that FDP flexes the DIP joint while FDS flexes the PIP joint.

Dynamic EMG with wire electrodes helps distinguish behavior of FDS and FDP during voluntary tasks such as reaching. Dynamic EMG is also useful in determining intrinsic muscle behavior, especially when the stronger extrinsics dominate the clinical picture; wire electrode recordings reveal voluntary behavior of EDC. When selective voluntary extension of the fingers falls short of the available passive range, flexor overactivity and weakness of EDC are likely. Contracture of finger flexors is also common. When a patient is able to do alternating voluntary flexion and extension, timing and amplitude asymmetries can be identified. When extension movements are visibly longer in time than flexion movements, overactivity of flexors is likely, but EDC weakness is typical and flexor stiffness may be a factor. Amplitude asymmetries have similar implications. In addition, contracture may limit extension amplitude.

Findings and Treatment Options

Consider chemodenervation with botulinum toxin for overactive finger flexors without significant contracture. When contracture and muscle overactivity limit range, chemodenervation followed by aggressive ranging and serial splinting may be considered. FDS can be chemodenervated separately from FDP. Individual muscle slips of FDS and FDP can be identified by electrical stimulation through the injecting hypodermic needle. We use electrical stimulation to guide chemodenervation of FDS and FDP because EMG guidance is less certain for these deep muscles. Ultrasound guidance is also useful. When additional neurological recovery is not expected, consider tendon lengthenings. A superficialis to profundus transfer is considered for a nonfunctional hand with major hygiene problems.

The Thumb-in-Palm Deformity

Description, Functional Consequences, and Penalties

Signs and Symptoms: Thumb is flexed into the palm at rest or with effort (Figure 50-16); thumbnail digs into skin.

Passive Function: Impaired access to palm for washing, nail clipping, donning gloves; psychologically bothersome appearance.

Active Function: Impaired 3 jaw chuck, key pinch, other types of grasp; small web space limits size of objects that can be acquired by the radial side of the hand.

Differential Diagnosis and Diagnostic Workup

Muscles that may contribute: Flexor pollicis longus (FPL) and flexor pollicis brevis (FPB), adductor pollicis (AP), first DI. Thumb range of motion and tone are examined with wrist extended and flexed; thumb intrinsics are examined with wrist flexed. Flexion of DIP suggests FPL involvement; carpometacarpophalangeal joint flexion with a flexed wrist points to potential involvement of FPB; a narrowed web space and adducted thumb suggests potential

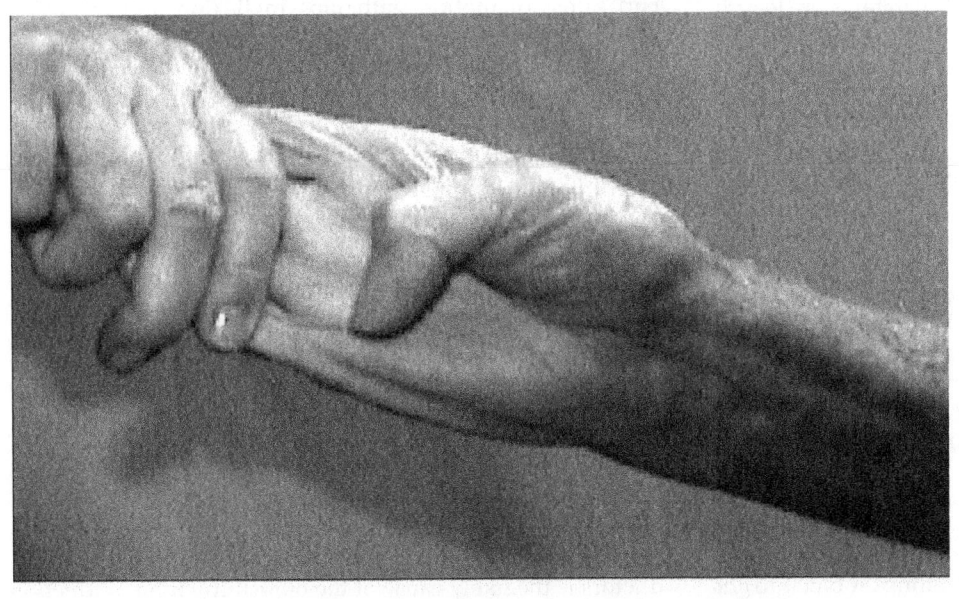

THUMB-IN-PALM WITH WRIST IN NEUTRAL POSITION

FIGURE 50–16 Example of a thumb-in-palm deformity. Flexor pollicis longus is clearly involved. Flexor pollicis brevis must also be considered because of flexion of the metacarpophalangeal joint.

involvement of AP and/or first DI. Voluntary thumb extension is tested with the wrist flexed to minimize FPL tightness. Ulnar nerve block in Guyon canal eliminates overactivity in AP and first DI, opening the web space. If the web space remains narrow, muscle contracture is suggested; examine for skin contracture as well. Median nerve block in the carpal tunnel eliminates median innervated intrinsics of the thenar eminence. Dynamic EMG of thumb intrinsics and extrinsics may be useful in localizing muscle overactivity.

Findings and Treatment Options

If diagnostic block of ulnar nerve in Guyon canal opens the web space, muscle overactivity without contracture is the likely cause of an adducted thumb. Consider botulinum toxin for muscle overactivity without contracture. If web space remains tight after block, muscle contracture is likely; examine for joint contracture as well.

During early recovery, stretching exercises, dynamic splinting, and serial casting may be considered. If FPL is overactive, consider botulinum toxin injection; stretch FPL contracture after toxin injection. When further neurological recovery is not expected, skin, muscle, and joint contractures may be handled surgically. When thumb flexion is weak, fusion of the DIP joint may enhance pinch power. When thumb flexion is adequate, thumb extension by an orthosis with elastic properties is theoretically desirable but often difficult to fabricate. Chemical or surgical relief of the thumb-in-palm (TIP) deformity can enhance "hand as a holder" function, that is, the insertion of objects into the TIP hand for useful holding (without manipulation).

The Flexed Hip Deformity

Description, Functional Consequences, and Penalties

Flexed hip deformity during stance phase with forward flexed trunk. Other findings include compensatory knee flexion during stance phase and relative leg length discrepancy with increased energy consumption. Limited hip extension with shortening of the contralateral step length. Hyperlordosis present in an attempt to keep upright posture.

Differential Diagnosis and Diagnostic Workup

Muscles that can contribute to this deformity: Iliopsoas, rectus femoris, and in some cases, the hip adductors and pectineus. Hip range of motion should be examined with the Thomas test reducing spine motion. The Eli test will help elucidate the contribution of the rectus femoris to the deformity. The hip flexion may be caused as a compensation for equinus deformity and will be evident only during walking but not confirmed by passive range of motion examination of the hip. Involvement of the rectus femoris may be clinically elucidated by observation of gait with knee extension and hip flexion occurring always together.

Dynamic EMG is helpful in clarifying the contribution of rectus femoris vs hip adductors and iliopsoas. Radiographs should be obtained to rule out bony deformity of the hip. Obturator nerve block or a motor branch block to the rectus femoris with local anesthetic can help differentiate the

role of the hip adductors vs iliopsoas or rectus femoris vs iliopsoas. Increase stance phase hip extension following a diagnostic block helps to determine contribution from other muscles. Persistent hip flexion postblock will point to the iliopsoas as the deforming force. Hip adduction deformity may be present in conjunction with flexion.

Findings and Treatment Options

If a temporary nerve or motor branch block results in increased hip extension, spasticity without contracture of the hip adductors or rectus femoris is the likely cause of the deformity. If the hip flexion persists and no radiographic evidence of boney involvement is evident, iliopsoas is the source of the deficit. Botulinum toxin could then be injected to the iliacus followed by stretching. If there is no change in the hip range of motion a contracture is determined. In the early period of recovery, stretching and botulinum toxin to control hip flexion is considered. If EMG studies or blocks demonstrate static origin to the deformity or sufficient time has elapsed for further neurological recovery, surgical intervention should be considered. Stretching of the hip flexors and strengthening of the hip extensors should be undertaken.

The Adducted Hip Deformity

Description, Functional Consequences, and Penalties

Adducted hip deformity during swing phases with narrow base of support (Figure 50-17). Other findings may include associated hip flexion and relative leg length discrepancy with decrease stability in stance phase. Limited hip extension with shortening of the contralateral step length and difficulty with limb advancement in swing phase.

Differential Diagnosis and Diagnostic Workup

Muscles, which can contribute to this deformity, include the adductor magnus, adductor brevis, and adductor longus; in some cases, the iliopsoas and pectineus may be involved. Hip range of motion with hips in flexion and extension should be examined. Limitation in hip extension may be secondary to the limitation in hip abduction. Dynamic EMG is helpful in clarifying the contribution of the adductor magnus, adductor brevis, and adductor longus and the lack of activation of the gluteus medius. Radiographs should be obtained to rule out bony deformity of the hip.

Diagnostic obturator nerve block with local anesthetic can help differentiate spasticity or muscle overactivity from contracture. Increase hip abduction with widening of the base of support following a diagnostic block helps to differentiate muscle overactivity from contracture.

Persistent hip flexion postblock will point to the pectineus or iliopsoas as deforming forces. Hip flexion deformity may be present in conjunction with adduction.

Findings and Treatment Options

If a temporary nerve block results in increased hip abduction, muscle overactivity without contracture of the hip adductors is the likely cause of the deformity. If hip adduction persists and no bone problems are seen on imaging, then

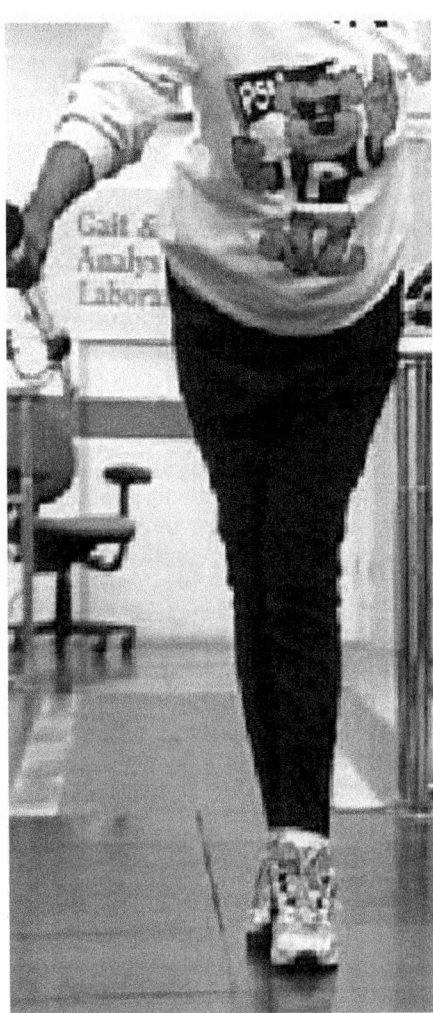

FIGURE 50–17 The consequence of an adducted hip is a narrow base of support.

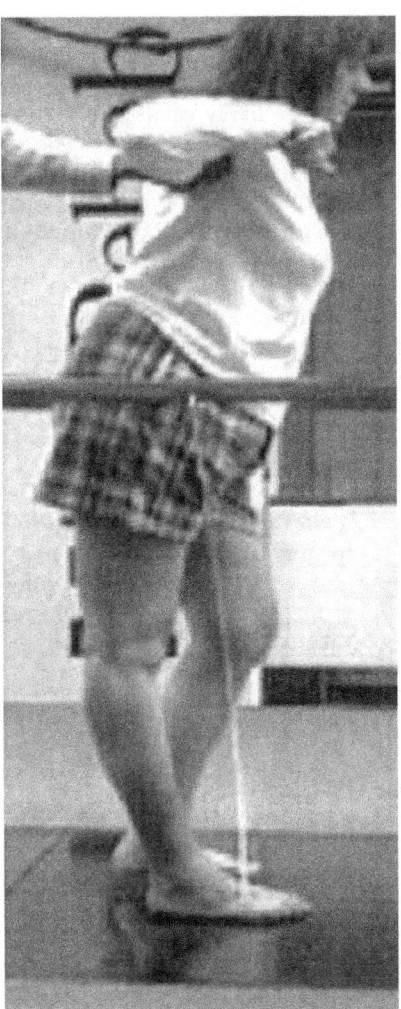

FIGURE 50–18 This patient has plantarflexor overactivity and contracture leading to hyperextension of the knee with recurvatum thrust and impaired forward progression of the body over the stance phase limb.

contracture is the likely source of deformity. Phenol or botulinum toxin can be used to achieve longer term relief of overactivity in the early period of recovery, stretching of the hip adductors and strengthening of the abductors should follow these interventions. If overactivity is severe, obturator neurectomy can be entertained. If blocks demonstrate a static origin of the deformity or neurological recovery has lapsed, hip adductor tenotomy should be considered. Stretching of the hip flexors and strengthening of the hip extensors should be undertaken.

The Stiff Knee Deformity

Description, Functional Consequences, and Penalties
Stiff knee deformity is present during swing phase with impairment of limb clearance (Figure 50-18). Limited limb advancement in swing phase also occurs. Other findings include pelvic hike, trunk lean during stance phase, and relative leg length discrepancy with increased energy consumption. Ipsilateral circumduction and contralateral vaulting as compensatory mechanisms can be seen in swing phase.

Differential Diagnosis and Diagnostic Workup
Muscles that can contribute to this deformity: The quadriceps, hamstrings, iliopsoas, and gastrocnemius. Knee range of motion should be examined with the hip extended and flexed. The knee extension caused by the quadriceps is often noted by inspection during ambulation. Hip extension reduces the stiff knee deformity. Dynamic EMG is helpful in differentiating the contribution of muscles such as the vastii from the rectus femoris. Radiographs should be obtained to rule out bony deformity at the knee or hip.

Femoral nerve motor branch block in the anterior thigh with local anesthetic can help differentiate the role of overactive knee extensors vs hip extensors. Increase swing phase knee flexion following a diagnostic block helps to determine potential for ambulation. Persistent knee extension after femoral motor branch block will point to the hip extensors or ankle plantar flexors as the deforming force. Ankle plantar flexion deformity may be present in conjunction with stiff knee.

Findings and Treatment Options

If a temporary diagnostic femoral nerve motor branch block results in increased knee flexion, muscle overactivity without contracture is the likely cause of the deformity. If the knee extension persists, hip extensors may be the cause of the deformity. If EMG studies or blocks demonstrate dynamic origin to the deformity, botulinum toxin injection or motor branch block with phenol should be considered. Botulinum toxin injection of the hip extensors should be considered. Stretching of the knee extensors and strengthening of the knee flexors should be undertaken. Surgery in the form of a transfer of the rectus to the gracilis and lengthening of the vastii is considered in late recovery.

The Flexed Knee Deformity

Description, Functional Consequences, and Penalties

Flexed knee deformity during stance phase with knee instability with weight bearing (Figure 50-19). Limited knee extension in the terminal swing phase. Other findings include pelvic drop and trunk lean during stance phase and relative leg length discrepancy with increased energy consumption. Limited knee extension with shortening of the step length.

Differential Diagnosis and Diagnostic Workup

Muscles that can contribute to this deformity: The hamstrings, gracilis, gastrocnemius, and adductor longus. Knee range of motion should be examined with the hip extended and flexed. The knee flexion caused by the hamstrings is often noted by inspection during ambulation. Hip extension reduces the flexed attitude of the knee. Dynamic EMG is helpful in clarifying the contribution of muscles such as the medial vs lateral hamstrings or the

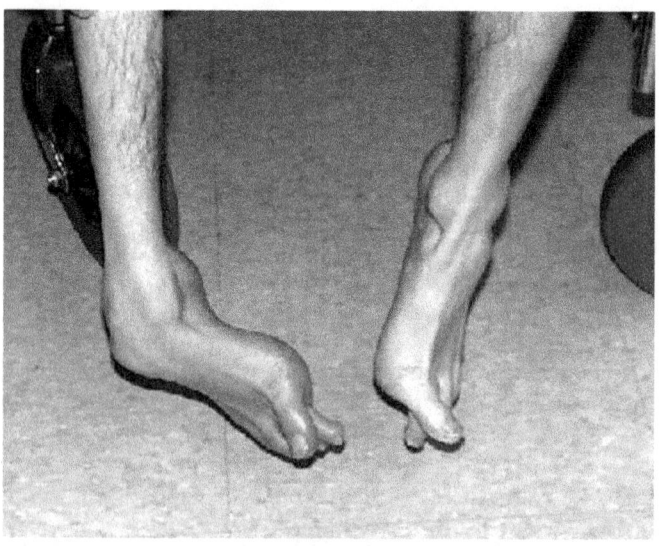

FIGURE 50–19 Two feet with equinovarus deformities in the same patient. As confirmed electromyographically, left foot varus was attributable to tibialis anterior overactivity. Right foot varus was driven by tibialis posterior overactivity. Note bilateral great toe hyperextension, variously termed "striatal toe or hitchhiker's toe."

adductor longus. Radiographs should be obtained to rule out bony deformity at the knee.

Sciatic nerve motor branch block in the gluteal fold with local anesthetic can help differentiate the role of dynamic spasticity with respect to contracture in this deformity. Increase stance and swing phase knee extension following a diagnostic block helps to determine ambulatory potential. Persistent knee flexion post-sciatic nerve block will point to the hip adductors as the deforming force. Hip adduction deformity may be present in conjunction with flexion.

Findings and Treatment Options

If a temporary diagnostic sciatic nerve motor branch block results in increased knee extension, spasticity without contracture is the likely cause of the deformity. If the knee flexion persists, hip adduction may be the cause of the deficit. If there is no significant change in the knee range of motion after a sciatic nerve block, a static deformity, that is, knee contracture is determined. In the early period of recovery, orthotic management to control knee flexion is considered. If EMG studies or blocks demonstrate dynamic origin to the deformity, botulinum toxin injection or motor branch block with phenol should be considered. Stretching of the knee flexors and strengthening of the knee extensors should be undertaken. Surgery in the form of distal hamstrings lengthening is considered for a static deformity in late recovery. A capsular release is considered if knee flexion is present while under general anesthesia.

The Equinovarus Foot Deformity

Description, Functional Consequences, and Penalties

Abnormal base of support during stance phase with weight bearing applied to the lateral border of the foot with pain and ankle instability with antalgic gait pattern. Equinovarus posturing is seen in swing phase. Other findings include hyperextension at the knee with recurvatum thrust (Figure 50-18), impaired forward progression of the center of gravity, and relative leg length discrepancy with increased energy consumption.

Differential Diagnosis and Diagnostic Workup

Muscles that can contribute to this deformity: The gastrocnemius, soleus, tibialis anterior, tibialis posterior, extensor hallucis longus, extensor digitorum, flexor digitorum, and foot intrinsics (Figure 50-19). Ankle range of motion should be examined with the knee extended and flexed. Curl toes and claw toes, subset deformities of equinovarus, are typically generated by overactivity of flexor digitorum longus and the foot intrinsics (short toe flexors), respectively.

The inversion pull of tibialis anterior is often noted by inspection during ambulation. Hind foot inversion is often generated by an overactive tibialis posterior. Dynamic EMG is helpful in clarifying the contribution of muscles such as the tibialis posterior and anterior. Radiographs should be obtained to rule out bony deformity at the ankle.

Tibial nerve block in the popliteal fossa with local anesthetic can help differentiate the role of dynamic spasticity with respect to contracture in this deformity. An improved base of support following a diagnostic block helps to determine ambulatory potential. Persistent ankle inversion post-tibial nerve block will point to the tibialis anterior as the deforming force. Curled toes may be associated with an equinovarus deformity and worsened by increase ankle dorsiflexion.

Findings and Treatment Options

If a temporary diagnostic tibial nerve block results in increased ankle dorsiflexion, muscle overactivity without contracture is the likely cause of the deformity. If varus persists in swing phase, the most likely cause is tibialis anterior and/or extensor hallucis longus. If there is no significant change in the range of motion after a tibial nerve block, a static deformity, that is, contracture is determined.

In the early period of recovery, orthotic management to control equinus is considered, with appropriate components to control ankle inversion and toe flexion. If EMG studies or blocks demonstrate dynamic origin for the deformity, botulinum toxin injection or percutaneous MP blocks with phenol should be considered. Stretching of the ankle plantar flexors and strengthening of the ankle dorsiflexors should be undertaken. The pain generated by curl toes and claw toes can be handled effectively with botulinum toxin injections. Surgery in the form of Achilles tendon lengthening or intramuscular lengthening is considered for a static deformity in late recovery. An split anterior tibialis tendon transfer (SPLATT) is considered if ankle inversion is present during swing phase and is caused by tibialis anterior. If inversion is caused preferentially by tibialis posterior, a lengthening of this muscle is indicated.

Concepts in Pharmacological Intervention

Pharmacological reduction of involuntary muscle overactivity may be beneficial for selected clinical problems. However, drug treatment of muscle overactivity is often a trade off between a decrement in overactivity against side effects (51). Several drugs including dantrolene sodium, baclofen, TZD, and diazepam are frequently used to treat muscle overactivity in various diagnostic conditions. Their use in TBI must be considered carefully because the side effect of sedation, although typically different for each drug, can prove to be quite problematic in patients with TBI who have arousal or cognitive dysfunction. It is both ironic and sobering that patients with TBI, who often need help for muscle overactivity more than most, are also among the most sensitive to the side effects of these agents with respect to the mental functions of attention and cognition.

Dantrolene Sodium

In contrast to centrally acting drugs such as diazepam and baclofen, dantrolene sodium exerts its effect directly on skeletal muscle fibers. Physiologically, a neural signal to a muscle triggers a motor unit action potential that causes release of calcium from storage sites in the sarcoplasmic reticulum within the muscle fiber itself. Calcium ions initiate cross bridging of myofilaments and the subsequent build up of contractile muscle tension. By influencing the release of calcium from the sarcoplasmic reticulum, dantrolene sodium reduces the force of muscle contraction and, thereby, has the potential for reducing tension in contractile muscles. It should be noted that tendon jerk response and electrically induced twitch tensions of muscle are reduced much more effectively than tetanic stimulation or sustained volitional contraction. In the latter conditions, the amount of calcium released into the sarcoplasmic reticulum over the course of continued stimulation of muscle by nerve activity (whether through volition or through electrical stimulation) tends to accumulate and overcome the inhibitory effects of the drug. This latter observation is important in understanding the use and limitations of dantrolene sodium as a clinical agent.

Dantrolene sodium may be useful in treating short duration, low-frequency spastic phenomena, such as clonus or brief spasms (52) (Figure 50-4). Phasic, small tension spasticity rather than tonic, large tension spasticity is favored for treatment with dantrolene sodium. Patients with TBI who have severe muscle overactivity are not typically responsive to dantrolene sodium. Although its influence on treating muscle overactivity is peripheral, dantrolene sodium apparently has a number of side effects that are central in nature, and it can be sedating to patients with arousal dysfunction. Nevertheless, it may be a reasonable choice for mild-to-moderate spasticity, especially for clonus involving many different muscles. Clonus often remits at a dose level of 50 mg, 4 times daily, although doses of up to 400 mg a day may be used. Cases of hepatotoxicity have been reported, and liver function tests should be monitored, especially in those at risk for liver toxicity for other reasons.

Diazepam

This agent, centrally acting and highly sedating, increases the central inhibitory effects of gamma-aminobutyric acid (GABA) (53). Diazepam appears to bind to receptors located at GABAergic synapses and increases GABA-induced inhibition at those sites. The characteristics of diazepam appear to arise from GABA-related inhibitory effects on alpha motoneuron activity in the spinal cord. Because diazepam also exerts sedative effects in the brain, some of its muscle relaxant properties may be caused by diazepam's ability to produce a more generalized state of sedation. Although it is often successful in reducing muscle overactivity, the primary problem with diazepam is the sedation it fosters. In general, diazepam is not a suitable drug for persons with TBI who have attention or cognitive dysfunction. For patients who have persistent phasic flexor spasms that disturb ADLs or nighttime sleep, small doses of diazepam may be effective in reducing the frequency and intensity of these spasms with tolerable sedation.

Baclofen

This drug, a derivative of GABA, appears to act as a GABA agonist inhibiting transmission at specific synapses within the spinal cord (54). When used as an antispastic agent, baclofen ultimately appears to have an inhibitory effect on alpha motoneuron activity. It is unclear whether this inhibition is presynaptic (through inhibition of other excitatory neurons that synapse with the alpha motor neuron), or whether it is postsynaptic on the alpha motoneuron itself. Nevertheless, the net result of baclofen's action is to inhibit the firing pattern of the alpha motoneuron pool in the spinal cord with subsequent reduction of muscle overactivity in skeletal muscles.

Clinical research studies using baclofen for muscle overactivity have primarily addressed the problems of patients with multiple sclerosis or spinal cord injury who have enhanced flexor reflex afferent activity (55). Baclofen has been effective in these populations, especially when the clinical problem has related to flexor spasms. Oral baclofen is generally initiated at 10 mg a day in divided doses and increased to 80 mg or more as needed. Such high doses will invariably lead to side effects in many patients that can overshadow any benefits. In patients with TBI who are in a persistent vegetative state and are not expected to recover, high doses may be considered because cognitive and arousal functions are not an issue. Nevertheless, on the remote possibility that the patient might be making some recovery, it might be wise to taper the drug periodically and observe.

Oral baclofen has been little studied in spasticity of cerebral origin. Meythaler et al. (56) performed a retrospective review of 35 adult patients with acquired brain injury (ABI) before and after starting treatment with oral baclofen. Twenty-two patients had TBI and were found to have a change in Ashworth grade and deep tendon reflexes in the lower limbs. For the upper limbs, no significant change in Ashworth grade, deep tendon reflexes, or spasm frequency in upper or lower limbs. The average dosage at follow-up was 57 mg baclofen (range: 15–120 mg/day). For the group as a whole, a 17% incidence of somnolence limited the maximum daily dosage. The authors speculated that the lack of effect of oral baclofen on Ashworth scores and tendon reflexes may have been related to their observation that systemic delivery may have profound central side effects at brain level before it reaches adequate concentrations at cervical cord level necessary for affecting upper limb spasticity. Drowsiness, confusion, and memory impairment are known side effects of oral baclofen and can be particularly troublesome for patients with TBI who already have impairments of arousal, attention, and cognition (54,57).

A potential method for reducing central side effects is the intrathecal delivery of baclofen (ITB) (58), an approach for controlling hypertonia in ABI that has more extensive literature than oral ingestion. A drug pump is implanted subcutaneously to infuse baclofen into the lumbar subarachnoid space. Compared with oral administration, the pump allows much smaller doses of baclofen to be used (59–61). Side effects are reduced and effectiveness in refractory cases is enhanced. The pump has an 18 mL reservoir, connected to an intrathecal catheter that is refilled periodically by percutaneous puncture. The rate of baclofen infusion is adjusted by an external computer. The most common adverse effects of ITB include hypotonia, drowsiness, dizziness, nausea, vomiting, hypotension, and headache (62,63). Life-threatening complications have occurred, associated with overdose or withdrawal of medication and often linked to mechanical failure or human error (64–68). Intrathecal overdose can cause coma and respiratory depression. Sudden withdrawal of the drug (e.g., by unrecognized pump failure) can cause an exaggeration of spasticity along with hallucinations and seizures. The system is expensive and potentially hazardous

when technical problems arise. However, the pump system may be useful for patients who have regional muscle overactivity distributed across many lower extremity muscle groups, especially bilateral hip flexor, adductor, and hamstrings groups. Most studies with ITB (as with oral baclofen) have focused on the evaluation of stretch reflexes and spasms while active function has not been systematically investigated (69). In a pilot study, Francisco and Boake (70) reported an improvement in walking speed in 10 patients with poststroke spastic hemiplegia after ITB in combination with physical therapy.

Tizanidine

TZD has muscle relaxant properties, acting as an agonist at alpha-2 adrenergic receptor sites both spinally and supraspinally. Placebo-controlled studies have shown that TZD reduces muscle response to passive stretch in both the spinal and cerebral forms of spasticity, including patients with TBI (71–73). TZD does not appear to confer functional changes (71,74). Adverse effects have included hypotension, sedation, generalized fatigue, falls, dry mouth, reduced renal clearance, and the potential for hepatotoxicity and hypotension (75). In a recent randomized, double-blind, placebo-controlled trial that compared injection of onabotulinumtoxinA into spastic upper limb muscles vs oral TZD or placebo, in subjects with upper limb spasticity caused by brain injury (76), onabotulinumtoxinA produced greater tone reduction than TZD or placebo in finger and wrist flexors at week 3 and 6 and greater improvement in the cosmesis domain of the Disability Assessment Scale (DAS) at that point in time. TZD was not superior to placebo in tone reduction at either time point, and the incidence of adverse events (AE) related to study treatment was higher with TZD than in the onabotulinumtoxinA or placebo groups. They concluded that onabotulinumtoxinA is safer and more effective than TZD in reducing tone and disfigurement in upper extremity spasticity and may be considered as first-line therapy for this disorder.

Sedation, a particular problem for patients with TBI, is the most common adverse effect occurring in almost 50% of patients who use it (76). The amount of TZD that a clinician can use for patients with TBI is necessarily curtailed by its side effects, particularly drowsiness. Hence, its therapeutic effect for muscle overactivity is often limited. In addition to spastic stretch reflexes, TZD has been shown to have a physiologic effect on co-contraction, a common positive sign of UMN activity that hampers voluntary movement (31).

Botulinum Neurotoxin

Pharmacological management of muscle overactivity often requires a balance between acceptable reduction in overactivity and acceptable side effects (77). From this perspective, botulinum neurotoxin (BoNT) is an excellent therapeutic agent because of its focal action without significant side effects (78). In the United States, there are 3 approved formulations of commercially available BoNT-A. They are different and distinct in their formulation, purification, and dosing, and to avoid potential errors in dosing, the US Food and Drug Administration (FDA) has assigned specific identifying names for each agent: abobotulinumtoxinA (Dysport) produced by Ipsen, incobotulinumtoxinA (Xeomin) produced by Merz, and onabotulinumtoxinA (BOTOX) from Allergan. BOTOX is the only product approved at the current time by the US FDA for the treatment of upper limb spasticity, and several clinical trials are ongoing in an attempt to expand their clinical indications. BoNT-B is identified as rimabotulinumtoxinB and branded as Myobloc (Solstice) and is only approved for the treatment of cervical dystonia in the United States. BOTOX and Dysport are approved in multiple countries for the management of spasticity in both children and adults. Xeomin has limited approval for this last indication in a handful of countries at this time.

A recent evidence-based review Report of the Therapeutics and Technology Assessment Subcommittee of the American Academy of Neurology on BoNT for the treatment of spasticity recommended BoNT-A as a class A intervention for reduction of tone and spasticity management and class B for improvement of function (79). A more recent international consensus statement was published and further expanded these recommendations to children and adults with upper and lower limb spasticity (80). A number of double-blind, placebo-controlled studies have reported significant reductions in muscle tone for patients with ABI, primarily stroke (81–83). Yablon et al. (84) performed an open-label study of 21 patients with TBI who had severe wrist and finger flexor spasticity. Improvements were seen in range of motion at the wrist, and in the modified Ashworth Scale, there were no significant side effects. Esquenazi and collaborators (85) reported significant improvement in walking velocity in patients with brain injury after treatment of the upper limb (elbow and wrist flexors) with onabotulinumtoxinA. Brashear et al. (86) performed a large scale multicenter trial of onabotulinumtoxinA that was randomized, double blind, and placebo controlled in persons with spasticity of the wrist and finger flexors after a stroke. The study assessed efficacy and safety of onabotulinumtoxinA in 126 subjects who received a one-time injection of 200–240 units. The primary outcome measure was self-reported targets in 4 areas: personal hygiene, dressing, pain, and limb position at 6 weeks. At baseline, each subject selected one of these areas as the principal target of treatment. Based on Ashworth scores, they found significantly greater improvement in subjects treated with onabotulinumtoxinA in wrist and finger flexor tone at all follow-up visits for 12 weeks than did for subjects who received placebo. In addition, subjects treated with onabotulinumtoxinA had greater improvement in the principal target of treatment at weeks 4, 6, 8, and 12. There were no major adverse events associated with injection of the neurotoxin. Brashear et al. (87) demonstrated interrater and intrarater reliability for the disability assessment scale, based on the 4 targets, as well as for the Ashworth Scale applied to elbow, wrist, finger, and thumb flexors of poststroke patients. Brashear et al. (88) have reported results of an open-label, single-treatment session using rimabotulinumtoxinB in 10 patients with upper limb spasticity (elbow, wrist, fingers). Improvements in Ashworth scores as well as global assessment changes by investigators and patients were obtained. Nine of ten subjects reported dry mouth at week 4 of the study with resolution by week 12. No changes were seen on functional measures. Several scientific studies have demonstrated the efficacy and safety of abobotulinumtoxinA in the management of spasticity (89–91) and some case reports (92) supporting the use of incobotulinumtoxinA at this writing.

BoNT is injected directly into affected muscle groups, usually under EMG, electrical stimulation, or ultrasound guidance causing reversible, dose-dependent muscle relaxation by blocking acetylcholine release at the neuromuscular junction (Figures 50-20 and 50-21).

The purpose of toxin injection is to reduce force generated by UMN muscle overactivity to create a more favorable net balance of forces acting across joints (Figures 50-22 and 50-23).

When target muscles are identified, the toxin's localized inhibitory effect makes it a very useful agent for carrying out focal strategies for managing muscle overactivity. A reduction in excessive tension can lead to improvement in passive and active range of motion and allows for more successful stretching of dynamically and statically tight musculature. More subtly, and more importantly, a patient's improved control over movement and posture may allow for compensatory behaviors during functional activities that rely on active as opposed to passive movement. A reduction in muscle overactivity in one muscle group may have consequences for tone in other muscle groups of the limb through a reduction in the overall effort required to perform movement and/or possibly through changes in sensory information going to the central nervous system from that limb.

In contrast to phenol or alcohol, exposure to the toxin causes reversible denervation atrophy without fibrosis. There are 7 serologically distinct toxins produced by *Clostridium botulinum* that are potent neuroparalytic agents, and these are designated as BoNT A, B, C, D, E. F, and G. Only 2 types (A and B) are available for therapeutic human use. BoNT type A is synthesized as single-chain polypeptides with a molecular mass of approximately 150 kDa. Neurotoxin activation requires a 2-step modification in the structure of the protein. In the first step, the parent chain is cleaved. The result is the formation of a heavy chain tethered by a disulfide bond to a light chain that is associated with 1 atom of zinc. The second activation step, disulfide reduction, requires internalization by the target cell. The toxin must enter the endplate zone to exert its effect. The process is partially dependent on nerve stimulation and independent of Ca^{2+} concentration. Patients typically experience benefits 3–7 days after injection. The duration of action in the management of muscle overactivity is about 3 months, after which reinjection is indicated. Reported adverse events have included excessive weakness of injected muscles, pain at the injection site, nausea, headache, fatigue, and flu-like symptoms. Weakness of adjacent nontargeted muscles can be seen and may vary on the basis of dilution, number of sites injected in a particular muscle, dose, and the ability of the specific toxin used to diffuse. Treatment success, in part, depends on the skill of the injector. Muscle selection, injection technique, and dose must be individualized (see Table 50-2 subsequently).

Nerve Blocks

Nerve and MP blocks are very useful in targeting specific muscles or muscle groups for diagnostic and therapeutic maneuvers. The purpose of the nerve or MP block is to reduce force produced by an overactive muscle or muscle group. A reduction in tension can lead to improvement in passive and active range of motion and allows for more successful stretching of tight musculature. More subtly, and more importantly too, a patient's improved control over movement

Rapid passive stretch & stretch & hold : session 2

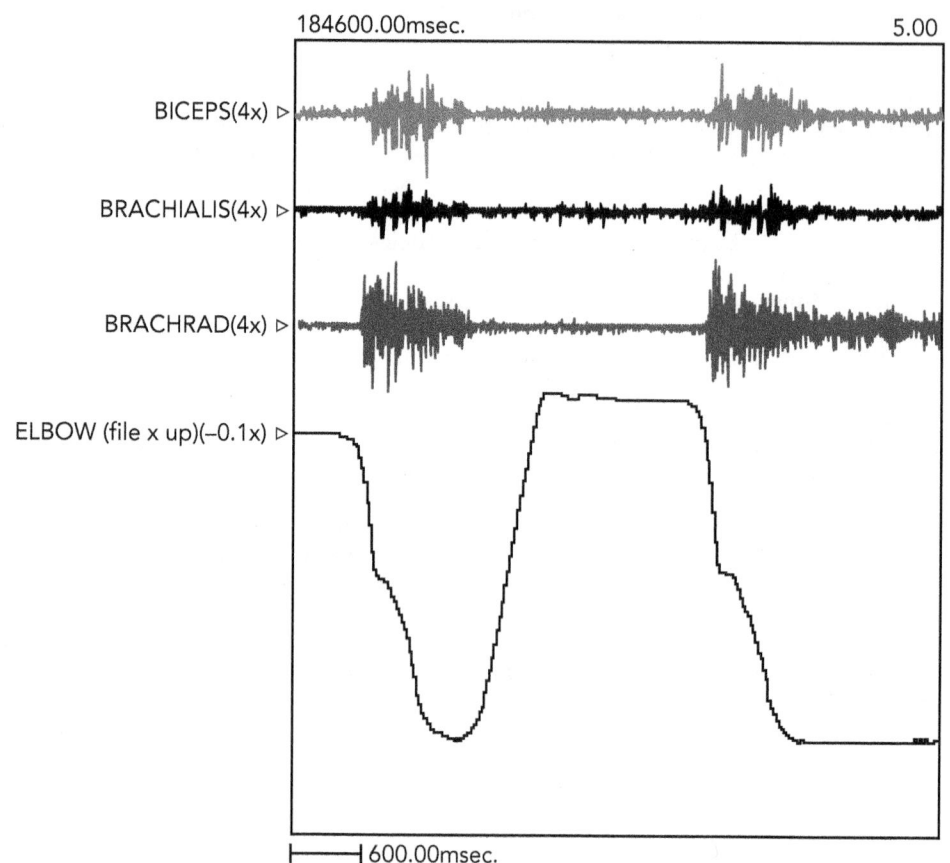

FIGURE 50–20 Prior to injection of botulinum neurotoxin (BoNT) A, rapid passive stretch of elbow flexors followed by rapid passive stretch and hold in a patient with traumatic brain injury (TBI) and hemiparesis reveals spastic reactivity in all 3 elbow flexors during dynamic stretch. Tonic activity is also seen in brachioradialis (BRACH-RAD) during static stretch ("hold" phase). Bottom movement trace shows a "spastic catch" midway during displacement.

and posture may allow for compensatory behaviors during functional activities. A reduction in muscle overactivity in one muscle or muscle group may have consequences for tone in other muscle groups of the limb through a reduction in the overall effort required to perform movement and/or through changes in sensory information going to the central nervous system from that limb. Finally, the application of external devices, such as braces, casts, and even shoes, can be facilitated by nerve and MP blocks.

Blocks may be classified broadly as diagnostic or therapeutic in nature. Diagnostic blocks are typically performed with short-acting local anesthetics such as lidocaine or bupivacaine. These quick-acting, short-duration agents allow the examiner to evaluate factors described earlier such as passive range of motion, muscle stiffness unrelated to overactivity, changes in active range of motion when dynamic resistance is blocked, and enhanced motor control during functional movements. For example, a patient with overactive adductors causing scissoring during gait may be prone to fall because of the narrow base of support. A temporary block of the obturator nerve with 2% lidocaine will allow the examiner to observe whether the base of support widens and stability improves. The key to understanding the use of a diagnostic nerve block is that it is used to test a hypothesis. In the given example, the hypothesis behind the obturator nerve block is that the base of support was narrowed by excessive adduction of the leg caused by spastic adductors. It was further postulated that a wider base of support would lead to greater stability during dynamic gait. After the nerve

block is performed with a quick-acting local anesthetic, the patient is ambulated to test the hypotheses about widening the base of support and improving stability during ambulation. If improved ambulation results, then more permanent (i.e., less reversible) types of intervention may be contemplated with a greater sense of outcome prediction. Therefore, the prediction of a likely outcome for an intervention is an important feature of temporary nerve or MP blocks. In the given example, it is possible that the base of support might not widen. For example, a severe adductor contracture will not remit after a nerve block. However, this information is useful in designing the next step in the treatment program. Similarly, it is possible that the nerve block may be physiologically successful, spasticity of the adductors are blocked, and the base of support widens. Yet, the overall gait pattern is only partially improved because instability was coming from other sources of neuromuscular neurological impairment. Again, this kind of information can lead to further diagnostic testing of other hypotheses relevant to why the patient has an ambulation dysfunction.

Therapeutic nerve and MP blocks are primarily performed with aqueous solutions of phenol. When it is injected in or near a nerve bundle, phenol denatures protein in the myelin sheath or cell membrane of axons with which it makes contact. When administered in the operating room under direct nerve visualization, phenol is instilled directly into the nerve bundle in a glycerin solution to minimize leakage. Related to this technique, the desired motor nerves are identified by electrical stimulation prior to injection,

Rapid passive stretch & stretch & hold : session 3

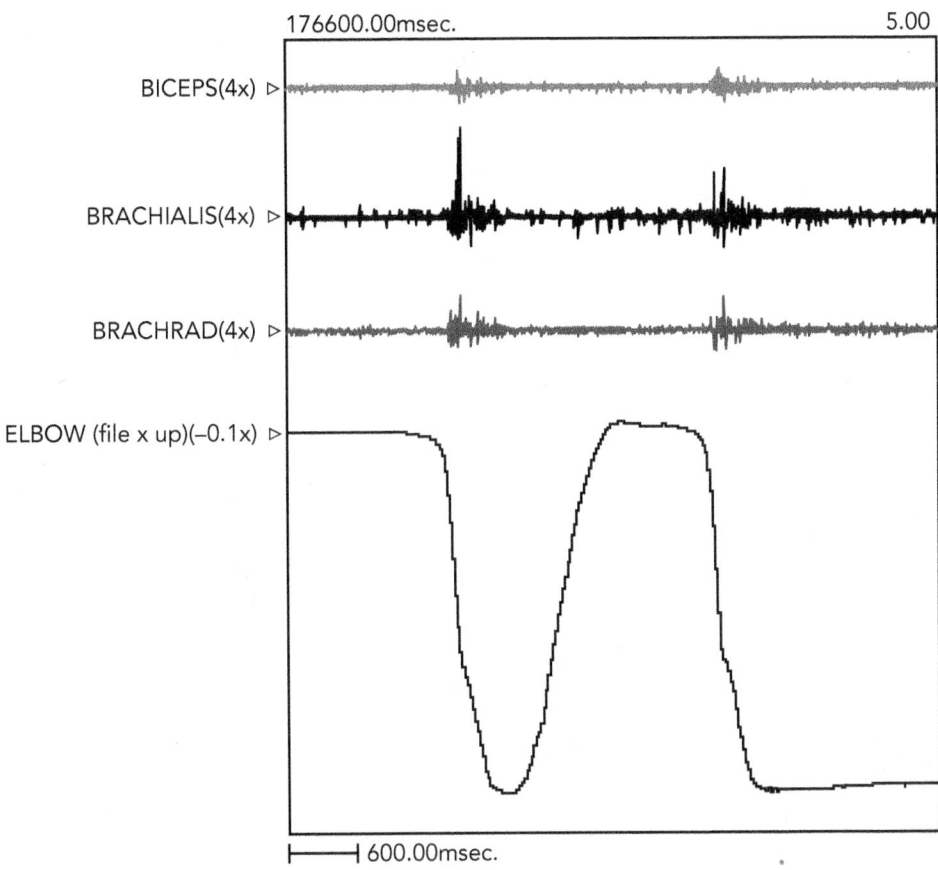

176600.00msec.   5.00

BICEPS(4x) ▷

BRACHIALIS(4x) ▷

BRACHRAD(4x) ▷

ELBOW (file x up)(–0.1x) ▷

├──┤ 600.00msec.

FIGURE 50–21 Biceps was injected with 120 U botulinum neurotoxin (BoNT) A (Botox); brachioradialis was injected with 80 U. This figure is a 22 day follow-up study. Note marked reduction in stretch reflex activity and absence of "spastic catch" in the movement trace. As reflected in electromyography (EMG) of all flexors during stretch, BoNT A inhibits muscle contraction by blocking acetylcholine release at the neuromuscular junction.

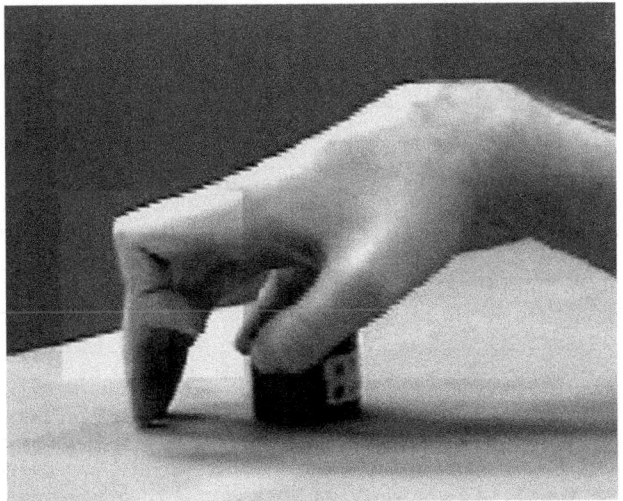

FIGURE 50–22 Flexed index finger during reach to grasp in a 22-year-old woman 2 years after traumatic brain injury (TBI). Muscle overactivity on the radial side of the hand impairs access of objects into the web space of the hand.

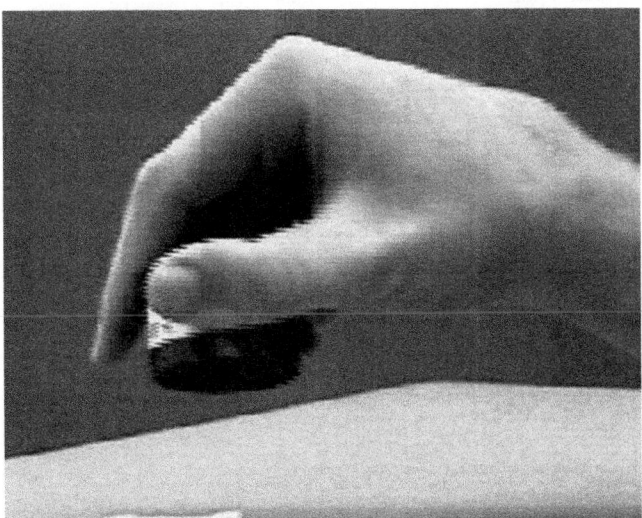

FIGURE 50–23 Twenty-two days after injection of 20 U of botulinum neurotoxin (BoNT) A (Botox) into isolated muscle fascicles of flexor digitorum profundus and flexor digitorum sublimis. Access to the web space was improved and objects were more easily grasped.

TABLE 50-2 Suggested Adult Dosing

CLINICAL PATTERN	POTENTIAL MUSCLES INVOLVED	ONABOTULINUMTOXINA BOTOX DOSE UNITS PER VISIT	ABOBOTULINUMTOXINA DYSPORT DOSE UNITS PER VISIT	NO. OF INJECTION SITES
Upper limb				
Adducted/internally	Pectoralis major	60–140	150–300	3
Rotated shoulder	Latissimus dorsi	80–160	150–300	3–4
	Teres major	25–50	100	1
	Subscapularis	25–50	100–150	1
Flexed elbow	Brachioradialis	40–80	100–150	2
	Biceps	60–120	200–300	3–4
	Brachialis	30–60	150–200	1–2
	Pronator teres	25–50	100–200	1
Pronated forearm	Pronator teres	25–50	100–200	1
	Pronator quadratus	20–40	100–200	1
Flexed wrist	Flexor carpi radialis	40–70	100–200	1–2
	Palmaris longus	30–40	100–175	1
	Flexor carpi ulnaris	20–30	100–150	1
	Extrinsic finger flexors	40–80	100–150	4
Thumb-in-palm	Flexor pollicis longus	20–30	100–150	1
	Flexor pollicis brevis	10–20	50–100	1
	Adductor pollicis	10–20	50–100	1
Clenched fist	Various muscle slips FDP	20 U/slip, (total 80U)	100–200	4
	Various muscle slips FDS	20 U/slip, (total 80U)	100–200	4
Intrinsic plus hand	Dorsal interossei (with diffusion to palmer interossei)	10 U/site, (total 40U)	NDA	4
	Lumbricales (rarely injected; marked atrophy seen at surgery by Dr. Mary Ann Keenan, personal communication)	5–10 U/muscle slip	NDA	4
Lower limb				
Flexed hip	Iliacus	50–100	200–400	1
	Rectus femoris	75–150	NDA	3
Flexed knee	Medial hamstrings	50–150	200–400	2
	Lateral hamstrings	50–150	200–400	2
Adducted thighs	Adductor longus	50–100	500–750	2
	Adductor magnus	50–100	500–750	2
Stiff (extended) knee	Rectus femoris	50–150	NDA	3
	Vastus lateralis	25–50	150	1
	Vastus medialis	25–50	150	1
	Vastus intermedius	25–50	1500	1
Equinovarus foot	Medial gastrocnemius	25–75	150–400	2
	Lateral gastrocnemius	25–75	150–400	2
Curl toes	Flexor digitorum longus	50	150	1
Claw toes	Foot intrinsics (Short toe flexors)	50	100	1

Abbreviations: FDS, Flexor digitorum sublimis; FDP, flexor digitorum profundus; NDA, no dose assigned.

mixed nerves with sensory and motor fibers are avoided because of consequent dysesthesias, and the duration of effect is often 6 months or more because the injection of the nerve is so direct. An aqueous solution of phenol, on the other hand, is the medium used for percutaneous injection in the laboratory or at the bedside, and the location of the nerve is approximated by an electrical stimulation technique that typically results in variable contact of phenol with axons (Figure 50-24). This variability is a key factor in the duration of effectiveness of a percutaneous phenol nerve or MP block. As Glenn (93) has indicated, a peripheral nerve block is more

likely to last longer than a block of a MP (a motor nerve branch located much closer to a muscle than the more proximal peripheral nerve). Phenol neurolysis of peripheral nerve may result in Wallerian degeneration. Reinnervation probably takes longer for the proximally blocked peripheral nerve because it has a longer distance for axoplasm to advance to reach muscle compared with the reinnervation distance of nerve blocked at the more distal MP. The smaller size of the nerve involved in a MP block may also make it harder to localize percutaneously. In addition, if a mixed sensorimotor nerve is selected for phenolization (typically in a low-level

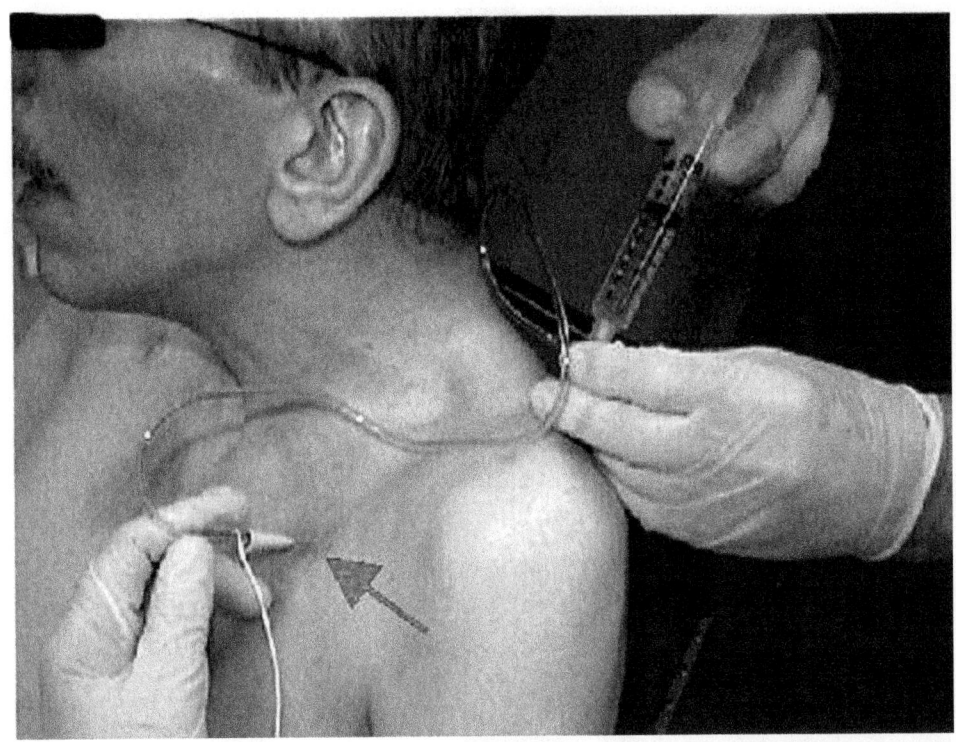

FIGURE 50–24 Phenol injection into a motor point of pectoralis major. A motor point is defined electrophysiologically rather than by anatomy. It is the most distal location of a motor nerve at which electrical current produces a visible or palpable contraction of muscle. The hypodermic needle in the photo is insulated on the outside and has a conductive core on the inside. When connected to an electrical stimulator, the needle is used to find a motor point and, when found, to inject phenol into the region of the motor point.

patient where there is less concern about consequent dysesthesia), a reduction in afferent drive of spasticity may add to the effectiveness of the block as well. It is our impression that a MP block with phenol can influence overactivity for 3–5 months. Nevertheless, reports on duration effectiveness in the literature have varied over a very broad range from several days to 3 years. The reader should glean from this that phenol blocks are temporizing measures and are most effectively used in the period of expectant neurological recovery. The rationale for the other injectable agents such as alcohol and botulinum toxin is, in our view, essentially the same.

The strategy of performing a block is as follows: a surface stimulator is used to locate the selected peripheral nerve or MP. The skin is then prepared with an antiseptic iodine solution, swabbed with alcohol, and subcutaneously anesthetized with lidocaine prior to insertion of the teflon-coated, 22-gauge injecting needle (see Figure 50-24). The electrically conductive inner core of the tip of the needle is used to pass current to the tissues. As the needle is advanced closer to the nerve, less current is required to produce similar amounts of muscle contraction. When a minimal current producing a visible or palpable muscle contraction is reached, we typically inject 3–5 mL of aqueous phenol in concentration of 7%. When injecting multiple nerves or MPs, we usually do not exceed a total volume of 15 mL, and we generally avoid injecting patients taking anticoagulants where the risk of systemic absorption of phenol is greater. (In very large quantities, systemically absorbed phenol can cause seizures, central nervous system depression, and cardiovascular collapse). The essence of the technique is in the clinical manipulation of needle advancement toward the nerve. Depth of penetration and directional orientation of the needle tip require a steady hand, competent knowledge of anatomy, and

a good assistant. Morbidity is typically benign. Local irritation at the site of the block is treated symptomatically with ice, compression, or mild analgesics. We avoid mixed sensorimotor nerves so as not to induce painful dysesthesias, and we substitute MP blocks that involve motor branches only. The injection technique is a good temporizing measure during the period of expectant neurological recovery and facilitates serial casting, range of motion exercises, passive ADL functions, and active movements and function as well.

Some studies have compared phenol and botulinum toxin injections (94–97). Borg-Stein and Stein (94) indicated that a reduction in overactivity after phenol MP block tends to diminish after several months but may last as long as several years. The effect of botulinum toxin appears to last for about 3–4 months with a more complete return to baseline than is generally seen after phenol injection. Botulinum toxin is not associated with dysesthesia but neither is MP block with phenol. Only injection of phenol into a mixed sensorimotor nerve may produce such an effect. The cost of the toxin compared with the cost of phenol is large, and the cost will escalate if multiple injections are required to titrate a desired clinical effect. Also, it is not clear how to control the titration process for an overactive muscle that also has volitional capacity. An ideal agent would eliminate a muscle's overactivity while preserving its voluntary capacity. Moreover, the technique for injecting deeper muscles with toxin requires electrical stimulation to verify the muscle's identity. This requires searching skill akin to the skill of advancing toward a motor nerve using the phenol technique. For deep muscles, EMG guidance does not really specify which muscle is being injected. Such a technique may be useful in dystonia but is riskier in UMN muscle overactivity. Phenol has local anesthetic properties so that one can see an immediate result after injection (Figures 50-25 and 50-26).

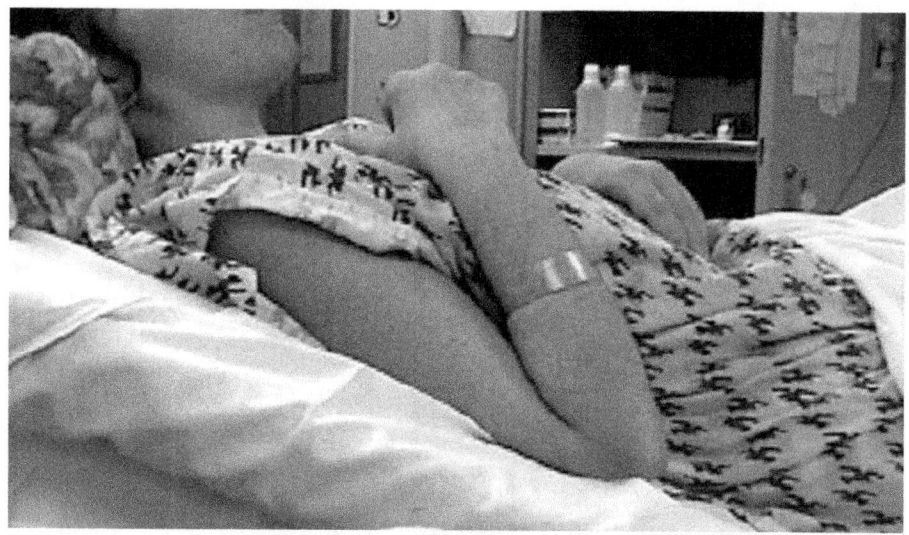

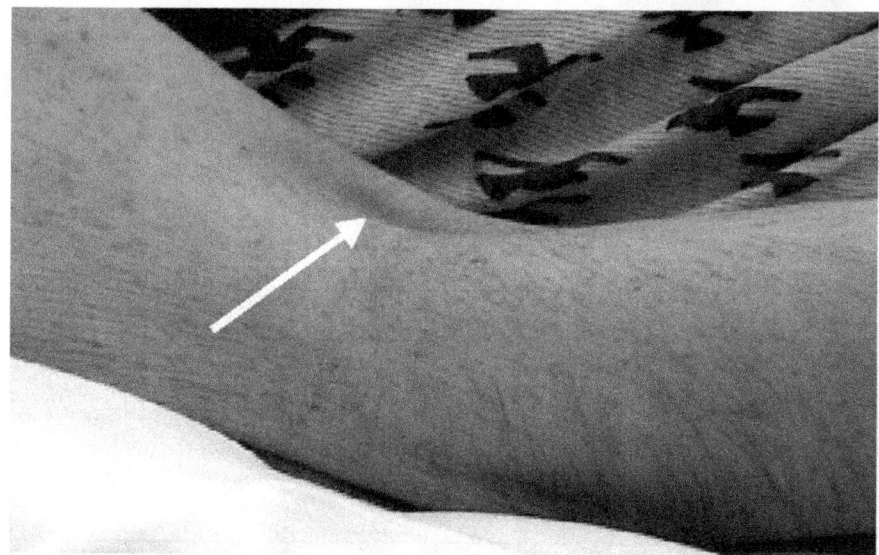

FIGURE 50–25 Phenol has local anesthetic properties so that one can see an immediate result after injection. In this photo, a prominent biceps tendon is observed when the biceps is stretched.

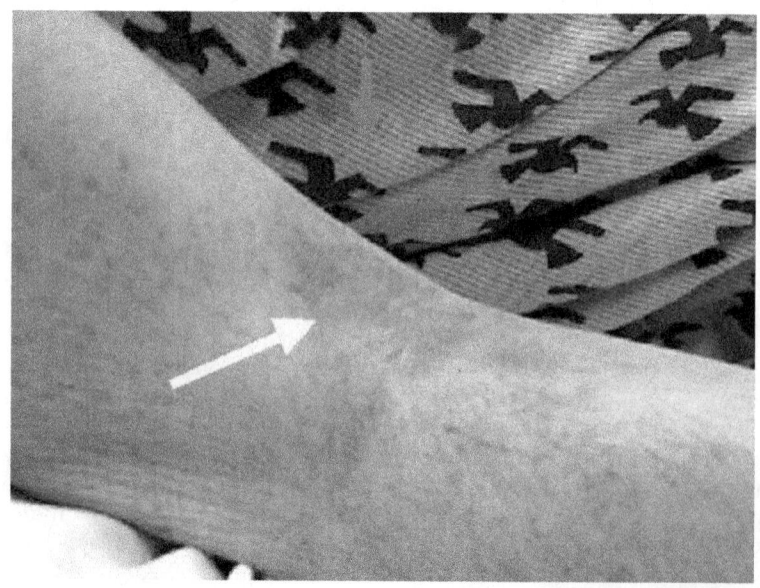

FIGURE 50–26 This photo was taken 5 minutes after phenol block of the musculocutaneous nerve was performed with 4mL of 7% aqueous phenol. The biceps tendon is no longer prominent because the local anesthetic effect of phenol has eliminated stretch reflex activity in the biceps (and brachialis). Beginning of the longer term denaturation effect of phenol is not expected for 48–72 hours after phenol injection.

Botulinum toxin effects are variably seen after 5–14 days. On the whole, injecting botulinum toxin into a single superficial muscle under EMG guidance is quicker than injecting phenol but more individual muscles are injected with the toxin so that total work time may turn out to be a wash. To inject phenol, we typically use an assistant. Botulinum toxin can be managed entirely by the physician. Finally, BoNT and phenol can be used together in situations where large proximal muscles receive phenol blocks and smaller distal muscles receive toxin. Because the current upper range of onabotulinumtoxinA is 600 units, large muscles would absorb most, if not all, of the prescribed toxin leaving little left over for many smaller distal muscles. Hence, phenol applied to proximal musculature spares toxin for use elsewhere.

CONCLUSION

Involuntary muscle overactivity generated by a UMN lesion contributes to the development of typical UMN patterns, such as the clenched fist and the equinovarus foot. Induced by a UMN lesion to contract involuntarily, individual muscles become units of maladaptive structure and function (98,99). Chemoneurolytic agents are able to target such muscles individually, offering focal relief without adverse systemic effects. Future research would do well to improve identification of the best loci of injection to gain maximum physiologic effectiveness while minimizing dosing. In addition, the development of shorter and longer acting agents would allow clinicians to strategize their treatment protocols more effectively.

KEY CLINICAL POINTS

1. Positive behaviors of the UMN syndrome refer to stretch sensitive and nonstretch sensitive involuntary motor behaviors. Stretch sensitive behaviors include tonic and phasic spasticity, clonus, spastic dystonia, and co-contraction generated supraspinally with volitional effort, which may have a superimposed spastic component added to it. Nonstretch sensitive behaviors include increased flexor reflex afferent activity (such as flexor and extensor spasms and the Babinski response) and associated reactions generated supraspinally.
2. Muscle overactivity is the general term used for positive behavior of individual muscles described by each source of involuntary behavior namely stretch or nonstretch generated motor behaviors.
3. The interaction between positive and negative signs results in a net balance of forces that favors the development of typical UMN patterns (postural configurations) such as the flexed elbow, the equinovarus foot, and others described in Table 50-1 of this chapter.
4. Oral medications are often referred to as "antispastic medications." Ironically, most antispastic (stretch sensitive) agents such as baclofen, diazepam, and TZD are most effective against exaggerated flexor reflex afferent activity—a nonstretch sensitive (hence nonspastic) phenomenon of the UMNS.
5. Because many muscles cross individual joints of the upper and lower limbs, clinical evaluation focuses on determining which of those muscles are involuntarily overactive and contribute to the observed UMN pattern and its associated clinical problems. Accordingly, successful

treatment of focal problems with neurotoxin chemodenervation and phenol neurolysis depends on proper muscle selection. Marketing propaganda aside spasticity, a clinical finding is not in and of itself an indication for treatment. Rather, it is the maladaptive skin, musculoskeletal, and movement consequences of UMNS that serve as indications warranting treatment.

KEY REFERENCES

1. Esquenazi A, Mayer NH. Clinical experience and recent advances in the management of gait disorders with botulinum neurotoxin. In: Jankovic J et al., eds. *Botulinum Toxin Therapeutic Clinical Practice & Science*. Philadelphia, PA: Saunders Elsevier; 2009:192–203.
2. Mayer NH, Esquenazi A. Upper limb skin and musculoskeletal consequences of the upper motor neuron syndrome. In: Jankovic J et al., eds. *Botulinum Toxin Therapeutic Clinical Practice & Science*. Philadelphia, PA: Saunders Elsevier; 2009:131–147.
3. McCrory P, Turner-Stokes L, Baguley IJ, et al. Botulinum toxin A for treatment of upper limb spasticity following stroke: a multi-centre randomized placebo-controlled study of the effects on quality of life and other person-centred outcomes. *J Rehabil Med*. 2009;41(7):536–44.
4. Sheean GL. Neurophysiology of spasticity. In: Barnes MP, Johnson GR, eds. *Upper Motor Neuron Syndrome and Spasticity, Clinical Management and Neurophysiology*. Cambridge, UK: Cambridge University Press; 2001:12–78.
5. Yelnik AP, Simon O, Parratte B, Gracies JM. How to clinically assess and treat muscle overactivity in spastic paresis. *J Rehabil Med*. 2010;42(9):801–807.

References

1. Lewis SL. An approach to neurologic symptoms. In: Weiner WJ, Goetz CG, eds. *Neurology for the Non-Neurologist*. 4th ed. Philadelphia, PA: Lippincott Williams & Wilkins; 1999:17–18.
2. Olney RK, Aminoff MJ. Weakness, myalgias, disorders of movement, and imbalance. In: Braunwald E, Fauci AS, Kasper DL, Hauser SL, Longo DL, Jameson JL, eds. *Harrison's Principles of Internal Medicine*. Vol. 1. 15th ed. New York, NY: McGraw-Hill; 2001: 118–120.
3. Whitlock JA. Neurophysiology of spasticity. In: Glen MB, Whyte J, eds. *The Practical Management of Spasticity in Children and Adults*. Philadelphia, PA: Lea & Febiger; 1990:8–33.
4. Yelnik AP, Simon O, Parratte B, Gracies JM. How to clinically assess and treat muscle overactivity in spastic paresis. *J Rehabil Med*. 2010; 42(9):801–807.
5. Herman R. The myotatic reflex. Clinico-physiological aspects of spasticity and contracture. *Brain*. 1970;93(2):273–312.
6. Dietz V, Trippel M, Burger W. Reflex activity and muscle tone during elbow movements in patients with spastic paresis. *Ann Neurol*. 1991;30(6):767–779.
7. O'Dwyer N, Ada L, Neilson PD. Spasticity and muscle contracture following stroke. *Brain*. 1996;119(pt 5):1737–1749.
8. Aida L, O'Dwyer N, Green J, et al. The nature of the loss of strength and dexterity in the upper limb following stroke. *Hum Mov Sci*. 1996;15:671–687.
9. Nathan P. Some comments on spasticity and rigidity. In: Desmedt JE, ed. *New Developments in Electromyography and Clinical Neurophysiology*. Vol. 3. Basel, Switzerland: Karger; 1973:13–14.
10. Burke D. Spasticity as an adaptation to pyramidal tract injury. In: Waxman SG, ed. *Functional Recovery in Neurological Disease, Advances in Neurology*. New York, NY: Raven Press: 1988; 47:401–23.
11. Burke D, Gillies JD, Lance JW. The quadriceps stretch reflex in human spasticity. *J Neurol Neurosurg Psychiatry*. 1970;33(2): 216–223.

12. Sherrington CS. Decerebrate rigidity and reflex coordination of movements. *J Physiol* . 1898;22(4):319–322.

13. Sherrington CS. On plastic tonus and proprioceptive reflexes. *Quart J Exp Physiol*. 1909;2:109–156.

14. Burke D. Critical examination of the case for or against fusimotor involvement in disorders of muscle tone. In: Desmedt JE, ed. *Motor Control Mechanisms in Health and Disease*. New York, NY: Raven Press; 1983:133–50.

15. Sheean GL. Neurophysiology of spasticity. In: Barnes MP, Johnson GR, eds. *Upper Motor Neurone Syndrome and Spasticity, Clinical Management and Neurophysiology*. Cambridge, UK: Cambridge University Press; 2001:12–78.

16. Nielsen JB, Crone C, Hultborn H. The spinal pathophysiology of spasticity—from a basic science point of view. *Acta Physiol (Oxf)*. 2007;189(2):171–80.

17. Delwaide PJ. Pathophysiological mechanisms of spasticity at the spinal cord level. In: Thilmann AF, Burke DJ, Rymer WZ, eds. *Spasticity: Mechanisms and Management*. Berlin, Germany: Springer-Verlag; 1993:296–308.

18. Veale JL, Rees S, Mark RF. Renshaw cell activity in normal and spastic man. In: Desmedt JE, ed. *New Developments in Electromyography and Clinical Neurophysiology*. Vol. 3. Basel, Switzerland: Karger; 1973:523–537.

19. Jankowska E, Läckberg ZS, Dyrehag LE. Effects of monoamines on transmission from group II muscle afferents in sacral segments in the cat. *Eur J Neurosci*. 1994;6(6):1058–1061.

20. Lance JW. Symposium synopsis. In: Feldman RG, Young RR, Koella WP, eds. *Spasticity: Disordered Motor Control*. Chicago, IL: Yearbook Medical; 1980:485–494.

21. Gracies JM, Wilson L, Gandevia SC, Burke D. Stretch position of spastic muscles aggravates their co-contraction in hemiplegic patients. *Ann Neurol*. 1997;42(3):438–439.

22. Miglietta O. Effect of dantrolene sodium on muscle contraction. *Am J Phys Med*. 1977;56(6):293–299.

23. Pedersen E. Clinical assessment and pharmacological therapy of spasticity. *Arch Phys Med Rehabil*. 1974;5(8):344–354.

24. Rack PMH, Ross HF, Thilmann AF. The ankle stretch reflexes in normal and spastic subjects. The response to sinusoidal movement. *Brain*. 1984;107(pt 2):637–654.

25. Dimitrijevic MR, Nathan PW, Sherwood AM. Clonus: the role of central mechanisms. *J Neurol Neurosurg Psychiatry*. 1980;43(4):329–332.

26. Humphrey DR, Reed DJ. Separate cortical systems for control of joint movement and joint stiffness: reciprocal activation and coactivation of antagonist muscles. In: Desmedt JE, ed. *Motor Control Mechanisms in Health and Disease*. New York, NY: Raven Press; 1983:347–372.

27. Delwaide PJ, Olivier E. Pathophysiological aspects of spasticity in man. In: Benecke R, Conrad B, Marsden CD, eds. *Motor Disturbances I*. London, UK: Academic Press; 1987:153–168.

28. Crone C, Nielsen J, Petersen N, Ballegaard M, Hultborn H. Disynaptic reciprocal inhibition of ankle extensors in spastic patients. *Brain*. 1994;117(pt 5):1161–1168.

29. Okuma Y, Lee RG. Reciprocal inhibition in hemiplegia: correlation with clinical features in recovery. *Can J Neurol Sci*. 1996;23(1):15–23.

30. Fellows SJ, Klaus C, Ross HF, Thilmann AF. Agonist and antagonist EMG activation during isometric torque development at the elbow and spastic hemiparesis. *Electroencephalogr Clin Neurophysiol*. 1994;93(2):106–112.

31. Delwaide PJ, Pinnisi G. Tizanidine and electrophysiologic analysis of spinal control mechanisms in humans with spasticity. *Neurology*. 1994;44(11)(suppl 9):S21–S28.

32. Lance JW. Pyramidal and extrapyramidal disorders. In: Shahani DT, ed. *Electromyography in CNS Disorders: Central EMG*. Boston, MA: Butterworth; 1984:1–19.

33. Denny-Brown D. *The Cerebral Control of Movement*. Springfield, IL: Thomas Publisher; 1966.

34. Gracies JM, Elovic E, McGuire JR, Simpson DM. Traditional pharmacologic treatments for spasticity. Part I: Local treatments. In: Mayer NH, Simpson DM, eds. *Spasticity Etiology, Evaluation, Management and the Role of Botulinum Toxin*. New York, NY: WE MOVE; 2002:44–64.

35. Walshe FMR. "On certain tonic or postural reflexes in hemiplegia, with special reference to the so-called associated movements". *Brain*. 1923;46:1–37.

36. Bourbonnais D. *Quantification of upper limb synkinesis in hemiparetic subjects. Rehabilitation R & D Progress Report 1994*. Department of Veterans Affairs; 1995:118–119 [issue no. 32].

37. Dewald JPA, Rymer WZ. Factors underlying abnormal posture and movement in spastic hemiparesis. In: Thilmann AF, Burke DJ, Rymer WZ, eds. *Spasticity: Mechanisms and Management*. Berlin, Germany: Springer-Verlag; 1993:123– 138.

38. Palmeri A, Weisendanger M. Concomitant depression of locus coeruleus neurons and of flexor reflexes by an alpha-2 adrenergic agonist in rats: a possible mechanism for an alpha-2 mediated muscle relaxation. *Neuroscience*. 1990;34(1):177–187.

39. Thilmann AF, Fellows SJ, Ross HF. Biomechanical changes at the ankle joint after stroke. *J Neurol Neurosurg Psychiatry*. 1991;54(2):134–139.

40. Hufschmidt A, Mauritz KH. Chronic transformation of muscle in spasticity: a peripheral contribution to increased tone. *J Neurol Neurosurg Psychiatry*. 1985;48(7):676–685.

41. Akeson WH, Woo SLY, Amiel D, Coutts RD, Daniel D. The connective tissue response to immobility: biochemical changes in periarticular connective tissue of the immobilized rabbit knee. *Clin Orthop*. 1973;(93):356.

42. Gossman MR, Rose SJ, Sahrmann SA, Katholi CR. Length and circumference measurement in one-joint and multijoint muscles in rabbits after immobilization. *Phys Therapy*. 1986;66(4):516–520.

43. Herbert R. The passive mechanical properties of muscle and their adaptations to altered pattern of use. *Austral J of Physiotherapy*. 1988;34:141–149.

44. Carey JR, Burghardt TP. Movement dysfunction following central nervous system lesions: a problem of neurologic or muscular impairment? *Phys Therapy*. 1993;73:538–547.

45. Tabary JC, Tabary C, Tardieu C, Tardieu G, Goldspink J. Physiological and structural changes in the cat's soleus muscle due to immobilization at different lengths by plaster casts. *J Physiol*. 1972;224(1):231–244.

46. Williams PE, Goldspink G. Changes in sarcomere length and physiological properties in immobilized muscle. *J Anat*. 1978;127(pt 3):459–468.

47. Witzmann FA, Kim DH, Fitts RH. Hindlimb immobilization: length-tension and contractile properties of skeletal muscle. *J Applied Physiol*. 1982;53(2):335–345.

48. Tardieu C, Huet de la Tour E, Bret MD, Tardieu G. Muscle hypoextensibility in children with cerebral palsy: I. Clinical and experimental observations. *Arch Phys Med Rehabil*. 1982;63(3):97–102.

49. Fridén J, Lieber RL. Spastic muscle cells are shorter and stiffer than normal cells. *Muscle & Nerve*. 2003;26(2):157–164.

50. Brooks N, Campsie L, Symington C, Beattle A, McKinlay W. The five year outcome of severe blunt head injury: a relative's view. *J Neurol Neurosurg Psychiatry*. 1986;49(7):764–770.

51. Rekand T. Clinical assessment and management of spasticity: a review. *Acta Neurol Scand Suppl*. 2010;(190):62–66.

52. Mayer N, Necomber SA, Herman R. Treatment of spasticity with dantrolene sodium. *Am J Phys Med*. 1973;52(1):18–29.

53. Davidoff RA. Pharmacology of spasticity. *Neurology*. 1978;28(9, pt 2):46–51.

54. Whyte J, Robinson KM. Pharmacologic management. In: Glenn MB, Whyte J, eds. *The Practical Management of Spasticity in Children and Adults*. Philadelphia, PA: Lea & Febiger; 1990:201–226.

55. Young RR, Delwaide PJ. Spasticity. *N Engl J Med*. 1981;304:28–33, 96–99.

56. Meythaler JM, Clayton W, Davis LK, Guin-Renfroe S, Brunner RC. Orally delivered baclofen to control spastic hypertonia in acquired brain injury. *J Head Trauma Rehabil*. 2004;19(2):158–165.

57. Sandy KR, Gillman MA. Baclofen-induced memory impairment. *Clin Neuropharmacol*. 1985;8(3):294–295.

58. Penn RD, Kroin JS. Continuous intrathecal baclofen for severe spasticity. *Lancet*. 1985;2(8447):125–127.

59. Meythaler JM. Pharmacology update: intrathecal baclofen for spastic hypertonia in brain injury. *J Head Trauma Rehabil*. 1996;12:87–90.

60. Meythaler JM, Guin-Renfroe SG, Grabb PA, Hadley MN. Long-term continuously infused intrathecal baclofen for spastic-dystonic hypertonia in traumatic brain injury: 1-year experience. *Arch Phys Med Rehabil*. 1999;8(1):13– 19.

61. Francisco GE, Kothari S, Huls C. GABA agonists and gabapentin for spastic hypertonia. *Phys Med Rehabil Clin N Am.* 2001;12(4): 875–888.

62. Gilmartin R, Bruce D, Storrs BB, et al. Intrathecal baclofen for management of spastic cerebral palsy: multicenter trial. *J Child Neurol.* 2000;15(2):71–77.

63. Loubser PG, Narayan RK, Sandin KJ, Donovan WH, Russell KD. Continuous infusion of intrathecal baclofen: long-term effects on spasticity in spinal cord injury. *Paraplegia.* 1991;29(1):48–64.

64. Armstrong RW, Steinbok P, Cochrane DD, Kube SD, Fife SE, Farell K. Intrathecally administered baclofen for treatment of children with spasticity of cerebral origin. *J Neurosurg.* 1997; 87(3):409–14.

65. Meinck HM, Tronnier V, Rieke K, Wirtz CR, Flügel D, Schwab S. Intrathecal baclofen treatment for stiff-man syndrome: pump failure may be fatal. *Neurology.* 1994;44(11):2209–2210.

66. Levin AB, Sperling KB. Complications associated with infusion pumps implanted for spasticity. *Stereotact Funct Neurosurg.* 1995; 65(1–4):147–151.

67. Saltuari L, Kronenberg M, Marosi MJ, et al. Indication, efficiency and complications of intrathecal pump supported baclofen treatment in spinal spasticity. *Acta Neurol (Napoli).* 1992;14(3):187–194.

68. Haranhalli N, Anand D, Wisoff JH et al. Intrathecal baclofen therapy: complication avoidance and management. *Childs Nerv Syst.* 2011;27(3):421–427.

69. Vanschaeybroeck P, Nuttin B, Lagae L, Schrijvers E, Borghgraef C, Feys P. Intrathecal baclofen for intractable cerebral spasticity: a prospective placebo-controlled, double-blind study. *Neurosurgery.* 2000;46(3):603–612.

70. Francisco GC, Boake C. Improvement in walking speed in poststroke spastic hemiplegia after intrathecal baclofen therapy: a preliminary study. *Arch Phys Med Rehabil.* 2003;84(8):1194–1199.

71. Smith C, Birnbaum G, et al. Tizanidine treatment of spasticity caused by multiple sclerosis: results of a double-blind, placebo controlled trial. US Tizanidine Study Group. *Neurology.* 1994;44(suppl 9):34–44.

72. Meythaler JM, Gun-Renfroe S, Johnson A, Brunner RM. Prospective assessment of tizanidine for spasticity due to acquired brain injury. *Arch Phys Med Rehabil.* 2001;82(9):1155–1163.

73. Nance TW, Bugaresti J, Shellenberger K, Sheremata W, Martinez-Arizala A. Efficacy and safety of Tizanidine in the treatment of spasticity in patients with spinal cord injury. North American Tizanidine Study Group. *Neurology.* 1994;44(suppl 9):44–53.

74. Bes A, Eyssette M, Pierrot-Deseilligny E, Rohmer T, Warter JM. A multi-center, double-blind trial of tizanidine as anti-spastic agent, in spasticity associated with hemiplegia. *Curr Med Res Opinion.* 1988;10(10):709–718.

75. Taricco M, Adone R, Pagliacci C, Telaro E. Pharmacological interventions for spasticity following spinal cord injury. *Cochrane Database Syst Rev.* 2000; (2):CD001131.

76. Simpson DM, Gracies JM, Yablon SA, Barbano R, Brashear A. Botulinum neurotoxin versus tizanidine in upper limb spasticity: a placebo-controlled study. *J Neurol Neurosurg Psychiatry.* 2009;80(4): 380–385.

77. Gracies JM, Elovic E, McGuire JR, Nance P, Simpson DM. Traditional pharmacologic treatments for spasticity. Part II: systemic treatments. In: Mayer NH, Simpson DM, eds. *Spasticity Etiology, Evaluation, Management and the Role of Botulinum Toxin.* New York, NY: WE MOVE; 2002:65–93.

78. Wissel J, Ward AB, Erztgaard P, et al. European consensus table on the use of botulinum toxin type A in adult spasticity. *J Rehabil Med.* 2009;41(1):13–25.

79. Simpson DM, Gracies JM, Graham HK, et al. Assessment: botulinum neurotoxin for the treatment of spasticity (an evidence-based review): report of the Therapeutics and Technology Assessment Subcommittee of the American Academy of Neurology. *Neurology.* 2008;70(19):1691–1698.

80. Esquenazi A, Novak I, Sheean G, Singer BJ, Ward AB. International consensus statement for the use of botulinum toxin treatment in adults and children with neurological impairments—introduction. *Eur J Neurol.* 2010;17(suppl 2):1–8.

81. Bhakta BB, Couzens JA, Chamberlain MA, Bamford JM. Impact of botulinum toxin type A on disability and carer burden due to arm spasticity after stroke: a randomized double blind placebo controlled trial. *J Neurol Neurosurg Psychiatry.* 2000;69(2):217–221.

82. Simpson DM, Alexander DN, O'Brien CF, et al. Botulinum toxin type A in the treatment of upper extremity spasticity: a randomized double blind placebo controlled trial. *Neurology.* 1996;46: 1306–1310.

83. Bakheit AM, Thilman AF, Ward AB, et al. A randomized, double-blind, placebo- controlled dose-ranging study to compare the efficacy and safety of three doses of botulinum toxin type A (Dysport) with placebo in upper limb spasticity after stroke. *Stroke.* 2000; 31(10):2402–2406.

84. Yablon SA, Agana BT, Ivanhoe CB, Boake C. Botulinum toxin in severe upper extremity spasticity among patients with traumatic brain injury: an open-labeled trial. *Neurology.* 1996;47(4):939–944.

85. Esquenazi A, Mayer N, Garreta R. Influence of botulinum toxin type A treatment of elbow flexor spasticity on hemiparetic gait. *Am J Phys Med Rehabil.* 2008;87(4):305–311.

86. Brashear A, Gordon MF, Elovic E, et al. Intramuscular injection of botulinum toxin for the treatment of wrist and finger spasticity after a stroke. *N Engl J Med.* 2002;347(6):395–400.

87. Brashear A, Zafonte R, Corcoran M, et al. Inter-and intrarater reliability of the Ashworth Scale and the Disability Assessment Scale in patients with upper-limb poststroke spasticity. *Arch Phys Med Rehabil.* 2002;83(10):1349–1354.

88. Brashear A, McAfee AL, Kuhn ER, Ambrosius WT. Treatment with botulinum toxin type B for upper-limb spasticity. *Arch Phys Med Rehabil.* 2003;84(1):103– 107.

89. McCrory P, Turner-Stokes L, Baguley IJ, et al. Botulinum toxin A for treatment of upper limb spasticity following stroke: a multi-centre randomized placebo-controlled study of the effects on quality of life and other person-centred outcomes. *J Rehabil Med.* 2009; 41(7):536–544.

90. Bakheit AM, Fedorova NV, Skoromets AA, Timerbaeba SL, Bhakta bb, Coxon L. The beneficial antispasticity effect of botulinum toxin type A is maintained after repeated treatment cycles. *J Neurol Neurosurg Psychiatry.* 2004;75(11):1558–1561.

91. Bakheit AM, Pittock S, Moore AP, et al. A randomized, double-blind, placebo-controlled study of the efficacy and safety of botulinum toxin type A in upper limb spasticity in patients with stroke. *Eur J Neurol.* 2001;8(6):559–565.

92. Kanovsk P, Slawek J, Denes Z, et al. Efficacy and safety of botulinum neurotoxin NT 201 in poststroke upper limb spasticity. *Clin Neuropharmacol.* 2009;32(5):559–565.

93. Glenn MB. Nerve blocks. In: Glenn MB, Whyte J, eds. *The practical management of spasticity in children and adults.* Philadelphia, PA: Lea and Febiger; 1990.

94. Borg-Stein J, Stein J. Pharmacology of botulinum toxin and implications for use in disorders of muscle tone. *J Head Trauma Rehabil.* 1993;8(3):103–106.

95. Kirazli Y, On AY, Kismali B, Aksit R. Comparison of phenol block and botulinus toxin type A in the treatment of spastic foot after stroke: a randomized, double-blind trial. *Am J Phys Med Rehabil.* 1998;77(6):510–515.

96. Sheean G. Botulinum toxin treatment of adult spasticity: a benefit-risk assessment. *Drug Saf.* 2006;29(1):31–48.

97. Wong AM, Chen CL, Chen CP, Chou SW, Chung CY, Chen MJ. Clinical effects of botulinum toxin A and phenol block on gait in children with cerebral palsy. *Am J Phys Med Rehabil.* 2004;83(4): 284–291.

98. Mayer NH, Esquenazi A. Upper limb skin and musculoskeletal consequences of the upper motor neuron syndrome. In: Jankovic J et al., eds. *Botulinum Toxin Therapeutic Clinical Practice & Science.* Philadelphia, PA: Saunders Elsevier; 2009:131–147.

99. Esquenazi A, Mayer NH. Clinical experience and recent advances in the management of gait disorders with botulinum neurotoxin. In: Jankovic J et al., eds. *Botulinum Toxin Therapeutic Clinical Practice & Science.* Philadelphia, PA: Saunders Elsevier; 2009:192–203.

Neuro-Orthopedics

Harish Hosalkar, Nirav K. Pandya, Keith Baldwin, and Mary Ann Keenan

INTRODUCTION

Orthopedic rehabilitation involves the care of patients with complex musculoskeletal problems, which are global in nature rather than having pathology limited to 1 or 2 anatomic locations. It is a specialty that combines biomechanics and biology in a unique manner with an approach that focuses on improving the functional outcome for individuals with musculoskeletal disability through surgical and nonsurgical management (1–5).

This specialty encompasses patients of all ages, a broad range of anatomic locations, and a variety of musculoskeletal dysfunctions. Orthopedic rehabilitation comprises all of the traditional orthopedic subspecialties, including amputation surgeries, prosthetic and orthotic management, neuromuscular diseases, and the variety of other neurologic disorders, with focus on the musculoskeletal system as a whole as well as on the linkages and couplings between bones, joints, muscles, and the nervous system (2,3).

PRINCIPLES OF NEURO-ORTHOPEDIC MANAGEMENT

It is important to employ a systematic approach to the evaluation, diagnosis, and treatment of extremity deformities and dysfunction in persons with upper motor neuron syndromes from brain injuries. It is important to be as aggressive as possible in diagnosing and treating fractures, dislocations, and peripheral nerve injuries during the period of acute trauma. During the period of physiologic recovery from the brain injury, close collaboration between physicians and therapists yields the optimal result for the patients. During this time, the use of physical and occupational therapies, oral medications, splinting, nerve blocks, and chemodenervation are all helpful to prevent or minimize joint subluxation, contractures, and heterotopic ossification (HO) (2) (also refer to Chapter 50).

Generally, the patient is neurologically stable and most motor recovery has occurred after 6 months. Decisions can then be made regarding neuro-orthopedic surgery to correct limb deformities and rebalance the muscle forces. This is the time of greatest contribution by the neuro-orthopedic surgeon (3).

When evaluating patients with brain injury, questions commonly arise regarding the indications for surgery, the cost, what outcome to expect, and the practicality of this approach. These issues should be considered on an individual basis for each patient. General principles that can serve as guidelines for decision making are outlined.

A. Operate early – before deformities are severe and fixed. Orthopedic surgery is a powerful rehabilitation tool. It is often the only treatment that will correct a limb deformity or improve function. Surgery should not be considered a treatment of last resort when "conservative" measures have failed. The choice of treatment technique—surgical or nonsurgical—should be predicated on which one will provide the most optimal result (3).

B. Better underlying motor control means better function for the extremity. Orthopedic surgery cannot impart control to a muscle. Lengthening a spastic muscle can improve its function by diminishing the overactive stretch response and uncovering any control that was present. Successful surgery depends on a careful evaluation preoperatively to determine the amount of volitional control present in each individual muscle that is affecting limb posture and movement.

C. Distinguish between the function of the extremity and the function of the individual. One should consider *active function* and *passive function of the extremity*. These terms refer to the expected outcomes for a limb but do not indicate the outcome for the person as a whole. Surgical releases of an arm contracted in a flexed and internally rotated position in a hemiplegic patient often allows the person to become independent in dressing even though the arm itself does not have volitional movement (3).

D. Consider the cost of not correcting limb deformities. Allowing limb deformities to occur or persist is detrimental to well-being and quality of life of the person with brain injury. Likewise, the cost of laboratory-based motor control evaluation using dynamic electromyography (EMG); video and motion analysis is relatively modest for the benefits it provides. Dynamic EMG is a one-time expense. The cost of performing an incorrect surgical procedure that fails to correct or worsens a limb deformity is much greater. The cost of performing a surgical procedure is likewise limited when compared to a lifetime of attendant care, spasticity medications, repeated blocks, orthotics to control limb position, complications such as skin ulceration and infection, and lost productivity for the patient and caretakers (3).

SHOULDER

The paretic shoulder is a common source of pain and impairment in patients with traumatic brain injury (TBI). A variety of different factors contribute to the painful, immobile shoulder (also refer to Chapter 49): complex regional pain syndrome; brachial plexitis; inferior subluxation; spasticity with adduction, internal rotation contracture; adhesive capsulitis; spastic abduction; HO, and traumatic lesions such as rotator cuff tears or fractures and dislocations.

Shoulder problems are most often the result of a combination of both neurogenic and mechanical factors. The mechanical problems include fracture malunions, joint subluxation, adhesive capsulitis, HO, and soft tissue contractures. Together, these cause the static component of the deformity. The dynamic component of the deformity or dysfunction is the result of neurogenic factors such as weakness, spasticity, rigidity, impaired motor control, and spastic reactions triggered by distant stimuli. Extremity impairments are also classified whether they cause problems of active function or passive function. Active function implies that the person has some capacity or potential to move the extremity volitionally. Passive function indicates that there is no active movement of the extremity possible. Problems of passive function in an immobile extremity include pain, skin maceration, malodor, ulceration, and contractures, which impair passive mobility needed for hygiene, dressing, and comfortable positioning (1,6–9) (also refer to Chapter 49).

Fracture Malunion

Fracture malunions are common in the patient with TBI. Trauma concurrent with the brain injury may cause complex fractures, which are predisposed to malunion. Shoulder girdle injuries (scapula, clavicle, and acromioclavicular joint) are the most common upper extremity injuries in TBI. Frequently, these injuries can be treated nonoperatively; however, patient agitation and muscle spasticity may necessitate open reduction and internal fixation. Malunion of the proximal humerus may result from inadequate closed reduction or failed internal fixation. These are difficult to treat because of excessive scar formation, HO, and retraction of the humeral tuberosities (9). Treatment of malunited tuberosity fractures is similar to acute injuries, with open reduction of the tuberosity to prevent subacromial impingement. In 3- and 4-part fracture malunions, where the humeral head, shaft, and tuberosities are separated from one another, prosthetic replacement is generally indicated. If there is no evidence of avascular necrosis of the head and a congruent joint in a 3-part fracture, osteotomy and internal fixation may be considered.

Because of the high risk of HO in patients with TBI with fractures (Figure 51-1), stable internal fixation should be obtained so that early motion may be initiated. Prophylaxis for HO should also be considered in the acute injury phase when performing internal fixation in patients with brain injury. The drug therapy we employ is oral diphosphonate 20 mg/kg/day for 6 weeks. Low-dose radiation—single dose 9 Gy limited field—can also be employed. Although this is a common practice in trauma centers; there are no published studies of the effectiveness of prophylaxis of HO in patients with TBI with extremity trauma (10).

On rare occasions, an untreated dislocation of the shoulder is encountered. This is problematic because long-standing dislocation leads to loss of the articular surface of the joint. In this situation, an arthrodesis of the shoulder may be the only surgical option.

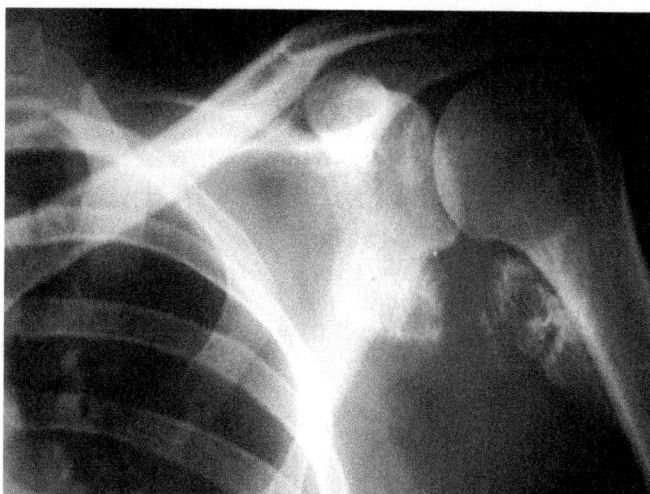

FIGURE 51-1 AP radiograph of the left shoulder demonstrating heterotopic bone formation on the medial aspect of the bone.

Rotator Cuff Tears

When there is weakness of shoulder abduction and pain with shoulder motion, a tear of the rotator cuff should be suspected. The cuff tear may have been present prior to the TBI or may have occurred as a consequence of the traumatic event. The clinical examination is often difficult in patients with brain injury because of their spasticity and inability to cooperate. Patients with spinal cord injury also have an increased rate of rotator cuff tears compared to the general population because of their usage of wheelchair ambulation (11). Definitive diagnosis of a torn rotator cuff is made by magnetic resonance imaging (MRI).

Elimination of pain, reducing abnormal muscle tone, and maximizing joint mobility and strength are of critical importance in restoring function to persons with TBI. A partial thickness tear is treated with oral nonsteroidal anti-inflammatory drugs (NSAIDs) and therapy. Small cuff tears can be repaired arthroscopically. Larger tears with retraction of the rotator cuff may require an open surgical repair. Any surgery done in a patient with an upper motor neuron (UMN) syndrome will result in a significant increase in muscle tone during the perioperative period. This increase in spasticity must be anticipated and treated aggressively (also refer to Chapter 50). Oral antispasmodic medications are often very helpful in reducing spasticity, but their use may be limited by the cognitive side effects of these drugs. Preoperative chemodenervation of the supraspinatus with botulinum toxin is also very helpful. Because the onset of action of botulinum toxin is delayed, the injection should be given 2 weeks prior to surgery.

Heterotopic Ossification

HO of the shoulder is seen in approximately 5% of patients with brain injury (12). When shoulder HO is extensive and limits the mobility and function (active or passive) of the shoulder, surgical resection is indicated. The HO should be mature at the time of surgical resection to prevent recurrence. Maturity of the HO is determined by seeing a well-defined cortical edge on radiographs (Figure 51-1). Serum alkaline phosphatase levels and technetium bone scans are not accurate indicators of the maturity of HO (12).

Shoulder HO radiographically appears to form infero-medial to the joint. Because of the inability to move the shoulder and obtain multiple views, radiographs can be deceiving. Computed tomography is needed to carefully localize the abnormal bone. Surgical approach must be planned depending on the location of the lesion. Following HO resection, active and passive range of motion exercises are begun immediately even if the internal rotators have been released. Strengthening exercises are done in persons with active shoulder function.

Prophylaxis for recurrent HO should also be considered, although no studies have been done to establish the effectiveness of this treatment. The drug therapy we employ is oral diphosphonate 20 mg/kg/day for 6 weeks. In our program, low-dose radiation of a single dose of 9 Gy is reserved only for those patients with very extensive shoulder HO (12).

Inferior Subluxation of the Shoulder

Inferior subluxation of the shoulder is a common occurrence in patients with flaccid paralysis of the shoulder girdle. The patients typically have little or no use of the extremity (also refer to Chapter 49). They complain of greater pain when sitting or standing if the arm is not supported (13). The pain may be caused by chronic stretch on the shoulder capsule, trapezius muscle, or from traction on the brachial plexus. When the pain is lessened by manually reducing the subluxation, it can be assumed to be mechanical in nature and amenable to treatment aimed at reducing the subluxation.

Several procedures have been described to treat paralytic inferior subluxation of the shoulder but none has gained widespread acceptance. Braun has advocated using the coracoacromial ligament to suspend the humeral head. Garland described detaching the proximal end of the long head biceps tendon and looping the tendon over the clavicle and securing it back on itself. With time the paretic biceps muscle tends to stretch and the humerus once again subluxates inferiorly. Shoulder arthrodesis has also been performed but is not well accepted by the patient because it produces a rigid joint, which interferes with passive positioning, hygiene, and nursing care.

The preferred procedure is to convert the long head biceps tendon to a proximally based suspensory ligament (13). This preserves passive shoulder motion while correcting the subluxation. Because only the tendon is being used, there is no opportunity for paretic muscle to develop laxity and for the deformity to recur (Figure 51-2).

Laboratory Assessment of Motor Control

Clinical examination, supported by laboratory studies, is the mainstay of evaluation. The clinical questions of interest regarding a given muscle, which might be targeted for localized intervention, include the following: (a) Does the patient have selective voluntary control over the given muscle? (b) Is the muscle activated dyssynergically (i.e., in antagonism to movement) when the patient attempts to move the relevant joint? (c) Is the muscle resistive to passive stretch? (d) Does the muscle have fixed shortening (i.e., contracture: limited range of motion that is attributed, in large measure, to fixed shortening of the given muscle crossing its joint)?

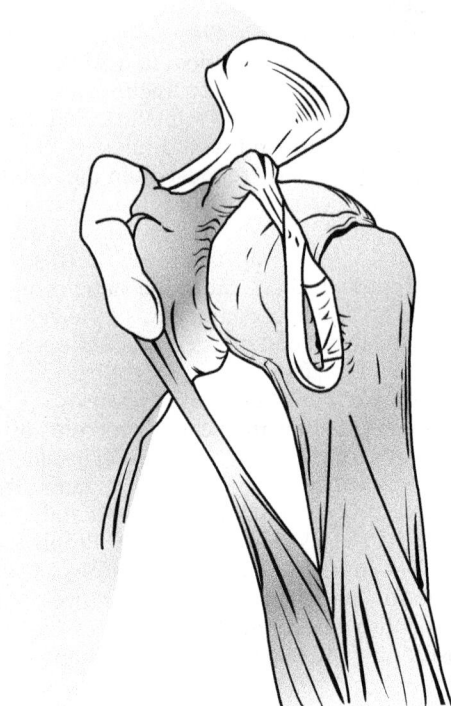

FIGURE 51-2 The biceps suspension procedure.

Laboratory assessments that include dynamic EMG studies and nerve blocks are helpful (also refer to Chapter 50). Dynamic multichannel EMG is acquired with simultaneous measurements of joint motion (kinematics) in the upper extremity (14). Motion and dynamic EMG data (Figure 51-3) assist the clinician in interpreting whether voluntary function (effort-related initiation, modulation, and termination of activity) is present in a given muscle and whether that muscle's behavior is also dyssynergic (also called "out of phase" behavior). In addition, responses to different rates of passive stretch of muscle before and after local anesthetic nerve block can help the clinician distinguish between the dynamic, velocity-sensitive reflex resistance of spasticity vs passive muscle tissue stiffness and contracture. Combined with clinical information, laboratory measurements of muscle function provide the degree of detail and confidence necessary for making conservative and surgical treatment decisions.

The Adducted/Internally Rotated Shoulder

The arm is adducted tightly against the lateral chest wall and shoulder internal rotation causes the forearm to lie against the middle of the chest. Although the tendon of the pectoralis major is prominent with attempts to abduct and externally rotate the shoulder, other muscles routinely contribute to the deformity as well. Shoulder adduction and internal rotation can lead to problems of active or passive function. When patients attempt to reach forward, spastic adductors and internal rotators can severely restrict acquisition of targets in the environment and on the body. The patient's ability to stabilize, push, or apply force to an object is compromised. From the perspective of passive function goals such as skin care and axillary hygiene, spastic adduc-

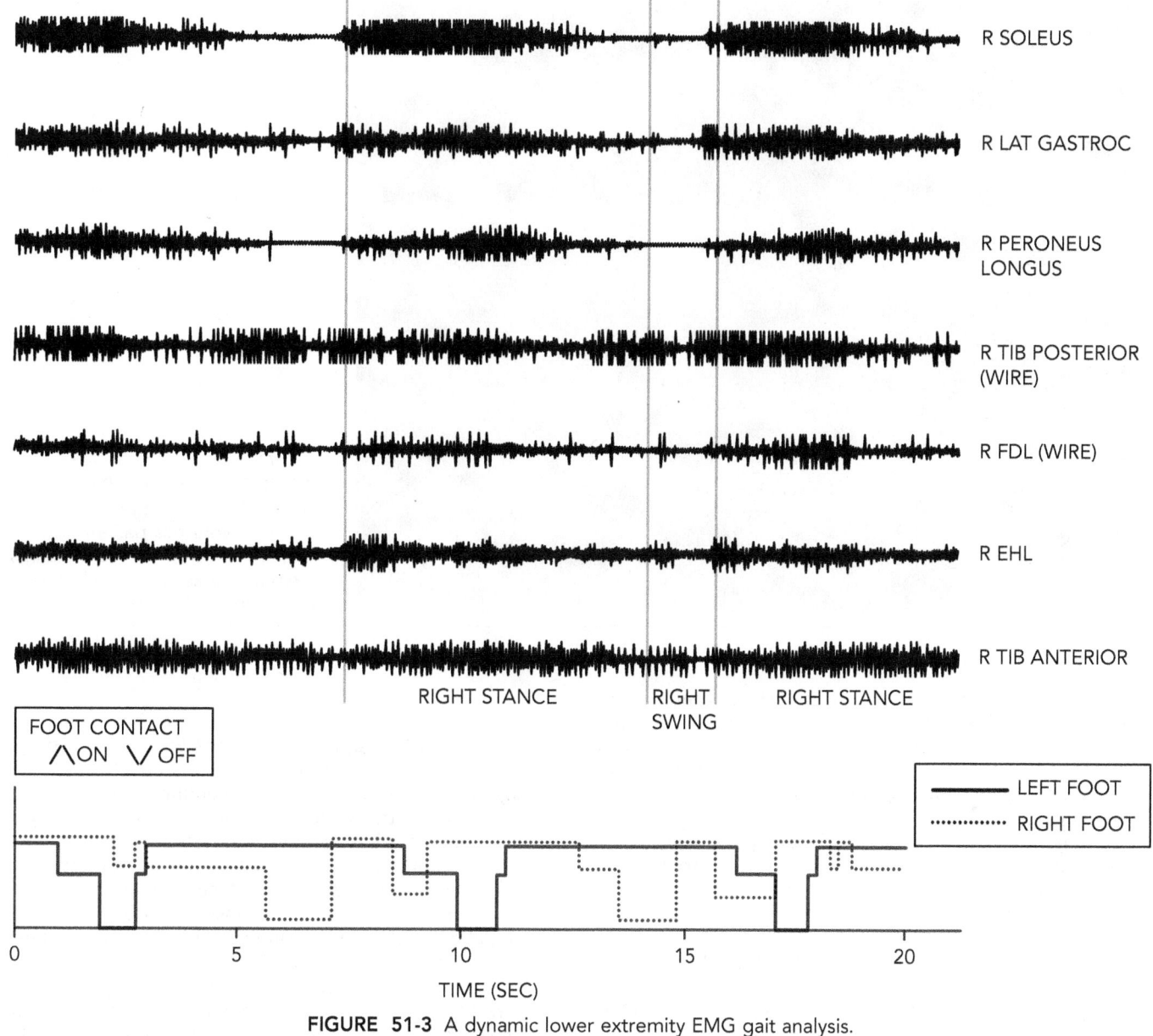

FIGURE 51-3 A dynamic lower extremity EMG gait analysis.

tors and internal rotators hinder efforts of caregivers to gain access to the axilla to provide needed care (Figure 51-4) (also refer to Chapter 49). Restricted motion may impair dressing, washing, and bathing and promote skin irritation and maceration. Passive manipulation of the shoulder during personal care may cause pain when motion and contact trigger spastic resistance in reactive muscles.

Muscles that often contribute to spastic adduction/internal rotation dysfunction of the shoulder include latissimus dorsi, teres major, the clavicular and sternal heads of pectoralis major, and subscapularis. The clinical question is whether the limited forward flexion is a result of weakness of the shoulder muscles or the result of inappropriate activity of the shoulder extensor muscles during forward reach. If the limitation of forward reach is caused by restriction of movement by the posterior muscles, then these muscles can be selectively lengthened. In patients with shoulder contractures who do not have volitional control of their muscles,

release of the pectoralis major, latissimus dorsi, subscapularis, and teres major muscles is usually required to relieve the contractural deformity.

Technique of Anterior Shoulder Release for Contracture

An incision is made on the anterior shoulder beginning at the coracoid process and extending distally. The tendinous insertion of the pectoralis major tendon is identified and released near its insertion with electrocautery. The subscapularis is exposed and isolated from the shoulder capsule near its insertion on the humerus. Release of the subscapularis muscle is performed without violating the glenohumeral joint capsule. The joint capsule should not be opened because instability or intra-articular adhesions may result. The latissimus dorsi and teres major muscles are identified through

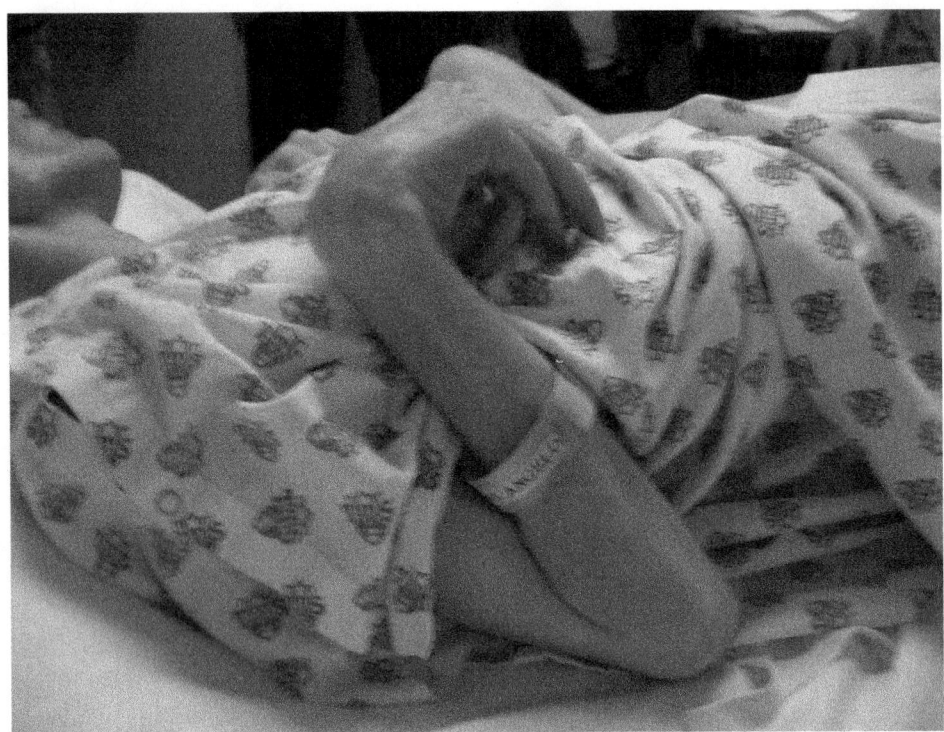

FIGURE 51-4 Spastic adduction and internal rotation contractures at the shoulder. Note this patient also has elbow and wrist flexion contractures, a common presentation with upper motor neuron disease.

the interval between the short head of the biceps and deltoid musculature. Release of these deforming muscles can then be performed in a nonfunctional extremity. A drain is placed deep into the wound prior to closure. Postoperatively, an aggressive mobilization program is instituted following skin healing. Gentle range of motion exercises are employed to correct any remaining contracture. Careful positioning of the limb in abduction and external rotation is necessary for several months to prevent recurrence.

Technique of Selective Shoulder Lengthening

An incision is made on the anterior shoulder beginning at the coracoid process and extending distally. The tendinous insertion of the pectoralis major tendon is identified. The pectoralis is lengthened by transecting the tendon where it overlaps with the muscle belly. This junction can be found on the undersurface of the muscle. The tendon must be transected proximally to avoid complete rupture of the muscle tendon unit. The amount of spasticity in the muscle ultimately determines the amount that the muscle tendon unit will lengthen. A new tendon forms within 3 weeks of the surgery. The latissimus dorsi and teres major muscles are identified through the interval between the short head of the biceps and deltoid musculature and lengthened at the musculotendinous junction (6). When the long head of the triceps is dyssynergic, it is also lengthened. The long head of the triceps can be exposed and lengthened through the same incision.

After surgery, the patient does not need immobilization. Therapy is started on the first postoperative day and consists of active and active-assisted movement of the shoulder. No passive stretching or resistive exercises are permitted until 3 weeks after surgery to avoid overlengthening or rupture of the lengthened muscles (6).

Spastic Abduction

Overactivity of the supraspinatus muscle can cause spastic abduction posturing (Figure 51-5). The contracture may be fixed, but is more often dynamic, becoming more prominent with ambulation, transfers, or other attempted activities. The affected arm is held in an abducted posture making balance while ambulating difficult. Patients complain that their balance is thrown off because of bumping into furniture, doorways, and people in crowds. Diagnosis requires examination of the patient at rest and during a variety of activities (also refer to Chapter 50). It is also helpful to elicit from caretakers or family members any history of activities that trigger this posture. Dynamic electromyography is necessary to confirm that spasticity of the supraspinatus muscle is causing the deformity.

Technique of the Supraspinatus Slide

Although most shoulder muscles are not amenable to lengthening procedures that subserve active movement, it is possible to effectively lengthen the supraspinatus by means of a slide procedure. The patient is placed in the lateral decubitus position with the affected extremity uppermost. An incision is made parallel to the scapular spine. The trapezius insertion is detached from the spine of the scapula, leaving a cuff of fascia for later reattachment. The deltoid is retracted laterally. Using a small periosteal elevator, the origin of the supraspinatus is elevated subperiosteally from the medial border of the scapula. The dissection is continued laterally, with care being taken to avoid injury to the neurovascular pedicle at the suprascapular notch. The muscle is then allowed to slide laterally. The trapezius is then reattached to the scapular spine. The remainder of the closure is per-

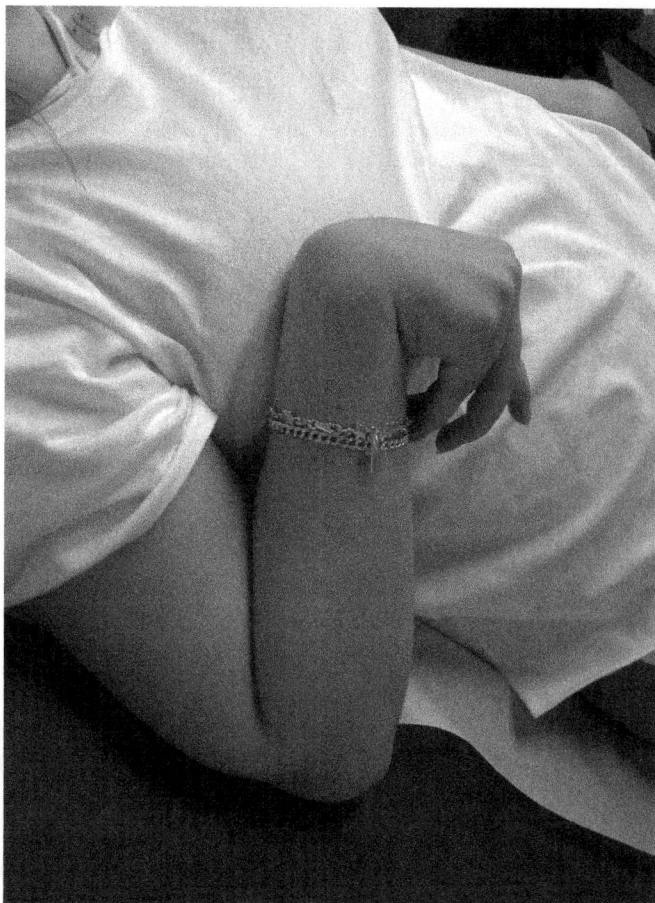

FIGURE 51-5 A patient with spastic adduction contracture of the arm.

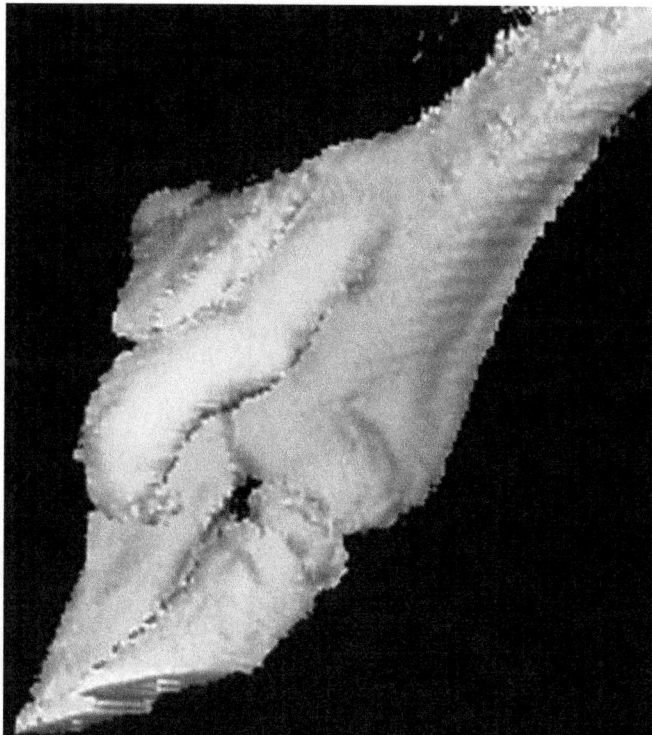

FIGURE 51-6 Anterior heterotopic ossification about the elbow that bridges the humerus and ulna.

formed in routine fashion. The patient is allowed full, unrestricted postoperative motion.

ELBOW

Heterotopic Ossification

At the elbow, HO forms anteriorly and posteriorly. Anteriorly, it forms from the humeral shaft to the ulna with no involvement of the radial head (Figure 51-6) and may involve neurovascular structures. Posteriorly, it forms from the humeral shaft to the olecranon. Ankylosis and ulnar nerve entrapment are common with HO at the elbow (Figure 51-7). Involvement of the radial head is not seen unless there has also been a fracture or dislocation. Therefore, even when there is complete loss of elbow flexion and extension, forearm rotation is commonly preserved. Surgical with transposition of the nerve is necessary to reestablish motion. Following HO resection, active and passive range of motion exercises are begun immediately (15).

Spastic Flexion

Control of limb placement depends on both shoulder and elbow control. Smooth control of elbow flexion and exten-

sion is frequently impaired. This limits the patient's ability to perform activities of daily living.

Elbow extension range is often limited with a very prolonged period of extension. Elbow flexion is relatively normal. Laboratory examination using dynamic EMG helps to confirm the presence of volitional capacity as well as dyssynergy during movement for each of the elbow flexors (16). Dynamic recordings are obtained from biceps, brachialis,

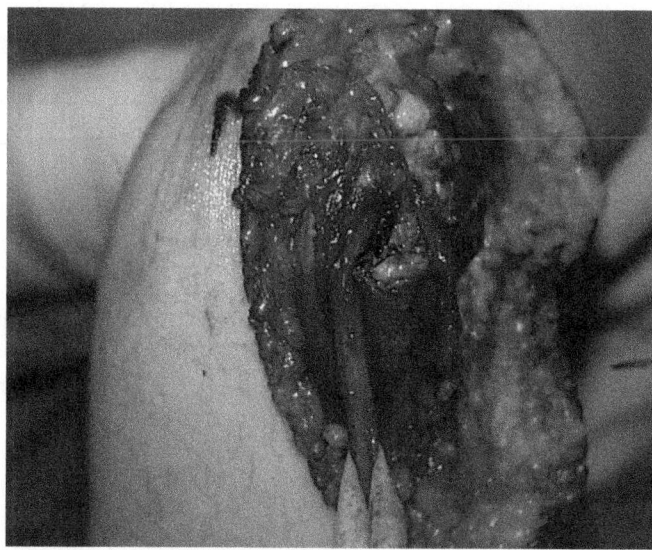

FIGURE 51-7 Interoperative photo that shows the ulnar nerve encased in heterotopic bone.

brachioradialis, lateral, medial, and long head of the triceps. Dynamic electromyography combined with electrogoniometric measurement of elbow motion of patients with stroke and TBI has revealed a consistent pattern of muscle activity responsible for this clinical picture (also refer to Chapter 50). The pattern most commonly seen is that all 3 heads of the triceps muscle are operating in a normal phasic pattern. The brachioradialis muscle most frequently shows continuous spastic activity. One or both heads of the biceps muscle is also spastic. Less frequently, some spasticity is observed in the brachialis muscle. This pattern of muscle activity is also common in patients with cerebral palsy. Armed with this information a rational surgical plan can be devised to improve elbow control.

The Elbow With Active Function: Technique of Selective Flexor Lengthening

Beginning with the biceps, a longitudinal incision is made over the proximal anterior arm starting at the lower edge of the pectoralis major tendon. The muscle tendon junctions of both the long and short heads of the biceps are exposed. The tendons are then sharply transected directly overlying the muscle belly, which allows the muscle tendon unit to lengthen. Next, an incision is made on the lateral aspect of the elbow. The brachialis muscle is exposed and lengthened over its broad muscle tendon junction. Through a separate incision on the radial aspect of the forearm, the myotendinous junction of the brachioradialis is identified and lengthened using the same technique (8).

The Elbow With Passive Function: Technique of Elbow Flexor Release

Persistent spasticity of the elbow flexors causes a myostatic contracture and flexion deformity of the elbow. This results in skin maceration and breakdown of the antecubital space. This position of severe elbow flexion also predisposes the ulnar nerve to an acquired compression neuropathy by increasing the vulnerability to direct pressure and decreasing the cross-sectional area of the cubital tunnel. Surgical release of the biceps tendon and brachioradialis muscles and lengthening or release brachialis is performed depending on the severity of the contracture (8). The joint capsule is not released. Gradual extension of the elbow with serial casting or physical therapy corrects the preoperative deformity and decreases the ulnar nerve compression.

Spastic Elbow Extension

Spastic extension of the elbow is much less common than spastic flexion. These patients have frequently had a brain stem infarct or injury. They complain of difficulty reaching their face for activities of daily living (also refer to Chapter 50). A lengthening of the triceps tendon distally allows improved flexion range of motion (8).

Ulnar Neuropathy

Prolonged elbow flexion with traction on the nerve can lead to decreased volume of the cubital tunnel resulting in nerve compression. Support of the torso by leaning on a chronically flexed elbow may result in direct compression of the nerve (17). The patients are often limited in their ability to complain about ulnar nerve symptoms because of limited cognitive and communicative abilities. The diagnosis is usually suspected because of intrinsic atrophy and confirmed using nerve conduction studies. A 2.5% incidence has been shown in patients with TBI. Treatment is ulnar nerve transposition, often at the same time as elbow flexor lengthening or flexor releases. Subcutaneous transposition is preferred.

FOREARM

Supination and pronation deformities are associated with upper motor neuron syndromes. Pronation deformities are much more common. These deformities are most often treated together with the associated deformities, seldom requiring treatment by themselves (8).

Spastic Pronation

Pronation deformity of the forearm in an upper motor neuron lesion is more common than supination deformity. Pronation bias makes it difficult for a person to reach for a target underhand whereas supination deformity impairs reaching for targets that require overhand reach (8). Many activities of daily living depend on active supination. The use of feeding and grooming utensils and clothes fasteners becomes problematic when supination is restricted by spastic or contracted pronators. Muscles that potentially contribute include pronator teres and pronator quadratus. Dynamic EMG studies of pronator teres, pronator quadratus, and biceps greatly augment clinical examination (also refer to Chapter 50).

Technique of Fractional Lengthening of the Forearm Pronators

The pronator teres is approached in the interval between the mobile wad and the flexor carpi radialis (FCR) in the mid forearm. Myotendinous lengthening is then performed by cutting the tendinous fibers of the musculotendinous junction and allowing the tendon fibers to slide on the muscle belly thereby lengthening the muscle tendon unit.

The pronator quadratus is approached via an incision over the volar aspect of the forearm just proximal to the wrist crease. The finger flexor tendons are retracted radially to expose the broad myotendinous junction of the pronator quadratus. The tendon fibers are transected, leaving the underlying muscle fibers intact. The arm is then supinated, separating the ends of the tendon fibers and lengthening the pronator quadratus (8).

Spastic Supination

Spastic supination is a far less common deformity but is also associated with elbow flexion deformities (also refer to Chapter 50). Correction of the supination deformity is performed in conjunction with correction of the elbow flexion deformity (8).

Technique of Biceps Rerouting

Correction of a supination contracture is done by rerouting the course of the biceps tendon distally around the radius to reposition the forearm in neutral rotation. A step cut is made in the biceps tendon as is done for a Z-plasty. The distal end of the tendon is then passed around the neck of the radius to rotate the forearm to the desired position. The tendon is then repaired using nonabsorbable sutures. It is necessary to protect the repair with a long arm cast for 6 weeks to allow the biceps tendon to fully heal (8).

WRIST

A flexed wrist is common after TBI, but hyperextension deformity may also be seen. Patients complain of difficulty inserting their hand into shirts, jackets, and other narrow openings, and they frequently have pain on passive motion. They may also have symptoms of carpal tunnel syndrome secondary to compression of the median nerve against the transverse carpal ligament by taut flexor tendons. In severe cases, wrist subluxation may be present. Radial or ulnar deviation and a clenched fist are often present as well.

Spastic Flexion

Muscles that potentially contribute to wrist flexion include FCR, flexor carpi ulnaris (FCU), palmaris longus (PL), flexor digitorum sublimis (FDS), and flexor digitorum profundus (FDP). Singly or in combination, these muscles may have variable features of spasticity, contracture, and voluntary control. Because they have a larger cross-sectional area, wrist flexor muscles are generally stronger than their extensor counterparts. Despite a net balance of forces favoring flexion, the extent to which a patient may have voluntary control over wrist extensors should be investigated. Dynamic EMG studies and temporary diagnostic motor point blocks are helpful in this regard (also refer to Chapter 50).

When a patient has underlying voluntary control, the surgical treatment for wrist flexion is usually myotendinous lengthening of the wrist flexors. Selective muscle releases, wrist fusion, proximal row carpectomy, and superficialis-to-profundus (STP) tendon transfer may be considered when the goal is to improve passive function only (18).

Technique of Fractional Wrist Flexor Lengthening

In an extremity with documented volitional control, fractional lengthening of the appropriate wrist flexors is performed. This is done in conjunction with lengthening of the extrinsic finger flexors when indicated. A longitudinal incision is made on the volar surface of the forearm. This incision is extended distally if a carpal tunnel release is necessary. The PL tendon is divided if tight. Lengthening is performed by transecting the tendinous portion overlying the myotendinous junction.

Technique of Wrist Flexor Release and Wrist Fusion

When wrist flexion deformities are severe and there is little or no active function seen in the hand, release of the wrist flexors is performed. A proximal row carpectomy may be needed in some patients to correct a severe deformity. The wrist is then stabilized with a wrist fusion to eliminate the need for a wrist orthosis after surgery (19). Splints tend to be lost by these patients and their caretakers. Gravity alone can cause a recurrence of the flexion deformity. Unopposed wrist or finger extensor tone can result in a hyperextension deformity. Because the median nerve compresses against the proximal transverse carpal ligament causing a painful neuropathy, a carpal tunnel release is performed as well.

A volar forearm incision is made extending to the transverse carpal ligament. The tendons of the PL, FCR, and FCU are identified and transected. A carpal tunnel release is performed. If wrist fusion is to be performed, the forearm is then supinated, and a longitudinal dorsal incision is made to expose the wrist joint. Using a high-speed burr, the articular cartilage and subchondral bone of the radiolunate, radioscaphoid, scaphocapitate, lunocapitate, and capitate-third metacarpal joints are removed. The wrist is then stabilized using a prebent titanium wrist fusion plate fixed distally to the third metacarpal and proximally to the radius. The wrist is then placed in a well-padded splint or cast for 6 weeks until the fusion has healed.

Spastic Extension

Extension deformity of the wrist cause hygiene problems and may prevent release in patients with poor digital extension (also refer to Chapter 49). Median nerve compression may also be caused by prolonged extension. If median nerve compression is diagnosed, carpal tunnel release is performed. When wrist hyperextension deformity is present, wrist extensors are typically volitional and spastic, wrist flexors are often poorly volitional and mildly spastic, and the fingers are tightly clenched into the palm (8) (also refer to Chapter 50).

Technique of Wrist Extensor Lengthening

When volitional control has been demonstrated in the dyssynergic wrist extensors, myotendinous lengthening of the extensor carpi ulnaris is performed through a short longitudinal incision on the ulnar border of the forearm. The myotendinous junction is identified and the tendinous portion transected, allowing the muscle to stretch. The extensor carpi radialis longus and brevis are then identified in a separate longitudinal incision on the radial side of the forearm. Again, the myotendinous junction is identified and the tendinous portion cut, allowing the muscle to lengthen. The incisions are closed in routine fashion. Active motion is begun immediately after surgery (8).

Technique of Wrist Extensor Release

When no volitional activity is seen in the wrist extensor muscle by clinical examination and dynamic EMG, tendon release with wrist fusion with or without proximal row carpectomy is performed. A midline dorsal incision is made. Dissection is carried out medially and laterally, exposing the distal extensor carpi radialis longus and brevis and the distal extensor carpi ulnaris. These tendons are transected proximal to their insertions. Wrist fusion with or without proximal row carpectomy is performed as described previously.

HAND

Spastic Clenched Fist

The spastic clenched fist deformity is common in brain injury or stroke involving the upper extremity. This pattern results from unmasking of the primitive grasp reflex. The fingers are typically clasped into the palm. Fingernails may dig into palmar skin and access to the palm for washing may be compromised. When access is chronically restricted, skin maceration, breakdown, and malodor occurs (also refer to Chapter 49). Patients may complain of pain when they or their caregivers attempt to pry fingers open in order to gain palmar access. Some relaxation of finger tightness may occur if the wrist is positioned by the examiner in extreme flexion. The deformity, however, is often accompanied by wrist flexion as well.

Muscles that contribute to the clenched fist deformity include FDS and FDP. If the proximal interphalangeal (PIP) joints flex while the distal interphalangeal (DIP) joints remain extended, spasticity of FDS rather than FDP may be suspected. Dynamic electromyographic studies have shown that the flexor digitorum superficialis muscles exhibit a marked degree of spasticity, whereas the FDP muscles are often normal or minimally spastic. Despite the marked increase in tone, it often has some underlying volitional control. The flexor profundus has less spasticity and better volitional control. Volitional control of the finger extensors is present in 50% of patients with spastic flexion deformities.

The intrinsics may also be spastic along with the extrinsics but an intrinsic plus posture (i.e., combined metacarpophalangeal (MCP) flexion and PIP extension) is not seen because spastic extrinsic flexors dominate by flexing the PIP joints. Some degree of contracture of the extrinsics is typical of the chronically clenched fist. From the perspective of active functional potential, some degree of volitional control may also be present in either or both sets of extrinsic finger flexors. Spastic finger flexors may override and mask the patient's potential to extend the fingers (also refer to Chapter 50). Sometimes, a patient presents with spasticity in just 1 or 2 muscle slips of either FDP or FDS. During the period of residual deficits/remediable function, a variety of orthopedic options are available.

Technique of Fractional Lengthening of Extrinsic Finger Flexors

The surgery is performed through a longitudinal incision on the volar surface of the forearm, commonly at the same sitting with wrist flexor lengthenings. The PL tendon is divided. The lengthening of the individual flexor digitorum superficialis and FDP tendons is performed by sharply incising the tendon fibers as they overlay the muscle belly at the musculotendinous junction, allowing the tendon to slide distally. The flexor pollicis longus (FPL) tendon is lengthened in an identical manner. This technique allows the tendons to lengthen with minimal scarring. By transecting the tendon over the muscle belly, no sutures are needed. This eliminates scarring from foreign body reaction to suture material. The underlying support and vascularity of the muscle provides an optimal environment for the tendons to heal and reconstitute themselves.

Superficialis-to-Profundus Tendon Transfer

In a hand with skin maceration and malodor from a clenched fist deformity in which no volitional movement is detected, more significant lengthening of the flexor tendons is required. In this situation, an STP tendon transfer is performed (20,21). This provides a more cosmetically pleasing hand position, aids in hygiene by getting the fingers out of the palms, and provides, at best, a mass action grasp pattern, and at least a passive restraint to extension.

The STP tendon transfer is performed through a longitudinal volar incision, which may be extended distally to allow release of the carpal tunnel and access to Guyon canal. The PL tendon is identified and transected. The 4 superficialis tendons are sutured together distally and then transected for the en masse transfer. The profundus tendons are sutured together proximally and then cut. The fingers are extended and the distal end of the superficialis tendons is then sutured en masse to the proximal end of the profundus tendons.

Several other surgical procedures are routinely done in combination with the STP tendon transfer to treat the concurrent deformities. A neurectomy of the motor branch of the ulnar nerve is needed to prevent an intrinsic plus deformity from developing. If an intrinsic contracture is seen at the time of surgery following the STP lengthening, then release of the intrinsics is also performed. A carpal tunnel release is done to decompress the median nerve. To prevent a recurrent wrist flexion deformity from occurring secondary to passive wrist flexion, the wrist must be stabilized. A fusion of the wrist in 15° angle of extension provides the most reliable means of maintaining hand position and is now routinely performed. A proximal release of the thenar muscles is often needed to correct a thumb-in-palm deformity. Because the STP transfer and wrist fusion are extensive surgery, we prefer to perform the thenar slide procedure at a later time if it is indicated (22).

Spastic Thumb-in-Palm Deformity

The thumb-in-palm deformity is heterogeneous in appearance and may be secondary to spasticity of multiple muscles including the FPL muscle and the median and ulnar innervated thenar muscles. The thumb is held within the palm, the DIP joint of the thumb is commonly flexed, and the thumb is unable to function during key grasp or in 3-jaw chuck grasp (i.e., in opposition to the pads of the index and third fingers) (23) (also refer to Chapter 50). In addition, skin maceration and breakdown can occur as proper hygiene is prevented (also refer to Chapter 49).

Clinically, spasticity of the FPL is indicated by flexion of the interphalangeal joint. Some patients may be able to extend the thumb if the wrist is flexed; suggesting that a spastic FPL may be impeding active thumb extension when the wrist is more extended and FPL is tighter. The thumb-in-palm deformity may result from spastic activity in FPL, adductor pollicis (AP), and/or the thenar muscles (particularly flexor pollicis brevis). The adduction deformity may be caused by spasticity of muscles enervated by the ulnar nerve, median nerve, or, commonly, a combination of both. Adduction of the thumb metacarpal indicates spasticity of the AP muscle and possibly the first dorsal interosseous muscle. Contracture of the skin of the web space and interphalangeal joint contracture of the thumb may also develop over time (23) (also refer to Chapter 49).

In those cases with a fixed adduction contracture, surgical lengthening of the thenar muscles is indicated. Generally, all of the thenar muscles are spastic or contracted and a proximal myotomy is required to reposition the thumb and decrease the underlying tone in order to improve pinch function. Distal releases are to be avoided because these often result in a hyperextension deformity of the MCP joint of the thumb.

Technique of Thenar Muscle Slide

Under tourniquet control, an incision is made along the thenar crease on the palm. The origins of the flexor pollicis brevis, opponens pollicis, and abductor pollicis muscles are detached from their origins while protecting the recurrent branch of the median nerve. The thumb is extended allowing the released muscles to slide radially and reattach in an improved position preserving function and preventing a hyperextension deformity.

The origin of the AP muscle is released from the third metacarpal. Careful dissection to retract the digital neurovascular bundles and flexor tendons to the index and long digits is necessary. The deep palmar vascular arch and deep branch of the ulnar nerve are identified as they penetrate the AP muscle between its oblique and transverse heads prior to adductor muscle release. The neurovascular supply of the AP is preserved (23).

If the first dorsal interosseous muscle is contracted, a release is performed through a dorsal incision along the ulnar margin of the thumb metacarpal while protecting the radial sensory nerve. The origin of the first dorsal interosseous is released from its origin on the base of the first metacarpal. In persistent web space contractures, despite appropriate muscle releases, a Z-plasty of the thumb web space is indicated.

Finger Deformities From Intrinsic Spasticity

When spasticity of the extrinsic flexors is present, intrinsic spasticity should be expected, although intrinsic spasticity and contracture is frequently masked by the presence of extrinsic flexor spasticity or contracture (also refer to Chapter 50). Extension of the fingers at the MCP joints may be blocked by spasticity of the interossei and lumbrical muscles of the hand. Another manifestation of intrinsic spasticity is the tendency to swan-neck or boutonniere positioning of the fingers (Figure 51-8). When a release or tendon lengthening of the spastic extrinsic flexor muscles has already been done, an intrinsic positive deformity of the hand will be unmasked. These hand deformities can be painful and disfiguring. Such contractures often lead to maceration of the palmar skin and recurrent nail bed infections from poor hygiene (2) (also refer to Chapter 49).

Boutonniere deformities are commonly associated with intrinsic spasticity (Figure 51-8). They result from a combination of intrinsic spasticity combined with flexor digitorum superficialis tone. Swan-neck deformities may also result from increased intrinsic tone. The central extensor band is relatively shortened relative to the lateral bands because of tension exerted by the intrinsics and long extensor. In both of these cases, care must be taken to distinguish between deformities caused by the intrinsic spasticity that should improve with treatment and deformities resulting from the

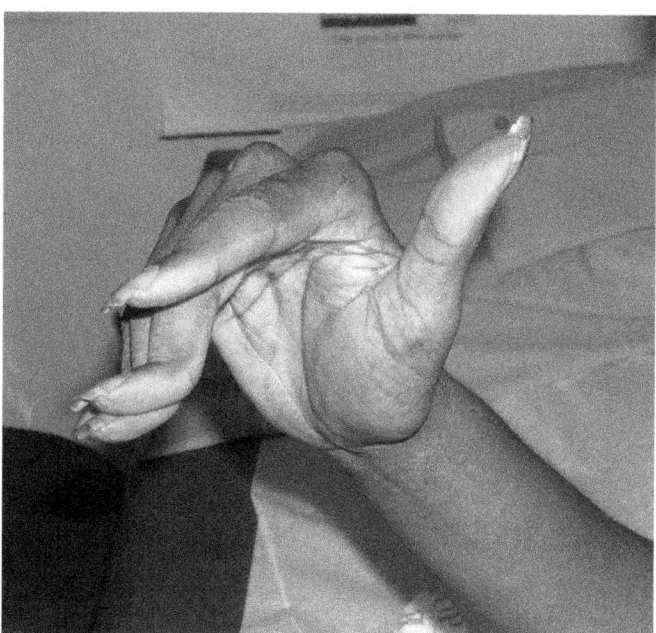

FIGURE 51-8 Spastic Boutonnière deformity of the digits.

more usual mechanisms such as traumatic central slip injury with lateral band subluxation or traumatic mallet finger because if not caused by spasticity, the deformity will not improve with treatment for spasticity.

Because it is impossible to fully delineate the relative contributions and balance of spasticity and contracture of the intrinsic and extrinsic muscles by clinical assessment alone, we routinely obtain dynamic EMG studies of the intrinsic muscles before embarking on treatment of hand deformities. This is especially important prior to considering any surgical intervention.

In the period of residual deficits/remediable function, 3 treatment options are available. The procedure chosen is based on considerations of contracture and the presence or absence of volitional activity in the intrinsic muscles. When no significant intrinsic contracture is present and dynamic EMG indicates that there is no volitional control in the intrinsic muscles, a neurectomy of the motor branches of the ulnar nerve in the palm is performed. The sensory branches are left intact to preserve protective sensation in the hand. When a contracture of the intrinsic muscles is present and the dynamic EMG study shows no volitional activity, a release is performed of the lateral bands of the extensor hood mechanism at the level of the proximal phalanx. In these cases, neurectomy of the motor branches of the ulnar nerve is done simultaneously to prevent recurrence of the intrinsic plus deformity from spasticity of the interosseous muscles. When there is either a dynamic or static intrinsic plus deformity, but the EMG demonstrates volitional control, the palmar interossei are lengthened. A static deformity is one in which a myostatic contracture is present. A dynamic deformity is one where the deformity results mostly from increased tone with little or no fixed contracture.

Technique of Ulnar Motor Neurectomy

The phenol block must be done surgically because of the close proximity of the sensory and motor branches of the nerve. An incision is made on the palmar surface of the hand radial to the pisiform bone and extended distally for 1 in. Care is taken to prevent harm to the ulnar artery. The ulnar nerve is exposed and the motor branches are identified using a nerve stimulator. Generally, 2 motor branches are seen. The main motor branch lies beneath the sensory branch and a smaller motor branch can be seen entering the hypothenar muscles. Once identified, the nerves are transected, with care taken to preserve the ulnar artery and the sensory branch of the ulnar nerve.

Technique of Intrinsic Release

In a hand in which a contracture of the intrinsic muscles is present and the dynamic EMG study shows no volitional activity, lateral band releases are performed. A midline longitudinal incision is made over the dorsum of the MCP joint and proximal phalanx of each finger. Dissection is carried out both on the ulnar and radial sides of the extensor mechanism. The palmar edge of the lateral bands is identified. The lateral band and oblique fibers of the extensor hood are transected on each side. Care is taken to preserve the transverse fibers of the sagittal extensor hood.

Recurrent intrinsic plus deformities are common. This is thought to be secondary to residual attachment of the interossei muscles to the base of the proximal phalanges. To prevent recurrent deformities, it is advisable to perform a concomitant neurectomy of the motor branches of the ulnar nerve in Guyon canal as described previously.

Technique of Interosseous Lengthening

In a hand with volitional control of the intrinsic musculature, intrinsic lengthening is performed. Under tourniquet control, 2 parallel palmar incisions are made over the distal metacarpals. The lumbrical muscles are very small and have a minimal muscle tendon overlap. They are left intact. Dissection is carried deep into the palm to expose the palmar interossei muscles. The interossei are substantial bipennate muscles that can be fractionally lengthened at the muscle tendon overlap.

Intrinsic Minus Deformities

A less common deformity pattern is the intrinsic minus hand. In these patients, the intrinsic muscles have normal or weakened tone, but there is spasticity of the extrinsic finger flexors. There may be increased tone in the extrinsic extensors as well. This pattern results in a claw hand posture, with hyperextension of the MCP joints and flexion of the proximal and distal interphalangeal joints. Ulnar neuropathy must be considered as a possible diagnosis. Hyperextension contracture of the MCP joint capsule is common. When present, the contractures require surgical release. Treatment of this deformity may also require lengthening of the extrinsic digital flexors or STP transfers as described earlier. Volar capsulodesis may also be required to restore MCP flexion and place the hand in a more functional and cosmetic position.

PELVIS AND HIP

Pelvic malunion can occur following unreduced unstable pelvic fractures. The need for surgical correction must be individualized to each patient's symptoms. For example, a small leg length discrepancy without pelvic pain may be best managed with a shoe lift.

Malunions of both intertrochanteric and subtrochanteric hip fractures can be seen in patients with TBI. They usually present with leg length discrepancy, gait abnormalities, and pain. These deformities can be managed with a corrective osteotomy after careful preoperative planning.

Most deformities can be managed with a corrective osteotomy and intramedullary fixation.

Heterotopic Ossification

Anterior Hip (Flexor)
After TBI, HO typically occurs along the lines of tension caused by the spastic muscles. Anterior HO is seen to follow the iliopsoas muscle. Anterior HO usually extends from the anterior superior iliac spine (ASIS) and inner aspect of the pelvis to the proximal femur in the region of the lesser trochanter. When resecting anterior hip HO, a standard anterior approach to the hip is performed, but the femoral triangle and its contents are also dissected. Care is taken to identify all major divisions of the femoral artery, nerve, and vein. It is prudent to place vascular loops around all major vessels proximally in order to assure easier control of bleeding should a major vessel be damaged during the procedure. A wide exposure and meticulous hemostasis are needed. Although all the neurovascular structures may be encased in HO, it is more common for the nerve to be entrapped. The femoral nerve is already dividing into its many branches within the femoral triangle. The motor branches are small in diameter and must be carefully identified. Because it is difficult to mobilize the neurovascular structures, the heterotopic bone must be removed in small segments. It is difficult to distinguish normal from abnormal bone. The morphology of the normal bone and the HO must be closely observed. Preoperative computed tomography scans with 3-dimensional reconstructions can be extremely helpful in understanding the morphology. Intraoperative radiographs should also be used to guide the resection (12).

Medial Hip (Adductor)
Heterotopic bone seen inferomedial to the hip joint follows the adductor muscles from the pubis and extends toward the medial aspect of the femur (Figure 51-9). A medial approach to the hip is used for resection. If there is a significant hip adduction contracture, release of the hip adductors may also be needed. Often, HO is seen both anterior and medial to the hip. In these cases, it is necessary to make 2 separate incisions and work between both (12).

Posterior Hip (Extensor)
Posterior HO lies immediately posterior to the femoral head and neck. Although posterior bone forms in conjunction with hip extensor spasticity, it is usually associated with a flexion contracture of the hip. A posterior approach to the hip is used for resection. The sciatic nerve is identified distally and dissected proximally. It is common for the sciatic nerve to be encased within the mass of heterotopic bone. Significant scarring is also seen around the sciatic nerve secondary to the intense inflammatory reaction that happen during the intermediate stages of bone formation. A neuroly-

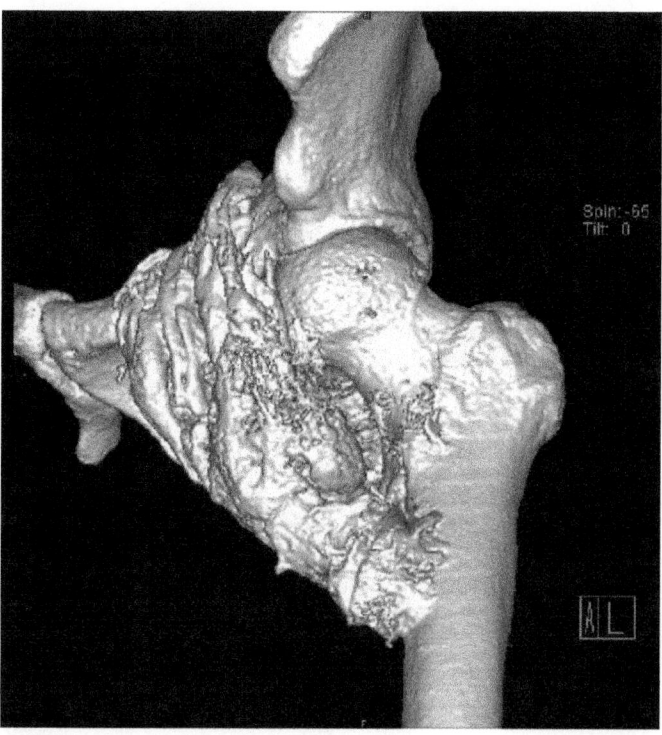

FIGURE 51-9 CT reconstruction demonstrating bridging heterotopic bone in the proximal medial compartment of the thigh.

sis of the sciatic nerve may be needed. Once the sciatic nerve is identified, a more aggressive resection of the bone is begun. If a significant hip flexion contracture persists after excision of the posterior HO, an anterior soft tissue release may then be necessary (12).

Lateral Hip (Abductor)

When HO is seen in the abductor region, it is usually a result of trauma or surgical stimulation. A straight lateral or posterior incision can be used. It is important to separate the heterotopic bone from the abductor muscles and preserve as much muscle function as possible. The abductor muscles are usually very atrophic (12).

Spastic Hip Adduction Deformity

Scissoring of the legs in an ambulatory patient gives the patient a narrow base of support while standing and results in poor balance. A preoperative obturator nerve block will eliminate the adductor spasticity and allow assessment of the adduction contracture (Figure 51-10) (also refer to chapter 50). Alternately, the patient can be examined at the time of surgery while under anesthesia to determine if a fixed myostatic contracture is present. When no fixed adduction contracture is present, transection of the anterior branches of the obturator nerve will denervate the adductors and allow the patient with a broader base of support. Commonly, a small contracture is found and the adductor longus muscle is released at the time of the obturator neurectomy.

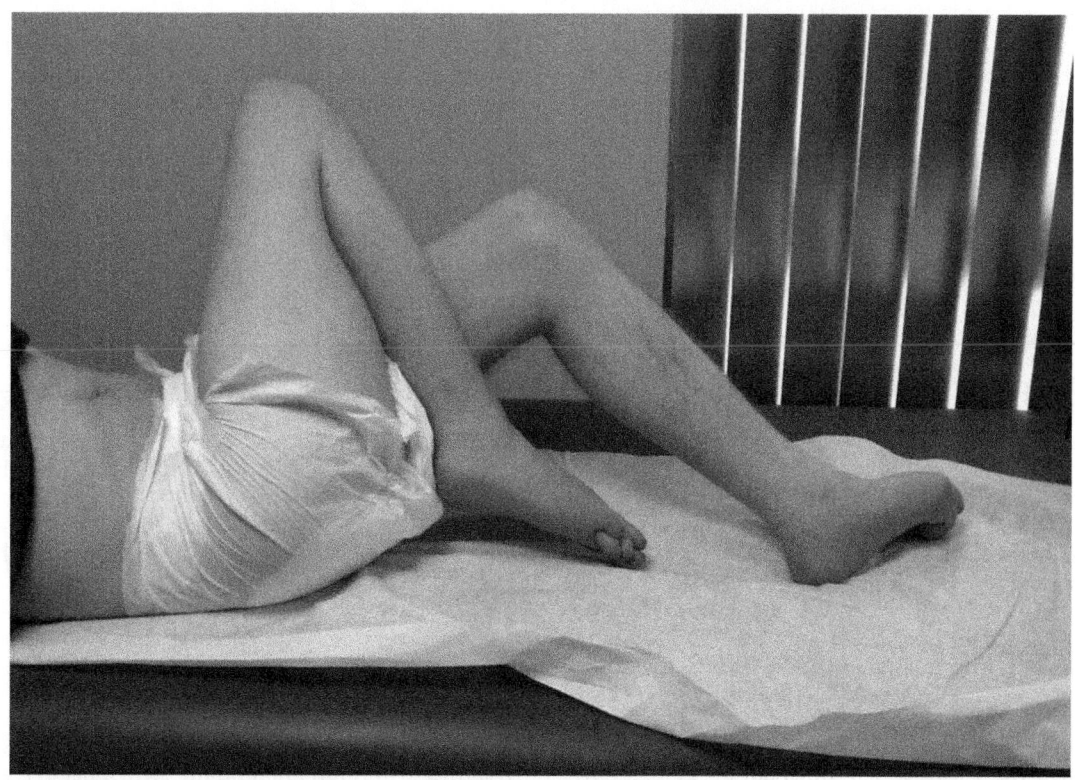

FIGURE 51-10 Flexion adduction contracture of the hip in a patient with brain injury.

Technique of Obturator Neurectomy

A longitudinal incision is made directly over the adductor longus muscle. The adductor longus muscle is released and retracted. The anterior branch of the obturator nerve is transected over the muscle belly of the adductor brevis. Early gait training with weightbearing as tolerated is instituted in the postoperative period.

Technique of Hip Adductor Tenotomy

A hip adduction contracture that interferes with nursing care and hygiene in a nonambulatory patient or excessive limb scissoring during attempted transfers and ambulation in a patient with active function are indications for surgical release.

In a severely spastic patient, a flexion contracture of the hip and knee commonly occur in conjunction with an adduction contracture. As with any contracture, preoperative radiographs should be obtained prior to performing soft tissue releases in order to rule out the presence of HO or an underlying bony deformity that would prevent correction.

With the patient in the supine position, a longitudinal incision is made over the adductor longus muscle. The incision is placed distal to the groin crease to position the incision in a more hygienic location. The adductor longus muscle is dissected free and transected using electrocautery. The anterior branches of the obturator nerve are identified and transected. The adductor brevis and gracilis are released close to their origin on the pubis. The wound is closed over a drain.

Hip Flexion Deformity

Spasticity of the hip flexors can result in a crouched gait with compensatory knee flexion to maintain balance. This is a very costly deformity because it requires constant use of the quadriceps, hip extensor, and calf muscles to maintain upright posture. The energy requirement for the continuous firing of these muscles is extremely high. Few patients are able to remain ambulatory with this deformity.

Technique of Functional Hip Flexor Release

The hip flexor muscles are needed to advance the limb during gait. Complete release of the hip flexors should be avoided in any patient with the potential to ambulate. Because the iliopsoas has capsular insertions, release of the iliopsoas tendon from the lesser trochanter of the femur does not provide a complete release. Release of the tendon from the lesser trochanter permits the iliopsoas to recess proximally, thereby diminishing its pull but retaining its function.

A medial approach to the hip is used. A longitudinal incision is made overlying the adductor longus tendon. The adductor longus is released because it contributes to hip flexion. The pectineus muscle is identified where it lies deep to the femoral vessels and medial to the adductor longus. The pectineus muscle is divided using electrocautery. The lesser trochanter of the femur can be palpated in the depth of the wound. The tendon of the iliopsoas is visualized by placing narrow reverse retractors above and below the lesser trochanter. The iliopsoas tendon is divided from the trochanter

and allowed to retract proximally. The wound is closed over a drain.

Technique of Nonfunctional Hip Flexor Release

A hip flexion contracture or severe spasticity in a nonambulatory patient causing poor hygiene or pressure sores that cannot be healed secondary to limited positioning of the patient are indications for surgical release (also refer to Chapter 49). When a severe adduction contracture of the hip is present, it may be necessary to perform a percutaneous release of the adductor longus tendon in the groin in order to position the patient adequately and prepare for further surgery. Any flexion contracture of the knee should be corrected simultaneously to prevent the leg from positioning in flexion and causing a recurrent and more resistant contracture.

With the patient in the supine position, an anterior incision is made beginning just below the ASIS and is carried distally following the sartorius muscle for a short distance. The lateral femoral cutaneous nerve is identified as it passes distal to the ASIS and is protected. The sartorius muscle is detached from its origin on the ASIS. The rectus femoris muscle is released from its origin on the anterior inferior spine of the pelvis. The femoral nerve and vessels are gently retracted medially to expose the iliopsoas muscle on the anterior aspect of the hip. The iliopsoas and pectineus muscles are carefully divided over the pelvic brim using the electrocautery to diminish postoperative bleeding. Because the iliopsoas has capsular insertions, release of the iliopsoas tendon from the lesser trochanter of the femur does not provide a complete release. The tensor fascia lata and the anterior portion of the gluteus medius and gluteal aponeurosis may be released from the iliac crest if necessary. The hip joint capsule is not released.

Regarding the release of other contracted joints, approximately 50% of the deformity will be corrected at the time of surgery (Figure 51-11). Daily wound care will help prevent infection in this area where bacterial contamination is likely and a large dead space remains following surgery. Placing the patient in a prone position 3 times a day for increasing periods and gentle stretching exercises will assist in correcting any residual hip flexion deformity. When a release of a knee flexion contracture has been performed simultaneously, the weight of the long leg cast will also provide a correcting force. Sitting in a wheelchair is allowed for short periods.

On occasion, a patient is seen with chronic hip subluxation or dislocation from severe and very long-standing hip flexion and adduction spasticity (also refer to Chapter 50. In these cases, it is usually necessary to resect the femoral head at the same time as performing a complete muscle release. After this surgery, it is very important to maintain the leg in a neutral position for at least 3 months while soft tissue healing occurs. This can be done with bilateral short leg casts connected with a bar to hold the legs in neutral rotation and slight abduction.

Extension Deformity

Following a severe brainstem injury, spasticity of the extensor muscles of the leg may result in a hip extension contracture. Although uncommon, an extension contracture will interfere with a person's ability to sit (also refer to Chapter

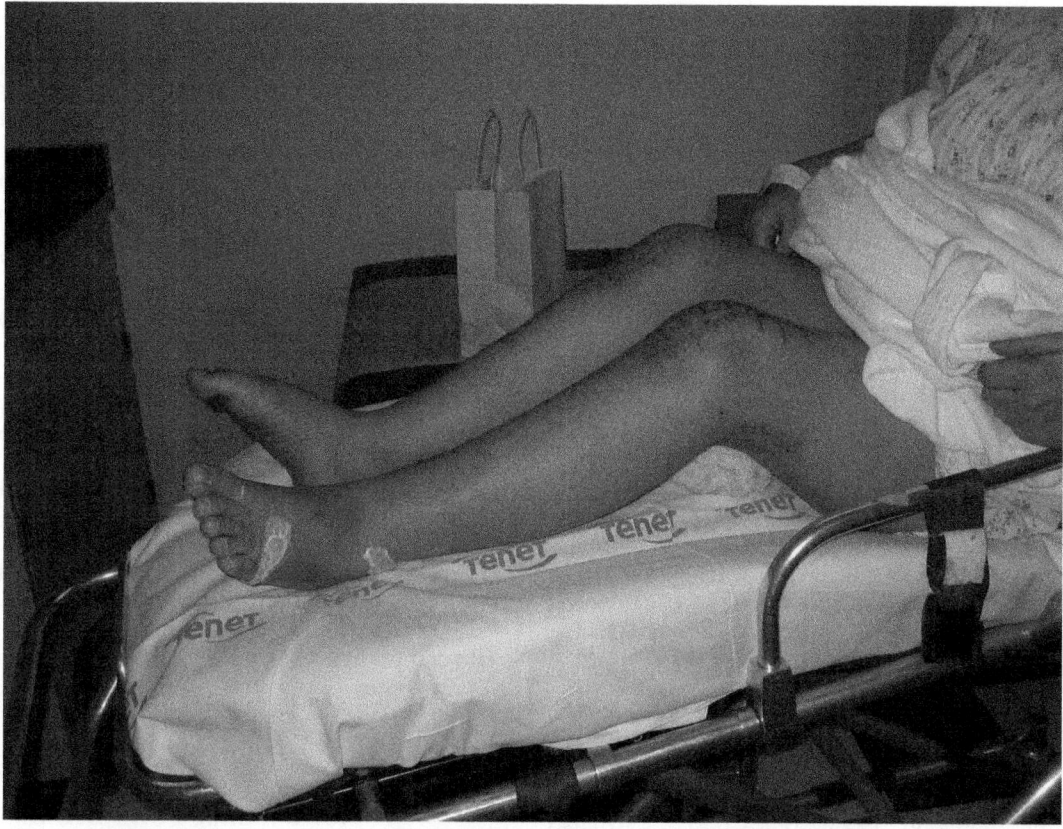

FIGURE 51-11 Partially corrected flexion contractures of the knee postoperatively.

49). When good sitting posture cannot be obtained, a release of the proximal origin of the hamstring muscles is indicated.

Technique of Proximal Hamstring Release

The patient is placed in the prone position for surgery. A longitudinal incision is made over the posterior thigh beginning at the gluteal fold. The posterior femoral cutaneous nerve is identified and protected. The distal edge of the gluteus maximus is lifted proximally to expose the underlying hamstring muscles. The biceps femoris, semimembranosus, and semitendinosus muscles are then detached from their origins on the ischial tuberosity and allowed to retract distally. Postoperatively, the patient is started on gentle passive range of motion exercises to regain hip flexion.

KNEE

Fracture Malunion

Tibial malunions can lead to abnormal stresses across the ankle and knee. This malalignment can lead to degenerative changes at both the knee and ankle. Like the femur, corrective osteotomies can be performed to restore balance. External fixators can be employed for more complex deformities if intramedullary fixation is not possible.

Heterotopic Ossification

HO is less common in the thigh and the knee compared to the region around the hip joint. When it does occur, it usually is seen medially and may appear as a Pellegrini-Stieda lesion. Even when the medial HO does not bridge the joint, it commonly will cause a knee flexion contracture by placing tension on the surrounding tissues. When there has been knee extensor spasticity, the HO can be found along the distal shaft of the femur beneath the quadriceps muscle. It often wraps around both the medial and lateral sides of the femur and greatly restricts knee motion. Posterior HO is uncommon after head injury but can occur in conjunction with hamstring spasticity.

Surgical resection of the HO should be done if knee motion is limited (24). The choice of the surgical approach depends on the location of the HO. Continuous passive motion devices are helpful postoperatively.

Spastic Knee Deformities

Knee Flexion Deformity

A knee flexion deformity is caused by overactivity of the hamstring muscles (also refer to Chapter 50). When the knee flexion deformity is less than 60° angle and the patient have documented volitional activity in the hamstring muscles, then a lengthening procedure is done. This will correct the flexion deformity while preserving the function of the hamstrings.

Technique of Distal Hamstring Lengthening

With the patient in the supine position, a longitudinal incision of approximately 8 cm is made on the lateral aspect of the distal thigh just proximal to the knee joint. The peroneal nerve is isolated and protected and the biceps femoris tendon is divided obliquely as it overlies the muscle belly. This allows the tendon to slide distally while still maintaining continuity of the muscle (25). The portion of the iliotibial band that is posterior to the axis of knee flexion is also divided transversely.

A longitudinal incision is then made on the medial aspect of the distal thigh. The tendons of the gracilis and semimembranosus are isolated and fractionally lengthened at the myotendinous junction by making an oblique cut in the tendon as it overlies the muscle belly. The semitendinosus tendon has a very short myotendinous junction that does not permit fractional lengthening. This tendon is simply transected.

Technique of Distal Hamstring Release

In a nonambulatory patient with a marked increase in hamstring muscle tone, knee flexion contractures result. Spasticity is frequently present. Distal release of the hamstring tendons does not prevent a patient from becoming ambulatory. If the hip flexion contracture or spasticity is not corrected at the same time as the hamstring release, a recurrent knee flexion contracture is likely to develop, which is very resistant to surgical correction (25).

With the patient in the supine position, a longitudinal incision is made on the lateral aspect of the distal thigh just proximal to the knee joint. The peroneal nerve is isolated and protected and the biceps femoris muscle and tendon are divided just proximal to its insertion using the electrocautery. The portion of the iliotibial band that is posterior to the axis of knee flexion is also divided transversely.

A longitudinal incision is then made on the medial aspect of the knee and the tendons of the gracilis, semimembranosus, and semitendinosus are isolated and divided. The semitendinosus tendon is usually surrounded by a layer of fat and can closely resemble the posterior tibial nerve. The fatty tissue should be dissected from the tendon to confirm its identity prior to transection. In severe contractures, release of the sartorius muscle is also performed. By using electrocautery, the procedure is easily performed without a tourniquet, which facilitates localization and protection of the posterior tibial artery, vein, and nerve. Following localization of the neurovascular bundle, any remaining restricting bands are divided as required. The posterior fascia at the knee is often thickened, limiting extension and may require release. The posterior joint capsule may need to be released in long-standing contractures. The joint capsule is stripped from the distal posterior femur using a periosteal elevator. The cruciate ligaments are not divided. If more correction is required, a closing wedge osteotomy can be performed. A closing wedge will allow for some shortening of the femur and release some tension from the neurovascular structures and posterior skin.

Knee Extension Deformity

Patients with a stiff knee gait are unable to flex the knee during the swing phase of gait. The deformity is a dynamic one, meaning that it only occurs during walking. There is no restriction of passive knee motion and the patient does not have difficulty sitting. Usually, the knee is maintained in extension throughout the gait cycle. Toe drag, which is likely in the early swing phase, may cause the patient to trip; thus, balance and stability are also affected. The limb appears to be functionally longer. Circumduction of the involved limb, hiking of the pelvis, and/or contralateral limb vaulting may occur as compensatory maneuvers.

A gait study with dynamic EMG should be done preoperatively to document the activity of the individual muscles of the quadriceps (also refer to Chapter 50). Dyssynergic activity is commonly seen in the rectus femoris from preswing through terminal swing throughout the gait cycle (26,27). Abnormal activity is also common in the rectus intermedius. If knee flexion is improved with a block of the rectus femoris or vastus intermedius, the rationale for surgical intervention is strengthened. Any equinus deformity of the foot should be corrected prior to evaluation of a stiff knee gait because equinus causes a knee extension force during stance. Because the amount of knee flexion during swing is directly related to the speed of walking, the patient should be able to ambulate with a reasonable velocity in order to benefit from surgery. Good hip flexion strength is also needed for improved knee flexion because it is the forward momentum of the leg that normally provides the inertial force to flex the knee. Transfer of the rectus femoris to a hamstring tendon not only removes it as a deforming muscle force; it also converts the rectus into a corrective flexion force.

Technique of Rectus Femoris to Gracilis Transfer for Dynamic Stiff Knee Gait

A longitudinal incision is made on the anterior thigh from mid-thigh to the middle of the patella. The rectus femoris muscle is dissected free from the other vasti muscles. Dissection is carried distally to the patella where a strip of periosteum is also removed from the patella to gain additional length. If significant, spasticity was seen in the vasti muscle on the dynamic EMG study, these muscles are fractionally lengthened by transecting their tendons as they overlay the muscle belly (27).

A second incision is made over the medial hamstrings just proximal to the knee. The gracilis tendon is identified and released proximally. This provides a distal length of tendon to attach to the transferred rectus femoris. A subcutaneous tunnel is then made between the 2 incisions and through the intermuscular septum. The distal end of the rectus femoris tendon is passed through the tunnel to the medial wound with the knee flexed 90° angle and the femur externally rotated. The rectus femoris tendon is sewn the gracilis tendon (27).

Technique of Selective Quadriceps Lengthening

After a brainstem injury, extensor spasticity can cause a knee extension contracture. This is usually seen in combination with a hip extension contracture. Both deformities result in problems with sitting. The knee extension deformity can be corrected by lengthening the quadriceps. Quadriceps weakness is not a problem in these patients because they are not ambulatory. This procedure is more easily performed and has less morbidity in the V–Y lengthening. It also does not cause a patella baja deformity. Even severe hyperextension knee deformities can be corrected with this procedure as long as there is some flexibility within the quadriceps muscles.

V–Y Quadriceps

When a severe extension contracture has been present for years, there is often thickening and scarring within the substance of the quadriceps muscle bellies (also refer to Chapter 49). In this situation, it is often not feasible to consider a fractional lengthening technique. A V–Y lengthening within the substance of the combined quadriceps tendon is then indicated.

A longitudinal incision is made over the distal thigh extending to the proximal patella. The deep fascia is incised and the rectus femoris tendon identified. A distally based inverted V portion of the rectus tendon is harvested in preparation for lengthening. The knee is flexed slowly to attain at least 90° angle of flexion and to release any intra-articular adhesions. The rectus tendon is sutured with the knee flexed to complete the V–Y lengthening. It is often necessary to remove the patella to gain sufficient knee flexion. The wound is closed over suction drainage.

FOOT AND ANKLE

Fracture Malunions

Ankle malunions can also be seen in the patient with TBI. The most common malunion of the ankle is shortening and malrotation of the fibula. A corrective osteotomy can be performed, which restores length and reestablishes alignment.

Equinus

Equinus is the most common spastic deformity causing gait difficulty (Figure 51-12) (also refer to Chapter 50). This defor-mity hinders both swing and stance phases of ambulation by making limb clearance difficult and preventing initial heel contact. Surgical lengthening of the Achilles tendon (TAL) is indicated when the patient's foot and ankle position is not adequately controlled by an orthosis or when attempting to make the patient brace free (28).

Technique of Achilles Tendon Lengthening

Adequate TAL can be performed using the Hoke triple hemi-section technique percutaneously (Figure 51-13). With the foot held in maximum dorsiflexion, 3 percutaneous hemi-transections of the Achilles tendon are made. If a varus de-formity of the foot is present, the proximal and distal cuts are made in the medial half of the tendon and the center cut is placed laterally. The foot is then pushed into dorsiflexion, allowing the tendon to lengthen.

Varus

Spastic varus deformity of the foot interferes with ambula-tion and renders brace wear difficult or impossible. Varus deformities most commonly occur as the result of increased and inappropriate activity of the tibialis anterior muscle. When dynamic EMG has documented the tibialis anterior to be the cause of varus, the deformity is corrected by a split anterior tibial tendon (SPLATT) transfer. The SPLATT maintains the half of the tendon on the medial aspect of the foot and transfers the other half of the tibialis anterior tendon to the lateral side of the foot (Figure 51-14). This deformity is usually accompanied by an equinus deformity of the foot

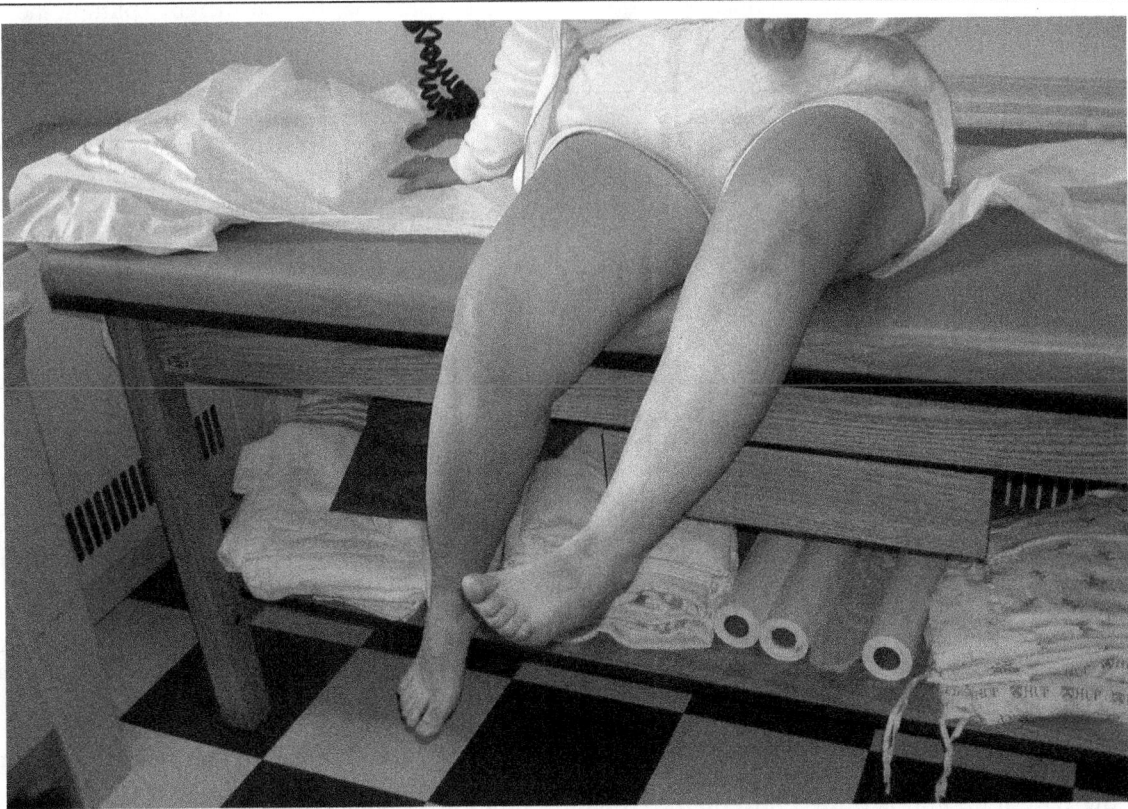

FIGURE 51-12 An equinovarus foot in an ambulatory patient.

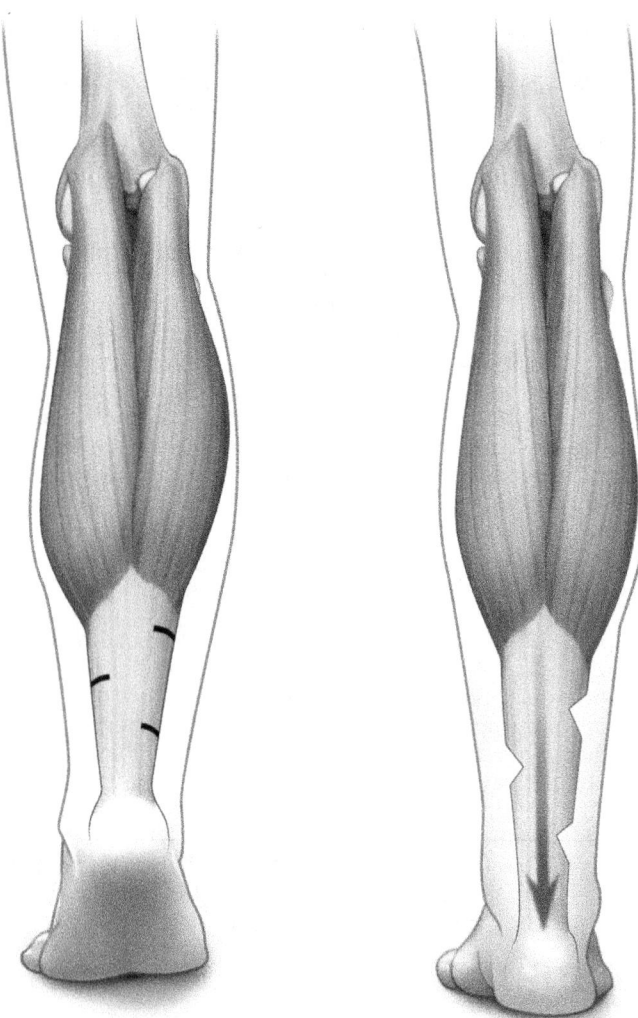

FIGURE 51-13 Technique of tendo-Achilles lengthening.

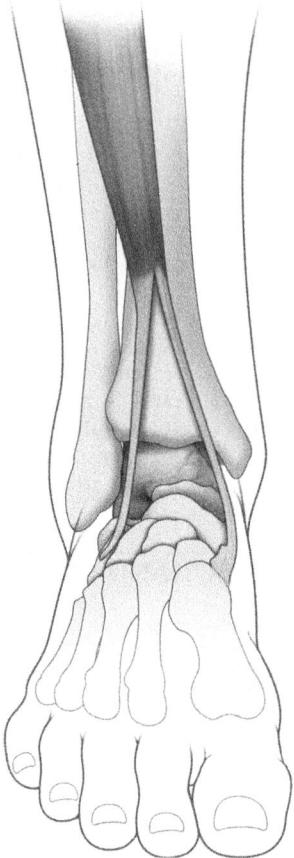

FIGURE 51-14 Split anterior tibialis tendon transfer.

secondary to spasticity of the gastrocnemius and soleus muscles, and toe curling secondary to spasticity of the extrinsic and intrinsic toe flexor muscle. Because equinus and toe curling usually accompany the varus deformity, a lengthening (28) of the Achilles tendon should be performed first and the toe flexor tendons divided.

Technique of Split Anterior Tibial Tendon Transfer

An incision is made over the distal insertion of the tibialis anterior tendon on the medial aspect of the foot. The lateral half of the tendon is sharply divided from its insertion. An absorbable suture is placed in the end of the tendon for ease of handling.

A second incision is made on the anterior distal third of the leg just lateral to the crest of the tibia over the tibialis anterior muscle. An opening is made in the fascia overlying the tibialis anterior. We use a long twisted wire loop as a tendon passer. The wire loop is passed under the fascia and follows the tibialis anterior tendon to the incision on the medial foot. The suture in the free end of the tendon is passed through the wire loop and is pulled into the proximal wound. This suture is used to pull the free end of the tendon

into the proximal wound thereby splitting the tibialis anterior tendon and a portion of the muscle belly.

A third incision is then made on the lateral aspect of the foot. The cuboid is exposed. A 5-mm drill is used to make a tunnel through the cuboid. The tibialis tendon is passed subcutaneously to the lateral foot incision. A straight needle is used to pull the suture and then the tibialis anterior tendon into the bony tunnel of the cuboid. With the foot held in a corrected position, the tendon is then secured in the cuboid by placing an absorbable 7-mm interference screw in the tunnel adjacent to the tendon (Figure 51-15). The free end of the suture is trimmed at skin level.

Technique of Tibialis Anterior Lengthening

Occasionally, a mild varus deformity is seen during walking that is caused by a moderate increase in tibialis anterior activity. In this situation, a myotendinous lengthening is sufficient to control the varus deformity. An incision is made over the tibialis anterior muscle approximately 10 cm proximal to the ankle joint. The fascial sheath of the tibialis anterior is opened and the tendon is transected over the muscle belly of the tibialis anterior, thereby allowing the muscle to lengthen fractionally (29). If this is the only procedure performed, no immobilization is needed after surgery. Full weightbearing ambulation is allowed immediately.

Technique of Tibialis Posterior Lengthening

In approximately 10% of patients with stroke and brain injury, the tibialis posterior muscle is also spastic and can peroneal sensory nerve. A bony tunnel is made through the cuneiform bone using a 5-mm drill. The EHL tendon is then identified through the same incision. The EHL tendon is transected and then pulled into the tunnel of the cuneiform using a suture and a straight needle. With the foot held in a corrected position, the tendon is secured in the tunnel using a 7-mm interference screw. Most commonly, the EHL is transferred in combination with a SPLATT procedure (29). The postoperative protocol of the SPLATT is followed.

Valgus

Spastic valgus foot deformities are less common in the population with stroke and brain injury. The deformity can result from overactivity of the peroneus longus, peroneus brevis, or both. Dynamic EMG is used to determine which muscles are causing the deformity. In the "spastic combination foot" deformity, equinovarus is observed during swing phase from premature and prolonged firing of the tibialis anterior and gastrocsoleus muscles. The planovalgus deformity occurs during stance from the inappropriate activity of the peroneus longus muscle. The pronation deformity may be accentuated (30) by a premorbid tendency to flat foot or by the presence of an equinus contracture.

Technique of Peroneal Lengthening

If the deformity is not severe, a myotendinous lengthening can be considered. An incision is made over the lateral leg

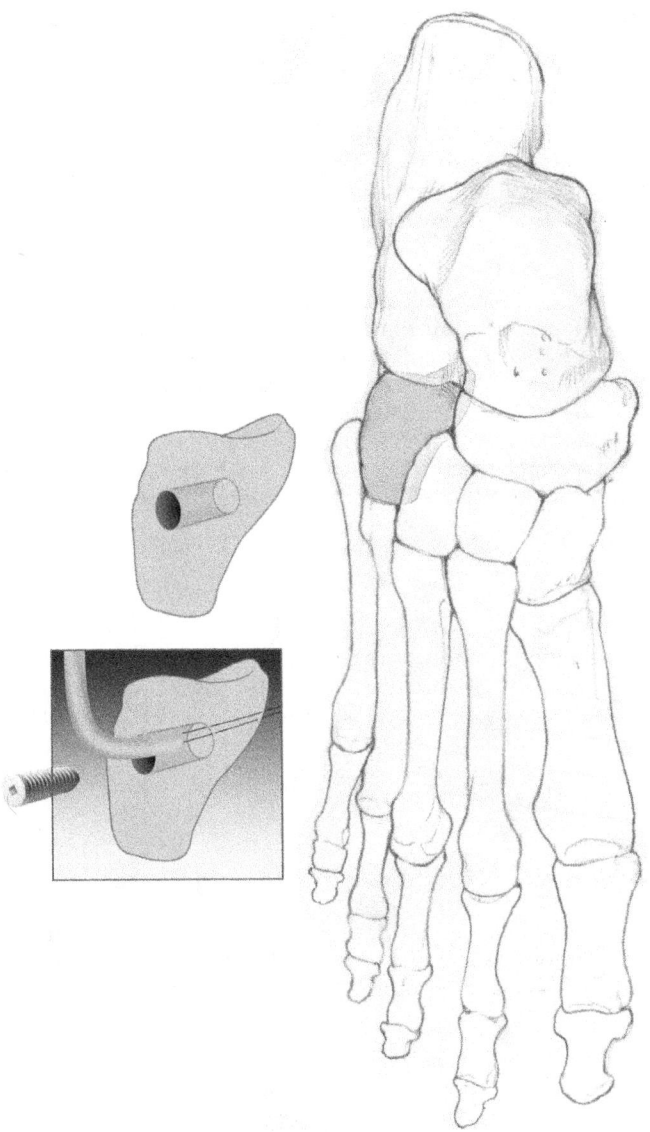

FIGURE 51-15 A bioabsorbable screw is placed in the cuboid to secure the SPLATT transfer.

contribute to the varus deformity. Clinically, this is evidenced by the increased heel varus in addition to the forefoot varus caused by the tibialis anterior muscle.

When spasticity of the tibialis posterior muscle is present, a myotendinous lengthening of the tendon is performed posterior and slightly proximal to the medial malleolus. Complete release of the tibialis posterior tendon is not recommended because a planovalgus deformity may occur secondarily (29).

Technique of Extensor Hallucis Transfer

With the equinovarus deformity, the patient may also have hyperextension of the great toe secondary to spasticity of the extensor hallucis longus (EHL) tendon. The EHL is easily transferred to the mid-dorsum of the foot to provide a more balance dorsiflexion force (Figure 51-16). A small incision is made over the middle cuneiform bone. Care must be taken to identify and protect the dorsalis pedis artery and the

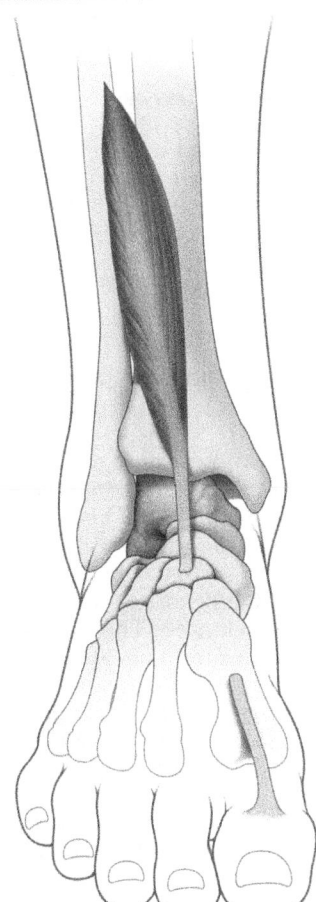

FIGURE 51-16 Extensor hallucis longus transfer to the midfoot.

approximately 10 cm above the ankle joint. The fascia of the lateral compartment is opened and the offending peroneal muscles are fractionally lengthened (30).

Technique of Peroneus Longus Transfer

When a severe spastic valgus occurs, the peroneus longus tendon is transferred through the interosseous membrane to the tarsal navicular bone to support the longitudinal arch of the foot during stance. A small incision is made on the lateral border of the foot just proximal to the base of the fifth metatarsal. The peroneus longus and brevis tendons are identified. The peroneus longus tendon is divided obtaining maximal length. A second incision is made over the lateral leg approximately 10 cm above the ankle. The peroneus longus muscle is identified and the distal end of the tendon is pulled proximally into this wound. A third incision is made over the anterior leg 10 cm proximal to the ankle. Dissection is carried down to expose the interosseous membrane. A window is made in the interosseous membrane and the peroneus longus tendon is passed through to the anterior leg wound. A final incision is made over the navicular bone on the medial side of the foot. A drill is used to create a tunnel through the navicular bone. The peroneus longus tendon is then passed subcutaneously to the medial foot using a long forceps. The end of the tendon is passed through the tunnel in the navicular and secured back with an interference screw. The tendon is secured to hold the foot in a neutral alignment.

When a combined deformity is present, a SPLATT is performed along with a TAL and toe flexor release (TFR) to correct the swing phase abnormalities.

Cavus

A *cavus deformity* is defined as an elevated arch that does not flatten with weightbearing. The deformity is probably a result of muscle imbalance of both the intrinsic and extrinsic muscles of the foot. If the foot is supple, a soft tissue procedure can be done; however, if the foot is rigid, a bony fusion must be done.

Technique of Steindler Stripping (Release of the Plantar Structures)

The plantar fascia is exposed through a medial foot incision. Care is taken to identify and preserve the medial calcaneal nerve branches to the heel pad. The origin of the fascia is released under direct vision. The origin of the abductor hallucis is identified and elevated from the tuberosity of the os calcis. The origin of the flexor brevis and intrinsic muscles of the foot are also released. The foot is then passively corrected and placed into a short leg cast for 2 weeks. Weightbearing can be started on the first postoperative day (29). Because this procedure is usually done in combination with the SPLATT operation, the SPLATT protocol is generally followed.

Technique of Triple Arthrodesis

For severe rigid bony deformities, a triple arthrodesis is done to correct the foot. Most commonly, this procedure is being done in combination with a plantar release and the SPLATT procedure (29).

An incision is made over the lateral foot from the tip of the fibula to the base of the fourth metatarsal. The extensor brevis and fat pad are elevated to expose the calcaneocuboid joint and the sinus tarsi. The superior process of the distal calcaneous is removed using an oscillating saw to facilitate exposure. The bone is saved to use as a graft later. A lamina spreader is inserted between the talus and calcaneous to further expose the joint surfaces. The posterior and middle facets of the subtalar joint are denuded of cartilage. The calcaneocuboid joint is also exposed and the cartilage is removed. The lateral talonavicular joint is exposed and prepared through the same incision. A small medial incision is made over the talonavicular joint and the remaining cartilage is removed. At this time, the 3 joints are fixed with 3 large-diameter cannulated screws confirmed by fluoroscopic guidance. The fusion is protected until full bony healing is seen.

Claw Foot

Toe clawing or curling is a common accompaniment of overactivity of the gastrocnemius muscles. Toe curling is caused by overactivity of the flexor hallucis longus (FHL) and flexor digitorum muscle as well as the short toe flexor and occasionally the intrinsic muscles of the foot (29) (also refer to Chapter 50).

Technique of Toe Flexor Release

A longitudinal incision is made on the plantar surface of each toe at the metatarsal phalangeal joint level (Figure 51-17). The flexor tendons are identified and released under

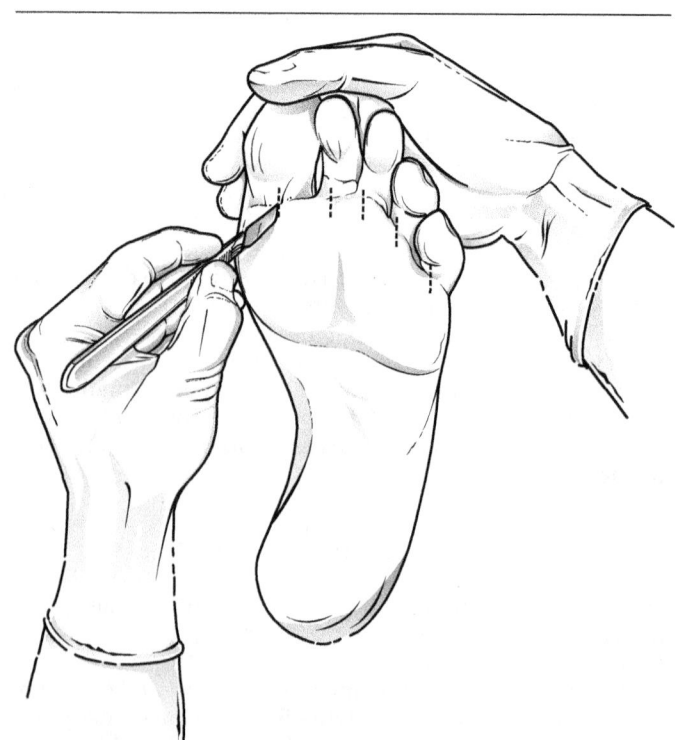

FIGURE 51-17 Toe flexor distal releases.

direct vision. This procedure is commonly done in combination with a TAL because bringing the foot into a plantigrade position will worsen the toe curling. When a TAL has been performed, the foot must be immobilized as described earlier (29).

Plantarflexion Weakness

Muscle paresis (weakness) is an integral part of upper motoneuron syndrome. Lengthening the Achilles tendon to correct an equinus deformity weakens the gastrocnemius-soleus muscle group, which was already weak as a consequence of the underlying upper motor neuron syndrome. This calf paresis generally results in the need of an ankle–foot orthosis (AFO) during ambulation. Thus, transfer of the digitorum longus muscle can be done in order to augment calf strength. With this transfer, more patients eventually achieve brace-free ambulation. In prior studies of treatment of a spastic equinovarus foot deformity, 30% of patients were able to walk safely without an AFO. When the gastrocsoleus strength is augmented (31) by transfer of the flexor digitorum longus (FDL) to the os calcis, 70% of patients achieve brace-free ambulation.

Technique of Transfer of the Flexor Digitorum Longus to Os Calcis

An incision is made on the medial border of the foot dorsal and parallel to the abductor hallucis muscle. The abductor hallucis is reflected plantarward from the base of the first metatarsal and the FHL and FDL are isolated through the deep fascia at the master knot of Henry. At this level, the FDL has not yet split into 4 tendons and the FHL is easily

dissected free. If the flexor brevis tendons are to be released simultaneously to correct toe curling, they are released prior to transecting the FDL tendon. The FHL and FDL are dissected at the knot of Henry.

A second incision is then made at the medial supramalleolar region where the muscle belly of the FDL is isolated with its tendon and delivered through the medial supramalleolar incision (Figure 51-18). A 1-cm incision is made over the medial posterior superior os calcis. A 5-mm drill is used to create a tunnel through the posterior superior calcaneous exiting on the lateral side. A suture ligature is placed in the FDL and the tendon is passed subcutaneously to the medial heel wound. The tendon is then passed through the tunnel created in the os calcis from medially to laterally using a straight needle attached to the tendon suture. With the foot held in maximum dorsiflexion, the tendon is secured in the bony tunnel using an interference screw. Holding the foot in maximum dorsiflexion while tensioning the transferred tendon prevents a recurrent equinus deformity (Figure 51-19 and 51-20).

Foot Deformities in the Nonambulatory Patient

Severe deformities of the feet are common in patients with spasticity (also refer to Chapter 50). Even in the nonambulatory patient, these deformities cause significant problems. The complications include pressure sores, inability to wear shoes or protective footwear, and difficulty positioning the feet on wheelchair supports for improved sitting balance (also refer to Chapter 49). These deformities should be surgically corrected to maintain a plantigrade foot.

The most common deformity is equinovarus with claw toes. As in the more functional patient, muscle balance must be achieved by performing the SPLATT, a TAL, and release

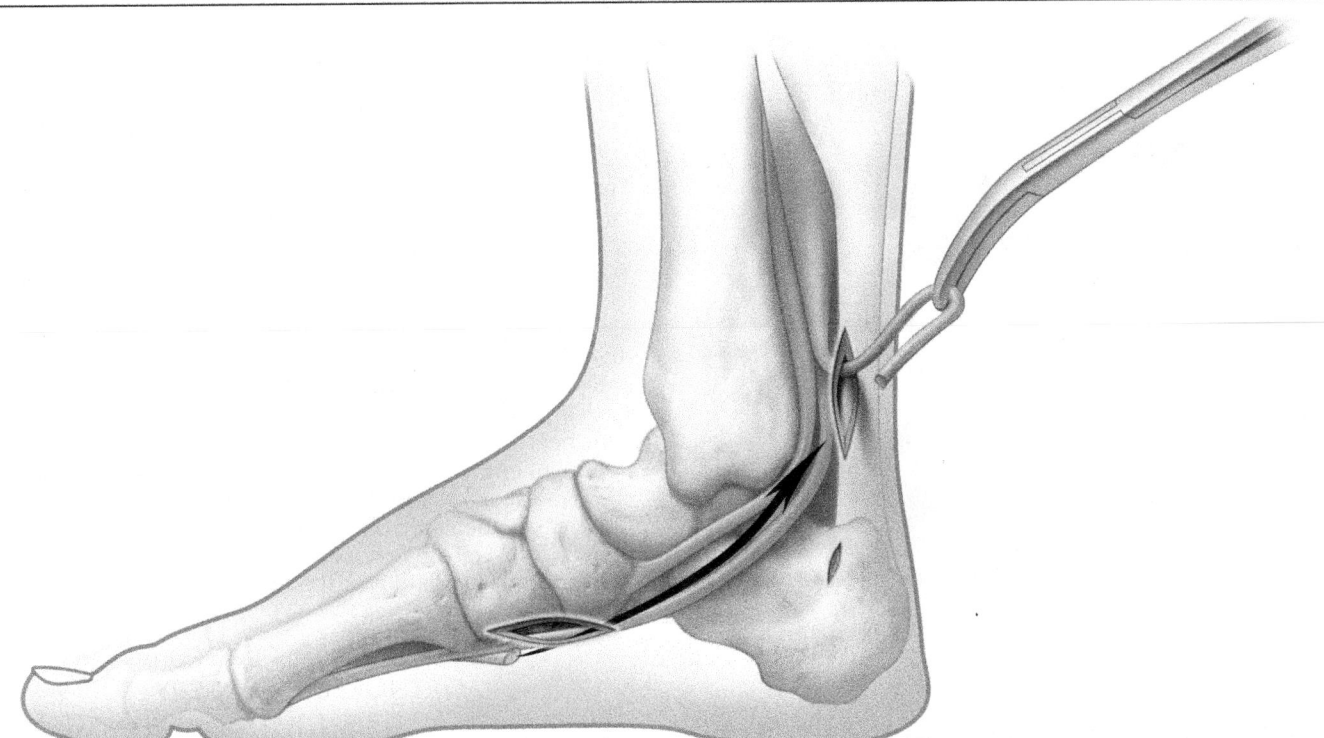

FIGURE 51-18 Flexor digitorum longus transfer to the os calcis.

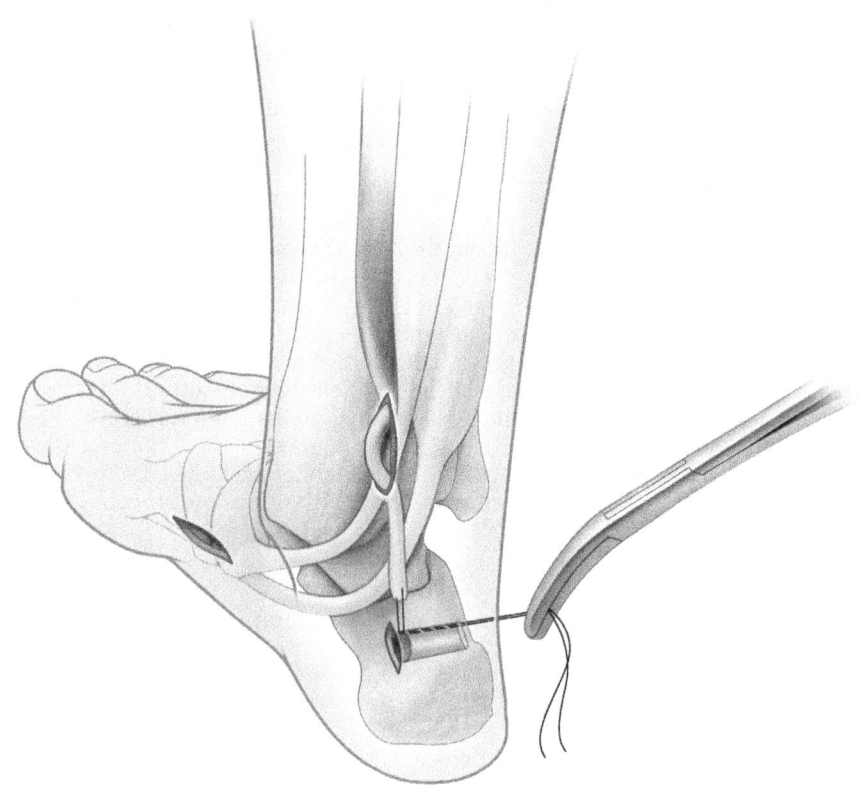

FIGURE 51-19 The FDL to heel is passed through a bone tunnel.

of the toe flexor tendons and lumbrical insertions. Because the spasticity is often extreme and of long duration, it is commonly necessary to perform a release of the plantar fascia to correct a cavus deformity as well as a triple arthrodesis in conjunction with the tendon transfer.

HETEROTOPIC OSSIFICATION IN THE POPULATION TBI: SYSTEMATIC REVIEW FINDINGS FROM THE ERABI GROUP

The ERABI group performed a systematic review comparing the HO treatment within the population with TBI and spinal cord injury (SCI) (32). Twenty-six studies (nTBI = 12; nSCI = 14) met inclusion criteria. Most studies (10/12) conducted in the population with TBI were surgical interventions. Studies conducted with the population with SCI investigated diverse pharmacological treatments including bisphosphonates, NSAIDs, and warfarin. Nonpharmacological studies investigated the benefits of pulse low-intensity electromagnetic field therapy, surgical excision, and radiotherapy in the treatment of HO. Within the SCI literature, NSAIDs showed the greatest efficacy in the prevention of HO when administered early after an SCI, and bisphosphonates were found to be the most effective treatment strategy. In the TBI population, surgical excision was the most effective treatment.

COMPLICATIONS IN NEURO-ORTHOPEDIC SURGERY

Complications in neuro-orthopedic surgery fall into 3 broad categories: complications resultant from surgery (such as

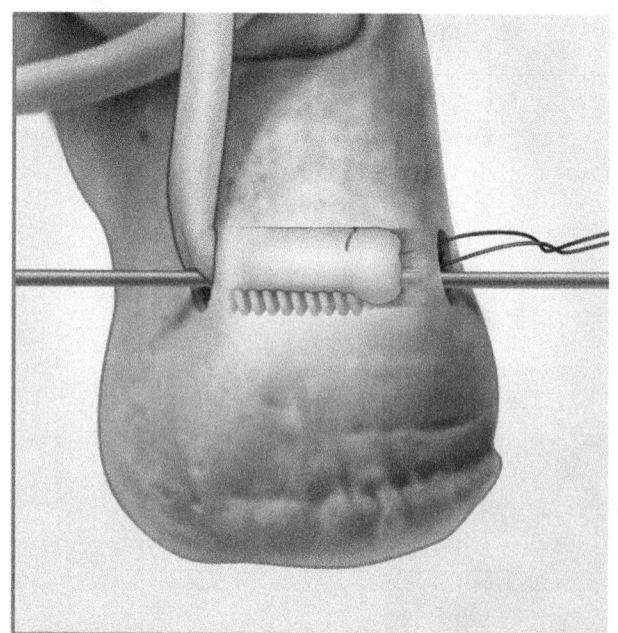

FIGURE 51-20 The FDL to heel transfer is secured with a bi-oabsorbable screw.

DVT, infection, recurrence, or failure of fixation), complications resultant from general medical condition (such as UTI, cardiac arrhythmia, or pneumonia), and complications resultant from exacerbation of medical condition by surgery (such as increased spasticity in the perioperative period).

Surgical complications are generally minimized by meticulous surgical planning and technique. For example, when a large piece of heterotopic bone is removed from the pelvis in the area of blood vessels, generally, it is our practice to alert vascular surgery, cross-match blood, and obtain preoperative 3-dimensional imaging of the heterotopic bone to avoid vascular injury. Deep vein thrombosis is relatively unusual in most surgeries outlined in this chapter. Many patients we care for fit in to the American Academy of Orthopaedic Surgeon's "high bleeding risk" category. We generally use 325 mg of enteric-coated aspirin twice daily to prophylax against pulmonary embolism in the perioperative period, unless a compelling reason exists to treat more aggressively. Infection is relatively rare. We have found that the higher risk procedures in terms of infection result from standard surgical issues, such as large dead spaces (in the case of heterotopic bone removal) or skin, which is in a difficult area (such as the proximal medial thigh). Recurrence of deformity is also relatively unusual—generally speaking—and we often treat residual deformity with bracing and serial splinting. Failure of fixation is also unusual owing to the strength of the interference screw fixation we use in many of our constructs. We have seen, on rare occasions, patients have reactions to the bioabsorbable material in the interference screw, which has necessitated debridement.

Medical complications in neurologically involved patients are not unusual. Many organ systems can be injured at the time of TBIs. As such, close care must be paid to other medical problems the patient has. We recommend liberal usage of consultants to assist in the perioperative care of these complicated patients. Care must also be taken to manage perioperative medications with the neurologic agents the patient already takes in mind.

Spasticity increases in the perioperative period. This is a response to the tissue injury, which increases the abnormal reflex arc, leading to increased muscle tone and pain. We routinely prescribe diazepam on a standing basis in the perioperative period to help offset this increased tone.

CONCLUSION

Musculoskeletal issues play a major role in determining the short- and long-term function of patients who have sustained brain injury. Orthopedic intervention is one component of a dedicated, multidisciplinary approach, which must be used to rehabilitate the musculoskeletal manifestations of neurologic compromise. Understanding the principles of current and expected function, structural deformities, and operative timing are critical. With these principles in mind, the ideal outcomes for the individual can be manifested.

Future research must focus on the long-term functional outcomes of the various surgical procedures, which are used in this patient population. This not only relates to both patient- and physician-centered outcomes but also on the biomechanical effects (via the use of motion analysis and EMG) of neurologic injury on the musculoskeletal system before and after intervention. Furthermore, the appropriate timing and role of nonsurgical interventions (i.e., antispasmodic modalities and bracing) both in combination with, and distinct from, surgical intervention must be explored. Finally, as may arise regarding the long-term degenerative effects of neurologic injury on the musculoskeletal system and the manner in which these issues can be addressed.

KEY CLINICAL POINTS

1. Patients with complex UMN disorders can initially be overwhelming to a clinician or treating surgeon. It is therefore important to understand that the care of these patients follows standard, well-known orthopedic principles. Considering the specific limb problems individually and then constructing a prioritization list is the most effective method of dealing with patients who have multiple problems.
2. It is helpful to start by considering problems in functional categories and next to consider whether or how correction of a specific limb deformity is likely to improve the function. Examples of functional categories include dressing, eating, transfers, and walking.
3. Limb function can be either active or passive. Passive function refers to problems of passive manipulation of limbs to achieve functional ends. Problems of passive function typically relate to activities such as dressing, bathing, sitting, or transfers. Problems of active function refer to a patient's direct use of a limb to carry out the functional activity. It is useful to categorize problems of function as being either passive or active in nature.
4. Walking is a commonly desired goal for patients and their caregivers. Realistic goals can be achieved by thorough assessment of patient's complete body involvement. For example, a patient with severe spastic equinovarus foot deformity may present with inability to walk. If the patient has some active hip flexion to provide limb advancement and good sitting balance, then the correction of the foot deformity is likely to make the patient ambulatory. In some cases, it may be necessary to correct a hand contracture for the patient to use a cane or a walker to achieve this goal. If the patient lacks active hip flexion and has poor trunk balance, then correction of the foot deformity will not allow walking. Correction of the foot deformity may still be indicated in this patient because it will be useful to allow shoe wear or to improve sitting balance with the foot resting on the leg support of a wheelchair.
5. By using a systematic approach and dividing problems into both functional and anatomic categories, it is easier to sort through the numerous musculoskeletal issues faced by persons with neurologic disorders. A major improvement in function and quality of life can be achieved in many patients, giving both the surgeon and the patient a feeling of satisfaction and accomplishment.

KEY REFERENCES

1. Chae J, Mascarenhas D, Yu DT, et al. Poststroke shoulder pain: its relationship to motor impairment, activity limitation, and quality of life. *Arch Phys Med Rehabil.* 2007;88(3): 298–301.
2. Esquenazi A, Mayer NH, Keenan MA. Dynamic polyelectromyography, neurolysis, and chemodenervation with

botulinum toxin A for assessment and treatment of gait dysfunction. *Adv Neurol*. 2001;87:321–331.

3. Keenan, MA. Management of the spastic upper extremity in the neurologically impaired adult. *Clin Orthop Relat Res*. 1988;(233):116–125.

4. Keenan MA. Surgical decision making for residual limb deformities following traumatic brain injury. *Orthop Rev*. 1988;17(12):1185–1192.

5. Keenan MA, Esquenazi A, Mayer NH. Surgical treatment of common patterns of lower limb deformities resulting from upper motoneuron syndrome. *Adv Neurol*. 2001;87:333–346.

Recommended E-Books

1. Vaccaro A, Fehlings M, Dvorak M. *Spine and Spinal Cord Trauma: Evidence Based Management*. New York, NY: Thieme; 2011.

2. Castro W, Jerosch J, Grossman TW. *Examination and Diagnosis of Musculoskeletal Disorders*. New York, NY: Thieme; 2001.

References

1. Keenan MA, Mehta S. Neuro-orthopedic management of shoulder deformity and dysfunction in brain-injured patients: a novel approach. *J Head Trauma Rehabil*. 2004;19(2):143–154.

2. Pill SG, Keenan MA. Neuro-orthpaedic management of extremity dysfunction in patients with spasticity from upper motor neuron syndromes. In: Mayer NH, Brashear A, eds. *Spasticity and other Forms of Muscle Overactivity in the Upper Motor Neuron Syndrome*. New York, NY: WE MOVE; 2008:119–141.

3. Garland DE, Keenan MA. Orthopedic strategies in the management of the adult head-injured patient. *Phys Ther*. 1983;63(12):2004–2009.

4. Keenan MA. Surgical decision making for residual limb deformities following traumatic brain injury. *Orthop Rev*. 1988;17(12):1185–1192.

5. Lusskin R, Grynbaum BB, Dhir RS. Rehabilitation surgery in adult spastic hemiplegia. *Clin Orthop Relat Res*. 1959;63:132–141.

6. Namdari S, Alosh H, Baldwin K, Mehta S, Keenan MA. Outcomes of tendon fractional lengthenings to improve shoulder function in patients with spastic hemiparesis [published online ahead of print June 28, 2011]. *J Shoulder Elbow Surg*. 2011.

7. Namdari S, Alosh H, Baldwin K, Mehta S, Keenan MA. Shoulder tenotomies to improve passive motion and relieve pain in patients with spastic hemiplegia after upper motor neuron injury. *J Shoulder Elbow Surg*. 2011;20(5):802–806.

8. Keenan MA. Management of the spastic upper extremity in the neurologically impaired adult. *Clin Orthop Relat Res*. 1988;(233):116–25.

9. Chae J, Mascarenhas D, Yu DT, et al. Poststroke shoulder pain: its relationship to motor impairment, activity limitation, and quality of life. *Arch Phys Med Rehabil*. 2007;88(3):298–301.

10. Chan KT. Heterotopic ossification in traumatic brain injury. *Am J Phys Med Rehabil*. 2005;84(2):145–146.

11. Akbar M, Balean G, Brunner M, et al. Prevalence of rotator cuff tear in paraplegic patients compared with controls. *J Bone Joint Surg Am*. 2010;92(1):23–30.

12. Cipriano CA, Pill SG, Keenan MA. Heterotopic ossification following traumatic brain injury and spinal cord injury. *J Am Acad Orthop Surg*. 2009;17(11):689–697.

13. Namdari S, Keenan MA. Outcomes of the biceps suspension procedure for painful inferior glenohumeral subluxation in hemiplegic patients. *J Bone Joint Surg Am*. 2010;92(15):2589–2597.

14. Kozin SH, Keenan MA. Using dynamic electromyography to guide surgical treatment of the spastic upper extremity in the brain-injured patient. *Clin Orthop Relat Res*. 1993;(288):109–117.

15. Baldwin K, Hosalkar HS, Donegan DJ, Rendon N, Ramsey M, Keenan MA. Surgical resection of heterotopic bone about the elbow: an institutional experience with traumatic and neurologic etiologies. *J Hand Surg Am*. 2011;36(5):798–803.

16. Keenan MA, Haider TT, Stone LR. Dynamic electromyography to assess elbow spasticity. *J Hand Surg*. 1990;15(4):607–614.

17. Keenan MA, Kauffman DL, Garland DE, Smith C. Late ulnar neuropathy in the brain-injured adult. *J Hand Surg*. 1988;13(1):120–124.

18. Pomerance JF, Keenan MA. Correction of severe spastic flexion contractures in the nonfunctional hand. *J Hand Surg*. 1996;21(5):828–833.

19. Rayan GM, Young BT. Arthrodesis of the spastic wrist. *J Hand Surg Am*. 1999;24(5):944–952.

20. Keenan MA, Korchek JI, Botte MJ, Smith CW, Garland DE. Results of transfer of the flexor digitorum superficialis tendons to the flexor digitorum profundus tendons in adults with acquired spasticity of the hand. *J Bone Joint Surg Am*. 1987;69(8):1127–1132.

21. Botte MJ, Keenan MA, Korchek JI, Waters RL. Modified technique for the superficialis-to-profundus transfer in the treatment of adults with spastic clenched fist deformity. *J Hand Surg Am*. 1987;12(4):639–640.

22. Pappas N, Baldwin K, Keenan MA. Efficacy of median nerve recurrent branch neurectomy as an adjunct to ulnar motor nerve neurectomy and wrist arthrodesis at the time of superficialis to profundus transfer in prevention of intrinsic spastic thumb-in-palm deformity. *J Hand Surg Am*. 2010;35(8):1310–1316.

23. Botte MJ, Keenan MA, Gellman H, Garland DE, Waters RL. Surgical management of spastic thumb-in-palm deformity in adults with brain injury. *J Hand Surg Am*.1989;14(2, pt 1):174–182.

24. Botte MJ, Keenan MA, Abrams RA, von Schroeder HP, Gellman H, Mooney V. Heterotopic ossification in neuromuscular disorders. *Orthopedics*. 1997;20(4):335–341.

25. Keenan MA, Ure K, Smith CW, Jordan C. Hamstring release for knee flexion contracture in spastic adults. *Clin Orthop Relat Res*.1988;(236):221–226.

26. Esquenazi A, Mayer NH, Keenan MA. Dynamic polyelectromyography, neurolysis, and chemodenervation with botulinum toxin A for assessment and treatment of gait dysfunction. *Adv Neurol*. 2001; 87:321–331.

27. Namdari S, Pill SG, Makani A, Keenan MA. Rectus femoris to gracilis muscle transfer with fractional lengthening of the vastus muscles: a treatment for adults with stiff knee gait. *Phys Ther*. 2010;90(2):261–268.

28. Namdari S, Park MJ, Baldwin K, Hosalkar HS, Keenan MA. Effect of age, sex, and timing on correction of spastic equinovarus following cerebrovascular accident. *Foot Ankle Int*. 2009;30(10):923–927.

29. Keenan MA, Esquenazi A, Mayer NH. Surgical treatment of common patterns of lower limb deformities resulting from upper motoneuron syndrome. *Adv Neurol*. 2001;87:333–346.

30. Young S, Keenan MA, Stone LR. The treatment of spastic planovalgus foot deformity in the neurologically impaired adult. *Foot Ankle*. 1990;10(6):317–324.

31. Keenan MA, Lee GA, Tuckman AS, Esquenazi A. Improving calf muscle strength in patients with spastic equinovarus deformity by transfer of the long toe flexors to the Os calcis. *J Head Trauma Rehabil*. 1999;14(2):163–175.

32. Aubut JA, Mehta S, Cullen N, Teasell RW; for ERABI Group and Scire Research Team. A comparison of heterotopic ossification treatment within the traumatic brain and spinal cord injured population: an evidence based systematic review. *NeuroRehabilitation*. 2011;28(2):151–160.

XI

AUTONOMIC AND OTHER ORGAN SYSTEM PROBLEMS

Autonomic Dysfunction

Ian J. Baguley and Melissa T. Nott

INTRODUCTION

The effects of traumatic brain injury (TBI) on the autonomic nervous system (ANS) are many and varied. This chapter will briefly review the anatomy and functions of the ANS before considering how TBI may affect ANS function. Although the ANS subserves a multitude of bodily functions, this chapter will predominantly focus on the cardiovascular changes that result from TBI. A practical approach toward interpreting and managing ANS abnormalities will be presented.

A BRIEF REVIEW OF AUTONOMIC ANATOMY AND PHYSIOLOGY

Basic Functions

The basic functions of the ANS are known to all trained health professionals. The ANS maintains homeostasis in the face of the body's daily challenges, without requiring the organism's direct conscious attention. Principally among these tasks, the ANS manages the body's power plant, distributing energy to all parts of the body, and organizing waste removal. It fulfills this maintenance role through 2 main subsystems: the sympathetic and the parasympathetic nervous systems. These 2 arms of the ANS provide complementary services, and the balance between the 2 is vital to accommodate normal homeostasis.

The actions of the sympathetic arm of the ANS are most easily remembered with consideration of the "flight or fight" response. Here, the classical effect of sympathetic efflux is to increase heart rate, increase cardiac ejection fraction, raise blood pressure, redirect blood flow from the gastrointestinal tract to skeletal muscle, tighten sphincters, dilate the pupils, and prime the body for sweating. Conversely, the parasympathetic arm is more concerned with vegetative functions: slowing heart rate, increasing blood flow to the gastrointestinal tract, contracting the pupils, modulating bladder wall compliance, and so on (1).

The ANS is normally visualized with the emphasis on the effector organs and the peripheral nerves. However, for the purposes of understanding how TBI may impact the ANS, it is more useful to consider the ANS at the level of its integration into the central nervous system (CNS). This has been termed the central autonomic network (CAN) (2), a model that describes a hierarchical approach to the control of the ANS, from the simplest components to the most complex interconnected pathways.

Working from the periphery, the first point of contact between the effector organ (such as arterial smooth muscle or the adrenal glands) and the ANS are the peripheral synapses. The axon from this synapse travels via a peripheral mixed nerve back toward the spinal cord where it enters via the vagus or sacral nerves for parasympathetic or T2-L2 levels for sympathetic pathways. Within the spinal cord, some autonomic pathways interact directly with somatic sensory nerves to establish spinal reflex centers. These distal reflex centers are then wired under the influence of brainstem centers, which in turn may be influenced by 1 or more hypothalamic centers, subcortical, and/or cortical centers. The pattern of organization within the CAN is such that each additional hierarchical level progressively "fine tunes" the relatively cruder responses of the levels below.

A well understood and practical example of CAN integration is the control of micturition. In this example, the effector organs are the detrusor muscle and the internal sphincter, which obtain innervation from parasympathetic and sympathetic neurons respectively. At the spinal level, parasympathetic centers control bladder muscle tone, whereas sympathetic centers control internal sphincter muscle tone. Coordination of these spinal centers is undertaken at the level of the pons, and lesions below this level will produce predictable patterns of lower motor neuron, upper motor neuron, or mixed type bladder dyscontrol. Acting independently, the pontine micturition center produces low pressure micturition at a bladder volume of around 150 mL. The pontine center is, in turn, under the control of frontal lobes via pathways developed during early childhood that allows a larger volume, low pressure bladder under volitional control (1).

At the highest conceptual levels of the CAN, information from multiple autonomic subsystems is integrated to produce a coordinated response to any event that upsets homeostasis. Eating a meal or undertaking vigorous exercise will set in motion a predictable pattern of ANS activation, effected through the balance of inhibitory and stimulatory influences over sympathetic and parasympathetic "lower" centers. In addition to physical stressors, purely psychological inputs can increase sympathetic efflux, for example, when encountering an anxiety-provoking situation, such as that seen in "white coat hypertension" (3).

The simultaneous presentation of multiple homeostatic challenges produces a series of competing agendas and urgencies that the ANS must negotiate automatically and in a way that maximizes survival. The ANS resolves the issue of competing interests via complex feedback loops that relay information within and between the various structures and levels of the CAN. The complexity of this system ensures that the human body can respond to multiple challenges appropriately, using flexible and finely balanced control between its sympathetic and parasympathetic arms.

The Pathophysiology of TBI and Its Impact on Autonomic Function

By definition, the effects of TBI will impact on neurological tissue above the level of the spinal cord. Therefore, TBI will not directly affect the integrity of the peripheral nerves or end organs controlling ANS function, such as the arterial smooth muscle. Similarly, TBI will not directly impact on ANS spinal cord reflex centers because their immediate structural integrity will be unimpaired. The possible exception to this scenario will be in patients with coincident TBI and spinal cord injury (SCI), estimated to occur in 6% of severe TBI presentations to emergency departments (4).

In severe TBI, the nature of the injury is such that both cortical and subcortical ANS control mechanisms are likely to suffer structural damage. The integrity of ANS responses in the first weeks post-TBI will, therefore, depend on a range of parameters: the overall severity of the injury, the relative contribution of diffuse, focal and/or hypoxic damage from the primary injury, and the extent of secondary postinjury brain damage. These will be examined in turn.

Focal injuries such as contusions or intracerebral hemorrhages carry the potential to produce localized damage to ANS control centers. It would be expected that focal injuries in the hypothalamus and brainstem would be particularly likely to affect midlevel CAN reflex centers. In contrast, diffuse axonal injury or axonal shear secondary to an extra-axial collection or intracerebral hemorrhage has the capacity to produce a relative de-afferentation between midlevel ANS control centers and mechanisms higher in the CAN hierarchy. This "disconnection" could hypothetically reduce integration of more complex homeostatic mechanisms. Severe hypoxia may have a preferential effect on grey matter (5), therefore making it likely to damage neuronal clusters rather than axonal connections. This is also true of many secondary brain injury mechanisms occurring at the cellular level (e.g., late neuronal death caused by apoptotic pathways, mitochondrial dysfunction, impaired glucose metabolism, and so on) (6). Interrelated with all of these potential injury modes are issues of raised intracerebral pressure (ICP) and secondary impairments of cerebral blood supply.

Considered in overview, the impact that severe TBI will have on ANS responsivity will be the result of cumulative damage from these various discrete pathological forms. Consequently, radiological investigations rarely assist in predicting the impact that TBI will have on ANS structures. Rather, the severity of ANS dysfunction is best inferred from monitoring physiological parameters in the intensive care unit (ICU). As a general rule, the greater the cumulative damage to cerebral ANS pathways, the cruder and less sophisticated the ANS response to homeostatic challenge is likely to be.

In the most severe form, damage to central ANS control systems following severe TBI will be incompatible with life. Indeed, aspects of failure of autonomic responses are used within the criteria for the diagnosis of brain death (7). Individuals with marginally less severe trauma may present with a variety of injuries that produce the net effect of a near-complete midbrain lesion. These injuries may be compatible with life in the controlled environment of the modern ICU but may be nonsurvivable outside of this setting. Such injuries have been hypothesized to release spinal cord ANS centers from higher level control (8).

The midrange of the ANS injury severity spectrum includes damage to the midlevel hypothalamic controls and/or less complete brainstem damage. These injuries may prevent the reception of peripheral stimuli or the appropriate response of autonomic reflexes. Such syndromes include conditions such as Cheyne-Stokes respiration, uncontrolled hypertension following spontaneous subarachnoid hemorrhage (SAH), primary vagal failure, orthostatic hypotension, or prolonged hyperthermia. Although these specific symptoms or deficits may be identifiable, it is common for such injuries to remain undiagnosed because of the comorbidities associated with brainstem injuries, such as severe physical disability, anarthria, and impaired arousal. Conversely, the mildest end of the spectrum is the most controversial, consisting of a range of conditions including subjective complaints of temperature dysregulation and excessive or gustatory sweating.

AUTONOMIC SYNDROMES ASSOCIATED WITH TBI

In acute physical trauma (that does not involve the CNS), sympathetic drive increases in proportion to the severity of the originating traumatic stimulus. In the immediate posttrauma period, the body responds with increased sympathetic drive, producing tachycardia, increased blood pressure, and a redirection of blood flow toward vital organs. Having survived the initial trauma, the body's challenge is to maintain homeostasis in response to secondary issues such as infection, fractures, postsurgical complications, drug withdrawal, and so on. The evolution of these homeostatic challenges should subtly alter the dynamic interaction of sympathetic and parasympathetic activation with increasing time postinjury.

A similar situation also occurs following severe TBI. Immediately postinjury, a hypersympathetic response with tachycardia, hypertension, and increased respiratory rate is common, occurring in between 62% (9) and 92% (10) of patients admitted to the ICU. The extent to which regulation of ANS function changes over time from this point will be influenced by the overall extent of brain damage and later by the effects of neural plasticity. In the early stages postinjury, continued failure of ANS control has the potential to exacerbate the cascade of secondary brain insults, increasing brain damage, and/or resulting in death (11). Ideally, neurological improvements in the weeks and months postinjury will result in normalization of CAN functions. However, in some situations, changes resulting from dysfunctional neuroplasticity have the potential to result in long-term ANS deficits (8).

TABLE 52-1 Main Classes of Autonomic Problems

SEVERITY	DESCRIPTION	EXAMPLES
Mild	Autonomic incoordination syndromes	Post-TBI heat intolerance, gustatory sweating
Moderate	Selective autonomic failure	Primary vagal dysfunction, abnormal GIT function, orthostatic hypotension
Severe	Widespread autonomic dysregulation	Hypertensive crisis in spontaneous subarachnoid hemorrhage, paroxysmal sympathetic hyperactivity

Abbreviation. GIT, gastrointestinal tract.

Based on these concepts, it is possible to categorize post-TBI autonomic abnormalities into 3 major groups based on their overall impact on ANS function (Figure 52-1). At the mildest end are high-level ANS "incoordination syndromes." Of greater importance are discrete failures of various midlevel ANS control centers. At the severe end of the spectrum are conditions that produce widespread dysregulation of autonomic functions. Although these issues will be addressed in turn, the impact and recent evidence for paroxysmal sympathetic hyperactivity (PSH) warrants greater discussion, and much of the remainder of this chapter will address this issue.

Autonomic Incoordination Syndromes

At the mildest end of the spectrum, it is possible to imagine scenarios where the midlevel and low-level controls of the CAN are intact, but where the highest levels, those that coordinate responses to multiple competing homeostatic challenges, may be adversely affected. By nature, this hypothetical situation could be expected to produce a collection of relatively ill defined, subtle, and nonspecific syndromes. Furthermore, because most TBI occurs in the mild or moderate severity categories, it could be expected that such mild syndromes could be a commonplace, but because of their nonspecific nature, objective data for the existence of these types of symptoms is lacking. For these reasons, it is possible that many of the ANS effects of brain injury may occur at this subtle and poorly investigated end of the spectrum. Furthermore, the subjective experience of the TBI survivor may be indistinguishable from psychological or anxiety-related phenomena in laboratory testing. As such, these injuries remain controversial but include subjective complaints of temperature dysregulation and excessive or gustatory sweating.

Clinical Example: Post-TBI Temperature Intolerance

A relatively common complaint in the postacute outpatient TBI setting is the subjective report of temperature intolerance. In this scenario, the patient will perceive recurrent sensations of altered temperature. Three main variations have been reported: a feeling of excessive body temperature, a marked sensation of cold, or a combination of both experiences at different times (12). Some patients may have outward signs of increased body temperature and sweating, irrespective of the prevailing temperature conditions. Indeed, the person may attend the clinic wearing a singlet and shorts, even though everyone else is wearing winter clothing. Another variant of these symptoms are patients with a self-perceived "poikilothermia," the sensation that their core temperature fluctuates in sync with prevailing environmental conditions. In this scenario, there will be some occasions where they report feeling excessively hot, whereas at other times, the sensation will be feeling of unable to warm up. When financially covered by an injury compensation system of some sort, this second group of patients often request temperature control systems to assist in managing the problem.

Because the sensation of temperature dysregulation is cortical in nature, the importance that the affected individual ascribes to the symptom complex is likely to be modified by personality variables. For example, individuals with a tendency toward excessive somatization (defined here as the overinterpretation of the importance of physical symptoms) will tend to be overly aware of the symptoms and believe they are of great importance. While the individual may be extremely concerned by their day-by-day symptoms, objective evidence is usually lacking. Even with access to appropriately equipped autonomic laboratories, investigation of such individuals may produce equivocal results.

Such heightened symptom awareness, often coupled with the lack of an adequate medical diagnosis, can contribute to chronically elevated anxiety in susceptible individuals. Such a situation will tend to exacerbate the problem by increasing sympathetic drive further. Any lack of concordance between the objective symptoms and the importance that affected person places on their significance could lead clinicians to treat the symptoms as fictitious. Sparse literature, coupled with lack of an accepted treatment paradigm, and absent evidence of organicity often results in increased anxiety and a significant reduction in the patient's quality of life. Perhaps, for these reasons, differentiating the actual importance from the perceived importance of the syndrome can be difficult, as is determining whether the observed psychological response is a cause or effect of the syndrome.

Selective Autonomic Failure

Damage to localized brainstem centers can produce long-term impairment of basic homeostatic functions. In many situations, the brainstem damage will be too diffuse to allow the individual mechanisms to be clearly delineated; however, in a minority of patients it is possible to identify discreet loss of autonomic control functions. There are large numbers of these syndromes affecting all areas of autonomic function, for example, increased vagal tone leading to impaired immune system function following TBI (13).

With reference to cardiovascular pathways, abnormal function can follow from failure of the afferent pathways, the brainstem reflex center, or efferent pathways. A good example of this class of disorders is those involving failures of baroreflex function. The baroreflex provides a feedback mechanism for blood pressure control. Receptors in the carotid sinus and other sites provide afferent information via the glossopharyngeal and vagal nerves. Centers in the brainstem then modulate sympathetic outflow based on whether the blood pressure is detected to be higher or lower than threshold. Failure of the baroreflex may lead to a number of different clinical situations including hypertensive crisis, volatile hypertension, orthostatic tachycardia, and malignant vagotonia depending on the location of the lesion/s (14). In postural tachycardia syndrome after TBI, subjects have reported dizziness, fatigue, and palpitations when challenged in a head up tilt table test, whereas most reported occasional syncope (15). Management of blood pressure improves outcomes in some but not all patients.

Although such midlevel ANS disorders are easy to understand in terms of their pathophysiology, the brainstem is relatively protected from all but the most severe injuries. As a consequence, it is uncommon for injuries to be constrained within a small enough area of the brainstem for discrete syndromes to be identified, making this group of disorders an interesting but relatively uncommon complication of TBI. Instead, the association of high-energy injuries (particularly where there are large rotational forces involved in the injury) and brainstem injury makes the likelihood of widespread autonomic dysregulation much more probable than selective lesions following severe TBI.

Widespread Autonomic Dysregulation

The clearest example of a widespread autonomic disorder is PSH. PSH shows similarities with other conditions such as the hypertensive crisis resulting from spontaneous SAH; however, the 2 conditions appear to have separate pathophysiological causes.

Paroxysmal Sympathetic Hyperactivity

The term PSH is used to identify a syndrome of simultaneous and paroxysmal sympathetic and muscle overactivity following acquired brain injury. Historically, the nomenclature for the condition has been very convoluted, with at least 31 different names used for the condition in published literature (16). The term PSH was coined in 2007 (17) and is increasingly being adopted to replace less specific terms such as sympathetic storming (18), autonomic dysfunction syndrome (19), dysautonomia (20), and paroxysmal autonomic instability with dystonia (21). Part of the confusion in nomenclature has stemmed from the use of generic terms such as dysautonomia, a term that is used in other contexts to identify different medical syndromes (22).

The hallmarks of PSH are presumed to be the result of excessive activation of the sympathetic arm of the ANS, often as an exaggerated response to physical or environmental stimuli. The hypersympathetic drive occurs over a range of severities but includes documented heart rates up to 190 beats per minute (bpm), respiratory rates up to 60 breaths per minute, core temperatures up to 42°C, and arterial blood pressures of 170/120 mm Hg (11). These sympathetic features are most often reported in association with sweating and motor overactivity, the latter presenting as decorticate or decerebrate posturing, muscle spasticity, and/or dystonias.

The most easily recordable features of PSH are the paroxysms of elevated blood pressure, heart rate, temperature, and respiratory rate. In a retrospective age-, sex-, and Glasgow Coma Scale (GCS)-matched case controlled series, TBI subjects with PSH showed clear differences in daily physiological maxima compared to controls (Figure 52-1) (11). Data for the 2 groups were similar until day 7 post-TBI, when the PSH group data diverged from the non-PSH group for each physiological variable; a differentiation that coincided with the withdrawal of regular sedation. The largest and most persistent differences were observed in heart rate, with blood pressure being the first variable where values normalized between groups.

In the early period following sedation withdrawal, individuals with PSH can display paroxysmal episodes that are frequent, prolonged, and intense. The extent of these changes can readily be observed via heart rate changes recorded from a 24-hour Holter monitor (Figure 52-2). In this example, the unmedicated patient was 28 days post-TBI and nursed supine for the period of data collection. Mean heart rate for the day was 129 bpm, ranging from a minimum of 67 bpm to a maximum of 182 bpm. The heart rate trace also provides an example of the variability of PSH, with a number of distinct paroxysmal episodes of differing severity lasting between 2 and 6 hours. Occasionally, the patient's heart rate rested at below 80 bpm (amounting to 11% of the day), consistent with normal expectations of a person lying supine in bed. Conversely, the patient experienced heart rates greater than 140 bpm for more than one-third of the day. Investigations failed to identify an alternative medical explanation for these observations.

The elevated cardiorespiratory parameters observed in patients with PSH are accompanied by sweating and assorted forms of motor overactivity, including decerebrate or decorticate posturing, dystonia, rigidity, and spasticity. Motor components are often exacerbated during paroxysms, are often asymmetrical (11,23), and can also show a degree of variability from one paroxysm to the next. The variability in motor overactivity is displayed in Figure 52-3, where the individual with PSH was nursed in a position of comfort between PSH episodes (Figure 52-3a) but variably showed extensor posturing (Figure 52-3b) or upper limb flexor posturing (Figure 52-3c) during paroxysms. Sweating (Figure 52-4) can also be dramatic, with 5 L/day of insensible fluid losses being reported (11).

Aside from the autonomic and motor parameters reported in PSH, authors have suggested a variety of additional features as being associated with the diagnosis. For example, elevated creatinine kinase levels have been identified wherever they have been assayed (11,24–28). Circulating sympathetic hormone levels have not been reported between and during paroxysms; however, catecholamine production is usually in the order of twice the normal upper limit when assayed (28,29). These markedly elevated circulating sympathetic hormones have been postulated as a cause of the poor gastrointestinal tract absorption observed following severe TBI (30). Less frequently reported PSH-related features include elevated white blood cell count in

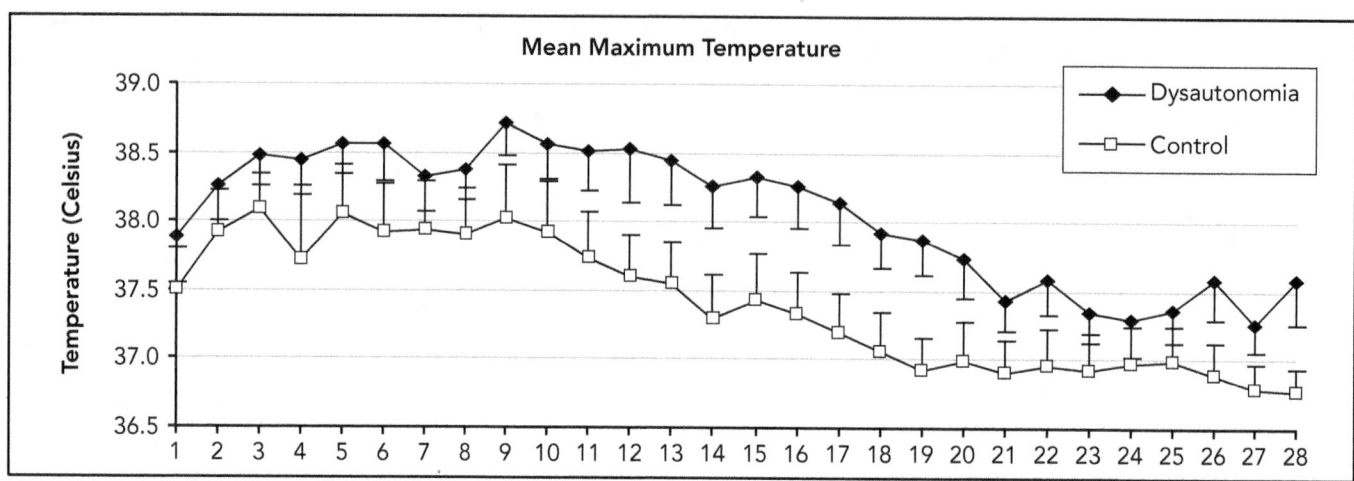

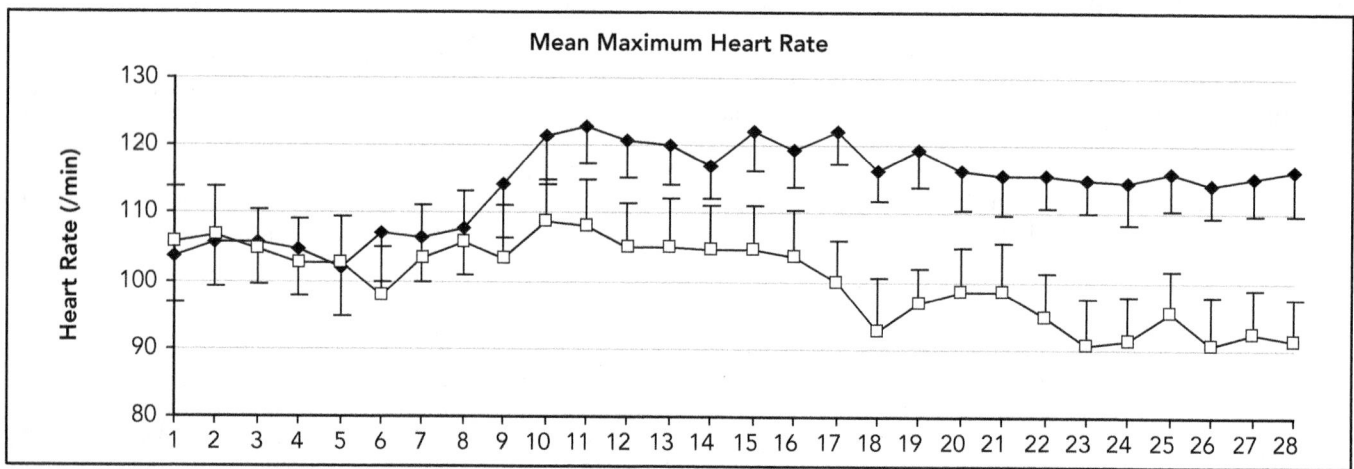

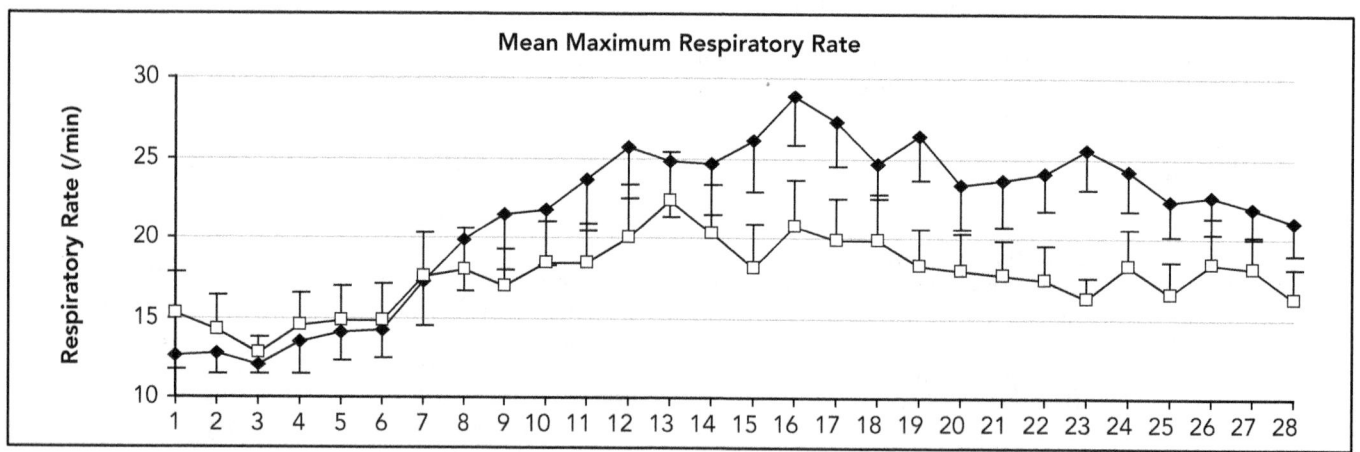

FIGURE 52-1 Daily physiological maxima by group. Adapted from Baguley et al (11) with permission.

the absence of microbial infection (11), asymptomatic arrhythmias and neurogenic lung disease (31), pupillary dilatation (32–34), excessive salivation (35), crying, hiccups, yawning, and sighing (19). However, not all subjects with PSH develop all features of the syndrome (10,36), and the importance of each individual symptom is unknown.

The clinical features of PSH vary between affected individuals with respect to severity and duration; therefore, it has been suggested that PSH should best be considered a spectral disorder (10). In this study, sympathetic hyperactiv-

ity lasting up to 7 days postinjury occurs in 25%–33% of survivors of severe TBI. A smaller group, estimated at 8%–14% of all severe TBI subjects, develop the more prolonged form of PSH (10). Although the clinical implications of short duration sympathetic hyperactivity are uncertain (37), most reports associate prolonged PSH following severe TBI with worse outcome (10,11,38,39), evidenced by prolonged swallowing abnormalities, longer coma (38), longer duration of post-traumatic amnesia (11), longer hospital admission (10,11), and greater overall health care costs (10).

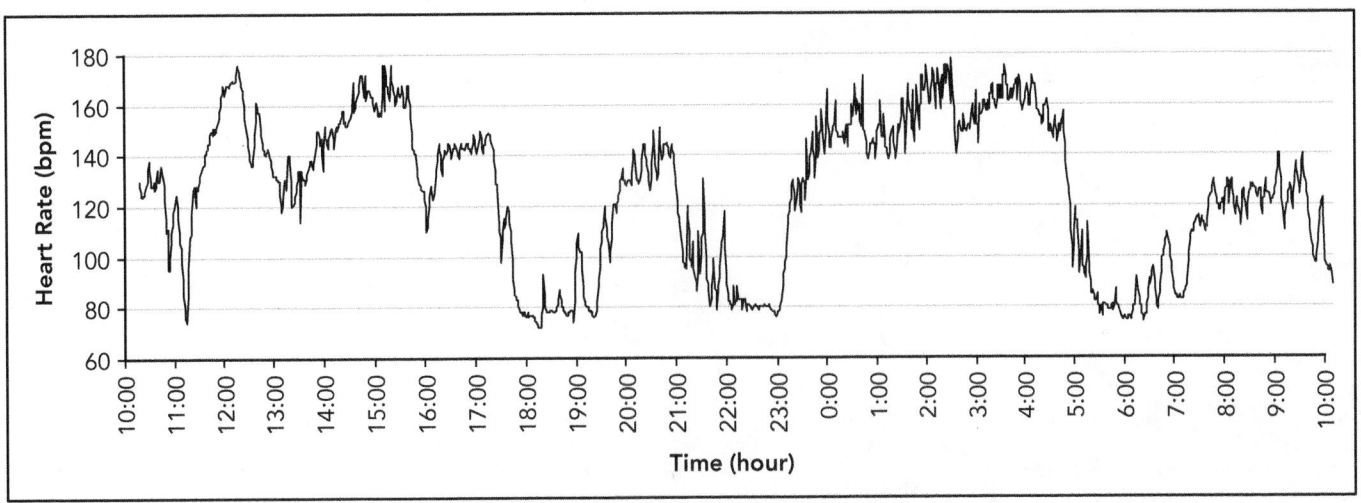

FIGURE 52-2 Minutely heart rate in an unmedicated patient with paroxysmal sympathetic hyperactivity, collected over a 24-hour period. Reproduced from Jaypee Brothers Medical Publishers Pty. Ltd., India with permission.

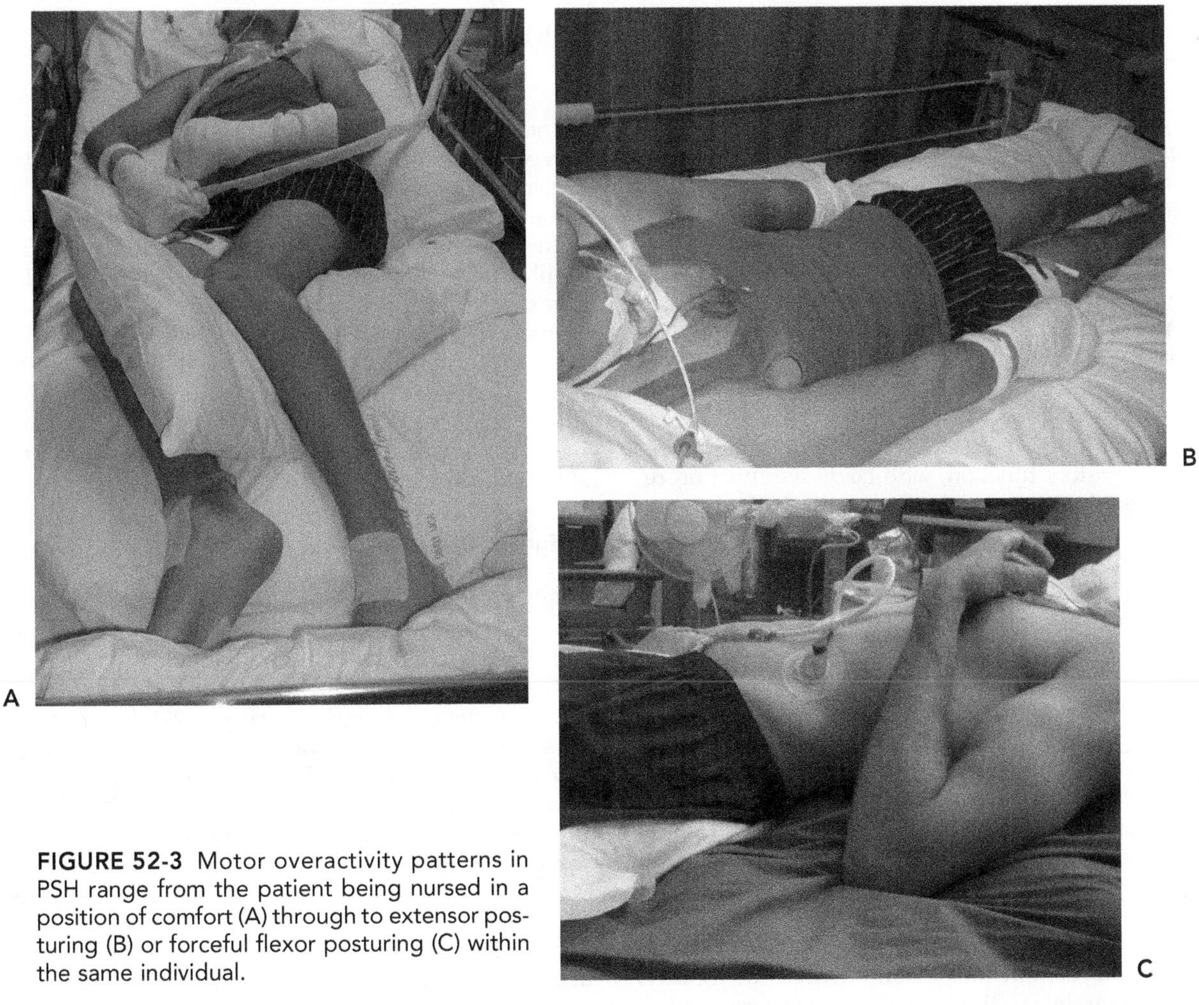

FIGURE 52-3 Motor overactivity patterns in PSH range from the patient being nursed in a position of comfort (A) through to extensor posturing (B) or forceful flexor posturing (C) within the same individual.

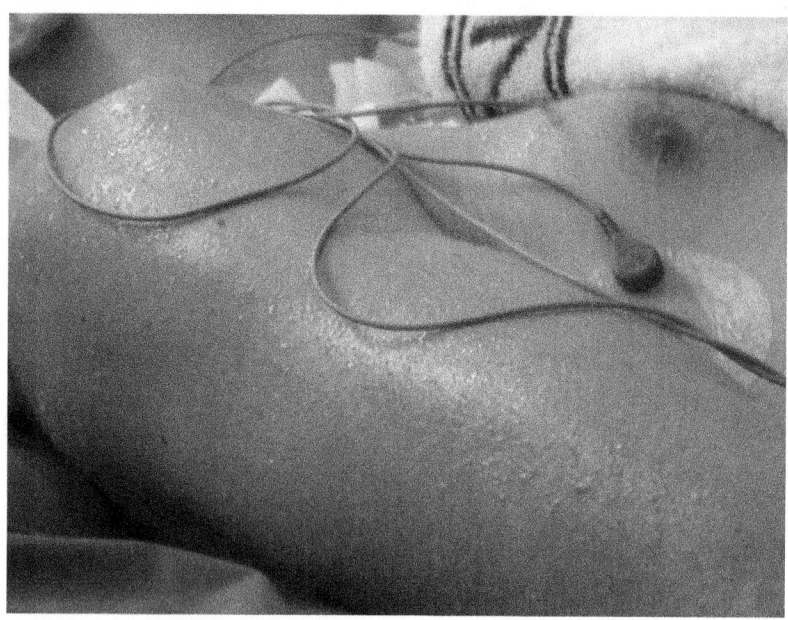

FIGURE 52-4 Severe sweating in a patient with PSH.

A smaller number of studies have not identified such an association (40,41).

In its most severe form, PSH continues after discharge from ICU and persists during the rehabilitation phase. For most patients, objective evidence of sympathetic arousal decreases with increasing time postinjury, although the timing of this progression differs from person to person. The progressive reduction and extinguishment of hypersympathetic episodes represents the chronic phase of PSH. In this stage, the paroxysmal increases in physiological parameters become less pronounced in duration, frequency, and severity. The observed improvement often coincides with improving neurological status (19), although it is unclear whether the 2 events are causally linked. When considering neurological status, it is important to note that the presence of PSH does not exclude cognitive function, with cognitive function reported to be evident *between* paroxysms (18,24,42) or even *during* paroxysms (34,43). Furthermore, there are case reports of subjects with PSH showing evidence of a "locked-in syndrome" (10,44,45), suggesting that the presence of PSH does not require catastrophic cerebral injury or preclude cognitive function in all individuals.

Along with other sympathetic variables, the intensity of sweating and the extent of the body surface involved reduces with increasing time postinjury (46). In a number of studies, the cessation of sweating has been used to mark the transition into the chronic PSH phase, occurring at 2.5 and 5.9 months postinjury respectively in 2 large cohort studies (11,39). In another study, sympathetic overactivity had settled by 6 months postinjury in 22 of 31 subjects with PSH (38).

Although hypersympathetic features abate, many patients continue to exhibit motor abnormalities of rigidity, dystonia, and muscle spasticity (11,18). As recovery continues, posturing may decrease, revealing an underlying spastic quadriparesis or a focal neurological deficit. Individuals with very severe PSH often experience a permanent degree of dystonia and muscle spasticity (10). In some cases, the

high degree of physical disability further limits the accuracy of cognitive assessment.

Diagnostic Criteria

A recent literature review identified 81 PSH-related articles, either published as case data or topic reviews (16). Most of these articles used anecdotal techniques to diagnose PSH, with only 27 (33%) employing diagnostic criteria from 1 of 9 published diagnostic criteria sets. Most of the 9 diagnostic sets showed a high degree of overlap in their core criteria (namely heart rate, blood pressure, respiratory rate, temperature, sweating, and motor hyperactivity) and used a polythetic diagnostic system (47). All but one indicated severity thresholds, for example, heart rate >120 bpm. An international consensus process is currently underway to establish standardized nomenclature and diagnostic criteria (48).

"Triggering" of Paroxysmal Sympathetic Hyperactivity Episodes

Applying the current definition of PSH (22), the first clearly reported case was reported by Wilder Penfield in 1954 (49). A 1929 article by Dr. Penfield is commonly reported to be the earliest case report; however, some features of the case do not meet current diagnostic criteria (22). In the 1954 article, Penfield reported an association between paroxysmal features and afferent stimuli. This association has continued to be reported intermittently, with "triggering" of episodes reported to follow pain, endotracheal tube (ETT) suctioning, passive movement (e.g., turning, bathing, and muscle stretching) (11,34,50–58), constipation or urinary retention (50,59), emotional stimuli (34), and even loud noises (18).

Empirical research has recently given support to these anecdotal observations, with exaggerated responsiveness to stimuli having been reported from day 7 to 5 years postinjury. In one prospective study, ETT suctioning was used to provide a semistandardized nociceptive stimulus (37). Using this as a trigger, heart rate data was recorded as a marker of sympathetic drive before and after application of the stimulus. In this study, subjects who went on to develop prolonged PSH showed markedly greater heart rate reactivity to the stimulus at 7 days postinjury compared to those whose sympathetic features settled prior to discharge from ICU.

Although the hypersympathetic drive is thought to "burn out" in the chronic phase of the disorder, evidence suggests that *subclinical* sympathetic overactivity in response to afferent stimuli persists long-term. An empirical study of subjects who had experienced prolonged PSH assessed heart rate variability (HRV) as a marker of neural heart rate control at least 14 months postinjury (60). In this study, HRV responses of PSH subjects remained abnormal well beyond the period when hypersympathetic drive was clinically evident. In a further study (61), prolonged PSH subjects were assessed a mean of 5 years postinjury using heart rate reactivity and HRV with botulinum toxin injections (for treatment of muscle spasticity) as the semistandardized nociceptive stimulus. PSH subjects continued to show immediate exaggerated responsiveness not seen in non-PSH groups, suggestive of persisting sympathetic overactivity. This overactivity was not associated with clinical evidence of PSH during the procedure and was not observed in non-PSH subjects under equivalent experimental conditions.

There are 2 conclusions to draw from these data: first, that excessive stimulus reactivity is a core feature of PSH, and second, that this overreactivity persists long-term in subjects whose PSH is otherwise subclinical in nature. For these reasons, it has been proposed that overreactivity to minor stimuli, the so-called "triggering" of paroxysms, should be added to the diagnostic criteria (8).

Pathophysiology

The pathophysiology of PSH remains open to conjecture, with an absence of definitive research. The first name given to the syndrome, "diencephalic epilepsy" (32), inferred an epileptogenic etiology. However, attempts to identify and/or treat epilepsy in individuals with PSH have not been successful (19,26,27,34,43,57,62).

Most authors currently infer a variety of "disconnection syndrome." This term is taken to mean that the usual balance of CNS excitatory and inhibitory drives become disordered in subjects with PSH, thereby and producing the observed autonomic disturbances. Although the details of the various disconnection syndromes vary, the general conclusion is supported by a small number of autopsy and pathophysiological studies, which suggest a relative disconnection of pathways at or around the level of the midbrain (reviewed in [63]). However, no single lesion or pattern of lesions has been identified, with cases also reported from a wide range of other causes of acquired brain injury, including hypoxia, stroke, hypoglycemic coma, carotid artery dissection, and cerebral infection (22). Thus, although most disconnection theories suggest that paroxysms follow from upper brainstem and diencephalon lesions, the details of how this might occur remain sketchy.

An additional clue to the pathophysiology of PSH comes from the "triggering" of paroxysms outlined previously. This evidence suggests that PSH results from changes occurring at the level of both the brain and spinal cord. Putatively, this scenario presents similarities with autonomic dysreflexia (AD) (50,54). AD is observed in SCIs above the T6 level and also presents with sympathetic hyperactivity following peripheral stimulation (64,65). In contrast to PSH, however, AD has been extensively studied at a physiological and anatomical level. In AD, the loss of supraspinal inputs to the distal spinal cord produces a variable period of "spinal shock," where the spinal cord is under responsive (65). With increasing time, dendritic rearborization occurs within the dorsal horn of the spinal cord, producing dysfunctional connections between afferent sensory neurons and the sympathetic lateral horn efferents. In the absence of descending supraspinal inhibitory influences, the net result is sympathetic hyperresponsiveness to otherwise benign afferent stimuli.

This "faulty rewiring" analogy presents a potential pathophysiological link between AD and PSH. A theoretical framework incorporating these 2 conditions and a range of other "overlap syndromes" has been put forward as the excitatory/inhibitory ratio (EIR) model (8). This model proposes that loss of inhibitory activation from centers above the level of the midbrain predisposes the distal spinal cord to rewire in a way that results in overactivity to afferent stimuli. Such a process is akin to that seen in allodynia, where nonpainful stimuli become perceived as nociceptive (68). The principal difference between AD and PSH then becomes the presence of functional brainstem reflexes in the spinally injured person, which produces vagally-mediated bradycardia to compensate for the hypersympathetic drive. The difference in response to nociceptive stimuli between AD and PSH are shown in the following diagram (Figure 52-5). In this diagram, a normally non-nociceptive stimulus was applied at beat zero. Control subjects show minor heart rate changes. In comparison, subjects with PSH produce a persistent reactive tachycardia, contrasting with an initial tachycardia leading to prolonged bradycardia in the SCI subject.

Clinical Management of Paroxysmal Sympathetic Hyperactivity

Given the limited understanding of the pathophysiology of PSH, the current approach to management is in its infancy. Despite the symptomatology of subjects with PSH, there is little literature available to guide management of the condition (54,67,68). As will be discussed, a wide range of medications have been used to treat the syndrome, and there are a few anecdotal treatment paradigms (18,67,68).

Given these limitations, management is probably best undertaken from first principles incorporating

- adequate examination and investigations,
- differential diagnosis, and
- appropriate management

Adequate Examination and Investigations

The limited data on the condition makes the process of confirming the diagnosis of PSH largely one of exclusion (18,31,69). The timing of the onset of paroxysms (i.e., within 7 days of the acute event) in a patient with a suitably severe injury should lead the clinician to have a high index of suspicion. Raising the possibility of the diagnosis is most important in patients with the most severe clinical features, where it is also important to exclude other diagnoses.

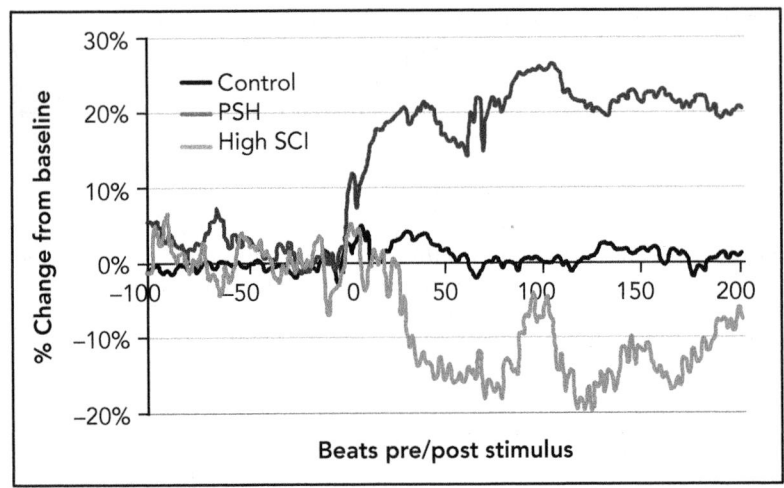

FIGURE 52-5 Event related heart rate changes following stimuli (occuring at beat zero) in PSH and control groups compared to a patient with high SCI. *PSH*, pararoxysmal sympathetic hyperactivity; *SCI*, spinal cord injury.

A careful physical examination for evidence of triggering is useful in this context. Empirical research suggests that a generalized overreactivity to afferent stimuli may be a hallmark of the syndrome (37). Careful physical examination may identify the presence of allodynia to light touch and "myodynia," taken to be neurologically derived pain related to muscle movement or deep pressure. The pattern of overreactivity is often asymmetrical, for example, affecting 1 upper limb and the contralateral leg. Although patterns differ from one patient to the next, they tend to be consistent over time within the same individual.

Assessing the patient for such overreactivity is a simple process in the ICU, where heart rate can be monitored during physical examination. Outside of ICU, the simplest way to achieve the same result is via the use of a pulse oximeter. This allows the patient to be examined for evidence of heart rate overresponsiveness to stimuli such as light touch, muscle stretch, and ETT suctioning. An example of heart rate "triggering" is shown in Figure 52-6. This example details

heart rate over a 90-minute period, with different patterns of heart rate elevation occurring depending on environmental considerations. For example, heart rate fluctuated while the patient had visitors who were talking among themselves more than interacting with the patient. When left alone, the patient's heart rate settled, although it remained hyperresponsive to environmental noise, akin to the prominent startle reflex seen in cerebral palsy. After each discrete stimulus, heart rate reduced in an asymptotic fashion to a baseline around 70 bpm. Heart rate again became markedly variable during a therapy session where custom made splints were being applied to joints affected by muscle spasticity.

Differential Diagnosis
The clinical features of PSH can mimic a variety of other conditions where hypersympathetic drive dominates. For example, there are a range of conditions that appear very similar to PSH but with differing etiologies. These so-called "overlap syndromes" (67) include conditions such as neuro-

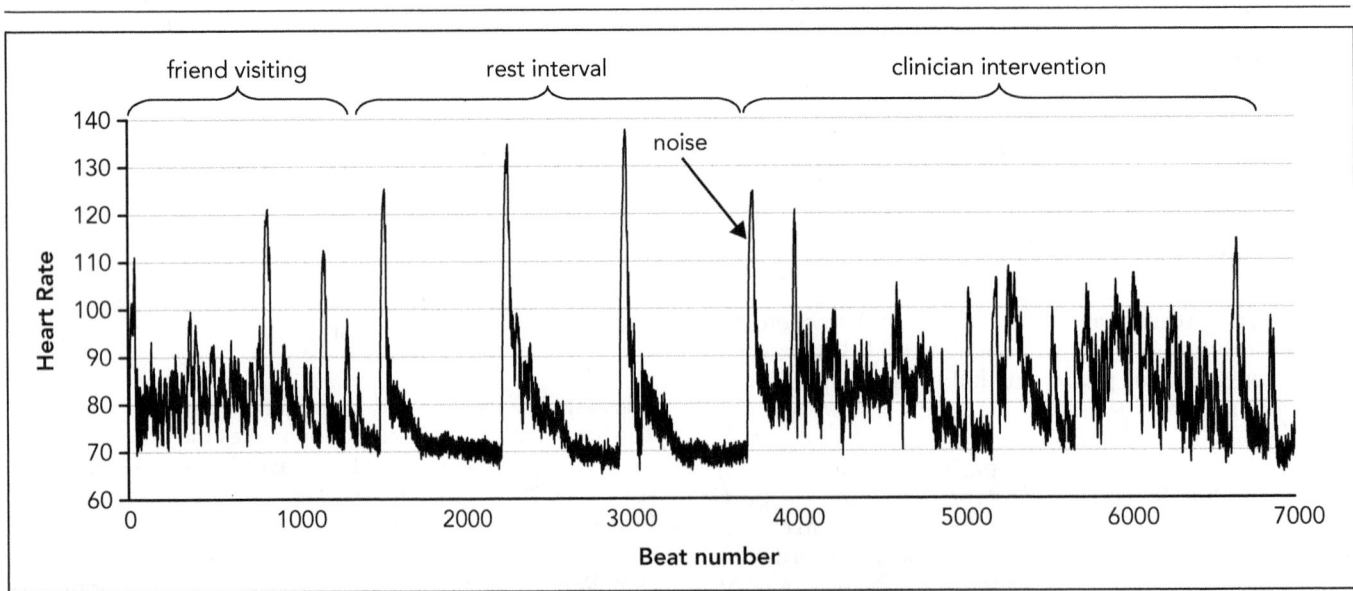

FIGURE 52-6 Beat-to-beat heart rate changes in patient with PSH. Note the exaggerated heart rate response to environmental noise and clinical intervention.

leptic malignant syndrome (NMS), malignant hyperthermia, opiate and other drug withdrawal, serotonin syndrome, and so on. In particular, NMS warrants careful consideration, particularly in an environment where dopamine blocking agents may have been used; a situation that may lower the threshold for NMS in people with widespread ANS dysfunction (67).

In addition, increased sympathetic drive could indicate another primary disease process such as acute hydrocephalus, sepsis, or untreated sources of pain, such as occult fractures, constipation, pressure areas, or heterotopic ossification (HO). HO is a particular consideration because the relative risk of developing HO in subjects with PSH is 55 times that seen in TBI patients without PSH (36). Post-SAH hypertensive crisis is another potential differential diagnosis, however, and will normally be seen in the immediate postinjury period and is of shorter duration than PSH. Where identified, other diagnoses require intervention but do not preclude a diagnosis of PSH, as suggested in some diagnostic criteria (21). Instead, the frequency or severity of paroxysms in patients with PSH is likely to be exacerbated in circumstances where there are additional sources of nociception (18,54).

Appropriate Management
In the first instance, management of PSH aims to minimize the occurrence of avoidable secondary morbidity (11,60,70). To do this, clinicians should target the drivers of paroxysms, hence ensuring appropriate positioning, constipation and pain management, preventing pressure areas, and so on. In spite of these possible interventions, conservative measures alone are rarely sufficient to control the paroxysmal sympathetic overactivity of severe PSH.

A large number of medications have been used to treat PSH, although reports are almost all anecdotal in nature (21,54,67,68). Accepting the limitations of current literature, a range of medications from many classes of neurologically active agents have been proposed to be beneficial. These medications are outlined in Table 52-2.

The management of PSH differs with increasing time postinjury. In the early postinjury phase, patients in ICU are managed in a manner that cannot be replicated during the rehabilitation phase. This is because of the presence of artificial ventilation, close physiological monitoring, and the relative under importance of reducing sedation in this setting (54). For these reasons, ICUs often focus on minimizing sympathetic hyperactivity through intravenous (IV) sedation with agents such as morphine, midazolam, or propofol.

Where "triggering" is identified in ICU, it has been suggested that patients with PSH receive "pretreatment" with an IV bolus of an analgesic or sedative prior to nociceptive procedures being undertaken to reduce paroxysms (18). This strategy is also relevant for rehabilitation practice, although it is more difficult to implement in this setting.

The intervention that appears to be the most effective is intrathecal baclofen (ITB), with all cases reporting a reduction in paroxysmal sympathetic overactivity (53,57,71–75). However, deciding when to use ITB is difficult because many patients will exhibit paroxysms for only a few months

TABLE 52-2 Number of Studies Reporting Paroxysmal Sympathetic Hyperactivity Medication Effects

NEUROTRANSMITTER CLASS	DRUG	UNHELPFUL	BENEFICIAL
Opiate agonist	Morphine	5	7
	Methadone	2	
GABA A agonist	Diazepam	3	2
	Midazolam	3	2
	Clonazepam		1
	Lorazepam		1
GABA B agonist	Baclofen (oral)	4	
	Baclofen (intrathecal)	7	
Alpha antagonist	Clonidine	5	3
Beta antagonist	Propanolol	4	8
	Labetalol	1	1
	Metoprolol	2	
Dopamine agonist	Carbidopa/levodopa	1	2
	Bromocriptine	4	7
Dopamine antagonist	Chlorpromazine		2
Other	Gabapentin		1
	Dantrolene	5	1
	Phenobarbital	4	
	Phenytoin	3	
	Carbamazepine	1	
	Propofol		1
	Acetaminophen	1	

Each report of a treatment as either helpful or unhelpful is indicative of the number of articles referencing the use and efficacy of each medication. Adapted from Baguley (67) with permission.

(11,36,38), the intervention is not always available, has a high cost, and is invasive. Additionally, ITB may be warranted as it is also highly effective for managing muscle spasticity that is a common sequela of PSH (76,77).

Gabapentin is hypothesized to reduce the frequency and severity of paroxysms by modifying the reactivity of neurological circuits in the spinal cord (57,78). Furthermore, gabapentin introduction allowed an overall reduction in other medications, including ITB, without a recurrence of symptoms (57). However, it has been suggested that the drug should be trialled at a low starting dose (100 mg) to minimize the risk of marked bradypnea or sedation, presumed to result from the sudden reduction in sympathetic drive (57).

Of the more traditional medications, beta-blockers have been suggested to improve survival post-TBI (79), with propanolol and labetalol potentially being more effective than metoprolol in reducing the severity of paroxysms. Propanolol has the added advantage that decreases catecholamine levels following TBI (80,81). Although clonidine also decreases post-TBI catecholamine levels (82,83), its ability to control PSH episodes appears to require high doses (e.g., 800 µg second hourly) that are more practically achieved in the ICU (84). Benzodiazepines also present a mixed picture, with anecdotal reports favoring diazepam and midazolam. Dopamine agonists (predominantly bromocriptine) have been very successful in isolated cases but relatively ineffective in others.

On this background it is difficult to provide a definitive order of treatment options; however, evidence would suggest gabapentin, propanolol/labetalol, and morphine/midazolam are the most appropriate medications in the first instance. Occasional reports of excellent efficacy with bromocriptine suggest that it may have a secondary role. Although effective, ITB is probably best suited to cases that are resistant to oral medication, are of greater severity or duration, and/or exhibiting a significant motor component.

CONCLUSION

Autonomic complications following TBI are a relatively common occurrence; however, the true incidence is unknown. It is thought likely that there will be many individuals with minor autonomic changes post-TBI who are not identifiable with current knowledge or investigations. Even at the most severe end of the autonomic injury spectrum, PSH remains underdiagnosed, and management options are not supported by a solid literature base. Current research suggests that the widespread autonomic dysregulation seen in PSH presents a considerable risk of potentially preventable additional cerebral and physical dysfunction in affected patients. How much of this morbidity may be preventable through better identification and more active treatment of the condition remains an area for additional research.

Promisingly, the awareness of and research into post-TBI autonomic abnormalities is improving, with a yearly increase in peer-reviewed publications on the condition. There is a current move toward the development of international consensus guidelines covering nomenclature and diagnostic criteria. These tools should become available in the near future. Furthermore, literature is beginning to emerge with the promise of providing new investigations and research tools that should improve specificity of diagnosis for the condition

and better evaluate treatment efficacy, for example, the empirical data supporting "triggering" of PSH episodes. These issues will be the focus of future research with the promise to improve care of this condition in future years.

KEY CLINICAL POINTS

1. Autonomic complications are common after TBI, although the true incidence is unknown.
2. The most severe form of autonomic abnormality following TBI is PSH, a spectral disorder with a reported incidence of 10%–25% of survivors of severe TBI in the ICU, falling to 5% with the most prolonged version of PSH.
3. Outcome data for those with prolonged PSH indicates a poorer outcome for this group; conversely, there is no evidence to suggest that short duration of PSH is associated for adverse outcomes.
4. The diagnosis of PSH is one of exclusion. Preliminary data suggests that the hallmark of the disease is sympathetic overactivity in response to routine physical or psychological stimuli (so-called "triggering" of paroxysms), irrespective of whether these stimuli would be nociceptive in an ordinary context.
5. Treatment paradigms for autonomic disorders are anecdotal in nature. In the absence of other physiological targets, the emphasis has been on minimizing the symptoms of the condition. Early and aggressive intervention is recommended, although it is recognized that there is no current empirical evidence to show clinical benefit from such management.

KEY REFERENCES

1. Baguley IJ, Nicholls JL, Felmingham KL, Crooks J, Gurka JA, Wade LD. Dysautonomia after traumatic brain injury: a forgotten syndrome? *J Neurol Neurosurg Psychiatry*. 1999; 67(1):39–43.
2. Baguley IJ, Nott MT, Slewa-Younan S, Heriseanu RE, Perkes IE. Diagnosing dysautonomia following acute traumatic brain injury: evidence for over-responsiveness to afferent stimuli. *Arch Phys Med Rehabil*. 2009;90(4): 580–586.
3. Baguley IJ, Slewa-Younan S, Heriseanu RE, Nott MT, Mudaliar Y, Nayyar V. The incidence of dysautonomia and its relationship with autonomic arousal following traumatic brain injury. *Brain Inj*. 2007;21(11):1175–1182.
4. Perkes I, Baguley IJ, Nott MT, Menon DK. A review of paroxysmal sympathetic hyperactivity after acquired brain injury. *Ann Neurol*. 2010;68(2):126–135.
5. Rabinstein AA, Benarroch EE. Treatment of paroxysmal sympathetic hyperactivity. *Curr Treat Options Neurol*. 2008;10(2):151–157.

References

1. Ganong WF. Central regulation of visceral function: Hypothalamus. In: *Review of Medical Physiology*. 21st ed. New York, NY:Appleton & Lange McGraw-Hill; 2003:236–254.
2. Benarroch EE. The central autonomic network: functional organization, dysfunction, and perspective. *Mayo Clin Proc*. 1993;68(10): 988–1001.

3. Verdecchia P, Angeli F, Gattobigio R, et al. The clinical significance of white-coat and masked hypertension. *Blood Press Monit.* 2007; 12(6):387–389.

4. Michael DB, Guyot DR, Darmody WR. Coincidence of head and cervical spine injury. *J Neurotrauma.* 1989;6(3):177–189.

5. Guo MF, Yu JZ, Ma CG. Mechanisms related to neuron injury and death in cerebral hypoxic ischaemia. *Folia Neuropathol.* 2011;49(2): 78–87.

6. Robertson CL, Scafidi S, McKenna MC, Fiskum G. Mitochondrial mechanisms of cell death and neuroprotection in pediatric ischemic and traumatic brain injury. *Exp Neurol.* 2009;218(2):371–380.

7. Gardiner D, Shemie S, Manara A, Opdam H. International perspective on the diagnosis of death. *Br J Anaesth.* 2012;108(suppl 1): i14–i28.

8. Baguley IJ. The excitatory: inhibitory model (EIR model): an integrative explanation of acute autonomic overactivity syndromes. *Med Hypotheses.* 2008;70(1):26–35.

9. Jennett B, Teasdale G, Galbraith S, et al. Severe head injuries in three countries. *J Neurol Neurosurg Psychiatry.* 1977;40(3):291–298.

10. Baguley IJ, Slewa-Younan S, Heriseanu RE, Nott MT, Mudaliar Y, Nayyar V. The incidence of dysautonomia and its relationship with autonomic arousal following traumatic brain injury. *Brain Inj.* 2007; 21(11):1175–1182.

11. Baguley IJ, Nicholls JL, Felmingham KL, Crooks J, Gurka JA, Wade LD. Dysautonomia after traumatic brain injury: a forgotten syndrome? *J Neurol Neurosurg Psychiatry.* 1999;67(1):39–43.

12. Childs C, Jones AK, Tyrrell PJ. Long-term temperature-related morbidity after brain damage: survivor-reported experiences. *Brain Inj.* 2008;22(7–8):603–609.

13. Kox M, Pompe JC, Pickkers P, Hoedemaekers CW, van Vugt AB, van der Hoeven JG. Increased vagal tone accounts for the observed immune paralysis in patients with traumatic brain injury. *Neurology.* 2008;70(6):480–485.

14. Ketch T, Biaggioni I, Robertson R, Robertson D. Four faces of baroreflex failure: hypertensive crisis, volatile hypertension, orthostatic tachycardia, and malignant vagotonia. *Circulation.* 2002;105(21): 2518–2523.

15. Kanjwal K, Karabin B, Kanjwal Y, Grubb BP. Autonomic dysfunction presenting as postural tachycardia syndrome following traumatic brain injury. *Cardiol J.* 17(5):482–487.

16. Perkes I, Menon DK, Nott MT, Baguley IJ. Paroxysmal sympathetic hyperactivity: the need for a single set of diagnostic criteria. *J Neurotrauma.* 2010;27(5):85.

17. Rabinstein AA. Paroxysmal sympathetic hyperactivity in the neurological intensive care unit. *Neurol Res.* 2007;29(7):680–682.

18. Lemke DM. Sympathetic storming after severe traumatic brain injury. *Crit Care Nurse.* 2007;27(1):30–37.

19. Rossitch E Jr, Bullard DE. The autonomic dysfunction syndrome: aetiology and treatment. *Br J Neurosurg.* 1988;2(4):471–478.

20. Fearnside MR, Cook RJ, McDougall P, McNeil RJ. The Westmead Head Injury Project outcome in severe head injury. A comparative analysis of pre-hospital, clinical and CT variables. *Br J Neurosurg.* 1993;7(3):267–279.

21. Blackman JA, Patrick PD, Buck ML, Rust RS Jr. Paroxysmal autonomic instability with dystonia after brain injury. *Arch Neurol.* 2004; 61(3):321–328.

22. Perkes I, Baguley IJ, Nott MT, Menon DK. A review of paroxysmal sympathetic hyperactivity after acquired brain injury. *Ann Neurol.* 2010;68(2):126–135.

23. Bricolo A, Turazzi S, Alexandre A, Rizzuto A. Decerebrate rigidity in acute head injury. *J Neurosurg.* 1977;47(5):680–698.

24. Figa-Talamanca L, Gualandi C, Di Meo L, Di Battista G, Neri G, Lo RF. Hyperthermia after discontinuance of levodopa and bromocriptine therapy: impaired dopamine receptors a possible cause. *Neurology.* 1985;35(2):258–261.

25. Lu CS, Ryu SJ. Neuroleptic malignant-like syndrome associated with acute hydrocephalus. *Mov Disord.* 1991;6(4):381–383.

26. Sneed RC. Hyperpyrexia associated with sustained muscle contractions: an alternative diagnosis to central fever. *Arch Phys Med Rehabil.* 1995;76(1):101–103.

27. Thorley RR, Wertsch JJ, Klingbeil GE. Acute hypothalamic instability in traumatic brain injury: a case report. *Arch Phys Med Rehabil.* 2001;82(2):246–249.

28. Wortsman J, Burns G, Van Beek AL, Couch J. Hyperadrenergic state after trauma to the neuroaxis. *JAMA.* 1980;243(14):1459–1460.

29. Leow MK, Loh KC, Kwek TK, Ng PY. Catecholamine and metanephrine excess in intracerebral haemorrhage: revisiting an obscure yet common "pseudophaeochromocytoma." *J Clin Path.* 2007;60(5):583–584.

30. Ott L, Young B, Phillips R, et al. Altered gastric emptying in the head-injured patient: relationship to feeding intolerance. *J Neurosurg.* 1991;74(5):738–742.

31. Strum S. Post head injury autonomic complications. 2002. Available at: http://emedicine.medscape.com/article/325994-overview. Accessed 8th April 2004.

32. Penfield W. Diencephalic autonomic epilepsy. *Arch Neurol Psychiatry.* 1929;22:358–374.

33. Talman WT. Cardiovascular regulation and lesions of the central nervous system. *Ann Neurol.* 1985;18(1):1–13.

34. Bhigjee AI, Ames FR, Rutherford GS. Adult aqueduct stenosis and diencephalic epilepsy. A case report. *J Neurol Sci.* 1985;71(1):77–89.

35. Strich SJ. Diffuse degeneration of the cerebral white matter in severe dementia following head injury. *J Neurol Neurosurg Psychiatry.* 1956;19(3):163–185.

36. Hendricks HT, Guerts AC, van Ginnekin BC, Heeren AJ. Brain injury severity and autonomic dysregulation accurately predict heterotopic ossification in patients with traumatic brain injury. *Clin Rehabil.* 2007;21(6):545–553.

37. Baguley IJ, Nott MT, Slewa-Younan S, Heriseanu RE, Perkes IE. Diagnosing dysautonomia following acute traumatic brain injury: evidence for overresponsiveness to afferent stimuli. *Arch Phys Med Rehabil.* 2009;90(4):580–586.

38. Krach LE, Kriel RL, Morris WF, Warhol BL, Luxenberg MG. Central autonomic dysfunction following acquired brain injury in children. *J Neurol Rehabil.* 1997;11(1):41–45.

39. Dolce G, Quintieri M, Leto E, et al. Dysautonomia and clinical outcome in vegetative state. *J Neurotrauma.* 2008;25:1079–1082.

40. Fernández-Ortega JF, Prieto-Palomino MA, Muñoz-Lopez A, et al. Dysautonomic seizures in patients admitted to an intensive care unit following severe traumatic brain injury. *Rev Neurol.* 2004;39(8): 715–718.

41. Fernández-Ortega JF, Prieto-Palomino MA, Muñoz-Lopez A, Lebron-Gallardo M, Cabrera-Ortiz H, Quesada-Garcia G. Prognostic influence and computed tomography findings in dysautonomic crises after traumatic brain injury. *J Trauma.* 2006;61(5):1129–1133.

42. Talman WT, Florek G, Bullard DE. A hyperthermic syndrome in two subjects with acute hydrocephalus. *Arch Neurol.* 1988;45(9): 1037–1040.

43. Do D, Sheen VL, Broomfield E. Treatment of paroxysmal sympathetic storm with labetalol. *J Neurol Neurosurg Psychiatry.* 2000; 69(6):832–833.

44. Scott JS, Ockey RR, Holmes GE, Varghese G. Autonomic dysfunction associated with locked-in syndrome in a child. *Am J Phys Med Rehabil.* 1997;76(3):200–203.

45. Baguley IJ. Nomenclature of "paroxysmal sympathetic storms." *Mayo Clin Proc.* 1999;74(1):105.

46. Bullard DE. Diencephalic seizures: responsiveness to bromocriptine and morphine. *Ann Neurol.* 1987;21(6):609–611.

47. Graham B. Diagnosis, diagnostic criteria, and consensus. *Hand Clin.* 2009;25(1):43–48.

48. Baguley IJ, Perkes IE. Paroxysmal sympathetic hyperactivity after acquired brain injury; a coming of age. 2011. Available at: http://www.internationalbrain.org/?q=node/16949. Accessed 20th Feb 2012.

49. Penfield W, Jasper H, eds. Somatic motor seizures, in epilepsy and the functional anatomy of the human brain. 1st ed. London, UK: J & A Churchill Ltd; 1954:350–358.

50. Sandel ME, Abrams PL, Horn LJ. Hypertension after brain injury: case report. *Arch Phys Med Rehabil.* 1986;67(7):469–472.

51. Boeve BF, Wijdicks EF, Benarroch EE, Schmidt KD. Paroxysmal sympathetic storms ("diencephalic seizures") after severe diffuse axonal head injury. *Mayo Clin Proc.* 1998;73(2):148–152.

52. Russo RN, O'Flaherty S. Bromocriptine for the management of autonomic dysfunction after severe traumatic brain injury. *J Paediatr Child Health.* 2000;36(3):283–285.

53. Cuny E, Richer E, Castel JP. Dysautonomia syndrome in the acute recovery phase after traumatic brain injury: relief with intrathecal baclofen therapy. *Brain Inj.* 2001;15(10):917–925.

54. Baguley IJ, Cameron ID, Green AM, Slewa-Younan S, Marosszeky JE, Gurka JA. Pharmacological management of dysautonomia following traumatic brain injury. *Brain Inj.* 2004;18(5):409–417.

55. Lemke DM. Riding out the storm: sympathetic storming after traumatic brain injury. *J Neurosci Nurs.* 2004;36(1):4–9.

56. Diesing TS, Wijdicks EF. Arc de cercle and dysautonomia from anoxic injury. *Mov Disord.* 2006;21(6):868–869.

57. Baguley IJ, Heriseanu RE, Gurka JA, Nordenbo A, Cameron ID. Gabapentin in the management of dysautonomia following severe traumatic brain injury: a case series. *J Neurol Neurosurg Psychiatry.* 2007;78(5):539–541.

58. Tong C, Konig MW, Roberts PR, Tatter SB, Li X. Autonomic dysfunction secondary to intracerebral haemorrhage. *Anesth Analg.* 2000;91(6):1450–1451.

59. Srinivasan S, Lim CCT, Thirugnanam U. Paroxysmal autonomic instability with dystonia. *Clin Auton Res.* 2007;17(6):378–381.

60. Baguley IJ, Heriseanu RE, Felmingham KL, Cameron ID. Dysautonomia and heart rate variability following severe traumatic brain injury. *Brain Inj.* 2006;20(4):437–444.

61. Baguley IJ, Heriseanu RE, Nott MT, Chapman J, Sandanam J. Dysautonomia after severe traumatic brain injury: evidence of persisting overresponsiveness to afferent stimuli. *Am J Phys Medi Rehabil.* 2009;88(8):615–622.

62. Pranzatelli MR, Pavlakis SG, Gould RG, De Vivo DC. Hypothalamic-midbrain dysregulation syndrome: hypertension, hyperthermia, hyperventilation, and decerebration. *J Child Neurol.* 1991;6(2):115–122.

63. Baguley IJ, Heriseanu RE, Cameron ID, Nott MT, Slewa-Younan S. A critical review of the pathophysiology of dysautonomia following traumatic brain injury. *Neurocrit Care.* 2008;8:293–300.

64. Silver JR. Early autonomic dysreflexia. *Spinal Cord.* 2000;38(4):229–233.

65. Krassioukov AV, Furlan JC, Fehlings MG. Autonomic dysreflexia in acute spinal cord injury: an under-recognized clinical entity. *J Neurotrauma.* 2003;20(8):707–716.

66. Cervero F, Laird JM. Mechanisms of touch-evoked pain (allodynia): a new model. *Pain.* 1996;68(1):13–23.

67. Baguley IJ. Autonomic complications following central nervous system injury. *Semin Neurol.* 2008;28(5):716–725.

68. Rabinstein AA, Benarroch EE. Treatment of paroxysmal sympathetic hyperactivity. *Curr Treat Options Neurol.* 2008;10(2):151–157.

69. Oh SJ, Hong YK, Song E. Paroxysmal autonomic dysregulation with fever that was controlled by propanolol in a brain neoplasm patient. *Korean J Int Med.* 2007;22(1):51–54.

70. Rabinstein AA. Paroxysmal autonomic instability after brain injury. *Arch Neurol.* 2004;61(10):1625.

71. Senno RG, Anderson V, Ahmed G, Duraski SA. Intrathecal baclofen administration in the management of hyperadrenergic state in an adult with a severe anoxic brain injury: a case report. *Arch Phys Med Rehabil.* 2004;85(9):e15.

72. Francois B, Vacher P, Roustan J, et al. Intrathecal baclofen after traumatic brain injury: early treatment using a new technique to prevent spasticity. *J Trauma.* 2001;50(1):158–161.

73. Becker R, Benes L, Sure U, Hellwig D, Bertalanffy H. Intrathecal baclofen alleviates autonomic dysfunction in severe brain injury. *J Clin Neurosci.* 2000;7(4):316–319.

74. Anderson VL, Ahmed G, Duraski SA, Senno RG. Alternative treatment in the management of combined hyperadrenergia and spasticity in the adult with a severe traumatic brain injury: a case report. *Arch Phys Med Rehabil.* 2004;85(9):e15.

75. Turner MS. Early use of intrathecal baclofen in brain injury in pediatric patients. *Acta Neurochir Suppl.* 2003;87:81–83.

76. Ivanhoe CB, Tilton AH, Francisco GE. Intrathecal baclofen therapy for spastic hypertonia. *Phys Med Rehabil Clin N Am.* 2001;12(4):923–938.

77. Guillaume D, Van Havenbergh A, Vloeberghs M, Vidal J, Roeste G. A clinical study of intrathecal baclofen using a programmable pump for intractable spasticity. *Arch Phys Med Rehabil.* 2005;86(11):2165–2171.

78. Baguley IJ, Nott MT. Quantitating the efficacy of gabapentin in a novel case of dysautonomia. *Neurorehabil Neural Repair.* 2008;22(5):570–571.

79. Salim A, Hadjizacharia P, Brown C, et al. Significance of troponin elevation after severe traumatic brain injury. *J Trauma.* 2008;64(1):46–52.

80. Feibel JH, Baldwin CA, Joynt RJ. Catecholamine-associated refractory hypertension following acute intracranial hemorrhage: control with propranolol. *Ann Neurol.* 1981;9(4):340–343.

81. Robertson CS, Clifton GL, Taylor AA, Grossman RG. Treatment of hypertension associated with head injury. *J Neurosurg.* 1983;59(3):455–460.

82. Payen D, Quintin L, Plaisance P, Chiron B, Lhoste F. Head injury: clonidine decreases plasma catecholamines. *Crit Care Med.* 1990;18(4):392–395.

83. Metz SA, Halter JB, Porte D Jr, Robertson RP. Autonomic epilepsy: clonidine blockade of paroxysmal catecholamine release and flushing. *Ann Intern Med.* 1978;88(2):189–193.

84. Dunne SL. Clonidine for the treatment of paroxysmal autonomic instability with dystonia following traumatic brain injury. In: Neonatal & Paediatric Pharmacists Group Conference; November, 2007; Bournemouth, UK.

Neuroendocrine Dysfunction After Traumatic Brain Injury

Brent E. Masel

INTRODUCTION

Approximately two-thirds of patients who die from a severe traumatic brain injury (TBI) and come to autopsy have been found to have structural abnormalities in the pituitary stalk, pituitary, and/or hypothalamus (2). Therefore, any of the hormones produced from the pituitary or regulated by the pituitary axis can be affected by a TBI. The clinical manifestations of hormone deficiencies can be quite subtle or overtly obvious. The clinical consequences of these deficiencies may be minor, severe, or fatal, and they can be masked by the signs and symptoms from the injuries to other structures of the brain. Therefore, the diagnosis and treatment of post-traumatic hypopituitarism (PTH) may well play a significant role in the recovery from a brain injury.

The first clinical syndrome of hypopituitarism (then known as *hypophyseal cachexia*) was published in 1914 by Morris Simmonds, a pathologist at the University of Hamburg (3). Based on his autopsy findings, he described septic pituitary necrosis in a previously healthy young woman who developed severe postpartum (puerperal) sepsis. She eventually died while in coma but first developed menopause, dizziness, muscle weakness, anemia, and premature aging. Although it is no longer commonly used, the name "Simmonds disease" was given to hypopituitarism shortly thereafter. The first case of anterior hypopituitarism because of head trauma was described by Cyran in 1918 (4).

In 2000, Benvenga (5) added 15 new cases of PTH to the literature and performed a large review, citing 299 additional cases. Of those 15 new cases, 11 of the 12 who had imaging studies had an abnormal computed tomography (CT) or magnetic resonance imaging (MRI). Eight cases were diagnosed more than 10 years postinjury, and in several cases, the patients did not remember the history of a TBI. Only 3 cases had a history of a loss of consciousness. The authors suggested that many cases of previously diagnosed idiopathic hypopituitarism might really be caused by PTH from a forgotten brain injury.

In 1942, Escamilla and Lister (6) published a clinical review on Simmonds disease. They cited 595 cases, of which 101 were proven pathological. The cardinal features were described as marked weight loss, loss of sexual function, and a low basal metabolic rate (BMR). Only 4 of the 595 cases (0.7%) were caused by a head injury. However, because most moderate to severe TBIs in those days were fatal, and au-

topsy reports were not readily available for academic review, the number of cases of PTH may have been well understated. In 1961, Altman and Pruzanski (7) published a case report and an additional literature review, increasing the number of reported cases of hypopituitarism following TBI to 15. Twenty-five years later, Edwards and Clark (8) reviewed 47 cases of PTH in the literature and added 6 new cases of their own. They reported that skull fractures and prolonged unconsciousness were common; however, 8 cases had either no or brief loss of consciousness and therefore may have what is now considered to be a mild TBI (mTBI). Hypogonadism was the most common reported symptom, with amenorrhea, loss of libido, impotence, and loss of secondary sexual characteristics. They reported on specific endocrine testing in 20 cases. Only 1 patient had a normal cortisol response and none had a normal growth hormone (GH) response to the insulin tolerance test (ITT). Eighty-five percent were hypothyroid, and 40% had a history of diabetes insipidus (DI).

In 2000, Benvenga and colleagues (5) published a large review of PTH. They identified 299 additional cases and added 15 cases of their own. Fourteen had multiple hormonal deficits, and 11 of the 12 who had imaging studies had an abnormal CT or MRI. Although all of the 15 cases had a documented head injury, none had a skull fracture, and only 3 had a loss of consciousness. Therefore, 12 of the 15 patients probably had an mTBI. Eight cases were diagnosed over 10 years following their injury. The authors noted that in several cases, the patients failed to recount a history of a TBI, and the information was only obtained after detailed pointed questioning of patients and families. The authors related that the incidence of PTH is underestimated because many cases previously diagnosed as "idiopathic" hypopituitarism might really be caused by head trauma.

PREVALENCE STUDIES

Acute TBI

Data on acute anterior pituitary dysfunction after a TBI is limited. Agha and colleagues (9) studied 50 consecutive patients in the NICU with moderate to severe TBIs. The time from injury to testing ranged from 7 to 20 days. Gonadotropin deficiencies were the most common finding (80%). A low GH response to stimulation was present in 18%. A low peak cortisol was found in 16%, and 1 patient had thyroid stimulating hormone (TSH) deficiency. Tanriverdi et al. (10) followed 104 patients within 24 hours of their TBI. Eighty-four patients survived their injury. Gonadotropin deficiency was the most common finding (40%). GH deficiency to stimulation was present in 20% and a low cortisol response was found in 8.8%. There was no relationship of mortality to basal hormonal levels.

Wagner et al. (11) studied acute serum hormone levels in 117 adults for 7 days after a severe TBI. They found significantly increased estradiol levels in men and increased testosterone in women. These increased levels were associated with increased mortality and worse global outcome.

Chronic TBI

Kelly and colleagues (12) first studied the prevalence of PTH in 24 patients, including 2 patients who had sustained a nontraumatic subarachnoid hemorrhage. Fourteen of those subjects were enrolled or had been enrolled in observational studies and were therefore not selected on the basis of symptoms suggesting hypopituitarism. The mean interval from injury to study was 27 months. All had either Glasgow Comas Scale (GCS) scores of 3–12, or 13–15 with CT or MRI abnormalities. They found 8 patients with a TBI (36.4%) had a subnormal response in at least 1 hormonal axis, including 5 subjects (22.7%) who were deficient in 2 axes. GH deficiency (GHD) was seen in 4 (18%). Although all males had adequate testosterone levels, 4 of 18 males had an insufficient response to gonadotropin releasing hormone (GnRH) stimulation. One of the 4 females had a low serum estradiol level. Only 1 subject had an inadequate rise in TSH. None of the subjects had either an inadequate cortisol response or evidence of DI. They also found that all subjects with pituitary dysfunction had an initial GCS score of 10 or less and had diffuse swelling on the CT scan. Of the 8 patients, 7 had sustained a hypotensive and/or hypoxic insult. They concluded that hypopituitarism was common following a moderate to severe TBI and was most likely to occur with the more severe injuries.

Lieberman and colleagues (13) evaluated 70 adults with moderate to severe TBIs recruited from a residential post acute brain injury program. Forty-six males and 24 females were enrolled. The time from TBI was 49 ±8 months (median, 13 months). Of the 38 patients who had initial GCS scores in the records, 32 were lower than 8, indicating a severe injury. Because of concerns that the ITT might provoke seizures in an at-risk population, the glucagon stimulation test (GST) was performed to assess GH axis function.

Of those undergoing GST, 14.6% met the Growth Hormone Research Society criteria (maximum value <3 μg/L) for severe GHD. The mean insulinlike growth factor-1 (IGF-1) level was below normal in 4 of 7 (57.1%) patients with GHD, and in 5 of 41 (12.2%) patients without GHD. Although the GHD patients had a higher BMR than the non-GHD group, the differences in weight and height were not statistically significant. Eight patients (11%) had serum thyroxine (T_4) levels below normal, and 7 patients (10.1%) had normal T_4 levels with low TSH levels. Overall, 60 of 69 patients (87%) fell below the mid-normal value for both TSH and T_4. Basal morning cortisol levels were below the normal lower limit in 32 of 70 patients (45.7%). One man had a

history of antecedent testicular failure. None of the remaining male patients had low free or total testosterone levels. Of the 24 female patients, 2 had previous hysterectomies. All other females had normal menses.

Overall, 36 patients (51.4%) had a single abnormal axis and 12 subjects (17.1%) had 2 abnormalities. Twenty-two patients (31.4%) had no abnormalities. No patients had evidence of DI or syndrome of inappropriate antidiuretic hormone (SIADH). As opposed to the Kelly study (12), there was no relationship between hypopituitarism and GCS score.

Aimaretti and colleagues (14) published a multicenter study on hypopituitarism in acute (3 months postinjury) moderate to severe TBI. The patients were then reevaluated 1 year postinjury (15). Fifteen had a severe TBI, 22 had a moderate TBI, and 33 had an mTBI. At the 3-month interval, 32.8% had PTH. Panhypopituitarism (defined as deficiencies in all axes) were found in 5.7% with DI present in 4.2%. Of those deficient in at least 1 axis, 22.8% were defined as having severe GHD and 15.7% were classified as partial GHD.

At 1 year retesting, some degree of hypopituitarism was present in 22.7%. All subjects with panhypopituitarism at 3 months had panhypopituitarism at the 12-month follow-up. Seventy-five percent of the patients with single or multiple axis abnormalities at 3 months were normal at 12 months. Conversely, 2 of the 36 subjects who were normal at 3 months developed single axis hypopituitarism at the 12-month follow-up, and 2 of 15 who had single axis deficiencies at 3 months developed multiple deficiencies by 12 months.

They concluded that early isolated and multiple axis deficiencies may resolve over time; however, normal pituitary function shortly after TBI may become impaired by 12 months. They also concluded that early diagnosis of panhypopituitarism is always confirmed after 12 months. This important study suggested that early pituitary deficits may recover over time, and conversely, normal pituitary testing early after injury may become abnormal at 12 months, indicating a failure of pituitary reserve.

Bondanelli and colleagues (16) further addressed the issues of recovery from PTH by studying 50 individuals from 1 to 5 years following TBI. Of the 50 patients studied, 29 patients were more than 4 years from their TBI. Sixteen patients were classified based on the GCS score as having mTBIs, 7 moderates and 27 severe. Hypogonadotrophic hypogonadism was present in 7 (14%) and central hypothyroidism in 5 (10%). Partial GHD was present in 10 (20%) and severe GHD in 4 (8%). All subjects had normal corticotrophic and posterior pituitary function. MRI revealed pituitary abnormalities in only 2 patients, although PTH was present in 27 patients (54%). PTH was present in 37.5%, 57.1%, and 59.3% of the patients with mild, moderate, and severe TBI, respectively. There was no relationship of PTH to years since TBI, type of injury, or outcome from the TBI.

Krahulik et al. (17) followed a large group of patients with mild to severe TBI, testing acutely, and at 3, 6, and 12 months post-TBI. During the acute phase, 93 of 186 patients had PTH. Of the 54 who died in the acute phase, 32 had a hormonal disorder. At 3 months postinjury, 55% of the survivors who had PTH acutely had recovered normal function; however, 7 patients with normal function acutely had developed PTH. At 6 months, 10 patients had recovered hormonal function, but 3 patients had developed PTH. At 12

TABLE 53-1 Anterior Pituitary Dysfunction (%)

AUTHORS	GCS SCORES	INJURY TO TESTING TIMES (MONTHS)	TOTAL	GHD (SEVERE)	ACTHD	GnTD	TSHD	↑ PRL	ASSOCIATION WITH TBI SEVERITY
Kelly et al. n = 22	3–15	Median 26	36.4	18.2	4.5	22.7	4.5	0	Diffuse brain swelling
Lieberman et al. n = 70	N/A	Median 13	68.5	14.6	45.7	14.0	21.7	10.0	None
Agha et al. n = 102	3–13	Median 17	28.0	10.7	12.7	11.8	1.0	11.8	None
Aimaretti et al. n = 100	3–15	3	35.0	37.0	8.0	17.0	5.0	10.0	None
Bondanelli et al. n = 50	3–15	Range 12–64	54.0	28.0	0	14.0	10.0	8.0	Lower GCS scores
Popovic et al. n = 67	9–13	Median 44	34.0	15.0	7.0	9.0	4.0	3.5	None
Leal-Cerro et al. n = 170 (99 had biochemical testing)	<8	>12	24.7	5.8	6.4	17.0	5.8	N/A	None
Tanroverdi et al. n = 52	3–15	>12	50.9	37.7	19.2	7.7	5.8	3.8	None

GHD, growth hormone deficiency; ACTHD, adrenocorticotropic hormone deficiency; GnTD, gonadotrophins deficiency; TSHD, thyroid stimulating hormone deficiency; PRL, prolactin; GCS, Glasgow Coma Scale; TBI, traumatic brain injury. Reprinted from Agha and Thompson *Clinical Endo.* 2006;64,481–488.

months, 2 patients had now recovered function, but 1 patient had now developed PTH. Thus, 21% of those initially studied and had survived to 1 year had PTH. Imaging abnormalities in the hypothalamic-hypophyseal region were found in 21% of those with PTH. They also noted that the individuals with normal hormonal dysfunction had better GCS scores. Of note, the major changes in hormonal function appeared within 6 months of injury, with little change after that.

Tanriverdi et al. (18) studied pituitary dysfunction in 44 actively competing and 17 retired boxers of the Turkish National Boxing Team. They found 9 to have GHD and 5 to have adrenocorticotropin hormone (ACTH) deficiency. All boxers except for 1 who were found to have GHD were retired. In a novel approach, they measured pituitary volume in 38 of the cohort and found that the retired boxers with GHD had significantly lower pituitary volume than retired boxers with a normal GH axis.

As indicated in Table 53-1, several other studies have confirmed the findings in these initial reports (9,10,12,13, 15,16,19). Although there were differences in patient selection and diagnostic methodology, there was broad agreement that pituitary screening is indicated after a TBI because PTH is common in adults.

ANATOMY AND PHYSIOLOGY OF THE PITUITARY AND HYPOTHALAMUS

In an adult, the pituitary gland is a pea-sized structure that weighs approximately 600 mg and lies beneath the brain in the middle cranial fossa. The pituitary sits within a boney cave called the sella turcica ("Turk's saddle") because of its shape. It is connected to the hypothalamus by the slender pituitary stalk. The superior hypophyseal arteries branch from the internal carotid to supply the hypothalamus. The blood supply to the pituitary is from the long and short hypophyseal vessels that form the hypothalamic portal circulation. The long hypophyseal portal veins arise from the median eminence and free part of the stalk above the diaphragma sellae. They course downward along the anterior

portion of the stalk to penetrate the anterior lobe. The long portal veins provide the anterior pituitary with 70%–90% of its blood supply. The short portal veins arise below the diaphragma sellae and supply the anterior gland with less than 30% of its blood supply, predominantly to the medial portion. Severed portal vessels are capable of regeneration, and therefore permit some resumption of anterior pituitary function, although this process is likely to be quite slow and not always complete (20).

The pituitary gland is actually 2 closely associated anatomically and functionally distinct endocrine organs. The posterior lobe is actually an outgrowth from the floor of the hypothalamus. It is directly innervated by hypothalamic neurons that produce hormones that travel to the posterior

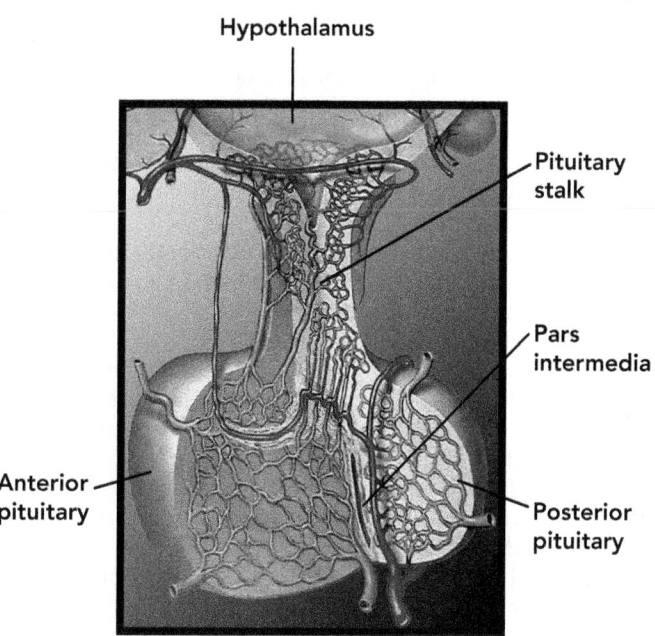

FIGURE 53-1 Hypothalamus and pituitary.

lobe via the pituitary stalk and receives its blood supply from the short hypophyseal vessels, which also supply the medial portion of the anterior lobe. The posterior lobe is responsible for the storage and release of oxytocin and vasopressin, also called antidiuretic hormone (ADH) into the surrounding capillary circulation. Vasopressin controls water secretion by the kidney and causes constriction of the arterioles with a subsequent rise in blood pressure. Oxytocin secretion causes contraction of the smooth muscle of the uterus and also causes lactation. The posterior lobe does not synthesize hormones; rather, they are produced in the nerve cells of the hypothalamus. These hormones then travel along the nerve fibers in the pituitary stalk and are released at the posterior lobe into the surrounding capillaries. There is also some release at the hypothalamus and the stalk itself. Vasopressin and oxytocin are therefore very sensitive to neuronal damage at the level of the hypothalamus and stalk as well as at the pituitary gland itself.

The structurally larger part of the pituitary, the anterior lobe, is more glandular than neuronal in appearance. Neural cells within the hypothalamus synthesize specific inhibiting and releasing hormones, which are then secreted directly into the portal vessels within the pituitary stalk. The portal vessels then carry these hormones to the secretory cells within the anterior lobe. The somatotrophs, responsible for the secretion of GH, are located predominantly in the lateral wings of the anterior lobe of the pituitary and constitute approximately 40% of the pituitary cells. The corticotrophs, responsible for ACTH, constitute approximately 20% of the anterior pituitary and are positioned mainly in the central median pituitary wedge. The thyrotrophs, which secrete TSH, constitute 5% of the anterior pituitary and are located in the anterior medial region of the gland. The gonadotrophs secrete follicle-stimulating hormone (FSH) and luteinizing hormone (LH) and constitute 10%–15% of the anterior pituitary. Like the somatotrophs, the gonadotrophs are also situated in the lateral wings of the anterior lobe. The lactotrophs, which secrete prolactin, constitute 15%–25% of the anterior lobe. They are scattered throughout the anterior lobe, but also clustered mainly in the median wedge and the lateral wings (21).

The vascular supply to the pituitary as well as the location of the secretory cells within the pituitary plays a key role in PTH. Only a thin layer of surface cells of the anterior lobe receive arterial blood. The overwhelming majority of blood supply to the anterior lobe is from the hypophyseal portal system of veins. Because the long portal veins arise within the subarachnoid space, and then travel through the diaphragma sellae, these vessels are extremely vulnerable to intracranial hypertension, direct mechanical trauma, direct brain and pituitary swelling, as well as low cerebral blood flow. The long portal veins supply 70%–90% of the anterior lobe, predominantly to the lateral wings. Because the short portal veins arise from capillaries in the lower part of the stalk below the diaphragma sellae, they are less vulnerable to trauma. The short portal vessels supply a layer of the medial anterior lobe adjacent to the posterior lobe. When the pituitary stalk (and subsequently the long portal vessels) is cut surgically, approximately 90% of the anterior lobe becomes infarcted (8).

Not only is the vascular supply to the pituitary tenuous following trauma, but confinement of the pituitary within

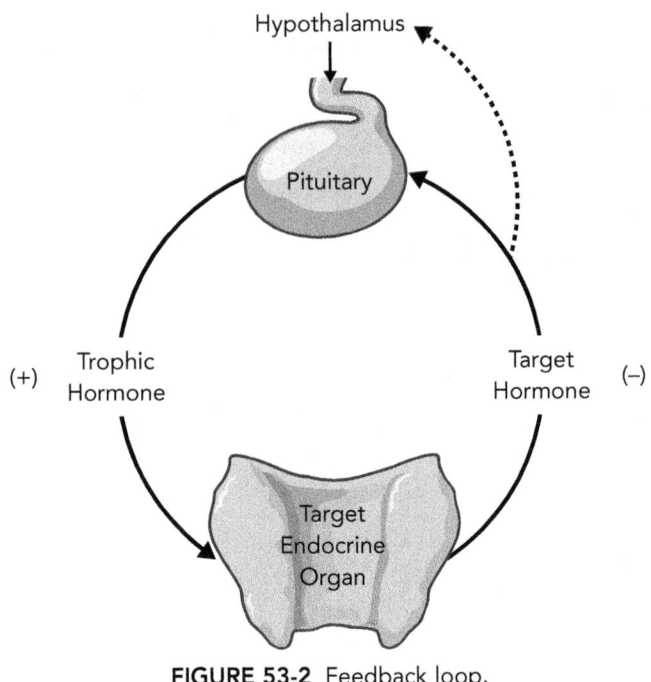

FIGURE 53-2 Feedback loop.

the sella turcica by the diaphragma sellae renders the infundibulum and stalk vulnerable to shearing. Also, swelling of the gland following trauma is limited by its boney encasement, therefore causing compression of the pituitary itself, as well as compression of the long portal vessels between the stalk and the free edge of the diaphragma sellae. The fragile vessels are also susceptible to pituitary stalk rupture or transaction as well as vasospasm and hypotension.

A fundamental feature of the endocrine system is negative and positive feedback control, a process that maintains hormone levels within a tight range. Releasing factors from the hypothalamus stimulate the trophic cells of the anterior lobe to release a particular hormone, which then acts on a target gland (Figure 53-2). The target gland then releases a hormone. If that hormone level is low, there is positive feedback to the hypothalamus to increase the releasing factors. If that level is too high, there is negative feedback to the hypothalamus to decrease the output of releasing factors.

PITUITARY HORMONES

Prolactin

Prolactin (PRL) induces and maintains lactation, suppresses sexual drive, and decreases reproductive function. It therefore ensures that maternal lactation is sustained and not interrupted by pregnancy. Prolactin is unique because its predominant central control mechanism is inhibitory. It blocks reproductive function by suppressing the release of GnRH from the hypothalamus. In the ovary, PRL blocks folliculogenesis and leads to anovulation. In males, low gonadotropin production leads to low testosterone levels, decreased libido, and decreased spermatogenesis (22).

Measurement of PRL is by a basal fasting morning level. Because the secretion of PRL (as well as many other pituitary hormones) is pulsatile, several different readings may be required. PRL levels may be increased because of many different factors, including exercise, surgery, trauma, chronic renal failure, and seizures. Many medications, including antihypertensives, oral contraceptives, neuroleptics, serotonin reuptake inhibitors, and dopamine antagonists, will also elevate PRL levels (22). Because PRL levels are sensitive to so many different disease states, some endocrinologists consider an elevated PRL level as a nonspecific indicator for the presence of disease.

Thyroid Hormone

The thyroid gland produces 2 related hormones: triiodothyronine (T_3) and its precursor, T_4. This axis operates in a classical feedback loop. The hypothalamus secretes thyroid releasing hormone (TRH), which then stimulates the thyrotrophs in the pituitary to release TSH, which in turn stimulates the synthesis and secretion of thyroid hormones. Negative feedback from the thyroid hormones inhibits both TSH and TRH production, although the major "set point" in this axis is TSH. Low levels of thyroid hormones will normally cause a rise in TSH. High levels of thyroid hormones will normally cause a decrease in TSH. Both T_3 and T_4 are highly protein bound. Because only the unbound portion is active, routine thyroid screening involves a TSH level and a free T_4 level. Symptoms of hypothyroidism are noted in Table 53-2. Replacement with T_4 is adjusted by measurement of the TSH level. In the presence of normal pituitary functioning, a high TSH indicates the need to increase the dose of replacement thyroid. The mean incidence of spontaneous hypothyroidism in females is approximately 3.5/1,000 females per year. The mean incidence in males is approximately 0.6/1,000 males per year (23).

Thyroid Hormone and Cognition

Although the literature on the cognitive and psychiatric effects of abnormal thyroid function from a TBI is sparse, there has been much written about the effects of thyroid dysfunc-

tion and replacement therapy in general. Some of the cognitive effects of thyroid dysfunction appear to mimic deficits seen following brain injury. Patients with hypothyroidism may demonstrate deficits in information processing speed, executive functioning, and some aspects of memory (24). In their comprehensive literature review, Davis and Tremont (25) concluded that "overall, hypothyroidism appears to be associated with neuropsychological deficits in attention, some aspects of executive functioning, and verbal and visual memory in both older and younger adults and across a spectrum of thyroid disease severity." Hypothyroidism has also been implicated in depressive symptomatology and has been described as a modifiable risk factor for depression (26). This relationship appears to be true for both clinical and subclinical hypothyroidism (27).

Thyroid replacement is most often achieved by administering synthetic T_4. The extent to which replacement improves psychiatric and cognitive symptoms is somewhat unclear and may well be dependent on the severity of hypothyroidism before treatment is started (e.g., subclinical vs clinical hypothyroidism). Davis and Tremont (25) also reviewed several studies of thyroid replacement for subclinical hypothyroidism, typically with most female patients. Results were generally positive with improvement in symptoms, at times to the point of performing equivalently to healthy controls. However, recent studies of overt hypothyroidism suggested that the recovery following treatment may be incomplete. Wekking (28) evaluated cognitive functioning and psychological well-being in 141 patients who had primary hypothyroidism that had been treated with T_4 for at least 6 months. These patients demonstrated decreased levels of psychological well-being as well as poor performance in several cognitive domains, particularly on tests of verbal memory and complex attention. Samuels (29) also found that patients with treated primary hypothyroidism reported more symptoms and poorer quality of life compared to euthyroid subjects and also demonstrated poorer performance on measures of working memory and motor learning.

The animal literature provides evidence for a possible mechanism linking thyroid function to cognition and also for the positive effects of thyroid hormone replacement on cognition in hypothyroidism following brain injury. There is some evidence that thyroid hormone can regulate neurogenesis in the rat hippocampus, therefore providing a logical role for thyroid hormone in learning and memory (30). Smith and colleagues (31) administered either T_4 or a placebo to rats prior to learning a water maze task. The T_4 was administered either subchronically (every day for 4 days) or chronically (every third day for 28 days). A cognitive deficit was then produced by scopolamine administration in half of the rats. Both of the treatment regimens facilitated the initial learning of the spatial task when compared to untreated controls.

Steroids

In response to ACTH stimulation, the adrenal cortex produces 3 major classes of steroids: mineralocorticoids, glucocorticoids, and adrenal androgens. The adrenal androgens are responsible for secondary sexual characteristics in females. The glucocorticoids modulate metabolism and the im-

---

TABLE 53-2 Signs and Symptoms of Hypothyroidism

SIGNS

Weight gain
Coarse hair and skin
Puffy face, hands, feet
Hypothermia
Bradycardia
Hoarse voice
Intellectual impairment
Delayed deep tendon reflex relaxation

SYMPTOMS

Tiredness and weakness
Hair loss
Constipation
Dyspnea
Dry skin
Feeling cold

mune responses. The mineralocorticoids are responsible for the modulation of blood pressure, vascular volume, and electrolytes and are also critical in the stress response.

The corticotrophs synthesize and secrete ACTH under the feedback control of hypothalamic corticotropin releasing hormone (CRH). Other factors including hypoglycemia, stress, the sleep–wake cycle, exercise, and free cortisol levels also are involved in ACTH regulation. ACTH is secreted in a pulsatile fashion and tends to follow the circadian rhythm. Levels are lowest just before sleep and highest just before awakening. The half-life of circulating ACTH is less than 10 minutes, and its actions are within minutes of its release (22). Basal plasma cortisols and free urinary cortisols are often used for diagnostic testing of the adrenal axis; however, even with proven disease, levels are frequently in the low normal range (21). The more definitive test is by stimulation with a low dose of ACTH (cosyntropin).

Because cortisol levels will normally increase in response to hypoglycemia, the ITT or the glucagon stimulation test can also be used for diagnosing secondary hypoadrenalism. Because hypoglycemia can induce seizures, most clinicians feel that these tests are relatively contraindicated in individuals with epilepsy. Common clinical signs and symptoms of cortisol deficiencies include fatigue, anorexia, weakness, nausea, and hypotension.

There is evidence suggesting that following a TBI, basal cortisol levels may be predictive of fatigue severity. Bushnik and colleagues (32) examined the relationship between neuroendocrine function and fatigue in 64 individuals greater than 1 year post-TBI. They found a trend between lower basal cortisol and greater fatigue severity on both the Global Fatigue Index and Fatigue Severity Scale.

Given its function as a stress hormone, the relationship between cortisol levels and psychiatric symptoms, particularly symptoms of anxiety, seems tenable. In fact, there is evidence in the literature for a complex relationship between postinjury cortisol levels and injury severity, in the development of anxiety. Tanriverdi and colleagues (33) measured pituitary functions within 24 hours of trauma in a sample of 104 patients with TBI. They found a positive correlation between cortisol levels and GCS, with the less severe injuries associated with higher cortisol levels. Flesher and colleagues (34) examined the relationship between serum cortisol levels, amnesia, and the development of post-traumatic stress disorder (PTSD) at 1 month post-TBI in 70 motor vehicle accident victims. Amnestic patients had lower norepinephrine/cortisol ratios than nonamnestics and were less likely to meet criteria for PTSD than those who were not amnesic. The results of these 2 studies suggest that the factors associated with injury severity are antagonistic to an elevated cortisol response. Perhaps the cortisol response is related to stressful recollections of the incident that caused the TBI. Factors such as loss of consciousness and post-traumatic amnesia may prevent injury awareness, thus precluding an associated response to the stress.

Because the short half-life of hydrocortisone is similar to the normal cortisol circadian rhythm, it is the preferred replacement therapy at a daily dose of 10–12.5mg/m². Hydrocortisone is also not associated with loss of bone density. Because of the short half-life, however, it must be given 2 or 3 times per day. Other glucocorticoids such as prednisone or dexamethasone can be administered with less frequent dosing (35).

Gonadotropins

The gonadotrope cells make up approximately 10% of the anterior pituitary. They produce 2 hormones: FSH and LH. Their synthesis and release are dynamically regulated by GnRH from the hypothalamus. GnRH is secreted in discrete pulses every 1–2 hours, which in turn results in discrete pulses of FSH and LH. In concert with peripheral hormones, FSH and LH initiate and regulate germ cell development and regulate gonadal steroid hormone biosynthesis (21). Testosterone and estrogen provide feedback to both the hypothalamus and the pituitary. Depending on the severity of the insult and the individual's stage of life, the symptoms of hypogonadism can present with varying degrees. Adult males may have decreased libido and fertility, decreased muscle mass and muscular weakness, and loss of secondary sexual characteristics. Women exhibit secondary amenorrhea, decreased libido and fertility, as well as decreased bone density.

Central hypogonadism is associated with low or inappropriately normal serum gonadotropin levels despite low testosterone in males and estradiol in females. Assessment of the axis is by measurement of the total serum testosterone, FSH, and LH. As they are secreted in a diurnal pulsatile fashion, FSH and LH are best measured in the morning by pooling 3 or 4 blood samples drawn 20 minutes apart. Dynamic testing involves intravenous (IV) injection of GnRH followed by measurement of FSH and LH. In females, a measurement of 17 beta estradiol-2 may be obtained. In the appropriate clinical setting, a history of normal menstrual cycles may also be considered adequate.

In the late 1980s, Stein observed that following a TBI, female rats tended to have a better recovery than males (36). This lead to a series of studies in which he discovered the female rats had a better recovery during the estrus phase of their cycle when the level of progesterone was highest (37). Later studies on progesterone-treated rats showed decreased cerebral edema and decreased axonal injury inversely proportional to the progesterone level (38,39). Rats treated with progesterone following a TBI also performed better in Morris water maze tasks than untreated rats, suggesting that there might be improved recovery with this treatment (40). Progesterone treatment initiated as long as 24 hours after the injury was felt to possibly provide neuroprotection by reducing glutamate toxicity and upregulating gamma-aminobutyric acid (GABA) (41). Wagner et al. (11) found reduced progesterone levels in a study of acute severe TBI suggesting that men and women might benefit from pharmacologic dosing in a clinical trial. A pilot study in 100 human subjects with acute TBI showed progesterone to be safe and produced a marginally significant improvement in 30-day survival (42).

Interestingly, testosterone levels may influence rehabilitation outcomes in males with brain injury. Young et al. (43) examined the relationship between serum testosterone, length of stay, and functional independence in 54 males with TBIs consecutively admitted to an inpatient rehabilitation setting. Low serum testosterone at the time of admission was associated with longer lengths of stay, lower functional independence ratings, and less improvement in functional independence over time. Individuals with low serum testosterone on admission stayed on average, 26 days longer than those with normal levels.

There are no large studies on the results of sex hormone replacement after TBI, and therefore any changes must be inferred from other disease states. It has been theorized that the age-related decline in cognitive functioning in males may be associated with the age-related decline in sex hormones. Muller and colleagues (44) found higher circulating levels of testosterone in the oldest age category studied to have better performance on visual memory, verbal memory, attention and visual-spatial rotation. They also found that lower testosterone levels were associated with an increased risk for Alzheimer disease. The results of testosterone supplementation in hypogonadal males (45) as well as in normal healthy males (46) have shown improvement in some domains of memory as well. Studies on cognitive improvement following estrogen supplementation in females have yielded conflicting results (47,48,49,50). Presently, the issue of cognitive changes with sex hormone supplementation or replacement remains unresolved.

Please also refer to Chapter 55 in this text on sexuality.

Growth Hormone

Located within the lateral wings, the GH secreting cells make up approximately 50% of the total anterior pituitary cell population. GH secretion declines throughout adulthood, paralleling the gradual age-related decline in slow-wave sleep. GH secretion is pulsatile, and occurs predominantly during the first epoch of slow-wave sleep, largely reflecting the interplay of 2 hypothalamic regulatory hormones—somatostatin (somatotropin release-inhibiting factor or SRIF) and growth hormone releasing hormone (GHRH)—also with modulation from peripheral factors. SRIF sets basal GH tone, whereas GHRH is secreted in discrete spikes that produce GH pulses (22). GH levels are increased with fasting, hypoglycemia, physical stress, and exercise. GH secretion is suppressed by obesity, hypothyroidism, hyperglycemia, and an elevated IGF-1.

Although GH has direct effects in target tissues, many of its physiologic and metabolic effects are mediated through the stimulation of the synthesis and release of IGF-1. Produced predominantly in the liver, IGF-1 levels are also significantly affected by age. Levels increase during puberty, peak at adolescence, and then gradually decline through middle age.

Isolated GH deficiency in children is characterized by short stature, increased fat, and a tendency toward hypoglycemia. Regardless of the cause, GHD in adults can produce many metabolic disturbances that may compromise the health and quality of life of the patients by increasing their risk for cardiovascular and cerebrovascular disease. This includes decreased lean body mass, decreased bone mass, and increased visceral fat and subcutaneous fat (51). As such, GHD in adults is associated with decreased life expectancy (52). GHD is also associated with impaired left ventricular ejection fraction as well as reduced left ventricular mass with subsequent decreased exercise capacity (53). GHD has been linked to a higher risk of bone fractures and increased lipid

TABLE 53-3 Signs and Symptoms of Growth Hormone Deficiency

SIGNS OF GROWTH HORMONE DEFICIENCY (GHD)
Abnormal lipid profile
increased cholesterol
increased LDL, VLDL, triglycerides
decreased HDL
Decreased bone density
Reduced strength
Altered body composition
decreased lean body mass
increased truncal fat

SYMPTOMS OF GROWTH HORMONE DEFICIENCY (GHD)
Fatigue
Impaired psychological function
poor memory
poor concentration
depression
anxiety
Reduced exercise performance
Increased abdominal fat

HDL, high density lipoprotein.
LDL, low density lipoproteins.
VLDL, very low density lipoproteins.

levels (54). GH is anabolic (55) and can cause an increase in muscle mass and fat mobilization with resultant decreased fat deposition. Replacement of GH in deficient adults will result in decreased lipids and decreased body fat. The signs and symptoms of GHD are listed in Table 53-3.

GH is known to promote angiogenesis (56) and may have an effect on neuroprotection, regeneration, and functional plasticity of the brain. IGF-1 has been regarded as a neurotrophic factor in experimental models and in human diseases such as vascular dementia and Alzheimer disease (57,58). IGF-1 has been shown to improve both neurologic, motor, and cognitive outcome following experimental brain injury (59). It appears that GH/IGF-1 may well be a part of a neurotrophic response to multiple types of injury to the CNS, including TBI (60). Whether the magnitude of the IGF-1 response is associated with the degree of recovery after a TBI has yet to be studied.

GH replacement in adults with nontraumatic GHD has been shown to improve exercise capacity, decrease fat mass, and increase lean body mass without altering carbohydrate tolerance (61,62,63). Casanueva and colleagues (64) reviewed parameters in the KIMS (a metabolic database maintained by Pfizer), comparing those with GHD from PTH to individuals whose GHD was caused by a nonfunctioning pituitary adenoma. The patients with TBI were significantly younger at date of entry into the database and also showed a significant delay in the time from injury to treatment. Patients with a TBI had a lower GH reserve and were significantly shorter (more than 4 cm) than the adenoma group, indicating a problem with delay in the diagnosis of PTH. After a year of treatment, the adenoma group had improvement in height, fat mass and lean body mass, quality of life scores, and lipoprotein reduction. There was improvement in these variables in the PTH group but not to significance, suggesting that the delay to treatment may adversely affect target outcomes.

Previous studies have shown that patients with hypopituitarism have a 1.5–6.7-fold increase in mortality from vascular disease (52). GH replacement has been shown to decrease the risk factors for atherosclerosis in GHD using intimal-media thickness as a marker for vascular disease. Pfeiffer and colleagues (65) evaluated intimal thickness in 11 males with nontraumatic GHD compared to matched controls and followed them over 18 months of treatment. At baseline, the GHD subjects had significantly greater intimal thickness when compared to controls, and with treatment, the early morphological and functional atherosclerotic changes were reversed. These findings suggest that treatment may reduce vascular morbidity and mortality for individuals with nontraumatic GHD.

Mossberg et al. (66) studied aerobic capacity in 35 individuals with moderate to severe TBI. Twelve had a normal GH axis, 11 were GH insufficient (GH response to glucagon of 3–8 ng/mL), and 12 were GH deficient (GH response <3 ng/mL). Although the GH normal group had a below normal aerobic capacity when compared to the non-TBI population, the GH insufficient and deficient groups performed even worse, raising the issue of whether GH replacement can improve cardiorespiratory fitness and prevent secondary disability in this population.

Cognitive Effects of Growth Hormone Deficiency

Although PTH may be included in study cohorts, published reports on GH replacement are predominantly from other disease entities such as radiation therapy, tumors, and vascular insults. GHD has been demonstrated to interfere with cognitive functioning in individuals with nontraumatic conditions. Falleti and colleagues (67) reviewed 5 cross-sectional studies investigating GHD. Patients studied included those presenting with either multiple or isolated pituitary deficiencies from pituitary tumors treated either surgically or with medication. Compared to matched controls, analysis of effect sizes revealed moderate to large impairments in attention, memory, and executive functioning. These symptoms are very similar to those seen in individuals who have sustained a TBI, further complicating attempts to separate the independent effects of brain injury and GHD on cognition.

Greater cognitive dysfunction has been reported in patients who have a TBI and GHD compared to those with normal GH levels. However, an important question is whether this observation reflects specific effects of GHD or simply a reflection of injury severity. León-Carrión and colleagues (68) examined cognitive and emotional functioning in 22 patients with severe TBI. Eleven had an isolated GHD and 11 had no pituitary deficiencies. The GH-deficient group showed greater deficits in simple attention, more intrusions and repetitions on a memory task, greater emotional disruption, and increased reaction time. The results were supportive of the notion that some deficits following TBI may be the direct result of GHD rather than being attributable more generally to the brain injury per se. These results must be interpreted with caution because there was no indication that injury severity was similar across groups.

Popovic and colleagues (19) evaluated the relationship of PTH to cognitive disabilities and mental distress in 67 survivors of moderate to severe TBI. They found a significant correlation with provocative testing of the peak GH response to short-term and long-term memory deficits as well as paranoid ideation and somatization. They also found that lower IGF-1 levels correlated significantly with impaired visual memory.

Kelly and colleagues (69) reviewed quality of life issues and neurobehavioral deficits in 44 patients with complicated mild, moderate, and severe TBI who were 6–9 months postinjury. When compared to individuals with normal pituitary function, those with deficits of the GH axis had higher rates of at least 1 marker of depression, and reduced quality of life relative to the domains of physical health, energy, fatigue, emotional well-being, pain, and general health. The authors noted a weak trend toward the GH deficient/insufficient group having a more severe injury as seen on CT scans.

Effects of Growth Hormone Replacement

The positive effects of GH and GHRH administration on cognitive functioning have been examined in adults with and without GHD. Vitiello and colleagues (70) administered growth hormone releasing hormone (GHRH) to 89 healthy older adults with normal pituitary functioning in a prospective randomized design. Following 6 months of treatment, there was significant improvement in nonverbal intellectual functioning, psychomotor speed, and working memory. These findings were independent of gender, estrogen status, or baseline cognitive abilities.

In a double-blind crossover treatment trial in nontraumatic GHD, Burman and colleagues (71) found that GH replacement improved quality of life measures, including energy and emotion. Gibney and colleagues (62) assessed psychological well-being in a 10-year double blind placebo-controlled study of 21 adults with nontraumatic GHD over using the Nottingham Health Profile. When compared to placebo, they found improvement in the overall score, energy levels, and emotional reaction. Arwert et al. (72) also followed 23 males over 10 years with nontraumatic GHD who were receiving replacement. Compared to baseline, there was improvement in mood and anxiety as well as short- and long-term memory. However, the results of a meta-analysis of 15 different studies on GH replacement and patient reported (subjective) outcomes suggested that no conclusion could be drawn on the impact of GH treatment on cognition (72). Oertel and colleagues (73) evaluated cognitive performance in a study using a double-blind treatment phase followed by an open-label treatment phase in 18 patients with nontraumatic GHD. GH replacement resulted in a significant improvement in attentional performance, but there was no change in nonverbal intelligence and long-term verbal memory. Arwert and colleagues (74) studied the effects of GH replacement in 13 childhood onset nontraumatic GHD adults in a double-blind placebo-controlled study using functional magnetic resonance imaging (fMRI). After 6 months of treatment, they found improved working memory as well as long-term memory. During working memory tasks, the fMRI showed activation in areas of the parietal, prefrontal, motor, and occipital cortex as well as in the anterior cingulate cortex and right thalamus. After GH treatment, decreased activation was seen in the ventrolateral prefrontal cortex when compared to their period following placebo treatment. This suggested decreased effort and more efficient recruitment of the involved neural system.

In 2010, High and colleagues (75) published the first double-blind placebo-controlled study on GH replacement in chronic moderate to severe TBI. Eighty-three subjects were screened for hypopituitarism, and 42 subjects were found to have either GHD (GH peak to glucagon stimulation <3 ng/mL) or GH insufficient (GH peak between 3 and 8ng/mL). Twenty-three subjects agreed to undergo a battery of neuropsychological tests and to be randomized to either a year of placebo (n = 11) or GH replacement (n = 12). The subjects were matched with respect to education, age, initial GCS score, level of disability, and level of supervision needed. No subjects reported any untoward side effects.

Because of the small "n," the growth hormone deficient/insufficient groups were combined for statistical analysis. The authors found improvement in the domains of dominant hand finger tapping, information processing speed, verbal learning, and executive functioning. The authors concluded that, possibly, some of the observed cognitive impairments following a moderate to severe TBI could be the result of GHD and therefore could perhaps be partially reversible with replacement therapy, and that the effects of GH replacement might be maximized if given during rehabilitation.

GH is presently made by recombinant DNA technology and is referred to as recombinant human growth hormone (rhGH). Because it is species-specific, GH from nonprimates can not be used in humans. GH is a protein and comes as a powder that must be liquefied for injection subcutaneously. It cannot be given orally in a pill or liquid form. Some brands must be kept refrigerated not only after it is mixed into a liquid form but before reconstitution as well. Any claims of supplements that stimulate GH secretion are pure bogus.

Although the circulating half-life is only 20 minutes, the biological half-life is 9–17 hours and therefore can be given once a day. There are presently no long-acting forms of rhGH, therefore daily injection is required. Children with GHD require 20–40 μg/kg daily, targeting a normal IGF-1 level for age and sex. There are varying protocols for adults as well. Adults are frequently started on 150–300 μg and then increased after 2–3 months if the IGF-1 level does not normalize when adjusted for age and sex. The dose is reduced if patient has any major side effects such as myalgias, hypoesthesias, arthralgias, peripheral edema, or paresthesias (76). Although the many of the effects of GH are mediated by IGF-1; however, as IGF-1 produces hypoglycemia, it is not used clinically. One of the biggest impediments to GH replacement is its cost, which can be as much as $15,000 per year. Some insurers require 2 confirmatory tests before approving payment for replacement.

Diagnosis and Treatment

There is no simple blood test for the diagnosis of GHD. Because of the pulsatile nature of GH secretion and the very short half-life (16–20 minutes), a random GH assay is inadequate. Random GH levels are undetectable in 50% of the samples taken from healthy adults and are undetectable in most obese and elderly subjects (21). Therefore, a random GH level is useless. The diagnosis of GHD is therefore established with the appropriate clinical history and a GH peak concentration of less than 5 μg/L after adequately produced hypoglycemia (<40 mg/dL). Because the rapid and marked hypoglycemia produced by ITT can be epileptogenic, and the TBI population has a greater incidence of seizures, there is reluctance on the part of many—if not most—endocrinologists to use that method of testing. Although the ITT remains the "gold standard," provocative testing with glucagon stimulation test (GST) (normal peak >5 μg/L), Arginine + GHRH (normal peak >16.5 μg/L), and Arginine + Growth Hormone Releasing Peptide-6 (normal peak >20 μg/L) have also been used (77). Because the latter 2 tests do not produce hypoglycemia, they are preferred by many endocrinologists. Unfortunately, Arginine may be difficult to obtain, and many endocrinologists are using the GST. An age-adjusted IGF-1 level can only be used merely as a rough measure of GH status because it only provides an integrated "average" measure of GH secretion. Moreover, in adults, a normal IGF-1 level does not necessarily exclude the diagnosis of GHD. As a rough rule of thumb, patients with an IGF-1 level more than 2 standard deviations below the norm for their age should be considered abnormal. By comparing the IGF-1 levels against the peak GH level by GST in 138 patients, Zgaljardic and colleagues (78) found that an IGF-1 cut-off value of 175 micrograms/L minimized the misclassification of GHD patients and GH-sufficient patients and provided a specificity of 40%, a sensitivity of 83%, as well as a negative predictive power of 90% considering a criterion for peak GH response of <3 ng/mL. Regardless of the IGF-1 level, provocative testing is also recommended when another pituitary deficit is identified because there is a significant likelihood of GHD as well.

PEDIATRIC TBI

Annually in the United States, approximately 475,000 children younger than 14 years of age are victims of a TBI. There are 37,000 hospitalizations and more than 2,500 deaths. On a yearly basis, more than 30,000 children become disabled from a TBI. This clearly affects their physical, cognitive, neuropsychological, and competitiveness. It is also estimated that annually, more than 900,000 children have mTBIs (79). Children are also at risk for PTH, which is known to lead to problems with physical and emotional maturation. Acerini and colleagues (80) published a review article of 20 cases of pediatric PTH. All except one had multiple pituitary deficiencies. Growth failure was the presenting symptom in 11 patients. Delayed or arrested puberty was the second most common symptom. Because PTH was not considered as a possible complication of TBI, delay of diagnosis was extreme in many cases.

Einaudi and colleagues (81) evaluated pediatric PTH in retrospective and prospective studies. The retrospective group had 22 patients recruited by a review of medical charts. Nine patients were prepubertal and 13 were pubertal or postpubertal. TBI classification was severe in 8, moderate in 6, and mild in 8 patients. PTH was diagnosed in 4 patients. The prospective group consisted of 30 patients who were screened acutely and then rescreened at 6 and 12 months. Twenty patients completed the study. Eighteen patients were prepubertal and 12 were pubertal or postpubertal. TBI was severe in 6, moderate in 9, and mild in 15 patients. Only

1 patient had PTH at 12 months. Overall, the incidence of PTH was in 10.4% in both studies. They theorized that the reason for a lower incidence of PTH than found in the adult population could be because of differences in neuronal plasticity, which might allow children and adolescents to recover without endocrine impairment.

Niederland and colleagues (82) studied 26 children 30.6 ± 8.3 months postinjury against 21 aged matched controls. The average age was 11.47 ± 0.75 years. Although there was no history of loss of consciousness in 7 children, all had abnormal CT scans. None had a history of DI. In addition to testing for thyroid, gonadal, and cortisol dysfunction, the patients with TBI underwent 2 separate provocative tests for GHD. Although the TSH, free thyroxine (FT_4), and T_3 concentrations were within normal limits, the peripheral thyroid levels were statistically lower in the TBI group when compared to the controls. Both basal cortisols and peak cortisols after ITT-induced hypoglycemia were also statistically lower in the TBI group when compared to the controls. Eleven of 26 patients with a TBI had below normal GH responses to both the levodopa (L-Dopa) and ITT. Basal cortisols were below normal in 9 patients with TBI. TSH stimulation produced abnormal results in 9 patients with TBI. As a group, the GHD subjects were slightly shorter than their chronological age when compared to the controls, although the difference was not statistically significant. Although counterintuitive, they found no correlation between the severity of the head injury and the incidence of hypopituitarism.

Aimaretti and colleagues (15) looked at PTH in adolescents and young adults (16–25 years). They studied 23 individuals at 3 and 12 months postinjury. The patients were classified as having mTBI (10), moderate (6), and severe (7) based on their initial GCS scores. At 3 months, PTH was found in 34.6%. Panhypopituitarism, multiple, and isolated deficits were present in 8.6%, 4.3%, and 21.7%, respectively. Secondary gonadal, adrenal, and thyroid deficits were present in 13.0%, 13.0%, and 8.6%, respectively. Severe GHD was found in 26%, and partial GHD was present in 4.3%. At 1 year post-TBI, hypopituitarism was found in 30.3%, with the same percentages of adrenal, gonadal, and thyroid deficits as noted previously at 3 months. Severe GHD was present in 21.7%, and partial GHD was present in 8.6%. All patients who had either panhypopituitarism or multiple deficits at 3 months had the same findings at 12 months. Notably, it was also found that individuals with isolated pituitary deficits may improve over time (21.7% at 3 months vs 17.4% at 12 months). They concluded that neuroendocrine testing in adolescents and young adults should be performed at 3 and 12 months post-TBI, and that multiple or total pituitary deficits at 3 months may be stable, and the damage irreversible.

POSTERIOR PITUITARY DYSFUNCTION

The posterior pituitary gland (the neurohypophysis) is formed by axons originating from large cell bodies in the paraventricular and supraoptic nuclei of the hypothalamus. As opposed to the anterior pituitary that releases hormones in response to releasing factors from the hypothalamus, cells in the neurohypophysis actually store and release hormones produced in the hypothalamus. The neurohypophysis releases 2 hormones. ADH, also known as arginine vasopressin

(AVP), acts on the renal tubules to reduce water loss by concentrating the urine. Oxytocin, the other hormone produced by the neurohypophysis, stimulates postpartum milk letdown in response to sucking.

Vasopressin

AVP is synthesized in the hypothalamus, then packaged in neurosecretory vesicles, and transported down the axon to the posterior pituitary to be stored until released into the peripheral blood in response to the osmotic pressure of body fluids. In response to an elevated plasma osmolarity, plasma AVP rises to affect an antidiuresis. AVP secretion may also be stimulated by nausea, glucocorticoid deficiency, acute hypoglycemia, and smoking (22). In response to a decreased plasma osmolarity, plasma AVP decreases to affect a diuresis.

Diabetes Insipidus
There are 2 types of DI. Malfunction or injury to the neurohypophysis may result in pituitary (or central) DI. The resultant pathologically decreased secretion of AVP usually results in the production of abnormally large volumes of dilute urine. Nephrogenic DI occurs with deficiencies in the antidiuretic actions of AVP and can be acquired, genetic, or caused by various drugs.

DI of either type is usually associated with hypernatremia and plasma hyperosmolarity. DI should be considered in the presence of urinary frequency and/or persistent thirst and should be verified by a 24-hour urine output of >50 mL/kg/day and a urine osmolarity of <300 mOsm/L (22). To differentiate the various causes of DI, a water deprivation test can be performed followed by a response to the administration of desmopressin (DDAVP) (a synthetic analog of AVP) (21).

Uncomplicated pituitary DI can be treated (but not cured) with DDAVP, which can be administered IV, subcutaneously, by nasal spray, or by pill. Nephrogenic DI does not respond to DDAVP, but the signs and symptoms may improve with thiazide diuretics or amiloride in conjunction with a low sodium diet (22).

Syndrome of Inappropriate Antidiuretic Hormone
SIADH results when plasma levels of AVP are elevated at times during which the secretion of vasopressin should be suppressed. The clinical hallmark is hypoosmolarity of body fluids and hyponatremia with the production decreased volumes of hyperosmolar urine. SIADH may be caused by neoplasms, infections, drugs, ischemia, and trauma. The diagnosis is one of exclusion based on history, physical, and laboratory findings. The treatment of acute SIADH is to reduce the fluid intake to less than urine output and insensible loss. The treatment for chronic SIADH is with either demeclocycline or fludrocortisone.

INCIDENCE OF POSTERIOR PITUITARY DYSFUNCTION

Chronic posterior pituitary dysfunction after a TBI has not received much attention. Bohnen and colleagues (83) found mild DI in 8 (21%) of 38 patients studied 5 weeks after an mTBI. Agha and colleagues (84) studied 102 individuals who were evaluated for posterior pituitary dysfunction at a median of 17 months (range 6–36 months) postinjury, using a retrospective review of their medical records from the immediate post-TBI period. All patients had moderate-to-severe TBIs. Twenty-two patients (21.6%) developed DI during the immediate post-TBI period, of which 7 patients (6.9%) were found to have permanent DI with later testing. The group with the acute DI, and ultimately permanent DI, had lower GCS scores and the presence of cerebral edema.

Of the study subjects, 13 patients (12.7%) had SIADH acutely. There was no relationship to GCS score or cerebral edema. Only 2 patients had permanent SIADH when tested during the chronic phase of their TBI. Because of different selection and diagnostic criteria, other studies have yielded conflicting data on the incidence of post-TBI SIADH. Figures have ranged from 2.3%–36.6% (85,86,87,88,89).

IMAGING IN NEUROENDOCRINE DISORDERS AFTER TBI

Very few systemic reviews of the pituitary and hypothalamus following TBI have been performed. In a study of women with transient amenorrhea after a TBI, normal pituitary CT scans were present in 10 of 11 cases with PTH (90). Bondanelli and colleagues (16) found abnormal pituitary–hypothalamic MRIs in only 2 of 27 cases of PTH. This contrasts with Benvenga and colleagues (5) who found abnormal pituitary/hypothalamic imaging (CT/MRI) in more than 90% in a clinical review of 76 patients, and in 10 of 13 patients in a later study (91). As noted previously, Tanriverdi et al. (18) found reduced pituitary volume in GH deficient boxers when compared to boxers with normal GH axis function.

In patients without imaging abnormalities, the functional damage at the hypothalamic–pituitary level could be caused by hypoxic insult. Axonal shearing could also cause pituitary–hypothalamic axis disruption. Such injuries might not be detectable by CT or MRI, especially during the immediate period after the trauma. In sum, normal imaging does not rule out PTH.

TREATMENT

When to Screen

Consensus guidelines on screening for hypopituitarism following moderate to severe TBIs were published in 2005 by a group of endocrinologists and rehabilitation specialists (77). Hormonal testing was recommended during hospitalization if clinically indicated. If studies were negative, follow-up evaluation was recommended at 3 months, and even if negative, again at 12 months. Patients with DI, one pituitary deficiency, or other symptoms of hypopituitarism were recommended to undergo testing of the entire pituitary axis immediately. For patients more than 12 months post-TBI who have not had previous screening, a baseline hormonal work-up was recommended. Subsequent to that publication,

Krahulik et al. (17) found little change in pituitary function between 6 and 12 months postinjury. Many specialists are now recommending screening and treating at 6 months. Because of the relative paucity of studies, there are no published guidelines for mTBI.

Who to Screen

The data is quite clear that PTH occurs in a very significant number of individuals with moderate to severe TBI, and therefore, the clinician should strongly consider screening all patients with TBIs in the moderate-to-severe category. Consensus guidelines suggested, however, that for individuals in a permanent vegetative state or at an extremely low level of functioning, the evaluation and treatment should be limited to hypoadrenalism, DI, SIADH, and thyroid dysfunction (77). Although PTH does occur in mTBIs, the incidence and prevalence is not clearly known, and there are no guidelines for pituitary screening of these individuals. Guerrero and Alfonso (92) addressed the issue of who to screen in the military population and generally endorsed the civilian guidelines regarding individuals in an extremely low level of functioning or in a vegetative state. Their recommendation went further, stating that all patients who had a TBI (including mTBI) should have baseline hormonal evaluation at 3–6 months following discharge from acute care, with repeat testing at 12 months if a deficiency is noted or if the patient developed symptoms of pituitary dysfunction. However, they had no recommendations regarding treatment, stating, "Patients who have positive screening test results for pituitary hormone deficiency should be referred to an endocrinologist for further evaluation and management."

How to Screen

Routine basal hormonal screening recommendations for PTH are in Table 53-4. As noted previously, GHD can be present despite a normal IGF-1 level. When GHD is suspected, that is, other pituitary deficits are present or there is a high index of suspicion, provocative testing should be conducted. Baseline screenings can be conducted and evalu-

TABLE 53-4 Routine Basal Hormonal Screening Tests for Post-Traumatic Hypopituitarism

BASAL HORMONE TEST	TEST TIME
Serum cortisol (morning)	0900 hrs
fT3*, free T$_4$, thyroid stimulating hormone (TSH)	0900 hrs
IGF-I	0900 hrs
Follicle stimulating hormone (FSH), luteinizing hormone (LH), testosterone (in men) or Estradiol (E2) (in women)	0900 hrs
Prolactin (PRL)	0900 hrs
Patients with polyuria: diuresis or Estradiol, urine density, Na^{++} and plasma osmolality	

*May be omitted per physician discretion
From Ghigo E, et al (3). Copyright 2005 by Informa Healthcare-Journals.

TABLE 53-5 How to Best Test Pituitary Function

TEST	CRITERIA FOR HORMONE DEFICIENCY[a]
Corticotropic function	
Morning cortisol	<100 nmol/L (or <30 µg/L): hypocortisolism; >500 nmol/L (or >180 µg/L): hypocortisolism excluded
Morning ACTH	Lower than the upper reference range: secondary adrenal insufficiency
Insulin tolerance test	Cortisol <500 nmol/L (or >180 µg/L)
250 µg ACTH test (or 1 µg ACTH test)	Cortisol <500 nmol/L (or >180 µg/L) after 30 min
Glucagon test	Cortisol <500 nmol/L (or >180 µg/L)
Thyrotrope function	
ƒT4	Low (<11 pmol/L)
TSH	Low or normal ("inappropriately" normal)
Gonadotropic function	
Women: clinic	Oligo-amenorrhea, oestradiol <100 pmol/L, LH and FSH inappropriately low
Postmenopause	LH and FSH inappropriately low
Men: testosterone	Low (<10–12 nmol/L), LH and FSH inappropriately low
Somatotropic function	
IGF-1	Lower or in the normal age-related range
Insulin tolerance test	GH < 3 µg/L
GHRH + arginine test	BMI-dependent cut-off; BMI < 25 kg/m² = GH< 11.5 µg/L; BMI ≥25 to <30 kg/m² = GH<8.0 µg/L; BMI ≥ 30 kg/m² GH < 4.2 µg/L
GHRH + GHRP-⌃test	Lean subjects GH <10 µg/L; BMI > 35 kg/m² GH <5.0 µg/L
Glucagon test	GH <3 µg/L
Posterior pituitary function	
Basal urine and plasma sample	Urine volume (≥40 mL/kg body weight/day) + urine osmolality <300 mosm/kg H₂O + hypernatriaemia
Water deprivation test	Urine osmolality <700 mosm/kg Ratio of urine to plasma osmolality <2

Abbreviations: ACTH, adrenocorticotropic hormone; fT4, free thyroxine; TSH, thyroid stimulating hormone; LH, luteinizing hormone; FSH, follicle stimulating hormone; GH, growth hormone; GHRH, growth hormone releasing hormone; BMI, body mass index.
[a] Hormone levels may differ to the one indicated, dependent on laboratory and assay used.
Reproduced with permission from Springer Science + Business Media. Gasco V, Prodam F, Pagano L, et al. Hypopituitarism following brain injury: when does it occur and how best to test? *Pituitary.* doi:10.1007/S11102-010-0235-6

ated by nonendocrinologists; however, patients should be referred to an endocrinologist for the evaluation and performance of provocative testing. A summary of suggested criteria for hormone deficiencies is listed in Table 53-5.

When to Treat

Previously noted studies have shown that some deficits of the hypothalamic–pituitary axis may be transient, or conversely, may develop as long as a year following a TBI. At present, there is no way to predict the future of an individual patient's hormonal integrity following a TBI. Nevertheless, immediate hormone replacement therapy should be instituted in patients with panhypopituitarism, DI, and adrenal insufficiency. All patients 6–12 months postinjury with isolated, multiple pituitary deficits or panhypopituitarism should also undergo immediate replacement of all pituitary deficiencies except for GH. Replacement of other pituitary deficits may restore a normal GH response to provocative testing. It is therefore recommended that appropriate replacement of other deficits be provided first to avoid unnec-

essary expensive GH therapy in patients with transient GHD that simply reflects other pituitary impairments.

As with GHD, gonadal deficits may be transient and merely a reflection of a stress-induced impairment. Because secondary hypogonadism does not represent a clinical emergency, it is recommended that patients with isolated gonadal deficits be retested before hormonal replacement is initiated. Because of the anabolic actions of testosterone, however, replacement therapy might be advantageous in males. In women, however, with secondary amenorrhea, it may be prudent to monitor menses over time to forestall hormone therapy. In the situation where the patient has multiple deficits or has panhypopituitarism, replacement of the gonadal hormones should be instituted because most likely, the patient has central hypogonadism.

The timing of when to treat GHD is controversial. As noted previously, GH is anabolic, may be neurotrophic, and promotes protein synthesis and angiogenesis. Therefore, some clinicians advocate for replacement (once other pituitary deficits have been corrected) sooner than 12 months postinjury. Because there is some evidence that IGF-1 may improve or enhance recovery (59,60) and there is only a small chance of spontaneous deficit resolution between 6 and 12 months (17), starting treatment at 6 months might be more prudent.

Individuals with PTH should be referred to an endocrinologist for treatment, monitoring and follow-up as defined by international guidelines (93). The objective is always to maximize benefits and minimize side effects following the adage of "start low and go slow."

CONCLUSION

Because the pituitary is vulnerable to trauma, PTH is clearly a common problem following moderate to severe TBI (94), PTH also occurs following mTBI, although the incidence has not yet been clearly identified. For acute TBI, screening and treatment should be accomplished whenever clinically indicated. For chronic moderate-to-severe TBI, screening and treatment should be initiated between 6 and 12 months postinjury because any pituitary deficits at that point are most likely permanent (17). GHD is the most common pituitary dysfunction following TBI with some evidence now that recombinant growth hormone (rhGH) replacement may have a positive effect on outcome (79). There are presently no studies on the effects of the replacement of the other pituitary hormones specifically in chronic brain injury, although replacement is recommended (77).

It is clear that the effects of untreated PTH can be both psychological and physical, as can the signs and symptoms of TBI. Many of those signs and symptoms previously attributed to the generalized effects of a TBI could be because of PTH. This suggests that those treating an individual with chronic unrelenting symptoms referable to TBI should have an elevated index of suspicion for the presence of PTH. A recent literature review on mTBI stated that "specific to drug interventions, this review has failed to produce solid evidence that any specific drug treatment is effective for one or more symptoms of mTBI" (95). By investigating for the presence of PTH instead of merely treating the symptoms, the health care provider has the opportunity to treat the underlying root cause of the problem, and potentially affecting a better outcome for individuals with a TBI.

KEY CLINICAL POINTS

1. The pituitary gland is very vulnerable to trauma.
2. Screening for pituitary dysfunction after moderate-to-severe TBIs is recommended if clinically indicated.
3. At present, no recommendation can be made for pituitary screening after mTBIs but should be considered in patients who remain symptomatic, especially if they complain of fatigue.
4. Screening and treatment for pituitary dysfunction immediately after the acute injury should be done if clinically indicated.
5. Screening for pituitary dysfunction for chronic TBI should occur at 6–12 months.
6. After a TBI, pituitary dysfunction can be transient; however, it is felt to be permanent at 12 months postinjury.

Therefore, although there is debate about when to start treatment, it can certainly begin at 12 months postinjury.
7. Growth hormone is the most common hormonal deficiency.
8. Post-traumatic hypopituitarism can negatively impact recovery from a TBI.

KEY REFERENCES

1. Agha A, Thornton E, O'Kelly P, Tormey W, Phillips J, Thompson CJ. Posterior pituitary dysfunction after traumatic brain injury. *J Clin Endocrinol Metab*. 2004;89(12): 5987–5992.
2. Aimaretti G, Ambrosio MR, Di Somma C, et al. Residual pituitary function after brain injury-induced hypopituitarism: a prospective 12-month study. *J Clin Endocrinol Metab*. 2005;90(11):6085–6092.
3. Ghigo E, Masel B, Aimaretti G, et al. Consensus guidelines on screening for hypopituitarism following traumatic brain injury. *Brain Inj*. 2005;19(9):711–724.
4. High WM Jr, Briones-Galang M, Clark JA, et al. Effect of growth hormone replacement therapy on cognition after traumatic brain injury. *J Neurotrauma*. 2010;27(9):1565–1575.
5. Schneider HJ, Kreitschmann-Andermahr I, Ghigo E, Stalla GK, Agha A. Hypothalamopituitary dysfunction following traumatic brain injury and aneurysmal subarachnoid hemorrhage: a systematic review. *JAMA*. 2007;298(12): 1429–1438.

References

1. Centers for Disease Control and Prevention. Facts about TBI. CDC Web site. http://www.cdc.gov/ncipc/tbi/SL/TBI/TBI777_files/textonly/slide7.html. Accessed October 22, 2007.
2. Gupta, N. Classification and features of closed head. NeuroReview. Online University of Chicago education resource Web site. http://www.ucsf.edu/nreview/08-CNSTrauma/HeadInjuryTypes.html. Accessed January 14, 2004.
3. Simmonds, M. Üeber Hypophysisschwund mit tödlichem Ausgang. *Dtsch Med Wochenschr*. 1914;40:322–323.
4. Cyran, E. Hypophysenschädigung durch Schädelbasisfraktur. *Dtsch Med Wochenschr*. 1918;44:1261–1270.
5. Benvenga S, Campenní A, Ruggeri RM, Trimarchi F. Clinical review 113: Hypopituitarism secondary to head trauma. *J Clin Endocrinol Metab*. 2000;85(4):1353–1361.
6. Escamilla RF, Lisser H. Simmonds disease. A clinical study with review of the literature. *J Clin Endocrinol Metab*. 1942;2(2):65–96.
7. Altman R, Pruzanski W. Post-traumatic hypopituitarism. Anterior pituitary insufficiency following skull fracture. *Ann Intern Med*. 1961;55:149–154.
8. Edwards OM, Clark JD. Post-traumatic hypopituitarism. Six cases and a review of the literature. *Medicine (Baltimore)*. 1986;65(5): 281–290.
9. Agha A, Rogers B, Mylotte D, et al. Neuroendocrine dysfunction in the acute phase of traumatic brain injury. *Clin Endocrinol (Oxf)*. 2004;60(5):584–591.
10. Tanriverdi F, Senyurek H, Unluhizarci K, Selcuklu A, Casanueva FF, Kelestimur F. High risk of hypopituitarism after traumatic brain injury: a prospective investigation of anterior pituitary function in the acute phase and 12 months after trauma. *J Clin Endocrinol Metab*. 2006;91(6):2105–2111.
11. Wagner AK, McCullough EH, Niyonkuru C, et al. Acute serum hormone levels: characterization and prognosis after severe traumatic brain injury. *J Neurotrauma*. 2011;28(6):871–888.

12. Kelly DF, Gonzalo IT, Cohan P, Berman N, Swerdloff R, Wang C. Hypopituitarism following traumatic brain injury and aneurysmal subarachnoid hemorrhage: a preliminary report. *J Neurosurg.* 2000; 93(5):743–752.

13. Lieberman SA, Oberoi AL, Gilkison CR, Masel BE, Urban RJ. Prevalence of neuroendocrine dysfunction in patients recovering from traumatic brain injury. *J Clin Endocrinol Metab.* 2001;86(6): 2752–2756.

14. Aimaretti G, Ambrosio MR, Di Somma C, et al. Traumatic brain injury and subarachnoid haemorrhage are conditions at high risk for hypopituitarism: screening study at 3 months after the brain injury. *Clin Endocrinol (Oxf).* 2004;61(3):320–326.

15. Aimaretti G, Ambrosio MR, Di Somma C, et al. Residual pituitary function after brain injury-induced hypopituitarism: a prospective 12-month study. *J Clin Endocrinol Metab.* 2005;90(11):6085–6092.

16. Bondanelli M, De Marinis L, Ambrosio MR, et al. Occurrence of pituitary dysfunction following traumatic brain injury. *J Neurotrauma.* 2004;21(6):685–696.

17. Krahulik D, Zapletalova J, Frysak Z, Vaverka M. Dysfunction of hypothalamic-hypophysial axis after traumatic brain injury in adults. *J Neurosurg.* 2010;113(3):581–584.

18. Tanriverdi F, Unluhizarci K, Kocyigit I, et al. Brief communication: pituitary volume and function in competing and retired male boxers. *Ann Intern Med.* 2008;148(11):827–831.

19. Popovic V, Pekic S, Pavlovic D, et al. Hypopituitarism as a consequence of traumatic brain injury (TBI) and its possible relation with cognitive disabilities and mental distress. *J Endocrinol Invest.* 2004; 27(11):1048–1054.

20. Daniel PM, Prichard MM, Treip CS. Traumatic infarction of the anterior lobe of the pituitary gland. *Lancet.* 1959;2(7109):927–931.

21. Larsen PR, Kronenberg HM, Melmed S, Polonsky KS, eds. *Williams Textbook of Endocrinology.* 10th ed. Philadelphia, PA: Saunders; 2007.

22. Kasper DL, Braunwald E, Fauci AS, Hauser SL, Longo DL, Jameson JL, eds. *Harrison's Principles of Internal Medicine.* 16th ed. New York, NY: McGraw-Hill Professional; 2004.

23. Vanderpump MP, Tunbridge WM, French JM, et al. The incidence of thyroid disorders in the community: a twenty-year follow-up of the Whickham Survey. *Clin Endocrinol (Oxf).* 1995;43(1):55–68.

24. Denicoff KD, Joffe RT, Lakshmanan MC, Robbins J, Rubinow DR. Neuropsychiatric manifestations of altered thyroid state. *Am J Psychiatry.* 1990;147(1):94–99.

25. Davis JD, Tremont G. Neuropsychiatric aspects of hypothyroidism and treatment reversibility. *Minerva Endocrinol.* 2007;32(1):49–65.

26. Haggerty JJ Jr, Stern RA, Mason GA, Beckwith J, Morey CE, Prange AJ Jr. Subclinical hypothyroidism: a modifiable risk factor for depression? *Am J Psychiatry.* 1993;150(3):508–510.

27. Davis JD, Stern RA, Flashman LA. Cognitive and neuropsychiatric aspects of subclinical hypothyroidism: significance in the elderly. *Curr Psychiatry Rep.* 2003;5(5):384–390.

28. Wekking EM, Appelhof BC, Fliers E, et al. Cognitive functioning and well-being in euthyroid patients on thyroxine replacement therapy for primary hypothyroidism. *Eur J Endocrinol.* 2005;153(6): 747–753.

29. Samuels MH, Schuff KG, Carlson NE, Carello P, Janowsky JS. Health status, psychological symptoms, mood, and cognition in L-thyroxine-treated hypothyroid subjects. *Thyroid.* 2007;17(3):249–258.

30. Desouza LA, Ladiwala U, Daniel SM, Agashe S, Vaidya RA, Vaidya VA. Thyroid hormone regulates hippocampal neurogenesis in the adult rat brain. *Mol Cell Neurosci.* 2005;29(3):414–426.

31. Smith JW, Evans AT, Costall B, Smythe JW. Thyroid hormones, brain function and cognition: a brief review. *Neurosci Biobehav Rev.* 2002;26(1):45–60.

32. Bushnik T, Englander J, Katznelson L. Fatigue after TBI: association with neuroendocrine abnormalities. *Brain Inj.* 2007;21(6):559–566.

33. Tanriverdi F, Ulutabanca H, Unluhizarci K, Selcuklu A, Casanueva FF, Kelestimur F. Pituitary functions in the acute phase of traumatic brain injury: are they related to severity of the injury or mortality? *Brain Inj.* 2007;21(4):433–439.

34. Flesher MR, Delahanty DL, Raimonde AJ, Spoonster E. Amnesia, neuroendocrine levels and PTSD in motor vehicle accident victims. *Brain Inj.* 2001;15(10):879–889.

35. Salvatori, R. Adrenal insufficiency. *JAMA.* 2005;294(19):2481–2488.

36. Stein, DG. Brain damage, sex hormones and recovery: a new role for progesterone and estrogen? *Trends in Neurosciences.* 2001;24(7): 386–391.

37. Roof RL, Duvdevani R, Stein DG. Gender influences outcome of brain injury: progesterone plays a protective role. *Brain Res.* 1993; 607(1–2):333–336.

38. Wright DW, Bauer ME, Hoffman SW, Stein DG. Serum progesterone levels correlate with decreased cerebral edema after traumatic brain injury in male rats. *J Neurotrauma.* 2001;18(9):901–909.

39. O'Connor CA, Cernak I, Johnson F, Vink R. Effects of progesterone on neurologic and morphologic outcome following diffuse traumatic brain injury in rats. *Exp Neurol.* 2007;205(1):145–153.

40. Roof RL, Duvdevani R, Braswell L, Stein DG. Progesterone facilitates cognitive recovery and reduces secondary neuronal loss caused by cortical contusion injury in male rats. *Exp Neurol.* 1994; 129(1):64–69.

41. Roof RL, Duvdevani R, Heyburn JW, Stein DG. Progesterone rapidly decreases brain edema: treatment delayed up to 24 hours is still effective. *Exp Neurol.* 1996;138(2):246–251.

42. Wright DW, Kellermann AL, Hertzberg VS, et al. ProTECT: a randomized clinical trial of progesterone for acute traumatic brain injury. *Ann Emerg Med.* 2007;49(4):391–402.

43. Young TP, Hoaglin HM, Burke DT. The role of serum testosterone and TBI in the in-patient rehabilitation setting. *Brain Inj.* 2007;21(6): 645–649.

44. Muller M, Aleman A, Grobbee DE, de Haan EH, van der Schouw YT. Endogenous sex hormone levels and cognitive function in aging men: is there an optimal level? *Neurology.* 2005;64(5):866–871.

45. Cherrier MM, Craft S, Matsumoto AH. Cognitive changes associated with supplementation of testosterone or dihydrotestosterone in mildly hypogonadal men: a preliminary report. *J Androl.* 2003; 24(4):568–576.

46. Cherrier MM, Matsumoto AM, Amory JK, et al. The role of aromatization in testosterone supplementation: effects on cognition in older men. *Neurology.* 2005;64(2):290–296.

47. Genazzani A, Pluchino N, Luisi S, Luisi M. Estrogen, cognition and female ageing. *Hum Reprod Update.* 2007;13(2):175–187.

48. Kampen DL, Sherwin BB. Estrogen use and verbal memory in healthy postmenopausal women. *Obstet Gynecol.* 1994;83(6):979–983.

49. Mitchell JL, Cruickshanks KJ, Klein BE, Palta M, Nondahl DM. Postmenopausal hormone therapy and its association with cognitive impairment. *Arch Intern Med.* 2003;163(20):2485–2490.

50. Sherwin BB. Estrogen and cognitive functioning in women. *Endocr Rev.* 2003;24(2):133–151.

51. Bengtsson BA, Edén S, Lönn L, et al. Treatment of adults with growth hormone (GH) deficiency with recombinant human GH. *J Clin Endocrinol Metab.* 1993;76(2):309–317.

52. Rosén T, Bengtsson BA. Premature mortality due to cardiovascular disease in hypopituitarism. *Lancet.* 1990;336(8710):285–288.

53. Colao A, Di Somma C, Cuocolo A, et al. The severity of growth hormone deficiency correlates with the severity of cardiac impairment in 100 adult patients with hypopituitarism: an observational, case-control study. *J Clin Endocrinol Metab.* 2004;89(12):5998–6004.

54. Colao A, Di Somma C, Pivonello R, et al. Bone loss is correlated to the severity of growth hormone deficiency in adult patients with hypopituitarism. *J Clin Endocrinol Metab.* 1999;84(6):1919–1924.

55. Mulligan K, Grunfeld C, Hellerstein MK, Neese RA, Schambelan M. Anabolic effects of recombinant human growth hormone in patients with wasting associated with human immunodeficiency virus infection. *J Clin Endocrinol Metab.* 1993;77(4):956–962.

56. Struman I, Bentzien F, Lee H, et al. Opposing actions of intact and N-terminal fragments of the human prolactin/growth hormone family members on angiogenesis: an efficient mechanism for the regulation of angiogenesis. *Proc Natl Acad Sci U S A.* 1999;96(4): 1246–1251.

57. Aberg ND, Brywe KG, Isgaard J. Aspects of growth hormone and insulin-like growth factor-I related to neuroprotection, regenera-

tion, and functional plasticity in the adult brain. *ScientificWorldJournal*. 2006;6:53–80.

58. Watanabe T, Miyazaki A, Katagiri T, Yamamoto H, Idei T, Iguchi T. Relationship between serum insulin-like growth factor-1 levels and Alzheimer's disease and vascular dementia. *J Am Geriatr Soc*. 2005;53(10):1748–1753.

59. Saatman KE, Contreras PC, Smith DH, et al. Insulin-like growth factor-1 (IGF-1) improves both neurological motor and cognitive outcome following experimental brain injury. *Exp Neurol*. 1997; 147(2):418–427.

60. Walter HJ, Berry M, Hill DJ, Logan A. Spatial and temporal changes in the insulin-like growth factor (IGF) axis indicate autocrine/paracrine actions of IGF-I within wounds of the rat brain. *Endocrinology*. 1997;138(7):3024–3034.

61. Whitehead HM, Boreham C, McIlrath EM, et al. Growth hormone treatment of adults with growth hormone deficiency: results of a 13-month placebo controlled cross-over study. *Clin Endocrinol (Oxf)*. 1992;36(1):45–52.

62. Gibney J, Wallace JD, Spinks T, et al. The effects of 10 years of recombinant human growth hormone (GH) in adult GH-deficient patients. *J Clin Endocrinol Metab*. 1999;84(8):2596–2602.

63. Bengtsson BA, Abs R, Bennmarker H, et al. The effects of treatment and the individual responsiveness to growth hormone (GH) replacement therapy in 665 GH-deficient adults. KIMS Study Group and the KIMS International Board. *J Clin Endocrinol Metab*. 1999; 84(11):3929–3935.

64. Casanueva FF, Leal A, Koltowska-Häggström M, Jonsson P, Góth MI. Traumatic brain injury as a relevant cause of growth hormone deficiency in adults: a KIMS-based study. *Arch Phys Med Rehabil*. 2005;86(3):463–468.

65. Pfeifer M, Verhovec R, Zizek B, Prezelj J, Poredos P, Clayton RN. Growth hormone (GH) treatment reverses early atherosclerotic changes in GH-deficient adults. *J Clin Endocrinol Metab*. 1999;84(2): 453–457.

66. Mossberg KA, Masel BE, Gilkison CR, Urban RJ. Aerobic capacity and growth hormone deficiency after traumatic brain injury. *J Clin Endocrinol Metab*. 2008;93(7):2581–2587.

67. Falleti MG, Maruff P, Burman P, Harris A. The effects of growth hormone (GH) deficiency and GH replacement on cognitive performance in adults: a meta-analysis of the current literature. *Psychoneuroendocrinology*. 2006;31(6):681–691.

68. León-Carrión J, Leal-Cerro A, Cabezas FM, et al. Cognitive deterioration due to GH deficiency in patients with traumatic brain injury: a preliminary report. *Brain Inj*. 2007;21(8):871–875.

69. Kelly DF, McArthur DL, Levin H, et al. Neurobehavioral and quality of life changes associated with growth hormone insufficiency after complicated mild, moderate, or severe traumatic brain injury. *J Neurotrauma*. 2006;23(6):928–942.

70. Vitiello MV, Moe KE, Merriam GR, Mazzoni G, Buchner DH, Schwartz RS. Growth hormone releasing improves the cognition of healthy older adults. *Neurobiol Aging*. 2006;27(2):318–323.

71. Burman P, Broman JE, Hetta J, et al. Quality of life in adults with growth hormone (GH) deficiency: response to treatment with recombinant human GH in a placebo-controlled 21-month trial. *J Clin Endocrinol Metab*. 1995;80(12):3585–3590.

72. Arwert LI, Deijen JB, Witlox J, Drent ML. The influence of growth hormone (GH) substitution on patient-reported outcomes and cognitive functions in GH-deficient patients: a meta-analysis. *Growth Horm IGF Res*. 2005;15(1):47–54.

73. Oertel H, Schneider HJ, Stalla GK, Holsboer F, Zihl J. The effect of growth hormone substitution on cognitive performance in adult patients with hypopituitarism. *Psychoneuroendocrinology*. 2004; 29(7):839–850.

74. Arwert LI, Veltman DJ, Deijen JB, van Dam PS, Drent ML. Effects of growth hormone substitution therapy on cognitive functioning in growth hormone deficient patients: a functional MRI study. *Neuroendocrinology*. 2006;83(1):12–19.

75. High WM Jr, Briones-Galang M, Clark JA, et al. Effect of growth hormone replacement therapy on cognition after traumatic brain injury. *J Neurotrauma*. 2010;27(9):1565–1575.

76. Parker KL, Schwimmer BP. Pituitary hormones and their hypothalamic releasing factors. In: Hardman JG, Limbird LE, eds. *Goodman and Gilman's: The Pharmacological Basis of Therapeutics*. 10th ed. New York, NY: McGraw-Hill Medical Publishing Division; 2001: 1541–1562.

77. Ghigo E, Masel B, Aimaretti G, et al. Consensus guidelines on screening for hypopituitarism following traumatic brain injury. *Brain Inj*. 2005;19(9):711–724.

78. Zgaljardic DJ, Guttikonda S, Grady JJ, et al. Serum IGF-1 concentrations in a sample of patients with traumatic brain injury as a diagnostic marker of growth hormone secretory response to glucagon stimulation testing. *Clin Endocrinol (Oxf)*. 2011;74(3):365–369.

79. Centers for Disease Control and Prevention. TBI in the United States Children (0–14 yrs.). CDC Website. http://www.cdc.gov/ncipe/tbi/SL/TBI/TBI777_files/txtonly/slide7.html. Accessed October 22, 2007.

80. Acerini CL, Tasker RC, Bellone S, Bona G, Thompson CJ, Savage MO. Hypopituitarism in childhood and adolescence following traumatic brain injury: the case for prospective endocrine investigation. *Eur J Endocrinol*. 2006;155(5):663–669.

81. Einaudi S, Matarazzo P, Peretta P, et al. Hypothalamo-hypophysial dysfunction after traumatic brain injury in children and adolescents: a preliminary retrospective and prospective study. *J Pediatr Endocrinol Metab*. 2006;19(5):691–703.

82. Niederland T, Makovi H, Gál V, Andréka B, Abrahám CS, Kovács J. Abnormalities of pituitary function after traumatic brain injury in children. *J Neurotrauma*. 2007;24(1):119–127.

83. Bohnen N, Twijnstra A, Jolles, J. Water metabolism and postconcussional symptoms 5 weeks after mild head injury. *Eur Neurol*. 1993;33(1):77–79.

84. Agha A, Thornton E, O'Kelly P, Tormey W, Phillips J, Thompson CJ. Posterior pituitary dysfunction after traumatic brain injury. *J Clin Endocrinol Metab*. 2004;89(12):5987–5992.

85. Becker RM, Daniel RK. Increased antidiuretic hormone production after trauma to the craniofacial complex. *J Trauma*. 1973;13(2): 112–115.

86. Born JD, Hans P, Smitz S, Legros JJ, Kay S. Syndrome of inappropriate secretion of antidiuretic hormone after severe head injury. *Surg Neurol*. 1985;23(4):383–387.

87. Dóczi T, Tarjányi J, Huszka E, Kiss J. Syndrome of inappropriate secretion of antidiuretic hormone (SIADH) after head injury. *Neurosurgery*. 1982;10(6, pt 1):685–688.

88. Twijnstra A, Minderhoud JM. Inappropriate secretion of antidiuretic hormone in patients with head injuries. *Clin Neurol Neurosurg*. 1980;82(4):263–268.

89. Vingerhoets F, de Tribolet N. Hyponatremia hypo-osmolarity in neurosurgical patients. "Appropriate secretion of ADH" and "cerebral salt wasting syndrome". *Acta Neurochir (Wien)*. 1988; 91(1–2):50–54.

90. Cytowic RE, Smith A, Stump DA. Transient amenorrhea after closed head trauma. *N Engl J Med*. 1986;314(11):715.

91. Benvenga S, Vigo T, Ruggeri RM, et al. Severe head trauma in patients with unexplained central hypothyroidism. *Am J Med*. 2004; 116(11):767–771.

92. Guerrero AF, Alfonso A. Traumatic brain injury-related hypopituitarism: a review and recommendations for screening combat veterans. *Mil Med*. 2010;175(8):574–580.

93. Growth Hormone Research Society. Consensus guidelines for the diagnosis and treatment of adults with growth hormone deficiency: summary statement of the Growth Hormone Research Society Workshop on Adult Growth Hormone Deficiency. *J Clin Endocrinol Metab*. 1998;83(2):379–381.

94. Schneider HJ, Kreitschmann-Andermahr I, Ghigo E, Stalla GK, Agha A. Hypothalamopituitary dysfunction following traumatic brain injury and aneurysmal subarachnoid hemorrhage: a systematic review. *JAMA*. 2007;298(12):1429–1438.

95. Comper P, Bisschop SM, Carnide N, Tricco A. A systematic review of treatments for mild traumatic brain injury. *Brain Inj*. 2005;19(11): 863–880.

Gastrointestinal and Nutritional Issues

Donald F. Kirby, Linda Creasey, and Keely R. Parisian

INTRODUCTION

Depending on the extent of neurological injury, the spectrum of gastrointestinal and nutritional ramifications can be vast. Often the patient who has suffered a traumatic brain injury (TBI) is well nourished prior to the injury; however, hypermetabolism resulting from an injury can quickly deplete nutritional stores, especially protein, resulting in a nitrogen death (1).

Many other gastrointestinal (GI) and nutritional problems are common and predictable. Knowledge of their occurrence and protocols for their prevention can help limit their impact on patients. This chapter discusses the GI and nutritional problems that can affect the patient with TBI in the acute and chronic phases of injury. Patients with spinal cord injury (SCI), in addition to TBI, may complicate the overall care; however, the care of patients with SCI will generally not be discussed in this chapter. Of note, older references may not have distinguished between the patient populations with TBI with and without SCI.

BACKGROUND

The interrelationships of gastrointestinal and nutritional reactions to TBI were not appreciated for many years. Although Drew et al. reported on the rapid nutritional deterioration after craniotomy in 1947, it was not until 1975 that hypermetabolism was correlated with TBI (2,3). It was noted that many patients tolerated gastric feeding poorly and widely regarded that hyperosmolar parenteral solutions could worsen cerebral edema (4). Thus, many patients succumbed to their neurological illness or injury, not so much from the initial insult, but from the lack of subsequent feeding during the hospitalization. Furthermore, it was not until 1983 that Rapp and colleagues showed that there was a higher survival rate in patients fed early by total parenteral nutrition (TPN) rather than by attempts at intragastric feeding (5). This was an important conceptual advance because it dispelled the myth that the hyperosmolar TPN solutions would exacerbate cerebral edema, and thereby increase morbidity and mortality.

The actual molecular and cytokine reactions to TBI are beyond the scope of this chapter. However, certain GI or nutritional problems may be associated with changes in hormonal actions that are important to recognize. These will be highlighted with their physiologic consequences.

GASTROINTESTINAL COMPLICATIONS

Gastrointestinal complications should be separated into conditions that are associated with acute injury and later events. There may also be some differences when there is an associated SCI, but the focus will be on TBI.

Gastritis or Erosions or Ulcers

Depending on the severity of the neurological damage, there appears to be an increased incidence of acute GI erosive lesions in the stomach. A prospective study by Kamada et al. demonstrated a higher rate of gastroduodenal lesions (6). Up to 75% of patients had lesions that were mostly in the stomach (78%). Erosive gastritis was the most common lesion and was often found in the first week after the injury. The use of steroids did not seem to affect the incidence of gastritis. However, it should be noted that this study was performed prior to the commonplace usage of H_2-receptor antagonists or proton pump inhibitors and the advent of early enteral feeding, all of which may ameliorate this type of injury. The risk of gastric ulceration from TBI has also been well described and may be the result of another mechanism unrelated to the high incidence of stress gastritis previously mentioned. It has been reported that there is gastric acid hypersecretion that can be the direct result of the elevated serum gastrin levels that have been seen in patients with head injury (7). Although gastric ulceration is well known after traumatic injuries, those associated with brain injury have been noted to be potentially severe and may progress to perforation. These have been referred to as Cushing ulcers (8). Because gastric acid hypersecretion can be controlled with either H_2-receptor antagonists or proton pump inhibitors, initial care protocols for the patient with TBI should include one of these classes of medications to control intragastric pH. A meta-analysis comparing the efficacy and safety of proton pump inhibitors vs H_2-receptor antagonists did not find significant differences between the 2 groups in terms of stress-related upper gastrointestinal bleeding, pneumonia, and mortality among patients in intensive care units (9). In addition to H_2-receptor antagonists and proton pump inhibitors, sucralfate is a cytoprotective agent that acts locally to protect gastric mucosa. A systematic review of patients in an intensive care unit compared H_2-receptor antagonists vs sucralfate and found no difference in effectiveness in treating gastrointestinal bleeding secondary to stress ulcers

TABLE 54-1 Prevention of Stress Gastritis/Erosions/Ulcers*

DRUG CLASS	ROUTE	MEDICATION	USUAL PROTOCOL
Histamine-2-receptor antagonists (H$_2$RA)	IV	**Cimetidine (Tagamet)	300 mg bolus, 50 mg/hr continuous infusion; creatinine clearance (CrCl) <30 mL/min reduce dose by 50%
	IV	Famotidine (Pepcid)	20 mg bolus, 40 mg every 24 hours continuous infusion (or 20 mg every 12 hours); CrCl <50 mL/min reduce dose by 50% or increase interval to every 36–48 hours
	IV	Ranitidine (Zantac)	50 mg bolus, 150–200 mg every 24 hours continuous infusion (or 50 mg every 8 hours); CrCl <50 mL/min give 50 mg every 18–24 hours
Proton pump inhibitors (PPI)	IV	Pantoprazole (Protonix)	40 mg every 12 hours (may bolus with 80 mg initially)
	IV	Esomeprazole (Nexium)	40 mg every 12 hours (may bolus with 80 mg initially)
	Enteral	Lansoprazole suspension (Prevacid)	30 mg every 12 hours
	Enteral	Omeprazole suspension (Prilosec)	40 mg bolus, repeat 40 mg dose in 6 hours, then 20 mg daily (or 40 mg daily or 20 mg every 12 hours)
	Enteral	Rabeprazole (Aciphex)	20 mg every 24 hours
	Enteral	Dexlansoprazole (Dexilant, Kapidex)	30 mg every 24 hours
Cytoprotective agents	Enteral	§Sucralfate (Carafate)	1 g every 6 hours

* Table created from references 9 to 16. (Trade name in parentheses)
**Currently the only FDA-approved agent for stress ulcer prophylaxis, often not preferred clinically as the first line H$_2$RA because of drug interactions.
§ Higher risk of clogging tubes if placed through an enteral feeding tube

(10). However, H$_2$-receptor antagonists showed a higher incidence of ventilator associated pneumonia and gastric colonization. Table 54-1 lists commonly used protocols; note that these may not be specifically approved by the Food and Drug Administration (FDA), but rather what is commonly used in clinical practice (9–16).

Delayed Gastric Emptying

Delayed gastric emptying or gastroparesis can occur either with isolated head injury, as previously mentioned, or with cervical SCIs (17,18). This has ramifications for both nutrition and general care because some patients may experience severe gastric stasis or dilatation that may require nasogastric decompression. Ileus is variably present, but appears more commonly in patients with spinal cord pathology (19). Because the enteric nervous system and smooth muscle layers are still intact, promotility agents should be useful. Unfortunately, because of concerns on cardiovascular side effects, cisapride has been removed from the market for common usage. Metoclopramide is presently the only FDA-approved promotility agent. Unfortunately, its use may be limited by its potential for central nervous system (CNS) side effects because of its central dopaminergic blocking activity and black box warning by the US FDA. The drug should not be used in epileptics because the severity and frequency of seizures may be increased. Also, patients taking medications that can increase the risk of extrapyramidal side effects should avoid this medication. Published experience with metoclopramide in TBI is limited and consists mostly of case reports (20).

Erythromycin is a macrolide antibiotic that is structurally similar to the GI hormone motilin. It has been used very effectively as a promotility agent, but as an off-label use and not as an FDA-approved indication. A retrospective study of patients with and without TBI admitted to a trauma or neurosurgical intensive care unit with gastric feeding intolerance showed efficacy rates for metoclopramide 10 mg, metoclopramide 20 mg, and metoclopramide-erythromycin of 55%, 62%, and 79%, respectively (21). Patients with gastric residual volume >200 mL or emesis were given 10 mg metoclopramide intravenously every 6 hours followed by a dose escalation to 20 mg every 6 hours if gastric residual volume did not improve. Combination therapy with metoclopramide and erythromycin 250 mg intravenously every 6 hours was instituted if increased gastric residual was observed after dose escalation of metoclopramide alone. TBI was defined as penetrating head injury or closed head injury and an initial Glasgow Coma Scale (GCS) score prior to sedation of <8. The study reported that metoclopramide failure occurred more frequently in patients with TBI compared to patients without TBI. Therefore, the authors recommend combination therapy with erythromycin as first-line therapy for patients with TBI with gastric feeding intolerance.

Domperidone is another promotility agent that is available outside the United States. It has not been approved for sale in the United States, but can often be obtained from pharmacies in Canada or Mexico or even as a compounded, unapproved medication from some pharmacies in America. Thus, inpatient use is unlikely, but it may be useful in carefully selected outpatients.

Initially, after a person experiences a TBI, a delay in gastric emptying may be suspected when there is feeding tube intolerance with high residuals. This is often dealt with clinically by feeding into the small bowel with or without the addition of prokinetics. After the transition from an ICU, the delay in emptying may continue depending on the severity of the TBI and if elevated intracranial pressure continues. In an alert patient who can swallow, a nuclear medicine scan can be useful in determining the severity of the problem. A solid phase study should be ordered first and if there is a severe delay, then consider following this with a liquid phase study. Antiemetics may be useful if patients are symptomatically nauseated. Low fat (<30%) meals are preferred for patients with delayed gastric emptying because high fat meals may further prolong gastric emptying.

Diarrhea and Constipation

Diarrhea is not a common finding in patients with TBI. Thus, patients who have diarrhea should be investigated like any other patient who presents with this symptom. Table 54-2 lists some of the key elements in investigating the cause of diarrhea. If the patient is hospitalized and/or has recently, up to 6 weeks, received antibiotics, then the standard

TABLE 54-2 Diarrhea

QUESTIONS TO CONSIDER

How is "diarrhea" being defined?
Is there a new fever?
Has the patient received antibiotics in the past 6 weeks?
Is the patient being tube-fed?
What medications are being given to the patient, are the medications in liquid form?
Does the patient have diabetes mellitus?
Are there any GI complications that could lead to diarrhea?
Does the patient have a malabsorptive disorder?
Is the diarrhea secretory or osmotic?
Is there visible or occult blood in the stool?
Is there a history of inflammatory bowel disease, radiation therapy, or ischemic bowel?
Is there a preexisting motility disorder?

STANDARD WORKUP—VARIES WITH THE CLINICAL SITUATION

Complete blood count (CBC), erythrocyte sedimentation rate (ESR)
Serum chemistries
Thyroid studies
Giardia antigen
Clostridium difficile toxin
Stool cultures, including *Shigella, Salmonella, Yersinia*
Stool for ova and parasites
Stool examination for blood

MORE INVOLVED WORKUP

Gastrointestinal consultation
Intake and output measurements
Endoscopic procedures
Radiologic investigations
Stool for osmolarity

workup should include stool for white blood cells, investigation for ova and parasites, and stool cultures that include testing for *Clostridium difficile*. Flexible sigmoidoscopy or colonoscopy may be required in some patients.

Other causes of diarrhea must also be considered. The administration of liquid versions of medications may contain sorbitol, which even in modest amounts can cause diarrhea. Antacids may contain magnesium and other medications, such as lactulose, are commonly used. Many other drugs may have diarrhea as a side effect, and medication profiles should be reviewed carefully for potential clues.

Diarrhea is the most common complication of enteral tube feeding; however, reports have varied in the incidence from 2.3% to 6.8% (22–24). Differences in definitions by various investigators make many studies difficult to compare or interpret. It may be that the actual genesis of diarrhea in these patients is multifactorial. Etiologies can include concurrent use of antibiotics or diarrhea-inducing medications, formula composition, rate of infusion, altered bacterial flora, enteral formula contamination, and hypoalbuminemia (25, 26). Additionally, it appears that the more critically ill patients seem to experience a higher incidence of tube feeding-related diarrhea (24). Initiation of feedings at slower rates until tolerance is seen can help limit this problem. Blood in the stool must also concern the clinician to look for inflammatory causes or ischemic bowel. Occult blood in the stool is a nonspecific finding, but may require a more thorough investigation and gastrointestinal consultation. Etiologies are numerous and are beyond the scope of this review.

Constipation can be a much more serious problem in the TBI/SCI patients. Patients who have spinal cord lesions above the fifth thoracic root can experience autonomic dysreflexia, which can be a life-threatening event. Either bladder distention or fecal impaction can precipitate this abnormal autonomic reflex that can lead to tachycardia and severe hypertension (27). Treatment must be prompt because subarachnoid hemorrhage, stroke, or seizures may result. These patients should be managed with prevention of constipation and routine bladder catheterization to avoid this complication. This will be discussed further in a later section on Bowel Regimens.

Gallbladder Disease

Acute acalculous cholecystitis is an often unrecognized and a potentially fatal complication that may develop among patients hospitalized for trauma. The cause, although not yet clearly defined, is believed to be multifactorial, resulting from bile stasis, ischemia, bacterial infection, sepsis, narcotics (opiates) that induce sphincter of Oddi spasticity, and the activation of factor XII (28). Mortality rates of 10%–75% have been reported. The high mortality is attributed to the fact that the gallbladder disease (i.e., necrosis, gangrene, or perforation) is frequently advanced by time of diagnosis. The symptoms and signs are not much different from those of cholecystitis with stones, the most common being right upper quadrant pain, fever, and leukocytosis. However, in the posttraumatic neurosurgical patient, obtundation or neurological deficits can make these valuable physical findings hard to detect (28,29). Most reports showed that symptoms usually begin between 1 and 4 weeks after the trauma. The most important factor in early diagnosis of this condition is the clinician's awareness of abnormal laboratory findings and any unexplained deterioration of a previously improving posttraumatic course. Suggestive laboratory findings include elevated serum bilirubin, alkaline phosphatase, liver enzymes, and leukocytosis; suggestive physical findings consist of fever, vomiting, abdominal distention, ileus, and in some cases palpable right upper quadrant mass (30,31).

Ultrasonography is the investigation of first choice and strongly recommended whenever acalculous cholecystitis is suspected. Additional radiologic studies should include plain abdominal x-ray, which is useful predominantly to exclude a perforated viscus, bowel ischemia, or renal stones. Another advantage of ultrasonography includes its ability to examine the liver, pancreas, kidneys, and bile ducts in addition to the gallbladder (32,33). Ultrasonographic features suggestive of acalculous cholecystitis may include the following: (*a*) absence of gallstones or sludge, (*b*) thickening of the gallbladder wall (>5 mm) with pericholecystic fluid, (*c*) a positive Murphy sign induced by the ultrasound probe, (*d*) failure to visualize the gallbladder, (*e*) emphysematous cholecystitis with gas bubbles arising in the fundus of the gallbladder (champagne sign), and (*f*) frank perforation of the gallbladder with associated abscess formation.

On the other hand, in a retrospective study, Puc and coworkers questioned the use of ultrasonography and found that abdominal ultrasound was sensitive only in 30% and specific in 93% of 62 trauma patients who underwent cholecystectomy for suspected acute acalculous cholecystitis (34). In stable patients in whom the diagnosis is unclear after ultrasonography, radioisotope hydroxyiminodiacetic acid (HIDA) scan may be useful. HIDA is an iminodiacetic acid derivative, which is given by intravenous injection, taken up by hepatocytes, and excreted into bile with concentration in the gallbladder. Failure to opacify the gallbladder is indicative of cystic duct obstruction or necrosis with very high sensitivity, 90%–100%. Leakage into the pericholecystic space suggests perforation. HIDA should not be recommended in critically ill patients in whom a delay in therapy can be potentially fatal (32,35). Treatment should be instituted promptly, intravenous broad spectrum antibiotics should be started, and emergent cholecystectomy is now believed to be the treatment of choice. Although cholecystostomy has been advocated, it should be only reserved for the sickest patients not tolerating surgery (28,29,36). In a series reported by DuPriest et al., a gangrenous gallbladder was found in 52% of cases (37).

Pancreatitis

Elevations of serum amylase and lipase have been described in patients in the neurointensive care setting. Hyperamylasemia has been observed in 19%–41% of patients with severe head injury and in 45%–60% of patients with intracranial bleeding from head trauma with no clinical signs or symptoms of pancreatitis (38,39). However, making the diagnosis of acute pancreatitis can be difficult in this patient population. These patients often suffer from altered mental status or require therapeutic sedation and/or paralysis to reduce intracranial pressure, so the clinical information obtained from the physical examination may not always be accurate. In addition, it is not clear whether this enzyme elevation is caused by head trauma itself, intracranial bleeding, or some

nonspecific intracranial event. Proposed causes include vagal stimulation, altered modulation of the central control of pancreatic enzyme release, and release of cholecystokinin from the brain (38,39). To investigate the role of intracranial events in patients with TBI, Justice et al. prospectively studied 38 patients admitted to their neurointensive care unit with traumatic intracranial bleeding for elevations of pancreatic enzymes (40). Twenty-five patients (66%) had elevated lipase enzyme activity, and 17 of the 25 also had elevated amylase without any evidence of clinical pancreatitis. Most lipase elevations occurred earlier than those of amylase, and there was a significant correlation between lipase elevation and decreasing GCS, indicative of increasing severity of intracranial bleeding. Similar findings were seen in a retrospective study by Liu and coworkers of 75 patients with TBI from Cook County Hospital where none of the patients with elevated serum lipase and amylase had any clinical or radiographic evidence of pancreatitis (39). In summary, because of the lack of their diagnostic value, routine pancreatic enzyme monitoring should not be performed in this patient population unless it is clinically indicated. Physician awareness of the association between intracranial bleeding and clinically insignificant elevations in pancreatic enzymes may save patients needless cost and manipulation.

Other Less Frequent Gastrointestinal Problems

There are several other GI problems that occur in patients with TBI, but they are less common than the other problems already discussed. The first two of these can be considered extensions of the altered bowel function that can occur with constipation and less commonly with TBI unless the patient is at a low level of function. Over time, diverticulosis can occur in these patients and lead to the usual complications of this disease: diverticulitis and/or diverticular hemorrhage (19). A diverticular bleed may be minor or cause hemodynamic compromise and potentially be life threatening. This argues for the adherence of a good bowel program to try and minimize the occurrence of these potential complications.

The superior mesenteric artery (SMA) syndrome has been reported in patients with neurological diseases. The syndrome occurs when the SMA that naturally crosses over the duodenum obstructs the duodenum, usually because of a more acute angle than usual. This can lead to dilatation of the proximal duodenum and stomach (41,42). Multiple precipitating factors can be seen in patients with TBI, including weight loss, prolonged bed rest, loss of tone in the abdominal wall musculature, previous abdominal surgery, and external compression from braces or body casts.

Once SMA syndrome is considered, a radiological study is usually confirmatory. The diagnosis can be made by an upper GI series, computed abdominal tomography, or rarely angiography. Management can include removal or reversal of a precipitating factor, nasogastric decompression, as well as intravenous hydration. Occasionally, patients receive tube feeds for a short period.

COMPLICATIONS OF BRAIN INJURY WITH NUTRITIONAL SIGNIFICANCE

Several other problems can be seen in patients with TBI that can have an impact on the patient's nutritional condition.

These include the following: hyperglycemia, syndrome of inappropriate antidiuretic hormone (SIADH), cerebral salt wasting, seizures, and the use of barbiturates. This chapter will only discuss hyperglycemia because the other topics are covered in different chapters.

Hyperglycemia

TBI is associated with an acute sympathoadrenomedullary response characterized by increased blood levels of norepinephrine, epinephrine, and dopamine. Catecholamine levels reflect the severity of head injury and appear to predict the neurological outcome in both the acute and chronic phases of TBI. This increase in circulating catecholamines seems to contribute to intracranial hypertension, hyperdynamic cardiovascular response, increase in brain oxygen requirements, and the rise in serum glucose levels (43,44). Rosner et al. showed that hyperglycemia occurred within minutes of experimental head injury in cats (45). In this animal model, hyperglycemia was related to severity of injury and was thought to be caused by catecholamine release. Similar results were also seen in rats (46). In another study in humans, Young et al. found that at the time of hospital admission, 48% of 59 brain-injured patients had a blood glucose concentration >200 mg/dL (47). Patients with peak 24-hour admission glucose >200 mg/dL had worse neurologic outcome at 18 days, 3 months, and 1 year than those with glucose levels ≤200 mg/dL. In a larger study of 169 patients who underwent surgery because of a traumatic intracranial hematoma, Lam and colleagues reported that glucose concentration at the time of hospital admission correlated with the initial GCS (48). Patients with a best Day-1 score of <8 had an admission serum glucose of 192 ± 7 mg/dL, compared with only 130 ± 8 mg/dL in patients with a score of 12–15. Patients who subsequently remained in a vegetative state or died had significantly higher glucose levels both on admission and postoperatively than patients with good outcome or moderate disability. Among the more severely injured patients (GCS score <8), a serum glucose level >200 mg/dL postoperatively was associated with a significantly worse outcome ($p < .01$) (48).

In summary, hyperglycemia is a common metabolic derangement seen early after both experimental and human TBI, and is a significant predictor of poor outcome. It is thought that high glucose levels enhance ischemia-mediated cell damage, probably through lactate accumulation (49). It has been shown that maintaining blood glucose at or <110 mg/dL reduces morbidity and mortality in critically ill patients in a surgical intensive care unit (50). In 2009, the American Diabetes Association recommended a target glucose level of 140–180 mg/dL in critically ill patients achieved by an approved insulin protocol (51). A randomized control trial of 97 patients with TBI (GCS score ≤8) compared an intensive insulin therapy (IIT) regimen with a target blood glucose of 80–120 mg/dL to a conventional insulin therapy regimen with a target blood glucose of 80–220 mg/dL (52). The incidence of hypoglycemic events was significantly increased among patients treated with IIT ($p < .0001$). The authors concluded that IIT was particularly dangerous in patients with TBI. Although serum glucose levels may be optimal in critically ill patients, they may lead to worsened neurologic outcome in neurocritical patients. As a result,

optimal blood glucose control in patients with TBI needs further data.

GOALS OF NUTRITION THERAPY

The first important goal of nutrition therapy is to decrease the incidence of mortality associated with previously mentioned difficulties in feeding patients with TBI. These patients exhibit hypermetabolism, increased protein breakdown, and turnover (53). Nutritional assessment is complicated by rapid volume shifts and fluid accumulation. Alterations in gut motility can also complicate the usual attempts to enterally feed patients.

Fortunately, most new patients with TBI are usually adequately nourished prior to their injury. The complex physiologic response to injury creates difficulty in estimating calorie and protein needs because these patients are often hypermetabolic (54). The hypermetabolic response can be prolonged and is usually inversely correlated with patient's GCS. Thus, patients with more severe brain injury have a higher measured resting energy expenditure (MREE) (55). Caloric estimation is often calculated by using a variety of predictive equations; however, these often underestimate energy expenditure in critically ill patients (56). When available, indirect calorimetry is a better means of estimating the resting energy expenditure. Makk and colleagues showed that predictive formulas, such as the Harris-Benedict equation, could only correctly estimate the measured values obtained by indirect calorimetry in about 56% of patients with TBI (57).

It is commonly believed that the protein losses in patients with TBI come from immobility and the mobilization of protein to meet increased protein needs. However, data from trauma patients have shown that there is both increased protein synthesis and catabolism (58). The amount of nitrogen loss is associated with increased hormone levels that are associated with hypermetabolism; namely epinephrine, norepinephrine, and glucagon (59). Immobility may exacerbate nitrogen losses, but steroid administration appears to have little effect (60). Trials that have attempted to correct negative nitrogen balance in the acute injury setting have had mixed results. Provision of high protein can help decrease nitrogen losses via protein synthesis, but high nitrogen excretion is not eliminated by simply increasing caloric intake (61). Recommendations for provision of protein in these patients will be discussed in more detail later. Although patients are in critical condition in an ICU, it is more important to provide "some" nutrition rather than trying to meet 100% of a patient's estimated nutritional needs. Once out of the ICU setting, the nutritional focus should be to provide sufficient calories for growth and repair of body stores and proper weight attainment depending on the patient's functional capacity. The provision of protein is important to decrease the amount of cannibalization of muscles as a source of protein because there is no distinct storage form for protein as there is for lipids, adipose tissue, or carbohydrate (glycogen in liver and muscle).

NUTRITION ASSESSMENT AND REQUIREMENTS

Predicting the nutritional needs of a patient with TBI is not a simple task because no single test can predict nutrition status. During recovery from TBI, nutrition status will not remain static, and therefore will require periodic reassessment and adjustments that are made depending on current weight and functional capability. Because many patients may be either comatose or confused and unable to provide accurate information, family members or caregivers should be contacted as part of an initial subjective global assessment.

Subjective Global Assessment

Subjective global assessment is well documented in the literature as a valid measure of nutritional status in hospitalized patients (62). It consists of five key areas from the medical history: (a) amount of weight loss over the previous 6 months; (b) usual dietary intake and if abnormal, length of time of abnormal intake; (c) gastrointestinal symptomatology (e.g., nausea, vomiting, diarrhea); (d) previous functional capacity (i.e., bedridden or independent); and (e) metabolic demands of current disease state(s). A physical examination should also be completed to assess for muscle wasting, ascites, and edema. These factors should give an overall assessment of the patient's prior status and ability to use nutrients (62).

In response to brain injury, the systemic inflammatory process characterized by the previously discussed hormonal response causes a shift from anabolism to catabolism (63). Hepatic glucose production leads to hyperglycemia in response to counterregulatory hormones. Despite exogenous insulin, resistance at the peripheral tissues makes glucose control difficult. Elevations in epinephrine and glucagon also increase lipolysis, which offers an additional fuel source. However, current data suggests that few lipids are oxidized and used for fuel (64). Therefore, protein is the major source of fuel following brain injury. Although the demand increases for acute-phase protein production by the liver, the liver is unable to keep up with urinary losses of nitrogen because protein is also used for gluconeogenesis. These losses contribute to further tissue breakdown and loss of muscle stores (63).

Severity of injury directly correlates with the degree of substrate mobilization. Therefore, a lower GCS leads to increased protein mobilization and calorie expenditure (65). Increased intracranial pressure is also associated with an increase in caloric expenditure (66).

In addition to severity of injury and intracranial pressure, motor activity, infection, fever, level of sedation, level of consciousness, and other trauma can also affect caloric expenditure. Ideally, indirect calorimetry is helpful in guiding nutritional care to assure adequate calories to allow protein synthesis and avoid overfeeding.

Calculating Protein and Calorie Requirements

Because indirect calorimetry may not always be available, several formulas have been published to estimate calorie needs. Estimated caloric requirements can vary from 140% to 200% higher than the normal. Studies have shown that this hypermetabolism can last from weeks up to 1 year postinjury, and is most significant in the first week in non-paralyzed patients (58,67). Current practice guidelines

recommend to provide 40–50 nonprotein kcal/kg/day for patients with a GCS <5 and 30–35 nonprotein kcal/kg/day for patients with a GCS 8–12 (68). Because severe brain injury is correlated with significant stress, one must be prudent not to provide large amounts of carbohydrate because this may exacerbate hyperglycemia and potentially complicate ventilator weaning (69).

Because many brain injuries do not occur in isolation, it is important to note if an SCI is present. Because caloric expenditure decreases in correlation with the degree of muscle immobility, this will alter feeding regimens. Estimated caloric needs for SCI may be as low as 28 kcal/kg for paraplegia, and 23 kcal/kg for quadraplegia (58).

Despite adequate calories, excessive nitrogen losses have been noted in patients with brain injury. Urinary nitrogen losses of up to 30 g/day have been documented in the acute course of injury. Nitrogen loss is well associated with epinephrine and glucagon levels (60). In addition, immobility can account for 25% of nitrogen losses (70).

Patients with TBI require 1.9–3.0 g of protein per kg of usual body weight daily while maintaining 20%–25% of total calories from protein. Despite providing adequate calories and protein, positive nitrogen balance is often unachievable in the early weeks after injury and may be difficult to achieve until the patient stabilizes medically (71).

Weight Loss Expectations

A secondary effect from hypermetabolism and hypercatabolism is weight loss. Loss of <10% of usual body weight is not considered significant. However, severe weight loss of up to 40% of usual body weight correlates with mortality. On average, patients lose 15.6 ± 0.9 pounds during their acute hospitalization despite the provision of adequate nutrition support (54). If the patient also has an SCI, another 5%–10% weight loss is expected because of muscle loss from immobility dependent on paraplegia or quadraplegia.

ENTERAL VS PARENTERAL NUTRITION SUPPORT

The use of enteral and parenteral nutrition has undergone significant changes over the past 3 decades. Initial fears about the use of hyperosmolar solutions in patients with TBI have been replaced with the aggressive use of TPN, but now attempts to use the GI tract as early as possible are commonplace.

Several studies have recently begun to address the role of enteral nutrition with hospital acquired infections and mortality. A recent retrospective study demonstrated that early enteral nutrition exhibited a protective effect against ventilator associated pneumonias (72). A cumulative negative energy balance in subarachnoid hemorrhage was found to be significantly associated with infectious complications (73). Lee et al. retrospectively reviewed patients with hypertensive intracerebral hemorrhage and concluded a decrease in pneumonia, critical care days, and in-hospital mortality (74). Hartl et al. prospectively analyzed 797 patients with severe TBI during the first 2 weeks and found that survival improved with early enteral nutrition when a focus was achieving targeted goal rates. Specifically, mortality increased by 30%–40% for every 10 calories per kg decrease in calorie intake. Patients not fed enterally in the first 5–7 days exhibited a twofold to fourfold increase in mortality (75). Additionally, one study demonstrated a high protein combination of parenteral and enteral nutrition yielded higher Glasgow Outcome Scores in a 3- to 6-month period after brain injury (76).

Gastric Feeding vs Intestinal Feeding

The decision about what form of nutritional support to choose for a new patient with a TBI is an important one, and it should be addressed shortly after the initial injury. As previously discussed, delays in providing nutrition increase the risk of mortality or at least could prolong rehabilitation time (5). For patients with TBI, the main question will be if there is an associated abdominal injury that requires laparotomy? If so, then a surgeon may place a jejunal feeding tube at the time of surgery, thereby providing small bowel access. This concept has been popular at many trauma centers around the country, and more importantly, early enteral feeding may limit the progression to multiple organ failure (77–81). For isolated brain injury, facial fractures and spinal injury must be detected and stabilized before decisions regarding enteral nutrition can be made. These issues are important because they guide clinical decisions regarding the initial blind passage of nasoenteric tubes and the possible use of either radiologic or endoscopic enteral access options.

Although providing parenteral nutrition may be easier than obtaining adequate enteral access, enteral nutrition has a decreased incidence of complications and cost compared to parenteral nutrition with no significant differences in measured nutritional parameters (77,79). Also, provision of fuel substrates to the intestine can stimulate gut immune function and limit deterioration of the intestinal mucosa with bacterial translocation and its potential for contributing to sepsis (82,83). It is known that attempts at bolus feeding (BF) in patients with TBI are associated with a high incidence of intolerance (84). It is believed that elevations in intracranial pressure delay gastric emptying. Also, BF can also be associated with gastric emptying delays. Rhoney and coworkers showed in a brain-injured population that continuous gastric feeding was significantly better tolerated than BF (85). Prokinetic agents were not found to be helpful, and medications such as propofol and sucralfate were associated with feeding intolerance.

Klodell and colleagues showed that after early percutaneous endoscopic gastrostomy (PEG) placement that intragastric feeding was well tolerated in their patients with TBI. Five of the 118 patients did experience aspiration but there was no evidence of intolerance prior to the aspiration (86).

In a related study, Neumann and DeLegge compared gastric vs small bowel feeding in an intensive care setting (87). They were also able to show that the gastric route was highly successful in feeding ICU patients without a marked increase in complications.

It is becoming clear that attempts at enteral therapy should be made before using parenteral nutrition. Protocols for feeding should be developed for individual intensive care areas that stress the available resources for that unit. Careful attention must be made so that pulmonary aspiration is limited. Taylor et al. showed that enhanced enteral nutrition (started feeding rate at estimated needs the first day of feeding) appeared to enhance neurological recovery, as well as postinjury inflammatory responses and incidence of major complications (88).

Our group has shown that it is possible to obtain early enteral access in patients with TBI (89–92). Our present protocol is to attempt gastric feeding, if it is deemed safe and feasible. Ideally, feeding may be started with a nasogastric tube, unless placement is contraindicated. If there are any signs of intolerance, then enteral feeding can be attempted with a nasoenteric tube placed by institutional ICU protocol or a PEG with a jejunal extension (called percutaneous endoscopic jejunostomy (PEJ) or Jejunal Extension Through-Percutaneous Endoscopic Gastrostomy (JET-PEG)) can be placed. Endoscopic, surgical or fluoroscopic tube placement is generally performed as soon as it can be arranged and is often defined by local expertise. In this way, patients are fed as quickly as possible.

When to Use Parenteral Nutrition

If the gut is nonfunctioning or safe enteral access cannot be achieved, then it is appropriate to fall back on the use of parenteral nutrition. Central venous access is necessary to infuse the hyperosmolar solutions, but the solutions are not dangerous as previously believed. More importantly, it is crucial to monitor electrolyte changes and glucose levels. It is known that hyperglycemia >220 mg/dL is associated with alterations in the immune system. Caution must be taken to prevent infection, particularly in patients receiving parenteral nutrition (93). Another common pitfall for the clinician is the concept that nutrition support must be "all or none." If the patient's nutritional needs cannot be met by enteral means alone, then it is acceptable to supplement this with intravenous nutrition to help approximate a patient's needs. Although overlap of enteral and parenteral nutrition is more common during the transition from parenteral to enteral therapy, trials of combination feeding are acceptable in an attempt to reach an individual patient goal.

Choosing an Appropriate Formula

Depending on calorie and protein needs, the clinician will need to use either a 1-kcal/mL high protein formula or a 2-kcal/mL formula. It has been our experience that most 2-kcal/cc formulas do not meet estimated protein requirements for this population. Therefore, most patients will initially require use of a protein supplement to meet needs. A calorie dense formula may also be warranted in instances of fluid restriction for control of the SIADH.

The use of fiber must be considered in light of the medical plan of care. Fiber is avoided in cases where paralytics or pressors are being used because they may aggravate constipation from either reduced peristalsis or reduced gut perfusion. Once these medications are discontinued, fiber should be a part of the bowel regimen. This is especially important for patients with TBI that are likely to have long-term immobility or in patients with associated SCI.

Monitoring the Effectiveness of the Care Plan

Daily assessment is critical in the intensive care unit to respond to changes in medical status. At a minimum, daily assessment should include an assessment of laboratory values, gastrointestinal function, tolerance to feedings, fluid balance, and medication changes. If intracranial pressure monitoring is present, it is helpful to know how frequently it is drained because this may correlate with feeding tolerance. Because feeding intolerance is noted, alternative recommendations should be made. Weekly, a prealbumin, nitrogen balance, subjective global assessment, and weight should be monitored for assessment of overall nutritional status because many of these parameters may be reflective of the patient's medical course and not solely of nutritional significance.

Once medically stable and transferred to a nonintensive care unit, feeding tolerance should be monitored daily. Laboratory values may be checked more infrequently as long as not medically indicated, and the patient continues to tolerate feedings. Weights and prealbumin remain important indicators in this population to monitor overall status and needs. As time progresses, a patient's metabolism may slow, requiring a change in feeding regimen to achieve weight maintenance or loss. Prealbumin is useful in determining if calories and protein intake are adequate to prevent skin breakdown while continuing to decrease overall calories. Feedback from physical and occupational therapists regarding mobility and skin breakdown is also helpful in estimating ongoing calorie and protein needs.

Micronutrient Supplementation

Vitamins and minerals should be supplemented if feeding volumes or oral intake does not meet the recommended dietary allowances. Antioxidants are felt to play a protective role in the recovery after brain injury. No significant changes in vitamin E levels have been observed in a recent study after brain injury. Therefore, it is felt that there is no benefit for additional supplementation (94).

Ascorbic acid is also known for its antioxidant properties. Polidori and coworkers demonstrated that ascorbic acid levels decreased during the first week after brain injury likely as a result of oxidative stress. These levels were inversely related to the GCS score and the major diameter of the lesion. Further studies are needed to see if vitamin C supplementation would be beneficial (95).

Zinc deficiency has been observed on admission and throughout the first 2 weeks of hospitalization (96). Adequate zinc status is necessary to minimize neuroimmune cell death in animal models. In addition, zinc supplementation has been used to treat deficiency and the severe protein turnover in patients with TBI (97). Daily supplementation of 12 mg of zinc is recommended (98). Losses can be substantial if patients have diarrhea or associated traumatic injury with a high-output enterocutaneous fistulas.

IMMUNE ENHANCING NUTRITIONAL SUPPORT ISSUES

The Role of Arginine

Arginine is a conditionally essential amino acid. Under normal circumstances, it is synthesized endogenously from L-citrulline. However, during stressful periods such as growth, illness, or metabolic stress, endogenous synthesis is unable to meet the increasing body demands, and a dietary source is required. On administration of pharmacologic doses, arginine stimulates the pituitary growth hormone, insulinlike growth factor, prolactin, insulin, and other hormones, resulting in net positive effect on wound healing and immune functions (99). It is also a precursor for growth substances like putrescine, spermine, and spermidine. Importantly, arginine is a precursor for nitrates, nitrites, and nitric oxide. Nitric oxide is particularly important as a vasodilator, but it also participates in immunologic reactions, including the ability of macrophages to kill tumor cells and bacteria. These and other functions of arginine are still being evaluated, but it is clear that supplementation of arginine can have a generally positive effect on immune system functions and wound healing in humans and animal (100,101). Numerous studies have demonstrated suppression of T-cell mediated immune function after major surgery or trauma. Daly et al. studied the effect of 30 g/day of arginine on patients undergoing elective surgeries compared to an isonitrogenous placebo (102). T-cell mediated immune function was evaluated preoperatively and 1, 4, and 7 days postoperatively. Patients who received arginine demonstrated a quicker return to normal T-cell function measured by in vitro mitogen proliferation assays. This study also revealed increases in the CD4 phenotype, which further suggests that supplemental level of arginine helps T-cell levels to recover faster (102).

The Role of Glutamine

Glutamine is also considered a conditionally essential amino acid. Of interest, it is the most abundant amino acid in the body. One of glutamine's major roles is as an oxidative fuel for rapidly replicating cells including gastrointestinal mucosal cells, enterocytes, and colonocytes, as well as immune cells, lymphocytes, and macrophages (99). Furthermore, glutamine appears to convey a protective or restorative influence on the GI tract, which may decrease translocation of enteric bacteria across the mucosal barrier. Perhaps the most compelling evidence for the immunomodulatory effects of glutamine comes from Ziegler et al. who studied 45 bone marrow transplant patients receiving either TPN supplemented with glutamine or an isonitrogenous, isocaloric control. Patients who received glutamine in their TPN demonstrated decreased incidence of infection and shorter hospital stay compared to the control group (103).

Unfortunately, the chemical structure of glutamine is relatively unstable in solution, unless the glutamine is bound to protein. Until recently, enteral formulas supplemented with glutamine were available only in powder form. Also, new technology using glutamine hydrolysate formulas and glutamine dipeptide has lead to the development of high glutamine liquid formulas that are compatible with TPN. It is important to note that there are no studies available that currently assess the direct effect of either glutamine or arginine in patients with TBI.

The Role of Vitamin D

Vitamin D has been known for its role in maintenance of serum calcium and phosphorus levels for bone calcification and neuromuscular function. Studies have documented vitamin D deficiency in institutionalized populations, such as the elderly, nursing home residents, and those with long hospitalizations. More recently, it has been studied for its anti-inflammatory properties in patients with cancer, autoimmune disease, heart disease, diabetes, and critical illness (104). In a retrospective study of 136 veterans, decreased vitamin D levels were associated with a twofold increased risk for increased ICU days and in-hospital mortality (105). In a prospective study of 1,100 ICU patients, levels of 25-hydroxyvitamin D associated with levels of ionized calcium and Simplified Acute Physiology Score II, but not with serum albumin. Those patients who were taking calcium and vitamin D supplements prior to admission were not protected for developing a deficiency during their critical care stay (106). Vitamin D is thought to augment the immune response by induction of cathelicidin, an antimicrobial peptide produced by macrophages and neutrophils. There exists limited research in critically ill patients. Jeng studied vitamin D, vitamin D-binding protein, and cathelicidin levels in medical ICU patients with and without sepsis and compared these to healthy controls. Critically ill patients were found to have significantly lower vitamin D and cathelicidin levels. Vitamin D binding protein levels were lower in septic patients than those without sepsis. Further studies are needed to ascertain the associations and appropriate interventions in this population (107). Traditionally, vitamin D adequacy is defined by levels of 25-hydroxyvitamin D, parathyroid hormone, and serum calcium. Monitoring only vitamin D status may be misleading because when serum calcium and phosphorus levels are depleted, parathyroid hormone is secreted to increase renal production of vitamin D in its active form (104).

Are Immune Enhancing Formulas Indicated in This Population?

There is sparse information available discussing immune enhancing diets and TBI. The first study was published in abstract form, patients with severe closed-head injury defined as GCS <8 with evidence of brain injury on imaging were randomized to an immune-modulated diet rich in glutamine, arginine, fish oil, and nucleotides (11 patients), Impact (Nestle Nutrition, Florham Park, NJ) or standard diet (9 patients), both via feeding tube (108). Patients were followed prospectively up to 1 week. In their findings, the infection rate was significantly lower in the enhanced diet group (9.1% vs 100%, $p < .0001$), there was also significant improvement in the total lymphocyte count and percentage of CD4 count in the study group (108). However, this study generated several areas of concern: the study is only available in abstract form and the sample size was too small to provide significant statistical analysis. Another paper addressing the use of immune enhancing formulas compared 2 immune diets: Crucial (Nestle Nutrition, Florham Park, NJ) and Impact (109). This study involved multiple trauma patients, but 9 of 13 patients had severe closed-head injury. This prospective study consisted of 13 patients randomized to receive, enterally, either Crucial or Impact. The randomized diet was given for 7 days with study measurements obtained at study entry and day 7. The feedings goals were calculated based on protein delivery of 1.5 g/kg body weight. Feedings were

started at 30 mL/hour and advanced 20 mL/hour every 4–8 hours until goal was met. The authors concluded that patients receiving Crucial had normalization of interleukin 1 (IL-1) release from peripheral monocytes incubated with lipopolysaccharide (LPS) in vitro, but no alteration was noted with Impact (109). This limited study did not lead to any concrete conclusions regarding these diets in patients with TBI.

Minard and colleagues studied immune enhancing diets in head injury and compared early enteral feeding to late enteral feeding with Impact in a prospective, randomized fashion (110). The early group received enteral feeding <72 hours after admission and the late group received feeding on resolution of the ileus from their head injury. The overall conclusion was that there was no significant difference between the 2 studied groups, but there was trend for higher mortality in the late group (4 of 15) (110).

Based on the available studies, very few conclusions on the use of immune modulated formulas in patients with TBI can be made. The single best conclusion is that these diets seem to be well tolerated. Further research, including larger randomized controlled trials, to compare the immune enhancing diets to isonitrogenous control are essential.

REHABILITATION ISSUES

Once the patient stabilizes and transfers to the rehabilitation service, the team's goals are to normalize the patient's care in a safe environment and provide education for postdischarge placement. Common nutritional problems faced include dysphagia, hydration, maintaining a realistic body weight, and bowel regimens.

Dysphagia

The treatment of dysphagia requires a team effort, including the speech-language pathologists, physiatrist, nursing staff, and dietitian. This important topic is covered in Chapter 65.

Maintenance of Realistic Body Weight

The hypercatabolism of brain injury that drives weight loss generally stops and plateaus at 2 months postinjury. In a multicenter retrospective study of severe TBI, 68% of patients exhibited severe weight loss of >10% through the second month, indicative of malnutrition, and often coinciding with admission to inpatient rehabilitation (111). Information regarding mobility, level of agitation, and progress in therapy and activities of daily living are useful in reassessing calorie needs. The more muscle groups used, the more muscle that is spared from disuse (112). Many patients have increased calorie needs during rehabilitation because of the calories spent during the work process of therapy. This increase can be 30%–60% higher than control groups. Assistive devices can ease this increase (113).

Weekly weights are very useful in monitoring for weight gain or loss. As medical status normalizes, calorie demands decrease. Of utmost importance for patients and their families is to understand that calorie needs are likely lower than normal in the setting of limited mobility or paresis. Indirect calorimetry was performed on nonambulatory tube-fed adults with neurologic disabilities. This study demonstrated an approximate 25% decrease in caloric needs for patients with fixed upper extremity contractures (114). Weight gain is also the result of altered food intake patterns. Some patients experience hyperphagia, which is compounded by a poor memory of when they last ate. Patients with brain injury are noted to consume larger meals and more calories per day than controls. This occurs without regard to premeal stomach contents (115).

These are important considerations regarding planning a diet for weight loss or weight maintenance. Behavior strategies should be employed to limit access to food and to schedule meals. Memory boards or diaries may be helpful in reminding individuals of the time and content of their last meal. Individuals should be discouraged from automatically eating because they think they are hungry, and food should not be used as a reward for participating in therapy or management programs.

Patients should be encouraged to follow a low-fat, well-balanced diet. The food guide pyramid is a starting resource for diet planning. In addition, they should consult a registered dietitian or recognized weight management center (e.g., Weight Watchers) for assistance with individualized dietary meal plans. A registered dietitian can also provide support to the caregiver, guidance to therapists, and assistance in monitoring the effectiveness of the weight loss plan.

Obesity and decreased mobility can precipitate pressure sore development in the chronic care setting (116,117). Therefore, all patients with brain injury with limited mobility should receive periodic routine skin assessments. If skin breakdown is noted, a further nutritional assessment is warranted.

Malnutrition can delay wound healing. It is important that deficiencies of protein, vitamins, and minerals be repleted to allow for tissue growth and repair. Frequently, a deficiency is not clinically noted; however, it has become a practice to provide daily supplementation of vitamins (118,119). In patients without significant liver or renal disease, a daily multivitamin and an additional 500 mg of ascorbic acid are recommended. Zinc should also be given if pressure sores do not heal or progress in staging (120). Clinicians should review dietary habits with patients to also ensure adequate calories and increased protein for wound healing (121).

Bowel Regimens

For nonambulatory patients, bowel programs are an essential part of their medical management. The chronic patient should eat a high-fiber diet of at least 30 g per day. Good sources of fiber include whole grains, bran products, leafy greens, and raw vegetables (122). It is important to investigate the patient's usual bowel habits. Often in the critical care environment, a bowel regimen may not be indicated or appropriate because of abdominal surgery, use of pressor agents, or medication-induced diarrhea. When a bowel program is initiated in either setting, it typically includes daily senna and a stool softener. Enemas, usually tap water, and magnesium citrate may be used when patients have not moved their bowels for a period longer than the institutional

protocol calls for. Close monitoring should be paid to the frequency of bowel movements on daily assessments, and further medications are ordered as necessary. Long-term use of senna products has been associated with melanosis coli. Thus, judicious intermittent usage should not become daily use. Polyethylene glycol 3350 (e.g., MiraLax [Schering-Plough, Kenilworth, NJ], et al.) may be useful long-term for improving bowel function. Often, the addition of a nighttime suppository, such as glycerin, may assist with regular bowel movements. However, in patients who experience prolonged constipation, a gastrointestinal motility workup may be appropriate and consultation may be required. Narcotic usage is a common cause of poor bowel function.

CONCLUSION

Care of patients with TBI can be complex yet rewarding. The gastrointestinal and nutritional ramifications of an individual's disease may be straightforward or require a specialist's input. Time should be taken to review the potential needs of each patient, and care plans should be created and implemented. Further understanding of the underlying disease will improve the delivery of comprehensive care to these afflicted patients. Additional research that is specific to persons with TBI is generally needed in most areas discussed in this chapter because the older literature may include other neurologically injured systems.

KEY CLINICAL POINTS

1. There are multiple gastrointestinal and nutritional complications associated with neurological injury.
2. The diagnosis and multidisciplinary approach to gastrointestinal and nutritional disorders is essential to the management of patients with traumatic brain injury.
3. Early nutritional assessment and therapy is important to decrease the incidence of mortality in patients with traumatic brain injury.

KEY REFERENCES

1. Idjadi F, Robbins R, Stahl WM, Essiet G. Prospective study of gastric secretion in stressed patients with intracranial injury. *J Trauma*. 1971;11(8):681–688.
2. Lin PC, Chang CH, Hsu PI, Tseng PL, Huang YB. The efficacy and safety of proton pump inhibitors vs histamine-2 receptor antagonists for stress ulcer bleeding prophylaxis among critical care patients: a meta-analysis. *Crit Care Med*. 2010;38(4):1197–1205.
3. Eisenberg PG. Causes of diarrhea in tube-fed patients: a comprehensive approach to diagnosis and management. *Nutr Clin Pract*. 1993;8(3)119–123.
4. Godoy DA, Di Napoli M, Rabinstein AA. Treating hyperglycemia in neurocritical patients: benefits and perils. *Neurocrit Care*. 2010;13(3):425–438.
5. Krakau K, Hansson A, Karlsson T, de Boussard CN, Tengvar C, Borg J. Nutritional treatment of patients with severe traumatic brain injury during the first six months after injury. *Nutrition*. 2007;23(4):308–317.

References

1. Cahill GF Jr. Starvation in man. *N Engl J Med*. 1970;282(12):668–675.
2. Drew JH, Koop CE, Grigger RP. A nutritional study of neurosurgical patients; with special reference to nitrogen balance and convalescence in the postoperative period. *J Neurosurg*. 1947;4(1):7–15.
3. Haider W, Lackner F, Schlick W, et al. Metabolic changes in the course of severe brain damage. *Eur J Int Care Med*. 1975;1:19–26.
4. White R. Aspects and problems of total parenteral alimentation in the neurosurgery patient. In: Manni C, Magalini SI, Scrascia E, eds. *Total Parenteral Alimentation*. Amsterdam, The Netherlands: Excerpta Medica; 1976:208–214.
5. Rapp RP, Young B, Twyman D, et al. The favorable effect of early parenteral feeding on survival in head-injured patients. *J Neurosurg*. 1983;58(6):906–912.
6. Kamada T, Fusamoto H, Kawano S, et al. Acute gastroduodenal lesions in head injury. An endoscopic study. *Am J Gastroenterol*. 1977;68(3):249–253.
7. Idjadi F, Robbins R, Stahl WM, Essiet G. Prospective study of gastric secretion in stressed patients with intracranial injury. *J Trauma*. 1971;11(8):681–688.
8. Cushing H. Peptic ulcers and interbrain. *Surg Gynecol Obstet*. 1932;55:1–34.
9. Lin PC, Chang CH, Hsu PI, Tseng PL, Huang YB. The efficacy and safety of proton pump inhibitors vs histamine-2 receptor antagonists for stress ulcer bleeding prophylaxis among critical care patients: a meta-analysis. *Crit Care Med*. 2010;38(4):1197–1205.
10. Huang J, Cao Y, Liao C, Wu L, Gao F. Effect of histamine-2-receptor antagonists versus sucralfate on stress ulcer prophylaxis in mechanically ventilated patients: a meta-analysis of 10 randomized controlled trials. *Crit Care*. 2010;14(5):R194.
11. Larson C, Cavuto NJ, Flockhart DA, Weinberg RB. Bioavailability and efficacy of omeprazole given orally and by nasogastric tube. *Dig Dis Sci*. 1996;41(3):475–479.
12. Chun AH, Shi HH, Achari R, Dennis S, Cavanaugh JH. Lansoprazole: administration of the contents of a capsule dosage formulation through a nasogastric tube. *Clin Ther*. 1996;18(5):833–842.
13. Balaban DH, Duckworth CW, Peura DA. Nasogastric omeprazole: effects on gastric pH in critically ill patients. *Am J Gastroenterol*. 1997;92(1):79–83.
14. Pisegna JR. Switching between intravenous and oral pantoprazole. *J Clin Gastroenterol*. 2001;32(1):27–32.
15. Morris J, Karlstadt R, Blatcher D, Field B, McDevitt M. Intermittent intravenous pantoprazole rapidly achieves and maintains gastric pH ≥4.0 compared with continuous infusion H2-receptor antagonist in intensive care unit patients. *Crit Care Med*. 2002;29(suppl 12):485,A147.
16. Cook DJ, Reeve BK, Guyatt GH, et al. Stress ulcer prophylaxis in critically ill patients. Resolving discordant meta-analyses. *JAMA*. 1996;275(4):308–314.
17. McArthur CJ, Gin T, McLaren IM, Critchley JA, Oh TE. Gastric emptying following brain injury: effects of choice of sedation and intracranial pressure. *Intensive Care Med*. 1995;21(7):573–576.
18. Segal JL, Milne N, Brunnemann SR. Gastric emptying is impaired in patients with spinal cord injury. *Am J Gastroenterol*. 1995;90(3):466–470.
19. Gore RM, Mintzer RA, Calenoff L. Gastrointestinal complications of spinal cord injury. *Spine(Phila Pa 1976)*. 1981;6(6):538–544.
20. Jackson MD, Davidoff G. Gastroparesis following traumatic brain injury and response to metoclopramide therapy. *Arch Phys Med Rehabil*. 1989;70(7):553–555.
21. Dickerson RN, Mitchell JN, Morgan LM, et al. Disparate response to metoclopramide therapy for gastric feeding intolerance in trauma patients with and without traumatic brain injury. *JPEN J Parenter Enteral Nutr*. 2009;33(6):646–655.
22. Cataldi-Betcher EL, Seltzer MH, Slocum BA, Jones KW. Complications occurring during enteral nutrition support: a prospective study. *JPEN J Parenter Enteral Nutr*. 1983;7(6):546–552.
23. Kelly TW, Patrick MR, Hillman KM. Study of diarrhea in critically ill patients. *Crit Care Med*. 1983;11(1):7–9.
24. Edes TE, Walk BE, Austin JL. Diarrhea in tube-fed patients: feeding formula not necessarily the cause. *Am J Med*. 1990;88(2):91–93.
25. Broom J, Jones K. Causes and prevention of diarrhoea in patients receiving enteral nutritional support. *J Hum Nutr*. 1981;35(2):123–127.
26. Eisenberg PG. Causes of diarrhea in tube-fed patients: a comprehensive approach to diagnosis and management. *Nutr Clin Pract*. 1993;8(3):119–123.
27. McGuire TJ, Kumar VN. Autonomic dysreflexia in the spinal cord-injured. What the physician should know about this medical emergency. *Postgrad Med*. 1986;80(2):81–84, 89.
28. Branch CL Jr, Albertson DA, Kelly DL. Post-traumatic acalculous cholecystitis on a neurosurgical service. *Neurosurgery*. 1983;12(1):98–101.
29. Okada Y, Tanabe R, Mukaida M. Postraumatic acute cholecystitis. Relationship to the initial trauma. *Am J Forensic Med Pathol*. 1987;8(2):164–168.
30. Orlando R III, Gleason E, Drezner AD. Acute acalculous cholecystitis in the critically ill patient. *Am J Surg*. 1983;145(4):472–476.
31. Romero Ganuza FJ, La Banda G, Montalvo R, Mazaira J. Acute acalculous cholecystitis in patients with acute traumatic spinal cord injury. *Spinal Cord*. 1997;35(2):124–128.
32. Kalliafas S, Ziegler DW, Flancbaum L, Choban PS. Acute acalculous cholecystitis: incidence, risk factors, diagnosis, and outcome. *Am Surg*. 1998;64(5):471–475.
33. Molenat F, Boussuges A, Valantin V, Sainty JM. Gallbladder abnormalities in medical ICU patients: an ultrasonographic study. *Intensive Care Med*. 1996;22(4):356–358.
34. Puc MM, Tran HS, Wry PW, Ross SE. Ultrasound is not a useful screening tool for acute acalculous cholecystitis in critically ill trauma patients. *Am Surg*. 2002;68(1):65–69.
35. Westlake PJ, Hershfield NB, Kelly JK. Chronic right upper quadrant pain without gallstones: does HIDA scan predict outcome after cholecystectomy? *Am J Gastroenterol*. 1990;85(8):986–990.
36. Heruti R, Bar-On Z, Gofrit O, Weingarden HP, Ohry A. Acute acalculous cholecystitis as a complication of spinal cord injury. *Arch Phys Med Rehabil*. 1994;75(7):822–824.
37. DuPriest RW Jr, Khaneja SC, Cowley RA. Acute cholecystitis complicating trauma. *Ann Surg*. 1979;189(1):84–89.
38. Bouwman DL, Altshuler J, Weaver DW. Hyperamylasemia: a result of intracranial bleeding. *Surgery*. 1983;94(2):318–323.
39. Liu KJ, Atten MJ, Lichtor T, et al. Serum amylase and lipase elevation is associated with intracranial events. *Am Surg*. 2001;67(3):215–220.
40. Justice AD, DiBenedetto RJ, Stanford E. Significance of elevated pancreatic enzymes in intracranial bleeding. *South Med J*. 1994;87(9):889–893.
41. Wilson-Storey D, MacKinlay GA. The superior mesenteric artery syndrome. *J R Coll Surg Edinb*. 1986;31(3):175–178.
42. Hines JR, Gore RM, Ballantyne GH. Superior mesenteric artery syndrome. Diagnostic criteria and therapeutic approaches. *Am J Surg*. 1984;148(5):630–632.
43. Flakoll PJ, Wentzel LS, Hyman SA. Protein and glucose metabolism during isolated closed-head injury. *Am J Physiol*. 1995;269(4, pt 1):E636–E641.
44. De Salles AA, Muizelaar JP, Young HF. Hyperglycemia, cerebrospinal fluid lactic acidosis, and cerebral blood flow in severely head-injured patients. *Neurosurg*. 1987;21(1):45–50.
45. Rosner MJ, Newsome HH, Becker DP. Mechanical brain injury: the sympathoadrenal response. *J Neurosurg*. 1984;61(1):76–86.
46. Cherian L, Goodman JC, Robertson CS. Hyperglycemia increases brain injury caused by secondary ischemia after cortical impact injury in rats. *Crit Care Med*. 1997;25(8):1378–1383.
47. Young B, Ott L, Dempsey R, Haack D, Tibbs P. Relationship between admission hyperglycemia and neurologic outcome of severely brain-injured patients. *Ann Surg*. 1989;210(4):466–472.
48. Lam AM, Winn HR, Cullen BF, Sundling N. Hyperglycemia and neurological outcome in patients with head injury. *J Neurosurg*. 1991;75(4):545–551.

49. Rovlias A, Kotsou S. The influence of hyperglycemia on neurological outcome in patients with severe head injury. *Neurosurgery*. 2000; 46(2):335–342.

50. van den Berghe G, Wouters P, Weekers F, et al. Intensive insulin therapy in critically ill patients. *N Engl J Med*. 2001;345(19): 1359–1367.

51. Kavanagh BP, McCowen KC. Clinical Practice. Glycemic control in the ICU. *N Engl J Med*. 2010;363(26):2540–2546.

52. Godoy DA, Di Napoli M, Rabinstein AA. Treating hyperglycemia in neurocritical patients: benefits and perils. *Neurocrit Care*. 2010; 13(3):425–438.

53. Young B, Ott L, Haack D, et al. Effect of total parenteral nutrition upon intracranial pressure in severe head injury. *J Neurosurg*. 1987; 67(1):76–80.

54. Young B, Ott L, Norton J, et al. Metabolic and nutritional sequelae in the non-steroid treated head injury patient. *Neurosurgery* 1985; 17(5):784–791.

55. Clifton GL, Robertson CS, Grossman RG, Hodge S, Foltz R, Garza C. The metabolic response to severe head injury. *J Neurosurg*. 1984; 60(4):687–696.

56. Frankenfield DC, Coleman A, Alam S, Cooney RN. Analysis of estimation methods for resting metabolic rate in critically ill adults. *JPEN J Parenter Enteral Nutr*. 2009;33(1):27–36.

57. Makk LJ, McClave SA, Creech PW, et al. Clinical application of the metabolic cart to the delivery of parenteral nutrition. *Crit Care Med*. 1987;13:818–829.

58. Sunderland PM, Heilbrun MP. Estimating energy expenditure in traumatic brain injury: comparison of indirect calorimetry with predictive formulas. *Neurosurgery*. 1992;31(2):246–252.

59. Birkhahn RH, Long CL, Fitkin D, Geiger JW, Blakemore WS. Effects of major skeletal trauma on whole body protein turnover in man measured by L-[1,14C]-leucine. *Surgery*. 1980;88(2):294–300.

60. Chioléro R, Schultz Y, Lemarchand T, et al. Hormonal and metabolic changes following severe head injury and noncranial injury. *JPEN J Parenter Enteral Nutr*. 1992;13(1):5–12.

61. Ott LG, Schmidt JJ, Young AB, et al. Comparison of administration of two standard intravenous amino acid formulas to severely brain-injured patients. *Drug Intell Clin Pharm*. 1988;22(10):763–768.

62. Detsky AS, McLaughlin JR, Baker JP, et al. What is subjective global assessment of nutritional status? *JPEN J Parenter Enteral Nutr*. 1987; 11(1):8–13.

63. Chioléro R, Revelly JP, Tappy L. Energy metabolism in sepsis and injury. *Nutrition*. 1997;13(suppl 9):45S–51S.

64. Clifton GL, Robertson CS, Choi SC. Assessment of nutritional requirements of head-injured patients. *J Neurosurg*. 1986;64(6): 895–901.

65. Robertson CS, Clifton GL, Grossman RG. Oxygen utilization and cardiovascular function in head-injured patients. *Neurosurg*. 1984; 15(3):307–314.

66. Bucci MN, Dechert RE, Arnoldi DK, et al. Elevated intracranial pressure associated with hypermetabolism in isolated head trauma. *Acta Neurochir (Wien)*. 1988;93(3–4):133–136.

67. Esper DH, Coplin WM, Carhuapoma JR. Energy expenditure in patients with nontraumatic intracranial hemorrhage. *JPEN J Parenter Enteral Nutr*. 2006;30(2):71–75.

68. Varella L, Jastremski C. Neurological Impairment. In: Gottschlich M, ed. *The Science and Practice of Nutrition Support: A Case-Based Core Curriculum*. Dubuque, IA: Kendall Hunt Publishing Company; 2001:421–444.

69. Ott L, Young B. Neurosurgery. In: Zaloga GP, ed. *Nutrition in Critical Care*. St. Louis, MO: Mosby; 1994:691–706.

70. Young B, Ott L. The neurosurgical patient. In: Rombeau JL, Caldwell MD, eds. *Clinical Nutrition: Parenteral Nutrition*. 2nd ed. Philadelphia, PA: W.B. Saunders Company; 1993:585–596.

71. Brain Trauma Foundation. Guidelines for the management of severe traumatic brain injury. XII. Nutrition. *J Neurotrauma*. 2007; 24(suppl 1):S77–S82.

72. Lepelletier D, Roquilly A, Demeure dit latte D, et al. Retrospective analysis of the risk factors and pathogens associated with early-onset ventilator-associated pneumonia in surgical-ICU head-trauma patients. *J Neurosurg Anesthesiol*. 2010;22(1):32–37.

73. Badjatia N, Fernandez L, Schlossberg MJ, et al. Relationship between energy balance and complications after subarachnoid hemorrhage. *JPEN J Parenter Enteral Nutr*. 2010;34(1):64–69.

74. Lee JS, Jwa CS, Yi HJ, Chun HJ. Impact of early enteral nutrition on in-hospital mortality in patients with hypertensive intracerebral hemorrhage. *J Korean Neurosurg Soc*. 2010;48(2):99–104.

75. Härtl R, Gerber LM, Ni Q, Ghajar J. Effect of early nutrition on deaths due to severe traumatic brain injury. *J Neurosurg*. 2008; 109(1):50–56.

76. Oertel MF, Hauenschild A, Gruenschlaeger J, Mueller B, Scharbrodt W, Boeker DK. Parenteral and enteral nutrition in the management of neurosurgical patients in the intensive care unit. *J Clin Neurosci*. 2009;16(9):1161–1167.

77. Moore EE, Jones TN. Benefits of immediate jejunostomy feeding after major abdominal trauma—a prospective, randomized study. *J Trauma*. 1986;26(10):874–881.

78. Adams S, Dellinger EP, Wertz MJ, Oreskovich MR, Simonowitz D, Johansen K. Enteral versus parenteral nutritional support following laparotomy for trauma: a randomized prospective trial. *J Trauma*. 1986;26(10):882–891.

79. Moore FA, Moore EE, Jones TN, McCroskey BL, Peterson VM. TEN versus TPN following major abdominal trauma—reduced septic morbidity. *J Trauma*. 1989;29(7):916–922.

80. Kudsk KA, Croce MA, Fabian TC, et al. Enteral versus parenteral feeding. Effects on septic morbidity after blunt and penetrating abdominal trauma. *Ann Surg*. 1992;215(5):511–513.

81. Moore FA, Feliciano DV, Andrassy RJ, et al. Early enteral feeding, compared with parenteral, reduces postoperative septic complications. The results of a meta-analysis. *Ann Surg*. 1992;216(2):172–183.

82. Alverdy J, Chi HS, Sheldon GF. The effect of parenteral nutrition on gastrointestinal immunity. The importance of enteral stimulation. *Ann Surg*. 1985;202(6):681–684.

83. Deitch EA, Winterton J, Li M, Berg R. The gut as a portal of entry for bacteremia. Role of protein malnutrition. *Ann Surg*. 1987;205(6): 681–692.

84. Clifton GL, Robertson CS, Contant CF. Enteral hyperalimentation in head injury. *J Neurosurg*. 1985;62(2):186–193.

85. Rhoney DH, Parker D Jr, Formea CM, Yap C, Coplin WM. Tolerability of bolus versus continuous gastric feeding in brain-injured patients. *Neurol Res*. 2002;24(6):613–620.

86. Klodell CT, Carroll M, Carrillo EH, Spain DA. Routine intragastric feeding following traumatic brain injury is safe and well tolerated. *Am J Surg*. 2000;179(3):168–171.

87. Neumann DA, DeLegge MH. Gastric versus small-bowel tube feeding in the intensive care unit: a prospective comparison of efficacy. *Crit Care Med*. 2002;30(7):1436–1438.

88. Taylor SJ, Fettes SB, Jewkes C, Nelson RJ. Prospective, randomized, controlled trial to determine the effect of early enhanced enteral nutrition on clinical outcome in mechanically ventilated patients suffering head injury. *Crit Care Med*. 1999;27(11):2525–2531.

89. Kirby DF, Clifton GL, Turner H, Marion DW, Barret J, Gruemer HD. Early enteral nutrition after brain injury by percutaneous endoscopic gastrojejunostomy. *JPEN J Parenter Enteral Nutr*. 1991; 15(3):298–302.

90. Duckworth PF Jr, Kirby DF, McHenry L, DeLegge MH, Foxx-Orenstein A. Percutaneous endoscopic gastrojejunostomy made easy: a new over-the-wire technique. *Gastrointest Endosc*. 1994; 40(3):350–353.

91. DeLegge MH, Duckworth PF Jr, McHenry L Jr, Foxx-Orenstein A, Craig RM, Kirby DF. Percutaneous endoscopic gastrojejunostomy: a dual center safety and efficacy trial. *JPEN J Parenter Enteral Nutr*. 1995;19(3):239–243.

92. Patrick PG, Marulendra S, Kirby DF, DeLegge MH. Endoscopic nasogastric-jejunal feeding tube placement in critically ill patients. *Gastrointest Endosc*. 1997;45(1):72–76.

93. Hennessey PJ, Black CT, Andrassy RJ. Nonenzymatic glycosylation of immunoglobulin G impairs complement fixation. *JPEN J Parenter Enteral Nutr*. 1991;15(1):60–64.

94. Paolin A, Nardin L, Gaetani P, et al. Oxidative damage after severe head injury and its relationship to neurological outcome. *Neurosurgery*. 2002;51(4):949–954.

95. Polidori MC, Mecocci P, Frei B. Plasma vitamin C levels are decreased and correlated with brain damage in patients with intracranial hemorrhage or head trauma. *Stroke*. 2001;32(4):898–902.

96. Ott L, Young B, McClain C. The metabolic response to brain injury. *JPEN J Parenter Enteral Nutr*. 1987;11(5):488–493.

97. Yeiser EC, Vanlandingham JW, Levenson CW. Moderate zinc deficiency increases cell death after brain injury in the rat. *Nutr Neurosci*. 2002;5(5):345–352.

98. Evans NJ, Compher CW. Nutrition and the neurologically impaired patient. In: Torosian MH, ed. *Nutrition for the Hospitalized Patient: Basic Science and Principles of Practice*. New York, NY: CRC Press; 1995:567–589.

99. Wesley AJ. Immunoenhancement via enteral nutrition. *Arch Surg*. 1993;128(11):1242–1245.

100. Kirk SJ, Hurson M, Regan MC, Holt DR, Wasserkrug HL, Barbul A. Arginine stimulates wound healing and immune function in elderly human beings. *Surgery*. 1993;114(2):155–159.

101. Barbul A, Sisto DA, Wasserkrug HL, Efron G. Arginine stimulates lymphocyte immune response in healthy human beings. *Surgery*. 1981;90(2):244–251.

102. Daly JM, Reynolds J, Thom A, et al. Immune and metabolic effects of arginine in the surgical patients. *Ann Surg*. 1988;208(4):512–523.

103. Ziegler TR, Young LS, Benfell K, et al. Clinical and metabolic efficacy of glutamine-supplemented parenteral nutrition after bone marrow transplantation. A randomized, double-blind, controlled study. *Ann Intern Med*. 1992;116(10):821–828.

104. Clark SF. Vitamins and trace elements. In: Gottschlich M, ed. *A.S.P.E.N. Nutrition Support Core Curriculum: A Case-Based Approach–The Adult Patient*. Silver Spring, MD: American Society for Parenteral and Enteral Nutrition; 2007:133–135.

105. McKinney JD, Bailey BA, Garrett LH, Peiris P, Manning T, Peiris AN. Relationship between vitamin D status and ICU outcomes in veterans. *J Am Med Dir Assoc*. 2011;12(3):208–211.

106. Lee P, Eisman JA, Center JR. Vitamin D deficiency in critically ill patients. *N Engl J Med*. 2009;360(18):1912–1914.

107. Jeng L, Yamshchikov AV, Judd SE, et al. Alterations in vitamin D status and anti-microbial peptide levels in patients in the intensive care unit with sepsis. *J Transl Med*. 2009;7:28.

108. Chendrasekkhar A, Fagerli JC, Prabhakar G, et al. Evaluation of an enhanced diet in patients with severe closed head injury. *Crit Care Med*. 1997;25(suppl 1):A80.

109. Jeevanandam M, Shahbazian LM, Petersen SR. Proinflammatory cytokine production by mitogen-stimulated peripheral blood mononuclear cells (PBMCs) in trauma patients fed immune-enhancing enteral diets. *Nutrition*. 1999;15(11–12):842–847.

110. Minard G, Kudsk KA, Melton S, Patton JH, Tolley EA. Early versus delayed feeding with an immune-enhancing diet in patients with severe head injuries. *JPEN J Parenter Enteral Nutr*. 2000;24(3):145–149.

111. Krakau K, Hansson A, Karlsson T, de Boussard CN, Tengvar C, Borg J. Nutritional treatment of patients with severe traumatic brain injury during the first six months after injury. *Nutrition*. 2007;23(4):308–317.

112. Janssen I, Heymsfield SB, Ross R. Low relative skeletal muscle mass (sarcopenia) in older persons is associated with functional impairment and physical disability. *J Am Geriatr Soc*. 2002;50(5):889–896.

113. Gonzalez EG, Edelstein JE. Energy expenditure during ambulation. In: Gonzalez EG, Myers SJ, Edelstein JE, Lieberman JS, Downey JA, eds. *Downey & Darling's Physiological Basis of Rehabilitation Medicine*. 3rd ed. Boston, MA: Butterworth Heinemann; 2001:417–448.

114. Dickerson RN, Brown RO, Hanna DL, Williams JE. Effect of upper extremity posturing on measured resting energy expenditure on nonambulatory tube-fed patients with severe neurodevelopmental disabilities. *JPEN J Parenter Enteral Nutr*. 2002;26(5):278–284.

115. Henson MB, De Castro JM, Stringer AY, Johnson C. Food intake by brain-injured humans who are in the chronic phase of recovery. *Brain Inj*. 1993;7(2):169–178.

116. Daniel RK, Priest DL, Wheatley DC. Etiologic factors in pressure sores: an experimental model. *Arch Phys Med Rehabil*. 1981;62(10):492–498.

117. Andersen KE, Jensen O, Kvorning SA, Bach E. Prevention of pressure sores by identifying patients at risk. *Br Med J*. 1982;284(6326):1370–1371.

118. ASPEN Board of Directors and the Clinical Guidelines Task Force. Guidelines for use of parenteral and enteral nutrition in adult and pediatric patients. *JPEN J Parenter Enteral Nutr*. 2002;26(suppl 1):51–89.

119. Salomon HK, McKnight LA. Management of a patient with severe burn injury and significant stress-induced weight loss: a case study. *Support Line*. 1999;21(4):11–20.

120. Flanigan KH. Nutritional aspects of wound healing. *Adv Wound Care*. 1997;10(3):48–52.

121. Guralnik JM, Harris TB, White LR, Cornoni-Huntley JC. Occurrence and predictors of pressure sores in the National Health and Nutrition Examination survey follow-up. *J Am Geriatr Soc*. 1988;36(9):807–812.

122. Cameron KJ, Nyulasi IB, Colier GR, Brown DJ. Assessment of the effect of increased dietary fibre intake on bowel function in patients with spinal cord injury. *Spinal Cord*. 1996;34(5):277–283.

Sexuality and Intimacy Following Traumatic Brain Injury

M. Elizabeth Sandel, Richard Delmonico, and Mary Jean Kotch

INTRODUCTION

Our understanding of human sexuality has evolved over the last century to a greater appreciation of the biological, cultural, and psychological factors that underpin sexual behavior. Biologists and ethnologists have studied animal models of sexual physiology and functioning, and these models have been important in advancing our understanding of human sexual behavior. These approaches have informed us that there is a wide range of variability in the expression of sexual and reproductive behaviors across species. In addition, anatomists and physiologists have further advanced our understanding of human reproduction and human sexuality. Social and cultural beliefs have also contributed to our evolving understanding of sexual behavior. Sociologists and anthropologists have studied broad variations in human behavior across cultures. Behaviors considered deviant in one culture might be accepted practices in another. Gender, gender roles, and sexual orientation are prime examples of differences that may be heavily influenced by cultural and political forces. Human sexual behavior is based on a complex interaction of biological, psychological, and cultural factors. Unfortunately, most of sexology research over the last few decades has focused on males and on heterosexual populations, although this bias is gradually being recognized and funding of research in the area has been more comprehensive in recent years. Research focused on women with traumatic brain injury (TBI) is sparse (1).

TBI profoundly affects every aspect of an individual's functioning. These injuries have an impact on physical, cognitive, emotional, behavioral, and social functioning. Physical disabilities may be caused by anatomic or physiologic changes as a result of the injury. Cognitive disabilities commonly include problems with concentration, learning, memory, information processing, language, problem solving, reasoning, planning, and organizational skills. Emotional difficulties are not only limited to psychological disorders, such as depression, but also difficulties that affect behavior and personality. Behavioral problems can include impulsivity, poor initiation, perseverative behaviors, and other frontal lobe disturbances. Interpersonal skills problems may significantly influence social and occupational functioning. The complexity of all of these factors and their interrelationships creates several methodological challenges for research in the area of sexuality and TBI.

SEXUAL RESPONSE MODELS AND SEXUAL DYSFUNCTION

According to the Masters and Johnson model of the 1960s, the sexual response cycle consists of 4 phases: excitement, plateau, orgasm, and resolution (2). A simplified model, described by Kaplan (3), included only desire, excitement, and orgasm. More recently described models take into account new perspectives and new research, suggesting that the genital focus of previous models and the linear sequence inherent to these models inaccurately reflects the cyclical nature of the interactions within the mind and between the mind and body during intimacy and sexual activity. Sexuality also includes personal factors such as self-image and desire for connection. However, context is also important and includes family, interpersonal relationships, society, and culture. Life stressors, including financial and health issues, also contribute to the sexual and intimate interactions between couples (4,5).

An alternative model described by Basson (6) takes into account other aspects of sexuality and intimacy: the desire to express affection and to share pleasure, a sense of being attracted to and attractive to another, and a sense of commitment. This model emphasizes that sexual experiences may begin with a nonsexual state of mind and take place within a much larger context of cognition and behavior, acknowledging the importance of the aspects of intimacy that contribute to both the nonsexual and the sexual state of mind. These factors include communication, respect, trust, vulnerability, and fear of loss.

Definitions and Epidemiology of Sexual Dysfunction

Sexual desire disorders include sexual aversion and hypoactive sexual desire. Sexual arousal disorders result in poor lubrication in women and erectile disorders in both men (penile) and women (clitoral). Orgasmic disorders include anorgasmia in men and women and premature ejaculation in men. Sexual pain disorders in women include dyspareunia and vaginismus. An international consensus development conference on female sexual dysfunction resulted in an expansion of these classifications.

The existing classification system for sexual dysfunction, based on the World Health Organization (WHO)'s *International Statistical Classification of Disease and Related Health Problems* (7) and the *Diagnostic and Statistical Manual of Mental Disorders 4th ed. Text Rev. (DSM-IV-TR)* (8), has been challenged by an interdisciplinary consensus conference panel consisting of 19 experts in female sexual dysfunction. The former classifications were expanded to include psychogenic and organic causes of desire, arousal, orgasm, and sexual pain disorders. A personal distress criterion has been added; this criterion specifies that a condition is considered a disorder only if it creates distress for the woman experiencing the condition. As noted by Sipski (9), patients with TBIs may lack awareness and appreciation of "personal distress." Definitions of sexual arousal and hypoactive sexual desire disorders were developed in this new classification system, and a category of noncoital sexual pain disorder was added (10).

Many psychological and biological factors influence the processing of sexual, sensual, or erotic stimuli. Psychological factors include past experiences (positive, affirming, negative, or traumatizing) and responses to the present sexual context. Inadequate or impaired emotional development may also influence openness to sexual experience and result in lack of sexual arousal or even impaired arousal in specific circumstances. Emotional intimacy and physical satisfaction with the sexual experience may not necessarily include orgasmic release. Biological factors that affect the processing of sexual stimuli include depression, medications that impair sexual function, fatigue, sleep disturbance, substance use, other medical conditions, and neuroendocrine factors. Individuals may also experience anxiety about intimacy, sexual performance, or consequences of sexual activity. This anxiety may be a primary or secondary factor in the development of sexual dysfunction. Anxiety may interfere with any stage of the sexual response cycle and commonly plays a role in arousal conditions, such as premature ejaculation, erectile dysfunction, and arousal dysfunction in women.

Studies suggest that sexual dysfunction is more prevalent in women than in men in the United States and several other countries. Prevalence data depend on the assessment techniques, which are variable (4). The Massachusetts Women's Health Study (11,12) documented decreased sexual desire among married women, those with psychological symptoms, cigarette smokers, and those in the perimenopausal state. However, of note, in healthy women, the prevalence of sexual dysfunction actually appears to decline with age, but frequency of sexual intercourse is not related to menopausal status (11–13).

There may be differences in sexual desire and drive between men and women, although this is still an area of considerable controversy (14). Male sex drive may be more urgent, less distractible, more goal oriented, and more focused on intercourse; female sex drive may be more diffuse, more distractible, more receptive, and more motivated by a desire for affection and emotional connection. Female desire may be more contextual, more aroused by words than images, more emotional than biological, more sensual than genital, more flexible and mutable. Men report more sexual fantasies and thoughts, and experience more spontaneous sexual desire, report having more desire for more sexual partners, masturbate at younger ages and with greater frequency, and become aware of their sexual drive earlier than women. Men also show a greater preference for sexual variety and novelty, have more favorable attitudes toward their genitals, and report higher and more consistent levels of desire across their lifetime (15,16). To what extent these differences are culturally driven or influenced by societal roles, teachings, and expectations is poorly understood (14–16).

Most studies of sexuality to date have focused on heterosexual populations. The research related to sexuality within gay, lesbian, and transgendered populations suggests that even more complexity is inherent in the study of human sexuality than has been formerly appreciated. As these topics are discussed and researched more widely, our understanding of human sexuality is evolving toward a greater awareness of how societal and cultural influences shape the understanding and expression of sexuality. This may, in fact, lead to more openness, acceptance, diversity of expression, and greater sexual health for everyone.

NEUROLOGICAL SYSTEMS AND SEXUALITY

The neurological aspects of sexuality include widespread and complex relationships among the neuroanatomic, neurochemical, neurophysiological, and neuropsychological systems that govern behavior, including what we define as emotional, physical, sensory, and cognitive components. The resulting sexual behaviors can be described more concretely as motivation, desire, arousal, genital responses, and orgasm. Our understanding of the brain–behavior relationships that are the basis for human sexuality is primarily derived from animal studies, and therefore, our conclusions must be tentative. The interrelationships among the systems that contribute to these concrete behaviors are not completely understood. However, the peripheral nervous system, including motor, sensory, and autonomic neurons and subcortical and cortical systems, contribute to sexual interest and responsiveness through an elaborate network. Lesions at any level may influence this behavior, although the actual effects of such lesions in humans are not fully established. Central nervous system control of sexual function is similarly organized in men and women (17).

Chemical Messengers

Neurotransmitters play a critical role in the physiological basis of sexual behaviors and sexual response. Spinal cord centers are under the control of brain regions that exert both excitatory and inhibitory influences. Sexual desire has been linked to activity of dopaminergic systems, including the mesolimbic and mesocortical systems. Serotonin may have an inhibiting effect on sexual function. Hypothalamic spinal pathways using oxytocin as a neurotransmitter have also been identified. Nitric oxide, crucial for sexual function at the genital level, may also be an important central nervous system messenger. Receptors for gonadal hormones include neurons in the midbrain, hypothalamus, and amygdala. The supraspinal sites involved in the sexual response network have both extensive interconnections and receive genital sensory input. There does not appear to be a strict division between reflexive and psychogenic erections given this organizational structure (17).

Spinal Systems

A coordinated system of sympathetic, parasympathetic, and somatic spinal outflow tracts are the basis for human sexual response. The spinal cord is "necessary and sufficient" to produce sexual responsiveness (17). Genital innervation is somatic, as well as autonomic (i.e., parasympathetic and sympathetic). Somatic sensory afferents, synapsing in the sacral spinal cord, induce local sexual responses and project sensory information to cortical regions resulting in sexual awareness and sexual excitation. Parasympathetic innervation originating at the sacral level, organized in the pelvic nerves, supply the neuronal inputs and outputs responsible for the initiation and maintenance of the erectile response. Erections are observed after lesions of sacral cord segments and pelvic nerves and the psychogenic erections in paraplegics with conus or cauda equina lesions may occur because of other noncerebral proerectile pathways operating via the hypogastric nerves (18). Psychogenic mechanisms of arousal may also be transmitted in sympathetic pathways. Sympathetic neurons from the thoracic cord, contained in the hypogastric plexus, provide efferent and afferent innervations to the internal genitalia; this system provides the neurological basis for emission. Ejaculation is a result of sympathetic outflow from T11 to L2 segments, including the sympathetic chain, the hypogastric plexus, and pelvic and pudendal nerve systems (19).

In women, these neurological connections are also the basis for sexual responses, including arousal, lubrication, and female ejaculation. Parasympathetic activity causes clitoral erection, engorgement of the labia, and vaginal lubrication. Orgasmic sympathetic activity results in contraction of pelvic structures, including uterus, fallopian tubes, paraurethral glands, and pelvic floor muscles (20).

The Brainstem and Related Structures

Brainstem centers that contribute to human sexual responses include the reticular activating systems of the pons and midbrain. These pathways, which provide input for initiation and maintenance of arousal and alertness, connect with limbic and other frontal structures, many of which play a role in sexual and sexually related behaviors, including affective responses. Brainstem regions connect with diencephalic structures and limbic and paralimbic structures, including the hippocampus, septal complex, cingulate gyrus, amygdala, and hypothalamus. Stimulation of these structures produces erection and in some cases, preorgasmic sensations of pleasure. Lesions of the piriform cortex, which is interconnected with the olfactory cortex, produce hypersexual responses in animals. The role of the basal ganglia in sexual function is not clear, although stimulation may result in species-specific sexual behaviors (21).

Subcortical Systems

The primary areas of the hypothalamus that contribute to sexual response are the paraventricular nucleus, tuberal region, medial preoptic area, and the dorsal hypothalamic area. These hypothalamic regions are likely involved in both sexual desire and sexual response. The basal hypothalamus is influenced by tissue levels of testosterone, dihydrotestosterone, and estradiol. The preoptic area has high concentrations of androgen and estrogen receptors and the enzyme that converts androgens to estrogens. Manipulating androgens and androgen receptors in this region affects sexual behavior. Lesions in the medial preoptic area of the hypothalamus reduce or eliminate sexual behavior. This area receives neuronal inputs from other brain regions, such as the olfactory system and the cerebral cortex, including the visual cortex (17,19,22).

The dorsomedial nucleus of the hypothalamus, when stimulated, produces ejaculation. This nucleus may receive input from the medial preoptic area and probably from other brain and body regions. The ventromedial nucleus of the hypothalamus appears to play a role in female sexual behaviors. This nucleus is also strongly influenced by sex hormones, in particular, estrogen and progesterone. The hypothalamus receives some of its information in the form of neuronal messages, but other information arrives in the form of chemical messages, including gonadal steroids. In addition, the hypothalamus synthesizes and secretes hormones of its own, many of which exert influences over sex and reproduction (22).

The pituitary hormones play a crucial role in the sexual and reproductive activity of humans. Gonadotropin-releasing hormone stimulates the release of follicle-stimulating hormone (FSH) and luteinizing hormone (LH), which regulates the menstrual cycle in women and testosterone secretion in men. Males with hypothalamo-pituitary disorders have decreased or absent sexual desire, and often, this is the first symptom to appear. In females with hypothalamo-pituitary disorders, two-thirds notice absence or a considerable decrease in sexual desire; lack of lubrication and anorgasmia are also very common (23).

Cortical Systems

The Klüver-Bucy syndrome results from injury or ablation to the anterior temporal poles, and the syndrome includes hypersexual and exploratory behaviors and hyperorality (24,25). Temporal lobe seizures may be manifested by genital sensation and other sexual phenomena, with hypersexual or hyposexual behavior during both ictal and interictal periods. Endocrine disturbances, which are common in both men and women with temporal lobe epilepsy, result in decreased libido, impotence, menstrual disturbances, and reproductive disorders (26–28).

The frontal lobes are clearly involved in the regulation of sexual behaviors. Injury to the orbitofrontal regions (limbic and paralimbic lesions) may produce hypersexual responses. Socially inappropriate behaviors are displayed more often than sexual behaviors. In the case of dorsolateral frontal injury, when attention and initiation impairments are primary, libido or sexual assertiveness may be impaired (29). Injury to these areas may also lead to an inability to fantasize (30). The role of the olfactory system is unclear, but recent research indicates that anosmia may not significantly affect sexual function. The hypothalamus is a crucial structure in the elaboration of the human sexual response. The supraoptic nucleus of the hypothalamus synthesizes *oxytocin*, a hormone involved in lactation, birthing, and orgasm. *Naloxone*, an opiate antagonist, prevents the release of oxytocin, suggesting that the release at orgasm is controlled, at least in part, by the endorphin system (31,32).

SEXUAL DYSFUNCTION AFTER BRAIN INJURY

People with brain injuries often experience changes in their relationships with others. Their intimate and sexual relationships are often affected by multiple, interrelated impairments that coexist after TBI. As with individuals without brain injuries, identification of the specific etiologies of sexual dysfunction following a TBI can present a diagnostic dilemma. This is in part because of the interactions among the physiological, psychological, behavioral, and cognitive changes that occur as a result of a TBI.

Much of the existing literature on TBI focuses on psychosocial consequences, and few studies have examined other causes of sexual dysfunction. Do impairments, such as communication, cognitive, or interpersonal deficits, have more impact on sexuality than physical deficits? What roles do depression or other psychological conditions play? What are the effects of medication? What interpersonal and relationship issues contribute to sexual dysfunction? What are the anatomic correlates of sexual dysfunction?

The impact of TBI on interpersonal relationships and more specifically on psychological adjustment in family and caregivers has been the focus of several studies. Thomsen (33) found that family members were more disturbed by intellectual than by physical impairments. Additionally, relationships were better between single adult survivors and their mothers than between survivors with TBI and their respective spouses. In Rosenbaum and Najenson's study (34) of veterans with brain injury in Israel, spouses' moods were associated with decreased sexual activity, and they viewed physical contact negatively. Lezak (35) emphasized that emotional adjustment for family members, including spouses, occurred only after detachment and acceptance of the permanence of deficits. This adjustment culminated in divorce, separation, and long-term placements for some partners. Bond (36) noted that the level of sexual activity among partners was not related to injury severity as measured by the duration of post-traumatic amnesia or level of cognitive or physical impairment.

Sexual function and marital adjustment were also examined among married couples (37). Frequency of intercourse declined for all couples but to a greater degree for couples in which the husband was brain-injured; orgasm in female spouses also showed a significant decline. Kreuter et al. (38) found 58% of their subjects with TBI had a stable partner relationship; 55% were postinjury relationships. Hibbard et al. (39) found that men with TBI were less sexually active, and fewer were involved in a relationship when compared with nondisabled controls. Interestingly, no significant differences between women with and without TBI were found on these same variables. In a study of older adults with TBI and their partners, Layman et al. (40) found that most respondents associated changes in sexuality postinjury with age-related factors rather than the TBI.

Kreuter and associates (41) also examined sexual adjustment following TBI. In a group of subjects who were sexually active prior to their injury, 30% of the men experienced erectile dysfunction and fewer ejaculations postinjury. Although

59% reported no changes in orgasm, 40% experienced orgasm difficulties. "Dissatisfaction with the frequency of sexual activity" was found in 56% of the subjects. This study found that approximately one-third of respondents had no intimate partner following the injury. However, they found that sexual dissatisfaction in individuals with partners was related to decreased interest, low self-esteem, partner's decreased interest (willingness to engage in sexual activity), "physical unattractiveness," and decreased sexual capacity. Kreutzer and Zasler (42) studied men with brain injury and noted declines in sex drive, erectile function, and frequency of intercourse. Although one-third of the married subjects reported their relationship as worse postinjury, 40% rated their relationships as good or very good when compared to their preinjury relationship status. The authors found no correlation between affect and sexual behavior.

Although Kreutzer and Zasler (42) and Zasler (43) found no association between affect and sexual dysfunction, O'Carroll et al. (44), using measures of anxiety and depression for both partners, found a significant level of psychiatric dysfunction. In addition, as time since injury increased, males with TBI became more sexually dissatisfied, and sexual communication became more problematic for their partners. Age and time since injury were related to measures of psychosexual dysfunction but severity of injury was not. Subjects with TBI in another study reported significant levels of anxiety and depression and found significant correlations between sexual adjustment and measures of psychosocial adjustment (38,41).

The negative impact of preinjury and/or postinjury substance use on physical, cognitive, and psychosocial functioning is clearly documented in the literature. The rates of preinjury and postinjury substance abuse in individuals with TBI are substantial. Approximately 16%–66% have chronic preinjury drinking problem, and 10%–50% continue to experience postinjury problems with alcohol (45–47). Problems include a higher incidence of medical and psychological complications during TBI recovery, poorer cognitive recovery, poorer long-term outcome, and exacerbation of cognitive and behavioral deficits. Most substances of abuse have been shown to adversely affect sexual functioning at some stage in the sexual response cycle in non-TBI subjects and have a substantial negative impact on sexual functioning in individuals with TBI (48).

Given that most injuries occur in individuals between the ages of 15 and 25, limitations in the person's preinjury sexual experience can influence postinjury sexual functioning. Individuals with limited sexual experience and knowledge often have significant deficits and experience in establishing and maintaining intimate relationships. These relationship deficits can greatly reduce their ability to meet people who may become potential intimate partners. In individuals who have an intimate relationship at the time of injury, cognitive, emotional, behavioral, physical impairments, and substance abuse postinjury can clearly have a negative effect on the quality of the relationship, as well as on the sexual functioning of partners. For individuals who have limited relationship skills prior to their injury, these problems are amplified.

The impact of TBI on the sexual response cycle has also been closely examined. In general, problems may occur at any stage (desire, excitement or arousal, orgasm, and resolution). Sexual difficulties are found in several areas, including decreased frequency of intercourse, decreased desire, impaired arousal, and orgasmic dysfunction (41,44,49). Aloni and Katz (50) reviewed the existing literature on the effects of TBI and the sexual response cycle. Although, significantly, more individuals with TBI experience decreased desire, some report increased desire. Although Kreuter et al. (41) found decreased desire, erectile dysfunction, and orgasmic dysfunction in many of their subjects, 59% reported no change in orgasm postinjury; and 50% noted no change in frequency of sexual intercourse postinjury.

Studies have also examined cognitive functioning and locus of injury. Although some studies (34) indicate no relationship between locus of lesion and sexual dysfunction, medial basal-frontal injury or diencephalic injury was associated with hypersexuality and limbic injury with changes in sexual orientation in a population of 8 patients (51). Sandel and associates (52) examined sexual functioning in a group of male and female outpatients with severe TBIs (average length of post-traumatic amnesia was 54 days). Sexual function was consistently lower than in the normal population but significantly only on the (*a*) orgasm and (*b*) drive and desire subscales of the Derogatis Interview for Sexual Functioning (53). Location of injury was relevant; patients with frontal lesions and right hemisphere lesions reported higher sexual satisfaction and higher function. No correlations were found with cognitive measures or clinical examination. Subjects with more recent injuries and subjects with right hemisphere injuries reported more levels of arousal.

Hibbard et al. (39) found men with TBI experienced significantly more difficulties on self-ratings of sexual energy, drive, ability to initiate sexual activity, ability to experience orgasm, and the ability to maintain an erection. Women with TBI experienced significantly more difficulties than women without TBI on self-ratings of sexual energy, drive, ability to initiate sexual activity, arousal, pain during sex, ability to masturbate, ability to experience orgasm, and with vaginal lubrication. This study found significant difficulties in both men and women with TBI in sexual positioning, sensation, and body image variables. These findings suggest the importance of interactions among cognitive, emotional, interpersonal, physical, and physiological functioning.

The etiologies of sexual dysfunction in TBI are complex and multifactorial. Sexual dysfunction following TBI are likely caused by 1 or more factors, including injury to specific brain regions, neurochemical changes related to this pathology, endocrinologic abnormalities, medications, secondary medical conditions, physical limitations, cognitive deficits, emotional difficulties, behavioral deficits, and interpersonal difficulties.

DISABILITY AND SEXUALITY

Individuals with disabilities are a diverse group of people reflecting a range of sexual expression and orientation, just as is the case in the population of individuals without disabilities. Providers often incorrectly assume that individuals with disability are sexually inactive or neglect to consider the issue of sexuality. In a recent study (54), 94% of the subjects with physical disabilities were found to be sexually active, a rate matching that of nondisabled individuals.

The paucity of information and biases that exist in the medical and scientific literature include myths that individuals with disabilities are asexual, lack sexual desire or attractiveness, are incapable of healthy sexual function, and lack the social and/or problem-solving skills necessary for sexual functioning. In addition, women with disabilities are viewed as being less affected in terms of their sexual function than men with disabilities. These myths are not based on scientific data and have been perpetuated by a general lack of knowledge about disability and sexual functioning, although they may still guide health care professionals' behavior (55,56).

The result of this general lack of awareness or bias is that individuals with disabilities may not receive adequate screening, education, or treatment for sexual dysfunction or reproductive health (56). Women with physical disabilities encounter serious barriers to receiving general, as well as reproductive health care, and have difficulty locating physicians who are knowledgeable about the disability to assist them in managing pregnancies (54).

For individuals with disabilities, the associated features of the disabling condition may adversely influence the assessment and treatment of sexual dysfunction. Incontinence may have a serious impact on sexual functioning (57). Intellectual or cognitive disabilities may present as an invisible disability. For this reason, health care professionals may not recognize the ways in which the disabling condition may affect sexuality and intimacy. Deficits in cognitive and social skills may have a serious effect on self-esteem and contribute to difficulties establishing and maintaining relationships. An individual with TBI may lack insight, judgment, self-awareness, and perception of others' needs or social cues. In other cases, the patient may not initiate conversation with the health care provider regarding issues related to sexuality. Individuals with TBI who have attention, memory, and judgment deficits may experience difficulties identifying and describing their symptoms. Conditions can be neglected or misdiagnosed.

For persons with TBI, a combination of cognitive and behavioral deficits may place them at increased risk for exposure to sexually transmitted diseases. Given the risk and potentially serious impact of sexually transmitted diseases and sexual victimization in persons with disabilities, it is extremely important for health care providers to be knowledgeable about sexuality and sexual functioning and to be prepared to open the discussion in the clinical setting. Professionals should perform a careful and comprehensive history and physical that includes information about all aspects of sexuality and sexual functioning as outlined in subsequent sections of this chapter. Cultural and religious beliefs and values can impact how open the patient will be to discussing sexuality and to accepting information. For example, in many Latino, Asian, and Native American cultures, women are not permitted to talk about their sexuality (58). Cultural awareness and cultural sensitivity are essential during any clinical encounter.

LESBIAN, GAY, BISEXUAL, AND TRANSGENDER AND INTERSEX INDIVIDUALS

Lesbian, gay, bisexual, transgender (LGBT), and individuals with sexual development disorders with TBI have received little attention in the literature. Given the diversity among these populations and issues related to stigma, estimates have been difficult to obtain. Prevalence estimates range from 5.5% to 20.8%, depending on definitions (58).

Sexual prejudice has led to homophobic, heterosexist attitudes, and heterosexual-centric attitudes in many areas of our culture, including health care (58–60). Having a disability and being in a sexual minority places one at risk for discriminatory behavior for multiple reasons. Individuals who are lesbian, gay, bisexual, transgender, and intersex (LGBTI) with TBI may not receive an optimal level of medical care or rehabilitation. For example, lesbian and gay sexuality issues may not be appropriately addressed in sexuality education, examinations, or treatment (60). Intersex or sexual development disorders are often poorly understood by medical professionals.

Sexual dysfunction may not be accurately identified because of a lack of knowledge or discomfort among health care professionals in dealing with these populations. Professionals lacking specific knowledge about LGBTI issues or holding certain biases may make incorrect conclusions or diagnoses based on inadequate information, especially if the patient feels threatened or lacks trust in the provider. The stress of sexual orientation disclosure and a fear about including partners in the treatment program may result in inadequate or inappropriate recommendations. Concerns regarding confidentiality may limit the amount of information the LGBTI individual and partner will disclose, particularly in an interdisciplinary setting, where a team of health care providers are providing care.

The incidence of TBI in adolescents and early adulthood is significant. During this stage of development, there is a developing awareness of sexuality, and TBI "can terminate such exploration" (61). Building a trusting and open relationship with LGBTI adolescent patients and using a nonjudgmental communication style will both facilitate discussion and identify if the adolescent should receive counseling to facilitate exploration of sexual orientation.

COMPREHENSIVE EVALUATION

Medical History

Evaluation of the patient begins with a careful history, including past illnesses, surgeries, and sexual activity and function (18). Many diseases and chronic conditions can influence sexual function (62). Whenever possible and with consent, information should be obtained from the current partner. Cultural aspects should be considered, and sensitivity to cultural differences is essential. Questions should focus on the following areas: (*a*) a review of neurologic, cardiovascular, endocrine, and urologic medical and surgical history; (*b*) preinjury and postinjury sexual functioning; (*c*) sexual orientation; (*d*) history of victimization, including sexual assault and domestic violence; (*e*) substance use and abuse history; (*f*) current medication; (*g*) safe sex practices; and (*h*) reproductive history and contraceptive practices.

The history should define the patient's expectations regarding sexual activity and functioning and through the course of the evaluation, information gaps, and misconceptions will become apparent. Dependency patterns, lack of self-esteem, and perceptions of unattractiveness should be identified. Education can be provided during the course of

the history-taking session, and written materials should be provided (63–65). The examiner must be comfortable discussing all aspects of sexuality, including alternative forms of sexual expression and alternative lifestyles (61). A nonjudgmental style is essential; staff training that focuses on attitudinal issues, as well as education, is recommended for physicians (66).

Regarding sexual functioning, the following areas should be further explored: (*a*) sexual desire; (*b*) sensory experience, as related to sexual arousal, including a history of painful experiences during sexual activity; (*c*) sexual response, including patterns of erections (penile or clitoral) and vaginal lubrication; (*d*) ejaculation (including forceful ejaculation of fluids from the urethra during orgasm in women); and (*e*) orgasmic sensations and experiences.

Psychological Evaluation

A comprehensive evaluation of sexual functioning includes a psychological evaluation. Establishing rapport with the client or with the couple is essential when discussing sexual issues. A widely used approach in the field of sexuality is the permission, limited information, specific suggestions, intensive therapy (PLISSIT) model (67). This approach emphasizes the importance of asking the client permission to discuss uncomfortable sexual issues and to facilitate comfort in the discussion of sexuality and intimacy. It is important for clinicians to remember that sexuality and relationship issues are often very difficult for clients and their partners to discuss. Increasing comfort will facilitate the client's ability to provide specific information, which is critical to identifying etiological factors in sexual dysfunction. Establishing the etiology of the sexual difficulty provides the basis for the development of an appropriate treatment plan. It is often more comfortable for clients if the interview begins with a review of nonsexual information, such as the medical history, demographic information, marital/relationship, and family history and then gradually begins to focus on emotional, relationship, intimacy, sexuality, and sexual dysfunction issues (68).

Although there are many different formats for organizing and conceptualizing information, the multiaxial problem-oriented system for sexual dysfunctions (69) is a useful guide. This approach assists the clinician in classifying sexual problems across several domains: desire, arousal, orgasm, coital pain, and frequency dissatisfaction. Another category labeled "qualifying information" includes sexual practices such as fetishism, exhibitionism, as well as other problems, which may interfere with sexual functioning, such as substance abuse and severe psychopathology. Problems are classified as lifelong vs not lifelong to more clearly identify individuals who have a history of relatively normal functioning followed by a period of sexual dysfunction. The circumstances under which the problems occur (global or in all situations vs specific situations) are also documented. This model provides the clinician with a framework in which to conceptualize the individual's sexual dysfunction as the basis for a problem-focused treatment plan. The *DSM-IV-TR* uses a similar model; subtypes of conditions are used to more clearly define the onset of sexual dysfunction (lifelong vs acquired), context (generalized vs situational), and presumed etiology (psychological vs combined factors) (8).

The sexual assessment and history should focus on identifying the sexual difficulties and how they function within the individual or the couple's relationship. LoPiccolo and Heiman (70) provided an outline for the interview and suggested using open-ended questions about the client and the primary partner (if one exists). It should include information about the client's/couple's life situation, adolescent and sexual development, attitudes, and values and beliefs toward sex (both past and current). Information about current behavior, including relationship issues, communication, displays of affection, intimacy, and sexual orientation, should also be obtained. The goal is obtaining specific information about the nature of the sexual difficulty, including onset, frequency, circumstances, treatment attempted, and both the client and partner's responses to the problem.

Current and past psychological symptoms must be examined, including anxiety, depression or other mood disorders, adjustment issues, psychotic behavior, personality disorders, use and abuse of substances, and any history of physical, emotional, and/or sexual abuse. In addition, it is important to obtain information about coping strategies, interpersonal communication skills, sexuality-specific anxieties (e.g., performance anxiety), and social support. Although most of this information can be obtained through an interview, some psychological assessment instruments, such as the Beck Depression Inventory-II (71), the Minnesota Multiphasic Personality Inventory-2 (72), and the Millon Clinical Multiaxial Inventory–III (73), may be helpful. When psychological disorders are identified, they must be treated because they are often significant contributing factors to sexual and relationship difficulties.

Cognitive difficulties can clearly impact the relationship. If the cognitive issues have not recently been assessed, a neuropsychological evaluation may be helpful. The neuropsychological evaluation may clarify the nature of the deficits, as well as compensatory strategies to lessen their impact on the person's functioning. The impact of these deficits can then be incorporated into the treatment plan for the sexual dysfunction.

Questionnaires

Several questionnaires have been developed to assess sexuality in more detail than in the usual history-taking session. The Derogatis Interview for Sexual Functioning (53) collects information by self-report in the 5 domains of fantasy, arousal, experience, orgasm, and drive and desire. A general sexual satisfaction score is obtained, as well as a total score. The Golombok-Rust Inventory of Sexual Satisfaction (GRISS) (74) is a 28-item self-report scale and provides male and female scores (2 versions) in the categories of vaginismus, anorgasmia, impotence, premature ejaculation, nonsensuality, avoidance, dissatisfaction, infrequency, and noncommunication, as well as a total score. This scale examines sexual functioning within the context of a relationship. Kreutzer and Zasler (42) developed an 11-item Psychosexual Assessment Questionnaire for patients with TBI. The items are grouped into 3 domains: sexual behavior, affect and self-esteem, and relationship issues with a focus on changes in functioning following a TBI. Another scale originally developed for use in spinal cord injury but modified and used in TBI is the Sexual Interest and Satisfaction Scale (SIS) (75). This scale examines sexual desire, satisfaction with sex before and after injury, and ability to satisfy a partner.

Several instruments have recently been developed for women with a history of sexual dysfunction. These include the Female Sexual Function Index (FSFI) (76), the Female Sexual Distress Scale (FSDS) (77), and the Sexual Function Questionnaire (SFQ) (78).

Physical Examination

A neurological and general physical examination should be completed, with a focused assessment to identify impairments that may influence communication, positioning, movement, oral ability, and sensory awareness. Aphasias, dysarthrias, aprosodias, and deficits in attention and concentration or memory should be noted. Facial scars, oral and facial movement, and visual and hearing impairments should be identified. Range of motion, especially in the proximal lower extremities, must be evaluated, along with movement of the limbs and trunk. Sensation is a crucial aspect of the examination. The genitalia, rectum, and the breasts should be examined. The bulbocavernosus muscles can be palpated in the male and tested for voluntary and reflex contraction. Anal sphincter tone should be assessed. The cremasteric reflex (L1) and the bulbocavernosus and anal reflex (S2–S5) should also be evaluated. In women, a Papanicolaou smear and pelvic examination are essential (43).

Medication Review

A thorough review of all medications is necessary. The most common cause of impotence in the general patient population is medication. Drug-related effects on sexual function are usually reversible after discontinuation of the drug. Frequently implicated are (a) antihypertensive agents, (b) antipsychotic drugs, (c) antidepressants, (d) anxiolytics, (e) sedatives, and (f) hormonal agents (including contraceptives and tamoxifen).

The most frequent adverse reactions with selective serotonic reuptake inhibitors (SSRIs) are decreased desire, anorgasmia, and ejaculatory delay (79). Impotence is less frequently reported with SSRIs than nonselective monoamine reuptake inhibitors. Trazadone has the highest number of reports of priapism of the antidepressants and has also been implicated in persistent sexual arousal syndrome in women. High-dose sildenafil may be effective in reducing ejaculatory latency (80).

Antihypertensive drugs may affect sexual function (libido and sexual response) through vascular or neurologic effects. Alpha- and beta-adrenoceptor blocking agents can cause ejaculatory failure. Antipsychotic agents may cause priapism, ejaculatory failure, and painful retrograde or spontaneous ejaculations (81).

In addition to the earlier mentioned medications, a large number of other agents have been implicated, including baclofen, cimetidine, clofibrate, cyproterone, digoxin, estrogen, indomethacin, lithium, metoclopramide, naproxen, phenoxybenzamine, prazosin, and progesterone, to name a few (82).

Laboratory Tests

Screening tests for sexual dysfunction include erythrocyte sedimentation rate, blood cell count, fasting blood sugar, serum lipids, urinalysis, hepatic function, kidney and thyroid function studies, and prolactin and testosterone levels (in both men and women).

Hypopituitarism may be manifested by low levels of growth hormone, thyroxine, or cortisol or by hypogonadism. In men, low sperm count, low serum levels of testosterone, and low levels of LH and FSH characterize hypogonadism. Because protein-bound testosterone may be increased by thyroid hormone therapy or cirrhosis and decreased by hypothyroidism or obesity, free testosterone levels or sex steroid-binding globulin may give a more accurate picture. In women, low serum levels of estradiol and low serum levels of LH and FSH characterize hypogonadism. Hypogonadism may be caused by primary gonadal failure, as well as secondary failure at a central level. Klinefelter syndrome, for example, which has an incidence of 1 in 500 men, may be an unrelated cause of low testosterone in a patient with brain injury. The gonadotropin-releasing hormone test is useful in distinguishing hypothalamic from pituitary causes of hypogonadism, although it is not infallible. The clomiphene citrate provocative test is also used to evaluate the gonadal axis. Single determinations of any of the above levels may not be accurate reflections of function (83).

Neurophysiologic and Vascular Evaluation

Spontaneous nocturnal penile tumescence and rigidity can be measured in the sleep laboratory using strain gauges, visual inspection, and other measures and is the most accurate technique for measuring erectile function. Rigidometers for evaluation at home have also been used (84–86). If no major vascular problem is present, intracorporeal injection (papaverine, papaverine/phentolamine, or prostaglandin E1) can be used as a diagnostic tool (87). If intracorporeal injection testing of penile tumescence is suggestive of a vascular etiology of sexual dysfunction, penile blood pressure using a Doppler method can be helpful to further evaluate (88).

Neurophysiological and vascular studies may further elucidate the pathophysiological underpinnings of the disorder. Somatic sensory, somatic motor, autonomic, and visceral sensory testing are available in some centers to further evaluate sexual dysfunction. These tests include dorsal penile nerve conduction studies, pudendal somatosensory evoked potential tests, pudendal motor latency, bulbocavernosus and anal reflex latency measurements, and electromyography (corpus cavernosum and somatic), cystometry, and anorectal manometry.

For women, magnetic resonance imaging (MRI) technology and vaginal photoplethysmograph devices are used for objective measurement of sexual response. Vaginal photoplethysmograph devices measure blood flow or engorgement following response to visual sexual stimulation (4,89,90).

PHARMACOTHERAPY

The following review of the literature focuses on medications that may have potential benefit because there are no well-controlled studies in patients with brain injury. Clearly, much more research is needed to understand the types of sexual disorders that occur in women, both disabled and nondisabled, and effective treatments for these disorders.

Women's sexuality has not been adequately addressed in research to date, but progress is being made. Recently the *Diagnostic and Statistical Manual of Mental Disorders-IV* (*DSM-IV*) classifications of female sexual dysfunction have been expanded to include psychogenic and organic causes of desire, arousal, orgasm, and sexual pain disorders that cause personal distress (8). The US Food and Drug Administration guidance paper (10) details the recommendations for the clinical development of pharmacologic interventions for female sexual dysfunction. Major pharmaceutical companies are now developing agents for female sexual disorders and or postmenopausal symptoms. These include dopaminergic agonists and related substances, melanocyte-stimulating hormones, adrenoceptor antagonists, nitric oxide delivery systems, prostaglandins, and androgens (4).

Phosphodiesterase Inhibitors

For men, major progress has been achieved in the development of medications for erectile dysfunction by the introduction of phosphodiesterase-5 (PDE5) inhibitors, and these agents have been used in a variety of populations with success (91–95). Phosphodiesterase enzymes are ubiquitous throughout the body and participate in a variety of functions. PDE5 is the predominant enzyme in the corpus cavernosum, and plays a significant role in penile erection. Sildenafil, tadalafil, and vardenafil are all potent inhibitors of PDE5. This class of medications is the most effective oral agents for the treatment of erectile dysfunction (96). These medications have led to a significant decrease in the use of other methods of treatment for erectile dysfunction. Side effects include flushing, headache, dyspepsia, and visual disturbances (91). These medications interact with nitrates and should not be given to patients on nitrates (97). Improved sexual function and sexual satisfaction appears to be well maintained over years following the initiation of treatment (98).

Antidepressant-associated (SSRI) or antipsychotic-associated sexual dysfunction may be effectively treated with sildenafil or other agents of this class (99,100).

Prostaglandin E₁

These agents are used topically for men with erectile dysfunction to maximize genital smooth muscle relaxation (101). Topical alprostadil (prostaglandin E₁) has been recommended for men with erectile dysfunction and appears to be well tolerated, with the most common adverse side effect being urogenital pain (102). Sildenafil combined with alprostadil administered via the intraurethal or intracavernous route was effective in some men with erectile dysfunction who failed other monotherapy (103). Topical administration of alprostadil has been used in the study of women with sexual arousal and orgasmic disorders, and ultrasound studies document clitoral cavernosal arterial changes that may be helpful in diagnosis of underlying pathology but is not recommended as an intervention at this time (104).

Dopaminergic Agents for Women and Men

Dopaminergic agents may be efficacious in the treatment of erectile dysfunction and may be an alternative to treatment with phosphodiesterase inhibitors. Because dopaminergic systems may be particularly vulnerable to TBI (especially mesocortical and mesolimbic systems), sexual dysfunction may be associated with decreases in dopaminergic activity. Levadopa (L-dopa) was investigated following the observation that patients with Parkinson disease who were treated with the drug reported increased sexual activity (105).

Apomorphine (a D2 greater than D1 dopamine receptor nonselective short-acting agonist) decreases secretion of prolactin, stimulates production of growth hormone, and induces erections. Apomorphine may act on neurons located within the paraventricular nucleus and the medial preoptic area of the hypothalamus (106). A MRI study (placebo-controlled) demonstrated frontal limbic area activity after administration of apomorphine (107). A positron emission tomography (PET) study has demonstrated cerebral activity in the right prefrontal cortex (108). Used in research to establish potential efficacy of longer acting agents (109,110), the drug is now licensed in some countries for the treatment of erectile dysfunction in a sublingual formulation. Side effects are nausea, dizziness, diaphoresis, syncope, and hypotension. The drug interacts with nitrates, increasing the risk of hypotension. Apomorphine combined with phentolamine was effective in 1 study, and this combination may prove to be an alternative to phosphodiesterase inhibitors (111).

Hormonal Agents for Women

O'Carroll reviewed the results of investigations of hypoactive sexual desire disorder in women and described it as "the major female psychosexual dysfunction" (112). However, little evidence suggests that the disorder can be traced to hormonal inadequacies in women. Women with hypogonadism (with androgen deficiency because of pathophysiologic problems that affect androgen production in the ovaries and/or adrenal glands) do demonstrate an increase in sexual interest after androgen replacement (113).

Androgen substitution should be administered as an adjuvant treatment to counseling in women with low libido, only when low androgen levels are caused by inadequate ovarian and/or adrenal function in the presence of normal estrogen levels. Administration of androgens to women without low androgen levels who complain of decreased sexual interest or desire is not recommended (114). The normal ranges for androgens and estrogens, especially as related to female sexual dysfunction, remain a subject of controversy (115). The possible adverse effects from testosterone therapy in women include breast cancer, fluid retention, masculinization (hirsutism, acne, temporal balding, voice deepening, clitoromegaly), and hepatocellular damage with high doses.

For women, intramuscular or subcutaneous injections, transdermal patches, or topical agents are available. However, the only clinical indications for testosterone replacement in women are symptomatic testosterone deficiency following natural menopause, surgical menopause, chemotherapy or irradiation, premature ovarian failure, or premenopausal loss of libido with diminished serum-free testosterone. Aging is associated with a decline in testosterone in normal premenopausal women (116).

Hormonal Agents for Men

Increasing age may result in a gradual hypogonadal state in men, referred to as *andropause*. The age of presentation for erectile dysfunction and andropause or "partial androgen deficiency in aging men" typically occurs in ages 50 and beyond, and these health issues may be harbingers for other related diseases, such as cardiovascular disease and depression (117). Treatment with hormone replacement is controversial, and a recent statement from Committee on Assessing the Need for Clinical Trials of Testosterone Replacement Therapy of the Institute of Medicine argues for caution. Testosterone can cause gynecomastia, testicular atrophy, congestive heart failure, and stroke and can accelerate the growth of prostate cancer (118).

For men, testosterone delivery systems include depotestosterone, patches (scrotal or nonscrotal), or a drying gel. Oral administration is associated with hepatic injury. Intramuscular injections, favored by bodybuilders and competitive athletes produce a fast rise and fall in levels. Testosterone injections biweekly for 6 weeks increased the frequency of sexual thoughts in a group of eugonadal men with low libido compared with placebo. However, no effect was observed in men with inhibited erectile dysfunction (119). Apparently, testosterone increases sexual interest in men with pretreatment levels in the normal range. This study also suggests that men with hyposexual desire disorder may benefit from testosterone injections even if serum levels are within the normal range. Additional research is needed, however, because the study included only 20 men.

Human chorionic gonadotropin was used as a treatment in 45 men with erectile failure and 6 men with lack of sexual desire (120). The treatment period was 1 month with twice weekly injections of 5,000 IU or placebo in a double-blind design. The investigators reported that 47% of treated patients had a "good result" compared with 12% of the placebo group; however, they did not separate the cases of erectile failure from the cases of low sexual interest or fully define "good result."

Antidepressants

Although many antidepressants (tricyclic antidepressants and monamine oxidase inhibitors) have been noted to cause a variety of sexual side effects, others have been noted to improve sexual functioning in patients without brain injuries, including both serotonin agents and buproprion, which inhibits reuptake of dopamine. Fluoxetine has been associated with orgasm dysfunction (121). Researchers postulate an excitatory mechanism for adrenergic systems and an inhibitory role for serotonergic systems but in view of reports of both increased and decreased sexual functioning, the neurochemical effects are unclear. Trazodone and fenfluramine have been associated with improvement in libido in several case reports (122–124), although both also have been reported to cause sexual dysfunction. Buproprion has also been shown to improve libido in individuals with hypoactive sexual desire disorders. In a study of 60 female and male outpatients with psychosexual dysfunction (sexual aversion, inhibited sexual desire, inhibited sexual excitement, and/or inhibited orgasm), 12 weeks of double-blind treatment with bupropion resulted in significantly greater improvements in sexual functioning among treated patients than in the placebo group. Only 3% of placebo-treated patients reported improvement compared with 63% of the medicated group (125).

Opiate Antagonists

Opioids have also been implicated in sexual function (159). In a small study involving 7 men, 25–50 mg/day led to full return of erectile function, as well as nocturnal penile tumescence in 6 patients (32). In a study of 30 men (age 25–50 years) with idiopathic impotence, naltrexone, an opiate antagonist, increased "sexual performance" (defined as intercourse) in 11 of 15 treated patients (31).

Natural Compounds

Several compounds from nature have been identified as treatments for erectile dysfunction. These include yohimbine, citrulline, pyrano-isoflavones, berberine, forskolin, and Korean red ginseng (126,127). Yohimbine, an alpha-adrenoceptor blocker, has been investigated in multiple studies of sexual dysfunction (128–133). Identifying the cause of impotence (arterial insufficiency) may also identify potential responders to yohimbine (133). Tobacco may negatively influence its effectiveness (129). Yohimbine administered with L-arginine glutamate (a nitric oxide precursor) resulted in substantially increased physiologic (vaginal pulse amplitude) responses in a group of women with female sexual arousal disorder (134). Similarly, this combination treatment was effective in improving erectile function in male patients with mild-to-moderate erectile dysfunction (135).

Other Treatments for Erectile Dysfunction

Intracavernosal injection (papaverine, phentolamine, prostaglandin E1, vasoactive intestinal peptide), transurethral vasoactive agents (prostaglandin E1), vacuum erection devices, vascular surgery, and penile prostheses are other therapeutic strategies for erectile dysfunction (136).

Self-injection of papaverine (a smooth muscle relaxant) or papaverine with phentolamine (an alpha-adrenergic blocker) is a treatment modality for impotence caused by neurological or vasculogenic causes. Nearly all patients with neurogenic impotence and 60%–70% of patients with vasculogenic impotence respond to intracavernous injections (137). Priapism, fibrosis of erectile tissues, hematomas, vasovagal reflex, and chemical hepatitis have been reported (138). Intracavernous injection of prostaglandin E1 is another approach, although painful erection occurs in up to 20% of patients, perhaps related to concentration and/or neuropathy (139,140). Papaverine (with or without phentolamine) and prostaglandin E1 acts by increasing arterial inflow through vasodilatation and decreasing venous outflow by occluding draining venules, probably through relaxation of smooth muscle in the corpus cavernosum. Unilateral injection results in bilateral effects through cross circulation.

Prosthetic surgery is less frequently chosen because other alternatives are available for men with erectile disor-ders. The 2 major categories of penile prostheses are the semirigid and the inflatable prosthesis. Complications include mechanical failure, infection, pain, and perforation, but the rate of complications is now lower because of technologic advances. Other alternatives include vacuum constriction devices, vascular reconstruction, and arterial and venous surgery. Nerve grafts, nerve growth factors, neuroprotection, and nerve regeneration explored at a basic science level may offer promise for the management of erectile dysfunction (141).

Other Alternatives for Women

Lubrication can be effective to promote sexual arousal in women with inadequate secretion and to treat dyspareunia and vaginismus. Some components of the sexual response continuum, including engorgement, elevation, and elongation of the vagina and clitoral erection, are not influenced by lubricants alone. Oral-genital stimulation and the use of vibrators may be helpful for some women.

Zestra (for women) is a botanical feminine massage oil (containing borage seed oil, evening primrose oil, special extracts of angelica, coleus forskolin, antioxidants, and vitamin E) formulated to enhance female sexual pleasure and arousal. The formulation has been shown to improve level of arousal, level of desire, satisfaction with arousal, genital sensation, ability to have orgasms, and sexual pleasure in a group of women with and without sexual arousal disorder in a randomized, placebo-controlled, double-blind, crossover design trial (142).

INTERVENTIONS FOR SEXUAL BEHAVIOR DISORDERS

Inappropriate sexual behaviors following TBI can be a significant challenge for the individual, their family/caregivers, and health care professionals. In some very limited cases, these problems can lead to sexually offending disorders. Unfortunately, the literature on inappropriate sexual behaviors is limited by lack of consensus in defining and delineating the boundaries of such behavior among researchers and clinicians (143,144). Documentation of sexual behavior disorders after TBI is recorded in surveys and case reports (51,145–149).

Johnson et al. (143) defined inappropriate sexual behavior as "a verbal or physical act of an explicit, or perceived, sexual nature, which is unacceptable within the social context in which it is carried out" (p. 688). The individual with brain injury may have reduced social skills, and this can be demonstrated in disinhibited interpersonal behaviors, which include sexual behaviors. When these behaviors occur in the presence of care providers, they may or may not be viewed as appropriate given the context of the situation and the subjective perception of the care provider. In addition, the sexual attitude or comfort level of the provider influences how these behaviors are classified and addressed. Sexual acting out can be a result of disinhibition, which creates a variety of inappropriate behaviors and social interactions with sexual implications (63). In addition, unwanted sexual advances may occur and require consistent redirection.

In many cases, disinhibition, associated with orbitofrontal injury, is the underlying force leading to hypersexual or inappropriate sexual behaviors. These behaviors are usually described in the context of interpersonal contact but also may manifest as perseverative self-directed behaviors, such as excessive masturbation. Such behaviors may represent response to injury, loss of self-esteem, or need to act out psychological conflict. Changes in sexual preference may represent release of inhibitions from frontal damage (51). Behavior modification techniques may be helpful in reducing the frequency of some of these behaviors (149). To increase the effectiveness of these approaches, the problematic behaviors need to be clearly described. In addition, the frequency of the behavior and the context in which it occurs are very important aspects of the assessment, as well as approaches attempted and how the behavior responded to the specific approaches. A behavior modification plan should include the approaches that led to a decrease in the problematic behavior, as well as ongoing assessment of their effectiveness.

Sexual offending disorders are defined as sexual acts against another person that cause affront or distress (144). These behaviors include touching (frotteurism, toucherism), exhibitionism, pedophilia, voyeurism, and sexual aggression or assault. In 1 study of 445 patients with TBI, 6.5% were identified as individuals who had committed some form of sexual offense. Alcohol was a factor in only 3. The most common offenses were inappropriate touching followed by exhibitionism and overt sexual aggression (142).

Sexual offenders have been treated with hormonal therapy, such as medroxyprogesterone and other antiandrogens (e.g., cyproterone) that are progesterone derivatives, and these agents have been used successfully in treatment of aggressive hypersexual behavior in patients with brain injury to decrease levels of serum testosterone (150,151). Such interventions have not been thoroughly studied in patients with brain injury, and violent sexual behaviors are rare in this population. Bezeau et al. (152) provide a detailed example of behavioral treatment for sexually intrusive behaviors. In contrast, most persons with brain injury are more likely to be victims of sexual abuse by others than perpetrators of violent crimes (153).

SEX THERAPY

Sex therapy focuses on various strategies to improve sexual functioning in both individuals and couples in which one or both partners may have some type of sexual dysfunction. Although sex therapy is more commonly conducted within the context of relationships, individuals without current partners may benefit from some of the techniques used. As previously mentioned, a thorough assessment of the problem(s) is essential to the development of a problem-oriented treatment plan. In this way, sex therapy focuses on the specific area of dysfunction. In addition, sex therapy often involves collaboration between the sex therapist and physicians (154). Therefore, treatment may include medication or change of medications and behavioral and cognitive psychotherapeutic techniques.

LoPiccolo (155) presented the concept of direct treatment of sexual dysfunction, which included some basic therapeutic principles, such as viewing sexual dysfunction within the context of the relationship, provision of basic sexual education and information, examination about sexual attitudes, addressing performance anxiety, improving sex-

ual communication, improving the partners' ability to use sexual techniques, prioritizing sexual activity, and providing specific techniques to change behavior. Therefore, in addition to common couples therapy, techniques, such as exploration of feelings and direct communication strategies and cognitive therapy techniques, such as reframing and coping skills development, are also used (156).

Behavioral strategies may include increasing affectionate behaviors, relaxation, behavioral rehearsal, and/or more sex-specific strategies, such as desensitization, nondemand pleasuring, directed masturbation, Kegel exercises, nondemand stimulation, start-stop techniques, the squeeze technique, and the quiet vagina exercise (18,157). Such techniques vary in effectiveness and require intervention by therapists with specific training in both sex therapy and experience in treating individuals with TBI. In this way, standard approaches to sex therapy can be appropriately modified to accommodate any physical, emotional, behavioral, or cognitive impairments that may be present. These techniques of sex therapy may be useful for persons with brain injury and their partners as they explore new ways of relating intimately and sexually to each other.

Treatment of premature ejaculation (PE) is an example of the usefulness of sex therapy techniques. PE is defined as "persistent or recurrent ejaculation with minimal sexual stimulation before, on, or shortly after penetration and before the person wishes it . . . the disturbance causes marked distress or interpersonal difficulty" (8). Estimates of incidence vary from 30% to 75% in men and suggest that it is a common problem (158). Given the demographics, cognitive, and behavioral characteristics of males with TBI, PE may be a common but unidentified problem. Treatment of PE can involve several components, including an exploration of early sexual or masturbatory experiences in adolescence or young adulthood that may have reinforced rapid arousal and ejaculation, as well as interactions within a sexual relationship that may be reinforcing or influencing decreased ejaculatory control. Specific information about the frequency of PE, sexual expectations and their negative effects, and the usefulness of improving communication during sex are also helpful. Treatment may also include masturbation exercises coupled with techniques, such as the squeeze technique, visualization or relaxation exercises, the start-stop technique, and graduated steps to increased stimulation. Using these approaches within the broader context of sex therapy can lead to good outcomes for these individuals and their partners (158).

PROFESSIONAL AND PATIENT EDUCATION

For many individuals and couples, the essential aspects of programs addressing sexuality are education and counseling. In both disabled and nondisabled populations, lack of education may result in problems establishing and maintaining healthy and intimate sexual relationships. Loss of sexual capacity may be related to failure of the rehabilitation program to address sexuality needs of clients (41). The goal of rehabilitation is to look holistically at the person with a disability, and this perspective includes sexuality (159). Quality of life is a goal of rehabilitation, and a commitment to including sexuality education as a component of information provided is essential. Education is an integral component of inpatient, outpatient, and residential programs.

Educational program development and implementation requires that health care professionals are knowledgeable and comfortable discussing the topic and value the importance of addressing sexuality. The health care professional must have an awareness of the perceptions and feelings that may influence communication of information to patients, partners, and families. Barriers identified that result in sexual education not being addressed in health care settings include inadequate knowledge, a perceived lack of time, an assumption that someone else is providing the education, and poor patient/family readiness to learn (160).

Staff education can be a method of exploring staff attitudes, awareness, and values. Key goals of education are to increase both the staff's comfort level and knowledge and to gain skills in communicating about sexuality with their peers, patients, and families. Discussions can explore the normal development of sexuality throughout the life cycle, human sexual response, cultural differences, and the impact of TBI on sexual function (161,162). In a recent study, results indicated that persons with TBI had more negative feelings about their sexuality and relationships than did participants without brain injury. Education in sexuality and ego adaptability for persons working with them is identified as a need (163).

Determining the best time for presenting information and education related to sexuality for the person with brain injury and partners and families is subject to debate but is probably best provided in the early phase after injury. Sexual dysfunction can develop later in recovery and follow-up with patients regarding sexual function, and integration of prevention programs is essential program components (164). Lack of awareness of the deficit can be prolonged, and education is helpful before and after return to the community (165). Nevertheless, learning readiness needs to be determined on an individual basis. The timing, topic areas, amount, and method of education should be individualized.

In some settings, sexuality is not addressed until socially inappropriate behavior occurs. Common behaviors seen in persons emerging from coma may be touching genitalia and self-stimulation, including masturbation. As the individual regains speech, verbal expression that includes sexual references may occur. Patients may be disinhibited and express sexual feelings to staff or family members. Privacy, safety for patients, and education and support are critical. It is important for partners and families to be prepared for such behaviors. Staff members are the most common targets for inappropriate social behaviors. Education is important for all members of the treatment team in inpatient and outpatient settings (144,166,167).

Health promotion and prevention is essential. Key topics to include in education of patients and family are potential changes after TBI that may impact sexuality. Of crucial importance is the provision of information about sexually transmitted diseases, including gonorrhea, chlamydial infections, herpes simplex viral infections, syphilis, parasitic infections, hepatitis, genital warts, urethritis, prostatitis, and acquired immunodeficiency syndrome. Safer sex practices include a careful selection of partners, mutual screening as necessary, and use of condoms and spermicides. Information on contraception should be provided, as well as strategies to address memory and compliance challenges because of cognitive impairments (63). Individuals with brain injury are at increased risk for sexual abuse (153).

Education to prepare the person with brain injury for optimal independent living, making informed choices, and socially appropriate behavior will facilitate a successful sexual adjustment (161). Addressing issues of self-esteem directly may be helpful (167). Social and communication skills, integral to initiating and sustaining relationships, should be included in education. Clinical practice guidelines for interventions may be helpful. Three psychosocial components of the guidelines are one-to-one verbal interpersonal skills, one-to-one nonverbal interpersonal skills, and strategies to deal with rejection. The guidelines provide specific interventions to foster the development of necessary social skills in long-term clients with TBI (168).

Education on psychosocial and sexual issues can be accomplished through group education meetings, social skills groups, family/patient meetings, community skills training, and individual or group counseling (165). Role-playing and more concrete and structured repetitive styles are better choices for presenting education (38). The group setting for patient education also provides experience with improving social skills. Treatment is adapted to the level of awareness of the individual (165). Identifying the person's preferred learning style is important, as well as combining various teaching methods to improve retention of the information. Providing written materials at an appropriate reading level and font size are particularly important when there are cognitive impairments. An interdisciplinary team approach, with all professional staff prepared to discuss sexuality issues in an atmosphere of permission is ideal. Leadership that fosters a team approach with the expectation that sexuality education is consistently delivered as part of the program will result in the best outcomes (161).

The PLISSIT model is a structure to guide interventions for sexual counseling and education. Permission (P) can be achieved by simply asking patients an open-ended question to identify concerns. This can be accomplished during the initial assessment and validates for the patient that you are open to discussing sexuality and lead to further questions and dialogue. Limited information (LI) may include factual information related to concerns, such as how the disability can affect sexual functioning. Specific suggestion (SS) may include information on problem solving or when to seek medical attention/intervention. Intensive therapy (IT) is individualized treatment provided by sex therapists and counselors. This model recognizes that there may be individual comfort levels and abilities among staff members (67,159,160).

A sexuality education program should include both professional and patient/family educational components and be integrated into the interdisciplinary rehabilitation programs in both inpatient and outpatient settings. A comprehensive sexuality education program, implemented in the Statewide Head Injury Program in Massachusetts, outlines both staff and patient education programs, implemented in residential and day treatment programs for adults with TBI. Components of the program include patient and staff needs assessments and evaluation measures, policies, and procedures. Sexuality education for staff occurs at the orientation level with advanced level workshops and professional readings programs. Patient education classes are presented in a style adapted to enhance learning, with various strategies in written question-and-answer format with prompt feedback and reinforcement, role-playing, and pre–post testing (169).

CONCLUSION

As noted in a recent qualitative study by Gill et al. (170), many factors remained strong among individuals with TBI and their intimate partners, including unconditional commitment, spending time together, open communication, a strong preinjury relationship, bonding through surviving the injury together, social support, family bonds, spirituality, experience with overcoming hardship, and coping skills. In this study, factors that were perceived as barriers to intimacy included injury-related changes, emotional reactions to changes, sexual difficulties, role conflict and strain, family issues, social isolation, and communication issues. The authors concluded that education regarding and sensitivity to the impact of TBI on intimacy should be an integral part of any rehabilitation program, which is a major conclusion of this chapter. Resources from both rehabilitation and community agencies can be particularly helpful (171). In some cases, complicated questions of ethics may arise and may require ethical or even judicial action as well (172).

The contributions of medical, psychological, social, and cultural factors to sexual functioning in diverse populations mandates individualized approaches to evaluation and treatment of sexual dysfunction. Further research is needed to further clarify the incidence and prevalence of these disorders and effective treatment approaches for optimal outcomes for men and women with TBI. In addition, attention to the needs of sexual minorities, including gay, lesbian, transgendered, and individuals with sexual development disorders, is required to further advance our understanding of sexuality across the entire disabled and nondisabled population. Despite gaps in our basic science and clinical knowledge base, major advances over the last decade have been made in the evaluation and treatment of sexual dysfunction that will be of benefit to our patients with TBI.

KEY CLINICAL POINTS

1. Consider sexual functioning and dysfunction in patients with TBI to be multifactorial
2. In clinical encounters, address issues of sexuality using the PLISSIT model and incorporate culturally competent approaches for diverse populations with TBI.
3. Be knowledgeable about how sexual minority status or disability may interact to affect both sexual functioning and clinical interactions with providers.
4. Understand the impact of pharmacologic agents on sexual function and adverse affects of medications during pregnancy.
5. Consider pharmacologic and other interventions for sexual dysfunction in patients with TBI, understanding the risks and potential benefits.

KEY REFERENCES

1. Aloni R, Katz S. *Sexual Difficulties After Traumatic Brain Injury and Ways to Deal With It.* Springfield, IL: Charles C. Thomas; 2003.
2. Basson R, Wierman M, van Lankveld J, Brotto LA. Summary of the recommendations on sexual dysfunctions in women. *J Sex Med.* 2010; 7(1, pt 2):314–326.

3. Gaudet L, Crethar HC, Burger S, et al. Self reported consequences of traumatic brain injury: a study of contrasting TBI and non TBI participants. *Sex Disabil.* 2001;9(2): 111–119.
4. Hibbard MR, Gordon WA, Flanagan S, Haddad L, Labinsky E. Sexual dysfunction after traumatic brain injury. *NeuroRehabilitation.* 2000;15(2):107–120.
5. Layman DE, Dijkers MP, Ashman TA. Exploring the impact of traumatic brain injury on the older couple: "yes, but how much of it is age, I can't tell you . . .". *Brain Inj.* 2005;19(11):909–923.
6. Rees PM, Fowler CJ, Maas CP. Sexual function in men and women with neurological disorders. *Lancet.* 2007; 369(9560):512–525.

References

1. Bell KR, Pepping M. Women and traumatic brain injury. *Phys Med Rehabil Clin N Am.* 2001;12(1):169–182.
2. Masters WH, Johnson VE. *Human Sexual Response.* Boston, MA: Little, Brown and Company; 1966.
3. Kaplan HS. Hypoactive sexual desire. *J Sex Marital Ther.* 1977;3(1): 3–9.
4. Fourcroy JL. Female sexual dysfunction: potential for pharmacotherapy. *Drugs.* 2003;63(14):1445–1457.
5. Levine SB. Erectile dysfunction: why drug therapy isn't always enough. *Cleve Clin J Med.* 2003;70(3):241–246.
6. Basson R. The female sexual response: a different model. *J Sex Marital Ther.* 2000;26(1):51–65.
7. World Health Organization. *International Statistical Classification of Diseases and Related Health Problems.* 10th Rev. Geneva, Switzerland: World Health Organization; 1992.
8. American Psychiatric Association. *Diagnostic and Statistical Manual of Mental Disorders.* 4th ed. Text Rev. Washington, DC: American Psychiatric Association; 2000.
9. Sipski ML. A physiatrist's views regarding the report of the International Consensus Conference on Female Sexual Dysfunction: potential concerns regarding women with disabilities. *J Sex Marital Ther.* 2001;27(2):215–216.
10. Basson R, Berman J, Burnett A, et al. Report of the international consensus development conference on female sexual dysfunction: definitions and classifications. *J Urol.* 2000;163(3):888–893.
11. Avis NE, Stellato R, Crawford S, Johannes C, Longcope C. Is there an association between menopause status and sexual functioning? *Menopause.* 2000;7(5):297–309.
12. Avis NE. Sexual function and aging in men and women: community and population-based studies. *J Gend Specif Med.* 2000;3(2): 37–41.
13. Laumann EO, Paik A, Rosen RC. Sexual dysfunction in the United States: prevalence and predictors. *JAMA.* 1999;281(6):537–544.
14. Baumeister RF, Catanese KR, Vohs KD. Is there a gender difference in the strength of sex drive? Theoretical views, conceptual distinctions, and a review of relevant evidence. *Pers Soc Psychol Rev.* 2001; 5(3):242–273.
15. Angier N. *Woman: An Intimate Geography.* New York, NY: Houghton Mifflin; 1999.
16. Leiblum SR. Sexual problems and dysfunction: epidemiology, classification, and risk factors. *J Gend Specif Med.* 1999;2(5):41–45.
17. McKenna K. The brain is the master organ in sexual function: central nervous system control of male and female sexual function. *Int J Impot Res.* 1999;11(suppl 1):S48–S55.
18. Allgeier WE, Allgeier AR. *Sexual Interactions.* 4th ed. Lexington, MA: DC Heath; 1995.
19. Giuliano FA, Rampin O, Benoit G, Jardin A. Neural control of penile erection. *Urol Clin North Am.* 1995;22(4):747–766.
20. Bérard EJ. The sexuality of spinal cord injured women: physiology and pathophysiology. A review. *Paraplegia.* 1989;27(2):99–112.
21. MacLean PD. Brain mechanisms of primal sexual functions and related behavior. In: Sandier M, Gessa GL, eds. *Sexual Behavior: Pharmacology and Biochemistry.* New York, NY: Raven Press; 1975.

22. Marson L, Platt KB, McKenna KE. Central nervous system innervation of the penis as revealed by the transneuronal transport of pseudorabies virus. *Neuroscience*. 1993;55(1):263–280.

23. Hulter B, Lundberg PO. Sexual function in women with hypothalamo-pituitary disorders. *Arch Sex Behav*. 1994;23(2):171–183.

24. Lilly R, Cummings JL, Benson DF, Frankel M. The human Klüver-Bucy syndrome. *Neurology*. 1983;33(9):1141–1145.

25. Góscínski I, Kwiatkowski S, Polak J, Orlowiejska M, Partyk A. The Kluver-Bucy syndrome. *J Neurosurg Sci*. 1997;41(3):269–272.

26. Herzog AG, Russell V, Vaitukaitis JL, Geschwind N. Neuroendocrine dysfunction in temporal lobe epilepsy. *Arch Neurol*. 1982;39(3):133–135.

27. Herzog AG, Seibel MM, Schomer DL, Vaitukaitis JL, Geschwind N. Reproductive endocrine disorders in men with partial seizures of temporal lobe origin. *Arch Neurol*. 1986;43(4):347–350.

28. Herzog AG, Seibel MM, Schomer DL, Vaitukaitis JL, Geschwind N. Reproductive endocrine disorders in women with partial seizures of temporal lobe origin. *Arch Neurol*. 1986;43(4):341–346.

29. Walker AE. The neurological basis of sex. *Neurol India*. 1976;24(1):1–13.

30. Horn LJ, Zasler ND. Neuroanatomy and neurophysiology of sexual dysfunction. *J Head Trauma Rehabil*. 1990;5(2):1–13.

31. Fabbri A, Jannini EA, Gnessi L, et al. Endorphins in male impotence: evidence for naltrexone stimulation of erectile activity in patient therapy. *Psychoneuroendocrinology*. 1989;14(1–2):103–111.

32. Goldstein JA. Erectile function and naltrexone. *Ann Intern Med*. 1986;105(5):799.

33. Thomsen IV. Late outcome of very severe blunt head trauma: a 10–15 year second follow-up. *J Neurol Neurosurg Psychiatry*. 1984;47(3):260–268.

34. Rosenbaum M, Najenson T. Changes in life patterns and symptoms of low mood as reported by wives of severely brain-injured soldiers. *J Consult Clin Psychol*. 1976;44(6):881–888.

35. Lezak MD. Living with the characterologically altered brain injured patient. *J Clin Psychiatry*. 1978;39(7):592–598.

36. Bond MR. Assessment of the psychosocial outcome of severe head injury. *Acta Neurochir (Wien)*. 1976;34(1–4):57–70.

37. Garden FH, Bonke CF, Hoffman M. Sexual functioning and marital adjustment after traumatic brain injury. *J Head Trauma Rehabil*. 1990;5(2):52–59.

38. Kreuter M, Sullivan M, Dahllöf AG, Siösteen A. Partner relationships, functioning, mood and global quality of life in persons with spinal cord injury and traumatic brain injury. *Spinal Cord*. 1998;36(4):252–261.

39. Hibbard MR, Gordon WA, Flanagan S, Haddad L, Labinsky E. Sexual dysfunction after traumatic brain injury. *NeuroRehabilitation*. 2000;15(2):107–120.

40. Layman DE, Dijkers MP, Ashman TA. Exploring the impact of traumatic brain injury on the older couple: "yes, but how much of it is age, I can't tell you . . .". *Brain Inj*. 2005;19(11):909–923.

41. Kreuter M, Dahllöf AG, Gudjonsson G, Sullivan M, Siösteen A. Sexual adjustment and its predictors after traumatic brain injury. *Brain Inj*. 1998;12(5):349–368.

42. Kreutzer JS, Zasler ND. Psychosexual consequences of traumatic brain injury: methodology and preliminary findings. *Brain Inj*. 1989;3(2):177–186.

43. Zasler ND, Horn LJ. Rehabilitative management of sexual dysfunction. *J Head Trauma Rehabil*. 1990;5(2):14–24.

44. O'Carroll RE, Woodrow J, Maroun F. Psychosexual and psychosocial sequelae of closed head injury. *Brain Inj*. 1991;5(3):303–313.

45. Corrigan JD. Substance abuse as a mediating factor in outcome from traumatic brain injury. *Arch Phys Med Rehabil*. 1995;76(4):302–309.

46. Kelly MP, Johnson CT, Knoller N, Drubach DA, Winslow MM. Substance abuse, traumatic brain injury and neuropsychological outcome. *Brain Inj*. 1997;11(6):391–402.

47. Sparadeo FR, Barth JT, Stout CE. Addiction and traumatic brain injury. In: Stout CE, Levitt JL, Ruben DH, eds. *Handbook for Assessing and Treating Addictive Disorders*. New York, NY: Greenwood Press; 1992.

48. Delmonico RL. Sexuality and substance abuse in traumatic brain injury independence. *Brain Inj Source*. 2001;5:24–26.

49. Kosteljanetz M, Jensen TS, Nørgård B, Lunde I, Jensen PB, Johnsen SG. Sexual and hypothalamic dysfunction in the postconcussional syndrome. *Acta Neurol Scand*. 1981;63(3):169–180.

50. Aloni R, Katz S. A review of the effect of traumatic brain injury on the human sexual response. *Brain Inj*. 1999;13(4):269–280.

51. Miller BL, Cummings JL, McIntyre H, Ebers G, Grode M. Hypersexuality or altered sexual preference following brain injury. *J Neurol Neurosurg Psychiatry*. 1986;49(8):867–873.

52. Sandel ME, Williams KS, Dellapietra L, Derogatis LR. Sexual functioning following traumatic brain injury. *Brain Inj*. 1996;10(10):719–728.

53. Derogatis LR. *The Derogatis Interview for Sexual Function (DISF)*. Baltimore, MD: Clinical Psychometric Research Inc.; 1987.

54. Center for Research on Women with Disabilities. National Study of Women with Physical Disabilities. Houston, Texas: Department of Physical Medicine and Rehabilitation; 1999. http://www.bcm.edu/crowd/national study/MAJORFIN.htm. Accessed July 28, 2002.

55. Olkin R. *What Psychotherapists Should Know About Disability*. New York, NY: Guilford Press; 1999:226–237.

56. Aloni R, Katz S. *Sexual Difficulties After Traumatic Brain Injury and Ways to Deal With It*. Springfield, IL: Charles C. Thomas; 2003:9–19.

57. Glass C, Soni B. ABC of sexual health: sexual problems of disabled patients. *BMJ*. 1999;318(7182):518–521.

58. Kaiser Permanente National Diversity Council, Kaiser Permanente National Diversity Department. *A Provider's Handbook on Culturally Competent Care: Lesbian, Gay, Bisexual and Transgendered Population*. 2nd ed. Oakland, CA: Kaiser Permanente; 2004.

59. Garnets LD. Sexual orientations in perspective. *Cultur Divers Ethnic Minor Psychol*. 2002;8(2):115–129.

60. O'Dell MW, Riggs RV. Traumatic brain injury in gay and lesbian persons: practical and theoretical considerations. *Brain Inj Source*. 2001;5(3):22–23.

61. Mapou R. Traumatic brain injury rehabilitation with gay and lesbian individuals. *J Head Trauma Rehabil*. 1990;5(2):67–72.

62. Sipski ML, Alexander CJ, eds. *Sexual Function in People With Disability and Chronic Illness: A Health Professionals Guide*. Gaithersberg, MD: Aspen; 1997.

63. Griffith ER, Lemberg S. *Sexuality and the Person With Traumatic Brain Injury: A Guide for Families*. Philadelphia, PA: FA Davis Co.; 1993.

64. Kroll K, Levy Klein E. *Enabling Romance: A Guide to Love, Sex, and Relationships for the Disabled*. New York, NY: Harmony Books; 1992.

65. Haseltine F, Cole SS, Gray DB. *Reproductive Issues for Persons With Physical Disabilities*. Baltimore, MD: Paul H. Brookes; 1993.

66. Ducharme S, Gill KM. Sexual values, training and professional roles. *J Head Trauma Rehabil*. 1990;5:38–45.

67. Annon J. The PLISSIT model: a proposed conceptual scheme for the behavioral treatment of sexual problems. *J Sex Ed Therapists*. 1976;5:1–15.

68. Schover LR. Sexual problems in chronic illness. In: Leiblum SR, Rosen RC, eds. *Principles and Practice of Sex Therapy*. 3rd ed. New York, NY: Guilford Press; 2000:398–422.

69. Schover LR, Friedman JM, Weiler SJ, Heiman JR, LoPiccolo J. Multiaxial problem-oriented system for sexual dysfunctions: an alternative to DSM-III. *Arch Gen Psychiatry*. 1982;39(5):614–619.

70. LoPiccolo L, Heiman JR. Sexual assessment and history interview. In: LoPiccolo J, LoPiccolo L, eds. *Handbook of Sex Therapy*. New York, NY: Plenum Press; 1978:103–112.

71. Beck AT, Steer RA, Brown GK. *Manual for the Beck Depression Inventory-II*. San Antonio, TX: The Psychological Corporation; 1996.

72. Butcher JN, Graham JR, Ben-Porath YS, Tellegen A, Dahlstrom WG, Kaemmer B. *MMPI-2 (Minnesota Multiphasic Personality Inventory-2): Manual for Administration, Scoring, and Interpretation*. Rev ed. Minneapolis, MN: University of Minnesota Press; 2001.

73. Millon T, Davis RD, Millon C. *Manual for the Millon Clinical Multiaxial Inventory–III (MCMI-III)*. 2nd ed. Minneapolis, MN: National Computer Systems Inc.; 1997.

74. Rust J, Golombok S. The Golombok-Rust Inventory of Sexual Satisfaction (GRISS). *Br J Clin Psychol*. 1985;24(pt 1):63–64.

75. Siösteen A, Lundqvist C, Blomstrand C, Sullivan L, Sullivan M. Sexual ability, activity, attitudes and satisfaction as part of adjustment in spinal cord-injured subjects. *Paraplegia*. 1990;28(5):285–295.

76. Rosen R, Brown C, Heiman J, et al. The Female Sexual Function Index (FSFI): a multidimensional self-report instrument for the as-

sessment of female sexual function. *J Sex Marital Ther*. 2000;26(2): 191–208.

77. Derogatis LR, Rosen R, Leiblum S, Burnett A, Heiman J. The Female Sexual Distress Scale (FSDS): initial validation of a standardized scale for assessment of sexually related personal distress in women. *J Sex Marital Ther*. 2002;28(4):317–330.

78. Quirk FH, Heiman JR, Rosen RC, Laan E, Smith MD, Boolell M. Development of a sexual function questionnaire for clinical trials of female sexual dysfunction. *J Womens Health Gend Based Med*. 2002;11(3):277–289.

79. Rosen RC, Lane RM, Menza M. Effects of SSRIs on sexual function: a critical review. *J Clin Psychopharmacol*. 1999;19(1):67–85.

80. Seidman SN, Pesce VC, Roose SP. High-dose sildenafil citrate for selective serotonin reuptake inhibitor-associated ejaculatory delay: open clinical trial. *J Clin Psychiatry*. 2003;64(6):721–725.

81. Sitsen JMA. Prescription drugs and sexual function. In: Money J, Musaph H, eds. *Handbook of Sexology*. Vol 6. Amsterdam/New York/London: Elsevier; 1988:425–461.

82. Drugs that cause sexual dysfunction. *Med Lett Drugs Ther*. 1983; 25(641):73–76.

83. Abboud CF. Laboratory diagnosis of hypopituitarism. *Mayo Clin Proc*. 1986;61(1):35–48.

84. Kaneko S, Bradley WE. Evaluation of erectile dysfunction with continuous monitoring of penile rigidity. *J Urol*. 1986;136(5): 1026–1029.

85. Morales A, Condra M, Reid K. The role of nocturnal penile tumescence monitoring in the diagnosis of impotence: a review. *J Urol*. 1990;143(3):441–446.

86. Thase ME, Reynolds CF III, Jennings JR, et al. Nocturnal penile tumescence is diminished in depressed men. *Biol Psychiatry*. 1988; 24(1):33–46.

87. Assessment: neurological evaluation of male sexual dysfunction. Report of the Therapeutics and Technology Assessment Subcommittee of the American Academy of Neurology. *Neurology*. 1995; 45(12):2287–2292.

88. Lundberg PO, Ertekin C, Ghezzi A, Swash M, Vodusk D. Neurosexology. Guidelines for neurology. *European*. 2001;8(supp 3):2–24.

89. Deliganis AV, Maravilla KR, Heiman JR, et al. Female genitalia: dynamic MR imaging with use of MS-325 initial experiences evaluating female sexual response. *Radiology*. 2002;225(3):791–799.

90. Sipski ML, Behnegar A. Neurogenic female sexual dysfunction: a review. *Clin Auton Res*. 2001;11(5):279–283.

91. Fink HA, Mac Donald R, Rutks IR, Nelson DB, Wilt TJ. Sildenafil for male erectile dysfunction: a systematic review and meta-analysis. *Arch Intern Med*. 2002;162(12):1349–1360.

92. Gans WH, Zaslau S, Wheeler S, Galea G, Vapnek JM. Efficacy and safety of oral sildenafil in men with erectile dysfunction and spinal cord injury. *J Spinal Cord Med*. 2001;24(1):35–40.

93. Padma-Nathan H, Steidle C, Salem S, Tayse N, Yeager J, Harning R. The efficacy and safety of a topical alprostadil cream, Alprox-TD, for the treatment of erectile dysfunction: two phase 2 studies in mild-to-moderate and severe ED. *Int J Impot Res*. 2003;15(1):10–17.

94. Porst H, Young JM, Schmidt AC, Buvat J; for International Vardenafil Study Group. Efficacy and tolerability of vardenafil for treatment of erectile dysfunction in patient subgroups. *Urology*. 2003; 62(3):519–524.

95. Sánchez Ramos A, Vidal J, Jáuregui ML, et al. Efficacy, safety and predictive factors of therapeutic success with sildenafil for erectile dysfunction in patients with different spinal cord injuries. *Spinal Cord*. 2001;39(12):637–643.

96. Carrier S. Pharmacology of phosphodiesterase 5 inhibitors. *Can J Urol*. 2003;10(suppl 1):12–16.

97. Herschorn S. Cardiovascular safety of PDE5 inhibitors. *Can J Urol*. 2003;10(suppl 1):23–28.

98. Gonzalgo ML, Brotzman M, Trock BJ, Geringer AM, Burnett AL, Jarow JP. Clinical efficacy of sildenafil citrate and predictors of long-term response. *J Urol*. 2003;170(2, pt 1):503–506.

99. Atmaca M, Kuloglu M, Tezcan E. Sildenafil use in patients with olanzapine-induced erectile dysfunction. *Int J Impot Res*. 2002;14(6): 547–549.

100. Nurnberg HG, Hensley PL, Gelenberg AJ, Fava M, Lauriello J, Paine S. Treatment of antidepressant-associated sexual dysfunction with sildenafil: a randomized controlled trial. *JAMA*. 2003;289(1): 56–64.

101. Yap RL, McVary KT. Topical agents and erectile dysfunction: is there a place? *Curr Urol Rep*. 2002;3(6):471–476.

102. Steidle C, Padma-Nathan H, Salem S, et al. Topical alprostadil cream for the treatment of erectile dysfunction: a combined analysis of the phase II program. *Urology*. 2002;60(6):1077–1082.

103. Steers WD. Viability and safety of combination drug therapies for erectile dysfunction. *J Urol*. 2003;170(2, pt 2):S20–S23.

104. Bechara A, Bertolino MV, Casabé A, et al. Duplex Doppler ultrasound assessment of clitoral hemodynamics after topical administration of alprostadil in women with arousal and orgasmic disorders. *J Sex Marital Ther*. 2003;29(suppl 1):1–10.

105. Benkert O, Crombach G, Kockott G. Effect of L-dopa on sexually impotent patients. *Psychopharmacologia*. 1972;23(1):91–95.

106. Montorsi F, Perani D, Anchisi D, et al. Apomorphine-induced brain modulation during sexual stimulation: a new look at central phenomena related to erectile dysfunction. *Int J Impot Res*. 2003;15(3): 203–209.

107. Montorsi F, Perani D, Anchisi D, et al. Brain activation patterns during video sexual stimulation following the administration of apomorphine: results of a placebo-controlled study. *Eur Urol*. 2003; 43(4):405–411.

108. Hagemann JH, Berding G, Bergh S, et al. Effects of visual sexual stimuli and apomorphine SL on cerebral activity in men with erectile dysfunction. *Eur Urol*. 2003;43(4):412–420.

109. Lal S, Ackman D, Thavundayil JX, Kiely ME, Etienne P. Effect of apomorphine, a dopamine receptor agonist, on penile tumescence in normal subjects. *Prog Neuropsychopharmacol Biol Psychiatry*. 1984; 8(4–6):695–699.

110. Lal S. Apomorphine in the evaluation of dopaminergic function in man. *Prog Neuropsychopharmacol Biol Psychiatry*. 1988;12(2–3): 117–164.

111. Lammers PI, Rubio-Aurioles E, Castell R, et al. Combination therapy for erectile dysfunction: a randomized, double blind, unblinded active-controlled, cross-over study of the pharmacodynamics and safety of combined oral formulations of apomorphine hydrochloride, phentolamine mesylate and papaverine hydrochloride in men with moderate to severe erectile dysfunction. *Int J Impot Res*. 2002;14(1):54–59.

112. O'Carroll RE. Sexual desire disorders: a review of controlled treatment studies. *J Sex Res*. 1991;28(4):607–624.

113. Sherwin BB, Gelfand MM. The role of androgen in the maintenance of sexual functioning in oophorectomized women. *Psychosom Med*. 1987;49(4):397–409.

114. Apperloo MJ, Van Der Stege JG, Hoek A, Weijmar Schultz WC. In the mood for sex: the value of androgens. *J Sex Marital Ther*. 2003; 29(2):87–102.

115. Anastasiadis AG, Davis AR, Salomon L, Burchardt M, Shabsigh R. Hormonal factors in female sexual dysfunction. *Curr Opin Urol*. 2002;12(6):503–507.

116. Zumoff B, Strain GW, Miller LK, Rosner W. Twenty-four-hour mean plasma testosterone concentration declines with age in normal premenopausal women. *J Clin Endocrinol Metab*. 1995;80(4): 1429–1430.

117. Tan RS. Novel treatment options for overlapping yet distinct erectile dysfunction and andropause syndromes. *Curr Opin Investig Drugs*. 2003;4(4):435–438.

118. Liverman CT, Blazer DG, eds. *Committee on Assessing the Need for Clinical Trials of Testosterone Replacement Therapy, Board of Health Sciences Policy, Institute of Medicine*. Washington, DC: The National Academies Press; 2003.

119. O'Carroll R, Bancroft J. Testosterone therapy for low sexual interest and erectile dysfunction in men: a controlled study. *Br J Psychiatry*. 1984;145:146–151.

120. Buvat J, Lemaire A, Buvat-Herbaut M. Human chorionic gonadotropin treatment of nonorganic erectile failure and lack of sexual desire: a double-blind study. *Urology*. 1987;30(3):216–219.

121. Zajecka J, Fawcett J, Schaff M, Jeffriess H, Guy C. The role of serotonin in sexual dysfunction: fluoxetine-associated orgasm dysfunction. *J Clin Psychiatry*. 1991;52(2):66–68.

122. Gartrell N. Increased libido in women receiving trazodone. *Am J Psychiatry*. 1986;143(6):781–782.

123. Mathews A, Whitehead A, Kellett J. Psychological and hormonal factors in the treatment of female sexual dysfunction. *Psychol Med*. 1983;13(1):83–92.

124. Stevenson RW, Solyom L. The aphrodisiac effect of fenfluramine: two case reports of a possible side effect to the use of fenfluramine in the treatment of bulimia. *J Clin Psychopharmacol.* 1990;10(1): 69–71.

125. Crenshaw TL, Goldberg JP, Stern WC. Pharmacologic modification of psychosexual dysfunction. *J Sex Marital Ther.* 1987;13(4):239–252.

126. Drewes SE, George J, Khan F. Recent findings on natural products with erectile-dysfunction activity. *Phytochemistry.* 2003;62(7): 1019–1025.

127. Hong B, Ji YH, Hong JH, Nam KY, Ahn TY. A double-blind cross-over study evaluating the efficacy of korean red ginseng in patients with erectile dysfunction: a preliminary report. *J Urol.* 2002;168(5): 2070–2073.

128. Danjou P, Alexandre L, Warot D, Lacomblez L, Puech AJ. Assessment of erectogenic properties of apomorphine and yohimbine in man. *Br J Clin Pharmacol.* 1988;26(6):733–739.

129. Guay AT, Spark RF, Jacobson J, Murray FT, Geisser ME. Yohimbine treatment of organic erectile dysfunction in a dose-escalation trial. *Int J Impot Res.* 2002;14(1):25–31.

130. Morales A, Condra M, Owen JA, Surridge DH, Fenemore J, Harris C. Is yohimbine effective in the treatment of organic impotence? Results of a controlled trial. *J Urol.* 1987;137(6):1168–1172.

131. Reid K, Surridge DH, Morales A, et al. Double-blind trial of yohimbine in treatment of psychogenic impotence. *Lancet.* 1987;2(8556): 421–423.

132. Sonda LP, Mazo R, Chancellor MB. The role of yohimbine for the treatment of erectile impotence. *J Sex Marital Ther.* 1990;16(1):15–21.

133. Susset JG, Tessier CD, Wincze J, Bansal S, Malhotra C, Schwacha MG. Effect of yohimbine hydrochloride on erectile impotence: a double-blind study. *J Urol.* 1989;141(6):1360–1363.

134. Meston CM, Worcel M. The effects of yohimbine plus L-arginine glutamate on sexual arousal in postmenopausal women with sexual arousal disorder. *Arch Sex Behav.* 2002;31(4):323–332.

135. Lebret T, Hervé JM, Gorny P, Worcel M, Botto H. Efficacy and safety of a novel combination of L-arginine glutamate and yohimbine hydrochloride: a new oral therapy for erectile dysfunction. *Eur Urol.* 2002;41(6):608–613.

136. Kalsi JS, Minhas S, Kell PD, Ralph DJ. Oral agents for erectile dysfunction. *Hosp Med.* 2003;64(5):292–295.

137. Sidi AA. Vasoactive intracavernous pharmacotherapy. *Urol Clin North Am.* 1988;15(1):95–101.

138. Levine SB, Althof SE, Turner LA, et al. Side effects of self-administration of intracavernous papaverine and phentolamine for the treatment of impotence. *J Urol.* 1989;141(1):54–57.

139. Ishii N, Watanabe H, Irisawa C, et al. Intracavernous injection of prostaglandin E1 for the treatment of erectile impotence. *J Urol.* 1989;141(2):323–325.

140. Stackl W, Hasun R, Marberger M. Intracavernous injection of prostaglandin E1 in impotent men. *J Urol.* 1988;140(1):66–68.

141. Burnett AL. Neuroprotection and nerve grafts in the treatment of neurogenic erectile dysfunction. *J Urol.* 2003;170(2, pt 2):S31–S34.

142. Ferguson DM, Steidle CP, Singh GS, Alexander JS, Weihmiller MK, Crosby MG. Randomized, placebo-controlled, double blind, cross-over design trial of the efficacy and safety of Zestra for women in women with and without female sexual arousal disorder. *J Sex Marital Ther.* 2003;29(suppl 1):33–44.

143. Johnson C, Knight C, Alderman N. Challenges associated with the definition and assessment of inappropriate sexual behaviour amongst individuals with an acquired neurological impairment. *Brain Inj.* 2006;20(7):687–693.

144. Simpson G, Blaszczynski A, Hodgkinson A. Sex offending as a psychosocial sequela of traumatic brain injury. *J Head Trauma Rehabil.* 1999;14(6):567–580.

145. Lusk MD, Kott JA. Effects of head injury on libido. *Med Aspects Hum Sex.* 1982;16(10):22–30.

146. Weinstein EA, Kahn RL. Patterns of sexual behavior following brain injury. *Psychiatry.* 1961;24:69–78.

147. Weinstein EA. Sexual disturbances after brain injury. *Med Aspects Hum Sex.* 1974;8(10):10, 16, 18 passim.

148. Weinstein EA. Effects of brain damage on sexual behavior. *Med Aspects Hum Sex.* 1981;15(11):158, 163–164.

149. Fyffe CE, Kahng S, Fittro E, Russell D. Functional analysis and treatment of inappropriate sexual behavior. *J Appl Behav Anal.* 2004; 37(3):401–404.

150. Britton KR. Medroxyprogesterone in the treatment of aggressive hypersexual behavior in traumatic brain injury. *Brain Inj.* 1998; 12(8):703–707.

151. Emory LE, Cole CM, Meyer WJ. Use of depo-provera to control sexual aggression in persons with traumatic brain injury. *J Head Trauma Rehabil.* 1995;10(3):47–58.

152. Bezeau SC, Bogod NM, Mateer CA. Sexually intrusive behaviour following brain injury: approaches to assessment and rehabilitation. *Brain Inj.* 2004;18(3):299–313.

153. Cole S. Facing the challenges of sexual abuse in persons with disabilities. *J Sex Disabil.* 1986;7(3–4):71–78.

154. Leiblum SR, Rosen RC. Introduction: sex therapy in the age of Viagra. In: Leiblum SR, Rosen RC, eds. *Principles and Practice of Sex Therapy.* 3rd ed. New York, NY: Guilford; 2000:1–13.

155. LoPiccolo J. Direct treatment of sexual dysfunction. In: LoPiccolo J, LoPiccolo L, eds. *Handbook of Sex Therapy.* New York, NY: Plenum Press; 1978:1–17.

156. Pridal CG, LoPiccolo J. Multielement treatment of desire disorders: integration of cognitive, behavioral, and systemic therapy. In: Leiblum SR, Rosen RC, eds. *Principles and Practice of Sex Therapy.* 3rd ed. New York, NY: Guilford; 2000:57–81.

157. Althof SE. Erectile dysfunction: psychotherapy with men and couples. In: Leiblum SR, Rosen RC, eds. *Principles and Practice of Sex Therapy.* 3rd ed. New York, NY: Guilford; 2000:242–275.

158. Polonsky DC. Premature ejaculation. In: Leiblum SR, Rosen RC, eds. *Principles and Practice of Sex Therapy.* 3rd ed. New York, NY: Guilford; 2000:305–332.

159. Duldt BW, Pokorny ME. Teaching communication about human sexuality to nurses and other healthcare providers. *Nurse Educ.* 1999;24(5):27–32.

160. Herson L, Hart KA, Gordon MJ, Rintala DH. Identifying and overcoming barriers to providing sexuality information in the clinical setting. *Rehabil Nurs.* 1999;24(4):148–151.

161. Hough S. Sexuality within the head-injury rehabilitation setting: a staff's perspective. *Psychol Rep.* 1989;65(3, pt 1):745–746.

162. Medlar TM, Medlar J. Nursing management of sexuality issues. *J Head Trauma Rehabil.* 1990;5(2):46–51.

163. Gaudet L, Crethar HC, Burger S, Pulos S. Self-reported consequences of traumatic brain injury: a study of contrasting TBI and non-TBI participants. *Sex Disabil.* 2001;19(2):111–119.

164. Aloni A, Keren O, Cohen M, Rosentul N, Romm M, Groswasser Z. Incidence of sexual dysfunction in TBI patients during the early post-traumatic in-patient rehabilitation phase. *Brain Inj.* 1999;13(2): 89–97.

165. Dombrowski LK, Petrick JD, Strauss D. Rehabilitation treatment of sexuality issues due to acquired brain injury. *Rehabil Psychol.* 2000;45(3):299–309.

166. Kotch MJ. Agitation: understanding and managing challenges on the nursing unit. *Brain Inj Source.* 2001;5(3):8–11.

167. Zencius A, Wesolowski MD, Burke WH, Hough S. Managing hypersexual disorders in brain-injured clients. *Brain Inj.* 1990;4(2): 175–181.

168. Gutman S, Deger D. Enhancement of one-on-one interpersonal skills necessary to initiate and maintain intimate relationships: a frame of reference for adults having sustained a traumatic brain injury. *Occup Ther Ment Health.* 1997;13(2):51–67.

169. Medlar T. The sexuality education program of the Massachusetts statewide head injury program. *Sex Disabil.* 1998;16(1):11–19.

170. Gill CJ, Sander AM, Robins N, Mazzei DK, Struchen MA. Exploring experiences of intimacy from the viewpoint of individuals with traumatic brain and their partners. *J Head Trauma Rehabil.* 2011; 26(1):56–68. PMID:21209563.

171. Simpson G, Long E. An evaluation of sex education and information resources and their provision to adults with traumatic brain injury. *J Head Trauma Rehab.* 2004;9(5):413–428.

172. Kirschner KL, Brashler R, Dresser R, Levine C. Sexuality and a severely brain-injured spouse. *The Hastings Center Report.* 2010; 40(3):14–16.

XII

POST-TRAUMA PAIN DISORDERS

Post-Traumatic Headache

Lawrence J. Horn, Benjamin Siebert, Neil Patel, and Nathan D. Zasler

INTRODUCTION

Headache (HA) (cephalalgia) is the most common physical complaint reported after traumatic brain injury (TBI)/concussion. In the past, the incidence was believed to be lower in severe brain injury (1), but more recent studies would indicate that it is also problematic for patients with moderate-to-severe TBI, corroborating the experience of clinicians working with these populations. The advent of craniectomy for the management of elevated intracranial pressure/focal swelling may in part explain the more recent increments in incidence in more severely injured populations (2,3). Post-traumatic headache (PTH), and in particular postconcussive HAs, seldom connote serious underlying neurological problems. However, clinicians should be aware of various significant clinical conditions that may be responsible for PTH requiring intervention, such as intracranial hematomas, cerebral venous sinus thrombosis, carotid cavernous fistula, or arterial dissection (4). In an effort to codify the types and etiologies of HA, the International Headache Society (IHS) has undertaken a monumental task in developing a classification system. Certain aspects of the IHS classification remain controversial, and this is particularly true because it relates to the descriptions and chronology of PTH. The IHS system does not specifically address the variety of PTHs and does little to guide the clinician in management strategies, other than with reference to "primary" HA types. A major goal of this chapter is to attempt to classify types of HA specifically encountered in association with TBI and provide a guide to expeditious and effective management strategies thereof.

In reviewing the pathobiology of PTH, there appears to be a finite number of peripheral nociceptors that may produce HA after trauma and considerable overlap between the receptive fields of their secondary projections within the central nervous system (CNS). As a result, there appears to be a relatively limited repertoire of HA responses. Thus, while attempting to address techniques to decipher the "primary" pain generators in PTH, a concurrent goal of this chapter is to emphasize the importance of multifaceted approaches to management of PTH, regardless of what is presumed to be the primary cause. Ultimately, PTH should not be thought of as a singular diagnosis but as a symptom of a potentially complex biopsychosocial interaction that may have more than one contributing pain generator.

EPIDEMIOLOGY

Civilian

It is very difficult to determine the prevalence of PTH in the civilian population because many people who experience mild TBI (MTBI) or concussion do not obtain medical attention. Although HA is the most common symptom after brain injury, there is wide variation in definitions so that the incidence ranges from 30% to 90% and historically has been considered more common in the population with MTBI. Further, it is believed that most patients with PTH have resolution within several weeks, yet 15%–42% complained of PTH at 3 months (5), and 36% at 6 months (6). Many patients show improvement in the first 3–6 months after injury, but then their pattern of symptom reporting appears to stabilize. HA reports span 32%–78% at 2–3 months, 8%–35% at 1 year, and 20%–24% at 2–4 years. Recent data would indicate, however, that between 40% and 50% of patients with brain injury admitted to a National Institute of Disability and Rehabilitation Research TBI model system, complained of HA at 3, 6, and 12 months, regardless of whether they were mild, moderate, or severe (although very few mild were enrolled in this study) (2). In contradistinction to previous studies that emphasized tension or musculoskeletal-type HA as the dominant phenotype (7), the dominant HA type was migraine or "probable migraine." In addition, 40%–50% of patients reported the HAs as having a severe impact on their functional status (2). As in previous studies, risk factors included being female and premorbid history of HA. Therefore, if HA is a presenting problem, particularly for patients with moderate and severe injury, there is a relatively high likelihood of persistence of this complaint. Migraine-type HA with or without aura clearly may be triggered by trauma or whiplash injury. Although some authors found cluster HAs occur in up to 10% of PTH patients (8), others have found them to be uncommon (9).

Military

There have been several studies in recent years directed toward determination of the prevalence of pain and HAs in the US soldiers and veterans after their return from active duty. Although brain injury management following war time is no novel practice, there has been an influx in data associating HA with TBI during combat and/or active duty.

Subsequently, there has been an increase in data to aid in identifying specific cases of migraine from the more generalized chronic PTH as defined by the IHS. In recent study by Theeler et al., 5,270 returning soldiers were evaluated, in which nearly 20% met criteria for "deployment-related concussion." Of those, approximately 98% subjectively reported having HA over the last 3 months of their deployment, 37% of which met criteria of PTH alone by the IHS criteria, and 58% met criteria for post-traumatic migraine (PTM). In short, more than 1 of every 3 soldiers who suffered concussion while deployed met criteria for PTH, with a majority being PTM (10,11). In a different study, Theeler et al. focused on prevalence of migraine in US Army soldiers who had returned from Operation Iraqi Freedom (OIF); it was found that approximately 19% of soldiers had screened positive for migraine, whereas an additional 17% screened positive for possible migraine (12). These results did not specifically designate the HAs as PTH or PTM, as trauma was not a required inclusion factor. Erickson reported in an observational study that triptans were found to be effective for aborting HA, and topiramate was an effective prophylactic agent, but tricyclic antidepressants (TCAs) appeared to have little efficacy in this population (see Treatment section) (13).

Gironda et al. reported that in a group of OIF and Operation Enduring Freedom (OEF) veterans who had recorded significant pain (a group of 100 veterans randomly selected from 219 that met the specified criteria), approximately 4.5% had HA as the primary condition (14).

A review of the epidemiology of deployment-related PTH was published by Neely et al., which reviews several studies in addition to the aforementioned. This data suggest that PTH and PTM may have a higher prevalence than previously seen in the military population (15). Schwab et al. found that 16% of veterans had sustained a MTBI, and of those, 36% reported HA (16), whereas in another study by Walker et al., it was reported that 38% of subjects with moderate-to-severe TBI developed acute PTH (3) (see Table 56-1).

A close association between TBI, post-traumatic stress disorder (PTSD), and HA has been reported, which is an important factor when evaluating the epidemiology of PTH. For example, a study in 2009 showed that PTSD and combat-related injury were related to higher rates of self-reported HA in veterans (17). An earlier study showed that approximately 1 out of 6 patients with tension-type headache (TTH) or migraine reports symptoms similar to PTSD (this was not specific for military personnel or veterans however) (18). Hoge et al. reported in their study that after adjustment for PTSD and depression, HA was the only physical symptom associated with MTBI (15% of subjects were positive for MTBI) (19). This showed that HA was more closely related to TBI than to PTSD but that health complaints in general may be more prevalent with PTSD. Although there is considerable recent information about the prevalence of deployment-related PTH, there is still much to be learned from this data. The information gathered presents a challenge to better identify the confounding environmental and situational factors, which may be contributing as to the subjective reporting of HA.

"Blast-Related" Headache

As mentioned earlier, there is a clear relationship between HA and TBI, particularly in military personnel and veterans. Modern warfare has led to increased use of improvised explosive devices (IEDs) and technology has brought improved body armor; thus, there has been a significant increase in both blast injury and survivors of blast injury (see Chapter 57). In the past few years, there has been an increase in research and reviews of blast-induced neurotrauma (BINT), but there is still much information lacking.

Cernak et al. have used animal models to observe physical changes to the brain secondary to blast injury. The rat models included head protection to account for protective equipment as worn by the soldiers in combat. They found that the rats had acquired cognitive impairment and bio-

TABLE 56–1 Overview Epidemiology of PTH in the Military

AUTHOR	DESCRIPTION	SUMMARY
Schneiderman et. al.	OIF/OEF veterans who left combat by October, 2004	275 report mild TBI: 35% of these report postconcussive symptoms. PTSD had a associated increase in symptoms. Headache recorded, but not isolated.
Theeler et. al.	US Army soldiers, post-deployment questionnaires	19% positive for PTM, 17% positive for possible migraine
Hoge et. al.	US Army soldiers post-deployment screenings	15% positive for mild TBI, with adjustment for PTSD and depression; headache was only symptom associated with mild TBI
Walker et. al.	Veterans with mod-severe TBI	Acute PTH in 38%. Delayed onset headache in approximately 25% at 6 months (and subsequently almost all of these at 1 year).
Schwab et. al.	Validation study of soldiers after return from Iraq/Afghanistan	16% positive for mild TBI; 36% of these report injury-related headache

Abbreviation: OIF, Operation Iraqi Freedom; OEF, Operation Enduring Freedom; TBI, traumatic brain injury; PTSD, post-traumatic stress disorder; PTH, post-traumatic headache.
Adapted from Neely ET, Midgette LA, Scher AI. Clinical review and epidemiology of headache disorders in US service members: with emphasis on post-traumatic headache. *Headache.* 2009;49(7):1089–1096.

chemical changes (measured by oxidative stress and anti-oxidant enzyme defense) in the hippocampus, which were correlated with the severity of blast injury (20). Several other studies have looked at animal models in the ensuing years to obtain more information on BINT. Blast injuries are categorized as follows:

- Primary – injuries as a direct result of overpressure blast waves,
  - This leads to a local, systemic, and cerebral response.
- Secondary – injuries from shrapnel or other projectiles as a result of the blast,
- Tertiary – injuries as a result of the body being thrown caused by displacement of air from blast (e.g., thrown against wall, ground, or in vehicle), or
- Quaternary – injuries caused by other results of the blast not listed in the first 3 types (21).

Brain injuries acquired from explosions often lead to brain swelling and cerebral vasospasm, even with continuous monitoring. The initial BINT symptoms may be delayed up to months or years after the initial injury, which then are considered secondary brain injuries. These symptoms may include retrograde amnesia for the time frame surrounding the blast, HA, and impaired cognition (22). There are different theories on pressurization of the brain from blast exposure, which has been of debate since World War II (23). Importantly, however, there is evidence in animal models simulating overpressurization from the blast injury that the *rate* of the stress caused by the blast leads to greater cellular damage than simply the total amount (24).

The HA associated with blast injury or BINT has not been well defined or isolated. What is known about BINT and understanding of PTH indicates that there may be both a neurovascular component, as well as a structural component to the HA. With blunt neurotrauma, it is known that there is an initial mechanical insult, followed by cellular responses, including gene expression. In BINT, the aforementioned stress to cells leads to vast immediate cell death and a cascade of cellular responses. Desmoulin and Dionne reviewed several studies that showed increased glial cell activation, as well as endogenous nitric oxide (NO) production. Glial cell activity was found to be prominent initially (first 1–7 days postinjury) but may be within normal limits within 3–4 weeks. It was noted that with microglial cells, although the increase activation was located throughout the brain, there was more prominence in the cerebral and cerebellar cortices, indicating that the blast pressure was likely more intense on the surface of the brain. With astrocytes (macroglial), it is hypothesized that the changes were caused by disruption of the blood-brain barrier. Inducible nitric oxide synthase (iNOS) gene expression is known to be increased in TBI, leading to increased glutamate activity. The subsequent cognitive deficits may be seen as early as 3 hours postblast exposure (23,25). This increase in glutamate activity is likely associated to the onset of HA as the excitatory neurotransmitters affect the trigeminal afferent system. This phenomenon is discussed further in conjunction with the section on migraine pathophysiology.

All of the earlier mentioned research must be considered in the context of the methodological challenges to studying the disorder of HA in patients with post-trauma. This is particularly true given that the etiology of the "disorder" is multifactorial and certainly influenced by a plethora or other factors aside from the nature of the brain injury itself.

NEUROBIOLOGY OF HEADACHE

Sources of Head Pain

Potential sources of head pain that may be relevant in the assessment of a patient presenting with PTH include intracranial, cranial, and cervical structures. The dura and venous sinuses are the most pain-sensitive intracranial structures. The skin, nerves, muscles, periosteum of the head, and cranial cavities (including the sinuses, eye socket, ear, nasal, and oral pharynx) are also pain sensitive. Cervical/cranial joint capsules (including the temporomandibular joint [TMJ]), cervical facets/zygapophyseal joints, cranial, and cervical autonomic nervous systems may all be primary nociceptive pain generators that produce local or referred head pain (26,27). Another common primary or contributing source of PTH is the musculature or the head and neck, including referred pain from any of the 4 layers of the posterior cervical musculature that is often injured in acceleration/deceleration injury (28,29) (see Figures 56-1–56-6).

Peripheral Nociception

External pain receptors of the head and neck are sensitive to mechanical, toxic, metabolic, and thermal injury. The afferent neurons are primarily unmyelinated C and myelinated Aδ neurons, with the cell bodies located in the dorsal root ganglia, entering the dorsal horn (DH) of the upper 3 cervical segments of the spinal cord or may travel with the trigeminal system to synapse in the spinal tract (nucleus caudalis) of the trigeminal nerve. They may be activated by the same processes of tissue injury and inflammation as described in Chapter 57 on pain and can produce peripheral sensitization. Peripheral nociceptive chemical mediators include bradykinin, serotonin, substance P, histamine, leukotrienes, cytokines, and prostaglandins. Second-order ascending systems in the spinal cord may follow the neospinothalamic tract, crossing over in the cord to the contralateral ventroposterolateral (VPL) nucleus of the thalamus, where a third-order neuron projects to the sensorimotor cortex of the parietal lobe. This system appears to be involved in the fine discrimination and localization of the nociceptive input. A second polysyn-

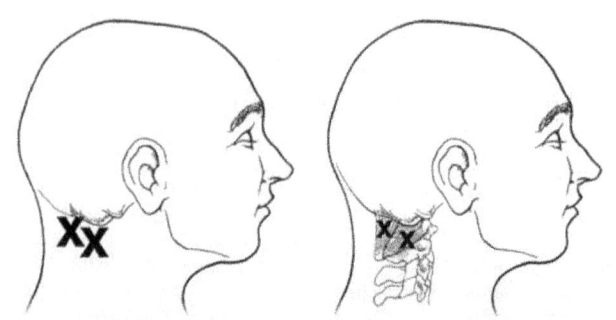

FIGURE 56-1 Sub-occipital muscle trigger points.

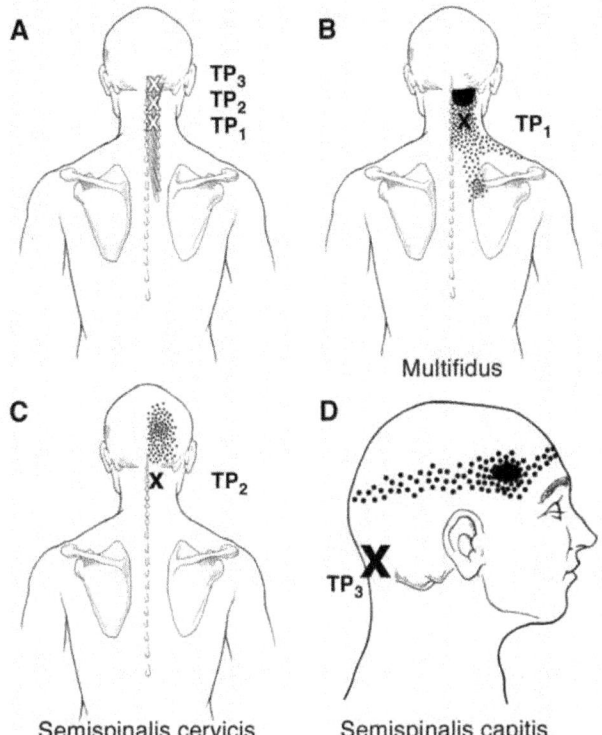

FIGURE 56-2 Posterior cervical muscles prone to development of trigger points producing referred pain perceived as cervicalgia and/or cephalalgia.

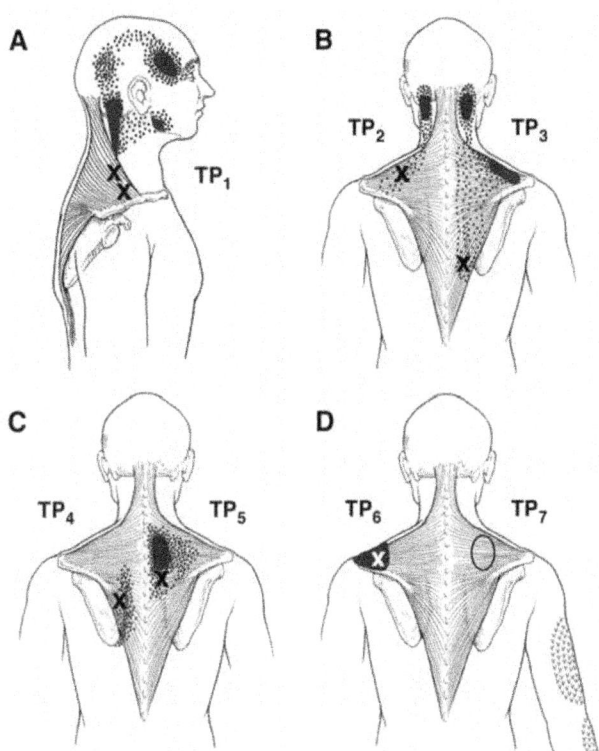

FIGURE 56-4 Trapezius muscle trigger point referral patterns.

aptic system (paleospinothalamic) has greater bilateral representation and projects to the insula and limbic system, including the anterior cingulate gyrus. It mediates the autonomic, endocrine, and emotional aspects of pain perception. This ascending system synapses at the reticular formation, midline, dorsomedial, and intralaminar nuclei of the thalamus. There are also projections to the periaqueductal gray of the mesencephalon. In both systems, there are both nociceptive-specific neurons and "wide dynamic range" neurons; the latter respond to both nociceptive and non-nociceptive affer-

ents. These systems are also subject to "windup" and central sensitization discussed in Chapter 57 on pain. Results of these processes may include allodynia—the perception of pain from otherwise neutral stimuli or hyperalgesia. In the region of the DH, glutamate, substance P, neurokinin A, and calcitonin gene-related peptide (CGRP) are considered pronociceptive chemical mediators.

Primary nociceptive afferents for the front of the scalp and face comprise the trigeminal sensory system. Afferents

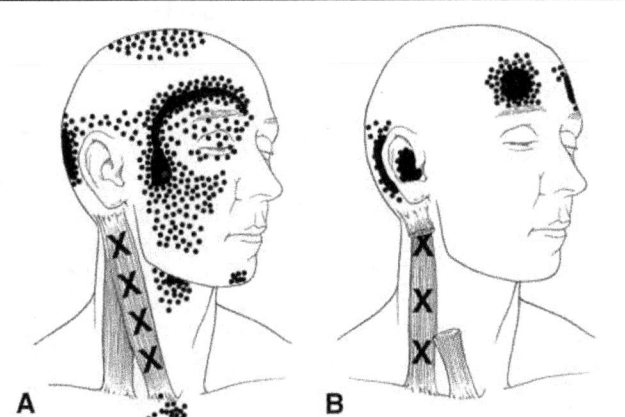

FIGURE 56-3 Referred pain patterns for sternocleidomastoid muscle trigger points, sternal division **(A)** and clavicular division **(B)**.

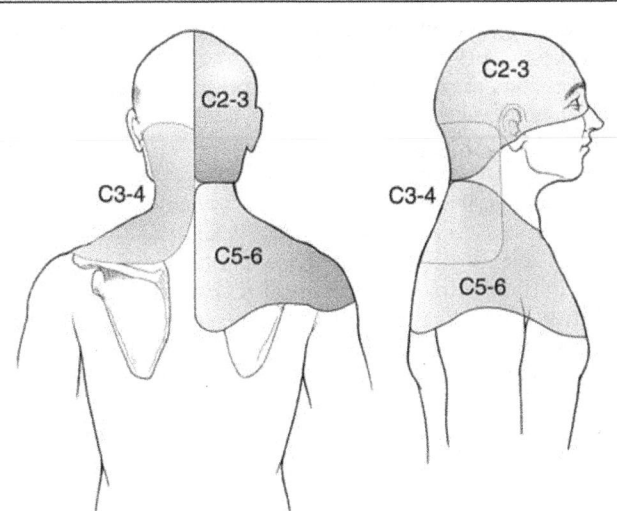

FIGURE 56-5 Cervical sensory dermatomes for sensory roots C2-6.

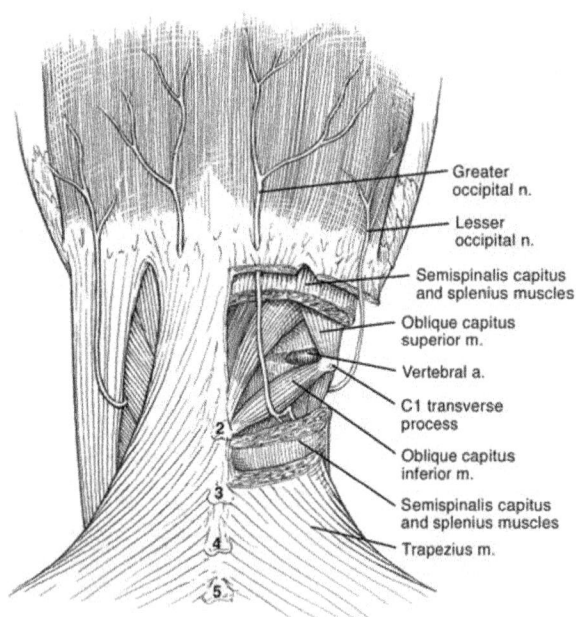

FIGURE 56-6 Anatomy of upper posterior cervical region with specific reference to C2 terminal branches of the lesser and greater occipital nerves.

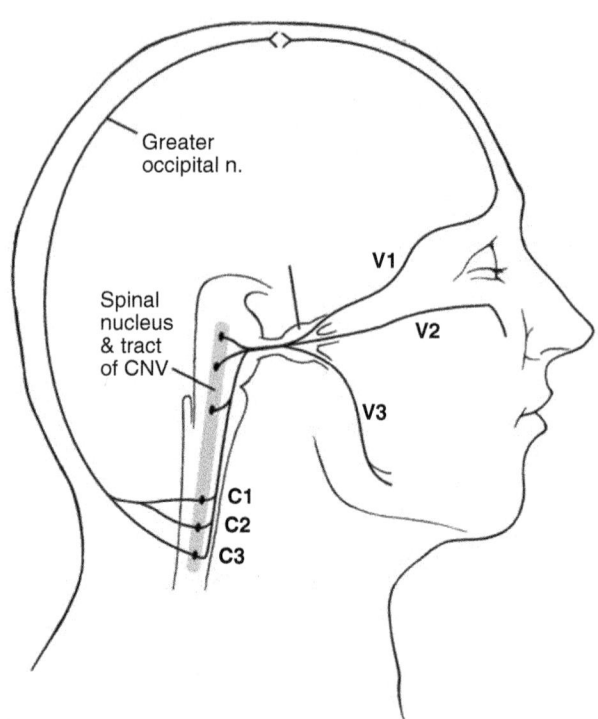

FIGURE 56-7 Schematic representation of interconnectivity between the spinal nucleus and tract of cranial nerve V, upper three cervical roots and the ophthalmic branch of the fifth cranial nerve through the gasserian ganglion.

from the meninges travel with the ophthalmic division (V_1). The area around the ear and the external auditory canal has sensory afferents from cranial nerves IX and X (although these, too, enter the spinal tract of the trigeminal nerve). The posterior scalp and upper neck give rise to sensory afferents to the upper 3 cervical segments, in part, mediated by the greater occipital nerve (GON) (C2) and lesser occipital nerve (LON) (C3). In the spinal tract of the trigeminal nerve, the most rostrally innervated structures are topographically most caudal; the superior sagittal sinus is represented most caudally in the nucleus at the level of C3 or C4. The upper cervical DH and the spinal tract of the trigeminal nerve are contiguous and overlap (30). There is also overlap of the second-order neurons in this region as well, so that central sensitization and expansion of receptive fields by second-order neurons may lead to the perception of pain in the occiput or neck when the primary nociceptive generator is subserved by the trigeminal system and vice versa. It is well established that a primary nociceptive generator in the cervical spine, musculature, or occipital nerves could activate the trigeminoneurovascular system (31,32). Central afferent convergence and sensitization of afferent second-order neurons may underlie the spread of pain and referral from supratentorial dura to areas innervated by cervical afferents. This would be the basis of 1 theory of referred pain: the "convergence projection" theory, whereby pain originating from an affected tissue (primary pain generator) is perceived as originating from a distant receptive field (33). As an example, in true migraine, sensitization of trigeminal meningeal neurons leads to central sensitization causing hemicranial allodynia (34). Stimulation of the occipital nerve activates the spinal nucleus caudalis in the same distribution as when the meninges or V_1 innervated structures are stimulated (i.e., cat

model) (31). Given the finite neurochemical and physiological responses to nociceptive stimuli, this overlap in receptive fields between the trigeminal system and somatic systems in the upper cervical area may obscure the principle pain generators in PTH. Hence, treatment approaches typically reserved for certain primary HAs may prove effective in phenotypes for which they might not typically be prescribed; this also underscores the potential for multimodality therapeutic approaches to provide optimized treatment. (see Figure 56-7)

CLINICAL EVALUATION OF POST-TRAUMATIC HEADACHE

The distinction between various types of PTH may be a challenging task and is often unclear in some scientific literature (i.e., PTH may be treated as if it were 1 clinical phenotype). Defining variables used in HA classification and for clinical purposes often overlap HA types. This is, in part, understandable because of the presence of primary and secondary sensitization, windup, expanded and overlapping receptive fields, and the theory of "convergence projection." In some respects, a fine distinction may be moot from a clinical perspective because it is important to treat the primary and secondary generators to reduce the disabling consequences of PTH (4).

Historical information regarding the mechanism of injury can help provide clues to distinguish types of PTH. The physical forces involved in PTH include impact and/or acceleration/deceleration (inertial) loading; the latter typically involves "whiplash" type injury to the neck. Blast injury in our military personnel may preferentially injure those anatomical areas and tissues exposed to external air pressure—such as the sinuses, eyes, and ears or produce a transient although severe increase in intracranial pressure or otherwise activate the excitatory neurochemical cascade of TBI (see "Blast-related" HA). Neurosurgical intervention provides yet another "external physical force" that may, in and of itself, produce structural changes that lead to head pain.

On review of systems, it is useful to use the acronym "COLDER."

- Character: dull, throbbing, lancinating, sharp, and so forth
- Onset: any precipitants, relationship to menses, time of day, temporal relationship to injury, and so forth
- Location: unilateral, bilateral, occipital, vertex, radiating
- Duration and frequency: length of time the HA has been present, onset relationship to trauma, frequency during the week.
- Exacerbation: physical activity, stooping, valsalva, bending, touch (allodynia), stress, poor sleep, menses, weather changes, and so forth
- Relief: medications that work, how frequently they are taken, response to rest, dark or quiet

The patient should also be asked about severity (0 is *none* and 10 is the *worst imaginable*), associated symptoms (nausea, vomiting, photophobia, visual changes, phonophobia), presence of aura, and the degree of functional disability associated with HA episodes, including vocational impact (e.g., how many days of work missed per month) (4,27). Other relevant historical information should include the circumstances of injury, whether the patient is actively engaged in litigation, previous history of head injury or premorbid history of HA, history of psychiatric illness, and other symptoms related to postconcussion syndrome or impairments from a more severe TBI.

The physical examination should include observation (for obvious traumatic changes, asymmetries, and general posture), neurological examination, cervical range of motion (ROM), palpation of cervical and cranial musculature, palpation for "clicking" in the TMJ, palpation of the GON and LON egress points and along the nuchal ridge, ocular examination and auscultation for carotid, mastoid, temporal, and ocular bruits. Although an in-depth discussion of myofascial pain is beyond the scope of this chapter, the reader is referred to other more extensive resources (27,28,35). Myofascial pain is very common in the sternocleidomastoids, trapezius, and other cervical musculature after whiplash or inertial injury. It is interesting to note that the zone of referred pain for the sternocleidomastoid extends to retro-orbital and periorbital areas; associated "autonomic" symptoms include vertigo, tinnitus, and a sense of fullness in the ear, as well as ear pain (commonly confused for otitis externa). These symptoms may be explained by convergence-projection theory in that there is overlap in the sensory dermatomes for the sternocleidomastoid muscle (SCM) and the trigeminal tract as discussed earlier; the second-order nociceptive neurons for the somatic afferents from cranial nerves VII, IX, and X are also located nearby in the nucleus caudalis of cranial nerve V.

The cervical musculature is also a major source of afferents to the vestibular systems integrating eye, head, and neck movement, thereby making dizziness a common complaint in the patient population (so-called cervical vertigo). The zone of referred pain to the ear overlaps the sensory area for the vagus. Theoretically, peripheral sensitization in the SCM could, therefore, lead to central sensitization within the vestibular and vagal systems (4). (see Figures 56-1–56-4)

CLASSIFICATION OF HEADACHE

International Headache Society

The IHS classification system is an internationally recognized tool to code and identify clinical presentations of head pain (11,36). The system is reliant primarily on history and to a limited extent on physical examination. It does not consistently address etiology in the sense of primary pain generators, treatment, or prognosis. HAs are divided into the major primary HAs (no other causative etiology), secondary HAs (a causative etiology is established by history or other means), and "cranial neuralgias, central and primary facial pain, and other disorders." (see Table 56-2)

The primary HAs include migraine, tension type, cluster, and "other primary HAs." Chronic daily HA or chronic types of HA as mentioned earlier are defined as HAs occurring for more than 15 days/month and for a period longer than 3 months not explained by medication overuse or withdrawal. PTHs and whiplash HAs are considered secondary HAs and are categorized in Table 56-3.

Acute and chronic HA are distinguished from one another by a 3-month threshold of duration: acute PTH is less than 3 months; chronic is more than 3 months. PTH is further subdivided into those attributed to MTBI or those attributed to moderate-to-severe injury. In all cases, the HA begins within 7 days of injury or "regaining consciousness." These definitions are controversial from several perspectives. The time to onset and the 3-month distinctions between acute and chronic may be considered arbitrary (3,37,38) and inconsistent with recent literature. Further, these classifications do not address the pathophysiology and presumably consequent treatment approaches (39). Another criticism of the IHS classification is that it is unclear about the pathobiology of many types of HA; as an example, TTH appears to be a common clinical presentation for PTH. Yet, in IHS literature, muscular pain and cervical pain are described as *associated* with TTH but never defined as the most likely pain generator. In addition, there is a separate classification for cervicogenic HA.

Clinical Classification of Post-Traumatic Headache

A clinical classification system for PTH also relies on history and physical examination but would emphasize the identification of primary (as well as associated) pain generators to better guide the clinician in management strategies. Historically, the major clinical classifications of PTH have, in order of prevalence, included musculoskeletal PTH, "vascular" or migraine-like HA, neuralgia/neuritic HA, and "other" PTH, including dysautonomic HAs (40,41). More recently, probable migraine or migraine HA has been reported as a domi-

TABLE 56–2 International Headache Society Classification: Primary Headaches

1. **Migraine**
   - 1.1 Migraine without aura
   - 1.2 Migraine with aura
     - 1.2.1 Migraine with typical aura
     - 1.2.2 Migraine with prolonged aura
     - 1.2.3 Familial hemiplegic migraine
     - 1.2.4 Basilar migraine
     - 1.2.5 Migraine aura without headache
     - 1.2.6 Migraine with acute onset aura
   - 1.3 Ophthalmoplegic migraine
   - 1.4 Retinal migraine
   - 1.5 Childhood periodic syndromes that may be precursors to or associated with migraine
     - 1.5.1 Benign paroxysmal vertigo of childhood
     - 1.5.2 Alternating hemiplegia of childhood
   - 1.6 Complications of migraine
     - 1.6.1 Status migrainous
     - 1.6.2 Migrainous infarction
   - 1.7 Migrainous disorder not fulfilling above criteria

2. **Tension-type headaches**
   - 2.1 Episodic tension-type headache
     - 2.1.1. Episodic tension-type headache associated with disorder of pericranial muscles
     - 2.1.2. Episodic tension-type headache unassociated with disorder of pericranial muscles
   - 2.2 Chronic tension-type headache
     - 2.2.1. Chronic tension-type headache associated with disorder of pericranial muscles
     - 2.2.2. Chronic tension-type headache unassociated with disorder of pericranial muscles
   - 2.3 Headache of the tension-type not fulfilling above criteria.

3. **Cluster headache and chronic paroxysmal hemicrania**
   - 3.1 Cluster Headache
     - 3.1.1. Cluster headache periodicity undetermined
     - 3.1.2. Episodic cluster headache
     - 3.1.3. Chronic cluster headache
       - 3.1.3.1. Unremitting from onset
       - 3.1.3.2. Evolved from episodic
   - 3.2 Chronic paroxysmal hemicrania
   - 3.3 Cluster headache-like disorder not fulfilling above criteria

4. **Miscellaneous headaches unassociated with structural lesion**
   - 4.1 Idiopathic stabbing headache
   - 4.2 External compression headache
   - 4.3 Cold stimulus headache
     - 4.3.1 External application of a cold stimulus
     - 4.3.2 Ingestion of a cold stimulus
   - 4.4 Benign cough headache
   - 4.5 Benign exertional headache
   - 4.6 Headache associated with sexual activity
     - 4.6.1 Dull type
     - 4.6.2 Explosive type
     - 4.6.3 Postural type

nant phenotype, especially among military personnel with blast injury (2,42). A clinical classification specific to PTH (albeit not all inclusive) is suggested in Table 56-4. Of course, there are other HAs within the IHS classification system not specific to PTH that are also potentially relevant. Perhaps, chief among these are HAs attributed to substances or their withdrawal, especially medication-overuse headaches (MOH).

CLINICAL APPROACH TO POST-TRAUMATIC HEADACHE

Tension Type/Musculoskeletal

TTH is the most common form of primary HA and historically, is the dominant type in PTH (43). It is also an ill defined and heterogeneous type of HA, which can be problematic for diagnosis (44). The IHS classifies TTH into 4 types:

1. infrequent episodic TTH,
2. frequent episodic TTH,
3. chronic tension-type headache (CTTH), and
4. probable TTH (as opposed to MOH, or other type of HAs)

The pathophysiology of TTH is controversial in its connection to head trauma. Unlike migraine, it tends to be the least addressed type of by health professionals and researchers. This is especially true for episodic tension type headaches (ETTH), where pain is typically mild to moderate, and there may be insufficient associated impairment for the patient to consider medical attention. CTTH, however, defined as 15 days/month or more of TTH, tend to cause more debilitation and therefore are addressed more frequently by health professions (11).

The typical presentation of TTH is as bilateral head pain of pressing quality (i.e., like a tight hat) and mild-to-moderate intensity. Notably, there is a lack of symptoms more commonly associated with other types of HAs, such as nausea and vomiting. TTH also does not appear to be aggravated by routine physical activity, nor does it appear to be associated with photophobia or sensitivity towards sound. Pericranial tenderness also appears characteristic in TTH and more prominent and sustained in CTTH than in ETTH.

When diagnosing TTH, one of the challenges that health professionals face is the difficulty in differentiating it from other types of HAs. Many patients classified with ETTH may actually have a mild form of a migraine HA without the aura. In children, the symptoms associated with both TTH and migraine tended to occur simultaneously (45). In the Spectrum Study, undertaken to determine the efficacy of sumatriptan for different types of HAs, 71% of patients initially diagnosed with TTHs had their diagnosis changed to migraine after a review of HA diaries (46). The diagnosis of CTTH is more straightforward because patients tend to have the HA for much longer periods without migraneous features, although this may not always be the case. MOH can also be misconstrued as CTTH. Typically, if a patient presents with the criteria of CTTH with simple analgesic use more than 15 days/month for more than 3 months, or ergotamine, opioid, triptans, or any other combination of medications for more than 10 days/month for more than 3 months, they may have MOH. CTTH and MOH must both be consid-

TABLE 56–3 Treatment of PTH

HEADACHE SUBCLASS	PHARMACOLOGICAL TREATMENT (EPISODIC)	PHARMACOLOGICAL PROPHYLAXIS	OTHER THERAPIES

Migraine	**Abortive**
	APAP/ASA/Caffeine 325/325/65
	• Naproxen 250–500 mg
	• Ibuprofen 200–800 mg
	Triptans
	• Almotriptan 6.25 to 12.5 mg orally
	• Eletriptan 20 to 40 mg orally
	• Frovatriptan 2.5 mg orally
	• Naratriptan 1 to 2.5 mg orally
	• Rizatriptan 5 to 10 mg
	• Sumatriptan
	  • Intranasal 5 to 20 mg
	  • Oral 25 to 100 mg
	  • Subcutaneous 4 to 6 mg
	• Zolmitriptan
	  • intranasal 5 mg
	  • Oral 1.25 to 2.5 mg
	Combo triptan and NSAIDs
	• Sumatiptan/Naproxen 85/500 mg
	Antiemetic
	• Metoclopramide 10 mg IV every 8hrs
	• Prochlorperazine 10 mg IV
	Dexamethasone 4 to 10 mg IV one time
	  8 to 24 mg oral one time
	Ergotamine
	• DHE
	  • Intranasal 1 spray in nostril
	  • IV 0.5 to 1 mg
	  • SubQ 1 mg every hr.
	Midrin 1 to 2 capsules every 4 hrs
		TCA's
		• Amitriptyline 10–75 mg
		• Nortriptyline 10–75 mg
		SSRI
		• Fluoxetine 20–60 mg
		SNRI
		• Duloxetine 30–90 mg daily
		Beta-Blockers
		• Propranolol
		• Nadolol 40–120 mg daily
		• Metoprolol 35–100 mg
		CCB
		• Verapamil 180–360 mg
		• Amlodipine 5–10 mg
		Anticonvulsants
		• Valproic Acid 500–1500 mg
		• Topriamate 75–100 mg
		• Gabapentin 900–3600 mg
		• Zonisamide 300–500 mg
		• Magnesium 600 mg divided daily
		• Vitamin B complex dosages vary
		• Cyproheptadine 4–12 mg daily
		• Tizanidine 4–16 mg daily
		• Onobotulinum A toxin injections 100–150 Units (for chronic type migraine headaches)
			Acupuncture
			Sphenopalatine block

Cervicogenic	TCA's Anticonvulsants Muscle relaxants NSAIDS		Manual therapy Occipital Nerve blocks/ liberation Radiofrequency Neurotomy
Tension	NSAIDS, Acetaminophen	TCA's Topiramate, Ononbotulinum A toxin injections for Chronic type headaches (questionable)	Low load Crainocervical mobilization
Trigeminal Neuralgia	Carbamazepine 200–400 mg bid Baclofen		Microvascular decompression Partial trigeminal rhizotomy
Medication-Overuse Headache		Topiramate	Abrupt withdrawal when using NSAID Triptans Gradual withdrawal when using opioids
Cluster Headache	SubQ or nasal administered Triptans Verapamil	Verapamil Prednisone Valproic Acid Topiramate Melatonin Ergotamine	Nasal-cannula Oxygen

Abbreviation: APAP, N-Acetyl-Para-Amino-Phenol (acetaminophen); ASA, acetylsalicylic acid (aspirin); IV, intravenous; TCAs, tricyclic antidepressants; SSRI, selective serotonin reuptake inhibitor; SNRI, serotonin norepinephrine reuptake inhibitor; CCB, calcium channel blocker.

TABLE 56–4 Clinical Classification System Specific to Post-Traumatic Headaches

1. Musculoskeletal PTH
   a. Tension-Type
   b. Myofascial
   c. Cervicogenic PTH
   d. Craniomandibular PTH
2. Post-traumatic Migraine/Probable Migraine
3. Neuralgias/Neuritic
   a. Certain cranial neuralgias
4. PTH from intracranial pressure abnormalities
   a. High intracranial pressure including tension pneumocephalus
   b. Low intracranial pressure
   c. Syndrome of the Trephined including post-craniectomy headache
5. Dysautonomic Headaches
6. Blast Injury Headaches

Abbreviation: PTH, post-traumatic headache.

ered for at least 2 months while reduction of pain medication use is undertaken. MOH is delineated from CTTH by improvement of HA by decrease in medication use (for more information, see Medication-Overuse Headache section in this chapter) (47).

Epidemiology

Population based studies suggest 1-year prevalence rates of 38.3% for episodic TTH and 2.2% for CTTH (48). Women have a higher prevalence than men, but this disparity is not as great as in migraine and tends to diminish with age.

Pathophysiology

The mechanism by which TTH generates pain is complex, as is the understanding of how ETTH evolves to CTTH. Recent investigations have began to clarify the role of activated peripheral nociception from pericranial myofascial tissues, related to episodic TTH, leading to central sensitization of the spinal dorsal sensory afferent nerves and trigeminal nucleus caudalis, producing CTTH. Human and animal models have confirmed this anatomical convergence of dorsal nerve roots and trigeminal afferents to the trigeminal caudate nucleus, which appears to be a culprit in different types of HAs, not just CTTH. It was also found that patients with CTTH tended to have decreased pressure pain thresholds in the shoulder, neck and trapezius regions, in comparison to patient without CTTH (49). Bendtsen (50) established a TTH pain model in which the progression of ETTH to CTTH is caused by the activation of dormant central pathways because of prolonged peripheral nociceptive inputs, possibly provoked by the liberation of algogenic substances at the periphery, such as bradykinin and substance P from pericranial myofascial tender points. The presence of prolonged peripheral inputs is considered to be a mechanism of major importance for the conversion of ETTH into CTTH.

Muscle pain either because of injury or strain is produced mainly by noxious stimuli that lead to increased synthesis and release of endogenous algogenic substances, such as serotonin, bradykinin, histamine, or prostaglandins. Such stimuli may cause the antidromic release of neuropeptides

from the pain nerve endings C fibers, such as CGRP, substance P, or neurokinin A (51). Liberation of algogenic substances would lower tissue pH and then activate the arachidonic acid cascade leading to further peripheral nociceptive sensitization. Sensitization of peripheral nociceptors would cause spontaneous neuronal discharge and a lowered threshold to stimuli that normally provoke pain, as well as increased firing in response to non-noxious stimuli that are not ordinarily perceived as painful. It also appears that there is an activation of silent peripheral nociceptors that might result in a change in the stimulus response system. This abnormal pain stimulus response is seen in both patients with chronic myofascial pain syndrome and in patients with CTTH (52). Patients with CTTH have increased peripheral nociceptive sensitization, as well as central sensitization, as opposed to ETTH where central sensitization does not play a role.

This prolonged peripheral nociceptive input leads to central sensitization, which can alter pain perception significantly. In this sensitized state, previously ineffective low threshold Aδ fibers input to nociceptive DH neurons may become effective. Pain then could be generated by the low-threshold Aβ fibers. In addition, the response to activation of high-threshold afferents would be exaggerated. These afferent Aβ fibers, which normally inhibit Aδ and C fibers by presynaptic mechanisms in the DH, will, on the contrary, stimulate the nociceptive second-order neurons. Therefore, the effect of Aδ and C fiber stimulation of the nociceptive DH neurons will be promoted, and the receptive fields of the DH neurons will be expanded (53).

When testing Bendsten's pain model, Ashina et al. found no difference in change in interstitial concentration of adenosine-5'-triphospate (ATP), glutamate, bradikinin, prostaglandin E$_2$, glucose, pyruvate, and urea from baseline to exercise and postexercise periods between nonspecific tender points of CTTH subjects and controls (54). Authors of that study concluded that *tender points* in CTTH subjects are not responsible for liberation of algogenic substances in the periphery. On the other hand, in a similar study, significantly higher levels of algogenic substances have been found in active myofascial *trigger points* of patients with CTTH (55). This led to an updated pain model by Fernández-de-las-Peñas et al. for TTH based on peripheral sensitization of muscle nociceptors provoked by myofascial trigger points, not tender points, leading to central sensitization and CTTH (56).

Simons et al. described the referred pain patterns from different trigger points in several head and neck muscles, which have the potential to refer pain to the head. These include upper trapezius, temporalis, sternocleidomastoid, splenius capitis, and suboccipital muscles (28). Tender points typical cause regional tenderness with irritation and palpation but not referred pain. Trigger points are hyperirritable areas that illicit pain with palpation and cause referred pain beyond the region of point of palpation (see Figures 56-1–56-4).

A recently described pain model suggests that trigger points located in head and neck muscles innervated by C1–C3 including upper trapezius, sternocleidomastoid, suboccipital muscles, or by the trigeminal nerve, such as the temporalis and masseter, are responsible for the peripheral nociceptive input and could produce a continuous afferent barrage into the trigeminal nerve nucleus caudalis. Connections between afferents innervating deep structures and second-order neurons could be altered by these nociceptive afferent inputs from muscle trigger points. Convergent synaptic connections on DH neurons, which are not usually functional, could be activated if nociceptive input reaches the DH. Changes in size and shape of peripheral receptive fields and the formation of new receptive fields would occur if nociceptive barrage from muscle trigger points is maintained during time. This would result in temporal and spatial integration of neuron signals and might be one of the reasons for the central sensitization in CTTH (56).

Trigger points are common in both patients with ETTH and CTTH, but central sensitization is not seen in ETTH, especially if they are infrequent. Central sensitization of DH and trigeminal nucleus, which is associated with CTTH, is believed to be caused by active trigger points. It is also believed that patients with ETTH have more latent than active myofascial trigger points, which do not lead to central sensitization. However, it was found that there were an equal number of active trigger points in the temporalis muscle and trapezius mucles of those who had classifications for both ETTH and CTTH (57). This suggests that active trigger points are not a consequence of central sensitization. These findings call into question whether central sensitization plays a role in ETTH and to what extent. After injections of algogenic substances into the trapezius muscles, patients with ETTH report substantially more local pain than healthy controls did, but none of the patients with ETTH developed HA (54).

The underlying mechanism for central sensitization still remains unclear. Magnesium levels have been noted to be abnormal not only in migraine HA, but also in CTTH, as well as which may contribute to central sensitization by facilitation of N-Methyl-D-aspartate (NMDA) receptor function (43). NO has also been thought to play a role in TTH, possibly contributing to sensitization of perivascular sensory afferent nerves. Trials of CTTH patients have shown reductions of HA and pericranial tenderness when L-NG methylarginine hydrochloride, an inhibitor of NO synthase, was given (58).

CGRP is associated with migraine-type and cluster-type HA but is typically not elevated in CTTH; however, in patients with CTTH with pulsating pain, they were (59). This suggests that patients who fulfill the criteria of TTH with an additional symptom of pulsating pain may also have pathophysiological criteria for migraine HA.

Diagnosis

As mentioned earlier in this chapter, there are various forms of TTH as listed in the IHS criteria; however, none of the criteria are mandatory in establishing the diagnosis of TTH. Typically, TTH is diagnosed by the absence of other symptoms that are characteristic of other primary HAs. TTH, especially ETTH, can share the same symptomology of other types of HAs, such as mild migraine without aura and cervicogenic HA. TTH is a clinical diagnosis without an approved laboratory, electrodiagnostic, or imaging study to confirm its existence. (see Table 56-5)

Treatment

CTTH, as well as frequent ETTHs, are difficult to treat given the different possible pathophysiological causes. Thus, these different types of HAs may require different types of thera-

TABLE 56–5 Derived From International Headache Society for Tension Headache

2.1. Infrequent episodic tension-type headache
   2.1.1. Infrequent episodic tension-type headache associated with pericranial tenderness
   2.1.2. Infrequent episodic tension-type headache not associated with pericranial tenderness

   Diagnostic criteria:
   A: At least 10 episodes occurring on <1 day per month on average (<12 days per year)
   B: Headache lasting from 30 minutes to 7 days
   C: Headache has at least two of the following characteristics:
     • bilateral location
     • pressing/tightening (non-pulsating) quality
     • mild or moderate intensity
     • not aggravated by routine physical activity such as walking or climbing stairs
   D: Both of the following:
     • no nausea or vomiting (anorexia may occur)
     • no more than one of photophobia or phonophobia
   E: Not attributed to another disorder

2.2. Frequent episodic tension-type headache
   2.2.1. Frequent episodic tension-type headache associated with pericranial tenderness
   2.2.2. Frequent episodic tension-type headache not associated with pericranial tenderness

   Diagnostic Criteria: At least 10 episodes occurring on ≥1 but <15 days per month for at least 3 months (≥12 and <180 days per year) and fulfilling criteria B-D

2.3. Chronic tension-type headache
   2.3.1. Chronic tension-type headache associated with pericranial tenderness
   2.3.2. Chronic tension-type headache not associated with pericranial tenderness

   Diagnostic Criteria: Headache occurring on ≥15 days per month on average for >3 months (≥180 days per year) and fulfilling criteria B-D

2.4. Probable tension-type headache. Please see IHHS-classification.org for criteria, for purposes of time and space was not placed in here
   2.4.1. Probable infrequent episodic tension-type headache
   2.4.2. Probable frequent episodic tension-type headache
   2.4.3. Probable chronic tension-type headache

pies and modalities in succession or in combination. Ideally, management of ETTH should be aimed at preventing them from converting to CTTH. Nonsteroidal anti-inflammatory drugs (NSAIDs) have historically been the drug of choice in treating all subtypes of TTH. Aspirin (500 mg or 1,000 mg) is more effective than placebo for the relief of acute TTH; the efficacy of aspirin is comparable to that of Tylenol (500 mg or 1,000 mg). In most trials, however, simple analgesics were inferior to NSAIDs (60). Ibuprofen is typically favored over naproxen given that it has fewer gastrointestinal (GI) side effects. Lumiracoxib, a cyclooxygenase (COX)-2 inhibitor, was efficacious in patients with TTH at 200 mg and 400 mg doses in a double-blind, double-dummy, placebo-controlled trial (61). Toradol was also noted to be effective in acute treatment of TTH.

Prophylactic Pharmacotherapy

TCAs have historically been used for CTTH prophylaxis, but there are very few methodologically sound studies to support this therapy. There are few clinical trials with TCAs, and not all of them showed superiority over placebo (62). Nevertheless, in clinical practice, TCAs are typically a first-line medication for CTTH and frequent ETTH. Amitriptyline, 25mg at bedtime, is typically used. Nortriptyline has fewer side effects than amitriptyline, and clomipramine has even more side effects associated with its degree of anticholinergic activity. Tricyclic treatment takes time, and an interesting trial was done wherein a 3-week boost course of tizanadine 4 mg daily with amitriptyline 20 mg/day. This trial revealed a beneficial effect with 52% vs 40% improvement of HA frequency at 3 months (63). Selective serotonin reuptake inhibitors (SSRIs) have *not* been proven to be effective in the treatment of TTH; however, mirtazapine was noted to be effective in TTH at 15–30 mg, but side effects included weight gain and fatigue. (64). These results may suggest the mechanism by which TCAs treat TTH may be related to inhibition of norepinephrine (NE) reuptake and/or NMDA antagonism, rather than the inhibition of serotonin reuptake. Topiramate, an anticonvulsant used in migraine prophylaxis, has also shown to be effective in CTTH (65) but requires confirmation in a randomized clinical trial (RCT) and may produce intolerable cognitive side effects. Recently, botulinum toxin type A injections have been used in the treatment of CTTH; however, they appear to play no role in treating ETTH. (66). Cognitive behavioral exercises and relaxation therapies have shown to be effective in treating CTTH, especially in combination with pharmacotherapy (67).

A systematic review of RCTs with physiotherapy and spinal manipulation in patients with TTH showed insufficient evidence to support or refute the effectiveness of such techniques (68). In a study by Boline et al., spinal manipulation therapy in patients with CTTH was as effective as or more effective in treating CTTH than treatment with amitriptyline (69). However, in an article establishing chiropractic guidelines and recommendations for treating HAs, these results were refuted noting the trial was inadequately controlled with imbalances in the number of subject clinician encounters between study groups, and results from manipulative therapy group were hard to interpret in isolation because premanipulative soft tissue therapy (70). The article suggested, according to their review, that low-load craniocervical mobilization (e.g., Thera-Band, resistive exercise systems) was better and therefore recommended for longer term (i.e., 6 months) management of patients with ETTH or CTTH.

In examining acupuncture, most trials had small samples sizes with questionable results. One trial showed clinically relevant results when comparing acupuncture to patients who had not been treated; interestingly, those in the placebo group who had sham acupuncture also had beneficial effects (71).

Cervicogenic Headache

Cervicogenic HA is defined as head pain referred from the spine. In terms of anatomical and physiological properties,

it may be the most well understood form of HA. The pathophysiology is well understood and has been induced in otherwise healthy patients. This pathophysiology involves the convergence of between cervical and trigeminal afferents in the trigeminal-cervical nucleus. (see Figures 56-5 and 56-7)

Pathophysiology

Nociceptive afferents from the C1, C2, and C3 spinal nerves converge onto second-order neurons that also receive afferents from adjacent cervical nerves and from the first division of the trigeminal nerve (V), via the spinal tract of V (75). Pain from the lateral atlanto-axial joint (C1–C2) tends to be focused on the occipital and suboccipital regions and tends to be referred to the vertex, orbit, and ear. Pain from the C2–C3 zygapophyseal joint also occurs in the occipital region and spreads across the parietal region to the frontal region and orbit. Pain from the C3–C4 joint can be referred to the head but is more commonly focused in the upper and lateral cervical region (72).

Diagnosis

There are 2 points of view as to how to properly diagnose cervicogenic HA. Physicians in Europe support the diagnosis by clinical criteria alone, but the North American and Australian view has fostered the belief that the diagnosis can only be established with application of controlled diagnostic blocks. The clinical criteria for diagnosis of cervicogenic HA consists of a unilateral HA associated with evidence of cervical involvement in the form of provocation of pain by movement of the neck or by pressing the neck and concurrent pain in the neck, shoulder, and arm, as well as reduced ROM of the neck (73). One concern about diagnosis with clinical criteria alone is that it may not effectively differentiate HAs of cervical origin from TTH, myofascial pain, and migraine. The diagnostic criterion proposed by the IHS reflects this and supports the assertion that a confirmed cervical source must be found, which can done with full reliability.

Treatment

No pharmacological therapies have been effective in treating cervicogenic HA. Manual therapy articles regarding treatment of cervicogenic HA have shown inconsistent results. One article noted that manual therapy was not efficacious even in conjunction with exercise (74,75).

Occipital nerve injections and liberations have also been seen as therapeutic but only for the short term because pain returned after 6 months (76). Another approach is radiofrequency neurotomy. The rationale for this procedure is that if HA can be relieved temporarily by controlled diagnostic blocks of the nerve (or nerves) that innervate a particular cervical joint, then interrupting the pain signal along that nerve, by coagulating it, should provide long-lasting relief. It appears that this procedure is most effective when addressing the C2–C3 zygapophyseal region as opposed to lower regions of the cervical spine where trials have been found it to be ineffective (77). For patients in whom effects of diagnostic blocks indicate that the C2–C3 zygapophyseal joint is the source of pain, that joint can be denervated percutaneously by radiofrequency neurotomy of the third occipital nerve. The procedure involves placing an electrode parallel close to the nerve where it crosses the joint and using the electrode to disrupt the nerve. Under these conditions, complete relief of pain was achieved in 88% of patients, with a median duration of relief of 297 days (78).

Craniomandibular Headache

TMJ or craniomandibular syndrome may be considered a variant of musculoskeletal or tension HA and is almost always seen in conjunction with direct trauma to the craniomandibular complex. This type of HA is also frequently overlooked as a primary or contributory cause for PTH. Other nontraumatic etiologies of TMJ disorder must be investigated. These include stress or tension, dental malocclusion, and/or psychosexual abuse, the latter being a more common cause of the condition in women than in men.

There may be internal derangement of the TMJ and there is almost always a myofascial component related to the muscles of mastication (temporalis, pterygoids, or masseter). Hypothetically, there may be a biomechanical relationship between the craniocervical region, the dynamics of the TMJ, and trigeminal nociceptive processing in different craniocervical postures (79).

Often, intervention is supplemented by the use of intraoral appliances, such as occlusal splints (bite blocks) (80) and dietary changes relative to softer food consistency and jaw exercises. Nonsurgical treatment is effective in managing more than 80% of patients with craniomandibular disorders. Joint pathology may be identified with magnetic resonance imaging (MRI) and may require arthroscopic surgical intervention. Open arthrotomy or arthroplasty is rarely needed and is often associated with suboptimal outcomes (81).

Migraine/Trigemino-Neurovascular Headache

Introduction

PTM, also known as neurovascular HA or vascular HA, has become a more commonly recognized complication of TBI. As mentioned previously, Theeler et al. found that nearly 1 in 3 soldiers returning from Iraq or Afghanistan who sustained concussion during deployment met the criteria for PTH. Of these, 58% were considered migraine (10). There is still some disparity between chronic and severe PTH and when it is considered PTM because there is no specific IHS classification for PTM. Therefore, a thorough understanding of the primary HA migraine phenotype is vital to be able to appropriately diagnose and treat PTM. Patients with PTM may have a genetic predisposition to the development of migraine following trauma to either the head, brain, and/or neck (82).

Clinical Presentation

Other than by patient history, there are no other significant clinical findings that differentiate PTM from migraine as a primary HA as classified by the IHS. Migraine is defined as a primary disabling HA disorder, which is characterized by episodic attacks of HAs and associated symptoms, including possible autonomic dysfunction with or without an aura (11). There are 4 principle phases of the migraine attack, including a prodrome or premonitory phase, aura, HA, and postdrome or hangover phase (83). This section will focus primarily on the HA phase of migraine.

The HA of migraine is most likely to be described as throbbing, typically unilateral, and exacerbated by coughing, bending over, or other physical exertion. They tend to occur most often in the morning; however, can be present at any time. Although typically unilateral, it may be bilateral in as many as 40% of patients and persistently located on the same side in approximately 20% of patients (84). There may be associated nausea, vomiting, or anorexia.

Typical progression of the HA is a gradual rise and fall of the pain that usually subsides within 24 hours. The duration of HA in adults ranges from 4 to 72 hours; however, it is typically of shorter duration in children, with ranges from 4 to 48 hours.

The pain associated with these HAs may in some instances have a radiating quality. Cold may help, but heat usually makes the pain worse. Patients will typically prefer a dark and quiet environment because photophobia and phonophobia may be present (this may be associated with the prodrome). Raskin et al. found that in approximately 42% migraneurs, there may also be short bouts of sharp pain, which are described as "icepick like" and may be a manifestation of migraine (85).

Patients with basilar migraine, also known as Bickerstaff syndrome (86), usually present with symptoms of vertebrobasilar insufficiency (VBI), which may precede the classic bi-occipital headache (BM) (although BM may be ancephalgic). The most common symptoms are dizziness and vertigo, although ataxia, tinnitus, decreased hearing, nausea and vomiting, dysarthria, diplopia, loss of balance, bilateral paresthesias or paresis, altered consciousness, syncope, and sometimes loss of consciousness may also be observed (87). This migraine variant is observed most frequently in adolescent girls and young women and has been reported following cervical whiplash injury (88).Vasoconstrictive medications, such as triptans, are contraindicated in such patients.

Proposed Pathophysiology

The precise trigger for migraine (or vascular/neurovascular) HA remains obscure and controversial; this is especially true in relation to PTM. The title of vascular HA stems from the vascular theory of pathophysiology of migraine. In the first edition of the classic publication, *Headache and Other Head Pain* by Wolff in 1948, the vascular theory was arguably best explained. He described 3 observations: (*a*) distension of extracranial vessels that became pulsatile during migraine attacks, (*b*) stimulation of intracranial vessels induced a HA, and (*c*) vasoconstrictor treatments improved the HA while vasodilators induced it (89,90). Over several years, however, the use of modern imaging technology, such as single-photon emission computed tomography (SPECT), has allowed researchers to identify that there were not consistent blood flow patterns (among other findings, such as regional cerebral blood flow [rCBF]), thus making this vascular theory alone inconsistent as the sole pathophysiological process of migraine (90). This led to further theories including that of neurovascular origin.

Another theory introduced by Leão in 1944 involves the association of the aura to the HA of migraine and is referred to as *cortical spreading depression* (91). This theory is said to be a spreading depolarization of glial and neuronal origin across the cortex, which has been stated to initiate the aura (92), induce matrix metallopeptidase 9 (MMP-9) activation, and upregulation leading to change in blood-brain barrier permeability (93) and ultimately activate the trigeminal afferent nerves (94,95).

In PTM following the injury, the trigeminal afferent system eventually becomes sensitized by a sterile inflammatory "soup" that includes excitatory neurotransmitters, NO, histamine, and prostaglandin E_2. This sensitization then produces vasodilatation of extracerebral vessels, including those in the meninges, and accentuates the inflammatory response. The pounding HA of migraine appears to originate from dilatation of large cranial vessels innervated by the trigeminovascular system and the associated release of CGRP, substance P, and neurokinin A from trigeminal neurons (sensory C fibers). Sensitized trigeminal afferents may provide nociceptive input from simple mechanical stimulation of the dilated vessels, akin to a vascular allodynia. Hemicranial allodynia may occur after central sensitization takes place. This aforementioned sterile inflammation and compounded inflammatory response also leads to plasma extravasation.

Plasma extravasation is inhibited by multiple agents, including but not limited to vessel constrictors, such as ergots, sumatriptan, and other selective 5-hydroxytryptamine $_{1B/D}$ (5-HT$_{1B/D}$) agonists. It is suggested that the serotonin (5-HT$_1$) agonists are one of the most important receptors in this pathway as recognized in the late 1980s (96,97). Whereas stimulation of 5-HT$_{1B}$ and 5HT$_{1D}$ receptors abort acute migraine (e.g., triptans), 5-HT$_{2A}$ stimulation increases neuronal excitability and potentiates nociceptive transmission. The increased density of 5-HT$_{2A}$ receptors could lead to an "excitable brain," a hyperalgesic state, with increased HA frequency and severity. It also underscores the antagonism of 5-HT$_2$, which is a common mechanism underlying preventative medications in migraine management (98). 5-HT$_{1B}$ receptors are also located in the trigeminal nucleus caudalis, which when stimulated (by 5-HT$_{1B}$ agonists or triptans), may decrease the HA by inhibiting the trigeminal nociceptive mechanism (99).

Diagnosis

The diagnosis of PTM depends on a thorough patient history and concise clinical findings. Once this information is obtained, the patient may be matched to the classification criteria as published by the aforementioned IHS. At this time, there remained no specific diagnostic tests available for migraine, but it must be carefully distinguished from other types of HA as described in this chapter. In this regard, there are several overlapping findings between TTH and migraine, but some characteristics that are more predictive of migraine include nausea/vomiting, phonophobia, photophobia, and exacerbation with physical activity, as stated in a comprehensive review of features of primary HA syndromes by Smetana (100).

Because there are no specific diagnostic tests available, the use of neuroimaging is crucial in determining acute pathologic findings in the setting of sudden onset. Although clinical findings and history may point to a classification of migraine, there are specific situations that may warrant neuroimaging. From this standpoint, migraine is not necessarily a diagnosis of exclusion, but other etiologies must be excluded. These situations include, but are not limited to, sudden severe onset of HA (potential for subarachnoid hemorrhage), atypical findings that complicate classification, or abnormal/focal neurological findings (101).

Treatment

The aim of treatment of migraine is to prevent or reduce the frequency of the onset of HA (prophylactic treatment) and/or to abort a HA rapidly should it occur (as well as sustain the HA relief once aborted). To effectively manage migraines, it is important to assess the impact that this migraine has on the daily living of the individual and the frequency of migraines that the individual sustains. With this information, it will be easier to determine the most appropriate treatment.

Pharmacologic treatment of migraine is divided into abortive and prophylactic medications for the migraine itself and symptomatic treatment for associated complaints, such as nausea and vomiting. In many cases, particularly in those patients with more frequent and severe HAs, a combination of these medications may be necessary. Abortive or acute treatment should only be used at maximum of 2–3 days/week (102). There have been many different pharmacologic approaches used throughout history; thus, this section will focus primarily on more modern, common place treatments in practice today.

Abortive medications may include NSAIDs, ergot derivatives (including dihydroergotamine or DHE), triptans, parenteral atypical antipsychotics (103), and/or narcotics, among other drugs. Many of the drugs are used for their vasoconstrictive properties (ergot derivatives) even though extracerebral vasodilation is a secondary phenomenon in migraine. It is important to note they have significant systemic or cardiac side effects. If patients experience chronic daily HA and use abortive analgesics, they are at risk for developing rebound HA or MOH. Caffeine overuse may also contribute to patients becoming refractory to abortive medications containing this substance.

NSAIDs may be beneficial for the treatment of acute nondisabling migraine. Studies indicate that ibuprofen, aspirin, and COX-2 inhibitors are more effective than placebo for acute migraine but not as effective as the combination of aspirin, acetaminophen, and caffeine (AAC) (104–108). Several other NSAIDs have been studied, with similar efficacy. The U.S. Headache Consortium recommendations indicate that several options exist with the analgesics. Aspirin, naproxen sodium, ibuprofen, and diclofenac-K are appropriate for a nondisabling migraine. If parenteral administration is required, then intravenous (IV) or intramuscular (IM) ketorolac may be used. AAC should be given for acute migraine (102).

Next, selective serotonin (5-HT$_1$) agonists continue to be used widely because they hold several advantages for treatment of the acute migraine. Lipton et al. demonstrated in a review that through multiple studies, the oral triptans have more advantages because of selective pharmacology, evidence-based dosing recommendations, and well-established efficacy (109). There are 7 triptans that have been reviewed and recommended for the treatment of acute migraine by the U.S. Headache Consortium. Those include the first developed 5-HT$_{1B/1D}$ inhibitor, sumatriptan, followed by the second generation triptans: almotriptan, eletriptan, frovatriptan, naratriptan, rizatriptan, and zolmitriptan.

These are all 5-HT$_{1B}$/$_{1D}$ agonist but differ in pharmacokinetics. However, triptans, as a class, may be ineffective if their use is delayed and allodynia develops (110). Stimulation of various analgesic receptors in the brainstem affects 5-HT. Short-term use (including acetaminophen) increases 5-HT release from raphe spinal pathways and has a therapeutic effect. However, long-term use may lead to 5-HT depletion and upregulation of 5-HT$_{2A}$ receptors, particularly. Triptans block the release of CGRP at 5-HT$_{1B}$ and 5-HT$_{1D}$ receptors. However, as mentioned previously, stimulation of 5-HT$_{2A}$ receptors may promote migraine. TCAs may block these receptors (111).

Preventative

TCAs are considered a prophylactic migraine treatment. They inhibit the high-affinity reuptake of NE and/or 5-HT and decreased 5-HT$_2$ receptor binding without affecting the 5-HT$_1$ binding sites (102,112). However, there is a propensity for TCAs to cause adverse effects because of their multiple interactions with other neurotransmitters. Particularly in PTM, caution should be observed because of the TCAs ability to lower the seizure threshold. Thus using TCAs may require individualized dosing and treatment plans.

Another preventative medication that fairly and widely used is topiramate. This drug was originally used as an anticonvulsant but is approved for treatment of migraine. In a study by Storer and Goadsby, it was shown to inhibit neuronal firing within the trigeminocervical complex, thus preventing migraine initiation (113). Topirimate has the potential to produce significant cognitive impairments; hence, it must be used with considerable circumspection in TBI. Other prophylactic migraine medications include some NSAIDs, beta-blockers, calcium channel blockers, and depakote as more traditional treatments. Naturopathic agents, such as butterbur and feverfew can also be considered, as can nutritional therapies, such as B-complex vitamins and magnesium supplementation (114).

Again, because of central overlap of primary nociceptive afferents involved in true vascular HA and those related to cervical sensory nerves, the patient may present with a combination of vascular, neuralgic, and/or musculoskeletal HA, all of which may require treatment. Cervical nociceptive input may also promulgate migraine through the trigeminocervical complex (115) and therefore must be addressed as part and parcel of comprehensive migraine assessment and treatment (116).

Botulinum toxin has also been used to treat migraine HA (117). Botulinum toxin may exert this effect not only through muscle relaxation but through inhibiting release of sensitizing neurotransmitters, such as glutamate and substance P. Current research with botulinum toxin seems to be focusing on specific HA subtypes specifically chronic daily HA (118). There was, however, a large study recently known as the Phase 3 REsearch Evaluating Migraine Prophylaxis Therapy trial (PREEMPT), which was a multicenter 24-week randomized, double-blind phase followed by a 32-week open-label phase focused on onabotulinumtoxinA (Botox) as HA prophylaxis in adults with chronic migraine. The primary endpoint was a change in the frequency of the HAs over the 24-week period. The results indicate that onabotulinumtoxinA is an effective prophylactic treatment (118).

There is clearly some relative crossover of treatment modalities between different types of PTH. In 1909, Greenfield Sluder published reported unilateral facial pain and overactivity of parasympathetics with the sphenopalatine ganglion (SPG), which was termed sphenopalatine neuralgia (or Meckel neuralgia) (120). Since that was published, there have been multiple associations with this neuralgia, including HA. In 1927, Sluder proposed a treatment of an intranasal SPG block, which involved intranasal local anaesthetic followed by injection of silver nitrate, formaldehyde, and phenol (121). This treatment was shown to have several risks, which has led to modification of the techniques and solutions by multiple clinicians still being used today.

The SPG (one of the parasympathetic ganglia) is located rather superficially in the pterygopalatine fossa just anterior to the pterygoid canal. Blockade of the SPG is thought to inhibit the inhabiting cell bodies of postganglionic parasympathetic neurons, as well as postganglionic sympathetic neurons and sensory afferent branches of the trigeminal nerve (V$_2$), which pass through the ganglion (122). Anatomically, these specific neurons supply parasympathetic outflow to the eye and sinuses. Overactivity of these, as well as the traversing sympathetics, has been thought to be contributory to the manifestation of cluster headaches (CHs). The efferents from the SPG are thought to supply the meninges and dura and subsequently play a role in vasodilatation and inflammation, leading to the initiation of migraine (123).

Multiple studies have shown efficacy in resolution of CHs. Devoghel reported up to 85% resolution of associated pain and parasympathetic symptoms (124). Other approaches/techniques have been proposed as well, such as a transoral approach, endoscopic approach, and lateral infratemporal approach, as well as blocking via ablation instead of solely chemical neurolysis and/or anaesthetic.

Although no data have shown any isolated study of PTHs, there was a case report by Shah and Racz showing long-term relief of PTH in a patient following pulsed radiofrequency lesioning of the SPG. This suggests potential similarity of effectiveness in treatment of primary HA and PTH (125).

In addition to SPG blocks, there has been data published to indicate that SPG stimulation (using electrical stimulation) has had some efficacy in resolution of chronic cluster headache (CCH) and migraines (for acute attacks), although current available data are limited (123).

SPG blockade is not a new treatment, but its efficacy in HA management, particularly CH and migraine, is still controversial.

Neuralgias/Neuromas

With injury to the head, whether traumatic or surgical, there may be associated injury to the nerves innervating the scalp, musculature, and periosteum. The injured nerve may be a small extension of a larger nerve and may be trapped in scar tissue, such as is a characteristic of a neuroma. In this case, the pain is very localized and sensitive to pressure. It is characterized by the patient as stinging, sharp, or lancinating. Examination of the scalp may reveal the specific site. The diagnosis of a neuroma is confirmed by palpatory exam; it may be further confirmed by elimination of the discomfort through site specific injection of local anaesthetic. Care must be taken in areas adjacent to craniectomy or near major blood vessels. Treatment may be effected through the use of modalities, most specifically cold (icing of the area) or through pharmacological means. Systemic medications that impact peripheral neuralgias include NSAIDs, TCAs, other antidepressants (serotonin-norepinephrine reuptake inhibitors [SNRIs] > SSRIs), or anticonvulsants, especially carbamazepine, gabapentin, or pregabalin. Topical treatments include anaesthetic ointments or creams or the use of pepper-based counter irritants. Topical agents for neuropathic pain may include TCAs, local anesthetic, NSAIDs, antiepileptic drugs (AEDs), such as gabapentin, clonidine, and ketamine hydrochloride, among other agents. (For information on local and/or regional compounding pharmacies see http://www.pcab.info/find-a-pharmacy.shtml) Finally, injection with local anaesthetics and steroids may be of benefit.

In addition to neuroma, cranial neuralgias may be a cause of PTH. Pain in the distribution of the GON is unilateral and described as paroxysmal and stabbing, radiating in the distribution of the nerve from the back of the head/upper cervical area near the sagittal midline to midcranium. The lesser occipital distribution is more lateral in its distribution above the ear. Certainly, either nerve could be injured in whiplash injury or direct trauma (i.e., falls onto the back of the head). The concept that either nerve may be irritated by muscle spasm or where it crosses the nuchal ridge is controversial (72). Furthermore, injury or dysfunction in the upper cervical joints may mimic the distribution of greater or lesser occipital neuralgia (cervicogenic HA), although the pain in this situation is typically described as deep and aching. Certain posterior neck muscles may also have referred pain patterns similar to GON referred pain. GON blocks have been used in the adjunctive treatment of other HA types, such as migraine and CH (29,126,127). It is conjectured that this may relate to the overlap in receptive fields for different peripheral afferents in the "dorsal horn" area of the upper cervical spinal cord and the spinal tract of the trigeminal nerve. Pain from GON may also radiate behind the ipsilateral eye. Treatment of GON or LON may include myofascial release techniques in the upper cervical musculature or pharmacological intervention. NSAIDs, TCAs, SNRIs, and anticonvulsants may be of benefit as described for neuroma. Injection of local anaesthetic with or without steroid may be of benefit. There are different techniques championed by different authorities. Injection of medication at the egress through the fascia above the splenius may also result in a trigger point injection in that muscle. "Purists" may prefer injection along the nuchal ridge to produce an isolated nerve block. GON or LON injection may be less effective if there is a concomitant MOH. Care must be taken to avoid vascular injection or other unintended injury. If repeated blocks produce only temporary relief, consideration could be given to cryoablation or radiofrequency ablation of the nerve. A final treatment consideration is the use of occipital nerve stimulators. CH, occipital neuralgia and other HA phenotypes have been treated effectively with this form of neuromodulation (128–131). In a recent systematic review of the literature, Jasper and Hayek found that there was only limited Level IV support for the use of these devices, yet concluded occipital nerve stimulation was a "useful tool" in the treatment of chronic, severe, and presumably refractory HAs. Based on their review, it would seem that one should expect significant and expeditious reduction in pain in transformed migraine or occipital neuralgia, but the reduction in pain in CH may take several months and may be less robust. A potential for infection or lead displacement exists for this treatment modality (131). (see Figures 56-5 and 56-6).

Headache Due to Intracranial Pressure Abnormalities

Any disruption to the normal flow of cerebral spinal fluid (CSF) may produce HA. In addition, lesions causing distortion of the meninges or ventricles may have HA as a symptom. If a patient is conscious, epidural and subdural hematomas may have HA as a presenting symptom. Both may lead to raised intracranial pressure or produce traction on the meninges. Clinicians should be aware that patients who are scanned early and show no significant findings may subsequently develop HA because of extra-axial collections that produce HA because of slow venous bleeds.

Headache Due to Raised Intracranial Pressure or Distortion of Meninges

Acute obstructive hydrocephalus is unusual in TBI but occurs occasionally because of large blood clots or fragments within the cranium. In this scenario, a major pathway for CSF flow is obstructed; most commonly this is the aqueduct of Sylvius or the foramen of Luschka or Magendie. Clinically, the patient presents as acutely ill with marked change in sensorium, papilledema, nausea, and vomiting. Progressive enlargement of the blind spot may also occur, as well as sixth nerve palsies. Treatment is surgical and emergent.

Much more common is "normal pressure" hydrocephalus (NPH). Rather than an obvious obstruction, the absorption of CSF is impeded. This may be secondary to blood, infection, direct injury, or scarring reducing the capacity of the arachnoid villi to drain CSF. The clinical presentation may be insidious and is characterized by gait disturbance, cognitive decline, and incontinence. HA is typically a late symptom. The HA is often progressive, occurs on a daily basis, worse in the morning, is diffuse and constant (not pulsating), and is aggravated by coughing or straining. Treatment is via drainage of the ventricular system, typically with a shunt. Even after shunt placement, shunt under drainage may produce high pressure HAs; this fact may make the argument for using programmable shunts to allow for postinsertion adjustments in the opening pressure of the shunt.

Tension pneumocephalus may be a complication of trauma, neurosurgical intervention (including placement of a shunt or pressure monitor), or a dural tear. It is caused by entry of air into the cranium, more specifically air entering the subdural space. There may be an associated ball-valve phenomenon allowing air into the subdural space but no egress. The result is compression of the underlying parenchyma, most typically in the frontal lobes. Presumably, the pressure of the accumulated air is greater than that of the CSF in the frontal horns. Unlike nontension pneumocephalus, tension pneumocephalus is often a neurosurgical emergency. Computer tomography (CT) may demonstrate a characteristic "Mount Fuji" sign. (132,133)

Headache Due to Low CSF Pressure

The average volume of CSF is 210 ml (134). CSF formation occurs at a rate of approximately 500 ml/day. In the supine position, lumbar and cisternal pressures are essentially equal, 60–180 mm H$_2$O. In the upright position, the vertex pressure decreases and becomes negative. HA may be produced with the removal of 10% of the estimated total volume of CSF, with concomitant further reduction in the already negative vertex pressure. Symptoms of low pressure HA include the following: worse within 15 minutes of sitting or standing, improved with lying down. It is also characterized as dull, typically not lateralized. Associated symptoms may include neck stiffness, tinnitus, hyperacusis, photophobia, and nausea.

In TBI, common causes of low CSF pressure and volume include CSF leaks, shunt over drainage, lumbar puncture HA, and the syndrome of the trephined. Shunt over drainage can lead to orthostatic HA and pachymeningeal enhancement on MRI with gadolinium. CSF leaks may occur with fracture at the base of the skull and have associated rhinorrhea or otorrhea; they may also occur after neurosurgical intervention. Treatment is predicated on identifying the source of the leak and surgical patch, although some may heal spontaneously. Lumbar puncture HAs can occur in up to one-third of patients undergoing the procedure. The HA is characteristic of most low CSF volume/pressure HAs; it may be throbbing or dull, with onset usually within 2 days. The HA is clearly positional, relieved with recumbency. They may be located anywhere on the cranium, usually symmetrically, and may involve the whole head. Typically, lumbar puncture HA resolves spontaneously but may require an epidural blood patch.

Although CSF leakage typically produces a lingering HA, in the case of intermittent CSF leakage, HAs and any associated symptoms may come and go. Associated symptoms may include neck pain, nausea/vomiting, diplopia, or tinnitus/dizziness. Postulated mechanisms for the HAs include stretch of the pain sensitive suspending structures of the brain and meninges and potentially stretching of the cranial nerves. Associated vascular congestion or engorgement of venous sinuses may occur. Although serious complications of CSF leaks are unusual, in addition to the obvious risk of infection, subdural hematoma and cerebral venous sinus thrombosis have been reported.

The syndrome of the trephined merits special discussion, given the prevalence of craniectomy as a management strategy for raised intracranial pressure after TBI. Up to 13% of patients may experience this syndrome typically in the post-acute phase of recovery (in rehabilitation or thereafter). The syndrome consists of postural headache, dizziness, fatigue, and cognitive and mood changes. There is typically a postural sinking of the skin flap. Some authors report more severe neurological and hemodynamic alterations (135). It is postulated that mechanically, the exposure of the intracranial contents to atmospheric pressure alters CSF dynamics that often leads to brain deformation and reduces cerebral perfusion. Many patients show an incremental functional improvement after cranioplasty, and there is coincident evidence of associated improvement in cerebral blood flow (136–139).

Although cranioplasty is the definitive intervention for the disorder, Bijlenga et al. described the use of a custom suction cup helmet pending definitive cranioplasty secondary to recurrent infection at the surgical site (135) . Concern has also been raised about the use of decompressive craniectomy. Recent studies comparing the Polin technique to non-surgically managed patients with diffuse traumatic TBI and raised intracranial pressures demonstrated that while the intracranial pressure was controlled, outcomes on the extended Glasgow Outcome Scale were worse for the surgery group compared to conservatively managed controls (140). However, the technique in question (involving a large bifrontotemporal resection) may be less commonly employed than a focal temporoparietal bone resection in most civilian and military trauma centers.

Other Trauma-Related Headaches

Various "dysautonomic" HAs have been reported after trauma. These are rare, and their existence remains controversial. They are described as unilateral episodic throbbing pain and are associated with hyperactive sympathetic signs involving the ipsilateral face during the attack (miosis, hyperhidrosis) but between attacks, a mild Horner syndrome. Theoretically, this is caused by injury of the sympathetic chain in proximity to the carotid sheath. (141). Other HAs with an autonomic component have also been reported, including trigeminal autonomic HA (142), paroxysmal hemicrania (143), and CH (144). The relationship between trauma and these rare HAs has not been clearly established.

Carotid carvernous fistulas (CCFs) may occur in association with trauma (145). A CCF is an abnormal communication between the cavernous sinus and the carotid arterial system. A CCF can be caused by a direct connection between the cavernous segment of the internal carotid artery and the cavernous sinus, or a communication between the cavernous sinus, and one or more meningeal branches of the internal carotid artery, external carotid artery, or both. These fistulas may be divided into spontaneous or traumatic in relation to cause and direct, or dural in relation to angiographic findings. The dural fistulas usually have low rates of arterial blood flow and may be difficult to diagnose without angiography. Patients with CCF may present with decreased vision, conjunctival chemosis, external ophthalmoplegia and proptosis. Radiological features may be helpful in confirming the diagnosis and determining possible intervention. Based on the patient's signs and symptoms, is timely intervention mandatory to prevent morbidity or mortality. The conventional treatments include carotid ligation and embolization, with minimal significant morbidity or mortality. CCFs may also be associated with HA (146).

Cavernous sinus thrombosis (CST) may also occur after trauma. The early signs and symptoms of CST may not be specific. A patient who presents with HA and any cranial nerve findings should be potentially evaluated for CST. The most common signs of CST are related to the anatomical structures affected within the cavernous sinus. Patients generally have sinusitis or a midface infection (most commonly a furuncle) for 5–10 days. In as many as 25% of cases in which a furuncle is the precipitant, it will have been manipulated in some fashion (e.g., squeezing, surgical incision). The clinical presentation is usually because of the venous obstruction, as well as impairment of the cranial nerves that are near the cavernous sinus. HA is the most common presentation symptom and usually precedes fever, periorbital edema, and cranial nerve signs. The HA is usually sharp, increases progressively, and is usually localized to the regions innervated by the ophthalmic and maxillary branches of the fifth cranial nerve. Without effective therapy, signs appear in the contralateral eye by spreading through the communicating veins to the contralateral cavernous sinus. Eye swelling begins as a unilateral process and spreads to the other eye within 24–48 hours via the intercavernous sinuses. This is pathognomonic for CST. The patient rapidly develops mental status changes, including confusion, drowsiness, and coma from central nervous system (CNS) involvement and/or sepsis. Death follows shortly thereafter (147).

Carotid artery dissection (CAD) may occur in association with TBI related trauma and is a potentially disabling and probably underdiagnosed post-traumatic sequelae. CAD mainly affects young to middle age people. Neck and facial pain, HA, unilateral pulsatile tinnitus, partial Horner syndrome (or oculosympathetic palsy), amaurosis fugax, retinal infarction, and anterior circulation brain ischemia may all occur in isolation or in various combinations. Medical imaging plays a pivotal role in making the right diagnosis. Clinical vigilance is of utmost importance because early diagnosis and timely treatment favor long-term prognosis and even prevent ischemic complications (148).

Epilepsy may also manifest as HA and when it occurs, although rare, can be confused with migraine or CH. Ictal HAs occur in association with seizure activity. They may occur either before (preictal) or after (postictal) a seizure and in rare circumstances during a seizure. Ictal HAs may be centrally situated or cover the entirety of the head (149–151).

Post-traumatic sinus HAs may be steady or have a throbbing quality. They may be seasonal or associated with allergic symptoms. A history of sinus or facial fractures is relevant. The daily pattern of sinus HAs may relate to drainage angles; frontal and ethmoid sinus HAs are often worse with recumbency at night and are better during the day when upright, whereas maxillary and sphenoid sinus HA improves with recumbency at night. Risks to sinus fracture include abscess formation and chronic cellulitis (152). Patients may respond to decongestants, NSAIDs, or steroid sprays. In severe cases, surgical intervention may be required to repair the mucosa or remove a mucocoele.

Medication-Overuse Headache

Analgesic rebound HA may be seen from overuse of a variety of analgesic and/or abortive HA agents, including ergotamines, opiates, caffeine, triptans, NSAIDS and/or barbiturates. Overuse of these medications may lead to the evolution of migraine or TTHs into their respective chronic phenotypes. Overuse of drugs intended to abort episodic HAs may cause the patient to become refractory to the effects of prophylactic medications. Drug withdrawal normally results in worsening of HA; this is particularly noted when medication is stopped suddenly as opposed to slowly weaned with concurrent alternative HA management options prescribed. HA medication overuse may also make HAs refractory to prophylactic HA medication. Recently the International Classification of Headache Disorder (ICHD)-11 implemented a new subform (8.2.6 MOH attributed to combination of acute medications) that takes into account patients overusing medica-

tions of different classes but not any single class (36). Typically, if a patient presents with the criteria of CTTH with simple analgesic use more than 15 days/month for more than 3 months of ergotamine, opioid, triptan, or any combination of medications for more than 10 days/month for more than 3 months, CTTH and MOH must both be considered. Previously, MOH was distinguished from CTTH by improvement of HA by decrease in medication used after 2 months; however, the resolution of HA or resumption of previous HA pattern is no longer requisite in the diagnosis of MOH. (153) MOH is more commonly seen in conjunction with overuse of short-acting analgesics than longer acting medications. (see Table 56-6)

Medications that include caffeine could cause rebound HA when discontinued. (154). Overuse, however, will vary depending on the offending medication. This has less to do with the amount in milligrams of a given substance but rather with the frequency it is consumed. Ergotamine or opioid use more than 2 days a week, triptans, barbiturates, or caffeine use more often than 3 days a week and simple analgesics taken more than 5 days a week may lead to MOH. Caution must be exercised in patients with HA when analgesics are used to treat non-HA symptoms because this practice may precipitate MOH. Finally, patients may use analgesics in a dysfunctional manner to "manage" other emotional or psychological problems.

Ultimately, the treatment of MOH relies on the gradual weaning of the patient from the offending agent. This process could obviously result in a worsening of the HA. Although a washout period may take 3–10 weeks, some patients require hospitalization for the process. Patients with

---

TABLE 56–6 IHS Classification of MOH

8.2 Medication-overuse headache (MOH)
Diagnostic criteria:
A. Headache present on ≥15 days/month fulfilling criteria C and D
B. Regular overuse for >3 months of one or more drugs that can be taken for acute and/or symptomatic treatment of headache
C. Headache has developed or markedly worsened during medication overuse
D. Headache resolves or reverts to its previous pattern within 2 months after discontinuation of overused medication

> **8.2.1 *Ergotamine-overuse headache***
> **8.2.2 *Triptan-overuse headache***
> **8.2.3 *Analgesic-overuse headache***
> **8.2.4 *Opioid-overuse headache***
> **8.2.5 *Combination analgesic-overuse headache***
> **8.2.6 *Medication-overuse headache attributed to combination of acute medications***
> **8.2.7 *Headache attributed to other medication overuse***
> **8.2.8 *Probable medication-overuse headache***

Diagnostic criteria:
A. Headache fulfilling criteria A and C for 8.2 *Medication-overuse headache*
B. Medication overuse fulfilling criterion B for any one of the subforms 8.2.1 to 8.2.7
C. One or other of the following:
  1. overused medication has not yet been withdrawn
  2. medication overuse has ceased within the last 2 months but headache has not so far resolved or reverted to its previous pattern

a long history of MOH may never become fully responsive to abortive or preventative medication. Consideration should also be given to replacing short-acting analgesics with long-acting substitutes during the weaning process.

PROGNOSIS IN POST-TRAUMATIC HEADACHE

For the purposes of prognosticating recovery from PTH, it is beneficial to identify both the severity of the brain injury and, whenever possible, the primary pain generator for the HA, as well as any secondary pain generators. Indeed, the IHS classification system divides PTH not only by chronicity (acute duration < 3 months, chronic > 3 months) but also as to whether it is associated with "significant" head trauma or minor head trauma. In the case of minor head trauma, the HA begins within 7 days of injury but "disappears" within 12 weeks by the IHS definition. Difficulties with these narrow definitions have been identified by several investigators. HAs that may be considered late onset are more common than in the general population. Brenner and Friedman determined that 6% of patients with MTBI had HAs that began within 16 months (155); in later studies, 12% of patients after MTBI showed late HA at 6 and 12 months (156). Head injury may also be a risk factor for the transition of episodic HA to chronic HA (157).

Because HA is also the most common physical complaint in MTBI, prognosis for this symptom may be specifically tied to the prognosis for the postconcussive syndrome. Factors influencing the time course and quality of recovery may include premorbid intellectual status, presence of litigation, socioeconomic status, and any mental health comorbidities. An interesting point in this regard is that most military personnel with TBI also have PTSD (unlike the civilian population). Effective treatment of postconcussive syndrome under these circumstances may be dependent on the results of interventions for PTSD. However, Hoge et al. found that HA was an independent variable from PTSD unlike other symptoms of MTBI (19). Additional findings in returning soldiers demonstrate that many had symptomatic HA prior to TBI. This underscores the critical point that HA may be an independent symptom from any TBI per se and may, in fact, not be causally related to the brain injury but to other injury-related factors.

MOH is common in patients with PTH (158,159) and may perpetuate HA after trauma even if the primary pain generator is no longer contributing to head pain. To summarize, PTH associated with MTBI generally has a good prognosis in the civilian population; the patient may be assured that in the "majority" cases, there is progressive improvement to complete resolution within a few months. However, there remains a sizeable minority of patient with PTH and MTBI that have a more prolonged course of improvement, sometimes without complete resolution, and this may be more common in military populations. Forty percent to 50% of patients with moderate-to-severe TBI who develop HAs may have them as a persistent problem.

Controversies in Post-Traumatic Headache

Many of the issues surrounding the nature and prognosis for PTH are similar to those related to postconcussive disorder.

Debate regarding the role of litigation and the quest for compensation influencing the manifestation of HA continues. In 1961, Miller opined that chronic postconcussion disorder was most likely because of a desire for compensation and disability from work (160–162), yet many patients do not recover after settlement of their case (163). A frequently quoted study in Lithuania failed to demonstrate any increase in reports of HA or neck pain years after injury; this was attributed to the lack of insurance and compensation in that country (164). However, a subsequent study in Sweden with a similar lack of injury related compensation, demonstrated a significant increase in reports of HA compared to controls up to 7 years after injury (165).

Other factors influencing outcome include sex (women have a 2-fold increased risk of PTH) (166) and age. Children may develop acute PTH but seldom develop the chronic varieties. The severity of injury does not appear to be correlated to duration of PTH; indeed, there is some suggestion that more severely injured patients are less likely to report persistent HA. On the other hand, those individuals reporting multiple symptoms within 7 days of injury have a greater likelihood of having symptoms 2 years after injury (167, 168). Preexisting HA or genetic predisposition for HA may increase the risk of PTH, particularly with reference to migraine-type HAs (169). In a recent review by Evans (170), factors that may influence the persistence of postconcussive syndrome include poor social support, base rate misattribution, litigation, and malingering. It has also been suggested that part of the increased prevalence in military personnel may be related to a generic response to stress; there is ample evidence that most military personnel with a diagnosed brain injury are also experiencing PTSD. Although this may appear to corroborate the stress or psychological perpetuation of PTH, it also underscores the need to address this comorbidity in military service personnel.

That being said, psychological and social factors do influence HA frequency and effectiveness of treatment interventions. The neural circuitry involved in emotional and psychological functions is interwoven with that of nociceptive systems (171); this provides an explanation for "stress" as a HA trigger. Cognitive/behavioral strategies (see chapter 57) and other counseling techniques may help to modify counterproductive psychological responses or behaviors, so that overall HA management is more effective.

KEY CLINICAL POINTS

1. The IHS classification system as it currently exists for PTH appears to be arbitrary from the perspective of defining acute vs chronic in relation to time of onset after brain injury. Neither does it identify clinical subtypes of PTH, and thus guide treatment.
2. If one uses the IHS HA classification system for primary types of HA, historically, tension or musculoskeletal HA has been the dominant type followed by neuralgia and migraine/probable migraine. More recent studies in the civilian and military populations would indicate that migraine/probable migraine is the most common phenotype. This may not be true for civilians with MTBI/postconcussive HA in whom tension/musculoskeletal HA may still be the dominant phenotype.

3. Careful history taking is imperative to correctly diagnosing the responsible pain generators for PTH in a given patient; more than one primary pain generator may be present.

4. A thorough physical examination should incorporate palpation of the head, neck, and shoulders, specifically looking for sensitive areas (neuromas, myofascial trigger points) and positive provocative tests for cervical pathology.

5. Treatment should be multimodal. Given the overlap of nociceptive systems,

   a. pharmacological intervention should be dictated by the clinical subtype of PTH but may likely incorporate the use of triptans as abortive therapy if there are any clinical elements of migraine. Antidepressants, anticonvulsants, beta-blockers, and calcium channel blockers should be considered for prevention if the HAs occur at high frequency, or if the patient has chronic daily HA.

   b. Long-acting medications are less likely to contribute to MOH; this includes opioid preparations and NSAIDs.

   c. Physical therapy/manual medicine to the upper cervical spine and associated musculature may be a useful adjunctive (if not primary) treatment modality for most types of PTH.

   d. Consideration should be given to local nerve block, particularly to the GON.

   e. Cognitive-behavioral therapy and biofeedback techniques are useful adjunctive therapies for many types of PTH if the patient's cognition permits these interventions to be effective.

KEY REFERENCES

1. Headache Classification Committee of the International Headache Society. International Classification of Headache Disorders: 2nd edition. *Cephalalgia*. 2004;24(suppl 1): 1–151.

2. Hoffman J, Lucas S, Dikmen S, et al. Natural history of headache following traumatic brain injury. *J Neurotrauma*. 2011. Accepted for publication July 2011.

3. Lipton RB, Scher AI, Silberstein SD, Bigal ME. Migraine diagnosis and comorbidity. In: Silberstein SD, Lipton RB, Dodick DW, eds. *Wolff's Headache and Other Pain*. 8th ed. New York, NY: Oxford University Press; 2008:153–175.

4. Theeler BJ, Flynn FG, Erickson JC. Headaches after concussion in US soldiers returning from Iraq or Afghanistan. *Headache*. 2010:50(8):1262–72.

5. Zasler N, Martelli M. Post-traumatic headache: Practical approaches to diagnosis and treatment. In: RB Weiner, ed. *Pain Management: A Practical Guide for Clinicians*. 6th ed. Boca Raton, FL: St. Lucie Press; 2002:313–344.

References

1. Yamaguchi M. Incidence of headache and severity of head injury. *Headache*. 1992;32(9): 427–431.

2. Hoffman J, Lucas S, Dikmen S, et al. Natural history of headache following traumatic brain injury. *J Neurotrauma*. 2011;28(9):1719–1725. http://www.liebertonline.com/doi/pdfplus/10.1089/neu.2011.1914. Accessed 7/1/2011.

3. Walker WC, Seel RT, Curtiss G, Warden DL. Headache after moderate and severe traumatic brain injury: a longitudinal analysis. *Arch Phys Med Rehabil*. 2005;86(9): 1793–1800.

4. Zasler N, Martelli M. Post-traumatic headache: practical approaches to diagnosis and treatment. In: RB Weiner, ed. *Pain Management: A Practical Guide for Clinicians*. 6th ed. Boca Ratan, FL: St. Lucie Press; 2002:313–344.

5. Ingebrigtsen T, Waterloo K, Marup-Jensen S, Attner E, Romner B. Quanitification of post-concussion symptoms 3 months after minor head injury in 100 consecutive patients. *J Neurol*. 1998;245(9): 609–612.

6. Kraus J, Schaffer K, Ayers K, Steneheim J, Shen H, Afifi AA. Physical complaints, medical service use, and social and employment changes following mild traumatic brain injury: a 6-month longitudinal study. *J Head Traum Rehabil*. 2005;20(3):239–256.

7. Haas DC. Chronic post-traumatic headaches classified and compared with natural headaches. *Cephalalgia*. 1996;16(7):486–493.

8. Evans RW. The postconcussion syndrome and the sequelae of mild head injury. *Neurol Clin*. 1992;10:815–847.

9. Packard R, Hamm L. Incidence of cluster-like posttraumatic headache: an inconsistency. *Headache*. 1996;7:139–141.

10. Theeler BJ, Flynn FG, Erickson JC. Headaches after concussion in US soldiers returning from Iraq or Afghanistan. *Headache*. 2010: 50(8):1262–1272.

11. Headache Classification Committee of the International Headache Society. International Classification of Headache Disorders: 2nd edition. *Cephalalgia*. 2004;24(suppl 1):1–151.

12. Theeler BJ, Mercer R, Erickson JC. Prevalence and impact of migraine among US Army soldiers deployed in support of Operation Iraqi Freedom. *Headache*.2008;48(6):876–882.

13. Erickson JC. Treatment outcomes of chronic post-traumatic headaches after mild head trauma in US soldiers: an observational study. *Headache*. 2011;51(6):932–944.

14. Gironda RJ, Clark ME, Massengale JP, Walker RL. Pain among veterans of Operation Enduring Freedom and Iraqi Freedom. *Pain Medicine*. 2006;7(4): 339–343.

15. Neely ET, Midgette LA, Scher AI. Clinical review and epidemiology of headache disorders in US service members: with emphasis on post-traumatic headache. *Headache*. 2009;49(7):1089–1096.

16. Schwab KA, Ivins B, Cramer G, et al. Screening for traumatic brain injury in troops returning from deployment in Afghanistan and Iraq: initial investigation of the usefulness of a short screening tool for traumatic brain injury. *J Head Trauma Rehabil*. 2007;22(6): 377–389.

17. Afari N, Harder LH, Madra NJ, et al. PTSD, combat injury, and headache in Veterans returning from Iraq/Afghanistan. *Headache*. 2009;49(9):1267–1276.

18. de Leeuw R, Schmidt JE, Carlson CR. Traumatic stressors and post-traumatic stress disorder symptoms in headache patients. *Headache*. 2005;45(10):1365–1374.

19. Hoge CW, McGurk D, Thomas JL, Cox AL, Engel CC, Castro CA. Mild traumatic brain injury in U.S. soldiers returning from Iraq. *N Engl J Med*. 2008;358(5):453–463.

20. Cernak I, Wang Z, Jiang J, Bian X, Savic J. Ultrastructural and functional characteristics of blast injury-induced neurotrauma. *J Trauma*. 2001;50(4):695–706.

21. Warden D. Military TBI during the Iraq and Afghanistan wars. *J Head Trauma Rehabil*. 2006;21(5):398–402.

22. Cernak I, Noble-Haeusslein LJ. Traumatic brain injury: an overview of pathobiology with emphasis on military populations. *J Cereb Blood Flow Metab*. 2010;30(2):255–266.

23. Desmoulin GT, Dionne JP. Blast-induced neurotrauma: surrogate use, loading mechanisms, and cellular responses. *J Trauma*. 2009; 67(5):1113–1122.

24. Doukas AG, McAuliffe DJ, Lee S, Venugopalan V, Flotte TJ. Physical factors involved in stress-wave-induced cell injury: the effect of stress gradient. *Ultrasound Med Biol*. 1995;21(7):961–967.

25. Cernak I, Wang Z, Jiang J, Bian X, Savic J. Cognitive deficits following blast injury-induced neurotrauma: possible involvement of nitric oxide. *Brain Inj*. 2001;15(7):593–612.

26. Packard RC. Epidemiology and pathogenesis of post-traumatic headache. *J Head Trauma Rehabil*. 1999;14(1):9–21.

27. Zafonte R, Horn L. Clinical assessment of post-traumatic headache. *J Head Trauma Rehabil.* 1999;14(1):22–33.

28. Travell JG, Simons D. *Myofascial Pain and Dysfunction. The Trigger Point Manual.* Vol 1. Baltimore, MD: Williams & Wilkins; 1992.

29. Hecht J. Occipital nerve blocks in postconcussive headaches: a retrospective review and report of ten patients. *J Head Trauma Rehabil.* 2004;19(1):58–71.

30. Bartsch T, Goadsby P. Increased responses in trigeminocervical nociceptive neurons to cervical input after stimulation of the dura mater. *Brain.* 2003;126(pt 8):1801–1813.

31. Goadsby P, Knight Y, Hoskin K. Stimulation of the greater occipital nerve increases metabolic activity in the trigeminal nucleus caudalis and cervical dorsal horn of the cat. *Pain.* 1997;73(1):23–28.

32. Shevel E, Speirings EH. Cervical muscles in the pathogenesis of migraine headache. *J Headache Pain.* 2004;5:12–14.

33. Arendt-Nielsen L, Laursen R, Drewes A. Referred pain as an indicator neural plasticity. *Prog Brain Res.* 2000;129:343–356.

34. Burstein R, Goor-Aryeh I, Jakubowski M. Migraine, sensitization of trigeminovascular neurons and triptan therapy. *Headache Currents.* 2004;1(2):25–32.

35. Russell IJ, Bieber CS. Myofascial pain and fibromyalgia syndrome. In: SB McMahon & M Koltzenburg, eds. *Wall and Melzack's Textbook of Pain.* 5th ed. Philadelphia, PA: Elsevier/Churchill Livingstone. 2006;669–682.

36. Silberstein SD, Olesen J, Bousser MG, et al. The International Classification of Headache Disorders, 2nd Edition (ICHD-II)—revision of criteria for 8.2 Medication-overuse headache. *Cephalalgia.* 2005; 25(6):460–465.

37. Couch JR, Lipton R, Stewart WF. Is post-traumatic headache classifiable and does it exist? *European J Neurol.* 2009;16(1):12–13.

38. Lenaerts ME. Post-traumatic headache: from classification challenges to biological underpinnings. *Cephalalgia.* 2008;28(suppl 1): 12–15.

39. Linder SL. Post-traumatic headache. *Curr Pain Headache Rep.* 2007; 11(5):396–400.

40. Lew HL, Lin PH, Fuh JL, Wang SJ, Clark DJ, Walker WC. Characteristics and treatment of headache after traumatic brain injury: a focused review. *Am J Phys Med Rehabil.* 2006;85(7):619–627.

41. Haas DC. Chronic post-traumatic headaches classified and compared with natural headaches. *Cephalalgia.* 1996;16(7): 486–493.

42. Bekkelund S, Salvesen R. Prevalence of head trauma in patients with difficult headache: the North Norway Headache Study. *Headache.* 2003;43(1):59–62.

43. Schoenen J, Fumal A. Tension-type headache: current research and clinical management. *Lancet Neurol.* 2008;7(1):70–83.

44. Lenaerts M, Newman L. Tension-type headache. In: Silberstein SD, Lipton RB, Dodick DW, eds. *Wolff's Headache and Other Pain.* 8th ed. New York, NY: Oxford University Press; 2008:293–315.

45. Turkdogan D, Cagirici S, Soylemez D, Sur H, Bilge C, Turk U. Characteristic and overlapping features of migraine and tension-type headache. *Headache.* 2006;46:461–468.

46. Lipton RB, Cady RK, Stewart WF, Wilks K, Hall C. Diagnostic lessons from the spectrum study. *Neurology.* 2002;58(suppl 6): S27–S31.

47. Headache Classification Committee, Olesen J, Bousser MG, et al. New appendix criteria open for a broader concept of chronic migraine. *Cephalalgia.* 2006;26(6):742–746.

48. Schwartz BS, Stewart WF, Simon D, Lipton RB. Epidemiology of tension-type headache. *JAMA.* 1998;279(5):381–383.

49. Christensen MB, Bendtsen L, Ashina M, Jensen R. Experimental induction of muscle tenderness and headache in tension-type headache patients. *Cephalalgia.* 2005;25(11):1061–1067.

50. Bendtsen L. Central sensitization in tension-type headache—possible pathophysiological mechanisms. *Cephalalgia.* 2000;20(5):486–508.

51. Mense S. Nociception from skeletal muscle in relation to clinical muscle pain. *Pain.* 1993;54(3):241–289.

52. Mørk H, Ashina M, Bendtsen L, Olesen J, Jensen R. Experimental muscle pain and tenderness following infusion of endogenous substances in humans. *Eur J Pain.* 2003;7(2):145–153.

53. Coderre TJ, Katz J, Vaccarino AL, Melzack R. Contribution of central neuroplasticity to pathological pain: review of clinical and experimental evidence. *Pain.* 1993;52(3):259–285.

54. Ashina M, Stallknecht B, Bendtsen L, et al. Tender points are not sites of ongoing inflammation -in vivo evidence in patients with chronic tension-type headache. *Cephalalgia.* 2003;23(2):109–116.

55. Shah JP, Phillips TM, Danoff JV, Gerber LH. An in vivo microanalytical technique for measuring the local biochemical milieu of human skeletal muscle. *J Appl Physiol.* 2005;99(5):1977–1984.

56. Fernández-de-las-Peñas C, Cuadrado LM, Arendt-Nielsen L, Simons DG, Pareja JA. Myofascial trigger points and sensitization: an updated pain model for tension-type headache. *Cephalalgia.* 2007;27:383–393.

57. Fernández-de-las-Peñas C, Alonso-Blanco C, CuadradoML, Pareja JA. Myofascial trigger points in the suboccipital muscles in episodic tension-type headache. *Man Ther.* 2006;11(3):225–230.

58. Ashina M, Bendtsen L, Jensen R, Olesen J. Nitric oxide-induced headache in patients with chronic tension-type headache. *Brain.* 2000;123(pt 9):1830–1837.

59. Ashina M, Bendtsen L, Jensen R, Schifter S, Jansen-Olesen I, Olesen J. Plasma levels of calcitonin gene-related peptide in chronic tension-type headache. *Neurology.* 2000;55(9):1335–1340.

60. Schoenen J. Guidelines for trials of drug treatments in tension-type headache. First edition: International Headache Society Committee on Clinical Trials. *Cephalalgia.* 1995;15(3):165–179.

61. Packman E, Packman B, Thurston H, Tseng L. Lumiracoxib is effective in the treatment of episodic tension-type headache. *Headache.* 2005;45(9):1163–1170.

62. Diamond S, Baltes BJ. Chronic tension headache—treated with amitriptyline—a double-blind study. *Headache.* 1971;11(3):110–116.

63. Bettucci D, Testa L, Calzoni S, Mantegazza P, Viana M, Monaco F. Combination of tizanidine and amitriptyline in the prophylaxis of chronic tension-type headache: evaluation of efficacy and impact on quality of life. *J Headache Pain.* 2006;7(1):34–36.

64. Bendtsen L, Buchgreitz L, Ashina S, Jensen R. Combination of low-dose mirtazapine and ibuprofen for prophylaxis of chronic tension-type headache. *Eur J Neurol.* 2007;14(2):187–193.

65. Lampl C, Marecek S, May A, Bendtsen L. A prospective, open-label, long-term study of efficacy and tolerability of topiramate in the prophylaxis of chronic tension-type headache. *Cephalalgia.* 2006; 26(10):1203–1208.

66. Evers S, Rahmann A, Vollmer-Haase J, Husstedt IW. Treatment of headache with botulinum toxin A—a review according to evidence-based medicine criteria. *Cephalalgia.* 2002;22(9):699–710.

67. Holroyd KA, Labus JS, O'Donnell FJ, Cordingley G. Treating chronic tension-type headache not responding to amitriptyline hydrochloride with paroxetine hydrochloride: a pilot evaluation. *Headache.* 2003;43(9):999–1004.

68. Lenssinck ML, Damen L, Verhagen AP, Berger MY, Passchier J, Koes BW. The effectiveness of physiotherapy and manipulation inpatients with tension-type headache: a systematic review. *Pain.* 2004;112(3):381–388.

69. Boline PD, Kassak K, Bronfort G, Nelson C, Anderson AV. Spinal manipulation vs. amitriptyline for the treatment of chronic tension-type headaches: a randomized clinical trial. *J Manipulative Physiol Ther.* 1995;18(3):148–154.

70. Bryans R, Descarreaux M, Duranleau M, et al. Evidence-based guidelines for the chiropractic treatment of adults with headache. *J Manipulative Physiol Ther.* 2011;34(5):274–289.

71. Melchart D, Streng A, Hoppe A, et al. Acupuncture in patients with tension-type headache: randomised controlled trial. *BMJ.* 2005;331(7513):376–382.

72. Bogduk N, Bartsch T. Cervicogenic headache. In: Silberstein SD, Lipton RB, Dodick DW, eds. *Wolff's Headache and Other Head Pain.* 8th ed. New York, NY: Oxford University Press; 2008:551–570.

73. Sjaastad O, Fredriksen TA, Pfaffenrath V. Cervicogenic headache: diagnostic criteria. The Cervicogenic Headache International Study Group. *Headache.* 1998;38(6):442–445.

74. Jull G, Trott P, Potter H, et al. A randomized controlled trial of exercise and manipulative therapy for cervicogenic headache. *Spine (Phila Pa 1976).* 2002;27(17):1835–1843.

75. Gross A, Hoving J, Haines T, et al. A Cochrane review of manipulation and mobilization for mechanical neck disorders. *Spine.* 2004; 29(14):1541–1548.

76. Bovim G, Fredriksen TA, Stolt-Nielsen A, Sjaastad O. Neurolysis of the greater occipital nerve in cervicogenic headache. A follow up study. *Headache.* 1992;32(4):175–179.

77. van Suijlekom HA, van Kleef M, Barendse GA, Sluijter ME, Sjaastad O, Weber WE. Radiofrequency cervical zygapophyseal joint neurotomy for cervicogenic headache: a prospective study of 15 patients. *Funct Neurol.* 1998;13(4):297–303.

78. Govind J, King W, Bailey B, Bogduk N. Radiofrequency neurotomy for the treatment of third occipital headache. *J Neurol Neurosurg Psychiatry.* 2003;74(1):88–93.

79. La Touche R, París-Alemany A, von Piekartz H, et al. The influence of cranio-cervical posture on maximal mouth opening and pressure pain threshold in patients with myofascial temporomandibular pain disorders. *Clin J Pain.* 2011;27(1):48–55.

80. Forssell H, Kalso E, Koskela P, Vehmanen R, Puukka P, Alanen P. Occlusal treatments in temporomandibular disorders: a qualitative systematic review of randomized controlled trials. *Pain.* 1999;83(3):549–560.

81. Hersh EV, Balasubramaniam R, Pinto A. Pharmacologic management of temporomandibular disorders. *Oral Maxillofac Surg Clin N Am.* 2008;20(2):197–210.

82. Weiss HD, Stern BJ, Goldberg J. Post-traumatic migraine: chronic migraine precipitated by minor head or neck trauma. *Headache.* 1991;31(7):451–456.

83. Lipton RB, Scher AI, Silberstein SD, Bigal ME. Migraine diagnosis and comorbidity. In: Silberstein SD, Lipton RB, Dodick DW, eds. *Wolff's Headache and Other Pain.* 8th ed. New York, NY: Oxford University Press; 2008:153–175.

84. Selby G, Lance JW. Observations on 500 cases of migraine and allied vascular headache. *J Neurol Neurosurg Psychiatry.* 1960;23:23–32.

85. Raskin NH, Schwartz RK. Icepick-like pain. *Neurology.* 1980;30(2):203–205.

86. Bickerstaff ER. Basilar artery migraine. *Lancet.* 1961;1:15–17.

87. Evans RW, Linder SL. Management of basilar migraine. *Headache.* 2002;42(5):383–384.

88. Jacome DE. Basilar artery migraine after uncomplicated whiplash injuries. *Headache.* 1986;26(10):515–516.

89. Wolff HG. *Headache and Other Head Pain.* New York, NY: Oxford University Press; 1948.

90. Chawla J. Migraine headache. Available at http://www.iranneurology.com/Downloads/articles/Migraine%20Headache.pdf. Accessed 7/1/2011.

91. Leão AAP. Pial circulation and spreading depression of activity in the cerebral cortex. *J Neurophysiol.* 1944;7:391–396.

92. Hadjikhani N, Sanchez Del Rio M, Wu O, et al. Mechanisms of migraine aura revealed by functional MRI in human visual cortex. *Proc Natl Acad Sci USA.* 2001;98(8):4687–4692.

93. Gursoy-Ozdemir Y, Qiu J, Matsuoka N, et al. Cortical spreading depression activates and upregulates MMP-9. *J Clin Invest.* 2004;113(10):1447–1455.

94. Moskowitz MA, Nozaki K, Kraig RP. Neocortical spreading depression provokes the expression of c-fos protein-like immunoreactivity within trigeminal nucleus caudalis via trigeminovascular mechanisms. *J Neurosci.* 1993;13(3):1167–1177.

95. Curter FM, Bajwa ZH, Sabahat A. Pathophysiology, clinical manifestations, and diagnosis of migraine in adults. Available at: http://www.uptodate.com/contents/pathophysiology-clinical-manifestations-and-diagnosis-of-migraine-in-adults?source=search_result&selectedTitle=1%7E150. Updated February 2011.

96. Doenicke A, Brand J, Perrin VL. Possible benefit of GR43175, a novel 5-HT1-like receptor agonist, for the acute treatment of severe migraine. *Lancet.* 1988;1(8598):1309–1311.

97. Saxena P, Ferrari MD. 5-HT(1)-like receptor agonists and the pathophysiology of migraine. *Trends Pharmacol Sci.* 1989;10(5):200–204.

98. Lake A III, Saper JR. Chronic headache: new advances in treatment strategies. *Neurology.* 2002;59(5)(suppl 2):S8–S13.

99. Cumberbatch MJ, Hill RG, Hargreaves RJ. Rizatriptan has central antinociceptive effects against durally evoked responses. *Eur J Pharmacol.* 1997;328(1):37–40.

100. Smetana GW. The diagnostic value of historical features in primary headache syndromes: a comprehensive review. *Arch Intern Med.* 2000;160(18):2729–2737.

101. Silberstein SD. Practice parameter: evidence-based guidelines for migraine headache (an evidence-based review): report of the Quality Standards Subcommittee of the American Academy of Neurology. *Neurology.* 2000;55(6):754–762.

102. Silberstein SD, Freitag FG, Bigal ME: Migraine treatment. In: Silberstein SD, Lipton RB, Dodick DW, eds. *Wolff's Headache and Other Pain.* 8th ed. New York, NY: Oxford University Press; 2008:177–292.

103. Siow HC, Young WB, Silberstein SD. Neuroleptics in headache. *Headache.* 2005;45(4):358–371.

104. Matchar DB, Young WB, Rosenberg JA, et al. Evidence-based guidelines for migraine headache in the primary care setting: pharmacologic management of acute attacks. *Neurology.* 2000. Available at: http://www.aan.org. Accessed 7/1/2011.

105. Misra UK, Jose M, Kalita J. Rofecoxib versus ibuprofen for acute treatment of migraine: a randomised placebo controlled trial. *Postgrad Med J.* 2004;80(950):720–723.

106. Saper J, Dahlof C, So Y. Rofecoxib in the acute treatment of migraine: a randomized controlled clinical trial. *Headache.* 2006;46(2):264–275.

107. Diener HC, Bussone G, de Liano H, et al. Placebo-controlled comparison of effervescent acetylsalicyclic acid, sumatriptan and ibuprofen in the treatment of migraine attacks. *Cephalalgia.* 2004;24(11):947–954.

108. Goldstein J, Silberstein SD, Saper JR, Ryan RE Jr, Lipton RB. Acetaminophen, aspirin, and caffeine in combination versus ibuprofen for acute migraine: results from a multicenter, double-blind, randomized, parallel-group, single-dose, placebo-controlled study. *Headache.* 2006;46(3):444–453.

109. Lipton RB, Bigal ME, Goadsby PJ. Double-blind clinical trials of oral triptans vs other classes of acute migraine medication—a review. *Cephalalgia.* 2004;24(5):321–332.

110. Burstein R, Goor-Aryeh I, Jakubowski M. Migraine, sensitization of trigeminovascular neurons, and triptan therapy. *Headache Currents.* 2004;1(2):25–32.

111. Waeber C, Moskowitz MA. Therapeutic implications of central and peripheral neurologic mechanisms in migraine. *Neurology.* 2003;61(8)(suppl 4):S9–S20.

112. Heninger GR, Charney DS. Mechanism of action of antidepressant treatments: implications for the etiology and treatment of depressive disorders. In: Meltzer HY, ed. *Psychopharmacology: The Third Generation of Progress.* New York, NY: Raven Press; 1987:535–544.

113. Storer RJ, Goadsby PJ. Topiramate inhibits trigeminovascular traffic in the cat: a possible locus of action in the prevention of migraine. *Neurology.* 2003;60:A238.

114. Schiapparelli P, Allais G, Castagnoli Gabellari I, et al. Non-pharmacological approach to migraine prophylaxis: part II. *Neurol Sci.* 2010;31(suppl 1):S137–S139.

115. Goadsby PJ. Primary neurovascular headache. In: McMahon SB, Koltzenburg M, eds. *Wall and Melzack's Textbook of Pain.* 5th ed. Philadelphia, PA: Elsevier/Churchill Livingstone; 2006:851–874.

116. Knight Y. Brainstem modulation of caudal trigeminal nucleus: a model for understanding migraine biology and future drug targets. *Headache Currents.* 2005;2(5):108–118.

117. Aoki K. Evidence for antinociceptive activity of botulinum toxin type A in pain management. *Headache.* 2003;43(suppl 1):S9–S15.

118. Silberstein SD, Stark SR, Lucas SM. Botulinum toxin type A for the prophylactic treatment of chronic daily headache: a randomized, double-blind, placebo-controlled trial. *Mayo Clin Proc.* 2005;80(9):1119–1121.

119. Dodick DW, Turkel CC, DeGryse RE, et al.; for PREEMPT Chronic Migraine Study Group. OnabotulinumtoxinA for treatment of chronic migraine: pooled results from the double-blind, randomized, placebo-controlled phases of the PREEMPT clinical program. *Headache.* 2010;50(6):921–936.

120. Sluder G. The anatomical and clinical relations of the sphenopalatine ganglion to the nose. *NY State J Med.* 1909;90:293–298.

121. Sluder G. *Nasal Neurology, Headaches and Eye Disorders.* St. Louis, MO: CV Mosby; 1927.

122. Windsor RE, Jahnke S. Sphenopalatine ganglion blockade: a review and proposed modification of the transnasal technique. *Pain Physician*. 2004;7(2):283–286.

123. Jenkins B, Tepper SJ. Neurostimulation for primary headache disorders, part 1: pathophysiology and anatomy, history of neuromodulation in headache treatment, and review of peripheral neuromodulation in primary headaches. *Headache*. 2011;51(8):1254–1266.

124. Devoghel JC. Cluster headache and sphenopalatine block. *Acta Anaesthesiolgica Belgica*. 1981;32(1):101–107.

125. Shah RV, Racz GB. Long-term relief of posttraumatic headache by sphenopalatine ganglion pulsed radiofrequency lesioning: a case report. *Arch Phys Med Rehabil*. 2004;85(6):1013–1016.

126. Young WB. Blocking the greater occipital nerve: utility in headache management. *Curr Pain Headache Rep*. 2010;14(5):404–408.

127. Weiner RL, Reed KL. Peripheral neurostimulation for control of intractable occipital neuralgia. *Neuromodulation*. 1999;2(3):217–221.

128. Johnstone CS, Sundaraj R. Occipital nerve stimulation for the treatment of occipital neuralgia—eight case studies. *Neuromodulation*. 2006;9(1):41–47.

129. Kapural L, Mekhail N, Hayek SM, Stanton-Hicks M, Malak O. Occipital nerve electrical stimulation via the midline approach and subcutaneous surgical leads for treatment of severe occipital neuralgia: a pilot study. *Anesth Analg*. 2005;101(1):171–174.

130. Fredriksen TA. Cervicogenic headache: invasive procedures. *Cephalalgia*. 2008;28(suppl 1):39–40.

131. Jasper JF, Hayek SM. Implanted occipital nerve stimulators. *Pain Physician*. 2008;11(2):187–200.

132. Ishiwata Y, Fujitsu K, Sekino T, et al. Subdural tension pneumocephalus following surgery for chronic subdural hematoma. *J Neurosurg*. 1988;68(1):58–61.

133. Michel SJ. The Mount Fuji sign. *Radiology*. 2004;232(2):449–450.

134. Hogan QH, Prost R, Kulier A, Taylor ML, Liu S, Mark L. Magnetic resonance imaging of cerebrospinal fluid volume and the influence of body habitus and abdominal pressure. *Anesthesiology*. 1996;84(6):1341–1349.

135. Bijlenga P, Zumofen D, Yilmaz H, Creisson E, de Tribolet N. Orthostatic mesodiencephalic dysfunction after decompressive craniectomy. *J Neurol Neurosurg Psychiatry*. 2007;78(4):430–433.

136. Sakamoto S, Eguchi K, Kiura Y, Arita K, Kurisu K. CT perfusion imaging in the syndrome of the sinking skin flap before and after cranioplasty. *Clin Neurol Neurosurg*. 2006;108(6):583–585.

137. Akins PT, Guppy KH. Sinking skin flaps, paradoxical herniation, and external brain tamponade: a review of decompressive craniectomy management. *Neurocrit Care*. 2008;9(2):269–276.

138. Mokri B. Orthostatic headaches in the syndrome of the trephined: resolution following cranioplasty. *Headache*. 2010;50(7):1206–1211.

139. Joseph V, Reilly P. Syndrome of the trephined. *J Neurosurg*. 2009;111(4):650–652.

140. Cooper D, Rosenfeld J, Murray L, et al. Decompressive craniectomy in diffuse traumatic brain injury. *N Engl J Med*. 2011;364(16):1493–1502.

141. Vijayan N. A new post-traumatic headache syndrome; clinical and therapeutic observations. *Headache*. 1977;17(1):19–22.

142. Putzki N, Nirrko A, Diener HC. Trigeminal autonomic cephalalgias: a case of post-traumatic SUNCT syndrome? *Cephalalgia*. 2005;25(5):395–397.

143. Matharu MJ, Goadsby PJ. Post-traumatic chronic paroxysmal hemicrania (CPH) with aura. *Neurology*. 2001;56(2):273–275.

144. Turkewitz LJ, Wirth O, Dawson GA, Casaly JS. Cluster headache following head injury: a case report and review of the literature. *Headache*. 1992;32(10):504–506.

145. Chaudhry IA, Elkhamry SM, Al-Rashed W, Bosley TM. Carotid cavernous fistula: ophthalmological implications. *Middle East Afr J Ophthalmol*. 2009;16(2):57–63.

146. Yamada SM, Masahira N, Shimizu K. A migraine-like headache induced by carotid-cavernous fistula. *Headache*. 2007;47(2):289–293.

147. Heckmann JG, Tomandl B. Cavernous sinus thrombosis. *Lancet*. 2003;362(9400):1958.

148. Schelfaut D, Dhondt E, De Raedt S, Nieboer K, Hubloue I. Carotid artery dissection: three cases and a review of the literature. *Eur J Emerg Med*. 2011. [Epub ahead of print].

149. http://professionals.epilepsy.com/page/migraine_headache.html

150. Belcastro V, Striano P, Kasteleijn-Nolst Trenité DG, Villa MP, Parisi P. Migralepsy, hemicrania epileptica, post-ictal headache and "ictal epileptic headache": a proposal for terminology and classification revision. *J Headache Pain*. 2011;12(3):289–294.

151. HELP Study Group. Multi-center study on migraine and seizure-related headache in patients with epilepsy. *Yonsei Med J*. 2010;51(2):219–224.

152. Sivori LA II, de Leeuw R, Morgan I, Cunningham LL Jr. Complications of frontal sinus fractures with emphasis on chronic craniofacial pain and its treatment: a review of 43 cases. *J Oral Maxillofac Surg*. 2010;68(9):2041–2046.

153. Silberstein SD, Lipton RB, Saper J. Chronic daily headache including transformed migraine, chronic tension-type headache, and medication-overuse headache. In: Silberstein SD, Lipton RB, Dodick DW, eds. *Wolff's Headache and Other Head Pain*. 8th ed. New York, NY: Oxford University Press; 2008:330–335.

154. Silverman K, Evans S, Strain E, Griffiths RR. Withdrawal syndrome after the double-blind cessation of caffeine consumption. *N Eng J Med*. 1992;327(16):1109–1114.

155. Brenner C, Friedman A, Merritt HH, Denny-Brown DE. Posttraumatic headache. *J Neurosurg*. 1944;1:379–391.

156. Cartlidge NE, Shaw DA. *Head Injury*. London, UK: WB Saunders; 1981.

157. Scher A, Lipton R, Stewart W. Risk factors for chronic daily headache. *Curr Pain Headache Rep*. 2002;6(6):486–491.

158. Warner JS. Posttraumatic headache—a myth? *Arch Neurol*. 2000;57(12):1778–1780.

159. Baandrup L, Jensen R. Chronic post-traumatic headache—a clinical analysis in relation to the International Headache Classification 2nd Edition. *Cephalalgia*. 2005;25(2):132–138.

160. Miller H. Accident neurosis: lecture I. *BMJ*. 1961;1(5230):919–925.

161. ller H. Accident neurosis. *Br Med J*. 1961;1(5231):992–998.

162. Binder LM, Rohling ML. Money matters: a meta-analytic review of the effects of financial incentives on recovery after closed-head injury. *Am J Psychiatry*. 1996;153(1):7–10.

163. Packard R. Posttraumatic headache: permanency and relationship to legal settlement. *Headache*. 1992;32(10):496–500.

164. Obelieniene D, Bovim G, Schrader H, et al. Headache after whiplash: a historical cohort study outside the medico-legal context. *Cephalalgia*. 1998;18(8):559–564.

165. Berglund A, Alfredsson L, Jensen I, Cassidy JD, Nygren A. The association between exposure to a rear-end collision and future health complaints. *J Clin Epidemiol*. 2001;54(8):851–856.

166. Jensen O, Nielsen F. The influence of sex and pre-traumatic headache on the incidence and severity of headache after injury. *Cephalalgia*. 1990;10(6):285–293.

167. Radanov B, Sturzenegger M, Di Stefano G. Long-term outcome after whiplash injury. A 2-year follow-up considering features of injury mechanism and somatic, radiologic, and psychosocial findings. *Medicine*. 1995;74(5):281–297.

168. De Kruijk J, Leffers P, Menheere P, Meerhoff S, Rutten J, Twijnstra A. Prediction of post-traumatic complaints after mild traumatic brain injury: early symptoms and biochemical markers. *J Neurol Neurosurg Psychiatry*. 2002;73(6):727–732.

169. Weiss HD, Stern BJ, Goldberg J. Post-traumatic migraine: chronic migraine precipitated by minor head or neck trauma. *Headache*. 1991;31(7):451–456.

170. Evans RW. Persistent post-traumatic headache, postconcussion syndrome, and whiplash injuries: the evidence for a non-traumatic basis with an historical review. *Headache*. 2010;50(4):716–724.

171. Nicholson RA, Houle TT, Rhudy JL, Norton PJ. Psychological risk factors in headache. *Headache*. 2007;47(3):413–426.

Post-Traumatic Pain Disorders: Medical Assessment and Management

Nathan D. Zasler, Michael F. Martelli, Keith Nicholson, and Lawrence J. Horn

INTRODUCTION

The medical management of pain in persons with traumatic brain injury (TBI) is fraught with challenges that are multidimensional in nature. The co-occurrence of pain with TBI has been found to be a common phenomenon (1,2). Clinicians evaluating patients with TBI with comorbid pain complaints need to be aware of the types of neurological, both peripheral and central, as well as orthopedic injuries that may result in post-traumatic pain disorders in this patient population. Adequate assessment and optimal treatment will typically require a multidisciplinary neuromedical and an interdisciplinary rehabilitation approach (see Chapters 56 and 58).

NEUROANATOMY AND NEUROBIOLOGY OF PAIN

The neuroanatomical systems involved in pain perception are complex and dynamic (i.e., plastic) and differ in many ways between acute and chronic pain states (3). The nociceptive system is now recognized as a sensory system in its own right. There are multiple redundancies and feedback loops for both ascending and descending inhibition and facilitation. Important structures include the peripheral afferents, the dorsal horn (DH) (replete with its complex interneuronal pool), ascending spinal tracts, descending spinal tracts, brain stem structures (including the periaqueductal gray [PAG], pontine, and mesencephalic reticular centers), thalamus, primary sensorimotor cortex, and paralimbic and limbic structures (4). Much of the cerebral cortex is involved with processing different aspects of pain.

Pain receptors are located throughout the peripheral somatic and visceral systems. They are sensitive to almost any mechanical, toxic, metabolic, and/or thermal injury. Peripheral afferents are unmyelinated C and myelinated A delta neurons with cell bodies in the dorsal root ganglia. These enter the spinal cord at the DH. Pain receptors and the primary afferent neurons are also affected by peripheral inflammatory processes and chemical mediators released during tissue injury. These mediators may lower the threshold for firing of the primary afferent neurons, perpetuating or augmenting peripheral pain input to the central nervous system (CNS). This process is called peripheral sensitization. The nociceptors themselves may release bradykinin, serotonin, substance P, and histamine that, in turn, increase the sensitivity of the receptor. In addition, inflammatory mediators such as leukotrines, cytokines, prostaglandins, and potassium from injured cells or via the inflammatory cascade contribute to increased sensitization of the nociceptors and peripheral afferents (5).

Traditionally, the ascending systems of the CNS begin in the DH of the spinal cord. The direct pathway, also referred to as the lateral pathway or neospinothalamic tract, begins in the nucleus proprius (lamina III and IV) of the DH, where the second-order neuron crosses over in the anterior white commissure to the lateral funiculus of the opposite side, forming or joining the spinothalamic tract. This crossover occurs over 1–3 levels above the afferent spinal level. The second-order neuron ascends to the ventroposterolateral (VPL) nucleus of the thalamus where a third-order neuron projects to the primary sensorimotor cortex of the parietal lobe and likely mediates fine discrimination of nociceptive input type and location.

There are also other more polysynaptic ascending pain systems referred to as *indirect pathways*, which comprise a medial pain system. These principally mediate the autonomic, endocrine, arousal, and emotional aspects of pain perception. Unlike the lateral system, these ascend bilaterally, have poor somatotopic organization, and synapse over multiple levels of the neuroaxis. The paleospinothalamic tract leaves the DH and ascends bilaterally in the ventrolateral spinal cord to synapse in the reticular formation, the midline, and intralaminar nuclei of the thalamus (including the dorsal medial nucleus) and then projects diffusely to limbic structures including the anterior cingulate gyrus. Associated tracts include the spinoreticular tract that ascends in the anterior white matter of the spinal cord to synapse in the medullary and pontine reticular nuclei, which then project to the midline and intralaminar nuclei of the thalamus and then project on to the cortex and limbic structures. The other major paleospinothalamic tract is the spinomesencephalic that projects from the DH to the PAG of the mesencephalon, then to the midline and intralaminar nuclei, and on to the cortex and limbic system. Both the PAG and the reticular nuclei generate important descending modulatory tracts to the DH and its interneuronal pool.

The DH is the origin of second-order neurons, which ascend to multiple levels of the CNS and synapse with various interneurons as well as primary peripheral afferents. The synapse between the first- and second-order nociceptive neurons is subject to both facilitory and inhibitory inputs from these interneurons as well as descending influences from the brain. Ascending neurons largely consist of nociceptive specific neurons and "wide dynamic range" (WDR) neurons that receive input from both nociceptive and non-nociceptive afferents (6). There is substantial local (perisegmental) interconnectivity via interneurons, accounting for spinal motor reflexes; whereby, a noxious input causes withdrawal via anterior horn (motor) neurons.

Two important functional classes of neurons are frequently described: nociceptive specific and WDR, the latter as noted earlier. Nociceptive specific neurons are typically lamina I neurons, which tend to receive predominantly high-threshold (small afferent) input. Starting at relatively high stimulus intensities, these cells begin to show a threshold increase in discharge that is proportional to an increasingly aversive range of stimulus intensities. WDR neurons are found in the nucleus proprius and have 3 noteworthy functional characteristics. First, given their connectivity (high-threshold small afferents on the distal terminals and low-threshold large afferents on their ascending dendrites and soma), these neurons display excitation driven by low- and high-threshold afferent input. Second, they demonstrate what has been termed *organ convergence*, that is, depending on the spinal level, a neuron in the nucleus proprius may be activated by both somatic stimuli and activation of visceral afferents. This convergence results in an admixture of excitation for a visceral organ and a specific area of the body surface and leads to referral of input from that visceral organ to that area of the body surface. These viscerosomatic and musculosomatic convergences onto DH neurons underlie the phenomenon of referred visceral or deep muscle or bone pain to particular body surfaces. Third, low frequency, repetitive stimulation of C fibers, but not A fibers, produces a gradual increase in the frequency discharge until the neuron is in a state of virtually continuous discharge (so-called wind-up).

As discussed earlier, the primary peripheral nociceptive neuron may become sensitized by a local tissue injury. It may also begin to develop spontaneous ectopic discharges that may also appear in a region near the dorsal root ganglia (7). Wind-up refers to a progressive increase in magnitude of C fiber evoked responses in the DH neurons produced by repetitive firing of the C fibers and the dorsal root ganglia. This process does not persist after a stimulus ceases and seems to be related to the activation of N-methyl-D-aspartate (NMDA) receptors and is akin to kindling in some forms of epilepsy. Wind-up is theorized to occur when successive synaptic depolarizations of the voltage dependent NMDA receptor lead to magnesium depletion, thereby allowing an influx of intracellular calcium, which in turn activates protein kinases and ultimately causes further amplification of nociceptive responses to stimuli (see Figures 57-1 and 57-2).

Ectopic impulse generation after a nerve injury is associated with increased expression of messenger RNA for certain voltage-gated sodium channels leading to increased accumulation of sodium channels at the sites of ectopic impulse generation, decreasing the neuron's threshold for firing (7).

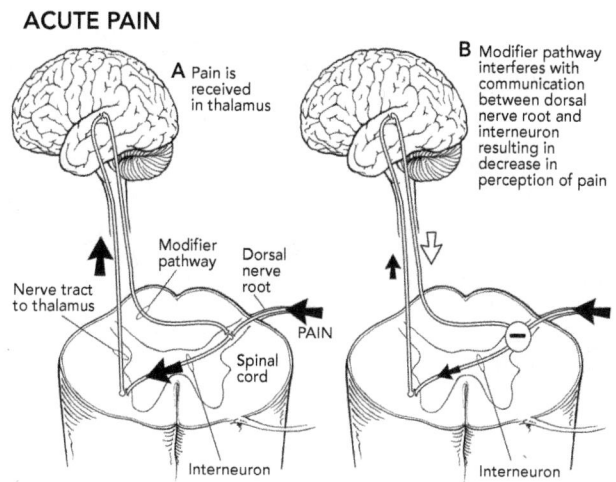

FIGURE 57-1 Proposed pathways for acute pain transmission.

Central sensitization is a related phenomenon which, at the spinal level, refers to an increased excitability of DH neurons associated with increased spontaneous activity and decreased firing thresholds in response to primary afferent inputs. It is thought to play a major role in the development of neuropathic pain syndromes. The receptive field for the involved DH neuron also expands. Sensitization of DH neurons may persist after a stimulus stops, often occurs after tissue injury, and contributes to secondary hyperalgesia (i.e., increased sensitivity to pain, which may be caused by damage to nociceptors or peripheral nerves), whereby there is an increased excitability of nociceptive spinal cord neurons to stimuli outside of the injured area (8). Different mechanisms have been theorized to be responsible for immediate/early central sensitization vs late central sensitization (see Figures 57-3 and 57-4).

Both wind-up and central sensitization contribute to allodynia (i.e., the perception of pain from otherwise neutral

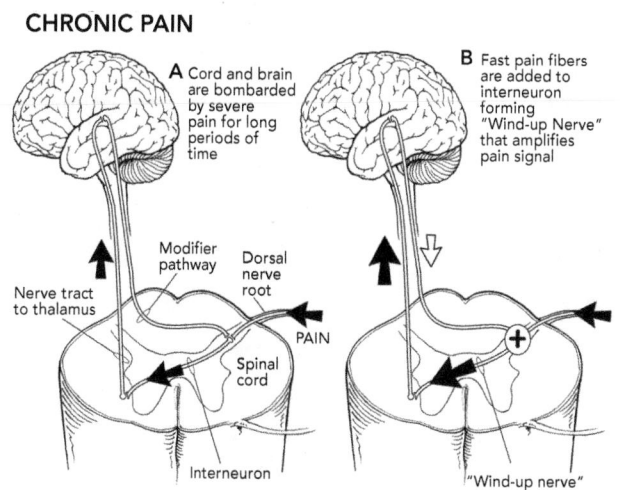

FIGURE 57-2 Proposed pathways for chronic pain transmission.

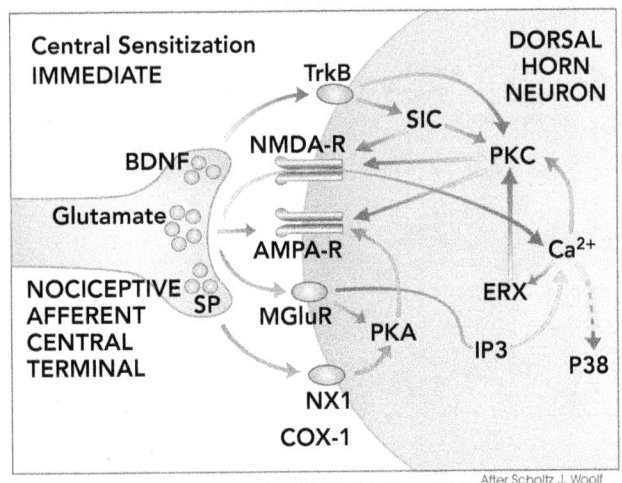

FIGURE 57-3 Theorized mechanisms of immediate central sensitization.

stimuli), particularly when the wide dynamic range neurons are affected. Furthermore, both peripheral and central sensitization may contribute to sympathetically mediated complex regional pain syndromes. The clinical implications for wind-up and central sensitization are that they can be minimized by early and appropriately comprehensive pain management (5,9). For example, in treating patients with chronic migraine, it is imperative that attacks be aborted early. Triptans may not be effective once cranial allodynia has occurred (10). Current belief is that sensitization phenomena, both peripheral and central, are likely involved in a wide variety of chronic pain conditions such as complex regional pain syndrome (CRPS), tension headache, and fibromyalgia, among other conditions.

The neurochemical milieu of the DH is no less complex than the anatomy. Of the neurotransmitters that can be manipulated through prescription medication, all have receptor sites throughout the pain neuroaxis. Although some are pri-

marily pronociceptive or antinociceptive, some have mixed effects depending on the site of action and the subtype of receptor present. Several neurotransmitters may be released from a single neuron or neuronal system. At the synapse between the peripheral afferent fiber and the nociceptive or wide dynamic ranger neuron in the DH, the presynaptic primary afferent may corelease glutamate, substance P, neurokinin A, and calcitonin gene-related peptide (CGRP). These neurotransmitters are all stimulatory to the DH neuron and are largely considered pronociceptive. The presynaptic afferent terminal also has opiate mu-receptors and alpha-2 noradrenergic receptors that are inhibitory to the release of the aforementioned neurotransmitters and are considered antinociceptive. In addition, the presynaptic terminal has 5-hydroxytryptamine$_3$ (5-HT$_3$) serotonin receptors that facilitate the release of substance P.

The DH neurons themselves are influenced by neurotransmitters released by cells other than the peripheral afferent fibers (PAF). Gamma-aminobutyric acid (GABA) interneurons (A and B) inhibit the firing of the DH cells. The 5-HT$_3$ also facilitates the GABA interneurons. Stimulation of alpha-2, mu-opiate, and 5-HT$_{1A}$ receptors on the DH cell also inhibit its firing. Some of these chemicals originate from descending inhibitory pathways in the dorsal lateral pontine (DLP) catecholamine cell groups or the rostral ventromedial medulla (RVM). Therefore, within the DH, alpha-2, mu-opiates, 5-HT$_{1A}$, and, GABA receptors are all antinociceptive; 5-HT$_3$ has mixed effects, not only facilitating the release of pronociceptive transmitter from the peripheral afferent neuron but also facilitating release of GABA. Glutamate, substance P, neurokinin A, and CGRP are all pronociceptive (11). Therefore, from the perspective of clinical pharmacologic interventions, those agents that result in net stimulation of mu-opiate, alpha-2, GABA, or 5-HT$_{1A}$ receptors, or that block substance P, glutamate, or neurokinin receptors, should all have analgesic properties.

The second-order neurons that ascend via the lateral spinothalamic tract primarily carry pain and temperature sensation from the contralateral body. Visceral pain is largely transmitted via the medial pain system. A lesion of the spinal cord involving the spinothalamic tract, therefore, will produce loss of pain and temperature over the surface of the body contralateral to the lesion, beginning 1 or 2 segments below the injury level. Incomplete lesions of the neospinothalamic tract may produce spinal generated central pain syndromes. Similarly, lesions of the thalamus may produce "thalamic pain" over the contralateral body and face because of abnormal firing in the VPL nucleus.

The paleospinothalamic system carries nociceptive information from the body viscera and is bilaterally represented in the spinal cord and above. Second-order neurons synapse rostrally in the PAG of the mesencephalon and the parabrachial nucleus of the pons; these pathways then project to thalamic and limbic structures and appear to be involved in the motivational and affective elements of pain and associated dysphoria. They also have extensive interconnectivity with hypothalamic, limbic, and brain stem structures related to autonomic control. They are closely linked, regionally and functionally, to the nucleus solitarius and afferent nuclei of the trigeminal nerve, which is implicated in vascular headache (see Chapter 56) (11,12).

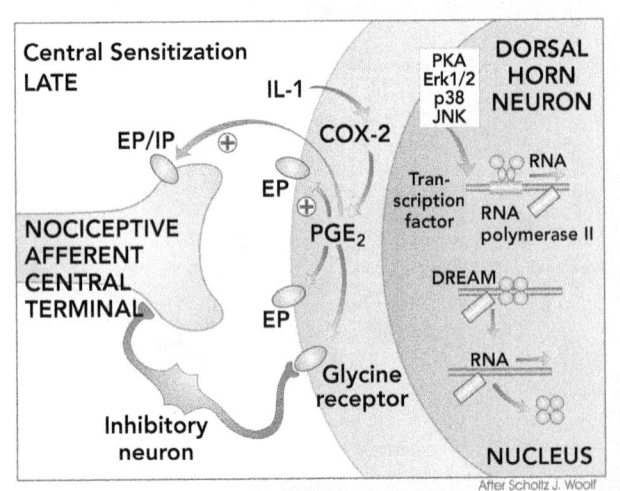

FIGURE 57-4 Theorized mechanisms of late central sensitization.

Projections from the PAG and parabrachial region ascend rostrally to thalamic nuclei and then to cortex, anterior cingulate gyrus, insular cortex, and/or directly to the amygdala. The PAG appears to be the center of the most powerful antinociceptive neuromodulator system in the brain (13). There is also an extensive interconnectivity between the PAG and orbitofrontal cortex. The aforementioned system may be critical to behavioral responses to threat and stress, switching attention away from pain when survival is essential. NMDA receptors in the anterior cingulate and insular cortices enhance persistent chronic behavioral responses to tissue injury and inflammation without affecting acute nociception in the spinal cord (12). The anterior cingulate gyrus is intimately involved with affective responses to pain. There is some evidence to support overlap of emotional pain (social rejection) with somatic pain in this region on functional magnetic resonance imaging (fMRI) (14). The nondominant ventral prefrontal cortex appears to dampen emotional distress caused by pain through its limbic and anterior cingulate connections. Positron emission tomography (PET) and fMRI studies have demonstrated that regional cerebral blood flow (rCBF) increases to noxious stimuli are almost constantly seen in the secondary somatosensory cortex (SSC), insular regions, and anterior cingulate cortex with slightly less consistency in the contralateral thalamus and primary SSC. Activation of the lateral thalamus, SSCI and SSCII, and insula are thought to be related to the sensory-discriminative aspects of pain processing. Bilateral thalamic responses may be related to the generalized arousal from pain. The anterior cingulate does not appear to be involved in coding intensity or location but rather in the affective, attentional, and response selection behavioral aspects of pain. Allodynia is associated with amplification of thalamic, insular, and SII (second somatosensory area) responses with a paradoxical decrease in rCBF in the cingulated region. The anterior cingulate may both respond to pain and participate in endogenous pain control circuitry (15). PET studies of 6 healthy volunteers with intravenous (IV) fentanyl showed selective increases in rCBF in the cingulated, orbitofrontal, and medial prefrontal cortices; all areas responsive to nociceptive stimuli that are involved in avoidance learning, reward, addiction, visceromotor control, mainternance of attention, and pain-related affective behavior (16).

Given the susceptibility of the aforementioned structural and neurochemical pain matrix to damage consequential to TBI, it would seem likely that pain perception and its emotional concomitants could be disturbed. Lesions of the primary and secondary tactile sensory cortex, which receives input from lateral spinothalamic projections, as well as the medial system, may produce a cortical loss of tactile sensation not confined to pain and temperature or disturbances in tactile/pain localization.

As indicated earlier, there are reciprocal connections between cortical, thalamic, and limbic structures and the brain stem regions intimately involved in pain transmission. The PAG appears to occupy a pivotal function in this regard, influencing other brain stem structures that in turn modulate DH nociceptive transmission. Stimulation of the PAG leads to inhibition of DH neurons, an effect mediated by PAG connections to structures in the RVM (nucleus magnus raphe, reticular formation) that provide the primary source of spinal 5-HT (and inhibitory influences on nociception).

The RVM has a somewhat complex internal relationship between "on" cells and "off" cells; however, the net descending effect is antinociceptive via 5-HT. Glutamate from the PAG facilitates this outflow, as do intrinsic opioids receptors. Finally, the RVM serotoninergic outflow is also facilitated by norepinephrine (NE) from the DLP catecholamine cell groups.

The DLP is also facilitated by the PAG. Its primary outflow is alpha-2 adrenergic and is antinociceptive not only at the RVM but also through direct NE influences on the DH through its descending pathways. The major descending noradrenergic axons originate in the locus ceruleus, subceruleus, and the Kölliker-Fuse nucleus. These nuclei are also the source of much of the adrenergic innervation to the cortex, cerebellum, and limbic system. Whereas approximately 50% of patients with intractable pain can be helped with chronic electrical stimulation of the PAG and thalamic relay nuclei, additional patients have reportedly been helped by stimulation of the Kölliker-Fuse nucleus (17).

In addition to classical neurotransmitters, prostaglandins also increase sensitivity of peripheral nociceptors and are also present in the DH and CNS. Cyclooxygenases (COXs) are enzymes that are produced during any inflammatory process. They convert arachidonic acid to prostaglandins. Peripheral inflammation increases COX-2 activity in the CNS. In the DH, prostaglandins produced by COX-2 cause increased release of pronociceptive neurotransmitters by primary nociceptive afferents and directly depolarize DH neurons. They also inhibit glycine release, which is typically antinociceptive.

A special consideration in TBI is the anatomical and functional associations related to post-traumatic head pain (cephalalgia) and neck pain (cervicalgia). Primary nociceptive afferents for the front of the scalp and face compose the trigeminal sensory system. Afferents from the meninges travel with the ophthalmic division of the fifth cranial nerve. The brain parenchyma itself does not appear to have any nociceptive afferent fibers. The area around the ear and the external auditory canal gives rise to sensory afferents to the ninth and tenth cranial nerves. Finally, the posterior scalp and upper neck are innervated by the upper 3 cervical dorsal roots, the greater occipital nerve C_2 and the lesser occipital nerve C_3. Nociceptive afferents from cranial nerves V, IX, and X travel to second-order neurons in the spinal tract and nucleus of the trigeminal nerve, which extend from the medulla to at least C_2 and at times to C_4. The V1, or ophthalmic division, is most caudal. The upper cervical DH and the spinal tract of the trigeminal nerve are contiguous and overlap (18). It appears that there is also an overlap between the second-order neurons in this region as well, so that central sensitization and expansion of receptive fields by second-order neurons may lead to perception of pain in the occiput or neck when the primary nociceptive generator is trigeminal and vice versa. Therefore, a primary nociceptive generator in the cervical musculature and/or occipital nerves could also activate the trigeminovascular system through central sensitization (19,20). Stimulation of the occipital nerve in animals activates the spinal nucleus caudalis of V in the same distribution, as when the meninges or cranial nerve V innervated structures are stimulated (19). Central afferent convergence and sensitization of afferent second-order neurons may underlie the spread of pain and referral from supratentorial dura to areas innervated by cervical afferents (muscles and joints of the head and neck). The "convergence-projection" theory stipulates that pain originating from an affected tissue (primary nociceptive generator) can be perceived as originating from a distant receptive field (21). Migraine appears to cause unique activation of the brain stem PAG as well as the dorsal raphe nuclei, which provide diffuse serotonin projections to cortex and blood vessels (22).

As with somatic nociceptive inputs, the PAG seems central to pain mediated by the trigeminal system (as in migraine) (23). PET studies demonstrate activation of the PAG, dorsal raphe nucleus, and locus ceruleus on the contralateral side to the headache (24). Capsaicin trigeminal stimulation in rats results in neuronal activation of the trigeminal nucleus, area postrema, solitary tract, reticular nucleus, locus ceruleus, parabrachial nucleus, raphe nucleus, PAG, intralaminar thalamic nucleus and various hypothalamic nuclei, as well as the amygdala (25).

The nociceptive systems in the peripheral nervous system (PNS) and CNS are both complex and dynamic, and the interplay of PNS and CNS in pain mechanisms is complex. Modulatory effects on pain transmission occur in the spinal cord, brain stem, and thalamus and occur via interconnections with limbic and frontal structures, especially those with relevance to the affective or attentional aspects of nociceptive processing. Many of the aforementioned sites, as previously noted, are susceptible to the pathology of TBI. The neurochemistry, and hence the neuropharmacology, of pain transmission and perception in the CNS often overlaps that of other disorders related to TBI such as depression, spasticity, and cognitive deficits, making any effort to treat these problems in isolation, without diligent awareness of the impact on the neurochemistry of associated conditions, ill advised. The plasticity of nociceptive transmission accounts for central sensitization and may also explain the neurological basis for referred pain.

Although on the one hand, the pain practitioner may wish to eliminate or control central sensitization; it is possible that the chemical and cytological architecture underlying central pain may also provide the structure for other important "plastic" processes in the CNS, such as motor recovery, learning, and memory. It is not clear at this time whether effective treatment of central pain (when available) will benefit or impede these other neuroplastic processes.

The neuroanatomical pathways associated with pain perception are clearly complex and not completely understood. Readers are referred to more in-depth sources for further detail (26–28). Cortical pain centers include the somatosensory cortex that receives input from the thalamus, which in turn receives its input from the midbrain nociceptive centers via input from brain stem nociceptive neuraxis. Input to the brain stem occurs through the spinothalamic tract, which derives its input through both wide dynamic range neurons and nociceptive specific neurons, which both compromise second-order afferents (4).

The lateral and medial pain systems should also be further considered, given the importance of these tracts in mediation of pain processing (27). Vogt and colleagues (29) considerably extended the concept of the medial pain system by demonstrating projections of the medial thalamic nuclei to area 24 of the anterior cingulate cortex. The anterior cingulate cortex is an extensive area of the limbic cortex overlying the corpus callosum and is involved in the integration of cognition, affect, and response selection. The descending connections of the anterior cingulate cortex to the medial thalamic nuclei and to the PAG in the brain stem suggest that this system may also be involved in the modulation of reflex responses to noxious stimuli. Partly because of the differences in latency of responses and their respective connections, researchers have suggested that the lateral and medial pain systems are predominantly responsible for processing acute and chronic pain, respectively (30). However, it is evident that these systems are highly interconnected and parallel; only at the level of the cortex do they become less obviously interrdependent. The intensity of sensation and pain perception is directly related to the energy level at the pain location.

Primary afferents comprise of A delta fibers and C fibers. A delta fibers are small, thin, and myelinated neurons, 1–5 μm in diameter with conduction velocities in the range of 5–30 m/s. Pain mediated by A delta fibers tends to be fast, sharp, localized, and well defined. These fibers have small receptive fields and tend to be modality specific. They are divided into thermoresponsive and mechanoresponsive subgroups. C fibers are small unmyelinated afferent fibers with diameters of 0.25–1.5 μm and conduction velocities from 0.5–2.0 m/s. Pain mediated by C fibers tends to be slow, diffuse, poorly localized, and of a burning, throbbing, or gnawing nature. These polymodal fibers subserve noxious nociceptive input from thermal, mechanical, and chemical stimuli, as well as non-noxious, low-intensity stimulation. Input to the primary afferents is provided through nociceptors, which ultimately are the first step in the sensory pathway of transduction of a painful stimulus to a relevant neural signal. Nociceptors occur in cutaneous, muscular, and visceral structures (30).

Pain may be triggered by sensory inputs, especially when acute, but may also be generated independently, especially when chronic. Sensitization effects represent hyperresponsiveness in either the peripheral or central components of the nervous system. Supraspinal sensitization effects associated with the medial pain system (27) and related limbic structures (31,32) seem to mediate the pain response. Thus, pain could be produced by the output of a widely distributed neural network in the brain rather than directly by nociceptive stimuli. Importantly, the central pain control processes seem to encompass the cognitive-evaluative, motivational-affective, and sensory-discriminative systems (33) that characterize the pain response. Functional brain imaging techniques, among other methods, have demonstrated that chronic pain, unlike acute pain, results in anatomical and functional reorganization of the brain and that brain regions involved in the former are distinct from the latter. Additionally, chronic pain, as noted, seems to preferentially activate prefrontal, paralimbic, and limbic areas in the brain, resulting in decreased gray matter density and disrupt gray and white matter interrelationships (34–36).

PAIN ASSESSMENT

Pain is a subjective experience, and therefore, a patient's self-report of pain is in actuality the cornerstone of pain assessment. There are several important aspects of the experience of pain that should be assessed. Pain character, onset, location, duration, and factors that exacerbate or relieve the pain should be explored. The clinician should also query about pain frequency and intensity and interference with everyday activities. Two useful methods of assessing pain intensity in adults are the Visual Analogue Scale (VAS) (37) and the Verbal Analogue Scale. The VAS is a 10-cm line with anchors of "no pain" and "the most pain imaginable," whereas the Verbal Analogue Scale solicits rating of pain on a 0–10 scale with the same anchors. The scale appears to be sensitive to treatment changes and is widely used in clinical settings. Pain is a complex perceptual process composed of behavioral, affective, cognitive, and sensory components, thereby requiring evaluation of not only the patient's medical findings but also physiological, behavioral, and cognitive-affective functioning, including vulnerabilities and strengths. A thorough review of the most useful pain assessment instruments, along with a model and methods of pain assessment, can be found in Chapter 58 of this text.

A comprehensive, multimodal, biopsychosocial assessment becomes even more critical when pain is chronic and should address beliefs about the individual's pain condition, pain coping strategies, psychological adjustment, activity level, and quality of life (38,39) (also see Chapter 58 in this text). The impact of various cognitive processes on the subjective perception of the patient's pain must be considered in the context of a comprehensive pain assessment. Turk (40) has emphasized the importance of understanding and addressing the important role of patient's pain appraisals, beliefs, and expectancies. In this latter context, clinicians must consider pain response biases as well as characterological traits that may "color" the patient's subjective reporting of his or her pain experience (see Chapters 58 and 85 in this text).

Components of emotion that are relevant to the pain experience include the subjective experience of how the pain feels, autonomic arousal associated with bodily reactions to pain, cognitive appraisal(s) of the painful experience as related to the personal meaning of the pain or the learned responses to pain and injury, nonverbal behaviors including facial expressions and body language associated with pain, and lastly, affective reactions to pain including anxiety (more typical acutely) and depression (more typical chronically) (38). People who have chronic pain have a much higher predilection and incidence of depression, anxiety, as well as anger. Diathesis-stress models have been proposed to explain the higher rate of depression in this patient population; however, the implications are likely applicable to other psychoemotional responses to chronic pain as well (41). Finally, psychological assessment is now a required element of pain treatment programs accredited by the Commission on Accreditation of Rehabilitation Facilities (42) as well as several managed care companies.

Adequate pain assessment requires a blinders-off approach and a search for the presumptive pain generator(s). The examining clinician must therefore take a relevant and focused pain history and perform a detailed pain exam in an attempt to identify any organic contributors to the patient's pain complaints. An adequate history should include at a minimum addressing factors expressed in the mnemonic "COLDER," that is, the *character, onset, location, duration,* as well as, *exacerbating* and *relieving factors.* A detailed pain medication history can also avoid unnecessary medication

trials and/or direct appropriate reconsideration of medications if dosing and/or trial duration was inadequate. It is not acceptable to just prescribe pain medications without an adequate attempt at the differential diagnosis of the pain generators responsible for the patient's subjective complaints. Abnormal pain exam findings including pertinent negatives and positives should be noted as observed including pathologic physical exam findings noted on observation, palpation, percussion, and/or auscultation, as well as pain behaviors, affect, and mood. Clinicians often do not spend enough examination time addressing inspection of the patient and the palpatory exam . . . these are key elements of the pain exam that should not be ignored. The physical exam should to a great extent be guided by the pain history. As clinically indicated, the exam would likely include an elemental neurological examination as well as a peripheral neurological examination and/or musculoskeletal medicine assessment based on the information elicited during the pain interview (43). A mental status exam should be performed on all patients with chronic pain, including assessment of cognitive status and psychoemotional state. Only through a detailed understanding of the myriad etiologies of post-traumatic pain following TBI can the examining clinician expect to be able to selectively and appropriately treat the relevant pain generators including ones that have become centrally sensitized, as is often the case in patients with chronic pain (44).

It is critical in the context of assessment to take an adequate pain history for the clinician to provide an adequate foundation for identifying possible or probable pain generators. Clinicians are cautioned against assumptions that commonly reported pain symptoms are caused by the brain injury itself (e.g., post-traumatic headache [PTHA]) when pain is more commonly produced by extracerebral injury. Evaluating clinicians should be familiar with both the broad array of pain symptoms that may be reported by patients with post trauma as well as assessment methodologies for the various types of pain seen in this population. Clinicians are referred to various other sources for a more detailed description of patient assessment methodologies for persons with pain disorders, including dual diagnoses of TBI and pain for more in-depth discussions of this topic (44,45).

PAIN MANAGEMENT STRATEGIES

The management of pain represents a significant public health issue in the United States. It is both costly to our health care system and devastating to the patient's quality of life. The goal of pain management is to modulate and ideally negate the associated physical and psychological symptoms of pain, prevent chronicity, and reduce functional disability. Realistic end points of pain relief consistent with the clinical situation should be established. Pain management methods include both nonpharmacologic and/or pharmacologic methods and are optimized when provided in a coordinated interdisciplinary and multidisciplinary fashion (see Chapter 58). Clinicians should strive to identify pain generators and treat them as directly as possible rather than simply treating the symptom of pain with pharmacological agents, such as opiates. Ideally, the simplest, least invasive, lowest risk, and most cost-effective management approaches that allow for optimization of patient compliance and maximal functional restoration should be used whenever possible. When pharmacologic agents are used, analgesia should be delivered with minimal adverse effects and inconvenience to the patient, with concurrent appropriate monitoring and clearly defined treatment expectancies, all of which will optimize compliance.

Medical Management: General Considerations

In the acute care setting, already compromised neurological status may limit the array of pharmacotherapeutic agents that might be appropriate to use in a patient whose neurosurgical and neurological status is either stabilized and/or static. Medications that potentially alter any aspect of the neurological assessment should be used with caution in the acute care setting if there is a more significant brain injury and/or neurologic instability. Additionally, consideration should be given to medications with reversible effects (e.g., opiate reversal with naltrexone) whenever there is question of medication effect vs ongoing deterioration of neurological status.

During the acute care phase, the primary pain generators in patients with trauma will typically be associated with fractures, intra-abdominal injuries, soft tissue injuries, and invasive procedures. Pain treatment should be tailored to the degree of pain observed and/or reported, the latter via metric (e.g., VAS) or qualitative (e.g., mild, moderate, severe, and excruciating) descriptors (assuming the patient is functional enough to engage in such feedback). For patients who are neurologically compromised and with response limitations, prophylactic pain management should be practiced based on injuries sustained and clinical presentation (44,45).

Pharmacologic prophylaxis of pain should be considered in patients with disorders of consciousness (DOC), given that (a) the difficulty in assessment of pain in this patient subgroup as well as controversies regarding pain appreciation and suffering in patient's whose awareness of pain may be difficult if not impossible to confirm and (b) the negative impact of pain (even in patients in a vegetative state [VS]) related to subcortical physiologic responses to nociceptive stimuli, including increased tone/posturing, tachycardia, tachypnea, and diaphoresis in addition to other adverse effects. The understanding of the neural correlates of pain in persons with DOC has grown substantively in the last decade. Prior to work by Schnakers and Zasler (46), the issue of pain assessment in persons with DOC had received minimal to no attention. There is now an actual validated pain scale for use with persons with DOC called the Nociception Coma Scale (47). Pain often affects functional assessment in patients with more severe impairments of consciousness and must be adequately assessed and treated. This includes pain associated with spasticity, posturing, fractures, pressure sores, peripheral nerve changes, CRPS, and postsurgical incisional pain.

In the subacute setting, many of the same issues present in the acute care setting will continue to serve as pain generators. As patients are weaned from general pain medication prescribed early on for prophylactic purposes, pain severity can increase along with subjective complaints and/or pain behaviors (i.e., increased agitation and fitful sleep, among the 2 most common in more persons who are severely injured with TBI). Acute pain generators can certainly then evolve into subacute pain generators. Ongoing attention to pain management must be continued, as patients are moved to neurosurgical step-down units and/or inpatient rehabilitation units. Changes in patient status in the subacute setting may reflect underlying neural changes that are adaptive or maladaptive. Maladaptive changes can result in additional pain generators (e.g., progression and/or increase of tonal abnormalities resulting in hypertonicity and/or rigidity) as well as central pain phenomena.

Chronic pain has many elements of acute and subacute pain but is generally promulgated by additional factors, including psychological ones. Current evidence strongly supports mechanisms of central sensitization in chronic pain phenomena that are not present in the acute and subacute periods (48). The patient suffering from chronic pain should be treated just as aggressively as a patient with acute or subacute pain. With chronic pain, biopsychosocial models for assessment and management are indicated to optimize treatment and outcomes (44,45) (also see Chapter 58 in this text).

Pharmacological Management

Mild pain medicines that should be considered for pain management in persons after TBI include aspirin, acetaminophen, and nonsteroidal anti-inflammatory drugs (NSAIDs). For moderate pain, the following may be considered: high-dose aspirin or acetaminophen, oral NSAIDs, newer generation NSAIDs such as COX-2 inhibitors (now limited to the single agent—celecoxib), injectable NSAIDs, mixed opiate analgesics with aspirin or acetaminophen (with or without caffeine), and tramadol. For severe pain, medications to consider would include parenteral narcotics (morphine sulfate = standard), mixed agonists/antagonists (pentazocine, nalbuphine), partial agonist narcotics (buprenorphine), antidepressants, anticonvulsants, and/or atypical agents (49). Stimulants, such as methylphenidate, can be used with opioid analgesics as an adjuvant analgesic and to help manage opioid-induced sedation and cognitive impairment. (see Tables 57-1 and 57-2)

Adjuvant analgesics are drugs that are analgesic in specific circumstances but have primary indications other than for pain management. Adjuvant analgesics are usually combined with analgesics. Corticosteroids, such as prednisone, are commonly used as short-term therapy to decrease pain and nausea and improve mood, appetite, and general sense of well-being. Adverse effects of short-term corticosteroid use include edema, dyspepsia, and neuropsychiatric changes. Patients with diabetes should be counseled about careful blood glucose monitoring while taking corticosteroids because of their hyperglycemic effect.

Antidepressants and anticonvulsants are used to manage various neuropathic pain states. Tricyclic antidepressants (TCAs), particularly amitriptyline, have shown efficacy in the management of diabetic neuropathy and are used for other neuropathic states. TCAs can also manage underlying depression in pain states. Other TCAs such as nortriptyline, imipramine, and desipramine can also be used; however, they should be used at low antinociceptive doses to avoid more significant anticholinergic effects. Agents that are serotonin-norepinephrine reuptake inhibitors (SNRIs), such as venlafaxine (Effexor) and duloxetine (Cymbalta), have also

TABLE 57-1 Medications for Pain

ANTIDEPRESSANTS		ANTICONVULSANTS	
Bedtime dose helps sleep & pain		Especially for lancinating pain	
	Typical dose		**Typical dose**
Amitriptyline	75 mg qhs	Carbamazepine	200 mg q8h
Desipramine	75 mg qhs	Valproic acid	250 mg q8h
Nortriptyline	75 mg qhs	Phenytoin	100 mg q8h
Fluoxetine	20 mg qd	Clonazepam	0.5 mg q8h
Venlafaxine	25 mg q8h	Gabapentin	600 mg q8h
Paroxetine	20–40mg qd	Lamotrigine	100–200 mg q12
		Pregabalin	50 mg tid
		Local anesthetics and miscellaneous agents	
Analgesics			**Typical dose**
	Typical dose	Lidocaine	1.5 mg/kg IV
Acetaminophen	650 mg q4–6h	Mexiletine	225 mg q8h
		Flecainide	150 mg q12h
Ibuprofen	400–800 mg q8h	Fluphenazine	40 mg/day
Aspirin	650 mg q4–6h	Ketamine—NMDA antagonist	150 mg IV test and 250 mg/day
Steroids		**Topical**	
	Typical dose		**Typical dose**
Prednisone	20–80 mg qd	Capsaicin	Topical qid
Dexamethasone	4–16 mg qd	Speed gel	Topical tid–qid

Abbreviations: IV, intravenous; NMDA, N-methyl-D-aspartate; qd, every day; qhs, every night at bedtime; qh, every hour; qid, 4 times a day; tid, 3 times a day.

been found effective in certain pain conditions because of apparent antinociceptive properties (50,51). TCA adverse effects include anticholinergic effects (dry mouth, sedation), weight gain, orthostatic hypotension, and cardiac arrhythmias. Secondary amines, such as nortriptyline and desipramine, have fewer adverse effects and should be used in patients, such as the elderly, when there is concern for anticholinergic effects, sedation, and orthostatic hypotension. Antidepressants generally should be initiated at a low dosage and titrated up slowly based on pain relief and patient tolerance.

Anticonvulsants, such as carbamazepine and gabapentin, can be effective for the management of neuropathic pain, particularly lancinating or paroxysmal pain. Clinicians should be familiar with which patients to screen for potential drug treatment contraindications (e.g., Asians for human leukocyte antigen-B [HLA-B] to avoid potentially fatal dermatological reactions). Carbamazepine-related compounds can cause hepatotoxicity, aplastic anemia, thrombocytopenia, and/or hyponatremia. Patients prescribed on this parent drug class should have complete blood counts performed at initiation of therapy and as clinically indicated, although there is no good evidence-based recommendations for same from the manufacturer relative to frequency (52). Gabapentin has shown efficacy in diabetic neuropathy and postherpetic neuralgia, and generally has a milder adverse effect profile consisting of sedation, ataxia, and does not require routine lab work. A Cochrane review examining the role of

TABLE 57-2 Opioid Analgesics

SHORT-ACTING OPIOIDS			LONG-ACTING OPIOIDS		
Drug	**Equivalent Doses**		Drug	**Equivalent Doses**	
	Oral	Parenteral		Oral	Parenteral
Morphine	30 mg q3–4h	10 mg q3–4h	MS-Contin	90–120 mg q12h	
Hydromorphone	7.5 mg q3–4h	1.5 mg q3–4h	Levorphanol	4 mg q6–8h	2 mg q6–8h
Codeine	200 mg q3–4h		Methadone	20 mg q6–8h	10 mg q3–6h
Hydrocodone	30 mg q3–4h		Oramorph SR	90–120 mg q12h	
Tramadol	50–100 mg q4–6h (max. 400 mg/day)				

Opioid-naive adults and children ≥ 50 kg body weight.
The above mentioned drugs are only a partial list of available opiate medications.
Abbreviations: max, maximum; MS, morphine sulfate; qh, every hour; SR, sustained release.

antiepileptic drugs (AEDs) for acute and chronic pain noted that although they are widely used for chronic pain, surprisingly, few trials have shown analgesic effectiveness. They noted that there was no evidence for anticonvulsant effectiveness in acute pain; however, in chronic pain syndromes, it was suggested that aside from treatment of trigeminal neuralgia, AEDs must be relegated to basically third-line treatment. Lastly, it was noted that there was no evidence to support the contention that gabapentin was superior to other AEDs in neuropathic pain management (53). As with the antidepressants, one should institute treatment at a low dosage and titrate the dose up slowly to improve tolerance and optimize compliance. Valproate, oxcarbazepine, lamotrigine, topamax, levetiracetam, phenytoin, and clonazepam are other anticonvulsants that also have been used for neuropathic pain with variable reports of efficacy. AEDs, such as pregabalin, an alpha-2 delta ligand, which have been found efficacious in certain types of neuropathic pain may also prove useful in the management of certain post-traumatic pain conditions (54,55). Animal derived toxins, such as ziconotide (Prialt), a synthetic neuronal N-type calcium channel blocker, have received recent Food and Drug Administration (FDA) approval and may also offer a promise for treatment of intractable severe chronic pain in patients intolerant of or refractory to other forms of treatment (56). This agent, such as other intraspinal (intrathecal or epidural) analgesics, should only be tried when other standard treatments have failed and must be administered via a programmable implanted microinfusion device for long-term users.

Implanted intrathecal drug delivery systems are widely used in the treatment of chronic pain when conservative therapies have failed and surgery is not a viable option; however, they have not been systematically evaluated in persons with acquired brain injury of any type. The current FDA-approved intrathecal medications include baclofen, morphine, and ziconotide. Other pharmacological agents are used off label (i.e., not FDA approved in this application) including bupivicaine, buprenorphine, clonidine, fentanyl, hydromorphone, ketamine, midazolam, ropivacaine, and sufentanil. Such therapies are not without potential complications, however, and prescribing physicians should remain current on the pain literature relevant to this class of interventions. There are many complexities associated with intrathecal drug prescription and maintenance, including issues germane to spinal drug safety. Intrathecal use of spinal drugs, particularly off label, cannot be presumed to be safe because they are used "safely" via other routes of administration (57).

Other agents that have more recently been recognized as adjuvants in the pharmacologic management of pain include tizanidine (Zanaflex) and sodium amobarbital (Amytal). Tizanidine has been shown to be effective in various pain conditions including fibromyalgia, as well as tension type headache, possibly on the basis of modulation of substance P and/or owing to its alpha-adrenergic effects (58). Mailis and Nicholson (59) have provided an excellent review of the use of sodium amytal infusion in the assessment and treatment of chronic pain (and functional disorders), and a recent, soon to be published, review article on sodium amytal discusses the history and neurorehabilitative applications of this agent including its use in a number of different pain disorders (60).

Capsaicin can be used topically to help decrease pain associated with peripheral neuropathies (61). It is also available commercially as a high-dose dermal patch (trade name—Qutenza) for peripheral neuropathic pain (62). It may be used in concentrations of between 0.025% and 0.075%. It may be used as a cream for the temporary relief of minor aches and pains of muscles and joints associated with arthritis, simple backache, strains, and sprains. Capsaicin depletes peptides such as substance P that mediate nociceptive transmission. Application of capsaicin is associated usually with a burning sensation, which may be severe enough to require premedication with either an oral analgesic or a topical lidocaine cream or ointment. The treatment typically involves the application of a topical anesthetic until the area is numb, then the capsaicin is applied wearing rubber gloves and a face mask. The capsaicin remains on the skin until the patient starts to feel the "heat," at that point, it is promptly removed. Patients should be counseled not to touch mucous membranes after applying capsaicin.

Compounded agents typically formulated through "compounding pharmacies" may also play a role in pain management of the patient after TBI. Agents that have been used in topical formulations for pain include local anesthetics, antidepressants, alpha-2 agonists, opioids, and glutamate antagonists such as gabapentin, calcium channel blockers, skeletal muscle relaxants, capsaicin, ketamine, menthol, and NSAIDs. Standard topical formulas such as "speed gel," which contains amitriptyline, lidocaine, guaifenesin, and ketoprofen, can work quite well for neuropathic/neuralgic scalp pain, scar pain, and post-traumatic myalgias. Similarly prepared compounded topicals with varying ingredients such as gabapentin, ketamine, and clonidine may be more helpful as adjuvants for CRPS-related pain (63). Many clinicians are unfamiliar with the concept of compounded medications and/or with compounding pharmacies. In the United States, there are agencies such as the Pharmacy Compounding Accreditation Board (PCAB) that aim to promote high quality in pharmacy compounding through a voluntary accreditation program that recognizes adherence to established principles, policies, and standards (64).

Surgery produces pain by releasing pain and inflammatory mediators via damaged tissue. This pain is acute pain and will improve as the wound heals and the patient convalesces. The goal of postoperative pain management is to provide continuous and effective analgesia with minimal adverse effects. NSAIDs, such as parenteral ketorolac, are used both intraoperatively and postoperatively to decrease the production of inflammatory prostaglandins released at the site of injury. The ketorolac dose is dependent on route, patient age, and weight and should only be continued at the appropriate dosage for 5 days because of the development of renal dysfunction and gastrointestinal (GI) toxicity. Opioid analgesics are the most commonly used medications for acute and subacute postoperative pain, usually administered intramuscularly or intravenously on an as needed basis. This approach can lead to delays in the patient receiving adequate analgesia because of medication administration delays and intramuscular route absorption. Patients should be switched to oral opioid analgesics when oral administration is tolerated. Patient-controlled analgesia (PCA) is a process where the patient is allowed to self-administer low doses of IV opioid analgesics to maintain analgesia (64). To use PCA, a patient should be sufficiently cognizant to understand the goals of PCA and understand the use of the equipment. Patients who are confused or cognitively impaired are not good candidates for PCA. The number of injections and attempted injections can be monitored for efficacy and adverse effects in addition to the patient's report of pain. Opioid analgesics can also be administered into the epidural or intrathecal space combined with local anesthetics, such as bupivacaine or ropivacaine, for postoperative pain management. Patient-controlled epidural analgesia should be considered in specific circumstances but obviously must consider the orientation level and cognitive status of the patient being treated.

Opioid analgesics stimulate the opioid receptors (mu, kappa, and delta subtypes) that are widely distributed throughout the brain, spinal cord, and PNS (65). The opiate receptors appear to function at presynaptic potassium channels and indirectly affect voltage-gated sodium channels to reduce the release of excitatory amino acids and substance P. Analgesia occurs primarily via action at the mu receptors and less so at the kappa and delta receptors. Mu receptor stimulation is also responsible for some other opiate effects such as miosis, depressed gastric motility, and respiratory depression. Kappa stimulation does influence spinal analgesia and also causes miosis and respiratory depression. Stimulation of delta receptors seems to account for hallucinations, confusion, and stimulation of respiratory and vasomotor centers (66).

The use of opiates in chronic nonmalignant pain management remains controversial. Poppy derivatives and opioid medications have demonstrated "proven" pain relieving properties for hundreds of years. It has only been in the last century that a significant social stigma has been attached to the use or prescription of opiates for chronic pain treatment. Now, the pressures from agencies such as the Joint Commission on Accreditation of Healthcare Organizations (JCAHO) to provide appropriate and thorough pain management appear to be at odds with legislative and legal considerations imposed by State Boards of Medicine and the Drug Enforcement Agency (DEA). Physicians and patients are concerned about addiction, tolerance, and side effects from opiates. Recent work has noted that the prescription of opioids for chronic noncancer pain (CNCP) has continued to escalate in the United States, although there is a continued lack of evidence supporting long-term effectiveness with commensurate increasing levels of abuse and diversion along with an uncertainty about the incidence and salience of a plethora of potential adverse side effects. The evidence base on opioid use in CNCP is limited by the short time frame of clinical trials, insufficient comprehensive outcome assessment, and incomplete categorization and quantification of adverse side effects (67). Others have advocated similarly, noting that the rise in opioid prescribing has outpaced the evidence regarding this practice. Increased opioid availability has been accompanied by an epidemic of opioid abuse and overdose with the rate of opioid addiction in long-term users unclear but clearly not a rare phenomenon. The risks for serious adverse events including fractures, cardiovascular events, and bowel obstruction (see the following text for further discussion) may be both dose related and underappreciated. By limiting long-term opioid therapy to patients for whom it provides decisive benefits could also reduce long term risks. Many clinicians and researchers are now taking the stance that until stronger evidence becomes available, clinicians should err on the side of caution when considering treatment with this class of drugs (68,69).

Tolerance to side effects develops fairly rapidly as compared to analgesic effects. Tolerance is simply a shift in the dose-response curve to achieve a desired therapeutic effect—one needs to either increase the dose or shorten the dosing interval. This phenomenon is not unique to opiates and occurs with various medications. Physical dependence refers to a state resulting from chronic use of a drug that has produced tolerance and where negative physical symptoms of withdrawal result from abrupt discontinuation or dosage reduction. In the case of opiates, abstinence syndrome symptoms may include lacrimation, diaphoresis, nausea, and vomiting and typically does not persist for more than 72 hours; however, associated sleep disturbances and depression can last several weeks. Tolerance and physical dependence are simply physiologic responses to opioid exposure and do not imply aberrant drug use. Addiction is a complex set of maladaptive behaviors resulting in physical, psychological, or social harm. There is an alteration in CNS function that the affected individual finds desirable, resulting in a craving for the drug in question, often associated with tolerance for the nonanalgesic and desired effect, resulting in unsanctioned dose escalation and preoccupation with acquisition of the drug and resultant adverse psychosocial consequences. The term *pseudoaddiction* refers to behaviors similar to those in addiction but more specific to desired analgesic affects. The behaviors cease when appropriate analgesic management leads to adequate pain control (in other words, the physician has failed to provide sufficient medication or alter dosing in response to expected physiologic tolerance) (66,67).

"Cognitive" and affective side effects can occur with opiate medications. Euphoria or dysphoria, sedation, hypnagogic, or hypnopompic hallucinations may appear and typically do so within 3–7 days of dose initiation or escalation but abate within the same time frame (67). Any worsening of cognitive performance occurs within the first few days of use or the first few hours after a dose, but tolerance develops to this phenomenon. There are relatively few differences found in cognitive performance in patients taking opioids compared to their performance before opioids or with the performance of a comparable pain population who are not taking opioids (70). Desirable clinical effects of opioid analgesics clearly include analgesia and reduced anxiety. Common side effects include constipation (the most common) and nausea, and tolerance to the aforementioned does not frequently develop. Drug development has led to agents such as Targin (available in Europe and Australia) that combines an opiate agonist with an antagonist (the latter in the form of naloxone) to prevent opiate-induced constipation because of the high-binding infinity of naloxone in the intestine and its additional high first-pass hepatic metabolism (71). Other well-established side effects include sedation, dizziness, vomiting, physical dependence, tolerance, respiratory, and cough depression, and less commonly, delayed gastric emptying, hyperalgesia, immunological and hormonal dysfunction, muscle rigidity, and myoclonus (72). Confusion, hallucinations, delirium, urticaria, hypothermia, bradycardia/tachycardia, orthostatic hypotension, headache, urinary retention, ureteral or biliary spasm, myoclonus (with high doses), and flushing (because of histamine release, except fentanyl and remifentanil) may also occur.

Opioid-induced hyperalgesia occurs when individuals using opioids to relieve pain may paradoxically experience more pain as a result of their medication. This phenomenon, although uncommon, is seen in some palliative care patients, most often when dose is escalated rapidly. If encountered, rotation between several different opioid analgesics may mitigate the development of hyperalgesia. Both therapeutic and chronic use of opioids can compromise the function of the immune system. Opioids have been shown to decrease the proliferation of macrophage progenitor cells and lymphocytes and affect cell differentiation. Opioids may also inhibit leukocyte migration. However, the relevance of this in the context of pain relief is unknown. Men who are taking moderate-to-high doses of an opioid analgesic in long-term are likely to have subnormal testosterone levels, which can lead to osteoporosis and decreased muscle strength if left untreated. Therefore, total and free testosterone levels should be monitored in these patients; if levels are suboptimal, testosterone replacement therapy, preferably with patches or transdermal preparations, should be given. Also, prostate-specific antigen levels should be monitored (72).

Overall, there is no strong evidence that there are any long-term significant cognitive side effects from opiates, and adequate pain control may enhance cognitive performance (66,73–75); although as with most things in science, there are examples to the contrary. As noted earlier, long-term data on the efficacy and safety of chronic opioid use are lacking; however, there is an anecdotal evidence that they can be safely administered, even in relatively high doses for many years (74). Over the last decade, various safeguards have been put in place in the United States to improve decision making, monitoring, and ultimately patient safety associated with opiate prescription including FDA stipulation that Risk Evaluation and Mitigation Strategy (REMS) would be required with extended-release and long-acting opiates (76). Institution of prescription drug monitoring programs or PDMPs has allowed multiple states in the United States to develop and maintain a database of prescribed controlled substances and in doing so facilitates efforts to track such medications to improve patient care, assure patients are not "drug seeking" from other physicians, and identify those individuals who might be acquiring medications for abuse or diversion (77).

A TBI clinician must also consider other factors when considering opiate prescription for pain-related issues, including the fact that the opiate system is intimately involved in learning and reward. In the rodent model, genetic absence of the mu receptor, but not the kappa receptor, resulted in severe impairments in spatial learning (78). Therefore, the possibility exists that opiate use after TBI may promote certain cognitive or affective improvements. However, practitioners must be aware that there may be adverse cognitive effects in those persons taking undue/excessive amounts of opioid medications, either because of inappropriate physician prescribing practices or patient noncompliance. Other potential reasons for occurrence of opioid-related cognitive impairment include drug sensitivity, concurrently use of other substances (e.g., alcohol), or temporary impairment associated with increasing of opioid dose.

There are various derived and synthetic opiates available, each with different potencies and properties. Meperidine, and to a lesser extent, propoxyphene have mixed opioid agonist and antagonist properties and may cause severe cognitive problems in the elderly, including hallucinations as with opiates in general. Neither drug should be used with monoamine oxidase (MAO) inhibitors secondary to a risk of hypertensive crisis or autonomic dysregulation. Moderate potency opiates (hydrocodone and oxycodone) are metabolized by liver P450 enzymes into morphine, and if given with other drugs that inhibit metabolism via this enzyme (e.g., selective serotonin reuptake inhibitors [SSRIs]), a given dose of these opiates may produce less than optimal pain relief. Similarly, the low potency synthetic opiate-like drug tramadol should be used with caution with SSRIs and other antidepressants secondary to increased seizure risk (more likely a function of its agonistic properties on NE and 5-HT receptors, which may also be desirable in dampening central sensitization) (79).

Most patients taking long-acting opioids should be supplied with a fast-acting rescue opioid to treat breakthrough pain. Oral rescue medicine may be needed every 2–4 hours. The usual dose is the analgesic equivalent of 5%–15% of the 24-hour baseline dose of the scheduled long-acting opioid analgesic. As with any pain medication and/ or intervention, the prescribed agent should be titrated to achieve optimal pain relief with minimal side effects. Clinicians should discuss treatment expectancies prior to issuing prescriptions for any pain medication (80).

Clinicians treating patients with TBI may be especially concerned about cognitive side effects and slowing of cognitive recovery; again, a concern that may be overemphasized. Indeed, for patients with polytrauma without brain injury with multiple fractures, physicians would have no qualms about administering opiates, especially in the acute care setting. Yet in the acute and subacute phases of brain injury, when the patient may be unable to communicate or have severely altered consciousness, physicians are reticent to provide adequate analgesia with opiates. From a practical perspective, it would be appropriate to use opiates for analgesia if the physician can reasonably assume that a patient with brain injury has opiate responsive sources of pain, even if he or she has limited ability to communicate. In fact, as previously noted in this chapter, a common contributor to "agitation" in the acute care or rehabilitation setting may be inadequate analgesia. On the other hand, there is an evidence that patients in a VS do not have conscious awareness of nociceptive stimuli; specifically, there is an activation of brainstem, thalamic, and primary somatosensory cortices but not of secondary association cortex (45,81). The implication is that patients who are truly in a VS (i.e., arousal without awareness) and not minimally conscious state (MCS) may in fact be incapable of "suffering" (in line with historical neurological dogma that persons in VS do not feel pain). However, it is also now known that the bedside clinical presentation of VS may not always be an accurate reflection of whether a given patient is in fact vegetative; specifically, there are now cases that have been shown via functional brain imaging protocols to be aware even though by clinical criteria that they meet standards for a VS diagnosis. Opioid analgesic treatment should therefore be considered in any patient, given the limitations of the bedside clinical exam and the potential benefits of not only modulating comfort level in those patients able to be aware of their pain but also decreasing aberrant physiological responses associated with pain in those who were not with the caveat that every attempt to modulate and/or minimize nociceptive stimuli should be made before using opiate analgesics.

Clinicians should be familiar with important documents concerning the use of controlled substances such as opiate medications. In 2004, the Federation of State Medical Boards of the United States published a *Model Policy for the Use of Controlled Substances for the Treatment of Pain*, which was developed in collaboration with pain experts around the country to provide guidance to state medical boards in developing state pain policies and regulations. Written in the form of a model policy document, the guidelines provided model language that may be used by states to clarify their positions regarding the use of controlled substances to treat pain, to alleviate physician uncertainty about such practice, and to encourage better pain management. In 2004, the Federation's House of Delegates adopted recommendations and revised the pain policy to reflect new medical insights in pain treatment, particularly regarding the undertreatment of pain (82). As prescribers, professionals should also be aware of the myriad issues that may confront both the clinician and the patient when opiate medications are used for chronic pain management (83). One must also remain aware of the current evidence-based medicine regarding the use of chronic opioid therapies in specific types of pain conditions, such as chronic, nonmalignant, and neuropathic pain (84,85).

Current consensus among pain specialists dictates that concerns regarding addiction are generally not a contraindication to opioid treatment for otherwise intractable pain, although the possible problems associated with inappropriate opioid treatment should be kept in mind. In particular, the need and efficacy of opioids in patients with chronic pain having prior drug abuse histories or addiction prone personalities should be carefully assessed and monitored. The effectiveness of opioids with respect to both reduction in pain severity ratings as well as effect on functional capacity should be considered. Practitioners should also be intimately familiar with the clinical features of opiate withdrawal and methodologies for tracking same (see Appendix I). Clinicians should always use a "controlled-substance agreement" when using such agents for pain management to protect not only the patient's safety but also his or her own given the litigious nature of our society (86) (see Appendix II). Ultimately, clinicians must have insight into the fact that chronic pain should be managed in a rational manner via integration of pharmacological approaches with behavioral and traditional rehabilitation interventions (87).

General Guidelines for Pain Pharmacotherapy

The physician should aim for drug prescriptions that optimize compliance and minimize potential side effects. Particularly in patients with cognitive impairments, physicians should aim for once- to twice-a-day drug dosing. Patients should be counseled on the goals of treatment and what to expect regarding adverse effects, especially constipation with opioid analgesics or GI side effects with NSAIDs. As possible, significant others should also be informed of treatment regimen and possible complications.

Depending on the severity of the pain and the patient's pain tolerance, consider a trial of acetaminophen as an initial management strategy. If prescribing a nonselective NSAID for more than 10–14 days then consider coadministration of a mucoprotectant agent such as a proton pump inhibitor and/or misoprostol. For elderly patients, a gastroprotectant should be used regardless of the duration of NSAID therapy. Only proceed to opiate-like and/or opiate medications when the pain level and functional disability associated with the pain are moderate to severe (80,84).

When using opioid analgesics, fears regarding dependence should be openly discussed as should other potential side effects, particularly when use may likely be longer term, including cognitive, GI, and sexual effects. Ideally, the clinician should aim for decreasing polypharmacy; however, when appropriate, combination drug regimens should be considered. It is also critical to ascertain whether patients are taking their medicine correctly (e.g., taking scheduled medicine on a as needed basis) and /or supplanting their prescribed medications with over-the-counter (OTC) products.

Nonpharmacologic Medical Management

A wide variety of medical rehabilitative interventions focusing on physical modalies (e.g., physiotherapy, exercise, chiropractic, massage, etc.), as well as other nonpharmacological medical interventions for chronic pain may be helpful in ameliorating pain complaints and suffering following TBI (88,89). However, more recent evidence suggests that many such treatments may be of questionable value relative to placebo or no treatment. Depending on the etiology of the pain generator in question, numerous nonpharmacologic medical and psychological approaches may be considered in the management of pain conditions including use of physical agents and modalities, injection therapies, exercise, biofeedback, adaptive equipment, and/or psychological interventions. These treatment modalities should all be given adequate consideration in conjunction with possible pharmacologic alternatives if physicians are to develop adequate functionally oriented treatment regimens for addressing chronic pain issues in persons with TBI. Readers are referred to Chapter 58 for details regarding the behavioral and psychological management of pain following TBI.

Physical Modalities

Physical agents used to modulate pain may include superficial heat and cold. The most common modalities used are hot/cold packs, heat lamps (incandescent or infrared), paraffin baths, and cryotherapy. Hydrotherapy interventions for pain management may involve prescription of whirlpool or contrast baths. Various diathermy techniques may also be used to facilitate pain control, including ultrasound, phonophoresis as well as short-wave and microwave diathermy. There are also a number of electrical stimulation techniques used in pain management such as transcutaneous electrical stimulation (TENS) and iontophoresis that are commonly employed as adjuvants for pain control. Although historically used for chronic pain modulation, a Cochrane (90) review examining the efficacy of TENS in the aforementioned application found inconclusive results with published trials not providing information on the stimulation parameters that are most likely to provide optimum pain relief or the effectiveness of long-term treatment. More recent reviews including an updated Cochrane review and a Veterans Administration Technology Assessment Program (91,92) have concluded that the current medical literature is inconclusive regarding the effectiveness of TENS for pain management. The quality and scope of the evidence is generally insufficient, or results with TENS were equivocal with respect to alternative modalities. A 2005 study (93) found that evidence was lacking, limited, or conflicting for efficacy in mechanical neck disorder management for electrotherapy interventions, including pulsed electromagnetic field (PEMF) therapy, galvanic current, iontophoresis, TENS, diadynamic current, and electrical muscle stimulation. Cranial electrical stimulation (CES) is a treatment for pain reduction that, unlike TENS, targets CNS function (see Chapter 17 in this text). The technique involves attachment of electrodes carrying microcurrent across the scalp and induces an approximate 15Hz cortical rhythm. Controlled studies support that it is a safe and useful treatment for pain, especially chronic pain and its associated symptoms of anxiety, depression, and insomnia (94); although truth be told, much of this literature is methodologically weak.

Physical modalities tend to play a more predominant role in the treatment of pain complaints of musculoskeletal origin and may include traction, manual medicine techniques (e.g., joint manipulation, myofascial release techniques, and strain counterstrain), as well as massage (95). Post-traumatic upper shoulder girdle and cervical myofascial pain are often seen in this patient population and may contribute not only to localized pain complaints but also to referred pain, including headache. Clinicians should be intimately familiar with both assessment and management of myofascial pain (96). Body-work techniques and bioenergetics, although not well studied aside from acupuncture, are 2 additional classes of intervention that may also be used as adjuvants in chronic pain management (e.g., Reiki, Alexander, Trager and meridian, acupuncture, and polarity, respectively). Injection techniques including intra-articular, periarticular, peritendinous, ligamentous/fibrous tissue (i.e., prolotherapy and plate rich plasma), and trigger point can all be used in various types of musculoskeletal pain disorders (95,97). Axial injections such as epidurals, zygapophyseal joint, and sympathetic blocks may all be relevant considerations for pain treatment in this population depending on the presumptive pain generators (97).

Exercise is an underappreciated and therefore underprescribed treatment intervention in persons with post-TBI or for that matter, many other patients with pain complaints. Exercise can play a significant role in controlling pain at both central and peripheral level, concurrently improving weight control, affect, general state of health, and well-being (98,99). Exercise has also been shown to elevate beta-endorphin levels, decrease stress, and enhance object recognition memory as well as upregulate brain-derived neurotrophic factor (BDNF) (the latter phenomena indicating that it may play a role in promoting neural repair and enhancement of learning and memory by increasing neurotrophic support) (100,101). Of course, the benefits of exercise are dependent on the patient taking an active role in his or her own rehabilitation and therapists such as recreational therapists (RTs) facilitating involvement through recommendations for adaptive exercise and sporting equipment as well as referral to appropriate adaptive sports programs (see Chapter 82 in this text).

Adaptive equipment such as reachers, sock aide, long-handled scrubbers, and/or brushes, as well as ergonomically modified task analyses for activities of daily living (ADLs), mobility, and work environments are few of the many different interventions that may also facilitate greater pain modulation and tolerance. Appropriate education regarding pacing and energy conservation techniques may also add to further improvement in functional status depending on the type of chronic pain condition being treated (see Chapter 58 in this text).

SPECIAL TOPICS IN PAIN MANAGEMENT IN PERSONS WITH TBI

Post-Traumatic Headache

Headache (e.g., cephalalgia) is the most common physical complaint reported after mild brain injury/concussion and cranial (i.e., head) trauma, and recent literature suggests it may also be more common than previously thought after moderate-to-severe TBI (see Chapter 56 in this text). Headache is also very frequently associated with cervical injuries and post-traumatic cervicalgia. Historically, head pain or headache was believed to be reported far less commonly in more severe injuries (102). More recent research suggests that even persons status post moderate-to-severe TBI suffer from acute headache symptoms, most often on a daily basis and in a frontal location and tended to improve in time with recovery generally leveling off by 6 months postinjury (103). The general experience, however, continues to indicate a trend toward greater levels of subjective complaints of headache among those individuals with milder brain injuries as opposed to more severe ones including as noted in military personnel injured during active duty (see Chapter 55 in this text). Zasler (104) has speculated that the primary cause for such headaches is in fact related to cervical injury and that early treatment rendered to persons with more severe TBI, such as chemical paralysis and protracted bedrest, may actually be therapeutically, albeit inadvertently, prophylaxing against the development of PTHA.

PTHA, and in particular post-concussive headaches, seldom connote serious underlying neurological problems. Clinicians should be aware, however, of various significant clinical conditions that may be responsible for PTHA and therefore should always appropriately consider the differential diagnosis of this condition including late extra-axial hematomas, tension pneumocephalus because of dural leaks, carotid artery dissection, communicating hydrocephalus, and ventriculoperitoneal shunt malfunction resulting in low- or high-pressure headaches, post-traumatic epilepsy (whether convulsive or nonconvulsive), syndrome of the trephined, post-traumatic sinus headache, cavernous sinus thrombosis, and carotid-cavernous fistulas (105) (also see Chapter 56 in this text).

There continue to be significant disparities in classification and nomenclature regarding PTHA, often because these are arbitrary and not predicated on physiology or established time courses for symptom manifestation (104). The classification, etiology, course, pathophysiology, and treatment remain poorly understood and controversial (106–108). One particularly pertinent issue is the use of opioids in patients with migraine, given recent literature indicating that such use leads to decreased gray matter, release of CGRP, dynorphin, proinflammatory peptides, and activation of excitatory glutamate receptors. Opioids have also been shown to be pronociceptive, prevent reversal of migraine central sensitization, interfere with triptan effectiveness, and can precipitate transformation to daily headache (109). The readers are referred to Chapter 56 for an in-depth discussion of important topics in PTHA.

Neuropathic Pain

Neuropathic pain is defined as a chronic pain condition that occurs or persists after a primary lesion or dysfunction of the PNS or CNS. Traumatic injury of peripheral nerves also increases the excitability of nociceptors in and around nerve trunks and involves components released from nerve terminals (neurogenic inflammation) and immunological and vascular components from cells resident within or recruited into the affected area. Action potentials generated in nociceptors and injured nerve fibers release excitatory neurotransmitters at their synaptic terminals such as L-glutamate and substance P and trigger cellular events in the CNS that extend over different time frames (110).

Neuropathic pain has been shown to be mediated by both PNS and CNS phenomena. In the PNS mechanisms that have been posited to be involved with neuropathic pain include, but are not necessarily limited to, spontaneous ectopic discharges, neuroimmune factors such as inflammatory cytokines, and sympathetic sensory coupling. CNS mechanisms that are theorized to be involved with neuropathic pain include central sensitization, disinhibition, as well as astrocyte and microglia activation (111,112).

Short-term alterations of neuronal excitability reflected, for example, in rapid changes of neuronal discharge activity are sensitive to conventional analgesics, and do not commonly involve alterations in activity-dependent gene expression. Novel compounds and new regimens for drug treatment to influence activity-dependent long-term changes in pain transducing and suppressive systems (pain matrix) are emerging. At present, therapeutic options are largely limited to drugs approved for other conditions, including anticonvulsants (carbamazepine, gabapentin, pregabalin), antidepressants (TCAs, venlafaxine, duloxetine), antiarrhythmics (e.g., mexiletine and flecainide), topical agents including transdermal lidocaine, NMDA receptor blockers such as ketamine and dextromethorphan, tramadol, and opioid analgesics as well as systemic local anesthetics (86,113).

Treatment based on the underlying disease state may be less than optimal, in that 2 patients with the same neuropathic pain syndrome may have different symptomatologies and thus respond differently to the same treatment. Increases in our understanding of the function of the neurologic system over the last few years have led to new insights into the mechanisms underlying pain symptoms, especially chronic neuropathic pain.

Neurosurgical options may need to be considered when enteral pharmacotherapeutic options fail or produce subop-

timal pain control. Surgical options include modulative techniques, such as neurostimulation or implanted drug delivery systems and ablative procedures such as rhizotomies (97).

Central Pain Syndromes

Central pain is defined as "pain associated with lesions of the central nervous system." Evident from the discussion of the anatomy and neurochemistry of nociceptive transmission, multiple systems contribute to the development of central pain. People with TBI may experience central pain akin to that recognized as poststroke pain but may also have associated spinal cord injury (SCI) with spinal pain. Sixty to seventy percent of patients with SCI have pain that is often chronic in nature (115). Diffuse pain below the level of the lesion may be caused by involvement of the posterior spinal tracts, there may be a band-like pain at the transitional zone, or pain developing late after injury; the source may be a syrinx (116). Brain-related central pain develops in about 8% of patients with stroke, although its incidence and prevalence following TBI are unclear (117). Probably the best study to date on central pain after TBI was conducted by Ofek and Defrin (118) and found that pain was developed at a relatively late onset and was almost exclusively unilateral. It was typically described as pricking, throbbing, and burning. Painful regions also exhibited very high rates of allodynia, hyperpathia, and exaggerated wind-up. Central pain following brain lesions has been hypothesized to be related to central disinhibition, imbalance of stimuli, and/or central sensitization phenomena (117). It is classically seen with lesions of the thalamus, particularly the ventrocaudal nuclei. It is generally acknowledged that lesions involving dissociated spinothalamic loss have a higher risk for developing central pain. Such lesions are typically located in the posterior insula and parietal operculum. Rates of central pain following spinal and brainstem spinothalamic lesions range from 30% to 70%. The pain syndrome associated with opercular-insular lesions has commonly been called *pseudothalamic*. Changes in thalamocortical processing may include loss of inhibition or sensitization. Allodynia and dysesthesias, sometimes involving the entire hemicorpora, are hallmarks of brain-related pain. Central pain syndromes have often been very challenging for both the treating physician and the patient (27,119).

It is prudent to be cautious in medication and other treatment choices, given the overlap in plasticity mechanisms subserving central sensitization and more positive dynamic neurological functions such as learning, memory, and motor recovery. However, it would also be clinically appropriate to consider combinations of medications with different mechanisms of action (whether in the same or different "class" of drug) in an effort to effectively treat pain syndromes after TBI. IV morphine and IV lidocaine may be effective for treatment. Enteral opioid pain medications may be effective but are sometimes poorly tolerated on a chronic treatment basis. Similarly, oral mexilitine does not seem to be as effective as its IV counterpart—lidocaine (120,121). TCAs have been used for decades, but particular caution must be observed in older patients because of increased sensitivity to anticholinergic side effects aside from the potential cognitive side effects of this class of medications when given at higher doses (122). Anticonvulsants have also been used, but the preferred agent(s) for this condition remain(s) debated, although some older research indicates that lamotrigine may be a reasonable choice (123). Gabapentin may also be effective (124), but topiramate does not seem to have clinical benefit (125). When drugs fail, which is often the case, neuromodulation, either chemical or electrical, can provide substantive relief in selected patients (126). Neurosurgical interventions can also be considered, including stereotactic lesioning of deep subparietal white matter (127).

Complex Regional Pain Syndrome

CRPS remains a much debated clinical condition with perhaps as much misinformation as information (128). The latest research developments suggest that this condition is multidimensional with neuropathic, nociceptive, and inflammatory components with associated sympathetic system dysfunction (129,130). Current consensus opinion also indicates that CRPS is likely associated with central sensitization phenomena as well as motor abnormalities. Treatments that have been shown to be efficacious include a gamut of physical interventions, pharmacotherapeutic measures, and interventional treatments. In general, the World Health Organization (WHO) analgesic ladder, with the exception of opioids, have been recommended for pharmacological management of CRPS type I with neuropathic pain elements best addressed by anticonvulsants and TCAs and inflammatory pain symptoms by free radical scavengers. Peripheral vasodilatation may be accomplished through the use of oral medications and when these are ineffective through the use of percutaneous sympathetic blockade (130).

Research has suggested that interdisciplinary programs emphasizing functional restoration may offer the optimal treatment paradigm. As noted by Harden (131), "Functional restoration should provide different interventional and noninterventional modalities in a timely manner to facilitate reanimation and normalization of use and movement of the affected limb." Pharmacotherapeutic interventions for CRPS pain can be considered as either "maintenance" or "rescue/abortive" and include such diverse drug classes as TCAs, opioids, anticonvulsants, NSAIDs, clonidine, nifedipine, alpha-adrenergic antagonists (e.g., phenoxybenzamine and phentolamine), biphosphonates, calcitonin, among the most well studied (131). Interventional treatments that have shown benefit include both sympathetic and epidural blocks.

CONCLUSIONS

Pain clearly is a complex clinical phenomena (132,133). Treatment of post-traumatic pain conditions associated with TBI is even more multidimensional whether in the acute or chronic phase postinjury. Judicious use of medical interventions must rely not only on sound medical knowledge that remains up-to-date with current accepted practice but also on keen observational, interview, and examination skills. A sound familiarity with the pain literature including current practice guidelines such as those published by major medical specialty groups (134) as well as a knowledge of the myriad conditions that can be seen following multitrauma and/or

TBI (43,135) is paramount to recognizing these clinical conditions when they present and provide optimal and timely treatment to mitigate injury-related impairment and disability as well as improve the quality of life.

KEY CLINICAL POINTS

1. Clinicians should have an understanding of the neuroanatomy and neurobiology of pain processes if treating pain disorders in persons with TBI.
2. Practitioners treating persons with pain and TBI should understand the impact of CNS and polytrauma injury on the development of pain generators including the primary, secondary, and tertiary aspects of pain development and promulgation inclusive of peripheral and central sensitization, wind-up, and psychoemotional responses to impairment and disability associated with pain.
3. Clinicians should ideally avoid treating the symptom of pain and seek the primary pain generators to optimize treatment outcomes.
4. Acquisition of a relevant and detailed pain history is paramount to focusing the pain physical exam and guiding identification of pain generators.
5. A thorough and focused pain physical examination takes time and an understanding of appropriate examination techniques of the multiple body systems that may be impacted by not just by TBI but, more broadly, by polytrauma.
6. Clinicians should be intimately familiar with current literature, including evidence-based medicine relative to pain treatment interventions, and understand the nuances of choosing interventions as germane to issues specific to persons with TBI.
7. Practitioners should be educated in and proficient at medication prescription, including having an understanding of drug mechanisms of action, drug side effects, and drug–drug interactions to optimize treatment outcomes.
8. Treating professionals should understand the treatment hierarchy relative to the appropriate role of certain drug clasess vs the role of nonpharmacological treatment approaches.
9. Pain management of persons with TBI can be challenging from multiple perspectives; however, there is much that can be offered to patients and their families if the evaluating professionals have been appropriately trained and educated in pain assessment and management within a holistic and functionally oriented biopsychosocial framework.

KEY REFERENCES

1. Nampiaparampil DE. Prevalence of chronic pain after traumatic brain injury: a systematic review. *JAMA*. 2008; 300(6):711–719.
2. Schnakers C, Zasler ND. Pain assessment and management in disorders of consciousness. *Curr Opin Neurol*. 2007;20(6):620–626.
3. Waldman SD, ed. *Pain Management*. 2nd ed. Philadelphia, PA: Elsevier/Saunders; 2011.

4. Zasler ND, Martelli MF. Chronic pain. In: Silver JM, McAllister TW, Yudofsky SC, eds. *Textbook of Traumatic Brain Injury.* 2nd ed. Arlington, VA: American Psychiatric Publishing, Inc; 2011:375–396.

5. Zasler ND, Martelli MF, eds. Pain management. *J Head Trauma Rehabil.* 2004;19(1):10–28

References

1. Lahz S, Bryant RA. Incidence of chronic pain following traumatic brain injury. *Arch Phys Med Rehabil.* 1996;77:889–891.

2. Nampiaparampil DE. Prevalence of chronic pain after traumatic brain injury: a systematic review. *JAMA.* 2008;300(6):711–719.

3. Apkarian AV, Bushnell MC, Treede RD, Zubieta JK. Human brain mechanisms of pain perception and regulation in health and disease. *Eur J Pain.* 2005;9:463–484.

4. Walker W. Pain pathoetiology after TBI: neural and non-neural mechanisms. *JHTR.* 2004;19(1):72–81.

5. McMahon SB, David LH, Bevan S. Inflammatory mediators and modulators of pain. In: McMahon SB, Koltzenburg M, eds. *Wall and Melzack's Textbook of Pain.* 5th ed. Philadelphia, PA: Elsevier/Churchill Livingstone; 2006:49–72.

6. Yaksh TL, Luo ZD. Anatomy of the pain processing system. In: Waldman SD, ed. *Pain Management.* 2nd ed. Philadelphia, PA: Elsevier/Saunders; 2011:10–18.

7. Yaksh TL, Luo ZD. Dynamics of the pain processing system. In: Waldman SD, ed. *Pain Management.* 2nd ed. Philadelphia, PA: Elsevier/Saunders; 2011: 19–30.

8. Li J, Simone D, Larson A. Windup leads to characteristics of central sensitization. *Pain.* 1999;79:75–82.

9. Tetzlaff J. Treatment of acute pain in the orthopedic patient. *Pain Management.* 2004 July;:12–24.

10. Burstein R, Goor-Aryeh I, Jakubowski M. Migraine, sensitization of trigeminovascular neurons and triptan therapy. *Headache Currents.* 2004;1(2):25–32.

11. Almeida TF, Roizenblatt S, Tufik S. Afferent pain pathways: a neuroanatomical review. *Brain Res.* 2004;1000(1–2):40–56.

12. Bolay H, Moskowitz M. Mechanisms of pain modulation in chronic syndromes. *Neurology.* 2002;59(5)(suppl 2):S2–S7.

13. Welch KM. Contemporary concepts of migraine pathogenesis. *Neurology.* 2003;61(suppl 4):S2–S8.

14. Eisenberger NI, Lieberman MD, Williams KD. Does rejection hurt? An FMRI study of social exclusion. *Science.* 2003;302(5643):237–239.

15. Peyron R, Laurent B, Garcia-Larrea L. Functional imaging of brain responses to pain. A review and meta-analysis. *Neurophysiol Clin.* 2000;30(5):263–288.

16. Firestone, L. Gyulai F, Mintun M, et al. Human brain activity response to fentanyl imaged by positron emission tomography. *Anesth Analg.* 1996;82:1247–1261.

17. Young RF, Tronnier V, Rinaldi PC. Chronic stimulation of the Kölliker-Fuse nucleus region for relief of intractable pain in humans. *J Neurosurg.* 1992;76(6):979–985.

18. Bartsch T, Goadsby P. Increased responses in trigeminocervical nociceptive neurons to cervical input after stimulation of the dura mater. *Brain.* 2003;126:1801–1813.

19. Goadsby P, Knight Y, Hoskin K. Stimulation of the greater occipital nerve increases metabolic activity in the trigeminal nucleus caudalis and cercial dorsal horn of the cat. *Pain.* 1997;73:23–28.

20. Shevel E, Speirings E. Cervical muscles in the pathogenesis of migraine headache. *J Headache Pain.* 2004;5:12–14.

21. Calvino B, Grilo RM. Central pain control. *Joint Bone Spine.* 2006; 73(1):10–16.

22. Lake A, Saper J. Chronic headache: new advances in treatment strategies. *Neurology.* 2002;59(suppl 2):S8–S13.

23. Knight Y. Brainstem modulation of caudal trigeminal nucleus: a model for understanding migraine biology and future drug targets. *Headache Currents.* 2(5):108–118.

24. Weiller C, May A, Limmroth V, et al. Brain stem activation in spontaneous human migraine attacks. *Nature Med.* 1995;1:658–660.

25. Terhors G, Meijler W, Korf J, Kemper R. Trigeminal nociception-induced cerebral Fos expression in the conscious rat. *Cephalalgia.* 2001;21:963–975.

26. Schnitzler A, Ploner M. Neurophysiology and functional neuroanatomy of pain perception. *J Clin Neurophysiol.* 2000;17(6):592–603.

27. Garcia-Larrea L. Insights gained into pain processing from patients with focal brain lesions [published online ahead of print May 10, 2012]. *Neurosci Lett.*

28. Willis WD, Westlund, KN. Neuroanatomy of the pain system and of the pathways that modulate pain. *J Clin Neurophysiol.* 1997;14: 2–31.

29. Vogt, BA, Sikes, RW, Vogt, LJ. Anterior cingulate cortex and the medial pain system. In BA Vogt and M Gabriel, eds., *Neurobiology of cingulate cortex and limbic thalamus: A comprehensive handbook.* 1993; 313–344.

30. Pain. http://courses.washington.edu/conj/sensory/pain.htm.

31. Chapman CR. Limbic processes and the affective dimension of pain. In: Carli G, Zimmerman M, eds. *Progress in Brain Research.* Vol 10. Amsterdam, The Netherlands: Elsevier; 1996:63–81.

32. Gabriel M. The role of pain in cingulate cortical and limbic thalamic mediation or dance learning. In: Besson JM, Guilbaud G, Ollat H, eds. *Forebrain Areas Involved in Pain Processing.* Paris, France: John Libbey Eurotext; 1995:197–211.

33. Ianetti GD, Mouraux A. From the neuromatrix to the pain matrix (and back). *Exp Brain Res.* 2010;205(1):1–12.

34. Apkarian AV, Hashmi JA, Baliki MN. Pain and the brain: specificity and plasticity of the brain in clinical chronic pain. *Pain.* 2011; 152(suppl 3):S49–S64.

35. Apkarian AV. The brain in chronic pain: clinical implications. *Pain Management.* 2011;1(6):577–586.

36. Baliki MN, Schnitzer TJ, Bauer WR, Apkarian AV. Brain morphological signatures for chronic pain. *PLoS ONE.* 2011;6(10):e26010.

37. Galer BS, Jensen MF. The development and preliminary validation of a pain measure specific to neuropathic pain: the Neuropathic Pain Scale, *Neurology.* 1997;48:332–338.

38. McCarberg BH, Stanos S, Williams DA. Comprehensive chronic pain management: improving physical and psychological function (CME Multimedia Activity). *Am J Med.* 2012;125(6):S1. www.cmeaccess.com/AJM/ChronicPain02.

39. Gatchel RJ, Lou L, Kishino N. Concepts of multidisciplinary pain management. In: Boswell MV, Cole BE, eds. *Weiner's Pain Management: A Practical Guide for Clinicians (Am. Acad. of Pain Management).* New York, NY: Taylor & Francis Group; 2006:1501–1508.

40. Turk DC. Understanding pain sufferers: the role of cognitive processes. *Spine J.* 2004;4:1–7.

41. Gonzales VA, Martelli MF, Baker JM. Psychological assessment of persons with chronic pain. *NeuroRehabilitation.* 2000;14(2):69–83.

42. CARF International. http://www.carf.org/home/. Accessed April 2, 2012.

43. Donohue CD. History and physical examination of the pain patient. In: Waldman SD, ed. *Pain Management.* 2nd ed. Philadelphia, PA: Elsevier/Saunders; 2011:36–49.

44. Zasler ND, Martelli MF, eds. Pain management. *J Head Trauma Rehabil.* 2004;19(1):10–28.

45. Zasler ND, Martelli MF. Chronic pain. In: Silver JM, McAllister TW, Yudofsky SC, eds. *Textbook of Traumatic Brain Injury.* 2nd ed. Arlington, VA: American Psychiatric Publishing, Inc; 2011: 375–396.

46. Schnakers C, Zasler ND. Pain assessment and management in disorders of consciousness. *Curr Opin Neurol.* 2007;20(6):620–626.

47. Schnakers C, Chatelle C, Vanhaudenhuyse A, et al. The Nociception Coma Scale: a new tool to assess nociception in disorders of consciousness. *Pain.* 2010;148(2):215–219.

48. Woolf CJ. Pain hypersensitivity. http://www.wellcome.ac.uk/en/pain/microsite/science4.html. Accessed April 2, 2012.

49. Singh MK. Chronic pain syndrome. http://emedicine.medscape.com/article/310834-overview. Accessed April 2, 2012.

50. Häuser W, Wolfe F, Tölle T, Uçeyler N, Sommer C. The role of antidepressants in the management of fibromyalgia syndrome: a systematic review and meta-analysis. *CNS Drugs.* 2012;26(4): 297–307.

51. Alba-Delgado C, Mico JA, Sánchez-Blázquez P, Berrocoso E. Analgesic antidepressants promote the responsiveness of locus coeruleus neurons to noxious stimulation: implications for neuropathic pain [published online ahead of print May 14, 2012]. *Pain.*

52. Novartis. Tegretol®. http://www.pharma.us.novartis.com/product/pi/pdf/tegretol.pdf. Accessed April 2, 2012.

53. Wiffen P, Collins S, McQuay H, Carroll D, Jadad A, Moore A. Anticonvulsant drugs for acute and chronic pain. *Cochrane Database Syst Rev.* 2005;(3):CD001133.

54. Shneker BF, McAuley JW. Pregabalin: a new neuromodulator with broad therapeutic indications. *Ann Pharmacother.* 2005;39(12):2029–2037.

55. Baidya DK, Agarwal A, Khanna P, Arora MK. Pregabalin in acute and chronic pain. *J Anaesthesiol Clin Pharmacol.* 2011;27(3):307–314.

56. Greenberg EN. Ziconatide. *J Pain Palliat Care Pharmacother.* 2011;25(4):380–381.

57. Hughes D. Challenges in using intrathecal medications for the treatment of chronic pain. 2012. http://www.empr.com/challenges-in-using-intrathecal-medications-for-the-treatment-of-chronic-pain/article/229487/. Accessed April 2, 2012.

58. Malanga G, Reiter RD, Garay E. Update on tizanidine for muscle spasticity and emerging indications. *Expert Opin Pharmacother.* 2008;9(12):2209–2215.

59. Mailis A, Nicholson K. The use of sodium amytal in the assessment and treatment of functional or other disorders. In: Zasler ND, Martelli MF, eds. *Functional Medical Disorders, State of the Art Reviews in Physical Medicine and Rehabilitation.* Philadelphia, PA: Hanley & Belfus; 2002:131–146.

60. Nichols L, Zasler ND, Martelli MF. Sodium amobarbital: historical perspectives and neurorehabilitation clinical caveats. *NeuroRehabilitation.* In press.

61. Flores MP, Castro AP, Nascimento Jdos S. Topical analgesics. *Rev Bras Anestesiol.* 2012;62(2):244–252.

62. Qutenza®. http://www.qutenza.com. Accessed April 2, 2012.

63. Argoff CE. Topical treatments for pain. *Curr Pain Headache Rep.* 2004;8:261–267.

64. http://www.pcab.org/about

65. Wikipedia. Patient-controlled analgesia. http://en.wikipedia.org/wiki/Patient-controlled_analgesia. Accessed April 2, 2012.

66. Leong M, Royal M. Opioid therapy in chronic non-cancer pain management. *Practical Pain Management.* 2004 August;:43–47.

67. Chapman CR, Lipschitz DL, Angst MS, et al. Opioid pharmacotherapy for chronic non-cancer pain in the United States: a research guideline for developing an evidence base. *J Pain.* 2010;11(9):807–829.

68. Von Korff M, Kolodny A, Deyo RA, Chou R. Long-term opioid therapy reconsidered. *Ann Intern Med.* 2011;155(5):325–328.

69. Rhodes C. Opioids: is it time to change? *The Pain Practitioner.* 2012;22(1):43–46.

70. Hewitt DJ, Chapman SL. Chronic pain. In: Rizzo M, Eslinger PJ, eds. *Principles and Practice of Behavioral Neurology and Neuropscyhology.* Philadelphia, PA: W.B. Saunders; 2004;737–776.

71. Wikipedia. Oxycodone/naloxone. http://en.wikipedia.org/wiki/Oxycodone/naloxone. Accessed April 2, 2012.

72. Benyamin R, Trescot AM, Datta S, et al. Opioid complications and side-effects. *Pain Physician.* 2008;11:S105–S120.

73. Chapman S. Effects of intermediate and long term use of opioids on cognition in patients with chronic pain. *Clin J Pain.* 2002;18:S83–S90.

74. Jamison R. Neuropsychological effects of long-term opioid use in chronic pain patients. *J Pain Symptom Manage.* 2003;26(4):913–921.

75. Sjøgren P, Christrup LL, Petersen MA, Højsted J. Neuropsychological assessment of chronic non-malignant pain patients treated in a multidisciplinary pain centre. *Eur J Pain.* 2005;9(4):453–462.

76. U. S. Food and Drug Administration. Postmarket drug safety information for patients and providers. http://www.fda.gov/Drugs/DrugSafety/PostmarketDrugSafetyInformationforPatientsandProviders/ucm111350.htm. Accessed April 2, 2012.

77. Department of Justice Drug Enforcement Administration Office of diversion Control. State prescription drug monitoring programs. http://www.deadiversion.usdoj.gov/faq/rxmonitor.htm. Accessed April 2, 2012.

78. Jamot L, Matthes H, Simmonin F, et al. Differential involvement of the mu and kappa opioid receptors in spatial learning. *Genes Brain Behav.* 2003;2(2):80–92.

79. Taghaddosinejad F, Mehrpour O, Afshari R, Seghatoleslami A, Abdollahi M, Dart RC. Factors related to seizure in tramadol poisoning and its blood concentration. *J Med Toxicol.* 2011;7(3):183–188.

80. Chou R, Fanciullo GJ, Fine PG, Adler JA, et al. Clinical guidelines for the use of chronic opioid therapy in chronic non-cancer pain. *J Pain.* 2009;10(2):113–130.

81. Schnakers C, Chatelle C, Demertzi A, et al. What about pain in disorders of consciousness? [published online ahead of print April 18, 2012]. *The AAPS Journal.*

82. Federation of State Medical Boards of the United States, Inc. *Model Policy for the Use of Controlled Substances for the Treatment of Pain.* 2004.

83. Anderson AV, Fine PG, Fishman SM. Opioid prescribing: Clinical tools and risk management strategies. http://www.state.mn.us/mn/externalDocs/BMP/New_Article_on_Pain_Management_020110034248_monograph_dec_07_final.pdf. Accessed Dec. 31, 2009.

84. Chou R. Drug class review on long acting opioid analgesics. Oregon evidence based practice center [published online ahead of print April 2004]. *OHSU.*

85. Eisenberg E, McNicol ED, Carr DB. Efficacy and safety of opioid agonists in the treatment of neuropathic pain of non-malignant origin. Systematic review and meta-analysis of randomized controlled trials. *JAMA.* 2005;293:3043–3052.

86. Hansen H, Jordan A, Bolen J. Controlled substances and risk management. In: Boswell MV, Cole BE, eds. *Weiner's Pain Management: A Practical Guide for Clinicians (Am. Acad. of Pain Management).* New York, NY: Taylor & Francis Group; 2006:1417–1455.

87. Gallagher RM. Rational integration of pharmacologic, behavioral, and rehabilitation strategies in the treatment of chronic pain. *Arch Phys Med Rehabil.* 2005;84(suppl 3):64–76.

88. Waldman SD, Kidder KA, Waldman HJ. Physical modalities in the management of pain. In: Waldman SD, ed. *Pain Management.* 2nd ed. Philadelphia, PA: Elsevier/Saunders; 2011;978–986.

89. Walsh NE, Maria DS, Eckmann M. Treatment of the patient with chronic pain. In: Frontera WR, DeLisa JA, Gans BM, Walsh NE, Robinson LR, eds. *DeLisa's Physical Medicine & Rehabilitation: Principles and Practice.* 5th ed. Philadelphia, PA: Wolters Kluwer/Lippincott Williams & Wilkins; 2010:1291–1295.

90. Carroll D, Moore RA, McQuay HJ, et al. Transcutaneous electrical nerve stimulation (tens) for chronic pain (Cochrane review). *Cochrane Database Syst Rev.* 2001;(3).

91. Nnoaham KE, Kumbang J. Effectiveness of transcutaneous electrical nerve stimulation (TENS) alone in the management of chronic pain. 2010.http://summaries.cochrane.org/CD003222/effectiveness-of-transcutaneous-electrical-nerve-stimulation-tens-alone-in-the-management-of-chronic-pain. Accessed April 2, 2012.

92. Department of Veterans Affairs Technology Assessmnt Program, Office of Patient Care Services. Bibliogrpahy: Transcutaneous electrical nerve stimulation. http://www.va.gov/VATAP/docs/TranscutaneousElectricalNerveStimulation2001tm.pdf. Accessed April 2, 2012.

93. Kroeling P, Gross AR, Goldsmith CH; for Cervical Overview Group. A cochrane review of electrotherapy for mechanical neck disorders. *Spine.* 2005;30(21):E641–E648.

94. Kirsch DL, Smith RB. The use of cranial electrotherapy in the management of chronic pain: a review. *NeuroRehabilitation.* 2000;14(2):85–94.

95. Hammer WI. *Functional Soft Tissue Examination and Treatment by Manual Methods.* 3rd ed. Norwalk, CT: Hands on Therapeutics; 2007.

96. Annaswamy TM, De Luigi AJ, O'Neill BJ, Keole N, Berbrayer D. Emerging concepts in the treatment of myofascial pain: a review of medications, modalities, and needle-based interventions. *PM R.* 2011;3:940–961.

97. Waldman SD, ed. *Pain Management.* 2nd ed. Philadelphia, PA: Elsevier/Saunders; 2011.

98. Frontera W. Exercise in physical medicine and rehabilitation. In:

Grabois M, Garrison SJ, Hart KA, Lehmkuhl LD, eds. *Physical Medicine and Rehabilitation. The Complete Approach.* London, United Kingdom: Blackwell Science; 2000:487–503.

99. Hoffman MD, Shepanski MA, Mackenzie SP. Experimentally induced pain perception is acutely reduced by aerobic exercise in people with chronic low back pain. *J Rehabil Res Dev.* 2005;42(2): 183–190.

100. Hopkins ME, Davis FC, Vantieghem MR, Whalen PJ, Bucci DJ. Differential effects of acute and regular physical exercise on cognition and affect. *Neuroscience.* 2012;215:59–68.

101. Vaynman S, Gomez-Pinilla, F. License to run: exercise impacts functional plasticity in the intact and injury central nervous system by using neurotrophins. *Neurorehabil Neural Repair.* 2005;19: 283–295.

102. Yamaguchi M. Incidence of headache and severity of head injury. *Headache.* 1992;32(9):427–431.

103. Walker WC, Seel RT, Curtiss G, Warden DL. Headache after moderate and severe traumatic brain injury: a longitudinal analysis. *Arch Phys Med Rehabil.* 2005;86(9):1793–1800.

104. Zasler ND, ed. Posttraumatic tension pneumoencephalus. *J Head Trauma Rehabil.* 1999;14(1):81–84.

105. Zasler ND, Martelli MF. Post-traumatic headache: practical approaches to diagnosis and treatment. In: Weiner RB, ed. *Pain Management: A Practical Guide for Clinicians.* 6th ed. Boca Raton, FL: St. Lucie Press; 2002;313–344.

106. Evans RW Post-traumatic headaches. In: Evans RW, ed. *Neurologic Clinics.* 22(1), 237–249. Philadelphia, PA: Saunders, 2004.

107. International Headache Society. The International Classification of Headache Disorders. 2nd Edition. *Cephalalgia.* 2004;24(suppl 1); 9–160.

108. Watanabe TK, Bell KR, Walker WC, Schomer K. Systematic review of interventions for post-traumatic headache. *PM R.* 2012;4:129–140.

109. Tepper SJ. Opioids should not be used in migraine. *Headache.* 2012; 52:(suppl 1):30–34.

110. Devor M. Response of nerves to injury in relation to neuropathic pain. In: Waldman SD, ed. *Pain Management.* 2nd ed. Philadelphia, PA: Elsevier/Saunders; 2011:905–928.

111. Harvey VL, Dickenson AH. Mechanisms of pain in non-malignant disease. *Curr Opin Support Palliat Care.* 2008;2(2):133–139.

112. Costigan M, Scholz J, Woolf CJ. Neuropathic pain: a maladaptive response of the nervous system to damage. *Annu Rev Neurosci.* 2009;32:1–32.

113. Backonja M, Rowbotham MC. Pharmacological therapy for neuropathic pain. In: McMahon SB, Koltzenburg M, eds. *Wall and Melzack's Textbook of Pain.* 5th ed. Philadelphia, PA: Elsevier/Churchill Livingstone; 2006:1075–1083.

114. Zhou Y. Principles of pain management. In: Daroff RB, Fenichel GM, Jankovic J, Mazziotta JC. *Bradley's Neurology in Clinical Practice.* 6th ed. Philadelphia, PA: Elsevier/Saunders; 2012:783–801.

115. Nicholson K. Pain associated with lesion, disorder or dysfunction of the central nervous system. *NeuroRehabilitation.* 2000;14(1):3–14.

116. Nicholson BD. Evaluation and treatment of central pain syndromes. *Neurology.* 2004;62(5)(suppl 2):S30–S36.

117. Kumar B, Kalita J, Kumar G, Misra UK. Central post-stroke pain: a review of pathophysiology and treatment. *Anesth Analg.* 2009; 108(5):1645–1657.

118. Ofek H, Defrin R. The characteristics of chronic central pain after traumatic brain injury. *Pain.* 2007;131(3):330–340.

119. Borsook D. Neurological diseases and pain. *Brain.* 2012;135(2): 320–344.

120. Attal N, Gaude V, Brasseur L, et al. Intravenous lidocaine in central pain: a double blind placebo controlled, psychophysical study. *Neurology.* 2000;54:564–574.

121. Attal N, Guirimand F, Brasseur L, et al. Effects of IV morphine in central pain: a randomized placebo-controlled study. *Neurology.* 2002;58:554–563.

122. Leijon G, Boivie J. Central post-stroke pain—a controlled trial of amitriptyline and carbamazepine. *Pain.* 1989;36:27–26.

123. Finnerup NB, Gottrup H, Jensen TS. Anticonvulsants in central pain. *Expert Opin Pharmacother.* 2002;3(10):1411–1420.

124. Tai QQ, Kirshblum S, Chen B, et al. Gabapentin in the treatment of neuropathic pain after spinal cord injury: a prospective randomized double-blind cross-over trial. *J Spinal Cord Med.* 2002;25: 100–105.

125. Canavero S, Bonicalzi V, Paolotti R. Lack of effect of topiramate for central pain. *Neurology.* 2002;58,831–832.

126. Son BC, Lee SW, Choi ES, Sung JH, Hong JT. Motor cortex stimulation for central pain following a traumatic brain injury. *Pain.* 2006; 123(1–2):210–216.

127. Canavero S, Bonicalzi V. Central pain syndrome: elucidation of genesis and treatment. *Expert Rev Neurotherapeutics.* 2007;7(11): 1485–1497.

128. Pearce JMS. Chronic regional pain and chronic pain syndromes. *Spinal Cord.* 2005;43:263–268.

129. Turner-Stokes L, Goebel A. Complex regional pain syndrome in adults: concise guidance. Guideline Development Group. *Clin Med.* 2011;11(6):596–600.

130. Perez RS, Zollinger PE, Dijkstra PU, et al. Evidence based guidelines for complex regional pain syndrome type 1. *BMC Neurology.* 2010;10:20

131. Harden N. Pharmacotherapy of complex regional pain syndrome. *Arch Phys Med Rehabil.* 2005;84(suppl 3):17–28.

132. Miller L. Neurosensitization: a model for persistent disability in chronic pain, depression and post-traumatic stress disorder following injury. *Neurorehabilitation.* 2000;14(1):25–32.

133. Nicholson, K, Martelli MF, Zasler ND. Myths and misconceptions about chronic pain: the problem of mind body dualism. In: Weiner RB, ed. *Pain Management: A Practical Guide for Clinicians.* 6th ed. Boca Raton, FL: St. Lucie Press; 2002:465–474.

134. American Society of Anesthesiologists Task Force on Chronic Pain Management; American Society of Regional Anesthesia and Pain Medicine. Practice guidelines for chronic pain management: an updated report by the American Society of Anesthesiologists Task Force on Chronic Pain Management and the American Society of Regional Anesthesia and Pain Medicine. *Anesthesiology.* 2010; 112(4):810–833.

APPENDIX I Clinical Features of Opioid Withdrawal

Physical Signs/Symptoms

Lacrimation, rhinorrhea, yawning
Dilated pupils, nausea/vomiting
Diaphoresis, chills, piloerection, mild tachycardia, and/or hypertension
Myalgias, abdominal cramps, diarrhea

Psychological Symptoms

Anxiety and dysphoria
Craving for opioids
Restlessness, insomnia, fatigue

Onset and Duration of Symptoms

Beginning < 8 hours from last opioid use (peak within 36–72 hours):
Anxiety, fear of withdrawal, craving for drug, diaphoresis, chills, lacrimation, rhinorrhea, yawning
Beginning 12 hours from last opioid use (peak at 72 hours):
Piloerection, anorexia, dilated pupils, anxiety, irritability dysphoria, restlessness, mild-to-moderate insomnia, tremor, mild tachycardia, hypertension, and/or abdominal cramps
Beginning 24–36 hours from last opioid use (Peak at 72 hours):
Abdominal cramps, diarrhea, myalgias, muscle spasms (especially in lower extremities), nausea, vomiting, diarrhea, severe insomnia, violent yawning

NOTE: Physical withdrawal symptoms generally resolve by 5–10 days. Psychological withdrawal symptoms (dysphoria, insomnia) may last weeks to month.

APPENDIX II Controlled Prescription Medication Agreement (Private)

Controlled medication(s) (e.g., opiates, tranquilizers, benzodiazepines, barbiturates, and psychostimulants) are potentially useful but may be misused and are, therefore, closely controlled by local state and federal authorities as well as by Dr. Zasler. These medications are intended to facilitate improved function and/or quality of life. Your compliance with any controlled medication prescriptions is essential if you wish to continue to receive care through this office.

The purpose of this agreement is to protect your access to controlled medication(s) as well as protect our ability to prescribe them to you. Because these drugs have the potential for abuse and/or diversion, strict accountability is necessary. In order for Dr. Zasler to consider, or continue, prescribing controlled medication(s), you must agree to the following:

1. I am responsible for the controlled medication(s) prescribed to me. I am responsible for taking the medication(s) in the dose prescribed and for keeping track of the amount of medication(s) remaining.
2. I will take my medication(s) as prescribed and not take additional doses without first having it approved by Dr. Zasler. I understand that misuse could result in serious medical complications, including my death.
3. Refills of controlled medication(s):
   - Must be requested *at least 48 hours in advance of pick-up*, only during the regular office hours of Monday–Friday, 9:00 AM–4:00 PM and picked up *by the patient or their guardian only*, once per month, and/or during a scheduled clinic visit, unless otherwise agreed to.
   - Will *not* be made at night, on weekends, or during holidays. Phone-in refills on most controlled medications are *not* legally permissible.
   - May *only be prescribed by Dr. Zasler* unless otherwise discussed with him.
4. I will establish an ongoing relationship with *1* pharmacy where I agree to fill *all* of my medication(s). I understand that the Prescription Monitoring Program will be used to keep track of my controlled medication(s). I waive any applicable privilege or right to privacy and give permission for my provider and pharmacy to cooperate fully with any city, state, or federal law enforcement.
5. It may be deemed necessary by my doctor that I see another specialist for a second opinion controlled medication(s) consult if Dr. Zasler has concerns about the appropriateness of continued treatment with a controlled medication or medications as part of my care. I understand that if I do not attend such an appointment, my medication(s) may be discontinued or may not be refilled beyond a tapering dose to completion. I understand that if the specialist feels that I am at risk for psychological dependence (addiction), my medication(s) will no longer be refilled.
6. I will comply with random urine, blood, saliva, and/or breath testing, documenting the proper use of my medication(s) as well as confirming compliance and absence of use of alcohol and/or other drugs including illicit medication or medications (e.g., marijuana, cocaine, etc.) and/or any drugs that may interact in a dangerous manner with the controlled medication or medications Dr. Zasler is prescribing. In addition, I agree to abstain from illicit (illegal) drugs, as it *will* be reported to my other treating physicians, medical facilities, and/or appropriate authorities, including the police. I understand that I am ultimately responsible for the costs associated with such testing if my insurance denies the claim for reimbursement or does not cover the said testing.
7. I understand that driving a motor vehicle may not be allowed while taking controlled medication(s) (i.e., impairment of driving skills while on a controlled medication(s) and that it is my responsibility to comply with the laws of the state in which I am in while taking the prescribed medication(s).
8. I will not to share, sell, or trade my prescribed medication(s) for money, goods and/or services, or obtain controlled medication(s) from another individual. I agree to also safeguard my medication(s) from theft, loss, or potential misuse (i.e., using a medication(s) lock box or a safe, and keeping medication(s) out of the reach of children).
9. I will comply with the treatment plan as prescribed by Dr. Zasler. I understand that a successful treatment outcome will be further optimized by following a healthy lifestyle such as engaging in regular exercise, weight control, and avoidance of the use of tobacco and alcohol, as the main treatment goal is to improve my ability to function and/or work.
10. I understand that the long-term advantages, disadvantages, and unknown risks of long-term controlled medication use have yet to be scientifically determined, and my treatment may change at any time. I understand that Dr. Zasler will advise me of any advances in this field and make treatment changes as needed.
11. I have been fully informed by Dr. Zasler and his staff regarding the rare occurrence of psychological dependence (addiction) to controlled medication(s) and agree that when I am advised to stop taking the medication(s), I will do so slowly and under medical supervision to reduce/eliminate withdrawal symptoms.
12. I agree to be treated with alternative methods, either medication(s) or nonmedication(s) in nature, as they become available, and at the recommendation of Dr. Zasler, even if my condition is positively modulated by the use of the controlled medication(s).
13. I have been informed that the Virginia Prescription Monitoring Program is being used regularly by Dr. Zasler's office. I understand that this means my controlled medication(s) prescription history is available to any of my treating physicians. If it is evident that I am not complying by this agreement, I understand that my controlled medication(s) may be discontinued and potential discharge from Dr. Zasler's care.

I have read this document and I fully understand its content and the consequences of violating the terms of this agreement, including the discontinuation of prescriptions for controlled medication(s) and/or discharge from Dr. Zasler's care.

Patient Name (printed): _____   Date of Birth: _____

Patient Signature: _____   Date: _____

The above terms and conditions have been discussed with, and understood by, the above named patient.

_____

Nathan D. Zasler, MD

Medical Director, CCCV and TOLS

Date: _____

58

Psychological Assessment and Management of Post-Traumatic Pain

Michael F. Martelli, Keith Nicholson, and Nathan D. Zasler

INTRODUCTION

The purpose of this chapter is to provide readers with an understanding of the psychological approaches to assessment and management of pain in persons with traumatic brain injury (TBI). It is not intended as a substitute for the necessary training and experience that is prerequisite to optimizing assessment and treatment of pain in persons with TBI.

Pain is defined by the International Association for the Study of Pain (1) as a "psychological state" characterized by "an unpleasant sensory and emotional experience associated with actual or potential tissue damage or described in terms of such damage." An important distinction relates to chronicity. Acute pain, usually occurring in response to identifiable tissue damage or a noxious event, has more clearly identifiable triggers and neuroanatomical pathways and communicates useful information that provokes adaptive responses. It has a time-limited course during which treatment is aimed at providing relief, as well as promoting resolution or correction of underlying pathophysiological processes.

As time passes without resolution of an acute pain problem, subjective components may become more pronounced, identifiable triggers and neuroanatomic pathways can become obscure, and behavioral responses can become more disproportionate to underlying pathophysiology and even obstructive to resolution and adaptation of pain-related impairments. *Chronic pain* is defined as pain persisting beyond 6 months postinsult or injury that may or may not be associated with any obvious tissue damage or pathological process. Concomitants of chronic pain include maladaptive protective responses or pain behaviors, protracted courses of medication use (oftentimes without tested proven efficacy for the pain condition in the particular patient being treated) and often suboptimally effective medical services (sometimes with associated iatrogenic complications), and functionally disabling behavioral or emotional changes including restrictions in daily activities. Pain-related avoidance behaviors and reduced activity are likely to result in a cyclic disability-enhancing pattern. The longer pain persists, the more recalcitrant it becomes, and the more treatment goals focus on improved coping with pain and its concomitants (2). Finally, persistent pain is often associated with peripheral or central sensitization effects in which hyperresponsiveness or spontaneous discharge of components of the pain system develops (3–5). Numerous functional imaging studies have documented the interaction of psychological and neurobiological processes in chronic pain conditions (3–12).

Pain is best conceptualized as a multidimensional subjective experience mediated by emotion, attitudes, and other perceptual influences. Variability in pain response is the rule rather than the exception and appears to reflect complex biopsychosocial interactions between genetic, developmental, cultural, environmental, psychological, and injury-/illness-related factors (13). Important distinctions between pain and suffering (14), sensory and affective experience, and impairment and disability (15) reflect the variability in response to pain problems. Although some patients with pain appear to present with unusual and possibly exaggerated suffering or disability, others present with a kind of "la belle indifference" in which extremely high reported pain severity may be associated with no apparent affective distress, pain behavior, or interference in many life activities. In some cases, the onset, maintenance, severity, or exacerbation of pain is primarily associated with psychological factors and may warrant a *Diagnostic and Statistical Manual of Mental Disorders, Fourth Edition, Text Revision (DSM-IV-TR)* (16) diagnosis of pain disorder associated with psychological factors. If both biomedical and psychological factors are deemed important in the presentation, then a *DSM-IV-TR* diagnosis of pain disorder associated with both psychological factors and a general medical condition would be indicated. In this regard, it has been noted that there is an association between post-traumatic stress reactions and development of chronic pain (17,18), with uncontrollable pain following physical injury potentially representing the core trauma resulting in post-traumatic symptomatology (19). However, it is cautioned that one should avoid the pitfalls of mind-body dualism and always consider both psychological and organic factors in the presentation of any patient with chronic pain (20). For example, fear of recurrent and unpredictable pain following physical injury is a core trauma that can produce dysregulation of the hypothalamic-pituitary-adrenocortical axis that significantly contributes to the central sensitization phenomenon often seen in patients with chronic pain (21).

The importance of assessing and managing pain has been incorporated into the prevailing standards of health care practice in the United States. The Joint Commission on Accreditation of Healthcare Organizations (JCAHO) acknowledges that pain coexists with a number of diseases and injuries, but it requires explicit attention in itself (22). Overall, the standards require organizations to (a) recognize individual's rights to appropriate pain assessment and management; (b) identify persons with pain in initial and ongoing assessments; and (c) educate patients, residents, clients, and families about pain management.

TRAUMATIC BRAIN INJURY AND PAIN

There is a very high comorbidity of chronic pain problems with cranial or other trauma whether or not there is a TBI. Indeed, headache is the primary complaint in virtually all surveys of the postconcussive syndrome (23). The frequency of post-traumatic headache (PTH) in the immediate postaccident period has been estimated to be as high as 90%, with problems continuing beyond 6 months in as many as 44% (3), although there is generally poor understanding of the incidence, etiology, or many other aspects of PTH (24).

In addition to headache, many other pain problems may follow trauma, including neck and back pain, complex regional pain syndrome, and fibromyalgia, among others. Curiously, most studies report that pain problems are much more common in less severe as compared with more severe TBI (2,23,25), although pain problems clearly also occur in the latter (26). Importantly, more severe brain injuries may result in reduced sensitivity to pain because of lesions in the central nervous system (CNS) structures involved in processing pain as observed in some dementias (4). It has also been suggested that there is an increased likelihood for developing central sensitization or neurosensitization effects (17,23) after milder injuries.

Traumatic Brain Injury, Pain, and Neuropsychological Function

There is an increasing awareness of the role that pain may play in symptom presentation following TBI, especially regarding cognitive complaints. Reviews (21,23,27,28) strongly support the conclusion that chronic pain, especially head and/or neck pain, as well as pain-related symptomatology, independent of TBI severity, can and often do produce impairment of cognitive functioning. A brief summary of the converging evidence that supports this conclusion (29–31) is presented in Table 58-1. Attentional capacity, processing speed, memory, and executive functions as assessed on neuropsychological tests are the cognitive domains most likely to be affected in patients with pain.

Many studies indicate that the concomitants of chronic pain may be as or more important than pain itself in producing cognitive impairment. Specifically, cognitive impairment in patients with chronic pain has been associated with mood change/emotional distress, somatic preoccupation and pain catastrophization, sleep disturbance, fatigue, and perceived interference with daily activities that are all potential sources of chronic stress. For example, major depression, frequently found following mild TBI, is associated with higher postconcussion symptom endorsement, poorer functional outcome, as well as higher distress levels, disability, and cognitive impairment, which all typically improve after effective treatment for depression (32). In a meta-analytic review, Pilcher

TABLE 58-1 Representative Summary of Evidence of Negative Effects of Pain on Cognition and Psychophysiological Function in Animals and Humans

Considerable replicated experimental animal and human studies showing that pain disrupts information processing/attentional capacity and performance.

Experimental mammalian and human studies showing improved information processing/performance after discontinuation of pain stimulus, including administration of opioid pain relievers that typically impair cognitive function.

Animal studies showing that persistent stress (including persistent pain) is associated with hippocampal damage, inhibition of neurogenesis, and memory and learning impairment.

Evidence of neuroendocrine and hypothalamic pituitary adrenal (HPA) perturbation in chronic pain that is associated with decreased attention and memory function in humans.

Evidence that experimental, chronic, and neuropathic pain across neurophysiological and neuropsychological measures and reward designs produce at least attentional interference effects.

Review and meta-analytic evidence that the concomitants of chronic pain alone may account for observed cognitive and psychomotor disruption (e.g., partial sleep deprivation, pain medications, depression, and anxiety) and suggestion that combinations are additive.

Neurophysiologic studies showing very specific effects (e.g., anterior cingulate cortex [ACC]) associated with chronic pain and attentional disruption, often coexisting with other defined patterns associated with cognitive impairments and neurophysiologic expressions (e.g., hypofrontality and depression).

Evidence of neural plasticity/cerebral reorganization/functional cerebral changes associated with chronic pain: (a) expansion of sensory cortex and (b) decreased prefrontal thalamic gray matter density.

Neurophysiologic evidence of central sensitization and disrupted pain inhibitory mechanisms associated with dysfunctional anterior/ventral and posterior/dorsal ACC quadrants (associated with cognitive and affective regulation, respectively) plus evidence that less severe/disruptive chronic pain is associated with a greater habituation vs sensitization response and not associated with cognitive disruption.

Biopsychosocial evidence linking an interaction of genetics, learning history, and psychological variables (especially anxiety, avoidance conditioning) to produce a pain-arousal pattern mimicking obsessional, depressive, and post-traumatic anxiety patterns with pain, obsessional thoughts, anxiety, somatic concerns, intrusive associations/memories, and disrupted allocation of attentional resources.

Adapted from Martelli, Nicholson, and Zasler (31) with permission.

and Huffcutt (33) found that partial sleep deprivation impairs cognitive and motor performance. In a review of experimental human and animal studies, Kundermann et al. (34) found that sleep deprivation produces hyperalgesic changes and can counteract analgesic medication effects via disruption of both serotonergic and opioidergic processes. Mahmood et al. (35) observed that measures sensitive to executive functioning and information-processing speed were associated with sleep quality scores. Consistent with these findings, Mooney, Speed, and Sheppard's (32) review of poor recovery following mild TBI found that most of the

TABLE 58-2 Recommendations for Assessing and Minimizing the Confounding Effects of Pain During Neurocognitive Examination

1. Always assess pain when present, especially when post-traumatic adaptation seems compromised by pain and related symptomatology, or limitations in daily functioning, and decrements in test performance seem atypical. Clarify frequency, intensity, character of pain during examination, and general characteristics of the chronic pain experience and related problems.

2. Assess problems commonly associated with chronic pain that have potential to disrupt cognitive function (e.g., sleep disturbance, pain medications, fatigue, somatic preoccupation, anxiety, depression).

3. Repeat measures sensitive to fatigue effects (e.g., sustained, attention-demanding, and timed tests) to help identify or corroborate fatigue-related deficits.

4. Always assess effort, motivation, and response bias during examination, especially regarding symptom complaints.

5. Consider postponing cognitive assessment in cases where pain and related symptomatology have not been appropriately or aggressively treated.

6. Use accommodating procedures during examinations when possible, for example, optimizing comfort, providing frequent breaks, allowing frequent position changes and use of personal orthotics (cushions, heating or ice pads, etc.), modifying lighting and sound, and so forth.

variance in recovery of mild TBI compensation seekers seemed to be explained by depression, pain, and response bias vs brain injury variables.

Chronic pain and associated problems can complicate the symptom picture after TBI. Especially in cases of persistent sequelae following mild TBI, increasing evidence suggests that chronic headache and other pain can present a differential diagnostic challenge and contribute to or maintain symptoms. This evidence provides strong support for the argument that resolution of postconcussive symptoms frequently relies on successful coping with post-traumatic pain and associated symptomatology.

Because pain and associated symptoms can have a disruptive effect on everyday function, including neuropsychological performance, special efforts are required to minimize the potential confounding effects. Some recommended procedures for conducting neuropsychological assessment of persons when pain is a significant complaint have been included in Table 58-2.

PAIN ASSESSMENT

Pain is a complex and subjective perceptual process comprised of behavioral, affective, cognitive, and sensory components. Especially when chronic, it often has no clear objective pathophysiological correlates. The complexity of this multidimensional experience is highlighted by functional imaging studies showing that the anticipation of painful stimulation produces similar activation of cortical networks to actual delivery of noxious stimulation (7,12,36). Biopsychosocial models can direct effective interventions for challenging

chronic health care situations, including chronic pain rehabilitation (37).

A comprehensive biopsychosocial assessment should be considered as the standard of care when pain is chronic (38, 39). As thorough a biomedical understanding of the patient as possible should be pursued. History from the patient, with information also obtained from relevant others as possible, regarding the presentation of the pain problem is as important as examination results and should include inquiry and questions about onset and course (e.g., when, where, how; sudden or progressive; fluctuating or steady, etc.); duration; pain severity levels and whether these appear concordant with known biomedical causes or pain behaviors; beliefs about the pain condition including understanding of the underlying biomedical cause; aggravating and relieving factors including activities preceding an exacerbation; stress-related effects; variability across the day and night; effect of movement and posture change; medications employed and effects; current activities and pain-related activity changes; level of function/disability and quality of life; specific effect of pain on mood, activity, cognition, affect, sleep, appetite, and more general effects of pain in the person's life; coping strategies and effectiveness; whether there are pain avoidance behaviors that may be perpetuating disability; pain behaviors and environmental effects/responses (e.g., whether there may be some solicitous reinforcement of pain behaviors); psychosocial context (e.g., whether pain is allowing the person to avoid work or responsibilities); and underlying personality and how this may be affecting presentation. Importantly, special assessment procedures are indicated in cases of persons with response limitations or significant cognitive impairments. These include special versions of instruments and reliance on observation and structured interview of relevant others and observers and integration of this information with physical examination procedures (see [48] for an extensive review of self-report, observational, and physiological measures used in pain assessment of adults with impaired communication abilities).

General Classes and Instruments Commonly Included in an Assessment of Pain and Psychological Variables Relevant to Adjustment and Coping

A brief survey of general classes and useful instruments for inclusion in a comprehensive biopsychosocial pain assessment, updated from previous work (40), is included in this section. A review of measures of specific pain report, including intensity and location, is included in Table 58-3.

Additional instruments have been designed for special application to children and adults with significant cognitive impairment. Some of the most common instruments include the following:

- Family Adaptability and Cohesion Evaluation Scale (FACES) (42) is designed for young children and consists of 6 cartoon faces ranging from a smiling face for "no pain" to a tearful face for "worst pain." Versions have been adapted for cognitively impaired adults.
- Face, Legs, Activity, Cry, Consolability (FLACC) Scale is a standardized rating composite measure of observed physical indicators of pain in infants and preverbal chil-

TABLE 58-3 Specific Pain Domain Instruments: Self-Reported Pain Intensity and Location

- *Visual Analogue Scale* (VAS) (41,42): a brief graphical non-psychometric measure of subjective pain intensity represented by a straight line with typical endpoints of no pain and worst possible pain. It is widely used to quickly assess pain report, track changes during treatment, and assess outcome (41).

- *Verbal Rating Scale* (VRS): a similar measure where pain intensity is indicated on a linear scale with verbal anchors ranging from "no pain" to "worst possible pain" and including mild, moderate, severe, and very severe (41).

- *Numeric Rating Scale* (NRS): a similar measure where pain intensity is indicated verbally or by pointing at a number from 0 or 1 to 10 with typical anchors of 0 (*no pain*) and 10 (*the worst that pain could ever be*) (41).

- *Pain drawing* (43): the most common instrument for measuring the location aspect of pain. It is the most common instrument used for this type of self-report (41).

- *McGill Pain Questionnaire*, short form (SF-MPQ) (44): designed to measure descriptive aspects of pain via selection of adjectival pain descriptors for 3 classes of pain—sensory (burning, sharp, sore), affective (e.g., exhausting, punishing), and intensity (e.g., intense, excruciating). Different combination of descriptors may be associated with different nociceptive or psychological factors.

- *Pain diaries*: temporal measures of frequency, duration, and intensity of pain episodes (45). They typically ask subjects to self-report, in a journal for several days or weeks, when and in what situations pain increases or decreases. More complete versions typically assess areas such as location, intensity, onset (e.g., sudden or progressive, fluctuating or steady, etc.), characteristics (e.g., throbbing, dull aching), duration, preceding activities, stress, effects of pain on activities, cognition, affect, sleep, appetite, and factors affecting pain mitigation or exacerbation (e.g., weather, activity, stress, medications, distraction).

dren who are unable to provide verbal report. It can also be used in children and adults with severe cognitive impairments (46).

- Observational Pain Scale (47) is a standardized rating measure for estimating pain level in patients who are cognitively impaired who can't respond to Visual Analogue Pain Scale (VAS), Numeric or Oucher Scales. It produces a composite pain score based on observation of facial expressions, verbalizations/vocalizations, and body movements; changes in interpersonal interactions; changes in activity patterns or routines; changes in mental status; and/or physiologic changes.

- Oucher Scale (48) consists of sequenced pictures of a child's face, ranging from "no hurt" to "the biggest hurt you could ever have"; these are shown and explained to a child who selects the one exemplifying current pain level. It is designed for children but can be used with adults with significant cognitive problems (49). Versions are available for most ethnicities.

Specific measures of pain functioning are critical to a competent biopsychosocial assessment. These measures examine pain quality, affect, behavioral, cognitive/attitudinal, and emotional coping. Some commonly employed instruments will be presented, ranging from more specific mea-

sures to more comprehensive batteries. More comprehensive biopsychosocial assessment batteries include the following:

The Battery for Health Improvement (BHI) assessment (50) is a dual-normed (community samples and pain patients) instrument designed for multidimensional assessment and computerized progress tracking to identify affective, characterological, psychophysiological, and social factors that affect pain, recovery and rehabilitation progress, vocational training or job placement readiness, and impairment and disability. It can contribute useful information regarding psychosocial factors underlying pain reports, perceived disability, somatic preoccupation, design for interventions, and outcome. A recent revision, the BHI-2, offers expanded national norms and multiple reference groups, along with expanded and updated scales.

The Multidimensional Pain Inventory (51) employs a biopsychosocial conceptualization to assess relevant psychosocial, cognitive, and behavioral aspects of responses to pain. This well-researched instrument has 61 items, includes 13 scales and measures pain severity, patient-perceived pain interference, affective distress, life control, social support, response from others, and disability. It includes specific norms for different statistically derived chronic pain subtypes: interpersonally distressed with inadequate social support, globally dysfunctional coping, and adaptive coping. An inexpensive software scoring program is available. This multiaxial classification system is a psychometrically sound and objective method of evaluating patients with chronic pain, may be integrated with useful psychological information from multiple other sources, and offers benefit for matching patients to types of pain management interventions.

The Profile of Chronic Pain: Extended Assessment Battery (PCP: EA) (52) is an 86-item instrument with (*a*) 33 items assessing pain location and severity, pain characteristics (e.g., worst daily pain), medication use, health care status, the identity of the most important person in the patient's life, and functional limitations in 10 areas of daily living; (*b*) 13 multi-item subscales addressing aspects of coping (guarding, ignoring, task persistence, and positive self-talk), catastrophizing, pain attitudes and beliefs (including disability beliefs, belief in a medical cure for pain, belief in pain control, and pain-induced fear); and (*c*) positive (tangible and emotional) and negative (insensitivity and impatience) social responses. National stratified samples across 3 age groups, 2 survey studies providing strong evidence for the hypothesized factor structure, internal consistency, independence from response bias and validity, and the presence of normative data suggest good diagnostic and prescriptive use.

The Psychosocial Pain Inventory (PPI) (53) is a 25-item, 8-page structured interview designed to assess the influence of psychosocial factors in chronic pain syndromes in 10 areas: (*a*) pain behavior (e.g., waking time, time in bed), (*b*) social reinforcement, (*c*) life changes, (*d*) litigation, (*e*) financial status, (*f*) use of alcohol, (*g*) medication use, (*h*) coping strategies, (*i*) social environment, and (*j*) environmental stress. In also includes questions concerning personal and family histories, past and current medical histories, and reactions and adjustments to the pain and medical treatments.

Measures of more specific aspects of chronic pain experience include the following:

The Chronic Pain Acceptance Questionnaire (CPAQ) revised version (54) is a measure of acceptance of pain. The 20-item revised form has 2 empirically derived subscales: activity engagement (i.e., degree to which respondents are living a normal life despite pain) and pain willingness (i.e., degree to which respondents have pain experiences without avoidance or control efforts). In a very recent large sample (55), the CPAQ scale was a reliable stronger predictor of distress and disability compared with coping variables, suggesting that pain management efforts can benefit from shaping a more accommodating view of pain experience for certain individuals or circumstances.

The Chronic Pain Coping Inventory (CPCI) (56) is a 65-item measure of strategies used by patients to cope with chronic pain across 11 pain-coping dimensions. In a cross-validational studies, 4 scales (guarding, resting, asking for assistance, and task persistence) reliably predicted patient and significant other and reported patient adjustment. Eight scales (guarding, opioid medication use, nonsteroidal anti-inflammatory drug [NSAID] use, sedative-hypnotic medication use, resting, asking for assistance, and exercise/stretch) demonstrated moderate-to-strong consistency between patient and significant other versions.

The Cogniphobia Scale (C-Scale) (57), adapted from the Kinesiophobia-Scale (K-Scale), quickly screens unreasonable or irrational fear of headache or painful reinjury on cognitive effort/exertion. The C-Scale is designed to assess anxiety-based avoidant behavior regarding cognitive exertion. Such as the K-Scale, this instrument measures anxiety-based avoidant behavior and offers information about the need for combination therapies that include such anxiety-reduction procedures.

The Cognitive Coping Strategies Inventory (58) assesses the degree to which patients engage in adaptive and maladaptive cognitive coping strategies. The Coping Strategies Questionnaire (59) is a 48-item scale that rates the frequency of engagement in 8 different behavioral and cognitive coping strategies in response to pain or physical symptom experience.

The K-Scale (60) is a quick screening measure of unreasonable or irrational fear of pain and painful reinjury on physical movement. It assesses pain phobias or avoidance-conditioned pain-related disability (i.e., unhealthy pain-maintaining habits that are major contributors to pain-related disability) and correlates highly with similar measures. High scores, once malingering factors are ruled out, signal the need for combination therapies with emphasis on reeducation, countering maladaptive phobic responses, and promoting adaptive attitudes and treatment participation/cooperation (e.g., graduated exposure, cognitive reinterpretation, and systematic desensitization). Recently, a version has been adapted for use in the general population (61).

The VAS can also be used to quickly assess affective pain distress (62) vs sensory intensity and similarly offers use for assessing treatment changes and outcome.

The Pain Anxiety Symptoms Scale (PASS) (63) is a measure of fear of pain across cognitive, overt behavioral, and physiological domains. It has good correlations with related measures of anxiety and disability and has been found to predict disability and interference because of pain when controlling for emotional distress and pain.

The Pain Catastrophizing Scale (PCS) (64) is a brief, well-researched measure of the negative mental set in the presence or anticipation of pain marked by magnification, rumination, and helplessness. Pain catastrophizing is a robust predictor of analgesic use, distress, psychosocial dysfunction and disability, and superior in comparisons to disease severity, pain levels, age, sex, depression, or anxiety. It also demonstrates benefit as a therapeutic measure of cognitive restructuring as a therapeutic tool (65). A child version is also available (66).

The Pain Patient Profile (P3) (67) is a screening measure for depression, anxiety, and excessive somatization in patients with pain. It is a double-normed (both healthy controls and patients with chronic pain) screening test developed to measure psychological factors related to chronic pain conditions to help identify those who would likely to benefit from mental health treatment as part of their treatment plan.

The Pain Stages of Change Questionaire (PSOCQ) (68) has a good demonstrated reliability and validity in predicting patient's readiness to adopt new beliefs and coping responses to pain. More recent research (69,70) suggests some use in identifying patient cluster types that differentially respond to specific multidisciplinary or cognitive-behavioral pain treatments consistent with a self-management approach to chronic pain problems.

The Profile of Chronic Pain: Screen (PCP: S) (71) is a brief 15-item measure designed to identify individuals who merit more detailed psychosocial evaluation. It assesses the psychological impact of chronic pain in terms of pain severity, functional interference, and pain-related emotional burden. Random national sample data were employed to demonstrate good validity and minimal social desirability response. National norms are available by gender for 3 age groups.

The Survey of Pain Attitudes (SOPA-R-35) (72) is a well-researched instrument that assesses patient's feelings about pain control, solicitude (solicitous responses from others in response to one's pain), medication (as appropriate treatment for pain), pain-related disability, pain and emotions (the interaction between emotions and pain), medical cures for pain, and pain-related harm (pain as an indicator of physical damage or harm).

The headache disability rating procedure of Packard and Ham (73) is a scale that estimates impairment from headache rated on frequency, severity, and duration of attacks and how activities impact on functional skills and activities of daily living. Importantly, it includes a modifier variable for rating motivation (i.e., treatment motivation, exaggeration/overconcern, and legal interest) that is used to adjust the total impairment rating.

The Oswestry Low Back Pain Disability Questionnaire (74) assesses the amount of restriction pain imposes on functional levels. Assessment areas include intensity, personal care, lifting, walking, sitting, standing, sleeping, sex life, social life, and traveling. The percentage of endorsed items gives an indication of the amount of disability. It has been proposed that up to 20% indicates minimal disability, 20%–40% indicates moderate disability, 40%–60% indicates severe disability, and more than 60% indicates very severe disability.

The Vanderbilt Pain Management Inventory (75) measures chronic pain coping strategies (e.g., active, passive) and provides useful information for treatment planning and recommendations.

TABLE 58-4 Measures of General Health Functioning and Behavior

- *Millon Behavioral Health Inventory* (MBHI) and its recent upgrade, the *Millon Behavioral Medicine Diagnostic test* (MBMD) (76) is one of the most frequently used health inventories for medical populations in the United States. The MBHI provides information across 4 broad categories: basic coping styles, psychogenic attitudes, specific disease syndromes, and prognostic indices. It has good psychometric properties, a large normative database of representative medical patients, and with specific disease scales developed for specific patient groups. The MBMD has updated and expanded the research base and clinical scales (165 items, 38 scales, 3 validity scales). The MBMD assists with identification of significant psychiatric problems, making specific recommendations; pinpointing personal and social assets to facilitate adjustment; identifying medical regimen compliance problems; and structuring post-treatment plans and self-care responsibilities in the patient's social network. Computerized scoring and an interpretive report facilitate use.

- *The SF-36 Health Survey* (SF-36) (77) surveys general health status in terms of physical and mental health and functional status. Widely used in research, and as an outcome measure (95), it assesses 8 areas, including limitations in physical functioning and social functioning and roles and activities, pain, mental health, vitality, and health perceptions.

- *The Neurobehavioral Functioning Inventory* (NFI) (78). The NFI is a multipurpose inventory designed to measure current cognitive, physical, and emotional functioning in persons with traumatic brain injury or other neurobehavioral disorders. It is comprised of 6 independent scales reflecting problems frequently experienced by persons with neurobehavioral disorders: depression, somatic, memory/attention, communication, aggression, and motor functioning. This well-researched instrument includes separate forms for patient and family, demonstrates concurrent validity with neuropsychological test data and objective personality inventory profiles, and can assist with treatment planning and allows measurement of change over time.

- *The Sickness Impact Profile* (SIP) (79) is a behaviorally based measure of health status designed to assess both psychosocial and physical dysfunction. It has sound psychometric properties, is used widely with patients with chronic pain, and can provide relevant information regarding degree of functional limitation in daily activity.

- *The Illness Behavior Questionnaire* (IBQ) (80, 81) provides useful information about attitudes, perceived reactions of others, and psychosocial variables. It delineates 7 factors that include general hypochondriasis, disease conviction, psychological vs somatic focusing, affective disturbance, affective inhibition, denial, and irritability. In addition, it has value in identifying patients who rely on illness behaviors as a coping style for need procurement.

Relevant measures of general health functioning and behavior are also an important part of a biopsychosocial pain assessment. Some common general measures are included in Table 58-4.

More general measures of mood, anger, and anxiety are also typically employed and commonly include the following:

- The Beck Depression Inventory-2 (BDI-2) (82) is a common self-report measure of depressive symptomatology that differentiates patients with chronic pain with and without major depression (optimal cutoff score of 21) (83) with well-documented predictive validity.

- The Zung Self-rating Depression Scale (SDS) (84) is especially well suited for medical settings; it is short, simple to read, administer, use as interview, understand, and score and fits well with medical and injury situations. Self-rating items (1 to 4, from "not at all" to "most or all of the time") are scored in the direction of increased depressive symptomatology; a raw score cutoff of 40 points suggests mild depression (40,83).

- The State-Trait Anger Expression Inventory-2 (STAXI-2) (85) is a reliable well-normed instrument for assessing the experience, expression, and control of both state and trait anger. Four relatively independent anger-related traits (anger expression outward, anger in, controlling outward expression, and controlling internal angry feelings) provide information regarding (*a*) contribution to psychophysiologic arousal and symptoms and risk for developing somatic symptoms and medical problems and (*b*) inferential suggestions for appropriate interventions. Importantly, anger is a frequent concomitant of chronic pain that has been underappreciated (45).

- The Beck Anxiety Inventory (BAI) (86) is a screening measure of anxiety severity (physiological and cognitive components, 21 items) describing subjective, somatic, or panic-related symptoms; it differentiates well between anxious and nonanxious groups in a variety of clinical settings.

- The Perceived Stress Scale (PSS) (87) measures degree to which life situations are appraised as stressful, including how unpredictable, uncontrollable, and overloaded respondents find their lives; higher scores are associated with more physical and psychological symptoms following stressful life events.

More comprehensive personality assessment measures are also typically employed. Some commonly used ones are included in Table 58-5.

These instruments should be integrated with information gathered through thorough history taking and psychological interview/assessment, patient and corroboratory interviews, the latter as possible, examination of relevant medical and allied health records, and physical assessment findings. The understanding derived from a comprehensive biopsychosocial pain assessment provides the framework for designing individually tailored treatment interventions and recommendations. Examining the impact of various cognitive processes on the subjective perception of the patient's pain and related disability is a critical component of this comprehensive assessment. Turk (95) has emphasized the importance of understanding and addressing the important role of patients' pain appraisals, beliefs, and expectancies. He and others (96) noted that patients with chronic pain resulting from traumatic events are predisposed to experiencing physical sensations as harmful and noxious, which increases both anxiety and subjective pain perceptions. This, in turn, leads to further activity avoidance and functional limitations that block recovery and facilitate increased deconditioning, creating increased risk for developing chronic and disabling pain.

Important psychoemotional components relevant to the assessment of chronic pain include the subjective experience

TABLE 58-5 Comprehensive Personality Assessment Instruments

- *The Minnesota Multiphasic Personality Inventory* (MMPI) (88) or (MMPI-2) (89) is the most widely used psychological assessment instrument in the United States. The MMPI is a 567-item (true or false) objective measure of personality function and emotional status with 10 clinical and 3 (7 in revised version) validity scales that were derived through empirical discrimination. Its predictive abilities are based on more than 50 years of actuarial data collection and analysis. It is a very sensitive measure of psychological states, traits, and styles (e.g., excessive anxiety, tension, depression, hostility and problematic anger, somatization tendencies, sociopathy, substance abuse, deviant thinking and experience, social withdrawal, etc.). Through configural interpretation of the relative scale elevations, tentative hypothesis regarding personality and coping style and relative degree of particular types of psychological disturbance can be gleaned. Importantly, although the MMPI can and is frequently misused and misinterpreted (e.g., application of psychiatric norms to medical patients tends to beg psychiatric interpretations), it represents one of the most useful adjuncts to personality assessment and treatment planning.

  A cursory summary of potential use of MMPI profile interpretation for assessing psychological reactions and contributions to physical conditions was offered by Fordyce (90) and roughly includes configural guidelines for interpreting (a) willingness to display physical symptom behaviors, (b) distress/discomfort about illness ("How comfortably sick?"), (c) poor general coping skills, (d) depression complicating physical symptoms, (e) tension (and sympathetic arousal) contributing to physical symptoms (high back pain, head, neck, shoulder, etc.), and (f) treatment outcome issues. Several subtypes of chronic pain have been identified by other researchers, although, as with other measures, it remains unclear to what extent results may inform the degree to which complaints are associated with organic (especially peripheral pathology) vs psychological contributions to patient presentation (91,92).

- *The Personality Assessment Inventory* (PAI) (93) is a measure of general psychopathology that can identify a wide variety of risk factors that could adversely affect adjustment. It has good psychometric properties and contains 340 items, with 22 scales, including 4 validity scales. As with most other general psychological assessment measures, it has no norms for chronic pain and tends to overpathologize this group.

- *Millon Clinical Multiaxial Inventory*, 3rd edition (MCMI-III) (94) includes scales assessing *DSM-IV*-based psychiatric disorders, including affective, personality and psychotic disorders, somatization, and others. It is useful for the differential diagnosis of personality disorders and psychological vulnerabilities for adaptation to pain. Such as other psychiatric measures, it has limited pain group norms and may be prone to overpathologizing rehabilitation in patients with pain.

of pain, autonomic arousal associated with bodily reactions to pain, cognitive appraisal(s) of the painful experience as related to the personal meaning of the pain or the historically learned responses to pain and injury, nonverbal behaviors including facial expressions and body language associated with pain, and affective reactions to pain including anxiety and depression. Persons with chronic pain have a much higher predilection and incidence of depression and anxiety, as well as anger. A diathesis-stress model has been proposed

to explain the higher rate of depression in this patient population and likely applies to other psychoemotional responses to chronic pain (97).

Finally, pain assessment and treatment strategies are best conceptualized in terms of suitability to a multidimensional process that evolves significantly as it persists over time. The stages of pain processing model (98) is an illustrative model that distinguishes the sensory, affective, cognitive-evaluative, and behavioral dimensions of pain as it changes with increasing chronicity. The first 2 stages involve sensory discrimination and associated affective responses. The former is commonly assessed by ratings of pain intensity and location, whereas the latter is assessed by ratings of pain unpleasantness. The third stage involves the meaning and implications of pain for the patient and associated emotional suffering and is commonly assessed by measuring pain-related emotional states (e.g., depression, anxiety, frustration) and beliefs (e.g., perceived ability to control or endure pain). The fourth stage refers to illness behavior (e.g., lifestyle and role disruption, avoidance) and can be assessed through self and collaborated ratings and observation (e.g., pain behaviors manifested at home, work, clinical interview). As pain persists, there is a transition of the focus of assessment from the first 2 stages to the latter 2.

Response Bias Assessment

As with any other human behavior, pain report can involve a response bias to report problems. This may involve an underreporting or overreporting of pain and related problems, with the latter commonly of greater concern, although both present inaccurate appraisals of the pain reality the particular patient is experiencing (99). It is very difficult to assess response bias with pain because there is no "gold standard" or unambiguous objective indicator of the pain subjective experience. One important consideration is whether there is a discrepancy from expectation based on underlying biomedical factors, for example, very high pain severity ratings or exhuberant pain behavior but little discernible biomedical pathology. This requires familiarity not only with how underlying biomedical conditions may present but also an understanding that there is often no discernible or identifiable biomedical condition to account for the presentation in chronic pain. It is also important to note any discrepancies between self-report of pain severity, pain behavior, pain-related disability, and affect, for example, if there are very high pain severity ratings but the person appears in no distress or in very good spirits and presents with circumscribed disability within the context of an otherwise comfortable lifestyle.

Much of the difficulty in assessing response bias in pain revolves around the distinction between the medial and lateral pain systems, that emotional or cognitive or attentional factors may be influencing the perception of pain and pain behavior, and that central sensitization effects may have resulted in the maintenance of a pain problem despite expected resolution of underlying biomedical causes (99). It is often important to determine how much any self-report of pain or pain behavior and related disability is caused by conscious vs unconscious exaggeration or malingering. Diagnosis and treatment is the usual reason for assessment of chronic pain, along with impairment and disability evaluation in compensation situations. Assessments can involve contexts with strong financial, personal, social, and/or other incentives. The assessment of deliberate and conscious exaggeration of problems for the purposes of secondary gain or outright malingering of nonexistent problems vs some exaggeration or accentuation of the pain experience and related disability associated with other psychosocial factors can be very difficult. Some assistance is offered through several pain assessment measures that include built-in response bias indicators. For example, the Millon Behavioral Medicine Diagnostic (MBMD) test (76) includes 3 built-in validity scales. In addition, Main and Spanswick (100) have outlined several factors that increase the suspicion of significant exaggeration, illness behavior, or malingering. These include

- failure to comply with reasonable treatment,
- report of severe pain with no associated psychological effects,
- marked inconsistencies in effects of pain on general activities,
- poor work record and history of persistent appeals against awards, and
- previous litigation.

Chapter 85 of this book is specifically devoted to the assessment of response bias. It provides background, relevant measures, and a general model for assessment with cautionary caveats including assessments conducted by persons without specialized chronic pain training and experience, which likely violates professional ethical standards (101,102).

PAIN MANAGEMENT

Early after the emergence of pain, treatment interventions invariably address amelioration of distress, correction of underlying pathophysiology, and promotion of healing. Inherent in all pain management interventions should be the prevention of chronicity. Chapter 57 of this book addresses the medical approaches involved in assessment and treatment of post-trauma pain. The importance of effective and timely assessment and treatment through a multipronged approach aimed at restoring function and minimizing disability is emphasized. Although acute pain management interventions are usually primarily medical in nature, behavioral, psychological, and other nonmedical pain management interventions still play an important role in cases where (a) associated psychological factors are significant, (b) medical interventions do not produce expected pain relief, and/or (c) where traditional medical interventions have not been successful or cannot be employed.

Although the goals of comprehensive chronic pain management interventions can vary with individuals and settings, they can generally be summarized as addressing the following areas:

- Modulation and reduction of intensity, frequency, and duration of sensory, as well as cognitive, evaluative, and affective distress responses related to pain experience.
- Modulation and reduction of associated physical and psychological symptoms and concomitants of pain, especially as they relate to mood and emotions, cognition,

energy, sleep, eating, physiological arousal, and general physical and emotional health.
- Reduction of functional disability, maladaptive avoidance and illness behavior, and interference with regular and preferred activities, including regular daily activities and preferred family, social, avocational, vocational, and recreational function and activities.
- Increasing self-management to actively use available strategies to minimize pain-related distress, functional disability, and life interference.

Persistent pain may be associated with a combination of physical and psychological factors; therefore, combination treatments and a multidisciplinary approach to chronic pain management consisting of pain specialists in medicine, psychology, physical therapy, occupational and/or vocational, and/or other allied health professions are logically indicated to optimize treatment efficacy and outcome. This approach is widely accepted as the most clinically successful and cost-effective process in treating chronic pain (103–106) and is best conducted and can usually only be effectively accomplished within the context of a specialty pain clinic. Specialty pain clinics are the treatment of choice for chronic pain conditions, with clinical efficacy supported by several recent reviews (103–110). Referral to pain management specialists and specialty pain clinics should be considered the standard of care for the treatment of persons with chronic pain.

When the person with pain has also sustained a TBI, additional recommendations are warranted. In persons with TBI and pain, there is evidence that pain is more difficult to manage (26), takes longer to complete a pain management program (111), and special attention is required because of cognitive difficulties (23). Hence, referral to specialty pain programs with experience in treating persons with TBI, and/or consultation with such providers to allow expectation of extended treatment periods and incorporation of cognitive compensatory strategies, is indicated.

Model for Conceptualizing Chronic Pain Treatments

There is considerable evidence and growing acceptance that many or most forms of chronic pain involve central and/or peripheral sensitization in which hyperresponsiveness or spontaneous discharge of components of the pain system develop (3–12). Conceptually, the thrust of current efforts in chronic pain management seem to be toward "desensitization" of the CNS and normalization of function through combination treatments. In addition, multidisciplinary, multicomponent, or combination treatment packages represent the most effective treatments in chronic pain, especially when comorbid with brain injury (3,17,30). A preliminary classification model for planning and conceptualizing chronic pain management interventions has been proposed (30,112) and is summarized in Table 58-6. The model facilitates the classification of currently available and potentially useful chronic pain treatment approaches according to specific area and manner of desensitization targeted.

It should be noted that Tyrer and Lievesley (113), among others, recommended the development of pain management facilities specifically designed for persons with brain injuries. The emotional disturbances associated with pain are also

TABLE 58-6 A Desensitization Model for Chronic Pain Treatment Interventions

Desensitizing peripheral CNS procedures

- EMG and temperature biofeedback, various relaxation and imagery procedures, transcutaneous electrical nerve stimulation (TENS)

Desensitizing CNS medications

- Antiepileptic drugs, tizanidine HCL, amytal (sodium amobarbital) intervention, neuroimmunomodulators, SSRIs, etc.

Desensitizing behavioral activity procedures

- Operant behavioral activity programs; graduated exposure/graduated activity programs; relaxation, imagery, refocusing; cognitive behavioral reinterpretive strategies

Desensitizing psychotherapeutic procedures

- Emotional desensitization of catastrophic reaction to injury and pain and other fears and trauma, splinting of emotional reactions and calming of catastrophic reactions and hypervigilance to pain, specific formal pain and fear desensitization procedures, pain graduated exposure/desensitization procedures, cognitive behavioral reinterpretive strategies, cognitive behavioral acceptance strategies, and meditative and mindfulness strategies.

Desensitizing neurophysiologic procedures

- Cranioelectrotherapy stimulation (CES). Consider EEG biofeedback or other potentially helpful adjunctive relaxation procedures such as sound and light (audio-visual stimulation [AVS]) and transcranial magnetic stimulation (TMS) and brain electrical stimulation (BES).

Abbreviations. CNS, central nervous system; EEG, electroencephalography; EMG, electromyography; HCL, hydrochloride; SSRIs, selective serotonin reuptake inhibitors.

frequently comorbid with TBI, highlighting the importance of a biopsychosocial perspective. Such perspective allows for a holistic conceptualization of the patient, incorporating multimethod, multimodal assessments that facilitate individualized treatment planning. Treatment goals include not only the reduction/relief from pain but also increased self-control, increased adaptation to life changes secondary to pain and brain injury, and improved functioning and quality of life.

Behavioral and Psychological Management

Behavioral and psychological services are important components of comprehensive pain management services. A review by McCracken and Turk (114) in 2002 identified more than 200 studies confirming that behavioral medicine interventions such as cognitive-behavioral therapy (CBT), biofeedback, and relaxation are effective in reducing pain and pain-related distress. The following text summarizes some of the most frequently used and empirically supported strategies. This discussion follows from the review by Martelli et al. (3), but readers are referred to additional reading for more comprehensive evidence-based summaries (115) and reviews of evidence-based recommendations for management of chronic nonmalignant pain (e.g., American Society of Anesthesiologists Task Force on Chronic Pain Management and the Ameri-

can Society of Regional Anesthesia and Pain Medicine) (116) or the many systematic reviews prepared for the Cochrane Collaboration (117). Although there is a paucity of studies examining pain management specific to persons with TBI, increasing studies are appearing, especially regarding PTH. In general, the interventions used are the same, qualified by understanding that treatment may take somewhat longer and require cognitive compensatory strategies and commensurate with cognitive impairments to assist with learning.

When persons with TBI initially present to psychologists for pain management services, the initial assessment process is always benefited by establishment of a therapeutic rapport. This includes countering any patient resistances or misconceptions (e.g., that pain must be in "their head" because they are seeing a psychologist) and engendering accurately informed and hopeful expectancies. Psychological management of persons with pain and TBI begins with an assessment that identifies all variables relevant for treatment. In addition to areas such as personality and emotional status, coping style and strategies, social support, and pain-specific factors (see preceding pain assessment section), evaluation must also include specific sequelae associated with brain injury. An integration of this information is necessary to ensure that the full constellation of residual sequelae and strengths are considered to optimize an individually designed treatment plan that anticipates and implements compensatory strategies for all potential obstacles to benefit from behavioral interventions. For example, deficits in memory, attention, or executive functioning might be addressed through task-analytic instruction and compensatory memory notebooks with provision of external reminders for completion of at-home assignments. The patients' specifically tailored treatment plan should provide a framework and outline for treatment, define goals and patient/therapist expectations and sequences, and provide psychoeducational information about the particular type of chronic pain and rationale for treatment.

In cases of post-traumatic pain, the severity and frequency of pain attacks or exacerbations and chronic pain-related sequelae, such as coping abilities, depression, and anxiety, are significantly improved by combined psychological treatment protocols (59,118–121). Supportive counseling that begins early after trauma and is continuous results in better patient response (59). A summary of useful behavioral treatments for chronic pain follows this paragraph. Nonetheless, readers are again referred to additional reading for more comprehensive summaries (e.g., 115–121).

Patient education: The most conspicuous and malleable factor that contributes to psychophysiologic arousal and stress responding is patient expectancy and knowledge about symptom management. For example, Ham and Packard (73) found that patients with headache desired an explanation of their headache at least as much as pain relief. In the case of mild TBI, education about expected symptoms and course has been shown to reduce the anxiety and selective attention and misattribution that can unnecessarily prolong symptoms (122). The best education treatment packages generally contain elements targeting numerous factors. Accurate information and expectancies help with this and also assist in coping with pain more adaptively. Stress management information and strategies can assist with reducing sympathetic arousal/discharge that exacerbates pain, whereas specific postural training and sleep hygiene can assist with postural rehabilitation and normalizing sleep patterns.

Biofeedback: Extensive research supports the use of electromyography (EMG) or thermal biofeedback for headache pain and chronic musculoskeletal pain disorders more generally (123). The forehead, trapezii, frontal-posterior neck, and neck areas are frequent EMG feedback sites. Patterns of pathophysiologic neuromuscular activity that underlie pain complaint and functional limitations, which can be remediated through feeding back physiologic information to allow self-correction, include (a) stress-related hyperarousal in musculoskeletal or other physiologic systems; (b) postural dysfunction; (c) hypertonicity or hypotonicity induced by reflex systems activated by inflammation, active trigger points, and cumulative strain or recurrent trauma; (d) learned guarding or bracing to mitigate anticipated pain or injury; (e) learned inhibition or avoidance of muscle activation/activity; (f) chronic muscular compensation for joint hypermobility/hypomobility associated with ligamentous injury; and (g) faulty motor schema and muscle imbalance reflecting development of 1 or more of the preceding syndromes, resulting in the lack of coordination and stability between typically coordinated muscle groups. Recently, data are emerging, which indicates that electroencephalography (EEG) biofeedback and associated EEG-driven stimulation offers efficacy in treatment of some persistent pain and persistent postconcussive symptoms (124,125). Finally, evidence has been reported that individuals can gain specific voluntary control over rostral anterior cingulate activation to directly control pain perception in severe chronic clinical pain (126).

Relaxation training: Progressive muscle relaxation (PMR) is the most studied relaxation procedure (115). PMR involves the systematic tensing and relaxing of various muscle groups to elicit a deepening relaxation response, usually with combination of muscle groups and addition of diaphragmatic breathing to shorten the protocol. Meta-analytic reviews generally conclude that relaxation training and biofeedback training are equally effective. Relaxation training presumably serves to (a) reduce proprioceptive input to the hypothalamus, thereby decreasing sympathetic nervous system activity (120,123) and (b) directly reduce muscle tension or preheadache vasoconstriction (127).

Behavioral treatments: Two major behavioral interventions include operant and graded exposure/activity strategies (115,119). Operant-based treatment strategies require altering environmental contingencies to eliminate reinforcement of pain and illness behaviors (e.g., verbal complaints, inactivity, avoidance) while rewarding "well" behaviors (e.g., incrementally increased exercise, activity level, involvement, and participation). Graded exposure/activity strategies involve graded increases in safe but feared activities that help resolve anxiety and distress. They promote increased activity through graded increases in safe but feared activities, which help reduce both fear of activity and experience of acute increases in pain, emotional distress, and avoidant responses.

Cognitive-behavioral treatments (CBTs): Cognitive-behavioral approaches incorporate the physical, psychological, and behavioral aspects of the pain experience in promoting patient's self-management of pain. They typically emphasize learning of self-regulation and self-control skills and taking more personal responsibility for lifestyle habit change, especially regarding identifying and replacing maladaptive beliefs about pain. Specific training is provided in cognitive strategies and skills to replace such inappropriate negative expectations and beliefs such as catastrophization and associated magnification, rumination, and helplessness that maintain physiologic arousal and maladaptive avoidance and illness behaviors that complicate symptom resolution (95). Specific cognitive strategies can range from very active (e.g., disputational cognitions and behaviors) to passive (e.g., mindfulness meditation and acceptance and commitment [ACT]) (128). A comprehensive multimodal approach should include education, skills acquisition, cognitive and behavioral rehearsal, homework, and generalization and maintenance (129) (Note that this approach incorporates most or all of the other supported behavioral interventions outlined in this section) in a manner that is tailored to the individual.

Social and assertiveness skills training: Skills training may help some patients with more effective communication of needs. Increased need fulfillment decreases distressful emotions, which reduces physiological arousal that contributes to pain experience (130).

Imagery and hypnosis: Using some combination of autohypnosis, suggestions of relaxation, and visual imagery, patients are generally instructed to visualize the pain (i.e., give it form) and focus on altering the image to reduce the pain. Imagery-based treatment is most effective following establishment of a good therapeutic alliance to facilitate compliance (131).

Notably, several authors have systematically reviewed evidence supporting the efficacy of behavioral interventions for chronic pain that includes chronic headache as well as PTH. A review by Kern, Sellinger, and Goodin (115) confirmed efficacy of psychological treatment outcomes for across various chronic pain groups. Branca and Lake (103) found that controlled studies of CBTs for migraine, such as biofeedback and relaxation therapy, had a prophylactic efficacy of about 50%, roughly equivalent to propranolol, whereas the combination of behavioral therapies greatly increased efficacy. Andrasik and colleagues (120,121,123) noted that meta-analytic reviews have consistently shown behavioral interventions (relaxation training, biofeedback, CBT, and stress-management training) to yield 35%–55% improvements in migraine and tension-type headache.

Finally, supportive evidence now increasingly includes randomized clinical trials (e.g., 65,105) and the interesting finding of Ruff, Ruff, and Wang (132) that a combined behavioral (sleep hygiene counseling) and pharmacologic (prazosin) treatment effectively improved sleep and decreased average frequency and intensity of PTH by 66% and improved cognitive assessment scores with results maintained at 6 months.

CONCLUSION

Chronic pain is a frequent concomitant of TBI; however, the assessment and treatment of persons with pain is a complicated and challenging process. Pain, by itself, can have a more disabling effect across a wider range of functions than brain or many other types of injuries. Associated symptoms such as sleep disturbance/deprivation, mood change, anxiety, somatic preoccupation and fear of pain, fatigue, perceived interference with activities, and medications may be as or more important than pain in producing chronic stress and peripheral or central sensitization effects with hyperresponsiveness in components of the pain processing system.

There have been long-standing problems and misconceptions regarding the assessment and monitoring of pain. The need for specialty expertise has been undervalued and appears to be essential for maximizing appropriate, timely, and cost-effective assessment and management. When specialty expertise is unavailable, clinicians should defer care to others with specialized knowledge and expertise. Recent advances in chronic pain assessment and treatment can be attributed to adoption of a biopsychosocial perspective. The most promising current treatment interventions are combination treatments that are holistic and include psychological interventions that target the patient's reaction to pain within his or her daily life and ability to exercise self-control. Multicomponent combination treatments are currently the preferred intervention for addressing chronic pain, especially when it accompanies TBI.

As part of the future research agenda, there is a need to better define the neuroanatomy and neurophysiology of pain processes to better inform understanding of pain disorders after TBI. Future efforts should focus on establishing specific treatment protocols for persons with dual diagnoses of pain and TBI, ideally demonstrated through randomized and controlled studies that consider the myriad types of pain conditions seen in this patient population and the impact of preinjury vulnerabilities and strengths in coping and adjustment.

KEY CLINICAL POINTS

1. Chronic pain is a frequent concomitant of TBI and can complicate the post-TBI clinical presentation and resolution of injury-related symptoms.
2. Special procedures are indicated for neuropsychological assessment and treatment of persons with pain after TBI; treatment may be more complex and may take longer because of associated cognitive-behavioral impairments that may require use of compensatory strategies.
3. Chronic pain, which is often not associated with obvious pathophysiology, is often associated with multiple phenomena including sleep disturbance/deprivation, mood changes such as depression, anxiety and irritability, as well as somatic preoccupation and fear of pain, fatigue, medication overuse, and perceived interference with activities, which in turn can produce chronic stress and central sensitization with hyperresponsiveness in components of the pain processing system.
4. The longer pain persists, the more likely the development of maladaptive protective and avoidant pain behavior responses, protracted and potentially inappropriate medication use, functionally disabling behavioral or emotional changes, and the more important it becomes for treatment goals to focus on improved pain coping.
5. Prevailing stands of international health care practice have emphasized the importance of assessing and managing pain.

6. A comprehensive biopsychosocial assessment should be considered as the standard of care when pain is chronic and should employ relevant instruments and procedures for integrating these findings with other data to generate individually tailored treatment interventions and recommendations.
7. Combination treatments that include psychological interventions are the treatment of choice. Multidisciplinary, multicomponent, or combination treatment packages represent the most effective treatments in chronic pain, especially when comorbid with brain injury.
8. Specialty pain experience should be considered prerequisite for clinical management of persons with TBI and pain disorders.
9. The ultimate goal of pain management of persons with TBI should be to facilitate early effective intervention aimed at restoring function, enhancing coping/adaptation, and minimizing functional disability through evidence-based practice.

KEY REFERENCES

1. Gatchel RJ, Peng YB, Peters ML, Fuchs PN, Turk DC. The biopsychosocial approach to chronic pain: scientific advances and future directions. *Psychol Bull.* 2007;133(4):581–624.
2. Kerns RD, Sellinger J, Goodin BR. Psychological treatment of chronic pain. *Annu Rev Clin Psychol.* 2011;7:411–434.
3. Martelli MF, Zasler ND, Nicholson K, Bender MC. Psychological, neuropsychological and medical considerations in the assessment and management of pain. *J Head Trauma Rehabil.* 2004;19(1):10–28.
4. Nicholson K, Martelli MF. The problem of pain. *J Head Trauma Rehabil.* 2004;19(1):2–9.
5. Tyrer S, Lievesley A. Pain following traumatic brain injury: assessment and management. *Neuropsychol Rehabil.* 2003;13(1–2):189–210.

References

1. Merskey H, Bogduk N, eds. *Classification of Chronic Pain.* 2nd ed. Seattle, WA: International Association for the Study of Pain Press; 1994.
2. Kulich RJ, Baker WB. A guide for psychological testing and evaluation for chronic pain. In: Aranoff GM, ed. *Evaluation and Treatment of Chronic Pain.* Baltimore, MD: Williams & Wilkins; 1999:301–312.
3. Martelli MF, Zasler ND, Nicholson K, Bender MC. Psychological, neuropsychological and medical considerations in the assessment and management of pain. *J Head Trauma Rehabil.* 2004;19(1):10–28.
4. Nicholson K. An overview of pain associated with lesion, disorder or dysfunction of the central nervous system. *NeuroRehabilitation.* 2000;14(1):3–14.
5. Nicholson K. At the crossroads: pain in the 21st century. *NeuroRehabilitation.* 2000;14(2):57–68.
6. Apkarian AV, Bushnell MC, Treede RD, Zubieta JK. Human brain mechanisms of pain perception and regulation in health and disease. *Eur J Pain.* 2005;9(4):463–484.
7. Wager TD, Rilling JK, Smith EE, et al. Placebo-induced changes in FMRI in the anticipation and experience of pain. *Science.* 2004;303:1162–1167.
8. Apkarian AV, Hashmi JA, Baliki MN. Pain and the brain: specificity and plasticity of the brain in clinical chronic pain. *Pain.* 2011;152(3)(suppl):S49–S64.
9. asser DS. Chronic pain: a neuroscientific understanding. *Med Hypotheses.* 2012;78(1):79–85.

10. Giesecke T, Gracely RH, Grant MA, et al. Evidence of augmented central pain processing in idiopathic chronic low back pain. *Arthritis Rheum.* 2004;50(2):613–623.

11. Apkarian AV, Baliki MN, Geha PY. Towards a theory of chronic pain. *Prog Neurobiol.* 2009;87(2):81–97.

12. Porro CA. Functional imaging and pain: behavior, perception, and modulation. *Neuroscientist.* 2003;9(5):354–369.

13. Gatchel RJ, Peng YB, Peters ML, Fuchs PN, Turk DC. The biopsychosocial approach to chronic pain: scientific advances and future directions. *Psychol Bull.* 2007;133(4):581–624.

14. Fordyce WE. Pain and suffering: a reappraisal. *Am Psychol.* 1988; 43(4):276–283.

15. World Health Organization. *International Classification of Functioning, Disability and Health.* Geneva, Switzerland: World Health Organization; 2001.

16. American Psychiatric Association. *Diagnostic and Statistical Manual of Mental Disorders.* 4th ed., text rev. Washington, DC: American Psychiatric Association; 2000.

17. Miller L. Neurosensitization: a model for persistent disability in chronic pain, depression, and posttraumatic stress disorder following injury. *NeuroRehabilitation.* 2000;14(1)25–32.

18. Sharp TJ, Harvey AG. Chronic pain and posttraumatic stress disorder: mutual maintenance? *Clin Psychol Rev.* 2001;21(6):57–877.

19. Schreiber S, Galai-Gati T. Uncontrolled pain following physical injury as the core-trauma in post-traumatic stress disorder. *Pain.* 1993;54(1):107–110.

20. Nicholson K, Martelli MF, Zasler ND. Myths and misconceptions about chronic pain: the problem of mind body dualism. In: Weiner RB, ed. *Pain Management: A Practical Guide for Clinicians.* 6th ed. Boca Raton, FL: St. Lucie Press; 2002:465–474.

21. Hart RP, Wade JB, Martelli MF. Cognitive impairment in patients with chronic pain: the significance of stress. *Curr Pain Headache Rep.* 2003;7(2):116–226.

22. Joint Commission on Accreditation of Healthcare Organizations. Pain management standards. 2001. Available at: www.jcaho.org/standard/pain_hap.html. Accessed January 28, 2012.

23. Nicholson K, Martelli MF. The problem of pain. *J Head Trauma Rehabil.* 2004;19(1):2–9.

24. Evans RW. Post-traumatic headaches. In: Evans RW, ed. *Neurologic Clinics.* Philadelphia, PA: Saunders; 2004:237–249.

25. Zasler ND, Martelli MF. Post-traumatic headache: practical approaches to diagnosis and treatment. In: Weiner RB, ed. *Pain Management: A Practical Guide for Clinicians.* 6th ed. Boca Raton, FL: St. Lucie Press; 2002.

26. Nampiaparampil DE. Prevalence of chronic pain after traumatic brain injury: a systematic review. *JAMA.* 2008;300(6):711–719.

27. Hart RP, Martelli MF, Zasler ND. Chronic pain and neuropsychological functioning. *Neuropsychol Rev.* 2000;10(3):131–149.

28. Nicholson K, Martelli MF. The confounding effects of pain, psychoemotional problems or psychiatric disorder, premorbid ability structure, and motivational or other factors on neuropsychological test performance. In: Young G, Kane A, Nicholson K, eds. *Psychological Knowledge for Court: PTSD, Chronic Pain and TBI.* New York, NY: Springer; 2006:335–351.

29. Moriarty O, McGuire BE, Finn DP. The effect of pain on cognitive function: a review of clinical and preclinical research. *Prog Neurobiol.* 2011;93(3):385–404.

30. Zasler ND, Martelli MF, Nicholson K. Chronic pain (and traumatic brain injury). In: Silver JM, McAllister TW, Yudofsky SC, eds. *Textbook of Traumatic Brain Injury.* 2nd ed. Washington, DC: American Psychiatric Publishing, Inc; 2011:375–396.

31. Martelli MF, Nicholson K, Zasler ND. Psychological approaches to comprehensive pain assessment and management following TBI. In: Zasler ND, Katz DI, Zafonte RD, eds. *Brain Injury Medicine: Principles and Practice.* New York, NY: Demos Medical Publishing; 2007:723–742.

32. Mooney G, Speed J, Sheppard S. Factors related to recovery after mild traumatic brain injury. *Brain Inj.* 2005;19(12):975–987.

33. Pilcher JJ, Huffcutt AL. Effects of sleep deprivation on performance: a meta analysis. *Sleep.* 1996;19(4):318–326.

34. Kundermann B, Krieg JC, Schreiber W, Lautenbacher S. The effect of sleep deprivation on pain. *Pain Res Manag.* 2004;9(1):25–32.

35. Mahmood O, Rapport LJ, Hanks RA, Fichtenberg NL. Neuropsychological performance and sleep disturbance following traumatic brain injury. *J Head Trauma Rehabil.* 2004;19(5):378–390.

36. Porro CA, Baraldi P, Pagnoni G, et al. Does anticipation of pain affect cortical nociceptive systems? *J Neurosci.* 2002;15;22(8): 3206–3214.

37. Martelli MF, Zasler ND, MacMillan P. Mediating the relationship between injury, impairment and disability: a vulnerability, stress and coping model of adaptation following brain injury. *NeuroRehabilitation.* 1998;11(1):51–66.

38. Gatchel RJ, Howard K, Haggard R. The biopsychosocial perspective of pain. In: Contrada RJ, Baum A, eds. *The Handbook of Stress Science: Biology, Psychology and Health.* New York, NY: Springer; 2010.

39. Gatchel RJ, Kishino HD. Managing pain. In: Thomas JC, Hersen M, eds. *Handbook of Clinical Psychology Competencies.* New York, NY: Springer; 2012.

40. Martelli MF, Zasler ND. Useful psychological instruments for assessing persons with functional medical disorders. In: Zasler ND, Martelli MF, eds. *Functional Medical Disorders, State of the Art Reviews in Physical Medicine and Rehabilitation.* Philadelphia, PA: Hanley and Belfus; 2002:147–162.

41. Jensen MP, Karoly P. Self-report scales and procedures for assessing pain in adults. In: Turk DC, Melzack R, eds. *Handbook of Pain Assessment.* 2nd ed. New York, NY: Guilford Press; 2001:15–34.

42. Whaley LF, Wong DL. *Nursing Care of Infants and Children.* 3rd ed. St. Louis, MO: Mosby; 1987.

43. Rainsford AO, Cairns D, Mooney V. The pain drawing as an aid to the psychologic evaluation of patients with lower back pain. *Spine.* 1974;1:127–134.

44. Melzack R. The short-form McGill Pain Questionnaire. *Pain.* 1987; 30:191–197.

45. Turk DC, Burwinkle TM. Assessment of chronic pain in rehabilitation: outcomes measures in clinical trials and clinical practice. *Rehabil Psychol.* 2005;50(1):56–64.

46. McGrath PA, Gillespie J. Pain assessment in children and adolescents. In: Turk DC, Melzack R, eds. *Handbook of Pain Assessment.* 2nd ed. New York, NY: Guilford Press; 2001:97–118.

47. Gagliese L. Assessement of pain in elderly people. In: Turk DC, Melzack R, eds. *Handbook of Pain Assessment.* 2nd ed. New York, NY: Guilford Press; 2001:119–133.

48. Knott C, Beyer J, Villarruel A, Denyes M, Erickson V, Willard G. Application of the oucher in practice: a developmental approach to pain assessment in children. *MCN Am J Matern Child Nurs.* 1994; 19(6):314–320.

49. Hadjistavropoulos T, LaChapelle DL. Extent and nature of anxiety experience during physical examination of chronic low back pain. *Behav Res Ther.* 2000;38(1)13–18.

50. Bruns D, Disorbio JM, Copeland-Disorbio J. *Battery for Health Improvement (BHI).* Minneapolis, MN: National Computer Systems; 1996.

51. Rudy TE, Turk DC. *Multiaxial Assessment of Pain: Multidimensional Pain Inventory Computer Program User Manual Version 2.1.* Pittsburgh, PA: University of Pittsburgh; 1989.

52. Ruehlman LS, Karoly P, Newton C, Aiken LS. The development and preliminary validation of the profile of chronic pain: extended assessment battery. *Pain.* 2005;118(3):380–389.

53. Heaton RK, Lehman RAW, Getto CJ. *Psychosocial Pain Inventory.* Odessa, FL: Psychological Assessment Resources; 1985.

54. McCracken LM, Vowles KE, Eccleston C. Acceptance of chronic pain: component analysis and a revised assessment method. *Pain.* 2004;107:159–166.

55. McCracken LM, Eccleston C. A comparison of the relative utility of coping and acceptance-based measures in a sample of chronic pain sufferers. *Eur J Pain.* 2006;10(1):23–29.

56. Jensen MP, Turner JA, Romano JM, Strom SE. The Chronic Pain Coping Inventory: development and preliminary validation. *Pain.* 1995;60(2):203–216.

57. Todd DD, Martelli MF, Grayson, RL. *The Cogniphobia Scale (C-Scale): A Measure of Headache Impact.* Glen Allen, VA: Concussion Care Centre of Virginia (Test in the public domain); 1998.

58. Butler R, Damarin F, Beaulieu C, Schwebel A, Doleys D. Assessing cognitive coping strategies for acute post-surgical pain. Psychological assessment. *J Consult Clin Psychol.* 1989;1:41–45.

59. Rosensteil AK, Keefe FJ. The use of coping strategies in chronic low back pain patients: relationship to patient characteristics and current adjustment. *Pain.* 1983;17:33–44.

60. Todd DD, Kinesiophobia: the relationship between chronic pain and fear-induced disability. *The Forensic Examiner.* 1998;7(5–6): 14–20.

61. Houben RM, Leeuw M, Vlaeyen JW, Goubert L, Picavet HS. Fear of movement/injury in the general population: factor structure and psychometric properties of an adapted version of the Tampa Scale for kinesiophobia. *J Behav Med.* 2005;28(5):415–424.

62. Gracely RH, McGrath P, Dubner R. Ratio scales of sensory and affective verbal pain descriptors. *Pain.* 1978;5(1):5–18.

63. McCracken LM, Zayfert C, Gross RT. The Pain Anxiety Symptoms Scale: development and validation of a scale to measure fear of pain. *Pain.* 1992;50(1):67–73.

64. Sullivan MJL, Bishop S, Pivik J. The Pain Catastrophizing Scale: development and validation. *Psychol Assessment.* 1995;7:524–532.

65. Thorn BE, Pence LB, Ward LC, et al. A randomized clinical trial of cognitive behavioral treatment targeted at the reduction of catastrophizing in chronic headache sufferers. *J Pain.* 2007;68(12): 938–949.

66. Crombez G, Bijttebier P, Eccleston C, et al. The child version of the Pain Catastrophizing Scale (PCS-C): a preliminary validation. *Pain.* 2003;104(3):639–646.

67. Tollison CD, Langley JC. *Pain Patient Profile (P3).* Minneapolis, MN: National Computer Systems; 1992.

68. Kerns RD, Rosenberg R, Jamison RN, Caudille MA, Haythornthwait J. Readiness to adopt a self-management approach to chronic pain: the Pain Stages of Change Questionnaire (PSOCQ). *Pain.* 1997;72(1–2):227–234.

69. Burns JW, Glenn B, Lofland K, Bruehl S, Harden RN. Stages of change in readiness to adopt a self-management approach to chronic pain: the moderating role of early-treatment stage progression in predicting outcome. *Pain.* 2005;115(3):322–331.

70. Kerns RD, Wagner J, Rosenberg R, Haythornthwaite J, Caudill-Slosberg M. Identification of subgroups of persons with chronic pain based on profiles on the pain stages of change questionnaire. *Pain.* 2005;116(3):302–10.

71. Ruehlman LS, Karoly P, Newton C, Aiken LS. The development and preliminary validation of a brief measure of chronic pain impact for use in the general population. *Pain.* 2005;113(1–2):82–90.

72. Jensen MP, Turner JA, Romano JM, Lawler BK. Relationship of pain-specific beliefs to chronic pain adjustment. *Pain.* 1994;57(3): 301–309.

73. Packard RC, Ham LP. Impairment rating for posttraumatic headache. *Headache.* 1993;33(7):359–364.

74. Fairbank JC, Mbaot JC, Davies JB, O'Brien JP. The Oswestry low back pain and disability questionnaire. *Physiotherapy.* 1980;66(8): 271–273.

75. Brown GK, Nicassio PM. The development of a questionnaire for the assessment of active and passive coping strategies in chronic pain patients. *Pain.* 1987;31(1):53–65.

76. Millon T. The MBHI and the MBMD. In: Strack S, ed. *Interpretive Strategies for the Millon Inventories.* New York, NY: Wiley; 1999.

77. Ware JE, Kosinski M, Gandek B. *SF-36 Health Survey: Manual and Interpretation Guide.* Lincoln, RI: QualityMetric, Inc; 2000.

78. Kreutzer JS, Marwitz JH, Seel R, Serio CD. Validation of a neurobehavioral functioning inventory for adults with traumatic brain injury. *Arch Phys Med Rehabil.* 1996;77(2):116–124.

79. Bergner M, Bobbitt RA, Carter WB, Gilson BS. The sickness impact profile: development and final revision of a health status measure. *Med Care.* 1981;19(8):787–805.

80. Pilowsky I, Spence ND. Patterns of illness behavior in patients with intractable pain. *J Psychosom Res.* 1975;19(4):279–287.

81. Pilowsky I, Spence ND. Illness behavior syndromes associated with intractable pain. *Pain.* 1976;2(1):61–71.

82. Beck AT, Ward CH, Mendelson M, Mock J, Erbaugh J. An inventory for measuring depression. *Arch Gen Psychiatry.* 1961;4:561–571.

83. Turner JA, Romano JM. Self-report screening measures for depression in chronic pain patients. *J Clin Psychol.* 1984;40(4):909–913.

84. Zeigler DK, Paolo AM. Headache symptoms and psychological profile of headache-prone individuals: a comparison of clinic patients and controls. *Arch Neurol.* 1995;52(6):602–606.

85. Spielberger CD. *State-Trait Anger Expression Inventory, Research Edition: Professional Manual.* Odessa, FL: Psychological Assessment Resources; 1999.

86. Beck AT. *Beck Anxiety Inventory (BAI).* San Antonio, TX: Harcourt Assessment, Inc; 1993.

87. Cohen S, Kamarck T, Mermelstein R. A global measure of perceived stress. *J Health Soc Behav.* 1983;24(4):385–396.

88. Dahlstrom WG, Welsh GS, Dahlstrom LE. *An MMPI Handbook: Research Applications.* Vol 2. Minneapolis, MN: University of Minnesota Press; 1975.

89. Butcher JN, Dahlstrom WG, Graham JR, Tellegren A, Kaemmer B. *MMPI-2: Manual for Administration and Scoring.* Minneapolis, MN: University of Minnesota Press; 1989.

90. Fordyce WE. Use of the MMPI in the assessment of chronic pain. In: Butcher J, Dahlstrom G, Schofield W, eds. *Clinical Notes on the MMPI. Number three in the series.* Seattle, WA: University of Washington Press; 1983:1–18.

91. Keller LS, Butcher JN. *Assessment of Chronic Pain Patients With the MMPI-2. MMPI-2 Monographs.* Minneapolis, MN: University of Minnesota Press; 1991.

92. Vendrig AA. The Minnesota Multiphasic Personality Inventory and chronic pain: a conceptual analysis of a long-standing but complicated relationship. *Clin Psychol Rev.* 2000;20(5):533–559.

93. Morey LC. *Personality Assessment Inventory—Professional Manual.* Florida, USA: Psychological Assessment Resources, Inc; 1991.

94. Millon T. *MCMI-II Manual.* Minneapolis, MN: National Computer Systems; 1977.

95. Turk DC. Understanding pain sufferers: the role of cognitive processes. *Spine J.* 2004;4(1):1–7.

96. Asmundson GJ, Nicholas Carleton R. Fear of pain is elevated in adults with co-occurring trauma-related stress and social anxiety symptoms. *Cogn Behav Ther.* 2005;34(4):248–255.

97. Banks SM, Kerns RD. Explaining high rates of depression in chronic pain: a diathesis-stress framework. *Psychol Bull.* 1996;119 (1):95–110.

98. Price DD, Riley JL, Wade JB. Psychosocial approaches to measurement of the dimensions and stages of pain. In: Turk DC, Melzack R, eds. *Handbook of Pain Assessment.* New York, NY: Guilford Press; 2001:53–75.

99. Nicholson K, Martelli MF. Section III: malingering in psychological injury: TBI, chronic pain and PTSD. In: Young G, Kane A, Nicholson K, eds. *Causality of Psychological Injury: Presenting Evidence in Court.* New York, NY: Springer; 2007:374–516.

100. Main CJ, Spanswick CC. "Functional overlay," and illness behaviour in chronic pain: distress or malingering? Conceptual difficulties in medico-legal assessment of personal injury claims. *J Psychosom Res.* 1995;39(6):737–753.

101. Martelli MF. Ethical challenges in the neuropsychology of pain, part 1. In: Bush SS, ed. *A Casebook of Ethical Challenges in Neuropsychology.* New York, NY: Swets & Zeitlinger; 2005:113–123.

102. Nicholson K. Ethical challenges in the neuropsychology of pain, part 2. In: Bush SS, ed. *A Casebook of Ethical Challenges in Neuropsychology.* New York, NY: Swets & Zeitlinger; 2005:124–130.

103. Branca B, Lake AE. Psychological and neuropsychological integration in multidisciplinary pain management after TBI. *J Head Trauma Rehabil.* 2004;19(1):40–57.

104. Gatchel RJ, Lou L, Kishino N. Concepts of multidisciplinary pain management. In: Boswell MV, Cole BE, Weiner SR, eds. *Weiner's Pain Management: A Practical Guide for Clinicians..* New York, NY: Taylor & Francis Group; 2006:1501–1508.

105. Lemstra M, Stewart B, Olszynski WP. Effectiveness of multidisciplinary intervention in the treatment of migraine: a randomized clinical trial. *Headache.* 2002;42(9):845–854.

106. Jeffery MM, Butler M, Stark A, Kane RL. Multidisciplinary pain programs for chronic noncancer pain. Technical brief no. 8. (Prepared by Minnesota Evidence-based Practice Center under contract no. 290-07-10064-I.). Rockville, MD: Agency for Health-

care Research and Quality; 2011. AHRQ Publication No. 11-EHC064-EF.

107. Campbell A, Cole BE. Interdisciplinary pain management programs: the American Academy of Pain Management Model. In: Boswell MV, Cole BE, Weiner SR, eds. *Weiner's Pain Management: A Practical Guide for Clinicians.* New York, NY: Taylor & Francis Group; 2006:1517–1530.

108. Scascighini L, Toma V, Dober-Spielmann S, Sprott H. Multidisciplinary treatment for chronic pain: a systematic review of interventions and outcomes. *Rheumatology (Oxford).* 2008;47(5):670–678.

109. Okifuji A, Turk DC, Kalauokalani D. Clinical outcome and economic evaluation of multidisciplinary pain centers. In: Block AR, Kremer EF, Fernandez E, eds. *Handbook of Pain Syndrome.* Mahwah, NJ: Lawrence Erlbaum Associates; 1999:77–97.

110. Recla JM. Recent developments in the management of post-traumatic pain. *ENJ.* 2010;2(1):73–82.

111. Andary MT, Crewe N, Ganzel SK, et al. Traumatic brain injury/chronic pain syndrome: a case comparison study. *Clin J Pain.* 1997;13(3):244–250.

112. Martelli MF, Grayson R, Zasler ND. Post-traumatic headache: psychological and neuropsychological issues in assessment and treatment. *J Head Trauma Rehabil.* 1999;1:49–69.

113. Tyrer S, Lievesley A. Pain following traumatic brain injury: assessment and management. *Neuropsychol Rehabil.* 2003;13(1–2):189–210.

114. McCracken LM, Turk DC. Behavioral and cognitive behavioral treatment for chronic pain: outcome, predictors of outcome, and treatment process. *Spine.* 2002;27(22):2564–2573.

115. Kerns RD, Sellinger J, Goodin BR. Psychological treatment of chronic pain. *Annu Rev Clin Psychol.* 2011;7:411–434.

116. American Society of Anesthesiologists Task Force on Chronic Pain Management, American Society of Regional Anesthesia and Pain Medicine. Practice guidelines for chronic pain management: an updated report by the American Society of Anesthesiologists Task Force on chronic pain management and the American Society of Regional Anesthesia and Pain Medicine. *Anesthesiology.* 2010;112(4):810–833.

117. Cochrane Collaboration. *The Cochrane Library.* 2010. Available at: http://www.thecochranelibrary.com/view/0/index.html. Accessed January 28, 2012.

118. Jensen MP, Turner JA, Romano JM. Self-efficacy and outcome expectancies: relationship to chronic pain coping strategies and adjustment. *Pain.* 1991;44(3):263–269.

119. Macedo LG, Smeets RJEM, Maher CG, Latimer J, McAuley JH. Graded activity and graded exposure for persistent nonspecific low back pain: a systematic review. *Phys Ther.* 2010;90(6):860–879.

120. Andrasik F. Biofeedback in headache: an overview of approaches and evidence. *Cleve Clin J Med.* 2010;77(suppl 3):S72–S76.

121. Nestoriuc Y, Martin A, Rief W, Andrasik F. Biofeedback treatment for headache disorders: a comprehensive efficacy review. *Appl Psychophysiol Biofeedback.* 2008;33(3):125–140.

122. Mittenberg W, Trement G, Zielinski RE, Fichera S, Rayls KR. Cognitive-behavioral prevention of postconcussion syndrome. *Arch Clin Neuropsychol.* 1996;11(2):139–145.

123. Andrasik F. Relaxation and biofeedback self management for pain. In: Boswell MV, Cole BE, Weiner SR, eds. *Weiner's Pain Management: A Practical Guide for Clinicians.* New York, NY: Taylor & Francis Group; 2006:697–710.

124. DeVore JR. Applied psychophysiology: state of the art. In: Zasler ND, Martelli MF, eds. *Functional Medical Disorders, State of the Art Reviews in Physical Medicine and Rehabilitation.* Philadelphia, PA: Hanley and Belfus; 2002:21–36.

125. Othmer S, Other S. Efficacy of neurofeedback for pain management. In: Boswell MV, Cole BE, Weiner SR, eds. *Weiner's Pain Management: A Practical Guide for Clinicians.* New York, NY: Taylor & Francis Group; 2006:719–739.

126. Decharms RC, Maeda F, Glover GH, et al. Control over brain activation and pain learned by using real-time functional MRI. *Proc Natl Acad Sci USA.* 2005;102(51):18626–18631.

127. Auerbach SM, Gramling SE. *Stress Management: Psychological Foundations.* New York, NY: Prentice-Hall, Inc; 1998.

128. Chiesa A, Serretti A. Mindfulness-based interventions for chronic pain: a systematic review of the evidence. *J Altern Complement Med.* 2011;17(1):83–93.

129. Brown KS, DeCarvalho LT. Psychotherapeutic approaches in pain management. In: Boswell M V, Cole BE, Weiner SR, eds. *Weiner's Pain Management: A Practical Guide for Clinicians.* New York, NY: Taylor & Francis Group; 2006:685–704.

130. Miller L. *Psychotherapy of the Brain Injured Patient.* New York, NY: WW Norton & Company, Inc; 1993.

131. Martin PR. *Psychological Management of Chronic Headaches.* New York, NY: Guilford Press; 1993.

132. Ruff RL, Ruff SS, Wang XF. Improving sleep: initial headache treatment in OIF/OEF veterans with blast-induced mild traumatic brain injury. *J Rehabil Res Dev.* 2009;46(9):1071–1084.

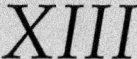

XIII

COGNITIVE PROBLEMS

59

Cognitive Impairments

Paul J. Eslinger, Giuseppe Zappalà, Freeman Chakara, and Anna M. Barrett

INTRODUCTION

Traumatic brain injury (TBI) causes several types of damage to the brain that affect the cerebral cortex, subcortical nuclear structures, and their widespread white matter connections. The resulting cascade of pathological events impairs neural functioning at multiple levels from altered cellular and neurotransmitter activity to vascular changes and disruption of the larger brain networks that mediate cognition (see Figure 59-1). This rapid deformation of brain anatomy and physiology leads to clinical impairments that affect cognition, sensorimotor, and somatic-vegetative functions, as well as social and emotional adjustment (1). This chapter is organized to provide an overview and synthesis of the cognitive impairments that are commonly associated with TBI in adults. Cognitive and behavioral symptoms are often major concerns in all types of TBI as indicated by the many other chapters relating to cognition and behavior in this volume. The importance of cognitive diagnosis and treatment stems from the fact that rehabilitation outcomes and long-term effects of TBI on personal, social, and occupational functioning can often be related to the integrity of cognitive abilities along with behavioral and emotional adjustment. Indeed, cognitive measures are among the most important predictors of patients' return to work and independent living, even among those with good medical recoveries (2).

TBI and postconcussion symptoms occur along a spectrum recognized as *mild to severe*. Clinical presentations are increasingly recognized as a predictable but somewhat variable hierarchy or cluster of symptoms that are determined by the intensity, severity, and location of the injury in the brain. The acute brain-behavioral effects of TBI can range from brief alteration of consciousness to coma. Clinical studies have further revealed that many complicating medical and psychological conditions can contribute to the nature and severity of post-TBI cognitive impairments. These include preexisting conditions such as learning disabilities, attention deficit hyperactivity disorder, substance abuse, and prior head trauma, as well as comorbid conditions such as seizures, major depression, chronic pain, sleep disturbance, and medication side effects underscoring the potentially complex nature of TBI (3,4). Hence, a multidisciplinary and comprehensive approach to TBI and specifically to cognitive and behavioral impairments is necessary for best treatment outcomes. From a lifespan perspective, this is particularly important because TBI has been identified as a risk factor for diseases causing dementia (5,6).

Neuropsychological assessment encompasses clinical and psychometric testing procedures that survey and objectively measure the effects of cerebral damage on cognition, behavior, and social-emotional functioning (7). These procedures help identify and define the nature and extent of TBI effects using standardized cognitive tests and survey instruments, together with comprehensive interview and clinical assessment. Neuropsychological test scores can change in different ways depending on TBI pathophysiology (8). To this end, a variety of specific assessment techniques have been developed to evaluate a patient's relative strengths and weaknesses in multiple domains such as memory, speech and language, attention concentration, spatial cognition, executive functions (EFs), and social cognition (see Chapter 60 for further details). Scores are then interpreted in reference to available normative data that provide the typical range and variation in test performance.

Interpretation of neuropsychological test scores is meant to identify the type and severity of cognitive impairments that, in turn, can reflect general location and severity of brain injury. Most clinicians employ a flexible battery approach that focuses on specific problem areas identified through clinical exam and observation. The flexible battery approach emphasizes on evaluating the patient's *pattern* of performance including the possible causes for their impaired test score. For example, impaired memory test scores may reflect attentional and encoding deficiencies, working memory (WM) limitations, memory consolidation deficits, poor access to and retrieval of information, or some combination of these underlying cognitive difficulties. Delineating specific processing impairments can potentially provide a more direct and efficient approach to cognitive remediation services that target impaired processes. Therefore, neuropsychological assessment, along with assessments provided through related medical and therapy services, is geared toward identifying how best to detect, characterize, and intervene in remediation of the cognitive and related behavioral, social, and emotional impairments that are caused by TBI.

The types of possible cognitive impairment caused by TBI are nearly as broad and challenging as cognition itself. This is because virtually any region of the brain potentially can be affected by TBI through primary injury or secondary pathophysiology effects. It is also important to realize, however, that TBI damage is not evenly distributed throughout

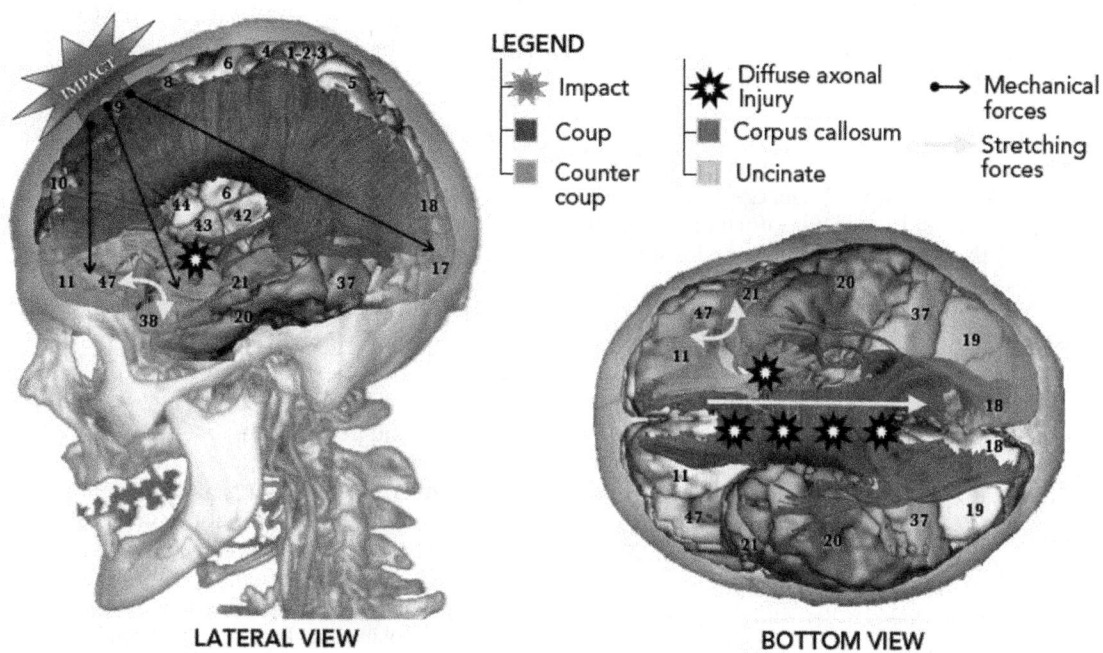

FIGURE 59-1 *See color insert.* Lateral and horizontal view of the mechanisms damaging the brain in TBI.

the brain. The manner in which the brain is encased within bony structures and the diverse lesions associated with different TBI causes comprise some of the factors that predispose certain regions of the brain to relatively greater damage. Subsequently, large sample studies have identified more frequent and proportionately greater deficits in certain domains of cognition than others, such as processing speed, attention, memory, and EFs. This chapter is organized into 2 major sections to provide a critical overview of cognitive impairments caused by TBI. First, deficits in fundamental processes that support most domains of cognition will be summarized. These include reaction time, attention, WM, and self-awareness. Second, the major domains of cognition will be examined, ranging from general intelligence, memory, and spatial cognition through EFs and social cognition (see Table 59-1 for summary).

FUNDAMENTAL PROCESSES OF COGNITION

Reaction Time

Reaction time measures are designed to determine the speed and accuracy of basic sensory-perception and perceptual-motor responses. These processes are mediated by dedicated cortical and subcortical regions along with white matter connections that are vulnerable to TBI-related damage. TBI may alter reaction time capacities in several ways. For example, Sarno et al. (9) demonstrated that severe TBI was associated with prolonged simple and choice reaction times to visual, auditory, and tactile stimuli. In this study, tactile stimuli presented particular difficulty in comparison to vision and audition (i.e., a sensory-specific deficit) as well as in combination with those modalities (i.e., cross-modal deficits). Moreover, reaction time studies have revealed that TBI slows the typical sensory detection and integration processes that are critical

TABLE 59-1 Cognitive Impairments Associated With TBI

IMPAIRMENTS IN FUNDAMENTAL PROCESSES SUPPORTING COGNITION	IMPAIRMENTS IN MAJOR DOMAINS OF COGNITION
Reaction time (particularly with increasing task difficulty, more informational load, and fatigue)	**General intelligence** Verbal intelligence Nonverbal intelligence
Attention-concentration (alertness, sustained attention, selective attention, and divided attention)	**Learning and memory** Post-traumatic amnesia Short-term, long-term, and procedural memory systems Confabulations and delusions
Working memory (tracking and manipulation of changing information during problem solving)	**Spatial cognition** Environmental navigation Mental maps and directions Object locations Spatial memory
Self-awareness (denial or lack of concern about symptoms)	**Executive functions** Orbital prefrontal network Medial prefrontal network Dorsolateral prefrontal network Decision making Emotional decision making Cognitive organization
	Social cognition Theory of mind Socio-moral judgment Emotional intelligence Social adaptation

for timely and consistent responses within stimulating and changing environments. Investigators have confirmed that reaction time can also be compromised after mild TBI (10), particularly as task difficulty increased and when interhemispheric transfer of information was required. Even when simple reaction time tasks are completed in normal fashion after TBI, deficits have been found to emerge under conditions of increasing task difficulty, greater informational load, and even fatigue (11) that lead to inconsistent, slowed, and erroneous responses.

Attention and Working Memory

Attention and WM problems after TBI are among the most common cognitive impairments reported by patients, family members, and clinicians constituting a significant limitation in speed and efficiency of cognitive processing (12). Attention and WM are sometimes considered to be overlapping processes, although most investigators separate them based on theoretical terms or differences in specific task requirements. For example, many tests of attention are externally directed (e.g., detection of stimuli, repeating increasing digits, or tap sequences), whereas many WM measures depend on an additional internally-directed dimension such as holding a rule in mind or manipulating presented materials in the midst of problem solving or completion of an action (such as in dual-task, n-back, and calculation paradigms). Several kinds of attention and WM components have been identified and examined in TBI, with troubling deficits often found to pose serious threats to everyday cognitive functions. In clinical practice, these deficits can be evident on specific tests of attention and WM (e.g., digit span, letter-number sequencing, continuous performance measures, n-back, and go/no-go tasks) as well as on tests where attention and WM are important components (e.g., Trail Making Test Part B, Stroop Test, Wisconsin Card Sorting, etc.).

Zoccolotti and colleagues (13) compared multiple attention and WM measures in 106 patients with generally more severe TBI drawn from multiple European sites. The sample was tested at least 5 months after injury (allowing for recovery of acute effects), and 80% of participants suffered coma ≥ 8 days. Four computerized tasks were compared. The first 2 tasks required rather straightforward or *intensive attention* and included measures of (*a*) alertness (reaction time with and without a tonal warning) and (*b*) sustained attention to horizontal bar movements. The final 2 tasks were considered measures of *selective attention* (i.e., WM) based on keeping certain rules in mind and allocating attentional resources between dual tasks. These were hypothesized to be more problematic after TBI and included (*c*) selective attention on go/no-go and design detection tasks, and (*d*) divided attention to simultaneous visual and auditory tasks, each to detect a specific pattern during continuous stimulus presentations. Results confirmed that patients showed considerably more difficulty in the selective attention tasks requiring go/no-go responding (combining WM with inhibitory control) and divided attention (increasing the WM load) with up to one-half of the sample demonstrating deficits. Some difficulties were also evident in the more straightforward intensive attention conditions varying between 9%–33% of patients. Analyses also indicated considerable variability in performance among patients. This is not unexpected given the diverse trauma and personal characteristics of the sample. At least 3 subgroups were identified:

- A severely impaired subgroup (comprising nearly 50% of the sample) with a similar attention deficit profile as the overall sample (greater impairment in selective and divided attention tasks). This subgroup suffered more severe trauma and longer length of coma. Although all patients with mild and moderate levels of coma completed the divided attention task, 5% of severe and 26% of very severe coma patients were unable to complete the task.
- A less impaired subgroup (nearly 44% of the sample) with a large dissociation between normal alertness scores and poor divided attention scores. This prevalent pattern of performance argued against a nonspecific or generalized slowing of performance and supported the possibility of a specific divided attention and WM-related deficit. We have encountered such deficits commonly in clinical practice, where the complaints can be described as disorganized behavior, inability to multitask, losing track of objects, paperwork and activities, and being able to undertake "only one activity or task at a time".
- A third subgroup (only 7% of the sample) included those with very long reaction times in both alertness and divided attention tasks suggesting slowed psychomotor speed.

Given their fundamental and widespread role in cognition, attention, and WM deficits essentially constrain the breadth and depth of intelligent and adaptive human behavior and hence can have pervasive effects within home, community, and occupational settings.

Functional magnetic resonance imaging (fMRI) have used WM tasks in the magnet as a measure of the functional activity of the brain after TBI. These experiments have been particularly important because structural imaging is not always revealing after TBI. In most studies, fMRI activation patterns appear to be different after TBI, revealed often by abnormally increased activation in expected WM-related brain areas and/or activation in additional brain regions, even when task performance is similar to controls. Abnormal fMRI responses have been found to be correlated with symptom severity in concussed athletes (14) and to be associated with longer recovery times (15). These results raise the possibility that patients with TBI generate greater neural activity in cognitive tasks that may have been managed more easily prior to injury as a type of compensatory response. This alteration may lead to increased physical and mental fatigue, even muscle tension and headaches that may be mistaken for simple stress effects. In these cases, a reduced work load and schedule is usually recommended. In some TBI cases, the degree of attentional change is sufficient to warrant evaluation of attention deficit-type symptoms (3). This is typically undertaken with a combination of standardized tests of attention (such as the Working Memory Index from the Wechsler Adult Intelligence Scale and continuous performance tasks) and behavioral survey of attentional behaviors (such as the Brown Adult Attention Deficit Disorder [ADD] Scale). Treatment of adult patients with TBI with low-dose stimulants and alternatives can be of significant benefit to their occupational and daily functioning, particularly when combined with cognitive compensatory strategies.

Unawareness of Deficits (Anosognosia)

Anosognosia (meaning, literally, "without knowledge of disease") is characterized by reduced awareness or frank denial of neurological symptoms after TBI that can include memory and cognitive deficits, hemiparesis, visual and other sensory disturbances, gait disorder, and deficits of naturalistic action (16,17). Patients' inability to recognize their functional limitations poses a significant safety risk and is known to be a major barrier to effective TBI rehabilitation (18). Disavowal of neurological impairment can take several forms including (a) lack of emotional concern for acknowledged deficits (anosodiaphoria), (b) conscious denial of deficits that are implicitly acknowledged (e.g., patients claim that they can walk but never actually attempt to get out of bed), (c) combined explicit and implicit denial of deficits, (d) denial of ownership of an impaired body part (asomatagnosia or somatoparaphrenia), and at the far end of the continuum, (e) dislike or hatred of a dysfunctional body part (misoplegia) (16,19). Patients with this disorder can evidence dramatic abnormalities in behavior, such as throwing themselves from their beds "to get rid of that awful leg." Although often occurring in conjunction with other clinical deficits associated with frontal, parietal, and subcortical lesions, anosognosia is currently characterized as an independent behavioral syndrome without a single etiology or neuroanatomic basis.

Although there are no formal studies of the contribution of anosognosia to delay in seeking medical attention after TBI, numerous anecdotal reports suggest that unawareness of deficits (sometimes theorized to be partly because of a functional adaptation, e.g., "shock") may keep patients from presenting promptly for medical evaluation, especially if patients lack other bodily injuries. Currently, no treatments for TBI are available that depend critically on initiation within a short period after the injury occurs, but this remains a real possibility within the near future, similar to acute thrombolytic therapies after stroke.

The most relevant impact of anosognosia on cognitive and clinical outcomes after TBI is thought to occur in the hesitant acceptance of rehabilitation services and inconsistent participation in them (16,19). It is reasoned that anosognosia may cause patients to put forward inadequate or erratic efforts, preventing gains in strength and endurance. Although anosognosia and decreased motivation has not been universally associated with a poorer rehabilitation outcome in formal studies (20), the scope of rehabilitation may be more limited because of safety and supervision needs, and fewer challenging tasks may be attempted to ensure that patients will not expose themselves to further harm or attempt to perform tasks of which they are incapable. Although large controlled trials of specific management and treatment methods for subjects with anosognosia after TBI are not yet available, a number of clinical approaches are reported to be symptomatically useful. These include both *explicit and implicit* techniques to improve self-monitoring and increase awareness of their functional abilities and deficits (21). From a clinical research perspective, anosognosia presents somewhat of a barrier to studying certain TBI outcomes because such patients may report better cognitive,

physical, and emotional outcomes than do caregivers and clinicians (22). This creates problems in interpretation of patient self-report data, which might under other circumstances be considered to be of greater validity than that of external observers.

Mechanisms of Anosognosia

Weinstein and Kahn (23) first proposed that psychological denial may produce inability to acknowledge neurological deficits after stroke such as hemiparesis. Important clinical observations, however, are inconsistent with the psychological defense mechanism hypothesis. A coping strategy should be more used as recovery progresses, cognition improves, and chronic losses become apparent. Anosognosia is most apparent immediately postinjury and gradually improves (16,18,19,21). A denial syndrome should be most severe for deficits posing the greatest potential ego threat and less marked for deficits not likely to produce disability. However, modular dissociations in anosognosia not clearly based on subjective deficit severity (e.g., unawareness of visual problems but awareness of gait problems) are reported after head injury (19,24). In subjects without brain injury, anosognosia can be induced by selective hemispheric anesthesia (16), but in the same individuals, this occurs more commonly after right-sided than left-sided injection. This asymmetry is difficult to explain on a psychological basis. Most critically, in patients who are brain injured, it is unclear that anosognosia confers even temporary functional advantage, either in reducing subjective distress or in improving function, which is central to the concept of a psychological defense.

MAJOR DOMAINS OF COGNITION

General Intelligence

Measures of intelligence are employed in the cognitive examination of patients who are brain injured to assess a broad range of cognitive abilities that underlie many daily living skills and adaptation (25). Because intelligence can be affected by TBI, it is important to consider both unusual variations in the profile of subtest scores and deviations from the patient's baseline or estimated premorbid intellectual ability. Such estimates can be obtained through standardized word reading tests (e.g., Wechsler Test of Adult Reading), multifactorial demographic formula such as the Barona Index, and less frequently from employment or educational records (26,27). Although several instruments have been designed for evaluating aspects of intelligence, the Wechsler scales are favored by most clinicians. In its most updated versions, the Wechsler Adult Intelligence Scale [WAIS-III and IV] has several important features:

- Survey of a broad range of verbal and nonverbal cognitive abilities with standardized instructions and materials.
- Test items are presented in order of ascending difficulty and are usually discontinued after a certain number of incorrect responses, allowing for the flexible assessment of many levels of ability without undue frustration for patients. Such scores across a variety of cognitive tasks help determine patient functioning relative to others

and their age and relative to the varying demands of different cognitive processes (e.g., attention span, mental arithmetic, spatial problem solving). These measures may also shed some light on the consistency of patient efforts in testing.

■ Interpretation of multiple subtest and composite index scores (i.e., full scale, general ability, verbal comprehension, perceptual organization/reasoning, WM, processing ppeed) is possible through extensive normative data that provide statistical comparisons, enhancing the strong reliability and validity indicators of the scale.

Interpretation of IQ tests requires highly trained clinical expertise particularly because there is no single or specific profile of intellectual impairment that results from brain damage (28). From available studies, however, it is possible to identify several common patterns associated with TBI effects (see Table 59-2).

Clinicians engaged in assessing intellectual functioning among patients with TBI use the principles summarized in Table 59-1 to guide interpretation and hypotheses about related functional deficits, their causes, and their remediation. Similarly, the cognitive strengths observed in IQ testing may point clinicians in the direction of harnessing intact patient abilities to compensate for acquired limitations. In our clinical experience, we do not rely on 1 cognitive measure, sign, or symptom of TBI as being sufficient for rendering diagnosis and understanding of the patient's complaints. Similarly, the presence of atypical IQ scores by itself should not be assumed to reflect cerebral impairment without further investigation. For individuals with unusual IQ profile scores, review of their health history, development, and school testing records may disclose significant preexisting discrepancies in their abilities. Competent neuropsychological evaluations take such factors into account as part of understanding TBI effects. IQ scores, moreover, should not be considered an isolation from measures of attention, memory, language, and other cognitive domains or not from the patient medical history, neurological evaluation, and related data from other service providers.

Learning and Memory

Learning and memory are among the most fundamental and important cognitive capacities that underlie human adaptation. The biological bases of neural plasticity and how we acquire and subsequently retain vast amounts of information and experiences remain enigmatic, although there is increasing understanding of the neural structures and processes that mediate functional memory systems. In scientific and clinical studies of TBI, there is an increasing evidence for anatomic damage to primary memory structures and for physiological disruption of memory processing.

The effects of TBI-related memory impairments can be disabling and significantly limit an individual's ability to live independently, handle a job, and interact productively with others (2). Subjective memory complaints after TBI are quite common, even among those with mild TBI and good medical recovery (31). Studies of TBI, however, reveal a broad range of measured learning/memory effects that makes it difficult to articulate a single dominant clinical pattern. The controversy arises in part from the wide variability

TABLE 59-2 Summary of Effects of TBI on Measures of General Intelligence (IQ)

1. A generalized pattern of intellectual decline is most likely to be observed in patients whose TBI is at least moderate to severe (29).

2. The Wechsler Working Memory and Processing Speed indexes are comparatively more sensitive to TBI effects than measures of crystallized knowledge and reasoning-based measures such as Vocabulary, Similarities, and Matrix Reasoning (29,30).

3. A large discrepancy between index scores is not always synonymous with brain damage, nor does it necessarily imply damage to one hemisphere vs the other. For example, a lower Perceptual Reasoning Index score may be related to slowed visuomotor processing speed rather than right hemisphere damage per se, and a lower Working Memory Index score may be related to impaired attention and concentration rather than specific left hemisphere damage. Large discrepancies have been identified among some non-TBI "normal" adults (32), though the frequency is low. Discrepancies of 15 points or more deserve close scrutiny for acquired cognitive dysfunction and possible relationship to neurological variables such as length of coma and post-traumatic amnesia, brain imaging, and electroencephalography as well as other premorbid or concurrent causes of test impairment.

4. In reasoning about and explaining any left vs right hemisphere disparities in intellectual processing, investigators have emphasized that the left hemisphere tends to fundamentally process information in more sequential and component fashion (e.g., mental arithmetic, digit span, vocabulary) whereas the right hemisphere engages in more simultaneous and holistic information processing (e.g., block design, matrix reasoning, picture completion). Thus, on the WAIS-III for example, left vs right hemisphere deficits, at least as expressed through verbal vs performance IQ score differences, should not be interpreted as simply verbal vs visuospatial differences; rather, they may reflect different levels and cognitive approaches to information processing.

5. Impairment on the block design subtest has been associated with damage to the parietal lobes regardless of the side of cerebral dysfunction (31).

6. Vocabulary and picture completion subtests have been employed in estimating premorbid intellectual functioning because of their robust resistance to the effects of most brain injuries.

7. Deficits on the similarities subtest have been associated predominantly with left frontal injury because of its reliance on verbal concept formation and abstraction.

8. In interpreting intellectual test scores and patterns, the important contributions of unique personal attributes must be assessed including educational level, premorbid functioning, learning disability, cultural/linguistic factors and others that are likely to affect IQ test scores.

in the effects of TBI on brain networks, in the different criteria for memory impairment across studies, and in the broad spectrum of memory demands the individuals face. For example, differences in patient sampling (e.g., consecutive series vs selected patients referred for assessment), in the specific tests of learning and memory employed, and in TBI-related factors (e.g., the length of time postinjury, age of injury, and severity of TBI) can contribute to different study findings. There are also complicating effects of TBI that include chronic pain, sleep disturbance, depression, stress because of loss of income, and so forth, which are known to negatively affect learning and memory capacities, and must be considered in both etiology and treatment plans. Despite these many cautions, several reliable correlations have been reported between memory impairments and TBI pathophysiology. Specifically, decreased hippocampal and temporal white matter volumes after mild TBI in adults were found to be significantly related to measured memory impairments (33). Despite normal MRI or computed tomography (CT) imaging in 15 of 20 patients with mild TBI, Umile et al. (34) discovered that dynamic brain imaging (i.e., single photon emission computed tomography [SPECT] and positron emission tomography [PET]) detected abnormalities in 18 of the 20 patients, with 15 of the 20 having abnormalities in the temporal lobe, primarily the hippocampal region. There are also important functional imaging data suggesting that the brain activity patterns of patients with TBI are abnormal during tasks of memory retrieval. Specifically, patients engaged increased levels of frontal, anterior cingulate, and occipital lobe activity during memory tasks while showing reduced right dorsomedial thalamic activation and attenuated hemispheric asymmetry that was a characteristic of healthy controls (35). Hence, although detection of learning and memory impairments after TBI is common, the specific characteristics underlying the deficits require careful and comprehensive evaluation.

Post-Traumatic Amnesia

Post-traumatic amnesia (PTA) refers to the immediate and dramatic loss of memory that TBI can cause. PTA is defined as the period during which patients are unable to effectively encode and retain new information and experiences, which can extend from a few moments after TBI to several weeks and even months later. There is often a period of retrograde amnesia as well, which can extend from a few moments before the accident to weeks and months previously. In addition to repeating questions and being disoriented in this acute/postacute phase, patients can be confused, unaware of their injuries, agitated, and even combative. Hence, some clinicians have suggested that the phase currently described as PTA may also encompass characteristics of a confusional state or delirium in some patients (36,37). Although patients are awake and alert during this period, they subsequently recall little to no information regarding the accident and post-traumatic events such as transportation to the hospital, medical evaluation, and even visits of family members. Patients may subsequently report that they were knocked out during this time and can be surprised to learn that they were awake, alert, and conversant.

PTA is variable in extent of amnesia, cognitive and behavioral deficits, and pattern of recovery. It is considered a general marker of neurological impairment and in most cases gradually improves. PTA can be assessed with standardized instruments such as the Galveston Orientation and Amnesia Test (38) and the Orientation Log (39). Recovery of orientation and short-term memory can be reliably predicted from early daily screening and is a moderately strong indicator of length of stay and functional independence on discharge (39,40). It is important during this early recovery period to rule out exacerbating effects of sleep disturbance, pain medications, alcohol and drug withdrawal, and other complicating factors on post-traumatic memory and behavioral deficits.

An interesting implication of PTA concerns its relationship to post-traumatic stress disorder (PTSD). That is, does loss of consciousness and memory after TBI protect against the development of PTSD symptoms that typically involve the reexperiencing of the traumatic events as well as heightened emotion with anxiety and avoidance behaviors? If the event cannot be remembered, can PTSD symptoms still be possible? PTSD symptoms were surveyed in 53 TBI respondents (out of a sample of 371 cases) and compared to their TBI trauma memories. Results indicated that those with traumatic memories of the TBI event (n = 26) reported the highest and most intrusive psychological distress followed by those with no traumatic memories at all (n = 14; although the most severe TBI cases overall) who reported less severe PTSD symptoms that were generally nonintrusive. Those with nontraumatic memories (n = 13) did not report any PTSD symptoms. Reviews by Bryant (41) and Harvey et al. (42) have generally favored the view that PTA and PTSD can coexist, although in ways may be different than in PTSD cases not related to TBI. The latter review underscored a number of caveats to the view that PTSD occurs after TBI despite loss of consciousness and PTA issues, related either to imprecise criteria for TBI and/or limited assessment of stress-related symptoms (PTSD and acute stress disorder). Further research is needed to clarify the causes and management of these comorbid conditions (see Chapter 33 on Military TBI: Special Considerations, for further discussion).

Multiple Memory Systems

There are multiple systems of memory that have been described along different axes such as declarative and procedural, short-term and long-term, anterograde and retrograde, as well as material-specific divides such as verbal and visuospatial, semantic and autobiographical (43). There is a strong scientific and clinical support for examining these diverse aspects of memory because they are usually affected in different ways and to varying extents after TBI. In this chapter, we will focus specifically on learning and short-term memory as well as the distinction between declarative and procedural memory systems.

For many aspects of everyday learning and short-term memory, information processing approaches have identified 3 principal aspects: *encoding, consolidation,* and *retrieval.* Encoding typically refers to learning processes that underlie the acquisition of new information and experiences through sensory-perceptual, cognitive, and attentional mechanisms. Encoding is thought to be mediated by subcortical-cortical sensory-perceptual systems together with prefrontal attentional/executive resources that are allocated according to the load of information, its difficulty, prior knowledge, interest in the material, and so forth. Thus, *how information is processed* (e.g., in shallow, brief fashion vs more in depth) has considerable influence on its subsequent activity in the brain. Consolidation pertains to those biological mechanisms that are necessary to establish and maintain a memory trace, thought to involve interactive processing between cortical sensory association areas where new information is perceived, and limbic system structures, particularly the hippocampus and its other limbic connections. Binding refers to the specific linking of different aspects of new information and events in relationship to time, place, and other contextual factors and appears to rely critically on hippocampal mediation. Retrieval refers to the access and recovery of memory traces either through recall or recognition processes. The neural basis of retrieval remains unclear but has been associated with executive search processes mediated by the prefrontal cortex as well as comparison of perceptual familiarity. Given this model of learning and memory and the evident diversity of neural structures and connections that subserve memory, it is somewhat clearer why memory complaints may be so common after TBI. That is, large scale coordination of cortical, subcortical, and limbic system structures is usually required to mediate the attentional, sensory-perceptual, cognitive, and executive processing underlying the multiple memory systems. When these systems are impaired, the behavior of patients typically regresses to a default mode, whereby they act on previous knowledge and habits without incorporating new information, events, and contingencies. Hence, patients may be quite capable in routine situations because of well-learned habits and behaviors but comparatively limited in their new current circumstances because personal and situational information is not updated and retained.

Studies investigating TBI and memory continue to show diverse results. Although some reports have identified principally encoding deficits, others have identified consolidation and retrieval deficits (44,45). It is more likely the case that there are identifiable subgroups of patients with memory impaired TBI that can present with mainly consolidation or retrieval deficits (46). Hence, it is important to assess sufficient aspects of memory to identify when impairments occur and what contributes to the deficiencies. This includes varying the difficulty of the task. For example, in patients with mild TBI, memory impairments may not be apparent on some standardized testing but do become evident under certain conditions such as when patients must divide their attention during the encoding phase, manage an increasing load of information, and maintain their learning over the course of a meeting, class, or nonroutine assignment (47). This can give rise to greater *variability* in learning and memory—a more subtle form of memory impairment. There are a number of other cognitive parameters that can affect learning and memory efficiency, such as attention, depth of information processing, and organization. For example, strategies of clustering similar semantic information (e.g., chunking of words or objects that naturally go together) require more effort during learning but once acquired can noticeably improve verbal retention, whereas the spaced repetition of words that need to be retained can contribute to more effective retention. An important clinical guideline that is emerging from extant literature is the realization that there are interactive effects of processing speed, WM, and EFs on episodic memory impairments that may combine to influence functional levels of learning and memory capacities in naturalistic settings (48). Such analyses will increase the options for developing effective memory remediation strategies as well as medication treatments (49,50).

Studies of human learning and memory have identified an important distinction between declarative and procedural systems (also referred to explicit vs implicit memory). Declarative memory refers to consciously and intentionally acquired factual and event knowledge that is typically assessed through tests of recall and recognition and depends on cortical-hippocampal mediation. In contrast, procedural memory refers to the skills and habits acquired by prior exposure and experience, such as learning to ride a bike and swim as well as learning perceptual-motor skills pertinent to sports and music. These abilities appear to be mediated through diverse cortical association regions in concert with the basal ganglia, cerebellum, and motor-related cortices. Patterns of declarative-procedural memory impairment in TBI support these distinctions and have shown clear preservation of procedural memory abilities, whereas declarative memory is frequently impaired. This dissociation was even evident during the period of PTA and later showed carryover of procedural learning after the PTA had resolved (51). The preservation of procedural learning and memory is an important asset during neurorehabilitation because it confirms that patients can progressively acquire new skills and habits, even though their conscious awareness and recollection of them may be very limited.

Confabulations and Delusions

TBI can cause both confabulations and delusions. These disorders lie at the interface of impaired memory, self-awareness, visual perception, and EFs and can occur as direct effects of TBI. Confabulations are defined as false beliefs that are context dependent and associated with significant amnesia. Patients attempt to fill in gaps of their memory loss with other overlearned knowledge about themselves and others. This kind of confabulation is thought to involve a combination of amnesia and disinhibited responding and is usually associated with temporal and frontal lobe dysfunction. In contrast, delusions are defined as fixed false beliefs that are not related to amnesia. Several delusional misidentification syndromes have been described after TBI. These center around altered ability to recognize persons well known to the patient as well as the false belief that strange people are disguising themselves in some way to look like the patient's spouse or other family member. These unusual symptoms have been associated with combined damage to frontal (usually bilateral frontal) and right posterior cortical regions. Examples include Capgras syndrome, defined as the false belief that someone well known to the patient has been replaced with a look-alike imposter (also described as reduplicative paramnesia) (52) and Fregoli syndrome in which the patient believes that a stranger, sometimes another patient or a staff member, is actually disguised and acting as a familiar person such as their mother (53). Confabulations and delusions generally resolve over time but are also known to persist chronically. Challenging a patient's false belief is often not helpful in recovery. Family members as well as providers often passively accommodate to these persisting symptoms. A single delusion can occur, or there may be several cooccurring delusions not necessarily interrelated. Misidentification and delusional syndromes can occur after TBI without other features of psychosis. Curiously, patients often do not appear distressed by these symptoms or do they act on them in any real way.

Spatial Cognition

Spatial cognition subserves a variety of adaptive behaviors from navigation within diverse environments and learning spatial maps to spatial-related attention, directional memory, and problem solving. Spatial cognition is critical to safety and execution of many daily activities such as ambulation, dressing, self-care, driving, and keeping track of items maintained in home and work settings. TBI infrequently causes the striking hemispatial neglect syndrome often associated with right parietal lobe damage. However, careful examination can reveal deficits in attention to spatial cues, visuomotor scanning that underlies reading, and other spatial search tasks within the environment, constructional praxis, visual and tactile perception of objects, spatial patterns and movement in space, and learning, as well as memory of new places (45,54). Spatial exploratory deficits and other motor-intentional spatial disorders commonly occur after TBI associated with medial frontal cortical dysfunction and hypokinesia (55). Most often, spatial cognitive deficits associated with TBI are not singled out per se but rather discussed within the context of safety and efficacy of daily living skills as well as attention, memory, and problem solving. Spatial-representational and spatial-motor dysfunction after TBI have been less fully investigated.

Executive Functions

EFs encompass cognitive, behavioral, and emotional processes that underlie decision making, psychosocial adjustment, and human achievements. These processes have often been defined in terms of complex cognitive functions such as planning, organization, judgment, problem solving, and anticipation that require the coordination of multiple subprocesses to orchestrate cognition and behavior from one action to another in pursuit of pertinent goals. Associated cognitive operations in EF include WM, prospective memory, strategic planning, cognitive flexibility, relational reasoning, and self-monitoring. EFs have also been implicated in the goal-directed regulation of attention, cognitive resources, and actions to manage transitions from one activity to another throughout the day, over extended intervals of time, and across diverse settings (1,6,56–59). The neural systems involved in EFs include the prefrontal cortex most

prominently, which is interconnected with other cortical and subcortical structures to form large neural networks. Several of these networks have been described under the terms *orbital*, *medial*, and *dorsolateral* (8,60,61).

Orbital Prefrontal Network

In minor and moderate TBI, the traumatic forces are frequently localized to the *orbitofrontal* and *temporal polar* zones including the amygdala and anterior hippocampus (see Figure 59-2 for underlying anatomy). These regions are closely interconnected via the uncinate fasciculus. The clinical manifestations of traumatic damage to these are often a mixture of behavioral, cognitive, and affective symptoms that include personality change, psychosocial coping disturbances, and impulsive behavior besides the more easily recognizable attentional impairments and EF deficits. Even minor or moderate TBI cases can manifest a distinctive pattern of symptoms referred to as "disinhibited" and "pseudopsychopathic" behavior that has characteristics of egocentrism, childishness, stubbornness, as well as tactless, aggressive, and abusive behaviors. Many of these symptoms are difficult to measure with precision. Usually, a combination of behavioral examinations and clinical analysis of real-world functioning is required. The orbital prefrontal region has been implicated mainly in social and emotional aspects of behavior including certain kinds of value-driven decision making, theory of mind, reward-based learning, and social judgment.

Medial Prefrontal Network

The medial prefrontal circuit has been related to social cognition, motivational, and attentional processes including social judgment, self-other evaluations, initiation, inhibition, and maintenance of motivated behavior. In studies of TBI-related pathology, both orbital and medial regions of the prefrontal cortex have been found to be especially vulnerable to damage by mechanisms of shearing and stretching of fibers as

ORBITOFRONTAL PARALIMBIC DIVISION

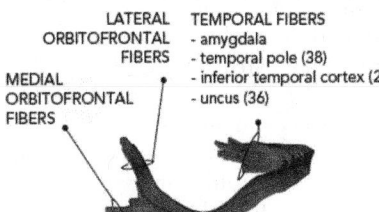

LATERAL ORBITOFRONTAL FIBERS

MEDIAL ORBITOFRONTAL FIBERS

TEMPORAL FIBERS
- amygdala
- temporal pole (38)
- inferior temporal cortex (20)
- uncus (36)

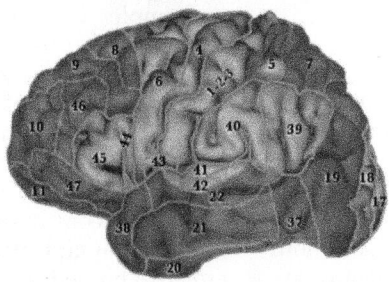

24, 32, 33, 36, 21, 22, 11, 47

Phylogeny and cytoarchitectonic
Paleocortical
granule cell

Anatomy
Amygdala, anterior parahippocampal, insula, temporal pole, subcallosal cingulate

Functions
Implicit processing, visceral integration, visual features analysis, appetite drives, social awareness, mood

FIGURE 59-2 *See color insert*. The orbital prefrontal network encompasses the close anatomical and functional relationships between orbital frontal areas (Brodmann's areas *11, 12, 25*) and the anterior temporal poles (Brodmann's areas *38, 36, 34, 28, anterior 20*) shown here using modern MRI tractography
Reprinted from Catani M, Thiebaut de Schotten M, in press with permission.

well as direct injury from impact against the irregular base of the skull. Applied force vectors and tissue compliance influence the intensity of the coup, countercoup, angular, and rotational forces that stretch and lacerate brain tissue centrifugally from midline sagittal aspects (i.e., medial and orbital prefrontal cortex impacting against the lamina cribrosa and the roof of the orbit as well as against the wing of the sphenoid bone) toward the surface of the cortex (dorsolateral prefrontal cortex) and the deep connections with the striatum, thalamus, and other subcortical nuclei such as the amygdala. As injury becomes more severe, patients are more likely to have an abulic syndrome in which the traumatic brain damage can extend toward more superior medial and subcortical frontal areas involving the anterior cingulate, supplementary area, corpus callosum, and the brain stem. These lesions often lead to disinterest, lethargy, reduced drive, and lack of initiative, clinically resembling an abulic, amotivational, or pseudodepressed state.

Dorsolateral Prefrontal Network

When traumatic lesions involve dorsolateral prefrontal cortex, disruptions can occur to corticocortical (such as frontal-parietal) and cortical-subcortical (such as frontal-striatal) connections. Patients may show significant impairments of EFs, including WM deficits, lack of insight, reduced relational reasoning and set shifting, poor divided attention, and defective discourse abilities (60,62). The dorsolateral prefrontal network mediates many higher cognitive aspects of behavior such as abstract reasoning, planning, and WM. Some clinical disorders such as distractability and impulsivity have been found to be related to measured attentional and EF deficits (61,63). Significant correlations between measures of EFs and regional cerebral glucose metabolism have been found in the medial and dorsolateral prefrontal regions and the cingulate gyrus. Interestingly, the correlations were evident, despite the absence of detectable structural lesions on brain MRI. These findings extended prior report by Goldenberg et al. (64) who reported correlation of executive measures with reduced blood flow in the thalamic region. Hence, impairments of EFs may be related not only to focal traumatic lesions of the prefrontal cortex but also to white matter disconnection (i.e., traumatic axonal injury) of prefrontal-related networks that link to the thalamus, basal ganglia, and other important cortical and subcortical regions. White matter damage, as well as the interruption of white matter tracts, has been frequently shown to be directly associated with cognitive-behavioral sequelae in TBI. Diffusion tensor imaging tractography is extremely sensitive to white matter changes following TBI including changes in the microstructure of white matter fibers and represents a promising methodology for studying TBI (65).

Decision-Making Tasks Requiring Emotional Processing

Some behavioral disorders after TBI have been linked to alterations in emotion-related processing in contrast to primary cognitive deficits. For example, Rolls et al. (66) reported that patients with ventral frontal damage after TBI had particular difficulty in reward-based contingency learning. That is, after successfully learning an initial stimulus-reward association, they were impaired in reversal learning (i.e., switching the association so that the stimulus that did not signal reward now does) and in extinction learning (i.e., when the stimulus no longer signal a reward). This flexibility in reinforcement-related associative learning is critical to adaptive behavior in changing environment and circumstances. The impairments were found to be correlated with behavioral deficits of disinhibition, social difficulties, lack of initiative, and perseveration. Interestingly, the deficits were not correlated with cognitive measures such as verbal IQ, verbal paired-associate learning or Tower of London problem solving.

Emotion processing may also be an integral part of value-driven decision-making capacities when one must rely on judgment of chance and probability of consequences such as applying for and taking a new job, prioritizing most important tasks, financial decisions, and gambling. This has been operationalized into a standardized task (The Iowa Gambling Task) in which subjects must learn to choose cards from stacks that are rigged to have different levels of risk and reward, varying from high-risk choices that led to occasional high payoffs (but also high losses) to low-risk choices that led to low but frequent rewards (67). Patients with TBI performed poorly on this task more so when they suffered large frontal lobe lesions (68), choosing the high-risk options that ultimately led to large losses. Such deficits may lead patients to make hasty decisions with little anticipation of the potential negative outcomes and support the role of the prefrontal cortex in integrative cognitive-emotional processing. Recent review has suggested that such value-driven probability decision-making deficits are largely unrelated to typical intelligence and cognitive EF measures (69). Hence, certain patients may appear normal on standard neurocognitive exam but are impaired in daily decision making that entails contingency learning and consideration of potential positive and negative outcomes (70).

From Single Deficits to Impaired Cognitive Organization

Both focal and diffuse frontal lesions after TBI disrupt activities of daily living (ADL) with associated EF impairments representing a main component of ADL failure (71). In particular, EF resources such as planning, WM, self-monitoring, and decision making are considered critical for independent and adaptive functioning within home, community, and occupational settings (72). The impact of EF impairments is best viewed not as a single deficit but as a damaging, complex, cognitive-emotional macrostructure of the brain or *managerial knowledge unit* that underlies most multistep requirements of daily life, such as meal preparation or a recreational activity (71,73). Meal preparation or going to a movie may be as difficult, if not more difficult, than many cognitive tasks presented during a formal clinical testing session. This is because the former situations require a patient to develop and implement a plan and invest executive resources in accomplishing the many aspects of the task (56,57,73,74), whereas in formal cognitive testing, the patient typically is administered a single task with instructions provided by the examiner; learning trials may be short, response initiation is prompted, and feedback may be given at the end of the task. Certainly, it is not the same in real-world settings where situational constraints, priorities, and requirements are not always clear and success depends on timely, internally generated, and self-monitored actions without the benefit of feedback. Moreover, most neuropsychological tests do not specifically explore strategic planning, competitive skills, thinking ahead, or prospective memory. A notable exception is the experimental strategic management simulation (SMS) technology that has shown promise in detecting executive impairments in patients with TBI with good medical recovery and few measured neuropsychological test deficits, as well as in remediation of persisting EF deficits (75,76). Although the SMS lays out a general scenario, it is up to the patient to research and organize specific resources in solving problems and then modifying those decisions when circumstances change. An important priority in both EF assessment and linkage to cognitive remediation is the development of further paradigms that tap multiple problem-solving variables in real time and with varying degrees of structure and feedback.

Social Cognition and Behavior

Humans are naturally social creatures born to live and thrive within social settings with many complex forms of interaction that have emotional coloring and context. Hence, this important facet of human behavior extends well beyond strictly cognitive endeavors to domains such as metacognitive thinking, social skills, moral beliefs, personality traits, and theory of mind (i.e., a special faculty of the human brain that mediates interpretation and appreciation of other people's feelings and mental states) (77). Frontotemporal damage from TBI can lead to dramatic alterations of conduct, personality, and psychosocial integration, at times leaving many cognitive and sensorimotor functions relatively intact. From a clinical standpoint, there is often a spectrum of social behavioral symptoms associated with TBI rather than definite syndromes. Some patients become puerile, profane, facetious, irresponsible, irascible, and aggressive as forms of social disinhibition. Others lose spontaneity, initiative, curiosity, and develop mental and behavioral inertia as forms of abulia and apathy (78). Still, others develop lack of awareness and insight, as well as loss of creativity and emotional vitality. Some of these deficits are expressed as pragmatic communication deficits, loss of empathy, and inability to understand and appreciate sarcasm, jokes, irony, and other vital social communication tools (79,80). Another facet of social-related processing involves recognition of common forms of emotional expressions. Hornak, Rolls, and Wade (81) showed that ventral frontal damage from head trauma and other etiologies was associated with impaired recognition of emotional facial expressions and correlated with subjective emotional change and social behavior of patients. Although many of these social-emotional deficits are difficult to objectively evaluate and measure with current instruments, some progress has been made in developing tests of social judgment, theory of mind, emotional intelligence, and social adaptation. These are important and problematic sequelae of TBI that must be examined clinically and managed with a combination of patient and family interventions. The combined use of clinical interview with patient and family members and behavioral inventories can uncover many of these deficits. Experimental measures of social judgment, theory of mind abilities, social knowledge, and emotion-related processing are beginning to shed light on deficits underlying these real-life problems and are increasingly targeted in experimental intervention programs.

CONCLUSION

Cognitive impairments after TBI present significant challenges for recovery and return to premorbid levels of occupational and social functioning. In early stages, patients' lack of awareness of their deficits (anosognosia), impaired self-regulation, and PTA constitute major limitations to participation in rehabilitation services and safety. Often, there is a combination of cognitive impairments that affects attention, memory, sensory perception, mental and motor processing speed, EF, and social processes that require multimodal therapy services and a gradual return to independent daily activities. Cognitive and social-emotional deficits are frequently slower to recover than physical injuries. Hence, outpatient cognitive therapy services can extend for 1–2 years after moderate-to-severe TBI. Education of caregivers is particularly important for monitoring and continued remediation of such impairments within home and community settings. When cognitive deficits remain persistent, longer term individualized therapy is usually required, combining aspects of skill retraining, compensatory strategies, and environmental supports to optimize functional cognitive capacities. Advances in treatment research, availability of cognitive therapy services, use of smart electronic and other adaptive devices, and public awareness of TBI will continue to reduce the burden of cognitive impairments.

 KEY CLINICAL POINTS

1. TBI is associated with often persisting cognitive deficits that interfere with return to school, occupational, and social roles.
2. Common areas of cognitive deficit include attention, WM, EFs, word retrieval, learning, memory, and social cognition.
3. In addition to cognitive deficits, patients may lack awareness of their deficits and functional limitations (i.e., anosognosia), further compounding their adjustment to injury and recovery.
4. Cognitive, behavioral, and emotional deficits after TBI are related to the underlying damage to the brain, including cortical, subcortical, limbic, and brainstem regions.
5. In cases of mild TBI, deficits may become evident mainly under conditions of time pressure, fast processing speed, multiple tasks requiring divided attention, consistent accuracy in responding, WM load, and need to monitor errors.
6. Cognitive difficulties are more common in nonroutine situations that require novel problem-solving approaches and are less common in routine actions and situations.
7. Cognitive deficits often require continued rehabilitation services that extend from acute and postacute care to extended follow-up outpatient care.

 KEY REFERENCES

1. Giacino JT, Cicerone K. Varieties of deficit unawareness after brain injury. *J Head Trauma Rehabil.* 1998;13(5):1–15.
2. Levine B, Dawson D, Boutet I, Schwartz ML, Stuss DT. Assessment of strategic self-regulation in traumatic brain

injury: its relationship to injury severity and psychosocial outcome. *Neuropsychology.* 2000;14(4):491–500.

3. Mathias JL, Beall JA, Bigler ED. Neuropsychological and information processing deficits following mild traumatic brain injury. *J Int Neuropsychol Soc.* 2004;10(2):286–297.

4. Pardini JE, Pardini DA, Becker JT, et al. Postconcussive symptoms are associated with compensatory cortical recruitment during a working memory task. *Neurosurgery.* 2010;67(4):1020–1027.

5. Satish U, Streufert S, Eslinger PJ. Simulation-based executive cognitive assessment and rehabilitation after traumatic frontal lobe injury: a case report. *Disabil Rehabil.* 2008;30(6):468–478.

References

1. Zappalà G. The frontal lobes: executive and behavioural control of human reasoning. Implications for understanding brain injury. *Riv Neurobiol.* 2008;54:195–202.

2. Drake AI, Gray N, Yoder S. Pramuka M, Llewellyn M. Factors predicting return to work following mild traumatic brain injury: a discriminant analysis. *J Head Trauma Rehabil.* 2000;15(5):1103–1112.

3. Levin H, Hanten G, Max J, et al. Symptoms of attention deficit/hyperactivity disorder following traumatic brain injury in children. *J Dev Behav Pediatr.* 2007;28(2):108–118.

4. Rapoport MJ, McCullagh S, Shammi P, Feinstein A. Cognitive impairment associated with major depression following mild and moderate traumatic brain injury. *J Neuropsychiat Clin Neurosci.* 2005;17:61–65.

5. Costanza A, Weber K, Gandy S, et al. Review: contact sport-related chronic traumatic encephalopathy in the elderly: clinical expression and structural substrates. *Neuropathol Appl Neurobiol.* 2011; 37(6):570–584.

6. Johnson VE, Stewart W, Smith DH. Traumatic brain injury and amyloid-β pathology: a link to Alzheimer's disease? *Nat Rev Neurosci.* 2010;11(5):361–370.

7. Jones RD, Anderson SW, Cole T, Hathaway-Nepple J. Neuropsychological sequelae of traumatic brain injury. In: Rizzo M, Tranel D, eds. *Head Injury and Postconcussive Syndrome.* New York, NY: Churchill Livingstone; 1996:395–414.

8. Eslinger P, Grattan L, Geder L. Neurologic and neuropsychologic aspects of frontal lobe impairments in postconcussive syndrome. In: Rizzo M, Tranel D eds. *Head Injury and Postconcussive Syndrome.* New York, NY: Churchill Livingstone; 1996:415–440.

9. Sarno S, Erasmus LP, Lipp B, Schlaegel W. Multisensory integration after traumatic brain injury: a reaction time study between pairings of vision, touch, and audition. *Brain Inj.* 2003;17(5): 413–426.

10. Mathias JL, Beall JA, Bigler ED. Neuropsychological and information processing deficits following mild traumatic brain injury. *J Intl Neuropsychol Soc.* 2004;1:286–297.

11. Stuss DT, Stethern LL, Hugenholtz H, Picto T, Pivik J, Richard MJ. Reaction time after head injury: fatigue, divided and focussed attention and consistency of performance. *J Neurol Neurosurg Psychiatry.* 1989;52(6):742–748.

12. McAllister TW, Flashman LA, Sparling MB, Saykin AJ. Working memory deficits after traumatic brain injury: catecholaminergic mechanisms and prospects for treatment—a review. *Brain Inj.* 2004; 18(4):331–350.

13. Zollolotti P, Matano A, DeLoche G, et al. Patterns of attentional impairment following closed head injury: a collaborative European study. *Cortex.* 2000;36(1):93–107.

14. Pardini JE, Pardini DA, Becker JT, et al. Postconcussive symptoms are associated with compensatory cortical recruitment during a working memory task. *Neurosurgery.* 2010;67:1020–1028.

15. Lovell MR, Pardini JE, Welling JS, et al. Functional brain abnormalities are related to clinical recovery and time to return to play in athletes. *Neurosurgery.* 2007;61:352–360.

16. Adair JC, Schwartz RL, Barrett AM. Anosognosia. In: Heilman KM, Valenstein E, eds. *Clinical Neuropsychology.* 4th ed. New York, NY: Oxford University Press; 2003:185–214.

17. Hart T, Giovannetti T, Montgomery MW, Schwartz MF. Awareness of errors in naturalistic action after traumatic brain injury. *J Head Trauma Rehabil.* 1998;13:16–28.

18. Prigatano GP, Schacter DL. *Awareness of Deficit After Brain Injury: Clinical and Theoretical Issues.* New York, NY: Oxford University Press; 1991.

19. Giacino JT, Cicerone K. Varieties of deficit unawareness after brain injury. *J Head Trauma Rehabil.* 1998;13:1–15.

20. Fleming JM, Strong J, Ashton R. Cluster analysis of self-awareness levels in adults with traumatic brain injury and relationship to outcome. *J Head Trauma Rehabil.* 1998;13:39–51.

21. Sohlberg MM, Rawlings-Boyd J. *Picture This! Strategies for Assessing and Increasing Awareness of Memory Deficits.* San Antonio, TX: Psychological Corporation; 1996.

22. Powell JM, Machamer JE, Temkin NR, Dikmen SS. Self-report of extent of recovery and barriers to recovery after traumatic brain injury: a longitudinal study. *Arch Phys Med Rehabil.* 2001;82: 1025–1030.

23. Weinstein EA, Kahn RL. *Denial of Illness: Symbolic and Physiological Aspects.* Springfield, IL: Charles C. Thomas; 1955.

24. Dalla Barba G, Bartolomeo P, Erigs AM, Boisse MF, Bachoud-Levi AC. Awareness of anosognosia following head trauma. *Neurocase.* 1999;5:59–67.

25. Fisher DC, Ledbetter MF, Cohen NJ, Marmor D, Tulsky DS. WAIS-III and WMS-III profiles of mildly to severely brain-injured patients. *Appl Neuropsychol.* 2000;7:126–132.

26. Green REA, Melo B, Christensen B, Ngo L, Monette G, Bradbury C. Measuring premorbid IQ in traumatic brain injury: an examination of the Wechsler Test of Adult Reading (WTAR). *J Clin Exp Neuropsychol.* 2008;30(2):163–172.

27. Barona A, Reynolds CR, Chastain R. A demographically based index of premorbid intelligence for the WAIS-R. *J Consult Clin Psychol.* 1984;52:885–887.

28. Lezak MD. *Neuropsychological Assessment.* 3rd ed. New York, NY: Oxford University Press; 1995.

29. Axelrod BN, Fichtenberg NL, Liethen PC, Czarnota MA, Stucky K. Performance characteristics of postacute traumatic brain injury patients on the WAIS-III and WMS-III. *Clin Neuropsychol.* 2001;15: 516–520.

30. Brooks BL, Strauss E, Iverson GL, Slick DJ, Sherman EMS. Developments in clinical neuropsychological assessment: refining psychometric and clinical interpretive methods. *Can Psychol.* 2009;50(3): 196–209.

31. Rimel RW, Giordani B, Barth JT, Boll TJ, Jane JA. Disability caused by minor head injury. *Neurosurgery.* 1981;9:221–228.

32. Martin TA, Donders J, Thompson E. Potential of and problems with measures of psychometric intelligence after traumatic brain injury. *Rehabil Psychol.* 2000;45:402–408.

33. Bigler ED, Anderson CV, Blatter DD. Temporal lobe morphology in normal aging and traumatic brain injury. *AJNR Am J Neuroradiol.* 2002;23(2):255–266.

34. Umile EM, Sandel ME, Alavi A, Terry CM, Plotkin RC. Dynamic imaging in mild traumatic brain injury: support for the theory of medial temporal vulnerability. *Arch Phys Med Rehabil.* 2002;83: 1506–1513.

35. Levine B, Carbeza R, McIntosh AR, Black SE, Grady CL, Stuss DT. Functional reorganisation of memory after traumatic brain injury: a study with H(2)(15)O positron emission tomography. *J Neurol Neurosurg Psychiatry.* 2002;73(2):173–181.

36. Stuss DT, Binns MA, Carruth FG, et al. The acute period of recovery from traumatic brain injury: posttraumatic amnesia or posttraumatic confusional state? *J Neurosurg.* 1999;90(4):635–643.

37. Nakase-Thompson R, Sherer M, Yablon SA, Nick TG, Trzepacz PT. Acute confusion following traumatic brain injury. *Brain Inj.* 2004; 18(2):131–142.

38. Levin HS, Benton AL, Grossman RG. *Neurobehavioral Consequences of Closed Head Injury.* New York, NY: Oxford University Press; 1992.

39. Frey KL, Rojas DC, Anderson CA, Arciniegas DB. Comparison of the O-Log and GOAT as measures of posttraumatic amnesia. *Brain Inj.* 2007;21(5):513–520.

40. Alderso AL, Novack TA. Measuring recovery of orientation during acute rehabilitation for traumatic brain injury: value and expectations of recovery. *J Head Trauma Rehabil.* 2002;17:210–219.

41. Bryant RA. Post-traumatic stress disorder and traumatic brain injury: can they co-exist. *Clin Psychol Rev.* 2001;21:931–948.

42. Harvey AG, Brewin CR, Jones C, Kopelman MD. Co-existence of post-traumatic stress disorder and traumatic brain injury: towards a resolution of the paradox. *J Intl Neuropsychol Soc.* 2003;9:663–676.

43. DeLuca J, Lengenfelder J, Eslinger PJ. Memory and learning. In: Rizzo M, Eslinger PJ eds. *Principles and Practice of Behavioral Neurology and Neuropsychology.* Philadelphia, PA: Elsevier; 2004:247–266.

44. DeLuca J, Schultheis MT, Madigan NK, Christodoulou C, Averill A. Acquisition versus retrieval deficits in traumatic brain injury: implications for memory rehabilitation. *Arch Phys Med Rehabil.* 2000;81:1327–1333.

45. Vanderploeg RD, Curtiss G, Schinka JA, Lanham RA. Material-specific memory in traumatic brain injury: differential effects during acquisition, recall, and retention. *Neuropsychology.* 2001;15(2): 174–184.

46. Curtiss G, Vanderploeg RD, Spencer J, Salazar AM. Patterns of verbal learning and memory in traumatic brain injury. *J Intl Neuropsychol Soc.* 2001;7:574–585.

47. Mangels JA, Craig FI, Levine B, Schwartz ML, Stuss DT. Effects of divided attention on episodic memory in chronic traumatic brain injury: a function of severity and strategy. *Neuropsychologia.* 2002; 40(13):2369–2385.

48. Perbal S, Couillet J, Azouvi P, Pouthas V. Relationships between time estimation, memory, attention, and processing speed in patients with severe traumatic brain injury. *Neuropsychologia.* 2003; 41:1599–1610.

49. Griffin SL, van Reekum R, Masanic C. A review of cholinergic agents in the treatment of neurobehavioral deficits following traumatic brain injury. *J Neuropsychiat Clin Neurosci.* 2003;15(1):17–26.

50. Morey CE, Cilo M, Berry J, Cusick C. The effect of Aricept in persons with persistent memory disorder following traumatic brain injury: a pilot study. *Brain Inj.* 2003;17:809–815.

51. Ewert J, Levin HS, Watson MG, Kalisky Z. Procedural memory during posttraumatic amnesia in survivors of severe closed head injury. Implication for rehabilitation. *Archiv Neurol.* 1989;46: 911–916.

52. Alexander MP, Stuss DT, Benson DF. Capgras syndrome: a reduplicative phenomenon. *Neurology.* 1979;29(3):334–339.

53. Box O, Laing H, Kopelman M. The evolution of spontaneous confabulation, delusional misidentification and a related delusion in a case of severe head injury. *Neurocase.* 1999;5:251–262.

54. Skelton RW, Bukach CM, Laurance HE, Thomas KG, Jacobs JW. Humans with traumatic brain injuries show place-learning deficits in computer-generated space. *J Clin Exp Neuropsychol.* 2000;22(2): 157–175.

55. Heilman KM. Intentional neglect. *Front Biosci.* 2004;9:694–705.

56. Shallice T, Burgess PW. Deficits in strategy application following frontal lobe damage in man. *Brain.* 1991;114:727–741.

57. Levine B, Dawson D, Boutet I, Schwartz ML, Stuss DT. Assessment of strategic self-regulation in traumatic brain injury: its relationship to injury severity and psychosocial outcome. *Neuropsychology.* 2000; 14(4):491–500.

58. Eslinger PJ. Conceptualizing, describing, and measuring components of executive function. In: Lyon GR, Krasnegor NA, eds. *Attention, Memory, and Executive Function.* Baltimore, MD: Paul H. Brookes; 1996:367–396.

59. Andres P, Van der Linden M. Are central executive functions working in patients with focal frontal lesions? *Neuropsychologia.* 2002; 40(7):835–845.

60. Allegri RF, Harris P. Prefrontal cortex in memory and attention processes [in Spanish]. *Rev Neurol.* 2001;32:449–453.

61. Baddeley A, Della Sala S, Papagano C, Spinnler H. Dual task performance in dysexecutive and nondysexecutive patients with a frontal lesion. *Neuropsychol* 1997;11:187–94.

62. Grafman J, Jones B, Salazar A. Wisconsin Card Sorting performance based on location and size of neuroanatomic lesion in Vietnam veterans with penetrating head injury. *Percept Mot Skill.* 1990;74(3, pt 2):1120–1122.

63. Burgess PW, Alderman N, Evans J, Emslie H, Wilson BA. The ecological validity of tests of executive function. *J Intl Neuropsychol Soc.* 1998;4(6):547–558.

64. Goldenberg G, Oder W, Spatt J, Podreka I. Cerebral correlates of disturbed executive function and memory in survivors of severe closed head injury: a SPECT study. *J Neurol Neurosurg Psychiatry.* 1992;55(5):362–368.

65. Zappalà G, Thiebaut de Schotten M, Eslinger PJ. Traumatic brain injury and the frontal lobes: what can we gain from diffusion tensor imaging? *Cortex.* 2012;48(2):156–165.

66. Rolls ET, Hornak J, Wade D, McGrath J. Emotion-related learning in patients with social and emotional changes associated with frontal lobe damage. *J Neurol Neurosurg Psychiatry.* 1994;57(12): 1518–1524.

67. Bechara A, Tranel D, Damasio H, Damasio AR. Failure to respond autonomically to anticipated future outcomes following damage to prefrontal cortex. *Cereb Cortex.* 1996;6(2):215–225.

68. Levine B, Black SE, Cheung G, Campbell A, O'Toole C, Schwartz ML. Gambling task performance in traumatic brain injury: relationships to injury severity, atrophy, lesion location, and cognitive and psychosocial outcome. *Cogn Behav Neurol.* 2005;18(1):45–54.

69. Toplak ME, Sorge GB, Benoit A, West RF, Stanovich KE. Decision-making and cognitive abilities: a review of associations between Iowa Gambling Task performance, executive functions, and intelligence. *Clin Psychol Rev.* 2010;30(5): 562–581.

70. Eslinger PJ, Damasio AR. Severe disturbances of higher cognition after bilateral frontal lobe ablation: patient EVR. *Neurology.* 1985; 35(12):1731–1741.

71. Fortin S, Godbout L, Braun CMJ. Cognitive structure of executive deficits in frontally lesioned head trauma patients performing activities of daily living. *Cortex.* 2003;39:273–291.

72. Acker MBA. Review of ecological validity of neuropsychological tests. In: Tupper DE, Cicerone KD, eds. *The Neuropsychology of Everyday Life: Assessment and Basic Competencies.* Boston, MA: Klucer Academic Publishing; 1990:19–55.

73. Grafman J. Similarities and distinctions among current models of prefrontal cortical functions. *Ann NY Acad Sci.* 1995;769:337–368.

74. Channon S, Crawford S. Problem-solving in real-life type situations: the effects of anterior and posterior lesions on performance. *Neuropsychologia.* 1999;37:757–770.

75. Satish U, Streufert S, Eslinger PJ. Measuring executive function deficits following head injury: an application of SMS simulation technology. *Psychol Rec.* 2006;56:181–190.

76. Satish U, Streufert S, Eslinger PJ. Simulation-based executive cognitive assessment and rehabilitation after traumatic frontal lobe injury: a case report. *Disab Rehabil.* 2008;30: 468–478.

77. Stuss DT, Gallup GG Jr, Alexander MP. The frontal lobes are necessary for "theory of mind." *Brain.* 2001;124:279–286.

78. Trexler LT, Zappalà G. Neuropathological determinants of acquired attention disorders in traumatic brain injury. *Brain Cogn.* 1988;8:291–302.

79. Eslinger PJ. Neurological and neuropsychological bases of empathy. *Eur Neurol.* 1998;39:193–199.

80. McDonald S, Flanagan S. Social perception deficits after traumatic brain injury: interaction between emotion recognition, mentalizing ability, and social communication. *Neuropsychology.* 2004;18:572–579.

81. Hornak J, Rolls ET, Wade D. Face and voice expression identification in patients with emotional and behavioral changes following ventral frontal lobe damage. *Neuropsychologia.* 1996;34:247–261.

Neuropsychological Assessment and Treatment Planning

Nancy H. Hsu, Emilie E. Godwin, Kathryn Wilder Schaaf, Stephen W. Smith, Laura A. Taylor, and Jeffrey S. Kreutzer

INTRODUCTION

Neuropsychology is a subspecialty in the field of clinical psychology that focuses on brain-behavior relationships. As such, clinical neuropsychologists have expertise in assessing, diagnosing, and treating problems of cognitive skills, psychological functions, and behaviors because they relate to the brain structures and systems. According to the National Academy of Neuropsychology (NAN) definition (1), clinical neuropsychologists use "psychological, neurological, cognitive, behavioral, and physiological principles, techniques, and tests to evaluate patients' neurocognitive, behavioral, and emotional strengths and weaknesses and their relationship to normal and abnormal central nervous system functioning." Consequently, individuals with neurologic conditions, health problems, neurodevelopmental disorders, cognitive problems, learning disorders, and psychiatric conditions are often referred for comprehensive neuropsychological assessment. Using the results from the assessments, clinical neuropsychologists can identify and diagnose neurobehavioral disorders, address prognosis, and formulate treatments plans to assist in the rehabilitation process. Clinical neuropsychologists can also be involved in the development and implementation of individual, group, and marital/family therapy, as well as education programs.

This chapter will review the role of clinical neuropsychologists in the assessment and treatment of individuals with traumatic brain injury (TBI), process of neuropsychological assessment and report writing, and use of the findings to develop treatment recommendations. The role of clinical neuropsychologists in rehabilitation and treatment, and a holistic approach to patient care will also be explored.

PRINCIPLES GUIDING THE PRACTICE OF CLINICAL NEUROPSYCHOLOGY

Neuropsychologists play an important role in the assessment and treatment of individuals with TBI. Although assessment of cognitive and functional skills remains an important component of neuropsychologists' work, many clinicians have taken a more holistic approach to treatment. Therefore, when working with patients with TBI, a neuropsychologist's re-

sponsibilities may vary to include traditional assessment, individual psychotherapy, couples/family therapy, psychoeducation, and functional skills building. For example, a neuropsychologist may help patients adjust to postinjury changes and make decisions regarding family and work responsibilities.

A set of guiding principles has been developed to help neuropsychologists develop a more holistic approach to clinical practice. Consideration of the following principles can help clinicians achieve more positive outcomes and greater levels of patient satisfaction:

- Empower patients and their families to take an active role in the evaluation and treatment process.
- Believe that people with neurological disabilities are more like people without neurological disabilities.
- Convey honesty and caring in personal interactions to form an adequate foundation for a strong therapeutic relationship.
- Develop practical plans for rehabilitation and explain rehabilitation techniques in language that patients, families, and interdisciplinary professionals are likely to understand.
- Help patients and their families understand the common neurobehavioral sequelae of brain injury and the typical recovery course.
- Recognize that change is inevitable and help the patients and their families develop plans to deal with changes as they arise over time.
- Remember that every patient is important and deserves to be treated with respect.
- Remember that patients and their families often have different perspectives; consider their individuality when formulating treatment approaches.
- Be willing to refer to other professionals if a case extends beyond personal areas of expertise.

COMPREHENSIVE NEUROPSYCHOLOGICAL ASSESSMENT

Comprehensive neuropsychological assessment typically involves clarification of the referral question(s), review of pertinent records, clinical interview, behavioral observations, and administration of standardized measures. Standardized measures that are valid and reliable are used to assess cognitive, academic, neurobehavioral, and emotional functioning. The impact of TBI on the family dynamic, pain, substance abuse, vocational and academic potential, motivation and effort, judgment, and safety are also areas of emphasis in neuropsychological assessment. The following sections will describe each step and assessment techniques in more detail.

Referral Question(s)

The first step in neuropsychological assessment is identifying issues of concern and clarifying referral question(s). This process allows for selection of relevant assessment methods. Referral sources often request information in 3 areas: (*a*) information pertaining to diagnosis, prognosis, and neuropsychological, neurobehavioral, and emotional functioning; (*b*) information about functional abilities, including level of independence and academic and vocational functioning; and (*c*) information about treatment and rehabilitation needs.

The diversity of referral questions highlight a variety of complex issues and questions, which neuropsychologists are often asked to address in their assessments. Answering these questions appropriately necessitates comprehensive, holistic approach. They also provide insight into potential recommendations and treatment needs. Directly answering referral sources' questions and addressing their concerns is a hallmark of a beneficial neuropsychological report.

Although the referral sources may ask about one direct issue, neuropsychologists are encouraged to identify concerns of the patients. Often, the referral sources may be unfamiliar with the process and purpose of neuropsychological testing. Thus, it is not uncommon for a neuropsychological report to answer the referral question(s) and address other areas of deficit or need for a patient.

Records Review

Obtaining relevant records pertaining to medical, psychological, criminal, academic, and vocational history is a necessary step in preparing for a neuropsychological assessment. Prior to meeting and interviewing the patient and family members, it is pertinent to thoroughly review the records. The neuropsychologist is then able to formulate relevant questions and communicate to the patient that he or she is well prepared and interested in the patient's well-being. Familiarity with the records also helps guide test selection and treatment planning.

Thorough review of records is a methodical data collection process. Culmination of data provides insight into a patient's functioning preinjury and postinjury, and comparisons can be made regarding the extent the injury has affected the patient's life. Data collection begins with reviews of relevant injury-related medical information, including mechanism of injury, injury severity, and injury-related cognitive and physical sequelae. Treatment records to pay attention to include rehabilitation therapies, psychological services, and pharmacological interventions. Other medical records provide information regarding preinjury health problems and treatments, as well as elucidate etiology. For example,

preinjury mental health records document presence of existing emotional issues and substance misuse, whereas postinjury records might suggest emotional, neurobehavioral, and personality changes. Review of psychological treatment history also provides valuable information about what has been effective. Positive criminal records history may illuminate difficulties with authority, antisocial behavior, mental health issues, substance abuse problems, and litigation history.

Academic records provide information about history of learning difficulties, need for remediation and accommodations, academic potential, and the patient's strengths and weaknesses. From examination of job descriptions, attendance records, performance reviews, promotions, and disciplinary actions, the neuropsychologist is able to ascertain work experience, habits, attitudes, and accomplishments. Vocational records also provide information about the patient's ability to function within structured environments, response to authority figures, and interpersonal skills.

Review of academic and vocational records assists with establishing the patient's preinjury or expected level of functioning, which provides the basis for judging current levels of impairment. Academic and vocational history also provides the basis for making recommendations about vocational and academic potential, optimal work/school settings, and appropriate remediation and/or accommodations.

Behavioral Observations

Careful observation during the course of interview and testing provides neuropsychologists with the opportunity to assess behaviors not measured by quantitative assessment instruments. Table 60-1 shows information that is typically gathered through behavioral observations. When possible, observation across different settings, by different observers, and at different times is ideal. Further, interviewing patients in their homes or current living situations provides opportunity to observe behaviors that may be missed in a clinical setting. If home-based observation is not possible, family members or caregivers should be asked to provide additional information about behaviors in home and community settings. Neuropsychologists should also gather information about behaviors from members of the interdisciplinary team who may have the opportunity to observe the patient in other settings.

Clinical Interview

The clinical interview is an opportunity to gather needed information, observe patient behaviors, and build rapport. Information is obtained in a variety of ways during the interview session. The primary intention of the clinical interview is to gather directed information about the patient's presenting issue and background history (see Table 60-2). The clinical interview is also a chance to gather behavioral data. The neuropsychologist has an opportunity to take note of the patient's reactions to questions, interpretation of questions, and general style. In addition, the neuropsychologist can use the clinical interview as an opportunity to educate the patient and assess for symptoms at the same time. For example, a clinician can talk about typical symptoms of brain injury, such as memory problems, word finding difficulty, problems

TABLE 60–1 Behavioral Observations Relevant to Neuropsychological Assessment

GENERAL OBSERVATION AREA	SPECIFIC AREAS TO ASSESS	GENERAL OBSERVATION AREA	SPECIFIC AREAS TO ASSESS
Appearance	• Dress • Physical condition • Hygiene • Eye contact		derailment, paraphasia, clanging, neologisms, blocking, perseveration) • Flexibility or rigidity in thinking • Appropriateness of responses
Motor abilities and stamina	• Gait/ambulation • Reaction time • Quality of gross motor and fine motor movements • Signs of restlessness/agitation • Fatigue and stamina • Signs of pain or discomfort	Attitude toward examiner and testing	• Cooperation and interest level • Consistency of effort • Persistence • Openness to questions • Ability to inhibit negative emotional reactions • Level of comfort in social interactions • Willingness to engage in conversation
Affect	• Range • Appropriateness to situation and content • Consistency with reported mood • Level of frustration tolerance • Signs of anxiety, grief, depression, euphoria, irritability, or emotional withdrawal • Emotional lability	Attitude toward self/ level of self-awareness	• Level of self-confidence • Awareness of errors and error correction • Reaction to successes and failures • Accuracy of performance rating • Insight and level of awareness • Attainability of goals
Communication	• Speech quality (e.g., rate, volume, tone, prosody) • Fluency, articulation, intelligibility, and spontaneity of speech • Word finding problems/anomia • Grammar and vocabulary • Auditory comprehension/receptive language abilities • Ability to understand questions and instructions	Reactions to test items	• Level of frustration tolerance • Expressed concern about task difficulty • Increase or decrease in effort with increasing task difficulty • Persistence
Thought patterns	• Organization of thoughts • Evidence of hallucinations, delusions, or paranoia • Difficulty remaining on topic or other unusual thinking patterns (e.g., tangentiality, circumstantiality,	Work habits and approach to testing	• Response rate, response latency, and processing speed • Deliberate vs impulsive responding • Planning and organization abilities • Problem-solving approach to tasks • Flexibility in shifting between tasks • Handwriting accuracy • Reaction to praise

focusing, and mood or personality changes, while assessing the patient's experience with each symptom.

An interview typically takes place between the patient and the neuropsychologist; however, the primary caregiver or a family member is encouraged to participate in the process. The caregiver or the family member may be interviewed together with the patient or individually, either in person or through telephone interview. Families provide an alternative vantage point on problems and behaviors pertaining to the patient and can be helpful in identifying inconsistencies with the patient's self-report. Further, a family member may elicit a different personality style from the patient that can enrich behavioral observations.

Rapport Building: Using the Clinical Interview as an Intervention

The clinical interview is typically the first face-to-face interaction a clinician and patient have. Patients may be nervous about undergoing a neuropsychological assessment for a variety of reasons. The interview is an opportunity to build rapport with the patient and help him or her feel as comfortable as possible with the testing process. The following suggestions are provided for rapport building during the clinical interview:

1. Take time to orient the patient to the purpose of the exam. Explain the scope of the process, including an estimate of time needed for the exam and opportunity for feedback to be scheduled at a later date. Review the questions being asked in the referral, and talk to the patient about how you will go about answering those questions.
2. Patients may get frustrated by being asked questions that they feel have been previously answered by records or questionnaires. Let the patient know that you understand that the clinical interview may feel repetitive but you want to ensure all the information is correct in the evaluation.
3. Start the interview with "easy" questions. Based on your knowledge of the patient after record review, ask ques-

TABLE 60–2 Pertinent Information Gathered During Clinical Interview

TOPICS TO ADDRESS	
Injury information	• First recall before injury • First recall after injury • Duration of loss of consciousness (if any) • Hospitalization course • Current and previous treatments
Presenting symptoms and problems	• Onset, intensity, frequency, and duration • Progression of symptoms (better, worsened) • Mood • Sleep • Fatigue • Changes in appetite, sense of smell, vision, or hearing • Sexuality issues
Pain	• Onset, intensity, frequency, and duration • Impact on daily functioning • Treatment history • What has and has not worked to reduce pain • Refer to pain chapter for formal assessment (see Chapter 57)
Education	• Highest grade completed • Preexisting learning disability, specify • Average grades/GPA • Favorite and least favorite classes
Vocational	• Most recent job and previous work history/injury • Reasons for job changes • Job descriptions • Safety issues • Vocational goals/interest
Current daily living situation	• Daily activities, including changes since injury • Ability to carry out daily self-care activities and safety concerns • Financial and medication management • Driving and safety issues related to driving
Family and social functioning	• Relationship status and interpersonal relationships • Current living situation, social activities, and support • Changes since injury
Medical and psychological	• Current and previous medical conditions unrelated to injury • Current providers and treatments • History of psychological diagnoses and interventions, including inpatient treatment
Substance use/abuse	• Current and preinjury alcohol and illicit substance use • History of legal, social, marital, or vocational problems from alcohol and substance use • Treatment history • Refer to substance abuse chapter for formal assessment (see Chapter 79)

Abbreviation: GPA, grade point average.

tions that help relax the patient and feel more comfortable with the process. Validate that some questions asked are difficult or uncomfortable. If needed, clarify why difficult questions are helpful for the purpose of providing a complete picture in the report.

Assessing Self-Awareness During the Clinical Interview

Self-awareness is a pinnacle issue in patients with TBI and can often affect the process and content of a clinical interview. Issues with self-awareness are sometimes clear at the onset of the interview, but the subtleties with a patient's awareness should also be assessed. Using family members, friends, teachers, or employer feedback can be an effective means of understanding a patient's capacity for self-awareness. Nevertheless, it is also important to directly ask the patient the following questions:

1. What do you know about your condition?
2. How is your condition affecting your life (socially, academically, vocationally, etc.)?
3. Do you feel like your problems are an issue for you? Others?

The answers to these questions, combined with knowledge of the patient's academic or work history, relationship status, and general well-being can provide the neuropsychologist with important information regarding the patient's current capacity for self-awareness.

Quantitative Assessment

Quantitative neuropsychological assessment findings provide a useful complement to data gathered through behavioral observations and clinical interview. Quantitative assessment provides the opportunity to gather data about neuropsychological functioning in a standardized way, allowing neuropsychologists to make comparisons to normative data and to make comparisons over time with repeated testing (2). In determining which assessment instruments to use, neuropsychologists consider several factors. First, comprehensive assessment is multidimensional and multimethod, covering a range of functioning areas using a variety of measures to assess each area. Second, tests are selected with emphasis placed on problem areas endorsed by the patient, his or her family members, and the referral source. Third, measures are chosen based on ease of completion and administration time whenever possible. Finally, in determining which tests to use, neuropsychologists consider the tests' reliability and validity, normative samples, and research findings specific to brain injury.

This section is not meant to provide encyclopedic knowledge about the function and process of quantitative neuropsychological assessment. On the contrary, the section purport to offer a broad overview of the topic emphasizing the importance of evaluating patients as multifaceted beings with significant preinjury histories, interpersonal relationships, emotional reactions to injury, and so forth. Readers interested in comprehensive reviews of this subject are encouraged to peruse Lezak's text, *Neuropsychological Assessment* (3); Strauss, Sherman, and Spreen's text, *A Compendium of Neuropsychological Tests* (2); and the chapter entitled, "Neuropsychological Examination of the Patient With Traumatic Brain Injury" in *Rehabilitation of the Adult and Child With Traumatic Brain Injury* (4).

Assessment of Cognitive and Academic Functioning

Because patients with TBI commonly experience cognitive and academic impairments, assessment of functioning is often performed to elucidate deficits. Areas typically assessed in comprehensive neuropsychological assessment include academic skills, attention and concentration, motor abilities, sensation, learning and memory, visuoperception, visuoconstructional abilities, language, and reasoning. Test selection should be based on referral questions, patient's concerns, location of injury, and functional status. Table 60-3 depicts specific tests and the corresponding areas of functioning assessed. Some instruments measure various functional domains, whereas others measure only 1. The readers are referred to Lezak's (3) and Strauss, Sherman, and Spreen's (2) texts for a thorough review of neuropsychological tests and their functions.

Assessment of Emotional, Personality, and Neurobehavioral Functioning

Neurobehavioral and personality changes are common following TBI. In addition, patients with TBI typically have difficulty adjusting to injury-related changes, increasing the risk of emotional difficulties. As such, comprehensive neuropsychological assessment involves assessment of neurobehavioral, emotional, and personality functioning. Table 60-4 describes measures that are commonly administered to assess these areas of functioning.

Concern has been expressed that traditional measures of emotional and personality functioning have limited use for patients with TBI. First, many instruments were developed specifically for people with psychiatric difficulties, not for those with neurological disorders. Many individuals with TBI may be diagnosed with psychiatric disorders secondary to the overlap between sequelae of TBI and psychiatric symptoms. Witol and colleagues (19) caution clinicians to consider the contributions of TBI when interpreting the results of measures of emotional and personality functioning. The Neurobehavioral Functioning Inventory (NFI) (17) and the Neurobehavioral Rating Scale (NBRS) (18) were developed for use with TBI populations and may be good alternatives. Second, reliance on self-report is difficult following TBI secondary to difficulties with self-awareness. As such, neuropsychologists seek out corroborating information from family members and records review. Finally, many measures are long and require at least a sixth grade reading level. Injury-related sequelae, such as reading comprehension problems, visual disturbances, pain, and attention and concentration problems, can negatively impact patients' abilities to respond to questionnaires. If concerns about a patient's ability to respond to the questionnaire emerge, neuropsychologists may wish to consider clinician-rated measures such as the Hamilton Depression Rating Scale (HAM-D) (9) or the structured clinical interview for *Diagnostic and Statistical Manual of Mental Disorder* (*DSM-IV*) Axis I (SCID) (22).

Assessment of Judgment and Safety

Caregivers, family members, and referral sources often express concerns about the judgment and safety of patients with TBI in the home and community environments. Questions arise about the patient's ability to travel, manage finances and medications, prepare foods, use appliances and tools, handle emergencies, and maintain home security. One study that examined caregivers' concerns about judgment and safety revealed that driving and financial management are key areas (30). The investigators noted that many of caregivers' concerns were related to inadequate memory functioning. Consequently, neuropsychologists are asked to assess the patient's ability to make sound decisions and safely carry out daily activities. Results of neuropsychological assessment can reveal significant impairments in areas of memory, attention, and reasoning skills that would interfere with ability to safely carry out daily activities.

The Judgment and Safety Screening Inventory (31) was designed to assess judgment and safety concerns in the following areas: travel; financial management; interpersonal functioning; food and kitchen; use of appliances, tools, and utensils; household issues; medications and alcohol; fire safety; and firearm safety. Respondents are asked to identify their concern level (none, little, much, or very) about different aspects of each functioning area. Space is provided for open-ended responses from patients and other informants. Patient and informant versions allow for comparisons between respondents. Interview and written versions are also available.

Assessing patients' judgment is critical in the process because, often times, patients exhibit impaired self-awareness as a result of TBI and misperceive their limitations and capabilities. Using information collected during clinical interview and results of neuropsychological assessment, issue of judgment and safety can be addressed. During interview, the neuropsychologist may ask the patients and their family members about daily functioning. For example, inquiry can be made about adherence to medication regimen, recent traffic violations or accidents, missing due date to pay bills, and incidence of leaving appliances unattended. Both the patients' and family members' concerns should be collected when possible to make comparisons.

Assessment of Pain

Pain, a common complaint of individuals who have sustained TBI, often contributes to cognitive deficits and negatively impacts quality of life secondary to activity restrictions. Patients' response to pain varies significantly based on the meaning of pain to the individuals and the impact of pain on their lives. Thorough pain assessment may include administration of standardized measures, such as the McGill Pain Inventory (32) and visual analog scales (33). Information is gathered about pain intensity, frequency, duration, quality, location, date of onset, history of pain problems, family history, and treatments and their effectiveness. In addition, behaviors that exacerbate and improve pain are important to assess. Patients are often asked to rate their pain on a 1 (*no pain*) to 10 (*extreme pain*) scale throughout the assessment to establish if poor performances are related to pain. During the evaluation, neuropsychologists are alert to pain behaviors (e.g., shifting in seat, rubbing areas of pain focus, frequent request for breaks) and to medication

TABLE 60–3 Tests and Their Corresponding Areas of Function

FUNCTIONING AREA	TESTS
ACADEMIC SKILLS	
Arithmetic calculation	Calculation (Woodcock-Johnson III Tests of Achievement [WJ III ACH]); math computation (Wide Range Achievement Test-Fourth Edition [WRAT4]); numerical operations (Wechsler Individual Achievement Test-Third Edition [WIAT-III])
Arithmetic reasoning	Mathematics reasoning (WIAT-III); applied problems (WJ III ACH)
Reading comprehension	Gray Oral Reading Tests-Fourth Edition (GORT-4); passage comprehension (WJ III ACH); reading comprehension (WIAT-III); sentence comprehension (WRAT4); Test of Reading Comprehension-Fourth Edition (TORC-4)
Word reading	Pseudonym decoding and word reading (WIAT-III); word reading (WRAT4)
Spelling	Spelling (WIAT-III); spelling (WJ III ACH); spelling (WRAT4)
Writing	Writing samples (WJ III ACH); written expression (WIAT-III)
ATTENTION AND CONCENTRATION	Conners' Continuous Performance Test II; Dementia Rating Scale-Second Edition (DRS-2) (attention scale); digit span (Wechsler Adult Intelligence Scale-Fourth Edition [WAIS-IV]); letter-number sequencing (WAIS-IV); Paced Auditory Serial Addition Test (PASAT); spatial span (Wechsler Memory Scale-Fourth Edition: WMS-IV); Speech Sounds Perception Test and Rhythm Test, and Trail Making Test (TMT): Parts A and B (Halstead-Reitan Battery [HRB]); Stroop Color Word Test; Symbol Digit Modalities Test (SDMT)
MOTOR AND SENSORY FUNCTIONS	
Speed and dexterity	Finger tapping test (HRB); Lafayette grooved pegboard
Grip strength	Hand dynamometer (HRB)
Coordinated bilateral movement	Luria Motor Tests
Hand-eye coordination	Coding (WAIS-IV); Grooved pegboard; Luria Motor Tests; SDMT (written); TMT Parts A and B (HRB)
Sensory and sensorimotor	Tactile perception, Tactile Performance Test (TPT), tactile form recognition, tactile localization, and fingertip writing (HRB)
NONVERBAL MEMORY	
Immediate	Benton Visual Retention Test; DRS-2, (memory scale); designs and visual reproduction (WMS-IV); Motor-Free Visual Perception Test
Delayed	DRS-2 (memory scale); designs delayed and visual reproduction delayed (WMS-IV); Recognition Memory Test; Rey Complex Figure Test (RCFT)
Learning	Coding (WAIS-IV); SDMT; TPT
VERBAL MEMORY	
Immediate	California Verbal Learning Test-Second Edition; logical memory and verbal paired associates (WMS-IV); Rey Auditory Verbal Learning Test
Delayed	CVLT-II (delay and recognition); logical memory and verbal paired associates delay (WMS-IV); RAVLT (delay and recognition)
Remote memory and fund of information	Information (WAIS-IV)
Learning	CVLT-II; RAVLT
VISUAL BASED SKILLS	
Visuoperception and visual reasoning	Culver Right-Left Orientation Test; cancellation, figure weights, matrix reasoning, picture completion, and symbol search (WAIS-IV); Hooper Visual Organization Test; Judgment of Line Orientation Test; Line Bisection Test; MVPT; SDMT (oral & written); Visual Form Discrimination Test
Visuomotor and visuoconstruction	Block design and coding (WAIS-IV); RCFT; SDMT; TMT Parts A and B

(Continued)

TABLE 60–3 Tests and Their Corresponding Areas of Function (*Continued*)

FUNCTIONING AREA	TESTS
LANGUAGE SKILLS	
Vocabulary	Clinical interview; vocabulary (WAIS-IV)
Oral Fluency	Controlled Oral Word Association Test
Naming	Boston Naming Test
Expressive language	Aphasia Screening Test (HRB); Boston Diagnostic Aphasia Examination; clinical interview; oral expression (WIAT-III)
Receptive language	Behavioral observation of instruction following; clinical interview; listening comprehension (WIAT-III); token test; oral comprehension and understanding directions (WJ III ACH)
REASONING AND JUDGMENT	
Verbal reasoning	Comprehension and similarities (WAIS-IV)
Nonverbal reasoning	Category test (HRB); visual puzzles (WAIS-IV); Raven's Progressive Matrices; TMT Part B (HRB); Wisconsin Card Sorting Test
Judgment of safety	Comprehension (WAIS-IV); Independent Living Scales; Judgment and Safety Screening Inventory (JASSI)–patient and informant versions
Self-awareness	Clinical interview; JASSI, comparison of patient and family responses; NFI, comparison of patient and family responses

side effects (e.g., fatigue). Additionally, consideration should be given to the impact that pain has on neurocognitive outcomes. Patients with chronic pain tend to demonstrate impairments on measures assessing attention, processing speed, as well as psychomotor speed. Overall, clinicians should assess for and consider pain when interpreting test data, especially when results are not consistent with the patient's neurological impairment (34). The readers are referred to Chapter 57 in this book entitled, "Post-Traumatic Pain Disorders: Medical Assessment and Management" for detailed information about the assessment and treatment of pain among individuals with TBI.

Assessment of Motivation and Effort

Comprehensive neuropsychological assessment typically incorporates evaluation of patients' motivation and effort. As Bush and colleagues (35) indicated in the NAN position paper on symptom validity assessment, a determination of the examinee's level of effort and honesty in responding is necessary to "place maximal confidence in the ability to interpret accurate results" from the evaluation. As a general practice, patients are encouraged to exert maximum effort during the testing process to reduce concerns about malingering (35–39). When there is a question of response bias and/or inadequate effort relative to the neuropsychological presentation, clinicians have several techniques to identify such activity. Neuropsychologists look for the following: consistency in self-reported and documented history; consistency in self- and collateral-reported information about presenting problems; consistency in performance across tests; consistency of test performance and presenting complaints with those expected given injury severity; and consistency between presenting complaints, observed behaviors, and test performance (35–38). Secondary gain issues are important to consider, including revenge, attention seeking, escape from responsibility, and pending lawsuits, worker's com-

pensation hearings, or disability benefit hearings. History of litigation and benefit seeking should be ascertained during clinical interview and records review.

Neuropsychological and psychological tests may be used to assess legitimate vs malingered memory impairments or exaggerated symptoms. Performance may be evaluated using embedded effort measures within ability tests or stand-alone tests of cognitive effort (36). Symptom validity tests are designed to measures exaggeration of deficits. On these tests, scores that fall below cut-off scores are suggestive of insufficient effort. Forced-choice tests are designed to assess for biased reasoning and performance that falls below chance at a statistically significant level and raises concerns about the validity of responses (35). Specialized tests developed specifically for detection of response bias are available for inclusion in neuropsychological test batteries, including the Portland Digit Recognition Test (40), Recognition Memory Test (41), Test of Memory Malingering (42), and the Word Memory Test (43). Multiple symptom validity measures may be administered over the course of the evaluation (36,39), without providing redundant data (44). Many self-report measures assessing psychological functioning include validity scales, which provide helpful information. For example, normative data on the F(p) Scale of the Minnesota Multiphasic Personality Inventory-2nd Edition (MMPI-2) aids in the identification of unusual response patterns suggestive of insufficient effort or symptom exaggeration (45).

The readers are referred to Chapter 85 in this book entitled, "Assessment of Response Bias in Clinical and Forensic Evaluations of Impairment" for a thorough review of assessment techniques for evaluating motivation and effort. The readers are also referred to the NAN position paper on symptom validity assessment by Bush and colleagues (35). This position paper provides definitions of terminology used in validity assessment, methodologies, evaluation contexts, procedures, interpretation, cultural factors, and information about purpose and medical necessity of this assessment.

TABLE 60–4 Tests and Their Corresponding Areas of Function

MEASURE	BRIEF DESCRIPTION
Beck Depression Inventory-Second Edition (BDI-II)	The BDI-II is a 21-item self-report measure designed to detect the presence and severity of depression symptoms (5). The multiple-choice format requires a sixth grade reading level. Repeated administrations permit monitoring of treatment effects. Notably, factor analysis of the BDI-II with a TBI population produces a unique factor structure that includes vegetative symptoms of depression factor. This additional factor may be measuring symptoms of depression, TBI, or a combination of the 2 (6).
Brief Symptom Inventory (BSI)	The BSI, a shortened version of the Symptom Checklist-90-R, is a 53-item self-report measure, which is designed to evaluate the severity of psychiatric symptoms (7). A sixth grade reading level is required. Although the BSI was initially developed for psychiatric populations, it has been evaluated with several medical populations. The BSI is purported to be an effective and accurate screening tool to inform further evaluation and intervention with TBI populations. Slaughter and colleagues (8) recommend the BSI as a measure of general distress and caution using the subscales of the measure.
Hamilton Rating Scale for Depression (HRSD; HAM-D)	The HRSD is a 17-item screening instrument, which was designed to assess the severity of cognitive, emotional, and physical symptoms of depression (9). The measure is completed by the clinician during the clinical interview with the patient and family and records review. As such, the measure is useful for screening depression in individuals who have limited reading abilities or vision problems which preclude reading. Witol and colleagues (10) expressed concern that many of the items are consistent with neurobehavioral sequelae of TBI.
Hospital Anxiety and Depression Scale (HADS)	The HADS is a 14-item self-report measure designed for use with a medical population (11). The 7-item subscale measuring depression reflects anhedonia, and the 7-item subscale measuring anxiety largely focuses on affective and cognitive symptoms. Technical data from the manual supporting the reliability of the measure are limited (12). A recent study examining the validity of the HADS with a TBI population recommended using the measure to monitor symptoms rates rather than for clinical diagnosis (13)
Minnesota Multiphasic Personality Inventory-2nd Edition (MMPI-2)	The MMPI-2 is a 567-item, self-report measure of personality and emotional functioning in adults (14). A sixth grade reading level is required, but audiotaped versions are available. Concern has been expressed about elevated profiles of individuals with TBI on the MMPI-2. Clinicians should examine how a patient's neurological complaints and perceptual competency may affect a profile when interpreting the results of the MMPI-2 (15).
Minnesota Multiphasic Personality Inventory-2nd Edition-Restructured Form (MMPI-2-RF)	The MMPI-2-RF is a self-report measure of personality and emotional functioning in adults. The restructured form has 338 items that were drawn from the original 567 items on the MMPI-2. Norms for the MMPI-2-RF are based on the MMPI-2 pool (16). Limited research has been conducted on this revised version of the MMPI-2-RF. Arbisi and colleagues (17) found that a group of National Guard soldiers who screened positive for a mTBI diagnosis did have significantly different MMPI-2-RF mean scale scores from a control group of National Guard peers.
Neurobehavioral Functioning Inventory (NFI)	Developed for use with a TBI population, the NFI is an 83-item measure that was designed to examine the frequency of neurobehavioral difficulties postinjury (18). The measure can be administered in a self-report format or orally. Patient and family versions are available, allowing for comparison of responses. Normative data, based on age and injury severity, is available. Information is gathered about functioning in 6 domains: depression, somatic symptoms, memory/attention, communication, aggression, and motor abilities.
Neurobehavioral Rating Scale (NBRS)	Adapted from the Brief Psychiatric Rating Scale, the NBRS was designed to assess behavioral and emotional symptoms, which are commonly exhibited post-TBI (19). The 27-item scale is completed by a clinician based on observations during an interview. Items are rated on a scale from 1 (*not present*) to 7 (*extremely severe*). Witol and colleagues (10) assert that the NBRS is a useful tool for assessing neurobehavioral functioning acutely.
Patient Health Questionnaire-9 (PHQ-9)	The PHQ-9 is a 9-item self-report screening measure for major depressive disorder (20). This tool parallels the diagnostic symptoms in the *DSM-IV*, and was developed for use with a medical patient population (21). Fann and colleagues (21) reported acceptable reliability and validity for use of the PHQ-9 with a TBI population, and provide recommendations for items to focus on for optimal screening.
Personality Assessment Inventory (PAI)	The PAI is a 344-item self-report measure of adult psychopathology (14). This objective inventory of adult personality assesses psychopathological syndromes and provides information for clinical diagnosis, treatment planning, and screen for psychopathology. Advantages over the MMPI-II include: a fourth grade reading level is required, shorter administration time, and the scales do not overlap. Limited research has been conducted with the TBI population, although most findings support the PAI as a useful measure of psychiatric and emotional disturbance among persons with TBI (22–24).
Structured Clinical Interview for *DSM-IV* Axis I Disorders (SCID)	The SCID is a semistructured interview designed to guide trained clinicians to make *DSM-IV* Axis I diagnoses (25). This assessment has been used in a number of studies assessing psychiatric disorders after TBI (26–28). The SCID is an effective tool for assessing the broad range of disorders that occur in patients with TBI (29). However, the length of time required to administer the SCID, 45–90 minutes, could prove to be difficult for some patients with TBI.

Abbreviations: *DSM-IV*, Diagnostic and Statistical Manual of Mental Disorders; TBI, traumatic brain injury.

Vocational Assessment

Research suggests that most persons with moderate or severe TBI are unable to sustain employment (46–52). Vocational issues are a primary concern for patients and their families, and referral sources frequently list return to work among their primary concerns for patients. Referral questions often focus on the patient's readiness to return to work, potential work capacity, obstacles to employment that need to be addressed, and needed rehabilitation services and workplace accommodations and supports. Prognostication about vocational potential should be based on thorough return to work and comprehensive neuropsychological assessments revealing strengths and limitations. Comprehensive assessment reveals potential obstacles to successful return to work, including cognitive deficits, emotional issues, interpersonal difficulties, transportation issues, stress tolerance, anger management problems, self-awareness problems, and pain and other physical symptoms. The readers are referred to Chapter 81 in this book entitled, "Returning to Work" for additional information.

Family and Caregiver Assessment

As the length of hospital and rehabilitation stays decrease (53,54), family members often have had to take on the principal caretaking role soon after injury. Caregiving places significant burden on the family. Research reveals that caregiving family members are at risk for emotional difficulties (55–63). Given the importance of the family's role in caring for the patient, assessment of the impact of injury on the family members is critical to ensure they have the support needed to continue performing their vital role. Family and caregiver assessment should center around gaining an understanding of the impact of injury on emotional functioning, relationship quality, financial situation, life plans, quality of life, and daily responsibilities (e.g., work, childcare, household responsibilities).

Approaching assessment by addressing the patient and family system allows the clinician to provide more effective treatment and intervention recommendations. According to Kreutzer and colleagues (64), an underlying tenant of effective approaches to working with families in brain injury is recognizing that every family member's voice or opinion should be heard and respected. One approach for including multiple family members in the assessment process is collaborative self-examination. During collaborative self-examination, each family member is asked to address the same question relating to thoughts, perceptions, and issues that arise from injury. The process of each family member sharing his or her answers not only facilitates reflecting and self-awareness, but also helps family members to speak up, share their points of view, and discuss relevant issues. Using collaborative self-examination, the clinician can introduce an area of assessment (e.g. impact of injury on emotional functioning) and gain multiple perspectives on that topic. If time allows, the clinician can guide the family in the process of discussing these reactions and perceptions to improve communication and enhance cohesion (64). This type of feedback can further inform the feedback and invention recommendation section.

An additional area of focus for family system-oriented assessment includes exploration of existing supports and consideration of additional support needs. Written recommendations that include options for increasing supports for family members are extremely beneficial. Special care should be taken to help the caregiving family members understand that they will be unable to support the survivors if they do not take care of themselves and seek assistance in managing their increasing responsibilities. The readers are referred to Chapter 80 in this book entitled, "Family Assessment and Intervention" for further information regarding issues related to assessment and treatment of family members and caregivers.

Comparison to Premorbid Functioning

Neuropsychologists are frequently asked to determine whether or not the injury resulted in cognitive, academic, neurobehavioral, or emotional impairments. Determining deficits requires comparison of current functioning to premorbid functioning. Four methods may be employed to estimate premorbid functioning. First, several indicators are highly correlated with intelligence and as such, provide an estimate of premorbid functioning. These indicators include academic grades, scores on standardized testing, and educational and vocational attainment. Review of records and clinical interview are avenues of gathering this information. Second, some measures of cognitive functioning (e.g., single-word reading) are highly correlated with intelligence and are typically not affected by TBI (2,65–67). Scores on these standardized measures will likely be comparable to premorbid levels of functioning. Third, regression-based models combining demographic variables or demographic variables with test scores are also used to estimate premorbid functioning (2,68,69). Finally, within the "best performance method," the highest test scores obtained during comprehensive neuropsychological assessment are considered in the estimation of preinjury abilities (2). In addition, consideration of change and acquired impairments mentioned by the patient and family members is important.

PROGNOSTICATION AND TREATMENT PLANNING

Prognostication

Questions about prognosis are typically among the primary questions posed by referral sources. As such, neuropsychologists are often called on to provide information about long-term academic, vocational, and independent living potential. In addition, questions are often posed about a patient's likelihood of benefiting from rehabilitation services and potential treatment benefits. Thorough review of the research literature on outcomes following TBI provides the foundation for prognostic estimation. Several factors need to be considered when making predictions about a patient's outcome, including age; premorbid level of functioning; injury type and severity; additional injuries (e.g., orthopedic); preexisting medical, psychological, or substance abuse issues; premorbid educational attainment and employment status; extent and chronicity of deficits; postinjury psychological functioning; daily functioning; and availability of support services and interventions (2,70–76). Repeated testing is a helpful avenue for accurate prognostication. The number and type of areas of impairment are important predictors.

Recommendations and Treatment Planning

Comprehensive neuropsychological assessment culminates in the development of practical, feasible recommendations and treatment plans, which will enhance patients' and families' well-being and optimize functioning. Referral for medical follow-up, psychological services, psychiatric intervention, support, vocational/academic assistance, and other rehabilitation services in the community are commonly included. Compensatory strategies to address impairments are also typically provided. Repeated neuropsychological testing is frequently suggested to monitor progress or deterioration. Based on findings from reassessment, amendments may be made to the existing treatment plan. Table 60-5 depicts recommendations that may be provided to address problems in a variety of functional areas.

DIFFERENTIAL DIAGNOSIS

Neuropsychologists are frequently asked to clarify the overall picture of patients with TBI who present with myriad of cognitive, behavioral, emotional, and somatic symptoms. The patient's clinical presentation and presenting symptoms can reflect overlapping of medical and psychological disorders, exacerbation of preexisting conditions, or presence of comorbid conditions that are psychological or somatic in nature. Differential diagnosis is often the crucial part of comprehensive neuropsychological assessment. Having a breadth of knowledge about the spectrum of the *DSM-IV* (77) conditions and proficient interviewing skills are the foundation to conducting differential diagnosis.

Unstructured, semistructured, or structured interviews are used to gather pertinent information for the process of differential diagnosis. Glenn (78) advised conducting a structured search to best discover etiology and recommended the following information be ascertained: preinjury diagnosis, neuropsychological disorders, sensorimotor disorders, medical disorders, adverse effects of medication, reactive mood and anxiety disorders, and sleep disorders. The *Structured Clinical Interview for DSM-IV Axis I Disorders: Clinician Version (SCID-CV)* (79) is an assessment tool available to practitioners for determining preinjury and postinjury psychological difficulties.

A comprehensive approach to neuropsychological assessment consisting of a thorough records review, interviewing the patient and family members, incorporating behavioral observation, and combining all the data with test results provides insight into presenting conditions. Neuropsychologists attempt to tease out premorbid problems from current injury-related complications and sequelae. To assist the neuropsychologists in differentiating between premorbid problems and postinjury complications, Table 60-6 provides questions to consider during the neuropsychological assessment. Premorbid psychological or personality disorders, learning disabilities, drug or alcohol problems, and medical conditions (e.g., cerebrovascular disease, hypertension, diabetes, epilepsy, prior TBI) are potential mediating variables that commonly influence the course of a TBI.

Differentiation between the etiologies of cognitive impairments may be challenging. Cognitive impairments are typical consequences of neurological conditions, such as frontotemporal dementia, Parkinson disease, and epilepsy.

Impairments in cognition are also often evident in individuals with psychiatric disorders, including depressive and anxiety disorders, and schizophrenia. Furthermore, neuropsychological impairments are common sequelae of TBI. Therefore, identifying the onset, nature, intensity, and duration of symptoms also contribute to formulating a diagnosis.

Identification of comorbid conditions is one of the principal aims of comprehensive neuropsychological assessment. Psychological comorbidities are quite common after a TBI because the risk of developing psychiatric disorders increase following the injury (80–82). Researchers have found that between 44% and 65% of the individuals with TBI received at least 1 Axis I diagnosis postinjury. Depression and anxiety disorders (e.g., post-traumatic stress disorder [PTSD], obsessive–compulsive disorder, panic disorder, generalized anxiety disorder) were the most frequently cited postinjury affective problems of this population. Specifically, the researchers have found that approximately 45%–60% of individuals meet criteria for major depression at some point after a brain injury. Research indicated the frequency of reported emotional difficulties is directly proportional to injury severity, except in the most severe cases of TBI (83). Common psychological comorbidities encountered in the clinical practice of patients with TBI include adjustment disorder with anxiety or depressed mood, adjustment disorder with mixed emotional features and disturbed conduct, major depressive disorder (MDD), mood disorder due to general medical condition, personality change secondary to general medical condition, substance use disorders, and PTSD. It is important to keep in mind that a number of psychiatric disorders, including MDD and PTSD, have overlapping symptoms including cognitive complaints with TBI.

Mild traumatic brain injury (mTBI) offers unique challenges to neuropsychologists in terms of differential diagnosis than moderate and severe neurological damage. Clear physiological consequences of serious brain injury are unquestionable, such as positive computed tomography (CT) or magnetic resonance imaging (MRI) findings. For mTBI, however, hard neurological signs of injury may not be present. In most cases, symptoms of mTBI resolve within 3–6 months at most. Some cases that are described as complicated mTBI can have longer persisting symptoms. Comorbid problems with affective and somatic functioning may be contributing factors. It is important to keep in mind that chronic pain, fatigue, psychological, and somatic issues when interpreting neuropsychological test results in this population. Clinicians are encouraged to be familiar with difficulties associated with somatic problems. According to the *DMS-IV-TR* (77), there are a number of distinct disorders with a physical presentation, including pain disorder, hypochondriasis, somatization disorder, and conversion disorder that must also be considered in the differential diagnostic assessment of persons following traumatic injuries who present with cognitive behavioral complaints.

Neuropsychologists also consider the impact of comorbidities such as mood disorders or psychosis on patients' assessment findings. For example, conditions that alter mental status (e.g., delirium, vegetative states, or active hallucinations) may invalidate results of assessment. Screening with measures such as the Mini-Mental State. Examination (84) or the MMPI-2 (85) is recommended. These instruments help to rule out potentially confounding factors of dimin-

TABLE 60–5 Postinjury Problem Areas and Sample Recommendations

FUNCTIONAL AREA	RECOMMENDATIONS
Arithmetic	Use a calculator for all but the most basic mathematical operations; check work carefully; rely on family for assistance with financial management.
Reading and reading comprehension	Use chapter headings to outline material; take notes and highlight or underline key words while reading; use self-sticking notepaper to create indexes in the reading material to facilitate reviewing information; use the PQRST method (preview, question, read, study, test); turn chapter headings into questions to focus reading; after reading a section, paraphrase and review main points; use a reading pen.
Spelling	Use an electronic spelling aid, word processing spell checker, or portable electronic spell checker; spell the word out loud or mouth each letter as you spell the word to help focus your attention as you write; keep a small speller's dictionary near where you write; use index cards to make flash cards of words you find yourself missing often and test yourself; play Scrabble; work crossword and other puzzles.
Writing and written expression	Focus on quality vs quantity; allow ample time for task completion; dictation software; keyboarding; use grammar and spell check; remedial training; reduction in written work; audiotape meetings and classes; notetaker; read written material aloud to catch errors.
Attention and concentration	Reduce distractions (e.g., wear ear plugs or headphones, use white noise machine, sit facing wall, clear desk before beginning work); avoid interruptions (e.g., use "do not disturb" sign); self-coaching to stay on task; schedule breaks throughout the day; avoid multitasking; before changing tasks, note stopping point.
Motor/sensory functioning	
Coordination and motor slowing	Occupational and physical therapy, fitness training, sports and recreational activities; pace tasks; allow adequate time for task completion and transition between tasks; organize environment for efficiency (e.g., gather all needed materials prior to initiating project); set realistic timelines for task completion.
Vision	Neuro-ophthalmologic evaluation, corrective lenses, vision therapy; use large print reading materials and thick pen when writing notes to be read by client; audiotaped instructions/reading material; make sure there is appropriate light; avoid glare; screen and text-reader software.
Hearing	Audiology examination; ask others to speak loudly and enunciate clearly; hearing aids
Smell	Smoke detectors; label and date perishable foods.
Learning and memory	Present information in many forms (e.g., auditory, visual, kinetic); use to-do lists, calendars, memory notebook, timers, PDA's, handheld tape recorders, and other assistive devices; repeat information; develop context (e.g., mnemonics, imagery, scaffolding); demonstrate tasks; record and replay information; break tasks down into small steps and introduce new steps as earlier steps are accomplished; verbally mediate tasks in event of visual memory problems; designate specific location for items that can easily be misplaced.
Visually-based skills	Use a blank piece of paper or fold the sheet to mask extraneous details on a page; use a straight edge, ruler, or finger to follow a line of text; always check work in the same order; describe a design or task in words rather than rely on a mental image; take part in activities that require hand-eye coordination.
Language	
Receptive language and instruction following	Improve instructional format (e.g., short, simple sentences); reduce distractions; provide instructions in multiple formats; repeat or write down key information; repeat back instructions to allow for clarification; shaping
Expressive language	Allow extra time for conveying information; with word-finding difficulties, individuals may benefit from talking about the word, describing it, or using similar words; speech therapy; use gestures.
Executive functioning	Delay starting a task until you have mapped out a plan for its completion and considered possible outcomes; schedule planning sessions each morning to map out the day's activities; develop a schedule for completing tasks; prioritize tasks according to their level of urgency; break down large or overwhelming projects into smaller, manageable steps; use a large calendar to provide a visual image of short- and long-term projects; develop specific locations to keep important information; attend to filing important information on a daily basis; maintain a well-organized location to complete mentally challenging tasks.
Judgment and safety	
Judgment and safety issues	Consider supervised living situations; 24-hour supervision; respite for family; seek feedback from others before beginning a task.
Problem solving	Teach structured problem solving; develop and maintain mentor relationship; ask client how they plan to approach task prior to beginning.

(Continued)

TABLE 60–5 Postinjury Problem Areas and Sample Recommendations (*Continued*)

FUNCTIONAL AREA	RECOMMENDATIONS
Driving	Take precautions to maximize safety (e.g., avoid driving in inclement weather or traffic, drive with licensed driver, take breaks on long trips, drive familiar routes, drive only when well rested, reduce distractions, leave safe following distance between vehicles); driving evaluation; driver's training; training in use of public transportation; exploration of other transportation options (family, friends, neighbors, and area resources).
Financial management	Rely on family to assist with financial management; use an organizer with dated slots and place bills in slots 1 week before they are due; record due dates for bills in a calendar or planner; use a calculator; check work carefully; take care of challenging tasks only when well rested and distractions are minimized.
Medication management	Use a compartmentalized medication box, distributing medication in appropriate compartments at the beginning of the week; set an alarm to cue when to take medication.
Fatigue/sleep problems	Promote sleep hygiene (e.g., regular sleep schedule, limit caffeine/exercise before bed); relaxation strategies before bed (i.e., progressive muscle relaxation); medication consultation (stimulants and sleep medication); consider sleep study; adjust work schedule; schedule breaks; schedule most challenging tasks at times of peak energy level.
Emotional issues	
Depression	Supportive psychotherapy, medication management, enhance support network, increase activity level and participation in pleasant activities, encourage focus on progress, avoid comparisons to the past, monitor sources of stress, support group.
Frustration, irritability, and anger problems	Stress management and relaxation training; anger management; assertiveness, conflict resolution, and social skills training; medication management.
Feeling misunderstood by others	Communication and social skills training; educate client about how to discuss injury with others; education of coworkers, employers, and families; supportive psychotherapy; support group; enhance social support.
Anxiety	Development of anxiety management strategies, including thought stopping; relaxation training; remember anxiety can inhibit ability to attend to and learn information, taking deep breaths and making positive self-statements can be beneficial; medication management.

ished consortium or significant affective disturbance, respectively. Table 60-7 provides a list of test measures least and most susceptible to the affect slowed mental processing and/or psychomotor performance often observed with certain mood disorders.

NEUROPSYCHOLOGICAL REPORT WRITING

Effectively communicating neuropsychological assessment results to referral sources, treatment providers, patients, and

families is an essential component of the assessment process. Because a neuropsychologist's report may be read by individuals with differing backgrounds and expertise, it is important that the information is presented in a way that is informative, yet easily understandable. Further, reports must be both comprehensive and concise. If test results are not communicated effectively, the use of the entire assessment process may be called into question.

TABLE 60–6 Questions to Facilitate Differentiation Between Premorbid Problems and Injury-Related Sequelae

- Did the patient have preexisting learning difficulties?
- When did emotional difficulties or substance use issues arise?
- Was the patient receiving mental health treatment for a mood disorder or other psychological problem before the injury?
- Were pain or sleep problems apparent prior to the patient having a TBI?
- How was the patient's daily functioning prior to the injury? Explore areas such as relationships, occupational or educational pursuits, and recreational activities.
- Have others noticed a change in the patient's functioning since the injury?
- Did the patient have a preinjury personality disorder?

Abbreviation: TBI, traumatic brain injury.

TABLE 60–7 Tests Least and Most Susceptible to Affect of Mood Disorders

LESS SUSCEPTIBLE	MORE SUSCEPTIBLE
Category Test	Symbol Digit Modalities Test
WAIS Verbal Subtests Vocabulary Comprehension Similarities	WAIS Performance Subtests Block Design Digit Symbol-Coding
Rey-Osterrieth Complex Figure Test	Trail Making Test: Parts A and B
Wide Range-Achievement Test Reading Spelling	Grooved Pegboard Test
Token Test	Controlled Oral Word Association Test

In creating a report, neuropsychologists should consider the following:

1. Review records thoroughly to ensure that historical information, preexisting conditions, and injury severity are understood and considered in formulating impressions and recommendations.
2. Be sure to address the referral questions, as well as the patient's concerns.
3. In formulating diagnostic impressions, consider the affect of preexisting conditions, psychological and emotional issues, motivation, effort, self-awareness, and pain.
4. Write reports in a language that patients and lay people can understand, avoiding jargon.
5. Tailor reports to each specific patient rather than being generic.
6. Write and disseminate reports in a timely fashion. Review test results with the patient and discuss findings in a meaningful way. Encourage the patient and his or her family to ask questions.
7. Consider the patient's and family's concerns and the meaning of the injury to the patient during report development.
8. Consider the patient's reactions to test findings and impressions, and take special care to ensure the presentation of the findings and conclusions will be palatable to the patient.
9. Highlight strengths as well as deficits.
10. Translate test results into recommendations which will make the patient's life better.

Although it is important that clinicians develop unique reports specific to each patient, structure is a useful way of providing a familiar framework for referral sources. Placing information in similar sections with distinct headings allows readers to locate information quickly. Structured report formats also provide a way to organize large amounts of information and make writing more efficient. Table 60-8 depicts important sections that may be included in comprehensive neuropsychological reports.

NEUROPSYCHOLOGICAL REHABILITATION

Neuropsychologists specialize in the assessment and treatment of neurobehavioral disorders encountered across the lifespan. As treatment providers, neuropsychologists offer invaluable expertise in developing compensatory strategies and identifying resources to help patients cope with disruptions in their daily functioning. Neuropsychological treatments and interventions are ideally created with appreciation of individuals' unique characteristics and needs. Treatment plans aim to accentuate patients' strengths to help them address neurocognitive and behavioral challenges identified by assessment and to maximize coping. Staples of neuropsychological rehabilitation include education and referral, individual and family psychotherapy, support groups, behavior management, cognitive remediation, and job advocacy and planning.

Education and Referral

Research has found that family members of patients with TBI most frequently cited health information as an important need (86). As such, rehabilitation professionals strive to provide reliable and accurate information about TBI to patients, family members, friends, teachers, employers, and other treatment providers. Bibliotherapy is chosen by many professionals to facilitate communication of vital medical knowledge. Patients may also be provided with written material for review and discussion. For example, *Getting Better and Better After Brain Injury: A Guide for Families, Friends, and Caregivers* by Kreutzer and Kolakowsky-Hayner (87) offers pertinent information about consequences of TBI and the recovery process. Rehabilitation specialists may also be called on to provide referral sources along with information about the common manifestations of TBI. Providers of adjunctive therapies are likely to profit from understanding an individual patient's neurobehavioral or cognitive postinjury difficulties.

Patients often demonstrate needs outside the realm of a neuropsychologist's expertise. Treatment providers are encouraged to be mindful of adjunctive treatments that may prove beneficial to patients. Appropriate and timely referrals to alternative treatment professionals are encouraged. The identification of services likely to be helpful to patients is the first step. Rehabilitation professionals may consider patients' abilities and willingness to fully participate and make use of additional treatments. Examples of adjunctive services include substance abuse treatment, psychotropic medication, vocational rehabilitation, clubhouse programs, support groups, or comprehensive driver's evaluation.

Individual Psychotherapy

Individual Psychotherapy With Traumatic Brain Injury Survivors

Psychotherapy is considered an essential component of holistic treatment for patients with TBI by many rehabilitation professionals (88–91). Qualified neuropsychologists play a vital role in providing psychotherapy for patients with TBI (89). Individual therapy with both patients and family members is a useful and commonly practiced mode of inpatient and outpatient rehabilitation. Patients may benefit from attending sessions without their family members present for private discussions of personal issues.

Psychotherapy further offers patients the opportunity to learn skills to better cope with dramatic life changes encountered after a TBI. Clinicians and patients with TBI determine mutually acceptable therapy goals to address areas of deficiency. Improving emotional adjustment, communication skills, and symptom management are examples of typical therapy goals. Training in anger or stress management, social skills, and strategies to manage depression or anxiety are therapeutic strategies often employed with patients following a TBI. Individual psychotherapy with TBI survivors often employs a cognitive-behavioral therapy (CBT) framework to achieve these therapeutic goals.

Individual Psychotherapy With Caregivers and/or Family Members

Research supports the need for interventions following TBI for family members (86,90–94). Researchers have found that 9 out of 10 patients are discharged to home after inpatient rehabilitation (53). Family members of patients have an un-

TABLE 60–8 Report Structure and Content

REPORT SECTION	CONTENT OF SECTION
Confidentiality statement	• Include statement indicating that report contents are "strictly confidential" and should not be disseminated or reproduced without the patient's explicit permission
Agency contact information	• Include agency name, complete mailing address, telephone number, fax number.
Demographic information and referral source	• Include patient's name, address, race, marital status, handedness, date of birth, medical record number, age, current medications, date of injury, and referral source.
Presenting problem and reason for referral	• Highlight presenting problems, including injury date, etiology, and injury specifics. • Identify specific referral questions.
Basis of evaluation	• Provide sources of interview information. • Identify records which were reviewed. • Provide checklist of tests administered in the appendices.
Behavioral observations	• Describe behavioral observations during the testing process, including information presented in Table 60-4 (general behavioral observations included in "Behavioral Observations" section and specific test related behaviors included in "Test Results" section).
Current symptoms	• Identify current problems reported by the patient family members. • Include current neurobehavioral symptoms endorsed on the NFI, listing specific items endorsed in a table. • Highlight changes in functioning compared to preinjury.
Historical information	• Include information about the following: • academic/vocational history • family/social history • medical/mental health history and current treatment • preinjury and postinjury substance use • criminal history
Summary of medical records Daily living abilities	• Provide summary of principal medical and mental health records reviewed. • Identify current living situation, daily activities, and ability to perform activities independently and safely (e.g., hygiene, driving, medication compliance, financial management). • Note any postinjury change in living situation, daily activities, and independence. • Highlight judgment and safety issues, with table depicting responses on the Judgment and Safety Screening Inventory.
Test results	• Provide behavioral observations pertaining to approach to testing and reaction to testing. • Note level of motivation and effort. • Estimate preinjury abilities (impaired to high average). • Describe of test performance in each functional area. • Provide table comparing test data to preinjury estimates, prior tests, and normative data. • Provide graphical depictions of selected test results in appendices (e.g., performance across trials on verbal learning tasks, figure depicting MMPI-2 results).
Impressions	• Integrate information from various report sections. • Note and discuss consistencies between various information sources. • Provide diagnostic formulation and support for each diagnosis. • Provide table depicting *DSM-IV* and ICD diagnoses. • Respond to referral questions clearly. • Highlight interactions between cognitive, emotional, neurobehavioral, pain, and medical factors. • Provide conclusions about prognosis for improvement and future academic and vocational functioning.
Recommendations	• Provide practical, feasible recommendations that address cognitive, neurobehavioral, and emotional issues. • Provide recommendations regarding judgment, safety, and daily living activities. • Provide referrals for services which may improve functioning (e.g., medical follow-up, evaluation, therapy, support group).

Abbreviations: *DSM-IV*, Diagnostic and Statistical Manual of Mental Disorders; MMPI-2, Minnesota Multiphasic Personality Inventory-2nd Edition.

derstandably difficult time coping with role changes, increased responsibilities, and stress associated with TBI (e.g., insurance issues, financial strain, and medical appointments). Despite the efforts of rehabilitation staff to prepare families for patients' discharge, many family members report feeling overwhelmed and ill equipped to manage the long-term needs of survivors (95,96).

Most family members do not receive professional emotional support following the TBI of a family member (86). Research on caregiver burden revealed that more than one-third of caregivers endorsed clinically significant levels of depression and anxiety (60). Emotional reactions of families following the brain injury of a loved one may also include intense feelings of anger, blame, and guilt. Reassuring family members that these reactions are normal responses to a tragic event can enhance long-term functioning.

Family interventions not only provide a valuable means for improving emotional support, but also may help with symptom reduction and coping skills enhancement. Some family members receive individual therapy as an adjunct to or as a substitution for family therapy. Neuropsychologists are often proactive in recommending and implementing treatments tailored for the needs of a family or an individual family member.

Family and Couples Intervention

Family therapy provides patients and their families the opportunity to share their feelings of grief, loss, and helplessness in a supportive and understanding environment. Treatment providers also impart information regarding the patients' neurological condition through patient-family education. Information commonly shared with the family includes the effects of brain injury, the process of recovery from TBI, and compensatory strategies. Whole family involvement in the psychoeducation process creates improved likelihood that intervention strategies will be implemented outside of therapy (97).

The family members who attend family therapy vary according to treatment goals. Clinicians trained in marital and family interventions may provide therapy to all members of a household as a method for improving daily family functioning and reducing heightened emotionality. Therapy may also incorporate extended family members to develop an educated and emotionally responsive family support network. Couples who are struggling to adjust to role changes and shifting relationship dynamics may benefit from intervention targeted to improve their relationship.

Marital/couples counseling is an approach often incorporated to improve interfamilial support and enhance quality of life following brain injury. Both survivors and caregiving spouses may struggle to communicate effectively with one another. Intervention strategies include improving communication patterns, enhancing connectivity, clarifying roles and responsibilities, and building on family strengths (98). Additionally, dysfunction in sexuality may be addressed as a component of therapy. Psychosocial treatment approaches are associated with helping survivors and their families cope with postinjury issues, such as impaired sexual performance or disinhibition (99). Readers interested in additional information about families of patients with TBI are referred to Chapter 80 in this book entitled, "Family Assessment and Intervention."

Support Groups

Support groups for survivors of TBI and their family members or friends provide a number of benefits to participants. Community-based support programs offer survivors of brain injury and their family members or friends help in managing a wide range of disability-related stressors. For example, support groups are a source of emotional support, education, and social networking. Participants in peer-oriented groups for survivors report having increased knowledge about TBI, enhanced quality of life, improved general outlook, and better emotional coping (100). Patients and their families often benefit emotionally from the shared experiences of others. Support group members commonly disclose information regarding resources or coping strategies they have found useful in recovering from TBI. People are given the opportunity to extend their social connections within the community through their participation in support groups. Additionally, survivors and caregivers may develop self-confidence and an improved sense of purpose by taking on a mentoring role for new group members (100).

Organizations such as the Brain Injury Association of America, Inc. (BIAA) and affiliated state-based advocacy groups provide referral services and information about local support groups for interested parties. Common objectives of a group for survivors with TBI and/or their family members may include discussing needs of survivors and families, sharing information, identifying local resources, and networking. Rehabilitation specialists are encouraged to maintain familiarity with such organizations and groups in their area and to provide patients and families with contact information and dates and times of local meetings.

Behavior Management

Behavior management is another tool available to treatment professionals for patients demonstrating disruptive or dangerous behavior. Problems such as impulsivity and aggressiveness can greatly interrupt patients' social functioning at work, home, or in treatment facilities. Behavior management strategies are designed to reduce the number of negative or aggressive behaviors displayed by the patient.

Researched and validated behavioral management strategies demonstrating efficacy fall into 3 broad categories: traditional contingency management, positive behavior interventions and supports, and a combination of these 2 approaches (101). Implementation of behavior management plans also often incorporates aspects of cognitive remediation. Regardless of structure, behavioral approaches providing emotional support and maintaining sensitivity to the contextual environment of the patient are recommended (102). Carnavale and colleagues (103,104) advocate for behavior management programs applying individualized behavior modification programs tailored to meet specific behavioral challenges and administered in a patient's natural setting. In addition to the stated benefit of developing skills in the environment in which they will need to be used, application within a home setting promotes whole family involvement in behavior modification strategies. Reduction in caregiver distress and burden has been suggested as a potential added benefit. For more information on behavior management strategies, the readers are referred to Chapter 63 in this book entitled, "Principles of Behavioral Analysis and Modification."

Cognitive Remediation

Direct intervention to address cognitive deficits incurred as a result of a TBI may be obtained through cognitive retraining/remediation (105). Interventions designed to improve cognitive functioning following brain injury are situated in 5 treatment domains: attention/executive functioning, visiospatial, language, memory, and comprehension (106). Meta-analytic review by Rohling and colleagues reveals a small but significant treatment effect for interventions designed to improve cognitive processes. Cicerone et al. (107) reported that therapies for skill acquisition and domain-specific knowledge demonstrate benefit for individuals with moderate-to-severe memory impairments. Research suggests that enhancement of specific skills areas may account for most noted benefits observed from cognitive retraining in such domains as attention (108).

Cognitive rehabilitation typically includes training patients in compensatory strategies to enhance functioning compromised by neurological damage. Patients' strengths and skills are often emphasized in attempts to overcome areas of relative neurocognitive weakness. For example, rehabilitation specialists train patients in the effective use of memory logs, checklists, mnemonic devices, and self-monitoring to compensate for cognitive deficits. Mateer and colleagues (109) suggest that neuropsychologists employing cognitive rehabilitation strategies combine these approaches with interventions designed to address emotionality. The authors indicate that successful integration maximizes treatment effect. For a more thorough coverage of this topic, the readers are referred to Chapter 61 in this book entitled, "Cognitive Rehabilitation."

Job Advocacy and Planning

As TBI frequently occurs to young people in the most productive years of their working lives, employment is an especially important issue (110). A common goal for adults who have experienced a TBI is employment or return to work (111). Following comprehensive assessment, neuropsychologists often advocate for services their patients need to successfully return to work. Specific cognitive skills (i.e., concept formation, cognitive flexibility, and problem solving) are cornerstones of functional recovery and successful rehabilitation (110). These skill sets are often disrupted following TBI, and deficits are identified during assessment.

Persons recovering from brain injury often require additional programs and supports to supplement traditional models of vocational rehabilitation. Wehman and colleagues (112) conducted a study about the efficacy of a supported employment program for survivors of severe brain injury. Findings concluded that helping survivors find financially and socially rewarding jobs and appropriate vocational supports enhances the probability patients will experience a suc-

cessful return to work after a TBI. In another study, Wehman and colleagues (113) investigated the long-term follow-up of persons with TBI after being involved in supported employment. Findings suggested that supported employment was cost-effective for individuals with TBI. A 2005 review of the literature by Wehman et al. (114) summarizes 20 years of findings with respect to TBI and employment. The authors provide a series of recommendations for future research and public policy. For additional information about issues related to vocation following TBI, the readers are referred to Chapter 81 in this book entitled, "Returning to Work."

CONCLUSION

Traditionally, neuropsychologists were involved in quantifying cognitive abilities and endeavoring to localize brain dysfunction. Over the past several decades, however, many neuropsychologists working in rehabilitation settings have expanded their practice to address the diverse and long-term needs of patients with TBI and their family members. With larger numbers of people surviving TBI, neuropsychologists have had an opportunity to play an increasingly vital role within the rehabilitation team. They help with addressing issues relating to behavioral management, emotional adjustment, substance abuse, driving, marital and family functioning, and return to work or school. Undoubtedly, many patients with TBI face long-term difficulties adjusting and returning to productive lives. Neuropsychologists are well qualified to help the patients and their families, and many have chosen to expand their roles far beyond that of a cognitive evaluator.

Future research direction for neuropsychologists in the field of TBI will be focused on the ecological validity of neuropsychological assessment. As the specialty shifts from diagnostic to functional implications and treatment planning, it will be important to develop ecologically valid instruments. Patients want to know how the test results are relevant in their daily functioning and how to incorporate the findings into their everyday life. Instead of providing a list of deficits, neuropsychologists would be able to make practical recommendations to help improve their patient's quality of life. The instruments would also help determine the extent an intervention improves patient's performance on everyday cognitive tasks.

KEY CLINICAL POINTS

1. Comprehensive neuropsychological assessment helps identify cognitive, academic, emotional, and neurobehavioral sequelae post-TBI.
2. Comprehensive neuropsychological assessment also assists in ascertaining etiology and differential diagnosis.
3. A beneficial neuropsychological report that addresses the referral questions and patient's concerns is written without jargons, identifies both strengths and weaknesses, and provides meaningful recommendations.
4. Clinical neuropsychologists play an important role in treatment planning post-TBI.
5. Establishing a baseline with repeat neuropsychological assessments allows the clinicians and patients to track changes over time.

KEY REFERENCES

1. American Psychiatric Association. *Diagnostic and Statistical Manual of Mental Disorders.* 4th ed. Washington, DC: American Psychiatric Press; 2000.
2. Hebben N, Milberg W. Essentials of neuropsychological assessment. 2nd ed. New Jersey: John Wiley & Sons; 2009. Available at: http://books.google.com/books?id=UOrO PZR_tfkC&lpg=PP1&dq=neuropsychological%20assessment&pg=PP1#v=onepage&q&f=false. Accessed 14 March 2012.
3. Lezak MD, Howieson DB, Loring DW, Hannay HJ, Fischer JS. *Neuropsychological Assessment.* 4th ed. New York, NY: Oxford University Press; 2004.
4. Putnam S, Fichtenberg N. Neuropsychological examination of the patient with traumatic brain injury. In: Rosenthal M, Kreutzer J, Griffith E, Pentland B, eds. *Rehabilitation of the Adult and Child With Traumatic Brain Injury.* Philadelphia, PA: FA Davis: 1999:147–166.
5. Strauss E, Sherman E, Spreen O. *A Compendium of Neuropsychological Tests.* 3rd ed. New York, NY: Oxford University Press; 2006.

References

1. Barth JT, Pliskin N, Axelrod B, et al. Introduction to the NAN 2001 definition of a clinical neuropsychologist. NAN Policy and Planning Committee. *Arch Clin Neuropsychol.* 2003;18(5):551–555.
2. Strauss E, Sherman EMS, Spreen O. *A Compendium of Neuropsychological Tests.* 3rd ed. New York, NY: Oxford University Press; 2006.
3. Lezak MD, Howieson DB, Loring DW, Hannay HJ, Fischer JS. *Neuropsychological Assessment.* 4th ed. New York, NY: Oxford University Press; 2004.
4. Putnam S, Fichtenberg N. Neuropsychological examination of the patient with traumatic brain injury. In: Rosenthal M, Kreutzer J, Griffith E, Pentland B, eds. *Rehabilitation of the Adult and Child with Traumatic Brain Injury.* Philadelphia, PA: FA Davis; 1999:147–166.
5. Beck AT, Steer RA, Brown, GK. *BDI-II: Beck Depression Inventory Manual.* 2nd ed. San Antonio, TX: The Psychological Corporation; 1996.
6. Rowland SM, Lam CS, Leahy B. Use of the Beck Depression Inventory-II (BDI-II) with persons with traumatic brain injury: analysis of factorial structure. *Brain Inj.* 2005;19(2):77–83.
7. Derogatis LR. *Brief Symptom Inventory.* Baltimore, MD: Clinical Psychometric Research; 1975.
8. Slaughter J, Johnstone G, Petroski G, Flax J. The usefulness of the Brief Symptom Inventory in the neuropsychology evaluation of traumatic brain injury. *Brain Inj.* 1999;13(2):125–130.
9. Hamilton M. Development of a rating scale for primary depressive illness. *Br J Soc Clin Psychol.* 1967;6(4):278–296.
10. Zigmond A, Snaith RP. The hospital anxiety and depression scale. *Acta Psychiatr Scand.* 1983;67(6):361–370.
11. Campbell MH. The hospital anxiety and depression scale with the irritability-depression-anxiety scale and the Leeds situational anxiety scale. In: Plake B, Impara JC, Spies R, eds. *The Fifteenth Mental Measurements Yearbook.* 2003.
12. Whelan-Goodinson R, Ponsford J, Schonberger M. Validity of the hospital anxiety and depression scale to assess depression and anxiety following traumatic brain injury as compared with the structured clinical interview for DSM-IV. *J Affect Disord.* 2009;114: (1–3)94–102.
13. Butcher JN, Dahlstrom WG, Graham JR, Tellegen A, Kaemmer B. *Minnesota Multiphasic Personality Inventory-2 (MMPI-2): Manual for Administration and Scoring.* Minneapolis, MN: University of Minnesota Press; 1989.
14. Lezak MD, Howieson DB, Loring DW, eds. Tests of personal adjustment and emotional functioning. *Neuropsychological Assessment.* 4th ed. New York, NY: Oxford University Press; 2004:738–754.
15. Tellegen A, Ben-Porath YS. *MMPI-2-RF (Minnesota Multiphasic Personality Inventory-2 Restructured Form): Technical Manual.* Minneapolis, MN: University of Minnesota Press; 2008.
16. Arbisi PA, Polusny MA, Erbes CR, Thuras P, Reddy MK. The Minnesota Multiphasic Personality Inventory-2 Restructured Form in National Guard soldiers screening positive for posttraumatic stress disorder and mild traumatic brain injury. *Psychol Assess.* 2011;23(1): 203–214.
17. Kreutzer J, Seel RT, Marwitz JH. *The Neurobehavioral Functioning Inventory.* San Antonio, TX: Psychological Corporation; 1999.
18. Levin HS, High WM, Goethe KE, et al. The Neurobehavioral Rating Scale: assessment of the behavioral sequelae of head injury by the clinician. *J Neurol Neurosurg Psychiatry.* 1987;50(2):183–193.
19. Witol AD, Kreutzer JS, Sander AM. Emotional, behavioral, and personality assessment after traumatic brain injury. In: Rosenthal M, Griffith ER, Kreutzer JS, Pentland B, eds. *Rehabilitation of the Adult and Child With Traumatic Brain Injury.* Philadelphia, PA: FA Davis; 1999:167–182.
20. Spitzer RL, Kroenke K, Williams JB. Validation and utility of a self-report version of PRIME-MD: the PHQ primary care study. Primary care evaluation of mental health disorders. Patient health questionnaire. *JAMA.* 1999;282(18):1737–1744.
21. Fann JR, Bombardier CH, Dikmen S, et al. Validity of the patient health questionnaire-9 in assessing depression following traumatic brain injury. *J Head Trauma Rehabil.* 2005;20(6):501–511.
22. Demakis GJ, Hammond F, Knotts A, et al. The Personality Assessment Inventory in individuals with traumatic brain injury. *Arch Clin Neuropsychol.* 2007;22(1):123–130.
23. Kurtz JE, Shealy SE, Putnam SH. Another look at paradoxical severity effects in head injury with the Personality Assessment Inventory. *J Pers Assess.* 2007;88(1):66–73.
24. Till C, Christensen BK, Green RE. Use of the Personality Assessment Inventory (PAI) in individuals with traumatic brain injury. *Brain Inj.* 2009;23(7):655–665.
25. First MB, Spitzer RL, Gibbon M, Williams JBW. *Structured Clinical Interview for DSM-IV-TR Axis I Disorders, Clinician Version (SCID-CV).* Washington, DC: American Psychiatric Press; 1996.
26. Hibbard MR, Uysal S, Kepler K, Bogdany J, Silver J. Axis I psychopathology in individuals with traumatic brain injury. *J Head Trauma Rehabil.* 1998;13(4):24–39.
27. Levin HS, Brown SA, Song JX, et al. Depression and posttraumatic stress disorder at three months after mild to moderate traumatic brain injury. *J Clin Exp Neuropsychol.* 2001;23(6):754–769.
28. Rapoport MJ, McCullagh S, Streiner D, Feinstein A. The clinical significance of major depression following mild traumatic brain injury. *Psychosomatics.* 2003;44(1):31–37.
29. Whelan-Goodinson R, Ponsford J, Johnston L, Grant F. Psychiatric disorders following traumatic brain injury: their nature and frequency. *J Head Trauma Rehabil.* 2003;24(5):324–332.
30. Kreutzer JS, Livingston LA, Everley RS, et al. Caregivers' concerns about judgment and safety of patients with brain injury: a preliminary investigation. *PM R.* 2009;1(8):723–728.
31. Kreutzer JS, West DD, Marwitz JH. *Judgment and Safety Screening Inventory: Administration Manual.* Richmond, VA: National Resource Center for Traumatic Brain Injury; 2001.
32. Melzack R. The McGill pain questionnaire: major properties and scoring methods. *Pain.* 1975;1(3):277–299.
33. Huskisson EC. Visual analogue scales. In: Melzack R, ed. *Pain Measurement and Assessment.* New York, NY: Raven Press; 1985:33–37.
34. Hart RP, Martelli MF, Zasler ND. Chronic pain and neuropsychological functioning. *Neuropsychol Rev.* 2000;10(3):131–149.
35. Bush SS, Ruff RM, Tröster AI, et al. Symptom validity assessment: practice issues and medical necessity. *Arch Clin Neuropsychol.* 2005; 20(4):419–426.
36. Heilbronner RL, Sweet JJ, Morgan JE, Larrabee GJ, Millis SR; for Conference Participants. American Academy of Clinical Neuropsychology Consensus Conference statement on the neuropsychological assessment of effort, response bias, and malingering. *Clinical Neuropsychol.* 2009;23(7):1093–1129.
37. Kreutzer J, Harris-Marwitz J, Myers S. Neuropsychological issues in litigation following traumatic brain injury. *Neuropsychology.* 1990;4(4):249–260.

38. Board of Directors, American Academy of Clinical Neuropsychology. American Academy of Clinical Neuropsychology (AACN) practice guidelines for neuropsychological assessment and consultation. *Clin Neuropsychol.* 2007;21(2):209–231.

39. Iverson GL. Ethical issues associated with the assessment of exaggeration, poor effort, and malingering. *Appl Neuropsychol.* 2006; 13(2):77–90.

40. Binder LM. *Portland Digit Recognition Test Manual.* 2nd ed. Portland, OR: Binder LM; 1993.

41. Warrington EK. *Recognition Memory Test Manual.* Windsor, UK: NFER-Nelson; 1984.

42. Tombaugh TN. *Test of Memory Malingering.* Toronto, Canada: Multi-Health Systems, Inc; 1996.

43. Green P, Allen LM, Astner K. *The Word Memory Test: A User's Guide to the Oral and Computer-administered Forms, US Version 1.1.* Durham, NC: CogniSyst; 1996.

44. Nelson NW, Boone K, Dueck A, Wagener L, Lu P, Grills C. Relationship between eight measures of suspect effort. *Clin Neuropsychol.* 2003;17(2):263–272.

45. Rothke SE, Friedman AF, Jaffe AM, et al. Normative data for the F(p) scale of the MMPI-2: implications for clinical and forensic assessment of malingering. *Psychol Assess.* 2000;12(3):335–340.

46. Brooks N, McKinlay W, Symington C, Beattie A, Campsie L. Return to work within the first seven years of severe head injury. *Brain Inj.* 1987;1(1):5–19.

47. Gollaher K, High W, Sherer M, et al. Prediction of employment outcome one to three years following traumatic brain injury. *Brain Inj.* 1998;12(4):255–263.

48. Jacobs HE. The Los Angeles head injury survey: procedures and findings. *Arch Phys Med Rehabil.* 1988;69(6):425–431.

49. Kreutzer JS, Marwitz JH, Walker W, et al. Moderating factors in return to work and job stability after traumatic brain injury. *J Head Trauma Rehabil.* 2003;18(2):128–138.

50. Machamer J, Temkin N, Fraser R, Doctor JN, Dikmen S. Stability of employment after traumatic brain injury. *J Int Neuropsychol Soc.* 2005;11(7):807–816.

51. Gary KW, Arango-Lasprilla JC, Ketchum JM, et al. Racial differences in employment outcome after traumatic brain injury at 1, 2, and 5 years postinjury. *Arch Phys Med Rehabil.* 2009;90(10): 1699–1707.

52. Van Velzen JM, van Bennekom CA, Edelaar MJ, Sluiter JK, Frings-Dresen MH. How many people return to work after acquired brain injury?: a systematic review. *Brain Inj.* 2009;23(6):473–488.

53. Harrison-Felix C, Newton CN, Hall K, Kreutzer J. Descriptive findings from the traumatic brain injury model systems national database. *J Head Trauma Rehabil.* 1996;11(5):1–14.

54. Kreutzer JS, Kolakowsky-Hayner SA, Ripley D, et al. Charges and lengths of stay for acute and inpatient rehabilitation treatment of traumatic brain injury 1990–1996. *Brain Inj.* 2001;15(9):763–774.

55. Gervasio A, Kreutzer J. Kinship and family member's psychological distress after traumatic brain injury: a large sample study. *J Head Trauma Rehabil.* 1997;12(3):14–26.

56. Harris JK, Godfrey HP, Partridge FM, Knight RG. Caregiver depression following traumatic brain injury (TBI): a consequence of adverse effects on family members? *Brain Inj.* 2001;15(3):223–238.

57. Kreutzer JS, Gervasio AH, Camplair PS. Primary caregivers' psychological status and family functioning after traumatic brain injury. *Brain Inj.* 1994;8(3):197–210.

58. Kreutzer JS, Gervasio AH, Camplair PS. Patient correlates of caregivers' distress and family functioning after traumatic brain injury. *Brain Inj.* 1994;8(3):211–230.

59. Livingston MG, Brooks DN, Bond MR. Three months after severe head injury: psychiatric and social impact on relatives. *J Neurol Neurosurg Psychiatry.* 1985;48(9):870–875.

60. Marsh NV, Kersel DA, Havill JH, Sleigh JW. Caregiver burden at 1 year following severe traumatic brain injury. *Brain Inj.* 1988;12(12): 1045–1059.

61. Oddy M, Humphrey M, Uttley D. Subjective impairment and social recovery after closed head injury. *J Neurol Neurosurg Psychiatry.* 1978;41(7):611–616.

62. Panting A, Merry PH. The long term rehabilitation of severe head injuries with particular reference to the need for social and medical support for the patient's family. *Rehabilitation.* 1972;38:33–37.

63. Perlesz A, Kinsella G, Crowe S. Psychological distress and family satisfaction following traumatic brain injury: injured individuals and their primary, secondary, and tertiary carers. *J Head Trauma Rehabil.* 2000;15(3):909–929.

64. Kreutzer JS, Marwitz JH, Godwin EE, Arango-Lasprilla JC. Practical approaches to effective family intervention after brain injury. *J Head Trauma Rehabil.* 2010;25(2):113–120.

65. Bright P, Jaldow E, Kopelman MD. The National Adult Reading Test as a measure of premorbid intelligence: a comparison with estimates derived from demographic variables. *J International Neuropsychol Soc.* 2002;8(6):847–854.

66. Green RE, Melo B, Christensen B, Ngo LA, Monette G, Bradbury C. Measuring premorbid IQ in traumatic brain injury: an examination of the validity of the Wechsler Test of Adult Reading (WTAR). *J Clin Exp Neuropsychol.* 2008;30(2):163–172.

67. Stebbins GT, Wilson RS. Estimation of premorbid intelligence in neurologically impaired individuals. In: Snyder PJ, Nussbaum PD, eds. *Clinical Neuropsychology: A Pocket Handbook for Assessment.* Washington, DC: American Psychological Association; 1998:76–87.

68. Griffin SL, Mindt MR, Rankin EJ, Ritchie AJ, Scott JG. Estimating premorbid intelligence: comparison of traditional and contemporary methods across the intelligence continuum. *Arch Clin Neuropsychol.* 2002;17(5):497–507.

69. Powell BD, Brossart DF, Reynolds CR. Evaluation of the accuracy of two regression-based methods for estimating premorbid IQ. *Arch Clin Neuropsychol.* 2003;18(3):277–292.

70. Draper K, Ponsford J, Schönberger M. Psychosocial and emotional outcomes 10 years following traumatic brain injury. *J Head Trauma Rehabil.* 2007;22(5):278–287.

71. Husson EC, Ribbers GM, Willemse-van Son AHP, Verhagen AP, Stam HJ. Prognosis of six-month functioning after moderate to severe traumatic brain injury: a systematic review of prospective cohort studies. *J Rehabil Med.* 2010;42(5):425–436.

72. Ponsford J, Draper K, Schönberger, M. Functional outcome 10 years after traumatic brain injury: its relationship with demographic, injury severity, and cognitive and emotional status. *J Int Neuropsychol Soc.* 2008;14(2):233–242.

73. Senathi-Raja D, Ponsford J, Schönberger M. Impact of age on long-term cognitive function after traumatic brain injury. *Neuropsychology.* 2010;24(3):336–344.

74. Senathi-Raja D, Ponsford J, Schönberger M. The association of age and time postinjury with long-term emotional outcome following traumatic brain injury. *J Head Trauma Rehabil.* 2010;25(5):330–338.

75. Willemse-van Son AHP, Ribbers GM, Verhagen AP, Stam HJ. Prognostic factors of long-term functioning after traumatic brain injury: a systemic review of prospective cohort studies. *Clin Rehabil.* 2007; 21(11):1024–1037.

76. Willemse-van Son AHP, Ribbers GM, Hop WCJ, Stam HJ. Community integration following moderate to severe traumatic brain injury: a longitudinal investigation. *J Rehabil Med.* 2009;41(7):521–527.

77. American Psychiatric Association. *Diagnostic and Statistical Manual of Mental Disorders.* 4th ed., text rev. Washington, DC: American Psychiatric Press; 2000.

78. Glenn MB. A differential diagnostic approach to the pharmacological treatment of cognitive, behavioral, and affective disorders after traumatic brain injury. *J Head Trauma Rehabil.* 2002;17(4):273–283.

79. First MB, Spitzer RL, Gibbon M, Williams JBW. *Structured Clinical Interview for DSM-IV Axis I Disorders: Clinician Version (SCID-CV).* Washington, DC: American Psychiatric Press; 1997.

80. Whelan-Goodinson R, Ponsford J, Johnston L, Grant F. Psychiatric disorders following traumatic brain injury: their nature and frequency. *J Head Trauma Rehabil.* 2009;24(5):324–332.

81. Rogers JM, Read CA. Psychiatric comorbidity following traumatic brain injury. *Brain Inj.* 2007;21(13–14):1321–1333.

82. Hibbard MR, Uysal S, Kepler K, Bogdany J, Silver J. Axis I pathology in individuals with traumatic brain injury. *J Head Trauma Rehabil.* 1998;13(4):24–39.

83. Golden Z, Golden CJ. Impact of brain injury severity on personality dysfunction. *Int J Neurosci.* 2003;113(5):733–745.

84. Folstein MF, Folstein SE, McHugh PR. "Mini-mental state": a practical method for grading the state of patients for the clinician. *J Psychiatr Res.* 1975;12(3):189–198.

85. Ben-Porath Y, Butcher J, Dahlstrom WG, Graham J, Tellgan A. *Minnesota Multiphasic Personality Inventory-II.* 2nd ed. Minneapolis, MN: University of Minnesota Press; 2001.

86. Kolakowsky-Hayner SA, Miner KD, Kreutzer JS. Long-term life quality and family needs after traumatic brain injury. *J Head Trauma Rehabil.* 2001;16(4):374–385.

87. Kreutzer J, Kolakowsky-Hayner S. *Getting Better (and Better) After Brain Injury: A Guide for Family, Friends, and Caregivers.* Richmond, VA: The National Resource Center for Traumatic Brain Injury; 1999.

88. Butler RW, Satz P. Individual psychotherapy with head injured adults: clinical notes for the practitioner. *Prof Psychol Res Pr.* 1988; 19(5):536–541.

89. Prigatano GP. Psychotherapy after brain injury. In: Prigatano GP, Fordyce DJ, Zeiner HK, Roueche JR, Pepping M, Wood BC, eds. *Neuropsychological Rehabilitation After Brain Injury.* Baltimore, MD: The John Hopkins University Press; 1986:67–95.

90. Prigatano G. Disordered mind, wounded soul: the emerging role of psychotherapy in rehabilitation after brain injury. *J Head Trauma Rehabil.* 1991;6(4):1–10.

91. Prigatano G, Ben-Yishay Y. Psychotherapy and psychotherapeutic interventions in brain injury rehabilitation. In: Rosenthal M, Kreutzer J, Griffith E, Pentland B, eds. *Rehabilitation of the Adult and Child With Traumatic Brain Injury.* Philadelphia, PA: FA Davis: 1999: 271–282.

92. Moules S, Chandler BJ. A study of the health and social needs of carers of traumatically brain injured individuals served by one community rehabilitation team. *Brain Inj.* 1999;13(12):983–993.

93. Serio CD, Kreutzer JS, Gervasio AH. Predicting family needs after brain injury: implications for intervention. *J Head Trauma Rehabil.* 1998;10(2):32–45.

94. Rotondi AJ, Sinkule J, Spring M. An interactive web-based intervention for persons with TBI and their families: use and evaluation by female significant others. *J Head Trauma Rehabil.* 2005;20(2): 173–185.

95. Hall KM, Karzmark P, Stevens M, Englander J, O'Hare P, Wright J. Family stressors in traumatic brain injury: a two-year follow-up. *Arch Phys Med Rehabil.* 1994;75(8):876–884.

96. Gillen R, Tennen H, Affleck G, Steinpreis R. Distress, depressive symptoms, and depressive disorder among caregivers of patients with brain injury. *J Head Trauma Rehabil.* 1998;13(3):31–43.

97. McFarlane W, Dixon L, Lukens E, Lucksted A. Family psychoeducation and schizophrenia: a review of the literature. *J Marital Fam Ther.* 2003;29(2),223–245.

98. Walsh F. *Strengthening Family Resilience.* 2nd ed. New York, NY: Guilford Press; 2006.

99. Dombrowski LK, Petrick JD, Strauss D. Rehabilitation treatment of sexuality issues due to acquired brain injury. *Rehabil Psychol.* 2000;45(3):299–309.

100. Hibbard M, Cantor J, Charatz H, et al. Peer support in the community: initial findings of mentoring program for individuals with traumatic brain injury and their families. *J Head Trauma Rehabil.* 2002;17(2):112–131.

101. Ylvisaker M, Turkstra L, Coehlo C, et al. Behavioural interventions for children and adults with behaviour disorders after TBI: a systematic review of the evidence. *Brain Inj.* 2007;21(8):769–805.

102. Ylvisaker M, Jacobs H, Feeney T. Positive supports for people who experience behavioral and cognitive disability after brain injury: a review. *J Head Trauma Rehabil.* 2003;18(1):7–32.

103. Carnevale G, Anselmi V, Johnston M, Busichio K, Walsh V. A natural setting behavior management program for persons with acquired brain injury: a randomized controlled trial. *Arch Phys Med Rehabil.* 2006;87(10):1289–1297.

104. Carnevale G, Anselmi V, Busichio K, Millis S. Changes in ratings of caregiver burden following a community-based behavior management program for persons with traumatic brain injury. *J Head Trauma Rehabil.* 2002;17(2):83–95.

105. Sohlberg M, Mateer C. *Introduction to Cognitive Rehabilitation.* New York, NY: Guilford Press; 1989.

106. Rohling M, Faust M, Beverly B, Demakis G. Effectiveness of cognitive rehabilitation following acquired brain injury: a meta-analytic re-examination of Cicerone et al.'s (2000, 2005) systematic reviews. *Neuropsychology.* 2009;23(1):20–39.

107. Cicerone K, Dahlberg C, Kalmar K, et al. Evidence-based cognitive rehabilitation: recommendations for clinical practice. *Arch Phys Med Rehabil.* 2000;81(12):1596–1615.

108. Park NW, Ingles JL. Effectiveness of attention rehabilitation after acquired brain injury: a meta-analysis. *Neuropsychology.* 2001;15(2): 199–210.

109. Mateer CA, Sira CS, O'Connell ME. Putting Humpty Dumpty together again: the importance of integrating cognitive and emotional interventions. *J Head Trauma Rehabil.* 2005;20(1):62–75.

110. Doninger N, Heinemann A, Bode R, Sokol K, Corrigan J, Moore D. Predicting community integration following traumatic brain injury with health and cognitive status measures. *Rehabil Psychol.* 2003; 48(2):67–76.

111. Vandiver V, Johnson J, Christofero-Snider C. Supporting employment for adults with acquired brain injury: a conceptual model. *J Head Trauma Rehabil.* 2003;18(5):457–463.

112. Wehman P, West M, Kregel J, Sherron P, Kreutzer J. Return to work for persons with severe traumatic brain injury: a data-based approach to program development. *J Head Trauma Rehabil.* 1995; 10(1):27–39.

113. Wehman P, Kregel J, Keyser-Marcus L, et al. Supported employment for persons with traumatic brain injury: a preliminary investigation of long-term follow-up costs and program efficiency. *Arch Phys Med Rehabil.* 2003;84(2):192–196.

114. Wehman P, Targett P, West M, Kregel J. Productive employment for persons with traumatic brain injury: what have we learned after 20 years? *J Head Trauma Rehabil.* 2005;20(2):115–127.

Cognitive Rehabilitation

Keith D. Cicerone

INTRODUCTION

Cognitive impairments are often the most persistent and prominent sequelae of brain injury in patients with moderate or good neurologic recovery. Interventions designed to promote the recovery of cognitive functioning and reduce cognitive disability are an integral aspect of brain injury rehabilitation programs after traumatic brain injury (TBI) (1). Despite this, as many as 80% of persons who have sustained a TBI believe that their need to improve their cognition had not been met at 1 year postinjury (2). The growth in clinical services directed at the rehabilitation of cognitive impairments has recently been matched by efforts to establish the empirical basis for cognitive rehabilitation (3). This chapter is intended to integrate some of the clinical issues involved in the remediation of cognitive impairments after TBI, with a discussion of the empirical literature. The discussion of the literature relies primarily on studies that provide evidence for the "best available practices" in cognitive rehabilitation but includes some discussion of clinically important or innovative therapies.

RECOVERY OF NEUROCOGNITIVE FUNCTIONS

In a seminal text on the *Restoration of Function after Brain Injury*, Luria (4) described several different mechanisms to support the reorganization of higher cortical functions after brain injuries. This description rests on the distinction between the 2 meanings of "function." The concept of function may be used to refer to the specific activity performed by a tissue or organ; however, in relation to the physiology of higher nervous activity and the psychology of higher cognitive processes, function refers to a complex adaptive activity consisting of a group of multistage representations, which are organized in a dynamic relationship, and directed toward performance of a particular task. This conceptualization of function might be better described as a "functional system," similar to the current concept of distributed cortical networks (5). A fundamental characteristic of a functional system is that different processes may be used to carry out a given task under different conditions, a property which increases the adaptability of higher cognitive functions. The mechanisms for recovery of function follow a similar evolution from simple to complex. In cases of damage to the primary cerebral areas serving sensory and motor functioning, reorganization after injury may take place through (a) the

ability of intrasystemic processes to take over role of damaged tissue, and (b) the intact influence of higher cortical centers on lower levels of function. At the highest levels of cerebral functional systems, recovery takes place through a process of intersystemic reorganization, which may include completely different components that formerly served widely different functions.

Luria (4) was eloquent in relating these principles of recovery to specific methods of rehabilitation. He also identified several factors considered to moderate recovery, such as the extent of neurologic damage and the developmental level and premorbid integrity of the disturbed function. One of the principle factors determining the success of restoration of higher cognitive functioning is the patient's level of motivation (or "capacity for mental tension") because recovery at this level requires active, effortful, and conscious compensation.

The neurological mechanisms underlying recovery have continued to receive attention with several attempts to apply these principles to neurorehabilitation (6,7). However, few interventions for cognitive impairment after TBI have been derived explicitly from such principles. For example, the therapeutic approach can be "bottom-up," based on the sequential building from elementary to complex skills, or "top-down" via the application of superordinate controls over subordinate processes. There is a tendency to associate "plasticity-based cognitive rehabilitation" with direct stimulation, drill, and practice on tasks, which is expected to foster the redistribution of functional activations (8) although with little direct evidence for this. In contrast, there is considerable evidence that remediation alters activation in frontal association cortices, associated with a qualitative shift, or functional reorganization, of the "strategic" cognitive processes associated with task performance (8,9). Perhaps most importantly, neuroplasticity neither appear to be a passive process nor is it associated with sensory experience alone, but it is highly use-dependent and requires active feedback and learning (10).

Process-Specific Remediation

Skill-specific or process-specific models of cognitive remediation assume that specific interventions can impact differentially on component neurocognitive deficits (see Eslinger et al., this volume). Sohlberg and Mateer (11) developed an influential, process-specific approach to cognitive rehabilitation in which treatments are directed, in highly targeted manner, at specific cognitive areas. The process-specific approach is based on the assumption that direct retraining of specific cognitive processes, through multiple repeated trials of stimulation and activation of the targeted cognitive process, can lead to the reorganization of higher level neurologic and cognitive processes. Treatments are provided in accordance with a hierarchical model of cognitive functioning from lower to higher components of cognitive functioning to provide continuous stimulation and activation of the cognitive process. It is assumed that improvements in functioning at the process-specific level will generalize to tasks that contain similar cognitive requirements, and eventually to improvements in everyday functioning.

Gordon and colleagues (12) also combined specific, well-controlled training procedures in basic scanning, somatosensory stimulation and size estimation, and visual-spatial organization into a comprehensive perceptual remediation program. The training program was effective in promoting improvement on psychometric measures closely related to the training areas. Limited generalization of improvements to measures not specifically related to the training tasks occurred, although the investigators noted more time spent in recreational reading after treatment.

Functional Skills Training

Functional skills training concentrates on the patient's ability in domain-specific, context-specific areas of functioning and the retraining of "competencies of daily life" (13) rather than the putative underlying deficits. Mayer et al. (13) suggested several approaches to training, such as (*a*) repetition of a whole skill in a natural context (e.g., drinking from a cup during breakfast), (*b*) training of component parts (e.g., looking for the cup, reaching, grasping, etc.) followed by whole-skill training, and (*c*) various attempts to substitute new procedures to perform the desired activity. Although conceptualizing behavior and presumable interventions according to a hierarchy of preskills, individual skills, and routine and activity patterns, this approach did not consider the cognitive task attributes distinct from the functional skills being trained. Following Tsvetkova's (14) notion of retraining within the context of a broader function, they suggest that the remediation of cognitive impairments should not address specific components through training exercises in memory, attention, reasoning, and so on but to address these impairments only in so far as they are embedded within functional activities (see Toglia and Golisz, this volume).

Although the work of Glisky and Schacter (15) is derived from neurocognitive-oriented work on spared memory abilities after brain injury, their training approach is very functionally oriented in its emphasis on the acquisition of domain-specific knowledge by patients with impaired memory. They used a method of "vanishing cues" to teach 4 patients with brain injury and amnesia computer-related vocabulary words. Consistent with a functional approach, the training was intended to provide the patients with specific knowledge in an area important to the patient's everyday lives (computer terms) rather than produce general improvements in memory function. Glisky and Schacter (15) suggested that the same procedure might be applied toward the acquisition of complex forms of knowledge by patients with brain injury, as well as the possibility of training patients to become expert in specific, defined content areas. In each of these functional approaches, the patient is trained on the same task that he or she is expected to perform in the context of daily activities, and training is specific to that situation. Generalization to other related situations is not expected as a consequence of the initial training. Thus, the necessity of training a wide range and number of specialized, context-specific skills and routines is characteristic of the functional model.

Metacognitive Remediation

Metacognition refers to the subjective knowledge and experience of one's own cognitive processes, which can be used to guide cognitive activity (16). Metacognitive training therefore places its major emphasis on increasing awareness of deficits, self-monitoring of errors, and self-regulation to improve the ability to independently recognize or anticipate the need for compensatory strategies and use those strategies in the appropriate situations. Shallice's (17) neuropsychological model distinguishes between the cognitive levels of *processing structures* and 2 levels of *cognitive control*. Processing structures consist of special-purpose cognitive subsystems such as object recognition, semantic comprehension, spatial orientation, and so on that can be analyzed by fractionation of the subsystems into the involved components. These cognitive subsystems can also be organized into relatively invariant functional routines or schema, such as eating breakfast or driving home from work. *Routine* control of activity is accomplished through relatively automatic and rapid selection of habitual schemata and the inhibition of weaker competing schemata. However, an additional level of voluntary, strategic, and *nonroutine* control is required when planning is required, when the correction of unexpected errors is required, when the required response is novel or not well-learned, or when habitual responses need to be inhibited. Reliance on the underlying assumption that patients will be able to develop sufficient awareness and insight to apply strategies in various situations is a distinctive aspect of the metacognitive approach.

Crosson et al. (18) has distinguished between intellectual, emergent, and anticipatory levels of awareness after brain injury. Different degrees of compensation may be available to patients depending on their degree of awareness deficit. For example, patients with marked deficits of intellectual awareness may require external, task-specific compensation, whereas patients with minimal awareness deficits may compensate by recognition or anticipation of problems while moving from 1 environment to another several times in the course of their daily functioning. (see Table 61-1)

REMEDIATION OF SPECIFIC AREAS OF IMPAIRMENT

Remediation of Attention Deficits

Various components of attention have been identified and related to different cerebral networks. Posner and Rothbart (19) identified 3 different attention networks. The posterior

TABLE 61-1 Empirically Supported Interventions for Cognitive Impairment After Traumatic Brain Injury

AREA OF INTERVENTION	INTERVENTION APPROACH	EMPIRICALLY SUPPORTED INTERVENTIONS	REFERENCES
Attention	Direct attention training	Attention process training	Sohlberg et al., 2000 Tiersky et al., 2005
		Working memory training	Cicerone, 2002 Serino et al., 2007
Memory	Compensatory memory training	Various mnemonic techniques	Ryan and Ruff, 1988 Berg et al., 1991 Thickpenny-Davis and Barker-Collow, 2007
		Visual imagery mnemonics	Kaschel et al., 2002
Attention Memory Executive functioning	External aides	Memory notebook	Schmitter-Edgecome et al., 1995 Ownsworth and McFarland, 1999 Sohlberg and Mateer, 1989
		External cuing	Wilson et al., 2005 Evans et al., 2003 Kime and Lamb, 1996
Executive functioning Social pragmatics	Social communication skills training	Social communication skills training groups	Dahlberg et al., 2007
Attention Memory Executive functioning Social pragmatics	Metacognitive regulation	Self-instructional training	Fasotti et al., 2000 Ownsworth and McFarland, 1999
		Error management training	Cheng et al., 2006 Goverover et al., 2007 Ehlhardt et al., 2005 Ownsworth et al., 2000 Ownsworth et al., 2006
		Problem solving training	Rath et al., 2003 Levine et al., 2000 Cicerone et al., 2008
		Emotional regulation training	Rath et al., 2003 Cicerone et al., 2008 Medd and Tate, 2000
Attention Memory Executive functioning Social pragmatics	Comprehensive–holistic neuropsychological rehabilitation	Integrated use of individual and group cognitive, psychological, and functional interventions	Cicerone et al., 2008 Rattok et al., 1992 Sarajuri et al., 2005 Goranson et al., 2003

attention network involves the parietal cortex, pulvinar and reticular thalamic nuclei, and superior colliculus and is involved in orienting to and locating sensory stimuli in space. The anterior attention network involves the anterior cingulate gyrus and supplementary motor area and appears active in the detection and selection of target stimuli and inhibition of responses to irrelevant stimuli. Although selectivity may occur on an automatic or unconscious level, situations that are novel or complex will require conscious and strategic control over attention. The vigilance network involves the locus coeruleus and brainstem reticular connections with cerebral cortex, especially lateral frontal cortex. This system may be responsible for maintaining alertness and vigilance. Whyte (20) also reviewed evidence suggesting that attention was not a single cognitive process controlled by a focal brain region and indicated that the neural control of attention was mediated by various structures including the brainstem, subcortical structures, and cerebral cortex, which interact in a richly interconnected network. Whyte (20) suggested that the distribution of attention across this dense neural network had 2 important clinical implications. First, he suggested that different brain lesions could produce qualitatively different attention deficits because of disruption of distinct aspects of the attentional network. Second, lesions to different brain regions could produce similar attentional impairments because of the distributed and integrative nature of the attentional system. The effectiveness of remedial interventions would, in principle, depend on providing treatment directed at the precise nature of the attentional deficit.

Impairments of attention are common after TBI and include reductions of processing speed, difficulty sustaining the focus of attention (e.g., maintaining concentration or a train of thought), and limitations in the ability to regulate the allocation of attention in complex situations (e.g., shifting attention to multiple speakers or between several ongoing tasks). Therefore it is not surprising that some of the earliest formal attempts at cognitive remediation after TBI were directed at deficits of attention. In an early study of attention process training (APT), Sohlberg and Mateer (21) provided the training to 4 patients and compared it with training for visual perceptual abilities using a multiple baseline across subjects design. The patients were all at least 1 year, and up to 6 years, after injury, so it is likely that their deficits were stable. All 4 subjects demonstrated gains on a single attentional-outcome measure following APT, but not after the visual perceptual treatment.

A controlled study of APT (22) used a randomized crossover design to compare APT with a "placebo" condition that consisted of education and support. The 14 patients with acquired brain injury were again all at least 1 year postinjury, ranging as far as 22 years postinjury. Most of the patients had sustained severe TBI including positive neuroimaging, and they all exhibited impairments of attention on neuropsychological evaluation and subjective report by the participant and/or a significant other. The APT tasks were again administered in accordance with a hierarchical approach, although the training exercises were selected for each of the patients based on their specific profiles of attention deficits. Treatment effects in this study were evaluated on a range of outcome measures, including neuropsychological measures intended to reflect specific components of attention, standardized questionnaires, and structured interviews. Significant benefits of APT, compared with therapeutic support, were most apparent in patients' self-reported changes in attention and memory functioning. Improvements in cognitive functioning on neuropsychological measures intended to assess the anterior attentional network for the regulation of attention (but not measures of spatial orienting or vigilance) were also greater following APT, and paralleled the patients' self-reports of improved functioning. The specificity of improvements on an aspect of attention related to the regulation of attention and relationship of these improvements to patients' subjective improvements in their daily functioning argues against the interpretation that the benefits of treatment were caused either by generalized stimulation or task-specific practice effects. These findings also suggest that the benefits of training are caused by patients' improved ability to control their attention, rather than restoration of more basic attentional processes.

A more recent, controlled study (23) investigated the effectiveness of APT as part of a program of cognitive remediation and cognitive-behavioral psychotherapy for participants with persisting complaints after mild or moderate TBI. The cognitive remediation consisted of direct attention training along with training in use of a memory notebook and problem-solving strategies. Cognitive-behavioral therapy was used to increase coping behaviors and reduce stress. Unlike the earlier study, this study combined APT with compensatory strategy training and psychotherapeutic treatment. Although it is therefore not a pure test of APT, it is representative of clinical practice. Participants demonstrated improved performance on a measure of complex attention and reduced emotional distress compared with a wait-list control group, although there was no effect on community integration. This study supports the beneficial effects of APT when incorporated with metacognitive strategy training.

Metacognitive strategy training has served as the basis for an intervention that was intended specifically to teach patients with TBI to compensate for the experience of "information overload" because of their slowed information processing during the performance of daily tasks (24,25). Twenty-two patients with TBI, most of whom were more than 6 months postinjury, received either Time Pressure Management (TPM) training or generic instructions to improve their concentration. The TPM was intended to increase patients' awareness of errors and use of strategies to manage demands under distracting conditions that were likely to be encountered in their everyday lives. Participants receiving TPM showed significantly greater use of self-management strategies during task performance, particularly on more complex tasks that allowed them to adjust their approach to the task but not on basic reaction time tasks in which such a strategy could not be applied. Similar beneficial effects have been demonstrated for TPM on mental slowness following a stroke (26).

Difficulties with multitasking and attending to more than 1 thing at a time are common after TBI. Couillet and colleagues (27) conducted a randomized controlled trial (RCT) to evaluate a rehabilitation program for divided attention after severe TBI, compared with nonspecific cognitive exercises that did not incorporate divided attention demands. The objective was to train patients to perform 2 concurrent tasks simultaneously. Each of the 2 tasks was first trained as a single task, then both tasks were given simultaneously. A progressive hierarchy of task difficulty was used by increasing time pressure and/or executive demands and/or working memory load based on each patient's individual improvement. The experimental treatment produced beneficial effects specific to measures of divided attention and patients' ratings of divided attention difficulties in their everyday functioning.

Patients with mild TBI often complain of difficulties with the more complex aspects of attention, and are likely to exhibit selective impairments of attention functioning in the context of generally intact cognitive functioning (see Iverson and Zasler, Zasler and Iverson, this volume). One small, observational study (28) has evaluated the effectiveness of an intervention intended to improve "working attention" in 4 patients with mild TBI compared with 4 patients who did not receive treatment. The intervention emphasized the use of strategies to allocate attention resources and manage the rate of information during task performance. The patients receiving attention treatment demonstrated "clinically significant gains" on objective measures of attention and significant reductions of self-reported attentional difficulties in their daily functioning.

Overall, these studies suggest that significant benefits can be obtained by patients with attentional difficulties during the postacute period of recovery from TBI. Gains on objective measures of attention are related to subjective improvements in patients' everyday functioning. Finally, these benefits appear to be related to patients' abilities to apply compensatory strategies in their daily functioning, even for relatively basic deficits such as reduced processing speed, rather than by restoration of the underlying attention processes. The evidence for generalized, functional improvements in attention functioning after treatment in the previously cited studies rests primarily on patients' subjective report. However, 1 single-subject study has reported beneficial effects of an intervention intended to facilitate control over attention during functional activities, such as decreasing the frequency of lapses in attention while the patient was reading novels and texts (29).

Remediation of Memory Deficits

Memory complaints are ubiquitous after brain injury. However, the memory difficulties seen after TBI typically do not reflect a classic amnesic disorder. Instead, memory difficulties are likely to be caused by several different factors, and are unlikely to represent a unitary deficit. For example, attention deficits such as distractibility or slowed processing are commonly believed to cause impairments in the acquisition of information, and executive impairments may cause memory failures because of the failure to adequately organize material or initiate efficient memory retrieval processes (30).

One of the first descriptions of remediation for memory deficits after brain injury (31) presented 2 case studies on the use of semantic elaboration and visual imagery techniques to improve the encoding of information. After the effectiveness of these techniques was demonstrated in the laboratory, they were applied to the patient's presenting problem of reduced academic performance. The success of treatment was assessed by the patient's improved subjective ratings of her memory functioning and reduction of negative self-statements, and her ability to remain in her academic classes with less subjective difficulty. Review of her academic performance suggested that she was able to apply the procedure in her everyday life, although the effects were not as great as were seen in the laboratory situation.

Ryan and Ruff (32) examined the general effectiveness of compensatory memory remediation by combining several strategies for improving verbal and nonverbal memory capacities in a comprehensive remediation program. Treatment was provided to 10 patients with TBI who exhibited persistent mild to moderate memory deficits. Interventions included instruction and practice in the use of rehearsal, elaborative semantic encoding, and associative strategies, imagery construction, "personalized emotional techniques," external memory strategies, and group education and practice with the various memory compensations. Individualized cuing procedures were developed for each patient and practiced on a daily basis. Control patients participated in recreational activities and psychosocial support.

At the completion of the treatment, both groups demonstrated significant improvement on memory measures, without any apparent specific benefits from the specialized memory remediation program. Subsequent analysis did suggest that the patients with relatively milder cognitive deficits showed greater benefit from the memory remediation strategies, whereas those with moderate residual impairments did not benefit from treatment. This study is important for several reasons. First, the treatment more closely resembled a multidimensional, clinical protocol than in many experimental studies. Second, the study evaluated the differential effectiveness of treatment in relation to the severity of cognitive impairment. Finally, the study provided an explicit comparison between active, specialized memory remediation and a nonspecific intervention.

Kaschel and colleagues (33) conducted a prospective, controlled study of a visual imagery technique for the rehabilitation of participants with mild memory impairment after acquired brain injury. The intervention consisted of a standardized imagery-acquisition procedure to promote imagery-generation, overlearning, and automatization, and included an individually tailored training period directed at the transfer of the strategy to everyday relevant materials. Visual imagery was compared with "pragmatic memory training" that included practical guidelines to improve memory and the use of notebooks and calendars. Twenty-four patients with TBI had initially been referred for memory rehabilitation, and memory problems were considered to be of primary importance, although patients with severe memory impairment were excluded. Significant improvement was apparent only for the imagery condition on the recall of verbal material, consistent with the expected effects of treatment. The improvements associated with visual imagery training were paralleled by positive changes in relatives' ratings of patients' memory functioning and were maintained at 3-month follow-up.

Another RCT (34) has specifically compared "repetitive drill and practice" on memory tasks with training in cognitive strategies to improve memory functioning after TBI. Cognitive strategies to improve memory functioning were explained, demonstrated, and practiced 3 times a week for 6 weeks, and patients received daily homework stressing the importance of application of memory strategies in everyday life. Intervention was highly individualized, with the specific memory problems selected for training based on the subjects' report of difficulties experienced in their daily functioning. Patients in both the strategy training and "drill and practice" groups reported subjective improvements in memory functioning but significant effects on objective memory performance could only be demonstrated in the strategy training group, and this difference was maintained at 4-month follow-up.

In a follow-up study 4 years after the initial training (35), subjective memory and objective memory performance were the same for both patient groups and equivalent to a no-treatment brain injury control group (and still well lower than the level of normal control subjects). Of note, several subjects in the strategy training group showed a decline in their performance, whereas the "pseudotreatment" group showed continued, significant improvements despite the fact that patients were between 5 and 25 years postinjury at the time of follow-up. In contrast with this study, Wilson (36) evaluated 26 patients with traumatic head injury who had been referred for memory therapy 5 to 10 years earlier. On standardized memory testing, most patients remained stable and 8 patients showed improved performance. It was noted that many subjects were using more memory aids and strategies at the time of follow-up assessment than they were at the completion of their initial memory rehabilitation, which may have accounted for the positive findings (37).

Prospective Memory

The ability to remember to do something at some future time, referred to as prospective memory, appears to be one of the most common memory problems for patients with acquired brain injury (38). Prospective memory interventions may be based on modifications of other memory interventions, such as space-retrieval and distributed practice techniques or use of elaborative encoding strategies. A series of case studies (39,40) described a specific prospective memory training procedure in 5 patients with severe TBI.

Training consisted of giving the patients simple, repetitive, 1-step prospective memory tasks to be carried out at increasingly longer time intervals following instructions, ranging from 2 to 10 minutes. The patients all improved with practice on the prospective memory tasks, with some evidence of improvement on neuropsychological measures and observations of daily memory functioning. However, the limited time between the assignment of tasks and their execution, lack of intervening or complex tasks, and degree of therapist control all limit the relevance of the training to real-life demands.

Errorless Learning

A preliminary study suggested that errorless learning can be used to teach compensatory strategies for specific memory problems, such as taking medications at mealtime or keeping keys in a consistent location (41). In a subsequent controlled study (42), adults with chronic TBI were trained to use compensatory strategies for personally relevant memory problems through errorless learning or didactic strategy instruction. Participant trained with errorless learning reported greater use of strategies after training, with limited generalization of strategy use. There was no difference between treatments in generalized strategy use or frequency of memory problems reported by participants or caregivers.

These studies support potential benefits of errorless learning for treatment for teaching new knowledge, including knowledge of compensatory strategies, to people with severe memory deficits resulting from TBI. Errorless learning techniques appear to be effective for teaching specific information and procedures to patients with mild executive disturbance as well as memory impairment, but the presence of severe executive dysfunction may limit effectiveness of this form of memory rehabilitation (43).

External Memory Compensations

Patients with memory impairments after TBI are commonly taught to use a memory notebook or diary to compensate for their difficulties in spontaneous or unassisted recall of information. One RCT (44) has compared notebook training with supportive therapy for 8 patients with TBI, all more than 2 years postinjury. The treatment consisted of teaching a specific protocol for use of a memory notebook, and individualized modifications to address the subjects' personal needs and application to novel settings. Patients who received the notebook training reported fewer observed everyday memory failures than the supportive therapy subjects. Three of the subjects who received the memory remediation were still actively using the memory notebook to assist with their daily activities at 6-month follow-up. In this study, and in the studies described earlier using some form of strategy training, the patients who benefited from treatment all exhibited relatively mild memory difficulties. In contrast, patients with severe memory deficits after TBI appear more likely to require training in the use of specific compensations that can be applied to specific tasks, rather than attempts to remediate their underlying memory deficits through the use of strategies. For example, the use of a memory notebook has been shown to be superior to verbal rehearsal strategies when patients are required to remember specific information, particularly for patients with more severe memory impairments (45).

Although external memory compensations such as memory notebooks are commonly employed in cognitive rehabilitation, patients with severe memory difficulties are likely to require an extended period of training to ensure the practical application of a memory notebook (46,47).

External Cuing and Environmental Compensations

In the last several years, there has been increased development of external cuing and assistive technologies as a compensation for memory impairments after TBI. For example, 3 studies have described the use and effectiveness of a portable voice organizer to help patients to recall their therapy goals (48) or to prospectively remember to perform relevant everyday tasks (49,50). The use of existing technologies to assist people with memory deficits will typically require additional training, and consideration of multiple factors that influence the selection of an external cuing system (e.g., the patient's cognitive strengths and weaknesses, knowledge and familiarity with specific technologies, and the necessary resources and "user friendliness" to support programming and maintenance of the assistive device) (51,52).

Several assistive devices have been developed specifically with the intent of improving the cognitive functioning of people with acquired neurocognitive impairments, such as the "Essential Steps" cognitive orthotic system (53), the ISAAC cognitive prosthetic system (54), and the NeuroPage paging service (55–57). Initial evidence for the effectiveness of these systems is limited to descriptive case studies (53–55). More recently, Wilson and colleagues (56) examined the results for 63 people with chronic TBI with memory and/or planning problems. A randomized crossover design was used to examine the impact of pager use on successful achievement of target behaviors. Results demonstrated significantly increased task behavior in each group when using the pager, indicating that the paging system was effective in reducing everyday memory and planning problems experienced by individuals with TBI.

Fish and colleagues (57) analyzed the effectiveness of this same paging system for 36 participants with stroke. As with participants with TBI, introduction of the paging system produced immediate benefits in compensating for memory and planning deficits. Unlike participants with TBI, the behavior of participants with stroke returned to baseline levels after removal of the pager. Further analyses suggested that maintenance of treatment benefits was associated with executive functioning, and the participants with stroke had poorer executive functioning.

Along these same lines, promising results have also been obtained suggesting that the use of a simple "content-free" alerting system can improve patients' prospective memory and attention to task. (58,59)

Remediation for Deficits in Executive Functioning

Disturbances in executive functioning are prevalent after acquired brain injury and represent significant obstacles to social functioning, work, and rehabilitation. Disorders of executive functioning may affect the ability to anticipate the effects of our actions, appreciate alternative perspectives, and to recognize other people's reactions to our behavior and modify our actions accordingly. Disturbances of executive functioning may be apparent after various types of cortical or subcortical damage, but are often associated with damage to the frontal lobes. The dorsolateral frontal cortex has extensive connections with polysensory posterior association areas (60) and appears to be related to deficits in complex discrimination and association (61). The medial prefrontal cortex has been implicated in the processes of motor initiation and motor regulation and also appears to play a role in tasks requiring complex attention and planning (60). The orbitofrontal cortex is part of paralimbic cortex (60) and has been related to disturbances of complex social and emotional behavior in humans (62,63).

Patients with frontal lobe damage may exhibit dissociation between the relative preservation of verbal knowledge and the failure of this knowledge to guide behavior in pursuit of the appropriate goals and actions. This tendency to disregard the requirements of a given task, even when these are verbally appreciated, represented a fundamental aspect of executive dysfunction, referred to as *goal neglect* (64). Levine and his colleagues (65) developed a formalized intervention for executive dysfunction referred to as goal management training (GMT) based on the theory of goal neglect. The process of GMT involves 5 discrete stages of what is essentially a general purpose, problem-solving algorithm starting with an evaluation of the relevant goals in a situation, through the selection of subgoals, and then monitoring the results of one's attempts at a solution; in the event of a mismatch, the entire process is repeated. Thirty patients with mild-to-severe TBI were randomly assigned to receive either GMT or an alternative treatment of motor skills training. GMT consisted of a single session in which participants were instructed to apply the problem-solving algorithm to 2 functional tasks. Patients in the motor skills training condition practiced reading and tracing mirror-reversed text and designs. Treatment effectiveness was assessed on several paper-and-pencil tasks that resembled the training tasks and were intended to simulate the kind of unstructured everyday situations, which might elicit goal management deficits. Participants who received GMT demonstrated significant reduction in errors and prolonged time to task completion (presumably reflecting increased care and attention to the tasks) on 2 of the 3 outcome measures following the intervention. The entire treatment in this study consisted of a 1 hour intervention, which may be adequate to suggest the potential efficacy of GMT but provides little evidence of its clinical effectiveness.

Another prospective randomized controlled study (66) used a problem-solving intervention intended to facilitate patients' ability to reduce the complexity of a multistage problem by breaking it down into manageable subgoals. Training was provided 37 patients who were identified as poor problem solvers on formal tests of planning and response regulation. Twenty participants received an intervention directed at remediation of executive function deficits, whereas 17 participants received an alternative intervention consisting of memory retraining. Patients who received the problem-solving training demonstrated significant gains on neuropsychological measures of planning ability as well as improvement on behavioral ratings of executive dysfunction, such as awareness of cognitive deficits, goal-directed ideas, and problem-solving ability.

Rath and his colleagues (67) evaluated the effectiveness of an "innovative" treatment for problems-solving deficits compared with a "conventional" neuropsychological group treatment for patients with TBI. The patients were described as being "higher functioning" but with documented, persistent impairments in social and vocational functioning (e.g., job loss, marital difficulties) with an average of 4 years postinjury. The conventional treatment consisted of group exercises intended to improve cognitive skills and provide support for coping with emotional reactions and changes after injury. The innovative problem-solving intervention focused on the development of emotional self-regulation strategies as the basis for maintaining an effective problem-orientation, along with a "clear thinking" component that included training in problem-solving skills using role-plays of real-life examples of problem situations. Both groups showed significant improvement of their memory functioning after treatment. Only the problem-solving group treatment resulted in significant beneficial effects on measures of executive functioning, self-appraisal of "clear thinking," self-appraisal of emotional self-regulation, and objective observer ratings of interpersonal problem solving behaviors in naturalistic simulations.

These 3 randomized controlled studies demonstrate that training patients with TBI to use formal problem-solving methods can be an effective intervention. The study by Rath et al. (67) suggests that the development of strategies to improve emotional self-regulation may be particularly relevant to the clinical treatment of patients with executive functioning deficits after TBI, and provides the clearest evidence that this intervention may improve patients' performance in everyday situations.

Several studies have attempted to remediate executive function impairments through the development and internalization of strategies for effective self-regulation. According to Luria (68), self-regulation is achieved through the covert, verbal mediation ("inner speech") of purposeful activity. However, simply having the patient repeat the task instruction is insufficient to reestablish self-regulation (69). Cicerone and Wood (70) used a self-instructional training procedure to encourage planning and self-monitoring while inhibiting inappropriate behaviors. The training procedure included 3 stages of self-verbalization, progressing from overt verbalization, through faded verbal self-instruction, to covert verbal mediation of appropriate responses. Over the course of training, there was a dramatic reduction in task-related errors as well as more gradual reduction and eventual cessation of off-task behaviors. Generalization to his functional, real-life behaviors were observed only with additional instruction and practice in the application and self-monitoring of the verbal mediation strategy to his everyday behaviors. A subsequent study (71) replicated this finding with 6 patients who exhibited impaired planning and self-monitoring after frontal lobe injury. Five of the 6 patients showed marked reduction of task-related errors and perseverative responses suggesting that the effectiveness of training was related to the patients' improved ability to inhibit inappropriate responses.

There also is continued evidence that the incorporation of interventions that include training in metacognitive strategies can facilitate the treatment of attention (24–26,72), memory (43,73–75), language deficits (76), and social skills (77,78) after TBI or stroke.

There is a potential paradox in attempts to remediate disorders of executive functioning in that these disorders affect the processes of self-monitoring and self-regulation that are an inherent aspect of remedial compensations. Successful compensation appears to require some residual capacity to deliberately and consciously apply strategies. Two controlled studies (79,80) have compared interventions protocols that were specifically developed to address patients' poor awareness and self-regulation skills during performance of functional tasks, compared with conventional occupational therapies, after TBI or stroke.

In 1 of these studies (80), the awareness-training protocol incorporated feedback to increase participants' awareness of their abilities, with experiential exercises requiring participants to predict, self-monitor, and self-evaluate their performance. Improvements in awareness, performance of instrumental activities of daily living (IADL), and overall function were evident for both groups. The awareness intervention was associated with greater increase in self-awareness of deficits after treatment but not with better performance of IADLs. The other study (79) employed self-awareness and verbal self-regulation strategies during performance of IADL tasks. Participants were asked to define their performance goals, predict task performance, anticipate difficulties, select a strategy to circumvent difficulties, assess the amount of assistance required to successfully perform the task, and self-evaluate performance. Participants who received conventional treatment performed the same IADL tasks as the treatment group without the awareness intervention. Participants who received the awareness intervention demonstrated significant improvements in self-regulation skills and cognitive aspects of IADL performance compared with participants receiving conventional therapy, whose performance either did not improve or declined.

A single-group study (81) of patients with documented frontal lobe damage, severe cognitive impairments, and poor self-awareness has demonstrated improvements after 4 months of treatment in patients' knowledge and use of self-regulatory strategies and the self-rated effectiveness of strategies in their daily functioning. Several case studies have also described interventions that improved the patients' ability to self-monitor their behavior (82,83). In each of these studies, the goal of cognitive remediation was not the training of task-specific performance but the training and internalization of regulatory cognitive processes. In contrast, limited success was observed in 2 descriptive case studies of patients with orbitofrontal damage that resulted in social cognition and affective regulation. In both cases, the patients were able to improve specific behaviors in the situations in which they had been trained but could not effectively modify their problematic social and emotional responses in novel, real-life situations, despite extensive treatment (84,85).

Remediation of Pragmatic Communication Deficits

Deficits in executive functioning may be expressed as a disturbance of the social, affective, and pragmatic aspects of communication. Thus, although classic neurologic syndromes of language impairment are not commonly seen after TBI, patients with TBI frequently exhibit impairments of pragmatic communication. These may include the loss of coherence and cohesiveness during narrative discourse, difficulty interpreting subtle, contextual aspects of communica-

tion (e.g., humor, sarcasm, irony), and failure to interpret or respond to nonverbal cues in the context of social communications (see Coelho, this volume).

Dahlberg and colleagues (86) investigated the efficacy of social communication skills training for people who had sustained a TBI at least 1 year earlier. A group of patients who received the social skills training were compared with a matched group of patients as wait-list control participants. Social skills training incorporated pragmatic language skills, social behaviors, and cognitive abilities required for successful social interactions. Between-group analyses demonstrated a significant treatment effect on 7 of 10 scales on the Profile of Functional Impairment in Communication and on the Social Communication Skills questionnaire, as well as improved quality of life at 6-month follow-up. Another study (78) has investigated social communication skills training among 51 participants with acquired brain injury, predominantly TBI, who were at least 12 months postinjury and residing in the community. Participants received either social skills training, an equivalent amount of group social activities (e.g., cooking, board games), or no treatment. The social skills training was devoted to pragmatic communication behaviors (listening, starting a conversation) and social perception of emotions and social inferences along with psychotherapy for emotional adjustment. Social communication skills training produced significant improvement in participants' ability to adapt to the social context of conversations compared with both control conditions. A subsequent study compared errorless learning and self-instructional training strategies for treating emotion perception deficits (77). Both interventions resulted in modest improvements in judging facial expressions and drawing social inferences, with some advantage for self-instructional training.

Several uncontrolled group studies (87,88) and single-case studies (89,90) have reported improved pragmatics and conversational skills following treatment that included systematic feedback and self-monitoring of interpersonal communications. The focus of the group-based treatment was to improve patients' communication competence in social contexts, including initiation, topic maintenance, turn taking, and active listening. Within each of these skill areas, treatment addressed the subjects' awareness of obstacles to effective communication, practice of effective communication, and generalization to natural contexts. The goal of the generalization phase was to apply the trained skills to relevant activities and settings in each individual's particular community, incorporating practice with parents and peers (72).

INTENSIVE-HOLISTIC COGNITIVE REHABILITATION

Cognitive rehabilitation of TBI may best be achieved through a comprehensive, *holistic* approach to the treatment of cognitive, emotional, and functional impairments and disability (see Malec, this volume). Comprehensive-holistic neuropsychological rehabilitation is centered around the goals of fostering patients' awareness of their functional potential and adapting to the chronic limitations imposed by their injury to alleviate disability in everyday, social functioning. Ben-Yishay was perhaps the first clinician to delineate and advocate the need for a holistic approach to the neuropsychological rehabilitation of individuals with brain injury (91). In discussing the rationale for the holistic or therapeutic milieu approach to neuropsychological rehabilitation, Ben-Yishay and Gold (92) emphasized that the neurobehavioral manifestations after TBI are dynamic and multidetermined. They suggest that "it is meaningless to make rigid distinctions between higher- and lower-level cognitive functions or between physiogenic and psychogenic factors in emotional disturbances" after brain injury (p. 194). Thus, neither isolated cognitive remedial exercises to improve attention, memory, and/or other "fragmentary" deficits nor a focus exclusively on traditional psychotherapeutic interventions are likely to be effective. Instead, an effective rehabilitation program must systematically integrate interventions directed at the remediation of cognitive deficits, functional skills, and interpersonal functions. Improvements in functioning are typically accomplished by an improvement in the effective functional application of residual cognitive abilities rather than restoration of the underlying cognitive deficits, per se.

An early study of the relationship between holistic cognitive rehabilitation and employability (93) evaluated the effectiveness of a clinical program consisting of 3 phases. The first phase consisted of individual modules of cognitive remediation and group treatments to improve interpersonal communication, social competence, and awareness and acceptance of the consequences of brain injury. Treatment was provided within the model of a "therapeutic community" which included the engagement of family members and significant others in the treatment process. The second phase of treatment was devoted to structured work trials, and the third stage involved actual work placements. Employability ratings suggested that 84% of the previously unemployed patients were able to engage in some form of productive activity following the neuropsychological rehabilitation program. A subsequent study (94) suggested that patient characteristics related to motivation, affective regulation, and accurate self-appraisal were more closely related to effective functioning after treatment than neurologic or neuropsychological characteristics.

The relative contributions of individualized cognitive remedial interventions and small-group based exercises in interpersonal communication within the context of a holistic neuropsychological rehabilitation program have been explicitly evaluated (95). One group of patients received a mixture of cognitive and interpersonal interventions. A second group of patients received the individualized cognitive remedial interventions but did not receive interpersonal communication training. The third group received the initial, basic attentional training followed by the interpersonal remediation, whereas the individualized cognitive interventions were withheld. Only the 2 groups receiving the individualized cognitive remediation showed improvement on near transfer measures of cognitive functioning, which may have reflected practice effects as these measures were similar to the tasks used in treatment. There was a tendency for patients receiving the interpersonal training to show improvement on measures of affect regulation, self-appraisal, and self-esteem. These findings are consistent with the holistic approach to treatment, indicating that the greatest gains in functioning may be achieved through the integrated treatment of both cognitive and interpersonal functioning.

Cicerone and colleagues (96) conducted an RCT to evaluate the effectiveness of comprehensive-holistic neuropsychological rehabilitation compared with standard, multidisciplinary rehabilitation for 68 participants with TBI. Most participants (88%) had sustained moderate or severe TBI and more than half were more than 1 year postinjury. Standard neurorehabilitation consisted primarily of individual, discipline specific therapies (physical therapy [PT], occupational therapy [OT], and speech therapy [ST]) along with 1 hour of individual cognitive rehabilitation. The holistic neuropsychological intervention included individual and group therapies that emphasized metacognitive and emotional regulation for cognitive deficits, emotional difficulties, interpersonal behaviors, and functional skills. Neuropsychological functioning improved in both conditions, but the holistic neuropsychological rehabilitation produced greater improvements in community functioning and productivity, self-efficacy, and life satisfaction. In an earlier nonrandomized study comparing these interventions for clinical referrals (97), participants receiving comprehensive-holistic rehabilitation were twice as likely to make clinically significant gains in community functioning than those receiving conventional rehabilitation, despite being more severely disabled and further postinjury. Several additional observational studies of comprehensive-holistic rehabilitation have demonstrated reductions in symptoms, improvements in community functioning, and better quality of life compared with conventional treatment (98) or no treatment (99,100).

These clinical studies support the effectiveness of a programmatic approach to cognitive rehabilitation for people with TBI, including those who have been unable to resume effective functioning several years after injury.

CONCLUSION

Cognitive rehabilitation is an integral part of the neurorehabilitation of TBI. Recent increases in our understanding of adult neuroplasticiy have raised hope regarding the potential to remediate cognitive deficits after acquired brain injury but have not yet been translated into clinical interventions. Changes in functional activation and structural connectivity appear to reflect the "strategic" reorganization of cognitive aspects of task performance (see Ricker et al., this volume). In light of these findings, we need to consider the roles of practice, feedback, learning, and metacognitive regulation in designing our clinical intervention.

Most studies of interventions for specific cognitive functions have been limited to assessing the effectiveness of treatment at the impairment level, although several recent studies have demonstrated clinically meaningful improvements in community integration following comprehensive-holistic cognitive rehabilitation. In clinical practice, there is general consensus that cognitive rehabilitation (regardless of the specific approach taken) should be directed at improving patients' everyday functioning and quality of life. This will require that these interventions be assessed with an appropriate range of relevant health-outcome measures (e.g., functional limitations, community integration, subjective well-being).

Efforts to provide patients with the best available treatment, and to evaluate the effectiveness of cognitive rehabilitation, need to consider the complex nature of the interventions, the heterogeneity of patients with TBI, and the need to individualize treatment according to the unique and varied demands of patients' lives (see Kreutzer et al.; Ponsford et al.; Malec; this volume). For these reasons, the practice of cognitive rehabilitation will continue to rely on clinical judgment and experience. Cognitive rehabilitation is not a distinct form of service, or the purview of any single discipline, but a specialized form of rehabilitation that requires adequate professional training in the nature of brain-behavior relationships, the neurologic basis of intact and impaired cognitive function, and the rehabilitation of cognitive disorders. It is also essential for clinicians who practice cognitive rehabilitation to maintain their knowledge of the literature and the empirical basis for the effectiveness of interventions as a means of guiding treatment selection and implementation. The increasing emphasis on evidence-based (cognitive) rehabilitation is not intended to supplant clinical judgment but to inform it through the best available scientific evidence.

From a scientific perspective, the evaluation of the effectiveness of cognitive rehabilitation is, of course, a continuous and ongoing process (Wagner, Hart, and Maas, this volume). There continues to be some debate regarding the most appropriate methodology for conducting research on cognitive rehabilitation. Well-designed single-case studies can provide important information, especially regarding novel or innovative interventions. Highly controlled clinical trials remain the surest way to subject an intervention to rigorous confirmation of its efficacy. The selection of an appropriate research methodology will depend on multiple considerations, including the state of the already existing evidence, the ability to standardize the intervention across subjects or settings, and the availability of resources required to conduct the study. Perhaps the most compelling need in this area is the establishment of sustained programs of research that develop and evaluate the effectiveness and utility of an intervention through increasingly rigorous and practical methods, including the replication of findings across settings. It is only through a sustained program of research that cognitive rehabilitation will fulfill its clinical and scientific promise to improve the quality of lives for people with neurocognitive disability.

KEY CLINICAL POINTS

1. The "best practice" of cognitive rehabilitation relies on a theoretical model of neurocognitive function, understanding the neurologic mechanisms of recovery, a conceptual approach to interventions, and use of empirically supported treatments.
2. The remediation of attention deficits should rely on a combination of direct attention training and metacognitive (compensatory) strategy training.
3. The approach to remediation of memory deficits (internal compensations vs external aides) should be based on the severity of the patient's memory deficits as well as the presence of other cognitive problems (e.g., executive dysfunction).
4. The remediation of executive functioning should incorporate metacognitive strategy training (awareness, self-monitoring, and self-regulation), formal problem-solving intervention, and strategies for emotional regulation.

5. The treatment of cognitive-communication deficits after TBI should include social skills training that addresses pragmatic language skills, social behaviors, and cognitive abilities required for successful social interactions.
6. Whether provided through individual therapy or a comprehensive multidisciplinary program, the cognitive rehabilitation of TBI should relay on a holistic approach to the treatment of cognitive, emotional, and functional impairments and disability.
7. Cognitive rehabilitation (regardless of the specific approach taken) should be directed at improving patients' everyday functioning and quality of life. The "ecological validity" of cognitive rehabilitation relies on therapists' active attempts at instruction that illustrates and promotes the application of strategies in patients' daily lives.

KEY REFERENCES

1. Cicerone KD, Mott T, Azulay J, et al. A randomized controlled trial of holistic neuropsychologic rehabilitation after traumatic brain injury. *Arch Phys Med Rehabil.* 2008; 89:2239–2249.
2. Dahlberg CA, Cusick CP, Hawley LA, et al. Treatment efficacy of social communication skills training after traumatic brain injury: a randomized treatment and deferred treatment controlled trial. *Arch Phys Med Rehabil.* 2007;88: 1561–1573.
3. Kaschel R, Della Sala S, Cantagallo A, Fahlbock A, Laaksonen R, Kazen M. Imagery mnemonics for the rehabilitation of memory: a randomised group controlled trial. *Neuropsych Rehab.* 2002;12:127–153.
4. Rath JF, Simon D, Langenbahn DM, Sherr RL, Diller L. Group treatment of problem-solving deficits in outpatients with traumatic brain injury: a randomized outcome study. *Neuropsychol Rehabil.* 2003;13:461–488.
5. Sohlberg MM, Mateer CA. Training use of compensatory memory books: a three stage behavioral approach. *J Clin Exp Neuropsychol.* 1989;11:871–891.
6. Sohlberg MM, McLaughlin KA, Pavese A, Heidrich A, Posner MI. Evaluation of attention process training and brain injury education in persons with acquired brain injury. *J Clin Exp Neuropsychol.* 2000;22:656–6762.
7. Winkens I, Van Heugten CM, Wade DT, Fasotti L. Training patients in time pressure management, a cognitive strategy for mental slowness. *Clin Rehabil.* 2009;23:79–90.

References

1. Mazmanian PE, Kreutzer JS, Devany CW, Martin KO. A survey of accredited and other rehabilitation facilities: education, training and cognitive rehabilitation in brain-injury programmes. *Brain Inj.* 1993;7:319–331.
2. Corrigan JD, Whiteneck G, Mellick MA. Perceived needs following traumatic brain injury. *J Head Trauma Rehabil.* 2004;19:205–216.
3. Cicerone KD, Dahlberg C, Kalmar K, et al. Evidence-based cognitive rehabilitation: recommendations for clinical practice. *Arch Phys Med Rehab.* 2000;81:1596–1615.
4. Lura AR. *Restoration of Function after Brain Injury.* Oxford, NY: Pergamon Press; 1963.
5. Mesulam MM. *Principles of Behavioral and Cognitive Neurology.* 2nd ed. New York, NY: Oxford University Press; 2000.
6. Roberson IH, Murre JM. Rehabilitation of brain damage: brain plasticity and principles of guided recovery. *Psych Bull.* 1999;125: 544–575.

7. Bach-y-Rita P. Theoretical basis for brain plasticity after a TBI. *Brain Inj.* 2003;17(8):643–651.

8. Kelly C, Foxe JJ, Garavan H. Patterns of normal brain plasticity after practice and their implications for neurorehabilitation. *Arch Phys Med Rehabil.* 2006;87(12)(suppl 2):S20–S29.

9. Strangman G, O'Neil-Pirozzi TM, Burke D, et al. Functional neuroimaging and cognitive rehabilitation for people with traumatic brain injury. *Am J Phys Med Rehabil.* 2005;84:62–75.

10. Blake DT, Heiser MA, Caywood M, Merxenich MM. Experience-dependent adult cortical plasticity requires cognitive association between sensation and reward. *Neuron.* 2006;52:371–381.

11. Sohlberg MM, Mateer CA. *Introduction to Cognitive Rehabilitation: Theory and Practice.* New York, NY: Guilford Press; 1989.

12. Gordon WA, Hibbard MR, Egelko S, et al. Perceptual remediation in patients with right brain damage: a comprehensive program. *Arch Phys Med Rehabil.* 1985;66:353–359.

13. Mayer NH, Keating DJ, Rapp D. Skills, routines and activity patterns of daily living: a functional nested approach. In: Uzzell B, Gross Y, eds. *Clinical Neuropsychology of Intervention.* Boston, MA: Martinus Nijhoff; 1986:205–222.

14. Tsvetkova LS. Basic principles of a theory of reeducation of brain-injured patients. *J Spec Educ.* 1972;6:135–144.

15. Glisky EL, Schacter DL. Acquisition of domain-specific knowledge in organic amnesia: training for computer-related work. *Neuropsychologia.* 1987;25:893–906.

16. Flavell JH. Metacognition and cognitive monitoring: a new area of psychological inquiry. *Am Psychol.* 1979;34:906–911.

17. Shallice T. Neurologic impairment of cognitive processes. *Br Med Bull.* 1981;37:187–192.

18. Crosson B, Barco PP, Velozo CA, et al. Awareness and compensation in post-acute head injury rehabilitation. *J Head Trauma Rehabil.* 1989;4(3),46–54.

19. Posner MI, Rothbart MK. Attentional mechanisms and conscious experience. In: AD Milner, MD Rugg, eds. *The Neuropsychology of Consciousness.* New York, NY: Academic Press; 1992:91–111.

20. Whyte J. Neurologic disorders of attention and arousal: assessment and treatment. *Arch Phys Med Rehabil.*1992;73:1094–1103.

21. Sohlberg MM, Mateer CA. Effectiveness of an attentional training program. *J Clin Exp Neuropsychol.* 1987;9:117–130.

22. Sohlberg MM, McLaughlin KA, Pavese A, Heidrich A, Posner MI. Evaluation of attention process training and brain injury education in persons with acquired brain injury. *J Clin Exp Neuropsychol.* 2000; 22:656–676.

23. Tiersky LA, Anselmi V, Johnston MV, et al. A trial of neuropsychologic rehabilitation in mild-spectrum traumatic brain injury. *Arch Phys Med Rehabil.* 2005;86:1565–1574.

24. Fasotti L, Kovacs F, Eling PATM, Brouwer WH. Time pressure management as a compensatory strategy training after closed head injury. *Neuropsychol Rehabil.* 2000;10:47–65.

25. Winkens I, Van Heugten CM, Wade DT, Fasotti L. Training patients in time pressure management, a cognitive strategy for mental slowness. *Clin Rehabil.* 2009;23:79–90.

26. Winkens I, Van Heugten CM, Wade DT, Habets EJ, Fasotti L. Efficacy of time pressure management in stroke patients with slowed information processing: a randomized controlled trial. *Arch Phys Med Rehabil.* 2009;90:1672–1679.

27. Couillet J, Soury S, Lebornec G, et al. Rehabilitation of divided attention after severe traumatic brain injury: a randomized trial. *Neuropsychol Rehabil.* 2010;20:321–339.

28. Cicerone KD. Remediation of "working attention" in mild traumatic brain injury. *Brain Inj.* 2002;16:185–195.

29. Wilson B, Robertson IH. A home based intervention for attentional slips during reading following head injury: a single case study. *Neuropsychol Rehabil.* 1992;2:193–205.

30. DeLuca J, Schultheis MT, Madigan NK, Christodoulou C, Aver-ill A. Acquisition versus retrieval deficits in traumatic brain injury: implications for memory rehabilitation. *Arch Phys Med Rehabil.* 2000;81:1327–1333.

31. Glasgow RE, Zeiss RA, Barrera M, Lewinsohn PM. Case studies on remediating memory deficits in brain damaged individuals. *J Clin Psychol.* 1977;33:1049–1054.

32. Ryan TV, Ruff RM. The efficacy of structured memory retraining in a group comparison of head trauma patients. *Arch Clin Neuropsychol.* 1988;3:165–179.

33. Kaschel R, Della Sala S, Cantagallo A, Fahlbock A, Laaksonen R, Kazen M. Imagery mnemonics for the rehabilitation of memory: a randomised group controlled trial. *Neuropsychol Rehabil.* 2002;12: 127–153.

34. Berg I, Konning-Haanstra M, Deelman B. Long term effects of memory rehabilitation. A controlled study. *Neuropsychol Rehabil.* 1991;1:97–111.

35. Milders MV, Berg IJ, Deelman BG. Four-year follow-up of a controlled memory training study in closed head injured patients. *Neuropsychol Rehabil .*1995;5:223–238.

36. Wilson B. Recovery and compensatory strategies in head injured memory impaired people several years after insult. *J Neurol Neurosurg Psychiatry.* 1992;55:177–180.

37. Evans JJ, Wilson B, Needhan P, Brentnall S. Who makes good use of memory aids? Results of a survey of people with acquired brain injury. *J Int Neuropsych Soc.* 2003;9:925–935.

38. Mateer CA, Sohlberg MM, Crinean J. Perceptions of memory function in individuals with closed head injury. *J Head Trauma Rehabil.* 1987;2(3):74–84.

39. Sohlberg MM, White W, Evans E, Mateer C. An investigation of the effects of prospective memory training. *Brain Inj.* 1992;6:139–154.

40. Raskin SA, Sohlberg MM. The efficacy of prospective memory training in two adults with brain injury. *J Head Trauma Rehabil.* 1996;11(3):32–51.

41. Melton AK, Bourgeois MS. Training compensatory memory strategies via the telephone for persons with TBI. *Aphasiology.* 2005;19: 353–364.

42. Bourgeois MS, Lenius K, Turkstra L, Camp C. The effects of cognitive teletherapy on reported everyday memory behaviors of persons with chronic traumatic brain injury. *Brain Inj.* 2007;21: 1245–1257.

43. Pitel AL, Beaunieux H, Lebaron N, Joyeux F, Desgranges B, Eustache F. Two case studies in the application of errorless learning techniques in memory impaired patients with additional executive deficits. *Brain Inj.* 2006;20:1099–1100.

44. Schmitter-Edgecombe M, Fahy J, Whelan J, Long C. Memory remediation after severe closed head injury. Notebook training versus supportive therapy. *J Consult Clin Psychol.* 1995;63:484–489.

45. Zencius A, Wesolowski MD, Burke WH. A comparison of four memory strategies with traumatically brain-injured clients. *Brain Inj.* 1990;4:33–38.

46. Burke J, Danick J, Bemis B, Durgin C. A process approach to memory book training for neurological patients. *Brain Inj.* 1994;8:71–81.

47. Sohlberg MM, Mateer CA. Training use of compensatory memory books: a three stage behavioral approach. *J Clin Exp Neuropsychol.* 1989;11:871–891.

48. Hart T, Hawkey K, Whyte J. Use of a portable voice organizer to remember therapy goals in traumatic brain injury rehabilitation: a within-subjects trial. *J Head Trauma Rehabil.* 2002;17:556–570.

49. van den Broek MD, Downes J, Johnson Z, Dayus B, Hilton N. Evaluation of an electronic memory aid in the neuropsychological rehabilitation of prospective memory deficits. *Brain Inj.* 2000;14: 455–452.

50. Yasuda K, Misu T, Beckman B, Watanabe O, Ozawa Y, Nakamura T. Use of an IC recorder as a voice output memory aid for patients with prospective memory impairment. *Neuropsychol Rehabil.* 2002; 12:1155–1166.

51. O'Connel ME, Mateer CA, Kerns KA. Prosthetic systems for addressing problems with initiation: guidelines for selection, training and measuring efficacy. *NeuroRehabilitation.* 2003;18:9–20.

52. LoPresti EL, Mihailidis A, Kirsch N. Assistive technology for cognitive rehabilitation: state of the art. *Neuropsychol Rehabil.* 2004;14: 5–39.

53. Bergman MM. The Essential Steps cognitive orthotic. *NeuroRehabilitation.* 2003;18:31–46.

54. Gorman P, Dayle R, Hood CA, Rumrell L. Effectiveness of the ISAAC cognitive prosthetic system for improving rehabilitation outcomes with neurofunctional impairment. *NeuroRehabilitation.* 2003;18:57–67.

55. Wilson BA, Emslie H, Quirk K, Evans J. George: learning to live independently with NeuroPage. *Rehabil Psychol*. 1999;44:284–296.

56. Wilson BA, Emslie H, Quirk K, Evans J, Watson P. A randomized control trial to evaluate a paging system for people with traumatic brain injury. *Brain Inj*. 2005;19:891–894.

57. Fish J, Manly T, Emslie H, Evans JJ, Wilson BA. Compensatory strategies for acquired disorders of memory and planning: differential effects of a paging system for patients with brain injury of traumatic versus cerebrovascular etiology. *J Neurol Neurosurg Psychiatry*. 2008;79:930–935.

58. Fish J, Evans JJ, Nimmo M, et al. Rehabilitation of executive dysfunction following brain injury: "content-free" cueing improves everyday prospective memory performance. *Neuropsychologia*. 2006;1318–1330.

59 Manly T, Heutink J, Davison B, et al. An electronic knot in the handkerchief: "content free cueing" and the maintenance of attention control. *Neuropsychol Rehabil*. 2004;14:89–116.

60. Barbas H, Pandya DN. Patterns of connections of the prefrontal cortex in the rhesus monkey associated with cortical architecture. In: Levin HS, Eisenberg HM, Benton AL, eds. *Frontal Lobe Function and Dysfunction*. New York, NY: Oxford University Press; 1991: 35–58.

61. Rezai K, Andreasan NC, Alliger R, Cohen G, Swayze V, O'Leary DS. The neuropsychology of the prefrontal cortex. *Arch Neurol*. 1993;50:636–642.

62. Lhermitte F. Human autonomy and the frontal lobes. Part II: patient behavior in complex and social situations: the "environmental dependency syndrome." *Ann Neurol*. 1986;19:335–343.

63. Eslinger PJ, Damasio AR. Severe disturbance of higher cognition after bilateral frontal ablation: patient EVR. *Neurology*. 1985;35: 1731–1741.

64. Duncan J, Emslie H, Williams P, Johnson R, Freer C. Intelligence and the frontal lobe: the organisation of goal-directed behaviour. *Cognit Psychol*. 1996;30:2257–2303.

65. Levine B, Robertson IH, Clare L, et al. Rehabilitation of executive functioning: an experimental-clinical validation of goal management training. *J Int Neuropsychol Soc*. 2000;6(3):299–312.

66. von Cramen DY, Mathesvon Cramen, Mai N. Problem solving deficits in brain injured patients. A therapeutic approach. *Neuropsychol Rehabil*. 1991;1:45–64.

67. Rath JF, Simon D, Langenbahn DM, Sherr RL, Diller L. Group treatment of problem-solving deficits in outpatients with traumatic brain injury: a randomized outcome study. *Neuropsychol Rehabil*. 2003;13:461–488.

68. Luria AR. *Higher Cortical Functions in Man*. New York, NY: Basic Books; 1980.

69. Luria AR, Pribram KH, Homskaya ED. An experimental analysis of the behavioral disturbance produced by a left frontal arachnoidal endothelioma. *Neuropsychologia*. 1964;2:257–280.

70. Cicerone KD, Wood JC. Planning disorder after closed head injury: a case study. *Arch Phys Med Rehabil*. 1987;68:111–115.

71. Cicerone KD, Giacino JT. Remediation of executive function deficits after traumatic brain injury. *NeuroRehabilitation*. 1992;2(3): 12–22.

72. Webster JS, Scott RR. The effects of self-instructional training of attentional deficits following head injury. *Clin Neuropsychol*. 1983; 5:69–74.

73. Ownsworth TL, McFarland K. Memory remediation in long-term acquired brain injury: two approaches in diary training. *Brain Inj*. 1999; 13:605–626.

74. Ehlhardt LA, Sohlberg MM, Glang A, Albin R. TEACH-M: a pilot study evaluating an instructional sequence for persons with impaired memory and executive functions. *Brain Inj*. 2005;19:569–583.

75. McKerracher G, Powell T, Oyebode J. A single case experimental design comparing two memory notebook formats for a man with memory problems caused by traumatic brain injury. *Neuropsychol Rehabil*. 2005;15(2):115–128.

76. Fillingham JK, Sage K, Ralph MAL. Treatment of anomia using errorless versus errorful learning: are frontal executive skills and feedback important? *Int J Lang Comm Dis*. 2005;40:505–523.

77. Bornhofen C, McDonald S. Comparing strategies for treating emotion perception deficits in traumatic brain injury. *J Head Trauma Rehabil*. 2008;23:103–115

78. McDonald S, Tate R, Togher L, et al. Social skills treatment for people with severe, chronic acquired brain injuries: a multicenter trial. *Arch Phys Med Rehabil*. 2008;89:1648–1659.

79. Goverover Y, Johnston MV, Toglia J, DeLuca J. Treatment to improve self-awareness in persons with acquired brain injury. *Brain Inj*. 2007;21:913–923.

80. Cheng SKW, Man DWK. Management of impaired self-awareness in persons with traumatic brain injury. *Brain Inj*. 2006;20:621–628.

81. Ownsworth TL, McFarland K, Young RmcD. Self-awareness and psychosocial functioning following acquired brain injury: an evaluation of a group support programme. *Neuropsychol Rehabil*. 2000; 10:465–484.

82. Sohlberg MM, Sprunk H, Metzelaar K. Efficacy of an external cuing system in an individual with severe frontal lobe damage. *Cog Rehabil*. 1988;6:36–41.

83. Alderman N, Fry RK, Youngson HA. Improvement of self monitoring skills, reduction of behaviour disturbance and the dysexecutive syndrome. *Neuropsychol Rehabil*. 1995;5:193–222.

84. von Cramen DY, Matthes-von Cramen G. Back to work with a chronic dysexecutive syndrome? (A case report). *Neuropsychol Rehabil*. 1994;4:399–417.

85. Cicerone KD, Tanenbaum LN. Disturbance of social cognition after traumatic orbitofrontal brain injury. *Arch Clin Neuropsychol*. 1997; 12:173–188.

86. Dahlberg CA, Cusick CP, Hawley LA, et al. Treatment efficacy of social communication skills training after traumatic brain injury: a randomized treatment and deferred treatment controlled trial. *Arch Phys Med Rehabil*. 2007;88:1561–1573.

87. Wiseman-Hakes C, Stewart ML, Wasserman R, Schuller R. Peer group training of pragmatic skills in adolescents with acquired brain injury. *J Head Trauma Rehabil*. 1998;13(6):23–38.

88. Ehrlich J, Sipes A. Group treatment of communication skills for head trauma patients. *Cognit Rehabil*. 1985;3:32–37.

89. Gajar A, Schloss PJ, Schloss CN, Thompson CK. Effects of feedback and self-monitoring on head trauma youths' conversational skills. *J App Beh Anal*. 1984;17:353–358.

90. Giles GM, Fussey I, Burgess P. The behavioral treatment of verbal interaction skills following severe head injury: a single case study. *Brain Inj*. 1988;2:75–79.

91. Ben-Yishay Y, Rattok J, Lakin P, et al. Neuropsychologic rehabilitation: quest for a holistic approach. *Semin Neurol*. 1985;5:252–259.

92. Ben-Yishay Y, Gold J. Therapeutic milieu approach to neuropsychological rehabilitation. In: Woods RL, ed. *Neurobehavioral Sequelae of Traumatic Brain Injury*. New York, NY: Taylor & Francis; 1990:194–215.

93. Ben-Yishay Y, Silver SM, Piasetsky E, Rattok J. Relationship between employability and vocational outcome after intensive holistic cognitive rehabilitation. *J Head Trauma Rehabil*. 1987;2(1):35–48.

94. Ezrachi O, Ben-Yishay Y, Kay T, Duller L, Rattok J. Predicting employment in traumatic brain injury following neuropsychological rehabilitation. *J Head Trauma Rehabil*. 1991;6(3):71–84.

95. Rattok J, Ben-Yishay Y, Ezrachi O, et al. Outcome of different treatment mixes in a multidimensional neuropsychological rehabilitation program. *Neuropsychology*. 1992;6(4):395–415.

96. Cicerone KD, Mott T, Azulay J, et al. A randomized controlled trial of holistic neuropsychologic rehabilitation after traumatic brain injury. *Arch Phys Med Rehabil*. 2008;89:2239–2249.

97. Cicerone KD, Mott T, Azulay JA, Friel J. Community integration and satisfaction with functioning after intensive cognitive rehabilitation for traumatic brain injury. *Arch Phys Med Rehabil*. 2004;85: 1643–1650.

98. Sarajuuri JM, Kaipio ML, Koskinen SK, et al. Outcome of a comprehensive neurorehabilitation program for patients with traumatic brain injury. *Arch Phys Med Rehabil*. 2005;86:2296–2302.

99. Goranson TE, Graves RE, Allison D, La Freniere R. Community integration following multidisciplinary rehabilitation for traumatic brain injury. *Brain Inj*. 2003;17:759–774.

100. Svendsen HA, Teasdale TW. The influence of neuropsychological rehabilitation on symptomatology and quality of life following brain injury: a controlled long-term follow-up. *Brain Inj*. 2006;20: 1295–1306.

XIV

BEHAVIORAL IMPAIRMENTS

Emotional and Behavioral Sequelae of Traumatic Brain Injury

Thomas W. McAllister

INTRODUCTION

Many functional domains can be altered after a traumatic brain injury (TBI). However, changes in emotional regulation, behavior, and "personality" often cause the most distress to survivors and their family/caregivers (1–9). Changes in these domains can disrupt a survivor's core sense of self, and fundamentally alter how loved ones, friends, and colleagues view the individual. The result can be devastating to all involved and can limit rehabilitation progress, interfere with return to work, and negatively impact achievement of maximum quality of life. The cost in care expenditures, lost productivity, and family disruption is staggering (7).

The overarching theme of this chapter is that understanding the epidemiology, pathophysiology, and clinical presentation of the emotional and behavioral sequelae of TBI is critical to the holistic treatment and rehabilitation of individuals with TBI. Furthermore, the clinical manifestations of these sequelae follow logically from the neuropathophysiology of TBI. Thus it is helpful to examine the emotional and behavioral changes in the context of the neuropathophysiology of TBI in general.

NEUROPATHOPHYSIOLOGY OF EMOTIONAL AND BEHAVIORAL SEQUELAE

Relationship of Structural Injury to Neurobehavioral Sequelae

Much progress has been made in the understanding of the neuropathophysiology of TBI (see 10 and Chapters 11 and 12). Certain aspects are helpful to highlight in that they explain the special vulnerability to neurobehavioral challenges seen in TBI survivors.

In brief, most injuries result from the brain coming into contact with an object (which might include the skull or some external object) or from rapid acceleration or deceleration of the brain. Contact mechanisms often result in damage to scalp, skull, and brain surface (e.g., contusions, lacerations, intracerebral hematomas) (10). Inertial forces generated by rapid acceleration or deceleration of the brain are associated with shear, tensile, and compression forces that have maximum impact on axons and blood vessels resulting in axonal

injury, tissue tears, and intracerebral hematomas. Injury from both mechanisms occurs immediately (referred to as primary injury) and may also evolve over time because of a variety of factors including massive release of neurotransmitters with subsequent triggering of excitotoxic injury cascades, and other injury-related factors such as hypoxia, edema, and elevated intracranial pressure (referred to as secondary injury).

Contact mechanisms tend to produce surface contusions and lacerations where the swirling motion of the brain comes into contact with bony protuberances on the interior of the skull. Frequent sites of such injury are the anterior temporal poles, the lateral and inferior temporal cortices, the frontal poles, and the orbital frontal cortices. Inertial forces produce more widespread injury to white matter. Although referred to as diffuse axonal injury, it is more helpfully viewed as multifocal with particular areas of vulnerability including the corpus callosum, the rostral brainstem, and subfrontal white matter (10).

Secondary injury is initiated by the mechanical distortion of the neurons with resultant widespread release of neurotransmitters including excitatory amino acids such as glutamate. The mechanical disruption and depolarization of neuronal membranes results in an influx of $Ca++$ and other ions into the cell, release of intracellular $Ca++$ stores, and subsequent triggering of several complex cascades (e.g., free radical generation, inflammatory cascades, apoptotic and necrotic cascades) that can damage or kill the cell (see 11–13). Although this probably occurs throughout the brain, the excitotoxic cascades and other forms of secondary injury such as hypoxia/ischemia have a disproportionate effect on certain brain regions such as the hippocampus, even in the context of an otherwise fairly mild injury (14).

Thus the typical profile of injury involves a combination of primary injury (occurs at time of application of force) and secondary injury (evolves over time subsequent to the primary injury) as well as a combination of focal and diffuse injury. Furthermore, certain brain regions are highly vulnerable to injury and account for the challenging behaviors and increased rates of psychiatric illness that are associated with TBI. These include the frontal cortex and subfrontal white matter, the deeper midline structures including the basal ganglia, the rostral brainstem, and the temporal lobes including the hippocampi (see Figure 62-1).

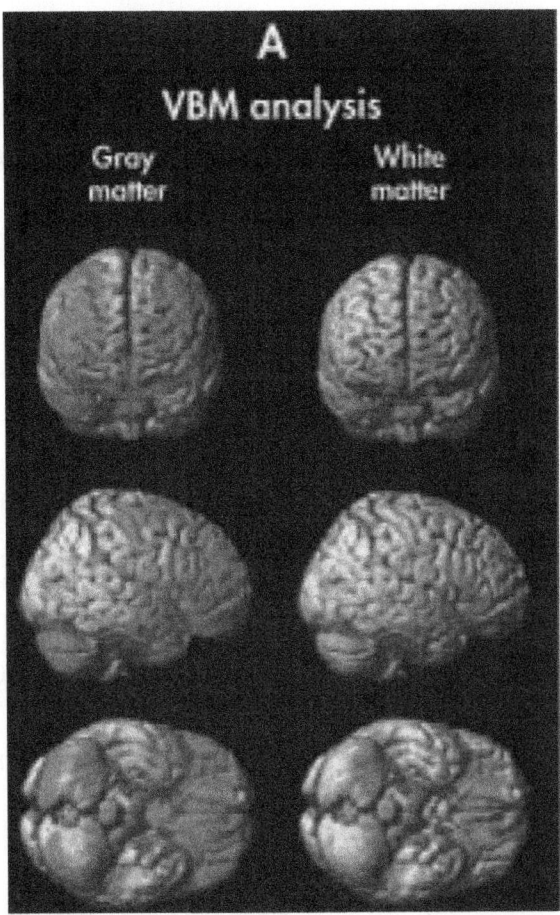

FIGURE 62-1 *See color insert.* Results of voxel-bashed morphometry demonstrating areas of reduced gray and white matter density in individuals with TBI compared to controls. Red areas show frontal and temporal abnormalities. Reprinted from Bigler E. Structural imaging. In: Silver JM, McAllister TW, Yudofsky SC, eds. Textbook of Traumatic Brain Injury. Washington, DC: American Psychiatric Press; 2005:87.

Relationship of Neurotransmitter Change to Neurobehavioral Sequelae

In addition to the profile of regional brain injury described earlier, there is evidence that neurotransmitters with important roles in modulating common neurobehavioral sequelae of TBI (such as regulation of mood, anxiety, motivation, impulse control, and aggression) are altered in TBI. This evidence is briefly summarized to set the stage for rational psychopharmacological interventions for these sequelae (see Chapter 74 for additional details and psychopharmacological applications).

Catecholaminergic System Changes

The catecholaminergic systems (epinephrine, norepinephrine, dopamine) are altered in TBI (15–17). Animal studies suggest that changes in dopamine, norepinephrine, and epinephrine levels can be prolonged after TBI, associated with alterations in catecholaminergic receptors in damaged cortical areas, and can impair catecholaminergic function after trauma (15,18). Administration of certain catecholaminergic

agonists may enhance recovery from brain injury (19–21), even after single doses (19,22–24). Conversely, catecholaminergic *antagonists* can slow rate of recovery from certain types of brain injury (25). Altered catecholaminergic function after TBI is of some interest because the catecholamines play critical roles in behavioral homeostasis including modulation of arousal, cognition, reward behavior, and mood regulation (26–28). Deficits in central adrenergic tone are associated with deficits in arousal, attention, memory, motivated behavior (apathy), and mood regulation. Dopaminergic tone and proper dopamine signaling are particularly important in the modulation of motivated behavior, attention, and working memory (see 17,29, and 30 for reviews).

Cholinergic System Changes

Cerebral cholinergic neurons and their ascending projections are vulnerable to trauma (see 31 for review). Acutely, cholinergic neurons release large amounts of acetylcholine with subsequent long-term reductions in acetylcholine levels (32). The release of acetylcholine at the time of injury may facilitate the excitotoxic cascades. In fact, cholinergic antagonists can be neuroprotective in some models of TBI (see 31 for review). Damage to the nucleus basalis of Meynert, as well as reduced levels of choline acetyltransferase (a marker of cholinergic afferents), have been shown in brain regions vulnerable to trauma in humans who died within several weeks of injury (31,33–35). Postsynaptic muscarinic and nicotinic receptors remained intact (33–35), suggesting cholinergic agonists as a potential point of intervention for cognitive deficits (31). Central cholinergic tone is critical to the modulation of most cognitive and behavioral domains, appearing to facilitate signal to noise ratios. It is of particular importance however with respect to attention and memory (36). Alterations in central cholinergic tone may also play a role in the genesis of mood disorders, particularly depression (see 37).

Serotonergic System Changes

The serotonergic system may also be affected after TBI, although the evidence is less robust than that for catecholamines and acetylcholine. For example, increased levels of serotonin are evident in areas of significant tissue damage associated with TBI, and in association with lowered regional cerebral glucose utilization (10,18,38,39). Central serotonergic tone is important in the modulation of normal mood states and aggression. Medications that increase serotonergic function are effective antidepressants and anxiolytics, and can reduce the frequency and intensity of aggressive behavior.

Circuitry of Altered Emotion and Behavior

The brain regions vulnerable to contact and inertial forces as well as the neurochemical vulnerabilities in TBI have been described. However, the substrate of complex emotional expression and behavior altered by TBI is best understood neither in terms of discrete modules ("this brain region does this" or "this region is the impulse control center") nor as a system in which each transmitter modulates a specific function (e.g., serotonin as the "mood" neurotransmitter or acetylcholine as the "memory" neurotransmitter). Rather it is more helpfully viewed as a carefully orchestrated, overlapping neural circuitry in which a particular behavior is the product of regionally distributed neurons connected to each other by white matter tracts that "communicate", often through complex positive and negative feedback loops employing multiple neurotransmitters. These circuits are not thoroughly understood; however, 3 major circuits that span large areas of frontal-subcortical regions have been identified as playing significant roles in nonmotor forms of behavior (see 40,41 for reviews). The brain regions traversed by these circuits overlap with brain regions vulnerable to TBI, making them of interest in the understanding of emotional and behavioral disturbances after injury.

Each circuit is named for its site of origin in the frontal cortex (e.g., the dorsolateral frontal-subcortical circuit, the lateral orbitofrontal-subcortical circuit, and the anterior cingulate-subcortical circuit) (see Figure 62-2). Each circuit follows a similar path starting from the site of origin in the frontal cortex projecting in sequence to the striatum, the globus pallidus, thalamus, and back to the frontal cortex. Each circuit is thought to be a more or less closed loop with some additional input from other functionally related brain regions. The circuits differ from each other with respect to exact pathways through the key nodal points. Thus, for example, the dorsolateral frontal circuit projects to the dorsal caudate, the lateral orbitofrontal circuit to the ventral caudate, and the anterior cingulate to the medial striatum/nucleus accumbens, respectively. Similar topographic differences can be traced through the global pallidus and the thalamus as well.

Damage to the dorsolateral prefrontal circuit impairs executive functions such as working memory, decision making, problem solving, and mental flexibility. Damage to the lateral orbitofrontal cortex and related circuitry impacts intuitive, reflexive, social behaviors, and the capacity to self-monitor and self-correct in real time within a social context. Damage to anterior cingulate and related circuitry impairs motivated and reward-related behaviors. Injury to medial temporal regions further impairs other aspects of memory and the smooth integration of emotional memory with current experience and real-time assessment of stimulus salience. In short, the profile of injury vulnerability predicts the neuropsychiatric sequelae of injury (see Figure 62-3).

Summary

Several cortical regions including frontal cortex, temporal cortex, and hippocampus are particularly vulnerable to TBI. Furthermore, subcortical white matter, particularly in frontal regions and the corpus callosum, are often damaged. In addition, catecholaminergic, cholinergic, and serotonergic systems are vulnerable to disruption, acutely and chronically, in TBI. These brain regions and neurotransmitter systems are critical components of at least 3 major frontal subcortical circuits that modulate complex human emotional expression and behavior. This profile of structural and neurochemical injury plays a direct role in the common neurobehavioral sequelae associated with TBI. With this as a context, common emotional and behavioral changes associated with TBI are reviewed.

CHANGES IN PERSONALITY

Survivors and family/caregivers frequently describe the effects of the injury as "changes in personality." Lifelong

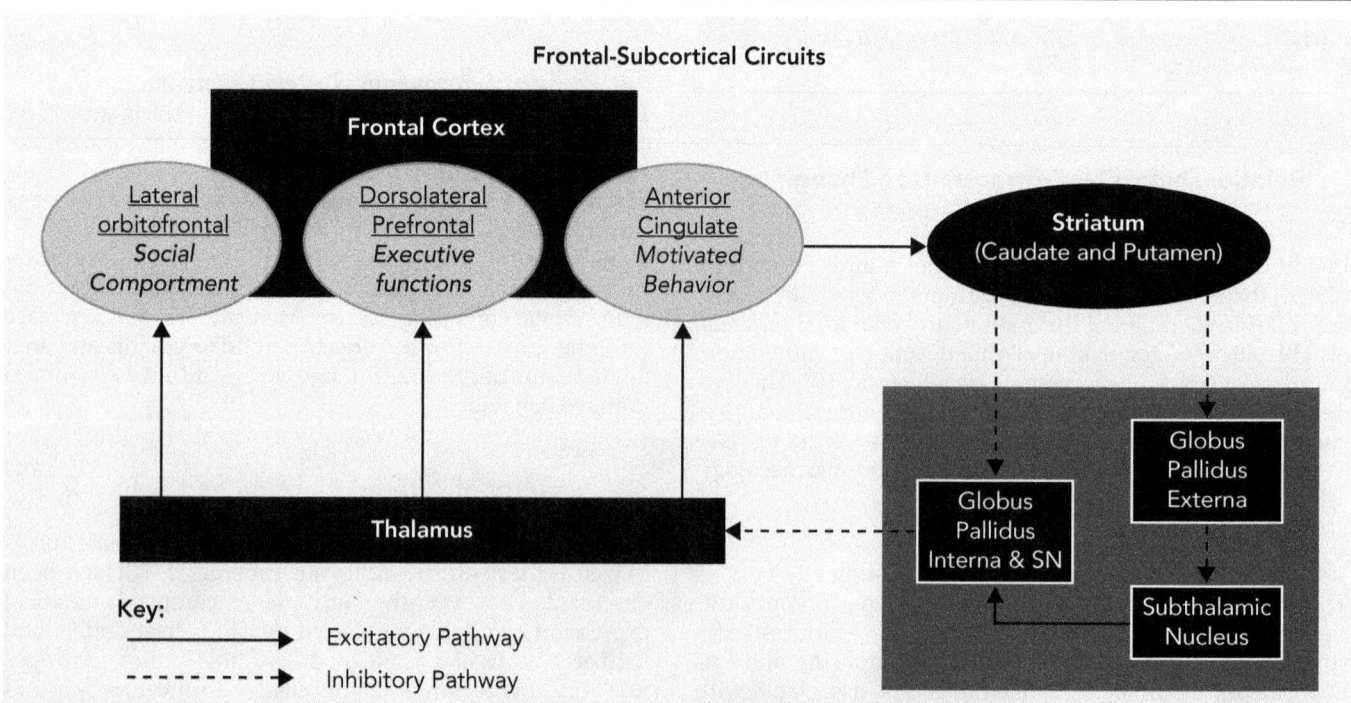

FIGURE 62-2 Outline of key nodal points in the 5 major frontal-subcortical circuits. Reprinted from Arciniegas DB, Beresford T. *Principles of Neuropsychiatry: An Introductory Approach.* Cambridge, United Kingdom: Cambridge University Press; 2001.

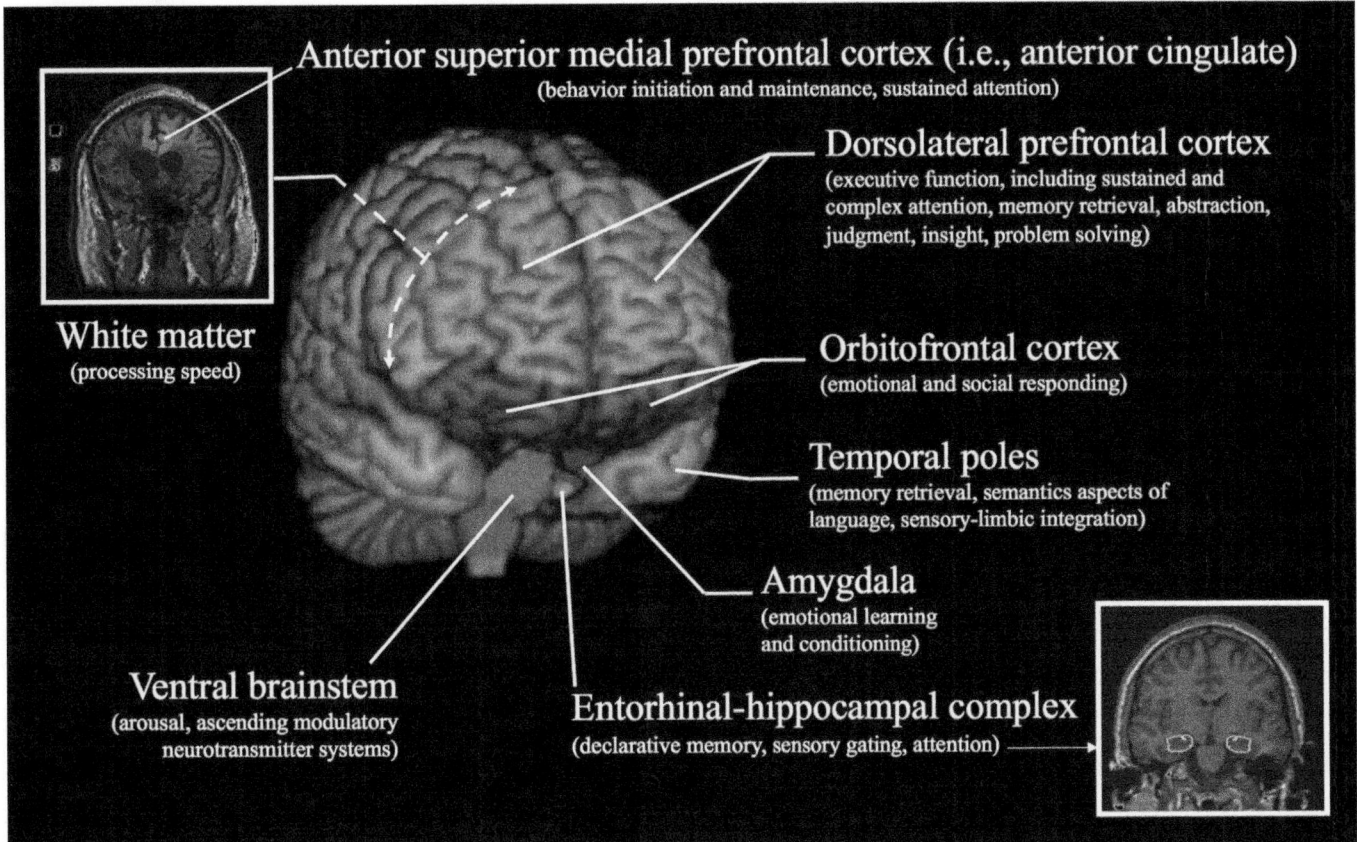

FIGURE 62-3 A three-dimensional reconstruction of the brain highlighting regional vulnerability to TBI and describing relevant brain-behavior relationships. Shaded areas represent brain regions that are especially vulnerable to TBI. The names of the cognitive, emotional, and behavioral functions with which they are most closely associated are labeled. Coronal T1-weighted magnetic resonance images of the brain (acquired at 1.5 Tesla) are inserted; at the top left, diffuse (multifocal) axonal injury is demonstrated; at the bottom right, the entorhinal-hippocampal complex is identified (outlined within image). From Arciniegas and Silver (2012) in Chapter 73 of this volume.

patterns of responding to external cues, situations in the environment, and internal drives or motivations, can be significantly altered with either exaggeration of preinjury traits or fundamental changes in response patterns. Much of the altered and distressing changes in personality after TBI can be subsumed under the rubric of impaired executive function (or "dysexecutive syndromes") (see 42 and Chapter 59 for review). Three broad (and somewhat overlapping) categories of executive functions are typically identified and correspond roughly to the 3 frontal subcortical circuits described earlier:

- *higher order cognitive function* (including mental flexibility, problem solving, set-shifting),
- *social comportment* (including context specific awareness of one's behavior relative to past individual and societal norms, self-monitoring and self-correction), and
- *motivated/reward-related behavior* (including initiation, sequencing, achieving/consuming).

As noted, these are not fully distinct domains but rather are more interactive and overlapping. This complex relationship is apparent clinically in that one can see individuals with prominent deficits in 1, 2, or all 3 domains to varying degrees. From the clinical standpoint, the prominent chal-

lenging behaviors brought to the clinician's attention flow from these domains and can be usefully grouped into the following categories.

Cognitive Syndromes

Cognitive deficits after TBI are covered in greater detail in Chapter 59. It is worth highlighting that initial and persistent cognitive deficits are the most common complaints after TBI (43,44) and the major hindrance to normalization in the areas of independent living, social readaptation, family life, and vocational endeavors (45,46). There are several predictable areas of impairment including short-term memory, speed of information processing, and attention (47–57). Many higher order cognitive functions such as judgment, problem solving, set shifting, and complex attention require intact function of the dorsolateral prefrontal subcortical circuit described earlier. It is important to point out that many challenging behaviors after TBI may flow from cognitive deficits. Impulsive behavior may reflect poor judgment as well as deficits in problem solving or set shifting (i.e., inability to conceptualize the effects of one's actions, or difficulties in imagining alternative responses). Individuals may respond with anger when confronted with memory deficits or the realization that they cannot perform tasks that were easy prior to their injury.

Social Comportment

Several aspects of social comportment are frequently disrupted after TBI.

Impulsivity

One of the more common concerns of patients and family/caregivers alike is that survivors have difficulty with impulse control. This can be manifested in verbal utterances, physical actions, snap decisions, and poor judgment flowing from the failure to fully consider the implications of a given action. This is closely related to the concept of stimulus boundedness in which the individual responds to the most salient cue in the environment or attaches exaggerated salience to a particular cue without regard to previously determined foci of attention or priorities.

Irritability

Another common concern of patients and family/caregivers pertains to the modulation of anger. Survivors describe themselves as more irritable or more easily angered. Although a particular cue might be perceived as a legitimate aggravation of some sort, the response is characteristically out of proportion to the precipitating stimulus. Responses can range from verbal outbursts to dangerous aggressive and assaultive behavior. This modulatory deficit differs in intensity, onset, and duration from the preinjury pattern for any given individual.

Affective Instability

Survivors and family/caregivers frequently describe a change in affective stability characterized by exaggerated displays of emotional expression that seem out of proportion to both the precipitating stimulus and the preinjury range of responses to similar stimuli. Cues or events that previously might have elicited momentary sadness may now precipitate weeping or crying. Events that in the past might have provoked modest irritation may now result in loud angry verbal outbursts associated with marked sympathetic arousal. The hallmarks of this instability typically include a paroxysmal onset, brief duration, and an exaggerated intensity of response out of proportion to the precipitating stimulus. This phenomenon is common to a variety of disorders affecting the central nervous system (CNS) and has been given a variety of terms including pathological affect, affective lability, pseudobulbar affect, and affective incontinence (see 58 for review).

Awareness Deficits

The burden of the earlier mentioned changes in personality and behavior is often complicated by a surprising and at times devastating lack of awareness of these changes (see 59,60 for reviews). The injured individual may be unable to appreciate that their behavior is different since the injury, in stark contrast to family/caregivers and providers who may be painfully aware that the injured individual has changed in fundamental ways and can often provide detailed lists of these changes.

Alternatively, an individual with TBI may have a vague sense that he or she is different or "not who I used to be" and yet struggle to define the specific ways in which their behavior or personality differs from prior to the injury. Of particular interest is that individuals with TBI are less likely to be aware of changes in behavior and executive function than changes in more concrete domains such as motor function (61). Even when the individual admits to some difficulties, he or she is often unable to predict the implications of these deficits in current or future social situations. Furthermore, the degree of awareness has been found to correlate with functional and vocational outcome in many (62–64), although not all, studies (65).

As is the case with disorders of affective stability, problems with awareness of deficits are not unique to individuals with TBI but rather occur in a broad range of disorders of the CNS including severe and persistent mental disorders such as schizophrenia (59). The literature suggests that lack of awareness of illness is not simply a function of global cognitive deficits but perhaps is more related to frontal-executive dysfunction (66–72). In individuals with TBI, this dimension is frequently the focus of family/caregiver concern yet is often not recognized by individuals with TBI (5,73–77).

Disorders of Motivation (Apathy)

Apathy reflects a deficit in motivated behavior (78). Although not as threatening or alarming as some of the other changes in personality described earlier, it can be disturbing to family/caregivers, and is frequently the reason that injured individuals fail to progress in rehabilitation programs. Furthermore, it is often misinterpreted as laziness or depression and may be paradoxically linked to aggression when for attempts to engage the individual in activities in which they have little interest precipitate assaultive behavior (28).

Apathy is quite common after TBI. Kant et al. (79) found that apathy (mixed with depression) occurred in 60% of their sample of individuals with TBI. Andersson et al. (80) found that almost half of their sample of individuals with TBI had significant degrees of apathy. Deficits in motivated behavior can occur in association with injury to the circuitry of "reward" which includes behavior specific (thirst, sex, hunger) hypothalamic centers (28,81), and a more general reward system linking the forebrain to the midbrain. Key nodal points in this circuitry include the amygdala, hippocampus, caudate, entorhinal and cingulate cortices, the ventral tegmental area, and the medial forebrain bundle. Catecholaminergic systems, particularly the mesolimbic dopaminergic system appear to play critical roles in the modulation of the reward system (see 28,81 for reviews).

RELATIONSHIP OF TBI TO PSYCHIATRIC DISORDERS

In addition to the changes in cognition, behavior, and personality described earlier, TBI results in an increased relative risk of developing psychiatric disorders including mood and anxiety disorders, and psychotic syndromes (82–86) (see Table 62-1). However there are certain challenges that should be noted when considering the complex relationship between TBI and psychiatric illness.

TABLE 62-1 Representative Summary of Relationship of TBI to Axis I Psychiatric Disorders

DISORDER	REPRESENTATIVE RATES (REFERENCES)	COMMENT
Preinjury psychiatric disorders	52% (Whelan-Goodinson et al., 2009) 51% (Hibbard et al., 1998) 20% dep, 32% SUD (Ashman et al., 2004)	Depression and SUD most common Preinjury rates consistently exceed community base rates
Any postinjury psychiatric disorders	65% (Whelan-Goodinson et al., 2009) 80% (Hibbard et al., 1998)	Higher in those with preinjury disorders Depression and anxiety most common
Novel postinjury psychiatric disorders	48% (Koponen et al., 2002) ~40% (Whelan-Goodinson et al., 2009)	Depression, SUD, anxiety most common
Depression	27%–61% (Rapoport 2010; Jorge and Starkstein, 2005)	Studies that used standardized diagnostic criteria
Anxiety disorders	48% (Hibbard et al., 1998) 38% (Whelan-Goodinson et al. 2009) 35% (Koponen et al., 2002)	Includes generalized anxiety disorder, panic, and phobic disorders
Substance use disorders	28% (Hibbard et al., 1998) 21% (Whelan-Goodinson et al., 2009) 22% (Koponen et al., 2002)	Typically most common preinjury disorder. Less frequent de novo after injury
Psychotic syndromes	3% (Whelan-Goodinson et al., 2009) 7% (Koponen et al., 2002)	Occur at higher rates postinjury than general population, less frequently than mood, anxiety, and substance use disorders
PTSD	19% (Hibbard et al., 1998) 14% (Whelan-Goodinson et al., 2009)	More common after mild TBI Common cause of persistent symptoms after mild TBI

SUD, substance use disorder; PTSD; post-traumatic stress disorder; TBI, traumatic brain injury.

Symptoms vs Disorder: Regarding any potentially disabling condition, individuals with TBI report a variety of symptoms in a variety of domains (discouragement, frustration, fatigue, anxiety, etc.). Not all of these symptoms will rise to the level of a disorder. However, symptoms that are consistent and sustained over time (usually weeks), and that are of sufficient severity to interfere with social or occupational function or quality of life, are legitimately considered disorders.

Labeling Issues: Many individuals, including some with TBI, resist the idea that they have a psychiatric illness. In some instances this reflects an unwillingness to be labeled as a psychiatric patient. Some individuals prefer to see their behavioral and emotional struggles as a product of their injury rather than "being crazy" or having mental illness. Alternatively, deficits in awareness may prevent accurate self-appraisal and make it difficult for an injured person to conceptualize him or herself as having a psychiatric disorder.

Use of Diagnostic and Statistical Manual of Mental Disorders

Nomenclature: The use of standardized phenomenological criteria in the *Diagnostic Statistical Manual* (*DSM*) has been an important advance in the categorization of idiopathic psychiatric disorders. It is less helpful when approaching diagnosis in neuropsychiatric populations, including those with TBI. In the *DSM*, psychiatric disorders in the context of brain disease or injury can be coded as "secondary to a general medical condition," implying that it is possible to assess causality when, for example, a depressive syndrome follows a TBI by some time interval. Although this may be true (and probably often is the case), proof is lacking and thus such a label reflects the impression or bias of the clinician.

Perhaps, most importantly, the current schema does not allow for the alteration of syndromic presentations by brain injury. The question of how to diagnose depression in a nonverbal individual, for example, is not addressed in the *DSM*. The idea that depression can be expressed in other ways is not reflected directly in the menu of symptom options. For example, so called "depressive equivalents" must be inferred by creative clinicians.

With these caveats in mind, current knowledge of the association of TBI and psychiatric disorders is reviewed.

Relationship of TBI to Risk of Psychiatric Illness in General

Several groups have explored links between sustaining a TBI and the relative risk of developing psychiatric illness. For example, in an ongoing longitudinal cohort study, Koponen et al. (84) reported on 60 individuals 30 years after their TBI and found that almost half (48%) developed a new Axis I psychiatric disorder after their injury. The most common diagnoses were depression, substance abuse, and anxiety disorders. Rates of lifetime and current depression (26%, 10%), panic disorder (8%, 6%), and psychotic disorders (8%, 8%) were significantly higher than base rates found in the Epidemiologic Catchment Area (ECA) study (87).

Hibbard et al. (83) studied 100 adults, on average, 8 years after TBI. A significant number of individuals had Axis I disorders prior to injury. After TBI, the most frequent Axis I diagnoses were major depression and anxiety disorders (i.e., post-traumatic stress disorder [PTSD], obsessive–compulsive disorder [OCD], and panic disorder). Almost half (44%) of individuals had 2 or more disorders. More recently (88), this group reported a longitudinal study of 188 individuals enrolled within 4 years of injury and assessed at yearly intervals on at least 2 occasions. Once again they found elevated rates of psychiatric disorders prior to injury. Subsequent to TBI, there were increased rates of depression, PTSD, and other anxiety disorders. This was particularly true of those with preinjury psychiatric disorders. Furthermore, the rates were greatest at the initial assessment point after injury and stabilized or decreased over time. Van Reekum et al. (82) carefully reviewed the literature on the relationship of TBI to a variety of psychiatric disorders and using the ECA data for baseline rates concluded that TBI was associated with an increase in the relative risk for several psychiatric disorders.

More recently, Whelan-Goodinson et al. (89) have published their investigation of the relationship of TBI and psychiatric illness, as well as the effect of psychiatric illness on outcome after TBI (90). One hundred patients with TBI selected from a database of former patients with TBI at a rehabilitation hospital were assessed with a standardized psychiatric diagnostic interview for both preinjury and postinjury psychiatric disorders. Participants were injured 6 months to 5 years prior to participation. Prior to injury, half of the patients (52%) had a psychiatric illness, most commonly a substance abuse disorder. After injury, two-thirds (65%) of the participants had a psychiatric illness. The most common post-TBI diagnoses were depression (45%) and anxiety (38%). Of note is that two-thirds of the postinjury diagnoses of depression and anxiety occurred in individuals without such a history. Rates of depression and anxiety in the TBI cohort were higher than in the base population. Furthermore, the presence of current depression and anxiety were strongly predictive of poor outcome (90).

Using a different approach, 2 groups examined large insurance databases to examine the association between TBI and indicators of mental illness. Fann et al. (91) studied a cohort of about 1,000 health maintenance organization (HMO) members who sustained a TBI classified as either mild (loss of consciousness [LOC] < 1 hour) or moderate to severe, and followed for 3 years. Compared to noninjured controls, the individuals with TBI had increased indicators of psychiatric illness, especially in the first year after injury, and there was some evidence of a biologic gradient (49% in the moderate-to-severe group, 34% in the mild group, 18% in the noninjured comparison group). In injured individuals without history of psychiatric illness, the odds ratio of developing psychiatric illness in the first 6 months was 4.0 in the moderate-to-severe group.

Wei et al. (92) in a study of Medicaid beneficiaries in 4 states found that 18% of ~3,600 individuals diagnosed with TBI suffered severe mental illness, and another 16.5% had other mental disorders. Those with mental illness had significantly higher expenditures.

In addition to studies of increased rates of psychiatric disorders in general, there is data on the relationship of TBI to specific disorders (see Table 62-1).

Mood Disorders

Depression
Depression after brain injury is common, although exact estimates vary significantly ranging from 27% to 61% of individuals with TBI when structured diagnostic criteria are used (93–95). These rates do not take into account individuals who have depressive (94) symptoms but who fail to meet

DSM-IV diagnostic criteria. Regardless of the exact rates, depression occurs more commonly than in the general population and is associated with poorer cognitive, social, functional, and quality of life outcome (90,94–97) and can act as an amplifier of other neurobehavioral challenges including anxiety and aggression (7,83,94,96). Given the common cooccurrence of TBI and depression, it is worth commenting on some of the factors thought to drive this association. One such factor is that brain regions thought to be involved in the pathophysiology of depression overlap with the areas vulnerable to the typical TBI (see 98–100). For example, functional imaging studies (see 98,101 for thorough discussion) that have indicated metabolic abnormalities in dorsolateral prefrontal cortex (DLPFC), anterior cingulate (reduced activity), and ventrolateral prefrontal cortex (increased activity) are associated with depression. Although there is some variability of findings, other regions including temporal lobe and basal ganglia have also been found to have reduced activity (98). Studies using induced mood state changes such as sleep deprivation and tryptophan depletion, or before and after induced sadness in healthy individuals, also implicate altered activity in DLPFC, anterior cingulate, and ventrolateral prefrontal cortex (see 98). Taken together, this evidence suggests that the 2 frontal-striatal-thalamocortical circuits originating in the orbitofrontal and DLPFC function abnormally in depression. It may be that the orbitofrontal circuit with its limbic connections is the substrate of disordered emotional processing and vegetative symptoms common in depression, whereas dysfunction in the dorsolateral circuit may result in the cognitive deficits associated with depression (98,100,101). Thus the brain regions and circuitry implicated in the genesis of depression overlap to a great extent with those regions at greatest risk for damage in the typical TBI. Furthermore, the major neurotransmitter systems felt to play key modulatory roles in the regulation of mood and affect are the same as those known to be altered by TBI (i.e., adrenergic, dopaminergic, cholinergic, and serotonergic systems).

In addition to the overlapping neurobiology of TBI and depression, other factors—no doubt—play an important role. Preinjury depression and other psychiatric disorders including substance abuse greatly increase the risk of postinjury depression (91,94). Increased age and female gender are also associated with increased risk of depression after TBI even when adjusting for other factors (102,103). When one considers the additional roles of stress, loss, social isolation, and other psychosocial insults common in TBI, it is not surprising that the frequency of depression following TBI is increased.

From a clinical perspective, depression does not always present in classic *DSM* fashion in someone with TBI (see 103 for discussion). Many of the factors previously mentioned, including difficulties with self-monitoring and awareness, deficits in memory which make it hard for someone to have an ongoing sense of how they are doing or what their mood has been like over the recent past, as well as struggles with complex constructs and abstractions, can conspire to make it hard for someone with TBI to paint a clear picture of a depressive episode. Clinicians need to look at other indicators of depression including loss of sleep, loss of appetite, and, perhaps most helpful, descriptions from family/caregivers of anhedonia (the individual derives little pleasure from things they previously enjoyed). There is a complex link between depression and aggression as well, and an increase in the frequency or intensity of angry, irritable, or assaultive behavior should alert clinicians to look carefully for other indicators of depression.

Manic Syndromes

Mania is characterized by episodes of sustained (longer than 1 week) changes in mood (euphoria or irritability) and increased psychomotor activity. It may be associated with increased energy, decreased need for sleep, and a penchant for dangerous behavior (reckless activities, increased spending, increased sexual activity). Some manic episodes can be accompanied by psychotic symptoms such as grandiose delusions or thought process disturbances such as loosened associations or flight of ideas. Mania is a well-described complication of many disorders of the CNS including TBI (104,105). Robinson et al. (105) found 6 of 66 (9%) carefully characterized patients with TBI developed manic episodes. In these patients, mania was not associated with severity of injury, post-traumatic epilepsy, family or past personal history of mania. It was associated with lesions in the temporal and orbitofrontal cortices. Shukla et al. (106) reported on 20 individuals with TBI and mania and found that 9 of their patients had epileptogenic activity on electroencephalography (EEG). Irritable mood, not euphoria, was more commonly observed. Van Reekum et al. (82) reviewed the literature and suggested that TBI was associated with a 5-fold increase in relative risk of developing bipolar disorder relative to base rates in the population, although some studies have not found an increased rate of bipolar illness (107) after TBI. The role of genetic loading in the etiology of mania after TBI is not clear.

It is difficult to determine the exact role that profile of injury plays in mania as the underlying circuitry of this disorder is less well-established than that for depression. In mania occurring after CNS disorders (not solely TBI), there is a marked preponderance of right frontotemporal and basal ganglia injury (5,105,108). As with depression, location and profile of injury (in the case of mania more severe injury and injury to right hemispheric regions including basoventral, temporal, orbitofrontal areas) may play more of a role in genesis of manic episodes within weeks or the first few months after injury, whereas other factors, particularly psychosocial stressors, may be more important factors further out from the injury (97,104,108,109). However, the literature on this is scarce, at least in part because mania is a less common complication of brain injury than is depression.

Psychotic Syndromes

The term psychosis refers to a cluster of symptoms, which includes problems in both thought content and thought process. Delusions and hallucinations typically characterize disorders of thought content. Alterations in the structure and flow of speech and language such as loosening of associations, flight of ideas, thought blocking, and production of nonsense words or neologisms, are characteristic of disordered thought process. Psychosis is often equated with schizophrenia but is more accurately viewed as a syndrome that

can accompany many neuropsychiatric conditions, including depression, bipolar affective disorder, delirium, and dementia, to name a few.

Although psychosis is a relatively rare complication of TBI, it does occur more frequently than in the general population and is a good example of a low-frequency, high-impact complication of TBI, causing enormous distress to individuals and their caregivers. There are several contexts in which psychotic syndromes following TBI can occur including during the period of post-traumatic amnesia (PTA), as a complication of post-traumatic epilepsy, in the context of TBI-related mood disorders, or associated with a chronic, schizophrenia-like syndrome. It is necessary to distinguish these different contexts, in so far as it is possible, to guide appropriate interventions (86,110–112).

Relatively few studies directly address the association and causal connections between TBI and psychosis. Davison and Bagley (113) summarized the results of 8 long-term (15–20 years) follow-up studies of individuals with brain injuries published between 1917 and 1960. Across these studies, the percentage of patients with TBI developing a schizophrenia-like psychosis varies from 0.7% to 9.8%, suggesting an observed incidence of schizophrenia-like psychosis that is 2–3 times greater than that expected by chance in the TBI population. Van Reekum et al. (82) reviewed the literature and found a more modest relative risk associated with TBI. The role of genetic vulnerability is also not clear. Davison and Bagley found no evidence of increased genetic loading for schizophrenia in patients with TBI who developed psychotic symptoms. Malaspina and colleagues (114), however, studied 1,830 individuals who were first-degree relatives of people with schizophrenia or bipolar disorder, looking for a relationship between these illnesses and TBI. Compared to other first-degree relatives with similar genetic vulnerabilities, those with a history of TBI were at significantly greater risk to develop schizophrenia. The authors proposed a synergistic effect between TBI and genetic risk in families with 2 or more members with schizophrenia.

Based on the studies to date, it seems reasonable to conclude that psychotic disorders do occur in individuals with a TBI at rates greater than in the noninjured population. The more severe the injury, the greater is the likelihood of psychosis. Psychotic syndromes may occur soon after the TBI, or after a delay of months to many years (see Table 62-3). In cases with delayed onset, the injury is almost certainly not the only etiologic factor, although it is interesting to note the high rate of previous TBI in patients with schizophrenia. Furthermore, it appears that TBI can interact with genetic vulnerability to greatly increase the risk of developing illnesses such as schizophrenia.

In addition to chronic psychotic syndromes resembling schizophrenia, psychotic symptoms can occur in several other contexts after TBI including mood disorders (psychotic depression or manic pychoses), as a component of the confusional state associated with the period of PTA and in association with post-traumatic seizure disorders. The latter context deserves some further comments.

A relationship between seizures and mental disorders, particularly psychotic syndromes, has been commented on for centuries (115) and is the subject of a somewhat confusing literature. In a comprehensive review of studies looking at the prevalence of psychosis in epileptic populations, McKenna and colleagues (116) found prevalence rates ranging from 0% to 27% in small clinic-based studies and rates of 2.8%–3.2% in larger surveys of patients attending epilepsy clinics. Two large-scale Scandinavian community surveys of individuals with epilepsy found prevalence rates for psychosis of 2% (117) and 7.1% (118), both of which are higher than prevalence rates in individuals without epilepsy.

Epileptic psychosis is overwhelmingly associated with complex partial seizures, occurring 4–12 times more frequently in temporal lobe epilepsy than in other types of epilepsy. Psychotic syndromes are most likely to occur in conjunction with left-sided temporal lobe lesions (119–122). This is particularly the case for schizophrenia-like syndromes and paranoid syndrome.

Psychotic syndromes associated with post-traumatic epilepsy can occur in the peri-ictal period (either during seizures or in the immediate postictal period), or interictally, in which case the psychotic symptoms are more commonly chronic rather than episodic (123). Most commonly seen is a postictal acute confusional state characterized by disorientation, fluctuating sensorium, agitation, hallucinations, and delusions, which is similar to the post-traumatic delirium described earlier. This condition generally resolves within a few hours of the seizure, although rarely it may persist for several days.

Less commonly psychotic symptoms occur as part of the seizure ictus. The clinical picture is one of paroxysmal onset of psychotic symptoms which can include auditory, visual or somatosensory hallucinations, delusions (often paranoid, grandiose, or religious), as well as alterations in thought process (loosened associations, flight of ideas, cognitive disorganization). As with other seizure phenomena, these symptoms usually recede quickly (over several minutes) unless they are associated with repetitive seizures of a more prolonged interictal psychotic syndrome. The most useful clue clinically is the time course of the psychotic symptoms, characterized by the paroxysmal onset, rapid resolution (most commonly), and relative absence of such symptoms in between events (124).

Although treatment is not the focus of this chapter it is worth highlighting that because of the multiple contexts in which psychosis can be seen after TBI (seizure and mood disorders, post traumatic amnesia, etc.) a critical first step in informing treatment is to determine what is the cause of the psychotic syndrome.

Neural Substrate of Psychosis After TBI

No single brain region has been identified as the site or cause of schizophrenia, rather several brain regions appear to play important roles in the genesis and phenomenology of this disorder. These regions overlap with those vulnerable to injury in the typical TBI. Neuroimaging studies of patients with schizophrenia have identified enlarged lateral and third ventricles (125,126), reduced frontal and temporal lobe volumes (127), reduced thalamic volumes (128), and enlargement of basal ganglia, particularly the caudate and globus-pallidus (129–131). Functional imaging studies have also focused on frontal, temporolimbic, and basal ganglia areas. Positron emission tomography (PET) studies of drug-free

schizophrenics have suggested reduced metabolism in the cingulated gyrus and hippocampus, (132,133) and reduced metabolism in the basal ganglia (134,135). Some patients with schizophrenia have abnormal patterns of frontal activation when engaged in cognitive tasks that require frontal function (132,135).

Recent neuropathological studies of patients with schizophrenia have suggested abnormalities in regions of the DLPFC and the hippocampus (136–138). Dysfunction of the prefrontal cortex is also implicated in delusion formation. The temporal lobes, particularly the left temporal lobe and the hippocampal formation appear to play a role in auditory hallucinations and in delusions of passivity and control. Thus there is significant overlap between the regions implicated in the etiology of schizophrenia and its prominent symptoms, and those regions which are commonly affected in TBI, including the frontal lobes (both dorsolateral cortex and orbitofrontal cortex), temporal lobes, basal ganglia, and thalamus. In some respects, it is surprising that psychotic syndromes are not seen more commonly after TBI.

Anxiety Disorders

Anxiety is a common complaint in injured and noninjured populations alike. Anxiety can present in several different patterns including generalized anxiety, panic disorder, phobic disorders, OCD, and PTSD. There are relatively few studies however addressing the incidence of these disorders after TBI and even fewer studies addressing treatment options (see 139 for review).

Generalized Anxiety Disorder

Van Reekum et al. (82) reported a 2.3 fold increase in relative risk for generalized anxiety disorder (GAD) based on 5 studies that met their inclusion criteria. For example, in a study by Fann et al. (7), 24% of their sample (most of whom had mild TBI [MTBI]) evaluated 2–3 years after injury met criteria for generalized anxiety disorder. Many had comorbid depression and many had symptoms that predated their TBI. Robinson and Jorge (140) also found high rates of comorbid anxiety and depression. The 76% of their sample of depressed patients with TBI also met criteria for GAD. The 22% of the nondepressed group also met GAD criteria.

Hibbard et al. (83) also found high rates of several different anxiety disorders (PTSD, 19%; OCD, 15%; panic disorder, 14%; GAD, 9%) in their sample of 100 individuals with mixed injury severity studied an average of 8 years after injury. Deb et al. (85) found a high rate of panic disorder (7%) but no change in rates for GAD or OCD relative to the general population. More recently, Whelan-Goodinson et al. (89) found that 35% of their cohort had some form of anxiety disorder other than PTSD.

The question of anxiety symptoms and their link to postconcussive symptoms is an important one. There is a significant overlap between many postconcussive symptoms and core symptoms in GAD. Thus, many patients endorse complaints of headache, dizziness, blurred vision, irritability, and sensitivity to noise or light after mild brain injury (57,141,142). It is less clear how many patients actually experience anxiety and how many have diagnosable anxiety disorders. Although 55% of Dikmen's group (141) of 20 patients with mild brain injury complained of subjective anxiety, 45% of the matched control subjects had similar complaints (a statistically nonsignificant difference). Schoenhuber and Gentilini (143) were unable to find a significant difference in mean anxiety scores in their study of 35 patients with mild brain injury and matched control subjects.

Obsessive-Compulsive Disorder

Three studies (82,83,144) assessed their TBI populations for OCD. As pointed out by Van Reekum et al. (82), these studies represent a combined sample of 282 subjects followed for a maximum of 7.5 years. The 6.4% had OCD, which represents about a 2-fold increase in relative risk compared to the general population.

Post-Traumatic Stress Disorder

There is an emerging literature on the complex relationships between psychological and biomechanical trauma, driven in part by the recent conflicts in Iraq and Afghanistan (e.g., see 145–147). In the past it was assumed that the presence of PTA prevented the development of PTSD by preventing the formation of what was felt to be a core component of the syndrome—vivid memories and reexperiencing of the traumatic life-threatening event. There is some evidence that individuals with LOC, particularly 15 minutes or more, do have reduced rates of PTSD (139,148,149). However, this is by no means an absolute rule. McMillan (150) reported on 10 individuals who met criteria for PTSD despite amnesia for the traumatic event and several others have reported similar findings (151–153). McMillan (151) described PTSD symptoms in a woman with a severe brain injury despite amnesia for the event itself and a PTA of approximately 6 weeks.

However it is more common to see PTSD and PTSD-like syndromes in individuals with mild brain injury and at least partial recall of the events. In this group PTSD may be quite common in some populations. Symptoms may include sleep disturbance, recurrent nightmares, exaggerated startle responses, daytime flashbacks, and avoidant behaviors such as refusing to drive or leave home. Driving phobias may become prominent.

Several recent studies highlight their complex interaction. In civilian populations, Bryant and Harvey have reported a series of studies of individuals hospitalized after motor vehicle accidents, some with and some without TBI (usually MTBI). They have shown that rates of acute stress disorder 1 month after an accident are comparable in the 2 groups, and that acute stress disorder is a good predictor of those who go on to develop PTSD 6 months after injury (154–156). For example, they studied 46 individuals admitted to a hospital after an MTBI (LOC with PTA < 24 hours) and 59 survivors of motor vehicle accidents without evidence of TBI 6 months after their accidents (152,157). Twenty percent of the TBI group and 25% of the non-TBI group had PTSD. The TBI group had more postconcussive symptoms than did the non-TBI group. Furthermore, the TBI group with PTSD was significantly more symptomatic than the TBI without PTSD group. This suggests that, like other psychiatric disorders such as depression, PTSD can amplify postconcussive symptoms after an MTBI and complicate recovery.

In the recent study by Whelan-Goodinson et al. (89), 14% of the TBI cohort had PTSD.

Similar findings have been reported in military populations. Hoge et al. (158) found that higher rates of Iraq war returnees reporting a TBI with LOC met criteria for PTSD, relative to those reporting only altered mental status, other injuries, and or no injury. Much of the variance across these groups with respect to physical health outcomes and symptoms could be accounted for by the presence of PTSD and/or depression. Participants were assessed 3–4 months after deployment and thus reflect individuals with persistent symptoms. Schneiderman et al. (159) found that combat-incurred MTBI approximately doubled the risk for PTSD and that a PTSD diagnosis was the strongest factor associated with persistent postconcussive symptoms. Belanger et al. (160) studied patients with mild and moderate-to-severe TBI and found, as expected, that MTBI was associated with higher levels of postconcussion complaints approximately 2 years after injury. However, after adjusting for PTSD symptoms, these between-group differences were no longer significant. These studies are consistent with the literature cited earlier that suggests that MTBI may increase the relative risk for psychiatric disorders, and that these disorders can interfere with recovery from the TBI.

There is reason to believe that part of the explanation for the complex interaction between biomechanical and psychological trauma relates to overlap in the neural substrates of both conditions (see 145–147,161 for discussion). For example, mesial temporal structures are vulnerable in TBI from both contact/impact forces, as well as increased sensitivity to excitotoxic injury. Hippocampal and amygdala injury are common. Both of these regions play key roles in PTSD as well, both in terms of contextual memory consolidation and fear conditioning. The hippocampus is also felt to be vulnerable to the effects of chronic stress presumably through the mediating effects of the hypothalamic-pituitary-adrenal (HPA) axis. Thus biomechanical and neurochemically mediated damage could conceivably interact with neurohumoral dysregulation to create a milieu that lends itself to the development of PTSD. Orbitofrontal cortex is also vulnerable to TBI through impact forces as well as frontal subcortical axonal injury.

Substance Abuse

Use of alcohol and other substances can play an important role in TBI including etiology, neuropathophysiology, recovery, and functional outcome (see Chapter 79). For example, about half of all TBIs involve the use of alcohol, and about one-half of these individuals are intoxicated at the time of injury (162). Most of these individuals have preinjury patterns suggestive of addictive drinking (alcohol dependence) (163). In fact, alcohol use is the single greatest risk factor for TBI, and TBI is often an irreversible consequence of alcohol and drug abuse (163). The presence of alcohol at the time of injury predicts longer durations of unconsciousness (164), increased challenging behaviors during the acute hospitalization (165), cognitive outcome (166), and overall outcome including mortality (167).

Individuals with preinjury substance abuse problems often continue to struggle with these issues after their injury.

Ashman et al. (88) found that their TBI population had an almost 2-fold increased rate of substance use disorders (drug/alcohol abuse/dependency) relative to the general population (32% vs 17%) *prior* to injury. Subsequent to injury the rates went down initially probably reflecting enforced abstinence related to hospitalization and rehabilitation stays. However, by the third assessment point the rate was identical to that seen in the general population (17%). In an earlier study of 100 individuals studied at least 1 year (mean 7.6 years) after injury, 28% of the sample struggled with substance use disorders (83).

Dementia

Dementia is a syndrome characterized by impairment in memory and at least 1 other domain of higher cognitive function ("memory plus") that is of sufficient severity to interfere with social and or occupational function. Although progression is often inferred this need not be the case. Thus many individuals with TBI who have significant impairments in memory and executive function meet this definition of dementia. However the larger issue is whether exposure to a TBI increases the risk of a progressive dementing disorder such as senile dementia of the Alzheimer type (SDAT) later in life (see Chapter 44 for discussion of the full scope of late complications of TBI). Several studies have raised a concern about the relationship of TBI to progressive dementia (168). For example, TBI-associated disruption of axonal transport results in the rapid accumulation of amyloid precursor protein (APP) in animals (168,169) and humans (170,171). APP, Abeta, and other proteins associated with Alzheimer and other neurodegenerative disorders accumulate rapidly after a TBI (172–174). Some—but not all—autopsy studies have shown increased amyloid plaques and neurofibrillary tangles in individuals with TBI (174,175). This variation has prompted exploration of the role of genetic factors in modulating risk for Alzheimer disease (AD) after TBI. For example, Mayeux et al. (176) retrospectively studied 113 older adults with AD, comparing them with a control group of 123 healthy older individuals. They found that the combination of apolipoprotein E4 (*APOEE4*) and history of TBI increased the risk of AD by a factor of 10. However, not all studies have found such a relationship. A large, prospective population-based study of 6,645 individuals 55 years and older and free of dementia at baseline found that mild brain trauma was not a major risk factor for the development of AD. Moreover, brain trauma did not appear to increase the risk of developing AD in people carrying the APOEE4 (177). One possibility is that diminished cognitive reserve associated with TBI facilitates earlier manifestation of dementia symptoms in individuals already at risk for AD (178). Therefore, although there are some compelling scientific reasons to consider the relationship of TBI to Alzheimer and other neurodegenerative disorders, and some strong evidence suggesting clinical associations, the relationship between TBI and dementia needs further study.

ASSESSMENT OF EMOTIONAL AND BEHAVIORAL DISTURBANCES

It is clear from the earlier discussion that a careful assessment of neurobehavioral concerns should be an important component of the evaluation and rehabilitation of individuals with TBI. A full discussion of all the dimensions of a neuropsychiatric assessment will not be attempted (see 179 for review). However, it is worth highlighting several points.

Need for Multiple Sources of Information

The cognitive deficits that frequently accompany a TBI alter the neuropsychiatric assessment, particularly the history taking. The presence of short-term memory deficits, problems with sequencing events in time, and difficulties with self-monitoring and self-awareness can make it very challenging for an individual to give a clear and consistent history. This puts the onus on the clinician to identify other sources of information (family members, friends, employers, primary medical/school/vocational records) that can help clarify the history and current clinical picture. The clinician must also obtain permission from the injured individual and work hard to explain the need for others to be involved in the treatment as observers and sources of critical information.

Assessment of Preinjury Baseline

Assessment of the effects of an injury must start with a thorough understanding of what the individual was like prior to the injury. Absent such information, there is a significant risk of misattributing life-long traits, characteristics, and behaviors to the brain injury. The following domains should be carefully explored and efforts made to gain primary records and reliable history with respect to

- *medical history,*
- *neurobehavioral traits and characteristics* (e.g., history of psychiatric illness),
- *intellectual capacity* (indicators include educational history, vocational history, parental education),
- *functional performance* (profile of personal, professional, and vocational accomplishments), and
- *personality style* (indicators include patterns of coping with stress, stability of key relationships).

Such information helps to paint a picture of life before the injury. Ideally, such information is obtained shortly after the injury. The more time that passes from the point of injury, the greater the tendency to attribute/misattribute more issues and life events to the injury. It is important to not simply take the word of injured individuals and their family/caregivers that "he was always perfectly normal" but make an effort to get primary documentation, not just "hearsay."

Assessment of Postinjury Change

Once the baseline picture is complete, the clinician is positioned to accurately assess the changes that have occurred since the time of the injury. It is important to carefully review the functional domains that are frequently affected by injury including cognition, personality, mood regulation, speech/language, mobility, and higher order domains such as vocational performance, major role performance within the family or equivalent context. It can be helpful to use standardized assessment scales and tools that serve to sample the full array of common problems such as the Neurobehavioral Rating Scale-Revised (180) or the Neuropsychiatric Inventory (181). Alternatively, one can use scales and instruments that offer a more detailed approach to a given problem area specific to the individual being assessed such as the Overt Aggression Scale (182) or Apathy Evaluation Scale (183). For bedside assessment of cognition, it is helpful to supplement a standardized instrument such as the Mini Mental Status Exam (184) with something that helps to assess frontal executive functions such as the Frontal Assessment Battery or the Behavior Rating Inventory of Executive Function (BRIEF) (185,186).

Attribution of Etiology

It is important to emphasize that temporal association does not guarantee causality. There are several ways that neurobehavioral change can be associated with brain injury. Change may be a direct effect of the insult to neural tissue with subsequent disruption of the functions subserved by the damaged tissue. For this to be properly assessed requires accurate, sometimes fine-grained knowledge of the profile of regional brain injury and the relationship of the related circuitry to the functional change in question (the "neural component").

Alternatively the change may reflect the development of a new illness or disorder that is the driving force behind the behavioral change. For example, an individual may develop various endocrine complications of their brain injury related to pituitary damage, chronic pain from orthopedic injuries, or depression that more reasonably explains the behaviors in question (the "biological component"). It is equally plausible that behavioral change could be caused by the meaning of the accident or injury, a reaction to a loss of self-esteem because of disfiguring injury, loss of mobility, or unemployment (the "psychological component"). Finally, changes in environment such as living situation, change in caregivers, or change in routine or flow of daily life can have an enormous impact on the behavior and adaptation of an individual with brain injury (the "social component").

Formulation and Interpretation

All of the earlier mentioned factors can reasonably be attributed to the event of the injury. For example, the individual would not have endocrine abnormalities save for the injury-related pituitary damage, or may have not developed depression absent the injury. However, the degree of linkage to neural tissue damage varies across these factors. An individual showing new, aggressive outbursts associated with a change in residential care providers may be better served by working to further train the residential provider rather than by the aggressive use of medications. On the other hand, if this patient has clear evidence of lateral orbitofrontal damage, it may be that their threshold for tolerating frustration is so lowered that treatment will require both medication approaches and environmental manipulation.

The proper assessment and formulation of the relative weighting or contribution of each of these factors to the genesis of the challenging behaviors frames what can be termed a neurobiopsychosocial paradigm. It differs from more traditional psychiatric assessments with respect to the critical importance placed on understanding the profile of regional brain injury, and the array of complex behavioral circuitry that this profile would reasonably disrupt. Thus the work of the neuropsychiatric assessment can be summarized as the process of matching the profile of brain injury with the changes that have occurred in cognition, behavior, and overall function, and gauging the "goodness of fit" between predicted and actual outcomes. Signs and symptoms that are not accounted for by the profile of injury must be explained on another basis or the profile of injury should be reassessed. The clinical picture should make sense in the context of the brain damage.

This is followed by an interpretative process whereby the clinician assigns relative weights to the various contributions made by the neural, biological, psychological, and social components. Treatment interventions should flow logically from this formulation. It is important to point out that even experienced clinicians can make mistakes in this process because of the complexity of clinical presentations and the incomplete data available. The final critical component to this process is the regular reevaluation of intervention efficacy. Essentially, each formulation should be hypothesis driven and each intervention flow logically and in an empirically testable fashion (e.g., "I believe the increase in aggression is caused by depression, thus I will prescribe antidepressants"). Poor or incomplete response to the intervention should prompt a reevaluation and formulation of a new and testable hypothesis. It is acceptable to be wrong; it is not acceptable to engage in sloppy thinking.

PRINCIPLES IN TREATMENT

A detailed approach to specific syndromes and disorders can be found in Chapters 63, 64, 73, and 74. However, several general treatment principles are worth emphasizing.

Variability in Presentation

It is important to be aware that the presentation of emotional and behavioral syndromes in individuals with TBI may differ from the presentation in the noninjured population. In general, the more mild the TBI, the more similar the presentation is. However, special challenges arise in more severely injured individuals with cognitive, motor, and speech/language deficits. There are 3 broad factors that contribute to variability in clinical presentation.

Mood Instability and Affective Lability

Because of the instability in mood and affect accompanying disruption of the aforementioned frontal-subcortical circuits, it is necessary to pay attention to an extended baseline of behavior. Individuals with TBI are subject to more rapid fluctuation in mood and affect and this overall instability should not be equated with the more sustained alteration in mood that is the hallmark of depression. Attributing internal feelings to external behavior is more difficult because of the frequent presence of pathological or "pseudobulbar" affect (58,187).

Alterations in Speech and Language Function

Varying degrees of speech/language impairment are commonly seen following TBI, particularly in individuals with more severe injuries. These changes can range from subtle problems with naming and word finding to global aphasia. Dysarthria and articulation problems can be seen. The ability to modulate the prosody of speech can also be altered (188). This is manifested by difficulties in modulating speech tone, pitch, and amplitude (expressive aprosody), or in decoding and interpreting these components in the speech of others (receptive aprosody). The result of these deficits is an uncoupling of the content or propositional component of speech from the emotional valence and related nonverbal components of language. Patients with receptive dysprosody may have difficulty reading social cues and this may contribute to problems in social comportment. Those with expressive dysprosody may express distressing thought content without seeming to have appropriate accompanying affect (e.g., "I am depressed and suicidal" expressed in a flat monotone without depth of feeling) leading the clinician to be somewhat confused about the clinical significance of what is being expressed.

Effects of Associated Neurological Impairments

One must also consider the effect that injury-related neurological deficits may have on clinical symptoms of psychiatric disorders. For example, how will depression be expressed or manifested in nonverbal patients? How will delusions and hallucinations be evident in these same patients? In an individual with quadriplegia, what does manic hyperactivity look like? How will PTSD present in someone with amnesia for the event? Thus the clinician must become adept at envisioning what the psychiatric illness would look like if expressed through the filter of the individual's neurological and functional deficits.

Effects of Cognitive Impairment

Individuals with poor self-monitoring, impaired memory, distorted sense of time, or time-sequencing deficits will have significant problems presenting an accurate history. The clinician must rely not only on what the individual reports but must strive to get additional information from family/caregivers.

Heightened Vulnerability to Medication Side Effects

Individuals with TBI as well as other neuropsychiatric disorders often manifest an increased sensitivity to medication side effects. This may take several forms. The first is a ten-dency to develop typical side effects associated with the given medication at a lower than usual dose. The second is a lowered threshold at which the individual develops a delirium or toxic encephalopathy. The third is a worsening of the neurological deficits associated with the TBI. For example, it is not uncommon to observe worsening of tremor or gait problems, increased emotional lability, or increased slowing of speed of information processing associated with psychotropic drug use. In other words, the very symptoms the clinician is treating may be made worse by the medications prescribed. This highlights the need to take a careful medication history encompassing not only the current medications but medications used in the past as well as the response to those agents. Furthermore it is important to clarify whether a history of "that medicine didn't help" reflects a true lack of response or more a manifestation of the heightened vulnerability to side effects just described.

The above issues contribute to diagnostic and treatment challenges that can be outlined as follows:

1. *Atypical Clinical Presentations* – As noted earlier, clinical presentations of common psychiatric disorders may not meet standard diagnostic criteria as outlined in the *DSM*. Thus, it is reasonable to employ a "relaxed fit" criteria when approaching diagnoses in individuals with TBI.

2. *Trait vs State Presentations* – It is important to point out that there are 2 broad factors that contribute to the neurobehavioral sequelae of TBI; the injury induced changes in personality, and the increased rate of psychiatric disorders. A problem arises when the latter presents as a heightening or worsening of the former. For example, it is quite common for an individual with TBI to have a baseline of increased irritability or lowered frustration tolerance. It is also quite common for these traits to be exaggerated in the presence of a superimposed episode of depression or mania (or some other psychiatric disorder). If the clinician does not carefully tease out the postinjury baseline and clearly ascertain whether there is a change in the frequency and/or intensity of the challenging behaviors, it is easy to misattribute challenging behavior to a dysexecutive syndrome only, as opposed to a dysexecutive syndrome exacerbated by the presence of an Axis I psychiatric disorder.

3. *Treat syndromes or disorders not symptoms (diagnosis before treatment)* – It goes without saying that it is best to have a clear sense of what is causing the challenging behavior before designing a treatment plan. Yet many clinicians are inclined to prescribe antipsychotics or selective serotonin reuptake inhibitors (SSRIs) without formulating a hypothesis for what they are treating. This is a symptomatic approach—similar to treating a fever associated with a bacterial infection with acetaminophen but not antibiotics. In the neuropsychiatric arena, the symptomatic approach should be a last resort after having carefully ruled in or out an Axis I disorder (e.g., depression, mania, psychosis), neuromedical conditions that would account for the behavior (e.g., complex partial seizures, pain, iatrogenic complications, medication side effects), or factors in the environment that are causing the change in behavioral symptoms. Again it is important to emphasize that being wrong sometimes is unavoidable, but sloppy diagnostic thinking is avoidable.

TABLE 62-2 Examples of Behavioral Metaphors

TYPE	BEHAVIOR	INITIAL TREATMENT
Depressive	Negativistic, lack of interest in activities, weepy, aggressive or self-injurious behavior	SSRI's or other antidepressants
Manic	Increased level of arousal and activity, irritability, decreased need for sleep, increased sexual activity	Mood stabilizers or anti-cycling agents (e.g., anticonvulsants, lithium)
Psychotic	Consistent misinterpretation of environment in a paranoidfashion, apparent response to internal stimuli, aggression that "comes out of nowhere" but may flow out of paranoid misinterpretation of events	Antipsychotics (e.g., low dose risperidone)
Anxiolytic	Challenging behaviors most apparent in setting of anticipation of events, change in routine, consistently difficult, or novel situations	Anxiolytics

Abbreviation: SSRI, selective serotonin reuptake inhibitor. Reprinted from Ryan JM, Kidder SW, Daiello LA, Tariot PN. Psychopharmacologic interventions in nursing homes: what do we know and where should we go? *Psychiatr Serv.* 2002;53(11):1407–1413.

4. *Role of behavioral metaphors* – There are times, especially when data is difficult to obtain or when the neurological deficits through which challenging behaviors are being expressed are severe, that one is at a loss to account for the etiology of a given behavior or behaviors, and thus not clear about a treatment strategy. A fallback position is to attempt to conceptualize the cluster of behaviors as if they were a particular syndrome or as if they represented what Tariot et al. (189,190) have termed a "behavioral metaphor." For example, an individual expressing increased negativism, loss of interest in activities, and/or self-destructive or self-injurious behavior might be conceptualized as having a depressive syndrome (see Table 62-2) and thus could reasonably be prescribed an antidepressant regimen. An individual with increased irritability, increased arousal and activation, and a significant reduction in sleep might be conceptualized as having an irritable manic-like syndrome and thus be started on an anticycling regimen or mood stabilizers. The critical issue is that these are testable hypotheses and should be treated as such. Target behaviors and baseline frequencies should be identified prior to treatment and an adequate but time-limited trial prescribed. It should be clearly decided what the endpoint is and if the desired goal is not attained, the medication should be discontinued and an alternative conceptual scheme considered.

Role of Behavioral and Environmental Interventions

It is important to point out that individuals with cognitive impairment of all kinds, including individuals with TBI, have a heightened sensitivity not only to medications but also to the environment in which they live. This is related to several factors.

Stimulus Boundedness
As mentioned earlier, one of the characteristics of damage to frontal-subcortical circuits with attendant problems in executive function and social comportment is that individuals have great difficulty with components of attention including complex, selective, and sustained attention. This results in difficulty with prioritization of incoming stimuli and the gating out of stimuli that would ordinarily be deemed of secondary importance. At its essence, this may be a problem assigning or decoding proper salience to the constant influx of environmental cues and stimuli. In any event, the result is that the individual becomes hostage for at least very sensitive to, events in their immediate environment.

Fondness for Routine
Individuals with cognitive deficits are often quite sensitive to changes in routine or schedule. This may relate to the aforementioned deficits in executive function in which problems with problem solving and mental flexibility can be quite apparent. Over time, individuals (injured or noninjured) develop routines that tend to maximize predictability and efficient function, and minimize stress. Changes in these routines call for mental flexibility and problem solving skills to maintain environmental homeostasis. Individuals challenged in these domains will often respond with anxiety, irritability, or even catastrophic reactions to these changes in routine. This tendency can be apparent in response to both changes in people in their environment or changes in time or schedule. The latter may relate to basic impairments in both sense of time and memory, resulting in ongoing anxiety and perseverative requests for information or reassurance with respect to upcoming events or activities. Family/caregivers and staff often function as cognitive prosthetic devices that the individual relies on to supply ongoing memory for events, maintenance of schedule, and overall sense of time. Being deprived of these human prosthetic devices is a frightening experience and can result in appearance of some very challenging behaviors.

Predictability of Response
Injured and noninjured individuals alike base much of minute-to-minute and long-term decisions and actions on predictions of the response a given action will produce. Increasing the probability of favorable responses and decreasing the likelihood of undesirable responses are powerful forces in shaping behavior. However, certain executive deficits such as inferential reasoning, self-monitoring, self-correction, and

episodic memory are critical to the successful application of these experiences to shaping behavior. In this context, predictability of response becomes even more critical to maximize contextual learning and generalize these lessons to other novel settings. Individuals existing in an environment in which the same behaviors elicit different responses from different people at different times can become confused, anxious, and agitated.

Thus it is critical to carefully consider these factors when performing a neuropsychiatric assessment. To ignore the environment and factors that may be provoking challenging behaviors will greatly reduce the efficacy of any prescribed medication even if it is the proper medication. On the other hand, without the properly prescribed medication, even massive efforts at applied behavioral analysis and environmental manipulation may be in vain. The therapeutic issue should not be "do we prescribe a drug, or write a behavioral plan?" Rather the question is better framed as "which medicine prescribed in the context of what changes in environment and strategies for shaping behavior has the best potential for success?"

CONCLUSION

Attention to the diagnosis and management of the emotional and behavioral sequelae of TBI can serve a critical role in advancing the rehabilitative process. It requires a knowledge and understanding of the profile of regional structural and neurochemical injury associated with the typical TBI and how that profile predicts the common neurobehavioral sequelae. Careful assessment requires an accurate description of the individual's functional and neurobehavioral status prior to the injury, and how that has changed subsequent to the injury. It is helpful to be aware of the problems in diagnosis in individuals who have a fluctuating behavioral baseline, who may have significant cognitive deficits, or in whom the usual connection between internal feeling state and external behaviors may be uncoupled. Treatment should follow from a clearly articulated diagnostic scheme and should be time-limited and reevaluated in the presence of poor or incomplete response.

KEY CLINICAL POINTS

1. Emotional and behavioral changes are extremely common sequelae of TBI and are often the most disabling challenges faced by survivors and family/caregivers.
2. The nature of the common emotional and behavioral sequelae follow predictably from the typical neuropathological profile of TBI, including vulnerability of the frontal cortex and subfrontal white matter, the deeper midline structures including the basal ganglia, the rostral brainstem, and the temporal lobes including the hippocampi to damage. Regions that are the site of origin of neurons of the catecholaminergic, cholinergic, and sertonergic systems are also commonly injured.
3. Changes in "personality" after TBI usually reflect varying degrees of dysexecutive syndromes resulting from damage to frontal subcortical circuitry with cells of origin in (*a*) the lateral orbitofrontal cortex (social comportment), (*b*) the dorsolateral frontal cortex (higher order cognitive functions), and (*c*) the anterior cingulate (alterations in motivated behavior).
4. TBI neuropathology is associated with significantly increased relative risk of developing a variety of psychiatric disorders, most notably depression and anxiety. The presentation of these psychiatric disorders can be somewhat atypical reflecting the characteristic deficits in cognition, impulse control, and speech and language that can also accompany TBI.
5. Assessment of emotional and behavioral challenges in an individual with TBI requires some adjustments on the part of the clinician including need for additional sources of information beyond the patient, clear assessment of preinjury baseline traits and behaviors, clarification of what has changed as a result of the injury, and careful appraisal of the profile of injury in a given individual. Neuropsychiatric appraisal involves a thoughtful synthesis of these factors in the context of the individual's psychosocial environment and the role the injury has played in altering this environment.

KEY REFERENCES

1. Bombradier CH, Fann JR, Temkin NR, Esselman, PC, Barber J, Dikmen SS. Rates of major depressive disorder and clinical outcomes following traumatic brain injury. *JAMA.* 2010;303(19):1938–1945.
2. Cummings JL. Frontal-subcortical circuits and human behavior. *Arch Neurol.* 1993;50(8):873–880.
3. Farkas O, Povlishock JT. Cellular and subcellular change evoked by diffuse traumatic brain injury: a complex web of change extending far beyond focal damage. *Prog Brain Res.* 2007;161:43–59.
4. Kim E, Lauterbach EC, Reeve A, et al; for ANPA Committee on Research. Neuropsychiatric complications of traumatic brain injury: a critical review of the literature (a report of the ANPA Committee on Research). *J Neuropsychiatry Clin Neurosci.* 2007;19:106–127.
5. McAllister TW. Neurobiological consequences of TBI. *Dialogues Clin Neurosci.* 2011;13(3):287–300
6. Smith C. Neuropathology. In: Silver J, McAllister T, Yudofsky S, eds. *Textbook of Traumatic Brain Injury.* 2nd ed. Washington, DC: American Psychiatric Publishing; 2011: 23–35.
7. Whelan-Goodinson R, Ponsford J, Johnston L, Grant F. Psychiatric disorders following traumatic brain injury: their nature and frequency. *J Head Trauma Rehabil.* 2009; 24(5):324–332.

References

1. Lishman WA. The psychiatric sequelae of head injury: a review. *Psychol Med.* 1973;3:304–318.
2. McKinlay WW, Brooks DN, Bond MR, Martinage DP, Marshall MM. The short term outcomes of severe blunt head injury as reported by relatives of the injured persons. *J Neurol Neurosurg Psychiatry.* 1981;44(6):527–533.
3. Oddy M, Humphrey M, Uttley D. Subjective impairment and social recovery after closed head injury. *J Neurol Neurosurg Psychiatry.* 1978;41(7):611–616.
4. Goethe KE, Levin HS. Behavioral manifestation during the early and long-term stages of recovery after closed head injury. *Psychiatr Ann.* 1984;14:540–546.

5. McAllister TW. Neurobiological consequences of traumatic brain injury. *Dialogues Clinical Neurosci.* 2011;13(3):287–300.

6. Arciniegas D, Topkoff J. The neuropsychiatry of pathological affect: an approach to evaluation and treatment. *Semin Clin Neuropsychiatry.* 2000;5(4):290–306.

7. Fann JR, Katon WJ, Uomoto JM, Esselman PC. Psychiatric disorders and functional disability in outpatients with traumatic brain injuries. *Am J Psychiatry.* 1995;152(10):1493–1499.

8. Sorenson SB, Kraus JF. Occurrence, severity, and outcome of brain injury. *J Head Trauma Rehabil.* 1991;5:1–10.

9. Levin HS, Gary HE, Eisenberg HM, et al. Neurobehavioral outcome 1 year after severe head injury. Experience of the traumatic coma data bank. *J Neurosurg.* 1990;73(5):699–709.

10. Smith C. Neuropathology. In: Silver J, McAllister T, Yudofsky S, eds. *Textbook of Traumatic Brain Injury.* 2nd ed. Washington, DC: American Psychiatric Publishing; 2011:23–35.

11. Friedlander RM. Apoptosis and caspases in neurodegenerative diseases. *N Engl J Med.* 2003;348(14):1365–1375.

12. Raghupathi R. Cell death mechanisms following traumatic brain injury. *Brain Pathol.* 2004;14(2):215–222.

13. Farkas O, Povlishock JT. Cellular and subcellular change evoked by diffuse traumatic brain injury: a complex web of change extending far beyond focal damage. *Prog Brain Res.* 2007;161:43–59.

14. Umile EM, Sandel ME, Alavi A, Terry CM, Plotkin RC. Dynamic imaging in mild traumatic brain injury: support for the theory of medial temporal vulnerability. *Arch Phys Med Rehabil.* 2002;83(11):1506–1513.

15. McIntosh TK. Neurochemical sequelae of traumatic brain injury: therapeutic implications. *Cerebrovasc Brain Metab Rev.* 1994;6:109–162.

16. McIntosh TK, Juhler M, Wieloch T. Novel pharmacologic strategies in the treatment of experimental traumatic brain injury: 1998. *J Neurotrauma.* 1998;15(10):731–769.

17. McAllister TW, Flashman LA, Sparling MB, Saykin AJ. Working memory deficits after mild traumatic brain injury: catecholaminergic mechanisms and prospects for catecholaminergic treatment-a review. *Brain Inj.* 2004;18(4):331–350.

18. Prasad MR, Tzigaret CM, Smith D, Soares H, McIntosh TK. Decreased alpha 1-adrenergic receptors after experimental brain injury. *J Neurotrauma.* 1992;9(3):269–279.

19. Feeney DM, Boyeson MG, Linn RT, Murray HM, Dail WG. Responses to cortical injury. I. Methodology and local effects of contusions in the rat. *Brain Res.* 1981;211:67–77.

20. Feeney DM, Hovda DA. Amphetamine and apomorphine restore tactile placing after motor cortex injury in the cat. *Psychopharmacology* (Berl). 1983;79(1):67–71.

21. Feeney DM, Sutton RL. Pharmacotherapy for recovery of function after brain injury. *Crit Rev Neurobiol.* 1987;1987(3):135–197.

22. Boyeson MG, Feeney DM. The role of norepinephrine in recovery from brain injury. *Soc Neurosci Abstr.* 1984;10:68.

23. Romhanyi R, Tandian D, Hovda DA, et al. Catecholaminergic stimulation enhances recovery of function following concussive brain injury. *J Neurotrauma.* 1990;9:164.

24. Tandian D, Romhanyi R, Hovda DA, et al. Amphetamine enhances both behavior and metabolic recovery following fluid percussion brain injury. *J Neurotrauma.* 1990;9:174.

25. Sutton RL, Feeney DM. α-Noradrenergic agonists and antagonists affect recovery and maintenance of beam-walking ability after sensorimotor cortex ablation in the rat. *Restor Neurol Neurosci.* 1992;4:1–11.

26. Smeets WJ, González A. Catecholamine systems in the brain of vertebrates: new perspectives through a comparative approach. *Brain Res Brain Res Rev.* 2000;33(2–3):308–379.

27. Charney DS. Monoamine dysfunction and the pathophysiology and treatment of depression. *J Clin Psychiatry.* 1998;59(suppl 14):11–14.

28. McAllister TW. Apathy. *Semin Clin Neuropsychiatry.* 2000;5(4):275–282.

29. Arnsten AFT. Catecholamine modulation of prefrontal cortical cognitive function. *Trends Cogn Sci.* 1998;2(11):436–447.

30. McAllister TW. Evaluation and treatment of neurobehavioral complications of traumatic brain injury—have we made any progress? *NeuroRehabilitation.* 2002;17:263–264.

31. Arciniegas DB. The cholinergic hypothesis of cognitive impairment caused by traumatic brain injury. *Curr Psychiatry Rep.* 2003;5(5):391–399.

32. Dixon CE, Liu SJ, Jenkins LW. Time course of increased vulnerability of cholinergic neurotransmission following traumatic brain injury in the rat. *Behav Brain Res.* 1995;70:125–131.

33. Dewar D, Graham DI. Depletion of choline acetyltransferase but preservation of M1 and M2 muscarinic receptor binding sites temporal cortex following head injury: a preliminary human postmorten study. *J Neurotrauma.* 1996;13:181–187.

34. Murdoch I, Perry EK, Court JA, Graham DI, Dewar D. Cortical cholinergic dysfunction after human head injury. *J Neurotrauma.* 1998;15(5):295–305.

35. Murdoch I, Nicoll JA, Graham DI, Dewar D. Nucleus basalis of Meynert pathology in the human brain after fatal head injury. *J Neurotrauma.* 2002;19:279–284.

36. Perry EK, Perry RH. Neurochemistry of consciousness: cholinergic pathologies in the human brain. *Prog Brain Res.* 2004;145:287–299.

37. Shytle RD, Silver AA, Sheehan KH, Sheehan DV, Sanberg PR. Neuronal nicotinic receptor inhibition for treating mood disorders: preliminary controlled evidence with mecamylamine. *Depression Anxiety.* 2002;16(3):89–92.

38. Pappius HM. Local cerebral glucose utilization in thermally traumatized rat brain. *Ann Neurol.* 1981;9(5):484–491.

39. Tsuiki K, Takada A, Nagahiro S, Grdisa M, Diksic M, Pappius HM. Synthesis of serotonin in traumatized rat brain. *J Neurochem.* 1995;64(3):1319–1325.

40. Cummings JL. Frontal-subcortical circuits and human behavior. *Arch Neurol.* 1993;50(8):873–880.

41. Bonelli RM, Cummings JL. Frontal-subcortical circuitry and behavior. *Dialogues in Clinical Neuroscience.* 9(2):141–151, 2007.

42. McDonald BC, Flashman LA, Saykin AJ. Executive dysfunction following traumatic brain injury: neural substrates and treatment strategies. *NeuroRehabilitation.* 2002;17:333–344.

43. Lovell M, Franzen M. Neuropsychological assessment. In: Silver JM, Yudofsky S, Hales RE, eds. *Neuropsychiatry of Traumatic Brain Injury.* Washington, DC: American Psychiatric Press Inc; 1994:133–160.

44. Whyte J, Polansky M, Cavallucci C, Fleming M, Lhulier J, Coslett HB. Inattentive behavior after traumatic brain injury. *J Int Neuropsychol Soc.* 1996;2:274–281.

45. Ben-Yishay Y, Diller L. Cognitive remediation in traumatic brain injury: update and issues. *Arch Phys Med Rehabil.* 1993;74(2):204–213.

46. Cicerone K, Dahlberg C, Kalmar K, et al. Evidence-based cognitive rehabilitation: recommendations for clinical practice. *Arch Phys Med Rehabil.* 2000;81:1596–1615.

47. Binder LM. A review of mild head trauma 2: clinical implications. *J Clin Exp Neuropsychol.* 1997;19(3):432–457.

48. Binder LM, Rohling ML, Larrabee J. A review of mild head trauma. Part I: meta-analytic review of neuropsychological studies. *J Clin Experimental Neuropsychol.* 1997;19(3):421–431.

49. Cripe LI. The neuropsychological assessment and management of closed head injury: general guidelines. *Cogn Rehabil.* 1987;5:18–22.

50. Gentilini M, Nichelli P, Schoenhuber R. Assessment of attention in mild head injury. In: Levin H, Eisenberg H, Benton A, eds. *Mild Head Injury.* New York, NY: Oxford University Press; 1989:163–175.

51. Gronwall D. Cumulative and persisting effects of concussion on attention and cognition. In: Levin H, Eisenberg H, Benton A, eds. *Mild Head Injury.* New York, NY: Oxford University Press; 1989:153–162.

52. Gronwall D. Minor head injury. *Neuropsychol.* 1991;5(4):253–265.

53. Leininger BE, Gramling SE, Farrell AD, Kreutzer JS, Peck EA III. Neuropsychological deficits in symptomatic minor head injury patients after concussion and mild concussion. *J Neurol Neurosurg Psychiatry.* 1990;53(4):293–296.

54. Levin HS, Grossman RG. Behavioral sequelae of closed head injury. *Arch Neurol.* 1978;35:720–727.

55. Levin HS, Amparo EG, Eisenberg HM, et al. Magnetic resonance imaging and computerized tomography in relation to the neurobehavioral sequelae of mild and moderate head injuries. *J Neurosurg.* 1987;66:706–713.

56. Levin HS, Goldstein FC, High WM, Eisenberg HM. Disproportionately severe memory deficit in relation to normal intellectual functioning after closed head injury. *J Neurol Neurosurg Psychiatry.* 1988; 51:1294–1301.

57. Binder LM. Persisting symptoms after mild head injury: a review of the postconcussive syndrome. *J Clin Exp Neuropsychol.* 1986;4: 323–346.

58. Arciniegas DB, Lauterbach EC, Anderson K, et al. The differential diagnosis of pseudobulbar affect (PBA): distinguishing PBA from disorders of mood and affect. Proceedings of roundtable meeting. *CNS Spectr.* 2005;10(5):1–14.

59. Flashman LA, McAllister TW. Lack of awareness and its impact in traumatic brain injury. *Neurorehabilitation.* 2002;17(4):285–296.

60. Flashman LA, Amador X, McAllister TW. Awareness of Deficits, in Silver JM, McAllister TW, Yudofsky SC (eds). Textbook of Traumatic Brain Injury. Second Edition, American Psychiatric Press, Inc. Washington D.C. 2011;307–323.

61. Fahy TJ, Irving MH, Millac P. Severe head injuries. A six-year follow-up. *Lancet.* 1967;2:475–479.

62. Ezrachi O, Ben-Yishay Y, Kay T, Diller L, Rattok J. Predicting employment in traumatic brain injury following neuropsychological rehabilitation. *J Head Trauma Rehabil.* 1991;6:71–84.

63. Sherer M, Bergloff P, Levin E, High WM Jr, Oden KE, Nick TG. Impaired awareness and employment outcome after traumatic brain injury. *J Head Trauma Rehabil.* 1998;13(5):52–61.

64. Sherer M, Boake C, Levin E, Silver BV, Ringholz G, High WM Jr. Characteristics of impaired awareness after traumatic brain injury. *J Int Neuropsychol Soc.* 1998;4(4):380–387.

65. Cavallo MM, Kay T, Ezrachi O. Problems and changes after traumatic brain injury: differing perceptions within and between families. *Brain Inj.* 1992;6:327–335.

66. Cuesta MJ, Peralta V. Lack of insight in schizophrenia. *Schizophr Bull.* 1994;20:359–366.

67. Cuesta MJ, Peralta V, Caro F, de Leon J. Is poor insight in psychotic disorders associated with poor performance on the Wisconsin Card Sorting Test? [erratum appears in *Am J Psychiatry.* 1996;153(2):270.]. *Am J Psychiatry.* 1995;152(9):1380–1382.

68. David A, Van Os J, Jones P, Harvey I, Foerster A, Fahy T. Insight and psychotic illness: cross-sectional and longitudinal associations. *Br J Psychiatry.* 1995;167:621–628.

69. Lysaker P, Bell M. Insight and cognitive impairment in schizophrenia: performance on repeated administrations of the Wisconsin Card Sorting Test. *J Nerv Ment Dis.* 1994;182(11):656–660.

70. McEvoy JP, Apperson LJ, Applebaum PS, et al. Insight into schizophrenia: its relationship to acute psychopathology. *J Nerv Ment Dis.* 1989;177:43–47.

71. Mohamed S, Fleming S, Penn DL, Spaulding W. Insight in schizophrenia: its relationship to measures of executive functions. *J Nerv Ment Dis.* 1999;187(9):525–531.

72. Young DA, Davila R, Scher H. Unawareness of illness and neuropsychological performance in chronic schizophrenia. *Schizophr Res.* 1993;10:117–124.

73. Ford B. Head injuries—what happens to survivors. *Med J Aust.* 1976;1:603–605.

74. Miller H, Stern G. The long-term prognosis of severe head injury. *Lancet.* 1965;1:225–229.

75. Oddy M, Coughlan T, Tyerman A, Jenkins D. Social adjustment after closed head injury: a further follow-up seven years after injury. *J Neurol Neurosurg Psychiatry.* 1985;48:564–568.

76. Ota Y. Psychiatric studies on civilian head injuries. In: Walker AE, Caveness WF, Critchley M, eds. *The Late Effects of Head Injury.* Springfield, IL: C. C. Thomas; 1969:110–119.

77. Prigatano GP. Disturbances of self-awareness of deficit after traumatic brain injury. In: Prigatano GL, Schacter DL, eds. *Awareness of Deficit After Brain Injury.* New York, NY: Oxford University Press; 1991:111–126.

78. Marin RS. Apathy: a neuropsychiatric syndrome. *J Neuropsychiatry Clin Neurosci.* 1991;3(3):243–254.

79. Kant R, Duffy JD, Pivovarnik A. Prevalence of apathy following head injury. *Brain Inj.* 1998;12(1):87–92.

80. Andersson S, Krogstad JM, Finset A. Apathy and depressed mood in acquired brain damage: relationship to lesion localization and psychophysiological reactivity. *Psychol Med.* 1999;29(2):447–456.

81. Chau DT, Roth RM, Green AI. The neural circuitry of reward and its relevance to psychiatric disorders. *Curr Psychiatry Rep.* 2004;6: 391–399.

82. van Reekum R, Cohen T, Wong J. Can traumatic brain injury cause psychiatric disorders? *J Neuropsychiatry Clin Neurosci.* 2000;12: 316–327.

83. Hibbard MR, Uysal S, Kepler K, Bogdany J, Silver J. Axis I psychopathology in individuals with traumatic brain injury. *J Head Trauma Rehabil.* 1998;13(4):24–39.

84. Koponen S, Taiminen T, Portin R, et al. Axis I and II psychiatric disorders after traumatic brain injury: a 30-year follow-up study. *Am J Psychiatry.* 2002;159(8):1315–1321.

85. Deb S, Lyons I, Koutzoukis C. Neuropsychiatric sequelae one year after a minor head injury. *J Neurol Neurosurg Psychiatry.* 1998;65(6): 899–902.

86. Kim E, Lauterbach EC, Reeve A, et al; for ANPA Committee on Research. Neuropsychiatric complication of traumatic brain injury: a critical review of the literature (a report of the ANPA Committee on Research). *J Neuropsychiatry Clin Neurosci.* 2007;19:106–127.

87. Bourdon KH, Rae DS, Locke BZ, Narrow WE, Regier DA. Estimating the prevalence of mental disorders in U.S. adults from the Epidemiologic Catchment Area Survey. *Public Health Rep.* 1992;107(6): 663–668.

88. Ashman TA, Spielman LA, Hibbard MR, Silver JM, Chandna T, Gordon WA. Psychiatric challenges in the first 6 years after traumatic brain injury: cross-sequential analyses of Axis I disorders. *Arch Phys Med Rehabil.* 2004;85(suppl 2):S36–S42.

89. Whelan-Goodinson R, Ponsford J, Johnston L, Grant F. Psychiatric disorders following traumatic brain injury: their nature and frequency. *J Head Trauma Rehabil.* 2009;24(5):324–332.

90. Whelan-Goodinson R, Ponsford J, Schönberger M. Association between psychiatric state and outcome following traumatic brain injury. *J Rehabil Med.* 2008;40:850–857.

91. Fann JR, Burington B, Leonetti A, Jaffe K, Katon WJ, Thompson RS. Psychiatric illness following traumatic brain injury in an adult health maintenance organization population. *Arch Gen Psychiatry.* 2004;61(1):53–61.

92. Wei W, Sambamoorthi U, Crystal S, Findley PA. Mental illness, traumatic brain injury, and medicaid expenditures. *Arch Phys Med Rehabil.* 2005;86(5):905–911.

93. Jorge RE, Starkstein SE. Pathophysiologic aspects of major depression following traumatic brain injury. *J Head Trauma Rehabil.* 2005; 20(6):475–487.

94. Rapoport M. Depression complicating traumatic brain injury. *Psychiatr Ann.* 2010;40(11):581–587.

95. Bombradier CH, Fann JR, Temkin NR, Esselman PC, Barber J, Dikmen SS. Rates of major depressive disorder and clinical outcomes following traumatic brain injury. *JAMA.* 2010;303(19):1938–1945.

96. Jorge RE, Robinson RG, Moser D, Tateno A, Crespo-Facorro B, Arndt S. Major depression following traumatic brain injury. *Arch Gen Psychiatry.* 2004;61(1):42–50.

97. Jorge RE, Robinson RG, Arndt S, Forrester AW, Geisler FH, Starkstein SE. Depression following traumatic brain injury: a 1 year longitudinal study. *J Affect Disord.* 1993;27:233–243.

98. Brody AL, Barsom MW, Bota RG, Saxena S. Prefrontal-subcortical and limbic circuit mediation of major depressive disorder. *Semin Clin Neuropsychiatry.* 2001;6(2):102–112.

99. Drevets WC, Raichle ME. Neuroanatomical circuits in depression: implications for treatment mechanisms. *Psychopharmacol Bull.* 1992; 28(3):261–274.

100. Liotti M, Mayberg HS. The role of functional neuroimaging in the neuropsychology of depression. *J Clin Exp Neuropsychol.* 2001;23(1): 121–136.

101. Drevets WC. Functional anatomical abnormalities in limbic and prefrontal cortical structures in major depression. *Prog Brain Res.* 2000;126:413–431.

102. Guillamondegui OD, Montgomery SA, Phibbs FT, et al. Traumatic Brain Injury and Depression: Comparative Effectiveness Review No. 25 (Prepared by the Vanderbilt Evidence-based Practice Center under Contract No. 290-2007-10065-I). AHRQ Publication No. 11-EHC017-EF. Rockville, MD: Agency for Healthcare Research and Quality; April 2011.

103. Seel R, Macciocchi S, Kreutzer JS. Clinical considerations for the diagnosis of major depression after moderate to severe TBI. *J Head Trauma Rehabil.* 2010;25(2):99–112.

104. Starkstein SE, Boston JD, Robinson RG. Mechanisms of mania after brain injury: 12 case reports and review of the literature. *J Nerv Ment Dis.* 1988;176:87–100.

105. Robinson RG, Boston JD, Starkstein SE, Price TR. Comparison of mania and depression after brain injury: causal factors. *Am J Psychiatry.* 1988;145(2):172–178.

106. Shukla S, Cook BL, Mukherjee S, Godwin C, Miller MG. Mania following head trauma. *Am J Psychiatry.* 1987;144:93–96.

107. Silver JM, Kramer R, Greenwald S, Weissman M. The association between head injuries and psychiatric disorders: findings from the New Haven NIMH Epidemiologic Catchment Area Study. *Brain Inj.* 2001;15(11):935–945.

108. Starkstein SE, Mayberg HS, Berthier ML, et al. Mania after brain injury: neuro-radiological and metabolic findings. *Ann Neurol.* 1990;27:652–659.

109. Starkstein SE, Pearlson GD, Boston JD, Robinson RG. Mania after brain injury: a controlled study of causative factors. *Arch Neurol.* 1987;44(10):1069–1073.

110. McAllister TW. Traumatic brain injury and psychosis: what is the connection? *Semin Clin Neuropsychiatry.* 1998;3(3):211–223.

111. McAllister T, Ferrell R. Evaluation and treatment of psychosis after traumatic brian injury. *NeuroRehabilitation.* 2002;17:357–368.

112. Arciniegas DB, Harris SN, Brousseau KM. Psychosis following traumatic brain injury. *Int Rev Psychiatry.* 2003;15(4):328–340.

113. Davison K, Bagley CR. Schizophrenia-like psychosis associated with organic disorders of the central nervous system. *Br J Psychiatry.* 1969;114(suppl 4):113–184.

114. Malaspina D, Goetz RR, Friedman JH, et al. Traumatic brain injury and schizophrenia in members of schizophrenia and bipolar disorder pedigrees. *Am J Psychiatry.* 2001;158(3):440–446.

115. Trimble MR. The psychoses of epilepsy. *Clin Neuropharmacol.* 1985; 8:211–220.

116. McKenna P, Kane J, Parish K. Psychotic syndromes in epilepsy. *Am J Psychiatry.* 1985;142:895–904.

117. Krohn W. A study of epilepsy in northern Norway, its frequency and character. *Acta Psychiatr Neurol Scand Suppl.* 1961;36(150): 215–225.

118. Gudmundsson G. Epilepsy in Iceland. A clinical and epidemiological investigation. *Acta Neurol Scand.* 1966;43(suppl 25):1–124.

119. Sherwin I, Peron-Magnan P, Bancaud J, Bonis A, Talairach J. Prevalence of psychosis in epilepsy as a function of the laterality of the epileptogenic lesion. *Arch Neurol.* 1982;39(10):621–625.

120. Toone BK, Dawson J, Driver MV. Psychoses of epilepsy: a radiological evaluation. *Br J Psychiatry.* 1982;140:244–248.

121. Trimble MR, Perez M. The phenomenology of the chronic psychosis of epilepsy. In: Koella W, Trimble MR, eds. *Temporal Lobe Epilepsy, Mania, and Schizophrenia.* Basle, Switzerland: Karger; 1982: 98–105.

122. Flor-Henry P. Psychosis and temporal lobe epilepsy: a controlled investigation. *Epilepsia.* 1969;10:363–395.

123. Trimble MR. Interictal psychoses of epilepsy. *Adv Neurol.* 1991;55: 143–152.

124. Tucker G, Price T, Johnson V, McAllister T. Phenomenology of temporal lobe dysfunction: a link to atypical psychosis—a series of cases. *J Nerv Ment Dis.* 1986;174(6):348–356.

125. Waldman AJ. Neuroanatomic/neuropathologic correlates in schizophrenia. *South Med J.* 1992;85(9):907–916.

126. Waldman AJ. Neuroanatomic/neuropathologic correlates in schizophrenia. *South Med J.* 1992;85(9):907–916.

127. Stevens JR. Anatomy of schizophrenia revisited. *Schizophr Bull.* 1997;23(3):373–383.

128. Turetsky B, Cowell PE, Gur RC, Grossman RI, Shtasel DL, Gur RE. Frontal and temporal lobe brain volumes in schizophrenia. Relationship to symptoms and clinical subtype. *Arch Gen Psychiatry.* 1995;52(12):1061–1070.

129. Andreasen NC, Arndt S, Swayze V II, et al. Thalamic abnormalities in schizophrenia visualized through magnetic resonance image averaging. *Science.* 1994;266:294–298.

130. Buchanan RW, Breier A, Kirkpatrick B, et al. Structural abnormalities in deficit and nondeficit schizophrenia. *Am J Psychiatry.* 1993; 150(1):59–65.

131. Jernigan TL, Zisook S, Heaton RK, Moranville JT, Hesselink JR, Braff DL. Magnetic resonance imaging abnormalities in lenticular nuclei and cerebral cortex in schizophrenia. *Arch Gen Psychiatry.* 1991;48(10):881–890.

132. Swayze VW II, Andreasen NC, Alliger RJ, Yuh WT, Ehrhardt JC. Subcortical and temporal structures in affective disorder and schizophrenia: a magnetic resonance imaging study. *Biol Psychiatry.* 1992;31(3):221–240.

133. Tamminga CA. Neuropsychiatric aspects of schizophrenia. In: Yudofsky SC, Hales RE, eds. *The American Psychiatric Press Textbook of Neuropsychiatry.* 3rd ed. Washington, DC: American Psychiatric Press; 1997:855–882.

134. Tamminga CA, Thaker GK, Buchanan R, et al. Limbic system abnormalities identified in schizophrenia using positron emission tomography with fluorodeoxyglucose and neocortical alterations with deficit syndrome. *Arch Gen Psychiatry.* 1992;49(7):522–530.

135. Buchsbaum MS, Haier RJ, Potkin SG, Nuechterlein K, et al. Frontostriatal disorder of cerebral metabolism in never-medicated schizophrenics. *Arch Gen Psychiatry.* 1992;49(12):935–942.

136. Selemon LD, Rajkowska G, Goldman-Rakic PS. Abnormally high neuronal density in two widespread areas of the schizophrenic cortex: a morphometric analysis of prefrontal area 9 and occipital area 17. *Arch Gen Psychiatry.* 1995;52:805–818.

137. Akbarian S, Kim JJ, Potkin SG, et al. Gene expression for glutamic acid decarboxylase is reduced without loss of neurons in prefrontal cortex of schizophrenics. *Arch Gen Psychiatry.* 1995;52(4):258–266.

138. Akbarian S, Kim JJ, Potkin SG, Hetrick WP, Bunney WE Jr, Jones EG. Maldistribution of interstitial neurons in prefrontal white matter of the brains of schizophrenic patients. *Arch Gen Psychiatry.* 1996;53(5):425–436.

139. Warden D, Labatte L. Posttraumatic stress disorder and other anxiety disorders. In: Silver J, McAllister T, Yudofsky S, eds. *Textbook of Traumatic Brain Injury.* Arlington, VA: American Psychiatric Publishing, Inc.; 2005:231–244.

140. Robinson RG, Jorge RE. Mood disorders. In: Silver J, Yudofsky SC, Hales RE, eds. *Neuropsychiatry of Traumatic Brain Injury.* Washington, DC: American Psychiatric Press; 1994:219–250.

141. Dikmen S, McLean A, Temkin N. Neuropsychological and psychosocial consequences of minor head injury. *J Neurol Neurosurg Psychiatry.* 1986;49(11):1227–1332.

142. Levin HS, Mattis S, Ruff RM, et al. Neurobehavioral outcome following minor head injury: a three-center study. *J Neurosurgery.* 1987;66(2):234–243.

143. Schoenhuber R, Gentilini M. Anxiety and depression after mild head injury: a case control study. *J Neurol Neurosurg Psychiatry.* 1988;51:722–724.

144. Deb S, Lyons I, Koutzoukis C. Neurobehavioural symptoms one year after a head injury. *Br J Psychiatry.* 1999;174:360–365.

145. Stein MB, McAllister TW. Exploring the convergence of posttraumatic stress disorder and mild traumatic brain injury. *Am J Psychiatry.* 2009;166(7):768–776.

146. McAllister T. Psychopharmacological issues in the treatment of tbi and ptsd. *Clin Neuropsychol.* 2009;23(8):1338–1367.

147. Vasterling JJ, Verfaellie M, Sullivan KD. Mild traumatic brain injury and posttraumatic stress disorder in returning veterans: perspectives from cognitive neuro-science. *Clin Psychol Rev.* 2009;29: 674–684.

148. Sbordone RJ, Liter JC. Mild traumatic brain injury does not produce post-traumatic stress disorder. *Brain Inj.* 1995;9(4):405–412.

149. Mayou RA, Black J, Bryant B. Unconsciousness, amnesia and psychiatric symptoms following road traffic accident injury. *Br J Psychiatry.* 2000;177:540–545.

150. McMillan TM. Post-traumatic stress disorder following minor and severe closed head injury: 10 single cases. *Brain Inj.* 1996;10(10): 749–758.

151. McMillan TM. Post-traumatic stress disorder and severe head injury. *Br J Psychiatry.* 1991;159:431–433.

152. Bryant RA, Harvey AG. The influence of traumatic brain injury on acute stress disorder and post-traumatic stress disorder following motor vehicle accidents. *Brain Inj.* 1999;13(1):15–22.

153. King N. Mild head injury: neuropathology, sequelae, measurement and recovery. *Br J Clin Psychol.* 1997;36(pt 2):161–184.

154. Bryant RA, Harvey AG. Relationship between acute stress disorder and posttraumatic stress disorder following mild traumatic brain injury. *Am J Psychiatry.* 1998;155(5):625–629.

155. Harvey AG, Bryant RA. Acute stress disorder after mild traumatic brain injury. *J Nerv Ment Dis.* 1998;186(6):333–337.

156. Harvey AG, Bryant RA. Predictors of acute stress following mild traumatic brain injury. *Brain Inj.* 1998;12(2):147–154.

157. Bryant RA, Harvey AG. Postconcussive symptoms and posttraumatic stress disorder after mild traumatic brain injury. *J Nerv Ment Dis.* 1999;187(5):302–305.

158. Hoge C, McGurk D, Thomas J, Cox A, Engel C, Castro C. Mild traumatic brain injury in U.S. soldiers returning from Iraq. *N Engl J Med.* 2008;358(5):453–463.

159. Schneiderman A, Braver E, Kang H. Understanding sequelae of injury mechanisms and mild traumatic brain injury incurred during the conflicts in Iraq and Afghanistan: persistent postconcussive symptoms and posttraumatic stress disorder. *Am J Epidemiol.* 2008; 167:1446–1452.

160. Belanger HG, Kretzmer T, Vanderploeg RD, French LM. Symptom complaints following combat-related traumatic brain injury: relationship to traumatic brain injury severity and posttraumatic stress disorder. *J Int Neuropsychol Soc.* 2010;16(1):194–199.

161. McAllister TW, Stein MB. Effects of psychological and biomechanical trauma on brain and behavior. *Ann N Y Acad Sci.* 2010;1208: 46–57.

162. Sparadeo FR, Strauss D, Bartels JT. The incidence, impact, and treatment of substance abuse in head trauma rehabilitation. *J Head Traum Rehabil.* 1990;5:108.

163. Miller N, Adams J. Alcohol and drug disorders. In: Silver J, McAllister T, Yudofsky SC, eds. *Text Book of Traumatic Brain Injury.* Arlington, VA: American Psychiatric Publishing, Inc.; 2005:509–532.

164. Edna TH. Alcohol influence and head injury. *Acta Chir Scand.* 1982; 148(3):209–212.

165. Sparadeo F, Gill D. Effects of prior alcohol use on head injury recovery. *J Head Trauma Rehabil.* 1989;4:75–82.

166. Brooks N, Symington C, Beattie A, Campsie L, Bryden J, McKinlay W. Alcohol and other predictors of cognitive recovery after severe head injury. *Brain Inj.* 1989;3(3):235–246.

167. Ruff RM, Niemann H. Cognitive rehabilitation versus day treatment in head-injured adults: is there an impact on emotional and psychosocial adjustment? *Brain Inj.* 1990;4(4):339–347.

168. Van Den Heuvel C, Thornton E, Vink R. Traumatic brain injury and Alzheimer's disease: a review. *Prog Brain Res.* 2007;161:303–316.

169. Van Den Heuvel C, Blumbergs PC, Finnie JW, et al. Upregulation of amyloid precursor protein messenger RNA in response to traumatic brain injury: an ovine head impact model. *Exp Neurol.* 1999; 159:441–450.

170. Blumbergs PC, Scott G, Manavis J, Wainwright H, Simpson DA, McLean AJ. Topography of axonal injury as defined by amyloid precursor protein and the sector scoring method in mild and severe closed head injury. *J Neurotrauma.* 1995;12(4):565–572.

171. Graham DI, Gentleman SM, Lynch A, Roberts GW. Distribution of beta-amyloid protein in the brain following severe head injury. *Neuropathol Appl Neurobiol.* 1995;21:27–34.

172. Uryu K, Chen X, Martinez D, et al. Multiple proteins implicated in neurodegenerative diseases accumulate in axons after brain trauma in humans. *Exp Neurol.* 2007;208(2):185–192.

173. Uryu K, Chen XH, Graham DJ. Short-term accumulation of beta-amyloid in axonal pathology following traumatic brain injury in humans. *Neurobiol Aging.* 2004;25(suppl 1):P2–P250.

174. Chen X, Johnson V, Uryu K, Trojanowski J, Smith D. A lack of amyloid beta plaques despite persistent accumulation of amyloid beta in axons of long-term survivors of traumatic brain injury. *Brain Pathol.* 2009;19(2):214–223.

175. Braak H, Braak E. Frequency of stages of Alzheimer-related lesions in different age categories. *Neurobiol Aging.* 1997;18(4):351–357.

176. Mayeux R, Ottman R, Maestre G, et al. Synergistic effects of traumatic head injury and apolipoprotein-epsilon 4 in patients with Alzheimer's disease. *Neurology.* 1995;45(3, pt 1):555–557.

177. Mehta K, Ott A, Kalmijn S, et al. Head trauma and risk of dementia and Alzheimer's disease: the Rotterdam Study. *Neurology.* 1999;53: 1959–1962.

178. Starkstein SE, Jorge R. Dementia after traumatic brain injury. *Int Psychogeriatr.* 2005;(17, suppl 1):S93–S107.

179. Ovsiew F, Bylsma FW. The three cognitive examinations. *Semin Clin Neuropsychiatry.* 2002;7(1):54–64.

180. McCauley S, Levin H, Vanier M, et al. The neurobehavioural rating scale-revised: sensitivity and validity in closed head injury assessment. *J Neurol Neurosurg Psychiatry.* 2001;71:643–651.

181. Cummings JL, Mega M, Gray K, Rosenberg-Thompson S, Carusi DA, Gornbein J. The Neuropsychiatric Inventory: comprehensive assessment of psychopathology in dementia. *Neurology.* 1994; 44(12):2308–2314.

182. Yudofsky S, Silver J, Jackson W, Endicott J, Williams D. The overt aggression scale for the objective rating of verbal and physical aggression. *Am J Psychiatry.* 1986;143:35–39.

183. Marin RS, Biedrzycki RC, Firinciogullari S. Reliability and validity of the Apathy Evaluation Scale. *Psychiatry Res.* 1991;38(2):143–162.

184. Folstein MF, Folstein SE, McHugh PR. "Mini Mental State": a practical method for grading the cognitive state of patients for the clinician. *J Psychiatry Res.* 1975;12:189–198.

185. Gioia GA, Isquith PK, Guy SC, Kenworthy L. *BRIEF: Behavior Rating Inventory of Executive Function.* Odessa, FL: Psychological Assessment Resources Inc; 2000.

186. Roth RM, Isquith PK, Gioia GA. *Behavioral Rating Inventory of Executive Function-Adult Version.* Lutz, FL: Psychological Assessment Resources Inc; 2005.

187. Arciniegas DB, Lauterbach EC, Anderson K, et al. The differential diagnosis of pseudobulbar affect (PBA): distinguishing PBA from disorders of mood and affect. *CNS Spectr.* 2005;10(5):1–4.

188. Ross DA, Olsen WL, Ross AM, Andrews BT, Pitts LH. Brain shift, level of consciousness, and restoration of consciousness in patients with acute intracranial hematoma. *J Neurosurg.* 1989;71(4):498–502.

189. Tariot PN, Loy R, Ryan JM, Porsteinsson A, Ismail S. Mood stabilizers in Alzheimer's disease: symptomatic and neuroprotective rationales. *Adv Drug Deliv Rev.* 2002;54(12):1567–1577.

190. Tariot PN. The older patient: the ongoing challenge of efficacy and tolerability. *J Clin Psychiatry.* 1999;(60, suppl 23):29–33.

Principles of Behavioral Analysis and Treatment

Robert L. Karol

INTRODUCTION

Behavioral dyscontrol after brain injury can take many forms and present with a multitude of patterns: physical aggression, verbal aggression, sexual inappropriateness, elopement, wandering, self-injurious behavior, suicide attempts, hoarding, stealing, nonadherence, demanding/manipulating, poor safety judgment, social inappropriateness, somatization, social withdrawal, unawareness of deficit, and so on. The spectrum of behaviors is broad, and there is no conclusive list. Behavioral challenges are common after brain injury (1–5). Apart from being problematic themselves, these behaviors interfere with the treatment of other brain injury sequela and increase disability (6).

Behavioral issues exist on a continuum, ranging from the merely troublesome to the outright dangerous. Some behaviors are only self-defeating, and others can place the person with brain injury or other people at risk. The armamentarium for treatment is the same across the range of behaviors, although the intensity and urgency of treatment may vary.

Some persons with brain injury who exhibit many of these behaviors may not get appropriate care. They may be placed in mental health units or prisons or may end up homeless. Persons with brain injury ought not to receive care for behavioral dyscontrol on generic mental health units where (*a*) the impact of cognitive deficits (and strengths) on behavior is poorly understood, (*b*) counseling is not adjusted for cognitive functioning, (*c*) staff usually are addressing different adjustment issues than those faced by people after brain injury, (*d*) the response to medication is different than that observed following brain injury, (*e*) team design fails to optimize care for persons with brain injury, and (*f*) discharge planning for persons with brain injury vexes traditional systems (7).

There is a high incidence of prior history of traumatic brain injury (TBI) in persons who are incarcerated, although the crime for which they were incarcerated may or may not be related to their brain injury. Still, some research shows that at least about 80% of inmates have had prior brain injuries (8,9). Many received no medical care even if there was loss of consciousness (10). If the goal of prison is to alter behavior, it is unclear how the punishment of incarceration or contingencies once incarcerated interacts with brain injury sequela to improve behavior nor are peer role models while incarcerated likely to be therapeutic.

Finally, brain injury is relatively common among the homeless, although obviously most persons with brain injury do not become homeless. Still, one report, for example, found that 32% of homeless people had received a blow to the head hard enough to knock them out or make them see stars. The problems they had thereafter included difficulty getting along with people. More than half of these people had their injuries before becoming homeless (55%), whereas some had injuries the same year (8%—it was unclear if the injury was before or after becoming homeless), and only 38% had their injury after becoming homeless (11).

Behavioral issues after brain injury can spill over from rehabilitation and brain injury treatment providers into other systems. The clinical presentations of persons with brain injury in mental health, correctional, and homelessness programs likely include behavioral challenges. Even when persons with brain injury are in appropriate treatment settings, behavioral dyscontrol interferes, leading to staff injuries and injuries to persons with brain injury, unless staff are well trained (12).

Hence, this chapter will address behavioral care. The intent of this chapter is to provide an overview of assessment and intervention methods related to behavioral treatment and highlight selected applications regardless of setting or severity. Two case vignettes are included at the end of the chapter.

BEHAVIORAL ASSESSMENT AND INTERVENTION

Assessment

Introduction to Assessment
Behavioral treatment is predicated on a thorough assessment. Assessment primarily covers three domains: emotional, behavioral, and cognitive functioning. Behavioral intervention risks being unsuccessful if there is inadequate evaluation of emotional, behavioral, and cognitive variables.

The *Diagnostic and Statistical Manual of Mental Disorders, Fourth Edition, Text Revision* (DSM-IV-TR) (13) inadequately describes the variations in disturbances related to brain injury (14). It is of limited value in providing guidance in assessing behavioral dyscontrol after brain injury. Its use often leads to a failure to consider how etiology (i.e., brain injury) impacts diagnoses (i.e., the presence of symptoms that would otherwise be evidence of a mental health condition may reflect brain injury and not a mental health diagnosis).

This can lead to persons with brain injury accumulating mental health diagnoses during their lives because aspects of their post-brain injury behavior present at various times, representing fluctuating behavioral symptoms of brain injury. Also, brain injury symptoms may not fit diagnostic categories (6,15,16); moreover, the diagnoses are insufficiently fine grained to determine behavioral intervention after brain injury. Nevertheless, persons with brain injury may have actual comorbid mental health issues (17,18). Because mental health conditions such as mood disorders, anxiety disorders, psychotic disorders, and so on have behavioral components, it is important to be aware of the behavioral presentation of comorbid mental health conditions.

Assessment of Emotional Status

Emotional disturbance is a significant component of brain injury and a critical determinant of behavior. The National Institute of Health Consensus Statement (19) states, "Mood disorders, personality changes, altered emotional control, depression, and anxiety are also prevalent after TBI" (p. 12). Because the brain regulates emotional functioning (20,21), organic damage can cause direct emotional changes. There is a documentation of the emotional sequela of brain injury (14,22), and researchers have paid particular attention to grief as distinct from depression (23). Brain lesions can alter emotional processing (24). There is also the emotional adjustment to having and living with a disability.

Both clinical acumen and psychometric assessment are useful to determine emotional functioning. Clinical assessment of emotional functioning occurs through a combination of diagnostic interview and observation. Interview can provide insight into what persons with brain injury are experiencing. How persons with brain injury express emotions can provide knowledge about their coping abilities. Observation when persons with brain injury demonstrate emotional dyscontrol provides clues as to what they are feeling. Knowledge of the antecedents and the consequences of emotions, as well as the qualitative and quantitative aspects of those emotions leads to a more complete understanding of the behavioral expression of emotions.

In the case of psychometric assessment, there is an unending array of published psychological test instruments for the determination of emotional functioning. These range from measures of particular emotional variables (e.g., Beck Depression Inventory-II) (25–28) to broader inventories (e.g., Minnesotta Multiphasic Personality Inventory-2 Restructured Form [MMPI-2-RF], Personality Assessment Inventory [PAI], Millon Clinical Multiaxial Inventory-III [MCMI-III]). Measures of particular emotional variables can give perspective on immediate drivers of behaviors. They can help inform short-term clinical decision making. They may be useful for determination of progress along specific lines. Broad measures of adjustment can be valuable for determining patterns of adjustment. They may reveal longer standing personality characteristics, and they can help identify important coping variables that may influence behavior.

For both measures of particular emotions and broader instruments, there may be limited norms for rehabilitation and neurological populations, cognitive deficits may impair the ability to take the tests, and somatic complaints may distort the results (29). Regarding cognitive deficits, the neurological experiences of persons with brain injury are unique

contaminants to the assessment of emotional status. Self-report by persons with brain injury can be distorted because of the injury. Memory deficits, in particular, can be a barrier to psychometric assessment of coping. Finally, cognitive deficits can impair the ability of persons with brain injury to complete the tests or they can lead to misinterpretation of the results because the findings are affected by cognitive deficits during test administration.

The application to the treatment of particular behaviors may require a significant degree of inference from measures of emotional states and coping to specific behaviors. These tests usually fail to point to particular behavioral intervention techniques. Hence, in many applied settings, specific instruments assessing particular behavioral functions may be more directly applicable.

Assessment of Behavior

It is essential that the formulation of any intervention program for behavioral problems be based on sound behavioral assessment. The principles of behavioral analysis and assessment have been long established (30,31). Furthermore, their application to brain injury care has been detailed for some time (32,33). Individualized behavioral assessment routinely begins with decisions about which behaviors to assess. The behavior is defined in operational terms, and determination is made of how it will be evaluated. Then observation of frequency, severity, duration, and so on of the behaviors can proceed.

Standardized rating of behavior is an alternative to individualized assessment of operationally defined target behaviors unique for each person. In this approach, behaviors are rated using predefined definitions. Ratings can be completed by professionals, families, persons with brain injury, or someone else. There are a myriad of rating scales, questionnaires, and interview formats that include behaviorally pertinent variables (34,35). Some of these are specific to particular types of behaviors (e.g., Overt Behavior Scale—verbal aggression, physical aggression, sexual behavior, wandering, etc. [36,37]). Other instruments include various aspects of functioning (e.g., Neurobehavioral Functioning Inventory—depression, communication, aggression, etc. [34, 35,38]; Neurobehavioral Rating Scale-Revised—behavioral regulation, emotional state, etc. [39,40]). Other measures are broader still and touch on behavioral issues in the context of wider rehabilitation issues (e.g., Mayo-Portland Adaptability Inventory—expressions of anger, social inappropriateness, legal violations, etc. [41–43]).

One challenge in the use of these measures is that the way the behavior is defined by the instrument may not match the behavior as observed. When using scales to rate a given behavior, it is essential to have awareness of how a scale is defining a behavior, what is included and what is not, and the impact that can have on ratings. There may be considerable behavior, but if the instrument defines the labeled behavior differently than what is necessary to measure, the instrument will insufficiently capture the behavior. Hence, clinical observation during behavioral performance can provide essential information (44). Also, these assessment tools may not point to intervention strategies or help formulate behavioral etiologies, but they do provide a standardized measure of the occurrence, and sometimes severity, of behaviors.

Assessment of Cognition

A keystone for successful behavioral treatment of persons with brain injury is evaluation of their cognitive functioning. For example, cognitive difficulties can trigger agitation when the environment fails to take into account cognitive problems or when performance requirements exceed cognitive abilities (45). Cognitive disturbance has far-reaching implications. It affects emotional coping, behavioral dyscontrol, participation in physical and medical care, and return to independence and productivity. The foundation of cognitive assessment is neuropsychological evaluation. Neuropsychological evaluations are beyond the scope of this chapter (see Chapter 60); however, there are two aspects of cognitive evaluations that are particularly pertinent to a discussion of behavioral dyscontrol.

The first aspect is the use of neuropsychological information to help formulate the treatment of emotional issues and behavioral dysfunction (46). Neuropsychological data greatly facilitates the treatment of emotional and behavioral problems (47), although care must be taken to not rely solely on neuropsychological data (48). Still, many emotional and behavioral problems are partially based on cognitive difficulties. For example, paranoia can be a reflection, in part, of attentional and memory deficits when persons with brain injury have perceptions of other people that are inaccurate because of a failure to attend to and recall all of the elements of an interaction. Similarly, speed of processing deficits can cause behavioral issues when persons with brain injury are unable to keep up in conversations, leading to frustration with getting their needs heard.

Second, the importance of clinical observation for the determination of cognitive deficits should not be understated. Observation of cognitive deficits is a crucial adjunct to testing. Also, sometimes issues of injury severity or nonadherence render formal neuropsychological testing impractical, forcing reliance on observation of cognition.

Intervention

Operant Conditioning

Operant conditioning entails both the setting of stimuli before a behavior occurs to signal the likelihood of particular consequences and the application of contingencies afterwards. The principles of operant conditioning are well delineated (30). These procedures can be applied for the treatment of behavioral dyscontrol after brain injury.

Stimulus Control

The use of contingencies is best applied simultaneously with the setting of stimuli that signals what contingency conditions are present. Stimuli can signal whether a behavior ought to occur, or not, to get a reward or earn a punishment, or even which behavior ought to occur. For example, a staff places a stop sign in a doorway signaling a person not to leave the room. A reward is earned when this cue is followed by remaining in the room while the sign is in place. Stimuli may consist of physical signals (e.g., objects, signs), places, events, or people. The person learns when, where, and by whom, selected behaviors will be rewarded or punished. Intentional control of these stimuli allows the gradual increase in desired behaviors in the presence of certain stimuli or the inhibition of unwanted behaviors through the antici-

pation of punishment in the presence of other stimuli. When contingencies are applied without attention to control of signaling stimuli, people may link contingencies to erroneous cues and develop inappropriate or even superstitious behavior. Intentionally linking contingencies to signaling stimuli makes the world more predictable for people with brain injury.

Rewards and Punishments

Technically, a reward is something that increases a behavior, and a punishment is something that decreases a behavior. There is a wide range of rewards and punishments (e.g., social, tangible, tokens/points) (49). Unfortunately, sometimes there is an independent belief that something should be a reward or a punishment, and then it is applied to change the behaviors of a particular person. This is problematic because the consequence may not be a reward or a punishment for that individual. Observation of behaviors and discussion of rewards or punishments with the person before plan implementation can facilitate accurate understanding of what is rewarding and punishing. Also, it can be helpful to use access to naturally occurring behavior as a reward for the performance of lower probability behaviors that professionals want to encourage (50).

A positive reinforcer, when *presented*, increases a behavior; a negative reinforcer, when *removed*, increases a behavior. Both positive and negative reinforcement are rewarding and can be used to teach appropriate behavior because they work to increase behavior. Punishment also can occur in two ways: the *application* of something unpleasant (positive punishment) or the *removal* of something pleasant (negative punishment) (50). Both forms of punishment decrease behavior.

Punishment will not increase a desired behavior, and punishment cannot teach correct behavior. Moreover, punishment typically suppresses a behavior but can be impermanent; when the punishment stops, the behavior may return (30). Also, as punishment begins, behavior may worsen. There may be significant emotional responses, and punishment may lead to aggression (50). After a period of worse behavior, persistent application of punishment may eventually suppress behavior. However, the severity of aggression or other behaviors in response to punishment may exceed what most programs are willing to tolerate.

Punishment can be detrimental to the process of treatment. It can impair rapport. Persons receiving punishment may avoid those people who are administering the punishment (50). At the same time, persons with brain injury receiving punishment may learn to use punishment to change the behavior of other people. The use of punishment may be seen as a model for how to act (50).

Punishment carries with it a numerous significant ethical and moral concerns beyond its ineffectiveness in teaching adaptive compensation strategies. In addition, there are regulatory standards regarding the use of aversive or psychologically risky procedures (51). It is also easy to slip into punitive paradigms. Punitive acts may include discharge from treatment when persons with brain injury are labeled as dishonest or unmotivated (52).

Schedules of Reinforcement

The pattern of reinforcement influences how subsequent behavior occurs. There are four primary schedules of reinforcement. The first pattern is "fixed ratio." The frequency of responses required to achieve reinforcement is set, and reinforcement occurs based on that frequency (e.g., every fourth time). For example, a person earns a reward each time the person puts a dirty dish from the table in the dishwasher. Fixed ratio schedules encourage fast bursts of responding because the faster people perform, the more reinforcement they receive. However, there tends to be behavioral pauses after reinforcement. Typically, reinforcement is given every time (continual reinforcement) at the start of treatment and faded over time to a less frequent rate (intermittent reinforcement).

The second schedule of intermittent reinforcement is called "variable ratio." Reinforcement occurs on a schedule with an average frequency of required responses (e.g., on average of every fourth time), but with random variation around the average. This produces a higher rate of responding with more uniformity than fixed ratio schedules.

The third intermittent schedule is "fixed interval." In this schedule, reinforcement happens after a set interval of time. For example, group home staff provide rewards at the end of their 8-hour shift. This schedule can cause a "scallop" effect in which appropriate behavior increases as the time for reinforcement approaches and then declines after reinforcement.

The fourth intermittent schedule is known as "variable interval." Variable interval schedules eliminate the scallop effect because reinforcement happens after the passage of an average amount of time, but not an uniform amount of time. Learning with variable intervals of reinforcement is fairly resistant to extinction (the cessation of a desired behavior during periods of lack of reinforcement). Variable interval schedules produce a more uniform response than fixed interval schedules.

There are also other schedules of reinforcement. These include conjunctive schedules that require adherence to two or more performance requirements to receive reinforcement or the chaining together of different schedules (50). The use of such schedules can become burdensome to apply and monitor in complex real-world settings, however.

Problems surface when there is inconsistency in reinforcement. Reinforcement will fail when there is inconsistency across professionals or between professionals and families. Inconsistency will decrease treatment effectiveness, induce confusion or anger in persons with brain injury, and may puzzle family members. Inconsistency may lead to staff splitting by persons with brain injury. Also, social attention can be a positive reinforcement and may be inadvertently provided for inappropriate behavior. Moreover, behavior can be unintentionally reinforced by removal from therapeutic activity that the person with brain injury wants to avoid (negative reinforcement).

Application of reinforcement may drift from treatment plan design. For example, suppose staff are to encourage a person with brain injury whenever the person attempts a desirable behavior or coping strategy (fixed ratio/continual reinforcement). Instead, encouragement happens at the end of the workday in the late afternoon for efforts during that shift (fixed interval). Chart entries note better behavior in the afternoon with gradual improvement as time passes (scallop effect). This is occurring because of the inadvertent change in the schedule of reinforcement.

Prompts, Generalization, and Extinction

Behavior must first occur to be reinforced. Prompts using cues and instruction can help initiate behaviors; once behaviors have begun, reinforcement can ensue. For example, reminders could be provided to a person to clean a room, and then rewards could be given for cleaning the room. Thereafter, prompts can gradually be discontinued. Also, desirable behaviors may begin in rudimentary forms. Behavior can be shaped by reinforcing successive approximations of the behavior, progressively requiring more sophisticated approximations of the final behavior before reinforcement occurs. Behaviors can also be chained together requiring a sequence of behaviors to obtain reinforcement.

Generalization occurs when behaviors learned in a particular setting occur in other settings, even without reinforcement of the behaviors in the new setting. Prompting and initial reinforcement can encourage generalization. Response generalization occurs when there is generalization of the behavior to similar behaviors; learning a behavior influences the frequency of similar behaviors. For example, increased willingness to take a shower may generalize to increased dental hygiene.

Extinction is an additional tool. Failure to provide reinforcement following behaviors is an extinction paradigm. Ignoring an unwanted behavior on the part of a person with brain injury helps extinguish the behavior. As powerful as extinction can be, there are crucial factors in its use. Often, after extinction begins, there is a surge in the undesirable behavior. There may also be periods of spontaneous recovery; after the behavior declines or stops, it may temporarily reappear. It is essential to avoid unintentionally reinforcing either a surge or spontaneous recovery of the behavior. Also, the schedules of reinforcement under which behaviors were acquired influence their resistance to extinction. Finally, extinction is best paired with reinforcement of alternative behaviors.

Selective Reinforcement

Behaviors often must be situation specific. As well as learning what to do, persons with brain injury must learn where and when to act. Reinforcement in certain settings and not in others teaches when and where behaviors ought to occur. Persons with brain injury often need instruction in reading social cues and context. Otherwise, they may do behaviors appropriate for home, for example, in other settings or they may attempt conversations acceptable with intimate friends when they are with strangers.

Contingency use can be selective. There are at least four useful procedures: differential reinforcement of other behavior (DRO), differential reinforcement of incompatible behavior (DRI), differential reinforcement of alternative behavior (DRA), and differential reinforcement of low-rate behavior (DRL) (53). In DRO, reinforcement is given when an identified undesirable behavior does not occur (e.g., rewards for not yelling). Using DRI, reinforcement occurs when a behavior happens that interferes with or prohibits an undesirable behavior (e.g., rewards for sitting down to talk instead of standing too close during conversation). For DRA, reinforcement is provided for a desirable behavior while ignoring an unwanted behavior (e.g., rewards for making a bed while ignoring complaining about having to do so). Lastly, in DRL, reinforcement takes place in response to the reduction of an unwanted behavior (e.g., rewards for yelling less frequently).

Token Economies

Token economies are a special format for the implementation of contingency management treatment and can be helpful for behavioral issues arising from brain injury. In token economies, explicit rules exist for the delivery, withholding, or debiting of tokens (or some other accounting system, such as points) based on the performance or absence of delineated behaviors. These tokens can be exchanged by persons with brain injury for specified reinforcing items, activities, and so on. In essence, the tokens substitute for money in a real economy (31). Tokens serve as conditioned (or secondary) generalized reinforcers (31,50). They are conditioned or secondary because people learn to associate them with things that are reinforcing (i.e., tokens by themselves have little inherent value without a relationship to what one can exchange for them). They are generalized because one can exchange them for several sources of reinforcement. Of course, unlike money, tokens can only be redeemed within the closed token economy of defined rewards. A token economy can be implemented in a programmatic fashion (30), but individualization of treatment remains important.

Token economies have a number of advantages over simpler contingency management efforts (30). There may be less satiation than would occur with a set reward because a variety of reinforcers may be purchased with the tokens. As an example, tokens could be exchanged for more access to television, an extra outing, special foods, and so on. For persons with brain injury, this can also provide a sense of choice. They may choose diverse rewards or settle on particularly desirable ones. The flexibility may help persons with brain injury feel engaged with the process of behavioral change, although persons with brain injury should be similarly involved in the selection of reinforcers in even simpler contingency management plans.

Because persons with brain injury can accumulate tokens toward a valuable or large reinforcer, their use can permit a measured acquisition of a valuable reinforcer. A corollary of this is the specification that a person can choose to save tokens, as permitted by the economy rules, or to spend the tokens shortly after they earn them. Still, tokens can prove to be strong reinforcers because of their power to translate into significant rewards. Also, tokens can decrease the delay between behavior and reinforcement because their provision can be expeditious. Rather than disrupting the flow of behavior by immediately giving a reinforcing item or event, tokens are easy to provide. However, tokens can become a stimulus for when to perform well, and behavior may be different when they are not available (30).

A token economy is an *actual* economy. In the real economy, people sometimes underperform and expect to be paid, use legalistic arguments regarding precise procedural concerns to reduce debits for improper behavior (e.g., financial penalties for crime), seek ambiguities in the specification of permissible behavior (e.g., analysis of tax code loopholes) to retain more money, commit theft to increase funds, hide inappropriate behavior, blame other people for their own acts, and so on. In a token economy, persons with brain injury may also attempt to outfox the rules through procedural challenges, loopholes, theft, hiding behavior, blaming oth-

ers, and so on. For example, they may seek tokens for behaviors close to those behaviors specified as due reinforcement, or they may claim that certain behaviors do not warrant a debit because the behaviors are not exactly the behaviors listed in the token economy behavioral descriptions (e.g., touching someone's hair does not count as touching the *person*, or standing 3 inches away from someone does not count as *touching* them).

Use of Operant Conditioning

There is no practical cookbook about which procedure to use with which brain injury symptom or person with brain injury. Because treatment must be founded on individual, multifaceted symptom patterns and causes, any predetermined treatment recipes will fail to capture the extraordinary diversity of clinical presentations and etiological variables on which to base treatment. Moreover, as has been reviewed in the preceding discussion, operant conditioning encompasses a breadth of actual procedures that are highly intricate. Still, operant conditioning is likely to work best when three conditions are met.

First, they are more effective when persons with brain injury accept the idea of explicitly receiving reinforcement to alter their behavior. Many persons with brain injury reject the idea of intentional reinforcement of their behavior. They dislike the manipulative feeling that apparent contingency procedures engender. Although adults may use consequences to alter the behavior of children, adults resist the idea that other people may attempt to apply contingencies to their own behavior. Persons with brain injury feel similar regarding any other adults and may resist contingency paradigms that remind them of being treated as if they are children whose behavior is to be controlled by others.

Second, when persons with brain injury act in their own best interests, contingency management is more effective. Some persons with brain injury fail to do so because of their cognitive impairments, even when they understand and recall the likely consequences. Despite their awareness, factors such as lability, rigidity, nonverbal processing deficits, impulsivity, and executive dysfunctions lead to the failure of consequences to change behavior. Persons with brain injury may act and later acknowledge having had awareness of the consequences, but they still proceeded. These persons may report either they could not stop themselves or could not think about the consequences quick enough to change their behavior. Sometimes they will state that the need for emotional release overrode their reflections about consequences.

Third, these techniques are likely to be more useful when memory difficulties do not interfere. Many persons with brain injury forget their own behavior before there is the opportunity to respond with consequences. This defeats the purpose of linking behavior with consequences. Some persons with brain injury, when they are in a situation where they might choose a behavior that was previously reinforced, forget the previous event. Because they forget that there were consequences last time, the previous consequences have no influence. Both of these scenarios can defeat the use of consequences. Moreover, consequence-oriented behavior management outside of controlled environments can be relatively ineffective (54).

Skill Building and Errorless Learning

The errors people make at the start of learning are additional concerns in the use of contingency techniques. There are potential cognitive (e.g., interference with acquisition) and emotional (e.g., frustration, self-esteem) issues that arise with persistent errors. In contrast, errorless learning provides structure and cues, with initial performance demands set at an achievable level, so that as task complexity increases, persons with brain injury perform correctly at each step. Correct responses can be provided to ensure avoidance of errors. When applied to cognitive learning tasks, there is evidence of the benefit of errorless learning procedures (55,56). Errorless learning procedures can be applied to behavioral concerns (57). Doing so ensures that the situations that persons with brain injury confront are of a type and level of complexity they can handle, with adequate prompts and training, before proceeding to more difficult emotional and behavioral challenges. For example, skill building could be applied to instruction in making appropriate rudimentary social statements in low-key situations one-on-one before eventually training social discourse in complex stressful situations with multiple speakers. Of course, operant conditioning techniques, including reinforcement, stimulus fading, and cueing, can be incorporated into errorless protocols. When contingencies are used, it is best to use the ones that are natural and related to the behavior (2).

Modeling and Learning

People receive vicarious reinforcement from observing other people receiving contingencies (58). Therefore, persons with brain injury may benefit from their observations of other people receiving reinforcement. Seeing other people obtaining desirable consequences for certain actions may encourage imitation in anticipation of obtaining the same results. Moreover, persons with brain injury may determine that certain behaviors are socially acceptable on observing the results of those behaviors for other people. For example, one person may dress less slovenly after observing another person receive social approval for dressing more neatly.

Modeling effects engender two issues. First, in some instances, one person with a brain injury may receive an award for a particular behavior when doing so is part of the treatment plan, but the same behavior from another person does not result in a reward. A particular reward may be given to someone who achieves a relatively low behavioral milestone, but one that is difficult for that person to reach. A second person, who is capable of much better behavior, demands a reward for identical behavior, despite that behavior being well below the second person's capabilities. Individualized treatment plans based on ability and goals are essential, but astute application must occur to avoid cross contamination.

Second, there must be cognizance of the modeling effect of staff behaviors (59). Staff are powerful role models. It can prove difficult to teach physical boundaries when persons with brain injury observe staff patting each other on the back, staff who are heard telling each other off-color jokes may struggle to teach sound sexually appropriate behavior, and staff who make an offhand comment about teammates may contribute to staff splitting and nonadherence by persons with brain injury.

Environmental Intervention

Environmental change strives to influence behavior by alteration of antecedent conditions. In general, how other people act toward persons with brain injury and physical elements in the environment comprise the antecedent conditions. Of the two, how other people act is probably the more crucial. In one estimate, 95% of maladaptive behaviors were felt to be a function of how staff act (60).

Environmental control emphasizes the establishment of environments conducive to appropriate behavior. The correct environment will vary for persons with brain injury depending on their cognitive and emotional functioning. Attention to neuropsychological and psychosocial factors permits the creation of a "neuropsychosocial environment," (47) one based on the etiological "phenomenology of dyscontrol" (47) of each person. In "neuropsychosocial intervention," all of the elements that contribute to the occurrence of behaviors constitute the phenomenology of dyscontrol, including the obvious—cognition and emotions, the discoverable—self-image, values, family influences, expectations, premorbid personality, and the subtle—noise tolerance, privacy needs, responses to others' appearance, sleep cycle effects, professionals' attitudes, and so on. Comprehensive consideration of the factors that determine the occurrence of each behavior facilitates formulation of the neuropsychosocial environment, a psychological and physical "world" for each person; this world interferes with the occurrence of behavioral dyscontrol or obviates the need for undesirable behaviors achieving "functional equivalence" (61) in which persons with brain injury can get their needs met, reaching the same ends, but without behavioral dyscontrol. Behavioral dyscontrol declines when the physical plant and the people one interacts with provide the right individualized support and avoid the person's behavioral triggers.

The assessment task is to determine the drivers of behavior: Why is the person doing the behavior? Comprehensively understanding all of the current and past social, cognitive, and emotional determinants of a behavior informs environmental changes that eliminate the need for the behavior. Two people might act the same for very different reasons. Rewards and punishments treat the actions; in contrast, environmental approaches determine *why* someone acts and treats the reasons. Typically, the reasons are the behavior, mood, and attitude of other people that interface with the person with brain injury's cognitive and emotional history and current status. The goal is to create a world—it can be thought of as cognitive, emotional, and behavioral terraforming—consisting of the behavior, mood, and attitude of others and physical plant elements that match the capabilities of each person (47). In essence, persons with brain injury encounter only situations they can handle.

There are two challenges in the environmental approach: the need for careful observation and generalization (62). Systematic observational assessment is necessary to precisely determine the antecedent conditions leading to behavioral dyscontrol. Behavioral triggers can be difficult to decipher in a complex social world for persons with impairment in cognitive and emotional functioning. When treatment does not work, either the treatment was poorly implemented or there was insufficiently understood drivers of the behavior (i.e., the hypothesized phenomenology of dyscontrol was erroneous). This view is in contrast to the assumption that the treatments are correct and that the person's behavior is intractable—essentially blaming the person with brain injury. Instead, treatment plans are a hypothesis testing of the understanding of the person and modifications of the plan should ensue. Treatment implementation is essentially "patient-specific hypothesis testing" (63). Second, because the approach is not skill building but environmental engineering, generalization can be a concern. Plans should be effective, transferable to additional settings, and doable by core people constituting the natural environment.

Environmental change is useful on its own or as an adjunct to other treatment. For example, it can be beneficial until skill building can take place (57). Positive behavioral supports (54,64) designed to organize antecedent conditions combine skill building with environmental structuring. Moreover, specific environments can be arranged that match the abilities of persons with brain injury and then modified as they can tolerate changes (65).

In general, an environmental approach is proactive (before an episode of behavioral dyscontrol happens) in contrast to contingency management, which is reactive (after behavior occurs). Treatment plans describe how other people should act before behavioral dyscontrol occurs, not merely how they should act afterwards (64). Traditional treatment plans tend to make statements such as "The person will curse less than 5 times per day in the next 2 weeks down from a level of 10 times per day and if they do so, they will receive the scheduled reward." In contrast, in an environmental approach, a plan might say, for example, "Staff will provide the person an opportunity every 2 hours to privately disclose their feelings about any recent events and staff will offer to help solve any frustrating problems." Implicit in this is that such intervention will lead to decreased cursing (assuming the phenomenology of dyscontrol analysis in this example determined that frustration with events that the person cannot independently problem solve is a contributor to cursing). This simple example captures the difference between contingency-based plans and environmentally-based plans. Persons with brain injury encounter a positive world, one that they can handle, individualized for each person.

Once the phenomenology of dyscontrol is accurately determined, treatment plans explicitly specify environmental antecedents for target behaviors and how they should be modified. Target behaviors will change implicitly. If they do not, either the understanding of the phenomenology of dyscontrol was incompletely understood, or the plan was poorly implemented.

It should be noted that similar planning is quite applicable to children and adolescents post-brain injury, including in school settings. There is a tendency to use contingencies with younger people because of the degree of control adults have over them, in contrast to adults who have more sophisticated tools to rebel against consequences (e.g., treatment nonadherence, legal action, etc.). However, a more comprehensive approach than contingencies alone is advisable with younger people, too, and environmental approaches can be particularly crucial when behavior is frequent, dangerous, or unpredictable (61).

Counseling for Behavioral Change

Counseling is an additional intervention for behavioral issues (18). Advising the person who exhibits behavioral dyscontrol is a common first step. Counseling can be used to prompt and teach appropriate behaviors. Skill building can be a corollary of counseling. Skill sets may range from cogni-

tive compensation techniques that lessen behavioral dyscontrol to anger management skills to social skills that decrease frustration, improve communication, enhance life satisfaction, and thereby decrease behavioral dysfunction. Counseling can facilitate persons with brain injury in learning to assert their desires in an effective manner and thereby decrease inappropriate behaviors. Finally, counseling can build rapport and provide rationales for treatment decisions. (See Chapters 62 and 64 for a more comprehensive discussion of adjustment and treatment issues.)

Pharmacotherapy for Behavioral Change

Medication management can be an effective component of a comprehensive treatment plan. It is essential that behavioral plans be coordinated with the prescription, administration, and monitoring of medications. A team effort is essential to ensure adequate communication. Knowledge of medication therapeutic effects and side effects can help with understanding what behavioral changes, positive and negative, are taking place as a function of medications (see Chapters 72, 73, and 74).

FAMILIES, TEAMS, AND BEHAVIORAL TREATMENT PLANNING

It is important to recognize that behavioral assessment and treatment planning does not take place in a vacuum. It takes a comprehensive team effort, and it is crucial to include family members and, whenever possible, the person with brain injury (66). Family members are special members of the team. They bring insight about the person from before the injury; are trusted by the person with a brain injury more than new, unknown professionals; and are likely to be involved for years (unlike transitory professionals) and across progressive settings (unlike organizationally bound professionals). Moreover, returning to family is a common goal of many people following brain injury. Of course, family members may have their own emotional and behavioral issues that they are dealing with and there ought to be care for them as well (67–69) (see Chapter 80 for further insight into family assessment and intervention).

Incorporation of family members as well as members of multiple disciplines strengthens behavioral planning. Family members and members of multiple disciplines bring a diversity of insights into the determination of behavioral etiology and treatment design, as well as being essential for intervention implementation. This is the nature of "supradisciplinary teams" (7)—teams that work *across* disciplines. In this model, everyone contributes to behavioral management; all parties—families and diverse professionals—are seen as having valuable input into behavioral issues.

TREATMENT DECISIONS

The integration of available treatment options and the complexities of designing treatment can appear overwhelming. Following the algorithms in Figures 63-1 and 63-2 can guide professionals. In Figure 63-1, after assessment, the crucial step is the formulation of the phenomenology of dyscontrol and its reformulation if treatment is unsuccessful. Figure 63-2

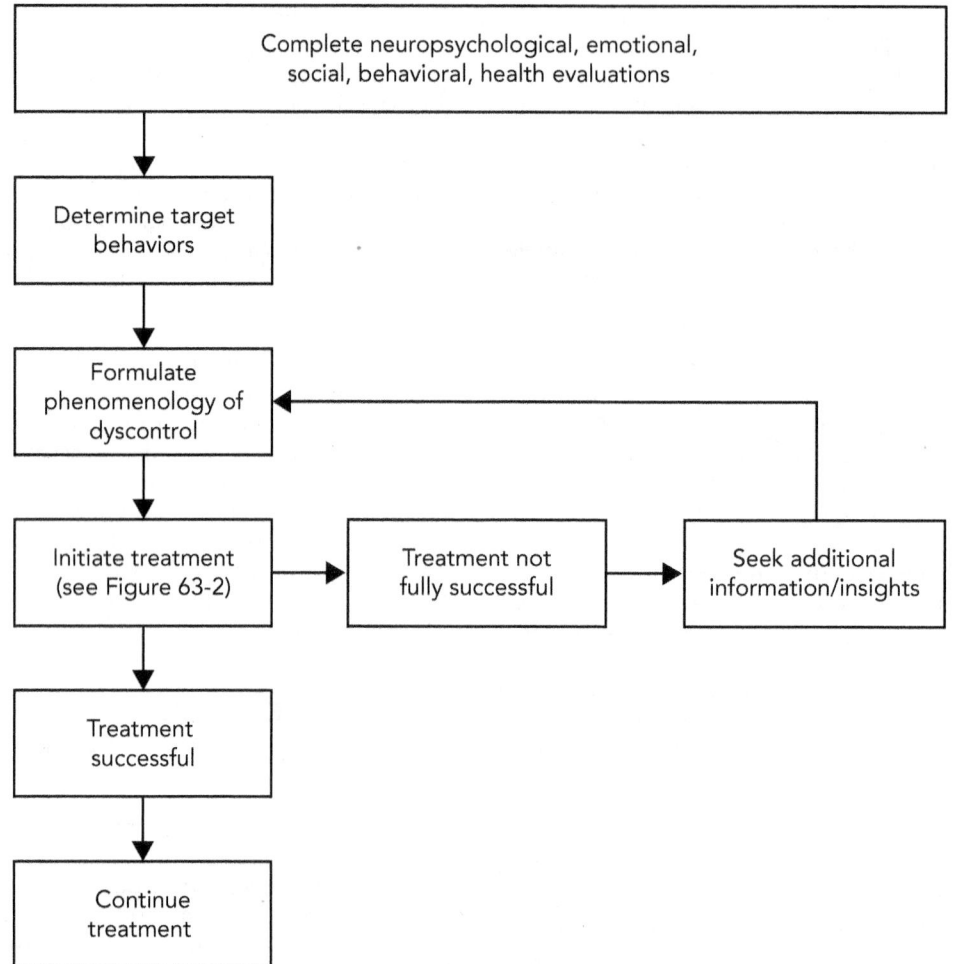

FIGURE 63-1 Treatment formulation algorithm.

provides a sequence of treatment options: counseling, skill building, operant conditioning, and neuropsychosocial intervention. This sequence progresses, in general, from treatment requiring the highest cognitive skill to the lowest cognitive ability. That is, counseling, at one end, although relatively straightforward to initiate, demands the greatest cognitive sophistication by people with brain injury and neuropsychosocial intervention, at the other end, although requiring the most of staff, can be implemented for anyone regardless of his or her cognitive ability, high or low. Of course, integration of all approaches may be the most powerful treatment.

SELECTED APPLICATIONS

The need to assess and treat some issues seems to arise repeatedly. A comprehensive review of all behavioral difficulties is unfeasible here, but selected topics are worthy of mention. These are aggression, nonadherence, impulsivity, and social skills.

Aggression

Verbal and physical aggression may be the most distressing of all brain injury symptoms to other people. People will

tolerate memory problems, depression, or the need for a wheelchair, but they will not permit nonverbal posturing, verbal threats, or physical acts against people or objects. When aggression occurs, it commands attention.

As the severity of aggression increases, it requires an increasingly comprehensive approach. Environmental change can address the antecedents of aggression. The main variable to manipulate is the behavior of other people. As already noted, their behavior often proves to be the primary antecedent for aggression. Contingency techniques can be used after aggression, although they may prove more useful as an adjunct to antecedent control. It is important to avoid the temptation to be punitive.

It is important to recognize the value of counseling as an adjunct to treatment for aggression. Counseling with persons with brain injury can be essential to facilitate interpretation of antecedent and contingency changes, use of skill-based techniques for anger management, cognitive restructuring of frustrating events, and preparation for future stressful events. Counseling can decrease errors and enhance errorless learning.

It is essential that there be attention to variables that influence the expression of aggression. Treatment is less likely to be successful if different people who exhibit the same behavior receive the same treatment without an under-

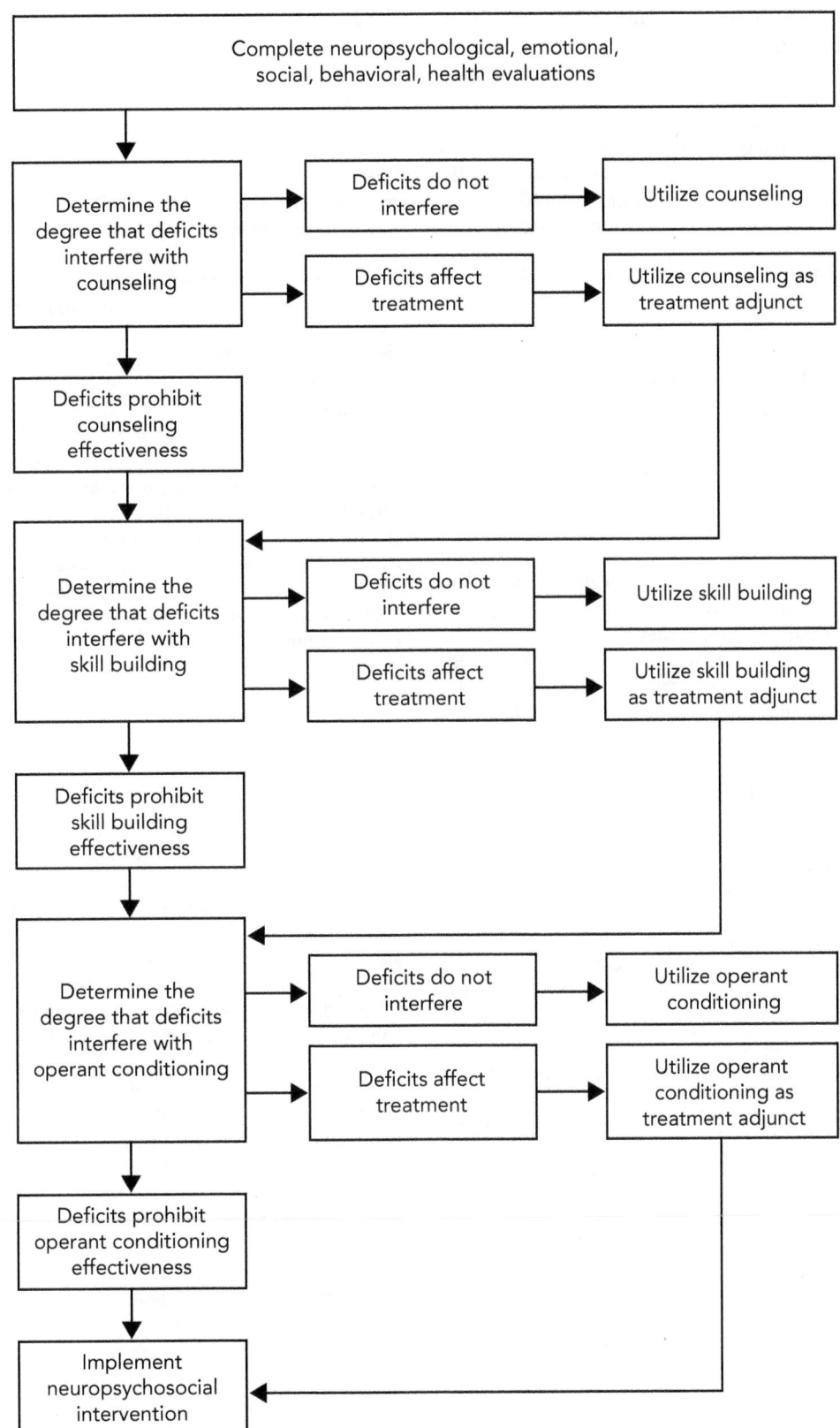

FIGURE 63-2 Treatment selection algorithm.

standing of the behavioral etiology. The focus needs to be, in part, on the contribution of emotional variables leading to aggression, not just on superficial behavioral symptoms of aggression. Similarly, cognitive processing often plays a crucial role in the expression of aggression.

Families need particularly attentive support when there is aggression. Aggression may embarrass or frighten family members, especially when it is directed at the family. There may need to be encouragement for family members to consider their own safety. Alternatively, families may need assistance regarding their own stimulus value and behavior as an environmental antecedent.

Nonadherence

Nonadherence with treatment recommendations is a difficult problem. The obstacle to avoid is the automatic assumption that nonadherence is an intentional challenge to authority. Nonadherence can be caused by a variety of factors. These include, among other factors, true dyscontrol (in which refusal is based on post-onset organic difficulty with acquiescence), manipulation for secondary gain, communication or memory deficits, premorbid oppositional personality, or attempts to reassert self-determination. It is also easy to miss the contribution to nonadherence of fatigue and poor sleep, depression, and initiation or impulsivity problems. As with all behaviors, determination of behavioral etiology is paramount for intervention. Intervention may be multifaceted. Avoidance of power struggles is important. Education about the implications of nonadherence can be useful, particularly when unawareness is present. Sometimes negotiation can determine alternatives and achieve creative solutions. Alterations in schedules or the use of reminders, as well as other environmental changes, can be successful.

Unfortunately, nonadherence can lead to paradoxical outcomes for persons with brain injury. Other people may view nonadherence as evidence for the need to restrict independence, despite its occurrence as an effort by persons with brain injury to expand their choices. They want the freedom to choose, and other people want to control poor choices. Treatment of nonadherence requires a careful balance of necessary rules and maximization of personal choice.

Finally, it is valuable to recognize that the behaviors of persons with brain injury are "adherent" with whatever variables are determining it. People behave in response to internal and external variables (70). The task is to ferret out those variables so as to help people act in an appropriate fashion. The focus should be on the alteration of the factors that drive self-defeating behavior and on program variables that facilitate persons with brain injury achieving their goals and maximizing their successes.

Impulsivity

Impulsivity can be a particularly frustrating behavior. Impulsivity is difficult to address because it crosses other behaviors (e.g., social inappropriateness, risk to elope, suicidal ideation, nonadherence, hoarding, physical and verbal aggression) causing a worsening of symptoms. For persons with brain injury, impulsivity can be embarrassing if there is sufficient self-awareness because they act contrary to how

they might otherwise behave. Oftentimes, on post hoc guided reflection, persons with brain injury will express regret regarding impulsive behavior.

Two scenarios exist regarding impulsivity. First, persons with brain injury may act too intensely or prematurely. The resulting behavior appears as "too much, too soon." The behavior is too much of a good thing. Treatment tries to modulate behavior that would be acceptable if performed in a different setting, more slowly, or less intensely. Second, persons with brain injury may fail to stop inappropriate behavior, acts that ought not to occur at all. There is a failure to inhibit impulses. Behavior in the first scenario appears as overly activated responses; behavior in the second situation presents as uncontrolled behavior. Persons with brain injury find themselves being told to slow down in the first instance and stop in the second case. Impulsivity, therefore, may represent over activation or under control (47).

Disinhibition would appear to be a prominent component of the complaint of personality change (e.g., irritability) after brain injury (14). It is likely to contribute to some of the more troublesome behaviors of aggression, sexual acting out, verbal abuse, and so on. Moreover, the negative consequences associated with such behaviors tend not to alter their occurrence when impulsivity is a factor. (64) As such, environmental changes, decreasing stimuli associated with impulsive responding, and skill building, when appropriate, may be more effective.

Social Skills

Social skills are a broad set of human interaction variables. They range from relatively narrow elements, such as eye contact or gestures, to broader factors including sensitivity to context and language communication skills. It can help to address social self-regulation (e.g., disinhibition, inertia), social self-awareness (i.e., knowledge of one's impact on other people), social insensitivity (i.e., understanding another person's perspective or emotions), and social problem solving (i.e., interpersonal issue resolution) (71). Without social skill competency, brief, seemingly simple, everyday exchanges become episodes of miscommunication, sources of frustration, and behavioral dyscontrol. Worse, the lack of proficiency in social skills impairs the establishment or maintenance of ongoing supportive relationships.

It is important to recognize that social skill enhancement is challenging for a number of reasons. First, underlying cognitive deficits can impair learning new skills or remembering to apply them. Second, emotional factors, such as anger or frustration, or social pressure, such as the desire to perform in a certain fashion to impress someone else, can distort how persons with brain injury perform skills. Third, persons with brain injury may relapse back to older, more overlearned, dysfunctional skills.

A prime example of skill building can be seen in comprehensive programs for the enhancement of social skills. There is a considerable work being done to develop and evaluate such programs (72,73). Moreover, comprehensive programs can be built around errorless learning that adopts a holistic approach (74). Facility with social skills should help address many behavioral issues. When behavioral dyscontrol has resulted in the attainment of desirable goals in the past, then training in socially acceptable alternative methods to reach the same goal can mitigate behavioral problems (57).

CASE VIGNETTES

Case 1: Irritability During Care at a Group Home

"Tom Johnson" had been living at various group homes following his TBI after a motor vehicle crash about seven years ago. Although dysarthric, he usually presented as sociable and engaging. His parents were his guardians. There was no evidence of hallucinations or thought disturbances. Unfortunately, he had behavioral dyscontrol exhibiting nonadherence and aggression. Recently, he had been brought to an emergency department after an aggressive episode, but after more than 15 sites refused to take him, he was placed in a short-term inpatient facility. Thereafter, he was tried at another group home at which time his behaviors resumed. He was apologetic during and after he exhibited behavioral dyscontrol. Staff could not identify the etiology of his behaviors.

Staff noted that his primary time for agitation appeared to be during their care of him and during transfers from his bed to his wheelchair—he needed assistance because of only partial use of one arm. However, because of his instantaneous behavior (he would suddenly lash out when all seemed fine), it was difficult to identify antecedents. His behavior analyst and psychologist could not be present all of the time to observe his behavior and when they were present, he seemed to do better.

Agreement was obtained from Tom and his parents to tape record his room whenever staff entered his room to care for him. Staff were consulted, so they understood that the intent was not to catch them doing something wrong. Hours of tape were collected and these were studied by his behavior analyst and psychologist. Based on exhaustive study of the tapes, the triggers for his behavior became apparent.

The first indicator was that frequently in mid-transfer, when all was fine, he would suddenly appear afraid, tense his body, and then lash out. Staff could not see this sequence because they were bent over transferring him. In addition, one staff, one time without being particularly aware of having made a change, altered the usual procedure (and common technique among staff in many settings) from counting down out loud readying him for a transfer ("3, 2, 1, go") to having *him* count down. This allowed him to know and control *precisely* when the transfer would occur because *he* was the one counting; it seemed to relax him. Together, these observations generated the hypothesis that anxiety was a major behavioral driver for him.

Next, it was noted that he appeared tense whenever staff were talking to each other preparing to care for him or to transfer him. In fact, his stress seemed to worsen as multiple people entered his room. Although staff wanted more people present, doing so seemed to increase the risk of dyscontrol. It was also noted that he calmed when one staff stroked his arm while looking him right in the eye reassuring him. Finally, it was noted that he struck out with his good hand but that if one had him grab the handrail from underneath it, that hand became unavailable; staff could lightly rest a hand on top of his to hold it there if he tensed it to let go.

The treatment plan therefore was as follows: One staff entered alone and talked to him. That staff got an agreement from him to have another staff enter who did not talk but followed directions. He grasped the handrail from underneath, and a staff rested a hand on his; in fact, he became so accustomed to this that he automatically placed his hand there during care without direction to do so. Staff stroked an arm and made a close eye-to-eye contact. The lead staff, the first one who entered his room and who was the designated speaker, provided reassurance while he was being cared for and during transfers. He counted down for procedures, such as transfers.

With this plan in place, his physical aggression dropped from about 145 episodes per month to 14 episodes per month. Simultaneously, his nonadherence as scored by staff dropped from 62 episodes per month to 1 or 2 episodes. Interestingly, his basal level of anxiety had remained fairly consistent, but because of how he was cared for, it no longer increased during staff care of him and was not triggering dyscontrol. Staff liked working with him, and his placement was secure. He loved the group home, and his family was very satisfied.

This case demonstrates the importance of a comprehensive approach. It entailed family support, detailed observational data, attendance to emotional variables that drive behavior, and the importance of treating the etiology of behavior. Also, it was essential to provide emotional support for staff and obtain their wholehearted participation in assessment (being taped) and treatment (how to interact with him).

Case 2: Unprovoked Aggressive Behavior

"Joe Smith" had been dismissed from various residential placements (group homes) because of "unprovoked behavior." Attempts also had been made at vocational training, but he was similarly asked to leave after he exhibited "acting out." Records indicated a consistent pattern of acting out behavior without any apparent provocation. The staff's response to him across settings had been to clamp down on him and place restrictions on him. He was threatened with locked placement when punishment did not work.

He had a history of TBI from a motor vehicle crash a few years previously. Prior to onset, he had not had behavioral problems. He had no past legal problems, and he was viewed by his family and friends as an independent, somewhat assertive individual who took pride in his work. He was a high school graduate with fair grades, but no learning disability or attention deficit hyperactivity disorder (ADHD) history. There was no history of alcohol abuse or illicit drug use. His history was fairly benign.

He presented as pleasant but quiet. He did not appear depressed or anxious, and there was no evidence of comorbid mental health issues. The problem was that he exhibited periodic episodes of acting out. Study of antecedents left staff perplexed as to what the triggers were for his episodic loss of control.

The first clue was that he had a delayed latency to his oral responses to questions. Examination of his neuropsychological data revealed that he tended to be slow in his information processing in the context of relatively strong memory functioning. He had a lowered vocabulary. When asked how he felt, he had difficulty identifying his emotions and also lacked the vocabulary to identify and communicate his mood.

One day, he was observed frowning while leaving a conversation with staff. Four days later, he was observed lashing out at the same staff. Observation of both events led to a hypothesis about his behavior. He had been angered by the conversation but did not immediately identify the feeling and certainly had not said how he felt. Because his processing speed was slow, he went off to think about the interaction. His good memory functioning allowed him to remember the event and so he pondered it for 4 days. When he finally resolved what he felt, he took action.

The final piece that contributed to understanding his behavior was that he had been raised in a family in which men did not discuss their feelings. They took action to solve problems. Physical displays of assertiveness were an acceptable solution to disagreements.

Treatment was multi-pronged. First, his family was engaged. The psychologist provided a hypothesis about the etiology of his behavior and enlisted their support for him to talk about his feelings. The family strongly communicated to him the pride they would all have in him if he would talk to staff about his feelings; they communicated their universal blessing to do so. In addition, they supported his working with staff to resolve problems as opposed to taking action on his own. Second, was a skill-building intervention. The speech language pathologist taught him words that described various emotions and helped him identify what they meant and how they felt to him. Third, were frequent, brief counseling contacts—typically twice daily—in which his ruminations and emotional status were checked. The information sought was what he was thinking about and whether anything had annoyed him or was bothering him. If he answered negatively, he was reminded of the teachings from speech pathology and the support from his family to encourage disclosure. If there was something that was concerning him, he went with the staff to resolve the problem. His unprovoked behavior ceased with this treatment plan.

This case highlights the integration of observational data, neuropsychological data, and social history with family participation and a team approach. Moreover, it entailed skill building and targeted counseling and eliminated punishment. As with the first case, a comprehensive approach was important.

CONCLUSION

Behavioral treatment works best when it is based on a solid assessment. This can include clinical observation, interview, and psychometric assessment of cognitive, behavioral, and emotional functioning. There is an array of possible intervention strategies. Treatment techniques include operant conditioning, modeling, environmental manipulation, skill building with errorless learning, and counseling. Family involvement is crucial, and pharmacological intervention is a powerful adjunct to behavioral management. Throughout behavioral care, during every type of evaluation and treatment for all behavioral problems, the unique nature of brain injury must be kept in the forefront of decision making.

KEY CLINICAL POINTS

1. Thorough assessment is the key to behavioral treatment. This should include cognitive, emotional, and behavioral evaluation. The goal is to fully comprehend the phenomenology of dyscontrol.
2. Cognitive, emotional, and behavioral evaluation must consider the unique nature of brain injury, and specialized assessment procedures or instruments should be used.
3. Operant conditioning can be an effective intervention for behavioral difficulties but must be predicated on cognitive functioning, and designing contingency management strategies is exceedingly complicated.
4. Operant conditioning interventions should include stimulus control procedures.
5. Token economies can be a successful strategy when there is a considerable investment in designing and implementing the economy.
6. Strategies such as skill building through errorless learning and modeling should be part of the armamentarium.
7. Modeling can help teach appropriate behavior and may provide vicarious reinforcement. Staff must also maintain awareness of their own stimulus value as a model.
8. Counseling is a valuable treatment in light of behavioral dyscontrol, and rapport is essential for all behavioral interventions.
9. Environmental intervention and the formation of a neuropsychosocial environment is a crucial intervention strategy to ameliorate behavioral dyscontrol.

KEY REFERENCES

1. Feeney TJ. There's always something that works: principles and practices of positive support for individuals with traumatic brain injury and problem behaviors. *Semin Speech Lang.* 2010;31(3):145–161.
2. Karol RL. *Neuropsychosocial Intervention: The Practical Treatment of Severe Behavioral Dyscontrol after Acquired Brain Injury.* Boca Raton, FL: CRC Press LLC; 2003.
3. Niemeier J, Karol RL. *Overcoming Grief and Loss After Brain Injury.* New York, NY: Oxford University Press; 2011.
4. Slifer KJ, Amari A. Behavior management for children and adolescents with acquired brain injury. *Dev Disabil Res Rev.* 2009;15(2):144–151.
5. Tate RL. *A Compendium of Tests, Scales, and Questionnaires: The Practitioner's Guide to Measuring Outcomes After Acquired Brain Injury.* New York, NY: Psychology Press; 2010.

ACKNOWLEDGMENTS

Grateful acknowledgment is due to Gwendolyn Barnes-Karol, Karen Brudvig, and Sharon Miller.

References

1. Ylvisaker M, Turkstra LS, Coelho C. Behavioral and social interventions for individuals with traumatic brain injury: a summary of the research with clinical implications. *Semin Speech Lang.* 2005; 26(4):256–267.
2. Feeney TJ. There's always something that works: principles and practices of positive support for individuals with traumatic brain

injury and problem behaviors. *Semin Speech Lang.* 2010;31(3): 145–161.

3. Baguley IJ, Cooper J, Felmingham K. Aggressive behavior following traumatic brain injury: how common is common? *J Head Trauma Rehabil.* 2006;21(1):45–56.

4. Rao V, Rosenberg P, Bertrand M, et al. Aggression after traumatic brain injury: prevalence and correlates. *J Neuropsychiatry Clin Neurosci.* 2009;21(4):420–429.

5. Ashman TA, Gordon WA, Cantor JB, Hibbard MR. Neurobehavioral consequences of traumatic brain injury. *Mt Sinai J Med.* 2006; 73(7):999–1005.

6. Vaishnavi S, Rao V, Fann JR. Neuropsychiatric problems after traumatic brain injury: unraveling the silent epidemic. *Psychosomatics.* 2009;50(3):198–205.

7. Karol RL, Sevenich R. Neurobehavioral crisis hospitalization: on the need to provide specialized hospital brain injury crisis programming. *Brain Inj Prof.* 2008;5(4):16–21.

8. Wald MM, Helgeson SR, Langlois JA. Traumatic brain injury among prisoners. *Brain Inj Prof.* 2008;5(1):22–25.

9. Slaughter B, Fann JR, Ehde D. Traumatic brain injury in a county jail population: prevalence, neuropsychological functioning and psychiatric disorders. *Brain Inj.* 2003;17(9):731–741.

10. Bogner J, Corrigan JD. Reliability and predictive validity of the Ohio State University TBI identification method with prisoners. *J Head Trauma Rehabil.* 2009;24(4):279–291.

11. Wilder Research. Homelessness in Minnesota 2009: results of the Wilder statewide survey. St Paul, MN: Wilder Research; 2010.

12. Stubbs B, Alderman N. Physical interventions to manage patients with brain injury: an audit on its use and staff and patient injuries from the techniques. *Brain Inj.* 2008;22(9):691–696.

13. American Psychiatric Association. *Diagnostic and Statistical Manual of Mental Disorders.* 4th ed., text rev. Washington, DC: American Psychiatric Association; 2000.

14. Prigatano GP, Maier F. Neuropsychiatric, psychiatric, and behavioral disorders associated with traumatic brain injury. In: Grant I, Adams KM, eds. *Neuropsychological Assessment of Neuropsychiatric and Neuromedical Disorders.* 3rd ed. New York, NY: Oxford University Press; 2010:618–631.

15. Warriner EM, Velikonja D. Psychiatric disturbances after traumatic brain injury: neurobehavioral and personality changes. *Curr Psychiatry Rep.* 2006;8(1):73–80.

16. Ciurli P, Formisano R, Bivona U, Cantagallo A, Angelelli P. Neuropsychiatric disorders in persons with severe traumatic brain injury: prevalence, phenomenology, and relationship with demographic, clinical, and functional features. *J Head Trauma Rehabil.* 2011;26(2):116–126.

17. Rogers MJ, Read CA. Psychiatric comorbidity following traumatic brain injury. *Brain Inj.* 2007;21(13–14):1321–1333.

18. Rusin MJ, Uomoto JM. Psychotherapeutic interventions. In: Frank RG, Rosenthal M, Caplan B, eds. *Handbook of Rehabilitation Psychology.* 2nd ed. Washington, DC: American Psychological Association; 2010:259–271.

19. Rehabilitation of persons with traumatic brain injury. *NIH Consens Statement.* 1998;16(1):1–41.

20. Beatty J. *The Human Brain: Essentials of Behavioral Neuroscience.* Thousand Oaks, CA: Sage Publications, Inc.; 2001.

21. McGee JM. Insight—neuroanatomy of behavior after brain injury or you don't like my behavior? You'll have to discuss that with my brain directly. *Premier Outlook.* 2004;4(2):24–32.

22. Rapoport MJ, McCullagh S, Streiner D, Feinstein A. The clinical significance of major depression following mild traumatic brain injury. *Psychosomatics.* 2003;44(1):31–37.

23. Niemeier JP, Kennedy RE, McKinley WO, Cifu DX. The loss inventory: a measure of emotional and cognitive responses to disability. *Disabil Rehabil.* 2004;26(10):614–623.

24. Jorge RE. Emotional awareness among brain-damaged patients. In: Prigatano GP, ed. *The Study of Anosognosia.* New York, NY: Oxford University Press; 2010:333–355.

25. Beck AT, Steer RA, Brown GK. *Manual for the Beck Depression Inventory-II.* San Antonio, TX: Psychological Corporation; 1996.

26. Rowland SM, Lam CS, Leahy B. Use of the Beck Depression Inventory-II (BDI-II) with persons with traumatic brain injury: analysis of factorial structure. *Brain Inj.* 2005;19(2):77–83.

27. Siegert RJ, Walkey FH, Turner-Stokes L. An examination of the factor structure of the Beck Depression Inventory-II in a neurorehabilitation inpatient sample. *J Int Neuropsychol Soc.* 2009; 15(1): 142–147.

28. Siegert RJ, Tennant A, Turner-Stokes L. Rasch analysis of the Beck Depression Inventory-II in a neurological rehabilitation sample. *Disabil and Rehabil.* 2010;32(1):8–17.

29. Johnson-Greene D, Touradji P. Assessment of personality and psychopathology. In: Frank RG, Rosenthal M, Caplan B, eds. *Handbook of Rehabilitation Psychology.* 2nd ed. Washington, DC: American Psychological Association; 2010:195–211.

30. Kazdin AE. *Behavior Modification in Applied Settings.* 6th ed. Belmont, CA: Wadsworth/Thomson Learning; 2001.

31. Pierce WD, Cheney CD. *Behavior Analysis and Learning.* 3rd ed. Mahwah, NJ: Lawrence Erlbaum Associates; 2004.

32. Ashley MJ, Krych DK, Persel CS, Persel CH. *Working With Behaviour Disorders. Strategies for Traumatic Brain Injury Rehabilitation.* San Antonio, TX: Communication Skill Builders, Psychological Corporation; 1995.

33. Wesolowski MD, Zencius AH. *A Practical Guide to Head Injury Rehabilitation: A Focus on Postacute Residential Treatment.* New York, NY: Plenum Press; 1994.

34. Tate RL. *A Compendium of Tests, Scales, and Questionnaires: The Practioner's Guide to Measuring Outcomes After Acquired Brain Injury.* New York, NY: Psychology Press; 2010.

35. The center for outcome measurement in brain injury. Available at: http://www.tbims.org/combi/. Accessed September 29, 2010.

36. Kelly G, Todd J, Simpson G, Kremer P, Martin C. The Overt Behaviour Scale (OBS): a tool for measuring challenging behaviours following ABI in community settings. *Brain Inj.* 2006;20(3):307–19.

37. Kelly G, Brown S, Todd J, Kremer P. Challenging behaviour profiles of people with acquired brain injury living in community settings. *Brain Inj.* 2008;22(6):457–470.

38. Kreutzer JS, Marwitz JH, Seel R, Serio CD. Validation of the neurobehavioral functioning inventory for adults with traumatic brain injury. *Arch Phys Med Rehabil.* 1996;77(2):116–124.

39. Vanier M, Mazaux JM, Lambert J, Dassa C, Levin HS. Assessment of neuropsychologic impairments after head injury: interrater reliability and factorial and criterion validity of the Neurobehavioral Rating Scale-Revised. *Arch Phys Med Rehabil.* 2000;81(6):796–806.

40. McCauley SR, Levin HS, Vanier M, et al. The Neurobehavioral Rating Scale-Revised: sensitivity and validity in closed head injury assessment. *J Neurol Neurosurg Psychiatry.* 2001;71(5):643–651.

41. Bohac DL, Malec JF, Moessner AM. Factor analysis of the Mayo-Portland Adaptability Inventory: structure and validity. *Brain Inj.* 1997;11(7):469–482.

42. Malec JF, Moessner AM, Kragness M, Lezak MD. Refining a measure of brain injury sequelae to predict postacute rehabilitation outcome: rating scale analysis of the Mayo-Portland Adaptability Inventory. *J Head Trauma Rehabil.* 2000;15(1):670–682.

43. Malec JF, Thompson JM. Relationship of the Mayo-Portland Adaptability Inventory to functional outcome and cognitive performance measures. *J Head Trauma Rehabil.* 1994;9(4):1–15.

44. Votruba KL, Rapport LJ, Vangel SJ Jr, et al. Impulsivity and traumatic brain injury: the relations among behavioral observation, performance measures, and rating scales. *J Head Trauma Rehabil.* 2008;23(2):65–73.

45. Flanagan SR, Elovic EP, Sandel E. Managing agitation associated with traumatic brain injury: behavioral versus pharmacologic interventions? *PM R.* 2009;1(1):76–80.

46. Franzen MD. Neuropsychological assessment in traumatic brain injury. *Crit Care Nurs Q.* 2000;23(3):58–64.

47. Karol RL. *Neuropsychosocial Intervention: The Practical Treatment of Severe Behavioral Dyscontrol After Acquired Brain Injury.* Boca Raton, FL: CRC Press LLC; 2003.

48. Sbordone RJ. Limitations of neuropsychological testing to predict the cognitive and behavioral functioning of persons with brain injury in real-world settings. *NeuroRehabil.* 2001;16(4):199–201.

49. Fasotti L, Spikman J. Cognitive rehabilitation of central executive disorders. In: Brouwer W, van Zomeren E, Berg I, Bouma A, de Haan E, eds. *Cognitive Rehabilitation: A Clinical Neuropsychological Approach.* Amsterdam: Boom Publishers; 2002:107–123.

50. Powell RA, Symbaluk DG, MacDonald SE. *Introduction to Learning and Behavior.* 2nd ed. Belmont, CA: Wadsworth/Thomson Learning; 2005.

51. Joint Commission on Accreditation of Healthcare Organizations. *Comprehensive Accreditation Manual for Hospitals: The Official Handbook.* Oakbrook Terrace, IL: Joint Commission Resources; 2004.

52. Pepping M, Prigatano GP. Psychotherapy after brain injury: costs and benefits. In: Prigatano GP, Plishkin NH, eds. *Clinical Neuropsychology and Cost Outcome Research: A Beginning.* New York, NY: Psychology Press; 2003:313–328.

53. Beatty C. Perception and reality: interventions for behavioral problems after brain injury. *Premier Outlook.* 2004;4(2):4–12.

54. Feeney TJ, Ylvisaker M, Rosen BH, Greene P. Community supports for individuals with challenging behavior after brain injury: an analysis of the New York state behavioral resource project. *J Head Trauma Rehabil.* 2001;16(1):61–75.

55. Kessles RP, de Haan EH. Implicit learning in memory rehabilitation: a meta-analysis on errorless learning and vanishing cues methods. *J Cl Exp Neuropsych.* 2003;25(6):805–814.

56. Tailby R, Haslam C. An investigation of errorless learning in memory-impaired patients: improving the technique and clarifying theory. *Neuropsychologia.* 2003;41(9):1230–1240.

57. Ducharme JM. Treatment of maladaptive behavior in acquired brain injury: remedial approaches in postacute settings. *Clin Psychol Rev.* 2000;20(3):405–426.

58. Bandura A. *Principles of Behavior Modification.* New York, NY: Holt, Rinehart & Winston, Inc.; 1969.

59. Mattheis BK, Kreutzer JS, West DD. *The Behavior Management Handbook: A Practical Approach to Patients With Neurological Disorders.* San Antonio, TX: Therapy Skill Builders, Psychological Corporation; 1997.

60. Yody BB, Schaub C, Conway J, Peters S, Strauss D, Helsinger S. Applied behavior management and acquired brain injury approaches and assessment. *J Head Trauma Rehabil.* 2000;15(4):1041–1060.

61. Slifer KJ, Amari A. Behavior management for children and adolescents with acquired brain injury. *Dev Disabil Res Rev.* 2009;15:144–151.

62. Ducharme JM. A conceptual model for treatment of externalizing behaviour in acquired brain injury. *Brain Inj.* 1999;13(9):645–668.

63. Turkstra LS. The positive behavioral momentum of Mark Ylvisaker. *Semin Speech Lang.* 2010;31(3):162–167.

64. Ylvisaker M, Jacobs HE, Feeney TJ. Positive supports for people who experience behavioral and cognitive disability after brain injury: a review. *J Head Trauma Rehabil.* 2003;18(1):7–32.

65. Hayden ME, Moreault AM, LeBlanc J, Plenger PM. Reducing level of handicap in traumatic brain injury: an environmentally based model of treatment. *J Head Trauma Rehabil.* 2000;15(4):1000–1021.

66. Burton GU. Psychosocial aspects of adaptation and adjustment during various phases of neurological disability. In: Darcy AU, ed. *Neurological Rehabilitation.* 4th ed. St. Louis, MO: Mosby; 2001:178–199.

67. Kreutzer JS, Marwitz JH, Godwin EE, Arango-Lasprilla JC. Practical approaches to effective family intervention after brain injury. *J Head Trauma Rehabil.* 2010;25(2):113–120.

68. Niemeier J, Karol RL. *Overcoming Grief and Loss After Brain Injury.* New York, NY: Oxford University Press; 2011.

69. Niemeier J, Karol RL. *Therapists Guide to Overcoming Grief and Loss After Brain Injury.* New York, NY: Oxford University Press; 2011.

70. Jacobs H. Ain't misbehaving! *Brain Inj Prof.* 2008;5(4):8–10.

71. Grattan LM, Ghahramanlou M. The rehabilitation of neurologically based social disturbance. In: Eslinger PJ, ed. *Neuropsychological Interventions – Clinical Research and Practice.* New York, NY: The Guilford Press; 2002:266–293.

72. Driscoll DM, Monte OD, Grafman J. A need for improved training interventions for the remediation of impairments in social functioning following brain injury. *J Neurotrauma.* 2011;28(2):319–326.

73. Cattelani R, Zettin M, Zoccolotti P. Rehabilitation treatments for adults with behavioral and psychosocial disorders following acquired brain injury: a systematic review. *Neuropsychol Rev.* 2010;20(1):52–85.

74. Martelli MF, Zasler ND, Tiernan PR. Skill acquisition and automatic process development after brain injury: a holistic habit retraining (HHR) model for community reentry. *Brain Inj Prof.* 2005;2(1):10–16.

Psychological Interventions for Emotional and Behavioral Problems Following Traumatic Brain Injury

Jennie Ponsford and Ming-Yun Hsieh

INTRODUCTION

Traumatic brain injury (TBI) results in complex and variable psychological consequences. Cognitive impairments are common, most often in the domains of attention, processing speed, memory, and executive function (e.g, poor planning, inflexible thinking) (1), as well as diminished self-awareness (2,3). Emotional disturbances such as irritability, reduced frustration tolerance, impaired emotion perception, mood and anxiety disorders, and affective instability also are common (see Chapter 62). Behavioral disturbances are among the most challenging consequences of TBI and include disinhibited, impulsive, aggressive, or other socially inappropriate behaviors, as well as reduced drive or initiative (i.e., apathy).

As a result of these problems, many individuals with TBI are unable to be independent in daily activities, to study, work, or pursue leisure activities. Disturbances of personality and behavior may place stress on personal relationships and affect social interactions (4–9). Outcome studies have shown that with increasing time postinjury many people with TBI become socially isolated and develop poor self-esteem (10–13). The experience of such changes caused by a sudden injury, often sustained in the prime of life, can have a devastating psychological impact. The manner in which a person responds to such changes is determined by various factors. These include the circumstances and severity of the injury, the person's recollection and interpretation of the injury, age and developmental stage, and preinjury psychosocial adjustment. For instance, a combination of factors, including history of risk-taking behavior, substance use, previous head injury, and/or poor psychosocial attainment, is likely to place the individual at greater risk of negative psychiatric consequences following a TBI. Postinjury factors, including the availability of social support and of rehabilitation and long-term health care supports, may also play a role.

TBI occurs most frequently in young males aged 15–25 years (14,15). Individuals in this age range are in the process of becoming independent of their parents and establishing their identity. They may be studying or training toward their employment future. Forming social networks and intimate relationships is an important part of this life phase. TBI may significantly disrupt any or all of these processes, preventing the attainment of important life goals. This, in turn, may result in low self-esteem and other negative changes in self-concept. Such responses may be associated with the development of psychiatric disorders, including depression, anxiety, and substance abuse. As Fryer (16) has observed, the inability to resolve adolescent issues can result in "lack of purpose, inability to find intimacy with others, and self-defeating behavior (i.e., substance abuse)." All of these behaviors may also result directly from the brain injury. Changes in personality and behavior may limit friendships and place significant stress on relationships with partners/spouses, parents, and children (17–21).

Epidemiological studies also suggest that TBI is more frequently sustained by individuals who engage in risk-taking behavior. These people are more likely to come from socially disadvantaged backgrounds, have lower education, learning difficulties, unemployment, previous head injury, drug or alcohol abuse or other psychiatric disorders prior to injury, and have dysfunctional family relationships (22,23). These factors place the individual at greater risk of experiencing negative psychiatric consequences following an injury (22,24–26).

There is some evidence that depression and anxiety may occur as a direct result of frontal systems injury, which disrupts the neural networks (e.g., frontal-striatal-thalamo-cortical circuits) and neurotransmitter systems important in the regulation of emotional states (27–30) (see Chapter 62). However, findings have not always supported this contention (31,32). Depression and anxiety developing later may occur as a consequence of experience of symptoms and their impact on the individual's lifestyle. A number of recent studies have provided evidence suggesting this is the most common pattern seen in individuals without a preinjury history of anxiety or depression (33–37).

Another factor associated with higher rates of depression and anxiety following TBI is the use of nonproductive coping styles, such as worry, wishful thinking, self-blame, and substance use (25,38–40). Nonproductive coping style has emerged as a factor in the experience of both depressive and anxiety disorders at 1 year postinjury (25). The presence of this relationship is consistent with previous findings (40–42) and argues for incorporation of coping skills training into rehabilitation programs. This is particularly important because many individuals have a preinjury history of using maladaptive coping strategies, which they may continue to employ postinjury. It has been postulated that nonproductive coping may be exacerbated by cognitive impairments. However, Spitz, Ponsford, and Schönberger (43) did not find this. They found that poorer cognitive function was directly associated with higher levels of depression and anxiety. Nevertheless, they did find that the use of productive coping strategies by individuals with slowed information processing could alleviate depression. This highlights the potential benefit of training effective coping skills.

Gould et al. (25) also identified the presence of limb injuries as a predictor of development of psychiatric disorders in the first year after injury. Pain was a concurrent factor significantly associated with depression, anxiety, and poorer functional outcome at 12 months postinjury. Pain further interferes with return to occupational and leisure activities. This highlights the importance of considering pain and pain coping as contributing factors in psychiatric disorders in individuals with TBI and addressing it accordingly.

Studies of psychiatric disorders following TBI, which have surveyed the full range of disorders, suggest that around 50% have had a psychiatric disorder at some time in their life preinjury. Substance use disorders, depression, and anxiety disorders are the most common preinjury psychiatric conditions. Gould et al. (33) found that during the first year following moderate-to-severe TBI, psychiatric disorders were diagnosed in 61% of participants. Postinjury patterns included a decline in substance use disorders, most likely because of hospital recommendations for abstinence for 1 year postinjury and a significant increase in frequency of major depressive disorder and anxiety disorders, which are often comorbid. The most common anxiety disorders included generalized anxiety disorder (GAD), post-traumatic stress disorder (PTSD), specific phobia, panic disorder (PD), social phobia, and relatively low rates of obsessive–compulsive disorder (OCD), and agoraphobia (33,44–47). Studies show a steady increase in onset of disorders up until 2–3 years postinjury, when the rate tends to plateau (44,48), but high rates of depression are still reported between 10 and 30 years postinjury (4,46,49). Although substance use declines in the first year after injury, studies have found that it tends to climb back toward preinjury levels thereafter (50). The reported frequency of psychiatric disorders is generally higher in groups with moderate-to-severe injuries than in groups with predominantly mild injuries (45). Thus, depression, anxiety, and substance use as well as poor self-awareness and self-esteem, anger management problems, and lack of initiative or apathy are amongst the most common psychological issues arising following TBI (51). Psychological approaches to managing these problems will be discussed in this chapter. Substance use issues are dealt with in details in Chapter 79, and behavioral issues are addressed in details in Chapter 63.

THE ROLE OF PSYCHOLOGICAL INTERVENTION AFTER BRAIN INJURY

It is not necessary to have a psychiatric disorder to benefit from psychological therapy. As Prigatano (52) has noted, most people who experience a brain injury feel stress and ask why the brain injury occurred, whether their lives are going to change and for how long, and whether their lives are going to be worth living. Psychotherapy may assist them

in managing this sense of loss and the associated emotions and is an important aspect of the rehabilitation process.

A multimodal approach needs to be taken to address emotional or behavioral problems following TBI. Intensive interdisciplinary rehabilitation is important in maximizing physical and cognitive recovery. It supports the development of strategies and external supports to minimize disability and maximize participation in desired life roles over time. Indeed, whoever is delivering psychological therapy needs to work closely with other therapists to achieve client goals. This approach promotes consistency and a comprehensive and mutual understanding of the most effective ways of supporting and maximizing improvement in the person with TBI, within the bounds of confidentiality. It is important to take a long-term view because some people might require some "booster therapy" months or years after postacute rehabilitation as they encounter new life challenges.

Pharmacological interventions are also relevant and useful in many cases (see Chapter 74 for detailed discussion). If a person was having pharmacological treatment for a psychiatric disorder prior to injury, following medical review this should, in many cases, be continued. Medications may be necessary as the first line of treatment to alleviate symptoms, particularly when these are severe (47,53). However, people with TBI are at risk of side effects with psychotropic medications, and no pharmacological intervention has been shown to consistently alleviate anxiety or depression without significant side effects in individuals with TBI (54,55) (see Chapter 74). More importantly, pharmacological treatments are not usually the most desirable long-term options. They cannot address the psychosocial factors, including use of nonproductive coping, inability to engage in meaningful vocational and recreational activities, and reduced social integration, which contribute to psychological distress following brain injury. Psychological treatments potentially equip people with TBI and/or family with strategies to be applied to search for a new meaning in their lives. Such strategies may increase their adaptive coping skills and enable them to manage problems independently in the longer term, thus strengthening their self-efficacy and offering potentially more durable effects. As a consequence, psychological interventions are frequently the preferred mode of treatment (55–57).

Psychotherapy is a term used to describe "the interactive/relational process between the therapist and the client based upon a wide range of differing theoretical frameworks of therapy. . . .The aim is to help troubled individuals reduce their distress and enjoy greater life satisfaction through changing their thoughts, feelings, and behavior" (58) (p. 438). Despite the high frequency of psychological problems following TBI, understanding of what brain injury means to the survivor from a psychological perspective lags far behind neuropsychological understanding, and availability of psychological therapy services both within and outside rehabilitation settings remains very limited. This is due, in part, to the view that the presence of injury-related cognitive impairments precludes benefit from psychological therapy.

It is true that cognitive difficulties present an impediment to benefiting from traditional psychotherapy for many individuals with TBI. Psychotherapy relies on self-awareness, verbal communication skills, and a capacity to pay attention to and remember the content of therapy from one session to the next. Difficulties with executive control of thinking and behavior may make it difficult to generalize and implement strategies in everyday life. It is, therefore, usually necessary to adapt psychological therapy methods to minimize the impact of these problems on potential benefit from therapy. Moreover, some individuals with severe impairments in these domains may be unable to benefit from such psychological interventions. For such cases, implementing changes to the environment or behavioral or pharmacological interventions as discussed in Chapters 63 and 74 will be more appropriate.

The first step in psychotherapy is the establishment of a therapeutic alliance. Judd and Wilson (58) highlight the importance of therapeutic alliance in building a strong and effective therapeutic relationship between therapist and client. A survey of psychologists treating clients with TBI identified impaired memory as the most common impediment to the establishment of a therapeutic alliance and progress in therapy (58). Written summaries and visual cues were used to overcome this problem. Inflexible thinking and lack of insight also presented challenges. Behavioral experiments in reality testing were used to enhance self-awareness and build a collaborative understanding. Goal setting and review also aided the process of self-reflection and sense of achievement. Not denying clients a sense of hope was seen as important. This has also been recognized by Klonoff (59). Therapists commonly experienced negative emotions toward the challenges of establishing therapeutic alliance—general frustration over cognitive difficulties or occasional fear over disinhibited behavior.

In light of the likely influence of cognitive impairments on response to psychological therapy, it is particularly important to communicate with clients in writing as well as orally. Written summaries of the assessment, agreed goals of therapy, number and timing of sessions, homework, procedures for cancelling or changing appointments, and payment, if relevant, need to be prepared and reviewed on a regular basis. The person with TBI should be encouraged to use a notebook to record important points made in therapy and agreed strategies and assisted in recording things in a clear and logical fashion. If writing in a notebook is not feasible because of physical, visual, or language problems or poor literacy, video or audio recording of sessions for subsequent review may be possible. Handouts using simple language and pictures to illustrate concepts are helpful, and these should be compiled in an organized fashion with the client's notes in the therapy workbook. Use of catchy phrases as prompts for adaptive behavior may be helpful. These may be written on cue cards or noteboards placed strategically around the home or workplace. Mobile phones or handheld computers also serve as useful prompting devices. Metaphors may be helpful as long as these are personally meaningful to the client. Drawings can also be used to illustrate points or processes in a concrete fashion, along with lists of positives and negatives or pros and cons (60). Because of the client's executive and memory problems, booster sessions are likely to be needed to maintain therapy gains.

ASSESSMENT FOR PSYCHOLOGICAL INTERVENTION

A comprehensive assessment needs to be made to determine suitability for and approaches to psychological therapy. Use of a case formulation and hypothesis testing approach is recommended (61,62). This considers the factors, which may have predisposed, precipitated, and perpetuated the psychological problems, as well as the individual's strengths that may promote change. Therefore, a detailed history is important. As discussed in Chapter 62, the history needs to be gathered from multiple sources, including the patient, family, and medical records, given the potential unreliability of the patient's awareness levels. It should cover all potential etiological or contributory factors. These include factors relating to the injuries sustained, including the brain injury and other injuries, to the person, their family, and to social or environmental factors or events since the injury. The relative contribution of each of these factors provides the basis of the formulation of treatment.

It is important to document physical injuries, which may be exacerbating distress or hampering recovery by, for example, causing pain and incapacity. Information regarding the nature, cause, and severity of the brain injury from the medical file, including scan results and results of neuropsychological assessments, will provide important background to assist in determining the likely contribution of the injury to the psychological problem. Is there evidence of fronto-limbic injury? Are there neuroendocrine abnormalities? Reference to a neuropsychological assessment report is important to understand the person's cognitive strengths and weaknesses, specifically their capacity to pay attention; remember new material in various modalities; and to initiate, plan, and follow through with their intentions, their verbal interaction skills, and above all, their degree of self-awareness of their problems. It is necessary to consider the extent to which the person with TBI is likely to be able to engage verbally with a therapist or a group of people, remember the content of therapy, and/or use and carry over strategies into their lives. This will aid in the decision as to what treatment approach to take and underpin the nature of the strategies employed. Severe impairments in these domains may preclude the use of psychological therapy and would certainly point to the need for a very structured approach to therapy. Such therapy would need to incorporate repetition and use of written aids and consideration of involvement of a family member as a cotherapist. In some cases, it may be more productive to guide other health professionals to engage clients better in other therapies or adapt the environment.

It is also vital to document the nature of the cognitive and behavioral changes observed by the person with TBI and significant others, how these have changed over time, and how they are impacting on the person's participation in life roles. Reports from and observations of other therapists working with the person with TBI are also helpful in providing a picture of how much awareness the person with TBI and family members have of on injury-related changes and their implications. This will influence the decision as to whether and how psychological therapy might proceed.

Regarding personal factors, it is important to consider the person's age, developmental stage, and social roles. What were they doing and what were their goals prior to injury and how has the injury disrupted these? How does the person with TBI feel about this? What is their motivation to return to various aspects of their lifestyle? How have their upbringing and family relationships been? What cultural influences are relevant to their responses to injury? Saltapidas and Ponsford (63,64) found that individuals from culturally and linguistically diverse backgrounds showed generally higher levels of emotional distress over injury-related changes, were less likely to have internal locus of control beliefs, and showed greater distress about changes in their ability to perform certain life roles postinjury, such as to work to support the family or be a homemaker. Thus, cultural views need to be taken into account in case formulation. The individual's premorbid intellectual ability, educational and occupational background, personality style, and previous and current methods of coping with stress need to be documented, along with the individual's lifetime history of psychiatric disorders, including substance use. Any previous trauma and their response to this should be recorded. If there have been previous psychiatric disorders, identify what treatment have they had in the past, how successful has this been, and what has been their experience with therapists. Do they have positive self-efficacy regarding therapy? Has medication been helpful, and is medication still being taken? It is also necessary to assess the extent to which the person with TBI and/or family members are willing or able to engage verbally with a therapist about psychological issues individually or to participate in group therapy. Sometimes information will only be divulged after a period of time has elapsed and the client with TBI trusts the therapist.

There is evidence that family functioning both before and after injury influences the psychosocial adjustment of the person with TBI (65–68). Sander and colleagues (69) have provided evidence to suggest that families of those with TBI may have had higher rates of preinjury stress and/or unhealthy family functioning, meaning they are less well equipped to cope with the impact of an injury in a family member. Families with preexisting problems may become more dysfunctional. Approximately 25%–30% of family members, predominantly caregivers, also exhibit clinically significant anxiety and/or depression 1–5 years following injury (70,71). Therefore, as outlined in Chapter 80, it is important to consider the family as an important focus of the assessment process. This is necessary, both in terms of understanding the psychological state of the person with TBI and also as a focus of intervention in itself as a means of maximizing their capacity to provide support for the person with TBI. The preinjury psychiatric state of family members and general family functioning should be documented, as well as responses of the family since the injury. The presence of other social supports and networks available to the person with TBI and family and how have these changed since the injury also need to be investigated. The willingness of family members to engage in discussion of psychological or adjustment issues, as well as the availability of a family member or close other to act as a cotherapist should be canvassed, if appropriate. It may be that in some cases, psychological interventions are not deemed appropriate for the person with TBI by virtue of their cognitive impairments, but they may be more appropriately directed toward the family. In other cases, it may not be in the interests of the person with TBI to have their family involved in therapy.

It is also important to assess the impact of events that may have occurred since the injury. Are there issues relating to the circumstances of the accident, including symptoms of post-traumatic stress, grief or guilt over death, or injury to another person involved? Is there pain or other disabilities resulting from other bodily injuries? How are they coping with these? Are there other life stressors, such as financial problems or legal issues? Has there been a lack of support from family or friends or funding bodies? Have significant relationships been disrupted by the injury and its effects? Have other environmental factors exacerbated the problems? Have cultural factors impacted on the local community's response to the injury?

SUPPORTIVE THERAPY AND EDUCATION

The experience of TBI is extremely stressful, even for those individuals with TBI and families who had healthy psychological functioning prior to injury. Provision of educational materials and supportive therapy may assist them to adjust to the effects of the injury. Ponsford and colleagues (72) demonstrated in a mild TBI sample that provision of an information booklet regarding symptoms and management strategies reduced psychological distress. Multimedia, such as storybooks (73) and short films (74) are also available to illustrate the consequences of brain injury.

Supportive therapy should provide an opportunity for both the person with TBI and family members to express and work through their emotional responses at different stages, including feelings of anxiety, helplessness, hope, denial, depression, guilt, anger, loss and grief. Ideally, the therapist is a psychologist or social worker. If the allied health team does not include members with these professional backgrounds, then another therapist or caseworker may need to provide this type of support. Alternatively, any team member with whom the person with TBI and/or family develops a trusting relationship may provide supportive therapy. However, these individuals need to be clear with the person and family about the limits of their time and expertise.

Supportive therapy is generally delivered in a nondirective way, using nonstrategic reflective listening (75,76). The client is invited to discuss their feelings or problems in an open-ended way, and thus the content is determined by the client. The therapist seeks to understand the client's feelings and thoughts without judging or criticizing and reflects these back to the client in an empathic way. Each individual experiences different responses at a given point in time. Many will not be ready to talk about their feelings until long after they or their relative have been discharged from hospital or rehabilitation. Some will never wish to do so, and this should be respected. Supportive therapy also provides a forum in which to provide information and education about the short- and long-term effects of TBI. This may be conveyed verbally in a manner appropriate to each case. It should be supported with written information provided at a level consistent with the person's cognitive functioning. The opportunity should be provided to ask questions about cognitive and behavioral changes observed and raise practical problems. These are most likely to become apparent after hospital discharge. The person may be connected with resources toward solving these problems. For family members, it also provides an opportunity to discuss their concerns regarding management of the newly acquired disabilities of the individual with TBI.

INDIVIDUAL PSYCHODYNAMIC PSYCHOTHERAPY: REESTABLISHING IDENTITY

Improved self-awareness commonly emerges after the individual with TBI has returned to the community and had more direct experience of injury-related changes, which affect their participation in independent living, work or study, leisure activities, and relationships (77). This growing awareness may precipitate the onset of anxiety and depression and possibly a catastrophic reaction (33,37). Ideally, psychological therapy should be available to support the process of developing a realistic self-appraisal of injury-related changes while minimizing loss of self-esteem. The work of Yehuda Ben-Yishay (78), George Prigatano (52), Pamela Klonoff (60) and others has contributed enormously to understanding of these issues. They view the restoration of the impaired identity or self as a central goal in rehabilitation following brain injury, to be achieved by bridging the gap between the person's ideal self and their actual postinjury self (52,79). Prigatano (52) posits that the therapist and client need to see the whole picture of the person's life and elicit their inner experience through words, poetry, or artwork. He sees it as important to guide the person with brain injury through discussion of the symbols of work, love, and play as important aspects of the human identity to be explored because these existed prior to injury and because they are likely to exist in the future.

Gracey and colleagues (80–83) suggest that participation in activities that were valued prior to injury, ideally within the safe context of a rehabilitation program, can assist in the process of reducing the sense of threat experienced over the discrepancy between the preinjury and postinjury self. This allows the person to slowly update their self-identity and develop a more realistic self-image. Through their use of metaphoric identity mapping, Ylvisaker and Feeney (84) have engaged and motivated clients with brain injury by guiding them to identify their own role model and adopt the positive qualities of that person. The ultimate goal of such therapy is the attainment of some acceptance of the new "postinjury" self and defining of new roles.

For adolescents and young adults in particular, the therapist needs to be attuned to the impact of the injury on pertinent developmental issues. These include body image and forming intimate relationships, having friends and feeling accepted, moving out of home and achieving independence, and having a job. Such factors are likely to be central to the building of the new identity. These approaches are central in the implementation of acceptance and commitment therapy (discussed later in this chapter). Some individuals may even come to view the injury as a catalyst for positive psychological changes, including an enhanced sense of self and more positive relationships (85–86).

GROUP THERAPY

In those individuals who have sufficient language, memory skills, and behavioral control, individual therapy may be supplemented with group therapy. This is exemplified by the closed group meeting daily in a "therapeutic milieu" at the Rusk Institute of Rehabilitation Medicine in New York, developed by Yehuda Ben-Yishay and colleagues (78,79, 87,88). This provides an opportunity to share with others the effects of the injury on key aspects of life, how they are perceived and affect others and hear others' experiences. This potentially improves awareness within a supportive environment and reduces the sense of isolation. Self-esteem may be enhanced by activities requiring them to identify their positive attributes or accomplishments. According to Ben-Yishay (79), participants in a therapeutic milieu progress through a hierarchy of 6 stages: engagement, awareness, mastery, control, acceptance, and identity, with the extent of progress determined by certain premorbid personality qualities. Following participation in the group program the focus moves to developing suitable vocational activities and community engagement. While these programs have been emulated by other eminent clinicians (52,78), there has been no specific experimental study of the impact of these methods on the development of self-awareness and identity after brain injury, in particular which aspects of the therapy are effective and in whom. Furthermore, for individuals with very severe memory, attentional and executive problems, and poor behavioral inhibition, neither individual nor group therapy aimed at developing realistic self-appraisal is likely to be successful. Nevertheless, their emotional responses deserve respect and consideration, and they should be given opportunities to ventilate feelings on a regular basis. In most cases, group therapy would need to be backed up with individual therapy.

In another intervention designed to enhance self-awareness and self-regulation, Ownsworth, McFarland, and Young (89) conducted a 16-week group program in a group of 21 individuals with chronic acquired brain injury of mixed etiology. Activities included training in problem solving and compensatory strategies, as well as role-plays. Participants showed improved knowledge and use of self-regulatory strategies to control emotional and behavioral problems. Their self-reported psychosocial function improved immediately postgroup, although these gains were not maintained at 6-month follow-up.

FAMILY SUPPORT

As noted in Chapter 80, because they provide the most long-term support for people with severe TBI, families need to be actively involved in all therapeutic processes. This includes those focused on psychological issues because these pertain to the person with brain injury—themselves as individuals or the family system. Family members may be invaluable cotherapists. However, they also have their own psychological needs. These may be addressed by provision of information and proactive support (90), social work liaison (91), individual therapy, or family support groups. Where there are preexisting problems in the family, or where family reactions to the injury are considered to be maladaptive, formal family therapy may be appropriate.

Family Groups

It is likely to be helpful to enable families to share information and emotional support during and after the rehabilitation phase. Although many families are not ready to discuss their own emotional responses to trauma, they may benefit from educational input regarding brain injury and resources for assistance. Different types and amount of education may need to be provided according to their stage of readiness. Over time, they may be more willing and able to discuss emotional issues and may benefit from hearing that others are having similar experiences. This may provide the opportunity to discuss responses that they may not feel comfortable discussing within their own families. The issues of importance to spouses of individuals with TBI may be somewhat different from those of parents of adolescents or adults with TBI. They may feel uncomfortable about discussing relationship issues or their feelings about changes in behavior and personality. It is, therefore, useful to enable spouses to talk with one another, providing relief from the guilt, which many experience regarding their negative feelings about their partner with TBI.

A few studies have evaluated educational interventions for carers. A small randomized controlled trial (RCT) comparing education alone with education combined with education in behavior management obtained no significant differences on the measures used (92). However, in another study, home-based problem-solving training reduced depression and health complaints and dysfunctional problem-solving styles in family caregivers of people with TBI relative to general education (93). Systems of web-based information and online support for family carers are also useful for providing social support, information, and guidance (94). The Brain Injury Family Intervention (BIFI; 95) is a manualized intervention comprising sessions in the home with the person with TBI and caregiver discussing injury consequences, ways of coping with change and managing stress, problem solving, and looking after one's self. This intervention has been shown to result in fewer reported unmet needs and obstacles to obtaining services but no changes in family functioning, satisfaction, or caregiver distress. A version of this intervention for families of adolescents with TBI has also been developed (96). There is a need for more controlled studies of such interventions.

Singer et al. (97) found that training in coping skills to manage stress and sharing of methods of coping reduced anxiety and depression symptoms more in parents of children and adolescents than an informational support group. This suggests that training in adaptation and coping skills may be a worthwhile focus of family support groups. Sander (98) evaluated a 6-session cognitive behavior therapy (CBT) intervention group aimed at reducing caregiver distress after TBI in 16 caregivers. It included general education of TBI; training in management of physical, cognitive, and emotional consequences of stress; discussion of relationship changes and strategies for improvement; training in stress management; and provision of community resources and support. Preliminary results revealed a significant reduction in anxiety and escape-avoidance coping pretest to posttest and a trend toward improved family functioning. This study did not include a control group, however.

A multifamily group approach, which focuses on psychoeducation and problem solving in groups involving both individuals with TBI and their family members, has been evaluated in 2 recent intervention studies. Rodgers et al. (99) conducted such a group over 12–18 months with 27 survivors of brain or spinal cord injury and 28 caregivers. They found a decrease in depressive symptoms and anger toward others, an increase in life satisfaction in those injured, and

a reduction in burden for caregivers. Themes emerging from a qualitative evaluation of this group included normalization of the caregiving experience, socialization, enhancement of coping skills, and education about the injuries. Findings from a more recent study involving 32 individuals with severe brain injury and their families revealed a significant improvement in family members' ratings of general family functioning on the Family Assessment Device and improved social integration reported by relatives in response to participation in a 3-month multifamily group program (100).

COGNITIVE BEHAVIOR THERAPY

Evidence regarding the effectiveness of specific psychological therapies following brain injury is scant. CBT appears to be among the most frequently used forms of psychotherapy in this population (58). In the general clinical population, CBT is the recommended choice of psychological treatment for a range of psychological disorders, including depression and anxiety disorders (101–105). CBT is based on the premise that emotional problems can be effectively managed using adaptive thinking and behavioral strategies (106). Therapy involves the client and therapist working collaboratively to identify current problems and develop a case formulation of factors underpinning the development and maintenance of the presenting problem. They may also engage in active problem solving using practical strategies and homework exercises, with the aim of equipping the client to manage their own problems (62,107). CBT is derived from both the cognitive model of psychological disorders and learning behavior theory. The cognitive model considers that people make sense of the world, and plan and evaluate behavior according to "core belief" systems. These belief systems are influenced by early experience and significant others, and operationalized as conditional assumptions, for example, "To be worthwhile I must be successful at work, have many friends, have a stable relationship." When a critical incident such as a brain injury occurs, the person with TBI may be unable to keep up with the standards set by the conditional assumptions. This triggers the production of "negative automatic thoughts", which are negative self-talk associated with unpleasant affect, behaviors, and physiological responses. These have a bidirectional relationship with the environment. CBT aims to break into the negative cycle that maintains depression or anxiety (106).

The structured nature of CBT allows for the delivery of therapy while making allowances for the effects of TBI. Written aids, cues, and repetition are components of CBT that can be extended for people with TBI. CBT can also be adapted to reduce the emphasis on abstract concepts and increase focus on behavioral strategies, such as exposure to feared situations or systematic desensitization and the achievement of concrete behavioral goals (109). It is important at the outset to make a careful assessment of the limitations the person with TBI is likely to have in such a therapy situation and to adapt the prescribed techniques as needed. For individuals with impaired attention, memory, and/or executive function, it is necessary to keep sessions short, focusing on just 1 or 2 rather than several issues or goals in a given session, to build repetition into therapy, to write all important points down in the person's diary or in a "therapy diary," and to use handouts and pictorial aids. The therapist will usually need to focus on very concrete personally relevant examples and behaviors, and may need to be quite directive.

If the client agrees, involvement of a family member or close friend as a "cotherapist" may facilitate the therapy processes. Once they have been made aware of the aims and processes of therapy, family members may be able to assist in describing the behavioral and emotional responses of the person with TBI in different situations, as well as their precipitating circumstance and consequences. They may provide assistance or reminders to carry out homework exercises, including monitoring thoughts and behavior and prompting adherence to strategies discussed in therapy sessions. This family member may also provide feedback in familiar situations and prompt more adaptive responses. They can assist in maintaining the use of strategies taught in therapy into the future and provide ongoing feedback as to their success. It may not always be appropriate to involve a family member in the therapy process, however. This may be the case in instances when family or marital conflict appears to be contributing to the problem, where family members are not able to give realistic, constructive, or appropriate feedback or input, or where there are issues of control or overprotectiveness.

CBT has shown demonstrated efficacy in the treatment of a range of psychiatric and psychological problems following TBI, including depression (108), anxiety (109–112), emotional distress (113), and anger (114), as well as poor psychosocial functioning (89), self-esteem, problem solving (115), and adaptive coping (116). However, most of the CBT research within the TBI population has been based on case studies and a few group studies involving small samples of persons with mild-to-moderate injuries. There is relative little evidence regarding its efficacy in people with severe TBI (117).

Group Cognitive Behavior Therapy Intervention Studies

CBT may also be applied in a group context. Several studies have evaluated the application of CBT in groups to facilitate adaptive coping skills, psychosocial functioning, and problem solving (89,115,116). Anson and Ponsford's (116) coping skills group consisted of 10 biweekly sessions, which aimed to enhance adaptive coping following TBI. The group focused on understanding the association between thoughts, feelings, and bodily sensations; developing strategies for managing anxiety, depression, and anger; for solving problems; and for maximizing use of adaptive coping strategies. Participants reported increased use of adaptive coping strategies on completion of the group, but this was not necessarily maintained over time. Levels of anxiety and depression did not change in the group as a whole. There was, however, some individual variability in response to this therapy. Further analysis revealed that participants who showed a reduction in depressive symptoms following the group tended to have higher premorbid intellectual function, less severe injuries, higher anxiety, and greater self-awareness on commencement of treatment (118).

More recently, Backhaus and colleagues (119) evaluated the efficacy of a 12-session manualized coping skills group using CBT principles to provide psychoeducation, support,

and coping skills training aimed at helping both survivors with TBI and their caregivers manage dysfunctional cognitive and behavioral patterns. Participation in the group resulted in significantly improved positive self-efficacy, assessed in terms of mastery over the topics presented in the group sessions compared with the control group immediately posttreatment and maintained this over time. Posttreatment positive self-efficacy was associated with global distress at 3-month follow-up. There were no group effects on psychological distress as measured on the Brief Symptom Inventory. However, the control group showed increased emotional distress at 3-month follow-up, whereas that of the coping skills group remained stable over time.

Overall, the evidence to date suggests that participation in group interventions using CBT methods, for either individuals with brain injury or their families, will result in participants reporting that they have learned the information and strategies that has been taught in the group. This may prevent or curtail the development of emotional distress in the future in individuals who do not already have clinically significant psychological problems. However, there is limited evidence that this is making a significant long-term impact on their psychological state. Anson and Ponsford (116) concluded that individual therapy, tailored to address individual issues and needs, may be more appropriate for clients with TBI.

Individual Cognitive Behavior Therapy

The efficacy of individual CBT has been evaluated in several studies (110,113,120) with encouraging results but involving small samples. At present, there is insufficient evidence to make a gold standard recommendation for the treatment of anxiety and depression following TBI, thus highlighting the need for more research.

Individual Cognitive Behavior Therapy for Depression
Following assessment and formulation of factors that need to be addressed and goals for therapy, the therapist introduces the cognitive model, outlining the association between thoughts, mood, behavior, and physiological changes in the body to the client. To illustrate this, the client may be encouraged, perhaps with the assistance of a relative, to monitor their moods, rate their intensity, and identify and document the thoughts, which accompany negative emotions. This may be done through innovative methods and technology (e.g., mobile, iPhone applications). The therapist may assist the client to understand the link between these thoughts and their emotions. The therapist may also engage the client in the process of cognitive restructuring, where the client learns to explore the assumptions and core beliefs that underlie unhelpful thoughts and to develop alternative constructive thinking patterns. Cue cards or mobile phone reminders may be used to prompt more adaptive thinking. The person with TBI is encouraged to look forward rather than backward and to focus on what is within his or her control. He or she learns to view his or her new postinjury self in a more realistic and positive light and begins to measure himself or herself by achievements since the injury rather than by preinjury achievements. The use of adaptive coping strategies such

as solving problems, working hard, using humor, physical recreation, and seeking relaxing diversions is encouraged, whereas nonproductive strategies such as worry, wishful thinking, self-blame, and substance use are discouraged.

Behavioral activation may be particularly helpful for individuals with TBI because it involves monitoring of activity levels and facilitating the person's engagement in personally meaningful and enjoyable activities. Targets may be set for gradually increasing such involvement. In this respect, the therapist may need to work with other members of the rehabilitation team in exploring appropriate options. Further detail regarding the use of CBT in the management of depression may be obtained from sources including Beck et al. (106).

There have been no published group studies evaluating the use of individual CBT specifically for depression following TBI. Montgomery (121) reported success in a single case intervention, focused on cognitive reframing, activity scheduling, time management, and relaxation skills training. Topolovec-Vranic and colleagues (122) evaluated a web-based CBT program and found significantly reduced depressive symptoms on treatment completion and at 12-month follow-up. However, only 62% of participants completed the whole program, highlighting the challenges in conducting clinical trials within a TBI population. Bradbury and colleagues (123) developed a pilot CBT program for emotional distress and coping skills and tested its effectiveness in a nonrandomized trial involving 20 participants with brain injury of mixed etiologies (50% with TBI). A comprehensive baseline assessment was performed, and the treating clinician was provided with a report, which documented participants' cognitive limitations and recommended ways of adapting CBT (e.g., repetition, slower rate of delivery, reduced complexity) to maximize treatment effectiveness. Participants who received CBT reported a significant decrease in overall psychological distress and showed a trend toward a reduction in escape-avoidance coping style. Additionally, treatment gains were maintained at 1-month follow-up.

Individual Cognitive Behavior Therapy for Anxiety
CBT for anxiety aims to give the client control over the anxiety. An important component of this process is the education of the client about the physiology of the anxiety response and the role that thoughts and avoidant behavior can play in perpetuating that response. This understanding will be enhanced if the person with TBI keeps a record (on paper or electronically), noting circumstances in which they feel anxious, including the thoughts, feelings, bodily sensations, and behaviors that accompany the anxiety response, monitoring and rating its severity. These records provide useful evidence for challenging irrational thinking, which may underpin the anxiety. By jointly reflecting on these situations with the client, the therapist can encourage alternative interpretations of situations and help the client to develop more coping statements, which may be recorded on cue cards to support the implementation of coping strategies. Repetition is needed to implement and monitor the use of such strategies. It can also be very useful to elicit and highlight adaptive coping statements that the client may already be using. These coping statements are easier to implement therapeutically, thereby enhancing the client's chance of success.

Use of muscle relaxation may provide a distraction from anxious thoughts, as well as decrease bodily symptoms, such as muscle tension. Slow breathing is one method of facilitating relaxation that can be applied in everyday situations. It is a "portable" technique that can be used in anxiety-provoking situations without drawing attention to the person. Some injured individuals may have difficulty focusing their attention sufficiently to engage in progressive muscle relaxation (PMR) or may fall asleep during relaxation sessions, so a brief, shortened version of PMR may be more practical than the traditional method. Making changes to positioning, lighting and timing of sessions, and getting a comfortable chair/couch in the office may be necessary. Additional adjustments may be required for those with pain conditions. Taped relaxation instructions using the same voice and sequence should be made available for practice at home. There are also applications available on smart phones for clients to practice relaxation techniques in their own time between therapy sessions. Emphasis needs to be placed on teaching the person with TBI to detect the signs and triggers of anxiety early, so that they can apply relaxation techniques before the anxiety has built up. In those who have poor self-monitoring, this will be difficult and this is one way in which a family member may be of assistance. A great deal of practice (e.g., mental imagery, role-plays) will be necessary to build the clients' skills in applying relaxation in stressful situations. .

For individuals who cannot apply relaxation techniques to reduce anxiety, a useful alternative may be physical exercise. It is also important to devote time to the development of concrete strategies or routines for refocusing thoughts onto the immediate situation or onto some simple statements, a poem or a list. Avoidance (which may be in the form of "safety behavior") needs to be tackled early in the therapy process. Depending on the situations, which are provoking the anxiety, it will be important to work with the client to develop a graded approach to those activities. For example, if anxiety in social situations were a problem, establishing a hierarchy of situations in which to practice strategies would be important, beginning with practice with the therapist, then extending to one-on-one social engagements, and progressing gradually toward a party situation, at the same time monitoring anxiety levels and use of designated coping strategies. Assistance from a relative or friend may facilitate this, as long as the client does not become dependent on another person to act on his or her behalf. Another important aspect of this process is likely to be the integration of therapeutic assistance in the development of conversational or social skills, assertiveness skills, or problem-solving skills in naturalistic contexts.

Given the role that cognitive difficulties have in contributing to anxiety, a vital aspect of therapy is empowering the client with strategies to manage these difficulties. For people with memory difficulties it will be important to review previous and current methods of recording things and work on a more systematic use of these methods. These might include strategies for remembering peoples' names in social situations, use of a diary or electronic organizer or other organizational system to deal with unexpected demands, note taking or tape recording of meetings or telephone conversations, asking questions to slow down the delivery of information in conversations, and other time pressure management strategies as suggested by Winkens et al. (124). Changes may also be made to the demands of work or study, for example, making the environment less distracting, altering work duties or hours, reducing or altering the subjects being studied to focus more on the strengths of the person with TBI, or providing assistance in planning or time tabling to reduce cognitive demands and hence anxiety.

There have been few studies evaluating the impact of interventions for anxiety in individuals with TBI. Hodgson and colleagues (110) conducted a RCT of a CBT intervention for managing social anxiety in a group of 12 individuals with predominantly mild brain injury of mixed etiology. Their CBT program included components such as relaxation training, cognitive restructuring, assertiveness skills, and graded exposure. Participants' cognitive limitations were accommodated using various strategies including the use of external aids, repetitions of treatment materials, and shorter sessions. They reported a significant improvement on measures of general anxiety, depression, and transient mood for the treatment group compared to wait-list control, which was maintained at 1-month follow-up. Tiersky et al. (125) described a RCT for treatment of anxiety in general, in which 20 participants with mild-to-moderate TBI received 2, 50-minute individual CBT sessions per day, 3 days a week over 11 weeks. CBT was integrated with cognitive remediation as part of a rehabilitation program. Participants reported significant reduction in anxiety and depression as measured by the Symptom Checklist-90-Revised. However participants' symptom ratings were still not within normal limits, suggesting a need to adjust expectations about treatment prognosis and to provide ongoing monitoring and assistance. The generalizability of the findings may be limited due with the exclusion of subjects with current behavioral or substance use disorders, as well as those with histories of psychotic disorders. These people represent a significant proportion of those who experience anxiety and depression following brain injury (33). Further studies are required to examine the impact of CBT in larger samples and in people with more severe injuries.

A more recent pilot study by Hsieh and colleagues (112,126) focused on reducing anxiety in patients with moderate-to-severe TBI using an adapted manualized form of CBT. This was organized around 5 core treatment modules: psychoeducation, anxiety management, cognitive therapy, graded exposure, and relapse prevention, with optional modules on pleasant event scheduling, mindfulness, and problem solving. There was an emphasis on accommodating participants' cognitive difficulties using concrete objectives and examples, checklists, record sheets, pictorial aids, and repetition, as well as cue cards, modeling, and/or role-plays. This therapy was more successful in reducing anxiety symptoms at posttreatment than treatment as usual in 27 patients with moderate-to-severe TBI.

Cognitive Behavior Therapy for Post-Traumatic Stress Disorder

Use of CBT techniques to treat PTSD involves use of graded exposure to assist the person to gradually process their memory and interpretation of the traumatic event and confront the stimuli that they are seeking to avoid. The aim is to extinguish the conditioned aversive arousal response via habituation, thereby reducing post-traumatic reactions, such as flashbacks, intrusive memories, and startle responses. Systematic desensitization may be implemented by use of imagination in relaxation exercises or through graduated exposure to real-life situations. Cognitive therapy is used to assist in reconstructing and integrating memories of the

event into autobiographical memory and promoting more adaptive appraisal of the trauma. CBT, which includes education about trauma reactions, progressive muscle relaxation training, imaginal exposure to trauma memories, cognitive restructuring, and graded in-vivo exposure to avoided situations, is an effective treatment for acute stress disorder and reduces the risk of PTSD following general trauma (127–129). This therapy also may be delivered effectively over the Internet (130). Evidence regarding the differential efficacy between cognitive therapy and exposure therapy for PTSD has been mixed, suggesting the need to use both treatment modalities (131).

Recent studies have shown that exposure using computer-generated virtual reality exposure therapy (VRET) is effective in reducing PTSD symptoms in military personnel (132,133). VRET has also demonstrated clinically significant effectiveness in a small sample of survivors of road traffic accidents (134). The use of VRET in addressing PTSD in individuals with TBI is worth exploring because the simulation reality technology may circumvent the impact of cognitive impairment on an individual's ability to fully engage in imaginal exposure (135).

A therapy that involves both exposure and cognitive structuring is eye movement desensitization and reprocessing (EMDR). This treatment focuses attention on a traumatic memory while visually tracking the therapist's finger, followed by restructuring of the memory with the therapist, applying more adaptive thoughts. It also has demonstrated effectiveness in treating PTSD (136). Another form of this therapy with established efficacy is cognitive processing therapy (CPT). The patient writes a detailed account of the trauma and relates this to the therapist who guides him to reframe unrealistic beliefs about safety, trust, control, esteem, and intimacy (137).

It is possible to develop PTSD in the absence of explicit memories of the event that caused the injury, as is generally the case in TBI. Memories may be reconstructed based on fleeting but painful memories of events after the accident, or of photographs, or police or media reports. Therapy needs to be adapted accordingly. Imaginal exposure should focus on these aspects of the trauma memory that are recalled and represent the source of fear, rather than reconstructing the entire event. In vivo exposure should focus on the triggers of anxiety (e.g., hearing a siren or seeing an accident on television) in the absence of actual memories. Cognitive restructuring may be used to assist the person with TBI to accept that they will never regain recall of the injury circumstances. It should focus on helping them to reconstruct the experience more adaptively, for example, to reduce catastrophizing or a sense of guilt relating to the accident. It may also be used to alter maladaptive thinking about the source and severity of symptoms, emphasizing that injury-related problems with concentration and irritability are likely to be exacerbated by post-traumatic stress (138).

Evidence in support of the efficacy of CBT in individuals with mild TBI and PTSD comes from a study by Bryant et al. (139), who ran a 5-week group CBT program to treat acute stress disorder in 24 participants with mild TBI. On treatment completion, fewer participants in the CBT group (17%) still met the diagnostic criteria for PTSD compared to participants who received nondirective supportive counseling (58%), and treatment gains were maintained at 6-month follow-up. However, treatment of PTSD in TBI remains an under researched area, especially for people with more severe injuries. Williams, Evans, and Wilson (140) reported 2 single cases with severe TBI who received CBT to treat PTSD symptoms in the context of a general rehabilitation program. In addition to group therapy, individual CBT sessions were held twice weekly over 14 weeks, incorporating exposure, relaxation training, reality testing, and cognitive compensatory strategies (e.g., a handheld computer to monitor mood and thoughts). Both participants reported improvement of PTSD symptoms following the intensive treatment program.

There is increasing interest in the development of methods of treating PTSD in the military, at least some of whom may also have had exposure to head trauma and may have experienced 1 or more TBIs. The overlap of PTSD symptoms with postconcussive symptoms has led to some controversy as to the most effective ways of managing these symptoms. Recent and current trials are focusing on the use of VRET to reduce symptoms (132,133) and use of CPT for combat-related PTSD (STRONG STAR Multidisciplinary Research Consortium). The extent to which such therapies are effective in TBI cases has yet to be documented.

Cognitive Behavior Therapy for Other Anxiety Disorders

OCD is less commonly documented following brain injury (33,44). However, Williams, Evans, and Fleminger (141) have described the successful treatment of a client with OCD who was 2 years post-severe TBI using CBT. Components of the treatment offered to this client included exposure, response, prevention, and management of intrusive thoughts, as well as cognitive remediation strategies to help overcome the client's cognitive impairments. Arco (142) treated a young man with severe TBI who presented with repetitive checking and voiding behavior. CBT strategies used included self-monitoring (of counting behavior), cue cards with coping instructions, response prevention, stimulus control, and social reinforcement for generalization and maintenance of behavior. The CBT program was supplemented with an errorless learning approach to facilitate the client's relearning of desired behavior.

For treatment of panic disorder, use of CBT and environmental manipulation of stimuli that induce panic are recommended (143). There is no evidence of differential effectiveness of cognitive vs exposure therapy (131). Self-help interventions may also be effective (144). However, there is a lack of research evidence to guide practice among clients with TBI. There have been case reports of psychological treatment of panic disorder supplemented by medication (109). The evidence regarding treatment of specific phobia is also limited to case reports. Kneebone and Al-Daftary (145) described the treatment of a female with severe TBI and with Down syndrome who developed a phobia of having her feet touched during physiotherapy. One session of flooding treatment reportedly reduced her display of distress significantly, such that she could be reengaged in physiotherapy. In the case of social phobia, cognitive therapy has demonstrated efficacy over exposure-based therapies in the general population (131). Self-help therapies are also superior to no therapy, although not as effective as those delivered by a therapist (144). The aforementioned study by Hodgson et al. (110) is the only study to date focused on social phobia

following acquired brain injury (ABI), however. There is a significant need for more trials evaluating the application of CBT methods for the broad range of anxiety disorders in individuals with moderate-to-severe TBI.

Cognitive Behavior Therapy for Anger Management

CBT can also be useful in managing anger following brain injury using methods outlined by Novaco (146). It is important to thoroughly document the ways in which the anger manifests preinjury behavior patterns, the nature of the brain injury, mood changes, and other stressors to identify potential contributing factors. Education regarding the effects of TBI and on control of mood and behavior should be provided to the person with TBI and close others. In applying CBT, a cognitive model is presented, showing how an angry response may be triggered and the ways in which thoughts during the decision phase can influence the anger response. This is followed by exploration and monitoring of the cognitive, physical, and emotional changes that occur at the beginning, during, and after the angry outburst.

The person with TBI is encouraged, ideally with the support of a family member, to monitor and record angry outbursts, their precipitating circumstances and the accompanying thoughts, feelings, and bodily sensations over a designated period. This record can be used as the basis for identifying factors that provoke anger, which may be addressed in therapy. This may involve, for example, minimizing fatigue, avoiding noisy or crowded situations, or the consumption of alcohol. Identifying the signals of impending anger may provide cues for using strategies to counter it, such as deep breathing or other relaxation strategies or removing themselves from the situation. Significant others may assist by removing triggers or prompting the use of coping strategies. The person with brain injury may also be supported in developing self-talk, cognitive challenging strategies, or assertiveness skills for use in anger-provoking situations. Coping skills may be practised using role-play techniques.

McKinlay and Hickox (147) have summarized the steps involved in this anger management process with the acronym ANGER, which stands for: anticipating the trigger situations (A); noticing the signs of rising anger (N); going through "temper routine" (G), which includes relaxation or breathing exercises and finding an alternative way of handling the situation; extracting oneself from the situation (E), if all else fails; and recording how one coped (R), as well as the lessons learned that will be used the next time one becomes angry.

A number of studies conducted on singles cases and in groups have shown successful application of CBT methods to reduce anger problems in people with TBI (114,147–150). CBT for anger management may be delivered in a group setting. Walker and colleagues (148) conducted an uncontrolled trial, reporting the success of 12 weekly sessions based on a modified CBT model, as shown by a decrease in anger frequency and increase in attempts at anger control. Changes were maintained at follow-up assessment.

MOTIVATIONAL INTERVIEWING

CBT requires active involvement of the client to have maximum benefit. Low motivation and engagement can prevent this involvement. Motivational interviewing (MI) has been used increasingly in recent years to enhance engagement in therapy and motivation to change. MI is a client-centered, goal-directed therapy, which uses specific strategies to explore and resolve ambivalence to change (151). It explores the pros and cons of change but leaves it up to the client to make the decision to engage in therapy. MI aligns well with the self-determination theory, which recognizes the importance of intrinsic motivation (152–154). It also complements the transtheoretical model of behavioral change (155).

Core principles of MI include collaboration (respecting clients' worldviews and perspectives and viewing them as the expert of their own lives), evocation (eliciting intrinsic motivation to change by building on clients' goals and values), and autonomy (empowering clients to make informed decisions). In CBT, clients are taught how to behave and think differently, whereas MI focuses on why and how they might want to change (156). The methods chosen by the therapist will differ depending on the therapeutic interactions, and the core strategies are open-ended questions, affirmation, reflective listening, and summarizing. To explore and resolve ambivalence about change, the therapist selectively reinforces and highlights the discrepancy between the client's current functioning and goals/aspirations, thus facilitating his or her own arguments for change. The therapist also facilitates the client's commitment to change, supports his or her self-efficacy, and emphasizes the client's own responsibility to carry out an agreed action plan (151,157,158).

The efficacy of MI has been demonstrated as a stand-alone treatment and as a motivational enhancement therapy prior to formal treatment (159,160). Although it was first developed for addiction treatment (151), it has been used in a range of behavior change contexts. MI can be applied to resolve ambivalence about the need to continue with treatment or fully engage in a challenging therapeutic task (e.g., exposure) (161). MI has been used to enhance engagement in CBT for anxiety disorders (161–164). Westra and Dozois (162,163,165) found that use of MI pretreatment resulted in a higher CBT completion rate, an increase in self-efficacy, more active involvement in CBT and homework compliance, and a reduction in anxiety symptoms.

It may be argued that neurologically based motivational deficits cannot be addressed through the use of MI. Considering that the delivery and interaction of MI involves a large language component (166), cognitive limitations may limit the capacity of individuals with severe TBI to benefit from MI, especially if the client has significant difficulty with verbal expression or is unable to respond to reflections (167). However, empathy and respecting a client's personal choice and autonomy can be demonstrated in nonverbal language, so reduced verbal skills do not necessarily preclude the use of MI. In addition, the bulk of MI studies involve clinical populations who are likely to have cognitive deficits (e.g., long-term substance abuse, severe psychiatric disorders, and health problems) (160). This provides implicit support for the applicability of MI to engage individuals with TBI (168–170). The use of summaries and worksheets is encouraged because these tools help the person with brain injury make concepts concrete and provide him or her with written reminders. The decisional balance exercise (a strategy to explore clients' perceived advantages and disadvantages of the status quo and the possibility of change) can be simplified with the use of stickers and visual scales to illustrate how the benefits and costs weigh up (171).

Several studies have used MI in TBI groups (172–177). In a study focused on substance use, Bombardier and Rimmele (172) demonstrated in a case series the potential benefit of MI in preventing alcohol use following TBI. In Cox and colleagues' (174) group treatment study, MI participants showed an increase in motivation and commitment to change, as well as a reduction in negative emotions and substance use, when compared with a nontreatment group. Therapists further noted that the use of MI strategies enhanced their understanding of clients' emotional and motivational needs. This facilitated their ability to individualize treatment delivery.

Motivational Interviewing for Anxiety

Hsieh and colleagues (178) developed a 3-session brief preparatory program based on the principles of MI as a way of engaging clients with TBI and preparing them for a CBT program for anxiety. The MI sessions focused on helping each client to develop more realistic goals while also supporting his or her self-efficacy about his or her ability to cope with anxiety. Specific strategies were used to accommodate the client's cognitive limitations, including the use of personally meaningful metaphors and role-plays, achieving positive outcomes in the single case described. The use of MI as a prelude to 9 sessions of CBT resulted in a significantly greater response to CBT in terms of reduction in anxiety, stress, and nonproductive coping when compared to outcome in participants who received 3 sessions of nondirective counseling (126). This program is now being applied to treat depression as well as anxiety using a similar protocol. An examination of the impact of cognitive function and other factors on treatment response revealed that greater injury severity and poorer memory were associated with poorer response to intervention (179).

Motivational Interviewing for Depression

Bell, Bombardier, and colleagues (175,176) developed a telephone intervention program consisting of MI, problem solving, and behavioral activation for individuals with mild-to-severe TBI. Emotional outcome assessed in the group as a whole on the Brief Symptom Inventory was not significantly better in the intervention group. However, when focusing only on individuals identified as depressed at baseline, those receiving the telephone intervention reported significantly fewer depressive symptoms than those receiving usual care at 1-year follow-up (176). Although it was not clear which were the effective elements of this intervention, the researchers noted that MI may have been helpful in addressing depression and TBI-related behavioral and executive deficits (e.g., apathy, reduced initiation). They also recommended future studies to incorporate standardized diagnostic interviews at baseline and follow-up assessments and explore active ingredients in treatment.

TREATMENT OF APATHY

Apathy is defined by Lane-Brown and Tate (180) as "a deficiency in overt behavioral, emotional, and cognitive components of goal-directed behavior." It is otherwise known as lack of drive or initiative. There have, according to Lane-Brown and Tate's (180) Cochrane review, been relatively few evaluative psychological intervention studies focused on treatment of apathy, with most studies conducted having been pharmacological interventions, as discussed in Chapter 74 using dopamine agonists (181), acetylcholinesterase inhibitors (182), or psychostimulants (183). Various psychological approaches have been taken to dealing with this problem, generally reported in case studies. These have included the successful use of checklists (184) and paging devices to provide external prompting (185). For individuals with TBI with sufficient self-awareness, there is some evidence to support the use of strategies to guide goal-directed behavior using overt and then covert guidance to follow steps of setting a goal, planning a solution, implementing it, and checking that it has been carried out as planned and making necessary adjustments (186–102).

In a single case study, Lane-Brown and Tate (177) evaluated treatment for apathy in a young man with severe TBI. The therapy comprised 28 weekly sessions. These sessions aimed to increase initiation and sustained activity toward 3 specific behavioral goals, which were set collaboratively. These related to tidying his room and improving his general fitness. Treatment incorporated MI and external compensatory strategies to assist in initiating and sustaining cumulative goal-directed activity. MI included developing awareness of the discrepancy between the client's desired state and current state (e.g., his desire to keep track of important financial documents vs haphazardly placing documents in his room). It also supported self-efficacy (e.g., by encouraging his self-belief in his capabilities by reviewing previously successful methods of filing financial documents and his current capability to file documents in this manner). MI also expressed empathy and explored reasons for resistance (e.g., diminished concern). Therapy sessions involved reviewing weekly progress toward goals, defining activities for the next week, and discussing how to overcome barriers. External compensation was a reminder alert set into his mobile device, providing daily reminders of planned activities toward goals. Daily recordings of the time spent on goals were made over 7.5 months. The researchers demonstrated a clinically and statistically significant reduction in apathy, measured by time spent working toward goals and goal attainment, and this was maintained at 1-month follow-up.

MINDFULNESS-BASED THERAPIES: ACCEPTANCE AND COMMITMENT THERAPY

Mindfulness-based psychotherapies have also been used in the treatment of anxiety and depressive disorders following TBI, including mindfulness-based cognitive therapy, dialectical behavioral therapy, and acceptance and commitment therapy (ACT) (193). ACT encourages the individual to accept their inner psychological and emotional experiences, identify the values that they wish to guide their life, and commit to act in a way that leads in the direction of fulfillment of those values. In the general population, it has been used with success to treat a variety of psychological disorders, including anxiety and depression (193–196). Although CBT therapies focus on altering psychological events (thoughts, beliefs, perceptions), mindfulness-based interventions aim to change the function of those events and

the individual's relationship with their psychological experiences, that to change functioning rather than reduce symptoms.

ACT has been suggested as a useful approach for enhancing emotional adjustment in individuals with brain injury. ACT encourages these individuals to engage in a life that has purpose and meaning for them, despite their disabilities or symptoms, and avoids the need to apply strategies to reduce symptoms, which may be difficult for those with cognitive impairments (194,197,198). Wong (198) reported successful treatment of depression in a man with TBI, reflected in improved mood ratings, reduced feelings of hopelessness and worthlessness, and increased achievement of goals. Bédard et al. (197) conducted a pilot study investigating the effectiveness of a 12-week mindfulness-based group support intervention for 10 individuals with mild-to-moderate TBI but no major mental health disorders. This emphasized developing present moment awareness, as well as acceptance by using insight meditation, breathing exercises, guided visualization, and group discussion encouraging patients to see injury-related disabilities from a new perspective. This reportedly resulted in improved quality of life and a reduction in cognitive-related mood symptoms relative to 3 people who dropped out of the group. There were no changes in overall daily function.

The importance of promoting acceptance of injury-related changes is a key feature of rehabilitation programs advocated by Prigatano (199), Ben-Yishay et al. (79), Gracey et al. (80), and Cantor et al. (83). However, no controlled studies have used ACT in treatment of psychological problems following brain injury. As in the application of CBT and MI, therapy delivery would need to accommodate cognitive limitations, including an increased focus on concrete behavioral strategies and goals, written aids, repetition, and so on. As suggested by Soo et al. (196), the choice of CBT or ACT may depend on the personal preferences of the client. Alternatively, it may be that elements of both therapies may be combined (200).

COMPASSION-FOCUSED THERAPY

Compassion-focused therapy (CFT) draws on attachment theory and the neurophysiology of affective regulation, positing that attachment and affiliative behaviors, such as kindness, care, support, encouragement, and validation serve to regulate threat-based emotions (201). The focus of therapy is on the development of these emotions to cope with or eliminate negative thoughts. A recent case study by Ashworth and colleagues (202) has applied CFT to enhance psychological adjustment in a girl with TBI. The girl had low self-esteem and symptoms of anxiety, depression, and anger following her injury, having grown up with an abusive father. She found that the application of CBT strategies was not effective in improving her mood and remained very self-critical. Through CFT she learned to apply self-soothing imagery to counter her overactive threat system. This involved identifying a "perfect nurturer," developing the image with associated soothing emotions and practising self-soothing by bringing this image to mind repeatedly. She achieved a significant reduction in anxiety and depression symptoms and increased self-esteem. These therapies represent examples of the application of positive psychology principles to

TABLE 64-1 Application of Therapeutic Approaches to Psychological Problems Following TBI

THERAPY APPROACH	MODE		RECIPIENT		PSYCHOLOGICAL PROBLEM			
	Individual	Group	TBI individual	Family	Anxiety	Depression	Anger	Apathy
Support and education	✕	✕	✕	✕	✕	✕	✕	
Psychodynamic psychotherapy	✕	✕	✕	✕	✕	✕		
CBT	✕	✕	✕	✕	✕	✕	✕	✕
MI	✕		✕		✕	✕		✕
ACT	✕		✕		✕	✕		
CFT	✕		✕		✕	✕		

Abbreviations: ACT, acceptance and commitment therapy; CBT, cognitive behavior therapy; CFT, compassion-focused therapy; MI, motivational interviewing; TBI, traumatic brain injury.

enhance mental health after brain injury, a trend that will hopefully continue but requires much more rigorous evaluation (203).

CONCLUSION

Psychological interventions potentially have a very significant role in the management of emotional and behavioral problems associated with TBI. They avoid the side effects of pharmacological treatments and potentially result in more enduring gains. Education and supportive therapy are most commonly offered to people with TBI and their families in the context of acute and postacute treatment, although formal evaluation of their effectiveness has been limited. Psychological therapy is offered to a smaller proportion of individuals, sometimes because of very severe cognitive impairments but often because of the lack of funding or access to a psychologist. Psychological interventions form an important part of holistic rehabilitation, aiming to support the person with TBI to search for meaning in their new life. They are also important for the significant proportion of individuals who develop anxiety, depression, and behavioral problems following TBI.

Cognitive impairments place some limitations on the capacity to benefit from psychological therapies. Therapy generally needs to be adapted to overcome these limitations. There is some evidence supporting the efficacy of cognitive-behavioral interventions for anger management and for the treatment of anxiety and depression, particularly in people with mild-to-moderate injuries. However, there is a need for more comprehensive studies assessing the efficacy of CBT in people with severe TBI. In particular, the impact of specific adaptations (e.g., session frequency, use of visual aids, involving a family member) or modes of therapy delivery (e.g., group, individual, Internet based, virtual reality vs in vivo) needs to be evaluated systematically. Engagement of the person with TBI is important to increase their readiness for formal treatment. MI is one of the many ways to do this. Other techniques such as ACT and CFT offer potentially useful alternatives depending on the person's preferences and psychological history. However, the evidence supporting these approaches is limited to single case studies and uncontrolled case series. Group therapy offers the opportunity to share experiences, but most likely needs to be backed up with individual therapy to achieve more sustainable gains. Families

have a significant influence on the psychological adjustment of the person with TBI. They, therefore, need to receive education and be involved in the therapeutic process, both that focused on the person injured and their own psychological responses. Potential applications of various psychological therapies following TBI are summarized in Table 64-1.

There are many challenges in performing evaluative research in this field. Patients are extremely heterogeneous in terms of their brain injuries, other system injuries, preinjury, psychiatric and social histories, developmental life stages, and life goals. This makes it difficult to match groups and determine inclusion criteria. The presence of cognitive impairments may limit motivation for and ability to benefit from therapy. Interventions are generally being delivered alongside a range of other therapies and supports, which may also impact the injured person's psychological state and make it difficult to evaluate the "pure" effects of any intervention. All these factors limit the conduct of RCTs, which remain the gold standard of evidence. It will only be with development of more extensive international collaborative efforts that the evidence base can be significantly advanced. Much further research is required to establish the most effective ways of achieving this. Efforts also need to be made to translate the research evidence into clinical practice. Open discussions will be required to facilitate collaboration between clinicians and researchers and to achieve a balance between the reality of clinical settings and the quality of research.

The greatest challenge, however, lies in making changes to our health care systems and to public awareness to allow for greater access to psychological therapy following TBI. Ultimately, individuals with TBI are likely to progress better when various forms of rehabilitation (e.g., psychology, social work, physiotherapy, occupational therapy, speech pathology) are integrated and when they are provided with timely support.

 KEY CLINICAL POINTS

1. A comprehensive assessment must precede and will determine the choice of psychological intervention.
2. Therapy should only be offered when the person with TBI is willing and able to cope with it, from both a cognitive and emotional point of view.

3. The approach to intervention should be selected on the basis of the level of cognitive function, behavioral control, and self-awareness of the person with TBI, as well as their personal preferences.

4. It is important to set goals collaboratively, to proceed slowly, and assist the person with TBI to develop realistic expectations. Collaboration with other team members is also crucial in order to facilitate generalization of new coping skills.

5. Flexibility, ingenuity, empathy, and persistence on the part of health professionals are generally required to achieve change.

6. Use concrete and personally relevant examples, a notebook, handouts, and visual and written cues and build in repetition, reminders, and booster sessions.

7. It is essential to assess the effectiveness of interventions using ecologically valid measures taken before, during, and following treatment.

8. Group therapy offers the opportunity to share problems and coping strategies and realize others have similar experiences, but should be backed up with individual therapy wherever possible.

9. Family members also deserve to be engaged in these processes, not only to assist the person with TBI but also to assist family to cope with and adjust to the consequences of the injury.

KEY REFERENCES

1. Anson K, Ponsford J. Evaluation of a coping skills group following traumatic brain injury. *Brain Inj*. 2006;20(2):167–178.
2. Bryant RA, Moulds M, Guthrie R, Nixon RD. Treating acute stress disorder following mild traumatic brain injury. *Am J Psychiatry*. 2003;160(3):585–587.
3. Hodgson J, McDonald S, Tate R, Gertler P. A randomised controlled trial of a cognitive behavioral therapy program for managing social anxiety after acquired brain injury. *Brain Impair*. 2005;6:169–180.
4. Hsieh M, Ponsford J, Wong D, Schönberger M, Taffe J, McKay A. Motivational interviewing and cognitive behavior therapy for anxiety following traumatic brain injury: A pilot randomized controlled trial. *Neuropsychol Rehabil*. In press.
5. Klonoff PS. *Psychotherapy After Brain Injury: Principles and Techniques*. New York, NY: Guilford Press; 2010.

References

1. Dikmen SS, Corrigan JD, Levin HS, Machamer J, Stiers W, Weisskopf MG. Cognitive outcome following traumatic brain injury. *J Head Trauma Rehabil*. 2009;24(6):430–438.
2. Hart T, Seignourel PJ, Sherer M. A longitudinal study of awareness of deficit after moderate to severe traumatic brain injury. *Neuropsychol Rehabil*. 2009;19(2):161–176.
3. Sherer M, Hart T, Nick TG, Whyte J, Thompson RN, Yablon SA. Early impaired self-awareness after traumatic brain injury. *Arch Phys Med Rehabil*. 2003;84(2):168–176.
4. Draper K, Ponsford J, Schönberger M. Psychosocial and emotional outcome following traumatic brain injury. *J Head Trauma Rehabil*. 2007;22(5):278–287.
5. Machamer J, Temkin N, Fraser R, Doctor JN, Dikmen S. Stability of employment after traumatic brain injury. *J Int Neuropsychol Soc*. 2005;11(7):807–816.
6. Ponsford J, Draper K, Schönberger M. Functional outcome 10 years after traumatic brain injury: its relationship with demographic, injury severity, and cognitive and emotional status. *J Int Neuropsychol Soc*. 2008;14(2):233–142.
7. Dikmen SS, Machamer JE, Powell JM, Temkin NR. Outcome three to five years after moderate to severe traumatic brain injury. *Arch Phys Med Rehabil*. 2003;84(10):1449–1457.
8. Tate RL, Broe GA, Cameron ID, Hodgkinson AE, Soo CA. Pre-injury, injury and early post-injury predictors of long-term functional and psychosocial recovery after severe traumatic brain injury. *Brain Impair*. 2005;6(2):75–89.
9. Ponsford JL, Olver JH, Curran C. A profile of outcome: 2 years after traumatic brain injury. *Brain Inj*. 1995;9(1):1–10.
10. Tyerman A, Humphrey M. Changes in self concept following severe head injury. *Int J Rehabil Res*. 1984;7(1):11–23.
11. Goodinson R, Ponsford J, Johnston L, Grant F. Psychiatric disorders following traumatic brain injury: their nature and frequency. *J Head Trauma Rehabil*. 2009;24(5):324–332.
12. Gouick J, Gentleman D. The emotional and behavioral consequences of traumatic brain injury. *Trauma*. 2004;6(4):285–292.
13. Cooper-Evans S, Alderman N, Knight C, Oddy M. Self-esteem as a predictor of psychological distress after severe acquired brain injury: an exploratory study. *Neuropsychol Rehabil*. 2008;18(5–6):607–626.
14. Kraus JF, McArthur DL. Incidence and prevalence of and costs associated with traumatic brain injury. In: Rosenthal M, Griffith ER, Kreutzer JS, Pentland B, eds. *Rehabilitation of the Adult and Child With Traumatic Brain Injury*. Philadelphia, PA: FA Davis; 1999:3–17.
15. O'Rance L. *Disability in Australia: Acquired Brain Injury*. Canberra, Australia: Australian Institute of Health and Welfare; 2007.
16. Fryer J. Adolescent community integration. In: Bach-y-Rita P, ed. *Traumatic Brain Injury*. New York, NY: Demos Publications; 1989:255–286.
17. Wood RL, Yurdakul LK. Change in relationship status following traumatic brain injury. *Brain Inj*. 1997;11(7):491–502.
18. Winstanley J, Simpson G, Tate R, Myles B. Early indicators and contributors to psychological distress in relatives during rehabilitation following severe TBI: findings from brain injury outcomes study. *J Head Trauma Rehabil*. 2006;21(6):453–456.
19. Bracy CA, Douglas JM. Comparison of a group of long-term TBI marital dyads with a control group of orthopaedic marital dyads, on measures of marital satisfaction, marital coping, and perception of husbands' communication skills. *Brain Impair*. 2002;3(1):71.
20. Willer BS, Allen KM, Liss M, Zicht MS. Problems and coping strategies of individuals with traumatic brain injury and their spouses. *Arch Phys Med Rehabil*. 1991;72(7):460–464.
21. Burridge AC, Williams WH, Yates PJ, Harris A, Ward CD. Spousal relationship satisfaction following acquired brain injury: the role of insight and socio-emotional skill. *Neuropsychol Rehabil*. 2007;17(1):95–105.
22. Robinson RG, Jorge RE. Longitudinal course of mood disorders following traumatic brain injury. *Arch Gen Psychiatry*. 2002;59(1):23–24.
23. Kraus JF, Sorenson SB. Epidemiology. In: Silver JM, Yudofsky SC, Hales RE, eds. *Neuropsychiatry of Traumatic Brain Injury*. Washington, DC: American Psychiatric Press; 1994:3–41.
24. Bombardier CH, Fann JR, Temkin NR, Esselman PC, Barber J, Dikmen SS. Rates of major depressive disorder and clinical outcomes following traumatic brain injury. *JAMA*. 2010;303(19):1938–1945.
25. Gould KR, Ponsford JL, Johnston J, Schönberger M. Predictive and associated factors of psychiatric disorders after traumatic brain injury: a prospective study. *J Neurotrauma*. 2011;28(7):1149–1154.
26. Whelan-Goodinson R, Ponsford J, Schönberger M. Validity of the hospital anxiety and depression scale to assess depression and anxiety following traumatic brain injury as compared with the structured clinical interview for DSM-IV. *J Affect Disord*. 2009;114(1):94–102.
27. Bryant RA. Disentangling mild traumatic brain injury and stress reactions. *N Engl J Med*. 2008;358(5):525–527.
28. Bryant RA, Creamer M, O'Donnell M, Silove D, Clark CR, McFarlane AC. Post-traumatic amnesia and the nature of post-traumatic stress disorder after mild traumatic brain injury. *J Int Neuropsychol Soc*. 2009;15(6):862–867.

29. Jorge RE, Robinson RG, Moser D, Tateno A, Crespo-Facorro B, Arndt SV. Major depression following traumatic brain injury. *Arch Gen Psychiatry*. 2004;61(1):42–50.

30. Schönberger M, Ponsford J, Reutens D, Beare R, Clarke D, O'Sullivan R. The relationship between mood disorders and MRI findings following traumatic brain injury. *Brain Inj*. 2011;25(6):543–550.

31. Salmond CH, Menon DK, Chatfield DA, Pickard JD, Sahakian BJ. Cognitive reserve as a resilience factor against depression after moderate/severe traumatic brain injury. *J Neurotrauma*. 2006;23(7): 1049–1058.

32. Koponen S, Taiminen T, Kurki T, et al. MRI findings and Axis I and II psychiatric disorders after traumatic brain injury: a 30-year retrospective follow-up study. *Psychiatry Res*. 2006;146(3):263–270.

33. Gould KR, Ponsford JL, Johnston L, Schönberger M. The nature, frequency and course of psychiatric disorders in the first year after traumatic brain injury: a prospective study. *Psychol Med*. 2011; 41(10):2099–2109.

34. Fedoroff JP, Starkstein SE, Forrester AW, et al. Depression in patients with acute traumatic brain injury. *Am J Psychiatry*. 1992; 149(7):918–923.

35. Pagulayan KF, Hoffman JM, Temkin NR, Machamer JE, Dikmen SS. Functional limitations and depression after traumatic brain injury: examination of the temporal relationship. *Arch Phys Med Rehabil*. 2008;89(10):1887–1892.

36. Jorge RE, Robinson RG, Arndt SV, Forrester AW, Geisler F, Starkstein SE. Comparison between acute- and delayed-onset depression following traumatic brain injury. *J Neuropsychiatry Clin Neurosci*. 1993;5(1):43–49.

37. Schönberger M, Ponsford J, Gould KR, Johnston L. The temporal relationship between depression, anxiety, and functional status after traumatic brain injury: a cross-lagged analysis. *J Int Neuropsychol Soc*. 2011;17(5):1–7.

38. Curran CA, Ponsford JL, Crowe S. Coping strategies and emotional outcome following traumatic brain injury: a comparison with orthopaedic patients. *J Head Trauma Rehabil*. 2000;15(6):1256–1274.

39. Anson K, Ponsford J. Coping style and emotional adjustment following traumatic brain injury. *J Head Trauma Rehabil*. 2006;21(3): 248–259.

40. Wolters G, Stapert S, Brands I, van Heugten C. Coping following acquired brain injury: predictors and correlates. *J Head Trauma Rehabil*. 2011;26(2)150–157.

41. Kortte KB, Wegener ST, Chwalisz K. Anosognosia and denial: their relationship to coping and depression in acquired brain injury. *Rehabil Psychol*. 2003;48(3):131–136.

42. Anson K, Ponsford J. Coping and emotional adjustment following traumatic brain injury. *J Head Trauma Rehabil*. 2006;21(3):248–259.

43. Spitz G, Schönberger M, Ponsford J. The relationship between cognitive impairment, coping style, and emotional adjustment following traumatic brain injury [published online ahead of print April 10, 2012]. *J Head Trauma Rehabil*.

44. Whelan-Goodinson R, Ponsford J, Johnston L, Grant F. Psychiatric disorders following traumatic brain injury: their nature and frequency. *J Head Trauma Rehabil*. 2009;24(5):324–332.

45. Deb S, Lyons I, Koutzoukis C, Ali I, McCarthy G. Rate of psychiatric illness 1 year after traumatic brain injury. *Am J Psychiatry*. 1999; 156(3):374–378.

46. Koponen S, Taiminen T, Portin R, et al. Axis I and II psychiatric disorders after traumatic brain injury: a 30-year follow-up study. *Am J Psychiatry*. 2002;159(8):1315–1321.

47. Hibbard MR, Uysal S, Kepler K, Bogdany J, Silver J. Axis I psychopathology in individuals with traumatic brain injury. *J Head Trauma Rehabil*. 1998;13(4):24–39.

48. Ashman TA, Spielman LA, Hibbard MR, Silver JM, Chandna T, Gordon WA. Psychiatric challenges in the first 6 years after traumatic brain injury: cross-sequential analyses of axis I disorders. *Arch Phys Med Rehabil*. 2004;85(4)(suppl 2):S36–S42.

49. Hoofien D, Gilboa A, Vakil E, Donovick PJ. Traumatic brain injury (TBI) 10–20 years later: a comprehensive outcome study of psychiatric symptomatology, cognitive abilities, and psychosocial functioning. *Brain Inj*. 2001;15(3):189–209.

50. Ponsford J, Whelan-Goodinson R, Bahar-Fuchs A. Alcohol and drug use following traumatic brain injury: a prospective study. *Brain Inj*. 2007;21(13–14):1385–1392.

51. Lezak MD, Howieson DB, Loring DW, Hannay HJ, Fischer JS. *Neuropsychological Assessment*. 4th ed. New York, NY: Oxford University Press; 2004.

52. Prigatano GP. *Principles of Neuropsychological Rehabilitation*. Oxford, United Kingdom: Oxford University Press; 1999.

53. Fournier JC, DeRubeis RJ, Hollon SD, et al. Antidepressant drug effects and depression severity: a patient-level meta-analysis. *J Am Med Assoc*. 2010;303(1):47–53.

54. Warden DL, Gordon B, McAllister TW, et al. Guidelines for the pharmacologic treatment of neurobehavioral sequelae of traumatic brain injury. *J Neurotrauma*. 2006;23(10):1468–1501.

55. Hiott D, Labbate LA. Anxiety disorders associated with traumatic brain injuries. *NeuroRehabilitation*. 2002;17(4):345–355.

56. Dobson KS, Hollon SD, Dimidjian S, et al. Randomized trial of behavioral activation, cognitive therapy, and antidepressant medication in the prevention of relapse and recurrence in major depression. *J Consult Clin Psychol*. 2008;76(3):468–477.

57. Fann JR, Hart T, Schome KG. Treatment for depression after traumatic brain injury: a systematic review. *J Neurotrauma*. 2009;26(12): 2383–2402.

58. Judd D, Wilson SL. Psychotherapy with brain injury survivors: an investigation of the challenges encountered by clinicians and their modifications to therapeutic practice. *Brain Inj*. 2005;19(6):437–449.

59. Klonoff PS. Individual and group psychotherapy in milieu-oriented neurorehabilitation. *Appl Neuropsychol*. 1997;4(2):107–118.

60. Klonoff PS. *Psychotherapy After Brain Injury: Principles and Techniques*. New York, NY: Guilford Press; 2010.

61. Persons JB. Empiricism, mechanism, and the practice of cognitive-behavior therapy. *Behav Ther*. 2005;36(2):107–118.

62. Persons JB. *The Case Formulation Approach to Cognitive-behavior Therapy (Guides to Individualized Evidence-based Treatment)*. New York, NY: Guilford Press; 2008.

63. Saltapidas H, Ponsford J. The influence of cultural background on motivation for and participation in rehabilitation and outcome following traumatic brain injury. *J Head Trauma Rehabil*. 2007;22(2): 132–139.

64. Saltapidas H, Ponsford J. The influence of cultural background on experiences and beliefs following traumatic brain injury and their association with outcome. *Brain Impair*. 2008;9(1):1–13.

65. Curtiss G, Klemz S, Vanderploeg RD. Acute impact of severe traumatic brain injury on family structure and coping responses. *J Head Trauma Rehabil*. 2000;15(5):1113–1122.

66. Kozloff R. Networks of social support and outcome from severe head injury. *J Head Trauma Rehabil*. 1987;2(3):14–23.

67. Perlesz A, Kinsella G, Crowe S. Impact of traumatic brain injury on the family: a critical review. *Rehabil Psychol*. 1999;44(1):6–35.

68. Yeates KO, Taylor HG, Drotar D, et al. Preinjury family environment as a determinant of recovery from traumatic brain injuries in school-aged children. *J Int Neuropsychol Soc*. 1997;3(6):617–630.

69. Sander AM, Sherer M, Malec JF, et al. Preinjury emotional and family functioning in caregivers of persons with traumatic brain injury. *Arch Phys Med Rehabil*. 2003;84(2):197–203.

70. Ponsford JL, Olver JH, Ponsford M, Nelms R. Long-term adjustment of families following traumatic brain injury where comprehensive rehabilitation has been provided. *Brain Inj*. 2003;17(6): 453–468.

71. Ponsford J, Schönberger M. Long-term family functioning following traumatic brain injury. *J Int Neuropsychol Soc*. 2010;16:1–12.

72. Ponsford J, Willmott C, Rothwell A, Cameron P, Kelly AM, Nelms R. Impact of early intervention on outcome following mild head injury in adults. *J Neurol Neurosurg Psychiatry*. 2002;73(3):330–332.

73. Field K. *My Dad's had a Head Injury*. Nottingham, United Kingdom: Headway United Kingdom; nd.

74. Troynar M, ed. *Goodbye Hello* [short film]. Melbourne, Australia: Victoria College of the Arts, University of Melbourne; 2010.

75. Bower P, Byford S, Sibbald B, et al. Randomised controlled trial of non-directive counselling, cognitive-behaviour therapy, and usual general practitioner care for patients with depression. II: cost effectiveness. *BMJ*. 2000;321(7273):1389–1392.

76. Friedli K, King M, Lloyd M, Horder J. Randomised controlled assessment of non-directive psychotherapy versus routine general-practitioner care. *Lancet*. 1997;350 (9092):1662–1665.

77. Dirette D, Plaisier BR. The development of self-awareness of deficits from 1 week to 1 year after traumatic brain injury: preliminary findings. *Brain Inj*. 2007;21(11):1131–1136.

78. Ben-Yishay Y. Post-acute neuropsychological rehabilitation. In: Christensen A, Uzzell B, eds. *International Handbook of Neuropsychological Rehabilitation*. New York, NY: Kluwer Academic/Plenum Publishers; 2000:131–139.

79. Ben-Yishay Y. Foreward. *Neuropsychol Rehabil*. 2008;18(5–6):513–521.

80. Gracey F, Palmer S, Rous B, et al. "Feeling part of things": personal construction of self after brain injury. *Neuropsychol Rehabil*. 2008;18(5–6):627–650.

81. Yeates P, Henwood K, Gracey F, Evans J. Awareness of disability after acquired brain injury (ABI) and the family context. *Neuropsychol Rehabil*. 2007;17(2):151–173.

82. Dewar BK, Gracey F. "Am not was": cognitive-behavioural therapy for adjustment and identity change following herpes simplex encephalitis. *Neuropsychol Rehabil*. 2007;17(4–5):602–620.

83. Cantor JB, Ashman T, Schwartz ME, et al. The role of self-discrepancy theory in understanding post-traumtic brain injury affective disorders. *J Head Trauma Rehabil*. 2005;20(6):527–543.

84. Ylvisaker M, Feeney TJ. Construction of identity after traumatic brain injury. *Brain Impair*. 2000;1:12–28.

85. Ownsworth T, Fleming J. Growth through loss after brain injury. *Brain Impair*. 2011;12(2):79–81.

86. Silva J, Ownsworth T, Shields C, Fleming J. Enhanced appreciation of life following acquired brain injury: posttraumatic growth at 6 months postdischarge. *Brain Impair*. 2011;12(2):83–104.

87. Daniels-Zide E, Ben-Yishay Y. Therapeutic milieu day program. In: Christensen A, Uzzell B, eds. *International Handbook of Neuropsychological Rehabilitation*. New York, NY: Kluwer Academic/Plenum Publishers; 2000:183–193.

88. Ben-Yishay Y, Piasetsky EB, Rattock J, Cohen H, Diller L. *Developing a Core "Curriculum" for Group-exercises Designed for Head Trauma Patients Who Are Undergoing Rehabilitation. Working Approaches to Remediation of Cognitive Deficits in Brain Damaged Persons (Rehabilitation Monograph No 61)*. New York, NY: New York University Medical Centre, Institute of Rehabilitation Medicine; 1980:175–234.

89. Ownsworth TL, McFarland K, Young RM. Self awareness and psychosocial functioning following acquired brain injury: an evaluation of a group support program. *Neuropsychol Rehabil*. 2000;10(5):465–484.

90. Kreutzer JS, Kolakowsky-Hayner SA, Demm SR, Meade MA. A structured approach to family intervention after brain injury. *J Head Trauma Rehabil*. 2002;17(4):347–369.

91. Albert SM, Im A, Brenner L, Smith M, Waxman R. Effect of social work liaison program on family caregivers to people with brain injury. *J Head Trauma Rehabil*. 2002;17(2):175–189.

92. Carnevale GJ, Anselmi V, Buischio K, Millis S. Changes in ratings of caregiver burden following a community-based behavior management program from persons with traumatic brain injury. *J Head Trauma Rehabil*. 2002;17(2):83–95.

93. Rivara PA, Elliott TR, Berry JW, Grant JS. Problem-solving training for family caregivers of persons with traumatic brain injuries: a randomized controlled trial. *Arch Phys Med Rehabil*. 2008;89(5):931–941.

94. Rotondi AJ, Sinkule J, Spring M. An interactive web-based intervention for persons with TBI and their families: use and evaluation by female significant others. *J Head Trauma Rehabil*. 2005;20(2):173–185.

95. Kreutzer JS, Stejskal TM, Ketchum JM, Marwitz JH, Taylor LA, Menzel JC. A preliminary investigation of the brain injury family intervention: impact on family members. *Brain Inj*. 2009;23(6):535–547.

96. Gan C, Gargaro J, Fkreutzer JS, Boschen KA, Wright FV. Development and preliminary evaluation of a structured family system intervention for adolescents with brain injury and their families. *Brain Inj*. 2010;24(4):651–663.

97. Singer GHS, Glang A, Nixon C, et al. A comparison of two psychosocial interventions for parents of children with acquired brain injury: an exploratory study. *J Head Trauma Rehabil*. 1994;9(4):38–49.

98. Sander AM, ed. Intervening With Caregivers to Improve the Outcome of Persons With Traumatic Brain Injury. In: 15th Annual Mayo Clinic Brain Injury Conference; 2008; Rochester, MN.

99. Rodgers ML, Strode AD, Norell DM, Short RA, Dyck DG, Becker B. Adapting multiple family group treatment for brain and spinal cord injury: intervention development and preliminary outcomes. *Am J Phys Med Rehabil*. 2007;86(6):482–492.

100. Couchman G, Ponsford J, Kelly A, McMahon G. Impact of of a multi-family group intervention on family functioning and community integration following traumatic brain injury. *J Head Trauma Rehabil*. In press.

101. Covin R, Ouimet AJ, Seeds PM, Dozois DJA. A meta-analysis of CBT for pathological worry among clients with GAD. *J Anxiety Disord*. 2008;22(1):108–116.

102. Butler AC, Chapman JE, Forman EM, Beck AT. The empirical status of cognitive-behavioral therapy: a review of meta-analyses. *Clin Psychol Rev*. 2006;26(1):17–31.

103. National Institute for Health and Clinical Excellence. *Clinical Guideline 22 Anxiety: Management of Anxiety (Panic Disorder, With or Without Agoraphobia, and Generalised Anxiety Disorder) in Adults in Primary, Secondary and Community Care*. London, United Kingdom: National Institute for Health and Clinical Excellence; 1991. Available at: http://www.nice.org.uk/nicemedia/pdf/CG022quickref-guideamended.pdf. Accessed December 14, 2007.

104. Parikh SV, Segal ZV, Grigoriadis S, et al. Canadian Network for Mood and Anxiety Treatments (CANMAT) clinical guidelines for the management of major depressive disorder in adults. II. Psychotherapy alone or in combination with antidepressant medication. *J Affect Disord*. 2009;117(suppl 1):S15–S25.

105. Stewart RE, Chambless DL. Cognitive-behavioral therapy for adult anxiety disorders in clinical practice: a meta-analysis of effectiveness studies. *J Consult Clin Psychol*. 2009;77(4):595–606.

106. Beck AT, Rush AJ, Shaw BF, Emery G. *Cognitive Therapy of Depression*. New York, NY: Guilford Press; 1979.

107. Kinney A. Cognitive therapy and brain-injury: theoretical and clinical issues. *J Contemp Psychother*. 2001;31(2):89–102.

108. Khan-Bourne N, Brown RG. Cognitive behaviour therapy for the treatment of depression in individuals with brain injury. *Neuropsychol Rehabil*. 2003;13(1–2):89–107.

109. Scheutzow MH, Wiercisiewski DR. Panic disorder in a patient with traumatic brain injury: a case report and discussion. *Brain Inj*. 1999;13(9):705–714.

110. Hodgson J, McDonald S, Tate R, Gertler P. A randomised controlled trial of a cognitive behavioural therapy program for managing social anxiety after acquired brain injury. *Brain Impair*. 2005;6:169–180.

111. Tiersky LA, Anselmi V, Johnston MV, et al. A trial of neuropsychologic rehabilitation in mild-spectrum traumatic brain injury. *Arch Phys Med Rehabil*. 2005;86(8):1565–1574.

112. Hsieh M, Ponsford J, Wong D, Schönberger M, McKay A, Haines K. Development and preliminary evaluation of a cognitive behaviour therapy (CBT) programme for anxiety following moderate–severe traumatic brain injury (TBI): two case studies. *Brain Inj*. 2012;26(2):126–138.

113. Bradbury CL, Christensen BK, Lau MA, Ruttan LA, Arundine AL, Green RE. The efficacy of cognitive behavior therapy in the treatment of emotional distress after acquired brain injury. *Arch Phys Med Rehabil*. 2008;89(12)(suppl):S61–S68.

114. Medd J, Tate R. Evaluation of an anger management therapy programme following acquired brain injury: a preliminary study. *Neuropsychol Rehabil*. 2000;10(2):185–201.

115. Rath JF, Simon D, Langenbahn DM, Sherr RL, Diller L. Group treatment of problem-solving deficits in outpatients with traumatic brain injury: a randomised outcome study. *Neuropsychol Rehabil*. 2003;13(4):461–488.

116. Anson K, Ponsford J. Evaluation of a coping skills group following traumatic brain injury. *Brain Inj*. 2006;20(2):167–178.

117. Soo C, Tate R. Psychological treatment for anxiety in people with traumatic brain injury. *Cochrane Database Syst Rev*. 2007;(3):CD005239.

118. Anson K, Ponsford J. Who benefits? Outcome following a coping skills group intervention for traumatically brain injured individuals. *Brain Inj*. 2006;20(1):1–13.

119. Backhaus SL, Ibarra SL, Klyce D, Trexler LE, Malec JF. Brain injury coping skills group: a preventative intervention for patients with brain injury and their caregivers. *Arch Phys Med Rehabil* 2010;91(6):840–848.

120. Bryant RA, Moulds M, Guthrie R, Nixon RDV. Treating acute stress disorder following mild traumatic brain injury. *Am J Psychiatry.* 2003;160:585–587.

121. Montgomery GK. A multi-factor account of disability after brain injury: implications for neuropsychological counselling. *Brain Inj.* 1995;9(5):453–469.

122. Topolovec-Vranic J, Cullen N, Michalak A, et al. Evaluation of an online cognitive behavioural therapy program by patients with traumatic brain injury and depression. *Brain Inj.* 2010;24(5):762–772.

123. Bradbury CL, Christensen BK, Lau MA, Ruttan LA, Arundine AL, Green RE. The efficacy of cognitive behavior therapy in the treatment of emotional distress after acquired brain injury. *Arch Phys Med Rehabil.* 2008;89(12)(suppl 1):S61–S68.

124. Winkens I, Van Heugten CM, Wade DT, Fasotti L. Training patients in time pressure management, a cognitive strategy for mental slowness. *Clin Rehabil.* 2009;23(1):79–90.

125. Tiersky LA, Anselmi V, Johnston MV, et al. A trial of neuropsychologic rehabilitation in mild-spectrum traumatic brain injury. *Arch Phys Med Rehabil.* 2005;86(8):1565–1574.

126. Hsieh M, Ponsford J, Wong D, Schönberger M, Taffe J, McKay A. Motivational interviewing and cognitive behavior therapy for anxiety following traumatic brain injury: A pilot randomized controlled trial. *Neuropsychol Rehabil.* In press.

127. Bryant RA, Sackville T, Dang ST, Moulds M, Guthrie R. Treating acute stress disorder: an evaluation of cognitive behavior therapy and supportive counselling techniques. *Am J Psychiatry.* 1999;156(11):1780–1786.

128. Roberts NP, Kitchiner NJ, Kenardy J, Bisson JI. Early psychological interventions to treat acute traumatic stress symptoms. *Cochrane Database Syst Rev.* 2010;(3):CD007944.

129. Roberts NP, Kitchiner NJ, Kenardy J, Bisson JI. Systematic review and meta-analysis of multiple-session early interventions following traumatic events. *Am J Psychiatry.* 2009;166(3):293–301.

130. Spence J, Titov N, Dear BF, et al. Randomized controlled trial of Internet-delivered cognitive behavioral therapy for posttraumatic stress disorder. *Depress Anxiety.* 2011;28(7):541–550.

131. Ougrin D. Efficacy of exposure versus cognitive therapy in anxiety disorders: systematic review and meta-analysis. *BMC Psychiatry.* 2011;11(1):200.

132. McLay RN, Wood DP, Webb-Murphy JA, et al. A randomized, controlled trial of virtual reality-graded exposure therapy for post-traumatic stress disorder in active duty service members with combat-related post-traumatic stress disorder. *Cyberpsychol Behav Soc Netw.* 2011;14(4):223–229.

133. Wood DP, Webb-Murphy J, McLay RN, et al. Reality graded exposure therapy with physiological monitoring for the treatment of combat related post traumatic stress disorder: a pilot study. *Stud Health Technol Inform.* 2011;163:696–702.

134. Beck JG, Palyo SA, Winer EH, Schwagler BE, Ang EJ. Virtual reality exposure therapy for PTSD symptoms after a road accident: an uncontrolled case series. *Behav Ther.* 2007;38(1):39–48.

135. Wiederhold BK, Wiederhold MD. Virtual reality treatment of post-traumatic stress disorder due to motor vehicle accident. *Cyberpsychol Behav Soc Netw.* 2010;13(1):21–27.

136. Spates CR, Koch E, Cusack K, Pagoto S, Waller S. Eye movement desensitization and reprocessing. In: Foa EB, Keane TM, Freidman MJ, Cohen JA, eds. *Effective Treatments for PTSD: Practice Guidelines From the International Society for Traumatic Stress Studies.* New York, NY: Guilford Press; 2009:279–305.

137. Resick PA, Galovski TE, O'Brien Uhlmansiek M, Scher CD, Clum GA, Young-Xu Y. A randomized clinical trial to dismantle components of cognitive processing therapy for posttraumatic stress disorder in female victims of interpersonal violence. *J Consult Clin Psychol.* 2008;76(2):243–258.

138. Bryant RA, Litz BT. Treating Posttraumatic stress disorder following mild traumatic brain injury. In: Vasterling J, Bryant R, Keane T,

eds. *PTSD and Mild Traumatic Brain Injury.* New York, NY: Guilford Press; 2012:219–234.

139. Bryant RA, Moulds M, Guthrie R, Nixon RD. Treating acute stress disorder following mild traumatic brain injury. *Am J Psychiatry.* 2003;160(3):585–587.

140. Williams W, Evans J, Wilson B. Neurorehabilitation for two cases of post-traumatic stress disorder following traumatic brain injury. *Cognit Neuropsychiatry.* 2003;8(1):1–18.

141. Williams W, Evans J, Fleminger S. Neurorehabilitation and cognitive-behaviour therapy of anxiety disorders after brain injury: an overview and a case illustration of obsessive-compulsive disorder. *Neuropsychol Rehabil.* 2003;13(1–2):133–148.

142. Arco L. Neurobehavioural treatment for obsessive-compulsive disorder in an adult with traumatic brain injury. *Neuropsychol Rehabil.* 2008;18(1):109–124.

143. Newburn G. Psychiatric disorders associated with traumatic brain injury: optimal treatment. *CNS Drugs.* 1998;9(6):441–456.

144. Lewis C, Pearce J, Bisson JI. Efficacy, cost-effectiveness and acceptability of self-help interventions for anxiety disorders: systematic review. *Br J Psychiatry.* 2012;200(1):15–21.

145. Kneebone II, Al-Daftary S. Flooding treatment of phobia to having her feet touched by physiotherapists, in a young woman with Down's syndrome and a traumatic brain injury. *Neuropsychol Rehabil.* 2006;16(2):230–236.

146. Novaco R. *Anger Control: The Development and Evaluation of an Experimental Treatment.* Lexington, MA: Lexington Books; 1975.

147. McKinlay WM, Hickox A. How can families help in the rehabilitation of the head injured? *J Head Trauma Rehabil.* 1988;3(4):64–72.

148. Walker AJ, Nott MT, Doyle M, Onus M, McCarthy K, Baguley IJ. Effectiveness of a group anger management programme after severe traumatic brain injury. *Brain Inj.* 2010;24(3):517–524.

149. Lira FT, Carne W, Masri AM. Treatment of anger and impulsivity in a brain damaged patient: A case study applying stress inoculation. *Clin Neuropsychol.* 1983;5:159–160.

150. Uomoto JM, Brockway JA. Anger management training for brain injured patients and their family members. *Arch Phys Med Rehabil.* 1992;73(7):674–679.

151. Miller WR, Rollnick S. *Motivational Interviewing: Preparing People for Change.* 2nd ed. New York, NY: Guilford Press; 2002.

152. Deci EL, Ryan RM. The "what" and "why" of goal pursuits: human needs and the self-determination of behavior. *Psychol Inq.* 2000;11(4):227–268.

153. Markland D, Ryan RM, Tobin VJ, Rollnick S. Motivational interviewing and self-determination theory. *J Soc Clin Psychol.* 2005;24(6):811–831.

154. Vansteenkiste M, Sheldon KM. There's nothing more practical than a good theory: Integrating motivational interviewing and self-determination theory. *Br J Clin Psychol.* 2006;45(1):63–82.

155. DiClemente CC, Velasquez MM. Motivational interviewing and the stages of change In: Miller WR, Rollnick S, eds. *Motivational Interviewing:Preparing People for Change.* New York, NY: Guilford Press; 2002:201–216.

156. Arkowitz H, Westra HA, Miller WR, Rollnick S, eds. *Motivational Interviewing in the Treatment of Psychological Problems.* New York, NY: Guilford Press; 2008.

157. Moyers TB, Rollnick S. A motivational interviewing perspective on resistance in psychotherapy. *J Clin Psychol.* 2002;58(2):185–193.

158. Moyers TB, Miller WR, Hendrickson SML. How does motivational interviewing work? Therapist interpersonal skill predicts client involvement within motivational interviewing sessions. *J Consult Clin Psychol.* 2005;73(4):590–598.

159. Burke BL, Dunn CW, Atkins DC, Phelps JS. The emerging evidence base for motivational interviewing: a meta-analytic and qualitative inquiry. *J Cogn Psychother.* 2004;18(4):309–322.

160. Lundahl BW, Kunz C, Brownell C, Tollefson D, Burke BL. A meta-analysis of motivational interviewing: twenty-five years of empirical studies. *Res Soc Work Pract.* 2010;20(2):137–160.

161. Westra HA, Dozois DJA. Integrating motivational interviewing into the treatment of anxiety. In: Arkowitz H, Westra HA, Miller WR, Rollnick S, eds. *Motivational Interviewing in the Treatment of Psychological Problems.* New York, NY: Guilford Press; 2007:26–56.

162. Arkowitz H, Westra HA. Integrating motivational interviewing

and cognitive behavioral therapy in the treatment of depression and anxiety. *J Cogn Psychother*. 2004;18(4):337–350.

163. Westra HA, Dozois DJ. Preparing clients for cognitive behavioral therapy: a randomized pilot study of motivational interviewing for anxiety. *Cognit Ther Res*. 2006;30(4):481–498.

164. Westra HA. Managing resistance in cognitive behavioural therapy: The application of motivational interviewing in mixed anxiety and depression. *Cogn Behav Ther*. 2004;33(4):161–175.

165. Westra HA, Arkowitz H. Combining motivational interviewing and cognitive behavioral therapy to increase treatment efficacy for generalized anxiety disorder. In: Sookman D, Leahy RL, eds. *Resolving Treatment Impasses With Resistant Anxiety Disorders*. New York, NY: Routledge; 2009:199–232.

166. Amrhein PC. How does motivational interviewing work? What client talk reveals. *J Cogn Psychother*. 2004;18(4):323–336.

167. Carey KB, Leontieva L, Dimmock J, Maisto SA, Batki SL. Adapting motivational interventions for comorbid schizophrenia and alcohol use disorders. *Clin Psychol*. 2007;14(1):39–57.

168. Manchester D, Wood RL. Applying cognitive therapy in neurobehaivoural rehabilitation. In: Wood RL, ed. *Neurobehavioral Disability and Social Handicap Following Traumatic Brain Injury*. New York, NY: Oxford University Press; 2001:157–174.

169. Medley AR, Powell T. Motivational interviewing to promote self-awareness and engagement in rehabilitation following acquired brain injury: a conceptual review. *Neuropsychol Rehabil*. 2010;20(4):481–508.

170. Giles GM, Manchester D. Two approaches to behavior disorder after traumatic brain injury. *J Head Trauma Rehabil*. 2006;21(2):168–178.

171. Mendel E, Hipkins J. Motivating learning disabled offenders with alcohol-related problems: a pilot study. *Br J Learn Disabil*. 2002;30(4):153–158.

172. Bombardier CH, Rimmele CT. Motivational interviewing to prevent alcohol abuse after traumatic brain injury: a case series. *Rehabil Psychol*. 1999;44(1):52–67.

173. Bombardier CH, Heinemann AW. The construct validity of the readiness to change questionnaire for persons with TBI. *J Head Trauma Rehabil*. 2000;15(1):696–709.

174. Cox WM, Heinemann AW, Miranti SV, Schmidt M, Klinger E, Blount J. Outcomes of systematic motivational counseling for substance use following traumatic brain injury. *J Addict Dis*. 2003;22(1):93–110.

175. Bell KR, Temkin NR, Esselman PC, et al. The effect of a scheduled telephone intervention on outcome after moderate to severe traumatic brain injury: a randomized trial. *Arch Phys Med Rehabil*. 2005;86(5):851–856.

176. Bombardier CH, Bell KR, Temkin NR, Fann JR, Hoffman J, Dikmen S. The efficacy of a scheduled telephone intervention for ameliorating depressive symptoms during the first year after traumatic brain injury. *J Head Trauma Rehabil*. 2009;24(4):230–238.

177. Lane-Brown A, Tate R. Evaluation of an intervention for apathy after traumatic brain injury: a multiple-baseline, single-case experimental design. *J Head Trauma Rehabil*. 2010;25(6):459–469.

178. Hsieh M, Ponsford J, Wong D, Schönberger M, McKay A, Haines K. Development of a motivational interviewing program as a prelude to CBT for anxiety & depression following traumatic brain injury. *Neuropsychol Rehabil*. In press.

179. Hsieh MY, Ponsford J, Wong D, McKay A. Exploring variables associated with change in cognitive behaviour therapy (CBT) for anxiety following traumatic brain injury. *Disabil Rehabil*. 2012;34(5):408–415.

180. Lane-Brown A, Tate R. Interventions for apathy after traumatic brain injury. *Cochrane Database Syst Rev*. 2009;(2):CD006341.

181. Kant R, Smith-Seemiller L. Assessment and treatment of apathy syndrome following head injury. *NeuroRehabilitation*. 2002;17(4):325–331.

182. Tenuvuo O. Central acetylcholinesterase inhibitors in the treatment of chronic traumatic brain injury—clinical experience in 111 patients. *Prog Neuropsychopharmacol Biol Psychiatry*. 2005;29(1):61–67.

183. Deb S, Crownshaw T. The role of pharmacotherapy in the management of behaviour disorders in traumatic brain injury. *Brain Inj*. 2004;18(1):1–31.

184. Burke WH, Zenicus AH, Wesolowski MD, Doubleday F. Improving executive function disorders in brain-injured clients. *Brain Inj*. 1991;5(3):241–252.

185. Evans JJ, Emslie H, Wilson BA. External cueing systems in the rehabilitation of executive impairments of action. *J Int Neuropsychol Soc*. 1998;4(4):399–408.

186. Levine B, Robertson IH, Clare L, et al. Rehabilitation of executive functioning: an experimental-clinical validation of goal management training. *J Int Neuropsychol Soc*. 2000;6(3):299–312.

187. Turkstra LS, Flora TL. Compensating for executive function impairments after TBI: a single case study of functional intervention. *J Commun Disord*. 2002;35(6):467–482.

188. Dawson DR, Gaya A, Hunt A, Levine B, Lemsky C, Polataiko HJ. Using the cognitive orientation to occupational performance (CO-OP) with adults with executive dysfunction following traumatic brain injury. *Can J Occup Ther*. 2009;76(2):115–127.

189. Grant M., Ponsford, J., & Bennett, P. C. (in press) The application of Goal Management Training to aspects of financial management in individuals with traumatic brain injury. *Neuropsychological Rehabilitation*, Accepted 3 May 2012.

190. Miotto E, Evans JJ, Souza de Lucia MC, Scaff M. Rehabilitation of executive dysfunction: a controlled trial of an attention and problem-solving treatment group. *Neuropsychol Rehabil*. 2009;19(4):517–540.

191. Spikman JM, Boelen DHE, Lamberts KF, Brouwer WH, Fasotti L. Effects of a multifaceted treatment program for executive dysfunction after acquired brain injury on indications of executive functioning in daily life. *J Int Neuropsychol Soc*. 2010;16(1):118–129.

192. Kennedy MRT, Coelho C, Turkstra L, et al. Intervention for executive functions after traumatic brain injury: a systematic review, meta-analysis and clinical recommendations. *Neuropsychol Rehabil*. 2008;18(3):257–299.

193. Hayes SC, Luoma JB, Bond FW, Masuda A, Lillis J. Acceptance and commitment therapy: model, processes and outcomes. *Behav Res Ther*. 2006;44(1):1–25.

194. Kangas M, McDonald S. Is it time to act? The potential of acceptance and commitment therapy for psychological problems following acquired brain injury. *Neuropsychol Rehabil*. 2011;21(2):250–276.

195. Ruiz FJ. A review of accpetance and commitment therapy (ACT) empirical evidence: correlational, experimental psychopathology, component and outcome studies. *Int J Psychol Psychol Ther*. 2010;10(1):125–162.

196. Soo C, Tate RL, Lane-Brown A. A systematic review of acceptance and commitment therapy (ACT) for managing anxiety: applicability for people with acquired brain injury? *Brain Impair*. 2011;12(1):54–70.

197. Bédard M, Feleau M, Mazmamian D, et al. Pilot evaluation of a mindfulness-based intervention to improve quality of life among individuals who sustained traumatic brain injuries. *Disabil Rehabil*. 2003;25(13):722–731.

198. Wong D. Acceptance and commitment therapy following acquired brain injury: a useful alternative? *Brain Impair*. 2008;9(1):70.

199. Prigatano GP, Fordyce DJ, Zeiner HK, Rouche JR, Pepping M, Wood BC. *Neuropsychological Rehabilitation After Brain Injury*. Baltimore, MD: Johns Hopkins University Press; 1986.

200. Orsillo SM, Roemer L, Barlow DH. Integrating acceptance and mindfulness into existing cognitive-behavioral treatment for GAD: a case study. *Cogn Behav Pract*. 2003;10:222–230.

201. Gilbert P. *Compassion: Conceptualisation, Research and Use in Psychotherapy*. Hove, United Kingdom: Routledge; 2005.

202. Ashworth F, Gracey F, Gilbert P. Compassion focused therapy after traumatic brain injury: theoretical foundations and a case illustration. *Brain Impair*. 2011;12(2):128–139.

203. Evans J. Positive psychology and brain injury rehabilitation. *Brain Impair*. 2011;12(2):117–127.

XV

SPEECH, LANGUAGE, AND SWALLOWING PROBLEMS

Assessment and Treatment of Speech and Language Disorders in Traumatic Brain Injury

Bruce E. Murdoch, Fiona M. Lewis, and Christina Knuepffer

COMMUNICATION DISORDERS FOLLOWING TRAUMATIC BRAIN INJURY: AN INTRODUCTION

Traumatic brain injury (TBI) represents the effectuation of impact-induced biomechanical forces on neural tissue, including compression, acceleration–deceleration, and rotational acceleration (1,2). Associated neurological injuries may be focal, multifocal, or diffuse, involving direct trauma, as well as tension-related tearing of tissue and/or shearing as a consequence of rotational force (1). In relation to communication skills, the potentially wide-ranging and heterogeneous nature of TBI accommodates an infinite compendium of prospective motor speech and language disturbances via the implication of cortical, subcortical, bulbar, and/or cerebellar systems.

Of particular note, the integrity of an individual's communication skills subsequent to TBI has been depicted as a critical factor in determining postinjury quality of life (3). Indeed, it has been recognized that speech and language deficits manifesting as a result of TBI may impose substantial social (4,5) and vocational (4,6) ramifications. Relative to adults, the speech and language corollary of TBI has been held accountable for social segregation, academic failure, and/or vocational demotion following injury (1,2). In the case of children, TBI has been documented to invoke immediate communication deficits, as well as a potential predisposition to speech and/or language impediments evident during the formative years, whereby infants fail to meet milestones as they proceed along an anticipated motor-cognitive developmental continuum (2,4). Until recently, the remediation of communication sequelae associated with TBI has been considered somewhat subordinate to the management of related medical conditions (7). In light of the potentially adverse psychosocial impact communicative compromise may impose on individuals with TBI, however, it must be emphasized that effective speech–language rehabilitation can no longer be perceived as an ancillary treatment objective.

Dysarthria represents a frequently documented sequela of TBI, reportedly constituting greater than one-third of the communication deficits manifesting within this population (8). Furthermore, a diverse range of dysarthric subtypes has been observed in individuals subsequent to TBI (8), and within these subtypes, reported levels of motor speech dysfunction have been documented to vary from mild articulatory imprecision to nonfunctional speech intelligibility (9). In contrast, apraxia of speech constitutes a rarely documented motor speech anomaly associated with TBI (10–12), however, it has been reported to manifest in tandem with dysarthria and aphasic symptoms in some cases (11). The limited amount of research available pertaining to apraxia in TBI and the frequently encountered diagnostic conundrum faced by clinicians with respect to delineating between the symptomatology of co-occurring motor programming and muscular control deficits preclude further discourse pertaining to this motor speech anomaly within this chapter.

Another communication disorder rarely exhibited by individuals subsequent to TBI is the onset of stuttering (for a recent review see Lundgren et al. [13]), which may occur in association with either dysarthria or language impairment. Although this condition, referred to as acquired neurogenic stuttering, may be seen in association with several different neurogenic disorders (e.g., stroke, Parkinson disease, senile dementia, seizure disorder), it has also been reported to occasionally manifest in individuals with TBI (14–17). To date, however, many aspects of the condition remain controversial and in doubt. For instance, it is not clear whether acquired neurogenic stuttering is a distinct disorder or an epiphenomenon of other motor speech disorders such as apraxia of speech. Further, characterization of the speech output in this condition has proven challenging with few comprehensive descriptions of the speech patterns being reported and a lack of agreement regarding the specific features of the condition that distinguish it from developmental fluency disorders (17). No single neuropathological correlate of acquired neurogenic stuttering has been determined with various reports implicating brain regions as diverse as the right parietal lobe and the mesial aspect of the left parietal lobe (15), the corpus callosum, and the basal ganglia (16). Magnetic resonance imaging (MRI) of a woman who developed stuttering following closed head injury demonstrated right frontoparietal brain lesions in addition to diffuse axonal injury (DAI) (14). In cases of TBI, identification of the causative lesion of acquired neurogenic stuttering is made more difficult given that DAI is superimposed on multiple focal lesions. Adding even further to this complexity is the recognition that some cases of acquired stuttering may have a psychological or neuropsychiatric genesis rather than a neuropathological basis. Overall, factors such as rarity of the condition, the lack of agreement regarding its characteristic features, and the absence of a clear understanding of its neuropathological basis preclude further discussion of acquired neurogenic stuttering in this chapter.

Current knowledge pertaining to the impact of TBI on linguistic function is somewhat secondary to that respecting influences on motor speech control. This discrepancy may be attributed to the fact that individuals with TBI have been historically reported to perform within normal limits on assessments of primary language function (i.e., early emerging language skills such as semantics, syntax, use of morphological markers, etc.) (18), largely resulting in the exclusion of this population from supplemental linguistic analysis. Using appropriately sensitive measures of higher order, in addition to primary language function, deficits at the cognitive-linguistic interface have been identified in TBI subjects (19). Similar to motor speech sequelae, the nature of linguistic impairments resulting from head injury has been reported as variable (18). Incidence rates with respect to language dysfunction, however, have been documented as high as 100% in some research (20), highlighting patients with TBI as a clinically viable population for language screening and intervention.

The following sections of this chapter are subsequently devoted to contemporary maxims underlying the assessment and treatment of motor speech and language impairments resulting from TBI, including those communication deficits potentially affiliated with mild head injury. Mild TBI (mTBI) has received recent attention in the popular media as a public health concern (21,22). Despite the fact that most neurobehavioral alterations imposed as a result of mTBI have been documented to resolve within months of the related trauma, recent evidence suggests that premorbid levels of functioning may never be salvaged subsequent to injury (21). Of note, speech and language constitute neurobehavioral domains implicated within this population (23). Evidently, TBI encompassing the full spectrum of severity levels has the capacity to impact on communicative proficiency. It was the aim of this chapter, therefore, to delineate the speech and language deficits that may manifest in individuals with TBI, as well as to provide a summary of applied assessment and treatment techniques that may be readily integrated within contemporary rehabilitation programs.

ASSESSMENT AND TREATMENT OF MOTOR SPEECH DISORDERS IN TBI

The variable nature of the neuropathology resulting from TBI prognosticates the potential implication of isolated or manifold motor speech subsystems. Consequently, emergent motor speech profiles in TBI subjects may encompass articulatory, velopharyngeal, laryngeal, and/or respiratory deficiencies. A characteristic common to the dysarthria associated with TBI, however, is its intractable nature (8). Of note, it has been documented that although frequently presenting in tandem with language impairments at onset, the dysarthria of TBI endures long after initial linguistic deficits have resolved (3,24,25). Recent outcome studies, however, have indicated that the dysarthria of TBI may respond effectively to a range of treatment techniques, documented to facilitate improvements in clinical speech features, functional commu-

nication skills, and physiological substrates (26–33). The ensuing section subsequently outlines the nature of motor speech impairments associated with TBI, suitable assessment techniques, and relevant treatment approaches.

The Dysarthria of TBI: Neuroanatomical Classification and Clinical Features

As mentioned previously, the precise nature of the dysarthria that manifests as a consequence of TBI is governed by the location and scope of neural damage endured (8). The inherently diffuse nature of TBI, however, typically accommodates potential disruption at exponential loci along the neural axis, implicating upper as well as lower motor neuron systems. Indeed, classifications of spastic (34), hyperkinetic/hypokinetic (35,36), flaccid (37,38), ataxic (32,39,40), and mixed (34,41) dysarthria have been reported within the TBI literature (42), however, spastic (42) and more recently mixed (i.e., spastic-ataxic) (41) subtypes have been highlighted as the most prevalent motor speech disturbances in this population. This motor speech profile is consistent with diffuse bilateral hemispheric damage following head injury (42), potentially implicating terminal loci of the neural fulcrum, such as the frontal lobes (43–45) and cerebellum, as the neuropathological substrates of the dysarthria of TBI.

Spastic Dysarthria

Spastic dysarthria, resulting from upper motor neuron damage implicating cortical motor areas and/or associated descending motor tracts (46), reportedly manifests as a result of wide-ranging disturbance across the motor speech subsystems, characterized by hypertonicity of the muscles and reduced range, speed, and strength of muscle excursion (47). Perceptually, this physiological symptom complex is typically characterized by strained-strangled vocal quality, as well as reduced alternate motion and speech rates (47).

Hyperkinetic and Hypokinetic Dysarthria

Although less common than spastic dysarthria, upper motor neuron damage as a consequence of TBI has also been reported to result in hypokinetic or hyperkinetic dysarthric subtypes (42). Neuropathologically defined within extrapyramidal nuclei such as the basal ganglia and divisions of the brain stem, hyperkinetic motor behavior denotes aberrantly excessive movement and hypokinesia (diminished and decelerated movement) (1). Clinically, hyperkinetic dysarthria is characterized by disturbances in the rhythm and rate of oromotor movements as a consequence of involuntary motor actions and variability in muscle tone (48,49). Perceptually, this profile is most often distinguished by prosodic deviations including impairments in pitch and volume control, stress, rate, phrase, as well as interword and phoneme duration, but may also include additional aberrant speech features such as sudden respiratory inhalations and exhalations, vocal arrest, strained-strangled vocalization, articulatory imprecision, and hypernasality (48–51).

In contrast, the clinical characteristics of hypokinetic dysarthria embody oromotor deviations associated with rigidity, diminished range, as well as force of movement and variations in movement velocity (52,53). Perceptually, these neuromuscular disturbances commonly manifest as monopitch, monoloudness, reduced stress, festinatory speech (i.e., short rushes), hoarse and/or breathy vocal quality, articulatory imprecision, phoneme repetition, low pitch, overall increased but variable speech rate, and diminished volume control (52–54).

Flaccid Dysarthria

In keeping with the inherently heterogeneous nature of neurological damage associated with TBI, motor speech disturbances consistent with lower motor neuron lesions have also been observed within this population. Resulting from damage to the motor cranial and/or spinal nerves, flaccid dysarthria is characterized by muscular weakness, absent or reduced reflexes, muscle atrophy, and fasciculations (1). Clinically, the motor speech deficits associated with this neurological profile may vary, dependent on the specific cranial nerves implicated (55,56). A common assemblage of deviant speech features, however, has been observed in flaccid dysarthric populations including breathiness, audible inspiration, hypernasality, nasal emission, reduced phrase length, consonant imprecision, vocal harshness, monopitch, and monoloudness (50). Of particular note, the resonatory and phonatory deficiencies frequently seen in flaccid dysarthria have been described as largely unique to this dysarthric subtype (55).

Ataxic Dysarthria

Extending further along the neural axis, cerebellar damage has also been reported as a possible outcome of TBI (8). Ataxic dysarthria constitutes the resultant motor speech deficit and is typically characterized by articulatory and prosodic insufficiencies (57). Perceptually, these insufficiencies translate as articulatory imprecision (encompassing both consonants and vowels), articulatory breakdowns, excess and equal stress, prolongation of phonemes and interword intervals, diminished speech rate, monopitch, monoloudness, and harsh vocal quality (58). This motor speech profile has been reported to specifically represent the neuromuscular effects of reduced tone and coordination, affecting slow and inaccurate motor behaviors relevant to the force, range, timing, and direction of speech musculature movement (57,59).

Mixed Dysarthria

The heterogeneous and often pervasive nature of TBI, respecting lesion location, has also been associated with the clinical presentation of mixed dysarthria, concomitantly encompassing the motor speech deviations of several dysarthric subtypes (1,42,60). Notably, a recent body of research identified mixed dysarthria as the most prevalent form of motor speech impairment in a cohort of TBI subjects, including spastic-ataxic, spastic-hypokinetic, spastic-flaccid, flaccid-ataxic, and spastic-flaccid-ataxic subtypes (8,41). Of further interest, within this group, individuals classified with mixed dysarthric subtypes demonstrated the most

qualitatively severe motor speech disturbances, suggesting that more diffuse brain damage may correlate with more severe speech disturbances.

Dysarthria Acquired During Childhood

The aforementioned neuroanatomical classification of dysarthric subtypes and associated clinical features largely relate to motor speech anomalies acquired in adulthood or at neurodevelopmentally stable life stages. Historically, this taxonomy has been adopted as a frame of reference to classify dysarthria resulting from TBI in childhood, however, not without recognized limitations (61–63). Previously, it has been assumed that the physiologic impairment underlying dysarthria in children is the same as in adults and, consequently, the adult classification of dysarthria correlating with the pathophysiology of the motor systems has usually been applied to describe childhood dysarthria. More recently, it has been suggested that acquired dysarthria occurring in children requires its own classification system (62), given that there are several reasons why the physiologic manifestation of dysarthria in children with TBI may differ from that in adults with TBI. Indeed, TBI in childhood has been documented to recover more rapidly than that endured in adulthood, as a consequence of distinctive neuroplasticity mechanisms (62). Furthermore, children have been reported to predominantly endure brain injuries as a result of low-speed motor vehicle accidents or falls, in opposition to adolescents and adults commonly involved in high-speed collisions (4,62). These factors suggest that the mechanisms of child vs adult TBI may be incongruent, with greater rotational acceleration effects and consequently more diffuse brain damage expected in adult populations (61,62).

Until recently, the perceptual and physiological features of dysarthria resulting from TBI in childhood have been relatively unexplored (4,63). Contemporary research, however, has revealed similar dysarthric profiles in children as compared to adults following TBI, with respect to the presentation of a variable array of disturbances in prosodic, resonatory, phonatory, and articulatory aspects of speech production (61). Despite these clinical parallels, future research investigating the nature of interactions between developmental and acquired factors is considered critical to the better elucidation of mechanisms underpinning dysarthrias contracted in childhood (64). In particular, resultant motor speech impairments may represent a maturation-sensitive consequence of head injury within the context of developmental neurological systems. As such, longitudinal monitoring of motor speech abilities in children with TBI is considered pivotal to the prompt identification and remediation of speech deficits that may potentially manifest at any point during the course of motor development.

The Dysarthria of TBI: Perceptual, Acoustic, and Physiological Evaluation

Conventionally, perceptual speech analysis has provided the mainstay of dysarthria assessment (4,61). Despite offering qualitative insights into the audible deviations apparent in dysarthric speech, these methods proffer little with respect to empirically identifying the neuromuscular locus or neurophysiological basis of the presenting deficits. Recently, advancements in technology have catalyzed the development of more objective motor speech assessment tools, affording the compilation of quantitative acoustic and physiological profiles by way of state-of-the-art instrumentation. Notwithstanding the value of the data generated via instrumental assessments, speech is, by its very nature, an audible entity, its "normalcy" considered by some to be most efficiently judged by the human ear. To this end, perceptual and instrumental techniques combined have been recommended as the most effective means of evaluating motor speech dysfunction (61), taking into consideration relevant pathophysiological substrates as well as deviant perceptual features impacting on functional communication proficiency. The proceeding summary of assessment methods used in the evaluation of dysarthria is largely applicable to both adult and pediatric populations. Recommendations have been made, however, with respect to the screening of developmental articulatory or phonological processes, and/or accommodating literacy-related limitations in children.

Perceptual Assessment

Comprehensive perceptual evaluations of motor speech function have been described as those that evaluate the five major elements of speech production, including respiration, phonation, resonance, articulation, and prosody (4,61). The perceptual motor speech assessment battery used in our research laboratory adheres to this recommendation, providing qualitative judgments pertaining to deviant speech dimensions (i.e., speech feature analysis [60], Fisher-Logemann Test of Articulation Competence [66]), speech intelligibility (i.e., Assessment of Intelligibility of Dysarthric Speech [60]), and subsystem dysfunction (i.e., Frenchay Dysarthria Assessment [67]). For a more detailed summary of specific assessments applicable to TBI, refer to Table 65-1.

Instrumental Assessment

The instrumental evaluation of dysarthria encompasses both acoustic and physiological assessment techniques. Acoustic assessment is specifically dedicated to the evaluation of voice; providing measures of frequency, amplitude, perturbation, and signal noise; as well as temporally constrained aspects of phonation (e.g., maximum phonation time and voice onset time) (68) and is certainly applicable to TBI populations. Several acoustic analysis systems are available commercially, including the Computerized Speech Lab® (CSL) (Kay Elemetrics Corp.), VisiPitch® (Kay Elemetrics Corp.), CSpeech®, the Canadian Speech Research Environment® (CSRE), MacSpeech Lab II®, and Dr. Speech Science for Windows® (Tiger Electronics) (69,70). The CSL and VisiPitch, however, represent the most commonly employed acoustic analysis programs, rated as user-friendly via the provision of real-time visual displays of acoustic parameters and the facility to store and analyze data (68).

Physiological assessments represent a corpus of instrumentation dedicated to the evaluation of the neuromuscular control mechanisms underlying speech. Available physiological apparatus not only evaluate phonatory aspects of speech production but also extend to the assessment of articulation, resonance, and respiration, including devices such as the Laryngograph®, Electromagnetic Articulograph®, Na-

TABLE 65-1 Comprehensive Perceptual Motor Speech Assessment Battery Applicable to TBI

- Assessment of Intelligibility of Dysarthric Speech (60)
  - □ Standardized assessment of severity of dysarthric speech.
  - □ Incorporates measures of speech intelligibility at both single word and sentential levels, overall speech rate, rate of intelligible speech, and a ratio of communication efficiency.
- Frenchay Dysarthria Assessment (67)
  - □ Standardized assessment of neuromuscular systems associated with motor speech production, including reflexive, respiratory, articulatory, resonatory, and phonatory mechanisms.
  - □ Provides composite profile relative to status of motor speech subsystem functioning.
- Speech Feature Analysis (65)
  - □ Following reading aloud of a standard citation such as "The Grandfather Passage" (45) or in the case of children who may not be able to read—an oral picture description task—speech samples are analyzed and rated according to the presence and severity of 33 possible deviant speech dimensions.
  - □ Relevant dimensions encompass five domains of speech production, namely: prosody (i.e., pitch, loudness, phrasing, rate, stress), respiration (i.e., breath support for speech), resonance (i.e., nasality), phonation (i.e., vocal quality), and articulation (i.e., consonant precision, length of phonemes, precision of vowels).
  - □ Also provides an overall rating of speech intelligibility
- Fisher-Logemann Test of Articulation Competence (66)
  - □ *Relevant to childhood TBI*, this assessment generates an articulatory profile that may be further analyzed relating to the nature of deviant speech productions within the context of developmental articulatory and phonological errors.

someter®, and Respitrace®. Refer to Table 65-2 for a summary of physiological instrumentation that may be used in the assessment of individuals with TBI.

Physiological Measures of Laryngeal Function
In relation to the physiological assessment of laryngeal function, electroglottography (EGG) and measures of laryngeal aerodynamics represent 2 of the most commonly applied

TABLE 65-2 Physiological Instrumentation Used in the Assessment of Dysarthria Following TBI

Laryngeal function	□ Electroglottographic assessment (Laryngograph®)
	□ Aerodynamic assessment (Aerophone II®)
Respiratory function	□ Spirometric assessment
	□ Kinematic assessment (Respitrace®)
	□ Aerodynamic assessment (Aerophone II®)
Articulatory function	□ Lip and tongue pressure transduction systems
	□ Electropalatography (EPG)
	□ Electromagnetic articulography (EMA)
Velopharyngeal function	□ Nasometer® (Kay Elemetrics)
	□ Accelerometric assessment

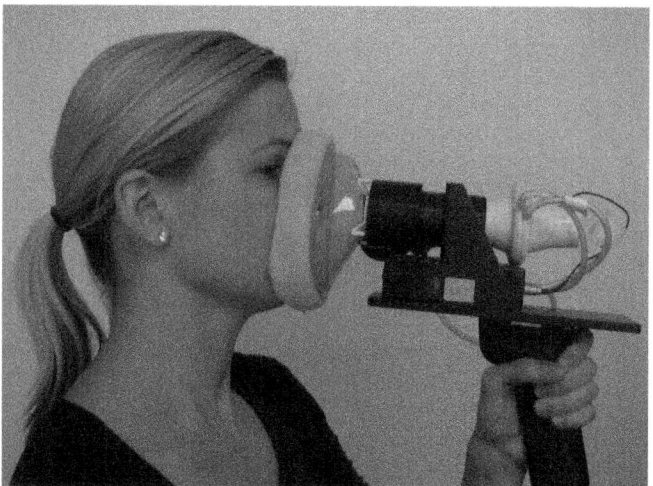

FIGURE 65-1 Aerophone II® airflow measurement system.

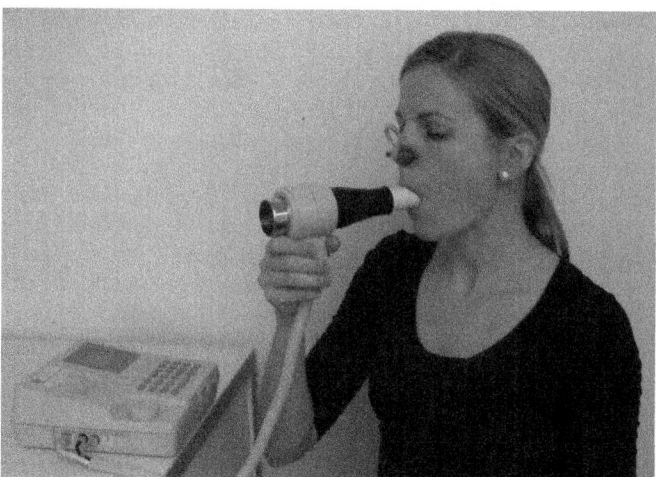

FIGURE 65-2 Respiratory spirometer.

physiological tools in the clinical assessment of voice (68). EGG provides a means of representing vocal fold vibratory patterns (71,72) and aerodynamic measures generate information pertaining to the interaction of various phonatory parameters. Waveforms generated via electroglottographic methods (e.g., Fourcin® Laryngograph) correspond to the opening and closing phases of the glottal cycle, and the velocity at which the vocal folds adduct (70). Measures of laryngeal aerodynamics such as the Aerophone II® (see Figure 65-1) provide indices relating to the interplay of various laryngeal mechanisms in the production of voice, such as subglottal pressure, phonatory air flow, sound pressure level, and laryngeal airway resistance (68). In addition to the parameters mentioned earlier, the Aerophone II® is also capable of measuring vocal fold adduction-abduction rates (73). Of note, high variability rates in performance have been reported in studies of aerodynamic laryngeal function (68). To counteract these variability effects, it has been recommended that the average of at least five repetitive samples should be established as a representative illustration of laryngeal function on such measures (74). Within the context of TBI, however, fatigue effects as a result of effortful or repetitive physiological assessment tasks must also be considered in the interpretation of such data (68).

Physiological Measures of Respiratory Function
Assessments of laryngeal function routinely co-occur with an evaluation of respiratory mechanisms underlying speech production (68). Physiological measures of speech breathing may be divided into two broad categories: (*a*) spirometric (i.e., direct measures of lung volume and capacity) and (*b*) kinematic (i.e., indirect measures of lung function by way of monitoring chest wall activity during breathing cycles and speech production tasks). Dry spirometers (see Figure 65-2) provide a means of measuring a range of respiratory parameters, including vital capacity, inspiratory capacity, expiratory and inspiratory reserve volumes, forced expiratory volume, respiration rate, tidal volume, and volume or flow relationships. Furthermore, each of the parameters obtained may be compared to predicted age, height, and sex-based values by way of formulae weighted for age and/or height (75,76).

Kinematic measures of speech breathing provide independent yet simultaneous recordings of alterations in rib cage and abdomen volumes during speech and nonspeech tasks. A range of kinematic instrumentation has been applied to the study of speech breathing in neurologically impaired populations (73), including magnetometers, strain-gauge belt pneumographs, and inductance plethysmography (77–79). Respitrace® (see Figure 65-3), an inductance plethysmographic measure of respiratory function, is the instrument of choice in our research laboratory. This instrument monitors changes in chest wall circumference via electrical inductance. Wires contained within elasticized straps placed around the chest and abdomen register dimensional alterations during specified tasks. A visual display signal is generated for analysis purposes and may also function as a biofeedback tool during therapy.

Physiological Measures of Articulatory Function
In relation to the evaluation of articulatory function, pressure transduction systems are commonly employed to measure lip and tongue strength, endurance, velocity of movement, and fine force control. Within our research laboratory, a miniaturized pressure transducer (Entran Flatline®, Entran Devices Inc., Model EPL 20001-10) with factory calibration, mounted on an aluminium strip, is used to measure interlabial pressures during speech and nonspeech tasks, resembling that initially described by Hinton and Luschei (80). Similarly, a rubber-bulb pressure transduction system is used to evaluate tongue function (81,82).

Electropalatography (EPG) and electromagnetic articulography (EMA) represent measures of dynamic articulatory function. More specifically, EPG provides a means of evaluating the positioning and timing of tongue to hard palate contacts during speech via a thin acrylic palate studded with miniature sensory electrodes, fitted within a subject's oral cavity (see Figure 65-4). Contact patterns during speech are subsequently acquired and stored in an external processing unit for analysis. By way of transmitter and receiver coil systems generating electromagnetic fields, the Electromagnetic Articulograph® (EMA) AG-500 (Carstens Medizinelektronik, Germany) provides a three-dimensional

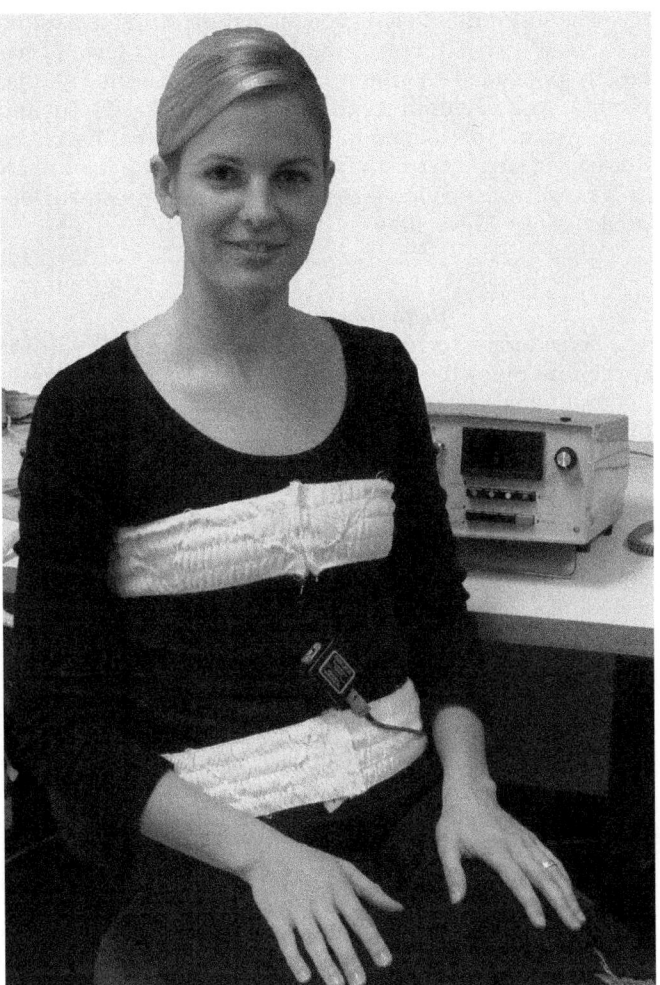

FIGURE 65-3 Respitrace® system for kinematic assessment of speech breathing.

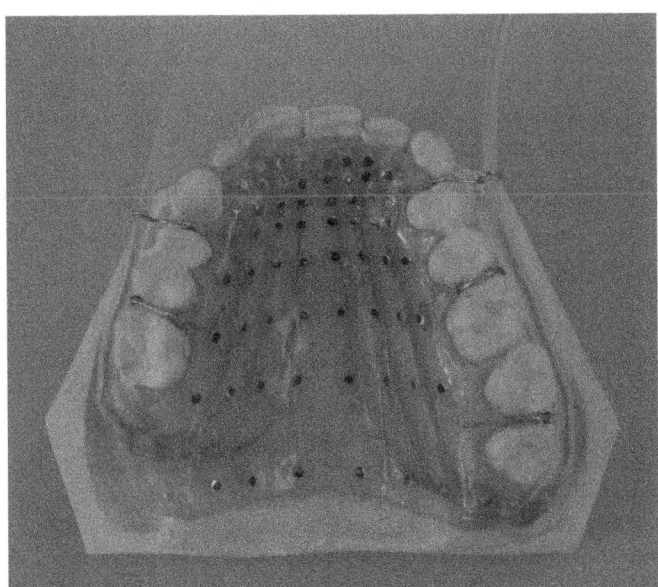

FIGURE 65-4 Acrylic electropalatography palate with imbedded touch sensors.

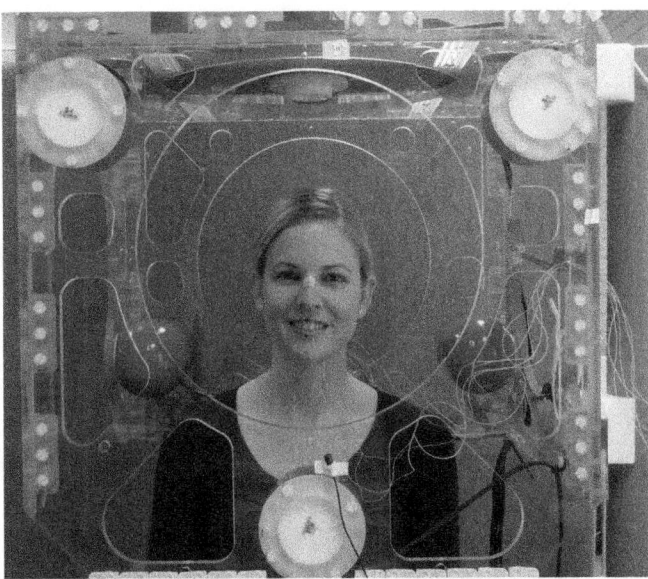

FIGURE 65-5 AG-500 electromagnetic articulograph.

representation of articulatory movements (83) (see Figure 65-5). More specifically, the EMA has the capacity to generate kinematic articulatory parameters, including trajectory, velocity, duration, and acceleration, via the tracking of displacement relative to receiver coils positioned on the tongue, upper and lower lips, velum, and mandible.

Physiological Measures of Velopharyngeal Function
Measures of nasal airflow, air pressure, vibration, and oronasal acoustic output offer noninvasive, clinically viable methods of assessing velopharyngeal competence (84). Nasal accelerometry and measures of oronasal acoustic output ratios represent the assessments of velopharyngeal function used routinely within our research laboratory. Nasal accelerometry involves the placement of miniature, vibration-sensitive accelerometers on the lateral nasal cartilage and thyroid lamina, which detect nasal and laryngeal vibrations during speech. The magnitudes of vibration detected are then used to calculate a ratio of nasal to laryngeal vibration, providing an index of nasality, the Horri Oral Nasal Coupling (HONC) index (85,86). High HONC indices are considered representative of velopharyngeal incompetence.

The Nasometer® (Kay Elemetrics) (see Figure 65-6) offers a measure of nasality via the generation of oronasal acoustic output ratios (87–89). Two directional microphones separated by a sound-separating plate are positioned anterior to the nose and mouth that record acoustic output signals. Accompanying software calculates nasalance scores that effectively represent nasal to oral acoustic output ratios during various speech tasks. High scores are considered representative of velopharyngeal dysfunction.

Neuroradiological Assessment

In addition to the perceptual, acoustic, and physiological assessments outlined earlier, recently introduced neuroradiological techniques also have added to the battery of procedures available to determine the pathophysiological basis of communication impairments seen in individuals post-TBI.

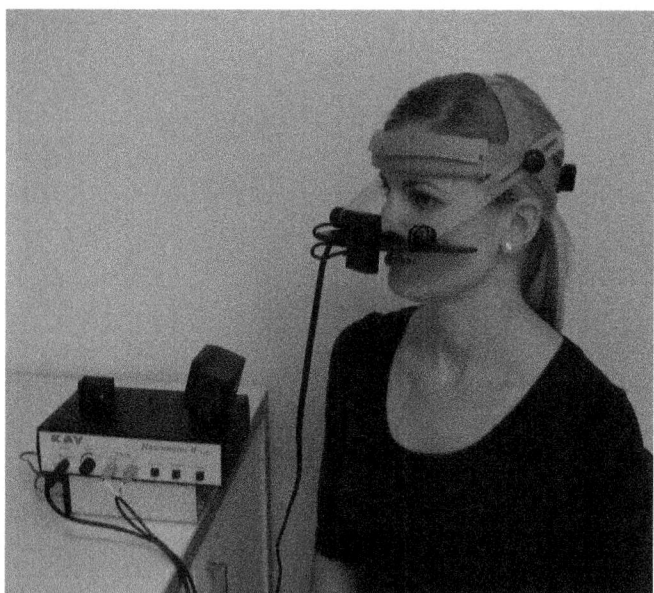

FIGURE 65-6 Nasometer.

Communication deficits subsequent to TBI are the products of induced brain pathologies, in particular DAI (1). DAI disrupts fiber tracts connecting different parts of the brain leading to the production of speech and language deficits. A powerful emerging imaging technique to visualize white matter integrity and any axonal damage sustained is the acquisition of diffusion magnetic resonance images based on tensor or higher order models and the subsequent tractography analysis of white matter pathways (diffusion MRI tractography). This technique allows the virtual in vivo dissection of white matter fasciculi in the brain providing measures of location and integrity of speech and language fiber tracts (90). Recent studies relating measures of fiber integrity in the brain to neurobehavioral outcomes following TBI consistently report high correlations between the two (91,92). In addition, alteration of cerebral blood flow assessed by functional MRI (fMRI) may aid our understanding of the neuropathophysiology of speech and language disorders subsequent to TBI.

The Dysarthria of TBI: Treatment Approaches

The treatment of the dysarthria of TBI in both child and adult populations has been described as a convoluted and protracted process, necessitating consideration of individual deficits within the context of functional communication requirements (93). The International Classification of Functioning, Disability and Health (ICF) offers a widely accepted framework for intervention relative to domains of health (94), which encompass communication skills. Within this model, the treatment of dysarthria is viewed from a three-tiered perspective, including (*a*) integrity of body function and structure, (*b*) associated activity limitations and participation restrictions, and (*c*) contextual factors facilitating functional improvements or reduction in disability.

The inherently heterogeneous nature of the dysarthria associated with TBI respecting lesion site and severity has largely precluded the reporting of group outcome studies relative to individual treatment techniques (95). By and large, research pertaining to treatment effects has been conducted via single case study designs, reporting the impact of a range of behavioral, instrumental, and prosthetic approaches (27–31,96–104).

Behavioral Approach
The behavioral approach to the rehabilitation of dysarthric speech involves the teaching of compensatory strategies via traditional methods, which encompass the presentation of therapeutic stimuli and the establishment of response contingencies (105). Historically, traditional or behavioral techniques have provided the mainstay of dysarthria therapy, given their economic viability and wide-ranging environmental utility (106). Although failing to constitute an unabridged stockpile of behavioral dysarthria therapy techniques, Table 65-3 represents several commonly used traditional approaches in the remediation of phonatory, respiratory, resonatory, articulatory, and prosodic deficits.

Instrumental Approach
The instrumental therapeutic approach incorporates techniques that offer direct physiological or biofeedback pertaining to motor speech subsystem function during therapy tasks. Biofeedback tools provide a means of reestablishing motor control patterns by way of unconventional or adjunct sensory channels (107). Sensory channels may incorporate auditory, visual, or tactile modalities, however, visual feedback signals have been documented as the most effective in the remediation of dysarthria (108–110). Table 65-4 highlights a range of biofeedback techniques currently used in the treatment of respiratory, phonatory, resonatory, articulatory, and prosodic disorders.

Prosthetic or Surgical Approach
Prosthetic and/or surgical interventions, which effectively modify the physical configuration of specific motor speech subsystems (105), are commonly employed in the remediation of severe dysarthria (106). Table 65-5 summarizes a range of prosthetic/surgical techniques used in the treatment of motor speech impairments, usually employed subsequent to an ineffective trial of more traditional therapeutic approaches.

Case Reports: Clinical Management of Dysarthria Following TBI

The ability to apply the previously highlighted principles of dysarthria assessment and treatment to the management of a clinical caseload represents a requisite skill for any clinician. Within the context of the framework for intervention outlined in the ICF (94), the following vignettes constitute proposed clinical management plans relevant to the treatment of dysarthria following TBI, in a 26-year-old adult and a 14-year-old child.

TABLE 65-3 Behavioral Therapeutic Approaches in the Treatment of Dysarthria Following TBI

TARGETED MOTOR SPEECH SUBSYSTEM	METHOD
• Phonation	□ *Hyperadduction reduction techniques* aim to alleviate excessive vocal fold adduction by way of tension reduction techniques such as *chewing* (111), *yawn-sigh*, and *gentle voice onset* methods (112).
	□ *Hypoadduction reduction techniques* aim to achieve effective vocal fold adduction and effective phonation in dysphonic patients via the application of *push/pull* (113), *hard glottal attack* (114), and *increased phonatory effort* (115) methods.
• Respiration	□ *Manipulating posture* to maximize respiratory control (116) via the provision of visual, tactile, and/or auditory cues.
	□ *Inspiratory checking* (117) technique aims to increase breath support and enhance respiratory control during exhalation via drills that encourage the regulation of air flow and volume during vocalization.
• Resonance	□ Exercises aimed at increasing range of movement and strength of velum including *blowing*, *gagging*, and *sucking* (106), as well as palatal awareness via *visual feedback* (106), *palatal massage*, (118) and *icing/brushing* (119) techniques.
• Articulation	□ Aim to normalize function of the articulators (i.e., lips, tongue, and jaw) via the *modification of muscle tone* (e.g., hypertonia vs hypotonia), *maximizing muscle strength* (i.e., isotonic and isometric oromotor exercises [118]), and *articulation/speech drills* of increasing complexity (105).
• Prosody	□ Methods aimed at remediating stress patterning (e.g., *contrastive stress drills* [118]), intonation (e.g., *altering respiratory capacity and patterning* [120]), and rate (e.g., *intersystemic reorganization* [118] involving therapist-directed pacing of speech).

TABLE 65-4 Instrumental Therapeutic Approaches in the Treatment of Dysarthria Following TBI

TARGETED MOTOR SPEECH SUBSYSTEM	METHOD
• Phonation	□ Use of apparatus with the facility to display vocal parameters such as pitch, intensity, and duration during speech output (e.g., *Vocalite* [121], *Visipitch* [120], *Visispeech* [122], *Speech Viewer* [98], *storage oscilloscope* [123]).
• Respiration	□ *U-tube manometer* requires patient to maintain specific water level over a designated time via controlled exhalation (118).
	□ *Kinematic instrumentation* (e.g., *Respitrace*®) provides visual representation of chest wall movements during speech tasks. Feedback shown to be effective in increasing lung volumes, increasing abdominal contributions to breathing, as well as enhancing coordination of speech breathing (102,124).
• Resonance	□ *Endoscopy* and *flexible fiber nasopharyngoscopy* provides direct visual feedback pertaining to velar and posterior pharyngeal wall excursion during speech (125,126).
	□ *Velograph* provides real time representation of velar movement via an oscilloscope (127).
	□ *Nasometer*® provides bar graphs and/or real time visual displays of nasalance during speech (106).
• Articulation	□ *Electromyography (EMG)* represents a biofeedback tool with applications for altering labial and lingual muscle tone and strength (31,99,128–130).
	□ *Electropalatography (EPG)* may be used as a biofeedback device to alter lingual postures during speech (131,132).
• Prosody	□ *Speech Viewer* (133) provides both visual and auditory feedback pertaining to fundamental frequency and vocal intensity; documented as a successful device in improving pitch, intonation, and rate of speech (134).
	□ Modification of speech rate during reading via *PACER computerized rhythmic cueing* (135)
	□ *Delayed Auditory Feedback (DAF)* documented as useful biofeedback device in reducing rate, increasing vocal intensity, and enhancing overall speech intelligibility (136–138).

Case 1 (Adult): Moderate Spastic-Ataxic Dysarthria

Case History

Jacob is a 26-year-old male who sustained a TBI as the result of a motor vehicle accident. On admission to hospital, a Glasgow Coma Scale score of 5 was reported, indicative of severe head injury. MRI investigations revealed bilateral subcortical hemorrhages and multiple contusions. At the time of his accident, Jacob was married and working as a practicing accountant. His family and employer were reportedly committed to his rehabilitation and return to the work force.

Motor Speech Profile: Moderate Spastic-Ataxic Dysarthria
Perceptual assessment results revealed reduced speech intelligibility, consonant imprecision, reduced breath support for speech, hypernasality, strained-strangled vocal quality, reduced pitch and loudness control, reduced speech rate, and impaired stress patterning. Physiological assessment revealed wide-ranging motor speech subsystem dysfunction, incorporating reduced respiratory support for speech, hyperfunctional laryngeal activity, velopharyngeal insufficiency, and reduced range and speed of labial and lingual movement.

TABLE 65-5 Prosthetic and/or Surgical Approaches in the Treatment of Dysarthria Following TBI

TARGETED MOTOR SPEECH SUBSYSTEM	METHOD
• Phonation	▫ *Voice amplifiers*—electronic device aimed at increasing voice volume (120,139)
	▫ *Botox injections* (140), *laryngeal nerve resections* (141) in the treatment of hyperadduction
	▫ *Reinnervation of paralyzed vocal folds* (142), *collagen/Teflon implants* (143, 144), and *arytenoid adduction* (145) in the treatment of hypoadduction
• Respiration	▫ *Abdominal muscle girdling* by way of elasticized bandages (118) enhances expiratory control during speech by facilitating recoil of the abdominal musculature.
	▫ Postural enhancement by use of *overhead slings* (118) provides surface on which individuals may bear down to establish expiratory force for speech.
• Resonance	▫ *Palatal lift prosthesis* aims to achieve palatopharyngeal closure (146).
• Articulation	▫ *Bite block* to increase jaw stability and maximize function of other articulators (147).
• Prosody	▫ *Pacing* (148) or *alphabet board* (149) encourages speech rate reduction.

Clinical Management Plan

A multisystem approach was adopted in the rehabilitation of Jacob's speech, involving a combination of behavioral and instrumental treatment techniques. Consistent with the ICF, his presenting motor speech deficit was considered in relation to structural and functional impairments, imposed activity limitations, and participation restrictions as well as manipulable contextual factors. Refer to Table 65-6 for the proposed rehabilitation schedule.

Case 2 (Child): Moderate Spastic Dysarthria

Case History

Max is a 14-year-old male who sustained a TBI following a pedestrian or motor vehicle accident. On admission to hospital, a Glasgow Coma Scale score of 5 was reported, indicative of severe head injury. Computed tomography (CT) scan revealed soft tissue hematoma over right temporal and left zygomatic regions as well as an area of high attenuation in the left lentiform nucleus and additional foci scattered over peripheral gray or white region anteriorly and superiorly. No significant mass effect was observed. At the time of his accident, Max was a high-achieving year 9 high school student with a range of extracurricular interests, including debating, football, and tennis.

Motor Speech Profile: Moderate Spastic Dysarthria

Subsequent to TBI, Max endured a 5-month period of mutism. Perceptual assessment of speech function following this period revealed severely reduced range and speed of lingual movement, moderately reduced range and speed of labial movement, consonant imprecision, strained-strangled vocal quality, hypernasality, reduced breath support for speech, slow speech rate, monopitch, and moderately reduced speech intelligibility.

Physiological assessment also revealed wide-ranging motor speech subsystem dysfunction, incorporating reduced lung volumes and capacities as well as reduced abdominal excursion during speech, laryngeal hyperfunction, velopharyngeal insufficiency, and reduced labial and lingual strength and endurance.

Clinical Management Plan

A multisystem approach was again adopted in the rehabilitation of Max's speech, involving a combination of behavioral and instrumental treatment techniques. Consistent with the ICF, his presenting motor speech deficit was considered in relation to structural and functional impairments, imposed activity limitations and participation restrictions as well as manipulable contextual factors. Refer to Table 65-7 for the proposed rehabilitation schedule. Furthermore, longitudinal monitoring of Max's speech and language abilities was considered pivotal in maximizing educational and, subsequently, vocational potential as he continued to mature from adolescence into adulthood.

ASSESSMENT AND TREATMENT OF LANGUAGE IMPAIRMENTS IN TBI

In addition to impairments in motor speech functioning, TBI during adulthood or childhood can affect language functioning by disrupting the established or emerging neural structures underpinning proficient cognitive-linguistic processing or the future development thereof. Among the most influential developments that changed how language outcomes following TBI are investigated today have been publications highlighting the unique characteristics of language breakdown in the TBI population (150). It is now widely accepted that language deficits following TBI cannot be reliably assessed using traditional aphasia test batteries that focus on the form of language rather than providing data on an individual's overall communicative competence in real life (151,152). Consequently, there is an ongoing trend to explore novel assessment methods that are sensitive to the unique language impairments that can arise following TBI. This includes dynamic and ecologically valid behavioral techniques as well as neuroimaging and neurophysiological methods.

Language Impairments in TBI: Characteristics and Clinical Features

Most people who sustain TBI have residual communication problems that can occur irrespective of the severity of the injury (153). Although primary language skills are generally intact, more complex language processes requiring a high level of cognitive manipulation are frequently impaired (19). Competence in communication is achieved by a complex interplay between effortless cognitive and linguistic processing, social perception, and executive functions such as planning, initiating, organizing, self-monitoring, and directing

TABLE 65-6 Multisystem Approach to the Rehabilitation of Moderate Spastic Dysarthria Following TBI in an Adult: Jacob

TREATMENT GOAL	METHOD

• *Reducing impairment in body structure and function*
Remediate physiological dysfunction within motor speech sub-systems
   ○ Enhance coordination of chest wall movements during speech
   ○ Remediate hyperadduction of vocal folds
   ○ Increase velopharyngeal competence
 	
   ○ Increase strength and range of labial and lingual movements
	➤ Kinematic instrumentation to offer visual feedback of chest wall movement
	➤ Chewing/yawn-sigh, gentle voice onset techniques
	➤ Use of Nasometer® to provide visual feedback of nasalance during speech
	➤ Isometric and isotonic lip and tongue exercises

• *Reducing activity limitations and participation restrictions*
Enhance speech intelligibility
   ○ Modify stress and intonation patterns
   ○ Increase speech rate
   ○ Enhance articulatory precision
Maximizing communicative success across a range of communication environments
   ○ Increasing communication partner awareness of conversational topics and contextual cues
   ○ Repairing communication breakdowns
 	
   ○ Capitalizing on situational and environmental recompense to maximize effectiveness of communication
	➤ Contrastive stress and intonation drills
	➤ PACER technique
	➤ Articulation drills
	
	➤ Practice routinely identification of contextual cues and establishment of topic of conversation.
	➤ Clarify if communication partner has comprehended intended message and provide strategies for communication partners to request clarification.
	➤ Limit communicative interactions when fatigued and maximize interaction when energy levels are at their peak; avoid noisy environments.

• *Manipulating contextual factors* *Enhancing opportunities for participation across social and vocational contexts* ○ Providing information to family/friends/workmates pertaining to nature of communicative disability and strategies to enhance communicative effectiveness within social and vocational environments.	➤ Provide resources outlining the cause and nature of presenting communication deficit; strategies to maximize communicative success with unfamiliar communication partners (e.g., sitting in front of partner, requesting clarification in the event of a misunderstood message). ➤ Provide assistance in communicatively taxing situations (e.g., board meetings, face to face client contact).

Note: References pertaining to individual treatment techniques may be located in Tables 65-3, 65-4, and 65-5.

attention (154). All of these factors contribute to the human ability to use language flexibly to meet the demands of a given situation. To varying degrees, all of the factors contributing to competent language use have been shown to be vulnerable to the neuropathology caused by TBI (e.g., 155,156), resulting in a pronounced heterogeneity of language outcomes.

Interactions with adults following TBI often leave communicative partners with the feeling that they are tangential, disorganized, off-target, unable to understand social cues, humor, irony, figurative language, to get the "gist" out of a story, and to grasp the intentionality of others (18,19, 157,158). Further characteristics include inappropriate levels of self-disclosure, prosody, affect, topic selection and maintenance, perseveration, self-focus, difficulties with the generation of comments and questions to promote conversation, and tactlessness (159,160). Difficulties are evident in everyday social situations because the individual who lacks communication skills also lacks the tools necessary for effective interpersonal behavior, which is a crucial prerequisite for academic achievement, social integration, and good quality of life (4,160).

These functional deficits are recognized as significant factors in determining the resumption of former life roles, interests, employment, and daily activities at the same functional level (161) because they may reduce the individual's ability to establish and maintain interpersonal relationships (162). In addition, concrete thinking reflecting difficulties with using language flexibly and inefficient learning of new language result in impaired abstract language comprehension and interpretation of ambiguity (151,163), which may lead to frequent misunderstandings and socially unskilled behavior (164).

It is now widely established, therefore, that rather than presenting with specific impairments in primary language skills, adults who sustain TBI typically encounter disruptions to a wide range of social, cognitive, and executive functions (152,165). Proficient language use is dependent on the interplay between these functions, and minor breakdowns in a combination of these components or even a single component can pervasively influence communicative competence. The exact relationship between structural pathology and behavioral outcome is yet to be fully established.

TABLE 65-7 Multisystem Approach to the Rehabilitation of Moderate Spastic Dysarthria Following TBI in a Child: Max

TREATMENT GOAL	METHOD
• *Reducing impairment in body structure and function* *Remediate physiological dysfunction within motor speech subsystems* ○ Increase strength, range, and speed of labial and lingual movements ○ Increase breath support for speech ○ Remediate hyperadduction of vocal folds ○ Enhance velopharyngeal closure	➤ Isometric and isotonic lip and tongue exercises; timed alternate motion exercises ➤ Inspiratory checking technique ➤ Chewing, yawn-sigh, and gentle voice onset techniques ➤ Use of accelerometer to provide visual biofeedback during nasal/nonnasal contrasts
• *Reducing activity limitations and participation restrictions* *Enhance speech intelligibility* ○ Enhance articulatory precision ○ Increase speech rate and enhance pitch variation	➤ Articulation drills ➤ Speech Viewer® to provide auditory and visual feedback, rate and pitch parameters during speech tasks
Maximizing communicative success across a range of communication environments ○ Increasing communication partner awareness of conversational topics ○ Repairing communication breakdowns ○ Capitalizing on situational and environmental recompense to maximize effectiveness of communication	➤ Max to consistently orient communication partner to topic of conversation and to maximize use of contextual cues (e.g., environmental props) ➤ Clarify if communication partner has comprehended intended message and offer revisions when needed ➤ Write message if not understood ➤ Avoid noisy environments; utilize friends and family to assist in communicative interactions with unfamiliar partners or in unfamiliar environments
• *Manipulating contextual factors* *Enhancing opportunities for participation across social and educational contexts* ○ Providing information to family or friends or teachers pertaining to nature of communicative disability and strategies to enhance communicative effectiveness within social and educational environments	➤ Provide resources outlining: the cause and nature of presenting communication deficit; strategies to maximize communicative success with unfamiliar communication partners (e.g., ask for clarification if Max's speech is unable to be understood, ask him to write messages in the event of communication breakdown, move to a quiet environment, affirm comprehension of conversational topic with close friends) ➤ Oral assessment items/debating (e.g., English orations may be written by Max and tape recorded by family member/friend for class presentation) ➤ Usage of flash cards for scoring when umpiring a game of tennis

Note: References pertaining to individual treatment techniques may be located in Tables 65-3, 65-4, and 65-5.

Terminology Associated With Language Impairment in TBI

In addition to the realization that traditional aphasia language test batteries fail to reliably assess an individual's overall functional communicative competence following TBI, there is the acknowledgement that traditional aphasia terminology likewise fails to adequately describe the functional communication deficits following injury. Thus, the term cognitive-communication impairment has recently been advocated to describe the unique communication profile observed in individuals after injury (166). The application of this term reflects the interplay between linguistic aspects of communication such as semantics, syntax, and metalinguistic awareness, and nonlinguistic cognitive functions such as attention, memory, perception, and executive skills (166).

Assessment of Language Skills in TBI

Although primary language skills typically present with minor or no impairment post-TBI, deficits often become apparent on more complex language skills, which are more demanding of metalinguistic skill, controlled processing, and semantic manipulations (18,19,167). Adults with a history of TBI tend to display difficulties when performing tasks requiring controlled word retrieval, lexico-semantic manipulations, the comprehension of complex auditory information, the interpretation of figurative language, and pragmatic language use (18). In some cases, nonetheless, primary functions such as word retrieval during confrontation naming have also been found to be susceptible to impairment (19,23).

Consequently, language assessment batteries need not only to include tests that evaluate primary language processes but also tests designed to examine the integrity of linguistic skills during complex and linguistically demanding tasks (19). Table 65-8 provides an overview of currently employed primary and high-level language tests—standardized and nonstandardized—that research has proven to be sensitive in discriminating between TBI and control research participants and/or have been recommended by the Academy of Neurologic Communication Disorders and Sciences Practice Guidelines Group (ANCDS) (151). For an in-depth evaluation of language functioning following TBI, it is recommended that 1 or more tests from each of the language domains listed be included because all of these domains have been found to be susceptible to impairment in the TBI population. Some of the listed tests provide assessment of multiple cognitive-linguistic domains that are susceptible to impairment post-TBI.

Although standardized tests are suitable for the assessment of single word and sentence processing, by design, many of these tests are limited in their strength to provide information on real-life language functioning (ecological validity), which is based on effortless discourse comprehension and production during oftentimes challenging conditions (e.g., background noise, changes in prosody) that differ from the structured, supportive environment established during testing (151,168). An accumulating body of evidence has highlighted that TBI can lead to disruptions in all aspects of discourse processing and production, such as story grammar, coherence, thematic unity, amount and accuracy of information or content, and propositional analyses (see 152 for a review). Thus, in line with recent guidelines published by the ANCDS (151), it is recommended that dynamic measures of discourse processing (152,168) and social skills (169) using a combined approach involving standardized and nonstandardized procedures be included. Formal, standardized measures are recommended for the identification of strengths and weaknesses at the level of impairment (151,170), whereas informal, nonstandardized measures are recommended for the evaluation of proficiency of language use in challenging real-world settings beyond what contemporary standardized tests allow to assess (151,152,170).

Additionally, although still in its infancy, it is safe to assume that the application of advanced neuroimaging and neurophysiological techniques will play an important role in the future assessment of language functioning, as well as in the monitoring of outcomes following intervention. By implementing novel and established techniques to map neural correlates of intact or impaired language functioning, these techniques have the potential to facilitate the identification of subtle deviations in neural language structures and their functioning. Thus, they might prove to be applicable as sensitive biomarkers of immediate and long-term language functioning, providing powerful tools to complement behavioral language assessment information.

Advances in Neuroimaging Techniques Following TBI: Investigating Early Biomarkers of Later Language Outcomes

As outlined earlier, recent advances in neuroimaging techniques have led to an increased understanding of the neural correlates of language functioning in typically developing individuals (90) and in individuals who have sustained TBI (181). Although conventional neuroimaging methods such as routine MRI and CT scans lack the sensitivity to detect the microscopic white matter lesions that are the hallmark pathology of closed head injuries (182), diffusion MRI tractography methods allow the sensitive quantification and lo-

TABLE 65-8 Recommended Linguistic Assessment Battery: Adult TBI

TYPE OF TEST	ASSESSMENT TOOL	ASSESSMENT DOMAIN
Standardized tests of primary language functioning	□ Neurosensory Comprehensive Examination for Aphasia (NCCEA) (171) □ Western Aphasia Battery—Revised (WAB-R) (172) □ Boston Naming Test—Second Edition (173)	Comprehensive batteries Word retrieval
Standardized tests of high-level cognitive-linguistic skills and pragmatics	□ NCCEA Verbal Fluency subtest (171) □ The Word Test 2 (TWT-2) (174) □ Test of Language Competence—Expanded (TLC-E) (175) □ WAB-R (172) □ The Revised Token Test (176) □ Wiig and Semel Test of Linguistic Concepts (177)	Verbal fluency lexico-semantic manipulation Comprehension of complex auditory information
	□ Communication Activities of Daily Living—Second Edition (CADL-2) (178) □ TLC-E (175) □ The Right Hemisphere Language Battery (179) □ The American Speech Language Hearing Association Functional Assessment of Communication Skills in Adults (180) □ CADL-2 (178)	Nonliteral language skills Social language skills
Nonstandardized assessment methods of discourse and pragmatic skills	□ Assessing monologic and conversational discourse measures including productivity, efficiency, story grammar, content accuracy and organization, coherence, and topic management (152) □ Interpreting videotaped conversational exchanges: judging speakers' emotions, beliefs, intentions, and identifying sarcasm and lies (154)	Discourse skills Pragmatic skills

calization of disruptions in the neural language pathways and thus link structural outcomes in these pathways to behavioral profiles (181).

Because of the potential of this technique to detect white matter lesions that would previously be overlooked, and the relatively short amount of time required to acquire diffusion MRI data, diffusion MRI tractography has become a highly popular tool in the investigation of clinical populations such as individuals with TBI (181). For example, in mTBI, diffusion MRI tractography has been reported to reveal disruptions in callosal white matter that were correlated with the severity of postconcussion symptoms, whereas conventional MRI scans and CT scans did not indicate any anomalies (e.g., 183).

Among the neural pathways, the corpus callosum, which allows information exchange between the two brain hemispheres, is selectively vulnerable to the impact of TBI, especially in children and adolescents (91). With recent findings highlighting the importance of efficient interhemispheric communication during complex linguistic processes such as metaphor interpretation (184), future research investigating how corpus callosum white matter integrity correlates with high-level linguistic skills holds potential to identify structural biomarkers of behavioral language performance. The same rationale underlies the need to investigate this link throughout the entire neural language network, such as frontotemporoparietal structures, which are significantly involved in language processing (90,185) and which, like the corpus callosum, are particularly vulnerable to the insults associated with TBI.

An improved understanding of how the structural presentation of a given language pathway correlates with immediate and long-term language outcomes will be particularly beneficial in the early detection of neural insults that might put children at risk for later language impairments. A recent study has highlighted that proficient adult language use is associated with the recruitment of the later maturing dorsal pathway connecting Broca's pars orbitalis Brodmann Area (BA) 44 to superior temporal areas, rather than the reliance on the earlier-maturing ventral pathway connecting Broca's pars triangularis (BA 45) to superior temporal regions seen in children (186). Thus, as an example, the early detection of diffuse axonal damage sustained to the dorsal frontotemporal connections might aid in identifying children whose neural disposition might prevent them from switching to the use of those neural pathways associated with proficient language use. It has been reported that following TBI, children tend to employ lower level strategies when summarizing or condensing information (187), which might be indicative of a persisting reliance on early-maturing strategies and a failure to switch to proficient levels—structurally and functionally. In addition to these benefits, diffusion MRI tractography also holds significant potential as an objective, sensitive marker of speech therapy–induced plasticity in the neural language pathways (188).

FMRI research has provided support for the hypothesis that a breakdown in higher level linguistic processing is associated with a disruption in frontal lobe functioning. FMRI investigations during strategic clustering for verbal recall (156) and novel metaphor processing (155) have shown that individuals who have sustained TBI fail to activate dorsolat-eral-prefrontal (156) and left inferior frontal (155) areas to the extent observed in healthy control participants. These findings were congruent with behavioral deficits in TBI participants reported for both tasks, and the authors concluded that a functional decoupling of frontal structures from other active brain regions during language tasks that require strategic and abstract thinking might be present.

One of the few studies investigating neural activation patterns during language processing in children following TBI reported a significant association between the fMRI blood-oxygen-level dependent (BOLD) signal in perisylvian language areas and performance on language-specific neuropsychological tests (189), even after controlling for potential confounders such as level of executive functioning. Future fMRI research will be helpful in investigating more specifically how TBI affects neural processing characteristics during various language tasks in children and adults and how activity patterns are related to immediate and later behavioral language outcomes. Furthermore, recent findings by Laatsch and colleagues (190) showed that fMRI provides a sensitive neurobiological measure of change following therapy for mTBI, highlighting its potential as a tool for monitoring neural changes associated with language intervention programs.

Although diffusion MRI tractography and fMRI are ideally suited to the detection and localization of structural and functional deviations in the neural language networks, the recording of event-related potentials (ERPs) during language processing using electroencephalography (EEG) provides a powerful tool for the sensitive detection of language processing deviations following TBI. ERP recordings allow the online mapping of neural language processing within the millisecond range, thereby outperforming the temporal resolution of fMRI. Considering the fact that ERP recordings have played a major role in advancing scientific insight into neural language processing characteristics in typically developing individuals (e.g., 191) or clinical populations, such as dyslexic (192) or aphasic (193) individuals, it is surprising that very few studies have implemented this technique in the investigation of neural language processing characteristics following TBI to date.

By comparing the N400 ERP component involved in semantic processing, Münte and Heinze (194) showed that 2 years after a severe closed head injury, patients with TBI exhibited deviations in the timing and amplitude of their N400 response to terminal words of true sentences, semantically primed words, and recognized words in comparison to a group of matched-control participants. The authors suggested that the language processing deviations in former patients with TBI might result from difficulties in integrating incoming linguistic stimuli with the previous context. The N400 component has long been established as a sensitive measure of semantic memory use during language comprehension, providing insight into the efficiency of language processes relying on widespread multimodal networks within the millisecond range (see 195 for a review). In the face of the often widespread, diffuse axonal damage caused by closed head injuries, ERP recordings might prove to be a sensitive measure to map subtle changes in the efficiency of language processing that might not have been discovered using behavioral methods.

From a developmental perspective, an increased understanding of how pediatric TBI can affect neural language processing and how subsequent language development relates to early ERP findings holds the potential to provide a sensitive tool for the timely identification of children whose neural activity during language processing indicates a risk for later language impairment. In their landmark study on the link between early N400 characteristics and later language functioning in children, Friedrich and Friederici (196) showed that age-adequate expressive language skills at the age of 30 months were present in children who had shown an N400 effect during a semantic integration task completed at the age of 19 months. In contrast, children with later poor expressive language skills who have an increased risk for the development of specific language impairment did not show an N400 at the age of 19 months.

Future research is needed to establish the specific link between early ERP findings post-TBI and later language development. Friedrich and Friederici's (196) findings warrant the inclusion of ERP recordings to the neuroimaging techniques that have the potential to improve current language assessment sensitivity and, ultimately, to improve future rehabilitative care for individuals following TBI. Findings by Popescu and colleagues (197) showing that N400 effects were modified from deviant to typical activation following a 5-week narrative-based language intervention in children with primary language disorder additionally highlights the potential of ERP recordings to be used as a sensitive biomarker of intervention outcomes.

Cognitive-Communication Impairments in TBI: Approaches to Treatment

Although cognitive-communication impairment is unique to the TBI population, homogeneity is not a feature of the TBI population's communicative abilities (198). Preinjury communication skill, learning style, the personality of the individual (199), and sociocultural background (200) highlight the need to tailor programs to the individual's needs (see e.g., 190) and also present challenges for the clinician in developing effective interventions for individuals with TBI (201).

Considering the heterogeneous presentation of communicative outcomes post-TBI, the ICF (94) is ideally suited to investigating key issues in the rehabilitative needs of individuals with cognitive-communication impairment because it uses a framework suitable for approaching intervention planning for the functional alleviation of the difficulties. Within the context of cognitive-communication impairment, the ICF framework allows an investigation of the influence of capacity, performance, and context such as the environmental and personal factors that influence the individual's ability to undertake activities (150). Relevant personal treatment goals are subsequently devised to reduce impairment in body function and structure resulting from the injury, increase activity and participation in life situations and maximize skills across a range of environments by exploiting successes and reducing barriers through the manipulation of the environment (e.g., family, friends, employment) (94).

Given the reciprocal interactions between communication, cognition and the psychosocial factors resulting from TBI, a comprehensive and integrated program of rehabilitation that includes intensive individual and group therapy is necessary. Interventions embedded into meaningful activities and settings are a prerequisite as decontextualized interventions may have limited generalization to the changing demands of day-to-day interactions (150). Interventions delivered in various relevant contexts, such as the individual's home, school, workplace, and community, will optimize functional gains in active participation in daily encounters. As engagement in life's activities in terms of number of activities, and the range of communicative activities, and the number of communicative partners is often limited, intervention should focus on increasing participation.

Cognitive Rehabilitation for Cognitive-Communication Impairment

Cognitive rehabilitation is a standard component of medical care subsequent to TBI (202) and requires an integrated approach comprised of individually tailored interventions delivered with multidisciplinary support (203). Cognitive rehabilitation aligns with the ICF framework (94) to decrease the impact of impairment, increase everyday functional abilities, and reduce barriers to participation. Rather than focusing on discrete impairments, this approach targets specific behaviors and activities as well as the factors that influence performance (204). Intervention typically involves 2 basic approaches, that is, direct restoration and compensation strategy training. Both approaches are used simultaneously in rehabilitation (205).

Direct restoration is believed to be associated with restitution/restoration of function via reconnection of pathways. This approach is based on the assumption that damaged neural circuits can be retrained if they have been partially or substantially spared after injury. In direct restoration, the effect of the deficit following injury is reduced through systematic exposure to specific cognitive activities targeting specific neural processes (206).

Compensation strategy training, in contrast, is thought to be associated with the reorganization, redistribution, and use of adjacent and remote neural circuits following injury (190). This approach is based on the assumption that the individual will learn to compensate for deficits via the acquisition of newly learned strategies using retrained cognitive skills and functional reorganization of the brain. Compensation strategy training involves the substitution of a function through the development of new compensatory skills in order to enhance participation in everyday tasks and activities (207).

Communicative abilities are influential in determining the success of social and vocational reintegration subsequent to TBI (208), hence speech-language pathology rehabilitation programs focus on decreasing the effect of identified impairments, often through the inclusion of social skill training (209). Interventions should be integrated and directed toward achieving goals in school (210), workplaces (211), community (212), and family and social engagement (213) because individuals receiving an integrated therapy composed of individually tailored interventions achieve the greatest overall improvements in functioning (214). Speech-language pathology rehabilitation may include direct restoration, compensatory strategy training, process-specific intervention, behavioral approaches, pharmacological, and multimodal programs that are delivered through a range of service delivery models (see 210,212,213,215,216). Advances in technology have introduced the potential for computer-based interventions (217) and telerehabilitation with TBI (218). The ultimate goal of all intervention approaches is the highest level of communicative participation in everyday living (150). Tables 65-9 and 65-10 provide examples of restorative and compensatory intervention approaches used by speech-language pathologists with TBI clients.

There is no consensus regarding the timing and duration of rehabilitation sessions. Some argue that intervention should be instigated as soon as medical stability is achieved (206). But Kennedy and Turkstra (204) concluded there was no evidence of treatment efficacy for interventions delivered during the acute stage postinjury. Delaying the provision of

TABLE 65-9 Restorative Treatment of Cognitive-Communication Impairment Following TBI

DEFICIT	THERAPY TASK
Difficulties with word retrieval	➤ Phonetic and semantic word retrieval tasks (219)
Difficulties with lexico-semantic manipulation	➤ Generating synonyms and antonyms (220) ➤ Word-definition matching (220) ➤ Semantic categorization activities (220) ➤ Elaborative encoding (221)
Difficulties with comprehension of complex linguistic information	➤ Interpreting abstract expressions (220) ➤ Proverb/metaphor explanation (220) ➤ Interpreting figurative expressions (222) ➤ Predicting outcomes (222) ➤ Discriminating between fact and opinion (222) ➤ Following instructions of increasing length and complexity (220)
Disorganization of verbal expression	➤ Sequencing tasks (220) ➤ Story retelling (220) ➤ Development of story grammars establishing relationships between characters and events (222) ➤ Narrative production using specified schemas (220) ➤ Scripting of social interactions (152)
Social skill deficits	➤ Decoding facial expressions ➤ Increasingly complex guided tasks to shape social behavior ➤ Greetings and topic selection ➤ Develop self-awareness skills although videotape viewing/reviewing ➤ Problem solving ➤ Community practice (Replicable program: Group Interactive Structured Treatment for Social Competence [GIST] [209], formerly known as Social Skills and Traumatic Brain Injury: A Workbook for Group Treatment [223–225])

TABLE 65-10 Compensatory Strategy Training for the Treatment of Cognitive-Communication Impairment Following TBI

DEFICIT	STRATEGY
Word/name retrieval problems	➤ Development of cueing strategies (e.g., assistive devices) (226) ➤ Organizational strategies to facilitate retrieval (227)
Word retrieval problems with natural tendency to circumlocute	➤ Use circumlocution as a means of facilitating word retrieval (220)
Verbosity with good insight into maladaptive behavior	➤ Frequent clarification with communication partner that they are following conversation (220) ➤ Cueing and monitoring using assistive technology for cognition (216) ➤ Video training for functional verbal tasks (228) ➤ Development of internal cueing and self-monitoring skills (152,209,223) ➤ Internal and external cues (e.g., requests for repetition of information) (158)
Verbosity with poor insight into maladaptive behavior	➤ Obtain assistance of external communication partner regarding relevance of verbal output (220)
Ineffective functional communication	➤ Identify where communication breakdowns occur (i.e., in what environments), formulate communication strategies for use in those environments, and develop skills by way of functional therapy tasks (e.g., role playing) (220) ➤ Strategies to assist with planning and monitoring behavior (e.g., **WSTC: W**hat am I doing? What's the best **S**trategy? **T**ry it. **C**heck it out) (225) ➤ Develop strategies with communicative partners to facilitate effective communication (213)

intervention may be preferable because the individual may, over time, develop insight and awareness of their communicative difficulties (229). Arousal, attentional capacity, and fatigue (230,231) will dictate duration of therapy sessions. Pharmacological boosting of arousal (206) and increasing inhibitory control of perseverative behaviors may be instigated (232) to optimize participation.

Clinicians must avail themselves to empirical research to support their clinical decision making in determining interventions for the patient with TBI (233). The heterogeneity of the TBI presentation, however, prevents the application of a generic approach to intervention (234) and population-based intervention standards hold little validity for the individual clinician making decisions about which therapy approach to implement (235).

Although randomized controlled trials offering supporting evidence of efficacy are needed to make clinical judgments for the selection of interventions, a broad definition of evidence, including for instance case studies and single case experimental designs, may need to be adopted. There is, however, no substitute for clinical judgment in determining the appropriate assessment and interventions for an individual presenting with communication deficits following TBI (236). Ultimately, the speech-language pathologist's decision will be based on evidence-based clinical practice, combined with clinical judgment, anecdotal evidence from colleagues' opinions and experiences, and from their own personal experiences of what has been successfully implemented previously with other similar presentations (237).

Several features judged to contribute to the efficacy of cognitive rehabilitation for cognitive-communication impairment have been identified through a randomized controlled trial of a replicable social skills intervention program (see 209,223). The use of interdisciplinary co-group leaders; an emphasis of self-awareness and self-assessment; individual goal setting; the use of the group to foster interaction, feedback, and problem solving; and a focus on generalization of skills through the involvement of family, friends, and multisite activities were integral to successful outcomes as measured by improved communication skills and self-rated quality of life measures that were maintained at 6 months follow-up (208).

Outcome following interventions may be tempered by physical, cognitive and emotional factors, educational level, IQ, attentional control deficits, and awareness of deficits (205). Outcome measures, nonetheless, should be a core component of interventions (205) and should include behavioral outcome measures that reveal the effectiveness of intervention regarding maintenance and generalization of treatment. Such measures should not be restricted to performance indicators from neuropsychological tests and formal language assessments but need to include functional outcomes such as quality of life measures or indicators of everyday skills (190,208,238). Additionally, considering the trends toward involving neuroimaging and neurophysiological techniques in the assessment and monitoring of clinical populations, these techniques have the potential to provide sensitive complementary outcome measures for the future monitoring of neural changes post-intervention (188,190).

Language Outcomes Following Mild TBI

The identification of mTBI as an ongoing health issue has been triggered by the impairments reported in veterans who have experienced mTBI during recent wars in Iraq and Afghanistan (e.g., 239,240) and by accumulating evidence for negative sequelae resulting from single and repeated sports-related concussions (241). It is now well understood that even people who have sustained mTBI and are rendered unconscious for as little as 5 minutes after injury can have some degree of brain damage (242). Many of these individuals have DAI (182), suggesting that mTBI may, fundamentally, not be that different to more severe TBI presentations (243). mTBI may therefore have the potential to affect the neural structures underlying competent communication

(23). Indeed, several studies addressing language skills following mTBI have reported residual deficits in lexical access and complex lexico-semantic manipulation at 6 months (23) and 22 months (157) post-mTBI, which were hypothesized to result from underlying damage to the neural connectivity of the frontal lobe. The identification of higher order language deficits reflecting cognitive-communication impairment suggests the impact of mTBI on language functions may indeed be similar to that of more severe injuries.

The reliable assessment of language impairments following mTBI provides a major challenge to speech-language pathologists because of the often subtle nature of the impairment (244). Overall, the currently available literature and assessment methods in language outcomes following mTBI are limited in their ability to reliably describe and assess the language profiles of this unique population. A recent study by Docking and Murdoch (245) presenting preinjury and postinjury language skills in an adolescent indicated a declining trend in expressive and higher level language skills even though norm-referenced postinjury scores remained within the normal range. Their findings highlight the need for informed assessments in this population because their subclinical language deficits often remain undetected. Further research addressing language outcomes, rehabilitative needs, and the feasibility of intervention programs in mTBI is needed to identify those who are at risk for ongoing impairments and to provide informed speech pathology care for individuals following mTBI (244).

Current research in sports-related mTBIs, encompassing preinjury and postinjury measures, is applying innovative techniques to assess the risk for chronic traumatic encephalopathy posed by repetitive mild injury, where several variables including the location of impact, magnitude of the injury, and the frequency of the injuries are analyzed through on-field monitoring during high-impact sports such as football (246), with the potential for application in other high-impact sports such as boxing.

It is anticipated that speech-language pathologists have a potentially valuable role in the future educational and/or vocational rehabilitation of individuals with mTBI because the precise nature of the neurocognitive sequelae associated with the presentation continue to be unravelled. Furthermore, ascertaining whether or not the communicative sequelae of mTBI are responsive to traditional cognitive rehabilitation techniques is yet to be determined.

Pediatric Considerations

Children who sustain TBI present a particular clinical challenge compared to adults with comparable injury because an early brain injury can affect the delicate, emerging brain structures that are essential for the future development of proficient language skills. In contrast to the long-held view that an early age at injury is associated with more preferable outcomes, young children who sustain TBI have been reported to be particularly vulnerable to impairments at basic linguistic functions, discourse skills (for review on language outcomes following pediatric TBI, see 247), and communicative competence (see 248). Outcomes following TBI in adolescents, on the other hand, typically resemble the higher order linguistic and discourse deficits reported in adults (187,249), leaving primary skills largely intact.

The diffuse injuries associated with TBI have the capacity to disrupt widespread neural networks, which, in the maturing brain, might lead to a disruption of skills that emerge during a rapid stage of development (250,251). Skills established at the time of injury, however, tend to be resilient to disruption. Children may fail to make age-appropriate gains in developmental skills following injury (198), suggesting an inability to acquire new skills following pediatric TBI (250). The inability to acquire new knowledge at an age-appropriate rate is possibly caused by the presence of consolidation deficits in verbal learning following TBI (252). Other issues, such as the possible coexistence of developmental learning problems are peculiar to the pediatric population and further influence the long-term outcome profile of the child with TBI (220).

The evaluation of language skills subsequent to pediatric TBI requires the careful consideration of the current developmental state and preinjury level of functioning as reported by teachers and family members. The aim of the assessment should be the early identification of language deficits, which, if left untreated, might impact on a child's progression through later developmental milestones. Contemporary research is emphasizing the use of discourse measures when evaluating communicative competence in children, following the same reasoning that has led adult TBI research to explore novel, dynamic discourse-based methods, rather than relying on word or sentence-level-based standardized tests. The work of Chapman and colleagues (253,254) has shown that children with a history of TBI have difficulties in identifying the central meaning out of a story and organizing narrative summaries. Similar to the presentation of adults, these findings suggest impairment in executive functions involved in organizing and planning verbal output, which might be caused by disruptions in frontal lobe connectivity to proximate and distant brain regions involved in cognitive-linguistic processing (154).

Consequently, language comprehension and production following pediatric TBI should be assessed at the level of primary and high-level language functioning, including measures of complex language skills that challenge the child beyond the single-word level. Table 65-11 provides an overview of standardized and nonstandardized tests that have been reported to be sensitive to the communication impairments resulting from pediatric TBI and/or have been recommended by the ANCDS (151,170).

By and large, the same cognitive rehabilitation intervention approaches may be applied to the rehabilitation of communication deficits as a consequence of TBI sustained during the developmentally formative childhood years. Nonetheless, therapeutic hierarchies must focus not only on the remediation of skills already established at the time of injury, but also take into account the future acquisition of developmental language processes in order to permit the prompt identification and remediation of potential difficulties.

The risk of later emerging difficulties throughout adolescence and adulthood on tasks that draw on higher order cognitive skills (264,199) offers strong support for the long-term evaluation of developmental trajectories and management by speech-language pathologists following pediatric TBI. Liaison with teachers or school-based intervention programs provides the platform for the promotion of an individualized educational and vocational plan (270). Final conclusions about the impact of the TBI on language and general cognitive functioning can only be drawn once children enter adulthood (271).

TABLE 65-11   Recommended Linguistic Assessment Battery: Pediatric TBI

TYPE OF TEST	ASSESSMENT TOOL	ASSESSMENT DOMAIN
Standardized tests of primary language functioning	□ Clinical Evaluation of Language Fundamentals—Fourth Edition (257)	Comprehensive battery
	□ Peabody Picture Vocabulary Test—Fourth Edition (258)	Receptive language skills
	□ Expressive One-Word Picture Vocabulary Test (259)	Expressive language skills
	□ The Hundred Pictures Naming Test (260)	Word retrieval
Standardized tests of high-level cognitive-linguistic skills and pragmatics	□ Controlled Oral Word Association Test (261)	Verbal fluency
	□ TLC-E (175)	Lexico-semantic manipulation
	□ TWT-2 (174)	
	□ Test of Auditory Comprehension of Language—Third Edition (262)	Comprehension of complex auditory information
	□ TLC-E (175)	Nonliteral language skills
	□ The Bus Story Test (263)	Discourse skills
	□ Test of Problem Solving (265,266)	Verbal problem solving
Nonstandardized assessment methods of discourse and pragmatic skills	□ Assessing cohesion and coherence using a rating scale for well-formedness of narrative summaries (253–256,264)	Discourse comprehension and production
	□ Storytelling task: "The Lobster and the Crab Story" (267)	
	□ Assessing the ability to link events with outcomes in common social situations (268)	Pragmatic skills
	□ Answering questions about beliefs and first- and second-order intentionality (269)	
	□ Choosing one explanation out of three that explains why a given scene or sentence is funny (249)	

Case Reports: Clinical Management of Cognitive-Communication Impairments Following TBI

The following vignettes present clinical management plans relative to the rehabilitation of cognitive-communication impairment following TBI in a 30-year-old adult and a 7-year-old child.

Case 1: Cognitive-Communication Impairment Following TBI Sustained in Adulthood

Case History

Greg is a 30-year-old hotel concierge who sustained a TBI as the result of a motor vehicle accident. He experienced loss of consciousness for less than 30 minutes at the scene of the accident. He was oriented to place and time, but complained of dizziness for approximately 20 minutes following the incident. He was taken to the Department of Emergency Medicine (DEM) and monitored. CT scan failed to identify any focal neurological damage, and he was discharged into the care of his wife within 6 hours of the accident. At the routine postinjury Rehabilitation Medicine follow-up phone call the next day, his wife reported he was fully recovered, had not complained of headaches, but was excessively fatigued.

Greg returned to work 2 weeks after the accident. His work entails answering the phone, taking bookings, greeting guests, providing local information to tourists, and settling accounts. Greg reported that his previously enjoyable job has become difficult to complete, his wife has complained of his forgetfulness with names and words, and his work supervisor has noted a decrease in performance and suggested Greg consider changing to a behind-the-scene job at the hotel—something Greg is not willing to consider. Greg, with his wife's support, requested a speech-language pathology assessment.

Language Profile

Greg's primary level language was found to be largely intact but with evidence of word retrieval deficits. He exhibited a natural inclination to use circumlocution as a means of facilitating word retrieval. High-level language deficits were evident, with particular difficulties noted with humor appreciation. Greg often demonstrated overfamiliarity and inappropriate communicative behaviors with unfamiliar communication partners, but had some insight pertaining to these character traits.

Clinical Management Plan

Based on the previous information and directed by Greg's expressed personal and vocational needs and goals, a functional plan for his rehabilitation was devised 3 months subsequent to injury. The therapy plan—based on the ICF framework and aimed at increasing functional abilities and reducing barriers to participation—encompassed a range of service delivery models including individual-, group-, and community-based therapy sessions as well as training of communicative partners (Table 65-12). Greg's next performance review at work was established as a functional outcome measure to monitor his progress through therapy.

Case 2: Cognitive-Communication Impairment Following TBI Sustained in Childhood

Case History

Suzannah is a 7-year-old primary school student who sustained a TBI as the result of a fall from a tree onto the ground. According to a witness, Suzannah was unresponsive for about 1 minute following the fall. On arrival of the paramedics, she was responsive but disorientated. A CT scan at the DEM showed a small, uncomplicated occipital fracture with no cerebral anomalies. Suzannah was admitted to the hospital for monitoring and treatment of her skull fracture. She

---

TABLE 65-12 Rehabilitation Plan for Cognitive-Communication Impairment Following Adult TBI: Greg

GOAL	METHOD
• To develop and automatically apply strategies to assist with name and word retrieval to reduce frustration experienced by Greg and his wife	➤ Phonetic and semantic word retrieval tasks ➤ Train to use his circumlocutionary skills as a means of facilitating retrieval
• Develop appropriate conversational style with unfamiliar communication partners with particular reference to hotel guests	➤ Discuss various communication contexts, appropriate and inappropriate communication styles ➤ Group therapy for role-playing, video analysis to judge appropriateness of conversational style ➤ Provide opportunities for role-playing and video feedback to enhance self-monitoring skills
• Reduce verbosity in conversation at home with wife and at work with colleagues and hotel guests	➤ Discuss content categories such as relevant, irrelevant, and embellishment. ➤ Discuss narrative structure. ➤ Identify presence and absence of content within conversations. ➤ Establish self-initiated cues to reduce verbosity. ➤ Develop the strategy of thinking in bullet-points to effectively impart requested behavior succinctly. ➤ Train communicative partners (wife, work colleagues) to provided external feedback, cueing, and topic focus. ➤ Provide opportunities for role-playing, video feedback, and group therapy.

could not remember the events leading up to her hospitalization and remained disorientated and irritable for the following 2 days with occasional vomiting. She recovered well and was discharged 2 weeks following the incident. Suzannah's parents received an information brochure about the impact of a head injury on a child's behavior and were invited to contact the rehabilitation team should they notice any changes in her behavior.

Upon return to school, anecdotal teacher reports praised Suzannah's overall functioning, yet a decline in her previously superior ability to tell stories was noted. This decline was most evident during oral presentations, where the teacher noticed a breakdown in her ability to sequence the order of her thoughts, which led to considerable personal frustration. The teacher also reported that Suzannah's ability to follow verbal instructions and to remember the task at hand was inferior to her previous levels. To help reduce Suzannah's frustration and to seek guidance about how to help their daughter, her parents sought formal language assessment with a speech-language pathologist. The evaluation was completed 3 months following the injury.

Language Profile

Suzannah's primary level language was largely intact and her use of pragmatic language skills was appropriate. However, her conversational and narrative discourse was marked by disorganized sequencing during story recall and describing familiar procedures. Her ability to comprehend auditory instructions of increasing length and complexity was found to be within the low average range.

Clinical Management Plan

Guided by the assessment results and directed by the need to optimize Suzannah's classroom performance, a functional plan aligned with the framework for intervention promoted by the ICF was devised. This plan included a teacher resource kit to foster appropriate classroom strategies and the provision of parent training in the delivery of a home program (Table 65-13). Suzannah's next 2 school reports were agreed upon as the measure to evaluate her functional outcome. Ongoing monitoring and support of Suzannah's further development by teachers and parents was recommended in order to facilitate her progression through milestones of later language development.

KEY CLINICAL POINTS

1. TBI of various severities is frequently associated with motor speech and language impairments that can have a debilitating impact on an individual's social functioning and reintegration into former life roles.
2. Motor speech impairments can affect all aspects of speech production, which warrants the inclusion of comprehensive perceptual, physiological, and acoustic assessment methods prior to determining treatment priorities and the individual tailoring of treatments designed for a given individual.
3. Effective treatment of motor speech impairments can involve a combination of behavioral, instrumental, and, in some cases, prosthetic or surgical approaches.
4. Language deficits post-TBI are unique to the TBI population and differ from the impairments seen in focal lesions (e.g., stroke), whereby primary language skills remain relatively intact and impairments manifest in higher order language functions and the pragmatic use of language in social situations.
5. Appropriate evaluation of language skills post-TBI necessitates a combination of sufficiently sensitive standardized, nonstandardized, and neuroimaging or neurophysiological techniques allowing the identification of strengths and weaknesses, an evaluation of real-world language functioning in discourse processing and comprehension and the mapping of neural correlates of language functioning to complement behavioral techniques.
6. Treatment of communication deficits post-TBI should focus on functional aspects of communication and include patient-directed functional outcome measures.

TABLE 65-13 Rehabilitation Plan for Cognitive-Communication Impairment Following Pediatric TBI: Suzannah

GOAL	METHOD
• Reduce discourse sequencing difficulty and relieve resulting frustration	➤ Encouragement and rewarding of retelling past events such as weekend activities or holidays
	➤ Story retell/story construction tasks using pictures to facilitate sequencing of events
	➤ Training sequencing when recounting simple and complex stepwise activities, such as getting ready for school in the morning, or steps involved in a crafting project
• Enhance comprehension of complex auditory instructions	➤ Proverb/metaphor explanation
	➤ Following instructions of increasing length and complexity
	➤ Provide opportunities to request repetition of information when information is not understood (e.g., role-play in classroom environment)
	➤ Provide classroom strategies: request teachers to write complex instructions down when not understood, provide written summary of each class, engage in tutorials at the end of a lesson to ensure Suzannah has understood the main concepts, regular contact with parents and monitoring of academic progress.

KEY REFERENCES

1. Catroppa C, Anderson V. Recovery and predictors of language skills two years following pediatric traumatic brain injury. *Brain Lang.* 2004;88(1):68–78.
2. Coelho C, Ylvisaker M, Turkstra LS. Nonstandardized assessment approaches for individuals with traumatic brain injuries. *Semin Speech Lang.* 2005;26(4):223–241.
3. Larkins B. The application of the ICF in cognitive-communication disorders following traumatic brain injury. *Semin Speech Lang.* 2007;28(4):334–342.
4. Murdoch BE. Acquired childhood aphasia subsequent to childhood traumatic brain injury. In: Murdoch BE, ed. *Handbook of Acquired Communication Disorders in Childhood.* San Diego, CA: Plural Publishing; 2011:65–103.
5. Murdoch BE. Speech-language disorders associated with traumatic brain injury. In: Murdoch BE, ed. *Acquired Speech and Language Disorders: A Neuroanatomical and Functional Neurological Approach.* 2nd ed. Oxford, UK: Wiley-Blackwell; 2010:118–152.

References

1. Murdoch BE. *Acquired Speech and Language Disorders: A Neuroanatomical and Functional Neurological Approach.* 2nd ed. Oxford, UK: Wiley-Blackwell; 2010.
2. Murdoch BE, Theodoros DG. Introduction: epidemiology, neuropathophysiology, and medical aspects of traumatic brain injury. In: Murdoch BE, Theodoros DG, eds. *Traumatic Brain Injury: Associated Speech, Language and Swallowing Disorders.* San Diego, CA: Singular Thomson Learning; 2001:1–23.
3. Najenson T, Sazbon L, Fiselzon J, Becker E, Schechter I. Recovery of communicative functions after prolonged traumatic coma. *Scand J Rehabil Med.* 1978;10(1):15–21.
4. Murdoch BE. *Handbook of Acquired Communication Disorders in Childhood.* San Diego, CA: Plural Publishing Inc.; 2011.
5. Malkmus DD. Community re-entry: cognitive-communication intervention within a social skill context. *Topics Lang Disord.* 1989;9(2):50–66.
6. Brooks N, McKinlay W, Symington C, Beattie A, Campsie L. Return to work within the first seven years of severe head injury. *Brain Inj.* 1987;1(1):5–19.
7. Murdoch BE, Theodoros DG, eds. *Traumatic Brain Injury: Associated Speech, Language and Swallowing Disorders.* San Diego, CA: Singular Thomson Learning; 2001.
8. Theodoros DG, Murdoch BE, Goozée JV. Dysarthria following traumatic brain injury: incidence, recovery and perceptual features. In: Murdoch BE, Theodoros DG, eds. *Traumatic Brain Injury: Associated Speech, Language and Swallowing Disorders.* San Diego, CA: Singular Thomson Learning; 2001:27–52.
9. Sarno MT, Buonaguro A, Levita E. Characteristics of verbal impairment in closed head injury patients. *Arch Phys Med Rehabil.* 1986;67(6):400–405.
10. Ewing-Cobbs L, Fletcher JM, Levin HS. Neurobehavioural sequelae following head injury in children: educational implications. *J Head Trauma Rehabil.* 1986;1:57–65.
11. Yorkston KM, Beukelman DR. Motor speech disorders. In: Beukelman DR, Yorkston KM, eds. *Communication Disorders Following Traumatic Brain Injury.* Texas: Pro-Ed; 1991:251–315.
12. Dworkin JP, Abkarian GG. Treatment of phonation in a patient with apraxia and dysarthria secondary to severe closed head injury. *J Med Speech Lang Pathol.* 1997;4:105–115.
13. Lundgren K, Helm-Estabrooks N, Klein R. Stuttering following acquired brain damage: a review of the literature. *J Neurolinguistics.* 2010;23(5):447–454.
14. Helm-Estabrooks N, Hotz G. Sudden onset of "stuttering" in an adult: neurogenic or psychogenic? *Semin Speech Lang.* 1998;19(1):23–29.
15. Lebrun Y, Bijleveld H, Rousseau JJ. A case of persistent neurogenic stuttering following a missile wound. *J Fluency Disord.* 1990;15:251–258.
16. Ludlow C, Rosenberg J, Salazar A, Grafman J, Smutok M. Site of penetrating brain lesions causing chronic acquired stuttering. *Ann Neurol.* 1987;22(1):60–66.
17. Jokel R, De Nil LF, Sharpe AK. Speech disfluencies in adults with neurogenic stuttering associated with stroke and traumatic brain injury. *J Med Speech Lang Pathol.* 2007;15(3):243–261.
18. Hinchliffe FJ, Murdoch BE, Theodoros DG. Linguistic deficits in adults subsequent to traumatic brain injury. In: Murdoch BE, Theodoros DG, eds. *Traumatic Brain Injury: Associated Speech, Language and Swallowing Disorders.* San Diego, CA: Singular Thomson Learning; 2001:199–222.
19. Hinchliffe FJ, Murdoch BE, Chenery HJ. Towards a conceptualization of language and cognitive impairment in closed-head injury: use of clinical measures. *Brain Inj.* 1998;12(2):109–132.
20. Sarno M. The nature of the verbal impairment after closed head injury. *J Nerv Ment Dis.* 1980;168(11):685–692.
21. Lustig AP, Tompkins CA. An examination of severity classification measures and subject criteria used for studies on mild paediatric traumatic brain injury. *J Med Speech Lang Pathol.* 1998;6:13–25.
22. Ferguson RJ, Mittenberg W, Barone DF, Schneider B. Postconcussion syndrome following sports-related head injury: expectation as etiology. *Neuropsychology.* 1999;13(4):582–589.
23. Wong MN, Murdoch BE, Whelan BM. Language disorders subsequent to mild traumatic brain injury (mTBI): evidence from four cases. *Aphasiology.* 2010;24(20):1155–1169.
24. Levin HS. Aphasia in closed head injury. In: Sarno M, ed. *Acquired Aphasia.* New York, NY: Academic Press; 1981:427–463.
25. Sarno M, Levin HS. Speech and language disorders after closed head injury. In: Darby JK, ed. *Speech Evaluation in Neurology: Adult Disorders.* New York, NY: Grune and Stratton; 1985:323–339.
26. Aten JL. Spastic dysarthria: revising understanding of the disorder and speech treatment procedures. *J Head Trauma Rehabil.* 1988;3(2):63–73.
27. Brand HA, Matsko TA, Avart HN. Speech prosthesis retention problems in dysarthria: case report. *Arch Phys Med Rehabil.* 1988;69(3, pt 1):213–214.
28. Enderby P, Crowe E. Long-term recovery patterns of severe dysarthria following head injury. *Br J Disord Commun.* 1990;25(3):341–354.
29. Kuehn DP, Wachtel JM. CPAP therapy for treating hypernasality following closed head injury. In: Till JA, Yorkston KM, Beukelman DR, eds. *Motor Speech Disorders: Advances in Assessment and Treatment.* Baltimore, MD: Paul H. Brookes Publishing; 1994:207–212.
30. Light J, Beesley M, Collier B. Transition through multiple augmentative communication systems: a three year case study of a head injured adolescent. *Aug Alternat Commun.* 1988;4:2–14.
31. Nemec RE, Cohen K. EMG biofeedback in the modification of hypertonia in spastic dysarthria: case report. *Arch Phys Med Rehabil.* 1984;65(2):103–104.
32. Simmons N. Acoustic analysis of ataxia dysarthria: an approach to monitoring treatment. In: Berry W, ed. *Clinical Dysarthria.* San Diego, CA: College-Hill Press; 1983:283–294.
33. Workinger M, Netsell R. Restoration of intelligible speech 13 years post-head injury. *Brain Inj.* 1992;6(2):183–187.
34. Groher M. Language and memory disorders following closed head trauma. *J Speech Hear Res.* 1977;20(2):212–223.
35. Kent RD, Netsell R, Bauer L. Cineradiographic assessment of articulatory mobility in the dysarthrias. *J Speech Hear Disord.* 1975;40(4):467–480.
36. Lehiste I. Some acoustic characteristics of dysarthric speech. *Bibl Phonet.* 1965;2:1–124.
37. Netsell R, Daniel B. Dysarthria in adults: physiologic approach in rehabilitation. *Arch Phys Med Rehabil.* 1979;60(11):502–508.
38. von Cramon D. Traumatic mutism and the subsequent reorganization of speech functions. *Neuropsychologia.* 1981;19(6):801–805.
39. Yorkston KM, Beukelman DR. Ataxic dysarthria: treatment sequence based on intelligibility and prosodic considerations. *J Speech Hear Disord.* 1981;46(4):398–404.

40. Yorkston KM, Beukelman DR, Minifie FD, Sapir S. Assessment of stress patterning in dysarthric speakers. In: McNeil MR, Aronson AE, Rosenbeck JC, eds. *The Dysarthrias: Physiology, Acoustics, Perception, Management*. San Diego, CA: College-Hill Press; 1984: 131–162.

41. Theodoros DG, Murdoch BE, Chenery HJ. Perceptual speech characteristics of dysarthric speakers following severe closed head injury. *Brain Inj*. 1994;8(2):101–124.

42. Marquardt TP, Stoll J, Sussman H. Disorders of communication in traumatic brain injury. In: Bigler ED, ed. *Traumatic Brain Injury: Mechanisms Damage, Assessment, Intervention, and Outcome*. Austin, TX: Pro-Ed; 1990:181–205.

43. Langfitt TW, Obrist WD, Alavi A, et al. Computerized tomography, magnetic resonance imaging, and positron emission tomography in the study of head trauma. Preliminary observations. *J Neurosurg*. 1986;64(5):760–767.

44. Netsell R, Lefkowitz D. Speech production following traumatic brain injury: clinical and research implications. *American Speech-Language-Hearing Association Special Interests Division: Neurophysiology and Neurogenic Speech and Language Disorders*. 1992;2:1–8.

45. Wilson JT, Hadley DM, Weidmann KD, Teasdale GM. Intercorrelations of lesions detected by magnetic resonance imaging after closed head injury. *Brain Inj*. 1992;6(5):391–399.

46. Thompson-Ward EC. Spastic dysarthria. In: Murdoch BE, ed. *Dysarthria: A Physiological Approach to Assessment and Treatment*. Cheltenham, UK: Stanley Thornes Ltd; 1998:205–241.

47. Duffy JR. Spastic dysarthria. In: Duffy JR, ed. *Motor Speech Disorders: Substrates, Differential Diagnosis, and Management*. St. Louis, MO: Mosby; 1995:128–144.

48. Duffy JR. Hyperkinetic dysarthria. In: Duffy JR, ed. *Motor Speech Disorders: Substrates, Differential Diagnosis, and Management*. St. Louis, MO: Mosby; 1995:189–221.

49. Theodoros DG, Murdoch BE. Hyperkinetic dysarthria. In: Murdoch BE, ed. *Dysarthria: A Physiological Approach to Assessment and Treatment*. Cheltenham, UK: Stanley Thornes Ltd; 1998:314–336.

50. Darley FL, Aronson AE, Brown JR. *Motor Speech Disorders*. Philadelphia, PA: W.B. Saunders Company; 1975.

51. Zraick RI, LaPointe LL. Hyperkinetic dysarthria. In: McNeil MR, ed. *Clinical Management of Sensorimotor Speech Disorders*. New York, NY: Theime; 1997:249–260.

52. Duffy JR. Hypokinetic dysarthria. In: Duffy JR, ed. *Motor Speech Disorders: Substrates, Differential Diagnosis and Management*. St. Louis, MO: Mosby; 1995:166–188.

53. Theodoros DG, Murdoch BE. Hypokinetic dysarthria. In: Murdoch BE, ed. *Dysarthria: A Physiological Approach to Assessment and Treatment*. Cheltenham, UK: Stanley Thornes Ltd; 1998:266–313.

54. Darley FL, Aronson AE, Brown JR. Clusters of deviant speech dimensions in the dysarthrias. *J Speech Hear Res*. 1969;12(3):462–496.

55. Duffy JR. Flaccid dysarthria. In: Duffy JR, ed. *Motor Speech Disorders: Substrates, Differential Diagnosis, and Management*. St. Louis, MO: Mosby; 1995:99–127.

56. Murdoch BE, Thompson-Ward EC. Flaccid dysarthria. In: Murdoch BE, ed. *Dysarthria: A Physiological Approach to Assessment and Treatment*. Cheltenham, UK: Stanley Thornes Ltd; 1998:176–204.

57. Duffy JR. Ataxic dysarthria. In: Duffy JR, ed. *Motor Speech Disorders: Substrates, Differential Diagnosis, and Management*. St. Louis, MO: Mosby; 1995:145–165.

58. Brown JR, Darley FL, Aronson AE. Ataxic dysarthria. *Int J Neurol*. 1970;7(2):302–318.

59. Murdoch BE, Theodoros DG. Ataxic dysarthria. In: Murdoch BE, ed. *Dysarthria: A Physiological Approach to Assessment and Treatment*. Cheltenham, UK: Stanley Thornes Ltd; 1998:241–265.

60. Yorkston KM, Beukelman DR. *Assessment of Intelligibility of Dysarthric Speech*. Austin, TX: Pro-Ed; 1981.

61. Cahill LM, Murdoch BE, Theodoros DG. Dysarthria following traumatic brain injury in childhood. In: Murdoch BE, Theodoros DG, ed. *Traumatic Brain Injury: Associated Speech, Language, and Swallowing Disorders*. San Diego, CA: Singular Thomson Learning; 2001: 121–153.

62. Morgan AT, Liégeois F. Re-thinking diagnostic classification of the dysarthrias: A development perspective. *Folia Phoniatr Logop*. 2010; 62(3):120–126.

63. van Mourik M, Catsman-Berrevoets CE, Paquier PF, Yosef-Bak E, van Dongen HR. Acquired childhood dysarthria: review of its clinical presentation. *Pediatr Neurol*. 1997;17(4):299–307.

64. Murdoch BE, Hudson-Tennent LJ. Speech disorders in children treated for posterior fossa tumours: ataxic and developmental features. *Eur J Disord Commun*. 1994;29(4):379–397.

65. FitzGerald FJ, Murdoch BE, Chenery HJ. Multiple sclerosis: associated speech and language disorders. *Aust J Hum Commun Disord*. 1987;15:15–33.

66. Fisher HB, Logemann JA. *The Fisher-Logemann Test of Articulation Competence*. Boston, MA: Houghton Mifflin Co.; 1971.

67. Enderby P. *Frenchay Dysarthria Assessment*. San Diego, CA: College-Hill Press; 1983.

68. Theodoros DG, Murdoch BE. Laryngeal dysfunction following traumatic brain injury. In: Murdoch BE, Theodoros DG, eds. *Traumatic Brain Injury: Associated Speech, Language and Swallowing Disorders*. San Diego, CA: Singular Thomson Learning; 2001:89–109.

69. Thompson-Ward EC, Theodoros DG. Acoustic analysis of dysarthric speech. In: Murdoch BE, ed. *Dysarthria: A physiological Approach to Assessment and Treatment*. Cheltenham, UK: Stanley Thornes Ltd; 1998:102–129.

70. Colton R, Casper JK. The voice history, examination and testing. In: Colton R, Casper JK, eds. *Understanding Voice Problems: A Physiological Perspective for Diagnosis and Treatment*. 2nd ed. Baltimore, MD: Williams & Williams; 1996:186–240.

71. Colton R, Conture EG. Problems and pitfalls of electroglottography. *J Voice*. 1990;4:10–24.

72. Hanson DG, Gerratt BR, Karin RR, Berke GS. Glottographic measures of vocal fold vibration: an examination of laryngeal paralysis. *Laryngoscope*. 1988;98(5):541–548.

73. Theodoros DG, Murdoch BE. Laryngeal dysfunction in dysarthric speakers following severe closed-head injury. *Brain Inj*. 1994;8(8): 667–684.

74. Hammen V, Yorkston KM. Effect of instruction on selected aerodynamic parameters in subjects with dysarthria and control subjects. In: Till JA, Yorkston KM, Beukelman DR, eds. *Motor Speech Disorders: Advances in Assessment and Treatment*. Baltimore, MD: Paul H. Brookes Publishing; 1994:161–173.

75. Boren HG, Kory RC, Synder JC. The Veterans-Administration Army cooperative study of pulmonary function. II. The lung volume and its subdivisions in normal men. *Am J Med*. 1966;41:96–114.

76. Kory RC, Callahan R, Boren HG. The Veterans Administration-Army cooperative study of pulmonary function. I. Clinical spirometry in normal men. *Am J Med*. 1961;30:243–258.

77. Hoit JD, Hixon TJ. Body type and speech breathing. *J Speech Hear Res*. 1986;29(3):313–324.

78. Solomon NP, Hixon TJ. Speech breathing in Parkinson's disease. *J Speech Hear Res*. 1993;36(2):294–310.

79. Stathopoulos ET, Sapienza C. Respiratory and laryngeal function of women and men during vocal intensity variation. *J Speech Hear Res*. 1993;36(1):64–75.

80. Hinton VA, Luschei ES. Validation of modern miniature transducer for measurement of interlabial contact pressure during speech. *J Speech Hear Res*. 1992;35(2):245–251.

81. Murdoch BE, Attard MD, Ozanne AE, Stokes PD. Impaired tongue strength and endurance in developmental verbal dyspraxia: a physiological analysis. *Eur J Disord Commun*. 1995;30(1):51–64.

82. Robin DA, Somodi CB, Luschei ES. Measurement of tongue strength and endurance in normal and articulation disordered subjects. In: Moore CA, Yorkston KM, Beukelman DR, editors. *Dysarthria and Apraxia of Speech: Perspectives on Management*. Baltimore, MD: Paul H. Brookes Publishing; 1991:173–184.

83. Murdoch BE. Physiological assessment. In: Lowit A, Kent R, eds. *Assessment of Motor Speech Disorders*. San Diego, CA: Plural Publishing Inc.; 2011:39–74.

84. Theodoros DG, Murdoch BE. Velopharyngeal dysfunction following traumatic brain injury. In: Murdoch BE, Theodoros DG, eds. *Traumatic Brain Injury: Associated Speech, Language and Swallowing Disorders*. San Diego, CA: Singular Thomson Learning; 2001:75–88.

85. Horri Y. An accelerometric approach to nasality measurement: a preliminary report. *Cleft Palate J*. 1980;17(3):254–261.

86. Horri Y. An accelerometric measure as a physical correlate of perceived hypernasality in speech. *J Speech Hear Res.* 1983;26(3): 476–480.

87. Dalston RM, Seaver EJ. Relative values of various standardized passages in the nasometric assessment of patients with velopharyngeal impairment. *Cleft Palate Craniofac J.* 1992;29(1):17–21.

88. Dalston RM, Warren DW, Dalston ET. A preliminary investigation concerning the use of nasometry in identifying patients with hyponasality and/or nasal airway impairment. *J Speech Hear Res.* 1991; 34(1):11–18.

89. Nellis JL, Neiman GS, Lehman JA. Comparison of nasometer and listener judgments of nasality in the assessment of velopharyngeal function after pharyngeal flap surgery. *Cleft Palate Craniofac J.* 1992; 29(2):157–163.

90. Glasser MF, Rilling JK. DTI tractography of the human brain's language pathways. *Cereb Cortex.* 2008;18(11):2471–2482.

91. Ewing-Cobbs L, Prasad MR, Swank P, et al. Arrested development and disrupted callosal microstructure following pediatric traumatic brain injury: relation to neurobehavioral scores. *Neuroimage.* 2008; 42(4):1305–1315.

92. Levin HS, Wilde EA, Chu Z, et al. Diffusion tensor imaging in relation to cognitive and functional outcome of traumatic brain injury in children. *J Head Trauma Rehabil.* 2008;23(4):197–208.

93. Theodoros DG, Murdoch BE. Treatment of dysarthria following traumatic brain injury. In: Murdoch BE, Theodoros DG, eds. *Traumatic Brain Injury: Associated Speech, Language and Swallowing Disorders.* San Diego, CA: Singular Thomson Learning; 2001:155–196.

94. World Health Organization. International classification of functioning, disability and health (ICF). Geneva, Switzerland: WHO; 2001.

95. Yorkston KM. Treatment efficacy: dysarthria. *J Speech Hear Res.* 1996;39(5):S46–S57.

96. Bellaire K, Yorkston KM, Beukleman DR. Modification of breath patterning to increase naturalness of a mildly dysarthric speaker. *J Commun Disord.* 1986;19(4):271–280.

97. Beukleman DR, Yorkston K. A communication system for the severely dysarthric speaker with an intact language system. *J Speech Hear Disord.* 1977;42(2):265–270.

98. Bouglé F, Ryalls J, Le Dorze G. Improving fundamental frequency modulation in head trauma patients: a preliminary comparison of speech-language therapy conducted with and without IBM's Speech Viewer. *Folia Phoniatr Logop.* 1995;47(1):24–32.

99. Draizar D. Clinical EMG feedback in motor speech disorders. *Arch Phys Med Rehabil.* 1984;65(8):481–484.

100. Goldstein P, Ziegler W, Vogel M, Hoole P. Combined palatal-lift and EPG-feedback therapy in dysarthria: a case study. *Clin Linguist Phonet.* 1994;8(3):210–218.

101. Murdoch BE, Pitt G, Theodoros DG, Ward EC. Real-time continuous feedback in the treatment of speech breathing disorders following childhood traumatic brain injury: report of one case. *Pediatr Rehabil.* 1999;3(1):5–20.

102. Murdoch BE, Sterling DK, Theodoros DG. Physiological rehabilitation of disordered speech breathing in dysarthric speakers following severe closed head injury. In: Fourez J, Page N, eds. *Treatment Issues and Long-term Outcomes. Proceedings of the 18th Annual Brain Impairment Conference, Hobart.* Brisbane, Australia: Australian Academic Press; 1995:137–146.

103. Stewart DS, Rieger WJ. A device for the management of velopharyngeal incompetence. *J Med Speech Lang Pathol.* 1994;2(2):149–155.

104. Stringer AY. Treatment of motor aprosodia with pitch biofeedback and expression modelling. *Brain Inj.* 1996;10(8):583–590.

105. Kearns KP, Simmons NN. The efficacy of speech-language pathology intervention: motor speech disorders. *Semin Speech Lang.* 1990; 11:273–295.

106. Theodoros DG, Thompson-Ward EC. Treatment of dysarthria. In: Murdoch BE, ed. *Dysarthria: A Physiological Approach to Assessment and Treatment.* Cheltenham, UK: Stanley Thornes Ltd; 1998: 130–175.

107. Volin RA. Clinical applications of biofeedback. *Am Speech Hear Assoc.* 1993:43–51.

108. Garber SR, Burzynski CM, Vale C, Nelson R. The use of visual feedback to control vocal intensity and nasalization. *J Commun Disord.* 1979;12(5):399–410.

109. Prosek RA, Montgomery AA, Walden BE, Schwartz DM. EMG biofeedback in the treatment of hyperfunctional voice disorders. *J Speech Hear Disord.* 1978;43(3):282–294.

110. Rubow R. Role of feedback, reinforcement, and compliance on training and transfer in biofeedback-based rehabilitation of motor speech disorders. In: McNeil MR, Rosenbeck JC, Aronson AE, eds. *The Dysarthrias: Physiology, Acoustics, Perception, Management.* San Diego, CA: College-Hill Press; 1984:207–230.

111. Froeschels E. Chewing method as therapy; a discussion with some philosophical conclusion. *Arch Otolaryngol.* 1952;56(4):427–434.

112. Boone DR. *The Voice and Voice Therapy.* 2nd ed. Englewood Cliffs, NJ: Prentice Hall; 1977.

113. Froeschels E, Kastein S, Weiss DA. A method of therapy for paralytic conditions of the mechanisms of phonation, respiration, and glutination. *J Speech Hear Disord.* 1955;20(4):365–370.

114. Boone DR, McFarlane SC. *The Voice and Voice Therapy.* 4th ed. Englewood Cliffs, NJ: Prentice Hall; 1988.

115. Ramig LO, Bonitati CM, Lemke JH, Horri Y. Voice treatment for patients with Parkinson's disease: development of an approach and preliminary efficacy data. *J Med Speech Lang Pathol.* 1994;2: 191–209.

116. Netsell R, Rosenbeck JC. Treating the dysarthrias. In: Darby JK, ed. *Speech and Language Evaluation in Neurology: Adult Disorders.* Orlando, FL: Grune and Stratton; 1995:363–392.

117. Netsell R, Hixon TJ. Inspiratory checking in therapy for individuals with speech breathing dysfunction. *J Am Speech Hear Assoc.* 1992; 34:152.

118. Rosenbeck JC, LaPointe LL. The dysarthrias: description, diagnosis and treatment. In: Johns D, ed. *Clinical Management of Neurogenic Communication Disorders.* Boston, MA: Little, Brown & Co.; 1991: 97–152.

119. Dworkin JP, Johns DF. Management of velopharyngeal incompetence in dysarthria: a historical review. *Clin Otolaryngol Allied Sci.* 1980;5(1):61–74.

120. Yorkston KM, Beukelman DR, Bell KR. *Clinical Management of Dysarthric Speakers.* Boston, MA: Little, Brown & Co.; 1988.

121. Scott S, Caird FI. Speech therapy for Parkinson's disease. *J Neurol Neurosurg Psychiatry.* 1983;46(2):140–144.

122. Johnson JA, Pring TR. Speech therapy and Parkinson's disease: a review and further data. *Br J Disord Commun.* 1990;25(2):183–194.

123. Berry WR, Goshorn EL. Immediate visual feedback in the treatment of ataxia dysarthria: a case study. In: Berry WR, ed. *Clinical Dysarthria.* San Diego, CA: College-Hill Press; 1983:253–265.

124. Thompson EC, Murdoch BE. Treatment of speech breathing disorders in dysarthria: a biofeedback approach. In: Conference proceedings of Australian Association of Speech and Hearing; 1995; Brisbane, Australia. Melbourne, Australia: Australian Association of Speech and Hearing; 1995.

125. Siegel-Sadewitz VL, Shprintzen RJ. Nasopharyngoscopy of the normal velopharyngeal sphincter: an experiment of biofeedback. *Cleft Palate J.* 1982;19(3):194–200.

126. Witzel MA, Tobe J, Salyer K. The use of nasopharyngoscopy biofeedback therapy in the correction of inconsistent velopharyngeal closure. *Int J Pediatr Otorhinolaryngol.* 1988;15(2):137–142.

127. Künzel H. First applications of a biofeedback device for the therapy of velopharyngeal incompetence. *Folia Phoniatr.* 1982;34(2):92–100.

128. Hand CR, Burns MO, Ireland E. Treatment of hypertonicity in muscles of lip retraction. *Biofeedback Self Regul.* 1979;4(2):171–181.

129. Booker HE, Rubow RT, Coleman PJ. Simplified feedback in neuromuscular retraining: an automated approach using electromyographic signals. *Arch Phys Med Rehabil.* 1969;50(11):621–625.

130. Gallegos X, Medina R, Espinoza E, Bustamante A. Electromyographic feedback in the treatment of bilateral facial paralysis: a case study. *J Behav Med.* 1992;15(5):533–539.

131. Gibbon F, Dent H, Hardcastle W. Diagnosis and therapy of abnormal alveolar stops in speech-disordered child using electropalatography. *Clin Linguist Phonet.* 1993;7(4):247–267.

132. Hardcastle WJ, Morgan Barry RA, Clark CJ. Articulatory and voicing characteristics of adult dysarthric and verbal dyspraxic speakers: an instrumental study. *Br J Disord Commun.* 1985;20(3):249–270.

133. International Business Machines. *Speech Viewer: Guide de l'Utilisateur.* Paris, France: IBM; 1989.

134. Le Dorze G, Dionne L, Ryalls J, Julien M, Oullet L. The effects of speech and language therapy for a case of dysarthria associated with Parkinson's disease. *Eur J Disord Commun.* 1992;27(4):313–324.

135. Beukelman DR, Yorkston KM, Tice B. *Pacer/Tally.* Tucson, AZ: Communication Skill Builders; 1988.

136. Downie WW, Low JM, Lindsay DD. Speech disorder in parkinsonism—usefulness of delayed auditory feedback in selected cases. *Br J Disord Commun.* 1981;16(2):135–139.

137. Hanson WR, Metter EJ. DAF as instrumental treatment for dysarthria in progressive supranuclear palsy: a case report. 1980;45(2):268–276.

138. Hanson WR, Metter EJ. DAF speech rate modification in Parkinson's disease: a report of two cases. In: Berry WR, ed. *Clinical Dysarthria.* San Diego, CA: College-Hill Press; 1983:231–251.

139. Allan CM. Treatment of non fluent speech resulting from neurological disease—treatment of dysarthria. *Br J Disord Commun.* 1970;5(1):3–5.

140. Blitzer A, Brin MF, Fahn S, Lovelace RE. Localized injections of botulinum toxin for the treatment of focal laryngeal dystonia (spastic dysphonia). *Laryngoscope.* 1988;98(2):193–197.

141. Dedo HH. Recurrent laryngeal nerve section for spastic dysphonia. *Ann Otol Rhinol Laryngol.* 1976;85(4, pt 1):451–459.

142. May M, Beery Q. Muscle-nerve pedicle laryngeal reinnervation. *Laryngoscope.* 1986;96(11):1196–1200.

143. Ford CN, Martin DW, Warner TF. Injectable collagen in laryngeal rehabilitation. *Laryngoscope.* 1984;94(4):513–518.

144. Hammarberg B, Fritzell B, Schiratzki H. Teflon injection of 16 patients with paralytic dysphonia: perceptual and acoustic elevations. *J Speech Hear Disord.* 1984;49(1):72–82.

145. Isshiki N, Tanabe M, Sawada M. Arytenoid adduction for unilateral vocal cord paralysis. *Arch Otolaryngol.* 1978;104(10):555–558.

146. Gonzalez JB, Aronson AE. Palatal lift prosthesis for treatment of anatomic and neurologic palatopharyngeal insufficiency. *Cleft Palate J.* 1970;7:91–104.

147. Netsell R. Construction and use of bite-block for the evaluation and treatment of speech disorders. *J Speech Hear Disord.* 1985;50(1):103–106.

148. Helm NA. Management of palilalia with a pacing board. *J Speech Hear Disord.* 1979;44(3):350–353.

149. Beukelman DR, Yorkston K. Communication options for patients with brain stem lesions. Arch Phys Med Rehabil. 1978;59(7):337–340.

150. Larkins B. The application of the ICF in cognitive-communication disorders following traumatic brain injury. *Semin Speech Lang.* 2007; 28(4):334–342.

151. Turkstra L, Ylvisaker M, Coelho C. Practice guidelines for standardized assessment for persons with traumatic brain injury. *Journal of Medical Speech-Language Pathology.* 2005;13(2):ix–xxxviii.

152. Coelho CA. Management of discourse deficits following traumatic brain injury: progress, caveats, and needs. *Semin Speech Lang.* 2007; 28(2):122–135.

153. Kraus MF, Susmaras T, Caughlin BP, Walker CJ, Sweeney JA, Little DM. White matter integrity and cognition in chronic traumatic brain injury: a diffusion tensor imaging study. *Brain.* 2007;130(pt 10):2508–2519.

154. McDonald S. Frontal lobes and language. In: Stemmer B, Whitaker HA, eds. *Handbook of the Neuroscience of Language.* Oxford, UK: Elsevier; 2008:289–297.

155. Yang FG, Fuller J, Khodaparast N, Krawczyk DC. Figurative language processing after traumatic brain injury in adults: a preliminary study. *Neuropsychologia.* 2010;48(7):1923–1929.

156. Strangman GE, Goldstein R, O'Neil-Pirozzi TM, et al. Neurophysiological alterations during strategy-based verbal learning in traumatic brain injury. *Neurorehabil Neural Repair* 2009;23(3):226–236.

157. Whelan BM, Murdoch BE, Bellamy N. Delineating communication impairments associated with mild traumatic brain injury: a case report. *J Head Trauma Rehabil.* 2007;22(3):192–197.

158. Body R, Parker M. Topic repetitiveness after traumatic brain injury: an emergent, jointly managed behaviour. *Clin Linguist Phon.* 2005; 19(5):379–392.

159. Moran C, Gillon G. Inference comprehension of adolescents with traumatic brain injury: a working memory hypothesis. *Brain Inj.* 2005;19(10):743–751.

160. Kilov AM, Togher L, Grant S. Problem solving with friends: discourse participation and performance of individuals with and without traumatic brain injury. *Aphasiology.* 2009;23(5):584–605.

161. Ylvisaker M, Turkstra LS, Coelho C. Behavioral and social interventions for individuals with traumatic brain injury: a summary of the research with clinical implications. *Semin Speech Lang.* 2005; 26(4):256–267.

162. Ponsford J, Olver J, Ponsford M, Nelms R. Long-term adjustment of families following traumatic brain injury where comprehensive rehabilitation has been provided. *Brain Inj.* 2003;17(6):453–468.

163. King KA, Hough MS, Walker MM, Rastatter M, Holbert D. Mild traumatic brain injury: effects on naming in word retrieval and discourse. *Brain Inj.* 2006; 20(7):725–732.

164. Ylvisaker M, Szekeres SF, Feeney T. Communication disorders associated with traumatic brain injury. In: Chapey R, ed. *Language Intervention Strategies in Aphasia and Related Neurogenic Communication Disorders.* 4th ed. Philadelphia, PA: Lippincott Williams & Wilkins; 2001:745–808.

165. de Sousa A, McDonald S, Rushby J, Li S, Dimoska A, James C. Understanding deficits in empathy after traumatic brain injury: the role of affective responsivity. *Cortex.* 2011;47(2):526–535.

166. American Speech-Language-Hearing Association. Position statement: the role of speech-language pathologists in the identification, diagnosis, and treatment of individuals with cognitive-communicative impairments. *ASHA.* 1988;30(3):79.

167. Hanten G, Dennis M, Zhang L, et al. Childhood head injury and metacognitive processes in language and memory. *Dev Neuropsychol.* 2004;25(1–2):85–106.

168. Coelho C, Ylvisaker M, Turkstra LS. Nonstandardized assessment approaches for individuals with traumatic brain injuries. *Semin Speech Lang.* 2005;26(4):223–241.

169. McDonald S, Flanagan S. Social perception deficits after traumatic brain injury: interaction between emotion recognition, mentalizing ability, and social communication. *Neuropsychology.* 2004;18(3):572–579.

170. Turkstra LS, Coelho C, Ylvisaker M. The use of standardized tests for individuals with cognitive-communication disorders. *Semin Speech Lang.* 2005;26(4): 215–222.

171. Spreen O, Benton AL. *Neurosensory Centre Comprehensive Examination for Aphasia: Manual for Directions.* Victoria, BC: University of Victoria; 1969.

172. Kertesz A. *Western Aphasia Battery—Revised.* San Antonio, TX: Psychological Corporation; 2006.

173. Goodglass H, Kaplan E, Barresi B. *Boston Diagnostic Aphasia Examination.* 3rd ed. Austin, TX: Pro-Ed.; 2000.

174. Huisingh R, Bowers L, LoGiudice C, Orman J. *The Word Test 2.* East Moline, IL: LinguiSystems; 2005.

175. Wiig EH, Secord W. *Test of Language Competence—Expanded Edition.* San Antonio, TX: Psychological Corporation; 1989.

176. McNeil MM, Prescott TE. *The Revised Token Test.* Baltimore, MD: University Park Press; 1978.

177. Wiig EH, Semel E. Development of comprehension of logical grammatical sentences by grade school children. *Percept Mot Skills.* 1974; 38(1):171–176.

178. Holland A, Frattali C, Fromm D. *Communication Activities of Daily Living.* 2nd ed. Austin, TX: Pro-Ed; 1999.

179. Bryan K. *The Right Hemisphere Language Battery.* Southampton, UK: Far Communications; 1989.

180. Frattali CM, Holland AL, Thompson CK, Wohl C, Ferketic M. *The American Speech Language Hearing Association Functional Assessment of Communication Skills in Adults.* 2nd ed. Rockville, MD: American Speech Language Hearing Association; 2003.

181. Mao H, Polensek SH, Goldstein FC, Holder CA, Ni C. Diffusion tensor and functional magnetic resonance imaging of diffuse axonal injury and resulting language impairment. *J Neuroimaging.* 2007;17(4):292–294.

182. Gennarelli TA. Cerebral concussion and diffuse brain injuries. In: Cooper PR, ed. *Head Injury.* 2nd ed. Baltimore, MD: Williams and Wilkins; 1987:108–124.

183. Wilde EA, McCauley SR, Hunter JV, et al. Diffusion tensor imaging of acute mild traumatic brain injury in adolescents. *Neurology.* 2008; 70(12):948–955.

184. Schmidt GL, Seger GA. Neural correlates of metaphor processing: the roles of figurativeness, familiarity and difficulty. *Brain Cogn.* 2009;71(3):375–386.

185. Catani M. The connectional anatomy of language: recent contributions from diffusion tensor tractography. In: Johansen-Berg H, Behrens TE, eds. *Diffusion MRI: From Quantitative Measurement to In vivo Neuroanatomy.* Boston, MA: Academic Press; 2009:403–414.

186. Brauer J, Anwander A, Friederici AD. Neuroanatomical prerequisites for language functions in the maturing brain. *Cereb Cortex.* 2011;21(2):459–466. doi:10.1093/cercor/bhq108.

187. Dennis M, Barnes M. Comparison of literal, inferential, and intentional text comprehension in children with mild or severe closed head injury. *J Head Trauma Rehabil.* 2001;16(5):456–468.

188. Schlaug G, Marchina S, Norton A. Evidence for plasticity in white-matter tracts of patients with chronic Broca's aphasia undergoing intense intonation-based speech therapy. *Ann NY Acad Sci.* 2009; 1169:385–394.

189. Karunanayaka PR, Holland SK, Yuan W, et al. Neural substrate differences in language networks and associated language-related behavioral impairments in children with TBI: a preliminary fMRI investigation. *NeuroRehabilitation.* 2007;22(5):355–369.

190. Laatsch LK, Thulborn KR, Krisky CM, Shobat DM, Sweeney JA. Investigating the neurobiological basis of cognitive rehabilitation therapy with fMRI. *Brain Inj.* 2004;18(10):957–974.

191. Byrne JM, Connolly JF, MacLean SE, Dooley JM, Gordon KE, Beattie TL. Brain activity and language assessment using event-related potentials: development of a clinical protocol. *Dev Med Child Neurol.* 1999;41(11):740–742.

192. Bonte ML, Blomert L. Developmental dyslexia: ERP correlates of anomalous phonological processing during spoken word recognition. *Brain Res Cogn Brain Res.* 2004;21(3):360–376.

193. Kawohl W, Bunse S, Willmes K, Hoffrogge A, Buchner H, Huber W. Semantic event-related potential components reflect severity of comprehension deficit in aphasia. *Neurorehabil Neural Repair.* 2010; 24(3):282–289.

194. Münte TF, Heinze HJ. Brain potentials reveal deficits of language processing after closed head injury. *Arch Neurol.* 1994;51(5): 482–493.

195. Kutas M, Federmeier KD. Thirty years and counting: finding meaning in the N400 component of the event-related brain potential (ERP). *Annu Rev Psychol.* 2011;62:621–647.

196. Friedrich M, Friederici AD. Early N400 development and later language acquisition. *Psychophysiology.* 2006;43(1):1–12.

197. Popescu M, Fey ME, Lewine JD, Finestack LH, Popescu EA. N400 responses of children with primary language disorder: intervention effects. *NeuroReport.* 2009;20(12):1104–1108.

198. Catroppa C, Anderson V. Recovery and predictors of language skills two years following pediatric traumatic brain injury. *Brain Lang.* 2004;88(1):68–78.

199. Brenner LA, Dise-Lewis JE, Bartles SK, O'Brien SE, Godleski M, Selinger M. The long-term impact and rehabilitation of pediatric traumatic brain injury: a 50-year follow-up case study. *J Head Trauma Rehabil.* 2007;22(1):56–64.

200. Faleafa M. Community rehabilitation outcomes across cultures following traumatic brain injury. *Pac Health Dialog.* 2009;15(1):28–34.

201. Fager S, Hux K, Beukelman DR, Karantounis R. Augmentative and alternative communication use and acceptance by adults with traumatic brain injury. *Augment Altern Commun.* 2006;22(1):37–47.

202. McCrea M, Pliskin N, Barth J, et al. Official position of the Military TBI Task Force on the role of neuropsychology and rehabilitation psychology in the evaluation management, and research of military veterans with traumatic brain injury. *Clin Neuropsychol.* 2008;22(1): 10–26.

203. Cicerone KD, Azulay J, Trott C. Methodological quality of research on cognitive rehabilitation after traumatic brain injury. *Arch Phys Med Rehabil.* 2009;90(suppl 11):S52–S59.

204. Kennedy MR, Turkstra L. Group intervention studies in the cognitive rehabilitation of individuals with traumatic brain injury: challenges faced by researchers. *Neuropsychol Rev.* 2006;16(4):151–159.

205. Cicerone KD, Dahlberg C, Malec JF, et al. Evidence-based cognitive rehabilitation: updated review of the literature from 1998 through 2002. *Arch Phys Med Rehabil.* 2005;86(8):1681–1692.

206. Robertson IH, Murre JM. Rehabilitation of brain damage: brain plasticity and principles of guided recovery. *Psychol Bull.* 1999; 125(5):544–575.

207. Vanderploeg RD, Collins RC, et al. Practical and theoretical considerations in designing rehabilitation trials: the DVBIC cognitive-didactic versus functional-experiential treatment study experience. *J Head Trauma Rehabil.* 2006;21(2):179–193.

208. Dahlberg C, Hawley L, Morey C, Newman J, Cusick CP, Harrison-Felix C. Social communication skills in persons with post-acute traumatic brain injury: three perspectives. *Brain Inj.* 2006;20(4): 425–435.

209. Hawley L, Newman J. *Group Interactive Structured Treatment—GIST: For Social Competence.* Denver, CO: Author; 2008.

210. Feeney TJ. Structured flexibility: the use of context-sensitive self-regulatory scripts to support young persons with acquired brain injury and behavioral difficulties. *J Head Trauma Rehabil.* 2010;25(6): 416–425.

211. Dodson MB. A model to guide the rehabilitation of high-functioning employees after mild brain injury. *Work.* 2010;36(4):449–457.

212. McCormack E, Liddiard H. Home or away? Community rehabilitation following traumatic brain injury: a case report. *Physiother Res Int.* 2009;14(1):66–71.

213. Togher L, McDonald S, Code C, Grant S. Training communication partners of people with traumatic brain injury: a randomised controlled trial. *Aphasiology.* 2004;18(4):313–335.

214. Cicerone KD, Dahlberg C, Kalmar K, et al. Evidence-based cognitive rehabilitation: recommendations for clinical practice. *Arch Phys Med Rehabil.* 2000;81(12):1596–1615.

215. Luton LM, Reed-Knight B, Loiselle K, O'Toole K, Blount R. A pilot study evaluating an abbreviated version of the cognitive remediation programme for youth with neurocognitive deficits. *Brain Inj.* 2011;25(4):409–415.

216. Kirsch NL, Shenton M, Spirl E, Simpson R, Lopresti E, Schreckenghost D. An assistive-technology intervention for verbose speech after traumatic brain injury: a single case study. *J Head Trauma Rehabil.* 2004;19(5):366–377.

217. Egan J, Worrall L, Oxenham D. An internet training intervention for people with traumatic brain injury: barriers and outcomes. *Brain Inj.* 2005;19(8):555–568.

218. Brennan DM, Georgeadis AC, Baron CR, Barker LM. The effect of videoconference-based telerehabilitation on story retelling performance by brain-injured subjects and its implications for remote speech-language therapy. *Telemed J E Health.* 2004;10(2):147–154.

219. Thomas-Stonnell N, Johnson P, Schuller R, Jutai J. Evaluation of a computer-based program for remediation of cognitive-communication skills. *J Head Trauma Rehabil.* 1994;9(4):25–37.

220. Hinchliffe FJ, Murdoch BE, Theodoros DG. Treatment of cognitive-linguistic communication disorders following traumatic brain injury. In: Murdoch BE, Theodoros DG, eds. *Traumatic Brain Injury: Associated Speech, Language and Swallowing Disorders.* San Diego, CA: Singular Publishing; 2001:273–309.

221. Oberg L, Turkstra LS. Use of elaborative encoding to facilitate verbal learning after adolescent traumatic brain injury. *J Head Trauma Rehabil.* 1998;13(3):44–62.

222. Cannizzaro MS, Coelho CA. Treatment of story grammar following traumatic brain injury: a pilot study. *Brain Inj.* 2002;16(12): 1065–1073.

223. Hawley L, Newman J. *Social Skills and Traumatic Brain Injury: A Workbook for Group Treatment.* Denver, CO: Author; 2006.

224. Braden C, Hawley L, Newman J, Morey C, Gerber D, Harrison-Felix C. Social communication skills group treatment: a feasibility study for persons with traumatic brain injury and comorbid conditions. *Brain Inj.* 2010;24(11):1298–1310.

225. McDonald S, Tate R, Togher L, et al. Social skills treatment for people with severe, chronic acquired brain injuries: a multicenter trial. *Arch Phys Med Rehabil.* 2008;89(9):1648–1659.

226. Burke R, Beukelman DR, Hux K. Accuracy, efficiency and preferences of survivors of traumatic brain injury when using three organization strategies to retrieve words. *Brain Inj.* 2004;18(5):497–507.

227. Manasse NJ, Hux K, Snell J. Teaching face-name associations to survivors of traumatic brain injury: a sequential treatment approach. *Brain Inj.* 2005;19(8):633–641.

228. Helffenstein D, Wechsler R. The use of interpersonal process recall (IPR) in the remediation of interpersonal and communication skill deficits in the newly brain injured. *Clin Neuropsychol.* 1982;4(3):139–143.

229. Raymer AM, Beeson P, Holland A, et al. Translational research in aphasia: from neuroscience to neurorehabilitation. *J Speech Lang Hear Res.* 2008;51(1):S259–S275.

230. Ziino C, Ponsford J. Selective attention deficits and subjective fatigue following traumatic brain injury. *Neuropsychology.* 2006;20(3):383–390.

231. Hicks EJ, Larkins BM, Purdy SC. Fatigue management by speech-language pathologists for adults with traumatic brain injury. *Int J Speech Lang Pathol.* 2010;13(2):145–155.

232. Frankel T, Penna C. Perseveration and conversation in TBI: response to pharmacological intervention. *Aphasiology.* 2007;21(10/11):1039–1078.

233. McLennan JD, Wathen CN, MacMillan HL, Lavis JN. Research-practice gaps in child mental health. *J Am Acad Child Adolesc Psychiatry.* 2006;45(6):658–666.

234. Clay DL, Hopps JA. Treatment adherence in rehabilitation: the role of treatment accommodation. *Rehabil Psychol.* 2003;48(3):215–219.

235. Ylvisaker M, Coelho C, Kennedy M, et al. Reflections on evidence-based practice and rational clinical decision making. *J Med Speech Lang Pathol.* 2002;10:xxv–xxxiii.

236. Karthikeyan G, Pais P. Clinical judgement and evidence-based medicine: time for reconciliation. *Indian J Med Res.* 2010;132(5):623–626.

237. Perdices M, Schultz R, Tate R, et al. The evidence base of neuropsychological rehabilitation in acquired brain impairment (ABI): how good is the research? *Brain Impair.* 2006;7(2):119–132.

238. Demir SO, Altinok N, Aydin G, Köseoğlu F. Functional and cognitive progress in aphasic patients with traumatic brain injury during post-acute phase. *Brain Inj.* 2006;20(13–14):1383–1390.

239. French LM, Spector J, Stiers W, Kane RL. Blast injury and traumatic brain injury. In: Kennedy CH, Moore J, eds. *Military Neuropsychology.* New York, NY: Springer; 2010:101–125.

240. Parrish C, Roth C, Roberts B, Davie G. Assessment of cognitive-communication disorders of mild traumatic brain injury sustained in combat. *Perspect Neurophysiol Neurogenic Speech Lang Disord.* 2009;19(2):47–57.

241. Echemendia RJ. *Sports Neuropsychology: Assessment and Management of Traumatic. Brain Injury.* New York, NY: Guilford Press; 2006.

242. Zhang K, Johnson B, Pennell D, Ray W, Sebastianelli W, Slobounov S. Are functional deficits in concussed individuals consistent with white matter structural alterations: combined FMRI & DTI study. *Exp Brain Res.* 2010;204(1):57–70.

243. Hammond-Tooke GD, Goei J, du Plessis LJ, Franz EA. Concussion causes transient dysfunction in cortical inhibitory networks but not the corpus callosum. *J Clin Neurosci.* 2010;17(3):315–319.

244. Duff MC, Proctor A, Haley K. Mild traumatic brain injury (MTBI): assessment and treatment procedures used by speech-language pathologists (SLPs). *Brain Inj.* 2002;16(9):773–787.

245. Docking KM, Murdoch BE. Mild traumatic brain injury (mTBI) and language in childhood: pre- and postinjury trends. *Brain Lang.* 2007;103:236–237.

246. Guskiewicz KM, Mihalik JP. Biomechanics of sport concussion: quest for the elusive injury threshold. *Exerc Sport Sci Rev.* 2011;39(1):4–11.

247. Sullivan JR, Riccio CA. Language functioning and deficits following pediatric traumatic brain injury. *Appl Neuropsychol.* 2010;17(2):93–98.

248. Lundy CT, Woodthorpe C, Heederly TJ, Chandler C, Lasoye T, McCormick D. Outcome and cost of childhood brain injury following assault by young people. *Emerg Med J.* 2010;27(9):659–662.

249. Docking K, Murdoch BE, Jordan FM. Interpretation and comprehension of linguistic humour by adolescents with head injury: a group analysis. *Brain Inj.* 2000;14(1):89–108.

250. Ewing-Cobbs L, Barnes M. Linguistic outcomes following traumatic brain injury in children. *Semin Pediatr Neurol.* 2002;9(3):209–217.

251. Hebb DO. The effect of early and late brain injury upon test scores, and the nature of normal adult intelligence. *Proc Amer Philos Soc.* 1942;85:275–292.

252. Vanderploeg RD, Crowell TA, Curtiss, G. Verbal learning and memory deficits in traumatic brain injury: encoding, consolidation, and retrieval. *J Clin Exp Neuropsychol.* 2010;23(2):185–195.

253. Chapman SB, Gamino JF, Cook LG, Hanten G, Li X, Levin, HS. Impaired discourse gist and working memory in children after brain injury. *Brain Lang.* 2006;97(2):178–188.

254. Chapman SB, Sparks G, Levin HS, et al. Discourse macrolevel processing after severe pediatric traumatic brain injury. *Dev Neuropsychol.* 2004;25(1–2):37–60.

255. Chapman SB, Levin HS, Matejka J, Harward H, Kufera JA. Discourse ability in children with brain injury: correlations with psychosocial, linguistic, and cognitive factors. *J Head Trauma Rehabil.* 1995;10(5):36–54.

256. Chapman SB, Culhane KA, Levin HS, et al. Narrative discourse after closed head injury in children and adolescents. *Brain Lang.* 1992;43(1):42–65.

257. Semel E, Wiig EH, Secord WA. *The Clinical Evaluation of Language Fundamentals.* 4th ed. San Antonio, TX: The Psychological Corporation; 2003.

258. Dunn LM, Dunn DM. *Peabody Picture Vocabulary Test.* 4th ed. Circle Pines, MN: American Guidance Service; 2007.

259. Gardner M. *Expressive One-Word Picture Vocabulary Test (2000 edition).* Novato, CA: Academic Therapy Publications; 2000.

260. Fisher J, Glenister JM. *The Hundred Pictures Naming Test.* Hawthorn, Victoria: Australian Council for Educational Research; 1992.

261. Benton AL, Hamsher K, Sivan AB. *Manual for the Multilingual Aphasia Examination.* 3rd ed. Iowa City, IA: University of Iowa; 1994.

262. Carrow-Woolfolk E. *Test of Auditory Comprehension of Language.* 3rd ed. Austin, TX: DLM Teaching Resources; 1999.

263. Renfrew C. *Renfrew Bus Story Manual: A Test of Narrative Speech.* 3rd ed. Oxford, UK: C.E. Renfrew; 1995.

264. Chapman SB, McKinnon L, Levin HS, Song J, Meier MC, Chiu S. Longitudinal outcome of verbal discourse in children with traumatic brain injury: three-year follow-up. *J Head Trauma Rehabil.* 2001;16(5):441–455.

265. Bowers L, Huisingh R, LoGiudice C. *Test of Problem Solving 2—Adolescent.* East Moline, IL: LinguiSystems; 2007.

266. Bowers L, Huisingh R, LoGiudice, C. *Test of Problem Solving 3—Elementary.* East Moline, IL: LinguiSystems; 2005.

267. Brookshire BL, Chapman SB, Song J, Levin HS. Cognitive and linguistic correlates of children's discourse after closed head injury: a three-year follow-up. *J Int Neuropsychol Soc.* 2000;6(7):74–751.

268. Dennis M, Barnes MA. Knowing the meaning, getting the point, bridging the gap, and carrying the message: aspects of discourse following closed head injury in childhood and adolescence. *Brain Lang.* 1990;39(3):428–446.

269. Dennis M, Purvis K, Barnes MA, Wilkinson M, Winner E. Understanding of literal truth, ironic criticism, and deceptive praise following childhood head injury. *Brain Lang.* 2001;78(1):1–16.

270. Szekeres SF, Meserve NF. Collaborative intervention in schools after traumatic brain injury. *Top Lang Disord.* 1994;15(1):21–36.

271. Horneman G, Emanuelson I. Cognitive outcome in children and young adults who sustained severe and moderate traumatic brain injury 10 years earlier. *Brain Inj.* 2009;23(11):907–914.

Evaluation and Treatment of Swallowing Problems

Jeri A. Logemann

INTRODUCTION

Traumatic brain injury (TBI) in children or adults can affect swallowing in a variety of ways (1–4). It is important for the clinician to investigate the history of the patient's original injury and acute care for that injury in order to understand the type(s) of swallowing disorders that may be present. The neural damage resulting from TBI and the incident causing the injury can vary tremendously from patient to patient. There is rarely a direct relationship between the location of the trauma and the nature of the swallowing disorders. The clinician should learn the locus of the direct injury and results of any other testing of neural function to identify other areas of damage (5). In addition to the neural damage, there is potential structural damage during the injury that could affect swallowing. For example, if the patient's neck is broken as his or her head is injured, he or she may exhibit problems in swallowing related to cervical spine injury (6). If the patient is ejected from a motor vehicle and lands on a foreign body such as a stick or a piece of metal, there may be penetrating wounds into the neck that affect swallowing. Thus, the exact nature of the patient's damage at the scene of the accident is quite important. Another factor in identifying swallowing disorders in the patient who has suffered a TBI is to define any emergency medical care that could affect swallowing (7) such as an emergency tracheostomy, which might be placed higher in the neck than normal and damage laryngeal function. If there is a traumatic intubation to establish an airway, there can be dislocation of 1 or both arytenoid cartilages or damage to the larynx, particularly the true vocal folds. Understanding the nature of the patient's injuries and the medical care that he or she received is important in accurately assessing dysphagia in the patient with brain injury. The key to successful recovery/rehabilitation of dysphagia after TBI is to define the exact structural or physiologic abnormalities in the swallow and to design the therapy program to address these disorders.

SWALLOWING DISORDERS

A broad range of swallowing disorders is seen in patients after TBI, probably because of the wide range of damage that can cause dysphagia in these patients. If the patient exhibits upper motor neuron damage with high muscle tone, there may be difficulty in opening the mouth and in controlling the tongue and the soft palate. Most commonly, there is a delay in triggering the pharyngeal swallow or even an absent pharyngeal swallow. There may be reduced motor control of the pharyngeal stage of swallowing when it triggers, involving reduced movement of the tongue base to generate pressure to move the food into the pharynx; reduced laryngeal elevation because of scar tissue, tracheostomy, and so forth; or there may be reduced pharyngeal wall contraction resulting in reduced pressure generation. Dysfunction in the airway protection provided by the larynx does not occur frequently in individuals with brain injury. Dysfunction at the upper esophageal sphincter (UES) at the entrance of the esophagus. However, patients with structural damage can have scar tissue in place that affects either airway closure or opening of the UES. Myoclonus may occur in any oral or pharyngeal structure, including the tongue, tongue base, soft palate, pharyngeal walls, and larynx, and completely discoordinate the swallow. The speech-language pathologist must characterize the exact nature of the patient's swallowing disorder(s) to delineate appropriate therapy/management for the patient's swallowing problem(s).

Counseling the Patient's Family

In a patient who has suffered a severe brain injury, swallowing is often one of the last things to be evaluated. Sometimes, patients are allowed to eat because they do not exhibit external symptoms of a swallowing disorder such as coughing or choking. Then, as recovery progresses, the patient begins to exhibit some signs of dysphagia while swallowing particular types of food. It is important that the clinician working with the patient's swallowing counsel the physician and family as soon as possible regarding the possibility of swallowing disorders and the potential need to evaluate it. Families often think that if the patient is not visibly struggling to eat, coughing, and choking, their swallowing is fine. If the patient is allowed to eat and then later has an assessment that identifies a significant swallowing impairment, families and patients can become very angry, complaining that they were allowed to eat at an earlier stage in recovery sometimes at another institution, but now the clinician is "making them go backward" and delaying their recovery. Because of this reaction, it is important that clinicians introduce the possibility of a swallowing impairment early, even if evaluation is not possible immediately because of the patient's medical status.

EVALUATION OF DYSPHAGIA: WHEN AND HOW

The evaluation of dysphagia in patients following brain injury should begin when they are admitted to the acute care hospital. However, in some situations, the patient receives a severe enough injury that swallowing evaluation is not even considered until the patient has been stabilized and life is no longer threatened. For some patients, this may be days or weeks. The initial screening assessment may simply indicate that the patient is not ready for a full swallowing assessment. Many patients are initially in a coma. A small amount of data point to the fact that the longer the coma, the more severe the swallowing problems are likely to be (3). When the patient is consistently awake and exhibits some level of alertness, dysphagia assessment should begin at the bedside.

General factors such as body habitus, drooling, and mental status should be noted. Voice quality (e.g., a wet sounding voice suggesting pooling of secretions) should be assessed as well as wheezing or labored breathing and any cranial nerve impairments. Inspection or palpation of the tongue and tongue strength may unmask fibrillation or fasciculation of one or both sides. The oropharynx should be inspected for palatal elevation, posterior pharyngeal motion on phonation, and/or palatal myoclonus. Lateral movement of the mucosa of the posterior pharynx typically indicates weakness on the opposite side. Laryngeal examination is important but can be made difficult by the presence of pooled secretions. The nature of a patient's secretions can provide clues to the nature of the disorder, with thick mucoid secretions being associated with standing accumulation such as paralysis or adynamic motor dysfunction and foamy secretions in the pyriform sinus or laryngeal vestibule indicating turbulence secondary to anatomic obstruction such as a non-relaxing cricopharyngeal muscle or stricture. Vocal fold movement during variable pitch phonation, whispering, loud voicing, and during inspiration should be observed. Arytenoids should be inspected for immobility if the interarytenoid mucosa is erythematous and edematous in gastroesophageal reflux disease.

Formal swallowing evaluation and therapy have been found to improve dysphagia outcomes in patients after brain injury (8). Bedside assessment usually includes an oral motor assessment of the face, lips, tongue, palate, pharynx, and larynx; a review of receptive and expressive language and ability to understand direction; history of medications used since the injury; and oral sensory testing to identify any abnormal oral reflexes or postural abnormalities (9). The major purpose of the bedside clinical assessment is to identify oromotor difficulties in the face, lips, tongue, palate, pharynx, and larynx and to determine whether there is significant risk of a pharyngeal stage swallowing impairment. Pharyngeal stage swallowing impairments cannot be diagnosed at the bedside and require an instrumental assessment to define the exact nature of the swallowing problem and its sequelae such as inefficient swallow or aspiration. A review of the patient's medications may identify medications that could negatively affect swallowing including tranquilizers, psychotropics, and medications that cause xerostomia (10). Oral sensory assessment examining 2-point discrimination and light touch sensitivity is important in determining the patient's ability to recognize where food is located in the mouth

and whether or not all of the food has been cleared in any swallowing attempt. Some individuals following brain injury exhibit severely slowed oromotor control such that opening the mouth can take 3–5 minutes. In this situation, there is generally significant hypertonicity in facial musculature that requires rotary massage on 1 cheek while digital pressure downward is applied firmly to the chin and the patient is given repeated directions to try to open his or her mouth. Even with this assist to heighten sensory awareness, the patient may take 3–5 minutes to open his or her mouth. In such a patient, who may also be nonverbal, an instrumental swallowing assessment must be delayed until he or she is able to open his or her mouth in less than 10 seconds. The rotary massage and continuous digital pressure to the chin will facilitate faster oral opening, as well as an understanding of the patient's neural and structural damage causing the swallowing problem. Family members should be counseled regarding the fact that the patient is not yet ready to have an instrumental swallowing assessment but rather needs to build control over his or her oral mechanism instead. The patient's ability to manage his or her own saliva and awareness of his or her saliva is also an important component of the bedside assessment.

At the end of a bedside assessment, the clinician should be able to describe the patient's level of alertness, his or her ability to follow direction, behavior control, oral motor function, and saliva control, as well as understand the patient's neural and structural damage causing the swallowing problem. Patients should also be assessed for their ability to vocalize and to coordinate respiratory and laryngeal function. If the patient has been given food or is eating, the clinician should observe the patient swallowing to identify any dysphagic symptoms. Unfortunately, the bedside clinical examination cannot define pharyngeal physiology or pharyngeal symptoms of swallowing disorders such as the presence and cause of aspiration (11).

Instrumental Assessments

Instrumental assessments may include a radiographic evaluation, often known as the modified barium swallow, fiberoptic endoscopic examination of swallowing (FEES), or manometric assessment. Radiographic assessment is the simplest for the patient who has sustained a brain injury because no tube or other instrumentation must be placed into his or her nose or mouth. During the radiographic assessment, the patient must be able to be positioned into the fluoroscopy equipment so that the head and neck can be viewed in the lateral plane (Figures 66-1 and 66-2). Even this can be difficult for some lower functioning patients; however, in many instances the patient can be moved into the equipment and positioned between the fluoroscopy tube and the table on a cart or gurney, thus requiring no voluntary motor control on his or her part.

The radiographic study is designed to define the anatomy and physiology of the oral preparatory, oral, and pharyngeal phases of swallowing and to identify therapy procedures to improve dysphagia. The goal of the test is to find ways for the patient to swallow successfully, not to keep them from eating (12). The patient is given measured volumes of thin liquids, pudding, and, if the patient is capable of chewing, a material requiring mastication, generally a

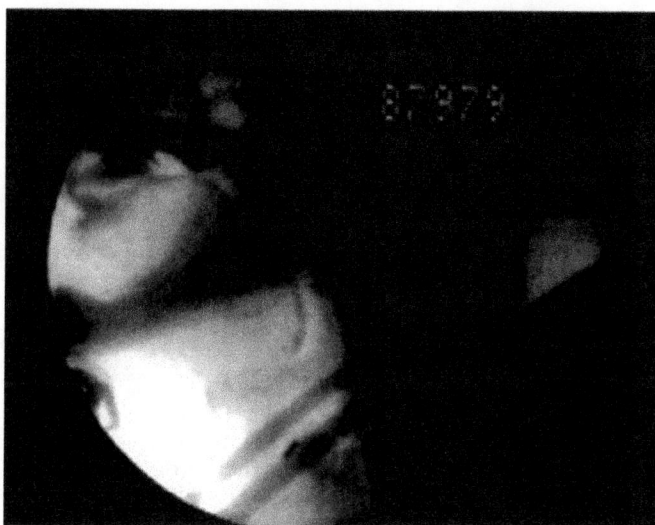

FIGURE 66–1 Lateral radiographic view of the oral cavity and pharynx after a swallow in a patient with brain and spinal cord injury and is wearing a neck brace. There is significant residue in the mouth and the tongue base is also coated with material.

piece of Lorna Doone cookie coated with barium pudding. Other foods coated with barium can be given as needed. The patient is presented with measured volumes of thin liquid beginning with a small amount (1 mL) and asked to swallow it. The material is a flavored barium. The patient is given 2 swallows of each bolus volume or food type and the swallow is observed fluoroscopically. In total, the patient should receive 2 swallows each of 1, 3, 5, and 10 mL of thin liquids; cup drinking of thin liquids; pudding; and masticated material. The bolus volumes of thin liquid are increased sequentially as long as the patient swallows the smaller volume

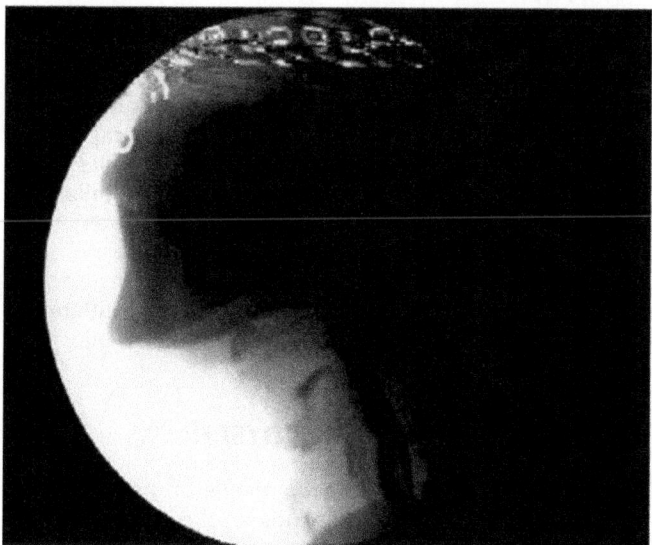

FIGURE 66–2 Lateral radiographic view of the oral cavity and pharynx at mid-swallow in a patient post brain injury. The airway should be completely closed at this time but there is penetration and aspiration present.

successfully, that is, without aspiration or large amounts of residual food left in the mouth or pharynx. If the patient exhibits a significant swallowing impairment that results in aspiration or large amounts of oral or pharyngeal residue, the patient should be given treatment strategies during the x-ray study to improve swallowing and eliminate these sequelae of swallowing disorders.

Generally, when selected treatment techniques are introduced during the radiographic study, 3 types of techniques are attempted in the following order: (a) postural change, (b) heightening sensory awareness, and (c) voluntary swallow maneuvers. The specific postural techniques, sensory enhancements, and voluntary swallow maneuvers to be introduced with a particular patient will depend on the nature of his or her swallowing disorders revealed by the diagnostic portion of the test and the level of his or her ability to follow direction. The purpose of introducing therapy strategies into the radiographic diagnostic study is to determine which procedures are the most efficacious for the patient and to do so in a way that documents their effectiveness. If none of these strategies improve the safety or efficiency of swallowing, the clinician can introduce other food consistencies such as nectar- or honey-thickened liquids to determine whether or not the patient can gain a safe and fairly efficient swallow with a diet change.

At the end of the radiographic study, the clinician should be able to define the patient's swallow physiology and safety, the best treatment procedures for the patient's swallowing disorder(s), and the optimal diet as well as safety of the swallow. The report provided after the study should provide this information in a concise and accurate format. Because the clinician is directly observing the details of the oral and pharyngeal swallow during videofluoroscopy, the damaged muscle function and structural movements can be easily related to the abnormal movement of food or liquid. The videofluoroscopy exam also allows for assessment of intraoral, laryngeal, and/or pharyngeal residue, as well as aspiration and help guide treatment strategies. Glottal dysfunction is a rare cause of aspiration unless the patient with brain injury has suffered laryngeal trauma.

The interpretation of aspiration requires an understanding of the fact that occasional aspiration can occur in people without brain injury. Clinically, one must look at the age and medical history of the patient in question, as well as their pulmonary and mobility status. Because patients with brain injury are frequently young, they can often tolerate some levels of chronic aspiration for 1–2 years or longer before developing pneumonia. Patients with brain injury regularly are found to have variable levels of aspiration than other types of patients and can often tolerate chronic aspiration for many years, especially if they have good pulmonary function. Young patients with brain injury can, at times, tolerate chronic liquid aspiration for 2–5 years without pulmonary problems. The dysphagia team must take this information into consideration when deciding whether to allow the patient to eat or drink. Unfortunately, little research has examined this problem.

Another instrumental assessment is the FEES, which involves the nasal insertion of a fiberoptic tube to view the pharynx from above. This procedure does not enable observation of the oral preparatory or oral phases of swallowing and it does not permit assessment of the pharyngeal stage

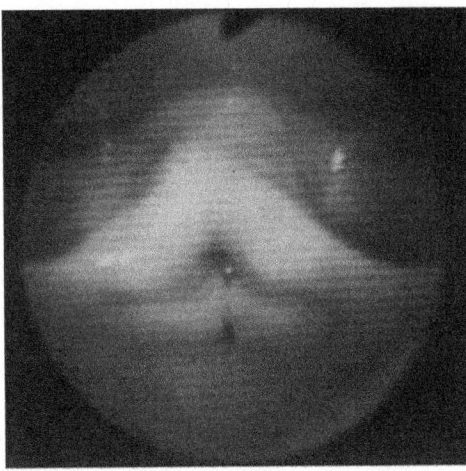

FIGURE 66–3 A superior endoscopic view of the larynx and the pharynx with the false vocal folds closely approximated prior to swallow. The arytenoids and pyriform sinuses are also in view. The UES is located at the top of the image behind the arytenoids and is closed. Opening of the UES is not usually visible during endoscopy because the endoscopic image disappears as the larynx elevates during the first third of the pharyngeal swallow (17,18).

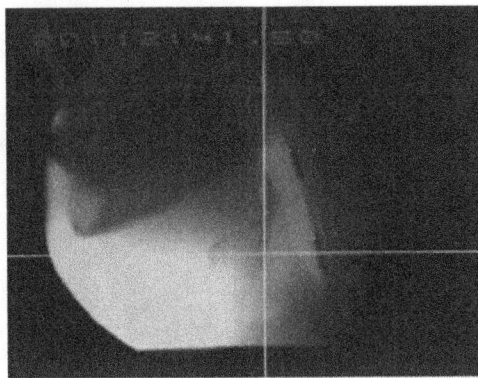

FIGURE 66–4 Lateral radiographic view of the oral cavity and pharynx prior to a swallow with a solid-state manometric catheter in place prior to swallow. The manometric catheter is a 3-mm diameter flexible tube containing the solid state pressure sensors represented by the *dark elongated rectangles* resting on the pharyngeal wall first at the level of the tongue base and second at the level of the laryngeal entrance.

of swallowing during the moment of laryngeal elevation, tongue base retraction, and UES opening (6,13–14). It does enable observation of the bolus entering the pharynx over the base of the tongue, the initial movements of the pharyngeal stage of swallowing, and any aspiration that may occur as the bolus appears in the pharynx. It also enables viewing of the pharynx after the swallow when any bolus residual may be aspirated. In summary, endoscopy provides a superior view of the pharynx and enables the clinician to observe selected aspects of the oropharyngeal swallow (see Figure 66-3). Endoscopy has the advantage of involving no radiographic exposure and enabling the clinician to bring the equipment to the patient's bedside (15). The question that the clinician must answer is whether the endoscopic examination will provide the information needed for the management of the patient's swallowing disorder(s).

If the question the clinician needs answered in the swallowing assessment is whether the pressure generated during swallowing is adequate, then manometry may be the appropriate procedure to be used. Many swallowing disorders—including difficulties with the tongue, tongue base, or pharyngeal wall—lead to reduced pressure generation in the pharynx including reduced movement of the base of tongue, reduced movement of the pharyngeal walls, and reduced laryngeal elevation and forward movement. Although the radiographic study or the fiberoptic endoscopic study can give a perception of reduced pressure to clear food through the pharynx, actual measurements of pressure can only be made with manometry. Manometry, too, involves placement of a tube transnasally into the pharynx and the top of the cervical esophagus. Generally, this is done under fluoroscopy to assure where the pressure sensors in the manometric tube are located (see Figure 66-4) and to determine what structures are touching the manometric tube that may create pressure changes (16).

Before scheduling the instrumental assessment, the patient should be screened for his or her readiness for an instrumental assessment. If the patient is unable to control his or her behavior or tolerate leaning against the back of a cart during a radiographic study, then he or she is not ready for that assessment. Similarly, if the patient is easily upset or will not tolerate a tube placed in his or her nose, he or she is not ready for an endoscopic or manometric study in many cases.

Other procedures can be used in the assessment of dysphagia in persons following brain injury including the use of ultrasound and electromyography. These procedures are not frequently used in the evaluation of swallowing function in the individual with brain injury because the information that they can provide has limited clinical use. Ultrasound is an imaging procedure using high frequency sound waves that enables examination of tongue motion in the mouth but does not visualize the pharynx. Because many of the greatest concerns in the patient with dysphagia resulting from a brain injury are pharyngeal concerns, ultrasound will not provide the requisite information. Similarly, electromyography is a procedure that shows electrical activity in the muscles being used during swallowing, but does not enable visualization of oral and oropharyngeal structures or their movement.

In summary, a radiographic study, that is, the modified barium swallow, is the most commonly used instrumental assessment to evaluate oropharyngeal swallowing abnormalities in the patient who has sustained a brain injury.

MANAGEMENT OF DYSPHAGIA

The initiation of treatment for dysphagia in the individual with brain injury generally depends on the outcome of the detailed physiologic assessment. In some cases, treatment may begin immediately with exercise programs to facilitate improved swallowing motor control. Or, treatment may involve compensatory postural strategies or diet changes in an attempt to direct the flow of food in a more safe or efficient manner. Exercises to reestablish a coordinated swallowing may also be appropriate. Each of these will be discussed subsequently.

Compensatory Treatments

Compensatory strategies to manage swallowing disorders typically involve changes in head or body postures. There are 5 different head and body positions that have known effects on pharyngeal dimensions, the bolus, and structural movements during the oropharyngeal swallow: (a) chin down, (b) chin up, (c) head rotated, (d) head tilted, and (e) lying down. Table 66-1 presents these 5 postures and their known effects on the anatomic relationships of structures in the pharynx and also on the oropharyngeal swallowing. Postural techniques are usually attempted first because they are relatively easy for most patients to achieve and can have dramatic effects on the oropharyngeal swallow (19–21). Table 66-1 presents a list of swallowing disorders and appropriate postural techniques along with the effects of the posture on swallow function.

Enhancing Sensory Input

Another set of management procedures involves enhancing sensory input in the patient's oral cavity prior to the attempt to swallow (22–24). Generally, these procedures include thermal tactile stimulation and enhancing the bolus taste, texture, volume, carbonation, or viscosity. The sensory enhancements are appropriate for patients with sensory swallowing disorders, which are (a) a delay in recognition of food in the mouth resulting in a delay in the oral onset of the swallow and (b) a delay in triggering the pharyngeal

swallow. Both of these disorders must be identified in the careful swallowing assessment. Sensory treatment procedures such as intensifying or changing bolus taste or presenting carbonation have not been adequately studied in the patient with a brain injury. The small amount of available data indicates that such procedures are variably effective in patients with impairment in motor control of the oral or pharyngeal stages of swallowing.

Swallow Maneuvers

Swallow maneuvers are voluntary controls applied to selected motor characteristics of the oropharyngeal swallowing. There are 4 voluntary swallow maneuvers that have known effects during the motor control of swallow: (a) supraglottic swallow, (b) super-supraglottic swallow, (c) effortful swallow, and (d) the Mendelsohn maneuver. The supraglottic swallow involves a voluntary light breath hold before and during the oropharyngeal swallow. This closes the airway at the level of the true vocal folds. The super-supraglottic swallow closes the airway entrance between the arytenoids, base of epiglottis, and false vocal folds, thus closing the entrance to the airway. This is done by breath holding with effort. The effortful swallow increases the known pressure exerted during swallowing by the tongue and tongue base. The patient is instructed to squeeze hard with all of their muscles during swallowing. This improves tongue base and tongue action and the resultant pressures during swallow. The Mendelsohn maneuver is designed to increase laryngeal elevation and forward movement during the swallow and thereby to increase opening of the UES. The sphincter is controlled by hyolaryngeal movement. The patient is told to swallow normally and as he or she swallows, feel his or her "voice box" or "Adam's apple" elevate. When he or

TABLE 66-1 Postural Techniques Generally Most Appropriate for Each Swallowing Disorder and the Physiologic/Anatomic Effect(s) of the Posture on Pharyngeal Dimensions or Bolus Flow

DISORDER OBSERVED ON FLUOROSCOPY	POSTURE APPLIED	PHYSIOLOGIC/ANATOMIC EFFECT OF POSTURE
Inefficient oral transit (reduced posterior propulsion of bolus by tongue)	Head back	Uses gravity to clear oral cavity
Delay in triggering the pharyngeal swallow (bolus past ramus of mandible but pharyngeal swallow is not triggered)	Chin down	Widens valleculae to prevent bolus entering the airway and narrows airway entrance
Reduced tongue base retraction (residue in valleculae)	Chin down	Pushes tongue base backward toward pharyngeal wall
Unilateral laryngeal dysfunction	Chin down	Places epiglottis in a more posterior, protective position
Aspiration during swallow	Head turned to damaged side	Pushes damaged side toward midline
Reduced laryngeal closure (aspiration during the swallow)	Head rotated to damaged side and chin down	Increases vocal fold closure by applying extrinsic pressure; narrows laryngeal entrance. Places epiglottis in a more protective position
Reduced pharyngeal contraction (residue spread throughout pharynx)	Lying down on one side	Eliminates gravitational effect on pharyngeal residue
Unilateral pharyngeal paresis	Head rotated to damaged side	Eliminates damaged side from bolus path
Cricopharyngeal dysfunction (residue on one side of the pharynx; residue in pyriform sinuses)	Head rotated	Pulls cricoid cartilage away from posterior pharyngeal wall, reducing resting pressure in cricopharyngeal sphincter

she can feel his or her larynx elevate, he or she should grab the larynx with his or her muscles in the neck and hold the larynx up. The effort of holding the larynx up extends its elevation and increases opening of the UES. These maneuvers can be used during eating or as an exercise. There is another swallow maneuver, the tongue-holding maneuver, which is an exercise maneuver and cannot be used to eat. During the tongue-holding maneuver, the patient holds his or her tongue tip between his or her teeth to stabilize it, thereby pulling the tongue base forward and putting extra pull on the glossopharyngeal muscle which contracts the pharynx at the tongue base level and pulls the tongue base backward.

All of these maneuvers require the ability to follow direction and thus may not be appropriate for the most severely impaired individuals after TBI. Data on the nature of swallowing disorders among individuals with brain injury indicates that disorders of airway closure or upper sphincter opening occur relatively infrequently (3). When these disorders do occur among patients with brain injury, swallow maneuvers can be very helpful if the patient is able to follow the directions necessary.

Exercise Programs

Exercise programs can also be very helpful to improve structural range of motion, muscle strength, and coordination (22). Range of motion exercises can be very helpful in patients with neurologic or structural damage to the brainstem or to the periphery and are available for the facial muscles, tongue, laryngeal elevation, and laryngeal adduction (22). Strengthening or resistance exercises for the tongue can result in significant improvements (17,25) in tongue function for swallowing. Swallow maneuvers can be used as exercises to improve swallowing coordination (18,26). An increasing published amount of data supports the efficacy of exercise in improving tongue strength (27,28). When prescribed, these exercises should be done for short periods (5 minutes, 10 times per day). These exercises can be difficult for patients with language or cognitive deficits who may not be able to follow directions. Such patients may more successfully use postural changes, sensory enhancements, or diet change.

Diet Change

Sometimes, patients can only swallow safely on a particular viscosity of food such as thin liquid, nectar-thick liquids, honey-thick liquids, pudding, and so forth. Limiting a patient's diet should be the clinician's last choice in management because most patients dislike diet changes such as thickened liquids. However, there are patients for whom there is no other feasible management and diet change is necessary. Or, the patient is recovering and can, initially, only swallow safely and efficiently on a particular food consistency. Table 66-2 presents food consistencies that are particularly helpful for patients with various oropharyngeal swallowing disorders.

Surgical Management of Dysphagia

Generally, there are few surgical procedures that have proven consistently successful in treating oropharyngeal

TABLE 66-2 Bolus Consistencies and the Swallowing Problems for Which They Are Usually Most Appropriate. The Patient Should Be Tested Radiographically With Each Bolus Type to See Which Can Be Most Efficiently and Safely Swallowed

FOOD CONSISTENCIES	CORRESPONDING DISORDERS
Thin liquids	Reduced tongue base retraction[a] Reduced pharyngeal wall contraction[a] Reduced laryngeal elevation[a] Reduced cricopharyngeal opening Tongue dysfunction[a]
Thickened liquids (nectar and/or honey), purees, and thick foods	Delayed pharyngeal swallow Reduced laryngeal closure at the entrance Reduced laryngeal closure throughout the larynx

[a]All of these disorders affect generation of pressure to drive the bolus through the oral cavity and/or pharynx. Thinner foods (liquids) require less pressure to swallow.

dysphagia after TBI. Studies of cricopharyngeal myotomy have shown inconsistent ability to improve cricopharyngeal problems. Use of botulinum toxin injection into the UES has been effective in some patients (22). Generally, any surgical procedure is only used after spontaneous neurological recovery and behavioral therapy have been given adequate time to improve the swallowing impairment.

Experimental Treatment Procedures

There are several treatment procedures currently being discussed in the area of dysphagia therapy that are experimental in nature because these procedures have no published efficacy data to support them (29,30,31,32,33). They should be used carefully and only with a very strong rationale. These procedures include neuromuscular electrical stimulation to various points on the neck, deep pharyngeal neuromuscular stimulation (DPNS), vital stimulation, myofascial release, and feeding patients with reflexive swallows. None of these procedures have been identified as effective with any specific swallowing impairment or with patients with a specific diagnosis. Additionally, none of these procedures have been studied in clinical trials or have taken spontaneous recovery into account in their design. Therefore, clinicians should approach their clinical application with care, particularly in patients with seizures or muscular hypertension in the head or neck.

SHORT-TERM AND LONG-TERM FOLLOW-UP

It is important that patients who have sustained a TBI are regularly seen after discharge if therapy has not returned their swallowing to a functional status, that is, no aspiration and only minimal residual food left in the mouth or pharynx after swallowing (30,35). There are numerous instances in which patients, after TBI, have received swallowing therapy and shown improvement in dysphagia but ultimately plateaued and have not been able to return to full oral intake yet subsequently develop functional swallowing 3, 6, or 9 months later. We do not know enough about recovery from swallowing disorders caused by TBI and, as a consequence, it is best to reassess the patient's function at periodic intervals (i.e., 6 months or a year post discharge from treatment) if the patient is left nonoral. Several studies emphasize the importance of continuing to follow-up the patient with a brain injury (34–36) in order to return them to oral feeding if or when their swallowing function returns.

CONCLUSION

TBI and the circumstances under which they occur can cause problems with oropharyngeal swallowing. In general, the more severe the injury, the more severe the swallowing problem and the longer postinjury for the patient to return to safe and efficient oral feeding. It is critical to evaluate the patient's oropharyngeal swallowing physiology—if at all possible—during acute care. This evaluation should be a radiographic (videofluoroscopic) study—the modified barium swallow—to identify the anatomy and physiology of the patient's swallowing, best treatment strategies, and need to limit oral feeding. Waiting to evaluate a patient's oropharyngeal swallowing until the rehabilitation phase may be extremely upsetting to the patient and his or her family because the patient's oral feeding may be restricted. The patient may not understand the feeding restriction and may feel as if he or she is moving backward in his or her recovery. Regular swallowing therapy by the swallowing therapist (usually a speech-language pathologist) should be provided after the evaluation. Although most patients with brain injury recover safe and efficient swallowing with therapy, there are a few, generally severely injured patients, who will need maintenance therapy or remain on nonoral feeding.

There is a great deal of more research needed in the area of TBI and dysphagia to assist clinicians in establishing evidence-based assessment and management guidelines. The pattern of recovery of swallowing disorders after TBI has not been clearly defined, although it is clear that most patients do recover swallowing abilities over the first 3–5 months postinjury (37–40). There are some patients, however, who do not achieve functional and safe swallowing or who require much longer rehabilitation to do so (41). The exact nature of their neural damage or resulting swallowing disorders in comparison to individuals who have achieved faster recovery of swallowing function have not been defined. There have been no clinical trials in the comparative effectiveness of specific strategies for swallowing therapy in patients following TBI. One reason for this is the wide variety and high variability between patients in this population with dysphagia, making the research more methodologically challenging. There are certainly numerous patient characteristics that must be controlled for and such research is very much needed to establish better evidence-based guidelines for this condition. The relationship between injury severity and type (traumatic axonal injury [TAI], focal vs mixed) as well as the neuroanatomical correlates of TBI in relation to the nature of swallowing disorders and their recovery patterns also deserve further research attention. Novel treatment strategies incorporating pharmacological as well as neurotechnological strategies also warrant further exploration. Issues of feeding patients at various levels of conscious-

ness must be further resolved (42). Factors associated with the development of pneumonia after severe TBI with and without dysphagia need to be examined further although at least 1 study found that a Glasgow Coma Scale (GCS) score < 5, evidence of swallowing disorder, aspiration, and/or field intubation were risk factors for early pneumonia in persons with TBI (43). This area of swallowing dysfunction following TBI, therefore, remains a potentially furtive area for basic science and clinical research. In general, because it relates to post-TBI dysphagia, there is a need for further research to drive evidence-based assessment and treatment guidelines.

KEY CLINICAL POINTS

1. Swallowing problems occur frequently after brain injury. A physiologic swallowing assessment such as the modified barium swallow should be used when oropharyngeal dysphagia is suspected.
2. The physiologic swallowing assessment should include assessment of treatment strategies to improve swallowing.
3. Therapies should have treatment efficacy data or be considered experimental.
4. Patients with brain injury on nonoral feeding should be scheduled in a long-term follow-up (1–2 years) to identify any improvements in their swallowing that might enable oral feeding.

KEY REFERENCES

1. Halper AS, Cherney LR, Cichowski K, Zhang M. Dysphagia after head trauma: the effect of cognitive–communicative impairments on functional outcomes. *J Head Trauma Rehabil.* 1999;14(5):486–496.
2. Lazarus C, Logemann JA. Swallowing disorders in closed head trauma patients. *Arch Phys Med Rehab.* 1987;68:79–87.
3. Logemann JA. *Evaluation and Treatment of Swallowing Disorders.* 2nd ed. Austin, TX: Pro-Ed Publisher; 1998.
4. Logemann JA. *A Manual for Videofluoroscopic Evaluation of Swallowing.* 2nd ed. Austin, TX: Pro-Ed Publisher; 1993.
5. Terré R, Mearin F. Prospective evaluation of oropharyngeal dysphagia after severe traumatic brain injury. *Brain Inj.* 2007;21(13–14):1411–1417.

References

1. Cherney LR, Halper AS. Swallowing problems in adults with traumatic brain injury. *Semin Neurol.* 1996;16(4):349–353.
2. Field LH, Weiss CJ. Dysphagia with head injury. *Brain Inj.* 1989; 3(1):19–26.
3. Lazarus C, Logemann JA. Swallowing disorders in closed head trauma patients. *Arch Phys Med Rehab.* 1987;68:79–87.
4. Morgan A, Ward E, Murdoch B, Bilbie K. Acute characteristics of pediatric dysphagia subsequent to traumatic brain injury: videofluoroscopic assessment. *J Head Trauma Rehabil.* 2002;17(3):220–241.
5. Rowe LA. Studies in dysphagia after pediatric brain injury. *J Head Trauma Rehabil.* 1999:14(5):497–504.

6. Logemann JA, Rademaker AW, Pauloski BR, Ohmae Y, Kahrilas PJ. Normal swallowing physiology as viewed by videofluoroscopy and videoendoscopy. *Folia Phoniatr*. 1998;50:311–319.

7. Morgan AS, Mackay LE. Causes and complications associated with swallowing disorders in traumatic brain injury. *J Head Trauma Rehabil*. 1999;14(5):454–461.

8. Schurr MJ, Ebner KA, Maser AL, Sperling KB, Helgerson RB, Harms B. Formal swallowing evaluation and therapy after traumatic brain injury improves dysphasia outcomes. *J Trauma*. 1999; 46(5):817–823.

9. Halper AS, Cherney LR, Cichowski K, Zhang M. Dysphagia after head trauma: the effect of cognitive-communicative impairments on functional outcomes. *J Head Trauma Rehabil*. 1999;14(5):486–496.

10. Sliwa JA, Lis S. Drug-induced dysphagia. *Arch Phys Med Rehabil*. 1993;74(4):445–447.

11. Splaingard ML, Hutchins B, Sulton LD, Chaudhuri G. Aspiration in rehabilitation patients: videofluoroscopy vs bedside clinical assessment. *Arch Phys Med Rehabil*. 1988;69(8):637–640.

12. Logemann JA. *A Manual for Videofluoroscopic Evaluation of Swallowing*. 2nd ed. Austin, TX: Pro-Ed Publisher; 1993.

13. Logemann JA, Rademaker AW, Pauloski BR, Ohmae Y, Kahrilas PJ. Normal swallowing physiology as viewed by videofluoroscopy and videoendoscopy. *Folia Phoniatr Logop*. 1998;50:311–319.

14. Logemann JA, Rademaker AW, Pauloski BR, Ohmae Y, Kahrilas PJ. Interobserver agreement on normal swallowing physiology as viewed by videofluoroscopy and videoendoscopy. *Folia Phoniatr Logop*. 1999;51:91–98.

15. Leder SB. Fiberoptic endoscopic evaluation of swallowing in patients with acute traumatic brain injury. *J Head Trauma Rehabil*. 1999;14(5):448–453.

16. Ergun GA, Kahrilas PJ, Logemann JA. Interpretation of pharyngeal manometric recordings: limitations and variability. *Dis Esophagus*. 1993;6:11–16.

17. Robbins JA, Levine R, Wood J, Roecker EB, Luschei E. Age effects on lingual pressure generation as a risk factor for dysphagia. *J Gerontol A Biol Sci Med Sci*. 1995;50A:M257–M262.

18. Lazarus C, Logemann JA, Gibbons P. Effects of maneuvers on swallowing function in a dysphagic oral cancer patient. *Head Neck*. 1993; 15:419–424.

19. Drake W, O'Donoghue S, Bartram C, Lindsay J, Greenwood R. Eating in side-lying facilitates rehabilitation in neurogenic dysphagia. *Brain Inj*. 1997;11(2):137–142.

20. Logemann JA, Rademaker AW, Pauloski BR, Kahrilas PJ. Effects of postural change on aspiration in head and neck surgical patients. *Otolaryngol Head Neck Surg*. 1994;110:22–27.

21. Rasley A, Logemann JA, Kahrilas PJ, Rademaker AW, Pauloski BR, Dodds WJ. Prevention of barium aspiration during videofluoroscopic swallowing studies: value of change in posture. *Am J Roentgenol*. 1993;160:1005–1009.

22. Logemann JA. *Evaluation and Treatment of Swallowing Disorders*. 2nd ed. Austin, TX: Pro-Ed Publisher; 1998.

23. Logemann JA, Pauloski BR, Colangelo L, Lazarus C, Fujiu M, Kahrilas PJ. Effects of a sour bolus on oropharyngeal swallowing measures in patients with neurogenic dysphagia. *J Speech Hear Res*. 1995;3:556–563.

24. Bülow M, Olsson R, Ekberg O. Videoradiographic analysis of how carbonated thin liquids and thickened liquids affect the physiology of swallowing in subjects with aspiration on thin liquids. *Acta Radiol*. 2003;44:366–372.

25. Lazarus CL, Logemann JA, Huang CF, Rademaker. Effects of two types of tongue strengthening exercises in young normals. *Folia Phoniatr Logop*. 2003;55(4):199–205.

26. Logemann JA, Kahrilas PJ. Relearning to swallow post-CVA: application of maneuvers and indirect biofeedback: a case study. *Neurology*. 1990;40:1136–1138.

27. Robbins J, Gangnon RE, Theis SM, Kays SA, Hewitt AL, Hind JA. The effects of lingual exercise on swallowing in older adults. *J Am Geriatr Soc*. 2005;53(9):1483–1489.

28. Robbins J, Kays SA, Gangnon RE, et al. The effects of lingual exercise in stroke patients with dysphagia. *Arch Phys Med Rehabil*. 2007; 88(2):150–158.

29. Ashford J, McCabe D, Wheeler-Hegland K, et al. Evidence-based systematic review: oropharyngeal dysphagia behavioral treatments. Part III—Impact of dysphagia treatments on populations with neurological disorders. *J Rehabil Res Dev*. 2009;46(11):195–204.

30. Clark H, Lazarus C, Arvedson J, Schooling T, Frymark T. Evidence-based systematic review: effects of neuromuscular electrical stimulation on swallowing and neural activation. *Am J Speech Lang Pathol*. 2009;18(11): 361–375.

31. Reddy NP, Simcox DL, Gupta V, et al. Biofeedback therapy using accelerometry for treating dysphagic patients with poor laryngeal elevation: case studies. *J Rehabil Res Dev*. 2000:37(5/6):361–372.

32. Xia W, Zheng C, Lei Q, et al. Treatment of post-stroke dysphagia by vitalstim therapy coupled with conventional swallowing training. *J Huazhong Univ Sci Technolog Med Sci*. 2011;31(1):73–76.

33. Shaw GY, Sechtem PR, Searl J, Keller K, Rawi TA, Dowdy E. Transcutaneous neuromuscular electrical stimulation (vitalstim) curative therapy for severe dysphagia: myth or reality? *Ann Otol Rhinol Laryngol*. 2007:116(1):36–44.

34. Terré R, Mearin F. Prospective evaluation of oropharyngeal dysphagia after severe traumatic brain injury. *Brain Inj*. 2007;21(13–14): 1411–1417.

35. Terré R, Mearin F. Evolution of tracheal aspiration in severe traumatic brain injury-related oropharyngeal dysphagia: 1-year longitudinal follow-up study. *Neurogastroenterol Motil*. 2009;21(4): 361–369.

36. Leder SB, Suiter DM, Lisitano Warner H. Answering orientation questions and following single-step verbal commands: effect on aspiration status. *Dysphagia*. 2009;24(3):290–295.

37. Yorkston KM, Honsinger MJ, Mitsuda PM, Hammen V. The relationship between speech and swallowing disorders in head injured patients. *J Head Trauma Rehabil*. 1989;4(4):1–16.

38. Ward EC, Green K, Morton AL. Patterns and predictors of swallowing resolution following adult traumatic brain injury. *J Head Trauma Rehabil*. 2007;22(3):184–191.

39. Hansen TS, Larsen K, Engberg AW. The association of functional oral intake and pneumonia in patients with severe traumatic brain injury. *Arch Phys Med Rehabil*. 2008;89(11):2114–2120.

40. Hansen TS, Engberg AW, Larsen K. Functional oral intake and time to reach unrestricted dieting for patients with traumatic brain injury. *Arch Phys Med Rehabil*. 2008;89(8):1556–1562.

41. Burke D, Alexander K, Baxter M, et al. Rehabilitation of a person with severe traumatic brain injury. *Brain Inj*. 2000;14(5):463–471.

42. Brady SL, Darragh M, Escobar NG, O'Neil K, Pape TL, Rao N. Persons with disorders of consciousness: are oral feedings safe/effective? *Brain Inj*. 2006;20(13–14):1329–1334.

43. Woratyla SP, Morgan AS, Mackay L, Bernstein B, Barba C. Factors associated with early onset pneumonia in the severely brain-injured patient. *Conn Med*. 1995;59(11):643–647.

Cognitive-Communication Deficits Following Traumatic Brain Injury

Carl A. Coelho

INTRODUCTION

Cognitive-communication disorders encompass difficulty with any aspect of communication that is affected by disruption of cognitive processes (e.g., attention, memory, organization, executive function). Communication includes listening, speaking, gesturing, reading, and writing in all areas of language (phonology, morphology, syntax, semantics, and pragmatics). Cognitive impairments impact activities of daily living, behavioral self-regulation, social interaction, and academic and vocational performance (1,2).

Human communication involves the sharing and exchange of information between people. Language use is frequently displayed through speech. Speech has developed into a highly efficient system for the exchange of even the most complex ideas. However, speech is the end product of a multifaceted cognitive process. For example, in a situation in which 2 people are interacting; the speaker has to organize his thoughts, decide what he wants to say, and put what he wants to say into an appropriate linguistic form. This occurs through the selection of appropriate words and phrases to express the intended meaning, and then accurately sequencing these words as specified by grammatical rules of the language. The next stage involves the formulation of motor commands necessary for programming the speech mechanism (i.e., the neural and muscular activities for activating respiration, phonation, resonance, articulation, and prosody) to produce an acoustic signal that accurately represents the words selected to communicate the speaker's intent. The final step in this process is the execution of the commands resulting in the production of speech (3).

Brain injuries may disrupt the process of communication at a variety of levels. Speech disorders (e.g., apraxia of speech or the dysarthrias) will not be discussed in this chapter. The reader is referred to Chapter 65 for a thorough discussion of that topic. Rather, this chapter will focus on language disorders following traumatic brain injury (TBI).

LANGUAGE IMPAIRMENTS FROM A SITE OF LESION PERSPECTIVE

The nature of a brain injury will, in large, measure determine the characteristics of the subsequent language disorder. For example, strokes are typically associated with focal lesions to either hemisphere or subcortical structures, resulting in fairly predictable deficit patterns. By contrast, TBI may result in focal injury to specific regions of the brain (e.g., coup and contrecoup sites of impact), diffuse axonal injury (i.e., stretching, tearing, shearing of nerve fibers), or a combination of both. This mechanism of injury yields a far less homogenous array of deficits. Language disorders resulting from lesions to the left hemisphere, right hemisphere, subcortical regions, and diffuse damage are reviewed separately afterward.

Focal Left Hemisphere Damage

McKinley and colleagues (4) have noted that language is disturbed in 75% or more of individuals with TBI. However, for most, the nature of this language disturbance is not consistent with aphasia. *Aphasia* is defined as an acquired impairment of language processes underlying receptive and expressive modalities caused by damage to areas of the brain that are primarily responsible for language function (5). Aphasia is characterized by grammatical disturbances, deficits of word retrieval, auditory comprehension, reading, and writing in the presence of relatively intact cognitive abilities (e.g., orientation, attention, memory). Lesions associated with aphasia are usually located in the left hemisphere in the region of the posterior frontal lobe, anterior temporal lobe, and/or inferior parietal lobe (i.e., usually along the distribution of the left middle cerebral artery). The incidence of aphasia secondary to TBI reported in the literature varies greatly. Reports range from approximately 2% (6,7) to nearly 50% (8,9). Sarno, Buonaguro, and Levita (10) reported on a group of 125 individuals with closed head injuries admitted to a rehabilitation center. The individuals studied fell into 3 groups: those with classic aphasia (30%), those with dysarthria accompanied by subclinical aphasia (34%), and those with subclinical aphasia (36%). The authors classified individuals as aphasic if their use of speech for expression and/or reception was impaired. Subclinical aphasia referred to evidence of linguistic processing deficits on formal testing in the absence of clinical manifestations of linguistic impairment. The apparent discrepancies regarding the incidence of aphasia following TBI are difficult to resolve because of the lack of consistency in the descriptions of the individuals with TBI studied, the different aphasia assessment tools employed, as well as the varied definitions of aphasia applied. An examination of specific linguistic deficits following TBI reported in the literature indicates that anomia, difficulty retrieving words (6,8,10–14), and impaired auditory comprehension (7,9) are the most commonly observed symptoms. Holland (15) noted that there is overlap in these deficit areas between individuals with aphasia and those with TBI, as well as in the associated reading and writing deficits both groups often demonstrate. However, it is the qualitative differences in the naming errors between the 2 groups which may be most useful in distinguishing between aphasic and nonaphasic responses. Both individuals with aphasia and those with TBI (particularly those in the acute stages) produce circumlocutions and various paraphasias and have reduced fluency in the generation of category-specific words; individuals with TBI, however, demonstrate additional naming errors. For example, they may also produce naming errors related to their personal situations or make errors of confabulation (i.e., sometimes bizarre responses related to the individual's disorientation). Milton and colleagues (16) have described a system for qualitatively evaluating naming behavior for individuals with TBI. The system permits descriptions of correct responses, and, when responses are incorrect, descriptions of their semantic, phonemic, and other relationships to the target. For example, for the target stimulus "apple," semantically related responses might include such utterances as "fruit," "Granny Smith," or "pear." Phonemically related responses might include such utterances as "able" or "ubel." Other responses might include such things as "saw" or "we grew them in our backyard."

Focal Right Hemisphere Damage

As noted by Myers (17), it has only been in the last several years that the cognitive and communicative deficits associated with the right hemisphere have been considered. As was the case for left hemisphere damage, most instances of focal lesions to the right hemisphere are the result of cerebrovascular accidents (CVA). Localization of specific functions related to language processing in the right hemisphere has been a confusing endeavor. Some investigators have observed that the difficulty localizing the component processes involved in maintaining semantic information may be attributable to the involvement of both anterior and posterior cerebral regions and their interconnections (18). Generally speaking, the range of deficits linked to rheumatic heart disease right hemisphere damage (RHD) may be placed into 5 broad categories (17). The first is attentional deficits, which includes problems with arousal, orientating, vigilance, sustained, and selective attention. The next category is neglect, which involves a reduction of attention to left-sided input, use of left limbs, awareness and recognition of left-sided body parts, and awareness of illness. The third category involves visuoperceptual deficits including visual attention, integration, memory, spatial, and topographical orientation. A fourth category is affective and emotional deficits including reductions in the use of facial expression to convey emotion, sensitivity to facial expressions of others, use of prosody to convey emotion, and comprehension of emotional prosody. The final category is cognitive and communicative deficits; included here are reduced discourse comprehension

and production, communicative efficiency and specificity, processing of complex inferences as well as alternative and ambiguous meanings, sensitivity to contextual information, and appreciation of shared knowledge.

Regarding specific linguistic impairments, individuals with RHD typically perform adequately on language tasks that involve convergent processing (i.e., those requiring a limited number of responses and familiar word meanings) such as confrontation naming, yes/no questions, and providing definitions. Divergent language tasks (i.e., those involving a wide range of meanings which diverge from a single semantic concept such as verbal fluency, open-ended questions, or resolving ambiguities) present more difficulty for this group. They often have trouble understanding intended meanings because of a decreased ability to generate, maintain, or inhibit additional, alternate, and related meanings when the dominant meaning is inappropriate to the context (17).

Focal Subcortical Damage

There is a growing body of literature which documents that right-handed individuals who sustain damage to the left basal ganglia or left thalamus can also develop aphasia (19–21). Three subcortical aphasia syndromes have been described by Naeser and associates. The first—anterior syndrome—results from damage in the internal capsule, lenticular nucleus, and anterior white matter. This syndrome is characterized by hemiplegia; slow, dysarthric speech with near normal phrase length and prosody; poor confrontation naming; good repetition; good comprehension; and poor oral reading and writing. The second is posterior syndrome, which is associated with damage in the putamen and internal capsule, and the posterior white matter. Features of this syndrome are hemiplegia, fluent speech without dysarthria, good single word repetition but poor sentence repetition, impaired confrontation naming, poor comprehension, reading, and writing. The third pattern described—anterior–posterior syndrome—results from capsular-putamenal damage with anterior and posterior white matter involvement. Characteristics include a combination of symptoms seen in both Broca's and Wernicke's aphasias. Robin and Scheinberg (22) have cautioned that aphasia caused by lesions in the basal ganglia result in a variety of speech and language impairments that are not all accounted for by the 3 syndromes described by Naeser and associates.

Aphasia resulting from damage to the left thalamus is typically characterized by hemiplegia and difficulty initiating spontaneous speech. In addition, speech may be echolalic and contain neologistic errors. Fairly good auditory comprehension and reading are usually noted, whereas writing and word retrieval are impaired. These individuals have also been observed to be perseverative with fluctuating performance moment to moment (23).

Focal Damage to Prefrontal Cortex

Focal injury to the prefrontal cortex (PFC) is a relatively common consequence of TBI. Although the frontal lobes have long been implicated in language functions, relatively little is known about the specific contribution of the PFC. It has been suggested that the right PFC is the center for slower processing of implicit information such as themes and morals (24), and specific coding of immediate and obvious connections ascribed to the left PFC (25). Specific language functions of the PFC have been examined in a variety of lesion studies. Localized frontal lesions diminished complex propositional language while basic language skills were preserved. Impairments in spontaneous discourse were observed regardless of side of the lesion (26). Chapman (27) has noted that children with frontal lobe injuries demonstrate a higher incidence of discourse deficits than those with brain injury not involving the frontal lobes.

Lateralized functions have been reported in adults and children with brain injury. For example, individuals with anterior right brain damage have been noted to embellish their narratives and have difficulty selecting critical story elements (28). They also displace propositions and incorrectly interpret pictures (29). Narratives of children with right frontal lesions are characterized by reduced content with adequate grammatical complexity, whereas those with left frontal lesions produce simplified narratives at the sentential and discourse levels (27,30). Similarly, adults with left dorsolateral PFC (LDLPFC) lesions produced fewer complex sentences and had difficulty developing narratives, often perseverating on the first proposition. Narratives of those with left orbitofrontal lesions were characterized by more complex grammar but frequent digressions; these individuals had an apparent inability to regulate their verbalizations (29).

Other research on frontal language processes has focused on the distinctions between the PFC and traditional language regions. Sirigu and colleagues (31) presented 2 tasks to individuals with lesions to either Broca's or left dorsolateral areas. In the first task, participants were required to sequence words to form syntactically well-formed sentences and, in the second task, to group words to form logical action sequences. Participants with lesions to Broca's area had little difficulty sequencing the words into appropriate action sequences but were severely impaired in their ability to sequence the words to form grammatical sentences. Conversely, those individuals with dorsolateral lesions demonstrated no difficulty generating grammatical word sequences and a pronounced deficit producing temporally coherent sequences of actions. This double dissociation of syntax- and script-level abilities highlights an important characteristic of the PFC and the dorsolateral region in particular.

Diffuse Axonal Damage

Although individuals with TBI may incur focal lesions, a far more common type of brain pathology following TBI, and specifically closed head injury, is diffuse axonal injury. This pattern of injury is typically associated with what has been termed confused language (11,32–34). Confused language is described as receptive/expressive language that may be phonologically, syntactically, and semantically intact, yet lacking in meaning because responses are irrelevant, confabulatory, circumlocutory, or tangential in relation to a specific topic and lacking a logical sequential relationship between thoughts (35). Such language dysfunction may be mistaken for a fluent aphasia but is more appropriately considered cognitive in nature as opposed to linguistically based; that

is, as a symptom of cognitive rather than linguistic deficits. TBIs frequently result in significant disruption of cognitive processes such as attention, memory, and executive functions. More recent considerations of language disruption following TBI have suggested use of the term cognitive-communicative disorders as being a more accurate description of these impairments. Some individuals with TBI exhibit language disorders most consistent with aphasia, some with communicative deficits comparable to those seen in RHD, and some particularly in the acute stages of recovery from TBI demonstrate language behavior consistent with confused language. Regardless, a primary component of language dysfunction in most TBI survivors pertains to disordered language use (i.e., pragmatics). Pragmatics refers to the set of rules that govern the use of language in context (36). Sohlberg and Mateer (37) observed that whereas individuals with aphasia may communicate better than they talk, individuals with TBI appear to talk better than they communicate. Pragmatic deficits are probably most prevalent in those individuals with frontal lobe injuries. Although the frontal lobes are not thought to be responsible for primary cognitive functions, it appears they are involved in coordinating and actualizing many functions involved in cognitive processing such as attention, motivation, regulation, and self-monitoring (38).

CHARACTERIZING LANGUAGE IMPAIRMENTS SUBSEQUENT TO TRAUMATIC BRAIN INJURY

Just as predominant impairments of language caused by focal lesions may mask subtle cognitive disturbances, primarily cognitive disturbances resulting from diffuse brain injury may mask subtle language deficits (39). Such deficits typically go undetected or are incompletely delineated by the traditionally used language assessment tools such as aphasia batteries (see 40 for a review of standardized assessment tools for TBI including language batteries). In an effort to document such language deficits, many investigators of verbal communicative ability following TBI have chosen to analyze *discourse* (27,41–51). Discourse is a series of related linguistic units that convey a message. The length of a given discourse is determined by the communicative function of the message. There are various types of discourse and each type has different cognitive and linguistic demands (51). It has been suggested that discourse is the most natural and basic unit of normal verbal communication (52). Furthermore, accurate production or comprehension of a narrative requires a complex interaction of linguistic, cognitive, and social abilities (i.e., language use) that are sensitive to the particular disruption following TBI.

Discourse analyses begin with the elicitation of a spoken *narrative*, minimally 5 sentences in length. A variety of types of discourse may be studied including *procedural* (e.g., describing how to change a tire), *descriptive* (e.g., describing a favorite activity), *story narratives*, and *conversational*. The discourse samples are audiotaped and transcribed verbatim. Once transcribed, the narratives are divided into basic units for analysis, such as T-units (i.e., an independent clause plus any dependent clauses associated with it). A T-unit is similar to a sentence but is more reliably identified. Segmenting narratives into sentences is often problematic because of the tendency of some speakers to link sentences of a narrative

TABLE 67-1 Various Levels in the Analysis of Narrative Discourse Production

GENERAL LEVELS	SUBLEVELS	EXAMPLES OF MEASURES
Within-sentence microlinguistic	Lexical Syntactic Semantic	Lexical errors Completeness Complexity Analysis
Between-sentence macrolinguistic	Local (microstructure)	Cohesion Local coherence
	Global (macrostructure)	Global coherence story grammar

with conjunctions such as *and, or,* and *then,* making it difficult to delineate sentence boundaries (53). Depending on the type of discourse and the focus of the analysis, the actual discourse analysis may be done at a variety of levels (see Table 67-1). For example, in a narrative story—at the sentence level—the number of T-units may be tallied as a measure of narrative length, or the number of subordinate clauses may be counted as a measure of grammatical complexity. Across-sentence analyses may involve examining how speakers link meaning units across several sentences (e.g., counting complete or incomplete ties) referred to as *intersentential cohesion.* In story narrative analysis, episodes may also be examined. Episode components are defined as information units pertaining to stated goals, attempts at solutions, and consequences of these attempts. Additional analyses include productivity measures such as total words produced or total speaking time, content measures such as accurate or irrelevant content units, and measures of conversational speech, for example, appropriateness of an utterance or topic maintenance.

DISCOURSE DEFICITS FOLLOWING TRAUMATIC BRAIN INJURY

Functional communication requires language competence in a variety of settings ranging from informal social interactions to formal educational or work-related tasks (49). Findings of recent investigations have demonstrated that individuals with TBI experience difficulty with communicative effectiveness across several discourse genres (see 54–56 for reviews). What follows is a summary of several studies of discourse in individuals with TBI. Throughout the review that follows, the generic term TBI will be used because in many instances, authors have not specified whether the individuals with brain injuries studied had a penetrating or closed head injury. This review is organized by the level analysis. The most basic distinction in the analysis of discourse is whether the discourse genre of interest involves a monologue (narratives such as telling a story) or is interactive in nature (such as participating in a conversation). At the most general level, analyses of narrative discourse are focused on within-sentence processes, termed microlinguistic; or between-sentence processes, referred to as macrolinguistic. Under each of these broad categories are sublevels such as, lexical, syntactic, and lexico-semantic for the within-sentence analyses, and under the between-sentence analyses are the sublevels of local (microstructure) and global (macrostructure). Each of the sublevels has corresponding measures or analyses (see Table 67-1). Conversational analyses can be broken

down in terms of the role of the participant during an interaction, that is, whether the individual functions as an initiator or as a responder. In each role, there are sublevels again with corresponding measures in the analysis.

Narrative Discourse

For each of the levels of analysis for narrative discourse, a brief description is provided of each analysis followed by a summary of the findings from the TBI discourse literature. Examples of some of the more commonly used narrative analyses appear in Table 67-2. This will be followed by a comparable discussion of the analyses of conversational discourse.

Microlinguistic Analyses

Lexical Production
Examinations of lexical production typically involve measures such as lexical diversity (i.e., number of different words produced) and the occurrence of paraphasic errors. The literature on lexical problems in discourse following TBI has been somewhat equivocal. For example, some authors have reported a reduction in the number of different words produced (57) or a greater frequency of verbal paraphasias (58) following TBI, whereas others have noted that lexical production was not a problem for the individuals with TBI that they studied (59,60). Difficulties with verbal fluency and word retrieval following TBI reported in the discourse literature must be interpreted cautiously. Some of these studies have included, within their participant groups, individuals with TBI who were aphasic (e.g., 44,58).

Syntax
Syntactic aspects of discourse have been examined in several studies with mixed findings. Syntactic complexity—as measured by percentage of T-units containing dependent clauses (58), embeddedness of subordinate clauses (61), subordinate clauses per T-unit (62), and words per T-unit (54)—was comparable to that of normal controls. Further, syntactic complexity was not judged as being a primary deficit when rated on various pragmatic rating scales (59,60,63). By contrast, other investigators have reported syntactic impairments in the discourse of individuals with TBI. For example, Campbell and Dollaghan (57) noted that syntactic complexity, as measured by percentage of utterances containing 2 or more lexical verbs, was decreased in 6 of 9 participants that they studied. In addition, an increased incidence of grammatical

TABLE 67-2 Examples of Narrative Story Analyses

DISCOURSE MEASURES	DESCRIPTION	EXAMPLE
Sentence Production		
Words per T-unit	Total words in story divided by number of T-units	118 words/6 T-units = 19.7
Subordinate clauses per T-unit	Number of subordinate clauses in story divided by number of T-units	3 subordinate clauses/6 T-units = 0.5
Cohesion		
Cohesive adequacy– Percentage complete ties of total ties	Each occurrence of a cohesive tie judged regarding its adequacy. Number of complete ties in story divided by total number of cohesive ties.	**Complete tie**—The girl was hungry. *She* ate her lunch. **Incomplete tie**—The boys walked home from the mall. *They* stopped at his house for a snack. **Erroneous tie**—Dave and Joe drove to the game. *He* forgot the tickets.
Story Grammar		
Number of total episodes	Total number of complete and incomplete episodes in a story.	**Complete episode**— **(Initiating event)** and this fly comes in. and the Father's bothered by this. **(Attempt)** so he decides to swat or hit the fly. And he hits his wife. **(Direct consequence)** and she goes down. **Incomplete episode**— **(Attempt)** and he hits his daughter **(Direct consequence)** and the daughter goes down to the floor.
Proportion of T-units within episode structure	Number of T-units in episode structure divided by total number of T-units in a story.	10 T-units in episodes/16 total T-units = 0.62

From Coelho (71).

errors (e.g., omissions of the subject, main verb and other required grammatical morphemes, word order transpositions, verb tense and agreement errors) have also been noted for participants with TBI vs normal controls (58,64). A recent study examined pause time and verbal initiation time during reading and repetition of sentences varying in syntactic complexity in 2 groups: TBI and matched comparison. Significant group differences were noted in pausing in both tasks. Pausing patterns of the participants with TBI were strongly correlated with syntactic complexity, suggesting that these individuals may also demonstrate difficulties with sentence planning (65).

Lexico-Semantic
The contradictory findings noted for lexical production and syntax have prompted other investigators to examine the microlinguistic dysfunction in the discourse of individuals with TBI through semantic analyses, specifically propositional analysis. The advantage of propositional analysis is that it permits the examination of semantic complexity of an utterance apart from sentence structure and grammaticality (66). Propositions are meaning units identified with respect to a predicate (i.e., verb, modifier) and its arguments (i.e., agent, instrument). Any sentence may contain several propositions (67). Using a measure of words per proposition, Chapman and colleagues (27) did not find deficiencies in information flow for a group of adolescents with TBI. However, McDonald (46) tallied unspecified propositions in explanations of a board game by 2 individuals with TBI and found that 1 participant provided less detail than the non–brain-injured (NBI) controls. Another study that applied propositional analyses noted that individuals with TBI appeared to have difficulty with the planning and organization of language (68). Similarly, individuals with TBI were noted to produce significantly fewer propositions per T-unit than normal controls. In other words, they demonstrated a decreased ability to insert multiple ideas into single sentences. By contrast, the NBI participants' appeared to chunk information, and that appeared to be a mechanism for linking propositions together, which increased the likelihood that the listener might understand multiple ideas as a connected semantic unit. The participants with TBI appeared less adept at applying this strategy to facilitate discourse organization.

Macrolinguistic Analyses
Continuing with the review of narrative discourse analyses, the focus now shifts to the macrolinguistic analyses that examine discourse performance between or across sentences.

Cohesion
Sentences are connected by various kinds of meaning relations described as cohesive markers or ties. A word is considered a cohesive marker if its meaning cannot be adequately interpreted without the listener searching the text—beyond that sentence—for the completed meaning. Cohesional analyses, as described by Halliday and Hasan (52), have been

undertaken in several studies of discourse and TBI. Discourse samples of individuals with TBI have been described as lacking continuity as evidenced by their production of fewer cohesive ties than normal controls in both narrative and procedural discourse tasks (44,47). However, other investigators have reported that individuals with TBI produced a comparable number of cohesive ties as NBI participants in narrative discourse (46,58,61,69). Differences in the proportional use of ties across discourse tasks have been reported for individuals with TBI (47,61). Mentis and Prutting observed that their TBI participants used different cohesional patterns that appeared to be related to their reduced linguistic processing abilities, their reduced pragmatic abilities, as well as their attempts to compensate for the linguistic deficits. Liles and colleagues noted that, in a story retelling task, similar proportions of referential (e.g., *Tom is an engineer. **He** works in Ohio.*), lexical (e.g., *I gave Frank our tickets. The **idiot** lost them all.*), and conjunctive (e.g., *Bill worked all night. **And** his hammering kept the rest of us awake.*) markers occurred for both the TBI and NBI groups. In the story generation task, however, a distinction between the groups appeared in which the individuals with TBI showed a reversal of the pattern used in the story retelling task. In story generation, all of the TBI participants decreased the proportional use of reference and increased the proportion of lexical ties. This shift in the proportional use of types of cohesive ties across the story tasks was attributed to the TBI groups' apparent direct reference to the stimulus picture. These direct references were characterized as interjected descriptors of the picture that were unrelated to the rest of the text. The individuals with TBI rarely integrated these lexical items into the text structure and, consequently, they were often judged to be incomplete ties. The TBI participants' tendency to refer outside their texts suggested that they were unable to detach themselves from the perceptual salience of the stimulus picture to organize their language for story development. In a final study, Coelho and colleagues (42) examined cohesion in discourse samples from a story generation task gathered longitudinally from 2 individuals with TBI. One individual demonstrated poor cohesive adequacy with meaningful content, as measured by story structure; and the second, fair-to-good cohesion with poor content. These findings emphasize the clinical utility of monitoring discourse abilities longitudinally and of employing a multilevel analysis procedure.

Coherence

Coherence refers to the conceptual organization of discourse. The coherence of a text depends on the speaker's ability to maintain thematic unity (70). Coherence is typically considered from 2 perspectives: global and local. Global coherence pertains to how discourse is organized with respect to a general goal, plan, or topic. Local coherence refers to the maintenance of meaningful conceptual links between individual sentences within a text. Coherence has been specifically examined in the narrative discourse of individuals with TBI (46,58,69) and the findings have been mixed. With the exception that the participants with TBI produced more unexplained references, McDonald (46) noted that their texts were as coherent as those of the normal controls. Similarly, Van Leer and Turkstra (69) found no differences in the coherence ratings for their groups of TBI and NBI participants. How-

ever, Glosser and Deser (58) reported that the individuals with TBI that they studied were significantly impaired relative to the normal controls in measures of local and global coherence, with global coherence most impaired. These authors suggested that coherence depends on intact access to semantic memory representations of real-world knowledge, as well as perceptual and conceptual integration necessary to maintain the plan and overall organization of discourse. In addition, the ability to produce discourse coherently perceived because coherent requires simultaneous attention and mental manipulation of several bits of information including integration of the speaker's plan and the listener's perspective. The TBI participants' greater impairment with the maintenance of global vs local coherence suggested that their discourse impairment was more related to a disruption of macroorganizational abilities as opposed to problems with meaning relationships between contiguous concepts (58).

Story Grammar

Story grammar pertains to the purported regularities in the internal structure of stories that direct an individual's comprehension and production of the logical relationships between people and events. Story grammar knowledge is typically measured by complete episodes. An episode consists of (*a*) an initiating event that prompts a character to formulate a goal-directed behavior, (*b*) an action, and (*c*) a direct consequence marking attainment or nonattainment of the goal. An episode is considered complete only if it contains all 3 components (71). A variety of difficulties with story grammar has been reported for individuals with TBI. For example, Chapman and colleagues (27) noted that their severely impaired group of individuals with TBI demonstrated a reduction in the number of essential story components, failed to signal new episodes with setting information, and often omitted essential action information. These authors commented that it was unclear whether this difficulty was a reflection of an underlying impairment of the internal story schema or difficulty implementing story schema during discourse production. In another study, NBI participants and those with TBI produced comparable numbers of complete episodes in a story retelling task but 3 of the 4 individuals with TBI produced no episodes in story generation (61). The TBI participants' apparent inability to use episode structure in the story generation task, in spite of having been able to produce complete episodes in the story retelling task, suggested that the story generation task required an interaction of cognition and language use in which the TBI participants could not consistently engage. A reduction in the number of total episodes produced was also noted in a later study by the same authors (42). Finally, Coelho (71) noted that a group of 55 TBI participants produced fewer T-units within episode structure (i.e., the proportion of total T-units that contributed to episodic structure) than did a group of 47 NBI individuals. Although the TBI and NBI participants were not different in terms of the number of total episodes produced, which had been reported in previous studies (42,61), the NBI participants produced more T-units within the structure of episodes. In other words, the NBI group produced fewer extraneous T-units—that is, T-units that did not contribute to episodic structure. This measure was considered to be an indication of participants' ability to use story grammar as an organizational plan for language.

Miscellaneous Measures

Informativeness

The measurement of informativeness in discourse production has focused on 3 primary aspects: amount of information communicated, quality of information (encompassing such descriptors as irrelevant, redundant, off topic, over personalized, etc.), and efficiency of information (72). The discourse output of TBI participants has been described as reduced in several studies as measured by number of words (and/or meaningful words), utterances, or sentences; mean length of utterance in morphemes or communication units (comparable to T-units); or some combination of these measures such as number of words per T-unit or syllables per story grammar element, and percentage of syllables or utterances in mazes (27,44,49,57,62,71,73). Individuals with TBI have also been described as comparable to normal controls in terms of the amount of pertinent content expressed and in narrative length but significantly slower in the rate of information produced (43,62). These individuals appeared to "talk past the point of diminishing returns," their oral narratives were lengthier and slower relative to the amount of content provided (43, p. 6). Other investigators have reported normal productivity for individuals with TBI in terms of the number of T-units or sentences in narrative tasks (47,61). Other indices of informativeness have included such measures as number of essential steps included in a description of a procedure (49); amount of pertinent content (43); content units (44); amount of essential information, accuracy of story, and implied meanings (74); and number of concepts introduced (62). In general, mixed findings have been noted with essential steps and pertinent content the TBI participants being comparable to the normal controls (43,49), but in other studies, the individuals with TBI produced fewer content units and concepts and demonstrated some difficulty with implied meanings (44,62,74). Recently, a new measure of story narrative completeness was described in which the presence of 5 key content components was tallied. When the completeness and story grammar measures were plotted using a 2-coordinate grid system, "goodness" of the story was quantified. Plotting the 2 sets of scores into quadrants discriminated the comparison group from the group with TBI (75).

Summary of Findings on Narrative Discourse

Numerous investigations have illustrated the clinical utility of narrative discourse analyses with the TBI population (27,41–44,46–49,57,58,61,62,69,71,73–76). In terms of microlinguistic processes, findings on lexical production and syntactic aspects of discourse have been noted to be somewhat ambiguous. Some investigators have reported difficulties in these areas for individuals with TBI, and others have observed that these abilities remain intact following injury. Results from these studies have been difficult to compare because of the varied analysis techniques employed. When microlinguistic processes are examined by means of semantic analyses, the findings are more straightforward. Individuals with TBI demonstrate consistent problems with the planning and organization of language as reflected in their difficulties inserting multiple ideas into single sentences (69,76).

Narrative discourse performance has also been evaluated extensively in terms of macrolinguistic processes,

namely cohesion, coherence, and story grammar. Cohesion has been noted to be an area of inconsistent impairment and performance may vary considerably depending on the discourse elicitation task presented (47,61). For example, the cohesive adequacy of individuals with TBI has been reported to be comparable to that of normal speakers in story retelling but impaired for story generation (64). Similarly, the proportion of types of cohesive ties used by participants with TBI changed from story retelling to story generation, which was not the case for the normal speakers (47,61). Similar to cohesion, TBI participants' ability to generate complete episodes was frequently affected by the nature of the task, with story retelling being easier than story generation. Story generation required a complex interaction of language and various cognitive abilities that were difficult for even mildly impaired individuals with TBI (61,71). It has also been noted that TBI participants produced more T-units that did not contribute to episodic structure. It appears that these individuals have difficulty using story grammar to organize language (71). Along similar lines, conceptual organization of discourse (i.e., coherence) has also been noted to be problematic for individuals with TBI. Specifically, their greater difficulty with the maintenance of global (i.e., general plan or goal) vs local (i.e., conceptual links between sentences) coherence suggests a disruption of macro-organizational processes for discourse (58). Analyses of story grammar (i.e., the generation of episodes) and cohesion enable discourse samples to be examined at multiple levels allowing for the delineation of distinct discourse patterns (42).

Finally, the applicability of findings on narrative discourse productivity and content analysis of individuals with TBI have also been limited by the inclusion of individuals with aphasia and dysarthria in the groups studied. However, in general terms, the TBI participants studied demonstrated decreased discourse efficiency, generating information at a slower rate in lengthier utterances than controls (42,62,75).

Conversational Discourse

The analysis of conversational discourse is of particular interest for the study of the TBI population because of its importance in the process of socialization. The development and maintenance of social relationships has been noted to be challenging for survivors of TBI. The consequences of this difficulty are social isolation, increased reliance on family for social support, and significant problems returning to work, school, and premorbid avocations. It has been suggested that these interactional problems are the result of social skills deficits, and that these deficits in social skills are felt to be a reflection of subtle impairments in pragmatic language use during conversation (77,78). There have been numerous reports pertaining to the analysis of conversational discourse following TBI. These reports are summarized afterward by type of analysis.

Response Appropriateness

The appropriateness of TBI participants' utterances within conversations utilizing procedures specified by Blank and Franklin (79) has been described (80,81). A greater number of turns per conversation were noted for the participants with TBI than for the normal controls. This increased number of turns resulted from their shorter length of utterance per turn and their conversational partner's higher percentage of oblige production (i.e., utterances for which a response is expected, as in a question) (80). In a follow-up to the original study, which involved 5 individuals with TBI, Coelho and colleagues (81) studied 32 individuals with TBI, all of whom had recovered a high level of functional language, and were all rated as Rancho Los Amigos Level of Cognitive Functioning (82) VII (automatic-appropriate) or above. As a group, the individuals with TBI did not initiate a great deal and appeared dependent on the examiner to maintain the momentum of the interaction. They produced fewer spontaneous obliges and comments (i.e., utterances for which a response is not required) than did the NBI controls and functioned primarily as "responders." Further, when they did respond, they provided more information than was requested. Although this extra information was not inappropriate or bizarre, it did not facilitate disclosure on the part of the conversational partner. The function of disclosure in social interaction is to allow the opportunity to talk about oneself or subjects of interest to oneself in order to establish, sustain, and enjoy social interaction (77). Youse and colleagues (83) have recently described an elaborated version of Blank and Franklin's response appropriateness rating schema, which appears to be more sensitive to the nuances of conversation and may facilitate in treatment planning.

Analysis of Topic

The proficiency by which participants manage conversational topics is critical to the success of an interaction. Topic management pertains to how participants in a conversation extend or maintain a given topic, as well as how discussion of a topic is discontinued, and how and when participants change topics (84). The specific contribution of speakers and their conversational partners to topic maintenance and development through analysis of ideational intonation units has been examined (85). Ideational describes a concept borrowed from Halliday (86) and pertains to the idea that discourse is about something or contributes some content. Therefore, ideational units can be assumed to represent what speakers contribute to topic maintenance and development, and to exist as a function of cognitive processes. For example, there are categories of ideational units for new information appropriate to the topic contributed by a speaker and categories representing no new information but still maintaining a topic. Thus, it is reasonable to assume that production of ideational intonation units is likely to be disrupted in persons with brain injuries and cognitive impairments. Mentis and Prutting (85) found differing patterns of production between an adult with TBI and an NBI control in their intonation unit analysis across unspecified, concrete, and abstract conversational contexts. The individual with TBI produced fewer units containing novel information not specifically requested, fewer clarification and confirmation requests, and more agreement and acknowledgement units. In a follow-up study, this analysis procedure was applied to conversational samples of a group of 10 individuals with TBI and 10 NBI controls (87). The intonation unit analysis did not distinguish high-functioning individuals with TBI from controls matched for age, gender, and socioeconomic status. The method of eliciting conversation, with the examiner directing the conversation, may have constrained the context and, thereby, masked deficits commonly attributed to this population's difficulty in social interchanges.

Other approaches to the analysis of topic management have involved the examination of how topics are introduced and changed during a conversation (81,88). Any participant in a conversation may introduce topics. Topics are changed in 1 of 3 ways: (a) at the beginning of the conversation, or by ending discussion of one topic and initiating another, referred to as a novel introduction; (b) by means of a smooth shift, in which discussion of one topic is subtly switched to another; or (c) by means of a disruptive shift, in which discussion of one topic is abruptly or illogically switched to another topic. Findings on this measure have been mixed. Coelho et al. (88) observed that 5 individuals with TBI demonstrated difficulty initiating and sustaining topics compared to 5 matched controls. However, when a group of 32 individuals with TBI were compared to an NBI group of 43 individuals, the group with TBI produced comparable numbers of novel introductions and smooth shifts as the NBI group during their conversations with an examiner. Neither group produced many disruptive shifts (81).

Consideration of Communicative Context

The potential influence of various dimensions of the communicative context on conversational performance has been studied by Togher and colleagues (50,89–91). As described by these authors, context is a combination of 3 components: field, mode, and tenor. Field pertains to the nature of the social interaction taking place (e.g., a formal presentation vs a conversation with friends). Mode refers to the modality by which the discourse is produced (e.g., written vs oral). Tenor describes those who are involved in the interaction, their relationship to each other, and their roles or status (e.g., teacher and student, 2 strangers, clerk and customer) (50). Two additional components are genre, which pertains to the influence of culture on language (i.e., the step-by-step structure that is followed to achieve goals), and ideology, which is the participants' biases and personal perspectives. As a speaker produces an utterance, he or she makes choices about what is to be said and how it is to be said, and this is influenced by the listener and situation. Togher and colleagues stress that these contextual factors should be considered in analyses of conversational exchanges.

Conversation Analysis

Other highly structured analyses have also been applied to conversational samples. One such system is conversation analysis (CA), which was developed to delineate the structural organization and sequential ordering of talk. Friedland and Miller (92) have applied CA to conversational samples of an individual with TBI. The authors commented that CA was sensitive for identifying pragmatic deficits in this individual. Specifically, it identified the precise locale of conversational breakdowns and hoe these were repaired or not. Further, it demonstrated how one conversational partner adapted to these breakdowns and was successful during interactions with the TBI participant and another was not.

Pragmatic Rating Scales

In contrast to the very structured analysis procedures of CA, several investigators have utilized pragmatic rating scales to investigate conversational abilities (63,93–98). Some scales rate both nonverbal (e.g., intonation, facial expression, eye contact, gesture) and verbal (conversation initiation, turn taking, topic maintenance, response length, presupposition and referencing) communication (95). Although others focus on specific aspects of the verbal message such as intelligibility, sentence formation, and coherence of narrative story(63). Some theoretically based scales focus on aspects of pragmatics such as utterance acts (e.g., vocal intensity, voice quality, prosody), propositional acts (e.g., lexical selection, word order, stylistic variations), and illocutionary and perlocutionary acts (e.g., speech acts, topic, turn taking) (96). Other scales are questionnaires completed during an observation or from personal knowledge that deal with such issues as, "Does client: make rapid and inappropriate changes in conversational topic without clues to the listener? Or fail to attend to cues for conventional turns, interrupting frequently or failing to hold up his or her end of the conversation?" (95,99). Observations on the use of such pragmatic rating scales for assessing individuals with TBI have been generally positive. The scales are not labor intensive, which is the case for most of the other formal analysis procedures, and they are useful for assessing selected communicative behaviors unobtrusively—in real-world settings. Although various pragmatic rating scales have face validity, these assessments have not been carefully studied and findings should be interpreted with caution (100).

Social Information Processing

A final category of analysis views communication as an integral aspect of social pragmatic skills. A universally accepted definition of social skills is absent from the enormous literature on this topic. Similarly, numerous conceptual models of social skills have been described (101). The ability to communicate effectively is the basis of socially skilled behavior, and in humans, language is the primary method of communication. Ylvisaker, Urbanczyk, and Feeney (102) suggested a conceptualization of social skills following TBI that specifically incorporated the dimension of communication. Five components are included: (a) the individual's knowledge of self, (b) the extent to which an individual attends to their personal appearance, (c) social cognition (i.e., social perception, social knowledge, and social decision making), (d) communication, and (e) the social environment (i.e., significant people in the individual's natural environment). Analysis procedures pertaining to social cognition have examined such skills as cooperation, turn taking, politeness, negotiation, topic management, and sensitivity to role and status of all participants. For example, McDonald (46) studied 2 individuals with TBI and 12 NBI participants explaining a novel procedure to a blind-folded third person. The productions of the TBI participants were rated as disorganized, confusing, and ineffective as compared to the controls. The disorganization was attributed to errors in sequencing and inclusion of irrelevant propositions. In a second study, individuals with TBI and NBI controls participated in a barrier task, which required that the participants explain a board game to a listener not present in the room (103). The authors noted that the TBI participants appeared to be bound to the physical properties of the stimulus before them, and omitted important details from their explanations that the listener needed to understand the game. Similar findings were noted for adolescents using the same task (104). The investigators concluded that overall performance was limited by the TBI participants' decreased ability at role taking, which in turn was associated with frontal lobe damage. In a final study, Turkstra and colleagues (105) studied social cognition of 10 adolescents with TBI and 60 NBI peers. Two tasks were presented: emotion recognition and conversation judgment. In the emotion recognition task, the participants were asked to identify the emotion depicted by an actor (happy, sad, peeved, angry, disgusted). For the conversation judgment task, 6 conversation skills were depicted: (a) attentive listening, (b) perception of nonverbal cues, (c) detection of sarcasm, (d) sharing the conversational burden, (e) humility, and (f) speaking at the listener's level. Each participant was asked to make judgments about the actor during videotaped vignettes (e.g., "Is the person a good listener?," "What makes you think so?"). Results indicated that the TBI group differed significantly from the NBI group for both recognition of emotion and the conversational judgments. Most of the errors on the conversation skills task were related to the detection of sarcasm and the feelings it might evoke in a listener. This finding was consistent with those of McDonald (106), which demonstrated impaired understanding of sarcasm and other forms of social inference in adults with TBI.

Summary of Findings on Conversational Discourse

The analysis of conversational discourse has been conducted from a variety of perspectives and the procedures applied have ranged from rating scales or checklists to highly structured analysis protocols. Although not entirely consistent, results from various pragmatic rating scales, and analyses of response appropriateness and topic management suggest that individuals with TBI experience difficulty when called on to function as a partner in communicative dyads, whether in conversation or referential communication. These individuals demonstrate problems initiating and sustaining topics in conversation and frequently rely on their discourse partner to assume a greater proportion of the communicative burden to ensure a successful interchange of information (46,63,80,81,85,99). The role of individuals with TBI as participants in conversational dyads will vary according to the tenor relationships. In addition, the factors of familiarity and status appear to influence the language choices made by conversational partners during these interactions. These language choices are the result of the different roles the conversational participants assume and how conversational partners respond to the disability of the participant with TBI (50).

Finally, when conversation is considered as a component of social skills or social cognition, a decreased ability for role taking has been identified as a primary deficit for individuals with TBI. Problems with the recognition of emotion and interpretation of sarcasm and inference also compromise their social functioning (105,106).

INTERPRETATIONS OF DISCOURSE DEFICITS FOLLOWING TBI

This review has indicated that individuals with TBI frequently demonstrate a variety of subtle language impairments best categorized at cognitive-communication deficits. These difficulties can be characterized by a variety of discourse analyses. This chapter has focused primarily on descriptions of narrative and conversational discourse deficits.

If it is assumed that these types of discourse are different in terms of underlying requisite processes, what follows are interpretations of narrative and conversational discourse impairments following TBI.

Narrative Discourse Impairments

A recent investigation of individuals with penetrating head wounds illustrates the value of discourse analyses for delineating the nature of language impairments. Story retelling narratives were elicited from 3 participant groups; 2 with focal damage to the dorsolateral prefrontal cortex (DLPFC) left (LDLPFC) and right (RDLPFC) and a non-injured comparison cohort. None of the dorsolateral (DLPFC) participants were aphasic, but all were classified as having a cognitive-communication disorder. The discourse samples were analyzed at microlinguistic and macrolinguistic levels. Results indicated that the discourse performance of the LDLPFC group was characterized by difficulty with local and global coherence as well as completeness (all scores were significantly different from those of the comparison group). Although the RDLPFC group's performance on those same measures was better than that of the LDLPFC group and worse than the comparison group, those differences were not significant (107).

Global coherence refers to how discourse is organized with respect to an overall goal, plan, or topic. Local coherence pertains to conceptual links between adjacent sentences, which maintain the meaning of the text. Difficulty with global and local coherence has been reported to be characteristic of individuals with diffuse brain dysfunction such as Alzheimer disease or closed head injuries (58). However, impairments of coherence have also been reported to occur following focal perisylvian lesions (108). Discourse organization necessary for story retelling may involve a dynamic interaction between linguistic and other cognitive processes, which are diffusely represented. Macro-organizational dysfunction might then result from either focal, as in the case of the LDLPFC participants or diffuse brain pathology.

The measure of completeness involved a tally of the predetermined critical components or events from the story that were produced by the DLPFC participants. Although the story retelling was requested immediately following the visual presentation of the story, successful completion of this task undoubtedly involved various aspects of memory. Presumably, an individual with difficulty recognizing associations among the critical components of the story would have a greater load on working memory than one who was able to integrate and organize the components into a meaningful synopsis of the story. Therefore, a high score on the completeness measure would require intact elements of both memory and organizational processes.

The notion that discourse impairments may be attributed to specific cognitive dysfunction is consistent with the definition of cognitive-communication deficits. The scores for local and global coherence of the LDLPFC group were significantly correlated with a nonverbal measure of working memory but not the completeness score. This is consistent with a previous report of discourse performance being correlated with working memory (109). Interestingly, none of those scores for the RDLPFC group were correlated with working memory.

The relationship between executive functioning and discourse would appear to be quite logical. It has been suggested that discourse proficiency involves an interaction of cognitive and linguistic organizational processes, which requires executive control (110). Recent findings have demonstrated several significant but modest correlations between measures of executive functions and story narratives (71,74, 111,112).

Conversational Discourse Impairments

The complexities of conversational discourse have been well described in several studies (50,56,113–115). Effective participation in a conversation is dependent on a variety of factors such as topic maintenance, turn taking, appropriate referencing, sensitivity to the conversational partner, and general cognitive abilities such as attention, vigilance, and memory. Social cognition (i.e., social perception, knowledge, and decision making) will also have important influences on conversational skill. Galski and colleagues (116) have commented that the success of an individual's social, vocational, familial, and academic integration rests on the recovery of effective communication.

Although individuals with TBI demonstrate difficulty with many narrative discourse tasks, conversational discourse appears to be more difficult for this population. This may be attributed to the interactive nature of conversation. Consistent with this explanation is the report that individuals with TBI produced more discourse errors in conversation than in a structured referential communication task. The authors suggested that conversations are more complex because of social aspects such as the relationship between conversational partners—that is, familiarity, status, and role—as well as the face-saving strategies used for politeness when communication breakdowns occur (117). Such factors, typically, are not at issue in noninteractive types of discourse. Additional support for the contention that conversation may be more challenging than narrative discourse for individuals with TBI comes from a study that entered measures of both narrative and conversational discourse into a discriminant factor analysis (DFA). The goal was to determine which type of discourse analysis would best discriminate TBI from NBI participants. Results of the DFAs run with both sets of discourse data indicated that the conversational measures were most accurate in discriminating the groups (118). It appears that because the conversational measures were pragmatic in nature and more sensitive to the communicative dysfunction displayed by individuals with TBI than the more structurally focused narrative measures.

An additional explanation pertains to the potential cognitive factors that have been suggested to be important for meaningful participation in conversation. For example, topic maintenance and appropriate referencing requires both selective and sustained attention. Further, functional memory is required to recall what the speaker has said as well as the listener (116). Social competence requires the ability to apply social skills flexibly in accordance with the rules of an interaction. It has been argued that the inability to flexibly apply behavior according to rules, which entails executive functioning, may account for conversational difficulty following TBI (77). Support for the notion that executive functioning may be an important factor in conversational proficiency comes from findings of significant correlations between measures of conversational performance and executive functions (119). Finally, comprehension of sarcasm and implicit language may also influence the effectiveness of a conversational participant (106).

CONCLUSION

This chapter has reviewed the nature of language dysfunction following TBI. Although some individuals with TBI will demonstrate aphasia, most will present with language deficits that are cognitively based vs linguistic, referred to as cognitive-communicative impairments. Most of these individuals will present with pronounced difficulties with pragmatics, that is, with the use of language in context. These pragmatic deficits are not readily apparent when the assessment of language is focused on single words or isolated sentences. Rather, language should be evaluated in terms of discourse. Discourse permits the analysis of language at multiple levels (i.e., microlinguistic and macrolinguistic, microprocessing and macroprocessing), which may be differentially impaired after TBI. Further, the analysis of interactive discourse (i.e., conversation) will reveal difficulties with social cognition that cannot be observed in the typical noncontextual assessment settings.

Most survivors of TBI will demonstrate a variety of narrative and conversational discourse deficits. The underlying bases for these impairments are probably different but in many ways similar as well. Problems with narrative discourse are attributed to disruption of macrolinguistic processes involved in the organization of semantic information. This organizational process more than likely involves executive control. Meaningful interactions involve the flexible application of social rules, which is also associated with executive functions. Future research should focus on the delineation of the processes that subserve discourse. Findings will provide important treatment implications for cognitive-communicative impairments.

KEY CLINICAL POINTS

1. Impairments of social cognition are a source of long-term disability, and tools are needed to assess such deficits.
2. Aphasia batteries, typically used to assess communication after TBI, assess language at the single word or sentence level.
3. Individuals with TBI struggle with the organization of complex language.
4. There is substantial evidence to support the assessment of communication beyond levels of lexicon and grammar typically included in standardized aphasia batteries.
5. Individuals with damage of the prefrontal cortex demonstrate difficulties with formulation of complex language. These deficits are not attributable to aphasia.

6. Discourse (narrative and conversational) analyses are useful for delineating these difficulties.
7. Discourse impairments have been documented in individuals 30-35 years post TBI.

KEY REFERENCES

1. Coelho C, Ylvisaker M, Turkstra L. Nonstandardized assessment approaches for individuals with traumatic brain injuries. *Semin Speech Lang.* 2005;26(4):223–41.
2. Galski T, Tompkins C, Johnston MV. Competence in discourse as a measure of social integration and quality of life in persons with traumatic brain injury. *Brain Inj.* 1998; 12(9):769–782.
3. Lê K, Coelho C, Mozeiko J, Grafman J. Measuring goodness of story narratives. *J Speech Lang Hear Res.* 2011;54(1): 118–126.
4. Sirigu A, Cohen L, Zalla T, et al. Distinct frontal regions for processing sentence syntax and story grammar. *Cortex.* 1998;34(5):771–778.
5. Togher L, Hand L, Code C. Exchanges of information in the talk of people with traumatic brain injury. In: S McDonald, L Togher, C Code, eds. *Communication Skills Following Traumatic Brain Injury.* Hove, UK: Psychology Press; 1999;113–145.

References

1. American Speech-Language-Hearing Association. Roles of speech-language pathologists in the identification, diagnosis, and treatment of individuals with cognitive-communication disorders. Position statement. (ASHA Supplement No. 25). Rockville, MD: American Speech-Language-Hearing Association; 2005.
2. Kennedy MR, Avery J, Coelho C, et al. Evidence-based practice guidelines for cognitive-communication disorders after traumatic brain injury: initial committee report. *J Med Speech Lang Path.* 2002; 10(2):ix–xiii.
3. Denes PB, Pinson EN. *The Speech Chain.* Baltimore, MD: Williams & Wilkins; 1964.
4. McKinlay WW, Brooks DN, Bond MR, Martinage DP, Marshall MM. The short-term outcome of severe blunt head injury as reported by the relatives of the injured persons. *J Neurol Neurosurg Psychiatry.* 1981;44(6):527–533.
5. Davis A. *A survey of adult aphasia and related language disorders.* Englewood Cliffs, NJ: Prentice Hall Inc; 1993.
6. Heilman KM, Safran A, Geschwind N. Closed head trauma and aphasia. *J Neurol Neurosurg Psychiatry.* 1971;34(3):265–269.
7. Schwartz-Cowley R, Stepanik MJ. Communication disorders and treatment in the acute trauma center setting. *Top Lang Disord.* 1989; 9:1–9.
8. Levin HS, Grossman RG, Kelly PJ. Aphasic disorder in patients with closed head injury. *J Neurol Neurosurg Psychiatry.* 1976;39(11): 1062–1070.
9. Thomsen IV. Evaluation and outcome of aphasia in patients with severe closed head trauma. *J Neurol, Neurosurg Psychiatry.* 1975; 38(7):713–718.
10. Sarno MT, Buonaguro A, Levita E. Characteristics of verbal impairment in closed head injured patients. *Arch Phys Med Rehabil.* 1986; 67(6):400–405.
11. Levin HS, Grossman RG, Rose JE, Teasdale G. Long-term neuropsychological outcome of closed head injury. *J Neurosurg.* 1979; 50(4):412–422.
12. Levin HS, Benton AL, Grossman RG. *Neurobehavioral Consequences of Closed Head Injury.* New York, NY: Oxford University Press; 1982; 140–161.

13. Sarno MT. The nature of verbal impairment after closed head injury. *J Nerv Ment Dis*. 1980;168(11):685–692.

14. Thomsen IV. Evaluation and outcome of traumatic aphasia in patients with severe verified lesions. *Folia Phoniatr*. 1976;28(6): 362–377.

15. Holland AL. When is aphasia aphasia? The problem of closed head injury. In: Brookshire RH, ed. *Clinical Aphasiology Conference Proceedings*. 1982;12:345–349.

16. Milton SB, Turnstall C, Wertz RT. Dysnomia: a rose by any other name may require elaborate description. In: Brookshire RH, ed. *Clinical Aphasiology Conference Proceedings*. 1983;14:114–123.

17. Myers PS. *Right Hemisphere Damage*. San Diego, CA: Singular Pub; 1999.

18. Molloy R, Brownell HH, Gardner H. Discourse comprehension by right-hemisphere stroke patients: deficits of prediction and revision. In: Joanette Y, Brownell HH, eds. *Discourse ability and brain damage: Theoretical and Empirical Perspectives*. New York, NY: Springer-Verlag; 1990:113–130.

19. Crosson B, Nadeau SE. The role of subcortical structures in linguistic processes: recent developments. In: Stemmer B, Whitaker HA, eds. *Handbook of neurolinguistics*. San Diego, CA: Academic Press; 1998:431–445.

20. Nadeau SE, Rothi LG. Rehabilitation of subcortical aphasia. In: Chapey R, ed. *Language intervention strategies in aphasia and related neurogenic communication disorders*. 4th ed. Philadelphia, PA: Lippincott Williams & Wilkins; 2001:457–470.

21. Naeser MA, Alexander MP, Helm-Estabrooks N, Levine HL, Laughlin SA, Geschwind N. Aphasia with predominantly subcortical lesion sites: description of three capsular putaminal aphasia syndromes. *Arch Neurol*. 1982;39(1):2–14.

22. Robin DA, Scheinberg S. Subcortical lesions and aphasia. *J Speech Hear Disord*. 1990;55(1):90–100.

23. Brookshire RH. *Introduction to Neurogenic Communication Disorders*. 7th ed. St. Louis, MO: Mosby; 2007.

24. Beeman M. Course semantic coding and discourse comprehension. In: Beeman M, Chiarello C, eds. *Right Hemisphere Language Comprehension*. Mahway, NJ: Lawrence Erlbaum; 1998;255–284.

25. Grafman J. The structured event complex and the human prefrontal cortex. *Principles of Frontal Lobe Function*. New York, NY: Oxford University Press; 2002;292–310.

26. Barbizet J, Duizabo P, Flavigny R. [Role of the frontal lobes in language. (A neuropsychological and experimental study)] [in French]. *Rev Neurol*. 1975;131(8):525–544.

27. Chapman S, Culhane K, Levin H, et al. Narrative discourse after closed head injury in children and adolescents. *Brain Lang*. 1992; 43(1):42–65.

28. Wapner W, Hamby S, Gardner H. The role of the right hemisphere in the apprehension of complex linguistic materials. *Brain Lang*. 1981;14(1):15–33.

29. Kaczmarek BL. Neurolinguistic analysis of verbal utterances in patients with focal lesions of frontal lobes. *Brain Lang*.1984;21:52–58.

30. Chapman SB, Levin HS, Wanek A, Weyrauch J, Kufera J. Discourse after closed head injury in young children. *Brain Lang*. 1998;61(3): 420–449.

31. Sirigu A, Cohen L, Zalla T, et al. Distinct frontal regions for processing sentence syntax and story grammar. *Cortex*. 1998;34(5):771–778.

32. Groher M. Language and memory disorders following closed head trauma. *J Speech Hear Research*. 1977;20(2):212–223.

33. Halpern H, Darley F, Brown JR. Differential language and neurologic characteristics in cerebral involvement. *J Speech Hear Disord*. 1973;38(2):162–173.

34. Prigatano G. *Neuropsychological rehabilitation after brain injury*. Baltimore, MD: Johns Hopkins University Press; 1986.

35. Hagan C. Language disorders in head trauma. In: Holland A, ed. *Language Disorders in Adults: Recent Advances*. San Diego, CA: College-Hill Press; 1984:245–282.

36. Newhoff M, Apel K. Impairments in pragmatics. In: LaPointe LL, ed. *Aphasia and Related Neurogenic Language Disorders*. 2nd ed. New York, NY: Thieme; 1997.

37. Sohlberg MM, Mateer CA. *Introduction to Cognitive Rehabilitation: Theory and Practice*. New York, NY: Guilford Press; 1989.

38. Stuss DT, Benson DF. *The Frontal Lobes*. New York, NY: Raven Press; 1986.

39. Adamovich BLB. Cognition, language, attention, and information processing following closed head injury. In: Kreutzer JS, Wehman PH, eds. *Cognitive Rehabilitation for Persons with Traumatic Brain Injury*. Baltimore, MD: Paul H. Brookes; 1991.

40. Turkstra L, Ylvisaker M, Coelho C, Kennedy M, Sohlberg MM, Avery J. Practice guidelines for standardized assessment for persons with traumatic brain injury. *J Med Speech Lang Pathol*. 2005; 13(2):ix–xxxviii.

41. Coelho CA, Liles BZ, Duffy RJ. The use of discourse analyses for the evaluation of higher level traumatically brain-injured adults. *Brain Inj*. 1991;5(4):381–392.

42. Coelho CA, Liles BZ, Duffy RJ. Discourse analyses in closed head injured adults: evidence for differing patterns of deficits. *Arch Phys Med Rehabil*. 1991;72(7):465–468.

43. Ehrlich JS. Selective characteristics of narrative discourse in head-injured and normal adults. *J Commun Disord*. 1988;21(1):1–9.

44. Hartley LL, Jensen PJ. Narrative and procedural discourse after closed head injury. *Brain Inj*. 1991;5(3):267–285.

45. Hartley LL, Jensen PJ. Three discourse profiles of closed-head-injury speakers: theoretical and clinical implications. *Brain Inj*. 1992;6(3):271–282.

46. McDonald S. Pragmatic language skills after closed head injury: ability to meet the informational needs of the listener. *Brain Lang*. 1993;44(1):28–46.

47. Mentis M, Prutting CA. Cohesion in the discourse of normal and head-injured adults. *J Speech Hear Res*. 1987;30(1):88–98.

48. Snow P, Douglas J, Ponsford J. Discourse assessment following traumatic brain injury: a pilot study examining some demographic and methodological issues. *Aphasiology*. 1995;9(4):365–380.

49. Snow P, Douglas J, Ponsford J. Procedural discourse following traumatic brain injury. *Aphasiology*. 1997;11:947–967.

50. Togher L, Hand L, Code C. Exchanges of information in the talk of people with traumatic brain injury. In: S McDonald, L Togher, C Code, eds. *Communication Skills Following Traumatic Brain Injury*. Hove, UK: Psychology Press; 1999;113–145.

51. Cherney LR. Pragmatics and discourse: an introduction. In: Cherney LR, Shadden BB, Coelho CA, eds. *Analyzing Discourse in Communicatively Impaired Adults*. Gaithersburg, MD: Aspen; 1998;1–8.

52. Halliday MAK, Hasan R. *Cohesion in English*. London, UK: Longman; 1976.

53. Hughes D, McGillivray L, Schmidek MA. *Guide to Narrative Language: Procedures for Assessment*. Eau Claire, WI: Thinking Publications; 1997.

54. Coelho CA. Discourse production deficits following traumatic brain injury: a critical review of the recent literature. *Aphasiology*. 1995;9(5):409–429.

55. Snow PC, Douglas JM. Conceptual and methodological challenges in discourse assessment with TBI speakers: towards an understanding. *Brain Inj*. 2000;14(5):397–415.

56. Togher L. Discourse sampling in the 21st century. *J Commun Disord*. 2001;34(1–2):131–150.

57. Campbell TF, Dollaghan CA. Expressive language recovery in severely brain-injured children and adolescents. *J Speech Hear Disord*. 1990;55(3):567–581.

58. Glosser G, Deser T. Patterns of discourse production among neurological patients with fluent language disorders. *Brain Lang*. 1991; 40(1):67–88.

59. Milton SB, Prutting CA, Binder GM. Appraisal of communicative competence in head injured adults. In: Brookshire RH, ed. *Clinical Aphasiology Conference Proceedings*; 1984;14:114–123.

60. Penn C, Cleary J. Compensatory strategies in the language of closed head injured patients. *Brain Inj*. 1988;2(1):3–17.

61. Liles BZ, Coelho CA, Duffy RJ, Zalagens MR. Effects of elicitation procedures on the narratives of normal and closed head-injured adults. *J Speech Hear Disord*. 1989;54(3):356–366.

62. Stout CE, Yorkston KM, Pimentel JI. Discourse production following mild, moderate, and severe traumatic brain injury: a comparison of two tasks. *J Med Speech Lang Path.* 2000;8:15–25.

63. Ehrlich J, Barry P. Rating communication behaviors in the head-injured adult. *Brain Inj.* 1989;3(2):193–198.

64. Peach RK, Schaude BA. Reformulating the notion of "preserved" syntax following closed head injury. Paper presented at: The Annual Convention of the American Speech-Language-Hearing Association; November 1986.

65. Ellis C, Peach RK. Sentence planning following traumatic brain injury. *NeuroRehabilitation.* 2009;24(3):255–266.

66. Kamhi AG, Johnston JR. Semantic assessment: determining prepositional complexity. In Secord WE, Damico JS, eds. *Best practices in school speech-language pathology: descriptive/non-standardized language assessment.* New York, NY: The Psychological Corp. Harcourt Brace Jovanovich; 1992;99–105.

67. Kintsch W. The psychology of discourse processing. In: Gernsbacher MA, ed. *Handbook of Psycholinguistics.* San Diego, CA: Academic Press; 1994;721–740.

68. Coelho CA, Grela B, Corso M, Gamble A, Feinn R. Microlinguistic deficits in the narrative discourse of adults with traumatic brain injury. *Brain Inj.* 2005;19:1139–1145.

69. Van Leer E, Turkstra L. The effect of elicitation task on discourse coherence and cohesion in adolescents with brain injury. *J Commun Disord.* 1999;32(5):327–349.

70. Glosser G. Discourse production patterns in neurologically impaired and aged populations. In: Brownell HH, Joanette Y, eds. *Narrative Discourse in Neurologically Impaired and Normal Aging Adults.* San Diego, CA: Singular; 1993;191–212.

71. Coelho CA. Story narratives of adults with closed head injury and non-brain-injured adults: influence of socioeconomic status, elicitation task, and executive functioning. *J Speech Lang Hear Res.* 2002; 45(6):1232–1248.

72. Shadden BB. Information analyses. In: Cherney LR, Shadden BB, Coelho CA, eds. *Analyzing Discourse in Communicatively Impaired Adults.* Gaithersburg, MD: Aspen; 1998;85–114.

73. Snow P, Douglas J, Ponsford J. Narrative discourse following severe traumatic brain injury: a longitudinal follow-up. *Aphasiology.* 1999;13(7):529–552.

74. Tucker FM, Hanlon RE. Effects of mild traumatic brain injury on narrative discourse production. *Brain Inj.* 1998;12(9):783–792.

75. Lê K, Coelho C, Mozeiko J, Grafman J. Measuring goodness of story narratives. *J Speech Lang Hear Res.* 2011;54(1):118–126.

76. Biddle KR, McCabe A, Bliss LS. Narrative skills following traumatic brain injury in children and adults. *J Commun Disord.* 1996; 29(6):447–469.

77. Bond F, Godfrey HPD. Conversation with traumatically brain-injured individuals: a controlled study of behavioural changes and their impact. *Brain Inj.* 1997;11(5):319–329.

78. Godfrey HPD, Shum D. Executive functioning and the application of social skills following traumatic brain injury. *Aphasiology.* 2000; 14(4):433–444.

79. Blank M, Franklin E. Dialogue with preschoolers: a cognitively-based system of assessment. *Appl Psycholinguist.* 1980;1(2):127–150.

80. Coelho CA, Liles BZ, Duffy RJ. Analysis of conversational discourse in head injured adults. *J Head Trauma Rehabil.* 1991;6(2): 92–99.

81. Coelho CA, Youse KM, Le KN. Conversational discourse in closed-head-injured and non-brain-injured adults. *Aphasiology.* 2002; 16(4–6):659–672.

82. Hagan C, Malkmus D, Durham P. Levels of cognitive functioning. In: *Rehabilitation of the Head Injured Adult: Comprehensive Physical Management.* Downey, CA: Professional Staff Association of Rancho Los Amigos Hospital; 1980.

83. Youse KM, Gathof M, Fields RD, Lobianco TF, Bush HM, Noffsinger JT. Conversational discourse analysis procedures: a comparison of two paradigms. *Aphasiology.* 2011;25(1):106–118.

84. Brinton B, Fujiki M. *Conversational management with language-impaired children.* Rockville, MD: Aspen; 1989.

85. Mentis M, Prutting CA. Analysis of topic as illustrated in a head-injured and normal adult. *J Speech Hear Res.* 1991;34(3):583–595.

86. Halliday MAK. *An Introduction to Functional Grammar.* London, UK: Edward Arnold; 1985.

87. Wozniak RJ, Coelho CA, Duffy RJ, Liles BZ. Intonation unit analysis of conversational discourse in closed head injury. *Brain Inj.* 1999; 13(3):191–203.

88. Coelho CA, Liles BZ, Duffy RJ, Clarkson JV, Elia D. Conversational patterns of aphasic, closed head injured, and normal speakers. *Clinical Aphasiology.* 1993;12:145–155.

89. Togher L, Hand L, Code C. Measuring service encounters in the traumatic brain injury population. *Aphasiology.* 1997;11(4–5):491–505.

90. Togher L, Hand L, Code C. Analyzing discourse in the traumatic brain injury population: telephone interactions with different communication partners. *Brain Inj.* 1997;11(3):169–189.

91. Togher L, Hand L. Use of politeness markers with different communication partners: an investigation of five subjects with traumatic brain injury. *Aphasiology.* 1998;12(7–8):755–770.

92. Friedland D, Miller N. Conversation analysis of communication breakdown after closed head injury. *Brain Inj.* 1998;12(1):1–14.

93. Damico J. Clinical discourse analysis: a functional language assessment technique. In: Simon CS, ed. *Communication Skills and Classroom Success: Assessment of Language-Learning Disabled Students.* San Diego, CA: College-Hill; 1985;165–106.

94. Gerber S, Gurland G. Interactive Analysis of Pragmatic-Linguistic Abilities in Acquired Aphasia. Paper presented at: The annual convention of the American Speech-Language-Hearing Association; November 17, 1990; Seattle, WA.

95. Halper AS, Cherney LR, Burns MS, Mogil SI. *Clinical Management of Right Hemisphere Dysfunction.* 2nd ed. Gaithers-berg, MD: Aspen; 1996.

96. Prutting C, Kirchner D. Applied pragmatics. In: Gallagher TM, Prutting CA, eds. *Pragmatic assessment and intervention issues in language.* San Diego, CA: College-Hill; 1983;29–64.

97. Roth F, Spekman N. Assessing the pragmatic abilities of children: Part I. Organizational framework and assessment parameters. *J Speech Hear Disord.* 1984;49(1):2–11.

98. Roth F, Spekman N. Assessing the pragmatic abilities of children: Part II. Guidelines, considerations, and specific evaluation procedures. *J Speech Hear Disord.* 1984;49(1):12–17.

99. Snow P, Douglas J, Ponsford J. Conversational discourse abilities following severe traumatic brain injury: a follow-up study. *Brain Inj.* 1998;12(11):911–935.

100. Coelho C, Ylvisaker M, Turkstra L. Nonstandardized assessment approaches for individuals with traumatic brain injuries. *Semin Speech Lang.* 2005;26(4):223–41.

101. Marsh NV. Social skill deficits following traumatic brain injury: assessment and treatment. In: McDonald S, Togher L, Code C, eds. *Communication Disorders Following Traumatic Brain Injury.* New York, NY: Psychology Press; 1999.

102. Ylvisaker M, Urbanczyk B, Feeney SF. Social skills following traumatic brain injury. *Semin Speech Lang.* 1992;13:308–322.

103. McDonald S, Pearce S. The 'dice' game: a new test of pragmatic language skills after close-head injury. *Brain Inj.* 1995;9(3):255–271.

104. Turkstra LS, McDonald S, Kaufman P. Assessment of pragmatic communication skills in adolescents after traumatic brain injury. *Brain Inj.* 1996;10(5):329–345.

105. Turkstra LS, McDonald S, DePompei R. Social information processing in adolescents: data from normally-developing adolescents and preliminary data from their peers with traumatic brain injury. *J Head Trauma Rehabil.* 2001;16(5):469–483.

106. McDonald S. Differential pragmatic loss after closed head injury: ability to comprehend conversational implicature. *Appl Psycholinguist.* 1992;13:295–312.

107. Coelho C, Le K, Mozeiko J, Krueger F, Grafman J. Discourse impairments following lesions to the dorsolateral prefrontal cortex. In: *Federal Interagency Conference on Traumatic Brain Injury;* June 13–15, 2011; Washington, DC.

108. Coelho CA, Flewellyn L. Longitudinal assessment of coherence in an adult with fluent aphasia: a follow-up study. *Aphasiology.* 2003; 17(2):173–182.

109. Youse KM, Coelho CA. Working memory and discourse production abilities following closed-head injury. *Brain Inj.* 2005;19(12): 1001–1009.

110. Ylvisaker M, Szekeres SF, Feeney T. Communication disorders associated with traumatic brain injury. In: Chapey R, ed. *Language Intervention Strategies in Aphasia and Related Neurogenic Communication Disorders.* Philadelphia, PA: Lippincott, Williams & Wilkins; 2001:745–800.

111. Coelho CA, Liles BZ, Duffy RJ. Impairments of discourse abilities and executive functions in traumatically brain injured adults. *Brain Inj.* 1995;9(5):471–477.

112. Mozeiko J, Le K, Coelho C, Krueger F, Grafman J. The relationship of story grammar and executive function following TBI. *Aphasiology.* In press.

113. Doyle PJ, Goda AJ, Spencer KA. The communicative informativeness and efficiency of connected discourse by adults with aphasia under structured and conversational sampling conditions. *A J Speech Lang Pathol.* 1995;4(4):130–134.

114. Mackenzie C. Adult spoken discourse: the influences of age and education. *Int J Lang Commun Disord.* 2000;35(2):269–285.

115. Wilkinson R. Sequentiality as a problem and a resource for intersubjectivity in aphasic conversation: analysis and implications for therapy. *Aphasiology.* 1999;13(4):327–343.

116. Galski T, Tompkins C, Johnston MV. Competence in discourse as a measure of social integration and quality of life in persons with traumatic brain injury. *Brain Inj.* 1998;12(9):769–782.

117. Prince S, Haynes WO, Haak NJ. Occurrence of contingent queries and discourse errors in referential communication and conversational tasks: a study of college students with closed head injury. *J Med Speech Lang Pathol.* 2002;10:19–39.

118. Coelho CA, Youse KM, Le KN, Feinn R. Narrative and conversational discourse of adults with closed head injuries and non-brain-injured adults: a discriminant analysis. *Aphasiology.* 2003;17(3): 499–510.

119. Coelho CA, Youse KM. Conversational abilities and executive functions following closed head injury. Paper presented at: International Neuropsychological Society Conference; February 3, 2004; Baltimore, MD.

XVI

FUNCTIONAL MOBILITY AND ADL'S

Neuroscientific Basis for Occupational and Physical Therapy Interventions

Randolph J. Nudo and Numa Dancause

INTRODUCTION

The field of neurorehabilitation is currently undergoing a fundamental change in approach to therapy after central nervous system (CNS) injury. In the past, occupational and physical therapies after brain injury were based almost exclusively on empirical data and without a full understanding of the neural processes or correlates of recovery mechanisms. Since the early 1980s, experimental data has been accumulating to provide compelling evidence that the adult brain is capable of significant anatomical and physiological plasticity. These data have contributed to a renewal of the long-debated theory of vicariation or the taking over of function of damaged brain regions by spared healthy regions. It has become clear that in both humans and in experimental animal models, the injured brain compensates in a variety of ways that contribute to the return of function and that behavioral interventions are powerful modulators of postinjury plasticity supporting recovery.

Based on this growing evidence for behaviorally driven neural plasticity after brain injury and the increasing number of scientists and clinicians who are now designing therapeutic approaches grounded in the latest neuroplasticity principles, some have suggested that we are fast approaching an impending paradigm shift in neurorehabilitation therapy. In the coming years, advances in behavioral principles, robotics, pharmacotherapeutics, brain imaging, genetics, genomics, nanoelectronics, and neural prosthetics are likely to change the landscape of functional restoration after brain injury. The purpose of this chapter is to introduce the reader to the underlying principles of functional brain plasticity and how they may be applied to restoration of function after brain injury. What circumstances gave rise to the fundamental changes in emerging therapeutic principles? What factors modulate brain structure and function in the healthy and injured brain? How can contemporary therapeutic interventions be improved based on principles of neural plasticity? What does the future hold for further development of therapeutic approaches? Although the answers to these questions are still fragmentary, it is hoped that this chapter will help to prepare students and practitioners of neurorehabilitation for the paradigm shift that is already in progress.

It is important to note that most of the clinical examples and animal models of plasticity are based on recovery after ischemic infarct rather than on traumatic brain injury (TBI) per se. This is primarily because most of the literature on postinjury plasticity associated with recovery focuses on stroke or ischemia. In many ways, poststroke plasticity, at least in animal models, is an easier phenomenon to investigate and understand. The injury is typically focal and well circumscribed. The surviving cortical and subcortical tissue is often undamaged. In TBI, injuries may be diffused or multifocal; axonal shearing of corticocortical fibers may occur. Thus, even with the same lesion volume, the severity of deficits in TBI models may be greater (1). The same plasticity principles based on poststroke recovery generalized to TBI is still unknown because direct comparisons have not been made. The neurophysiological mapping studies that have formed the basis for many of the plasticity principles in this chapter have been infrequent in the TBI literature. However, the description of the various modulators of poststroke plasticity and their neuroanatomical and neurophysiological bases provide a fundamental understanding of the potential for the role of neuroplasticity in post-TBI recovery.

MATURATION OF OUR UNDERSTANDING OF BRAIN PLASTICITY AND RECOVERY PRINCIPLES

The modern era of the application of brain plasticity principles to recovery after injury began in the mid-1980s with a series of experiments demonstrating use-dependent modulation of the functional organization of somatosensory cortex (2–6). These studies demonstrated that after amputation of a digit or transection of a peripheral nerve in experimental animals, the deafferented cortex quickly became responsive to inputs from adjacent skin surfaces. Although later studies eventually showed that these functional alterations could be attributed, in part, to modulation of preexisting divergent connections in the lemniscal pathway (such as diverging thalamocortical arbors), other changes such as alterations in local cortical circuits and long-term anatomical changes have also been reported within the cortex. It is, thus, clear that the functional organization observed in the adult cerebral cortex is supported, at least in part, by cortical plasticity (Figure 68-1).

Results demonstrating use-dependent (and skill-dependent) modulation of auditory cortex, visual cortex, and

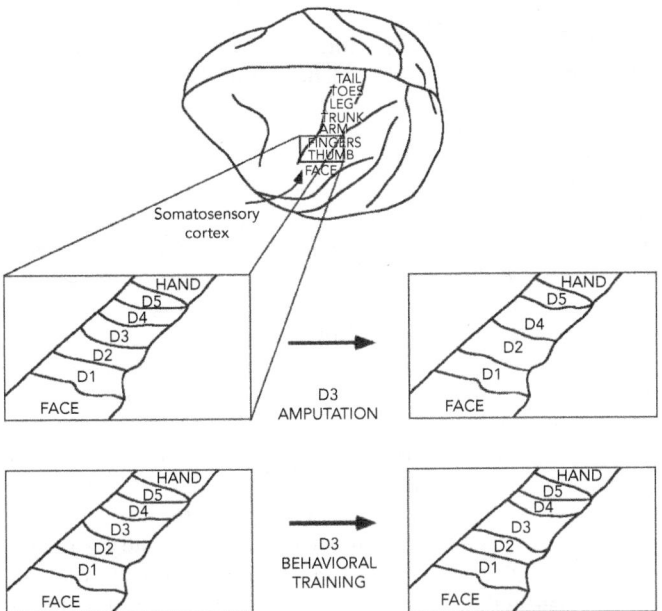

FIGURE 68-1 Classic neurophysiological studies in primary somatosensory cortex (area 3b) of nonhuman primates demonstrating that the functional topography of cerebral cortex is modifiable after peripheral injury and after repetitive use. Top experiment shows the area 3b hand map before and a few months after amputation of a single digit. Prior to the amputation, area 3b displays the normal topographic pattern with neurons responding to light touch on individual digits progressing from ulnar to radial aspects of the hand as a microelectrode is introduced from more medial to more lateral locations. Each digit's representational territory in cortex is demarcated by a sharp border. After a digit 3 amputation, neurons in the former digit 3 cortical territory become responsive to stimulation of skin surfaces adjacent to the missing digit, that is, to stimulation of digits 2 and 4. Bottom experiment depicts changes in the digit 3 representation in area 3b following several weeks training on a sensorimotor task in which digit 3 is repetitively stimulated. The representation of the stimulated digit expands, and receptive field sizes become smaller (7). Adapted from Kaas et al. (2), Killackey et al. (3), Merzenich et al. (4), Merzenich et al. (5), and Merzenich et al. (6) with permission.

motor cortex eventually erased any lingering doubts that topographic plasticity may be a methodological epiphenomenon, or specific to only certain portions of the cerebral cortex. Behavioral improvement correlates with neurophysiologic map plasticity, suggesting that these changes are an adaptive response of the cerebral cortex to novel behavioral requirements.

However, even in the early 19th century, clinicians and scientists began to ask specific questions regarding brain plasticity, although their knowledge of underlying neuronal mechanisms was rudimentary. Although better known for his study of phrenology (with Gall), Johann Spurzheim wrote that brain and muscles can increase with exercise "because the blood is carried in greater abundance to the parts which are excited and nutrition is performed by the blood." In the mid-19th century, Jean-Pierre Flourens, one of the first experimental brain researchers, asserted that after restricted lesions of the cerebellum, recovery could occur as the result

of compensation by other brain areas. This view was later to be incorporated in Lashley's principle of equipotentiality that states that all parts of the neocortex (or at least, all parts within a localized functional area such as visual cortex or somatosensory cortex) play an equal role in memory storage or in a particular physiological function (8).

Several other investigators took up the question of brain recovery mechanisms throughout the first half of the 20th century, including Sherrington, Franz, Glees, Denny-Brown, Kuypers, and others using behavioral and neurophysiological techniques (9–14). But it was in the final 2 decades of the century when solid evidence from experimental animal models accumulated to give adequate credence to the notion that cortical functions are not static in adulthood (15). Parallel human neuroimaging studies confirmed that these same processes could probably be generalized to humans (16).

Thus, the recent intensive interest in recovery after brain injury has come about as a result of 2 nearly simultaneous events: (a) the maturation of our understanding of brain plasticity principles and (b) the rapid development of sophisticated neuroimaging techniques. In addition, interest has been spurred by the initial effectiveness of pharmacologic and physiotherapeutic interventions introduced during the acute or chronic stages after brain injury (i.e., thrombolytic agents poststroke, amphetamine, constraint-induced movement therapy [CIT]) (17–19). These recently developed interventions were largely based on neuroscientific and behavioral principles developed from animal models of postinjury recovery.

Although results demonstrating neuroplasticity in healthy brains as a result of experience and in injured brains as a result of trauma or stroke were largely phenomenological in the initial stage of discovery, the molecular and cellular mechanisms regulating these events are now intensively investigated. The coming decade will be important in defining which of the many potential features of neuroplasticity represent adaptive mechanisms, which represent maladaptive mechanisms, and which are epiphenomenal.

NEURAL CORRELATES OF SKILLED MOTOR CONTROL

Because many of the same underlying adaptive neurological processes are thought to occur in both normal and injured brains, to appreciate the events that shape anatomical and physiological plasticity and promote functional motor recovery after brain injury, it is first necessary to understand how repetitive use and motor skill acquisition modulate the structure and function of the normal uninjured brain. In this section, the organization of the motor cortex will be reviewed briefly. Then, the modulatory role of sensorimotor behavior will be discussed.

Organization of Motor Cortex

The motor cortex is composed of several interconnected cortical regions that are distinguishable from surrounding areas primarily on the basis of cytoarchitecture, thalamocortical and intracortical connectivity (hodology), and electrophysiological properties. In addition to the extensively studied primary motor cortex (M1) located in the precentral gyrus, there

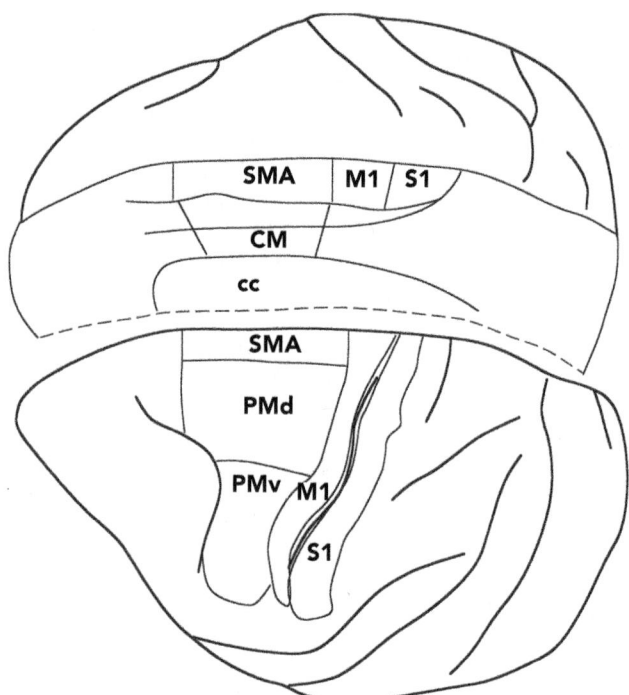

FIGURE 68-2 Location of motor areas in the cerebral cortex of a macaque monkey. At least 5 subdivisions can be recognized on the basis of structural and functional properties. These include the primary motor cortex (M1) located in the precentral gyrus, the dorsal and ventral premotor cortex located anterior to M1 (PMd and PMv, respectively), the supplementary motor area (SMA) located medial to PMd on the medial aspect of the cortex, and the cingulate motor areas (CM) located in the cingulate gyrus on the medial wall. Each of these main motor areas can be subdivided further based on cytoarchitectonic, neurophysiologic, and chemoarchitectonic criteria. Note that much of the M1 representation is buried in the central sulcus (i.e., on the anterior bank of the perceptual gyrus) in most primates (including humans). Thus, access for detailed neurophysiological mapping studies is limited. Certain nonhuman primate species (e.g., squirrel monkeys, marmoset monkeys) possess a relatively shallow central sulcus allowing more access to the caudal aspect of M1. cc, corpus callosum; S1, somatosensory cortex.

are several other motor areas that play important roles in motor control. These include the premotor cortex (dorsal and ventral premotor cortex or PMd and PMv, respectively), the supplementary motor area (SMA), and the cingulate motor cortex (CM). Each of these motor regions can be further subdivided based on histochemical, hodological, and neurophysiological properties (Figure 68-2) (20).

The primary pathway through which the motor cortex directs motor commands to the spinal cord motor neurons is the corticospinal tract. Corticospinal neurons originate from each of the cortical motor regions in the frontal cortex, that is, from CM, PMv, PMd, SMA, and from M1. Additional corticospinal neurons originate from parietal cortex, although their precise function in motor control is still unclear. Monosynaptic corticomotoneuronal projections (i.e., from neurons with somata located in cerebral cortex with fibers terminating directly onto motoneurons in the spinal cord)

are thought to originate primarily from M1 and terminate almost exclusively in the contralateral cord (21). Although approximately 10% of the corticospinal fibers remain uncrossed, modulation of motor neurons via the ipsilateral corticospinal tract is thought to be weak and indirect, at least in the healthy brain (22).

Each of the cortical motor areas is reciprocally interconnected with the others, although to varying degrees (20). Thus, M1 receives input from premotor, supplementary motor, and cingulate motor areas, and emanates corticocortical axons to terminate in these same regions. In addition, cortical motor areas receive substantial input from parietal cortex, specifically from somatosensory regions. Thus, the motor cortex cannot be considered strictly as a motor structure, but instead, is a site of somatosensory-motor integration with a primarily motor output function based on its corticospinal connections, in particular its monosynaptic connections with contralateral motor neurons. In fact, when focal ischemic lesions are made in either the primary somatosensory cortex (S1) or M1 of nonhuman primates, deficits are quite similar when performance on sensorimotor tasks is assessed (23,24). For example, in addition to a decrement in manual skill, monkeys with lesions in either S1 or M1 display a type of sensory agnosia. The sensory agnosia eventually subsides, possibly because of the use of visual guidance to compensate for deficits in somatosensory-motor integration.

The functional organization of the skeletal motor apparatus is represented in cortical motor areas in a topographic fashion with the contralateral leg represented more medially and the hand and face represented more laterally in M1. However, because of anatomical divergence of corticospinal neurons, a strict topography is not apparent when the spatial organization is examined on a more refined scale. It has been estimated that each corticomotoneuronal cell innervates about 4 or 5 separate motor neuron pools (25). Further, neurons originating corticomotoneuronal fibers innervating a single motor neuron pool are located in multiple sites within a topographic region in M1 (Figure 68-3). This anatomical divergence and convergence of corticospinal fibers, along with a dense network of local intracortical connections within M1, results in a substrate that provides a great deal of flexibility in its functional arrangement. In other words, it appears that motor cortex is expressly designed to allow for plastic reorganization of its local circuitry and ultimately of its functional outputs.

Use-Dependent and Skill-Dependent Modification of Motor Cortex Topography

A common technique for demonstrating the detailed topography of cortical motor areas in experimental animals is known as intracortical microstimulation (ICMS) (30). Based on ICMS results in nonhuman primates, the general topographic representation of specific body parts is quite consistent in M1, but substantial individual variability exists in the detailed topography on a more refined level, for example, within the hand representation (Figure 68-4). The size of the hand representation can vary by more than 100% in different monkeys, a difference that cannot be accounted for on the basis of the animal's size alone. It has been hypothesized that individual variation in motor maps is a result of each

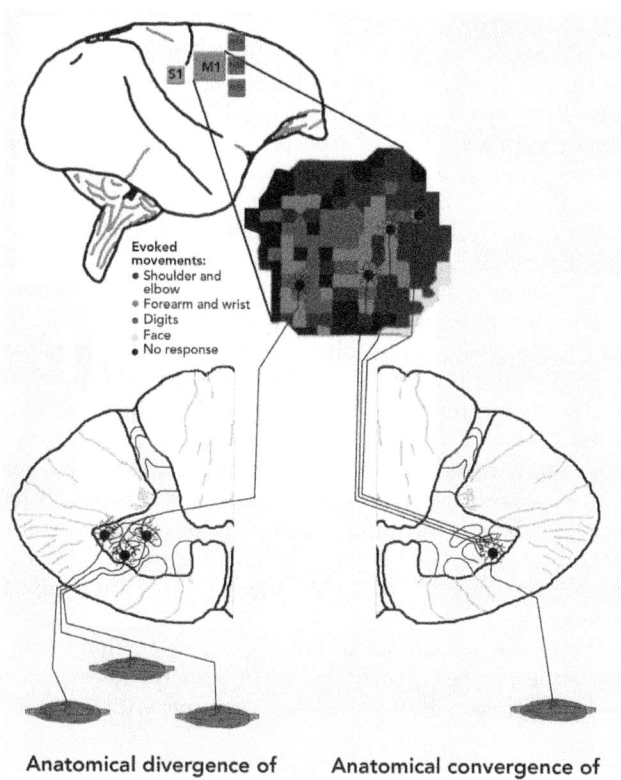

Anatomical divergence of
corticospinal neurons

Anatomical convergence of
corticospinal neurons

FIGURE 68-3 Anatomical divergence and convergence of corticospinal neurons. *Upper:* Example of a motor map of evoked movements in the primary motor cortex (M1) derived from intracortical microstimulation techniques. The map shows the intermingling of evoked digits, wrist and forearm movements clustered in the middle of more proximal (elbow and shoulder) movements. *Lower left:* Corticospinal divergence. One cell located in the digit representation of M1 projects to several motoneuronal pools in the spinal cord that, in turn, project to different arm muscles. This result has been demonstrated using both axonal tracing and spike-triggered averaging techniques (26,27). Functionally, this illustrates that one very small area of the motor map can have a very widely distributed influence on the musculature of the arm. *Lower right:* Corticospinal convergence. Several cells located at various locations within the wrist and forearm representations in M1 all project to the same motoneuronal pool in the spinal cord, which then projects to a single muscle of the arm. This has been demonstrated using both intracortical microstimulation and stimulus-triggered averaging techniques (28,29). Functionally, this illustrates that a wide surface area of the motor map can have a very focal influence on the musculature of the arm.

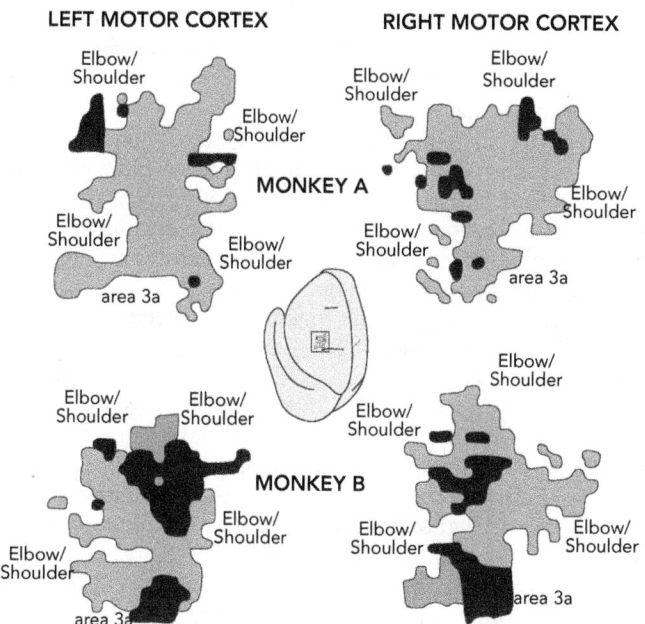

FIGURE 68-4 Individual variability in primary motor cortex (M1) maps in nonhuman primates. When the M1 maps of the hand representation are compared between hemispheres of the same animal, the mosaical patterns are similar on the 2 sides. For example, in both Monkeys A and B, the pattern of digit flexion representations (black) in the left motor cortex is roughly a mirror image of the pattern in the right motor cortex. However, when the digit flexion representation is compared between Monkeys A and B, the patterns are strikingly different, if not complementary. This high degree of individual variability in motor maps may result from the differential motor experiences of the animals prior to the mapping experiment. Gray denotes nondigit distal forelimb areas, and black is digit movement areas. Adapted from Hess and Donoghue (31) with permission.

individual's sensorimotor experiences leading up to the motor mapping procedure (31).

The modifiability of the motor map has now been studied extensively in M1 of humans and nonhuman primates and in the caudal forelimb area (CFA) of rodents (32,33). Soon after the learning of a new fine motor skill, the representations of the movements involved in the skilled task are enlarged. At least in experimental animals, specific combinations of movements used in the task emerge in ICMS maps (34). Presumably, local functional networks are established within the reorganized cortex, potentially reflecting the emergence of muscle and movement synergies within M1. Long-term potentiation of intracortical connections is likely to play a role in the emergent properties of reorganized cortex (35,36). Plasticity in motor maps resulting from the acquisition of motor skills is both progressive and reversible.

Plasticity in motor cortex organization as a result of motor skill learning has also been shown in humans using functional magnetic resonance imaging (fMRI) techniques (37). Although neuroimaging results represent a very different form of data in comparison to ICMS, skill-dependent changes can be demonstrated during the acquisition of motor tasks. However, the timing of the learning events may be critical to the particular changes that are observed (38). Although the relationship between acquired skills and the size of motor representations holds for M1, the story may be more complex for other motor areas or for simpler motor tasks. For example, during the sequential learning of foot movements, cerebral blood flow was increased bilaterally in the PMd and cerebellum during the execution of the movement. After a 1-hr training session, blood flow in these regions was no longer increased during foot movement (39). As the authors suggest, these areas may be involved in cognitive strategies and motor routines to execute the foot movements but are no longer involved once the sequence of movements is learned. Motor skill learning is now typically divided into 2 stages: fast and slow (37).

More recent fMRI studies of motor learning have demonstrated specific neural correlates of off-line learning, presumably involved in motor skill consolidation (40,41). Although this subject is beyond the scope of the current chapter, these neuroimaging studies may provide important clues regarding optimal schedules for motor retraining after brain injury.

Structural changes in motor cortex also occur during the acquisition of motor skills. In rodents assigned to a skilled-reaching task, reaching accuracy increased significantly at 3, 7, and 10 days of training. However, synaptogenesis (synapses per neuron) increased after 7 or 10 days of training, but not after 3 days of training. Motor map plasticity occurred at 10 days of training only. Motor learning-dependent synaptogenesis is localized only to those motor regions undergoing the motor map changes (42) (Figure 68-5). Thus, structural and functional changes in motor cortex are colocalized and are evident only in late stages of training, possibly related to the consolidation of motor skills rather than their initial acquisition (43). This late change in motor maps and motor cortex synaptogenesis is important in interpreting differ-

ences between fMRI results in human motor learning studies with electrophysiological and anatomical results in animal studies. The typical human studies are conducted over relatively short time intervals (minutes to hours), and thus, may be reflecting very different aspects of motor learning-dependent neuroplasticity. However, a more recent study has demonstrated in mouse motor cortex that the learning of novel motor skills leads to formation of dendritic spines within 1 hr (44).

In human neuroimaging studies, structural plasticity has typically been associated with the slow stage of motor skill learning (45). The results reflect increased gray matter volume in various cortical locations. More recent fMRI studies have shown relatively brief motor skill training sessions (30-min sessions, 4 times) resulted in increased gray matter in premotor cortical areas that paralleled increased functional interactions between cortex and striatum (46). It has been speculated that rapid remodeling of dendritic spines and axonal terminals, as well as glial hypertrophy and synaptogenesis, may contribute to the increased gray matter volume.

From the standpoint of developing new rehabilitative interventions based on neuroplasticity principles, it is important to contrast the effects of skill learning with repetitive

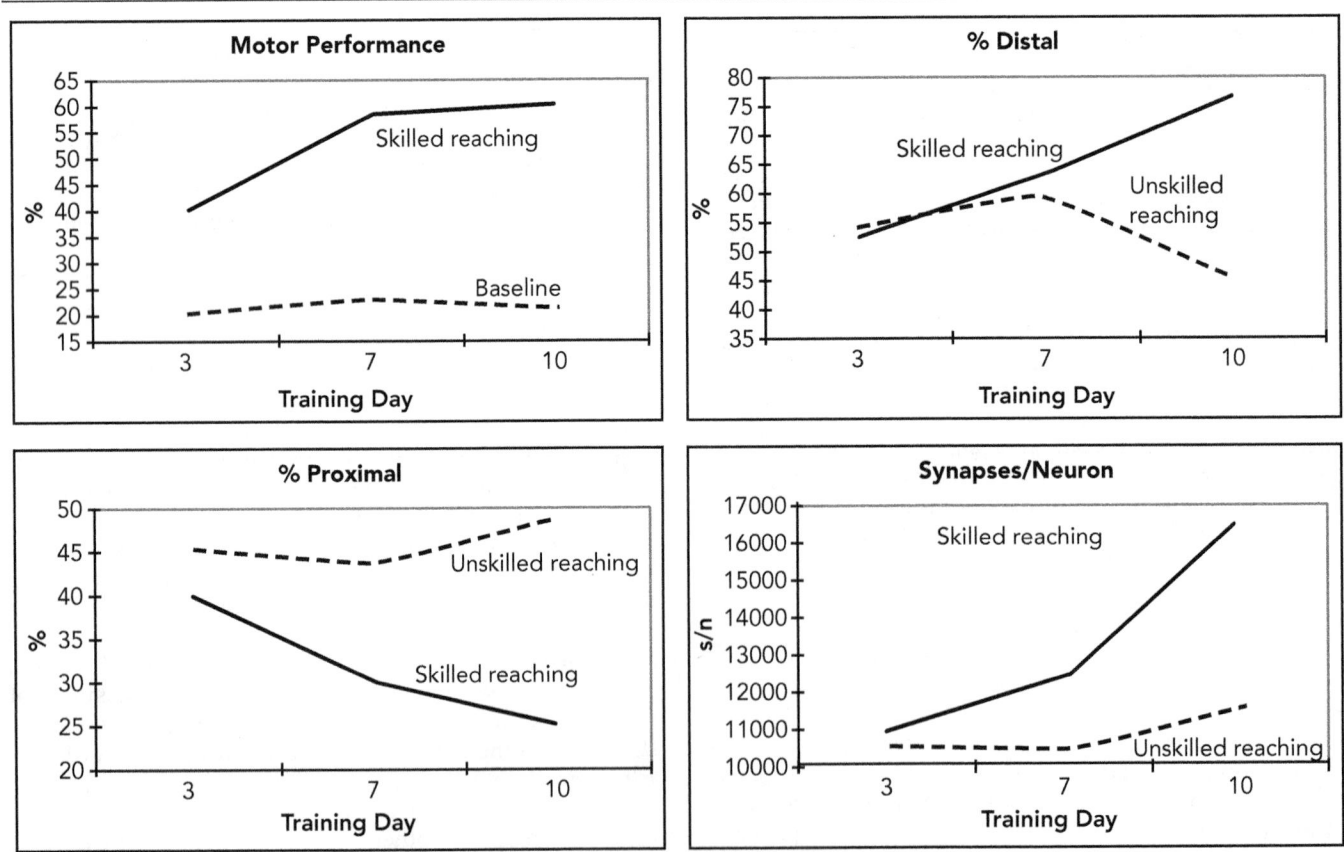

FIGURE 68-5 Functional and structural changes in motor cortex related to improvements in motor skill. As rats develop skill at a reach and retrieval task (upper left), distal representations occupy a progressively greater portion of the forelimb area (upper right), whereas proximal representations occupy a progressively smaller portion (lower left). In addition, synaptogenesis occurs during motor skill acquisition, especially during the later phases of motor learning (i.e., mostly at 10 days, but not substantially at 3 or 7 days; lower right). Simple repetitive tasks that do not require acquisition of new motor skills result in non-neurophysiological map changes or synapse changes. Adapted from Kleim et al. (43) with permission.

but nonskilled motor activity (Figure 68-5). In experimental animals, repetitive motor activity that does not induce improvements in motor skill or motor learning fail to alter motor map topography or synapse number (42,47,48) albeit induces angiogenesis (49,50). Also, the rapid formation of dendritic spines associated with motor skill learning only occurs if the tasks are novel and not with previously learned tasks (44). This phenomenon has not yet been extensively studied but may play a very important role in recovery at particular stages after brain injury.

ACUTE AND CHRONIC CHANGES IN PERILESIONAL AND REMOTE REGIONS AFTER BRAIN INJURY

Following injury to the brain, a cascade of molecular and cellular events is set into motion in the surrounding tissue that results in both temporary and permanent changes in the anatomy and physiology of the affected structures (51). Many of these changes are pathological consequences of the injury (e.g., edema) and have potentially damaging results. However, many adaptive processes may begin early in the postinjury stage and result in reduction of pathophysiological events or in neuroplastic changes leading to at least some restoration of function (52,53) (Figure 68-6). Although a thorough understanding of these processes at the molecular, cellular, and network levels is just beginning, sufficient knowledge is now available to begin testing hypotheses about the effects of specific postinjury interventions on functional recovery and its underlying neuroanatomical and neurophysiological bases.

Theories of Recovery

At least 3 general theories have been proposed to explain the substantial recovery that often follows brain injury, referred to here as reversal of diaschisis, compensation, and adaptive plasticity (or vicariation of function) (Figure 68-6). As early as 1914, von Monakow discussed the role of diaschisis, or the temporary reduction in function of structures interconnected with an injured brain region, in the acute stages after injury (54). It is well known that both cerebral blood flow and metabolism are decreased in the region immediately adjacent to the injured tissue. Further, structures anatomically connected with the injured region undergo similar reductions in blood flow and metabolism. Gradually, blood flow and metabolism returns to the connected regions. Because this disruption is temporary, functional recovery is likely to be related, in part, to a gradual reduction in diaschisis.

Compensation in motor behavior is a common consequence of brain injury, as the individual attempts to supplant lost functions with alternative strategies. As an extreme example of compensatory behavior, an individual with brain injury may begin to use the less-impaired limb for completing common tasks. However, more subtle changes in movement patterns occur even during use of the impaired limb. Individuals with impaired function of the arm and hand may use proximal musculature in compensatory strategies to propel the limb forward (55). Depending on the specificity of the motor endpoint that is assessed, such compensatory behavior could be missed, leading to the suggestion that motor performance has normalized. Even with the smallest experimental ischemic infarcts that can be made reliably in experimental monkeys, subtle changes in the kinematics of motor strategies take place, leading to the question of whether "true recovery," that is, return to normal, prelesion behavior, ever occurs (56). This is an extremely important but often overlooked aspect of recovery that is critical for interpreting studies of neuroplasticity mechanisms after injury. Since use- and learning-dependent changes are observable in the anatomy and physiology of normal intact brains, it must be presumed that the development of compensatory motor patterns postinjury also alters brain structure and function.

A third general theory posits that functional recovery is largely dependent on adaptive plasticity of intact remaining brain structures. Various alternative terms have also been used to describe this theory, including "vicariation of function" and "neural compensation." Although this theory is

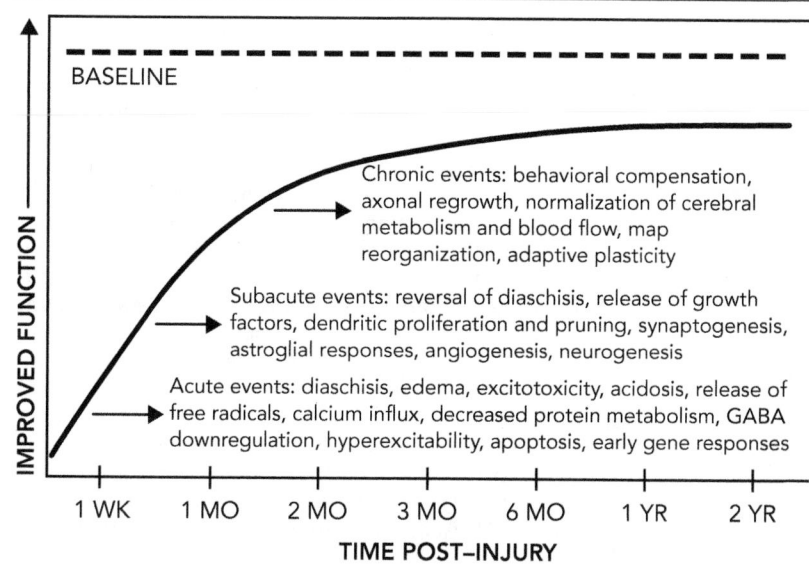

FIGURE 68-6 Cascade of acute, subacute, and chronic events that are triggered by cortical injury. As acute pathogenesis subsides, improved sensorimotor function occurs. During the subacute phase, presumed restorative mechanisms are set in motion, such as dendritic arborization, release of growth factors, and angiogenesis. Finally, functional and structural changes are consolidated in chronic phases, as evidenced by alterations in axonal pathways and functional map configuration.

also at least a century old, it has received considerable support in the past 2 decades from correlative studies in both experimental animals and in humans after brain injury. Underlying mechanisms thought to be involved in adaptive plasticity include unmasking of existing connections, long-term potentiation, long-term depression, axonal sprouting, dendritic sprouting, synaptogenesis, and angiogenesis. Also, although the role of neurogenesis after brain injury is still controversial, some studies now suggest that brain injury can induce this process at least in some regions, and that neurogenesis may contribute to functional recovery (57).

Neurophysiologic Alterations in Intact Structures After Brain Injury

Focal injury to the cerebral cortex does not simply result in a ''hole'' in the affected structure. Adjacent intact cortical regions, as well as more remote cortical regions interconnected with the damaged area, undergo substantial physiological and anatomical changes. A well-orchestrated cascade of molecular events influences these changes (58). As early as 1950, Glees and Cole (11), using cortical surface stimulation techniques, demonstrated that if the motor representation of the thumb in M1 was destroyed in experimental monkeys, it reappeared in the adjacent intact motor cortex. Later, it was demonstrated that a focal ischemic infarct in the primary S1 that eliminated the sensory representation of a single digit resulted in the eventual reemergence of the digit representation in the adjacent tissue (59). These results would seem to support the adaptive plasticity or vicariation hypothesis. However, when the newer ICMS techniques were applied to M1, the vicariation phenomenon could not be replicated (34). Instead, when small focal infarcts were made in the digit representation of M1, a further loss in digit representation occurred in the adjacent M1. Although it may be tempting

to dismiss the earlier results of Glees and Cole based on the spatially crude surface mapping techniques that were used, another important factor was found to contribute to the findings. This factor—the postinjury motor experience of the animal—has a great impact on the ultimate chronic condition of the motor map and very likely on the ultimate motor performance that can be achieved.

To determine the effects of postinjury experience on reorganization of motor maps, Nudo and colleagues (60) encouraged the use of the impaired limb by placing a restrictive jacket on experimental monkeys. The jacket contained a long sleeve that extended the length of the less impaired forelimb and ended in a soft mesh mitt on the hand. The restricted hand could still be used for climbing but was ineffective for grasping small objects, a task that was difficult to perform with the affected hand. Beginning about 5 days postinjury, 2 half-hour sessions of reach/grasp training were conducted each day. Several days to weeks were required to retrain skilled use of the affected hand, but eventually, motor performance on the experimental task was similar to prelesion levels. Following this recovery period, the ICMS-derived motor maps revealed that the digit representations in the intact areas were maintained. In some cases, they expanded into regions where prior mapping revealed proximal representations (60). Thus, motor experience after injury can drastically alter the ultimate functional organization of motor cortex (Figure 68-7).

This phenomenon is not limited to the adjacent cortex. In other nonhuman primate experiments employing slightly larger lesions encompassing the entire M1 hand area, hand representations in the premotor cortex were enlarged several months later, even in the absence of postinjury training. Further, the magnitude of the premotor enlargement was directly related to the size of the injury in M1 (61,62) (Figure 68-7). Because premotor cortex has reciprocal connections with M1, it is not surprising that this region is altered. But the

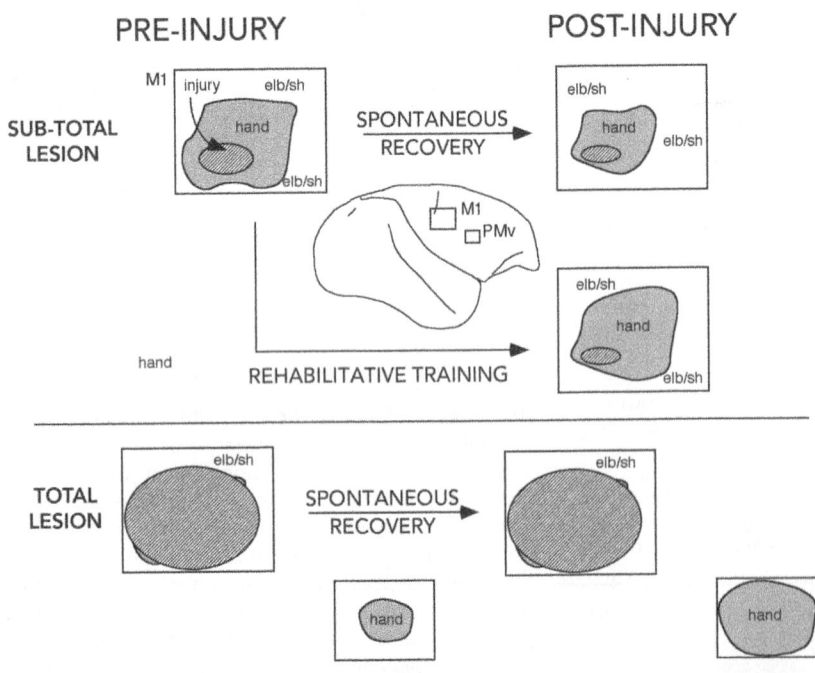

FIGURE 68-7 Functional alteration of local and distant cortical organization following focal injury. Subtotal lesion: if the injury is small enough, reorganization is primarily confined to the local adjacent tissue. For example, a subtotal injury to the primary motor cortex (M1) hand area results in changes in representational maps in the spared hand area adjacent to the injury. Postinjury rehabilitative training can have a profound influence on the inevitable map configuration. Total lesion: after a total lesion of the M1 hand area, other motor regions interconnected with M1 are stimulated to reorganize. For example, the hand representation in the ventral premotor cortex (PMv) enlarges. This premotor area normally has reciprocal connections with the injured M1. Adapted from Frost et al. (62) with permission.

enlarged representation related to the size of the M1 injury suggests that it may play a significant vicarious role in recovery. This enlargement in secondary cortical representations has also been demonstrated in the supplementary motor area in nonhuman primates (63). Importantly, after controlled cortical impact in the rat homolog of M1 (caudal forelimb area), the secondary motor area (rostral forelimb area) was reduced in size (1). The representations that remained suggested that the reorganization was related to compensatory motor behaviors.

Anatomical Alterations in Intact Cortical Structures After Brain Injury

In concert with behavioral recovery and neurophysiological remodeling, injured brains undergo significant anatomical plasticity in neuronal and nonneuronal structures. In experimental animals, small ischemic lesions result in a time-dependent alteration of structure and function in the peri-infarct territory. In an elegant series of 2-photon imaging studies by Murphy and colleagues (64), some of the details of this early process have now been elucidated. During the first hours to days following injury, neurons in the peri-infarct region lose dendritic spines. Sensory responses become less specific, and neurons are generally hypoexcitable. Over the ensuing weeks, growth processes are upregulated. Axons begin to sprout and migrate. Dendritic spine turnover and synaptogenesis increases. Neurons then begin to become responsive once again and may become hyperexcitable. A great deal of attention is now being paid to the balance between excitability states after injury, and whether pharmacological agents can improve function by rebalancing neuronal activity (65).

In rat motor cortex, intracortical fibers in the bordering intact tissue display orientations different from those seen in normal animals (66). Arteriolar collateral growth and new capillaries also form in the ischemic border (67). Significant neuroanatomical changes also occur in the contralesional (intact) motor cortex, but the role of this cortex in functional recovery of the affected limb is still a subject of debate. Recent results from animal studies suggest that the neuroanatomical changes in the intact cortex occur as a use-dependent or skill-dependent change because of increased use of the less-affected limb (68).

The latent potential for enhancing neuroanatomical plasticity mechanisms after brain injury has been demonstrated by the use of mutant mouse strains that lack the neurite outgrowth inhibitor (Nogo) receptor. Nogo is a protein involved in the inhibition of axonal growth. Mice lacking the Nogo receptor recover motor function after injury better than controls. Further, rats subjected to anti-Nogo antibody treatment initiated 1 week after injury resulted in better behavioral recovery compared with controls. Further, sprouting of contralateral corticorubral and ipsilateral corticospinal fibers was observed (69). However, in another rat study using a specific antagonist of Nogo-66 action at Nogo-66 receptor 1 (NgR1) (Nogo-66 receptor antagonist peptide [NEP1-40]), recovery was improved only when NEP1-40 was paired with rehabilitative training and not when given alone (70). Pharmacologic treatment with dexthroamphetamine (D-amphetamine) after brain injury has also been shown to enhance neocortical sprouting, synaptogenesis and behavioral recovery (71).

PHYSIOTHERAPEUTIC TREATMENT FOR MOTOR DISABILITY AFTER BRAIN INJURY: CURRENT PRACTICE

Because it is now clear that certain types of behavioral and pharmacologic interventions have the potential to alter neurophysiological activity and neuroanatomical structure, it may be helpful to examine the various therapeutic approaches used in postinjury rehabilitation and consider their potential for maximization of recovery based on neuroplasticity principles. This discussion may lead to a better understanding of the underlying mechanisms of rehabilitative therapy by pointing out the current gaps in our basic knowledge. It also may help us to refine therapeutic interventions to take advantage of the modulatory role that specific behavioral and pharmacological therapies play.

The Maximization of Motor Recovery Through Diverse Approaches

Treatment of upper limb impairments following brain injury follows either (*a*) principles of neurofacilitation or (*b*) principles of functional retraining. Traditionally, the choice between these rehabilitation strategies has been based on the phase of recovery. Whereas in the acute/subacute phase, therapy typically focuses on the prevention of maladaptive compensatory strategies while promoting the recovery of normal function; in the chronic phase, the emphasis is placed on maximizing function, often through the teaching of compensatory strategies (72).

Principles of Neurofacilitative Approaches
Neurofacilitative approaches, such as Rood, Brunnstrom, Bobath, proprioceptive neuromuscular facilitation (PNF) and sensory integration (SI) therapy, are usually used in early postinjury stages to favor motor recovery when most of the recovery seems to occur (73). These approaches focus on the recovery of normal movement. Unwanted movements and spasticity are inhibited, and normal patterns are facilitated under the assumption that regaining of voluntary control over key movements will transfer to functional improvement. These approaches are based on empirical assumptions that motor impairments are a consequence of a disruption of CNS hierarchical and reflex motor control (74–78). In the traditional view of these approaches, recovery of motor function follows the same chronology that is observed in neurodevelopmental stages, supposedly reflecting the CNS efforts to reestablish its internal hierarchical order that was disrupted by the neuronal loss consequent to the injury. Therefore, these approaches use neurophysiological phenomena (e.g., reflex pathways) to favor "normal" motor behaviors and are largely based on neurodevelopmental knowledge (79). Whereas largely used and trusted by therapists (80,81), in general, they have not resulted in substantial impact on patients' recovery when examined in controlled trials (82–85) and seem to result in similar behavioral outcomes when compared to each other (86–88).

Currently, to our knowledge, no studies have explored physiological or morphological effects of neurofacilitative approaches on the CNS. This contrasts with the large number of mechanistic studies that are related to approaches based on movement repetition and retraining. However, it should be noted that the current absence of basic research investigating the effects of these approaches may be caused by technical challenges rather than a weaker scientific rationale. Among the technical difficulties, because the Neuro-Developmental Treatment (NDT) approach is specifically adapted for the individual's particular needs and because it involves a high level of therapist manual expertise, inter-subject and intertherapist variability is very high, making it quite difficult to standardize protocols. It is hoped that in the near future, the mechanisms of action of these approaches will be investigated. Currently, the urge for experimental support for the widely used clinical practice is felt and underlined by the NDT community (89). The desire to provide an evidence-based practice is supported by the NDT Association, which is currently providing financial support for research and favoring the development of a consistent knowledge base among therapists.

Principles of Functional Retraining

Recently, studies evaluating the mechanisms underlying motor acquisition and motor control have resulted in the elaboration of behavioral treatment approaches based on practice (72,86,90,91). In these approaches, it is believed that the hemiparetic subject has distorted central motor programs resulting from CNS cell death. Based on the assumption that repetition of movements has the same effects as the ones reported for normal individuals (92), it is believed that practice establishes novel motor plans for the resolution of encountered motor problems (93). Additionally, it is taught that movement repetition improves behavior by affecting muscle weakness, an important problem affecting upper limb function (94–96).

Initial evaluations of the efficacy of repetition of movement to improve motor outcomes following brain injury have provided encouraging results. Several studies have shown that repetitive concentrated practice improves motor outcomes (15,97–101). Additionally, diverse practice approaches have been explored to maximize retention and transferability (91,102–108). At this point, whereas it is well established that practice improves motor outcomes and function following brain injury, currently, a consensus on a precise and consistent protocol to use to maximize the recovery is far from established. The elaboration of standardized training protocols based on principles of motor learning, retention, and transferability specific to the hemiparetic population is one of the most urgent needs for patient management.

Although animal models have frequently been used to optimize basic therapeutic strategies in preclinical drug trials, their use has been underappreciated. Surely, animal research allows investigation of mechanisms through which practice favors recovery and the identification of morphological and physiological processes that accompany improved motor performances. Whereas physiological changes at the level of the motor cortex induced by practice following brain injury has been shown (60), the impact of diverse types of practice, intensity, or even the time at which practice is most

beneficial for the modulation of adaptive physiological and/or morphological changes has yet to be investigated. For example, it was recently shown that rats undergoing training consisting of repetitive movements demonstrated functional and structural plasticity within the same cortical regions (42). This study provides strong evidence that synapse formation and physiological expansion of cortical representation of movement are concomitant and probably interdependent adaptive processes playing important roles in learning. Knowing that learning and practice are so influential in the recovery from brain injury, the investigation of the parallel changes of dendritic arbors and physiological reorganization of motor maps in M1 or in premotor cortex will be of great interest. In the near future, the choice of treatment, intensity, and schedule of therapy at different stages of recovery (e.g., acute, chronic) could be directed to take advantage of the most prolific stages of morphological and physiological reorganization.

Although it is a long-held belief that most of the rehabilitation of motor function in individuals with brain injury occurs in the first few weeks to months following injury (68), until recently, there was little evidence available indicating that physical rehabilitation is effective for patients in chronic phases of recovery (109,110). However, the fact that some patients with a given extent and locus of lesion recover more movement than others suggests that additional factors may be involved. Taub and colleagues (109) suggested that some motor abilities were possible but were not reinforced. In the vernacular of classical conditioning, these behaviors were extinguished or actively inhibited. From this assumption, it was stipulated that function could be improved months or years after injury. In particular, this group has developed an innovative approach known as CIT that has received a great deal of attention in the last decade. The idea behind the application of CIT originates from fundamental experiments conducted in nonhuman primates following peripheral deafferentation (111). In these experiments, disuse of the affected upper limb was observed following the injury. This maladaptive behavior persisted if no manipulation was introduced, even after 3–6 months of spontaneous recovery period. At that point, the function of the deafferented limb could be greatly enhanced by forcing its use by restraining the nonaffected limb (112). This led to the "learned nonuse" hypothesis, which stipulates that nonuse or less than maximal use of the deafferented limb results from negatively reinforced attempts to use the affected limb. This negative feedback would consist of unsuccessful behavioral consequences of attempts to use the affected upper limb (e.g., absence of reward for goal-directed activity or painful execution). After the initial recovery period, when the ability to use the affected limb is stable, behavioral squeal caused by the learned nonuse remain. Therefore, because of the phenomenon, the actual use of the affected limb is much less than its true potential (113–115). Strong support for the learned nonuse formulation came from a study where restraint was applied directly following the deafferentation of the upper limb of an animal for a 3-month duration, therefore preventing the learned nonuse phenomenon to occur (116). When the restraint was removed, the animals used their deafferented limb. Also, when deafferented prenatally, animals exhibited purposive use of the deafferented limb from the first day of extrauterine life (117,118). In that experimental paradigm, the use of the upper limb following the lesion was also restricted because of the limited intrauterine space, thus preventing the negative feedback from unsuccessful usage of the limb and supposedly the learned nonuse phenomenon from developing.

Physiologically, it can be assumed that deafferentation is a lesion which, such as potentially many others, such as TBI or stroke, creates a disruption of sensorimotor integration loops. By this logic, disruption would result in initial poor motor behavior. The progressive reestablishment of sensorimotor integration loops through motor behavior favoring CNS adaptive mechanisms may underlie a substantial amount of spontaneous recovery from these lesions. However, during the adaptive period, the learned nonuse phenomenon would negatively intervene, making the subjects subconsciously or consciously learn that the use of the affected limb results in poor behavioral outcomes. The negative feedback from these outcomes would reinforce preferential usage of the nonaffected limb. In that view, the learned nonuse phenomenon would not only be present following deafferentation but also following any injury disrupting sensorimotor integration loops. Therefore, the application of a restraint on the unaffected limb to force the use of the affected limb should result in improvement of motor outcomes in numerous neurologic, and even orthopedic, conditions (119).

In the original application of the learned nonuse hypothesis to the hemiparetic population, a simple arm restraint was employed (120). In that study, patients with brain injury were required to keep their uninvolved upper extremities within a hand-enclosed sling during waking hours over a 2-week interval. Functional improvements in diverse tasks and in force were reported, and most of them were maintained when examined in a 1-yr follow-up assessment. The results supported the hypothesis that learned nonuse occurs in selected patients with neurological disorders, and that this maladaptive behavior can be reversed through application of a forced-use paradigm. In a second experiment (121), use of the sling for 14 days was combined with 6-hr practice of functional movements with the impaired limb for 10 of those days. The behavioral training paradigm consisted of operant conditioning (122). Patients demonstrated improvements beyond what had been reported with the sole use of the sling, and improvements in motor performance were maintained during a 2-year period of follow-up. The increase of motor improvements obtained from the combination of behavioral training with the wearing of the sling is a strong indication that, in addition to reversal of learned nonuse, additional factors may be involved in the recovery in chronic stages.

Positive results using the CIT paradigm have been reported in several experiments (109,115,123) and by unrelated research groups (124,125), repeatedly demonstrating large effect sizes for the Motor Activity Log (MAL) and for the Wolf Motor Function Test (WMFT). A subsequent multisite clinical trial with 222 ischemic stroke survivors confirmed efficacy for CIT on the WMFT (126). In addition, other studies using a modified CIT demonstrate that upper extremity function can be improved after TBI (127,128). Most importantly, improvement in motor skill made by the patients has been shown to be transferable to other activities in their daily lives. It should be pointed out that the constraint increases the time of treatment up to 90% of waking hours of the subject. Thus, it imposes a discipline that might otherwise be difficult to achieve in practice. It can be argued that it probably is the simplest and most reliable way to reach such a high level of intensity for a clinical intervention. In the absence of constraint, if a task introduces too many obstacles to execute with the affected limb, the subject will naturally have the tendency perform it with the other limb, therefore limiting the learning experience with the impaired limb. The constraint forces the patient to immediately apply the motor skills he or she is learning during daily treatment in a natural and very significant location: at home. Learning is context dependent, meaning that an important factor in the retention of motor skills is the relationship between the context of practice and the context of application (129). Therefore, the level of intensity of intervention and direct context-dependent application of the learned motor patterns during the day might explain why the therapy has such a high impact on the performance level on tests evaluating functional motor state of the patient (e.g., MAL, WMFT).

The paradigm used in nonhuman primate experiments is strikingly similar to CIT. Monkeys wore a jacket with a long sleeve restricting fine control by the less affected limb. Thus, these animal experiments may be very useful for evaluating various aspects of the CIT protocol (e.g., timing, intensity, specific behavioral factors, etc.). From the monkey studies, it would appear that the repetitive behavior is the more important factor in CIT rather than the presence of the constraint device. Recovery of hand representations in M1 is very rapid when the use of the restraint jacket is combined with repetitive training. However, when the restraint device is the sole source of motivation to use the impaired limb, normalization of motor maps occurs extremely slowly, if at all. Monkeys that wore a restraint jacket for up to 1 year did not display as much map recovery as to monkeys engaged in repetitive training for only 2 weeks (130).

A series of experiments to evaluate the presence of cortical representation changes, paralleling the behavioral changes resulting from CIT, has also been performed (131, 132). These studies reported increased cortical representation areas of the affected arm following treatment, an upper limb representational map size that was similar in both affected and less affected hemispheres at 6 months follow-up, and shifts of the center of the output map, suggesting recruitment of adjacent brain areas examination. This last result has been related by the authors to the phenomenon that has been reported in monkeys undergoing repetition of movement therapy following a cortical ischemic lesion (60). Therefore, human studies now support the hypothesis that CIT modulates recovery through processes that are similar to the ones that are known to occur following motor learning through practice and repetition.

As previously mentioned, one of the interesting results that came from these studies was that, in addition to the reversal of the learned nonuse phenomena, other factors appeared to be involved in the motor recovery in chronic stages. In fact, it was even shown that subjects that were undergoing intensive physical therapy consisting of aquatic therapy, neurophysiological facilitation, and task practice showed a level of improvement similar to that of sling restraint of the less affected arm, combined with intensive task practice or shaping (99,110). However, in these experiments, the intensive therapy control groups showed higher levels of decrement of arm use at the 2-year follow-up in comparison to the CIT group. Therefore, it appears that one of the advantages of the usage of a sling is the higher retention of use of the affected limb at the 2-year follow-up and that the common factor in all techniques producing an equivalently large treatment effect is repeated use of the more affected upper extremity (114). It, thus, can be suggested that patients with chronic hemiparesis have the capacity for functional motor learning and that they have not maximized their motor potential after traditional acute care.

In conclusion, we would tend to consolidate the preceding literature into one treatment hypothesis: intensive treatment based on repetition creates plastic changes that are associated with learning (which might include reversal of learned nonuse). This probably acts through positive behavioral conditioning of the use of the impaired limb resulting in learning and amelioration of the general motor schema of the upper limb.

Too Much, Too Early?

After injury to the sensorimotor cortex in rats, extreme use of the affected limb can result in an enlargement of the lesion and further motor impairment (133). If the unimpaired limb is placed in a restrictive cast after cortical injury, rats must rely heavily on the impaired limb for posture and locomotion. Forced overuse of the impaired limb during the first week after injury results in expansion of the injury and poorer motor performance (134). Forced overuse during the next 7 days does not result in injury expansion but nonetheless resulted in poorer motor performance. It has also been shown that after TBI in rats, neuroplasticity-related intracellular signaling proteins are disrupted if voluntary exercise is provided within the first week postinjury (135). These studies strongly suggest that there are specific vulnerable periods for maladaptive effects of use after injury. Timing of these maladaptive effects must be considered along with timing of adaptive effects in any rational therapeutic design for treatment of motor deficits after injury.

Assessment of Efficacy

The assessment of efficacy of clinical approaches is an important issue not only for brain injury recovery but also for the entire field of neurorehabilitation in general. One important question surrounding this topic is: should we focus on the return of "normal" movement (true recovery) or just on return of function at any cost (i.e., compensatory strategies)? This question extends beyond the clinical field and is also debated in the literature discussing animal models of brain injury (55,56,136). It also raises the question of evaluative tools. Obviously, very different tools are needed to evaluate the divergence from "normality" of movement and functional capacities of a patient. Whereas evaluation tools focusing on the "abnormalities" of movements are much more useful and appropriate to the practice of neurodevelopmental approaches, newer, strictly functional scales are used in several research protocols to measure the impact of movement repetition based treatments. Particularly, in the cases of CIT, the validity of the clinical tests they traditionally use to assess motor recovery has been questioned (123,137,138). These tests only evaluate function and use, and do not evaluate the use of compensatory strategies. In fact, the treatment

effects become much more uncertain when using evaluation tools monitored by trained therapists, such as the Fugl-Meyer (139) or the Barthel Index (138). It can be argued that the WMFT and MAL are self-reports that could circumvent the blinding process (138); familiarizing patients with the MAL questions on a daily basis may permit recollection of previous responses, thereby narrowing the choice points on the MAL. This effectively reduces the variability and enhances the effect size (139). On the other hand, it can also be argued that the ultimate goal of therapy, specifically at a chronic stage, is to improve function and use of the affected limb and that the WMFT and MAL are specifically designed and were shown to do this well (137). Alternatively, for the validation and evaluation of learning processes, movement kinematics could be assessed. One showed that in chronic patients, when immobilizing the trunk, the subjects use their shoulder and elbow joints in a more normal way (140). The use of the trunk helps patients to create end-point trajectories that are more similar to healthy subjects. This study underlines that compensatory behavior can potentially be detrimental to maximization of function, in this case, limiting the range of reaching. Whereas maximization of function is the goal of rehabilitative approaches, the identification of these detrimental compensatory strategies is necessary to achieve this goal. Novel evaluation scales are being developed (141) and will hopefully help clinicians in that task.

Treatment Groups and Valid Controls

It now seems obvious that the evaluation of treatment outcomes must take into consideration the type of treatment and the initial level of function of the targeted population (73,142). Intrinsic, nontreatment-related elements are key determinants in the level of potential benefits a patient derives from a particular treatment. Whereas the initial level of function (as reflected by clinical assessments such as the Fugl-Meyer) has traditionally been used as the main predictor for recovery, other factors are now identified as better predictors. The initial grade of paresis appears to be the most important clinical predictor for motor recovery (147). Additionally, motor-evoked potentials (MEP) seem to be highly predictive for the occurrence of motor recovery (144–146). It was shown to be a much better predictor than clinical examination, infarct size and location, age, and gender. Also, preservation of the corticospinal tract with magnetic resonance imaging (MRI) was found to correlate with good recovery, confirming the transcranial magnetic stimulation (TMS) studies (147). This confirms that studies evaluating the efficacy of different clinical approaches need to have stringent selection criteria for their subjects. Recovery after brain injury can vary largely between individuals. For example, individuals with purely cortical injury recover better than purely subcortical or mixed cortical-subcortical injuries. Decreases in the level of recovery can be observed from cortex, corona radiata, and posterior limb of internal capsule (148). This suggests that recovery of upper limb movement is heavily dependent on the preservation of corticofugal fibers (148,149). Also, the recovery period is approximately twice as long for patients with severe paresis (15 weeks) compared to patients with mild paresis (6.5 weeks) (150). Therefore, to truly evaluate the impact of a treatment on individuals with brain injury, studies should be designed to include patients with similar predicted outcomes in each experimental group. Additionally, if some subjects have intrinsic conditions rendering them unable to benefit from a certain approach, they should be studied separately to identify the substrate of this failure and the potential alternative approaches from which they could benefit more. Such results raise questions concerning the use of movement repetition in this particular population of patients with hemiparesis.

CONCLUSION

Our understanding of recovery from damage to the CNS has evolved tremendously in the last few decades. Fundamental research on the diverse physiological, morphological, molecular, and genetic changes resulting from ischemic damage and the association of certain phenomena to behavioral recovery has drastically impacted patient management. Evolving knowledge of plastic changes accompanying functional recovery coming from both animal studies and technological advancements in humans (e.g., fMRI) might create an entire new set of outcome predictors and/or surrogate markers of recovery states useful for both study design and patients' treatment choices. These novel indicators might also direct the type, intensity, and duration of treatments. For example, cortical representation of body segments evaluated with TMS could become a means to identify the endpoint for treatment. When patients demonstrate a plateau in physiological reorganization, this could imply that most of the adaptive changes have already taken place. Whereas much work has been done, obviously, many questions are still unanswered. Most of the experiments that have been performed so far have included only subjects with high functional scores. Unfortunately, a large proportion of patients with hemiparesis show mild improvements with currently available treatments. Surely, significant work in both animals and humans needs to be accomplished to better understand and provide more efficient treatments to individuals with brain injury.

KEY CLINICAL POINTS

1. Intense interest in recovery mechanisms after brain injury has come about as a result of (a) the maturation of our understanding of brain plasticity principles and (b) the rapid development of sophisticated neuroimaging techniques. Clinical trials employing pharmacological, physiotherapeutic (e.g., CIT), and device-based interventions are now largely based on neuroscientific and behavioral principles of neuroplasticity.

2. Both physiological and structural plasticity occurs during the learning of motor tasks in normal brains. Correlated phenomena include motor map reorganization, remodeling of dendritic spines and axonal terminals, as well as glial hypertrophy and synaptogenesis. These events are evident in human neuroimaging studies as gray matter volume increases. It is likely that similar phenomena are associated with relearning after brain injury.

3. Although known for decades, 3 general principles of brain recovery still guide our thinking regarding brain repair processes and the effects of interventions. These are the reversal of diaschisis, behavioral compensation, and neural plasticity. The notion that vicarious functions emerge

in undamaged regions now has support from animal models and human neuroimaging studies.

4. Following a focal ischemic or traumatic injury, a cascade of time-dependent molecular events is triggered in the perilesion area. Importantly, neurons are initially hypoexcitable but then become hyperexcitable at late time points. Maintaining balance in neuronal excitability may be an important factor in developing therapeutic inteventions.

5. The "learned nonuse" hypothesis and its reversal via repetitive training techniques predicts both outcomes in individuals with brain injury as well as motor map changes in animal models of brain injury.

KEY REFERENCES

1. Carmichael ST. Brain excitability in stroke: the yin and yang of stroke progression. *Arch Neurol.* 2012;69(2): 161–167.
2. Carmichael ST. Cellular and molecular mechanisms of neural repair after stroke: making waves. *Ann Neurol.* 2006;59(5):735–742.
3. Murphy TH, Corbett D. Plasticity during stroke recovery: from synapse to behaviour. *Nat Rev Neurosci.* 2009;10(12): 861–872.
4. Nudo RJ, Wise BM, SiFuentes F, Milliken GW. Neural substrates for the effects of rehabilitative training on motor recovery after ischemic infarct. *Science.* 1996; 272(5269):1791–1794.
5. Wolf SL, Winstein CJ, Miller JP, et al. Effect of constraint-induced movement therapy on upper extremity function 3 to 9 months after stroke: the EXCITE randomized clinical trial. *JAMA.* 2006;296(17):2095–2104.

References

1. Nishibe M, Barbay S, Guggenmos D, Nudo RJ. Reorganization of motor cortex after controlled cortical impact in rats and implications for functional recovery. *J Neurotrauma.* 2010;27(12):2221–2232.
2. Kaas JH, Merzenich MM, Killackey HP. The reorganization of somatosensory cortex following peripheral nerve damage in adult and developing mammals. *Annu Rev Neurosci.* 1983;6:325–356.
3. Killackey HP, Gould HJ III, Cusick CG, Pons TP, Kaas JH. The relation of corpus callosum connections to architectonic fields and body surface maps in sensorimotor cortex of new and old world monkeys. *J Comp Neurol.* 1983;219(4):384–419.
4. Merzenich MM, Kaas JH, Wall J, Nelson RJ, Sur M, Felleman D. Topographic reorganization of somatosensory cortical areas 3b and 1 in adult monkeys following restricted deafferentation. *Neuroscience.* 1983;8(1):33–55.
5. Merzenich MM, Kaas JH, Wall JT, Sur M, Nelson RJ, Felleman DJ. Progression of change following median nerve section in the cortical representation of the hand in areas 3b and 1 in adult owl and squirrel monkeys. *Neuroscience.* 1983;10(3):639–665.
6. Merzenich MM, Nelson RJ, Stryker MP, Cynader MS, Schoppmann A, Zook JM. Somatosensory cortical map changes following digit amputation in adult monkeys. *J Comp Neurol.* 1984;224(4):591–605.
7. Jenkins WM, Merzenich MM, Ochs MT, Allard T, Guic-Robles E. Functional reorganization of primary somatosensory cortex in adult owl monkeys after behaviorally controlled tactile stimulation. *J Neurophysiol.* 1990;63(1):82–104.
8. Finger S. *Origins of Neuroscience.* New York, NY: Oxford University Press; 1994.
9. Denny-Brown D. Motor mechanisms—introduction: the general principles of motor integration. In: Field J, ed.*Handbook of Physiology, Section I: Neurophysiology.* Vol 2. Washington, DC: American Physiological Society; 1960:781–796.

10. Franz SI. Variations in distributions of the motor centers. *Psychol Monogr.* 1915;19:80–162.

11. Glees P, Cole J. Recovery of skilled motor functions after small repeated lesions in motor cortex in macaque. *J Neurophysiol.* 1950; 13:137–148.

12. Lashley KS. Temporal variation in the function of the gyrus precentralis in primates. *Am J Physiol.* 1923;65:585–602.

13. Lawrence DG, Kuypers HG. The functional organization of the motor system in the monkey. I. The effects of bilateral pyramidal lesions. *Brain.* 1968;91(1):1–14.

14. Sherrington CS. *The Integrative Action of the Nervous System.* New York, NY: C. Scribner and Sons; 1906.

15. Bach-y-Rita P, Wood S, Leder R, et al. Computer-assisted motivating rehabilitation (CAMR) for institutional, home, and educational late stroke programs. *Top Stroke Rehabil.* 2002;8(4):1–10.

16. Chollet F, DiPiero V, Wise RJ, Brooks DJ, Dolan RJ, Frackowiak RS. The functional anatomy of motor recovery after stroke in humans: a study with positron emission tomography. *Ann Neurol.* 1991;29(1): 63–71.

17. Feeney DM, Gonzalez A, Law WA. Amphetamine, haloperidol, and experience interact to affect rate of recovery after motor cortex injury. *Science.* 1982;217(4562):855–857.

18. Papadopoulos SM, Chandler WF, Salamat MS, Topol EJ, Sackellares JC. Recombinant human tissue-type plasminogen activator therapy in acute thromboembolic stroke. *J Neurosurg.* 1987;67(3): 394–398.

19. Walker-Batson D, Smith P, Curtis S, Unwin H, Greenlee R. Amphetamine paired with physical therapy accelerates motor recovery after stroke. Further evidence. *Stroke.* 1995;26(12):2254–2259.

20. Dancause N, Barbay S, Frost SB, et al. Ipsilateral connections of the ventral premotor cortex in a new world primate. *J Comp Neurol.* 2006;495(4):374–390.

21. Rathelot JA, Strick PL. Subdivisions of primary motor cortex based on cortico-motoneuronal cells. *Proc Natl Acad Sci U S A.* 2009;106(3): 918–923.

22. Soteropoulos DS, Edgley SA, Baker SN. Lack of evidence for direct corticospinal contributions to control of the ipsilateral forelimb in monkey. *J Neurosci.* 2011;31(31):11208–11219.

23. Friel KM, Barbay S, Frost SB, et al. Dissociation of sensorimotor deficits after rostral versus caudal lesions in the primary motor cortex hand representation. *J Neurophysiol.* 2005;94(2):1312–1324.

24. Xerri C, Merzenich MM, Peterson BE, Jenkins W. Plasticity of primary somatosensory cortex paralleling sensorimotor skill recovery from stroke in adult monkeys. *J Neurophysiol.* 1998;79(4):2119–2148.

25. Cheney PD, Fetz EE, Palmer SS. Patterns of facilitation and suppression of antagonist forelimb muscles from motor cortex sites in the awake monkey. *J Neurophysiol.* 1985;53(3):805–820.

26. Cheney PD, Fetz EE. Comparable patterns of muscle facilitation evoked by individual corticomotoneuronal (CM) cells and by single intracortical microstimuli in primates: evidence for functional groups of CM cells. *J Neurophysiol.* 1985;53(3):786–804.

27. Shinoda Y, Yokota J, Futami T. Divergent projection of individual corticospinal axons to motoneurons of multiple muscles in the monkey. *Neurosci Lett.* 1981;23(1):7–12.

28. Donoghue JP, Leibovic S, Sanes JN. Organization of the forelimb area in squirrel monkey motor cortex: representation of digit, wrist, and elbow muscles. *Exp Brain Res.* 1992;89(1):1–19.

29. Park MC, Belhaj-Saif A, Gordon M, Cheney PD. Consistent features in the forelimb representation of primary motor cortex in rhesus macaques. *J Neurosci.* 2001;21(8):2784–2792.

30. Asanuma H, Rosen I. Topographical organization of cortical efferent zones projecting to distal forelimb muscles in the monkey. *Exp Brain Res.* 1972;14(3):243–256.

31. Nudo RJ, Jenkins WM, Merzenich MM, Prejean T, Grenda R. Neurophysiological correlates of hand preference in primary motor cortex of adult squirrel monkeys. *J Neurosci.* 1992;12(8):2918–2947.

32. Donoghue JP. Plasticity of adult sensorimotor representations. *Curr Opin Neurobiol.* 1995;5(6):749–754.

33. Nudo RJ. Adaptive plasticity in motor cortex: implications for rehabilitation after brain injury. *J Rehabil Med.* 2003;(41)(suppl):7–10.

34. Nudo RJ, Milliken GW. Reorganization of movement representations in primary motor cortex following focal ischemic infarcts in adult squirrel monkeys. *J Neurophysiol.* 1996;75(5):2144–2149.

35. Flynn C, Monfils MH, Kleim JA, Kolb B, McIntyre DC, Teskey GC. Differential neuroplastic changes in neocortical movement representations and dendritic morphology in epilepsy-prone and epilepsy-resistant rat strains following high-frequency stimulation. *Eur J Neurosci.* 2004;19(8):2319–2328.

36. Hess G, Donoghue JP. Long-term potentiation of horizontal connections provides a mechanism to reorganize cortical motor maps. *J Neurophysiol.* 1994;71(6):2543–2547.

37. Dayan E, Cohen LG. Neuroplasticity subserving motor skill learning. *Neuron.* 2011;72(3):443–454.

38. Karni A, Meyer G, Rey-Hipolito C, et al. The acquisition of skilled motor performance: fast and slow experience-driven changes in primary motor cortex. *Proc Natl Acad Sci U S A.* 1998;95(3):861–868.

39. Lafleur MF, Jackson PL, Malouin F, Richards CL, Evans AC, Doyon J. Motor learning produces parallel dynamic functional changes during the execution and imagination of sequential foot movements. *Neuroimage.* 2002;16(1):142–157.

40. Wymbs NF, Grafton ST. Neural substrates of practice structure that support future off-line learning. *J Neurophysiol.* 2009;102(4): 2462–2476.

41. Debas K, Carrier J, Orban P, et al. Brain plasticity related to the consolidation of motor sequence learning and motor adaptation. *Proc Natl Acad Sci U S A.* 2010;107(41):17839–17844.

42. Kleim JA, Barbay S, Cooper NR, et al. Motor learning-dependent synaptogenesis is localized to functionally reorganized motor cortex. *Neurobiol Learn Mem.* 2002;77(1):63–77.

43. Kleim JA, Hogg TM, VandenBerg PM, Cooper NR, Bruneau R, Remple M. Cortical synaptogenesis and motor map reorganization occur during late, but not early, phase of motor skill learning. *J Neurosci.* 2004;24(3):628–633.

44. Xu T, Yu X, Perlik AJ, et al. Rapid formation and selective stabilization of synapses for enduring motor memories. *Nature.* 2009; 462(7275):915–919.

45. Draganski B, May A. Training-induced structural changes in the adult human brain. *Behav Brain Res.* 2008;192(1):137–142.

46. Hamzei F, Glauche V, Schwarzwald R, May A. Dynamic gray matter changes within cortex and striatum after short motor skill training are associated with their increased functional interaction. *Neuroimage.* 2012;59(4):3364–3372.

47. Plautz EJ, Milliken GW, Nudo RJ. Effects of repetitive motor training on movement representations in adult squirrel monkeys: role of use versus learning. *Neurobiol Learn Mem.* 2000;74(1):27–55.

48. Remple MS, Bruneau RM, VandenBerg PM, Goertzen C, Kleim JA. Sensitivity of cortical movement representations to motor experience: evidence that skill learning but not strength training induces cortical reorganization. *Behav Brain Res.* 2001;123(2):133–141.

49. Black JE, Isaacs KR, Anderson BJ, Alcantara AA, Greenough WT. Learning causes synaptogenesis, whereas motor activity causes angiogenesis, in cerebellar cortex of adult rats. *Proc Natl Acad Sci U S A.* 1990;87(14):5568–5572.

50. Kleim JA, Cooper NR, VandenBerg PM. Exercise induces angiogenesis but does not alter movement representations within rat motor cortex. *Brain Res.* 2002;934(1):1–6.

51. Farooqui AA, Haun SE, Horrocks LA. Ischemia and hypoxia. In: Siegel GJ, Agranoff B, Albers RW, Molinoff PB, eds. *Basic Neurochemistry.* New York, NY: Raven Press; 1994:867–883.

52. Cramer SC, Bastings EP. Mapping clinically relevant plasticity after stroke. *Neuropharmacology.* 2000;39(5):842–851.

53. Witte OW, Buchkremer-Ratzmann I, Schiene K, et al. Lesion-induced network plasticity in remote brain areas. *Trends Neurosci.* 1997;20(8):348–349.

54. Finger S, Koehler PJ, Jagella C. The Monakow concept of diaschisis: origins and perspectives. *Arch Neurol.* 2004;61(2):283–288.

55. Cirstea MC, Levin MF. Compensatory strategies for reaching in stroke. *Brain.* 2000;123(pt 5):940–953.

56. Friel KM, Nudo RJ. Recovery of motor function after focal cortical injury in primates: compensatory movement patterns used during rehabilitative training. *Somatosens Mot Res.* 1998;15(3):173–189.

57. Zhang R, Zhang Z, Wang L, et al. Activated neural stem cells contribute to stroke-induced neurogenesis and neuroblast migration toward the infarct boundary in adult rats. *J Cereb Blood Flow Metab.* 2004;24(4):441–448.

58. Carmichael ST. Cellular and molecular mechanisms of neural repair after stroke: making waves. *Ann Neurol.* 2006;59(5):735–742.

59. Jenkins WM, Merzenich MM. Reorganization of neocortical representations after brain injury: a neurophysiological model of the bases of recovery from stroke. *Prog Brain Res.* 1987;71:249–266.

60. Nudo RJ, Wise BM, SiFuentes F, Milliken GW. Neural substrates for the effects of rehabilitative training on motor recovery after ischemic infarct. *Science.* 1996;272(5269):1791–1794.

61. Dancause N, Barbay S, Frost SB, et al. Effects of small ischemic lesions in the primary motor cortex on neurophysiological organization in ventral premotor cortex. *J Neurophysiol.* 2006;96(6):3506–3511.

62. Frost SB, Barbay S, Friel KM, Plautz EJ, Nudo RJ. Reorganization of remote cortical regions after ischemic brain injury: a potential substrate for stroke recovery. *J Neurophysiol.* 2003;89(6):3205–3214.

63. Eisner-Janowicz I, Barbay S, Hoover E, et al. Early and late changes in the distal forelimb representation of the supplementary motor area after injury to frontal motor areas in the squirrel monkey. *J Neurophysiol.* 2008;100(3):1498–1512.

64. Murphy TH, Corbett D. Plasticity during stroke recovery: from synapse to behaviour. *Nat Rev Neurosci.* 2009;10(12):861–872.

65. Carmichael ST. Brain excitability in stroke: the yin and yang of stroke progression. *Arch Neurol.* 2012;69(2):161–167.

66. Carmichael ST, Wei L, Rovainen CM, Woolsey TA. New patterns of intracortical projections after focal cortical stroke. *Neurobiol Dis.* 2001;8(5):910–922.

67. Wei L, Erinjeri JP, Rovainen CM, Woolsey TA. Collateral growth and angiogenesis around cortical stroke. *Stroke.* 2001;32(9):2179–2184.

68. Bury SD, Jones TA. Facilitation of motor skill learning by callosal denervation or forced forelimb use in adult rats. *Behav Brain Res.* 2004;150(1–2):43–53.

69. Lee JK, Kim JE, Sivula M, Strittmatter SM. Nogo receptor antagonism promotes stroke recovery by enhancing axonal plasticity. *J Neurosci.* 2004;24(27):6209–6217.

70. Fang PC, Barbay S, Plautz EJ, Hoover E, Strittmatter SM, Nudo RJ. Combination of NEP 1–40 treatment and motor training enhances behavioral recovery after a focal cortical infarct in rats. *Stroke.* 2010;41(3):544–549.

71. Stroemer RP, Kent TA, Hulsebosch CE. Enhanced neocortical neural sprouting, synaptogenesis, and behavioral recovery with D-amphetamine therapy after neocortical infarction in rats. *Stroke.* 1998;29(11):2381–2393; discussion 2393–2385.

72. Shumway-Cook A, Woollacot M. *Motor Control: Theory and Practical Applications.* Baltimore, MD: Williams & Williams; 1995.

73. Duncan PW, Lai SM. Stroke recovery. *Top Stroke Rehabil.* 1997;4:51–58.

74. Bobath B. *Adult Hemiplegia: Evaluation and Treatment.* 3rd ed. Oxford, UK: Heinemann Medical Books; 1990.

75. Bobath K, Bobath B. The neurodevelopmental treatment. In: Scrutton D, ed. *Management of Motor Disorders of Children with Cerebral Palsy. Clinics in Developmental Medicine, No. 90.* London, UK: Heinemann Medical Books; 1984:16–18.

76. Brunnstrom S. *Movement Therapy in Hemiplegia: a Neuropsychological Approach.* New York, NY: Harper & Row; 1970.

77. Montgomery P. Neurodevelopmental treatment and sensory integrative theory. *II Step Conference.* Alexandria, VA: American Physical Therapy Association; 1991.

78. Voss D, Ionata M, Myers B. *Proprioceptive Neuromuscular Facilitation: Patterns and Techniques.* 3rd ed. Philadelphia, PA: Harper & Row; 1985.

79. Gordon J. Assumptions underlying physical therapy intervention: theoretical and historical perspectives. In: Carr JH, Shepherd RB, Gordon J, Andal E, eds. *Movement Sciences: Foundations for Physical Therapy in Rehabilitation.* Rockville, MD: Aspen; 1987:1–30.

80. Lennon S. Physiotherapy practice in stroke rehabilitation: a survey. *Disabil Rehabil.* 2003;25(9):455–461.

81. Lennon S, Baxter D, Ashburn A. Physiotherapy based on the Bobath concept in stroke rehabilitation: a survey within the UK. *Disabil Rehabil.* 2001;23(6):254–262.

82. Basmajian JV, Gowland CA, Finlayson MA, et al. Stroke treatment: comparison of integrated behavioral-physical therapy vs traditional physical therapy programs. *Arch Phys Med Rehabil.* 1987;68(5, pt 1):267–272.

83. Dickstein R, Hocherman S, Pillar T, Shaham R. Stroke rehabilitation. Three exercise therapy approaches. *Phys Ther.* 1986;66(8):1233–1238.

84. Logigian MK, Samuels MA, Falconer J, Zagar R. Clinical exercise trial for stroke patients. *Arch Phys Med Rehabil.* 1983;64(8):364–367.

85. Wagenaar RC, Meijer OG, van Wieringen PC, et al. The functional recovery of stroke: a comparison between neuro-developmental treatment and the Brunnstrom method. *Scand J Rehabil Med.* 1990;22(1):1–8.

86. Crow JL, Lincoln NB, Nouri FM, De Weerdt W. The effectiveness of EMG biofeedback in the treatment of arm function after stroke. *Int Disabil Stud.* 1989;11(4):155–160.

87. Paci M. Physiotherapy based on the Bobath concept for adults with post-stroke hemiplegia: a review of effectiveness studies. *J Rehabil Med.* 2003;35(1):2–7.

88. Woldag H, Hummelsheim H. Evidence-based physiotherapeutic concepts for improving arm and hand function in stroke patients: a review. *J Neurol.* 2002;249(5):518–528.

89. Howle JM, ed. *Neuro-Developmental Treatment Approach: Theoretical Foundations and Principles of Clinical Practice.* Laguna Beach, CA: NeuroDevelopmental Treatment Association; 2002.

90. Horak FB, Shumway-Cook A. Clinical implications of postural control in research. In: Duncan PW, ed. *Balance.* Alexandria, VA: American Physical Therapy Association; 1990:105–111.

91. Schmidt RA. *Motor Control and Learning.* 2nd ed. Champaign, IL: Human Kinetics; 1988.

92. Gottlieb GL, Corcos DM, Jaric S, Agarwal GC. Practice improves even the simplest movements. *Exp Brain Res.* 1988;73(2):436–440.

93. Whiting HTA. Dimensions of control in motor learning. In: Stelmach GE, Requin J, eds. *Tutorials in Motor Behavior.* New York, NY: North Holland; 1980:537–550.

94. Bogousslavsky J, Van Melle G, Regli F. The Lausanne Stroke Registry: analysis of 1,000 consecutive patients with first stroke. *Stroke.* 1988;19(9):1083–1092.

95. Bourbonnais D, Vanden Noven S. Weakness in patients with hemiparesis. *Am J Occup Ther.* 1989;43(5):313–319.

96. Gillen G, Burkhard A. *Stroke Rehabilitation: A Function-based Approach.* St. Louis, MO: Mosby; 1998.

97. Balliet R, Blood KM, Bach-y-Rita P. Visual field rehabilitation in the cortically blind? *J Neurol Neurosurg Psychiatry.* 1985;48(11):1113–1124.

98. Basmajian JV, Gowland C, Brandstater ME, Swanson L, Trotter J. EMG feedback treatment of upper limb in hemiplegic stroke patients: a pilot study. *Arch Phys Med Rehabil.* 1982;63(12):613–616.

99. Butefisch C, Hummelsheim H, Denzler P, Mauritz KH. Repetitive training of isolated movements improves the outcome of motor rehabilitation of the centrally paretic hand. *J Neurol Sci.* 1995;130(1):59–68.

100. Langhammer B, Stanghelle JK. Bobath or motor relearning programme? A comparison of two different approaches of physiotherapy in stroke rehabilitation: a randomized controlled study. *Clin Rehabil.* 2000;14(4):361–369.

101. Sunderland A, Tinson DJ, Bradley EL, Fletcher D, Langton Hewer R, Wade DT. Enhanced physical therapy improves recovery of arm function after stroke. A randomised controlled trial. *J Neurol Neurosurg Psychiatry.* 1992;55(7):530–535.

102. Adams JA. A closed-loop theory of motor learning. *J Mot Behav.* 1971;3(2):111–149.

103. Gentile AM. Skill acquisition: action, movement, and neuro-motor processes. In: Carr JH, Shepherd RB, Gordon J, Gentile AM, Held JM, eds. *Movement Science: Foundations for Physical Therapy in Rehabilitation.* Rockville, MD: Aspen; 1987:93–154.

104. Kottke FJ. From reflex to skill: the training of coordination. *Arch Phys Med Rehabil.* 1980;61(12):551–561.

105. Shea CH, Shebilske W, Worchel S. *Motor Learning and Control.* Englewood Cliffs, NJ: Prentice Hall; 1993.

106. Smyth MM. Memory for movements. In: Smyth MM, Wing AM, eds. *The Psychology of Movement*. San Diego, CA: Academic Press; 1984:83–117.

107. Stallings LM. Retention and transfer. In: Stallings LM, ed. *Motor Learning: From Theory to Practice*. St. Louis, MO: Mosby; 1982: 197–218.

108. Winstein CJ. Motor learning considerations in stroke rehabilitation. In: Duncan P, Badke M, eds. *Stroke Rehabilitation: The Recovery of Motor Control*. Chicago, IL: Year Book Medical Publishers, Inc; 1987: 109–134.

109. Taub E, Crago JE, Uswatte G. Constraint-induced (CI) therapy: a new approach to treatment in physical rehabilitation. *Rehabil Psychol*. 1998;43:152–170.

110. Taub E, Morris DM. Constraint-induced movement therapy to enhance recovery after stroke. *Curr Atheroscler Rep*. 2001;3(4):279–286.

111. Taub E, Uswatte G, Morris DM. Improved motor recovery after stroke and massive cortical reorganization following constraint-induced movement therapy. *Phys Med Rehabil Clin N Am*. 2003; 14(1)(suppl):S77–S91, ix.

112. Knapp HD, Taub E, Berman AJ. Movements in monkeys with deafferented forelimbs. *Exp Neurol*. 1963;7:305–315.

113. Andrews K, Stewart J. Stroke recovery: he can but does he? *Rheumatol Rehabil*. 1979;18(1):43–48.

114. Taub E, Uswatte G, Pidikiti R. Constraint-induced movement therapy: a new family of techniques with broad application to physical rehabilitation—a clinical review. *J Rehabil Res Dev*. 1999;36(3): 237–251.

115. Taub E, Wolf SL. Constraint-induced movement techniques to facilitate upper extremity use in stroke patients. *Top Stroke Rehabil*. 1997;3:38–61.

116. Taub E. Movement in nonhuman primates deprived of somatosensory feedback. *Exercise and Sports Sciences Reviews*. 1977;4:335–374.

117. Taub E, Goldberg IA, Taub P. Deafferentation in monkeys: pointing at a target without visual feedback. *Exp Neurol*. 1975;46(1):178–186.

118. Taub E, Perrella P, Barro G. Behavioral development after forelimb deafferentation on day of birth in monkeys with and without blinding. *Science*. 1973;181(103):959–960.

119. Catania AC. *Learning*. 4th ed. Upper Saddle River, NJ: Prentice Hall; 1998.

120. Wolf SL, Lecraw DE, Barton LA, Jann BB. Forced use of hemiplegic upper extremities to reverse the effect of learned nonuse among chronic stroke and head-injured patients. *Exp Neurol*. 1989;104(2): 125–132.

121. Taub E, Miller NE, Novack TA, et al. Technique to improve chronic motor deficit after stroke. *Arch Phys Med Rehabil*. 1993;74(4): 347–354.

122. Taub E. Overcoming learned nonuse: a new approach to treatment in physical medicine. In: Carlson JG, Seifert AR, Birbaumer N, eds. *Clinical Applied Pathophysiology*. New York, NY: Plenum; 1994: 185–220.

123. Kunkel A, Kopp B, Müller G, et al. Constraint-induced movement therapy for motor recovery in chronic stroke patients. *Arch Phys Med Rehabil*. 1999;80(6):624–628.

124. Levy CE, Nichols DS, Schmalbrock PM, Keller P, Chakeres DW. Functional MRI evidence of cortical reorganization in upper-limb stroke hemiplegia treated with constraint-induced movement therapy. *Am J Phys Med Rehabil*. 2001;80(1):4–12.

125. Miltner WH, Bauder H, Sommer M, Dettmers C, Taub E. Effects of constraint-induced movement therapy on patients with chronic motor deficits after stroke: a replication. *Stroke*. 1999;30(3):586–592.

126. Wolf SL, Winstein CJ, Miller JP, et al. Effect of constraint-induced movement therapy on upper extremity function 3 to 9 months after stroke: the EXCITE randomized clinical trial. *JAMA*. 2006;296(17): 2095–2104.

127. Page S, Levine P. Forced use after TBI: promoting plasticity and function through practice. *Brain Injury*. 2003;17(8):675–684.

128. Shaw SE, Morris DM, Uswatte G, McKay S, Meythaler JM, Taub E. Constraint-induced movement therapy for recovery of upper-limb function following traumatic brain injury. *J Rehabil Res Dev*. 2005;42(6):769–778.

129. Hochstenbach J, Mulder T. Neuropsychology and the relearning of motor skills following stroke. *Int J Rehabil Res*. 1999;22(1):11–19.

130. Friel KM, Heddings AA, Nudo RJ. Effects of postlesion experience on behavioral recovery and neurophysiologic reorganization after cortical injury in primates. *Neurorehabil Neural Repair*. 2000;14(3): 187–198.

131. Liepert J, Bauder H, Wolfgang HR, Miltner WH, Taub E, Weiller C. Treatment-induced cortical reorganization after stroke in humans. *Stroke*. 2000;31(6):1210–1216.

132. Liepert J, Miltner WH, Bauder H, et al. Motor cortex plasticity during constraint-induced movement therapy in stroke patients. *Neurosci Lett*. 1998;250(1):5–8.

133. Kozlowski DA, James DC, Schallert T. Use-dependent exaggeration of neuronal injury after unilateral sensorimotor cortex lesions. *J Neurosci*. 1996;16(15):4776–4786.

134. Humm JL, Kozlowski DA, James DC, Gotts JE, Schallert T. Use-dependent exacerbation of brain damage occurs during an early post-lesion vulnerable period. *Brain Res*. 1998;783(2):286–292.

135. Griesbach GS, Gomez-Pinilla F, Hovda DA. The upregulation of plasticity-related proteins following TBI is disrupted with acute voluntary exercise. *Brain Res*. 2004;1016(2):154–162.

136. Roby-Brami A, Feydy A, Combeaud M, Biryukova EV, Bussel B, Levin MF. Motor compensation and recovery for reaching in stroke patients. *Acta Neurol Scand*. 2003;107(5):369–381.

137. Morris DM, Taub E. Constraint-induced therapy approach to restoring function after neurological injury. *Top Stroke Rehabil*. 2001; 8(3):16–30.

138. Dromerick AW, Edwards DF, Hahn M. Does the application of constraint-induced movement therapy during acute rehabilitation reduce arm impairment after ischemic stroke? *Stroke*. 2000;31(12): 2984–2988.

139. Van der Lee JH, Wagenaar RC, Lankhorst GJ, Vogelaar TW, Deville WL, Bouter LM. Forced use of the upper extremity in chronic stroke patients: results from a single-blind randomized clinical trial. *Stroke*. 1999;30(11):2369–2375.

140. Michaelsen SM, Luta A, Roby-Brami A, Levin MF. Effect of trunk restraint on the recovery of reaching movements in hemiparetic patients. *Stroke*. 2001;32(8):1875–1883.

141. Levin MF, Desrosiers J, Beauchemin D, Bergeron N, Rochette A. Development and validation of a scale for rating motor compensations used for reaching in patients with hemiparesis: the reaching performance scale. *Phys Ther*. 2004;84(1):8–22.

142. Lincoln NB, Parry RH, Vass CD. Randomized, controlled trial to evaluate increased intensity of physiotherapy treatment of arm function after stroke. *Stroke*. 1999;30(3):573–579.

143. Hendricks HT, van Limbeek J, Geurts AC, Zwarts MJ. Motor recovery after stroke: a systematic review of the literature. *Arch Phys Med Rehabil*. 2002;83(11):1629–1637.

144. Escudero JV, Sancho J, Bautista D, Escudero M, Lopez-Trigo J. Prognostic value of motor evoked potential obtained by transcranial magnetic brain stimulation in motor function recovery in patients with acute ischemic stroke. *Stroke*. 1998;29(9):1854–1859.

145. Heald A, Bates D, Cartlidge NE, French JM, Miller S. Longitudinal study of central motor conduction time following stroke. 2. Central motor conduction measured within 72 h after stroke as a predictor of functional outcome at 12 months. *Brain*. 1993;116(pt 6): 1371–1385.

146. Pennisi G, Rapisarda G, Bella R, Calabrese V, Maertens De Noordhout A, Delwaide PJ. Absence of response to early transcranial magnetic stimulation in ischemic stroke patients: prognostic value for hand motor recovery. *Stroke*. 1999;30(12):2666–2670.

147. Binkofski F, Seitz RJ, Hacklander T, Pawelec D, Mau J, Freund HJ. Recovery of motor functions following hemiparetic stroke: a clinical and magnetic resonance-morphometric study. *Cerebrovasc Dis*. 2001;11(3):273–281.

148. Shelton FN, Reding MJ. Effect of lesion location on upper limb motor recovery after stroke. *Stroke*. 2001;32(1):107–112.

149. Werring DJ, Clark CA, Barker GJ, et al. The structural and functional mechanisms of motor recovery: complementary use of diffusion tensor and functional magnetic resonance imaging in a traumatic injury of the internal capsule. *J Neurol Neurosurg Psychiatry*. 1998;65(6):863–869.

150. Jorgensen HS, Nakayama H, Raaschou HO, Olsen TS. Recovery of walking function in stroke patients: the Copenhagen Stroke Study. *Arch Phys Med Rehabil*. 1995;76(1):27–32.

Movement Rehabilitation

Katherine J. Sullivan and Karen McCulloch

INTRODUCTION

Innovative approaches in neurorehabilitation continue to evolve as advances in neuroscience and cognitive neuroscience unravel the physiologic events that occur with brain injury and recovery. Neuroplasticity is the remarkable capacity of the nervous system to respond and adapt to behavioral experience and change throughout one's life or after brain injury. Principles of neuroplasticity provide the scientific foundation for therapeutic strategies that facilitate recovery or slow the progression of degenerative disease or the natural consequences of aging (1). Survival from a traumatic event usually results in complex behavioral, personality, or cognitive impairment that may or may not be accompanied by physical disability. Currently, models of disablement applied to rehabilitation are moving away from the medical model as the exclusive approach to health and are moving toward a biopsychosocial model of disablement and ablement. Today, there is building evidence that psychological, social, and environmental determinants of health are important modulators that are associated with well-being and quality of life for the person who survives the traumatic event but lives with brain damage (2).

The biological events at injury onset and behavioral interventions during the early phases of recovery affect later phases of recovery. The potential for neurorecovery and the success of rehabilitation are associated with the survival of functional brain tissue and interventions that improve cognitive and motor function (see chapter 68) (3). Because of the complex postinjury physical and psychological impairments, optimal recovery after brain injury is best for those that receive a structured rehabilitation program from health care professionals that specialize in acute care management and skillfully guide the long-term recovery process. Recovery is marked by distinct temporal stages that are associated with changing health priorities that differ for each phase of care postinjury.* The early, hyperacute phase of recovery is highly weighted toward the biological health dimensions; thus, medical interventions focused on survival and decreasing morbidity receive the highest priority. The acute and subacute phases of rehabilitation include the rapid change in motor and cognitive capacity that occurs as a person passes through the periods of spontaneous physiologic recovery. During this phase, experience-dependent rehabilitation interventions are designed to optimize neural recovery and repair. However, for the person with disability and the family who cares for them, the road to long-term recovery and adjustment is just the beginning.

PHYSICAL DISABLEMENT AFTER TRAUMATIC BRAIN INJURY

Disablement after brain injury is a complex, multifactorial process that is not determined by the level of ability or disability at the time of discharge from acute or subacute rehabilitation. *The International Classification of Functioning Disability and Health* (ICF) is a widely accepted framework to categorize the biopsychosocial dimensions of health (4); the ICF model is particularly useful for understanding the multidimensional aspects of disability after traumatic brain injury (TBI). The levels of function within the ICF model (body function and structure, activity, participation) have both a negative dimension (i.e., abilities lost) and a positive dimension (i.e. abilities retained) so that equal emphasis is placed on abilities and not just on disabilities associated with a health condition such as TBI (see Table 69-1 in the e-book).

A person is considered to have a physical disability if he or she is unable to perform age-expected basic activities of daily living (ADLs) (i.e., the ability to walk or dress) or more complex instrumental ADL (i.e., the ability to live at home unassisted, manage money, or drive). Physical disability that limits functional mobility combined with cognitive impairment can seriously restrict participation in age-expected life activities, such as the ability to play, go to school, raise a family, work, or live alone.

Current rehabilitation approaches for acquired traumatic or nontraumatic brain damage are beginning to move toward a greater appreciation that health and health outcomes are

---

*Temporal phases of neural recovery and neurorehabilitation: (a) hyperacute period, minutes to hours—brain injury onset through emergency, early medical management, and transfer to intensive care unit (ICU); (b) acute period, 24 hours to 5–7 days—time of physiologic responses to acute injury; (c) subacute phase, 1 week to 3–4 months—time of rapid neurorecovery and functional improvements because of combined effects of spontaneous physiologic recovery and therapeutic interventions; and (d) chronic phase, 4 months to years—neurorecovery and functional recovery associated with activity-dependent neuroplasticity.

BIOPSYCHOSOCIAL MODEL OF HEALTH AND HEALTH STATUS

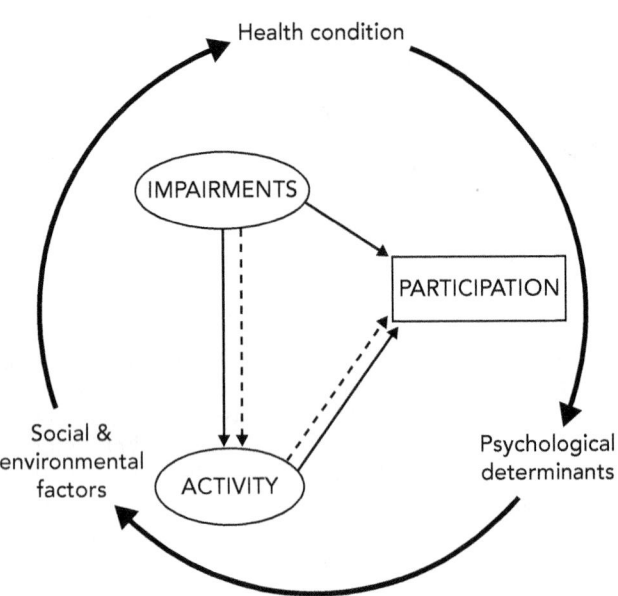

FIGURE 69-1 Biospychosocial model of health status.

Health Status: Figure 69-1 illustrates the dynamic relationships between the biologic determinants of health (*inner circle*) and the biopsychosocial factors that affect health and well-being (*outer circle*). Trauma or an acute disease-related event results in a sudden and drastic change in health status. The consequences of disease or injury impact the ability to participate in socially expected life activity. Each health professional on the rehabilitation team provides specialized expertise to address the health-related problems that are specific to the person with brain damage.

Biological Determinants

Physical disability level is influenced by the following:

1. Impairment severity (*solid arrow, impairment to participation*)
2. Inability to complete basic or instrumental activities of daily living (i.e., greater assistance needed by another person) (*solid arrow, activity to participation*).
3. Limitations in the physiologic capacity needed to meet task demands (*dotted arrow, impairment to activity to participation*) (i.e., lack of capacity in motor control, postural control, strength, endurance, and joint mobility restricts capability to perform activities).

Psychosocial Determinants

The level of ability or recovery after brain injury is not predicted by the biologic or medical management of damaged body systems and functions alone; rather, recovery is a multifactorial process affected by the personal and environmental factors that affect health and health outcomes (i.e., the psychological and social determinants of health).

---

modulated by both biological and social determinants of health (Figure 69-1). Thus, rehabilitation is most effective when the biological (i.e., physiological health condition/current health status), psychological (lifelong emotional health), and environmental (social and environmental facilitators and barriers) factors that affect health status and health outcomes are specific to the needs of the person with acquired brain injury and the family that cares for them at each phase along the recovery and adjustment process (see Table 69-2 in the e-book).

This chapter will focus on current evidence-based approaches to physical rehabilitation that are based on therapeutic principles from neuroscience, exercise science, and movement science. Motor skill acquisition drives neuroplasticity in cortical and subcortical brain structures (3); thus, principles of motor learning applied to task-specific practice will be discussed. Additionally, trauma to body structures and functions can affect limb alignment or motor control needed to complete functional tasks because of impaired or abnormal movement. Therapeutic interventions that improve movement control and prevent complications associated with immobility will be described. This chapter will end with 3 case studies to illustrate a biopsychosocial approach to health, recovery, and rehabilitation after brain injury.

MOTOR SKILL ACQUISITION: THE CONTROL AND LEARNING OF MOVEMENT

Motor skill acquisition is the process by which an individual learns a purposeful movement. As with other cognitive pro-

cesses such as learning language or developing declarative memories, various cortical and subcortical structures of the brain interact during motor learning. For movements that require speed and accuracy, a motor program develops over multiple repetitions so that a movement pattern can be executed with the correct timing and spatial location to meet the task goal (5). For example, a child learning to hit a baseball has to develop the strength and coordination to swing a bat with the appropriate speed and location to meet the ball as it passes over the plate. This type of motor skill is called coincident timing. Coincident timing tasks are one of multiple classifications of purposeful movements that require cognitive processing so that the correct response is executed between a stimulus or desire to move and the successful achievement of a task goal. The cortical representation of an action plan develops within networks of neurons that functionally link occipital and parietal sensory cortices that identify and locate a stimulus to move, prefrontal cortices that initiate the desire to move, and the secondary and primary motor cortices that program and execute the action.

The development and storage of motor memories is similar yet fundamentally different from the storage and retention of declarative memories (6). Declarative memory relies on a specific area—the hippocampus—to encode visual, auditory, and verbal stimuli into a short-term memory representation. Long-term storage and retention that is required to recall learned declarative memories occurs within dorsal lateral prefrontal cortical areas. In contrast, short-term motor representations do not rely on one specific functional cortical area but rely on networks of neurons that are specific to the action and parameters of the task. Motor memory is encoded during task practice; thus, motor performance during a practice session is similar to a short-term test of declarative memory. Motor representations are strengthened when the practice is active, goal directed, motivating, and effortful. Motor learning is evident when movements or actions are performed accurately, consistently, and are retained over time. The retention and retrieval of motor memories rely on cortical and subcortical networks that include the dorsal lateral prefrontal cortex, the basal ganglia, and the cerebellum (7).

Motor skill learning requires cortical processing to develop accurate effective motor plans; however, the final common pathway for all actions is the corticospinal tract where neurons that originate in the primary motor cortices descend to the convergent or divergent motor neuron pools within the spinal cord (8). Movement speed and accuracy during movement execution are modulated according to the demands of the task. Fine, coordinated movements rely on convergent motor neuron pools to generate discrete fractionated movements, sometimes described as isolated control. Coordinated forceful movements, such as throwing a baseball to a target, rely on divergent motor neuron pools. Motor units are recruited between the muscles of a functional movement synergy so that each muscle is activated with sufficient amplitude and timing needed to complete the motor task.

The corticospinal tract is the direct pathway for forces generated to support voluntary movements; however, the basal ganglia and cerebellum exert indirect influences on the corticospinal tract. Thus, normal movement relies on voluntary action modulated by the basal ganglia and cerebellum so that optimal postural and limb control are coordinated with the command to move (7,9). After brain injury, damage in the cortical areas that modulate the response, planning, and execution of movement can interfere with information processing demands needed for motor learning. In addition, motor control needed for limb movement, postural control, or locomotion can be impaired because of the damage within the direct and indirect motor pathways that control force production (i.e., corticospinal tract), coordination (i.e., cerebellum), and postural control (i.e., basal ganglia).

Motor Learning Is a Cognitive-Motor Process

Motor learning is the ability to acquire, retain, and retrieve movement plans so that actions are executed with the speed, accuracy, coordination, and consistency to achieve task goals (10). Motor learning is a cognitive process because information processing across cortical areas in occipital, parietal, temporal, and frontal areas is engaged during the process of skill acquisition. Motor learning involves both conscious and unconscious cognitive processing across declarative and nondeclarative areas of the brain (5,7).

The explicit learning system uses the declarative memory system to encode the visual, verbal, and auditory attributes that comprise the observable aspects of the task. The brain areas that process information regarding task goals, procedural steps, and analysis of outcome are processed by the conscious, aware, and explicit learning systems of the brain (11). The implicit learning systems do not rely on declarative memory and comprise the components of movement that are not under conscious awareness. Studies that use the serial reaction time task demonstrate that learners improve reaction time to embedded serial sequences without

having any conscious awareness that repeated sequences exist. Functional magnetic resonance imaging (fMRI) studies reveal that the more rapid yet unconscious awareness of motor performance is caused by synaptic efficacy within neural networks engaged during task practice (1). The implicit system is nondeclarative; improvements in performance such as faster reaction time or movements with greater speed and accuracy emerge from neural networks that are more responsive with each successive movement or practice repetition. Implicit learning is evident in other forms of nondeclarative learning, such as procedural learning, habit formation, priming and perceptual learning, classical conditioning, and nonassociative learning (7).

The distinction between explicit and implicit learning is especially important in the treatment of individuals with TBI or other forms of brain damage when there is declarative memory impairment (12). Because the declarative and procedural learning systems are neuroanatomically and functionally distinct, a person with short-term declarative memory impairment because of damaged hippocampus may not be able to describe the explicit dimensions of the motor task (e.g., goals, procedural steps, outcome analysis) but is likely to improve motor performance without conscious awareness. Clinically, this dissociation is significant because it reveals that there is no direct relationship between the ability to learn new declarative information and the ability to learn motor skills. Thus, a patient during the period of post-traumatic amnesia can improve motor performance with repetition, even though there is no conscious awareness or declarative memory of the task components or practice experience. For individuals with declarative memory impairments, improvements in the ability to complete a task accurately or to perform the task in a shorter amount of time are indications of procedural learning, even if there is no declarative recall.

Task-specific training is a clinical strategy used by physical therapists during movement rehabilitation that focuses on the direct acquisition of skills through structured practice that does not rely on declarative memory ability. Often, task-specific training requires extensive practice; thus, task practice is most effective if practiced in the functional environment where the skill is needed. Perceptual cues that are implicitly associated with the environment are reinforced and become habitual if the task practice occurs in the environment where the person needs to function without declarative recall. Memory cues such as prearranged functional setups, pictures, or other declarative memory aids are very useful for habit formation and procedural learning because the declarative cue is recognized, but recall is not needed.

Motor Learning Requires Practice

The acquisition and retention of motor skills requires practice. In the 1970s, cognitive psychologists Fitts and Posner (13) described 3 phases that a learner passes through from the early phases of motor learning to the later phases of high-level skilled performance. The *cognitive* phase is the initial phase of learning where the learner develops the execution requirements of the skill to be learned. During the cognitive phase, the learner makes frequent errors and demonstrates variable performance as he or she develops an understanding of what to do. The learner is dependent on visual, verbal, and environmental cues to organize the movement. As errors decrease, other forms of feedback, such as kinesthetic, will be used for error detection and correction. In this early stage of learning, therapists serve as important sources of augmented verbal, visual, or tactile feedback.

Knowledge of results (KRs) is a postresponse feedback that provides information about movement outcome; knowledge of performance (KP) is a postresponse feedback about movement error (10). For example, following a 10-m walk test, the physical therapist can provide feedback to the person about the time it took to walk 10 m (KR) or the stance and swing gait deviations that are observed during the walk (KP). Both forms of performance feedback can be used by the therapist to enhance the motor learning of functional mobility tasks. With more severe cognitive impairment, such as slowed information processing, attention deficits, and high distractibility, practice environments with fewer distractions are preferred during the early stages of motor learning when cognitive demands are high.

With additional practice, the learner shifts to the second phase of motor learning—the *associative* phase. In this phase, the learner shifts from "what to do" to "what is the best way" to complete the action. The learner begins to rely less on visual and verbal cues and attends to kinesthetic cues to develop an internal reference of correctness for the motor skill. As kinesthetic awareness develops, the learner has a greater ability to detect and correct movement errors without augmented feedback.

After extended practice, the learner shifts to the third phase—the *autonomous* phase. In this phase, motor tasks are performed more automatically and with less error, cognitive effort is less, and attentional demands directed to the explicit dimensions of the task are reduced. In the later stages of motor learning, the person with brain injury should be introduced to more environmental complexity and distraction that is most similar to real-life conditions. There is fluidity between the 3 stages of skill acquisition; thus, the performance proficiency (i.e., cognitive, associative, autonomous) will vary with the complexity of the task and environmental demands. In other words, a functional task such as a wheelchair transfer to a firm treatment mat may be performed at an autonomous level in the structured and quiet atmosphere of a therapy room. However, on the nursing unit where environmental demands are different (e.g., transfer to a higher compressible bed) or during a car transfer where task demands are more challenging, performance proficiency may regress to a lower level until sufficient practice with these additional challenges has occurred.

Summary

Motor skill learning is a purposeful, problem-solving, cognitive-motor process. The learner develops the coordination of perception and action to perform motor skills efficiently and effectively. Task-specific practice is one of the most effective intervention strategies to develop the motor skills that are needed to learn the movements and tasks needed in everyday life. Understanding that motor learning occurs in stages that have varying cognitive demands is especially important when planning a therapeutic session for someone with brain injury. In addition, it is important to be aware that the level of performance proficiency (i.e., cognitive, associative, autonomous) will vary with the task and environmental demands.

MOTOR LEARNING PRINCIPLES APPLIED TO PRACTICE

Motor learning is a process associated with practice or experience that leads to a relatively permanent change in the ability to produce skilled movements (14). Learning is not directly observable because learning occurs in the cortical and subcortical neural networks that modulate movement execution and retention. Physical therapists use movement analysis to observe and analyze how a patient moves during functional task performance. Through movement observation and analysis, the physical therapist determines whether a movement resulted in a successful task completion. In addition, the therapist assesses the actual movement performance to determine the level of skill (i.e., speed, accuracy, consistency) and the nature of the movement pattern during movement execution.

Movement observation is observation of motor performance. Motor learning is not directly observable but is inferred when movement performance becomes more skillful (i.e., improved speed, accuracy, consistency), is sustained over time, and can be transferred to a similar but different condition. Retention or transfer tests are used to determine if motor learning has occurred. Retention is the ability to retrieve and execute an action at a later time; transfer is the ability to generalize the movement execution to a similar but different condition. The distinction between motor performance and changes in performance over time and motor learning is important because the structure of practice and feedback can either strengthen or interfere with the cognitive processing during skill acquisition.

How would a therapist determine if the patient learned the motor task? A retention test applied to the clinical setting would be to observe the patient as they perform a previously practiced functional task with no feedback or cueing provided. The observed performance would indicate what was retained from the previous practice session. In contrast, a transfer test would be to observe task performance in a condition different than the practice environment to determine the patient's ability to generalize to a similar but different condition. Some tasks used during a therapy session can be retained but cannot transfer well to real-world conditions. For example, in studies of individuals with walking impairment after chronic stroke, static balance practice on a force plate with center of mass feedback did not transfer to the balance requirements needed during walking (15). In contrast, walking on a treadmill at speeds closer to normal walking speeds did transfer well to overground walking ability (16). Thus, specificity of training during practice is an important factor that drives skill acquisition and learning for those with or without brain injury.

Practice and feedback are 2 of the most important training variables that can affect motor performance and learning. The challenge point hypothesis, proposed by Guadagnoli and Lee (17), is a theoretical framework that can be used to illustrate how motor learning is a cognitive and motor process. According to the challenge point hypothesis, challenge during motor learning depends on the skill of the learner, the information processing capacity of the person, and the cognitive demands of practice. Learning requires the ability to attend to movement information but will be delayed if overloaded with too much information. Practice and feedback are modifiable and can be structured to affect the amount of cognitive demand that is needed during motor skill learning. The challenge point hypothesis proposes that motor learning is optimal when information processing demands imposed during task practice are sufficient to create a cognitive challenge that is effortful but does not exceed the cognitive capacity of the learner.

Conditions of Practice

Practice conditions can be manipulated to vary the presentation of tasks (i.e., practice schedule) across a training session or the presentation of feedback within a training session of a particular task. Conditions of practice or feedback that invoke greater cognitive effort appear to be more effective for motor learning (17). Cognitive effort involves the perceptual, motor, and decision-making processes that occur during skill acquisition. When cognitive effort is high during task practice, performance may be degraded; however, retention performance is better compared to task practice with less cognitive effort. How does greater cognitive effort during practice affect the ability to learn motor skills for a person with impaired cognitive function?

One way that practice can be structured in the clinical environment is to determine if a task should be practiced as a whole or broken into less complicated parts of the task. The literature consistently demonstrates that the effectiveness of whole-task or part-task practice is associated with task demands. Tasks are characterized as being either serial or continuous.

Serial tasks are discrete task units that are sequenced together to result in a meaningful functional outcome. For example, a patient learning to brush his or her teeth in the morning must learn to unscrew the toothpaste and apply it to the brush, move the brush to clean his or her teeth, and reach for a glass to rinse his or her mouth. Each discrete component of this functional task sequence can be practiced individually, then sequenced together to be practiced as a whole.

Continuous tasks are tasks where the movement is not defined by a described set of units. Tasks such as walking, driving a car, and interacting with others in a basketball game require both motor control to make appropriate adjustments for movement speed and accuracy and cognitive control to respond to environmental cues for safe and effective movement.

Movements that are continuous do not respond well to part-task practice. Thus, rising to stand from the edge of the bed to walk to the bathroom may include practice of sit to stand or stand to walk, but breaking up walking into discrete units is not consistent with how the nervous system responds to afferent and efferent information needed for locomotion.

Practice conditions can be structured to be variable or constant. Variable practice is practice of a movement pattern within a class of actions where the temporal or spatial parameters of the action are varied; constant practice is practice repeated along one dimension. For example, walking can be varied by walking at various speeds or by taking steps of various distances. In a study of treadmill training for walking impairment severity after stroke, training at constant fast speeds (2.0 mph) was more effective than walking at variable speeds (0.5, 1.0, 1.5, 2.0 mph) or at a constant slow speed (0.5 mph) (16). However, it could be argued that walking at very slow speeds is a different class of action compared to walking at normal age-expected speeds. In a more recent study, speeds that varied around more normal walking speeds (1.5–2.5 mph) proved to be effective (18). Although the exact mechanism is not fully explained, it appears that for continuous tasks such as walking, the nervous system responds to the practice conditions where the practice parameters are within the expected range of normal human performance.

Random-ordered practice is a practice schedule in which the order of multiple tasks is scheduled throughout a therapy session. Blocked practice is when a task is repeatedly practiced prior to moving to practice of a different task. For example, a therapy session could include 3 tasks that need to be practiced: coming to sit, sit to stand, and reaching to place books on a high shelf. A blocked practice schedule would be a repeated practice of coming to sit, followed by sit to stand practice, then reaching. Random-scheduled practice would order the tasks differently throughout the therapy session. Random-ordered practice is usually more effective than block-ordered practice because of a cognitive process called the *contextual interference effect* (10). During random ordered practice, greater cognitive effort is needed because each change in task induces a form of forgetting that requires the learner to reconstruct the motor memory from a previous, but not immediately preceded, practice trial.

Dual-task practice is a practice where 2 tasks (typically a motor and cognitive task) are performed at the same time. Cognitive load is higher during dual-task practice, which increases contextual interference. For example, a secondary cognitive task performed during walking may elicit slower and more variable walking. Training with dual-task conditions is one way to increase task complexity and higher information processing demands. Dual-task training is ecologically valid because the cognitive and motor challenge of dual-task practice can be increased in complexity to simulate motor performance demands with higher cognitive challenge as would be experienced in real-world environmental conditions.

Most of our current understanding of the cognitive-motor processing that is critical for motor learning has been derived from the study of young healthy adults. However, there is growing evidence that conditions of practice with high information processing demands that are within the capacity of young healthy adults is too high for an individual with impaired cognitive function. In other words, for a person with impaired cognitive function, such as declarative memory ability, task shifting, or rate of information processing, the use of blocked practice rather than random or constant practice rather than variable will be more effective for the learner who may need less cognitive challenge during task practice to focus on the motor demands during practice (19,20). The optimal scheduling of task practice for a person after TBI has not been well studied. However, the most effective practice for a person with cognitive impairment after TBI is practice that is structured, gradated to provide an appropriate level of challenge that is effortful but does not exceed cognitive capacity, and emphasizes implicit (e.g., task-practice) rather than explicit (e.g., direction driven) strategies.

Scheduling of Feedback

Feedback has a powerful influence on motor performance. During skill learning, visual, auditory, and proprioceptive systems provide intrinsic feedback regarding the movement and outcome of the task. For a person with brain injury, impaired sensory systems are less reliable sources of information during skill acquisition. Therapists provide augmented feedback by using verbal, visual, or tactile information during functional training session. Because augmented feedback can be both beneficial and detrimental to motor learning, the skilled therapist gradates the amount and type of feedback based on patient response.

Continuous or frequent feedback "guides" the patient to the optimal response and interferes with the problem-solving thought processes that should occur during practice (21). Feedback that is effortful but does not exceed the cognitive capacity of the learner is more effective than feedback that is too guiding or not of sufficient frequency to be meaningful. Concurrent feedback is a feedback that is provided continuously during the practice session. Consistently, it has been demonstrated that concurrent feedback degrades learning compared to less frequent feedback (10). Therapeutic interventions that use biofeedback, computer-generated feedback, or continuous physical guidance by a therapist are examples of concurrent feedback often observed in a clinical environment. In contrast, feedback that is reduced in its relative frequency of presentation across practice is more effective than feedback provided after every trial. For example, 100% relative feedback is feedback about the outcome of the movement (i.e., KR) or the action (i.e., KP) provided after every practice attempt. However, feedback provided after every other trial would be an example of a 50% relative frequency rate. Feedback that is delayed, postresponse, and faded from high frequency during early practice to lower frequency during later practice are associated with better motor learning (10).

How can feedback be manipulated in the clinical situation? There is growing evidence that children who have age-related differences in information processing rate compared to adults or adults with cognitive impairment because of a disease or injury may respond differently to feedback or practice conditions with high-information processing demands compared to age-matched controls (22). During the early cognitive stages of learning, the learner may rely on frequent feedback to learn what to do and how to do it; however, over practice, the learner becomes less reliant on external feedback sources. A therapist can manipulate feedback provided in the clinic by using a faded-feedback schedule, which reduces the relative frequency of feedback within or between practice sessions. As with practice, feedback can be manipulated by the therapist to create a challenging learning environment that encourages active cognitive processing, such as problem solving and error detection and correction without providing all of the feedback and cues that make learning a more passive process.

Summary

The use of practice and feedback during motor learning are essential elements in the recovery of movement after brain injury. Skill acquisition requires sufficient effortful practice for motor memory representations to be encoded and consolidated to be accessed for later retrieval. It is the process of motor skill acquisition that induces neuroplasticity in functionally related cognitive and motor neural networks; the process of skill acquisition is also associated with neural recovery and repair after brain injury.

CURRENT APPROACHES TO MOVEMENT REHABILITATION AFTER ACQUIRED BRAIN INJURY

Disease or injury of the brain that results in primary impairment of motor, sensory, and executive function affects functional mobility. Acquired brain damage can result in focal impairments of movement, vision, auditory, tactile/sensory perception, or high-order cognitive functions such as speech, reasoning, or motor planning. Reduced information processing capacity occurs with impaired cortical function. Typically, information processing occurs within modules of functionally connected neural networks that are linked spatial within and between hemispheres and across time as skill evolves with practice (23). However, after TBI or other conditions with focal or diffuse brain damage, motor performance can be negatively affected by (a) damage to primary motor areas that control the execution of fractionated, coordinated, fast, and accurate movements; or (b) secondary effects of impaired information processing capacity or other multimodal cognitive and executive functions that are needed for motor learning and to perform the functional movements needed to complete the tasks of daily life. Figure 69-2 shows how motor recovery and cognitive recovery can occur along different trajectories after brain injury.

Movement rehabilitation interventions provided by physical therapists include strategies to build capacity in impaired neuromuscular and cognitive-motor systems. In addition, physical therapists are particularly concerned with the development of functional capacity needed to perform mobility tasks such as sitting, standing, walking, running, throwing, and lifting. For the person with movement dysfunction after acquired brain injury, each treatment session is individualized to create the appropriate challenge point relative to the person's cognitive capacity and ability to execute fractionated movements.

Traumatic or nontraumatic brain injury results in a sudden and drastic change in health status. Physical and emotional health is a dynamic interplay of the biologic and social determinants that affect health and well-being. This section will focus on interventions that build capacity of sensorimotor and cognitive systems and capability in the tasks needed for age-expected participation. (Figure 69-1, *inner circle*, relationship between impairment severity, activity limitations, and participation ability).

Building Capacity in Impaired Body Systems

Body function and structure impairments such as impairments of voluntary movement, abnormal tone, and balance are primary impairments because of damage to functionally specific neural structures. Immobility results in secondary impairments of musculoskeletal and cardiovascular systems such as muscle contracture, joint mobility restriction, disuse weakness, and reduced endurance. Both neural and musculoskeletal impairments can be major contributors to func-

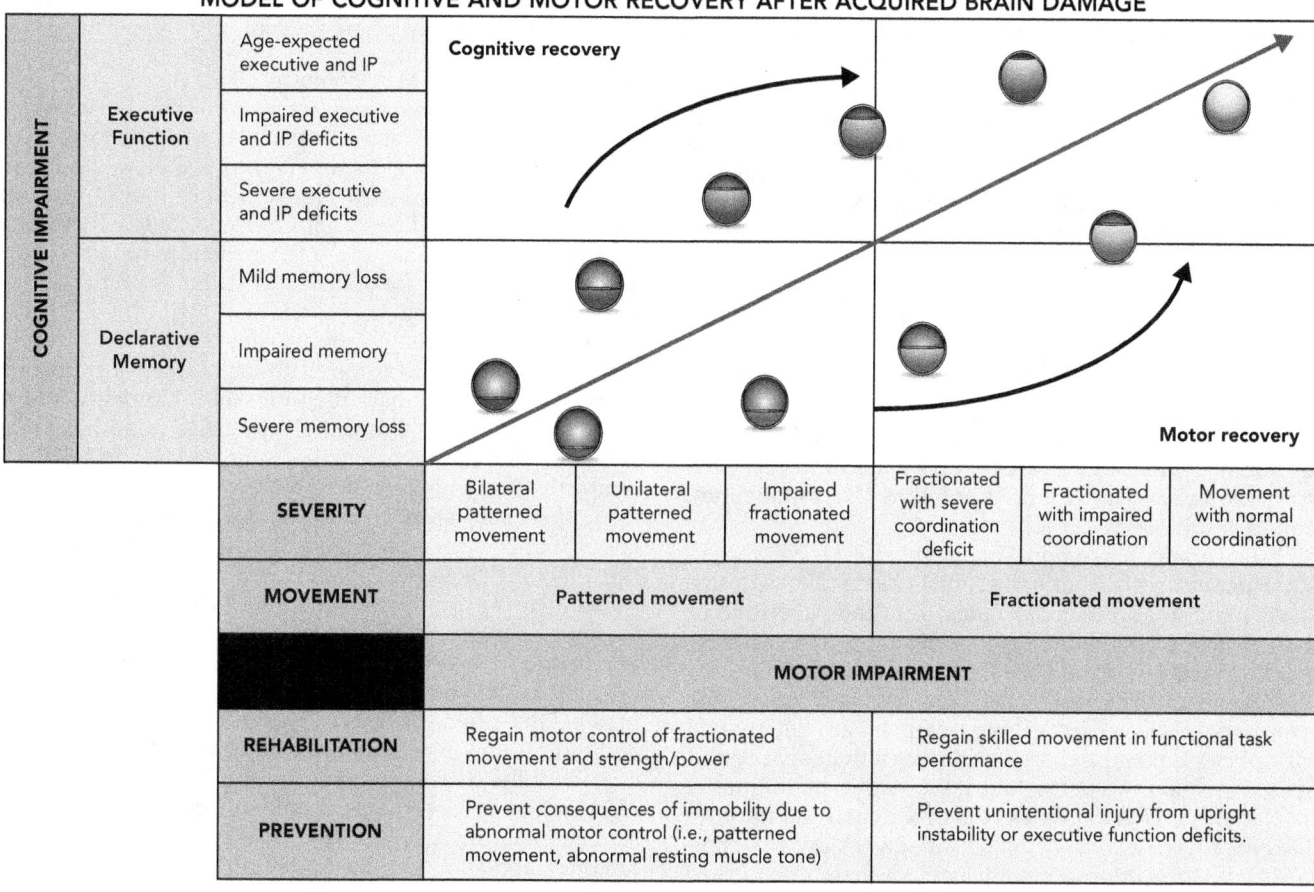

FIGURE 69-2 Relative change in cognitive capacity during cognitive recovery (*Y axis, spheres above the diagonal arrow*) from the relative change in motor capacity during motor recovery (*X axis, spheres below the diagonal arrow*). IP, information processing.

Explicit and implicit learning are modulated in functionally distinct neural networks; thus, cognitive capacity can recover along a trajectory that is independent from the recovery of motor capacity. Cognitive capacity can range from unconscious awareness with complete loss of explicit declarative memory systems to the highest level of age-expected executive function. Motor capacity can range from complete loss of corticospinal tract function with inability to generate voluntary fractionated movement to the highest level of skill with fast, accurate, and coordinated movements.

After TBI, damage to cortical or subcortical motor systems can vary substantially. For example, after diffuse axonal injury, a person could have high-motor capacity (voluntary control, fractionated movement with impaired coordination, *X axis* of Figure 69-2) with low cognitive capacity because of post-traumatic amnesia (severe declarative memory loss, *Y axis* of Figure 69-2). A patient with mild diffuse axonal injury after trauma but vertebral artery dissection with pontine and cerebellar infarcts may present with low-motor capacity (bilateral patterned movement), but cognitive capacity is relatively high because of minimal damage to explicit cortical learning systems (impaired executive and information processing deficits, *Y axis* of Figure 69-2).

For the person with post-traumatic amnesia but higher motor function, rehabilitation would focus on the development of functional mobility in higher level balance and coordinated skill tasks with preventive measures for safety given the executive and memory deficits. For the person with vertebral artery dissection, greater emphasis would be on motor recovery to damaged corticospinal and cerebellar tracts of the ventral pons and cerebellum.

tional deficits after brain injury. The following section provides a brief overview of current therapeutic strategies to address these problems.

Management of Impaired Cognitive, Behavioral, and Emotional Systems

In the days, weeks, and months after TBI, patients present with a variety of potential behavioral disorders that may affect their ability to participate in therapy. Organic impairments in cognition may compound behavioral issues further because the patient may not have the cognitive ability to accurately perceive and understand events or people involved in their care. Cognitive deficits may include confusion and disorientation, lack of ability to maintain alertness, inability to focus and sustain attention, decreased short-term memory, decreased problem solving and reasoning ability, delayed information processing, motor and verbal disinhibition, and lack of initiative and concrete reasoning. Perceptual disorders may also reduce the patient's ability to understand the environment (e.g., visual, auditory, tactile hypersensitivity or hyposensitivity, neglect, visual field deficits, right-left discrimination problems). Communication may be limited because of expressive aphasia, decreased comprehension, or delayed responsiveness that can limit the ability to interact with others. Emotional responses to the injury and disability can be manifested by outbursts of anger and frustration, or depression.

Individuals with prefrontal cortex damage may also demonstrate limited self-awareness of deficits and capabilities. This lack of insight may be especially challenging clinically because the presence of limitations and safety concerns may not be recognized by the patient. Without this awareness of a limitation in balance ability, for instance, a patient may attempt activities that are beyond to his or her capability, not see a need to ask for help, or follow safety guidelines, creating additional risk.

After serious TBI or non-TBI, the therapist is confronted with a patient who is, at some point, along the cognitive recovery continuum that can range from the vegetative or minimally conscious state to profound confusion and amnesia to the postconfusional state (24,25) (see also chapter 1 for a discussion of the natural history of recovery after TBI). Performance expectations during treatment are determined by the physical therapist based on the cognitive capacity and physical mobility of a person along the recovery continuum. The Rancho Los Amigos Levels of Cognitive Function (LOCF) Scale is the most common framework used by clinicians to describe the cognitive behaviors that are observed in the clinical environment during the cognitive recovery process (26). Table 69-3 describes common therapeutic strategies by low-, mid-, and high-level cognitive as defined by the Rancho LOCF. Physical therapists adapt the therapeutic learning environment so that the optimal challenge point

is provided based on the level of consciousness or confusion and the motor ability of the person.

Low-Level Cognitive Management
Patients who are considered within the LOCF Levels of I, II, and III have low levels of responsiveness that range from unresponsive (LOCF I) to generalized responses (increased breathing rate or stereotypic movement responses to stimulation) that is limited and nonpurposeful (LOCF II) to localized responsiveness in which the patient may localize to a stimulus (e.g., reach for an aversive stimulus on the arm) or follow simple commands (LOCF III).

Decreased levels of responsiveness are often accompanied by severe postural tone and lack of active movement that can lead to secondary musculoskeletal impairments, including contracture. Preventive strategies to address these secondary impairments will be discussed later. In collaboration with other team members, therapists usually begin some form of sensory stimulation program to encourage arousal and responsiveness. Once the patient is medically stable, upright mobility activities are initiated progressing from bed mobility to upright postures in a wheelchair or tilt table. Changes in posture and upright positions may be effective in evoking increased levels of responsiveness including eye opening in patients in the lower levels. Even as responsiveness begins, often, there is a low level of consistency in the ability to follow a command or move purposefully.

Since the development of Rancho LOCF, additional categorization of lower level cognitive function has been described including the vegetative state, where a patient's eyes are open and some routine body functions resume, and the minimally conscious state, where some degree of response to external stimuli is observable, although often is inconsistent (27). These disorders of consciousness are delineated by the type and consistency of responses to external stimuli and can be detected with the use of structured evaluation tools such as the "Coma Recovery Scale-Revised" (28). This measure allows therapists to carefully evaluate responses for purposefulness. Once the ability to follow commands is present, the patient can use that ability to engage in rehabilitation more actively and may begin to communicate basic needs and preferences (see chapter 32 for further discussion of patients at this level of recovery).

Mid-Level Cognitive Management
The transition from unresponsiveness to LOCF IV is accompanied by confusion and agitation in a range of 11%–50% of patients with brain injury (29). A patient at this level is easily confused and disoriented and may present with aggressive and inappropriate behavior. Agitated responses during this phase appear to be caused by internal confusion. The patient with agitation may not readily engage in self-care activity, and episodes of incontinence are frequent because of the lack of internal and external awareness. The therapeutic strategy at this phase is to provide a structured environment with minimal distraction that can allow the patient some freedom to move about while maintaining safety. Within this structured environment, brief directed activity can be introduced. Frequent short treatments that are interspersed across the day are the ideal therapy schedule for a patient in this phase.

Patients at LOCF V and VI are not agitated but continue to present with confusion and profound declarative memory

---

TABLE 69-3 Behavioral Treatment Strategies

LOCF	RECOVERY PHASE	APPROACH
I, II, III	Minimal response	Sensory stimulation Preventive maintenance Monitoring response to early mobilization
IV	Confused, agitated	Structured environment Directed activity Monitor response to stimulation Brief, frequent activity changes
V, VI	Confused	Structured environment Directed activity Consistent approach Complexity of tasks progressed gradually Environmental distractions progressed gradually
VII, VIII	Automatic	Reduce structure Greater self-monitoring Progressively challenging tasks

Abbreviation: LOCF, Levels of Cognitive Functioning. Reprinted from Hagen (26) with permission.

deficits. At LOCF V, the patient responds to commands and is more alert but is easily distractible with difficulty concentrating on tasks. Agitated outbursts and inappropriate verbal responses may still occur when the patient is frustrated. At LOCF VI, the patient has more consistent goal-directed behavior but needs cuing. Greater participation in ADLs is evident as the individual is developing greater awareness of self and others.

Cognitive Levels IV–VI are associated with post-traumatic amnesia in which the ability to develop new declarative memories is seriously impaired, so learning new information may be difficult. However, the distinction between the explicit (declarative) and implicit (nondeclarative) memory systems would suggest that patients during post-traumatic amnesia do have the capability to learn new motor skills and in fact, has been demonstrated in individual's post-TBI with post-traumatic amnesia.

Effective therapeutic strategies during this mid-level phase include the use of task-specific training in structured environments, encouraging adaptive task practice in which tasks chosen are challenging but allow for success. The expectation is that repetitive task practice will lead to a gradual improvement in motor performance. Acquisition of motor skill may be independent of any verbal recollection of the task training, using implicit memory systems. Patients with confusion benefit from a consistent approach to the daily schedule, treatment environment, choice of activities, mode of instruction, and familiar team members. Task complexity and changes in the structure of practice (i.e., increased variability) and feedback (i.e., decreased frequency) can progress as the patient's cognitive status improves.

High-Level Cognitive Management

The progression from the previous levels to LOCF VII and VIII is marked by improvements in short-term memory with more appropriate and purposeful behavior. During this phase, there is less confusion, better recall, and increased self-awareness and interaction with others and the environment. However, limitation in insight, abstract reasoning, and problem solving can still exist, particularly for those in LOCF VII. At this level, it is realistic to expect the completion of ADLs with relative independence. Therapy focuses on the tasks and skills needed to facilitate community integration. This phase is primarily focused on skill acquisition in the tasks that will assist the individual to participate in their desired self-care, social, educational, occupational, and recreational goals.

Management of Impaired Body Function and Structures

Optimal age-expected movement performance depends on the capacity of the (a) neuromuscular system to generate forces needed to control body movements, (b) musculoskeletal system to support the biomechanical requirements to meet task demands, and (c) cognitive system to generate actions that result in meaningful outcomes. This section will review therapeutic strategies that are designed to facilitate the recovery of voluntary purposeful movement, prevent the secondary consequences associated with immobility or impaired motor control, and develop motor performance capability in tasks that enhance participation.

Voluntary and Purposeful Movement

Impairments in voluntary movement associated with TBI can be caused by an upper motor neuron weakness syndrome that includes inability to activate selective joint movements out of synergy, decreased force production, and impaired initiation of purposeful voluntary movement. The primary mechanisms for these movement deficits post-TBI can be attributed to diffuse axonal injury because of scatted white matter disruptions in the descending motor pathways, focal cortical contusions, or deep cerebral hemorrhage. Direct damage to the corticospinal tract can occur as it passes through the striatocapsular region, and transtentorial herniation with compression of motor pathways in the upper brainstem can occur (30). Diffuse axonal injury and/or major brainstem contusion can result in low levels of consciousness in which reflexive movement patterns within decorticate and decerebrate postures can result from motor output of subcortical motor brainstem systems that include the rubrospinal, reticulospinal, and vestibulospinal systems (25).

In contrast to stroke where 70% of all stroke survivors will present with a motor hemiparesis, only 17% of patients post-TBI will have arm/hand paresis with synergistic movement and of these individuals, motor recovery is good such that only 3% will have synergistic hemiparesis at 4 months postinjury (31). The predominant motor deficit in patients post-TBI is impaired force production leading to decreased power generation and strength and impaired integration of voluntary movement with the other cortical, subcortical, and cerebellar motor systems involved in the planning, initiation, completion, and retention of accurate and consistent goal-directed movement (30). Weakness and impaired power generation can be a major factor along with sensory integration and cognitive deficits that interfere with performance of mobility tasks.

Appropriate therapeutic strategies to address neural motor control deficits after TBI vary according to the level of consciousness and ability to engage in activity-based interventions. In the acute care phase, patients are not always able to actively engage in therapy so treatment may involve therapist-driven interventions (i.e., stretching, sensory stimulation) to prevent secondary complication that can result from immobility (see chapter 49). In later recovery phases, task-specific training strategies are used to improve movement ability and increase functional mobility skills.

Abnormal Muscle Tone

Clinically, therapists are confronted with 2 major problems related to the impaired regulation of muscle tone: (a) abnormal muscle tone problems includes problems with velocity-dependent increases in phasic stretch reflexes associated with the upper motor neuron syndrome (i.e., spasticity) and (b) abnormal postural control interferes with the ability to maintain upright head, neck, and trunk postures against gravity. A wide range of clinical assessment tools (i.e., modified Ashworth Scale, modified Tardieu Scales) are used to assess abnormal tone, particularly spasticity (32,33). Although commonly used, the reliability and validity of spasticity assessments is poor, suggesting that further work is needed to develop more objective measures that capture the real-world impact of abnormal tone on function.

The approach to abnormal tone management is twofold. First is to address the spasticity and abnormal postural control with therapeutic interventions that decrease tone or increase upright control in functional postures such as sitting and standing. The second approach is to address the secondary musculoskeletal impairments that can occur when severe and unrelenting increases in abnormal muscle tone cause muscle contracture and joint deformity.

Botulinum toxin injections are more commonly used to target muscles that are overly active, which prevents muscle coordination between agonist and antagonists needed for functional movement. A recent study of 100 individuals with muscle spasticity because of motor control problems after stroke, cerebral palsy, and TBI demonstrated that targeted botulinum toxin injections followed by physical therapy was most effective (34). Muscle reeducation after injection is essential. The temporary benefit of reducing excessive motor unit recruitment in spastic muscles after botulinum toxin injection can be coupled with movement training so that more normal patterns of muscle activation needed for functional movement develop.

Balance and Vestibular Disorders

After head injury, gait instability is a major movement problem that contributes to increased risk for falls. Balance deficits can be a result of the combined effects of visual, somatosensory, and vestibular impairments as well as motor control deficits that result in weakness and incoordination. The vestibular system is a critical sensory system for postural control and balance so specific assessment of vestibular function is important (see chapter 47).

Vestibular disorders after TBI may occur with damage of the peripheral vestibular sensory apparatus or central structures that respond to the vestibular sensory inputs such as the vestibular nuclear complex, central pathways of the vestibulo-ocular and vestibulospinal reflexes, the brainstem, and the cerebellum. Peripheral vestibular dysfunction after TBI may result in unilateral hypofunction with symptoms of dizziness, disequilibrium, and impaired gaze stability. If peripheral damage is bilateral, complaints of vertigo or dizziness may be less severe, but the presence of severe disequilibrium and gait ataxia is often present. Trauma to the head can also result in benign paroxysmal positional vertigo (BPPV) caused when otoconia are displaced in the semicircular canals floating in the endolymph. BPPV results in distorted perceptions triggered by head position changes with brief episodes of severe vertigo and positional nystagmus.

Central vestibular disorders can commonly occur as a result of diffuse damage to white matter tracts that interact with vestibular areas of the brainstem and the cerebellum. A person after severe or even mild brain trauma can have complaints of a wide range of symptoms, but typically, vestibular dysfunction as a result of trauma to central vestibular structures will report a constant feeling of vertigo that is often accompanied by nausea, nystagmus, ataxia, or disequilibrium. It is now evident that vestibular dysfunction is a common problem after brain injury from repeated concussive blows to the head during sports-related activity (35) or as a result of blast exposure in military conflicts (36,37).

In addition to the measures of vestibulo-ocular function, such as oculomotor control, vestibular ocular reflexes, dynamic visual acuity, gaze stability, and positional testing, functional measures of balance should be assessed. Vestibular rehabilitation is specific to the type, severity, and functional deficits of a person post-TBI. Dependent on the physi-

cal therapist's assessment interventions can include vestibular adaptation exercises such as gaze stabilization exercises, balance retraining, sensory organization exercises with progressively more difficult static and dynamic activity, and canalith repositioning maneuvers.

There is a good evidence that vestibular rehabilitation that incorporates various balance retraining strategies that are designed to address specific patient problems can be effective (38) and is also beneficial for patients with TBI (39). It is beyond the scope of this chapter to discuss the appropriate evaluation and treatment of vestibular dysfunction. Excellent sources are available to provide greater background in this rehabilitation specialty area (40).

Muscle Contracture and Joint Mobility

Impaired voluntary motor control and spasticity are the primary cause of muscle contracture and joint deformity after TBI. Hypertonia, in combination with immobility because of lower levels of responsiveness and altered mechanical properties of muscle and connective tissues from disuse, can result in severe deformity of the upper and lower extremities. In addition, heterotopic ossification can further complicate joint mobility management. Common patterns of deformity that result from spastic motor patterns include shoulder adduction; internal rotation; elbow flexion; forearm pronation; wrist and finger flexion contractures of the upper limb and equinovarus foot with clawed toes, valgus foot, stiff or flexed knee; and hip adductor and flexor contractures of the lower limb. Spastic deformities interfere with bed positioning, sitting and standing, transfer and walking, as well as self-care activities such as hygiene and dressing. In addition to interfering with function, spastic deformities can be a major source of pain. The cumulative effect of these secondary musculoskeletal impairments can seriously reduce quality of life and the potential for recovery, especially for individuals who have been in coma for a long time.

The primary therapeutic goal is to prevent or correct muscle contractures. Various preventive methods are employed in the acute care setting immediately postinjury such as performing passive range of motion and stretching or using preventive bed positioning with wedges, splints, and pillows to improve limb alignment. Therapeutic interventions that are effective to increase passive range of motion or prevent its loss include stretching, serial casting, dynamic splinting, orthotic management, and, in combination with these types of physical approaches, pharmacologic management such as motor point blocks and intrathecal baclofen. In severe cases, when more conservative management has not been effective, surgical management for tendon lengthening or releases may be indicated.

Weakness and Deconditioning

One area that is beginning to receive more study is the effect of immobility on work capacity in individuals with brain injury. Individuals after brain injury have a reduction in peak aerobic capacity of 25%–30% compared with healthy sedentary persons (41). It is common in the acute phase that patients with TBI are confined to bedrest for days, weeks, or months depending on the initial brain injury severity. The adverse effects of prolonged bedrest are well documented in humans, but little attention has been given to the additive effects of immobility to chronic disease or injury. Immobility because of bedrest with a reduction in physical activity results in decreased muscular strength and aerobic capacity that leads to reduced work capacity. Prolonged immobility can also result in osteopenia, which can interfere with fracture healing for patients who may also present with multiple fractures in addition to the brain injury (see chapter 49 on Immobility).

The prevalence of fatigue at 43%–73% following brain injury is significant (42). Problems with fatigue are commonly multifactorial but could be accentuated by the injury itself (e.g., pituitary damage) as a result of increased cognitive effort that occurs because of changes in attention, sometimes referred to as the "coping hypothesis," or a result of other psychological, sleep, or physiological factors. Analysis of factors that may contribute to fatigue is necessary to determine most appropriate interventions to reduce feelings of fatigue. (see chapter 42 on Fatigue)

Building Capacity in Functional Activity

Mobility problems after brain injury include impaired limb and trunk movements and activity limitations in tasks such as sitting, standing, and walking. Exercise is used as a therapeutic modality to build capacity in weak muscles or to increase capability in functional motor performance. Traditionally, therapeutic exercise programs have been designed to remediate impairment-specific mobility problems. As discussed in the previous section, impairment-specific interventions are used to prevent complications of immobility, facilitate motor recovery, and address the combined behavioral cognitive-motor interactions that affect movement, speed, and accuracy.

Task-Specific Training

A comprehensive movement rehabilitation program for a person recovering from brain injury is one that builds capacity in impaired motor and cognitive systems as well as capability in the functional activities needed to fully participate in age-expected social roles such as going to school, working, or taking care of a family (43). Task-specific training is one of the most effective therapeutic approaches used to increase skill in functional tasks (44). A comprehensive systematic review compiled by Van Peppen et al. (45) on physical therapy interventions poststroke demonstrated that repetitive task-oriented practice is effective for improvements in functional limb movements and mobility tasks such as walking. Even though methodologically sound clinical trials in TBI are lacking (46), it is likely that therapeutic strategies that have been shown to be effective in brain injury because of stroke will be effective for those with traumatic forms of brain injury.

Training Intensity

Training intensity can be modulated by longer duration of time spent in exercise training or by increased difficulty or physiologic demands of the exercise session. Exercise dosing can be varied by time in the activity (minute per day), frequency of sessions (times per week), and the duration of training (weeks of training) (47,48). Incremental increases in task difficulty that increase physiologic demand of the exercise are additional methods to manipulate training intensity. Adaptive task practice is a form of task practice where the therapist grades task difficulty and feedback so that the patient is practiced at the optimal challenge point

and adjusted such that the patient experiences progressive challenge across training.

Summary

Task specificity and intensity are important principles of exercise that can be applied to the treatment of individuals with brain injury. There is strong evidence that intensive functional task training is effective in individuals with stroke-related brain damage; however, there is limited (yet developing) evidence in populations with TBI. Most likely, principles of exercise incorporated into therapeutic interventions will extend to other populations with brain damage such as those with TBI. It is unknown if cognitive and behavioral problems, common post-TBI, will interfere with the adherence needed to achieve the desired training effect. The "challenge point hypothesis" is a theoretical approach, which suggests that higher levels of motor skill acquisition are, in fact, a cognitive-motor process. Thus, intensity of training can be modulated by increasing the motor, cognitive, or motor/cognitive demands of tasks beyond the motor control needed for the execution of limb movements or postural control.

BIOPSYCHOSOCIAL MODEL OF REHABILITATION APPLIED TO PRACTICE

Models of ablement or disablement, such as the ICF model, are reminders that rehabilitation, which focuses only on the biologic determinants of health (43), does not fully address recovery after brain injury for the survivor or their family. This chapter has focused primarily on the biological and physiological aspects of movement rehabilitation. However, health after acquired brain injury is not a stepwise linear progression from survival to well-being. Rather, the road to recovery and the rehabilitation process is a dynamic interplay between the complications and comorbid conditions that result from trauma, severity of primary sensorimotor and cognitive system impairments, secondary impairments that are common after prolonged coma or lack of access to specialized care, level of assistance to perform functional activities, and the influence of personal and environmental contextual factors that affect participation and quality of life.

We end this chapter with 3 case studies (available in the e-resource material) to illustrate how the goals and priorities of movement rehabilitation evolve over a life course of recovery. When physical mobility is limited, physical therapy interventions address the physiologic consequences of trauma or disease on body functions and structures needed to move; however, each intervention provided by a physical therapist, *at any point along the recovery continuum*, is an element of a progressive program along a recovery path toward increased ability and optimal function for the person with brain injury (Figure 69-3).

Therapists use objective measures of movement dysfunction to assess the biological/physical consequences of brain injury. Therapists integrate these findings with equal consideration to the social and psychological factors that interact to influence health outcomes. Recovery from severe brain injury is a lifelong process. Early after injury, biological health takes priority; mobility goals are to prevent the complications of immobility. As the time line postinjury extends, high priority is placed on rapid discharge from the rehabili-

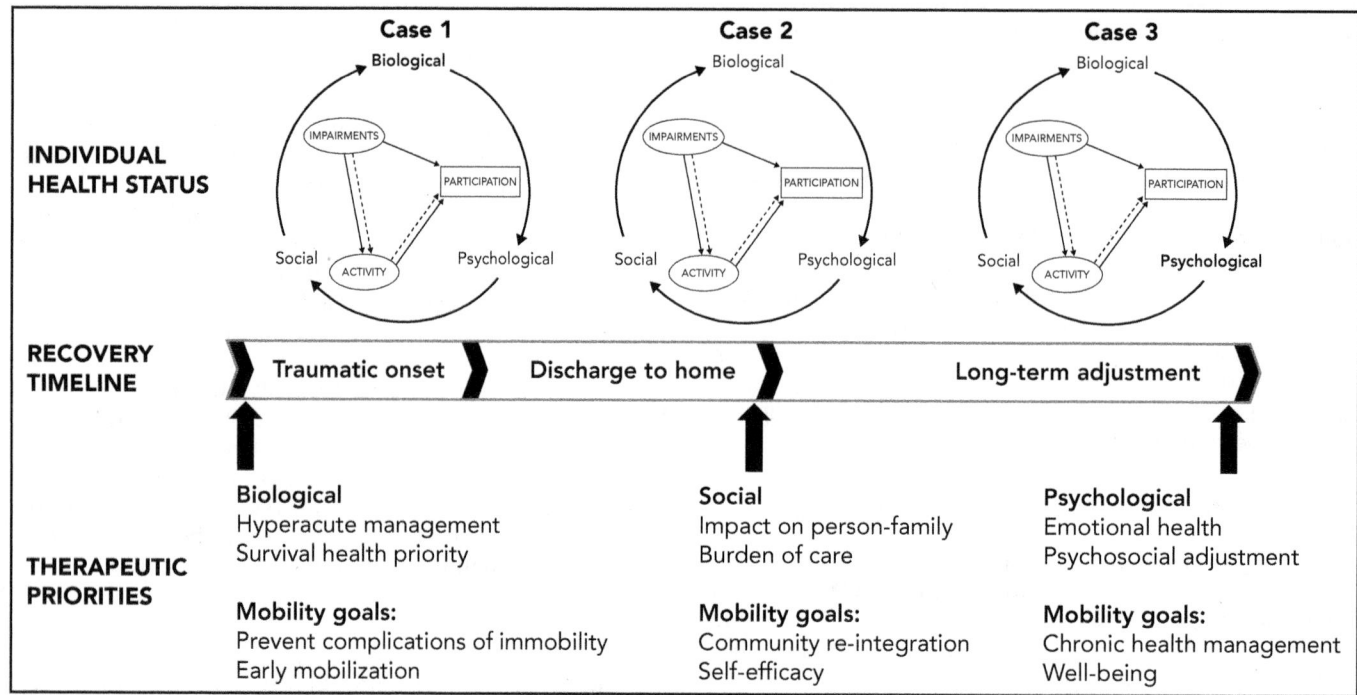

FIGURE 69-3 Movement rehabilitation priorities by phase of recovery. The individual case studies that correspond to each time point on the recovery timeline are provided in the supplemental on-line material.

tation center to home with caregivers. The success of community reintegration is often dependent on the intrinsic or extrinsic resources of a family. Social and environmental factors are powerful predictors of successful transition to community life. For those who progress to independent function, psychological adjustment and personal resilience drive continued long-term recovery. Unfortunately, long-term chronic care for physical and behavioral health needs of the person with brain injury is limited in today's health care environment.

CONCLUSION

We are just beginning to understand the brain-behavior relationships of motor skill learning. Skill acquisition is a cognitive-motor process; thus, further research is needed to understand how the type of therapeutic exercise, the time postinjury, and the intervention dose affects motor learning after brain injury. In addition, further research is needed to understand how motor recovery is affected by damage to the white matter tracts of the descending motor systems in combination with damage to cortical areas needed during the processing of skill learning.

 KEY CLINICAL POINTS

1. Neuroplasticity is the remarkable capacity of the nervous system to respond and adapt to behavioral experience and change throughout one's life or after brain injury.
2. Movement recovery after brain injury is associated with the survival of functional brain tissue and rehabilitation interventions that improve cognitive and motor function.

3. Health status for the person with acquired brain injury and the family who cares for them is the dynamic interaction of the biologic determinants of health and the psychological and environmental factors that affect health and well-being.
4. Motor learning is the ability to acquire, retain, and retrieve movement plans so that actions are executed with speed, accuracy, coordination, and consistency to achieve task goals.
5. Task-specific practice is one of the most effective movement rehabilitation strategies for a person with TBI to learn and execute motor skills needed in everyday life.
6. Recovery from brain injury is a lifelong process.

KEY REFERENCES

1. Bassett DS, Wymbs NF, Porter MA, Mucha PJ, Carlson JM, Grafton ST. Dynamic reconfiguration of human brain networks during learning. *Proc Natl Acad Sci U S A.* 2011; 108(18):7641–7646.
2. Dimyan MA, Cohern LG. Neuroplasticity in the context of motor rehabilitation after stroke. *Nat Rev Neurol.* 2011; 7(2):76–85
3. Guadagnoli MA, Lee TD. Challenge point: a framework for conceptualizing the effects of various practice conditions in motor learning. *J Mot Behav.* 2004;36(2):212–224.
4. McCulloch K. Attention and dual-task conditions: physical therapy implications for individuals with acquired brain injury. *J Neurol Phys Ther.* 2007;31(3):104–118.
5. Sullivan KJ, Cen SY. Model of disablement and recovery: knowledge translation in rehabilitation research and practice. *Phys Ther.* 2011;91(12):1892–1904.

References

1. Cramer SC, Sur M, Dobkin BH, et al. Harnessing neuroplasticity for clinical applications. *Brain.* 2011;134(pt 6):1591–1609.
2. Yeates GN, Gracey F, McGrath JC. A biopsychosocial deconstruction of "personality change" following acquired brain injury. *Neuropsychol Rehabil.* 2008;18(5–6):566–589.
3. Warraich ZK, Kleim JA. Neural plasticity: the biological substrate for neurorehabilitation. *PM R.* 2010;2(12)(suppl 2):S208–S219.
4. World Health Organization. *International Classification of Functioning, Disability and Health: ICF.* Geneva, Switzerland: World Health Organization; 2001.
5. Yarrow K, Brown P, Krakauer JW. Inside the brain of an elite athlete: the neural processes that support high achievement in sports. *Nat Rev Neurosci.* 2009;10(8):585–596.
6. Kantak S, Sullivan K, Fisher B, Knowlton B, Winstein C. Neural substrates of motor memory consolidation depend on practice structure. *Nat Neurosci.* 2010;13(8):923–925.
7. Doyon J, Bellec P, Amsel R, et al. Contributions of the basal ganglia and functionally related brain structures to motor learning. *Behav Brain Res.* 2009;199(1):61–75.
8. Dimyan MAC, Cohen LG. Neuroplasticity in the context of motor rehabilitation after stroke. *Nat Rev Neurol.* 2011;7(2):76–85.
9. Shadmehr R, Smith MA, Krakauer JW. Error correction, sensory prediction, and adaptation in motor control. *Annu Rev Neurosci.* 2010;33:89–108.
10. Schmidt R, Lee T. *Motor Control and Learning: A Behavioral Emphasis.* 5th ed. Champaign, IL: Human Kinetics; 2011.
11. Squire LR. Declarative and nondeclarative memory: multiple brain systems supporting learning and memory. *J Cogn Neurosci.* 1992; 4:232–243.
12. McCulloch K. Attention and dual-task conditions: physical therapy implications for individuals with acquired brain injury. *J Neurol Phys Ther.* 2007;31(3):104–118.
13. Fitts PM, Posner MI. *Human Performance.* Belmont, CA: Brooks/Cole; 1967.
14. Schmidt PL. *Medicare and the Patient Protection and Affordable Care Act. Health Care Issues, Costs, and Access.* Hauppauge, NY: Nova Science Publishers; 2011.
15. Winstein CJ, Gardner ER, McNeal DR, Barto PS, Nicholson DE. Standing balance training: effect on balance and locomotion in hemiparetic adults. *Arch Phys Med Rehabil.* 1989;70(10):755–762.
16. Sullivan K, Knowlton B, Dobkin B. Step training with body weight support: effect of treadmill speed and practice paradigms on poststroke locomotor recovery. *Arch Phys Med Rehabil.* 2002;83(5): 683–691.
17. Guadagnoli MA, Lee TD. Challenge point: a framework for conceptualizing the effects of various practice conditions in motor learning. *J Mot Behav.* 2004;36(2):212–224.
18. Sullivan K, Brown D, Klassen T, et al. Effects of task-specific locomotor and strength training in adults who were ambulatory after stroke: results of the STEPS randomized clinical trial. *Phys Ther.* 2007;87(12):1580–1602.
19. Lin C, Sullivan K, Wu A, Kantak S, Winstein C. Effect of task practice order on motor skill learning in adults with Parkinson disease: a pilot study. *Phys Ther.* 2007;87(9):1120–1131.
20. Kantak SS, Sullivan KJ, Fisher BE, Winstein CJ. Role of primary motor cortex in motor memory consolidation: effect of practice conditions. *J Sport Exerc Psychol.* 2009;31:S74–S74.
21. Winstein CJ, Schmidt RA. Reduced frequency of knowledge of results enhances motor skill learning. *J Exp Psychol Learn Mem Cog.* 1990;16:677–691.
22. Sullivan K, Kantak S, Burtner P. Motor learning in children: feedback effects on skill acquisition. *Phys Ther.* 2008;88(6):720–732.
23. Bassett DS, Wymbs NF, Porter MA, Mucha PJ, Carlson JM, Grafton ST. Dynamic reconfiguration of human brain networks during learning. *Proc Natl Acad Sci USA.* 2011;108(18):7641–7646.
24. Katz DI, Polyak M, Coughlan D, Nichols M, Roche A. Natural history of recovery from brain injury after prolonged disorders of consciousness: outcome of patients admitted to inpatient rehabilitation with 1–4 year follow-up. *Prog Brain Res.* 2009;177:73–88.
25. Bruno MA, Vanhaudenhuyse A, Thibaut A, Moonen G, Laureys S. From unresponsive wakefulness to minimally conscious PLUS and functional locked-in syndromes: recent advances in our understanding of disorders of consciousness. *J Neurol.* 2011;258(7): 1373–1384.
26. Hagen C, Malkmus D, Durham P. *Levels of cognitive functioning. Rehabilitation of the Head Injured Adult: Comprehensive Management.* Downey, CA: Rancho Los Amigos Hospital; 1979.
27. Giacino JT, Kalmar K. Diagnostic and prognostic guidelines for the vegetative and minimally conscious states. *Neuropsychol Rehabil.* 2005;15(3–4):166–174.
28. Kalmar K, Giacino JT. The JFK coma recovery scale—revised. *Neuropsychol Rehabil.* 2005;15(3–4):454–460.
29. American Congress of Rehabilitation Medicine, Brain Injury-Interdisciplinary Special Interest Group, Disorders of Conciousness Task force, et al. Assessment scales for disorders of consciousness: evidence-based recommendations for clinical practice and research. *Arch Phys Med Rehabil.* 2010;91(12):1795–1813.
30. Choi GS, Kim OL, Kim SH, et al. Classification of cause of motor weakness in traumatic brain injury using diffusion tensor imaging. *Arch Neurol.* 2012;69(3):363–367.
31. Katz DI, Alexander MP, Klein RB. Recovery of arm function in patients with paresis after traumatic brain injury. *Arch Phys Med Rehabil.* 1998;79(5):488–493.
32. Platz T, Eickhof C, Nuyens G, Vuadens P. Clinical scales for the assessment of spasticity, associated phenomena, and function: a systematic review of the literature. *Disabil Rehabil.* 2005;27(1–2): 7–18.
33. Malhotra S, Pandyan AD, Day CR, Jones PW, Hermens H. Spasticity, an impairment that is poorly defined and poorly measured. *Clin Rehabil.* 2009;23(7):651–658.
34. Bergfeldt U, Borg K, Kullander K, Julin P. Focal spasticity therapy with botulinum toxin: effects on function, activities of daily living and pain in 100 adult patients. *J Rehabil Med.* 2006;38(3):166–171.
35. Register-Mihalik JK, Mihalik JP, Guskiewicz KM. Balance deficits after sports-related concussion in individuals reporting posttraumatic headache. *Neurosurgery.* 2008;63(1):76–80; discussion 80–82.
36. Scherer MR, Schubert MC. Traumatic brain injury and vestibular pathology as a comorbidity after blast exposure. *Phys Ther.* 2009; 89(9):980–992.
37. Weightman MM, Bolgla R, McCulloch KL, Peterson MD. Physical therapy recommendations for service members with mild traumatic brain injury. *J Head Trauma Rehabil.* 2010;25(3):206–218.
38. Herdman SJ, Schubert MC, Tusa RJ. Strategies for balance rehabilitation: fall risk and treatment. *Ann N Y Acad Sci.* 2001;942:394–412.
39. Maskell F, Chiarelli P, Isles R. Dizziness after traumatic brain injury: overview and measurement in the clinical setting. *Brain Inj.* 2006;20(3):293–305.
40. Herdman S. *Vestibular Rehabilitation.* 3rd ed. Philadelphia, PA: F.A. Davis; 2007.
41. Mossberg KA, Amonette WE, Masel BE. Endurance training and cardiorespiratory conditioning after traumatic brain injury. *J Head Trauma Rehabil.* 2010;25(3):173–183.
42. Belmont A, Agar N, Hugeron C, Gallais B, Azouvi P. Fatigue and traumatic brain injury. *Ann Readapt Med Phys.* 2006;49(6):283–288.
43. Sullivan KJ, Cen SY. Model of disablement and recovery: knowledge translation in rehabilitation research and practice. *Phys Ther.* 2011;91(12):1892–1904.
44. Foley NT, Bhogal S. Mobility and the lower extremity. In: Teasell RFN, Salter K, Bhogal S, Jutai J, Speechley M, eds. *Evidence-Based Review of Stroke Rehabilitation.* Ontario, CA: Canadian Stroke Network; 2007.
45. Van Peppen RP, Kwakkel G, Wood-Dauphinee S, Hendriks HJ, Van der Wees PJ, Dekker J. The impact of physical therapy on functional outcomes after stroke: what's the evidence? *Clin Rehabil.* 2004;18(8):833–862.
46. Bragge P, Chau M, Pitt VJ, et al. An overview of published research about the acute care and rehabilitation of traumatic brain injured and spinal cord injured patients [published online ahead of print March 2, 2012]. *J Neurotrauma.*
47. Kwakkel G. Impact of intensity of practice after stroke: issues for consideration. *Disabil Rehabil.* 2006;28(13–14):823–830.
48. Eng JJ, Rowe SJ, McLaren LM. Mobility status during inpatient rehabilitation: a comparison of patients with stroke and traumatic brain injury. *Arch Phys Med Rehabil.* 2002;83(4):483–490.

Therapy for Activities of Daily Living: Theoretical and Practical Perspectives

Joan Toglia and Kathleen Golisz

INTRODUCTION

The activities that we do on a daily basis provide a sense of coherence and meaning to life. Our lives are organized around daily routines, roles, responsibilities, and goal directed pursuits that are comprised of multiple tasks and activities. These individual daily tasks or "everyday occupations" form patterns of activities that provide structure and meaning to our lives. The term "occupations" is used broadly by occupational therapists to include all the daily tasks that are part of a person's lifestyle (1).

A traumatic brain injury (TBI) can disrupt everyday occupations such as looking after oneself; fulfilling household, family, and work responsibilities; enjoying and participating in life activities; and contributing socially and economically to one's community. Everyday activities can become a major struggle because of physical, sensory, behavioral, or cognitive-perceptual changes. Persistent cognitive and behavioral symptoms are among the most frequent and disabling symptoms that interfere with long-term functional outcomes. The pattern and extent of daily life limitations depends on the nature and severity of the TBI, but even mild injuries can restrict the ability to participate in personally meaningful and valued activities. Life plans and future goals may need to be put on hold or revised, and the person may feel as though they have lost their "sense of place within the world" (2). Engagement in life activities is important to one's sense of accomplishment, self-esteem, self-confidence, and overall health and identity (3).

Activities of daily living (ADLs) need to be considered and understood within the broader context of a person's life context; including their culture, living environment, and lifestyle. There are wide variations in the activities that people do and value in their lives. The process of improving function goes far beyond improving performance in specific daily life tasks. It involves helping a person get back *into* their life. This requires understanding how specific tasks fit within a person's daily activity patterns, roles, and life context as well as identifying and prioritizing activities that are most important and meaningful to the person and his or her family.

The intent of this chapter is to provide an overview of assessment and intervention approaches addressing limitations in ADL. Types of ADL assessments will be discussed along with challenges to assessing function. Intervention approaches and strategies that address everyday activities will be highlighted.

THE OCCUPATIONAL PROFILE

The first step in assessment is obtaining an understanding of the client's concerns and identifying the activities that are most important and meaningful to the person's everyday life. This includes gathering information on the person's previous lifestyle such as the context of the person's previous function (e.g., home, work and community environments, social supports, and past experiences), as well as the person's previous roles, interests, activities, and daily routines. It also involves understanding the person's cultural beliefs that can influence how independence is defined and how activities are chosen, prioritized, and organized (4,5). This background information helps to provide a broad lens from which to understand who the person is, what they value, what they need and want to be able to do in their lives, and what their preinjury life was like. If the person is unable to provide this information because of cognitive or language deficits, the information can be obtained from close relatives or friends.

EVERYDAY OCCUPATIONS AND ACTIVITIES

The broad range of everyday activities that people engage in can be divided into different areas and includes ADLs as well as major life areas such as work, school, social, community, and leisure activities. ADLs can be subdivided into personal activities of daily living (PADLs) and instrumental activities of daily living (IADLs). PADLs are also referred to as basic activities of daily living (BADLs) and are those activities related to taking care of one's self such as personal hygiene and grooming, bowel and bladder management, bathing, showering, dressing, eating, and feeding.

Within the framework of the International Classification of Functioning, Disability and Health (ICF) (6), difficulties in PADLs and specific IADLs are described as activity limitations, whereas difficulties in major life areas such as work, social, and community activities are considered participation restrictions. The ICF model emphasizes the role of the environment and personal context and identifying the gap between actual performance and capacity to perform. Thus, in addition to specific activities, enhancing everyday function requires analyzing patterns of desired activities, and understanding how one spends a day in one's life context and how the environment facilitates or challenges performance of daily activities.

The ability to engage in life activities and daily occupations after a TBI can be affected by a wide array of impairments in physical, sensory, cognitive, perceptual, language, behavioral, or psychosocial skills. Different types, patterns, and levels of severity of impairments can limit performance of PADLs. For example, a person may need assistance or supervision with feeding because of physical limitations in vision, tactile sensation in the hands, or coordinated movement. Perceptual impairments may cause the person to inappropriately select or use feeding utensils, miscalculate the distance when reaching for objects, or neglect half the food on the plate. Cognitive symptoms may result in perseveration on the same food item without switching between foods, impulsive shoveling of food into one's mouth thereby creating a risk for choking, or an inability to recall a recent meal or sustain attention needed for meal completion.

PADLs are performed more routinely, automatically, and consistently across the life span than IADLs and rely heavily on physical abilities and procedural or implicit memory. Difficulties in PADLs occur most frequently in the early stages of recovery from a TBI and generally improve over time in most persons. Persons with severe injuries, however, may continue to demonstrate persisting challenges in PADLs. Data from the Traumatic Brain Injury Model Systems centers (TBIMS) (https://www.tbindsc.org) shows that although 50%–65% of individuals with TBI initially required assistance with bathing, only 10%–18% continue to require assistance at 1 year postinjury. Similar improvements were observed for other PADLs as measured by the Functional Independence Measure (FIM) (7).

IADLs are activities that support daily life within the home and community and typically require more complex skills and interactions than PADLs (4). Examples of IADLs include meal preparation, household tasks and maintenance, communication management such as writing, using everyday technologies, shopping, financial management, community mobility, care of others, safety, and health management and maintenance. Physical IADL tasks such as sweeping the floor or taking out the garbage are sometimes distinguished from cognitive IADL tasks or tasks that primarily involve application of cognitive skills such as paying bills, planning activities, or managing medications. Although this division is useful, it is not always that simple as many tasks (e.g., shopping) involve an integration of higher level cognitive, perceptual, physical, and communication skills. Limitations in IADL therefore, can occur for many different reasons. IADLs often require the person to deal with unstructured or novel situations, plan and organize, multitask, make decisions, and problem solve on the spot. Therefore, they are easily affected by cognitive deficits, particularly executive functioning.

Persisting difficulties in IADL activities contribute to long-term disability, restricted participation in one's home and community, impaired overall health, and increase caregiver burden in persons with TBI (8,9). Approximately 60% of persons continue to experience IADL difficulties several years post-TBI (9,10). Colantonio et al. (9) found that the most

IADL limitations were in the areas of money management, financial management, and community mobility in persons who were an average of 14 years post-TBI. Important predictors of long-term activity limitations and participation restrictions following TBI include greater functional limitations at rehabilitation admission, preinjury unemployment, longer post-traumatic amnesia, cognitive deficits, and preinjury substance abuse (11,12). Severity of injury and age at time of injury has also been associated with functional outcome (13).

Because performance of functional everyday activities may be limited by multiple factors, functional assessment requires carefully observing and analyzing those factors interfering with performance as well as identifying individual variations in styles of performance and available supports to foster greater independence.

Challenges to Addressing Function

The person's functional skills will evolve over the course of a client's recovery from TBI. Fluctuations in the ability to perform functional tasks may be observed because of changes in the environment, the task demands, or the personal characteristics and abilities of the individual.

Within a hospital setting, the ability to observe and fully assess functional performance of PADLs and IADLs can be limited. The hospital environment provides structure to the task and sequencing of functional activities. The person is told when to get up, when and what to eat, when to go to appointments, and when to take their medications. The person's functioning may appear adequate and the full extent of functional difficulties can be masked (i.e., hidden). As a person returns home and is expected to initiate activities on their own or resume former responsibilities, different types of problems can emerge that were not previously observed.

A person's ability to perform a given activity successfully can easily change depending on the degree of environmental distractions and predictability, the number of items or information presented, and the degree of structure present within the task or environment. Observation of performance should analyze the task and environmental conditions that influence performance. For example, a person asked to make a specific snack may appear more functional than when generally asked to make themselves something to eat. In the latter example, the person needs to generate ideas and make decisions themselves. The familiarity of materials can also impact performance. Improved performance may be observed if the therapist engages the client in a budgeting activity that uses real bills and their personal checkbook register and checks. PADLs completed with the client's own clothing and grooming supplies in their home environment may tap into overlearned skills and habits. Comparison of function in familiar and unfamiliar situations is needed because both are required for independent functioning.

Inconsistencies in functional performance can be observed because of mental or physical fatigue or fluctuations in mood, dizziness, medication levels, headaches, or pain (see Chapters 42, 47, 57, and 62). At certain times of the day, or after periods of sustained activities, the person may have greater difficulty with activities that were completed earlier with ease. Functional performance therefore needs to be observed across multiple periods throughout the day. Emotional response to functional limitations can interact with cognitive symptoms and further complicate the clinical picture.

One of the major challenges in rehabilitation is that persons with TBI may not recognize the changes that have occurred. Self-awareness is an important consideration during assessment of function because diminished self-awareness may lead to unrealistic personal goals, decreased persistence, and use of compensatory strategies (14–16). Persons with TBI have been found to consistently rate their ability to perform PADL and IADL tasks higher than their actual ability as judged by experienced clinicians (17).Decreased recognition of limitations can compromise safety because the person may try to attempt activities that are beyond their current abilities.

Impaired self-awareness is commonly assessed by structured or semi-structured interviews. There may be a disassociation, however, between the ability to acknowledge difficulties in an interview and the ability to anticipate, recognize, and monitor errors within the context of a functional activity. Awareness may vary across different functional tasks depending on familiarity and level of task difficulty. It is important to examine the person's perception of their performance throughout functional assessment and treatment (18). This includes asking clients to judge task difficulty, anticipate challenges or the need for assistance, and self-assess performance within the context of various functional activities. Fleming and Strong (19) found that self-awareness varied across different functional tasks in persons with severe TBI. In the early phases of the injury, participants were more aware of difficulties with PADL tasks such as dressing and personal hygiene, and were less aware of limitations in IADL tasks such as preparing meals, doing laundry, and scheduling appointments. Over 12 months, self-awareness improved across most functional tasks, suggesting that as a person returns home and directly experiences IADL tasks, self-awareness gradually develops.

ASSESSING FUNCTIONAL PERFORMANCE

A full understanding of everyday function requires analysis of the fit between the person's abilities, functional tasks, and the environment in which the tasks will be performed. The process of assessment involves a synthesis of data from each of these areas. Multiple assessment methods may be needed to gain a complete profile of the client's functional performance and rehabilitative needs. These methods include interviews of the client and others, direct observation and rating of functional performance, evaluation of underlying impairments that appear to contribute to the client's performance, and exploration of environmental supports or barriers to functional performance (20). Both standardized and nonstandardized assessments may be employed to provide a comprehensive view of the client's abilities.

It is important to identify the goal of assessment or why the assessment is being done and what information is needed from the assessment (2). Various methods and types of assessments have different aims and provide different kinds of information about everyday function (21). For example, if the goal is to identify those activities the client can and cannot perform independently, an assessment with broad and dichotomous ratings is sufficient. On the other hand, if the goal is to determine the amount of help a person needs,

an assessment that rates levels of assistance is needed. Finally, if the goal is to provide information related to intervention planning, assessments that analyze types of errors or identify underlying factors contributing to difficulties in functional performance may be most useful (see Table 70-1).

When selecting a functional assessment, therapists must consider the content or type of tasks included in the assessment (i.e., PADL, IADL, or both). Some functional assessments focus on PADLs whereas others focus on IADLs and participation. The therapist needs to determine if the functional tasks contained within the assessment are relevant to the client's culture and life roles and if the data provided by the assessment will meet the information needs of the team.

Informal Observation

In the early phase of recovery, a person may not be able to participate in standardized PADL assessments because of altered levels of consciousness, limited attention, or agitated behaviors. In acute settings, or as a person emerges from a coma, therapists can systematically observe if the client is able to recognize common objects, perform basic movements, and appropriately sequence PADL task components. Frequency counts, such as the number of times that a client chooses the correct object for a task, initiates actions, or sustains task engagement, can be measured and documented. Inability to perform tasks during this early phase of recovery may or may not indicate lasting problems with functional performance. Repeated assessment of PADL skills is needed because the client's alertness, attention, and ability to follow instructions improve.

Performance Based Assessments vs Functional Rating Scales

Some functional rating scales use self-report or surrogate report rather than direct observation of ADL performance. Indirect ratings of functional performance may lead to either overestimation or underestimation of the client's abilities. Persons with deficits in self-awareness may have difficulty accurately rating their performance, and perceptions of others may be biased by caregiver burden, expectations, and emotional response (22). Performance based ratings of PADLs and IADLs require additional time, space, and staff resources, but they offer the advantage of providing reliable and valid data quantifying the client's performance. These assessments require the therapist to rate what a client *does*, not what a client *could* do, and allows one to observe and identify the factors that might be interfering with performance. Documented changes in observed performance can denote progress in the client's recovery providing justification for continued services and information on the efficacy of the interventions.

Rating Functional Performance

Direct performance assessments vary in the operational definition of the task (e.g., self-feeding vs cutting, using fork, and placing food in mouth) and levels of assistance that are specified and rated. Some assessments broadly rate func-

TABLE 70-1 Selected Functional Performance Assessments

ASSESSMENT AND CATEGORY	DESCRIPTION	COMMENTS (RELIABILITY AND VALIDITY)
Measuring Competency		
Barthel Index (115) [PADL]	Measures functional independence in feeding, wheelchair transfer, self-bathing, dressing, sphincter control, stairway navigation, toileting, personal hygiene, ambulation, and wheelchair propulsion. Scores range from 0 to 100; higher scores indicate greater independence.	Dichotomized scoring reduces outcome information, is insensitive, and has ceiling and floor effects. Most items are included in the FIM.
Katz ADL Index (116) [PADL]	Assesses the degree of dependence using an 8-point ordinal scale in six areas: bathing, dressing, toileting, transfers, feeding, and continence.	Good content validity with low interrater reliability.
Klein-Bell Activities of Daily Living Scale (117) [PADL]	The 170 items divided into mobility, emergency communication, dressing, elimination, bathing/hygiene, and eating. Scored as achieved (without physical or verbal assistance) or unable (required assistance). Raw scores converted to percentages.	Good interrater reliability, construct validity, and responsiveness.
Measuring Assistance Required		
Assessment of Living Skills and Resources (118) [IADL]	Assesses performance of 11 IADL tasks by rating skill and availability and consistent use of resource (i.e., human or technical, formal or informal support for task completion) for each task. Interview, supplemented with observation of skills when possible.	Internally consistent with moderate to good interrater reliability and concurrent validity.
Functional Assessment Measure (FAM) (119) [IADL]	Expansion of the FIM to include 12 items related to community functioning (e.g., car transfers, employability, adjustment to limitations, swallowing function). Often used in conjunction with the FIM as the FIM + FAM.	Training and decision trees increase the interrater reliability of the measure.
Functional Independence Measure (FIM) (120) [PADL]	Measures functional performance in 18 areas of self-care, sphincter control, transfers, locomotion, communication, and social cognition. Uses 7-level scale of disability from "total assist" to "complete independence."	Proven reliability and validity enhanced by decision trees and training. Subtle changes expected after acute inpatient rehabilitation discharge may not be measured by FIM.
Kettle Test (121) [IADL]	Assesses assistance needed to prepare two hot drinks. Scores 13 indices of performance. A 4-point scale based on the need for general or specific cues, approach to task (i.e., slow, trial and error), completeness of performance, and need for physical demonstration or assistance.	Excellent test–retest and interrater reliability. Concurrent validity established with elderly and stroke populations.
Performance Assessment of Self-Care Skills, Version 3.1 (122) [PADL and IADL]	Assesses 26 core tasks in areas of functional mobility, personal self-care tasks, and IADLs with a cognitive or physical emphasis. Performance rated for type and amount of assistance required, risks to safety, and specific point of task breakdown. Hierarchical sequence of prompts/cue provided when performance breaks down. Forms are available for both clinic and home-based assessment.	Good to excellent test–retest and interrater reliability. Construct validity and sensitivity to change demonstrated in several studies.
Observing Factors Interfering with Performance		
Analysis of Cognitive Environmental Support (32) [IADL]	Assesses supports and barriers to cognitive performance of everyday tasks within rooms in the home environment. Notes client's awareness, who introduced the support/barrier, effectiveness, and used/present prior to TBI. The 27 items in support domain categories (e.g., home arrangement, home aids, and person aids); 29 items in the barrier domain categories (i.e., safety and environment).	Content validity verified through expert opinion. Concurrent validity and interrater reliability studies currently show mixed results and authors are revising the assessment to improve its psychometric qualities.
Arnadóttir OT-ADL Neurobehavioral Evaluation (28,123) [PADL]	Standardized and structured observation of functional performance. Comprised of a Functional Independence Scale and a Neurobehavioral Impairment Scale (hypothesizes localization of cerebral dysfunction) with two subscales.	Good interrater reliability. Limited ability to differentiate between left and right hemisphere lesions (28).

(Continued)

TABLE 70-1 Selected Functional Performance Assessments   *(Continued)*

ASSESSMENT AND CATEGORY	DESCRIPTION	COMMENTS (RELIABILITY AND VALIDITY)
Observing Factors Interfering with Performance *(Continued)*		
Assessment of Motor and Process Skills (30) [IADL]	Observational measure of the quality of functional performance (more than 100 standardized tasks).Rates effort, efficiency, safety, and independence of 16 motor and 20 process skill items. Requires therapist certification to administer.	Proven reliability and validity. Numerous calibrated tasks enables selection of culturally relevant and appropriately challenging ADL tasks.
Executive Function Performance Task (23) [IADL]	Identifies the real-world tasks (e.g., preparing cooked oatmeal or managing medication) requiring executive skills. Uses standardized progressive cueing. Task components and total scores are calculated.	Construct, criterion, and discriminant validity established in the stroke population.
IADL Profile (124) [IADL]	Performance-based measure of independence in IADLs based on executive functioning (i.e., goal formulation, planning, carrying out the task, and/or attaining the initial task goal). Administered in client's home and community environment.	Moderate to good interrater agreement (improved with training) and criterion related validity with relation to TBI injury severity, education, planning, and working memory.
Performance Assessments Measuring Error Patterns		
Naturalistic Action Test (33) [IADL]	Assesses learned, sequential, object-oriented behavior using three functional tasks (e.g., gift-wrapping a present) under standardized conditions. Scores accuracy of steps performed and a variety of error types (e.g., omissions, perseveration, spatial estimation, reversals, substitutions, quality, etc.). Comprehensive error and lateralized attention error scores can be generated.	High interrater reliability. Acceptable internal consistency. Robust concurrent validity with the FIM.
Multiple Errands Test (34,125) [IADL]	Assesses executive function skill of multitasking requiring completion of several tasks while adhering to specific rules. Conducted in a shopping mall or a hospital environment. Errors recorded include inefficiencies, rule breaks, interpretation failures or misunderstanding task requirements, and task failures. Several variations of test available.	Interrater reliability, validity in differentiating between individuals with TBI and healthy controls, and concurrent validity with other measures of executive functions have all been demonstrated.

Additional reviews of the aforementioned assessments can be found in Asher IE. *Occupational Therapy Assessment Tools: An Annotated Index.* 3rd ed. Bethesda, MD: American Occupational Therapy Association; 2007.

Meta-OT: Tools & Discussion of Occupational Therapy. OT Assessments and Outcome Measures. http://metaot.com/ot-assessments-outcome-measures.

Rehabilitation Measures Database. Rehabilitation Institute of Chicago. http://rehabmeasures.org.

tional performance for the entire task whereas others define and rate specific task components separately. Assessments that break functional tasks down into fine subcomponents may detect small changes in function that could be missed with broader assessments.

In addition to differences in the specification of task components, there are also differences in level of assistance rated. Some assessments rate performance grossly on 2- or 3-point scales, whereas others differentiate the amount of assistance needed using finer 7- or 9-point scales. Conventional ADL assessments tend to focus heavily on PADL tasks and physical levels of assistance. Newer assessments that include functional activities with higher level cognitive requirements such as the Executive Function Performance Task (23) and the Kettle Task (24) distinguish between levels of verbal or cognitive assistance.

Outcome measures that only quantify independence by rating levels of assistance may not capture improvements in speed and qualitative improvements in efficiency of func-

tional performance. For clients with moderate to severe disability who continue to need lifelong assistance in PADLs and IADLs, performing everyday activities more efficiently and quickly may have a significant impact on quality of life because more time and energy are available to engage in other meaningful activities (25). This may be equally meaningful to the client's caregiver. IADL assessments that focus on time required to complete tasks have been used within older adult populations experiencing reduced processing speed (26) and visual impairments (27).

Observing Factors Contributing to Functional Performance

Several assessments take a "top down" approach to understanding the underlying factors interfering with performance of functional tasks by simultaneously rating activity performance and underlying skills or impairments using standardized and structured observations.

The Arnadóttir Occupational Therapy–Activities of Daily Living (OT-ADL) Neurobehavioral Evaluation (A-ONE) (28) rates the level of independence in PADLs as well as observed neurobehavioral impairments such as motor apraxia, spatial relations, or perseveration. The Executive Function Performance test (29) rates the degree of verbal assistance needed for executive function skills within functional tasks. The Assessment of Motor and Process Skills (AMPS) (30) separately rates 16 motor and 20 process skills or observable actions (e.g., searching and locating tools and materials, or sequencing task steps logically) within the context of IADL tasks. A pilot study has found this tool to be sensitive in measuring functional change in persons with severe TBI (31). The AMPS and A-ONE assessments require training courses to be certified in proper administration and use.

Factors within the environment that may support or hinder functional performance can be assessed with structured checklists or more standardized assessments. Current assessments tend to focus on physical elements of the environment influencing performance and safety. The Analysis of Cognitive Environmental Support (32) is an in-home assessment—currently under development—that focuses on environmental factors supporting or hindering cognitive skills related to functional performance. The authors plan to validate this assessment on the TBI population.

Examining Error Patterns Observed Within Functional Activities

Another group of IADL assessments provides the clinician with information on the pattern of errors observed within performance of functional activities. Analysis of error patterns is particularly important for treatment approaches that focus on helping clients use strategies to monitor and control task errors. The Naturalistic Action Test (33) uses functional tasks such as making toast and coffee or packing a child's lunchbox and backpack under standardized conditions to assess accuracy and types of error patterns made (e.g., omissions, perseveration, spatial estimation, reversals, substitutions, quality, etc.). The Multiple Errands Test (MET) (34,35) has several variations that can be completed in either a hospital environment or community setting such as a shopping mall. The MET requires the client to use multitasking skills (i.e., executive functions) to complete several functional tasks while adhering to specific rules. The evaluator or observer notes the types of errors made by the individual with TBI (e.g., inefficiencies, rule breaks, interpretation failures or misunderstanding task requirements, and task failures).

Observational, task-based assessment approaches such as the Perceive, Recall, Plan and Perform (PRPP) System of Task Analysis can be used with clients who are unable to participate in standardized language based assessments because of agitation or post-traumatic amnesia. The PRPP system is a process oriented, criterion-referenced assessment (36). The system begins with selection of a targeted functional task, such as upper body dressing or simple meal preparation, and analysis of the sequence of task components. Observed errors are analyzed and classified into categories (i.e., perceive, recall, plan, or perform) and type (e.g., omission, repetition, accuracy, or timing). The PRPP system can detect changes in functional task behavior over time (36) and has demonstrated good reliability across raters and within the assessment process (37).

Assessments using a dynamic assessment method, such as the Contextual Memory Test (38), Toglia Category Assessment (39), or the Dynamic Lowenstein Occupational Therapy Cognitive Assessment (40), can also provide information about error patterns and strategy use as well as the ability to change the client's performance with cues, strategies, feedback, or task modifications. The goal of dynamic assessment methods is to systematically measure how and to what extent task errors can be decreased with guidance or task alterations as a foundation for intervention planning (41,42).

Assessing Impairments That May Interfere With Function

Greater specification and understanding of underlying impairments that may be contributing to difficulties in functional performance is sometimes needed to guide treatment planning. Assessment of specific skills may be helpful in sorting out the underlying difficulties and confirming identification of impairments that were observed during functional task performance (see Chapters 40 and 59).

Assessments such as the Action Research Arm Test (43), Fugl-Meyer Motor Assessment (44), or the Wolf Motor Function Test (45) look at physical impairments in strength, sensation, or coordination of the upper extremities using simple motor actions or components of functional tasks such as griping everyday objects. Other assessments such as the Arm Motor Ability Test evaluate motor recovery using standardized functional tasks and scoring (46). These assessments require the therapist to make a hypothesis about the client's abilities to perform functional tasks.

Cognitive impairments may be assessed more specifically with assessments such as the Test of Everyday Attention (47), Rivermead Behavioural Memory Test (48,49), the Lowenstein Occupational Therapy Cognitive Assessment (50), and the Behavioural Assessment of Dysexecutive Syndrome (51). Perceptual impairments may be explored by using assessments such as the Occupational Therapy Adult Perceptual Screening Test (52), the Behavioral Inattention Test (53), or the Brain Injury Visual Assessment Battery for Adults (54). These assessment results need to be compared to performance on PADL or IADL tasks that require use of the same cognitive perceptual skills to verify the effect of the impairment on function.

INTERVENTION: GOAL SETTING STRATEGIES

Early in the intervention phase, information gathered from interviews, direct observation of performance, and formalized assessment of functional skills is synthesized and used to collaborate with the client and significant others on selecting goals and creating an intervention plan to address functional limitations. Goals that are meaningful and chosen by the client are most likely to enhance participation and motivation, however, decreased understanding of one's strengths and limitations can negatively impact the goal setting process and result in conflicts between the goals embraced by the client and goals identified by significant others or clinicians.

Persons with TBI often need assistance and structure to break down their long-term goals into smaller, achievable components. Cognitive impairments can compromise the ability to set priorities, estimate time frames, understand cause and effect, or comprehend how subgoals are connected to larger goals and to each other. For example, if the person's goal is to return to living independently or driving, a picture representing a ladder illustrating a stepwise, progressive set of task components can be used to assist the person in seeing and understanding connections between smaller, immediate tasks and larger functional goals (41). A chart or goal mapping process can also be used to help the person formulate a vision of what they are working towards. Once smaller attainable goals are identified, a goal attainment method can be used to rate performance and measure progress (55). Achievement of small daily or weekly goals focused on the "here and now" can help build motivation, self-confidence, and self-esteem.

Involving the Family

It is essential for rehabilitation professionals to collaborate with families across all phases of recovery. In the early phases of rehabilitation, communication systems can be set up to include family members in the rehabilitation process. Family members can be asked to write observations or questions in a journal to which the rehabilitation team members respond. Often, family members are first to observe signs of improvement, but they may be confused or frightened about changes in behavior or the person's inability to complete simple activities. It is important to help family members understand the factors that might be interfering with the ability to do everyday tasks and how they can help.

Limitations in functional abilities of the person with TBI can create additional burden and responsibilities for others. Spouses or close family members may have to take on additional household, family, or work activities that can strain relationships and create tensions within the family. It is important to carefully listen to the needs and goals of family members and work with them collaboratively in setting functional goals and planning intervention activities (56). A client-centered problem solving approach to working with significant others as co-partners to identify the main functional problem, brainstorm solutions, critique the solutions, choose and implement a solution, and assess the outcome has been found to alleviate stress in caregivers (57).

The family's ability to provide appropriate structure and assistance to enhance functioning and participation is critical to the TBI survivor's success. Consistency among all team members, including family or significant others, is key in enhancing function. It is important to recognize signs of stress and caregiver burden. If family members are feeling completely exhausted and overwhelmed, it can reduce their ability to carryover strategies and support the person with TBI. In these situations, the family may need additional resources, counseling, or assistance themselves before they are capable of fully supporting and enhancing function of the person with TBI.

ACTIVITIES OF DAILY LIVING INTERVENTION: BRINGING MEANING BACK TO LIFE

There are several methods that can be used to optimize functional performance in PADL and IADL activities. Interven-

tions can be aimed at increasing the ability to perform a specific functional task or routine, or toward special methods, strategies, or skills that can be used across different functional activities. Improvements in specific daily tasks are easier to achieve than approaches that require generalization of skills across different situations.

Specific tasks or routines such as getting ready in the morning or doing the laundry may be broken into smaller physical or cognitive task components or adapted with the goal of improving the ability to complete specific activities with less physical or cognitive assistance. Modifications in task methods or use of adaptive equipment may be recommended to compensate for physical, visual, or perceptual impairments, however, this requires new learning and may be confounded by cognitive impairments that limit the client's ability to remember, learn, and generalize new methods to novel situations.

Task-specific training methods such as errorless learning or vanishing cues are often used when learning, and carryover from day-to-day is significantly limited. These methods involve "learning by doing" and repeated systematic practice of the same functional task with gradually decreasing prompts or assistance. The aim is to increase specific functional skills by relying on procedural memory or implicit learning integrating experiences unconsciously. Task-specific training methods have been shown to be effective with persistent functional deficits in PADL and IADL even 10 years after the TBI (58).

Functional activities can also be used as a means to improve underlying skills by manipulating aspects of the activities to place gradual demands on specific physical, perceptual, or cognitive skills. This approach can serve a dual purpose of improving underlying impairments as well as functional performance, resulting in the use of functional activities as both an "end" and a "means" of intervention. For example, if a person has decreased active movement, functional activities can be set up so the person has to repeatedly use their affected extremity in activities such as folding laundry, washing a table, and removing items from a shelf. Similarly, if the person has a left-sided spatial neglect, functional activities such as finding items from a list on shelves or in a room can be used to have the person repeatedly scan toward the left side. Functional activities that focus on improving underlying skills are often included in interventions within the early stages of rehabilitation to optimize recovery, however, concentrated, intense, and repetitive practice that is focused directly on the person's area of difficulty has been found to lead to significant, clinically meaningful improvements in motor and language function in some persons with chronic stroke (59) and TBI (60–62). Finally, functional activities can be embedded within a structured problem solving or metacognitive framework to enhance self-awareness, self-monitoring skills, strategy use, and functional performance across a variety of situations. This approach is typically used within the context of IADL activities that are often limited by executive dysfunction. This approach requires generalization of learning and systematic practice of the same strategies across varied activities. Several studies have documented effectiveness of strategy training within the context of functional activities (63–67).

The following section provides examples of how these different intervention techniques can be used to optimize performance in PADLs and then IADLs.

Optimizing Personal Activities of Daily Living Performance

Interventions for PADLs such as dressing, eating, bathing, and toileting are often emphasized in acute care settings or early phases of recovery. Even within the intensive care unit, PADL tasks may be introduced by providing the client with a wet washcloth to wash their face, body lotion to moisturize their skin, lipstick or balm to apply, or simple soft foods to self-feed if permitted by physician order. Presenting the client with familiar objects such as a spoon or toothbrush can stimulate purposeful movement, alertness, and attention.

Improving Underlying Skills

Underlying impairments may express themselves in various manners during the performance of PADL tasks providing the opportunity to address the impairments while improving functional performance. Functional activities may be gradually increased in difficulty to require greater motor skills (see Chapters 68 and 69) and increased number of step or tools and materials needed to complete the task. For example, in dressing, the client may first be asked to don an overhead shirt. The shirt might be presented in the correct orientation on the person's lap limiting motor and perceptual skills needed. As the client improves, additional pieces of clothing and those requiring more complex sequencing and motor skills (e.g., a button-down shirt) are presented. Clothing may be placed on the bed or in the closet to encourage reaching patterns or scanning to a spatially neglected side. All the clothing needed to dress can be presented simultaneously; challenging the person's need to perceptually identify clothing items, sequence their donning, and maintain adequate energy to complete the entire dressing task. Gradually, fewer cues are provided for initiation and an increased number of clothing items can be positioned in closets and drawers to encourage walking, reaching, standing, bending, and selection of appropriate clothing items. Balance demands can be challenged by changing the client's position from sitting to standing. Assistance and cues are lessened as skills improve and more complex tasks are introduced. Thus, the same task (e.g., dressing) can be manipulated to place varying demands on different underlying skills. This requires careful task analysis as well as in depth understanding of the components of motor, perceptual, and cognitive skills.

Although functional tasks such as self-feeding offer naturally occurring practice sessions throughout the day, therapists may also work on subcomponents of the underlying impairments interfering with PADL performance during scheduled therapy sessions. For example, to address underlying impairments affecting self-feeding, grip strength, hand-to-mouth movement patterns, and opening of food containers may be completed using functional items in simulated settings. Clients' oral motor control may be practiced in a dysphagia-based program carried out by the occupational therapist or speech language pathologist (see Chapter 66). Changes in the consistency of food are presented as the person's oral–motor skills improve. Gradually, adaptations and techniques may be applied to the task to compensate for underlying impairments.

Adapting the Task

Adaptations to task structure and materials or the environment may facilitate functional performance. Cognitive impairments interfering with PADLs may require modifications to the task by others, particularly if the client's awareness is limited. Directions to complete a functional task can be provided one step at a time. Clients with physical impairments such as weakened grasp may require built-up handles on eating utensils and grooming tools. Fine motor or sensory issues interfering with dressing may require Velcro closures on clothing and elastic shoelaces. Visual impairments may require increased contrast or color coding to distinguish objects. For example, a razor handle can be wrapped in red tape to help the client distinguish the razor from the toothbrush. Placing food on a high-contrast plate and/or placemat may help clients with low-contrast sensitivity distinguish the food and utensils from the background. A brightly colored napkin or food item (e.g., red apple or can of soda) can be placed on a spatially neglected side. This may draw attention to that side of the table or tray reducing the need for a caregiver to cue the client or periodically rotate their plate. Clients with distractibility may initially eat meals in their room rather than the rehabilitation unit dining room; only joining the more stimulating environment as their attention improves.

Environmental adaptations for physical impairments interfering with PADLs can involve adaptive equipment such as a raised toilet seat, tub bench, grab bars, or a hand-held shower (see Chapter 71) or rearranging items within the environment (e.g., positioning items on lower shelves or within reach) to place less demands on motor skills. Occupational and physical therapists may need to collaborate to identify modifications to standardized durable medical equipment to address cognitive/perceptual impairments. Placing bright tape on the wheelchair brake on the left may assist the client with spatial neglect, locate the brake, and improve safety in wheelchair transfers during functional tasks.

Environmental adaptations that involve ongoing implementation require caregiver training to understand the purpose of the adaptations and process of setting up the environment to facilitate performance. For example, a caregiver may need to organize clothing items together in a designated place to facilitate sequencing of dressing. This organizational task would need to be completed weekly by a caregiver.

Teaching Compensatory Skills

Compensatory methods require the client to learn and initiate the compensation themselves. Self-awareness is needed to understand when and how to apply the compensation. Techniques can be specific to a task or can be general and used across situations. Consider the task of self-feeding, clients with severe visual impairments (e.g., cortical blindness) can be taught the clock method of locating food items and utensils on the food tray or table and taught to monitor the amount of beverage poured into a glass using a liquid sensors or their finger. Clients demonstrating impulsivity may be taught to monitor the pacing of their food intake to minimize the risk of choking. Clients with hemiplegia can be taught one-handed dressing techniques.

Clients can also be taught more general compensatory strategies that may be used in various tasks to improve functional performance. A client who is distracted and overwhelmed by a cluttered environment might be taught the strategy of reducing or covering elements in the environment to only those needed to complete the task. During feeding, the client might set aside items from the tray or table, cover them with a napkin, or remove items once they are finished.

Errorless Learning

Cognitive impairments may limit the client's ability to learn and remember new compensatory methods and generalize these methods to novel situations. Several case studies have demonstrated that performance on specific PADL tasks can be improved in persons with moderate and severe TBI several years postinjury, with task specific training methods including errorless learning (58,68,69).

PADL tasks rely on "habit" or procedural memory and are well suited to approaches that incorporate vanishing cues and errorless learning involving repetition and practice of tasks with gradually fading assistance or cues. Errorless learning techniques involve prevention or elimination of errors in the learning process (68) and capitalize on procedural or implicit memory. A therapist applying the neurofunctional approach (70) to a client's morning grooming routine might engage the client in completing the tasks in the exact same sequence each morning at the same time and place. Using chaining techniques and errorless learning, the therapist would provide prompts or cues to facilitate performance. Gestural prompts might include pointing to the toothbrush, tapping the client's hand, or looking toward an item (e.g., toothpaste) needed in the task. Visual cues could include pictures or written cue cards, or a real-time video clips showing the toothbrushing task sequence that can be played on an electronic aid. Physical prompts might include touching the client's hand or completing hand-over-hand movements to facilitate the motor component of the task. Prompts are initiated to prevent the client from making errors during the learning phase of the task, then are graduated, reduced, or faded as the client demonstrates consistent performance of that task component. This type of approach to retraining specific PADL tasks focuses on improving functional performance without improving the underlying impairments that may be limiting performance.

Optimizing Function in Instrumental Activities of Daily Living Activities

IADL activities are typically introduced during inpatient rehabilitation once the person is able to perform most of their PADLs. Intervention directed at IADLs (e.g., money management, banking, budgeting, meal planning and prepara-

tion, crossing the street, taking the bus, or shopping) become a greater focus as a person progresses to outpatient, home, or community rehabilitation. Although training within one's actual home or community environment is ideal, this is not always feasible and training is often addressed in clinic-based settings. This requires the need to transfer skills learned in a rehabilitation setting to natural environments such as the person's home and local community.

To enhance carryover of skills, rehabilitation environments should be set up to look like the environment in which the skills will be needed. Occupational therapy departments within inpatient rehabilitation units often include a mock apartment area with a kitchen, bedroom, and living room so that patients can practice performing household tasks. In addition to an apartment area, the rehabilitation unit might have a real car to practice getting in and out of a vehicle. An area with open shelves containing items with different prices could be created to simulate shopping. Different types of flooring and walking surfaces can be installed as well as different types of doors, handles, and locks to simulate a variety of physical demands.

Some clinics have Easy Street Environments, which replicate real world settings such as a movie theater, restaurant, grocery store, bank or automated teller machine (ATM), gas pump, and a bus. Simulated environments can be very engaging for patients because they help them connect therapy experiences with everyday life and provide a controlled and safe environment to practice and regain confidence in daily life skills (2). Therapists can also set up tasks that require use of natural environments such as the hospital lobby, gift shop, public rest rooms, cafeteria, or vending machines. A client may be asked to find and purchase items that meet specific criteria in the gift shop or order a lunch in the cafeteria. These activities involve interacting with others, handling money, and dealing with unexpected problems that may arise. High-level balance, visual, and cognitive difficulties may be observed when the person is required to negotiate new environments, scan for information, calculate prices of items, or keep track of previous task steps.

As the person progresses to outpatient or day programs, real world and natural environments should be used in intervention. This can include visits to local stores, malls, banks, post offices, restaurants, bus or train stations, and other public areas. Treatment environments can be gradually increased in complexity from a quiet controlled clinic setting to busy or crowded environments with multiple distractions. Persons with TBI often have more difficulty functioning in these types of environments and can become easily anxious, irritable, or overwhelmed. They may be hypersensitive to sensory stimuli such as sounds and lights or have difficulty filtering out irrelevant information. Strategies such as stress reduction, mental rehearsal, or adaptations such as sunglasses or earphones may be needed.

Along with considering the variety and complexity of different environments, it is important to use an assortment of everyday materials and tasks that are relevant to a person's lifestyle and interests that can be used during treatment. Whenever feasible, it is helpful to have family members bring in examples of the person's bills, work related tasks or samples of previous work materials, as well as the everyday technologies that the person used prior to their TBI (e.g., mobile phone or iPad). Multiple-step activity kits can be organized in a clinic for tasks such as making flight reservations, uploading digital photography, shopping online for specified items, taking inventory, setting a table for 10 people, or caring for pets. In addition, activities that involve following a simulated list of errands, using a map to find locations within the building, or obtaining specified information from different offices or locations around the facility can be used to approximate real life situations. It is important to consider the demographics, general interests, and occupations of the population being served so that activities and materials can be relevant to the lifestyles and cultures within the community of practice. Prevocational activities can be used along with IADL activities depending on the person's goals and priorities. For example, if the clinic includes persons that work in construction or manual labor jobs, activities might include assembling pipe fittings, putting together a car engine, or refinishing a wooden chair. Clients who work in primarily professional settings may engage in tasks in a simulated office station such as listening to an answering machine, collating documents and filing, putting appointments in calendars, or completing a computerized excel budget. Leisure activities may be simulated based on the intervention location with some areas needing fishing rods, golf clubs, or gardening equipment, and other areas needing schedules of theaters, museums, and take-out restaurant menus. These IADL, leisure, or prevocational activities can be used with any of the approaches and techniques described subsequently.

Techniques such as adaptations of the task or environment, compensatory methods, use of of electronic devices, and errorless learning can be used alone or in combination to reduce physical, cognitive, or perceptual demands and improve performance in specific tasks.

Compensatory Methods and Adaptation of the Task or Environment

IADL activities such as cooking, shopping, medication management, money management, household tasks, or scheduling activities can be adapted by changing the task or environmental demands, rather than the person's skills. The pattern of underlying difficulties guides the type of adaptation or compensation that is needed. The following are illustrations of how these methods can be applied to two IADL tasks: cooking and financial management.

Cooking

Prior to cooking activities, the kitchen environment may need to be analyzed and adapted. For example, supplies and ingredients may need to be reorganized or arranged differently so that they are easier to reach or find. Lighting may need to be changed to improve vision and/or attention (see Chapter 45). The height of the microwave oven may need to be adjusted to decrease reaching and a stove top that is wheelchair-accessible may be recommended if mobility is decreased. Timers and safety features such as automatic appliance shut off devices (e.g., gas on stove) can be effective for persons with decreased memory. Clearly written labels, color codes, or pictures can be placed on the stove or stove knobs or outside draws and cabinets to help a person locate the correct burner or items easily (71). To reduce executive functioning demands, menus can be preplanned or set for

the week and meals that are familiar or require the least number of steps and ingredients to prepare can be selected. A simplified checklist that can be used to guide meal preparation can decrease cognitive load and further enhance performance.

Financial Management

A talking calculator or a calculator with large buttons can be used to assist calculation and compensate for decreased vision, attention to details, or impaired fine motor coordination. Use of magnifiers or page blockers can enhance the ability to read bills or complete banking forms if there are visual impairments. Methods such as highlighting the balance due on each bill, reorganizing filing systems and calendar systems, or switching to electronic or telephone payment methods may be recommended to decrease cognitive demands. In these situations, modifications of the computer including a filter to reduce glare on the screen, changes in contrast and size of print, adaptations of the key board, or use of voice activation may be recommended depending on the pattern of impairments. Electronic calendars or preprogrammed text messages can be used to remind a person with memory problems when bills are due. A checklist of steps may be helpful in use of an ATM or in navigating a bank. If the person has difficulty in tolerating complex environments, careful selection of banking locations or times that are least busy may be recommended.

Electronic Aids

In addition to adaptive techniques, a variety of everyday technologies including mobile phones, iPads, and internet site calendars with reminder capabilities can help to support everyday functioning. For example, there are several internet sites that can send preprogrammed text messages or e-mails at specified times to mobile phones to remind persons about appointments, tasks, or upcoming events. Low-technology devices, internet sites, and application programs (i.e., apps) are available, which can assist with task organization, time management, and reminders. Care needs to be taken to match the person's skills, abilities, and needs with the characteristics of the device. Electronic aids may be more easily integrated into the client's everyday occupations when the person used technology prior to their injury. Higher rates of task completion have been demonstrated for persons with TBI when using electronic devices such as mobile phones, portable voice organizers, computers, personal data assistants, or pagers (72,73). Systematic reviews have supported use of electronic aids for improving participation in everyday activities (74–76). As a result, training in external compensations including electronic aids has been recommended as a practice guideline for people with moderate or severe memory impairment following TBI or stroke to facilitate participation in functional activities (64,72,75,77–81).

The Errorless Learning Approach

Errorless learning may be used to train clients in the operation and use of electronic devices (82) or memory notebooks (83) as well as to address persistent difficulties in IADLs. Parish and Oddy (84) describe an 11-month training program using errorless learning to increase independence in doing the laundry for persons 17 years post-TBI. Initiation and independence in this task was still maintained after 2 years. Similar results have been reported for meal preparation (69,85), banking and budgeting (69), awareness of traffic in the community (69), and caring for a pet (83).

Metacognitive and Strategy Training

Systematic reviews support use of strategy training and structured metacognitive frameworks as a means of improving functional outcomes for persons with TBI (77,86). Metacognition involves self-awareness of cognitive abilities as well as the ability to self-monitor and regulate ongoing activities. These approaches can be used across a wide range of IADL activities as a means of enhancing self-awareness, self-monitoring, and strategy use to improve functional performance.

Increases in self-awareness have been related to strategy use and improvements in functional performance (14,67,87). Strategies can include external compensatory methods such as using a checklist, a daily planner, highlighting details, or removing and rearranging task materials as well as internal strategies such as self-cues or instructions, mental rehearsal, or visual imagery.

Self-awareness is most likely to emerge within the context of daily tasks because these activities are familiar and inherently provide concrete feedback (e.g., food burns in oven if forgotten). Several case studies (67,85,88) and a pilot randomized study in persons with TBI (89), describe use of structured activity experiences that incorporate techniques such as prediction and self-evaluation of performance within everyday activities including bill paying, budgeting, cooking activities, leisure, prevocational activities, and vocational activities (90). For example, a randomized pilot study ($n = 20$) compared persons with TBI who received IADL practice to those who received IADL practice plus metacognitive training including self-prediction and self-evaluation. The ADL metacognitive intervention significantly improved IADL performance on untrained tasks as well as selective aspects of awareness compared to the control group (89).

Other metacognitive techniques that have been studied within the context of IADL activities include role reversal and use of video for feedback, modeling, and problem solving (91–93). For example, video scenarios of everyday activities such as preparing fruit, handling money transactions, washing dishes, or forgetting to pay bills has been used to help clients identify difficulties and generate alternative strategies (66,93).

Several case studies describe use of generic problem solving frameworks such as goal management training (94) and the Cognitive Orientation to Occupational Performance (Co-Op) (95) approach within the context of functional activities. For example, the Co-Op approach uses a global problem solving strategy, Goal-Plan-Do-Check within a client-centered framework that has been applied to persons with TBI, showing improvement on both trained and untrained functional goals. In this approach, clients identify functional goals and engage in a combination of IADL, leisure, and prevocational activities to practice the Goal-Plan-Do-Check strategy. Other strategies that have been studied within simulated daily life activities include a time pressure management strategy (96), mental imagery (92), self-generation strategies, and spacing techniques (97,98).

Toglia (67,99) has proposed a multi-context framework that provides broad guidelines for strategy training with a focus on promoting generalization across functional activities. Intervention activities are embedded within a metacognitive framework and involve repeated practice of the same strategies across a wide range of activities and contexts that are systematically varied to help persons connect activity experiences. Toglia et al. (67) described the application of the multi-context approach using a single-subject design with repeated measures for four persons with TBI 3–5 years post-injury. All clients learned to use targeted strategies such as a checklist across different IADL tasks.

Resuming Daily Routines and Roles

It is important to keep in mind that a person may be able to perform individual IADL activities but may have difficulty initiating and organizing these activities during a day or carrying out multiple activities across a week. TBI symptoms can be cumulative and emerge with sustained activities or after performing several activities because of physical and cognitive fatigue or experiences of "overload." As the person attempts to increase their activity level or resume other roles and responsibilities, the ability to manage and coordinate IADL activities may diminish.

Analysis of daily activity patterns and routines is an important component of outpatient and community rehabilitation. In addition to the frequency and quantity of activities a person participates in during the day, the type and combination of activities that the person engages in as well as perceived satisfaction needs to be analyzed. Activities that are more physically or cognitively challenging may need to be balanced with those that are less demanding. Establishment of a productive routine may be difficult for persons who are transitioning from a highly structured inpatient rehabilitation program to an unstructured home environment. A person who is unable to resume former work and leisure activities may tend to spend their days unproductively watching television (100). Idle time and decreased engagement in meaningful activities can create boredom and a decreased sense of competence that can contribute to functional decline and decreases in life satisfaction, quality of life, and overall health (8,101).

A goal directed and problem oriented approach that helps the person self-select goals and activities, identify daily life challenges, and generate possible solutions with guidance can be used to enhance activity participation. Goals focused on increasing daily activity level, decreasing idle time, or increasing participation in meaningful activities can be established in collaboration with the client and rated on a weekly basis. A journal of daily activities that includes time spent on each activity, level of satisfaction, and descriptions of challenges or problems encountered can be useful in monitoring and increasing overall activity level and perceived satisfaction as well as helping a person identify new activities, interests, and goals.

Therapy for improving ADLs needs to be combined with increasing participation in meaningful activities. This may involve exploring new leisure and social activities or developing new interests, particularly if the person is unable to resume work, school, or other activities that previously occupied most of their time. For some persons, the main reason for discontinuing leisure and social activities may be inability to drive or financial limitations related to inability to work (102). Resumption of preinjury roles as parent, student, or worker may require driving. Approximately half of individuals who sustain a TBI return to the task of driving and experience more positive community reintegration (103). Other individuals will require training in the use of alternative transportation methods to participate in community activities.

The areas of work, leisure, driving, and community integration are discussed in detail in other chapters within this book (see Chapters 77, 78, 81, and 82). The same treatment approaches described earlier in this chapter can be applied to work, school, or leisure activities including training or adapting specific tasks, using task specific compensatory methods, or incorporating electronic or assistive devices.

Emerging Role of Technology in Functional Training

Virtual Reality
Virtual reality (VR) is a novel modality that allows people to view, navigate, or interact with a computer-generated environment that simulates real world environments. VR offers the opportunity for intensive repetition and practice with everyday tasks under a variety of simulated and controlled (i.e., safe) conditions. Several virtual reality programs have been developed and tested with persons with TBI or stroke including a virtual shopping mall (104), supermarket (105), office (106), a wheelchair driving environment (107), street crossing program (108,109), ATM (110), and a community skills program (111). For example, a supermarket VR system has been developed where users see themselves navigating in the supermarket and are required to locate, select, and reach for virtual food items on shelves of different heights. VR can provide precise, objective, and sophisticated measures of a range of physical and cognitive performance components. This technology, however, is not yet widely accessible and may be contraindicated in persons with vestibular or visual difficulties.

Technology and Adaptation
Smart House technology has been developed to provide automated task cueing and safety monitoring (112,113). Monitoring systems can track patterns of activity within a home or room and provide prompts or sound an alarm if a problem is detected. For example, sensors located in the bathroom can help determine how long patients spend shaving and prompt them to finish and move on if they're taking too long. Presently, smart house technology that includes task prompts and safety monitoring is being tested for persons with TBI and dementia.

Intervention Summary

Factors Influencing Selection and Combination of Treatment Approaches
Several different approaches to increase ADL were reviewed in this chapter. Some intervention techniques focus on modi-

fying the task or environment, whereas others focus on improving the person's skills or strategies. In clinical practice, several different approaches to improving function are often used simultaneously. Successful functional performance requires a match between the person's abilities and the task and environmental demands. As the person progresses through recovery, the treatment approaches, methods, and activities used changes. The focus of intervention and methods selected to enhance ADLs vary depending on injury severity; type of impairments; time postinjury; length of treatment; the person's priorities, interests, and goals; as well as level of awareness and motivation. Emotional and behavioral responses of the client, such as anxiety, depression, perceived stress, frustration, and anger, can impact functional outcome and require an interdisciplinary team approach.

There is increasing evidence supporting the efficacy of approaches that enhance functional performance—even many years after the injury. Methods to improve performance in specific tasks using errorless learning and adaptations by others has promise to improve ADL performance in persons with severe or chronic TBI. A growing body of evidence supports the use of electronic aids to support daily functioning in persons with moderate to severe deficits, whereas training of strategies embedded within IADL activities and a metacognitive framework appears to have promise for persons with mild to moderate deficits. Emerging technologies such as virtual reality and smart houses show great promise in improving functional skills. Finally, methods to increase participation, including coordinating and balancing life tasks, roles, and activities, are needed as a person returns to their communities.

Regardless of the adaptations, strategies, or approaches used, treatment is most successful when the client, family, or support persons are involved as co-partners in identifying the problems, selecting goals, and collaborating in the solutions. Consistency and reinforcement from others is a key component of intervention success. Persistent deficits in ADLs require others to take over tasks or provide supervision and assistance, thereby creating a long-term burden for others and for society.

LONG-TERM ACTIVITIES OF DAILY LIVING NEEDS

New roles and environments, or changes in social networks and supports that naturally evolve across time can be expected to alter the value and types of meaningful tasks and IADLs in which a person engages. Individuals with TBI and persisting physical and/or cognitive difficulties face new challenges as life circumstances change, resulting in the need for periodic rehabilitation to maintain or improve functional performance and participation in life roles.

Consider the young adult who sustained a TBI during their high school years. Rehabilitation provided at the time of injury may focus on skills needed to return to school or home. However, as the individual ages and assumes new life roles, intermittent rehabilitation may be required to help the person adapt to new expectations, demands, and environments. Changes in social support of the family and a familiar home environment may result in the breakdown of existing strategies used to aid performance. A person that was previously functioning independently may decline with changes in living situations or life roles. New strategies may need to be taught or adapted to meet the life demands and changes in IADLs. Long-term supports, resources, and intermittent rehabilitation periods are needed to maintain and maximize participation in the community and society.

OCCUPATIONAL THERAPY'S ROLE IN TBI REHABILITATION

The occupational therapist is the team member that is primarily involved in addressing ADLs. The core philosophy and approach of occupational therapy focuses on the ability of individuals with TBI to engage in meaningful daily occupations using the client's occupations or activities as the therapeutic change agent and the ultimate goal of therapy (114). Occupational therapy intervention focuses on those PADLs and IADLs the client needs and wants to be able to do, and the factors that either support or interfere with the desired performance (4). Occupational therapy practitioners commonly bill for skilled activity-based interventions addressing PADLs and IADLs using billing codes related to self-care or home management training and community or work reintegration training in addition to codes addressing cognitive rehabilitation and therapeutic activities to develop underlying motor skills.

The comprehensive entry-level educational preparation of occupational therapists, typically at the master's level, is based on the biological, physical, social, and behavioral sciences. Educational preparation to practice the profession includes content related to the relationship between cognitive processes and performance in daily life occupations (20), motor recovery (see Chapters 68 and 69), home and environmental adaptation, activity analysis, and use of assistive devices and technology to promote independence. The American Occupational Therapy Association has published practice guidelines (75) that provide an overview of the occupational therapy process for adults with TBI using an evidence-based perspective and key concepts from the *Occupational Therapy Practice Framework* (4). As members of the interdisciplinary team providing rehabilitation, occupational therapists can contribute science-driven, evidence-based intervention to address the occupational performance needs of the client with TBI to support their health and participation in life through engagement in meaningful occupations.

CONCLUSION

Performance of daily life tasks, often taken for granted, can suddenly become a major struggle after a TBI. Inability to perform life tasks can impact one's sense of self-confidence and competence. Functional performance can continue to improve for years after a TBI. Therapists and the entire rehabilitation team are challenged to engage in client-centered care that addresses the everyday activities that client wants and needs to do to fulfill life roles and find satisfaction in

daily life. Conceptualizing participation as an interaction between the person, activity, and environment can aid the rehabilitation team in thinking beyond the restrictions of the current intervention environment and client abilities to foster greater independence and community engagement. Working with clients with TBI and their families on self-selected functional performance goals can bring meaning back to the client's life.

 KEY CLINICAL POINTS

1. Occupations or everyday activities provide meaning to life and can be disrupted when a person sustains a TBI.
2. Successful functional performance involves a match between the person's skills and the demands of the task and environment.
3. PADLs and IADLs assessments can focus on measuring competency, needed assistance, factors interfering with performance, or patterns of errors.
4. Persisting difficulties in IADLs because of cognitive and behavioral symptoms restricts one's participation in the home and community and increases caregiver burden.
5. Intervention approaches may address underlying skills, adapt the task or environment, teach compensatory skills, or train the individual in applying strategies to improve functional performance.
6. Individuals who sustained TBIs may need periodic intervention to help adjust to new roles, environments, and tasks required for independence. Evidence supports the potential for continued functional improvements even years after the injury.

WEBSITES:

- Brainline.org is a comprehensive website for TBI survivors, families, and professionals. http://www.brainline.org/
- Working with TBI. http://www.tbistafftraining.info includes a module on independent living skills and toolkit to promote independence.
- AbleData provides information about assistive technology products and rehabilitation equipment. http://www.abledata.com.

 KEY REFERENCES

1. Baum CM, Katz N. Occupational therapy approach to assessing the relationship between cognition and function. In: Marcotte TD, Grant I, eds. *Neuropsychology of Everyday Functioning*. New York, NY: The Guilford Press; 2010: 62–90.
2. Golisz KM. *Occupational Therapy Practice Guidelines for Adults with Traumatic Brain njury*. Bethesda, MD: American Occupational Therapy Association; 2009.
3. Katz N, ed. *Cognition and Occupation Across the Life Span*. Bethesda, MD: American Occupational Therapy Association; 2004.

4. Radomski MV. Traumatic brain injury. In: Radomski MV, Trombly Latham CA, eds. *Occupational Therapy for Physical Dysfunction*. 6th ed. Baltimore, MD: Lippincott Williams & Wilkins; 2008:1042–1078.

5. Roley SS, DeLany JV, Barrows CJ, et al. Occupational therapy practice framework: domain & practice. 2nd ed. *Am J Occup Ther*. 2008;62(6):625–683.

References

1. Hasselkus BR. The world of everyday occupation: real people, real lives. *Am J Occup Ther*. 2006;60(6):627–640.

2. McNeny R. Therapy for activities of daily living: theoretical and practical perspectives. In: Zasler ND, Katz DI, Zafonte RD, eds. *Brain Injury Medicine: Principles and Practice*. 1st ed. New York, NY: Demos Medical Publishing; 2007.

3. Christiansen CH. The 1999 Eleonor Clarke Slagle lecture. Defining lives: occupation as identity: an essay on competence, coherence, and the creation of meaning. *Am J Occup Ther*. 1999;53(6):547–558.

4. Roley SS, DeLany JV, Barrows CJ, et al. Occupational therapy practice framework: domain & practice, 2nd edition. *Am J Occup Ther*. 2008;62(6):625–683.

5. Royall DR, Lauterbach EC, Kaufer D, Malloy P, Coburn KL, Black KJ. The cognitive correlates of functional status: a review from the Committee on Research of the American Neuropsychiatric Association. *J Neuropsychiatry Clin Neurosci*. 2007;19(3):249–265.

6. World Health Organization. *International Classification of Functioning, Disability, and Health*. Geneva, Switzerland: World Health Organization; 2001.

7. National Institute on Disability and Rehabilitation Research. The Traumatic Brain Injury Model Systems of Care. Englewood, CO: National Data and Statistical Center; 2011. https://www.tbindsc.org/Documents/2011%20TBIMS%20Slide%20Presentation.pdf. Accessed August 15, 2011.

8. Andelic N, Sigurdardottir S, Schanke AK, Sandvik L, Sveen U, Roe C. Disability, physical health, and mental health 1 year after traumatic brain injury. *Disabil Rehabil*. 2010;32(13):1122–1131.

9. Colantonio A, Ratcliff G, Chase S, Kelsey S, Escobar M, Vernich L. Long-term outcomes after moderate to severe traumatic brain injury. *Disabil Rehabil*. 2004;26(5):253–261.

10. Dikmen SS, Machamer JE, Powell JM, Temkin NR. Outcome 3 to 5 years after moderate to severe traumatic brain injury. *Arch Phys Med Rehabil*. 2003;84(10):1449–1457.

11. Devitt R, Colantonio A, Dawson D, Teare G, Ratcliff G, Chase S. Prediction of long-term occupational performance outcomes for adults after moderate to severe traumatic brain injury. *Disabil Rehabil*. 2006;28(9):547–559.

12. Ownsworth T, McKenna K. Investigation of factors related to employment outcome following traumatic brain injury: a critical review and conceptual model. *Disabil Rehabil*. 2004;26(13):765–783.

13. Schönberger M, Ponsford J, Olver J, Ponsford M, Wirtz M. Prediction of functional and employment outcome 1 year after traumatic brain injury: a structural equation modelling approach. *J Neurol Neurosurg Psychiatry*. 2011;82(8):936–941.

14. Dirette D. The development of awareness and the use of compensatory strategies for cognitive deficits. *Brain Inj*. 2002;16(10):861–871.

15. Fischer S, Gauggel S, Trexler LE. Awareness of activity limitations, goal setting and rehabilitation outcome in patients with brain injuries. *Brain Inj*. 2004;18(6):547–562.

16. Ownsworth T, Clare L. The association between awareness deficits and rehabilitation outcome following acquired brain injury. *Clin Psychol Rev*. 2006;26(6):783–795.

17. Abreu BC, Seale G, Scheibel RS, Huddleston N, Zhang L, Ottenbacher KJ. Levels of self-awareness after acute brain injury: how patients' and rehabilitation specialists' perceptions compare. *Arch Phys Med Rehabil*. 2001;82(1):49–56.

18. Toglia J, Kirk U. Understanding awareness deficits following brain injury. *NeuroRehabilitation*. 2000;15(1):57–70.

19. Fleming J, Strong J. A longitudinal study of self-awareness: functional deficits underestimated by persons with brain injury. *Occup Ther J Res*. 1999;19(1):3–17.

20. Commission on Practice. Cognition, cognitive rehabilitation, and occupational performance. *Am J Occup Ther*. In press.

21. Baum CM, Katz N. Occupational therapy approach to assessing the relationship between cognition and function. In: Marcotte TD, Grant I, eds. *Neuropsychology of Everyday Functioning*. New York, NY: The Guilford Press; 2010: 62–90.

22. Goverover Y. Categorization, deductive reasoning, and self-awareness: association with everyday competence in persons with acute brain injury. *J Clin Exp Neuropsychol*. 2004;26(6):737–749.

23. Baum CM, Morrison T, Hahn M, Edwards DF. *Test Manual: Executive Function Performance Test*. St. Louis, MO: Washington University; 2008.

24. Hartman-Maeir A, Harel H, Katz N. Kettle test—a brief measure of cognitive functional performance. Reliability and validity in stroke rehabilitation. *Am J Occup Ther*. 2009;63(5):592–599.

25. Waehrens EE, Fisher AG. Improving quality of ADL performance after rehabilitation among people with acquired brain injury. *Scand J Occup Ther*. 2007;14(4):250–257.

26. Owsley C, Sloane M, McGwin G Jr, Ball K. Timed instrumental activities of daily living tasks: relationship to cognitive function and everyday performance assessments in older adults. *Gerontology*. 2002;48(4):254–265.

27. Owsley C, McGwin G Jr, Sloane ME, Stalvey BT, Wells J. Timed instrumental activities of daily living tasks: relationship to visual function in older adults. *Optom Vis Sci*. 2001;78(5):350–359.

28. Gardarsdóttir S, Kaplan S. Validity of the Arnadóttir OT-ADL Neurobehavioral Evaluation (A-ONE): performance in activities of daily living and neurobehavioral impairments of persons with left and right hemisphere damage. *Am J Occup Ther*. 2002;56(5): 499–508.

29. Baum CM, Connor LT, Morrison T, Hahn M, Dromerick AW, Edwards DF. Reliability, validity, and clinical utility of the Executive Function Performance Test: a measure of executive function in a sample of people with stroke. *Am J Occup Ther*. 2008;62(4):446–455.

30. Fisher AG. *Assessment of Motor and Process Skills*. 3rd ed. Fort Collins, CO: Three Star; 1999.

31. Lange B, Spagnolo K, Fowler B. Using the assessment of motor and process skills to measure functional change in adults with severe traumatic brain injury: A pilot study. *Aust Occup Ther J*. 2009;56(2):89–96.

32. Ryan JD, Polatajko HJ, McEwen S, et al. Analysis of Cognitive Environmental Support (ACES): preliminary testing. *Neuropsychol Rehabil*. 2011;21(3):401–427.

33. Schwartz MF, Segal ME, Veramonti T, Ferraro M, Buxbaum LJ. The naturalistic action test: a standardized assessment for everyday-action impairment. *Neuropsychol Rehabil*. 2002;12(4):311–339.

34. Alderman N, Burgess PW, Knight C, Henman C. Ecological validity of a simplified version of the multiple errands shopping test. *J Int Neuropsychol Soc*. 2003;9(1):31–44.

35. Knight C, Alderman N, Burgess PW. Development of a simplified version of the multiple errands test for use in hospital settings. *Neuropsychol Rehabil*. 2002;12(3):231–255.

36. Nott MT, Chapparo C. Measuring information processing in a client with extreme agitation following traumatic brain injury using the Perceive, Recall, Plan, and Perform System of Task Analysis. *Aust Occup Ther J*. 2008;55(3):188–198.

37. Nott MT, Chapparo C, Heard R. Reliability of the Perceive, Recall, Plan, and Perform System of Task Analysis: a criterion-referenced assessment. *Aust Occup Ther J*. 2009;56(5):307–314.

38. Toglia JP. *Contextual Memory Test*. San Antonio, TX: Psychological Corporation; 1993.

39. Josman N. Reliability and validity of the Toglia Category Assessment Test. *Can J Occup Ther*. 1999;66(1):33–42.

40. Katz N, Golstand S, Bar-Ilan RT, Parush S. The Dynamic Occupational Therapy Cognitive Assessment for Children (DOTCA-ch): a new instrument for assessing learning potential. *Am J Occup Ther*. 2007;61(1):41–52.

41. Toglia JP. A dynamic interactional model to cognitive rehabilitation. In: Katz N, ed. *Cognition and Occupation Across the Life Span*. 2nd ed. Bethesda, MD: American Occupational Therapy Association; 2005: 29–72.

42. Toglia J, Cermak SA. Dynamic assessment and prediction of learn-

ing potential in clients with unilateral neglect. *Am J Occup Ther.* 2009;63(5):569–579.

43. Lyle RC. A performance test for assessment of upper limb function in physical rehabilitation treatment and research. *Int J Rehabil Res.* 1981;4(4):483–492.

44. Fugl-Meyer AR, Jääskö L, Leyman I, Olsson S, Steglind S. The post-stroke hemiplegic patient. 1. a method for evaluation of physical performance. *Scand J Rehabil Med.* 1975;7(1):13–31.

45. Wolf SL, Catlin PA, Ellis M, Archer AL, Morgan B, Piacentino A. Assessing Wolf motor function test as outcome measure for research in patients after stroke. *Stroke.* 2001;32(7):1635–1639.

46. O'Dell MW, Kim G, Finnen LR, Polistena C. Clinical implications of using the arm motor ability test in stroke rehabilitation. *Arch Phys Med Rehabil.* 2011;92(5):830–836.

47. Robertson IH, Ward T, Ridgeway V, Nimmo-Smith I. *The Test of Everyday Attention.* Bury St. Edmunds, UK: Thames Valley Test; 1994–1999.

48. Wilson B, Cockburn J, Baddley A. The Rivermead Behavioral Memory Test. Reading, UK: Thames Valley Test; 1985.

49. Hartman-Maeir A, Katz N. Validity of behavioral inattention test (BIT): relationships with functional tasks. *Am J Occup Ther.* 1995; 49(6):507–516.

50. Katz N, Itzkovich M, Averbuch S. The Loewenstein Occupational Therapy Cognitive Assessment. *Arch Phys Med Rehabil.* 2002;83(8): 1179.

51. Wilson B, Alderman N, Burgess PW, Emslie H, Evans JJ. *Behavioural Assessment of the Dysexecutive Syndrome (BADS).* Bury St. Edmonds, UK: Thames Valley Test; 1996.

52. Cooke DM, McKenna K, Fleming J, Darnell R. Construct and ecological validity of the Occupational Therapy Adult Perceptual Screening Test (OT-APST). *Scand J Occup Ther.* 2006;13(1):49–61.

53. Wilson B, Cockburn J, Halligan P. *The Behavioural Inattention Test Manual.* Fareham, UK: Thames Valley Test; 1987.

54. Warren M. *Brain Injury Visual Assessment Battery for Adults.* Lenexa, KS: visAbilities Rehab Services; 1998.

55. Doig E, Fleming J, Cornwell PL, Kuipers P. Qualitative exploration of a client-centered, goal-directed approach to community-based occupational therapy for adults with traumatic brain injury. *Am J Occup Ther.* 2009;63(5):559–568.

56. Toglia JP, Golisz KM. Traumatic brain injury and the impact on daily life. In: Chiaravalloti ND, ed. *Changing Brain, Changes in Daily Life.* New York, NY: Springer Publishing; In press.

57. Rivera PA, Elliott TR, Berry JW, Grant JS. Problem-solving training for family caregivers of persons with traumatic brain injuries: a randomized controlled trial. *Arch Phys Med Rehabil.* 2008;89(5): 931–941.

58. Parish L, Oddy M. Efficacy of rehabilitation for functional skills more than 10 years after extremely severe brain injury. *Neuropsychol Rehabil.* 2007;17(2):230–243.

59. Meinzer M, Elbert T, Djundja D, Taub E, Rockstroh B. Extending the constraint-induced movement therapy (CIMT) approach to cognitive functions: constraint-induced aphasia therapy (CIAT) of chronic aphasia. *NeuroRehabilitation.* 2007;22(4):311–318.

60. Cho YW, Jang SH, Lee ZI, Song JC, Lee HK, Lee HY. Effect and appropriate restriction period of constraint-induced movement therapy in hemiparetic patients with brain injury: a brief report. *NeuroRehabilitation.* 2005;20(2):71–74.

61. Page SJ, Levine P, Khoury JC. Modified constraint-induced therapy combined with mental practice. thinking through better motor outcomes. *Stroke.* 2009;40(2):551–554.

62. Shaw SE, Morris DM, Uswatte G, McKay S, Meythaler JM, Taub E. Constraint-induced movement therapy for recovery of upper-limb function following traumatic brain injury. *J Rehabil Res Dev.* 2005;42(6):769–778.

63. Dawson DR, Gaya A, Hunt A, Levine B, Lemsky C, Polatajko HJ. Using the cognitive orientation to occupational performance (CO-OP) with adults with executive dysfunction following traumatic brain injury. *Can J Occup Ther.* 2009;76(2):115–127.

64. Fish J, Manly T, Wilson BA. Long-term compensatory treatment of organizational deficits in a patient with bilateral frontal lobe damage. *J Int Neuropsychol Soc.* 2008;14(1):154–163.

65. Fleming JM, Lucas SE, Lightbody S. Using occupation to facilitate

self-awareness in people who have acquired brain injury: a pilot study. *Can J Occup Ther.* 2006;73(1):44–55.

66. Shum D, Fleming J, Gill H, Gullo MJ, Strong J. A randomized controlled trial of prospective memory rehabilitation in adults with traumatic brain injury. *J Rehabil Med.* 2011;43(3):216–223.

67. Toglia J, Johnston MV, Goverover Y, Dain B. A multicontext approach to promoting transfer of strategy use and self regulation after brain injury: an exploratory study. *Brain Inj.* 2010;24(4): 664–677.

68. Clare L, Jones RS. Errorless learning in the rehabilitation of memory impairment: a critical review. *Neuropsychol Rev.* 2008;18(1): 1–23.

69. Cohen M, Ylvisaker M, Hamilton J, Kemp L, Claiman B. Errorless learning of functional life skills in an individual with three aetiologies of severe memory and executive function impairment. *Neuropsychol Rehabil.* 2010;20(3):355–376.

70. Giles GM. A neurofunctional approach to rehabilitation following severe brain injury. In: Katz N, ed. *Cognitive and Occupation Across the Lifespan: Models for Intervention in Occupational Therapy.* Bethesda, MD: American Occupational Therapy Association; 2005: 139–166.

71. Kiser L, Zasler N. Residential design for real life rehabilitation. *NeuroRehabilitation.* 2009;25(3):219–227.

72. Dowds MM, Lee PH, Sheer JB, et al. Electronic reminding technology following traumatic brain injury: effects on timely task completion. *J Head Trauma Rehabil.* 2011;26(5):339–347.

73. Wilson BA, Emslie HC, Quirk K, Evans JJ. Reducing everyday memory and planning problems by means of a paging system: a randomised control crossover study. *J Neurol Neurosurg Psychiatry.* 2001;70(4):477–482.

74. Cappa SF, Benke T, Clarke S, Rossi B, Stemmer B, van Heugten CM. EFNS guidelines on cognitive rehabilitation: report of an EFNS task force. *Eur J Neurol.* 2005;12(9):665–680.

75. Golisz KM. *Occupational Therapy Practice Guidelines for Adults with Traumatic Brain Injury.* Bethesda, MD: American Occupational Therapy Association; 2009.

76. Cappa SF, Benke T, Clarke S, Rossi B, Stemmer B, van Heugten CM. Cognitive rehabilitation. In: Gilhus NE, Barnes MP, Brainin M, eds. *European Handbook of Neurological Management.* Vol 1. 2nd ed. Oxford, UK: Blackwell Publishing Ltd; 2011:545–567.

77. Cicerone KD, Langenbahn DM, Braden C, et al. Evidence-based cognitive rehabilitation: updated review of the literature from 2003 through 2008. *Arch Phys Med Rehabil.* 2011;92(4):519–530.

78. de Joode E, van Heugten C, Verhey F, van Boxtel M. Efficacy and usability of assistive technology for patients with cognitive deficits: a systematic review. *Clin Rehabil.* 2010;24(8):701–714.

79. Fish J, Manly T, Emslie H, Evans JJ, Wilson BA. Compensatory strategies for acquired disorders of memory and planning: differential effects of a paging system for patients with brain injury of traumatic versus cerebrovascular aetiology. *J Neurol Neurosurg Psychiatry.* 2008;79(8):930–935.

80. Gentry T, Wallace J, Kvarfordt C, Lynch KB. Personal digital assistants as cognitive aids for individuals with severe traumatic brain injury: a community-based trial. *Brain Inj.* 2008;22(1):19–24.

81. Stapleton S, Adams M, Atterton L. A mobile phone as a memory aid for individuals with traumatic brain injury. *Brain Inj.* 2007;21(4): 401–411.

82. Evans JJ, Wilson BA, Schuri U, et al. A comparison of "errorless" and "trial and error" learning methods for teaching individuals with acquired memory deficits. *Neuropsychological Rehabilitation.* 2000;10(1):67–101.

83. Campbell L, Wilson FC, McCann J, Kernahan G, Rogers RG. Single case experimental design study of carer facilitated errorless learning in a patient with severe memory impairment following TBI. *NeuroRehabilitation.* 2007;22(4):325–333.

84. Parish L, Oddy M. Efficacy of rehabilitation for functional skills more than 10 years after extremely severe brain injury. *Neuropsychol Rehabil.* 2007;17(2):230–243.

85. Ownsworth T, Quinn H, Fleming J, Kendall M, Shum D. Error self-regulation following traumatic brain injury: a single case study evaluation of metacognitive skills training and behavioural practice interventions. *Neuropsychol Rehabil.* 2010;20(1):59–80.

86. Kennedy MR, Coelho C, Turkstra L, et al. Intervention for executive functions after traumatic brain injury: a systematic review, meta-analysis, and clinical recommendations. *Neuropsychol Rehabil.* 2008; 18(3):257–299.

87. Goverover Y, Johnston MV, Toglia J, Deluca J. Treatment to improve self-awareness in persons with acquired brain injury. *Brain Inj.* 2007;21(9):913–923.

88. Fleming JM, Lucas SE, Lightbody S. Using occupation to facilitate self-awareness in people who have acquired brain injury: a pilot study. *Can J Occup Ther.* 2006;73(1):44–55.

89. Goverover Y, Johnston MV, Toglia J, Deluca J. Treatment to improve self-awareness in persons with acquired brain injury. *Brain Inj.* 2007;21(9):913–923.

90. Ownsworth T. A metacognitive contextual approach for facilitating return to work following acquired brain injury: three descriptive case studies. *Work.* 2010;36(4):381–388.

91. McGraw-Hunter M, Faw GD, Davis PK. The use of video self-modelling and feedback to teach cooking skills to individuals with traumatic brain injury: a pilot study. *Brain Inj.* 2006;20(10): 1061–1068.

92. Liu KP, Chan CC, Lee TM, Hui-Chan CW. Mental imagery for relearning of people after brain injury. *Brain Inj.* 2004;18(11): 1163–1172.

93. Liu KP, Chan CC, Lee TM, Li LS, Hui-Chan CW. Self-regulatory learning and generalization for people with brain injury. *Brain Inj.* 2002;16(9):817–824.

94. Levine B, Robertson IH, Clare L, et al. Rehabilitation of executive functioning: an experimental-clinical validation of goal management training. *J Int Neuropsychol Soc.* 2000;6(3):299–312.

95. Dawson DR, Gaya A, Hunt A, Levine B, Lemsky C, Polatajko HJ. Using the cognitive orientation to occupational performance (CO-OP) with adults with executive dysfunction following traumatic brain injury. *Can J Occup Ther.* 2009;76(2):115–127.

96. Winkens I, Van Heugten CM, Wade DT, Fasotti L. Training patients in time pressure management, a cognitive strategy for mental slowness. *Clin Rehabil.* 2009;23(1):79–90.

97. Goverover Y, Chiaravalloti N, DeLuca J. Pilot study to examine the use of self-generation to improve learning and memory in people with traumatic brain injury. *Am J Occup Ther.* 2010;64(4): 540–546.

98. Goverover Y, Arango-Lasprilla JC, Hillary FG, Chiaravalloti N, Deluca J. Application of the spacing effect to improve learning and memory for functional tasks in traumatic brain injury: a pilot study. *Am J Occup Ther.* 2009;63(5):543–548.

99. Toglia JP. A dynamic interactional approach to cognitive rehabilitation. In: Katz N, ed. *Cognition and Occupation Across the Life Span: Models for Intervention in Occupational Therapy.* 2nd ed. Baltimore, MD: American Occupational Therapy Association; 2005:5–50.

100. Turner B, Ownsworth T, Cornwell P, Fleming J. Reengagement in meaningful occupations during the transition from hospital to home for people with acquired brain injury and their family care-givers. *Am J Occup Ther.* 2009;63(5):609–620.

101. Cicerone KD, Azulay J. Perceived self-efficacy and life satisfaction after traumatic brain injury. *J Head Trauma Rehabil.* 2007;22(5): 257–266.

102. Fleming J, Braithwaite H, Gustafsson L, Griffin J, Collier AM, Fletcher S. Participation in leisure activities during brain injury rehabilitation. *Brain Inj.* 2011;25(9):806–818.

103. Rapport LJ, Bryer RC, Hanks RA. Driving and community integration after traumatic brain injury. *Arch Phys Med Rehabil.* 2008;89(5): 922–930.

104. Rand D, Basha-Abu Rukan S, Weiss PL, Katz N. Validation of the virtual MET as an assessment tool for executive functions. *Neuropsychol Rehabil.* 2009;19(4):583–602.

105. Rand D, Weiss PL, Katz N. Training multitasking in a virtual super-market: a novel intervention after stroke. *Am J Occup Ther.* 2009; 63(5):535–542.

106. Logie RH, Trawley S, Law A. Multitasking: multiple, domain-specific cognitive functions in a virtual environment. *Mem Cognit.* 2011;39(8):1561–1574.

107. Spaeth DM, Mahajan H, Karmarkar A, Collins D, Cooper RA, Boninger ML. Development of a wheelchair virtual driving environment: trials with subjects with traumatic brain injury. *Arch Phys Med Rehabil.* 2008;89(5):996–1003.

108. Katz N, Ring H, Naveh Y, Kizony R, Feintuch U, Weiss PL. Interactive virtual environment training for safe street crossing of right hemisphere stroke patients with unilateral spatial neglect. *Disabil Rehabil.* 2005;27(20):1235–1243.

109. Kim DY, Ku J, Chang WH, et al. Assessment of post-stroke extra-personal neglect using a three-dimensional immersive virtual street crossing program. *Acta Neurol Scand.* 2010;121(3):171–177.

110. Fong KN, Chow KY, et al. Usability of a virtual reality environment simulating an automated teller machine for assessing and training persons with acquired brain injury. *J Neuroeng Rehabil.* 2010;7:19.

111. Yip BC, Man DW. Virtual reality (VR)-based community living skills training for people with acquired brain injury: a pilot study. *Brain Inj.* 2009;23(13–14):1017–1026.

112. Gentry T. Assistive technology for people with neurological disability. *NeuroRehabil.* 2011;28(3):181–182.

113. VA rolls out 'smart home' project to rehabilitate brain injury patients. Washington, DC: National Journal Group, Inc.; 2010. http://www.nextgov.com/nextgov/ng 20101214 7113.php?oref=topstory. Updated December 14, 2010. Accessed August 10, 2011.

114. The philosophical base of occupational therapy. Bethesda, MD: American Occupational Therapy Association; 2011. http://www.aota.org/Practitioners/Official/Statements/41098.aspx?FT=.pdf. Updated 2011. Accessed August 15, 2011.

115. Mahoney FI, Barthel DW. Functional evaluation: the barthel index. *Md State Med J.* 1965;14:61–65.

116. Katz S, Akpom CA. A measure of primary sociobiological functions. *Int J Health Serv.* 1976;6(3):493–508.

117. Klein RM, Bell B. Self-care skills: behavioral measurement with Klein-Bell ADL scale. *Arch Phys Med Rehabil.* 1982;63(7):335–338.

118. Clemson L, Bundy A, Unsworth C, Singh MF. Validation of the modified assessment of living skills and resources, an IADL measure for older people. *Disabil Rehabil.* 2009;31(5):359–569.

119. Hall KM, Mann N, High WM, Wright J, Kreutzer JS, Wood D. Functional measures after traumatic brain injury: ceiling effects of FIM, FIM+FAM, DRS, and CIQ. *J Head Trauma Rehabil.* 1996;11: 27–39.

120. Granger CV, Brownscheidle CM. Outcome measurement in medical rehabilitation. *Int J Technol Assess Health Care.* 1995;11(2): 262–268.

121. Hartman-Maeir A, Harel H, Katz N. Kettle test—a brief measure of cognitive functional performance. Reliability and valdity in stroke rehabilitation. *Am J Occup Ther.* 2009;63(5):592–599.

122. Holm MB, Rogers JC. Performance assessment of self-care skills. In: Hemphill-Pearson BJ, ed. *Assessments in Occupational Therapy Mental Health.* Thorofare, NJ: Slack; 1999:117–124.

123. Arnadóttir G, Fisher AG. Rasch analysis of the ADL scale of the A-ONE. *Am J Occup Ther.* 2008;62(1):51–60.

124. Bottari CL, Dassa C, Rainville CM, Dutil E. The IADL profile: development, content validity, intra- and interrater agreement. *Can J Occup Ther.* 2010;77(2):90–100.

125. Knight C, Alderman N, Burgess PW. Development of a simplified version of the multiple errands test for use in hospital settings. *Neuropsychol Rehabil.* 2002;12(3):231–255.

Assistive Technology for People With Traumatic Brain Injuries

Rory A. Cooper, Michael McCue, Richard M. Schein, Rosemarie Cooper, Michelle L. Sporner, Matthew B. Dodson, Amanda M. Reinsfelder, Arthur F. Yeager, Andrew Jinks, Edmund LoPresti, Laura McClure, Hongwu Wang, Jennifer L. Collinger, Shivayogi Hiremath, Dan Ding, and Allen Lewis

INTRODUCTION

Technology can be of tremendous benefit to people with brain injuries and facilitate greater independence and community participation. Mobility, communication, computer usage, and assistance with cognitive functioning can all be supported with the appropriate usage of technology. The delivery of assistive technologies for people with brain injuries mandates a team approach involving therapists, counselors, physicians, engineers, and most importantly the person with a brain injury (and the person's family). Brain injury can affect many aspects of functioning, and therefore, a thorough assessment of the individual's abilities, his or her understanding of technology, and his or her interaction with other people and various environments is needed. Unfortunately, there is a shortage of health care professionals with the expertise to provide and train individuals with brain injuries in the application and usage of assistive technology (AT). This need is in part beginning to be addressed using telerehabilitation, which is expected to grow because remotely programmable devices such as smart phones, smart pads, and remotely controllable software become ubiquitous. This should have the benefit of addressing geographical barriers to access to expertise and lower the cost of some technologies as the hardware becomes more mainstream and the adaptive component are largely software applications.

TELEREHABILITATION

Telerehabilitation may be defined as the delivery of rehabilitation services via information and telecommunication technologies (i.e., assessment, monitoring, intervention, supervision, education, consultation, and counseling) (1) in an emerging field incorporating advanced technologies while improving quality of life and leading to a more efficient use of health care resources (2–4). Primarily, the development of telerehabilitation has been driven by the need to provide equitable access to rehabilitation services for individuals who are geographically remote from rehabilitation special-

ists. The long-term rehabilitation requirements for individuals as a result of traumatic brain injury (TBI), neurological disorder, orthopedic, and developmental diagnoses are frequently unmet because of limited resources or expertise; however, the use of telerehabilitation allows the individual a mechanism for an alternative model to promote his or her quality of life within his or her home setting or at a remote clinical site.

Assessing Telerehabilitation

Since the late 1950s, technologists and clinicians have explored the use of advanced information technologies as a way of bridging the gap between individuals with specialized medical needs living in remote areas and the source of specialty care (5–6). The field of telerehabilitation exists under the assumption that the barrier of distance can be minimized to enhance access that will open new possibilities for delivering intervention strategies across the continuum of care (7). The telecommunication tools that assist with rehabilitation services offer advantages and disadvantages. Technology affects the access, quality, and cost of care, and because these aspects are interconnected, a comprehensive assessment should incorporate all the 3 (8). The rehabilitation field has been gradually integrating telecommunication tools into clinical practice. The benefits of using telerehabilitation include (a) decreased travel between rural communities and specialized urban health centers, (b) better clinical support in local communities, (c) improved access to specialized services, (d) delivery of local health care in rural communities, (e) indirect educational benefits for remote clinicians, (f) reduced feelings of isolation for rural clinicians, and (g) improved service stability in regions with high staff turnover (9). In addition, it has been proposed that telerehabilitation has the potential to deliver more effective rehabilitation services because it is able to incorporate contextual factors from the environment into the rehabilitation intervention. Acknowledging that the social and physical environment can be facilitative (or inhibitory), rehabilitation that can occur within the individual's natural setting has greater relevance. For individuals with brain injury, cognitive rehabilitation that occurs in the natural setting and within the context of everyday interaction and demand domains is more relevant to the individual (10). There has emerged considerable evidence to support the value of conducting TBI rehabilitation within the natural environment (4). Such naturalistic treatment has been shown to increase functional outcomes, address problems with generalizability of rehabilitation gains, and enhance consumer satisfaction and self-direction. Therefore, telerehabilitation can play a key role in the accessibility and implementation of naturalistic and in vivo treatment.

Technology Used for Current Developments

The format currently most applicable to telerehabilitation is videoconferencing where there is an interaction between service providers to an individual at a remote site (i.e., clinic or home). Telecommunication technologies supporting the remote service provision have changed dramatically including broad bandwidth Internet connections, virtual reality, wireless devices, remote monitoring devices, and wearable sensors.

Two different models of telerehabilitation applications predominately are in use today. The first, store and forward or asynchronous, is used for transferring digital data from 1 location to another. Common tools include discussion boards, blogs, shared calendars, and narrated slideshows. These tools allow people to connect together at each person's own convenience and own schedule. The other widely used technology, real time or synchronous, is used when a "face-to-face" encounter is necessary. It is usually between the client, his or her provider, and a specialist but may be any combination of the 3. Videoconferencing equipment at both locations allows a real-time encounter to take place. The technology has decreased in price and complexity over the past years, and many rehabilitation programs now use desktop videoconferencing systems. There are also many peripheral devices or instruments that can be connected to computers to transmit heart sounds, blood pressure, and outcome measurements that assist with interactive assessment and evaluation. Although video conferencing is the most popular synchronous rehabilitation technology, other technologies such as chat, short message service (SMS) text messaging, and audio telephony have been applied in real-time rehabilitation applications. Many rehabilitation and AT professionals involved in telerehabilitation are becoming increasingly creative with available technology. For instance, it is not unusual to use store and forward, interactive audio, and video still images in a variety of combinations and applications. Use of the Internet to transfer clinical information and data is becoming more prevalent.

Although it is outside the scope of this chapter to provide a description of every possible clinical application of telerehabilitation, the following are specific reviews that exemplify telerehabilitation for a diverse group of diagnoses. Remote assessment of rehabilitation needs has been described for neuropsychological status (11), apraxia (12), motor speech disorders (13), and wheeled mobility and seating (14) among numerous other applications. There is also

sufficient evidence to support the use of telerehabilitation in individuals with brain injury (15).

The University of Pittsburgh's Rehabilitation Engineering Research Center on Telerehabilitation has developed Versatile and Integrated System for Telerehabilitation (VISYTER)—a software platform that combines both synchronous and asynchronous activity into 1 integrated system for telerehabilitation services (16). As part of the center's state of the science, Schmeler et al. (17) detailed the use of telerehabilitation for clinical and vocational applications for various ATs. The center is currently implementing VISYTER for various cognitive and vocational rehabilitation (VR) applications such as testing the reliability and validity of a remote neuropsychological assessment, augmentative communication device evaluations and training, developing mobile telerehabilitation applications, and testing of the cognitive skills enhancement program.

Intervention in the home environment has been provided remotely for numerous needs including cognitive rehabilitation over the Internet (18–19) while the University of Medicine and Dentistry of New Jersey designed the remote console that uses virtual reality to guide patients through exercise programs (20). In collaboration with virtual reality, Zheng et al. (21) provides an overview of current sensor technologies from position and motion sensing technologies that can be incorporated into telerehabilitation systems. Finally, the growth of Internet services and wireless communications offer a wide range of general information and other services to be shared with one another or to a group with the use of a computer. For instance, social networking sites provide wide-ranging benefits from improved communication skills and a more intuitive way of understanding technology and establishing better relationships. In addition, access to the Internet enables individuals to take a more active role in their health care by editing and saving information into a personal health record portal system.

Telerehabilitation Resources

In the United States since 1998, the National Institute on Disability and Rehabilitation Research has funded a Rehabilitation Engineering Research Center (RERC) Telerehabilitation that supports research and the development of methods, systems, and technologies that support telerehabilitation. Other funders of research include the Federal Communications Commission, the United States Department of Agriculture-Rural Access, and the Department of Defense and Veterans Affairs (VA). Outside the United States, clinical research and funding opportunities are being conducted in both Australia and Europe. The predominant professional organization of telerehabilitation is the American Telemedicine Association (ATA), where their official journal *Telemedicine and e-Health* and supporting journal *Telemedicine and Telecare* provide direct relevance to the topic. In addition to the ATA, several other professional organizations or departments have produced position papers on the use of telerehabilitation applications, including the American Occupational Theory Association (AOTA) (22), American Social Health Association (ASHA) (23), and VA (24). Policy implications such as reimbursement, privacy and security, and cost are supported by the Center for Telemedicine and e-Health Law (CTeL). Additional information on the practice of telerehabilitation can be found in the *Blueprint for Telerehabilitation Guidelines*, published by the ATA's special interest group on telerehabilitation (1). Information on the evidence for telerehabilitation is found in the 3 recent review articles on telerehabilitation (15,25,26).

WHEELCHAIR USAGE IN POPULATIONS WITH BRAIN INJURY

After sustaining a TBI, wheeled mobility may become necessary because of impaired balance and coordination, abnormal muscle tone, or a decrease in strength. Safety is a top priority and an important consideration when prescribing a device. Common symptoms associated with TBI including excessive sleepiness, inattention to tasks, difficulty concentrating, impaired memory, faulty judgment, irritability, and slowed thinking (27), all of which can interfere with a person's ability to safely use a wheeled mobility device. If a client is using an independent form of mobility, the user needs to prove to the clinician that he or she can safely, effectively, and consistently use the device.

Because each person with a TBI presents in a unique manner, a wheelchair evaluation may be an extensive process, and the most effective equipment may not be obvious. Several different devices should be tried. To prevent the client from being overwhelmed, the evaluation may need to be broken into several sessions. Clinicians should first evaluate and instruct the client how to use a wheelchair in a quiet and controlled environment. Once the client becomes familiar with the device, the user's ability should be evaluated in everyday situations, such as noisy, crowded, and distracting public areas. A variety of devices may be used that range from attendant-propelled manual wheelchairs (MWCs) to power wheelchairs (PWCs) with multiple seat functions.

Attendant-Propelled Manual Wheelchairs

If a person has a very severe TBI, he or she may not be able to independently use a wheelchair or ambulate. An attendant-propelled MWC (Figure 71-1) may be appropriate for an individual who is unable to follow even very basic commands or consistently attend to tasks. Because the user will be completely dependent on an attendant, frequent evaluations should be performed to determine if the user is able to transition to some type of independent device. When prescribing the device, the comfort of both the rider and assistant must be considered because the wheelchair is propelled solely by the attendant. The rider should be positioned in a comfortable position and be afforded sufficient ability to change position. Attendant-propelled MWCs often have the option of manual tilt in space and manual recline. Some chairs can accommodate a power module to allow the rider to independently change his or her position with a switch. To make the attendant comfortable, the wheelchair should be kept as light as possible, be easy to push, and have ergonomically designed and placed push handles.

Self-Propelled Manual Wheelchairs

If a person is able to follow commands and has a reasonable attention span, he or she should use a device that affords

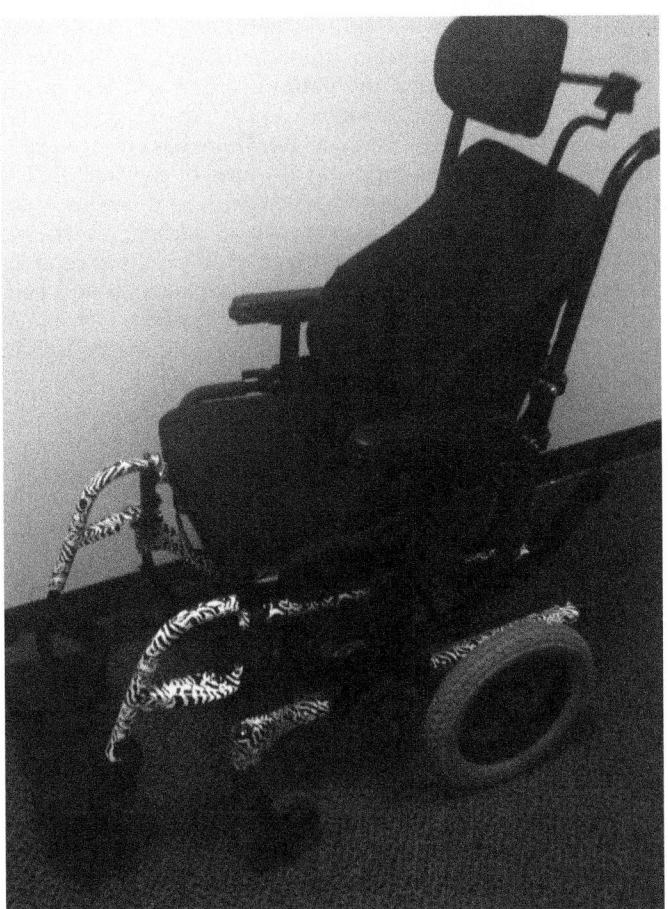

FIGURE 71-1 An attendant-propelled manual wheelchair.

independent mobility. A MWC may be an appropriate device for a person who has good and equal upper extremity strength, reasonable coordination, and good activity tolerance. (Persons with other comorbid factors, such as cardiac or respiratory impairments, may not be able to tolerate propelling a MWC over longer distances.). A clinician should carefully evaluate coordination because this will be a key factor in a person's ability to effectively propel a MWC. If a MWC is determined to be the most appropriate device, the team should strive to make the chair as light as possible to prevent repetitive strain injuries of the upper extremity. *The Clinical Practice Guidelines for Preservation of Upper Limb Function Following Acute Spinal Cord Injury* (28) provides a detailed description of the proper MWC setup and selection and is available at http://www.pva.org. Although this guideline is focused on spinal cord injury, many of the recommendations are appropriate for all people using wheelchairs full time, including those affected by TBI. MWCs are typically categorized by their weight. If the person will be using the device full time, an ultralight wheelchair (see Figure 71-2 in the e-book) is the most appropriate. Ultralight weight chairs weigh < 30 lbs, are made of high quality materials (often titanium or aluminum), and provide a high degree of adjustability. Before the chair is ordered, the person should be carefully measured for the most appropriate size. Although the chair should be comfortable, it should not have a lot of extra room. A properly fitting MWC keeps the user's upper limb in neural alignment during propulsion and does not force the shoulder into excessive abduction (28).

Rear axle position has a large impact on preservation of the upper limb. In the horizontal direction, the axle should be moved as anterior as possible to allow maximum contact with the large rear wheels (29). The user, however, must be careful not to move the axle too far forward because the stability of the chair will decrease. When the chair is first ordered, the clinician should not only set the chair up to allow sufficient wheel contact but also to allow for stability. As the user becomes more comfortable, the rear axle should be progressively moved forward. In the vertical direction, the axle should be placed high enough so the user has sufficient contact with the wheel but not too high that the shoulder is in extreme abduction. A simple way to check for correct position is to have the user sit upright in the chair and drop his or her arm downward. The user's finger tips should be at the level of the rear axle (28) (Figure 71-3). Achieving the ideal setup is an ongoing process, and it may take several weeks before the user feels comfortable.

If the user has sufficient strength in the lower extremities, foot propulsion may be an effective method of mobility. If the person is using his or her feet, the seat to floor height of the wheelchair should be lowered to allow the foot to contact the floor.

Pushrim-activated power-assisted wheels (PAPAW) (see Figure 71-4 in the e-book) are motorized wheels that can be fitted on a MWC frame. PAPAW can decrease the forces needed for propulsion but can be difficult to use if the user has even mild coordination impairments. If the device is chosen, extensive training may be necessary.

Power Wheelchair Options

If the user is not able to effectively use a MWC, a power mobility device can serve as an excellent solution. A power operated vehicle (POV), more commonly called a scooter, (Figure 71-5) is a potential option but should be extensively evaluated to determine if the device serves all of the client's needs. A POV typically has 3–4 small wheels, is driven by a tiller system, and has little or no adjustability. Power seat functions, such as tilt in space and recline, cannot be added to manage some common symptoms of TBI, such as an individual's pain or spasticity. To drive the POV, the user must coordinate both arms to control the device, which may be difficult for a user with impaired coordination. The POV, however, can be easily transported unlike a PWC.

A PWC allows for independent mobility even in the presence of weakness, spasticity, and impaired coordination. Such impairments may be compensated with joystick placement and programming. There are many options available,

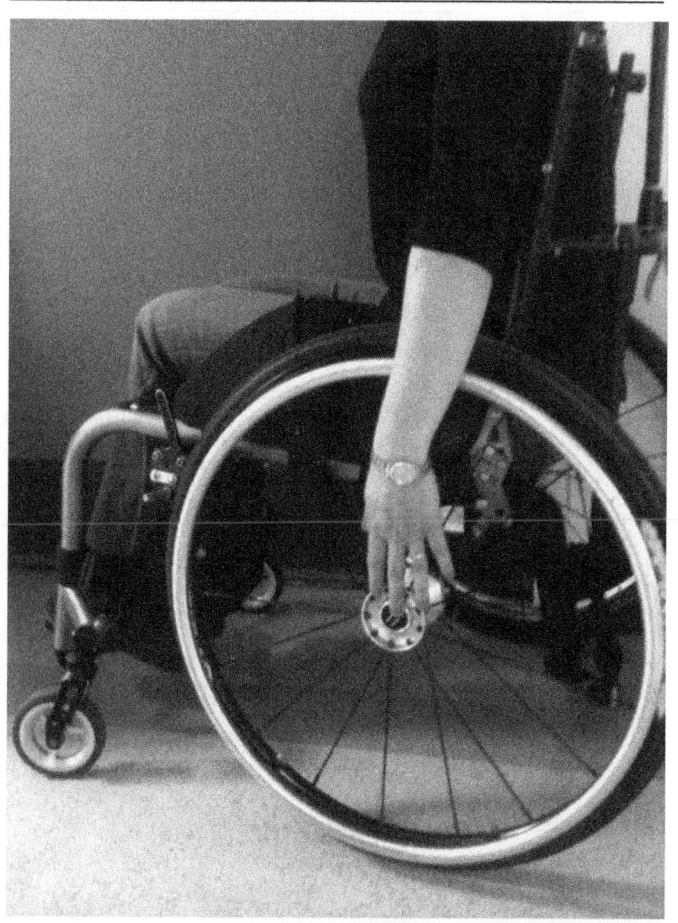

FIGURE 71-3 Correct vertical positioning of the wheelchair: the user's fingertips reach the rear axle.

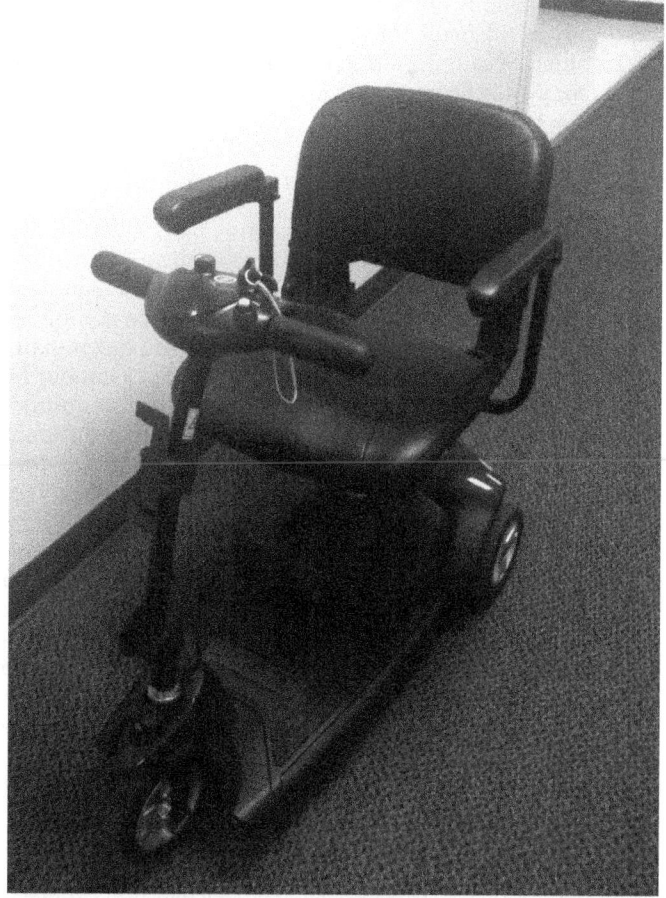

FIGURE 71-5 A power operated vehicle (POV), a.k.a. scooter.

and a potential PWC user should spend time working with a knowledgeable team when choosing a device.

Important to the success of a PWC is finding the right base. The "base" is the portion of the chair that contains the motors, batteries, wheels, casters, and components to control the power seat functions. Most PWCs have 1 of 3 basic wheel configurations: front wheel drive (FWD), midwheel drive (MWD), and rear wheel drive (RWD). The user should try out each base to see what works best for him or her. RWD (Figure 71-6 in the e-book) is the classic PWC configuration. The drive wheels are located behind the user that provides good stability, is intuitive to drive, and can be driven at high speeds. Unfortunately, RWD chairs do not maneuver well in tight areas such as homes or schools. Because of lack of maneuverability, many manufactures have limited production of RWD chairs, thus there are few options available.

MWD chairs (Figure 71-7 in the e-book) have increased in popularity in the past several years. The drive wheel is in the center of the chair, leading to superior maneuverability and ease of use in tight spaces. Driving is also more intuitive, especially for clients with cognitive or spatial impairments. Because of wheel placement, a MWD chair can be less stable and is not able to obtain the high speeds of a RWD chair, although manufactures are working to eliminate such problems. Because of increased popularity, there are also several different types of MWD chairs to choose from.

A FWD power base (Figure 71-8 in the e-book) has the large drive wheel in the front of the chair. This design allows the chair to traverse many obstacles, have fair maneuverability indoors, and be driven at higher speeds. This type of chair, however, is not as intuitive to drive as a MWD chair and may be difficult for an individual who has impaired perception. Because brain injuries affect people differently, different power bases should be tried to determine which is most appropriate.

Control Mechanisms

The user must work with the clinical team to decide how to control the mobility device. A joystick is the standard method of control and may be programmed to accommodate for spasticity, tremors, or any perceptional impairments that affect driving. If a standard joystick cannot be used, alternative input devices are available. The alternative device may be as simple as a handle with a different shape to accommodate range of motion or strength limitations. If a more complex system is necessary, the user should work with a clinician who has several demonstration devices available. Some options that are available include mini joysticks (Figure 71-9) in which the user has to use only a very small range of motion to control the chair, head array systems (Figure 71-10) in which the user controls switches and sensors mounted on the headrest to drive the chair, or newly developed tablet joysticks (Figure 71-11) in which the user moves his or her hand across a flat surface with sensors to drive the chair.

Standing Options

Another option that is beneficial to wheelchair users affected by TBI is the use of a standing device. Standers can be inte-

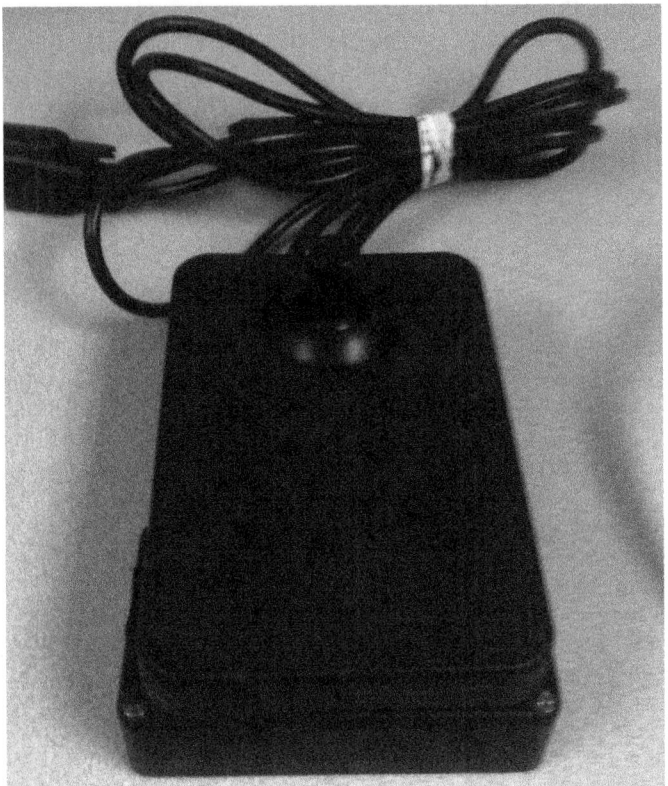

FIGURE 71-9 Controlling mechanism option: a mini-joystick.

grated into the wheelchair or be a free-standing device, either manual or powered. Regardless of the setup, standing has many physiological benefits including prevention of bone mineral density (30–34) loss, reduction in the frequency of urinary tract infections (35), increased vital organ capacity (35–38), improved circulation (36), increased passive range of motion, decreased tone (39) and spasticity (40), and decreased risk of pressure sores (41). In addition, standing can

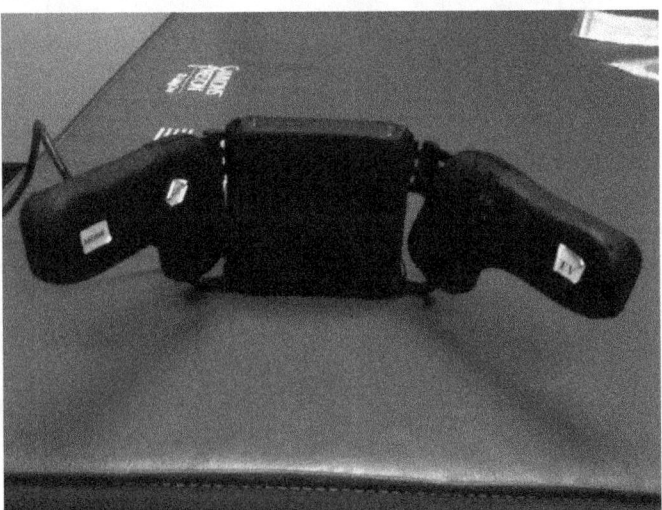

FIGURE 71-10 Controlling mechanism option: a head-array system.

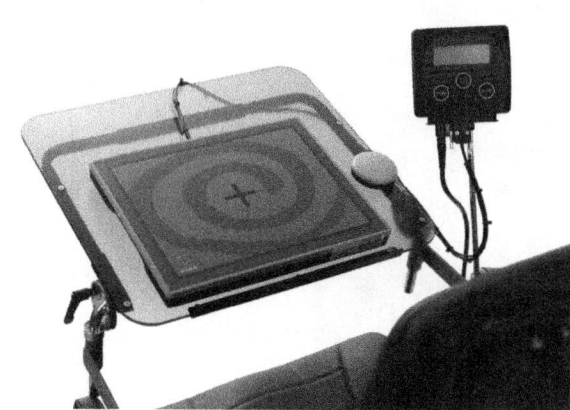

FIGURE 71-11 Controlling mechanism option: a tablet joystick.

be psychologically beneficial, can improve activity of daily living (ADL) performance, and increase functional mobility. The Rehabilitation Engineering Society of North America (RESNA) (42) has published a position paper on wheelchair standing devices that provides an in-depth description of the benefits of standing. As with any accessory, care must be taken when recommending standers. A licensed medical professional (physical or occupational therapist) must be involved with assessment, prescription, trials, and training in the use of the equipment (42). The clinician should carefully evaluate the user's blood pressure to prevent a hypotensive episode and bone density to prevent fractures. An individual may also have range of motion limitations that may make standing painful. With proper setup and precautions, standing can be very beneficial.

Robotics

For many people with disabilities using electric powered wheelchairs (EPW), essential tasks such as dressing, preparing food, shopping, or taking medications require the assistance of a caregiver. The use of a device that provides independent mobility and assistance with personal tasks could have a large impact on activity, participation, and quality of life and may reduce reliance on caregivers (43). Technology that aids in these tasks must allow the user to independently control mobility and manipulation work within real-world environments (44). The need for integrated AT systems is steadily growing. In the 2005 US Census, more than 11 million people reported a problem reaching overhead and an equal number needed assistance with ADLs or instrumental ADLs (45). Almost 16 million people had difficulty with lifting grocery bags, and 7 million had problems grasping a drinking glass (45). Most of these individuals had concomitant mobility impairments (45). More than 27 million Americans reported difficulty with ambulation, and about 3.3 million individuals used wheelchairs (45). Even if initially independent with self-care, most wheelchair users will likely develop chronic pain and shoulder pathology that can limit these tasks (46). Robotic systems have emerged as a rehabilitation engineering solution to ameliorate disabling conditions. A survey study by Prior (47) showed that 84% of EPW users would purchase a robotic arm if it were available.

Prototype robotic arms have been proposed in the literature (48,49) but until now have not been fully developed. An emerging area of technology to help people with disabilities is to seamlessly combine mobility and manipulation. Some EPW users cannot retrieve a remote control, book/magazine, or drink if not placed in their immediate proximity. Frequently, people with disabilities will have a family member or assistant pre-prepare their meals and place them in their refrigerator, thus requiring only reheating or simply removing and eating. Work is being done to develop symbiotic systems to retrieve real-life objects through user, remote, and autonomous methods in a time-efficient, safe, acceptable, and reliable manner (50–57).

One novel approach is to use a remote caregiver to provide assistance with operating a robotic device remotely to perform such difficult or unique tasks (58). This would help to address the shortage of skilled and dedicated caregivers and ease the strain on family caregivers (44).

Personal mobility and manipulation appliance (PerMMA) Generation I is a human-centered intelligent system that aims to provide users with assistance to perform ADLs in their homes as well as in the community (Figure 71-12). Because PerMMA Gen I is a complex system integrating intelligent mobility and dexterous manipulation, there are several fundamental barriers that must be overcome. First of all, safety and reliability are of utmost importance, paramount to all other functions, especially when PerMMA Gen I allows an off-site caregiver to remotely provide assistance to the local user who is seated in the smart base. Because the remote user can only obtain limited perception and awareness in unstructured and possibly unknown environments, the problems faced in ensuring safety are substantial.

Several researchers have developed EPWs with the ability to climb steps. Nagasaki University designed an 8-wheel wheelchair with an extendable rear arm to reach high steps (59). A similar concept was used by Politecnico di Torino, which developed a chair that had 3 wheels in each corner of the base (60). The University of La Castilla-La Mancha developed a climbing wheelchair, which deployed a foot onto the step to push the wheelchair up and drag the casters forward to the next step (61,62). However, these systems either have not been evaluated by wheelchair users or have not reported their results for the International Organization for Standardization (ISO) or RESNA standard wheelchair tests. The commercially available TopChair is a climbing EPW only available in the European market and includes the same features as an EPW with the addition of a track under the base activated only during a climbing sequence. However, the TopChair is heavier than standard EPW and does not support seating functions (63). In addition, its design is useful for stair climbing but does not compensate for posture when driving on uneven terrains.

PerMMA Generation II mobile robotic wheelchair base is designed as a power mobility mobile base with enhanced mobility and safety for EPW users (Figure 71-13). PerMMA Gen II is an advanced robotic mobile base with reconfigurable driving wheels and positioned caster wheels. It will allow users to drive through challenging terrains such as steep slopes, 8-inch curbs, and stairs that they might not be able to overcome with current commercially available PWCs, thus increasing users' opportunities for outdoor activities and community participation. It will allow users to drive under-

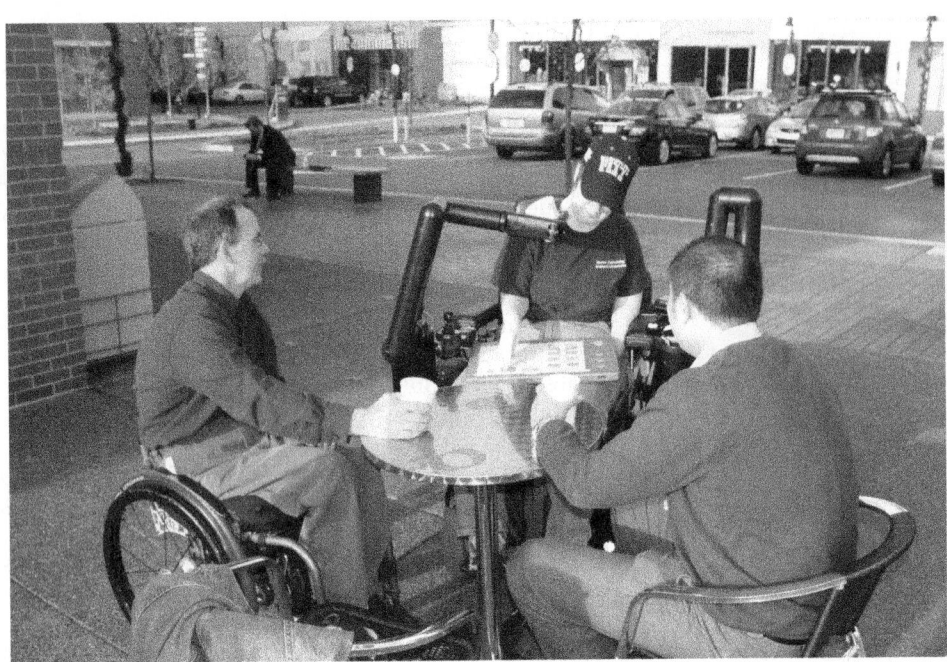

FIGURE 71-12 Robotic arm systems are currently being developed to provide users with greater lifting and handling abilities. The Personal Mobility and Manipulation Appliance (PerMMA), seen in this photo, can be controlled either locally by the user or remotely by an assistant.

neath regular 26-inch high office desks, which may lead to more working opportunities for PWC users and reduce the costs to employers of rebuilding the working environment. It will keep the seat in the most comfortable and safe position selected by the user when driving on uneven surfaces. It will also support lateral tilt power seating functions that will reduce the risk of pressure ulcers and increase the quality of life of PWC users.

The Future of Wheeled Mobility

The future of wheeled mobility is progressing quickly with many new designs coming on the market everyday to facilitate stair climbing, traversing over uneven terrain, and allowing wheelchair users to perform activities that once seemed impossible. Several new wheelchair designs are integrating gyroscope technology to allow a wheelchair to traverse rough terrain and navigate stairs. Other experimental chairs are being designed with "smart" technology to avoid obstacles and remind the user to use pressure-relief technology, key features that would benefit individuals affected by TBI. Clinicians need to be aware of the new technology by attending conferences, workshops, and reading papers related to wheelchair technology.

SEATING FOR PEOPLE WITH BRAIN INJURY

When faced with the decision of recommending an appropriate seating system, it is important to understand that AT for seating and positioning for a person with a TBI can vary

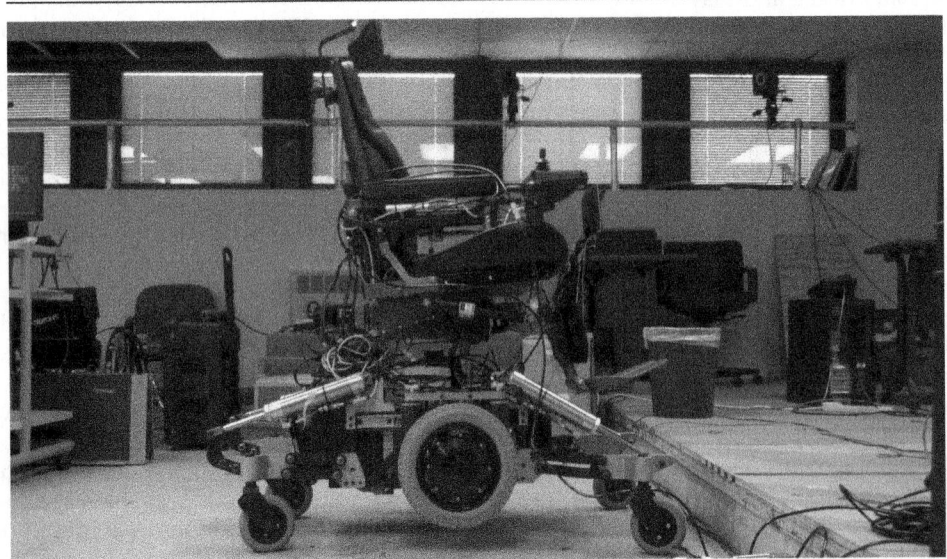

FIGURE 71-13 Driving over steps and difficult terrains are challenges for users of electric powered wheelchairs (EPWs). PerMMA Generation II, currently under development, hopes to overcome these challenges by sensing the terrain and automatically adapting to it.

according to the individual's needs and that clinicians will encounter several seating challenges depending on the severity of the injury as well as physical residual recovery following a TBI. Understanding the physical presentation and its progression will allow the clinician to determine the selection of the wheelchair base and frame on the seating system where it will be mounted, either to be a "static" frame, meaning all seat angles of the system are fixed, or a "dynamic" seat frame with adjustable seating features such as tilt, backrest recline, and elevating leg rests. The dynamic seat features can be manually or power adjusted and will be addressed later within this section.

For the person with a TBI to be considered a dynamic sitter, he or she has to be able to conduct independent, functional, and safe transfers and independent and effective weight shifts for positioning, pressure relief, and comfort. For a dynamic person, a static seat frame such as a MWC, a scooter, or power base with a captain style seat would be appropriate (64).

For a person with a TBI to be considered a static sitter, he or she is no longer able to conduct independent transfers and independent weights shifts. Losing the ability to conduct independent weight shifts compromises and limits effective pressure relief and exposes the person at increase risk for pressure sores and skin break down. For a static sitter, a dynamic seat frame, for example, a PWC base with power seating system to include power tilt, recline, seat elevator, and leg rests would be indicated if the person is cognitively able to independently operate and safely control a PWC; if not, then the alternative would be a manual tilt in space with manual recline and elevating leg rests (65) (Figure 71-14).

Several residuals from the TBI can affect the person's ability to complete many daily tasks he or she was able to previously perform. These residuals include impairments

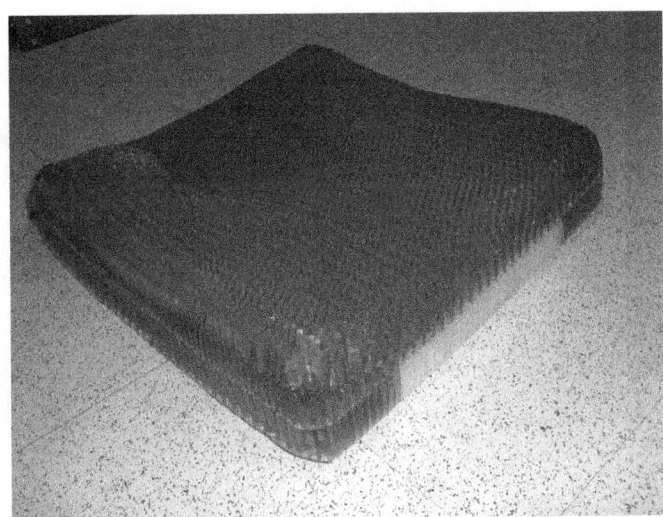

FIGURE 71-15 A contoured wheelchair seat cushion.

with motor skills, cognition, and vision. The individual requiring the use of a mobility device must become more functionally independent with their ADL needs while seated in the wheelchair (66). A key to functional seating involves stabilizing the pelvis. In seating, the pelvis may be referred to as the foundation of the house. Therefore, it is important to make sure that the seating system provides a stable support for the pelvis to enhance trunk balance and allow for improved upper trunk mobility, thus increased ability to perform ADL skills (66).

There are several seat cushions available on the market, which include both solid and contoured bases. The contour of the base aids in maintaining the pelvis, hips, and lower extremities in neutral alignment (67). The degree of the contour depends on the amount of support the individual needs to maintain the position. Most contoured cushions (Figure 71-15) will have integrated raised elevation in the midfrontal section of the cushion for lower extremity alignment to prevent abduction and internal rotation of the hip.

Having a good understanding of the person's skin integrity is crucial to cushion selection because external factors such as heat, moisture, pressure, and shearing may contribute to skin ulceration. Understanding the effect of cushion material and design will aid in the selection of the appropriate cushion to enhance sitting tolerance and comfort. Various densities and types (polyurethane, urethane, T-Foam, Sun-Mate) of foam are commonly used in linear seating systems. Foam has been shown to offer the lowest maximum pressure over the seating surface when the appropriate densities and contours are used. Air floatation cushions do an excellent job of distributing the pressure over the entire seating area. To better control interface pressure, many air floatation cushions use multiple compartments, contouring, and baffling.

Viscous fluid cushions use an electrolyte fluid mixture in a closed plastic or latex pocket. The viscous fluid conforms to the body and provides a nearly even pressure distribution. Viscous fluid cushions work much like air to equalize pressure over the entire seating surface. This is because the viscous fluid moves to come to a constant pressure within its container. Baffles can be used to control the flow of the viscous fluid just as with air cushions. The pressure distribution

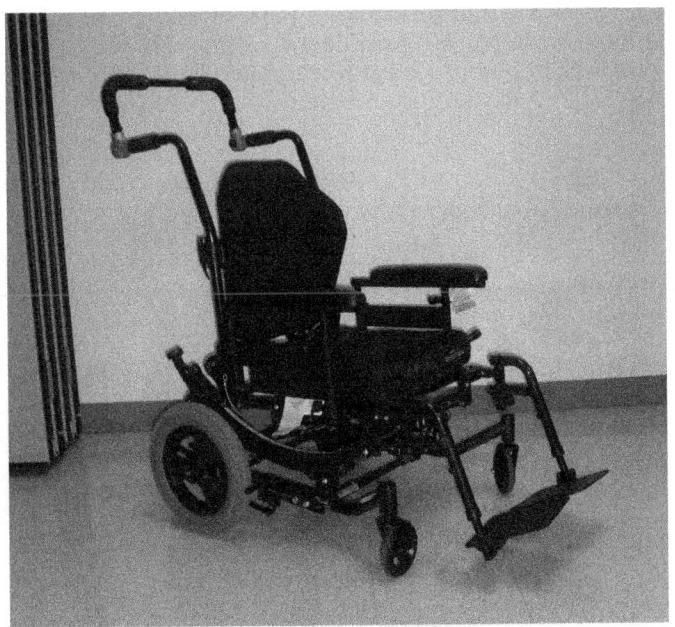

FIGURE 71-14 Individuals who are unable to control a power wheelchair safely may be better suited to using a manual tilt in space wheelchair with manual recline and elevating leg rests, as seen here.

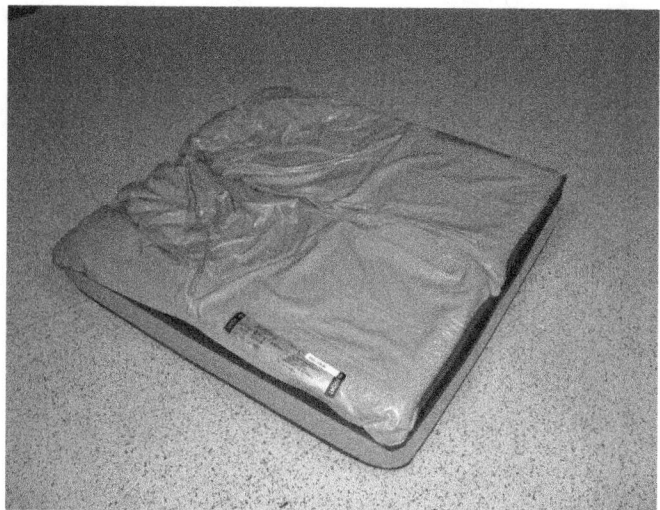

FIGURE 71-16 A viscous fluid gel wheelchair seat cushion.

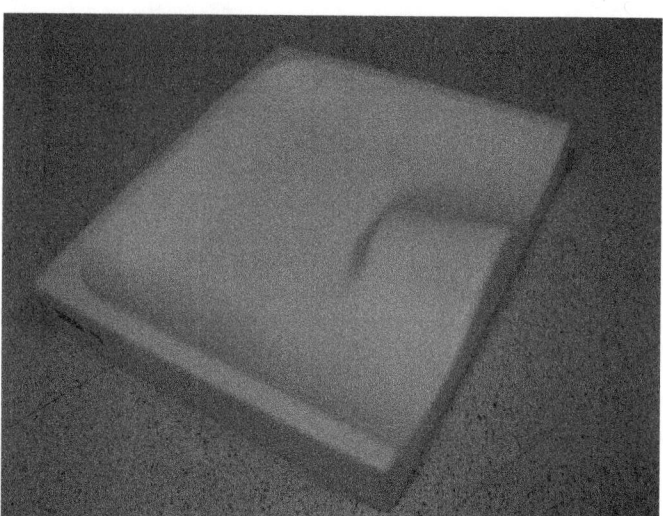

FIGURE 71-18 A foam wheelchair seat cushion.

can be altered by using a stiff base (e.g., plastic or foam) to provide some contouring.

If heat and moisture are the main culprit for skin breakdown, thermal characteristics of the cushion material are important and conductive cushion material such as "honeycomb," "air," or "air foam" should be considered over "viscous fluid" or "gel" with insulating characteristics. If pressure management is an issue, cushions that allow for pressure relief through immersion and custom contour should be selected. These cushions are viscous fluid gel (Figure 71-16), "air floatation," (Figure 71-17) or simply just foam (Figure 71-18) or any combination of all 3. Foam-based cushions are appropriate; however, they need to be replaced frequently because foam has a tendency to deteriorate at an undesirable rate (68).

The addition of thigh guides along the lateral aspect of the upper portion of the lower extremity will provide lower extremity support and alignment to reduce the risk of external rotation and abduction of the hip joint (Figure 71-19).

Pelvic support and positioning can be achieved using a pelvic belt, lap belt, subasis bar, or antithrust cushion. Pelvic support for minor cases can be provided by using a seat belt and an antithrust seat cushion. The antithrust seat helps to maintain posture by positioning the ischial tuberosities. The pelvic belt or subasis bar must be positioned snugly (e.g., about 2 adult fingers should be able to fit between the belt and abdomen). The pelvic belt or subasis bar should prevent the person from sliding forward on the seat even when the occupant wiggles or squirms.

Lower extremity alignment and support is critical in maintaining pelvic stability. It is necessary that the individual achieves full foot contact and placement on the footplates (66). Without foot support, the individual will slide and shift on the seat. The hanger angle of the wheelchair frame is an important part of achieving foot placement. A range of motion assessment will provide information needed to determine the appropriate leg rest hanger configuration. When using elevating leg rests, the individual should maintain foot

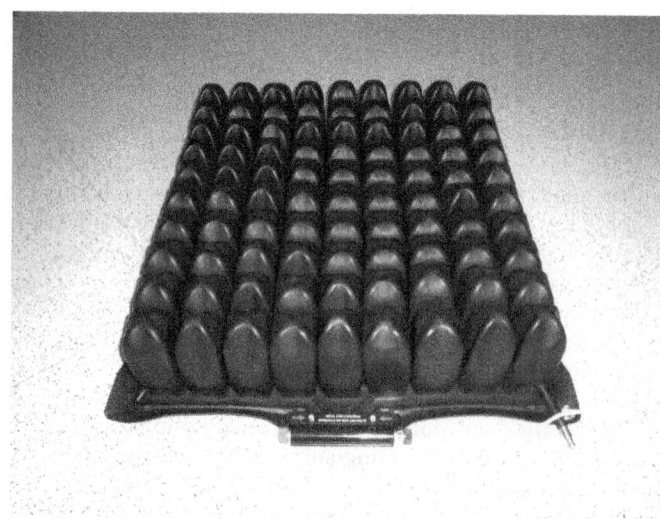

FIGURE 71-17 An air-floatation wheelchair seat cushion.

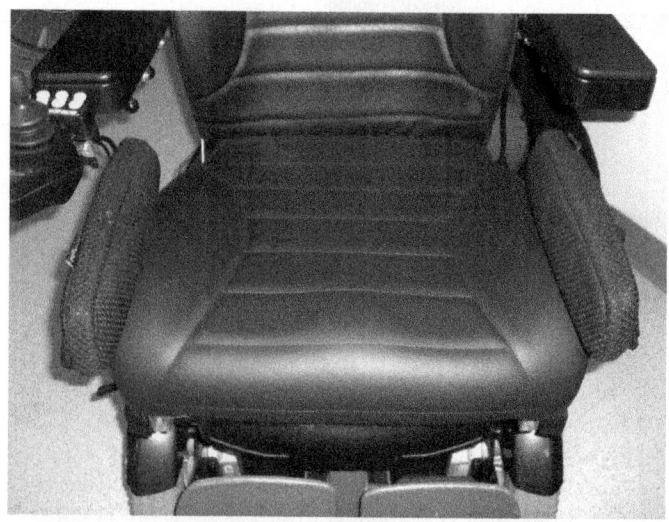

FIGURE 71-19 Thigh guides added to a wheelchair seat.

contact as well as knee extension throughout the elevation process. Angle adjustable footplates can be adjusted to assure foot contact in the event of decreased ankle range of motion or ankle instability at neutral posturing.

When selecting the appropriate back support, it is important to consider that the design and shape of the system will provide stability not only to the upper trunk but also has to work in combination with the seat cushion to provide stability to the posterior pelvis. The selection of an appropriate back support depends largely on trunk balance and whether the person is a dynamic or static sitter.

The simplest form of backrest is linear sling back and adjustable tension back upholstery that provide upper trunk stability without the need to use a solid support. The adjustable tension may also be contoured to provide additional support for those people who need it. This will aid in keeping the overall weight of the wheelchair down for the individual that is a self-propeller. For people who use MWCs, the backrest should follow the individual's frontal contour, and the height should not extend above 4 cm below the scapula (Figure 71-20).

Solid back supports are typically made of a "hard" aluminum shell, and the shape of the shell—flat or mildly, moderately, or deeply contoured—determines the level of support. The contoured back support provides for lateral stability of the upper trunk. The amount of contour depends on the amount of support the individual requires to remain upright. Two common approaches used are a flat back base with additional supports or a back base with curved sides. The width and height of the back base should be determined based on the user's mode of mobility (e.g., manual, attendant propelled, power) and postural support needs. The height

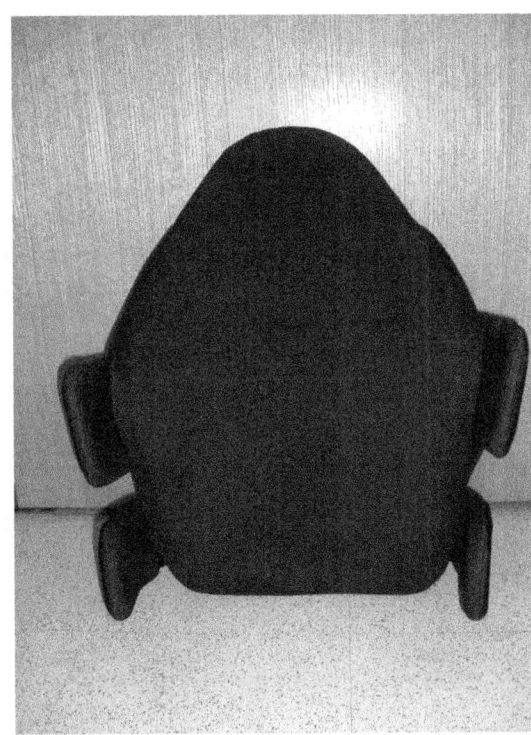

FIGURE 71-21 Lateral trunk supports for a wheelchair backrest.

should be sufficient to provide comfortable support and to provide a base to push against (67). Generally, the higher the degree of impairment, the taller the backrest must be to provide adequate support. Contour can be added to backrests via carved foam, foam in place, standard contours, or custom molded/carved contours. People with significant loss of lateral stability may benefit from fixed or adjustable lateral trunk supports (Figure 71-21). Lateral trunk supports attached to the side frame of the wheelchair provide stability and support of the upper trunk. Placement of the support is also crucial because it should not be placed directly under the axilla because it may cause nerve impingement.

A lumbar support (Figure 71-22) can be added to the backrest, or a rigid backrest can be used on many wheelchairs for people who have difficulty maintaining the natural curvature of the spine. Rigid backrests for lumbar support are becoming widely used among people who use wheelchairs. Lumbar support can improve balance with added comfort and mobility. Other seating features that can be incorporated into the frame of the wheelchair are tilt in space (Figure 71-23), and recline (Figure 71-24). For a person identified as a static sitter, the feature of tilt in space will provide gravity-assisted positioning to stabilize and improve sitting and will also provide pressure relief used in combination with power function to independently change position and shift the weight for effective pressure relief maneuvers. When using a tilt seating system, it is recommended to add a headrest (see Figure 71-25 in the e-book) for cervical support and stability.

The benefits of a dynamic seating system such as tilt and recline will allow the static sitter to change seating position while remaining safely seated in the system. Changing

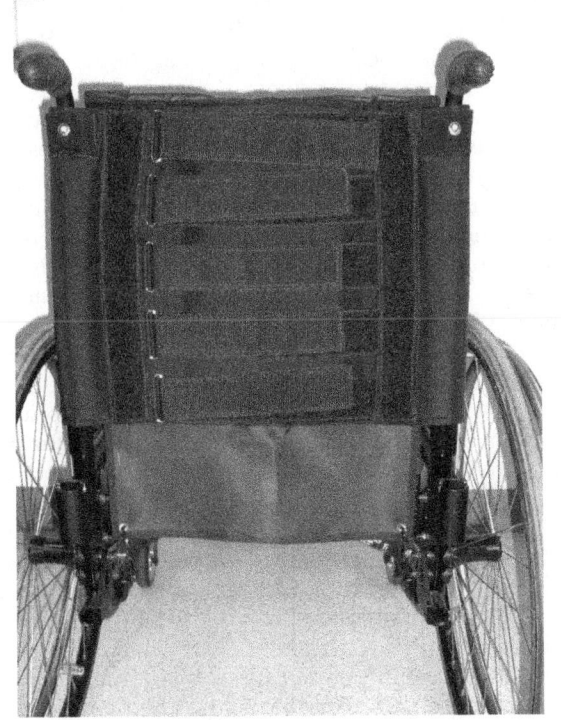

FIGURE 71-20 A linear sling wheelchair backrest with adjustable tension back upholstery.

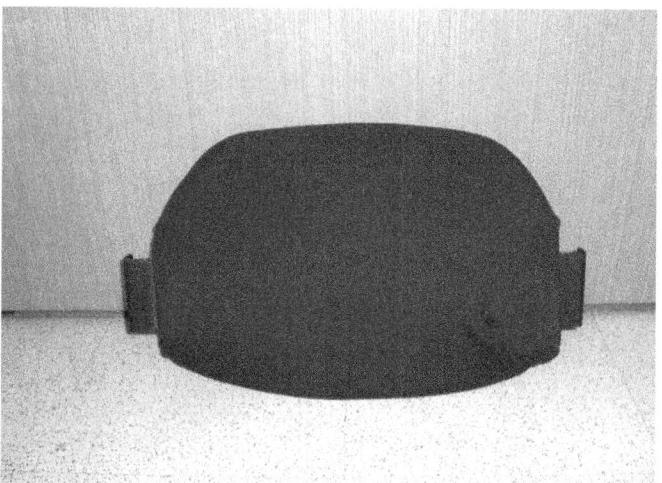

FIGURE 71-22 A lumbar support cushion for a wheelchair backrest.

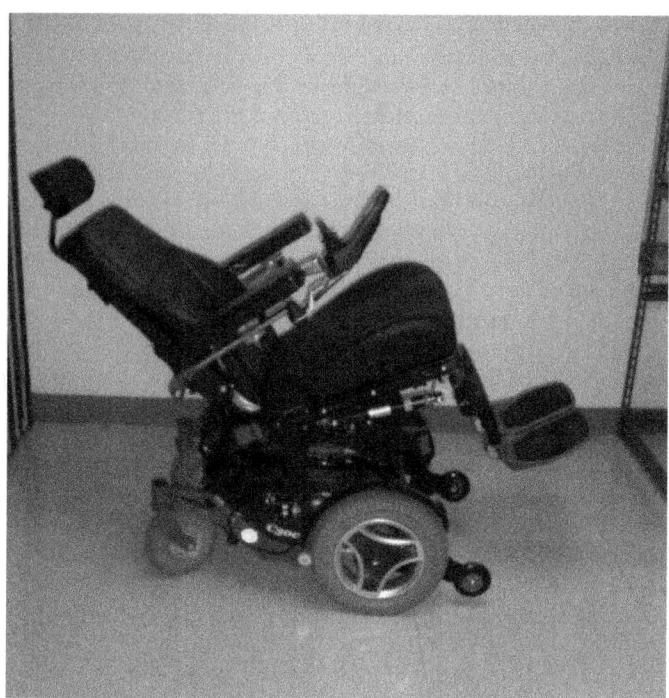

FIGURE 71-24 Recline feature in an EPW.

seating position redistributes pressure on weight-bearing surfaces, alters the load on postural musculature, and changes circulation (69). Changing position can also facilitate respiration. Caution is given to recline-only feature because it opens the hip angle, thus decreases the stability of the pelvis. The lack of control of the pelvis can lead to poor support and alignment of the upper and lower trunk. It is recommended to use recline always in combination with tilt in space to reduce the risk of posterior rotation of the pelvis and skin break down as result of sliding and shearing (66). Elevating the legs while lowering the torso can improve venous return and decrease fluid pooling in the lower extremities.

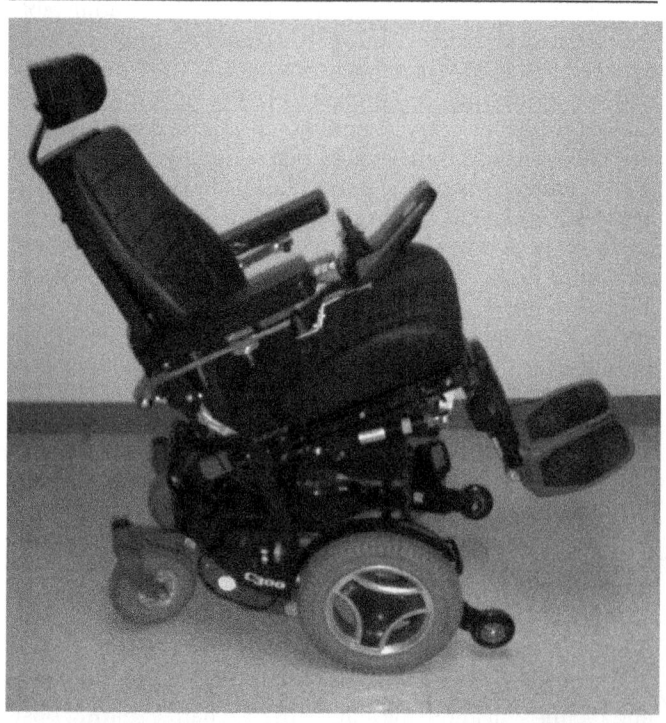

FIGURE 71-23 Tilt in space feature in an EPW.

SMART HOME TECHNOLOGY FOR BRAIN INJURY

People with brain injury usually have difficulties with their ADLs because of associated physical and/or cognitive impairments. Over the past decade, smart home technology has emerged as a potential solution to assist individuals with disabilities in completing ADLs independently. Two key supporting features of a smart home are its ability to monitor ADL performance and safety of its resident and to provide appropriate assistance. Most of the smart home technology has been developed to showcase technological capabilities of sensors, actuators, and algorithms rather than addressing specific needs of a particular population. As a result, the field is currently lacking an extensive body of evidence on the appropriateness, usefulness, and effectiveness of smart home technology (70,71). There has also been little research on smart home technology for individuals with brain injury.

Gentry (70) reviewed the state of the art of smart home technology for people with neurological disability. The article pointed out that smart home technology such as any environmental adaptations that allow remote control of home appliances, electronic communication, safety monitoring, and automated task cueing could prove useful for people with neurological disability. The article also suggested that more outcome-based research and collaboration among stakeholders is necessary for designing, selecting, and implementing smart home technology for people with neurological disability. Giroux et al. (72) provided a comprehensive review of the research on smart home technology for people with cognitive impairments at DOMUS laboratory. The article presented the infrastructure of their smart home and discussed how cognitive assistance was implemented to address 4 kinds of cognitive deficits including initiation, attention, planning, and memory.

Most recently, the Tampa Smart Home project was launched, which aims to create a pervasive supportive environment to assist cognitive rehabilitation in patients with TBI (73). The project, supporting 10 veterans with TBI, involves modifying residential facilities with advanced tracking and locating systems, environmental sensors, and interactive liquid crystal display (LCD) panels throughout the facilities. To track the staff and patients, a commercial real-time location system (Ubisense Ltd., Cambridge, United Kingdom) is used where each individual wears a wrist tag that transmits ultra-wideband radio signals to a network of fixed sensors embedded in the wall. The tag position is determined based on the time delay of arrival and angle of arrival of signals. The environmental sensors, such as a pressure sensor or a light sensor, are connected to a microcontroller that, in turn, is connected to an Ubisense Tag Module for data transmission. Such sensors are used to monitor appliance and object use, for example, pill boxes, garbage cans, and laundry machines. The locating system and the environment sensors also enable the delivery of customized prompts at the most opportune moments through the LCD panels. The Tampa Smart Home is different from many research smart homes in veterans with TBI that live in the facility. As a result, the project will be able to collect outcome measures including all clinical assessment of patient progress and staff assessment as well as the data generated by the location and environment sensors.

In the Quality of Life Technology Engineering Research Center in Pittsburgh (where several of this chapter's authors are affiliated), there is a smart home-related project on developing a research kitchen that can detect user actions and provide appropriate assistance to guide people with cognitive impairments, including those with brain injury, to complete common kitchen tasks. The kitchen is equipped with low-level sensors (e.g., contact switches, current sensors, temperature sensors, and pressure sensors) to monitor the cabinet status, appliance use, user presence at key locations, and water use. The kitchen can also deliver different types of cues for task guidance including device-mediated cues in the form of verbal or nonverbal audio, texts, pictures/graphics, video footage, and environment-mediated cues such as illuminating cabinet/drawer handles. One ongoing project in the kitchen is to evaluate the usability, usefulness, acceptance, and preference of different types of cues for assisting persons with TBI in locating items for a recipe, using appliances, and cleaning up the kitchen. Our goal is to develop guidelines regarding how different types of cues, encompassing both the level of information and modality of presentation, can be tailored to the individual's level of cognitive, sensory, and physical impairments. Another ongoing project in the kitchen is to evaluate a semiautomatic prompting strategy based on sensed user actions and minimal user inputs against the conventional prompting strategy based on task analysis and user inputs at each step. The former strategy is expected to reduce user cognitive loads and unnecessary prompts.

In general, smart home technology could potentially provide an answer to relieve the demanding workload of care from family caregivers and health care providers and support independent living of individuals with brain injury. However, it is important to ensure the design and implementation of smart home technology are not determined simply by technological advances but by the actual needs of this population. More research on evaluating the usefulness of smart home technology could contribute to its successful integration into people's actual homes or clinical environments.

ALTERNATIVE AND AUGMENTATIVE COMMUNICATION

It is beneficial for patients with TBI who experience moderate-to-severe speech, language, and/or cognitive deficits to be evaluated by speech-language pathologists with specialization in augmentative communication. Individuals who experience TBI can present with speech disability (dysarthria), language deficit (aphasia), or cognitive-communicative deficits. Each of these disabilities can occur individually or in combination. Beyond speech and language impairments, concomitant deficits in memory, initiation, new learning, or executive functioning are often present in patients who suffer from TBI. These associated deficit areas must be taken into account when selecting an augmentative and alternative communication (AAC) system. The level of impairment of speech, language, and/or cognitive deficits can be broad, from mild word retrieval deficits interfering with high level communication skills to severe, receptive, and expressive aphasia rendering an individual nonverbal without the ability to read or write.

Low-Tech Augmentative and Alternative Communication Approaches for Traumatic Brain Injury

Individuals who experience dysarthria with primary vocal intensity deficits may benefit from portable amplification systems. These wearable devices include small headset, lapel, or handheld microphones coupled with pendant or belt mounted speakers. Some individuals will chose writing or printing in lieu of impaired speech production. Alphabet or communication boards (picture symbols representing messages) can provide a means of conveying information that must be read or interpreted by communication partners. Letter arrangement (alphabetical vs standard QWERTY keyboard arrays) can also be critical for patients with TBI who may or may not be familiar with standard typing keyboards (74).

Dedicated Versus Nondedicated Devices

Augmentative communication device manufacturers choose to either dedicate their devices to only serve as communication systems or provide nondedicated options incorporating all aspects of computer operations (applications, games, Internet access, etc.). This distinction is important because many patients with TBI use third-party funding sources to pay for their systems. Because insurers will not fund computers, only dedicated devices can be considered for funding assistance by third-party insurance companies.

Types of High-Tech Augmentative and Alternative Communication Devices

There are 3 general types of high-technology AAC devices: (*a*) single-message picture displays, (*b*) text-to-speech keyboard spelling, and (*c*) sophisticated symbolic coding-based display devices.

Single-Message Picture-Based Devices

Individuals who suffer severe language and cognitive deficits secondary to TBI may be best served by picture message digitized speech devices. These provide a set of prerecorded messages and can be especially helpful in intensive care unit (ICU), acute care, or long-term care settings. For individuals whose memory and cognitive impairments are of such severity that they will not regain spelling skills, digitized speech output devices are recommended. Fixed display devices use a printed overlay to cover mechanical buttons. By depressing a picture symbol or printed word on the overlay, a prerecorded message is produced. Dynamic display devices with digitized speech feature a LCD with many types of visual images. Symbols may include cartoon drawings, digital photographs, or printed words to represent messages. These symbol locations, referred to as on-screen "buttons," can be arranged in a symmetrical array or in variable-sized grids. Using an onboard or external microphone, recorded messages are assigned to each button. With both fixed and dynamic displays, single word productions can be strung together to form simple sentences. Fixed display devices require the removal of a paper overlay and placement of a new overlay. A dial or key is used to switch the level or set of recorded messages assigned to each page. The benefit of dynamic displays is the linking of "pages" of symbols. This allows the user to rapidly access tens or hundreds of words/messages.

Keyboard-Based Devices

If an individual has good spelling and typing skills, then a text-to-speech keyboard is optimal for facilitating speech-synthesized voice output. Keyboard-based devices come in different sizes based on access capabilities of the user. Smaller keyboards may be accessed by single-finger typists, whereas oversized keyboards can be beneficial for users with motor impairments. Text-to-speech devices can also provide rate enhancement features, such as abbreviation expansion through which programmed key sequences can produce complete sentences, memory keys that toggle key functions from letters to messages, or word prediction features that can aid spelling skills.

Symbolic Coding-Based Devices

Devices that employ symbolic coding systems and speech synthesizers permit the user to spell unique words and messages that can be assigned to icon buttons. Icons can represent different words based on their sequence of use. Multiple screens of icons or word labels permit rapid access to spoken words or sentences. The use of visual scenes (full screen pictures with hidden buttons) can serve to provide a context for the user and communication partner. Significant improvement in variety and quality of speech synthesizers have occurred in the past decade. Augmentative communication device manufacturers offer 1 or more of these current popular speech synthesizers: DecTalk, VeriVox, AT&T Natural Voices, NeoSpeech, Acapela, Real Speak, and Loquendo. Samples of the AT&T Natural Voices can be heard at http://www2.research.att.com/~ttsweb/tts/demo.php.

Augmentative and Alternative Communication Device Access

AAC device selection is also based on access potential. For patients with more severely involved TBI, control of upper extremities and fingers may be impaired. These individuals will require an AAC system that provides access through alternative devices such as a switch, joystick, trackpad, mouse, head pointer, or eye gaze system. Use of mounting systems is required to stabilize devices for access from a chair, wheelchair, or bed. Types of device and accessory mounts include switch mounts; rigid, folding, or swing-away wheelchair mounts; table top mounts; lap trays; and rolling floor mounts.

Augmentative and Alternative Communication Device Features

Devices come in various shapes and sizes providing enhanced portability and acceptability. Individuals with accompanying visual impairments often require a large display or full size screen. These can range from 11–14 in diagonally. A tablet-size device averages 7–10 in, whereas a handheld device display is in the 3–5 in range. The quality of speech output clarity is often dependent on the speech synthesizer and speaker size. To provide speech output that can be heard over background noise and across a room, larger speakers are used than what are supplied with standard laptop or netbook computers. A number of AAC devices are designed to last 8–10 hours on a single battery charge so consumers may use it throughout a day of work. This additional time requires increases in battery size and weight.

Nondedicated Handhelds

The introduction of iDevices (i.e., iTouch, iPhone, and iPad) provides low cost options of augmentative communication applications for individuals with TBI. Although acceptability, portability, and cost are primary features of iDevices that appeal to patients and family members, the initial release of these first-generation devices have provided limited access options, weak volume of speaker output, and limited language representation systems. Additional hardware resources (i.e., add-on speakers, positioning platforms, switch access modules) and new applications are providing means for iDevices to become mainstream AAC options (75).

Supplementary Features

Devices that can serve as both augmentative communication and reminding systems may be optimal for individuals with TBI. Some AAC devices permit time-based messages to be stored and alarmed during device use. Devices also can include navigational systems, remote environmental control, adapted on-screen computer keyboards, cell phone capability, and e-mail.

Challenges for Communicators With Augmentations

All AAC systems pose challenges for acceptance and use for consumers who must rely on them as their primary means of vocal communication. Rate of communication will always be significantly slower than natural English speech (180 words or more per minute). Expert AAC users often struggle to communicate at more than 30 words per minute (76). Although speech synthesizer quality has improved considerably in the past few years, the artificial voice is not easily accepted by individuals who once were able to speak naturally. Use of a speech generating device also changes the pragmatics of communication because users are unable to maintain consistent eye contact with their communication partners. The cognitive load of learning device operations, communication strategies, and rate enhancement techniques can also be challenging for individuals with TBI (74).

COMPUTER ACCESS

Individuals with TBI may face barriers to independent computer use because of physical, sensory, and/or cognitive impairments. Access to computer technology has become critical for enhancing the vocational, educational, and recreational opportunities of people with disabilities while also providing access to health information, reducing social isolation, and providing a forum for the exchange of information (77–81). However, people with disabilities have reduced access to computers. Although 85% of working age adults without disabilities use computers, computer usage is 80% among those who have mild impairments and is 63% among individuals who have severe disabilities (83). Among working age individuals with severe disabilities who use computers, only 24% use AT for computer access, only 20% are aware that alternative methods of computer access were available, and only 36% are aware of free accessibility options available within the Windows and Macintosh operating systems (82). Lack of access to adaptive computer interfaces leads to inefficient or nonfunctional computer use (83).

Choosing the most appropriate computer access equipment is a collaborative decision-making process involving the consumer, clinician(s), and third-party payers (84). The challenges involved in a successful computer access intervention include (*a*) evaluating and documenting client abilities and specific difficulties with the standard computer interface (85), (*b*) choosing the most appropriate AT to address these difficulties, (*c*) configuring the technology to the user's needs, (*d*) training the user in appropriate use of their system (86), and (*e*) providing continuous follow-up to ensure that the interface remains well suited to the user (87).

Some barriers to computer use can be alleviated by configuring the computer using freely available accessibility options. The Windows, Macintosh, and Linux operating systems all include accessibility tools that address physical and sensory difficulties (82,88,89). Some settings affect keyboard response such as reducing unwanted key repeats and supporting the use of modifier keys when typing with 1 finger. Other settings affect the physical response of the cursor to a mouse or other pointing device, such as slowing down cursor movement or providing more time to double click. Other settings affect the visibility of the cursor or the visibility of other on-screen objects. Recent versions of these operating systems include built-in on-screen keyboards, screen readers, and voice control capabilities. Although these built-in options offer limited features compared to dedicated assistive software, they provide many adjustments that can be made for free.

Beyond these built-in accessibility features, many hardware options are available to provide an alternative to the mouse for physical access to the computer cursor (77). The simplest and least expensive include trackballs, which allow the pointing device to remain stationary (unlike the mouse that must physically be moved) while the user manipulates a ball with the thumb or finger. The ball can be very small or quite large, and various button arrangements are available for performing clicks. Joysticks and trackpads provide other alternatives to the mouse for hand operation of the cursor. If use of the upper extremities is impossible or uncomfortable, other options include head-operated pointing devices, eye gaze, or single-switch interfaces (91). If an individual can control a pointing device but has difficulty executing mouse button operations (i.e., clicking, double clicking, dragging, etc.), there are software programs available that allow a time delay or "dwell" to perform these operations.

Similarly, there are multiple alternatives to the standard keyboard for text entry (77). In some cases, software modifications may allow someone to continue using a standard keyboard. However, if a standard keyboard will not suffice, there are a wide variety of enlarged or reduced size keyboards that may be a better option. Some reduced-size keyboards are available on the mainstream market, whereas others are specifically designed for one-handed or one-finger typists. Enlarged keyboards can assist with low vision (by making the keys easier to see) as well as physical access. There are also software alternatives to a physical keyboard. An on-screen keyboard allows someone to "type" by clicking keys on a virtual keyboard, which inserts the typed characters into another application (such as a word processor or e-mail program) as if they were typed on a physical keyboard. Voice recognition software has made significant improvements in recent years. Voice recognition can benefit a wide range of individuals, especially when there is a need to enter large amounts of text.

Many people with TBI require access to multiple devices, such as wheelchairs, computers, AAC devices, and electronic aids to daily living (EADLs). Often, each device has a separate input method. However, a person may have a limited ability to physically operate these devices and may only be able to achieve reliable and effective control at a single site (91). An alternative is to use an integrated control system, which allows a person to operate several pieces of assistive equipment through a single universal input device (92). Mouse operations can be executed through the electronics available on most new PWCs, and many AAC devices offer mouse and/or keyboard emulation.

Various alternatives exist for computer users with low vision (77). For some, a larger monitor and/or adjusted resolution display may be sufficient to improve visibility. For others, software options include applications that magnify the screen or provide an auditory description of objects on the screen.

Individuals with cognitive impairments because of TBI may find traditional computer interfaces difficult to learn and navigate or visually distracting. It is often desirable to provide a clean user interface with a minimum icons and buttons (93). Sometimes this can be achieved through the arrangement of icons and system configuration settings, although other times, it is desirable to obtain software that is designed with a simpler interface (94–97).

COGNITIVE ASSISTIVE TECHNOLOGY

The rehabilitation field has made significant advances in serving individuals with cognitive deficits through AT. Cognitive dysfunction can significantly impact an individual's quality of life and his or her educational and vocational outcomes (98). Cognitive assistive technology (CAT) devices, sometimes called cognitive orthotics, are designed to be used as a means to support weakened or poor cognitive functions (99). Specifically, the goal of CAT is to reinforce an individual's residual abilities, provide alternative means for completing a desired activity, and/or serve as an extrinsic support to performance (93). The use of CAT devices has gained popularity as a way to compensate for cognitive impairments following TBI and other injury etiologies, including stroke, cancer, multiple sclerosis, encephalitis, mental illness, and learning disorders.

CAT not only compensates for what are traditionally referred to as "memory deficits" but is also used to compensate for limitations in higher level of cognitive functions such as decreased working memory capacity, task prioritization, decision making, complex information processing, and self-monitoring of specific behaviors.

Such as any AT device, CAT should be recommended to meet the complex needs of individuals with cognitive loss and not be considered an "off the shelf" fix. Cole (95) defined a cognitive prosthetic as a device that uses computer technology, is designed specifically for rehabilitation purposes, directly assists the individual in performing daily activities, and has a high ease of customization to the specific needs of the individual. Customizable AT readily available to and designed for the general public may at first appear to be a panacea for all cognitive limitations but may not be appropriate for individuals with cognitive deficits (100). For example, advances in smart mobile telephones have increased access for the general population to features once reserved for personal digital assistants (PDAs). However, simple design factors such as screen/display size, outdoor glare, or the level of intuitivism greatly impact the intended benefits for users with cognitive loss. Recommending technology used in the general population may reduce stigma associated with a rehabilitation device. However, proper training is essential to ensure effective use and improved functional outcomes. Eventually, both the advancements in technology and the abilities of the person change, present a need to reevaluate the efficacy of the current solution. At a minimum, a provider must ensure that the current solution is still in good working condition (condition of the battery, brightness of the screen, etc.).

Navigation Aids

Decreased community mobility can significantly degrade an individual's quality of life. Although physically mobile, cognitively impaired individuals with difficulties in way finding are seriously challenged regarding work and productive activities outside home. Because of differing etiologies and the actual locations of trauma to the brain, preexisting skills with technology and varying functional limitations will help determine the use of assisted cognitive devices (101). AT needs to address the unique needs of each individual, considering both low-tech and high-tech solutions (102). Further, Kirsch et al. (102) identified 2 categories of interventions that can be used independently from each other or together: person-oriented (internal) interventions or environmentally oriented (external) interventions. Person-oriented interventions use strategies or alternative neurological systems to accomplish a goal. Environmentally oriented interventions can assist individuals who are unable to benefit from compensatory strategies without external compensation; navigation aids are a prime example of environmentally oriented interventions.

AT devices are best when an ideal intervention is minimally intrusive, provides assistance without assuming unnecessary control, and does not demand an uncharacteristic level of comfort with technological aids (103). Clearly, the graphic user interface (GUI) of any navigational aid is the portal for the AT with an opposing correlation between the complexity and the practicality of such devices. Too much information can lead to confusion.

It is important to explore different methods of portraying information, based on user preference, learning style, and accurate assessment of current abilities. People's spatial abilities depend mainly on perceptual capabilities, fundamental information-processing capabilities, previously acquired knowledge, and motor capabilities (104). There are 3 critical points to a route: the origin, choice points, and the destination, and there are 3 types of orientation directions for proceeding on that route: landmarks, cardinal directions (north, south, east, west), and left/right directions (105). A study by Lemoncello et al. (105) discusses the orientation of travelers at the origin of the trip and found that using landmarks resulted in the highest rate of success. Once a person has begun to travel his or her walking route, it has been suggested that the aerial map view was the least helpful, and simple audio (speech-based) prompts were the most successful means of assistance during an active route (106). Other literature has suggested that geographic information systems (GIS) (such as Google's Street View) be integrated in the traveler's route where it is feasible, and accessibility to this feature may improve as technology improves (107). When directions fail, it is suggested that a GIS be used with a global positioning system (GPS). The Lemoncello et al. (107) study indicates that navigational devices for individuals with brain injuries should not only provide directions but also provide reassurance when they are on the correct path.

Technology for Attention and Memory Impairments

It is not uncommon for individuals who report difficulty with "remembering things" to actually have shortfalls in their attention (or encoding) systems rather than memory systems. Regardless of the system negatively affecting their recall or ability to attend to tasks, both can be compensated with the use of CAT.

In the course of cognitive rehabilitation, intervention strategies or "internal supports" are often provided to support functional performance. However, because of injury or illness, an individual may be unable to reliably use these internal techniques and instead must rely on CAT to help meet his or her performance goals ("external supports").

External supports can consist of low- or high-tech CAT. Both approaches can assist individuals track and record prospective tasks (such as appointments, money management) as well as semantic information such as names, numbers, and groceries to buy. Low-tech CAT for cognitive deficits can be as simple as desk or paper planners, timers, post-it notes, preorganized/labeled books or folders, or even a decorative box by the front door for one's wallet, keys, and phone upon entering the home. High-tech examples include smart phones with PDA calendar functions and automatic reminder alarms, automatic bill paying software, paging systems/services, "digital leashes" with Bluetooth technology, or automated medication dispensers.

Technology for Processing Impairments

In addition to compensating for deficits in subcomponents of cognitive processing, CAT for impairments in information processing can focus on compensation for the context of sensory processing and compensation for social and behavior issues (93). Examples of low-tech devices include alarms and timers, preorganized books and folders, and color coding for tasks, objectives, and/or subjects. Typically, high-tech options are items that require more training or customization. In some cases, these can include the use of PDAs or cell phones. A number of software programs are available with the options for word prediction, thought organization (guiding from graphics to text), grammar assistance, and spelling assistance. Other programs may read to the user, helping the user to hear possible mistakes and providing the opportunity for self-correction. In some cases, speech recognition software options may also be used to assist with composition.

Wearable Devices

Advancements in the fields of electronics, mobile computing, and manufacturing have led to the development of miniaturized electronic devices that can be handheld or worn on one's body to assist persons with TBI with daily activities. ATs for persons with TBI include PDAs, smartphones, pocket-sized and handheld computers, paging systems, programmable wristwatches, and wearable devices. Many of these AT devices contain sensors that detect a particular activity or context, a keyboard or touch screen to input the information, electrical stimulators to stimulate muscles and nerves, microprocessors to analyze and process the information, and LCDs to provide feedback to the user. Some of the applications of the wearable ATs include cognitive aids, way finders, and stimulators for nerves and brain.

Hart et al. (108) have indicated that the areas with the most potential for AT devices in persons with TBI include learning/memory, planning/organization, and initiation; on the other hand, the least potential areas seem to be social/interpersonal or behavioral difficulties. Multiple research studies have shown how programmable paging systems, PDAs, mobile phones, and portable voice recorders can help people with TBI to complete assignments independently, keep appointments, and perform time-related tasks (98,109–112). The paging systems send preprogrammed messages regarding events and assignments to complete. The mobile phones function as task reminders reportedly achieved 100% success with activities such as taking medication. DePompei et al. (112) have indicated that the factors influencing the success of the PDAs and smartphones include user motivation, audible beep of the device, support for programming and troubleshooting, alteration of functions, and selection of features to motivate. Overall, current CATs address memory, attention, planning, and task completion areas by helping individuals organize their schedule, plan reminders, and concentrate on a particular task. However, research has also indicated that the portable electronic memory devices for persons with TBI may be underused, and there is a need for ongoing clinician training to maximize clinician confidence using these devices in TBI rehabilitation (113).

In addition, wearable devices have been used as rehabilitation systems for the hand (114) and foot (115) in persons with TBI. Wearable rehabilitation devices are functional electrical stimulation (FES) systems that incorporate an orthosis with electrodes and a control unit. The electrodes provide mild electronic impulses to stimulate nerves and muscles, thus allowing the hand or foot to move without spasms. The H200 Hand Rehabilitation System allows the user to reach, grasp, open, and close his or her hand. The NESS L300 Foot Drop System provides knee flexion and extension, in addition to ankle dorsiflexion during gait. An individual wearing such a device on his or her foot can walk more safely and easily; the device also facilitates muscle reeducation, prevents muscle atrophy, maintains or increases the range of motion, and increases local blood flow. The foot system also includes a wireless gait sensor that detects gait events while the user is navigating uneven surfaces, changes in elevation, and walking speeds that are then communicated to a handheld control unit. Further, the control unit offers the user the possibility to select appropriate operating modes and stimulation parameters. Recent research found that persons with TBI using the NESS L300 neuroprosthesis increased their walking speed and improved their gait rhythmicity and steadiness (116). Future applications of wearable devices include providing magnetic stimulations to cortical, deep brain, vagus nerve, and transcranial regions (117).

A new emerging research area is the rehabilitation of persons with TBI using ubiquitous computing. Static home and wearable wireless sensors have been used to detect in-home activities of persons with TBI. These systems use statistical machine learning algorithms that use time-domain and frequency-domain characteristic features from the accelerometer data to detect various activities in home (118). Information regarding the current activity being performed can then be seamlessly integrated with rehabilitation systems and CATs to provide a holistic rehabilitation of persons with TBI.

Efficacy of Cognitive Assistive Technology

Evidence suggests that the use of PDAs and personal mobile cellular telephones result in functional performance and community participation improvements for those with a TBI (98,119,120). Gentry et al. (19) conducted a study with 23 community-dwelling individuals who sustained a TBI to determine the efficacy of PDAs. Participants were trained to use a PDA and instructed to use the PDA for 8 weeks, with measurements pretraining and after the 8 weeks. Individuals with TBI reported improvements in performance of everyday life tasks. This study also found that the provision of a PDA in conjunction with training and follow-up resulted in the improvements in performance of everyday life tasks (119). Gillette and Depompei (120) found that students with intellectual disabilities and TBI were significantly more likely to be on time more frequently while using a PDA as compared to a "times and tasks" list and with a paper planner. Mobile phones are becoming more popular with increases in applications and functions available to users and have similar capacities to PDAs. Wade and Troy (98) found mobile phones are effective strategies for increasing self-initiated behaviors and memory (98). Wilson et al. (110) conducted a 16-week crossover design randomized control trial designed to evaluate a paging system to improve independence in individuals with limitations in memory and executive functions (110). All individuals in the study had some degree of memory, planning, attention, and/or organization problems and received a pager. More than 80% of the participants had significant increases in their ability to participate in everyday activities after the 16-week trial compared to their baseline measurements. The results indicate that a paging system may be beneficial in reducing memory and planning problems for individuals with memory and executive functioning problems.

Direct Brain Interfaces

Mobility impairments after TBI may limit a person's ability to use traditional control interfaces such as switches, joysticks, AAC interfaces, or a keyboard and mouse. Direct brain interfaces (DBIs) have been proposed as an alternative access strategy for computers, wheelchairs, and other AT (121–123). A DBI records neural signals and decodes a user's intention to operate a device and also provides feedback to the user about his or her brain activity. This feedback could be visual such as the movement of a computer cursor, auditory, or even tactile. Over time, the user learns to control his or her brain activity to improve performance of the DBI. To date, there has been little investigation about whether or not DBIs would be appropriate for individuals with TBI. As with wheeled mobility, cognitive impairments commonly associated with TBI may impair a user's ability to use a DBI effectively and safely. Screening and practice with a DBI in a safe and supervised environment should be conducted to ensure that the technology is appropriate for a given client. It may be possible to augment DBI with additional safety mechanisms such as obstacle avoidance for PWCs. DBIs should be considered when they offer additional functional benefit over simpler control interfaces and when they can be operated consistently and safely by the user.

Various sensors can be used to record neural activity from the brain (124,125). Electroencephalography (EEG) electrodes are placed on the scalp and can record brain activity noninvasively. Research has demonstrated that many users are able to use an EEG DBI to operate a speller for communication or to control a cursor on a computer screen (126–128). Performance is slower than operating an AAC or computer through traditional interfaces; however, DBI makes communication technology accessible to individuals who are unable to use direct input devices. EEG DBIs can be run with a laptop computer, but they do require daily set up and calibration, which can take up to 30 minutes and likely requires the assistance of another individual.

Electrocorticography (ECoG) uses electrodes placed directly on the surface of the brain to record electrical activity from the cortex. These electrodes are often use for mapping seizure foci and eloquent cortical areas in patients with intractable epilepsy prior to surgical resection of cortical tissue. Although these patients are undergoing clinical monitoring, researchers have been able to investigate the potential of ECoG electrodes for DBI control (129–131). Another type of implanted electrode, typically called an intracortical electrode, penetrates a small distance into the cerebral cortex and can record activity from single neurons. Limited clinical trials of these devices have occurred in individuals with tetraplegia (132,133). These invasive methods of neural recording record more detailed information from the cortex because of higher spatial resolution and proximity to the neural sources. However, drawbacks include the need for implantation surgery, cost, and increased system complexity. To make implanted DBIs available for widespread clinical use, additional technical development is needed (134). Currently, researchers are working to improve the chronic recording quality for these implanted sensors and also to develop fully implantable wireless systems.

Until very recently, DBIs have been used primarily in a research setting, but a few EEG-based DBIs are now on the market for in-home use. These devices are most commonly used for computer access, to operate electronic spellers, or to interface with environmental control units. Performance depends on a number of factors including the extent of cortical damage, motivation, gender, mood, and age (135,136). To date, most research with DBIs has been conducted with able-bodied individuals or people with spinal cord injury or locked-in syndrome. Additional research is need to determine if DBIs are appropriate for people with TBI and to develop appropriate screening and training paradigms to test the capacity for DBI on an individual basis. Rehabilitation engineers will need to work with the client to ensure that the DBI interfaces with other assistive devices to provide the maximal functional benefit.

CHALLENGES IN THE USE OF ASSISTIVE TECHNOLOGY

In this second decade of the 21st century, the application of AT to persons with TBI and all disabilities should be commonplace. After all, we now live in a technology-driven era. In the field of rehabilitation, there has been an emphasis on the usage of AT to improve the quality of life of persons with disabilities for the past 25 years as evidenced by the passage of AT legislation in 1988, 1994, 1998, 2004, and 2010.

Some research maintains that AT is serving a growing role in many lives in the United States (137). The challenges in the use of AT for individuals with TBI are not significantly different from the generic ones that prohibit the widespread use of AT for most disabilities. The major challenges are lack of awareness of AT options, adjustment and cultural barriers, and funding.

The first challenge is lack of awareness, and it has 2 components. First, many providers of rehabilitative services to individuals with TBI and other disabilities are typically not sufficiently prepared to facilitate the augmentation of an individual's functioning with AT. This deficiency primarily has to do with the fact that many graduate trained VR providers have minimal exposure to the knowledge base needed to demonstrate a keen understanding of the full array of AT options. Evidence of this deficiency can be seen in the fact that few council on rehabilitation education-accredited graduate programs in the United States have a curriculum-anchored requirement that VR counselors in training (i.e., graduate students) be exposed to this area in a substantive manner (138). Secondly, it is not clear if persons with disabilities are assertive in addressing the need for AT when they believe that it may be indicated, but the topic has not been introduced for discussion by the rehabilitation provider. The goal would be for self-advocacy related to AT to routinely occur when needed and initiated by individuals with disabilities. This, of course, assumes that service recipients would have adequate familiarity with the positive benefits of AT on functionality and quality of life. Therefore, more education is needed of all involved stakeholders (e.g., counselors and persons with disabilities).

There are also some adjustment challenges that can impede the use of AT by persons with TBI and other disabilities. To fully actualize the use of AT, a person with a disability has to not only be able to engage in self-advocacy if the involved VR counselor is not broaching a discussion of AT options but also, the person must devote time toward mastery of the AT application once obtained and trained on the device. This is a skill and competency-based task that will take time and effort to achieve. In addition, the individual must exhibit a beginning acceptance of the new identity as a user of the AT along with the improved functioning that goes with it. Further, the AT user's family must also be supportive of AT usage for true integration of the device and the accompanying new identity to occur. Once this integration occurs, and there exists an optimal person-environment fit, then the person with TBI or other disability will be on the way toward full adjustment with the help of AT.

Similar to adjustment challenges, cultural issues can surface in the use of AT as well. Despite mixed findings in the literature about the role of culture as indicated by race and ethnicity in AT usage, it is clear that culture plays a role. For example, African Americans typically use smaller more portable AT devices, whereas European Americans tend to make use of larger devices such as those associated with home modification (139). Not surprisingly, income or ability to pay tends to be more of an issue for groups such as African Americans because they typically have a disproportionately high representation of individuals who live below the poverty line. Just as the existence of disability disparities related to service access, participation and outcomes has been attributed to cultural orientation (i.e., race and ethnicity) by the

rehabilitation literature as well as section 21 of the Rehabilitation Act Amendments of 1992; there may also be disparities related to the deployment of AT in the population of people with TBI.

Arguably, the most significant challenge in the use of AT is securing funding to pay for it. Funding for AT as applied to TBI is not specific to this disability. That is, the funding options are the same ones that usually apply to all disabilities. The options for funding AT include Medicare (coverage is usually limited) and Medicaid (AT must meet the definition of medical necessity and definitions vary by state), private health or disability insurance (difficult to know what is covered without in-depth knowledge of the policy), workers' compensation when the disability results from an on-the-job injury, state VR agencies (if AT increases return-to-work probability), the Veterans' Administration for veterans, the Plan to Achieve Self-Support Program offered by the Social Security Administration for recipients of Supplemental Security Income (SSI) or Social Security Disability Insurance (SSDI), local community-based service entities, national disability organizations, federally funded state AT projects, state-based alternative financing programs (i.e., AT loan programs) as per federal AT legislation, school systems for individuals still in grade school, state disability rights networks, as well as private agencies and foundations (140,141).

Finally, the topic of AT has been discussed internationally. There are 4 organizations that have provided direction and guidance on this matter. They are the United Nations Convention on the Rights of People with Disabilities, the World Health Organization, the ISO, and the World Bank (138). The efforts of these organizations related to AT on the global stage can be thought of as embracing 3 strategies: policy guidance, harmonization across organizations for a unified voice, and the offering of recommendations around approaches to implement AT in developing countries. Given the existence of this broader global discussion of AT, we can expect more recommendations and strategies forthcoming on how AT can optimize outcomes for all people with disabilities.

FUTURE DIRECTIONS

It is difficult to predict the future with any certainty; however, there are some indicators that emerging technologies and practices may contribute greatly to improving the lives of people with TBI in the future. Although therapeutic robots are becoming increasingly used clinically, assistive robots are just approaching the point where they can be applied in homes and communities. The potential of assistive robots widely defined (e.g., hardware and software) has the potential to increasing independence and community reintegration. Cueing environments and CATs are becoming more intelligent and benefitting from the explosion in handheld connected devices (e.g., smart phones) and sensors networks (e.g. energy and security monitoring) to the point where they can be truly effective as therapies and compensatory strategies. Service delivery models also need to be better understood. Ideally a face-to-face team approach would be available to all, but this is unlikely in the near future because of the shortage of clinical expertise and the dispersion of people with TBI. Technologies such as virtual environments and telerehabilitation may serve as tools to extend the reach of clinical expertise, if only policy barriers can be overcome. It is apparent that technology is making a difference in the lives of people with TBI and their families and will likely to play an even greater role in the future.

CONCLUSION

AT and telerehabilitation are emerging as methodologies that have the potential to address obstacles facing people with brain injuries and to rehabilitation, although cost-effective alternatives to face-to-face and clinic-based care. In addition, AT and telerehabilitation have been demonstrated as an effective and satisfactory (from both the consumer and clinician perspective) means of promoting independence, augmenting caregivers, and accessing necessary services in rural areas where specialized brain injury services and resources have not been available. Telerehabilitation offers a unique clinical advantage of enabling intervention and support to take place within the natural context of the individual's home, workplace and community setting, and applying technical interventions. This potential for "in vivo" intervention is of particular value in addressing the needs of individuals with TBI.

KEY CLINICAL POINTS

1. The development of telerehabilitation has been driven by the need to provide equitable access to rehabilitation services for individuals who are geographically remote from rehabilitation specialists, and the field of telerehabilitation exists under the assumption that the barrier of distance can be minimized to enhance access that will open new possibilities for delivering intervention strategies across the continuum of care.
2. Individuals affected by TBI need to be frequently reevaluated for the proper wheeled mobility device because of the frequently changing nature of their injury.
3. AT for seating and positioning for a person with a TBI can vary according to the individuals needs and that clinicians will need to understand the physical presentation and its progression to determine the selection of the wheelchair base and frame on the seating system where it will be mounted.
4. Smart home technology, such as any environmental adaptations that allow remote control of home appliances, electronic communication, safety monitoring, and automated task cueing, could prove useful for people with neurological disability.
5. Augmentative communication applications for individuals with TBI should include both low- and high-technology approaches. Low-technology augmentative communication systems include portable amplification systems, writing or printing, gestures, and alphabet/communication boards. High-technology augmentative communication systems are designated as single-message picture displays, text-to-speech keyboard spelling devices, and sophisticated symbolic coding-based devices.
6. Alternative computer access can address barriers to computer use because of physical, sensory, and/or cognitive impairments.

7. The goal of CAT is to reinforce an individual's residual abilities, provide alternative means for completing a desired activity, and/or serve as an extrinsic support to performance. Such as any AT device, CAT should be recommended to meet the complex needs of individuals with cognitive loss and not be considered an "off the shelf" fix.
8. CAT compensates for what are traditionally referred to as memory deficits as well as limitations in higher level cognitive functions such as decreased working memory capacity, task prioritization, decision making, complex information processing, and self-monitoring of specific behaviors.
9. DBIs have been proposed as an alternative access strategy for computers, wheelchairs, and other AT.
10. Evaluation of persons with TBI for the application of AT should be routine. Efforts to improve adjustment to AT for persons with TBI must proactively address the change domains of basic awareness of AT options, skill and competency in the use of AT, full integration of AT into one's new identity as an adjusted individual, and building support from significant others for full AT usage within the natural environments within which the person with TBI functions.

KEY REFERENCES

1. Beukelman D, Garrett K, Yorkston K. *Augmentative Communication Strategies for Adults With Acute or Chronic Medical Conditions*. Baltimore, MD: Paul H. Brookes; 2007.
2. Cook AM, Hussey SM, Sasser M. *Assistive Technologies: Principles and Practice*. St. Louis, MO: Mosby-Year Book, Inc; 1995.
3. Koontz AM, Ding D, Spaeth DM, Schmeler MR, Cooper RA. Prescription of wheelchairs and seating systems. In: Braddom RL, ed. *Physical Medicine and Rehabilitation*. 3rd ed, London, UK: Elsevier Limited; 2007:381–411.
4. Scherer MJ, Galvin JC. *Evaluating, Selecting and Using Appropriate Assistive Technology*. Gaithersburg, MD: Aspen Publication; 1996:1–26.
5. Addressing the Assistive Technology Needs of Individuals With Disabilities Through Financial Loans, October 2006. Report on the Fourth and Fifth Years of Operation of the Alternative Financing Program for Individuals With Disabilities. Arlington, VA: Rehabilitation Engineering Society of North America; 2006. Available at: http://www.resna.org/AFTAP/library/afp/report1006.pdf.

References

1. American Telemedicine Association, Special Interest Group on Telerehabilitation. *A Blueprint for Telerehabilitation Guidelines*. Washington, DC: American Telemedicine Association; 2010.
2. Krupinksi E, Nypaver M, Poropatich R, Ellis D, Safwat R, Sapci H. Telemedicine/telehealth: an international perspective. Clinical applications in telemedicine/telehealth. *Telemed J E Health*. 2002; 8(1):13–34.
3. Rosen MJ. Telerehabilitation. *NeuroRehabilitation*. 1999;3:3–18.
4. McCue M, Fairman A, Pramuka M. Enhancing quality of life through telerehabilitation. *Phys Med Rehabil Clin N Am*. 2010;21(1): 195–205.
5. Heinzelmann PJ, Lugn NE, Kvedar JC. Telemedicine in the future. *J Telemed Telecare*. 2005;11(8):384–390.

6. Ricker J, Rosenthal M, Garay E, et al. Telerehabilitation needs: a survey of persons with acquired brain injury. *J Head Trauma Rehabil.* 2002;17(3):242–250.

7. Winters JM. Telerehabilitation research: emerging opportunities. *Annu Rev Biomed Eng.* 2002;4:287–320.

8. Bashshur RL. Telemedicine effects: cost, quality, and access. *J Med Syst.* 1995;19(2):81–91.

9. Lemaire ED, Boudrias Y, Greene G. Low-bandwidth, Internet-based videoconferencing for physical rehabilitation consultations. *J Telemed Telecare.* 2001;7(2):82–89.

10. Ylvisaker M. Context-sensitive cognitive rehabilitation after brain injury: theory and practice. *Brain Impair.* 2003;1:1–16.

11. Girard P. Military and VA telemedicine systems for patients with traumatic brain injury. *J Rehabil Res Dev.* 2007;44(7):1017–1026.

12. Hill AJ, Theodoros D, Russell T, Ward E. Using telerehabilitation to assess apraxia of speech in adults. *Int J Lang Commun Disord.* 2009;44(5):731–747.

13. Hill A, Theodoros D, Russell T, Ward E, Wooton R. The effects of severity of aphasia upon the ability to assess language disorders via telerehabilitation. *Aphasiology.* 2008;5:627–642.

14. Schein RM, Schmeler MR, Holm MB, Saptono A, Brienza DM. Telerehabilitation wheeled mobility and seating assessments compared to in person. *Arch Phys Med Rehabil.* 2010;91(6):874–878.

15. Hailey D, Roine R, Ohinmaa A, Dennett L. *Evidence on the Effectiveness of Telerehabilitation Applications.* Helsinki, Finland: Institute of Health Economics and Finnish Office for Health Technology Assessment; 2010.

16. Parmanto B, Saptono A, Pramana G, et al. VISYTR: versatile and integrated system for telerehabilitation. *Telemed J E Health.* 2010; 16(9):939–944.

17. Schmeler MR, Schein RM, McCue MP, Betz K. Telerehabilitation and clinical applications: research, opportunities, and challenges. *Int J Telerehabil.* 2009;1:59–72.

18. Bernquist T, Gehl C, Mandrekar J, et al. The effect of internet-based cognitive rehabilitation in persons with memory impairments after severe traumatic brain injury. *Brain Inj.* 2009;23(10): 790–799.

19. Forducey PG, Ruwe WD, Dawson SJ, Scheideman-Miller C, McDonald NB, Hantla MR. Using telerehabilitation to promote traumatic brain injury recovery and transfer of knowledge. *NeuroRehabilitation.* 2003;18(2):103–111.

20. Lewis JA, Deutsch JE, Burdea G. Usability of the remote console for virtual reality telerehabilitation: formative evaluation. *Cyberpsychol Behav.* 2006;9(2):142–147.

21. Zheng H, Black ND, Harris ND. Position-sensing technologies for movement analysis in stroke rehabilitation. *Med Biol Eng Comput.* 2005;43(4):413–420.

22. American Occupational Therapy Association. Telerehabilitation. *Am J Occup Ther.* 2010;64(6)(suppl):S92–S102.

23. American Speech Language and Hearing Association. Speech language pathologists providing clinical services via telepractice: Position statement. 2005. Available at: http://www.asha.org/docs/html/PS2005-00116.html. Accessed February 28, 2011.

24. Veterans Health Administration. *VHA Telerehabilitation Toolkit.* Washington, DC: Veterans Administration; 2005.

25. Rogante M, Grigioni M, Cordella D, Giacomozzi C. Ten years of telerehabilitation: a literature overview of technologies and clinical applications. *NeuroRehabilitation.* 2010;27(4):287–304.

26. Kairy D, Lehoux P, Vincent C, Visintin M. A systematic review of clinical outcomes, clinical processes, healthcare utilization, and costs associated with telerehabilitation. *Disabil Rehabil.* 2008;31(6): 427–447.

27. Model Systems Knowledge Translation Center. Available at: http://msktc.washington.edu/index.asp. Accessed January 13, 2011.

28. Consortium for Spinal Cord Medicine. *Preservation of Upper Limb Function Following Spinal Cord Injury: A Clinical Practice Guideline for Healthcare Professionals.* Washington DC: Paralyzed Veterans of America; 2005.

29. Boninger ML, Baldwin MA, Cooper RA, Koontz AM, Chan L. Manual wheelchair pushrim biomechanics and axle position. *Arch Phys Med Rehabil.* 2000;81(5):608–613.

30. Hangartner TN. Osteoporosis due to disuse. In: Matkovic V, ed. *Physical Medicine and Rehabilitation Clinics of North America.* Philadelphia, PA: WB Saunders Company; 1995:579–594.

31. Kaplan PE, Gandhavadi B, Richards L, Goldschmidt J. Calcium balance in paraplegic patients: influence of injury duration and ambulation. *Arch Phys Med Rehabil.* 1978;59(10):447–450.

32. Kaplan PE, Roden W, Gilbert E, Richards L, Goldschmidt JW. Reduction of hypercalciuria in tetraplegia after weight-bearing and strengthening exercises. *Paraplegia.* 1981;19(5):289–293.

33. Goemaere S, Van Laere M, De Neve P, Kaufman JM. Bone mineral status in paraplegic patients who do or do not perform standing. *Osteoporos Int.* 1994;4(3):138–143.

34. Kunkel CF, Scremin AM, Eisenberg B, Garcia JF, Roberts S, Martinez S. Effect of "standing" on spasticity, contracture, and osteoporosis in paralyzed males. *Arch Phys Med Rehabil.* 1993;74(1):73–78.

35. Dunn RB, Walter JS, Lucero Y, et al. Follow-up assessment of standing mobility device users. *Assist Technol.* 1998;10(2):84–93.

36. Eng JJ, Levins SM, Townson AF, Mah-Jones D, Bremner J, Huston G. Use of prolonged standing for individuals with spinal cord injuries. *Phys Ther.* 2001;81(8):1392–1399.

37. Stainsby K, Thornton H. Justifying the provision of a standing frame for home use—a good case to quote. *Synapse.* 1999;3–5.

38. Hoening H, Murphy T, Galbraith J, Zolkewitz M. Case study to evaluate a standing table for managing constipation. *SCI Nurs.* 2001;18(2):74–77.

39. Odéen I, Knutsson E. Evaluation of the effects of muscle stretch and weight load in patients with spastic paraplegia. *Scand J Rehabil Med.* 1981;13(4):117–121.

40. Bohannon RW. Tilt table standing for reducing spasticity after spinal cord injury. *Arch Phys Med Rehabil.* 1993;74(10):1121–1122.

41. Hobson DA. Comparative effects of posture on pressure and shear at the body-seat interface. *J Rehabil Res Dev.* 1992;29(4):21–31.

42. Arva J, Paleg G, Lange M, et al. RESNA position on the application of wheelchair standing devices. *Assist Technol.* 2009;21(3):169–171.

43. Hoenig H, Taylor DH, Sloan FA. Does assistive technology substitute for personal assistance among the disabled elderly? *Am J Public Health.* 2003;93(2):330–337.

44. Platts RG, Fraser MH. Assistive technology in the rehabilitation of patients with high spinal cord lesions. *Paraplegia.* 1993;31(5): 280–287.

45. McNeil JM. Americans With Disabilities: 2005. Household Economic Studies. Current Population Reports. Washington, DC: U.S. Government Printing Office; 2008: 70–117.

46. Curtis KA, Drysdale GA, Lanza RD, Kolber M, Vitolo RS, West R. Shoulder pain in wheelchair users with tetraplegia and paraplegia. *Arch Phys Med Rehabil.* 1999;80(4):453–457.

47. Prior SD. An electric wheelchair mounted robotic arm—a survey of potential users. *J Med Eng Technol.* 1990;14(4):143–154.

48. Farahmand F, Pourazad M, Moussavi Z. An intelligent assistive robotic manipulator. *Conf Proc IEEE Eng Med Biol Soc.* 2005;5: 5028–5031.

49. Galindo C, Gonzalez J, Fernàndez-Madrigal JA. Control architecture for human-robot integration: application to a robotic wheelchair. *IEEE Trans Syst Man Cybern B Cybern.* 2006;36(5):1053–1067.

50. Tsui K, Yanco H, Kontak D, Beliveau L, eds. *Development and Evaluation of a Flexible Interface for a Wheelchair Mounted Robotic Arm.* Amsterdam, The Netherlands: Association for Computing Machinery; 2008.

51. Ha Q, Tran T, Dissanayake G. A wavelet-and neural network-based voice interface system for wheelchair control. *IJISTA.* 2005;1(1–2): 49–65.

52. Pineau J, Atrash A, eds. *Smartwheeler: A Robotic Wheelchair Test-Bed for Investigating New Models of Human-Robot Interaction.* Montreal, Canada: McGill University; 2007.

53. Bien Z, Kim DJ, Chung MJ, Kwon DS, Chang PH. Development of a Wheelchair-based Rehabilitation Robotic System (KARES II) with various human-robot interaction interfaces for the disabled. In: *IEEE/ASME International Conference Proceedings on Advanced Intelligent Mechatronics.* 2003;2:92–97.

54. Jia P, Hu HH, Lu T, Yuan K. Head gesture recognition for hands-free control of an intelligent wheelchair. *J Ind Robot.* 2007;34(1): 60–68.

55. Matsumotot Y, Ino T, Ogsawara T. Development of intelligent wheelchair system with face and gaze based interface. In: *10th IEEE International Workshop Proceedings on Robot and Human Interactive Communication*. 2001:262–267.

56. Moon I, Joung S, Kum Y. Safe and reliable intelligent wheelchair robot with human robot interaction. In: *IEEE International Conference Proceedings on Robotics and Automation*. 2002;4:3595–3600.

57. Yanco HA. Wheelesley: a robotic wheelchair system: indoor navigation and user interface. *Assistive Technology and Artificial Intelligence*. 1998:256–268.

58. Edwards J. Robotic "doctors" bring a personal touch to automated healthcare. Mobile video platforms extend physician's reach. *Robotic Trends*. 2011;9:9–12.

59. Lawn M, Ishimatsu T. Modeling of a stair-climbing wheelchair mechanism with high single-step capability. *IEEE Trans Neural Syst Rehabil Eng*. 2003;11:323–332.

60. Quaglia G, Franco W, Oderio R. Wheelchair.q, a mechanical concept for a stair climbing wheelchair. In: *Robotics and Biomimetics (ROBIO) IEEE International Conference Proceedings*. 2009;800–805.

61. Morales R, Feliu V, Gonzales A, Pintado P. Kinematic model of a new staircase climbing wheelchair and its experimental validation. *Int J Rob Res*. 2006;25:825–841.

62. Morales R, Gonzalez A, Feliu V, Pintado P. Environment adaptation of a new staircase-climbing wheelchair. *Auton Rob*. 2007;23:275–292.

63. Souza A, Kelleher AR, Cooper RM, Cooper RA, Ienozzi LI, Collins DM. Multiple Sclerosis and mobility related assistive technology: systematic review of literature. *J Rehabil Res Dev*. 2010;47:213–224.

64. Dicianno BE, Arva J, Lieberman JM, et al. RESNA position on the application of tilt, recline, and elevating legrests for wheelchairs. *Assist Technol*. 2009;1:13–22.

65. Rehabilitation Engineering & Assistive Technology Society of North America. *RESNA Position on the Application of Tilt in Space, Lateral /Rotation Tilt, Reclining Backrest and Elevating Legrests for Wheelchair Users*. Arlington VA: Rehabilitation Engineering & Assistive Technology Society of North America; 2008.

66. Engstroem B. *Ergonomic Seating: A True Challenge. Wheelchair Seating and Mobilty Principles*. Stockholm, Sweden: Posturalis Books; 2002.

67. Koontz AM, Ding D, Spaeth DM, Schmeler MR, Cooper RA. Prescription of wheelchairs and seating systems. In: Braddom RL, ed. *Physical Medicine and Rehabilitation*. 3rd ed. London, UK: Elsevier Limited; 2007:381–411.

68. Cooper RA, Cooper RM, Boninger ML. Wheelchair design and seating technology. In: Selzer M, Clarke S, Cohen L, Duncan P, Gage F, eds. *Textbook of Neural Repair and Rehabilitation*. Cambridge, MA: Cambridge University Press; 2006:147–164.

69. Ding D, Leister E, Cooper RA, et al. Usage of tilt-in-space, recline, and elevation seating functions in natural environment of wheelchair users. *J Rehabil Res Dev*. 2008;45(7):973–983.

70. Gentry T. Smart homes for people with neurological disability: state of the art. *NeuroRehabilitation*. 2009;25(3):209–217.

71. Frisardi V, Imbimbo BP. Gerontechnology for demented patients: smart homes for smart aging. *J Alzheimers Dis*. 2011;23(1):143–146.

72. Giroux S, Leblanc T, Bouzouane A, Bouchard B, Pigot H, Bauchet J. The praxis of cognitive assistance in smart homes. In: Gottfried B, Aghajan H, eds. *Behavior Monitoring and Interpretation—BMI—Smart Environments*. Vol 3. Amsterdam, The Netherlands; 2009:183–211.

73. Jasiewicz J, Kearns W, Craighead J, Fozard JL, Scott S, McCarthy J. Smart rehabilitation for the 21st century: the Tampa Smart Home for veterans with traumatic brain injury. *J Rehabil Res Dev*. 2011:48(8):vii–xvii.

74. Beukelman D, Garrett K, Yorkston K. *Augmentative Communication Strategies for Adults With Acute or Chronic Medical Conditions*. Baltimore, MD: Paul H. Brookes; 2007.

75. Mobile Devices and Communication Apps: An AAC-RERC White Paper. Available at: http://aac-rerc.psu.edu/index.php/pages/show/id/46. Accessed March 22, 2011.

76. Beukelman D, Mirenda P. *Augmentative and Alternative Communication*. Baltimore, MD: Paul H. Brookes; 2003.

77. Anson DK. *Alternative Computer Access: A Guide to Selection*. Philadelphia, PA: F.A. Davis; 1997.

78. Madara E. The mutual-aid self-help online revolution. *Soc Policy*. 1997;27:20–26.

79. Drainoni M, Houlihan B, Williams S, et al. Patterns of Internet use by persons with spinal cord injuries and relationship to health-related quality of life. *Arch Phys Med Rehabil*. 2004;85(11):1872–1879.

80. Morahan-Martin J, Schumacher P. Loneliness and social use of the Internet. *Comp Human Behav*. 2003;19:656–671.

81. Dobransky K, Hargittai E. The disability divide in Internet access and use. *Inf Commun Soc*. 2006;9(3):313–334.

82. Stevenson B, McQuivey JL. *Examining Awareness, Use, and Future Potential*. Cambridge, MA: A Research Study Commissioned by Microsoft Corporation and Conducted by Forrester Research; 2003.

83. Trewin S, Pain H. Keyboard and mouse errors due to motor disabilities. *Int J Hum Comp Stud*. 1999;50:109–144.

84. Simpson R, Koester HH, LoPresti E. Research in computer access assessment and intervention. *Phys Med Rehabil Clin N Am*. 2010; 21(1):15–32.

85. Hazell G, Colven D. *ACE Centre Telesupport for Loan Equipment*. Oxford, UK: Aiding Communication in Education Centre Advisory Trust; 2001:35.

86. Scherer MJ, Galvin JC. *Evaluating, Selecting and Using Appropriate Assistive Technology*. Gaithersburg, MD: Aspen Publication. 1996: 1–26.

87. Phillips B, Zhao H. Predictors of assistive technology abandonment. *Assist Technol*. 1993;5(1):36–45.

88. Koester HH, LoPresti EF, Simpson RC. Toward automatic adjustment of keyboard settings for people with physical impairments. *Disabil Rehabil Assist Technol*. 2007;2(5):261–274.

89. LoPresti EF, Koester HH, Simpson RC. Toward automatic adjustment of pointing device configuration to accommodate physical impairment. *Disabil Rehabil Assist Technol*. 2008;3(4):221–235.

90. LoPresti EF, Brienza DM, Angelo J. Evaluation of computer head control software to compensate for neck movement limitations. *Interact Comput*. 2002;14(4):359–379.

91. Angelo J, Trefler E. A survey of persons who use integrated control devices. *Assist Technol*. 1998;10(2):77–83.

92. Guerette P, Sumi E. Integrating control of multiple assistive devices: a retrospective review. *Assist Technol*. 1994;6(1):67–76.

93. LoPresti EF, Mihailidis A, Kirsch N. Technology for cognitive rehabilitation and compensation: state of the art. *Neuropsychol Rehabil*. 2004;14(1–2):5–39.

94. Cole E, Dehdashti P. Interface design as a prosthesis for an individual with a brain injury. *SIGCHI Bull*. 1990;22(1):28–32.

95. Cole E. Cognitive prosthetics: an overview to a method of treatment. *NeuroRehabilitation*. 1999;12(1):39–51.

96. Davies DK, Stock SE, Wehmeyer ML. Enhancing independent Internet access for individuals with mental retardation through use of a specialized web browser: a pilot study. *Educ Train Ment Ret*. 2001;36(1):107–113.

97. Stock SE, Davies DK, Davies KR, Wehmeyer ML. Evaluation of an application for making palmtop computers accessible to individuals with intellectual disabilities. *J Intellect Dev Disabil*. 2006;31(1): 39–46.

98. Wade TK, Troy JC. Mobile phones as a new memory aid: a preliminary investigation using case studies. *Brain Inj*. 2001;15(4):305–320.

99. Bergman MM. The benefits of a cognitive orthotic in brain injury rehabilitation. *J Head Trauma Rehabil*. 2002;17(5):431–445.

100. Kim HJ, Burke DT, Dowds MM, Boone KAR, Park GJ. Electronic memory aids for outpatient brain injury: follow-up findings. *Brain Inj*. 2000;14(2):187–196.

101. Liu AL, Hile H, Kautz H, et al. Indoor wayfinding: developing a functional interface for individuals with cognitive impairments. *Disabil Rehabil Assist Technol*. 2008;3(1):69–81.

102. Kirsch NL, Shenton M, Spirl E, et al. Web-based assistive technology interventions for cognitive impairments after traumatic brain injury. *Rehabil Psychol*. 2004;49(3):200–212.

103. Kirsch NL, Shenton M., Rowan J. A generic, "in-house", alphanumeric paging system for prospective activity impairments after traumatic brain injury. *Brain Inj*. 2004;18(7):725–734.

104. Chang Y, Peng S, Wang T, Chen S, Chen Y, Chen H. Autonomous indoor wayfinding for individuals with cognitive impairments. *J Neuroeng Rehabil.* 2010;7:45.

105. Lemoncello R, Moore-Sohlberg M, Fickas S. How best to orient travelers with acquired brain injury: a comparison of three directional prompts. *Brain Inj.* 2010;24(3):541–549.

106. Sohlberg MM, Fickas S, Hung PF, Fortier A. A comparison of four prompt modes for route finding for community travelers with severe cognitive impairments. *Brain Inj.* 2007;21(5):531–538.

107. Lemoncello R, Sohlberg MM, Fickas S. When directions fail: investigations of getting lost behavior in adults with acquired brain injury. *Brain Inj.* 2010;24(3):550–559.

108. Hart T, O'Neil-Pirozzi T, Morita C. Clinician expectations for portable electronic devices as cognitive-behavioural orthoses in traumatic brain injury rehabilitation. *Brain Inj.* 2003;17(5):401–411.

109. Hart T, Hawkey K, Whyte J. Use of a portable voice organizer to remember therapy goals in traumatic brain injury rehabilitation: a within-subjects trial. *J Head Trauma Rehabil.* 2002;17(6):556–570.

110. Wilson BA, Emslie HC, Quirk K, Evans JJ. Reducing everyday memory and planning problems by means of a paging system: a randomised control crossover study. *J Neurol Neurosurg Psychiatry.* 2001;70(4):477–482.

111. Wilson BA, Emslie H, Evans JJ, Quirk K, Watson P, Fish F. The NeuroPage system for children and adolescents with neurological deficits. *Dev Neurorehabil.* 2009;12(6):421–426.

112. DePompei R, Gillette Y, Goetz E, Xenopoulos-Oddsson A, Bryen D, Dowds M. Practical applications for use of PDAs and smartphones with children and adolescents who have traumatic brain injury. *NeuroRehabilitation.* 2008;23(6):487–499.

113. O'Neil-Pirozzi TM, Kendrick H, Goldstein R, Glenn M. Clinician influences on use of portable electronic memory devices in traumatic brain injury rehabilitation. *Brain Inj.* 2004;18(2):179–189.

114. Bioness LiveOn. The NESS L300 Foot Drop System. Available at: http://www.bioness.com/L300_for_Foot_Drop.php. Accessed February 3, 2012.

115. Bioness LiveOn. The NESS H200 Hand Rehabilitation System. Available at: http://www.bioness.com/H200_for_Hand_Paralysis .php. Accessed February 3, 2012.

116. Hausdorff JM, Ring H. The effect of the NESS L300 neuroprosthesis on gait stability and symmetry. *J Neurol Phys Ther.* 2006;30(4):198.

117. Center for Integration of Medicine & Innovative Technology. Traumatic brain injury: Clinical trials from the past to the future. Available at: http://www.cimit.org/forum/forum-trauma-04.01.08.Za fonte.html. Accessed February 3, 2012.

118. Ince NF, Min C-H, Tewfik A, Vanderpool D. Detection of early morning daily activities with static home and wearable wireless sensors. *EURASIP J Adv Signal Process.* 2008.

119. Gentry T, Wallace J, Kvarfordt C, Lynch KB. Personal digital assistants as cognitive aids for individuals with severe traumatic brain injury: a community-based trial. *Brain Inj.* 2008;22(1):19–24.

120. Gillette Y, Depompei R. Do PDAs enhance the organization and memory skills of students with cognitive disabilities? *Psychol Sch.* 2008;45(7):665–677.

121. Wolpaw JR. Brain-computer interfaces as new brain output pathways. *J Physiol.* 2007;579(pt 3):613–619.

122. Birbaumer N, Cohen LG. Brain-computer interfaces: communication and restoration of movement in paralysis. *J Physiol.* 2007;15(pt 3):621–636.

123. Millán JD, Rupp R, Müller-Putz GR, et al. Combining brain-computer interfaces and assistive technologies: State-of-the-art and challenges. *Front Neurosci.* 2010;4:161.

124. Schwartz AB, Cui XT, Weber DJ, Moran DW. Brain-controlled interfaces: movement restoration with neural prosthetics. *Neuron.* 2006;52(1):205–220.

125. Moran D. Evolution of brain-computer interface: action potentials, local field potentials and electrocorticograms. *Curr Opin Neurobiol.* 2010;20(6):741–745.

126. Kleih SC, Kaufmann T, Zickler C, et al. Out of the frying pan into the fire—the P300-based BCI faces real-world challenges. *Prog Brain Res.* 2011;194:27–46.

127. Zickler C, Riccio A, Leotta F, et al. A brain-computer interface as input channel for a standard assistive technology software. *Clinical EEG Neurosci.* 2011;42(4):236–244.

128. McFarland DJ, Sarnacki WA, Wolpaw JR. Electroencephalographic (EEG) control of three-dimensional movement. *J Neural Eng.* 2010; 7(3):036007.

129. Vinjamuri R, Weber DJ, Mao ZH, et al. Toward synergy-based brain-machine interfaces. *IEEE Trans Inf Technol Biomed.* 2011;15(5): 726–736.

130. Blakely T, Miller KJ, Zanos SP, Rao RP, Ojemann JG. Robust, long-term control of an electrocorticographic brain-computer interface with fixed parameters. *Neurosurg Focus.* 2009;27(1):E13.

131. Schalk G, Miller KJ, Anderson NR, et al. Two-dimensional movement control using electrocorticographic signals in humans. *J Neural Eng.* 2008;5(1):75–84.

132. Hochberg LR, Serruya MD, Friehs GM, et al. Neuronal ensemble control of prosthetic devices by a human with tetraplegia. *Nature.* 2006;442(7099):164–171.

133. Simeral JD, Kim SP, Black MJ, Donoghue JP, Hochberg LR. Neural control of cursor trajectory and click by a human with tetraplegia 1000 days after implant of an intracortical microelectrode array. *J Neural Eng.* 2011;8(2):025027.

134. Gilja V, Chestek CA, Diester I, Henderson JM, Deisseroth K, Shenoy KV. Challenges and opportunities for next-generation intracortically based neural prostheses. *IEEE Trans Biomed Eng.* 2011; 58(7):1891–1899.

135. Allison B, Luth T, Valbuena D, Teymourian A, Volosyak I, Graser A. BCI demographics: how many (and what kinds of) people can use an SSVEP BCI? *IEEE Trans Neural Syst Rehabil Eng.* 2010;18(2): 107–116.

136. Nijboer F, Birbaumer N, Kubler A. The influence of psychological state and motivation on brain-computer interface performance in patients with amyotrophic lateral sclerosis—a longitudinal study. *Front Neurosci.* 2010;4:55.

137. Carlson D, Ehrlich N, Berland BJ, Bailey H. Assistive technology survey. 2001. Available at: http://www.ncddr.org/products/ researchexchange/v07n01/atpaper/. Accessed September 9, 2011.

138. Lewis AN, Cooper RA, Seelman KD, Cooper RM, Schein RM, Assistive technology in rehabilitation: Improving impact through policy. *J Rehabil Res Policy Educ.* In press.

139. Rubin RM, White-Means SI. Race, disability and assistive devices: sociodemographics or discrimination. *Int J Soc Econ.* 2001;28: 927–941.

140. ABLEDATA Informed Consumer's Guide to Funding Assistive Technology. Available at: http://www.abledata.com/abledata docs/funding.htm. Accessed February 17, 2012.

141. Funding for Assistive Technology: Who Pays? Available at: http:// www.rehabtool.com/forum/discussions/95.html. Accessed February 17, 2012.

XVII

NEUROPHARMACOLOGY, NEUROTECHNOLOGY, AND ALTERNATIVE TREATMENT

Neuropharmacology: A Rehabilitation Perspective

Jay M. Meythaler and Ross D. Zafonte

INTRODUCTION

Traumatic brain injury (TBI) is not a homogenous entity. Rather, it encompasses a series of mechanisms that may each have a preferential effect on different regions of the brain and/or effect preferentially specific types of neuronal populations (1). One needs to consider the mechanism of TBI whether it is blunt trauma to the outer cortex, diffuse axonal injury (DAI), induced intracerebral hemorrhage (as well as the type of hemorrhage), or complicating factors such as anoxia and secondary ischemia when considering injury, prognosis, and treatment (1–4). Each has unique biochemical consequences on prognosis and recovery. Consequently, it is unrealistic that one approach will fit persons with TBI. This is likely the case on both a mechanical as well as person specific (gender, genetic) plane. It is most important to stress that there is no "silver bullet" that will treat each area of the brain and its specific cell types with equal efficacy. TBI and its subsequent recovery are a continuum of events that are spread out over several months or years.

A second principle that has become quite evident is that what may be useful early in TBI will not be useful later in the recovery stage and may be detrimental. The very time course of injury cascades suggests that some mechanisms that enhance injury in the acute period encourage recovery in the postacute period. This fact leads to some of the clinical controversies that shape the rehabilitation perspective of neuropharmacology. Furthermore, what may be neuroprotective or enhance recovery of one cell type may not have any effect on another type of neuronal cell population or even may be detrimental to that cell population (1). There is a complex interaction between the various neuronal populations and their associated glial cells that scientists are only just beginning to understand.

Despite the fact that TBI is the number 1 cause of disability and comprises 12% of all hospital admissions in the United States (5–13), the current state of research funding in TBI has traditionally been abysmal especially for postacute TBI. This fact is compounded by professional perceptions, and the limited funding for trauma research. Thus much opportunity exists to understand the role of rehabilitation neuropharmacology in the recovery process and how pharmacology can interact with recovery programs.

There have been some advances in our understanding of the mechanisms of injury and the following physiologic processes in TBI. This has resulted in some general principles that have evolved regarding the mechanism of injury, the location of injury, the cell types involved and the various neurotransmitters that may be affected following TBI. All of this leads one to consider the utilization of medications that may affect the neurotransmitter systems of the brain following TBI. This chapter will serve to outline some theoretical principles of rehabilitation neuropharmacology; these principles of injury and neurotransmitter function will be highlighted by their role in the acute injury and recovery process. This chapter will also focus on the controversy these principles raise that help to shape the clinician perspective of neuropharmacology. This is not an all-inclusive discussion because it is beyond the scope of a chapter, but it should aid in the readers' understanding of various chapters in this book.

MEDICATION PRINCIPLES

Early Versus Late Effects

Acute TBI is really a series of mechanical events that affects the physical structure of the brain followed by a series of physiological and biochemical responses. When mechanical energy is applied to a substance it is deformed as defined by its mechanical property interrelations (elastic, viscous, or plastic response). The deformation response is time-dependent, and dependent on the amplitude of the impact energy wave. When some of the energy is transmitted from the deformed structure to the structures it contacts, there are forces deforming these structures as well (1). If the elastic limit of a structure, such as the cell membrane, the neural filaments, and other intra-axonal organelles, is exceeded then there will be a permanent physical deformation to this structure (1). These factors are often referred to as the primary injury and reflect clinical processes such as contusion, intra- and extra-axial lesions.

This is followed by a series of biochemical of events. After the initial period of injury, there is a prolonged progression of secondary events that may ultimately result in neuronal and/or glial cell death. Maxwell et al. summarized this theorized sequence of events (14). After injury, there is a depolarization followed by a focal loss of axonal transport as a result of disruption of the cellular organelles. One of the consequences of DAI is direct intracellular injury from direct mechanical displacement of the cytoskeleton and cytoplasm (15). The cascade of biochemical events that leads to further neuronal cell injury and axonotmesis likely exacerbates cellular injury and death. This injury process may involve the neuron cell body and even the glial cells. The sequence of events involves the depletion of adenosine-5'-triphosphate (ATP), intracellular calcium overload, and the production of strong oxidants, resulting in oxidative stress (1,16). The energy failure mechanism is key to the injury process. Clearly, injury to the mitochondria results in a decrease in the local production of ATP within the cell (17). Without ATP, the ion pumps that maintain Na^+, K^+, and Ca^{++} homeostasis within the axon begin to fail (1,18) (Figure 72-1).

Neuronal cell death as a result of neuronal and glial cell injury is in part mediated by the secondary release of glutamate activating N-methyl-D-aspartate (NMDA) channels and α-amino-3-hydroxy-5-methylisoxazole-4-propionate (AMPA) receptors on the neuronal cell body (1,18,19). After neuronal cells start to die and their membrane integrity is breached, more glutamate, free radicals, and strong oxidants are released and the cycle repeats itself (1,15). The influx of calcium through voltage-gated calcium channels may cause further cellular death and the release of more glutamate and inflammatory substances resulting in the activation of more NMDA receptors (1,18).

Except for the secondary ischemia and anoxia complications, it appears this whole process is a much more prolonged series of events than noted to occur in ischemic stroke. Animal and basic science data indicates that hours after acute TBI as much as 50%–60% of the neurons affected could potentially be saved via intervention. This is very different than that noted with ischemic stroke where perhaps only 15% of the neurons might be salvageable after 4 hours or more after the event. This fact raises potential clinical concerns regarding early activation and intervention. The reason for this is that the penumbra of secondary biochemical affects that can cause cellular death is quite large in trauma vs that noted in ischemic stroke (1). These principles are well established when one compares a stroke caused by an intracerebral hemorrhage to a stroke caused by ischemia (1–4). Magnetic resonance imaging has only recently been able to evaluate the extent of injury because of DAI (traumatic axonal injury) (20). However, there is great potential in evaluating neural-chemical pathways in acute injury (19). Newer methods may allow the separate evaluation of various neurochemical pathways.

The timing of various interventions may be key, as certain early treatments may be detrimental later. One prominent example is that seizure prophylaxis with phenytoin during the first week following injury may help prevent seizures, but that treatment prophylaxis for up to 6 months may slow recovery (21). Yet it has been suggested that phenytoin may actually be neuroprotective and prevent further damage as it acts as a sodium channel blocker during the first week after injury (22). This is the oldest example of a medication that is useful early after injury and is detrimental during the later stages of recovery following TBI. This discovery resulted in the early practice guidelines originating from the Brain Trauma Foundation and American Academy of Physical Medication and Rehabilitation (21,23).

Neuroprotective Agents

Recently, there has been considerable focus on agents that may block excitatory neurotransmitters that can cause cellular

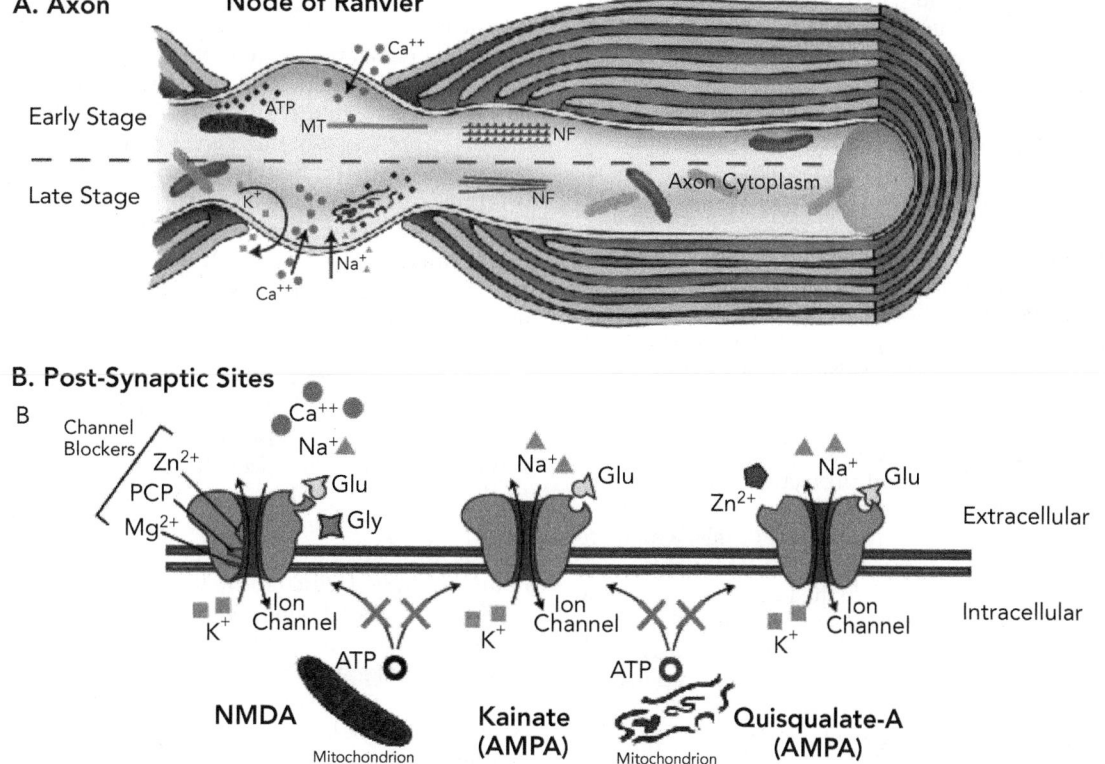

FIGURE 72-1 Axonal Injury. (From *Archives of Physical Medicine & Rehabilitation*, V82. Copyright © 2001 American Congress of Rehabilitaion Medicine and the American Academy of Physical Medicine and Rehabilitation. Reprinted with permission.)

death in already injured and susceptible neurons (24). Drugs that block NMDA channels, AMPA channels, as well as the cytokines that are increased after TBI have been the focus of much research (14). Over the first few hours following TBI, there is compaction of the neurofilaments and collapse of their side arms as well as a loss of axonal microtubules (1,14,25). The changes in the neurofilaments correspond with an influx of extracellular calcium resulting from the altered membrane pump Ca-ATPase and ecto-Ca-ATPase activity (25). High levels of calcium also activate several lipases that results in the production of arachidonic acid leading to inflammatory eicosanoids that promote neutrophil, macrophage invasion, and the production of more strong oxidants (26–28). In other words, those cells that have been injured but have enough metabolic capability to "hold on" are pushed over the edge to cell death by secondary factors that increase calcium influx into the cell. The cycle repeats itself as the calcium/sodium influx reaches a critical level in the adjacent cells; there is more cellular necrosis and apoptosis (29). The prolonged period of elevated intracellular Ca^{++} activates the calcium-dependent neutral cysteine proteases such as caspase-3 and calpains, which hydrolyze proteins resulting in more cellular necrosis and apoptosis (16,30,31). The slow progression of neuronal injury may suggest that apoptosis may be occurring with this type of injury because of the oxidative stress that accompanies reduced-glutathione depletion (32).

Secondary biochemical pathways, particularly those focused on the reduction of sodium and calcium influx into neuronal cells following TBI, eventually activate the apoptotic pathways. These 4 have also been the focus of considerable scrutiny (1,2). Glutamate is often mentioned as the mediator of the final common pathway in part because of microglial activation (1–4), quickly followed by caspase 1-activated apoptosis (4), increases in the activity of inducible nitric oxide synthase and p38 mitogen-activated protein kinase (33) as well as pathways that increase the activity of cysteine proteases (34) and the matrix metalloproteinases (35). Additionally, in the cerebral vasculature, it has been shown that initial increases in neural growth factors such as epidermal growth factor (EGF) and fibroblast growth factor (FGF), which are implicated in recovery, may work as cofactors increasing inflammation and damage in the first few days (36).

It is also clear that glutamate and other excitatory neurotransmitters are required if one is to learn to adapt and take advantage of the neuroplasticity that is present in all human brains (1). Without a release of glutamate one cannot learn. Thus, long-term glutamate suppression is not optimal during the rehabilitation process.

It is likely that those treatments that treat more than 1 pathway may be the most effective. More importantly, it may be that there will be neural protective agents that are cell specific for various neural transmitter systems. There are new treatments that are currently in clinical trials, which are working on these various pathways. Some treatments, such as cyclosporine, intend to modulate the neural immunologic response to trauma (37). Other trials using drugs that affect many of the aforementioned pathways simultaneously, such as minocycline, are currently undergoing clinical trials.

Enhancing Neuroplasticity

It may be just as detrimental to use those drugs or treatments that may enhance neuroplasticity too early in the recovery process. This includes medications that enhance excitatory neurotransmitters as well as therapy interventions that may increase these same processes. It has been recently established in animal models that rehabilitative physical or cognitive therapy started too early after neuronal injury may increase damage (38). Furthermore, over stimulating the neuronal process to fatigue may also cause cell death. Understanding this process further has important implications for rehabilitation.

Although neural recovery may occur over a lifetime, it is clear that the first 6 months are the most important because this is where the most recovery will occur. It is likely that in TBI, similarly to stroke, that the first 6 months where intensive therapy of at least 3 hours per day may be the most important for recovery (39). After the initial phase of injury, focused therapy has been able to improve functional recovery and to affect outcome in TBI (40).

NEUROTRANSMITTER SYSTEMS

Cholinergic System

The cholinergic system is intimately involved in the pathways associated with memory as well as in patterned motor movements. A lack of cholinergic neurons has been implicated in Alzheimer disease. Over activity of the cholinergic system regarding a balanced affect from the dopaminergic system has also been implicated in the development of tardive dyskinesia, and other associated movement disorders (41–43).

The hippocampal pathways have been considerably implicated in the development of antegrade memory loss associated with TBI. This is particularly true of DAI, which may be a factor in more than half of all TBI. Secondarily, it is well-established that anoxia preferentially affects these areas. This region is rich in cholinergic pathways. Within 10–13 minutes of induced anoxia there is calcium influx into the neurons of the hippocampus, which is followed by cellular loss (44). Antegrade post-traumatic amnesia (PTA) is one of the most profound developments of TBI. Preserving and subsequently enhancing these pathways may be of paramount importance.

Acetylcholine receptors are classified as either nicotinic, muscarinic, or activate alpha-Latrotoxin. Acetylcholine receptors are ligand-gated cation units composed of several different polypeptide groups (45). The activation of acetylcholine receptors leads to an influx of Na^+ and an efflux of K^+ thus resulting in cellular depolarization. Naturally occurring or synthetic compounds affect cholinergic neurons either positively or negatively. Muscarinic receptors employ a G-protein activation system whereas nicotinic receptors do not; their effector mechanism is shown in Table 72-1 (46). Cholinergic neurons can be facilitated by the administration of cholinesterase inhibitors. Cholinesterase inhibitors have also been employed as nerve gases and have a clinical role in the treatment of myasthenia gravis. Several antagonists of acetylcholine receptors exist and may be clinically useful in the acute care period following brain injury. Atropine blocks acetylcholine receptors at muscarnic receptors only, whereas botulinum toxin inhibits the release of acetylcholine (47). (see also Table 72-2)

TABLE 72-1 Acetylcholine-Muscarinic

RECEPTOR	G-PROTEIN	EFFECTOR MECHANISM
M_1, M_3, M_5	G_q G_i, G_o	↑PLC, ↑ phosphinositide hydrolysis; ↑IP_3; ↑
M_2, M_4		[Ca^{2+}]I
		↓adenylyl cyclase;
		↓cAMP; ↓Ca^{2+} influx/ ↑K^+ efflux

Acute Injury

In the first week following injury, it has been postulated agents that can protect these neurons may be quite useful. Cannabinoids—naturally occurring (marijuana), endogenous, or synthetic (dexanabinol)—have been theorized to be useful in TBI where this region is susceptible to injury (48). Studies with the synthetic cannabinoid dronaxinabol have improved TBI patient outcomes as measured by the Galveston Orientation and Amnesia Test (GOAT). However, they did not improve other outcome measures that may be more dependent on other neuronal cell types. A multicenter trial sponsored by Pharmos has reported a negative for the primary outcome measure (47).

Recovery

On the other hand the neuroscience literature is replete with examples of medications and substances that block these cholinergic pathways and accelerate the processes noted with memory loss or inhibit the recovery of memory (49,50). This needs to be kept in mind when treating patients following TBI. Profound and long-term blockade of the muscarinic system can worsen the Alzheimer pathology associated with Parkinson disease (49–51). Furthermore, long-term use of cannabinoids can be detrimental to memory pathways in otherwise healthy individuals (49).

These drugs and substances should be evaluated in the recovering person with TBI. At the very least they likely will impede recovery in a TBI patient. On the other hand, it has been suggested that donepizil, an acetylcholinesterase inhibitor, improves memory disorders following TBI (52–55).

Controversy

The level of evidence to support the use of cholimemetic agents after TBI is not robust (56). The use of citicoline (a phosphosphingolipid) is purported to have both neuroprotective and neurofacilitatory properties (57,58). The acetylcholinesterase inhibitors have been studied in a limited fashion in the brain injury population (59,60). The effects of cholinergic augmentation with donepezil on short-term memory and sustained attention have been examined in one randomized, double-blind, placebo-controlled trial. Zhang studied 20 patients with TBI who were randomized from 2 postacute rehabilitation clinics; 18 completed the trial. During the donepezil phase, the drug was administered at 5 mg/day for the first 2 weeks and 10 mg/day for the remaining 8 weeks of the trial. Group analysis showed significant benefits of donepezil on neuropsychological functioning (60). Benefits of donepezil were sustained after the washout period. An early case series found that this medication did help in self-reported improvement of memory in two persons with acute TBI, yet this series was problematic in its design and control (55). In an open label trial of 10 subjects with TBI treated with donezepil, patients noted a clinical global improvement (53). These agents have not yet been shown to assist in emergence from PTA despite the number of open label trials and small randomized trials.

Dopamine Pathways

Dopamine neurons are generally located in the midbrain in the periventricular areas of lateral ventricles, including in the very well-known substantia nigra pathways. The most important dopaminergic pathways are the nigtostriatal, tuberoinfundibular, mesolimbic and mesocortical pathways (61,62). Dopamine receptors exist as families of receptors with their designation in part being determined by their ability to activate adenyl cyclase (D_1, D_2, D_3, D_4, D_5) (see Table 72-3 and Figure 72-2) (62). The D_1 and D_5 family of receptors activate adenyl cyclase whereas the D_2, D_3, and D_4 family of receptors inhibit adenyl cyclase. These receptors all employ G-proteins to inhibit or activate processes (62). Dopamine is associated with motor movement and possibly arousal. The pathways project to the hypothalamus and are associated with autonomic functions and hormone levels.

In acute injury, a vast excitotoxic cascade occurs. It has been well-established that the increases in dopamine are correlated with increased cell death in the regions where dopamine acts as a neurotransmitter (63). Furthermore, medications that block dopamine release or receptors have been implicated in slowing neuronal recovery (43,64–68). These agents may affect hormone levels through their effects on the hippocampal releasing hormones, and cause dysautonomia. Deficits associated with decreased dopamine such as movement disorders and neuroleptic malignant syndrome are associated with blockade of the dopamine pathways as well (43).

Recovery

Patients who have had profound disruption of the dopamine pathways as noted in DAI and anoxic injury may forever be

TABLE 72-2 Acetylcholine-Nicotinic

RECEPTOR	G-PROTEIN EFFECTOR MECHANISM
α4β2, α7, α3β4NA	Ligand-gatedion channel; Na^+/Ca^{2+} influx; K^+ efflux

TABLE 72-3 Dopamine

RECEPTOR	G-PROTEIN	EFFECTOR MECHANISM
D_1, D_5, D_2,	G_s, G_i, G_o	↑adenylyl cyclase; ↑cAMP adenylyl cyclase
D_3, D_4		↓cAMP; Ca^{2+}/K^+ channels

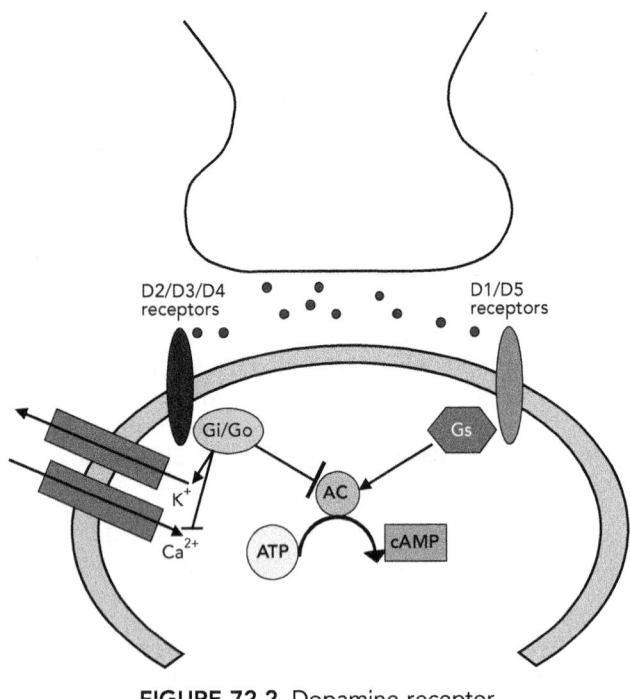

FIGURE 72-2 Dopamine receptor.

susceptible to the side effects of medications that block the D_1-D_5 pathways (42,43). These medications need to be judiciously used with preference to medications that block as few of these pathways as possible. The administration of typical and atypical antipsychotic agents can cause symptoms that include fever, leukocytosis, and muscle stiffness; this entity carries a potential mortality of 10% (69). The source of these adverse events appears to be the typical antipsychotic medications, particularly those with an affinity for the D_2 dopamine receptor. Atypical antipsychotic agents have less D_2 activity (as well as D_1–D_5 in general) and are more 5-HT_{2A} activating thus theoretically reducing some of the undesirable effects and adrenergic blockade (67). Clinical concerns with cardiac dysfunction have been raised in the dementia population with the use of atypical and typical antipsychotic agents (70).

Controversy

Typical antipsychotics and atypical antipsychotics carry varying degrees of dopamine blockade. Typical antipsychotics exist along a spectrum carrying various degrees of dopamine blockade (mostly D_2) and anticholinergic activity (67). Atypical antipsychotics have activity not only via dopamine blockade but also on the serotonin system (67). Typical antipsychotics have been used for the immediate control of aggression or agitation in TBI (68). There is concern that these agents can potentially lower seizure threshold and cloud sensorium. As with other patient groups, neuroleptic malignant syndrome has been reported.

Although numerous studies have been done in animal models, there is a lack of clarity in optimal timing and in human data. Animal models of recovery after TBI consistently demonstrate a negative impact of dopamine blockers on recovery in the postacute period (65,71). Yet not all animal models are clear on this issue. In an animal study evaluating

the effects of antipsychotics on cognitive function after TBI, haloperidol was demonstrated to be harmful while olanzapine was not (72). There are reports of the development of neuroleptic malignant syndrome with haloperidol in patients with TBI using standard dosing (43).

Although most rehabilitation clinicians treating those with TBI would attempt to avoid dopamine blockade, the actual human evidence for this is rather weak. Rao et al. studied the impact of haloperidol in a rehabilitation setting and noted no change in outcome but a longer length of PTA in the haloperidol group (73). Maryinak et al. demonstrated the successful use of the older antipsychotic methotrimeprazine in persons with TBI admitted to a rehabilitation unit (74). The authors noted that those treated with the antipsychotic had a longer length of PTA that likely reflects a greater injury severity (74). Other authors have noted that weaning antipsychotics in the chronic setting results in improved neuropsychological test scores (75). Of interest is a recent study suggesting a benefit to the use of haloperidol in the intensive care unit (ICU) setting. Milbrandt and colleagues examined a total of 989 persons with ICU stays and mechanical ventilation of greater than 48 hours (76). Haloperidol use was associated with lower hospital mortality. Although this retrospective study has limitations, this data appeared to remain consistent for those with trauma and neurological dysfunction. The authors postulated that, at least acutely, haloperidol inhibits the secretion of proinflammatory cytokines.

Medications that may increase dopamine have been postulated to enhance recovery from TBI (77,78). The most studied of these medications is amantadine, which also may have effects on various neuronal growth factors (79). Other medications such as bromocriptine that demonstrate specific D_1-D_2 receptor pathway activity have also been useful (79).

The disruption of the dopaminergic pathways has also been implicated in the development of psychiatric disorders following TBI (42,43). Delusions, hallucinations, and various behavioral dyscontrol syndromes have been implicated with TBI (43).

The role of dopamine enhancing medications in the potential recovery of persons with TBI remains an issue of great interest. These agents have been employed for aphasia, hemineglect, arousal, agitation, and dysautonomic syndromes. Dixon and Klein have demonstrated the role of amantadine in the treatment of a laboratory model of chronic TBI (80). Bromocriptine has also been shown to improve lipid peroxidation after TBI (81). Other agents such as selegiline have shown promise in the laboratory (82). Potential side effects of these medications include dyskinesia, hypotension, lowered seizure threshold, hallucinations, and behavioral dysfunction.

Many clinicians use neurostimulant medications for the treatment of hypoarousal in persons with TBI; unfortunately, the literature to support their use is sparse (47). Amantadine has both pre- and post-dopaminergic activity and functions as a NMDA antagonist (78). In a case report by Zafonte and colleagues, a male patient in a minimally conscious state regained full consciousness when placed on the dopaminergic agent amantadine but subsequently experienced a significant decline when the medication was withdrawn (83). A double-blind placebo cross over study by Meythaler and colleagues, showed significant improvements in Disability Rating Scale (DRS) scores and Functional Independence

Measure (FIM)-cognitive scores in groups taking amantadine, regardless of when it was started (78). The findings were similar in a study by Whyte et al. (79). Additionally, amantadine has shown promising results when given in the acute phase of TBI. Saniova et al. found decreased mortality rates and improved GCS scores in a small group of persons admitted to the ICU after severe TBI who were given a 3-day course of amantadine (84). Recently, Giacino and colleagues demonstrated an improved rate of recovery with amantadine while the therapy was being administered among those with disorders of consciousness (85).

McDowell tested a group of 24 subjects with TBI using a double-blind, placebo-controlled crossover trial (86). Bromocriptine was found to improve performance on some tasks served by prefrontal function, but not others. Dobkin had previously shown improvement in antegrade amnesia in a woman with TBI (87). Substantial work is needed to identify the specific syndromes and characteristics of persons who respond to these medications.

Serotonergic Pathways

The serotonin pathways are found predominately in the midbrain and brainstem but are distributed diffusely throughout the central nervous system (CNS). They have profound projections throughout the brain including to the frontal lobes and the hippocampus (88,89). It has been theorized that these pathways are most disrupted by DAI (90). Serotonin (5-hydroxytryptamine or 5-HT) is likely the most phylogenetically ancient of currently known neurotransmitter molecules. Serotonergic neuronal cell bodies are organized in 2 distinct groups (89): caudal (in the medulla oblongata and the caudal half of the pons) and rostral (in the midbrain and rostral pons) (89). The rostral 5-HT neuron axons ascend toward the forebrain, whereas those from the caudal group descend to brainstem structures and the spinal cord. Numerous serotonin receptor types have been identified (91,92) (Table 72-4). The current classification system takes into account drug related properties as well as information about amino acid sequencing of the receptor. It is the receptor interaction with the G-protein that permits the particular receptor to modulate the activity of different effector systems such as ion channels, substances like adenyl cyclase. The 5-HT$_1$ family and 5-HT$_2$ family represent the major classes of serotonin receptors, but this family also includes the 5-HT$_4$, 5-HT$_6$, and 5-HT$_7$ receptors all of which are G-protein dependent (92,93). The 5-HT$_3$ receptor system is a gated ion channel dependent system and represents a separate functional family of receptors. These receptor differences create opportunities and hazards in drug development as well as clinical utility.

These widely distributed serotonergic pathways are involved in diverse cognitive functions. Data suggests that serotonergic neurotransmission plays a major role in stabilizing and modulating brain function (93,94). The rostral part of the serotonergic raphe system consists of the caudal linear nucleus (in the midbrain), the dorsal raphe nucleus (extending from the caudal midbrain to rostral pontine levels), and the median raphe nucleus (superior central raphe nucleus found in the rostral pons) (78,79). In the caudal division there are descending serotonergic neuronal projections found in the raphe magnus nucleus, raphe pallidus nucleus, and raphe obscurens nucleus. In addition, there are serotonergic neuronal cell bodies present in the medullary reticular formation (involved in alertness and wakefulness) and other non-raphe regions such as the hippocampus (involved in memory functions) and the substantia nigra (involved with motor control) (88,89) (see Table 72-4).

Acute Injury

Increasing the levels in the first week following injury is hypothesized to have the same effect of causing increased neuronal cell death as with other excitatory neurotransmitters.

Unfortunately, projections of the serotonin system—including the forebrain, limbic areas, and hippocampus—are prime sites of direct or secondary injury resulting from TBI. There is ample evidence that TBI impacts levels of serotonin in the CNS, but whether there is an elevation or depletion of serotonin is a matter of some debate. Several studies have documented elevations of serotonin in the CNS during the hours immediately after CNS injury, possibly extending for several days (90,94–96). Markianos et al. found a significant negative correlation between CNS level of serotonin and the Glasgow Coma Scale score obtained at the time of assay, as well as an association of high serotonin levels with subsequent death (97). Under these conditions, serotonin has been suspected of worsening edema and contributing to vascular spasm (90,94–96). On the other hand, there are also studies that indicate diminished CNS serotonin levels within the first 24 hours after TBI (96–99), even in cases of mild injury (100). The decrease in serotonin level has been documented up to 60 days following TBI (68), suggesting a chronic downregulation of the serotonergic system. In addition, there is evidence that serotonin may assist in controlling edema, and serotonin receptor agonists may diminish the excitotoxic effects of glutamate release or secondary inflammatory factors after neurotrauma (101,102). Disruption of normal serotonin functioning has been documented on a chronic basis after even milder injury, based on a diminished prolactin response to buspirone, which activates serotonin receptors under normal conditions and results in prolactin release (98). Animal models also suggest that neuronal synthesis of serotonin may be inhibited even though extracellular levels of the substance may be high (103).

Recovery

Damaged serotonergic neurons can survive an injury and in time reenervate target regions, reestablishing synaptic and

---

TABLE 72-4 Serotonin

RECEPTOR	G-PROTEIN	EFFECTOR MECHANISM
5-HT$_{1A, 1B, 1D, 1E, 1F}$	G$_i$, G$_o$	↓adenylyl cyclase; ↓cAMP; ↓Ca$_2^+$ influx/↑K$^+$ efflux
5-HT$_{2A, 2B, 2C}$	G$_q$, G$_1$	↑PLC, ↑ phosphinositide hydrolysis; ↑IP$_3$; ↑[Ca^{2+}]i
5-HT$_3$	N$_A$	Ligand-gated ion channel; Na$^+$/Ca^{2+} influx; K$^+$ efflux
5-HT$_{4, 6, 7}$	G$_s$	↑adenylyl cyclase; ↑cAMP
5-HT$_5$	Unknown	Poorly Characterized

neurotransmitter function and restoring behavior (1,103–105). Mature adult neural circuitry can be remodeled and affected by the use of neurotrophic or neurotoxic factors (104). Serotonin facilitation may be involved in controlled neurogenesis. Pharmacological manipulation of neurotransmitter levels, including serotonin, may aid in the repair and reestablishment of useful neural pathways. Serotonin also plays a key role in sleep initiation.

Controversy

Animal data has suggested that 5HT agonist medications may be both helpful and harmful. Repinotan hydrochloride (repinotan) is a highly potent and selective 5-HT$_{1A}$ full receptor agonist. This agent has shown rapid uptake and a broad spectrum of neuroprotection in stroke and TBI (105). Kline has reported that 5-HT$_{1A}$-receptor agonist 8-hydroxy-2-(di-n-propylamino) tetralin (8-OH-DPAT) attenuated TBI-induced cognitive deficits and histopathology (104). However, Wilson studied the selective serotonin 5HT$_{1A}$ receptor agent fluoxetine in a chronic administration and it did not impact motor or cognitive recovery (106). Boyeson's team observed that high dose of the phenylpiperazine agents trazodone-induced deficits in an animal model of TBI (107,108). Studies in TBI have failed to establish any connection between serotonin and negative motor recovery and indicated that sertraline is safe regarding deleterious effects on cognitive or motor recovery (109–111). However, recent studies in ischemic stroke have made a connection between increased serotonin and motor recovery (112).

Thus, there may be a period when introduction of serotonin agonist agents might be beneficial to recovery of the normal serotonin response. Selective serotonin reuptake inhibitors (SSRIs) are among the most used medications in North America.

These agents have been suggested to enhance arousal, improve behavior, and treat depression and emotional liability. A recent randomized trial indicated that the use of sertraline prevents the onset of organic depression in acute TBI with little effect on cognitive or motor recovery (111). It has been theorized that disruption of these pathways is one of the causes of increased depression following TBI (113,114). A single blind placebo run-in trial by Fann et al. demonstrated the potential utility of the SSRI Zoloft in the treatment of depression following mild TBI in those patients who have depression more than 1 year out (110). These pathways have also been implicated in the development of the emotional liability and emotional incontinence noted to follow TBI (111,113–115). The use of SSRI antidepressants has become common during the rehabilitation phase following brain injury because of either stroke or TBI. SSRI antidepressants were shown to aid in the management of behavioral disturbance. Kant and colleagues gave sertraline for 8 weeks to 13 patients with TBI, resulting in decreased outbursts and irritability yet this study failed to clarify this issue (114). Bupropion, a dopaminergic and serotonergic agonist, was reported to improve psychomotor agitation and participation in therapies in a 20-year-old woman with TBI who had failed treatment with several other medications (115).

Trazodone, a triazolopyridine antidepressant, is a selective 5-HT reuptake inhibitor and 5-HT$_2$ receptor antagonist and has been frequently used for its sedating effects. Used as an antidepressant, doses of up to 500 mg/dL are commonly required; however, at lower doses its sedative properties likely result from its antagonistic effect of the 5-HT$_2$ receptors (116,117). The effects of trazodone on sleep have been shown to occur after the first dose (117,118). It has been found to closely mimic the natural sleep cycle by increasing the amount of total sleep, increasing the percentage of deep sleep (stages 3 and 4) and decreasing the number of intermittent awakenings (116,118–124). Trazodone in 1 dose of 50–100 mg nightly showed improvements in early sleep wakening, lack of sound sleep, and difficulty in initiating sleep at 2 weeks and 6 weeks with significant increases in total sleep time (121).

Mirtazapine is an alpha$_2$-adrenoceptor antagonist as well as an indirect 5-HT agonist, increasing both synaptic norepinephrine (NE) and serotonin. Mirtazapine has been found to improve sleep continuity and increase latency to rapid eye movement (REM) sleep, which may in part be caused by its antihistamine properties (125). Concerns regarding rapid weight gain have been noted. Further studies evaluating the role of mirtazapine in sleep disorders in the TBI population are warranted to evaluate potential cognitive sequelae.

Despite the absence of studies examining the role of buspirone for imbalance in persons with TBI, this HT$_3$ agonist has been used to treat imbalance and ataxia in a fashion that parallels its use in other ataxic disorders (126,127). However, despite these studies, none have been performed in TBI induced cerebellar ataxia.

These studies need to be expanded upon and several are currently underway. Whether increases in serotonin at specific receptors or in general will improve functional status following TBI, beyond that associated with affective disorders is not well understood. Just as important is a clearer understanding of the risks of these agents and their effectiveness in this population.

Norepinephrine Pathways

The excitatory norepinephrine pathways are widely distributed in the brain. However, they are most predominant in the neocortex. From a small cluster of neurons in the locus coeruleus axons project to vast areas diffusely throughout the CNS including the spinal cord, cerebellum, thalamus, and cerebral cortex (117), these pathways have profound effects on behavior, affect, motor function, and attention to name just a few of the wide effects of NE. As an example of the critical interactions between neurotransmitters, a reduction of NE in the frontal cortex has been associated with attention deficits related to new learning (120). Hence, memory deficits may be related to reduced attention without deficits in the acetycholine pathways. (see Table 72-5)

TABLE 72-5 Norepinephrine

RECEPTOR	G-PROTEIN	EFFECTOR MECHANISM
αdA, αlB, αlD	G$_q$	↑PLC, ↑ phosphinositide hydrolysis; ↑IP$_3$; ↑ [Ca^{2+}]i
α2A, α2B, α2C	G$_i$, G$_o$	↓adenylyl cyclase; ↓cAMP; ↓Ca^{2+} influx/↓K$^+$ efflux
β31, β32, β33	G$_s$	↑adenylyl cyclase; ↑cAMP

Acute Injury

Increases of NE are discouraged in the first minutes, hours, and days following TBI because the increase alone has been linked to increased neuronal cell death (101,128). These increases play into the secondary injury cascade and appear to exacerbate other pathways. Indeed, blockade of some NE adrenergic pathways has been hypothesized to be useful in the first few days after injury (91,94,95).

Recovery

Long-term reductions have been associated with an acquired attention deficit syndrome in TBI. This chronic decrement in response has been demonstrated in animal models (90,129). Consequently, there has been research on the use of agents to increase NE in the weeks following TBI (130,131).

Controversy

D-amphetamine enhances NE release and has been demonstrated to show benefits in dorsal frontal injury. Kline has demonstrated that chronic methylphenidate treatment enhances water maze performance in animal models of TBI (129).

The most commonly used medication to enhance NE in humans is also methylphenidate (130–132). Methylphenidate is believed to impact its action at least in part by activity at the dopamine transporter (DAT) (133). One group of investigators has conducted 2 randomized, double-blind, placebo-controlled trials using crossover designs to evaluate the effects of methylphenidate on various aspects of attention after TBI (130). Methylphenidate's potential utility was demonstrated in a study of 34 adults with TBI and persistent deficits in attention (130). Significant benefits of methylphenidate were seen on speed of information processing but not on divided attention, sustained attention, or susceptibility to distraction. This well-designed study suggests the potential beneficial effects of methylphenidate on specific aspects of attention after TBI. Although its role in arousing patients is not clear, methylphenidate does appear to improve attention and processing speed. In a study of ICU persons with TBI, early use of methylphenidate was associated with reductions in ICU and hospital length of stay by 23% in patients with severe TBI (134). There are concerns on the proper timing of such therapies, as early methylphenidate therapy has the potential of increasing the excitability cascade.

Recently, modafinil has been reported to decrease daytime sleepiness in patients with TBI (135). Other medications such as amphetamine, dextroamphetamine, modafinil, atomoxetine, and armodafinil have been used in an off label fashion in patients with TBI to improve attention and processing speed in those patients with documented deficits. Clinical trials of such medications among those with TBI have been either inconclusive or not performed. Because attention is related to so many neurocognitive functions, there is a significant need to perform further research in this area to evaluate benefits as well as side effects.

Gamma-Aminobutyric Acid Pathways

Gamma-aminobutyric acid (GABA) is one of the most widespread neurotransmitters in the CNS. It invariably acts as an

TABLE 72-6 Gamma-Aminobutyric Acid

RECEPTOR	G-PROTEIN	EFFECTOR MECHANISM
GABA$_A$ GABA$_C$	NA	Cl- channel
GABA$_B$	G$_i$, G$_o$	↓adenylyl cyclase; ↓cAMP; ↓Ca2$^+$ influx/↑K$^+$ efflux

Abbreviation: NA, not applicable.

inhibitory neurotransmitter on excitatory neurotransmitters such as acetylcholine, dopamine, glutamate, and NE. GABA pathways are distributed throughout the brain (117,134).

GABA receptors have been classified into subtypes A, B, and more recently C. The GABA$_A$ receptor is the best understood and has three distinct subunits (117,134,136). GABA has been implicated in the inhibition of dopamine, NE, and cholinergic pathways in the brain. It also modulates the excitotoxicity of glutamate (117). More recently, GABA has been implicated in the release of serotonin via GABA$_B$ receptor inhibition (137). (see Table 72-6)

Acute Injury

GABA mediates its effects via the G$_1$ protein at glutamate activated channels. It has been considered to be a potentially neuroprotective agent in the first minutes, hours, and days following TBI (117,138,139). Unfortunately, GABA is completely hydrophilic and does not cross membranes. Medications that indirectly increase its release or act on subtype receptors to indirectly increase its release from GABA neurons should be considered.

One potential mechanism has been linked to the neuroprotective effects of GABA. Acute ethyl alcohol (ETOH) exposure following CNS injury may improve recovery via blocking the effects of glutamate by activating G-protein ligand activated NMDA channels (140). However, chronic use of ETOH may actually down regulate these receptors thereby reducing the brain's ability to protect itself from excitatory neurotransmitters (141–145).

Recovery

Use of GABA agonists has been implicated to reduce the rate of recovery following brain injury (146). This includes medications such as benzodiazepines and baclofen (147). The benzodiazepines are termed sedative hypnotics because they induce amnesia and/or sleep (146,147). Both conditions are not conducive to recovery. It is felt that the first 6 months after injury from TBI are most critical to recovery. This means that these medications—often used for seizure prophylaxis, spasticity management, and behavioral control—should be restricted as much as possible.

Controversy

Bennzodiazepines, antiepileptic drugs (AEDs), and antispasticity agents act via GABA, yet their long-term impact of these agents is not well understood (146). Benzodiazepines are the oldest family of medications used for spasticity. Diazepam, the most commonly used agent, acts near the GABA$_A$ receptor to hyperpolarize the cellular membrane, and thus increases presynaptic inhibition (148,149). Work on the use of diazepam in spinal cord injury, cerebral palsy, and multiple sclerosis demonstrated its efficacy in the treatment of spasticity over placebo (150,151). Diazepam has not shown functional improvement. Diazepam's major limitation is in its rather significant side effect profile, such as sedation, has limited its use in the TBI population (146,148).

Baclofen is active at the GABA$_B$ receptor both presynaptically and postsynaptically. It has been employed for the treatment of spasticity in persons with spinal cord injury (SCI), cerebral palsy, multiple sclerosis, stroke, and brain injury (146). Enteral baclofen therapy may be warranted for those with severe spasticity of cerebral origin who cannot tolerate dantrolene sodium and face the risk of severe contracture or loss of range of motion (148).

Baclofen has been noted to produce sedation, especially among those with cerebral disorders. Concerns with the use of this medication include asthenia, depression, hallucinations, nausea, dizziness, and paresthesias. Attention and memory induced deficits have been raised in animal models and observed with humans. GABA facilitory agents may impair recovery (152,153). Memory dysfunction has been associated with baclofen therapy in both animals and humans (152–154). Additional concerns with baclofen include lowered seizure threshold, and withdrawal syndrome (152,154). Rapid withdrawal from baclofen therapy should be avoided and can induce seizures, altered mental status, hallucinations, hyperthermia, and rigidity (146,152). Therefore concerns are raised regarding potential negative impact on neurorecovery. One implication of this concept is the long-term use of AEDs, particularly those that may function via GABA, are discouraged in the long-term prophylaxis of seizures following TBI. There is considerable evidence that they may impede recovery. Finally, inhibiting the effects of excitatory neurotransmitters such as glutamate via GABA invariably affects our ability to learn and adapt. Glutamate is necessary for neuroplasticity and learning and blockade invariably has the potential to reduce the rate and end-point of recovery. The timing of dosing of GABA agonists (early may be better than late) and amount of blockade by the various drugs may be critical.

CONCLUSION

Although this is a brief discussion regarding some of the principles of neuropharmacology following TBI, there is much more to follow in the later chapters of the book. The primary purpose of this chapter is to give one a general outline of some of the major neurotransmitter systems that may affect the outcome from TBI. Therapeutic thresholds and toxicity levels for many of the medications have not been explored.

More research needs to be performed on the use of medications that modulate transmitter systems and the pharmacogenetics involved. When using medications, thought should be given to their profound effects, often beyond the intended results. Randomized placebo-controlled trials are needed to further define the potential benefits and risks of such therapy. In addition, a broad understanding of the "window of opportunity" for such medications is needed. As one reads further chapters in the textbook, consider the untoward side effects presented as well as the beneficial uses of medications that may affect the CNS.

1. Multiple neurotransmitter systems play dynamic and time-dependent roles after TBI.
2. Chronic changes in these neurotransmitter systems are believed to have a negative impact on cognition and motor recovery.
3. The most important dopaminergic pathways are the nigrostriatal, tuberoinfundibular, mesolimbic, and mesocortical pathways. Dopamine is associated with motor function and arousal.
4. The cholinergic system is intimately involved in the pathways associated with memory as well as in patterned motor movements.
5. Serotonergic pathways are involved in diverse cognitive functions. Data suggests that serotonergic neurotransmission plays a major role in stabilizing and modulating brain function.
6. GABA has been implicated in the inhibition of dopamine, NE, and cholinergic pathways in the brain. It also modulates the excitotoxicity of glutamate.
7. Evidence for clinical manipulation of the neurotransmitter system is minimal but growing, and 1 recent randomized controlled trial suggests an improved rate of recovery with amantadine among those with disorders of consciousness.

KEY REFERENCES

1. Giacino JT, Whyte J, Bagiella E, et al. Placebo-controlled trial of amantadine for severe traumatic brain injury. *N Engl J Med*. 2012;366(9):819–826.
2. Gordon WA, Zafonte R, Cicerone K, et al. Traumatic brain injury rehabilitation: state of the science. *Am J Phys Med Rehabil*. 2006;85:343–348.
3. Lombard L, Zafonte R. Agitation after traumatic brain injury: considerations and treatment options. *Am J Phys Med Rehabil*. 2005;84;797–812.
4. Meythaler JM, Kowalski S. Pharmacologic management of spasticity: oral medications. In: Brashear A, Elovic E, eds. *Spasticity: Diagnosis and Management*. New York, NY: Demos Medical; 2011:199–228.
5. Whyte J, Katz D, Long D, et al. Predictors of outcome in prolonged posttraumatic disorders of consciousness and assessment of medication effects: a multicenter study. *Arch Phys Med Rehabil*. 2005;86:453–462.

References

1. Meythaler JM, Peduzzi J, Eleftheriou E, Novack T. Current concepts: diffuse axonal injury-associated traumatic brain injury. *Arch Phys Med Rehabil*. 2001;82:1461–1471.
2. Graham DI. Neurpathology of head injury. In: Narayan RK, Wilburger JE, Povlishock JT, eds. *Neurotrauma*. New York, NY: McGraw-Hill; 1996:43–59.
3. Nelson JS, Parisi JE, Schochet SS. *Principles and Practice of Neuropathology*. St Louis, MO: Mosby; 1993.
4. Denny-Brown D, Russell WR. Experimental cerebral concussion. *Brain*. 1941;64:93–164.
5. Frankowski RF, Annegers JF, Whitman S. The descriptive epidemiology of head trauma in the United States. In: Becker DP, Povlishock JT, eds. *Central Nervous System Research Status Report*. Bethesda, MD: NINCDS; 1985:33–43.

6. Kraus JF. Epidemiology of head injury. In: Cooper PR, ed. *Head Injury*. 3rd ed. Baltimore, MD: Williams & Wilkins; 1993:1–25.

7. Horn J, Sherer M. Rehabilitation of traumatic brain injury. In: Grabois M, Hart KA, Lehmkuhl LD, eds. *Physical Medicine and Rehabilitation: The Complete Approach*. Malden, MA: Blackwell Science; 2000: 1281–1299.

8. Guerrero J, Thurman DJ, Sniezek JE. Emergency department visits association with traumatic brain injury: United States, 1995–1996. *Brain Inj*. 2000;14(2):181–186.

9. Thurman DJ, Guerrero J. Trends in hospitalization associated with traumatic brain injury. *JAMA*. 1999;282(10):954–957.

10. Unpublished data from Multiple Cause of Death Public Use Data from the National Center for Health Statistics, 1996. CDC Web site. http://www.cdc.gov/ncipc/dacrrdp/tbi.htm. Accessed January 12, 2012. Methods are described in Sosin DM, Sniezek JE, Waxweiler RJ. Trends in death associated with traumatic brain injury, 1979–1992. *JAMA*. 1995;273(22):1778–1780.

11. Analysis by the CDC National Center for Injury Prevention and Control, using data obtained from state health departments in Alaska, Arizona, California (reporting Sacramento County only), Colorado, Louisiana, Maryland, Missouri, New York, Oklahoma, Rhode Island, South Carolina, and Utah. Methods are described in:

   a. Centers for Disease Control and Prevention. Traumatic brain injury—Colorado, Missouri, Oklahoma, and Utah, 1990–1993. *MMWR Morb Mortal Wkly Rep*. 1997;46(1):8–11.

   b. Thurman DJ, Sniezek JE, Johnson D, Greenspan A, Smith SM. *Guidelines for Surveillance of Central Nervous System Injury*. Atlanta, GA: Centers for Disease Control and Prevention; 1995.

12. Thurman DJ, Alverson CA, Dunn KA, Guerrero J, Sniezek JE. Traumatic brain injury in the United States: a public health perspective. *J Head Trauma Rehab*. 1999;14(6):602–615.

13. Sandel ME, Finch M. The case for comprehensive residency training in traumatic brain injury: a commentary. *Am J Phys Med Rehabil*. 1993;72:325–326.

14. Maxwell WL, Povlishock JT, Graham DL. A mechanistic analysis of nondisruptive axonal injury: a review. *J Neurotrauma*. 1997;14: 419–440.

15. Povlishock JT. Pathobiology of traumatically induced axonal injury in animals and man. *Ann Emerg Med*. 1993;22:980–986.

16. Juurlink BH, Paterson PG. Review of oxidative stress in brain and spinal cord injury: suggestions for pharmacological and nutritional management strategies. *J Spinal Cord Med*. 1999;21:309–334.

17. Radi R, Rodriguez M, Castro L, Telleri R. Inhibition of mitochondrial electron transport by peroxynitrite. *Arch Biochem Biophys*. 1994;24:369–380.

18. Young WY. Death by Calcium: a way of life. In: Narayan RK, Wilburger JE, Povlishock JT, eds. *Neurotrauma*. New York, NY: McGraw-Hill; 1996:1421–1431.

19. Pike BR, Zhao X, Newcomb JK, Glenn CC, Anderson DK, Hayes RL. Stretch injury causes calpain and caspase-3 activation and necrotic and apoptotic cell death in septohippocampal cell cultures. *J Neurotrauma*. 2000;17:283–298.

20. Benson R, Meda S, Vasudevan S, et al. Global white matter analysis of diffusion tensor images is predictive of injury severity in TBI. *J Neurotrauma*. 2007;24:446–459.

21. Yablon SA, Meythaler JM, Englander J; for Brain Injury special Interest Group (AAPM&R-BI-SIG). A practice parameter recommendation of the American Academy of Physical Medicine and Rehabilitation. Antiepileptic drug (AED) prophylaxis of posttraumatic seizures (PTS). Approved by the Board of the American Academy of Physical Medicine and Rehabilitation. *Arch Phys Med Rehabil*. 1998;79(5):594–597.

22. Bullock MR, Lyeth BG, Muizelaar JP. Current status of neuroprotection trials for traumatic brain injury: lessons from animal models and clinical studies. *Neurosurgery*. 1999;45(2):207–217.

23. The Brain Trauma Foundation, The American Association of Neurological surgeons, The Joint Section on Neurotrauma and Critical care. Role of antiseizure prophylaxis following head injury. *J Neurotrauma*. 2000;17:549–553.

24. Meyer MJ, Megyesi J, Meythaler J, et al. Acute management of acquired brain injury part II: an evidence-based review of pharmacological interventions. *Brain Inj*. 2010; 24:706–721.

25. Povlishock JT, Christman CW. The pathobiology of traumatically induced axonal injury in humans and animals: a review of current thoughts. In: Bandak FA, Eppinger RH, Ommaya AK, eds. *Traumatic Brain Injury: Bioscience and Mechanics*. Larchmont, NY: Mary Ann Liebert Inc; 1996:51–60.

26. Bazan NG, Deturco EB, Allan G. Mediators of injury in neurotrauma: intracellular signal transduction and gene expression. *J Neurotrauma*. 1995;12:791–814.

27. Bates EJ. Eicosanoids, fatty acids and neutrophils: their relevance to the pathophysiology of disease. *Prostagland Leukotr Ess Fatty Acids*. 1955;53:75–86.

28. Henderson WR Jr. The role of leukotrienes in inflammation. *Ann Int Med*. 1994;121:684–697.

29. Fern R, Ransom BR, Waxman SG. Voltage-gated calcium channels in CNS white matter: role in anoxic injury. *J Neurophys*. 1995;74: 369–377.

30. Saido TC, Sorimachi H, Suzuki K. Calpain: new perspectives in molecular diversity and physiological-pathological involvement. *FASEB J*. 1994;8:814–822.

31. Campfl A, Posmanur RM, Zhao X, Schmutzhard E, Clifton GL, Hayes RL. Mechanisms of calpain proteolysis following traumatic brain injury: implications for pathology and therapy: review and update. *J Neurotrauma*. 1997;14:121–134.

32. Ratan RR, Murphy TH, Baraban JM. Macromolecular synthesis inhibitors prevent oxidative stress-induced apoptosis in embryonic cortical neurons by shunting cysteine from protein synthesis to glutathione. *J Neurosci*. 1994;14:4385–4392.

33. Tikka T, Fiebich BL, Goldsteins G, Keinanen R, Koistinaho J. Minocycline, a tetracycline derivative, is neuroprotective against excitotoxicity by inhibiting activation and proliferation of microglia. *J Neurosci*. 2001;21(8):2580–2588.

34. Imamura T, Matsushita K, Travis J, Potempa J. Inhibition of trypsin-like cysteine proteinases (gingipains) from Porphyromonas gingivalis by tetracycline and its analogues. *Antimicrob Agents Chemother*. 2001;45(10):2871–2876.

35. Machado LS, Kozak A, Ergul A, Hess DC, Borlongan CV, Fagan SC. Delayed minocycline inhibits ischemia-activated matrix metalloproteinases 2 and 9 after experimental stroke. *BMC Neurosci*. 2006;7:56.

36. Clark RS, Kochanek PM, Chen M, et al. Increases in Bcl-2 and cleavage of caspase-1 and caspase-3 in human brain after head injury. *Faseb J*. 1999;13(8):813–821.

37. Mazzeo AT, Brophy GM, Gilman CB, et al. Safety and tolerability of cyclosporine A in severe traumatic brain injury patients: results from a prospective randomized trial. *J Neurotrauma*. 2009;26(12): 2195–2206.

38. Schallert T, Fleming SM, Woodlee MT. Should the injured and intact hemispheres be treated differently during the early phases of physical restorative therapy in experimental stroke or parkinsonism? *Phys Med Rehabil Clin N Am*. 2003;14(1)(suppl):S27–S46.

39. Wang H, Camicia M, Terdiman J, Hung YY, Sandel ME. Time to inpatient rehabilitation hospital admission and functional outcomes of stroke patients. *PM R*. 2011;3(4):296–304.

40. Marshall S, Teasell R, Bayona N, et al. Motor impairment rehabilitation post acquired brain injury. *Brain Inj*. 2007;21:133–160.

41. Missal C, Nash SR, Robinson SW, Jaber M, Caron MG. Dopamine receptors: from structure to function. *Physiol Rev*. 1998;78:189–225.

42. Jaber M, Robinison SW, Missale C, Caron MG. Dopamine receptors and brain function. *Neuropharmacol*. 1996;35:1503–1519.

43. Wilkinson W, Meythaler JM, Guin-Renfroe S. Neuroleptic malignant syndrome induced by haloperidol following traumatic brain injury. *Brain Inj*. 1999;13:1025–1031.

44. Shkryl VM, Nikolaenko LM, Kostyuk PG, Lukyanetz EA. Highthreshold calcium channel activity in rat hippocampal neurons during hypoxia. *Brain Res*. 1999;833:319–328.

45. Okuda T, Haga T. High affinity choline transporter. *Neurochemical Res*. 2003;28:483–488.

46. Clader J, Wang Y. Muscarnic receptor agonists and antagonists in the treatment of Alzheimer's disease. *Curr Pharm Des*. 2005;11:3353–3361.

47. Gordon WA, Zafonte R, Cicerone K, et al. Traumatic brain injury rehabilitation: state of the science. *Am J Phys Med Rehabil*. 2006;85:343–348.

48. Narajan, RK, Michel ME, Ansell B. Clinical Trials in Head Injury. *J Neurotrauma*. 2002;19:503–557.

49. Solowij N, Stephens RS, Roffman RA, et al. Cognitive functioning of long-term heavy cannabis users seeking treatment. *J Am Med Assoc*. 2002;287:1123–1131.

50. Perry EK, Kilford L, Lees AJ, Burn DJ, Perry RH. Increased Alzheimer pathology in Parkinson's disease related to antimuscarinic drugs. *Ann Neurol*. 2003;54:235–238.

51. Levy AI. Chronically mad as a hatter: anticholinergic's and Alzheimer's disease pathology. *Annal Neurol*. 2003;54:144–146.

52. Morey CE, Cilo M, Berry J, Cusick C. The effect of Aricept in persons with persistent memory disorder following traumatic brain injury: a pilot study. *Brain Inj*. 2003;17:809–815.

53. Kaye NS, Townsend JB III, Ivins R. An open-label trial of donepezil (aricept) in the treatment of persons with mild traumatic brain injury. *J Neuropsychiatry Clin Neurosci*. 2003;15:383–384.

54. Blount PJ, Nguyen CD, McDeavitt JT. Clinical use of cholinomimetic agents: a review. *J Head Trauma Rehabil*. 2002;17:314–321.

55. Masanic CA, Bayley MT, VanReekum R, Simard M. Open-label study of donepezil in traumatic brain injury. *Arch Phys Med Reha-bil*. 2001;82:896–901.

56. Ballesteros J, Güemes I, Ibarra N, Quemada JI. The effectiveness of donepezil for cognitive rehabilitation after traumatic brain injury: a systematic review. *J Head Trauma Rehabil*. 2008;23:171–180.

57. Dempsey RJ, Raghavendra Rao VL. Cytidinediphosphocholine treatment to decrease traumatic brain injury-induced hippocampal neuronal death, cortical contusion volume, and neurological dysfunction in rats. *J Neurosurg*. 2003;98:867–873.

58. León-Carrión J, Dominguez-Roldán JM, Murillo-Cabezas F, del Rosario Dominquez-Morales M, Muñoz-Sanchez MA. The role of citicholine in neuropsychological training after traumatic brain injury. *NeuroRehabilitation*. 2000;14:33–40.

59. Taverni JP, Seliger G, Lichtman SW. Donepezil mediated memory improvement in traumatic brain injury during post acute rehabilitation. *Brain Inj*. 1998;12:77–80.

60. Zhang L, Plotkin RC, Wang G, Sandel ME, Lee S. Cholinergic augmentation with donepezil enhances recovery in short-term memory and sustained attention after traumatic brain injury. *Arch Phys Med Rehabil*. 2004;85:1050–1055.

61. Smythies J. Section II. The dopamine system. *Int Rev Neurobiol*. 2005;64:123–172.

62. Bonci A, Hopf F. The dopamine D2 receptor: new surprises from an old friend. *Neuron*. 2005;47:335–338.

63. Willis C, Lybrand S, Bellamy N. Excitatory amino acid inhibitors for traumatic brain injury. *Cochrane Database Syst Rev*. 2004;(1):CD003986.

64. Cardenas DD, McLean A. Psychopharmacologic management of traumatic brain injury. *Physical Med Rehabil Clinics N Am*. 1992;3:273–290.

65. Feeny DM, Gonzalez A, Law WA. Amphetamine, haloperidol and experience interact to affect rate of recovery after motor cortex surgery. *Science*. 1982;217:855–857.

66. Vasconcellos J. Clinical evaluation of trifluoperazine in maximum-security brain-damaged patients with an organic brain disorder. *JAMA*. 1978;240:380–382.

67. Elovic E, Lansang R, Li Y, Ricker J. The use of atypical antipsychotics in traumatic brain injury. *J Head Trauma Rehabil*. 2003;18:177–195.

68. Fugate L, Spacek L, Kresty L, Levy C, Johnson J, Mysiw W. Measurement and treatment of agitation following traumatic brain injury: II. A survey of the Brain Injury Special Interest Group of the American Academy of Physical Medicine and Rehabilitation. *Arch Phys Med Rehabil*. 1997;78:924–928.

69. Lombard L, Zafonte R. Agitation after traumatic brain injury: considerations and treatment options. *Am J Phys Med Rehabil*. 2005;84;797–812.

70. Bullock R. Treatment of behavioral and psychiatric symptoms in dementia: implications of recent safety warnings. *Curr Med Res Opin*. 2005;21:1–10.

71. Goldstein LB. Pharmacologic modulation of recovery after stroke: clinical data. *J Neuro Rehab*. 1991;5:129–140.

72. Wilson M, Gibson C, Hamm R. Haloperidol, but not olanzapine, impairs cognitive performance after traumatic brain injury in rats. *Am J Phys Med Rehabil*. 2003;82(11):871–879.

73. Rao N, Jellienk H, Woolston D. Agitation in closed head injury: haloperidol effect on rehabilitation outcome. *Arch Phys Med Rehabil*. 1985;66;30–34.

74. Maryniak O, Manchanda R, Velani A. Methotrimeprazine in the treatment of agitation in acquired brain injury patients. *Brain Inj*. 2001;15:167–174.

75. Stanislav SW, Childs A. Evaluating the usage of droperidol in acutely agitated persons with brain injury. *Brain Inj*. 2000;14:261–265.

76. Milbrandt E, Kersten A, Kong L, et al. Haloperidol use is associated with lower hospital mortality in mechanically ventilated patients. *Crit Care Med*. 2005;33;226–229.

77. Toide K. Effects of amantadine on dopaminergic neurons in discrete regions of the rat brain. *Pharm Res*. 1990;7:670–672.

78. Meythaler JM, Brunner RC, Johnson A, Davis L, Novack T. Amantadine to improve neurorecovery in traumatic brain injury associated diffuse axonal injury: a pilot double-blind randomized trial. *J Head Trauma Rehabil*. 2002;17:300–313.

79. Whyte J, Katz D, Long D, et al. Predictors of outcome in prolonged posttraumatic disorders of consciousness and assessment of medication effects: a multicenter study. *Arch Phys Med Rehabil*. 2005;86:453–462.

80. Dixon CE, Kraus MF, Kline AE, et al. Amanatadine improves water maze performance without affecting motor behavior following traumatic brain injury in rats. *Restor Neurol Neurosci*. 1999;14(4):285–294.

81. Kline AE, Massucci JL, Ma X, Zafonte RD, Dixon CE. Bromocriptine reduces lipid peroxidation and enahances spatial learning and hippocampal neuron survival in a rodent model of focal brain trauma. *J Neurotrauma*. 2004;21:1712–1722.

82. Zhu J, Hamm RJ, Reeves TM, Povlishock JT, Phillips LL. Postinjury administration of L-deprenyl improves cognitive function and enhances neuroplasticity after traumatic brain injury. *Exp Neurol*. 2000;166(1):136–152.

83. Zafonte RD, Watanabe T, Mann NR. Amantadine: a potential treatment for the minimally conscious state. *Brain Inj*. 1998;12:617–621.

84. Snaiova B, Drobny M, Kneslova L, Minarik M. The outcome of patients with severe head injuries treated with amantadine sulphate. *J Neural Transm*. 2004;111(4):511–514.

85. Giacino JT, Whyte J, Bagiella E, et al. Placebo-controlled trial of amantadine for severe traumatic brain injury. *N Engl J Med*. 2012;366(9):819–826.

86. McDowell S, Whyte J, D'Esposito M. Differential effect of a dopaminergic agonist of prefrontal function in traumatic brain injury patients. *Brain*. 1998;121(pt 6):1155–1164.

87. Dobkin BH, Hanlon R. Dopamine agonist treatment of antegrade amnesia from a mediobasal forebrain injury. *Ann Neurol*. 1993;33:313–316.

88. Azmitia EC. The serotonin-producing neurons of the midbrain median and dorsal raphe nuclei. In: Iverson I, Iverson S, Snyder S, eds. *Handbook of Pharmacology*. Vol 9. New York, NY: Plenum Press; 1978:233–314.

89. Jacobs BL, Fornal CA, Wilkinson LO. Neurophysiological and neurochemical studies of brain serotonergic neurons in behaving animals. *Ann N Y Acad Sci*. 1990;600:260–268.

90. van Woerkom T, Minderhoud J. Pharmacologic interventions. In: Sandel M, Ellis D, eds. *Physical Medicine and Rehabilitation State of the Art Reviews*. Philadelphia, PA: Hanley & Belfus Inc: 1990:447–464.

91. Nayak AK, Mohanty S, Singh RK, Chansouria JP. Plasma biogenic amines in head injury. *J Neurol Sci*. 1980;47:211–219.

92. Salzman SK, Hirofuji E, Llados-Eckman C, MacEwen GD, Beckman AL. Monoaminergic responses to spinal trauma. Participation of

serotonin in posttraumatic progression of neural damage. *J Neurosurg.* 1987;66:431–439.

93. Sharma HS, Dey PK, Olsson Y. Brain edema blood brain barrier permeability and cerebral blood flow changes following intracarotid infusion of serotonin: modification with cyproheptadine and indomethacin. In: Krieglstein J, ed. *Pharmacology of Cerebral Ischemia.* Boca Raton, FL: CRC Press; 1989:317–323.

94. Wester P, Bergström U, Eriksson A, Gezelius C, Hardy J, Winblad B. Ventricular cerebrospinal fluid monoamine transmitter and metabolite concentrations reflect human brain neurochemistry in autopsy cases. *J Neurochem.* 1990;54(4):1148–1156.

95. Karaküçük EI, Paşaoğlu H, Paşaoğlu A, Oktem S. Endogenous neruopeptides in patients with acute traumatic head injury. II: changes in the levels of cerebrospinal fluid substance P, serotonin and lipid peroxidation products in patients with head trauma. *Neuropeptides.* 1997;31(3):259–263.

96. Pellegrino TC, Bayer BM. Role of central 5-HT (2) receptors in fluoxetine-induced decreases in T-lymphocyte activity. *Brain Behav Immun.* 2002;16:87–103.

97. Markianos M, Seretis A, Kotsou S, Baltas I, Sacharogiannis H. CSF neurotransmitter metabolites and short-term outcome of patients in coma after head injury. *Acta Neurol Scand.* 1992;86:190–193.

98. Mobayed M, Dinan TG. Buspirone/prolactin response in post head injury depression. *J Affect Disord.* 1990;19:237–241.

99. Singh S, Singh PM, Prasad GC, Udupa KN. Response and action of 5-hydroxytryptamine in experimental head injury. *Indian J Exp Biol.* 1986;24:505–507.

100. Saran AS. Depression after minor closed head injury: role of dexamethasone suppression test and antidepressants. *J Clin Psychiatry.* 1985;46:335–338.

101. Zauner A, Bullock R. The role of excitatory amino acids in severe brain trauma: opportunities for therapy: a review. In: Bandak FA, Eppinger RH, Ommaya AK. *Traumatic Brain Injury: Bioscience and Mechanics.* Larchmont, NY: Mary Ann Liebert Inc; 1996:97–104.

102. Whitaker-Azmitia PM, Shemer AV, Caruso J, Molino L, Azmitia EC. Role of high affinity serotonin receptors in neuronal growth. *Ann N Y Acad Sci.* 1990;600:315–330.

103. Fuller R, Wong D. Serotonin reuptake inhibitors without affinity for neuronal receptors. *Biochem Pharmacol.* 1987;7:14–20.

104. Kline AE, Yu J, Massucci JL, Zafonte RD, Dixon CE. Protective effects of the 5-HT1A receptor agonist 8-hydroxy-2-(di-n-propylamino) tetralin against traumatic brain injury-induced cognitive deficits and neuropathology in adult male rats. *Neurosci Lett.* 2002; 333:179–182.

105. Mauler F, Horvath E. Neuroprotective efficacy of repinotan HCI, a 5-1A receptor agonist, in animal models of stroke and traumatic brain injury. *J Cereb Blood Flow Metab.* 2005;25:451–459.

106. Wilson M, Hamm R. Effects of fluoxetine on the 5HT1a receptor and recovery of cognitive function after TBI in rats. *Am J Phys Med Rehabil.* 2002;81;364–372.

107. Boyeson MG, Harmon RL, Jones JL. Comparative effects of fluoxetine, amitriptyline and serotonin on functional motor recovery after sensorimotor cortex injury. *Am J Phys Med Rehabil.* 1994;73: 76–83.

108. Boyeson MG, Harmon RL. Effects of trazodone and desipramine on motor recovery in brain-injured rats. *Am J Phys Med Rehabil.* 1993;72:286–293.

109. Meythaler JM, Depalma L, Devivo MJ, Guin-Renfroe S, Novack TA. Sertraline to improve arousal and alertness in severe traumatic brain injury secondary to motor vehicle crashes. *Brain Inj.* 2001;15: 321–331.

110. Fann J, Uomoto J, Katon W. Sertraline in the treatment of major depression following traumatic brain injury. *J Neuropsych Clin Neurosci.* 2000;12:226–232.

111. Novak TA, Baños JH, Brunner RC, Renfroe S, Meythaler JM. Impact of early administration of sertraline on depressive symptoms, in the first year after traumatic brain injury. *J Neurotrauma.* 2009;26: 1921–1928.

112. Chollet F, Tardy J, Albucher JF, et al. Fluoxetine for motor recovery after acute ischaemic stroke (FLAME): a randomised placebo-controlled trial [Erratum appears in *Lancet Neurol.* 2011;10:205]. *Lancet Neurol.* 2011;10:123–130.

113. Fann J, Uomoto J, Katon W. Cognitive improvement with treatment of depression following mild TBI. *Pscyhosom.* 2001;42:48–54.

114. Kant R, Smith-Seemiller L, Zeiler D. Treatment of aggression and irritability after head injury. *Brain Inj.* 1998;12:661–666.

115. Teng CJ, Bhalerao S, Lee Z, et al. The use of bupropion in the treatment of restlessness after a traumatic brain injury. *Brain Inj.* 2001;15:463–467.

116. Haffmans PM, Vos MS. The effects of trazodone on sleep disturbances induced by brofaromine. *Eur Psychiatry.* 1999;14:167–171.

117. Bear MF, Connors BW, Paradiso. Neurotransmitter systems. *Neuroscience Exploring the Brain.* 2nd ed. Philadelphia, PA. Lippincott Williams and Wilkins; 2001.

118. Maj J, Palider W, Rawlłów. Trazodone, a central serotonin antagonist and agonist. *J Neural Transm.* 1979;44:237–288.

119. Kaynak H, Kaynak D, Gözükirmizi E, Guilleminault C. The effects of trazodone on sleep in patients treated with stimulant antidepressants. *Sleep Med.* 2004;5:15–20.

120. Karli D, Burke D, Kim H, et al. Effects of dopaminergic combination therapy for frontal lobe dysfunction in traumatic brain injury rehabilitation. *Brain Inj.* 1999;13:63–68.

121. Mashiko H, Niwa S, Kumashiro H, et al. Effect of trazodone in a single dose before bedtime for sleep disorders accompanied by a depressive state: dose-finding study with no concomitant use of hypnotic agent. *Psychiatry Clin Neurosci.* 1999;53:193–194.

122. Ware JC, Pittard JT. Increased deep sleep after trazodone use: a double-blind placebo-controlled study in healthy young adults. *J Clin Psychiatry.* 1990;51(suppl):18–22.

123. Scharf MB, Sachais BA. Sleep laboratory evaluation of the effects and efficacy of trazodone in depressed insomniac patients. *J Clin Psychiatry.* 1990;51(suppl):13–17.

124. Mouret J, Lemoine P, Minuit MP, Benkelfat C, Renardet M. Effects of trazodone on the sleep of depressed subjects—a polygraphic study. *Psychopharmacology (Berl).* 1988;95(suppl):S37–S43.

125. Haddjeri N, Blier P, de Montigny C. Noradrenergic modulation of central serotonergic neurotransmission: acute and long-term actions of mirtazapine. *Int Clin Psychopharmacol.* 1995;(10)(suppl 4): 11–17.

126. Trouillas P, Xie J, Adeleine P, et al. Buspirone, a 5-hydroxytryptamine1A agonist, is active in cerebellar ataxia. Results of a double-blind drug placebo study in patients with cerebellar cortical atrophy. *Arch Neurol.* 1997;54:749–752.

127. Ogawa M. Pharmacological treatments of cerebellar ataxia. *Cerebellum.* 2004;3:107–111.

128. Hamill RW, Woolf PD, McDaonald JV, Lee LA, Kelly M. Catecholamines predict outcome in traumatic brain injury. *Ann Neurol.* 1987; 21:438–443.

129. Kline AE, Yan HQ, Bao J, Marion DW, Dixon CE. Chronic methylphenidate treatment enhances water maze performance following traumatic brain injury in rats. *Neurosci Lett.* 2000;280(3):163–166.

130. Whyte J, Hart T, Schuster K, Fleming M, Polansky M, Coslett HB. Effects of methylphenidate on attentional function after traumatic brain injury. *Am J Phys Med Rehabil.* 1997;76:440–450.

131. Evans RW, Gaultieri CT, Patterson D. Treatment of chronic closed head injury with psychostimulant drugs: a controlled case study and an appropriate evaluation procedure. *J Nerv Ment Disease.* 1987; 175:106–110.

132. Kaelin D, Whyte J, Sandel M. Methylphenidate effect on attention deficit in the acutely brain injured adult study. *Arch Phys Med Rehabil.* 1996;77(1):6–9.

133. Wagner AK, Chen X, Kline AE, Li Y, Zafonte RD, Dixon CE. Gender and environmental enrichment impact dopamine transporter expression after experimental traumatic brain injury. *Exp Neurol.* 2005;195:475–483.

134. Moein H, Khalili HA, Keramatian K. Effect of methylphenidate on ICU and hospital length stay in patients with sever and moderate traumatic brain injury. *Clin Neurol Neurosurg.* 2006;108:539–542.

135. Kaiser PR, Valko PO, Werth E, et al. Modafinil ameliorates excessive daytime sleepiness after traumatic brain injury. *Neurology.* 2010;75:1780–1785.

136. Francisco GE, Kothari, S, Huls C. GABA agonists and gabapentin for spastic hypertonia. *Phys Med Rehabil Clin N Am.* 2001;12(4): 875–888, viii.

137. Meythaler JM, Roper JF, Davis L, Brunner RC. Cyproheptadine in intrathecal baclofen withdrawal: a case series. *Arch Phys Med Rehabil.* 2003;84:638–642.

138. Kaplan JP, Raizon BM. New anitconvulsants: shiff bases of gamma-aminobutyric acid and gamma-aminobutyramide. *J Med Chem.* 1980;23:702–704.

139. Meythaler JM, Kowalski S. Pharmacologic management of spasticity: oral medications. In: Brashear A, Elovic E, eds. *Spasiticity: Diagnosis and Management.* New York, NY: Demos Medical; 2011: 199–228.

140. Kelly DF, Kozlowski DA, Haddad E, Echiverri A, Hovda DA, Lee SM. Ethanol reduces metabolic uncoupling following experimental head injury. *J Neurotrauma.* 2000;17:261–272.

141. Corrigan JD. Substance abuse as a medicating factor in outcome from traumatic brain injury. *Arch Phys Med Rehabil.* 1995;76: 302–309.

142. Jurkovich GJ, Rivara FP, Gurney JG, et al. The effect of acute alcohol intoxication and chronic alcohol abuse on outcome from trauma. *J Am Med Assoc.* 1993;270:51–56.

143. Zink BJ, Feustel PJ. Effects of ethanol on respiratory function in traumatic brain injury. *J Neurosurg.* 1995;82:822–828.

144. Yamakami I, Vink R, Faden AI, Gennarelli TA, Lenkinski R, McIntosh TK. Effects of acute ethanol intoxication on experimental brain injru in the rat: neurobehavioral and phosphorus-31 nuclear magnetic resonance spectroscopy studies. *J Neurosurg.* 1995;82: 813–821.

145. Bombardier CH, Thurber CA. Blood alcohol level and early cognitive status after traumatic brain injury. *Brain Inj.* 1998;12:725–734.

146. Zafonte R, Lombard L, Elovic E. Antispasticity medications: uses and limitations of enteral therapy. *Am J Phys Med Rehabil.* 2004; 83(10)(suppl):S50–S58.

147. Meythaler JM. Use of intrathecally delivered medications for spasticity and dystonia in acquired brain injury. In: Yaksh TL, ed. *Spinal Drug Delivery.* New York, NY: Elsevier; 1999:513–554.

148. Zafonte R, Elovic E, Lombard L. Acute management of post TBI spasticity. *J Head Trauma Rehabil.* 2004;18:403–407.

149. Kelley AE, Andrzejewski ME, Baldwin AE, Hernandez PJ, Pratt WE. Glutamate-mediated plasticity in corticostriatal networks. *Ann N Y Acad Sci.* 2003;1003:159–168.

150. Naftchi NE, Schlosser W, Horst WD. Correlation of changes in the GABA-ergic system with the development of spasticity in paraplegic cats. *Adv Exp Med Biol.* 1979;123:431–450.

151. Wilson LA, McKechnie AA. Oral diazepam in the treatment of spasticity in paraplegia a double-blind trial and subsequent impressions. *Scott Med J.* 1966;11:46–51.

152. Meythaler JM, Clayton W, Davis LK, Guin-Renfroe S, Brunner RC. Orally delivered baclofen to control spastic hypertonia in acquired brain injury. *J Head Trauma Rehabil.* 2004;19(2):101–108.

153. Terrence CF, Fromm GH, Roussan MS. Baclofen its effect on seizure frequency. *Arch Neurol.* 1983;40:28–29.

154. Sandyknb R, Gillman M. Baclofen induced memory impairment *Clin Neuropaharm.* 1985;8:294–299.

Pharmacotherapy of Cognitive Impairment

David B. Arciniegas and Jonathan M. Silver

INTRODUCTION

Cognitive impairments are among the most common neuropsychiatric sequelae of traumatic brain injury (TBI) (1). Event-related impairments of arousal, attention, processing speed, memory, and/or executive function that reflect biomechanically induced disruptions of brain function and/or structure define TBI (2–4). Many persons with TBI—especially those with mild injuries—experience substantial cognitive recovery in the weeks to months following injury (1,5,6). For some of these individuals, however, recovery is incomplete and cognitive impairments become persistent problems (1).

Environmental, behavioral, educational, supportive, and cognitive rehabilitative interventions contribute importantly to recovery and may mitigate the functional consequences of early and late cognitive impairments (7–13); these interventions are appropriately regarded as the first-line interventions for post-traumatic cognitive impairments. Pharmacotherapy may serve a useful adjunctive role to nonpharmacologic interventions (14–16) and offers promise of altering cerebral functioning in a manner that facilitates more effective engagement in other types of treatment.

Neurotrauma impairs cognition by disturbing the function and/or structure of cortical, subcortical, or brainstem areas; the axons connecting these areas; the ascending neurotransmitter systems that modulate their function; and/or the physiologic context in which all of these processes operate (17,18). Understanding the neuroanatomy and neurophysiology of both cognition and TBI is necessary for the development of rational pharmacotherapy of post-traumatic cognitive impairments. Clinicians working with persons with post-traumatic cognitive impairments are encouraged to remain apprised of important conceptual and scientific developments that inform decisions regarding the use, or the avoidance, of pharmacotherapies among persons with TBI.

This chapter addresses several such issues and then provides a brief review of pharmacotherapies for post-traumatic cognitive impairments. Because neurotransmitter systems are the principal targets of pharmacotherapy, the neuroanatomic and neurochemical consequences of TBI are considered first. Thereafter, pharmacotherapies for post-traumatic cognitive impairments are presented according to the cognitive domains to which they are most relevant. In light of the discussion regarding post-traumatic neurotransmitter disturbances, the time postinjury at which they are likely to be most beneficial also is discussed and practical recommendations regarding their use are offered.

NEUROBIOLOGY AND COGNITIVE PHARMACOTHERAPY

The types of cognitive deficits produced by TBI follow from the regional vulnerability of the brain to the combined effects of contact and inertial forces as well as the cytotoxic cascade that they incite (17–19). Focal structural injuries and large-magnitude contact forces produce immediate and, often, persistent cognitive impairments of types and severities that reflect the areas and volumes of injured brain tissue (1). The application of inertial forces also disrupts wider areas of brain structure, especially where movement within the intracranial space is less restricted (e.g., anterior frontal and temporal areas), at the junction between the supratentorial and infratentorial compartments (e.g., brainstemdiencephalic regions), and across white matter pathways within and between these areas (17,19–21) (see Figure 73-1). Cytotoxic processes such as calcium and magnesium dysregulation, free radical injury, neurotransmitter (especially glutamate and cholinergic) excitotoxicity, altered cellular energetics, and disturbances in autoregulation of cerebral blood flow also alter brain function and/or structure at the sites of focal injury as well as across wider areas of brain tissue, thereby contributing to the broad range of post-traumatic cognitive impairments (18,21–23). These processes reach their maxima in the minutes to hours following TBI and wane over the days to weeks following TBI (18,21,23). The time course of their resolution appears to vary with initial injury severity as well as the specific element of the cytotoxic cascade studied.

Experimental injury studies (24) and cerebrospinal fluid sampling studies of persons with severe TBI (18) demonstrate that biomechanical trauma induces cerebral neurotransmitter excesses in the immediate postinjury period; these include elevated levels of glutamate, L-aspartate, acetylcholine, dopamine, norepinephrine, serotonin, and gamma-aminobutyric acid (GABA), among others. This "neurotransmitter storm" not only produces cognitive dysfunction but also contributes to the cytotoxic cascade (18,23–25). Based on reviews of this literature (24), it appears likely that cognitive disturbances occurring at the time of

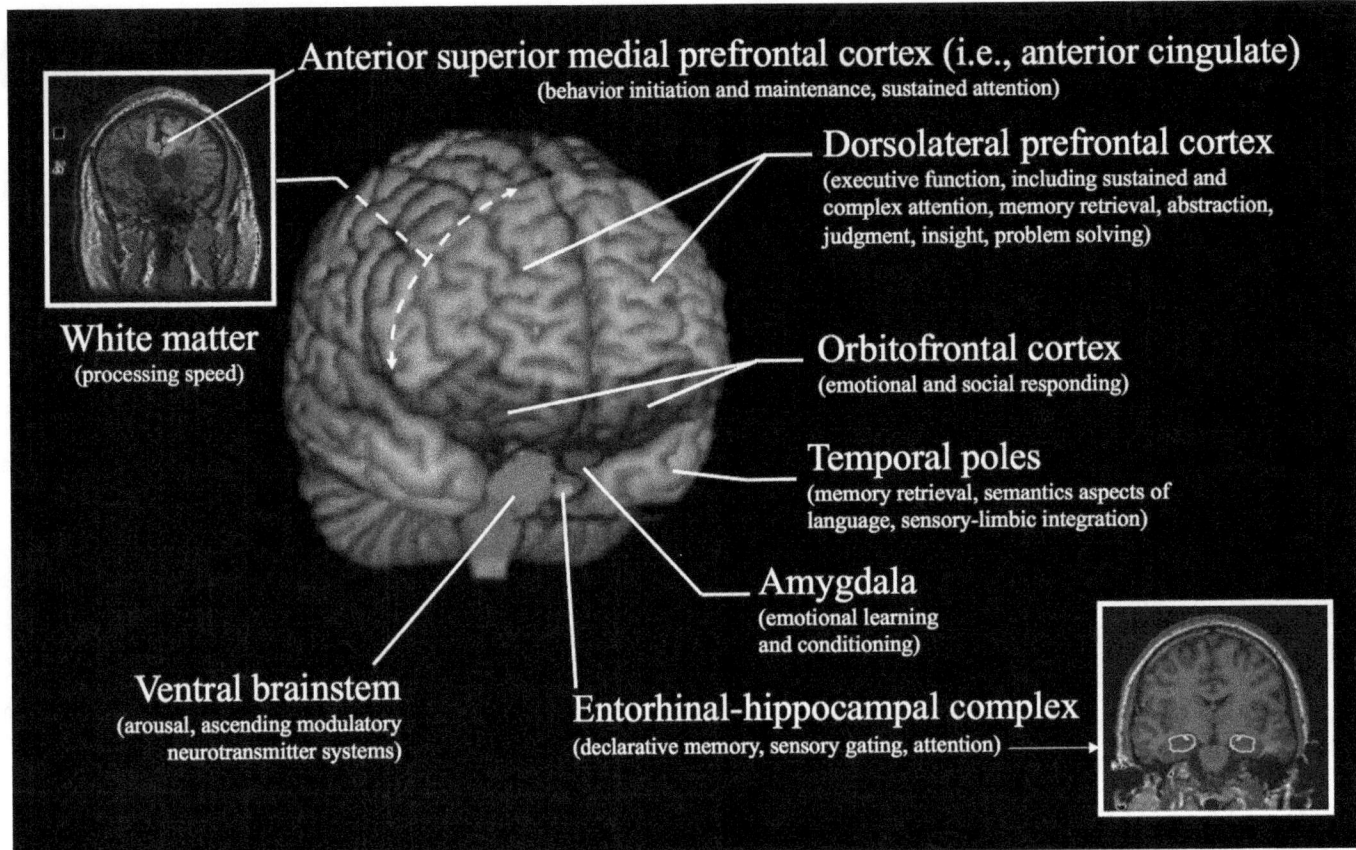

FIGURE 73-1 A three-dimensional reconstruction of the brain highlighting regional vulnerability to TBI and describing relevant brain-behavior relationships. Shaded areas represent brain regions that are especially vulnerable to TBI. The names of the cognitive, emotional, and behavioral functions with which they are most closely associated are labeled. Coronal T1-weighted magnetic resonance images of the brain (acquired at 1.5 Tesla) are inserted; at the top left, diffuse (multifocal) axonal injury is demonstrated; at the bottom right, the entorhinal-hippocampal complex is identified (outlined within image).

TBI are predicated at least in part on acute neurotransmitter excesses.

Cerebral neurotransmitter excesses abate over the first several weeks following severe TBI and may do so more rapidly after less severe injuries. In the late postinjury period, the cerebral levels of excitatory amino acids (e.g., glutamate, aspartate) and monoamine neurotransmitters (i.e., dopamine, norepinephrine, serotonin) are normal in most TBI survivors. However, early postinjury cholinergic excesses are followed by functionally important late cortical cholinergic deficits in a substantial subpopulation of patients (18). The evidence suggesting that catecholaminergic (i.e., dopaminergic, noradrenergic) function may be altered after TBI and contribute to post-traumatic cognitive impairments (25–27) does not necessarily imply that there are neurotrauma-induced losses of ascending catecholaminergic fibers; instead, this evidence appears more likely to reflect the consequences of genetically mediated individual differences in catecholamine metabolism that amplify the effects of modest injury-related structural deficits in these systems.

Unfortunately, pretreatment identification of individuals with functionally important cerebral neurotransmitter disturbances is not possible with presently available neuroimaging, neuropsychological, and clinical genetic assessments. The selection and timing of pharmacotherapies for post-traumatic cognitive impairments are therefore guided most usefully by an understanding of the course of post-traumatic neurotransmitter disturbances.

Normal cognition ultimately depends on a complex set of neurotransmitters, neuroactive peptides, neurohormones, second messenger system, and genetically regulated neurochemical processes and interactions (28–35). When cerebral neurotransmitter levels are excessive or deficient, cognition is affected adversely. The common approach of symptom-targeted pharmacotherapy—for example, treating early post-traumatic amnesia with an acetylcholinesterase inhibitor—is overly simplified and, in principle, potentially hazardous. Administering agents that augment cerebral neurotransmitter levels during the "neurotransmitter storm" (i.e., during the first few hours to weeks postinjury, depending on the severity of TBI) risks exacerbating and/or prolonging both cognitive impairments and the injurious neurobiology underlying them. Some elements of this cascade may be necessary for neuronal recovery and plasticity; accordingly, administering agents that robustly antagonize cerebral neurotransmitter receptors (e.g., potent dopamine receptor antagonists like haloperidol or risperidone) during the acute and subacute postinjury periods risks delaying clinical and neurobiological recovery (36–38).

Rational pharmacotherapy of post-traumatic cognitive impairments requires consideration of not only the intended cognitive targets of treatment but also initial TBI severity, the time postinjury at which the medication is administered (i.e., the phase of the cytotoxic cascade), the stage of post-traumatic encephalopathy during which the cognitive target symptom occurs, the influence and interactions between these and other factors (19,22). In the next section of this chapter, these considerations are applied to the pharmacotherapy of post-traumatic cognitive impairments.

PRETREATMENT CONSIDERATIONS

As noted earlier in this chapter, evaluation for and initiation of nonpharmacologic interventions for post-traumatic cognitive impairments takes precedence over pharmacotherapy in most circumstances (8–10,39,40). With rare exceptions, pharmacotherapy is adjunctive to nonpharmacologic cognitive treatments.

Prior to initiating any pharmacologic treatment for post-traumatic cognitive impairments, a thorough neuropsychiatric evaluation (22) is essential. In particular, the potential contributions of noncognitive neuropsychiatric, neurological, medical, substance use, and preinjury factors (e.g., premorbid cognitive baseline) to the patient's presenting complaints and/or impairments require consideration. When it is feasible to do so, it is advisable to address such problems prior to initiating cognition-specific treatments. In some cases (e.g., during inpatient rehabilitation in the early postinjury period), concurrent management of cognitive and noncognitive problems may be required.

When the decision is made to initiate pharmacotherapy for post-traumatic cognitive impairment, the presenting cognitive complaints and/or impairments require careful assessment. Obtaining and clarifying the patient's and/or caregiver's reports of cognitive and functional performance problems is undertaken in a manner that allows translation of those reports into clinical parlance (which often are framed as "memory" problems regardless of their true nature). Additionally, cognitive performance is assessed using objective measures appropriate to the stage of post-traumatic encephalopathy during which the patient is evaluated; see Arciniegas (41) for a detailed discussion of these issues.

The necessity, effectiveness, and possible contributions of other treatments to the patient's cognitive complaints and/or impairments also require consideration. Medications of particular concern include anticonvulsants (42), antipsychotic medications with potent antidopaminergic properties (38,43), benzodiazepines (38,44), anticholinergic agents (45), and opiates (38). When possible, eliminating or reducing the dose of these agents is encouraged before initiating treatment with medications aimed at improving cognition. It sometimes will not be possible to eliminate cognitively impairing medications; in such cases, it is important to recognize that cognition-enhancing medications may be treating the adverse cognitive effects of other agents as much, or perhaps more, than the cognitive consequences of TBI.

Pharmacotherapy of neuropsychiatric (i.e., cognitive, emotional, or behavioral) disturbances among persons with TBI follows the basic principles of pharmacotherapy (see Chapter 74). Advances in the science of TBI allow for the development a priori hypotheses regarding the potential benefits and side effects of pharmacotherapies. Such hypotheses have been used to guide some studies of medications for post-traumatic cognitive impairments (46–49). In the absence of hypothesis-driven evidence-based treatments, using agents that appear to improve cognitive impairments among persons with phenotypically similar but etiologically distinct neuropsychiatric disorders (e.g., attention-deficit hyperactivity disorder, multiple sclerosis, Alzheimer's disease) may be necessary. It is important to bear in mind that this is a relatively weak foundation for pharmacotherapy; and pathophysiologic, demographic, medical comorbidities, and other factors may limit the extent to which the beneficial effects in another population translate to the care of persons with TBI.

When pharmacotherapies are provided, we recommend regarding each medication prescription as "n-of-one" empiric trial in which modest treatment response expectations are established, vigilance for adverse effects is maintained, and consent to treatment with uncertain benefits and risks is obtained. At a minimum, the consent process includes: discussion of the published evidence for the treatment selected and/or the rationale for treatment-by-analogy; acknowledgement of "off-label" treatment (i.e., one lacking regulatory agency approval for the proposed use); the target symptom for which medication is prescribed; the side effects and risks of treatment; and the anticipated costs of treatment, especially those third-party payors are unlikely to cover financially.

Clinicians and patients should anticipate that cognitive improvements during the early or subacute postinjury periods (i.e., concurrent to spontaneous recovery) may or may not be attributable to medications administered. Time limited empiric trials therefore are necessary; whether they are based on clinical plateau, duration of treatment, or both, one or more medication discontinuation attempts should be undertaken after cognitive improvements plaeteau. Cognitive improvements (whether from spontaneous recovery, pharmacotherapy, or both) may be maintained after medication discontinuation (50). In such cases, additional pharmacotherapy is unnecessary. When treatment discontinuation is followed by cognitive decline, continued (and possibly chronic) pharmacotherapy may be required.

PHARMACOTHERAPIES

In the sections that follow, pharmacotherapies for post-traumatic cognitive impairments are presented according to the cognitive domains to which they are most relevant. In light of the discussion regarding post-traumatic neurotransmitter disturbances, the time postinjury at which they are likely to be most beneficial also is discussed. The studies reviewed include some double-blind placebo-controlled studies, uncontrolled open-label studies, and also case series or single-case reports. The strength of the evidence they provide for the use of these agents in clinical practice is debatable and can only be regarded as treatment options for post-traumatic cognitive impairments. Guided by the published literature and our own clinical experience, we offer a synthesis of this literature and preliminary recommendations regarding the pharmacotherapy of post-traumatic cognitive impairments. However, we suggest that clinicians consider reviewing the reviews and the primary articles cited herein prior to using these agents in their clinical practice.

Arousal

Arousal denotes a state of wakefulness that occurs along a continuum with pathological extremes at both ends. Coma is the extreme of the hypoarousal end of that continuum, and manic excitement, severe anxiety (including the hypervigilance and heightened reactivity of posttraumatic stress disorder), and agitated delirium represent conditions along the hyperarousal side of that continuum.

Based on the neurochemistry of arousal systems, glutamate-modulating, catecholamine-augmenting, and/or procholinergic agents might be useful treatments of hypoarousal, including disorders of consciousness (i.e., coma, vegetative states, minimally conscious state). Among medications with such properties, amantadine (an uncompetitive N-methyl-d-aspartate (NMDA) antagonist that also indirectly facilitates dopaminergic function) is regarded presently as the first-line treatment for disorders of consciousness (51–53). There are reports describing improvements among persons with disorders of consciousness in response to bromocriptine (54), levodopa (55), pramipexole (55), methylphenidate (56,57), lamotrigine (58), modafinil (59), and zolpidem (49,60,61), among others. The evidence supporting the use of these agents is limited, and the benefits and risks attendant to their use among persons with disorders of consciousness are uncertain. Nonetheless, these medications may be treatment options when amantadine is ineffective or when amantadine-induced side effects are intolerable.

The treatment of hyperarousal first requires clarification of its etiology. In some cases, post-traumatic delirium may involve sustained hyperarousal, restlessness, and agitation. Alternatively, hyperarousal may be the result of mania, severe anxiety, akathisia, medications (e.g., levetiracetam, corticosteroids, adrenergic agonists), substance withdrawal (e.g., alcohol, benzodiazepine, opiates) and other neuropsychiatric or medical conditions. In general, the treatment appropriate for hyperarousal is best directed at its underlying cause. When it is a manifestation of delirium caused by TBI, adjunctive treatment with an atypical antipsychotic (e.g., quetiapine, olanzapine), anticonvulsant, and/or acetylcholinesterase inhibitor may enhance the effectiveness of other environmental, behavioral, and supportive interventions (19,62).

Attention and Processing Speed

Attention refers to the ability to select targets for information processing, sustain focus on those targets, and, with executive control, to alternate between information processing targets. Processing speed denotes the rate at which an individual processes and reacts to stimuli or information and is usually described clinically as reaction time or response latency. Problems with attention and processing speed frequently co-occur, and their pharmacologic treatments overlap substantially. For these reasons, they are considered together here.

Attention and processing speed are highly sensitive to the effects of cerebral glutamatergic, GABAergic, catecholaminergic (i.e., dopamine, norepinephrine), and cholinergic function (14,28). Glutamate is the principal excitatory neurotransmitter in the central nervous system (CNS). Glutamatergic excesses produce significant neuronal dysfunction and, consequently, induce a broad range of cognitive impairments (14,30–32,63). GABA is the principal inhibitory neurotransmitter in the CNS, and excessive levels of GABA or agonism at GABA receptors reliably impairs a broad range of cognitive and motor functions. Catecholamines modulate signal-to-noise ratio in information processing systems quadratically. Midrange cerebral catecholamine levels optimize processing of "signal" within relevant cortical areas (i.e., information to which attention is directed), which actively inhibit processing in cortical areas unnecessary to that task (i.e., "noise"). When cerebral catecholamine levels are low, these areas do not generate maximal cortical "signal" or actively inhibit surrounding cortical areas, resulting in a low signal-to-noise ratio in information processing circuits and networks. When cerebral catecholamine levels are high, cortical "signal" is generated in both task-relevant and task-irrelevant (or unnecessary) cortical areas; persistent activity in cortical areas outside those necessary for attentional processing creates "noise" within information processing circuits, results in a low signal-to-noise ratio therein, and allows extraneous stimuli or information processing to compete for and compromise attention and processing speed. Acetylcholine also improves the efficiency of signaling across many cognitively salient cerebral circuits and networks (29). Like the catecholamines, acetylcholine modulates the function of these networks quadratically, and either deficits or excesses of acetylcholine compromise cognition.

Attention and processing speed impairments in the immediate postinjury period are likely to be polyetiological and contributed to by injury-induced neurotransmitter excesses (24). In general, supportive care and attempts to reduce risk of reinjury are the best interventions treatments of attention and processing speed impairments during this period (64). Pharmacotherapies directed specifically at disturbed attention—including antipsychotics or acetylcholinesterase inhibitors, which are often prescribed to persons with delirium, the characteristic feature of which is impaired selective and sustained attention—are of unproven benefit among persons with post-traumatic delirium, may complicate the course of neurotransmitter disturbances during the immediate postinjury period, and risk delaying recovery (38,43,65,66). Despite promising findings from experimental injury studies (67,68), antagonism of acetylcholine in the immediate postinjury period does not appear to be a useful neuroprotective or cognition-enhancing strategy among persons with TBI. When agents are necessary for the management of behavioral disturbances associated with post-traumatic delirium, use of the lowest effective dose for as short a time as possible is encouraged.

In the subacute (i.e., after the first several weeks) or late postinjury periods, attention and processing speed impairments are usually treated with medications that augment catecholaminergic function, cholinergic function, or both. Among the catecholamine-augmenting medications, the evidence is best developed for methylphenidate (14–16,69). This agent tends to improve processing speed more reliably than it does sustained attention, although the evidence and expert opinions on this point are mixed. It also is well tolerated among most persons with brain injuries (70–73) including older adults and those with cardiovascular problems. It does not appear to alter seizure frequency among persons with TBI including those with epilepsy (70,71,74,75). Nonetheless, performing baseline cardiovascular assessments, evaluating seizure risk, and monitoring assiduously for adverse events is encouraged when treatment with methylphenidate or similar medications is undertaken. Although tachyphylaxis to the beneficial effects of treatment and/or the development of methylphenidate abuse/dependence are of concern to some clinicians and patients, these are uncommon problems even among persons with histories of substance use disorders (76,77). Nonetheless, it is important to remain vigilant for signs of drug abuse, dependence, and/or diversion when this or any other stimulant medication is used to treat attention and/or processing speed impairments.

When methylphenidate is ineffective or tolerated poorly, other catecholamine-augmenting agents may be useful as well. These agents include dextroamphetamine, amantadine, bromocriptine, levodopa, bupropion (sustained-release formulation), atomoxetine, and modafinil (14–16). The literature describing their effects on attention and related problems among persons with TBI and other neurological disorders suggests that these agents vary with regard to effects on processing speed and attention (vigilance). This variance in part derives from individual differences in medication responsiveness. It also may reflect interindividual variability in the relevance of catecholaminergic dysfunction to post-traumatic cognitive impairments. Additionally, individual genetic differences in catecholamine metabolism (78–80) and their influence on medication effects may contribute to individual variability in response to treatment with these agents and the doses required to produce clinical responses.

Treatment using procholinergic agents (e.g., acetylcholinesterase inhibitors) may remediate attention and processing speed impairments to the extent that those impairments reflect cerebral cholinergic deficits (18,29). However, individual variability in the occurrence and severity of posttraumatic cerebral cholinergic deficits necessitates caution with respect to the use of medications that augment cerebral cholinergic function. Among patients who are normal cognitively (and, presumably, possess relatively normal cerebral acetylcholine levels), acetylcholinesterase inhibitors may impair cognition (81,82). The evidence describing the effects of acetylcholinesterase inhibitors (i.e., physostigmine, donepezil, rivastigmine) on attention and processing speed impairments after the immediate postinjury period are mixed (46,47,50,83,84). These agents appear to be most useful for individuals with post-traumatic declarative memory impairments (16,46,47,50). Among the acetylcholinesterase inhibitors, donepezil is used most commonly in light of its relative ease of use (once-daily dosing, one-step titration to maximal dose), favorable side effect profile, and limited drug–drug interactions. Galantamine, particularly in its extended-release formulation, and transdermal rivastigmine are similarly easy to use, but there are no published reports of their use for the treatment of post-traumatic attention and processing speed impairments. In general, these agents are second-line pharmacotherapies of impaired attention and/or processing speed.

In principle, agents that normalize glutamatergic signaling (e.g., uncompetitive NMDA receptor antagonists, sigma-1 agonists) also may improve attention and processsing speed. The uncompetitive NMDA receptor antagonists memantine and amantadine are not generally used as first-line treatments for attention and processing speed impairments. However, they may improve these problems among some persons with TBI (14–16,85). The beneficial effects of these agents derive normalizing glutamatergic signaling at NMDA receptors, indirectly facilitating dopaminergic function, and other mechanisms (14).

In contexts where hyperarousal interferes with attention (e.g., severe anxiety), augmentation of GABA function (e.g., with benzodiazepines) attenuates the activity of a broad range of neurobehaviorally salient networks and neurotransmitter systems. This, in turn, reduces hyperarousal and, in some instances, limits the adverse effects of these agents on selective and sustained attention. Among most persons with TBI, however, benzodiazepines concurrently inhibit information-processing networks involved in attention, processing speed, and motor performance and therefore tend to impair these functions (44).

Serotonergic augmentation may modulate attention and processing speed via alterations of emotional, motivational, and social cognition as well as through modulatory influences on other neurotransmitter systems (86,87). Agents that influence cerebral serotonergic systems, either through global increases in serotonin or receptor subtype-specific effects, thereby indirectly alter attention and processing speed through various mechanisms. At present, however, attention and processing speed impairments usually are not primary targets of serotonergic pharmacotherapies; exceptions to this rule are depressive, anxiety, or other psychiatric disorders for which agents of these types are used to treat emotional or behavioral symptoms and secondarily improve cognitive disturbances.

Partial responses to pharmacologic monotherapy of attention and processing speed are not uncommon. In some cases, it may be reasonable to augment partial responses with a second medication that enhances attention or processing speed. Because most medications used to treat attention and processing speed augmentation of cerebral catecholaminergic function, augmentation strategies are more likely to succeed when an agent with a complementary (rather than redundant) mechanism of action is used. For example, rational augmentation of a medication that enhanced cerebral catecholaminergic function (e.g., methylphenidate) might include the addition of a medication that augments cholinergic function (e.g., donepezil) but not one that directly or indirectly augments catecholaminergic function (e.g., amantadine, memantine, carbidopa-levodopa, bromocriptine, modafinil). When augmentation is undertaken and maximally tolerated and beneficial doses established, it is important to taper the dose of the primary medication in order to determine the necessity of its continued use.

Recognition (Gnosis)

Agnosia describes a sensory domain-specific inability to recognize objects resulting from impaired integration of sensory information at a cortical level (cortically based perception), impaired attachment of meaning to those percepts (association), or both. There also are no established pharmacotherapies for any of the agnosias. Educational, supportive, environmental, behavioral interventions as well as compensatory strategies may be provided. Although the benefits of these treatments are unproven, they may help patients and families adapt to agnosia-related functional limitations. However, it is prudent to maintain modest expectations about the likelihood of benefits afforded by any attempts to treat agnosia.

Memory

Memory refers to the ability to learn, store, and retrieve information. Memory is not a unitary cognitive function; it comprises multiple cognitive processes that are supported by multiple neuroanatomical networks and neurochemical processes (88,89). In clinical practice, the evaluation and treatment of memory disturbances is simplified by dividing them into three types: working memory, declarative memory, and procedural memory.

Working Memory

Working memory refers to the process of holding information in mind, or "on-line," for a brief period immediately after that stimulus leaves the sensory field. In effect, working memory is the process of sustaining attention to a stimulus when the stimulus itself is no longer present. Working memory is predicated on a complex set of bihemispheric cortical (especially frontoparietal) and subcortical structures that are supported by multiple neurotransmitter systems (89,90). The cortical, subcortical, and/or white matter elements of these networks are susceptible to disruption by a wide range of neurological and psychiatric disorders, including TBI.

In general, the pharmacologic treatments of working memory impairments are similar to those used to treat attention and processing speed impairments—both in type and in timing. In general, augmentation of cerebral catecholaminergic function, cholinergic function, or both appears most likely to improve working memory impairments after the early post-TBI "neurotransmitter storm" wanes. When working memory, attention, and/or processing speed impairments co-occur, augmenting cerebral catecholaminergic function using stimulant medications (e.g., methylphenidate, dextroamphetamine, mixed amphetamine salts), guanfacine (an agonist at adrenergic α2A receptors) (91), atomoxetine (92), or bromocriptine (an agonist at dopamine D2 receptors) (93) also may be useful. When working memory impairments co-occur with declarative memory impairments, acetylcholinesterase inhibitors may be useful (46,47). However, these agents do not appear to be particularly useful first-line treatments of working memory impairments (94–96).

Working memory impairments are not the primary targets of serotonergic pharmacotherapies, but impairments in this function produced by depressive, anxiety, and other psychiatric disorders; working memory and other cognitive disturbances associated with these conditions may improve secondarily during treatment with such agents (47). Additionally, preclinical evidence suggests that agents that agonize nicotinic α4β2 and/or α7 receptors (e.g., augment acetylcholinergic function and its secondary effects on other neurotransmitter systems) (97,98) or that antagonize histamine H3 receptors (e.g., secondarily increasing cerebral catecholamines, acetylcholine, and histamine) (99) may become useful treatments for these types of cognitive impairments as well.

Declarative Memory

Declarative memory describes the learning (encoding), storage (consolidation), and retrieval (recall) of semantic (facts), episodic (events), and autobiographical (personal) information. Acquiring, storing, and retrieving these types of information requires intact sensory-to-cortical pathways, primary and secondary association cortices, parietal heteromodal association cortices, entorhinal-hippocampal complex, frontal cortices, and white matter connections between these areas. It is dependent on the development of long-term potentiation (LTP), a glutamatergically mediated and cholinergically dependent process (100,101) that creates relatively stable large-scale representational networks, that is, the neural bases of "memory." Impaired declarative new learning is generally associated with dysfunction of the hippocampal-forniceal-mammillothalamic pathway, and impaired volitional retrieval of declarative information is associated with dysfunction of the frontal-subcortical systems necessary for reactivation of the neural network in which such information is represented (e.g., executive control of memory).

There are no pharmacotherapies that effectively attenuate the early adverse effects of neurotransmitter excesses on declarative memory. As noted earlier in this chapter, acute cholinergic excesses are followed, in a substantial subset of patients, by chronic cerebral cholinergic deficits (18,29). When patients present with memory impairments during the subacute and/or late postinjury periods, augmentation of cerebral cholinergic function with an acetylcholinesterase inhibitor may be useful (14–16,46,47,50,102). The benefits of these agents do not appear to depend on the type of declarative memory impairment (i.e., encoding deficits, retrieval problems, or both). In clinical practice, all of the agents in this class appear to be similarly effective but often differ in terms of their tolerability. Accordingly, donepezil is used most commonly in light of its relative ease of use (once-daily dosing, one-step titration to maximal dose), favorable side effect profile, and limited drug–drug interactions. Galantamine, particularly in its extended-release formulation, and transdermal rivastigmine are similarly easy to use. However, there are no published reports of their use for the treatment of post-traumatic declarative memory impairments. Because cerebral cholinergic deficits are produced invariably by TBI, not all persons with persistent posttraumatic memory impairments are expected to respond to treatment with acetylcholinesterase inhibitors.

There is a limited literature suggesting that catecholamine augmentation using methylphenidate or neurochemically similar compounds may improve declarative memory among persons with TBI and other acquired brain injuries (14–16). In light of the neurochemistry of declarative memory reviewed earlier in this section, it is likely that the effect of catecholamine augmentation on declarative memory is indirect and related primarily to improvements in arousal, sustained attention, processing speed, working memory, depression, and/or other affective disturbances. It is possible that catecholamine augmentation might improve declarative memory more directly, although the mechanisms of this effect are incompletely characterized (103).

Uncompetitive NMDA receptor antagonists (i.e., memantine or amantadine) also improve declarative memory function associated with TBI (85). However, additional evidence demonstrating the safety and tolerability of NMDA receptor antagonists is needed before recommending them as treatments for TBI-associated declarative memory impairments.

There also is evidence that citicholine (CDP-choline) may improve declarative memory impairments associated with various neurological and psychiatric conditions, including TBI (104–106). The available evidence suggests that this is a relatively safe agent. However, the minimal regulatory oversight of the production of citicholine and the limited data regarding its efficacy and safety suggest that any use of this agent be undertaken cautiously.

As noted earlier in this chapter, preclinical reports suggest that nicotinic α4β2 and/or α7receptor agonists or histamine H3 receptors antagonists also may be useful treatments for declarative memory impairments. However, additional clinical studies are needed to determine the role, if any, of these agents for this purpose among persons with TBI.

Procedural Memory

Procedural memory, a type of implicit memory, refers to the learning, storing, and retrieval of motor sequences (i.e., "how" to do tasks), and relies on the development and fine-tuning of sensorimotor-frontal-subcortical-cerebellar networks involved in skill acquisition and performance. Conceptually, procedural learning is related to praxis, which describes the performance of previously learned skilled purposeful movement on demand. Consolidation of procedural learning is facilitated by intensive, rather than temporally distributed, rehearsal (107,108) and by sleep (especially rapid eye movement or REM sleep) (109).

Although procedural and declarative memory sometimes are described as being cleanly dissociable from each other, recent evidence (107) suggests that episodic memory and executive function are involved in the learning phase of procedural memory. Accordingly, severe disturbances and/or comorbid impairments in all three of these cognitive domains, as well as those that do not provide for adequate REM sleep (or pharmacologically disrupt it), may attenuate the benefits of compensatory strategies that rely on intact procedural memory.

The pharmacologic treatment of procedural memory impairments more specifically is underdeveloped. It is plausible that medications that improve the functioning of the sensorimotor-frontal-subcortical-cerebellar networks involved in skill acquisition and performance might facilitate improvements in procedural memory, that is, agents that augment cerebral catecholamine and/or acetylcholine levels or that normalize glutamatergic signaling. However, the effects of medications with these properties on procedural memory impairments are not yet demonstrated, and any such treatment should be regarded as investigational.

Language

Language refers to any system of symbolic communication and includes the use of verbal, written, gestural, or other symbols to effect information transfer. In most adults, the left hemisphere is dominant for the syntactic and semantic aspects of language. Injury to language-related areas of the brain disturbs syntax and/or semantics, producing clinical problems that are described as aphasias. Even when frank aphasia is not produced by TBI, injury to or disturbances of brain areas that interact with those supporting language may impair the functional use of language.

The pharmacotherapies for aphasia and functional communication impairments associated with TBI are not established but may be informed by the stroke literature. Agents augmenting cerebral dopaminergic function and/or cholinergic function may improve aphasia in the subacute and late poststroke periods (110,111). Catecholaminergic augmentation strategies for poststroke aphasia, including bromocriptine and dexamphetamine, sometimes are useful for the treatment of nonfluent aphasias, but reports of their effectiveness are mixed (112,113). The benefits conferred by these agents are relatively modest, occur in a limited subset of patients, and may be attributable to concurrent effects on motor function and/or motivational systems. Combined memantine and constraint-induced aphasia therapy (114) and combining piracetam (115,116), mixed amphetamine salts (117), or bromocriptine (113,118) with poststroke language rehabilitation also may improve aphasia outcomes over rehabilitation or pharmacotherapies alone. Whether, or to what extent, these approaches will translate usefully to the treatment of TBI-related language and functional communication impairments requires investigation.

Prosody

Prosody refers to the melodic, affective, and kinesic components of language that add meaning and enhance communication. Aprosodia results from injury to or dysfunction of areas in the nondominant hemisphere neuroanatomic homologues of the language areas of the dominant hemisphere. At the present time, there are no established pharmacotherapies for the aprosodias.

Praxis

Praxis is the process by which a skill is enacted, and the use of this term in medicine generally is limited to its negative forms: apraxia (without praxis) or dyspraxia (poor praxis). These terms describe impaired ability to perform skilled purposeful movements that is not attributable to sensory, motor, or language deficits. The neuroanatomy of praxis closely approximates the neuroanatomy of language, reflecting defects in movement representations coded for in premotor association areas of the dominant hemisphere (119). Ideational praxis engages neural systems involved in routine movements and requires their sequencing into more complex routines; as such, this form of praxis requires executive control of complex motor programming (120) and often is comorbid with executive dysfunction.

There is very little evidence to guide the pharmacotherapy of apraxia associated with any neurological condition, including TBI. There are case reports describing lessening of neurodegenerative disease-related apraxias during treatment with levodopa (121), amantadine (122), acetylcholinesterase inhibitors (123,124), and/or memantine (125–127). As with the other pharmacotherapies discussed in this chapter, if time-limited empiric trials of catecholamine-augmenting agents (including indirect augmentation with amantadine or memantine) or acetylcholinesterase inhibitors for post-traumatic apraxias are considered, then they are best undertaken in the subacute or late postinjury period.

Visuospatial Function

Visuospatial function refers to collection of complex visual processing abilities, including spatial awareness and attention, awareness of self-other and self-object spatial relationships, visuospatial memory, and the ability to interpret and navigate the extrapersonal space. Visuospatial function is supported by a distributed neural network involving the reticular system, thalamus, superior colliculus, striatum, parietal cortex, and frontal eye fields (28). Right hemispheric specialization for this cognitive function is typical, and the right parietal cortex is a critical node in the extended bihemispheric network supporting spatial attention. Visuospatial memory also is relatively lateralized to the right hemisphere, and the parahippocampal gyrus is a critical node in the visuospatial memory network (128). Catecholamines and acetylcholine modulate visuospatial function (28), although the purported influences of these neurotransmitter systems on visuospatial function are based primarily on inferences drawn from the effects of pharmacotherapies in neurodegenerative dementias or stroke.

The pharmacotherapy of poststroke hemispatial neglect generally involves treatment with catecholamine-augmenting agents including bromocriptine or methylphenidate (129). Unfortunately, these agents not infrequently exacerbate hemispatial neglect by increasing information in the healthy cerebral hemisphere and thereby increase attention to the unaffected visual hemispace (130,131). Acetylcholinesterase inhibitors and uncompetitive NMDA receptor antagonists may improve visuospatial function among persons with neurodegenerative dementias (123) or stroke (132). Collectively, the available evidence suggests that there may be a role for pharmacotherapy in the treatment of TBI-related visuospatial dysfunction during the period following abatement of the "neurotransmitter storm." However, if medication is added to other rehabilitative interventions for this problem, assiduous monitoring for treatment-induced exacerbation of hemispatial inattention is essential.

Executive Function

Executive function refers to a broad set of cognitive processes needed to meet the demands of everyday life in a flexible and adaptive fashion. These processes are of two general types: executive control functions over the relatively more "basic" cognitive domains described in the preceding sections of this chapter and intrinsic executive functions such as categorization and abstraction, problem solving, behavioral planning and organization, and set shifting (133,134). Executive function relies on the dorsolateral prefrontal-subcortical circuits in both cerebral hemispheres and their connections to brain areas serving other sensory, motor, cognitive, emotional, and behavioral functions (135), and interacts with other prefrontal-subcortical circuits and limbic-subcortical circuits to provide executive control of motivation, social cognition, and emotion (135). Executive function is influenced by all of the major neurotransmitter systems, including glutamate, GABA, acetylcholine, dopamine, norepinephrine, serotonin, and histamine (135). Impairments in this cognitive domain may result from injury to or dysfunction of these circuits, their open-loop elements, or a broad range of neurotransmitter disturbances and is common among persons with TBI (136).

Despite the common occurrence of executive dysfunction in the early and late postinjury periods, few studies are available to guide the pharmacotherapy of this problem. The neuroanatomy and neurochemistry of executive function predict that problems in this cognitive domain are likely to be accompanied by other neuropsychiatric disturbances including other cognitive impairments, emotional and behavioral disturbances, motor dysfunction, and/or movement disorders. Identifying and treating such problems should precede attempts to pharmacologically remediate executive dysfunction specifically (133).

In general, pharmacotherapies for executive dysfunction are best reserved for the subacute (i.e., rehabilitation) and late postinjury periods. Treatment selection is most usefully guided by co-occuring types of cognitive dysfunction. For example, co-occurring impairments of attention, processing speed, working memory, and executive function suggest that the use of catecholamine augmentation (e.g., methylphenidate) is the best initial pharmacologic approach. When executive dysfunction co-occurs with declarative memory impairments, a cholinesterase inhibitor may be the most useful initial pharmacotherapy. Combination therapies, including catecholamine-augmenting agents, acetylcholinesterase inhibitors, and/or uncompetitive NMDA receptor antagonists may be needed in some cases (14,137).

CONCLUSION

Pharmacotherapy is one of several potentially useful strategies for the treatment of post-traumatic cognitive impairments. When medications are prescribed for post-traumatic cognitive impairments, they are most appropriately regarded as adjunctive to other interventions. Their use is guided by the principles of pharmacotherapy presented in Chapter 74.

Interindividual differences in TBI-induced abnormalities of brain structure, dysfunction of neurotransmitter systems, and genetically mediated neurotransmitter metabolism may offer some explanation for the variable benefits afforded by cognitive pharmacotherapies. Additionally, the effects of any given pharmacotherapy will vary with time postinjury at which treatment is undertaken, and few of the presently available treatments are likely to improve cognitive function in the midst of the "neurotransmitter storm" that develops in the immediate postinjury period.

The neurochemistry of cognition and the neurochemical consequences of TBI suggest that catecholaminergic, cholinergic, and glutamatergic systems are likely to be the most useful neurochemical targets of pharmacologic intervention among persons with cognitive impairments in the subacute and late postinjury periods. In the absence of cost-effective and widely available in vivo markers of neurotransmitter function with which to guide the selection of a class of medication, pharmacologic treatment of post-traumatic cognitive impairments in an individual patient remains a matter of clinical judgment and empiric trial. Some patients respond robustly to catecholaminergic agents, others to cholinesterase inhibitors or uncompetitive NMDA receptor antagonists, some require treatment with some combination of these agents, and others respond poorly to all presently available medications. Additional studies are needed to clarify which agents are most effective for which types of post-traumatic cognitive impairments, and better methods are needed to facilitate the identification of patients most likely to respond to cognitive pharmacotherapies.

KEY CLINICAL POINTS

1. Pharmacotherapy is a potentially effective element of a comprehensive treatment plan for post-traumatic cognitive impairments and is regarded most appropriately as adjunctive to other interventions.
2. The literature describing the benefits, risks, and side effects of medications used for this purpose is underdeveloped. Treatment selection therefore is guided by synthesizing information gleaned from studies of persons with TBI, patients with phenomenologically similar but etiologically distinct conditions, expert opinions, and consensus statements.
3. Rational pharmacotherapy requires consideration of the intended targets of treatment, initial TBI severity, time postinjury, and the stage of post-traumatic encephalopathy during which the cognitive target symptom occurs.
4. Effective interventions for cognitive impairments in the immediate postinjury period are predominantly nonpharmacologic. In the subacute and late postinjury periods, catecholamine augmentation (e.g., stimulants), cholinergic augmentation (e.g., acetylcholinesterase inhibitors), and glutamatergic stabilization (e.g., uncompetitive NMDA receptor antagonists) are the principal pharmacologic interventions for post-traumatic cognitive impairments.
5. Interindividual differences in TBI-induced abnormalities of brain structure, dysfunction of neurotransmitter systems, and genetically mediated neurotransmitter metabolism may offer some explanation for the variable benefits afforded by cognitive pharmacotherapies.

KEY REFERENCES

1. Arciniegas DB, Frey KL, Newman J, Wortzel HS. Evaluation and management of posttraumatic cognitive impairments. *Psychiatr Ann.* 2010;40(11):540–552.
2. Arciniegas DB, Silver JM. Pharmacotherapy of posttraumatic cognitive impairments. *Behav Neurol.* 2006;17(1): 25–42.
3. Bigler ED. Anterior and middle cranial fossa in traumatic brain injury: relevant neuroanatomy and neuropathology in the study of neuropsychological outcome. *Neuropsychology.* 2007;21(5):515–531.
4. Chew E, Zafonte RD. Pharmacological management of neurobehavioral disorders following traumatic brain injury—a state-of-the-art review. *J Rehabil Res Dev.* 2009; 46(6):851–879.
5. Jordan BD. Genetic influences on outcome following traumatic brain injury. *Neurochem Res.* 2007;32(4–5):905–915.
6. McAllister TW. Polymorphisms in genes modulating the dopamine system: do they influence outcome and response to medication after traumatic brain injury? *J Head Trauma Rehabil.* 2009;24(1):65–68.
7. Shaw NA. The neurophysiology of concussion. *Prog Neurobiol.* 2002;67(4):281–344.
8. Warden DL, Gordon B, McAllister TW, et al. Guidelines for the pharmacologic treatment of neurobehavioral sequelae of traumatic brain injury. *J Neurotrauma.* 2006; 23(10):1468–1501.

References

1. Dikmen SS, Corrigan JD, Levin HS, Machamer J, Stiers W, Weisskopf MG. Cognitive outcome following traumatic brain injury. *J Head Trauma Rehabil.* 2009;24(6):430–438.
2. Kay T, Harrington DE, Adams RE, et al. Definition of mild traumatic brain injury: Report from the Mild Traumatic Brain Injury Committee of the Head Injury Interdisciplinary Special Interest Group of the American Congress of Rehabilitation Medicine. *J Head Trauma Rehabil.* 1993;8(3):86–87.
3. Menon DK, Schwab K, Wright DW, Maas AI. Position statement: definition of traumatic brain injury. *Arch Phys Med Rehabil.* 2010; 91(11):1637–1640.
4. Management of Concussion/mTBI Working Group. VA/DoD Clinical Practice Guideline for Management of Concussion/Mild Traumatic Brain Injury. *J Rehabil Res Dev.* 2009;46(6):CP1–CP68.
5. Carroll LJ, Cassidy JD, Peloso PM, et al. Prognosis for mild traumatic brain injury: results of the WHO collaborating centre task force on mild traumatic brain injury. *J Rehabil Med.* 2004;(43 suppl): 84–105.
6. McCrea M, Iverson GL, McAllister TW, et al. An integrated review of recovery after mild traumatic brain injury (MTBI): implications for clinical management. *Clin Neuropsychol.* 2009;23(8):1368–1390.
7. Cicerone KD. Evidence-based practice and the limits of rational rehabilitation. *Arch Phys Med Rehabil.* 2005;86(6):1073–1074.
8. Cicerone KD, Dahlberg C, Kalmar K, et al. Evidence-based cognitive rehabilitation: recommendations for clinical practice. *Arch Phys Med Rehabil.* 2000;81(12):1596–1615.
9. Cicerone KD, Dahlberg C, Malec JF, et al. Evidence-based cognitive rehabilitation: updated review of the literature from 1998 through 2002. *Arch Phys Med Rehabil.* 2005;86(8):1681–1692.
10. Cicerone KD, Langenbahn DM, Braden C, et al. Evidence-based cognitive rehabilitation: updated review of the literature from 2003 through 2008. *Arch Phys Med Rehabil.* 2011;92(4):519–530.
11. Bell KR, Hoffman JM, Doctor JN, et al. Development of a telephone follow-up program for individuals following traumatic brain injury. *J Head Trauma Rehabil.* 2004;19(6):502–512.
12. Bell KR, Hoffman JM, Temkin NR, et al. The effect of telephone counselling on reducing post-traumatic symptoms after mild traumatic brain injury: a randomised trial. *J Neurol Neurosurg Psychiatry.* 2008;79(11):1275–1281.
13. Bell KR, Temkin NR, Esselman PC, et al. The effect of a scheduled telephone intervention on outcome after moderate to severe traumatic brain injury: a randomized trial. *Arch Phys Med Rehabil.* 2005; 86(5):851–856.
14. Arciniegas DB, Silver JM. Pharmacotherapy of posttraumatic cognitive impairments. *Behav Neurol.* 2006;17(1):25–42.
15. Chew E, Zafonte RD. Pharmacological management of neurobehavioral disorders following traumatic brain injury—a state-of-the-art review. *J Rehabil Res Dev.* 2009;46(6):851–879.
16. Neurobehavioral Guidelines Working Group, Warden DL, Gordon B, et al. Guidelines for the pharmacologic treatment of neurobehavioral sequelae of traumatic brain injury. *J Neurotrauma.* 2006;23(10): 1468–1501.
17. Bigler ED. Anterior and middle cranial fossa in traumatic brain injury: relevant neuroanatomy and neuropathology in the study of neuropsychological outcome. *Neuropsychology.* 2007;21(5):515–531.

18. Arciniegas DB. Cholinergic dysfunction and cognitive impairment after traumatic brain injury. Part 2: evidence from basic and clinical investigations. *J Head Trauma Rehabil.* 2011;26(4):319–323.

19. Arciniegas DB, McAllister TW. Neurobehavioral management of traumatic brain injury in the critical care setting. *Crit Care Clin.* 2008;24(4):737–765.

20. Meythaler JM, Peduzzi JD, Eleftheriou E, Novack TA. Current concepts: diffuse axonal injury-associated traumatic brain injury. *Arch Phys Med Rehabil.* 2001;82(10):1461–1471.

21. Povlishock JT, Katz DI. Update of neuropathology and neurological recovery after traumatic brain injury. *J Head Trauma Rehabil.* 2005;20(1):76–94.

22. Arciniegas DB, Frey KL, Newman J, Wortzel HS. Evaluation and management of posttraumatic cognitive impairments. *Psychiatr Ann.* 2010;40(11):540–552.

23. Giza CC, Hovda DA. The neurometabolic cascade of concussion. *J Athl Train.* 2001;36(3):228–235.

24. Shaw NA. The neurophysiology of concussion. *Prog Neurobiol.* 2002;67(4):281–344.

25. Bales JW, Wagner AK, Kline AE, Dixon CE. Persistent cognitive dysfunction after traumatic brain injury: a dopamine hypothesis. *Neurosci Biobehav Rev.* 2009;33(7):981–1003.

26. McAllister TW. Polymorphisms in genes modulating the dopamine system: do they influence outcome and response to medication after traumatic brain injury? *J Head Trauma Rehabil.* 2009;24(1):65–68.

27. Redell JB, Dash PK. Traumatic brain injury stimulates hippocampal catechol-O-methyl transferase expression in microglia. *Neurosci Lett.* 2007;413(1):36–41.

28. Mesulam M-M. Attentional networks, confusional states, and neglect syndromes. In: Mesulam MM, ed. *Principles of Behavioral and Cognitive Neurology.* 2nd ed. Oxford, UK: Oxford University Press; 2000:174–256.

29. Arciniegas DB. Cholinergic dysfunction and cognitive impairment after traumatic brain injury. Part 1: the structure and function of cerebral cholinergic systems. *J Head Trauma Rehabil.* 2011;26(1):98–101.

30. Rammsayer TH. Effects of pharmacologically induced changes in NMDA-receptor activity on long-term memory in humans. *Learn Mem.* 2001;8(1):20–25.

31. Rammsayer TH. Effects of pharmacologically induced changes in NMDA receptor activity on human timing and sensorimotor performance. *Brain Res.* 2006;1073–1074:407–416.

32. Parsons CG, Stöffler A, Danysz W. Memantine: a NMDA receptor antagonist that improves memory by restoration of homeostasis in the glutamatergic system—too little activation is bad, too much is even worse. *Neuropharmacology.* 2007;53(6):699–723.

33. Mehta MA, Riedel WJ. Dopaminergic enhancement of cognitive function. *Curr Pharm Des.* 2006;12(20):2487–2500.

34. Robbins TW, Roberts AC. Differential regulation of fronto-executive function by the monoamines and acetylcholine. *Cereb Cortex.* 2007;17(suppl 1):i151–i160.

35. Buhot MC, Martin S, Segu L. Role of serotonin in memory impairment. *Ann Med.* 2000;32(3):210–221.

36. Goldstein LB. Neuropharmacology of TBI-induced plasticity. *Brain Inj.* 2003;17(8):685–694.

37. Liepert J. Pharmacotherapy in restorative neurology. *Curr Opin Neurol.* 2008;21(6):639–643.

38. Mysiw WJ, Bogner JA, Corrigan JD, Fugate LP, Clinchot DM, Kadyan V. The impact of acute care medications on rehabilitation outcome after traumatic brain injury. *Brain Inj.* 2006;20(9):905–911.

39. Cappa SF, Benke T, Clarke S, Rossi B, Stemmer B, van Heugten CM. EFNS guidelines on cognitive rehabilitation: report of an EFNS task force. *Eur J Neurol.* 2003;10(1):11–23.

40. Cappa SF, Benke T, Clarke S, Rossi B, Stemmer B, van Heugten CM. EFNS guidelines on cognitive rehabilitation: report of an EFNS task force. *Eur J Neurol.* 2005;12(9):665–680.

41. Arciniegas DB. Addressing neuropsychiatric disturbances during rehabilitation after traumatic brain injury: current and future methods. *Dialogues Clin Neurosci.* 2011;13(3):325–345.

42. Schierhout G, Roberts I. Anti-epileptic drugs for preventing seizures following acute traumatic brain injury. *Cochrane Database Syst Rev.* 2001;(4):CD000173.

43. Rao N, Jellinek HM, Woolston DC. Agitation in closed head injury: haloperidol effects on rehabilitation outcome. *Arch Phys Med Rehabil.* 1985;66(1):30–34.

44. Bleiberg J, Garmoe W, Cederquist J, Reeves D, Lux W. Effects of dexedrine on performance consistency following brain injury: a double-blind placebo crossover case-study. *Neuropsy Neuropsy Be.* 1993;6(4):245–248.

45. Fortin MP, Rouch I, Dauphinot V, et al. Effects of anticholinergic drugs on verbal episodic memory function in the elderly: a retrospective, cross-sectional study. *Drugs Aging.* 2011;28(3):195–204.

46. Silver JM, Koumaras B, Chen M, et al. Effects of rivastigmine on cognitive function in patients with traumatic brain injury. *Neurology.* 2006;67(5):748–755.

47. Silver JM, Koumaras B, Meng X, et al. Long-term effects of rivastigmine capsules in patients with traumatic brain injury. *Brain Inj.* 2009;23(2):123–132.

48. Wheaton P, Mathias JL, Vink R. Impact of early pharmacological treatment on cognitive and behavioral outcome after traumatic brain injury in adults: a meta-analysis. *J Clin Psychopharmacol.* 2009;29(5):468–477.

49. Whyte J, Myers R. Incidence of clinically significant responses to zolpidem among patients with disorders of consciousness: a preliminary placebo controlled trial. *Am J Phys Med Rehabil.* 2009;88(5):410–418.

50. Zhang L, Plotkin RC, Wang G, Sandel ME, Lee S. Cholinergic augmentation with donepezil enhances recovery in short-term memory and sustained attention after traumatic brain injury. *Arch Phys Med Rehabil.* 2004;85(7):1050–1055.

51. Meythaler JM, Brunner RC, Johnson A, Novack TA. Amantadine to improve neurorecovery in traumatic brain injury-associated diffuse axonal injury: a pilot double-blind randomized trial. *J Head Trauma Rehabil.* 2002;17(4):300–313.

52. Giacino JT, Whyte J. Amantadine to improve neurorecovery in traumatic brain injury-associated diffuse axonal injury: a pilot double-blind randomized trial. *J Head Trauma Rehabil.* 2003;18(1):4–5.

53. Whyte J, Katz D, Long D, et al. Predictors of outcome in prolonged posttraumatic disorders of consciousness and assessment of medication effects: a multicenter study. *Arch Phys Med Rehabil.* 2005;86(3):453–462.

54. Passler MA, Riggs RV. Positive outcomes in traumatic brain injury-vegetative state: patients treated with bromocriptine. *Arch Phys Med Rehabil.* 2001;82(3):311–315.

55. Patrick PD, Buck ML, Conaway MR, Blackman JA. The use of dopamine enhancing medications with children in low response states following brain injury. *Brain Inj.* 2003;17(6):497–506.

56. Hornyak JE, Nelson VS, Hurvitz EA. The use of methylphenidate in paediatric traumatic brain injury. *Pediatr Rehabil.* 1997;1(1):15–17.

57. Worzniak M, Fetters MD, Comfort M. Methylphenidate in the treatment of coma. *J Fam Pract.* 1997;44(5):495–498.

58. Showalter PE, Kimmel DN. Stimulating consciousness and cognition following severe brain injury: a new potential clinical use for lamotrigine. *Brain Inj.* 2000;14(11):997–1001.

59. Rivera VM. Modafinil for the treatment of diminished responsiveness in a patient recovering from brain surgery. *Brain Inj.* 2005;19(9):725–727.

60. Clauss RP, Nel WH. Effect of zolpidem on brain injury and diaschisis as detected by 99mTc HMPAO brain SPECT in humans. *Arzneimittelforschung.* 2004;54(10):641–646.

61. Cohen SI, Duong TT. Increased arousal in a patient with anoxic brain injury after administration of zolpidem. *Am J Phys Med Rehabil.* 2008;87(3):229–231.

62. Arciniegas DB. Neuropsychiatric assessment of traumatic brain injury during acute neurorehabilitation. In: Miyoshi K, Morimura Y, Maeda K, eds. *Neuropsychiatric Disorders.* Tokyo, Japan: Springer; 2010:125–146.

63. van Wageningen H, Jørgensen HA, Specht K, Hugdahl K. Evidence for glutamatergic neurotransmission in cognitive control in an auditory attention task. *Neurosci Lett.* 2009;454(3):171–175.

64. Tabet N, Howard R. Non-pharmacological interventions in the prevention of delirium. *Age Ageing*. 2009;38(4):374–379.

65. Hoffman AN, Cheng JP, Zafonte RD, Kline AE. Administration of haloperidol and risperidone after neurobehavioral testing hinders the recovery of traumatic brain injury-induced deficits. *Life Sci*. 2008;83(17–18):602–607.

66. Tabet N, Howard R. Pharmacological treatment for the prevention of delirium: review of current evidence. *Int J Geriatr Psychiatry*. 2009;24(10):1037–1044.

67. Lyeth BG, Dixon CE, Jenkins LW, et al. Effects of scopolamine treatment on long-term behavioral deficits following concussive brain injury to the rat. *Brain Res*. 1988;452(1–2):39–48.

68. Saija A, Robinson SE, Lyeth BG, et al. The effects of scopolamine and traumatic brain injury on central cholinergic neurons. *J Neurotrauma*. 1988;5(2):161–170.

69. Whyte J, Hart T, Vaccaro M, et al. Effects of methylphenidate on attention deficits after traumatic brain injury: a multidimensional, randomized, controlled trial. *Am J Phys Med Rehabil*. 2004;83(6):401–420.

70. Willmott C, Ponsford J. Efficacy of methylphenidate in the rehabilitation of attention following traumatic brain injury: a randomised, crossover, double blind, placebo controlled inpatient trial. *J Neurol Neurosurg Psychiatry*. 2009;80(5):552–557.

71. Willmott C, Ponsford J, Olver J, Ponsford M. Safety of methylphenidate following traumatic brain injury: impact on vital signs and side-effects during inpatient rehabilitation. *J Rehabil Med*. 2009;41(7):585–587.

72. Alban JP, Hopson MM, Ly V, Whyte J. Effect of methylphenidate on vital signs and adverse effects in adults with traumatic brain injury. *Am J Phys Med Rehabil*. 2004;83(2):131–137.

73. Burke DT, Glenn MB, Vesali F, et al. Effects of methylphenidate on heart rate and blood pressure among inpatients with acquired brain injury. *Am J Phys Med Rehabil*. 2003;82(7):493–497.

74. Wroblewski BA, Leary JM, Phelan AM, Whyte J, Manning K. Methylphenidate and seizure frequency in brain injured patients with seizure disorders. *J Clin Psychiatry*. 1992;53(3):86–89.

75. Feldman H, Crumrine P, Handen BL, Alvin R, Teodori J. Methylphenidate in children with seizures and attention-deficit disorder. *Am J Dis Child*. 1989;143(9):1081–1086.

76. Castells X, Casas M, Pérez-Mañá C, Roncero C, Vidal X, Capellà D. Efficacy of psychostimulant drugs for cocaine dependence. *Cochrane Database Syst Rev*. 2010;(2):CD007380.

77. Castells X, Casas M, Vidal X, et al. Efficacy of central nervous system stimulant treatment for cocaine dependence: a systematic review and meta-analysis of randomized controlled clinical trials. *Addiction*. 2007;102(12):1871–1887.

78. Lipsky RH, Sparling MB, Ryan LM, et al. Association of COMT Val158Met genotype with executive functioning following traumatic brain injury. *J Neuropsychiatry Clin Neurosci*. 2005;17(4):465–471.

79. Jordan BD. Genetic influences on outcome following traumatic brain injury. *Neurochem Res*. 2007;32(4–5):905–915.

80. McAllister TW, Flashman LA, Sparling MB, Saykin AJ. Working memory deficits after traumatic brain injury: catecholaminergic mechanisms and prospects for treatment—a review. *Brain Inj*. 2004;18(4):331–350.

81. Beglinger LJ, Tangphao-Daniels O, Kareken DA, Zhang L, Mohs R, Siemers ER. Neuropsychological test performance in healthy elderly volunteers before and after donepezil administration: a randomized, controlled study. *J Clin Psychopharmacol*. 2005;25(2):159–165.

82. Beglinger LJ, Gaydos BL, Kareken DA, Tangphao-Daniels O, Siemers ER, Mohs RC. Neuropsychological test performance in healthy volunteers before and after donepezil administration. *J Psychopharmacol*. 2004;18(1):102–108.

83. Levin HS, Peters BH, Kalisky Z, et al. Effects of oral physostigmine and lecithin on memory and attention in closed head-injured patients. *Cent Nerv Syst Trauma*. 1986;3(4):333–342.

84. Tenovuo O, Alin J, Helenius H. A randomized controlled trial of rivastigmine for chronic sequels of traumatic brain injury-what it showed and taught? *Brain Inj*. 2009;23(6):548–558.

85. Kim YW, Shin JC, An YS. Changes in cerebral glucose metabolism in patients with posttraumatic cognitive impairment after memantine therapy: a preliminary study. *Ann Nucl Med*. 2010;24(5):363–369.

86. Fink KB, Göthert M. 5-HT receptor regulation of neurotransmitter release. *Pharmacol Rev*. 2007;59(4):360–417.

87. Canli T, Omura K, Haas BW, Fallgatter A, Constable RT, Lesch KP. Beyond affect: a role for genetic variation of the serotonin transporter in neural activation during a cognitive attention task. *Proc Natl Acad Sci USA*. 2005;102(34):12224–12229.

88. Aigner TG. Pharmacology of memory: cholinergic-glutamatergic interactions. *Curr Opin Neurobiol*. 1995;5(2):155–160.

89. Budson AE. Understanding memory dysfunction. *Neurologist*. 2009;15(2):71–79.

90. Schlösser RG, Wagner G, Sauer H. Assessing the working memory network: studies with functional magnetic resonance imaging and structural equation modeling. *Neuroscience*. 2006;139(1):91–103.

91. Gamo NJ, Arnsten AF. Molecular modulation of prefrontal cortex: rational development of treatments for psychiatric disorders. *Behav Neurosci*. 2011;125(3):282–296.

92. Hazell PL, Kohn MR, Dickson R, Walton RJ, Granger RE, van Wyk GW. Core ADHD symptom improvement with atomoxetine versus methylphenidate: a direct comparison meta-analysis. *J Atten Disord*. 2011;15(8):674–683.

93. Wallace DL, Vytlacil JJ, Nomura EM, Gibbs SE, D'Esposito M. The dopamine agonist bromocriptine differentially affects fronto-striatal functional connectivity during working memory. *Front Hum Neurosci*. 2011;5:32.

94. Sharma T, Reed C, Aasen I, Kumari V. Cognitive effects of adjunctive 24-weeks rivastigmine treatment to antipsychotics in schizophrenia: a randomized, placebo-controlled, double-blind investigation. *Schizophr Res*. 2006;85(1–3):73–83.

95. Stip E, Sepehry AA, Chouinard S. Add-on therapy with acetylcholinesterase inhibitors for memory dysfunction in schizophrenia: a systematic quantitative review, part 2. *Clin Neuropharmacol*. 2007;30(4):218–229.

96. Dyer MA, Freudenreich O, Culhane MA, et al. High-dose galantamine augmentation inferior to placebo on attention, inhibitory control and working memory performance in nonsmokers with schizophrenia. *Schizophr Res*. 2008;102(1–3):88–95.

97. D'Souza MS, Markou A. Schizophrenia and tobacco smoking comorbidity: nAChR agonists in the treatment of schizophrenia-associated cognitive deficits. *Neuropharmacology*. 2011; Epub ahead of print.

98. Wallace TL, Porter RH. Targeting the nicotinic alpha7 acetylcholine receptor to enhance cognition in disease. *Biochem Pharmacol*. 2011;82(8):891–903.

99. Brioni JD, Esbenshade TA, Garrison TR, Bitner SR, Cowart MD. Discovery of histamine H3 antagonists for the treatment of cognitive disorders and Alzheimer's disease. *J Pharmacol Exp Ther*. 2011;336(1):38–46.

100. Giovannini MG. The role of the extracellular signal-regulated kinase pathway in memory encoding. *Rev Neurosci*. 2006;17(6):619–634.

101. Kullmann DM, Lamsa KP. Long-term synaptic plasticity in hippocampal interneurons. *Nat Rev Neurosci*. 2007;8(9):687–699.

102. Kim YW, Kim DY, Shin JC, Park CI, Lee JD. The changes of cortical metabolism associated with the clinical response to donepezil therapy in traumatic brain injury. *Clin Neuropharmacol*. 2009;32(2):63–68.

103. Dujardin K, Laurent B. Dysfunction of the human memory systems: role of the dopaminergic transmission. *Curr Opin Neurol*. 2003;16(suppl 2):S11–S16.

104. Levin HS. Treatment of postconcussional symptoms with CDP-choline. *J Neurol Sci*. 1991;103(suppl):S39–S42.

105. Zafonte R, Friedewald WT, Lee SM, et al. The citicoline brain injury treatment (COBRIT) trial: design and methods. *J Neurotrauma*. 2009;26(12):2207–2216.

106. Leon-Carrión J, Dominguez-Roldán JM, Murillo-Cabezas F, del Rosario Dominguez-Morales M, Muñoz-Sanchez MA. The role of citicholine in neuropsychological training after traumatic brain injury. *NeuroRehabilitation*. 2000;14(1):33–40.

107. Beaunieux H, Hubert V, Witkowski T, et al. Which processes are involved in cognitive procedural learning? *Memory.* 2006;14(5):521–539.

108. Hauptmann B, Reinhart E, Brandt SA, Karni A. The predictive value of the leveling off of within session performance for procedural memory consolidation. *Brain Res Cogn Brain Res.* 2005;24(2):181–189.

109. Walker MP, Brakefield T, Morgan A, Hobson JA, Stickgold R. Practice with sleep makes perfect: sleep-dependent motor skill learning. *Neuron.* 2002;35(1):205–211.

110. Berthier ML, Green C, Higueras C, Fernandez I, Hinojosa J, Martín MC. A randomized, placebo-controlled study of donepezil in poststroke aphasia. *Neurology.* 2006;67(9):1687–1689.

111. Berthier ML, Hinojosa J, Martin Mdel C, Fernández I. Open-label study of donepezil in chronic poststroke aphasia. *Neurology.* 2003;60(7):1218–1219.

112. Whiting E, Chenery HJ, Chalk J, Copland DA. Dexamphetamine boosts naming treatment effects in chronic aphasia. *J Int Neuropsychol Soc.* 2007;13(6):972–979.

113. Ashtary F, Janghorbani M, Chitsaz A, Reisi M, Bahrami A. A randomized, double-blind trial of bromocriptine efficacy in nonfluent aphasia after stroke. *Neurology.* 2006;66(6):914–916.

114. Berthier ML, Green C, Lara JP, et al. Memantine and constraint-induced aphasia therapy in chronic poststroke aphasia. *Ann Neurol.* 2009;65(5):577–585.

115. Enderby P, Broeckx J, Hospers W, Schildermans F, Deberdt W. Effect of piracetam on recovery and rehabilitation after stroke: a double-blind, placebo-controlled study. *Clin Neuropharmacol.* 1994;17(4):320–331.

116. Huber W. The role of piracetam in the treatment of acute and chronic aphasia. *Pharmacopsychiatry.* 1999;32(suppl 1):38–43.

117. Spiegel DR, Alexander G. A case of nonfluent aphasia treated successfully with speech therapy and adjunctive mixed amphetamine salts. *J Neuropsychiatry Clin Neurosci.* 2011;23(1):E24.

118. Bragoni M, Altieri M, Di Piero V, Padovani A, Mostardini C, Lenzi GL. Bromocriptine and speech therapy in non-fluent chronic aphasia after stroke. *Neurol Sci.* 2000;21(1):19–22.

119. Leiguarda R. Limb apraxia: cortical or subcortical. *Neuroimage.* 2001;14(1, pt 2):S137–S141.

120. Shallice T. Fractionation of the supervisory system. In: Stuss DT, Knight RT, eds. *Principles of Frontal Lobe Function.* New York, NY: Oxford University Press; 2002:261–277.

121. Yamada S, Matsuo K, Hirayama M, Sobue G. The effects of levodopa on apraxia of lid opening: a case report. *Neurology.* 2004;62(5):830–831.

122. Yasuoka T, Ikeda M, Maki N, Hokoishi K, Komori K, Tanabe H. A case of corticobasal degeneration of which movemental disturbances were improved by administration of amantadine. *No To Shinkei.* 2001;53(8):781–785.

123. Kim E, Lee Y, Lee J, Han SH. A case with cholinesterase inhibitor responsive asymmetric posterior cortical atrophy. *Clin Neurol Neurosurg.* 2005;108(1):97–101.

124. Burns A, Bernabei R, Bullock R, et al. Safety and efficacy of galantamine (Reminyl) in severe Alzheimer's disease (the SERAD study): a randomised, placebo-controlled, double-blind trial. *Lancet Neurol.* 2009;8(1):39–47.

125. Schmitt FA, van Dyck CH, Wichems CH, Olin JT. Cognitive response to memantine in moderate to severe Alzheimer disease patients already receiving donepezil: an exploratory reanalysis. *Alzheimer Dis Assoc Disord.* 2006;20(4):255–262.

126. Emre M, Mecocci P, Stender K. Pooled analyses on cognitive effects of memantine in patients with moderate to severe Alzheimer's disease. *J Alzheimers Dis.* 2008;14(2):193–199.

127. Mecocci P, Bladstrom A, Stender K. Effects of memantine on cognition in patients with moderate to severe Alzheimer's disease: post-hoc analyses of ADAS-cog and SIB total and single-item scores from six randomized, double-blind, placebo-controlled studies. *Int J Geriatr Psychiatry.* 2009;24(5):532–538.

128. Epstein R, Kanwisher N. A cortical representation of the local visual environment. *Nature.* 1998;392(6676):598–601.

129. Mukand JA, Guilmette TJ, Allen DG, et al. Dopaminergic therapy with carbidopa L-dopa for left neglect after stroke: a case series. *Arch Phys Med Rehabil.* 2001;82(9):1279–1282.

130. Barrett AM. Dopamine agonists reorient visual exploration away from the neglected hemispace. *Neurology.* 1999;53(7):1610.

131. Barrett AM, Crucian GP, Schwartz RL, Heilman KM. Adverse effect of dopamine agonist therapy in a patient with motor-intentional neglect. *Arch Phys Med Rehabil.* 1999;80(5):600–603.

132. Paolucci S, Bureca I, Multari M, Nocentini U, Matano A. An open-label pilot study of the use of rivastigmine to promote functional recovery in patients with unilateral spatial neglect due to first ischemic stroke. *Funct Neurol.* 2010;25(4):195–200.

133. Royall DR, Lauterbach EC, Cummings JL, et al. Executive control function: a review of its promise and challenges for clinical research. A report from the Committee on Research of the American Neuropsychiatric Association. *J Neuropsychiatry Clin Neurosci.* 2002;14(4):377–405.

134. Royall DR, Lauterbach EC, Kaufer D, Malloy P, Coburn KL, Black KJ. The cognitive correlates of functional status: a review from the Committee on Research of the American Neuropsychiatric Association. *J Neuropsychiatry Clin Neurosci.* 2007;19(3):249–265.

135. Mesulam M-M. Behavioral neuroanatomy: large-scale networks, association cortex, frontal syndromes, the limbic system, and hemispheric specializations. In: Mesulam MM, ed. *Principles of Behavioral and Cognitive Neurology.* 2nd ed. New York, NY: Oxford University Press; 2000:1–120.

136. Cicerone K, Levin H, Malec J, Stuss D, Whyte J. Cognitive rehabilitation interventions for executive function: moving from bench to bedside in patients with traumatic brain injury. *J Cogn Neurosci.* 2006;18(7):1212–1222.

137. Silver JM, McAllister TW, Arciniegas DB. Depression and cognitive complaints following mild traumatic brain injury. *Am J Psychiatry.* 2009;166(6):653–661.

Pharmacotherapy of Neuropsychiatric Disturbances

David B. Arciniegas and Jonathan M. Silver

INTRODUCTION

The neuropsychiatric consequences of traumatic brain injury (TBI) include depression, mania, affective lability, anxiety, apathy, psychosis, aggression, fatigue, and sleep disturbances, among many others. Although each of these conditions may develop as an independent problem after TBI, they more commonly occur in combinations or in partial forms that cross conventional diagnostic boundaries. The occurrence of neuropsychiatric problems after TBI reflects the combined influences of preinjury vulnerability factors (i.e., preinjury psychiatric conditions, genetics, and psychosocial circumstances) and injury-related factors (i.e., anatomic location and/or severity of injury) on brain systems regulating cognition, emotion, and behavior. Additionally, the development and persistence of such problems is influenced by many postinjury factors, including psychological responses, coping styles, social and economic circumstances, and medicolegal issues.

The relationships between preinjury, injury-related, and postinjury factors as they contribute to post-traumatic neuropsychiatric disturbances are complex (Figure 74-1). Regardless of the mechanisms by which they develop, the neuropsychiatric consequences of TBI complicate recovery and neurorehabilitation, are substantial sources of suffering for those in whom they develop, and are important targets of treatment. A complete review of the epidemiology, pathophysiology, and phenomenology of post-traumatic neuropsychiatric disturbances is beyond the scope of this chapter, and readers are referred to Chapter 62 in this volume for additional information on these matters. In this chapter, such matters are reviewed only when they are directly relevant to neuropsychiatric pharmacotherapy. This approach should not be misconstrued as suggesting that a cursory consideration of these issues is acceptable in clinical practice; quite the contrary, clinicians are encouraged to perform a comprehensive evaluation of each individual for whom neuropsychiatric pharmacotherapy is considered.

Similar to the treatment of psychiatric disorders such as depression, panic disorder, and obsessive–compulsive disorder, a combination of therapeutic interventions (e.g., medications, rehabilitative therapies, psychotherapies) administered simultaneously to the person with neuropsychiatric disturbances after TBI is often more effective than an approach employing only 1 mode of treatment. Individual, cognitive, behavioral, and family therapy, as well as environmental accommodations, may alleviate neuropsychiatric disturbances and improve recovery from and/or adjustment to TBI. These and other nonpharmacologic interventions are reviewed in Chapters 60, 61, 63, 64, and 79 among others in this volume. Accordingly, the present chapter focuses narrowly on pharmacotherapy of neuropsychiatric disturbances following TBI.

PRETREATMENT EVALUATION

Prior to initiating any pharmacologic treatment, a comprehensive neuropsychiatric history (Table 74-1) and examination (Table 74-2) is required. Presenting complaints must be carefully assessed, defined, and operationalized, preferably through the use of clinician-administered rating scales (1,2) (Table 74-3) or, when clinically appropriate, self-report rating scales (3,4) (see Table 74-4). In addition to clarifying the types, frequencies, and severities of symptoms requiring treatment(s), serial administration of standardized scales and other structured assessment measures improves the accuracy and objectivity of neuropsychiatric diagnosis and the evaluation of treatment responses.

The use and effectiveness of all ongoing treatments also requires reevaluation before any new medications are prescribed, including prescribed and self-administered pharmacotherapies as well as nonpharmacologic treatments. Three key issues must be addressed: (a) the indications for all current treatments, (b) the rationale and continued need for their use, and (c) the potential side effects of current treatments and their possible contribution(s) to presenting symptoms. Consultation with other treating clinicians may be required to decide which, if any, current treatments should be continued and/or whether new medications may be helpful. Sometimes previously prescribed treatments have not been applied properly, for example, ongoing treatments may be predicated on misdiagnosis or duplicative as a result of poor communication between prescribing clinicians. In some cases, potentially effective medications are declared ineffective erroneously after being prescribed at doses that are too low and/or for an inadequately brief period of time. After a thorough consideration of these issues and performance of a comprehensive neuropsychiatric assessment, the most appropriate recommendation sometimes will be to eliminate 1 or more medications and to employ only nonpharmacologic interventions. When comprehensive neuropsychiatric

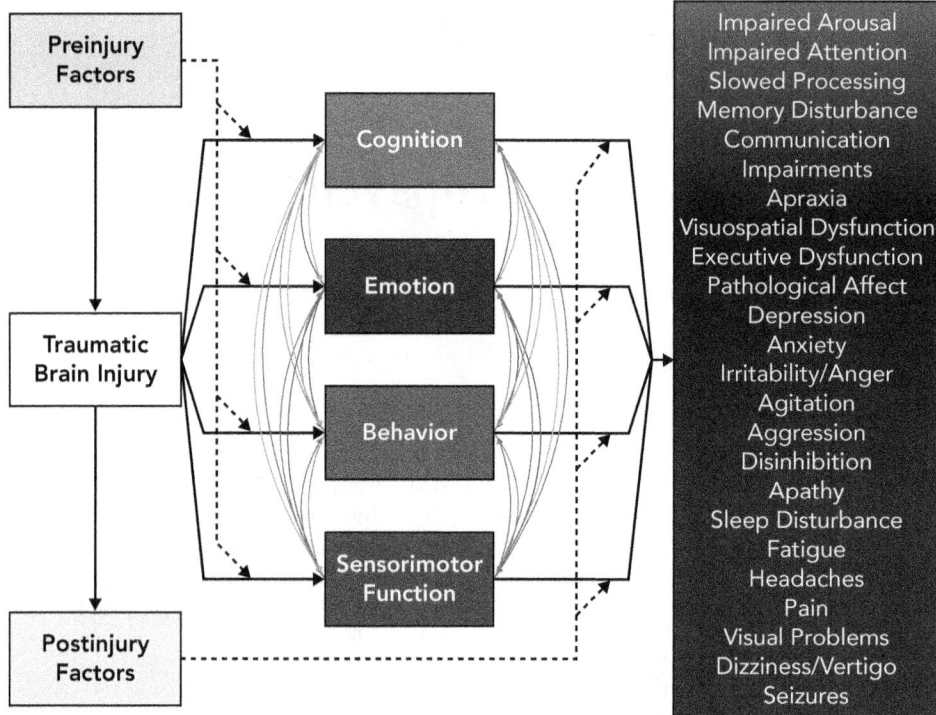

FIGURE 74–1 A model of the interactions between contributions of preinjury factors, injury factors, and postinjury factors to post-traumatic neuropsychiatric disturbances. Preinjury factors include age, gender, neurogenetics, baseline cognitive function, psychiatric conditions, substance abuse, socioeconomic environment, and risk-taking behaviors, among others. Injury factors include inertial forces, contact forces, cytotoxic processes, and secondary injury factors (e.g., increased intracranial pressure; subdural, epidural, and subarachnoid hemorrhage; hypoxia; hypovolemia) and the resulting locations, types, and severities of structural and functional disturbances of the brain. The type of brain injury (i.e., injury factors) and the brain that is injured (preinjury factors) individually and interactively affect the principal domains of neuropsychiatric function: cognition, emotion, behavior, and sensorimotor function. Disturbances in 1 of these domains affect function in 1 or more of the other domains. The expression and/or persistence of those disturbances are influenced by postinjury factors, including timely medical and rehabilitative treatments, social supports, socioeconomic status, and medicolegal entanglements. Collectively, these factors and the interactions between them produce post-traumatic neuropsychiatric symptoms (a partial list of which is presented on the right side of the figure) and influence their persistence and functional consequences.

assessment supports the decision to treat post-traumatic neuropsychiatric symptoms pharmacologically, applying the principles of pharmacotherapy is essential.

PRINCIPLES OF PHARMACOTHERAPY

There are relatively few controlled clinical trials of pharmacotherapies for post-traumatic neuropsychiatric disturbances, and most of these are single-site studies of relatively small numbers of participants (5,6). The pharmacotherapies of post-traumatic neuropsychiatric symptoms described in this chapter therefore represent, by necessity, a synthesis of the TBI-specific treatment literature, extensions of the medications used to treat phenotypically similar psychiatric populations, treatments for neuropsychiatric disturbances observed among persons with other types of brain injuries (e.g., stroke, multiple sclerosis, etc.), and the authors' opinions derived from careful review of these literatures and extensive clinical experience with this population. The intended product of this synthesis is practical guidance that may be applied immediately to the care of persons with post-traumatic neuropsychiatric disturbances. However, there are many limitations of this approach, and clinicians are encour-

aged to remain circumspect about the potential effectiveness and tolerability of the treatments discussed herein.

In light of the limited evidence base on which to base neuropsychiatric pharmacotherapies for persons with TBI, decisions regarding which medication (if any) to prescribe are guided by: hypotheses regarding the relationship between the neurobiology of TBI; neurobiologic bases of neuropsychiatric symptoms; a medication's purported mechanism(s) of action; analogies drawn from the treatment of persons with neuropsychiatric symptoms associated with other neurological or psychiatric conditions; current knowledge of the efficacy of those medications in other psychiatric disorders; side effect profiles of those medications; and the possibility of increased sensitivity to side effects among persons with TBI. When medications are prescribed, following the general principles of pharmacotherapy for post-traumatic neuropsychiatric symptoms and syndromes is encouraged (Table 74-5).

Persons with TBI may experience multiple concurrent neuropsychiatric symptoms that seem to suggest a single psychiatric condition (e.g., co-occurring depressed mood, irritability, impaired attention, fatigue, and sleep disturbances might suggest the presence of a major depressive episode). Nonetheless, it is not uncommon to observe persistence of

TABLE 74-1 Essential Elements of History-Taking in the Medical Evaluation of Persons With TBI

ELEMENT	COMMENTS
History of present illness	Obtain chief complaint(s) and characterize current cognitive, emotional, behavioral, and sensorimotor symptoms, as well as their effects on functional status.
	For each problem reported, assess onset and duration, quality, intensity, context in which it occurs, precipitating and palliating factors, and all prescribed and self-directed treatments.
	If other medical, neurological, psychiatric, and/or substance use disorders are present, note the temporal and contextual relationship of the presenting problems to these conditions.
Injury history	Ascertain whether a biomechanical (including blast-related) force was applied and whether it produced a loss of consciousness, period of amnesia, alteration of consciousness, and/or focal neurological signs (i.e., whether traumatic brain injury occured).
	When present, evaluate the duration and course of event-related disturbances of consciousness and/or neurological signs.
	Include patient account, witness account(s), description in medical record(s), and the relative contributions of which vary with the injury type and severity as well as the context of the evaluation and the time postinjury at which it is performed.
	Identify factors relevant to the differential diagnoses of event-related disturbances of consciousness and/or neurological signs, including head, neck, cervical adnexa, sensory organ, cranial nerve, peripheral nerve, and other bodily injuries as well as event-concurrent medical, neurological, and psychiatric conditions; substance use issues (acute intoxication or withdrawal, chronic abuse/dependence); and medications.
Preinjury and postinjury medical history	Identify all other medical conditions, neurological disorders, and injuries, as well as their treatment, courses, and outcomes.
Preinjury and postinjury mental health history	Identify all psychiatric conditions, including substance use disorders, as well as their treatments, courses, and outcomes; screen for episodes of psychiatric disturbance regardless of whether they were diagnosed and/or treated.
Treatments	Identify current medications (prescribed, over-the-counter, herbal products, nutritional supplements) and rehabilitative interventions, as well as their indications and effects.
	Review past medications, surgeries and other procedures, rehabilitative interventions, as well as their indications and effects; this serves as a second screening for past medical and mental health problems.
Allergies and sensitivities	Identify medication and other allergies.
	Identify medication side effects, drug–drug interactions, and idiosyncratic (i.e., rare) medication reactions, which are recorded as "sensitivities" rather than allergies.
Social history	At a minimum, include assessment of intellectual and social development, academic history and educational level, occupational history, place of residence, relationships and marital status, support network, financial status, health care insurance, military service (if any), legal history (including past and present civil and criminal matters, assignments of powers of attorney, guardianship, and/or conservatorship), and advanced directives.
Family history	At a minimum, identify medical, neurological, psychiatric, and substance use disorders in first-degree relatives.
Review of systems	If not otherwise addressed in the other elements of the medical history, review cognitive function, emotional status (e.g., mood and affect), behavior, self-awareness, sensorimotor function, and general health status.

some of these symptoms despite treatment of that condition. Although diagnostic parsimony should be sought, it is not always the best or the most accurate diagnostic approach in this population. The neuropsychiatric approach to evaluating and monitoring individual symptoms is often a more useful one, despite its divergence from the more typical "syndromal" approach to diagnosis and treatment used in conventional psychiatric practice. It also supports the common clinical observation that symptom-targeted treatments,

and, in some cases, polypharmacy, may be required to provide relief from multiple co-occurring post-traumatic neuropsychiatric symptoms.

EMOTIONAL DISTURBANCES

Emotional disturbances, including mood disorders and disorders of affect, are common consequences of TBI that inter-

TABLE 74-2 Essential Elements of the Medical Examination of Persons With TBI

ELEMENT	COMMENTS
Physical examination	Vital signs, height, weight, body mass index, musculoskeletal, and other relevant body areas/systems.
Neurological examination	Cranial nerves I–XII, reflexes, motor and sensory function, coordination, balance and gait, and subtle neurological signs (e.g., primitive reflexes).
	Detailed problem-focused examinations are performed on persons with headache, visual complaints, tinnitus, hyperacusis, hearing loss, chemosensory impairments, dizziness, and balance problems.
Mental status examination	General mental status examination focuses on appearance and behavior, mood and affect, communication, thought process and content, insight (self-awareness, social cognition), and judgment.
	Cognitive examination includes assessment of arousal, attention, processing speed, working memory, recognition, language and prosody, declarative memory, praxis, visuospatial function, calculation, and executive function.
Neurodiagnostic studies	Review previously performed structural neuroimaging (i.e., CT or MRI); obtain MRI of the brain if it has not been performed previously during postinjury period during which the evaluation occurs (i.e., acute, subacute, or late postinjury periods).
	Electrophysiologic assessment when clinically indicated (e.g., evaluation of persons with suspected post-traumatic epilepsy).
	Laboratory tests when clinically indicated (e.g., suspected endocrinopathy, encephalopathy not well explained by brain injury alone).
	Neuropsychological evaluation when clinically indicated and feasible.

Abbreviations: CT, computed tomography; MRI, magnetic resonance imaging.

fere with rehabilitation and recovery from TBI and contribute substantially to long-term disability and functional limitations (7–13). The most common types of emotional disturbances experienced by persons with TBI are mood disorders (i.e., depressive disorders, mania, or mixed mood states) and disorders of affect (i.e., pathological laughing and crying [PLC]), the treatments of which are considered here.

Depression

Although many factors may produce or contribute to apparent depressive symptoms among persons with TBI, when a patient presents with symptoms consistent with a major depressive episode, regardless of the possible causes of those symptoms, diagnosing and treating depression is appropriate (14). Depression after TBI is amenable to pharmacologic intervention (15–17) and such treatments alleviate not only the mood disturbance but also reduce the number and perceived severity of other symptoms that occur after a concussion (18).

Medications for depression following TBI include several classes of antidepressant medications (Table 74-6), including selective serotonin reuptake inhibitors (SSRIs), stimulants, tricyclic antidepressants (TCA), and tetracyclic agents (TeCA), dopamine-norepinephrine reuptake inhibitors (DNRI), serotonin-norepinephrine reuptake inhibitors (SNRI), and monoamine oxidase inhibitors (MAOIs).

The SSRIs include fluoxetine, sertraline, paroxetine, citalopram, escitalopram, and fluvoxamine. Given the relatively favorable efficacy and tolerability profiles of the SSRIs, this class is recommended as the first-line pharmacotherapy of depression following TBI (17,19). Among the SSRIs, the evidence is best developed for sertraline (18,20–22) and citalopram (23,24). These agents also are favorable in light of their beneficial effects, relatively limited side effects, few

drug–drug interactions, and short half-lives. In addition to improving depressed mood, treatment with these agents may improve cognitive performance and reduce both the number and perceived severity of other postconcussive symptoms (18).

Although used commonly in clinical practice, fluoxetine and paroxetine sometimes are problematic as a result of their adverse effects and drug–drug interactions. Fluoxetine robustly inhibits cytochrome P450 (CYP450) enzymes 2D6, 2C19, and 3A, thereby increasing the likelihood of drug–drug interactions during co-administration with a medication that is a substrate, inhibitor, or inducer of these enzymes. Fluoxetine also is metabolized to norfluoxetine; this is an active metabolite that also inhibits these P450 isoenzymes and whose average half-life is approximately 16 days. When patients develop problematic side effects or drug–drug interactions during treatment with fluoxetine, the metabolic profile and long half-life of its primary metabolite, norfluoxetine, may increase their duration substantially. Paroxetine also is a potent inhibitor of CYP450 2D6 and 2C19 and presents similar risks of clinically significant drug–drug interactions. Additionally, paroxetine commonly impairs cognitive function, even among healthy adults—an effect that most likely reflects its relatively potent anticholinergic properties (25). Collectively, these issues limit enthusiasm for, but do not preclude, treatment of depression after TBI with fluoxetine or paroxetine.

At present, there are no reports describing the use of either escitalopram or fluvoxamine for the treatment of depression following TBI. Our experience suggests that escitalopram is more effective for this purpose and is similar to citalopram with respect to efficacy, tolerability, and drug–drug interactions. However, these agents should be used with caution, pending further study of their effects and side effects among persons with depression following TBI.

TABLE 74-3 Examples of Clinician-Administered Scales That May Be Used to Characterize the Clinical Concerns of Persons With TBI or Their Caregivers

MEASURE	METHOD(S)	COMMENTS
Neurobehavioral Rating Scale-Revised	Structured clinical interview and observation	This instrument is used to evaluate a broad range of disturbances in cognition, emotion, behavior, and motor function associated with TBI; well suited to inpatient and outpatient evaluations.
Neuropsychiatric Inventory (NPI)	Structured informant interview	The original version is a structured clinical interview of a reliable informant assessing 10 domains of neuropsychiatric disturbances and caregiver distress; also available in 12-domain forms, as well as versions adapted for use in nursing homes (NPI-NH), response from caregivers by questionnaire (NPI-Q), and clinician input (NPI-C).
Hamilton Depression Rating Scale	Semistructured clinical interview and observation	Depression focused with questions about anxiety, general somatic symptoms, insight, depersonalization, paranoia, and obsessional thinking.
Young Mania Rating Scale	Semistructured clinical interview and observation	Assesses classically defined manic symptoms; a version based on interview of others (e.g., parents) is also available.
Pathological Laughing and Crying Scale (PLACS)	Structured clinical interview	Identifies the characteristics of pathological laughing and crying (PLC); affords a more thorough evaluation than the Center for Neurologic Study Lability Scale (CNS-LS).
Hamilton Anxiety Rating Scale	Semistructured clinical interview and observation	Assesses psychological symptoms of anxiety and physical complaints related to anxiety.
Agitated Behavior Scale	Clinical observation	Provides anchored ratings for agitation, including disinhibition, aggression, and affective lability.
Overt Aggression Scale	Clinical observation	Provides anchored ratings for verbal aggression, aggressive behaviors towards objects or other people, and self-directed aggression.
Overt Behavior Scale	Semistructured informant interview	Incorporates the four modified verbal and physical aggression subscales of the Overt Aggression Scale with five additional subscales focusing on inappropriate sexual behavior, perseveration/repetition, wandering/absconding, inappropriate social behavior, and lack of initiation.
Apathy Evaluation Scale	Semistructured clinical interview and observation, informant interview, and/or self-report	Three versions of this scale are available, the choice of which depends on a patient's ability to accurately self-report and/or the availability of a knowledgeable informant; each assesses cognitive, emotional, behavioral, and other manifestations of disorders of diminished motivation.
Awareness Questionnaire	Semistructured clinical interview and observation, informant interview, and/or self-report	Assesses self-awareness of deficits through comparisons of clinician ratings, informant ratings, and patient self-ratings of cognitive, behavioral, motor, and functional abilities.

Stimulants, more specifically methylphenidate, also may be useful treatments for depression following TBI (26,27). Although methylphenidate is an uncommon first-line intervention for depression after TBI in an outpatient setting, it may be a useful initial treatment of depression in an inpatient (including acute rehabilitation) setting or when rapidity of treatment response is essential (28,29). Early positive responses to methylphenidate in such circumstances are generally followed by a transition to maintenance therapy with an SSRI. Additionally, methylphenidate and other stimulants may be used to augment partial responses to SSRIs, especially when cognitive impairments and/or fatigue are residual symptoms during treatment with conventional antidepressants.

Subsequent to the development of the SSRIs, TCAs have been used less commonly for the treatment of depression. Among persons with TBI, the limited use of TCAs may reflect concerns regarding the possibility of increased side

TABLE 74-4 Examples of Self-Report Measures That Broadly Assess Symptoms and Signs Experienced Commonly by Persons With TBI

MEASURE	METHOD(S)	COMMENTS
Rivermead Post-Concussion Symptoms Questionnaire	Self-report	Inquires about the presence and severity of common physical, cognitive, and emotional symptoms experienced by persons with traumatic brain injuries.
Neurobehavioral Functioning Inventory	Self-report and/or family report	Symptoms assessed are organized into scales describing depression, somatic concerns, memory/attention problems, communication difficulties, aggression, and motor disturbances.
Neurobehavioral Symptom Inventory	Self-report	This scale assesses physical, cognitive, affective and sensory symptoms commonly experienced by persons with traumatic brain injuries; it is currently being used by the US Department of Defense and Department of Veterans Affairs as a part of the evaluation of persons with suspected postconcussive symptoms.
Cognitive Failures Questionnaire	Self-report	Asks questions about subjectively experienced failures in perception, memory, and motor function; although cognitively focused, responses to these questions tend to correlate highly with self-ratings of depression and other psychiatric symptoms.
Multiple Abilities Self-Report Questionnaire	Self-report	Asks questions about experiences of cognitive performance in five domains: attention, verbal memory, visuospatial memory, visual perception, and language.
Behavioral Rating Inventory of Executive Function-Adult Version	Self-report, informant report	Asks questions about executive function and self-regulation, responses to which comprise behavioral regulation, metacognition, and global executive composite indices.
Beck Depression Inventory-II	Self-report	Asks questions about depressive symptoms described in *DSM-IV-TR*.
Center for Neurologic Study-Lability Scale	Self-report	Asks a brief set of questions about symptoms of pathological laughing and crying.
Beck Anxiety Inventory	Self-report	Asks questions about current anxiety symptoms.
State-Trait Anxiety Inventory	Self-report	Asks questions about current anxiety (state) as well as the propensity to be anxious (trait).
PTSD Checklist (PCL)	Self-report	Asks questions about symptoms of post-traumatic stress disorder (PTSD) as defined in *DSM-IV-TR*; includes military (PCL-M), civilian (PCL-C), and event-specific (PCL-S) versions.
Epworth Sleepiness Scale	Self-report	Asks questions about the patient's tendency to fall asleep, or, conversely, the ability to maintain wakefulness in common situations.
Pittsburgh Sleep Quality Index	Self-report	Asks questions about sleep quality and disturbances.

DSM-IV-TR, Diagnostic and Statistical Manual of Mental Disorders, Fourth Edition, Text Revision.

effects associated with these agents, reports of more limited effectiveness of these agents among persons with TBI, waning familiarity with the use of these agents on the part of recently trained clinicians, or some combination of these factors (17). Nonetheless, TCAs and TeCAs may be useful as primary or adjunctive treatments for depression following TBI (30,31). The evidence with which to guide their use among persons with TBI is very limited and that which is available suggests lower response rates and higher adverse event rates (including seizures) that are associated with the use of SSRIs (17).

When a TCA is used to treat depression after TBI, nortriptyline or desipramine are preferable to other agents in this class based on their benefits, tolerability, and ease of use. Treatment with these agents proceeds slowly, with incremental dose increases made no more often than weekly. Complementing symptom reassessments with periodic measurements of TCA (parent compound and metabolite)

plasma levels is encouraged; beneficial effects generally require treatment with doses sufficient to develop plasma nortriptyline levels of 50–100 μg/mL and plasma desipramine levels more than 125 μg/mL. If side effects such as sedation, confusion, or symptomatic hypotension (orthostatic or otherwise) develop, dose reductions may alleviate these effects and/or allow time to accommodate to them before undertaking additional attempts at dose escalation. When these or other side effects limit TCA dosing to subtherapeutic levels, initiating an antidepressant augmentation strategy (e.g., addition of an SSRI or a stimulant) or switching to a different medication may be required.

Common clinical experience suggests that SNRIs and DNRIs may be useful in the treatment of depression following TBI. However, cautious use is advised, given the paucity of reports with which to inform pretreatment benefit/risk assessments. Among these agents, the relationship between bupropion and seizures merits specific comment (19). The

TABLE 74-5 General Principles of Pharmacotherapy for Neuropsychiatric Disturbances Among Persons With TBIs

Start low, go slow, but go	Initiate treatment at doses lower than those used in patients without brain injuries, and raise doses more slowly than in patients without brain injuries. Although patients with brain injuries may be more sensitive to the side effects of many medications, standard doses may be needed to treat adequately their neuropsychiatric disturbances.
Perform an adequate therapeutic trial	Gradually titrate each medication to a maximally tolerable dose and maintain that dose long enough to evaluate its effectiveness.
Continuously reassess treatment need	The need for continued treatment should be reassessed in an ongoing fashion. Dose reduction or medication discontinuation should be attempted after achieving remission of target symptoms. Spontaneous recovery occurs, and in such circumstances, continued pharmacotherapy is unnecessary. If medication tapering or discontinuation results in recurrent symptoms, then restart treatment and establish a date for another trial of treatment discontinuation.
Monitor drug–drug interactions	Patients with brain injuries are often sensitive to medication side effects and may require treatment with several medications; accordingly, heightened vigilance and assiduous monitoring for possible drug–drug interactions is a standard practice in this population.
Augment partial responses	Partial response to monotherapy is common. Adding a second medication with a different and/or complementary mechanism of action to the treatment regimen may afford additional improvements. In general, augmentation of partial responses is preferable to switching to a medication with an identical (or highly similar) pharmacologic profile to the one producing the partial response.
Initiate medications serially, not concurrently	It is prudent to initiate each treatment sequentially rather than concurrently to understand as clearly as possible both the beneficial and adverse effects of each medication prescribed.
Respond promptly to symptom intensification	If targeted psychiatric symptoms worsen soon after initiation of pharmacotherapy, lower the dose of the medication; if symptom intensification persists, discontinue the medication entirely.

immediate-release form of bupropion appears more likely to produce dose-related seizures than the sustained- or extended-release forms of this medication. It is not clear whether TBI, which also increases seizure risk (32), alters the dose at which bupropion-related seizures may occur. Eschewing immediate-release bupropion for depression following TBI is not justified; nonetheless, clinicians using this agent need to consider the possibility that the dose at which this increased risk emerges may be lower among persons with TBI than in the general population and to maintain heightened vigilance for treatment-related seizures during treatment initiation and dose escalation.

Depression among persons with TBI is treated infrequently with MAOIs. This practice pattern reflects challenges of ensuring patient adherence to the complex dietary restrictions required during use of these medications, especially among persons with significant post-traumatic cognitive impairments and/or behavioral disturbances. Additionally, the literature offers little support for the effectiveness of these medications in the TBI population (17). If treatment with an MAOI is considered, consultation with a neuropsychiatrist experienced in the use of these agents among persons with TBI is advised.

Mania

A broad range of medications may be used to treat secondary mania, idiopathic (or primary) mania, and mixed mood states among persons with TBI (5,11,33). Although the literature with which to assess the effectiveness and tolerability of treatments for mania after TBI is sparse, that which is available suggests that valproate, quetiapine, carbamazepine, and lithium are effective and reasonably well tolerated when used for this purpose (Table 74-7). In the absence of evidence demonstrating the clear superiority of one of these agents over the others, valproate (34–37) or quetiapine (11,38) are recommended as first-line treatments, given their effectiveness for acute mania, rapid-cycling bipolar disorder, and antimanic prophylaxis as well as their reasonable tolerability in persons with TBI. When these agents, alone or in combination, prove ineffective, then the use of one or more of the other agents presented in Table 74-7 may be required.

Several of the newer anticonvulsants (e.g., lamotrigine, oxcarbazepine) and the atypical antipsychotics (e.g., risperidone, olanzapine, ziprasidone, aripiprazole, etc.) also may be useful treatments for post-traumatic mania. However, there are few reports describing its use for this purpose among persons with post-traumatic mania. Clinicians using any of these medications to treat post-traumatic mania are advised to do so cautiously and to assiduously monitor their patients for treatment-related cognitive, motor, cardiac, and metabolic side effects.

Partial response, relapse of symptoms, and/or need for a second mood-stabilizing medication are common limitations of the use of these agents in this population. Additionally, treatment-limiting adverse cognitive and motor side effects occur commonly. Valproate appears less likely to pro-

TABLE 74-6 Medications Used to Treat Depression Following TBI

MEDICATION	CLASS	DAILY DOSE RANGE	COMMENTS
Citalopram	SSRI	5–40 mg	Relatively short half-life; few drug–drug interactions
Escitalopram	SSRI	5–30 mg	Relatively short half-life; few drug–drug interactions; may be modestly more anxiolytic than citalopram
Sertraline	SSRI	25–250 mg	Relatively short-half life; modest sexual dysfunction; increased serum carbamazepine levels
Fluoxetine	SSRI	10–60 mg	Long half-life of primary active metabolite, norfluoxetine; possible excessive activation; inhibits multiple cytochrome P450 enzymes; increased the risk of problematic drug–drug interactions
Paroxetine	SSRI	5–40 mg	Risk of discontinuation syndrome; anticholinergic effects; weight gain; inhibits multiple cytochrome P450 enzymes; increased risk of problematic drug-drug interactions; discontinuation syndrome may be worse than for other SSRIs
Methylphenidate	Stimulant	10–60 mg	Low but nontrivial risk of anorexia, insomnia, and dependence/abuse; may usefully augment partial responses to SSRIs.
Nortriptyline	TCA	25–150 mg	Relatively less anticholinergic than older TCAs
Desipramine	TCA	50–200 mg	Relatively less anticholinergic than older TCAs.
Mirtazapine	TeCA	15–45 mg	Initial dose may be sedating and is usually administered prior to sleep; may usefully augment partial responses to SSRIs
Venlafaxine XR	SNRI	37.5–225 mg	Hypertension may be treatment limiting for some patients; usual neurological symptoms ("twitching" or "shock-like" sensations) are sometimes reported; potentially difficult discontinuation syndrome
Bupropion XL or SR	DNRI	150–450 mg	Possible dose-related seizure risk; generally entails lower risk of treatment-related sexual dysfunction than SSRIs

Abbreviations: DNRI, dopamine-norepinephrine reuptake inhibitor; SNRI, serotonin-norepinephrine reuptake inhibitor; SR, sustained release; SSRI, selective serotonin reuptake inhibitor; TeCA, tetracyclic agents; TCA, tricyclic antidepressant; XL, extended release; XR, extended release.

SSRIs are first-line therapies for most outpatients; SSRIs or stimulants are first-line therapies for inpatients, particularly during the early postinjury period. With the possible exception of mirtazapine use to augment partial responses to SSRIs, the use of TCAs, TeCAs, and other antidepressants in this population is generally reserved for those in SSRIs and/or stimulants, alone or in combination, have been ineffective. Clinicians are encouraged to refer to each medication's product information sheet as well as other reference materials for complete reviews of dosing, side effects, drug–drug interactions, treatment risks, and treatment contraindications before prescribing these or any other medications.

duce cognitive impairments rather than carbamazepine or lithium (39–41). Quetiapine may also be cognitively neutral, or perhaps even cognitively enhancing, at doses used to effect behavioral improvements among persons with TBI (42). Carbamazepine commonly impairs cognition and motor function among persons with TBI (43), although these effects are generally modest. Lithium intolerance (e.g., nausea, tremor, ataxia, and lethargy) appears to develop at lower doses among persons with TBI than among those with primary mania or mixed mood states. Lithium also lowers seizure threshold—an effect that is particularly concerning given the increased risk of seizures associated with TBI more generally (32).

Regardless of potential differences in tolerability between these agents, the use of any antimanic medication among persons with TBI necessitates careful and continuous assessment. In particular, vigilant monitoring for treatment-related motor (e.g., tremor, incoordination, ataxia, gait disturbances) and cognitive impairments, as well as other adverse somatic side effects (e.g., weight gain, gastrointestinal problems/diarrhea, hematologic abnormalities, hepatotoxicity, alopecia, etc.), is required.

Pathological Laughing and Crying

PLC (also known as pseudobulbar affect, emotional incontinence, emotional lability, or involuntary emotional expres-

sion disorder) is a disorder of affect (see [44] for review). This condition is characterized by brief, involuntary, intense, and uncontrollable episodes of crying and/or laughing that may occur many times per day. These episodes are provoked by sentimental, trivially sentimental, and/or nonsentimental stimuli and tend to be stereotyped in their presentation. The expressed emotion in any given episode may or may not be accompanied by expression-congruent feelings; however, the occurrence of the laughing and/or crying episodes neither reflects nor produces a persistent change in the prevailing mood. PLC occurs in 5%–11% of patients during the first year following TBI (12,13); the frequency of this problem in the late postinjury period is uncertain.

There are several medications that effectively treat PLC after TBI (Table 74-8). Among these, serotonergically and noradrenergically active antidepressants are among the most effective, best tolerated, and simplest agents to use for this purpose (44). SSRIs with relatively short half-lives, limited drug–drug and CYP450 interactions, and the most favorable side effect profiles are the first-line treatments of PLC. This condition usually responds to relatively low doses of these agents (often below those required for the treatment of depression), and initial responses may be evident within the first few days of treatment. Achieving maximal treatment response, however, frequently requires several additional weeks of treatment.

TABLE 74-7 Medications Used to Treat Mania and/or Mixed Mood Episodes Among Persons With TBI

MEDICATION	STARTING DOSE	TARGET TOTAL DAILY DOSE	COMMENTS
Valproate	250 mg 3 times daily	1,500–4,500 mg	One of the best tolerated anticonvulsant mood-stabilizing agents; tremor and, rarely, extrapyramidal symptoms may occur; monitoring for hematologic and hepatic toxicity is necessary; risk of polycystic ovarian syndrome may prompt use of alternate agent in females; maximum dose is 60 mg/kg daily, and usual target serum concentrations is 50–125 µg/mL.
Quetiapine	25–50 mg daily	300–800 mg	In patients with acute mania, initial dose of 100 mg daily and increasing by 100 mg daily is appropriate; sedation and hypotension may be treatment limiting; monitoring for metabolic syndrome is essential.
Carbamazepine	100 mg daily	200–1,600 mg	Baseline and serial assessment of hematologic, hepatic, renal, and electrolyte indices is essential; significant risk for treatment-induced hyponatremia; cognitive and motor side effects may be treatment limiting; usual target serum concentration is 4–12 µg/mL.
Lithium	150 mg daily	300–1,500 mg	Most patients tolerate treatment best if initially daily dose is given at bedtime; baseline and serial monitoring of renal and thyroid function as well as lithium level monitoring is essential; side effects may be mitigated by dose reduction, use of slow-release formulations or bedtime dosing; cognitive and motor side effects may emerge at "therapeutic" serum lithium levels; lithium may lower seizure threshold; usual target serum level is 0.5–1.2 mEq/L.

Other medications may be used and may be informed by the American Psychiatric Association's *Practice Guideline for the Treatment of Patients with Bipolar Disorder*, 2nd edition. Additionally, each medication's product information sheet as well as other reference materials should be reviewed before prescribing these or any other medications for the treatment of manic or mixed mood episodes.

If SSRIs prove ineffective or are tolerated poorly, then consideration may be given to other treatment options including TCAs (usually nortriptyline), medications that directly or indirectly augment dopaminergic and/or noradrenergic function (e.g., stimulants), and uncompetitive *N*-methyl-D-aspartate (NMDA) antagonists (44). The latter category merits specific comment given the recent approval of the combination of dextromethorphan-quinidine (DM-Q) by the US Food and Drug Administration for the treatment of "pseudobulbar affect."

Both dextromethorphan (DM) and amantadine agents are classified as uncompetitive NMDA antagonists. Their neurochemical effects also include indirect facilitation of dopaminergic function (mediated by antagonism of NMDA receptors in the dopaminergic neurons of the ventral tegmental area) as well as agonism of sigma-1 receptors (45,46) and facilitation of serotonergic neurotransmission through sigma-1 agonist (47). The latency between treatment initiation and PLC improvement is often quite long for DM-Q (4–5 weeks); in contrast, amantadine tends to effect improvement as quickly as the SSRIs (2–5 days).

There is a substantial risk of nontrivial drug–drug interactions attendant to the use of DM-Q (see [44] for review), and this risk derives principally from the effects of quinidine (Q) on hepatic drug metabolism. The purpose of low-dose Q in this combination drug is to inhibit CYP450 2D6 metabolism of DM, thereby increasing the proportion of DM that enters the central nervous system in an unmetabolized and therapeutically effective state. Unfortunately, inhibition of the CYP450 2D6 pathway also elevates serum levels of all other medications metabolized by it. Clinicians electing to prescribe this agent, therefore, must review carefully all other concurrently prescribed medications and identify which, if any, are substrates of CYP450 2D6 to assess the risk

of DM-Q treatment-related drug–drug interactions. Additionally, all other clinicians contributing to the care of a patient receiving DM-Q must anticipate adjusting the dose of all medications metabolized by the CYP450 2D6 pathway.

Finally, neurological and neurobehavioral comorbidities also may influence the selection of treatments for PLC. Lamotrigine may be useful for PLC occurring in the context of comorbid TBI and epilepsy (48). When PLC is accompanied by episodic irritability/anger, aggressive and/or self-destructive behaviors, augmenting partial responses to SSRIs with anticonvulsants (e.g., valproate, lamotrigine) may be useful.

Anxiety Disorders

Anxiety disorders, including generalized anxiety disorder, panic disorder, phobias, obsessive–compulsive disorder, and/or post-traumatic stress disorder, may develop following TBI and are sources of substantial morbidity for persons with these problems (49). When any of these conditions are present, clinicians should carefully assess patients for other comorbid major psychiatric disorders, most notably depression as well as personality, medical, substance use, and/or iatrogenic (e.g., medication induced) contributors to anxiety symptoms. Treating these comorbid conditions may eliminate or reduce the drivers of anxiety, although it may not obviate the need for concurrent psychological and/or pharmacologic management of anxiety.

When anxiety symptoms are so severe that they require pharmacological intervention, treatment with SSRIs, benzodiazepines, or buspirone may be required. In general, SSRIs are the preferred treatments for post-traumatic anxiety disorders in light of their beneficial effects on a wide variety of

TABLE 74-8 Medications Used to Treat Pathological Laughing and Crying Because of TBI

MEDICATION	CLASS	DAILY DOSE RANGE	SPECIAL CONSIDERATIONS
Citalopram	SSRI	5–20 mg	Relatively short half-life; few drug–drug interactions.
Escitalopram	SSRI	5–30 mg	Relatively short half-life; few drug–drug interactions; may be modestly more anxiolytic than citalopram.
Sertraline	SSRI	25–150 mg	Relatively short-half life; modest sexual dysfunction; increased serum carbamazepine levels.
Fluoxetine	SSRI	10–30 mg	Long half-life of primary active metabolite—norfluoxetine; possible excessive activation; inhibits multiple CYP450 enzymes; increase the risk of problematic drug–drug interactions.
Paroxetine	SSRI	5–40 mg	Risk of discontinuation syndrome; anticholinergic effects; weight gain; drug interactions; discontinuation syndrome may be worse than for other SSRIs.
Nortriptyline	TCA	10–150 mg	Relatively less anticholinergic than older TCAs.
Impiramine	TCA	10–300 mg	Anticholinergic side effects and cardiac disease-related contraindications may limit the use of this agent, especially in older patients.
Amitriptyline	TCA	10–300 mg	Anticholinergic side effects and cardiac disease-related contraindications may limit the use of this agent, especially in older patients.
Methylphenidate	Stimulant	5–60 mg	Low but nontrivial risk of anorexia, insomnia, and dependence/abuse; may usefully augment partial responses to SSRIs.
Dextroamphetamine	Stimulant	5–60 mg	Low but nontrivial risk of anorexia, insomnia, and dependence/abuse; may usefully augment partial responses to SSRIs.
Carbidopa-levodopa	Dopamine agonist	25/100 mg, 1 to 2 tablets, 3–4 times daily	Tablets include carbidopa 25 mg and levodopa 100 mg; carbidopa doses of less than 75 mg are associated with nausea and vomiting; postural hypotension may occur when coadministered with antihypertensive agents; dose-related hallucinations and paranoia—dyskinesias.
Mirtazapine	TeCA	15–45 mg	Initial dose may be sedating and usually is administered prior to sleep; may usefully augment partial responses to SSRIs.
Venlafaxine XR	SNRI	37.5–225 mg	Hypertension may be treatment limiting for some patients; usual neurological symptoms ("twitching" or "shock-like" sensations) are sometimes reported; potentially difficult discontinuation syndrome.
Lamotrigine	Anticonvulsant	25–100 mg	Initial dose is maintained for 2 weeks, then increased to 50 mg daily for 2 weeks, then increased by 50 mg daily every 1–2 weeks to effective dose; coadministration of valproate necessitates slower titration (see manufacturer's product information sheet); coadministration of other anticonvulsants also alters rate of dose escalation; the risk of severe potentially life-threatening rash may be increased by coadministration with valproate or by exceeding either the recommended initial dose or rate of dose escalation.
Amantadine	Uncompetitive NMDA receptor antagonist	50–200 mg daily	The effects of anticholinergic agents and psychostimulants may be potentiated by amantadine; risk of treatment-related seizures is uncertain, and monitoring for their development is essential; psychosis and confusion may occur at high doses.
Dextromethorphan-quinidine (DM-Q)	Uncompetitive NMDA receptor antagonist	20 mg/10 mg capsule, once or twice daily	Treatment is initiated as DM-Q 20 mg/10 mg capsule once daily; after 7 days, dose may be advanced to DM-Q 20 mg/10 mg capsule twice daily; quinidine inhibits CYP450 2D6, necessitating dose adjustment of medications also metabolized through this pathway.

Abbreviations: CYP450, cytochrome P450; NMDA, N-methyl-D-aspartate; SNRI, serotonin-norepinephrine reuptake inhibitor; SSRI, selective serotonin reuptake inhibitor; TeCA, tetracyclic antidepressant; TCA, tricyclic antidepressant; XR, extended release.

Initiating treatment with relatively low doses of the medications in this table is encouraged; treatment effect is often obtained at total daily doses lower than those used to treat primary psychiatric disorders (e.g., depression, anxiety disorders). Clinicians are encouraged to refer to each medication's product information sheet as well as other reference materials for complete reviews of dosing, side effects, drug–drug interactions, treatment risks, and treatment contraindications before prescribing these or any other medications.

primary anxiety disorders in the general psychiatric population (50), as well as their relatively favorable efficacy and tolerability for other neuropsychiatric consequences of TBI. As noted earlier, the pharmacologic profiles of sertraline, citalopram, and escitalopram, as well as their efficacy in the treatment of anxiety disorders in persons with no brain injury, make these agents particularly attractive anxiolytics in this context (51).

Buspirone may be an effective alternative or adjunctive treatment to SSRIs for anxiety among persons with TBI (52). This medication appears to entail a lower risk of medication-induced cognitive dysfunction than benzodiazepines (53). Additionally, its use is not associated with medication abuse/dependence or discontinuation syndrome. Treatment is generally initiated with buspirone 5 mg two or three times daily; however, adequate and sustained anxiolysis often requires higher doses (e.g., 15 mg twice daily), and the latency between treatment initiation and response may be several weeks. This sometimes necessitates short-term treatment with another anxiolytic (e.g., a benzodiazepine) and/or relatively intensive supportive psychotherapy for patients to maintain engagement in treatment and confidence in the use of this medication.

When SSRIs and/or buspirone fail to afford the desired degree of anxiolysis, it may be necessary to effect short-term anxiolysis with a benzodiazepine, especially during the initial dose-titration period of treatment with an SSRI or buspirone or during the early period of psychological treatment. Although benzodiazepines offer the benefit of rapid anxiolysis, their use among persons with TBI entails a variety of potentially problematic side effects. These agents are sedating and, even with chronic use, impair memory and motor function (e.g., balance, coordination) (53–56). Additionally, TBI is not uncommonly associated with preinjury alcohol and/or drug problems; among patients with such problems, prescribing benzodiazepines risks the development of benzodiazepine dependence as well as relapse into alcohol abuse/dependence. This constellation of potential problems makes benzodiazepines undesirable treatments for anxiety among patients with TBI. If use of a benzodiazepine is necessary, then selecting one with a moderate half-life that is serum metabolized (i.e., lorazepam, oxazepam) is preferable to the use of agents with either very short half-lives (which are highly reinforcing and may produce rebound anxiety between doses) or very long half-lives (which may result in cumulative adverse effects when administered repeatedly).

APATHY AND RELATED DISORDERS OF DIMINISHED MOTIVATION

States of diminished motivation, including apathy, abulia and akinetic mutism, are characterized by decreased goal-directed cognition, emotion, and behavior, and are relatively common consequences of TBI (57–59). It is important to be clear that, in this context, the term "diminished motivation" does not connote poor effort or malingering, instead, it refers to a state of diminished function of the paralimbic cortical and subcortical structures required to generate and sustain goal-directed thought, feeling, and action. Apathetic states occur on a continuum of severity, with mildly diminished motivation at one end and akinetic mutism at the other. Apathy may be a feature of other neuropsychiatric conditions, most notably depression, and may occur as an independent clinical problem as well (60).

When apathy is a feature of depression, treatment of the underlying depression with agents such as the SSRIs may relieve both mood and apathy symptoms. When apathy occurs as an independent problem, that is, in the absence of depression, treatment with SSRIs not only fails to improve this problem but also may worsen it (61). Accordingly, careful distinction between depression, depression with apathy, and apathy alone is an essential prerequisite to the pharmacotherapy of any of these problems (58).

When apathy occurs as an independent clinical problem, it often is a difficult problem to treat effectively. Nonpharmacologic (i.e., environmental, behavioral) interventions are essential elements of treatment, but the evidence of their effectiveness is very limited (62). When apathy is severe, caregiver education and direct (i.e., "hands-on") facilitation of everyday activities are often required. Pharmacotherapies are adjunctive, at best, to these interventions. Agents that directly or indirectly augment cerebral catecholaminergic function (e.g., methylphenidate, dextroamphetamine, amantadine, bromocriptine) and medications that augment cerebral cholinergic function (e.g., donepezil, rivastigmine, galantamine) may modestly improve apathy (58,63). The available evidence suggests that either of these pharmacotherapeutic approaches may be useful. In clinical practice, however, catecholaminergic agents (64–75) are generally used as the first-line pharmacotherapies of apathy. When these interventions fail, combinations of catecholaminergic agents and cholinesterase inhibitors may be used (58) (Table 74-9).

Apathy also commonly co-occurs with behavioral dyscontrol (i.e., disinhibition, impulsivity, and aggression). This combination of behavioral problems presents substantial challenges to clinicians attempting to treat such problems; medications targeting apathy may worsen behavioral dyscontrol and those targeting for behavioral dyscontrol may worsen apathy. The combination of apathy and behavioral dyscontrol, therefore, poses one of the most difficult neuropsychiatric treatment dilemmas. After assessing the functional consequences of apathy and behavioral dyscontrol with a patient's and/or caregiver's tolerance for these problems, a more fully informed choice of neuropsychiatric treatment target and medication strategy, if any, may be made.

PSYCHOSIS

Hallucinations and delusions are typical psychotic symptoms. Hallucinations are sensory perceptions that occur in the absence of relevant external stimuli (i.e., seeing things that are not present, hearing voices or perceiving sounds, body sensations, odors, or tastes for which there are no sources), whereas an illusion is a misperception of an actual external stimulus (i.e., perceiving a coat draped on a chair as a person, hearing one's name in a ringing bell). Delusions are fixed false beliefs, that is, ideas that are factually or logically incorrect, which are consistently held even in the face of evidence that refutes them. Delusions sometimes derive from ordinary life experience (e.g., beliefs about theft, betrayal, power, wealth, or love) or instead may be entirely implausible and bizarre (e.g., logically impossible events such as thought broadcasting, thought insertion, thought control). By contrast, confabulation refers to incorrect ideas that are not fixed (i.e., temporally transient) and that usually

TABLE 74-9 Medications Used to Treat Apathy and Related Disorders of Diminished Motivation

MEDICATION	CLASS	DAILY DOSE RANGE
Amantadine	Uncompetitive NMDA receptor antagonist	50–200 mg
Methylphenidate	Stimulant	5–60 mg
Dextroamphetamine	Stimulant	5–60 mg
Modafinil	Stimulant-like agent	100–400 mg
Bromocriptine	Dopamine agonist	2.5–90 mg
Carbidopa-levodopa	Dopamine agonist	25/100 mg, 1–2 tablets, 3–4 times daily
Donepezil	AChEI	5–10 mg
Rivastigmine	AChEI	1.5–12 mg
Galantamine	AChEI	4–32 mg
Bupropion XL or SR	DNRI	150–450 mg
Venlafaxine XR	SNRI	37.5–225 mg
Protriptyline	TCA	20–60 mg

Abbreviations: AChEI, acetylcholinesterase inhibitor; DNRI, dopamine-norepinephrine reuptake inhibitor; NMDA, N-methyl-D-aspartate; SNRI, serotonin-norepinephrine reuptake inhibitor; SR, sustained release; SSRI, selective serotonin reuptake inhibitor; TCA, tricyclic antidepressant; XL, extended release; XR, extended release.

Clinicians are encouraged to refer to each medication's product information sheet as well as other reference materials for complete reviews of dosing, side effects, drug–drug interactions, treatment risks, and treatment contraindications before prescribing these or any other medications.

are associated with, and contributed to by, profound memory impairments.

Hallucinations and delusions (i.e., psychotic symptoms) developing during the early postinjury period may reflect post-traumatic delirium, delirium because of comorbid general medical conditions, active severe preinjury mood disorders (e.g., severe major depression, mania, or mixed mood states), active preinjury psychotic disorders (i.e., schizophrenia, schizoaffective disorder), severe early secondary depressive or manic episodes, or another TBI-related neuropsychiatric disorder (e.g., post-traumatic epilepsy). Less often, psychotic symptoms because of a new onset post-traumatic psychotic disorder (i.e., schizophrenia-like psychosis) may develop during the early or late post-injury periods (49,76). Regardless of their cause, these symptoms often require treatment with antipsychotics to reduce symptom-induced distress and behavioral disturbances.

The first-generation ("typical") or second-generation ("atypical") antipsychotics are similar in terms of efficacy; however, their side effect profiles are often quite different, and some are more likely to produce cognitive impairments or motor abnormalities than the others (77–82). In general, antipsychotics that robustly antagonize type 2 dopamine (D_2) receptors are most likely to produce cognitive and motor problems among persons with TBI (83–87). Examples of antipsychotics with these properties are high-potency typical antipsychotics (e.g., haloperidol, fluphenazine), even when used at relatively low doses; low-potency typical antipsychotics (e.g., chlorpromazine, thioridazine), especially when used at moderate-to-high doses; and some atypical antipsychotics (e.g., risperidone, paliperidone, olanzapine), also when used at moderate-to-high doses.

Antipsychotics with clinically important anticholinergic effects also may be cognitively impairing among some persons with TBI (88,89). This is a complicated issue, however, because some agents demonstrating potent antimuscarinic binding in vitro may promote cholinergic function in vivo via their effects at presynaptic muscarinic type 2 (M_2) autoreceptors and/or by antagonizing type 3 serotonin (5-HT_3)

receptors (90, 91). Accordingly, the purported "anticholinergic" effects of some antipsychotics, especially atypical antipsychotics such as olanzapine and clozapine, predicted by their in vitro receptor binding profiles are not borne out reliably as such in a clinical practice.

The motor side effects of first- and second-generation antipsychotics also may be treatment limiting. The adverse motor effects of these agents include tremor, dykinesia, dystonia, parkinsonism, and akathisia in their acute and tardive (late onset) forms (78,82,92). Among the second-generation antipsychotics, risperidone and ziprasidone are most likely to be problematic in these regards, whereas quetiapine and clozapine are least likely to produce such problems (78, 82,93).

Additionally, the metabolic (e.g., serum lipid and glucose) effects, weight gain, and potential cardiovascular risk profiles of the atypical antipsychotics are potentially treatment limiting, and all of the antipsychotics may cause neuroleptic malignant syndrome. Given the risks of such problems associated with the use of these medications and their relatively limited benefits on dementia-related psychosis or agitation (79,94,95), it is reasonable to remain circumspect about their use among persons with psychotic symptoms after TBI.

Nonetheless, persons with TBI who are experiencing psychotic symptoms may benefit from judicious treatment with antipsychotics, especially when nonpharmacologic interventions afford inadequate relief of those symptoms and/or fail to reduce dangerous psychosis-related behaviors. When antipsychotics are used to treat post-traumatic psychotic symptoms, second-generation agents are generally preferred over first-generation agents in light of the relatively lower risk of treatment-related cognitive and motor impairments (76,96–98). Regardless of the agent selected, starting doses of antipsychotic medications in these contexts generally are from one-third to one-half of those used among persons with primary psychotic disorders. Gradual titration to doses similar to those used for the treatment of psychotic symptoms among persons with schizophrenia, schizoaffective disorder, and/or psychotic manic or depressive episodes may be required to effect improvement in post-traumatic psychosis and psychosis-associated behavioral disturbances. Baseline assessment of and periodic monitoring for cardiac problems (i.e., prolonged corrected QT [QTc]) as well as metabolic parameters during treatment with any atypical antipsychotic medication is recommended. Additionally, vigilance for the development of treatment-emergent movement disorders such as dystonias, dyskinesias, akathisia, and neuroleptic malignant syndrome is particularly important in this population. Heightened vigilance for treatment-related seizures is also encouraged, especially during treatment with clozapine (96).

DISINHIBITION

Disinhibited behaviors are common among persons with TBI and include socially or contextually inappropriate nonaggressive verbal, physical, and sexual acts (57,99). Although disinhibition may reflect focal injury to lateral orbitofrontal-subcortical circuits involved in a rule-governed social behavior (100), disinhibition also may be a manifestation of another primary or secondary psychiatric disorder (e.g., anxiety, mania, psychosis). Compulsive, perserverative, and tic behaviors may be misunderstood as intrinsic disinhibition or impulsivity, especially among patients with severe cognitive-communication impairments. Cognitive impairments such as attentional impairments, working memory disturbances, and/or executive dysfunction may contribute to the development of disinhibited-appearing behaviors in a manner analogous to that observed among persons with attention deficit hyperactivity disorder. Considering the differential diagnosis for disinhibition is a prerequisite to its treatment. When disinhibited behaviors occur in the context of another primary or secondary psychiatric disorder, the most appropriate initial step in treatment is to treat that disorder rather than initiating pharmacotherapy for disinhibition specifically.

Pharmacotherapy is adjunctive to the nonpharmacologic management of disinhibition. As noted earlier, SSRIs and serotonergically active TCAs may decrease behavioral drive (i.e., induce apathy) and therefore may be useful pharmacotherapies of disinhibition inhibitors (61,101,102). When this approach is used, SSRIs are the preferred medication class, and treatment with relatively high doses of these medications may be required to reduce disinhibition. There are cardiac complications associated with the use of high-dose citalopram (i.e., total daily doses of more than 40 mg); these complications also may result from treatment with high-dose escitalopram. Other SSRIs are, therefore, preferred over citalopram and escitalopram for the pharmacotherapy of disinhibition when high-dose treatment is required. Anticonvulsant medications, including valproate and carbamazepine, may be used for this purpose as well. Effective doses are similar to those required to treat secondary mania or post-traumatic epilepsy. There are reports that antiandrogenic agents may reduce sexually impulsive or disinhibited behaviors (103), although this treatment approach is inconsistently effective and often entails complex proxy consent considerations. If all of these approaches fail partially or completely, then adjunctive or primary treatment with atypical antipsychotic agents may be necessary (104).

AGITATION, AGGRESSION, AND SELF-INJURIOUS BEHAVIORS

Agitated, aggressive, and self-injurious behaviors are major sources of stress to caregivers and families of persons with these problems. These behaviors can endanger the safety of not only patients and their families but also the professionals providing their care. A multimodal, multidisciplinary, collaborative approach to treatment is necessary in most cases. Concurrent and collaborative behavioral, environmental, psychotherapeutic, psychopharmacologic evaluations and interventions often are required to manage these problems effectively (5,105–108).

The neuroanatomy and neurochemistry of post-traumatic aggression are highly individual, and treatment response predictions based on current clinical and/or neurodiagnostic assessment techniques are frequently unreliable. Consequently, the pharmacotherapy of agitation, aggressive, and/or self-injurious behaviors usually requires a trial-and-error approach to identify a medication that is both effective and tolerable. Polypharmacy is often required to treat these behaviors effectively. The beneficial and adverse effects of medications used to treat agitation, aggression, and/or self-injurious behaviors vary with the presence of other pre- and post-TBI neuropsychiatric conditions as well as the time since injury at which treatment is initiated (with the latter variable serving as a proxy marker of the state of the post-TBI neurochemical cascade).

Pharmacotherapy of Acute Agitation, Aggression, and Self-Injurious Behaviors

Antipsychotics and benzodiazepines are the most commonly used medications in the treatment of acute aggressive, agitated, and self-injurious behaviors among persons with TBI (109–111). When these agents are used, they may decrease the rate of recovery following TBI (83,84). This possibility needs to be weighed against the risks of harm to self and others as well as the risk of reinjury or medical complications conferred by uncontrolled agitation, aggression, or self-injurious behaviors.

As noted earlier in this chapter, if an antipsychotic medication is used at all, then atypical (i.e., second generation) agents are the preferred type in this population in light of their relatively favorable adverse cognitive and motor side effect profiles. Atypical antipsychotic treatment of acute agitation, aggression, and/or self-injurious behavior is usually initiated using low doses given at frequent intervals until the target behavior abates. In some cases, repeated dosing up to the point of treatment-induced sedation may be required to reduce the risk of harm to self and to others associated with severe aggressive or self-injurious behaviors. If treatment with an atypical antipsychotic is not effective, then low-dose haloperidol prescribed according to a similar dose-escalation protocol is a reasonable alternative treatment (50). Unfortunately, tolerance to the sedating effects of these agents develops relatively rapid. Therefore, an alternate medication strategy is needed when acute agitation, aggression, and/or self-injurious behaviors become chronic problems. Additionally, treatment-related akathisia and extrapyramidal side effects are not infrequent and are easily misunderstood as (or, in fact, contribute to) increasing agitation, restlessness, and self-injurious behaviors. The development of akathisia and extrapyramidal side effects, when unrecognized as such, may set in motion a cycle of continued dose escalation and behavioral deterioration. Worsening behavior during treatment of acute agitation, aggression, or self-injurious behavior, therefore, should prompt consideration of treatment induced behavioral disturbances and use of a different pharmacotherapeutic approach.

When acutely dangerous behavior abates, antipsychotic doses should be decreased gradually to determine the minimal effective dose (if any) needed for their continued management. Chronic treatment with these agents is usually reserved for patients with persistent psychotic symptoms or disorders. As noted earlier in this chapter, long-term use of antipsychotics requires vigilance for treatment-related adverse events including metabolic syndrome, late-onset (tardive) movement disorders, seizures, and neuroleptic malignant syndrome.

Benzodiazepines also may be helpful in the management of acute agitation and aggression (50,109). However, these agents predictably impair memory, motor function, coordination, and balance, and their use may slow neurobehavioral recovery and increase the risk of fall-related reinjury. Benzodiazepines occasionally produce paradoxical agitation (112), the occurrence of which may set in motion a cycle of behavioral worsening and benzodiazepine dose escalation. If benzodiazepines must be used to treat acute agitation, aggression, or self-injurious behaviors, then using serum metabolized agents with short- or moderate-duration half-lives and no active metabolites (e.g., lorazepam, oxazepam) for as brief a period of time as possible is recommended.

Pharmacotherapy of Chronic Agitation, Aggression, and Self-Injurious Behaviors

Chronic agitation, aggression, and/or self-injurious behaviors may be manifestations of another neuropsychiatric syndrome (e.g., depression, anxiety disorders, psychosis). This possibility requires consideration before, or concurrent to, directing pharmacotherapies toward chronic agitation, aggression, and/or self-injurious behaviors more specifically. These behaviors also may be independent problems, that require long-term symptom-targeted pharmacotherapy. In this context, realistic treatment goals, analogous to those for the pharmacologic treatment of intractable epilepsy, is not eliminating them completely but instead, simply reducing their frequency and severity. Multiple empiric trials of potentially effective agents are often required to accomplish this goal. When a medication is ineffective or only partially effective, subsequent and/or adjunctive medications should be selected based on substantive differences in their pharmacologic profiles from those used previously (i.e., addition of an anticonvulsant to an atypical antipsychotic is preferred over the use of 2 atypical antipsychotics).

The Neurobehavioral Guidelines Working Group (with the support of the National Brain Injury Research Treatment and Training Foundation, Centers for Disease Control and Prevention, Defense and Veterans Brain Injury Center, and Neurotrauma Foundation) performed an evidence-based review of pharmacotherapies for aggression and other post-traumatic neuropsychiatric disturbances (5). Readers are encouraged to consider their findings when developing a treatment plan for post-traumatic aggression. This group concluded that the evidence is insufficient to support treatment standards (highest recommendation level) but does support treatment guidelines (intermediate level) and options (lowest level). The adrenergic receptor antagonists propranolol and pindolol were recommended as treatment standards, and SSRIs, TCAs, buspirone, methylphenidate, valproate, and lithium were recommended as treatment options.

From a practical standpoint, the selection of medications for chronic post-traumatic agitation, aggression, and/or self-injurious behavior is usefully guided by developing a hypothesis about the neurobiological bases of the target behavior, considering the tolerability and ease of use of a particular antiaggressive medication and the extent to which that medication's mechanism of action matches the hypothesized neurobiological bases of the target behavior. For example, behavioral dyscontrol may reflect decreased "top-down" regulation of temporolimbic activity because of damage to anterior and/or dorsolateral prefrontal circuits and networks. If this hypothesis is correct, then these behaviors might respond to treatment with agents that reduce limbic catecholaminergic function, that is, dopamine receptor antagonists (i.e., haloperidol), β-adrenergic receptor antagonists (i.e., propranolol), or to medications that augment limbic serotonergic function, that is, SSRIs, 5-HT$_{2A}$ receptors (i.e., atypical antipsychotics), anticonvulsants, or uncompetitive NMDA receptor antagonists (e.g., amantadine, memantine). Among patients with relatively preserved dorsal prefrontal and orbitofrontal circuits and networks, augmentation of their function might decrease aberrant limbic drive of aggressive behaviors. If this hypothesis is correct, then using agents that augment monoaminergic function (e.g., amantadine, methylphenidate, dextroamphetamine, bromocriptine) or agents that improve prefrontally mediated modulation of limbic activity (e.g., SSRIs, buspirone, atypical antipsychotics) might reduce agitated, aggressive, and/or self-injurious behaviors.

Whether agitation, aggression, and self-injurious behaviors arise as a result of failed top-down inhibition of limbic activity or aberrant limbic drive, the SSRIs may be useful. In clinical practice, these agents are reasonably effective and generally well tolerated initial and long-term pharmacotherapies for these challenging behaviors. When used for these purposes, doses are similar to those used to treat depressive disorders. Some patients respond to or tolerate one SSRI more favorably than another; it, therefore, often is worthwhile to perform empiric trials of more than one agent from this class before declaring this class of medication ineffective for a given patient and switching treatment to another type of serotonergically active medication (e.g., trazodone, TCAs, buspirone).

When serotonergically active antidepressants do not adequately reduce chronic agitation, aggression, and/or self-injurious behaviors, an empiric trial of adjunctive or primary treatment with a mood stabilizing anticonvulsant may be considered. Valproate often is used as a first-line treatment, given its effectiveness, tolerability, and relatively limited drug–drug interactions. Carbamazepine may also be effective, but its side effect profile and hepatic autoinduction complicate its use. Other mood-stabilizing anticonvulsants including oxcarbazepine, gabapentin, and lamotrigine are used commonly in clinical practice to treat agitated, aggressive, and/or self-injurious behaviors; anecdotal experience suggests that these may be useful but are probably best reserved for use when serotonergically active antidepressants, valproate, carbamazepine, and lithium are inadequately effective.

Lithium, β-adrenergic receptor antagonists, long-acting benzodiazepines (e.g., clonazepam), and, among persons with preserved ventral frontal-subcortical systems, catecholamine-augmenting agents such as methylphenidate and amantadine also may reduce chronic agitation, aggression, and/or self-injurious behaviors. The evidence suggests that the β-adrenergic receptor antagonists are the most effective antiaggressive agents, but they are used relatively infrequently for this purpose. Instead, they tend to be used after or adjunctively to treatment with serotonergically active antidepressants, mood-stabilizing anticonvulsants, and/or lithium. Concerns regarding the potential cardiovascular, hypotensive, tolerance-related exercise, and depressogenic effects of these agents are often voiced by clinicians inexperienced with their use in the treatment of aggression. Although these concerns are not appropriate to dismiss offhandedly, slow titration to antiaggressive doses is rarely complicated by these problems. Despite the complexity of the use of any of these agents, they are important to consider when other agents prove ineffective, partially effective, or intolerable at doses needed to reduce agitation, aggression, and self-injurious behaviors.

Finally, atypical antipsychotics also may be required to reduce chronic aggression (42,95,96, 113). When used as an adjunctive intervention, low doses of these agents may be effective. If adjunctive treatment with an atypical antipsychotic reduces chronic agitation, aggression, and/or self-injurious behavior, then an empiric trial of atypical antipsychotic monotherapy should be considered. Although there is evidence suggesting that clozapine may be a useful treatment for aggressive, agitated, or self-injurious behaviors among persons with TBI, its cumbersome administration and monitoring requirements, its tendency to lower seizure threshold, and its risk for potentially life-threatening blood dyscrasias render it a treatment of last resort. When any of the atypical antipsychotics are used long term either as monotherapy or an augmentation agent, performing baseline and serial reassessment for cardiac, metabolic, and other antipsychotic-induced adverse effects are essential.

OTHER CHALLENGES IN NEUROPSYCHIATRIC PHARMACOTHERAPY

Biases against the use of medications to treat neuropsychiatric symptoms among persons with TBI are commonly held by patients and families as well as some clinicians and brain injury treatment centers. These biases often reflect an extension of the stigma associated with mental illness and psychiatric treatment. Additionally, they sometimes are derived from previous personal or witnessed suboptimal experiences with psychotropic medications.

Another fear about medication is that it will interfere with a "natural healing process" that occurs after TBI. Animal and human studies suggest that agents that reduce cerebral dopaminergic and/or noradrenergic function may delay recovery from TBI (83,85–87,114). However, the evidence addressing this issue in humans is limited to retrospective uncontrolled observations. There are no prospectively acquired data demonstrating that treatment of persons with TBI using medications that reduce cerebral dopaminergic and/or noradrenergic function results in adverse long-term outcomes. Prospective studies of anticonvulsants used during the early postinjury period also demonstrate short-term treatment-induced cognitive and motor impairments (43,115). These observations, along with the failure of these agents to reduce the long-term risk of post-traumatic epilepsy, have led to recommendations against the use of prophylactic anticonvulsants after the first postinjury week (116,117). As with the agents that decrease cerebral catecholaminergic function, early postinjury use of anticonvulsants does not appear to adversely affect long-term outcomes in this population (118).

Addressing biases against neuropsychiatric pharmacotherapies is often challenging and may not be possible to overcome in some cases. Acknowledging such concerns without endorsing biases is an important first step in developing the type of therapeutic rapport needed to productively consider the full range of treatment options for post-traumatic neuropsychiatric disturbances. Providing education to persons with TBI and their families on the neuropsychiatric perspective on brain-behavior relationships and the manner in which those relationships are vulnerable to disruption by TBI is a useful way to destigmatize neuropsychiatric symptoms and their treatments. The neuropsychiatric paradigm, one that rejects the misleading demarcation between "brain" and "mind" and emphasizes the neurobiological bases of all cognitive, emotional, and behavioral problems regardless of the relationship of such problems to brain injury, is among the most clinically useful responses to stigma-related antimedication biases. Patients struggling to accept treatment in the face of old stigmas may benefit from an explanation of symptoms as the products of alterations in neurotransmitters, brain structures, brain networks, or some combination of these and from the presentation of treatments as designed to alleviate or compensate for such brain dysfunctions.

Acknowledging adverse pharmacologic experiences among patients (or family members) with a history of prior treatments with psychotropic medications is necessary. At the same time, it is important to provide education and counseling on pharmacotherapies and to communicate optimism that appropriate treatment can reduce distress, mitigate disability, and improve quality of life. Developing a collaborative empirical approach to treatment with patients and/or their medical decision makers also may overcome antitreatment biases and allow all parties to these treatments to assess realistically the effectiveness of neuropsychiatric pharmacotherapies.

CONCLUSION

In this chapter, the roles of medications in the treatment of post-traumatic neuropsychiatric disturbances were reviewed. It would be ideal if neuropsychiatric disturbances among persons with TBI were fully responsive to nonpharmacologic treatments alone. Unfortunately, this often is not the case. When administered with care and forethought, pharmacotherapies may contribute usefully to the treatment of post-traumatic neuropsychiatric disturbances and improve quality of life for persons with TBI and their families.

1. Pharmacotherapy is a potentially effective element of a comprehensive treatment plan for post-traumatic neuropsychiatric disturbances; it is most appropriately regarded as adjunctive to other rehabilitative, environmental, behavioral, and psychological interventions.

2. The literature describing the benefits, risks, and side effects of medications used for this purpose is underdeveloped. Treatment selection, therefore, is guided by synthesizing information gleaned from studies of persons with TBI and patients with phenomenologically similar but etiologically distinct conditions, expert opinions, and consensus statements.

3. Rational pharmacotherapy requires consideration of the intended targets of treatment, initial TBI severity, time postinjury, and the stage of post-traumatic encephalopathy during which the neuropsychiatric target symptom occurs.

4. SSRIs are useful initial treatments of depressive disorders, anxiety disorders, PLC, disinhibition, aggression, and self-injurious behaviors among persons with TBI.

5. Secondary mania as well as recurrent mania because of idiopathic bipolar disorder may respond to initial treatment with anticonvulsants (e.g., valproate) or atypical antipsychotics (e.g., quetiapine).

6. Atypical antipsychotics are appropriate initial treatments for psychosis following TBI and may be useful in some patients with severe disinhibition and chronic agitation, aggression, and/or self-injurious behaviors.

7. Identify fears and concerns about neuropsychiatric pharmacotherapy before initiating such treatments. Education of the persons requiring treatment as well as their families and care providers can then focus on setting realistic expectations about the effects of pharmacotherapy and create a context for ongoing therapeutic collaboration.

1. Chew E, Zafonte RD. Pharmacological management of neurobehavioral disorders following traumatic brain injury—a state-of-the-art review. *J Rehabil Res Dev.* 2009; 46(6):851–879.

2. Warden DL, Gordon B, McAllister TW, et al. Guidelines for the pharmacologic treatment of neurobehavioral sequelae of traumatic brain injury. *J Neurotrauma.* 2006; 23(10):1468–1501.

3. Wheaton P, Mathias JL, Vink R. Impact of pharmacological treatments on cognitive and behavioral outcome in the postacute stages of adult traumatic brain injury: a meta-analysis. *J Clin Psychopharmacol.* 2011;31(6):745–757.

References

1. McCauley SR, Levin HS, Vanier M, et al. The neurobehavioural rating scale-revised: sensitivity and validity in closed head injury assessment. *J Neurol Neurosurg Psychiatry.* 2001;71(5):643–651.

2. Cummings JL, Mega M, Gray K, Rosenberg-Thompson S, Carusi DA, Gornbein J. The Neuropsychiatric Inventory: comprehensive assessment of psychopathology in dementia. *Neurology.* 1994; 44(12):2308–2314.

3. Kreutzer JS, Marwitz JH, Seel R, Serio CD. Validation of a neurobehavioral functioning inventory for adults with traumatic brain injury. *Arch Phys Med Rehabil.* 1996;77(2):116–124.

4. Seel RT, Kreutzer JS, Sander AM. Concordance of patients' and family members' ratings of neurobehavioral functioning after traumatic brain injury. *Arch Phys Med Rehabil.* 1997;78(11):1254–1259.

5. Warden DL, Gordon B, McAllister TW, et al. Guidelines for the pharmacologic treatment of neurobehavioral sequelae of traumatic brain injury. *J Neurotrauma.* 2006;23(10):1468–1501.

6. Chew E, Zafonte RD. Pharmacological management of neurobehavioral disorders following traumatic brain injury—a state-of-the-art review. *J Rehabil Res Dev.* 2009;46(6):851–879.

7. Bombardier CH, Fann JR, Temkin NR, Esselman PC, Barber J, Dikmen SS. Rates of major depressive disorder and clinical outcomes following traumatic brain injury. *JAMA.* 2010;303(19):1938–1945.

8. Jorge RE, Robinson RG, Moser D, Tateno A, Crespo-Facorro B, Arndt S. Major depression following traumatic brain injury. *Arch Gen Psychiatry.* 2004;61(1):42–50.

9. Seel RT, Kreutzer JS, Rosenthal M, Hammond FM, Corrigan JD, Black K. Depression after traumatic brain injury: a National Institute on Disability and Rehabilitation Research Model Systems multicenter investigation. *Arch Phys Med Rehabil.* 2003;84(2):177–184.

10. Jorge RE, Robinson RG, Starkstein SE, Arndt SV, Forrester AW, Geisler FH. Secondary mania following traumatic brain injury. *Am J Psychiatry.* 1993;150(6):916–921.

11. Oster TJ, Anderson CA, Filley CM, Wortzel HS, Arciniegas DB. Quetiapine for mania due to traumatic brain injury. *CNS Spectr.* 2007;12(10):764–769.

12. Tateno A, Jorge RE, Robinson RG. Pathological laughing and crying following traumatic brain injury. *J Neuropsychiatry Clin Neurosci.* 2004;16(4):426–434.

13. Zeilig G, Drubach DA, Katz-Zeilig M, Karatinos J. Pathological laughter and crying in patients with closed traumatic brain injury. *Brain Inj.* 1996;10(8):591–597.

14. Cook KF, Bombardier CH, Bamer AM, Choi SW, Kroenke K, Fann JR. Do somatic and cognitive symptoms of traumatic brain injury confound depression screening? *Arch Phys Med Rehabil.* 2011;92(5): 818–823.

15. Alderfer BS, Arciniegas DB, Silver JM. Treatment of depression following traumatic brain injury. *J Head Trauma Rehabil.* 2005;20(6): 544–562.

16. Silver JM, McAllister TW, Arciniegas DB. Depression and cognitive complaints following mild traumatic brain injury. *Am J Psychiatry.* 2009;166(6):653–661.

17. Fann JR, Hart T, Schomer KG. Treatment for depression after traumatic brain injury: a systematic review. *J Neurotrauma.* 2009;26(12): 2383–2402.

18. Fann JR, Uomoto JM, Katon WJ. Cognitive improvement with treatment of depression following mild traumatic brain injury. *Psychosomatics.* 2001;42(1):48–54.

19. Alper K, Schwartz KA, Kolts RL, Khan A. Seizure incidence in psychopharmacological clinical trials: an analysis of Food and Drug Administration (FDA) summary basis of approval reports. *Biol Psychiatry.* 2007;62(4):345–554.

20. Ashman TA, Cantor JB, Gordon WA, et al. A randomized controlled trial of sertraline for the treatment of depression in persons with traumatic brain injury. *Arch Phys Med Rehabil.* 2009;90(5): 733–740.

21. Novack TA, Baños JH, Brunner R, Renfroe S, Meythaler JM. Impact of early administration of sertraline on depressive symptoms in the first year after traumatic brain injury. *J Neurotrauma.* 2009;26(11): 1921–1928.

22. Fann JR, Uomoto JM, Katon WJ. Sertraline in the treatment of major depression following mild traumatic brain injury. *J Neuropsychiatry Clin Neurosci.* 2000;12(2):226–232.

23. Lanctôt KL, Rapoport MJ, Chan F, et al. Genetic predictors of response to treatment with citalopram in depression secondary to traumatic brain injury. *Brain Inj.* 2010;24(7–8):959–969.

24. Rapoport MJ, Chan F, Lanctôt K, Herrmann N, McCullagh S, Feinstein A. An open-label study of citalopram for major depression following traumatic brain injury. *J Psychopharmacol.* 2008;22(8): 860–864.

25. Schmitt JA, Kruizinga MJ, Riedel WJ. Non-serotonergic pharmacological profiles and associated cognitive effects of serotonin reuptake inhibitors. *J Psychopharmacol.* 2001;15(3):173–179.

26. Lee H, Kim SW, Kim JM, Shin IS, Yang SJ, Yoon JS. Comparing effects of methylphenidate, sertraline and placebo on neuropsychiatric sequelae in patients with traumatic brain injury. *Hum Psychopharmacol.* 2005;20(2):97–104.

27. Gualtieri CT, Evans RW. Stimulant treatment for the neurobehavioural sequelae of traumatic brain injury. *Brain Inj.* 1988;2(4):273–290.

28. Rosenberg PB, Ahmed I, Hurwitz S. Methylphenidate in depressed medically ill patients. *J Clin Psychiatry.* 1991;52(6):263–267.

29. Rothenhäusler HB, Ehrentraut S, von Degenfeld G, et al. Treatment of depression with methylphenidate in patients difficult to wean from mechanical ventilation in the intensive care unit. *J Clin Psychiatry.* 2000;61(10):750–755.

30. Rush AJ, Trivedi MH, Stewart JW, et al. Combining medications to enhance depression outcomes (CO-MED): acute and long-term outcomes of a single-blind randomized study. *Am J Psychiatry.* 2011;168(7):689–701.

31. Fava M, Rush AJ, Wisniewski SR, et al. A comparison of mirtazapine and nortriptyline following two consecutive failed medication treatments for depressed outpatients: a STAR*D report. *Am J Psychiatry.* 2006;163(7):1161–1172.

32. Frey LC. Epidemiology of posttraumatic epilepsy: a critical review. *Epilepsia.* 2003;44(suppl 10):11–17.

33. American Psychiatric Association. Practice guideline for the treatment of patients with bipolar disorder (revision). *Am J Psychiatry.* 2002;159(4)(suppl):1–50.

34. Pope HG Jr, McElroy SL, Satlin A, Hudson JI, Keck PE Jr, Kalish R. Head injury, bipolar disorder, and response to valproate. *Compr Psychiatry.* 1988;29(1):34–38.

35. Kim E, Humaran TJ. Divalproex in the management of neuropsychiatric complications of remote acquired brain injury. *J Neuropsychiatry Clin Neurosci.* 2002;14(2):202–205.

36. Monji A, Yoshida I, Koga H, Tashiro K, Tashiro N. Brain injury-induced rapid-cycling affective disorder successfully treated with valproate. *Psychosomatics.* 1999;40(5):448–449.

37. Yassa R, Cvejic J. Valproate in the treatment of posttraumatic bipolar disorder in a psychogeriatric patient. *J Geriatr Psychiatry Neurol.* 1994;7(1):55–57.

38. Daniels JP, Felde A. Quetiapine treatment for mania secondary to brain injury in 2 patients. *J Clin Psychiatry.* 2008;69(3):497–498.

39. Dikmen SS, Machamer JE, Winn HR, Anderson GD, Temkin NR. Neuropsychological effects of valproate in traumatic brain injury: a randomized trial. *Neurology.* 2000;54(4):895–902.

40. Massagli TL. Neurobehavioral effects of phenytoin, carbamazepine, and valproic acid: implications for use in traumatic brain injury. *Arch Phys Med Rehabil.* 1991;72(3):219–226.

41. Hornstein A, Seliger G. Cognitive side effects of lithium in closed head injury. *J Neuropsychiatry Clin Neurosci.* 1989;1(4):446–447.

42. Kim E, Bijlani M. A pilot study of quetiapine treatment of aggression due to traumatic brain injury. *J Neuropsychiatry Clin Neurosci.* 2006;18(4):547–549.

43. Smith KR Jr, Goulding PM, Wilderman D, Goldfader PR, Holterman-Hommes P, Wei F. Neurobehavioral effects of phenytoin and carbamazepine in patients recovering from brain trauma: a comparative study. *Arch Neurol.* 1994;51(7):653–660.

44. Wortzel HS, Oster TJ, Anderson CA, Arciniegas DB. Pathological laughing and crying: epidemiology, pathophysiology and treatment. *CNS Drugs.* 2008;22(7):531–545.

45. Peeters M, Romieu P, Maurice T, Su TP, Maloteaux JM, Hermans E. Involvement of the sigma 1 receptor in the modulation of dopaminergic transmission by amantadine. *Eur J Neurosci.* 2004;19(8):2212–2220.

46. Werling LL, Keller A, Frank JG, Nuwayhid SJ. A comparison of the binding profiles of dextromethorphan, memantine, fluoxetine and amitriptyline: treatment of involuntary emotional expression disorder. *Exp Neurol.* 2007;207(2):248–257.

47. Narita N, Hashimoto K, Tomitaka S, Minabe Y. Interactions of selective serotonin reuptake inhibitors with subtypes of sigma receptors in rat brain. *Eur J Pharmacol.* 1996;307(1):117–119.

48. Chahine LM, Chemali Z. Du rire aux larmes: pathological laughing and crying in patients with traumatic brain injury and treatment with lamotrigine. *Epilepsy Behav.* 2006;8(3):610–615.

49. Kim E, Lauterbach EC, Reeve A, et al. Neuropsychiatric complications of traumatic brain injury: a critical review of the literature (a report by the ANPA Committee on Research). *J Neuropsychiatry Clin Neurosci.* 2007;19(2):106–127.

50. American Psychiatric Association. *Quick Reference to the American Psychiatric Association Practice Guidelines for the Treatment of Psychiatric Disorders: Compendium 2006.* Arlington, VA: American Psychiatric Association; 2006.

51. McAllister TW. Psychopharmacological issues in the treatment of TBI and PTSD. *Clin Neuropsychol.* 2009;23(8):1338–1367.

52. Gualtieri CT. Buspirone for the behavior problems of patients with organic brain disorders. *J Clin Psychopharmacol.* 1991;11(4):280–281.

53. van Laar MW, Volkerts ER, van Willigenburg AP. Therapeutic effects and effects on actual driving performance of chronically administered buspirone and diazepam in anxious outpatients. *J Clin Psychopharmacol.* 1992;12(2):86–95.

54. Angus WR, Romney DM. The effect of diazepam on patients' memory. *J Clin Psychopharmacol.* 1984;4(4):203–206.

55. Lucki I, Rickels K, Geller AM. Chronic use of benzodiazepines and psychomotor and cognitive test performance. *Psychopharmacology (Berl).* 1986;88(4):426–433.

56. Roth T, Hartse KM, Zorick FJ, Kaffeman ME. The differential effects of short- and long-acting benzodiazepines upon nocturnal sleep and daytime performance. *Arzneimittelforschung.* 1980;30(5a):891–894.

57. Ciurli P, Formisano R, Bivona U, Cantagallo A, Angelelli P. Neuropsychiatric disorders in persons with severe traumatic brain injury: prevalence, phenomenology, and relationship with demographic clinical, and functional features. *J Head Trauma Rehabil.* 2011;26(2):116–126.

58. Marin RS, Wilkosz PA. Disorders of diminished motivation. *J Head Trauma Rehabil.* 2005;20(4):377–388.

59. Andersson S, Gundersen PM, Finset A. Emotional activation during therapeutic interaction in traumatic brain injury: effect of apathy, self-awareness and implications for rehabilitation. *Brain Inj.* 1999;13(6):393–404.

60. Seel RT, Macciocchi S, Kreutzer JS. Clinical considerations for the diagnosis of major depression after moderate to severe TBI. *J Head Trauma Rehabil.* 2010;25(2):99–112.

61. Hoehn-Saric R, Lipsey JR, McLeod DR. Apathy and indifference in patients on fluvoxamine and fluoxetine. *J Clin Psychopharmacol.* 1990;10(5):343–345.

62. Lane-Brown AT, Tate RL. Apathy after acquired brain impairment: a systematic review of non-pharmacological interventions. *Neuropsychol Rehabil.* 2009;19(4):481–516.

63. Roth RM, Flashman LA, McAllister TW. Apathy and its treatment. *Curr Treat Options Neurol.* 2007;9(5):363–370.

64. Kraus MF, Maki P. The combined use of amantadine and l-dopa/carbidopa in the treatment of chronic brain injury. *Brain Inj.* 1997;11(6):455–460.

65. Kraus MF, Maki PM. Effect of amantadine hydrochloride on symptoms of frontal lobe dysfunction in brain injury: case studies and review. *J Neuropsychiatry Clin Neurosci.* 1997;9(2):222–230.

66. Van Reekum R, Bayley M, Garner S, et al. N of 1 study: amantadine for the amotivational syndrome in a patient with traumatic brain injury. *Brain Inj.* 1995;9(1):49–53.

67. Gualtieri T, Chandler M, Coons TB, Brown LT. Amantadine: a new clinical profile for traumatic brain injury. *Clin Neuropharmacol.* 1989;12(4):258–270.

68. Chandler MC, Barnhill JL, Gualtieri CT. Amantadine for the agitated head-injury patient. *Brain Inj.* 1988;2(4):309–311.

69. Nickels JL, Schneider WN, Dombovy ML, Wong TM. Clinical use of amantadine in brain injury rehabilitation. *Brain Inj.* 1994;8(8):709–718.

70. Powell JH, al-Adawi S, Morgan J, Greenwood RJ. Motivational deficits after brain injury: effects of bromocriptine in 11 patients. *J Neurol Neurosurg Psychiatry.* 1996;60(4):416–421.

71. Eames P. The use of Sinemet and bromocriptine. *Brain Inj.* 1989;3(3):319–322.

72. Lal S, Merbtiz CP, Grip JC. Modification of function in head-injured patients with Sinemet. *Brain Inj.* 1988;2(3):225–233.

73. Debette S, Kozlowski O, Steinling M, Rousseaux M. Levodopa and bromocriptine in hypoxic brain injury. *J Neurol.* 2002;249(12): 1678–1682.

74. Evans RW, Gualtieri CT, Patterson D. Treatment of chronic closed head injury with psychostimulant drugs: a controlled case study and an appropriate evaluation procedure. *J Nerv Ment Dis.* 1987; 175(2):106–110.

75. Glenn MB. Methylphenidate for cognitive and behavioral dysfunction after traumatic brain injury. *J Head Trauma Rehabil.* 1998;13(5): 87–90.

76. Arciniegas DB, Harris SN, Brousseau KM. Psychosis following traumatic brain injury. *Int Rev Psychiatry.* 2003;15(4):328–340.

77. Crossley NA, Constante M, McGuire P, Power P. Efficacy of atypical v. typical antipsychotics in the treatment of early psychosis: meta-analysis. *Br J Psychiatry.* 2010;196(6):434–439.

78. Rummel-Kluge C, Komossa K, Schwarz S, et al. Second-generation antipsychotic drugs and extrapyramidal side effects: a systematic review and meta-analysis of head-to-head comparisons. *Schizophr Bull.* 2012;38(1):167–177.

79. Gentile S. Second-generation antipsychotics in dementia: beyond safety concerns. A clinical, systematic review of efficacy data from randomised controlled trials. *Psychopharmacology (Berl).* 2010; 212(2):119–129.

80. Foussias G, Remington G. Antipsychotics and schizophrenia: from efficacy and effectiveness to clinical decision-making. *Can J Psychiatry.* 2010;55(3):117–125.

81. Saunders KE, Hawton K. The role of psychopharmacology in suicide prevention. *Epidemiol Psichiatr Soc.* 2009;18(3):172–178.

82. Volavka J, Citrome L. Oral antipsychotics for the treatment of schizophrenia: heterogeneity in efficacy and tolerability should drive decision-making. *Expert Opin Pharmacother.* 2009;10(12):1917–1928.

83. Mysiw WJ, Bogner JA, Corrigan JD, Fugate LP, Clinchot DM, Kadyan V. The impact of acute care medications on rehabilitation outcome after traumatic brain injury. *Brain Inj.* 2006;20(9):905–911.

84. Rao N, Jellinek HM, Woolston DC. Agitation in closed head injury: haloperidol effects on rehabilitation outcome. *Arch Phys Med Rehabil.* 1985;66(1):30–34.

85. Hoffman AN, Cheng JP, Zafonte RD, Kline AE. Administration of haloperidol and risperidone after neurobehavioral testing hinders the recovery of traumatic brain injury-induced deficits. *Life Sci.* 2008;83(17–18):602–607.

86. Kline AE, Hoffman AN, Cheng JP, Zafonte RD, Massucci JL. Chronic administration of antipsychotics impede behavioral recovery after experimental traumatic brain injury. *Neurosci Lett.* 2008; 448(3):263–267.

87. Kline AE, Massucci JL, Zafonte RD, Dixon CE, DeFeo JR, Rogers EH. Differential effects of single versus multiple administrations of haloperidol and risperidone on functional outcome after experimental brain trauma. *Crit Care Med.* 2007;35(3):919–924.

88. Stanislav SW. Cognitive effects of antipsychotic agents in persons with traumatic brain injury. *Brain Inj.* 1997;11(5):335–341.

89. Sandel ME, Olive DA, Rader MA. Chlorpromazine-induced psychosis after brain injury. *Brain Inj.* 1993;7(1):77–83.

90. Bymaster FP, Felder CC, Tzavara E, Nomikos GG, Calligaro DO, McKinzie DL. Muscarinic mechanisms of antipsychotic atypicality. *Prog Neuropsychopharmacol Biol Psychiatry.* 2003;27(7):1125–1243.

91. Johnson DE, Nedza FM, Spracklin DK, et al. The role of muscarinic receptor antagonism in antipsychotic-induced hippocampal acetylcholine release. *Eur J Pharmacol.* 2005;506(3):209–219.

92. Volavka J, Citrome L. All antipsychotics are equal, but some are more equal than others. *J Clin Psychiatry.* 2009;70(3):429–430.

93. Edwards SJ, Smith CJ. Tolerability of atypical antipsychotics in the treatment of adults with schizophrenia or bipolar disorder: a mixed treatment comparison of randomized controlled trials. *Clin Ther.* 2009;31(pt 1):1345–1359.

94. Mittal V, Kurup L, Williamson D, Muralee S, Tampi RR. Risk of cerebrovascular adverse events and death in elderly patients with dementia when treated with antipsychotic medications: a literature review of evidence. *Am J Alzheimers Dis Other Demen.* 2011;26(1): 10–28.

95. Ballard C, Corbett A, Chitramohan R, Aarsland D. Management of agitation and aggression associated with Alzheimer's disease:

96. Michals ML, Crismon ML, Roberts S, Childs A. Clozapine response and adverse effects in nine brain-injured patients. *J Clin Psychopharmacol.* 1993;13(3):198–203.

97. Burke JG, Dursun SM, Reveley MA. Refractory symptomatic schizophrenia resulting from frontal lobe lesion: response to clozapine. *J Psychiatry Neurosci.* 1999;24(5):456–461.

98. Schreiber S, Klag E, Gross Y, Segman RH, Pick CG. Beneficial effect of risperidone on sleep disturbance and psychosis following traumatic brain injury. *Int Clin Psychopharmacol.* 1998;13(6):273–275.

99. Tellier A, Marshall SC, Wilson KG, Smith A, Perugini M, Stiell IG. The heterogeneity of mild traumatic brain injury: where do we stand? *Brain Inj.* 2009;23(11):879–887.

100. Lichter DG, Cummings JL. *Frontal-subcortical Circuits in Psychiatric and Neurological Disorders.* New York, NY: Guilford Press; 2001.

101. Guay DR. Inappropriate sexual behaviors in cognitively impaired older individuals. *Am J Geriatr Pharmacother.* 2008;6(5):269–288.

102. Chow TW. Treatment approaches to symptoms associated with frontotemporal degeneration. *Curr Psychiatry Rep.* 2005;7(5): 376–380.

103. Guay DR. Drug treatment of paraphilic and nonparaphilic sexual disorders. *Clin Ther.* 2009;31(1):1–31.

104. Sink KM, Holden KF, Yaffe K. Pharmacological treatment of neuropsychiatric symptoms of dementia: a review of the evidence. *JAMA.* 2005;293(5):596–608.

105. Beaulieu C, Wertheimer JC, Pickett L, et al. Behavior management on an acute brain injury unit: evaluating the effectiveness of an interdisciplinary training program. *J Head Trauma Rehabil.* 2008; 23(5):304–311.

106. Kelly G, Brown S, Todd J, Kremer P. Challenging behaviour profiles of people with acquired brain injury living in community settings. *Brain Inj.* 2008;22(6):457–470.

107. Najdowski AC, Wallace MD, Ellsworth CL, MacAleese AN, Cleveland JM. Functional analyses and treatment of precursor behavior. *J Appl Behav Anal.* 2008;41(1):97–105.

108. Corrigan PW, Yudofsky SC, Silver JM. Pharmacological and behavioral treatments for aggressive psychiatric inpatients. *Hosp Community Psychiatry.* 1993;44(2):125–133.

109. Pabis DJ, Stanislav SW. Pharmacotherapy of aggressive behavior. *Ann Pharmacother.* 1996;30(3):278–287.

110. Hankin CS, Bronstone A, Koran LM. Agitation in the inpatient psychiatric setting: a review of clinical presentation, burden, and treatment. *J Psychiatr Pract.* 2011;17(3):170–185.

111. Allen MH, Currier GW, Carpenter D, Ross RW, Docherty JP. The expert consensus guideline series. Treatment of behavioral emergencies 2005. *J Psychiatr Pract.* 2005;11(suppl 1):5–108; quiz 110–112.

112. Smith VM. Paradoxical reactions to diazepam. *Gastrointest Endosc.* 1995;41(2):182–183.

113. Scott LK, Green R, McCarthy PJ, Conrad SA. Agitation and/or aggression after traumatic brain injury in the pediatric population treated with ziprasidone. Clinical article. *J Neurosurg Pediatr.* 2009; 3(6):484–487.

114. Liepert J. Pharmacotherapy in restorative neurology. *Curr Opin Neurol.* 2008;21(6):639–643.

115. Dikmen SS, Temkin NR, Miller B, Machamer J, Winn HR. Neurobehavioral effects of phenytoin prophylaxis of posttraumatic seizures. *JAMA.* 1991;265(10):1271–1277.

116. Bratton, SL, Chestnut, RM, Ghajar J, et al; for Brain Trauma Foundation, American Association of Neurological Surgeons, Congress of Neurological Surgeons, Joint Section on Neurotrauma and Critical Care, AANS/CNS. Guidelines for the management of severe traumatic brain injury. XIII. Antiseizure prophylaxis. *J Neurotrauma.* 2007;24(suppl 1):S83–S86.

117. Chang BS, Lowenstein DH. Practice parameter: antiepileptic drug prophylaxis in severe traumatic brain injury: report of the Quality Standards Subcommittee of the American Academy of Neurology. *Neurology.* 2003;60(1):10–16.

118. Schierhout G, Roberts I. Anti-epileptic drugs for preventing seizures following acute traumatic brain injury. *Cochrane Database Syst Rev.* 2001(4):CD000173.

Neurotechnology in Traumatic Brain Injury Rehabilitation

Paolo Bonato

INTRODUCTION

Over the past two decades, advances in electronics, robotics, and computer science have led to several new technologies that have enabled interventions relevant to traumatic brain injury (TBI) rehabilitation. Their impact on the clinical management of individuals with TBI far exceeds the content of this chapter, which is solely focused on neurotechnologies that have enabled new rehabilitation interventions. Technologies (such as new imaging techniques) that have provided, for instance, new diagnostic tools are not discussed in this chapter.

The chapter is organized into 5 main sections. The first section is devoted to neurotechnologies for brain stimulation. This section provides a short review of deep brain stimulation, cortical stimulation, transcranial magnetic stimulation, and transcranial direct current stimulation. It also provides some notes about the use of low-level laser therapy, transcranial Doppler sonography, and galvanic vestibular stimulation (GVS) for brain stimulation.

The second section of this chapter is focused on neurotechnologies for peripheral stimulation. It contains information about invasive and noninvasive technologies for vagus nerve stimulation (VNS), functional electrical stimulation (FES) of the upper and lower limbs, and electrical as well as mechanical subsensory stimulation of muscle spindles, Golgi tendon organs, and mechanoreceptors using a technique known as *stochastic resonance*.

Brain computer interfaces (BCIs) are discussed in the following section. This section is mostly focused on BCIs implemented by means of scalp recordings, but cortical and intracortical recording techniques are also discussed. This is a topic of growing interest and although there appear to be no published applications of BCIs in individuals with TBI, the potential for rehabilitation applications of BCIs in this patient population is significant and therefore discussed in this section. The section also mentions the potential implementation of BCIs using functional near-infrared spectroscopy.

Rehabilitation robotics has generated a great deal of attention among researchers and clinicians. Although further research is needed to develop clinical protocols for robotic-assisted rehabilitation and to assess their effectiveness, robotics has entered into the clinic. Therefore, a section of this chapter has been devoted to robotic technologies designed for upper- and lower-limb rehabilitation. The section provides an overview of the main technological aspects of rehabilitation robotics and discusses their potential clinical implications.

Finally, a section of this chapter is devoted to the use of virtual reality and interactive gaming in rehabilitation. The implementation of fully immersive virtual reality environments requires significant financial investments. Therefore, immersive virtual reality environments have been rarely adopted in the clinic. However, highly engaging interactive gaming platforms that have been recently developed for the consumer market have been adopted or modified for application in rehabilitation. A section of this chapter is devoted to virtual reality and interactive gaming technologies of interest in rehabilitation. The section discusses existing and potential future clinical applications of these technologies in individuals with TBI.

Whereas some of the technologies discussed in this chapter have witnessed broad clinical adoption, others are still undergoing development and clinical evaluation. An example of technology that has recently made it into the clinic is FES. Researchers started exploring the use of this technology about 4 decades ago, but at that time systems for FES were bulky and difficult to use. Recent advances in electronics have allowed manufacturers to redesign FES systems, thus making their use appealing to clinicians and patients. Products like the Bioness L300 (Bioness Inc, Valencia, CA) and the WalkAide (Innovative Neurotronics Inc, Austin, TX) are now commonly used in the clinic for the management of foot drop. Vice versa, technologies like BCIs are mostly of interest in a research context and have not seen broad clinical application as yet. BCIs (particularly systems implemented using scalp recordings of brain activity) have great potential in rehabilitation. However, a clear application in the clinic has not been identified as yet. Consequently, it is anticipated that, for a few years to come, their use will be limited to research studies. It is hoped that researchers will be able to make progress toward the development of clinical applications of relevance in the rehabilitation of individuals with TBI and patients with other neurological conditions. At the end of this chapter, the key current and future clinical applications of the technologies herein described are discussed.

BRAIN STIMULATION

Several invasive and noninvasive brain stimulation techniques have been used in individuals with TBI including deep brain stimulation, cortical stimulation, transcranial magnetic stimulation, and transcranial direct current stimulation. Other experimental techniques of brain stimulation are low-level laser therapy, transcranial Doppler sonography (TCD), and GVS. GVS is not applied directly to the brain. However, herein the technique is presented as a potential means to stimulate attentional networks via projections from the vestibular system to the perisylvian region (mediated by the ventral posterior subthalamic nucleus). Consequently, GVS is presented together with the above-mentioned brain stimulation techniques listed previously.

Deep brain stimulation has been used in patients in the minimally conscious state following severe TBI. Schiff et al. (1) recently presented a single-case study in which deep brain stimulation of the central thalamus was applied to an individual with TBI in the minimally conscious state showing preservation of large-scale cerebral networks as observed via functional magnetic resonance imaging (fMRI) (2). Deep brain stimulation was initially developed for Parkinson's control therapy, but more recently, it has been used for the clinical management of various neurological conditions by targeting appropriate brain regions (3). In the case reported by Schiff et al. (1), the authors implanted a Kinetra pulse generator (Medtronic, Minneapolis, MN) (shown in Figure 75-1) in the infraclavicular region and connected it to stimulation leads with electrodes positioned bilaterally in the central thalamus. The Kinetra pulse generator allows one to generate stimulation pulses with the following char-

acteristics: pulse width ranging from 60 μs to 450 μs, pulse amplitude ranging from 0.0 V to 10.5 V, and frequency ranging from 3 Hz to 250 Hz. Besides, the 2 sets (for bilateral stimulation) of 4 electrodes connected to the pulse generator can be used to deliver either unipolar or bipolar stimulation. Schiff and colleagues implemented an 18-week protocol to test a range of stimulation parameters and observed the effects of different stimulation settings on the behavioral responsiveness of the patient using the JFK Coma Recovery Scale-Revised (4) to determine optimal stimulation conditions. At conclusion of this 18-week titration period, the authors started a 6-month double-blinded crossover study to assess the responsiveness of the subject to deep brain stimulation. The patient, a 38-year-old male who had remained in a minimally conscious state for 6 years following a severe TBI, demonstrated an increase in behavioral responsiveness when subject to deep brain stimulation. Schiff and colleagues concluded that deep brain stimulation can have effects that compensate for the loss of arousal regulation controlled by the frontal lobe in the intact brain.

Prior to the study by Schiff et al. (1), Tsubokawa et al. (5) had explored the use of deep brain stimulation in 8 patients in a persistent vegetative state. These individuals were subject to deep brain stimulation for a period ranging between 3 and 6 months. Three of these patients emerged from the persistent vegetative state. One other patient showed signs of recovery. Four patients showed no response. A key difference between the study carried out by Schiff et al. (1) and the study performed by Tsubokawa et al. (5) is that Schiff and colleagues selected a candidate in the minimally conscious state showing preservation of brain structure and evidence of interactive behavior (6). Recently, Yamamoto et al. (7) also obtained encouraging results in patients in the vegetative state following a brain injury. The authors recruited 107 patients in the study, 21 of which were subject to deep brain stimulation. Interestingly, none of the patients in the control group (i.e., receiving no stimulation) recovered from the vegetative state. The stimulation was applied to the mesencephalic reticular formation (2 patients) and centromedian-parafascicularis nucleus complex (19 cases). Recovery from the vegetative state was found to be associated with specific characteristics of brain activity as detected using electroencephalographic (EEG) recordings.

Invasive cortical stimulation has also been used in individuals with TBI. Son et al. (8) reported the results of a single-case study in which cortical stimulation was used for pain management in an individual reporting severe spontaneous burning pain that affected the upper and lower limbs. The authors used the Itrel 3 neurostimulator (Medtronic, Minneapolis, MN) that delivers stimulation pulses with the following characteristics: pulse width ranging from 60 μs to 210 μs, pulse amplitude ranging from 0.0 V to 10.5 V, and frequency ranging from 2.1 Hz to 130.0 Hz. In addition, the stimulation can be delivered either continuously or in bursts (i.e., cycling mode). During a 7-day test period, the authors observed significant pain relief when the upper limb area was subject to stimulation with the following characteristics: 21 Hz, 210 μs, 0.8–1.2 V. Also, significant pain relief was observed when the lower limb area was subject to stimulation with the following characteristics: 30 Hz, 210 μs, 2.0–2.5 V. Adjustments in the stimulation settings were performed by relying on feedback concerning pain relief from the patient. This was the first

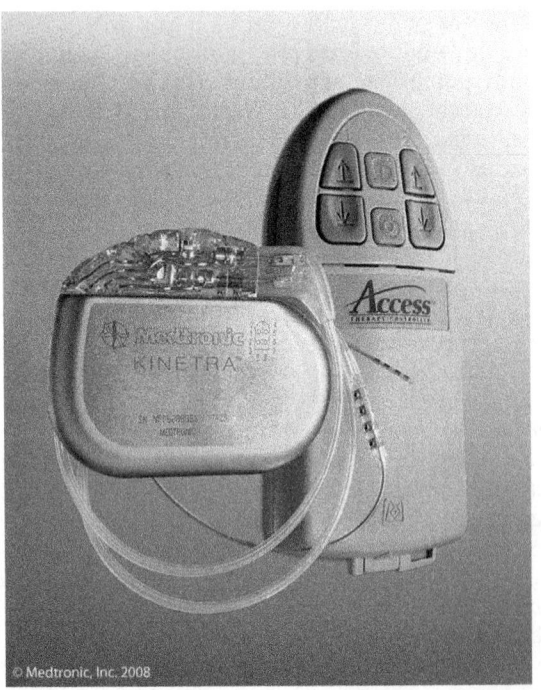

© Medtronic, Inc. 2008

FIGURE 75-1 The Kinetra system (Medtronic, Minneapolis, MN) for deep brain stimulation with stimulation leads and a handheld programming unit to set the stimulation parameters. Reproduced with permission, courtesy of Medtronic.

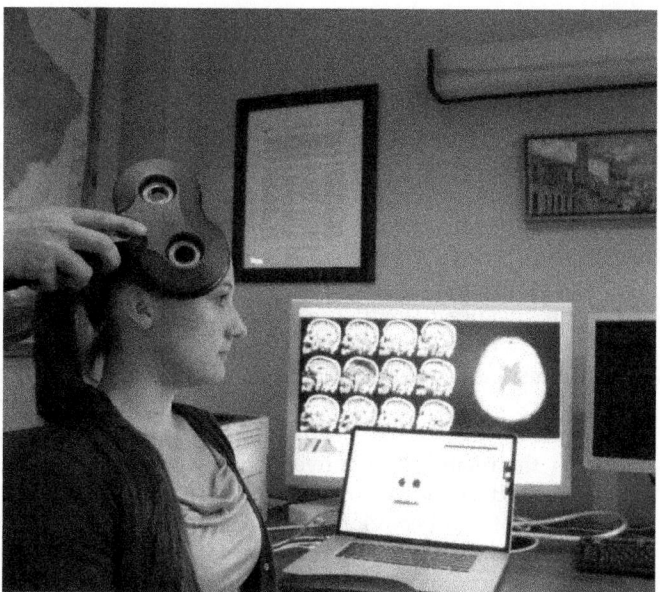

FIGURE 75-2 A subject receives transcranial magnetic stimulation (TMS) delivered using a figure-8 coil. Reproduced with permission, courtesy of Dr. Felipe Fregni, Spaulding Rehabilitation Hospital.

report of cortical stimulation for pain relief in a TBI survivor, but several studies had been previously performed in stroke (9–11) with positive results.

Brain stimulation can also be achieved via noninvasive techniques. Demirtas-Tatlidede et al. (12) recently reviewed 4 modalities of noninvasive brain stimulation and their potential use in TBI: transcranial magnetic stimulation (TMS), transcranial direct current stimulation (tDCS), low-level laser therapy, and transcranial Doppler sonography (TCD).

TMS is based on the induction of a current in a discrete area of the brain via an external coil that is positioned on the skull on top of the brain area of interest (Figure 75-2). The coil is used to generate a rapidly changing magnetic field that in turn causes the generation of a current in the brain. The strength of the generated field typically varies between 1 and 2 Tesla. The field is applied as a monophasic or biphasic waveform typically of about 1 millisecond in duration. Single-pulse TMS can be used to map brain areas leading to a given behavioral output. For instance, when TMS is applied to motor cortical areas, a motor response is induced (13). Paired-pulse TMS has also been extensively used. This technique has allowed researchers to study intracortical inhibitory/excitatory circuits and corticocortical connectivity (14). TMS could be used in TBI to assess the extent of the injury. It could also facilitate understanding of plasticity via mapping cortical areas as well as assessing changes in connectivity overtime.

Other TMS-based stimulation modalities have been developed to increase or decrease cortical excitability. Repetitive transcranial magnetic stimulation (rTMS) has been used in this context. Low-frequency rTMS (≤ 1 Hz) decreases excitability of cortical areas whereas bursts of intermittent high-frequency stimulation (≥ 5 Hz) increase excitability of targeted cortical areas. Additional ways to deliver rTMS have been explored. Researchers have experimented with a

subtype of rTMS known as theta burst stimulation (TBS). TBS consists of very short, high-frequency (50 Hz) trains of stimuli delivered intermittently or continuously. Intermittent TBS increases cortical excitability whereas continuous TBS decreases cortical excitability. The effects of rTMS outlast the duration of the stimulation. Therefore, many have looked into the potential therapeutic use of this technique. The prolonged effects of rTMS are thought to be caused by modulation of long-term depression (LTD) and long-term potentiation (LTP) between synaptic connections. Following diffuse damage after TBI, LTP and LTD may be abnormal because of cellular injury and altered connectivity. Therefore, rTMS could facilitate recovery after a TBI.

TMS is the only noninvasive stimulation technique among the ones discussed in this chapter that has been broadly used to study the altered neurophysiology of patients following a TBI (15–16) and to treat patients (17–18). The use of rTMS to achieve neurobehavioral gains has been explored in patients recovering from a coma following a TBI (17). It has also been used to treat depression (18). Side-effects include the following: transient headache, local pain, neck pain, toothache, paresthesias, transient hearing changes, transient changes in cognitive/neuropsychological functions, and syncope (as epiphenomenon). The most serious adverse event is induced seizure, but this is rare.

tDCS is another technique of noninvasive brain stimulation. tDCS is based on delivering a small constant level current (1–2 mA) to the brain. This is typically achieved via large sponge electrodes (approximately 35 cm^2 in size) positioned on the skull on top of the brain area of interest. The positive electrode provides anodal stimulation that has excitatory effect. The negative electrode provides cathodal stimulation that has inhibitory effect. For motor training purposes, this is typically done by application of the electrodes on M1. Encouraging preliminary results have been achieved in individuals with TBI (19) and several pilot studies have been performed in subjects with stroke (20–28) with potential applicability to motor training in individuals with TBI. Also, preliminary results indicate that tDCS has potential as a noninvasive brain stimulation technique for pain treatment (29). The application of tDCS is generally safe if proper attention is devoted to issues such as scalp defects and plates (30) as well as to avoid skin irritation. Skin irritation is the byproduct of the accumulation of ions because of the direct current nature of the stimulation. Patients have to be instructed to immediately report if they feel a warm "spot" under the electrodes typically corresponding to high current concentration. Other potential side effects are headache and nausea, but they are transitory and mild (12).

New modalities of application of tDCS are emerging. Researchers are considering the use of electrode arrays and electrodes of different shapes to improve the delivery of focal cortical stimulation (31–32). This is of interest, although recent work has questioned whether focal stimulation should be favored to a traditional stimulation modality (33). Another recent development is the use of alternating currents, which has been claimed to have similar effects to the ones observed when delivering direct current stimulation but without inducing skin irritation (34).

Low-level laser therapy and TCD are noninvasive brain stimulation techniques for which clinical application has not been pursued systematically as yet. So, they should be considered experimental techniques at this point in time. Preliminary studies have been performed to assess the potential benefits of low-level laser therapy (35) in several different clinical applications. The technique (also referred to as *photobiostimulation*) is based on the observation that laser light generated in a range of specific wavelengths can safely penetrate into the brain. Low-level laser therapy has been thought to facilitate cellular survival and promote neurogenesis. It has been suggested to improve outcomes following stroke and spinal cord injury (36–37). TCD has recently gained the interest of researchers and clinicians because of its potential use as an adjunct to thrombolytic therapy (tPA) or replacement of tPA in those cases in which tPA cannot be used (38). Other potential benefits of TCD such as its use as a noninvasive surrogate for measures of cerebral perfusion pressure and intracranial pressure (ICP) (39) and its hypothesized neuroprotective effects (40) are still under investigation and further evidence is needed before clinical adoption can be recommended.

Another emerging technique is GVS. GVS involves the delivery of small amounts of current to the left and right vestibular nerves which lie directly below the mastoid bones (Figure 75-3). GVS relies on the use of a low-level "noisy" current that is typically calibrated below the sensory threshold. This small current has a modulating effect on the vestibular neurons similar to that of natural head movements. It can increase or decrease the firing rates of vestibular neurons when positively or negatively charged. The vestibular system is made up of the semicircular canals and the otoliths, which help detect linear and angular acceleration of the head. Sensory afferent signals travel along the vestibular nerves to nuclei in the pons and medulla where they subsequently project to motor pathways that control ocular, axial, and limb muscles. Connections are also made via the ventral posterior thalamic nucleus to a cortical and subcortical neural network distributed along the perisylvian region. Functional imaging studies have shown that vestibular stimulation activates the cortical areas around the perisylvian region on the same side as the stimulation (41–43). These same right hemisphere regions have been shown to be selectively involved in target detection, sustained attention, and spatial attention. Thus, the effectiveness of GVS may be from stimulating a perisylvian right hemisphere attentional network. At this point in time, GVS has to be considered an experimental technique. Several aspects of the delivery of GVS still have to be studied. For instance, the relationship between the level of "noisy" current delivered to the vestibular system (Figure 75-3) and the magnitude of the behavioral response mediated by attentional networks is unclear. Further research is needed before clinical adoption may be recommended.

PERIPHERAL STIMULATION

Several peripheral stimulation techniques are relevant to the clinical management of individuals with TBI. In this section, we provide a short overview of 3 techniques: vagus nerve stimulation (VNS), FES, and mechanical as well as electrical stimulation delivered using a paradigm known as stochastic resonance (SR).

VNS has been of interest in TBI because vagal dysfunction is observed both in the acute and the chronic phases of TBI. In the acute phase of TBI, vagal activity is augmented (44) thus resulting in a shift in the sympathovagal balance, possibly as a consequence of increased ICP. The increased vagal tone has been associated with immune paralysis in patients with TBI (45). In the chronic phase of TBI, vagal output is decreased possibly because of damage to the brainstem and medulla oblongata thus resulting in impaired activity of the vagus nerve. Animal models have suggested that stimulation of the vagus nerve following TBI has potential for enhancing motor and cognitive recovery (46–48). Little evidence of the benefits of VNS following TBI has been obtained in human subjects but preliminary results are encouraging (49–50).

VNS can be delivered either via an implantable system or via a noninvasive stimulator. Cyberonics (Houston, TX) manufactures the only Food and Drug Administration (FDA)-approved implantable system for VNS. The device was originally designed for the treatment of drug-resistant epilepsy. Cyberonics' VNS device consists of a titanium-encased generator about the size of a pocket watch and electrodes that are anchored to the vagus nerve to deliver the stimuli. The device is usually implanted during an outpatient visit. Noninvasive stimulators are under development. An example is NEMOS (Figure 75-4), a device developed by Cerbomed (Erlangen, Germany). The stimulation is delivered using an earpiece that targets the auricular branch of the vagus nerve. The use of a noninvasive means to deliver VNS is very appealing, but evidence of its effectiveness is still lacking.

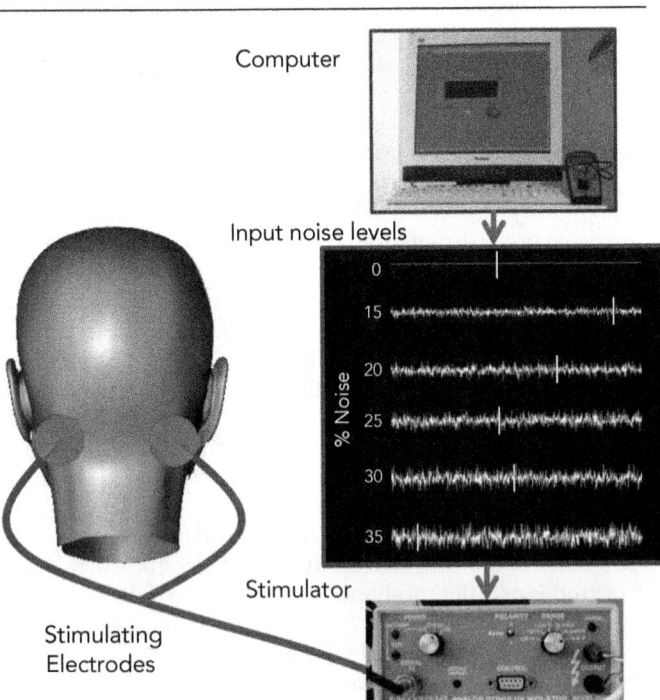

Computer

Input noise levels

% Noise

Stimulator

Stimulating Electrodes

FIGURE 75-3 Schematic representation of a system to deliver galvanic vestibular stimulation (GVS) whose effects on attention-related networks are currently under study. Studies are focused on establishing optimal levels of stimulation, namely the "amount of noisy current" that leads to significant effects on attentional networks.

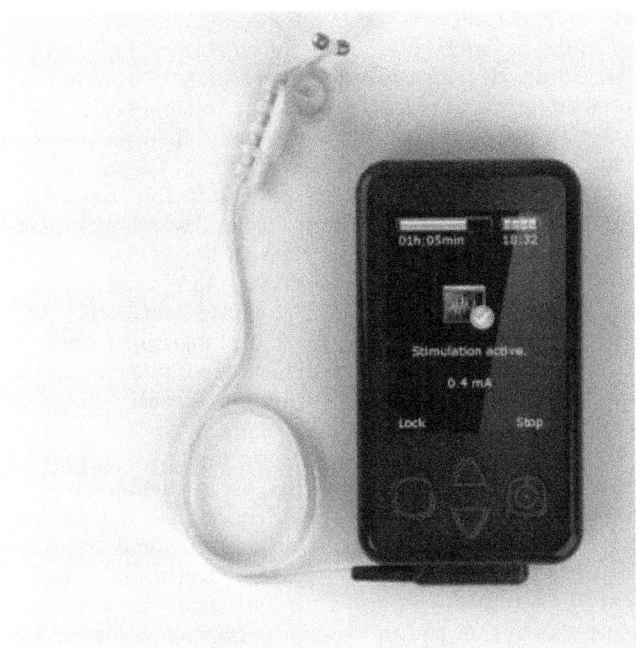

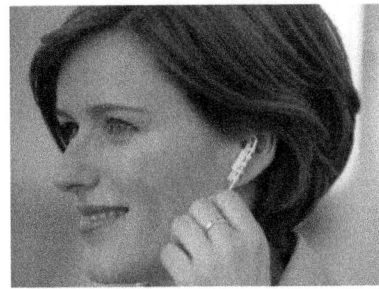

FIGURE 75-4 The NEMOS system (Cerbomed, Erlangen, Germany) is the first noninvasive system for vagus nerve stimulation (VNS). Reproduced with permission, courtesy of Cerbomed.

Another peripheral stimulation technique of interest in the clinical management of TBI is FES. The use of FES was first explored in the late 1970s (51) with main focus on FES of the lower limbs (e.g., for the correction of foot drop) and some but less emphasis on the use of FES to restore upper limb function (52–53). Research in this field eventually led to the development of FES products. The first product that, in this context, gained the interest of clinicians was a stimulator for the correction of foot drop. The most prominent among the systems developed in these early phases of the history of FES was the Dropped Foot Stimulator by Odstock Medical Limited (54) (Salisbury, United Kingdom). The original system consisted in a peroneal nerve stimulator and a foot switch, which was used to trigger the stimulation. The main benefit of the system was the perceived decreased effort during gait, but the system in its original configuration was not easy to use and patients encountered significant difficulties in, for instance, positioning properly the stimulation electrodes (55). To achieve ease of use of this technology, several companies have developed systems that are compact and ergonomic. The Bioness L300 (Bioness Inc, Valencia, CA) foot-drop system provides similar functions to the one originally provided by the Odstock Medical Limited (Salisbury, United Kingdom) system. However, the Bioness L300 system has no wires between the foot switch and the stimulator. These two components of the system communicate wirelessly. Another system for the correction of foot drop is the WalkAide system by Innovative Neurotronics Inc (Austin, TX) (see Figure 75-5). Its design went one step further by integrating the sensing technology into the stimulation unit. The movement of the unit triggers the stimulation with appropriate timing. The WalkAide system is theoretically less sensitive to the initiation of movement than the Bioness L300 system, but it is more "wearable" because the WalkAide requires the use of a single unit that integrates both the sensing components and the stimulator whereas the Bioness

L300 system requires the use of a stimulator and foot switches.

A recent generation of stimulators has totally bypassed the "wearability" problem by opting for an implantable solution. Finetech Medical (Hertfordshire, United Kingdom) was the first company to launch an implantable system for the management of foot drop. The system was called the StimuStep and was launched in 2004. More recently, Otto Bock's Neurodan unit (Aalborg, Denmark) launched the ActiGait. In both cases (i.e., for both the Finetech Medical's system and the Neurodan's system), the stimulator is implanted and equipped with leads that are used to deliver the stimulation directly to the peroneal nerve. These implantable systems have been shown to be effective in delivering the stimulation and suitable to achieve satisfactory clinical outcomes (56–57).

Clinical evidence indicates that FES of the peroneal nerve is effective in restoring gait function (58–59). Some evidence has also been produced in support of a potential therapeutic effect of FES of the peroneal nerve (60–61). However, the level of evidence supporting the hypothesized therapeutic benefits of FES of the peroneal nerve is weak even for implantable systems (62). Nonetheless, some authors believe that FES of the peroneal nerve is likely to provide therapeutic benefits (63). Following this theory, researchers have initiated the exploration of the use of peroneal nerve stimulation in the acute setting (64). Another interesting relatively recent development is the use of multichannel stimulation techniques to assist both dorsiflexion during swing and plantarflexion during stance (65–66). Also, recent work has explored the potential benefits of FES applied to proximal muscles, such as the gluteus medius (67). Preliminary results are encouraging. Other interesting applications of FES of the lower limbs are the combination of FES and body weight-supported gait training (68–69) and the combination of FES and robotic-assisted gait therapy (70–72). Finally, FES has

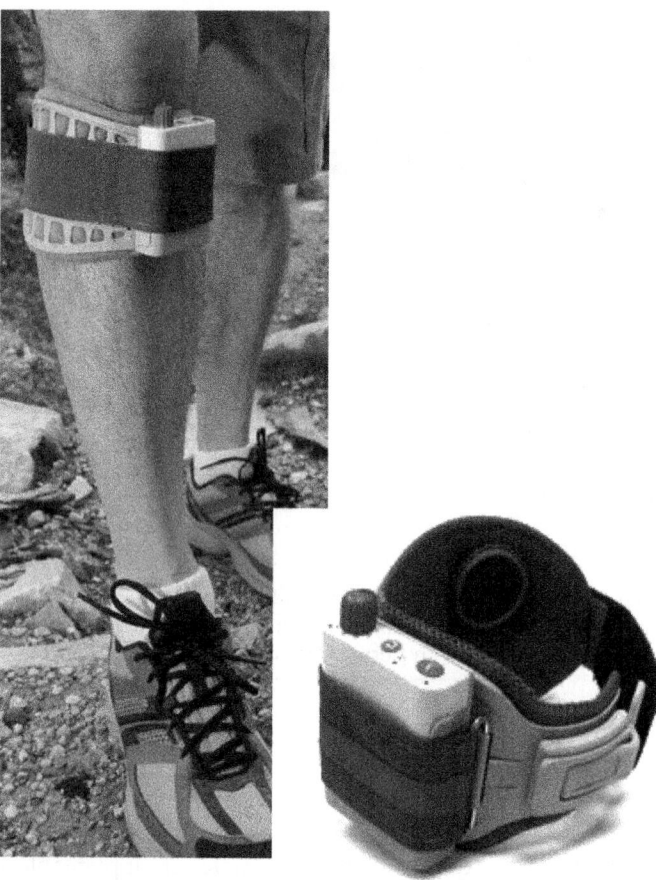

FIGURE 75-5 The WalkAide system (Innovative Neurotronics Inc, Austin, TX) for transcutaneous peroneal nerve stimulation is one of the products that leverage functional electrical stimulation (FES) to control foot drop.

been used to facilitate leg cycling (73–76). This technique has been found beneficial, for instance, in decreasing spasticity in the lower limbs.

The application of FES to the upper limbs has been also extensively studied. Nonetheless, delivering stimulation to the upper limbs is significantly more complicated than delivering stimulation to the lower limbs. One problem is, for instance, the sensitivity of the motor output to the correct positioning of the FES electrodes. In an attempt to address this matter, Freeman et al. (77) developed a model of the arm receiving stimulation and Goffredo et al. (78) developed smart algorithms to control the stimulation. Upper-limb FES has gone through tremendous transformations over the past few years. For instance, Mann et al. (79) developed an accelerometer-triggered stimulator for the upper limbs. Also, EMG-triggered methods have been proposed (80). The literature on upper-limb FES has stronger emphasis on the potential therapeutic effect of FES than the literature on lower-limb FES (81–82). Because of its hypothesized therapeutic effect, researchers have investigated the possibility of using FES as part of upper-limb therapy in the early stages of patient recovery from a TBI (83). The most prominent commercially available system for upper-limb FES is the Bioness H200 (Bioness Inc, Valencia, CA, USA). The system is designed to help wrist and finger extension movements.

To conclude, it is worth mentioning an emerging interest in the research community for combining FES and BCIs (84). Future developments in this research area are expected to facilitate the transition toward implantable solutions that leverage miniature sensing technology such as the bionic neuron (BION) (85).

An emerging technique of stimulation that aims at boosting proprioception either via mechanical stimulation (targeting mechanoreceptors such as the Pacinian corpuscles) or via electrical stimulation (targeting muscle spindles and Golgi tendon organs) is "stochastic resonance (SR)" stimulation. SR stimulation relies on "injecting" noise into the sensory system (86–87). By doing so, one can create a "pedestal" on top of which incoming stimuli will sit thus leading to increased sensory input.

Preliminary results concerning the application of SR stimulation to the upper limbs (88) are available, but results so far do not provide strong evidence of the hypothesized positive impact of SR stimulation on functional ability and motor recovery. Conversely, results concerning the application of SR to the lower limbs are consistently positive. It has been shown that proprioception is improved via electrical SR stimulation of the knee (89). Also, it has been shown that motor training enhanced by SR stimulation at the ankle improves postural control in subjects with functional ankle instability (90). Mechanical SR stimulation has been also extensively studied. This technique has been shown to be associated with reduced gait variability (91). Besides, mechanical SR stimulation has been shown to reduce postural instability (92–93).

There is no commercially available system as yet to deliver SR stimulation. Existing evidence does not appear to be sufficient to justify clinical recommendation of SR stimulation. However, it is expected that, as researchers continue to study SR, methodologies to effectively deliver SR stimulation will emerge and scientific evidence will be added to demonstrate the potential clinical relevance of SR stimulation.

BRAIN COMPUTER INTERFACES

BCIs are based on recording electrical signals from the brain and on using such information to provide subjects with real-time feedback or to enable real-time functions (e.g., controlling a computer screen or a robotic system) (94). Brain recordings in the context of BCIs are gathered using 3 different techniques: (*a*) scalp recordings (EEG-based BCIs) (see Figure 75-6), (*b*) cortical recordings (electrocorticogram [ECoG]-based BCIs), and (*c*) intracortical recordings (intracortical BCIs) .

The seminal work by Wolpaw et al. (95–96) provided the basis for current EEG-based BCIs. EEG-based BCIs are the ones of greatest interest in rehabilitation because they rely on a noninvasive technique to record brain activity. In contrast, ECoG-based BCIs and intracortical BCIs rely on invasive recordings. EEG-based BCIs have been implemented using a variety of electrode configurations, but most often by using dense electrode arrays with several channels typically ranging between 64 and 128. However, more traditional electrode configurations (i.e., fewer electrodes) have been used as well. Their software implementation varies according to the application at hand and the modality of data collection.

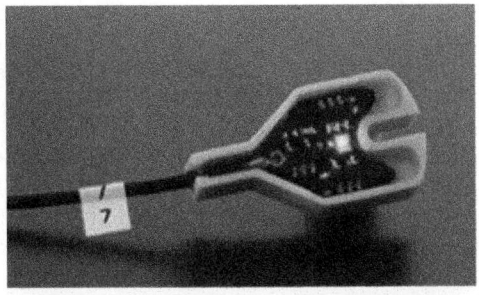

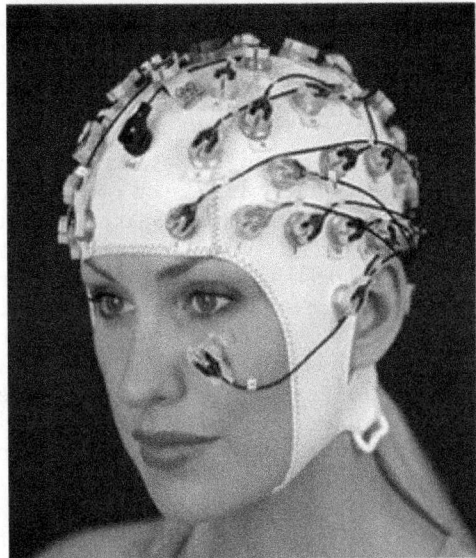

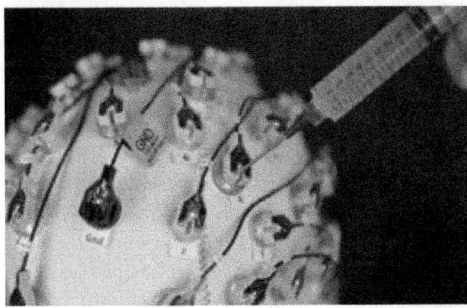

FIGURE 75-6 The actiCAP system (Brain Products GmbH, Gilching, Germany) is an example of dense electrode array used for the implementation of EEG-based brain computer interfaces (BCIs). Reproduced with permission, courtesy of Brain Products GmbH.

The first work in this field was focused on providing patients with simple control capability, such as choosing letters on a computer screen to enable communication in patients with locked-in syndrome (97). These early studies focused on using evoked responses by capturing a particular signature in the EEG recordings that is referred to as P300 (98). Relatively efficient computer-based systems to facilitate spelling were developed and tested in a variety of patient populations, including individuals with amyotrophic lateral sclerosis (99).

A second approach to the implementation of EEG-based BCIs relies on the analysis of sensorimotor rhythms, typically the μ-rhythm (i.e., data in the frequency range between 8 and 12 Hz) and the β-rhythm (i.e., data in the frequency range

between 18 and 26 Hz). These waveforms are detected from the sensorimotor cortices and change their characteristics with movement, sensation, and motor imagery (100–101). The interest for this approach originates from the observation that individuals can learn how to control the amplitude of μ-rhythm and β-rhythm waveforms in absence of movement and sensory inputs. This technique has been used mostly in relatively simple applications such as the control of a cursor on a computer screen (101).

A third technique used in the implementation of EEG-based BCIs relies on the identification of slow cortical potentials (SCPs) (102). This is also a technique that requires subject training. With training, subjects can achieve control of SCPs and in turn, control a cursor on a computer screen or a computer-based spelling system.

Over the past few years, several researchers and clinicians have been inspired by the earlier-mentioned research work and have pursued the implementation of EEG-based BCIs to enable rehabilitation interventions. For instance, Daly et al. (84) presented a single-case study in which an EEG-based BCI was used to facilitate training volitional motor control in a stroke survivor. The authors successfully used an EEG-based BCI to control FES to improve the performance of isolated finger movements. Do et al. (103) recently studied the use of an EEG-based BCI to control the delivery of FES to facilitate ankle movements. The authors achieved positive results. Also, positive results have been achieved toward the use of EEG-based BCIs to enable training using motor imagery (104). Finally, several researchers have started investigating the use of EEG-based BCIs to control robotic systems for rehabilitation (105). For instance, Ang et al. (106) combined an EEG-based BCI with robotics to enable motor imagery and facilitate upper-limb rehabilitation. Broetz et al. (107) also presented a single-case study in which an upper limb robot was controlled using an EEG-based BCI thus facilitating motor training. These studies have to be considered as preliminary and clinical adoption of this technique cannot be recommended as yet because of the limited results available at the moment. However, combining EEG-based BCIs and robotics for rehabilitation is a very intriguing concept because the robot allows for closing the loop by providing the "correct" sensory feedback in association with cortical activity that corresponds to a given movement (105). It is expected that further studies will clarify the clinical applicability and effectiveness of this approach.

The other two recording techniques that have been used in the implementation of BCIs are cortical recordings (ECoG) and intracortical recordings. Both techniques are invasive and therefore of difficult application, particularly in a rehabilitation context.

ECoG-based BCIs are somehow similar to EEG-based BCIs, but the invasiveness of the recording technique leads to data marked by higher signal-to-noise ratios, which is to say that "small signals" that cannot be identified by using EEG data can in fact be detected using ECoG data. For instance, when using ECoG recordings to identify rhythms, not only one can detect μ-rhythm and β-rhythm data (as observed in EEG recordings), but also higher frequency data (i.e., γ-rhythm, 30–200 Hz) that are typically nondetectable from scalp data (i.e., EEG recordings). ECoG recordings are fairly commonly used in patients with epilepsy and motor imagery experiments have been performed in this patient population (108). However, suitable commercially available systems to implement ECoG-based BCIs appear to be lacking at this time. This technique has to be considered experimental and it is unlikely that it will be adopted soon in rehabilitation.

Intracortical-based BCIs are also experimental. Data collections using this approach have been limited so far to a few studies. Experiments with intracortical arrays have been performed mostly in animal models (109–110) although a few studies have been recently performed in human subjects (111). However, this technique is highly invasive and currently of limited clinical interest.

New techniques are currently emerging that provide alternative means to gather brain activity data by using noninvasive recording techniques. Most notably, researchers and clinicians have demonstrated a growing interest for BCIs based on functional near-infrared spectroscopy (fNIRS) (112). fNIRS is an imaging technique based on the observation that infrared light can safely penetrate the scalp and is reflected back differently according to the oxygen level in blood vessels. However, contrary to other imaging techniques, fNIRS is relatively inexpensive and portable. Therefore, it lends itself to be used in rehabilitation more than other imaging techniques such fMRI. Although only preliminary results concerning the use of this technique are available at the moment (113), the technique has great potential (114). It is expected that future studies will clarify the clinical relevance of fNIRS in rehabilitation and assess its suitability to implement BCIs.

ROBOTICS

Over the past two decades, we have witnessed the development of several robotic systems for upper- and lower-limb rehabilitation. Key elements of the design of robotic systems are (a) the human machine interface, and (b) the methodology used to control the robot. Because of the paramount importance of these aspects of the design of robotic systems for rehabilitation the systems are often categorized according to the characteristics of the human machine interface and the main features of the adopted control methodology.

There are two types of human–machine interfaces, namely (a) end-effector based interfaces, and (b) exoskeleton-based interfaces. End-effector robotic systems are designed by relying on a single point of contact between the robotic components that deliver robotic-generated forces and the subject. Figure 75-7 shows examples of end-effector robotic systems for upper- and lower-limb rehabilitation (panels A and C). Figure 75-7A shows a graphic representation of the G-EO-System by Reha Technology AG (Olten, Switzerland) (115). The GE-O is a system for gait training with a human machine interface consisting of footplates where the subject stands on. The footplates are controlled in such a way as to achieve well-defined trajectories of movement of the feet. Figure 75-7C shows the MIT-Manus (116–117), a robotic system for upper-limb rehabilitation originally designed by Neville Hogan and Igo Krebs at MIT and eventually commercialized by Interactive Motion Technologies (Cambridge, MA). The MIT-Manus is also an end-effector system. The interaction between the robot and the subject takes place by using a single point of contact, that is, the "handle" the subject holds onto. Figure 75-7 also shows examples of exoskeleton-based

systems (panels B and D). Exoskeleton-based systems are robotic systems designed with multiple points of contact between the subject and the robot. This is achieved via robotic components in the shape of an artificial external supporting structure functioning like an "external skeleton." Figure 75-7B shows an exoskeleton-based system for gait training, namely the Lokomat system by Hocoma AG (Volketswil, Switzerland) (118–119). Robotic components are "attached" to the lower body thus providing interaction forces to control lower-limb movements during treadmill gait training. Figure 75-7D shows an exoskeleton-based system for upper-limb rehabilitation, namely the ArmeoPower also by Hocoma AG (Volketswil, Switzerland) (120–121). The human-machine interface consists of robotic elements that are "attached" to the upper limbs and deliver forces that "guide" upper-limb movements.

Theoretically, end-effector and exoskeleton systems are equivalent. However, there are 2 main considerations that make end-effector and exoskeleton systems rather different from a practical point of view. First of all, the patient set-up time for end-effector based human–machine interfaces is virtually zero, whereas the patient set-up time to use an exoskeleton system is significant because the length of the robotic elements of the exoskeleton must be adjusted before one can attach such elements to the subject's body segments. However, exoskeleton-based systems provide the advantage over end-effector systems of allowing clinicians to more easily control the motion at different joints. This is of paramount importance when one wants to avoid, for instance, exerting excessive loads on some joints. Controlling such forces is theoretically possible even if one uses an end-effector system. In fact, an appropriate set-up and the use of a biomechanical model of the subject could lead to indirectly controlling forces exerted on the joints. However, accomplishing this goal in a clinical environment is very challenging. It has to be acknowledged that appropriate control of joint movements via an exoskeleton can only be achieved if the exoskeleton's mechanical joints are properly aligned with the anatomical joints. This is also challenging, particularly for complex joints like the shoulder. Finally, it is worth keeping in mind that exoskeleton-based systems are typically more costly and more challenging to control than end-effector based systems. However, exoskeleton-based systems can be designed to be wearable and therefore potentially used during the performance of activities of daily living.

The second major characteristic of robotic systems for rehabilitation is the methodology used to control the robot. Several methodologies have been developed in the field of rehabilitation robotics. Such methods can be divided into 2 main categories: (a) methods aimed to provide assistance to the patient thus facilitating movement, and (b) methods aimed to "guide" limb motion for the purpose of achieving physiological patterns of movement.

These control methods are dramatically different. Methods aimed to provide assistance to the patient serve the purpose of augmenting function. In other terms, the robot makes up for the inability of the subject to produce appropriate muscle forces to achieve the desired movement trajectories. The amount of assistance provided by the robot is typically manually adjusted by the therapist on the basis of his or her assessment of the subject's motor performance. Technically speaking, this control modality is referred to as *position control*. In contrast, methods aimed to "guide" limb movements

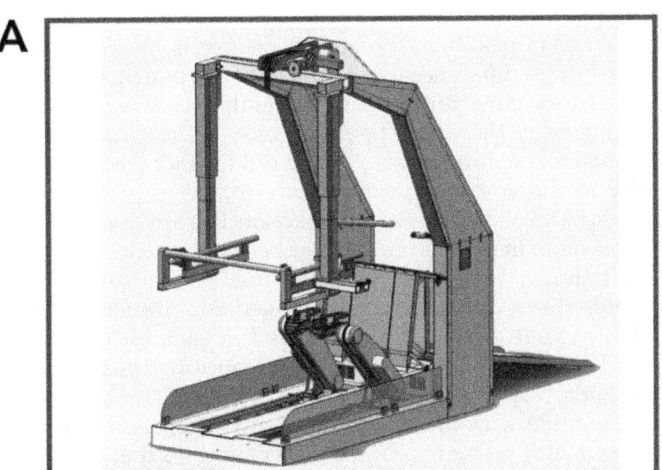
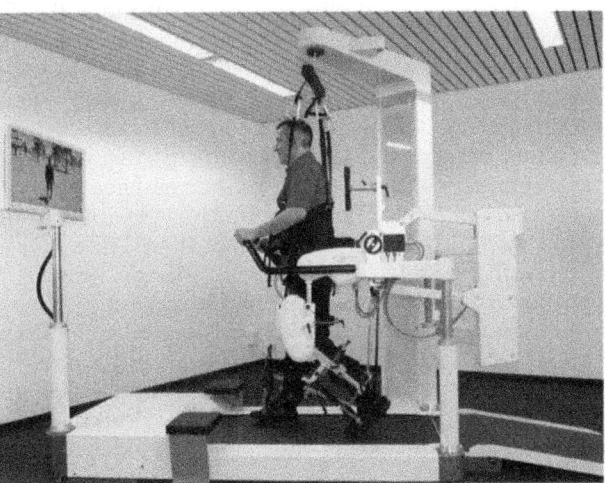
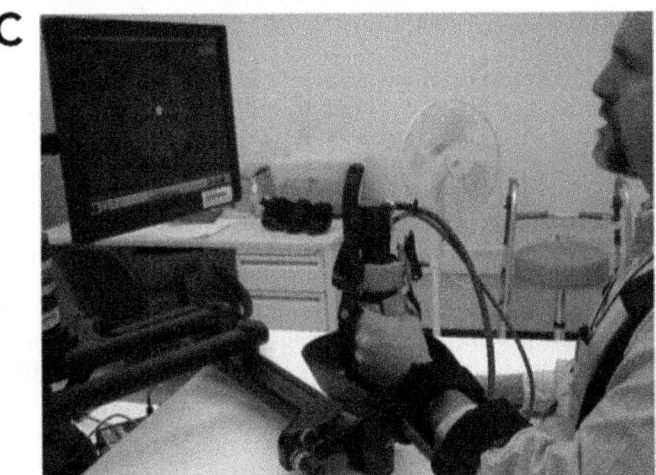
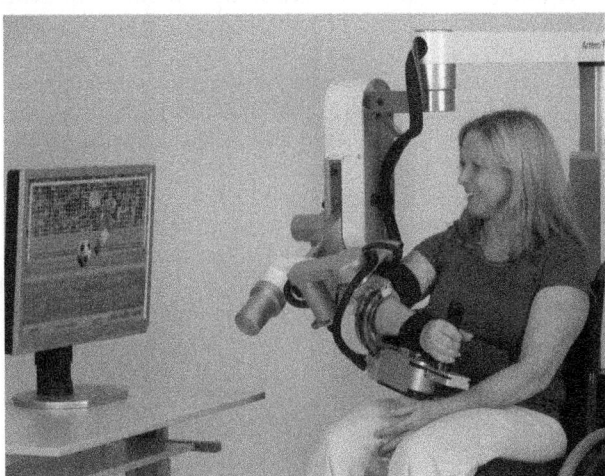

FIGURE 75-7 Examples of commercially available robotic systems for rehabilitation of the lower (A and B) and upper (C and D) limbs. The systems shown in panels A and C are end-effector systems, that is, systems equipped with a robotic component (referred to as "end effector") that constitute the sole point of interaction with the patient. The systems shown in panels B and D are exoskeleton systems, that is, systems equipped with an "external skeleton" consisting of mechanical components that provide multiple points of attachment to the body.

are based on generating robotic forces that are proportional to the distance between the actual subject's trajectory of movement and the desired trajectory of movement. This control strategy is typically referred to as *impedance control*. The forces generated by the robotic system around the target trajectory of movement are referred to as *force field*. Over the past few years, as clinical results have indicated that position control methodologies are not as effective as impedance control methods in fostering motor learning during training sessions, several research groups have developed several variations of the impedance control methodology. Recently, a set of control techniques inspired by such principles as the one that originated the use of impedance control methods in rehabilitation has emerged under the name of "patient-cooperative" control strategies (122). These new control methods should be considered an evolution of impedance control methods and their clinical relevance is currently undergoing assessment.

A recent review of the literature by Tefertiller et al. (123), focused on the efficacy of robot-assisted gait training in neu-

rological disorders, found that robot-assisted gait training is generally beneficial to patients with neurological conditions such as stroke and spinal cord injury. The review also found limited evidence of the efficacy of robot-assisted gait training in TBI, multiple sclerosis, and Parkinson's disease. However, the authors correctly emphasized the heterogeneity of the studies carried out by different research groups. Differences were noted among technologies used in different clinical studies, among protocols used to implement gait training interventions, and among inclusion/exclusion criteria used across studies. In contrast with previous reviews of the literature on robot-assisted gait training, the authors carefully attempted to analyze results obtained with different technologies thus acknowledging the significant differences among available robotic systems for rehabilitation. A rather complex picture emerges highlighting the challenges associated with assessing the efficacy of robotic technology in rehabilitation.

Tefertiller's review paper (123) appears to confirm a previously published review by Mehrholz et al. (124) supporting the statement that robot-assisted gait training in combination with conventional physical therapy is more likely to allow patients to achieve independent walking than conventional physical therapy alone. Nonetheless, the efficacy of robotic-assisted gait training is still questioned by many given that several studies have found conventional therapy to be either as effective as robotic-assisted therapy or, in some cases, more effective than robotic-assisted therapy. The virtual absence of any systematic work on robotic-assisted gait training in individuals with TBI makes it extremely challenging for clinicians to decide whether to adopt robotic therapy in this patient population.

As some of the systems for robotic-assisted gait training are based on treadmill training, some authors have looked at the literature to seek evidence that treadmill-based gait training is beneficial to patients with neurological conditions such as TBI and stroke. Unfortunately, the evidence in this regard is still questionable. A review paper by Moseley et al. (125) did not find any evidence of the superiority of treadmill-based gait training with or without weight support compared to other therapeutic modalities. This result appears to be consistent with the outcomes of the Locomotor Experience Applied Post-Stroke (LEAPS) study (126) that once again did not provide any evidence of the superior efficacy of treadmill-based gait training compared to other therapies. However, it should be emphasized that robotic-assisted gait training is not a simple robotic version of treadmill-based gait training. Although some of the initial work in rehabilitation robotics was in fact inspired by such a line of thought, recent findings have reoriented research in this field toward a human–machine interaction design that is based on motor control and motor learning principles. Clinical results obtained by using such advanced control strategies are still lacking. Therefore, making a decision concerning the clinical adoption of robotic-assisted gait training appears to be premature, especially in regards to individuals with TBI, a population in which only a handful of studies have been performed (127–128) and none with advanced robotic-based techniques.

There is a paucity of studies on upper-limb rehabilitation in individuals with TBI (129), not to mention on robot-assisted upper-limb rehabilitation. Therefore, clinical decisions concerning the use of robotic systems for upper-limb rehabilitation in TBI survivors are often made on the basis of stroke literature. In this context, the largest randomized control trial performed in the field is the 1 carried out by Lo et al. (130) using the MIT-Manus (Interactive Motion Technologies, Cambridge, MA). The authors recruited 127 patients with moderate-to-severe upper-limb impairment (i.e., Fugl-Meyer score in the 7–38 points range) 6 months or more after they suffered a stroke. Subjects were randomized to 1 of 3 groups: (*a*) receiving intensive robotic-assisted therapy, (*b*) receiving intensive comparison therapy, and (*c*) receiving usual care. Subjects in the first 2 groups received therapy over 36 sessions each of the duration of 1-hour during a period of 12 weeks. The usual care group received customary care available to all patients, which was not dictated by the protocol. Patients randomized to the robot-assisted therapy group used all robotic modules of the MIT-Manus system to progress from sessions focused on proximal joints to sessions devoted to improving distal function. Fugl-Meyer scores, Stroke Impact Scale scores, and Wolf Motor Function Test scores were compared in the 3 groups at 12 weeks and 36 weeks. Results in the group re-

ceiving robotic-assisted therapy were found to be generally better than results in the group of subjects receiving usual care but no difference was found between patients receiving robotic-assisted therapy and patients receiving intensive comparison therapy. The study received conflicting comments. Some individuals pointed out the fact that the intensity of therapy used in the study for the robotic therapy group and the intensive comparison therapy group is not achievable in the clinical settings because several outpatient visits typically reimbursed by insurance companies or the national health care system is limited to about one-third of the number of sessions performed in each patient in the study. Therefore, these individuals concluded that the only realistic way to deliver high-intensity rehabilitation that is compatible with the financial constraints of the health care system is by using robotics. Others countered that the results of the study point out the fact that "robots do not contribute anything special to rehabilitation" and that the main result of the study is that it is the intensity of the intervention that matters.

The question of whether robots can add anything to conventional therapy is one that has been raised several times. For instance, Kahn et al. (131) studied the effect of delivering therapy to stroke survivors by using a robot to facilitate completion of motor tasks when subjects were able to initiate but not complete a set of target movements. The authors showed no significant difference in outcomes achieved when the robot was programmed to facilitate completion of motor tasks vs when it was programmed to provide no assistance in completing the movement. Although the authors expressed confidence that using robots to guide movement is bound to eventually lead to better results than those achieved using traditional therapeutic approaches, their work raised the question as to whether robots can indeed improve upon results achieved using manual therapy delivered by therapists.

This question has not been fully addressed by any of the studies and review papers published over the past decade. Reviews of the literature have consistently indicated that insufficient evidence exists to make any conclusion about the potential superiority of robotic-assisted therapy for upper-limb rehabilitation compared to traditional therapy. Prange et al. (132) reviewed 8 clinical studies in stroke survivors focused on assessing robotics for upper-limb rehabilitation with emphasis on proximal function (i.e., shoulder and elbow control). They concluded that robotic-assisted therapy improves several aspects of the control of upper-limb motion such as speed of movement and leads to a normalization of the activation of muscles involved in the control of movement. They also concluded that robotic-assisted therapy has a positive impact on upper-limb impairments as shown by improvements in Fugl-Meyer scores. However, a trend was identified only on the basis of comparing studies of robotic-assisted training and conventional training. The results show larger improvements (trends) in short-term motor impairments and motor control characteristics. Insufficient data was found concerning long-term results and to assess the impact of robotic therapy on subacute vs chronic patients.

Another review paper by Kwakkel et al. (133) considered 10 studies on robot-assisted upper-limb therapy in subjects with stroke and showed (via a meta-analysis) a trend toward larger improvements (i.e., decrease in motor impairments) in patients undergoing robotic-assisted therapy compared to traditional therapy. Although, the authors pointed out that the heterogeneity of the studies considered in their meta-analysis might have made it difficult to identify significant differences between robotic-assisted and traditional therapy, the review appears to suggest that limited gains are associated with the use of robotic-assisted therapy compared to traditional therapy. So, as the authors had shown that, in the first 6 months after a stroke, the intensity of therapy is a key factor to achieve optimal clinical outcomes (134), many concluded that the main benefit of robots is that they facilitate the delivery of high-intensity and task-specific therapy (135).

These studies do not provide sufficient evidence to make a clinical decision concerning the suitability of robotic-assisted therapy to improve upper-limb function in individuals with TBI. However, trends identified in studies focused on stroke survivors suggest that robotic-assisted upper-limb therapy provides a tool to deliver high-intensity therapy and maximize clinical outcomes compared to traditional therapy.

VIRTUAL REALITY

Virtual reality (VR) tools have been used in the context of both motor and cognitive training. In this section, we provide a detailed overview of VR-based tools that have been combined with robotics to facilitate motor training and a summary of studies that have been focused on developing and testing the use of VR environments for cognitive assessment and training.

A wide variety of VR-based systems have been used in motor training. Their sophistication ranges from fully immersive systems such as the Computer Assisted Rehabilitation Environment (CAREN) system (136) to simple off-the-shelf interactive gaming systems like the Nintendo Wii (137–138) and the Microsoft Kinect (139). Off-the-shelf interactive gaming systems have received a lot of attention over the past few years, but not in combination with robotic systems for rehabilitation. Dedicated systems have been developed to combine VR and interactive gaming with rehabilitation robotics. This is not unexpected given that, to be meaningful, the integration of VR and interactive gaming in a robotic system requires that robotic components be programmed to control aspects of the virtual environment or the game thus encouraging the subject to achieve a target motor task. Such integration calls for ad-hoc solutions rather than off-the-shelf components. Besides, the needs of patients are different from those addressed by the entertainment industry and although a few off-the-shelf interactive gaming systems could be adapted for clinical use, the great majority of the interactive gaming systems are not suitable for application in rehabilitation. Herein, we present examples of VR and interactive gaming systems that have been integrated with robotic components in systems designed to facilitate either lower- or upper-limb rehabilitation.

Although the first systems for robotic-assisted rehabilitation were seldom combined with a VR system or an interactive gaming system, recently developed systems for robotic-assisted rehabilitation almost always include a VR or an interactive gaming component. This section provides examples of systems that integrate robotics and VR or interactive games.

Figure 75-8 shows examples of robotic-assisted gait training systems that integrate robotics and VR/interactive gaming. The Lokomat system (Hocoma AG, Volketswil,

Switzerland) shown in Figure 75-8A is perhaps the most prominent among all commercially available robotic systems for gait training that offer a VR/interactive gaming module. A large computer screen positioned in front of the subject shows an avatar of the subject and provides a virtual environment in which he or she can "walk." The system is referred to as *augmented feedback*. Currently available games are "navigation" games, namely games in which the subject is encouraged to walk in a virtual environment where, for instance, he or she is instructed to collect objects. By assigning a score to the objects retrieved in the virtual environment and calling his or her attention to the score achieved in the game, the system provides subjects with motivation.

The interactive games used with the Lokomat system are relatively simple and nonimmersive. The computer screen does not provide a strong sense of presence in the virtual environment. This is intended by design and many seem to think that this is a sensible approach to avoid that patients may feel disoriented as sometimes reported when fully immersive environments are used. However, others favor immersive environments. An example of an immersive system is shown in Figure 75-8B. The system was developed by Dr. Deutsch's team at UMDNJ (140). Movements of the lower limbs are guided by footplates that are controlled by a pneumatic system providing 6 degrees of freedom of movement. Virtual environments are shown on a large screen to convey a sense of presence in the virtual environment.

A fully immersive system is shown in Figure 75-8C. The subject is here surrounded by a screen covering the whole visual field thus providing a strong sense of presence. The system shown in the figure leverages the CAREN system to track subject's movements and to control the VR scene accordingly. This is perhaps the most advanced VR system used in rehabilitation so far.

Numerous systems combining VR/interactive games and robotics have also been developed to facilitate the implementation of protocols for upper-limb motor training. Figure 75-9 shows examples of such systems. Figure 75-9A shows the ArmeoSpring (141–142). The system is equipped with interactive games designed to encourage subjects to perform arm reaching and manipulation tasks. The system is programmed to remap the position of the arm in the virtual environment. In the games, subjects reach for objects and retrieve them or manipulate them. For instance, in one game, subjects pick up an apple from a shelf and move it to a basket. In another game, subjects pick up eggs from a basket and break them on top of a frying pan.

Slightly more complex VR solutions have been used in research platforms. Figure 75-9C shows an example of one such system, namely the New Jersey Institute of Technology Robot-Assisted Virtual Rehabilitation (NJIT-RAVR) (143). Originally designed for application in a pediatric population, the NJIT-RAVR system provides guidance to accomplish upper-limb movements using the Haptic Master. Three-dimensional (3D) vision is provided using a large screen and 3D glasses. The games require reaching and manipulating objects in the virtual environment. In one game, subjects are instructed to reach for bubbles that randomly appear on the video display and to explode them by touching them in the VR. In another game, subjects are instructed to catch falling objects on the visual display by moving a cursor representing the position of the hand in space.

A

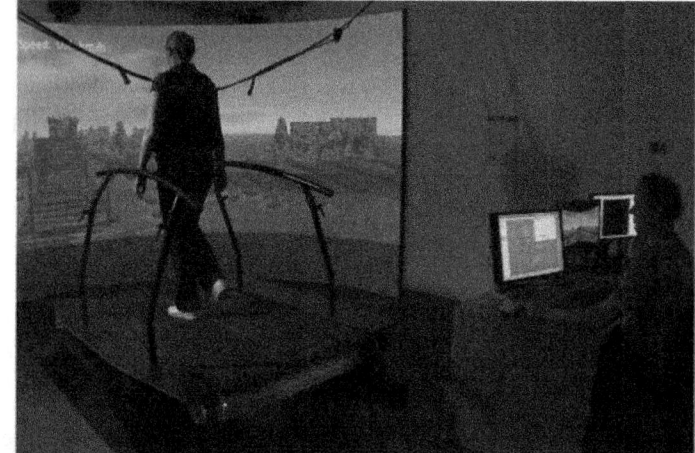

C

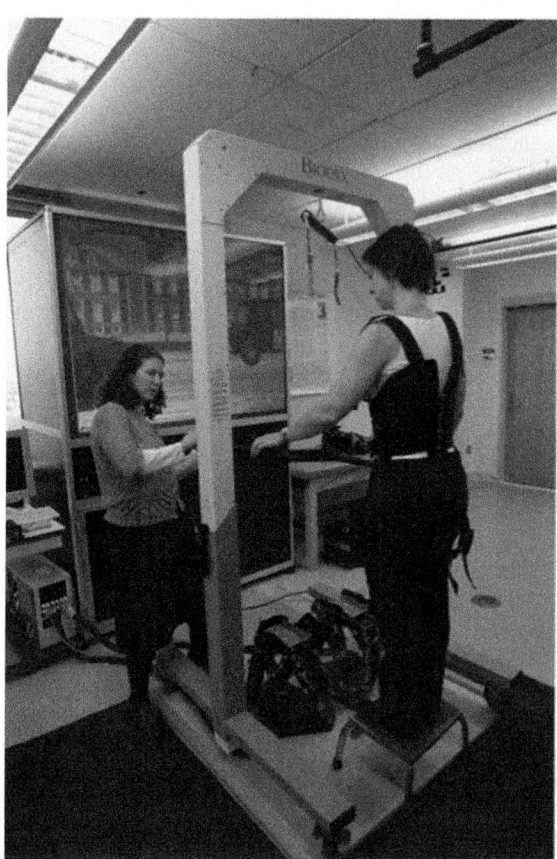

B

FIGURE 75-8 Examples of VR-based systems designed to enhance robotic platforms for gait training. Panel A shows the augmented feedback systems used with the Lokomat system for treadmill-based gait training. Panel B shows a VR-based system used in combination with a footplate-based system for gait training. Panel C shows a fully immersive VR system used in combination with a treadmill-based system for gait training.

A few systems for robot-assisted upper-limb training are designed to facilitate hand dexterity training. Figure 75-9B shows one such system (143). In this system, the CyberGlove (CyberGlove Systems LLC, San Jose, CA) is used to track movements of the hand whereas the CyberGrasp (CyberGlove Systems LLC, San Jose, CA) is used to provide haptic feedback. A computer display enables the use of computer games such as the Virtual Piano (shown in the figure).

The systems described earlier constitute a small but representative sample of the systems for upper- and lower-limb rehabilitation that combine VR/interactive gaming with robotics. The examples provided demonstrate the wide variety of approaches taken by different companies and research groups, mostly in regard to the complexity of the virtual environment used to implement the games. Some groups favor using a fully immersive virtual environment. Others have emphasized the fact that fully immersive VR environments are often confusing to patients. This appears to be the case for individuals with TBI where difficulties are apparent in maintaining a sufficient attention level, processing visual input, and integrating visual and somatosensory inputs. Consequently, several research groups have favored the use

of simple interactive games over complex VR environments. A systematic comparison of these 2 approaches is still lacking.

There is consensus around the need for designing games that are focused on a task rather than simply providing feedback on the biomechanical characteristics of movement. This principle is inspired by extensive work supporting the superiority of implicit learning compared to explicit learning (144). Accordingly, rather than providing feedback to the patient in the form of joint angles or movement trajectories, subjects are instructed to accomplish a motor task such as reaching for an object in space or negotiating an obstacle. Setting task-oriented goals has been shown to be more effective than setting "abstract" goals such as increasing knee flexion during stance (for gait training) or increasing elbow extension during the performance of arm reaching movements.

A limited number of studies have been performed to assess the suitability of VR technologies to implement motor training protocols in individuals with TBI. Mostly such studies have been focused on balance training. An example is the work by Sveistrup et al. (145) in which the authors demonstrated the suitability of the Interactive Rehabilitation Ex-

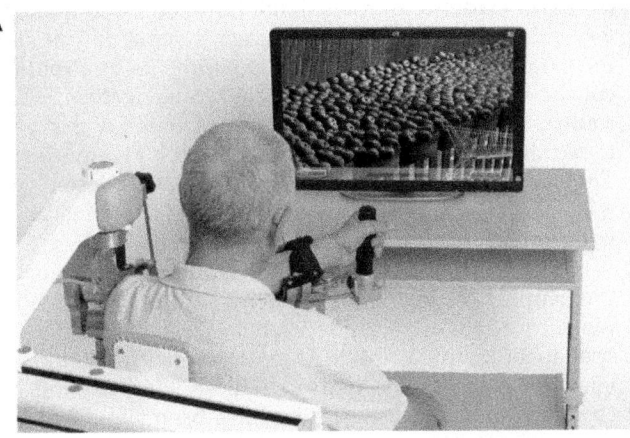

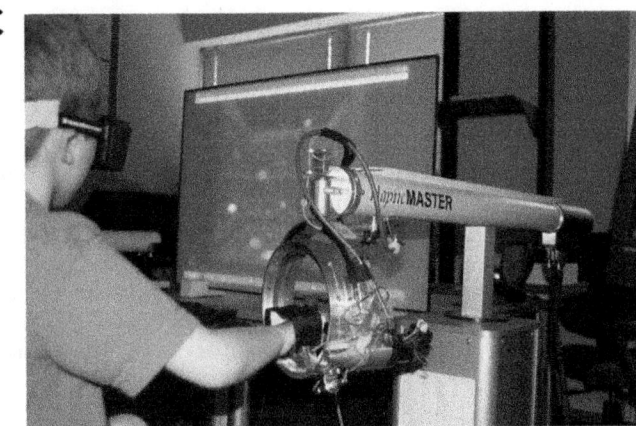

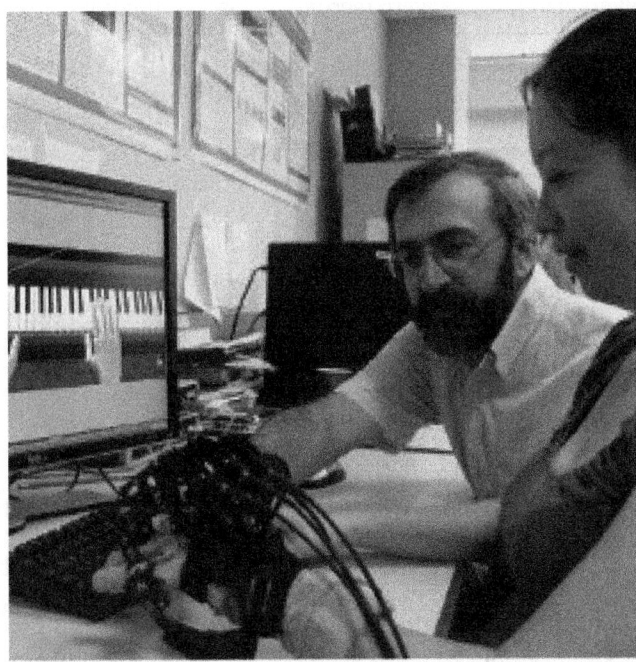

FIGURE 75-9 Examples of VR-based systems designed to enhance robotic platforms for upper limb motor training. Panel A shows the interactive gaming system used with the Armeo Spring. Panel B shows the HapticMaster system when combined with an immersive display. Patients are provided with 3D glasses when using the system in order to achieve 3D vision. Panel C shows an interactive gaming system used with a fully actuated system to guide movements of the hand and fingers.

ercise System (IREX) by GestureTek (Toronto, Canada) to perform balance training in subjects with moderate-to-severe TBI. The IREX system is similar in concept to the Microsoft Kinect system, but implemented with less advanced technology and marked by a simpler implementation of the computer games. When using the IREX system, the subject stands in front of a camera positioned on top of a large TV set. Behind the subject, a green drape is positioned to assure a uniform background thus making it easier to subtract the background and identify the subject standing in front of the camera. Therefore, the system captures the subject's movements in real time and projects the subject into a scene displayed on the TV set. Games are then enabled by overlaying the image of the subject and the images of objects the subject interacts with in the VR environment. Although surpassed by recently developed off-the-shelf interactive gaming products (such as the Nintendo Wii and the Microsoft Kinect), the IREX system anticipated future developments in the field of interactive gaming and provided a tremendous platform to demonstrate the effectiveness of VR-based rehabilitation. For instance, the work by Sveistrup et al. (145) showed greater improvements in individuals with TBI who received balance training using the IREX system compared to conventional therapy.

Following positive initial results concerning the assessment of VR-based rehabilitation in the context of balance training, several studies were performed to assess the use of VR tools in upper- and lower-limb motor training. The great majority of these studies were devoted to stroke rehabilitation. When a clinical decision has to be made concerning the suitability of VR-based rehabilitation protocols in individuals with TBI, the ample literature on VR in stroke rehabilitation should be considered as a reference point. Three major reviews (146–148) have been published over the past few years to summarize the studies in the field. Herein, we will report the conclusions of the most recent of these reviews, that is, the one by Laver et al. (148), which draws conclusions largely similar to those drawn by the other 2 reviews. The systematic review of the literature carried out by Laver et al. (148) showed that VR leads to better results than conventional therapy targeting upper-limb impairments and function, but with moderate effect size and with respect to only specific aspects of arm function. Insufficient evidence of the superiority of VR-based training was found for studies focused on lower-limb training. In general, the authors emphasized the heterogeneity of the reviewed studies. Only a few of the studies considered in these reviews combined VR/interactive gaming with robotics. However, because of the growing interest for integrating VR/interactive gaming and robotics and the availability now of systems for robotic-assisted training that leverage VR and interactive gaming, it is becoming more and more common that studies concerning the clinical assessment of robotic-assisted motor training include the use of VR and interactive gaming tools.

An example of work of this type is the one by Housman et al. (149) in which 28 stroke survivors with moderate-to-severe hemiparesis were recruited to assess motor gains associated with the use of the Therapy Wilmington Robotic Exoskeleton (T-WREX). The use of the exoskeleton was combined with that of interactive games shown on a computer screen in which the position of the arm used to play the game (and strapped onto the exoskeleton) was remapped in the virtual environment of the game to facilitate the performance of arm reaching and object manipulation tasks. The outcomes of the intervention were compared with the outcomes of a training protocol based on the use of a tabletop for gravity support (i.e., performing arm reaching movements using the surface of a table as support and positioning a towel between the arm and the table to minimize friction). The study showed better outcomes with the T-WREX system compared to the earlier-described conventional therapy.

Researchers are studying the effectiveness of using haptic feedback and the powerful combination obtained by utilizing both haptic feedback (as delivered by a robot) and visual feedback (as delivered using VR) (150). Besides, VR has been shown to be effective in providing motivation and encouraging active participation in therapy even among challenging populations such as the pediatric population (151). Furthermore, some studies have provided evidence that the combined use of VR and robotics offers a powerful tool to implement rehabilitation interventions and that the addition of VR/interactive gaming is not solely a means to motivate subjects to actively participate in the therapy, but also a way to challenge subjects with visuomotor integration tasks thus leading to better clinical outcomes (152–153).

Overall, studies combining VR/interactive gaming and robotics for motor training interventions show promising results. This is the case for both lower-limb training (154) and upper-limb training (143). So, although future studies would have to confirm trends identified in investigations conducted so far, it appears clinically justifiable to pursue the adoption of these technologies while taking a cautious approach in situations in which no solid evidence of the superiority of a particular method has been demonstrated as yet.

VR-based systems have been also used to implement cognitive assessments and training protocols (155–156). In this context, a primary area of interest has been the design of VR environments to test and train individuals with executive dysfunction, that is, impairments affecting the ability of an individual to achieve sequencing and organization of behaviors that are key for planning and strategy formation. In this context, Pugnetti et al. [157] developed a VR environment in which patients navigated through the rooms of a building. In the rooms, patients received clues about how to exit the building. Patients had to process the information gathered in the different rooms to find their way out. Elkind et al. (158) designed a VR environment based on a beach scene to test executive dysfunction. Patients were instructed to sell items to people in the beach scene. They received instructions about how to reach the umbrellas where they could find buyers for the items to be sold. Colors of umbrellas helped identifying the location of the buyers. These examples demonstrate that VR can provide an ecologically valid environment to test and train individuals with executive dysfunction.

Another area of interest has been the assessment of memory impairments. Seminal work by Brooks et al. (159)

provides evidence of the suitability of VR environments to test individuals with memory impairments and to implement training protocols. In the experiments by Brooks and colleagues, subjects were instructed to navigate a VR environment and, once they had completed their navigation task, to recollect objects that they had seen in the VR environment. The proposed methodology was extensively tested in patients with vascular brain injury (160) and shown to be effective for both testing and training purposes.

VR also provides tools to train prospective memory failure, namely the inability to remember to perform actions in the future (161). VR lends itself to train individuals with spatial ability impairments, attention deficits, and unilateral visual neglect. Besides, daily activities such as driving, street crossing, and food preparation have been simulated in VR environments for the purpose of testing and training patients (162–164).

CONCLUSION

Over the past two decades, the development of neurotechnologies has provided clinicians with new tools to implement clinical interventions in individuals with TBI. The development of invasive and noninvasive brain stimulation technologies have provided the opportunity to implement novel interventions such as facilitating the activation of cerebral networks via deep brain stimulation (1) and modifying the excitability of brain areas of interest (with techniques such as rTMS and tDCS) (12).

Advances in electronics and computer science have made it possible to manufacture compact and user-friendly devices that have enabled clinical adoptions of existing technologies such as FES (53). Researchers had experimented with the use of FES for decades, but only recently the availability of compact systems for FES of the upper and lower limbs has triggered clinical adoption of this technology. In the near future, it is expected that implantable FES systems will make it into the clinical environment.

Other technologies appear to be extremely promising but not ready as yet for clinical adoption. BCIs are an example of such technologies (94). EEG-based BCIs are of particular interest in rehabilitation. It is conceivable that, in the future, EEG-based BCIs will be broadly used in rehabilitation, most likely in combination with robots and/or systems for FES. Also, their use as a means to facilitate motor imagery is expected to grow rapidly in the next few years.

Significant technological advances have taken place in rehabilitation robotics. However, some fundamental aspects of the design of robotic systems for rehabilitation still has to be assessed. For instance, robotic-control strategies to achieve optimal clinical outcomes have not been clearly defined as yet. Patient-cooperative strategies appear to be particularly promising (122).

VR environments have been looked upon for some time as tools to facilitate the implementation of motor and cognitive training. Available evidence suggests that VR tools can be effective in both motor and cognitive training (148,155). Recently, researchers and clinicians have shifted their focus on the use of interactive gaming as a surrogate of VR environments. Preliminary results focused on the use of interactive gaming platforms are promising but also they show that adaptations of off-the-shelf gaming systems should be considered.

The large number of new technologies that are becoming available to clinicians to implement rehabilitation interventions are a cause of excitement. However, one should be cautious in assuming that clinical adoption will occur in a relatively short period of time. In fact, it has been the case in the past (for instance, for the adoption of FES systems) that clinical adoption follows research studies with a significant time lag.

KEY CLINICAL POINTS

1. TMS is the most broadly used among the techniques for brain stimulation that were considered in this chapter. The main clinical use of TMS is pain management. However, in the near future, it is expected that TMS will be used in the clinic for additional purposes such as priming cortical areas to facilitate plasticity effects during motor training and assessing plasticity effects in response to rehabilitation interventions.

2. tDCS is not yet as broadly used as TMS. However, it is expected that the clinical use of this technique will soon become significant. The interest for tDCS resides in the fact that it is an easy-to-use neuromodulation technique, that it is relatively inexpensive, and that it is compatible with the performance of rehabilitation protocols.

3. The development of compact systems for FES has made a tremendous difference in the clinical adoption of FES. Their use in the clinic is now routine. Positive outcomes have been shown in association with the use of FES in both upper- and lower-limb rehabilitation.

4. BCIs are very promising and one would anticipate that their adoption will take place within the next few years. However, at the moment, BCIs are not ready for clinical application.

5. The use of robotic systems in rehabilitation is still controversial. There is no good "general rule" to prescribe robotic-assisted training. Clinicians should decide on a case-by-case basis if the use of a robotic system is appropriate for the patient under consideration. Also, robotic-assisted therapy should be considered only 1 component of a comprehensive motor training intervention.

6. VR environments have shown to have a positive impact on rehabilitation outcomes for both motor and cognitive training.

7. The use of interactive gaming systems in rehabilitation is emerging because such systems are significantly less expensive than fully immersive VR environments but appear to achieve comparable clinical outcomes.

KEY REFERENCES

1. Daly JJ, Wolpaw JR. Brain-computer interfaces in neurological rehabilitation. *Lancet Neurol.* 2008;7:1032–1043.
2. Demirtas-Tatlidede A, Vahabzadeh-Hagh AM, Bernabeu M, Tormos JM, Pascual-Leone A. Noninvasive brain stimulation in traumatic brain injury [published online ahead of print June 17, 2011]. *J Head Trauma Rehabil.*

3. Laver KE, George S, Thomas S, Deutsch JE, Crotty M. Virtual reality for stroke rehabilitation. *Cochrane Database Syst Rev.* 2011;(9):CD008349.
4. Mehrholz J, Werner C, Kugler J, Pohl M. Electromechanical-assisted training for walking after stroke. *Cochrane Database Syst Rev.* 2007;(4):CD006185.
5. Ring H, Weingarden H. Neuromodulation by functional electrical stimulation (FES) of limb paralysis after stroke. *Acta Neurochir Suppl.* 2007;97(pt 1):375–380.

References

1. Schiff ND, Giacino JT, Kalmar K, et al. Behavioural improvements with thalamic stimulation after severe traumatic brain injury. *Nature.* 2007;448:600–603.
2. Schiff ND, Rodriguez-Moreno D, Kamal A, et al. fMRI reveals large-scale network activation in minimally conscious patients. *Neurology.* 2005;64:514–523.
3. Yamamoto T, Katayama Y, Kano T, Kobayashi K, Oshima H, Fukaya C. Deep brain stimulation for the treatment of parkinsonian, essential, and poststroke tremor: a suitable stimulation method and changes in effective stimulation intensity. *J Neurosurg.* 2004;101:201–209.
4. Giacino JT, Kalmar K, Whyte J. The JFK Coma Recovery Scale-Revised: measurement characteristics and diagnostic utility. *Arch Phys Med Rehabil.* 2004;85:2020–2029.
5. Tsubokawa T, Yamamoto T, Katayama Y, Hirayama T, Maejima S, Moriya T. Deep-brain stimulation in a persistent vegetative state: follow-up results and criteria for selection of candidates. *Brain Inj.* 1990;4:315–327.
6. Schiff ND, Giacino JT, Fins JJ. Deep brain stimulation, neuroethics, and the minimally conscious state: moving beyond proof of principle. *Arch Neurol.* 2009;66:697–702.
7. Yamamoto T, Katayama Y, Kobayashi K, Oshima H, Fukaya C, Tsubokawa T. Deep brain stimulation for the treatment of vegetative state. *Eur J Neurosci.* 2010;32:1145–1151.
8. Son BC, Lee SW, Choi ES, Sung JH, Hong JT. Motor cortex stimulation for central pain following a traumatic brain injury. *Pain.* 2006;123:210–216.
9. Nguyen JP, Keravel Y, Feve A, et al. Treatment of deafferentation pain by chronic stimulation of the motor cortex: report of a series of 20 cases. *Acta Neurochir Suppl.* 1997;68:54–60.
10. Katayama Y, Fukaya C, Yamamoto T. Poststroke pain control by chronic motor cortex stimulation: neurological characteristics predicting a favorable response. *J Neurosurg.* 1998;89:585–591.
11. Son UC, Kim MC, Moon DE, Kang JK. Motor cortex stimulation in a patient with intractable complex regional pain syndrome type II with hemibody involvement. Case report. *J Neurosurg.* 2003;98:175–179.
12. Demirtas-Tatlidede A, Vahabzadeh-Hagh AM, Bernabeu M, Tormos JM, Pascual-Leone A. Noninvasive brain stimulation in traumatic brain injury [published online ahead of print June 17, 2011]. *J Head Trauma Rehabil.*
13. Pascual-Leone A, Davey NJ, Rothwell J, Wasserman EM, Puri BK. *Handbook of Transcranial Magnetic Stimulation.* London, United Kingdom: Arnold; 2002.
14. Reis J, Swayne OB, Vandermeeren Y, et al. Contribution of transcranial magnetic stimulation to the understanding of cortical mechanisms involved in motor control. *J Physiol.* 2008;586:325–351.
15. Bernabeu M, Demirtas-Tatlidede A, Opisso E, Lopez R, Tormos JM, Pascual-Leone A. Abnormal corticospinal excitability in traumatic diffuse axonal brain injury. *J Neurotrauma.* 2009;26:2185–2193.
16. Nardone R, Bergmann J, Kunz A, et al. Cortical excitability changes in patients with sleep-wake disturbances after traumatic brain injury. *J Neurotrauma.* 2011;28:1165–1171.
17. Louise-Bender Pape T, Rosenow J, Lewis G, et al. Repetitive transcranial magnetic stimulation-associated neurobehavioral gains during coma recovery. *Brain Stimul.* 2009;2:22–35.
18. Fitzgerald PB, Hoy KE, Maller JJ, et al. Transcranial magnetic stimulation for depression after a traumatic brain injury: a case study. *J ECT.* 2011;27:38–40.

19. Chew E, Straudi S, Fregni F, Zafonte RD, Bonato P. Transcranial direct current stimulation enhances the effect of upper limb functional task training in neurorehabilitation. In: 5th World Congress of the International Society of Physical and Rehabilitation Medicine; June 13–17, 2009; Istanbul, Turkey. Abstract.

20. Edwards DJ, Krebs HI, Rykman A, et al. Raised corticomotor excitability of M1 forearm area following anodal tDCS is sustained during robotic wrist therapy in chronic stroke. *Restor Neurol Neurosci.* 2009;27:199–207.

21. Schlaug G, Renga V, Nair D. Transcranial direct current stimulation in stroke recovery. *Arch Neurol.* 2008;65:1571–1576.

22. Bolognini N, Pascual-Leone A, Fregni F. Using non-invasive brain stimulation to augment motor training-induced plasticity. *J Neuroeng Rehabil.* 2009;6:8.

23. Lindenberg R, Renga V, Zhu LL, Nair D, Schlaug G. Bihemispheric brain stimulation facilitates motor recovery in chronic stroke patients. *Neurology.* 2010;75:2176–2184.

24. Madhavan S, Weber KA II, Stinear JW. Non-invasive brain stimulation enhances fine motor control of the hemiparetic ankle: implications for rehabilitation. *Exp Brain Res.* 2011;209:9–17.

25. Tanaka S, Takeda K, Otaka Y, et al. Single session of transcranial direct current stimulation transiently increases knee extensor force in patients with hemiparetic stroke. *Neurorehabil Neural Repair.* 2011;25:565–569.

26. Bolognini N, Vallar G, Casati C, et al. Neurophysiological and behavioral effects of tDCS combined with constraint-induced movement therapy in poststroke patients. *Neurorehabil Neural Repair.* 2011;25:819–829.

27. Nair DG, Renga V, Lindenberg R, Zhu L, Schlaug G. Optimizing recovery potential through simultaneous occupational therapy and non-invasive brain-stimulation using tDCS. *Restor Neurol Neurosci.* 2011;29:411–420.

28. Lindenberg R, Zhu LL, Schlaug G. Combined central and peripheral stimulation to facilitate motor recovery after stroke: the effect of number of sessions on outcome. *Neurorehabil Neural Repair.* 2012;26(5):479–483.

29. Zaghi S, Heine N, Fregni F. Brain stimulation for the treatment of pain: a review of costs, clinical effects, and mechanisms of treatment for three different central neuromodulatory approaches. *J Pain Manag.* 2009;2:339–352.

30. Datta A, Bikson M, Fregni F. Transcranial direct current stimulation in patients with skull defects and skull plates: high-resolution computational FEM study of factors altering cortical current flow. *Neuroimage.* 2010;52:1268–1278.

31. Datta A, Bansal V, Diaz J, Patel J, Reato D, Bikson M. Gyri-precise head model of transcranial direct current stimulation: improved spatial focality using a ring electrode versus conventional rectangular pad. *Brain Stimul.* 2009;2(4):201–207, 207.e1.

32. Faria P, Hallett M, Miranda PC. A finite element analysis of the effect of electrode area and inter-electrode distance on the spatial distribution of the current density in tDCS. *J Neural Eng.* 2011;8(6):066017.

33. Boychuk JA, Adkins DL, Kleim JA. Distributed versus focal cortical stimulation to enhance motor function and motor map plasticity in a rodent model of ischemia. *Neurorehabil Neural Repair.* 2011;25:88–97.

34. Fedorov A, Chibisova Y, Szymaszek A, Alexandrov M, Gall C, Sabel BA. Non-invasive alternating current stimulation induces recovery from stroke. *Restor Neurol Neurosci.* 2010;28:825–833.

35. Chung H, Dai T, Sharma SK, Huang YY, Carroll JD, Hamblin MR. The nuts and bolts of low-level laser (light) therapy. *Ann Biomed Eng.* 2012;40:516–533.

36. Lampl Y, Zivin JA, Fisher M, et al. Infrared laser therapy for ischemic stroke: a new treatment strategy: results of the NeuroThera Effectiveness and Safety Trial-1 (NEST-1). *Stroke.* 2007;38:1843–1849.

37. Byrnes KR, Waynant RW, Ilev IK, et al. Light promotes regeneration and functional recovery and alters the immune response after spinal cord injury. *Lasers Surg Med.* 2005;36:171–185.

38. Eggers J, Seidel G, Koch B, Konig IR. Sonothrombolysis in acute ischemic stroke for patients ineligible for rt-PA. *Neurology.* 2005;64:1052–1054.

39. Bellner J, Romner B, Reinstrup P, Kristiansson KA, Ryding E, Brandt L. Transcranial doppler sonography pulsatility index (PI) reflects intracranial pressure (ICP). *Surg Neurol.* 2004;62:45–51.

40. Vykhodtseva N, McDannold N, Hynynen K. Progress and problems in the application of focused ultrasound for blood-brain barrier disruption. *Ultrasonics.* 2008;48:279–296.

41. Lobel E, Kleine JF, Bihan DL, Leroy-Willig A, Berthoz A. Functional MRI of galvanic vestibular stimulation. *J Neurophysiol.* 1998;80:2699–2709.

42. Lobel E, Kleine JF, Leroy-Willig A, et al. Cortical areas activated by bilateral galvanic vestibular stimulation. *Ann N Y Acad Sci.* 1999;871:313–323.

43. Stephan T, Deutschlander A, Nolte A, et al. Functional MRI of galvanic vestibular stimulation with alternating currents at different frequencies. *Neuroimage.* 2005;26:721–732.

44. Cernak I, Noble-Haeusslein LJ. Traumatic brain injury: an overview of pathobiology with emphasis on military populations. *J Cereb Blood Flow Metab.* 2010;30:255–266.

45. Kox M, Pompe JC, Pickkers P, Hoedemaekers CW, van Vugt AB, van der Hoeven JG. Increased vagal tone accounts for the observed immune paralysis in patients with traumatic brain injury. *Neurology.* 2008;70:480–485.

46. Smith DC, Modglin AA, Roosevelt RW, et al. Electrical stimulation of the vagus nerve enhances cognitive and motor recovery following moderate fluid percussion injury in the rat. *J Neurotrauma.* 2005;22:1485–1502.

47. Clough RW, Neese SL, Sherill LK, et al. Cortical edema in moderate fluid percussion brain injury is attenuated by vagus nerve stimulation. *Neuroscience.* 2007;147:286–293.

48. Neese SL, Sherill LK, Tan AA, et al. Vagus nerve stimulation may protect GABAergic neurons following traumatic brain injury in rats: an immunocytochemical study. *Brain Res.* 2007;1128:157–163.

49. Haig AJ, Ho KC, Ludwig G. Clinical, physiologic, and pathologic evidence for vagus dysfunction in a case of traumatic brain injury. *J Trauma.* 1996;40:441–444.

50. Corcoran C, Connor TJ, O'Keane V, Garland MR. The effects of vagus nerve stimulation on pro- and anti-inflammatory cytokines in humans: a preliminary report. *Neuroimmunomodulation.* 2005;12:307–309.

51. Vodovnik L, Kralj A, Stanic U, Acimovic R, Gros N. Recent applications of functional electrical stimulation to stroke patients in Ljubljana. *Clin Orthop Relat Res.* 1978;131:64–70.

52. Kralj A, Acimovic R, Stanic U. Enhancement of hemiplegic patient rehabilitation by means of functional electrical stimulation. *Prosthet Orthot Int.* 1993;17:107–114.

53. Ring H, Weingarden H. Neuromodulation by functional electrical stimulation (FES) of limb paralysis after stroke. *Acta Neurochir Suppl.* 2007;97:375–380.

54. Burridge JH, Taylor PN, Hagan SA, Wood DE, Swain ID. The effects of common peroneal stimulation on the effort and speed of walking: a randomized controlled trial with chronic hemiplegic patients. *Clin Rehabil.* 1997;11:201–210.

55. Taylor P, Burridge J, Dunkerley A, et al. Clinical audit of 5 years provision of the Odstock dropped foot stimulator. *Artif Organs.* 1999;23:440–442.

56. Van Swigchem R, Weerdesteyn V, van Duijnhoven HJ, den Boer J, Beems T, Geurts AC. Near-normal gait pattern with peroneal electrical stimulation as a neuroprosthesis in the chronic phase of stroke: a case report. *Arch Phys Med Rehabil.* 2011;92:320–324.

57. Van Swigchem R, van Duijnhoven HJ, den Boer J, Geurts AC, Weerdesteyn V. Effect of peroneal electrical stimulation versus an ankle-foot orthosis on obstacle avoidance ability in people with stroke-related foot drop. *Phys Ther.* 2012;92:398–406.

58. Kottink AI, Oostendorp LJ, Buurke JH, Nene AV, Hermens HJ, IJzerman MJ. The orthotic effect of functional electrical stimulation on the improvement of walking in stroke patients with a dropped foot: a systematic review. *Artif Organs.* 2004;28:577–586.

59. Robbins SM, Houghton PE, Woodbury MG, Brown JL. The therapeutic effect of functional and transcutaneous electric stimulation on improving gait speed in stroke patients: a meta-analysis. *Arch Phys Med Rehabil.* 2006;87:853–859.

60. Thrasher TA, Popovic MR. Functional electrical stimulation of walking: function, exercise and rehabilitation. *Ann Readapt Med Phys.* 2008;51:452–460.

61. Stein RB, Everaert DG, Thompson AK, et al. Long-term therapeutic and orthotic effects of a foot drop stimulator on walking performance in progressive and nonprogressive neurological disorders. *Neurorehabil Neural Repair.* 2010;24:152–167.

62. Kottink AI, Hermens HJ, Nene AV, Tenniglo MJ, Groothuis-Oudshoorn CG, IJzerman MJ. Therapeutic effect of an implantable peroneal nerve stimulator in subjects with chronic stroke and footdrop: a randomized controlled trial. *Phys Ther.* 2008;88:437–448.

63. Everaert DG, Thompson AK, Chong SL, Stein RB. Does functional electrical stimulation for foot drop strengthen corticospinal connections? *Neurorehabil Neural Repair.* 2010;24:168–177.

64. Dunning K, Black K, Harrison A, McBride K, Israel S. Neuroprosthesis peroneal functional electrical stimulation in the acute inpatient rehabilitation setting: a case series. *Phys Ther.* 2009;89:499–506.

65. Kesar TM, Perumal R, Reisman DS, et al. Functional electrical stimulation of ankle plantarflexor and dorsiflexor muscles: effects on poststroke gait. *Stroke.* 2009;40:3821–3827.

66. Embrey DG, Holtz SL, Alon G, Brandsma BA, McCoy SW. Functional electrical stimulation to dorsiflexors and plantar flexors during gait to improve walking in adults with chronic hemiplegia. *Arch Phys Med Rehabil.* 2010;91:687–696.

67. Kim JH, Chung Y, Kim Y, Hwang S. Functional electrical stimulation applied to gluteus medius and tibialis anterior corresponding gait cycle for stroke [published online ahead of print March 03, 2012]. *Gait Posture.*

68. Prado-Medeiros CL, Sousa CO, Souza AS, et al. Effects of the addition of functional electrical stimulation to ground level gait training with body weight support after chronic stroke. *Rev Bras Fisioter.* 2011;15:436–444.

69. Daly JJ, Zimbelman J, Roenigk KL, et al. Recovery of coordinated gait: randomized controlled stroke trial of functional electrical stimulation (FES) versus no FES, with weight-supported treadmill and over-ground training. *Neurorehabil Neural Repair.* 2011;25:588–596.

70. Ng MF, Tong RK, Li LS. A pilot study of randomized clinical controlled trial of gait training in subacute stroke patients with partial body-weight support electromechanical gait trainer and functional electrical stimulation: six-month follow-up. *Stroke.* 2008;39:154–160.

71. Dohring ME, Daly JJ. Automatic synchronization of functional electrical stimulation and robotic assisted treadmill training. *IEEE Trans Neural Syst Rehabil Eng.* 2008;16:310–313.

72. McCabe JP, Dohring ME, Marsolais EB, et al. Feasibility of combining gait robot and multichannel functional electrical stimulation with intramuscular electrodes. *J Rehabil Res Dev.* 2008;45:997–1006.

73. Lo HC, Tsai KH, Su FC, Chang GL, Yeh CY. Effects of a functional electrical stimulation-assisted leg-cycling wheelchair on reducing spasticity of patients after stroke. *J Rehabil Med.* 2009;41:242–246.

74. Yeh CY, Tsai KH, Su FC, Lo HC. Effect of a bout of leg cycling with electrical stimulation on reduction of hypertonia in patients with stroke. *Arch Phys Med Rehabil.* 2010;91:1731–1736.

75. Ambrosini E, Ferrante S, Pedrocchi A, Ferrigno G, Molteni F. Cycling induced by electrical stimulation improves motor recovery in postacute hemiparetic patients: a randomized controlled trial. *Stroke.* 2011;42:1068–1073.

76. Lo HC, Hsu YC, Hsueh YH, Yeh CY. Cycling exercise with functional electrical stimulation improves postural control in stroke patients. *Gait Posture.* 2012;35:506–510.

77. Freeman CT, Hughes AM, Burridge JH, Chappell PH, Lewin PL, Rogers E. A model of the upper extremity using FES for stroke rehabilitation. *J Biomech Eng.* 2009;131:031011.

78. Goffredo M, Bernabucci I, Schmid M, Conforto S. A neural tracking and motor control approach to improve rehabilitation of upper limb movements. *J Neuroeng Rehabil.* 2008;5:5.

79. Mann G, Taylor P, Lane R. Accelerometer-triggered electrical stimulation for reach and grasp in chronic stroke patients: a pilot study. *Neurorehabil Neural Repair.* 2011;25:774–780.

80. Chiou YH, Luh JJ, Chen SC, Chen YL, Lai JS, Kuo TS. Patient-driven loop control for hand function restoration in a non-invasive

81. functional electrical stimulation system. *Disabil Rehabil.* 2008;30:1499–1505.

81. Hughes AM, Freeman CT, Burridge JH, Chappell PH, Lewin PL, Rogers E. Feasibility of iterative learning control mediated by functional electrical stimulation for reaching after stroke. *Neurorehabil Neural Repair.* 2009;23:559–568.

82. Alon G, Levitt AF, McCarthy PA. Functional electrical stimulation (FES) may modify the poor prognosis of stroke survivors with severe motor loss of the upper extremity: a preliminary study. *Am J Phys Med Rehabil.* 2008;87:627–636.

83. Mangold S, Schuster C, Keller T, Zimmermann-Schlatter A, Ettlin T. Motor training of upper extremity with functional electrical stimulation in early stroke rehabilitation. *Neurorehabil Neural Repair.* 2009;23:184–190.

84. Daly JJ, Cheng R, Rogers J, Litinas K, Hrovat K, Dohring M. Feasibility of a new application of noninvasive brain computer interface (BCI): a case study of training for recovery of volitional motor control after stroke. *J Neurol Phys Ther.* 2009;33:203–211.

85. Popovic D, Baker LL, Loeb GE. Recruitment and comfort of BION implanted electrical stimulation: implications for FES applications. *IEEE Trans Neural Syst Rehabil Eng.* 2007;15:577–586.

86. Nozaki D, Collins JJ, Yamamoto Y. Mechanism of stochastic resonance enhancement in neuronal models driven by 1/f noise. *Phys Rev E Stat Phys Plasmas Fluids Relat Interdiscip Topics.* 1999;60:4637–4644.

87. Priplata A, Niemi J, Salen M, Harry J, Lipsitz LA, Collins JJ. Noise-enhanced human balance control. *Phys Rev Lett.* 2002;89:238101.

88. Stein J, Hughes R, D'Andrea S, et al. Stochastic resonance stimulation for upper limb rehabilitation poststroke. *Am J Phys Med Rehabil.* 2010;89:697–705.

89. Collins AT, Blackburn JT, Olcott CW, Dirschl DR, Weinhold PS. The effects of stochastic resonance electrical stimulation and neoprene sleeve on knee proprioception. *J Orthop Surg Res.* 2009;4:3.

90. Ross SE, Arnold BL, Blackburn JT, Brown CN, Guskiewicz KM. Enhanced balance associated with coordination training with stochastic resonance stimulation in subjects with functional ankle instability: an experimental trial. *J Neuroeng Rehabil.* 2007;4:47.

91. Galica AM, Kang HG, Priplata AA, et al. Subsensory vibrations to the feet reduce gait variability in elderly fallers. *Gait Posture.* 2009;30:383–387.

92. Priplata AA, Niemi JB, Harry JD, Lipsitz LA, Collins JJ. Vibrating insoles and balance control in elderly people. *Lancet.* 2003;362:1123–1124.

93. Priplata AA, Patritti BL, Niemi JB, et al. Noise-enhanced balance control in patients with diabetes and patients with stroke. *Ann Neurol.* 2006;59:4–12.

94. Daly JJ, Wolpaw JR. Brain-computer interfaces in neurological rehabilitation. *Lancet Neurol.* 2008;7:1032–1043.

95. Wolpaw JR, McFarland DJ, Neat GW, Forneris CA. An EEG-based brain-computer interface for cursor control. *Electroencephalogr Clin Neurophysiol.* 1991;78:252–259.

96. Wolpaw JR, McFarland DJ. Multichannel EEG-based brain-computer communication. *Electroencephalogr Clin Neurophysiol.* 1994;90:444–449.

97. Hinterberger T, Kubler A, Kaiser J, Neumann N, Birbaumer N. A brain-computer interface (BCI) for the locked-in: comparison of different EEG classifications for the thought translation device. *Clin Neurophysiol.* 2003;114:416–425.

98. Donchin E, Spencer KM, Wijesinghe R. The mental prosthesis: assessing the speed of a P300-based brain-computer interface. *IEEE Trans Rehabil Eng.* 2000;8:174–179.

99. Mak JN, McFarland DJ, Vaughan TM, et al. EEG correlates of P300-based brain-computer interface (BCI) performance in people with amyotrophic lateral sclerosis. *J Neural Eng.* 2012;9:026014.

100. Kostov A, Polak M. Parallel man-machine training in development of EEG-based cursor control. *IEEE Trans Rehabil Eng.* 2000;8:203–205.

101. Wolpaw JR, McFarland DJ. Control of a two-dimensional movement signal by a noninvasive brain-computer interface in humans. *Proc Natl Acad Sci U S A.* 2004;101:17849–17854.

102. Kubler A, Neumann N, Kaiser J, Kotchoubey B, Hinterberger T, Birbaumer NP. Brain-computer communication: self-regulation of

slow cortical potentials for verbal communication. *Arch Phys Med Rehabil.* 2001;82:1533–1539.

103. Do AH, Wang PT, King CE, Abiri A, Nenadic Z. Brain-computer interface controlled functional electrical stimulation system for ankle movement. *J Neuroeng Rehabil.* 2011;8:49.

104. Prasad G, Herman P, Coyle D, McDonough S, Crosbie J. Applying a brain-computer interface to support motor imagery practice in people with stroke for upper limb recovery: a feasibility study. *J Neuroeng Rehabil.* 2010;7:60.

105. Gomez-Rodriguez M, Peters J, Hill J, Scholkopf B, Gharabaghi A, Grosse-Wentrup M. Closing the sensorimotor loop: haptic feedback facilitates decoding of motor imagery. *J Neural Eng.* 2011;8: 036005.

106. Ang KK, Guan C, Chua KS, et al. A clinical study of motor imagery-based brain-computer interface for upper limb robotic rehabilitation. *Conf Proc IEEE Eng Med Biol Soc.* 2009;2009:5981–5984.

107. Broetz D, Braun C, Weber C, Soekadar SR, Caria A, Birbaumer N. Combination of brain-computer interface training and goal-directed physical therapy in chronic stroke: a case report. *Neurorehabil Neural Repair.* 2010;24:674–679.

108. Schalk G, Miller KJ, Anderson NR, et al. Two-dimensional movement control using electrocorticographic signals in humans. *J Neural Eng.* 2008;5:75–84.

109. Serruya MD, Hatsopoulos NG, Paninski L, Fellows MR, Donoghue JP. Instant neural control of a movement signal. *Nature.* 2002;416: 141–142.

110. Carmena JM, Lebedev MA, Crist RE, et al. Learning to control a brain-machine interface for reaching and grasping by primates. *PLoS Biol.* 2003;1:E42.

111. Hochberg LR, Serruya MD, Friehs GM, et al. Neuronal ensemble control of prosthetic devices by a human with tetraplegia. *Nature.* 2006;442:164–171.

112. Coyle SM, Ward TE, Markham CM. Brain-computer interface using a simplified functional near-infrared spectroscopy system. *J Neural Eng.* 2007;4:219–226.

113. Zimmermann R, Marchal-Crespo L, Lambercy O, et al. Towards a BCI for sensorimotor training: initial results from simultaneous fNIRS and biosignal recordings. *Conf Proc IEEE Eng Med Biol Soc.* 2011;2011:6339–6343.

114. Belda-Lois JM, Mena-del Horno S, Bermejo-Bosch I, et al. Rehabilitation of gait after stroke: a review towards a top-down approach. *J Neuroeng Rehabil.* 2011;8:66.

115. Hesse S, Kuhlmann H, Wilk J, Tomelleri C, Kirker SG. A new electromechanical trainer for sensorimotor rehabilitation of paralysed fingers: a case series in chronic and acute stroke patients. *J Neuroeng Rehabil.* 2008;5:21.

116. Aisen ML, Krebs HI, Hogan N, McDowell F, Volpe BT. The effect of robot-assisted therapy and rehabilitative training on motor recovery following stroke. *Arch Neurol.* 1997;54:443–446.

117. Krebs HI, Hogan N, Volpe BT, Aisen ML, Edelstein L, Diels C. Overview of clinical trials with MIT-MANUS: a robot-aided neurorehabilitation facility. *Technol Health Care.* 1999;7:419–423.

118. Colombo G, Joerg M, Schreier R, Dietz V. Treadmill training of paraplegic patients using a robotic orthosis. *J Rehabil Res Dev.* 2000; 37:693–700.

119. Jezernik S, Colombo G, Keller T, Frueh H, Morari M. Robotic orthosis lokomat: a rehabilitation and research tool. *Neuromodulation.* 2003;6:108–115.

120. Nef T, Mihelj M, Riener R. ARMin: a robot for patient-cooperative arm therapy. *Med Biol Eng Comput.* 2007;45:887–900.

121. Staubli P, Nef T, Klamroth-Marganska V, Riener R. Effects of intensive arm training with the rehabilitation robot ARMin II in chronic stroke patients: four single-cases. *J Neuroeng Rehabil.* 2009;6:46.

122. Duschau-Wicke A, Caprez A, Riener R. Patient-cooperative control increases active participation of individuals with SCI during robot-aided gait training. *J Neuroeng Rehabil.* 2010;7:43.

123. Tefertiller C, Pharo B, Evans N, Winchester P. Efficacy of rehabilitation robotics for walking training in neurological disorders: a review. *J Rehabil Res Dev.* 2011;48:387–416.

124. Mehrholz J, Werner C, Kugler J, Pohl M. Electromechanical-assisted training for walking after stroke. *Cochrane Database Syst Rev.* 2007;(4):CD006185.

125. Moseley AM, Stark A, Cameron ID, Pollock A. Treadmill training and body weight support for walking after stroke. *Cochrane Database Syst Rev.* 2005;(4):CD002840.

126. Duncan PW, Sullivan KJ, Behrman AL, et al. Body-weight-supported treadmill rehabilitation after stroke. *N Engl J Med.* 2011; 364:2026–2036.

127. Brown TH, Mount J, Rouland BL, Kautz KA, Barnes RM, Kim J. Body weight-supported treadmill training versus conventional gait training for people with chronic traumatic brain injury. *J Head Trauma Rehabil.* 2005;20:402–415.

128. Scherer M. Gait rehabilitation with body weight-supported treadmill training for a blast injury survivor with traumatic brain injury. *Brain Inj.* 2007;21:93–100.

129. Lannin NA, McCluskey A. A systematic review of upper limb rehabilitation for adults with traumatic brain injury. *Brain Impairment.* 2008;9:237–246.

130. Lo AC, Guarino PD, Richards LG, et al. Robot-assisted therapy for long-term upper-limb impairment after stroke. *N Engl J Med.* 2010; 362:1772–1783.

131. Kahn LE, Lum PS, Rymer WZ, Reinkensmeyer DJ. Robot-assisted movement training for the stroke-impaired arm: does it matter what the robot does? *J Rehabil Res Dev.* 2006;43:619–630.

132. Prange GB, Jannink MJ, Groothuis-Oudshoorn CG, Hermens HJ, Ijzerman MJ. Systematic review of the effect of robot-aided therapy on recovery of the hemiparetic arm after stroke. *J Rehabil Res Dev.* 2006;43:171–184.

133. Kwakkel G, Kollen BJ, Krebs HI. Effects of robot-assisted therapy on upper limb recovery after stroke: a systematic review. *Neurorehabil Neural Repair.* 2008;22:111–121.

134. Kwakkel G, van Peppen R, Wagenaar RC, et al. Effects of augmented exercise therapy time after stroke: a meta-analysis. *Stroke.* 2004;35:2529–2539.

135. Brochard S, Robertson J, Medee B, Remy-Neris O. What's new in new technologies for upper extremity rehabilitation? *Curr Opin Neurol.* 2010;23:683–687.

136. Lamontagne A, Fung J, McFadyen BJ, Faubert J. Modulation of walking speed by changing optic flow in persons with stroke. *J Neuroeng Rehabil.* 2007;4:22.

137. Saposnik G, Teasell R, Mamdani M, et al. Effectiveness of virtual reality using Wii gaming technology in stroke rehabilitation: a pilot randomized clinical trial and proof of principle. *Stroke.* 2010;41: 1477–1484.

138. Deutsch JE, Brettler A, Smith C, et al. Nintendo wii sports and wii fit game analysis, validation, and application to stroke rehabilitation. *Top Stroke Rehabil.* 2011;18:701–719.

139. Chang YJ, Chen SF, Huang JD. A kinect-based system for physical rehabilitation: a pilot study for young adults with motor disabilities. *Res Dev Disabil.* 2011;32:2566–2570.

140. Boian RF, Bouzit M, Burdea GC, Deutsch JE. Dual Stewart platform mobility simulator. *Conf Proc IEEE Eng Med Biol Soc.* 2004;7: 4848–4851.

141. Reinkensmeyer DJ, Kahn LE, Averbuch M, McKenna-Cole A, Schmit BD, Rymer WZ. Understanding and treating arm movement impairment after chronic brain injury: progress with the ARM guide. *J Rehabil Res Dev.* 2000;37:653–662.

142. Gijbels D, Lamers I, Kerkhofs L, Alders G, Knippenberg E, Feys P. The Armeo Spring as training tool to improve upper limb functionality in multiple sclerosis: a pilot study. *J Neuroeng Rehabil.* 2011;8:5.

143. Merians AS, Fluet GG, Qiu Q, et al. Robotically facilitated virtual rehabilitation of arm transport integrated with finger movement in persons with hemiparesis. *J Neuroeng Rehabil.* 2011;8:27.

144. Shumway-Cook A, Woollacott MH. *Motor Control: Translating Research into Clinical Practice.* Philadelphia, PA: Lippincott Williams & Wilkins; 2011.

145. Sveistrup H, McComas J, Thornton M, et al. Experimental studies of virtual reality-delivered compared to conventional exercise programs for rehabilitation. *Cyberpsychol Behav.* 2003;6:245–249.

146. Crosbie JH, Lennon S, Basford JR, McDonough SM. Virtual reality in stroke rehabilitation: still more virtual than real. *Disabil Rehabil.* 2007;29:1139–1152.

147. Saposnik G, Levin M. Virtual reality in stroke rehabilitation: a meta-analysis and implications for clinicians. *Stroke*. 2011;42: 1380–1386.

148. Laver KE, George S, Thomas S, Deutsch JE, Crotty M. Virtual reality for stroke rehabilitation. *Cochrane Database Syst Rev*. 2011;9: CD008349.

149. Housman SJ, Scott KM, Reinkensmeyer DJ. A randomized controlled trial of gravity-supported, computer-enhanced arm exercise for individuals with severe hemiparesis. *Neurorehabil Neural Repair*. 2009;23:505–514.

150. Koritnik T, Koenig A, Bajd T, Riener R, Munih M. Comparison of visual and haptic feedback during training of lower extremities. *Gait Posture*. 2010;32:540–546.

151. Brutsch K, Schuler T, Koenig A, et al. Influence of virtual reality soccer game on walking performance in robotic assisted gait training for children. *J Neuroeng Rehabil*. 2010;7:15.

152. Mirelman A, Bonato P, Deutsch JE. Effects of training with a robot-virtual reality system compared with a robot alone on the gait of individuals after stroke. *Stroke*. 2009;40:169–174.

153. Mirelman A, Patritti BL, Bonato P, Deutsch JE. Effects of virtual reality training on gait biomechanics of individuals post-stroke. *Gait Posture*. 2010;31:433–437.

154. Stoller O, Waser M, Stammler L, Schuster C. Evaluation of robot-assisted gait training using integrated biofeedback in neurologic disorders. *Gait Posture*. 2012;35(4):595–600.

155. Rose FD, Brooks BM, Rizzo AA. Virtual reality in brain damage rehabilitation: review. *Cyberpsychol Behav*. 2005;8:241–271.

156. Zhang L, Abreu BC, Masel B, et al. Virtual reality in the assessment of selected cognitive function after brain injury. *Am J Phys Med Rehabil*. 2001;80:597–605.

157. Pugnetti L, Mendozzi L, Motta A, Cattaneo A, Barbieri E, Brancotti A. Evaluation and retraining of adults' cognitive impairment: which role for virtual reality technology? *Comput Biol Med*. 1995; 25:213–227.

158. Elkind JS, Rubin E, Rosenthal S, Skoff B, Prather P. A simulated reality scenario compared with the computerized Wisconsin card sorting test: an analysis of preliminary results. *Cyberpsychol Behav*. 2001;4:489–496.

159. Brooks BM, Attree EA, Rose FD, Clifford BR, Leadbetter AG. The specificity of memory enhancement during interaction with a virtual environment. *Memory*. 1999;7:65–78.

160. Rose FD, Brooks BM, Attree EA, et al. A preliminary investigation into the use of virtual environments in memory retraining after vascular brain injury: indications for future strategy? *Disabil Rehabil*. 1999;21:548–554.

161. Brooks BM, Rose FD, Potter J, Jayawardena S, Morling A. Assessing stroke patients' prospective memory using virtual reality. *Brain Inj*. 2004;18:391–401.

162. Liu L, Miyazaki M, Watson B. Norms and validity of the DriVR: a virtual reality driving assessment for persons with head injuries. *Cyberpsychol Behav*. 1999;2:53–67.

163. Christiansen C, Abreu B, Ottenbacher K, Huffman K, Masel B, Culpepper R. Task performance in virtual environments used for cognitive rehabilitation after traumatic brain injury. *Arch Phys Med Rehabil*. 1998;79:888–892.

164. Zhang L, Abreu BC, Seale GS, Masel B, Christiansen CH, Ottenbacher KJ. A virtual reality environment for evaluation of a daily living skill in brain injury rehabilitation: reliability and validity. *Arch Phys Med Rehabil*. 2003;84:1118–1124.

Complementary and Alternative Medicine

Jacinta McElligott, Felise S. Zollman, and Sunil Kothari

INTRODUCTION

Traditional Whole Medical Systems

In Western societies, complementary and alternative medicine (CAM) is often defined as the use and practice of therapies or diagnostic techniques that are not part of the current Western health care system. Complementary medicine is used together with conventional medicine, and alternative medicine refers to an intervention used instead of conventional medicine. The term integrative medicine is used when complementary medicine is integrated with modern biomedical practice. In the mid-1800s, medical and health care in the United States included a rich tapestry of many different health care practices and philosophies from various cultures around the world. The development and increased understanding of the pathogenesis of disease and the scientific research and rigor that forms the foundation of the modern Western biomedical approach to medicine was only introduced in the latter part of the 19th century. The modern biomedical approach to medical practice is founded on an understanding of the pathophysiology of disease and scientific proof of the efficacy of an intervention. Nevertheless, traditional medical practices and CAM encompass a wealth of wisdom developed over centuries of human experience; in the preferential development of the biomedical approach, invaluable traditional practices may have been inadvertently left behind. This is especially true in Western societies because the success of and emphasis on the biomedical approach has predominated medical practice.

The World Health Organization (WHO) defines *traditional medicine* as "the sum total of knowledge, skills, and practices based on the theories, beliefs, and experiences indigenous to different cultures that are used to maintain health as well as to prevent, diagnose, improve, or treat physical or mental illness" (1). A traditional medical system is referred to as a "CAM" practice when it is adopted by other populations outside of indigenous culture. Unfortunately, although traditional medicine practices have been adopted in different cultures and regions, there has not generally been a parallel advance of international standards and methods of evaluation of CAM practices. According to the WHO (1), few countries have national policies for traditional medicine and regulation of traditional medical products, practices, and practitioners is difficult from a global perspective especially because the scientific evidence to evaluate the safety and effectiveness of traditional medicine products and practices is very limited. Nevertheless, despite this lack of scientific evidence, in some developed countries, 70%–80% of the population have reported use of some form of CAM interventions (e.g., acupuncture). Recognizing the reliance of underdeveloped countries on traditional medicine and the use of CAM practices in developed countries, the WHO promotes the use of traditional medicine for health care in a collaborative fashion that aims to

1. acknowledge traditional medicine as part of primary health care to increase access to care and preserve knowledge and resources;
2. support and integrate traditional medicine into national health systems in combination with national policy and regulation for products, practices, and providers to ensure safety and quality;
3. ensure patient safety by upgrading the skills and knowledge of traditional medicine providers; and
4. ensure the use of safe, effective, and quality products and practices based on available evidence.

There are many examples of whole traditional medical systems from ancient history. For instance, the practice of Chinese medicine has evolved more than thousands of years and Ayurvedic medicine—practiced in the Indian subcontinent—dates back more than 7,000 years. In its earliest forms (i.e., more than 5,000 years ago), traditional Chinese medicine (TCM) was handed down orally from practitioner to practitioner; TCM concepts first appear in written form in a text known as the *Nei Jing* (or *Yellow Emperor's Inner Classic*), written approximately 2,000 years ago. The practice of Chinese medicine evolved from observation of natural phenomena such as the life cycle, the cycle of the sun and moon, and the cycle of the seasons of the year. From these observations, a system of medicine evolved, which focuses on the harmonious flow of energy known as "Qi" (pronounced as "chee") within an organism as well as the interaction between the organism and the environment. Blockage of the smooth flow of Qi or imbalance in the flow or strength of Qi through some part of the body is seen as the cause of illness. Herbs and acupuncture is used to try to restore the harmonious, balanced flow of Qi, thereby restoring the individual to good health.

Ayurveda medicine uses an integrated approach to the prevention and treatment of disease with a healthy lifestyle of diet, herbs, exercise, and yoga (2). Ayurveda, with roots in the Indian subcontinent, is one of the oldest systems of medicine known with several sources dating as far back as 7,000 years. The term Ayurveda is an amalgamation of the root words "ayur" (meaning life) and "veda" (meaning science or knowledge), hence the meaning of Ayurveda as the knowledge of life. Ayurveda focuses on a holistic approach to care for patients in all aspects—physical, mental, emotional, and spiritual. Ayurveda is a multidisciplinary whole medical system that incorporates many methods for treatment including lifestyle modifications, yoga, meditation, and pranayama (deep breathing exercises) as well as herbal remedies. It should be noted that yoga and meditation are often used as general terms; there are many varieties and styles within each category. Yoga and meditation are also not necessarily independent practices because yoga incorporates many aspects of meditation as well.

Although traditional whole medical systems such as TCM and Ayurveda have evolved over thousands of years, the relatively more recent Western whole medical system is founded on a biomedical approach to health care and is based on an understanding of the pathophysiology of disease and scientific proof of the efficacy of an intervention. Some believe that this approach to medicine was established in the second century AD by Galen, a Greek physician (2). Galen published a guide to the evaluation and treatment of patients that focused on anatomical knowledge and the use of visual and physical objectivity. In the 1800s, scholars in China also sought to move away from speculation and root their studies in "hard facts" by practicing "kaozhang," translated as "practicing evidential research" (3). However, it was the development of the randomized controlled trial (RCT) that was the landmark in the evolution of evidential research in the 18th century. James Lind (1716–1794) (4) was a ship's surgeon in Britain, who is often cited as a pioneer of the effective use of evidential research with the development of the RCT and the use of evidential research to implement health care changes. In Lind's time, scurvy was a crippling and prevalent disease among sailors. In his meticulous observations, Lind included a simple account of what may have been the first prospective RCT ever undertaken in humans. With their full cooperation, Lind randomized sailors afflicted with scurvy into separate groups, each group receiving a different mode of treatment thought efficacious at that time. The results of the experiment were simply stated, "Of the 2 men who had received 2 oranges and 1 lemon daily, 1 was fit for duty at the end of 6 days and 1 recovered to the point of attending the rest of the sick patients in the other groups." (see Figure 76-1)

With this 1 concise clinical experiment, Lind established the clear superiority of citrus fruits above all other supposed antiscorbutic remedies. Lind's work ultimately led to a government ordinance requiring the provision of citrus fruits to all sailors, which in turn led to virtual eradication of this disease. (see Figures 76-2 and 76-3)

In the latter part of the 19th century, continued systematic development of scientific rigor in proving the efficacy of interventions resulted in an explosion of effective preventative, diagnostic, and therapeutic interventions, which form

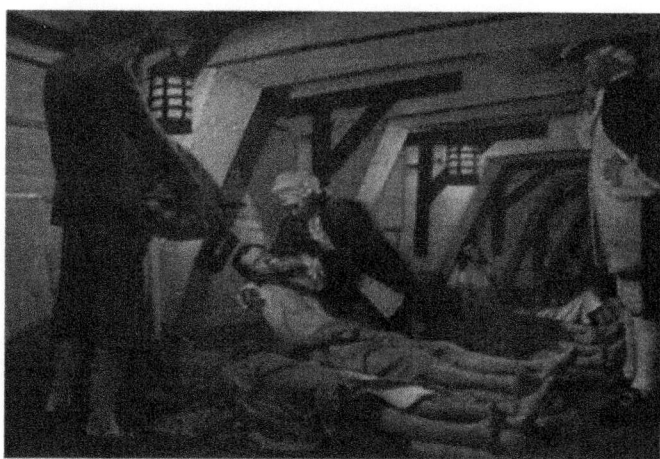

FIGURE 76-1 James Lind (1716–1794). Randomized control trial and the treatment of scurvy.

the basis for current medical practices and therapeutic interventions in Western societies at this time.

Practicing evidential (or evidence-based) medicine is the norm for physicians trained in the biomedical approach. It was the Evidence-Based Medicine Working Group at McMaster University in Canada who proposed a paradigm shift in health care called evidence-based medicine (EBM) (5,6). EBM is defined as the integration of best research evidence with clinical expertise and patient values (6). *Best research evidence* is the clinically relevant research from patient centered clinical research and/or from the basic sciences of medicine. Clinically relevant research includes clinical research into the accuracy and precision of procedural examinations or diagnostic tests, the power of prognostic markers, and the efficacy and safety or therapeutic, rehabilitative, and preventative regimens. *Clinical expertise* is the ability to use our clinical skills and past experiences to assess and identify each patient's unique health state and diagnosis, individual risks, and benefits of potential interventions as relates to their personal values and expectations. Finally, by *patient values* we refer to the unique preferences, concerns expectations each patient brings to a clinical encounter and which must be integrated into clinical decisions if they are to serve the patient (6). (see Figure 76-4)

EBM stresses the need for the clinician to examine the available information, or lack of information, from clinical

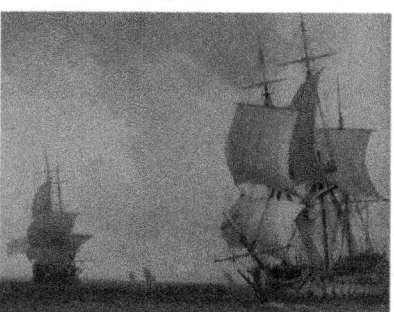

FIGURE 76-2 Ultimately, James Lind's experiment and treatise led to the virtual erradication of scurvy.

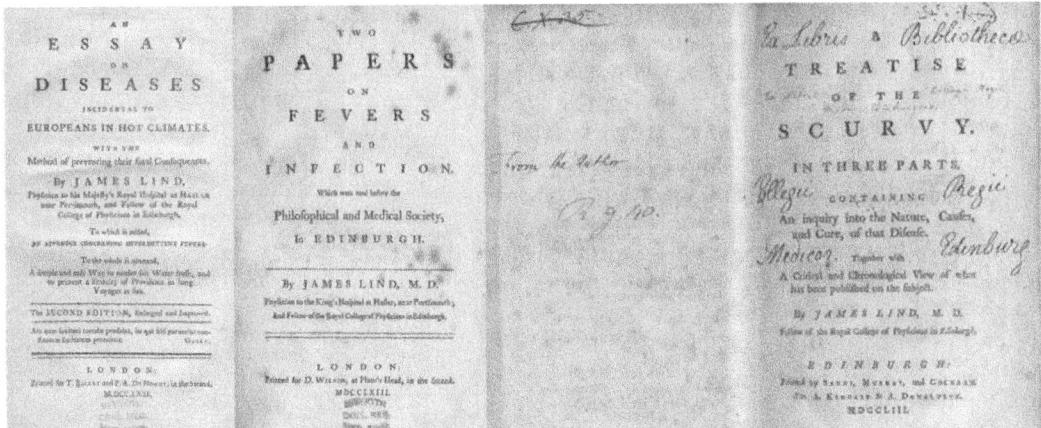

FIGURE 76-3 James Lind (1716–1794). Publications and treatise on scurvy.

research and to critically analyze the literature and incorporate the results of such analysis into clinical practice. Furthermore, with the expansion and development of research centers, internet access to libraries, and electronic databases, the evidence to support clinical diagnostic and therapeutic interventions is now more available than ever in real time to clinicians. The same principles of EBM is applicable to the use of CAM, and the expansion and availability of health sciences electronic databases and libraries has supported the access and availability of pertinent research on CAM in real time to clinicians. The development of research centers such as the National Center of Complementary Medicine in the United States along with the creation of electronic databases of systematic reviews of best evidence devoted to CAM interventions allows clinicians rapid access to current research and concise summaries and evaluations of the evidence to

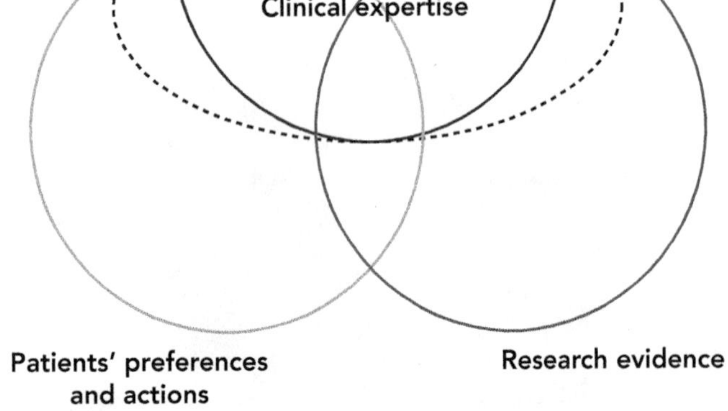

support the therapeutic and diagnostic practices of CAM. See Table 76-1 for electronic databases, which contain literature applicable to CAM.

The National Centre for Complementary and Alternative Medicine (NCCAM) is the federal government's lead agency for scientific research on CAM (7). The NCCAM is 1 of 27 institutes and centers that make up the National Institute of Health (NIH) within the US Department of Health and Human Services. The mission of the NCCAM is to explore complementary and alternative healing practices in the context rigorous research, train complementary and alternative medicine researchers, and disseminate authoritative information to the public and professionals. The division of intramural research within NCCAM has three main objectives: (*a*) Conduct clinical, translational, and basic research on the efficacy, safety, and mechanisms of action of diverse complementary and alternative modalities; (*b*) Facilitate the integration of effective CAM and conventional practices into interdisciplinary health care systems; and (*c*) Foster and develop research and training curricula about safe and effective CAM and conventional practices (7). In addition to the expansion of research related to CAM, libraries have also developed services and electronic access to CAM. For example, PubMed is a service of the National Library of Medicine (NLM) and CAM on PubMed was developed jointly by the NLM and NCCAM as a subset of the PubMed system.

Patient Preferences and Use of Complementary and Alternative Medicine in Western Societies

In December 2008, the NCCAM and the National Centre for Health Statistics released the findings of the 2007 National Health Interview Survey (NHIS), an annual in person health survey of Americans regarding their health- and illness-related experiences (8). The CAM section gathered information on 23,393 adults aged 18 years and older and 9,417 children aged 17 and younger. CAM therapies included in the 2007 NHIS are shown in Figure 76-5. In general, the NCCAM survey in 2007 noted an increase in CAM use by American adults from 36% in 2002 to 38.3% in 2007; the 2007 survey also identified that almost 12% of children in the

Clinical state and circumstances

Clinical expertise

Patients' preferences and actions

Research evidence

FIGURE 76-4 An updated model for evidence-based clinical decisions. Reprinted from *BMJ*. 2002;324(7350):1350.

TABLE 76-1 Evidence-Based Databases and Complementary and Alternative Medicine

- The Cochrane Library: http://www.cochrane.org/index0.htm
  - **CAM on PubMed:**
    Web site: www.ncbi.nim.nih.gov/sites/entrez
    Web site: www.ncbi.nim.nih.gov/sites/entreznccam.nih.gov/research/camonpubmed/
  - Cochrane Central Register of Controlled Trials: nccam.nih.gov/research/camonpubmed/
  - Cochrane Database of Systematic Reviews

  Published by Wiley InterScience with new and updated Cochrane Reviews every 3 months.
- ACP Journal Club: http://www.acpjc.org/
- PubMed:http://www.ncbi.nlm.nih.gov/entrez/query.fcgi (searchers can apply the limit ''Complementary Medicine'')[a]
- MD Consult-First Consult: http://www.mdconsult.com/offers/standard.html
- EMBASE: http://www.embase.com/
- Alt HealthWatch (via EBSCOhost): http://www.epnet.com/academic/althw.asp
  - MANTIS: http://www.healthindex.com/ MANTISDatabaseOverview.html
  - Natural Standard: http://www.naturalstandard.com/
- The TRIP Database: http://www.tripdatabase.com/
  - BMJ Clinical Evidence
- AMED—Allied and Complementary Medicine Database (produced by the Health Care Information Service of the British Library): http://www.bl.uk/collections/health/amed.html#net
- Herbs at a Glance http://nccam.nih.gov/research/results/spotlight/040310.htm[a]
  - Herbal database (an interactive, electronic herbal database—provides hyperlinked access to the scientific data underlying the use of herbs for health. Evidence-based information resource provided by the nonprofit Alternative Medicine Foundation, Inc.): http://www.herbmed.org/
- National Center for Complementary and Alternative Medicine
  - http://nccam.nih.gov/health
  - http://nccam.nih.gov/health/whatiscam

[a]Available without subscription

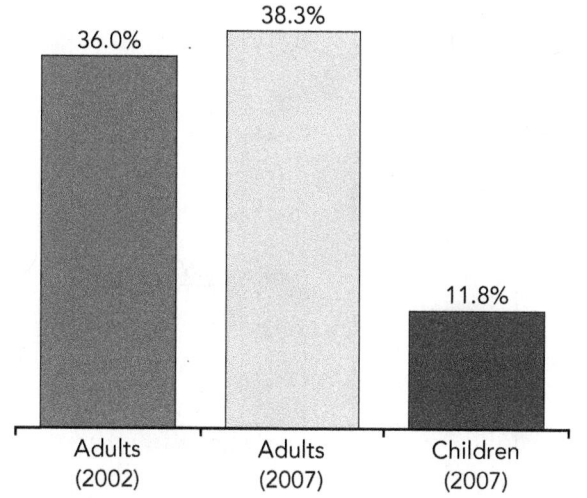

FIGURE 76-5 Complementary and alternative medicine use by US adults and children. Reprinted from *Natl Health Stat Report*. 2008;(12):1–23.

for which CAM interventions are sought out, however, CAM is also frequently used for treatment of anxiety, headaches, and insomnia. The 2007 survey also asked selected adult respondents about CAM use by their children (Figure 76-9). Most common therapies for children were natural products followed by osteopathic or chiropractic treatments. In the survey report, almost 24% of these children using CAM had 6 or more health conditions and a disturbing 17% of these families had delayed conventional care because of cost (9).

The remainder of this chapter will explore specific CAM practices in more detail, particularly with a view to gaining insights into some CAM practices currently in use, which may be relevant to brain injury (BI). We will use an EBM approach whenever possible to guide clinicians the evidence where available to support the potential benefit, no benefit, or indeed risk of some CAM practices for persons with BI.

United States use CAM (Figure 76-5). Figures 76-5–76-9 include data and information from the full 2007 NHIS on CAM use in the United States and the full 2007 NHIS report is available at http://nccam.nih.gov/news/camstats/2007/camsurveyfsl.htm (8).

In general, people of all ages (Figure 76-5) and backgrounds use CAM (Figure 76-6), however, CAM use is more prevalent among women and those with higher education and income. Nonvitamin, nonmineral natural products are the most commonly used CAM therapy among adults, followed by deep breathing, meditation, chiropractic and osteopathic, massage, yoga, diet-based therapy, progressive relaxation, guided imagery, and homeopathic treatment (Figure 76-7). The disease and conditions as identified by the NHIS for which CAM is used by adults and children in the United States is noted in Figure 76-8 and 76-9, respectively. Diseases and conditions for which CAM was most frequently used among adults are noted in Figure 76-8. Back pain and musculoskeletal conditions are the most frequent conditions

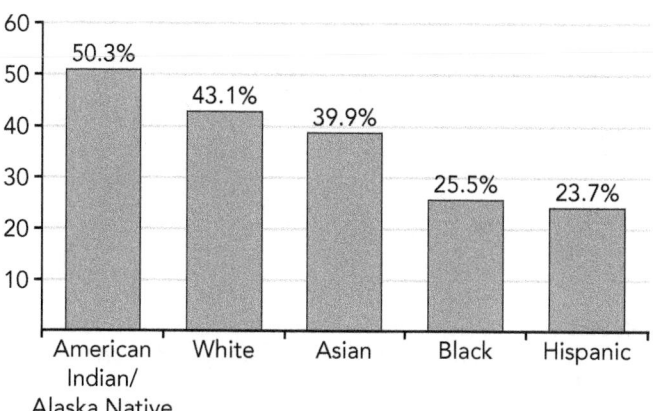

FIGURE 76-6 Complementary and alternative medicine use by race or ethnicity among adults–2007. Reprinted from *Natl Health Stat Report*. 2008;(12):1–23.

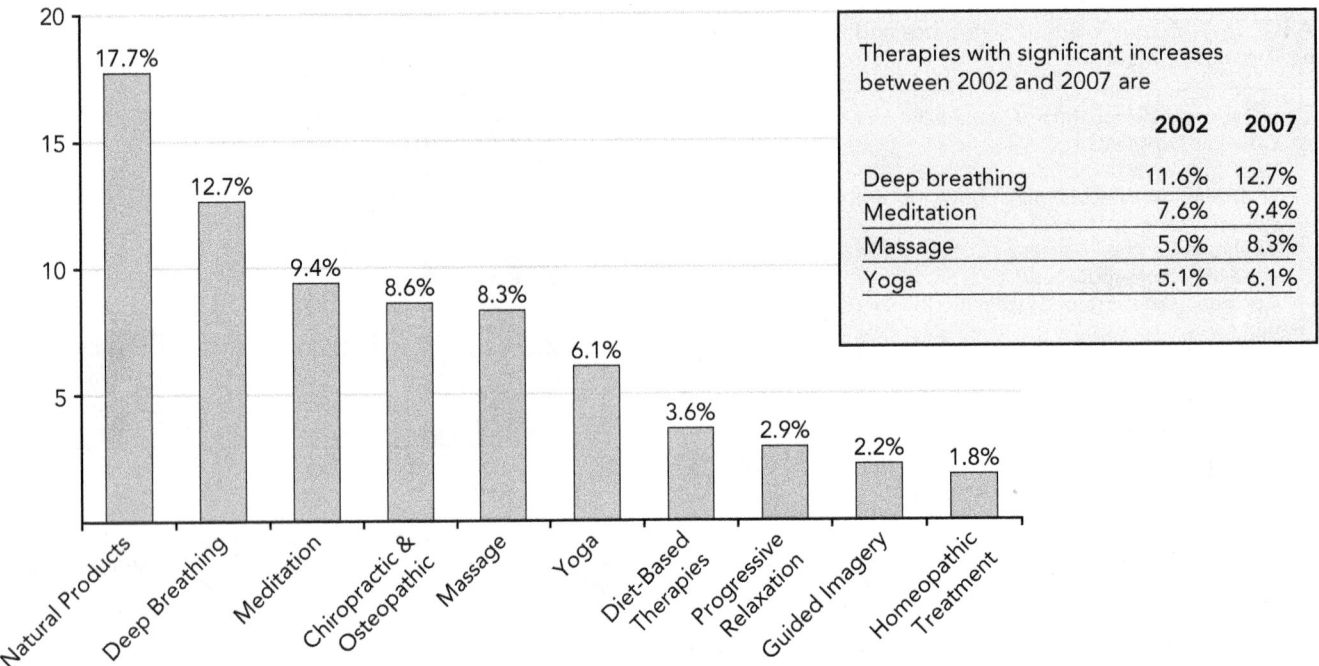

Therapies with significant increases between 2002 and 2007 are		
	2002	**2007**
Deep breathing	11.6%	12.7%
Meditation	7.6%	9.4%
Massage	5.0%	8.3%
Yoga	5.1%	6.1%

FIGURE 76-7 Ten most common complementary and alternative medicine therapies among adults–2007. Reprinted from *Natl Health Stat Report.* 2008;(12):1–23.

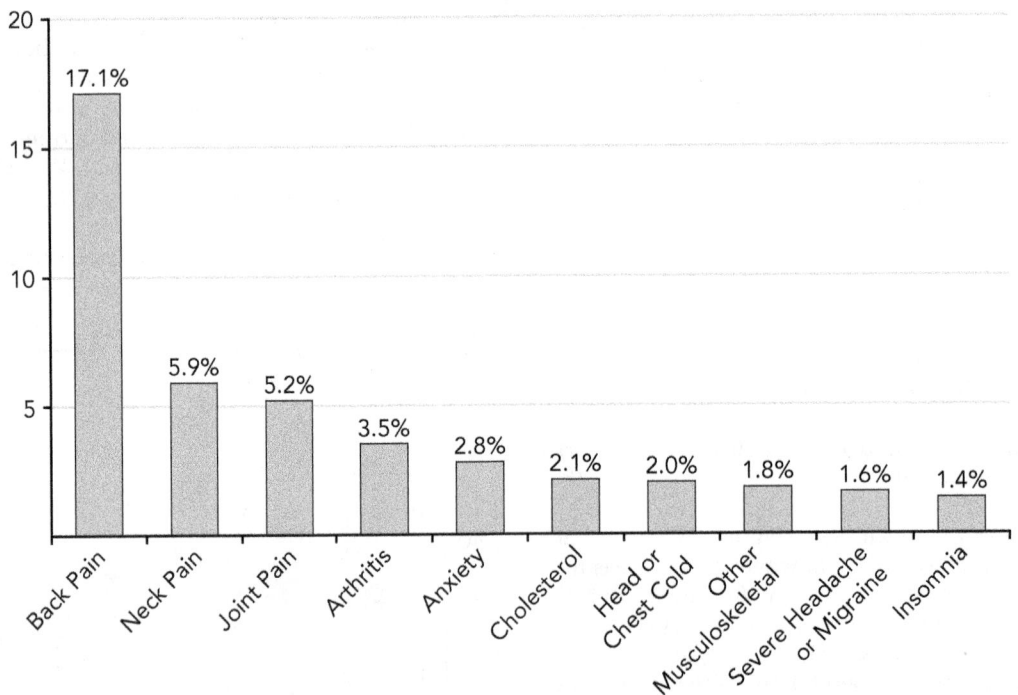

FIGURE 76-8 Diseases and conditions for which complementary and alternative medicine is most frequently used among adults–2007. Reprinted from *Natl Health Stat Report.* 2008;(12):1–23.

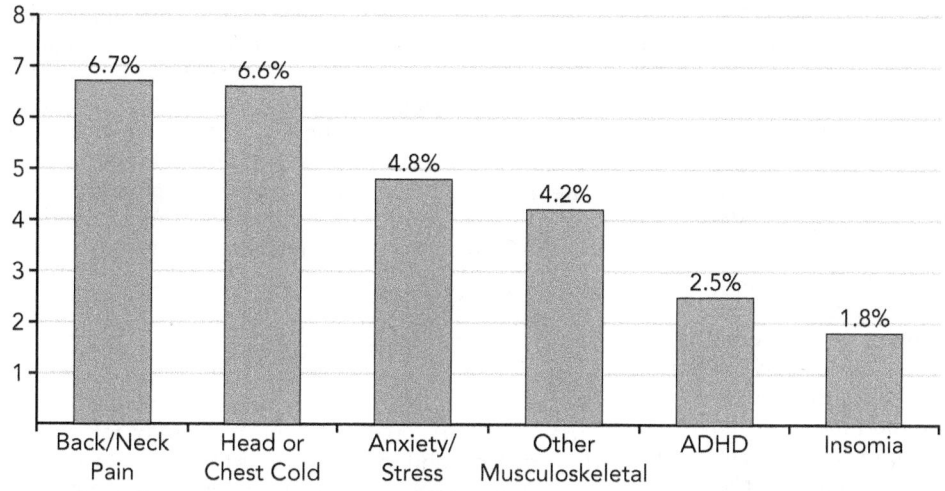

FIGURE 76-9 Diseases and conditions for which complementary and alternative medicine is most frequently used among children—2007. Reprinted from *Natl Health Stat Report*. 2008; (12):1–23.

NATURAL PRODUCTS

Herbal Medicines

In the 2007 NHIS, natural products were the most commonly sought CAM intervention and 17.7% of American adults had used a nonvitamin or nonmineral natural product (Figure 76-7). Herbal medicines may be the most lucrative form of traditional medicine, generating billions of dollars in revenue in the international market. In China, for example, the WHO reports sales of products totaled $14 billion in 2005 and in Western Europe sales reached $5 billion in 2003–2004. Herbal medicines include herbs, herbal materials, and herbal preparations that contain plants or other plant materials as active ingredients. The scientific evidence to support the quality, safety, and effectiveness of traditional medicine products is limited; many people may believe that because traditional medicines are herbal (natural)—they are safe. However, to the contrary, herbal and natural products can be unsafe and cause harmful and adverse reactions especially if the product is of poor quality and/or if taken with other medicines. Unfortunately, counterfeit, poor quality, or adulterated products in international markets can present a serious patient safety threat; very few countries have national policies for regulating traditional medicine products because regulation remains very difficult (1). The US Food and Drug Administration (FDA) regulates herbal and other dietary supplements differently from conventional medicines. The standards that apply to prescription and over-the-counter medications in the United States do not apply to supplements (9). The standards for supplements are found in the Dietary Supplement Health and Education Act (DSHEA), a federal law that defines and sets standards for product labeling and health claim limits. More information can be obtained regarding the DSHEA at the FDA Web site (10).

Herbal medicines have been used in traditional medical practices for thousands of years to treat or improve the human condition, and a large proportion of the world population relies on traditional medicines for their primary care. The use of natural or herbal products or Zhong Yao has been an integral part of Chinese culture for more than 1,600 years. The source of the Chinese materia medica includes plants, minerals, and animal parts. Classic Chinese herbal medicine uses a combination of various herbs in a formula. The earliest documented herbal formula can be traced back to the end of the third century BC when approximately 280 formulas for 52 different ailments were recorded in the Ma Wang Tui tomb manuscript. By the time of the Ming dynasty (1368–1644), more than 60,000 formulas had been recorded in the 1406 book of *Formulas of Universal Benefit (Pu Ji Fang)* (11). In Europe, by the Middle Ages, thousands of botanical products had been inventoried for their medicinal effects. The interest and current use of herbal or natural products continues to expand worldwide, and the WHO is concerned that the expanding herbal product market could drive overharvesting of wild plant populations and threaten biodiversity; there is, therefore, a recognized need to preserve both plant populations and the knowledge from traditional practices regarding how to use them. The scientific evidence to support the use of herbal or natural products is very limited; however, with the development and expansion of research centers specifically focused on CAM interventions, the evidence to support or refute the use of herbal products is growing. For example, chamomile, a herbal plant within the daisy family, has been widely used for thousands of years in a variety of conditions including insomnia, anxiety, and digestive disturbances such as upset stomach and diarrhea. One double-blind, placebo-controlled trial at the University of Pennsylvania funded through the NCCAM included a study on the effectiveness of chamomile (*Matricaria recutita*—German chamomile) on Generalized Anxiety Disorder (GAD) (12). For 8 weeks, 57 participants diagnosed with GAD were given either chamomile capsules containing 220 mg of pharmaceutical-grade extract from German chamomile, standardized to 1.2% of the constituent apigenin or chamomile-scented placebo capsules containing lactose. Dosages were increased incrementally based on the Hamilton Anxiety Rating (HAM-A) scores. Compared to placebo, chamomile was associated with a greater reduction in mean HAM-A scores and the difference was clinically meaningful and statistically significant. Chamomile was well tolerated by participants. Because this was the first RCT of chamomile extract for the use of anxiety, the authors note that additional studies using larger subject populations will be necessary. That said, this preliminary study seems to indicate that chamomile may have modest benefits for some people with mild to moderate GAD (12).

The NCCAM and the NIH have published a guideline for the public that includes an inventory of commonly used herbs and supplements in the United States. The guide *"Herbs at a Glance: A Quick Guide to Herbs and Supplements"* provides an outline of the use of the herbal product from a historical or traditional medicine perspective, the condition it treats, and precautions and risks (13). In this guideline, there is no category specific for BI; however, several herbal products are listed for the treatment of some common symptoms encountered in patients with BI including headaches, mental alertness, memory enhancement, tinnitus, insomnia, cognitive decline, anxiety, and depression. The NCCAM stresses that the index list is *not* an endorsement of the product. In addition to providing a basic understanding of some of the most common herbs and dietary supplements, their historical use and what they are used for now, side effects, and cautions, the guideline provides the public with an outline of the literature on scientific evidence available on the effectiveness of herbal remedies, including studies funded by NCCAM.

Homeopathy

Homeopathy is a 200-year-old therapeutic system that uses small doses of various substances to stimulate self-regulating and self-healing processes (13). Of the nearly 2.5 million patients using CAM in the United States in 1997, approximately 3.4% of patients used homeopathy and 0.7% used naturopathy (14). Homeopathy remains one of the most controversial CAM practices. *Similia similibus curentur* or treating "like with like" is the basis of homeopathy. Homeopathists believe that patients complaining of particular symptoms can be cured with substances that can produce the same symptoms in healthy individuals. In addition to matching the symptoms of the disease, a homeopathist will select remedies based on the constitutional factors of the individual patient such as the patients' psychological state, environmental reactions, and habitus. Of the large number of homeopathic medicines that have been described, approximately 200 are in regular use (15), about 60% of which are of plant origin. Animal products, minerals, chemical salts, and disease products also may be used. Homeopathists believe that remedies retain biological activity if they are serially diluted and agitated between each dilution. The dilution most frequently used is designated "6c," which is a 10^{-12} dilution of the original "mother tincture." It is likely that a 6c dilution will contain a few molecules of the initial substance. These dilutions are said to produce effects even when diluted beyond Avogadro number, at which point no original molecules of the starting substance remain. Many scientists believe that homeopathy violates natural laws and thus any effect must be a placebo effect (16). However, because of the high dilution, homeopathy appears to be very safe, which is an important motivating factor amongst its adherents.

The public's belief in the effectiveness of homoeopathy is widespread (17). In the United States, patients who seek homeopathic care are more affluent and younger (18). As with other diseases and syndromes, the effectiveness of homeopathy for BI is quite questionable and controversial. A small pilot research study suggested that homeopathy is efficacious for certain symptoms related to BI such as headache (19). There is, however, insufficient evidence to show that homoeopathy is clearly efficacious for any single clinical condition. Reviews on homeopathic clinical trials have found that most available studies have reported some positive results but the evidence is not convincing (20,21).

Naturopathy

There is no concise history of naturopathic medicine; the development of naturopathy has been strongly influenced by various cultures and religions and is therefore not a single discipline. Naturopathy and conventional medicine hold certain principles in common. Both emphasize disease prevention, patient education, seeking and treating the causes of disease, and both employ the therapeutic potential of the doctor–patient relationship. The basic principle of naturopathy dictates that nature acts powerfully through healing mechanisms in the body and mind to maintain and restore health. Naturopaths work to restore and support these inherent healing systems using noninvasive treatments believed to be in harmony with natural processes such as lifestyle modifications, nutrition, dietetics, herbs, education, and hydrotherapy. In addition, naturopaths may elect to use a variety of healing modalities including acupuncture, botanicals, homeopathy, massage, oriental medicine, and minor surgery (22). In general, naturopaths function as primary care providers with emphasis on prevention, education, and health maintenance (19,22). It is vital that conventional medical practices be incorporated into naturopathy where treatment that has been proven to be effective is available. For example, if a BI patient develops progressive hydrocephalus, a neurosurgical procedure may be appropriate to prevent further neural damage and facilitate functional recovery. It would not be appropriate to overemphasize natural healing and natural treatment modalities in such situations.

Most of the modalities applied by naturopathy are relatively safe; however, they are not without any risks (16,23). Naturopathy recommends administering vitamins and herbal medicines widely, even though more clinical trials are necessary to obtain evidence supporting their efficacy. For example, vitamins A, C, and E are considered necessary for protecting tissue from free-radical damage and are commonly used by naturopaths, however, there is not enough scientific data supporting their necessity in addition to what is consumed in a normal diet (16). Only a small fraction of the thousands of medicinal plants used worldwide have been tested rigorously in RCTs (24). Several clinical trials have shown that some herbal or natural medicines may have efficacy in BI-related symptoms, for instance, use of hypericum perforatum (St. John's Wort) for depression is supported by a significant amount of evidence (25–27). Results of RCTs also support the use of kava for anxiety and valerian root or melatonin for insomnia (28–31). Although evidence for the use of vitamins and amino acids as sole agents for BI-related neuropsychological symptoms is not strong, there is intriguing preliminary evidence for the use of folate, tryptophan, and phenylalanine as adjuncts to enhance the effectiveness of conventional antidepressants (28–31). Another product, S-adenosylmethionine, seems to have some antidepressant effects, whereas omega-3 polyunsaturated fatty acids, particularly docosahexaenoic acid, may have mood-stabilizing effects (32). It is important to note that scientific evidence is still lacking to support that natural methods serve any therapeutic purpose in a fashion that would be superior to conventional management. Potential side effects and drug–drug interactions should be considered when using naturopathy (27,33).

In summary, persons with BI who seek alternative medical management may do so because the available standard pharmacological treatments are not effective for their symptoms, however, the evidence on the effectiveness of homeopathy for post-BI patient is scant. Rehabilitation physicians should ask their BI patients about the "natural products" they take and discuss their use and potential risk, benefit, and nonbenefit if any in a frank and nonjudgmental manner; this will provide patients with the most up-to-date information and support informed choices.

Aromatherapy

Aromatherapy is the therapeutic use of aroma-producing oils (essential oils) extracted from organic materials (flowers, leaves, stalks, bark, rind, or roots) and used, typically, for relaxation. The oils are mixed with another substance such as an alcohol, oil, or a lotion and are then applied to the skin, sprayed in the air, or inhaled. The oils can also be poured into a soaking bath to derive the therapeutic effect. Originating in Europe in the early 1900s, the philosophy behind aromatherapy is that specific plant oils produce aromas and fragrances that stimulate or relax the body by acting on certain areas within the brain. Fragrances stimulate nasal nerves, which then send impulses to the areas of the brain controlling memory and emotion. The oils themselves are thought to interact with the body's own naturally occurring hormones and enzymes to cause changes to autonomically mediated reflexes including blood pressure and pulse. Theory suggests that a fragrance stimulates glands to produce analgesic substances, perhaps prostaglandin-stimulating substances, effecting relaxation and/or pain relief. Practitioners use essential oils to treat physical conditions including inflammation and infection. Aromatherapy is used to treat mental health conditions including anxiety, depression, and insomnia. Individuals with asthma, respiratory allergies, chronic lung disease, or certain skin allergies should use care participating in aromatherapy. Aromatherapy should be avoided in children younger than the age of 5 years because their immune systems are not yet fully competent.

Energy-Based Therapies

Bi-Aura Therapy

Bi-aura therapy is an energy-based therapy that works to seek out and remove energy blockages from within the body and from within the body's energy field (aura or biofield). Eastern medicine has long recognized the known energy and energy flow from the body, also known as Chi, Qi, and Prana. Bi-aura therapy is a therapy in which a practitioner, mostly through non-touch bi-aura techniques, removes imbalances in the body's energy field. These imbalances can occur from trauma, physical and emotional distress, and from physical illness. Bi-aura therapy seeks to locate energy imbalances, address them, and allow the body to return to health. Bi-aura therapy can also function to help balance the mental and emotional state of the individual by clearing these biofield blockages and restoring health.

Light Therapy

Light therapy, known also as phototherapy, involves the exposure to bright, non-full spectrum light. White light is considered preferable over narrow-band wavelengths or ultraviolet light, both of which have been demonstrated to be toxic to skin and internal organs. It is believed that light therapy has an antidepressant effect, that it may help balance certain brain chemicals, and that it may help reset proper circadian rhythms within the brain. Light therapy of 2,500–10,000 lux is generally considered safe and is considered one of the first lines of therapy for seasonal affective depression (SAD)—a transient affective disorder affecting many during the cold and shortened daylight periods found in more Northern latitudes in the winter. The side effects of light therapy include visual disturbances, eyestrain, headaches, or skin irritation (34–36).

Healing Touch Therapy

Healing touch therapy is an energy-based therapeutic approach to healing. Healing touch is viewed as influencing the energy system that is life itself. By assessing and treating the energy system, the practitioner helps the patient to self-heal. Healing touch begins with the thought that people are naturally healthy, and that physical and emotional stress disturbs the natural energy, thereby causing illness. The goal in healing touch is to restore wholeness through harmony and balance through the "centered heart." It is noninvasive and economical (38). Healing touch is not considered appropriate or safe for acute life-threatening situations.

Reflexology

Reflexology is a type of energy-based therapy that predates the discovery of the new world. Reflexology presumes that there are specific areas in the hands and the feet—reflex points—that correlate to analogous organ systems in the body. Manipulation of these reflex points is believed to promote mental and physical relaxation—relaxation that then promotes healing. Reflexology is used to treat 1 of 9 principle systems, each representing a major organ system, thereby aligning the harmony of the body.

Reiki

Reiki is an ancient healing method that uses a hands-on approach to manipulate energy flow throughout the body. Reiki means "universal life energy," and practitioners believe that there is an energy force in and around one's body, flowing between the person performing Reiki and the receiver of the treatment. It is thought that Reiki releases your own energy flow and allows your body's own natural healing ability to work. It is completely noninvasive; the Reiki practitioner will put his or her hands over the body of the recipient at one of the main energy centers called chakras. Reiki is occasionally used to assist sufferers with chronic pain.

MIND-BODY MEDICINE

Meditation

Meditation is the third most commonly used CAM practice in the NCCAM; 9.4% of adults surveyed reported using meditation (8). Meditation involves focusing one's attention on the present moment. The practice is often aided by assumption of specific postures, breathing techniques, and focusing on a specific object or phrase. Meditation is a complex mental process involving changes in cognition, sensory perception, affect, hormones, and autonomic activity (38). The health benefits of meditation have been recognized in Eastern philosophies for thousands of years with meditation now also widely practiced in the West. There are 2 meditation techniques most commonly used: concentrative and mindful. In concentrative meditation, one focuses on a single image, sound, mantra (words spoken or sung in a pattern), or one's own breathing. Mindful meditation does not focus on a single purpose; rather, one is aware of all thoughts, feelings, sounds, or images that pass through one's mind. Meditation is used to help treat a wide range of physical and mental problems, including addictive behaviors; immune system diseases; anxiety, stress, or depression; high cholesterol and high blood pressure; and pain. There are no believed negative side effects or medical complications of meditation when combined with conventional medical treatment. Meditation alone is not considered appropriate or safe for acute or life-threatening situations.

Ospina et al in 2007 (39) reviewed and synthesized the state of research on a variety of meditation practices. The authors included in their review the specific meditation practice examined, the research designs employed, the conditions and outcomes examined, the efficiency and effectiveness of different meditation practices for the 3 most common studied conditions, the role of modifiers and outcomes, and the effects of medication on physiological and neuropsychological outcomes. Five broad categories of meditation practices were identified (mantra meditation, mindfulness meditation, yoga, Tai Chi, and Qigong). Meta-analyses of results from 55 studies indicated that some meditation practices produced significant changes in healthy participants. The 3 most studied conditions were hypertension, other cardiovascular diseases, and substance abuse. Sixty-five intervention studies examined the therapeutic effect of meditation practices for these conditions. Meta-analyses based on low-quality studies and small numbers of hypertensive participants showed that TM(R), Qigong, and Zen Buddhist meditation significantly reduced blood pressure. Yoga helped reduce stress. Yoga was no better than mindfulness-based stress reduction at reducing anxiety in patients with cardiovascular diseases. The authors concluded that many uncertainties surround the practice of meditation. Scientific research on meditation practices did not appear to have a common theoretical perspective and was characterized by poor methodological quality. Unfortunately, firm conclusions on the effects of meditation practices in health care

could not be drawn based on the available evidence. In addition, future research on meditation practices must be more rigorous in the design and execution of studies and in the analysis and reporting of results (39).

Relaxation Techniques

Guided Imagery

Guided imagery is a relaxation technique where a series of thoughts or suggestions direct a person's imagination toward a relaxed and focused state. An instructor, in person or on recorded media, guides the individual through the process of imagery. Guided imagery is based on the concept that one's mind and body share a unique connection. Using the special senses, one's body seems to respond as though what one is imagining is indeed occurring. A relaxed state may be achieved when it is imagined in full detail. Guided imagery is especially useful in promoting relaxation. This relaxed state can lower blood pressure, reduce other stress-related problems, and enables one to reach other goals. Guided imagery is helpful in preparing for athletic events and for performance enhancement, including learning, weight loss, smoking cessation, and in pain management. Guided imagery is safe, with no known associated risks, and it can be performed in any circumstance where improved performance is desired.

Autogenic Training

Autogenic training is a relaxation technique that teaches your body to respond to your own verbal commands. Using certain commands, a practitioner of autogenic training is able to tell their own body to relax, thus controlling breathing, blood pressure, heart rate, and temperature. Autogenic training consists of 6 standard exercises. Each exercise has the individual assuming a simple posture, concentrating without goal, and then using visual imagery and verbal cuing to promote relaxation of the body in a specific way. The ultimate goal of autogenic training is to allow the individual to achieve a deep relaxation and stress reduction, the mechanism of action is not fully understood, but the effects on the body are measurable. Experts believe that autogenic training works similarly to hypnosis or self-hypnosis or biofeedback. Helpful with problems like generalized anxiety, fatigue, and irritability, some use autogenic training to manage pain, reduce sleep disorders, or increase their resistance to stress. Autogenic training has shown some effectiveness in addressing hyperventilation, asthma, gastrointestinal disorders, cardiovascular irregularities, autonomic dysfunction, headaches, and endocrine disorders. Some individuals have noticed a sharp change in their blood pressure when practicing autogenic training exercises; therefore, it is recommended that individuals with hypotension or hypertension have their physician's approval prior to participating in autogenic training. Autogenic training is not recommended for children younger than the age of 5 or in individuals with severe mental or emotional disorders (40).

Humor Therapy

Humor therapy, also known as therapeutic humor, is a relaxation method that uses the power of smile and laughter to help heal. Therapeutic humor or humor therapy simply means finding ways to make others or yourself smile and laugh more often. Laughter appears to actually change the brain chemistry, and it is thought to boost the immune system as well. Humor allows people to feel in greater control of their situations, can provide special perspective on problems, can allow the release of fear and anger, and it can reduce stress. Commonly, humor is used in the treatment of long-term and chronic diseases, especially those worsened by stress. Humor therapy is valuable as well as a preventative measure aiding the care partners of people with chronic illness or disease because they are at high risk of becoming ill themselves.

Music Therapy

Music therapy is a relaxation therapy used to promote physical and emotional healing and wellness. Generally, a trained and certified music therapist is able to offer therapy in a school, health care facility, hospice, mental health facility, or private practice setting. Sessions of therapy can involve passive listening, active music-making, or both. The rhythm and tone of music can stimulate or sedate; has positive effects on heart rate, oxygen saturation, blood pressure, and cognitive ability; and is a healthy, nonverbal mode of self-expression. It is socially connective and expressive, and it enhances verbal expression, fluency, and communication with self and with others. Sometimes music therapy, combined with movement therapy, such as dance, is used as a combined therapy. There are no known risks to music therapy; more information can be obtained by visiting the American Music Therapy Association website at www.music therapy.org (41).

Spiritual Healing

Many individuals respond to illness and impairment by turning to prayer and requests for spiritual healing. Traumatic brain injury (TBI) often occurs at a young age, and the consequences can be devastating for the patient and their family and social support network. Maintaining hope in spite of these challenges may be helpful to people. Prayer has been a traditional means of keeping a positive, constructive outlook in the face of despair. Prayer has an extensive literature that was reviewed in Larry Dossey's book *Healing Words* (42). In this book, the author demonstrates the positive effect of prayerful intention on health across several clinical conditions. He notes that prayer is both nonlocal and not bound by time. Effective prayer may cross great distances or incredible boundaries. The time of prayer may be unrelated to the time of its need by the individual receiving prayer.

In a review of more than 1,200 articles from the 20th century evaluating the association between religion and health, Harold Koenig found that most of them showed a positive association (43). Medical literature suggests that patients do want to discuss how their spirituality and beliefs play a role in the recovery from illness and relief from impairment (44). Koenig also wrote about spirituality and religion as a practical part of patient care (45). Three simple questionnaires discussed and in use today are the FICA spiritual assessment tool (46), the health outcome prevention evaluation (HOPE) questionnaire (47), and the ACP Spiritual History (48). These tools can be used as part of the psychosocial history during patient interviews. Collecting this information serves as a means to let the patient know that their beliefs are valued and may strengthen the therapeutic relationship between the clinician and the patient. If the patient desires, the information is used to refer the patient to the hospital chaplain, a pastoral counselor, a clergy, or another person within his or her spiritual or religious community.

The shaman, or community medicine man, probably represents the oldest spiritual healing tradition, dating back to prehistoric times. Historically, the shaman represents a cross-cultural approach to the diagnosis and treatment of illness. This has traditionally been a culturally bound practice. Western contemporary shamanic practitioners may practice without a culturally bound approach.

Alternative Movement Therapies

Alexander and Feldenkrais

The Alexander technique and Feldenkrais method are 2 popular contemporary movement therapies used by individuals with BI. Both techniques are active treatment programs usually learned from a certified practitioner and performed by the patient. Both focus on awareness of movement and the person's inner emotional state associated with it. Frederic Matthias Alexander was a 19th century actor who lost his voice and developed his technique in response to observing how his uncoordinated movements and posture led to his voice loss. Alexander therapy consists of evaluating how common functional activities such as sitting, standing, and walking have muscular tension associated with them and then learning how to avoid triggering the muscular tension with the old pattern of movement. Attention initially focuses the individual's inner sense of movement and then progresses to shifting that sense to discover the release of tension with awareness of proper posture. By inhibiting those postural elements leading to tension, the participant is able to recover greater fluidity of movement. No references were identified in a review of the medical literature specific to the application of Alexander technique to BI survivors. A randomized controlled clinical trial compared the Alexander technique, massage, and no intervention on disability, depression, and attitude toward self for patients with Parkinson disease (PD) (49). The study showed statistically significant improvement in all 3 categories only in those patients treated with the Alexander technique.

Moshe Feldenkrais, a physicist, initially developed the Feldenkrais method based on his personal experience with severe knee injury. The therapy has evolved to a series of mat exercises and some touch-guided movement that together raise the awareness of the patient to their own movement patterns. Unlike traditional physical therapy techniques that desire a specific movement pattern as the outcome and train the patient toward the desired pattern, Feldenkrais's method seeks to support change through the deepest inner sense of the client's actual movement. A review of the medical literature did not provide any references specific to the application of the Feldenkrais method to BI survivors. Both the Alexander technique and the Feldenkrais method use awareness-based learning rather than repetitive physical exercise. They seek to produce more fluid movement and more choices in movement with greater conscious awareness of the potential outcomes for chosen movement patterns. Patients with TBI using these therapies may report a greater sense of comfort during activity, more solidity in their standing and walking, and fewer complaints related to their neurologic compromise such as vestibular hyperreactivity and paresis. Based on the types of interventions and exercises applied, the mechanism could be postulated to result from greater body awareness of posture and movement. Through this awareness, the individual may inhibit muscular tension, poor posture, and gait abnormalities.

Tai Chi or Qigong

Tai Chi roughly translates as "great energy," it is recognized as both a healing art and martial arts discipline. Qigong means "energy work," it is characterized by generally slower movements and is considered easier to perform. Although both disciplines incorporate smooth, balanced movement with mindfulness, the specific focus of Qigong is on mindfulness and physical health. Specific "forms" are intended to promote the smooth flow of Qi along certain meridians and/ or (particularly with respect to Qigong) for the purpose of nourishing certain organs or organ qualities. Both practices are used in healthy populations to maintain balance, strength and flexibility, and in selected medical populations to restore impaired function. The present state-of-the-art pertaining to use of Tai Chi in TBI includes the following limited medical evidence: Shapira (50) and colleagues undertook a case series study at the Hadassah University Hospital in Jerusalem. They enrolled three subjects with severe TBI, all ambulatory, but with significantly impaired balance. Subjects were taught Tai Chi movements in a gradual progression from sitting to standing to movement. Training took place over 2–4 years. By study completion, all subjects were ambulating without assistance. Gemmell and Leatham (New Zealand) (51) published a case series with the "waiting list" group used as controls—the subjects were 18 participants with TBI (mild to severe), average of 8.7 years postinjury. The experimental group underwent a 6-week biweekly Tai Chi course. Investigators measured SF-36 (a life satisfaction scale), self-esteem, and eight mood states (via visual analog scales). They found improvement in mood and presession vs postsession anger scores decreased. No long-term carryover effect was noted, however. Blake and Batson (52) published a pilot randomized case or control study; 20 subjects with TBI (mild to severe) were randomized: 10 to the exercise group and 10 to the control group. Subjects in the exercise group underwent an 8-week course of Qigong. The exercise group showed improved mood and self-esteem postintervention. Although this limited published data is not conclusive, it does suggest that Qigong may be beneficial in addressing aspects of balance and motor impairment post-TBI.

Massage Therapy

Massage therapy comprises many varied forms from light touch to very deep massage. Like other consumers of massage therapy, individuals with BI seek relief of pain and musculoskeletal symptoms using massage. Massage therapy has been successfully used in several post-traumatic pain syndromes as well as chronic pain syndromes for patients both with and without BI. For example, massage therapy is often used by physical therapists for treatment of myofascial pain syndrome in conjunction with trigger point injections and stretching (53). In a survey of individuals with neck or back pain, 14% chose to use massage; 65% found it "very helpful," whereas 27% of those receiving conventional care found it to help (54). Massage has been applied to temporomandibular joint dysfunction (TMD). In a survey of CAM use by individuals with TMD, CAM with massage was the most frequently used, the most satisfactory, and the most helpful (55).

The literature specific to TBI is less substantial. Posttraumatic headache has been shown to respond to cervical massage more so than to cold packs in 1 prospective controlled study (56). A case report successfully used massage therapy for hypersexuality after TBI (57). In other patient populations, massage produces relaxation, decreases anxiety, and decreases pain (58). One mechanism of action that could account for better pain control, decreased anxiety, and the induction of relaxation could be increased parasympathetic activity. Parasympathetic activity can be assessed by analysis of heart rate variability. The respiratory sinus arrhythmia (the mild acceleration and deceleration of heart rate associated with breathing) has a parasympathetic component that can be isolated through analysis of heart rate variability. An RCT evaluating the short-term autonomic effects of massage to the back, neck, and shoulders on 30 healthy individuals noted significantly decreased systolic blood pressure and increased parasympathetic activity (59). Other possible mechanisms producing beneficial effects could be soft tissue mobilization with passive stretching, stimulation of circulation to remove accumulated metabolic products in chronically tense muscles, and the effect of touch itself.

In summary, the general literature supports the use of massage to reduce pain and anxiety in patients with post-traumatic pain syndromes such as neck and back pain, temporomandibular dysfunction, and myofascial pain syndrome. There is scant literature supporting its usefulness in other neurologic conditions. Massage also forms an adjunct to other therapeutic interventions provided by physical therapists, occupational therapists, massage therapists, and nonconventional body workers. The literature specific to BI is sparse, but for musculoskeletal post-traumatic pain syndromes, the demonstrated benefits of the use of massage may be generalized to brain-injured individuals.

Craniosacral Manipulation

William Garner Sutherland, DO, devised craniosacral manipulation, also known as osteopathy in the cranial field in 1939 (60). Practitioners palpate subtle movements of the cranial vault and other structures to assess the cranial rhythmic impulse and to prompt its balancing. From the standpoint of osteopathic philosophy, return of wholeness to the person is the ultimate goal of this therapy. The physiologic effects of this therapy have yet to be clearly elucidated in the medical literature.

Individuals using craniosacral therapy typically seek relief from pain and functional problems such as balance deficits. There is very limited medical literature on craniosacral therapy and only 1 study of craniosacral therapy for BI. Most of the studies look at interrater reliability and reproducibility as well as documenting an abnormal cranial rhythm (61,62).

Greenman et al. (63) studied the cranial rhythmic impulse in 55 patients with TBI as part of their assessment and treatment within an outpatient rehabilitation program. The author notes that cranial osteopathy has been empirically shown to be effective in the treatment of patients with TBI. The study documents that the cranial impulse is slower than is typically encountered with cranial strain patterns noted in 97% of the patients. Three of the patients (5%) seized during treatment. Other unlikely adverse reactions reported include mild headache, exacerbation of vertigo, and visceral symptoms. Because of this seizure risk and adverse reactions, consideration of the practitioner of the risk benefits and no benefit should include a fully informed patient and consent and preparedness for these events.

Both positive outcomes and adverse side effects suggest that cranial osteopathy affects the autonomic nervous system. Patients who have participated in this treatment commonly report profound relaxation, suggesting a parasympathetic activation. This was evaluated by Robbins (64) in a randomized controlled study of 6 normal individuals. Each subject underwent 4 interventions. The active treatments were cranial osteopathy on the head and on the sacrum. The control treatments were no touch and light touch to different areas of the body. The order of treatment and controls was randomized and each subject underwent the whole protocol twice with washout periods between interventions. Cranial therapy at the head, as opposed to treatment at the sacrum, produced significantly higher parasympathetic activity than no touch or light touch.

In conclusion, despite patient reports of osteopathic cranial therapy and its variations having effectiveness in post-traumatic headache, anxiety, and balance deficits, the paucity and quality of research on craniosacral therapy as reviewed by (65) Green do not support its effectiveness.

Acupuncture

Basic Principles

From a Chinese medicine perspective, the human body is viewed as a microcosmic reflection of the universe. The physician's role is to maintain the body's harmonious balance, both internally and in relation to the external environment. Vital energy, known as Qi, flows through meridians (a multilayered, interconnecting network of channels or energy pathways that establish an interface between an individual's internal and external environments), creating an interwoven network of circulation. These energy pathways are named for organs whose realms of influence are expanded from their conventional biomedical physiology to include functional, energetic, and metaphorical qualities. Pathology involves disharmony or disruption of energy flow (66).

Diagnosis in Chinese Medicine

Diagnostic systems are based on descriptors of natural phenomena. Two of the most frequently used systems involve the interrelationship of yin and yang and the 5-phase system.

The relationship of yin and yang to each other consists of four basic qualities (67):

1. Opposite stages: yin represents the material aspect of an entity; yang represents the immaterial or rarefied aspect. For example, yin = water, yang = steam.

2. Interdependent: yin and yang can be understood only in relation to one another. For example, a table is yang relative to the floor, but yin relative to the ceiling.
3. Mutual consumption: excess of yang consumes yin, resulting in yin deficiency.
4. Intertransformation: each transforms into the other, helping to maintain a balance of one to the other.

The 5-phase approach to diagnosis emerged from observation of relationships seen in nature, for example, water nourishes wood, wood fuels fire, and so forth. These observations led to the description of a dynamic energy balance amongst these elements, which can be viewed diagrammatically by arranging the elements as seen in Figure 76-10.

Body organs can be overlaid onto this paradigm in a specific pattern based on the understanding of the essential qualities and spheres of influence of these structures on various physiological and broad metaphorical qualities with which they are associated. The relationship between these organs and their broader spheres of influence is often represented via table of correspondences.

Any of the correspondences (e.g., emotions, organs) from Table 76-2 can be overlaid onto this 5-phase construct to understand the relative influence of one to the other. For example, the emotion of water is fear, the emotion of wood is anger or irritability, and the emotion of fire is joy or mania. The 5-phase relationship tells us that fear nourishes anger and controls (or mitigates) joy or mania.

Use of Acupuncture in TBI

TBI from a Chinese medicine perspective, 2 syndromes are typically recognized: *Qibi* (or blockage of Qi), presents with an agitated, hyperadrenergic state; and *Qituo* (or exhaustion of Qi), presents with unresponsiveness. Additional factors may include Kidney yin deficiency and Liver yin deficiency or Liver yang excess (capitalized organ names represent both associated characteristic energetic qualities and meridian pathway names). Although the data is scant, acupuncture has been reported to be of benefit in TBI, with respect to improvement in level of consciousness, as well as outcomes (68–70). One interventional controlled study of subjects in coma compared 17 subjects to 15 historical controls. Diagnoses included TBI and ruptured intracranial aneurysm. Subjects within 1 week of injury underwent four acupuncture treatments at 12-hour intervals: "A significantly greater number of patients in the acupuncture group (59%) had a >50% neurological recovery than the patients in the no acupuncture group (20%) ($p = .025$)." Study conclusion: early acupuncture intervention may be a reasonable adjunctive treatment for brain-injured patients (67). Another recently published study demonstrated that acupuncture has demonstrated efficacy in treating insomnia in TBI (70). Acupuncture treatment is designed to restore the smooth balanced flow of Qi through meridian channels and their associated organs. This is accomplished through the manipulation of acupuncture points, primarily via the use of needles. Acupuncture needles have unique bioelectrical characteristics, they are typically bimetallic (stainless steel shaft, copper or silver or bronze alloy handle) and therefore effectively create a battery. One needle inserted causes local agitation. Two or more needles cause a directional current flow. Current flow can

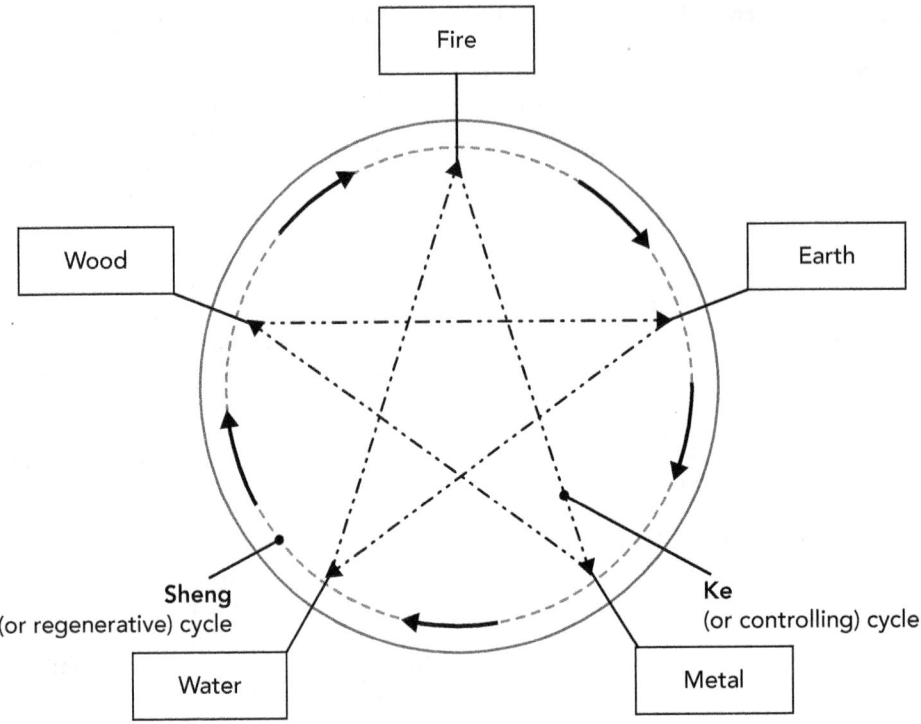

FIGURE 76-10 The 5 phase relationships.

be enhanced with the use of heat or electricity. Once needles are placed, they may be manipulated in one of the following ways: (*a*) no manipulation or neutral or dispersion, (*b*) manual tonification (manipulation), (*c*) heat, or (*d*) electrical stimulation, which facilitates the directed flow of Qi (electrons). Low frequency electrical stimulation results in an endorphin-mediated generalized effect. High-frequency stimulation results in a monoamine-mediated, more rapid onset, segmental response (66). Risks or side effects associated with acupuncture treatment include bleeding or bruising, infection, needle shock or fainting, nerve irritation, and puncture of an organ or vital structure, the latter of which is very rare, with a reported incidence of pneumothorax between 1 per 70,000 and 1 per 250,000 (71). In general, acupuncture is a very safe and well-tolerated procedure.

Electroencephalographic Biofeedback

Electroencephalographic biofeedback (EEG biofeedback) (also known as neurofeedback or neurotherapy) is a widely used alternative treatment for a variety of neurologic and nonneurologic conditions. Based on the same principles as conventional (somatic) biofeedback, EEG biofeedback teaches individuals to modify, through the use of computerized feedback, the electrical activity of their own brains (72). As in other biofeedback modalities, the goal is to make normally unconscious or involuntary bodily processes perceptible so that they can be manipulated consciously. In conventional biofeedback, targets include such somatic processes as muscle tension, heart rate, and skin temperature. In EEG biofeedback, on the other hand, the target processes

Table 76-2 Table of Correspondences

Element	Water	Wood	Fire	Earth	Metal
Season	Winter	Spring	Summer	Late Summer	Fall
Associated Pathogen	Cold	Wind	Heat	Damp	Dryness
Yin Organ	Kidney	Liver	Heart & SNS[a]	Spleen	Lung
Yang Organ	Bladder	Gallbladder	Small Intestine & PNS[b]	Stomach	Large Intestine
Primary Sense Organ	Ears	Eyes	Tongue	Mouth	Nose
Body Tissue	Bone	Ligaments &Tendons	Blood	Muscles	Skin
Emotion	Fear	Anger	Joy/Mania	Worry	Grief
Taste	Salty	Sour	Bitter	Sweet	Spicy
Color	Blue	Green	Red	Yellow	White

[a]Sympathetic Nervous System (also known as Pericardium or Master of the Heart)
[b]Parasympathetic Nervous System (also known as Triple Heater or Triple Burner)
Adapted from Beinfield, H and Korngold, E; *Between Heaven and Earth: A Guide to Chinese Medicine*

are certain characteristics of the patient's own EEG, such as frequency, amplitude, or cerebral localization.

During a typical EEG biofeedback session, the patient's brainwaves are recorded through scalp electrodes placed according to the "10–20" system used in traditional EEG recordings. The raw signal is amplified, filtered, and analyzed by specialized software that determines by how much the patient's EEG pattern deviates from target values (which have been determined ahead of time by the treating clinician). This information, in simplified form, is then communicated to the patient ("feedback"). Usually, the patient is only informed whether or not they are reaching their targets. This feedback can be delivered by something as simple as a light or sound that turns on only when patients are in the target range. Newer systems are characterized by more sophisticated and engaging modes of delivering feedback. For instance, 1 system uses a "Pacman-style" video game; the Pacman character only moves (and thus scores points) when the EEG pattern is in target range.

Although the scenario described previously represents the most basic (and common) of EEG biofeedback, there are increasing numbers of alternative methods and protocols that are being used (72). The costs of an EEG biofeedback session can range from $50 to $150 per session and most practitioners recommend an average of 40 (range 20–60) sessions for TBI, resulting in a total average cost of approximately $4,000 for a full course of treatment.

There are few, if any, dangerous side effects reported (73), although practitioners express concern about the possibility of triggering a seizure in patients with a known seizure disorder (despite the fact that EEG biofeedback is considered a treatment for epilepsy). In general, the reported side effects already assume that EEG biofeedback is efficacious. For instance, practitioners will report concerns about "overshooting" and agitating a person with reduced initiation or, conversely, causing someone who is restless and anxious to become too sedated. A recent case report described impaired memory and disorientation caused by EEG biofeedback (74). Obviously, whether or not these side effects actually occur depends on whether EEG biofeedback can actually modify neurological or psychological symptoms.

The proposed mechanism of action of EEG biofeedback rests on 2 assumptions. First, it is assumed that EEG patterns are correlated with neurological or psychological states. For instance, the EEG of someone with anxiety disorder is thought to differ in predictable ways from the EEG of someone with depression. There is a fair degree of empirical support for this claim (75–77). There is also evidence for the second assumption, namely that individuals can be trained to modify features of their own EEG (72). Indeed, this sort of control over the electrical activity of one's brain underlies the growing field of brain-computer interfaces. Furthermore, there is evidence from functional magnetic resonance imaging (fMRI) studies of changes in activation that occur after EEG biofeedback (78).

Given these empirically supported assumptions, one proposed explanation of how EEG biofeedback works is that patients are learning to "normalize" abnormal EEG patterns and that, as these patterns are normalized, the patient's symptoms improve or even resolve completely.

The FDA does not regulate either EEG biofeedback as a treatment modality or the equipment used (except generically as general biofeedback equipment). In addition, there are no locally or nationally mandated standards regulating the training or qualifications of those who provide this treatment. There are 2 national competency certifications offered by the Biofeedback Certification Institute of America as well as the Neurotherapy and Biofeedback Certification Board; however, these are strictly voluntary. Although anyone can provide these treatments, most providers tend to be professionals licensed in the fields of psychology, medicine, counseling, and so forth. There is a professional society entirely devoted to EEG biofeedback, International Society for Neuronal Regulation, as well as an EEG biofeedback section in the well-established Association for Applied Psychophysiology and Biofeedback. There are textbooks (71,79) and a professional journal (*Journal of Neurotherapy*) devoted to the field. In addition, there are a growing number of dissertations being written on the topic.

Finally, EEG biofeedback has become increasingly visible amongst consumers with TBI and their families. Over a decade ago, the Brain Injury Association of America published an article that discussed the modality in their national magazine (80). And there are an increasing number of books on neurofeedback that are addressed to the general public (81). Although the public visibility of neurofeedback has occurred primarily in the last 10 years, EEG biofeedback has been used for approximately 30 years to treat a variety of psychological conditions (including attention deficit disorders, depression, substance abuse, etc.) (82–87).

The earliest and strongest evidence for the efficacy of EEG biofeedback is in the treatment of epilepsy (88). The intuition behind this research was the recognition that epilepsy was, by definition, a condition characterized by disordered electrophysiology. The goal was to teach individuals to modify those aspects of their EEG that most strongly correlated with seizure risk. Since 1972, there have been more than 60 articles published on the use of EEG biofeedback to reduce seizure frequency in epilepsy; these have been recently summarized (89). Several of these articles reported the results of trials (including blinded, placebo controlled trials). The results were almost uniformly positive and supported the efficacy of EEG biofeedback in reducing seizure frequency. Indeed, even a recent review article that was skeptical of EEG biofeedback acknowledged its potential role in epilepsy (90).

Unfortunately, as noted by the same reviewer, the evidence of efficacy in the treatment of other neurological or psychological conditions is much more limited. Much of it has been in the form of case reports and case series (91). Although there were early trials, most had significant methodological weaknesses that limit the conclusions that can be drawn from them. These weaknesses include high risk of type I error caused by multiple outcomes and multiple statistical comparisons, small sample sizes, lack of blinded assessments, and lack of adequate controls (including the lack of blinded control groups) (90,92). Recognizing these methodological flaws, the 2 primary organizations in the field recently assembled a task force on "methodology and empirically supported treatments," which discussed some of the methodological problems unique to the field of EEG biofeedback (in contrast, for instance, to pharmaceutical research). These authors published a set of standards (93). These recommendations have been echoed by others (94). More recent studies have been methodologically stronger and have appeared to support the efficacy of EEG biofeedback for several different conditions such as attention deficit hyperactivity disorder (87,95,96).

The published literature on the use of EEG biofeedback in TBI is sparse. All of the published accounts reported positive results. However, the number of articles in the peer-reviewed literature is very small and consists primarily of case reports (97) and case series (98–101), although 2 prospective trials (102,103) have recently been published. Moreover, the published reports have almost exclusively involved individuals with mild TBI (82). There have been no published reports on individuals with primarily moderate or severe TBI.

The best designed prospective trial in TBI (103) still shares many of the methodological weaknesses of the studies discussed earlier. In this NIH funded study, 12 subjects with chronic, symptomatic, predominantly mild TBI were randomized into either an active treatment group or a wait-list control group. The treatment consisted of 25 sessions of neurotherapy over 8 weeks. Outcome measures, comprised of symptom rating scales and neuropsychological tests were administered at baseline, posttreatment, and at 3-month follow-up. Once the initial active treatment group finished treatment, the wait-list control underwent the same treatment protocol. At the conclusion of the study, 2 different types of statistical analyses were performed.

First, the results for the 2 different groups (active vs control) were compared in a "between-groups" analysis. Subsequently, the results of all subjects were pooled and their pretreatment and posttreatment outcomes were compared in a "within-groups" analysis. The analyses revealed that subjects experienced improvement in a variety of different domains (8 out of 26 measures in the between-groups analysis and 18 out of 26 measures in the within-groups analysis). The authors concluded that "taken as a whole, the findings of this study are strong enough to identify Flexyx Neurotherapy System as a promising new treatment for TBI, which merits further evaluation" (103).

Despite the promising results, there are several limitations of this study. These include a very small sample size ($n = 12$), heterogeneous sample composition (9 mild and 3 moderate TBI), no mention of issues of subject retention or drop out, lack of a placebo control group, unblinded outcome assessments, no correction for practice effects seen in the neuropsychological measures, and multiple outcomes or statistical testing. The authors of the study recognized many of these weaknesses and correctly point out that many of them are inherent in the exploratory nature of the study. However, they are all issues that any future study must address.

In summary, there is insufficient evidence currently to support the use of EEG biofeedback in the treatment of TBI. However, the evidence of efficacy in other conditions is promising and more studies are clearly warranted. In the meantime, clinicians may choose to discuss this option with their patients, especially when there seem to be no further conventional treatments for relevant applicable symptoms. The relatively low risk and costs associated with EEG biofeedback make EEG biofeedback one of the more attractive options in alternative medicine. However, the clinician should stress the lack of research evidence supporting its use in TBI.

Hyperbaric Oxygen Therapy

Hyperbaric oxygen therapy (HBOT) is an established medical therapy for certain conditions and is increasingly being advocated for the treatment of neurological disorders such as cerebral palsy, multiple sclerosis (MS), stroke, and TBI (104). HBOT delivers 100% oxygen under pressure, which increases the amount of oxygen dissolved in the blood, thereby increasing the oxygen delivered to the body's tissues. HBOT may also enhance the formation of new blood vessels, decrease inflammation, and increase the volume of blood flow (104,105). Treatment sessions occur inside a sealed, pressurized space known as a hyperbaric chamber. The oxygen is delivered either by mask or directly into the chamber. The pressures used are expressed in units of atmospheric pressure and commonly range from 1.5 to 3 atmospheres. The sessions, often referred to as "dives," usually last from 30 to 90 minutes. Many practitioners recommend an average of 100 sessions (range 80–150) for the treatment of chronic, severe BI (104). Because the cost ranges from approximately $200 to $400 per session, the total estimated cost of a full course of treatment is approximately $25,000. This amount is never covered by Medicare and rarely by commercial insurance. Moreover, the treatment of TBI is not recognized as an approved indication for HBOT.

Adverse events can be significant and are related to either the increased pressure or the high concentration of oxygen and include the possibility of seizures, pulmonary injury, and otic trauma. The incidence of seizures is thought to be about 1%–2% in the non-neurological population and is related to the duration of treatment as well as the pressures used (105). Pulmonary injury includes aspiration, infiltrates, or direct barotrauma and has a reported incidence of 10%–30% (106). Otic complications such as pain or rupture of the tympanic membrane have an incidence of 5%–10% (107) but may be prevented by temporary myringotomies. Additionally, there is concern that a prolonged course of HBOT may result in subtle, long-term neurological deficits, although this has not been established (107). A rare complication is tension pneumocephalus (106). Recently, protocols have been suggested that, reportedly, significantly decrease the risk of adverse events in acute TBI (108).

Although the FDA regulates the hyperbaric chambers themselves as medical devices, there are no mandated national or local standards for the staffing or training of personnel. Even less regulation governs freestanding facilities because they are not covered under the regulations for hospitals. These issues are partially being addressed by a recent program of voluntary accreditation administered through the Undersea and Hyperbaric Medical Society. Treatment with HBOT requires a prescription from a physician. However, prescribing HBOT for the treatment of BI would be considered an "off-label" use because BI, stroke, MS, and cerebral palsy are not FDA-approved indications for HBOT. In fact, there are only 15 FDA-approved indications for HBOT; among them are carbon monoxide poisoning, air embolism, selected wounds, and decompression sickness.

Although many of these conditions have been treated by HBOT for over 50 years, the use of HBOT has recently become even more common. There are more than 500 HBOT centers currently operating in the United States. In addition, there is a major professional organization devoted to HBOT—the Undersea and Hyperbaric Medicine Society, which also publishes *Undersea and Hyperbaric Medicine Journal*. This organization, founded in 1967, now has more than 2,500 members. Board certification is offered by passing a subspecialty examination offered by the American Board of Preventive Medicine or the American Board of Emergency Medicine. Finally, there are 2 main textbooks in the field (104,105).

The evidence for the efficacy of HBOT in the treatment of TBI, strokes, and cerebral palsy was extensively reviewed by the Agency for Healthcare Research and Quality (AHRQ) in 2003 (107). The main authors of this report also published a separate review specifically addressing the evidence in TBI (109). The conclusions of these reviews were endorsed by the Undersea and Hyperbaric Medicine Society in a position paper (110). In addition, a review of HBOT as a treatment for BI and stroke was also separately completed by an agency of the government of British Columbia (111). Finally, the Cochrane Database of Systematic Reviews has published their own reviews of the HBOT in TBI (112). All together, these reviews evaluated more than 100 papers that met their inclusion criteria.

In general, these reviews found that there was little evidence for the efficacy of HBOT for TBI. The position paper of the Undersea and Hyperbaric Medical Society concluded that "the weight of the currently available scientific literature is not felt to support an endorsement of HBOT for chronic brain injury" (110). Likewise, the evidence-based review by the government of British Columbia also concluded that "the scientific literature as reviewed up until August 2001 does not support the use of hyperbaric oxygen in the treatment of head injury or stroke" (111). The Cochrane Review concluded that the "routine application of HBOT to these patients cannot be justified from this review" (112). These conclusions are in accord with the findings of the AHRQ report (113). However, given the limited number of clinical trials as well as their methodological limitations, these reports concluded only that there was currently insufficient evidence of efficacy in these conditions (as opposed to evidence of lack of efficacy). Although there have been a handful of investigations on the use of HBOT after TBI published since these reviews, the small number and limitations of these recent studies, which are discussed subsequently, mean that the general conclusions of the earlier reviews are still valid.

In acute TBI, there has been 1 controlled study using clinical outcomes in the past 25 years (113). This trial was in the acute care setting and involved 168 patients with severe brain injury randomized to receive either HBOT or standard treatment. The treatments, begun within 24 hours of injury, were 60 minutes in length and at 1.5 atmospheres. They were administered every 8 hours for 2 weeks or until the patient was either brain dead or could follow simple commands. On average, patients received 21 treatments. After 1 year, patients who received HBOT treatment had an almost 50% reduction in mortality (17% vs 31%). However, the proportion of those who were dead or severely disabled was unchanged (approximately 50% in each group). Thus, although mortality decreased, the rate of a favorable outcome was

unchanged. This study was rated as "fair" by the AHRQ. The only other controlled trial using clinical endpoints in the acute care setting (114) was conducted in 1976. Unlike the later study, it did not find any statistically significant difference between the HBOT and control groups (although there was a trend toward better outcomes in the treatment group). This study was also rated as "fair" by the AHRQ task force. Unfortunately, it is difficult to apply the findings because the study was conducted when the care for TBI was substantially different than it is now.

There were also 2 uncontrolled acute care trials that reported on clinical endpoints (115,116). Both reported benefits to HBOT treatment; however, both had serious methodological flaws and were rated as "poor" quality by the task force. The remainder of the studies in acute TBI was all observational studies or case reports. Although promising, most of these studies used intermediate endpoints such as cerebral blood flow, cerebral metabolism, cerebrospinal fluid (CSF) biochemistry, and intracranial pressure, thereby limiting their clinical applicability. In subacute TBI (approximately 1 month after injury), there has been 1 recent trial (117). Although subjects were randomized to receive either HBOT or standard treatment, not enough information is available to fully assess the methodology. Nonetheless, the authors do report improvements in both the Glasgow Coma Scale (GCS) as well as the Glasgow Outcome Scale (GOS) 6 months after treatment.

In chronic TBI, there have been no HBOT trials with clinical endpoints in the past 20 years. In fact, there are only 5 case reports and 2 case series (excluding abstracts or conference proceedings) (118–124). One case series found no evidence of clinical benefit in chronic TBI (118), whereas a more recent series did (119). Of the case reports, 1 reported a benefit to HBOT treatment but involved a patient only 6 weeks postinjury, thus making it difficult to separate out the effects of natural recovery (120). Another case report involved a patient approximately 6 months after BI and reported a benefit to HBOT treatment. However, the patient was also receiving rehabilitative intervention, thus making it difficult to separate the contributions of HBOT treatment from that of rehabilitation and natural recovery (121). One case report noted no benefit of HBOT treatment, but the focus was only on measures of gait and postural stability (122). A more recent case report that studied neurocognitive functioning reported improvements; moreover, because the patient was more than a year postinjury, concerns about spontaneous recovery are not quite as salient as in the other case reports (123). Finally, a recent publication reports an apparent benefit of HBOT for 2 patients who sustained mild TBI from blast injuries (124).

In the summary, given the lack of clinical trials as well as the mixed results of the other studies, there is little evidence currently to support the use of HBOT as a treatment for chronic BI. This is an area that would benefit greatly from an appropriately powered trial of high methodological rigor. The evidence of benefit in acute BI is more suggestive but, as the reviews discussed earlier concluded, there is still insufficient evidence to recommend the routine use of HBOT in this setting. However, once again, it is noted that there is simply not enough evidence of efficacy now (as opposed to evidence of lack of efficacy). This situation makes advising patients about the use of HBOT more difficult.

Indeed, BI clinicians may be facing a difficult dilemma as consumer demand for HBOT increases in the BI community. This increase in demand may be fueled by several different trends including the general population's interest in alternative treatments, the continued lack of many effective treatments for chronic BI, and the aggressive marketing by many HBOT facilities. The fact that most families will have to pay for the treatments themselves (because of lack of coverage of HBOT for BI) further underscores the importance of advising patients and families appropriately. Recently, guidelines have been developed to help clinicians better address the ethical dilemmas this situation raises (125). In addition to supporting the evidence-based guidelines reviewed here, the authors also emphasize the importance of continued research to establish, definitively, the role of HBOT in the treatment of BI. Until definitive research is conducted, the authors recommend a full discussion with patients and families regarding the current lack of evidence of benefit as well as the risks, including the substantial financial commitment involved.

Electrical and Magnetic Therapies

The history of magnetic and electrical therapy dates back into early recorded medical history. Dr. Frank Krusen, in his classic *Physical Medicine and Rehabilitation* (126), notes the medical reference to electrical therapy dated to about 2000 years ago—electrotherapy was inaugurated in the reign of the Roman Emperor, Tiberius (14–37 CE). Anthero, a freedman, during a walk at the seashore, stepped on a torpedo (an electrified fish) and was thus "freed of gout." About 50 CE, the physician Scribonius Largus recommended repeated applications of the electric-ray fish for the treatment of headache and neuralgia. In 78 CE, Pedanius Dioscorides recommended shocks from the torpedo fish for intractable headache, a procedure echoed by Galen in 200 CE. Moving away from the fish itself, Aetius in 450 CE recommended that a patient with gout hold a magnet as a treatment. Paracelsus (before 1541 CE) observed that the magnet has "power over the matter of all diseases." It was William Gilbert, however, who became the father of magnetic therapy, Gilbert published *De Magnete* (Of the Magnet) in 1600 CE and was appointed "chief physician in personal attendance on Queen Elizabeth" the next year. Gilbert also coined the term "electric," derived from the Greek name for amber.

Magnetic Therapy

Magnets have been used in shoes and wristbands purportedly to help reduce pain. Electromagnetic fields are commonly used to facilitate bone healing in the setting of a nonunion, particularly of the tibia or spine. There is also limited research behind advocating magnets for various other medical conditions including wound healing, pain in the limbs, and muscle recovery after exercise (127). Unfortunately, numerous claims in the lay literature that magnetism promotes healing are not supported in the available scientific literature to date. The relevance of magnetism to health care is only recently being explored in a scientific manner as demonstrated by the expansion of magnetic resonance imaging technology over the last 20 years.

Functional Electrical Stimulation

Functional electrical stimulation (FES), sometimes referred to as functional neuromuscular stimulation (FNS) or neuromuscular stimulation (NMS), has both therapeutic and functional purposes. FES is used to stimulate nerves that innervate specific muscle groups to produce an effect similar to muscles in voluntary exercise. The clinical applications of FES in rehabilitation include muscle strengthening, improved range of motion, facilitation and reeducation of voluntary motor function in orthotic training, and inhibition of spasticity. It is believed that there are no absolute contraindications for FES; relative contraindications include cardiac arrhythmias, pregnancy, wounds that are healing (as stimulating muscle directly under healing tissues may be contraindicated), electrode sensitivity, or congestive heart failure. Occasionally, these devices are implanted in the body to provide long-lasting effects, usually with electrodes at or near the spinal cord itself. FES is known to benefit paralysis of spasticity (upper motor neuron [UMN] disorders) and is known to improve deconditioned cardiovascular patients, and facilitate improved limb movement. Neurogenic bowel and bladder have been shown to benefit from FES, as has sexual dysfunction resulting from spinal cord injury, stroke, MS, or closed head injury.

Transcutaneous Electrical Nerve Stimulation

Transcutaneous electrical nerve stimulation (TENS) is a therapy that uses electrical current, usually direct current, delivered through electrodes that have been placed on the skin. TENS is used for pain relief via encouraging the body to produce endorphins, which function to block the perception of pain, both centrally and peripherally. TENS is performed with a battery-powered device, attached to 2 or 4 electrodes by small-gauge insulated wires, which then conduct the electrical current from the TENS unit to the area of pain. The placement is frequently in a rectangle surrounding the painful area, and the current generated by the device creates a circuit of electrical impulses that travel along the nerve fibers—reducing pain. The machine can be set for various wavelengths and frequencies. The individual's physical therapist or physician usually determines the settings. Used most often to treat muscle, joint, and bone problems occurring with neuromuscular or musculoskeletal problems, TENS is often used for acute or chronic pain, including low back pain, neck pain, tendonitis, or bursitis. Although considered generally safe, the machine could cause harm if misused, so TENS use is currently restricted to application only after physician's prescription.

Cranial Electrical Stimulation

Cranial electrical stimulation (CES) is an experimental and an investigational therapy used for the treatment of neuropsychological disorders. CES uses microcurrent, pulsed high-frequency carrier waves (15,000 Hz) in a modulating action at low current levels to reestablish optimal neurotransmitter levels and functioning within the injured brain. The foundational theory behind CES therapy is conversion of amino acids to neurotransmitters, improving the quality of neurotransmission (128). Its particular mode of functioning is as a corrective measure for brain dysrhythmia. After placement of electrode clips on each earlobe, the microcurrent pulses are thought to reach the brain via a perineuronal or vascular pathway, coursing via the auditory meatus to the thalamus—the primary center of activity. Cell membrane interaction occurs in a manner which then produces modifications in information transduction (physical energy conversion into nervous signal energy), as is associated with classical second messenger pathways, calcium channels, and cyclic AMP (cAMP). Neuroleptic medication use in individuals with BI is decreased with CES therapies and the effects of general brain dysfunction and mood change subsequent to closed head injury appear responsive to CES (129). CES treatments are applied in the early hours, after awakening from sleep, avoiding use within 3 hours of scheduled sleep to avoid a stimulative effect. Generally, CES is well tolerated, with no known contraindications. Rare paradoxical events occur, such as hyperexcitement, although this is unusual.

Transcranial Magnetic Stimulation

Transcranial magnetic stimulation (TMS) is a widely available, painless, and safe technique with a good sensitivity for both corticospinal and corticobulbar tract abnormalities. Owing to the low sensitivity of clinical signs in assessing UMN disorders, there is a need for investigative tools capable of detecting abnormal function of the pyramidal tract. In TMS, an electromagnetic coil is placed on the scalp; high-intensity electrical current is rapidly turned on and off in the coil, through the discharge of capacitors, with the stimulation produced by this discharge of electromagnetic capacitors then causing either an increase or a decrease in the excitability of the affected brain structures. TMS may contribute to the diagnosis of motor neuron disorders by reflecting UMN dysfunction that is not clinically detectable (130–135).

Electrical stimulation was and is still used on the brain by psychiatrists (electroconvulsive therapy [ECT]) to treat intractable depression. It has been speculated that the pathophysiology of depression may include synaptic hypoactivity of the left prefrontal cortex (136). Recently, TMS has been used to treat depression as well. TMS has been shown to be effective in double-blind, placebo-controlled trials (137,38) and in a head-to-head comparison with ECT (39).

In 2001, a meta-analysis was conducted involving 12 published and unpublished sham-controlled studies of left or right prefrontal cortical repetitive transcranial magnetic stimulation (rTMS) in the treatment of depression (140). The study compared the decrease in Hamilton Depression Rating Scale (HDRS) achieved with rTMS and sham stimulation. The authors reported that rTMS was statistically superior to sham stimulation in the treatment of depression, showing a moderate to large effect size. However, the clinical significance of these results was modest, and the differences in response to rTMS across studies were not clearly explained (141).

In addition to its reported effect on mood, TMS has been studied in various types of motor pathology. Diseases for which TMS has been studied include PD, corticobasal degeneration, multiple system atrophy, progressive supranuclear palsy, essential tremor, dystonia, Huntington chorea, myoclonus, the ataxias, Tourette syndrome, restless legs syndrome, Wilson disease, Rett syndrome, and stiff-person (stiff-man) syndrome (141). In a controlled study from Spain, Gironell reported that TMS over the cerebellum is helpful in the treatment of essential tremor (142). From his Neuro Communication Research laboratory in Danbury, Connecticut, Sandyk has used TMS extensively in PD (143). Sandyk reported improvements with weak electromagnetic fields using TMS in PD patients with speech impairments (124, 132,133,143–145). Some would argue that his studies are quite controversial, however, because of their publication in non-refereed journals, the weakness of the employed magnetic fields (in picotesla), generalization from case studies of just 1 subject or a limited number of subjects, and the lack of any attempt at blinding the patient and observer.

Moser and others at the University of Iowa found improvements in cognition with use of TMS—reporting that rTMS improved executive functioning (135). In their study, the cognitive effects of active and sham rTMS were examined in 19 middle-aged and elderly patients with refractory depression. Patients received either active ($n = 9$) or sham ($n = 10$) rTMS targeted at the anterior portion of the left middle frontal gyrus. Patients in the active rTMS group improved significantly on a test of cognitive flexibility and conceptual tracking (Trail Making Test-B). Roth et al. studied rTMS on knowledge acquisition in 20 normal subjects and found no significant difference in a group of normal subjects treated with 25 minutes of high-frequency left dorsolateral prefrontal rTMS compared to a sham untreated group for any memory acquisition. In the area of motor functioning, Fraser et al. at the University Department of Gastroenterology in Salford, United Kingdom reported that TMS can improve motor recovery following BI and speculated that the mechanism is improved plasticity of the motor cortex (146). They studied a group of acute dysphagic stroke patients. TMS was used with varying patterns of input. They found that a specific pattern of magnetic stimulation induced the strongest cortical activation (and thus enhanced brain excitability) as measured by fMRI. This pattern was 5 Hz at 75% of the maximal tolerated intensity for 10 minutes. When this specific pattern of frequency, intensity, and duration of the magnetic stimulus was applied, a greater improvement in swallowing function was seen. This enhanced corticobulbar excitability was increased mainly in the undamaged hemisphere and correlated with recovery.

Others have likewise speculated on and studied the mechanism of TMS. Conforto reported that TMS speeds central motor conduction time (147). As noted earlier, 1 study found that TMS treatments were associated with significant decreases in motor-evoked potential threshold (136). Fraser and others speculated that TMS enhances plasticity of the motor cortex (146). From the Max Planck Institute of Psychiatry in Munich, Keck and others reported that rTMS increases the release of dopamine in the mesolimbic and mesostriatal systems. These authors speculated that this increase in dopaminergic neurotransmission may contribute to the beneficial effects of rTMS in the treatment of affective disorders and PD. From the Montreal Neurological Institute at McGill University, Strafella and others reported that rTMS of the dorsolateral prefrontal cortex, but not the left occipital cortex, in healthy human subjects induces dopamine release in the ipsilateral caudate nucleus (132). They used [^{11}C]raclopride and positron emission tomography to measure changes in extracellular dopamine concentration in vivo after rTMS. In this study, there were no dopaminergic changes in the putamen, nucleus accumbens, or right caudate.

Areas of greatest controversy regarding the use of TMS include the necessary intensity of the magnetic field for clinical effects to be seen and potential risks or side effects. One study reported 1 case of a "pseudoabsence seizure"(148). Another study specifically looking for complications found TMS had no adverse effects on neuropsychological performance (136). Regarding strength of the electromagnetic field, the FDA had ruled that a limit of 80% of the level, which would cause neuron depolarization, was the maximum level considered safe for application. It has been suggested that frequency and variation of the field is more important than its strength. These are both areas that need to be addressed with further research. It remains to be seen whether what appears to be promising technology will be proven to be useful in BI.

CONCLUSION

Although the use of CAM therapy is growing, and limited evidence does exist to support the value of some selected interventions for symptom relief (e.g. acupuncture guided imagery or meditation), there are limitations to the available scientific evidence to support the use of many CAM techniques to treat common associated sequelae of BI. BI survivors and their families will continue to seek CAM interventions to treat the multitude of symptomatic sequelae of BI, particularly where conventional medical practices may fail to provide effective relief.

In some African and Asian countries, 80% of the population rely on traditional medical practices for primary care, and in Western societies, consumer use of CAM continues to grow. The integration of some CAM practices into modern medical practices may be of benefit to Western populations especially with healthy lifestyle adaptations of diet, exercise, meditation, and yoga. In addition, the expanding research focus on CAM and with the further elucidation of the benefits and risks of CAM, the integration of evidence-based CAM interventions into conventional medical practices is inevitable. Although most CAM interventions are relatively safe, the risk associated with and potential adverse effects of certain CAM interventions such as HBOT and some electrical therapies can be significant. It is important for physicians to recognize that their patients may pursue CAM interventions and that knowledge of the potential benefits and risk is essential to provide patients with the information they need for effective and safe use of CAM within Western health care systems.

KEY CLINICAL POINTS

1. The National Centre for Complementary and Alternative Medicine (NCCAM) is the federal government's lead agency for scientific research on CAM.
2. In general the NCCAM survey in 2007 noted an increase in CAM use by American adults from 36% in 2002 to 38.3% in 2007; the 2007 survey also identified that almost 12% of children in the United States use CAM.
3. The United States Federal Drug and Administration regulates herbal and other dietary supplements differently from conventional medicines. The standards that apply to prescription and over the counter medications in the US do not apply to supplements. http://nccam.nih.gov/news/camstats/2007/camsurveyfsl.htm.
4. The public's belief in the effectiveness of homoeopathy may be widespread. As with other diseases and syndromes, the effectiveness of homeopathy for brain injury is quite questionable and controversial.
5. In a review of more than 1200 articles from the 20th century evaluating the association between religion and health, Harold Koenig found that the vast majority of them showed a positive association.
6. In general the weight of the currently available scientific literature does not support the use of hyperbaric oxygen therapy in brain injury.
7. Adverse events in HBOT can be significant and are related to either the increased pressure or the high concentration of oxygen and include the possibility of seizures, pulmonary injury, and otic trauma.
8. The earliest and strongest evidence for the efficacy of EEG biofeedback is in the treatment of epilepsy, literature review appears to support the efficacy of EEG biofeedback in reducing seizure frequency.
9. Areas of greatest controversy regarding the use of transmagnetic brain stimulation (TMS) include the necessary intensity of the magnetic field for clinical effects to be seen and potential risks or side-effects. It remains to be seen whether what appears to be promising technology will be proven to be useful in brain injury.

KEY REFERENCES

1. Agency for Healthcare Research and Quality. *Hyperbaric Oxygen Therapy for Brain Injury, Cerebral Palsy, and Stroke.* Rockville, MD: AHRQ Publications; 2003
2. Bennett MH, Trytko B, Jonker B. Hyperbaric oxygen therapy for the adjunctive treatment of traumatic brain injury. *Cochrane Database Syst Rev.* 2004;4:CD004C09.
3. http://nccam.nih.gov
4. Ospina MB, Bond K, Karkhaneh M, et al. Meditation practices for health: state of the research. *Evid Rep Technol Assess (Full Rep).* 2007;(155):1–263.
5. Tan G, Thornby J, Hammond DC, et al. Meta-analysis of EEG biofeedback in treating epilepsy. *Clin EEG Neurosci.* 2009:40(3):173–179.

References

1. Traditional Medicine. World Health Organization Web site. http://www.who.int/mediacentre/factsheets/fs134/en/.
2. Spencer JW, Jacobs JJ. *Complementary/Alternative Medicine: An Evidence-based Approach.* St. Louis, MO: Mosby; 1999.
3. Spence, JD. *Conquest and Consolidation: The Search For Modern China.* 1st ed. New York, NY: WW Norton & Co.; 1990.
4. Lind J. *A Treatise on the Scurvy.* London, UK: Crowder; 1772.
5. Evidence-Based Medicine Working Group. Evidence-based medicine. A new approach to teaching the practice of medicine. *JAMA.* 1992;268(147):2420–2425.
6. Sackett DL, Strauss SE, Richardson WS, Rosenberg W, Haynes RB. *Evidence-Based Medicine: How to Practice and Teach EBM.* 2nd ed. London, UK: Churchill Livingstone; 2000.
7. info@nccam.nih.gov
8. National Center for Complementary and Alternative Medicine. National Institutes of Health Web site. http://nccam.nih.gov/news/camstats/2007/camsurveyfsl.htm.

9. National Center for Complementary and Alternative Medicine. Statistics on Complementary and Alternative Medicine Use. National Institutes of Health Web site. nccam.nih.gov/news/camstats/.

10. US Food and Drug Administration Web site. www.fda.gov/RegulatoryInformation/Legislation/.

11. Zhu X, Teng S, Eds. *Formulas of Universal Benefit (Pu Ji Fang). 1406 A.D.* Beijing, China: People's Health Publishers; 1959.

12. US Department of Health and Human Services, a. N. I. o. H. a. N. C. f. C. a. A. M. (2010). Herbs, at a glance, a quick guide to herbal supplements. NIH publication no 10-6248 revised June 2010. N. I. o. H. a. N. C. f. C. a. A. M. US Department of Health and Human Services, National Institute of Health and National Centre for Complementary and Alternative Medicine.

13. National Center for Complementary and Alternative Medicine. Study Shows Chamomile Capsules Ease Anxiety Symptoms. National Institutes of Health Web site. http://nccam.nih.gov/research/results/spotlight/040310.htm.

14. Brazier NC, Levine MA. Drug-herb interaction among commonly used conventional medicines: a compendium for health care professionals. *Am J Ther.* 2003;10(3):163–169.

15. Chapman EH, Weintraub RJ, Milburn MA, Pirozzi TO, Woo E. Homeopathic treatment of mild traumatic brain injury: a randomized, double-blind, placebo-controlled clinical trial. *J Head Trauma Rehabil.* 1999;14(6):521–542.

16. Cohen MH, Eisenberg DM. Potential physician malpractice liability associated with complementary and integrative medical therapies. *Ann Intern Med.* 2002;136(8):596–603.

17. Dantas F, Rampes H. Do homeopathic medicines provoke adverse effects? A systematic review. *Br Homoeopath J.* 2000;89(suppl 1):S35–S38.

18. D'Huyvetter K, Cohrssen A. Homeopathy. *Prim Care.* 2002;29(2):407–418, viii.

19. Eisenberg DM, Davis RB, Ettner SL, et al. Trends in alternative medicine use in the United States, 1990–1997: results of a follow-up national survey. *JAMA.* 1998;280(18):1569–1575.

20. Linde K, Clausius N, Ramirez G, et al. Are the clinical effects of homeopathy all placebo effects? A meta-analysis of placebo-controlled trials. *Lancet.* 1997;350(9081):834–843.

21. Linde K, Hondras M, Vickers A, ter Riet G, Melchart D. Systematic reviews of complementary therapies—an annotated bibliography. Part 3: homeopathy. *BMC Complement Altern Med.* 2001;1:4.

22. Smith MJ, Logan AC. Naturopathy. *Med Clin North Am.* 2002;86(1):173–184.

23. Eliopoulos C. Using complementary and alternative therapies wisely. *Geriatr Nurs.* 1999;20(3):139–142.

24. Meyers DG, Maloley PA, Weeks D. Safety of antioxidant vitamins. *Arch Intern Med.* 1996;156(9):925–935.

25. Goldman P. Herbal medicines today and the roots of modern pharmacology. *Ann Intern Med.* 2001;135(8, pt 1):594–600.

26. Gupta RK, Möller HJ. St. John's wort. An option for the primary care treatment of depressive patients? *Eur Arch Psychiatry Clin Neurosci.* 2003;253(3):140–148.

27. Fugh-Berman A, Cott JM. Dietary supplements and natural products as psychotherapeutic agents. *Psychosom Med.* 1999;61(5):712–728.

28. Le Bars PL, Katz MM, Berman N, Itil TM, Freedman AM, Schatzberg AF. A placebo-controlled, double-blind, randomized trial of an extract of Ginkgo biloba for dementia. *JAMA.* 1997;278(16):1327–1332.

29. Lehmann E, Kinzler E, Friedemann J. Efficacy of a special kava extract (Piper methysticum) in patients with states of anxiety, tension, and excitedness of nonmental origin—a double-blind placebo-controlled study of four weeks treatment. *Phytomedicine.* 1996;2:113–139.

30. Zhdanove IV, Wurtman RJ, Regan MM, Taylor JA, Shi JP, Leclair OU. Melatonin treatment for age-related insomnia. *J Clin Endocrinol Metab.* 2001;86(10):4727–4730.

31. Stevinson C, Ernst E. Valerian for insomnia: a systematic review of randomized clinical trials. *Sleep Med.* 2000;1(2):91–99.

32. Volz HP, Kieser M. Kava-kava extract WS 1490 versus placebo in anxiety disorders—a randomized placebo-controlled 25-week outpatient trial. *Pharmacopsychiatry.* 1997;30(1):1–5.

33. Miller LG. Herbal medicinals: selected clinical considerations focusing on known or potential drug-herb interactions. *Arch Intern Med.* 1998;158(20):2200–2211.

34. Lam RW, Levitt AJ. *Canadian consensus guidelines for the treatment of seasonal affective disorder: a summary of the report of the Canadian Consensus Group on SAD.* Vancouver, BC: Clinical and Academic Publishers; 2000.

35. Lewy AJ, Bauer VK, Cutler NL, et al. Morning vs evening light treatment of patients with winter depression. *Arch Gen Psychiatry.* 1998;55(10):890–896.

36. Terman M, Terman JS, Ross DC. A controlled trial of timed bright light and negative air ionization for treatment of winter depression. *Arch Gen Psychiatry.* 1998;55(10):875–882.

37. Astin JA, Harkness E, Ernst E. The efficacy of "distant healing": a systematic review of randomized trials. *Ann Intern Med.* 2000;132(11):903–910.

38. Newberg AB, Iversen J. The neural basis of the complex mental task of meditation: neural transmitter and neurochemical considerations. *Med Hypotheses.* 2003;61(2):282–291.

39. Ospina MB, Bond K, Karkhaneh M, et al. Meditation practices for health: state of the research. *Evid Rep Technol Assess (Full Rep).* 2007;(155):1–263.

40. Davis M, Eshelman ER, McKay M. *The Relaxation and Stress Reduction Workbook.* 5th ed. Oakland, CA: New Harbinger; 2000.

41. American Music Therapy Association Web site. www.musictherapy.org.

42. Dossey L. *Healing Words: The Power of Prayer and the Practice of Medicine.* San Francisco, CA: Harper; 1993.

43. Koenig HG, McCullough ME, Larson DB. *Handbook of Religion and Health.* New York, NY: Oxford University Press; 2001.

44. Ehman JW, Ott BB, Short TH, Ciampa RC, Hansen-Flaschen J. Do patients want physicians to inquire about their spiritual or religious beliefs if they become gravely ill? *Arch Intern Med.* 1999;159(15):1803–1806.

45. Koenig HG. *Spirituality in Patient Care: Why, How, When and What.* Philadelphia, PA: Templeton Foundation Press; 2002.

46. Puchalski C, Romer AL. Taking a spiritual history allows clinicians to understand patients more fully. *J Palliat Med.* 2000;3(1):129–137.

47. Anandarajah G, Hight E. Spirituality and medical practice: using the HOPE questions as a practical tool for spiritual assessment. *Am Fam Physician.* 2001;63(1):82–88.

48. Lo B, Quill T, Tulsky J. Discussing palliative care with patients. *Ann Intern Med.* 1999;130(9):744–749.

49. Stallibrass C, Sissons P, Chalmers C. Randomized controlled trial of the Alexander technique for idiopathic Parkinson's disease. *Clin Rehabil.* 2002;16(7):695–708.

50. Shapira MY, Chelouche M, Yanai R, Kaner C, Szold A. Tai Chi Chuan practice as a tool for rehabilitation of severe head trauma. *Arch Phys Med Rehabil.* 2001;82(9):1283–1285.

51. Gemmell C, Leathem JM. A study investigating the effects of Tai Chi Chuan: individuals with traumatic brain injury compared to controls. *Brain Inj.* 2006;20(2):151–156.

52. Blake H, Batson M. Exercise intervention in brain injury: a pilot randomized study of Tai Chi Qigong. *Clin Rehabil.* 2009;23(7):589–598.

53. Rubin D. Myofascial trigger point syndromes: an approach to management. *Arch Phys Med Rehabil.* 1981;62(3):107–110.

54. Wolsko PM, Eisenberg DM, Davis RB, Kessler R, Phillips RS. Patterns and perceptions of care for treatment of back and neck pain: results of a national survey. *Spine (Phila Pa 1976).* 2003;28(3):292–298.

55. DeBar LL, Vuckovic N, Schneider J, Ritenbaugh C. Use of complementary and alternative medicine for temporomandibular disorders. *J Orofac Pain.* 2003;17(3):224–236.

56. Jensen OK, Nielsen FF, Vosmar L. An open study comparing manual therapy with the use of cold packs in the treatment of post-traumatic headache. *Cephalalgia.* 1990;10(5):241–250.

57. Zencius A, Wesolowski MD, Burke WH, Hough S. Managing hypersexual disorders in brain-injured clients. *Brain Inj*. 1990;4(2):175–181.

58. Ferrell-Torry AT, Glick OJ. The use of therapeutic massage as a nursing intervention to modify anxiety and the perception of cancer pain. *Cancer Nurs*. 1993;16(2):93–101.

59. Delaney JP, Leong KS, Watkins A, Brodie D. The short-term effects of myofascial trigger point massage therapy on cardiac autonomic tone in healthy subjects. *J Adv Nurs*. 2002;37(4):364–371.

60. Sutherland WG. *The Cranial Bowl*. Mankato, MN: Freeman Press; 1939.

61. Grietz D, Wirestam R, Franck A, Nordell B, Thomsen C, Ståhlberg F. Pulsatile brain movement and associated hydrodynamics studied by magnetic resonance phase imaging: the Monro-Kellie doctrine revisited. *Neuroradiology*. 1992;34(5):370–380.

62. Kostopoulos DC, Keramidas G. Changes in elongation of falx cerebri during craniosacral therapy techniques applied on the skull of an embalmed cadaver. *Cranio*. 1992;10(1):9–12.

63. Greenman PE, McPartland JM. Cranial findings and iatrogenesis from craniosacral manipulation in patients with traumatic brain syndrome. *J Am Osteopath Assoc*. 1995;95(3):182–8; 191–192.

64. Robbins H. Evaluating the short term effect of cranial osteopathy on spectral analysis of heart rate variability (unpublished data). Department of Physical Medicine and Rehabilitation. UMDNJ New Jersey Medical School (Newark). Medical Rehabilitation Fellowship; 1996.

65. Green C, Martin CW, Bassett K, Kazanjian A. A systematic review of craniosacral therapy: biological plausibility, assessment reliability and clinical effectiveness. *Complement Ther Med*. 1999;7(4):201–207.

66. Helms JM. *Acupuncture Energetics: A Clinical Approach for Physicians*. Berkeley, CA: Medical Acupuncture Publishers; 1995.

67. Maciocia G. *The Foundations of Chinese Medicine*. 1st ed. Edinburgh, UK: Churchill Livingstone; 1989: 5–7.

68. Frost EA. Acupuncture for the comatose patient. *Am J Acupuncture*. 1976;4(1):45–48.

69. Wang XM, Yang SL. The effect of acupuncture in 90 cases of sequelae of brain concussion. *J Tradit Chin Med*. 1988;8(2):127–128.

70. Zollman FS, Larson EB, Wasek-Throm LB, Cyborski CM, Bode RK. Acupuncture for treatment of insomnia in patients with traumatic brain injury: a pilot intervention study. *J Head Trauma Rehabil*. 2011.

71. Chung A, Bui L, Mills E. Adverse effects of acupuncture: which are clinically significant? *Can Fam Physician*. 2003;49:985–989.

72. Evans JR, Abarbanel AA, eds. *Quantitative EEG and Neurofeedback*. San Diego, CA: Academic Press; 1999.

73. Hammond DC, Kirk L. First do no harm: adverse effects and the need for practice standards in neurofeedback. *Journal of Neurotherapy*. 2008;12(1):79–88.

74. Todder D, Levine J, Dwolatzky T, et al. Case report: impaired memory and disorientation induced by delta band down-training over the temporal brain regions by neurofeedback treatment. *Journal of Neurotherapy*. 2010;14(2):153–155.

75. Hughes J, John ER. Conventional and quantitative electroencephalography in psychiatry. *J Neuropsychiatry Clin Neurosci*. 1999;11(2):190–208.

76. Thornton K. Electrophysiology of the reasons the brain damaged subject can't recall what they hear. *Arch Clin Neuropsychol*. 2002;17:1–17.

77. Thornton K. The electrophysiological effects of a brain injury on auditory memory functioning: the QEEG correlates of impaired memory. *Arch Clin Neuropsychol*. 2003;18(4):363–378.

78. Beauregard M, Lévesque J. Functional magnetic resonance imaging investigation of the effects of neurofeedback training on the neural bases of selective attention and response inhibition in children with attention-deficit/hyperactivity disorder. *Appl Psychophysiol Biofeedback*. 2006;31(1):3–20.

79. Demos J. *Getting Started with Neurofeedback*. New York, NY: W. W. Norton & Company; 2004.

80. Thatcher R. QEEG and traumatic brain injury: present and future. *Brain Injury Source*. 1999;3(4):28–32.

81. Albright C. *Neurofeedback: Transforming Your Life with Brain Biofeedback*. Kansas City, MO: Beckworth Publications; 2010.

82. Duff J. The usefulness of quantitative EEG (QEEG) and neurotherapy in the assessment and treatment of post-concussion syndrome. *Clin EEG Neurosci*. 2004;35(4):198–209.

83. Thatcher RW. EEG operant conditioning (biofeedback) and traumatic brain injury. *Clin Electroencephalogr*. 2000;31(1):38–44.

84. Rosenfeld JP. An EEG biofeedback protocol for affective disorders. *Clin Electroencephalogr*. 2000;31(1):7–12.

85. Moore NC. A review of EEG biofeedback treatment of anxiety disorders. *Clin Electroencephalogr*. 2000;31(1):1–6.

86. Sokhadze TM, Cannon RL, Trudeau DL. EEG biofeedback as a treatment for substance abuse disorders: review, rating of efficacy, and recommendations for further research. *Appl Psychophysiol Biofeedback*. 2008:33(1):1–28

87. Arns M, de Ridder S, Strehl U, Breteler M, Coenen A. Efficacy of neurofeedback treatment in ADHD: the effects on inattention, impulsivity and hyperactivity: a meta-analysis. *Clin EEG Neurosci*. 2009:40(3):180–189.

88. Sterman MB, Egner T. Foundation and practice of neurofeedback for the treatment of epilepsy. *Appl Psychophysiol Biofeedback*. 2006: 31(1):21–35.

89. Tan G, Thornby J, Hammond DC, et al. Meta-analysis of EEG biofeedback in treating epilepsy. *Clin EEG Neurosci*. 2009:40(3):173–179.

90. Lohr J. Neurotherapy does not qualify as an empirically supported behavioral treatment for psychological disorders. *Behavior Therapist*. 2001;24(5):97–104.

91. Comprehensive Neurofeedback Bibliography. International Society for Neurofeedback & Research Web site. www.isnr.org.

92. Kline J. A cacophony in the brainwaves: a critical appraisal of neurotherapy for attention-deficit disorders. *The Scientific Review of Mental Health Practice*. 2002;1(1):44–54.

93. LaVaque T. Task Force Report on methodology and empirically supported treatments. *Applied Psychophysiology and Biofeedback*. 2002;27(4):271–281.

94. Nelson L. Neurotherapy and the challenge of empirical support: a call for a neurotherapy practice research network. *Journal of Neurotherapy*. 2003;7(2):53–67.

95. Gevensleben H, Holl B, Albrecht B, et al. Is neurofeedback an efficacious treatment for ADHD? A randomised controlled clinical trial. *J Child Psychol Psychiatry*. 2009;50(7);780–789.

96. Gevensleben H, Holl B, Albrecht B, et al. Neurofeedback training in children with ADHD: 6-month follow-up of a randomised controlled trial. *Eur Child Adolesc Psychiatry*. 2010:19(9);715–724.

97. Byers A. Neurofeedback therapy for a mild head injury. *Journal of Neurotherapy*. 1995;v1(n1):22–37.

98. Bounias M, Laibow RE, Bonaly A, Stubblebine AN. EEG-NeuroBioFeedback treatment of patients with brain injury: part 1: typological classification of clinical syndromes. *J of Neurother*. 2001;5(4):23–44.

99. Thornton KE. The improvement/rehabilitation of auditory memory functioning with EEG biofeedback. *NeuroRehabilitation*. 2002; 17(1):69–80.

100. Thornton K. Improvement/rehabilitation of memory functioning with neurotherapy/QEEG biofeedback. *J Head Trauma Rehabil*. 2000;15(6):1285–1296.

101. Walker JE, Norman CA, Weber RK. Impact of QEEG guided coherence training for patients with a mild closed head injury. *J Neurother*. 2002;6(2):31–43.

102. Keller I. Neurofeedback therapy of attention deficits in patients with traumatic brain injury. *J Neurother*. 2001;5(1/2):19–32.

103. Schoenberger NE, Shif SC, Esty Ml, Ochs L, Mathies RJ. Flexyx Neurotherapy System in the treatment of traumatic brain injury: an initial evaluation. *J Head Trauma Rehabil*. 2001;16(3):260–274.

104. Jain KK, ed. *Textbook of Hyperbaric Medicine*. 5th ed. Cambridge, MA: Hogrefe & Huber; 2009.

105. Kindwall EP, ed. *Hyperbaric Medicine Practice*. 2nd ed. Flagstaff, AZ: Best Publishing; 2004.

106. Lee CH, Chen WC, Wu CI, Hsia TC. Tension pneumocephalus: a rare complication after hyperbaric oxygen therapy. *Am J Emerg Med*. 2009;27(2):257.e1–e3.

107. Agency for Healthcare Research and Quality. *Hyperbaric Oxygen Therapy for Brain Injury, Cerebral Palsy, and Stroke.* Rockville, MD: AHRQ Publications; 2003.

108. Rockswold SB, Rockswold GL, Defillo A. Hyperbaric oxygen in traumatic brain injury. *Neurol Res.* 2007;29(2):162–172.

109. McDonagh M, Helfland M, Carson S, Russman BS. Hyperbaric oxygen therapy for traumatic brain injury: a systematic review of the evidence. *Arch Phys Med Rehabil.* 2004;85(7):1199–1204.

110. Undersea & Hyperbaric Society. *Position Paper: Hyperbaric Oxygen Therapy for Chronic Brain Injury.* www.uhms.org. 2003.

111. Alternative Therapy Evaluation Committee for the Insurance Corporation of British Columbia. A review of the scientific evidence on the treatment of traumatic brain injuries and strokes with hyperbaric oxygen. *Brain Inj.* 2003;17(3):225–236.

112. Bennett MH, Trytko B, Jonker B. Hyperbaric oxygen therapy for the adjunctive treatment of traumatic brain injury. *Cochrane Database Syst Rev.* 2004;4:CD004C09.

113. Rockswold GL, Ford SE, Anderson DC, Bergman TA, Sherman RE. Results of a prospective randomized trial for treatment of severely brain-injured patients with hyperbaric oxygen. *J Neurosurg.* 1992; 76(6):929–934.

114. Artru F, Chacornac R, Deleuze R. Hyperbaric oxygenation for severe head injuries. *Eur Neurol.* 1976;14(4):310–318.

115. Ren H, Wang W, GE Z, Zhang J. Clinical, brain electric earth map, endothelin and transcranial ultrasonic Doppler findings after hyperbaric oxygen treatment for severe brain injury. *Chin Med J (Engl).* 2001;114(4):387–390.

116. Mogami H, Hayakawa T, Kanai N, et al. Clinical application of hyperbaric oxygenation in the treatment of acute cerebral damage. *J Neurosurg.* 1969;31(6):636–643.

117. Lin JW, Tsai JT, Lee LM, et al. Effect of hyperbaric oxygen on patients with traumatic brain injury. *Acta Neurochir Suppl.* 2008: 101:145–149.

118. Barrett K, Masel B, Patterson J, Scheibel RS, Corson KP, Mader JT. Regional CBF in chronic stable TBI treated with hyperbaric oxygen. *Undersea Hyperb Med.* 2004;31(4):395–406.

119. Golden Z, Golden CJ, Neubauer RA. Improving neuropsychological function after chronic brain injury with hyperbaric oxygen. *Disabil Rehabil.* 2006:28(22):1379–1386.

120. Eltorai I, Montroy R. Hyperbaric oxygen therapy leading to recovery of a 6-week comatose patient afflicted by anoxic encephalopathy and posttraumatic edema. *J Hyperbaric Med.* 1991;6(3):189–197.

121. Neubauer RA, Gottlieb SF, Pevsner NH. Hyperbaric oxygen for treatment of closed head injury. *South Med J.* 1994;87(9):933–936.

122. Wolley SM, Lawrence JA, Hornyak J. The effect of hyperbaric oxygen treatment on postural stability and gait of a brain injured patient. *Pediatr Rehabil.* 1999;3(3):81–90.

123. Hardy P, Johnston KM, De Beaumont L, et al. Pilot case study of the therapeutic potential of hyperbaric oxygen therapy on chronic brain injury. *J Neurol Sci.* 2007;253(1–2):94–105.

124. Wright JK, Zant E, Groom K, Schlegel RE, Gilliland K. Case report: treatment of mild traumatic brain injury with hyperbaric oxygen. *Undersea Hyperb Med.* 2009;36(6):391–399.

125. Chan EC, Brody B. Ethical dilemmas in hyperbaric medicine. *Undersea Hyperb Med.* 2001;28(3):123–130.

126. Krusen FH. *Physical Medicine: The Employment of Physical Agents for Diagnosis and Therapy.* Philadelphia, PA: WB Saunders; 1941.

127. Steizinger C, Yerys S, Scowcroft N, Wygand J, Otto RM. The effects of repeated magnet treatment on prolonged recovery from exercise induced delayed onset muscle soreness. *Med Sci Sports Exerc.* 1999; 31(5):S208.

128. Keck ME, Welt T, Müller MB, et al. Repetitive transcranial magnetic stimulation increases the release of dopamine in the mesolimbic and mesostriatal system. *Neuropharmacology.* 2002;43(1):101–109.

129. Strafella AP, Paus T, Barrett J, Dagher A. Repetitive transcranial magnetic stimulation of the human prefrontal cortex induces dopamine release in the caudate nucleus. *J Neurosci.* 2001;21(15):RC157.

130. Sandyk R. Reversal of visuospatial deficit on the Clock Drawing Test in Parkinson's disease by treatment with weak electromagnetic fields. *Int J Neurosci.* 1995;82(3–4):255–268.

131. Sandyk R. Weak electromagnetic fields reverse visuospatial hemi-inattention in Parkinson's disease. *Int J Neurosci.* 1995;81(1–2): 47–65.

132. Sandyk R. Reversal of cognitive impairment in an elderly parkinsonian patient by transcranial application of picotesla electromagnetic fields. *Int J Neurosci.* 1997;91(1–2):57–68.

133. Sandyk R. Improvement in short-term visual memory by weak electromagnetic fields in Parkinson's disease. *Int J Neurosci.* 1995; 81(1–2):67–82.

134. Heldmann B, Kerkhoff G, Struppler A, Havel P, Jahn T. Repetitive peripheral magnetic stimulation alleviates tactile extinction. *Neuroreport.* 2000;11(14):3193–3198.

135. Moser DJ, Jorge RE, Manes F, Paradiso S, Benjamin ML, Robinson RG. Improved executive functioning following repetitive transcranial magnetic stimulation. *Neurology.* 2002;58(8):1288–1290.

136. Triggs WJ, McCoy KJ, Greer R, et al. Effects of left frontal transcranial magnetic stimulation on depressed mood, cognition, and corticomotor threshold. *Biol Psychiatry.* 1999;45(11):1440–1446.

137. Klein E, Kreinin I, Chistyakov A, et al. Therapeutic efficacy of right prefrontal slow repetitive transcranial magnetic stimulation in major depression: a double-blind controlled study. *Arch Gen Psychiatry.* 1999;56(4):315–320

138. George MS, Nahas Z, Molloy M, et al. A controlled trial of daily left prefrontal cortex TMS for treating depression. *Biol Psychiatry.* 2000:48(10):962–970.

139. Dannon PN, Dolberg OT, Schrieber S, Grunhaus L. Three and six-month outcome following courses of either ECT or rTMS in a population of severely depressed individuals—preliminary report. *Biol Psychiatry.* 2002;51(18):962–970.

140. Holtzheimer PE III, Russo J, Avery DH. A meta-analysis of repetitive transcranial magnetic stimulation in the treatment of depression. *Pyschopharmacol Bull.* 2001;35(4):149–169.

141. Cantello R. Applications of transcranial magnetic stimulation in movement disorders. *J Clin Neurophysiol.* 2002;19(4):272–293.

142. Gironell A, Kulisevsky J, Lorenzo J, Barbanoj M, Pascual-Sedano B, Otermin P. Transcranial magnetic stimulation of the cerebellum in essential tremor: a controlled study. *Arch Neurol.* 2002;59(3): 413–417.

143. Sandyk R. Reversal of body image disorder (macrosomatognosia) in Parkinson's disease by treatment with AC pulsed electromagnetic fields. *Int J Neurosci.* 1998;93(1–2):43–54.

144. Sandyk R. Improvement in word-fluency performance in Parkinson's disease by administration of electromagnetic fields. *Int J Neurosci.* 1994;77(1–2):23–46.

145. Fraser C, Power M, Hamdy S, et al. Driving plasticity in human adult motor cortex is associated with improved motor function after brain injury. *Neuron.* 2002;34(5):831–840.

146. Conforto AB, Marie SK, Cohen LG, Scaff M. Transcranial magnetic stimulation [in Portugese]. *Arq Neuropsiquiatr.* 2003;61(1):146–152.

147. Conca A, König P, Hausmann A. Transcranial magnetic stimulation induces 'psuedoabsence seizure'. *Acta Psychiatr Scand.* 2000; 101(3):246–248.

XVIII

PSYCHOSOCIAL FUNCTIONING, COMMUNITY RE-ENTRY, AND PRODUCTIVITY

Posthospital Rehabilitation

James F. Malec

INTRODUCTION

Over the last 30 years, there has been a steady evolution of postacute or posthospital rehabilitation after acquired brain injury (ABI). Even the name has changed. Whereas postacute rehabilitation formerly referred to outpatient or residential rehabilitation that occurred after inpatient rehabilitation, the current terminology of health care reform describes any health care services after acute hospital care as *postacute* including inpatient rehabilitation. For this reason, the term *posthospital rehabilitation* will be used throughout this chapter to refer to the types of rehabilitation that occur outside of a traditional hospital setting and typically occur after initial acute brain injury medical care and inpatient rehabilitation.

Over the last 30 years, the nature of rehabilitation has also changed dramatically. Lengths of hospital stays (LOS) have decreased markedly for inpatients with brain injury and other disabilities (1,2). In general, LOS for inpatient rehabilitation after ABI has declined from 2–3 months in the 1980s to 2–3 weeks currently. Reduced LOS provides little opportunity for comprehensive rehabilitation. The focus of the inpatient rehabilitation has shifted to assuring medical stability and mobilizing self-care skills. It is not unheard of for patients to be discharged from inpatient rehabilitation before the period of post-traumatic amnesia has fully resolved.

Much of the rehabilitation that was accomplished in an inpatient setting during the 1980s can be accomplished in outpatient, day treatment, or residential settings. If posthospital rehabilitation were readily available to most patients, the decline in inpatient rehabilitation LOS would be justifiable, reasonable, and probably preferable to most patients. However, due to an absence of funding, the availability of posthospital rehabilitation has not increased concomitantly with the decrease in inpatient rehabilitation LOS. Most private and government insurance policies offer no or only very limited coverage for posthospital rehabilitation programming or specific services, such as cognitive rehabilitation.

The large amount of variability among posthospital rehabilitation programs frustrates precise classification of these programs (3,4). In 1996, Malec and Basford (5) attempted to describe the landscape of posthospital rehabilitation. They described *subacute rehabilitation* as residential care of individuals with ABI who are unable to participate in more intensive rehabilitation because of severe cognitive and behavioral impairments and described 2 types of programs

in this category: (*a*) coma management, that is, care of patients in minimally responsive states; and (*b*) behavioral management, that is, supportive environmental management for individuals with ABI whose behavioral problems preclude either independent living or participation in rehabilitation. They also described 4 types of specialized programs that provided more intensive rehabilitation with the expectation of more dramatic gains for participants in functional abilities and community reintegration: (*a*) *neurobehavioral programs*, that is, residential programs that provide intensive behavioral treatment to patients with ABI and severe behavioral disturbances; (*b*) *residential community reintegration programs* that provide integrated rehabilitation to patients who cannot participate in outpatient programs either because of severe cognitive and behavioral impairments or local unavailability of outpatient services; (*c*) *comprehensive (holistic) day treatment programs* that offer integrated, multimodal, milieu-oriented rehabilitation; and (*d*) *outpatient community reentry programs* that provide circumscribed rehabilitative treatment for community reintegration. Malec and Basford also commented on short- and long-term community supports that were available to individuals with ABI.

THE CURRENT LANDSCAPE

To some degree, descriptions offered by Malec and Basford still apply. Perhaps one of the most significant changes in the last 15 years has not been so much in the types of programs available but rather in a movement away from a "one size fits all" philosophy towards identifying specific programs and approaches that are most suitable for particular types of patients based on their disability profiles. There has also been an increase in the preponderance and availability of supportive programs, both residential- and community-based, whose goals are primarily to assist participants in maintaining stability rather than improving their adjustment and level of community integration. However, during this same period of time, the availability of holistic residential or day treatment programs has not increased and has probably declined primarily due to the difficulty in obtaining funding for this service. Although intensive rehabilitation may be of substantial benefit and even requisite for the successful community reintegration of individuals with pervasive disabilities and limited self-awareness after ABI, these programs are costly. Hence, funding for such programs must typically be negotiated on a case-by-case basis with third

TABLE 77-1 Supported Living Posthospital Rehabilitation Programs

PROGRAM TYPE	PATIENTS SERVED	GOALS	PRIMARY METHODS	PROVIDER COMPOSITION
Residential				
Slow-to-recover	Minimally responsive	Maintain health, physical status Improve responsiveness	Pharmacology Therapy for maintenance and stimulation	Interdisciplinary team directed by physician
Long-term residential	Chronic, stable Unable to live independently	Maintain health status Support community reintegration	Applied behavior analysis (ABA) Support Supervision	Professional/ paraprofessional team
Community				
Long-term community supportive	Chronic, stable Able to live independently with assistance	Maintain health status Support community reintegration	ABA Support Supervision	Professional/ paraprofessional team

party payers. Such negotiations represent a significant personnel expense to the provider which often is beyond the provider's capacity to assume.

In contrast, the availability of community-based rehabilitation in which rehabilitation services are provided in community and home settings has increased. Such programs are less costly because they do not require facility maintenance but nonetheless can be quite beneficial for appropriate participants. There has also been increasing interest in interventions, such as resource facilitation in which the target of the intervention is as much the participant's social environment as the participant. Tables 77-1 and 77-2 describe general program types in four major categories.

Supported Living (SL) Programs

Slow-to-Recover Programs

Issues and approaches regarding the care of individuals who remain for a prolonged period of time in a minimally responsive state are covered comprehensively elsewhere in this volume (see Giacino et al., Chapter 32). Programs designed for such patients may be seen as supportive in that a primary goal is to maintain health and avoid physical deterioration, such as decubitus ulcers or muscle contractures. However, these programs also typically include pharmacologic and behavioral stimulation interventions designed to increase responsiveness and normal awareness. There is some evidence of a positive effect of medications to increase the rate of recovery in this population as well as of stimulation therapies (6). In their systematic review of the efficacy of stimulation protocols, Vanier and colleagues (7) described the limitations in studies of the efficacy of stimulation programs to improve consciousness among patients in minimally responsive states. Noting that research is challenged in this area by the small numbers and heterogeneity of available subjects—as in much of interventional research in brain injury—these reviewers recommend alternative research strategies to the randomized controlled trial, such as single subject designs.

Long-Term Residential SL Programs

Data from the TBI model systems (8) suggest that a large majority of patients who survive moderate-to-severe brain injuries will return to independent living in the community with or without support from family or significant others (SO). However, a small percentage is unable to live without significant support and supervision. In cases in which such support and supervision cannot be provided by family or SO, supportive care may be available in residential facilities specifically designed for individuals with ABI.

In addition to supportive care, these programs typically offer limited rehabilitation and behavioral intervention and support services to assist residents in maintaining functional abilities and acceptable behavioral and emotional control. Medical and nutritional consultation is typically available to help support general health maintenance. With such support and services, residents in these programs can usually be involved in the larger community outside the residence for leisure and work. Leisure and work activities are also often available within the residential program. Professional services, such as the design of behavioral intervention strategies, medical care, nutritional programs, and rehabilitation are provided by staff with professional credentials in appropriate disciplines (i.e., psychologists, nurses and physicians, dieticians, and rehabilitation therapists, respectively). Activities to encourage community participation and implementation of behavioral plans are often provided by paraprofessionals who receive specific training in working with individuals with ABI and in the duties for which they are responsible. Specific academic credentials are not required for paraprofessional staff; however, certification through the Academy of Certified Brain Injury Specialists (ACBIS) is encouraged for paraprofessional staff by a growing number of providers.

Those admitted to long-term residential SL programs are believed to have reached their maximum recovery. Consequently, the goal of these programs is maintenance of gains rather than further improvement. Eicher and colleagues (9) reported that individuals involved in residential SL programs were able to maintain their functional status for at least the 6–9 months during the study period (see Figure 77-1). This uncontrolled study documents that the goal of maintained function was achieved.

TABLE 77-2 Intensive Post-hospital Rehabilitation Programs

PROGRAM TYPE	PATIENTS SERVED	GOALS	PRIMARY METHODS	PROVIDER COMPOSITION
Residential				
Neurobehavioral	Severely disorganized or dangerous behavior	Reduce/ eliminate/ replace severe behavior dysfunction	Phamacologic Applied behavior analysis (ABA)	Interdisciplinary team with emphasis on neuropsychiatry and ABA
Residential Treatment	Severe and pervasive cognitive and behavioral disabilities that preclude outpatient or community-based rehabilitation Impaired self-awareness Psychiatric/substance-related comorbidities	Increase independent living and community reintegration	Holistic milieu-oriented group and individual therapy Cognitive rehabilitation ABA Other therapies, medication as indicated Family involvement	Transdisciplinary team
Community				
Traditional outpatient	Isolated impairment(s) Reasonable awareness of disabilities	Impairment remediation to improve function	Medically-supervised physical, occupational, speech therapy as indicated	Multidisciplinary team
Home- and community-based	Strong potential for independent living and work Reasonable awareness of disabilities Social or family support	Increase independent living Community reintegration	Physical, occupational, speech therapy as indicated Psychological/family counseling Cognitive rehabilitation	Interdisciplinary team
Outpatient holistic day treatment	Severe and pervasive cognitive and behavioral disabilities Impaired self-awareness Psychiatric/substance-related comorbidities	Increase independent living Community reintegration	Holistic milieu-oriented group and individual therapy Cognitive rehabilitation ABA Other therapies, medication as indicated Family involvement	Transdisciplinary team

There is evidence that a percentage of individuals decline in functional abilities after brain injury (10–12). However, it cannot be assumed that individuals in programs like those studied by Eicher and colleagues would deteriorate without following a similar cohort who do not receive the intervention. Rigorous study of the effectiveness of these types of programs is challenged by a number of factors including the heterogeneity and limited availability of samples and difficulty in blinding both participant and provider to the experimental condition. Ethical and humanitarian concerns argue against conducting a randomized controlled trial because admission to such programs requires evidence and professional opinion that the individual admitted would indeed deteriorate without the benefit of supportive care. Future research may use quasi-experimental designs that examine the course of residents in such programs over longer periods of time and that examine dose-response relationships between level of services provided and functional outcome. Case-controlled studies in which individuals in residential support programs are compared to historical or concurrent controls with similar characteristics who do

not have access to such programs may also provide a more rigorous evaluation of these programs. However, as with all case-controlled studies, the comparability of treatment and control groups is open to challenge.

Long-Term Community SL Programs

An additional small percentage of individuals with severe and pervasive disabilities after ABI are able to live in community-integrated settings, such as family, group homes, or supported apartments but require ongoing supportive services in order to maintain their maximum level of health, functional ability, and community participation. The services provided by community SL programs are similar to those provided by residential SL programs but typically not as frequent or intensive. By definition, the degree of supervision and support required by those in community programs is less than for residential programs, with the exception of individuals who enter residential programs only because of a lack of availability of community-based programs in their local community. Community SL programs typically

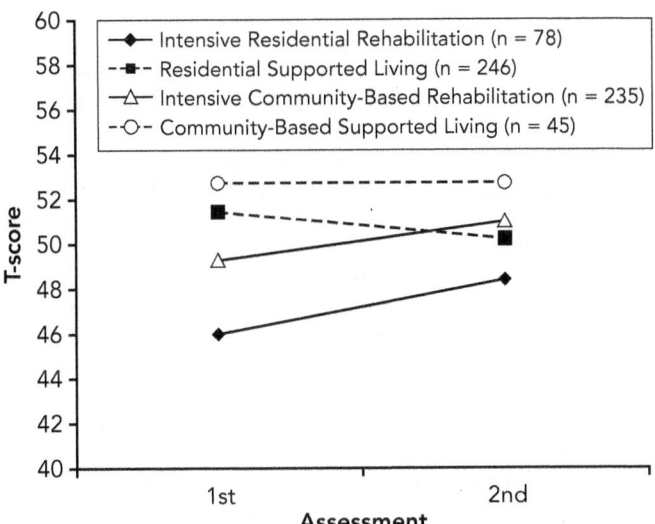

FIGURE 77-1 Changes in functional status as indicated by Mayo-Portland Adaptability Inventory (MPAI-4) total T-score by program type over time. From Meyer et al. (9).

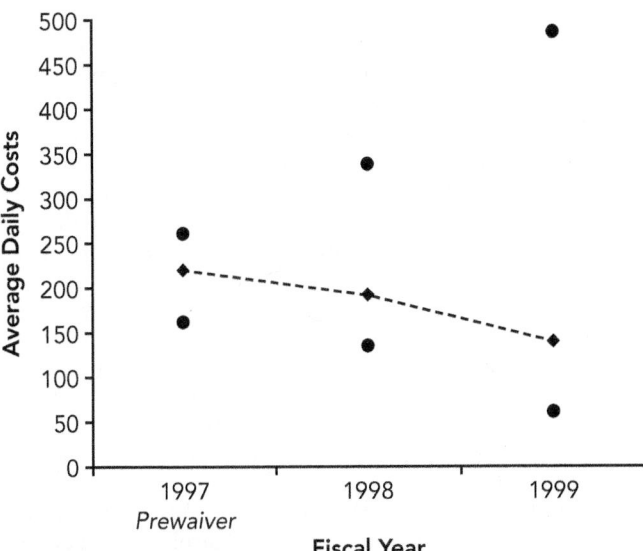

FIGURE 77-2 Prewaiver and postwaiver costs of care for 80 individuals with TBI and behavioral disturbance in New York state (13) dotted line shows average costs; circles bracket the range of costs.

focus on the maintenance of functional abilities, community participation, and health through a mixture of pharmacologic, behavioral, and health maintenance interventions. Services to encourage and support involvement in community-based social, leisure, and vocational activities are also characteristic of these types of programs. As in residential SL programs, these services are often provided by trained paraprofessional staff.

The Eicher et al. study mentioned earlier also investigated progress among a cohort of individuals involved in community SL programs (see Figure 77-1). These individuals demonstrated stable functional abilities over the period of time of this study, as did those in residential SL programs. Feeney and colleagues (13) took another approach to investigating the impact of community SL programs for individuals with ABI. These investigators examined the costs of care and services for 80 community-dwelling individuals with severe behavioral disturbance associated with ABI before and after the implementation of a *waiver* program in New York State. These individuals were able to access support services in the community more readily after the waiver program supplied funding for such services. Feeney's group found that overall costs of community services declined in the 2 years following implementation of the waiver program (see Figure 77-2). However, the variability of costs increased dramatically because individuals who needed more extensive services were able to obtain these services through the waiver program. The researchers concluded that providing adequate services reduces the overall cost of care and that, even when intensive services are needed, the cost-benefit ratio is positive.

Supportive community programs may take many forms. The Clubhouse model (14), originally developed in mental health, has been successfully applied in ABI. In the Clubhouse model, individuals with ABI work together to provide each other with necessary supports to maintain community participation with minimal staff assistance. Hibbard et al. (15) describe a peer mentoring program in which individuals with ABI and their families receive support and life coaching from other individuals who have made a successful

adjustment after ABI. Individuals receiving peer-mentoring services reported a positive impact on their quality of life. Heinemann, Corrigan, and Moore (16) describe positive effects on well-being, community integration, and employment for a comprehensive case management system for individuals with traumatic ABI and alcohol-related problems. Early intervention and employment at the time of recruitment to the program were associated with the largest gains for participants. The authors comment on the potential cost-benefit of comprehensive case management services.

Intensive Rehabilitation Programs

Neurobehavioral Programs

Neurobehavioral programs offer relatively short-term, very intensive interventions for individuals with extremely severe behavioral disorders. Treatment is delivered in a highly restricted and supervised inpatient or residential setting. The rational for placement in a highly restricted environment is that the maladaptive, often very aggressive, behavior of patients admitted to such programs puts them or others at risk for harm. Treatment that most often combines pharmacotherapy with Applied Behavioral Analysis (ABA, i.e., behavioral modification, or in more contemporaneous terms, behavioral intervention and support) is directed at reducing the frequency and intensity of maladaptive behaviors and replacing these maladaptive behaviors with more adaptive behaviors to a level where the patient can enter or resume life and rehabilitation in a less restrictive environment.

The treatment team is highly coordinated and interdisciplinary. With ABA playing a critical role in treatment, consistency in following the behavioral plan by all members of the team is essential. Although traditional rehabilitation interventions (e.g., physical therapy, occupational therapy) may be included, the treatment program is usually focused on reducing maladaptive behavior and developing more adaptive behavior. Consequently, the team often includes a neuropsychiatrist, neuropsychologist, behavior analysts, and psychiatric or behaviorally trained nursing staff. Another key component of these programs is training families and other care providers in behavioral techniques to support generalization of successful behavioral intervention beyond the treatment setting following discharge.

Braunling-McMorrow et al. (17) reported positive changes in functional status as a result of participation in a neurobehavioral treatment program for a group of 76 individuals with ABI. Functional status improved over the course of treatment (see Figure 77-3) and gains were maintained at 1-year follow-up. Time from injury or event to admission did not appear to affect outcome. Braunling-McMorrow's report also describes outcomes for 129 individuals with ABI who participated in an intensive residential treatment program and describes components of each of these types of programs.

Chapters in Section IV and XVII of this book provide more detailed information about pharmacologic and behavioral approaches to address dysfunctional and disruptive behavior. In their systematic review of nonpharmacologic treatments for behavioral disorders associated with ABI, Cattelani, Zettin, and Zoccolotti (18) found single-case evidence for the efficacy of ABA procedures that used contingency management or positive behavior interventions or combined these 2 approaches. Contingency management involves regulating the consequences of the patient's behavior so that desirable behaviors are rewarded and undesirable behaviors are not rewarded or are punished. Positive behavior interventions also involves designing contingencies to reward positive behaviors as well as antecedent interventions to encourage positive behaviors (e.g., modeling, prompting) and to prevent maladaptive behavior (e.g., stimulus control, environmental structuring).

Residential Treatment

Community reintegration is a goal for most residential brain injury rehabilitation programs. However, at the time of their admission, most patients in these programs require a supervised and supportive environment because of significant

cognitive and behavioral as well as physical impairments that serve as severe obstacles to successful independent living in more traditional community settings. In some cases, the primary reason for residential placement is that the family or SO is unable to provide adequate supervision and support for the patient in a community setting. Behavioral dysfunction among patients in residential programs is usually not sufficiently severe to put them at high risk of harm to self or others. The patient's environment and activities are usually supervised and monitored but not highly restricted. Rehabilitation is delivered by the full complement of rehabilitation disciplines (physical therapy, occupational therapy, speech therapy, recreational therapy, rehabilitation psychology or neuropsychology) and by other providers and medical consultants as required. The approach is typically transdisciplinary, that is, rehabilitation is delivered in a coordinated fashion by a team that communicates frequently and is able to assume each other's roles temporarily when the need arises. Pharmacologic treatment and ABA are frequently used to assist in addressing more severe behavioral and emotional dysregulation.

Although the setting is residential, these programs share many characteristics in common with outpatient holistic day treatment programs. Consequently, studies of holistic day treatment (reported subsequently) are relevant to some degree in evaluating the effectiveness of residential treatment. A difference between outpatient day treatment and residential programs is perhaps a greater emphasis on the use of ABA in residential programs. ABA programs can be applied more consistently in residential settings because of greater control over the patient's social environment. Pharmacologic treatment may also be more actively managed in residential settings because of increased opportunity to monitor the effects of medications and adjust judiciously. Another important difference is that residential programs can provide more structured learning opportunities directed by professional staff throughout the day (and night). For instance, in a residential setting, meals are an opportunity to teach food preparation, and community outings can be structured to train social skills and how to use of money and public transportation.

The Braunling-McMorrow study (17) described previously documented significant improvement in functional status as a result of residential treatment and maintenance of gains at 1-year follow-up (Figure 77-3). Further examination of Figure 77-3 reveals that the residential treatment group made greater gains than a group with greater behavioral and psychosocial dysfunction who were triaged to a neurobehavioral treatment program. Residential treatment appeared more effective with those admitted within 6 months post-ABI; however, time since injury did not impact the effectiveness of neurobehavioral treatment.

Seale and colleagues (19) reported that community integration as measured by the Community Integration Questionnaire (CIQ) improved significantly for a cohort of 87 individuals involved in a residential rehabilitation program. Improvement was greater for those admitted within 1 year of injury than for those admitted 1–5 years postinjury (see Figure 77-4). The Eicher study (9) described previously also included a cohort of 78 individuals who received intensive rehabilitation in residential treatment centers. Some of these programs may have more closely resembled neurobehavioral programs. Significant gains were made by the individu-

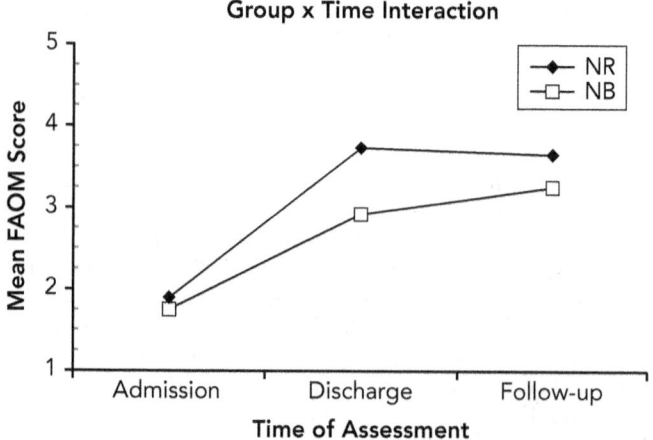

FIGURE 77-3 Changes in on the functional assessment outcome menu (FAOM) at admission, discharge, and 12-month follow-up for individuals in neurobehavioral (NB) and neurorehabilitation (NR) programs (17).

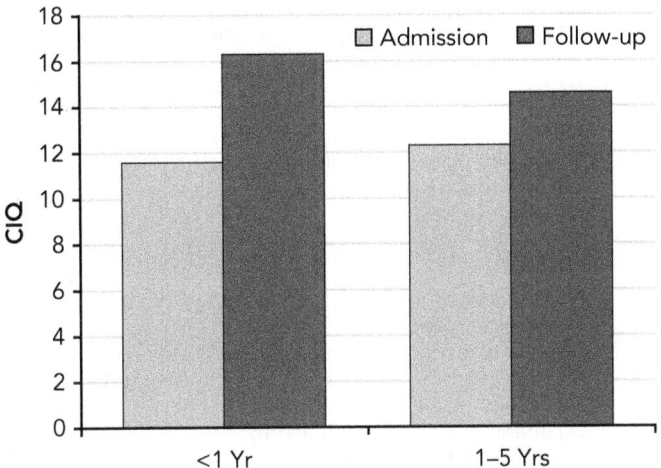

FIGURE 77-4 Community integration questionnaire (CIQ) at admission to residential rehabilitation and at 6-month follow-up for individuals admitted < 1 and 1–5 years postinjury (19).

als in this cohort even though many were admitted years after injury (See Figure 77-1). The average time postinjury for individuals included in the Eicher study was greater than 7 years.

Traditional Outpatient Rehabilitation

Delivered in a health care clinic or outpatient facility, traditional outpatient rehabilitation focuses on reducing impairment. It is a single discipline or multidisciplinary activity, that is, more than 1 discipline may work with the patient; however, each therapist addresses a specific set of impairments and does so in relative isolation with little or no cross-disciplinary consultation or coordination. For individuals with a small number of circumscribed impairments, reasonable self-awareness of their disabilities and the capacity to formulate reasonable goals in collaboration with their therapist(s), traditional outpatient rehabilitation is both appropriate and effective. Although data are not available to make a confident estimate, clinical experience suggests that a majority of individuals with ABI can benefit from such short term and focused rehabilitation. Research is not available regarding the effectiveness of traditional outpatient rehabilitation on a programmatic level. However, for example, an extensive literature demonstrates the efficacy of single modality cognitive rehabilitation interventions including specific treatments to improve language and social communication skills (20–22) (see also Cicerone, Chapter 61).

Home- and Community-Based Rehabilitation

Traditional outpatient rehabilitation focuses on reducing impairment with the expectation that improved functional abilities will transfer to the real world and translate into increased community participation. Although these expectations may be logical, they ignore the limitations in generalization of learning that are often present among most individuals with ABI. In contrast, home- and community-based rehabilitation (HCBR) attempts to enhance generalization of learning by providing training in the patient's real world environment. Providing rehabilitation in the same or similar environment to that in which the actual activity will take

place in real life reduces concern that skills learned in an artificial clinical setting will fail to transfer to the real world. Costs of care are also reduced by minimizing facility-related expenses. Along these same lines, the goals of HCBR are more often focused on directly increasing functional activities and community participation rather than on reducing impairment. Because goals are more directly linked to real world functioning, service provision tends to be interdisciplinary rather than multidisciplinary with therapists from various disciplines providing coordinated treatment linked to achieving real world, functional goals.

Patients appropriate for this type of program must be able to live in the community with, at most, partial supervision and thus are generally less severely and pervasively disabled than those admitted to residential or day treatment programs. With a transdisciplinary approach, impaired self-awareness on the part of the patient can be addressed in the context of HCBR. Therapy conducted in real life settings provides opportunities to demonstrate to the patient both the difficulties of which they are unaware as well as ways to overcome or work around these impairments. Nonetheless, some patients with very limited self-awareness may require residential or day treatment. Often key to the success of HCBR is family or SO who are actively engaged in the therapeutic process and assist the patient in continuing activities that will support the maintenance of gains after formal therapy has ended.

Altman and colleagues (23) described results of HCBR for a national sample of 489 individuals with TBI who completed the full rehabilitation program compared to 114 individuals who were precipitously discharged from the program. The sample included participants from seven programs in geographically distinct cities in the US within a privately owned rehabilitation system (Rehab Without Walls; RWW). The group that completed the full rehabilitation program made greater gains than the group who only completed a partial program (Figure 77-5). Although an unfortunately large percentage of both groups were lost to follow-up, available data at 3 months and 12 months postdischarge documents continued gains in functional status. Chronicity appeared to affect program outcome. Compared to the entire cohort, gains for a smaller group of participants completing the full treatment but admitted more than 1 year postinjury were not as great and appeared nonexistent for

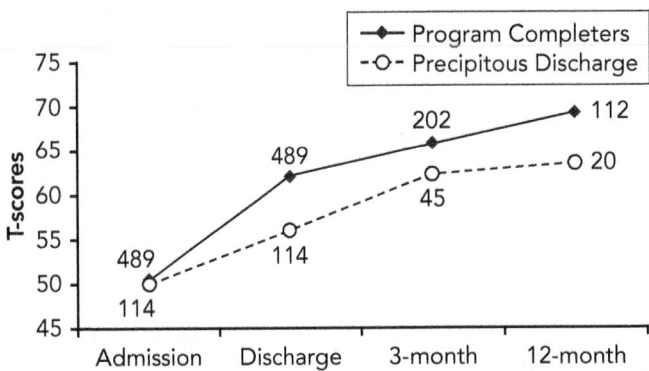

FIGURE 77-5 Mayo-Portland Adaptability Inventory (MPAI-4) participation index T-score by group on admission, discharge, 3- and 12-month follow-up (23); numbers in graph indicate numbers of participants at each time point.

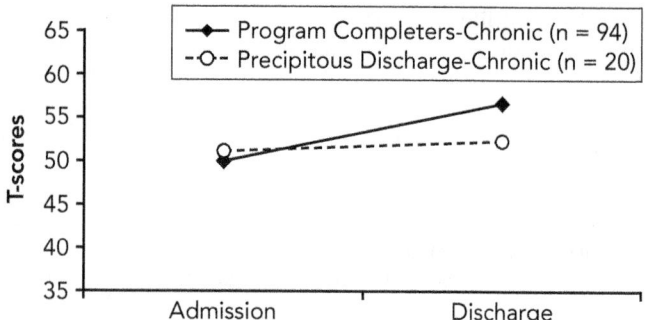

FIGURE 77-6 Mayo-Portland Adaptability Inventory (MPAI-4) total T-score score for chronic cases (time since injury > 1 year) by group at admission and discharge (23).

the precipitously discharged group admitted more than 1 year postinjury (Figure 77-6). The Altman study provides a description of the methods used by the RWW system in their HCBR programs.

The Eicher study (9) also reported on a cohort served in community-based rehabilitation programs. Participants in these programs made significant gains over the study period (Figure 77-1). Although gains were not as great as in the Altman study, participants in the Eicher study were generally more chronic (average time since injury > 7 years) than the Altman group most of whom entered HCBR within the first year of injury. The Eicher study also did not report final discharge status for all participants but rather looked at progress over a specified period of time (6–9 months) during which participants were engaged in various types of intensive and supportive rehabilitation programs.

Outpatient Holistic Day Treatment

Holistic day treatment (HDT) was originally developed by Yehuda Ben-Yishay and elaborated by George Prigatano (24–25). This approach emphasizes multimodality therapy that addresses the range of psychological, social, behavioral, physical, and cognitive disabilities that can occur after ABI. Therapy is delivered primarily in groups in a therapeutic environment (milieu) by a transdisciplinary team. Ben-Yishay's program in Manhattan was one of the first posthospital rehabilitation programs for ABI available in the US, and many of the methods developed in his program form the basis of approaches to brain injury rehabilitation that continue to be used in posthospital rehabilitation programs of all types. A recently published volume (26) by Ben-Yishay and Leonard Diller provides a very detailed description of these methods and includes examples of therapeutic interventions and activities on an accompanying set of DVDs. In 1994, Yehuda Ben-Yishay, Leonard Diller, Anne-Lise Christiansen, Pamela Klonoff (from George Prigatano's program) and others participated in a consensus conference convened by Lance Trexler in Zionsville, Indiana (27) and identified the key element of holistic day treatment (Table 77-3).

In this author's opinion, individuals best served through HDT are those with severe and pervasive disabilities due to ABI including impaired self-awareness which require the intensity of this form of treatment. The group milieu provides an opportunity to address impaired self-awareness through group process and peer feedback that cannot be

TABLE 77-3 Defining Features of Holistic Day Treatment

I. Neuropsychological orientation focusing on

   A. Cognitive and metacognitive impairments
   B. Neurobehavioral impairments
   C. Interpersonal and psychosocial issues
   D. Affective issues

II. Integrated treatment that includes

   A. Formal staff meetings with core team in attendance 4 times per week
   B. A team leader or manager for each patient
   C. A program leader or manager with at least 3 years experience in BI rehabilitation
   D. Integrated goal setting and monitoring
   E. Transdisciplinary staff roles

III. Group interventions that address

   A. Awareness
   B. Acceptance
   C. Social pragmatics

IV. Dedicated resources, including

   A. An identified core team
   B. Dedicated space
   C. A patient to staff ratio no greater than 2:1

V. A neuropsychologist is part of the treatment team, not just a consultant.

VI. Formal and informal opportunities for involvement of significant others including systematic inclusion of significant others on a weekly basis

VII. Inclusion of a dedicated vocational or independent living trial

VIII. Multiple outcomes are assessed, including

   A. Productive activity
   B. Independent living
   C. Psychosocial adjustment
   D. Emotional adjustment

From Malec and Basford (5), based on Trexler et al. (27).

replicated in HCBR or traditional outpatient treatment. In order to successfully reintegrate into work and community life, patients with severe and pervasive cognitive and behavioral disabilities including impaired self-awareness may require holistic treatment on a daily basis for 6 months or more. Although data are not available to accurately estimate the percentage of individuals with ABI who require this intensive form of treatment, clinical experience suggests that the percentage is relatively small (< 10%) of hospital admissions for ABI who experience persistent deficits. A small group of these will require similar treatment in a residential setting because of a higher need for supervision or safety concerns.

A number of uncontrolled and quasi-experimental studies reviewed by Cicerone and associates (20–22) have documented the benefits of HDT. Cicerone and his colleagues at the JFK Johnson Rehabilitation Center in New Jersey also reported a randomized controlled trial demonstrating superior outcomes for 22 participants in HDT compared to 22 patients participating in traditional outpatient rehabilitation

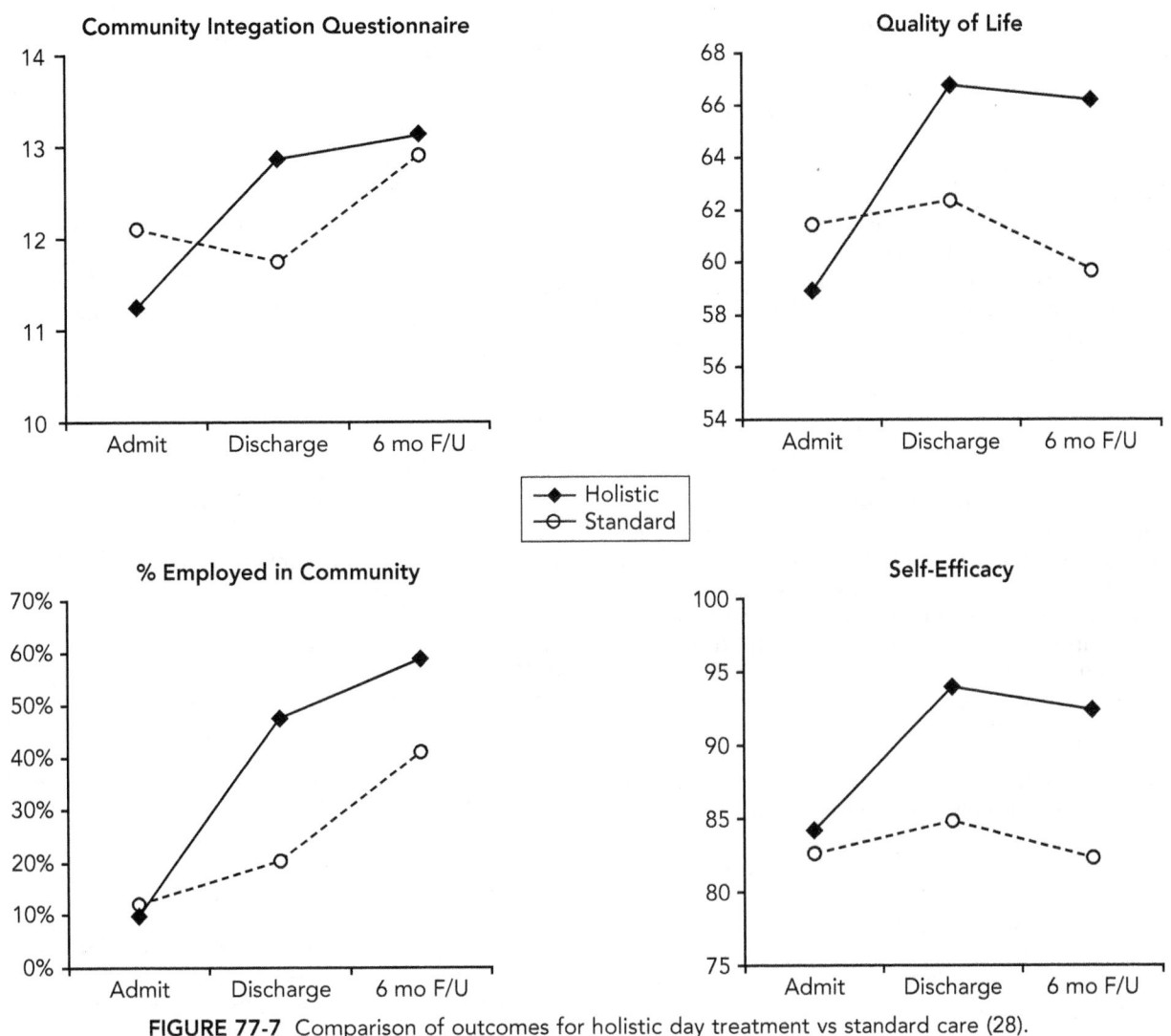

FIGURE 77-7 Comparison of outcomes for holistic day treatment vs standard care (28).

(28). Those in the HDT program showed more rapid gains in community integration on the CIQ than the control group. The control group (who continued to receive services and therapy after HDT was discontinued for the treatment group) achieved similar gains in community integration to the HDT group over the 6-month follow-up period. However, the HDT group showed greater quality of life, self-efficacy and vocational achievement both at discharge and follow-up (Figure 77-7).

Diversity Within Program Types

As Glenn and associates reported (3,4), there is great diversity among both residential- and community-based posthospital brain injury rehabilitation programs. Within any of the categories described previously and in Table 77-1 and 77-2, exist a wide variety of programs using a variety of methods. For instance, a typical Clubhouse program has been described as a community-based supportive rehabilitation program; however, participants in some Clubhouse programs may be actively engaged in intensive rehabilitation organized by the membership of the Clubhouse. Neurobehavioral programs differ widely in their use of pharmacology, ABA,

as well as family counseling and other social and psychological interventions. Some residential facilities involve their residents extensively in community activities and closely resemble HCBR programs in this regard, whereas some HCBR programs work with individuals with very severe and pervasive impairments who are more typically served in residential or day treatment programs. With this in mind, the broad categories of posthospital program types offered here should be considered an effort to "bring order out of chaos" which hopefully has some validity but also does not entirely capture the broad diversity of posthospital brain injury rehabilitation programs. Identification of the most beneficial programmatic approaches to achieve well-specified goals for well-specified patients remains a challenge to the field which, when achieved, will result in more consistent protocol-based posthospital rehabilitation care.

POSTHOSPITAL PROGRAM METHODS

Review of the various types of posthospital programs (Table 77-1 and 77-2) reveals specific methods that are used to a greater or lesser degree across many program types. Most programs use traditional rehabilitation therapies (i.e., physical, occupation, speech therapies) to some degree. Among intensive programs, those that are designed for patients with more severe cognitive impairment tend to rely, at least initially, on interventions that are managed external to the patient (e.g., pharmacology, ABA, family or SO training, other environmental interventions). Whereas, those programs in which patients have more intact cognitive abilities and greater self-awareness tend to rely more heavily on developing self-management skills through cognitive rehabilitation, cognitive-behavioral therapy, and group therapy. Many of these specific methods are discussed in detail elsewhere in this volume (for example, see chapters on pharmacology, ABA, cognitive rehabilitation). Two additional methods that are commonly used deserve further discussion: cognitive-behavioral therapy and group therapy.

Traditional **cognitive-behavioral* therapy (CBT)**, as described in the clinical psychology and psychiatry literature, is based on the observation that beliefs and internal (nonvocalized) statements have a primary effect on guiding human emotion and behavior (29). In other words, what human beings say to themselves about their immediate reality directly results in how they feel about and interact with that reality. Maladaptive behavior or emotions result from inaccurate or unconstructive cognitions. For instance, if a person with ABI consistently tells themselves that their life is "awful and intolerable" since their injury, they are likely to become depressed and even suicidal. A CBT therapist assists the patient in challenging these beliefs. In the example, both "awful and intolerable" are entirely subjective and relative appraisals. A CBT therapist engages the patient in considering ways in which their life could become less awful and intolerable. However, the CBT approach is not simply a process of focusing on the positive. Rather, CBT is training to identify subjective and relative statements like "awful and intolerable" as red flags that can prompt an effort to consider the situation more rationally and develop a plan to improve it. The plan for improvement begins the behavioral component of CBT, that is, not only is the patient involved in reappraising the distressing situation in a more rational and constructive way but then in planning how to take action to address the situation more adaptively. Because CBT is based on self-reflection and self-monitoring, it is probably not an appropriate intervention for individuals with severe cognitive impairments. However, recent studies suggest that CBT can be effective for some individuals with ABI (30–32).

Group Therapy

Therapy in groups is not the same as group therapy. Rehabilitation therapies of many types, including psychological therapy, can be delivered to 1 patient at a time in a group situation in which other members of the group observe and support. In contrast, group therapy is a process in which psychological adaptation and behavioral change is encouraged through group interaction and by expert therapeutic use of the group dynamic. For individuals with ABI, group therapy is particularly effective to address impaired self-awareness. Individuals with impaired self-awareness will

often deny and resist information given to them by doctors and therapists regarding their impairments and disabilities. However, these same individuals will often attend to similar feedback given to them from other individuals with brain injuries. Most of us listen most attentively to people whom we consider our peers, and people with ABI are no different.

For feedback from peers to be effective, however, typically requires that the feedback be given repeatedly from multiple sources and tied to behavioral examples that support the feedback. (For example, "I think you have a memory problem because you keep forgetting things that we schedule to do together.") Group therapy provides an ideal setting to provide such feedback if managed expertly by the therapist. Effectively managed group therapy also provides an ideal environment to balance feedback with support, for participants to share and, in this way, normalize intense emotional experiences, and for participants to observe, model and practice adaptive behaviors and emotional responses. Group therapy typically plays a significant role in holistic treatment programs and may underlie the success of these programs. Limited research in the use of group therapy with individuals with ABI supports its effectiveness in improving self-awareness and social communication skills (33,34). Backhaus and her colleagues (30) reported results of a group program that included participants with ABI and a family member or SO. Her program combined CBT and education with standard group therapy techniques and resulted in significant improvement in participants' self-efficacy which, in turn, appeared to prevent future emotional distress.

PROGRAM PHILOSOPHIES AND ORGANIZATION

In addition to diversity in the array and configuration of specific therapeutic methods and techniques employed, programs also differ in their treatment philosophy and organization.

Team Orientation

Almost all rehabilitation programs involve a team of treating providers. However, the team may be configured in several ways, each of which is appropriate to address a particular set of treatment goals.

A *multidisciplinary* team is one in which each of the treatment providers addresses a specific treatment goal consistent with their expertise with little or no interaction with other providers. Multidisciplinary treatment is appropriate for patients who have reasonable awareness of a small set of circumscribed problems. For instance, in a multidisciplinary treatment setting, an individual with mild memory impairment and gait instability in the absence of other significant associated impairments is treated by a physical therapist to improve gait and by another provider (e.g., occupational therapist, speech therapist, or psychologist) to develop memory compensation techniques.

An *interdisciplinary* team also addresses specific treatment goals consistent with disciplinary expertise but does so in a coordinated fashion in order to mutually reinforce progress. Treatment planning and coordination is accomplished through regular case conferences. An interdisciplinary approach is most appropriate and effective for patients with multiple problems and disabilities which can com-

---

* "Cognitive-behavioral" may have a different meaning in some rehabilitation circles where it is used to refer to interventions that combine cognitive rehabilitation with behavioral intervention and support.

pound each other. For instance, in an interdisciplinary treatment setting, a patient who has memory problems, gait instability, and depression is treated by (a) a physical therapist for gait instability and who also encourages the patient to use their memory notebook to keep track of their exercise compliance; (b) by a psychologist for depression who also assists the patient in focusing on reframing gait instability as a "problem to be overcome" rather than a frustrating and embarrassing disability; and (c) by an occupational therapist who is training the patient in memory compensation techniques and also prompts the patient to use cognitive-behavioral methods recommended by the psychologist to reduce self-criticism about memory impairment. Most intensive rehabilitation programs that admit complex patients use an interdisciplinary approach and many use a transdisciplinary model.

A *transdisciplinary* team is one in which providers from various disciplines not only provide treatment in a coordinated fashion but are also able to temporarily adopt each other's roles in treating the patient. This high level of coordination and mutual trust within the team requires frequent team communication. Each team member is not only aware of but is also sufficiently versed in the recommended treatment approach of other team members to be able to provide interventions at a fundamental level for which other team members are primarily responsible. A transdisciplinary approach is required for patients with severe cognitive impairment and impaired self-awareness who require an immediate and consistent response to critical behaviors in order to make progress. For instance, a patient with severe cognitive limitations and difficulty in anger management will not benefit from simply being told to "take it to the psychologist" when anger emerges. Rather, each team member must be sufficiently schooled in how to respond to the patient's anger to do so therapeutically. Similarly, some physical disabilities require a consistent approach to improve function whether the physical activity emerges during a memory group, a social skills group, or a community outing. Transdisciplinary teams are most common in intensive residential or day treatment programs. (This high level of team integration and role flexibility characterizes most high-performance teams. For instance, special forces military teams typically have well-defined roles but must be able to assume each other's roles at critical junctures when one or more members may be compromised.)

Treatment Milieu

To some degree, the social environment in which treatment is delivered varies with team orientation. For instance, programs provided by a transdisciplinary team also typically emphasize the importance of the *therapeutic milieu*. In a therapeutic milieu, an attempt is made to orchestrate all interactions in the treatment setting and design the interpersonal and physical environment in order to support patient progress and goal achievement. In a therapeutic milieu, therapists not only convey optimism, support, and task orientation but also consciously develop an integrative environment in which most interactions and activities have a therapeutic orientation. These transdisciplinary and interdisciplinary settings differ from a more focused, multidisciplinary setting in which any interactions beyond that between the patient and the treating therapist are considered irrelevant.

Explicit Development of Therapeutic Alliance

Therapeutic alliance refers to the positive relationship, characterized by mutual trust, positive regard, and shared goals between provider and patient in a treatment program. Therapeutic alliance has been identified as a significant variable in psychotherapy outcome and more recently has been found to significantly enhance outcomes in posthospital brain injury rehabilitation (35–37). In the psychotherapy literature, therapeutic alliance has been considered a "necessary but not sufficient" condition for positive behavioral change (38,39). In other words, a secure alliance between patient and therapist is required for therapeutic change but will not cause that change in and of itself. Additional specific procedures are required to effect behavior change and generalization. The same may be true in rehabilitation although this question has not been addressed in research to date. Most programs and therapists seek to develop a positive working relationship with their patients with varying degrees of success. A higher level of clinical sophistication characterizes programs in which the therapeutic alliance is explicitly monitored and interventions, including changing therapists, are implemented if a positive alliance is not developing.

Impairment Focus vs Outcome Focus

Traditional outpatient rehabilitation tends to be impairment focused. Patients are referred for specific therapies in order to address the remediation of specific impairments, or as a result of a multidisciplinary evaluation, an array of impairments are identified that become the targets of an array of multidisciplinary or interdisciplinary treatments. This same approach of developing a comprehensive problem list and a corresponding treatment plan to address each identified problem may also characterize some more integrated programs. However, more frequently, highly integrated, intensive treatment programs are outcome focused. That is, participation goals, such as independent living or return to work, are identified as the primary objectives of the program and the patient's strengths and weaknesses are assessed as they relate to these goals. Strengths that support goal achievement are further developed. Remediation procedures or training in compensation strategies are implemented to address weaknesses (i.e., impairments) that serve as obstacles to achievement of the identified participation goals. An outcome-focused model of rehabilitation does not address the patient's impairments that are not relevant to achievement of participation goals. The outcome-focused approach more closely resembles the pursuit of life goals during a normal transition into adulthood. Most successful people make a place for themselves in their communities in which they can capitalize on their strengths and minimize their weaknesses (although these weaknesses remain). In many ways, the outcome-focused approach follows Covey's (40) exhortation "to begin with the end in mind."

Inclusion of Adjunctive and Environmental Interventions

Programs also differ in their inclusion of interventions to address comorbidities as well as social and environmental factors that are relevant to participation goals. Examples of these are preventive and specific treatments for substance abuse; involvement of family and significant others; and development of a social resource network outside of the treatment setting. Some programs have admission criteria that require involvement of family or an SO or exclude patients with active substance abuse. Other programs include these issues in the treatment plan. If adjunctive treatment is required to address issues such as family problems or substance abuse, this may be done as (*a*) a requirement for admission to the rehabilitation program; (*b*) separately and in parallel with the rehabilitation program; or (*c*) in an integrated fashion with rehabilitation. HCBR programs are more likely than facility-based programs to assist patients and families or SO to develop support and service networks as part of the rehabilitation program—although not all make this an explicit goal of the program.

Adjunctive and environmental interventions may take many forms. A few of the most common forms are discussed in the next section.

Environmental and Adjunctive Interventions

Family or SO Involvement or Intervention. Family issues are discussed in depth in Chapter 38; consequently, only a few considerations specific to family involvement in posthospital rehabilitation programs will be reviewed here. Most programs provide opportunities for families or SO to learn more about brain injury and the treatment that is being provided to their loved one. In many cases, family support and education is provided through the program as well as through collaborations with state brain injury associations. In programs that emphasize external management of the participant's behaviors through ABA, understanding and consistency in following through with the behavior intervention plan outside of the treatment setting by family or SO is essential for maintenance of positive behavior changes achieved in the treatment setting.

Special considerations in involving families in the rehabilitation program include recognition that not all families or SO provide a positive influence on the patient's care. Although in the minority, some families or SO may reinforce excessive dependency, codependency, or maladaptive behavior. A percentage of individuals with ABI are injured at a time in life when they are transitioning out of the family structure and into independent adulthood. A brain injury can necessitate a return to dependence on the family for a period of time. However, at some point, movement back out of the family into a more independent lifestyle may be appropriate. Ideally, this is done with the support of the family. However, in some cases, the family may inappropriately resist the quest for adult independence of the individual with ABI, and the treatment team finds themselves in the uncomfortable but therapeutically necessary position of supporting the patient's wishes to exclude family or SO from their care and function independently.

Sander et al. (41) found that approximately one-fourth to one-third of families are experiencing some degree of unhealthy family functioning at the time that one of their members experiences a brain injury. Significant preinjury family pathology may escape notice by the rehabilitation team because the stress within the family is believed to be a reaction to the injury. No doubt the stress of brain injury intensifies family distress. However, in cases involving preinjury family pathology, a more intensive treatment approach provided by a specialist in family therapy may be required than the typical education and support that is offered to families as part of most rehabilitation programs. Ideally, these more intensive family services will be provided in collaboration with rehabilitation services. Providing this level of family therapy, however, is often challenging. A family specialist with an understanding of ABI who can collaborate with the rehabilitation team is often difficult to identify in a given community. Furthermore, even when family therapy services are available, funding for these services may not be. Consequently, many posthospital rehabilitation programs are unable to provide this level of service.

Alcohol and Other Substance Abuse Treatment. Identification, treatment, and prevention of alcohol and substance-abuse related problems are thoroughly discussed in Chapter 79 of this volume. A significant minority of individuals participating in posthospital rehabilitation programs will have a history of substance abuse or a current disorder. Most rehabilitation programs will not accept individuals with an active substance abuse disorder unless they agree to participate in treatment as part of the rehabilitation process and maintain sobriety. Some programs require a history of sobriety for a period of time (e.g., 6 months) prior to admission to the program, and this may be justified in cases of chronic or severe dependency in which the likelihood of relapse during program participation is very high. As with family services, substance abuse treatment, when provided simultaneously with posthospital rehabilitation, is ideally provided in collaboration with the rehabilitation program with regular communication between the providers of both types of services. Nonetheless, as with family services, it is often challenging to find substance abuse treatment providers who have experience or are willing to gain experience in working with individuals with ABI. In negotiating, such cooperative treatment arrangements, it may be useful for rehabilitation staff to increase substance abuse treatment staff's awareness that many of their typical clientele may have a history of at least mild brain injury that has previously gone unrecognized.

Vocational Services and Resource Facilitation. Many programs provide vocational services through referral to state vocational services. In most cases, this referral is not adequate to ensure sustained placement in community-based employment because most vocational counselors do not have adequate experience or resources to assist individuals with significant disabilities after ABI to obtain and sustain employment. Past studies suggest that less than 40% of individuals with significant ABI return to work (42–43). However, a number of research and demonstration projects have shown that, with specialized vocational services, a much higher percentage (70%–80%) can sustain employment in the community (42).

Fadyl and McPherson (44) identified 3 broad categories of specialized vocational services for individuals with ABI: (*a*) program-based, that is, specialized services, such as work trials, are provided in the context of a rehabilitation program; (*b*) supported employment, that is, on-the-job assistance, such as job coaching, is provided temporarily or long term; (*c*) case management, more currently termed *resource facilitation*, in which a designated individual assists the person with ABI to develop a network of medical and community-based supports for vocational and community reintegration. Fundamental features (44) a resource facilitation approach including the following:

(1) a resource facilitator to assist the individual with ABI to develop

    (a) a self-directed plan for vocational and community reintegration and

    (b) a network of medical center and community services and support;

(2) early medical, rehabilitative, independent living, and vocational intervention;

(3) work or independent living trials;

(4) temporary or long-term supports and coaching; and

(5) family or SO, employer and coworker education.

Two large cohort studies (45, 46) and a randomized controlled trial (47) have demonstrated the success of resource facilitation approach with up to 80% of the studied cohorts sustaining employment in the community for at least 1 year following placement. In addition to superior employment outcomes, Trexler et al. (47) demonstrated significantly better community integration and participation for the group receiving resource facilitation compared to controls.

OUTCOME MEASUREMENT

The accrediting agency for rehabilitation facilities (CARF International) mandates outcome measurement in all rehabilitation programs. There is general agreement that outcome measurement is essential in posthospital rehabilitation (*a*) to provide ongoing data for continuing quality improvement of programs and practices, (*b*) to inform prospective participants about the effectiveness of programs for individuals with specified problems and characteristics, and (*c*) to support advocacy for rehabilitation and rehabilitation funding generally and in the individual case. However, unlike inpatient rehabilitation in which the FIM™ (48) has become the gold standard for outcome evaluation, there is no clear consensus regarding the most appropriate measure(s) to be used to evaluate post-hospital rehabilitation.

This lack of consensus has resulted in a plethora of measures used including many "home grown" scales of uncertain validity, making it difficult for providers to identify industry benchmarks or to advocate in a unified manner for themselves and their patients. In recent years, there has been growing support of the use of the Mayo-Portland Adaptability Inventory, (now in its fourth edition; MPAI-4), as a posthospital assessment and outcome measure. The MPAI-4 has well-established, high-quality psychometric properties (49–51) and was recommended as a supplemental measure to the brief Core Battery endorsed by the NIH Common Data Elements consensus conference (52). The measure, a manual for its use, and non-English translations are available for download on the Center for Outcome Measurement website (53). Psychometric studies have shown the MPAI-4 to represent a unitary construct of outcome after acquired brain injury that can be reliably divided into correlated subcomponents for the measurement of physical and cognitive ability, psychological and interpersonal adjustment, and community participation (49–50). The measure is a rating scale that is ideally completed by consensus of an evaluating rehabilitation team but can be completed by a single provider who is knowledgeable about the patient. The measure can also be completed by the person with ABI and by a significant other for comparison. With funding from the National Insti-

tute for Neurological Disease and Stroke (NINDS) (54), a web-based outcome measurement system is under development in collaboration with Inventive Software Solutions (55). The MPAI-4 is the core measure of this system which allows providers to enter outcome data as well as demographic, medical, and other patient data into a HIPAA-compliant, secure national database. Reports can be generated from the database to assist in the evaluation of individual program participants and their progress, the rehabilitation program overall, and for anonymous comparison with other programs in the database that serve similar patients and use similar methods. As it develops, this national database should serve as a resource for rehabilitation researchers.

CONCLUSION

The current landscape of posthospital brain injury rehabilitation programs is characterized by a great deal of diversity in characteristics of these programs. In a general way, programs can be described as providing supportive services primarily designed to assist individuals with ABI to maintain their current status or as more intensive with goals of improving health, functional abilities, and community participation. Programs can be further characterized by the level of supervision, the level of medical or nursing care, whether services are provided in a facility or in home and community settings, whether the approach is milieu-oriented, and by the style of team function, that is, multidisciplinary, interdisciplinary, or transdisciplinary. The diversity of programs may reflect the heterogeneity of characteristics of individuals with ABI. The diversity of program structures is confusing to both consumers and payers who have no clear description of the nature of or options for posthospital rehabilitation. A goal for the field is to move toward more consistency and definition in service provision through specific arrays of protocol-based services.

Although differing in overall structure, most programs mix-and-match a small set of interventions (e.g., pharmacology, ABA, cognitive rehabilitation, traditional rehabilitation therapies, family or SO involvement and support) to provide a highly individualized program for each person served. The benefits of adjunctive and supportive services, such as family therapy, substance abuse interventions, and resource facilitation, have become increasingly apparent in the research and professional literature. However, such services delivered in a coordinated fashion with posthospital rehabilitation services, are not available in most communities.

Although there is no doubt that there is a period of readiness for rehabilitation that varies among individual patients, the literature is consistent in suggesting that early involvement in posthospital rehabilitation, that is, within the first year after injury, results in the greatest gains. To some degree, these greater gains may reflect continuing natural recovery and adjustment. However, individuals who do not have access to posthospital rehabilitation services early on typically develop a number of other problems that serve as obstacles to successful rehabilitation. In individuals with ABI who receive inadequate rehabilitation and follow along, common secondary complications include substance abuse, mood disorders, marital family problems, chronic unemployment, and social alienation.

Research generally supports the effectiveness of the various types of rehabilitation programs reviewed here to achieve stated goals of the program for most participants.

The methodology of reported studies, particularly at the programmatic level, rarely meets the gold standard in medicine of the randomized controlled trial. However, a number of factors (e.g., heterogeneous and small-numbered samples, ethical and humanitarian issues, difficulty in blinding) argue against the appropriateness of the randomized controlled trial for this type of research. Future research may more productively use alternative experimental and quasi-experimental designs ranging from n-of-1 and n-of-1 with multiple replications to large community-based observational studies that include examination of dose-response relationships between levels of rehabilitation provided and outcomes (56–57). In both research and practice, posthospital rehabilitation continues to evolve toward more clearly defined, evidence-based therapies and approaches that can be offered to more clearly characterized patients with increasing specificity.

KEY CLINICAL POINTS

1. Post-hospital brain injury rehabilitation programs are highly diverse and challenging to classify.
2. Very broadly, programs can be described as (1) supportive with goals of assisting individuals with ABI to maintain their current status or (2) more intensive with goals of improving health, functional abilities, and community participation.
3. Programs can be further distinguished by the (1) level of supervision and, (2) the level of medical/nursing care provided to those served, (3) setting, i.e., residential or outpatient facility or home and community-based services, (4) whether the approach is milieu-oriented, and (5) by style of team function, i.e., multi-, inter-, or transdisciplinary.
4. The diversity of programs mirrors the heterogeneity of individuals with ABI; currently most post-hospital programs mix-and-match interventions to provide a highly individualized program for each person served.
5. Program diversity can be confusing to both consumers and payers; offering more consistent and well-defined arrays of protocol-based services is a goal for the field.
6. Adjunctive and supportive services delivered in a coordinated fashion with post-hospital rehabilitation services are beneficial but unavailable in most communities.
7. Although patients vary in readiness for rehabilitation, early involvement in post-hospital rehabilitation, i.e., within the first year after injury, results in the greatest gains. Individuals with ABI who receive inadequate rehabilitation and follow-along, commonly develop secondary complications, such as, substance abuse, mood disorders, marital family problems, chronic unemployment, and social alienation.
8. Available research generally supports the effectiveness of posthospital rehabilitation; future research would benefit from employing a range of methodologies and designs.

KEY REFERENCES

1. Glenn MB, Goldstein R, Selleck EA, Rotman M. Characteristics of facility-based community integration programs for people with brain injury. *J Head Trauma Rehabil.* 2004; 19(6):482–493.

2. Glenn MB, Selleck EA, Goldstein R, Rotman M. Characteristics of home-based community integration programmes for adults with brain injury. *Brain Inj.* 2005;19(14): 1243–1247.
3. High WM, Sander AM, Struchen MA, Hart KA, eds. *Rehabilitation for Traumatic Brain Injury.* New York, NY: Oxford; 2005.
4. Malec JF, ed. *New Methodologies for Intervention and Outcome Measurement.* Hove and New York: Psychology Press; 2009.

ACKNOWLEDGMENT

The author is grateful to the following people for their careful review and suggestions for improvement of an earlier draft of this chapter. Irwin M. Altman, PhD, MBA, Area Executive Director, Rehab Without Walls®; Vicki Eicher, MSW, Director of Quality Management & Training and Mary Pat Murphy, MSN, CRRN, CBIST, Vice President of Clinical Services, ReMed; and Debra Braunling-McMorrow, PhD, Consultant, Carbondale, IL.

References

1. Kreutzer JS, Kolakowsky-Hayner SA, Ripley D, et al. Charges and lengths of stay for acute and inpatient rehabilitation treatment of traumatic brain injury 1990–1996. *Brain Inj.* 2001;15(9):763–774.
2. Ottenbacher KJ, Smith PM, Illig SB, Fiedler RC, Granger CV. Length of stay and hospital readmissions for persons with disabilities. *Am J Public Health.* 2000;90(12):1920–1923.
3. Glenn MB, Goldstein R, Selleck EA, Rotman M. Characteristics of facility-based community integration programs for people with brain injury. *J Head Trauma Rehabil.* 2004;19(6):482–493.
4. Glenn MB, Selleck EA, Goldstein R, Rotman M. Characteristics of home-based community integration programmes for adults with brain injury. *Brain Inj.* 2005;19(14):1243–1247.
5. Malec JF, Basford JS. Postacute brain injury rehabilitation. *Arch Phys Med Rehabil.* 1996;77(2):198–207.
6. Meyer MJ, Megyesi J, Meythaler J, et al. Acute management of acquired brain injury Part III: an evidence-based review of interventions used to promote arousal from coma. *Brain Inj.* 2010;24(5): 722–729.
7. Vanier M, Lamoureux J, Dutil E, Houde S. Clinical efficacy of stimulation programs aimed at reversing coma or vegetative state (VS) following traumatic brain injury. *Acta Neurochir Suppl.* 2002;79: 53–57.
8. Penna S, Novack TA, Carlson N, Grote M, Corrigan JD, Hart T. Residence following traumatic brain injury: a longitudinal study. *J Head Trauma Rehabil.* 2010;25(1):52–60.
9. Eicher V, Murphy MP, Murphy TF, Malec JF. Progress assessed with the Mayo-Portland Adaptability Inventory in 604 participants in 4 types of post-inpatient rehabilitation brain injury programs. *Arch Phys Med Rehabil.* 2012;93(1):100–107.
10. Hammond FM, Grattan KD, Sasser H, et al. Five years after traumatic brain injury: a study of individual outcomes and predictors of change in function. *NeuroRehabilitation.* 2004;19(1):25–35.
11. Hammond FM, Hart T, Bushnik T, Corrigan JD, Sasser H. Change and predictors of change in communication, cognition, and social function between 1 and 5 years after traumatic brain injury. *J Head Trauma Rehabil.* 2004;19(4):314–328.
12. Olver JH, Ponsford JL, Curran CA. Outcome following traumatic brain injury: a comparison between 2 and 5 years after injury. *Brain Inj.* 1996;10(11):841–848.
13. Feeney TJ, Ylvisaker M, Rosen BH, Greene P. Community supports for individuals with challenging behavior after brain injury: an analysis of the New York state behavioral resource project. *J Head Trauma Rehabil.* 2001;16(1):61–75.
14. International Brain Injury Clubhouse Alliance. Available at: http://www.braininjuryclubhouses.net/. Accessed May 15, 2011.
15. Hibbard MR, Cantor J, Charatz H, et al. Peer support in the community: initial findings of a mentoring program for individuals with

traumatic brain injury and their families. *J Head Trauma Rehabil.* 2002;17(2):112–131.

16. Heinemann AW, Corrigan JD, Moore D. Case management for traumatic brain injury survivors with alcohol problems. *Rehabil Psychol.* 2004;49(2):156–66.

17. Braunling-McMorrow D, Dollinger SJ, Gould M, Neumann T, Heiligenthal R. Outcomes of post-acute rehabilitation for persons with brain injury. *Brain Inj.* 2010;24(7–8):928–938.

18. Cattelani R, Zettin M, Zoccolotti P. Rehabilitation treatments for adults with behavioral and psychosocial disorders following acquired brain injury: a systematic review. *Neuropsychol Rev.* 2010; 20(1):52–85.

19. Seale GS, Caroselli JS, High WM Jr, Becker CL, Neese LE, Scheibel R. Use of community integration questionnaire (CIQ) to characterize changes in functioning for individuals with traumatic brain injury who participated in a post-acute rehabilitation programme. *Brain Inj.* 2002;16(11):955–967.

20. Cicerone KD, Dahlberg C, Kalmar K, et al. Evidence-based cognitive rehabilitation: recommendations for clinical practice. *Arch Phys Med Rehabil.* 2000;81(12):1596–1615.

21. Cicerone KD, Dahlberg C, Malec JF, et al. Evidence-based cognitive rehabilitation: updated review of the literature from 1998 through 2002. *Arch Phys Med Rehabil.* 2005;86(8):1681–1692.

22. Cicerone KD, Langenbahn DM, Braden C, et al. Evidence-based cognitive rehabilitation: updated review of the literature from 2003 through 2008. *Arch Phys Med Rehabil.* 2011;92(4):519–530.

23. Altman IM, Swick S, Parrot D, Malec JF. Effectiveness of community-based rehabilitation after traumatic brain injury for 489 program completers compared with those precipitously discharged. *Arch Phys Med Rehabil.* 2010;91(11):1697–1704.

24. Ben-Yishay Y, Prigatano GP. Cognitive remediation. In: Rosenthal M, Griffith ER, Bond MR, Miller JD, eds. *Rehabilitation of the Adult and Child with Traumatic Brain Injury.* Philadelphia, PA: FA Davis; 1990: 393–400.

25. Prigatano GP, Fordyce DJ, Zeiner HK, Roueche JR, Pepping M, Wood BC. *Neuropsychological Rehabilitation After Brain Injury.* Baltimore, MD: Johns Hopkins University; 1986.

26. Ben-Yishay Y, Diller L. *Handbook of Holistic Neuropsychological Rehabilitation Outpatient Rehabilitation of Traumatic Brain Injury.* New York, NY: Oxford University; 2011.

27. Trexler LE, Diller L, Gleuckauf R, Tomusk A, Anreiter B, Ben-Yishay Y. Consensus conference on the development of a multicenter study on the efficacy of neuropsychological rehabilitation. Zionsville, IN. June 1994.

28. Cicerone KD, Mott T, Azulay J, et al. A randomized controlled trial of holistic neuropsychologic rehabilitation after traumatic brain injury. *Arch Phys Med Rehabil.* 2008;89(12):2239–2249.

29. Greenberger D, Padesky CA. *Mind Over Mood: Change How You Feel by Changing the Way You Think.* New York, NY: Guilford Press; 1995.

30. Backhaus SL, Ibarra SL, Klyce D, Trexler LE, Malec JF. Brain injury coping skills group: a preventative intervention for patients with brain injury and their caregivers. *Arch Phys Med Rehabil.* 2010;91(6): 840–848.

31. Bradbury CL, Christensen BK, Lau MA, Ruttan LA, Arundine AL, Greene RE. The efficacy of cognitive behavior therapy in the treatment of emotional distress after acquired brain injury. *Arch Phys Med Rehabil.* 2008;89(suppl 12):S61–S68.

32. Tiersky LA, Anselmi V, Johnston MV, et al. A trial of neuropsychologic rehabilitation in mild-spectrum traumatic brain injury. *Arch Phys Med Rehabil.* 2005;86(8):1565–1574.

33. Dahlberg CA, Cusick CP, Hawley LA, et al. Treatment efficacy of social communication skills training after traumatic brain injury: a randomized treatment and deferred treatment controlled trial. *Arch Phys Med Rehabil.* 2007;88(12):1561–1573.

34. Lundqvist A, Linnros H, Orlenius H, Samuelsson K. Improved self-awareness and coping strategies for patients with acquired brain injury—a group therapy programme. *Brain Inj.* 2010;24(6):823–832.

35. Davis LC, Sander AM, Struchen MA, Sherer M, Nakase-Richardson R, Malec JF. Medical and psychosocial predictors of caregiver dis-

tress and perceived burden following traumatic brain injury. *J Head Trauma Rehabil.* 2009;24(3):145–154.

36. Evans CC, Sherer M, Nakase-Richardson R, Mani T, Irby JW Jr. Evaluation of an interdisciplinary team intervention to improve therapeutic alliance in post-acute brain injury rehabilitation. *J Head Trauma Rehabil.* 2008;23(5):329–338.

37. Klonoff PS, Lamb DG, Henderson SW. Outcomes from milieu-based neurorehabilitation at up to 11 years post-discharge. *Brain Inj.* 2001;15(5):413–428.

38. Cailhol L, Rodgers R, Burnand Y, Brunet A, Damsa C, Andreoli A. Therapeutic alliance in short-term supportive and psychodynamic psychotherapies: a necessary but not sufficient condition for outcome? *Psychiatry Res.* 2009;170(2–3):229–233.

39. Hewitt J, Coffey M. Therapeutic working relationships with people with schizophrenia: literature review. *J Adv Nurs.* 2005;52(5): 561–570.

40. Covey SR. *The Seven Habits of Highly Effective People.* Carlsbad, CA: Hay House, Inc; 2003.

41. Sander AM, Sherer M, Malec JF, et al. Preinjury emotional and family functioning in caregivers of persons with traumatic brain injury. *Arch Phys Med Rehabil.* 2003;84(2):197–203.

42. Malec JF. Vocational Rehabilitation. In: High WM, Sander AM, Struchen MA, Hart KA, eds. *Rehabilitation for Traumatic Brain Injury.* New York, NY: Oxford University Press; 2005.

43. van Velzen JM, Van Bennekom CA, Edelaar MJ, Sluiter JK, W. Frings-Dresen MH. How many people return to work after acquired brain injury?: a systematic review. *Brain Inj.* 2009;23(6): 473–488.

44. Fadyl JK, McPherson KM. Approaches to vocational rehabilitation after traumatic brain injury: a review of the evidence. *J Head Trauma Rehabil.* 2009;24(3):195–212.

45. Malec JF, Buffington AL, Moessner AM, Degiorgio L. A medical/vocational case coordination system for persons with brain injury: an evaluation of employment outcomes. *Arch Phys Med Rehabil.* 2000;81(8):1007–1015.

46. Malec JF, Moessner AM. Replicated positive results for the VCC model of vocational intervention after ABI within the social model of disability. *Brain Inj.* 2006;20(3):227–36.

47. Trexler LE, Trexler LC, Malec JF, Klyce D, Parrott D. Prospective randomized controlled trial of resource facilitation on community participation and vocational outcome following brain injury. *J Head Trauma Rehabil.* 2010;25(6):440–446.

48. Ottenbacher KJ, Hsu Y, Granger CV, Fiedler RC. The reliability of the functional independence measure: a quantitative review. *Arch Phys Med Rehabil.* 1996;77(12):1226–1232.

49. Kean J, Malec JF, Altman IM, Swick S. Rasch measurement analysis of the Mayo-Portland Adaptability Inventory (MPAI-4) in a community-based rehabilitation sample. *J Neurotrauma.* 2011;28(5): 745–753.

50. Malec JF, Kragness M, Evans RW, Finlay KL, Kent A, Lezak MD. Further psychometric evaluation and revision of the Mayo-Portland Adaptability Inventory in a national sample. *J Head Trauma Rehabil.* 2003;18(6):479–492.

51. Manual for the Mayo-Portland Adaptability Inventory. 2008. Available at: www.tbims.org/combi/mpai.

52. Wilde EA, Whiteneck GG, Bogner J, et al. Recommendations for the use of common outcome measures in traumatic brain injury research. *Arch Phys Med Rehabil.* 2010;91(11): 1650–1660.e17.

53. Center for Outcome Measurement in Brain Injury. National TBI Model System Data Center. Available at: www.tbims.org/combi/mpai. Accessed November 3, 2010.

54. Murphy T, Malec JF, Danaher B, Seeley J, Gau J. An Internet-Based Evaluation System for Postacute Acquired Brain Injury. In: *National Institute for Neurological Diseases and Stroke;* 2009–2010.

55. Inventive Software Solutions. Available at: www.inventivesoftware.net. Accessed May 31, 2011.

56. Malec JF, ed. *New Methodologies for Intervention and Outcome Measurement.* East Sussex, UK: Psychology Press; 2009.

57. Shadish WR, Cook TD, Campbell DT. *Experimental and Quasi-Experimental Designs for Generalized Causal Inference.* Boston, MA: Houghton Mifflin Harcourt; 2002.

Driving After Traumatic Brain Injury

Megan H. W. Preece, Carolyn A. Unsworth, and Morris Odell

INTRODUCTION

As standards of medical care improve, more individuals have been surviving traumatic brain injury (TBI) than ever before and hence fitness to drive has emerged as an important consideration for these individuals and their physicians. Many individuals with TBI have a strong desire to return to driving (1). Unsurprisingly, driving is a predictor of community reintegration, workforce participation, and psychosocial well-being after TBI (1–4). On the other hand, alternatives to driving, such as using public transport or reliance on family or friends for mobility, can often be viewed as inconvenient, unreliable, or burdensome (1), and may not be a realistic option for some (e.g., rural residents). However, driving a vehicle is a complex task requiring the driver to control the vehicle while interacting with the external environment at the same time (5). Safe driving requires simultaneous operation of motor coordination, visual perception, information processing, divided attention, and aspects of higher order cognition (particularly, self-awareness or insight), and persons with TBI often have marked impairments in these domains. The challenge for physicians in assessing fitness to drive is to balance the importance of driving in facilitating independence and community reintegration for a person with TBI while also considering the likely risks to the wider community posed by that individual being on the road.

Even though return to driving is of great concern to individuals with TBI (6), there is a considerable lack of knowledge regarding driving after TBI. Fisk et al. found that 18% of individuals with TBI received no advice about driving (7). Of concern was the finding that for individuals who did receive advice, the primary source was from family members, as opposed to physicians or other health professionals (7). Providing advice regarding fitness to drive can be a source of great anxiety for physicians (8). In the United Kingdom, a study of health professionals' attitudes toward giving advice about fitness to drive revealed that many physicians receive little formal training regarding their role in advising patients about driving (9). Although most respondents believed that it was their role to discuss driving with patients, 40% indicated that they did not have sufficient knowledge regarding fitness to drive (9).

This chapter reviews the research literature regarding driving after TBI. It also provides an overview of driver as-sessment and rehabilitation, highlighting the physician's role in this process. This chapter focuses on return to driving after TBI, as opposed to learning to drive after TBI. Similarly, this chapter limits its focus to car driving for private use; it does not discuss riding a motorcycle or driving a heavy or commercial vehicle. There are indications that individuals can learn to drive after TBI (7,10), and that individuals return to being commercial drivers (9,10), but there are few research reports and guidelines currently devoted to these special topics.[1] Finally, this chapter limits discussion to driving after moderate-to-severe TBI; although there is evidence suggestive of driving-related impairments immediately after mild TBI (12), mild TBI is usually a self-limiting condition that is not an issue for driver licensing (5).

PREVALENCE AND PREDICTORS OF DRIVING AFTER TBI

Incidence and Prevalence of Driving After TBI

Between 25% and 60% of individuals drive after TBI (1,7,13–18). Three studies that compared preinjury and postinjury driving status for their samples reported figures suggesting that between one- and two-thirds of people with TBI returned to driving (7,14,18). One longitudinal study showed that return to driving rates increased with time since injury; at 1 year postinjury, 42% of individuals with TBI reported driving, whereas at 5 years postinjury, 53% were driving (3). Therefore, it appears that many individuals with TBI do successfully return to driving even several years after an injury.

A few investigations have reported data on the frequency and extent of driving by persons with TBI. In the United States, research has reported that most individuals

---

[1] Note that the Federal Motor Carrier Administration has published the opinions of an expert panel regarding drivers with TBI driving for the purposes of interstate commerce (i.e., bus and truck drivers). Federal Motor Carrier Safety Administration. Opinions of expert panel: Traumatic brain injury and commercial motor vhicle driver safety: Federal Motor Carrier Safety Administration; 2009. Available at http://www.fmcsa.dot.gov/rules-regulations/TOPICS/mep/report/TraumaticBrainInjury_MEP_Opinion.pdf.

TABLE 78-1 Predictors of Driving After TBI

Less severe injury
- Drivers had higher Glasgow Coma Scale scores than nondrivers (1,3), but other investigations report no association (perhaps because of a restricted range of scores) (4,7,15,17).
- One study found that drivers had shorter coma duration than nondrivers (15), but another found no relationship (18).

No history or reports of epilepsy
- Drivers were less likely to have self-reported epilepsy than nondrivers; however, this does not exclude the possibility that they had epilepsy but chose not to report it (14).

No history or reports of vision problems
- Drivers were less likely to self-report vision problems than nondrivers; however, this does not exclude the possibility that they had unperceived visual problems or chose not to report them (14).

Greater functional independence
- Drivers' discharge Functional Independence Measure scores were higher than those of nondrivers (3,7).
- Drivers' current Functional Independence Measure and Functional Assessment Measure scores for driving-related items were higher than those of nondrivers (14).
- Drivers had lower Disability Rating Scale scores at discharge than nondrivers (3), but no association has also been reported in the literature (17).

Better performance on neuropsychological tests
- Drivers performed better on neuropsychological testing than nondrivers (1,17,18).

Formal driving assessment sought
- Drivers were more likely to have sought a formal driving assessment than nondrivers, even when costs were borne by the health system (1,4).
- Drivers were more likely to have been approved for driving following a formal driving assessment than nondrivers (7).

Higher levels of self-awareness
- Those with insight were more likely to be drivers than individuals with awareness of deficit problems (17).
- Drivers rated themselves more highly on driving ability than nondrivers' ratings (4,17).

Fewer social and resource-related barriers
- Drivers perceived fewer social and resource-related barriers to driving than nondrivers (1,4).

Caregiver's perception is that the person is fit to drive
- Drivers were seen as more functional in general than nondrivers by their caregivers (17).
- Drivers were rated more highly on driving ability than nondrivers by their caregivers (17).

Caregivers report more social support
- Drivers had caregivers who perceived that they had more social support than nondrivers' caregivers (17).

Certain personal characteristics at the time of injury
- One study found that drivers were more likely to be younger than nondrivers at the time of injury (3), but another study found no association (15).
- Drivers were more likely to have finished high school (3).
- Drivers were less likely to be unemployed or retired (3).
- Drivers were less likely to be living in a facility situation (3).

Caucasian ethnic background
- Caucasians were more likely to be driving compared with other ethnic groups (3).

drove every day and more than 50 miles per week (7,18), yet 30% of their sample drove less than 25 miles per week. In Norway, Schanke et al. surveyed drivers 6–9 years after injury (19). The findings were similar to those of Fisk et al., in that most individuals with TBI drove every day and about 100 miles per week on average.

Predictors of Driving After TBI

Table 78–1 lists the factors that have been found to predict driving after TBI. Perhaps unexpectedly, time since injury (1,15), and preinjury driving record (15,17) have not been found to predict resumption of driving. Other factors that have not been shown to predict driving status include gender (1,15,17), current age (1,4,15,17), current educational

level (1,4,15,17), occupation (1), relationship status (17), negative affect (1), and social support (1).

ROAD SAFETY OF DRIVERS WITH TBI

Crash Risk of Drivers With TBI

A key concern for physicians is to what extent individuals with TBI pose a risk to themselves or other road users if they resume driving. In the road safety literature, crash involvement is regarded as the key outcome measure for evaluating driver safety. However, crashes are rare events and are often caused by a confluence of individual factors. Furthermore, pure crash involvement may be an unreliable measure of an individual driver's true crash risk because another road user may be at fault. For example, a driver

TABLE 78–2 Summary of Studies Measuring Crash Risk After TBI

DATE, FIRST AUTHOR, LOCATION	PARTICIPANTS	DESIGN	MAIN FINDING
1998, Haselkorn (22) Washington state, US	• 896 drivers hospitalized for TBI of unknown severity in 1992 • 1625 age-, gender-, and postal code-matched nonhospitalized drivers	Retrospective study of officially documented crashes 12 months after hospitalization (adjusted for previous driving record)	Drivers with TBI were not at increased risk of crashing cf. nonhospitalized drivers (relative risk: 0.9)
2002, Schultheis (23) New Jersey, US	• 47 drivers with TBI of unknown severity, 0.50–22 years postinjury • 22 age-, gender-, education-, driving experience-matched healthy drivers	Retrospective study of self-reported and officially documented crashes up to 5 years after successfully completing a driver evaluation program	Drivers with TBI had a comparable rate of officially documented and self-reported crashes cf. healthy drivers (relative risk: 0.9 and 1.3, respectively)
2005, Formisano (16) Lazio, Italy	• 90 adults with severe brain injury (Glasgow Coma Scale score ≤8; 80% TBI), mean = 4.67 years postinjury ○ 29 had returned to driving	Retrospective study of caregiver-reported crashes for consecutive admissions to a rehabilitation unit	11 drivers (38%) were involved in at least 1 crash cf. 4.7 expected crash-involved drivers based on normative data (relative risk: 2.3)
2005, Pietrapiana (15) Piedmont, Italy	• 66 adults with severe TBI (Glasgow Coma Scale score ≤8), 1–16 years postinjury ○ 31 had returned to driving for at least 1 year	Retrospective study, which included significant other-reported crashes	11 drivers (36%) were involved in at least 1 crash, whereas 20 drivers were crash-free
2008, Schanke (19) Akershus, Norway	• 28 drivers with TBI of unknown severity assessed between 1997 and 2000	Retrospective study of self-reported and officially documented crashes after successfully completing a driver assessment	Drivers with TBI were at least 2 times more likely to have an officially documented crash cf. normative data for Norwegian drivers (15.0 vs 6.3 crashes per million km driven)

whose vehicle is struck by another driver running a red light would be categorized as "crash-involved," although the crash did not result from any action on the part of the driver. Conversely, an individual may cause several near miss events where other road users' quick reactions prevent a crash; such a person's crash record would not reflect their crash risk (20). Additionally, in the case of drivers with TBI, it may be difficult to establish the extent to which any impairments related to TBI contributed to a crash above any preexisting or coexisting conditions.

Table 78–2 summarizes the available evidence for the crash risk of drivers with TBI.[2] The evidence is not consistent across the 5 studies: 2 reported no increased crash risk, whereas 3 reported indications of increased crash risk for drivers with TBI. Two of the most recent studies suggested that drivers with TBI are twice as likely to crash compared to rates in the general population (16,19). However, this level of crash risk is similar to that posed by young or inexperienced male drivers, and similar to that posed by experienced drivers with a blood alcohol concentration of 0.050% to 0.079% (21). Further studies using larger samples and officially documented minor as well as major crashes are required to gain a clearer understanding of the relative crash risk of drivers following TBI.

Driving Violations by Drivers With TBI

Another important consideration for determining the safety of drivers with TBI is the extent to which they commit driving violations, which can be characterized as deliberate deviations from safe driving (e.g., speeding or driving while intoxicated). A large-scale investigation by Haselkorn et al. found that the relative risk of a traffic citation was not greater for unrestricted licensed drivers with TBI than for a matched group of nonhospitalized drivers in the 12 months after injury (23). However, after adjustment for previous driving record, there was a modest increase in traffic citations for drivers with TBI (relative risk: 1.3). Because there was also a similar increase in an isolated fracture (orthopedic) control group (relative risk: 1.2), the researchers argued that the findings could reflect the inability to completely account for driver characteristics (e.g., differences general risk-taking propensity) rather than being the direct result of TBI. In contrast, Schultheis et al. reported that drivers with TBI who had completed a driver evaluation program did not have more officially documented violations than a closely matched group of uninjured drivers over a 5–year period (23). Surprisingly, the uninjured drivers reported engaging in more unsafe driving situations than the drivers with TBI (23). This may signal that drivers with TBI are especially

---

[2] These studies were located through a Web site of Science database search using the terms traumatic brain injur*, crash* or accident*, and driving, for all years that the database covers (1898–2011). Relevant articles were manually searched for additional references.

cautious when it comes to avoiding driving violations, or that they may perhaps underreport violations.

Unlicensed Driving and Driving Against Medical Advice by Persons With TBI

Although licensed drivers with TBI seem to commit driving violations at no greater frequency than the general population, there are several reports that a subset of people with TBI may continue to drive despite being formally advised not to drive. Although there are no studies comparing rates of unlicensed driving in people with TBI compared to other vulnerable groups such as older drivers who have been advised to retire from driving, there are indications that up to a third of people with TBI may drive against clinical recommendations (14,15,24). In one study, upon commencing a daily rehabilitation program, 35% of the participants with severe TBI were driving against clinical recommendations and half of these patients went on to have a serious driving incident (24).

Overall, the indications are that licensed drivers with TBI commit driving violations at a similar rate to the general population of drivers. Generally, drivers with TBI who have been medically cleared or have been through a driver assessment process do not pose an unacceptable risk to road safety for driving violations. However, those with TBI who continue to drive despite professional recommendations likely constitute a high-risk group (24,25).

DRIVING ASSESSMENT AND TRAINING AFTER TBI

The previous section highlighted the safety of licensed drivers with TBI as a group. However, only a subset of people with TBI are able to return to driving (7,14), and it is important that each individual with TBI who wants to return to driving is thoroughly assessed. Driver assessment is important not just for "screening out" those unsafe for driving, it is also a process that allows a certified driving rehabilitation specialist (CDRS) to identify what supports, remedial training, or licensing conditions could enable individuals with TBI to continue to hold a driver's license safely. Furthermore, undertaking a driving assessment may make it easier for a person with TBI to accept that they may no longer be safe on the road (although, perhaps, only for those with an adequate degree of insight into their condition) rather than having to rely solely on the recommendations of their clinicians or family and friends.

This section outlines the most common forms of driver assessment and training available after TBI. First, the Comprehensive Driving Evaluation (CDE) is described as the "gold standard" form of driving assessment (26,27). The *Driver Fitness Medical Guidelines* that are jointly published by the National Highway Traffic Safety Administration and American Association of Motor Vehicle Administrators recommend that resumption of driving after TBI should not be attempted without a CDE, given the complicated and variable nature of TBI (28). Second, the effectiveness of other forms of assessment is considered. Finally, the evidence for driver training after TBI is outlined.

Comprehensive Driving Evaluation

The CDE is a functional assessment that comprises of an off-road clinical assessment, which is then followed by an on-road practical driving test. In some jurisdictions, it may be the role of the physician to decide whether or not to refer an individual for a CDE (i.e., deciding whether the individual meets relevant medical standards for driving) (29,30). The CDE is usually administered by an occupational therapist with postgraduate training in driving assessment of functionally impaired drivers. Other health professionals who are CDRS's and driver rehabilitation professionals with specialized training in determining how health-related changes can affect driving ability may also assess clients with TBI. In most regions, the outcome of the CDE is framed as a recommendation regarding an individual's license status, with the final decision then being made by a representative of the driver licensing authority (DLA) (28). In some jurisdictions, the DLA accepts the CDRS's report as a legal basis for issuing a license (31). The CDE is based on a theory now referred to as the Gadget Matrix (32). The Gadget Matrix, which is an extension of Michon's (1979) model, helps us understand driver behavior and guides the assessment and rehabilitation process (32).

The CDE is commonly cited as the gold standard for the assessment of functionally impaired drivers (26,27). The high ecological validity of the on-road portion of the CDE, and the appearance of face validity for individuals with TBI are advantages of this approach. However, a critical consideration for any driving assessment is its criterion validity or sensitivity (i.e., to what extent does a test identify unsafe driving behaviors leading to crash risk). Supporting the criterion validity of the CDE, Schultheis et al. found that 47 drivers with TBI who had successfully completed a CDE did not differ in self-reported or officially documented reports of crashes or violations over a 5–year period as compared to a matched uninjured group of drivers (23). Similarly, a study reporting on drivers with acquired brain injuries (of which drivers with TBI usually comprise a sizeable subgroup) showed that those who successfully completed a CDE did not differ in their driving safety profile from that of uninjured drivers (33). Furthermore, there is often a close correspondence between errors observed in CDEs and unsafe behaviors observed in real driving (34). For instance, older drivers tend to be over-involved in crashes at intersections (35), and poor intersection negotiation is frequently documented on CDRS reports (34).

Despite their efficacy, some controversy exists regarding the use of CDEs (27,36). CDEs are resource-intensive and expensive, and may not be widely available outside urban areas. Given their relatively recent and sometimes ad hoc development, normative data and psychometric properties may be lacking for individual tests administered as part of the CDE (36). However, researchers involved in driving assessment are addressing these weaknesses incrementally (37–39). More importantly, some CDEs are not standardized, and portions of the clinical assessment and on-road assessment often vary according to a client's profile of strengths and weaknesses and motivations for seeking a CDE (27,34).

Off-Road Clinical Assessment

Before the on-road evaluation, the client's motor, sensory, and cognitive capacities that are considered important to the driving task are assessed (30,40). The main aims of this assessment are to (a) determine if the client meets the criteria

TABLE 78–3 Off-Road Clinical Assessments Employed in a Comprehensive Driver Evaluation (40–42)

Client interview
- Written consent for the assessment is obtained.
- Provision of information regarding licensing authority regulations, assessment outcomes and reporting process
- Collection of information regarding
  - medical history and current medications
  - current license status and previous driving history
  - client's perception of strengths and weaknesses (establishing degree of insight)

Sensory assessment
- Vision (visual acuity, visual fields, depth perception, or contrast sensitivity)
- Hearing
- Proprioception and kinesthesis
- Pain

Physical assessment
- Range of motion (ROM)
- Muscle strength
- Muscle tone
- Balance and coordination
- Endurance
- Reaction time (speed of movement)

Cognitive and perceptual assessment
- Visual perception and attention
- Reaction time (information processing speed)
- Executive function
- Memory
- Unilateral spatial neglect screen (which precludes driving)
- Client's knowledge and application of road rules

set by the licensing authority for obtaining a driver's license and (b) develop a profile of the client's strengths and weaknesses in relation to driving (29). The clinical assessment commonly comprises an initial interview (sometimes with a family member present as well), sensory assessment, physical assessment, and cognitive assessment. Table 78–3 presents a list of commonly assessed capacities (41,42). The clinical assessment usually lasts between 1 and 2 hours (31). If the client cannot meet the criteria set by the licensing authority for obtaining a driver's license (e.g., visual acuity is too poor even with corrective lenses), then the off-road clinical assessments are discontinued.

After considering the results of the clinical assessment, the CDRS may take one of four courses of action. In most cases, the CDRS will proceed to the on-road evaluation. Second, the CDRS may refer the client to another health professional if particular tests uncover conditions requiring further assessment. For instance, uncertainties regarding the client's level of self-awareness may trigger a referral to a neuropsychologist for tests of executive functioning, or visual deficits may be followed-up with an appropriate professional. Third, if the client is revealed to have significant physical limitations, the CDRS may arrange for suitable vehicle modifications and training in their use before proceeding to the on-road evaluation (28). Finally, in a very small number of cases, the CDRS may decide that the client poses too great a risk to themselves and others to proceed to the on-road assessment (usually supported by indications of globally poor performance across the off-road assessments) (42).

Adaptations for Physical and Sensory Limitations

The CDRS will determine whether the client requires assistive technology or that modifications be made to their vehicle to compensate for certain physical and sensory limitations. Physical conditions can impact on an individual's ability to enter or exit their vehicle, sit comfortably, or safely use the vehicle's controls (40). Similarly, hearing or visual impairments can impact on an individual's ability to drive in a safe manner using the vehicle's controls. CDRSs are familiar with the types of assistive technology that are available and permissible in the client's jurisdiction. Commonly deployed modifications include mandating the use of a vehicle with automatic transmission (e.g., for a client with hemiparesis or for preventing fatigue), spinner devices attached to the steering wheel (e.g., for a client with unilateral hemiparesis affecting an arm), hand controls instead of foot pedals (e.g., for a client with no functional use of their lower limbs), or a more extensive mirror system (e.g., to eliminate blind spots for a client with limited neck or trunk rotation). Certain jurisdictions have detailed guidelines covering adaptations for physical and sensory limitations. The CDRS will recommend the most appropriate assistive technology or vehicle modifications to suit an individual client's circumstances, including consideration of whether the client can learn to use the additional devices or drive a modified vehicle (40). The CDRS or a driving instructor experienced in training drivers with functional impairments will train a client in the use of any assistive technology before the final on-road assessment (40).[3]

On-Road Practical Driving Test

The on-road assessment is usually undertaken in a dual-control vehicle with a driving instructor experienced in supervising functionally impaired drivers engaged to instruct and supervise the driver (26,40). The driving instructor's role is to maintain the safety of the vehicle and they can interact with the client and the CDRS as necessary during the assessment. This arrangement frees the CDRS (seated behind the driving instructor) to focus on observing the client's driving performance (26,40). The CDRS assesses the driver's performance and consults with the driving instructor on the conclusion of the drive to gain any additional information (5,30).

The on-road assessment is usually longer than an entry-level practical driving test, lasting between 40 and 120 minutes (37,40). Typically, the assessment commences on quiet residential roads or in a parking lot. Time is allowed for clients to familiarize themselves with vehicle handling and the testing environment and, importantly, to allow any test anxiety to subside (26,34,43). To achieve acceptable reliability, the on-road assessment is standardized in that the client follows a set route that has been designed to allow a driver to demonstrate common driving maneuvers several times (e.g., changing lanes, negotiating an uncontrolled intersection, etc.) (26,30). The set route also incorporates a variety of traffic conditions, allowing the driver to demonstrate the

---

[3] See the following sources for more information about assistive technology and vehicle modifications: Pellerito JM, ed. Driver Rehabilitation and Community Mobility: Principles and Practice. St Louis, MO: Elsevier Mosby; 2006. Redepenning S. Driver Rehabilitation Across Age and Disability: An Occupational Therapy Guide. American Occupational Therapy Associaton Press; 2006.

ability to match the vehicle's speed to traffic conditions, scan the road environment, and position the vehicle relative to other road users (e.g., gap selection and maintaining an appropriate distance from parked cars) (26). The CDRS scores the driver's behavior on explicit criteria at certain points along the route (e.g., whether the driver safely negotiated a particular intersection or not) (26,34,43). In this respect, the on-road assessment may be similar to an entry-level driving test. However, in an on-road assessment of a functionally impaired driver, the CDRS may also record additional qualitative observations of behaviors indicative of unsafe driving (e.g., confusion or aggression toward other road users) (34). The client may also be questioned about their driving performance (in order to gauge self-awareness) at certain points during the on-road assessment.

When undertaking the on-road assessment, the CDRS may monitor undesirable actions and behaviors (rather than fail the client outright as would occur in an entry-level driving test) and observe if the client can learn from the feedback provided. For example, a client may have previously developed bad habits such as rolling through stop signs or neglecting to complete over-shoulder head checks prior to lane changes. The CDRS observes if the client is able to use feedback about these problems for the remainder of the drive, and then determines if the recommendation should be for the client to continue to drive or if lessons and retesting are required. If the driving instructor intervenes during the assessment, a recommendation of "fail" is generally made, however, even in these circumstances, there are benefits to continuing with the assessment. Establishing patterns of errors may allow the CDRS to suggest specific remedial training to improve future performance (40).

The on-road assessment can also be tailored to a particular client's needs (34). For example, if fatigue is a concern, then the test may be lengthened to establish whether a client's driving deteriorates to unsafe levels after a certain time spent on the road (which can then result in the granting of a conditional license specifying that the driver is not to drive more than a specified number of hours in a 24–hour period). Another common variation is that testing may be relocated from a set route to the client's local area if the client is only seeking a conditional license to drive within a certain radius of their home (34,40). In some rare circumstances, the assessment might proceed in the client's vehicle rather than a dual-control vehicle such as when the client's vehicle has been modified to accommodate their physical disability, and the perceived risk of completing the assessment in this vehicle is judged as low (34,40).

On completion of the on-road assessment, the client is given immediate feedback regarding the overall outcome and specific information regarding their performance on the various skills assessed (26,34,40). Feedback is tailored to the client's level of understanding and their degree of insight. For some clients, it may be beneficial to involve their family members at this stage (34).

Outcomes of the Comprehensive Driving Evaluation

After considering the information from both the off- and on-road assessments, the CDRS makes a recommendation to the DLA regarding the client's license. The recommendation usually falls into 1 of 3 categories: (*a*) the client is fit to drive with no conditions (or to hold an unconditional license), (*b*)

the client is fit to drive with certain conditions (or to hold to a conditional license), or (*c*) the client is not fit to drive (and either ceases to drive, or undertakes a period of rehabilitation or lessons and is reassessed) (37). Where the client is found to be fit to drive with certain conditions or not fit to drive (i.e., driving is to be limited), the CDRS provides advice regarding alternative means of transport to maintain mobility in the community (40). In most jurisdictions, there is an established appeals process if the client is unsatisfied with the outcome of the CDE.

Conditional Licenses

Conditional licenses are an effective alternative to the withdrawal of an unconditional license. They allow the CDRS and DLA to mandate certain necessary restrictions to enable functionally impaired drivers to remain independent in their local area (accessing vital services such as the local physician and stores) while upholding community road safety standards (5). Examples of conditions that might be specified for drivers with TBI include wearing corrective lenses, daylight driving only, power steering, zero blood alcohol concentration, driving in off-peak only, passenger restriction, and not to drive more than a certain number of hours in a 24–hour period to assist in fatigue management (5). Conditions must be set with an eye to enforceability; for instance, proscriptions against driving in inclement weather are unacceptable because a driver might start out in fine weather and be stranded if they are not allowed to continue their journey in rain. Further, some conditions, such as requiring a copilot (which puts the other person at risk) or that certain routes be followed are inappropriate. If a driver's "allowed route" is unexpectedly diverted to different roads, the driver will be stranded or forced to disobey their licensing conditions. In such cases, it is more likely that the individual is in fact unsafe to drive independently. Lastly, clients with unrestricted or conditional licenses may be subject to periodic reviews (e.g., medical review or a full CDE is to be completed at prescribed intervals) in order to monitor client compliance with the conditions and to monitor the effect of the client's physical or cognitive impairment on their driving over time (40).

Successful Timing of the Comprehensive Driving Evaluation

Although there is scarce evidence regarding when is the best time to attempt a CDE after TBI, people with TBI cannot hold a driver's license unless they meet their local medical standards for driving. Additionally, it is prudent for an individual with TBI to begin the CDE process only when their physician and other health professionals involved in their care believe (e.g., on the basis of progress in occupational therapy) that the individual stands a good chance of being able to pass the CDE. Attempting a CDE too soon can result in a premature fail that is financially costly, personally devastating, and prompts the CDRS to delay reassessment for several months (40).

Other Options for Driver Assessment

Neuropsychological and Cognitive Tests

Many researchers have attempted to identify off-road tests that can predict on-road performance and thus vastly reduce the need for the costly (and potentially risky) on-road component of the CDE. There have been numerous attempts to validate various combinations of neuropsychological and cognitive tests as potential substitutes for on-road testing for persons with TBI. Tests found to predict on-road assessment results after TBI include choice reaction time tasks, the Color Trail Test, the Listening Span test, the Paced Auditory Serial Addition Test, the Rey Complex Figure Test recall, a perceptual speed task (matching symbolic figures), a time estimation task, the Simultaneous Capacity test, the Tactual Performance Test, the Trail Making Test, and the Useful Field of View Test (44–50). Similarly, batteries of tests, such as the Cognitive Behavioral Driver's Inventory and Neurocognitive Driving Test, have been found to be predictive of on-road driving assessment outcome (51,52). These findings show tests of attention, information processing speed, visual memory, and psychomotor skills may be of use in predicting on-road driving performance (20). However, because the predictive powers of many of these tests are modest, neuropsychological test performance cannot account for all the variance in such a complex task as driving (43). As shown in a study by Rapport et al., a driver who is sensitive to their cognitive difficulties can maintain their safety by adapting their driving to their cognitive profile to some extent (1). Conversely, a driver with reasonably intact cognitive abilities may still be an unsafe driver because of a lack of impulse control or excessive risk taking (15). More importantly, although neuropsychological test performance of a sample of TBI drivers has been shown to predict a composite measure of driver safety (17), it has not been shown to predict crash risk (53). Therefore, although neuropsychological testing is valuable as an information-gathering tool as part of the off-road assessment, it seems unlikely that it will ever be able to entirely replace the on-road portion of the CDE.

Hazard Perception Tests

Hazard perception is defined as a driver's ability to anticipate potentially dangerous traffic situations (54). In the field of traffic psychology, it is the only driving-specific ability that has been found to relate to drivers' crash records across studies (54–56). Because of their demonstrated efficacy, ecological validity, short duration, easy administration, and relative inexpensiveness, driver licensing authorities in Australia and the United Kingdom have incorporated hazard perception tests into their graduated licensing systems for novice drivers. A computer-based hazard perception test presents videos of real traffic scenes filmed from the driver's perspective, and the test-taker is required to indicate as soon as they anticipate a potential hazard in a scene (i.e., the response time from the onset of the hazard is measured) (12).

Recently, individuals with TBI have been found to be slower to anticipate traffic hazards in a hazard perception test than non–head-injured controls (12,57). Although hazard perception tests are not routinely incorporated into CDEs for drivers with TBI, inclusion of such tests could provide the CDRS with useful information, and is an area for further research investigation. Because hazards are relatively infrequent occurrences on the road, hazard perception tests are beneficial in that they allow for an individual to demonstrate anticipatory responses—or a lack thereof—to many hazards in a short space of time without the test-taker or CDRS being put at risk. Finally, hazard perception is not

only a skill that can be reliably assessed, but also a skill that can be improved through short, easily administered training interventions (58,59).

Driving Simulators

Driving simulators allow researchers and clinicians to quantitatively measure many aspects of driving performance while ensuring the safety of all involved (27). Driving simulators can range from a relatively simple setup involving a desktop PC with an attached steering wheel and foot pedals, to an actual vehicle mounted on a motion platform with a 180 degree field of view provided on a projector screen, LCD screens to simulate rear view mirror images, and surround sound. Similar to hazard perception tests, driving simulators can allow test-takers to respond to multiple high-risk situations in a short time. For instance, Cyr et al. were able to expose high-functioning drivers with TBI and uninjured controls to simulated high-crash-risk road events with an element of time pressure—with and without a dual task (which is when the driver must divide attention between two tasks). They found that drivers with TBI crashed significantly more than controls and that dual-task performance correlated with crash rate (60). Furthermore, driving simulators can be combined with other measurement tools (e.g., eye movement trackers) to further understand the processes underlying driving after TBI (61,62). For example, Charron et al. found that drivers with TBI were more reactive rather than anticipative in their visual scanning of the roadway in a driving simulator and less able to manage "secondary" tasks such as glancing at the mirror to monitor rearward traffic (61).

There are indications that driving simulators can accurately measure drivers' performance after TBI. Lew et al. reported that drivers with TBI's speed and steering control, crashes, and vigilance to a divided attention task in the Systems Technology Incorporated PC-based driving simulator correlated with their observed on-road driving performance 10 months afterward, demonstrating the predictive and ecological validity of this particular simulator (63). Furthermore, drivers with TBI (who were seeking driver assessment at the time of the study following moderate-to-severe TBI within the previous 2 years) performed worse on the driving simulator compared to uninjured controls. There was no significant correspondence between drivers with TBI's driving simulator performance and the results of a concurrent on-road assessment. In addition, the on-road assessment did not predict driving performance at the 10–month follow-up (suggesting that the simulator may have been more sensitive than the on-road assessment employed) (63). However, although the Systems Technology Incorporated simulator appears to capture some aspects of drivers with TBI's performance, it does not follow that all driving simulators are valid indicators of the performance of drivers with TBI. Each simulator type needs to have its validity established for specific groups of functionally impaired drivers.

Driving simulators are not without their disadvantages. The scenarios presented need to be realistic (perhaps recreating filmed traffic scenes that contain some degree of risk) and not present oversimplified representations of the traffic environment such as empty roads. A key concern is that drivers may behave differently in a driving simulator (where they know that dangerous driving will not result in negative consequences for them) (64). Also, some drivers experience "simulator sickness" (also known as Simulator Adaptation Syndrome) and cannot complete testing in the driving simulator because of symptoms such as motion sickness and headache (60). Moreover, certain driving simulators may be expensive to purchase and maintain (e.g., advanced high-fidelity simulators often require a full-time technician), and may not be widely available outside metropolitan areas. Driving simulators (especially high-fidelity simulators) are usually limited to being used as research tools after TBI. Research is required to investigate whether simulators have a role to play in driver rehabilitation. For example, in one study, a woman with TBI was given remedial driver training in a driving simulator, although there was no on-road transfer test (65).

Closed-Course Driving Assessment

Closed-course driving assessments usually evaluate basic vehicle operation skills such as steering through traffic cones, cued emergency braking, or parking (30). Drivers are judged on the accuracy of their performance or the time taken to complete various tasks. Although such resource-intensive assessments may serve certain practical objectives well, such as reacclimatizing a driver who has been away from driving for several years or testing the driver's mastery of certain vehicle modifications before an on-road assessment, closed-course driving provides no information on a driver's ability to safely interact with other road users or changing environmental demands and thus lacks ecological validity (20,30). Galski et al. found that closed-course driving behaviors did not explain much more variance in on-road performance beyond that explicable by neuropsychological assessment and simulator driving for people with acquired brain injury (66).

Event-Triggered Recorders to Monitor Driving

Recently, researchers have begun investigating the efficacy of commercially available event-triggered "black box" video recorders as an intervention to increase the monitoring and safety of novice drivers (67,68). Concurrently, driver fleet companies have installed event-triggered recorders in a bid to increase fleet driver awareness and safety, reduce crash rates, and reduce insurance costs. One study found that implementing event-triggered recorders in fleets significantly reduced crash rates by 20% (69).

An event-triggered recorder is mounted on the vehicle's windshield behind the rearview mirror and usually comprises two video cameras (capturing forward roadway and vehicle interior views), a microphone, and an accelerometer (67,68). The recorder is continually recording on a loop, but data are only recorded to internal memory when certain thresholds are breached (e.g., significant acceleration) or the driver manually initiates the "save" function (e.g., to capture an incident involving other road users). Following a trigger, video and sound for the 10 seconds preceding and the 10 seconds following the trigger are retained (67,68).

The authors are unaware of any investigations or interventions trialing the use of event-triggered recorders with drivers with TBI or drivers with functional impairments more generally. However, an event-triggered recorder could be used for a period of time after a CDE so that the CDRS can monitor a driver with TBI's solo driving to facilitate a more gradual progression to fully independent driving. Event-triggered recorders could even be used during a CDE so that any critical errors captured by the system can be replayed for the client to maintain safety and promote self-awareness. Finally, event-triggered recorders (potentially coupled with automated data logging of speed, distance travelled, and time of day) could be a powerful tool in research to increase our knowledge of driving after TBI, obviating the need for reliance on self-reported or officially documented crash rates.

Driver Training and Rehabilitation After TBI

As part of the CDE process, the CDRS may develop a plan for a client with TBI to undertake remedial driver training with an experienced driving instructor. Intuitively, this form of training would appear to be effective given its sensitivity to the variable needs of clients, but formal evaluations of such training for drivers with TBI or functionally impaired drivers in general have not yet been conducted. This on-road training may also be supplemented or replaced by less costly off-road training. The relative efficacy of these forms of training requires investigation.

There have been some attempts to establish the efficacy of various forms of off-road cognitive training for individuals with TBI. In the early 1980s, Sivak et al. demonstrated that 8–10 hours training in driving-related perceptual and cognitive skills (via paper-and-pencil tasks) after TBI or stroke resulted in improved driving performance (70,71). More recently, Klonoff et al. found that for individuals with acquired brain injury, better performance on cognitive re-training tasks (comprising remediation and compensatory training delivered during 40–minute sessions at least 4 times per week) was associated with subsequent clearance to drive (72). Similarly, investigations in older adult samples have found that computerized speed-of-processing training improved driving performance (including executing fewer dangerous maneuvers during an on-road driving test 18 months posttraining) and delayed driving cessation (73,74). Therefore, relatively simple forms of cognitive training appear to be effective in improving driving for clients with TBI and other functional impairments.

Newer forms of technology may also be effective in delivering off- and on-road driver training for persons with TBI. Driving video games are now approaching research simulators in realism and fidelity but at a much lower cost. There may be a role for such games in rehabilitation of persons with TBI before they progress to more formal training with a driving instructor. As mentioned earlier, driving simulators and computerized hazard perception packages may become effective means of providing off-road training for individuals with TBI (57,64,65). Event-triggered recorders could also be deployed as a training intervention. Adolescent drivers who were given immediate visual feedback and sent weekly reports based on events captured by such recorders (with reports also being sent to their parents) reduced their number of safety-relevant events by up to 76% over several months (67,68). Event-triggered recorders have obvious applicability beyond the novice driver population; drivers with TBI could be similarly coached to use such technology to increase their driver safety, perhaps in concert with a family member or friend taking on the important "driving mentor" role.

THE PHYSICIAN'S ROLE IN ASSESSING FITNESS TO DRIVE AFTER TBI

Legal and Ethical Considerations

In the United States, Australia, and elsewhere, most jurisdictions have regulations that require drivers to self-report to the DLA any change in their medical condition that could affect their driving, and a failure to do so may be grounds for suspension or criminal proceedings (5,8,28). Physicians and the DLA do not routinely communicate with each other, which maintains patient confidentiality. Nevertheless, physicians may communicate with the DLA in situations where patients known to be a risk to road safety continue to drive against repeated advice to stop (5). In some jurisdictions, physicians are protected from legal action if, acting in good faith, they report potentially unsafe drivers to the DLA. Additionally, certain jurisdictions may mandate reporting by physicians regarding unsafe drivers or drivers with specific medical conditions (75). However, physicians do not have a duty to physically prevent patients from driving, only to inform patients at risk to cease driving (36). For a state-by-state listing of driver licensing and reporting laws in the United States, see Chapter 8 of the American Medical Association's *Physician's Guide to Assessing and Counseling Older Drivers* (75). Physicians practicing in other jurisdictions can consult their regional or national transport authority for more information (e.g., in Australia, information about these laws can be found in *Assessing Fitness to Drive* published by Austroads) (5,8).

Even though it is expected that drivers self-report changes in their medical condition to the DLA, the law expects that physicians foresee the impact of a disabling medical condition on driver safety and counsel their patient accordingly (36). Physicians are regarded as experts in this matter and given the responsibility for determining whether a person is fit to drive, although physicians receive little formal training regarding driving assessment and generally do not have the knowledge and resources to conduct a CDE (9,36).

It is recommended that a physician who treats patients with TBI directly and comprehensively discuss driving and the local return-to-driving process early on in the recovery process, including the discussion of alternatives to driving. The discussion should include mention of concrete examples of how the patient's TBI is likely to impact on their driving. This avoids the situation that driving is only discussed in passing by the physician, and the patient is not made aware of the potentially dangerous consequences of returning to driving after TBI without proper evaluation and ongoing monitoring (5,36). Furthermore, the physician should inform their patient of any responsibility that the patient has to self-report their condition to the DLA and any mandatory reporting requirements that the physician is obliged to abide by. The physician should consider involving family members in such discussions, if the patient is willing (36). Such an approach can serve to demonstrate the importance and respect that the physician accords the patient's desire to return to driving (and perhaps making the delivery of advice to

stop driving more likely to be heeded by the patient). It is always good practice for all health practitioners including physicians and occupational therapists to thoroughly document any advice or recommendations given to patients in the clinical record. This can afford legal protection in the event of a crash or other adverse outcome involving the patient.

Assessing Medical Fitness to Drive

Physicians' main clinical role in driving after TBI is in determining individuals' medical fitness to drive, and referring the client for CDE with a CDRS if appropriate. Indeed, the *Driver Fitness Medical Guidelines* recommend that resumption of driving after moderate-to-severe TBI should not be attempted without a CDE, given the complicated and variable nature of TBI (28). Conversely, in many jurisdictions, a CDRS cannot undertake a CDE without clearance from a physician that the client is medically fit to drive. The website for the Association for Driver Rehabilitation Specialists is listed at the end of this chapter.[4] A physician may be requested to determine an individual's medical fitness to drive by the DLA or by the patient themselves (5). Similar to the off-road clinical assessment portion of the CDE, the physician undertakes a clinical examination to determine whether their patient has the requisite motor, sensory, and cognitive capacities for driving based on the relevant standards (usually, state or federal laws). A review of systems can show whether the patient's symptoms or conditions may impair driving performance (75). Also, an appraisal of the patient's medications can indicate if further action regarding driving assessment is necessary. Exemplar forms or reporting templates are sometimes available to facilitate the progress of the clinical examination (5,75).[5] As mentioned earlier, clients with conditional and unrestricted licenses may also need ongoing monitoring of fitness to drive at prescribed intervals through either medical reviews, CDEs, or both.

OTHER MEDICAL ISSUES FOR DRIVERS WITH TBI

Seizures and Epilepsy

If a patient with TBI is found to have epilepsy, then the physician should counsel the patient that they are also subject to the jurisdiction's regulations regarding seizures and epilepsy. Most jurisdictions have specific guidelines relating to driving following a seizure, a diagnosis of epilepsy, or while taking antiepileptic drugs (some antiepileptic drugs are known to cause side effects which affect driving in some patients) (28). Generally, persons with epilepsy who have been seizure-free for a certain time (varying between 3 and 12 months in most jurisdictions) are allowed to drive under certain conditions; for example, if their seizures are con-

---

[4] Physicians involved in the care of veterans in the United States may also refer patients to the Driver Rehabilitation for Veterans with Disabilities Program—a system-wide service that provides both driver assessment and rehabilitation for veterans.
[5] See http://www.transport.sa.gov.au/pdfs/forms/cert_fitness_light_712.PDF for an example form for South Australia.

trolled by medication, are simple partial seizures that do not interfere with consciousness or motor control, occur only during sleep, or can be predicted by the individual because of a prolonged and reliable aura (75,76). Drivers with epilepsy are usually legally required to self-report their condition to the relevant DLA, although some states also require mandatory reporting by physicians. The *Driver Fitness Medical Guidelines* recommend that drivers with epilepsy undergo an annual assessment with their treating physician, a requirement that may be relaxed over time in accordance with the physician's clinical judgment (28).

Dual Diagnosis

Other medical conditions, psychiatric conditions, or even advancing age may exert a cumulative or interactive effect on an individual with TBI's ability to drive safely (5,28). Examples include an individual who sustained TBI as a result of a motor vehicle crash with multiple disabling orthopedic injuries; a combat veteran with TBI and post-traumatic stress disorder which is exacerbated by certain elements of the traffic environment (77); or an individual with TBI who is also experiencing gradual age-related declines in the vision, motor, and cognitive domains. Furthermore, depression is commonly associated with TBI (78) and can result in cognitive impairment and psychomotor slowing (41). Although it is important for the physician to be aware of the patient's comorbidities, the presence of dual diagnoses does not change the functional focus of the clinical examination (i.e., the question is still whether the patient meets the criteria for driving) (5,28). It is important that the physician integrate all clinical information including the functional impact of impairments on driving and whether any comorbidities are stable, transient, or degenerative conditions, in order to determine the frequency of ongoing monitoring of the patient's driving capacity.

Medications

Many prescription and nonprescription medications have the potential to exert a harmful effect on an individual's fitness to drive. Persons with TBI often take medications to alleviate or prevent neurological and psychiatric sequelae (e.g., antiepileptic drugs as prophylaxis against seizures). Medications may impair driving by themselves or in combination with other drugs (75,79). All medications that may impair drivers of all ages are listed in Chapter 9 of the American Medical Association's *Physician's Guide to Assessing and Counseling Older Drivers* (75). Classes of medication associated with impaired driving or increased crash risk include but are not limited to hypnotics, antiepileptic agents, antiemetic agents, narcotics, barbiturates, benzodiazepines, antihistamines, antidepressants, antipsychotics, and muscle relaxants (75).

It is suggested that the physician prescribe medications that are least likely to impair driving whenever possible. Also, patients (especially those taking several medications) should be started on the lowest dosage possible. Patients should be fully informed of the likely side effects of any new prescriptions or dosage changes that have the potential to impair their driving (75). Ideally, the patient is recom-

mended to take the first few doses while refraining from driving in order to establish the extent of any side effects likely to impair driving. It can also be beneficial if a family member (someone who can observe the patient's behavior across several occasions) is informed of any medication changes, so that the patient's degree of insight into any side effects or impairments is corroborated. Physicians should also warn their patients of the risk of consuming alcohol and driving, particularly if the patient is taking other drugs that act on the central nervous system. Additionally, physicians should encourage their patients to disclose any over-the-counter or alternative medicines that they may be taking to avoid any adverse interactions.

WORKING WITH THE FAMILY OF A PERSON WITH TBI

Coordination of efforts with the family or support networks of the person with TBI is valuable in facilitating the individual's resumption of driving, or in supporting the person to access alternative forms of transportation (80). As highlighted at the beginning of this chapter, caregivers' perceptions of fitness to drive and a lack of social barriers have a measurable impact on persons continuing to drive after TBI (4,17,18). Families often have a vested interest in the outcome of the driving assessment process, and family support is often a critical factor in successful rehabilitation (79). For instance, if the driver with TBI must abide by the stipulations of a conditional license, family members can encourage adherence to such limits. Early in the process, family members can often supply additional or even contradictory information to health professionals regarding the person with TBI's driving history, degree of self awareness, or likely strengths and weaknesses (80). Occasionally, family opposition to driving must be overcome or explored in order to achieve greater independence for a person with TBI.

If family members or close friends are involved in the driving assessment process for a person with TBI, they can often be a source of practical and emotional support or provide additional guidance when the individual is found to be unfit to hold a driver's license (particularly if the person has limited insight into their impairments). Additionally, if a family member believes someone is unsafe to drive but continues to do so, some jurisdictions provide protection from legal action and anonymity for concerned family members who report such a driver to the DLA. Conversely, sometimes family denial of driving-related deficits or resistance to an unfavorable driving assessment outcome will need to be addressed. In such cases, family members may not wish to be burdened by having to provide transport, or a nondriver partner may also resist having to access alternate forms of transportation. However, such individuals can usually be counseled regarding their liabilities (e.g., by discussing that their relative will not likely gain motor vehicle insurance given the driving assessment outcome, and that family members enabling dangerous behavior may be at risk for civil court action in the event of a crash) (79).

CONCLUSION

Many individuals with TBI have a strong desire to resume driving, and between 25% and 60% of individuals with TBI will return to driving (1,7,13–18). Even though return to driving is of utmost importance to individuals with TBI, there still exists a considerable lack of knowledge regarding driving after TBI. This chapter has provided an overview of current driver assessment and rehabilitation practices after TBI, highlighting the physician's role in this process. However, there exist many avenues for future research regarding driving and TBI. First, this chapter has been limited to discussing return to driving after TBI because there is no research addressing learning to drive after (pediatric) TBI. Second, more studies using larger samples and officially documented minor as well as major crashes (perhaps via installing event-triggered recorders in the vehicles of drivers with TBI) are required to gain a clearer understanding of the relative crash risk of drivers with TBI. Third, and most importantly, more research is needed on the efficacy of both on- and off-road driver training after TBI. Newer testing and training paradigms (e.g., hazard perception testing) and newer technologies (e.g., driving simulators, event-triggered recorders, perhaps even driving video games) will undoubtedly have a role to play in driving rehabilitation in the future.

KEY CLINICAL POINTS

1. A key concern for physicians is the extent to which individuals with TBI pose a road safety risk if they resume driving. The evidence for increased crash risk for drivers who are able to resume driving post-TBI is equivocal and suggests modest increase in risk at best. Moreover, drivers with TBI commit driving violations at a comparable rate to the general population of drivers. However, those with TBI who continue to drive against professional recommendations are likely to be a high-risk group of drivers.
2. It is important that each individual with TBI who wants to return to driving is thoroughly assessed. Driver assessment is important not just for identifying those unsafe for driving, it is also a process that allows professionals to identify what supports, remedial training, or licensing conditions could enable individuals with TBI to continue to hold a driver's license safely. Because of its high ecological validity, the CDE is considered the gold standard form of assessment for drivers with TBI. It is a functional assessment, usually administered by a CDRS, which comprises of an off-road clinical assessment followed by an on-road practical driving test.
3. Physicians must be aware of the legal and ethical issues posed by driver assessment after TBI. Even though it is expected that drivers self-report changes in their medical condition to the DLA, the law expects that physicians foresee the impact of a disabling medical condition on driver safety and counsel their patient accordingly. Furthermore, physicians may be required to communicate with the DLA in situations where patients known to be a risk to road safety continue to drive.
4. It is suggested that physicians directly and comprehensively discuss driving and the local return-to-driving process early on in the recovery process from TBI, involving the family and support network whenever possible.
5. Physicians' main role in driving after TBI is in assessing a patient's medical fitness to drive (including consideration of the impact of seizures, dual diagnoses, or medica-

tions on driving). If the physician has any doubts about a patient's capacity to drive resulting from a clinical examination, then the physician may arrange a referral for the patient to undergo further assessment.

KEY REFERENCES

1. American Medical Association. *Physician's Guide to Assessing and Counseling Older Drivers.* 2nd ed. Chicago, IL: American Medical Association; 2010. http://www.ama-assn.org/ama/pub/physician-resources/public-health/promoting-healthy-lifestyles/geriatric-health/older-driver-safety/assessing-counseling-older-drivers.page. Accessed April 25, 2012.
2. Association for Driver Rehabilitation Specialists Web site. www.driver-ed.org. Accessed April 25, 2012.
3. Galski T, Ehle HT, McDonald MA, Mackevich J. Evaluating fitness to drive after cerebral injury: basic issues and recommendations for medical and legal communities. *J Head Trauma Rehabil.* 2000;15(3):895–908.
4. Pellerito JM, ed. *Driver Rehabilitation and Community Mobility: Principles and Practice.* St Louis, MO: Elsevier Mosby; 2006.
5. Schultheis MT, Matheis RJ, Nead R, DeLuca J. Driving behaviors following brain injury: self-report and motor vehicle records. *J Head Trauma Rehabil.* 2002;17(1):38–47.

References

1. Rapport LJ, Bryer RC, Hanks RA. Driving and community integration after traumatic brain injury. *Arch Phys Med Rehabil.* 2008;89(5): 922–930.
2. Kreutzer JS, Marwitz JH, Walker W, et al. Moderating factors in return to work and job stability after traumatic brain injury. *J Head Trauma Rehabil.* 2003;18(2):128–138.
3. Novack TA, Labbe D, Grote M, et al. Return to driving within 5 years of moderate-severe traumatic brain injury. *Brain Inj.* 2010; 24(3):464–471.
4. Rapport LJ, Hanks RA, Bryer RC. Barriers to driving and community integration after traumatic brain injury. *J Head Trama Rehabil.* 2006; 21(1):34–44.
5. Austroads. *Assessing Fitness to Drive.* Sydney, New South Wales, Australia: Austroads2003. Report No.: AP-G56/03.
6. Coleman Bryer R, Rapport LJ, Hanks RA. Determining fitness to drive: neuropsychological and psychological considerations. In: Pellerito JM Jr, ed. *Driver Rehabilitation: Principles and Practice.* St Louis, MO: Elsevier Mosby; 2006; 165–184.
7. Fisk GD, Schneider JJ, Novack TA. Driving following traumatic brain injury: prevalence, exposure, advice and evaluations. *Brain Inj.* 1998;12(8):683–695.
8. Brooks N, Hawley CA. Return to driving after traumatic brain injury: a British perspective. *Brain Inj.* 2005;19(3):165–175.
9. Hawley C. *The Attitudes of Health Professionals to Giving Advice on Fitness to Drive.* London, UK: Department for Transport, Local Government & the Regions; 2010. Road Safety Research Report No. 91.
10. van Zomeren AH, Brouwer WH, Rothengatter JA, Snoek JW. Fitness to drive a car after recovery from severe head injury. *Arch Phys Med Rehabil.* 1988;69(2):90–96.
11. Federal Motor Carrier Safety Administration. *Opinions of expert panel: Traumatic brain injury and commercial motor vhicle driver safety:* Federal Motor Carrier Safety Administration; 2009. Available from: www.fmcsa.dot.gov/rules-regulations/TOPICS/mep/report/TraumaticBrainInjury_MEP_Opinion.pdf.
12. Preece MH, Horswill MS, Geffen GM. Driving after concussion: the acute effect of mild traumatic brain injury on drivers' hazard perception. *Neuropsychology.* 2010;24(4):493–503.

13. Ponsford JL, Olver JH, Curran C. A profile of outcome: 2 years after traumatic brain injury. *Brain Inj.* 1995;9(1):1–10.
14. Hawley CA. Return to driving after head injury. *J Neurol Neurosurg Psychiatry.* 2001;70(6):761–766.
15. Pietrapiana P, Tamietto M, Torrini G, Mezzanato T, Rago R, Perino C. Role of premorbid factors in predicting safe return to driving after severe TBI. *Brain Inj.* 2005;19(3):197–211.
16. Formisano R, Bivona U, Brunelli S, Giustini M, Longo E, Taggi F. A preliminary investigation of road traffic accident rate after severe brain injury. *Brain Inj.* 2005;19(3):159–163.
17. Coleman RD, Rapport LJ, Ergh TC, Hanks RA, Ricker JH, Millis SR. Predictors of driving outcome after traumatic brain injury. *Arch Phys Med Rehabil.* 2002;83(10):1415–1422.
18. Priddy DA, Johnson P, Lam CS. Driving after a severe head injury. *Brain Inj.* 1990;4(3):267–272.
19. Schanke AK, Rike PO, Molmen A, Osten PE. Driving behaviour after brain injury: a follow-up of accident rate and driving patterns 6–9 years post-injury. *J Rehabil Med.* 2008;40(9):733–736.
20. Tamietto M, Torrini G, Adenzato M, Pietrapiana P, Rago R, Perino C. To drive or not to drive (after TBI)? A review of the literature and its implications for rehabilitation and future research. *Neuro Rehabilitation.* 2006;21(1):81–92.
21. Zador PL, Krawchuk SA, Voas RB. Alcohol-related relative risk of driver fatalities and driver involvement in fatal crashes in relation to driver age and gender: an update using 1996 data. *J Stud Alcohol.* 2000;61(3):387–395.
22. Haselkorn JK, Mueller BA, Rivara FA. Characteristics of drivers and driving record after traumatic and nontraumatic brain injury. *Arch Phys Med Rehabil.* 1998;79(7):738–742.
23. Schultheis MT, Matheis RJ, Nead R, DeLuca J. Driving behaviors following brain injury: self-report and motor vehicle records. *J Head Trama Rehabil.* 2002;17(1):38–47.
24. Leon-Carrion J, Dominguez-Morales MR, Martin JM. Driving with cognitive deficits: neurorehabilitation and legal measures are needed for driving again after severe traumatic brain injury. *Brain Inj.* 2005;19(3):213–219.
25. McCabe P, Lippert C, Weiser M, Hilditch M, Hartridge C, Villamere J. Community reintegration following acquired brain injury. *Brain Inj.* 2007;21(2):231–257.
26. Fox GK, Bowden SC, Smith DS. On-road assessment of driving competence after brain impairment: review of current practice and recommendations for a standardized examination. *Arch Phys Med Rehabil.* 1998;79(10):1288–1296.
27. Classen S, Levy C, McCarthy D, Mann WC, Lanford D, Waid-Ebbs JK. Traumatic brain injury and driving assessment: an evidence-based literature review. *Am J Occup Ther.* 2009;63(5):580–591.
28. United States National Highway Traffic Safety Administration, American Association of Motor Vehicle Administrators. *Driver Fitness Medical Guidelines.* Washington DC: U.S. Dept. of Transportation, National Highway Traffic Safety Administration; 2009.
29. Unsworth CA, Lovell RK, Terrington NS, Thomas SA. Review of tests contributing to the occupational therapy off-road driver assessment. *Aust Occup Ther J.* 2005;52(1):57–74.
30. Fox GK, Bashford GM, Caust SL. Identifying safe versus unsafe drivers following brain impairment: the Coorabel Programme. *Disabil Rehabil.* 1992;14(3):140–145.
31. Unsworth CA. Development and current status of occupational therapy driver assessment and rehabilitation in Victoria, Australia. *Aust Occup Ther J.* 2007;54(2):153–156.
32. Hatakka M, Keskinen E, Gregersen NP, Glad A. Theories and aims of educational and training measures. In: Siegrist SE, ed. *Driver Training, Testing and Licensing: Toward Theory-Based Management of Young Drivers' Injury Risk in Road Traffic.* Berne, Switzerland: Human Research Department, Swiss Council for Accident Prevention; 1999: 13–44.
33. Katz RT, Golden RS, Butter J, et al. Driving safety after brain damage: follow-up of twenty-two patients with matched controls. *Arch Phys Med Rehabil.* 1990;71(2):133–137.
34. Di Stefano M, Macdonald W, Baker PT, Huss CP. On-road driver evaluation and training. In: Pellerito JM Jr, ed. *Driver Rehabilitation and Community Mobility: Principles and Practice.* St Louis, MO: Elsevier, Mosby; 2006.
35. Clarke DD, Ward P, Bartle C, Truman W. Older drivers' road traffic crashes in the UK. *Accid Anal Prev.* 2010;42(4):1018–1024.
36. Galski T, Ehle HT, McDonald MA, Mackevich J. Evaluating fitness to drive after cerebral injury: basic issues and recommendations for medical and legal communities. *J Head Trama Rehabil.* 2000;15(3): 895–908.
37. Unsworth CA, Pallant JF, Russell KJ, Germano C, Odell M. Validation of a test of road law and road craft knowledge with older or functionally impaired drivers. *Am J Occup Ther.* 2010;64(2):306–315.
38. Kay LG, Bundy AC, Clemson LM. Predicting fitness to drive using the visual recognition slide test (USyd). *Am J Occup Ther.* 2008;62(2): 187–197.
39. Krishnasamy C, Unsworth CA. Normative data, preliminary inter-rater reliability and predictive validity of the Drive Home Maze Test. *Clin Rehabil.* 2011;25(1):88–95.
40. VicRoads, OT Australia (Victoria). *Guidelines for Occupational Therapy (OT) Driver Assessors.* Victoria, Australia: VicRoads; 2008.
41. Wheatley CJ, Pellerito JM Jr, et al. The clinical evaluation. In: Pellerito JM Jr, ed. *Driver Rehabilitation and Community Mobility: Principles and Practice.* St Louis, MO: Elsevier, Mosby; 2006.
42. Unsworth CA, Pallant JF, Russell KJ, Odell M. *Occupational Therapy Driver Off-Road Assessment (OT-DORA) Battery.* Baltimore, MD: AOTA Press; 2011.
43. Galski T, Ehle HT, Bruno RL. An assessment of measures to predict the outcome of driving evaluations in patients with cerebral damage. *Am J Occup Ther.* 1990;44(8):709–713.
44. Korteling JE, Kaptein NA. Neuropsychological driving fitness tests for brain-damaged subjects. *Arch Phys Med Rehabil.* 1996;77(2): 138–146.
45. Hartman-Maeir A, Erez AB, Ratzon N, Mattatia T, Weiss P. The validity of the Color Trail Test in the pre-driver assessment of individuals with acquired brain injury. *Brain Inj.* 2008;22(13–14): 994–998.
46. Lundqvist A, Alinder J, Alm H, Gerdle B, Levander S, Rönnberg J. Neuropsychological aspects of driving after brain lesion: simulator study and on-road driving. *Appl Neuropsychol.* 1997;4(4):220–230.
47. Brooke MM, Questad KA, Patterson DR, Valois TA. Driving evaluation after traumatic brain injury. *Am J Phys Med Rehabil.* 1992;71(3): 177–182.
48. Stokx LC, Gaillard AW. Task and driving performance of patients with a severe concussion of the brain. *J Clin Exp Neuropsychol.* 1986; 8(4):421–436.
49. Novack TA, Baños JH, Alderson AL, et al. UFOV performance and driving ability following traumatic brain injury. *Brain Inj.* 2006;20(5): 455–461.
50. Sommer M, Heidinger C, Arendasy M, Schauer S, Schmitz-Gielsdorf J, Häusler J. Cognitive and personality determinants of post-injury driving fitness. *Arch Clin Neuropsychol.* 2010;25(2):99–117.
51. Duquette J, McKinley P, Mazer B, et al. Impact of partial administration of the Cognitive Behavioral Driver's Inventory on concurrent validity for people with brain injury. *Am J Occup Ther.* 2010;64(2): 279–287.
52. Schultheis MT, Hillary F, Chute DL. The Neurocognitive Driving Test: applying technology to the assessment of driving ability following brain injury. *Rehabil Psychol.* 2003;48(4):275–280.
53. Lundqvist A, Alinder J, Rönnberg J. Factors influencing driving 10 years after brain injury. *Brain Inj.* 2008;22(4):295–304.
54. McKenna FP, Horswill MS. Hazard perception and its relevance for driver licensing. *J Int Ass Traffic Safety Sci.* 1999;23(1):26–41.
55. Horswill MS, Anstey KJ, Hatherly CG, Wood JM. The crash involvement of older drivers is associated with their hazard perception latencies. *J Int Neuropsychol Soc.* 2010;16(5):939–944.
56. Darby P, Murray W, Raeside R. Applying online fleet driver assessment to help identify, target and reduce occupational road safety risks. *Safety Sci.* 2009;47(3):436–442.
57. Preece MH, Horswill MS, Geffen GM. Assessment of drivers' ability to anticipate traffic hazards after traumatic brain injury. *J Neurol Neurosurg Psychiatry.* 2011;82(4):447–451.
58. Pradhan AK, Pollatsek A, Knodler M, Fisher DL. Can younger drivers be trained to scan for information that will reduce their risk in roadway traffic scenarios that are hard to identify as hazardous? *Ergonomics.* 2009;52(6):657–673.

59. Poulsen AA, Horswill MS, Wetton M, Hill A, Lim SM. A brief office-based hazard perception intervention for drivers with ADHD symptoms. *Aust N Z J Psychiatry.* 2010;44(6):528–534.

60. Cyr AA, Stinchcombe A, Gagnon S, Marshall S, Hing MM, Finestone H. Driving difficulties of brain-injured drivers in reaction to high-crash-risk simulated road events: a question of impaired divided attention? *J Clin Exp Neuropsychol.* 2009;31(4):472–482.

61. Charron C, Hoc JM, Milleville-Pennel I. Cognitive control by brain-injured car drivers: an exploratory study. *Ergonomics.* 2010;53(12):1434–1445.

62. Milleville-Pennel I, Pothier J, Hoc JM, Mathé JF. Consequences of cognitive impairments following traumatic brain injury: pilot study on visual exploration while driving. *Brain Inj.* 2010;24(4):678–691.

63. Lew HL, Poole JH, Lee EH, Jaffe DL, Huang H, Brodd E. Predictive validity of driving-simulator assessments following traumatic brain injury: a preliminary study. *Brain Inj.* 2005;19(3):177–188.

64. Lew HL, Rosen PN, Thomander D, Poole JH. The potential utility of driving simulators in the cognitive rehabilitation of combat-returnees with traumatic brain injury. *J Head Trama Rehabil.* 2009;24(1):51–56.

65. Gamache PL, Lavallière M, Tremblay M, Simoneau M, Teasdale N. In-simulator training of driving abilities in a person with a traumatic brain injury. *Brain Inj.* 2011;25(4):416–425.

66. Galski T, Bruno RL, Ehle HT. Prediction of behind-the-wheel driving performance in patients with cerebral brain damage: a discriminant function analysis. *Am J Occup Ther.* 1993;47(5):391–396.

67. Carney C, McGehee DV, Lee JD, Reyes ML, Raby M. Using an event-triggered video intervention system to expand the supervised learning of newly licensed adolescent drivers. *Am J Public Health.* 2010;100(6):1101–1106.

68. McGehee DV, Raby M, Carney C, Lee JD, Reyes ML. Extending parental mentoring using an event-triggered video intervention in rural teen drivers. *J Safety Res.* 2007;38(2):215–227.

69. Wouters IJ, Bos JM. Traffic accident reduction by monitoring driver behaviour with in-car data recorders. *Accid Anal Prev.* 2000;32(5):643–650.

70. Sivak M, Hill CS, Olson PL. Improving driving performance of persons with brain damage via perceptual/cognitive remediation. *Int J Rehabil Res.* 1982;5(4):551–552.

71. Sivak M, Hill CS, Henson DL, Butler BP, Silber SM, Olson PL. Improved driving performance folllowing perceptual training in persons with brain damage. *Arch Phys Med Rehabil.* 1984;65(4):163–167.

72. Klonoff PS, Olson KC, Talley MC, et al. The relationship of cognitive retraining to neurological patients' driving status: the role of process variables and compensation training. *Brain Inj.* 2010;24(2):63–73.

73. Edwards JD, Delahunt PB, Mahncke HW. Cognitive speed of processing training delays driving cessation. *J Gerontol A Biol Sci Med Sci.* 2009;64(12):1262–1267.

74. Roenker DL, Cissell GM, Ball KK, Wadley VG, Edwards JD. Speed-of-processing and driving simulator training result in improved driving performance. *Hum Factors.* 2003;45(2):218–233.

75. American Medical Association. *Physician's Guide to Assessing and Counseling Older Drivers.* 2nd ed. Chicago, IL: American Medical Association; 2010.

76. Krumholz A. Driving issues in epilepsy: past, present, and future. *Epilepsy Curr.* 2009;9(2):31–35.

77. Lew HL, Amick MM, Kraft M, Stein MB, Cifu DX. Potential driving issues in combat returnees. *Neuro Rehabilitation.* 2010;26(3):271–278.

78. Kreutzer JS, Seel RT, Gourley E. The prevalence and symptom rates of depression after traumatic brain injury: a comprehensive examination. *Brain Inj.* 2001;15(7):563–576.

79. Hopewell CA. Driving assessment issues for practicing clinicians. *J Head Trama Rehabil.* 2002;17(1):48–61.

80. Radomski MV, Davidson L, Voydetich D, Erickson MW. Occupational therapy for service members with mild traumatic brain injury. *Am J Occup Ther.* 2009;63(5):646–655.

Substance Misuse Among Persons With Traumatic Brain Injury

John D. Corrigan and W. Jerry Mysiw

INTRODUCTION

Clinicians working with people who have incurred a traumatic brain injury (TBI) cannot avoid the issue of alcohol and other drug use. Whether consumption of substances contributed to the cause of injury, or use after injury places the individual at risk for medical complications and poorer psychosocial outcomes, alcohol and other drug use must be addressed with adolescents and adults in rehabilitation for TBI. Studies of both brain structure and function indicate that substance misuse and TBI interact in an additive way, specifically, their co-occurrence results in more impairment than either one alone. In addition to the contribution to impairments, substance misuse after TBI can lower seizure thresholds, interact with prescribed medications and lead to additional injuries. Substance misuse also limits outcomes from TBI by undermining environmental supports such as familial care or access to services. The detriment to the person and family is reason enough to be concerned about substance misuse; however, as a field, we must also be concerned that the benefit to society of rehabilitation interventions is compromised when our patients misuse substances following their TBI. As we will describe later, the threat among adult rehabilitation patients with TBI is of sufficient frequency to jeopardize the perceived value of rehabilitation in any public policy equation that considers long-term costs to society.

This chapter provides a review of past and current research on TBI and the use of alcohol and other drugs. The scope of the problem of these co-occurring conditions is initially addressed in terms of etiology and prevalence. Injury-related characteristics with implications for later rehabilitation are described, including pertinence for prognostication. Research on TBI and substance misuse in rehabilitation patients is summarized and the impact on long-term outcomes is described. Finally, a brief summary of what is known about these co-occurring conditions in other treatment settings and populations concludes the discussion of scope of the problem. The second section of this chapter is focused on intervention. A review of treatment studies that have specifically addressed substance use following TBI is followed by presentation of a theoretical model for conceptualizing treatment goals based on severity of the conditions and settings for intervention. Using the model as a framework, best practices for clinical use in rehabilitation are discussed. The rehabilitation research literature continues to be characterized by having a significantly greater number of studies describing the problem of substance misuse and TBI than those investigating treatment approaches to ameliorate use-related disorders.

In this chapter we use the terms "substance use," "substance misuse," and "substance use disorder." In some instances, we will be more specific about the substance in question and may refer specifically to alcohol or other drug use or misuse or disorder. By "use," we mean the consumption of any amount of the substance. For alcohol and prescription drugs, any use is not illegal or by definition unhealthy; however, there are amounts of consumption that are considered risky if not unhealthy. The National Institute on Alcohol Abuse and Alcoholism (NIAAA) defines risky drinking as 15 or greater drinks per week and 5 or greater drinks on any day for men; and 8 or greater drinks per week and 4 or greater drinks on any day for women (http://rethinkingdrinking.niaaa.nih.gov Accessed May 28, 2011). For prescription drugs, use of someone else's prescribed medication or one's own in greater dose or frequency than prescribed is unhealthy and/or risky. For illicit drugs, use is by definition illegal and is presumed unhealthy. At the other end of the spectrum from use is the presence of a diagnosable substance use disorder—either in the form of abuse or dependence. The current *Diagnostic and Statistical Manual (DSM-IV-TR)* (1) distinguishes between these diagnoses, primarily on the basis of whether a person continues to use despite actual or imminent consequences (abuse), or if all of a person's behavior has come to center on the acquisition, consumption, and recovery from the use of the drug (dependence). As of this writing, the recommendation for the *DSM-V* (www.dsm5.org Accessed May 28, 2011) is that abuse and dependence for various substances be combined into the single category "substance use disorder." In this chapter, our use of the term "substance use disorder" is consistent with this recommendation. To avoid confusion, we have avoided the term "substance abuse" and instead referred to "substance misuse," that includes consumption that is unhealthy and/or risky as well as that which constitutes a diagnosable substance use disorder (SUD).

SCOPE OF THE PROBLEM OF SUBSTANCE MISUSE AND TBI

Patients who are known to have been intoxicated at time of injury often receive the most scrutiny of their substance use. However, persons with prior histories of SUD (who may or may not have been intoxicated at time of injury but often are), and those who use excessively after injury (who may or may not have had a prior SUD) may be at risk for the greatest functional impairment. There is considerable overlap among groups defined by intoxication at injury, prior history and postinjury misuse, although comprehensive epidemiologic data is still lacking. Existing studies suggest multiple long-term health and behavioral consequences, including greater vulnerability for morbidity experienced by members of special populations who have a prior history of TBI.

Cause and Effect

Several systematic reviews conclude that substance misuse is more likely to cause TBI than TBI is likely to cause SUD (2,3), whereas others have been more cautious citing insufficient evidence about the directionality of causal factors and risk factors associated with each condition (4,5). The causal relationship between TBI and SUD is further confused by the choice of injury used to ask the question. Both reviews that concluded SUD causes TBI relied on studies in which samples were captured in adult trauma or rehabilitation units. It is accurate to expect that a substantial proportion of subjects in such samples will have prior histories of substance misuse if not a diagnosable SUD. However, these studies do not take into account whether the TBI that has resulted in their inclusion in the cohort is indeed their first TBI, or if 1 or more earlier TBIs may have influenced the development of the substance misuse. Recent studies have raised concerns that childhood TBI may have long-term consequences that include the development of adolescent or adult behavioral health problems, including substance misuse (6–8). Particularly useful findings have resulted from the developmental perspective provided by birth cohort data (6,7).

Birth cohorts that have studied childhood TBI were conducted in Northern Finland (9) and Christchurch, New Zealand (7). The Northern Finland studies identified TBI from hospital records and death certificates; these data were supplemented by health, criminal, and other social service records, as well as survey data collected at age 14. Studies using the Northern Finland birth cohort have reported multiple risk factors associated with incurring a TBI, including that if parents misused alcohol, there was a two-fold greater chance of childhood TBI (10); and that an alcohol related, first injury after age 12 resulted in a four-fold greater risk of repeat injury by age 34 (11). Both studies suggested that early childhood substance-related history (parental or personal) was associated with later TBI. One study that examined TBI as a risk for developing behavioral health problems found that after controlling for potential confounders, including preinjury psychiatric disorders, children and adolescents who incurred a TBI before age 15 were twice as likely to be hospitalized for a psychiatric disorder by age 31; however, childhood TBI was not found to be an independent risk factor for late adolescence or early adulthood SUD (12).

The Christchurch birth cohort project conducted prospective interviews to identify health events, including medically treated TBI that were then verified via hospital, clinic, or doctors' office records. The contemporaneous collection of medically verified TBI's provides a unique and important resource for studying lifetime history of these injuries. In a series of analyses, the cohort was divided into those children who had experienced no TBI, those who experienced mild TBI (loss of consciousness for less than 20 minutes and no skull fracture) but received only outpatient treatment, and those who experienced mild TBI and were hospitalized 1 or 2 days only. Children with longer hospitalizations (presumably indicating more severe injuries) were not included in the analyses. Controlling for multiple demographic and developmental characteristics, those with preschool (before age 5) mild TBI requiring brief hospitalization were more likely to show symptoms of attention deficit or hyperactivity, conduct disorder or oppositional defiant behavior, SUD and mood disorder in adolescence (13). Only anxiety disorders were not different among the groups. The Christchurch studies imply greater than expected later consequences, including the development of SUD, from early life complicated but mild TBI.

Injury-Related Characteristics

Estimates of the percentage of TBIs that occur while intoxicated vary by population (e.g., country, year sampled) and method of capture, (e.g., emergency department admission, trauma center patients, rehabilitation admissions) but in all circumstances, it is reasonable to expect that a disproportionate number of adults treated for a TBI will have alcohol present in excess of the legal limit for driving and/or a positive screen for illegal drugs (4,14,15). Intoxication at time of injury is associated with the likelihood of incurring a TBI as a component of that injury (16); and persons intoxicated at time of TBI are more likely, young and have prior histories of misuse (14,15,17). A population-based study of intoxication at the time of hospitalization among patients 16 and older admitted with a diagnosis of TBI to hospitals in Colorado found 20.8% had a blood alcohol content above 80 mg/dL (18). In a metropolitan area, 9% of youth 12–18 years old who were hospitalized with blunt trauma were positive for alcohol or illicit drugs—cannabis was most frequent (40%) followed by alcohol (30%) (19). Based on TBI Model Systems data for the 75% of the cohort in which it was tested (almost 8,000 cases), 44% had a blood alcohol content equal to or greater than 100 mg/dL (http://www. tbindsc.org Accessed May 30, 2011). Studies consistently find higher rates of intoxication at time of injury for rehabilitation patients, which is likely due to a series of adverse selection factors (e.g., greater intoxication is involved in more severe injuries, prior history of misuse is associated with both greater intoxication and worse outcomes) that increase the likelihood of having a more severe TBI and, thus, greater likelihood that rehabilitation is necessary (14,15,20).

Intoxication at time of injury is important information for assessment of a patient's substance use; however, it is not sufficient for drawing conclusions or projecting prognosis. The circumstances around an injury that occurs while intoxicated may be a reflection of a person's habits with regard to use (e.g., substance and amount consumed, tolerance for alcohol, social setting, days of the week or risk-taking tendencies); however, the clinician must also explore these habits in the weeks, months, and years preceding the injury. Prior history of substance use is more important information than intoxication at time of injury for drawing conclusions about risk for postinjury use. Prior history has also been found to be associated with less favorable outcomes (5,14,15), although studies of the prognostic value of intoxication at time of injury have had mixed findings that include some researchers' speculation about a protective effect of alcohol. As described later, both postulations ("prior history of misuse results in poorer outcomes" and "alcohol has a protective effect on TBI outcome") are subject to confound that should suggest caution when drawing conclusions.

Corrigan summarized reports from the research literature indicating that those acutely intoxicated were more likely to have more severe injuries, require intubation, develop pneumonia and have other forms of respiratory distress; manifest greater neurologic impairment at discharge; have longer agitation and lower cognitive function at acute hospital discharge; and require greater time from admission to rehabilitation (14). Like adults, adolescents intoxicated at time of injury were more severely injured, required more procedures and longer hospitalizations, and had worse outcomes at discharge (19). However, in contrast to evidence for intoxication causing greater morbidity, some studies of cohorts drawn from trauma centers have found no difference in outcomes for those alcohol intoxicated and those who are not (21,22), or have observed better outcomes for the intoxicated group with comparable TBI severity (23–25). These findings have led to speculation that alcohol may have a neuroprotective effect; however, the results may also be due to a confound between intoxication and the determination of TBI severity whereby a less severe TBI appears more severe in the presence of intoxication. Because the alcohol can obtund alertness and responsiveness, measures such as the Glasgow Coma Scale (GCS) score or length of loss of consciousness can be artificially affected by intoxication. When TBI severity based on 1 of these measures is used as a mediating factor on outcomes assessed at a later point in time, the confounding effect can result in the intoxicated group appearing to have a better outcome, when in fact they may have had a less severe TBI. Schutte and Hanks found alcohol intoxication lowered GCS by an average of 1.9 points (26). Lange and colleagues did not observe an overall effect of intoxication on GCS but found an interaction between blood alcohol content and GCS severity for highly intoxicated patients with abnormal imaging findings (27).

There is also a potential confound when considering the influence of prior history of substance misuse on TBI outcome. Several studies have reported that patients with histories of SUD are more likely to be involved in injuries in which there is greater energy transfer (i.e., gun shot wounds, moving vehicle crashes, falls from greater heights, or violent assaults with a weapon) (28). High-velocity forces cause more brain damage, which in turn will result in poorer outcomes. This risk of artifact is further exacerbated by the likelihood that persons with more severe histories of SUD are also likely to have had a prior TBI and/or experienced other sources of CNS compromise (e.g., prenatal alcohol exposure, attention deficit disorder, history of drug overdose). These premorbid characteristics will affect the eventual outcome observed from a recent injury. Even though the association between prior history of substance misuse and poorer TBI

outcomes may not be straightforward (29,30), the consistency of the association suggests that prior history is still essential information for clinical inference and planning.

Among Adults in Acute Rehabilitation

Most studies that report preinjury substance misuse in TBI populations have either (a) not been limited to rehabilitation inpatients (e.g., trauma center or acute hospital cohorts) or (b) have collected the sample from outpatient or community-dwelling former inpatients. Both methods will underestimate rates for inpatient rehabilitation populations. The selection factors described earlier that affect who goes to acute rehabilitation result in lower prevalence rates among hospitalized patients or trauma center admissions when compared to rehabilitation cohorts. Samples captured from outpatient settings or community-living former inpatients underestimate the prevalence because those with prior histories are more likely to be lost to follow-up (31–33).

Based on studies that had used a prospective method of detection to evaluate rehabilitation populations with TBI, Corrigan concluded that approaching two-thirds of adolescents and adults treated in rehabilitation for TBI have prior histories of alcohol misuse or illicit drug use (14). There have been several studies since that provide a more precise estimate. For a prospective sample of 356 consecutive admissions to acute rehabilitation at the Ohio State University Medical Center, Corrigan and colleagues reported that 54% were identified as having preinjury alcohol misuse, and 34% were having preinjury other drug misuse (although this study analyzed patients for whom follow-up data were available, the aforementioned rates reflect the consecutive sample of inpatients from whom follow-up data were sought) (33). Due to the high rate of co-occurrence of alcohol and other drug use disorders, 58% of the sample showed 1 or the other or both. Bombardier, Rimmele, and Zintel reported very similar results for 142 consecutive admissions to acute rehabilitation at the University of Washington (34). In their sample, 58% misused alcohol, 39% had recently used illicit drugs, and 61% had either or both histories. Ponsford and colleagues reported preinjury alcohol misuse for 31% of a consecutive sample of acute rehabilitation patients treated at 1 center in Australia (35). The same sample had 34% reporting any illicit drug use and co-occurrence was high although not reported in a manner that provided a rate of any substance misuse. TBI Model Systems data for the 10-year period from 2001–2010 indicates 43% of adults in rehabilitation with a primary diagnosis of moderate or severe TBI had preinjury histories of any problem use; 21% had used illicit drugs (http://www. tbindsc.org Accessed May 30, 2011).

The results of the mentioned studies suggest high rates of premorbid problem use; however, because earlier studies (33,34) approached Corrigan's conclusion that two-thirds of adults in acute rehabilitation have prior histories of misuse, more recent results (35), and longitudinal findings from the TBI Model Systems (see Fig. 79-1) would suggest a lower estimate. The TBI Models Systems method of detection may be less sensitive than those used in the facility-specific studies, and the results for premorbid alcohol misuse reported by Ponsford and colleagues were substantially lower than North American studies, perhaps more reflective of alcohol use disorders and not including unhealthy or risky use.

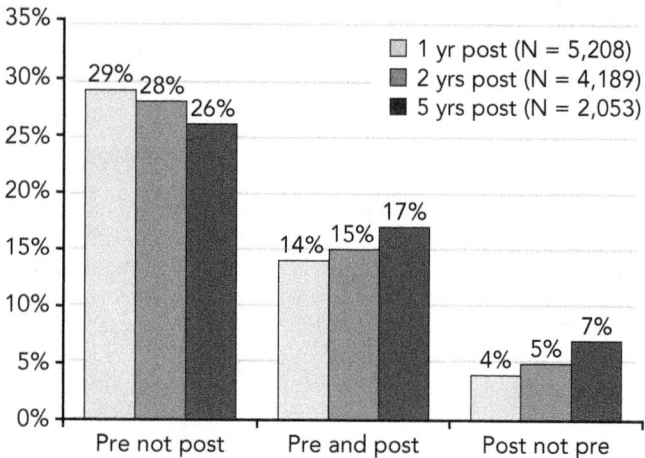

FIGURE 79-1 TBI model systems problem substance use at follow-up as a function of preinjury problem use and time post-injury.

When all factors are considered, it would appear reasonable to expect half of the adults under age 65 receiving inpatient rehabilitation for a primary diagnosis of TBI to have prior histories of either alcohol misuse or illicit drug use. A cluster analysis that examined both premorbid history and early postinjury attitudes toward use suggested that there may be some utility in further categorizing those with a positive preinjury history of alcohol use disorders by premorbid abuse, dependence in remission and dependence not in remission (36); however, there have been no subsequent studies demonstrating the utility of this recommendation. Furthermore, as addressed later, those at risk for future substance misuse include patients with no prior history.

The Extent of Misuse Following TBI

Like other patients hospitalized due to injury, patients who have incurred a TBI consume less alcohol and use fewer illicit drugs in the immediate postinjury period (35,37–39); however, there are also indications that a significant proportion eventually return to preinjury levels of use as time postinjury increases (35,38,40–42). Among persons hospitalized with mild-to-severe TBI, almost one-third appear to be misusing substances upon later follow-up. Horner and colleagues found that 1 year after hospitalization, 29% of South Carolina Traumatic Brain Injury Surveillance and Follow-up Registry survey respondents reported moderate or heavy drinking in the prior month (43). Although illicit drug use was not reported, the Colorado Follow Survey reported 10% of persons hospitalized with a TBI used an illicit drug in the first year after injury (18). Silver and colleagues found that approximately 25% of a population-based sample of persons with TBI also had alcohol use disorders (vs 10% for those without TBI); and 11% had other drug use disorders (vs 5% without TBI) (44). Assuming that most other drug misuse is engaged in by persons who are also misusing alcohol leads to the estimate that approximately one-third of persons hospitalized are misusing substances later. However, the South Carolina Traumatic Brain Injury Surveillance and Follow-up Registry findings also indicated that half of the cohort had

engaged in binge drinking during the past 30 days—the expected rate based on the general population of South Carolina would be 30%. Particularly given that the study participants were only a year posthospitalization for a TBI, one-third may be a conservative estimate of the proportion misusing substances after TBI.

For patients requiring inpatient rehabilitation, a similar proportion are estimated to be engaged in postinjury substance misuse. In an Australian cohort reported by Ponsford and colleagues, 25% were drinking alcohol at hazardous levels by 2 years postinjury (vs approximately 30% preinjury and for controls) and 9% had other drug use disorders. The same research group reported that 21% of the cohort in a cross-sectional follow-up study of patients 6 months to 5.5 years postinjury manifested an SUD (38). The inclusion of patients within a year postinjury would account in part for the lower rate. Fig. 79-1 shows problem substance use (alcohol misuse or illicit drug use) for the TBI Model Systems cohort as a function of both preinjury problem use and time postinjury. By 5 years postinjury approximately, 25% are misusing substances, which is somewhat lower than estimates for acute hospital patients; however, the methodology used by the TBI Model Systems tends to result in lower estimates.

It is difficult to estimate the proportion of patients who develop substance misuse only after an index injury. First, as described earlier, most studies have looked at a particular index injury and whether or not substance misuse preceded or not but have not considered whether the index injury was a person's first. This problem aside several studies report that a proportion of patients develop substance misuse for the first time after an injury in adolescence or adulthood (37,44–47). The TBI Model Systems data suggest that 25%–30% of those with postinjury substance misuse did not have these problems preinjury. Interestingly, the only 2 studies that concluded there are few patients with "novel" or new onset substance dependence also reported relatively high rates for new onset alcohol abuse. Whelan-Goodinson and colleagues reported that two-thirds of their participants who had a postinjury alcohol abuse disorder did not have a history preinjury (38). Koponen and colleagues reported that two-thirds of their sample who manifested an alcohol abuse disorder 30 years after an index injury developed their disorder postinjury (48). Confidence in the results from both studies are limited by their small sample size. Bjork and Grant speculated that dopaminergic disruption and/or executive dysfunction arising from orbital-frontal damage could increase the risk of substance misuse following TBI (4).

Regardless the level of hospitalization required following TBI, those who develop postinjury substance misuse are more likely young, single males with preinjury histories of misuse. Horner and colleagues' population-based study exemplifies this observation (43). These researchers found risk factors for heavy drinking included a preinjury history of SUD, a diagnosis of depression since the injury, better physical functioning, male gender, younger age, being uninsured or on Medicaid, and not being married. Similar associations were evident for moderate levels of drinking. There was no relationship between postinjury drinking patterns and TBI severity. The presence of co-occurring depression reported by Horner is also a consistent finding; indeed, the "triple threat" of TBI, SUD, and affective disorders is evident in both rehabilitation follow-up studies and reports of the prevalence of TBI among participants in SUD treatment.

Long-Term Consequences

There is growing evidence that the effects of TBI, including some that are less severe, persist long-term and may be exacerbated in conjunction with the normal aging process (3). Those who also misuse substances face additional complications, including they are less likely to be working (32,49–52), have lower subjective well-being (33,53,54), have an increased likelihood of suicide (55–59), have an increased likelihood of premature mortality due to any cause (60,61) and are at greater risk for seizure (62,63).

Numerous studies have observed that substance use problems preceding injury are often a significant predictor of postinjury unemployment. MacMillan and colleagues studied 45 adults 2 years after moderate or severe TBI (50). They found that both preinjury psychiatric and SUD histories predicted a lower likelihood of employment and that preinjury SUD also was associated with less independence in living situation. Sherer and colleagues studied 76 persons with moderate or severe TBI who received services through a specialized day treatment program (49). Employment status 3 months following discharge from this program was assessed; on average, 2 years postinjury. Predictors of employment status included severity of injury, premorbid education, preinjury substance misuse, and need for physical, cognitive, and behavioral supervision at discharge from acute rehabilitation. Multiple logistic regressions revealed that only level of preinjury substance use was predictive of later productivity. Subjects with no history of preinjury substance misuse were more than 8 times as likely to be employed at follow-up. Bogner and colleagues investigated the relative contribution of substance misuse and violent injury etiology in a sample of 351 consecutive admissions for acute brain injury rehabilitation (53). At 1 year following injury, prior history of SUD was a significant predictor of postinjury unemployment, as were age, preinjury unemployment and cognitive function at rehabilitation discharge. A review of 35 published articles describing 14 prospective cohorts concluded that preinjury history of substance misuse was associated with long-term disability and lack of productivity (51). Consistent with previous studies, preinjury unemployment, longer post-traumatic amnesia and more disability at rehabilitation admission were also important predictors of subsequent unemployment.

Despite the consistent finding that preinjury substance misuse is associated with postinjury unemployment, the relationship with postinjury use may be more complex. Jorge and colleagues studied 158 patients with TBI during the first year following injury (52). A history of SUD was associated with development of mood disorders and was more marked in those who resumed substance use. Both substance use and mood disorders postinjury were associated with poorer vocational outcomes. Volumetric studies of gray matter also found reduced frontal lobe volumes for those with a history of substance use disorder. Those who resumed alcohol abuse had decreased medial frontal gray matter volumes and impaired performance in executive tasks. These results suggest multiple possible relationships among substance misuse, TBI, and poor vocational outcomes. Sander, Kreutzer, and

Fernandez found that employed persons who had incurred moderate or severe TBI and were on the average 16 months postinjury reported consuming greater amounts of alcohol than similar subjects who were unemployed (64). This finding may be consistent with clinical observations that return to work can be a trigger for substance use because of having financial resources to purchase alcohol or other drugs, as well as increased stressors arising from the work environment.

Substance misuse and mood are highly related to subjective well-being. Corrigan and colleagues reported that a prior history of SUD was highly associated with subjective well-being both 1 and 2 years after injury (33). At year 1, prior substance misuse was the strongest independent predictor of life satisfaction and continued to be a significant predictor 2 years after injury, even after the effects of depressed mood, social integration, and employment had been accounted for. The complex relationship between mood and subjective well-being was evident in Bombardier and colleagues' study of major depressive disorder (MDD) following TBI (54). Among trauma center patients followed the first year after TBI, more than half met criteria for MDD at least once during follow-up. As would be expected, MDD was significantly associated with subjective well-being. Depressed mood results in lower life satisfaction, but its absence does not assure higher subjective well-being (33). Bombardier and colleagues also found a strong association with substance misuse—in addition to MDD presence at time of injury and history of MDD before TBI, lifetime alcohol dependence was the only other significant predictor of postinjury MDD onset (54). Finally, Bogner and colleagues identified that the relationship previously reported between violent etiology of injury and lower subjective well-being was better accounted for by substance misuse history than violent etiology of injury (53).

People who initially survive TBI are susceptible to premature mortality and substance misuse is associated with certain etiologies (61,65,66). Himanen and colleagues found age at injury and postinjury employment to be highly associated with premature death; employment, in turn, was predicted by age, severity of TBI and cognitive impairment, subsequent TBI, and alcohol abuse (61). Pentland and colleagues found substance misuse-related death was the most common etiology in deaths that occurred up to 20 years following hospitalization for TBI (60). Compared to the general population matched for age, gender, and race, persons who required rehabilitation for TBI were 37 times more likely to die of seizures (65,67). At least 2 studies have observed a relationship between late developing seizures and substance misuse following TBI. De Reuck compared patients with moderate TBI who developed seizures over the first 3 years postinjury to matched patients with TBI who did not (63). All participants had cerebral contusions but had not required neurosurgical intervention. In addition to vascular risk factors, the only other predictor of late onset seizures was the presence of alcohol abuse. Verma and colleagues examined the relationship between chronic alcohol abusers' withdrawal and the occurrence of a seizure episode (62). They separated a sample of 54 adult male alcoholics who had experienced seizures into 3 groups—those for whom there was always a clear relationship between withdrawal and the seizure episode (the last drink occurring between 6 and 96 hours prior to seizure), those for whom some but not all seizure episodes were associated with withdrawal, and a third group in which none of the seizure episodes were associated with withdrawal. They found that a history of severe TBI preceding the onset of a seizure disorder was present for none of the patients in the first group, approximately 40% of those in the second group, and more than 75% of those in the third. They concluded the lack of a consistent relationship between alcohol withdrawal and seizure precipitation for the second and third groups appears to be a result of the higher incidence of prior TBI in those subjects, and that this relationship may account for the previously observed heterogeneity in the relationship between alcohol withdrawal and seizure episodes.

Suicide is another source of premature mortality (55–59,68). There has been some indication of an independent relationship between substance misuse and the likelihood of suicide following TBI. Teasdale and Engberg examined suicide after TBI using the Danish population register for hospital admissions and found that the likelihood of suicide increased by a factor of 2.7 for concussions, 3.0 for cranial fractures, and 4.1 for intracranial hemorrhage compared to age- and gender-matched rates in the general population (55). When substance use diagnosis was combined with TBI diagnosis, standardized mortality ratios increased significantly. Silver, Kramer, Greenwald, and Weissman reported the relative risks of psychiatric problems for a randomly selected subgroup of the New Haven portion of the NIMH Epidemiologic Catchment Area study (44). Again, TBI alone significantly increased the risk of suicide by an odds ratio of 5.7. After controlling for alcohol use disorders, the likelihood of suicide attempt declined to 4.5, suggesting that alcohol use accounted for approximately 20% of the risk of suicide after TBI. Brenner and colleagues controlled for psychiatric disorders including substance abuse in examining hazard ratios for suicide among veterans who did and did not have histories of TBI (59). Among those with more severe injuries (i.e., cerebral contusions and traumatic intracranial hemorrhage), those who died by suicide were more likely to have a diagnosed SUD. Tsaousides and colleagues aggregated findings from 4 previous studies and found that 40%–50% of participants with diagnosed SUD endorsed suicidal ideation (68). Among all endorsing suicidal ideation, a significantly greater proportion had histories of SUD. Taken together these studies all suggest that SUD increases the already elevated risk of suicide following TBI.

Unique Populations

Negative effects of the co-occurrence of TBI and substance misuse or SUD have been reported among several populations that are known to have greater problems with substance use. In each case, the presence of TBI appears to exacerbate other consequences and/or comorbidities experienced by these cohorts.

There is growing evidence that the caseloads of SUD treatment providers include a substantial proportion of clients who have incurred a TBI. Alterman and Tarter found 53% of a sample of 76 male alcoholics had histories of TBI (69). Hillbom and Holm observed that 38% of a sample of 157 alcoholics had a history of TBI with loss of consciousness or hospitalization (70). Malloy and colleagues found 58% of a sample of 60 alcoholics had TBI marked by loss of con-

sciousness, hospitalization, or major neurological change (71). In a more recent study, Sacks reported finding 63% of 243 consecutive admissions to 13 publicly funded programs in upstate New York were positive for TBI, as were 48% of 404 clients screened in 12 facilities in New York City (72). Researchers at Ohio State University studied a sample of 119 clients receiving residential treatment, intensive outpatient, or ambulatory detoxification in a publicly funded SUD treatment facility (73). They found that 68% had at least 1 TBI with loss of consciousness $\geq$ 5 minutes or requiring emergency department care or hospitalization. Perhaps more remarkably, 35% of the entire sample had at least 1 TBI with 1 hour or longer loss of consciousness or requiring hospitalization. Furthermore, 53% of the sample had at least 1 TBI from which symptoms persisted at the time of screening. When considered together, it appears justified to expect as much as half of clients in SUD treatment to have histories of TBI.

Clients in SUD treatment programs with histories of TBI differ from those without histories in terms of the onset and course of the disease. Corrigan and colleagues found that substance dependent clients requiring more intensive levels of SUD treatment who also were positive for histories of TBI performed more poorly on tests of cognitive functioning and reported poorer emotional control when compared to clients without a history (73). Clients with a history of TBI have been found to experience their first use at an earlier age than those without (72,74) and are more likely to have co-occurring psychiatric disorders (72,74–78). Corrigan and Deutschle reported that both clients with and without histories of TBI showed a good treatment response to an intensive, coordinated approach to treating co-occurring SUD and severe mental illness (74). However, this study also found that staff unaware of whether clients had prior histories of TBI rated those with as having much poorer prognosis for long-term recovery due to a greater need for ongoing case management.

In studies of the prevalence of TBI and criminal activity and/or incarceration, there is evidence of a three-way co-occurrence of involvement with the criminal justice system, TBI, and substance misuse. A study of medical center patients with TBI found those who had preinjury histories of arrest were more likely to be males with lower education who were injured in assaults and had a history of SUD (79). Barnfield and Leathem studied persons with TBI and SUD in the New Zealand prison population and used a combination of reported loss of consciousness and frequency of injuries to derive a categorization system for severity that classified each subject as having none, light, mild, moderate, or severe TBI (80). Half of their sample incurred a TBI that was mild or worse, with 17% reporting moderate or severe injuries. Inmates with mild or worse TBI were approximately 17% more likely to have severe SUD. Greater cognitive problems were observed among those with both TBI and SUD.

It is well known that there is greater alcohol consumption, with consequent misuse and alcohol use disorders, among military personnel (81). The apparently high rate of TBI incurred during the wars in Iraq and Afghanistan have spawned interest in whether TBI exacerbates problems arising from this greater alcohol use. In 1 study of veterans of these conflicts who screened positive for potentially incurring a TBI while deployed were 2 times more likely to have an alcohol or drug diagnosis (82). Similarly, military personnel from the United Kingdom with a positive mild-TBI screen were 2.3 times more likely to report alcohol misuse (83). Among active duty personnel with past 12 months combat deployment, those self-reporting TBI were more likely to be heavy drinkers and have possible alcohol dependence (84). Because these early studies suggest that the rate of misuse or SUD may be increased among those with TBI, the relationship with additional consequences or the impact on treatment await further study.

INTERVENTION FOR CO-OCCURRING SUBSTANCE MISUSE AND TBI

Although descriptive information is beginning to accumulate about the scope and nature of substance misuse and TBI, research on interventions for these co-occurring conditions is sparse. In this section, we review studies of the prevalence of persons with TBI in SUD treatment programs, what is known about their success in treatment, and implications for referral of rehabilitation patients to existing SUD treatment programs. This discussion is followed by a review of treatment programs developed specifically for persons with TBI and SUD. Although residential treatment models for co-occurring TBI and SUD have been proposed, they have not been tested (85,86). Quasi-experimental studies have provided some support for motivational interviewing (87,88) and intensive case management (40,89,90). The only randomized controlled trials have tested methods for improving engagement and retention in treatment (91,92). In the context of this limited empirical evidence for specific interventions, we discuss best practices for treatment during and after rehabilitation. The chapter ends with a description of the 4-quadrant model for addressing co-occurring TBI and SUD in multiple health care venues.

Effectiveness of SUD Treatment for Persons With TBI

There is reason to suspect that persons with TBI present for treatment with characteristics unique enough that the effectiveness of proven SUD interventions should be evaluated specifically for efficacy in this population. Cognitive impairments arising from TBI may affect a person's learning style, making participation in didactic training and group interventions more difficult. Misinterpretation of attention or memory problems as resistance to treatment can undermine a treatment relationship. Damage to the frontal lobes affects executive thinking skills and promotes socially inappropriate behavior. It is easy to interpret these behaviors as intentionally disruptive, particularly when the individual with TBI shows no visible signs of disability (93). Even if different SUD treatments are not required for this population, it would be necessary to make accommodations to the way in which existing treatments are delivered such that cognitive and emotional sequelae of the TBI do not preclude a client with TBI experiencing the active ingredients of a clinical intervention.

One example of an intervention proven to work in the general population of persons misusing substances is Screening and Brief Intervention (SBI) (94) or Screening Brief Intervention, Referral and Treatment (SBIRT) (95). Corrigan and

colleagues reviewed the considerable efficacy and effectiveness studies for the use of these interventions in emergency departments and trauma centers to determine if the results could be confidently generalized to persons with TBI (96). Because the studies were conducted as research, patient consent was required, which in turn dictated that any patient exhibiting confusion or more severe levels of altered consciousness be excluded from the studies. Because patients with the mildest TBIs were likely included in this body of literature, the requirements for consent likely precluded participation by anyone with complicated mild or more severe TBI. Corrigan and colleagues conclude that adapted methods of providing SBI should be investigated to assure that patients with more serious TBI benefit from this type of intervention.

Studies of the effectiveness of both pharmacologic and behavioral interventions for persons with TBI are required. The greater the cognitive and emotional sequelae of the TBI, the more necessary this research becomes. There are approaches to treatment developed for special populations within the field of SUD treatment that merit further consideration for persons with TBI. For instance, several treatment models have been developed for persons with co-occurring SUD and mental illness (97). There are many parallels between these dually diagnosed clients and persons with TBI and SUD. Both populations have cognitive and emotional sequelae arising from their disorders; members of both groups report using substance to regulate emotional symptoms; and both groups often have multiple other psychosocial needs (e.g., housing, finances, transportation) that arise from or are interdependent with their treatment needs. Techniques developed and lessons learned in the treatment of persons with SUD and mental illness may be a fruitful source of ideas for addressing the needs of persons with SUD and TBI (74,97).

Treatment Interventions Specifically Designed for Persons With TBI

Although several models of how SUD treatment can be adapted to TBI rehabilitation have been proposed (40,85, 86,98), most presumed protracted inpatient or residential treatment that is no longer available to most persons with TBI. Bombardier and colleagues have promoted brief interventions based on motivational interviewing techniques for use during acute rehabilitation (87,99). Cox, Heinemann, and colleagues found some support for the efficacy of motivational counseling based on a quasi-experimental design using a nonrandom comparison group (88). In contrast, Corrigan and colleagues found a brief motivational intervention did no better than an attention control condition in terms of engaging clients with TBI and SUD in treatment (92). In contrast, a financial incentive condition and a condition in which logistical barriers were systematically addressed both resulted in significantly better engagement than the motivational interviewing and attention control conditions. However, the very brief duration of the intervention, delivered via telephone, may have served to undermine the effectiveness of the motivational interviewing.

Corrigan and colleagues have described a community-based model of care that uses intensive case management as its core intervention (40,89,90). Consumers and their families receive education and counseling, and interprofessional consultation and linkage is extended to all health care and social service professionals working with a client. An "ad hoc" community team of professional and natural supports is established whenever possible. The principles of the approach resemble those guiding Integrated Dual Diagnosis Treatment (IDDT) for SUD and mental illness, except the team is ad hoc rather than being employees of a single agency. Like IDDT, the focus is long term—the median length of stay for those discharged successfully is 18 months. Also like IDDT, embedded within the intensive case management is a supported employment program for those wanting to work. Although a randomized controlled trial of the supported employment component did not show it to be superior to case management alone in the intent to treat analyses, those who were actually engaged in treatment were more likely to be employed during the study than either those randomized to case management alone or those not engaged in the supported employment program (100). The employment program also tended to result in higher paying jobs and greater self-esteem, although improved self-esteem and more likely abstinence from substances was observed for all those employed regardless of treatment group.

Only quasi-experimental designs have been used to assess the effectiveness of the overall intensive case management approach used in this community-based program. Pre–postcomparisons of outcomes for those treated successfully and those who prematurely terminate support the effectiveness of the program for attaining abstinence, gaining employment, and experiencing better subjective well-being (40,45,89). Heinemann, Corrigan, and Moore used a quasi-experimental design to study initial progress in 2 programs using the model and a nonrandom, comparison group of persons with TBI and SUD who were not receiving treatment (90). Nine months after admission to treatment, actual use did not change for either the treatment or comparison groups; however, life and family satisfaction were significantly better for the treated group. Program referral earlier after injury was associated with larger gains in physical well-being, employment, and community integration. The authors concluded that change in substance use requires longer duration treatment and also noted the challenge of premature termination. If a case management model is found to be an efficacious treatment approach for this population, its effectiveness would be improved by determining better methods to engage and retain clients in treatment. Randomized controlled trials conducted subsequently have shown that engagement (92) and retention (91) in treatment can be significantly improved via reducing barriers to treatment participation and providing strategic financial incentives.

Best Practice in Rehabilitation Settings

The issues related to substance abuse inevitably affect therapeutic decisions during the medical rehabilitation of TBI survivors. First, the fact that substance abuse is both a risk factor for TBI and a predictor of suboptimal rehabilitation outcome underscores the importance of a comprehensive history that includes substance abuse. In addition, the medical rehabilitation of the neuropsychiatric consequences of TBI includes therapeutic interventions for cognitive, neurobehavioral, sensory, and somatic symptoms and impairments (101).

Therapeutic options for these sequelae often include pharmacologic interventions with risk for abuse such as opiates for acute and chronic pain secondary to trauma, stimulants for cognitive and neurobehavioral impairments, and benzodiazepines for neurobehavioral and sleep disturbances. Therefore, therapeutic interventions for the neuropsychiatric consequences of TBI require the usual risk to benefit analysis within the context of a heightened potential for substance abuse, the negative impact of substance abuse on rehabilitation outcome, and the increasing risk for liability associated with abuse of medical prescriptions. Finally, the neuropsychiatric impairments that frequently occur secondary to TBI—when left untreated due to the natural fluctuation in symptom severity or missed diagnoses due to the complexity of the medical comorbid conditions—increase that patient's risk for substance abuse should the patient attempt to self medicate. Therefore, all patients being followed for the chronic effects of TBI should periodically be rescreened for substance misuse. Those patients who misuse should be advised to stop due to the increased likelihood of negative consequences on recovery from the TBI. Also, those patients with a diagnosable SUD should be assisted to both access appropriate SUD treatment and receive more definitive treatment for comorbid conditions that place the patient at heightened risk.

Although evidence for effective treatment is scant, the scope and nature of the problem together with the increasing emphasis on risk assessment requires that substance use be addressed in TBI rehabilitation. Corrigan, Bogner, and Lamb-Hart have suggested that all rehabilitation centers provide patient and family education, screening, and, for those at greater risk, referral to community resources. Education should be provided for all patients and families independent of prior history (102). Although light or occasional alcohol use does not constitute a substance abuse problem in the general population of healthy adults, multiple factors necessitate different criteria for assessing substance use after TBI. There are several risk factors for development of substance use disorders, or complications accompanying them, applicable to the patients with TBI.

- young age
- high frequency of a prior history
- unknowns regarding effect on the recovery process
- decreased tolerance for any drugs
- interaction with prescribed medications
- potential to cause seizures
- exacerbation of sequelae of brain injury
- the stresses of prolonged recovery from serious brain injury

Although a "safe" amount to drink for the general population of healthy adults can be recommended, risk factors associated with brain injury make it difficult to identify a level of consumption, other than abstinence, that is certain to not be detrimental. However, abstinence recommendations for therapeutic interventions with known abuse risk such as stimulants, opiates, and benzodiazepines are mitigated by the potential consequences of inadequately treating the cognitive, neurobehavioral, and somatic impairments secondary to TBI (101,103). A palatable message for persons who have had a TBI is that no matter the extent of one's use before an injury, the occurrence of TBI dictates a reexamination of health factors associated with any substance use. Thus, every patient, regardless of the prior history or potential risk, should receive education regarding risks associated with substance use following TBI. The information provided should include the potential effects of alcohol and other drugs on recovery—the immediate and long-term detrimental impact on cognition, behavior, and physical function—as well as health risks associated with substance use. Families also need this information, as well as additional suggestions for supporting behavior change. Because education should be designed for all patients regardless of risk, it provides initial groundwork for those with prior substance use disorders who need to reconsider their use after TBI. A consistent message about substance use after TBI provided by the entire rehabilitation team creates dissonance between the desire to use and the desire to achieve an optimum recovery. Subsequent referral for treatment is more likely to be successful if the individual is beginning to consider consequences of substance use.

Screening should be conducted during rehabilitation to determine which patients have prior histories of substance abuse or dependence, and thus require referral for ongoing treatment. Laboratory tests for alcohol or other drugs are not adequate to determine which TBI patients' substance use is likely to interfere with their rehabilitation and long-term recovery. The presence or absence of drugs at any given point in time cannot confirm or rule out preexisting substance use disorders or the potential for them to emerge after discharge. Tests of liver function will be prone to false negatives. A prior history of substance use disorder is best determined from information provided by the patient or a knowledgeable family member. There are standardized measures for inquiring about alcohol abuse and dependence (e.g., the Brief Michigan Alcohol Screening Test [104], the Alcohol Use Disorder Identification Test [AUDIT] [105], or the CAGE [106]); as well as illicit drug use, the Drug Abuse Screening Test [DAST] [107] or the Simple Screening Instrument [SSI] [108]). However, standardized instruments may be compromised by cognitive impairments common in the acute phase of recovery. A sensitively conducted interview may be the most flexible way of gaining the information necessary to make a determination of prior history and future risk; however, a staff member must be adequately trained and comfortable with the subject matter and method.

Those patients at greater risk for substance abuse after discharge need additional attention. If specialized services are not available through the TBI rehabilitation program, then a referral to community resources needs to be made. Referral is not just providing a name and phone number, it is an intervention. Every TBI rehabilitation program should have a method for making a referral in such a way that patients will find the community resource accessible, acceptable, and useful. The program should develop a referral network of providers who, through experience and training, have some understanding of the unique issues of TBI. Potential referral sources near any rehabilitation facility or patient's home can be identified via the Substance Abuse Treatment Facility Locator (http://findtreatment.samhsa .gov) sponsored by the Substance Abuse and Mental Health Services Administration. This electronic database includes more than 11,000 addiction treatment programs, including types of drug addiction addressed, treatment setting, and

age group served. All information is completely updated each year based on facility responses to the National Survey of Substance Abuse Treatment Services (http://findtreat ment.samhsa.gov Accessed September 2, 2011).

Community providers can be most effective when they are adequately prepared for the client. The rehabilitation program should provide educational materials or in-service training regarding TBI in general, as well as common characteristics of persons who may be referred. Cultural congruence should play a role in choosing an appropriate resource, whether AA group, individual counselor, or culturally-specific treatment programs (if available) in the home community. When possible, staff should visit referral sources to gain a better appreciation of the program and facility. For instance, will there be issues of physical, cognitive, or financial access? Patients and family members should be prepared for the first meeting with a provider in order to increase the likelihood that they will accept the services offered. Furthermore, the rehabilitation program's responsibility for referral is not complete until it is determined that at least an initial contact occurred. Better yet, follow-up communication with either the person served or the provider should be undertaken to ascertain that premature termination did not result.

The absence of a definitive cure or treatment for substance abuse disorders, the need for ongoing supportive care, and the risk for recidivism has led to the increased application of chronic disease models in the treatment of people with a substance abuse history. As part of the chronic disease model of care, pharmacologic interventions are available and approved for the treatment of alcohol and opiate dependence (109). The acute and maintenance treatment of opioid dependence is outside the scope of care for the rehabilitation physician and will not be reviewed here other than mentioning that naltrexone, methadone, and buprenorphine are FDA-approved for the treatment of opioid dependence. However, naltrexone, acamprosate, and disulfiram are currently FDA-approved for the treatment of alcohol dependence, whereas topiramate is frequently used despite the fact that it is not approved for this indication. Table 79-1 shows the FDA-approved pharmacological treatments for alcohol and opioid dependence. Each of the 3 FDA-approved agents is safe and within the scope of care offered by a rehabilitation physician. All 3 agents should be introduced after 7–10 days of abstinence so as to not induce withdrawal, and all 3 agents require baseline assessment of kidney and liver function. Naltrexone is the only agent to have a Black Box Warning regarding hepatotoxicity despite no reported cases of liver failure and no clear data as to the incidence of elevated liver enzymes (110); thus, clinicians are encouraged to demonstrate additional caution with clinically appropriate interval liver function testing. Each of the 3 agents requires close, ongoing monitoring for depression and suicide risk.

These agents have been shown to help patients reduce drinking quantity, avoid relapse to heavy drinking, or achieve and maintain abstinence (111). The drugs are best used as adjuncts to behavioral treatment for alcohol dependence when a patient is intending to change behavior but struggling to sustain abstinence due to cravings. Also, the use of these medications as adjuncts in the behavioral treatment of alcohol dependence is particularly advocated for patients who previously failed to respond to behavioral approaches alone. In the general population, there are no clear

TABLE 79-1 FDA-Approved Pharmacotherapy for Alcohol and Opioid Dependence

DRUG	FDA INDICATION	CLINICAL BENEFIT	DOSE	WARNINGS
Naltrexone	Alcohol or opioid dependence	Decreases craving	380 mg IM q4 week; 50–100 mg qd	Opioid free for 7 days; depression; hepatotoxicity
Acamprosate	Alcohol dependence	Decreases craving	666 mg tid	Cr at baseline; depression
Disulfiram	Alcohol dependence	Aversive therapy	125–500mg qam	Contraindicated if intoxicated; monitor LFT, CBC, electrolytes
Methadone	Opioid dependence	Decreases craving	15–30 mg x1; max 40 mg day 1	Cr at baseline; respiratory suppression; depression
Buprenorphine	Opioid dependence	Decreases craving	Restricted distribution	Not for maintenance treatment

IM, intramuscular; Cr, creatinine; LFT, liver function test; CBC, complete blood count.

guidelines or advantages for any 1 of these medications over the other 2. Each drug has a different mechanism of action and therefore, failure to benefit from 1 agent may warrant additional trials with the others. If monotherapy fails, combinations of these drugs have been used effectively. However, the efficacies of these drugs have not been confirmed in a TBI population. Due to the potential for an adverse interaction of disulfiram with alcohol use, some caution may be needed if a patient's cognitive impairment limits his or her understanding of the need to abstain from alcohol.

Ultimately, the problem of substance abuse affects all aspects of a person's recovery and all staff members should be a part of the education, screening, and referral process. Attention should be given to the attitudes, beliefs, and knowledge of the entire professional, if not nonprofessional, treatment staff. A formal policy should be developed to identify which team members have responsibility for conducting patient and family education, compiling information regarding alcohol and other drug history and risk factors, and making referrals to outside resources. All treatment professionals should support the process, as relevant information or insights may come from statements expressed spontaneously during any staff members' interactions. Substance abuse is a complex behavior, and changing it is difficult. Although there are many issues to confront during rehabilitation, there is a unique opportunity to address substance use and abuse. The consequences of a TBI may cause a patient to question risky behavior. Detoxification has occurred by the time rehabilitation commences. Family members may be more willing to intervene after experiencing the emotional trauma of serious injury to a loved one. Acute rehabilitation following injury is an opportunity for substance abuse intervention that should not be squandered.

Four-Quadrant Model for Clinical Intervention

To help establish a context for a comprehensive research agenda, Corrigan and colleagues have proposed a model for venue-specific treatment of co-occurring TBI and SUD that is based on the severity of these co-occurring conditions. The starting point for the model was borrowed from the literature on persons with co-occurring SUD and mental illness (112). As shown in Figure 79-2, persons with SUD and TBI are assumed to vary according to the severity of each condition, arbitrarily categorized into low and high. When mapped orthogonally, 4 quadrants are defined by high or low severity of each condition. Although dichotomizing severity is arbitrary, it proves useful in considering the service venues where individuals are both likely to be found and there is an opportunity for intervention. For instance, persons with low severity substance misuse (i.e., unhealthy use) and low severity TBI are not found in treatment systems dedicated to SUD or TBI as often as they are found in primary care settings and treatment systems for injury (e.g., emergency departments or trauma centers). Only with more severe substance misuse (i.e., SUD) or TBI is a person likely to receive treatment in programs dedicated to chemical dependency or TBI rehabilitation, respectively. In our model, the co-occurrence of severe presentations of both conditions suggests the need for specialized treatment programs; however, given the essential absence of such services, this quadrant of the model is mostly hypothetical.

Differences in the venues where individuals are most likely to be identified dictate different treatment approaches.

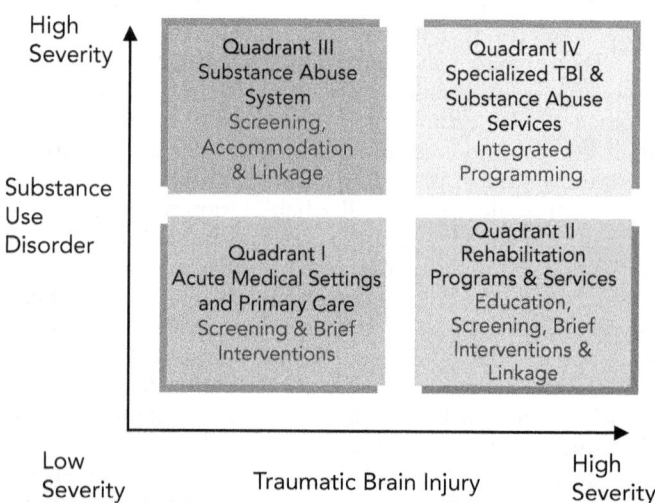

FIGURE 79-2 The Four-Quadrant Model of interventions for substance misuse intervention.

For instance, in quadrant I, the most effective interventions will need to be compact in order to accommodate the more pressing agenda of primary care or emergency treatment of an injury. Thus, SBI is the most likely services to be provided. There is a significant body of literature on SBI for both primary and emergent care (94,95), although its effectiveness for more serious TBI is not known (96). Similarly, quadrants II–IV dictate different service delivery opportunities, although in contrast to quadrant I, there is very little research to guide clinical practice. In quadrant II, rehabilitation settings, the best practices described earlier in this chapter are the primary basis for guiding clinical care. Whereas for quadrant III, screening for TBI and accommodating for neurological sequelae in existing treatment approaches and programs is the current best practice. We expect that an advantage of the 4-quadrant model is that research questions can be generated specific to each quadrant, which will narrow the scope of both the target population and proposed intervention. Significantly, more research is needed to provide guidance both to clinical practice and the configuration of health care delivery systems.

CONCLUSION

Rehabilitation professionals lack the empirically based evidence for treatment of persons who incur a TBI and experience SUD. There is considerable need for research to determine the extent to which interventions found effective with the general population are also effective with this group of patients. The anecdotal clinical experience from SUD treatment is that many approaches have to be adapted to engage and treat persons with TBI. In addition to research on interventions, the field would benefit from additional epidemiologic data about who is at risk for substance use and why. Some patients significantly reduce use after injury, whereas others start or resume. Furthermore, it would be very useful to know how neurobehavioral impairments that result from TBI differ from those that arise from chronic substance use, and whether and how such differences affect treatment.

For our health care systems to be more capable of addressing this population, we need evidence-based recommendations as to what methods of screening for SUD are the most effective in persons with TBI at different points in their recovery. Similarly, how do neurobehavioral impairments due to TBI interact or moderate the efficacy of brief interventions for substance use? Within the substance abuse system, we need to know the most effective methods for screening for TBI and to have evidence-based recommendations for how treatment can be adapted and impairments can be accommodated. As suggested by the 4-quadrant model, we are sorely in need of models for integrated treatment of those individuals with more severe manifestations of both TBI and SUD. Assuming effective models can be identified, we then need to determine how treatment can be made widely available to persons needing this level of care.

KEY CLINICAL POINTS

1. Rehabilitation professionals working with persons with TBI must take responsibility for anticipating and addressing substance misuse and substance use disorders.

2. All patients with brain injury should be screened for substance misuse or preexisting substance use disorder.

3. All patients, with or without prior histories, should be advised that substance use following TBI creates greater risks for consequences affecting brain functioning and long-term outcome.

4. Patients who misuse should be advised to stop using postinjury due to increased likelihood of consequences.

5. Patients with substance use disorders should be assisted in accessing treatment.

6. Patients being followed for chronic effects of TBI should periodically be rescreened for substance misuse.

KEY REFERENCES

1. Bogner JA, Corrigan JD, Spafford DE, Lamb-Hart G. Integrating substance abuse treatment and vocational rehabilitation after traumatic brain injury. *J Head Trauma Rehabil.* 1997;12(5):57–71.

2. Corrigan JD. Substance abuse as a mediating factor in outcome from traumatic brain injury. *Arch Phys Med Rehabil.* 1995;76(4):302–309.

3. Corrigan JD, Bogner J, Hungerford DW, Schomer K. Screening and brief intervention for substance misuse among patients with traumatic brain injury. *J Trauma.* 2010;69(3):722–726.

4. Draus JM Jr, Santos AP, Franklin GA, Foley DS. Drug and alcohol use among adolescent blunt trauma patients: dying to get high? *J Pediatr Surg.* 2008;43(1):208–211.

5. Horner MD, Ferguson PL, Selassie AW, Labbate LA, Kniele K, Corrigan JD. Patterns of alcohol use 1 year after traumatic brain injury: a population-based, epidemiological study. *J Int Neuropsychol Soc.* 2005;11(3):322–330.

References

1. American Psychiatric Association. *Diagnostic and Statistical Manual of Mental Disorders, Fourth Edition Text Revision (DSM-IV-TR).* Washington DC: American Psychiatric Association; 2000.

2. Rogers JM, Read CA. Psychiatric comorbidity following traumatic brain injury. *Brain Inj.* 2007;21(13–14):1321–1333.

3. IOM (Institute of Medicine). *Gulf War and Health, Volume 7: Long-term Consequences of Traumatic Brain Injury.* Washington DC: The National Academies Press; 2009.

4. Bjork JM, Grant SJ. Does traumatic brain injury increase risk for substance abuse? *J Neurotrauma.* 2009;26(7):1077–1082.

5. Graham DP, Cardon AL. An update on substance use and treatment following traumatic brain injury. *Ann N Y Acad Sci.* 2008; 1141:148–162.

6. Winqvist S, Jokelainen J, Luukinen H, Hillbom M. Adolescents' drinking habits predict later occurrence of traumatic brain injury: 35-year follow-up of the northern Finland 1966 birth cohort. *J Adolesc Health.* 2006;39(2):275.e1–275.e7.

7. McKinlay A, Grace RC, Horwood LJ, Fergusson DM, Ridder EM, MacFarlane MR. Prevalence of traumatic brain injury among children, adolescents and young adults: prospective evidence from a birth cohort. *Brain Inj.* 2008;22(2):175–181.

8. Corrigan JD, Bogner JA, Holloman C. Lifetime history of traumatic brain injury among persons with substance use disorders. *Brain Inj.* 2012.

9. Winqvist S, Lehtilahti M, Jokelainen J, Luukinen H, Hillbom M. Traumatic brain injuries in children and young adults: a birth cohort study from northern Finland. *Neuroepidemiology.* 2007;29(1–2): 136–142.

10. Winqvist S, Jokelainen J, Luukinen H, Hillbom M. Parental alcohol misuse is a powerful predictor for the risk of traumatic brain injury in childhood. *Brain Inj.* 2007;21(10):1079–1085.

11. Winqvist S, Luukinen H, Jokelainen J, Lehtilahti M, Näyhä S, Hillbom M. Recurrent traumatic brain injury is predicted by the index injury occurring under the influence of alcohol. *Brain Inj.* 2007; 21(10):1079–1085.

12. Timonen M, Miettunen J, Hakko H, et al. The association of preceding traumatic brain injury with mental disorders, alcoholism and criminality: the Northern Finland 1966 Birth Cohort Study. *Psychiatry Res.* 2002;113(3):217–226.

13. McKinlay A, Grace R, Horwood J, Fergusson D, MacFarlane M. Adolescent psychiatric symptoms following preschool childhood mild traumatic brain injury: evidence from a birth cohort. *J Head Trauma Rehabil.* 2009;24(3):221–227.

14. Corrigan JD. Substance abuse as a mediating factor in outcome from traumatic brain injury. *Arch Phys Med Rehabil.* 1995;76(4): 302–309.

15. Parry-Jones BL, Vaughan FL, Miles Cox W. Traumatic brain injury and substance misuse: a systematic review of prevalence and outcomes research (1994–2004). *Neuropsychol Rehabil.* 2006;16(5): 537–560.

16. Savola O, Niemelä O, Hillbom M. Alcohol intake and the pattern of trauma in young adults and working aged people admitted after trauma. *Alcohol Alcohol.* 2005;40(4):269–273.

17. Puljula J, Savola O, Tuomivaara V, Pribula J, Hillbom M. Weekday distribution of head traumas in patients admitted to the emergency department of a city hospital: effects of age, gender and drinking pattern. *Alcohol Alcohol.* 2007;42(5):474–479.

18. Whiteneck G, Melick D, Brooks C, Harrison-Felix C, Nobel K, Sendroy TM, eds. *Colorado Traumatic Brain Injury and Follow-up System.* Englewood, CO: Craig Hospital; 2001.

19. Draus JM Jr, Santos AP, Franklin GA, Foley DS. Drug and alcohol use among adolescent blunt trauma patients: dying to get high? *J Pediatr Surg.* 2008;43(1):208–211.

20. Taylor LA, Kreutzer JS, Demm SR, Meade MA. Traumatic brain injury and substance abuse: a review and analysis of the literature. *Neuropsychol Rehabil.* 2003;13(1–2):165–188.

21. Shandro JR, Rivara FP, Wang J, Jurkovich GJ, Nathens AB, MacKenzie EJ. Alcohol and risk of mortality in patients with traumatic brain injury. *J Trauma.* 2009;66(6):1584–1590.

22. Talving P, Plurad D, Barmparas G, et al. Isolated severe traumatic brain injuries: association of blood alcohol levels with the severity of injuries and outcomes. *J Trauma.* 2010;68(2):357–362.

23. Tien HCN, Tremblay LN, Rizoli SB, et al. Association between alcohol and mortality in patients with severe traumatic head injury. *Arch Surg.* 2006;141:1185–1191.

24. Berry C, Salim A, Alban R, Mirocha J, Marguiles DR, Ley EJ. Serum ethanol levels in patients with moderate to severe traumatic brain injury influence outcomes: a surprising finding. *Am Surg.* 2010; 76(10):1067–1070.

25. O'Phelan K, McArthur DL, Chang CW, Green D, Hovda DA. The impact of substance abuse on mortality in patients with severe traumatic brain injury. *J Trauma.* 2008;65(3):674–677.

26. Schutte C, Hanks R. Impact of the presence of alcohol at the time of injury on acute and one-year cognitive and functional recovery after traumatic brain injury. *Int J Neurosci.* 2010;120(8):551–556.

27. Lange RT, Iverson GL, Brubacher JR, Franzen MD. Effect of blood alcohol level on Glasgow Coma Scale scores following traumatic brain injury. *Brain Inj.* 2010;24(7–8):919–927.

28. Andelic N, Jerstad T, Sigurdardottir S, Schanke AK, Sandvik L, Roe C. Effects of acute substance use and pre-injury substance abuse on traumatic brain injury severity in adults admitted to a trauma centre. *J Trauma Manag Outcomes.* 2010;4:6.

29. Vickery CD, Sherer M, Nick TG, et al. Relationships among premorbid alcohol use, acute intoxication, and early functional status after traumatic brain injury. *Arch Phys Med Rehabil.* 2008;89(1): 48–55.

30. De Guise E, Leblanc J, Dagher J, et al. Early outcome in patients with traumatic brain injury, pre-injury alcohol abuse and intoxication at time of injury. *Brain Inj.* 2009;23(11):853–865.

31. Corrigan JD, Harrison-Felix C, Bogner J, Dijkers M, Terrill MS, Whiteneck G. Systematic bias in traumatic brain injury outcome studies because of loss to follow-up. *Arch Phys Med Rehabil.* 2003; 84(2):153–160.

32. Corrigan JD, Bogner JA, Mysiw WJ, Clinchot D, Fugate L. Systematic bias in outcome studies of persons with traumatic brain injury. *Arch Phys Med Rehabil.* 1997;78(2):132–137.

33. Corrigan JD, Bogner JA, Mysiw WJ, Clinchot D, Fugate L. Life satisfaction following traumatic brain injury. *J Head Trauma Rehabil.* 2001;16(6):543–555.

34. Bombardier CH, Rimmele CT, Zintel H. The magnitude and correlates of alcohol and drug use before traumatic brain injury. *Arch Phys Med Rehabil.* 2002;83(12):1765–1773.

35. Ponsford J, Whelan-Goodinson R, Bahar-Fuchs A. Alcohol and drug use following traumatic brain injury: a prospective study. *Brain Inj.* 2007;21(13–14):1385–1392.

36. Turner AP, Bombardier CH, Rimmele CT. A typology of alcohol use patterns among persons with recent traumatic brain injury or spinal cord injury: implications for treatment matching. *Arch Phys Med Rehabil.* 2003;84(3):358–364.

37. Bombardier CH, Temkin NR, Machamer J, Dikmen SS. The natural history of drinking and alcohol-related problems after traumatic brain injury. *Arch Phys Med Rehabil.* 2003;84(2):185–191.

38. Whelan-Goodinson R, Ponsford J, Johnston L, Grant F. Psychiatric disorders following traumatic brain injury: their nature and frequency. *J Head Trauma Rehabil.* 2009;24(5):324–332.

39. Kreutzer JS, Witol AD, Sander AM, Cifu DX, Marwitz JH, Delmonico R. A prospective longitudinal multicenter analysis of alcohol use patterns among persons with traumatic brain injury. *J Head Trauma Rehabil.* 1996;11(5):58–69.

40. Corrigan JD, Lamb-Hart GL, Rust E. A programme of intervention for substance abuse following traumatic brain injury. *Brain Inj.* 1995;9(3):221–236.

41. Corrigan JD, Smith-Knapp K, Granger CV. Outcomes in the first 5 years after traumatic brain injury. *Arch Phys Med Rehabil.* 1998; 79(3):298–305.

42. Kreutzer JS, Witol AD, Marwitz JH. Alcohol and drug use among young persons with traumatic brain injury. *J Learn Disabil.* 1996; 29(6):643–651.

43. Horner MD, Ferguson PL, Selassie AW, Labbate LA, Kniele K, Corrigan JD. Patterns of alcohol use 1 year after traumatic brain injury: a population-based, epidemiological study. *J Int Neuropsychol Soc.* 2005;11(3):322–330.

44. Silver JM, Kramer R, Greenwald S, Weissman M. The association between head injuries and psychiatric disorders: findings from the New Haven NIMH Epidemiologic Catchment Area Study. *Brain Inj.* 2001;15(11):935–945.

45. Corrigan JD, Rust E, Lamb-Hart GL. The nature and extent of substance abuse problems in persons with traumatic brain injury. *J Head Trauma Rehabil.* 1995;10(3):29–45.

46. Hibbard MR, Uysal S, Kepler K, Bogdany J, Silver J. Axis I psychopathology in individuals with traumatic brain injury. *J Head Trauma Rehabil.* 1998;13(4):24–39.

47. Fann JR, Burington B, Leonetti A, Jaffe K, Katon WJ, Thompson RS. Psychiatric illness following traumatic brain injury in an adult health maintenance organization population. *Arch Gen Psychiatry.* 2004;61(1):53–61.

48. Koponen S, Taiminen T, Portin R, et al. Axis I and II psychiatric disorders after traumatic brain injury: a 30-year follow-up study. *Am J Psychiatry.* 2002;159(8):1315–1321.

49. Sherer M, Bergloff P, High W Jr, Nick TG. Contribution of functional ratings to prediction of longterm employment outcome after traumatic brain injury. *Brain Inj.* 1999;13(12):973–981.

50. MacMillan PJ, Hart RP, Martelli MF, Zasler ND. Pre-injury status and adaptation following traumatic brain injury. *Brain Inj.* 2002; 16(1):41–49.

51. Willemse-van Son AH, Ribbers GM, Verhagen AP, Stam HJ. Prognostic factors of long-term functioning and productivity after traumatic brain injury: a systematic review of prospective cohort studies. *Clin Rehabil.* 2007;21(11):1024–1037.

52. Jorge RE, Starkstein SE, Arndt S, Moser D, Crespo-Facorro B, Robinson RG. Alcohol misuse and mood disorders following traumatic brain injury. *Arch Gen Psychiatry*. 2005;62(7):742–749.

53. Bogner JA, Corrigan JD, Mysiw WJ, Clinchot D, Fugate L. A comparison of substance abuse and violence in the prediction of long-term rehabilitation outcomes after traumatic brain injury. *Arch Phys Med Rehabil*. 2001;82(5):571–577.

54. Bombardier CH, Fann JR, Temkin NR, Esselman PC, Barber J, Dikmen SS. Rates of major depressive disorder and clinical outcomes following traumatic brain injury. *JAMA*. 2010;303(19):1938–1945.

55. Teasdale TW, Engberg AW. Suicide after traumatic brain injury: a population study. *J Neurol Neurosurg Psychiatry*. 2001;71(4):436–440.

56. Simpson G, Tate R. Clinical features of suicide attempts after traumatic brain injury. *J Nerv Ment Dis*. 2005;193(10):680–685.

57. Simpson GK, Tate RL, Whiting DL, Cotter RE. Suicide prevention after traumatic brain injury: a randomized controlled trial of a program for the psychological treatment of hopelessness. *J Head Trauma Rehabil*. 2011;26(4):290–300.

58. Mainio A, Kyllönen T, Viilo K, Hakko H, Särkioja T, Räsänen P. Traumatic brain injury, psychiatric disorders and suicide: a population-based study of suicide victims during the years 1988–2004 in Northern Finland. *Brain Inj*. 2007;21(8):851–855.

59. Brenner LA, Ignacio RV, Blow FC. Suicide and traumatic brain injury among individuals seeking Veterans Health Administration services. *J Head Trauma Rehabil*. 2011;26(4):257–264.

60. Pentland B, Hutton LS, Jones PA. Late mortality after head injury. *J Neurol Neurosurg Psychiatry*. 2005;76(3):395–400.

61. Himanen L, Portin R, Hämäläinen P, Hurme S, Hiekkanen H, Tenovuo O. Risk factors for reduced survival after traumatic brain injury: a 30-year follow-up study. *Brain Inj*. 2011;25(5):443–452.

62. Verma NP, Policherla H, Buber BA. Prior head injury accounts for the heterogeneity of the alcohol-epilepsy relationship. *Clin Electroencephalogr*. 1992;23(3):147–151.

63. De Reuck J. Risk factors for late-onset seizures related to cerebral contusions in adults with a moderate traumatic brain injury. *Clin Neurol Neurosurg*. 2011;113(6):469–471.

64. Sander AM, Kreutzer JS, Fernandez CC. Neurobehavioral functioning, substance abuse, and employment after brain injury: implications for vocational rehabilitation. *J Head Trauma Rehabil*. 1997;12(5):28–41.

65. Harrison-Felix CL, Whiteneck GG, Jha A, DeVivo MJ, Hammond FM, Hart DM. Mortality over four decades after traumatic brain injury rehabilitation: a retrospective cohort study. *Arch Phys Med Rehabil*. 2009;90(9):1506–1513.

66. Rutherford GW, Wlodarczyk RC. Distant sequelae of traumatic brain injury: premature mortality and intracranial neoplasms. *J Head Trauma Rehabil*. 2009;24(6):468–474.

67. Harrison-Felix C, Whiteneck G, Devivo MJ, Hammond FM, Jha A. Causes of death following 1 year postinjury among individuals with traumatic brain injury. *J Head Trauma Rehabil*. 2006;21(1):22–33.

68. Tsaousides T, Cantor JB, Gordon WA. Suicidal ideation following traumatic brain injury: prevalence rates and correlates in adults living in the community. *J Head Trauma Rehabil*. 2011;26(4):265–275.

69. Alterman AI, Tarter RE. Relationship between familial alcoholism and head injury. *J Stud Alcohol*. 1985;46(3):256–258.

70. Hillbom M, Holm L. Contribution of traumatic head injury to neuropsychological deficits in alcoholics. *J Neurol Neurosurg Psychiatry*. 1986;49(12):1348–1353.

71. Malloy P, Noel N, Longabaugh R, Beattie M. Determinants of neuropsychological impairment in antisocial substance abusers. *Addict Behav*. 1990;15(5):431–438.

72. Sacks AL, Fenske CL, Gordon WA, et al. Co-morbidity of substance abuse and traumatic brain injury. *J Dual Diagn*. 2009;5(3):404–417.

73. Corrigan JD, Lamb-Hart GL, Bogner JA. Detecting Traumatic Brain Injury in Clients Receiving Substance Abuse Treatment Services. Report to the Ohio Department of Alcohol and Drug Addiction Services.

74. Corrigan JD, Deutschle JJ Jr. The presence and impact of traumatic brain injury among clients in treatment for co-occurring mental illness and substance abuse. *Brain Inj*. 2008;22(3):223–231.

75. Walker R, Cole JE, Logan TK, Corrigan JD. Screening substance abuse treatment clients for traumatic brain injury: prevalence and characteristics. *J Head Trauma Rehabil*. 2007;22(6):360–367.

76. Walker R, Hiller M, Staton M, Leukefeld CG. Head injury among drug abusers: an indicator of co-occurring problems. *J Psychoactive Drugs*. 2003;35(3):343–353.

77. Felde AB, Westermeyer J, Thuras P. Co-morbid traumatic brain injury and substance use disorder: childhood predictors and adult correlates. *Brain Inj*. 2006;20(1):41–49.

78. Olson-Madden JH, Brenner L, Harwood JE, Emrick CD, Corrigan JD, Thompson C. Traumatic brain injury and psychiatric diagnoses in veterans seeking outpatient substance abuse treatment. *J Head Trauma Rehabil*. 2010;25(6):470–479.

79. Kolakowsky-Hayner SA, Gourley EV III, Kreutzer JS, Marwitz JH, Cifu DX, Mckinley WO. Pre-injury substance abuse among persons with brain injury and persons with spinal cord injury. *Brain Inj*. 1999;13(8):571–581.

80. Barnfield TV, Leathem JM. Incidence and outcomes of traumatic brain injury and substance abuse in a New Zealand prison population. *Brain Inj*. 1998;12(6):455–466.

81. Adams RS, Corrigan JD, Larson MJ. Alcohol use after combat-aquired traumatic brain injury: What we know and don't know. *Journal of Social Work Practice in Addictions*. 2011; in press.

82. Carlson KF, Nelson D, Orazem RJ, Nugent S, Cifu D, Sayer NA. Psychiatric diagnoses among Iraq and Afghanistan war veterans screened for deployment-related traumatic brain injury. *J Traumatic Stress*. 2010;23(1):17–24.

83. Rona RJ, Jones M, Fear NT, et al. Mild traumatic brain injury in UK military personnel returning from Afghanistan and Iraq: Cohort and cross-sectional analyses. *J Head Trauma Rehabil*. 2011; in press.

84. Adams RS. Examining alcohol use after combat-acquired TBI among active duty personnel. 2011.

85. Langley MJ, Lindsay WP, Lam CS, Priddy DA. A comprehensive alcohol abuse treatment programme for persons with traumatic brain injury. *Brain Inj*. 1990;4(1):77–86.

86. Blackerby WF, Baumgarten A. A model treatment program for the head-injured substance abuser: preliminary findings. *J Head Trauma Rehabil*. 1990;5(3):47–59.

87. Bombardier CH, Rimmele CT. Motivational interviewing to prevent alcohol abuse after traumatic brain injury: a case series. *Rehabilitation Psychology*. 1999;44(1):52–67.

88. Cox WM, Heinemann AW, Miranti SV, Schmidt M, Klinger E, Blount J. Outcomes of systematic motivational counseling for substance use following traumatic brain injury. *J Addict Dis*. 2003;22(1):93–110.

89. Bogner JA, Corrigan JD, Spafford DE, Lamb-Hart G. Integrating substance abuse treatment and vocational rehabilitation after traumatic brain injury. *J Head Trauma Rehabil*. 1997;12(5)57–71.

90. Heinemann AW, Corrigan JD, Moore D. Case management for TBI survivors with alcohol problems. *Rehabil Psychol*. 2004;49(2):156–166.

91. Corrigan JD, Bogner J. Interventions to promote retention in substance abuse treatment. *Brain Inj*. 2007;21(4):343–356.

92. Corrigan JD, Bogner J, Lamb-Hart G, Heinemann AW, Moore D. Increasing substance abuse treatment compliance for persons with traumatic brain injury. *Psychol Addict Behav*. 2005;19(2):131–139.

93. Center for Substance Abuse Treatment. Substance use disorder treatment for people with physical and cognitive disabilities. In: *Treatment Improvement Protocol (TIP) Series Number 29*. Washington, DC: U.S. Government Printing Office; 1998.

94. Hungerford DW, Pollock DA. *Alcohol problems among emergency department patients: proceedings of a research conference on identification and intervention*. Atlanta, GA: Centers for Disease Control and Prevention, National Center for Injury Prevention and Control; 2002.

95. Committee on Trauma. Screening and Brief Intervention Quick Guide. www.facs.org/trauma/publications/sbirtguide.pdf

96. Corrigan JD, Bogner J, Hungerford DW, Schomer K. Screening and brief intervention for substance misuse among patients with traumatic brain injury. *J Trauma*. 2010;69(3):722–726.

97. Corrigan JD, Cole TB. Substance use disorders and clinical management of traumatic brain injury and posttraumatic stress disorder. *JAMA*. 2008;300(6):720–721.

98. Hensold TC, Guercio JM, Grubbs EE, Upton JC, Faw G. A personal intervention substance abuse treatment approach: substance abuse treatment in a least restrictive residential model. *Brain Inj*. 2006; 20(4):369–381.

99. Bombardier CH, Ehde D, Kilmer J. Readiness to change alcohol and drinking habits after traumatic brain injury. *Arch Phys Med Rehabil*. 1997;78:592–596.

100. Corrigan JD. Efficacy of the individualized placement and support model for persons with TBI. Presentation at the 2009 ACRM-ASNR Joint Educational Conference; October, 2009; Denver, Colorado.

101. Halbauer J, Ashford JW, Zeitzer JM, Adamson MM, Lew HL, Yesavage JA. Neuropsychiatric diagnosis and management of chronic sequelae of war-related mild to moderate traumatic brain injury. *J Rehabil Res Dev*. 2009;46(6):757–796.

102. Corrigan JD, Bogner JA, Lamb-Hart GL. Substance abuse and brain injury. In: Rosenthal M, Griffith ER, Miller JD, Kreutzer J, eds. *Rehabilitation of the Adult and Child with Traumatic Brain Injury*. 3rd ed. Philadelphia, PA: FA Davis Co; 1999:556–571.

103. Nicholl J, Lafrance WC Jr. Neuropsychiatric sequelae of traumatic brain injury. *Semin Neurol*. 2009;29(3):247–255.

104. Pokorny AD, Miller BA, Kaplan HB. The brief MAST: a shortened version of the Michigan Alcoholism Screening Test. *A J Psychiatry*. 1972;129(3):342–345.

105. Babor TF, Higgins-Biddle JC, Saunders JB, Monteiro MG. *The Alcohol Use Disorders Identification Test: Guidelines for Use in Primary Care*. 2nd ed. Geneva Switzerland: World Health Organization; 2001.

106. Ewing JA. Detecting alcoholism. The CAGE questionnaire. *JAMA*. 1984;252(14):1905–1907.

107. Skinner HA. Early identification of addictive behaviors using a computerized life style assessment. In: Baer J, Marlett G, McMahon R, eds. *Addictive Behaviors Across the Lifespan: Prevention, Treatment and Policy Issues*. Newbury Park, CA: Sage; 1993:88–111.

108. Center for Substance Abuse Treatment. Simple screening instruments for outreach for alcohol and other drug abuse and infectious diseases. In: *Treatment Improvement Protocol (TIP) Series Number 11*. Washington, DC: U.S. Government Printing Office; 1994.

109. Dennis M, Scott CK. Managing addiction as a chronic condition. *Addict Sci Clin Pract*. 2007;4(1):45–55.

110. Yen MH, Ko HC, Tang FI, Lu RB, Hong JS. Study of hepatotoxicity of naltrexone in the treatment of alcoholism. *Alcohol*. 2006;38(2):117–120.

111. National Institute on Alcoholism and Alcohol Abuse. Helping patients who drink too much: a Clinician's Guide. U.S. Department of Health and Human Services National Institutes of Health Web site. http://www.niaaa.nih.gov/guide. Updated 2008. Accessed October, 2008.

112. Substance Abuse and Mental Health Services Administration. Report to Congress on the Prevention and Treatment of Co-Occurring Substance Abuse Disorders and Mental Disorders; 2002; Rockville, MD.

Practical Approaches to Family Assessment and Intervention

Emilie E. Godwin, Kathryn Wilder Schaaf, and Jeffrey S. Kreutzer

INTRODUCTION

Traumatic brain injury (TBI) is a leading cause of disability that involves cognitive, behavioral, emotional, and psychosocial sequelae (1,2,3). Because of frequent problems with executive functioning (4), learning and memory (5), and independently carrying out daily living activities, family members are often responsible for ensuring that a loved one with TBI is well cared for. The long-term effect of brain injury on family members has been well documented. Research has firmly established that brain injury is associated with several difficult outcomes including caregiver burden (6), problems with family functioning (7,8), unmet family needs, and adjustment to changed family roles (9). The following chapter will provide a background on the effects of brain injury on the family and a rationale for involving the patient and family system as a requirement for accurate assessment and effective intervention after TBI.

Caregiver Burden

Many caregivers report feeling ill-equipped for the challenge of caring for a loved one with a brain injury, even with rehabilitation care teams' efforts to prepare families for the return home. Estimations indicate that nearly 90% of caregivers of patients with TBI report significant caregiver burden (6). Caregiving for a TBI survivor often requires a significant life shift, and is associated with loss of social connections and increased social isolation (10) as well as increased depression, anxiety, and other forms of distress (11). In addition, many caregivers report having negative feelings about their ability to provide care, experiences with caregiving, and caregiving beliefs (6). Although patient-related factors such as level of disability, unemployment, and problems with alcohol abuse are associated with caregiver burden (11), effective coping strategies have been shown to decrease negative outcomes (12). That is, caregivers who are able to change their expectations and attitudes and rely on family typically feel better about their role as a caregiver. Research indicates a continued need to provide support and effective intervention for those who provide regular care to TBI survivors.

Family Functioning

Although caregivers are often responsible for the bulk of care after a brain injury, other members of the family also may be profoundly affected by changes associated with TBI. Family dysfunction is reported in 25%–74% of families after an injury (7,8), with research indicating that many families dealing with brain injury also report psychosocial problems preinjury. Communication problems are a prevalent issue reported by caregivers. Communication difficulties can include a variety of issues ranging from problems with a patient's altered linguistic abilities to caregivers' reluctance to speak about feelings of annoyance or grief (13). Additional issues include problems with affective functioning indicating that the survivor and other family members may be unaware or inattentive toward caregiver needs. The family's ability to distribute roles in an equitable way has also been shown to create concern. After an injury, family members are forced to compensate for the patient and redistribute responsibilities. In response, some family members often take on overwhelming responsibilities, and families may feel the need to adopt more rigid rules to respond to behavior (14). Families dealing with brain injury experience several significant long-term adjustments. Interventions that address the impact of this change with the family as a whole will provide key support needed by the family system.

Family Needs

Understanding family needs can assist departments in developing effective and utilized family support and education services. The Family Needs Questionnaire (FNQ) (15) has been widely used with a wide variety of samples of injury severity, injury acuity, geographical location, ethnicity, relationship between patient and family members, and family income. Despite both sample and methodological differences, brain injury FNQ studies have reported consistent findings. The reported need for health information is one of the most consistent findings (16–21). Items most frequently endorsed in the health information domain include the need for having questions answered honestly and the need for complete information about the patient. However, emotional needs and instrumental support needs are often cited as less important and least likely to be met (6,18–20). This finding indicates that family members do not see needs such as having help keeping the house clean, getting reassurance about negative feelings, and spending time with friends to be as important as needs that pertain to the patient (16,21).

Couples or Intimate Relationships

The unique loss a spouse or partner may experience after TBI has generated interest in studying couples' relationships after brain injury. Although most interpersonal relationships are affected by changes associated with brain injury, partners must live in limbo without the physical and emotional support they once enjoyed from their loved one (9). Although several studies have addressed issues pertaining to marital quality and stability after brain injury, outcomes are inconsistent (22). Reports of divorce or separation after brain injury range from 15% to 78% (23,24). Across studies, partners' report of factors such as sexual satisfaction (25,26.), marital satisfaction (25,27), and relational communication (27,28) vary. Factors such as injury severity, specificity of measures, and time since injury may help to explain the mixed findings. Despite the unclear picture of precisely how couples are affected by the consequences of brain injury, it is certain that many partners experience burden and distress as they adjust to the myriad of changes accompanying an injury (22,25, 27–29). Interventions should be sensitive to the unique challenges a spouse or partner faces after a loved one has sustained brain injury.

Additional Issues

Cultural Issues

Although some attention has been given to how caregiver characteristics such as relationship to patient influence the caregiving experience, little attention has been given to cultural factors. One study comparing African American and White caregivers indicates survivor functioning affects the emotional health of the caregiver, regardless of race. However, African American caregivers spend more hours per week caregiving, are at an increased risk for emotional distress, and are less likely to use community support available to alleviate distress (30). A study comparing reported needs from TBI caregivers in Columbia, South America to Anglo populations in the United States indicates that Columbian caregivers report a greater number of unmet needs, particularly in the emotional support domain. This lack of emotional support could have long-term consequences for caregiver's mental and physical health (31). Further studies of racial and ethnic differences are warranted to draw more complete conclusions and to better target interventions for different groups.

Substance Abuse

Substance abuse is an issue that commonly intersects with brain injury, creating complicated problems for both the survivor and the family. Among patients admitted to brain injury rehabilitation programs, more than 50% present with a history of substance abuse. In addition, one-fourth to one-third of individuals are intoxicated at the time the TBI is sustained (32). Research suggests a link between those patients who sustain a TBI while intoxicated and the likelihood of heavy drinking preinjury and postinjury (33). Although much research has focused on preinjury substance abuse, there is also evidence that incidence of brain injury, especially involving the orbitofrontal cortex, can increase risk of future substance abuse (34).

Although many individuals with brain injury are able to abstain from alcohol and drugs after their injury, 17% of individuals report drinking at hazardous levels 1 year postinjury and 25% at hazardous levels 2 years postinjury. Use of illicit drugs, although less frequent, has also been shown to be problematic with 8% of TBI survivors reporting a drug problem 2 years postinjury (35). Families often find themselves at the center of problems with both brain injury and substance abuse. As a result, families can become organized around the problem creating dysfunctional patterns of behavior such as codependency and overfunctioning or underfunctioning relationships (36). Although many interventions for treatment are patient centered, family members can play an important positive or negative role in the recovery process. Clinicians should elicit information about the frequency, quantity, and impact of substances in both the patient's and the family member's lives. In addition, family therapy should educate family members on strategies for providing reinforcement for behaviors that facilitate a substance-free life (37).

Military Families

Family members of veterans or military service members may face several unique challenges or circumstances. Understanding of the family's connection to the military culture can facilitate a more effective therapeutic relationship between the practitioner and the family. In addition, having a general understanding of the language and structure of the military while assessing why the patient joined and the general sacrifices the patient and family have made can aid the process of joining with each family member (38). Another factor to consider is the role of the conflicts in Iraq and Afghanistan. As a result of these wars, families have increasingly been required to deal with stressors arising from multiple deployments and extended separation from family members. Understanding the impact that this separation has had on both the marriage and the family is important to gain a complete picture of family functioning.

With military families, additional information pertaining to the injury is important to assess. First, the mechanism of injury may have added significance. As a result of use of improvised explosive devices (IEDs) and other explosive devices, military service members have sustained polytraumatic injuries. These injuries are complex and unpredictable and include conditions such as severe burns, traumatic amputations, psychological trauma, and other combat-related injuries (39). Family members are often tasked with caring for these patients and dealing with the difficult and complex sequela that accompany polytrauma. In addition, the complex relationship between post-traumatic stress disorder (PTSD) and mild traumatic brain injury (mTBI) is a signature issue of the current conflicts. A survey of returning service members from Iraq indicated that, of those reporting a loss of consciousness during their deployment, nearly 44% also met the criteria for PTSD (40). Given the overlap of symptoms between mTBI and PTSD, clinicians should be careful to evaluate and assess for each, in order to construct targeted and effective interventions.

APPLYING THEORY: DEVELOPING AND USING A THEORETICAL FOUNDATION

Working with families following brain injury is a hands-on art and science. The challenges that families face day-to-day, hour-to-hour, and minute-to-minute are ever-changing, alive, and present. Practitioners interested in assisting families to manage these challenges are often concerned with practical, immediate strategies to both help the family in facing these hurdles and improve the influence the family has on a survivor's course of treatment. As a result, the theoretical framework underlying best practice may often be overlooked. However, practice that is devoid of theory quickly becomes a rapid-fire reaction to crises rather than a planful approach to delivering services. Although theory is not practice, theory must guide practice, inform decisions, and drive patient and family care if clinicians are to have a sustainable impact on the course of recovery.

In addition to providing a broad scaffold for selecting and implementing treatment strategies, theory also aids brain injury professionals in understanding the importance of taking a systemic approach to individualized care. Patients do not exist in a vacuum. Inpatient treatment teams traditionally understand the systemic nature of medical services—how a physical therapy (PT) appointment at 11:00 AM can have a profound impact on a speech therapy session at 2:00 PM, and an even greater impact on the symptoms a patient or family reports to the attending physician at rounds the next morning. However, clinicians may stop short of recognizing the integral influence that family systems have on patient recovery. From the moment a brain injury survivor enters the hospital, the family members involved will exist as one of the most significant components of the pace, effectiveness, and sustainability of patient rehabilitation (41). Providers may be inclined to think only of the problematic families as exerting this influence, but systems-based theories reveal the pervasive impact of familial interactions and patterns on all human lives. Rather than expending futile energy to manage and quarantine families from the process of rehabilitation, brain injury providers who employ family systems theory (FST), cognitive behavioral family therapy (CBFT), and/or resilience theory (RT) will be able to work alongside families, with the ultimate aim of improving patient outcomes.

Family Systems Theory

Family systems theory is grounded in the notion that families are interlocking pieces of a puzzle. Take 1 puzzle piece away, and the picture is incomplete. Developed by psychiatrist Murray Bowen (42), FST explains the ways in which the interactions between individuals shape and guide the behaviors, thoughts, and feelings of individuals. Since the generation of systems theory, theorists have explored the application of basic principles of science to human systems (43). Extending these laws of natural science, FST postulates that just as there is no singularity in nature, human beings are no different. Given that a primary sphere of influence in the lives of most people is the family, people are believed to be guided and influenced by both conscious and subconscious forces that develop out of family interactions (44).

The application of FST to practice in brain injury medicine allows clinicians to understand the often puzzling and complex reactions of both patients and families to challenges in the rehabilitation process. Through uncovering the foundational concepts and the underlying principles of FST, practitioners may be better equipped to untangle and intervene on the interactive forces shaping patient recovery through family processes. Although FST is a broad and dynamic theory encompassing many conceptual components, there are 2 primary concepts that are crucial to an application of theory to practice: homeostasis and feedback loops (45).

The idea of homeostasis as applied to families states that families seek to maintain their customary organization styles and functioning and, therefore, are resistant to change (45). This desire to maintain balance is actively sought by all family members, and will protect both positive and negative behaviors in a family unit. Even families with highly dysfunctional behavior patterns, such as active alcoholism or patterns of abuse, will often subconsciously fight movement toward change, even when that change could be beneficial.

Feedback loops are the methods families use to maintain a homeostatic or stable environment (45). Families will initially engage in negative feedback loops, which are made up of the strategies family members use to enforce unwritten family rules, such as the way each family member is expected to behave. These strategies include tactics such as guilt and punishment, which family members will use whenever there is a threat to family balance. When negative feedback loops are not working, families will move into positive feedback loops. Positive loops are when one or more family members behave differently, either in a beneficial or detrimental way as a method to getting a different outcome for the family. Although positive feedback loops bring about change, which can be helpful for a family, families who are experiencing frequent positive loops will feel that their environment is chaotic, unstable, and emotionally charged.

Following brain injury, families are necessarily thrust out of homeostasis and into change processes. Often, family members will try to bring the family back to what feels comfortable and stable by striving to return to balance (46). Through the use of negative feedback loops, family members may attempt to get patients to behave like their "old selves" through shaming or by chastising behavior. However, after brain injury, negative feedback loops will not return the family to preinjury balance in the way they may have before. Therefore, most families move very quickly into a cycle of continuous positive feedback loops.

The experience of multiple family members changing their typical behaviors at once results in a very unpredictable family system. Although each family member is unconsciously attempting to spark positive feedback loops as a method for bringing about positive change, the result is that each member of the family is uncertain about the behaviors or actions of the other members of the family (47). Given that these loops occur when families are already in a crisis situation, this makes the unpredictability of the family and the nonhomeostatic tenor of the relationships particularly unsettling for each individual within the family. Although some families will respond to this intensity with heightened emotions and expression, others will withdraw and become overly deferent to authority. This unstable nature of inter-family relationships may result in poor decision making in the rehabilitation process (48).

The elemental components homeostasis and feedback loops can enable clinicians to better make sense of family and patient processes as rehabilitation progresses. Family systems theorists take a positive view of family functioning with the assumption that most families are not challenged to handle crises effectively, but rather are responding to change and disruption with methods for stabilization that have worked before (49). By recognizing that whether or not family members are present in the room, the disruption of the family system results in additional confusion and uncertainty for the patient, practitioners can identify treatment approaches designed to make the best use of unexpected family behaviors.

Cognitive Behavioral Family Therapy

Traditional cognitive behavioral therapy (CBT) is often employed by clinicians following brain injury as a process to spark positive change in patient lives (50). CBFT integrates the primary tenets of CBT while adopting a systems-based philosophy (51). Effective family intervention requires a theoretical foundation grounded in systems theory as a method for understanding and making use of familial interactions. Although inpatient settings allow clinicians to set the tone of the rehabilitation process and dictate the implementation of strategies or techniques aimed at enacting positive change, patients are ultimately discharged to a home environment. Once home, family members and caregivers will play a predominant role in determining how often a patient engages in the rehabilitation process. CBFT allows clinicians in inpatient rehabilitation settings to set the stage for positive family involvement and those in outpatient clinics to foster the application of therapy techniques in the home environment.

CBT—the guiding framework for CBFT—is based on the A-B-C philosophy of emotion and behavior process (52) and is structured around 5 primary underlying principles (53). The A-B-C philosophy suggests that humans (**A**) experience an **A**ctivating event, (**B**) use an existing **B**elief to draw conclusions about that event, and (**C**) experience emotions or enact behaviors as a **C**onsequence of that belief. CBT therapists operate with the premises that (a) we often *are not* in control of activating events, (b) we *are* in control of our beliefs about what events mean, and (c) changing belief structures will result in a change in emotions and/or behaviors. Following brain injury, clinicians adopting this theoretical frame may assume that patients and families were not in control of the event that caused the injury, nor are they in control of many events that occur in the rehabilitation process, however, the preinjury belief systems that they often use to make sense of events may be resulting in irrational or illogical consequential feelings and behaviors. Assisting patients and families in shifting their beliefs to be more in line with their postinjury lives may result in more productive feelings and behaviors.

CBT integrates the A-B-C philosophy with principles guiding therapeutic assessment and intervention: (a) another point of view always exists, (b) events are not responsi-ble for feelings, (c) feelings impact behavior, (d) each person's unique experiences shape their beliefs, and (e) thought patterns are developed when challenges to current ways of thinking occur (53). CBFT expands these principles with the assumption that families as a unit also hold unique belief systems (51). Both whole-family experiences and the interactions within a family between individuals result in family-wide belief patterns that guide both individual and familial interpretations of events. Additionally, competing belief systems within the family can result in misperceptions regarding the behaviors and feelings of other family members. CBFT applies the first CBT principle—another point of view always exists—when assisting families in identifying and accepting the beliefs of other family members.

CBFT compliments FST and RT by providing a technique-driven approach to therapy (51). Practitioners implementing CBFT practices use common CBT strategies but apply them to whole family systems. Primary techniques include disputing irrational beliefs, changing definitive language, assigning cognitive homework, and using humor while embracing a positive perspective. Families are often fraught with irrational beliefs in the process of rehabilitation. Practitioners applying CBFT assist families and patients in identifying whole family belief patterns that are founded on preinjury truths or misinformation and then slowly guide families to adopt more rational beliefs. Additionally, patients and families are often bound by definitive language such as, "He *has to* learn to dress himself before we leave or we'll never make it" or "I *must* get back to work within a month." When families use language such as this, clinicians can challenge them to explore what will happen if these "must's" and "have to's" are not realized. Allowing flexible definitions for success will permit the family to more readily see progress and adopt postinjury thinking. Finally, through homework and the use of humor, clinicians enable families to begin the process of reclaiming power over their lives.

Resilience Theory

As with the cognitive-behavioral theories, RT began as an outgrowth of investigation into the individual (54). Although psychology and corresponding psychotherapeutic approaches were constructed in a medical model looking for deficits within the individual, the birth of RT marked the movement of research away from a focus on pathology and toward a model of wellness. Early resiliency theorists wondered why it is that some people, despite an onslaught of adverse circumstances, are able to rise above their presumed destinies to find success, achievement, and happiness in their lives. By examining populations encumbered by a wide array of challenges and hurdles, researchers were able to identify and describe the traits associated with those people who "beat the odds."

Studies examining the traits shared by resilient individuals, regardless of the type of adverse circumstance(s), indicate resilience is primarily connected to an internal belief system defined by (a) a conviction that individuals can control or influence the events in their lives, (b) a sense of deep connectivity to the people and activities in one's life, and (c) the tendency to approach life changes with eager anticipation as a vehicle for personal growth (54–56). In addition to this core personal philosophy, resilient individuals also often have an easygoing temperament, are described as being inherently optimistic, and are willing to modify their own definitions of success. Further, although these personality characteristics and inner belief systems have long been thought of as being innate or inborn, research into resilience has countered this idea. In a longitudinal assessment of resiliency, Werner (57) followed 700 children born into extreme poverty on the island of Kauai for more than 30 years. Not only did children who shared the identified traits grow into functioning and happy adults, several of those who were faltering in their adolescence were able to develop the traits associated with resiliency to ultimately succeed in their adult lives.

Although these individual traits associated with success create a useful framework for clinicians working with survivors of brain injury, the more recent expansion of RT to include those qualities attributed to resilient families allows providers a broader understanding of how to integrate the family into effective rehabilitation. Researchers such as Froma Walsh (56) have identified characteristics of interaction that are shared by whole family systems that produce resilient individuals. Resilient families share 3 core components: (a) belief systems defined by an ability to make meaning out of adversity, a positive outlook, and an inherent spirituality; (b) organizational patterns that demonstrate the capacity to change, are integrally connected to one another in supportive ways, and make use of social resources; and (c) communication processes that are clear, emotionally open, and take a collaborative approach to problem solving.

Recent literature in RT has moved from descriptive portrayals of individuals and families to identification of the methods used to promote these characteristics. Walsh (56) suggests that practitioners infuse therapy with a 5-part framework designed to assist patients and families in becoming increasingly resilient. Clinicians are encouraged to (a) normalize family distress, (b) identify and affirm existing family strengths, (c) involve whole families in the recovery from individual trauma, (d) encourage families to adopt a positive, future-oriented focus, and (e) teach families to track both stressors and coping processes over time as a method for identifying progress. Application of these broad approaches to therapeutic intervention allows clinicians the flexibility to choose and integrate additional strategies such as CBT techniques, which can target specific challenges faced by families at different stages in the rehabilitation process.

ASSESSMENT AND INTERVENTION: COMPREHENSIVE WHOLE-FAMILY REHABILITATION

Psychotherapy or counseling with families following brain injury differs from other more traditional, patient-centered psychological services such as neuropsychological evaluation and cognitive rehabilitation in that assessment and intervention are fluidly interconnected processes. Although some approaches to treatment draw distinct boundaries between the process of assessing patient or family functioning and then intervening to enact positive change, the process of assessing families in counseling is often in and of itself an intervention. Likewise, ongoing interventions inherently encompass the process of assessing and modifying treatment approaches and strategies. For this reason, the delineation

between assessment and intervention can be seen as somewhat of a false distinction. Although some components of assessment such as the use of measurement instruments are more focused on evaluating families, clinicians should assume that assessment is a catalyst for change and intervention is an opportunity for appraisal.

The overlapping process of assessment and intervention that is a part of all counseling regardless of the presenting issue becomes even more ambiguous when working with families after brain injury. The developmental progression of emotional recovery for family systems following brain injury requires frequent reevaluation of family needs (16) and functioning (58). Timing and acuity are highly relevant with respect to which services families need or are ready to receive. Muriel Lezak (9) proposed a posthospitalization sequence of familial beliefs and expectations that follow a time line of 0–24 months postinjury. Family reactions are described sequentially, beginning with happiness and relief that the patient has survived, moving then through stages of limited awareness regarding recovery potential, to a period of grief and mourning, followed eventually by whole-family reorganization. Because families move tentatively into each new developmental stage of emotional recovery, clinicians must reassess and modify intervention strategies to match family needs.

PSYCHOTHERAPEUTIC ASSESSMENT OF FAMILIES AFTER BRAIN INJURY

Assessment of families following brain injury is a complex and multidimensional process. Although assessment begins and is often most substantial early in a clinician's interactions with a family, it remains interwoven with intervention throughout treatment. Primary components of assessment when working with families include the interview, therapeutic assessment strategies, formal and informal measurement instruments, and evaluation of referral needs. Within each of these, clinicians must approach their evaluation systemically and integrate a focus on strengths as well as deficits (59).

Traditional assessment and treatment approaches have used patient-centered models. Using this framework, the patient is the sole target of the rehabilitation process and the family members are a peripheral concern. However, by applying a family and patient-centered approach to care, clinicians have the opportunity to uncover multifaceted influences, needs, and resources that may have a profound impact on rehabilitation outcomes. Practically speaking, assessing a patient systemically means moving away from a focus on the "Identified Patient" or "I.P." Although the physical recovery components of a treatment plan will focus on the brain injury survivor, emotional rehabilitation should include all members of the family. This shift toward incorporating the whole family will enable practitioners to see an increase in the number of options for effective intervention.

With each new stage of assessment, practitioners should evaluate both the patient and the pertinent family members regarding symptoms, beliefs, skills, challenges, and complicating factors or concerns. Clinicians may choose to explain to the family that they are "the expert" on their family system (52) and that, combined with the clinician's status as "the expert" on brain injury, they can together develop the most comprehensive rehabilitation plan possible for the patient. Often, when families are enlisted as collaborating partners, reluctance to participate in the assessment process will dissipate (60).

In addition to broadening traditionally patient-centered assessment methods, practitioners working with families after brain injury should resist the temptation to solely focus assessment on deficits. A thorough assessment of patient and family strengths is a crucial part of developing a comprehensive, successful treatment plan (59). Including strengths-based assessment moves beyond simply identifying treatment progress. Practitioners should ask for family feedback on how and why they have been successful in avoiding or managing struggles often faced by other families. For example, when evaluating current family needs, if a family does not highlight the need for information about the patient's medical condition as a primary concern, the clinician should turn attention to how the family has managed to get that need met to their satisfaction. Has the family conducted their own research? Is there a member of the family who is comfortable in an assertive, questioning stance with the medical treatment team? Have the patient and family developed an effective method for asking each other about and answering questions regarding physical symptoms? A "yes" answer to any of these questions will give the clinician clues regarding existing family strengths. Each strength identified is 1 less strength that needs to be developed in the course of recovery, and 1 more tool to be integrated into achieving goals in the treatment plan.

The Interview

The first interview with families and patients demonstrates the interrelated nature of assessment and intervention. From the beginning, both statements and questions delivered by the clinician will spark reflection on the part of the patient and family. The function of this interview is to both construct a working alliance with the family (discussed in the section Intervention—Working with Families to Improve Overall Wellness) and to formulate hypotheses about goals for rehabilitation and processes for achieving those goals. Although the degree and type of information that clinicians will have access to prior to the first interview will vary based on time postinjury and treatment setting, the following interview segments should each be addressed fully in a first family interview and revisited in subsequent interviews.

Comprehensive Assessment of Injury

Practitioners should evaluate all available medical records to establish a clear picture of injury severity, client functioning preinjury and postinjury (preinjury when available), areas of progress and deficits, degree of current medical interventions, and anticipated outcomes. Additionally, clinicians are wise to investigate both patient and family beliefs and opinions about physical abilities and limitations. Although the degree to which medical services impact families' daily lives varies depending on the amount of time that has passed since the injury, clinicians should assess family feelings about medical care throughout rehabilitation.

Background Information

Within an FST framework, family beliefs and opinions are as instrumental to the progress and process of rehabilitation

as available medical information (61). Effectively gathering background information regarding the entire family system will enable clinicians to create a template for working with the family as a compliment to their strategies for overcoming obstacles. Practitioners vary regarding the degree of formality used when collecting a psychosocial history; some use standardized outlines whereas others allow the family to guide the discussion to pertinent events in family history. Although both approaches are acceptable, clinicians taking a less-structured approach should be careful to pointedly seek information that family members may not be comfortable with offering, such as whole family substance abuse patterns.

History of Challenges

Making use of background data in treatment planning is optimal when interviewers incorporate discussion about a variety of types of family challenges. In addition to challenges directly related to the injury, clinicians should explore other family illnesses or injuries, significant experiences of grief or loss, past patient difficulties with learning or learning environments, and additional events that have shaped the course of the family history. Practitioners may consider asking, "Before this injury, what are the significant struggles that your family has faced?" In addition to assisting in creating a therapeutic bond between clinician and family, this question may elicit information about how a family organizes at times of crisis and what types of challenges are perceived as the most overwhelming.

History of Successes

Equally as essential in the gathering of background data is gathering the history of family successes with respect to challenges (62). Although repetitive family challenges and/or marked catastrophic family events are crucial in understanding a family's reaction to crisis, selecting treatment strategies based on previous family successes is one method for making expedient progress in rehabilitation. Although many components of family and individual functioning change following brain injury, often basic family interactions and patterns about leadership, problem solving strategies, and pathways for support can be used to build a treatment plan. Previous family successes may also help practitioners to identify beneficial family traits such as flexibility or ingenuity, which may be crucial in the process of recovery. Clinicians may choose to be transparent in this process, telling families that previous successes can help the team to identify ways the family may succeed in rehabilitation. This can be followed by the question, "What times can you think of that your family has overcome a big challenge? How did you succeed?"

Family Needs

Research indicates after brain injury family members have substantial needs for health information regarding their loved one (17). This highlights the importance of incorporating a family needs assessment into initial and subsequent interviews. Clinicians are encouraged to ask family members specifically about the extent to which their needs have been met in additional areas as well, including emotional support, instrumental support (practical assistance with tasks and chores), professional support, and peer support (63). Although the FNQ (see Instruments & Measures) provides a categorical picture of family needs, clinicians can encourage families to provide a subjective assessment of the impact of unmet needs on rehabilitation through the interview. In addition, interviews should provide families the opportunity to identify additional, nontraditional needs with the use of open-ended questions such as, "What do you feel your loved one needs most? What does your family need most?"

Goals for Rehabilitation

Goals, like assessment itself, are an ever-evolving component of brain injury rehabilitation. When assessing family goals, it is essential to keep in mind where a family is with respect to their stage of emotional recovery (9). Early on in acute settings, family goals may be unrealistic and include vague statements such as, "We'd like to get back to normal." When families are transitioning from increasing awareness to a stage of grief and mourning, they may have trouble identifying consequential goals at all. Often, the most appropriate intervention identified by an assessment of existing family and patient goals involves assisting families in modifying their goals to be both realistic and meaningful. Still, initial goal assessment requires (*a*) assisting each member

of the family in identifying both conscious and unrecognized short-term goals, (*b*) clarifying with the family the short-term goals motivating the family as a whole, and (*c*) when participation by the patient is possible, distinguishing patient goals for the patient from family member goals for the patient. As recovery progresses, clinicians should regularly reassess each of these 3 components of goal formation. As families move into a stage of reorganization, practitioners must also incorporate discussions around long-term individual and family goals.

Additional Interview Components

Although family structure, family dynamics, precipitating events, level and significance of injury severity, and additional factors will make every family interview unique, there are also many areas of difficulty that are shared by most families after brain injury. Interviewing family members to assess areas of need, strength, and new challenges and to design appropriate treatment strategies is likely to be more effective if clinicians incorporate these shared topics into the interview. Table 80-1 provides a list of questions to guide clinicians. Some questions may be more appropriate in outpatient rehabilitation settings only, whereas others will be more universally appropriate. Additionally, some questions

TABLE 80-1 Invaluable Family Interview Questions

QUESTION	TIME FRAME FOR ASKING QUESTION: ANY TIME POSTINJURY OR OUTPATIENT ONLY	QUESTION AUDIENCE: WHOLE FAMILY WITH SURVIVOR OR CAREGIVING FAMILY MEMBERS ONLY
How did you feel when you first learned that your injured family member was hurt?	Any time postinjury	Caregivers only
How did you feel when you began to recognize that the brain injury might have long-term effects?	Outpatient only	Whole family
How have other family members reacted to the injury?	Any time postinjury	Whole family
Have you made yourself available to provide more emotional support to your family member and/or other family members? If yes, please explain.	Any time postinjury	Caregivers only
Before the brain injury, what were the most important plans you had for your future and your family's future?	Outpatient only	Whole family
How has the brain injury affected your plans for the future?	Outpatient only	Whole family
What responsibilities do you now have to care for your injured family member?	Any time postinjury	Caregivers only
Have you taken on new responsibilities since the injury? If yes, what new responsibilities do you have (caring for the house, maintaining car(s), working, paying bills, caring for children, etc.)? What responsibilities do you no longer have?	Any time postinjury	Whole family
Have you changed your work responsibilities or hours since the injury? Please explain.	Any time postinjury	Whole family
How has your family's income been affected?	Any time postinjury	Whole family
What new expenses are you facing because of the injury?	Any time postinjury	Whole family
How has your participation in social and recreational activities been affected by the injury?	Outpatient only	Whole family

Adapted from Kreutzer, Taylor (64).

are appropriate for the whole family including the survivor, whereas others are more appropriate for caregiving family members only. Questions should be revisited throughout the rehabilitation process because family members and patients are likely to have different responses at different points in their recovery.

Therapeutic Assessment Strategies

Schools of family therapy have a wide range of assessment strategies and techniques, dependent on the theoretical frame applied and the nature of the challenges and family structures to be assessed. When working with families after brain injury, 2 assessment strategies in particular may provide helpful information to clinicians. Although both the genogram and the family map can be used in either an acute or outpatient setting, neither is a crisis-oriented assessment technique. Therefore, both are tools that clinicians may want to use subsequent to the initial interview and background review as a method for creating a comprehensive picture of family structure and dynamics.

Genogram

The genogram is a method for uncovering, recording, and assessing family patterns and interactions over 3 or more generations (65). Originally developed by Family Systems Theorists, the genogram has now been widely employed by therapists and medical doctors alike to gather both psychosocial and medical family histories (66). Within a rehabilitation setting, the genogram allows clinicians to easily identify family patterns and relationship dynamics that may substantially impact the rehabilitation process.

Essentially, the genogram is a diagram of the family resembling a family tree. Clinicians employing this assessment strategy begin gathering and writing information about the identified patient and then branch out to the generations both above and, when present, below the patient. When relevant, information about the patient's grandparents and other members of a third or fourth generation may be included in the assessment as well.

Genogram assessment can be brief, focusing on only the most important and essential information or it can be broad and comprehensive in scope. Clinicians create symbols based on gender (see Table 80-2) to represent each family member and use different styles of lines—solid, dashed, zigzagged, etc.—to denote the type of relationship linking each family member to the others. Important dates—birth, death, divorce, marriage, etc.—are recorded, along with markers to indicate substance abuse, psychological and physical illnesses, family "secrets," and more. Once complete, a genogram can make family patterns readily and visibly apparent, and can quickly provide a visual picture of family functioning. Additionally, many clinicians work in concert with family members to develop the genogram, allowing family members the opportunity to uncover patterns of strength and limitations along with the clinician. For detailed instructions on the creation of genograms and the multidimensional applications of this assessment technique, see (65) McGoldrick, Gerson, and Petry's *Genograms: Assessment and Intervention, 3rd edition.*

Family Mapping

Although similar in design to the genogram, family mapping takes a slightly different approach to assessing families. Born out of structural family therapy, family maps are widely used in psychotherapy with families who have confused or inappropriate roles and boundaries (67). Following brain injury, family roles are frequently disrupted and old family relationship boundaries are discarded while new ones develop. The family map can enable practitioners to understand how these new roles and relationships are affecting a family. Additionally, the focus of the family map on the power structure within a family can give clinicians a very helpful tool. To effectively involve the family in the rehabilitation process, clinicians who understand the power dynamics within a family can work with that structure to enlist key family members as allies in the therapeutic process.

The family map begins with a power line (see Figure 80-1) (67). Practitioners draw a straight line through the center of a page and then use genogram gender symbols to place family members above or below the power line. The more power an individual has in a family, the farther above the power line their symbol is placed, whereas the reverse is true for individuals in a family with little power. Important relationships are also noted with the line markers used in genograms. Unlike genograms, family maps focus only on the immediately relevant family members.

A deviation of the standard family map that can be helpful following brain injury involves the creation of 2 maps—a preinjury and a postinjury map. Through the use of a nonjudgmental questioning stance, clinicians attempt to uncover the power structure of a family preinjury and create a map depicting those roles and relationships. To create a postinjury map, both interviews and clinician's observation are used. The comparison of these 2 maps allows clinicians to see how significantly power in the family has been disrupted as a result of the injury. For example, when a family map reveals a husband who, prior to his injury, held the highest position on the family map and then postinjury is represented well below the power line, the resultant power vacuum in the family is likely to affect decision making, the creation of a supportive environment, and the ability to effectively follow instructions in rehabilitation. Conversely, a family with a teenage daughter who is represented below the power line and parents who are squarely above the power line both preinjury and postinjury will likely retain the ability to function, but may struggle more with the emotional effects of injury. For more information on family mapping, see *Families and Family Therapy* by Salvador Minuchin (67).

Instruments and Measures

Assessment of families following brain injury requires a multifaceted approach incorporating a variety of strategies to create a whole picture of family needs, strengths, skills, and challenges. In addition to assessment techniques such as the interview, genograms, and family maps, which rely on the interpersonal interplay between clinician and family, tests and measures can provide valuable clinical insight for practitioners. Although many standardized assessments have been administered to rehabilitation populations demonstrating the applicability and usefulness with families after brain injury, studies rarely use appropriate family therapy ap-

Table 80-2 Genogram Symbol Meanings

Individual identifiers					
Male	Female	Age inside symbol (45)	Deceased	Death date (--- 2005)	Identified patient

Relationship connectors					
Married	Cohabitating couple	Separated	Divorced	Gay or lesbian couple	Cohabitating gay or lesbian couple

Children

55 ── 53

25 — Ann / Adopted / student at USC / Diabetic

1998–1998 — **Stillborn child**

2007 — **Miscarriage**

2008 — **Abortion**

15 15 — **Twins**

Due 10/2011 — **Pregnancy**

Physical / Psychological Identifiers (clinician notes types of illness or injury below the symbol)

TBI	Cocaine or alcohol	S	Marijuana	L
Physical or psychological illness	**Active substance abuse**	**Smoker**	**Suspected substance abuse**	**Language deficit**

Interaction pattern indicators

Good relationship	Distant relationship	Close relationship	Hostile relationship
Emotional abuse	**Distant & hostile**	**Close & hostile**	**Emotional cutoff**

Information included on a standard genogram:
1. Health and psychological characteristics, including substance abuse.
2. Names and/or titles, relational identifiers (e.g., adopted child, foster child).
3. Important dates: birth, death, illness/injury, marriage, separation, divorce.
4. Nature of interfamilial relationships (e.g., close, distant, hostile, abusive).
5. Interpersonal information that carries important meaning for the individual or family (e.g., occupation, geographic location, socioeconomic situation (SES), religious affiliation.

*Adapted from McGoldrick, Gerson, Petry (65) with permission.

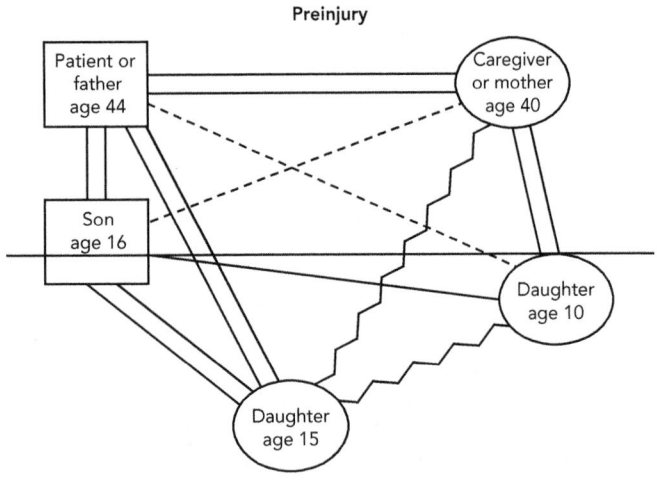

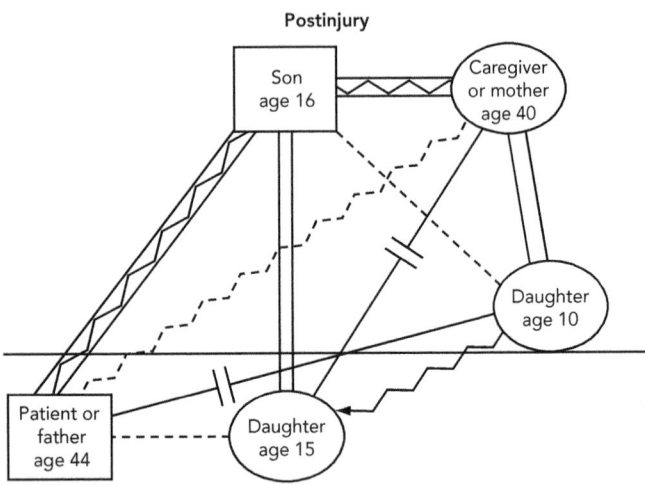

FIGURE 80-1 Family map. Significant family changes noted by family map as follows:

- Power shift; oldest child given parental level of power postinjury; father has lost family power status.
- Family members with most power postinjury have only one "close" family relationship each.
- Significant increase in number of hostile, distant, and/or cut-off family relationships; decrease in number of close relationships.
- Presence of emotional abuse between siblings postinjury.
- Middle daughter at significant emotional risk because of inadequate supportive interfamilial relationships postinjury.
- Father or patient no longer has any close interfamilial relationships.

proaches for administration (22). Researchers and clinicians in a rehabilitation setting have traditionally failed to give the instruments to more than 1 person in the family. Although in acute and subacute settings it may not be possible to include the brain injury survivor in the formalized assessment process, clinicians should strive to include as many family members as possible when using measures to assess a family. Scores can be interpreted conjointly (through averages), as well as in contrast to one another as a method for identifying interfamily discrepancies (68).

Both standardized and primarily therapeutic instruments are available for whole family assessment. Although standardized measures provide validated scores and the ability to juxtapose families with norms, therapeutic, non-standardized instruments are also valuable clinically. Unlike the available validated measures, many nonstandardized instruments have been designed specifically to assess the challenges families face after brain injury. The following tables detail both validated, standardized measures (Table 80-3) and available therapeutic measures (Table 80-4) that can assist clinicians when working with families in the rehabilitation process.

Referral Assessment

When available, case managers can be the ideal members of the treatment team to coordinate referrals (83). However, all clinicians have the responsibility when working with families to ensure a thorough assessment of referral needs is completed and contact with appropriate referral sources is made. Often times, families may not know enough about their current situation to know what questions they should ask or what services they may benefit from. The onus of responsibility falls to the treating practitioner and treatment team as a whole to evaluate how families might benefit from additional services. In addition to assessing standard referral needs such as ongoing outpatient rehabilitation, home health care, speech therapy, and so forth, clinicians should evaluate whole family psychosocial and daily living referral needs. In addition, all brain injury professionals should maintain an up-to-date referral list for services in and around their community. Table 80-5 describes some of the many areas that practitioners should assess to see if families could benefit from additional services.

INTERVENTION: WORKING WITH FAMILIES TO IMPROVE OVERALL WELLNESS

Because of the overlap between assessment and intervention, systemic treatment approaches must be constructed with astute intentionality. Without a firm foundation to guide treatment selection and intervention implementation, practitioners run the risk of continuously assessing families while failing to intervene. As such, brain injury professionals must solidly ground their work on principles of practice and then systematically build treatment plans within a structure which facilitates best practices. Practice principles—those beliefs that guide the work and decisions made by care providers on a daily basis—are often intuitive for clinicians, but rarely are they stated. Because these principles construct the foundation of the suggested pyramid for treatment implementation (see Figure 80-2), a lack of clarity regarding principle specifics can result in a treatment plan lacking specificity as well. This ambiguity has the potential to lead professionals to ask probing questions without a template for how to effectively respond to patient and family answers.

Although practice principles can vary in ways that are practitioner and facility specific or specific to the acuity and injury-severity needs of defined patient populations, it is a necessity to state practice principles. Much like the mission statements that guide organizations, these principles of prac-

TABLE 80-3 Family Instruments and Measures

MEASURE	BRIEF DESCRIPTION
Dyadic Adjustment Scale (DAS)	The DAS is a 32-item measure assessing relationship satisfaction (69). The scale provides a total adjustment score and 4 subscales scores: dyadic consensus, dyadic satisfaction, dyadic cohesion, and affectional expression. Several studies have supported the measure's internal consistency, concurrent and predictive validity, and reliability (70). Although not initially developed for a rehabilitation population, the DAS has been used with brain injury populations to examine couple functioning (71,72).
Family Adaptability and Cohesion Evaluation Scale (FACES IV)	The FACES IV is a self-report measure designed to assess family cohesion and flexibility based on the circumplex model of marital and family systems. The measure includes 42 items belonging to 6 subscales (cohesion, flexibility, chaotic, disengaged, enmeshed, and rigid) and can be completed by any family member older than than the age of 12 years (73). The FACES IV is a recently redeveloped version and has been tested with limited samples. However, previous iterations of the measure have been used with families in rehabilitation settings (74). The author's preliminary study indicates acceptable reliability and validity, but was tested on a convenience sample of nonclinical families (73).
Family Assessment Device (FAD)	The FAD is used to assess family functioning from the perspective of the caregiver. This 60-item self-report measure is based on the McMaster model of family functioning and has 6 subscales: problem solving, communication, roles, affective responsiveness, affective involvement, and behavior control. In addition, there is a general functioning subscale based on all items (75). The FAD has been used with families after TBI and has been shown to be sensitive to changes experienced after injury (14).
Family Needs Questionnaire (FNQ)	The FNQ is a frequently used 40-item self-report instrument intended to describe family members' perceived needs after brain injury (13,18,31,76). Items address commonly identified psychosocial and informational needs apparent after injury. Previous research indicates good content and construct validity as well as internal consistency (13). The measure contains 6 factor analytically derived scales: health information, emotional support, instrumental support, professional support, community support network, and involvement with care (63).
Neurobehavioral Functioning Inventory (NFI)	Developed for use with a TBI population, the NFI is an 83-item measure designed to examine the frequency of neurobehavioral difficulties postinjury (77). The measure can be administered in a self-report format or orally. Patient and family versions are available, allowing for comparison of responses. Normative data, based on age and injury severity, is available. Information is gathered about functioning in 6 domains: depression, somatic symptoms, memory or attention, communication, aggression, and motor abilities.
Service Obstacles Scale (SOS)	The SOS is a 6-item scale designed to solicit information regarding availability of and satisfaction with brain injury services. Items also address obstacles that might interfere with use of resources. Research has provided evidence for criterion-related validity and internal consistency of the measure when used with persons with brain injury and their caregivers (78).
Zarit Burden Interview (ZBI)	The ZBI is a self-administered scale consisting of 22 items regarding how the caregiver feels about their relationship with the patient, their health condition, finances, psychological well-being, and social life (79,80). The scale was originally developed for use with caregivers or family members of patients with dementia or elderly patients (80), but has also been used with brain injury samples (12). Despite criticism that the ZBI implicitly assumes the caregiver is stressed, reliability and validity of the scale are adequate (80).

tice should reflect the belief structure and objectives that underlie the work of individuals or entities. Clinicians who strive to take a family-inclusive approach to care are encouraged to make the construction of their own practice principles a priority, with the ultimate aim being widespread knowledge and implementation in daily treatment planning. The following principles guide the work of Kreutzer and colleagues (84), and can be used as a template from which practitioners can build their own core principles to guide intervention:

1. Brain injury often has a dramatic impact on the entire family in the long-term.
2. Most people would prefer to have their old lives back. This is often the driving force of most decisions and actions by patients and families.

3. People, in general, do best when they are well informed.
4. Each adult family member has a voice, deserves respect, and nearly all have the right to make their own decisions.
5. To be most helpful, caregivers must learn to make taking care of theirselves a priority.

Following development of a comprehensive list of practice principles, clinicians should build a treatment plan for each family based on the "treatment plan pyramid" presented in Figure 80-2. This foundation of principles is complimented by an integrated systemic theoretical framework. Although the supporting 2 structures of the pyramid—principles and theory—are static regardless of family being treated, the top portion of the pyramid is family and patient specific. For each clinical case, practitioners are to identify the primary challenges faced by the family, develop goals appropriate to each

TABLE 80-4 Qualitative Family Measures

MEASURE	DESCRIPTION
1. 13-Item Stress Test (64)	High levels of sustained stress that normally follow TBI typically have a detrimental impact on emotional well-being and relationships. The stress test helps family members be more self-aware of stress levels so they can more effectively manage stress. The test is used in the Brain Injury Family Intervention and consists of 13 true or false items. High levels of stress are indicated by a higher number of items marked as true. The measure is brief and easily readministered allowing assessment of change.
2. Brain Injury Problem Checklist (64)	The checklist was designed to help family members and survivors identify commonly reported injury-related changes. The 42 items are divided into 4 categories: (a) physical, (b) cognitive, (c) behavioral and emotional, and (d) communication and social. For the Brain Injury Family Intervention (BIFI), family members are asked individually to identify on paper the changes they have noticed. Afterward, the therapist facilitates family members' discussion of similarities and differences in their perceptions.
3. Change Recognition Questionnaire (81)	Ambiguous loss is commonly experienced after brain injury. Research suggests that diminishing ambiguity enables more effective coping. Developed by Kreutzer and colleagues in 1999, the Change Recognition Questionnaire helps family members appreciate how injury has affected their behavior, interactions, and feelings. The questionnaire consists of 10 open-ended questions that can be answered on paper or via interview with 1 or more family members. Sample items include, "What changes in the injured person are most upsetting?" and "How are you treating the injured person differently?"
4. Communication Questionnaire (64)	Many survivors and family members report feeling isolated, alone, and misunderstood. Although immediate family members may spend a considerable amount of time together, the quality of their relationships may suffer because effective communication is lacking. The Communication Question was designed as part of the BIFI to help family members appreciate their perceptions about obstacles to communication. Counselors can help families function more effectively by identifying obstacles and strategies to overcome them. The questionnaire consists of 16 true or false items such as, "Nobody understands what I am going through" and "I'm afraid to show my true feelings."
5. "Do I Have Mixed Feelings About the Person with the Injury?" Questionnaire (81)	Clinical experience has indicated family members can experience intense ambivalent feelings regarding the survivor. On one hand, family members may be deeply upset about the pain and disability experienced by the survivor. On the other hand, family members may also feel intimidated and appalled by neurobehavioral changes, especially anger, irritability, and lability. Consisting of 11 yes or no items, the mixed feelings questionnaire helps family members recognize and effectively address their ambivalence. Sample items include, "Sometimes I just feel sorry for him or her" and "I like my family member less now."
6. Family Change Questionnaire (FCQ) (64)	The FCQ was first developed to help all family members appreciate how brain injury often has a substantial impact on family members as well as the survivor. Respondents are asked a series of open-ended questions via interview or in writing. Items include, "How did you feel when you began to recognize that the brain injury might have long-term effects?" and "How has the brain injury affected your plans for the future?" The FCQ is available in 3 versions: a family member version, a survivor version, and a 5-item family or survivor version.
7. Feelings Questionnaire (64)	First developed for use in the BIFI, the Feelings Questionnaire consists of 20 items. Individual family members are asked to circle the items that describe how they have been feeling since the injury. Postinjury, many family members report feeling overwhelmed, emotionally drained, hopeless, and helpless. The questionnaire helps family members identify individual feelings experienced as a first step toward effectively mitigating distress. Items on the questionnaire include, "I often feel frustrated," "I get angry easily," and "I can't do much to make things better."
8. Guilty or Not Guilty? Checklist (81)	Guilt is commonly experienced by caregiving family members. The "Guilty or Not Guilty?" checklist was designed to help family members appreciate guilt relating to bad choices, causing or failing to prevent the injury, failing to help the patient get better, and causing new problems after the injury. The checklist is comprised of 9 items and respondents are asked to check off items relevant to their feelings and perceptions. Sample items include, "I can't let this happen again" and "Sometimes I wish I was the one who was hurt instead."
9. Healthy Marriage Quiz (82)	Designed for couples, the quiz contains 14 true or false items divided into 4 sections: (a) communication challenges, (b) changing responsibilities, (c) changing priorities, and (d) emotional and personality changes. Couples can review their individual responses in each section to identify areas of well functioning and areas that would likely benefit from improvement. Sample items include, "We are always arguing about something" and "My spouse gets upset at anything I say or do."

(Continued)

TABLE 80-4 Qualitative Family Measures (*Continued*)

MEASURE	DESCRIPTION
10. How Well Am I Taking Care of Myself Questionnaire (64)	The 17-item true or false questionnaire was designed as a first step toward helping family members more effectively take care of themselves. In particular, clinical research indicates that caregivers typically neglect their own personal needs to focus on the needs of the survivor and other family members. Respondents identify areas where they are doing well at taking care of themselves and areas where they are doing poorly. Sample items include, "I recognize my limits and adjust my activities accordingly" and "I take time out to rest and relax."
11. Obstacles to Problem Solving Questionnaire (64)	Postinjury, survivors and family members are often ineffective problem solvers. Kreutzer and colleagues developed the 17-item true or false questionnaire to help family members identify issues that limit the effectiveness of their problem solving skills. Items include, "I don't like talking to people about my problems" and "I am too depressed to do anything." The questionnaire was first developed and used as a tool in the BIFI to help therapists choose client-relevant cognitive behavioral and skill building strategies.
12. Problem Solving Personality Questionnaire (64)	Consisting of 20 true or false items, this questionnaire was developed for use in the BIFI as a complement to the Obstacles to Problem Solving Questionnaire. Ten of the items reflect personal characteristics that enable effective problem solving (e.g., "I carefully research my problems and possible solutions," "I try new approaches when old ones don't work"). The remaining 10 items reflect ineffective approaches (e.g., "Problems have to get really bad before I deal with them," "I tend to focus on what's wrong and why solutions won't work"). Therapists can use the questionnaire to help clients differentiate between personally effective and ineffective strategies, rely more on effective strategies, and diminish use of ineffective strategies.

challenge, and select both generalized and specific techniques to drive treatment.

Review of Existing Family Interventions

Although each family, as with each brain injury, is unique, researchers have developed a limited number of family-based interventions available for implementation by practitioners. However, intervention design and outcomes widely vary. Table 80-6 describes existing family interventions and established benefits and/or outcomes. Demonstration of significant positive outcomes is indicated in 4 studies. Interventions adopting a systemic, whole-family approach to treatment are limited to those designed by Carnevale et al. (85), Sinnakaruppan et al. (86), and Kreutzer et al. (87). Only 1 intervention, the Brain Injury Family Intervention (87) both provides whole family services and has demonstrable positive outcomes. Practitioners interested in implementing established inter-

ventions are encouraged to review the referenced manuscripts to learn more about implementation, limitations, and benefits of the intervention they would like to provide.

Constructing and Implementing Treatment Plans

Identifying Challenges

Whether or not brain injury professionals intend to implement existing interventions, every clinician should have the tools to develop comprehensive treatment plans that affect whole family involvement in rehabilitation. Following the establishment of practice principles and a complimentary theoretical framework, practitioners must use assessment techniques to establish the challenges most relevant to the family as a whole. Although each family will face unique struggles, there are also common challenges faced by many families after brain injury. In addition to those identified here, a more comprehensive list of common challenges is

TABLE 80-5 Areas for Potential Family Referral

• Whole family substance abuse treatment needs	• Psychotherapy for children or adolescents in the home	• Supportive therapy for caregivers or support groups	• Financial assistance (hospital or medical, TANIF, WIC, etc.)
• In-school support (school counselor or psychologist) for children	• Social support for survivors (support group, interest groups or meetup.com, etc.)	• Transportation assistance or accommodations assistance	• Vocational assistance for survivors and/or caregivers
• Legal services (patient = accident related, caregiver = power of attorney, etc.)	• Spiritual guidance	• Web-based support (online support groups, informational sites, etc.)	• Coordinating information for friends or family (caringbridge.org, yahoo groups, etc.)

WIC, Women, Infants and Children.

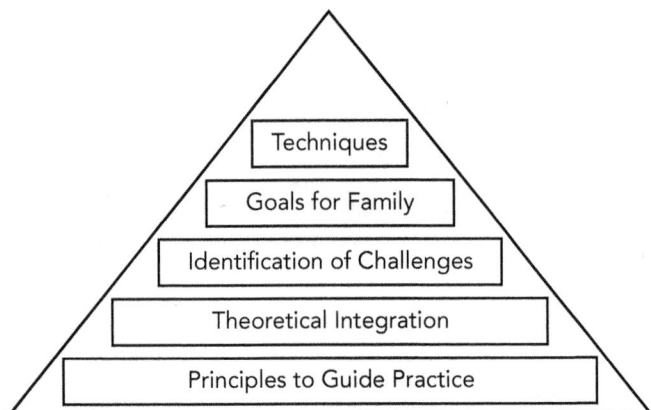

FIGURE 80-2 Treatment planning pyramid.

presented by Kreutzer and colleagues, in *Practical Approaches to Effective Family Intervention After Brain Injury* (84).

One of the most frequent hurdles faced by families is a feeling of confusion regarding patient neurobehavioral sequelae (84). Family members often attempt to make sense of patient behavioral changes without a base of knowledge regarding brain injury and typical outcomes. Additionally, family members may develop strong conflicting feelings regarding the person with the injury. Caregivers report vacillating between feelings of love and anger as they get to know their loved one anew, which often results in experiences of guilt and ambivalence. Another common experience is that of feeling trapped living with a stranger. This feeling is reported both by patients and by family members as all members of the family attempt to establish new relationships with one another. Rehabilitation itself can result in family frustration as the whole family moves from unbridled hope to disappointment in effectiveness and surprise that injury related problems do not end soon after hospital discharge. Finally, many times, both family members and patients fail to recognize the impact the injury has had on all members of the family.

Providers should familiarize themselves with these and other common challenges and use assessment strategies to ascertain how these hurdles may affect family recovery. Intervention strategies aimed directly at combating relevant challenges will help families to embrace the ideas presented in rehabilitation plans. Additionally, as clinicians identify ways in which both family members and survivors are struggling with similar challenges, albeit differently, the family will have the opportunity to form an empathic team rather than a splintered combative system.

Goal Identification

Following the identification of relevant challenges, practitioners are faced with the task of working with families to select appropriate goals for treatment. Goals should be developed through collaborative assessment with the family, combining family desires for change with clinical knowledge regarding best outcomes. The clinical knowledge component should draw from 2 parts: family and challenge—specific

goals and goals that are commonly beneficial to families following brain injury. When a common family challenge is identified as relevant, corresponding specific goals for treatment are suggested in Kreutzer et al (84). For example, when family members experience mixed feelings regarding the survivor, Kreutzer et al. suggests appropriate treatment goals could be (*a*) to help family members recognize their mixed feelings, (*b*) to normalize the discomfort that is associated with mixed feelings, (*c*) to educate family members on the negative outcomes associated with pervasive feelings of guilt, and (*d*) to build skills enabling family members to minimize feelings of guilt.

In addition to the development of challenge-specific goals, providers may wish to consider the inclusion of goals that are commonly beneficial for families after brain injury. Suggested goals that may benefit both family members and survivors include establishing a knowledge base regarding normal brain injury recovery patterns, developing effective problem solving skills, learning how to set postinjury goals that are realistic and achievable, learning how to talk to others about the injury, developing strategies to minimize guilt and blame, coping with losses and changes, managing stress and intense emotions, developing postinjury parenting skills, improving communication skills, and establishing hope-inspired and positive approaches to treatment and long-term recovery (87). Broad goals such as these can either compliment or be infused with challenge-specific goals as well as family-driven goals to create an approach to intervention that will help families in the short- and long-term.

Family Therapy Techniques

Achieving goals while working with families is a long-term process. Whole-family emotional recovery is tentative, lengthy, and involves multiple modifications of the term "success." A foundation of broadly applicable family therapy techniques will assist all brain injury professionals in creating a therapeutic environment, with an ultimate aim of allowing for the flexibility families need to achieve emotional health and wellness. The following are foundational techniques to be implemented regardless of identified challenges and corresponding goals. Although practitioners can and should incorporate additional techniques that are specific to family needs, these identified strategies will promote the success of all medical, occupational, recreational, and psychotherapeutic interventions.

Joining and Establishing a Working Alliance

The therapeutic relationship—e.g., "working alliance"—contributes to 30% of the change process in psychotherapy (60). In medical processes, the doctor–patient relationship has also been firmly established as a factor significantly contributing to overall patient outcome (93). Additionally, meta-analytic review found that within family therapy, the relationship between therapist and the family system is a dominant outcome factor, regardless of the developmental structure of the family seeking services (94). Therefore, in working with families following brain injury, providers are charged with establishing a working alliance with both the patient and the supporting family system.

TABLE 80-6 Summary of Family Intervention Research

AUTHOR/YEAR	N	INTERVENTION DELIVERY METHOD	RECIPIENT	INTERVENTION PURPOSE	CAREGIVER INTERVENTION BENEFITS
Acorn/1995 (88)	19	group; in person; three 5-hour sessions over 3 weekends; manualized	family members	psychological support, education	No significant changes in coping ability, self-esteem, or life-satisfaction.
Brown/1999[a] (89)	91	group; in person, on-site vs telephone; ten 1.5- to 2.0-hour session over 10 weeks; not manualized	family members	psychological support	Improvements in psychological distress for both treatment groups but no improvements in family functioning or burden for either.
Morris/2001 (90)	33	individual; off site; 2 follow-up telephone calls over 5 weeks; not manualized	family members	psychological support, education via information booklet	No improvements in psychological distress.
Albert/2002[a] (91)	56	individual; on-site, in person, and off-site; postdischarge by telephone; sessions varied in length for a period up to 16 months; not manualized	family members	psychological support, education	Intervention reduced burden levels, improved satisfaction with caregiving, and increased perceptions of caregiving competency.
Carnevale/2002 (85)[b]	27	individual; in person, home, and community setting; 2-hour education sessions provided weekly over 4 weeks to all participants; behavioral intervention group completed additional 2-hour sessions weekly for 8 weeks; not manualized	family members, survivors	behavioral management, problem solving skills training	No significant changes in perceived stress and psychological distress.
Sinnakaruppan/ 2005 (86)[b]	41	survivor and family member groups, in-person; eight 2.5-hour sessions over 8 weeks; not manualized	family members, survivors	education	No significant changes in psychological distress, coping, or self-esteem.
Rivera/2008[a] (92)	67	individual; 12 monthly sessions over 1 year, 4 in-home, 8 by telephone; not manualized	family members	problem solving skills training	Positive treatment impact on psychological distress or depression, health, dysfunctional problem solving styles. No impact on caregiver life satisfaction, burden, or constructive problem solving styles.
Kreutzer/2009[a,b] (87)	53	individual; on-site; five 1.5- to 2-hour sessions delivered over 10 weeks; manualized	family members, survivors	psychological support, education, skills training	Increased in met family needs and perceived access to services. No impact on psychological distress, family functioning, satisfaction with life.

[a]Interventions demonstrating significant positive outcomes
[b]Interventions taking a systemic approach, including both family members and survivors in treatment approaches
Table reprinted from Kreutzer, Stejskal, Ketchum, Marwitz, Taylor, Menzel (87) with permission.

The process of joining with a family is firmly rooted in a respectful, collaborative relationship between practitioner and each family member (60). Clinicians must straddle a line of providing expert knowledge and care while being respectful of family beliefs, opinions, concerns, and desires. Plainly stated, providers who work with family members from a humanistic perspective and treat each person as a valuable member of the rehabilitation process will be most successful in establishing an alliance. Practitioners should take an initial questioning stance, allowing each member of the family to contribute information with respect to family history, culture, concerns, and perspectives. Even beliefs that are in conflict with best medical practices should be treated with respect. Although clinicians have the responsibility of providing the best care possible, letting family members know that their concerns are valid and respected will create an atmosphere much more amenable to modification. A provider's professional identity may need to be reformulated. As professionals see themselves less as the omnipotent service provider and more as a collaborating team member who brings expert knowledge in a particular domain, relationships with families and patients will improve dramatically (95). Families who have an established working relationship with their care providers are much more likely to become invested in the rehabilitation process. Additionally, providers will establish treatment plans that are increasingly consistent with family and patient needs.

Active Listening

Although listening may seem to be an obvious component of intervention, practitioners must intentionally apply certain skills to convey effective, active listening when communicating with families. Active listening (96) involves first listening for the total meaning of what is being said. When suggesting strategies for change, providers must listen for family hesitation and/or resistance to ideas. Further, this hesitation should be explored—what are the reasons for the family's concern? When concerns are validated and acknowledged, families are much more likely to feel respected and included in the rehabilitation process. Additionally, responding to feelings in addition to content is an essential component of conveying interest and care. Particularly in the highly stressful, demanding context of brain injury recovery, family statements may sometimes seem difficult to make sense of. When practitioners listen for feelings such as fear, anger, frustration, and so forth rather than the content, they are likely to have increasingly empathic reactions to family statements. Finally, active listening involves looking for all cues, both verbal and physical, given when patients and family members are communicating. Voice inflection, body posture, and facial expressions may tell clinicians more about what family members wish to communicate than words will. When these underlying messages are responded to, families are likely to feel respected and included, and are much more likely to participate willingly in rehabilitation objectives.

Normalization

Normalization or "normalizing" family emotional responses is a fundamental part of therapeutic intervention. Particularly in situations that are outside a family's traditional life experiences, the process of normalizing responses can significantly reduce levels of anxiety and trepidation (97). Brain injury, although commonplace to practitioners working in the field, is an experience few families understand. Therefore, both the patient responses to injury and the family emotional reactions to the recovery process are often interpreted by family members as abnormal and/or concerning. By conveying to families that both patient sequelae and family responses are common and anticipated, family members can reduce fears that they may not be following a traditional brain injury recovery path.

Positive Reframing

As demonstrated by studies investigating resiliency, families who are able to embrace an optimistic approach to recovery are much more likely to experience positive outcomes. Clinicians can assist families in developing a hope-filled approach by using positive reframing skills throughout intervention. Reframing has been established as an effective interpersonal skill in hospital settings, particularly when patient prognosis is unlikely to change (98). Within the context of brain injury, reframing allows clinicians to begin to infuse expressions of hope into dominant family dialogues that may be filled with sadness and fear.

Clinicians implementing positive reframing must be cautious in their application. Reframing should simultaneously acknowledge a family member's negative emotions and experiences while offering hope that an alternate explanation is plausible (98). Therefore, when reframes are met with resistance, clinicians should explore family hesitation rather than persevering with a reframe. Wording and language is particularly important in reframes and providers should be careful to avoid use of contradictory statements such as "but" and/or language that questions an individual's perception of reality—that is, "I know you think he's getting worse, *but* our tests don't show that. You are probably just scared and things seem worse than they *really are.*" Instead, practitioners should strive to offer perspectives that can be both congruent with and supplemental to established ways of thinking—that is, "Seeing him get worse is frightening because you are wondering how bad things will get. The tests seem to show that he is stable, so I'm wondering if maybe its easier for you to see his challenges now that things have calmed down a bit and you have more energy to notice symptoms than you did early on? If what you're seeing has been there a while, that would mean both that things might not continue to get worse and that you can begin to trust your own observations more than you have been. What do you think?"

Collaborative Self-Examination

Developed by researchers at Virginia Commonwealth University, collaborative self-examination is a family therapy technique designed specifically for work with families following brain injury (87). This technique allows family members the opportunity to hear from and empathize with other members of their family regarding feelings and observations surrounding brain injury and brain injury recovery. Family members are asked to answer specific and direct questions in the presence of one another. Often, therapeutic measurement instruments and/or questionnaires are used to enhance this process (see Table 80-4). Practitioners then facilitate a respectful sharing of answers between family members, encouraging each family member to respond and react to the answers given by others. A clinician might ask, "Susan, what do you think about John's response to how his responsibilities at home have changed? What did you imagine he might say? How is what he said different or similar to what you expected?" Goals of collaborative self-examination may be to improve whole family awareness regarding the impact of injury on all family members, to improve survivor self-awareness, and/or to minimize family tendencies to dismiss or discount survivor input. This technique helps families to develop an empathic environment, improves family communication, and enhances family cohesion surrounding rehabilitation objectives.

Intervention Modality

Although therapy structure may sometimes be determined based on practical considerations such as family proximity to a facility and/or access to transportation, the intervention modality can have a significant impact on the course of rehabilitation. In addition to practical issues, clinicians should consider several variables when selecting the structure of intervention services. The primary consideration is ensuring a match with treatment plan goals and objectives. If family fragmentation or an unbalanced power structure is a primary challenge, full family therapy including the survivor would be an astute choice; whereas when caregiver burnout or frustration with the survivor is the dominant concern, individual therapy with the caregiver may be warranted. In addition, clinicians should consider patient and family preference. In medical processes, family members and patients may feel they have little control over the implementation of treatment. Offering the opportunity to have a substantial voice in the process of selecting therapy modality can give patients and family members an immediate sense of regaining control in their lives (99). Table 80-7 describes the more commonly implemented therapeutic modalities, who is served by each structure, and the function or objective of selecting each structure.

TABLE 80-7 Family Therapy Structure Options

THERAPY STRUCTURE	WHO IS INCLUDED	FUNCTION/OBJECTIVE
Individual therapy	Either the survivor or an individual family member	Allows the attending client to express concerns, fears, and frustrations that they may not feel comfortable or productive sharing with other family members. Therapist may infuse individual sessions throughout other modalities as well to understand individual points of view more completely. Individual sessions focus content on whole family, systemic concerns.
Family therapy	The whole family, including the survivor	Begins or facilitates the process of establishing the postinjury family system. This structure helps families to make sense of new roles and responsibilities, facilitates an empathic family environment, and provides skill building opportunities for whole family communication.
Family member therapy	All or some family members, not including the brain injury survivor	Provides an opportunity for family reorganization during the acute recovery phase. Also allows family members to identify their thoughts and feelings related to the injury prior to discussions with the survivor. Appropriate early in recovery, but should be implemented with reserve posthospital discharge because of the possibility of further alienation of the survivor within the family system.
Couples counseling	Survivor and spouse; parents of adult or minor children with TBI; coupled family members with caregiving responsibilities (e.g., married caregiving sister and her spouse)	Relationship-focused therapy often addressing issues related to connectivity, cohesion, stress-induced interpersonal anger, etc. For the survivor, provide an opportunity to establish new roles within the context of the committed relationship.
Group therapy: Caregiver or Survivor Groups	Caregiver(s), survivor, or other family members or friends	Typically structured as support groups, although may also be therapy groups, these meetings provide kinship, establish support networks, assist patients and family members in problem solving options, and offer a place to share feelings that individuals may not be comfortable sharing within the context of the family.
Group Therapy: Multifamily group structure	Whole family, including the survivor	Groups link families with other family units in the community who have experienced brain injury. Families often share whole-family challenges and find support and solutions through the responses of other members. One of the best therapeutic options for developing social networks and establishing connectivity within the family.
Variations to in person therapy (e.g., Web-based, telephone-based)	Varies	Although considered to be nontraditional, web-based (e.g., Skype, etc.) and telephone interventions offer patients who live in remote locations the opportunity to receive treatment from providers with expertise in brain injury. Challenges with billing, patient or family access to necessary technological resources, and confidentiality are often a concern.

CONCLUSION

The integration of theory, assessment, and intervention is a complicated yet integral component of working effectively with family members in the rehabilitative phase of recovery from TBI. Although the medical model of care stresses the importance of focusing on patient-centered treatment, the interactions between family members and patients as well as family members and hospital staff have a crucial role in the course of treatment. As a result, clinicians working with patients must also learn how to effectively incorporate families into the process of rehabilitation. Using a strengths-based, nonexpert stance, practitioners have the opportunity to enlist family assistance in rehabilitation. Further, once the patient leaves the hospital setting, families continue to need assistance and guidance in the long process of healing. Incorporating family needs into ongoing assessment and intervention enables clinicians to address concerns in a holistic manner.

KEY CLINICAL POINTS

1. Brain injury often affects the entire family. Be especially sensitive to the impact on younger children.
2. Recognize the need to focus on emotional as well as physical recovery.
3. Appreciate family member's unique reactions and perspectives.
4. Most families want their "old" lives back. The struggle for normalcy may take months, years, or longer.
5. Effective intervention requires a combination of approaches including psychological support, skill building, and education.
6. Helping family members take good care of themselves may be the greatest challenge faced by clinicians.
7. Family members are often overwhelmed by worry and negative perspectives. Help them focus on the positive and help them be hopeful.

ELECTRONIC RESOURCES

1. www.tbifamilyresearch.org
   Website designed for a clinical audience, providing multiple resources related to research and clinical practice with families after brain injury.
2. www.braininjuryeducation.org/Specific_population/Family_issues.aspx
   Consumer-focused website providing basic information, treatment strategies, and quizzes. A resource for patients and families.
3. www.msktc.washingon.edu/tbi/factsheets/index.asap
   TBI Consumer Information fact sheets—coming soon—on TBI and relationships to provide to patients and families.
4. Stejskal TM. *Evaluating an Evidence-based Intervention for Families and Survivors After Traumatic Brain Injury: The Brain Injury Family Intervention*. Ann Arbor, MI: ProQuest LLC; 2009.

KEY REFERENCES

1. Duncan B, Miller S, Wampold B, Hubble M. *The Heart and Soul of Change: Delivering What Works in Therapy*. 2nd ed. Washington, DC: American Psychological Association; 2009.
2. Kreutzer J, Taylor L. *Brain Injury Family Intervention: Implementation Manual*. Richmond, VA: The National Resource Center for Traumatic Brain Injury; 2004.
3. Lezak MD. Brain damage is a family affair. *J Clin Exp Neuropsych*. 1988;19:111–123.
4. Myers J. Coping with caregiving stress: a wellness-oriented, strengths-based approach for family counselors. *The Fam J*. 2003;11:153–161.
5. Witol AD, Sander AM, Kreutzer JS. A longitudinal analysis of family needs following traumatic brain injury. *NeuroRehabilitation*. 1996;7:175–187.

References

1. Draper K, Ponsford J, Schöberger M. (2007). Psychosocial and emotional outcomes 10 years following traumatic brain injury. *J Head Trauma Rehabil*. 2007;22(5):278–287.
2. Rao V, Rosenberg P, Bertrand M, et al. Aggression after traumatic brain injury: prevalence and correlates. *J Neuropsychiatry Clin Neurosci*. 2009;21(4):420–429.
3. Ruttan L, Martin K, Liu A, Colella B, Green RE. Long-term cognitive outcome in moderate to severe traumatic brain injury: a meta-analysis examining timed and untimed tests at 1 and 4.5 or more years after injury. *Arch Phys Med Rehab*. 2008;89(suppl 12):S69–S76.
4. Riggio S. Traumatic brain injury and its neurobehavioral sequelae. *Psychiatr Clin North Am*. 2010;33(4):807–819.
5. Mathias JL, Wheaton P. Changes in attention and information-processing speed following severe traumatic brain injury: a meta-analytic review. *Neuropsychology*. 2007;21(2):212–223.
6. Hanks RA, Rapport LJ, Vangel S. Caregiving appraisal after traumatic brain injury: the effects of functional status, coping style, social support, and family functioning. *NeuroRehabilitation*. 2007;22(1):43–52.
7. Ergh TC, Hanks RA, Rapport LJ, Coleman RD. Social support moderates caregiver life satisfaction following brain injury. *J Clin Exp Neuropsychology*. 2003;25(8):1090–1101.
8. Ponsford J, Olver J, Ponsford M, Nelms R. Long-term adjustment of families following traumatic brain injury where comprehensive rehabilitation has been provided. *Brain Inj*. 2003;17(6):453–468.
9. Lezak MD. Brain damage is a family affair. *J Clin Exp Neuropsych*. 1988;10(1):111–123.
10. Livingston LA, Kennedy RE, Marwitz JH, et al. Predictors of family caregivers' life satisfaction after traumatic brain injury at one and two years post-injury: a longitudinal multi-center investigation. *NeuroRehabilitation*. 2010;27(1):73–81.
11. Kreutzer JS, Rapport LJ, Marwitz JH, et al. Caregivers' well-being after traumatic brain injury: a multicenter prospective investigation. *Arch Phys Med Rehabil*. 2009;90(6):939–946.
12. Wells R, Dywan J, Dumas J. Life satisfaction and stress in family caregivers as related to specific behavioral changes after traumatic brain injury. *Brain Inj*. 2005;19(13):1105–1115.
13. Kreutzer JS, Gervasio AH, Camplair PS. Primary caregivers' psychological status and family functioning after traumatic brain injury. *Brain Inj*. 1994;8(3):197–210.
14. Ponsford J, Schönberger M. Family functioning and emotional state two and five years after traumatic brain injury. *J Int Neuropsychol Soc*. 2010;16(2):306–317.
15. Kreutzer JS. *Family Needs Questionnaire*. Richmond, VA: Rehabilitation Research and Training Center on Severe Traumatic Brain Injury, Medical College of Virginia; 1988.
16. Kolakowsky-Hayner SA, Miner KD, Kreutzer JS. Long-term life quality and family needs after traumatic brain injury. *J Head Trauma Rehabil*. 2001;16(4):374–385.

17. Kreutzer JS, Serio CD, Berquist S. Family needs after brain injury: a quantitative analysis. *J Head Trauma Rehabil.* 1994;9(3):104–115.

18. Moules S, Chandler BJ. A study of the health and social needs of carers of traumatically brain injured individuals served by one community rehabilitation team. *Brain Inj.* 1999;13(12):983–993.

19. Nabors N, Seacat J, Rosenthal M. Predictors of caregiver burden following traumatic brain injury. *Brain Inj.* 2002;6(12):1039–1050.

20. Serio CD, Kreutzer JS, Gervasio AH. Predicting family needs after brain injury: implications for intervention. *J Head Trauma Rehabil.* 1995;10(2):32–45.

21. Witol AD, Sander AM, Kreutzer JS. A longitudinal analysis of family needs following traumatic brain injury. *NeuroRehabilitation.* 1996;7(3):175–187.

22. Godwin EE, Kreutzer JS, Arango-Lasprilla JC, Lehan TJ. Marriage after brain injury: review analysis, and research recommendations. *J Head Trauma Rehabil.* 2011;26(1):43–55.

23. Thomsen IV. Late outcome of very severe blunt head trauma: a 10–15 year second follow-up. *J Neurol Neurosurg Psychiatry.* 1984; 47(3):260–268.

24. Wood RL, Rutterford, NA. Psychosocial adjustment 17 years after severe brain injury. *J Neurol Neurosurg Psychiatry.* 2006;77(1):71–73.

25. Gosling J, Oddy M. Rearranged marriages: marital relationships after head injury. *Brain Inj.* 1999;13(10):785–796.

26. Garden F, Bontke C, Hoffman M. Sexual functioning and marital adjustment after traumatic brain injury. *J Head Trauma Rehabil.* 1990;5(2):52–59.

27. Kreutzer JS, Zasler ND. Psychosexual consequences of traumatic brain injury: methodology and preliminary findings. *Brain Inj.* 1989;3(2):177–186.

28. Ponsford J. Sexual changes associated with traumatic brain injury. *Neuropsychol Rehabil.* 2003;13(1–2):275–289.

29. Machamer J, Temkin N, Dikmne S. Significant other burden and factors related to it in traumatic brain injury. *J Clin Exp Neuropsychol.* 2002;24(4):420–433.

30. Hart T, O'Neil-Pirozzi TM, Williams KD, Rapport LJ, Hammond F, Kreutzer J. Racial differences in caregiving patterns, caregiver emotional function, and sources of emotional support following traumatic brain injury. *J Head Trauma Rehabil.* 2007;22(2):122–131.

31. Arango-Lasprilla JC, Quijano MC, Aponte M, et al. Family needs in caregivers of individuals with traumatic brain injury from Columbia, South America. *Brain Inj.* 2010;24(7–8):1017–1026.

32. Corrigan JD. Substance abuse as a mediating factor in outcome from traumatic brain injury. *Arch Phys Med Rehabil.* 1995;76(4): 302–309.

33. Kreutzer JS, Witol AD, Sander AM, Cifu DX, Marwitz JH, Delmonico R. A prospective longitudinal multicenter analysis of alcohol use patterns among person with traumatic brain injury. *J Head Trauma Rehabil.* 1996;11(5):58–69.

34. Bjork JM, Grant SJ. Does traumatic brain injury increase risk for substance abuse? *J Neurotrauma.* 2009;26(7):1077–1082.

35. Ponsford J, Whelan-Goodinson R, Bahar-Fuchs A. Alcohol and drug use following traumatic brain injury: a prospective study. *Brain Inj.* 2007;21(13–14):1385–1392.

36. Seaton JD, David CO. Family role in substance abuse and traumatic brain injury rehabilitation. *J Head Trauma Rehabil.* 1990;5(3):41–46.

37. Taylor LA, Kreutzer JS, Demm SR, Meade MA. Traumatic brain injury and substance abuse: a review and analysis of the literature. *Neuropsychol Rehabilil.* 2003;13(1–2):165–188.

38. Hall LK. The importance of understanding military culture. *Soc Work Health Care.* 2011;50(1):4–18.

39. Friedemann-Sánchez G, Sayer NA, Pickett T. Provider perspectives on rehabilitation of patients with polytrauma. *Arch Phys Med Rehabil.* 2008;89(1):171–178.

40. Hoge CW, McGurk D, Thomas JL, Cox AL, Engel CC, Castro CA. Mild traumatic brain injury in U.S. soldiers returning from Iraq. *New Engl J Med.* 2008;358(5):453–463.

41. Sherer M, Evans C, Leverenz J, et al. Therapeutic alliance in post-acute brain injury rehabilitation: predictors of strength of alliance and impact of alliance on outcome. *Brain Inj.* 2007;21(7):663–672.

42. Bowen M. The use of family theory in clinical practice. *Compr Psychiatry.* 1966;7(5):345–374.

43. Umpleby S, Dent E. The origins and purposes of several traditions in systems theory and cybernetics. *Cybernet Syst.* 1999;30(2):79–103.

44. Dore M. *Family Systems Theory: Comprehensive Handbook of Social Work and Social Welfare.* Cambridge, MA: The Guidance Center; 2008.

45. Goldenberg H, Goldenberg I. *Family Therapy: An Overview.* 7th ed. Belmont, CA: Thomson Higher Education; 2007.

46. Verhaeghe S, Defloor T, Grypdonck M. Stress and coping among families of patients with traumatic brain injury: a review of the literature. *J Clin Nurs.* 2005;14(8):1004–1012.

47. Goff B, Smith D. Systemic traumatic stress: the couple adaption to traumatic stress model. Paper presented at: AAMFT Annual Conference; January 7, 2002; Cincinnati, OH.

48. Johnson J, McCown W. *Family Therapy of Neurobehavioral Disorders: Integrating Neuropsychology and Family Therapy.* Philadelphia, PA: The Haworth Press; 1997.

49. Walsh F. A family resilience framework: innovative practice applications. *Family Relations.* 2002;51(2):130–137.

50. Bradbury CL, Christensen B, Lau M, Ruttan LA, Arudine AL, Green RE. The efficacy of cognitive behavior therapy in the treatment of emotional distress after acquired brain injury. *Arch Phys Med Rehabil.* 2008;89(suppl 12):S61–S68.

51. Schwebel A, Fine M. Cognitive-behavioral family therapy. *J Fam Psychother.*1992;3:73–91.

52. Corey G. *Theory and Practice of Counseling and Psychotherapy.* 8th ed. Florence, KY: Cengage Learning; 2008.

53. Briers S. *Brilliant Cognitive Behavioral Therapy.* Philadelphia, PA: Trans-Atlantic Publications; 2009.

54. Richardson G. The metatheory of resilience and resiliency. *J Clin Psychol.* 2002;58(3):307–321.

55. Jacelon CS. The trait and process of resilience. *J Adv Nurs.* 1997; 25(1):123–129.

56. Walsh F. *Strengthening Family Resilience.* New York, NY: Guilford Publications; 2006.

57. Werner E. (1993). Risk, resilience, and recovery: perspectives from the Kauai longitudinal study. *Dev Psychopathol.* 1993;5(4):503–515.

58. Olver J, Ponsford J, Curran C. Outcome following traumatic brain injury: a comparison between 2 and 5 years after injury. *Brain Inj.* 1996;10(11):841–848.

59. Hodges T, Clifton D. Strengths-based development in practice. In: Linley PA, Joseph S, eds. *International Handbook of Positive Psychology in Practice: From Research to Application.* New York, NY: Wiley and Sons; In press.

60. Duncan B, Miller S, Wampold B, Hubble M. *The Heart and Soul of Change: Delivering What Works in Therapy.* 2nd ed. Washington, DC: American Psychological Association; 2009.

61. Madsen W. Problematic treatment: interaction of patient, spouse and physician beliefs in medical noncompliance. *Fam Syst Med.* 1992;10:365–383.

62. Myers J. Coping with caregiving stress: a wellness-oriented, strengths-based approach for family counselors. *The Fam J.* 2003; 11(2):153–161.

63. Serio CD, Kreutzer J, Witol A. Family needs after traumatic brain injury: a factor analytic study of the Family Needs Questionnaire. *Brain Inj.* 1997;11(1):1–10.

64. Kreutzer J, Taylor L. *Brain Injury Family Intervention: Implementation Manual.* Richmond, VA: The National Resource Center for Traumatic Brain Injury; 2004.

65. McGoldrick M, Gerson R, Petry S. *Genograms: Assessment and Intervention.* New York, NY: W.W. Norton & Company; 2008.

66. Jolly W, Froom J, Rosen M. The genogram. *J Fam Practice.* 1980; 10(2):251–255.

67. Minuchin S. *Families & Family Therapy.* Cambridge, MA: Harvard University Press; 1974.

68. Karney BR, Bradbury TN. The longitudinal course of marital quality and stability: a review of theory, methods, and research. *Psychol Bull.* 1995;118(1):3–34.

69. Spanier GB. Measuring dyadic adjustment: new scales for assessing the quality of marriage and similar dyads. *J Marriage Fam.* 1976; 38(1):15–30.

70. Budd KS, Heilman N, Stuart RB. Dyadic Adjustment Scale. In: *The Eighteenth Mental Measurements Yearbook* [Electronic Version]. Lin-

coln, NE: Buros Institute of Mental Measurement Yearbook Online database; 2010.

71. Peters LC, Stambrook M, Moore AD, Zubek E, Dubo H, Blumernschein S. Differential effects of spinal cord injury and head injury on marital adjustment. *Brain Inj.* 1992;6(5):461–467.

72. Charles N, Butera-Prinzi F, Perlesz A. Families living with acquired brain injury: a multiple family group experience. *NeuroRehabilitation.* 2007;22(1):61–76.

73. Olson D. FACES IV and the circumplex model: validation study. *J Marital Fam Ther.* 2011;37(1):64–80.

74. Perlesz A, Kinsella G, Crowe S. Impact of traumatic brain injury on the family: a critical review. *Rehabil Psychol.* 1999;44(1):6–35.

75. Epstein NB, Baldwin LM, Bishop DS. The McMaster family assessment device. *J Marital Fam Ther.* 1983;9:171–180.

76. Murray HM, Maslany GW, Jeffery B. Assessment of family needs following acquired brain injury in Saskatchewan. *Brain Inj.* 2006; 20(6):575–585.

77. Kreutzer J, Seel RT, Marwitz JH. *The Neurobehavioral Functioning Inventory.* San Antonio, TX: Psychological Corporation; 1999.

78. Kolakowsky-Hayner SA, Kreutzer JS, Miner KD. Validation of the Service Obstacles Scale for the traumatic brain injury population. *NeuroRehabilitation.* 2000;14(3):151–158.

79. Zarit SH, Reever KE, Bach-Peterson J. Relatives of the impaired elderly: correlates of feelings of burden. *The Gerontologist.* 1980; 20(6):649–655.

80. Kuhlenschmidt S, Wantz R, Barker BD. Memory and behavior problem checklist and the burden interview. In: *The Eighteenth Mental Measurements Yearbook* [Electronic Version]. Lincoln, NE: Buros Institute of Mental Measurement Yearbook Online database; 2010.

81. Kreutzer J, Kolakowsky-Hayner S. *Getting Better (and Better) After Brain Injury: A Guide for Families, Friends, and Caregivers.* Richmond, VA: The National Resource Center for Traumatic Brain Injury; 1999.

82. Kreutzer J, Godwin E. Healing your marriage after brain injury. *THE Challenge!* 2010;3:7–8.

83. Goering PN, Wasylenki DA, Farkas M, Lancee WJ, Ballantyne R. What difference does case management make? *Hosp Community Psychiatry.* 1988;39(3):272–276.

84. Kreutzer JS, Marwitz JH, Godwin EE, Arango-Lasprilla JC. Practical approaches to effective family intervention after brain injury. *J Head Trauma Rehabil.* 2010;25(2):113–120.

85. Carnevale G, Anselmi V, Busichio K, Millis S. Changes in ratings of caregiver burden following a community-based behavior man-

agement program for persons with traumatic brain injury. *J Head Trauma Rehabil.* 2002;17(2):83–95.

86. Sinnakaruppan I, Downey B, Morrison S. Head injury and family carers: a pilot study to investigate an innovative community-based educational programme for family carers and patients. *Brain Inj.* 2005;19(4):283–308.

87. Kreutzer JS, Stejskal TM, Ketchum JM, Marwitz JH, Taylor LA, Menzel JC. A preliminary investigation of the brain injury family intervention: impact on family members. *Brain Inj.* 2009;23(6): 535–547.

88. Acorn S. Assisting families of head-injured survivors through a family support programme. *J Adv Nurs.* 1995;21(5):872–877.

89. Brown R, Pain K, Berwald C, Hirschi P, Delehanty R, Miller H. Distant education and caregiver support groups: comparison of traditional and telephone groups. *J Head Trauma Rehabil.* 1999;14(3): 257–268.

90. Morris KC. Psychological distress in carers of head injured individuals: the provision of written information. *Brain Inj.* 2001;15(3): 239–254.

91. Albert S, Im A, Brenner L, Smith M, Waxman R. Effect of a social work liaison program on family caregivers to people with brain injury. *J Head Trauma Rehabil.* 2002;17(2):175–189.

92. Rivera PA, Elliott TR, Berry JW, Grant JS. Problem-solving training for family caregivers of persons with traumatic brain injuries: a randomized controlled trial. *Arch Phys Med Rehabil.* 2008;89(5): 931–941.

93. Ong LM, de Haes JC, Hoos AM, Lammes FB. Doctor-patient communication: a review of the literature. *Soc Sci Med.* 1995;40(7): 903–918.

94. Shirk S, Karver M. Prediction of treatment outcome from relationship variables in child and adolescent therapy: a meta-analytic review. *J Consult Clin Psychol.* 2003;71(3):452–464.

95. Waitzkin H. Medicine, superstructure and micropolitics. *Soc Sci Med Med Psychol Med Sociol.* 1979;13A(6):601–609.

96. Rogers C, Farson R. Active listening. In Newman R, Danziger M, Cohen M, eds. *Communication in Business Today.* Washington, DC: Heath and Company; 1987.

97. Geldard K, Geldard D. *Personal Counseling Skills: An Integrative Approach.* Springfield, IL: Charles C. Thomas Publisher Ltd.; 2008.

98. Eisendrath S. Reframing techniques in the general hospital. *Fam Syst Med.* 1986;4(1):91–95.

99. Herxheimer A. Communicating with patients about harms and risks. *PLoS Med.* 2005;2(2):e42.

Return to Work Following Traumatic Brain Injury

Michael D. West, Pamela S. Targett, Satoko Y. Crockatt, and Paul H. Wehman

INTRODUCTION

Vocational rehabilitation (VR) efforts in traumatic brain injury (TBI) have paralleled the increasing survival rate for those experiencing severe injury. Return to work (RTW) following TBI is increasingly viewed not only as worthwhile economically, but therapeutically as a means of cognitive and physical rehabilitation (1). Despite advances in critical care and rehabilitation methods, the research literature has consistently documented that RTW rates, particularly for those who sustain severe injuries, remain low (2–4).

In this chapter, we will focus not only on specific RTW issues, but also critical related factors such as career counseling in terms of work supports but community issues that affect employment. We begin with a review of the RTW literature, with emphasis on those who experience more significant TBI.

AN OVERVIEW OF THE RESEARCH ON RTW FOLLOWING TBI

Return to Work: Predictive Factors

TBI can result in variety cognitive deficits, impaired psychosocial functioning, and physical or sensory functioning (2–4). As a result, individuals with TBI often experience difficulty becoming competitively employed postinjury and maintaining employment for extended periods of time (5,6). RTW rates are highly variable across the literature; however, van Velzen and colleagues (4) conducted a systematic review of RTW studies and reported that on average, approximately 40% of individuals who sustain TBI have achieved RTW at both the 1- and 2-year milestones.

Shames and colleagues (7) recently conducted a review of the literature regarding predictive factors for successful RTW following TBI and current rehabilitation strategies for assisting them to achieve RTW. They note that prediction of RTW is a complex interaction of variables, including premorbid factors (i.e., age, education, employment history), injury-related factors (type, severity, location), postinjury impairments (cognitive, physical, behavioral, psychological), and personal and environment factors (marital status, alternative income sources, social support). Because of this complexity and the unique nature of each TBI patient, prediction of RTW for individual patient is not feasible. They note that the literature includes numerous examples of high-risk patients who did achieve successful RTW if given sufficient rehabilitation and support.

What are the RTW risk factors for individuals who sustain TBI? Research spanning several decades has generally found that the weight of evidence (there are studies with contradictory findings) indicates these factors are frequently found to contribute to poor employment outcomes:

- More severe injury (7–11), as measured by Glasgow Coma Scale scores, duration of coma or post-traumatic amnesia, duration of rehabilitation, or other means;
- Higher age at injury (5,7–9);
- Male (9,12);
- Lower levels of preinjury educational and/or occupational status (5,8,9,13–17);
- Less social support from friends, family, neighbors, church, and so forth. (14);
- Significant physical or psychosocial, or cognitive impairments (5,11,14,15,18);
- Minority group membership (9,16,19,20); and
- A history of substance abuse (11,21,22).

This list is far from exhaustive; many other factors have been studied. It illustrates the complex nature of RTW and the difficulty in applying a prediction model to individual cases. Moreover, synthesizing the research on RTW has long been complicated by differences across studies in such areas as defining what constitutes "work" (3,4). For example, studies have defined work to include full-time or part-time employment, sheltered work, engagement in education or training leading to employment, volunteerism, being a homemaker, and favorable ratings on employability scales. In addition, the research literature is international, which brings into consideration differences across economies, cultures, health care and rehabilitation systems, and national "landscapes" of disability and employment social and public policies.

Recent research in TBI RTW in the United States has been greatly enhanced by the funding of TBI Model Systems (TBIMS) beginning in 1987 by the U.S. Department of Education's National Institute on Disability and Rehabilitation Research (NIDRR). The 16 Model Systems projects contribute to a common longitudinal data system that tracks patients from emergency care, through postacute rehabilitation, to postinjury outcomes, including RTW. The TBIMS data system thus includes data on a large sample of TBI patients over an extended period of time from multiple locations, which may serve to reduce variability and bias. Perhaps equally important, each participating center uses common language and measures for assessing patients, treatments, and outcomes, including RTW.

Using the TBIMS data system, Arango-Lasprilla and colleagues (19) explored racial differences in RTW outcomes for 5,259 TBI patients, 34% of whom were minority group members, 1 year postinjury. After adjusting for other demographic, socioeconomic, and injury-related variables, they found that minority members were 2.17 times more likely to be unemployed at follow-up than were white patients. However, they did not find differences in occupational status of those who were employed. These findings were consistent with a TBIMS study by Sherer et al. (18) using a smaller sample, which found that whites were twice as likely to be employed as minority members.

Gary and colleagues (23), again using the TBIMS data system, examined employment outcomes for a smaller number of individuals (n = 2022, 30% minority) at 1, 2, and 5 years postinjury, and again with TBIMS cases who were 10 years postinjury (24). They found that minority members were significantly less likely to be employed at each of these milestones.

An area of great interest in TBI rehabilitation and RTW is substance abuse. Alcohol and drugs are often factors in automobile accidents leading to head injuries, and such problems can continue after the injury (22). Corrigan (22) estimated that up to two-thirds of rehabilitation patients had substance abuse problems which confound attempts at rehabilitation and RTW. Bogner and colleagues (21) found that substance abuse was a predictor of poor postinjury outcomes, including productivity, as did Jorge and colleagues (25).

Since the late 1970s and early 1980s, research has been devoted to identification of biomarkers, that is, objective, biological substances, or characteristics, for TBI. In recent years, however, there has been a focus on identifying biomarkers that are predictive of RTW and other outcomes following TBI. Berger (26) presented a review of the literature in this area and found that the most investigated biomarker related to post-TBI outcomes is Protein S100B, which has long been established as a serum marker for primary and secondary brain damage and stroke. Several studies (but not all) have found that elevated levels of S100B predict poor outcomes in terms of disability, cognitive functioning, and life satisfaction, but its predictive value for RTW has not been widely investigated.

In one such study, Stranjalis and colleagues (27), treating mild TBI patients at a hospital in Athens, Greece, examined levels of S100B within 3 hours of emergency room admission. They found that elevated levels of S100B were correlated with failure to return to work within a week. The RTW rate was 37.5% for those with normal levels, and 4.9% for those with elevated levels.

As noted by Berger (26) and others, S100B and other biomarkers have the potential to provide information that supplements clinical evidence in determining the extent and likely effects of the injury. This information will be useful in patient and family counseling, making clinical decisions, and providing appropriate levels of rehabilitation support.

Much of the prior research has focused on the symptoms and conditions of the individuals that influence retuning to work. It is becoming increasingly imperative to examine RTW after TBI as an interaction between the needs and motivations of the individuals with TBI and the supports available within vocational, social, and economic environments (8,28). Factors that lead to successful RTW included socially inclusive work environments, availability of health insurance, level of social interaction on the job, jobs with greater decision-making latitude, and environmental modifications and focusing on vocational strengths of the individual, in short, jobs that are worth getting and keeping.

It is important to realize that there are other influences on RTW that are often underestimated. Foremost among these is likely to be financial disincentives to RTW. In the United States and in many other countries, individuals with disabilities who are unemployed receive some type of public support. In other cases, the victim of a TBI may be pursuing a financial settlement. There is some evidence that individuals with TBI will intentionally forego RTW while awaiting or receiving disability benefits or settlements because they believe that working will negatively affect the financial well-being of themselves and their families (18).

In addition, a challenge that is common to many individuals across the range of disabilities is obtaining reliable and affordable transportation to and from work. This may be caused by physical problems (i.e., vision, movement, etc.) that may preclude driving, lack of public transportation or paratransit services, or economic limitations that come with long-term unemployment and high medical costs. Accommodations or alternative work arrangements, such as allowing the individual to telework from home, might be used to mitigate this barrier.

CAREER DEVELOPMENT OF PERSONS WITH TBI

Because of the myriad of cognitive, physical, and psychological problems that may result from TBI, and particularly severe TBI, many individuals who were employed at the time of the injury will be unable to return to their preinjury occupation (13). For these individuals, and for those who had little or no work experience preinjury, assistance may be needed to help the individual better learn or relearn their employment strengths and interests. This section will describe strategies to assist them through this experience.

Career Interest Assessment

Career assessment interventions are important tools that allow people with or without disabilities to take control of their career planning. The 1992 Amendments to the Rehabilitation Act emphasize consumer involvement in the rehabilitation process, including vocational assessment; self-rating instruments, and interviews appear to provide the individual with the disability with more involvement over the assessment process. In this section, we will review several types of career awareness assessments that would be applicable for people with TBI. Table 81-1 lists features of several career interest inventories available in paper format or on the internet.

Many career assessment tools are available on the Internet. One of the most popular career interest inventories is the Self-Directed Search (29) designed by John Holland. There are three versions: one for adults, one for college students, and one for secondary school students and adults with limited reading skills. It is based on Holland's theory that there are 6 basic personality types: creative, realistic, investigative, artistic, social, and enterprising. The theory assumes

TABLE 81-1 Details of Selected Career Interest Inventories

INTEREST INVENTORY	CHARACTERISTICS
Self-directed search	• Versions for secondary students, postsecondary students, and adults with limited reading abilities • Web access: www.self-directed-search.com • $4.95 per test • Purpose is to match career to personality type (Creative, Realistic, Investigative, Artistic, Social, and Enterprising)
Strong interest inventory	• Family of products designed for career counselors and educators • Some products require precertification • Paper products available at https://www.cpp.com (forms $8.95 ea., manual $89.50) • Online version available at www.discoveryourpersonality.com/Strong.html ($80)
DISCOVER	• Available from www.act.org/discover/ • Licensed to individuals or institutions • Individual 3-month license $19.95, 6-month $24.95
SIGI PLUS	• Career planning software • Licensed to educational or vocational institutions only • Information available at www.ets.org/sigi
Reading Free Vocational Interest Inventory	• Available from www.proedinc.com • $110 • Interest in 11 career areas • Select preferred activity from 55 sets of 3 pictures • 20 min
Yes! Your Employment Selections	• Reading free, video-based job preference program • Designed for individuals with disabilities • Videos for 120 jobs • Available on CD ($395) or web ($20 per person for 3 months) • www.yesjobsearch.com
Job Quest	• www.abledata.com • $199 • Specifically designed for individuals with cognitive disabilities • Watch videos, select preferred activity

that there are 6 corresponding work environments and that individuals will find "person-environment fit" in work environments that most closely match their personality (29).

The Strong Interest Inventory (30) may also be useful in assessing career interests of individuals from middle school through adulthood. The instrument reports a score for the 6 areas of interest described by John Holland, as well as 23 basic interest scales and 207 occupational scales. The Myers-Briggs Type Indicator (31) provides information on personality type and will give added perspective to self-exploration exercises.

Another popular career counseling strategy involves using computer-assisted systems. These systems are able to handle vast quantities of information and assist with integration of information. Many computer-assisted career guidance systems are available, such as SIGI PLUS (32) and DISCOVER (33). These interventions provide individuals

with current, accurate, locally relevant occupational, and educational information. DISCOVER is a computer program that assists people with self-assessment and provides information related to making career decisions. SIGI PLUS is similar; however, it does not provide information on postsecondary education.

Some persons with TBI may be able to use these tools without assistance, whereas others may need help with reading, writing and interpreting the results. Three of the assessments listed in Table 81-1 are reading free; users select favored career features from photos or videos. In addition to learning more about vocational interests and aptitudes, the opportunity to work through a career search exercise with a person with a TBI can also provide valuable information about current physical, cognitive, and social skills.

Several career planning books are available to assist persons with identifying their skills and abilities. For example, Melanie Witt's book *Job Strategies for People With Disabilities* (34) contains a wide range of self-assessment tools to help a person define their career direction. Another career-planning book, *Coming Alive From Nine to Five* by Betty Michelozzi (35) provides several self-assessment exercises that may be useful to person seeking a first job or switching career tracks. Again, some job seekers with TBI may require assistance with completing the assessments, as well as interpreting the results for useful career search information.

Experiential Assessment

Traditional evaluation practices that use aptitude batteries, work samples, and behavioral inventories have long been used in vocational evaluations of persons with disabilities. Since many persons with TBI or other severe disabilities enter the evaluation process with limited marketable skills, they are likely to be excluded from work. Instead, they may be told that they need a longer recovery period prior to seeking work or that they are not likely to ever work again. In the worst case scenario, they are advised to enter programs to "get ready" to work, offered preemployment training for menial jobs, or sent to nonwork day activity centers.

Traditional vocational evaluations occur in artificial and simulated environments, which are not reliable or valid indicators of what someone can do in the real world. There are several limitations in traditional approaches to vocational evaluation for persons with significant disabilities. A more fair and reliable way to assess a person's abilities is within the context of real work environments. And furthermore, they believe that the focus of a vocational assessment should be on interests, abilities, supports available, and supports needed to succeed at work.

Work experience and similar interventions like volunteering or job shadowing may be useful for some people with TBI. If an individual has very limited experiences from which to make an informed career decisions, a work experience may help the person choose a career direction (36). Volunteering in various work settings may give some individuals with TBI ideas on abilities, preferences, and support needs. Job shadowing (37) can also serve this purpose. This strategy typically involves observing or "shadowing" a person who is performing a job to obtain first-hand knowledge of what tasks the occupation entails. Some persons with TBI will need assistance with setting up and participating in either type of activity.

Closely related to job shadowing is situational assessment (38). The purpose is the same; but in the situational assessment, the individual with TBI is actively engaged in the work being performed. A VR specialist can assist an individual with contacting employers and making the necessary arrangements. Whereas the individual is engaged in work, the rehabilitation specialists makes systematic observations of (a) learning style; (b) performance, quality, consistency, and stamina; (c) skills that the individual is revealing that may be transferable to other occupations; (d) the individual's training needs for both hard and soft work skills and potential for success in that career; (e) any accommodations that may be needed; and (f) other occupational options that might better fit the individual's skills and needs.

This information can be very valuable in the future when the person is actively trying to determine an initial direction for the job search or making decisions about whether or not to accept a job offer. Please note that neither job shadowing nor situational assessment should be viewed as a prerequisite to going to work; they are time-limited career exploration activities that may be beneficial to individuals who have no employment history or who, because of their impairments, will need to explore other careers.

Home Visit

Whenever a VR specialist is involved with assisting a person with a TBI with locating work, a home visit can provide important vocational assessment and career search information. During the home visit, the individual with TBI is asked to share details on current abilities, work interests, and values. The individual is also observed performing various tasks in their home environment, which demonstrates current physical, cognitive, and social skills. In addition, casual conversations about activities of daily living, tasks completed around the house, and leisure pursuits can also lead to some ideas on vocational abilities and interests (39).

Career Information Interviews

Career information interviews (39) provide a valuable means for learning more about an occupation or industry. It involves setting up an appointment with someone in a particular field and interviewing the person to learn more about a specific occupation or industry. Some people with TBI may need assistance with setting up and conducting the interview. In such cases, a vocational specialist assists the person with determining the businesses to contact, making the contacts, coordinating interviews, formulating questions to ask, and actually conducting the interview. The individual with a TBI is encouraged to participate in each activity as much as possible. The vocational specialist should assist as needed and if present at the interview should take notes, as well as make observations of the individual's demeanor, social strengths and weaknesses, and personality. This type of exploratory interview offers the jobseeker information on minimal qualifications, education, or training needed, for certain types of work. Information on how a particular career choice might impact future earnings and quality of life can also be gleaned from an informational interview (39).

Accommodation and Support Needs

People with TBI who are returning to work may need to perform their job in a different way or require modified workstations, compensatory strategies, or other accommodations or supports (40). In this approach, a VR specialist works closely with both the employer and employee to assess the person's vocational abilities by taking data on some specific vocational skill and if warranted, recommend support strategies.

Once the person receives a release for RTW, the VR specialist (with the employer's permission) accompanies the employee with TBI back to work and makes observations on the person's ability to perform the essential job functions. This criterion-referenced assessment measures the individuals' ability to do a specified task by collecting data on the steps of that task. Depending on the nature and complexity of the job, other jobsite personnel may need to be involved in planning and implementing the assessment. If difficulties arise, the specialist makes recommendations on ways to remove barriers and enhance independent performance.

For example, the returning employee and employer may need assistance with identifying and implementing accommodations like compensatory memory strategies. The RTW assessment is not used to determine whether or not someone can return to work but instead can provide ideas on types of possible accommodations and supports needed to enhance successful RTW.

Residual Skills Assessment

Although some individuals who have sustained TBI may have work to which they can return to, others may not, but may have a keen interest in pursuing an employment opportunity that requires the use of his/her specialized skills, training, or educational background. To make an informed decision about whether or not to return to this type of occupation, the individual may need information on his or her current skills, abilities, and possible accommodations. A customized vocational assessment specifically designed to explore current level of functioning in a previous line of work and support needs may prove useful and instill the confidence the person needs to return to this type of work. Sometimes, the assessment may also relate to using one's educational background in the workplace and might help someone determine whether or not to pursue a career in a specific field.

Depending on the nature and complexity of the occupation in question, a consultant who is actively engaged in such work may be needed to assist with designing and implementing the assessment. The consultant should be someone who could be considered an expert in the field or area that is under exploration. The vocational specialist usually takes responsibility for locating and securing the consultant's service, coordinating the effort, assisting with the assessment design and tools, and writing a report. The specialist may also actively participate in the assessment process by making observations and collecting data on the individual's abilities and support needs.

STRATEGIES TO GAIN EMPLOYMENT

Career development and planning are necessary first steps toward going to work, and once a vocational direction has been established, the job search should begin. As the search unfolds, the direction should be modified based on any new information that surfaces during this process. This section will review some of the issues that impact the job search and suggest strategies that may be useful when assisting persons with TBI with going to work.

Disclosing Disability and Requesting Accommodations

In the United States, individuals with disabilities are protected from employment discrimination under the American's with Disabilities Act of 1990 (ADA). Similar legislation is in effect in the United Kingdom, Australia, India, Canada, and many other nations. These laws protect qualified applicants or employees with disabilities. However, an individual is only covered if he or she voluntarily discloses the disability to the employer. If an applicant or employee does not disclose the disability, then he or she is not entitled to protections. For individuals with hidden disabilities, this creates a conflict. He or she disclose their disability, and if so, when? Prior to the interview? After he or she is hired?

It is unfortunate that discrimination against individuals with disabilities continues to exist, but it does. In a study by Pearson and her colleagues (41) in Hong Kong, applications were sent in response to newspaper advertisements for open positions. Four applications with identical qualifications were sent for each position, with three disclosing a particular type of disability and the fourth not disclosing a disability. Positive responses, that is, offers to interview the applicants, were obtained for the nondisabled applications at more than twice the rate for the applications disclosing a disability.

It typically is the responsibility of the job applicant to best present his or her abilities to employers, and some people with TBI may have a difficult time doing so. Some individuals will not be able to explain to employers how their particular skills and abilities match the qualifications for the job. If the person is in need of an accommodation, he or she may experience difficulties explaining to the employer what is needed to allow him or her to succeed. Some persons with TBI may need to convince an employer to redesign task, location, or restructure a job that was originally designed with individuals without disabilities in mind. This may present difficulties for the applicant with a TBI if he or she has a myriad of cognitive difficulties and is unsure of what he or she may need to succeed on the job.

Sometimes, employers may not see a "new or different" way to get a task done or may see the request for change as bothersome. Instead, the company representative may simply choose to hire someone else who does not require any accommodation. On the other hand, many employers may be willing to hire individuals with TBI but may need support to determine how best to make reasonable accommodation. VR specialists can be a valuable resource for employers.

VR usually offers a range of job search and placement services, from the least to most intrusive approach. The approach selected generally depends on the individual's abilities and support needs. We will review a couple of these approaches and then focus in on what the author's view as the most favorable strategy for assisting persons with severe TBI with gaining employment; a customized and tailored approach to this process.

Minimal Intervention

The first approach generally involves a minimum amount of intervention from a VR specialist. For example, the jobseeker may simply need information on the labor market, insights concerning their interviewing skills, or leads on employment opportunities. Or perhaps the person simply needs information on adaptive aids or effective compensatory strategies. These individuals often know what they want but need specific information to put their plan into action. They may have pervious work history and have a good work ethic. These individuals are usually able to read, write, and can follow through on complex directives without assistance. They take the information given to them, generalize it, and apply it to their lives. Their need for vocational assistance is often minimal. Unfortunately, VR professionals, who are unfamiliar with TBI, may feel that a person with an injury is much more capable than he or she truly is and may only offer minimal job search and placement assistance. Afterwards, in instances where the person does not follow through on specific directives, this may be perceived by the VR provider as a lack of motivation to work on the part of the individual with TBI and in some instances may lead to termination of services.

Education and Preparation Approach

The second vocational placement approach is for those individuals who appear to need some type of intervention, but not an extensive intervention. Usually, these individuals do not assimilate information quickly and require assistance with carrying out a job search, but once employed may need no or limited assistance on the job. Often times, these individuals participate in classes designed to get ready or prepared for conducting either an independent job search or a job search with some limited assistance from a job placement specialist. This approach is usually not very effective for persons with significant TBI because most of the training takes place in a classroom type setting. Usually, classes are conducted to teach job seeking and maintenance skills. For instance, students learn about various occupations and how to analyze themselves and the job market to choose an appropriate career path or receive information on how to complete employment applications or learn how to interview for a job.

Sometimes, particularly for persons with severe TBI, an inordinate amount of time is spent trying to get the person ready to conduct a job search, when in reality it is highly unlikely that the learning that takes place in the classroom will ever generalize into the real world. Instead, the authors feel that time could be better expended by providing individualized job placement assistance that is tailored to each jobseekers' specific needs and abilities.

Advocacy Level Services

This approach can be helpful to anyone with a disability but is particularly useful for people with more severe disabilities such as severe TBI. Using this strategy, the type and intensity of services and supports are adapted to each individual's needs and under some circumstances involve extensive intervention. Generally, individuals with significant cognitive impairments need more assistance with obtaining employment than those who have moderate physical or sensory disabilities. These individuals tend to learn best in the milieu where they will be expected to perform instead of learning away from that environment. Generally, they need one-to-one assistance with identifying their vocational strengths, support needs, and conducting a job search. Once employed, they may need assistance on the job. One vocational service option that offers individualized and intensive support services for both gaining and maintaining employment is Supported Employment. A person does not have to get ready to work; instead, a vocational support person—sometimes called a job coach—provides assistance with helping the person identify his or her abilities and support needs, contacts employers to learn about business needs and as applicable represents the jobseeker and their support services, provides on the job site support to the new hire and ongoing long term support throughout employment.

WORKPLACE SUPPORTS

Individuals with TBI who are attempting to return to work will need supports that are customized to meet their individual needs at a specific workplace. The type, level, and intensity of support will vary depending on the person's abilities and the particular circumstances on hand. Some individuals with TBI may simply need information and guidance on how to conduct a job search or ways to compensate for memory deficits on the job, whereas others, particularly those with severe disabilities will need more intensive intervention and one-to-one assistance. Furthermore, the type, level, and intensity of support someone will need does not remain static, but changes over time. For example, after learning how to do a job task, the individual may need additional instruction when new duties are introduced. Individuals with TBI may benefit from a combination of workplace supports. Some examples follow. For example, someone who has a job to return to will not need assistance with locating a new occupation; however, once back to work, he or she may need assistance with learning how to get organized and manage their workload.

Accommodations

Because TBI may result in an array of physical, cognitive, and psychosocial problems, accommodation needs will need to be tailored to each individual's needs. Some will benefit from accessible building, particularly if the person has difficulty walking or uses a wheelchair for mobility. For example, a wheelchair lift was installed outside of the entrance of an inaccessible older historical building that allowed the employee who uses a wheelchair access. Those who have changes in vision postinjury may also benefit from access supports. For example, raised letter directional signs may be posted in a building to help an employee identify restrooms or elevator controls.

A modified work schedule that allows an employee to get to work on time may also be necessary. For example, a person may be allowed to work from 10 AM to 6 PM rather than from 9 AM to 5 PM because of limitations on the availability of transportation to and from work. In other instances, a person may need part-time work because of changes in stamina level or fatigue. Other people with TBI may be able to work full-time, but may need to have an opportunity to take additional scheduled breaks throughout the workday.

Job restructuring is another important accommodation. This involves having a nonessential (not major) work function or a marginal duty removed from an employee's job description or a difficult task that the employee cannot do is exchanged for one that can be done. For example, a general worker at a retail store is not able to climb ladders to change the light bulbs. Management agrees to allow another employee to do this, and in exchange, the worker is responsible for checking the parking lot and returning customer carts to the building.

Sometimes, particularly if the person has a physical disability or slowed movements postinjury, it will be useful to purchase assistive equipment or devices to improve their ability to get the job done. More often, existing items in the workplace may be modified or added on to accommodate the person. Assistive technology ranges from high tech to no tech and from costly to no cost. Fortunately, most auxiliary aids are not expensive.

For some individuals, a change in where their work is performed may be helpful. This may simply involve allowing the employee to move to a different workstation or in some instances and if applicable, allow telecommuting or working from home.

Some individuals with TBI may need support services. Examples of support services may include assisting the person with carrying out activities of daily living like eating or going to the restroom, having a "buddy" assigned to alert the worker to an emergency situation, or helping the individual take notes during an employee training or staff meeting.

Perhaps, one of the most useful accommodations for workers with a TBI is internal or external compensatory strategies. Internal strategies require the use of a mental support system and do not rely on external devices. Examples include making associations or drawings on analogies to remember how to do a task or using word mnemonics to remember a specific sequence. External strategies involve the use of objects like checklists or flowcharts to remember a sequence of steps to follow to complete a work activity. These strategies can serve multiple purposes. They not only promote learning, but can also serve as a reminder of what needs to be done and helps keep the worker organized so the job can be completed in a proper and timely manner.

Technology is advancing exponentially, with each day bringing new advances, products, and uses. Many products have been developed specifically for youth and adults with disabilities, but even those designed for the public at large can be used by individuals with TBI who require compensatory strategies. As examples, Depompei et al. (42) and Gentry et al. (43) describe practical applications of use of personal digital assistants (PDAs), smartphones, and other digital devices for students and adults with TBI that compensate for deficits in memory, concentration, and attention. Among those uses are

- personal calendars with alarms for reminders of important events, meetings, and so forth;
- contact lists with automatic dialing for reaching peers, family members, employers, and so forth;
- handy tools such as a calculator, clock, compass, and so forth;
- cameras for assigning a face with contacts to aid in recognition;
- games that can improve the student's memory, concentration, fine motor coordination, spatial relationships, and visual-perceptual skills; and

TABLE 81-2 Examples of Workplace Supports

POSITION TITLE	JOB-RELATED FUNCTIONAL LIMITATION	PRESENTING ISSUE	WORKPLACE SUPPORT
Receptionist at small business	No use of arms or hands, unable to walk	Taking messages on the telephone	Tape records voice messages then uses voice activated software to type messages
Garment bagger at dry cleaners	Unsteady gait, loss of balance while walking or standing; becomes tired easily	Pulling bags over cleaned garments from a standing position; maintaining stamina	Fabricated metal stand to maintain balance while standing; has flip down seat to rest on when tired
Inventory clerk/order puller for retail store	Becomes frustrated when interrupted and yells at others	Appears angry when new coworkers ask for instructions on how to do the job	Created oversized document to refer new employee's questions
File clerk at insurance company	Becomes defensive or denies having any difficulty when given personal feedback	Appears angry when given constructive feedback on job performance	Uses self-monitoring tool and discuss ways to improve performance
Cashier for fast food company	Socializing with strangers in an inappropriate manner	Asked customers for their telephone numbers	Posted reminder "Don't creep me out" with picture of unhappy looking female on the phone
Activities assistant at nursing home	Remembering sequence of things to be done throughout the day to complete normal routine	Could not remember what order to complete various job duties	Organized master schedule of various duties to complete on certain days and a list of things to do once duties are done
Plant installer at green house or plant retail store	Remembering how to complete a certain task	Could not remember how to clean and care for various types of plants	Created manual with instructions and cross referenced by plant typical and phylum name
Houseman at hotel	Remembering what to do outside of normal routine	Could not remember what tasks to do outside of normal work routine	Manager on duty writes daily list of things to do in order of occurrence

- a global positioning system (GPS) that can assist with wayfinding in the community.

Of course, one of the benefits of these devices is that they are ubiquitous—just about everyone has one—and they are relatively inexpensive compared to products developed exclusively for individuals with disabilities. Thus, they are far less likely to stigmatize the individual with TBI and are much more financially practical.

It is important to remember that all workplace supports and adaptive solutions that are used to compensate for functional limitations are highly individualized. In addition, the solution to the presenting problem will be highly dependent on the user's willingness to use a strategy, as well as the type of job tasks involved, the work environment, and the employers' consent to allow the use of the accommodation. Although these examples were presented in isolation, it is often the unique interplay and right combination of supports that will lead to success at work.

Table 81-2 subsequently provides some examples of the types of workplace strategies used by employees with TBI who used a Supported Employment approach to assist them with going to work postinjury.

Sometimes there are existing cues in the workplace that the new employee can learn to attend to that will promote successful job performance. Consider the following examples: A landscaper who is required to mow the lawn in a large office complex is given a diagram on a daily basis that illustrates what areas are to be cut that day; A patient transporter works in a hospital that has different colored signage

that helps him find his way to the correct destination; A medical supply order puller receives a printout indicating where in the warehouse the items needed are located.

In other instances, the necessary support will be simple ergonomic modifications to the workstation or a change in the way the work is performed. This might include adapting the layout of a workstation so that the task can be better sequenced, raising a worktable to accommodate a wheelchair or customized seat, or using jigs or adaptations to mitigate the employees limitations in vision, dexterity, judgment, and so forth.

Supported Employment

Most individuals with severe TBI will need assistance with locating work, as well as assistance learning how to perform the job. One approach that has successfully been used to assist people with TBI with going to work is supported employment (1,8). Using this approach, a VR specialist known as an "employment specialist" or "job coach" provides one-to-one individualized assistance to assist a person with a severe disability with finding a job, and once employed provides or facilitates the supports needed to help the person succeed at work. The type, level, and intensity of support varies depending on the newly hired employee's abilities, the job, the work environment, and existing supports in the workplace. Table 81-3 provides a brief overview of the role of the employment specialist, the person with a TBI, and other RTW process team members.

If a person is likely to return to his or her preinjury position, it is important that some member of the team or family member act as a liaison with the employer to keep them abreast of the individual's progress in rehabilitation. In some instances, the person may not be able to return to the same job, but there may be some other type of work within the organization. Some people may be able to begin to RTW while involved in day rehabilitation on a part-time basis. Some people will not have a job to return to or were unemployed at the time of injury. These individuals will need to seek new employment.

Again, the composition of the team will vary depending on several factors. For instance, if the person is involved in or has recently completed outpatient rehabilitation, the team is likely to be made up of the individual with a TBI, a physiatrist, an occupational therapist, a physical therapist, a neuropsychologist, a social worker, the parents or significant others, a state VR counselor, and if supported employment is being used, an employment specialist or job coach.

Over the years, businesses have become more confident in their ability to manage a diverse workforce and more cognizant of the abilities of workers with disabilities. Also, with the passage of the ADA, larger companies are more open to making reasonable accommodations in the workplace. Thus, individuals who lack access to Supported Employment may still be able to achieve success at work by simply working with the preinjury employer or by seeking out flexible and accommodating employers.

The importance of RTW after injury is being recognized, and these rehabilitation programs also offer similar types of vocational assistance such as work trials, training at workshops, or work training organized on the open job market. However, some programs limit the provision of VR to those who are eligible in terms of capabilities.

Other Promising Practices

The Virginia Department of Rehabilitative Services (DRS) funds 6 clubhouses for individuals with TBI across the state. The service model is loosely based on the clubhouse or Fountain House model that has long been a centerpiece of services for individuals with persistent mental illness (44). Clubhouses offer prevocational counseling and training, peer support, and social engagement. DRS added an additional component, the Vocational Transition Program (VTP), consisting of a 20-session standardized training program designed to build participants' knowledge and skills to enable them to enter the labor market.

Neimeier and colleagues (45) conducted a randomized clinical trial of the VTP program with 71 clubhouse members assigned to either the VTP (n = 39) or to a control group (n = 32). The treatment group was more likely to be competitively

TABLE 81-3 Overview of Supported Employment Services and Roles of Interdisciplinary Team Members

EMPLOYMENT SPECIALIST	INDIVIDUAL WITH TBI	OTHER TEAM MEMBER ROLES
Supported Employment Activity: Getting to know one another and establishing a direction for the job search		
• Conducts functional community-based activities to get to know the jobseeker and observe current skills, abilities, and potential support needs • Interviews those who know the person best to determine the above • Identifies jobseekers personal support network • Discusses impact of earnings on benefits • Discusses disclosure issues • Provides feedback to others (i.e. family, team, and funding source)	• Becomes familiar with service option • Gets to know the job coach • Participates in activities to learn more about self and job market • Expresses needs and wants related to employment • Decide who will disclose disability to potential employers	• Makes referral and introductions to Supported Employment • Advocates for Supported Employment services with funding source if needed • Shares information, current records, and insight on a person's abilities and support needs • If returning to preinjury job is liaison between employer and SE provider • Provides insight on family dynamics • Develops questions for neuropsychological evaluation and or assessment.
Supported Employment Activity: Conducting the job search, applying for jobs and interviewing		
• Locates work opportunities by tapping in to the hidden or unadvertised job market • Meets with employers to describe SE services and job seeker's desires and abilities • Analyzes workplace and job to determine pros and cons that may impact success at work and long-term job retention • Discusses above with job seeker • Practices interviewing skills • Arranges interviews • Helps negotiate accommodations • Provides feedback to others (i.e. family, team, and funding source) • Uses personal network and other resources to identify businesses to contact	• Decides whether or not to learn more about a work opportunity • Completes applications for employment • Attends job interviews • Decides whether or not to accept job offer	• Shares ideas on employers to contact • Provides ideas on types of tasks or jobs that may maximize use of personal strengths • Reviews job descriptions • Provide release for work if needed • Makes suggestions on types of accommodations or strategies that may prove useful

(Continued)

TABLE 81-3 Overview of Supported Employment Services and Roles of Interdisciplinary Team Members *(Continued)*

EMPLOYMENT SPECIALIST	INDIVIDUAL WITH TBI	OTHER TEAM MEMBER ROLES
Supported Employment Activity: Providing on the job site training and support • Supports the new hire during the employer's new employee orientation and training • Provides additional on the job skills training after the employer's training • Often helps ensure the work gets done while the new hire is learning how to do the job • Facilitates relationships with others on the job • Collects data to measure skill acquisition and productivity in order to measure the effectiveness of skills training • Designs and implements a process to fade presence from the job as the new hire shows proficiency in meeting the employer's performance standards.	• Asks for assistance if needed • Expresses job satisfaction • Helps problem solve • Helps develop compensatory strategies • Helps measure work performance • Expresses satisfaction with on the job support services and helps determine when job coach should fade assistance	• Helps problem solve • Helps problem solve issues related to performance problems on the job • Helps problem solve issues impacting job retention

Supported Employment Activity:

Providing long term support and case management services

- Stays in touch with employer and employee to assist with any additional training needs or help resolve difficulties in the workplace
- Collects data on performance levels
- Provides additional services as indicated
- Assists with problem solving issues outside of work that if left unaddressed could adversely effect work
- Makes referrals to other resources
- Identifying problems outside of work that are effecting performance
- Helps problem solve
- Provides resources
- Makes referrals to other resources

---

employed following completion of the program, but this finding was moderated by whether the member received disability income. In addition, participants overall thought the program were valuable and enjoyable to them.

A second promising practice in TBI RTW is the use of Resource Facilitator (RF), also referred to as brain injury information and referral, early referral, brain injury resource facilitation, service coordination, and case management (46). The first statewide RF program was established in 2003. RF is based on person-centered planning in which the individual with TBI and his or her family work collaboratively with the RF to identify personal goals and resource needs.

Trexler and colleagues (46) conducted a randomized controlled trial with 22 individuals with TBI. The dependent measures were participation and RTW as measured by the Participation Index of the Mayo-Portland Adaptability Index. There were no differences in Index scores or employment rates pretreatment. Following the treatment period, members of the treatment group had significantly higher ratings on the Participation Index items and also had higher posttreatment employment rates (64% compared to 36%). Although this was a small sample study and had associated limitations, it does suggest that the use of an improve RTW outcomes for individuals with TBI.

IMPROVING FUTURE OUTCOME THROUGH A TEAM APPROACH

TBI results in disability that requires comprehensive and often lengthy rehabilitation efforts. It is expensive from the standpoint of rehabilitation costs, lost earnings, and therefore, loss to the gross national product, but moreover, costly because of human suffering. Although health care and VR professionals are continually challenged in their efforts to return individuals with TBI to work, the likelihood of successful VR for persons with TBI can be enhanced by utilizing a team approach (55). Key members of the RTW team include the person with TBI; significant others; the employer; neuropsychologist; occupational, speech, and physical therapists; social worker; and VR counselor or specialist often under the leadership and direction of a physiatrist. Through interdisciplinary collaboration, the team can communicate frequently and set mutual treatment goals for recovery.

The task before the team is to maximize the potential of the individual with brain injury to return to as high a level of preinjury productivity as can be achieved. Further efforts related to RTW might focus on establishing new and different life goals and activities. The overall goal of rehabilitation, therefore, involves an enormous effort on the part of both the survivor and rehabilitation team.

Because there is no typical length of TBI rehabilitation, there is often a long and arduous process of treatment and therapies that assist the person with returning to preinjury lifestyles, including work. Much depends on the severity level of the TBI, the nature and extent of problems, availability of social support networks, accessible and available appropriate rehabilitation, and the circumstances surrounding reemployment and the current labor market. Fewer individuals return to work at the same level, for the same pay, and at the same number of hours per week as before the injury.

Some return to a similar job at a full- to part-time level, with a reduced rate of pay, others do not pursue competitive employment. Psychosocial outcomes encompass a similar range, from those being able to resume a familiar social and family life to those who become divorced, separated, or experienced shrinking social networks.

In the best case scenario, a psychiatrist will be integrally involved in and oversee the team efforts to assist the person with the returning to work (47). Once employed, the physiatrist and other team members continue to assist with either an advisory role or on an as needed basis.

As mentioned earlier, a neuropsychological evaluation is often used to assist in planning for employment or reemployment. A sound evaluation can provide valuable data to use when determining occupations or work settings that may be more suitable for the person with TBI to consider. The results of a good evaluation can help the person with TBI and team determine the best fit between cognitive assets and deficits, behavioral functioning, interpersonal propensities, overlearned skills or old learning ability, with specific job tasks and work environment for the person with TBI. The results can generate probability statements about the type of job, sort of tasks that may be most appropriate, as well as the types of environmental factors, and supports that may promote the person's success at work. However, the relationship between neuropsychological test scores and the demands of daily life can be weak. These is why the evaluation should include more than just testing, but also involve gathering other relevant historical, medical, psychosocial, and vocational information from the person, significant other, and team members.

The RTW team can make suggestions on what specific information needs to be obtained from the neuropsychological evaluation and provide other relevant information. For example, inquiring about the personal assets can often be more helpful than dwelling on what the person is unable to do, particularly when planning for an RTW. Also, whenever deficits are mentioned, asking what areas are amenable to remediation and to what extent training or supports can contribute to change is critical. For example, the neuropsychologist may be able to state functions that are expected to improve because of spontaneous recovery or can be assisted by compensatory strategies or other means like job restructuring or environmental modifications.

A TBI interferes with a person's identity and social roles. The results of the injury and particularly the inability to work often disrupt a person's sense of purpose, productivity, and self-worth. Therefore, counseling may prove beneficial and help a person with reestablishing a satisfactory level of self-sufficiency. Also, after returning to work, the individual may experience depression or increased frustration at not being able to do things as easy as preinjury levels. Furthermore, not being accepted by peers or rejection from coworkers can lead to problems. In some instances counseling may be warranted, in others medication may be helpful. The psychiatrist can recommend interventions to assist here. As illustrated, the role of the team, under the direction of a physiatrist, cannot be over emphasized (62). Unfortunately, in some instances, a physiatrist may not be accessible. In such an instance, a competent general medical practitioner, who is willing to consult with a physiatrist, can lead the team.

KEY CLINICAL POINTS

1. Because of the complexities of cognitive, physical, behavioral, and emotional impairments that can be caused by TBI, and the unique nature of each individual, prediction of RTW with individual patients is impossible.
2. Traditional vocational evaluation may underestimate the employment potential of individuals with severe TBI. Experiential assessments may better indicate residual work skills, interests, and aptitudes.
3. Career interest inventories can be useful in helping individuals with TBI identify the types of jobs that they would be interested in pursuing.
4. Aspects of the job and the workplace can also directly influence the employment success of individuals with TBI, such as employer-furnished health care, supportive work environment, and opportunities to engage with coworkers, in short.
5. Technology, job coaching, and accommodations can be very effective for enabling RTW following TBI.
6. Other promising practices include the use of an RF to help the patient and family members locate needed services and supports, and peer support and training as through a Clubhouse vocational model.
7. RTW is a team process that includes the individual with TBI, his or her psychiatrist and physiatrist, and the VR specialist or job coach.

KEY REFERENCES

1. Shames J, Treger J, Ring H, Giaquinto S. Return to work following traumatic brain injury: trends and challenges. *Disabil Rehabil.* 2007;29(17):1387–1395.
2. Tsaousides T, Ashman T, Seter C. The psychological effects of employment after traumatic brain injury: objective and subjective indicators. *Rehabil Psych.* 2008;53(4):456–463.
3. Wehman P. Traumatic brain injury (TBI) and return to work (video). http://www.worksupport.com.
4. Wehman P, Targett P, West M, Kregel J. Productive work and employment for persons with traumatic brain injury: what have we learned after 20 years? *J Head Trauma Rehabil.* 2005;20(2):115–127. Retrieved June 15, 2012.

ADDITIONAL RESOURCES

1. Arango-Lasprilla JC, Gary KW. Employment outcomes after traumatic brain injury: does race/ethnicity matter? Available online at http://www.worksupport.com/training/webcastDetails.cfm/154.
2. Arango-Lasprilla JC. Traumatic brain injury in Spanish-speaking individuals. Available online at http://www.worksupport.com/training/webcastDetails.cfm/172.
3. Traumatic Brain Injury Model Systems. 2011 TBIMS slide presentation. Available online at http://www.tbims.org.

References

1. Wehman P, West M, Johnson A, Cifu D. Vocational rehabilitation for individuals with traumatic brain injury. In: Rosenthal M, Griffith ER, Kreutzer JS, Pentland B eds. *Rehabilitation of the Adult and*

Child with Traumatic Brain Injury. 3rd ed. Philadelphia, PA: FA Davis; 1999; 326–341.

2. Colantonio A, Ratcliff G, Chase S, Kelsey S, Escobar M, Vernich L. Long-term outcomes after moderate to severe traumatic brain injury. *Disabil Rehabil*. 2004;26(5):253–261.

3. Langlois JA, Rutland-Brown W, Wald MM. The epidemiology and impact of traumatic brain injury: a brief overview. *J Head Trauma Rehabil*. 2006;21(5):375–378.

4. van Velzen JM, van Bennekom CA, Edelaar MJ, Sluiter JK, Frings-Dresen MH. How many people return to work after acquired brain injury?: a systematic review. *Brain Inj*. 2009;23(6):473–488.

5. Keyser-Marcus LA, Bricout JC, Wehman P, et al. Acute predictors of return to employment after traumatic brain injury: a longitudinal follow-up. *Arch Phys Med Rehabil*. 2002;83(5):635–641.

6. Curl RM, Fraser RT, Cook RG, Clemmons D. Traumatic brain injury vocational rehabilitation: preliminary findings for the coworkers as trainer project. *J Head Trauma Rehabil*. 1996;11(1):75–85.

7. Shames J, Treger I, Ring H, Giaquinto S. Return to work following traumatic brain injury: trends and challenges. *Disabil Rehabil*. 2007; 29(17):1387–1395.

8. Wehman P, Targett P, West M, Kregel J. Productive work and employment for persons with traumatic brain injury: what have we learned after 20 years? *J Head Trauma Rehabil*. 2005;20(2):115–127.

9. Kreutzer JS, Marwitz JH, Walker W, et al. Moderating factors in return to work and job stability after traumatic brain injury. *J Head Trauma Rehabil*. 2003;18(2):128–138.

10. Trexler LE, Trexler LC, Malec JF, Klyce D, Parrott D. Prospective randomized controlled trial of resource facilitation on community participation and vocational outcome following brain injury. *J Head Trauma Rehabil*. 2010;25(6):440–446.

11. Wagner AK, Hammond FM, Sasser HC, Wiercisiewski D. Return to productive activity after traumatic brain injury: relationship with measures of disability, handicap, and community integration. *Arch Phys Med Rehabil*. 2002;83(1):107–114.

12. Cifu DX, Keyser-Marcus L, Lopez E, et al. Acute predictors of successful return to work 1 year after traumatic brain injury: a multicenter analysis. *Arch Phys Med Rehabil*. 1997;78(2):125–131.

13. Walker WC, Marwitz JH, Kreutzer JS, Hart T, Novack TA. Occupational categories and return to work after traumatic brain injury: a multicenter study. *Arch Phys Med Rehabil*. 2006;87(12):1576–1582.

14. Yasuda S, Wehman P, Targett P, Cifu D, West M. Return to work for persons with traumatic brain injury. *Am J Phys Med Rehabil*. 2001;80(11):852–864.

15. Franulic A, Carbonell CG, Pinto P, Sepulveda I. Psychosocial adjustment and employment outcome 2, 5 and 10 years after TBI. *Brain Inj*. 2004;18(2):119–129.

16. Hart T, Whyte J, Polansky M, Kersey-Matusiak G, Fidler-Sheppard R. Community outcomes following traumatic brain injury: impact of race and preinjury status. *J Head Trauma Rehabil*. 2005;20(2):158–172.

17. Machamer J, Temkin N, Fraser R, Doctor JN, Dikmen S. Stability of employment after traumatic brain injury. *J Int Neuropsych Soc*. 2005;11(7):807–816.

18. McCrimmon S, Oddy M. Return to work following moderate-to-severe traumatic brain injury. *Brain Inj*. 2006;20(10):1037–1046.

19. Arango-Lasprilla JC, Ketchum JM, Williams K, et al. Racial differences in employment outcomes after traumatic brain injury. *Arch Phys Med Rehabil*. 2008;89(5):988–995.

20. Arango-Lasprilla JC, Rosenthal M, Deluca J, et al. Traumatic brain injury and functional outcomes: does minority status matter? *Brain Inj*. 2007;21(7):701–708.

21. Bogner JA, Corrigan JD, Mysiw WJ, Clinchot D, Fugate L. A comparison of substance abuse and violence in the prediction of long-term rehabilitation outcomes after traumatic brain injury. *Arch Phys Med Rehabil*. 2001;82(5):571–577.

22. Corrigan JD. Substance abuse as a mediating factor in outcome from traumatic brain injury. *Arch Phys Med Rehabil*. 1995;76(4):302–309.

23. Gary KW, Arango-Lasprilla JC, Ketchum JM, et al. Racial differences in employment outcomes after traumatic brain injury at 1,

2, and 5 years postinjury. *Arch Phys Med Rehabil*. 2009;90(10):1699–1707.

24. Gary KW, Ketchum JM, Arango-Lasprilla JC, et al. Differences in employment outcomes 10 years after traumatic brain injury among racial and ethnic minority groups. *J Voc Rehab*. 2010;33(1):65–75.

25. Jorge RE, Starkstein SE, Arndt S, et al. Alcohol misuse and mood disorders following traumatic brain injury. *Arch Gen Psychiatry*. 2005;62(67):742–749.

26. Berger RP. The use of serum biomarkers to predict outcome after traumatic brain injury in adults and children. *J Head Trauma Rehabil*. 2006;21(4):315–333.

27. Stranjalis G, Korfias S, Papapetrou C, et al. Elevated serum S-100B protein as a predictor of failure to short-term return to work or activities after mild head injury. *J Neurotrauma*. 2004;21(8):1070–1075.

28. West MD. Aspects of the workplace and return to work for persons with brain injury in supported employment. *Brain Inj*. 1995;9(3):301–313.

29. Holland J. *The Self-Directed Search*. San Antonio, TX: Psychological Corporation; 1994.

30. Harmon LW, DeWitt DW, Campbell DP, Hansen JC. *Strong Interest Inventory: Applications and Technical Guide*. Stanford, CA: Stanford University Press; 1994.

31. Myers IB, McCaulley MH. *Manual: A Guide to the Development and Use of the Myers-Briggs Type Indicator*. Palo Alto, CA: Consulting Psychologists Press; 1985.

32. Educational Testing Service. SIGI PLUS. Princeton, NJ: Educational Testing Service; 1987.

33. Rayman JR, Harris-Bolsbev J. DISCOVER: a model for a systematic career guidance program. *Voc Guid Qtly*. 1977;26(1):3–11.

34. Witt, MA. *Job Strategies for People with Disabilities*. Princeton, NJ: Peterson's Guides; 1992.

35. Michelozzi BN. *Coming Alive from Nine to Five: A Career Search Handbook*. 5th ed. Mountain View, CA: Mayfield Publishing Company; 1996.

36. Szymanski EM, Turner KD, Hershenson D. Career development of people with disabilities: theoretical perspectives. In: Rusch FR, DeStefano L, Chadsey-Rusch J, Phelps LA, Szymanski EM, eds. *Transition from School to Adult Life: Models, Linkages, and Policy*. Sycamore, IL: Sycamore; 1992:391–406.

37. Koch LC. Career development interventions for transition-age youths with disabilities. *Work*. 2000;14(1):3–11.

38. Parsons MB, Reid DH, Green CW. Situational assessment of task preferences among adults with multiple severe disabilities in supported work. *JASH*. 2001;26(1):50–55.

39. Targett PS, Witting KM. Functional vocational assessment. In: Wehman P, Targett PS. *Vocational Curriculum for Individuals with Special Needs*. Austin, TX: Pro-Ed; 1999:25–61.

40. Target P, Wehman P, Petersen R, Gorton, S. Enhancing work outcome for three persons with traumatic brain injury. *Int J Rehabil Res*. 1995;21(1):41–50.

41. Pearson V, Yip N, Lo E. To tell or not to tell: disability disclosure and job application outcomes. *J Rehabil*. 2003;69(4):35–8.

42. Depompei R, Gillette Y, Goetz E, Xenopoulos-Oddsson A, Bryen D, Dowds M. Practical applications for use of PDAs and smartphones with children and adolescents who have brain injury. *NeuroRehab*. 2008;23(6):487–499.

43. Gentry T, Wallace J, Kvarfordt C, Lynch KB. Personal digital assistants as cognitive aids for high school students with autism: results of a community-based trial. *J Voc Rehab*. 2010;32(2):101–107.

44. Beard JH, Propst RN, Malamud, TJ. The Fountain House model of psychiatric rehabilitation. *Psychosoc Rehab J*. 1982;5(1):47–53.

45. Niemeier JP, DeGrace SM, Farrar LF, et al. Effectiveness of a comprehensive, manualized intervention for improving productivity and employability following brain injury. *J Voc Rehab*. 2010;33(3):167–179.

46. Trexler LE, Trexler LC, Malec JF, Klyce D, Parrott D. Prospective randomized controlled trial of resource facilitation on community participation and vocational outcome following brain injury. *J Head Trauma Rehabil*. 2010;25(6):440–446.

47. Zasler ND. The role of medical rehabilitation in vocational reentry. *J Head Trauma Res*. 1997;12(5):42–56.

Lifelong and Therapeutic Recreation and Leisure

Anne M. Fenech and Kelly L. Shaw Fisher

INTRODUCTION

This chapter contains 4 sections including an introduction to recreation and leisure occupations and the costs of not engaging in them, recreation during rehabilitation, lifelong leisure, and funding. Engagement in occupations has been divided into self-care, productivity, and the theme of this chapter—recreation and leisure (1). All of these may be influenced by brain injury (2–5), which may lead to a "catastrophic reaction" (6), involving a steep decline in overall health, well-being, self-esteem, self-identity (7), and quality of life. These effects may result from a reduced ability to take part, perceptions about what is suitable for individuals with brain injury to do (8), or because leisure was not thought to have been earned (9,10). For individuals who face a lifestyle made up of free time resulting from being unable to return to work, leisure has been suggested to be of especial importance (11–15). Facilitating leisure engagement should therefore begin as soon as possible in order to begin to define the individual's sense of self, roles, and goals (16), and to avoid occupational deprivation.

Why Bother With Recreation and Leisure After Brain Injury?

Neurological disability is predicted to become the highest cause of disability globally, with satisfying free time use being the end goal of rehabilitation for many (17,18). This is noteworthy given that individuals have been described as being at their most human when engaged in occupations (19). As will be presented in the third part of the chapter, leisure may offer an experience of perceived freedom, competence, self-determination, and choice (20). Recreational interventions offer a holistic approach to enhancing functional ability, adaptation to life role changes (21), reducing stress (22), as well as enhanced physical fitness (23). The social benefits of leisure include the development and maintenance of social support networks (1), social identity, social interaction skills, and the expression of creativity (24,25). Leisure choices may be influenced by ability, and the cultural value judgments of the individual and those about them (26). They may support occupational balance and influence hope and optimism (27,28). An inability to maintain previous leisure occupations may reinforce uncertainty about the future (29), leading to redefinition of their sense of self, roles, goals, and

thus, requiring a new self-image (16,21,30). Therefore, leisure satisfaction may be a predictor of quality of life (24) and associated with adjustment to disability and to well-being (31).

Knowing that individuals with brain injuries may have more "free" time to fill (32), what is important about leisure is not only what is done but also why it was carried out (33) in association with the individual's personal background (34). Free time and leisure are different if free time was imposed, because of having nothing else to do to fill it (35,36), and it may feel unsatisfying in the wrong environment (35,36). Free time boredom, (even if chosen) or occupations imposed to fill free time cannot be defined as leisure (10,34). The gap between desired and experienced leisure may widen after brain injury (28). This may result from perceived constraint, loss of interest or motivation, lack of facilities, reduced ability, lack of time (37), or environmental obstacles (38). It may also be a consequence of reduced concentration, memory, initiative, viable transport, or compensatory strategies (20,28,39). However, the most harmful effect of not engaging in leisure may be occupational deprivation, which may result in longer periods of sleep, altered quality of life, lack of social acceptance and social status, diminished sense of self-efficacy, atrophied occupational capacities, loss of self-identity, social exclusion, altered occupational patterns and time use, enforced dependence, and/or limitations to hand or tool use (33). These will each be described later in the chapter.

Leisure has been defined as freely chosen and free from demands (8,40–42) but may overlap with self-care and paid employment (43). It has been described as an observable phenomenon (8), which uses time, and is a subjective and transitory experience (44,45) that may be relaxing and intrinsically rewarding (44). Additionally, only the individual may define what they consider to be leisure (41). *Recreation*, on the other hand, has been defined as refreshment by means of agreeable pastimes that may amuse, stimulate, restore, relax, and be enjoyable (46). Recreational occupations may be neither intrinsically rewarding nor freely chosen (44) because they resulted from the demands of the body. *Therapy*, alternatively, may include any form of healing treatment (47), the effects of which may carry over to other contexts or time (45). While *human occupations* include activities in which the individual is engaged (48), that is, everything that people do to occupy themselves (including looking after themselves), leisure, and contributing to the social and economic fabric of their communities (49). It should be noted that what is leisure to one individual could be work to another; and so it is the reason why, and the method in which, an occupation is carried out, that determines whether it is a leisure occupation (50).

GOAL PLANNING

Goal planning has been described as crucial (51) and may enable individual participation rather than imposing objectives in rehabilitation (52,53). Additionally, the provision of opportunities, rather than prescriptions, may facilitate self-determination, in turn positively affecting subjective well-being and health (54). Occupational prescriptions (54), or arranging for "things to do," may not offer opportunities for truly meaningful and engaging occupations (19,41,55). Whereas, leisure conducted in a relaxing, safe, and comfortable environment, may enable participants to become self-actualised by their accomplishments (54). Leisure has been portrayed as less important than self-care and returning to work oriented rehabilitation goals (8,56), as a luxury (38), and as self-indulgent and unproductive (57). Whereas, free time use may be an important concern after brain injury (58) because a lack of employment may decrease the opportunity for developing social contacts (15), thus further limiting leisure participation (28). Therefore, selecting, adapting (59,60), or learning new leisure occupations (61) and using them as therapeutic media (62) has been proposed as central to rehabilitation (7).

Leisure Role

Disability may decrease the number, frequency, and length of leisure opportunities and increase the level of support required because of their physical and cognitive demands, including rapid integration of balance, coordination, vision, and decision making (28). Therefore, individuals have been reported to withdraw from all but predominantly passive, solitary, home-based, casual leisure occupations (28,63), where they may be independent, rather than engaging in active leisure occupations that require support from others. However, passive occupations appear less satisfying than more active leisure roles (44,64). Leisure may require a serious or a casual approach (65) with each individual experiencing leisure in a unique way (66). Choice of the role undertaken (i.e., active participant or spectator) may affect satisfaction, motivation, and sense of identity (67). The role offered may also reflect supporter's perceptions about what may be considered suitable for them to undertake (8).

The Costs of Not Engaging in Leisure

Reduced leisure skills and opportunities to use then may eventually result in occupational deprivation (68). This "devastating and widespread" outcome may result in loss of roles and routines (68). Occupationally deprived individuals have been reported to spend longer periods sleeping, or being passive (32,69,70), which may be a response to boredom and a way of using time in the absence of meaningful occupations (71,72). Sleep may offer a way of withdrawing from the world and the new self-image (16) and enable the

individual to exercise some control over his or her life. A second cost of occupational deprivation is poor quality of life.

Occupationally deprived individuals may also experience compromised self-identity and reduced self-efficacy (72). Occupational limitation has been recognised as a measure of disability (73) and as an indicator of quality of life, perceived health, and adjustment to disability (32). Moreover, time spent inactive or carrying out passive occupations has been negatively linked to life satisfaction (74,75). Another cost of occupational deprivation is a lack of social acceptance and social status. Occupational deprivation and underemployment may affect social status (76,77), becoming a further barrier to community reintegration because the individual may become accustomed to low self-esteem and self-efficacy (72). Individuals who are unable to "do" are at risk of losing their roles and relationships based social identity (78). A diminished sense of self-efficacy is also thought to be a cost of occupational deprivation.

Self-efficacy involves a self-assessment of competence and influences the choices made, effort expended, and persistence. A diminished sense of self-efficacy, may lead to low expectations and feelings of futility, dissuading individuals from further attempts to participate (72), and influencing coping with disability, disease progression (79), and symptomatology (e.g., severity of pain) (80). Individuals with high support needs may prefer to be an independent spectator rather than a supported participant (66,81). This may be caused by the individuals' awareness of their occupational capacities and a wish to prevent further dependence on others (66). This choice may lead to further atrophied occupational capacity through lack of use.

Individuals with brain injuries may experience difficulty engaging in occupations because of altered ability and lack of opportunity, resulting in a spiral of skills degradation, diminished self-efficacy beliefs, and restricted role repertoires (72,82). A loss of role repertoires, in turn, may influence integration into the community, reducing opportunities to engage in occupations and thus compounding the skills degradation spiral which has been described as a "dehumanising phenomenon" (72). Another aspect of occupational deprivation is loss of identity.

A loss of self-identity may result from occupational deprivation (72,76), in turn influencing how the individual thinks, acts, and feels (83). The feedback from others (84), from a persistent lack of achievement (85) and the interrelationship between the individual and others (83) which result from leisure engagement, may also influence self-identity. Disability may present the individual with many challenges and lifestyle changes beyond the symptoms of the condition, including unemployment, altered social relationships, roles, and increased dependence on others (86), which may threaten the individual's sense of self and identity, and lead to identity alienation (a self-image that is not consistent with their current situation) (87). Another aspect of occupational deprivation is social exclusion.

Social interaction may offer feedback about how others perceive us (10,88), but may be restricted because of language, comprehension problems, or aphasia, and this may not provide a benchmark or a sense of social approval (10). Social exclusion and confinement may result in the person being uncreative, unmotivated, and fatigued (89), and be associated with feelings of powerlessness (90). Another aspect of occupational deprivation is altered patterns of occupational engagement.

Altered occupational patterns and time use may result from having more free time (32) but less energy or opportunities to use it after brain injury because of the individual's reliance on assistive technology and adaptation to the environment, resulting in occupational deprivation (91). Having less to do may also affect their perception of time passing (92). The resultant reduced performance and well-being (88) may in turn result in less time spent on productivity-related tasks and more time on personal care occupations, leaving more free time (32). This may be significant because a little time spent doing a satisfying occupation contributes to health and well-being more than a long time spent doing a minimally satisfying occupation (32). Another aspect of occupational deprivation is enforced dependence.

Lack of control over one's occupation (72,88) may influence an individual's sense of time passing and of time spent between occupations (93,94). Individuals' self-identity may be influenced if they depend on others to allow "choice" and "doing" their occupations (95). Therefore, limitations to control of occupational choice may lead to enforced dependence and an altered self-identity.

The loss of ability to use the tools to undertake occupations may be a cost of occupational deprivation (68) because a lack of opportunities for hand use may lead to a spiral of degrading occupational capacities (96). In addition, expert hand use involves the brain's ability to associate concepts, sensory perception, and communication (97), which may have been affected by the brain injury. Therefore, individuals with brain injuries appear to be more vulnerable to occupational deprivation than other clinical groups. The challenge, therefore, becomes one of limiting the costs of occupational deprivation through enabling leisure and recreational engagement as soon as possible.

RECREATION DURING REHABILITATION

Recreation and leisure as part of a rehabilitation process may influence multiple domains, including the psychosocial, physical, cognitive, and behavioural. The following will explore some examples of therapeutic recreational interventions, including community integration, leisure education, exercise regimens, adapted sports, therapeutic horseback riding, aquatics, music, art, and tai chi.

Community Integration

Definitions of community integration include 3 ideas: relationships with others, autonomy both at home and in the community, and the meaningful use of free time (98), which has been proposed to be a key aim of rehabilitation (99). This may include supporting and enabling independent productivity away from the home or rehabilitation environment. It has been suggested that social support moderates the effects of negative life events (39), so encouraging community reintegration and social participation may influence adjustment after brain injury. Community integration goals should be based on an understanding of the individual's appreciation about the concept of leisure and its relationship to quality

of life (20). Additionally, their preferences in relation to community based leisure resources and how to access them should be established.

Leisure Education

Leisure counseling involves assisting individuals to determine their leisure interests and locating opportunities in the home and community to meet those interests (23). The preparation of a prioritised and individualised leisure interest inventory might involve a combination of several baseline assessment techniques: observation, structured interviews, standardised recreation and leisure assessment instruments, and questionnaires and checklists (100). This may allow for consideration of financial resources, functional ability, accessibility, and related background experience, thus enabling a more targeted approach toward rehabilitation goals (23). Community-based assessment and interventions conducted in the context of everyday interactions and natural settings may ensure that rehabilitation is more effective (23,99) by overcoming the non-generalisation of skills that may occur in clinical environments (99). Additionally, consistency of feedback regarding goal performance is crucial and may require the use of behavioural interventions, as well as constructive feedback to encourage relearning and generalisation of community integration and social skills. It may be preferable to use protocols such as the Community Integration Program to help measure progress (101). The complexity, intensity, and length of time required before progress is recognised and makes community integration goals challenging to achieve, and may require significant adjustment and coping strategies for overcoming stress (102).

Exercise

Exercise may offer a wide range of benefits for individuals with brain injury (103). Possible consequences of lack of exercise may include increased body weight, decreased range of motion, and chronic illnesses such as diabetes and hypertension (23). Increases in anxiety and altered mood states such as depression, frustration, and challenging behaviour may result from brain injury (104). However, the implementation of a structured exercise regimen might reduce the severity of these symptoms (105). The effects of counseling alone may not be significant, whereas continued exercise might lead to significantly reduced depression (106). Aerobic exercise may encourage functional changes within the brain, producing an effect on specific areas and the associated cognitive domains, particularly attention, memory, and executive function (107). Additionally, consistent exercise may improve muscular strength, endurance, flexibility, optimal body composition, cardiovascular condition, and mental health (108). When incorporating exercise into the treatment of individuals with brain injury, it may be useful to emphasise the individual's abilities, as well as preference for occupations while still offering well-rounded and diverse methods of increasing activity level such as adapted sports, therapeutic horseback riding, or aquatics.

Clinic Based

Exercise plans may be structured to include aerobic and anaerobic exercises targeting muscular strength, muscular endurance, body composition, and cardiovascular fitness. When working with individuals with brain injury, the development of a plan with graduated, incremental, and specific guidelines is common. The multitude of fitness equipment available allows therapists to individualise programs, incorporating 3 basic principles: frequency, intensity, and duration of activity. *Frequency* refers to how often occupational participation occurs; *intensity* to the level of achieved maximal heart rate or perceived exertion; and *duration* refers to the amount of time exertion is sustained (109). In addition to frequency, intensity, and duration of exercise, *adherence* may influence the effectiveness of an exercise regimen (109). Using leisure to combine pleasurable experiences with exercise may have the greatest potential to enhance recovery by encouraging consistency and adherence to an intervention regimen (23). An exercise regimen provided at http://www.tree-of-life.com/documents/adapted-weight-regimen.pdf illustrates how frequency, intensity, and duration can be incorporated. This type of circuit format may allow for creative, innovative, and individualised design, while offering substantial cardio and muscular endurance training.

Given the motivational challenges encountered during rehab, therapists may vary a regimen without sacrificing opportunity for repetition and relearning. Timely implementation of novel challenges and techniques throughout the reconditioning process may combat apathy and encourage positive attitudes toward participation in fitness-related occupations.

Adapted Sports

The use of adapted sports may offer physical and psychological benefits (110) such as improved cardiorespiratory fitness, increased muscle strength, increased self-esteem, and enhanced functional independence (110,111). The use of sports and the structured physical training and skill development it offers may encourage the emergence of an "athletic identity" (109). This may ameliorate the effects of role loss, improve self-esteem, motivation, self-awareness, self-efficacy, and commitment to health and wellness goals (112). Additionally, increased opportunity for socialisation and identification with a peer group through sports participation may promote community integration and enhance quality of life (110). Community organisations that provide adapted sports programming may be a useful resource when identifying sports-related activities to integrate into the treatment of individuals with TBI. Adapted sports might include power wheelchair soccer, bocce, track and field events, kayaking, wheelchair softball, handcycling, rowing, snow skiing, wheelchair basketball, and wheelchair tennis as demonstrated in Figure 82-1.

There may be risks associated with sports participation after brain injury. Medical advice is imperative to avoid injury, including the use of protective equipment and close monitoring of thermoregulatory status and signs of autonomic dysreflexia (113). Although the implementation of sports-related activities may be complex because of the multiple deficits individuals with TBI might experience, the potential benefits of successful participation outweigh the challenges of adapting the sports in the authors' opinion.

Therapeutic Horseback Riding and Hippotherapy

Therapeutic horseback riding (THR) involves the use of horses to attain therapeutic goals, whereas *hippotherapy* (HT) is a therapist directed intervention using equine movement to achieve rehabilitation goals (114). The adaptability of THR and HT are central to their efficacy for individuals with brain injury. Additionally, THR and HT have the ability to stimulate multiple domains of functioning, including physical, cognitive, and social or emotional (115,116). Commonly associated with brain injury are problems with alignment, posture, mobility, and balance (117), which the passive influence of rhythmic equine movements during hippotherapy sessions may enhance, as well as encouraging the normalisation of muscle tone, posture, and balance (118). Sensory stimulation to the pelvis, lumbar region, and hip joints may result from the precise and repetitive movements of a walking horse (119,118). THR may occur on a group or individual basis. A cooperative horse that relates to people (120,121) may influence the development of mutual trust and acceptance, while concurrently building skills, self-esteem, and mastery through collaboration, thus enhancing the individual's ability to cope with their disability (121). THR and HT programs have been demonstrated to have a positive impact on quality of life (118) and should be incorporated into the rehabilitation process whenever possible.

Aquatic Therapy

Aquatic therapy (or Aquability) (121a) may be beneficial (122) because, in addition to promoting the attainment of physical rehabilitation goals, an aquatic environment may relieve stress, improve coping skills and increase self-efficacy (123). The aquatic environment—for example, density, hydrostatic pressure, viscosity, buoyancy, and thermodynamics—may account for the biological effects of immersion (122). *Thermodynamics* is the ability of water to retain heat and transfer heat energy and may be essential to the therapeutic use of water (122). The warm aquatic environment of 32°C–33°C reduces muscle tone, allowing for more productive movement and inducing a relaxed state potentially enhancing neuromuscular function (124,125). *Buoyancy* allows for a reduced gravity environment and potentially decreased weight-bearing difficulties (122), thus allowing individuals to engage in physical rehabilitation and exercise that would otherwise be impractical and ineffective because of gravity. Health-promoting behaviours may emphasise positive lifestyle practices that may have declined because of the stress experienced after brain injury. Participation in an aquatic exercise program may encourage health-promoting behaviours, thus improving self-efficacy and coping with stress (122). Some examples of aquatic exercise techniques and their descriptions are provided at http://www.tree-of-life.com/documents/aquatic-exercise-techniques.pdf.

Expressive Arts Based Modalities

Expressive arts based modalities may be used alongside allopathic medicine to provide a holistic approach to treatment of individuals with brain injury (126) in order to address the

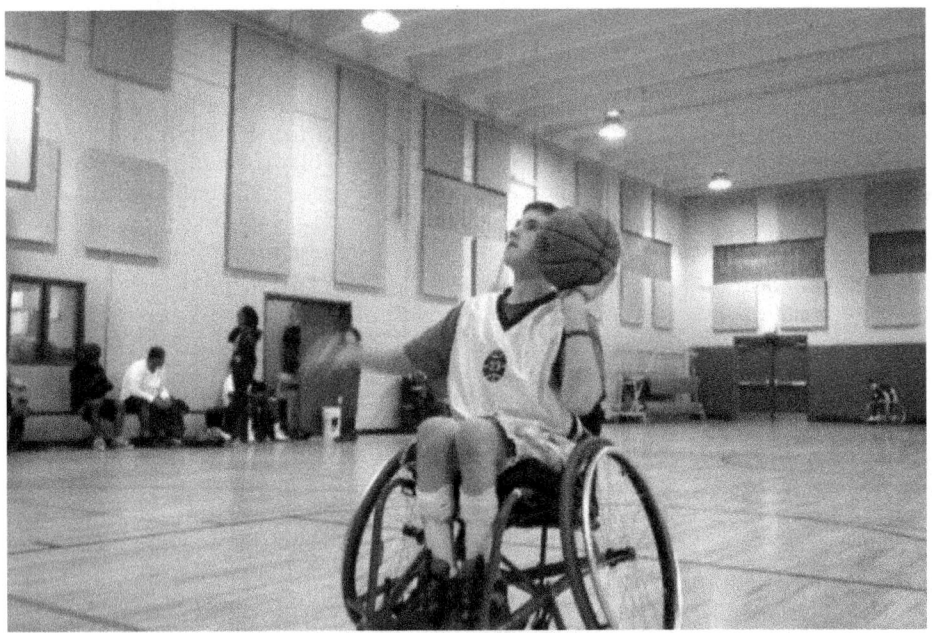

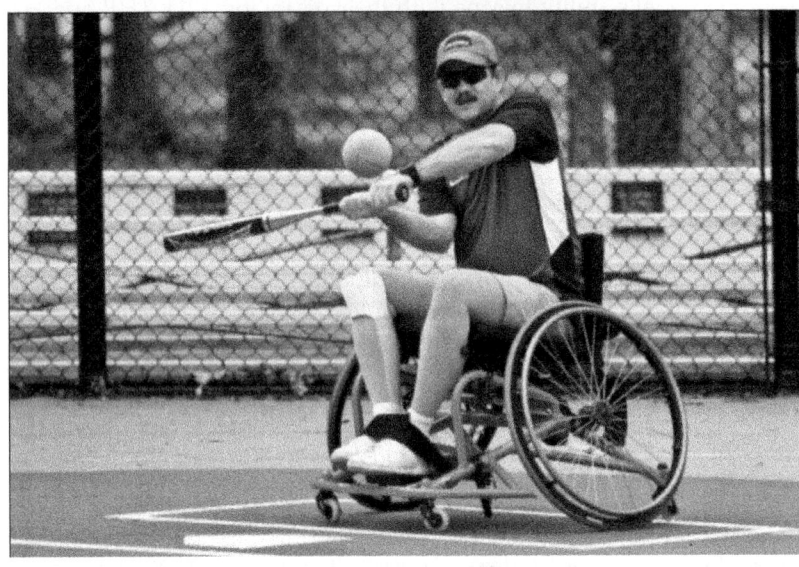

FIGURE 82-1 Adapted Sports.

complexity, severity, and chronic nature of neurobehavioural dysfunction sometimes present after injury. Music, art, and tai chi may be incorporated into the rehabilitation of individuals with brain injury (127). Collaboration with discipline specific trained professionals may ensure adequate assessment, goals, and treatment techniques are selected.

Music

Music, in conjunction with interpersonal skills, may contribute toward enhanced social, emotional, cognitive, and communication abilities, and thus health and well-being (128, 129). Listening to music has been reported to improve emotional and cognitive functioning; whereas practicing an instrument or singing may induce changes in the brain, as well as potentially aid in the establishment of alternative pathways (130). Music may encourage sharing of interests

with others and offer the opportunity for emotional and social connections and positive interactions (129). Additionally, recreational music may promote self-esteem, self-image and self-identity, emotional expression, social skills, and a reduction in depression (128). It may also enhance concentration, sequencing, motor planning, and self-initiation, resulting in reduced dressing times (128), while promoting generalisation of skills for other aspects of daily living (128). Concentration, autonomy, and motivation may be enhanced through the selection and experience of pleasurable and engaging music (127). In addition, communication, dysarthria, dysphasia, and both fluent and nonfluent aphasia may be influenced, as may expressive language (130), speech intelligibility, rate of speech, pitch range, speech intonation, breath capacity, and articulatory planning (128). Consideration of the management of the auditory environment is required (130) because the unstructured use of music may result in sensory overload. However, used appropriately, music may enable individuals who are minimally conscious to demonstrate awareness (129). Music may also influence a range of positive behavioural changes including arousal, purposeful response to stimuli, changes in respiration and heart rate, and communicative responses (131). Given the impact that communication, psychosocial, and cognitive deficits may have on quality of life, the inclusion of music as part of a recreational therapy program should be considered when treatment planning for individuals with brain injuries.

Art

The inclusion of art as a recreational intervention may generate positive physical, cognitive, and psychosocial goal outcomes (132). Brain injury survivors might experience multiple deficits leading to increased anxiety levels and even agitation or aggression when confronted with the challenge of rehabilitating multiple deficits. This may result in the individual withdrawing from their rehabilitation. Creative and artistic occupations may reinforce the individual's sense of autonomy, combating this loss of self-determination, offering a less structured, less confrontational environment that encourages individualism and creativity, consequently offering an autonomous experience (132). Recreational art may incorporate the use of a variety of artistic mediums ranging in complexity and skill requirements, all of which may promote improved fine motor function, hand-eye coordination, grip strength, range of motion (133), sequencing, problem solving, attention, concentration, memory, and organisation in individuals with brain injury (132,134). For those individuals with communication deficits, recreational art might offer the tools to convey stress and emotion (135). In addition, group-oriented expressive arts programming may improve psychosocial functioning (136), which in turn may be linked with increased life satisfaction and improved quality of life (136).

Tai Chi

The holistic and non-stressful nature of Tai Chi Chuan and Tai Chi Qigong involve soft flowing movements that may be practiced regardless of age, sex, and fitness level. Tai Chi may influence positive changes in physical and psychological responses (108,137), making it an ideal intervention for individuals with brain injury (138). The slow, gradual sequence of postures and movement in Tai Chi may influence the development of muscle tone control, muscular strength, kinesthetic sense, balance, and coordination (139). Further, Tai Chi has been revealed to reduce blood pressure, stress, fatigue, depression, and anger (137). Improving mood and self-esteem are valuable benefits because low mood and self-esteem may affect social adjustment and therefore overall quality of life (136). Tai Chi is a relatively low-cost and easy to participate in art form and requires no equipment (140). Once techniques and patterns have been learned, only space is required to perform the exercises.

LIFELONG LEISURE

This part of the chapter will present the voice of 50 individuals (selected from the original data because they had brain injuries) through secondary conceptual analysis. The original data about the leisure experienced by 228 neuropalliative individuals has been published separately (141,142). Ethical approval for the study was granted by the University of Roehampton School of Human and Life Sciences Ethics Committee on December 2, 2008 and by the facilities own research governance procedure on March 12, 2007. The aim of the secondary conceptual analysis was to portray the value and meaning of leisure to individuals with brain injuries once rehabilitation had ceased. It did this by clustering the words of participants, using as its deductive framework the facets which contribute meaning to occupations collated by one of the authors (141). It appears that the leisure occupations being discussed offered the participants many opportunities to experience meaningful occupations, each of which will be discussed subsequently.

Including an element of competition, personal challenge (143), or widening experience (62) may enhance the satisfaction being derived from goal achievement (directly or through others) (75). The leisure occupations engaged in may involve watching others participate rather than engaging in active leisure occupations that demand support from others (66,81,144). Participants have described a sense of "achievement & interest," "ability to keep still," and having "learned the story."

Belonging

Humans are a social species with a complex social structure, and so a sense of being "part of the group" (Participant 8) is an important benefit of participating in leisure. Sixty-eight percent of participants noted an increase in "team spirit" (Participant 9) and feeling a "good atmosphere" (Participant 2) among the participants, when engaging in social leisure. Participant who had been a performer described being able to "rejoined the performing community" (Participant 1), or reconnecting "with others in the same profession" (Participant 10) when involved in a drama project. This sense of bond between participants led one to describe the loneliness that results from disability especially when communication or behaviour was affected. Therefore "simply being in the company of others" (Participant 11), was a huge step toward a sense of belonging. Social occupations may involve coordination around the lives of others (145). The rituals, shared language, and sense of humour that may be part of a group, contributed to shared values and companionship, and may reflect the social status, beliefs, and *raison d'être* of a group (146), indicating that leisure in a social context may bring with it an implicit sense of belonging (however short-term). Altruism and social status beliefs may also influence feeling part of a group (69,146,147).

A Sense of Health, Well-Being, and Capability

Engagement in occupations (148) may influence perceptions of health and well-being (40,149,150,151). Their occupational choices may enable individuals to adapt their performance to cope with altered health, viewing the resumption of meaningful occupations as proof that they were capable and healthy individuals (152) with a sense of well-being (153). Several participants described their leisure as making them "feel full of life" (Participant 28), "healthier" (Participant 7), able to "forget my limitations" (Participant 7), and enjoy a sense of "freedom and escaping from my limitations" (Participant 47) or "freedom from the usual boundaries" (Participant 46). One participant reported that "this is me; I've escaped from my situation" (Participant 45). Engagement was described as "taking me away" (Participant 43). Similarly, social and achievement leisure may support mental health (143) while uninvolving or passive leisure may be significantly related to negative mental health outcomes because of lack of engagement (27).

Preventing Boredom

Boredom may result from insufficient complexity or challenge (94,154), limited opportunities to engage in occupation (91), or a mismatch between the challenge of the occupation and the individual's skill and motivations (155). The participants described leisure opportunities as a way of "avoiding boredom" (Participant 14) and as offering a "change from the boredom of everyday existence" (Participant 36). Boredom and being "bored" (Participant 14 and 36) were words that participants used frequently. This may be caused in part by their perception of what they may do with their time, for example, "I don't do anything apart from listen to music" (Participant 25). This is relevant because curiosity may result from insufficient stimulation, with learning, attitude change, and social interaction resulting from an optimal amount of novelty, unexpectedness, and complexity (156). Experience may result from change and consistency (157), with reduced awareness underpinning boredom (158,159). As a result, understimulated individuals may seek any kind of stimulation to achieve a balance. On the other hand, stimulation overload or an inability to process the stimulation may lead to boredom, inability to deal with distractions, and distress (160). This may demotivate the individual, dilute meaning, and reduce well-being (160).

Self-Expression or Creativity

The ability to express creativity (161), and to reinforce self-awareness and self-esteem through self-expression (162), may be linked to concentration and exhilaration (163). Creativity may also refresh (163), invigorate (164), and offer an outlet for self-expression (147,165). Self-expression and "being in touch with my creative side" (Participant 1) may result from occupations which are overtly creative, but also from those which require memory and association such as "discussions, puzzle solving, or cultural celebrations" (Participant 1). One participant commented that creativity is "another innate need that we all have regardless of ability; performing arts assist with enabling access to creative opportunities . . . and therefore meeting that need" (Participant 48). The participants appeared to value "getting the creative juices flowing" (Participant 7), "presenting a performance' (Participant 7), and a "dramatic expression" (Participant 1). A sense of freedom and enjoyment, leading to growth and legacy building may also have resulted (166,146), allowing others to see "who we really are" (Participant 48) (167, 162,161). Self-expression, satisfaction, and well-being have been described as the potential rewards of engagement in occupations (165,147,146).

Individual or Social Identity

Leisure may offer opportunities for experimentation, risk-taking, and challenge (10). Therefore, underoccupied individuals may feel socially excluded and demoralised, and use leisure as a coping or escaping strategy (10). Occupational performance may influence self-identity and well-being through reflection, goal orientation, and social approval (83). Likewise, internalisation of the perceptions of others may influence self-identity (168). Several of the participants interviewed reported "feeling valued" (Participant 7), being "treated like kings and queens for the day" (Participant 7), or made to "feel important and involved" (Participant 29), because "being treated as an individual with choices . . . promotes a sense of self worth" (participant 35). Moreover, restrictions to occupational participation may limit an individual's self and social identity (67). Additionally, the cultural, religious, or spiritual components of an occupation, and the feedback received influence self-esteem, social roles, approval, and values (10,83). When describing large seasonal events, several participants describe an opportunity for "interaction with others" (Participant 41). However, others explained their regret at having "no intimate relationships" (Participant 31) (169). Fifty-two percent of participants reported that the interactive drama project had increased social interaction among participants.

Challenge

Several leisure opportunities were reported as being those which encouraged participants to "be daring and take risks" (Participant 34) or "to be daring when I wouldn't have been before" (Participant 1) (142). Several participants actively welcomed the opportunity to "push the boat out" (Participant 24) or "stretch myself" (Participant 18), whereas others "wouldn't say no to a challenge" (Participant 24). One participant reported that "I had to use my limbs and memory" (Participant 17), another finding it "difficult having to learn the story, whilst having to act it" (Participant 2). A younger participant described how "it was a challenge to remember a bit more about the play" (Participant 18). Boredom may result from a lack of challenge, and may be experienced significantly more when an individual is engaged in passive leisure, or the challenge was perceived to be less than the skills brought to the occupation (71). Achievement may result from competition, personal challenge (10,71,143), widening experience (63), experimentation, or risk-taking (10). Occupational engagement may result from motivation to participate resulting from challenge (165), whereas meaningfulness, challenge, and satisfaction may compensate for occupational imbalance (32). Challenge was reported to be one of the salient motivating qualities of many leisure experiences, especially those of a more intense nature (170).

Links With Past Self

Leisure may link the individual with a past life (29,171), offering a buffer between the impact of negative life events and the reconstruction of a life story that is continuous with the past while generating optimism and sustaining coping with present circumstances (29). The occupation may have "reminded me of school days" (Participant 4) "and other links with my past life" (participant 6), enabling participants to remember things "from the past," setting off "tangential memories of the past" (Participant 1). Inevitably, memories that provoke links with the past bring up thoughts about how "life before was happy" (Participant 5) when participating in similar occupations.

Individual Growth and Life Satisfaction

A few participants were taking piano lessons; however, informal learning also occured, for example, I "learned about others, their sense of humor . . . their skills" (Participant 3) or "to be proud of myself" (Participant 6 and 11). In fact, 54% of participants reported discovering new things about themselves and others. Musical performances were described as "providing something entertaining and educational" (Participant 1). Learning (embedded in social relations) may be central to occupational engagement but not highly valued (172). The self-organisation and self-determination required enabled participants to aim for self-actualisation (173,174).

A Clear Sense of the Rhythm of Life

Everyday life is made up of a rhythm (150) of short- and long-term reality check occupations (day, week, season, year) (10), which may contribute to a social groups' values and beliefs about time use (145), influencing perceptions of time passing (145). The rhythm, whether internal (heartbeat or circadian rhythm) or social (meal times), balanced around "actual doing" may result in a sense of well-being (150). This sense of rhythm may also be derived from engagement in seasonal, monthly, weekly, or daily routines and occupations that follow themes and trends across the lifespan (69), for example, a play focused in childhood leading to a work focused in adulthood (69). The coordination of social occupations may involve an interweaving of the actions, schedules, and goals of participants and may engender a sense of belonging (145). Seasonal events remind participants of where they are in relation to the "passing weeks, months, seasons, or years" (Participant 7). This lets them "mark the passing of time rather than life passing us by" (Participant 7). Volunteers, performers, or facilitators from other communities and organisations provide residents "with the passing of time in the present world outside" (Participant 16) as do the TV and newspapers.

Goal Orientation or Aspiration or Anticipation

Self-selected occupations, may lead to pride in achievement (69,175) and a sense of well-being (148). A clear sense of individual purpose or goal orientation may influence occupational performance and result from reflection about how to achieve or contribute to a goal (176). Goal achievement may facilitate a positive reflection on accomplishment, or lead to frustration or lack of confidence (69). Repeated lack of success may motivate persistence (177), leading to redoubled effort or to withdrawal, depending on whether the effort required was realistic (178) and on the individual's optimism, resilience, and self-efficacy beliefs (177). Several participants expressed

having "looked forward to" (Participant 17) being part of the group, or "liked having something to aim for" (Participant 24). Participants' aspirations ranged from "I'd like to do another degree" (Participant 25) to wishing to "go out more" (Participant 26) or to be able to participate in "more of a range" (Participant 9) of leisure opportunities.

Self-Determination

Control and choice of occupations may influence perceptions of quality of life (19), act as an intrinsic motivator (179), and enhance the meaning of an occupation (67,161). Leisure, being self-determined and autonomous (179), may therefore promote curiosity (156), a sense of control (67), and adaptation to and coping with life (152). A synthesis of the meaning and context of an occupation may additionally support choice making and acceptance of the rules or norms of an occupation (153). This may in turn influence interest, excitement, and confidence, leading to enhanced performance, persistence, self-esteem, well-being (179), and engagement. In a residential care environment, there is a danger that participants experience little choice of location and timing for their occupations if they are organised on a group basis. Opportunities for self-determination may cushion the stress involved in disability (40,180). Sixty-four percent of participants felt able to choose whether to attend an interactive drama project, but 18% were not sure describing how "there was no where else to go" (Participant 11), which limited their perception of the choices available, or "the room was too crowded to leave once we were there" (Participant 13), others felt "expected to join in" (Participant 21), or had someone, for example, a spouse, who "makes choices for him in the belief that he would have come anyway" (Participant 12).

A Sense of Self-Efficacy

Self-efficacy is an individual's belief in his or her ability to succeed, which may determine how they thought, behaved, and felt (177) contributing to a sense of self-worth, creativity, and self-expression (181). Successful achievement, whether experienced or witnessed in others, may strengthen the individual's sense of self-efficacy; although a lack of success may undermine and weaken self-efficacy (177). Individuals may adapt their occupational participation to cope with altered health and reported the resumption of meaningful occupations to be taken as proof of capability and health (152,182). These findings equated doing with living, aiding adjustment to disability, or as participants put it, "It's not the end just because we are in wheel chairs" (Participant 1), and "this is who I am—a lady of leisure" (Participant 7). Two pleasantly surprised residents described how they "hadn't realised that I could act" (Participant 7) and "don't I look fine in my costume, I got my photo in the newspaper too" (Participant 9).

Transcendence to the "New Me" or Adjustment to Disability

Satisfaction with time use, especially productive and leisure may have a significant influence on adjustment to disability and life satisfaction (32). Having a satisfying leisure lifestyle may contribute to achieving and maintaining a sense of health and well-being (148), acknowledge social identity (67), and adjusting to disability (24). Leisure based social relationships with role models influence adjustment to a disability (25). The reconstruction of a leisure lifestyle may serve as a link between the present and previous identity and help the process of learning to live with a new self-identity (16,29), adjusting to a new self-image (27) and renovating the individual's life story beyond disability. A lack of leisure engagement may have a dramatic effect on the individual's experience of illness, offering insufficient diversion or leaving them vulnerable to stress. Solitary leisure may offer opportunities for self-reflection, problem solving, and relaxation, which may influence identity development and transcend negative life events (31).

FUNDING LEISURE AND RECREATION

The health care financing administrations responsible for defining "covered services" typically do not fund the recreational services offered in many treatment settings in the United States (183). Thus creativity is required to fund leisure and recreation interventions.

This portion of the chapter provides a very brief overview of some thoughts to working within funding constraints while still offering appropriate services. Further research is needed into service delivery models (184). Therapeutic leisure and recreational programs may be supported in many different ways. Funding may come from different revenue sources depending on the setting (i.e., government vs private pay).

Sponsorship and Contributions

Donations of expertise, materials, time, and equipment may come from individual, charitable, or commercial sources (185). Examples may include membership of a scrapstore scheme, which has been set up to support the reuse of unwanted resources for the benefit of the community. Other donations may include monetary donations or equipment loans or donations, time, experience, and knowledge offered by expert sports or craftsmen and volunteers to enable an individual to learn or progress their skills.

In exchange for the positive exposure that businesses may gain from association with support of a good cause, they may agree to sponsor tournaments and special events. Other donations may include time, experience, and knowledge offered by expert sports or craftsmen and volunteers who may assist with fundraising for or organising of an event or occupation. Donations and fundraising for special events or annual programs may include service users assisting in planning and execution of fundraising event such as race events (5k, 1 mile fun run/walk), sales of donated items, or manufacturing items to sell at a local farmer's market or craft fair. Collaborative working between a charity and a recreation and leisure service may lead to a pooling of ideas, staffing, facilities, and so forth to run a joint event which offers participants a wider social network and a wider range of leisure occupations. Other donations may include time given by 1:1 volunteers who build up a positive collaboration

with a specific participant or group of participants to support their leisure engagement. Similarly, volunteer donation may include offering to participate in a sponsored sports event on behalf of the donation recipient. Additionally, commercial companies may donate sponsorship for events, projects or award schemes, staff time, advice and expertise, products, training, research, materials or equipment, and use of company facilities out of enlightened self-interest. In addition, large not-for-profit agencies may see such donations as part of their community investment and responsibility. A service may alternatively be proactive and offer to pilot or showcase new or innovative equipment or invite professional performers to perform, both of which may generate press attention.

Partnerships

Partnerships may offer budgetary assistance through establishing connections with local individuals and agencies that support the mission and purpose of therapeutic leisure programs, and potentially generate income (186). Collaborative relationships may benefit both parties. Partnerships may prove an essential element in ensuring diverse recreational programming offering donations in many forms in return for enhanced exposure (186). Statutory facilities may offer grants or the use of their parks and recreation facilities to support an event. Additionally, grants may be sought from appropriate charities either brain injury related or related to the occupation and may be identified using a search engine such as http://www.trustfunding.org.uk.

Statutory Funding

Facility or departmental budgets tend to be used for in-house community-based activities for service users. In addition, pooling equipment with other similar organisations to offer a book/game/music/film library may expand the facilities available. A recreation and leisure service program should offer a range of leisure occupations, including those which are individual and social, physically active and spectator, and involve music, sport, and craft.

Government agencies may offer grant schemes linked to policy objectives or voluntary sector funding through relationships with specific organisations whose work matches their own interests. In addition, local government authorities may make grants to the local voluntary and community sector, using individual criteria, application procedures, and timescales. Devolution has meant that voluntary organisations should approach the relevant departments, who may offer time-limited local or regional program funding streams within their own country. Similarly, the European Union provides relatively little funding for voluntary and community sector, and this is channeled through the European Regional Development Fund (ERDF) and the European Social Fund (ESF).

Recreation on a Shoestring Budget

Although there may be multiple ways to enhance a limited budget, Leisure facilitators directors in various settings may also want to know how to optimise the resources that are readily available to them, including modest operating budgets. Methods may be very different from one facility to another; however, the principles may be similar.

Facility or departmental budgets tend to be used for in-house community-based activities for service users. Services with limited budgets may benefit from networking and requests for games, materials, and equipment from commercial and community budget streams. In addition, pooling equipment with similar organisations to offer a book/game/music/film library may expand the facilities available. In addition, individuals with brain injuries may contribute personal funds or time spent fundraising toward their own leisure occupations. This may be built into leisure education program budgeting that is, saving for leisure occupations and particular events.

KEY CLINICAL POINTS

1. Costs of not engaging in leisure may include longer periods of sleep, altered quality of life, lack of social acceptance and social status, diminished sense of self-efficacy, atrophied occupational capacities, loss of self-identity (individual or social), social exclusion, altered patterns of occupational engagement and time use, enforced dependence, and/or lack of opportunity to access the tools required to engage in occupations.
2. A rounded therapeutic recreation program should include community integration, leisure education, exercise, adapted sports, and/or expressive arts.
3. Lifelong leisure can offer the individual a sense of importance; purpose or meaning; goal orientation; a sense of achievement; a sense of being fully human; self-identity (individual or social); individual growth; a clear sense of the rhythm of life; a sense of belonging; opportunities for self-expression and creativity; a sense of health, well-being, and capability; preventing boredom through enablement; learning and discovery; control and choice of occupation or self-determination; a sense of engagement in the occupation; effects of an occupational environment which was conducive; acknowledgement of age/cultural/historical/gender identity; and/or a sense of self-efficacy.

KEY REFERENCES

1. Bier N, Dutil E, Couture M. Factors affecting leisure participation after a traumatic brain injury: an exploratory study. *J Head Trauma Rehabil.* 2009;24(3):187.
2. Caldwell LL. Leisure and health: why is leisure therapeutic? *Br Guid Counsell.* 2005;33(1):7–26.
3. Kleiber DA, Reel HA, Hutchinson SL. When distress gives way to possibility: the relevance of leisure in adjustment to disability. *NeuroRehabilitation.* 2008;23(4):321–328.
4. Phipps S, Richardson P. Occupational therapy outcomes for clients with traumatic brain injury and stroke using the Canadian Occupational Performance Measure. *Am J Occup Ther.* 2007;61(3):328.
5. Wise EK, Mathews-Dalton C, Dikmen S, et al. Impact of traumatic brain injury on participation in leisure activities. *Arch Phys Med Rehabil.* 2010;91(9):1357–1362.

References

1. Townsend E, Polatajko H. *Enabling Occupation II: Advancing an Occupational Therapy Vision for Health, Well-being & Justice Through Occupation.* Ottawa, ON: CAOT Publications ACE; 2007.
2. Colantonio A, Ratcliff G, Chase S, Kelsey S, Escobar M, Vernich L. Long-term outcomes after moderate to severe traumatic brain injury. *Disabil Rehabil.* 2004;26(5):253–261.
3. Gordon W, Safonte R, Cicerone K. Traumatic brain injury rehabilitation: state of the science. *Am J Phys Med Rehabil.* 2006;85:343–382.
4. Kozlowski O, Pollez B, Thevenon A, Dhellemmes P, Rousseaux M. Devenir et qualité de vie trois ans dans une cohorte de patients traumatisés cr niens graves [Outcome and quality of life after three years in a cohort of patients with severe traumatic brain injury]. *Ann Readapt Med Phys.* 2002;45(8):466–473.
5. Whiteneck GG, Gerhart KA, Cusick CP. Identifying environmental factors that influence the outcomes of people with traumatic brain injury. *J Head Trauma Rehabil.* 2004;19(3):191–204.
6. Martelli M, Zasler N, Tiernan P. Skill acquisition and automatic process development after brain injury: a holistic habit retraining model (HHR) for community re-entry. *Brain Injury/Professional.* 2009;2(2):10–16.
7. Reynolds F. Coping with chronic illness and disability through creative needlecraft. *Br J Occup Ther.* 1997;60(8):352–356.
8. Suto M. Leisure in occupational therapy. *Can J Occup Ther.* 1998;65(5):271–278.
9. Scanlan J, Bundy A, Matthews L. Investigating the relationship between meaningful time use and health in 18- to 25-year-old un/underemployed people in New South Wales, Australia. *J Community Appl Soc Psychol.* 2010;20(3):232–247.
10. Lobo F. The leisure and work occupations of young people: a review. *J Occup Sci.* 1999;6(1):27–33.
11. Hoofien D, Gilboa A, Vakil E, Donovick PJ. Traumatic brain injury (TBI) 10? 20 years later: a comprehensive outcome study of psychiatric symptomatology, cognitive abilities and psychosocial functioning. *Brain Inj.* 2001;15(3):189–209.
12. Eriksson G, Kottorp A, Borg J, Tham K. Relationship between occupational gaps in everyday life, depressive mood and life satisfaction after acquired brain injury. *J Rehabil Med.* 2009;41(3):187–194.
13. Steadman-Pare D, Colantonio A, Ratcliff G, Chase S, Vernich L. Factors associated with perceived quality of life many years after traumatic brain injury. *J Head Trauma Rehabil.* 2001;16(4):330.
14. Teasdale TW, Engberg A. Subjective well-being and quality of life following traumatic brain injury in adults: a long-term population-based follow-up. *Brain Inj.* 2005;19(12):1041–1048.
15. Wilson B. Neuropsychological rehabilitation. *Neuropsychol Rehabil.* 2008;4:141–162.
16. Jensen LA, Allen MN. A synthesis of qualitative research on wellness-illness. *Qual Health Res.* 1994;4(4):349–369.
17. World Health Organization. *Atlas: Country Resources for Neurological Disorders.* Geneva, Switzerland: World Health Organization; 2004.
18. Cicerone K, Azulay J. Perceived self-efficacy and life satisfaction after traumatic brain injury. *J Head Trauma Rehabil.* 2007;22:257–266.
19. Yerxa E, Clark F, Frank G, et al. An introduction to occupational science, a foundation for occupational therapy in the 21st century. *Occup Ther in Health Care.* 1990;6(4):1–17.
20. Peterson CA, Stumbo NJ, Lee S. *Therapeutic Recreation Program Design: Principles and Procedures.* Massachusetts, MA: Allyn and Bacon; 2000.
21. Kleiber DA, Hutchinson SL, Williams R. Leisure as a resource in transcending negative life events: self-protection, self-restoration, and personal transformation. *Leisure Sci.* 2002;24(2):219–235.
22. Sellar B, Stanley M. Leisure. In: Curtin M, Molineux M, Supyk J, eds. *Occupational Therapy and Physical Dysfunction: Enabling Occupation.* 6th ed. Oxford, United Kingdom: Elsevier; 2009:357–369.
23. Godbey G. *Leisure in Your Life.* 6th ed. Pennsylvania, PA: Venture Publishing Inc; 2003;357–369.
24. Kinney W, Coyle C. Predicting life satisfaction among adults with physical disabilities. *Arch Phys Med Rehabil.* 1992;73(9):863–869.
25. Lyons RF. Meaningful activity and disability: capitalizing upon the potential of outreach recreation networks in Canada. *Can J Rehabil.* 1993;6(4):256–265.

26. Larsson A, Nystrom C, Vikstrom S, Walfridsson T, Soderback I. Computer-assisted cognitive rehabilitation for adults with traumatic brain damage: four case studies. *Occup Ther Int.* 1995;2(3): 166–189.

27. Hutchinson SL, Loy DP, Kleiber DA, Dattilo J. Leisure as a coping resource: variations in coping with traumatic injury and illness. *Leisure Sci.* 2003;25(2):143–161.

28. Wise EK, Mathews-Dalton C, Dikmen S, et al. Impact of traumatic brain injury on participation in leisure activities. *Arch Phys Med Rehabil.* 2010;91(9):1357–1362.

29. Kleiber DA, Brock SC, Lee Y, Dattilo J, Caldwell L. The relevance of leisure in an illness experience: realities of spinal cord injury. *J Leisure Res.* 1995;27(3):283–299.

30. Swanson JM, Chenitz WC. Regaining a valued self: the process of adaptation to living with genital herpes. *Qual Health Res.* 1993;3(3): 270–297.

31. Kleiber DA, Reel HA, Hutchinson SL. When distress gives way to possibility: the relevance of leisure in adjustment to disability. *NeuroRehabilitation.* 2008;23(4):321–328.

32. Pentland W, Harvey AS, Walker J. The relationships between time use and health and well-being in men with spinal cord injury. *J Occup Sci.* 1998;5:14–25.

33. Fenech A. Inspiring transformations through participation in drama for individuals with neuropalliative conditions. *J Appl Arts Health.* 2010;1(1):63–80.

34. Stebbins RA. Leisure and its relationship to library and: information science: bridging the gap. *Libr Trends.* 2009;57(4):618–631.

35. Parry DC, Shinew KJ. The constraining impact of infertility on women's leisure lifestyles. *Leisure Sci.* 2004;26(3):295–308.

36. Russell RV, Stage FK. Leisure as burden: Sudanese refugee women. *J Leisure Res.* 1996;28(2):108–121.

37. Backman SJ. An investigation of the relationship between activity loyalty and perceived constraints. *J Leisure Res.* 1991;23:332–344.

38. Bier N, Dutil E, Couture M. Factors affecting leisure participation after a traumatic brain injury: an exploratory study. *J Head Trauma Rehabil.* 2009;24(3):187.

39. Douglas JM, Dyson M, Foreman P. Increasing leisure activity following severe traumatic brain injury: does it make a difference? *Brain Impairment.* 2006;7(2):107–118.

40. Iso-Ahola SE, Park CJ. Leisure-related social support and self-determination as buffers of stress-illness relationship. *J Leisure Res.* 1996;28(3):169–187.

41. Primeau LA. Work and leisure: transcending the dichotomy. *Am J Occup Ther.* 1996;50(7):569–577.

42. Kelly JR, Freysinger VJ. *21st Century Leisure: Current Issues.* Boston, MA: Allyn & Bacon; 2000.

43. Christiansen C, Townsend E. An introduction to occupation. In: Christiansen C, Townsend, E, eds. *Introduction to Occupation: The Art & Science of Living.* Upper Saddle River, NJ: Prentice Hall; 2003: 251–279.

44. Tinsley HEA, Tinsley DJ. A theory of the attributes, benefits, and causes of leisure experience. *Leisure Sci.* 1986;8(1):1–45.

45. Leng TR, Woodward MJ, Stokes MJ, Swan AV, Wareing LA, Baker R. Effects of multisensory stimulation in people with Huntington's disease: a randomized controlled pilot study. *Clin Rehabil.* 2003; 17(1):30–41.

46. Howell J, Pearce J. *Civil Society and Development: A critical Exploration.* Boulder, CO: Lynne Rienner Publishers; 2002.

47. Houghton Mifflin Company. *The American Heritage® Dictionary of the English Language.* 4th ed. Orlando, FL: Houghton Mifflin Company; 2009.

48. Merriam-Webster Inc. *Merriam-Webster Collegiate Dictionary.* 11th ed. Springfield, IL: HarperCollins Publishers Inc; 2003.

49. Canadian Association of Occupational Therapists. CAOT position statement: occupations and health. 2008. http://www.caot.ca/default.asp?pageid=2326. Accessed June 30, 2012.

50. Samuels T. What do occupations mean to people? *Occup Ther News.* 2007;16(8):28.

51. Barnes M, Ward A. *Textbook of Rehabilitation Medicine.* Oxford, FL: Oxford University Press; 2000.

52. Bergquist TF, Jackets MP. Awareness and goal setting with the traumatically brain injured. *Brain Inj.* 1993;7(3):275–282.

53. Carlson J. Evaluating patient motivation in physical disabilities practice settings. *Am J Occup Ther.* 1996;51(7):347–351.

54. Rebeiro KL, Cook JV. Opportunity, not prescription: an exploratory study of the experience of occupational engagement. *Can J Occup Ther.* 1999;66(4):176–187.

55. Wilcock A. A theory of the human need for occupation. *J Occup Sci.* 1993;1(1):17–24.

56. Specht J, King G, Brown E, Foris C. The importance of leisure in the lives of persons with congenital physical disabilities. *Am J Occup Ther.* 2002;56(4):436.

57. Dare B, Welton G, Coe W. *Concepts of Leisure in Western Thought: A Critical and Historical Analysis.* Dubuque, IA: Kendall/Hunt; 1987.

58. Institute of Medicine. *Long–Term Consequences of Traumatic Brain Injury. Gulf War and Health.* Washington, DC: National Academies Press; 2009.

59. Phipps S, Richardson P. Occupational therapy outcomes for clients with traumatic brain injury and stroke using the Canadian Occupational Performance Measure. *Am J Occup Ther.* 2007;61(3):328.

60. Turner BJ, Ownsworth TL, Turpin M, Fleming JM, Griffin J. Self-identified goals and the ability to set realistic goals following acquired brain injury: a classification framework. *Aust Occup Ther J.* 2008;55(2):96–107.

61. Jongbloed L, Morgan D. An investigation of involvement in leisure activities after a stroke. *Am J Occup Ther.* 1991;45(5):420–427.

62. Drummond A, Walker M. Generalisation of the effects of leisure rehabilitation for stroke individuals. *Br J Occup Ther.* 1996;59(7): 330–334.

63. Pollock N, Stewart D. A survey of activity patterns and vocational readiness of young adults with physical disabilities. *Can J Rehabil.* 1990;4(1):17–26.

64. Csikszentmihalyi M. Activity & happiness toward a science of occupation. *J Occup Sci.* 1993;1(1):38–42.

65. Stebbins RA. Casual leisure: a conceptual statement. *Leisure Stud.* 2001;16(1):17–25.

66. Lockwood R, Lockwood A. Recreation priorities for people with disabilities in Western Australia. *Aust J Leisure and Recreation.* 1991; 1(3):7–13.

67. Laliberte-Rudman D. Linking occupation and identity: lessons learned through qualitative exploration. *J Occup Sci.* 2002;9(1): 12–19.

68. Turner A. Occupation for therapy. In: Turner A, Foster M, Johnson S, eds. *Occupational Therapy and Physical Dysfunction: Principles, Skills and Practice.* 5th ed. Oxford, FL: Churchill Livingstone; 2002.

69. Minato M, Zemke R. Time use of people with schizophrenia living in the community. *Occup Ther Int.* 2004;11(3):177–191.

70. Weeder TC. Comparison of temporal patterns and meaningfulness of the daily activities of schizophrenic and normal adults. *Occup Ther Ment Health.* 1986;6(4):27–48.

71. Farnworth L. Doing, being, and boredom. *J Occup Sci.* 1998;5: 140–146.

72. Whiteford G. Occupational deprivation: global challenge in the new millennium. *Br J Occup Ther.* 2000;63(5):200–204.

73. World Health Organization. *International Classification of Impairments, Disabilities, and Handicaps.* Geneva, Switzerland: World Health Organization; 1980.

74. Larson K. Activity patterns and life changes in people with depression. *Am J Occup Ther.* 1990;44(10):902–906.

75. Passmore A. Does leisure support and underpin adolescents' developing worker role? *J Occup Sci.* 1998;5:161–165.

76. Home Office. The integration of refugees: positive practice for health professionals. 2006. http://www.nrif.homeoffice.gov.uk/Health/SpecialistSupport/ClinicalAreas/occupationaltherapy.asp?oi=06-04-18. Accessed April 15, 2011.

77. Whiteford G. Understanding the occupational deprivation of refugees: a case study from Kosovo. *Can J Occup Ther.* 2005;72(2):78–88.

78. Wilcock AA. Reflections on doing, being and becoming. *Aust Occup Ther J.* 1999;46(1):1–11.

79. Edwards R, Telfair J, Cecil H, Lenoci J. Self-efficacy as a predictor of adult adjustment to sickle cell disease: one-year outcomes. *Psychos Med.* 2001;63(5):850–858.

80. Schwartz CE, Coulthard-Morris L. Measuring self-efficacy in people with multiple sclerosis: a validation study. *Arch Phys Med Rehabil.* 1996;77(4):394–398.

81. Rosen JW, Burchard SN. Community activities and social support networks: a social comparison of adults with and adults without mental retardation. *Educ Train Ment Retard.* 1990;25(2):193–204.

82. Wilcock A. The occupational brain: a theory of human nature. *J Occup Sci.* 1995;2:68–73.

83. Christiansen CH. Defining lives: occupation as identity: an essay on competence, coherence, and the creation of meaning. *Am J Occup Ther.* 1999;53(6):547–558.

84. Unruh A. Reflections on: "So . . . what do you do?" occupation and the construction of identity. *Can J Occup Ther.* 2004;71(5):290.

85. Kleiber D, Kirshnit C. Sport involvement & identity formation. In: Diamant L, ed. *Mind-Body Maturity: Psychological Approaches to Sports, Exercise, and Fitness.* New York, NY: Hemisphere Pub. Corporation; 1991.

86. Reynolds F. Reclaiming a positive identity in chronic illness through artistic occupation. *OTJR.* 2003;23(3):118.

87. Charmaz K. The self as habit: the reconstruction of self in chronic illness. *OTJR.* 2002;22(1):31s–41s.

88. Whiteford G. When people cannot participate: occupational deprivation. In: Christiansen C, Townsend E, eds. *An Introduction to Occupation: The Art and Science of Living.* New Jersey, NJ: Prentice Hall; 2003:221–242.

89. Connors M, Harrison A, Akins F. *Living Aloft: Human Requirements for Extended Spaceflight. (NASA Special Publications No. 483).* Washington, DC: National Aeronautics & Space Administration; 1985.

90. Hammell KW. Reflections on well-being and occupational rights. *Can J Occup Ther.* 2008;75(1):61–64.

91. Whiteford G. Occupational deprivation and incarceration. *J Occup Sci.* 1997;4:126–130.

92. Zauberman G, Levav J, Diehl K, Bhargave R. 1995 feels so close yet so far: the effect of event markers on subjective feelings of elapsed time. *Psychol Sci.* 2010;21(1):133–139.

93. Christiansen CH. Three perspectives on balance in occupation. In: Zemke R, Clark F, eds. *Occupational Science: The Evolving Discipline.* Philadelphia, PA: F. A. Davis; 1996:431–451.

94. Farnworth L. Time use, tempo and temporality: occupational therapy's core business or someone else's business. *Aust Occup Ther J.* 2003;50(3):116–126.

95. Zemke R. The 2004 Eleanor Clarke Slagle Lecture—time, space, and the kaleidoscopes of occupation. *Am J Occup Ther.* 2004;58(6):608–620.

96. O'Sullivan G, Hocking C. Positive ageing in residential care. *N Z J Occup Ther.* 2006;53(1):17–23.

97. Wilcock AA. *An Occupational Perspective of Health.* Thorofare, NJ: Slack Inc; 2006.

98. McColl MA, Carlson P, Johnston J, et al. The definition of community integration: perspectives of people with brain injuries. *Brain Inj.* 1998;12(1):15–30.

99. Sloan S, Winkler D, Callaway L. Community integration following traumatic brain injury: outcomes and best practices. *Brain Impairment.* 2004;5(1):12–29.

100. Carter MJ, Van Andel GE, Robb GM. *Therapeutic Recreation: A Practical Approach.* Prospect Heights, IL: Waveland Press; 1995.

101. Armstrong M, Lauzen S. *Community Integration Program.* 2nd ed. Ravensdale, WA: Idyll Arbor; 1994.

102. Karlovitas T, McColl M. Coping with community reintegration after severe brain injury: a description of stresses and coping strategies. *Brain Inj.* 1999;13(11):845–861.

103. Gordon WA, Sliwinski M, Echo J, McLougbliu M, Sheerer M, Meili TE. The benefits of exercise in individuals with traumatic brain injury: a retrospective study. *J Head Trauma Rehabil.* 1998;13(4):58.

104. Driver S, Ede A. Impact of physical activity on mood after TBI. *Brain Inj.* 2009;23(3):203–212.

105. Hoffman JM, Bell KR, Powell JM, et al. A randomized controlled trial of exercise to improve mood after traumatic brain injury. *J Phys Med Rehabil.* 2010;2(10):911–919.

106. Passmore T, Lane S. Exercise as treatment for depression: a therapeutic recreation intervention. *J Sports Med.* 1994;17(2):108–116.

107. Lojovich J. The relationship between aerobic exercise and cognition: is movement medicinal? *J Head Trauma Rehabil.* 2010;25(3):184.

108. Broach E, Dattilo J, Loy D. Therapeutic use of exercise. In: Dattilo J, ed. *Facilitation Techniques in Therapeutic Recreation.* Pennsylvania, PA: Venture Publishing Inc; 2000;355–383.

109. Dattilo J, Loy D, Keeney R. Therapeutic use of sports. In: Dattilo J, ed. *Facilitation Techniques in Recreational Therapy.* Philadelphia, PA: Venture Publishing Inc; 2000;439–475.

110. Hanson CS, Nabavi D, Yuen HK. The effect of sports on level of community integration as reported by persons with spinal cord injury. *Am J Occup Ther.* 2001;55(3):332.

111. Goosey-Tolfrey V, Price M. Physiology of wheelchair sport. In: Goosey-Tolfrey J, ed. *Wheelchair Sport.* Champaign, IL: Human Kinetics; 2010:47–62.

112. Shearer D, Bressan E. Psychological aspects of wheelchair sport. In: Goosey-Tolfrey J, ed. *Wheelchair Sport.* Champaign, IL: Human Kinetics; 2010:99–114.

113. Dec K, Sparrow K, McKeag D. The physically challenged athlete: medical issues and assessment. *J Sports Med.* 2000;29(4):245–258.

114. American Hippotherapy Association. Hippotherapy as a treatment strategy. 2010. http://www.americanhippotherapyassociation.org/hippotherapy/hippotherapy-as-a-treatment-strategy. Accessed May 3, 2011.

115. Bass MM, Duchowny CA, Llabre MM. The effect of therapeutic horseback riding on social functioning in children with autism. *J Autism Dev Disord.* 2009;39(9):1261–1267.

116. Sausser C, Datillo J. Therapeutic horseback riding. In: Datillo J, ed. *Facilitation Techniques in Recreational Therapy.* Philadelphia, PA: Venture Publishing Inc; 2000;273–301.

117. Baker L. Brain injuries and therapeutic riding. *NARHA Strides.* 1996;2(2).

118. Lechner HE, Kakebeeke TH, Hegemann D, Baumberger M. The effect of hippotherapy on spasticity and on mental well-being of persons with spinal cord injury. *Arch Phys Med Rehabil.* 2007;88(10):1241–1248.

119. Meregillano G, Hippotherapy. *Phys Med Rehabil Clin N Am.* 2004;15(4):843–854.

120. Lentini JA, Knox MS. A qualitative and quantitative review of equine facilitated psychotherapy (EFP) with children and adolescents. *Int J Psychosoc Rehabil.* 2008;13(1):17–30.

121. Yorke J, Adams C, Coady N. Therapeutic value of equine human bonding in recovery from trauma. *Anthrozoos.* 2008;21(1):17–30.

121a. Fenech A. (2011). Aquatic Lesure satisfaction and engagement in Neuropalliative Disability Management. Scandinavian Journal of Caring Sciences. doi: 10.1111/j.1471-6712.2011.00958.x

122. Becker BE. Aquatic therapy: scientific foundations and clinical rehabilitation applications. *J Phys Med Rehabil.* 2009;1(9):859–872.

123. Driver S, Rees K, O'Connor J, Lox C. Aquatics, health-promoting self-care behaviours and adults with brain injuries. *Brain Inj.* 2006;20(2):133–141.

124. Getz M, Hutzler Y, Vermeer A. Effects of aquatic interventions in children with neuromotor impairments: a systematic review of the literature. *Clin Rehabil.* 2006;20(11):927–936.

125. Olson S. Get wet! How one PTA took the plunge to advance her career options. *Magazine of Physical Therapy.* March 2009:42–44.

126. Complementary Therapy. Therapy Courses & Training for Practitioners Web site. http://www.healthk.co.uk/holistic.htm. Accessed April 22, 2011.

127. Murrey GJ. Introduction and overview of brain injury in executive dysfunction. In: Murrey GJ, ed. *Alternate Therapies in the Treatment of Brain Injury and Neurobehavioral Disorders: A Practical Guide.* Philadelphia, PA: Haworth Press; 2006:1–5.

128. Magee W, Wheeler B. Music therapy for patients with traumatic brain injury. In: Murrey GJ, ed. *Alternative Therapies in the Treatment of Brain Injury and Neurobehavioral Disorders.* Philadelphia, PA: Haworth Press; 2000:51–65.

129. Magee WL, Bowen C. Using music in leisure to enhance social relationships with patients with complex disabilities. *NeuroRehabilitation.* 2008;23(4):305–311.

130. Wan C, Uber T, Hohmann A, Schlaug G. The therapeutic effects of singing in neurological disorders. *Music perception.* 2010;27(4):287–295.

131. Magee WL. Music as a diagnostic tool in low awareness states: considering limbic responses. *Brain Inj.* 2007;21(6):593–599.

132. Sell M, Murrey G. Art as a therapeutic modality with TBI populations. In: Murrey GJ, ed. *Alternate Therapies in the Treatment of Brain Injury and Neurobehavioral Disorders.* Philadelphia, PA: Haworth Press; 2006:29–49.

133. Alyami A. The integration of art therapy into physical rehabilitation in a Saudi hospital. *Arts Psychother.* 2009;36(5):282–288.

134. Pratt RR. Art, dance, and music therapy. *Phys Med Rehabil Clin N Am.* 2004;15(4):827–841.

135. Riley S. Art therapy with adolescents. *West J Med.* 2001;175(1):54.

136. Lynch RT, Chosa D. Group-oriented community-based expressive arts programming for individuals with disabilities: participant satisfaction and perceptions of psychosocial impact. *J Rehabil.* 1996; 62(3):4154–4160.

137. Blake H, Batson M. Exercise intervention in brain injury: a pilot randomized study of Tai Chi Qigong. *Clin Rehabil.* 2009;23(7): 589–598.

138. Gemmell C, Leathem JM. A study investigating the effects of Tai Chi Chuan: individuals with traumatic brain injury compared to controls. *Brain Inj.* 2006;20(2):151–156.

139. Shapira MY, Chelouche M, Yanai R, Kaner C, Szold A. Tai Chi Chuan practice as a tool for rehabilitation of severe head trauma: 3 case reports. *Arch Phys Med Rehabil.* 2001;82(9):1283–1285.

140. Wolf SL, Coogler C, Xu T. Exploring the basis for Tai Chi Chuan as a therapeutic exercise approach. *Arch Phys Med Rehabil.* 1997; 78(8):886–892.

141. Fenech A. Interactive drama in complex neurological disability management. *Disabil Rehabil.* 2009;31(2):118–130.

142. Fenech A. *Leisure satisfaction of residents at the Royal Hospital for neuro-disability: Audit report 2006.* Unpublished report, 2007.

143. Passmore A, French D. The nature of leisure in adolescence: a focus group study. *Br J Occup Ther.* 2003;66(9):419–426.

144. Dempsey I. Parental roles in the post-school adjustment of their son or daughter with a disability. *J Intellect Dev Disabil.* 1991;17(3): 313–320.

145. Larson EA, Zemke R. Shaping the temporal patterns of our lives: the social coordination of occupation. *J Occup Sci.* 2003;10(2):80–89.

146. Crombie IK, Irvine L, Williams B, et al. Why older people do not participate in leisure time physical activity: a survey of activity levels, beliefs and deterrents. *Age Ageing.* 2004;33(3):287–292.

147. Stebbins R. Fun, enjoyable, satisfying, fulfilling: describing positive leisure experience. *Leisure Stud Assoc Newsl.* 2004;69:8–11.

148. Wilhite B, Keller MJ, Hodges J, Caldwell L. Enhancing human development and optimizing health and well-being in persons with multiple sclerosis. *Ther Recreation J.* 2004;38:167–187.

149. Engelhardt H. Defining occupational therapy: the meaning of therapy and the virtues of occupation. *Am J Occup Ther.* 1977;31: 666–672.

150. Meyer A. The philosophy of occupational therapy. *Am J Occup Ther.* 1977;35(10):639–642.

151. Yerxa E. Authentic occupational therapy, 1966 Eleanor Clarke Slagle lecture. *Am J Occup Ther.* 1967;21(1):1–9.

152. Vrkljan B, Miller-Polgar J. Meaning of occupational engagement in life-threatening illness: a qualitative pilot project. *Can J Occup Ther.* 2001;68(4):237.

153. Bartalos MK. Work, health, and recreation: aspects of the total person. *Loss, grief & care.* 1993;6(4):7–14.

154. Mikulas WL, Vodanovich SJ. The essence of boredom. *Psychological Rec.* 1993.

155. Long C. On watching paint dry: an exploration of boredom. In: Molineux M, ed. *Occupation for Occupational Therapists.* Oxford, UK: Blackwell Publishing Ltd; 2004.

156. Berlyne D. Curiosity & exploration. *Science.* 1966;153(3731):25–33.

157. Cervone D. The architecture of personality. *Psychol Rev.* 2004; 111(1):183–204.

158. Zuckerman M. *Psychobiology of Personality.* Cambridge, MA: Cambridge University Press; 1991.

159. Zuckerman M. The psychophysiology of sensation seeking. *J Pers.* 1990;58(1):313–345.

160. Klapp OE. *Overload and Boredom: Essays on the Quality of Life in the Information Society.* Wesport, CT: Greenwood Press; 1986.

161. Molineux M, Whiteford G. Prisons: from occupational deprivation to occupational enrichment. *J Occup Sci.* 1999;6:124–130.

162. Reynolds F, Prior S. 'A lifestyle coat-hanger': a phenomenological study of the meanings of artwork for women coping with chronic illness and disability. *Disabil Rehabil.* 2003;25(14):785–794.

163. Reynolds F, Prior S. Creative adventures and flow in art-making: a qualitative study of women living with cancer. *Br J Occup Ther.* 2006;69(6):255–262.

164. Schmid T. *Promoting Health Through Creativity: For Professionals in Health, Arts and Education.* London, UK: Wiley Blackwell; 2005.

165. Tinsley H. I am wanting to tell you: reply to Borgen (1995) and Dawis (1995). *J Couns Psychol.* 1995;42(2):138–140.

166. Cohen G. *The Creative Age: Awakening Human Potential in the Second Half of Life.* New York, NY: Avon Books/ Harper Collins; 2000.

167. Markus HR, Kitayama S. Culture and the self: implications for cognition, emotion, and motivation. *Psychol Rev.* 1991;98(2):224.

168. Andersen SM, Chen S. The relational self: an interpersonal social-cognitive theory. *Psychol Rev.* 2002;109(4):619–645.

169. Prigatano GP. Work, love, and play after brain injury. *Bull Menninger Clin.* 1989;53:414–443.

170. Barnett LA. Measuring the ABCs of leisure experience: awareness, boredom, challenge, distress. *Leisure Sci.* 2005;27(2):131–155.

171. Caldwell LL. Leisure and health: why is leisure therapeutic? *Br J Guid Counsell.* 2005;33(1):7–26.

172. Dickie VA. The role of learning in quilt making. *J Occup Sci.* 2003; 10(3):120–129.

173. Lazzarini I. Neuro-occupation: the nonlinear dynamics of intention, meaning and perception. *J Occup Ther.* 2004;67(8):342–352.

174. Maslow AH. A theory of human motivation. *Psychol Rev.* 1943; 50(4):370–396.

175. Baxter R, Frel K, Mcatamney A, White B, Williamson S. *Leisure Enhancement Through Occupational Therapy.* London, United Kingdom: College of Occupational Therapists; 1995.

176. Nelson DL. Occupation: form and performance. *Am J Occup Ther.* 1988;42(10):633–641.

177. Bandura A. Cultivate self-efficacy for personal and organizational effectiveness. In: EA Locke, ed. *Handbook of Principles of Organization Behavior.* Oxford, UK: Blackwell; 2000:120–136.

178. Crocker J, Wolfe CT. Contingencies of self-worth. *Psychol Rev.* 2001; 108(3):593–623.

179. Ryan RM, Deci EL. Self-determination theory and the facilitation of intrinsic motivation, social development, and well-being. *Am Psychol.* 2000;55(1):68–78.

180. Coleman D, Iso-Ahola S. Leisure & health: the role of social support & self -determination. *J Leisure Res.* 1993;25(2):111–128.

181. Passmore A. The occupation of leisure: three typologies and their influence on mental health in adolescence. *OTJR.* 2003;23(2): 76–83.

182. Kagawa-Singer M. Redefining health: living with cancer. *Soc Sci Med.* 1993;37(3):295–304.

183. Passmore T. Coverage of therapeutic recreation in clinical settings. 2011. http://www.mendeley.com/research/coverage-not-reimbursement-recreational-therapy-four-primary-treatment-settings/ Accessed June 30, 2012.

184. Passmore T. Coverage, not primary reimbursement, of recreational therapy in the four primary treatment settings. *Am J Recreation Ther.* 2007;6(3):27–34.

185. Hannan M. Corporate connection. *Parks and Recreation.* 2011. http://www.nxtbook.com/nxtbooks/nrpa/201104. Accessed June 30, 2012.

186. Vance D. The value of partnerships: Kansas Recreation and Parks Association partners its way to success. *Parks and Recreation.* 2011; 46(2):14–16.

XIX

MEDICOLEGAL AND ETHICAL ISSUES

Ethics in Brain Injury Medicine

John D. Banja and Joseph J. Fins

INTRODUCTION

Epidemiologic data on the annual incidence of traumatic brain injury (TBI) in the United States suggest that more than 50,000 persons die from TBI every year; more than 1.3 million persons with head injuries are admitted to the emergency departments annually; medical costs and lost productivity costs consume about $60 billion a year; approximately 275,000 persons are hospitalized because of TBI every year; and, of that number, 60,000–80,000 sustain catastrophic life-long impairments (1,2). Thus, like "cancer survivors" or "air crash survivors," we speak of brain injury "survivors" to underline the extremely disturbing scope and gravity of serious brain injury.

What is perhaps ethically distinctive about brain injury is not simply the massive physical, psychological, and economic harm it wreaks but the way a serious brain injury causes massive disruption of "self" (3). If one understands the core function of self as "integrational,"—meaning the way the self integrates motor, cognitive, and behavioral activity into rational, goal-directed, and adaptive behavior—then serious brain injury disrupts the vital neural networks that enable those functions and their integration to occur (4). As other chapters in this volume show, the hallmark symptoms of serious brain injury such as impairments in attention, memory, language, emotional regulation, and executive function rob the individual of the ability to navigate his or her world effectively. He or she cannot engage or relate to the world and to others in an adaptive or productive way such that persons with serious brain injury commonly become socially and economically marginalized. Indeed, laypersons who are not acquainted with the physical and psychological manifestations of serious brain injury are often extremely uncomfortable being around persons with brain injury and so avoid them (5).

Ethical issues involving persons with brain injury occur in 2 major ways: The first involves difficulties in evaluating their ability (or inability) to behave in ways that are under their control, that are not unreasonably harmful to themselves or others, that comply with ethical and legal rules or expectations governing social behavior, and that are geared at producing benefits or desirable ends (6). Persons who cannot perform within the parameters that roughly define "acceptable" behavior will almost certainly face formal or informal attempts to restrict their freedoms, such as being prohibited from driving an automobile, running a business, or making decisions about their medical care. Consequently, a prominent ethical concern involves a plethora of issues connected with evolving and applying fair and just procedures and rules to persons with TBI when their individual freedoms and liberties are at stake.

The second ethical dilemma that persons with serious brain injury present challenges our moral intuitions about what we "owe" them (7). The social, economic, medical, physical, and psychological needs of such individuals can be considerable and even overwhelming. What kind of quality of life are they owed if they cannot provide such for themselves? What do we owe persons with disability in facilitating their "mainstreaming" into meaningful vocational and social life? To what extent should our society commit resources toward preventing brain injury given other competing health care priorities? How much care is owed to the person with serious brain injury if economic resources, such as the scope of that individual's insurance benefits, are extremely limited? Would certain persons with catastrophic brain injury be better off dead and how does one make and effect such determinations?

This chapter will survey certain dimensions of these problems. Space does not permit exploring any of them in the depth they deserve so the reader will be referred to some relevant literature. Nevertheless, the reader should be able to discern the enormous range of ethical dilemmas associated with brain injury, the difficulties they present, and the limited degree to which ethical theory, moral reasoning, and a nation's political will are capable of resolving them.

AUTONOMY

Concepts like individual freedom, liberty, and autonomy are at the heart of the sociopolitical ethos of America and other liberal democracies. Individuals are granted considerable leeway in exercising their self-determinative rights even to the point of self-harm as long as they are sufficiently aware of the nature and possible consequences of their behavior and desist from acting in ways that pose an unreasonable risk of harm to others (8,9). As virtually every health professional knows, respecting "patient autonomy" is a categorical moral obligation in clinical environments, which invites the question of what the term as well as what its moral requirements entail.

Aspects of Autonomy

A popular characterization of autonomy—whose Latin roots *auto* and *nomos* mean "self-rule"—understands it as consisting of 3 parts. The first aspect is that a decision or action made autonomously is "authentic" when it is congruent with one's "real" or true preferences and values. In explaining this, theorists like Gerald Dworkin and Harry Frankfurt have popularized the idea of first- and second-order beliefs and desires (10,11). A first-order desire is immediate and unreflective, whereas a second-order belief or desire reflects on the first-order and assesses it in light of its reasonableness or acceptability, as in "is this desire of mine really desirable?" or "is this belief, wish, or desire consistent with what I truly hold, or what I understand to be in my best interest? Is it consistent with whom I take myself to be?" Consequently, an individual who is excessively rash and impulsive; who is unable to impose rationally induced restraints on his or her first-order desires; who cannot envision the likely consequences of his or her decisions or behavior; or who simply cannot fashion a consistent and adaptive set of beliefs about and responses to the world could not be said to be acting autonomously (12).

The second aspect of autonomy, which is somewhat related to the first, is the capacity for rationality. Autonomous agents can envision the consequences of their behavior and assess whether or not those consequences have sufficient use to endorse or reject an associated behavioral plan. Importantly, they do not only understand the components of their action plans—why they are considering this or that plan, what it entails, what alternatives are available, and so forth—they are also able to identify and calculate the various burdens and benefits involved in the undertakings and their alternatives, and whether or not they will yield sufficient value or "net use." Consequently, an individual who cannot process the cognitive and affective variables affecting his or her decisions, who cannot use them to make utility determinations, who lacks insight into how an action or plan will ultimately affect him or her or other people, and who cannot remember lessons learned from previous experiences to fashion future adaptive decisions and action plans will fail this second aspect of autonomy (13).

The third aspect of autonomy is to exercise control or be free from factors that might unduly influence one's decisions or actions or that compromise or disrupt Frankfurt and Dworkin's second-order set of reflective capacities mentioned previously. The most obvious factors would be an oppressive government, group, or a significant other who unreasonably interferes with one's preferred choices and behaviors. Other factors might include irresistible temptations or coercions to choose or do what one normally wouldn't and shouldn't do. Thus, an individual might have a personality disorder marked by extremely brittle self-esteem and be easily manipulated to act in ill-advised ways to gain peer approval. Or an addictive disorder might diminish one's control over making choices that are conducive to his or her welfare. In these situations, one's control of oneself is being compromised by something that biases, alters, or "poisons" one's thinking, deciding, or acting and, hence, compromises one's autonomy (14).

Limiting Autonomy

Given autonomy's requiring a healthy or adaptive integration of rationality with one's deciding, choosing, and acting, the individual with brain injury can easily find his or her autonomy diminished. A substantive ethical challenge occurs when someone in authority, such as a health professional, perceives some kind of diminution of autonomy in the behavior of someone with brain injury and wonders about whether or not to intervene. Two questions immediately arise: whether or not that perceived loss of autonomy requires some kind of intervention—such as a "competency evaluation"—and, depending on the degree and nature of autonomy loss, how aggressive any intervention should be in view of the fact that the individual's rights are at stake. As will be discussed subsequently, the mere fact that some people make eccentric decisions or choices, not to mention very risky or ill-advised ones, does not necessarily imply that the individual lacks autonomy or capacity.

Consequently, although autonomy connotes a theoretical construct that speaks to an individual's right to his or her self-determinative interests and goals, determining that individual's "capacity" to exercise his or her presumptive autonomy constitutes the practical challenge of deciding whether or how much autonomy an individual can be allowed to retain (15). Thus, one might have the capacity and therefore be able to exercise his or her autonomy in raising children but not in managing a business. Or a person might have the capacity and be allowed to function autonomously in living alone but not be allowed to drive an automobile. Assessing capacity, or its legal designation "competency," is where the rubber of autonomy hits the road of rights.

COMPETENCE

Human life is replete with functional "domains." Consider an average day in the life of many adults. They rise from sleep and wash, groom, and dress themselves; help their children get ready for school; travel to work; perform their job responsibilities; eat, drink, and maintain personal hygiene; socially engage with numerous others; manage their money; spend meaningful and productive time with and help family members; maintain their homes; entertain themselves and others; pursue their hobbies; and take rest. Involved in each of these domains is an astonishing range of "know-how" skills requiring the mastery of a staggering array of cognitive, motor, affective, and relational behaviors. Consequently, whatever significantly affects their expression or adequate performance, such as a serious brain injury, will call attention to an individual's autonomous right to perform the associated acts. In resolving questions over one's autonomy, then, the individual's "capacity" to function adequately in the domain under question—for example, manage his or her finances, live alone, make medical decisions, drive, raise a family, and so forth—such that he or she does not constitute a harm to himself or herself or others, will be of signal concern.

Competence to Make Medical Decisions

A schema that is frequently used to determine whether or not a patient has the decisional capacity or "competence" to participate in decisions affecting his or her health care was developed by Paul Applebaum and Thomas Grisso (16). It consists of 4 critical domains:

- Can the patient *express a choice* or decision? Individuals who entirely lack communicative ability would fail this first test. Such persons might be in coma or a vegetative state, or they might be psychotic or delirious or babble incoherently.
- Can the patient *understand* whatever information is relevant and critical to his or her decision making? Individuals with serious attentional, memory, or comprehensional deficits might fail this test.
- Can the patient *reason* appropriately? Can the patient think logically, coherently, and abstractly? Given his or her comprehension of relevant information, can he or she make inferences and think in a way that indicates a sound enough ability to use and integrate cognitive materials and data (e.g., values, beliefs, factual information, opinions) such that his or her decision or choice appears authentic or sufficiently justified?
- Can the patient *appreciate* his or her circumstances, especially in recognizing that his or her choice making will directly impact him or her? This domain especially involves the capacity for being insightful and realistic. Patients who are in profound denial, who engage in magical thinking, or who cannot project consequences and imagine what those consequences would feel like would fail this domain.

In matters of informed consent, these 4 domains are tested against the patient's ability to process informed consent information and arrive at a justifiable decision (17). Informed consent information typically includes materials that explain why a patient might require a particular intervention, what that intervention will be like, what benefits might be expected from it, what risks are entailed by the procedure, the success probability of the intervention, the nature of alternative treatment, their associated risks and benefits, and the likely outcome if the patient decides on doing nothing (18).

The term "competency" is often used interchangeably with capacity, but its technical meaning is reserved for legal adjudications of a patient's decision making or functioning (6). In other words, if the patient fails a formal "competency assessment," then the courts will constrain his or her right to exercise whatever competency capacity or domain is in question. Most often, the court will appoint a proxy or surrogate to make decisions or choices on the patient's behalf (9). If, over time, the individual adequately regains his or her ability, the surrogate is morally obliged to surrender his or her authority to honor the return of the individual's autonomy. Doing so would require another appearance in court, however, which could be cumbersome and expensive (9,19).

Surrogacy

In practice, a court-authorized adjudication of an individual's competency and appointment of a proxy or surrogate occur less often than a more informal arrangement whereby a significant other, who is usually a family member, assumes the role of caretaker and authorizes decisions on the individual's behalf (6). Furthermore, in matters directly pertinent to one's capacity to participate in health care decision making, many states have statutes that list those individuals who can consent or refuse treatment for patients who cannot do so on their own (20). Frequently, those lists begin with granting decisional authority to a court-appointed individual such as a guardian, then recognize someone named in the patient's advance directive (such as in a living will or durable power of attorney for health care), then a spouse, adult child, parents, or next of kin.

Nevertheless, many individuals with serious neurological disorders and obviously diminished cognitive capacity might go years without a court-authorized decision maker because family members skillfully and lovingly take over the person's care. Problems, often heart-rending ones, emerge when circumstances force the legal appointment of a proxy or surrogate, such as when family members can no longer care for the individual, or when the individual has considerable wealth or property that he or she can no longer manage, or when the individual with brain injury receives a substantial amount of money from an inheritance or a legal settlement (perhaps occurring from a personal injury lawsuit) (21). At that point, the appointment of a surrogate or guardian might itself be fraught with problems, such as when no family member is available or willing to perform the role or when multiple people quarrel for the designation. Other cases have witnessed legally appointed surrogates, especially ones having authority for managing the individual's money, being accused of defrauding their ward by making off with his or her wealth (21). Fortunately, many states have enacted statutes that impose rigorous documentation and constraints on such financial guardians so that an opportunity to defraud their wards is virtually eliminated (21).

Along these lines, it should be noted that competency evaluations should be as "domain specific" as possible unless the individual is obviously globally incompetent (such as someone in coma or a vegetative state). This means that although a professional evaluating a patient's health care decision making will usually be a psychologist or psychiatrist, if the competency domain in question is driving, then a driving instructor or police officer might perform the evaluation; if the competency domain is living by oneself, then a home economist, occupational therapist, or recreational therapist might be the appropriate individual to perform the evaluation (17). In any case, an actual legal proceeding aimed at assessing someone's competency to make out a will, raise a family, or manage his or her money is do X is a very serious undertaking because it threatens to constrict an individual's legal right to do so (9).

Neurodiversity, Neurotypicality, and Competence

Disability and mental health activists have complained about a "neurotypicality" bias and charged that it unjustly oppresses many persons whose "neurodifferences" cause them to fall outside the boundaries of neurotypical functioning (22). These latter individuals constitute the "neurodiverse" population among us—persons who are easily recognized by their eccentric cognitive, behavioral, or affective presentations, but who might nevertheless, so the argument goes, have every right to exercise their choices and decisions. Robin Mackenzie and John Watts recently enumerated certain neurological disorders whose representatives might qualify as neurodiverse: autism spectrum disorder, attention deficit hyperactivity disorder (ADHD), Tourette syndrome, oppositional defiance disorder, dyspraxia, dyslexia, dyscalculia, bipolar disorder, schizophrenia, and Parkinson disease (23). Their point is that an individual might display these disorders or impairments but nevertheless be able to make authentic choices and decisions that should be honored and suffer no unreasonable interference.

Although Mackenzie and Watts do not put persons with brain injury on their list, certain ones could easily qualify as neurodiverse. Anyone who has been around persons with brain injury for any length of time will appreciate how some will present with odd or unusual behaviors that can easily be mistaken for impaired competency.

Affective Disorders and Neurodiversity

A matter of special and recent interest in the context of neurodiversity is how the presence of an *affective* disorder might impact someone's competence. For example, Applebaum and Grisso's template for assessing competence to consent to medical treatment has been criticized for its "cognitive bias" in terms of the emphasis they place on reasoning, understanding, communicating, valuing, and appreciating (22). Over the last 20 years and especially since the publication of Antonio Damasio's *Descartes' Error* (23), however, neuroscientists have underlined the critical role our *affective neural circuitry* plays in framing judgments and decisions. In contrast to Plato's or Kant's repeated cautions and worries about how feelings and emotions disturb rationality and reasoning, recent neuroscientific research indicates that "pure" reason unaided by feeling would be totally at a loss in assisting an individual to make adaptive decisions and be able to navigate his or her world (23). This body of research is too elaborate to survey here so the reader is directed to literature authored by Damasio (23), Charland (24), and Halpern and Arnold (25). Suffice to say, however, that feelings and emotions are thought to play utterly critical roles in directing attention, making valuative decisions, initiating actions, engaging socially, and pursuing and obtaining goals. They are also thought to be indispensable in learning and practicing moral behavior, as evidenced by fairly recent research on sociopathic and psychopathic behavior (23). Neurodiversity activists take this material, however, and turn it on its head: they argue that although impaired affect may indeed occasionally compromise the kinds of reasoning skills necessary for competent decision making, its appearance is sometimes *mistaken* as a frank lack of competence resulting in the individual's being deprived of his or her rights (22).

This discussion of neurodiversity, especially because it involves affective impairments, should be of keen interest to professionals who provide brain injury care. Persons with brain injury often present with a variety of affective impairments such as depression, anxiety, mania, flat or absent affect, or even altered personality. Perhaps the most obvious manifestation of their affective disorder is the difference between their expressions of feelings and the kinds of feelings "neurotypical" people commonly exhibit in a given situational context. Because feeling disorders can dramatically affect decisions and behaviors, brain injury clinicians must be keen to evaluate their interaction (26,27). To take only 1

example, consider how research on anxiety suggests how it can heighten one's aversion to risk—thus prompting an anxious individual to refuse a treatment he should have because he has unreasonably exaggerated its risks—vs how research on hypoemotionality shows how it can exacerbate risk taking because the individual's risk perception has been damaged (12).

The neurodiversity advocate would grant all this but might respond with the following challenge: suppose the individual *prior to his or her brain injury* was markedly risk-averse, was a risk-taker, or expressed little or exaggerated emotionality or feeling? In other words, suppose those behaviors were characteristic of his or her personality? If no one interfered with him or her *prior to injury* because his or her behavior was tolerable, it would seem a violation of this individual's rights to take advantage of his or her injury now in order to constrain a behavior we simply don't approve of. If authentic behavior implies behavior that is congruent and consistent with a person's identity over time, then the neurodiversity advocate would argue that we must honor that behavior despite its displeasing us as long as it doesn't unreasonably threaten the individual or others (28). Thus, it is morally interesting to review the list of neurodiversity candidates—for example, persons with autism, Tourette, ADHD, and so forth—because one might argue that their "disorders" are part of their identity or who they "authentically" are and which, sometimes, they wouldn't choose to give up, even if they could (29,30).

This discussion of neurodiversity brings us full circle to the previous problem of "assessing" capacity and competency in persons with acquired brain injury. The evaluation must ultimately be done not only with a view to whether or not the person can adequately exercise whatever skills are operationally at issue—for example, driving, managing money, consenting to medical treatment, and so forth—but must also factor in the individual's premorbid personality and decision making. The evaluator must not only ask himself or herself how much understanding, reasoning, imagination, and so forth are required to meet some capacity threshold but also be able to distinguish an odd, eccentric, or unorthodox decisional or behavior style from one that cannot reasonably be tolerated (22,31,32).

DISTRIBUTIVE JUSTICE AND THE MARKETPLACE

Most scholarly discussions about justice in health care focus on allocation problems, as in, "Who gets what and how much? Who pays? Who decides?" The American penchant for individualism and personal liberty has largely evolved a marketplace response to these questions—one that stands in marked contrast to other industrially advanced Western countries that have long opted for some form of government run universal access to health care subsidized by tax dollars (33). In the United States, the number of people with some form of health coverage currently stands at around 255 million, although more than 50 million Americans have chosen not to purchase coverage and so are without it (34). Obviously, these latter individuals particularly pose difficult problems about what they are "owed" when someone else has to pay, especially in the event of a catastrophic event like a serious brain injury.

It was of considerable historical moment then, when the Patient Protection and Affordable Care Act was passed in March of 2010 whose requirements are expected to result in as many as 97% of Americans having some kind of health insurance by 2016 and presumably much improved access to health care (35). Nevertheless, the continuing backlash to that legislation and the highly publicized avowals of the administration's opponents to overturn it indicate how unpopular universal health insurance continues to be among many Americans (36).

Access to health care coverage, which obviously facilitates access to care, is often understood as a privilege rather than a right, but that is incorrect. Depending on the circumstances of an individual's injury or on his or her personal characteristics, he or she might indeed enjoy access to health care as a right. The soldier who becomes ill or is injured in the line of duty, the employee injured in the line of work, or the older or impoverished citizen who becomes ill will unconditionally qualify for veteran's benefits, Workers' Compensation, Medicare, or Medicaid respectively. But in the absence of those benefits, most nonelderly Americans will have to purchase their health coverage either as individuals shopping in the insurance marketplace or by paying a premium for a benefits package offered by their employers (37).

The marketplace response to the allocational question of "who gets what and how much" largely looks to an ability to pay as a fundamental determinant of health care access. In addition to "ability to pay," justice theorists have proposed other distributional criteria such as "to each an equal share" or criteria that are based on a person's need, merit, or dessert. In 1985, Norman Daniels offered an intriguing argument to the effect that everyone living in a liberal society is owed the right to have a share in what Daniels called a "normal opportunity range"—which he characterized as "the array of life plans reasonable persons in (a given society) . . . are likely to construct for themselves." (p 33) (38). Daniels argued that citizens living in liberal societies which, of course, champion individual freedoms and liberties, have an inherent right to access health services necessary for exercising and enjoying their rights, especially if disease or disability prevents their accessing the "normal opportunity range." Thus, Daniels would argue that society has a duty to provide rehabilitation to individuals with significant disability if they have some reasonable prospects for improved function that would enable them to access the opportunity range. Similarly, John Rawls's distributional scheme—as captured by his famously speculating on the kinds of fundamental goods or benefits persons would desire if they designed a benefits distribution plan from behind a "veil of ignorance"—suggests the idea of health care as a basic social benefit (39). Readers interested in these proposals can study Daniels's *Just Health Care* (38) and Rawls's *Theory of Justice* (39).

Nevertheless, arguments that propose health care as a *basic* human good, and therefore access to it as a fundamental right, are keenly resisted by many Americans. The European penchant for government serving as a universal payer is resoundingly unpopular not only among the electorate but also among medical professionals, labor unions, and large and small employers (33). Not surprisingly, the 2010 Obama health plan duly respected the American tradition of a health insurance marketplace that is largely employer-subsidized and operated by private parties. Obama's plan requires employers to offer health insurance to employees as well as requiring citizens to purchase some level of coverage or else suffer fines (40). This has disturbed conservative thinkers, however, who argue that government's forcing citizens to purchase any kind of commodity is a violation of the 1st, 4th, 5th, and 10th amendments of the US constitution (41). Time will tell about how these debates will play out. What remains apparent is that the question regarding "who gets what and how much" continues in the United States to be answered *contractually*.

The Health Insurance Policy as a Contract

The primary contractual vehicle for health care delivery and reimbursement in the United States is the health insurance policy. What one is owed is largely defined by the nature and extent of whatever coverage he or she enjoys. As noted earlier, the individual might not explicitly pay for this coverage by way of a monthly premium—such as individuals covered under Medicare Part A, Workers' Compensation, Medicaid, and so forth—but more than 175 million Americans did purchase coverage in 2009, mostly by voluntarily purchasing it from their employers (34). If they become ill and require a professional's care, payment for that care will be determined by the benefits and exclusions of the coverage along with whatever amount the individual is contractually bound to pay out of his or her own pocket such as by way of deductibles or copayments. Of course, whatever the insurance plan has no obligation to pay for such as an experimental treatment, a treatment explicitly excluded in the coverage, or a treatment delivered in a manner that violates the coverage's terms becomes the individual's reimbursement responsibility.

Although this contractual arrangement of benefits determination often seems to work relatively well, it also leaves much to be desired especially in instances of catastrophic disability onset like TBI. An individual with TBI whose coverage is Medicaid, for example, may find little in the way of psychological services being covered in comparison to someone with a more generous array of benefits (42). Or 2 individuals who pay the same for coverage might find themselves with very different benefit packages especially in instances pertinent to catastrophic disability. Or the person with brain injury who successfully sues the party who injured himself or herself might receive a multimillion dollar award in contrast to someone who is uninsured and must exhaust his or her savings to become virtually indigent and qualify for Medicaid benefits.

Medical Necessity

Physicians note that "medical necessity" is not a clinical but a legal term because it primarily appears in legal instruments outlining reimbursement policies like state or federal regulations or health insurance policies (43). Because medical necessity is a key condition for allocating a third party payor's health care dollars, however, it will inevitably have ethical implications bearing on the distributive justice question "Who gets what and how much?"

Typically, health insurance policies contain medical necessity language that apply to situations wherein a clinically recognized malady or ailment exists that is known to be reasonably amenable to a treatment and delivered at an appropriate level of intensity (44). For example, the Centers for Medicare and Medicaid Services (CMS) have determined that an inpatient rehabilitation stay is medically necessary if (a) the patient requires and receives close medical supervision by a physician with specialized training or experience in rehabilitation; (b) the patient requires and receives 24-hour rehabilitation nursing as well as (c) a relatively intense level of rehabilitation services delivered by (d) a multidisciplinary rehabilitation team; (e) the patient's care program is coordinated; (f) the patient is likely to achieve a significant practical improvement; (g) the patient's goals are realistic; and (h) the patient's length of stay is reasonable. Each of these services must be "reasonable and necessary" per their efficacy, duration, frequency, and amount if they are to be reimbursed by Medicare (45).

On its face, the idea of coverage according to medical necessity determinations seems eminently reasonable. Its obvious ethical thrust is to discourage unnecessary, doubtful, or fraudulent practices. As practically implemented, however, medical necessity rules and regulations have proven remarkably difficult to operationalize and have particularly vexed rehabilitation providers. First of all, the language connected with medical necessity is inherently vague (46). The CMS medical necessity language for inpatient rehabilitation appearing earlier uses terms like "close medical supervision," "relatively intense level," "likely to achieve a significant practical improvement," "realistic," and "reasonable"—terms that predictably cause disputes over their interpretation at the practical, clinical level. For example, an American Hospital Association study of 72 inpatient rehabilitation facilities (IRFs) filing medical claims to CMS for services delivered between January and July of 2007 discovered that CMS's "fiscal intermediaries" (FIs)—which are business entities contracting with CMS to perform medical necessity determinations—*denied 80%* of the 2,200 claims that were studied. The usual reason given for the FIs' denials was that the service could have been delivered at a less intense level than inpatient rehabilitation (47).

The economic impact of these denials translated into more than $25 million being withheld from those IRFs (47). Many of them disputed the denials resulting in the appeals ultimately going to an administrative law judge (ALJ) for review. Of 652 claims that the courts evaluated, *63% were overturned in favor of the IRF*. Unfortunately, however, the appeals process was time-consuming, expensive, and disturbing for rehabilitation providers and their consumers. The average time involved in an appeal being adjudicated at the ALJ level was 12–24 months with IRFs' estimating their related costs at about $2,000 for each appeal. Not only did the facilities have to divert staff to work on these appeals, but some IRFs hired outside consultants and legal experts to help (47). Most problematic, perhaps, is that certain IRFs simply stopped admitting patients whose presenting symptoms resembled those that witnessed previous FI reimbursement denials. Yet, because of the unreliability of FI determinations themselves, the patient who is denied an IRF admission in one locality might be admitted to an IRF in another locale that is under a different IF who will approve the services (47).

Determining medical necessity thus presents a host of ethical problems. Although it plays a critical role in the distribution of rehabilitation benefits, it is nevertheless a term whose application is in sore need of reliable and consensually adopted specifications. Furthermore, it calls into question whether evidence-based practices, which should be able to resolve many of these disputes between physicians and CMS's FIs, have evolved to a point where they are all that reliable and useful (48). Medical necessity determinations also incur problems regarding who should ultimately make them. Decades ago, when payers and health professionals realized that whoever gained the upper hand in defining medical necessity would ipso facto direct the flow of health care dollars, the battle for definitional authority was on. Legal precedents like the 1978 case of *Blue Cross & Blue Shield v Smither* showed how insurers were writing policies with "sole judgment" or "sole discretion" language that attempted to give them a categorical right to reject claims (49). Alternatively, the 1986 court in *Cowan v Myers* scolded the plaintiffs for asserting that "the physician is the sole arbiter of what constitutes a medical necessity" noting that if such were allowed, "the State's requirement of reimbursement would be limited only by the imagination of physicians" (50).

The fact that the previous data show an FI-CMS rate of reimbursement denial at 80% coupled with a 63% reversal rate on appeal is ethically disturbing. Clearly and especially prior to the managed care era, health care charges based on a per service or per diem basis economically incentivized health professionals to treat as much as possible and hence, possibly provide "unnecessary" care. Today, however, suspicions run high that FIs base reimbursement denials on idiosyncratic interpretations of medical necessity as a way of conserving Medicare dollars and advancing their (i.e., the FIs') self-interests (43). Rehabilitation commentators complain that FI auditors provide little or no justification for their denials but that they are nevertheless compensated according to a percentage of the costs they recover for CMS (44). Contemporary attempts to resolve these problems have taken the form of an appeals process that most often terminates with the decision of an administrative law judge but could proceed to an appeals council review and even to a judicial review in US District Court (47).

Rehabilitation Research Informing Medical Necessity Determinations

As noted previously, rehabilitation research should be able to contribute substantially to the resolution of disputes over medical necessity. After all, that research should inform us about the outcomes of various interventions and their costs, which should, in turn, allow us to make valid comparisons among available treatments. Unfortunately, however, numerous problems related to rehabilitation research immediately present themselves. The first is that performing rehabilitation research according to the gold-standard model of randomized, double blinded trials is usually impossible (51). Providing rehabilitation treatment is not like evaluating a drug against a placebo or some other comparator. Unlike a placebo-control group, all rehabilitation patients get some kind of care. Furthermore, because inpatient rehabilitation patients present with disability, they receive treatments from a host of professionals whose goal is to help restore the patient's function, not necessarily rid him or her of a disease. This multidisciplinary approach to what are frequently multiple impairments that are sometimes synergistic—for example, the patient with brain injury who is profoundly emotionally dysregulated or who experiences considerable memory or attentional deficits will likely have poor employment prospects; the patient with visual field neglect will likely experience ambulation problems or difficulties affecting his or her performing activities of daily living—immensely complicates the assessment of a discrete rehabilitation treatment (52). Moreover, every neurological injury is unique and no 2 rehabilitation patients who enter a rehabilitation hospital are the same. In the parlance of research, it is next to impossible to "control for" the bewildering array of variables that can affect a rehabilitation outcome such as the individual's age, degree of neural plasticity, severity of injury, premorbid skill levels, degree of family support, coping skills, level of education, ability to pay for care, and so forth (52).

Furthermore, if a payor demands that a treatment be "beneficial and effective" to be deemed medically necessary, one can rightly ask about *the degree of benefit or effectiveness* the treatment should offer especially in comparison to alternative treatments. Obviously, rehabilitation treatments frequently do not eradicate functional impairments but rather diminish their handicapping effects. Thus, if a person with brain injury loses his temper 10 times a day but with some cognitive therapy can reduce that number to 3 times a day, should the treatment be considered "medically necessary"? Or, more generally, if the handicapping effects of a sensory or motor impairment can be reduced, at what point of functional improvement should a treatment be deemed medically necessary: If the treatment provides a 10% functional improvement? Or 30%? Or 50%? And if there is only a limited amount of money to spend, might some functional domains be valued over others? Is it more important to walk without assistance or improve one's memory and attentional skills than to be able to control one's temper?

The problem is that these are not empirical questions but valuative ones. Some payor of care must decide whether the intervention is "worth it." And because these questions are so ethically fraught, they are usually handled in the rehabilitation section of an insurance policy by the enumeration of specified benefits, such as 30 days of inpatient rehabilitative treatment or a particular number of treatments. Ultimately, "pure" ethical theory—because it might reveal the content of duty, human rights, and the essential natures of harm, burden, benefit, and fairness—seems entirely unable to resolve the practical, in-the-trenches problems of distributive justice. The latter are inevitably conditioned but also obscured by the real world phenomena of demand and supply, new technologies and their costs, inconclusive or limited knowledge, moral pluralism, unpredictable levels of economic resources, and self-interest. Although ethical theory can offer important insights about our moral obligations, it remains unable to reliably translate its theoretical principles and rules bearing on harms, benefits, and justice into concrete benefits allocations that might be included in health insurance policies. As is nicely illustrated by the near half century of debate on the phenomenon of medical necessity, humans tend to be in a continuous process of creating and recreating responses to their moral challenges rather than discovering timeless moral truths that provide morally conclusive solutions.

BRAIN DEATH

Societies need a coherent and consensually adopted notion of death. As scholars have pointed out, without a reliable concept of death, we would have enormous problems in regulating our grieving, discontinuing life-prolonging treatment, procuring organs, initiating funerals and burials, terminating insurance coverages, and dispersing life insurance benefits and other forms of property (53).

The Brain Death Criteria

Until the advent of intensive care units (ICUs) and life prolonging technologies like mechanical breathing machines, dialyzers, and sophisticated mechanisms for delivering medications, nutrition, and hydration, the irreversible cessation of respiration and circulation seemed a thoroughly adequate and obvious criterion for pronouncing someone dead. When sophisticated life prolonging technologies began appearing in the 1960s, however, the definition of death expanded to allow a second characterization. The new definition was triggered by patients who were on the verge of cardiopulmonary death that often resulted from traumatic injuries, but who were admitted to ICUs and placed on the earlier mentioned life prolonging interventions, especially artificial ventilation (54). Because the heart has an intrinsic activity that doesn't depend on the brain, some of these patients maintained circulation for prolonged periods even though they were entirely unresponsive to external stimuli and there was no clinical detection of any brain activity whatsoever including brainstem activity. These phenomena collectively encouraged the idea that "whole brain death" might serve as a second representation of death alongside the irreversible cessation of circulation and respiration (55). The idea eventually led to the development of the brain death tests listed in Table 83-1 that were first articulated in 1968 as the Harvard brain death criteria. Today, whole brain death appears to be legally accepted as death determinative in all 50 states and in many countries around the world (53). Two exceptions in the United States, however, are in New York and New Jersey which allow for "reasonable accommodation" of religious or moral objections in the former and outright rejection of the brain death criteria in favor of the traditional criteria in the latter. Cases in New York have typically involved some sects of Orthodox Jews but other groups have invoked this nod to moral pluralism in rejecting the use of these criteria (56,57).

In most jurisdictions, however, if a patient "fails" the brain death tests listed in Table 83-1, the patient is declared dead and life prolonging care is removed except if the patient is an organ donor. Indeed, the possibility of organ donation was a significant historical spur to developing the brain death construct because organ transplantation paradoxically requires both a *dead person* and a *living body*. The reason is that one cannot remove vital organs from a person and thereby cause his or her death because doing so would constitute homicide and violate what is understood as the "dead

TABLE 83-1 Brain Death Criteria in Adults

A. Prerequisites:
1. Clinical or neuroimaging evidence of an acute CNS catastrophe that is compatible with the clinical diagnosis of brain death
2. Exclusion of complicating medical conditions that may confound clinical assessment (no severe electrolyte, acid-base, or endocrine disturbance)
3. No drug intoxication or poisoning
4. Core temperature ≥ 32°C (90°F)
B. The 3 cardinal findings in brain death are coma or unresponsiveness, absence of brainstem reflexes, and apnea.
1. Coma or unresponsiveness—no cerebral motor response to pain in all extremities (nail bed pressure and supraorbital pressure)
2. Absence of brainstem reflexes
   a. Pupils
      i. No response to bright light
      ii. Size: midposition (4 mm) to dilated (9 mm)
   b. Ocular movement
      i. No oculocephalic reflex (testing only when no fracture or instability of the cervical spine is apparent)
      ii. No deviation of the eyes to irrigation in each ear with 50 mL of cold water
   c. Facial sensation and facial motor response
      i. No corneal reflex to touch with a throat swab
      ii. No jaw reflex
      iii. No grimacing to deep pressure on nail, nail bed, supraorbital ridge, or temporomandibular joint
   d. Pharyngeal and tracheal reflexes
      i. No response after stimulation of the posterior pharynx with tongue blade
      ii. No cough response to bronchial suctioning
3. Apnea: No spontaneous respirations should be evident on disconnection from the ventilator for a period long enough to allow the partial pressure of carbon dioxide in arterial blood to rise higher than 60 mm Hg and the pH to fall lower than 7.28 (usually 10 min)

Adapted from Lazar NM, Shemie S, Webster GC, Dickens BM. Bioethics for clinicians: 24. Brain death. *CMAJ.* 2001;164(6):833–836; American Academy of Neurology. Practice parameters: determining brain death in adults. American academy of Neurology Web site. http://www.aan.com/professionals/practice/guidelines/pda/Brain_death_adults.pdf. Accessed June 4, 2012.

donor" rule. Consequently, whole brain death proved an ideal construct for satisfying both the dead donor rule and the need for a living body because the life prolonging technology in the ICU could sustain many of the body's functions *without brain activity* such as circulation, digestion, food metabolism, excretory functions, hormonal balance, wound healing, growth and sexual maturation, and even, in rare cases, gestation of a fetus (58).

Multiple Meanings of Death

A heated and remarkably wide-ranging debate has ensued over the propriety of the brain death construct and its defining criteria, which in turn has generated even more controversy about the meaning and possibly *multiple* meanings of "death" (59,60,61). At one end of the debate are instances where families can invoke their religious beliefs to reject the whole brain death criterion outright. This position assumes the historically conservative tradition of insisting that a person be declared dead *only* when his or her respiration and circulation irreversibly cease. Thus, the 2008 case of 12-year-old Mordecai Brody made national news as he appeared to meet the brain death criteria, but his parents invoked their religious beliefs to argue that he could only be understood to be dead when his circulation and respiration irreversibly ceased (57). Their beliefs did not recognize whole brain death so that discontinuing Mordecai's intensive care measures would have been, according to his parents' view, homicide (57).

At the other end of the death definition spectrum are those commentators who hold that a "higher brain death" criterion including irreversible coma or persistent vegetative state could qualify as death defining as long as the individual had made declarations to that effect. Robert Veatch, for example, argues that once an individual is irreversibly unconscious and no longer enjoys a mind–body integration (or is no longer an "embodied consciousness"), he or she has lost what Veatch calls "moral standing," that is, the right to lay serious claim to health care entitlements (61). Veatch would argue that it is entirely reasonable for one to hold that his or her life ends with the irreversible loss of consciousness such as from irreversible coma or a vegetative state, and if that person wished to be declared dead—which would be known from an advance directive—that wish should be honored, all treatment should be stopped, and funereal plans should commence. Philosopher, lawyer, and ethicist William Winslade take the same position by privileging consciousness as the necessary criterion for moral standing (62).

Regardless of how this debate evolves, transparent communications must occur among the principal parties—not the least of whom are families who will need to be told about the nature of "brain death" in their consenting to discontinuing life prolonging treatment or donating their loved one's organs. Consensus among the various clinical and ethical voices will have to be achieved on (*a*) identifying the "facts" of the matter, such as the fact that with continued ICU treatment, the individual might still retain some brain activity and survive in a "dreamless sleep" for an indefinite time, (*b*) what the facts mean, such that the patient will never recover or regain any semblance of consciousness, and (*c*) how moral constraints should be applied, such as will be discussed subsequently. Given the moral pluralism that exists in the United States, these tasks will hardly be easy, but it is interesting to note that although robust scholarly controversies over defining death have endured for some years, they have not affected the public consciousness of brain death determination to any significant extent. Possibly, a deep but unspoken strain of pragmatism already exists among most people that intuitively recognizes when a person's life is spent or when his or her "right" to life is without the neurophysiological platform that supports it. At such a point and for most of us, it might seem the better course to direct our moral energies toward persons whose hold on life is far less problematic but challenge our moral obligations nevertheless. Essential to that redirection, however, is our confidence in the clinical judgment that determines this or that life as beyond clinical remedy. Recent research in disorders of consciousness has given considerable pause over that confidence, however, especially in cases of prognosticating someone as in an "irreversible" state of unconsciousness.

DISORDERS OF CONSCIOUSNESS

One of the most exciting areas in neurology, and perhaps medicine writ large, is that domain of research and practice addressing patients with disorders of consciousness—a range of conditions from coma onto the vegetative and minimally conscious states. It is an exciting and challenging topic because its history has been inextricably linked to important societal trends, such as the right-to-die movement, which have left a profound impact on clinical practice. These forces need to be understood, and indeed recast, in light of emerging knowledge about the diagnosis and even treatment of these conditions as illustrated in the following case.

Case Vignette

Consider the following hypothetical case:

A family has made a request to a hospital ethics committee to withdraw life-sustaining therapy from their loved one. The committee requires an expert assessment and turns to a neurologist for consultation (63). The neurologist finds a patient in the ICU on ventilatory support. A few days out from TBI, the patient is unresponsive and in an eyes closed state consistent with coma. A computed tomography (CT) scan shows significant bilateral injuries and some moderate degree of midline shift but no evidence of herniation.

The family is grief stricken by the suddenness of the injury and asks that life support be removed. The patient, they note, "never wanted to live like a vegetable." The neurologist presents his findings to the ethicist and reports with utmost confidence that there is "no hope for meaningful recovery." All involved agree that the best course of action would be to follow the family's earnest and heartfelt wishes to remove life support per the patient's preferences as expressed by his or her surrogates.

A Definitional Primer

Coma is a self-limited, eyes closed state of unresponsiveness (64). Comatose patients can proceed to brain death or cardiopulmonary death or to the vegetative and minimally conscious states or to complete recovery as would be the case for an anesthetized patient emerging from a drug-induced coma. From a coma, a patient can progress to the vegetative state (VS), which in contrast to a coma is an *eyes-open* state of unreponsiveness marked by sleep–wake cycles and an autonomic startle reflex. These latter changes reflect the partial recovery of the brainstem absent higher cortical function (65).

Under some classifications, a vegetative state lasting for at least a month is considered "persistent." After 3 months, it is deemed "permanent" if caused by anoxic brain injury. After a year, it is considered "permanent" if caused by a TBI. Before the vegetative state becomes permanent (a temporal marker linked to etiology of injury), the patient can move into the minimally conscious state (MCS).

MCS patients are conscious. As noted in Chapter 32, MCS patients have intention, attention, and memory. They may follow commands, reach for an object, or track a visitor (66). However, these manifestations of consciousness are episodic and intermittent. Their occurrence means that the pa-

tient is no longer vegetative but is in a state of higher level functioning. But because these manifestations are intermittent, it is easy to err and miss the behaviors that would lead to a diagnosis different from VS.

Furthermore, the diagnosis the patient carries can change as he or she progresses from hospital to nursing home to a rehabilitation center or to home. Patients may leave the hospital 2–3 weeks after an injury with an accurate diagnosis of "vegetative state." But over the ensuing weeks or months, they may morph surreptitiously into MCS without anyone noticing, or knowing to notice, or *caring to notice,* lest they contradict the "definitive academic" diagnosis made at the acute care hospital providing the initial care (67).

Studies have asserted that the degree of diagnostic error mistaking MCS for VS can be staggering (68,69,70). A more recent paper on this topic by Schnakers et al. (71) found that 18 of 44 patients (41%) with a consensus diagnosis of VS were found to be in MCS after evaluation using the Coma Recovery Scale-Revised evidence-based assessment (72). Patients who regain reliable functional communication are said to have *emerged* from MCS. The time plot on when and if emergence occurs is unpredictable and can be quite variable with late occurrences happening years and decades after the injury (73,74).

Case Vignette Reconsidered

At first glance, there might seem no cause for concern about the aforementioned withdrawal of life-sustaining therapy. The prognosis seemed grave, a consultation was obtained that confirmed it, and the patient's surrogate requested a withdrawal of life-prolonging treatment. But closer analysis, informed by emerging knowledge about severe brain injury and mechanisms of assessment and recovery, suggests a reconsideration of the process of decision making, if not the decision itself, to accommodate a growing evidentiary—and normative—position for the care of MCS patients.

To begin this reappraisal, consider the patient's prognosis. The patient described in the vignette is in a comatose state following TBI. Despite the decision to withdraw care while still in a coma, his prognosis might not be as dire as this rapid withdrawal suggests. Based on available data, patients in traumatic coma have about 50% chance of recovery to a moderate degree of impairment, if not better. Anoxic patients fare less well: 77% of anoxic comas result in death or permanent unconsciousness, whereas approximately 50% of comas resulting from TBIs have a similar outcome (75). Given these data, it is important to note the etiology of injury and avoid rapid judgments which reflect a degree of pessimism inconsistent with a more favorable prognosis (76).

It is also important to understand why decisions to withdraw care are often so precipitous instead of reflective and fully informed. One reason might be that the evolution of the right to die in the United States has been inextricably linked to patients with disorders of consciousness dating back to Karen Quinlan and continuing on to other notable cases like Nancy Cruzan and Terri Schiavo (77). All of these women were in the permanent vegetative state following anoxic brain injury.

The right to die gained legal standing in the Quinlan case in which the court invoked the "futility" of the vegetative state as the moral and legal warrant to allow Karen's parents to remove her ventilator (78). Based on the testimony of the court-appointed neurologist, Dr. Fred Plum—the cooriginator of the persistent vegetative state diagnosis with Scottish neurosurgeon Bryan Jennett (79)—Judge Hughes of the New Jersey Supreme Court permitted the withdrawal of life support (80). Ms. Quinlan survived because she had an intact brainstem and was able to breathe on her own.

The case gained national attention and launched the right-to-die movement, which has acculturated a generation of physicians to promote self-determination and patient autonomy at life's end. Obviously, the enfranchisement of patients and families to control their destinies in the face of grave injury is for the good. What has not been appreciated until recently, however, is the effect of this decision and others like it on cultural attitudes about patients with severe brain injury (81).

In achieving *and sustaining a right to die* from Quinlan to Schiavo, physicians have been trained to be receptive to families and other surrogates in instances of deciding whether to withhold or withdraw care. The false assumption that needs to be addressed, however, is *the implicit perception that all presentations of unconsciousness are prognostically the same and bespeak irretrievable injury.* This assumption extends back to Hippocrates but was countered by Galen who observed, "But I have seen a severely wounded brain healed" (82).

Galen's statement was so important to the famed neurosurgeon Wilder Penfield that he affixed it to the cathedral ceiling awaiting the visitor to the Montreal Neurological Institute which he founded (83). It is an orientation that all concerned with patients with head injury should adopt or at least entertain as a possibility, lest we fall prey to unintended negative biases that might preclude achievable recoveries. Nevertheless, it can be difficult for clinicians to overcome their assumptions and biases and prognosticate patients based on the etiology of their injury, the duration of the coma, and the time that has elapsed since the injury.

It is critical that the clinician carefully decouples his or her views about unconsciousness from an initial coma from the loss of consciousness which accompanies terminal illness and the dementing illnesses of old age. In most medical illnesses, a loss of consciousness is the sequelae, or "end game," of a degenerative process that leaves the patient unable to maintain himself or herself. It is also the occasion when a surrogate, rather than the patient, becomes the decision maker as evidenced by data which suggest that around 80% of do-not-resuscitate orders are consented to by surrogates, not patients. The upshot is that the patient's loss of consciousness and concomitant loss of capacity is taken as a dire negative prognostic sign, suggesting that a less aggressive therapeutic stance is indicated.

Although this practice pattern helpfully sets limits in most medical conditions, patients with acquired brain injury can represent a different clinical population. Their injury *and their recovery process begin with the loss of consciousness.* So in these contexts the loss of consciousness is not the end of a terminal process but potentially the start of a recuperative one.

These factors can coalesce in a fashion that can influence care decisions. Physicians acculturated both to respect the (post-Quinlan) right-to-die and influenced by their more general scope of practice outside of neurology may view the loss of consciousness that accompanies head trauma as akin to the encephalopathic coma that occurs in scenarios like the hepatorenal syndrome and view the condition as more grave than it actually is, thus leading to decisions to withhold or withdraw care which might be premature or precipitous.

Time-Delimited Assessment and Communication

Given the aforementioned caveats, clinicians should develop the aforementioned cases using a time-delimited approach to prognostication and communication previously developed by one of us (JJF) (84). This method parcelates assessment and communication into discrete periods following the trajectory of recovery after an injury and pays special attention to key temporal milestones which distinguish coma, the vegetative and minimally conscious states, and their emergence from each other. It avoids global and enduring comments like "there is no hope for meaningful recovery," except for those cases that are clearly dire and provides more nuanced and incremental information to families that tracks the course of the recovery process.

The process of time-delimitation is much like that used by meteorologists tracking a hurricane traveling across the South Atlantic to the Eastern seaboard of the United States from Africa. Although it is a tropical storm midway across the ocean, it is difficult to know whether the storm will result in a full-fledged hurricane and if it will make landfall. But that cone of uncertainty decreases with the march of time when prognostication can become more accurate.

Returning then to the *beginning* of the case while the patient is still in a coma, the first question that should be asked is whether we are "still at sea," to borrow from the previously mentioned metaphor. Are we sufficiently informed to make an irrevocable decision so early in the course of care? Or should we wait an interval to let the patient declare himself once out of coma? Should a family's request for a withdrawal be morally persuasive enough to allow that process to occur at whatever time the surrogate decision maker requests?

Because such judgments will be a mix of both the science underlying injury assessment and the values informing patient/family preferences, different family constellations will make different decisions in cases with the same fact patterns. Each will be a process of interpreting the facts against the patient's prior wishes and values. Although ethical principles dictate that deference should be given to the primacy of the family—and their expression of delegated patient self-determination—both for the decisions they make and their timing, decisions to accept or forgo treatment should nevertheless be as *informed* as possible.

Thus, decisions to withdraw care should be deferred until the patient has progressed beyond the coma stage unless there is an overwhelming structural injury, evidence of herniation, or other dire prognostic signs such as loss of visual evoked responses. These negative prognostic signs reflect a catastrophic outcome and delay is not necessary to determine the ultimate outcome. In patients who lack these dire tell-tale signs, it is often better to wait and see *how and when* the coma terminates.

How quickly the patient moves into the vegetative state can be a promising early sign of brainstem recovery. But even when the patient has emerged from coma, one needs to be cautious in speaking with families. A move into the vegetative state may be misunderstood and invariably viewed as a negative prognostic development even when it could be encouraging. Families need to be told that although a transition from coma to awareness is always preferable to a move from coma into the vegetative state, spending a shorter time in coma is a favorable prognostic sign. This transition reflects the early recovery of the brainstem and does not preclude additional function recovery.

The potential for additional recovery is an important point to communicate because families might view the transition to the vegetative state as being permanent and draw a potentially false analogy to prominent cases like Terri Schiavo who was in a *permanent* vegetative state (85,86). Although that outcome can await a patient, depending on etiology of injury and other factors, passage into the vegetative state may also be a temporary way-station or transitional state en route to MCS and additional recovery.

Once a patient has migrated from coma into the vegetative state, the next demarcation point at 1 month is designated in some classifications as "persistent" (85). For example a patient who rapidly moves from coma to VS but whose vegetative state lingers so it becomes persistent has a more favorable prognosis at the start of the month than at its end. Once the vegetative state has become persistent, the next marker is permanence at 3 months for anoxic injury and 12 moths for traumatic. It is important that families appreciate this outer limit of hope for additional recovery lest there evolve a futility dispute as occurred in the Schiavo case (86).

Although it is important to communicate about the possibility of a permanent vegetative state once the condition has become persistent, it is also important that clinicians *listen* to the observations of family members who might have noticed behaviors that might alter the patient's diagnosis from the vegetative to minimally conscious state. Because these behaviors are by definition intermittent and episodic, a diagnosis can be compromised from a sampling error and inadequate data be treated as definitive. Thus, it is essential that clinicians perform multiple examinations at multiple times of the day with the Coma Recovery Scale-Revised and also use the information and observations of families. Clinical staff should not simply attribute family members' claims to wishful thinking or psychological denial. Instead, they should seek to build a partnership and view their contributions to patient care as an essential supplement to the paucity of observations made by clinical staff who spend ever less time at the bedside.

A failure to note the movement from VS into MCS will mistakenly identify a conscious individual as an unconscious one. This is a clinical as well as an ethical omission because it excludes individuals from the human community who may have the ability to communicate and interact with others. Prognostically, it is especially difficult to predict the future of those who reach MCS. Being in MCS could represent a plateau of one's functional status or a transitional point, in additional, future recovery which at this time cannot be accurately predicted. Unlike the length of time in VS, which is a negative predictor for movement onto MCS, time spent in MCS does not correlate either positively or negatively with the likelihood of emergence out of MCS (73).

Technology and the Challenges of Differential Diagnosis

To date, no clinically reliable technologies are available to distinguish the vegetative from the minimally conscious state. All of these modalities remain investigational and a consensus report on this topic urges prudence in the use of neuroimaging methods in clinical practice until they are properly vetted (87). Premature dissemination outside the research context has the potential to confuse and mislead both patients and clinicians.

Consider, for example, the exciting neuroimaging work originating with the research of Hirsch, Schiff, and others (88,89) using functional MRI to assess passive and active language response,. Or consider Owen et al. report of a woman with TBI who was behaviorally in the vegetative state 5 months after an accident (90). An fMRI study demonstrated integrated neural networks in response to verbal stimuli that were indistinguishable from normal controls. As famously reported in the lay press, when the patient was asked to imagine herself playing tennis, there was activation in the supplementary motor areas; when she was asked to imagine walking in her home, there was activation in the parahippocampal gyrus, posterior parietal cortex, and the lateral premotor cortex; and when she was presented with ambiguous sentences to parse, there was activation in the middle and superior temporal gyrus bilaterally and the left inferior frontal region (90).

The case raised a host of nosological questions about her diagnosis. By established behavioral criteria she was in a vegetative state. But her response to language, as evidenced by neuroimaging, was inconsistent with the vegetative state. Although one of us (JJF) has suggested that patients like her who demonstrate responsiveness on neuroimaging without behavioral output should be described as being in a nonbehavioral MCS (91), the nomenclature for this state has yet to be agreed on, making this a challenge for clinical practice.

Subsequent work from the same group led by Monti used functional MRI to demonstrate that a patient previously thought to be vegetative could answer simple yes or no questions by volitional activation of regional networks in the brain. Although this patient was able to perform command following, a capability which changed his diagnosis from VS to nonbehavioral MCS, this report needs to be understood against the broader context of the entire study's cohort. Of 54 patients in either VS or MCS, 30 of the 31 MCS patients who were studied were found to be in MCS by the bedside Coma Recovery Scale-Revised tool developed by Giacino and Kalmar (72). This contrasts with 5 of the 54 patients found to be able to engage in command following, indicating the greater use of the bedside exam and the need for caution about the premature dissemination of neuroimaging tools for routine clinical assessment.

COMMUNICATING WITH FAMILIES

Anyone who is sensitive to the ethical dimensions of health care understands that communicating with patients and family members requires more than just securing their signature on some informed consent form. Indeed, not only is the ideal of informed consent not achieved by such a formality but a supportive health care relationship usually requires a good deal more than a patient's or the patient's representative consenting to some treatment intervention (92,93,94).

As discussed in the section on judgmental capacity and competency, an ideal of health care communications and relationships is honoring the patient's "autonomy." But doing so requires not only respecting his or her decisions but also facilitating the patient's understanding and reasoning such that his or her wishes truly express or derive from the patient's interests, needs, beliefs, and desires. Autonomous behavior is authentic behavior in that it proceeds from the patient's "real" self—namely, a self that is under the patient's rational and uncoerced control and will (22). Health professionals providing care for persons with serious brain injury must often wonder, however, how authentic or autonomous are their patients' and families' decisions and choices, given the way brain injury disturbs precisely those faculties necessary for autonomy. Family members who will usually function as the patient's representative may be so psychologically upset by their loved one's injury that they will be uncomprehending of the care that is required, in denial or in the grip of fantastical thinking, or be in the throes of disruptive emotions and feelings that compromise their thinking and deciding clearly (95). Some might also become difficult to manage because they might behave poorly or project feelings of rage, disbelief, misery, helplessness, and hopelessness onto staff (96).

Unfortunately, health care training programs sometimes fail to prepare students for managing these difficult patient and family encounters, so that once confronted with them, the professional can only resort to his or her (relatively untrained) communicative behaviors and hope for the best. Fortunately, though, some basic empathic skills are available for any health professional to learn that can prove enormously valuable in such situations. Learning these skills should be part and parcel of the professional's ethics skill set because clinical ethics is inevitably concerned with preserving and fostering healthy or benefits-generating relationships (97). Consequently, techniques that encourage the latter are ethically laudable and important to know, whereas behaviors that compromise trust or perceptions of integrity or caring are ethically problematic.

What follows will provide some basic insights on the psychological architecture of difficult communications—with anyone in fact, not just patients or families—and then provide recommendations on how professionals might empathically navigate the occasionally rough and choppy waters of health care communications.

Empathy and the Difficult Communication

The psychiatrist Meyer Gunther remarked about how "emotionally evocative" the onset of serious disability is (96). Typically, patients and their loved ones can feel overwhelmed, grief-stricken, profoundly depressed, utterly helpless, enraged, worthless, guilty, abandoned by God, and unloved. Although we might understand such feelings as ultimately unproductive, contemporary psychologists and neuroscientists underline the enormous importance that emotions and feelings play in our navigating our lives. Once thought to be counterproductive to thinking rationally and logically, emotions and feelings are now understood to be critical in our making sound, beneficial, or adaptive decisions (98). Emotions and feelings are now understood as neuroevolutionary products whose job is to reinforce adaptive behaviors and select against behaviors that are aversive; to channel behaviors in ways that maximize survival and reproduction; to prioritize response tendencies; and to regulate behavior in ways that foster adaptation (99).

Emotions and feelings have come to be thought of as not simply cognitional aids but as forms of cognition in themselves that assist in focusing a species' attention (such as on a predator or threat); in making appraisals, such as in these blue berries are good and desirable but those yellow berries are not; and to make contemplation and reflection more efficient by lessening the need to have to "think through" every action plan one considers (23). Thankfully, one's affects and feelings encode past plans that proved adaptive and successful in one's memory such one need not have to painstakingly analyze a plan or its alternatives step-by-step every time he or she encounters a situation. One simply executes the behavior that his or her unconscious sends up from memory as having previously been successful. Consequently, behavior becomes much more economical so that one's mental energies and "effortful" thinking can focus on matters that are truly perplexing but important.

Emotions and Feelings as a Window to the Self

The negative emotional displays that the health professional sometimes witnesses from patients and family members can actually constitute valuable information that he or she can use to help and support them. The patient's or family member's display of helplessness, anger, or bewilderment are windows into his or her feeling state, and *how we feel at any moment is how we are* at that moment (99). Indeed, such feeling displays should be expected in view of how disruptive, unjust, and horrid the onset of serious brain injury can be.

Nevertheless, the patient's or family member's displaying powerful emotions and feelings can make professionals feel uncomfortable because the latter will inevitably absorb or vicariously experience the other's feeling experience (100). Psychologists talk about how human beings "project" their feelings and emotions, meaning how we publicly exhibit them such that other people might not only sense how we are feeling but perhaps help us. In other words, visibly projecting one's feelings, that is, letting other people perceive or know how I feel, is actually a way of "sharing" them, such that perhaps something good will come out of it (100). A good example of projection is how a mother can take one look at her child and "know" how the child is feeling. Obviously, a species that has this ability to sense or infer how its conspecifics are faring will be much better poised to survive. But this only underlines the extraordinarily adaptive function of our affective architecture—how it is primarily informative and critical for meeting our survival objectives.

Persons with brain injury and their loved ones might wonder "How am I going to survive this?" and therefore might display various emotions and feelings that communicate their sense of loss and grief to the most salient individuals they now know: their health providers. Those moments of projection therefore take on high moral importance because they allow the professional a window into how the patient or family member can be helped and supported. They also offer an opportunity for the professional to learn more about the patient's condition in ways that can dramatically affect the care plan.

Empathy and the Temptation To Avoid It

The problem of projection, however, is that the health professional or the "projectee" may recoil from the experience. That should not be surprising. It can be very uncomfortable to absorb or vicariously feel the depths of another's suffering, so it is hardly uncommon for a health professional (or anyone) to occasionally lapse into a defensive posture, trying as much as possible to make uncomfortable feelings go away (101). For example, the professional might ignore the patient's or family member's feelings, distract them with a change of subject and hope for a change of feeling, or admonish them to feel differently. Professionals who are skilled at empathic communication are not only able to be with and tolerate their client's painful feelings, but they will go a step further and be *curious* about them. Whereas the professional unskilled in empathy may want to avoid situations that provoke uncomfortable feelings, the skilled "empathist" will be drawn to them. He or she will not only acknowledge the other's feelings—as in, "So, Mrs. Jones, you're obviously feeling very . . . (sad, lonely, angry, depressed)"—but he or she will want to know what the feeling is about, and what the listener wants done. The empathic communicator will resist judging the other's feelings but will instead understand them as anxious reactions to the situation at hand. Importantly, the empathic communicator will reflect his or her understanding back to the patient—not by saying "I know how you feel," but rather by saying, "So, that must make you feel . . . " or "So what you're saying is that . . . " (100).

Table 83-2 contains a list of empathic responses that can prove valuable in all sorts of uncomfortable communications. Their objective is to achieve rapport and communicate support and understanding. This is what listeners want from their health professionals: namely, signs that they care about them, are interested in them, and even worried about them. As noted earlier, the professional's keen display of curiosity about what the other is feeling cannot be overemphasized, such that the list of empathic responses ultimately represent that very kind of sensibility (26).

Furthermore, behavioral expressions of empathy such as sitting down, making good eye contact, using a gentle but firm tone of voice, and just being willing to listen and not speak are essential (100). Many health professionals mistakenly assume that if they simply convey treatment information to the patient and family, they are doing all that is necessary. And perhaps in most health communicational situations, information is what is being sought so that providing it is appropriate. Difficult conversations, however, are not primarily about information—even though they seem to be, such as when a family member screams at the therapist or nurse: "What did you say to her that made her so sad?"—but about the artful management of feelings. The health professional who has mastered a large body of clinical information and who takes great pride in that mastery might well be at a loss when feelings and emotions are at issue rather than information. Indeed, if the professional is not particularly

TABLE 83-2 Empathic Phrases and Responses

- "This must be . . . (dreadful, awful, depressing, frightening) . . . for you to hear."
- "This is obviously making you feel very . . . "
- "I hear you."
- "Tell me more about that."
- "And how did you experience (or feel about) that? What was that like?"
- "So, this must have caused/must be causing you a lot of . . . (heartache, sadness)."
- "I wonder what you're feeling right now."
- "What is it about that that . . . (worries, upsets) . . . you?"
- "What is it about talking about that . . . (you don't like, makes you anxious, makes you want to talk about something else?)"
- "What would you like to have happen from this?"
- "Anything else?"
- "Now let me make sure I'm understanding you. You're asking me . . . (whether or not, how it is that) . . . Is that correct?"
- "So, what you're saying is that . . . "
- Repeat the other's last 3 or 4 words.
- "It must be very hard for you to be here when you're so disappointed in me and in the care you've received."
- "Mr. Jones, I have a hunch that you're even more miserable (angry, distressed, sad) than you're letting on."
- "I'm wondering what it's like for you to be here."

Adapted from Halpern (26); Buckman, Kason (100) with permission.

good at understanding and managing his or her own feelings, or if projecting feelings make him or her uncomfortable, then it is quite likely that this kind of individual will not fare well when conversations take an emotionally challenging turn (102).

Ultimately, what empathic communication strategies aim at is maintaining an attentional and supportive focus on the needs and concerns of patients and their representatives (103). Like all good ethical behavior, empathy is profoundly "other regarding." Empathically artful professionals put their self-interests and self-regarding needs aside and focus intensely on the other. Not surprisingly, the other usually feels valued and supported so that it is hardly surprising that data indicate a correlation between improved clinical outcomes and patient compliance when empathy is present (104). Nevertheless, the health professional's occasional urge to distance himself or herself from emotionally painful situations is understandable, especially in a high "burnout" and stressful delivery system like providing brain injury services. The ability to understand and be able to "be with" the very painful feelings that are associated with catastrophic disability can require enormous maturity by way of a deep insight into and acknowledgement of life's fragility, unfairness, and brutality. It is not an exaggeration to say that achieving that professional sensibility can take a lifetime of work.

CONCLUSION

By way of a conclusion, consider that the lay public's reaction toward persons with brain injury is often uncaring and distancing. As was discussed in the section on competence and neurodiversity, because the behavior of persons with serious brain injury can be so dramatically different from what most people are accustomed to, persons with TBI may seem not only strange but also frightening. Perhaps it is not too surprising then that the public's common aversion toward persons with serious brain injury (and other kinds of disability) involves their blaming the individual for his or her injury or disability (104). This reaction might serve the purpose of relieving the blamer from feeling obligated to help the disabled individual get on with his or her life. In other words, thinking that persons with brain injury somehow "deserved" what happened to them justifies an impulse to distance oneself from them without feeling guilty. Indeed, the blamer might feel thoroughly entitled to his blaming by pointing out that so many persons with brain injury seemed to invite their injuries through irresponsible behavior. Failing to wear a seat belt or a motorcycle helmet, driving above the speed limit and/or under the influence of drugs or alcohol, using firearms, participating in gang violence, or simply taking foolish, juvenile risks may seem to vindicate what has been called the "just world" hypothesis: "You deserve what you get and you get what you deserve." (104)

But this invites a deeply disturbing consideration: Serious brain injury is an inevitable manifestation of certain societies' and especially America's values. Consider how poverty, drugs and alcohol, violent sports, love of speed and risk taking, aggressive driving and road rage, and the enthusiastic proliferation of firearms are part and parcel of American life and, simultaneously, are highly correlated with the occurrence of serious brain injury (62). We should be deeply disturbed over the fact that watching televised renderings of people sustaining head injuries—for example, football, professional boxing, and kick boxing—is a bona fide form of entertainment in the United States.

Of course, preventive measures have long been advocated in efforts to reduce the incidence of brain injury such as raising the driving age, mandatory motorcycle and bicycle helmet laws, severer penalties for drug and alcohol use, improved equipment—especially helmets—for youth athletes, and encouraging a greater political reluctance to wage war. But until Western societies begin seriously examining and revising the cultural values that encourage the very factors that heighten the risk of brain injury, it will remain a mainstay in Western life.

William Winslade, a bioethicist, law professor, psychoanalyst, and brain injury "survivor," has noted that "Doing what we know we must to halt the epidemic of traumatic brain injury should begin with redirecting our culture away from violence and selfishness and toward civility and empathy" (pp. 203–204) (62). Winslade's points are well worth pondering. Everyone takes risks, often very foolish ones, and everyone—even the most staunchly risk-averse—is vulnerable to the onset of serious disease, injury, and disability. It is remarkable how so many persons resist contemplating these unpleasant possibilities because their occurrence is so commonplace and their impact so devastating. In realizing a more disability-friendly society, our greatest challenge might be to exert a greater degree of compassion, kindness, charity, and humility in light of the inevitability of suffering. As Winslade implies, we need to redirect our attention away from self-interested concerns and more toward self-sacrificing and vigilance-inducing measures that reduce harms and suffering. How to achieve these objectives in a society that so champions individual liberties and self-reliance—virtually to the exclusion of admitting a responsi-

bility toward relieving another's suffering—will vex us for the foreseeable future. But it seems work well worth doing, given the burdens and miseries that await so many persons if we continue our blissfully self-interested and self-involved ways.

KEY CLINICAL POINTS

1. In assessing the judgmental ability of an individual with brain injury, professionals must be aware of the importance that is placed on individual freedoms and liberties, especially among Western societies, and therefore they must regard competency evaluations with the utmost seriousness.

2. Evaluations of judgmental ability or, in the legal context, competency must take into account the individual's ability to exert insight into his or her present interests, beliefs, and desires and whether or not they are consistent with those of his or her preinjury self. Evaluators must also insure that the individual's decisions are not unreasonably disturbed by an affective or mood disorder, fantastical or magical thinking, impaired memory, or attention. The individual being assessed must also be able to understand information and be able to rationally use that information, such as in performing benefits and burdens calculations.

3. A criterion that has long been used to justify restraining an individual's autonomy or liberty is the degree to which his or her behavior threatens harm to himself or herself or to others.

4. Evaluators must appreciate the fact that an individual might lack judgmental ability in one domain, such as managing a business, but retain it in others, such as living independently or raising children.

5. Oftentimes, patients who initiate queries and ask for more information can give the assessor an informal but excellent insight into those domains over which he or she can exercise adequate function and which ones not.

6. In assessing the ethical factors that affect health care distributional schemes in the United States, certain ones exerting considerable influence in public policy making include an American penchant for individual accountability and responsibility that rejects a welfarist or "brother's keeper" mentatility. There is also the historical tendency of health care spending to be inflationary, giving rise to the need to impose various constraints on public and private third-party coverage of health care services.

7. The obligation to reimburse health care costs was once understood to be informed by a patient's needs but more recently, and owing to the inflationary spiral of health care costs, has given way to criteria dictated by what are allowed or disallowed by an individual's health benefit policy. Consequently, the significance of medical necessity determinations and the associated need to consult evidence-based practice guidelines in determining what kinds of clinical interventions are reasonable and necessary have come to figure prominently in making allocational decisions by third-party payers.

8. Physicians must distinguish their roles as clinicians vs "stewards of societal resources" with the clinical relationship being held primary in the event of conflict.

9. Ethical considerations in treating low-level patients with brain injury, including those whose clinical course might be proceeding toward death, must consider the brain death criteria vs the opposing, more conservative viewpoint that understands death as the irreversible cessation of respiration and circulation (rather than whole brain death).

10. It is critical for health professional to distinguish the diagnostic terms of brain death, coma, vegetative state, and minimal responsiveness. Rehabilitationists should also be alerted to recent literature that has called attention to diagnostic cautions over mistaking someone who is actually minimally conscious as being in a vegetative state.

11. When communicating news to patients and family members that are unpleasant, professionals should realize that they will often have a natural urge to resist, defend, or protect themselves, especially in light of an emotionally distressed patient or family member's complaints or criticisms.

12. The literature on empathy recommends resisting the urge to react to a patient's or family member's complaints or distress and instead attempt to understand what it is like to be him or her.

13. Empathic responses especially exhibit a "curiosity" about what the other is feeling.

14. Appreciating the fact that many clients will feel better just by having someone available with whom they can share their grief or worries might help alleviate the health professional's discomfort in listening to their distress.

KEY REFERENCES

1. Banja J. *Medical Errors and Medical Narcissism*. Sudbury, MA: Jones & Bartlett; 2005.
2. Fins JJ. Rethinking disorders of consciousness: new research and its implications. *Hastings Cent Rep*. 2005;35(2): 22–24.
3. Grisso T, Appelbaum PS. *Assessing Competence to Consent to Treatment: A Guide for Physicians and Other Health Professionals*. New York, NY: Oxford University Press; 1998.
4. Halpern J. *From Detached Concern to Empathy: Humanizing Medical Practice*. Oxford, United Kingdom: Oxford University Press; 2001.
5. Mackenzie R, Watts J. Including emotionality in tests of competence: how does neurodiversity affect measures of free will and agency in medical decision making? *AJOB Neuroscience*. 2011;2(3):1–10.

References

1. Faul M, Xu L, Wald MM, Coronado VG. *Traumatic Brain Injury in the United States: Emergency Department Visits, Hospitalizations, and Deaths*. Atlanta, GA: Centers for Disease Control and Prevention, National Center for Injury Prevention and Control; 2010.
2. Centers for Disease Control and Prevention, National Center for Injury Prevention and Control. *Report to Congress on Mild Traumatic Brain Injury in the United States: Steps to Prevent a Serious Public Health Problem*. Atlanta, GA: Centers for Disease Control and Prevention; 2003.
3. Banja JD. Ethical dimensions of severe traumatic brain injury. In: Rosenthal M, Griffith E, Bond MR, Miller JD, eds. *Rehabilitation of the Adult and Child With Traumatic Brain Injury*. 3rd ed. Philadelphia, PA: F.A. Davis Company; 1999:413–434.
4. Hart T, Jacobs HE. Rehabilitation and management of behavioral disturbances following frontal lobe injury. *J Head Trauma Rehabil*. 1993;8(1):1–12.
5. Burleigh SA, Farber RS, Gillard M. Community integration and life satisfaction after traumatic brain injury: long term findings. *Am J Occup Ther*. 1998;52(1):45–52.
6. Kothari S, Kirschner K. Decision-making capacity after TBI: clinical assessment and ethical implications. In: Zasler ND, Katz DI, Zafonte RD, eds. *Brain InjuryMedicine*. New York, NY: Demos; 2007: 1205–1222.
7. Banja J. Patient advocacy at risk: ethical, legal, and political dimensions of adverse reimbursement practices in brain injury rehabilitation in the US. *Brain Inj*. 1999;13(10):745–758.
8. Hommel PA, Wang L, Bergman JA. Trends in guardianship reform: implications for the medical and legal professions. *Law Med Health Care*. 1990;18(3):213–226.
9. Buchanan AE, Brock DW. *Deciding for Others: The Ethics of Surrogate Decision Making*. Cambridge, United Kingdom: Cambridge University Press; 1989.
10. Dworkin G. *The Theory and Practice of Autonomy*. Cambridge, United Kingdom: Cambridge University Press; 1988.
11. Frankfurt H. Freedom of the will and the concept of a person. *J Philos*. 1971;68(1):5–20.
12. Bechara A, Tranel D, Damasio H. Characterization of the decision-making deficit of patients with ventromedial prefrontal cortex lesions. *Brain*. 2000;123(pt 11):2189–2202.
13. Bechara A, Damasio H, Tranel D, Damasio AR. Deciding advantageously before knowing the advantageous strategy. *Science*. 1997; 275(5304):1293–1295.
14. Caplan A. Denying autonomy in order to create it: the paradox of forcing treatment upon addicts. *Addiction*. 2008;103(12):1919–1921.
15. Janofsky JS, McCarthy RJ, Folstein MF. The Hopkins Competency Assessment test: a brief method for evaluating patients' capacity to give informed consent. *Hosp Community Psychiatry*. 1992;43(2): 132–136.
16. Grisso T, Appelbaum PS. *Assessing Competence to Consent to Treatment: A Guide for Physicians and Other Health Professionals*. New York, NY: Oxford University Press; 1998.
17. Auerbach VS, Banja JD. Assessing client competence to participate in rehabilitation decision making. *Neurorehabilitation*. 1996;6: 123–132.
18. Rozovsky F. *Consent to Treatment: A Practical Guide*. Boston, MA: Little Brown; 1984.
19. Wolf LR, Colenda CC III. The role of guardianship in the care and management of patients following head trauma. *Psych Med*. 1989; 7(1):51–58.
20. Auerbach VS, Banja JD. Competency determinations. In: Stoudemire A, Fogel BS, eds. *Medical-Psychiatric Practice*. Vol 2. Washington, DC: American Psychiatric Press; 1993:515–535.
21. Anderson TP, Fearey MS. Legal guardianship in traumatic brain injury rehabilitation: ethical implications. *J Head Trauma Rehabil*. 1989;4(1):57–64.
22. Mackenzie R, Watts J. Including emotionality in tests of competence: how does neurodiversity affect measures of free will and agency in medical decision making? *AJOB Neuroscience*. 2011;2(3): 1–10.
23. Damasio AR. *Descartes' Error: Emotion, Reason, and the Human Brain*. New York, NY: Avon Books; 1994.
24. Charland LC. Appreciation and emotion: theoretical reflections on the MacArthur Treatment Competence study. *Kennedy Inst Ethics J*. 1998;8(4): 359–376.
25. Halpern J, Arnold RM. Affective forecasting: an unrecognized challenge to making serious health decisions. *J Gen Internal Med*. 2008; 23(10):1708–1712.
26. Halpern J. *From Detached Concern to Empathy: Humanizing Medical Practice*. Oxford, United Kingdom: Oxford University Press; 2001.

27. Lee MA, Ganzini L. Depression in the elderly: effect on patient attitudes toward life-sustaining therapy. *J Am Geriatr Soc.* 1992; 40(10):983–988.

28. Meisel A, Roth LH, Lidz CW. Toward a model of the legal doctrine of informed consent. *Am J Psychiatry.* 1977;134(3):285–289.

29. Oliver Sachs. *The Man Who Mistook His Wife for a Hat and Other Clinical Tales.* New York, NY: Summit Books; 1985.

30. Templeton SK. Deaf demand right to designer deaf children. *The Sunday Times.* December 23, 2007. http://www.geneticsandsociety.org/article.php?id=3860. Accessed June 4, 2012.

31. *Vistica v. Presbyterian Hospital and Medical Center,* 432 P2d 193 (Cal 1967)

32. Sargent DA. Treating the condemned to death. *Hastings Cent Rep.* 1986;16(6):5–6.

33. Banja J. The improbable future of employment-based insurance. *Hastings Cent Rep.* 2000;30(3):17–25.

34. US Census Bureau. Health insurance highlights 2009. US Census Bureau Web site. http://www.census.gov/hhes/www/hlthins/data/incpovhlth/2009/highlights.html. Accessed June 4, 2012.

35. Patient Protection and Affordable Care Act Pub L No. 111–148, 124 Stat 119 (2010).

36. Herszenhorn DM, Pear R. House votes for repeal of health law in symbolic act. *The New York Times.* January 19, 2011: January 19, 2011. Available at http://www.nytimes.com/2011/01/20/health/policy/20cong.html. Accessed June 4, 2012.

37. Starr P. *The Social Transformation of American Medicine.* New York, NY: Basic Books; 1982.

38. Daniels N. *Just Health Care.* Cambridge, United Kingdom: Cambridge University Press; 1985.

39. Rawls J. *A Theory of Justice.* Cambridge, MA: Harvard University Press; 1971.

40. Wikipedia. Patient protection and affordable care act. Wikipedia Web site. http://en.wikipedia.org/wiki/Patient_Protection_and_Affordable_Care_Act. Accessed June 4, 2012.

41. Arts K, Erwin W. Legal challenges to health reform. Alliance for Health Reform Web site. http://www.allhealth.org/publications/Uninsured/Legal_Challenges_to_New Health_Reform_Law_97.pdf. Accessed June 4, 2012.

42. Bontke CF. Managed care in traumatic brain injury rehabilitation: physiatrists' concerns and ethical dilemmas. *J Head Trauma Rehabil.* 1997;12:37–43.

43. Granger CV, Carlin M, Diaz P, et al. Medical necessity: is current documentation practice and payment denial limiting access to inpatient rehabilitation? *Am J Phys Med Rehabil.* 2009;88(9):755–765.

44. Granger CV, Carlin M, Riggs RV, Roberts P. Medicare's recovery audit contractor program: inpatient rehabilitation facilities are taking back takebacks, but enough? *Am J Phys Med Rehabil.* 2011;90(5): 426–431.

45. Centers for Medicare and Medicaid Services. Medicare benefit policy manual, Chapter 1, Section 110—inpatient hospital stays for rehabilitation care (CMS Publication 100-02). Centers for Medicare and Medicaid Web site. http://www.cms.gov/manuals/downloads/bp102c01.pdf. Accessed June 4, 2012.

46. McClean K, Hanke CW. The medical necessity for treatment of port-wine stains. *Dermatol Surg.* 1997;23(8):663–667.

47. American Hospital Association, United BioSource Corporation. Limiting access to inpatient medical rehabilitation: A look at payment denials for Medicare patients treated in inpatient rehabilitation facilities. 2007. American Hospital Association Web site. http://www.aha.org/aha/content/2007/pdf/071003rehablcd.pdf. Accessed June 4, 2012.

48. Richter M. Symposium: evidence-based medicine: what is it and how should it be used? Is good outcomes research really better than personal experience and level V evidence? *Foot Ankle Int.* 2010; 31(11):1040–1042.

49. *Blue Cross and Blue Shield v Smither,* 573 SW2d 363, 365 (Ky App 1978).

50. *Cowan v Myers,* 484 U.S. 846, 108 S Ct 140.

51. Whyte J. Clinical trials in rehabilitation: what are the obstacles. *Am J Phys Med Rehabil.* 2003; 82(10)(suppl):S16–S21.

52. Whyte J. Distinctive methodologic challenges. In: Fuhrer M, ed. *Assessing Medical Rehabilitation.* Baltimore, MD: Paul H. Brookes; 1997:43–59.

53. Banja J. Are brain dead patients really dead? *J Head Trauma Rehabil.* 2009;24(2):141–144.

54. A definition of irreversible coma. Report of the Ad Hoc Committee of the Harvard Medical School to examine the definition of brain death. *JAMA.* 1968;205(6):337–340.

55. President's Commission for the Study of Ethical Problems in Medicine and Biomedical and Behavioral Research. *Defining Death: Medical, Legal and Ethical Issues in the Definition of Death.* Washington, DC: Government Printing Office; 1981.

56. Fins JJ. Approximation and negotiation: clinical pragmatism and difference. *Camb Q Healthc Ethics.* 1998;7(1):68–76.

57. Fins JJ. When brain death pulls at the heart strings. In: American Board of Internal Medicine. *Caring for the Dying, Identification and Promotion of Physician Competency: New Additions to Personal Narratives.* Philadelphia, PA: American Board of Internal Medicine; 1999.

58. Greenberg G. As good as dead. *The New Yorker.* 2001;77(23):36.

59. Laureys S, Fins JJ. Are we equal in death? Avoiding diagnostic error in brain death. *Neurology.* 2008;70(4):e14–e15.

60. Truog RD. Is it time to abandon brain death? *Hastings Cent Rep.* 1997;27(1):29–37.

61. Veatch RM. The death of whole-brain death: the plague of the disaggregators, somaticists, and mentalists. *J Med Philos.* 2005;30(4): 353–378.

62. Winslade WJ. *Confronting Traumatic Brain Injury: Devastation, Hope and Healing.* New Haven, CT: Yale University Press; 1998.

63. Fins JJ. Rethinking disorders of consciousness: new research and its implications. *Hastings Cent Rep.* 2005;35(2):22–24.

64. Giacino JT, Katz DI, Schiff N. Assessment and rehabilitative management of individuals with disorders of consciousness. In: Zasler ND, Katz DI, Zafonte RD, eds. *Brain Injury Medicine: Principles and Practice.* New York, NY: Demos; 2007:423–439.

65. Dubroja I, Valent S, Miklić P, Kesak D. Outcome of post-traumatic unawareness persisting for more than a month. *J Neurol Neurosurg Psychiatry.* 1995;58(4)465–466.

66. Giacino JT, Ashwal S, Childs N, et al. The minimally conscious state: definition and diagnostic criteria. *Neurology.* 2002;58(3): 349–353.

67. Fins JJ, Master MG, Gerber LM, Giacino JT. The minimally conscious state: a dagnosis in search of an epidemiology. *Arch Neurol.* 2007;64(10):1400–1405.

68. Childs NL, Mercer WN, Childs HW. Accuracy of diagnosis of persistent vegetative state. *Neurology.* 1993;43(8):1465–1467.

69. Andrews K, Murphy L, Munday R, Littlewood C. Misdiagnosis of the vegetative state: retrospective study in a rehabilitation unit. *BMJ.* 1996;313(7048):13–16.

70. Wilson FC, Harpur J, Watson T, Morrow JI. Vegetative state and minimally responsive patients—regional survey, long-term case outcomes and service recommendations. *NeuroRehabilitation.* 2002; 17(3):231–236.

71. Schnakers C, Vanhaudenhuyse A, Giacino J, et al. Diagnostic accuracy of the vegetative and minimally conscious state: clinical consensus versus standardized neurobehavioral assessment. *BMC Neurol.* 2009;9:35.

72. Giacino JT, Kalmar K, Whyte J. The JFK Coma Recovery Scale-Revised: measurement characteristics and diagnostic utility. *Arch Phys Med Rehabil.* 2004;85(12):2020–2029.

73. Lammi M, Smith VH, Tate RL, Taylor CM. The minimally conscious state and recovery potential: a follow-up study 2 to 5 years after traumatic brain injury. *Arch Phys Med Rehabil.* 2005;86(4): 746–754.

74. Schiff ND, Fins JJ. Hope for "comatose" patients. *Cerebrum.* 2003; 5(4):7–24.

75. Posner J, Saper C, Schiff ND, Plum F. *Plum and Posner's Diagnosis of Stupor and Coma.* 4th ed. New York, NY: Oxford University Press; 2007.

76. Fins JJ. Clinical pragmatism and the care of brain injured patients: toward a palliative neuroethics for disorders of consciousness. *Prog Brain Res.* 2005;150:565–582.

77. Fins JJ. *A Palliative Ethic of Care: Clinical Wisdom at Life's End.* Sudbury, MA: Jones & Bartlett Publishers; 2006.

78. *Matter of Karen Quinlan*, 70 NJ 10, 355 A2d 677 (1976).

79. Jennett B, Plum F. Persistent vegetative state after brain damage. A syndrome in search of a name. *Lancet.* 1972;1(7753):734–737.

80. Fins JJ. Minds apart: severe brain injury. In: Freeman M, ed. *Law and Neuroscience, Current Legal Issues.* Oxford, United Kingdom: Oxford University Press; 2010:367–384.

81. Fins JJ. Constructing an ethical stereotaxy for severe brain injury: balancing risks, benefits and access. *Nat Rev Neurosci.* 2003;4(4): 323–327.

82. Fins JJ. The ethics of measuring and modulating consciousness: the imperative of minding time. *Prog Brain Res.* 2009;177:371–382.

83. Penfield W. The significance of the Montreal Neurological Institute. In: Neurological Biographies and Addresses (Foundation Volume, Published for the Staff, to commemorate the Opening of the Montreal Neurological Institute, of McGill University). London, United Kingdom: Humphrey Milford/Oxford University Press; 1936.

84. Fins JJ. Ethics of clinical decision making and communication with surrogates. In: Posner J, Saper C, Schiff ND, Plum F, eds. *Plum and Posner's Diagnosis of Stupor and Coma.* 4th ed. New York, NY: Oxford University Press; 2007.

85. The Multi-Society Task Force on Persistent Vegetative State. Medical aspects of the persistent vegetative state (2) [published correction appears in *N Engl J Med.* 1995;333(2):130]. *N Engl J Med.* 1994; 330(22):1572–1579.

86. Fins JJ. Affirming the right to care, preserving the right to die: disorders of consciousness and neuroethics after Schiavo. *Palliat Support Care.* 2006;4(2):169–178.

87. Fins JJ, Illes J, Bernat JL, Hirsch J, Laureys S, Murphy E. Neuroimaging and disorders of consciousness: envisioning an ethical research agenda. *Am J Bioeth.* 2008;8(9):3–12.

88. Hirsch J. Functional neuroimaging during altered states of consciousness: how and what do we measure? *Prog Brain Res.* 2005; 150:25–43.

89. Schiff ND, Rodriguez-Moreno D, Kamal A, et al. fMRI reveals large-scale network activation in minimally conscious patients. *Neurology.* 2005; 64(3):514–523.

90. Owen AM, Coleman MR, Boly M, Davis MH, Laureys s, Pickard JD. Detecting awareness in the vegetative state. *Science.* 2006;313(5792): 1402.

91. Fins JJ, Schiff ND. Shades of gray: new insights from the vegetative state. *Hastings Cen Rep.* 2006;36(6):8.

92. Lo Bernard. *Resolving Ethical Dilemmas: A Guide for Clinicians.* 3rd ed. Philadelphia, PA: Lippincott Williams & Wilkins; 2005.

93. Jonsen AR, Siegler M, Winslade WJ. *Clinical Ethics.* 6th ed. New York, NY: McGraw Hill; 2006.

94. Beauchamp TL, Childress JF. *Principles of Biomedical Ethics.* 6th ed. New York, NY: Oxford University Press; 2009.

95. Maitz EA, Sachs PR. Treating families of individuals with traumatic brain injury from a family system perspective. *J Head Trauma Rehabil.* 1995;10:1–11.

96. Gunther M. Countertransference issues in staff caregivers who work to rehabilitate catastrophic-injury survivors. *Am J Psychother.* 1994;48(2):208–220.

97. Fiester A. Viewpoint: why the clinical ethics we teach fails patients. *Acad Med.* 2007;82(7): 684–689.

98. Damasio AR. *The Feeling of What Happens: Body and Emotion in the Making of Consciousness.* New York, NY: Harcourt Brace & Company; 1999.

99. Duncan S, Barrett L. Affect is a form of cognition: a neurobiological analysis.*Cogn Emot.* 2007;21(6):1184–1211.

100. Buckman R, Kason Y. *How to Break Bad News.* Baltimore, MD: The Johnson Hopkins University Press; 1992.

101. Gunther M. Catastrophic illness and the caregivers: real burdens and solutions with respect to the role of the behavioral sciences. In: Caplan B, ed. *Rehabilitation Psychology Desk Reference.* Rockville, MD: Aspen Publishers; 1987;219–243.

102. Banja J. *Medical Errors and Medical Narcissism.* Sudbury, MA: Jones & Bartlett; 2005.

103. Branch WT, Kern D, Haidet P, et al. The patient–physician relationship. Teaching the human dimensions of care in clinical settings. *JAMA.* 2001;286(9):1067–1074.

104. Scott C. Belief in a just world: a case study in public health ethics. *Hastings Cent Rep.* 2008;38(1):16–19.

Clinicolegal Issues

Arthur Ameis, Nathan D. Zasler, Michael F. Martelli, and Shane S. Bush

INTRODUCTION

For a clinician involved in the assessment and care of persons with a history of traumatic brain injury (TBI), requests to serve as an expert witness are common and should be considered routine and appropriate within the spectrum of professional demands. The legitimate needs of patients, insurers, and courts for expert advice may cover various topics with opinions being requested regarding numerous clinical aspects including, but not limited to, diagnosis, causation and apportionment, severity, prognosis, treatment (i.e., What is medically necessary and reasonable?), and delineation of impairment, disability, and handicap (i.e., Can the person live independently, work or drive again, manage finances, and make legal decisions?). These parties typically need education to delineate (a) science from pseudoscience, (b) the application of differential diagnosis, and (c) statistical properties and concepts (e.g., reliability, validity, sensitivity, specificity, positive predictive value, and negative predictive value) as applied to symptom lists and to clinical and neuropsychological tests. Services provided at the intersection of law and clinical practices are typically referred to as *clinicolegal, medicolegal,* or *forensic*; although, the terms are used interchangeably, the term *clinicolegal* will be used in this chapter.

Most of the Western world's professional organizations have set out policy statements supporting the importance to society of clinicians providing expert witness services to the courts, and numerous guidelines have been prepared to assist clinicians with providing such services in an ethical fashion. As noted in 2008 by the UK General Medical Council (1), *"Society needs doctors to act as expert witnesses; they are essential to our judicial and tribunal systems and help resolve disputes that require specialist medical knowledge."* This body noted that when expert witnessing, clinicians take on a different role from that of treatment provider and patient advisor/advocate. However, the same body went on to note the ongoing obligations for ethical practice, objectivity, and impartiality and stated that clinicians must avoid providing evidence that is misleading or which fails to disclose relevant information.

A similar declaration was recently made within the revised Rules of Evidence of the Province of Ontario (2), echoing the UK guidelines inasmuch as the clinician must (a) recognize an overriding duty to the court and to administration of justice, (b) give opinion evidence within the limits of scope of practice and professional competence, (c) keep up to date within one's scope of practice, (d) explain where there is a range of views, and (e) protect confidential information.

This chapter provides an overview of key issues and protocols relevant to clinicians who wish to provide ethical and useful expert witness services as well as become more knowledgeable regarding clinicolegal issues in general. Readers are encouraged to review the references provided, consult the guidelines of relevant professional organizations, and become familiar with local state laws and practices. Those so inclined should also strongly consider joining professional organizations involved in advising, mentoring, and creating continuing medical education (CME) opportunities for expert witnesses as well as for clinicians who find themselves being asked to provide clinicolegal testimony.

GENERAL CLINICOLEGAL PRECAUTIONS FOR PRACTITIONERS

Documentation Precautions

It is important for clinicians to be aware of the manner in which they document both clinical and clinicolegal contexts. Impartiality and expertise must be explicitly evident to the lay reader. In the clinical context, this means that clinicians should avoid using pejorative terminology in their patient notes, making judgmental statements, or coming to conclusions that may not be based on scientific evidence. In the clinicolegal context, it is essential that clinicians avoid opinions based on "suspicion" or "belief" that the patients are exaggerating symptoms or, worse yet, malingering, or alternatively, has a psychogenic basis for their condition.

Clinicians should also avoid creating documentation in which a pattern of emphasis may suggest examiner bias such as bolding, underlining, or italicizing only those positive or negative findings that are not supportive of the claimant's case. Offering opinions that are without scientific foundation, in either a clinical or clinicolegal context, increases the risk of legal action being pursued by patients/claimants and/or their legal representatives for slander or for unprofessional practices.

It is important to save material that may or did serve as the foundation of clinicolegal opinions so that there are ways to reference and confirm the source of information that examiners have put in their reports including exam findings and/or historical information that may support one's position(s). Selective inclusion of damaging information to the exclusion of information supportive of the examinee's or patient's claim would be considered unethical (3).

Requests for Records and Court-Ordered Subpoenas

It is important for clinicians to understand the nuances of responding to records requests as well as court-ordered subpoenas for either patients or claimants, the latter who may have been examined in an independent examination (IE) context. Clinicians must maintain adherence to general confidentiality guidelines and Health Insurance Portability and Accountability Act (HIPAA) regulations, the latter when governed by the laws of the United States of America (similar laws exist in Canada and most other Western nations). The HIPAA privacy rule does not apply to entities that are workers' compensation insurers, workers' compensation administrative agencies, or employers except to the extent that they may otherwise be covered entities. Because of the significant variability among such laws, the privacy rule permits disclosures of health information for workers' compensation purposes in a number of different ways including disclosure with and without authorization. Covered entities are required to reasonably limit the amount of protected health information disclosed to the minimum necessary to accomplish the workers' compensation purpose and/or in attempts to secure payment. Protected health information may be shared for such purposes to the full extent authorized by the state or other law (4).

Clinical care records should only be released by a health care professional on receipt of a duly executed subpoena that must be honored in the clinician's jurisdiction or by a signed declaration of release by the patient or a legal proxy (when the patient lacks decision-making capacity), which is relevant to the clinician or examiner to whom the release was sent. IE reports should not be released by an examiner to either opposing counsel or to the examinee unless there is a court-ordered subpoena. In most cases, such release should be handled directly by the party who retained the examiner to do the IE. The retaining party, rather than the examiner, is typically the holder of privilege, and thus should provide copies of reports or direct where the reports should be sent.

Ideally, internal flow sheets can be used to track and record subpoena requests and responses in an effort to ensure that all appropriate parties have been notified and that such requests are responded to in a timely fashion and within court-dictated timeframes (see Appendix I for a sample tracking sheet for subpoenas). It is important to follow court instructions closely. Only the specific records requested should be sent by an examiner in response to a court-ordered subpoena. On occasion, patients or examinees will not want their records to be released. If a subpoena has been issued, the patient/examinee and their lawyer will have to determine whether to make motions to the court to "quash" the request. In such circumstances, if clinicians are informed that an effort is to be made to block the subpoena, the clinicians should not proceed to release the records and should instead advise all parties that they will await further instructions.

If clinicians believe that the release of specific material would be materially harmful to their patients, then prior to complying with the subpoena, the patients' attorney should be so advised. Motions can then be made through the patients' attorney to quash the request entirely or to seal the documents of concern so that they cannot get into the public domain.

Professional Conduct

Examiners should always remain aware of both their staff's and their own conduct to avoid clinicolegal problems in daily practice. Clinicians and their staff should be as accommodating to claimants who are undergoing IEs as they are to their own patients. Such courtesy should include prior communication with the retaining party to let the claimants know to bring their medications (particularly medications for pain or seizures), reading glasses, and any snacks that they want to or need to consume during their examination. During the examination, the examinee should be allowed reasonable opportunities to take rest breaks, have access to drinks, and to have breaks for lunch, medication, and/or use the restroom facilities.

At the conclusion of examination, examiners should consider giving the examinee a simple feedback form (see Appendix II) in which they can rate the quality of the examination relative to thoroughness, accommodations, the courtesy of the examining clinicians and staff, and/or note any problems encountered during the examination. The examiners should review the feedback form before the examinees leave. If aspects were not rated optimally, then examiners should try to intervene in a constructive and supportive manner to correct the perception while the examinees/claimants are still in their office. If it is not possible to address the issue fully at that time, the examiners should strive to address the issue to the extent possible, document any relevant facts, and of course attempt to ensure that the difficulty does not present itself on future occasions. Such practices can actually help with shaping improved clinicolegal practice as well as potentially protect the examiners from later criticism about how the exam was conducted.

Clinicolegal Terminology

Clinicians need to be familiar with common clinicolegal terminology including such terms as (a) discovery vs de bene esse ("of well-being") deposition, (b) probability vs possibility, (c) medical probability vs medical certainty, (d) causality and apportionment, (e) aggravation vs exacerbation of a condition, and (f) medical maloccurrence vs medical malpractice or negligence. When clinicians are asked to testify, the triers of fact are only interested in opinions that can be stated probabilistically, which is with greater than 50% statistical likelihood. When lawyers ask if something is "possible," it is because experts' answers will generally be given no weight in the proceeding and will not be considered unless they can be stated with "a reasonable degree of medical or clinical probability." Occasionally, expert witnesses are asked if their opinions are being stated with "a reasonable degree of medical or clinical certainty." Based on common word usage, it would seem apparent that the latter phraseology implies a higher degree of statistical likelihood, yet, lawyers cannot, as a rule, define the numerical percentage difference between "probability" and "certainty" and traditionally use these terms analogously.

Causality opinions focus on whether the condition in question was a consequence of the claimed event or not. If the event was only part of the cause, then examiners are generally charged with examining the degree to which the event contributed to the ultimate impairment or disability (so-called apportionment). For example, if there were 3 ultimate reasons why the claimant was depressed and one of them was his or her TBI, the examiner might opine that the resultant depression was 40% apportionable (5) to the TBI and 60% apportionable to other issues. Although examiners refer to *exacerbation* of an impairment when a prior condition is temporarily worsened by the event under litigation, *aggravation* of an impairment is applicable only when the injury is determined to have permanently worsened a condition that already existed prior to the event being litigated. Clinicians who serve as examiners should also be aware of the differences between medical *malpractice* and medical *maloccurrence*. Malpractice applies when the advice or care given by a clinician can be shown to have fallen below the applicable standard of care. This is usually determined through reference to the level of care that was considered appropriate for that clinician's specialty and geographic locale during the time period in question. Maloccurrence refers to complications that (a) may be associated with a particular procedure or event, (b) are known to occur, and/or (c) were conveyed to the claimant prior to the procedure occurring but do not fall below the standard of care and/or meet negligence criteria.

Malpractice Coverage Issues

Clinicians need to be aware of malpractice policy stipulations regarding providing expert witness services. In this context, clinicians will often find that professional liability/malpractice insurance policies only cover them for practice within their own state and/or states with licensure reciprocity. Many clinicians inaccurately assume that providing medicolegal examinations or expert testimony are not part of the practice of medicine and/or does not fall under the purview of their professional board or college. In fact, at least in the United States and Canada, most state/provincial professional boards or colleges consider medicolegal examination and expert witness testimony, including the provision of opinions in court regarding diagnosis, prognosis, and/or treatment recommendations, to fall under the rubric of clinical practice and professionalism. Clinicians who provide clinicolegal services commonly travel across state lines to conduct examinations and/or provide expert witness testimony; however, failing to comply with the temporary practice requirements of that jurisdiction places them in potential jeopardy of being charged with practicing health care (medicine, psychology, nursing, etc.) without a license.

The expert witnesses are not absolutely immune from liability. Expert witnesses are and should be held accountable for the veracity of their testimony. An expert witness who states untruths while testifying under oath may be held in contempt of court and charged with perjury. Risks associated with expert testimony include civil liability, criminal liability, discipline by licensing boards, and discipline by professional associations (6).

Marketing Expert Witness Services

The topic of marketing one's expert witness services can be controversial. Some clinicians who do not primarily provide clinicolegal services assume that marketing oneself for expert witness work potentially stains one's professional reputation. Others do not hesitate to market their services by placing ads in one or more publications aimed at attorneys and insurance adjustors. Most professional organizations have guidelines for marketing as well as rules that dictate that persons who serve as expert witnesses should continue to be involved in clinical practices. Expert witnesses should be familiar with the guidelines and ethics codes of their professional organizations so that they can make informed decisions and promote their professional activities in an accurate and appropriate manner. As with any other business, there is nothing inherently wrong with marketing a professional practice or a medicolegal service if it is done professionally and ethically (7).

GENERAL GUIDELINES FOR CLINICOLEGAL EXPERT TESTIMONY

General Principles

Expert witnesses must testify honestly, impartially, and completely concerning their qualifications (5). They should testify honestly, fully, and impartially regarding the clinical information involved in the case. They should review standards of practice applicable at the time of the alleged occurrence if there is a question of malpractice. They should be prepared to state whether the testimony presented is based on specific evidence-based medicine, generally accepted consensus opinion in the field, and/or personal clinical experience. Expert witnesses should be able to testify on the validity and reliability of their examination results including whether and to what extent there was inclusion of effort and response bias testing (8) (also refer to chapter 85 in this volume).

Compensation and Fees

Compensation of the expert witnesses should be commensurate with qualifications and reputation as well as time dedicated to the case and such considerations as special circumstances and accommodations, exposure to unusual risk, and other considerations. Examiners must not accept payment terms based on contingency in which fees are based on the outcome of the case. Examiners are typically entitled to be paid at higher rates for clinicolegal work than for routine clinical services, owing to factors such as (a) requirements for an expanded and specialized scope of knowledge and assessment skills; (b) special stressors and exceptional rigor required in maintaining the standards and following guidelines associated with the litigation process; (c) the exceptional impact of such work on clinical responsibilities, including detraction from normal patient scheduling, and need for arranging clinical coverage under circumstances of deadlines and unpredictable scheduling, and so forth.; (*d*) requirements for careful reading and note taking of substantial amounts of material; and (*e*) special precision in note taking and record keeping, report structure and preparation, proofing, correction, issuance, privacy issues, and so forth. The creation of differential fee structures can also create potential ethical concerns. Differential fees can introduce at least an appearance of financial incentives exerting an influence on assessment process and ultimately on clinicolegal opinions.

Accountability for how charges are determined is essential and should be based on both internal consistency within one's own practice and general consistency to the practices of one's ethical colleagues. In the latter context, ethical standards for examiners can be expressed in terms of reasonableness and consistency of fees. In this case, "reasonableness" can be defined as the degree of similarity to fees charged by other examiners in similar specialties and locales, whereas "consistency" is defined as the degree to which fees are compatible with other medical or clinical procedures of similar type provided by the clinicians or by his peer group and/or the time spent on them (3,8).

Court-Selected and Court-Hired Experts

The use of court-nominated examiners is a potential solution to systemic problems of partiality and advocacy. In jurisdictions as disparate as England, Quebec, and Virginia, the courts have begun playing an increased role in the selection of experts for IEs. Specifically, the presiding trier of fact may solicit a list or panel of examiners from one or both counsel from which the judge, alone or in collaboration with opposing counsel, selects the professional to perform the IE. Although initially applied in situations where opposing counsel protested or attempted to block usage of a particular examiner, this practice seems to be expanding to other contexts.

So-called "hot tubbing" has become popular in Australia as a means of overcoming seemingly irreconcilable differences in expert opinions. In hot tubbing, opposing examiners are asked to sit down together to discuss their findings and to provide a joint report in which all areas of agreement are outlined, and differences are either resolved or explained in detail. In Ontario, pretrial mediation with participation of experts is being tried out in the hope that trial can be avoided entirely, or at least rendered less costly and time consuming, by identifying in advance all issues that examiners agree upon and the nature and extent of disagreement of residual outstanding issues.

Qualifying as an Expert Witness and Testimony Admissibility

The issue will often arise as to whether a given "expert" meets the qualifications of the court to testify as an expert witness. Based on traditional legal nomenclature, in most jurisdictions, expert witnesses are individuals who have spe-

cial knowledge or skill gained by education, training, or experience. Such individuals may be asked to appear at trial to provide expert opinions and/or evidence. The type of testimony that is admissible in court depends on the type of professional role that the experts play in a given case (e.g., treating clinician/fact witness or expert witness) (4,9). The aforementioned roles are expounded on in the next section.

The interpretation and enforcement of rules governing the admissibility of expert testimony is the domain of the trial judge and case law. The admissibility of the expert evidence is predicated on the experts having knowledge and experience that is beyond that of the ordinary citizen and is applicable to the matter before the court. Traditionally, there are several rules that have entered into the US judicial system that address the admissibility of the scientific evidence based on Daubert (10,11) and subsequent case law. In Canada, similar rules have entered into provincial courts on the basis of the Mohan, Resurfice, and other rulings as well as legislated rules of evidence. The expert witness (in federal court and those state courts that adopted the Daubert standard) may be held to that standard, which requires that the scientific strategy or procedure on which testimony is based has been tested, published under peer review, and is well accepted in the scientific community. Because the skills that make a good expert witness are not always consistent with reliance on "good science," the Daubert ruling seems to offer attorneys and the court a useful strategy for evaluating the merit of expert testimony. Given the complexity of many diagnostic questions and procedures, particularly in TBI cases, scrutiny of the scientific methodology on which diagnoses are based is warranted and is indeed essential.

The treating clinician, sometimes called to testify as a fact witness (see next section), is permitted to present information related to clinical assessment and treatment conducted based on medical judgment of necessity and reasonableness. In contrast, the expert witnesses are generally held to a higher scientific level of scrutiny regarding their testimony and may be held to the Daubert standard. Several organizations have published white papers on standards for expert witness testimony that clinicians should be familiar with as relevant to their specialty (12,13).

In an attempt to reduce "battles of experts" that prolong trials and compound costs, a new set of rules of evidence (2) was implemented in January 2010 in Ontario, Canada. The new rules require the courts to assert themselves in the role of gatekeepers, ensuring that experts testify only within their scope of practice, using scientific principles, carefully explaining the range of opinions in the case and where the expert opinion lies in that range, and addressing matters that the courts could not otherwise ascertain. The expectation is that the courts will actively exclude unqualified, biased, or otherwise unhelpful experts from taking up critical court time and resources.

Expert Versus Fact Witness

Clinicians need to appreciate the differences between the fact witnesses and expert witnesses in the context of how they may be summoned to testify at a deposition or in court. On occasion, lawyers will attempt to subpoena clinicians (whether expert witness or not) to trial as fact witnesses to testify as to what happened in the context of their interactions with the patient, rather than retain clinicians to serve specifically as expert witnesses. Frequently, this is done to save attorneys and their clients from paying large fees because fact witnesses fees are often fixed by the court (in some jurisdictions) or are otherwise lower than those for expert witnesses. In such contexts, clinicians are not obliged to provide "expert witness" opinions on matters that would fall outside of traditional fact witness testimony. For example, they should not be asked to provide opinions about proximate cause of deficits unless they have performed examinations sufficient to substantiate such opinions (in which case they are acting as expert witnesses and should be treated as such). If lawyers want such testimony, then they should be willing to pay clinicians as experts and not as fact witnesses. Even then, the potential advocacy position of treating clinicians would need to be carefully considered for possible bias in favor of the patient.

Calling clinicians to be fact or "lay" witnesses precludes asking "why" type question or departing from straightforward fact questions about what they observed or did. In US federal court, there are federal rules of evidence, including Rule 702, which refers to testimony by experts and stipulates as follows:

> If scientific, technical, or other specialized knowledge will assist the trier of fact to understand the evidence or to determine a fact in issue, a witness qualified as an expert by knowledge, skill, experience, training, or education may testify thereto in the form of an opinion or otherwise if (1) the testimony is based upon sufficient facts or data, (2) the testimony is the product of reliable principles and methods, and (3) the witness has applied the principles and methods reliably to the facts of the case (14)(p. 30)

Some comprehensive examinations performed in clinical contexts by treating clinicians would seem to meet those criteria; however, the tendency of treating clinicians, in general, to want the best for their patients could color testimony and should, therefore, be considered when they are asked to testify.

Testimony Preparation and Caveats

When clinicians get involved in clinicolegal work, they are often surprised about both the scope of questions that may be asked in depositions and/or courtroom testimony and the stress inherent in fielding the questions. Questions can concern topics such as whether the examiners have ever (*a*) been convicted of a crime, (*b*) been sued for malpractice or had professional board actions against them, (*c*) not paid their taxes, (*d*) gotten a divorce, and/or (*e*) used illicit drugs. These and other personal inquiries make some clinicians reticent to enter the clinicolegal arena. Some of these questions may be "allowable" by the court, whereas others will be routinely considered excessively intrusive and inappropriate/irrelevant. When providing testimony, expert witnesses are not obliged to answer every question, and it is perfectly acceptable to either assert their fifth amendment privilege (referencing the fifth amendment to the US constitution that addresses self-incrimination), or assert that they will not answer be-

cause they fail to see the question's relevance. Occasionally, a judge may rule that a question must be answered if it is deemed appropriate and relevant regardless of the expert witnesess' belief. Importantly, expert witnesses should talk to retaining attorneys to disclose any "skeletons in one's closet" before going to court or sitting for a deposition to allow preparation for addressing such issues if and when they arise.

It is always prudent to pause before answering questions presented during cross-examination to give the attorney who called the expert witness time to object to the other attorney's question. The court will then rule on whether the expert witness should try to answer or not. Expert witnesses are never obligated to try to answer questions for which they do not have sufficient knowledge. It is instead entirely proper and reasonable to state, "I don't know" (15).

Typically, expert witnesses have the option of either attending a deposition or trial voluntarily or by court order. The distinction between the two is not insignificant. Testifying voluntarily raises the specter of supporting the party who asked the witness to attend and, therefore, may leave the perception of a bias on the part of the expert witness. A subpoena or summons compels the expert witness to attend and testify at the order of the court without the same potential appearance of bias.

When preparing for a deposition or courtroom trial, it is recommended that expert witnesses fully review their records and decide which, if any, are necessary to take to court. Typically, when subpoenaed to court, if counsel requires the expert to bring records, it will be noted in the subpoena and should be explicitly followed. If nothing is noted, the best advice is to bring as little as possible and only what is needed for testimony purposes. Bringing extraneous information may lead to a request by opposing counsel to look at or even copy it, and this may become "fodder" for further examination by counsel or the court. Notes or documents prepared at the time of the examination have more evidentiary value than those made later based on memory. Expert witnesses should be aware that prior transcripts of depositions are generally public record and subject to independent peer review, either external or internal, and available to lawyers who may want to use them to "impeach" testimony in subsequent cases (16–18).

Expert witnesses should also consider the types of evidentiary illustrations or other demonstrative evidence that they may want to use to supplement testimony, such as brain models or medical illustrations. They must take care to not testify outside the scope of their expertise and to clarify, precisely, what type of testimony is to be expected of them. The earlier this is done, the better for both the examiner and the retaining party. Generally, written reports form the foundation of pretrial preparation, settlement negotiations, and testimony during trial. Some attorneys do not request written reports. However, having reports allows better consolidation of information and integration and elucidation of opinions by the clinicolegal expert. In some jurisdictions, an expert will only be permitted to testify to findings and opinions already committed to written reports, and thus available to all attorneys involved in the case.

When a deposition testimony—whether discovery or *de bene esse*—is requested, expert witnesses should request that their schedules be optimally accommodated. Otherwise, lawyers may schedule trial without first confirming the date and time, which can lead to an inability to attend because of schedule conflicts. When expert witnesses are not able to attend trials and are still being asked to provide testimony, de bene esse depositions may need to be scheduled (this can be done with or without video). If the expert witness is not a "strong" witness, the retaining attorney will likely opt for a nonvideo deposition where manner of presentation and delays in response time are "invisible" in court deposition transcripts. Attorneys generally want a "good" expert witness to appear in court and not by videotaped or transcripted deposition. It is typically beneficial for expert witnesses to request a predeposition or pretrial meeting with the retaining attorney to review the case issues of concern, including potential approaches and questions by the opposing counsel. As a rule, testifying successfully in a deposition or courtroom primarily occurs through adequate preparation.

When preparing for deposition or trial, expert witnesses should update their curriculum vitae (CV). An accurate up-to-date CV is critical to credibility. In the United States, when testifying in a federal case, clinicians are required to submit a list of cases in which they have testified as an expert witness over the preceding 4 years.

During a deposition or courtroom testimony, questions should be answered directly. Taking a "professional educator/teacher approach" allows expert witnesses to convey information in a manner that informs the trier of fact. If testimony is objected to, the court will then instruct the expert witness whether or not to answer the inquiry and in what manner. If technical jargon is used by the expert witness, it should be accompanied by explanations that are understandable to the lay person. Attempts should be made to keep testimony as simple and straightforward as possible. Expert witnesses should be precise about what they say and how they say it and think about this before they say it. Expert witnesses should make sure that they understand the question before answering it. For unclear or compound questions, expert witnesses have the right as deponents to ask for clarification. Expert witnesses should remember to answer only what is asked and to never try to "make a case" by expounding on an answer or going off on a tangent. Frequently, *yes* or *no* responses are requested. If the question cannot be answered with a simple *yes* or *no*, expert witnesses should state so before, rather than after, answering *yes* or *no*. Otherwise, they may be asked to cease testimony and then will not have an opportunity to expound. Expert witnesses should also be alert to questions that set out a hypothetical set of facts, as opposed to the facts that underpin the case in question (16–18).

Expert witnesses should not attempt to justify comments unless asked to do so. Expert witnesses should not respond to objections, argue about a comment if they disagree, or lose their temper during testimony. If expert witnesses want to use demonstrative aids or leave the witness stand, they should turn to the judge and ask permission to do so, rather than just get up from their seat. It is the judge who calls the witness to the stand and excuses the witness after testimony is complete. Generally, witnesses may stay in the courtroom or leave following their testimony; however, depending on whether they will be called back for rebuttal purposes, they may not be allowed to remain in the court-

room. Witnesses are often called to court at specific times but may end up waiting for significant periods of time and may not even have the opportunity to testify because of judicial process delays, having to be recalled on another day. Such occurrences are not uncommon, and preparation should be made for accommodating these possibilities (18).

When clinicians are subpoenaed to appear for a deposition, whether discovery or de bene esse, or required to appear via subpoena for courtroom testimony, knowing the exact testimony location ahead of time is required to ensure timely arrival. Trial schedules are typically posted on bulletin boards or video screens outside courtroom areas. Expert witnesses will be asked by an officer of the court to enter the courtroom when it is time to testify. When expert witnesses enter the courtroom, they should do so confidently. The witness stand is traditionally to either side of the judge and will generally have a microphone already mounted on it. There will typically be a glass of water at the witness stand, but if there is not, and a drink is desired, it can be requested.

Expert witnesses should dress professionally and arrive well groomed for any trial. For men, this generally implies a dark suit, white shirt, and conservative matching tie; for women, either a pantsuit or conservative dress, also dark in color, with a contrasting blouse. Expert witnesses who are unkempt tend not to present as "professional" to the triers of fact. If expert witnesses need corrective lenses, prescription glasses tend to project a more professorial and educated image for both the jury and the judge than contact lenses or squinting myopically. The common adage to "not judge a book by its cover" is usually not applicable to expert witnesses in the context of a deposition or trial.

Before providing testimony, expert witnesses take an oath to tell the truth. Typically, this no longer requires a bible and involves simply raising the right hand and agreeing to tell the whole truth and nothing but the truth. In some jurisdictions, such as the province of Ontario, a special form (i.e. Ontario Expert Witness Form 53) must be completed at the time the experts prepare their report; within the form, the experts declare that they are aware of an overriding obligation to the court. Nevertheless an oath is required before testifying. After being introduced, expert witnesses' credentials are usually reviewed. Qualifications can sometimes be challenged, as might an expert witnesses' ability to testify in an expert capacity. Expert witnesses should be prepared to respond to such challenges and ensure that the information in their CV is both accurate and current. The court will then make a determination about the expert witnesses' ability to testify in an expert capacity.

Expert witnesses should try and present as relaxed and animated, rather than "stiff," while testifying. Use of hands while testifying, at least to some extent, can augment and enhance narrative presentations. Educational aids for the judge and jury can also be very helpful. During testimony, the expert should not sigh, grunt, be obscene in any manner, or get frustrated (17). When asked, "Doctor, is this book authoritative?" it may be preferable to answer "no" inasmuch because there is no publication of any type (article, treatise, or textbook) that should ever be considered absolutely authoritative because science changes on a daily basis. Expert witnesses may be asked if they agree with specific quotes. For those experts who have written extensively, it important to know when a lawyer is actually quoting the expert's own work in an attempt at ambush. If an expert witness previously wrote something or testified to something with which they now disagree, it is proper to state so with an explanation. Science evolves, and a thoughtful and honest expert witnesses' view should evolve with it (5,17).

Testimony tends to be most effective when the retaining attorney permits expert witnesses to "tell a story" in their own words. In that way, the judge and jury can more fully understand the case, particularly when it is complex and/or catastrophic. This section of testimony (direct) is then followed by the opposing attorney doing a cross-examination, that is, either asking expert witnesses questions that might support their contentions in the case or challenging contrary opinions. Gaze should always be directed to the triers of fact (i.e., the judge and the jury). Ideally, eye contact should be fixed intermittently with different persons in the jury stand; in the absence of a jury, it should be intermittently shifted to the judge. Altering voice tone and avoiding a monotone presentation is recommended to keep the attention of the judge and jury. Humor should be used very cautiously and to a very limited extent, if at all, during testimony. Expert witnesses should testify dynamically and present as approachable, trustworthy, knowledgeable, and empathetic. It is acceptable to say "I don't know" if done appropriately and not too frequently because this can raise credibility with the triers of fact (5,17,18).

Occasionally, during cross-examination, expert witnesses will be presented with information which they were not aware of and which genuinely challenges their opinion. It is proper and necessary to acknowledge such circumstances, and their implication, rather than adamantly persisting to defend the prior opinion. After cross-examination, the lawyer who retained the expert witness will potentially ask further questions (redirect) but can only do so as related to information that arose in the cross-examination for clarification purposes. There can then be further questioning by the opposing counsel, specifically, a recross, but only about the information that arose in the redirect examination. This can potentially go back and forth for a while (16–19).

The judge then has the opportunity to directly question the expert witnesses, although this generally does not happen. It is important to carefully respond to any such question because they will reflect the court's difficulties with understanding certain points raised or their implications. The judge then thanks the expert witness for attending; whereupon, the expert witness may leave the court. If the expert witness looks satisfied with his or her testimony, it gives others the impression that the testimony was sound and reinforces an air of professionalism.

Generally, a discovery deposition is conducted to determine what expert witnesses understand about the case and their medically probable opinions. However, depositions are also used to determine abilities regarding performance under pressure and presentation to the triers of fact. Attorneys often push expert witnesses on certain topics to test tolerance for being challenged and/or irritated. Typically, in a courtroom context, this occurs much less frequently, but there are exceptions. A potentially significant adverse event occurs, for both the expert and the case, when the expert

witness become angry or uncooperative while testifying, as such behavior can discredit both the expert and his or her testimony (16–19).

Business Issues in Expert Witness Work

It is sound business and professional practice for expert witnesses to make clear and comprehensive contractual agreements with retaining parties in advance of starting to perform a service. In the context of any expert witness agreement, it is critical to stipulate what one will charge for various services. Expert witnesses should carefully think through the real cost of travel (portal to portal), attendance at court and other considerations,such as multiple follow-up requests for supplemental reports or addendums, teleconferences, repeat examinations, and so forth. In addition, there may be a need to consider additional charges for special requests involving urgency, night or weekend work, special risks, and/or multiple day court attendance, among other atypical demands compared to regular clinical practice (20–22).

It can be argued that expert witnesses should charge for their time without differences relative to tasks. It would then follow that fees should be based on a flat hourly rate that is set based on a published professional guideline (should one exist) or on a rate commensurate with nonmedical experts of equal standing (i.e., legal, tax accountant, engineer). In either case, the rate should be adjusted according to the expert witnesses' standing within the clinicolegal community, driven in part by clinical and forensic reputation and accomplishments within the profession. Generally, expert witness agreements should have a retainer fee that is nonrefundable and paid before services are provided. Other points that are commonly found in agreements include payment requirements regarding timing of bill payment, interest on late charges, and stipulation as to whether interest would be compounded (20–22). (See sample agreement in Appendix III).

Cancellation fees should also be clear, as should payment for any related expenses such as travel expenses (including gas and mileage and parking, food, hotel, etc.) and other costs that the expert witnesseses should not be expected to absorb as a "cost of doing business." Generally, the party retaining the expert witnesses should agree to pay for any and all preparation time for depositions or trial regardless of who requests the testimony. Additionally, expert witnesses should never waive their right to read deposition transcripts, and the retaining party should be agreeable to reimbursing the expert witnesses for time to read depositions and correct deposition transcript errors (21–23).

It can also be helpful to include a clause to cover expert witnesses in a situation where the opposing side refuses payment for services for a deposition and/or invokes rules of civil procedure regarding setting of "reasonable fees" that are open to the discretion of the court. These "reasonable fees" may, in fact, be significantly lower than the fees charged by the expert witnesses; therefore, the expert witnesses being hired would want the retaining party to guarantee payment of normal fees or the difference between the experts' fees as defined by the court and their standard fee for expert witness work. Some states in the United States have set predetermined rates for clinicolegal fees for expert witnesses such as New York.

PRACTICAL ASPECTS OF CONDUCTING A CLINICOLEGAL EXAMINATION

Screening and Accepting Cases and Establishing Ground Rules

Most commonly, referrals of a strictly clinicolegal nature come from attorneys, insurance companies, and other third-party payers and are clearly intended for use in facilitating either settlement negotiations or litigation. Clinicians have a clear opportunity to accept or decline involvement in such cases. By contrast, clinical referrals from clinicians or other referral sources may start out as requests for consultation or for participation in care giving, with the clinicians' caregiver involvement making some linkage to any subsequent litigation process inevitable. Indeed, a "Trojan horse" phenomenon is sometimes encountered in which the clinical referral for consultation is, in fact, instigated or influenced by a plaintiff lawyer whose intent is either to later obtain a relatively inexpensive expert clinicolegal report (by way of the clinical consultation report) or to ensure the expert witness' involvement in an eventual trial. There is even a rather Machiavellian twist that may occur in which a clinician may be retained with the sole intent of ensuring that no other party in the case can obtain that clinician's services as expert witness in the case.

Sometimes, the referral source will expect advice and ongoing care for the client. Indeed, some referrals are made by lawyers who, acting out of compassion, literally try to assume a care giving role by unilaterally determining what consulting, treatment, or investigative services the client needs or in an effort to facilitate the client's own wishes to see a specialist or out of a very real concern over apparent inadequacies in the client's current health care.

When clinicolegal referrals are made, it is important for examiners to proceed carefully and deliberately through a systematic checklist before acceptance. Examiners must clearly understand the basis of the referrals and the parameters of anticipated or permissible interaction with the examinees. It is important to ensure that referral sources appreciate that, within the context of clinicolegal examinations, no therapeutic relationship of advice or care will exist. Referral sources and examinees must understand in advance that (*a*) the examiners will not provide direct advice or care to examinees at the time of the examination or at any time thereafter, and (*b*) there will be no ongoing relationship or obligation to the examinees beyond normal ethical and professional behavior (21–23).

Avoiding or otherwise managing incorrect expectations is a critical aspect of clinicolegal work. Many patients fail to appreciate this critical distinction leading to possible resentment that may precipitate active complaints to regulatory boards about perceived failure to give the expected advice or care. The recent widespread development of web-based blog sites and clinician rating sites may provide still further opportunities for such expressions of resentment. The need to ensure that examinees understand these "ground rules" is particularly important when they suffer from severe pain and are actively seeking relief or an additional source of prescription medication. Ensuring understanding of IE ground rules, including that advice and care will not be provided, is made additionally challenging when one is dealing with a claimant who may have impairments of cognition, making it critical to also discuss such issues with the guardian of record. The informed consent process should clearly address the distinctions between the role of a treating clinician and an independent examiner and clearly define the examiner's role (6,7,13). The National Academy of Neuropsychology (NAN) provided a sample consent form that includes such language (5,24).

As a clear corollary, it is improper for examiners to offer direct advice or any form of care in the context of an IE and/or as long as they are involved as IE examiners in a particular case. Such actions create a therapeutic relationship with its associated obligations and responsibilities and generally will place the examiners in an advocacy position for the person in question. This negates their clinicolegal position of neutrality. Moreover, such actions carry the implication that the examiners have found inadequate current care. Advice given outside of the treatment team context can potentially disrupt existing therapeutic relationships, which is unethical and, thus, unprofessional (3,8). Of course, if examinees report or demonstrate intent to harm themselves or others, examiners have an overarching professional responsibility (the specifics of which may vary by jurisdiction) to promote safety and inform appropriate authorities.

The source and quantum of available funding for referrals must be carefully established at the outset. Seeking concurrent fees from both clinicolegal referral sources and any other party, such as a health care insurer, has been referred to as "double billing" or "double dipping" and is unethical, potentially illegal, and unacceptable. Some referral sources may not have adequate or guaranteed funding, or payment may be delayed on the basis of the referring party needing to complete the litigation. In such cases, examiners must carefully consider whether they wish to participate in "financing" the case and working on a lien basis.

A particularly serious ethical challenge may arise when examiners agree to conditional terms concerning payment such as the stipulation that payment will depend on "the proceeds of settlement if any." Not only will the clinician be "self-financing" his or her work but also there is a real prospect that the professional fee may not be paid, in full or even in part, if the settlement is not adequate. In such circumstances, examiners must, therefore, consider whether they are prepared to provide their services on a purely *pro bono* basis. Having payment for testimony contingent on the success of the case in such a scenario naturally presents incentive for experts to present information in a manner that supports the case because the expert now has a "stake" in the outcome, which will also greatly undermine the extent to which the expert will be perceived as capable of impartiality and primary loyalty to assisting the court. In general, therefore, clinicians who choose to serve as expert witnesses should not accept cases on a contingency or lien basis because of the inherent potential for bias, perceived or otherwise. Also, if expert witnesses choose to accept liens as a method of ensuring payment for clinical services not covered by third-party payers such as no fault or workers' compensation, any outstanding balances tied to the lien should be settled (i.e., paid) prior to testimony to eliminate that potential source of bias (25,26).

In some jurisdictions, as previously noted, clinicolegal fees may be regulated or "capped." This may also be the case with some payers who will insist on paying a flat rate for an IE, imposing a fee schedule, and/or cap their fees at a certain ceiling amount—irrespective of complexity, file size, risk, expertise, and so forth. Examiners must carefully consider whether they can complete a comprehensive examination within imposed fee guidelines and particularly with respect to not exceeding a maximum fee. If examiners believe that they will in any manner be compromising the quality of their work by accepting a controlled or capped rate, they should refuse to take the case.

Acceptance of a referral should also be preceded by a consideration of whether adequate time can be devoted to a methodical and complete examination. From a practical perspective, it is also helpful to consider past experiences with referral sources. If the referring counsel has not respected the examiners' circumstances, not paid their bills in a timely fashion or in full, and/or has made intolerably frequent or otherwise unreasonable or disproportionate demands of the examiners, they are likely to repeat the same pattern. It is wise and not inappropriate or unprofessional to be selective in accepting referrals on the basis of efficient and respectful prior working relationships.

Examiners must always ensure that referred cases fall squarely within their scope of practice and experience. They should consider their competence and confidence with the illness or injury and other circumstances of the case outlined by the referral source. It is equally important to consider whether there will be significant difficulty in performing a critical review of the case if the final opinion may be unsupportive of the claimant's legal case and/or critical of the clinical opinions or care given by other professionals (21–23).

Concerning this last point, it is not uncommon for legal counsel to make a referral strictly to determine if the case merits the legal as well as expert time and resources that will need to be devoted in preparation for negotiated settlement or litigation. In such circumstances, a candid opinion by a knowledgeable examiner may save both counsel and claimant unnecessary stress and cost. It is, thus, helpful to clarify with counsel, at the case outset, whether this is one of the considerations in making the referral.

Communicating Ground Rules to the Examinee

Having accepted a referral, the examiners have the obligation to ensure that in each encounter, the examinees are treated in a dignified and respectful manner. This is not always simple. Examinees very often present for IEs with ambivalence, anxiety, or even distrust (5,8,26). Seeing examiners for a purpose other than caregiving falls outside normal experience and expectations of most persons who are injured, and many examinees have difficulty with the concept. By extension, there is the inference that they, and their own clinicians, have been deemed lacking in credibility by the opposing insurance or legal party. Hostility and manipulation are not entirely uncommon, particularly when the examinees are aware that the outcome of the examination may have important implications for the parameters of settlement of the case. For the examinees, such psychoemotional states may be superimposed on (a) neurological impairments in cognition, language and/or behavior; (b) physical impair-

ments; and/or (c) financial, vocational, and/or interpersonal difficulties that are the reasons for the examination. Apprehension may be partly because of inaccurate or incomplete information provided to them by their attorney, family members, treating health professionals, or others regarding the purpose and nature of the IE.

Not uncommonly, referrals by insurance companies for clinicolegal examinations are interpreted by examinees as hostile in nature, implying or even seeming to overtly accuse the examinees of unreliability or deception or the attending clinicians of incompetence. The lack of proper understanding of the nature of independent clinicolegal examinations readily translates into regulatory body complaints. This is particularly likely when examinees perceive the absence of any offer of advice or prescription as improper professional behavior, even more so a refusal in response to a direct request by the examinees (26).

Recognizing the potential for anxiety that is inherent in such assessments and emphasizing the objective nature of the examination should serve to increase the examinees' comfort levels and perception of fairness while fostering reliable performance. Clearly, as Binder and Thompson (7) noted in the context of neuropsychology but with general applicability, examiners must attempt to minimize any potential discomfort associated with such examinations.

A standard protocol in which examinees are provided clear and accurate information about the purpose of the examination and the procedures to be employed at the outset of the examination helps to reduce anxiety and distrust and increase cooperation. Invariable usage of a standard protocol is a valuable defense, should there be any later accusation by examinees.

The Canadian Society of Medical Evaluators (CSME) (20) developed and provided educational pamphlets specifically for dissemination by examiners or insurers to the examinees. Separate pamphlets were prepared to meet the somewhat differing circumstances of physical medicine and psychiatric IEs. By anecdotal reports, the use of the pamphlets by CSME members has been associated with a marked decrease in regulatory body complaints and/or facilitation of complaint resolution.

It bears repeating that not only the examiners but also each member of their staff and the office environment itself must simultaneously project an unambiguous message of clinical professionalism along with complete absence of opportunity for care and advice to examinees. (9). The message must be projected proactively in word, gesture, and signage. Failure to ensure that examinees do not expect advice or care is unacceptable. Lack of a clear message leads by default to an expectation of care and advice.

Examinees must also understand certain "rules of engagement." Their full cooperation is essential; lack of full effort, withholding of information, or other action/inaction raises questions about effort and honesty and may be noted in the report and treated as a negative aspect to issues of severity or credibility. Cooperation not only means being forthright with responses to the examiners but also the examinees must be prepared to respond to the examiners with adequate detail. It is not acceptable for examinees to later claim that gaps in history fell under such rubrics as "he didn't ask, and I didn't offer" or "it's not my place to correct her."

Examinees need to understand that examiners typically do not discuss findings or opinions with them. Provocation of discomfort or pain may be necessary in physical examinations but strictly to the extent necessary for a clear understanding of the location, nature, and extent of the problem. Examinees are always free to ask for a pause or a break or to terminate an examination; however, if the examiner does not accept the reason for the pause, break, or termination and instead finds such requests unnatural, excessive, manipulative, or otherwise inappropriate, such information may be noted in the report as lack of reasonable cooperation.

It is appropriate to routinely explain to each examinee that the expert has a defined protocol in the event that any finding is made that is unexpected or otherwise of concern with respect to the examinee's immediate state of health. For example, the examiner might advise the examinee that he or she would be well advised to arrange an appointment with his or her own clinician but may not give further details; however, with consideration of and adherence to privacy and confidentiality agreements, the examiner will separately communicate the finding or concern promptly to the examinee's attending clinician and/or the retaining party (the latter who, in turn, has an obligation to report the same to the examinee's lawyer and that person, in turn, to the examinee's treating clinician) (3). Some examiners would take the position that the only recourse when there is a clinical concern requiring medical follow-up would be to inform the retaining party and request that they immediately convey the information to the examinee's attorney or health provider so as not to establish a physician-patient relationship in the context of the independent medical evaluation (IME) that would create a potential medicolegal and ethical morass.

"Trust But Verify" as a Fundamental Element of the Clinicolegal Examination

Barsky (27) was one of the first to point out the need for caution, special skills, and independent corroboration of the narrative history obtained during the clinical interview. This need for independent corroboration is particularly important when somatization or response bias is evident or suspected. Simply put, even the most well-intentioned person is capable of inadvertent but significant errors of recall and/or distortions of data presentation because of misunderstanding, personal perspective, prioritization, emphasis, emotional significance, fatigue, anxiety, and other factors unrelated to dissimulation. Examiners must not underestimate the importance of the very human social attribute of wanting to be seen in a favorable light by others.

In working with persons with a history of TBI, examiners are confronted with several special challenges. In addition to examinees' distinct financial motivation to secure or even enhance the legal claim by emphasizing certain complaints or shaping test responses, the nature of the brain injury may affect recall, insight, stamina, and motivation. Neuropsychiatric impairment may aggravate or create impulsivity, anxiety, distrust, paranoia, apathy, and/or other cognitive, emotional, and behavioral symptoms.

Don and Carragee (28), studying the self-reported history of persistent axial pain in vehicular trauma, found a significant lack of validity. Some 50% of claimants who had reported no previous axial pain problems did, in fact, have a documented history of such problems. Indeed, some 75% failed to report one or more preexisting comorbid conditions such as alcohol abuse, illicit drug use, and psychological diagnosis. These authors also noted that the disparity was more likely when patients perceived the motor vehicle accident (MVA) to have been the fault of another person, as opposed to their own fault, or no one's fault.

Response bias is a type of cognitive bias that can affect the results of the interview, physical examination, and certain testing results in terms of either underreporting or overreporting problems. There are several reasons that persons can demonstrate response bias above and beyond issues of secondary gain. In litigation, the literature shows that such behavior is not at all uncommon (29,30). Response bias is encountered in many routine clinical settings. For example, the elderly person who fears losing independence may attempt to minimize visual, auditory, or balance problems. A patient who is ill may overemphasize symptom severity or duration to be taken seriously. Response bias in clinicolegal circumstances is merely an extension of this common phenomenon and may be innocent, representing a sincere "cry for help" or an effort to ensure the injury claim is taken seriously. Of course, it may also reflect a desire to manipulate the examiners' perceptions, sympathies, and opinions. Owing to the latter, response bias must always be carefully considered in clinicolegal circumstances. It must be assessed and then commented on because it might pertain to the examination findings and their interpretation.

Response bias may involve misrepresentation by commission: a symptom may be fabricated or exaggerated/magnified. It may involve misrepresentation by omission: a critical piece of information may be withheld. Response bias may be subtle, sophisticated, and well rehearsed, or it may be blatant, naive, and impulsive. Cardinal signs include implausibility, unusual gaps in information recall, exceptional vagueness, contradictions in statements, and/or inconsistency. Despite the expertise of examiners in assessing human behavior, the preponderance of evidence indicates that examiners do not have the ability to make highly accurate determinations regarding symptom validity based on clinical judgment alone. However, the ability of examiners to make such determinations improves significantly when empirically based measures (e.g., symptom validity tests) are used (31) (see chapter 85 in this volume).

Employing formal and informal means of assessing response bias, followed by formal structured reporting of related findings is a critically important component of a comprehensive TBI examination. The official position paper of the NAN on symptom validity assessment posits that both response bias assessment and any specific symptom validity tests deemed necessary for examination of symptom validity are clinically necessary (31). However, examiners should exercise great caution regarding going further by inferring motivation—the intent and goal of the examinees. In the absence of performance significantly below chance on forced-choice symptom validity tests, thus demonstrating a deliberate and consistent effort at deception, examiners may be well served by avoiding speculation on whether response bias is inadvertent or deliberate and purposeful. Examiners should instead discuss the differential diagnostic list of potential sources of the unreliability detected. Such possible reasons for improbable performance or invalid responding may include inadvertency, medication, pain, fatigue, personality traits, pathopsychoemotional mechanisms (as might be seen with denial, repression, or somatoform disorders), symptom amplification/exaggeration, and deliberate deception or fabrication (the latter occurring in either malingering or factitious disorder). There is a considerable literature supporting the need for cautious consideration of response bias during the examination process (32–36) (also refer to chapter 85 in this text). Use of known group comparisons (i.e., comparing a given examinees' scores on symptom validity tests to groups of subjects known to have various diagnoses or to be simulating impairment) increases examiners' confidence in diagnostic impressions. A seminal paper on test effort was published by Rohling and colleagues (33) who looked at the effects of effort in patients involved in compensation claims. They concluded that for most exaggerating patients, neuropsychological test scores are *underestimates* of true ability.

A careful and complete explanation of the assessment of response bias provides the report's readers with a reference point as to how fairly and competently this confounding element was evaluated, what finding was made, and whether the implications were considered and applied to the balance of the report. It is reasonable to extend that commentary toward the impairment findings made by other examiners because it may serve to provide a basis of understanding for some differing clinical opinions. As a corollary of a careful assessment for response bias, the examiner will be in an enhanced position to consider the reliability and validity of the apparently abnormal findings of those examiners who did not look for inconsistencies or otherwise consider response bias or who chose to ignore any and all such matters. Diagnosis of *malingering*, when supported by a convergence of objective evidence, should be made using appropriate probabilistic language (32,37). (See chapter 84 in this volume).

As a further quality control measure, prior to examination, examinees should be given an explanation of the anticipated examination process. As a component of this description, examiners should emphasize the importance of examinee's displaying their real capacities, including consistently being honest and putting forth their best efforts throughout the examination. It should also be explained that the consistency and extent of the examinees effort and degree of disclosure will be assessed and may impact on the examiners' rating of reliability.

It is ethically necessary to give the examinees notice, before the actual examination, that response bias and effort will be tested (38). However, it is equally inappropriate to disclose to examinees or their advocates the nature of the symptom validity assessments including the specific tests that may be used. It is not necessary to inform the examinee of the results of response bias assessment. Such discussions can be highly confrontational and counterproductive unless carried out in a sophisticated manner and for a specific purpose such as giving the examinees an opportunity to try to reduce response bias behaviors during the balance of the examination. However, such efforts may serve only to create more sophisticated dissimulation. It is imperative that examinees also understand that pain, fatigue, confusion, memory lapses, or other neurological impairments will not be automatically and unreasonably deemed to be evidence of lack of cooperation or effort. In clinical (vs. clinicolegal) examination contexts, discussions of symptom validity assessment results between clinicians and patients are common. To facilitate that process, Carrone and colleagues (39) provided a symptom validity feedback model that promotes the exchange of information without confrontation.

Perceived Control and Quality Assurance

It is important for examinees undergoing clinicolegal examinations to retain a sense of personal safety, including some control over the proceedings. Examinees have, to a reasonable extent, the right to share control of the examination pace and the right to ask why a particular question is being posed or test procedure performed. It may be reasonable for examinees to ask why certain topics or tests, commonly encountered in interactions with attending clinicians, were omitted. Examiners must use their judgment regarding how best to respond to specific questions. Examinees have an absolute right to decline to proceed with a given question, exam procedure, and/or the examination itself. (In some forensic, typically criminal, contexts in which examinations are mandated, examinees may face significant adverse consequence for failing to comply with the process so they should understand the consequences when making decisions about participation). Within reason, accommodations should be made for breaks to use the restroom or to rest because of fatigue and/or the need to take medication. Examinees should also be informed of the importance of reporting any sense of difficulty or distress to the examiners in "real time" and not later. It is also often instructive to encourage examinees to comment during, and particularly toward the end of the examination if any element of questioning or testing was new, unfamiliar, and/or omitted relative to prior assessment either in a clinical or clinicolegal context (e.g., "Is there anything I neglected to ask you about your condition?" or alternatively, "Is there anything that I did not do on your physical exam that you think is important for me to look at?"). The absence of mention of such concerns may reduce or remove the ability of examinees to later complain about the examination. However, some examinees may maliciously attempt, from the beginning, to excessively control key aspects of the assessment (e.g., pace, direction of questioning, degree of detail) and/or to intimidate the examiners; such behavior is, of course, unacceptable. Examiners should never provide answers to test questions after examinees have offered an incorrect response because doing so may invalidate interpretation as well as potential future reexamination.

While it is appropriate and even necessary to notify examinees of "zero tolerance" rules regarding inappropriate verbal or physical behavior directed against the examiners and their staff and potential negative inferences from lack of cooperation or from premature termination of the examination, expert examiners should consider the possibility that in such examinations, there may be inconsistent cooperation or problematic verbal or physical behaviors related to direct TBI sequelae such as neurogenic fatigue, seizures, dysarthria, dyslexia, impulse control, perseveration, and inability to sustain attention, among other issues and/or other post-trauma impairments secondary to medications, pain, and/or psychological issues such as post-traumatic stress disorder (PTSD) or depression.

Confidentiality Issues

The clinicolegal examination is one in which a limited duty of confidentiality is owed to examinees. The referring party is entitled to full disclosure of anything learned by the examiner at any time during the examination. Examinees should be under no misapprehension that the examiners will suppress information disclosed under the proviso of "I tell you this in strict confidence," including disclosures involving sexual orientation; sexual, physical or substance abuse history; sexually transmitted disease (STDs); or abortion. When examinees begin a statement with something along the lines of the above proviso, or "Off the record. . .," examiners should quickly clarify the limits to confidentiality, typically stating that everything that the examinees say or do are considered to be "on the record."

The absence of a therapeutic relationship does not prevent the examiners from communicating verbally or in writing with a treating clinician, regarding any concerns or suggestions, particularly emerging issues such as suicidal rumination or inappropriate regimen or dose of medication. Examiners must have possession of appropriate releases signed by the holder of privilege, giving the examiners legal right to exchange information with treating clinicians, family members, employers, or others. A memo must be made of the date, name of person contacted, and content of any verbal communication. Written communication by mail, fax, or e-mail must be retained with the file. The appropriate means of communication will depend on the nature and priority of the circumstance. A note to a treating clinician or other person should not be entrusted to the examinee if there is any doubt as to whether and when it will be delivered or if there is concern about the examinee reading the contents. Another option in such a scenario is for the examiners to document the finding in writing, contact the retaining party, and request that the information be conveyed to the examinee's lawyer immediately.

Informed Consent

Once examinees understand the purpose of the examination, process of the examination, rules of disclosure, expectations for cooperation and effort, examinee rights, and the extent of feedback regarding the results of the examination, examiners should invite questions and provide further clarification as needed. A summary or overview sheet can be helpful in orienting the examinee to what will occur during their IME (see Appendix IV). Only after these issues are clearly understood should the informed consent to participate be sought. A consent or IME agreement form is necessary to document the examinee's understanding of the nature of the examination and their willingness to participate within the framework and conditions stipulated (see Appendix V). In addition, consent forms can facilitate communication between examiners and examinees. A checklist can be incorporated into the consent form, allowing examinees to systematically consider, seek clarification if necessary, and then indicate their understanding of each major point by initialing each point on the list and/or signing with a witness the bottom of the form. Informed consent cannot be obtained and should not be sought directly from examinees with marked cognitive or communication disorders or from minor children but rather from their legal guardians. In some circumstances examiners may need to seek written proof of guardianship. For examinees who have legal guardians that provide informed consent on their behalf, their consent to participate should nevertheless be sought and the response be recorded. In some criminal forensic contexts, or when the examination is ordered by the court, however, informed consent is not needed; rather, the examiners provide notification of purpose.

It cannot be emphasized enough that unless consent is freely and fully given within the context of being fully informed, examiners should not proceed and instead should allow the legal parties and claimants to settle any issues before proceeding or rescheduling. Expediency, sympathy, or urgency should never be the basis for disregarding prudence concerning informed consent. If examinees refuse to sign the consent form, then no examination should be conducted, and examiners should consult with the party that retained them (3).

Third Party Observers—Direct and Indirect

The issue of allowing a person other than the examiners and examinees into the examination session is complicated. Examiners should consider using a staff person as chaperone, to assist as necessary, as well as be able to attest that no inappropriate conversation or action took place. Examinees should never be asked or permitted to decide about the presence of a chaperone assigned at the request of the examiners because this is a nonnegotiable element that serves to protect the examiners from potential subsequent charges of inappropriate interactions or actions, among other benefits of same.

In many jurisdictions, it is the right of examinees to designate a suitable third party to be present for their comfort and/or as an observer, which means a passive witness to what transpires. Where the examiners retain a veto right, persuasive pro and con arguments can be considered. A "pro" argument for allowing a third party to be present may exist when examinees can be expected to be exceptionally apprehensive unless accompanied. In fact, the issue often benefits from avoiding the polarization of the "either/or" proposition, and instead, an office protocol should exist, which provides clarification of who should be able to observe, in which settings observation is permissible, and with what relative benefit to examiner or examinee. The examiner should, however, bear in mind that, frequently, skilled third-party witnesses such as nurses are specifically designated by the examinees' counsel, owing to the likelihood that they will be deemed to be credible observers about what happened during the examination, and their observations and notes given equal weight to those of the examiner.

Examiners should always keep in mind that they almost always retain the option of declining the referral if any of the imposed conditions of examination appear unacceptable, including designation of a third-party observer. A claimant-designated third party is, ideally, a passive witness to the procedural events, with no role beyond reassurance of the claimant. No third party should ever be permitted to participate, advise, or interfere unless invited to do so, and no third-party disruption that compromises the quality of the examination should ever be tolerated.

In contrast to third-party presence during physical examinations, such presence is clearly inappropriate during examinations that include standardized cognitive or behavioral testing (40,41). Several authors have presented reasons why the presence of a third party may be contraindicated during examinations in which standardized tests are used. These reasons include (*a*) compromise of test security and subsequent misuse of tests, (*b*) invalidation of results because of tests not having been standardized for third-party presence, and (*c*) invalidation of results because of social facilitation (42,43). A NAN policy statement, published in 2000, distinguished between settings with third-party observers being acceptable in clinical settings for training purposes but unacceptable in forensic settings (42). Issues of observer training, observer involvement, and examination context have all been considered relevant in the debate on the appropriateness of having a third party present during neuropsychological examinations. Guidelines that exist for in-person observation are also applicable to electronic observation (e.g., audio or video recording) (44). A policy statement from the American Academy of Clinical Neuropsychology made the distinction between involved observers and uninvolved observers (45). An involved third-party observer is someone who has some investment in the outcome of the examination (e.g., a family member or attorney), whereas an uninvolved third party has no stake in the outcome and instead is strictly a source of emotional or physical support to the examinees (e.g., a health care professional). The issues of third-party observers are just as relevant to clinician examinations as neuropsychological ones (46), although much less has been published in the extant medical forensic literature than one would expect to see on this topic relative to the neuropsychological literature.

The CSME developed and provided guidelines (47) for assisting in the determination of "who and when" for the presence of a third party where there is a choice. The CSME recommends that its members maintain a written protocol that details their policy on third-party presence not only to assist them but also to demonstrate to others the rational basis and consistency of their decisions. The protocol might explain that a chaperone will always be present. In addition, a first-order family member is mandatory when examining any minor. The CSME noted that a medical professional such as a nurse is preferable to a nonfamily lay third party as an examinee-designated observer owing to insight into what constitutes acceptable questions and routine examination practices. Any third party must agree to be placed outside the visual field of the examinee to prevent any cueing or other interaction.

There is both extensive experience and new scientific literature (48–51) to support the position that despite best intentions and circumstances, examinee performance may be adversely affected by observers, even or especially, when they are with their own family, friend, or case representative (e.g., case manager or lawyer). Negative consequences of third-party observers become difficult, if not impossible, to factor out when considering apportionment of suboptimal or otherwise misleading performance. Videotaping and audiotaping are seemingly less intrusive means of monitoring the examination process. However, these methods of observation can also introduce atypical dynamics into the examination process and affect examinees performance. Test security issues also remain problematic when examinations are recorded. Examiners, too, may experience alteration of well-established, efficient, and effective routines when third-party observation, in any form, is present because of inadvertent effects on body language, tonality, questioning style, or pace (unnaturally slow or hurried). Examination settings, too, are usually not ideal for recording.

Studies revealed that formal testing results can be negatively affected by the presence of observers or recording devices in a selective nonuniform fashion. In one study, audio recording appeared to negatively affect verbal learning and recall, but not motor performance (50). In another, video recording negatively affected immediate and delayed memory performance, but not motor performance or recognition memory (51). Such studies indicate that both direct observation and indirect observation via recording devices may have a negative effect on psychological test results posing a threat to the validity of tests developed without scrutiny for such variables, and placing in jeopardy the reliability of the test results and the relevance to the specific examinee of subsequent interpretations of test results.

Telemedicine is emerging as a mainstream form of clinical service delivery for remotely situated patients. The success of telemedicine is based on the common experience that an examination conducted in a telemedical setting does not significantly diminish the validity and reliability of the routine psychiatric interview and that age or severity of impairment should not be considered automatic confounding factors (52,53). However, examiners' familiarity and expertise in using telemedicine is necessary (53), and clearly, there are limitations to what can be done in this context vs an in-person examination.

In summary, examiners have an obligation to themselves and to the referring parties to ensure that the quality of the work product is not diminished by any intrusion into the routine examination setting. It is appropriate to carefully consider reasonable requests while at the same time asking whether the accommodation will be beneficial or at least neutral to the work product and whether the accommodation will prove costly, stressful, or otherwise overly onerous to the examiners and other office staff. Third-party presence, in any form, should not be allowed during cognitive or behavioral testing. Examiners should never lose sight of the fact that they hold an absolute right to decline to take any referred clinicolegal case and should do so if the demands of the case are inconsistent with their understanding of best practices.

Selection of Assessment Procedures

Routinely, clinicolegal assessment reports are closely scrutinized by all parties and are actively critiqued, particularly by opposing counsel who may retain professionals for that sole purpose. Examiners should be aware that every aspect of the assessment process including the selection of questions and tests, the method of carrying out the tests, the findings, and their interpretation will potentially be subject to retrospective analysis and possibly to aggressive criticism. Clinicolegal examiners, unlike treating clinicians, do not have the option of citing as excuses the practical exigencies of daily practice. Clinicolegal examiners are expected to devote as much time as necessary to carry out all relevant interviewing and testing and to review all potentially significant documentation before formulating opinions.

Even the most thorough and methodical approach is not safe from criticism. Because of differences of opinion regarding optimal methods of investigation, no set of medical, psychological, or neuropsychological test procedures is beyond the critic's reach. However, criticism is far less successfully applied to tests and assessment procedures that are standardized, psychometrically sound, well accepted, commonly taught, and widely used within the profession for the same general or specific purpose; a history of acceptance in the courts may also be relevant. To further ensure the perception of evenhandedness, examiners may benefit from consistently applying the same test protocols to all examinees seen with the same condition. For example, a medical examination of functional recovery for all claimants with TBI whose residual symptoms include excess daytime fatigue might routinely include an Epworth Sleepiness Scale (54) for severity quantification and a differential diagnostic screening for comorbid but nontraumatic nocturnally disruptive conditions such as obstructive sleep apnea.

"Cherry picking" applies to circumstances in which a less than comprehensive or fully balanced battery of tests is used to (a) reduce the examination time and effort, (b) support a "foregone conclusion" when there is no perceived need to explore other possibilities, or (c) deliberately control the findings to ensure that test results support a specific outcome. A comprehensive holistic approach to assessment with flexible protocols that are driven by clinical presentation indicates and ensures impartiality and thoroughness.

In balance, it is appropriate to omit or take particular precautions with administering, considering, and reporting tests that have poor psychometric properties despite widespread usage. To a reasonable extent, examiners may need to explain why commonly used tests were not employed, describe the other tests that were substituted, and discuss advantages of the tests selected.

Increasingly, evidence-based protocols for diagnosis and severity examination are becoming available. These protocols have the distinct advantage of quantification of validation and reliability as well as increasing clinical efficiency. Building routine protocols around peer-reviewed evidence-based methodology that the examiners fully understand is a sound practice.

Not uncommonly, rather than developing and defending their own protocols, some examiners rely reflexively on published authorities without ensuring familiarization with both strengths and weaknesses of the protocols for a given patient population. As an example, one widely used reference is the American Medical Association (AMA) Guides to the Examination of Permanent Impairment (GEPI) (55). The AMA GEPI, throughout its 6 editions, has provided, in substantial detail, sets of standardized measurement procedures. The GEPI describes means of determining the intraobserver variability and offers alternative methods to direct measurements, such as diagnosis related estimates (DRE). However, the GEPI do have numerous limitations (56) including (a) overreliance on consensus-based guidelines; (b) the dearth of strictly validated sets of test processes for impairment measurement in the various bodily systems; (c) the lack of specific identification, correlation, and weighting of impairments to various instrumental and per-

sonal activities of daily living (ADLs); and (d) the perpetuation of confusion regarding such terms as impairment and disability.

Examiners should acknowledge limitations in current scientific knowledge regarding aspects of their cases. Moreover, if, under special circumstances, experimental procedures or normative data not representative of the examinees' conditions are used, test results must be interpreted cautiously, and clear documentation of the procedures and the rationale for their use and potential for erroneous labeling (e.g., selectivity and specificity) should be provided. Caution should be employed in the use of tests that may be well accepted in certain domains of impairment examination but have no known reliability or usefulness in other domains. For example, Jamar grip testing is routinely employed in functional capacity testing for chronic pain and orthopedic impairment cases; consistent full effort is required for the results to be valid for peak strength. Falsification is a serious concern. The rapid exchange grip (REG) test (rapidly alternating right and left hand grips) has been found to be more difficult to falsify; therefore, when used with the typical examinee with soft tissue injury, REG results may be a more valid measure of whether full effort was consistently exerted, and thus whether the measurements obtained on routine Jamar grip testing were representative of peak strength. However, the typical examinee has no neurological impairment of coordination, pace, proprioception, or motor tone. The validity and reliability for applying the REG to patients with TBI who may have hemiparetic deficits, spasticity, or apraxia remains insufficiently tested and thus unknown.

Wood (57) noted that the general structure of a neuropsychological assessment has changed little over the past 3 decades and instead continues to focus mainly on assessment of cognitive constructs such as intelligence, memory, attention, and perception. However, cognitive neuroscience during the same time period has focused on integrative systems largely controlled by frontal mechanisms that allow cognitive functions to be used in an adaptive way, especially in novel or stimulus-ambiguous situations. Wood (57) reported that this has created a gap that places conventional neuropsychological methods in doubt with respect to use in the courtroom. However, Wood's perspective is not universally accepted and is not supported by statistics. As Kaufmann (58) summarized, neuropsychological evidence is being used by courts with increasing frequency. Of 3,492 cases identified in a Lexis search that had the root "neuropsycholo," 74% were adjudicated in the last decade. Additionally, the scope of forensic neuropsychological consulting has expanded into a wide range of civil, administrative, and criminal contexts. Neuropsychology, while continuing to evaluate core cognitive domains, emotional state, personality traits, and behavioral functioning, has progressed substantially in the past 30 years in terms of statistical methods, psychometric methods, neuropathological patterns on tests, symptom validity determinations, and diagnostic accuracy. Neuropsychological methods and opinions are widely accepted by courts. Admissibility of neuropsychological examinations and opinions under Daubert and the federal rules has been accepted for fixed and flexible neuropsychological batteries but not always for the Boston Process Approach (58).

The rules of evidence that flow from the Daubert decision make it imperative for examiners to be candid and clear with respect to the relevance, if any, of radiological testing in mild TBI (MTBI). Wortzel (59) noted the critical importance of properly presenting radiological information arising from single photon emission computed tomography (SPECT) scanning, particularly when there is civil litigation involving MTBI. Although cerebral SPECT is relatively sensitive to the metabolic changes produced by TBI, the changes are not specific to TBI, and findings do not *confirm* findings of brain damage. In parallel, absence of findings, while potentially of prognostic value, nevertheless does not exclude a diagnosis of TBI. A TBI *diagnosis* is generally based on characteristics of the injury (i.e., loss of consciousness, post-traumatic amnesia) and symptoms immediately following the injury (e.g., headache, dizziness, nausea). The length of post-traumatic amnesia and loss of consciousness and the presence of positive neuroimaging findings are used to determine TBI severity. There is no demonstrated consistency of relationship between SPECT images, neuropsychiatric symptoms, and neuropsychological test results. Hence, examiners should not cite SPECT results as stand-alone diagnostic data confirming a TBI diagnosis, but instead, only indicate how the testing may support history (e.g., injury characteristics), neuropsychological test results, and structural radiology.

Similar reservations were expressed in a commentary to the previous by Granacher (60). Noting the current trend by the legal profession to use functional neuroimaging such as SPECT or positron emission tomography (PET) as a sole imaging modality being used to prove MTBI at trial, Granacher observed that the current weak scientific evidence simply cannot meet the Daubert standard. He stated that "at the present time, there is a clear lack of clinical correlation between functional neuroimaging of MTBI and behavioral, neuro-psychological or structural neuroimaging deficits." In more general terms, examiners should tread carefully when advocating for the use of various neurodiagnostic tests that remain unproven, investigational and/or provide nonspecific or nonpathognomonic findings for confirming or refuting a diagnosis of TBI. Such tests would include SPECT, PET, functional magnetic resonance imaging (fMRI), diffusion tensor imaging on magnetic resonance imaging (DTI on MRI), magnetic resonance spectroscopy (MRS), and quantitative electroencephalography (QEEG), among others.

A widespread but potentially dangerous practice involves using test procedures that are anecdotal in origin (and thus not standardized or validated) such as those that some examiners might develop over the years within their own practices or might casually acquire from mentors and colleagues (without knowing whether the procedures are valid and reliable). Examiners are best served by using standardized, widely accepted, commercially available methods and procedures.

Delegation in Testing

Although common in clinical practice, delegation of testing to subordinates must be understood to be a source of potentially critical flaws and/or criticism within the clinicolegal context. Delegation may be found in certain procedures such as electromyography, neuropsychology, interview taking, test administration, and/or physical examinations. Argu-ably it is preferable in litigated contexts for the clinicolegal expert to do as much of the aforementioned testing and testing observation as possible; however, delegation of interpretation is never acceptable, and there is no argument that can support it in this context. Standardizing methods, choosing and ordering procedures, ensuring training and maintenance of competence, and minimizing or excluding subjective input are all elementary requirements of appropriate delegation.

Delegation of interviewing not only reduces examiners' total contact time with the examinees (contact time should be recorded somewhere in the expert report) but also reduces the dynamic interview element of following leads created by hesitation, special comment, facial expression, body language, vagueness, contradiction, implausibility, and/or ambiguity. Conversely, the accusation that the examiners rushed the interview or selected questions that precluded the examinees from providing complete or balanced information is offset when an assessment is allotted a standard amount of time using a standardized methodology. Although there is no "right" procedure applicable to all examiners or all circumstances, the general principles are consistently applicable: examiners are ultimately responsible for the comprehensiveness and validity of all data collection and for data interpretation. When it can be demonstrated that more direct examination or testing time, with either a more standardized or a more dynamic, responsive approach, would have led to a better outcome, then valid criticism can be applied, and the weight given to the examiners' opinion is proportionately diminished.

PREPARING THE CLINICOLEGAL REPORT

Critical Components

The reports of comprehensive independent examinations typically should include, in addition to typical medical components, some or all of the following medicolegally relevant information: referral source; date of retention; nature of the referral request; basis of report (i.e., file review vs direct examination); date, place, and duration of examination and persons present; date of report issuance; and documents unavailable at time of evaluation (3,9,25,61). Additionally, any special instructions provided by the referral source should be noted. When presenting findings and opinions, it is relevant to list all tests done, reasons for any test omissions, and all pertinent negative and positive findings. It may be relevant to comment on the reliability of key findings, including results of response bias and effort assessments. Causality and apportionment should be discussed with reference to principles of causation analysis (62). Referral sources commonly request that one or more clinical or clinicolegal components not be included and/or that additional information be included, but ultimately, additions or omissions should be at the discretion of the examiners whose credibility is "on the line."

It should be noted that expressions of degree of certainty should be consistent with legal definitions (e.g., likelihood with more than 50% confidence is termed "probable," whereas 50:50 or less is termed "possible"). Strong qualifiers of confidence in common clinical use include "balance of probabilities" and "reasonable medical certainty." Although there is no reference source that clearly distinguishes the terms "medical probability" from "medical certainty" on a statistical basis, the latter is commonly used to imply a higher degree of statistical likelihood, although most lawyers use the phrases analogously.

Review of Documentation

An important component of the clinicolegal report is the thoughtful review of specific findings and opinions from medical records, as well as accident-related records such as police reports. Although some readers with access to all medical records may find this integration of information to be repetitive, the IE report is sometimes the only place where a comprehensive integration of the totality of relevant information can be found. A review of background information and medical opinions serves to (*a*) demonstrate that the records were reviewed; (*b*) establish the temporal relationship of complaints to the reported injury; (*c*) facilitate an analysis of the symptom profile in relation to the type of injury being claimed; (*d*) evaluate the consistency of symptom reporting over time and across contexts; (*e*) evaluate indicators suggestive of recovery, if present, over time; and (*f*) provide clear delineation of the inferential reasoning process employed.

The clinicolegal report should contain an explanation of the potential relevance of any materials or other sources of information not available to examiners for review. Not uncommonly in TBI case work, this unavailable information may include records of fetal problems, birth trauma, childhood trauma (physical, sexual, and/or emotional), or infection. Similarly, school records of achievement and behavior, including learning disorders, intellectual functioning, and personality or aptitude test results, can all be of enormous value when determining whether and to what extent there are later acquired deficits. Prior workers' compensation records and legal records can also be an important source of information. Military records, which often are not provided for review, can also be an excellent source of baseline information (3,9). Of note is the fact that any person can obtain a veteran's military records from the National Archives in St. Louis, Missouri through the Freedom of Information Act.

There may be situations in which examiners are not provided all consultant, treatment, or investigative records related to a case. Such restrictions limit the confidence that examiners can place in their findings. Of course, the same shortcomings of database were likely in effect when other professionals reviewed the case, and the same reservations can be fairly applied to the balance of opinions already advanced by others. Materials not provided can be ranked on potential importance to report completion. Material may be deemed either "critically required" for a competent examination or merely of "potential value" for clarification or confirmation of existing evidence.

Critically required documentation is expected to contain important data, without which it would be impossible and improper for the ethical examiner to reach informed and authoritative final conclusions. Certain past medical records may contain information critical to establishing date of onset or other causation-related facts. Disinterested clinical or other observer records may enhance examiners' understanding of the nature and sequence of events or provide independent sources of information about daily function to supplement the narrative interview of the examinees or family members.

For example, when a student suffers a TBI and claims subsequent impairment of academic abilities, corroboration or clarification may be critically influenced by a direct review of prior and subsequent academic records of attendance, behavior, and grades. Similarly, a proper understanding of medication use and the presence of side effects may require not only the medical prescription record but also a pharmacy record (3,9,25,61).

Materials of *potential value* include documents whose review would be prudent to ensure thoroughness. For example, one or more "silent periods" in which there are no entries in either preinjury or postinjury medical records, out of keeping with established care-seeking patterns, and/or spanning long periods of time might well be corroborative of claims of interim good health or stoic self-reliance. Alternatively, such chronological "black holes" may reflect undisclosed health care in the same or another community or even episodes of hospitalization or incarceration. Review of health care records may reveal premorbid or comorbid social, familial, legal, vocational, financial, psychiatric, or physical problems, including instances of prior traumatic, vascular, infectious, or other brain injury. It may also be valuable, and sometimes it is important for examiners to request (where appropriate to scope of practice) raw data from certain testing procedures or hard copies of pertinent radiologic studies and to consider seeking corroboratory interviews of collateral sources (e.g., treating clinicians, family members) to round out information collection from other sources.

Regarding the overall analysis of assembled information, including examination findings documented in prior records, it is reasonable for examiners to comment on the appropriateness of any diagnostic procedures and processes employed. Such comments should address the reliability and validity of the findings, including estimation of the degree to which the measures used were specific and sensitive to the condition being examined and the degree of confidence that can be placed in the interpretations and opinions presented. Many examiners feel uncomfortable commenting on the methods and/or conclusions of their colleagues, especially in the absence of the raw data. However, balanced, expert, critical reviews are essential to promotion of thoroughness and objectivity and thus are essential to quality assurance in examinations in clinicolegal settings. Examiners have a responsibility to educate referral sources and triers of fact about questionable or insufficient procedures used by other examiners. However, critical reviews of the work of colleagues should be done in an objective, open-minded, professional manner with personal attacks avoided. Although colleagues should not be held to an unreasonable or arbitrary standard, each step in the examination process should be open to critical examination in the context of the case and the research literature.

Reviewers can critique the choice and administration of tests, and comment on whether the report offers a proper and balanced interpretation of all of the test data, appropriate data assembly, and sufficient and unbiased reporting of all data. In the absence of required raw data, informed critical review may not be possible, and report completion may have to be suspended.

Laypersons (e.g., jury members, family members), when reading clinicolegal reports from different experts, naturally attempt comparisons and query differences in protocols, findings, and conclusions. It is appropriate, and at times, even necessary to assist lay readers by describing the spectrum of findings or conclusions that are present within the entire body of documentation, including, but not limited to, the examiner's own report. Examiners may also discuss the reasons that they have for believing that their own report should be given precedence, such as breadth and/or depth of inquiry, consideration of response bias, validity and reliability of testing, recency of examination, clinical experience, or supportive scientific literature.

Completeness of Testing, Record Keeping, and Disclosure of Findings

Clinicolegal examinations require complete documentation of all procedures conducted and results obtained. Examiners must create appropriate documentation in the expectation that their records will be critically reviewed by independent professionals both within and outside of their professional specialty. In addition to formal reports, all information generated during an examination, including handwritten notes and test protocols, may be subject to review by others. Some examiners advocate for inclusion of all handwritten notes as part of their final report, including copies of all testing results (sans any copyrighted materials).Examiners who dispose of their original notes may be seen as disingenuous regarding the validity of any documentation noted in their final reports because there would be no "source" to confirm that what was stated in the report was, in fact, found. Notes must be legible and abbreviations universal or otherwise unequivocal in interpretation (3).

Many examiners use a recording and/or reporting methodology in which omission is understood to default to "testing successfully done, results within normal limits." Although routinely used and accepted in clinical practice, these omissions can be highly problematic within the clinicolegal context. It is necessary to list within clinicolegal reports each region, system, or function that was examined, along with explanations for any region, system, or function that might fall within the scope of practice of the examiners and might reasonably have been but was not tested. This description allows the examiners and even the lay readers to do a point-by-point comparison of differences in methodology and thoroughness between examiners' reports.

It is not necessary or even advisable to fill a report with details of all normal findings. A general statement of normality is appropriate, provided it applies to all specific elements of testing for a given domain. For example, examiners might state that "reflexes, sensation, strength, muscle tone, and bulk were examined proximally and distally in all limbs, and results were symmetrical and within normal limits." This statement precludes any doubt on persistence of hypertonicity after a spinal cord injury or calf atrophy after a radiculopathy but does not mire readers in details that they may not understand or find meaningful.

Examiners must be careful, however, to ensure that there will be no misinterpretation of sweeping statements. A declaration that "all cranial nerves were found normal" would entitle the readers to assume that all 12 cranial nerves were examined in detail and that olfaction, vision, hearing, balance, and taste were individually and thoroughly tested. Similarly, it is not acceptable to use vague terms such as "general neurological examination normal" or "a neurological system screen proved unremarkable"

unless the examiners append a detailed outline of the contents of the "general" or "screening" examination protocol (3,9).

Drafts and Final Reports

Ethical practice requires that examination findings be presented objectively, fully, and carefully in reports. No inaccurate documentation should be generated, especially for information not obtained or findings not made. Similarly, no salient information should be excluded. Notably, distinct from internal drafts, some professionals will release *preliminary reports* prior to preparing a final report. Such as most other areas of practice, the reasons for such procedures and the manner in which they are handled determine the degree to which these preliminary reports may potentially challenge ethical principles. Certainly, offering the referring party one or more drafts and soliciting "feedback" will introduce potential for perception of, as well as actual, biasing of the final report. Reports released to referral sources or others should be considered final for the purposes for which they were written (63). If additional information is later obtained or additional procedures are performed, examiners should draft addenda to the original report or draft updated reports that are numbered or dated accordingly (3).

Distinct from these general practices, circumstance may arise in which a preliminary report is released to apprise the parties of the status of a continuing examination, including justification for requests for further visits, tests, or documents. Similarly, a preliminary draft may be released to the referring party along with a specific request for confirmation that all issues of concern have been addressed and that the discussion is sufficiently detailed and clear from the layperson's perspective. It follows that no material alteration in the findings or conclusions reflecting the referring party's censorial or advocatorial preferences should appear in the subsequent final report. All copies of drafts should be retained and be produced if subpoenaed or questioned during testimony.

A report may be released in stages, reflecting completion of independent components. Any released report component should be considered final for its purpose. Thus, although pending neuropsychological testing or current school year marks prevents completion of a report on spectrum and severity of impairment from TBI, an initial report may be released in which the examiners address questions of causation, injury mechanism, and diagnosis.

The temptation to request "tweaking" (alteration to enhance value) of the final report can be irresistible to advocatorial referring/paying parties. Once a final report is issued, examiners must carefully consider whether and how to respond to any subsequent requests for alterations by the referring party, examinee, or others. Examiners should insist on receiving any such request in writing. If the requesting party is not prepared to put the request in writing, which would permit scrutiny by other parties or a trier of fact, then the examiners should not comply. Some requests for changes are fully justifiable, including typographical, chronological, or factual errors. It is also appropriate to respond to requests for clarification or amplification of points or requests of a similarly constructive nature while avoiding altering or debating the findings or opinions. Common appropriate requests for changes to reports include requests for clarification of technical terms or of reasoning for the court.

Another reasonable request involves the need for the examiners' opinion to be stated in accordance with the formulaic language of regulation or legislation. For example, it may be required that the report unequivocally establish whether impairments meet a verbal threshold such as "substantial," "permanent," or "severe." Also, an opinion regarding a treatment may require specific reference to whether it is both "necessary and reasonable." Similarly, a conclusion of disability may require qualification such as "disabled for the essential tasks of the prior work," "unable to return safely and productively to the workplace even within the framework of the accommodations that the employer has offered within the letter dated. . .," or "disabled for all forms of work for which the person is otherwise suited by education, training, or experience."

Options for rectification of factual errors include (a) attaching an amended page to the report, (b) marking through the incorrect portion of the report by putting a single line through the incorrect material so that the original can still be read and then writing (and initialing) the correction in the space above the line, or (c) producing a corrected version of the report and documenting the rationale within a cover letter (while keeping the original)..

All draft and amended versions of reports, other than those that fall under lawyer-expert privilege (such as notes and other work products made solely for purposes of discussion with the referring party), should be maintained and produced upon request as a proof of credibility. Outcome-oriented self-tweaking of an unsupported initial draft conclusion to improve the level of support in the final report release is not ethical; the examiner's final report should closely correspond to and logically flow from his/her written records. When requests or subpoenas for records, including reports, are received, all versions of previously released reports should be provided.

Use of Disclaimer Statements

It is often beneficial for examiners to provide a disclaimer at the beginning or end of their reports reiterating the basis of the report and the opinions, as related to their qualifications. The disclaimer should state that all opinions were provided with a degree of clinical/medical probability unless otherwise indicated. Examiners should also include a statement noting that their conclusions are based, in part, on the assumption that the materials provided for review are complete and correct and that if any additional information becomes available at a later date, opinions may be subject to change. Some referral sources provide wording for disclaimer statements in which examiners can accept or modify as appropriate (3,9).

It is relevant to state, in the case of file reviews, whether the opportunity for direct clinical assessment was offered and to what extent such an opportunity might have resulted in a different set of conclusions and recommendations. Some examiners will not provide testimony based on chart or peer review because they have not actually evaluated the injured party, which they consider essential for making clinicolegal determinations.

It is relevant to declare the absence of any known conflict of interest or to explain how any potential conflicts were identified and addressed. For example, when 2 clinicians work in an assessment center and one has been a treating clinician, the second—in the role of independent examiner—should state that (a) the case was never discussed between them, (b) the provision of a second opinion is common in medical practice, and (c) the examiner felt no reservations about discussing in the report any area of disagreement with the colleague over such medical opinions as diagnosis or prognosis.

MONITORING BIAS: EXAMINERS AND EXAMINEES

In the context of personal injury examinations, clinical *attribution bias* refers to the consistent and predictable tendency to incorrectly attribute current symptoms to the allegedly injurious event in question. Examiners' attribution bias typically results in a confounding of accurate diagnosis and appropriate treatment. Examinees demonstrate inadvertent attribution bias when they incorrectly interpret periodic, common cognitive inefficiencies as being pathological and entirely attributable to an event of perceived significance such as a resolved concussion. Attribution bias may interact with true neurogenic symptoms to increase the perception of neurogenic impairment. Attribution bias can be influenced by others (e.g., family, attorneys, or health care professionals) and can be intentional.

An examinees' presentation and approach to test taking exists on a continuum ranging from clearly reliable to clearly unreliable. Because of financial incentives for examinees to misrepresent their optimal abilities during examinations in clinicolegal contexts, assessment of symptom validity is a necessary examination component. Examiners must ensure that assessments, recommendations, reports, and diagnostic or evaluative statements are substantiated by sufficient information and techniques. Formal assessment of both response bias and effort is essential to increase the likelihood that interpretation of test data will be based on reliable and valid results, that is, the results will reflect the examinees' true abilities and deficits. Methodologies have been proposed to provide feedback to examinees regarding invalid test performance (64).

Examiners' misattribution bias represents a problematic source of error that can violate the core ethical principle of avoiding harm. Clinicians sensitized to the signs and symptoms of the patients they treat clinically, from the perspective of their unique specialty, may misdiagnose or overdiagnose problems with inadequate attention to competing explanations. For example, a neurologist and a psychiatrist, when confronted with the same symptom set, may be prone to specialty-specific diagnoses of, respectively, either brain injury or psychosocial distress (65). Inadequate rigor in developing an appropriate diagnosis causes increased medical costs, inappropriate treatment, treatment failures, and even chronic disability in the injured person. These errors can be prevented for patients or claimants with a history of TBI by comprehensive assessment that integrates data from observation, history, examination, radiological, and neuropsychological testing and collateral sources with a critical appraisal of base rates of relevant symptoms (25,26,61,65) and careful differential diagnosis of all possible explanations for symptoms. Examiners may benefit from asking questions of themselves, such as "what would an expert retained by the opposing side think?" or "what would a colleague from a different specialty think?"

Chapman and Elstein (66) discussed how biases can occur in the face of uncertainty in medical decision making. Examiners can signal decision bias through any predictable tendencies such as consistently discounting certain complaints as either not credible or unimportant, or to the contrary, consistently accepting all complaints uncritically, as being self-validating (67). Compelling evidence of perceived expert witness bias is offered from a Federal Judiciary Committee sanctioned study by Johnson, Krafka and Cecil (68) of active federal judges and lead attorneys who presented the docket cases before them. From 1991 to 1998, the primary problem with expert testimony was expert witnesses who "abandon objectivity and become advocates for the side that hired them" (68) (p. 5). Mean rating of partisan bias of experts on a 1–5 Likert rating scale was approximately 3.7.

There is a need for development, dissemination, and universal acceptance of bias avoidance guidelines and of active promotion of objectivity and ethical conduct in clinicolegal contexts (69). However, when serious ethical violations are observed in colleagues, carefully deliberated action is indicated. In most instances, such action should only be taken following adjudication of the case. Waiting for the case to be resolved gives examiners time to consider whether reporting of the ethical violation is needed once the emotional aspect of involvement in the case has passed or it avoids the appearance of having filed a complaint for the sole purpose of trying to discredit the opposing examiner. Filing of specious complaints is itself unprofessional and inappropriate (70).

Several professional associations, including the American Association of Neurological Surgeons (AANS) and AMA as well as the American Association for Psychiatry and Law (AAPL) and NAN have developed rules of professional conduct pertaining to expert testimony (13,71,72). There are several challenges when discussing how professionals and in particular professional organizations (61), the legal system, consumers, and society at large should deal with health professionals who conduct themselves unethically in the context of providing clinicolegal services. Resnick (73) noted that in dealing with unethical or incompetent expert witness testimony, some fundamental issues of law, ethics, and public policy were raised including, but not limited to, the following:

1. What are the current legal procedures or strategies for dealing with incompetent or unethical expert testimony?
2. Is expert testimony legally privileged? Aside from liability for perjury, do witnesses have immunity from civil or criminal liability resulting from their testimony in court?
3. Is expert testimony constitutionally protected free speech? Under what conditions could the state proscribe, restrict, or control expert testimony?
4. Are existing ethical rules and policies pertaining to expert testimony so vague that using them to sanction an individual would violate that individual's rights to due process? How should rules be formulated so that they avoid this problem?
5. Is it unfair to take away an expert witness' license to practice medicine for unethical or incompetent expert testimony? Is this form of punishment excessive?
6. Does sanctioning expert witnesses undermine access to the courts for plaintiffs?
7. Does sanctioning expert witnesses undermine scientific freedom?

The answers to many of these questions remain pending and controversial. Furthermore, honest discussion by all parties involved in the process is clearly warranted to not only set performance expectations but also consistent and hopefully national, if not international, standards for expert witness testimony in health care related fields. Ultimately, if health care professionals do not advocate for better monitoring of their own performance and are unwilling to report concerns regarding the clinicolegal practices of their peers, little would be expected to change given the current incentives for clinicolegal practice and disincentives associated and perceived with reporting fellow health care professionals.

CONCLUSION

Clinicians who are prepared to take on the role of clinicolegal examiner and expert witness have much to offer persons who are injured, courts, and other parties interested in establishing or clarifying the nature and extent of impairments reportedly resulting from compensable brain injuries. Competence in the clinical assessment of persons who have sustained brain injuries is essential, but not sufficient, for successful clinicolegal practice. Clinicians who perform clinicolegal services must strive for clinicolegal competence by understanding the unique requirements of the adversarial judicial process, including the need to maintain the highest degrees of thoroughness and rigor with examination procedures, methods, analysis, and documentation. Adherence to the highest professional standards for examinations lays the foundation for testimony to assist triers of fact or administrative decision makers with their determinations. If more clinicians become competent in clinicolegal examination and expert witnessing, parties will be increasingly able to identify those clinicians and reports that lack such attributes; more cases will reach early and fair settlement; and dispute resolution mechanisms such as mediation, arbitration, tribunal and the courts will be more effectively used.

KEY CLINICAL POINTS

1. Be aware of professional policy statements and/or white papers relevant to your specialty as related to expert witness testimony.
2. Clinicians should be fully cognizant of how to document in both clinical and medicolegal situations to avoid legal repercussions, negate impressions of bias, and provide valid scientific foundations for any opinions expressed.
3. Familiarity with clinicolegal terminology, subpoena protocols, as well as deposition and courtroom conduct are all paramount elements of knowledge for any clinician interested in serving as an expert witness.
4. As with clinical practice, clinicolegal practice has a business element, the dynamics of which must be understood in the context of optimizing one's standing in this arena of practice and protecting one's self relative to payment, liability, and ethical reputation.

5. IME practice is full of with potential pitfalls if examiners do not approach such assessments in a standardized, ethical, and professional manner using unbiased, scientific, and validated methods for both assessment and interpretation of findings.

6. Conducting peer reviews and IMEs of persons following brain injury is generally time consuming, labor intensive, and requires an eye to detail as well as an extensive knowledgebase on the part of the expert witness.

7. Clinicians must understand that engaging in clinicolegal work and expert witness testimony requires a very different set of skills than normal clinical practice, is potentially stressful, and yet can provide multiple benefits to the clinician, litigant, triers of fact, and society as a whole.

8. Expert witnesses, and those wanting to serve as expert witnesses, must remember that the expert is there to advocate for only one thing and that is the truth; anything other than that deters from the core principles of professional practice and ethics. The agenda of the plaintiff and defense counsel as well as the examinee may or may not be parallel to the aforementioned for a variety of reasons and incentives.

9. Health care practitioners involved in clinicolegal practice should be responsible for monitoring not only the competency and ethics of their own practices but also those of their peers through interactions on a peer-to-peer, institutional, as well as professional society level.

KEY REFERENCES

1. Ameis A, Zasler ND. The independent medical examination. *Phys Med Rehabil Clin of North Am.* 2002;13(2): 259–286.

2. Bush SS, Heilbronner RL. The neuropsychological IME. In: Bush SS, Iverson GL. eds. *Neuropsychological Assessment of Work-related Injuries.* New York, NY: Guilford Press.

3. Bush SS; for NAN Policy and Planning Committee. Independent and court-ordered forensic neuropsychological examinations: official statement of the National Academy of Neuropsychology. *Arch Clin Neuropsych,* 2005;20(8): 997–1007. http://nanonline.org/NAN/Files/PAIC/PDFs/NANIMEpaper.pdf.

4. Granacher R. *Traumatic Brain Injury: Methods for Clinical and Forensic Neuropsychiatric Assessment.* Boca Raton, FL: CRC Press; 2003.

5. Martelli MF, Zasler ND. Ethics and objectivity in clinicolegal contexts: recommendations for experts. In: Wiener RB, ed. *Pain Management: A Practical Guide For Clinicians.* 6th ed. Boca Raton, FL: St. Lucie Press; 2002:895–908.

References

1. Catto G. Acting as an expert witness. *BMJ.* 2008;337:a933.
2. *Rules of Civil Procedure, Amendments Bulletin, Rule 53.03—Expert Witnesses, Rule 4.1—Duty of Expert.* Ontario, Canada: 2010.
3. Brodsky SL. *Testifying in Court: Guidelines and Maxims for the Expert Witness.* Washington, DC: American Psychological Association; 1991.
4. Disclosure for Workers' Compensation Purposes. http://www.hhs.gov/ocr/privacy/hipaa/understanding/coveredentities/workerscomp.html. Accessed December 2, 2012.
5. Bush SS, Heilbronner RL. The neuropsychological IME. In Bush SS, Iverson GL eds. *Neuropsychological Assessment of Work-Related Inju-*

ries. New York, NY: Guilford Press. http://nanonline.org/NAN/Files/PAIC/PDFs/NANIMEpaper.pdf. Accessed October 3, 2011.
6. Official Position of the American Academy of Clinical Neuropsychology on ethical complaints made against clinical neuropsychologists during adversarial proceedings. *Clin Neuropsychol.* 2003;17(4): 443–445.
7. Binder LM, Thompson LL. The ethics code and neuropsychological assessment practices. *Arch Clin Neuropsychol.* 1995;10(1):27–46.
8. Merten T, Krahl G, Krahl C, Freytag HW. Base-rate estimates for negative response bias in a workers' compensation claim sample [in German]. *Versicherungsmedizin.* 2010;62 (3):126–131.
9. Ameis A, Zasler ND. The independent medical examination. *Phys Med Rehabil Clin North Am.* 2002;13(2):259–286.
10. *Daubert v. Merrell Pharmaceutical,* 61 USL W 4805 (US June 29, 1993).
11. Wikipedia. Daubert standard. http://en.wikipedia.org/wiki/Daubert_standard. Accessed July 3, 2009.
12. American Academy of Physical Medicine and Rehabilitation. Ethics. http://www.aapmr.org/practice/resources/positionpapers/ethics/Pages/Expert-Witness-Testimony.aspx. Accessed May 11, 2011.
13. Bush SS; for NAN Policy and Planning Committee. Independent and court-ordered forensic neuropsychological examinations: official statement of the National Academy of Neuropsychology. *Arch Clin Neuropsychol.* 2005;20(8):997–1007.
14. Federal Rules of Evidence 2012. http://federalevidence.com/downloads/rules.of.evidence.pdf. Accessed December 23, 2011.
15. Babitsky S, Mangraviti JJ. *Cross Examination: The Comprehensive Guide for Experts.* Falmouth, MA: SEAK Inc; 2003.
16. Miller L. May it please the court: Testifying tips for expert witness. http://www.doereport.com/article_testifying_tips.php. Accessed October 13, 2009.
17. Trial Skills Live. How to survive a deposition: Eight great tips. http://www.trialskillslive.com/law-tips-of-the-week/2009/8/2/how-to-survive-a-deposition-eight-great-tips.html. Accessed 29, 2011.
18. Stump E. The trials of providing expert witness testimony: what you need to know. *Neurology Today.* 2009;9(17):23,26–27.
19. Babitsky S, Mangraviti JJ. *How to Become a Dangerous Expert Witness.* Falmouth, MA: SEAK, Inc; 2005.
20. College of Physicians and Surgeons of Ontario. Third party reports: reports by treating physicians and independent medical examiners. Policy Statement #3–09. *Dialogue.* 2010;1:1–7.
21. Babitsky S, Mangraviti JJ. *Expert Witness Retention Contract.* Falmouth, MA: SEAK, Inc; 2008.
22. Hamilton R. *The Expert Witness Marketing Book: How to Promote Your Forensic Practice in a Professional and Cost-Effective Manner.* Dallas, TX: Expert Communications; 2003.
23. Murray J. Sixteen tips on testifying in court. http://www.pimall.com/nais/n.testify.html. Accessed September 15, 2011.
24. National Academy of Neuropsychology, Inc. Independent and court-ordered forensic neuropsychological examinations. (Appendix). http://nanonline.org/docs/PAIC/PDFs/NANIMEpaper.pdf. Accessed January 3, 2012.
25. Martelli MF, Zasler ND. Ethics and objectivity in clinicolegal contexts: recommendations for rxperts. In: RB Wiener, ed. *Pain Management: A Practical Guide for Clinicians.* 6th ed. Boca Raton, FL: St. Lucie Press; 2002:895–908.
26. Martelli MF, Zasler ND, Grayson R. Ethical considerations in impairment and disability evaluations following acquired brain injury. In: RV May, MF Martelli, eds. *Guide to Functional Capacity Evaluation With Impairment Rating Applications.* Richmond, VA: NADEP Publications; 1999:1–42.
27. Barsky AJ, Kazis LE, Freiden RB, Goroll AH, Hatem CJ, Lawrence RS. Evaluating the interview in primary care medicine. *Soc Sci Med Med Psychol Med Sociol.* 1980;14A(6):653–658.
28. Don AS, Carragee EJ. Is the self-reported history accurate in patients with persistent axial pain after a motor vehicle accident? *Spine J.* 2009;9(1):4–12.
29. Feinstein A, Ouchterlony D, Somerville J, Jardine A. The effects of litigation on symptom expression: a prospective study following mild traumatic brain injury. *Med Sci Law.* 2001;41(2):116–121.
30. Meyers JE, Volbrecht M, Axelrod BN, Reinsch-Boothby L. Embedded symptom validity tests and overall neuropsychological test performance. *Arch Clin Neuropsychol.* 2011;26(1):8–15.
31. Bush SS, Ruff RM, Tröster AI, et al. Symptom validity assessment:

practice issues and medical necessity. Official position of the National Academy of Neuropsychology. *Arch Clin Neuropsychol.* 2005; 20(4):419–426.

32. Carone DA, Bush SS, Iverson GL. Providing feedback on symptom validity, mental health, and treatment in mild traumatic brain injury. In: DA Carone DA, SS Bush, eds. *Mild Traumatic Brain Injury: Symptom Validity Assessment and Malingering.* New York, NY: Springer Publishing; In press.

33. Rohling ML, Allen LM, Green P. Who is exaggerating cognitive impairments and who is not? *CNS Spectr.* 2002;7(5):387–395.

34. Martelli MF, Zasler ND, Bush S. Assessment of response bias in impairment and disability evaluations following brain injury. In: J Leon-Carrion, G Zitnay eds. *Practices in Brain Injury.* Philadelphia, PA: Hanley & Belfus, Inc; 2006:354–384.

35. Guilmette T. The role of clinical judgment in symptom validity assessment. In: DA Carrone, SS Bush eds. *Mild Traumatic Brain Injury: Symptom Validity Assessment and Malingering.* New York, NY: Springer Publishing; In press.

36. Greiffenstein MF, Baker WJ. Validity testing in dually diagnosed post-traumatic stress disorder and mild closed head injury. *Clin Neuropsychol.* 2008;22(3):565–582.

37. Binder LM, Rohling ML. Money matters: a meta-analytic review of the effects of financial incentives on recovery after closed head injury. *Am J Psychiatry.* 1996;153(1):7–10.

38. Slick DJ, Sherman EMS, Iverson GL. Diagnostic criteria for malingered neurocognitive dysfunction: proposed standards for clinical practice and research. *Clin Neuropsychol.* 1999;13:545–561.

39. Carone DA, Iverson GL, Bush SS. A model to approaching and providing feedback to patients regarding invalid test performance in clinical neuropsychological evaluations. *Clin Neuropsychol.* 2010;24: 759–778.

40. Pascetta J, Samuel S, Michals TJ, Mandel S. Reflections on third party observers in neurologic forensic examinations. *Practical Neurology.* 2009.

41. Constantinou M, Ashendorf L, McCaffrey RJ. When the 3rd party observer of a neuropsychological evaluation is an audio-recorder. *Clin Neuropsychol.* 2002;16(3):407–412.

42. Binder JT, Johnson-Greene D. Observer effects on neuropsychological performance: a case report. *Clin Neuropsychol.* 1995;9:74–78.

43. Constantinou M, Ashendorf L, McCaffrey RJ. Effects of a third party observer during neuropsychological assessment: when the observer is a video camera. *J Forensic Neuropsychol.* 2005;4:39–48.

44. Howe L, McAffrey RJ. Third party observation in neuropsychological evaluation: an update on the literature, practical advice for practitioners, and future directions. *Clin Neuropsychol.* 2010;24:518–537.

45. Hamsher K, Baron IS, Lee GP. *Policy Statement* on for the presence of third party observers in neuropsychological assessment. American Academy of Clinical Neuropsychology. *TCN.* 2011;15(4):433–439.

46. American Bar Association Accredited Education. http://www.independent-medical-examination.com/american-bar-association-accredited-education.html. Accessed December 12, 2011.

47. College of Physicians and Surgeons of Ontario. Third party reports: Reports by treating physicians and independent medical examiners. http://www.cpso.on.ca/uploadedFiles/policies/policies/policyitems/ThirdParty.pdf. Accessed December 2, 2011.

48. McCaffrey RJ, Fisher JM, Gold GA, Lynch JK. The presence of third parties during neuropsychological evaluations: who is evaluating whom? *Clin Neuropsychol.* 1996; 10(40):435–449.

49. McCaffrey RJ, Lynch JK, Yantz CL. Third party observers: why all the fuss? *J Forensic Neuropsychol.* 2005;4:1–16.

50. National Academy of Neuropsychology, Policy, and Planning Committee. Presence of third party observers during neuropsychological testing: official statement of the National Academy of Neuropsychology. *Arch Clin Neuropsychol.* 2000;15(5):379–380.

51. Eastvold AD, Belanger HG, Vanderploeg RD. Does a third party observer affect neuropsychological test performance? It depends. *Clin Neuropsychol.* 2012;26(3):520–541.

52. Grady B, Myers KM, Nelson EL, et al.; for American Telemedicine Association Telemental Health Standards and Guidelines Working Group. Evidence-based practice for telemental health. *Telemed J E Health.* 2011;17(2):131–148.

53. Sharp IR, Kobak KA, Osman DA. The use of videoconferencing with patients with psychosis: a review of the literature. *Ann Gen Psychiatry.* 2011;10(1):14.

54. Johns MW. A new method for measuring daytime sleepiness: the Epworth Sleepiness Scale. *Sleep.* 1991;14(6):540–545.

55. American Medical Association. *American Medical Association Guides to the Evaluation of Permanent Impairment.* 6th ed. Chicago, IL: American Medical Association; 2008.

56. Rondinelli RD. Changes for the new AMA guides to impairment rating, 6th edition: implications and applications for physician disability evaluations. *PM R.* 2009;1(7):643–656.

57. Wood RL. The scientist-practitioner model: how do advances in clinical and cognitive neuroscience affect neuropsychology in the courtroom? *J Head Trauma Rehabil.* 2009;24(2):88–99.

58. Kaufmann PM. Admissibility of neuropsychological evidence in criminal cases: Competency, insanity, culpability, and mitigation. In: R Denney, J Sullivan, eds. *Criminal Forensic Neuropsychology.* New York, NY: Guilford Press; 2008:55–90.

59. Wortzel HS, Filley CM, Anderson CA, Oster T, Arciniegas DB. Forensic applications of cerebral single photon emission computed tomography in mild traumatic brain injury. *J Am Acad Psychiatry Law.* 2008;36(3):310–322.

60. Granacher RP Jr. Commentary: applications of functional neuroimaging to civil litigation of mild TBI. *J Am Acad Psychiatric Law.* 2008; 36(3):323–328.

61. Martelli MF, Zasler ND, Johnson-Greene D. Promoting ethical and objective practice in the clinicolegal arena of disability evaluation. *Phys Med Rehabil Clin N Am.* 2001;12(3): 571–584.

62. Freeman MD, Kohles SS. Application of the Bradford-Hill Criteria for assessing specific causation in post-traumatic headache. *Brain Inj Prof.* 2011;8(1):26–28.

63. Babitsky S, Mangraviti JJ, Melhorn JM. *Writing and Defending Your IME Report. The Comprehensive Guide.* Falmouth, MA: SEAK, Inc; 2004.

64. Bush SS, Connell MA, Denney RL. *Ethical Issues in Forensic Psychology: A Systematic Model for Decision Making.* Washington, DC: American Psychological Association; 2006.

65. Sweet JJ, Moulthrop MA. Self-examination questions as a means of identifying bias in adversarial assessments. *J Forensic Neuropsychol.* 1998;1:73–88

66. Chapman GB, Elstein AS. Cognitive processes and biases in medical decision making. In: GB Chapman, FA Sonnenberg, eds. *Decision Making in Health Care: Theory, Psychology, and Applications. Cambridge Series on Judgment and Decision Making.* New York, NY: Cambridge University Press; 2000:183–210.

67. Granacher R. *Traumatic brain injury: Methods for Clinical and Forensic Neuropsychiatric Assessment.* Boca Raton, FL: CRC Press; 2003.

68. Kratka C, Dunn MA, Treadway Johnson M, Cecil JS, Miletich D. Judge and attorney experiences, practices, and concerns regarding expert testimony in federal civil trials. Federal Judicial Center. *Psychol Public Pol L.* 2002;8(3):309–341.

69. Martelli MF, Bush SS, Zasler ND. Identifying, avoiding, and addressing ethical misconduct in neuropsychological medicolegal practice. *Int J Forensic Psychol.* 2003;1 (1):26–44.

70. Grote CL, Lewin JL, Sweet JJ, van Gorp WG. Responses to perceived unethical practices in clinical neuropsychology: ethical and legal considerations. *Clin Neuropsychol.* 2000;14(1):119–134.

71. American Academy of Neurology. Qualifications and guidelines for the physician expert witness. Preamble. 2005. http://www.aan.com/globals/axon/assets/2687.pdf. Accessed January 20, 2012.

72. Goldrich MS. Report of the council on ethical and judicial affairs. American Medical Association. *CEJA Report 12-A-04.* 2004;1–9.

73. Resnik DB. Punishing medical experts for unethical testimony: a step in the right direction or a step too far? *J Philo Sci Law.* 2004; 4(7).

Appendix I Sample Subpoena Checklist

Subpoena Protocol

_____ Date completed

_____ Document the date subpoena is received.

_____ Call or e-mail client's counsel (if subpoena is from opposing counsel) or client (if not legally represented) to notify them of subpoena.

Name of person notified _____

_____ Copy subpoena for client's file, as well as for Mr. Zasler, and give Emily the original to file in legal file.

Number of copies made _____

Cost (0.25¢ per page) _____

_____ Date records were sent.

_____ Sent certified AND regular mail letter to client confirming that we have sent the records.

Appendix II Sample Independent Medical Evaluation Examinee Feedback Form

Examinee Questions (Please mark an "X" in the appropriate box)	Totally Agree	Slightly Agree	Neutral	Slightly Disagree	Totally Disagree
The facilities at Dr. Zasler's clinic were comfortable and clean.					
Dr. Zasler's staff treated me politely and with respect.					
I was given reasonable opportunities for bathroom breaks and refreshments.					
Dr. Zasler told me to be honest in all my responses.					
Dr. Zasler told me to make my best effort during all parts of the IME.					
I was instructed to neither exaggerate nor underreport problems.					
I was treated in a respectful manner by Dr. Zasler during the IME					
I was instructed to report pain on exam so Dr. Zasler could change his approach.					
Dr. Zasler was thorough in terms of the interview and evaluation of my problems.					

<u>**Appendix III** Sample Retention Agreement</u>

Consultative Services Contract

Charge Description

Consultant witness **RETAINER FEE** (MINIMUM/NONREFUNDABLE)	$__,000.00
Clinical evaluation, phone conference, research, record review, preparation, reports, deposition (discovery or *de bene esse*), courtroom testimony, travel (portal-to-portal), and waiting time	$____.00/hr.
Auto mileage expenses related to personal travel by car to courtroom, deposition site, or evaluation location	$0.50/mile
Administrative time (obtaining and/or organizing records)	$100.00/hr.

1. **Payment due upon receipt.** All charges are hourly and prorated by the quarter hour and billed biweekly. An interest charge of 2% per month (24% APR) with interest compounded will be levied for accounts 60 days past due. All fees for clinical care will be billed separately.

2. **If bills are more than 60 days delinquent, all work on the case will be stopped until the outstanding balance is received.**

3. Should legal recourse be necessary to secure outstanding payment, said party agrees to pay all legal fees associated with collections not limited to court costs but including reasonable attorney's fees of 33.33%. All accounts more than 120 days will be turned over for collection.

4. The party (as well as their client[s]) requesting the consultative services agree(s) to release, indemnify, and hold harmless Dr. Zasler and/or Concussion Care Centre of Virginia from any claimed liability including error, omission, or negligence that is alleged to have resulted from Dr. Zasler's opinions, actions, and/or services provided in this case.

5. If reserved time is canceled inside of *1 week* of the scheduled date, the party requesting the IME and/or trial testimony will still be charged for the time set aside. For purposes of an IME, if the claimant is more than 30 min late, the payer will be charged for the time set aside, and the claimant will need to be rescheduled.

6. All travel-related expenses including airline, hotel, food, taxis, parking, and so forth are to be paid by the party requesting the consultative service(s).

7. Should opposing counsel refuse payment for services (e.g., deposition) and/or invoke Rules of Civil Procedure regarding setting of "reasonable fees" and a dispute occurs resulting in the court setting said fees lower than the aforementioned quoted rate, the party hiring Dr. Zasler will agree to guarantee payment of his normal fees and/or the difference between Dr. Zasler's fee and the court set fee.

8. The party hiring Dr. Zasler agrees to pay for any and all preparation time for depositions and/or trial.

9. Dr. Zasler's policy is *not* to waive his right to read his deposition transcript. The retaining party agrees to reimburse Dr. Zasler for time allotted to the reading and correcting of deposition transcripts.

10. Dr. Zasler *must* examine the claimant in question *prior* to providing any testimony.

11. If Dr. Zasler is retained for purposes of a peer review (no claimant exam), no testimony will be provided (with the potential exception of death cases).

IMPORTANT NOTE: IN RESPONSE TO SERVICES RENDERED, THE PARTY REQUESTING THE CONSULTATION IS EXPECTED TO PAY ALL BILLS FOR THEIR CLIENT AS INCURRED. THE FEES BILLED SHALL NOT BE DEPENDENT ON THE OUTCOME OF THE CASE, WHETHER IN OBLIGATION, AMOUNT, TIME, OR PAYMENT.

I, (Payor/Retaining Party), _____ **(Please Print),** have read the above terms and agree to abide by the policies, rates, and procedures set forth herein by Nathan D. Zasler, MD, of Concussion Care Centre of Virginia, Ltd. with regard to his involvement in this consultation.

Case

Name: _____ **(Please Print)**

_____   _____

Legible signature of retaining party   **Date**

_____   _____

                                                Phone number of retaining party

_____

Address of retaining party

Please make checks payable to:

Concussion Care Centre of Virginia, Ltd: EIN 00-1111111

Appendix IV Sample Independent Medical Evaluation Information and Instructions Form

Information and Instructions About Your IME

I, Nathan D. Zasler, MD am seeing you for an independent medical evaluation (IME). I am a board certified physician specialized in physical medicine and rehabilitation (PM&R) (also known as physiatry) and fellowship trained in brain injury medicine. I am a Fellow of the American Academy of Disability Evaluating Physicians and a Diplomate of the American Academy of Pain Management. I pledge to be both thorough and impartial during your assessment. In my capacity as an examiner, I am not an employee of any party involved with your current case (e.g., insurance company, third-party administrator, attorney, governmental agency, or employer).

No treating physician-patient relationship will be established in the context of this evaluation. In this context, you will not be provided with advice, opinions, or treatment, and in this context, I do not order tests as part of the IME, although I may recommend them. This IME is *not* a comprehensive medical examination geared to assess all aspects of your general health. The purpose of this visit is to answer specific questions concerning your case posed by the retaining party and potentially to prepare a report. The information that you share with me will be included in the report. Please understand that anything discussed with you or anyone else or otherwise documented may be included in the IME report.

I always request that a copy of my evaluation be provided to your primary treating clinician. During the visit, I will review your history, both preinjury and postinjury illness as well as perform a physical examination. If you have any difficulties whatsoever during the assessment, you should let me know immediately. Please understand that in an IME, because no treating physician-patient relationship is established, there is no physician-patient privilege/confidentiality associated with the evaluation. The purpose of the IME is to provide a thorough objective evaluation of the specific condition(s) related to your injury or illness that is/are in question as well as to assess how, if at all, prior or subsequent conditions might affect your injury or illness. I will also likely be asked to comment on your prognosis and provide treatment recommendations as well as opinions regarding your ability to work if you are not already doing so.

Appendix V Sample Independen Medical Evaluation Consent/Agreement Form

Examinee Pledge and Agreement to IME Terms

I understand that I am expected to give my best effort on all aspects of the evaluation; however, I need not perform any maneuver that I feel might cause injury or worsening of my symptoms. I will immediately inform the examiner if anything he does causes excessive discomfort. The IME is not intended to cause injury or excessive pain. I understand that to avoid any problems of the aforementioned nature, I must fulfill my responsibility to inform Dr. Zasler if there is something I cannot do, if a certain test is causing too much discomfort or if I am uncomfortable with any aspect of the exam.

I will inform Dr. Zasler, immediately, if there is anything limiting my ability to answer all questions accurately to the best of my knowledge or anything besides my condition for which I am being seen that limits my ability to put forth my best effort. I agree to not covertly (i.e., in secret) record any part of the IME without prior consent of Dr. Zasler and/or make any record of the exam (recordings, copies of tests, etc.) without first discussing with Dr. Zasler and getting consent.

I will make every effort to cooperate fully with the exam, to be honest, and exert my best effort during the entire assessment. I, hereby, authorize Dr. Zasler to release the results of this IME verbally and/or in writing to the party who has requested the IME.

I, hereby, acknowledge my willingness to participate in the IME assessment that involves taking a history from me as well as conducting various examinations including a physical exam. Dr. Zasler will also ask me for other people he might talk to in an effort to best understand the condition for which I am being seen. Lastly, if there is ever a time during the assessment when I am not satisfied with the manner in which I am being treated, I will let Dr. Zasler or one of his staff know immediately. By my signature below, I agree to the above terms and conditions of the IME being conducted today.

_____	_____	_____
Signature of Examinee	**Printed Name**	**Date**

_____	_____
Nathan D. Zasler, MD	**Witness**
Medical Director, CCCV, Inc	

_____	_____
Date	**Date**

Assessing and Addressing Response Bias

Michael F. Martelli, Keith Nicholson, Nathan D. Zasler, and Mark C. Bender

INTRODUCTION

Evaluation of neurologic impairments and associated disability presents a significant diagnostic challenge. In this chapter, impairment refers to alterations in cognitive or physical structure or function, whereas disability refers to the resulting alterations in functional activity performance. Although the evaluations and opinions of different practitioners are often fairly consistent for more catastrophic or functionally disabling injuries clearly associated with biomedical causes, in other cases they can vary widely.

Impairment and disability evaluation following neurologic injury typically involves such contexts as social security disability application, personal injury litigation, worker's compensation claims, disability insurance policy application, other health care insurance policy coverage, and determination of competence to handle finances or other important life functions (e.g., parenting) or decisions. These evaluations have traditionally fallen within the purview of the general fields of physical medicine and rehabilitation, neurology, neurosurgery, psychiatry, psychology, and neuropsychology. Recently and especially in cases of less catastrophic and more subtle cognitive impairment and disability, there is increasing reliance on specialists in brain injury evaluation and treatment.

Impairment and disability evaluation may be one of the more misunderstood areas because it applies to assessment and treatment of persons with injury related residua and/or associated functional limitations. The task of making determinations regarding impairment and disability in persons with neurologic impairment and injury is fraught with numerous challenges. These include the frequently subtle and complex nature of the deficits involved; the lack of formal, scientifically validated "rating systems" for many associated deficits; and the multiple possible types of problems associated with brain or other neurologic injury that can include, among other problems, chronic pain and psychoemotional problems. Disentangling the multiple contributors to cognitive dysfunction and to impairment and disability presents a diagnostic challenge that requires careful scrutiny (1).

IMPORTANCE OF RESPONSE BIAS ASSESSMENT IN BRAIN INJURY EXAMINATION

Persons with brain injury may present with some response bias regarding report or demonstration of impairment and related disability. Response bias is defined as a class of behaviors that reflect less than fully truthful, accurate, or valid symptom report and presentation. Response bias is a ubiquitous phenomenon affecting almost any domain of human self-report. Some forms of response bias may be associated with conscious manipulation or deceit but many, or most, are not (2–4).

In the context of impairment, disability, and insurance related evaluations, the importance of conscious or other bias becomes more acute (2–4). Accurate diagnosis is prerequisite to providing appropriate and timely treatment, promoting optimal recovery, appropriate legal compensation decisions, and preventing iatrogenic impairment and disability reinforcement. Ensuring accuracy of functional status evaluations requires consideration of the validity of observed impairment and disability, symptomatology displayed during the examination, sensitivity and specificity of assessment measures, and generalizability of test findings to functioning in everyday life. This is equally true for situations involving bias to overreport or underreport symptoms and impairment as discussed subsequently.

Blau (5) has expounded on the importance of determining response biases to measuring true levels of impairment in medicolegal situations. Medicolegal determinations depend on an alleged victim (of wrongful act or omission) establishing (a) causality to demonstrate entitlement to compensation based on (b) level of damages suffered. In cases of less obvious, clear cut and significant trauma with psychological, neurologic, or soft tissue damage, causality and level of current and future damages are more difficult to prove and rely heavily on expert evaluation and opinion for making legal determinations. Parallel insurance situations involve attempts to access entitlements to health care treatment and disability benefits with policy determinations relying on expert evaluation and opinion. In both cases, financial and other incentives represent motivational factors that increase the likelihood of response bias including symptom exaggeration/amplification as well as feigning.

RESPONSE BIAS ASSESSMENT

Examinee Response Biases

Examinee response bias can take several forms, ranging from symptoms that are denied or minimized to exaggerated or feigned. Symptom exaggeration (accentuation, magnification, etc.) is usually associated with psychological factors such as catastrophizing and less often with conscious deception (i.e., feigning or malingering) for financial or other compensation purposes. Symptoms may be accurately or inaccurately attributed to different events. For instance, pre-existing symptoms may be misattributed to an accident suddenly given more prominence because of attention, anxiety, and other psychological factors (see subsequently), for example, an accident or injury may result in heightened perception of symptoms problems associated with stress or age related problems that were previously minimized, ignored, or of subthreshold level. Increased awareness of these symptoms or difficulties that may be "normal" or generally common can be temporally related to an accident or injury and misattributed to such an event. Social and external reinforcement clearly influence response to symptoms. Aging and cancer, for example, produce vastly different consequences than mild traumatic brain injury (MTBI) or back injury. Although the latter can result in some desirable consequences (e.g., monetary compensation, avoidance of stressful work demands, accommodations), the former are usually associated with undesirable consequences and greater tendency to be minimized.

Martelli and colleagues (6) reviewed the literature and found several injury context variables associated with poorer postinjury adaptation and recovery and increased likelihood of response bias. These are listed in Table 85-1.

These variables represent vulnerability factors that can reduce effective coping with postinjury impairments and increase the likelihood of maladaptive coping and response bias. They are not mutually exclusive and, as with the variables presented subsequently, more than 1 can contribute to symptom report and presentation. Additional review of the literature (7–15), combined with clinical experience indicate several other sources of poor postinjury adaptation and increased likelihood of significant response bias that may be encountered during examinations. These are included in Table 85-2. A frequently overlooked form of bias is that which is iatrogenic and occurs because of an increasingly restrictive insurance and adversarial medicolegal system. In an exploratory convenience study, Martelli and colleagues

(6,16) conducted a convenience attitudinal survey of injured workers, rehabilitation, and worker's compensation case managers and the professionals who evaluate and treat them. They found an overall 25% estimate of exaggerating or malingering Worker's Compensation (WC) patients, with highest estimates from WC case managers (29%) suggesting a general skepticism and distrust faced by injured workers. Furthermore, most professionals and case managers filling out the survey believed that they would personally be treated unfairly by the WC system if they were injured, suggesting an even stronger general skepticism and distrust of the extant systems that fund evaluation and treatment of injury and disability. In other words, there may be bias of persons conducting an evaluation or responsible for a claim. These preliminary data reflect the characteristic levels of diffuse distrust often observed by the authors in impairment and disability evaluation situations across the United States and Canada. These findings highlight the importance of considering the motivational factors that operate on examinees that present for impairment and disability evaluations.

In an interesting conceptualization of a major type of response bias in chronically disabled workers, Matheson (7,10–12) defined symptom magnification as a conscious or unconscious self-destructive and socially reinforced pattern of behavior or symptom production intended to control life circumstances, but which impedes health care efforts. He defined 3 major subtypes. The Type I "refugee" displays illness behavior that reflects escapist or avoidant responses to situations perceived as unsolvable. It can include somatization, conversion, psychogenic pain, and hypochondriacal disorders as extreme responses. The Type II "game player" employs symptoms for positive gain; symptom magnification is considered the most frequent response and is seen as a treatable self-destructive syndrome. The Type III "identified patient" is motivated by maintenance of the patient role as a means of ego and life survival (e.g., factitious disorder).

Main and Spanswick (15) examined the response bias of simulated or exaggerated incapacity in persons claiming physical disability. A list of features they found associated with and suggestive of simulated or exaggerated incapacity associated with chronic pain included failure to comply with

---

TABLE 85-1 Variables Associated With Poor Postinjury Adaptation and Response Bias

• Anger, resentment, or perceived mistreatment	• Fear of losing disability status, benefits, and safety net
• Fear of failure or rejection (e.g., damaged goods; fear of being fired after injury)	• Perceptions of high compensability for injury
• Loss of self-confidence and self-efficacy associated with residual impairments	• Preinjury job (task, work environment) dissatisfaction
• External (health, pain) locus of control	• Collateral injuries (especially if "silent")
• Irrational fear of injury extension, reinjury, or pain	• Inadequate and inaccurate medical information
• Discrepancies between personality/coping style and injury consequences (e.g., highly physically active person with few intellectual resources who has a back injury)	• Misdiagnosis, late diagnosis, or delays in instituting treatment
• Insufficient residual coping resources and skills	• Insurance resistance to authorizing treatment or delays in paying bills
• Prolonged inactivity resulting in disuse atrophy	• Retention of an attorney
• Greater reinforcement for "illness" vs "wellness" behavior	

TABLE 85-2 Additional Variables Associated With Poor Post Injury Adaptation and/or Response Bias

Cultural differences. For example, different cultures mix emotional and physical pain and symptoms at a conceptual and phenomenological level in different ways. Also, some cultures see failure to impose severe penalty/extract significant compensation for harm as a sign of weakness and disgrace in God's eyes.

Conditioned avoidance pain related disability (CAPRD). CAPRD represents phobic reactions associated with fear of pain wherein behavior, either gross motor activity (kinesiophobia) or cognitive exertion (cogniphobia), is avoided because of fear of exacerbation of pain. True conditioned behavioral reactions are typically beyond or minimally within the realm of conscious awareness and control.

Desperation induced malingering/symptom exaggeration. Individuals that are particularly prone to these types of response bias may include the following: workers insecure about work changes, aging workers, tired workers; workers fearing their own limited or declining abilities; workers whose premorbid coping was tenuous and who feel too overwhelmed and unable to cope with an additional stress; those with real or imagined abuse from others (employers, family, etc.); and immigrants workers who attempt cultural assimilation but feel resentful that they were not rewarded and/are psychoemotionally insecure and/or feel rejected and/or disillusioned by the new culture and may feel entitled. A second group of patients represented by this category may be making desperate pleas for help and reduce their effort (especially on seemingly easy tests) in order to ensure their perceived problems are detected and not missed.

Sociopathic, manipulative, and opportunistic personality traits. These personality traits can be found in all groups, but may be associated with a greater incidence of conscious dissimulation.

Passive-aggressive, impatient, or rebellious personality traits. Such individuals tend to resent others when perceived to not unconditionally believe them or impose evaluations or doctor's visits, especially ones that examine psychological function or motivation. They may play games with doctors by withholding or undermining procedures or treatments, and may especially alter performance on tests that seem nonchallenging or do not appear face valid.

Factitious and somatoform disorders. Individuals with factitious disorder and somatoform disorders (i.e., conversion disorders including nonepileptic seizures [pseudo-seizures], somatoform pain disorder, somatization disorder, and undifferentiated somatoform disorder) may present symptoms that represent a combination of several items in this table or other factors.

Psychological decompensation. These individuals usually display conspicuous psychological distress and pathology that differentiates them from others.

Skepticism. Some individuals are very skeptical of doctors, examinations and examination procedures, and may be poorly motivated to comply with the conditions required for valid assessment.

Diagnosis threat. This refers to the effect of negative expectations on cognitive test performance. Subjects with a history of mild head injury perform significantly worse on general intellectual and memory measures and rate themselves as putting forth less effortful performance (13,14) when attention was called to their head injury ("diagnosis threat"). This effect may play an important role in many situations where response bias and poor adaptation are noted. Closely related is the concept of nocebo effect, or negative effects caused by the suggestion or belief that something is harmful.

Iatrogenic bias. A frequently overlooked form of bias is that which is a reaction to the nature of the insurance and adversarial legal system. As discussed in the preceding text, preliminary attitudinal data gathered from injured workers and the individuals who treat and case manage them (6,16) indicates a strong and prevalent skepticism and distrust faced by injured persons in the extant insurance systems. Mistrust and expectation of unfair treatment from employers, doctors, and insurance companies can produce a deliberate reactive magnification of symptoms. The presence of other variables listed in this table and in Table 85-1 will likely amplify the likelihood of this type of response bias.

reasonable treatment, report of severe pain with no associated psychological effects, marked inconsistencies in effects of pain on general activities, poor work record, and previous litigation. Features not found primarily suggestive of response bias included mismatch between physical findings and reported symptoms, report of severe or continuous pain, anger, poor response to treatment, and behavioral signs/symptoms.

Attribution and Bias

There are several sources of attribution bias and misattribution of symptoms that require assessment during evaluation of physical, sensory, and neurocognitive impairments.

Examinee attribution biases can include mistaking physical, cognitive, and motivation problems associated with depression and sleep disturbance for neurologic injury or sequelae. This can occur because of misattribution, overattribution, retrospective attribution, illusory correlation, or heightened awareness because of vigilance biases. Importantly, the previously mentioned conditions (e.g., depression, sleep disturbance) are reversible and may have been present prior to the injury without producing significant limitations. Furthermore, the emotional states or fatigue may be interacting with actual physical injury symptoms to increase impairment.

Examiner misattribution can occur when methodical neurologic, psychologic, and other assessments are not used to differentiate sequelae secondary to brain injury from factors with overlapping presentations (e.g., cranial/cranial adnexal and cervical trauma impairments, chronic pain, motivational factors, and/or other psychological sequelae or other nonneurologic factors). Tendencies toward "overdiagnosis" of neurologic disorders, such as MTBI, when "abnormal" neurocognitive findings and/or nonspecific somatic complaints are obtained, can only be avoided through careful differential diagnosis. Brain injury specialists sensitized to neurologic symptoms have been observed by the authors to misdiagnose chronic pain sequelae as postconcussive symptoms, which may result in an escalation of medical costs, prolongation of inappropriate treatment, and eventual treatment failure that may contribute to a sense of helplessness and chronic disability in the injured person. Conversely, similar observations have been made for psychiatrists and psychologists prone to infer psychiatric or psychological etiologies for all pathology, including brain injury or actual physical injury (1,6,17).

Response Bias Assessment

Formal response bias assessment procedures should be employed in order to increase the probability that clinical examination findings are an accurate and valid reflection of impairment. Response bias exists on a continuum that extends through denial and unawareness of impairments, symptom minimization, to no bias, to symptom magnification and malingering. Although many examinees approach testing in a forthright and adequately motivated manner without significant response bias, it is necessary to examine the potential for response bias with each patient.

Anosognosia or unawareness of deficits is a neurologic phenomenon owing to dysfunction of brain operations subserving awareness (6,17). Usually more pronounced early after injury and associated with more significant neurologic insults, it can lead to chronic under appreciation of deficits.

Symptom minimization may be consciously or unconsciously motivated. It is usually motivated by either a desire to engage in activities that might otherwise be restricted or to maintain a positive view of oneself and ones life (e.g., high "social desirability"). *Denial* is a psychological defense employed unconsciously to protect against painful and overwhelming realizations about losses or other psychological issues that may threaten the integrity of oneself.

Although this chapter focuses primarily on negative response bias and symptom exaggeration, detection of positive response bias is equally important and unfortunately too often neglected. In addition to the more to less conscious intention to protect against painful realizations of loss, impairment and decrements in self-integrity and functional status, there are a class of situations where highly desired or privileged activity may be restricted by symptom presence. These situations present a strong incentive to minimize impairments and/or inflate abilities. Some of these many common situations include maintaining or regaining desired driving privileges, maintaining or returning to desired work and/or other physical and cognitive activity, returning to game play in sports, and return to combat on the battlefield.

The task of detection of positive response bias can be equally or more challenging than the detection of negative response bias. Some highly motivated clients may prepare for and inflate neuropsychological test performance by doing internet searches, studying, making cheat sheets for common tests, and even asking others which tests will be performed by the examiner. Moreover, several recent news reports include video and audiotapes of the most talented football and hockey players in the United States reporting that they underperformed on baseline screening cognitive tests to reduce chances that postconcussion test results could keep them from playing.

Failure to detect such positive response biases (from unawareness, through minimization to denial) can result in fail-

ure to identify important impairments and produce an overestimation of abilities that could potentially endanger the welfare of the examinee and others. Because most assessment begins with interview, vigilance is required to prevent uncritical acceptance of minimization or injury and symptoms, especially when inconsistent with medical or other information or when additional screening will be based only on subjective symptom report. Special attention should be paid to observational, descriptive, and test measure signs of positive response bias. These include inconsistencies (e.g., between injury severity and expected impairments, between record of injury and denied or minimized report, and/or between self-report vs corroboratory report) (Table 85-3) and test measures (e.g., elevations on personality measures such as Minnesota Multiphasic Personality Inventory-Lie [MMPI-L] scale and Personality Assessment Inventory [PAI]–Positive Impression Management [PIM] scale) (Table 85-7) that suggest positive symptom impression management.

Symptom magnification refers to accentuation or exaggeration of impairment. This can occur in relation to multiple factors, can represent an attempt to inflate financial compensation, or can serve a wide range of psychological needs. Some examples include efforts to legitimize latent dependency needs, resolve preexisting life conflicts, retaliate against employer or spouse or other, reduce anxiety, fulfill self-denigrating or self-abasement personality patterns, exert a "plea for help," or solicit acknowledgment of perceived difficulties. Symptom exaggeration can also occur in patients with premorbid histories of psychiatric-psychoemotional problems who "latch on" to a specific diagnosis that not only becomes responsible for all life problems, but also promotes passivity, helplessness, and an external locus of control. When patients are assessed for claims of major disability following uncomplicated mild and often even more significant brain injury, nonneurologic contributors should be

TABLE 85-3 Waddell's Nonorganic Signs

Overreaction	Guarding/limping, bracing, rubbing affected area, grimacing, sighing
Tenderness	Widespread sensitivity to light touch of superficial tissue)
Axial loading	Light pressure to skull of standing patient should not significantly increase low back symptoms
Rotation	Back pain reported when shoulders and pelvis are passively rotated in the same plane
Straight leg raising	Marked difference between leg raising in the supine and seated position
Motor and sensory	Giving way or cog wheeling to motor testing or regional sensory loss in a stocking or nondermatomal distribution (with peripheral nerve dysfunction ruled out)

Additional nonorganic signs that have been considered have included lower extremity give-away, no pain-free spells in the past year, intolerance of treatments, and emergency admissions to hospital with back trouble (15,21,24). Adapted from Waddell et al. (24) and Fishbain et al. (25).

closely scrutinized. Depression, post-traumatic stress disorder and other anxiety conditions or other psychiatric syndromes or psychological processes such as catastrophizing can produce symptoms that are mistaken for neurologic impairment. Misdiagnosis of these conditions serves to promulgate misperceptions and amplify functional disability and health care costs.

Malingering is deliberate symptom production for purposes of secondary gain, especially financial compensation or avoidance of undesirable situations or responsibilities. Malingering in the examination setting will often be associated with unexpectedly poor performance (6). Measures of response bias should be administered in all contexts, but this is especially imperative in cases of medicolegal presentation or suspicion of any incentive to make less than fully effortful or accurate presentation.

Importantly, the identification of unambiguous cases of malingering is difficult. The most convincing evidence of certain or definite malingering is a confession or admission, but this seldom occurs and may not be truthful. A secondary form of evidence is when the person or examinee is detected, via surveillance, performing an act that they reported they could not do. This can be unreliable because a persons' report that they are unable to do certain things can represent, for example, a response bias to report problems or exaggerate, negative self-evaluations, poor self-judgment, or overgeneralization. A third form of evidence comes from corroboratory report, that is, a third party contradicts what the examinee claims. There are also various problems associated with this evidence as is true of many situations when there is a discrepancy between reports of 2 parties. Finally, a variety of instruments and examination procedures are available as indicators of response bias. Any of several measures designed to assess atypical, worse than chance performance, or nonorganic responses can be employed to assess response bias in cognitive, motor, sensory or physical performances, or self-report. However, again, most of these measures also require careful clinical interpretation because there may be several possible alternative explanations for performance.

Importantly, the presence of response bias, although required, is not sufficient evidence of malingering as this is a probabilistic evaluation predicated on converging evidence from a thorough analysis and integration of history, contextual information, behavioral observation, interview data, examination and test data, collaborative data, and personality and emotional status data. It requires thoughtful analysis of all data (e.g., consideration of both secondary gain and secondary losses) as well as competent differential diagnosis to consider alternative explanations (17). It also requires cautious and critical consideration of the probability of malingering vis-à-vis the limitations of the assessment and response bias measures and the potential consequences of incorrect impressions. *Measures of response bias provide valuable information for estimating the degree to which a person was presenting accurately and/or exerting full effort and the degree to which test results are reliable and valid and reflect actual abilities. They do not provide reliable evidence of malingering.*

Moreover, when lower than chance or below cutoff performance is observed on symptom validity testing (SVTs), the interpretation that conscious dissimulation is present should not be absolute. Probabilistically (at $P <.05$), 1 in 20

findings can be expected to be caused solely by chance. Given that a large number of SVTs are usually administered, some failures can be expected because of chance alone. In addition, reported samples have also demonstrated higher than expected failure rates in persons with no reason or even with disincentive to perform poorly. Finally, numerous other factors, including pain, psychiatric disorder, sleep disturbance, and motivational factors have been shown to contribute to poor performances on neuropsychological tests (2). This is discussed in later paragraphs in this text and in more detail in Chapter 58 in this text.

Evaluating clinicians should be familiar with psychological syndromes that may present as organic disorders that are important in the differential diagnosis of symptom exaggeration or malingering. These include factitious disorder and somatoform disorders (e.g., conversion disorders including nonepileptic seizures [pseudo-seizures], somatoform pain disorder, somatization disorder, and undifferentiated somatoform disorder). Because the presence of a psychological syndrome and/or response bias does not necessarily exclude the diagnosis of an actual neurological syndrome or malingering, the process of disentangling multiple clinical entities that sometimes coexist is further complicated. Unfortunately, the art and science of methodical differential diagnosis is too often underappreciated in the evaluation process (1).

Examination Strategies

Professionals who specialize in brain injury medicine should be familiar with examination strategies designed to evaluate nonorganic musculoskeletal and neurologic disorders, including the use of specialized bedside examination techniques for physical and cognitive dissimulation as well as other types of nonneurogenic impairment. Examples include such strategies as Hoover's test for evaluation of malingered lower extremity weakness, sideways/backwards walking for assessment of feigned gait disturbance, and a positive Stenger's test on audiologic assessment for nonorganic hearing loss. Other tests that might be of value in the context of response bias detection on the physical examination include Mankopf's maneuver, strength reflex test, arm and/or wrist drop test, hip adductor test, axial loading test, Gordon-Welberry toe test, Bowlus and Currier test, Burns bench test, Magnuson's test, and others (1,18) (also see Table 85-8).

Examination findings that suggest a possible nonneurological basis for the observed impairments include patchy sensory loss, pain in an improbable nondermatomal distribution (e.g., midline sensory demarcation), nonpronator drift, and/or astasia-abasia (19). Motor and other impairment inconsistencies that fluctuate or disappear under hypnosis, drug assisted interviews, or "presumed" nonobservation may also suggest some psychophysiological or functional substrate and cast doubt on a hardwired or intractable organic deficit. Importantly, some nonorganic or nonneurologic signs such as hemisensory loss may be in response to central psychophysiological factors associated with actual changes in brain function (20). Both feigned and conversional hemiparesis are typically more common on the left side (19–21), perhaps because of the fact that most persons are right hand dominant. Consistency regarding laterality of symptoms, particularly with neurologic impairment and/or referred pain, should be evaluated.

When of central (vs peripheral) origin, pain complaints should be assessed, in part, by concurrently assessing temperature perception, given that the same neural pathways mediate these sensations. When temperature sensation is preserved in the presence of a loss of pain sensation after central nervous system (CNS) injury, the deficit is not likely to reflect direct CNS impairment (the loss should occur contralateral to and lower than the level of the lesion). This point also reinforces the need to understand the neuropathology/pathology of the lesion based on imaging studies and to appreciate the implications that these findings have for anticipated clinical exam findings. Alleged pain imperception can be evaluated, as can nearly any reported neurological impairment, with appropriately designed forced choice testing (22). Additionally, examiners should realize that alleged pain imperception or loss of sensation is difficult to fake on repeated bilateral stimulation. This is caused by the fact that examinees that exaggerate rely on subjective strategies rather than truly responding to the strength of the stimuli. Therefore, assessments with such techniques as Von Frey hairs could be used to provide further objective evidence of the validity of reported symptoms.

Defining pain and its possible deception is extremely challenging (2,9,23). Pain is usually described as an unpleasant sensory and emotional experience and associated with or described in terms of actual or potential tissue damage. When acute, there is identifiable tissue damage or noxious event and clearly defined assessment and treatment targets. When chronic, associated tissue damage or pathology is often obscure or absent vs increased expression of anxiety, maladaptive protective responses or pain behaviors, protracted medication use, minimally effective medical services, marked behavioral or emotional changes, and restrictions in daily activities (23). Hence, necessary differentiation between pain and suffering vs exaggeration in the context of an Independent Evaluation (IE) is complicated because these can be inextricably intertwined with each other as well as with affective conditions such as depression and anxiety.

A controversial procedure for screening psychological factors contributing to pain responses that is frequently employed by physical therapists, physicians, and chiropractors is the assessment for Waddell nonorganic signs (24,25); see Table 85-3 for description. See chapter 58 for a detailed discussion of pain assessment and management following brain injury.

Intended to indicate degree of nonorganic or psychological contribution to pain experience, these signs were not intended to exclude causal physical components or imply that psychological factors were a cause vs result of pain. More recent evidence indicates that the Waddell signs are not valid measures of nonorganicity. Fishbain (25), in the first structured, evidence-based review of available evidence, concludes that Waddell signs (a) are neither correlated with psychological distress or secondary gain, (b) do not discriminate organic from nonorganic problems, (c) may represent an organic phenomenon, and (d) are associated with greater pain levels and poorer treatment outcomes.

The demonstration of invalidity of one of the most heavily relied upon methods for making inferences and diagnostic impressions about pain nonorganicity calls into question the general diagnostic validity of many physical and medical evaluations. Moreover, it almost certainly limits the utility of commonly used psychological response bias and somatization predictor scales that were validated using these invalid measures or diagnostic impressions as criterion. Regarding assessment of psychological and neuropsychological impairments and chronic pain, response bias represents an especially important threat to validity. As these assessments usually begin with an interview about self-reported symptoms and subsequently rely heavily on standardized measures of performance on well-normed tests, the validity of the results requires the veracity, cooperation, and motivation of the patient. Recent evidence, however, suggests that some patients seen for presumptive brain injury–related impairments overreport preinjury functional status (25). This may be especially true with postconcussive deficits because these symptoms appear with similar frequency in the general population (27). In addition, the demonstrated ability of neuropsychologists to accurately detect malingering in test protocols has been less than impressive (e.g., 28,29,30,31). Finally, the common practice of using technicians to administer tests, as previously noted, has been called into question for reasons that include adequacy to detect and manage response bias issues (32). Nonetheless, various instruments, techniques, and strategies are available, which have demonstrated utility in detecting response bias, as a means of increasing confidence in the validity of assessment findings.

Table 85-4 presents what have often been considered hallmarks signs of response bias (29,33). The signs can be applied to most aspects of a medical examination, with noted caveats for most.

The evaluation of response bias and all aspects of preinjury and postinjury status can include the following investigative tools in conjunction with client interviews and testing (a) school records; (b) medical records; (c) driver records; (d) military records; (e) criminal records; (f) employment records; (g) evaluations from other psychologists; (h) interviews with family members, friends, teachers, employers, and so forth; and (i) all materials available to the attorney through formal discovery or otherwise.

These guidelines and strategies are presented as important possible indicators for interpreting patient examination data. Integrating contextual information, history, behavioral observation, interview data, collaborative data, and personality data with measures of effort and neuropsychological test data provides the best information for estimating both the degree of effort put forth and the degree to which test results are reliable and valid predictors of actual abilities.

The recent increase in attention to response bias assessment and malingering may reflect a pendulum-like reaction to earlier times when such issues were not properly appreciated and when excessive compensation packages or awards may have been made because of an assessment of disability that did not take into account response bias. In the current and increasingly restrictive health care environment where services and benefits are more critically evaluated and where legal and decision-making policies favor either/or, black or white conceptualizations, there are tendencies to consider response bias as dichotomous and synonymous with malingering. Response bias measures have often been erroneously referred to as "malingering measures" in many publications. This can contribute to what the authors note as too frequently haphazard and overzealous application of poorly validated

TABLE 85-4 Response Bias: Typical Hallmark Signs

I. Inconsistencies within and between:

1. Reported symptoms
2. Examination/test performance
3. Clinical presentation
4. Known diagnostic patterns
5. Observed behavior (in another setting)
6. Reported symptoms and exam/test performance
7. Measures of similar abilities (intertest scatter)
8. Similar tasks or items within the same exam or test (intratest scatter)—especially when difficult tasks are performed more easily than easy ones
9. Different testing sessions

Caveat: The potential contributions of significant psychiatric, attentional, comprehension, or other problems that often involve inconsistent presentations should be considered in evaluating inconsistency. In addition, the effect of the examiner on eliciting responses should be considered.

II. Overly Impaired Performance (vs Expected)

1. Very poor performance on easy tasks presented as difficult
2. Failing tasks that all but those with severe impairment perform easily
3. Poorer performance than normative data for similar injury/illness
4. Lower than chance level performance

Caveat: Unusually, poor level of performance may be caused by actual interference effects associated with various psychologic, sleep, or other disturbances; statistically significant levels of lower than chance performance may be expected in 1/20 cases with the usual significance levels.

III. Lack of Specific Diagnostic Signs of Impairment

Caveat: Many disorders do not have unambiguous diagnostic signs.

IV. Specific Signs of Response Bias on Psychological or Neuropsychological Tests

1. MMPI-2/MMPI-RF Scales: F, F-K, L, VRIN, TRIN, Fb, S, Fp, Fs, RBS
2. MMPI-2 "Fake Bad Scale" (FBS) (41)
3. Malingering detection tests
4. Actuarial formulas for clinical neuropsychological tests (e.g., Wisconsin Card Sorting Test [WCST], California Verbal Learning Test [CVLT])

Caveat: Many of these signs are not unambiguous or have not been thoroughly validated.

V. Interview Evidence

1. Atypical temporal relationship of symptoms to injury
2. Psychological symptoms, or symptoms that are improbable, absurd, overly specific or of unusual frequency or severity (e.g., triple vision)
3. Disparate examinee history or complaints across interviews or examiners
4. Disparate corroboratory interview data vs examinee report

Caveat: Other explanations are possible for disparate or atypical interview data.

VI. Physical Exam Findings

1. Nonorganic sensory findings
2. Nonorganic motor findings
3. Pseudoneurologic findings in the absence of anticipated associated pathologic findings
4. Inconsistent exam findings
5. Failure on physical exam procedures designed to specifically assess malingering

Caveat: As indicated earlier, nonorganic sensory findings may have a psychophysiological basis as may psychogenic movement disorders or other pseudoneurologic presentations.

procedures, failure to critically and objectively evaluate weaknesses as well as strengths, tendencies to overinterpret or overgeneralize, or failure to objectively integrate (vs selectively confirm test results) other relevant information.

Numerous reports illustrate how response bias and malingering are not synonymous (2,9,10–13,17,23,34). Psychiatric history and financial compensation seeking can produce similar increases in likelihood of invalid responding on neuropsychological and cognitive symptom validity measures (35). Characterologic/personality disorder factors have been shown to contribute to exaggerated results in a forensic setting (36). Negative expectancy (e.g., "diagnosis threat"), independent of impairment, can reduce cognitive performance (13,14). Ample other evidence indicates that psychiatric or functional disorders can produce response bias or actual performance deficits related to poor adaptation and maladaptive coping vs malingering (e.g., 37–40).

Based on a critical evaluation of the current state of the art, it appears necessary to caution that malingering (a) should not be considered dichotomous (i.e., present or not); (b) should not be considered something that can be reliably or validly assessed with a high degree of probability, even when serious efforts are made; and (c) should not be considered a discrete entity assessed by commonly used response bias measures. Further, it should not be assumed that response bias measures have a high degree of reliability and external validity in predicting valid examination performance on other measures or functional ability in other settings, or even that examinees take the examination process as seriously as examiners.

A summary of some of the major limitations with current response bias procedures include (8,9,16,19,31,42–44, 45,46)

1. psychometric research inadequacies (i.e., basic test construction issues such as reliability and validity, sensitivity, and specificity);
2. limited generalizability of analogue research (e.g., unknown differences between simulated and real malingerers);
3. Variable Group Membership (wide variability in samples for both simulators and symptom disorder groups);
4. differential vulnerability to response bias (some tests are more obvious or subtle, sensitive or specific);
5. questionable generalizability (e.g., from analogue simulation studies to real life situations, from one response bias measure to another, to other tests or test administrations, to actual symptoms, or across time);
6. absence of mutual exclusivity (poor effort can occur in presence of real disorders);

7. "Law of the Instrument" bias wherein "malingering" becomes what "malingering" tests measure (specifically, the definitions of "effort," and validation studies to examine the construct, are often lacking; further "effort" cannot be assumed uniform for individuals, individuals within or across diagnostic groups or for nonlitigating and litigating situations);
8. questionable specificity—the effects of fatigue, pain, disinterest, nonattended (e.g., computer) administration, mixing cognitive tests and SVTs in a battery with unknown validity, and other factors on response bias tests, are not understood and have not been addressed;
9. frequently high misclassification (i.e., false positive or false negative) rates, especially in the very few studies that examined ecological or real world validity (42,43); and
10. incautious use of most current SVT indices regarding diagnosis and decision making can potentially violate American Psychological Association (APA) ethics code and "APA Standards for Educational and Psychological Tests," given the aforementioned psychometric limitations.

These aforementioned limitations emphasize the importance of (a) applying caution regarding overinterpretation of response bias procedures and (b) employing multiple data sources and making thoughtful inferences only after integration of thorough historical information, interview, assessment, behavioral observations, collaborative interview, and data sources. Using the scientific method of attempting to disconfirm (vs selectively confirm) predictions from response bias measures may be a useful way of promoting objective test interpretation.

Table 85-5 presents an illustrative caution against simplistic and dichotomous diagnostic conceptualizations. For any given symptom, it represents 4 levels of actual structural impairment (none, clear, mixed, indeterminate) × 4 levels of injury related residual functional life impairment (present or not; distorted report [exaggerated or minimized] or not) × 4 levels of measurable impairment on examination (present or not; distorted or not). Some of the possibilities range from persons who are denying or minimizing clear impairments found on structural tests, functional status, and neurologic and neuropsychological exam; to uncomplicated disorders with structural, functional, and exam detected impairments with or without distortion, through persons with complicated presentations with mixed findings and distortion; and/ or to completed misattributed, exaggerated, or malingered presentation on functional status and exam performance. Observations by the authors in reading many reports consis-

---

TABLE 85-5 Diagnostic Possibilities in Brain Injury Assessment

BRAIN INJURY STRUCTURAL IMPAIRMENT	RESIDUAL FUNCTIONAL LIFE IMPAIRMENTS	RESIDUAL IMPAIRMENTS ON EXAMINATION
1. Yes	1. Yes and Distorted (exaggerated; or minimized)	1. Yes and Not Distorted
2. Mixed	2. Yes and Not Distorted	2. Yes and Distorted
3. Indeterminate	3. No and Exaggerated	3. No and Exaggerated
4. No	4. No and Not Exaggerated	4. No and Not Exaggerated

tently indicate a preponderance of conclusions reflecting only a few of these possibilities with mostly dichotomous (present or absent) diagnostic inferences regarding neurologic, physical dysfunction, and malingering.

A cautious approach is indicated with regard to estimating the probabilities regarding presence or absence of neurologic or physical impairment and response bias. In the case where both actual symptoms and exaggerating are present, inferences must be generated about the degree of deliberateness, degree of physical impairment, and degree of awareness of exaggeration on the part of the subject. Has the person adopted a sick role and talked themselves into believing they cannot perform certain tasks and lack certain abilities (e.g., somatoform disorder), with conscious withholding of effort because of intention of demonstrating what they believe to be true disabilities? Or, are they less conscious and aware, consistent with suspected conversion type disorder? Are they completely aware and demonstrating sociopathic tendencies? Are they aware but coping in a way that may be potentially adaptive; for example, an aging worker with a chronic history of back failures, low self-esteem, and a historically poor and stressful relationship with an imposing employer. This employee may believe that another back injury is inevitable, will be increasingly painful and disabling, require uncomfortable interactions with others, result in being fired by a company believed to have not make obvious safety precautions to prevent their injury, and that no other competitive job options are realistic.

SVT, or effort testing, is a process of determining the veracity of one's symptom complaint or dysfunction. As previously indicated the purpose of SVT or effort testing is to assist in determining whether the obtained test results reflect the individual's true abilities or clinical condition. Effort testing can take many forms and assess for various conditions; with the determination of psychopathology and/or cognitive impairment most commonly evaluated. The specific procedures and methods for determining the validity of one's complaints also vary and include tests specifically designed for measuring effort/symptom veracity, imbedded items in existing psychological or neuropsychological measures, or empirically derived indicators of symptom validity. Common paradigms for SVT of cognitive impairment include forced-choice testing, comparison to performance of known diagnostic groups (e.g., various severities of brain injury, groupings of individuals based on the time to follow commands, presumed or known malingers), or comparison to "coached" samples. The forced-choice approach is based on probability assumptions that performance at "chance" levels would be obtained from random guessing and that below chance performance likely involves conscious effort. Many measures also involve more complex means of determining diagnostic probability (e.g., Bayesian diagnostic probability values). Some measures also incorporate base rates determined from performance of various diagnostic groups and allow for adjustments in cut-off scores based on diagnostic population or assessment context (litigation vs clinical evaluation). Several measures used to assess effort and symptom validity can be found in Tables 85-6–85-8.

Tables 85-8 present three summaries of a broadly representative sample of response bias detection strategies and techniques that may suggest compromised validity of neuro-

psychological, psychoemotional, and medical examination data. These tables were prepared on the basis of a review of much of the established literature (see 6–15,16,18–22,24–30, 32–151). Multiple sources were used for most indicators and special attention was given to well accepted reviews of specific empirical indicators (47,52,63, etc.) as a model. This table illustrates the utility of a constellation or profiling approach to response bias detection. A multiaxial conceptual model is presented as a methodological approach for constructing a profile of motivation and response bias. It incorporates a wide array of findings from common evaluation instruments and indicators, each with empirical support indicating at least some utility in detecting suboptimal effort or other response bias (e.g., 47,51,52,64).

Review of original test manuals and associated studies should be conducted before employing any of these instruments. The tables are not intended as substitutes for understanding the individual measures and latest findings and recommendations. They are representative but not definitive. Although numerous conceptual and methodological pitfalls and limitations exist for each procedure, increasing evidence indicates improved discrimination and increased reliability when multiple measures are employed (60). The proposed conceptual approach integrates multiple factors as an optimal method for estimating the degree of effort and the degree of reliability and validity of examination findings. The "Motivational Assessment Profile" (MAP) model is a guide and procedure that economically incorporates many currently available instruments and methods and much available published research for direct and indirect measurement of effort and response bias. For review of these instruments and methods, the reader is referred to several good reviews in textbooks of neuropsychology or the many previous reports and reviews of this literature (e.g., 9,47,51,52,60, 62,110,143,149,150).

Most major objective personality measures and many neuropsychological measures include imbedded scales or indices (66,67) that provide performance data to detect simulators or those with some other response bias. Inherent advantages include reduced need for administering and charging for sometimes lengthy tests designed solely for detection of potential motivation problems (especially when absent), increasing available time for administering relevant clinical measures and conducting comprehensive interviews (examinee, collaborative others), and potential enhancement of face validity of measures.

The techniques or strategies suggested in Tables 85-6–85-8 are offered with the following caveats.

Probabilistically (at $P < .05$), 1 in 20 findings of suboptimal performance can be expected to be caused solely by chance. Also, higher than expected failure rates have been reported in persons with no reason or even with disincentive to perform poorly. Finally, numerous other factors, including pain, psychiatric disorder, sleep disturbance, and motivational factors have been shown to contribute to poor performances on neuropsychological tests (2,34). The potential contributions of significant psychiatric, attentional, comprehension, motivational, pain, sleep, or other disorders that often involve inconsistent presentations should be considered in evaluating inconsistency. Unusually poor level of performance may be caused by actual interference effects

TABLE 85-6 Motivation Assessment Profile—Brain Injury Evaluations (MAP–BI) Objective Neurocognitive Tests

I. Performance Patterns on Existing Neuropsychological Tests

Arithmetic, Orientation scale Performance	"Near-miss" (Ganser errors)
Category Test Performance	Rare or "spike three" errors; or > 1 error on Trials I or II
Digit Span (Floor Effect)	Age scale score < 5 years
Digit Span: Testing Limits with "Chunking" (grouping larger list into 2 smaller ones)	Nonimprovement with "chunking"
Finger Agnosia—Errors	> 3
Finger Tapping Test	Unusually low w/o gross motor deficit
Finger Tip Number Writing—Errors	> 5
Full Scale IQ	Low (vs expected, estimated, etc.)
General Neuropsych Deficit Scale (40)	GNDS score < 44
Grip Strength with Dynamometer	Unusually low w/o gross motor deficit
List Learning Serial Order Effects	Abnormal patterns
Seashore Rhythm Test Performance	> 8 errors (Poor)
Tactual Stimulation Performance	Errors bilaterally vs laterally
Wisconsin Card Sorting Test Errors	Discrepant number perseverative vs number category errors
Recognition memory (RAVLT)	< 6
Recognition memory (CVLT)	< 13
Rey Complex Figure Recognition Trial	Atypical recognition errors (> 2); recognition failure errors
Warrington Recognition Memory Test (RMT)	Score < 38 (RMW), < 26 (RMF)

II. Instruments Designed to Specifically Evaluate Level of Cognitive Effort/Response Bias

21-Item Test	< 5 on free recall, < 3 on free recall, < 13 on recognition, < 9 on recognition
Autobiographical Interview (16)	> 3 errors
Computer Assessment of Response Bias (CARB)	< 89% raises suspicion
Dot Counting Test (DCT)	Correct/incorrect responses
Forced Choice test of Nonverbal Ability (67)	Sig < 50% chance level responding
Memorization of 16 Items Test (MSIT)	> 8 Omissions, > 6 Omissions, < 6 Total Correct
Portland Digit Recognition Test (PDRT)	Sig less than chance responding
Rey Complex Figure Test Recognition Trial	Atypical recognition errors (> 2); recognition failure errors
Rey Memory for 15 Items Test (MFIT); Rey Memory 15 Items Recognition Trial (MFIT-R)	< 3 complete sets, < 9 items (42)
Memorization of 16 Items Test (MSIT)	> 8 Omissions, > 6 Omissions, < 6 Total Correct
Rey Word Recognition List (WRL)	< 6 correct, < 5 (total correct minus false positives)
Test of Memory Malingering (TOMM)	< 45 trial 2 or recognition
Victoria Symptom Validity Test (VSVT)	Sig < chance level responding, < 16 on easy and/or hard items
Word Completion Memory Test (WCMT)	R < 9 or inclusion < 15
Word Memory Test (WMT) Immediate Recall (IR), Delayed Recall (DR), Consistency	< 89% raises suspicion

CVLT, California Verbal Learning Test; DR, Delayed Recall; IR, Immediate Recall; RAVLT, Rey Auditory Verbal Learning Test; RMF, Recognition Memory - Faces; RMW, Recognition Memory - Words.

TABLE 85-7 Motivation Assessment Profile—Brain Injury Evaluations (MAP–BI) Objective Personality Instruments and Qualitative Measures

Personality Instruments With Built-in Detection Designs

Minnesota Multiphasic Personality Inventory (MMPI-2/MMPI-RF)	• Validity indices (L, F, Fb, Fp, Ds, K, VRIN, TRIN, F-K) (103,121) • The Fake Bad Scale (41,131) *Rogers (29)—cutoff scores:* *Liberal:* • *F-Scale raw score > 23* • *F-Scale T-Score > 81* • *F-K Index > 10* • *Obvious-subtle score > 83* *Conservative:* • *F-scale raw > 30* • *F-K index > 25*
Personality Assessment Inventory (PAI) (110)	Inconsistency (INC), Infrequency (INF), Positive Impression Management (PIM), and Negative Impression Management (NIM) scales. 8 score patterns thought to comprise a response bias or "Malingering Index." • > 2 patterns malingering suspected • > 4 patterns malingering likely
Millon Clinical Multiaxial Inventory-III (MCMI-III) (108)	Four modifying (response bias) indices: V scale (random responding); Disclosure Scale; Desirability Scale; Debasement Scale.

Qualitative Variables for Assessing Response Bias

Time/response latency comparisons across similar tasks	
Time/response latency comparisons across similar tasks	Inconsistencies across tasks
Performance on easy tasks presented as hard	Low scores or unusual errors
Remote memory report	Difficulties, especially if less than recent memory, or severely impaired in absence of gross amnesia
Personal information	Very poor personal information in absence of gross amnesia discrepancies
Comparison between test performance and behavioral observations	Inconsistencies
Inconsistencies in history and/or complaints, performance	Inconsistencies across time, interviewer, etc.
Comparisons for inconsistencies within testing session (quantitative and qualitative):	A. Within tasks (e.g., easy vs hard items) B. Between tasks (e.g., easy vs hard) C. Across repetitions of same/parallel tasks (R/O fatigue) D. Across similar tasks under different motivational sets
Comparisons across testing sessions (qualitative, quantitative)	Poorer/inconsistent performance on re-testing
Symptom self-report: complaints	High frequency of complaints; patient complaints > significant others'

Main and Spanswick Indicators (15)

• Failure to comply with reasonable treatment
• Report of severe pain with no associated psychological effects
• Marked inconsistencies in effects of pain on general activities
• Poor work record and history of persistent awards
• Previous litigation

Symptom self-report: early vs late symptom complaint
Early symptoms reported late

TABLE 85-8 Motivation Assessment Profile—Brain Injury Evaluations (MAP–BI) Qualitative Neuromedical Indicators

	MOTOR
Astasia-abasia	"Drunken type" nonorganic gait with near-falls but no actual falls to ground
Assistive device "wear and tear" signs	In any examinee using assistive devices for any period of time, for example, cane, crutches, there should be commensurate wear on the device consistent with their claimed impairment and disability.
Calluses on hands in "totally disabled" examinee	An examinee who is unable to work should not present with signs of ongoing evidence of physical labor
Gait discrepancies when observed vs not observed	If organic should be consistent regardless of whether observed or not.
Gait discrepancies relative to direction of requested ambulation	Gait should present with same impairments in all directions. Malingerers do not as a rule practice a feigned gait in all directions.
Grip strength testing via dynamometer (Jamar)[a]	• Three repetitions at any setting should not vary more than 20% and/or Bell shaped curve if all 5 positions tested • Full effort required for valid results for peak strength (seen at grip position 3 of 5).
Rapid Exchange Grip (REG) test[a]	More difficult to falsify and may be a more valid measure of degree of full effort than Jamar
Hip adductor test	Test for claimed paralysis of lower extremity, similar to Hoover's test yet looks for crossed adductor response
Hoover's test	Test for feigned lower extremity weakness associated with normal crossed hip extensor response
Lack of atrophy in a chronically paretic/paralytic limb	Lack of atrophy in a paralyzed/paretic limb suggests the limb is being used or is getting regular electrical stimulation to maintain mass.
Lack of shoe wear in presence of gait disturbance	An examinee with claimed longer term gait deviation because of orthopedic or neurologic causes should demonstrate commensurate wear on shoes (if worn with any frequency)
Object drop test	Examinee claims inability to bend down yet does so to pick up a light object "inadvertently" dropped by examiner
Straight leg raise (SLR) disparities dependent on examinee positioning	Differences in SLR between sitting, standing and/or bending may suggest a functional overlay to low back complaints
Sudden motor give-away or ratchitiness on manual strength testing	Considered to normally be a sign of incomplete effort or symptom exaggeration.
Weakness on manual muscle testing without commensurate asymmetry of Deep Tendon Reflexes or muscle bulk.	Suggests simulated muscle weakness if longstanding.
Arm drop test	An aware patient malingering profound alteration in consciousness or significant arm paresis will not let their own hand, when held over their head, drop onto their face when the arm is released by the examiner
Wrist drop test	In an examinee with claimed wrist extensor loss, have them pronate forearm, extend elbow and flex shoulder . . . if on making a fist in this position, they also extend wrist then nonorganicity should be suspected.
Nonneurologic upper extremity drift	Long tract involvement results in pronator type drift. Proximal shoulder girdle weakness and malingering typically present with nonpronator drift, typically downward.
Disparity between tested and observed range of motion of any joint	When ROM under testing is significantly disparate (e.g., less) from observed, spontaneous range of motion (ROM) suspect functional contributors
	SENSORY AND PAIN
Nonorganic sensory impairments	Patchy sensory loss, midline sensory loss, large scotoma in visual field, tunnel vision (Note: usually not, but sometimes, organic)
Forearm pronation, hand clasping, and forearm supination test for digit/finger sensory loss	Malingered finger sensory loss is difficult to maintain in this perceptually confusing, intertwined hand/finger position
Pain vs temperature discrepancies	Because both sensory modalities run in the spinothalamic tract, they should be found to be commensurately impaired contralateral to the side of the CNS lesion.

(Continued)

TABLE 85-8 Motivation Assessment Profile—Brain Injury Evaluations (MAP–BI) Qualitative Neuromedical Indicators (*Continued*)

SENSORY AND PAIN	
Tell me "when I'm not touching" responses	An examinee with claimed sensory loss who endorses that he does not feel you touch him when you ask him to tell you "if you do not feel this."
Sensory "flip" test	Sensory findings should be the same if testing upper extremity in supination or pronation or lower extremity in internal vs external rotation. Differences may suggest a functional overlay.
Stenger's test	Test for malingered hearing loss during audiologic evaluation.
Magnuson's test	Have examinee point to area several times over period of examination; inconsistencies suggest increased potential for nonorganicity.
Delayed response sign	Pain reaction temporally delayed relative to application of perceived nociceptive stimulus.
Mankopf's maneuver	Increase in heart rate commensurate with nociceptive stimulation during exam (there is some controversy on whether this always occurs).
Toe test for simulated low back pain	Flexion of hip and knee with movement only of toes should not produce an increase in low back pain.
Pinch test for low back pain	Pinching the lumbar fat pad should not reproduce pain because of axial structure involvement; if test is positive suspect a functional overlay.
GENERAL	
Impairment diminishes under influence of sodium amytal, hypnosis, or lack of observation	These observations may indicate a nonorganic presentation or a central functional etiology including conversion disorder.
Incongruence between neuroanatomical imaging and neurologic examination	Lack of any static imaging findings on brain computed tomography (CT) or magnetic resonance imaging (MRI) in the presence of a dense motor or sensory deficit suggests nonorganicity.
Presence of ipsilateral findings when implied neuroanatomy would dictate contralateral findings	An examinee claiming severe right brain damage who claims right eye blindness and right-sided weakness and sensory loss.

[a] Neither has been validated for persons with CNS related motor impairment
DTRs, Deep Tendon Reflexes.

associated with various psychologic, sleep, or other disturbances, especially heightened anxiety or fear of pain. Many disorders do not have unambiguous diagnostic signs. Many of these indicators are not unambiguous and have not been thoroughly validated. Nonorganic sensory findings may have a psychophysiological basis as may psychogenic movement disorders or other pseudoneurologic presentations. Other explanations distinct from nonorganic ones are possible for disparate or atypical interview or exam data.

Hence, the indicators should not be used singly or to equate response bias or other phenomena (e.g., actual interference effects associated with sleep disturbance, pain, psychoemotional distress, etc.) to malingering or to consider examinee responses as either accurate or malingered. Evidence of response bias on any one indicator does not imply invalidity of all other data or absence of impairment in real world abilities. It cannot be concluded that failure on specific indicators represents inadequate performance or response bias. Rather, the strategies are offered with the following guidelines:

1. Examination responses can be influenced by multiple factors affecting reliability and validity of presentations and performances (e.g., deliberate and nondeliberate effort, psychiatric disorders, sleep disorder).
2. The degree to which presentations and performances accurately reflect genuine functional abilities exists on a continuum (vs a dichotomy) estimable by the extent of observed response bias indicators.
3. The reliability and validity of interpretations and impressions is reduced to the extent that indicators of response bias are present, in addition to the strength of their demonstrated validity.

A practical flow chart approach to integrating presented indicators for deriving meaningful inferences regarding presence and extent of response biases on examination self-report and performance is presented in Figure 85-1.

The danger of attorney "coaching" based on utilization of material in this chapter is a danger that could represent a form of "stealth" threat to the validity of examination data. This threat is an expected consequence of the collision between disparate legal and scientific ethics. It has been documented in a publication noting a case of attorney-client coaching (147). However, compared to simpler models where only a couple of isolated response bias measures are used, it seems more unlikely that the multiple measures employed in the MAP approach could be understood and manipulated.

Enhancing response bias detection as a means of optimizing interpretability of examination results should not be considered a final step. Decreasing the potential for response bias is a more efficacious and economic approach to enhancing utility of assessment. Recommendations for enhancing

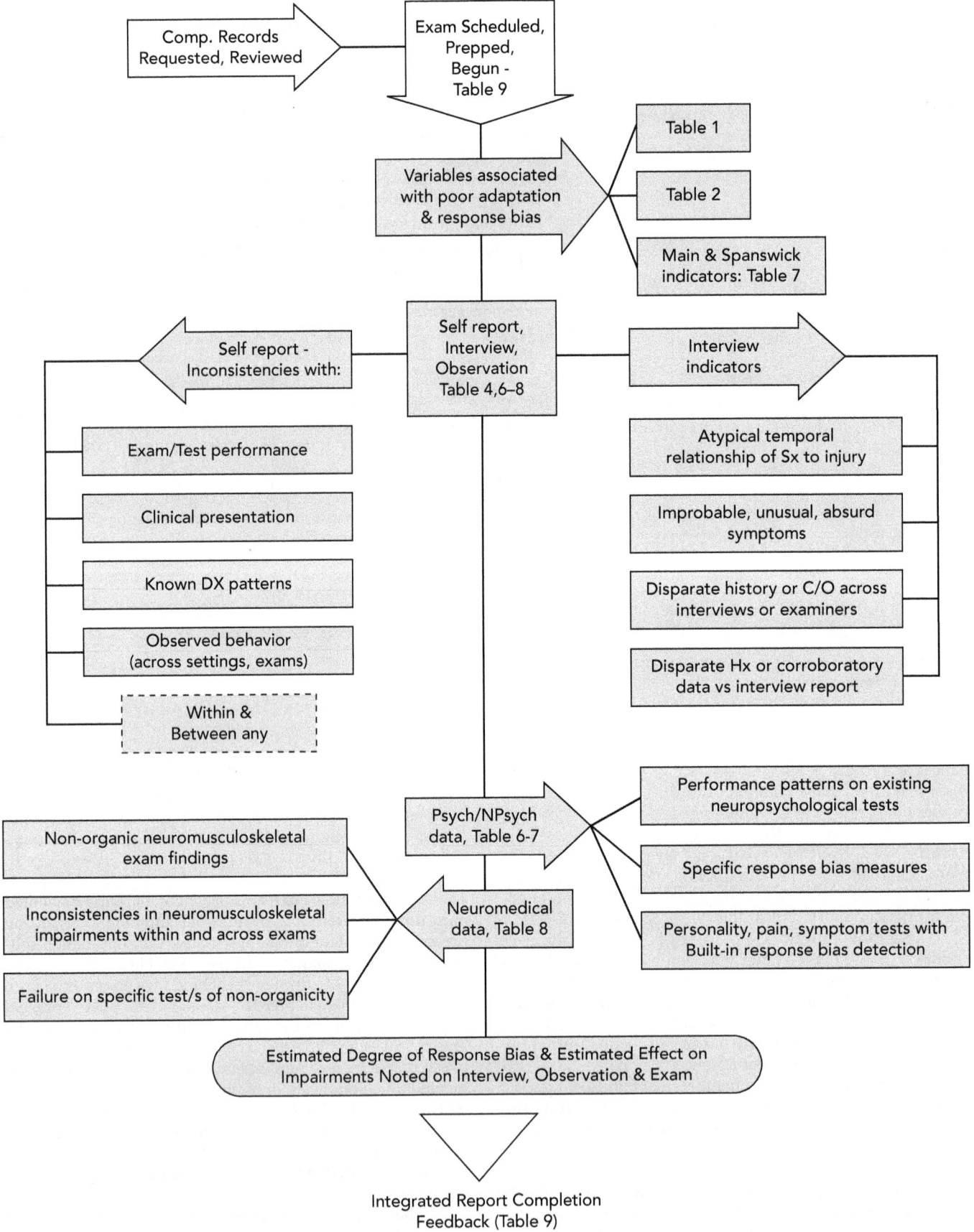

FIGURE 85-1 Flow chart for response bias assessment.

motivation, assessing response bias, and increasing efficiency, utility, and ecological validity of examination procedures are offered in following sections.

RECENT DEVELOPMENTS

Recent efforts to identify response bias and malingering have been problematic. Malingering, or the act of willful, deliberate, and fraudulent feigning, or gross exaggeration, is only one variant of response bias, and an extreme one. The presence of response bias is much more easily documented than malingering. As previously noted, the two are often confounded and used synonymously in publications and practice. Inferences about malingering, especially in a restrictive health care environment with strong gate keeping pressures, are inherently challenging. In the absence of dependent measures or clinical methods with demonstrated validity for assessment of malingering, inferences about malingering using current measures and procedures necessarily produce fallible judgments with unknown false-positive rates.

Two of the major obstacles to developing highly reliable and valid measures of malingering are (*a*) the absence of an accepted gold standard, which accounts for the absence of any blinded studies comparing malingerers and nonmalingerers; (*b*) and frequently exclusive reliance on simulation studies (i.e., noninjured persons instructed to feign deficits) for establishing reliability and validity (133). In one of the only large group studies that examined the validity of symptom validity instruments for identifying cognitive malingering, the results suggested high false-positive rates (42). A research design which attempts to circumvent obstacles relating to simulation studies and absence of a valid gold standard criterion for malingering is one that attempts to employ known groups. This design analyzes differences between criterion groups of patients and purported or assumed malingerers. This approach may benefit from recent proposals for specifying criteria for malingering (133).

Drawing on previous research, Slick et al. (152) have proposed diagnostic criteria for malingered neurocognitive dysfunction (MND), defined as volitional exaggeration or fabrication of cognitive dysfunction for the purpose of secondary environmental gain (e.g., compensation or avoidance of undesirable activities). The Slick et al. criteria allow for estimations of three probabilities of MND, including the following:

- Definite MND: presence of (*a*) substantial external incentive, (*b*) definite negative response bias on neuropsychological testing, and (*c*) definite negative response bias is not fully accounted for by psychiatric, neurological or developmental factors.
- Probable MND: presence of (*a*) substantial external incentive; (*b*) evidence from neuropsychological testing, excluding definite negative response bias, and one or more types of evidence from self-report; and (*c*) information or data utilized for criterion #2 are not fully accounted for by psychiatric, neurological or developmental factors.
- Possible MND: presence of (*a*) substantial external incentive, (*b*) evidence from self-report, and (*c*) information or data utilized for criterion #2 are not fully

accountable by psychiatric, neurological, or developmental factors.

Slick et al. (152) urge that inferences regarding malingering be preceded by thorough consideration of differential diagnostic considerations of other types of response bias and psychological, neurologic, and developmental contributors, and adoption of a "reasonable doubt" strategy that considers the limitations of assessment methodology, and the cost of false-positive errors.

The Slick et al. proposed diagnostic criteria for malingering are very helpful in delineating the need for multiple indicators for poor effort, and consideration of other non-SVT factors in reaching a somewhat less dichotomous diagnosis of definite, probable or possible malingered neurocognitive deficit. However, they still suffer from a somewhat limited consideration of factors (28,29,31,34) that can contribute to poor SVT scores, as well as most of the previously noted limitations of available symptom validity measures.

Regarding the latter, Ranks (153) examined a series of individual cases using detailed analysis of symptom validity measures that included the best currently available research support (e.g., Word Memory Test/WMT/MSVT). Willis et al. (104) conducted a similar analysis using the WMT. Their findings are consistent with the previous report of Vanderploeg et al. (42) and demonstrate the problems of assessing symptom validity and validity of neuropsychological test data in individual cases using instruments that appear much stronger when examining data from group studies. In findings from an investigation by Loring et al. (154), the Victoria Symptom Validity Test (VSVT) was found to identify cases of incomplete effort in patients being evaluated for strictly clinical purposes with no known external incentive to perform poorly, especially in older patients. An investigation of schizophrenia patients (155) concluded that suboptimal performances on SVTs reflected core components of that psychopathology. These and other findings (130) suggest that effort is a component of many neurologic disorders and false-positives can be expected on tests of effort and motivation, especially in the case of executive impairments.

Evidence from these and other studies and reviews (e.g., 2,29,31,33,42–44,86,91,92,94,104,136,151,153–156) indicate that true base rates for effort test scores (for which there may be a wide range of possible base rates) have not been established and that at least some reported sample norms are unlikely to be representative. One interesting study reports a base rate of effort test failure of 11% in the absence of any external incentive (91). These data argue against the assumption of a 0% failure rate effort or presumption that all failures can be attributed to feigning or intentional secondary gain pursuit (71). Hence, statements that anyone who is not severely demented can pass such tests if not motivated to fail appear overly exuberant and may be misleadingly presumptuous. The appearance of functional magnetic resonance imaging (fMRI) data on effort test performance adds further evidence that many assumptions about effort may be overly simplistic (92).

The search for simple solutions has a long and illustrious history in psychology and medicine where initially positive signs or tests are widely, prematurely and incautiously adopted. Examples such as using the MMPI "conversion V" (64) or the Waddell nonorganic physical signs

(1,2,24,106,158) to purportedly discriminate organic from nonorganic physical etiologies represent just 2 instances. In both cases, the professions have shown persistent recalcitrance in abandoning magic bullets and false safety blankets, despite proven invalidity and immense potential for negative consequences. A recent strong caution comes from a Psychological Bulletin critical review of the field of response bias assessment in psychology by McGrath et al (136). After reviewing studies that met stringent inclusion criteria, their controversial and challenged conclusion (137,141) was that, given the potentially high cost of false-positives, the amount and strength of the current evidence does not yet justify their continued use. Although the focus of this chapter does not endorse that conclusion, it certainly does endorse strong caution and consideration of the core bioethical principle of nonmaleficence (i.e., "First, do no harm") as prerequisite to sophisticated models and methods of response bias assessment.

Sreenivasan et al. (156) have recently proposed an impressive practical model for the assessment of amplified neuropsychological and psychiatric deficits in civil litigants in cases of MTBI. They offer a more comprehensive and detailed checklist that can assist with differentiating between subtle brain dysfunction, symptom amplification, psychological causes for cognitive and other deficits, and frank malingering. It includes examination and rating of patterns for greater consistency with either genuine injury or symptom exaggeration in the following areas:

1. Neuropsychological testing issues, including (a) base rates for brain injury, (b) testing consistency with severity of injury, and (c) findings on motivational tests.
2. Congruence of testing data and observed behavior during testing (within and between) with (a) CNS process, (b) across serial testing, (c) with medical reports, and (d) with occupational and/or or school functioning.
3. Congruence and consistency of symptoms or signs, clinical data, and clinical interview (within and between) with (a) clinical course, (b) past records, (c) physical exam, (d) objective laboratory and test findings, (e) collateral or surveillance data, (f) medication response for natural history of CNS disease, and (g) social, occupational, and/or school functioning.
4. Nonclinical factors, including whether there is (a) decline in income/business vs preinjury; (b) pending preinjury lawsuits; (c) preinjury work related burn out, job actions, coworker conflicts and skills problems; (d) compensation less than preinjury income; (e) repeated evaluations with same tests; (f) evaluation context impacting presentation; (g) reasonableness of expectations for recovery.

In addition, it allows for evaluation of the presence or absence of the following:

5. Psychiatric and other conditions that may contribute to amplified or atypical symptoms, including (a) depression/anxiety, (b) personality disorder, (c) conversion/somatization, (d) substance abuse, (e) cumulative concussion, (f) impact of chronic pain, (g) impact of medications, and (h) impact of medical comorbidities.
6. Miscellaneous history, including (a) prior history of litigation; (b) prior history of lying, malingering; (c) prior criminal activity; (d) prior job track record; and (e) prior responses to injury.

This model appears to warrant closer consideration, especially with regard to its attention to differential diagnosis and specification of the alternative contributors to failure on symptom validity measures. Future efforts to identify factors predictive of response bias and symptom invalidity should also pay more attention to not only indicators suggesting response bias, but also ones that are inconsistent with response bias and secondary gain, including secondary losses.

APPROACHING AND PROVIDING FEEDBACK ABOUT RESPONSE BIAS IN CLINICAL ASSESSMENTS

Because of many unique nuances of forensic examinations and separate coverage in Chapter 85, consideration in this section emphasizes clinical examinations. Notably, controversy and lack of consensus characterize efforts to both address and provide feedback about response bias. Despite this, proposed methods to address response bias have been offered (6,159,160) and essential elements from a comprehensive three-phase model are provided in Table 85-9. The ultimate goal of this model is to be able to engage in discussion with an individual about their apparent suboptimal effort.

Decreasing the potential for response bias may be the most intuitive and economic approach to enhancing utility of assessments (6). Hence, the first step in promoting valid assessment involves establishing rapport. The establishment of rapport through basic humanistic elements that communicate respect and a nonjudgmental interpersonal stance ideally promotes the establishment of a working relationship. The use of pejorative terms such as faking or lying are discouraged. As part of establishing rapport and to allow for an informed consent to the evaluation, it is recommended that clinicians describe the role of response bias assessment in the context of overall diagnostic assessment; and inform persons being tested about the potential adverse consequences of response bias on testing to the diagnostic and/or treatment process. In order to establish clear expectations for both the clinician and examinee, some (159) have even advocated that examinees complete a written consent form identifying that exaggeration of any kind will invalidate test results and that their best effort and honest responses should be provided at all times. Such information is intended to encourage forthrightness and optimal performance. Results are mixed however regarding the effects of warning patients prior to effort testing (161,162,163).

As a second and necessary step, response bias measures are included as an integral part of all assessments. During the evaluation evidence may begin to mount to suggest suboptimal effort and at such times a controversial step involves deciding whether to complete the evaluation or intervene and even stop further testing. Carone and colleagues (159) address pros and cons of intervening, which will be based on the context of the evaluation. Regardless of the decision to intervene or complete the evaluation, when there is clear evidence of suboptimal effort, the model encourages clinicians to determine whether a patient is willing to discuss and possibly acknowledge whether they put forth their best effort. The earlier establishment of rapport and use of non-

TABLE 85-9 Model for Approaching and Providing Feedback About Invalid Test Results

PHASE ONE (Preparation): BUILDING RAPPORT AND OBTAINING INFORMED CONSENT

- Establishing rapport;
- Providing information about the testing process and the role of response bias assessment in diagnostic assessment;
- Providing information about potential adverse consequences of response bias;
- Some clinicians use written consent forms that include agreement to be honest and put forth best effort

PHASE TWO: COMPLETING THE EVALUATION; PRELIMINARY DISCUSSIONS

- Gauge willingness to discuss sensitive topics, including response bias.
- Minimize stress, anxiety and/or confrontative responses via calmness, sensitivity, and empathy and adequate consideration of education, culture, personality and potential secondary gain motivations.
- Avoid judgmental and/or pejorative language (i.e. faking, malingering, exaggerating).
- Offer palatable topics such as possible lapses in energy, effort/ motivation or investment in the assessment process

PHASE THREE: THE FEEDBACK SESSION

- Thoroughly review all examination data prior to meeting
- Initiate feedback with inquiry about evaluation performance and easier vs challenging procedures.
- With effort at rapport and calm, discuss general evaluation conclusions. This should focus on how results may not fit with complaints or type of injury and developing willingness to discuss other explanations of performance patterns and results.
- Emphasize that the presence of response bias and/or less than full engagement, effort and motivation, an accurate assessment of presence and degree of neurological impairment is not possible.
- Request repetition of this feedback to ensure understanding.
- Be prepared for potential negative responses to feedback: defensiveness, aggression, denial, anger, crying, and others.
- The feedback process should ideally be documented including how findings were ultimately resolved.

Reprinted from Carone (159) with permission.

pejorative or threatening terms such as disengaged, not fully invested, difficulty mobilizing their effort are suggested as a way to initially address the findings.

Finally, when suboptimal behavior is identified, it must be reported, especially when it appears to have invalidated assessment results. It must also be addressed. The third and arguably most crucial phase of address response bias in clinical assessments involves the provision of feedback. A separate feedback session is recommended to allow for a thorough and complete review and integration of all available data. For numerous reasons (e.g., usual role as patient advocate, discomfort with creating a potentially conflictual interpersonal interaction, lack of consensus about how to address it), clinicians may have hesitancy in addressing negative response bias. Ideally, the examiner/clinician should approach such discussions with calmness, empathy and sensitivity with adequate consideration of their education and

cultural backgrounds, personality, and potential secondary gain motivations. Feedback should be initiated by inquiry from the patient on how they felt they did on the evaluation and requesting their feedback on what parts was easier vs more challenging. The more a calm rapport can be established up front the better for the ensuing discussion. A discussion of general conclusions from the evaluation and how the results may not fit with the injury along with other venues to explain the performance patterns/findings is recommended. Given the presence of response bias (however termed thus far to the patient), it is important to inform them that presence and degree of neurological impairment is not possible. The patient is encouraged to paraphrase information presented to them to ensure accurate comprehension of the feedback. Regardless of the care taken to establish rapport and maintain a professional, nonjudgmental stance, clinicians should be prepared to deal with negative responses to the aforementioned feedback. The feedback process should then ideally be documented including how findings were ultimately resolved. As previously indicated, a partial summary of the proposed model is in Table 85-9.

RECOMMENDATIONS FOR ENHANCING ASSESSMENT AND MANAGEMENT OF RESPONSE BIAS

1. Establish rapport and a basic working relationship with patients and examinees. Even in cases of independent or adversarial evaluations, valid data collection requires a collaborative effort. The possibility of dissimulation might be reduced given better rapport (6,9,34,134,159, 160), understanding of reported symptoms or complaints and communication of that understanding, as well as explanation, feedback, and clarification given any suggestion of uncertain motivation. Spending time with patients and getting to know a little about them as individuals may help them take our exams and procedures more seriously, be more interested and invested, and be more honest and effortful.

2. Ensure that emotional variables affecting motivation are adequately assessed during interviews before examination. Specifically, assess the impact of anger or blame and feelings of resentment or victimization (34,134), as well as the other variables associated with poor recovery and adaptation to impairment (6). Assess pain, fatigue and other factors that may interfere with optimal performance. Always assess interest/disinterest in the testing process and any obstacles or impediments to optimal effort and performance. Prepare patients/examinees before beginning testing. Employ understanding, as well as education to help prepare persons to perform to the best of their ability.

3. Make efforts to maximize validity of exam procedures. Where possible, use instruments with built-in symptom validity measures and utilize comparisons with published patterns and indices indicating suboptimal test performance for available tests with such data (e.g., hand dynamometer; finger tapping). Repeat testing with an instrument allows analysis of consistency of performance patterns across time, while measurement of completion time for similar tasks also allows analysis of consistency. Additionally, validity indicators should be

developed for existing assessment procedures and symptom validity measures should be built-in to newly developed cognitive assessment tests / procedures. Finally, most measures of symptom validity have limitations and caution is advised. Efforts should be made to avoid making strong inferences from instruments for which there are not available data regarding sensitivity and specificity in designated clinical samples. Instruments with disputed or disproved validity (e.g., Waddell signs) should not be employed or given credibility.

4. Employ shorter SVTs and tests with embedded response bias measures in order to minimize possibility of negative reactions to protracted participation in easy, boring, or atypical tasks. Where possible, employ procedures that both appear more credible and are not well-known. Vary measures and procedures that are employed in order to prevent discrimination of ability measures from symptom validity measures and to minimize recognition by attorneys, clients, support groups, internet groups, and so on. Finally, do not freely share information about symptom validity measures to nonmedical and related professionals. Some professionals adhere to a completely different set of professional ethics and recent law publications indicate a practice of preparing clients for testing by counseling them with this information (129,147).

5. Validity of examinations will likely be enhanced when conducted by clinicians who treat persons with brain injury. This helps to assure more adequate clinical skills for detecting and modifying suboptimal performance as well as allowing for tracking data to allow validation of previous inferences across time. More experienced brain injury clinicians are more capable of (a) integrating history, interview, corroboratory interview/reports, collateral data, test findings, and personality and emotional status data with more sophisticated clinical observations during examination; (b) adapting more creative modifications of exam procedures and instructions given suspicion of low motivation, to increase motivation and optimize effort; (c) benefiting from the probability that examinees will be more forthcoming, trusting and effortful with an experienced "doctor."

6. Remain aware that, in science and medicine, situations are rarely either-or, clear-cut, or one-dimensional. Avoid simplistic conceptual models that are compatible with dichotomous approaches to assessing effort and response bias. Such approaches usually rely on a couple of measures with cutoff scores that always entail judgment (151), inherently result in misclassification and impose an artificial dichotomy on essentially continuous variables. "True" cutoff scores do not exist. Employ sophisticated, continuous conceptualizations of effort and response bias by using multiple independent measures of estimated effort. Employ a model that conceptualizes motivation and effort as continuous variables that can vary across exam procedures, settings, and occasions.

7. Use and devise models that measure the degree of apparent motivation and effort, using multiple data sources, and estimate confidence levels of inferences, given consideration of the multiple factors that contribute to exam findings. Employ similarly sophisticated models for assessing persistent impairments, adaptation to impairments, and disability. Probability statements based on

multiple measures are the most appropriate. Integration of contextual information, history, behavioral observations, interview and collaborative data, personality and coping data with multiple measures of effort or performance and current tests exam and qualitative data provides the best information for estimating the degree of effort exerted, and the degree to which test results are reliable and valid.

8. Provide structured feedback in a manner that facilitates communication and provides therapeutic direction to the examinee in a sensitive, empathetic manner that takes into consideration the circumstances of that individual, education, cultural background, personality, and potential secondary gain motivations (6,159,160).

CONCLUSION

Evaluation of impairments following brain injury presents a significant challenge with numerous potential obstacles and confounding issues. In addition to frequently subtle and complex deficits, the lack of validated "rating systems" for many residual impairments, and the multiple potential contributors to impairment and disability, persons with brain injury may present with some bias to report or demonstrate impairment or related disability. Given the potential incentives to distort symptoms during examinations, assessment of examinee motivation is necessary in order to provide not only the most accurate diagnosis but the best estimates of true impairment level. This is prerequisite to provision of appropriate and timely treatment, promotion of optimal recovery, prevention of iatrogenic impairment and disability reinforcement, and appropriate legal compensation and treatment access decision making. In the current chapter, the importance of response bias was reviewed. Response bias assessment procedures relevant to brain injury assessment and treatment were considered and elucidated. Appropriate cautions were reviewed in detail with intention of avoiding oversimplification of concepts, measurement and conclusions. Finally, recommendations for enhancing validity in impairment and disability evaluations were offered, including two recommended models (MAP; Sreenivasan et al, 156). Future research should address establishment of appropriate base rates for response bias in different persons and situations. It should examine and aim to establish standardized assessment protocols that ideally use and integrate biopsychosocial concepts and consider the neural underpinnings of both effort and response biases. Investigation of strategies for optimizing accuracy and validity of symptom presentation and examination performance is also needed.

KEY CLINICAL POINTS

1. Valid assessment of impairment and disability is necessary to accurate diagnosis, appropriate treatment, recovery promotion, disability reinforcement, appropriate legal compensation and treatment need and access decision making.

2. Valid assessment requires efforts to assess response bias, ranging from examinee motivation to validity of responses to exam procedures. Preparation with rationale and emphasis for providing optimally accurate and ef-

fortful performance may be the most economical strategy for optimizing assessment validity.

3. Use multiple symptom validity methods (dedicated and built-in). Select for strong empirical support and published norms. Stay current with reading.

4. Ideally, use more credible appearing procedures, vary them and be careful about sharing information that could increase recognition by attorneys, clients, support groups, internet groups, and so forth.

5. Always evaluate for symptom minimization, especially in cases where internal and external reinforcers predispose underreporting of impairments (e.g., brain injured client wanting to drive or injured athlete wanting to return to play).

6. In addition to signs suggestive of response bias (e.g., secondary gain), always also assess for alternate contributors and for factors inconsistent with response bias (e.g., secondary losses).

7. Always assess for emotional and other variables that can affect motivation, recovery, adaptation to impairment and response bias. Interest/disinterest, pain, fatigue, and other factors that may interfere with optimal performance should always be assessed before and during evaluations.

8. Most measures of symptom validity have limitations and caution is advised. Avoid strong inferences without strong findings in several areas with good sensitivity and specificity in designated clinical samples. Consider the literature critical of the validity of response bias assessment when generating conclusions.

9. Always integrate history, interview, corroboratory interview/reports, collateral data, test findings, and personality and emotional status data with more sophisticated clinical observations and measures of symptom validity during examinations to reach conclusions about validity of assessments.

10. In science and medicine, situations are rarely clear-cut or black-white. Avoid simplistic conceptual models and dichotomous inferences.

11. The MAP approach attempts to provide a guide and procedure that incorporates many available instruments and methods and research for direct and indirect measurement of contextual response bias.

12. Models (e.g., 156) that offer an impressive practical model and methodology can assist with differential diagnosis. Comprehensive models that also include alternative contributors to symptom validity measures and factors inconsistent with response bias (e.g., secondary losses) warrant increased attention.

KEY REFERENCES

1. Larrabee GJ, ed. *Forensic Neuropsychology: A Scientific Approach.* New York, NY: Oxford University Press; 2011.

2. Martelli MF, Bush, SS, Zasler ND. Identifying and avoiding ethical misconduct in medicolegal contexts. *Int J Forensic Psychol.* 2003;1(1):26–44. http://ijfp.psych.uow.au/IJFPArticlesIssue1/Martelli.pdf. Accessed January 20, 2012.

3. Nicholson K, Martelli M. Section III: malingering in psychological injury: TBI, chronic pain and PTSD. In: Young

G, Kane A, Nicholson K eds. *Causality of Psychological Injury: Presenting Evidence in Court.* New York, NY: Springer Publishing; 2007:374–516.

4. Rogers R, ed. *Clinical Assessment of Malingering and Deception.* 3rd ed. New York, NY: Guilford Press; 2008.

5. Sreenivasan S, Eth S, Kirkish P, Garrick T. A practical method for the evaluation of symptom exaggeration in minor head trauma among civil litigants. *J Am Acad Psychiatry Law.* 2003;31(2):220–231.

References

1. Zasler ND, Martelli MF. Assessing Mild Traumatic Brain Injury. *AMA Guides Newsletter.* 1998; November/December:1–5.

2. Nicholson K, Martelli M. Section III: Malingering in psychological injury: TBI, chronic pain and PTSD. In: Young G, Kane A, Nicholson K, eds. *Causality of Psychological Injury: Presenting Evidence in Court.* New York, NY: Springer Publishing; 2007:374–516.

3. Samuel RX, Mittenberg W. Determination of Malingering in Disability Evaluations. *Prim Psychiatry.* 2005;12(12):60–68.

4. Binder LM, Rohling ML. Money matters: a meta-analytic review of the effects of financial incentives on recovery after closed-head injury. *Am J Psychiatry.* 1996;153:7–10.

5. Blau T. *The Psychologist as Expert Witness.* New York, NY: John Wiley & Sons; 1984.

6. Martelli MF, Zasler ND, Bush S. Assessment of Response Bias in Impairment and Disability Evaluations Following Brain Injury. In: Leon Carrion J, Zitnay G, eds. *Practices in Brain Injury.* Philadelphia, PA: Hanley & Belfus; 2006.

7. Matheson L. Symptom magnification syndrome: a modern tragedy and its treatment. Part one: description and definition. *Ind Rehabil Q.* 1990;3:1–23.

8. Hayes JS, Hilsabeck RC, Gouvier WD. Malingering traumatic brain injury: current issues and caveats in assessment and classification. In: Varney R, Roberts RJ, eds. *The Evaluation and Treatment of Mild Traumatic Brain Injury.* Mahwah, NJ: Lawrence Ehrlbaum and Associates; 1999:240–290.

9. Martelli MF, Zasler ND, Nicholson K, Pickett TC, May VR. Assessing the veracity of pain complaints and associated disability. In: Weiner RB, ed. *Pain Management: A Practical Guide for Clinicians.* 6th ed. Boca Raton, FL: St. Lucie Press; 2001:789–805.

10. Matheson L. Symptom magnification syndrome. In: Isernhagen S, ed. *Work Injury.* Rockville, MD: Aspen Publishers; 1988:48–91.

11. Matheson L. Symptom magnification syndrome: a modern tragedy and it's treatment. Part two: techniques of identification. *Ind Rehabil Q.* 1991;4;1:1–17.

12. Matheson L. Symptom magnification syndrome: a modern tragedy and it's treatment. Part three: techniques of treatment. *Ind Rehabil Q.* 1991;4:2:1–24.

13. Suhr JA, Gunstad J. Further exploration of the effect of "diagnosis threat" on cognitive performance in individuals with mild head injury. *J Int Neuropsychol Soc.* 2005;11(1):23–29.

14. Ozen, LJ, Fernandes MA. Effects of "diagnosis threat" on cognitive and affective functioning long after mild head injury. *J Int Neuropsychol Soc.* 2011;17,219–229.

15. Main CJ, Spanswick CC. "Functional overlay," and illness behaviour in chronic pain: distress or malingering? Conceptual difficulties in medico-legal assessment of personal injury claims. *J Psychosom Res.* 1995;39:737–754.

16. Martelli MF, Zasler ND, Nicholson K, Hart RP, Heilbronner RL. Masquerades of brain injury. Part III: critical examination of symptom validity testing and diagnostic realities in assessment. *J Controversial Med Claims.* 2002;9:19–21.

17. Martelli MF, Bush SS, Zasler ND. Identifying and avoiding ethical misconduct in medicolegal contexts. *International Journal of Forensic Psychology.* 2003;1(1):26–44. http://ijfp.psych.uow.au/IJFPArticlesIssue1/Martelli.pdf. Accessed January 20, 2012.

18. Babitsky S, Brigham CR, Mangraviti JJ. *Symptom Magnification, Deception and Malingering: Identification Through Distraction and Other Tests and Techniques* [VHS video]. Falmouth, MA: SEAK Inc; 2000.

19. Kaufman DM. *Clinical Neurology for Psychiatrists (Major problems in Neurology)*. Philadelphia, PA: WB Saunders; 2001.

20. Mailis A, Papagapiou M, Umana M, Cohodarevic T, Nowak J, Nicholson K. Unexplainable nondermatomal somatosensory deficits in patients with chronic nonmalignant pain in the context of litigation/compensation: a role for involvement of central factors? *J Rheumatol.* 2001;28:1385–1393.

21. Hall HV, Poirer JG. *Detecting Malingering and Deception: Forensic Distortion Analysis*. Delray Beach, FL: St. Lucie Press; 2000.

22. Ruchinskas R, Maitin I. The detection of exaggerated sensory symptoms. In: Zasler ND, Martelli MF, eds. *Physical Medicine and Rehabilitation: State of the Art Reviews Functional Disorders*. Philadelphia, PA: Hanley and Belfus; 2002:113–118.

23. Nicholson K, Martelli MF, Zasler ND. Myths and misconceptions about chronic pain: the problem of mind body dualism. In: Weiner RB, ed. *Pain Management: A Practical Guide for Clinicians*. 6th ed. Boca Raton, FL: St. Lucie Press; 2001:465–474.

24. Waddell G, Main CJ, Morris EW, Paola MD, Gray IC. Chronic low back pain, psychologic distesss, and illness behavior. *Spine.* 1984; 9:209–213.

25. Fishbain DA, Cole B, Cutler RB, Lewis J, Rosomoff HL, Rosomoff RS. A structured evidence-based review on the meaning of non-organic physical signs: waddell signs. *Pain Med.* 2003;4(2):141–81.

26. Lees-Haley PR, Williams CW, Zasler ND, Margulies S, English LT, Steven KB. Response bias in plaintiff's histories. *Brain Inj.* 1997;11: 791–799.

27. Faust D. *Coping with Psychiatric and Psychological Testimony*. 6th ed. New York, NY: Oxford University Press; 2011.

28. Boone, K. A reconsideration of the Slick et al. (1999) criteria for malingered neurocognitive dysfunction. In: Boone K. ed. *Assessment of Feigned Cognitive Impairment: A Neuropsychological Perspective*. New York, NY: Guilford; 2007:29–49.

29. Rogers R. *Assesssment of Malingering: Theory and Forensic Practice*. Paper presented at: The annual Forensic Mental Health Association of California; 2011.

30. Wedding D, Faust D. Clinical judgement and decision-making in neuropsychology. *Arch Clin Neuropsychol.* 1998;4(3)233–265.

31. Rogers R, Bender SD, Johnson SF. A critical analysis of the MND criteria for feigned cognitive impairment: implications for forensic practice and research. *Psychol Injury Law.* 2011;4:147–156.

32. Cummings JL, Therapeutics and Technology Assessment Subcommittee of the American Academy of Neurology. Report of the therapeutics and technology assessment subcommittee of the american academy of neurology: assessment: neuropsychological testing of adults. *Neurology.* 1996;47:592–599.

33. Rogers R, ed. *Clinical Assessment of Malingering and Deception*. 3rd ed. New York, NY: Guilford Press; 2008.

34. Nicholson K, Martelli M. The confounding effects of pain, psychoemotional problems or psychiatric disorder, premorbid ability structure, and motivational or other factors on neuropsychological test performance. In: Young G, Kane A, Nicholson K, eds. *Psychological Knowledge in Court: PTSD, Chronic Pain, and TBI*. New York, NY: Springer Publishing; 2006:335–351.

35. BA Moore, J Donders. Predictors of invalid neuropsychological test performance after traumatic brain injury. *Brain Inj.* 2004;18: 975–984.

36. Grillo J, Brown RS, Hilsabeck R, Price JR, Lees-Haley PR. Raising doubts about claims of malingering: implications of relationships between MCMI-II and MMPI-2 performances. *J Clin Psychol.* 1994; 50:651–655.

37. Heilbronner RL, Martelli MF, Nicholson K, Zasler ND. Masquerades of brain injury. Part IV: functional disorders. *J Controversial Med Claims.* 2002;9(3):1–7.

38. MacMillan PJ, Martelli MF, Hart RP, Zasler ND. Pre-injury status and adaptation following traumatic brain injury. *Brain Inj.* 2002; 16(1):41–49.

39. Martelli MF, Zasler ND, MacMillan P. Mediating the relationship between injury, impairment and disability: a vulnerability, stress & coping model of adaptation following–brain injury. *NeuroRehabilitation.* 1998;11(1):51–66.

40. Binder LM, Campbell KA. Medically unexplained symptoms and neuropsychological assessment. *J Clin Exp Neuropsychol.* 2004;26: 369–92.

41. Ben-Porath YS, Graham JR, Tellegen A. *The MMPI-2 Symptom Validity (FBS) Scale Development, Research Findings, and Interpretive Recommendations*. Minneapolis, MN: University of Minnesota Press; 2009.

42. Vanderploeg RD, Curtiss G. Malingering assessment: evaluation of validity of performance. *NeuroRehabilitation.* 2001;4:245–251.

43. Senior G, Douglas L. Misconceptions and misuse of the MMPI-2 in assessing personal injury claimants. *NeuroRehabilitation.* 2001;4: 203–214.

44. Williams AD. Psychometric concerns in neuropsychological testing. *NeuroRehabilitation.* 2001;4:221–224.

45. Allen MD, Bigler ED, Larsen J, Goodrich-Hunsaker NJ, Hopkins RO. Functional neuroimaging evidence for high cognitive effort on the Word Memory Test in the absence of external incentives. *Brain inj.* 2007;21(13–14):1425–1428.

46. Merten T, Bossink L, Schmand B. On the limits of effort testing: symptom validity tests and severity of neurocognitive symptoms in nonlitigant patients. *J Clin Exp Neuropsychol.* 2007;29(3):308–318.

47. Nies K, Sweet J. Neuropsychological assessment and malingering: a critical review of past and present strategies. *Arch Clin Neuropsychol.* 1994;9:501–552.

48. Simmonds MJ, Kumar S, Lechelt E. Psychosocial factors in disabling low back pain: causes or consequences? *Disabil Rehabil.* 1998; 18:161–168.

49. Martelli MF, Zasler ND. Assessment of motivation and response bias following acquired brain injury (ABI). *J Legal Nurse Consult.* 2002;13:7–14.

50. Bernard LC, McGrath MJ, Houston W. Discriminating between simulated malingering and closed head injury on the Wechsler Memory Scale-Revised. *Arch Clin Neuropsychol.* 1993;8:539–551.

51. Trueblood W. Qualitative and quantitative characteristics of malingered and other invalid WAIS-R and clinical memory data. *J Clin Exp Neuropsychol.* 1994;16:597–607.

52. Vickery CD, Berry DTR, Inman TH, Harris MJ, Orey SA. Detection of inadequate effort on neuropsychological testing: a meta-analytic review of selected procedures. *Arch Clin Neuropsychol,* 2001;16:45–73.

53. Strauss E, Spellacy F, Hunter M, Berry T. Assessing believable deficits on measures of attention and information processing capacity. *Arch Clin Neuropsychol.* 1994;9:483–490.

54. Martens M, Donders J, Millis SR. Evaluation of invalid response sets after traumatic head injury. *J Forensic Neuropsychol.* 2001;2: 1–18.

55. Mittenberg W, Theroux-Fichera S, Zielinski RE, Heilbronner RL. Identification of malingered head injury on the Wechsler Adult Intelligence Scale-Revised. *Prof Psychol.* 1995;26:491–498.

56. Mittenberg W, Arzin R, Millsaps C, Heilbronner R. Identification of malingered head injury on the Wechsler Memory Scale. *Psychol Assess.* 1993;5:34–40.

57. Curtis KL, Greve KW. The Wechsler Adult Intelligence Scale-III and malingering in traumatic brain injury classification accuracy in known groups. *Assessment.* 2009;16(4):401–414

58. Reitan RM, Wolfson D. Influence of age and education on neuropsychological test results. *Clin Neuropsychol.* 1995;9:151–158.

59. Millis SR, Putnam SH, Adams KM, Ricker JH. The California verbal learning test in the detection of incomplete effort in neuropsychological evaluation. *Psychol Assess.* 1995;7:463–471.

60. Nelson NW, Boone K, Dueck A, Wagener L, Lu P, Grills C. Relationships between eight measures of suspect effort. *Clin Neuropsychol.* 2003;17(2):263–272.

61. Greer S, Chambliss L, Mackler L. What physical exam techniques are useful to detect malingering? *J FamPrac.* 2005;54(8):719–722.

62. Lezak M. *Neuropsychological Assessment*. 4th ed. NewYork, NY: Oxford University Press; 2004.

63. Trueblood W, Schmidt M. Malingering and other validity considerations in the neuropsychological evaluation of mild head injury. *J Clin Exp Neuropsychol.* 1993;15:578–590.

64. Martelli MF, Zasler ND. Survey of indicators suggestive on nonorganic presentations and somatic, psychologic, and cognitive response biases. In: Zasler ND, Martelli MF, eds. *Physical Medicine and Rehabilitation: State of the Art Reviews Functional Disorders*. Philadelphia, PA: Hanley and Belfus; 2002:169–173.

65. Boone KB, Salazar X, Lu P, Warner-Chacon K, Razani J. The Rey 15-Item recognition trial: a technique to enhance sensitivity of the Rey 15-Item Memorization test. *J Clin Exp Neuropsychol.* 2002;24: 561–573.

66. Williams JM. *The Memory Assessment Scales.* Odessa, FL: Psychological Assessment Resources; 1992.

67. Meyers JE, Meyers KR. *Rey Complex Figure and Recognition Trial.* Odessa, FL: Psychological Assessment Resources; 1995.

68. Beetar JT, Williams JM. Malingering response styles on the memory assessment scales and symptom validity tests. *Arch Clin Neu-ropsy-chol.* 1995;10:57–65.

69. Allen LM, Cox DR. *Computerized Assessment of Response Bias: Revised edition.* Durham, NC: CogniSyst Inc; 1995.

70. Bigler ED. The lesion(s) in traumatic brain injury: implications for clinical neuropsychology. *Arch Clin neuropsychol.* 2001;6(2):95–131.

71. Green P. Welcoming a paradigm shift in neuropsychology. *Arch Clin Neuropsychol.* 2003;18(6):625–627.

72. Bernard LC. The detection of faked deficits on the Rey auditory verbal learning test: the effects of serial position. *Arch Clin Neuro-psychol.* 1991;6:81–88.

73. Sollman MJ, Berry DT. Detection of inadequate effort on neuro-psychological testing: a meta-analytic update and extension. *Arch Clin Neuropsychol.* 2011;26(8):774–789.

74. Delis D. *The California Verbal Learning Test.* San Antonio, TX: The Psychological Corporation; 1987.

75. Hurley KE, Deal WP. Assessment instruments measuring malingering used with individuals who have mental retardation: potential problems and issues. *Ment Retard.* 2006;44(2):112–119.

76. Green P. *Word Memory Test for Windows: User's Manual and Program.* Rev ed. Edmonton, Canada: Green's Publishing; 2005.

77. Allen LM, Iverson GL, Green P. Overview: computerized assessment of response bias in forensic neuropsychology. *Journal of Forensic Neuropsychology.* (2002);3(1–2):205–225.

78. Green P, Montijo J, Brockhaus R. High specificity of the Word Memory Test and Medical Symptom Validity Test in groups with severe verbal memory impairment. *Appl Neuropsychol.* 2011;18(2): 86–94.

79. Guilmette TJ, Hart KJ, Giuliano AJ. Malingering detection: the use of a forced-choice method in identifying organic versus simulated memory impairment. *Clin Neuropsychol.* 1993;7:59–69.

80. Iverson GL. Qualitative aspects of malingered memory deficits. *Brain Inj.* 1995;9:35–40.

81. Iverson GL, Franzen MD. The Recognition Memory Test, Digit Span, and Knox Cube Test as markers of malingered memory impairment. *Assessment.* 1994;1:323–334.

82. Lees-Haley PR, Green P, Rohling ML, Fox DD, Allen LM. The lesion(s) in traumatic brain injury: implications for clinical neuropsychology. *Arch Clin Neuropsychol.* 2003;18(6):585–594.

83. Iverson GL, Franzen MD, McCracken LM. Application of a forced-choice memory procedure designed to detect experimental malingering. *Arch Clin Neuropsychol.* 1994;9:437–450.

84. Iverson GL, Slick DJ, Franzen MD. Evaluation of a WMS-R malingering index n a non-litigating clinical sample. Paper presented at: the annual meeting of the National Academy of Neuropsychology; 1996; New Orleans, LA. November (Nov 18).

85. Frederick RI, Foster HG. Multiple measures of malingering on a forced-choice test of cognitive ability. *Psychol Assess.* 1991;3: 596–602.

86. Bigler ED, Green, RR, Millward JB. The rigor of research design and "forensic" publications in neuropsychological research. *Psychol Inj Law.* 2009.

87. Binder LM, Pankratz L. Neuropsychological evidence of a factitious memory complaint. *J Clin Exp Neuropsychol.* 1987;9:167–171.

88. Binder LM, Willis SC. Assessment of motivation after a financially compensable minor head trauma. *Psychol Assess.* 1991;3:175–181.

89. Binder LM. Forced-choice testing provides evidence of malingering. *Arch Phys Med Rehab.* 1992;73:377–380.

90. Binder LM. Assessment of malingering after mild head trauma with the Portland Digit Recognition Test [Erratum appears in *J Clin Exp Neuropsychol.* 1993;15(6):852]. *J Clin Exp Neuropsychol.* 1993;15: 170–182.

91. Hunt TN, Ferrara MS, Miller LS, Macciocchi S. The effect of effort on baseline neuropsychological test scores in high school football athletes. *Arch Clin Neuropsychol.* 2007;22:615–621.

92. Allen M, Wu T, Bigler E. Traumatic brain injury alters Word Memory Test performance by slowing response time and increasing cortical activation: an fMRI study of a symptom validity test. *Psychol Inj Law.* 2011:1–7.

93. Cliffe MJ. Symptom-validity testing of feigned sensory or memory deficits: a further elaboration for subjects who understand the rationale. *B J Clin Psychol.* 1992;31:207–209.

94. Bowden SC, Shores EA, Mathias JL. Does effort suppress cognition after brain injury? A re-examination of the evidence for the Word Memory Test. *Clin Neuropsychol.* 2006;20:858–872.

95. Daniel AE, Resnick PJ. Mutism, malingering, and competency to stand trial. *Bull Am Acad Psychiatry Law.* 1987;15:301–308.

96. Boone KB, Lu PH. Non-forced-choice effort measures.In: Larrabee GJ, ed. *Assessment of Malingered Neuropsychological Deficits.* New York, NY: Oxford University press; 2007:27–43.

97. Ensalada LH. Illness Behavior. *The AMA Guides Newsletter May/June.* 1998:4–6.

98. Faust D. The detection of deception. *Neurol Clin.* 1995;13:255–265.

99. Faust D, Guilmette TJ. To say it's not so doesn't prove that it isn't: research on the detection of malingering. Reply to Bigler. *J Consult Clin Psychol.* 1990;58:248–250.

100. Cullum C, Heaton R, Grant I. Psychogenic factors influencing neuropsychological performance: somatoform disorders, factitious disorders and malingering. In: Doerr HO, Carlin AS, eds. *Forensic Neuropsychol.* New York, NY: Guilford Press; 1991.

101. Braverman M. Post-injury malingering is seldom a calculated ploy. *Occup Health Saf.* 1978;47:36–40.

102. Franzen MD, Iverson GL, McCracken LM. The detection of malingering in neuropsychological assessment. *Neuropsychol Rev.* 1990; 1:247–279.

103. Frederick RI, Sarfaty SD, Johnston JD, Powel J. Validation of a detector of response bias on a forced-choice test of nonverbal ability. *Neuropsychology.* 1994;8:118–125.

104. Willis PF, Farrer TJ, Bigler ED. Are Effort Measures Sensitive to Cognitive Impairment? *Mil Med.* 2011;176(12):1426–1431.

105. Greiffenstein MF, Baker WJ, Gola T. Validation of malingered amnesia measures with a large clinical sample. *Psychol Assess.* 1994; 6:218–224.

106. Mailis-Gagnon A, Nicholson K. On the nature of nondermatomal somatosensory deficits. *Clin J Pain.* 2011;27:76–84.

107. Hiscock M, Hiscock C. Redefining the forced choice method for the detection of malingering. *J Clin Exp Neuropsychol.* 1989;11:967–974.

108. Millon T, Davis RD, Millon C. *MCMI-III Manual.* 2nd ed. Minneapolis, MN: National Computer Systems; 1997.

109. Tellegen A, Ben-Porath YS, McNulty JL, Arbisi PA, Graham JR, Kaemmer B. *The MMPI-2 Restructured Clinical Scales: Development, Validation, and Interpretation.* Minneapolis, MN: University of Minnesota Press; 2003.

110. Sweet JJ. Malingering: differential diagnosis. In: Sweet JJ, ed. *Forensic Neuropsychology: Fundamentals and Practice.* Lisse, The Netherlands: Swets & Zeitlinger; 1999:255–285.

111. Slick D, Hopp G, Strauss E, Hunter M, Pinch D. Detecting dissimulation: profiles of simulated malingerers, traumatic brain-injury patients, and normal controls on a revised version of His-cock and Hiscock's Forced-Choice Memory Test. *J Clin Exp Neuropsychol.* 1994;16:472–481.

112. Meyers JE, Volbrecht M. Detection of malingerers using the Rey Complex Figure and Recognition Trial. *App Neuropsychol.* 1999;6: 201–207.

113. Meyers JE, Galinsky A, Volbrecht M. Malingering and mild brain injury: how low is too low. *App Neuropsychol.* 1999;6:208–216.

114. Larrabee GJ. On modifying recognition memory tests for detection of malingering. *Neuropsychology.* 1992;6:23–27.

115. Lee GP, Loring DW, Martin RC. Rey's 15-item visual memory test for the detection of malingering: normative observations on patients with neurological disorders. *Psychol Assess.* 1992;4:43–46.

116. Sbordone RJ, Seyranian GD, Ruff RM. The use of significant others to enhance the detection of malingerers from traumatically brain injured patients. *Arch Clin Neuropsychol.* 2000;15:465–477.

117. Schacter DL. On the relation between genuine and simulated amnesia. *Behav Sci Law.* 1986;4:47–64.

118. Bigler ED. Effort—what is it, how should it be measured? *J Int Neuropsychol Soc.* 2011;17:751–752.

119. Iverson GL, Green P, Gervais R. Using the Word Memory Test to detect biased responding in head injury litigation. *J Cogn Rehabil.* 1999;2–6.

120. Jacobsen RR. The post-concussional syndrome: physiogenesis, psychogenesis and malingering. An integrative model. *J Psychosom Res.* 1995;39:675–693.

121. Lees-Haley PR, Brown RS. Biases in perception and reporting of following a perceived toxic exposure. *Percept Mot Skills.* 1992;75:533–544.

122. Pankratz L, Fausti SA, Peed S. A forced-choice technique to evaluate deafness in the hysterical or malingering patient. *J Consult Clin Psychol.* 1975;43:421–422.

123. Pankrantz L. Symptom validity testing and symptom retraining: procedures for the assessment and treatment of functional sensory deficits. *J Consult Clin Psychol.* 1979;47:409–410.

124. Lees-Haley PR, Brown RS. Neuropsychological complaint base rates of 170 personal injury claimants. *Arch Clin Neuropsychol.* 1993;8:203–210.

125. Lees-Haley PR, Brown RS. Biases in perception and reporting following a perceived toxic exposure. *Percept Mot Skills.* 1992;75:531–544.

126. Berry DT, Baer RA, Harris MJ. Detection of malingering on the MMPI: a meta-analysis. *Clin Psychol Rev.* 1991;11:585–591.

127. Whiteside DM, Galbreath J, Brown M, Turnbull J. Differential response patterns on the Personality Assessment Inventory (PAI) in compensation-seeking and non-compensation-seeking mild traumatic brain injury patients. *J Clin Exp Neuropsychol.* 2012;34(2):172–182.

128. Lees-Haley PR, English LT, Glenn WJ. A fake bad scale on the MMPI-2 for personal injury claimants. *Psychol Rep.* 1991;68:203–210.

129. Lees-Haley PR. Attorneys influence expert evidence in forensic psychological and neuropsychological cases. *Assessment.* 1997;4:321–324.

130. Thompson SB. *Effortless Effort: Current Views on Assessing Malingering Litigants in Neuropsychological Assessments.* WebmedCentral:REHABILITATION. 2011;2(7).

131. Lees-Haley PR, Iverson GL, Lange RT, Fox DD, Allen LM. Malingering in forensic neuropsychology: daubert and the MMPI-2. *J Forensic Neuropsychol.* 2002;3:167–203.

132. Axelrod B, Schutte C. Analysis of the dementia profile on the Medical Symptom Validity Test. *Clin Neuropsychol.* 2010;24(5):873–881.

133. Larrabee GJ. Assessment of malingering. In: Larrabee GJ, ed. *Forensic Neuropsychology: A Scientific Approach.* New York, NY: Oxford University Press; 2005.

134. Heilbronner R, Sweet J, Morgan J, Larrabee G, Millis S; for Conference Participants. American Academy of Clinical Neuropsychology Consensus Conference Statement on the neuropsychological assessment of effort, response bias, and malingering. *Clin Neuropsychol.* 2009;23(7):1093–1129.

135. May RV. Symptom magnification syndrome. In: May RV, Martelli MF, eds. *Guide to Functional Capacity Evaluation with Impairment Rating Applications.* Richmond, VA: NADEP Publications; 1998:21–22.

136. McGrath RE, Mitchell M, Kim BH, Hough GL. Evidence for response bias as a source of error variance in applied assessment. *Psychol Bull.* 2010;136(3):450–470.

137. Rohling ML, Larrabee GJ, Greiffenstein MF, et al. A misleading review of response bias: comment on McGrath, Mitchell, Kim, and Hough (2010). *Psychol Bull.* 2011;137(4):708–712.

138. Reznek L. The Rey 15-item memory test for malingering: a meta-analysis. *Brain Inj.* 2005;19(7):539–543.

139. Martelli MF, Zasler ND, Nicholson K, Hart RP, Heilbronner RL. Masquerades of brain injury. Part II: response bias assessment in medicolegal examinees and examiners. *J Controversial Med Claims.* 2001;8(3):13–23.

140. Gualtieri CT, Johnson LG. Reliability and validity of a computer-ized neurocognitive test battery, CNS vital signs. *Arch Clin Neuropsychol.* 2006;21(7):623–643.

141. McGrath RE, Mitchell M, Kim BH, Hough GL. Our main conclusion stands: reply to Rohling et al. (2011). *Psychol Bull.* 2011;137(4):713–715.

142. Larrabee GJ. Identification of malingering by pattern analysis on neuropsychological tests. In: Larrabee GJ, ed. *Assessment of Malingered Neuropsychological Deficits.* New York, NY: Oxford University press; 2007:80–99.

143. Bender SD, Rogers R. Detection of neurocognitive feigning: development of a multi-strategy assessment. *Arch Clin Neuropsychol.* 2004;9(1):49–60.

144. Teichner G, Wagner MT. The Test of Memory Malingering (TOMM): normative data from cognitively intact, cognitively impaired, and elderly patients with dementia. *Arch Clin Neuropsychol.* 2004;19(3):455–464.

145. Larrabee GJ. Detection of malingering using atypical performance patterns on standard neuropsychological tests. *Clin Neuropsychol.* 2003;17(3):410–425.

146. Rogers R, Harrell EH, Liff CD. Feigning neuropsychological impairment: a critical review of methodological and clinical considerations. *Clin Psychol Rev.* 1993;13:255–274.

147. Youngjohn JR. Confirmed attorney coaching prior to neuropsychological evaluation. *Assessment.* 1995;2:279–283.

148. Rutherford WH. Postconcussion symptoms: relationship to acute neurological indices, individual differences, and circumstances of injury. In: Levin HS, Eisenberg HM, Benton AL, eds. *Mild Head Injury.* New York, NY: Oxford University Press; 1989:229–244.

149. Hom J, Denney RL, eds. Detection of response bias in forensic neuropsychology: Part I. *J Forensic Neuropsychol.* 2002;2:1–166.

150. Larrabee GJ, ed. *Forensic Neuropsychology: A Scientific Approach.* New York, NY: Oxford University Press; 2011.

151. Dwyer CA. Cut scores & testing: statistics, judgment, truth, and error. *Psychol Assess.* 1996;8:360–362.

152. Slick DJ, Sherman EMS, Iverson GL. Diagnostic criteria for malingered neurocognitive dysfunction: proposed standards for clinical practice and research. *Clinical Neuropsychol.* 1999;13:545–561.

153. Ranks D. The problem of analyzing symptom invalidity. Presentation to the Reitan Society. June 2005.

154. Loring DW, Lee G P, Meador KJ. Victoria symptom validity test performance in non-litigating epilepsy surgery candidates. *J Clin Exp Neuropsychol.* 2005;27:610–617.

155. Gorissen M, Sanz JC, Schmand B. Effort and cognition in schizophrenia patients. *Schizophr Res.* 2005;78:199–208.

156. Sreenivasan S, Eth S, Kirkish P, Garrick T. A practical method for the evaluation of symptom exaggeration in minor head trauma among civil litigants. *J Am Acad Psychiatry Law.* 2003;31(2):220–231.

157. Merskey H, Bogduk N, eds. *Classification of Chronic Pain.* 2nd ed. Seattle, WA: IASP Press; 1994.

158. Ranney D. A proposed neuroanatomical basis of Waddell's nonorganic signs [Erratum appears in *Am J Phys Med Rehabil.* 2011;90(5):433]. *Am J Phys Med Rehabil.* 2010;89(12):1036–1042.

159. Carone DA, Iverson GL, Bush SS. A model to approaching and providing feedback to patients regarding invalid test performance in clinical neuropsychological evaluations. *Clinical Neuropsychol.* 2010;24(5):759–778.

160. Carone D, Bush S, Iverson GL. Providing feedback on symptom validity, mental health, and treatment in mild traumatic brain injury. In: Carone D, Bush S, eds. *Mild Traumatic Brain Injury: Symptom Validity Assessment and Malingering.* New York, NY: Springer; 2012.

161. Youngjohn JR, Lees-Haley PR, Binder LM. Comment: warning malingerers produces more sophisticated malingering. *Arch Clin Neuropsychol.* 1999;14:511–515.

162. Sullivan K, Richer C. Malingering on subjective complaint tasks: an exploration of the deterrent effects of warning. *Arch Clin Neuropsychol.* 2011;17:691–708.

163. Schenk K, Sullivan KA. Do warnings deter rather than produce more sophisticated malingering? *J Clin Exp Neuropsychol.* 2010;32(7):752–762.

Life Care Planning After Traumatic Brain Injury: Clinical and Forensic Issues

Roger O. Weed and Debra E. Berens

INTRODUCTION

This chapter presents an overview of the life care planning–related tenets, methodologies, topics, and issues to be considered when evaluating the future medical needs of the patient with acquired brain injury (ABI). Commonly known as a life care plan, the plan for someone with ABI can be relatively short, with very few "medical" needs, or very complex and detailed, with multiple medical and rehabilitation needs outlined. For example, a patient may or may not have experienced a loss of consciousness, yet still exhibit clinical signs and symptoms suggesting long-term follow-up that affect vocational and social functioning but require little or no physician or medical needs (1,2). Although information relating to a wide range of brain injury conditions is included in this chapter, most details will be geared toward the patient who has multiple future care needs that justify an assessment for life care plan development. A generally accepted and working definition for life care plan is as follows:

A *life care plan* is a dynamic document based upon published standards of practice, comprehensive assessment, data analysis and research, which provides an organized concise plan for current and future needs with associated costs, for individuals who have experienced catastrophic injury or have chronic health care needs.
Source: Combined definition of the University of Florida and Intelicus annual life care planning conference and the American Academy of Nurse Life Care Planners (now known as the International Academy of Life Care Planners) presented at the Forensic Section meeting, National Association of Rehabilitation Professionals in the Private Sector (NARPPS) annual conference, Colorado Springs, CO, and agreed upon April 3, 1998 (3).

As a "dynamic document," medication changes and other updates can be expected over time. As will be seen subsequently, however, life care plans, when completed according to established procedures, are a reliable document.

HISTORY

The concept of "life care planning" first appeared in the early 1980s in the legal publication, *Damages in Tort Action* (4), which established the guidelines for determining damages in civil litigation cases. By 1985, the life care plan was introduced to the health care industry in *A Guide to Rehabilitation* (5). One of the first professional rehabilitation training programs specific to the process of life care planning was organized by Dr. Paul Deutsch and offered on September 16–17, 1986, in Hilton Head, South Carolina, where more than 100 rehabilitation professionals from throughout the United States, including 1 of this chapter's authors, assembled to begin the process of setting standards for development of life care plans.

In the fall of 1992, 5 rehabilitation professionals— Richard Bonfiglio, MD; Paul Deutsch, PhD; Julie Kitchen, CDMS; Susan Riddick, RN; and Roger Weed, PhD met to discuss issues associated with the life care planning specialty practice. Concerned that fragmentation and lack of standardization would result in an overall decline of the industry, the group developed a concentrated training program representing the various aspects of life care planning (3).

After designing the program, a management company (Rehabilitation Training Institute) was contracted to set up training programs throughout the United States. Before the announcements were fully distributed, the first of the organized tracks was filled. It appeared obvious that there were several rehabilitation professionals interested in pursuing advanced education related to life care planning, and several participants requested official recognition for their educational efforts. Dr. Horace Sawyer of the University of Florida agreed to pursue an official certificate of completion through the University of Florida's Continuing Education Department. As a result, a private and public partnership between the Rehabilitation Training Institute and the University of Florida was formed and named Intelicus. The 5 founders donated the program content to Intelicus. Some even continue today as faculty of this original life care planning training program (which has since been merged and currently is solely managed by and within the University of Florida's Professional Development Program). Over the years, life care planning training courses have been adjusted to focus on the roles and responsibilities that more specifically identify with life care planners based on research and practitioner comments.

Although completion of the University of Florida training program added value to obtaining education specific to the specialty practice of life care planning, it did not provide the assurance of ethical practice or the professional identity desired by people who had invested thousands of dollars and many hours of their time in the training process. Ultimately, the International Commission on Health Care Certification (ICHCC), based in Midlothian, Virginia, and directed by V. Robert May, RhD, assumed the responsibility in leading the way to certification. Because of his efforts, the first national certification examination in life care planning (i.e., certified life care planner) was offered in 1996. A nurse-specific program leading to certification that was developed later is the certified nurse life care planner (CNLCP) designation. The nurses only certification was developed by Kelly Lance, RN, who was also the founder of the American Association of Nurse Life Care Planners (AANLCP). (For clarification, CLCP certification includes nurses as well as other qualified rehabilitation professionals, whereas the CNLCP is for nurses only). Currently, several organizations have approval of the ICHCC or AANLCP Boards to provide training leading to certification in life care planning and/or continuing education training for certification maintenance (i.e., Kaplan College on-line, University of Florida Professional Development, and Capital Law School, among others). Also in the 1990s, as part of the development of the specialty practice of life care planning, the International Academy of Life Care Planners (IALCP) was formed (previously known as the American *Academy* of Nurse Life Care Planners and is not to be confused with the American *Association* of Nurse Life Care Planners referenced previously) and is currently a specialty section within the International Association of Rehabilitation Professionals (IARP) professional organization. Additionally, in 2002, the *Journal of Life Care Planning* and the Foundation for Life Care Planning Research were launched. Professional Life Care Planning Summits also have been held biennially since 2000 to discuss and reach consensus on many topics of importance to ethical life care planning practice.

Over the years, life care plans have been expanding into various fields, including but not limited to, managed care, workers' compensation, civil litigation, mediation, reserve setting for insurance companies, estate trust fund planning, adoption for special needs of children, elder care, hospital discharge planning, and federal vaccine injury fund cases, all of which include individuals with brain injury in the patient population (3,6–11).

The range of future care needs for a patient with ABI can differ significantly depending on a mild, moderate, or severe brain injury. Individuals with mild brain injury, for instance, may not require a comprehensive life care plan and may be less likely to need all of the categories of care commonly considered for a life care plan. Nevertheless, there may be value in using the standardized approach in these cases to assure a comprehensive evaluation is done. For details regarding definitions and functional deficits for individuals with mild ABI, the reader is referred to Zasler's chapter in this book on Post-Concussive Disorders (Chapter 30).

Patients with mild or moderate brain injury can have few, if any, physical problems. Therefore, the physician or medical team may not be an integral part of the individual's future or life care planning. Instead, the case manager, neuropsychologist, vocational expert and, perhaps, the family or other support system, likely will be the most relevant participants in the life care planning process (12). However,

it is not uncommon for an individual with mild-to-moderate head injury to also have musculoskeletal problems including fractures, facial damage (which may or may not be repairable), seizures, and other physiological deficits (12). Conversely, patients with more severe brain injury often have multiple and obvious physical impairments as well as more severe cognitive deficits and require multiple physicians, lifelong medical care, and multiple supply, medication and equipment needs. Obviously, an effective life care plan will include items for all deficits that are related to or a result of the ABI.

In addition to an outline or delineation of the patient's life care needs, to assure that all appropriate issues for earning capacity analysis are addressed, it is helpful for a rehabilitation consultant to use a standard methodology such as RAPEL (2,3,8,9,13) to identify loss of earnings capacity as related to the brain injury. RAPEL is a mnemonic to help ensure the relevant ''damages'' of a case are evaluated. Adapted for pediatric cases, PEEDS-RAPEL expands the RAPEL method and analyzes relevant data specific to the child with a brain injury, that is, P (parental/family occupations), E (educational attainment), E (evaluation results), D (developmental stage), and S (synthesis). For further discussion on PEEDS-RAPEL for pediatric case evaluation, the reader is referred to Neulicht and Berens (14).

Although all sections of RAPEL will be discussed in this chapter, only 1 part, the Rehabilitation plan, is directly related to the life care plan.

RAPEL APPROACH

When developing a reasonable opinion for forensic cases, it is expected that the rehabilitation consultant follow a standardized assessment approach to provide the appropriate information for the patient, patient's family, attorney, and economist. Certain specific requirements are necessary to satisfy all of these issues and, although methods for determining the cost for future care as well as vocational and hedonic damages have been published (6,15,16), it appeared that a comprehensive ''common sense'' approach encompassing both needs was lacking. Therefore, the RAPEL method, representing 5 primary issues relating to future care needs and earnings capacity analysis (see Table 86-1), was designed to address rehabilitation needs and provide a ''road map'' of care, as well as generate a ''bottom line'' figure based on future care needs and earnings capacity analysis for persons with a catastrophic injury, including ABI.

The first of the RAPEL topics is as follows: **R = Rehabilitation plan**. The patient's vocational and functional limitations, strengths, emotional functioning, and cognitive capabilities are assessed using information gathered from treating professionals or other experts listed in this chapter. This may include additional future testing, counseling, training fees, rehabilitation technology, job analysis, job coaching, placement, and other needs for improving the patient's potential for employment. Future medical care also is addressed here, and typically is displayed in a life care plan for catastrophic injuries.

One commonly observed problem for forensic cases is the lack of complete data to probabilistically determine a complete lifetime cost. That is, many professionals who write reports expect that a reevaluation will take place in 1–2

TABLE 86-1 The Rapel Method: A Common Sense Approach to Future Care and Earnings Capacity Analysis

Rehabilitation plan	Determine the rehabilitation plan based on the patient's vocational and functional limitations, vocational strengths, emotional functioning, and cognitive capabilities. This may include testing, counseling, training fees, rehab technology, job analysis, job coaching, placement, and other needs for increasing employment potential. Also consider reasonable accommodation. A life care plan is appropriate for catastrophic injuries.
Access to the labor market	Determine the patient's access to the labor market. Methods include skillTRAN (www.skilltran.com) or various other computer programs, transferability of skills (or worker trait) analysis, disability statistics, and experience. This may also represent the patient's loss of choice and is particularly relevant if earnings potential is based on very few positions.
Placeability	This represents the likelihood that the patient could be successfully placed in a job. This is where the "rubber meets the road." Consider the employment statistics for people with disabilities, employment data for the specific medical condition (if available), economic situation of the community (may include a labor market survey), and availability (not just existence) of jobs in chosen occupations. Note that the patient's attitude, personality, and other factors will influence the ultimate opinion of outcome.
Earnings capacity	Based on the previous text, what is the preincident capacity to earn compared to the postincident capacity to earn? Methods include analysis of the specific job titles or class of jobs that a person could have engaged in preincident vs postincident, the ability to be educated (sometimes useful for people with ABI), family work capacity history, and computer analysis based on the individual's worker traits. Special consideration applies to children, women with limited or no work history, people who choose to work below their capacity (e.g., highly educated who are farmers), and military trained.
Labor force participation	This represents the patient's work life expectancy or ability to participate in the work force. Determine the amount of time that is lost, if any, from the labor force as a result of the disability. Issues include longer time to find employment, part-time vs full-time employment, medical treatment or follow up, earlier retirement, etc. Display data using specific dates or percentages. For example, an average of 4 hours a day may represent a 50% loss.

Reprinted from Weed, Field (12) with permission.

years, at which time additional recommendations will be made. However, in personal injury litigation, it is important to determine, as much as possible at the time of life care plan development, all of the issues that are expected to be addressed throughout the patient's lifetime. Generally, it is recommended that the rehabilitation consultant meet or communicate with the patient's treatment team (if able) or other appropriate experts associated with the case to discuss the case in detail, rather than completely rely on written reports or other records.

ELEMENTS OF THE LIFE CARE PLAN

First, it is important to understand that a variety of formats have been developed to display patient needs. In the original texts and books (4,5), the topics listed in the following text were recommended for consideration in development of life care plans and are still commonly used today. These categories have been accumulated through analysis of court requirements and decisions (4). The important aspect is to assure that all topics in the following text are considered, as appropriate, in effective life care planning.

1. *Projected Evaluations.* Intended to describe nonphysician evaluations that will occur on a periodic basis over the patient's lifetime. These may include evaluations in physical therapy, speech therapy, recreational therapy, occupational therapy, music therapy, dietary assessment, audiology, vision screening, swallow studies, and others. The information displays specific recommendations, frequency over lifetime, and expected costs.

2. *Projected Therapeutic Modalities.* After projected evaluations have been completed, recommendations for ongoing nonphysician treatment will be offered. With patients who have a catastrophic brain injury, it is common to include physical therapy, speech therapy, occupational therapy, family education, counseling, and so forth. This page identifies which nonphysician treatment is recommended, over a specific period of time, at what frequency, and what cost.

3. *Diagnostic Testing or Educational Assessment.* Generally speaking, individuals with a catastrophic brain injury will undergo a variety of diagnostic testing, including neuropsychological, psychological, vocational evaluation, and for children, psychoeducational testing. Often, evaluations will occur at specific points in a patient's life that would be identified by listing the years at which the evaluation would take place. For example, a child might be tested psychologically at ages that coincide with certain developmental stages or specific educational milestones. Such milestones may be the beginning of school, onset of puberty, beginning of high school, and entering employment or transitioning to adulthood. Consideration also should be given to additional evaluations that may be indicated as the patient ages, such as between ages 50 and 60.

4. *Wheelchair Needs.* This category includes recommendations for the type and configuration of wheelchairs the patient requires. For example, people with a dual diagnosis of brain injury and tetraplegia often require a power wheelchair that reclines or tilts in space (as 1 professional observed, "it is hard to break your neck

without hitting your head"). The individual accesses and controls the wheelchair in various ways, including joystick, sip and puff, head tilting, voice control, and others, and wheelchair specifications will allow the life care planner to research costs from various vendors (18). Some patients with hemiparesis may prefer a scooter for mobility assistance and some with less severe brain injuries may be ambulatory for short distances but need a light-weight manual wheelchair for longer distances.

5. *Wheelchair Accessories and Maintenance.* Each wheelchair requires certain accessories such as cushions for skin care, lap tables, carry bags, and other potential custom features. In addition, the wheelchair, depending on amount of use, requires maintenance. Maintenance can be very expensive for power wheelchairs, like the iBOT (which as of this writing is no longer manufactured, but those already purchased and owned or used by patients still need maintenance), or inexpensive for wheelchairs that are used only for back up purposes and are lightly used.

6. *Aids for Independent Function* (sometimes titled "assistive technology"). Many individuals with a brain injury have restricted ability to use their bodies and can make use of certain items for independence. A common example is the environmental control unit (ECU) or system that allows the patient to turn lights on and off, open and close doors, start and stop computers, turn on and off televisions, radios, fans, and so forth. Some less expensive adaptive aides may include reachers that will allow an individual to grasp items on a shelf or on the floor without having to stand up or bend over.

7. *Orthotics and Prosthetics.* Regarding significant brain injury, many patients will require braces or ankle-foot orthosis (AFO) to help with "drop foot," contractures, decrease spasticity, and so forth. Sometimes these braces, when custom designed, are costly and, over an individual's lifetime, can add up to a significant amount of money. Prosthetics generally are needed for individuals with 1 or more amputations. Prostheses also require accessories (e.g., socks, liners, cosmetic covers, etc.) and will need replacement and ongoing maintenance over the patient's lifetime. The cost for all of these items, as well as applicable maintenance and replacement schedules, will be included on this page.

8. *Home Furnishing and Accessories.* Often, a patient living at home will have need for a specialty bed and skin care mattress or powered lift and recline, portable ramps for accessibility, patient lift systems, and so forth. This section will require a specific inventory of the patient's needs at home or in their place of residence. Using a camera to document the needs can be useful.

9. *Drug and Supply Needs.* This page includes prescription and nonprescription medication and supplies as related to or a result of the brain injury. As an example, a patient who is in a persistent vegetative state will likely need catheters or adult diapers, skin care products, and medications for various injury-related problems or complications.

10. *Home Care and Facility Care.* Philosophically, it is more desirable to have a patient live in the least restrictive setting possible. This alternative also is a way to reduce complications from diseases or infections from other pa-

tients that are common in a facility setting, as well as to improve the emotional status of the patient by being in their home environment. However, this may not be the most cost-effective alternative nor, in some cases, the most medically appropriate. Facility care, generally, is not as responsive to an individual as a custom-designed home care program; however, some individuals have no capability of living at home, or their needs exceed those that are available in a home environment. In this situation, facilities for individuals with serious behavioral disorder or those in persistent vegetative state because of ABI may be the most appropriate. There also may be need for specialty programs such as yearly summer camps, especially for children and adolescents. The level of in-home care also should be identified. For example, some individuals need only occasional home care or a time specific amount each day (i.e., 4 hours per day), whereas other patients who, as an example, are ventilator dependent may need 24-hour, high-tech, nursing care. Some states and jurisdictions require a physician's prescription for attendant care, so the life care planner will advisedly seek information about the proper foundation for recommendations.

11. *Future Medical Care: Routine.* Probably the most common routine medical care for individuals with ABI is provided by a physiatrist (a specialist in physical medicine and rehabilitation). The frequency of visits will depend on the medications, complications, and severity of the injury. A person on antiseizure medication may be seen several times per year to evaluate the blood for toxicity level and efficacy of the drug. Routine medical care also may include annual evaluations by the various specialty/specialties that may be appropriate for the severity of the brain injury. For instance, in dual diagnosis cases where the individual has both a brain injury and a spinal cord injury, the patient may need a routine annual evaluation by physiatry, urology, orthopedics, neurology, and others, as well as x-rays and lab work or diagnostic tests (e.g., urodynamics). This category summarizes those routine future medical needs.

12. *Transportation.* Transportation needs vary substantially from patient to patient. Some individuals need little or no modification to their vehicles and may only require mileage reimbursement for injury-related appointments. Others may have a need for adding hand controls to their present vehicle so that they can drive. Yet other individuals may need a custom-designed van with lift and wheelchair tie-downs and rely on a driver for all driving activities, or be able to drive with highly sophisticated technology such as the Digi Drive system (19).

13. *Health and Strength Maintenance.* This category, titled Recreation and Leisure Time Activities in the original literature, is designed to identify specialty recreation needs, adaptive games, and devices that will allow patients to be as active as possible and engage in health improving therapeutic action. Activity is very important to the physical and emotional well-being of a patient and such activities are often adjunctive to, and less expensive than, hiring a physical or occupational therapist. Additionally, there are specialty cognitive retraining and socialization programs that are based in recreational activities that are designed to reteach socially appropriate

behaviors such as cooperation and community reintegration. Specialty sports-related wheelchairs (such as basketball, tennis, and other custom-designed chairs) should not go on this page, but instead should be placed on the wheelchair page. For more information on health and strength maintenance, see *Support for Recreation and Leisure Time Activities in Life Care Plans* (20).

14. *Architectural Renovations.* If the patient is to be cared for at home, significant and comprehensive architectural renovations often will be required depending on the extent of the injury and the patient's functional limitations. For example, a patient who uses a wheelchair for mobility will need ramps (preferably at 2 entries into the home), hallways and doorways may need to be widened, the kitchen may require modification, fire or smoke detection will be needed, specialized floor coverings may be installed, bathrooms may be enlarged, equipment and attendant rooms may be added, and an emergency exit out of or near the patient's bedroom may be added. Hablutzel and McMahon (21) published architectural renovation standards based on the Americans with Disability Act for those who wish to read more about this topic.

15. *Potential Complications.* Costs of potential complications are not included in the total cost of the life care plan, presumably because effective life care planning will reduce potential complications as it provides the structure for quality care. On the other hand, it is important for people to understand what common complications are involved with a particular disability (i.e., brain injury). In the case of people with significant ABI, they are at higher risk to reinjure themselves because of poor balance or judgment and lack of safety awareness (12). Also, individuals with severe brain injury or who are in a persistent vegetative state often have skin breakdown, cardiovascular difficulty, pulmonary diseases, and so forth. (12). Individuals on long-term Dilantin antiseizure medication often have gum disease or other dental problems (22). Poor psychological adjustment to the person's disability often is the direct result of poor environment, poor care, or inability to engage in meaningful activities (22).

16. *Future Medical Care and Surgical Intervention or Aggressive Treatment.* In some situations, the patient will have known needs for aggressive care. Commonly known problems for people with a brain injury include plastic surgery, dental restoration, time-limited rehabilitation programs, and short-term inpatient brain injury "tune-ups" (episodic 1–4 week rehabilitation programs). For recommendations or services to be placed on this page, it is expected that these services are more probable than not to occur and compose of occasional or time-limited treatment.

17. *Orthopedic Equipment Needs.* Some patients will need specific orthopedic equipment, such as body support equipment, walkers, or standing table. This is frequently termed "durable medical equipment."

18. *Vocational and Educational Plan.* This category was not specifically included in the original life care planning literature and was later added to specifically address future vocational and educational or training needs. The professional involved in developing the life care plan may not be responsible for addressing this portion of the patient's future care unless he or she is qualified to assess these issues. Additionally, other qualified professionals may choose to complete a narrative report and a specific rehabilitation plan that focuses on vocational issues in a separate document. In the same rationale, this category should be included in the life care plan in the same way that allied health recommendations are included, because overlap or "falling between the cracks" can otherwise result. This topic area obviously should include recommendations for vocationally related items such as job coaching, supported employment, vocational counseling, tuition or fees, books and supplies for training programs, rehabilitation technology, and/or specialized educational programs, as well as the cost of each item.

The Life Care Planning Team

In many ways, developing a comprehensive life care plan is much like completing a puzzle and making sure all the pieces fit together to complete the picture (11). The following individuals and professionals commonly have a role to play in the life care planning process and may or may not be involved in any given case. (Note 1: In forensic cases when retained by a defense attorney to develop a life care plan, the treating team, patient, and others involved in the patient's care may not be available to the life care planner. Note 2: The third edition of the *Life Care Planning and Case Management Handbook* [3] includes separate chapters for each typical professional involved.)

- **Patient or evaluee** (i.e., the person with the disability). (Also see discussion regarding who is the patient later in this chapter). Assuming that the person is accessible (i.e., legally permitted) and capable of appropriate interaction, interview and listen to him or her. Legally permitted in this context refers to the potential that defense experts in some states do not always have the "right" to interview patients and, therefore, do not have access to meet or talk with them (see also Note one previously). In cases where the patient is interviewed, the evaluee with a brain injury will often demonstrate deficits—or discuss their problems in reasonable detail. For cases where an interview does not occur, one possible alternative is to have the attorney ask standard interview questions via deposition. A videotaped "Day in the Life" of the patient also is helpful to review. An important point to make is that defense "consultants" (as compared to defense "testifying experts") are not disclosed and, therefore, will not interview patients. For those times when the patient is interviewed (regardless whether for defense or plaintiff retained experts), it is recommended that the patient interview take place in the person's residence (home or facility). When patients are interviewed in their residence, they are less inconvenienced and more comfortable. Secondly, for patients with numerous supplies, medications, and equipment requirements, this procedure for conducting the interview in the home maximizes the potential for a comprehensive assessment of needs, including a review of potential architectural needs.

- **Family members and caregivers.** Similar to the patient interview, life care planners commonly interview and listen to the family (if legally permitted) involved in the patient's care. It is not uncommon for patients with a brain injury to be unable to describe in adequate detail or accuracy the difficulties that they experience, and the family can help to "paint the picture." In addition, family support often is very important to ultimate outcome.
- **Medical evaluation.** Medical evaluation(s) with appropriate medical and allied health specialists should include an assessment of the patient's functional limitations, expected future medical treatment including referral to other specialties, a review of medications, supplies, and/or durable medical equipment, as well as related topics (see Table 86-2 for suggested questions). Again, for the person with a brain injury, the recommended resource is the physiatrist.
- **Physiatrist.** Some patients with mild-to-moderate brain injury will have few, if any, long-term *medical* needs. However, for brain injuries, a physiatrist who specializes in long-term brain injury rehabilitation can be designated the team leader for many of the specialties listed subsequently, and a team may be assembled that in-

cludes physicians who address specific areas, such as plastic surgery, pulmonology, orthopedics, and so forth. As cited in Weed and Berens (3), in general, the physiatrist will be the best physician to establish a medical foundation for a life care plan (23,24). As noted by Zasler (24), "All too often physicians may not be fully versed in life care planning. It is therefore critical that life care planners communicate in an appropriate and timely manner to assure that their role in a particular case is understood" (p. 57). One way to assure that future care information is properly solicited is to use the example questions checklist in this chapter. For physicians, if recommending a life care plan for a patient, or if meeting with an already assigned life care planner for one of his or her patients, it is recommended that the person conducting the life care planning assessment be asked if he or she is specifically qualified (by education, training, and experience) to develop life care plans that may include possessing certification as a life care planner (specifically if they are a CLCP or a CNLCP). The goal of this questioning is to increase the likelihood that the life care plan is developed according to peer-reviewed methodology and existing practice standards.

- **Neuropsychologist.** The neuropsychologist can play an invaluable role in evaluating the long-term effects of the brain injury on the patient's ability to function (25). It is within the role of the life care planner to refer a patient for a neuropsychological evaluation in cases where there is documented or suspected brain injury or impairment (26). To assure that the appropriate questions are asked during the evaluation, a specialized list of questions to help the life care planner prepare a life care plan, including addressing future vocational and educational issues, has been developed (see Table 86-3). Asking the right questions is important because many neuropsychological evaluations do not seem to be geared toward identifying long-term future care needs or rehabilitation strategies to maximize the patient's ability to function in society or participate in gainful work.
- **Occupational therapist.** The occupational therapist may be an appropriate referral for an assessment for seating and positioning, adaptive aids, safety in the residence, and other vocationally related issues (27). For some patients, activities of daily living (ADL) training, including household safety, would be included.
- **Speech and language pathologist** (may also be called communication disorders specialist). The qualified speech and language pathologist is instrumental in assessing augmentative communications for patients with more severe communications disorder, as well as assessing receptive or expressive speech and language abilities, and identifying cognitive remediation professionals to work with the patient (28).
- **Physical therapist.** A physical therapist is often the most appropriate referral to determine the patient's physical capabilities by compiling an objective functional capacity assessment that typically is more detailed than most physicians can report (29).
- **Educational consultant.** For the school-aged patient, an educational consultant can be very important to maximize the patient's educational potential. Under the fed-

---

TABLE 86-2 Example Questions for Physicians: Life Care Plan Only

1. Future care (Distinguish what is reasonable and appropriate vs medically necessary vs desirable.)
   - How long will the patient need follow-up?
   - When will the patient reach maximum medical improvement?
   - How long and how often will treatment be needed? (Include frequency and duration, e.g., every 6 months for 2 years then once per year thereafter, etc.)
   - What treatment is expected? (Follow-up visits, routine evaluations, etc.)
   - How much will each visit cost?
   - Are x-rays or lab work needed? If so, how often and how much will each cost?
   - Do you anticipate any further surgeries or aggressive medical treatment (e.g., several years from now because of complications)? If so, what, when, and how much will each cost?

2. Potential complications
   - What complications are possible or expected? (Traumatic arthritis, contractures, adverse reactions to medications, seizures, spasticity, earlier onset of aging-related dementia, maladaptive behaviors, additional injury because of reduced physical skills or poor judgment, etc.)

3. Recommended medical follow-up by other specialties
   - Orthopedist?
   - Neurology?
   - Physiatrist?
   - Cosmetic surgeon?
   - Dermatology?
   - Psychology or neuropsychology?
   - Occupational therapist, physical therapist, speech therapy, dietary, recreation therapy?
   - Other?

If you recommend any of the aforementioned, do you have an opinion regarding what treatment will be needed, how often it will be needed, and expected costs?

Partially adapted and reprinted from Weed (9) with permission.

TABLE 86-3 Neuropsychologist Questions (With credit to Robert Fraser, PhD)

In addition to the standard evaluation report, add the following as appropriate.

1. Please describe in lay terms the damage to the brain.
2. Please describe the effects of the brain injury on the patient's ability to function.
3. Please provide an opinion to the following topics:
   a. Intelligence level? (include preincident vs postincident if able)
   b. Personality style with regard to the workplace and home?
   c. Stamina level?
   d. Functional limitations and assets?
   e. Ability for education/training?
   f. Vocational implications—style of learning?
   g. Level of insight into present functioning?
   h. Ability to compensate for deficits?
   i. Ability to initiate action?
   j. Memory impairments (short-term, long-term, auditory, visual, etc.)?
   k. Ability to identify and correct errors?
   l. Recommendations for compensation strategies?
   m. Need for companion or attendant care?
4. What is the proposed treatment plan?
   a. Counseling? (individual and family)
   b. Cognitive therapy?
   c. Reevaluations?
   d. Referral to others? (e.g., physicians)
   e. Other?
5. How much and how long? (Include the cost per session or hour and reevaluations.)

Reprinted from Weed (9) with permission.

eral Individuals with Disabilities Education Act (IDEA), the public school system is responsible for providing specialized services to eligible school-age children with disabilities through age 21, if eligible. Additionally, each state offers early intervention programs for children from birth to age 3. However, many of these school-aged children are poorly served for various reasons. One may be that the child has not been adequately assessed to identify deficits that would meet the criteria for specialized education. Another is that the child may meet the eligibility requirements, but the school's funding is inadequate and the school fails to provide appropriate support. Another potential problem may be the school's contention that therapy is required for "medical" purposes rather than "educational" and the school, therefore, will not provide the services. Educational consultants who are familiar with the rules often can negotiate the appropriate education protocol, which would then be included in the life care plan.

- **Vocational evaluator** (if there is work potential). A vocational evaluator can establish standardized protocols for assessing the patient's vocational capabilities, including aptitudes, interests, temperaments, and other related information (25). For the patient with a brain injury, a "real work" situational assessment or on-the-job evaluation may be more appropriate than formal timed or time-limited testing. The evaluator should

have at least a master's degree and experience working with individuals with a brain injury. A certified vocational evaluator (CVE) is the recommended specialty for this assessment.

- **Rehabilitation counselor.** A rehabilitation counselor with a master's degree or higher from an accredited rehabilitation counselor training program should be involved to assist in arranging for a job analysis, labor market surveys, vocational guidance and counseling, selective job placement, and/or supported employment and is often the true coordinator of services (25,30). Indeed, for purposes of this chapter, the rehabilitation consultant for the patient with a mild-to-moderate brain injury is likely the prime candidate to take the information generated by the specialties listed previously and develop it into a rehabilitation plan and earnings capacity analysis. A certified rehabilitation counselor (CRC) is recommended, although a CVE (see previous text) may also have the expertise to provide this service.

- **Economist.** In most occasions, the life care planner or expert witness, in forensic cases, will work with an economist. The economist will rely on the base costs in the life care plan to project the cost of care throughout the patient's life expectancy (16). (Also see discussion regarding life expectancy in the Clinical and Forensic Issues section of this chapter, topic #11). This specialized practice is sophisticated and complex. The rehabilitation professional who does not have an education in economic forecasting is sometimes requested to project life care plan costs in personal injury litigation cases, and providing an economic evaluation is a dangerous practice in most instances. It is important to know, for example, what the different rates of inflation are for medical and nonmedical care, as well as discounts to present value methodologies. In most cases, the economist will be necessary as they are well-versed and educated in inflation rules and investment strategies. On the other hand, there are a few states that endorse the "Alaska Rule" that assumes that inflation and reasonable investment rates are essentially equal and "wash out" each other such that an economist may not be needed in those cases (9). In summary, it is strongly recommended that the life care planner defer to an economist or other trained and qualified professional for the ultimate cost of the life care plan, unless he or she has specific training in this specialized area.

As a general rule, in order for an economist to project the cost of care, certain details must be included within the life care plan. Many health care providers offer opinions that a patient will require follow-up services for "a long time;" however, it is not possible to identify specific costs for patient needs when the time frame is not quantified. To obtain a "bottom line" cost for the life care plan, the life care planning professional must obtain the following information:

a. expected type and amount of treatment (frequency)
b. date to start treatment
c. date to stop treatment
d. base cost of treatment (in today's dollars)

TABLE 86-4 Example Minimum Information Needed for Economist to Project Costs

- Psychological evaluation June 2011 at a cost of $600.
- Expect counseling to start July 2011, 1 time per week, 1-hour session each for 26 weeks at a cost of $100/hour.
- Expect group counseling 1 time per week for 2 years beginning January 2012 at a cost of $40/session.
- Expect medical follow-up 4 times by psychiatrist at a cost of $150 for the initial visit, then $75 each visit until January 2012.
- Medication prescribed is Prozac, one 20 mg/day, from July 2011 to January 2012, at a cost of $53.86 for 30 pills.
- Expect counseling to start July 2011, 1 time per week, 1-hour session each for 26 weeks at a cost of $100/hour.
- Expect group counseling 1 time per week for 2 years beginning January 2012 at a cost of $40/session.
- Expect medical follow-up 4 times by psychiatrist at a cost of $150 for the initial visit, then $75 each visit until January 2012.
- Medication prescribed is Prozac, one 20 mg/day, from July 2011 to January 2012, at a cost of $53.86 for 30 pills.

(See Table 86-4 for an example entry that contains the minimum required data for an economist to calculate future costs.)

Occasionally, identifying the frequency and duration of activities can be very complex. Pediatric brain injury cases often will include needs for periodic speech, occupational, and physical therapy that may begin and end at specific developmental periods in the child's life (27–29). Although these therapies may be provided through the school system while the child is in school, private or medically-based therapies often are indicated to address the child's needs outside the education setting for the following reasons: (*a*) to augment school-based services, (*b*) to address the child's needs at home and in the community, (*c*) to prevent or reduce medical complications or regression in functional abilities, and (*d*) to provide continuation of therapies throughout the summer to assure maintenance and carry over of skills into the next developmental stage. By knowing what services are provided by the school system, the life care planner can better determine what additional services the child needs outside the school environment to achieve short-term and long-term goals (31). For instance, occupational therapy may be needed for ADLs for a 6-year-old child and then be discontinued throughout school years until the patient is ready to enter the work world at which time an occupational therapist may rejoin the treatment team to furnish assistive devices for work-related activity as well as to enhance abilities for ADLs as an adult. A challenge for life care planning is that sometimes treatment team professionals fail to consider the lifetime needs of a patient, because they are most often involved in care lasting only 1–2 years.

To continue with an explanation of the RAPEL method previously described is as follows:

A = Access to labor market. In many cases involving individuals with ABI, the patient may very well be able to return to a job that is custom-designed around his or her disability or with an employer who is willing to hire an employee with mild-to-moderate cognitive deficits. However, the patient may not have access to the same number or level of vocational choices as he or she did prior to the injury. In essence, it may be that the patient would appear to have no particular loss of earnings capacity, but at the same time be at high risk for losing a job and then having a significant problem locating alternate suitable employment. Analysis of access to labor market following brain injury can be determined through the services of a qualified rehabilitation consultant and is beyond the scope of this chapter.

P = Placeability. Placeability represents the likelihood that the patient will be successfully placed in a job with or without rehabilitation or rehabilitation consultant assistance. One may need to conduct a labor market survey, job analysis, or, in pediatric cases, rely on statistical and family data to opine about ultimate placeability as an adult (17). In some situations, the economic condition of the community also may be a factor. It is important that the rehabilitation consultant recognize that the patient's personality, cognitive limitations, and other factors certainly influence the ultimate outcome. For adults, the rehabilitation consultant generally should include an opinion about jobs that are available (actual openings) in addition to jobs that exist but are not currently available to the patient.

E = Earnings capacity. Based on the rehabilitation or life care plan, access to the labor market, and placeability factors, the patient may or may not be employable in the labor market. If employment is likely, an estimate of the earnings potential is included as a mitigating factor in determining damages in forensic cases. In addition, identifying the preincident earnings capacity is a necessary element of determining what is included in the life care plan because jurisdiction "rules" will determine certain needs. For example, if the life care plan is being prepared for a patient related to a vaccine injury fund case, then general living costs (housing, food, transportation, etc.) will be part of the plan, whereas these costs generally are not included in personal injury cases when an argument for future lost earnings capacity is made.

L = Labor force participation. This category represents an opinion about the patient's expected work life expectancy or amount of time expected to be in the work force. Usually an individual who has a reduced life expectancy also will likely to have a reduced work life expectancy. At the other end of the spectrum, the patient's participation in the labor force may be unchanged after the brain injury. Or, an individual may have the capacity to work 6 hours/day after the brain injury rather than 8 hours/day, which represents a 25% loss of normal work life expectancy. Other patients may require a longer period of time to find a job or have longer time off between jobs as a result of the ABI and this could have an impact on their work life expectancy. Further, some patients, preinjury, may have demonstrated consistent extra income by working overtime hours or at a second job and this situation should be considered in the postinjury analysis as well.

In summary, the RAPEL method identifies the minimum data needed for determining damages in personal injury litigation and provides the data needed for economists to arrive at a bottom line figure.

GENERAL LIFE CARE PLANNING PROCEDURES

As a first step, the life care planner must request and receive all medical records and consultations (9,18,32,33). If the individual is involved in litigation, depositions of health care professionals often are available and useful to review as related to damages and/or future care needs. If information is unclear, confirmation of diagnosis is essential. As previously noted, if the patient resides at home or in a facility, it is recommended that the interview take place at the individual's place of residence rather than in an office or other location so that a complete inspection of the individual's needs can be completed. It is unlikely that the patient and/or family member(s) will remember all of the drugs and supplies, and an on-site inventory is the most effective way to determine the patient's current needs. In addition to an inventory of medications, supplies, and equipment during the initial interview, information is obtained with respect to the patient's preincident medical and social history, family history, current physical and emotional status (including limitations), medical treatment, socioeconomic status, employment history, and long-term plans. A thorough assessment usually requires several hours (3–5 hours average) to complete (for example, formats and checklists are useful for the interview, see reference 9).

Subsequent to the review of medical records and patient or family interview, the life care planner begins the process of identifying long-term care issues and options, including considerations for aging (32). If the care planner is retained by the plaintiff, the treatment team is usually consulted and is encouraged to take an active role in development of the life care plan. In fact, if the life care planner has access to relevant treatment members and fails to communicate with them, a serious breach of professional responsibility is likely. However, it is recognized that there are cases where it is not permissible to contact treatment team members. (For additional information on this topic, see 34). The life care planner acts to coordinate and communicate information to and from all members of the treatment team, patient, and family. Generally, the life care planner will be the author of the document, although many professionals involved or knowledgeable about the patient's care needs, including the patient and/or family, provide opinions and recommendations. The life care plan identifies the source of each recommendation(s), frequency, and treatment consistent with appropriate and reasonable care. To effectively participate in the planning process, the life care planner must have enough knowledge about the patient's disability and know which questions to ask, who to invite to participate, how to fill in gaps of information, and when participants' contributions are unreasonable (either excessive or deficient).

Similarly, the clinician on whom the life care planner relies needs to be competent and confident in their opinions regarding future needs as the reliability and validity of the life care plan rests on the foundation of each individual entry. The physiatrist or health care provider must know the patient's particular situation and the relevant literature regarding probable needs. For example, does a person with a brain injury really need EEGs every year to life and is there reasonable support, clinical practice guidelines, or other foundation for the recommendation? Obviously, there is a shared responsibility between the health care clinician and life care planner, and the life care planner must be acutely familiar with the patient and his or her disability to know if the clinician is offering recommendations that are reasonable and resemble an accepted standard of care. For example, 1 of the authors met with the treating physician for a patient with tetraplegia. After a few recommendations were elicited, it was obvious the doctor was not well-versed about the long-term implications of spinal cord injury as related to future care needs. It was eventually revealed that the physician had treated only 1 tetraplegic patient in his career, and he happily supported the author's recommendation to refer the patient to a specialty spinal center to obtain the required information. In this example, the life care planner had knowledge and experience working with individuals with spinal cord injury to appreciate that the treating physician was not in the best position to make recommendations for the life care plan. In addition, it is the physiatrist or health care professional's responsibility to make sure the life care planner is qualified with which to collaborate on development of the life care plan.

Once an initial life care plan is developed based on recommendations from the providers and adequate foundation for the entries, the life care planner begins an investigation into resources, cost research, and availability of services. The process of identifying resources can be a long and arduous task, involving research and personal contact with community and national resources, catalogs, and Internet databases. Upon a complete and thorough investigation, the life care plan is usually presented and reviewed by the patient and family (if clinically appropriate) and perhaps the treatment team or the providers most involved in the life care planning process. The plan can provide the patient, family, and treatment providers the opportunity to coordinate and execute effective care options with a clear understanding of the financial resources necessary for providing the service(s). Caveat: In the event the life care planner has solicited and received written recommendations from the medical or therapeutic providers, or consultation confirmation has been properly documented in the file, it may not be necessary to specifically send the life care plan back to the provider(s) for review. However, having the physiatrist or other physicians who participated in development of the plan review and sign off or endorse the relevant medically based recommendations as being a reasonable plan of care can be helpful and important for case documentation and treatment planning from a clinical perspective.

CLINICAL AND FORENSIC ISSUES

1. The rehabilitation expert or life care planner is expected to provide an opinion in personal injury cases about what is "more probable than not" within rehabilitation certainty, as represented by the standards of the profession (7,9,35,36). If a patient *might* need additional plastic surgery, then this does not represent what is more probable than not and cost for such surgery should not be included in the life care plan. It should not make a difference as to whether the expert is retained by the plaintiff or the defense because qualified professionals should arrive at similar conclusions if data are appropriately analyzed (37). However, there may be occasions where there are philosophical differences or, perhaps, an attorney has provided information that is biased, and it is within the rehabilitation consultant's ethics to attempt, to the best of his or her ability, to fairly and objectively develop a

plan that would accurately represent the patient's needs to help *resolve* litigation.

2. Replacement schedules for equipment can be dependent on various conditions (38). When possible, the source that supplied the product (assuming the patient already has it) should be contacted to obtain an opinion based on the individual patient. Contact with manufacturers also may be an acceptable source, although replacement schedules as promoted by the manufacturer may be less often than what it is in practical terms. Factors to consider include age, activity level, anticipated amount of use, patient's weight, quality of product, and some geographical considerations for beach or sandy environments, extremely cold or extremely hot environments, wet environments, and so forth. For example, a younger individual who requires the use of a wheelchair may be very active, participate in wheelchair sports, live in a rural area that is "hard" on wheelchairs, and so forth., and each of these factors must be considered. Another example may be that of a patient who is 70 years of age, very sedentary, and never leaves the residential facility where he or she lives. Replacement schedules based on the previous examples obviously differ for the reasons stated. An overview of basic guidelines to consider when determining replacement schedules can be reviewed in Amsterdam's chapter (38).

3. Items included in the life care plan should represent what is considered reasonable quality of care and presumes fewer complications than would otherwise be expected. The life care plan should identify potential complications based on research, patient's history of complications, records reviewed, or expert opinion. For example, as discussed earlier in this chapter, people with ABI commonly have a higher risk of reinjury because of poor judgment and/or reduced physical skills, among other factors. However, unless one can identify the nature of the complication, severity, frequency or duration, or the likelihood that reinjury has a better than 50% probability of occurrence, costs should not be included in the life care plan totals.

4. The life care plan generally should not include needs that are not directly related to the patient's disability (16) (Note: There are occasions where this rule does not apply, such as family trusts and vaccine injury fund cases). For example, a person with preexisting diabetes would not have the cost of medication, glucose monitor, or physician visits related to diabetes included in the plan. Assuming that damages related to earnings capacity is a part of the case, costs associated with normal living expenses also would be excluded. For example, the cost of an individual's vehicle would be deducted from the cost of a handicapped van so that the plan would only include those costs associated with the need to modify the van because of the injury. The additional costs associated with van maintenance (only for those parts that have been modified, that is, wheelchair lift, hand controls or other driving modifications, swivel seats, etc.), mileage to injury-related medical or therapy appointments, and increased insurance because of insuring a more costly, modified van would be included in the life care plan. Routine maintenance, fuel, and so forth would not be included in the plan as the patient

would have been expected to incur those costs associated with owning a regular vehicle had the injury not occurred (although an allowance for increased mileage may be added as appropriate). Similarly, the cost of home modifications because of the injury are reasonable to include in the plan, but the entire cost of a house is not (again, because the patient would have been expected to live somewhere had the injury not occurred, see 16 and 39 for details). In the event the existing home is not modifiable, the value of the existing home, or the average value of a comparable home in the local community should be deducted from the value of purchasing or building an accessible home. Another example is that individuals who reside in a facility usually receive food and housing as part of the per diem cost. If a part of the patient's damages includes earnings capacity, then the economist should be instructed to deduct the average yearly cost of food and housing that the patient would have expected to incur even without the injury. For patients who receive nutrition via enteral feeding, the average yearly cost of regular food should be deducted from the cost of their liquid nutrition. However, the life care planner must be cognizant of the nature of the case that may dictate what is properly included and accepted in the life care plan. As noted previously, special rules apply to litigation cases such as federal vaccine injury fund, Federal Employees Liability Act (FELA), or 1 of many other jurisdictions that may have special requirements.

5. For a child with a brain injury who attends public school, an individually designed educational program that includes occupational therapy, physical therapy, speech or language therapy, vision therapy, special education, and/or other resource services are available through the school by authority of the IDEA at no direct cost to the family. Typically, no cost for these school-based services should be included in the life care plan. However, what is defined as "educationally related" vs "medically related" can form the basis for conflict and may determine what or whether the child receives school-based services. As suggested previously in this chapter, it may be wise to include the services of an educational consultant or expert in the life care plan to help negotiate the most effective school-based program appropriate for the child's needs. In some rare situations, a private specialty school may clinically be the best option for the patient, in which event the costs for the private specialty school will be included in the life care plan.

6. Personal injury cases in some states have collateral source rules, which mean that certain patient needs, if covered by another entity, should not be a part of the life care plan cost. Procedurally, as well as for plan comprehensiveness, it may be appropriate to include services, supplies, products and such that are not permitted under the jurisdiction with a footnote to the economist to disregard for purposes of projecting the cost of the plan because the entries are either not permitted or will be paid by another entity. Although the life care planner must take this issue into account, the retaining attorney should be consulted to determine when or if this rule applies and should inform the expert about the proper format. For example, as noted earlier in this chapter, a

patient may have had preexisting diabetes and the medications, supplies, and medical follow up may be included in the life care plan but not compensable and should be noted as such.

7. The method for obtaining recommendations from treating professionals or other experts can take many forms. For life care planners who are retained by the plaintiff, direct contact with the treatment team is recommended. An in-person meeting with the physiatrist, for example, can assure that the life care planner has the full attention of the physician. Phone contact may also be a reasonable option, especially where distance and/or scheduling issues dictate alternate means of communication other than face-to-face. It is recommended that the life care planner take notes during such communications, then send the written notes back to the physician so that he or she can review, sign, and return them to the life care planner for documentation, along with any corrections or refinements that are indicated. Another method is to send the entire life care plan to the physician(s) for review, endorsement, and signature. A third approach is to submit a letter with specific questions on which the physician can handwrite recommendations or can dictate responses typed on the doctor's letterhead. The important factor is that written documentation from physicians and/or other health care providers verifies the medical foundation for life care plan entries.

8. For patients who require attendant care, the life care planner is expected to research agency costs (typically minimum of 3 sources are surveyed). Some experts assert that privately hired attendants are less expensive. However, the life care planner needs to be certain that the family infrastructure for private hiring is in place. Second, the costs associated with private hire are not as low as it may seem on the surface. Costs for advertising, interviewing, hiring, bonding, background checks, training costs, back up provision, insurance, payroll expenses, taxes, and so forth are in addition to the hourly rate paid to the private caregiver (see Kitchen & Brown, 40, for additional information).

9. The concept of "medically necessary" is one that the physician and allied health professionals are familiar. In general, a common tenet in personal injury cases is that the injured party has a "right" to be made whole (reasonably). So, what may be "medically necessary" in Medicare may not meet the same threshold in personal injury litigation. It behooves the life care planner to discuss this issue with the referral source to refine the definition and be sure all necessary and reasonable items are included in the life care plan.

10. *Qualified* life care planners are trained to conduct their assessments in the same manner (i.e., following the same methodology and procedures) regardless of who pays the bill. One test is to inquire about the percentage of plaintiff vs defense cases on which the professional has worked. Some life care planners are noted for providing close to 100% defense work, whereas others are close to 100% plaintiff work. One can easily assume there is a reason. It is recognized that there is no "law" that requires life care planners to be licensed or certified (unlike physicians), and that there are some experienced life care planners who are considered very good but who also

are not certified. However, certification or specific training and continuing education in life care planning at least assure that the life care planner has knowledge about standards and procedures generally accepted in the industry. As with most certifications, no competence can be assured, but minimum knowledge has been demonstrated in the testing process.

11. Life expectancy can be a significant factor for life care planning and controversy exists over who is qualified to render a life expectancy opinion. Additionally, there are specific terms and biostatistical concepts to understand as well as to have access to similar population-based data (41). It is clear that a life care plan is designed to provide the needs for the patient's life expectancy; however, for some children who are severely or significantly impaired, they may not live to be an adult. In these and other cases of individuals with a reduced life expectancy, the age of life expectancy becomes a critical point in assessing a patient's future. Typically, the life care planner will rely on a physician or medical expert to render the life expectancy opinion (23,41,42), and the life care plan needs will be adjusted accordingly. However, there are life expectancy experts who are not physicians or medical specialists who have been involved in research and have successfully been qualified in court to opine about how long a person will live (43–47). Obviously, this topic can be a battleground in forensic cases because each year that a person lives costs more. In some cases, an expert for the plaintiff may claim that a child would live to age 60 and the defense expert may opine to age 20, resulting in millions of dollars in differences. Also, in a few jurisdictions, a normal life expectancy table may be specifically required. The theory is that the defendant who is responsible for an injury that shortens one's life should not receive "credit" for the reduction and would therefore be required to pay for damages to a normal life expectancy.

12. The Health Insurance Portability and Accountability Act of 1996 (HIPAA) will have an effect on how health care providers, life care planners, insurance companies, law firms, and so forth interact with regard to medical information pertaining to an individual with a disability. Although details related to HIPAA considerations are beyond the scope of this chapter, many life care planners will need to sign business associate agreements with law firms and/or insurance companies and additional safeguards for "protected health information" will be required. Some life care planners have reported more difficulty interfacing with physicians and medical providers to access their patient's medical information and research their health care needs even with a properly signed and executed information release form. As an example, 1 of the authors researched a patient's medication costs to include in the life care plan and, as part of routine practice, asked the patient's pharmacist for a printout of the medications and supplies. Rather than complying as had been done numerous times in the past, the pharmacist informed the life care planner that the request and information release form signed by the patient had to be sent to an outside "HIPAA compliance vendor" for review and authorization before the pharmacy would release the information. Implications of this are that the

new procedure could potentially add weeks on the research portion of the life care plan and would delay obtaining the patient's actual medication history. In other instances, pharmacies have required that the patient or family personally pick up the medication history rather than send it directly to the life care planner. A more recent consideration is the effect of the 2010 Patient Protection and Affordable Care Act and the Health Care and Education Reconciliation Act of 2010 on the practice of life care planning.

BASIC ETHICAL ISSUES

The efficacy and value of the life care plan is dependent in large part on the ethics of the person developing the plan (48–50). Several common issues arise in this domain that deserve brief mention (Weed, Berens, 51, reprinted with permission).

Professional Preparation

The qualifications of professional rehabilitation practitioners depend on experience and academic preparation. It is imperative that one's credentials be represented accurately, and that current licensure and/or credentialing be maintained. Life care planning practitioners are held to the ethical standards of their professional discipline(s). Therefore, the life care planner should have specific training, belong to a relevant organization(s) that has ethics and standards of practice, and/or should be certified as a life care planner (see the International Academy of Life Care Planners at www.rehabpro.org/sections/ialcp, the International Commission on Health Care Certification at www.ichcc.org, or the Certified Nurse Life Care Planner Certification Board at www.cnlcpcertboard.org).

Who Is the Patient? (aka Client)

Common within rehabilitation service delivery, the patient or client is the person with an injury or disability for whom services are being provided. However, within the forensic arena, the person with the injury or disability is not the client per se as there is no expectation of an ongoing relationship with the life care planner (52). Life care planners who are current on terminology will likely use the term "evaluee" in their reports when referring to the person who has the disability. Regardless of whether the life care plan is developed for a forensic case or for a nonlitigated case, or whether the life care planner is retained by the plaintiff or defense (in a forensic case), the life care planner is expected to provide objective, independent opinions, limited to his or her field of expertise, and demonstrate no conflict of interest. It is important that the life care planner's contract for services clarifies the role, responsibilities, and duties of the life care planner. Ultimately, the goal is to develop a document that provides for the needs of the patient over his or her lifetime in a manner that preserves quality of life, reduces potential complications, and also provides quality, appropriate, efficient, and cost-effective services.

Informed Consent

In most cases, patient consent is required for the review of confidential medical records, for patient interviews, and communication with providers of goods and services. The patient or their legal representative must understand and consent to these services and he or she is free to withdraw consent from any or all portions of services at any time. For those cases where the life care planner is retained as a consultant to an insurance company or attorney, different rules may apply because direct contact with the patient or client may be limited or nonexistent. The life care planner must know which rules apply in the cases on which they provide services.

Confidentiality

Protection of patient confidentiality must be maintained at all times, within legal and ethical parameters. Life care planners may release records of their work with proper authorization from the patient or his or her legal representative. Written summaries and recommendations should be addressed to the referral source who can then be responsible for distribution of copies to insurers, the patient, and service providers. Special care should be taken with the use of computerized files, electronic mail, and facsimile transmission of information to protect confidentiality.

Written Reports

In personal injury litigation or forensic cases, especially when the life care planner is retained by the defense, it is not uncommon for the life care planner to defer providing written opinions, typically at the request of the attorney who retained their services. Obviously, written reports represent the most common way of expressing opinions and making recommendations in all rehabilitation industries and failure to do so in litigation-related cases is inviting criticism of the life care planning process as a whole. Based on training standards and practices, the life care planner should have some form of written documentation in their file representing conclusions and recommendations as well as foundation for such.

Use Existing Standards

Again, in personal injury litigation, certain trends are developing with regard to how life care plans are compiled. In the past, some life care planners have chosen to use their own "private logic" when outlining future care needs. Under the 1993 Daubert ruling (53), it is important for the expert to develop opinions subject to published and peer-reviewed methods, procedures, and standards. One publication that focuses exclusively on the Daubert topic as related to the practice of life care planning is the *Journal of Life Care Planning*, 2002, 1(1) (available through Elliott, Fitzpatrick, www.elliottfitzpatrick.com). The Standards of Practice for Life Care Planners (54) also is published in their entirely in the *Journal of Life Care Planning*. Additionally, another resource for consensus on life care planning issues is the 2000 Life Care Planning Summit Proceedings (55). The *Journal of*

Life Care Planning has also published proceedings from each of the biennial Life Care Planning Summits since 2000 (with exception of 2008 proceedings). (See above for publisher contact and website information.)

CONCLUSION

In general, determining lifetime future care needs for a patient with ABI can be a challenge. Oftentimes, deficits are subtle and require significant expertise to identify not only what the deficits are but also strategies to assist the patient with becoming as functional and independent as possible over his or her lifetime. These cases can require a remarkable amount of information gathering, records review, and diligent coordination among rehabilitation professionals as well as research of necessary items and services. If the evaluation is thorough, a life care plan with a reasonable estimate of financial damages can be attained and will assist in resolving the case (if in litigation), so the patient can "get on with his or her life" (i.e., have the services in the life care plan implemented). In all instances, a quality, reasonable life care plan can and should provide a "road map of care" for the patient with brain injury.

KEY CLINICAL POINTS

1. A Life Care Plan is a useful tool that identifies the long-term care needs, with associated costs of care, for individuals with ABI.
2. A Life Care Plan is a reliable document that is based on published and peer-reviewed standards of practice, established procedures and methodologies, and collaboration with the patient and his or her medical providers and experts.
3. Life Care Plans are applicable in a variety of settings, including but not limited to managed care, civil and personal injury litigation, workers' compensation, mediation/alternate dispute resolution, insurance reserve setting, estate planning, special needs trust planning, adoption for special needs children, elder care, hospital discharge planning, federal vaccine injury fund cases and other areas that include long-term services to individuals with ABI.
4. A Life Can Plan provides a holistic view of the patient and considers his or her comprehensive and lifelong needs; i.e., all of the issues that are expected to be addressed throughout the patient's lifetime as related to or a result of the ABI.
5. The comprehensive areas in which a Life Care Plan addresses include future medical care and evaluation, therapeutic care and evaluations, medications and supplies, wheelchairs and other DME, health and strength maintenance, braces/splints/orthotics/prosthetics, assistive devices/adapted aids, home accessibility, vehicle accessibility, school/educational/vocational needs, home care or facility care needs, and future surgical interventions or aggressive treatment.
6. The life care planner is the author of the Life Care Plan and acts to coordinate and communicate information to and from all members of the treatment team, patient, and patient's family.

7. In forensic or litigated cases, the Life Care Plan includes recommendations for services and items (with costs of such) that are considered "more probable than not" to be medically necessary.
8. The Life Care Plan also addresses "Potential Complications" that generally are based on the level of severity of ABI, the patient's actual history of complications related to the ABI, research regarding ABI, records reviewed, and/or expert opinions. Potential Complications are included for informational purposes only, and no cost of Potential Complications is included in the Life Care Plan.
9. Qualified Life Care Planners demonstrate training specific in the area of life care planning, clinical experience and expertise in the area, continuing education to stay current on trends in the industry, active membership in life care planning specific professional associations and, preferably, board certification as a life care planner.
10. Ethical practice among life care planners is imperative.

KEY REFERENCES

Foundation for Life Care Planning Research. http://www.flcpr.org (funds life care planning and related research)

International Academy of Life Care Planners. http://www.rehabpro.org/sections/ialcp (professional membership association; also offers continuing education)

Journal of Life Care Planning. http://www.elliottfitzpatrick.comp/ptfs.html and http://www.rehabpro.org/sections/ialcp

Riddick-Grisham S, Deming L. *Pediatric Life Care Planning and Case Management*, 2nd ed. 2011. http://www.CRCpress.com

Weed R, Berens D. *Life Care Planning and Case Management Handbook*, 3rd ed. 2010. http://www.CRCpress.com

References

1. Deutsch P, Fralish K. *Innovations in Head Injury.* New York, NY: Matthew Bender; 1989.
2. Weed, R. Life care planning and earnings capacity analysis for brain injured patients involved in personal injury litigation utilizing the RAPEL method. *J NeuroRehab.* 1996a;7(2):119–135.
3. Weed R, Berens D, eds. *Life Care Planning and Case Management Handbook.* 3rd ed. Boca Raton, FL: St. Lucie/CRC Press, LLC; 2010.
4. Deutsch P, Raffa J. *Damages in Tort Action.* Vol. 8 and 9. New York, NY: Matthew Bender; 1981.
5. Deutsch P, Sawyer H. *A Guide to Rehabilitation.* New York, NY: Matthew Bender; 1985.
6. Deutsch P, Sawyer H. *A Guide to Rehabilitation.* White Plains, NY: Ahab Press; 1994, 2003.
7. Weed RO. Life care plans as a managed care tool. *Med Interface.* 1995;8(2):111–114, 111–118.
8. Weed R. Life care planning: an overview. *Directions in Rehabilitation.* 1998;9(11): 135–147.
9. Weed R. Life care planning: past, present and future. In: Weed R, Berens P, eds. *Life Care Planning and Case Management Handbook.* 3rd ed. Boca Raton: CRC Press; 2010: 1–13.
10. Weed R, Riddick S. Life care plans as a case management tool. *The Individual Case Manager Journal.* 1992;3(1):26–35.
11. Riddick S, Weed R. The life care planning process for managing catastrophically impaired patients. In: Bancett S., Flarey D, eds. *Case Studies in Nursing Case Management.* Gaithersburg, MD: Aspen; 1996: 61–91.
12. Weed R, Field T. *Rehabilitation Consultant's Handbook.* 3rd ed. Athens, GA: Elliott & Fitzpatrick; 2001.

13. Weed R. Forensic rehabilitation. In: Dell Orto AE, Marinelle RP, eds. *Encyclopedia of Disability and Rehabilitation*. New York, NY: Macmillan; 1995: 326–330.

14. Neulicht AT, Berens DE. PEEDS-RAPEL: a case conceptualization model for evaluating pediatric cases. *Journal of Life Care Planning*. 2005;4(1):27–36.

15. Brookshire, M, Smith, S. *Economic/Hedonic Damages: The Practice Book for Plaintiff and Defense Attorneys*. Cincinnati, OH: Anderson Publishing Co.; 1990.

16. Dillman E. The role of the economist. In: Weed R, Berens D, eds. *Life Care Planning and Case Management Handbook*. 3rd ed. Boca Raton, FL: CRC Press, LLC; 2010: 303–317.

17. Weed R. Assessing the worth of a child in personal injury litigation cases. *The Rehabilitation Professional*. 2000;8(1):29–43.

18. Weed R. Life care plan development. *Topics in Spinal Cord Injury*. 2002;7(4):5–20.

19. Weed RO, Englehart LR. Factors affecting the cost of vehicle modifications: some considerations for life care planners. *Journal of Life Care Planning*. 2005;4(2):115–126.

20. Weed, R. Support for recreation and leisure activities in life care plans. *The Rehab Consultant*. 1991;3(1):1–3.

21. Hablutzel H, McMahon B. *The Americans With Disabilities Act: Access and Accommodations*. Orlando, FL: P. M. Deutsch Press; 1992: 129–138.

22. Blackwell T, Sluis-Powers A, Weed R. *Life Care Planning for the Brain Injured (Foreword by James S. Brady)*. Athens, GA: E & F Vocational Services; 1994.

23. Bonfiglio R. The role of the physiatrist in life care planning. In: Weed R, Berens D, eds. *Life Care Planning and Case Management Handbook*. 3rd ed. Boca Raton, FL: CRC Press, LLC; 2010: 17–25.

24. Zasler N. A physiatric perspective on life care planning. *Journal of Private Sector Rehabilitation*. 1994;9(2 & 3):57–61.

25. Berens D, Weed R. The role of the vocational counselor in life care planning. In: Weed R, Berens D, eds. *Life Care Planning and Case Management Handbook*. 3rd ed. Boca Raton, FL: CRC Press, LLC; 2010: 41–61.

26. Walker C. The role of the neuropsychologist in life care planning. In: Weed R, Berens D, eds. *Life Care Planning and Case Management Handbook*. 3rd ed. Boca Raton, FL: CRC Press, LLC; 2010:83–93.

27. Mitchell N. The role of the occupational therapist in life care planning. In: Weed R, Berens D, eds. *Life Care Planning and Case Management Handbook*. 3rd ed. Boca Raton, FL: CRC Press, LLC; 2010: 95–121.

28. Higdon C. The role of the speech language pathologist in life care planning. In: Weed R, Berens D, eds. *Life Care Planning and Case Management Handbook*. 3rd ed. Boca Raton, FL: CRC Press, LLC; 2010.

29. Peddle A. The role of the physical therapist in life care planning. In: Weed R, Berens D, eds. *Life Care Planning and Case Management Handbook*. 3rd ed. Boca Raton, FL: CRC Press, LLC; 2010: 123–138.

30. Blackwell T, Conrad D, Weed R. *Job Analysis and the ADA: A Step-by-Step Guide*. Athens, GA: E & F Vocational Services; 1992.

31. Neulicht AT, Berens DE. The role of the vocational rehabilitation consultant in life care planning. In: Riddick-Grisham S, Deming L, eds. *Pediatric Life Care Planning and Case Management*. Boca Raton, FL: CRC Press, LLC; 2011: 275–318.

32. Weed R. Future care planning for persons with acquired brain injury (feature article). *re-Learning* [Newsletter by Learning Services, Inc.]. 1996;3(4):5–6.

33. Weed R. Aging with a brain injury: the effects on life care plans

34. Weed R. The life care planner: secretary, know-it-all, or general contractor? One person's perspective. *Journal of Life Care Planning*. 2002;1(2):173–177.

35. Weed R. The role of the rehabilitation expert. In: PESI, ed. *Georgia Proof of Personal Injury Damages*. Eau Claire, WI: Professional Educational Systems; 1990.

36. Weed R. Presenting the rehabilitation consultant at trial. *Trial Diplomacy Journal*. 1990;13(4):212–226.

37. Sutton A, Deutsch P, Weed R, Berens D. Reliability of life care plans: a comparison of original and updated plans. *Journal of Life Care Planning*. 2002;1(3):187–194.

38. Amsterdam P. Medical equipment choices and the role of the rehab equipment specialist in life care planning. In: Weed R, Berens D, eds. *Life Care Planning and Case Management Handbook*. 3rd ed. Boca Raton, FL: CRC Press, LLC; 2010.

39. Karl J, Weed R. Home assessment in life care planning. *Journal of Life Care Planning*. 2007;5(4):159–171.

40. Kitchen J, Brown E. Life care planning resources. In: Weed R, Berens D, eds. *Life Care Planning and Case Management Handbook*. 3rd ed. Boca Raton, FL: CRC Press, LLC; 2010.

41. Weed R, Berens D. Ethics in life care planning. In: Weed R, Berens D, eds. *Life Care Planning and Case Management Handbook*. 3rd ed. Boca Raton, FL: CRC Press, LLC; 2010: 823–832.

42. Zasler ND. Long-term survival after severe TBI: clinical and forensic aspects. *Prog Brain Res*. 2009;177:111–125.

43. Winkler T, Weed R, Berens D. Life care planning for the spinal cord injured. In: Weed R, Berens D, eds. *Life Care Planning and Case Management Handbook*. Boca Raton, FL: CRC Press, LLC; 2010: 615–664.

44. Strauss DJ, DeVivo MJ, Shavelle RM. Long-term mortality risk after spinal cord injury. *Journal of Insurance Medicine*. 2000;32:11–16.

45. Shavelle R, Strauss D. Comparative mortality of adults with traumatic brain injury in California, 1988–97. *Journal of Insurance Medicine*. 2000;32:163–166.

46. Strauss DJ, Ashwal S, Day SM, Shavelle RM. Life expectancy of children in vegetative and minimally conscious states. *Pediat Neurol*. 2000;23(4):312–319.

47. Shavelle RM, Strauss D, Whyte J, Day SM, Yu YL. Long-term causes of death after traumatic brain injury. *Am J Phys Med Rehabil*. 2001; 80(7):517–519.

48. Weed RO. Ethics issues in expert opinions and testimony. *Rehabil Couns Bull*. 2000;43(4):215–218.

49. Weed R. Objectivity in life care planning. *Inside Life Care Planning*. 1995;1(1):1–5.

50. Weed R, Berens D, Pataky S. Malpractice and ethics issues in private sector rehabilitation practice: an update for the 21st century. *RehabPro*. 2003;11(1):47–54.

51. Weed R, Berens D. Ethics in life care planning. In: Deutsch P, ed. *The Expert's Role as an Educator Continues: Meeting the Demands Under Daubert*. White Plains, NY: Ahab Press; 2003: 59–67.

52. Barros-Bailey M, Carlisle J, Graham M, Neulicht A, Taylor R, Wallace A. Who is the client in forensics? *Journal of Life Care Planning*. 2008;7(3);125–132.

53. *Daubert v Merrell Dow*, 125 LEd2d 469 (1993).

54. International Academy of Life Care Planners. Standards of practice for life care planners. *Journal of Life Care Planning*. 2006;5(3): 123–129.

55. Weed R, Berens D, eds. *Life Care Planning Summit 2000 Proceedings*. Athens, GA: Elliott & Fitzpatrick, Inc.; 2000.

CASE STUDY*

*For purposes of this chapter, the below case study is in an abbreviated form.

Life Care Plan and Vocational Worksheet Using RAPEL Method and Approved by Physiatrist and Others Involved in Client's Treatment

Re: Sarah Bellum
Address: XXXX, Chicago, Illinois
Date of Report: 5/6/03
Date of Birth: 4/11/99
Date of Injury: 11/11/01

Description of Injury

Apparently, the patient was pulling on a chain when the counter to which the chain was attached fell on her. The mother states the counter weighed between 200 lbs and 300 lbs and required 2 men to pull it off. Reportedly, the patient was unconscious and had blood coming from her ears, mouth, and nose. She was diagnosed with severe closed head injury with multiple skull fractures and facial lacerations. She had a very good recovery based on the initial extent of injuries. However, several lifelong sequelae were expected and are outlined in the life care plan in the following text.

Rehabilitation Plan (see Life Care Plan)

Anticipated Length of Rehabilitation Program: Through childhood and potentially lifetime

RECOMMENDATION	DATES	FREQUENCY	EXPECTED COST
Comprehensive neuropsychological evaluation	2004 (age 5) through 2017	Once in 2004, then yearly through 2010 (age 11), 2013, 2017 (age 18)	$600 (2004) then $1,000 each
Psychological	2003–2005		$90–$110 per hour
a. Individual or couples therapy for parents		Expect once per week for 6–8 mos.	
b. Family and individual client counseling	Begin 2005	Once per week for 1 year, twice per week from ages 12 to14, twice per week from ages 16 to 18, once per week from ages 18 to 21	$90–$110 per hour
Physiatric evaluation	2003–2017	Yearly	$75–$100 each
Occupational therapy	To 2004 (age 5)	Once or twice per week	$100 each visit
Physical therapy evaluation	Est. September 2003	Once only (also see comprehensive eval.)	$100
Neurological evaluation	2003–2010	Yearly	$80 each (does not include EEG or CT scans or other diagnostic studies, if needed)
Ophthalmologic evaluation for strabismus related to ABI	June 2003 to life expectancy	Yearly	$35–$55 each (does not include dilation or corrective lenses, if necessary)
Speech or language evaluation	2003 and 2004 at age 5 (included in comprehensive evaluation)	Once in 2003, 2004	$100 (2003) 2004 cost included in comp. eval.

RECOMMENDATION	DATES	FREQUENCY	EXPECTED COST
Comprehensive team evaluation (include medical, physical therapist (PT), occupational therapist (OT), speech/language, etc.)	2004 (age 5)	Once only	$1,800
Special education Option 1: Private school for children with disabilities. Also consider summer education or camp. Option 2: Public school system covered by the Individuals with Disabilities Education Act (IDEA). Include 13 years of learning disability consulting, 3 days per week for school year and summer school.	2003–2017	36 weeks per year (40 weeks per year if summer school)	$10,000 per school year (recommended for maximum outcome) 4 weeks at $350–$1,000 per week (summer) $0 for public school. $40/hour learning disability consulting 36 weeks per year regular school or 40 weeks per year with summer school
Neurobehavior development consultant	2003–2017	3 contacts with school and patient per year to enhance educational achievement	Expect 2 hr per occasion at $100/hr (total 6 hr/year)
Health and strength maintenance (including pool therapy, walking, and recreational activities to encourage motor coordination, perceptual training, and strengthening)	2003 through entrance into school, 2004 (age 5)		No additional expected cost.
Driving evaluation	2014 (age 15)	Once only	$400
Vocational			
a. Prevocational evaluation	2015 (age 16)	Once only	$600
b. Vocational evaluation	2017 (age 18)	Once only	$600
c. Vocational counseling, guidance, placement assistance, and follow-up. (Note: Costs for job coaching and supported employment, which may be appropriate, are not included.)	2016–2019	150 hours over 3 years	$65/hour
d. Post-high school education or vocational-technical training			Unknown

Note. This plan does not include costs associated with the patient's case management services nor her reduced ability to work outside of the home.

Potential Complications

Potential complications include, but are not limited to:

1. Seizure disorder.
2. Risk of reinjury because of reduced judgment, intelligence, physical skills, and visual perception.
3. More significant psychological reaction to injury than expected.
4. Poorer educational or vocational achievement than expected.
5. Medical treatment and follow-up, which is more extensive than expected.

Access to the Labor Market

Vocational Considerations

The limitations listed subsequently are consistent with the US Department of Labor definitions:

Physical Demands

Jobs that require significant amounts of functioning in following categories:

Standing	Balancing
Reaching upward	Stooping
Crouching	Fingering
Sitting	Visual perception

Eye, hand, and foot coordination

Operating controls with right hand or arm or right foot or leg

Cognitive

Significant visual-spatial perception disturbance
Problems with attention, concentration, memory
Reduced frustration tolerance
Difficulties following through on tasks
Slowed thought process
Trouble following directions
Distractibility
Reduced intelligence
Reduced ability to be educated or trained (According to the neuropsychologist's report, auditory learning is recommended.)

Emotional

No current significant emotional difficulties noted. Expect moderate emotional difficulties on entrance into formal education program (2004, aged 5) and various developmental periods to adulthood.

Conclusion

The patient has experienced a mild to moderate impact on the range of job alternatives available to her and has reduced ability to be educated or trained. Her loss of access to the *competitive* labor market is expected to be in excess of 98%.

Placeability

The patient has experienced an impact on her ability to be placed in a job because of the ABI. Cognitive retraining and special educational services will be needed. Additionally, vocational guidance or career counseling, job skills training, and selective placement is expected to decrease the impact of the injury on the patient's ability to be placed in the *competitive* labor market. Job placement will depend to a large extent on the success of the patient's rehabilitation program and her ability to complete a minimum of a high school education. Employment, if likely, should maximize the patient's strength in auditory skills.

Earnings Capacity

Preincident	A review of the patient's family history suggests the capacity for college education or master's level education. Earnings potential to be determined by economist.
Postincident	High school or its equivalent and possibly technical school training. Earnings potential to be determined by economist.

Diminution of earnings capacity: To be computed by an economist.

Labor Force Participation (Work Life Expectancy)

Although clearly not employable in the manner as before the accident, the patient will have no reduction in labor force participation assuming no complications and excellent rehabilitation or education program. Expect entry into labor force at aged 20 (2019).

Index